Clinical Nursing Skills

BASIC TO ADVANCED SKILLS

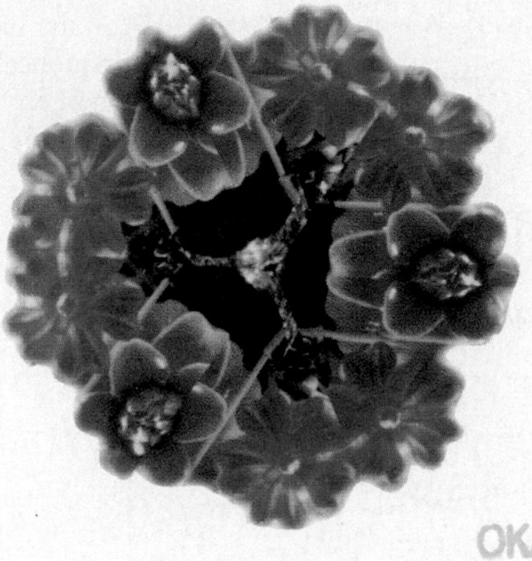

SANDRA F. SMITH, RN, MS, ABD
President, National Nursing Review
Los Altos, California

DONNA J. DUELL, RN, MS, ABD
Consultant to Deans
and Directors of Nursing
California

BARBARA C. MARTIN, MS, APRN, BC
Professor of Nursing
The University of Tulsa
Tulsa, Oklahoma

PEARSON
Prentice Hall

Upper Saddle River, New Jersey 07458

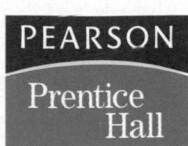

Library of Congress Cataloging-in-Publication Data
Smith, Sandra Fucci.
Clinical nursing skills: basic to advanced skills/Sandra F. Smith, Donna J. Duell, Barbara C. Martin.—6th ed.
p. cm.
Includes bibliographical references and index.
ISBN 0-13-049371-6
1. Nursing. I. Duell, Donna, 1938- II. Martin, Barbara, M.S. III. Title.
RT41.S5826 2004
610.73—dc21 2003048698

Publisher: Julie Levin Alexander
Assistant to Publisher: Regina Bruno
Editor-in-Chief: Maura Connor
Senior Acquisitions Editor: Nancy Anselment
Editorial Assistant: Gosia Jaros-White
Development Editor: Karen Hoxeng
Senior Marketing Manager: Nicole Benson
Product Information Manager: Rachele Strober
Director of Production and Manufacturing: Bruce Johnson
Managing Production Editor: Patrick Walsh
Manufacturing Buyer: Pat Brown
Production Liaison: Julie Li
Production Editor: Linda Begley
Manager of Media Production: Amy Peltier
New Media Project Manager: Stephen Hartner
Creative Director: Cheryl Asherman
Senior Design Coordinator: Maria Guglielmo Walsh
Interior Designer: Susan Walrath
Cover Designer: Mary Siener
Cover Photographer: Nick Rowe/Photodisc
Compositor: Rainbow Graphics
Printer/Binder: The Banta Company
Cover Printer: Lehigh Press

Pearson Education LTD.
Pearson Education Australia PTY, Limited
Pearson Education Singapore, Pte. Ltd
Pearson Education North Asia Ltd
Pearson Education Canada, Ltd
Pearson Educación de Mexico, S.A. de C.V.
Pearson Education—Japan
Pearson Education Malaysia, Pte. Ltd
Pearson Education, Upper Saddle River, NJ

PEARSON
Prentice Hall

10 9 8 7 6 5 4 3 2
0-13-049371-6

CONTRIBUTORS TO CURRENT AND PREVIOUS EDITIONS

Shirley S. Chang, RN, MS, PhD
Professor
Evergreen Valley College
San Jose, CA

Randy Caine, RN, MS, EdD
Associate Professor
California State University
Long Beach, CA

Janet W. Cook, RN, MS
formerly Assistant Professor
University of North Carolina
Greensboro, NC

Deborah Denham, RN, MS, PhD
Assistant Director, Nursing and Allied Health
Hartnell College
Salinas, CA

Jacqueline Dowling, RN, MS
Professor
University of Massachusetts
Lowell, MA

Lou Ann Emerson, RN, MSN
Assistant Professor
University of Cincinnati
Cincinnati, OH

Sally Talley, RN, ET
Specialist in Enterostomal Therapy
San Jose, CA

Jean O. Trotter, RN, C, MS
Assistant Professor
University of Maryland
Baltimore, MD

REVIEWERS

Sally Miller, RN, MS
Faculty, Cabrillo College
Aptos, CA

Lynette Hay, RN, MS
Nurse Manager, and staff of Orthopedic Department
Stanford University Medical Center
Stanford, CA

Nursing Management Team
Antelope Valley Hospital
Lancaster, CA

Michael Phillips, CRT, RCP
Respiratory Care
St. John Medical Center
Tulsa, OK

Victor C. Chiang, MD, MBA, FACS
Assistant Clinical Professor
Loma Linda School of Medicine
Loma Linda, CA

Rovilla Schell, MS, RD, LD, JD
Clinical Nutrition, St. John Medical Center
Adjunct Professor, School of Nursing
The University of Tulsa
Tulsa, OK

Kathy Mears, MS, RN
Director, Dialysis Services
St. John Medical Center
Tulsa, OK

PHOTO CONSULTANTS

Sherry DeHart, RN, MS
Donna Kirschner, RN, MS
Ann O'Neill, RN, MA
Laurie Phillips, RN, MS
Debbie Salerno, RN, MS
Constance Troolines, RN, BSN

PRENTICE HALL REVIEWER LIST

JoAnn Abegglen, APRN, MS, PNP
Brigham Young University

Marianne Adam, MSN, CRNP
St. Luke's SON at Moravian College

Stephanie S. Allen, MS, RN
Baylor University

Margaret W. Bellak, MN, BS, RN
Indiana University of Pennsylvania

Janet Witucki Brown, RN, PhD
University of Tennessee College of Nursing

Jeanie Burt, MA, RN
Harding University

Pam Cacchione, PhD, RN, GNP, BC
St. Louis University

Janis C. Childs, RN, PhD
University of Southern Maine

Pattie G. Clark, RN, MSN
Abraham Baldwin College

Gail DeLuca, CNP
Loyola University

Susan DeSanto-Madeya, RN, DNSc
St. Luke's SON at Moravian College

Nancy Duffy, RN, MSN
Presbyterian Hospital SON

Lisa M. Fiorentino, PhD, RN, CRNP
University of Pittsburgh

Rebecca Gesler, RN, MSN
St. Catharine College

Polly C. Haigler, PhD, RN, BC
University of South Carolina

Melanie Harrison, MSN, FNP
Indiana University East

Janice Hausauer, MS, RN
Montana State University

Susan P. Holmes, BSN, MSN, CRNP
Auburn University School of Nursing

Sylvia M. Kubsch, RN, PhD
University of Wisconsin – Green Bay

Chris Lafferty, RN
IVY State College

Patrica K. Leary, MS
MOISD and FSU

Peggy B. Lee, MSN
Arkansas Tech University

Karen Mastrippolito, RN, MS, BSN
University of Delaware

Kristen L. Mauk, PhD, BC
Valparaiso University

Carma Miller, RN, MSN
Brigham Young University

Margaret O'Hara, RN, MSN
Quincy College

Dr. C. Virginia Palmer, RN, DNSC
Millersville University

Alice Pappas, RN, PhD
Baylor University

Rhonda Reed, MSN, RN
Indiana State University

Mary Beth Reid, RN, MS, CNS, CCRN
TWU

Geneo A. Roberts, BSN, RNC
Odessa College

Sheryl K. Sommer, MSN, RN
Loyola University Chicago

RoxAnn Sparks, RN, MICN, AASN
Merced College

Linda Stevenson, PhD, RN
Baylor University

Donna Taliaferro, RN, PhD
Virginia Commonwealth University

Jana Doughty Taylor, RN, MS, HNC, CHTP
Linfield College

Sue G. Thacker, RNC, PhD
Wytheville Community College

Scott Thigpen, RN, MSN, CCRN, CEN
South Georgia College

Golden M. Tradewell, RN, PhD
McNeese State University

Sharon K. Vincent, EdD
Augusta State University

Carol Warner, RNC, CPN, CRNP-BC, MSN
St. Luke's School of Nursing

Jean C. Young, MS, RN, CNS
San Francisco State University

ACKNOWLEDGMENTS

The authors express their thanks to the many people who assisted with the editorial and production phases of this edition of *Clinical Nursing Skills,* with special thanks to Nancy Anselment, Nursing Editor, and Linda Begley, Project Coordinator at Rainbow Graphics. We especially wish to thank our Developmental Editor, Karen Hoxeng, for support, guidance, and editorial advice, and our photographer, Ron May. We also wish to thank our families and friends for their encouragement and support.

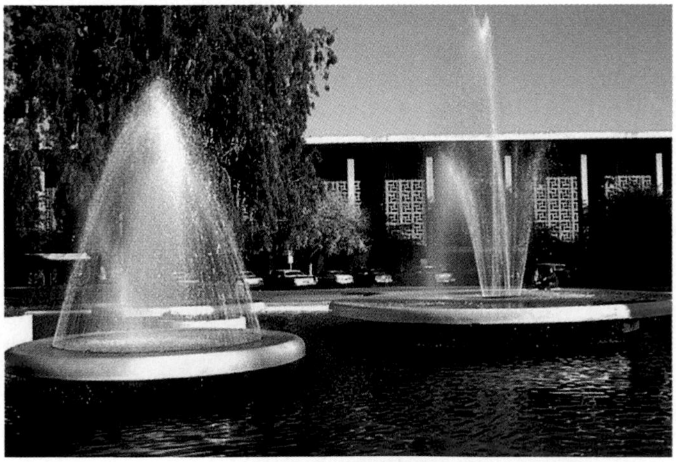

Stanford University Hospital

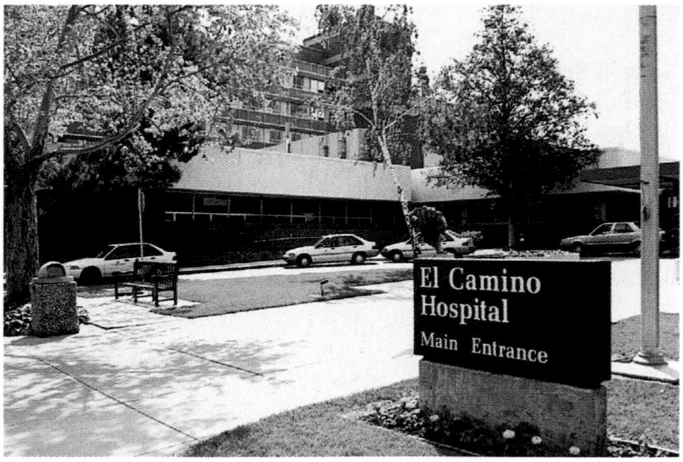

El Camino Hospital

The authors wish to express their appreciation to the hospitals and staff who so generously offered their assistance and support for our extensive photography in the appropriate clinical environment. We especially wish to thank Stanford University Medical Center, Stanford, California; El Camino Hospital, Mountain View, California; Regional Medical Center, San Jose, California; St. John Medical Center, Tulsa, Oklahoma; Sutter Hospital, Santa Cruz, California; and Watsonville Community Hospital, Watsonville, California.

PREFACE

The sixth edition of Clinical Nursing Skills continues its high standards for skill presentation. This new edition is expanded to include new chapters as well as new sections of material relevant for the twenty-first-century nurse.

The authors have strived to make this edition current, complete, and relevant for all nursing students, from those who are learning basic skills to senior students who are mastering critical care skills. The majority of skills in this text are also appropriate for the working clinical nurse. Because this text is so comprehensive, it has been adopted by many hospitals as their procedure manual.

Clinical Nursing Skills is a performance-based text written for all levels of nursing education: baccalaureate, associate degree, and diploma. New skills, new photos and illustrations, and new introductory material have been added throughout the text. Also, the text has expanded its very popular Critical Thinking Application at the end of each unit and added Critical Thinking Strategies, with scenarios based on chapter material to stimulate critical thinking ability.

Faculty feedback from prior editions confirms that the most effective way to utilize this text is to teach from the most basic to the more complex skills. The student will learn and perform each specific skill, while also learning how to assess the client, formulate nursing diagnoses, perform the procedure, evaluate the results, and document the pertinent data.

ORGANIZING FRAMEWORK

The Nursing Process continues to provide the organizing framework for this textbook. Within each of the 34 chapters, skills are grouped by unit. Nursing process data is then provided for each skill group or unit. Each procedure includes a list of equipment necessary to perform the skill, preparation, and step-by-step nursing interventions. Many steps include rationale for the nursing action. In order not to be redundant or repeat rationale time after time, we have limited these inserts to those most relevant.

The clear and concise format enables the student to easily access key material for immediate reference in the clinical area. Extensive color photographs and drawings within each unit illustrate the concepts presented and enable the student to visualize each step that must be performed.

NEW FEATURES

- **More than 650 skills,** new and updated, are included in this new edition, including basic, intermediate, and advanced skills. Presented in the Nursing Process framework, this text has **more than 1,100 pieces of art** to illustrate the skills.
- A new, extensive chapter entitled **"Bioterrorism—Disaster Nursing"** has been added to this edition. The impetus for including this material was a report by the American Hospital Association (AHA) entitled *Hospital Preparedness for Mass Casualties.* This report emphasized that a major barrier to developing and implementing a weapon of mass destruction (WMD) response training program is that most schools of nursing *do not* include this content in their basic curricula and do not prepare the graduating nurse to become a high-level participant in a WMD response team. The authors have included this chapter to assist schools of nursing to quickly add this important content to their curricula, with the hope that in the future, nurses will be prepared (with knowledge and skills) to participate on a professional level with a response team.
- **Two new sections, maternity and pediatrics,** have been added to the physical assessment chapter, which makes this chapter an all-inclusive reference. Selected pediatric and maternity skills have also been added.
- **Critical thinking** is found in two places throughout this edition. **Critical Thinking Strategies** in the form of case studies have been added at the end of each chapter to assist students to practice application of critical thinking principles to clinical situations. **Critical Thinking Application** sections, which include **unexpected outcomes and critical thinking options** are placed at the end of each unit. This section assists the student to apply the process of critical thinking when unexpected outcomes occur.
- **Cultural Competence and Evidence Based Nursing Practice** are adjunct data that have been added to this edition: *cultural competence* reminds students that cultural diversity principles play a major role in providing client care; and *evidence based nursing practice* demonstrates how to build a research base for specific interventions in client care.
- **Photos of newly introduced equipment** are included to denote advances in medical technology.
- **Management Guidelines** complete each chapter. This component includes **Delegation of Responsibilities** to teach the student nurse to make critical judgments when delegating tasks within the framework of legal, safe, and appropriate boundaries. It also includes a section on **Information Flow,** which assists the student to assume a management role by learning to prioritize and communicate relevant client data to members of the health care team.

HALLMARK FEATURES

Because each chapter "stands alone" and is consistently and independently structured, *Clinical Nursing Skills* can be adapted to all fundamental texts or any program curriculum. This feature allows faculty to use any conceptual model (Newman, Roy, Orem, Rogers, etc.) in the curriculum and to teach the material in any sequence. *Clinical Nursing Skills* remains the most complete and adaptable nursing skills text available.

- More than 1,100 full-color photographs, line drawings, charts, and tables depict step-by-step nursing procedures. These clear, specific, and up-to-date illustrations display new equipment and new procedures, as well as nurses performing basic to advanced skills.
- Each chapter's introductory material provides the basic theoretical foundation for the procedures that follow. Pedagogic features include **Learning Objectives** and **Terminology** pertinent to that chapter. **Nursing Diagnoses** (phrased in the latest terminology) are relevant to the chapter content and precede step-by-step procedures.
- Additional learning aids in each chapter will help the student assimilate the immense amount of nursing content. For example, **Rationale** for specific nursing actions assists the student to understand why certain actions are performed. Rationale is selective and pertinent to prevent overloading the student with too much data, which may occur if rationale is presented for every major step in each skill.
- **Clinical Alerts** throughout the skills call attention to safety issues, essential information, and actions that require critical decision making. Focus material in boxes and shaded areas emphasizes aspects of client care relevant to the skills.
- Frequent **Charts and Tables** supplement the procedures with useful information.
- For those schools using NIC and NOC, please note that **Expected Outcomes** continue to be found (and have been included in this book since the first, 1982, edition) in the Evaluation section of Nursing Process Data for each Unit. **Unexpected Outcomes** are presented in the **Critical Thinking Application** for each Unit.
- Two valuable sections are at the end of each chapter: **Gerontologic Considerations** present specific concepts that influence or affect care of the elderly; and **Management Guidelines,** as described above.

NCLEX RESOURCE

This text will effectively assist students to pass NCLEX. The national licensure examination for nurses (NCLEX) primarily focuses on decision-making and judgment in the clinical area. The *Practice Analysis of Newly Licensed Registered Nurses,* published by the National Council of State Boards of Nursing, lists 189 nursing activities performed by newly licensed nurses throughout the United States. These activities, many of which are nursing skills, comprise the framework for developing the NCLEX question pool. *Clinical Nursing Skills* includes all of these skills and 75% of the overall activities listed in the Job Analysis.

SUPPLEMENTAL MATERIALS

For faculty who adopt *Clinical Nursing Skills,* a valuable Instructor's Manual is available. Each chapter of the manual includes:

- Teaching/learning strategies
- Listings of reference and resource materials
- Critical thinking scenarios (originating in the text) and exercises with resolution suggestions
- Content exam questions with answers for a content review
- Checklists for all skills in printed form
- A CD-ROM, packaged with every textbook, contains checklists for all skills

WHAT DISTINGUISHES *CLINICAL NURSING SKILLS*

Its all-inclusive, clear, and concise format that teaches the student to:

- Learn each skill from basic to advanced in a contextual framework.
- Understand the theoretical concepts that serve as a foundation for skills.
- Apply this knowledge to a clinical situation with a "client need" focus.
- Use critical thinking to evaluate the outcome of the skill and consider unexpected outcomes.
- Appreciate cultural diversity principles as they apply to client situations.
- Validate clinical skills by applying evidence based nursing practice data and studies.
- Function in, and adapt to, the professional role by understanding management responsibilities.

Our primary goal in writing *Clinical Nursing Skills,* 6th edition, is to produce a relevant, useful, and comprehensive text that is adaptable to various programs and learning needs of students. Further, the authors hope that faculty will find this textbook a valuable teaching tool and reference for clinical practice.

CONTENTS IN BRIEF

CHAPTER 1 PROFESSIONAL NURSING 1

CHAPTER 2 NURSING PROCESS AND CRITICAL THINKING 21

CHAPTER 3 MANAGING CLIENT CARE: DOCUMENTATION AND DELEGATION 33

CHAPTER 4 COMMUNICATION AND NURSE–CLIENT RELATIONSHIP 65

CHAPTER 5 ADMISSION AND DISCHARGE 84

CHAPTER 6 CLIENT EDUCATION AND DISCHARGE PLANNING 105

CHAPTER 7 SAFE CLIENT ENVIRONMENT AND RESTRAINTS 128

CHAPTER 8 BATHING, BEDMAKING, AND MAINTAINING SKIN-INTEGRITY 159

CHAPTER 9 PERSONAL HYGIENE 194

CHAPTER 10 VITAL SIGNS 233

CHAPTER 11 PHYSICAL ASSESSMENT 272

CHAPTER 12 BODY MECHANICS AND POSITIONING 322

CHAPTER 13 EXERCISE AND AMBULATION 348

CHAPTER 14 INFECTION CONTROL 376

CHAPTER 15 BIOTERRORISM—DISASTER NURSING 413

CHAPTER 16 PAIN MANAGEMENT 465

CHAPTER 17 ALTERNATIVE THERAPIES AND STRESS MANAGEMENT 494

CHAPTER 18 MEDICATION ADMINISTRATION 515

CHAPTER 19 NUTRITIONAL MANAGEMENT AND NG INTUBATION 575

CHAPTER 20 SPECIMEN COLLECTION 624

CHAPTER 21 DIAGNOSTIC PROCEDURES 660

CHAPTER 22 URINARY ELIMINATION 698

CHAPTER 23 BOWEL ELIMINATION 755

CHAPTER 24 HEAT AND COLD THERAPIES 785

CHAPTER 25 WOUND CARE AND DRESSINGS 811

CHAPTER 26 RESPIRATORY CARE 870

CHAPTER 27 CIRCULATORY MAINTENANCE 932

CHAPTER 28 INTRAVENOUS THERAPY 993

CHAPTER 29 CENTRAL VASCULAR ACCESS DEVICES 1044

CHAPTER 30 ORTHOPEDIC INTERVENTIONS 1095

CHAPTER 31 PERIOPERATIVE CARE 1138

CHAPTER 32 END-OF-LIFE CARE 1183

CHAPTER 33 ADVANCED NURSING SKILLS 1205

CHAPTER 34 COMMUNITY-BASED NURSING 1245

CONTENTS

Acknowledgments iv

Preface v

CHAPTER 1

Professional Nursing 1

Learning Objectives 2
Professional Role 2
  Assuming the Nursing Role 2
  The Client Role 3
Standards and Statutes 4
  The Nurse Practice Act 4
  Nurse Licensure 4
  Standards of Clinical Nursing Practice 5
  Liability and Legal Issues 5
  Drugs and the Nurse 6
  Negligence/Malpractice 6
Clients' Rights 7
  HIPAA 7
  Consent to Receive Health Services 7
  Nurses' Responsibilities 8
  Patient Self-Determination Act 9
  Advance Medical Directives 9
  Do Not Resuscitate 10
Clinical Practice 10
  Guidelines for Clinical Practice 10
  Providing Client Care 11
  Client's Records 11
  Client's Chart 12
  Basic Nursing Assessment 13
Medical Asepsis Principles 14
  Handwashing 17
Protocol for Procedures 18
MANAGEMENT GUIDELINES 19
CRITICAL THINKING STRATEGIES 20

CHAPTER 2

Nursing Process and Critical Thinking 21

Learning Objectives 22
Nursing Process 22
  Assessment 22
  Nursing Diagnosis 23
  Outcome Identification and Planning 23
  Implementation 23
  Evaluation 24
Critical Thinking 24
Nurses Are Critical Thinkers 25
  Assessment in Critical Thinking 25
  Nursing Diagnosis in Critical Thinking 26
  Planning in Critical Thinking and Outcome Identification 26
  Implementation in Critical Thinking 27
  Evaluation in Critical Thinking 27
Nursing Diagnosis 27
  Types of Nursing Diagnoses 28
  Diagnostic Statement 29
  Components of Nursing Diagnosis 29
Evidence Based Nursing Practice 30
MANAGEMENT GUIDELINES 31
CRITICAL THINKING STRATEGIES 32

CHAPTER 3

Managing Client Care: Documentation and Delegation 33

Learning Objectives 34
Terminology 34
Client Care Plans 35
  Types of Plans 35
  Components of a Care Plan 35
  Critical Paths or Clinical Pathways 38
Charting 40
  Charting—A Method of Communication 40
  Charting Format 41
  Charting for Potential Legal Problems 41
  Forensic Charting 41
  Charting and the Nursing Process 42
  Charting Systems 42
  Computer-Assisted Charting 48
  Minimizing Legal Risks of Computer Charting 51
Legal Forms of Documentation 53

Unusual Occurrence, Variance, or Incident Report 53
Consent Forms 54
Reporting 56
Delegating Client Care 56
Client Acuity Systems 57
RN Delegation 57
Parameters of Delegation 58
Student Clinical Planning 59
Time Management 59
MANAGEMENT GUIDELINES 61
CRITICAL THINKING STRATEGIES 63

CHAPTER 4
Communication and Nurse–Client Relationship 65

Learning Objectives 66
Terminology 66
THEORETICAL CONCEPTS
Communication 67
Guidelines That Influence Effective Communication 67
Guidelines for Communicating with Clients 68
Therapeutic Communication Techniques 68
Blocks to Communication 69
Multicultural Health Care 70
Cultural Competence 70
Cultural Sensitivity 70
Cultural Assessment 71
Spiritual Assessment 71
Relationship Therapy 71
Relationship Principles 71
NURSING DIAGNOSES 73

UNIT ONE: Therapeutic Communication 74
Introducing Yourself to a Client 75
Beginning a Client Interaction 75
Assessing Cultural Preferences 75
Assessing Spiritual Issues 76
Assisting a Client to Describe Personal Experiences 76
Encouraging a Client to Express Needs, Feelings, and Thoughts 77
Using Communication to Increase a Client's Sense of Self-Worth 77
DOCUMENTATION 77
CRITICAL THINKING APPLICATION 78

UNIT TWO: Nurse–Client Relationship 79
Initiating a Nurse–Client Relationship 80
Facilitating a Nurse–Client Relationship 80
Terminating a Nurse–Client Relationship 80
DOCUMENTATION 81
CRITICAL THINKING APPLICATION 81
GERONTOLOGIC CONSIDERATIONS 81
MANAGEMENT GUIDELINES 82
CRITICAL THINKING STRATEGIES 83

CHAPTER 5
Admission and Discharge 84

Learning Objectives 85
Terminology 85
THEORETICAL CONCEPTS
Admission, Transfer, and Discharge 85
Admission to the Hospital 85
Admission to the Nursing Unit 86
Client Transfer 87
Discharge from the Agency 87
NURSING DIAGNOSES 89

UNIT ONE: Admission and Transfer 90
Admitting a Client 91
Transferring a Client 93
DOCUMENTATION 94
CRITICAL THINKING APPLICATION 94

UNIT TWO: Height and Weight 95
Measuring Height and Weight 96
DOCUMENTATION 97
CRITICAL THINKING APPLICATION 98

UNIT THREE: Discharge 99
Discharging a Client 100
Discharging a Client Against Medical Advice (AMA) 101
DOCUMENTATION 101
CRITICAL THINKING APPLICATION 102
GERONTOLOGIC CONSIDERATIONS 102

MANAGEMENT GUIDELINES 103
CRITICAL THINKING STRATEGIES 104

CHAPTER 6
Client Education and Discharge Planning 105

Learning Objectives 106
Terminology 106
THEORETICAL CONCEPTS
Client Education 107
  Readiness to Learn 108
  Resistance to Change 108
  Student Nurse's Role in Client Education 109
Discharge Planning 109
NURSING DIAGNOSES 112

UNIT ONE: Client Education 113
Collecting Data and Establishing Rapport 114
Determining Readiness to Learn 115
Assessing Learning Needs 115
Determining Appropriate Teaching Strategy 117
Selecting the Educational Setting 118
Implementing the Teaching Strategy 119
Evaluating Teaching and Learning 120
DOCUMENTATION 121
CRITICAL THINKING APPLICATION 121

UNIT TWO: Discharge Planning 122
Preparing a Client for Discharge 123
Completing a Discharge Summary 124
DOCUMENTATION 124
CRITICAL THINKING APPLICATION 124
GERONTOLOGIC CONSIDERATIONS 125
MANAGEMENT GUIDELINES 126
CRITICAL THINKING STRATEGIES 127

CHAPTER 7
Safe Client Environment and Restraints 128

Learning Objectives 129
Terminology 129
THEORETICAL CONCEPTS
Orientation to the Client Environment 130
  Maintaining Homeostasis 130
Characteristics that Influence Adaptation 130
  Age 130
  Mental Status 130
  States of Illness 131
Physical and Biological Dimensions 131
  Adequate Space 131
  Natural and Artificial Light 131
  Humidity and Temperature 131
  Ventilation 132
  Comfortable Sound Levels 132
  Furniture: Bed Safety 133
  Food and Water 133
  Hazardous Products and Waste Management 134
Sociocultural Dimensions 134
  Organization of Time 135
  Privacy 135
  Individualized Care 135
  Information and Teaching 135
A Safe Environment 136
  Safety Precautions 137
  Client Falls 138
  Guidelines for the Use of Restraints 138
  Restraint Guidelines 139
NURSING DIAGNOSES 139

UNIT ONE: A Safe Environment 140
Preventing Client Falls 141
Preventing Thermal/Electrical Injuries 142
Providing Safety for Clients During a Fire 143
Providing Safety for Clients Receiving Radioactive Materials 144
DOCUMENTATION 145
CRITICAL THINKING APPLICATION 145

UNIT TWO: Restraints 146
Managing Clients in Restraints 147
Applying Torso/Belt Restraint 148
Using Wrist Restraints 149
Using Mitt Restraints 150
Using Elbow Restraints 151

Applying a Vest Restraint 152
for Client in Bed 152
for Client in Wheelchair 153
Applying Mummy Restraints 154
DOCUMENTATION 155
CRITICAL THINKING APPLICATION 156
GERONTOLOGIC CONSIDERATIONS 157
MANAGEMENT GUIDELINES 157
CRITICAL THINKING STRATEGIES 158

CHAPTER 8
Bathing, Bedmaking, and Maintaining Skin-Integrity 159
Learning Objectives 160
Terminology 160
THEORETICAL CONCEPTS
Basic Health Care 162
Types of Beds 162
Support Surfaces 162
Specialty Beds 162
Bathing 162
Skin Conditions 163
NURSING DIAGNOSES 163

UNIT ONE: **Bedmaking** 165
Folding a Mitered Corner 166
Changing a Pillowcase 166
Making an Unoccupied Bed 166
Making a Surgical Bed 169
Changing an Occupied Bed 169
DOCUMENTATION 171
CRITICAL THINKING APPLICATION 171

UNIT TWO: **Bath Care** 172
Folding a Washcloth Mitt 173
Providing Morning Care 173
Bathing an Adult Client 174
for Female Client 176
for a Male Client 176
Bathing Using Disposable System 176
Bathing an Infant 177
Bathing in a Hydraulic Bathtub Chair 178
DOCUMENTATION 178
CRITICAL THINKING APPLICATION 179

UNIT THREE: **Skin Integrity** 180
Monitoring Skin Condition 181
Preventing Skin Breakdown 182
Preventing Skin Tears 183
Managing Skin Tears 184
Support Surfaces and Specialty Beds 184
DOCUMENTATION 185
CRITICAL THINKING APPLICATION 187

UNIT FOUR: **Evening Care** 188
Providing Evening Care 189
Providing Back Care 189
DOCUMENTATION 191
CRITICAL THINKING APPLICATION 191
GERONTOLOGIC CONSIDERATIONS 191
MANAGEMENT GUIDELINES 192
CRITICAL THINKING STRATEGIES 193

CHAPTER 9
Personal Hygiene 194
Learning Objectives 195
Terminology 195
THEORETICAL CONCEPTS
Hygienic Care 196
Oral Hygiene 196
Hair Care 196
Foot Care 196
Perineal and Genital Care 197
Eye Care 197
NURSING DIAGNOSES 197

UNIT ONE: **Oral Hygiene** 198
Providing Oral Hygiene 199
Flossing Client's Teeth 200
Providing Denture Care 201
Providing Oral Care for Unconscious Clients 202
DOCUMENTATION 203
CRITICAL THINKING APPLICATION 203

UNIT TWO: **Hair Care** 204
Providing Hair Care 205

for Routine Hair Care 205
for Tangled Hair 205
for Coarse or Curly Hair 205
Shampooing Hair 205
for Client in a Chair 206
for Client on a Gurney 206
for Client on Bed Rest 206
for Client Using Disposable System 206
Shaving a Client 207
DOCUMENTATION 208
CRITICAL THINKING APPLICATION 208

UNIT THREE: Pediculosis 209
Removing Lice and Scabies 210
for Using Lindane Lotion for Scabies 210
for Using Lindane Shampoo for Lice 210
for Using Permethrin (Nix) for Lice or Scabies 210
DOCUMENTATION 211
CRITICAL THINKING APPLICATION 212

UNIT FOUR: Foot Care 213
Providing Foot Care 214
Providing Nail Care 214
DOCUMENTATION 215
CRITICAL THINKING APPLICATION 215

UNIT FIVE: Bedpan, Urinal, and Commode 216
Using a Bedpan and Urinal 217
for Using a Bedpan 217
for Using a Urinal 217
Assisting Client to Commode 218
DOCUMENTATION 218
CRITICAL THINKING APPLICATION 219

UNIT SIX: Perineal and Genital Care 220
Draping a Female Client 221
Providing Female Perineal Care 221
Providing Incontinence Care 222
Providing Male Perineal Care 223
DOCUMENTATION 224
CRITICAL THINKING APPLICATION 224

UNIT SEVEN: Eye and Ear Care 225
Providing Routine Eye Care 226
Providing Eye Care for Comatose Client 226
Providing Postoperative Socket Care 226
Removing and Cleaning an Artificial Eye 227
for Heavy Mucus Deposit 228
Removing and Cleaning Contact Lenses 228
Cleaning and Checking a Hearing Aid 229
DOCUMENTATION 230
CRITICAL THINKING APPLICATION 230
GERONTOLOGIC CONSIDERATIONS 231
MANAGEMENT GUIDELINES 231
CRITICAL THINKING STRATEGIES 232

CHAPTER 10
Vital Signs 233

Learning Objectives 234
Terminology 234
THEORETICAL CONCEPTS
Vital Signs 235
Factors Influencing Vital Signs 236
Temperature 237
Regulatory Mechanisms 237
Measuring Body Temperature 238
Pulse 238
Circulatory System Control 238
Heart Rate and Rhythm 239
Evaluating Pulse Quality 239
Respiration 240
Evaluating Respirations 240
Blood Pressure 240
Measuring Blood Pressure 241
Pain 242
NURSING DIAGNOSES 242

UNIT ONE: Temperature 243
Using a Digital Thermometer 244
for Oral Temperature 244
for Axillary Temperature 245
Using an Electronic Thermometer 245
for Oral Temperature 245
for Rectal Temperature 246
Measuring an Infant or Child's Temperature 246
for Oral Route (only for child 3 years or older) 247

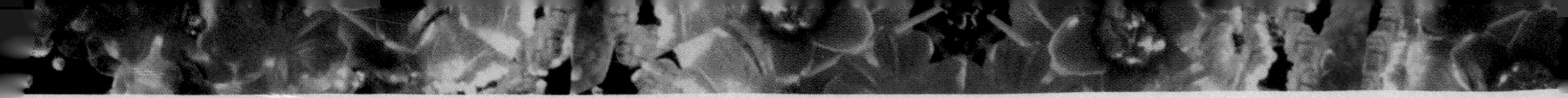

for Rectal Route 247
for Axillary Route 247
Using an Infrared Thermometer for Tympanic Temperature 247
Using a Heat-Sensitive Wearable Thermometer 248
DOCUMENTATION 248
CRITICAL THINKING APPLICATION 249

UNIT TWO: Pulse Rate 250
Determining a Radial Pulse 251
Taking an Apical Pulse 252
Taking an Apical–Radial Pulse 253
Palpating a Peripheral Pulse 254
Monitoring Peripheral Pulses with Doppler Ultrasound Stethoscope 255
DOCUMENTATION 256
CRITICAL THINKING APPLICATION 256

UNIT THREE: Respirations 258
Obtaining the Respiratory Rate 259
DOCUMENTATION 259
CRITICAL THINKING APPLICATION 260

UNIT FOUR: Blood Pressure 261
Measuring a Blood Pressure 262
Palpating Systolic Arterial Blood Pressure 265
Measuring Lower-Extremity Blood Pressure 265
Measuring Blood Pressure by Flush Method in Small Infant 266
Using a Continuous Noninvasive Monitoring Device 267
DOCUMENTATION 267
CRITICAL THINKING APPLICATION 268
GERONTOLOGIC CONSIDERATIONS 269
MANAGEMENT GUIDELINES 270
CRITICAL THINKING STRATEGIES 271
Cross Reference: Assessing Pain—Pain Management, Chapter 16

CHAPTER 11
Physical Assessment 272

Learning Objectives 273
Terminology 273
THEORETICAL CONCEPTS
Assessment 273
Equipment 273
Health History 273
Nurses' Role 273
Examination Techniques 274
Inspection 274
Palpation 274
Percussion 274
Auscultation 274
Focus Assessment 275
Physical Assessment 276
Assessment of the Head and Neck 282
Assessment of the Skin 286
Assessment of the Chest: Lungs, Breasts, and Heart 288
Assessment of the Abdomen, Liver, and Genitourinary Tract 295
Mental Health Assessment 299
Mental Status 299
Obstetrical Assessment 302
Newborn Assessment 308
Apgar Scoring 311
Pediatric Assessment 311
GERONTOLOGIC CONSIDERATIONS 317
MANAGEMENT GUIDELINES 320
CRITICAL THINKING STRATEGIES 321

CHAPTER 12
Body Mechanics and Positioning 322

Learning Objectives 323
Terminology 323
THEORETICAL CONCEPTS
Musculoskeletal System 324
Skeletal Muscles 324
Joints 324
Bones 324
System Alterations 324
Nursing Measures 324
Body Mechanics 324
NURSING DIAGNOSES 325

UNIT ONE: Proper Body Mechanics 326
Establishing Body Alignment 327
Maintaining Proper Body Alignment 328

Using Coordinated Movements 329
Using Basic Principles 329
DOCUMENTATION 331
CRITICAL THINKING APPLICATION 332

UNIT TWO: Moving and Turning Clients 333
Turning to Lateral Position 335
Turning to a Prone Position 335
Moving Client Up in Bed 336
Moving Client with Assistance 337
Transferring Client from Bed to Gurney 337
Moving Client Using Transfer Board 338
Dangling at the Bedside 339
Moving from Bed to Chair 340
Using a Hoyer (Sling) Lift 342
Logrolling the Client 343
Using a Footboard 344
Placing a Trochanter Roll 344
DOCUMENTATION 345
CRITICAL THINKING APPLICATION 345
GERONTOLOGIC CONSIDERATIONS 345
MANAGEMENT GUIDELINES 346
CRITICAL THINKING STRATEGIES 347

CHAPTER 13
Exercise and Ambulation 348

Learning Objectives 349
Terminology 349
THEORETICAL CONCEPTS
Rehabilitation Concepts 350
Musculoskeletal System 350
  Muscle Function 350
Joints 351
  Joint Movements 351
Exercise 351
Ambulation 352
Crutches 352
NURSING DIAGNOSES 353

UNIT ONE: Range of Motion 354
Performing Passive Range of Motion 355
Teaching Active Range of Motion 359
DOCUMENTATION 359
CRITICAL THINKING APPLICATION 359

UNIT TWO: Ambulation 360
Minimizing Orthostatic Hypotension 361
Ambulating with Two Assistants 361
Ambulating with One Assistant 362
Ambulating with a Walker 364
Ambulating with a Cane 364
DOCUMENTATION 366
CRITICAL THINKING APPLICATION 366

UNIT THREE: Crutch Walking 367
Teaching Muscle-Strengthening Exercises 368
Measuring Client for Crutches 368
Teaching Crutch Walking: Four-Point Gait 369
Teaching Crutch Walking: Three-Point Gait 369
Teaching Crutch Walking: Two-Point Gait 370
Teaching Swing-To Gait and Swing-Through Gait 370
Teaching Upstairs and Downstairs Ambulation with Crutches 371
Teaching Moving In and Out of Chair with Crutches 372
DOCUMENTATION 372
CRITICAL THINKING APPLICATION 372
GERONTOLOGIC CONSIDERATIONS 373
MANAGEMENT GUIDELINES 374
CRITICAL THINKING STRATEGIES 375
Cross reference: Continuous Passive Motion Machine, Chapter 30

CHAPTER 14
Infection Control 376

Learning Objectives 377
Terminology 377
THEORETICAL CONCEPTS
Chain of Infection 378
Barriers to Infection 379
  The Body's Natural Defenses 380
Conditions Predisposing to Infection 380
  Surgical Wounds 380
  Antibacterial Immune Mechanisms 380
  Respiratory Tract 381

Genitourinary Tract 381
Invasive Devices 381
Venipuncture Sites 381
Total Parenteral Nutrition Therapy 381
Implanted Prosthetic Devices 382
Nosocomial Infections 382
Standard Precautions 382
Acquired Immunodeficiency Syndrome 385
Epidemiology and Modes of Transmission 385
Definitions 385
Health Care Workers' Exposure to HIV 387
Other Infectious Diseases 387
Tuberculosis 387
Viral Hepatitis 388
Severe Acute Respiratory Syndrome (SARS) 388
NURSING DIAGNOSES 389

UNIT ONE: Basic Medical Asepsis 390
Handwashing (Medical Asepsis) 391
for Using Waterless Antiseptic Agents 393
Cleaning Washable Articles 393
Donning and Removing Clean Gloves 393
Managing Latex Allergies 395
DOCUMENTATION 396
CRITICAL THINKING APPLICATION 396

UNIT TWO: Standard Precautions (Tier One) 397
Donning Protective Gear Utilizing Standard Precautions 398
Exiting a Client's Room Utilizing Standard Precautions 399
DOCUMENTATION 400
CRITICAL THINKING APPLICATION 400

UNIT THREE: Isolation 402
Preparing for Isolation 403
Donning and Removing Isolation Attire 403
Using a Mask 405
Assessing Vital Signs 406
Removing Items from Isolation Room 406
Utilizing Double-Bagging for Isolation 406
Removing a Specimen from Isolation Room 408
Transporting Isolation Client Outside the Room 408
Removing Soiled Large Equipment from Isolation Room 409
DOCUMENTATION 410
CRITICAL THINKING APPLICATION 410
GERONTOLOGIC CONSIDERATIONS 410
MANAGEMENT GUIDELINES 411
CRITICAL THINKING STRATEGIES 412

CHAPTER 15
Bioterrorism–Disaster Nursing 413
Learning Objectives 414
Terminology 414
THEORETICAL CONCEPTS
Introduction 416
Disaster Defined 416
Public Policy 416
Mass Casualty Characteristics 416
Bioterrorism Response Act 416
Disaster Impact on the Infrastructure 417
Disaster Mitigation 417
Community Response Plan 417
Strategic Plan for Responding to Biological or Chemical Terrorism 417
JCAHO Standards 418
A Communication Network for Disaster Management 418
Internal (or In-Hospital) Communication 419
Triage 420
Triage Victim Flow 420
Field Triage 420
Catastrophic Triage 421
Triage and Decontamination 421
Post-Triage Organization 422
Weapons of Mass Destruction 422
Biological Agents 422
Chemical Agents 423
Radiation 424
Ethical Considerations 424
Diversity Considerations 425
Summary 425
NURSING DIAGNOSES 426

UNIT ONE: Bioterrorism Agents, Antidotes, and Vaccinations 427
Identifying Agents of Biological Terrorism 428
Prioritizing High-Risk Groups for Smallpox Vaccination 433
Reconstituting *Vaccinia* Vaccine for Smallpox 434
Administering Reconstituted Smallpox Vaccine 434
Understanding Post-Vaccination Reactions 436
Instructing Client in Post-Vaccination Evaluation 437
Identifying Indications for *Vaccinia* Immune Globulin (VIG) Administration 438
Collecting and Transporting Specimens 438
Identifying Chemical Agent Exposure 439
Triaging for Chemical Agent Exposure 440
Managing Care After Chemical Agent Exposure 441
Identifying Acute Radiation Syndrome 441
DOCUMENTATION 442
CRITICAL THINKING APPLICATION 443

UNIT TWO: Personal Protective Equipment and Decontamination 444
Implementing Hospital Infection Control Protocol 445
Decontaminating via Triage 447
Choosing Protective Equipment for Biological Exposure 448
Choosing Protective Equipment for Chemical Exposure 450
Choosing Protective Equipment for Radiological Attack 450
Decontaminating Victims Following a Biological Terrorist Event 451
Decontaminating Victims Following a Chemical Terrorist Event 451
Decontaminating Victims Following Radiation Exposure 452
Controlling Radiation Contamination 453
DOCUMENTATION 454
CRITICAL THINKING APPLICATION 454

UNIT THREE: Triage and a Communication Matrix 455
Establishing Triage Treatment Areas 456
Establishing Public Health Parameters 456
Developing a Communication Network 457
Establishing Viable Communication 458
Treating Life-Threatening Conditions 458
Assessing Victims Post-Triage 459
Caring for Those Who Died 460
Caring for Clients with Psychological Reactions 461
Identifying Post-Traumatic Stress Disorder 461
DOCUMENTATION 462
CRITICAL THINKING APPLICATION 462
GERONTOLOGIC CONSIDERATIONS 463
MANAGEMENT GUIDELINES 463
CRITICAL THINKING STRATEGIES 464

CHAPTER 16
Pain Management 465
Learning Objectives 466
Terminology 466
THEORETICAL CONCEPTS
Coping with Pain 467
Theories of Pain 468
The Discovery of Endorphins 469
Pain Pathways 470
The Pain Experience 470
Assessing Pain in a Cognitively Impaired or Nonverbal Client 470
JCAHO Standards for Pain Management 471
Noninvasive Pain Relief 471
The Nurse's Role 472
Techniques for Pain Control 473
Patient-Controlled Analgesia (PCA) 473
Epidural Pain Control 475
Direct IV Pain Control 475
Breakthrough Pain Control 475
NURSING DIAGNOSES 476

UNIT ONE: Nonpharmacological Pain Relief 477
Alleviating Pain Through Touch (Massage) 478
Using Relaxation Techniques 478
DOCUMENTATION 479
CRITICAL THINKING APPLICATION 479

UNIT TWO: Pharmacological Pain Management 480
Administering Pain Medications 481
Administering Epidural Narcotic Analgesia 481

for Bolus Injection 483
for Continuous Infusion 483
Qualifying the Client for PCA 483
Administering PCA 484
Terminating a PCA Infusion 487
Teaching PCA to a Client 487
DOCUMENTATION 489
CRITICAL THINKING APPLICATION 489
GERONTOLOGIC CONSIDERATIONS 491
MANAGEMENT GUIDELINES 492
CRITICAL THINKING STRATEGIES 493
Cross reference: End-of-Life Care, Chapter 32

CHAPTER 17

Alternative Therapies and Stress Management 494

Learning Objectives 495
Terminology 495
THEORETICAL CONCEPTS
Stress 496
The Effect of Stress 496
Individual Responses to Stress 497
Stress and Disease 499
Guidelines for Implementing Stress Objectives in Nursing 499
A New Paradigm for Health 501
A Holistic Approach to Health 501
Complementary and Alternative Medicine (CAM) 502
Legal Implications of Alternative Therapy 502
Alternative Treatment Methods 502
NURSING DIAGNOSES 506

UNIT ONE: Stress and Adaptation 507
Determining the Effect of Stress 508
Determining Response Patterns 508
Managing Stress 509
Manipulating the Environment to Reduce Stress 509
Teaching Coping Strategies 509
Managing Stress Using a Holistic Model 510
Teaching Controlled Breathing 510
Teaching Body Relaxation 511
Using Meditation as an Alternative Therapy 512
DOCUMENTATION 512
CRITICAL THINKING APPLICATION 512
GERONTOLOGIC CONSIDERATIONS 513
MANAGEMENT GUIDELINES 513
CRITICAL THINKING STRATEGIES 514

CHAPTER 18

Medication Administration 515

Learning Objectives 516
Terminology 516
THEORETICAL CONCEPTS
Pharmacologic Agents 517
Biologic Effects of Drugs 517
Administering Medications Safely 518
Safety Precautions 518
NURSING DIAGNOSES 519

UNIT ONE: Medication Preparation 520
Preparing Medications 521
Converting Dosage Systems 523
Calculating Dosages 523
Using the Narcotic Control System 524
Using an Automated Dispensing System 524
Administering Medication Protocol 526
CRITICAL THINKING APPLICATION 527

UNIT TWO: Oral Medications 528
Preparing Oral Medications 529
for Liquid Medications 529
for Crushing or Altering Medications 529
Administering Oral Medications to Adults 531
Administering Medications per NG or Enteral Tube 531
Administering Oral Medications to Children 532
for Liquid Medication 532
DOCUMENTATION 533
CRITICAL THINKING APPLICATION 533

UNIT THREE: Topical Medications 534
Applying Topical Medications 535
Applying Cream to Lesions 535
Applying Transdermal Medications 536
Instilling Ophthalmic Drops 537
Administering Ophthalmic Ointment 537

Irrigating the Eye 538
for Bilateral Irrigation 538
Adminstering Otic Medications 539
Irrigating the Ear Canal 539
DOCUMENTATION 540
CRITICAL THINKING APPLICATION 540

UNIT FOUR: Mucous Membrane Medications 542
Administering Sublingual Medications 543
Instilling Nose Drops 543
Administering Metered-Dose Inhaled (MDI) Medications 544
Using MDI with Spacer 545
Administering Medication by Nonpressurized (Nebulized) Aerosol (NPA) 546
Administering Rectal Suppositories 546
Administering Vaginal Suppositories 547
DOCUMENTATION 548
CRITICAL THINKING APPLICATION 548

UNIT FIVE: Parenteral Administration 549
Preparing Injections 550
for Withdrawing Medication from a Vial 550
for Combining Medications in One Syringe Using Two Vials 552
for Withdrawing Medications from an Ampule 553
for Combining Medications Using Alternative Method 553
for Preparing Prefilled Medication Cartridge Syringe 554
Administering Intradermal Injections 554
Administering Subcutaneous (Sub Q) Injections 555
Preparing Insulin Injections 556
for Newly Diagnosed Diabetic Client 556
for Two Insulin Solutions 559
Teaching Use of Insulin Pump 560
Administering Subcutaneous (Sub Q) Heparin 562
Administering Intramuscular (IM) Injections 563
Ventrogluteal Injection Site 564
Dorsogluteal Injection Site 565
Vastus Lateralus Injection Site 566
Using Z-Track Method 567
CRITICAL THINKING APPLICATION 569
GERONTOLOGIC CONSIDERATIONS 570
MANAGEMENT GUIDELINES 571
CRITICAL THINKING STRATEGIES 572

CHAPTER 19
Nutritional Management and NG Intubation 575

Learning Objectives 576
Terminology 576
THEORETICAL CONCEPTS
Nutritional Management 577
Essential Nutrients 577
Macronutrients 578
Carbohydrates 578
Fats 579
Proteins 579
Water 580
Micronutrients 580
Vitamins 580
Minerals 580
RDAs and DRIs 581
Nutritional Assessment 581
Assimilation of Nutrients 581
Gastrointestinal Tract 581
The Accessory Organs 584
Gastrointestinal Dysfunctions 584
Dysphagia 584
GI Hemorrhage 584
Intestinal Obstruction 584
Normal and Therapeutic Nutrition 585
Diet Related to Risk for Heart Disease 585
Nutritional Problems in the Hospital 585
Enteral Feeding for Nutritional Support 585
Therapeutic Management 586
NURSING DIAGNOSES 587

UNIT ONE: Modified Therapeutic Diets 588
Restricting Dietary Carbohydrates 589
Restricting Dietary Protein 589
Restricting Dietary Fat 589
Restricting Mineral Nutrients 590
Providing Nutrient Enhanced Diets 590

Providing Modified Diets 591
for Dietary Fiber 591
for Postoperative Diet Progression 591
Providing Consistency Diets 592
for Bland Diet 592
for Mechanical Soft Diet 592
for Pureed Diet 593
DOCUMENTATION 593
CRITICAL THINKING APPLICATION 593

UNIT TWO: Nutrition Maintenance 595
Serving a Food Tray 596
Assisting the Visually Impaired Client to Eat 596
Assisting the Dysphagic Client to Eat 597
DOCUMENTATION 598
CRITICAL THINKING APPLICATION 598

UNIT THREE: Gastrointestinal Intubation 599
Inserting a Large-Bore Nasogastric (NG) Tube 600
for Testing Blood in Gastric Specimen 601
for Decompressing the GI Tract 603
Irrigating/Maintaining a Nasogastric (NG) Tube 605
Performing Gastric Lavage 606
Administering Poison Control Agents 607
Removing an NG or Nasointestinal Tube 607
DOCUMENTATION 608
CRITICAL THINKING APPLICATION 609

UNIT FOUR: Enteral Tube Feedings 610
Giving an Intermittent Feeding via Large-Bore Nasogastric Tube 611
for Intermittent Feeding via Gastrostomy Tube 613
Dressing the Gastrostomy Tube Site 614
Inserting a Small-Bore Feeding Tube 615
Providing Continuous Feeding via Small-Bore Nasointestinal/Jejunostomy Tube 616
DOCUMENTATION 618
CRITICAL THINKING APPLICATION 618
GERONTOLOGIC CONSIDERATIONS 619
MANAGEMENT GUIDELINES 621
CRITICAL THINKING STRATEGIES 623
Cross reference: TPN and Lipids, Chapter 29

CHAPTER 20
Specimen Collection 624

Learning Objectives 625
Terminology 625
THEORETICAL CONCEPTS
Laboratory Tests 626
Nursing Responsibility 626
Urine Tests 626
Blood Tests 627
Test Tube Types for Specimen Collection 627
Cultures 627
NURSING DIAGNOSES 628

UNIT ONE: Urine Specimens 629
Collecting Midstream Urine 630
for a Male 630
for a Female 630
Collecting 24-Hour Urine Specimen 631
DOCUMENTATION 631
CRITICAL THINKING APPLICATION 632

UNIT TWO: Infant Urine Specimen 633
Collecting a Specimen from an Infant 634
DOCUMENTATION 634
CRITICAL THINKING APPLICATION 634

UNIT THREE: Stool Specimens 635
Collecting Adult Stool Specimen 636
Collecting Stool for Ova and Parasites 636
Collecting Infant Stool Specimen 637
Testing for Occult Blood 637
for gamma Fe-Cult Plus 637
for Hemoccult 638
for Gastroccult 638
Collecting Stool for Bacterial Culture 638
Teaching Parents to Test for Pinworms 638
DOCUMENTATION 639
CRITICAL THINKING APPLICATION 639

UNIT FOUR: Blood Specimens 640
Withdrawing Venous Blood (Phlebotomy) 641
Using Vacutainer System 641
Withdrawing Arterial Blood 643

Collecting a Specimen for Culture 644
Obtaining Blood Specimen for Glucose Testing (Capillary Puncture) 645
Measuring Blood Glucose Using Chemstrip 645
Measuring Blood Glucose Using a Glucometer 646
Monitoring Glucose: Sure Step FLEXX 646
for Quality Control 646
for Monitoring Blood Glucose 647
Measuring Blood Glucose Using Lifescan One-Touch II 647
DOCUMENTATION 649
CRITICAL THINKING APPLICATION 649

UNIT FIVE: Sputum Collection 650
Obtaining Sputum Specimen 651
Using Suction Trap 652
Collecting Specimen by Transtracheal Aspiration 652
DOCUMENTATION 653
CRITICAL THINKING APPLICATION 653

UNIT SIX: Throat and Wound Specimens for Culture 654
Obtaining a Throat Specimen 655
Obtaining Wound Specimen for Aerobic Culture 655
Obtaining Wound Specimen for Anaerobic Culture 656
DOCUMENTATION 657
CRITICAL THINKING APPLICATION 657
GERONTOLOGIC CONSIDERATIONS 657
MANAGEMENT GUIDELINES 658
CRITICAL THINKING STRATEGIES 659

CHAPTER 21
Diagnostic Procedures 660

Learning Objectives 661
Terminology 661
THEORETICAL CONCEPTS
Test Preparation 662
Instituting Standard Precautions 663
X-ray Studies 663
Ultrasound Studies 663
Nuclear Scanning 663
Microscopic Studies 664
Endoscopic Studies 664
Fluid Analysis Studies 664
Magnetic Resonance Imaging (MRI) 664
Assisting the Physician during Tests 664
NURSING DIAGNOSES 665

UNIT ONE: X-Ray Studies 666
Preparing for X-Ray Studies 667
for Oral Cholecystography 667
for Intravenous Pyelography (IVP) 668
for Myelography 668
for Arteriography 669
for Computed Tomography (CT Scan) 669
for Cardiac Catheterization 670
for Bone Densitometry 670
for Magnetic Resonance Imaging (MRI) 671
for Mammography 672
DOCUMENTATION 672
CRITICAL THINKING APPLICATION 673

UNIT TWO: Nuclear Scanning 674
Preparing for Nuclear Scans 675
for Bone Scan 675
for Lung Scan 675
for PET Scan 676
for Nuclear Cardiography 676
for Thyroid Scans 677
Teaching for Nuclear Scans 677
DOCUMENTATION 677
CRITICAL THINKING APPLICATION 678

UNIT THREE: Barium Studies 679
Preparing for Barium Studies 680
for Barium Enema 680
for Barium Swallow Study 680
for Small Bowel Follow-Through 681
DOCUMENTATION 681
CRITICAL THINKING APPLICATION 681

UNIT FOUR: Endoscopic Studies 682
Preparing for Endoscopic Studies 683
for Arthroscopy 683
for Bronchoscopy 683

for Colonoscopy 684
for Cystoscopy 684
for Gastrointestinal Tract Endoscopy 685
for Laparoscopy 685
for Sigmoidoscopy 685
DOCUMENTATION 686
CRITICAL THINKING APPLICATION 687

UNIT FIVE: Fluid Analysis and Microscopic Studies 688
Assisting with Lumbar Puncture 689
Assisting with Liver Biopsy 690
Assisting with Thoracentesis 691
Assisting with Paracentesis 692
Assisting with Bone Marrow Aspiration 693
Assisting with Vaginal Examination and Papanicolaou (Pap) Smear 693
Assisting with Amniocentesis 694
DOCUMENTATION 694
CRITICAL THINKING APPLICATION 695
GERONTOLOGIC CONSIDERATIONS 695
MANAGEMENT GUIDELINES 696
CRITICAL THINKING STRATEGIES 697

CHAPTER 22
Urinary Elimination 698

Learning Objectives 699
Terminology 699
THEORETICAL CONCEPTS
Urinary System 700
Urine Production 700
Micturition 701
Alterations in Urinary Elimination 702
Alterations Related to Fluids 702
Alterations Related to Obstructions 702
Alterations Related to Aldosterone and Antidiuretic Hormone 702
Alterations Related to Changes in Blood Volume 702
Alterations in Disease States 702
Alterations Related to End-Stage Renal Disease 703
Nursing Interventions 703
NURSING DIAGNOSES 703

UNIT ONE: Intake and Output 704
Measuring Intake and Output 705
DOCUMENTATION 706
CRITICAL THINKING APPLICATION 707

UNIT TWO: External Catheter System 708
Applying a Condom Catheter 709
Attaching Catheter to Leg Bag 709
DOCUMENTATION 710
CRITICAL THINKING APPLICATION 710

UNIT THREE: Catheterization 712
Draping a Female Client 713
Using a Bladder Scanner 713
Inserting a Straight Catheter (Female) 714
Inserting a Straight Catheter (Male) 716
Inserting a Retention Catheter (Female) 717
Inserting a Retention Catheter (Male) 721
Providing Catheter Care 722
Removing a Retention Catheter 723
DOCUMENTATION 724
CRITICAL THINKING APPLICATION 724

UNIT FOUR: Bladder Irrigation 726
Irrigating by Opening a Closed System 727
Irrigating a Closed System 728
Maintaining Continuous Bladder Irrigation 729
DOCUMENTATION 730
CRITICAL THINKING APPLICATION 730

UNIT FIVE: Suprapubic Catheter Care 732
Providing Suprapubic Catheter Care 733
DOCUMENTATION 734
CRITICAL THINKING APPLICATION 734

UNIT SIX: Specimens from Closed Systems 735
Collecting Specimen from a Closed System 736
DOCUMENTATION 736
CRITICAL THINKING APPLICATION 737

UNIT SEVEN: Urinary Diversion 738
Applying a Urinary Diversion Pouch 739
Obtaining Specimen from an Ileal Conduit 742
Catheterizing Continent Urinary Reservoir 742

DOCUMENTATION 743
CRITICAL THINKING APPLICATION 743

Unit Eight: Hemodialysis (Renal Replacement Therapy) 745
Providing Hemodialysis 746
for AV Fistula or Graft 747
Providing Ongoing Care of Hemodialysis Client 748
Terminating Hemodialysis 748
Maintaining Central Venous Dual-Lumen Catheter (DLC) 749
DOCUMENTATION 751
CRITICAL THINKING APPLICATION 751
GERONTOLOGIC CONSIDERATIONS 752
MANAGEMENT GUIDELINES 752
CRITICAL THINKING STRATEGIES 754
Cross reference: Urine Studies in Chapter 20; Peritoneal Dialysis (CAPD) in Chapter 34; Self-Catheterization (Male and Female) in Chapter 34; Suprapubic Catheter Care at Home in Chapter 34

CHAPTER 23
Bowel Elimination 755

Learning Objectives 756
Terminology 756
THEORETICAL CONCEPTS
Anatomy and Physiology 757
Defecation 758
Constipation 758
Alterations in Elimination 759
Changes in Motility 759
Obstruction of the Lumen of the Bowel 759
Circulatory Deficiencies 760
Surgically Induced Alterations in Bowel 760
NURSING DIAGNOSES 762

UNIT ONE: Bowel Evacuation 763
Removing a Fecal Impaction 764
Providing Digital Stimulation 764
Developing a Regular Bowel Routine 765
Administering a Suppository 766
DOCUMENTATION 767
CRITICAL THINKING APPLICATION 767

UNIT TWO: Enema Administration 768
Administering a Large-Volume Enema 769
Administering an Enema to a Child 771
Administering a Small-Volume Enema 772
Administering a Retention Enema 772
Administering a Return Flow Enema 773
DOCUMENTATION 774
CRITICAL THINKING APPLICATION 774

UNIT THREE: Fecal Ostomy Pouch Application 775
Applying a Fecal Ostomy Pouch 776
DOCUMENTATION 781
CRITICAL THINKING APPLICATION 781
GERONTOLOGIC CONSIDERATIONS 782
MANAGEMENT GUIDELINES 782
CRITICAL THINKING STRATEGIES 784
Cross reference: Colostomy Irrigation (*See* Home Care, Chapter 34); Bedpan (*See* Personal Hygiene, Chapter 9)

CHAPTER 24
Heat and Cold Therapies 785

Learning Objectives 786
Terminology 786
THEORETICAL CONCEPTS
Temperature Control 787
Adjustment Processes 787
Processes of Heat Transfer 788
The Inflammatory Process 788
Conditions That Affect Adaptive Processes 789
Hyperthermia (Body Temperature Exceeding 41.1°C) 789
Hypothermia (Body Temperature of 35°C) 789
Cold Therapies (Cryotherapies) 790
Heat Therapies (Thermotherapies) 790
NURSING DIAGNOSES 791

UNIT ONE: Heat Therapies 792
Applying a Commercial Heat Pack 793
Monitoring an Infant Radiant Warmer 793
Applying an Aquathermic Pad 794
Applying a Hot Moist Pack 795
Assisting with a Sitz Bath 796

DOCUMENTATION 797
CRITICAL THINKING APPLICATION 797

UNIT TWO: Cold Therapies 798
Applying an Ice Pack/Commercial Cold Pack 799
Applying a Disposable Instant (Chemical) Cold Pack 800
DOCUMENTATION 801
CRITICAL THINKING APPLICATION 801

UNIT THREE: Systemic Cooling Therapies 802
Providing a Tepid Bath 803
Using a Cooling Blanket 804
DOCUMENTATION 806
CRITICAL THINKING APPLICATION 807
GERONTOLOGIC CONSIDERATIONS 808
MANAGEMENT GUIDELINES 809
CRITICAL THINKING STRATEGIES 810

CHAPTER 25
Wound Care and Dressings 811

Learning Objectives 812
Terminology 812
THEORETICAL CONCEPTS
Wound Healing 813
 Inflammatory Phase 813
 Proliferative, or Granulation, Phase 813
 Maturation, or Wound-Remodeling, Phase 813
Wound Classification 814
Types of Wound Healing 814
 Primary Intention 814
 Secondary Intention 814
 Tertiary Intention 814
Major Factors Affecting Wound Healing 814
 Nutrition 814
 General Physical Health 814
 Medications 814
Goals of Wound Care 815
 Complications Associated with Wound Healing 815
Wound Infections 816
 Wound Specimens for Culture 816
 Wounds Caused by Vascular Insufficiency 816
 Venous Ulcers 816
 Arterial Ulcers 816
 Pressure Ulcers 816
Adjunctive Wound Care Therapy 817
NURSING DIAGNOSES 818

UNIT ONE: Measures to Prevent Infection 819
Completing a Surgical Hand Scrub 820
Donning Sterile Gloves 820
Pouring from a Sterile Container 822
Preparing a Sterile Field 822
 for Commercially Prepared Packages 823
 for Hospital-Wrapped Packages 823
Preparing a Sterile Field Using Prepackaged Supplies 824
Preparing for Dressing Change with Individual Supplies 824
DOCUMENTATION 825
CRITICAL THINKING APPLICATION 825

UNIT TWO: Dressing Change 826
Changing a Dry Sterile Dressing 827
Removing Sutures 828
Removing Staples 829
DOCUMENTATION 830
CRITICAL THINKING APPLICATION 830

UNIT THREE: Wound Care 831
Assessing a Wound 832
Changing a Wound Dressing 834
Packing a Wound 836
Changing a Dressing for a Venous Ulcer 837
Assessing Ankle–Brachial Index (ABI) 840
Caring for a Wound with a Drain 840
Applying an Abdominal Binder 842
Maintaining Wound Drainage System 842
Irrigating Wounds 844
DOCUMENTATION 845
CRITICAL THINKING APPLICATION 845

UNIT FOUR: Wet-to-Moist Dressings 847
Applying Wet-to-Moist Dressings 848
DOCUMENTATION 849
CRITICAL THINKING APPLICATION 849

UNIT FIVE: Pressure Ulcers 850
Preventing Pressure Ulcers 853

Applying Transparent Adhesive Film Dressing 854
Using Hydrocolloid Dressing 857
DOCUMENTATION 860
CRITICAL THINKING APPLICATION 860

UNIT SIX: Adjunctive Wound Care Therapy 861
Using Electrical Stimulation 862
Using Noncontact Normothermic Wound Therapy 863
for Using Warm-Up® Therapy System 863
for Changing Wound Cover 864
for Charging Batteries 864
Using Vacuum Assisted Closure (V.A.C.®) 865
for Removing Dressing 866
for Disconnecting V.A.C.® Unit 866
for Reconnecting V.A.C.® Unit 866
for Changing Canister 866
CRITICAL THINKING APPLICATION 867
GERONTOLOGIC CONSIDERATIONS 867
MANAGEMENT GUIDELINES 868
CRITICAL THINKING STRATEGIES 869
Cross reference: Chapter 8 for Special Beds

CHAPTER 26
Respiratory Care 870
Learning Objectives 871
Terminology 871
THEORETICAL CONCEPTS
The Respiratory System 872
Processes of Respiration 872
Alterations in Respiration 873
Alterations in Ventilation 873
Alterations in Diffusion 873
Alterations in Perfusion 873
Assessment of Respiratory Function 874
Nursing Interventions 874
NURSING DIAGNOSES 875

UNIT ONE: Respiratory Preventive and Maintenance Measures 876
Instructing Client to Deep Breathe 877
Instructing Client to Cough 877
Teaching Diaphragmatic Breathing 878
Teaching Use of an Incentive Spirometer (IS) 878
Teaching Peak Flow Measurement 879
Providing CPAP/BIPAP 880
Providing Bag–Valve–Mask Ventilation 881
DOCUMENTATION 882
CRITICAL THINKING APPLICATION 882

UNIT TWO: Chest Physiotherapy (CPT) 883
Preparing Client for CPT 884
Performing Postural Drainage 884
Performing Chest Percussion 885
Performing Chest Vibration 885
DOCUMENTATION 886
CRITICAL THINKING APPLICATION 886

UNIT THREE: Oxygen Administration 887
Monitoring Clients Receiving Oxygen 888
Using Pulse Oximetry 888
Using an Oxygen Analyzer 890
Using an Oxygen Cylinder 890
Using Nasal Cannula 891
Using an Oxygen Face Mask 892
Providing Oxygen Via a Pediatric Oxygen Tent 894
for Setting Up Pediatric Tent 894
for Monitoring Child in Tent 894
Using an Oxygen Hood 895
DOCUMENTATION 895
CRITICAL THINKING APPLICATION 895

UNIT FOUR: Artificial Intubated Airways 897
Inserting an Oropharyngeal Airway 898
Inserting a Nasopharyngeal Airway (Nasal Trumpet) 898
Assisting with Endotracheal Intubation 899
Providing Care for Client with Endotracheal Tube 900
Extubating an Endotracheal Tube 901
DOCUMENTATION 901
CRITICAL THINKING APPLICATION 902

UNIT FIVE: Suctioning 903
Suctioning Using Catheter and Gloves 904
Suctioning Using Catheter in Sleeve 906
Suctioning with In-Line Closed Suction System 907
DOCUMENTATION 908
CRITICAL THINKING APPLICATION 909

UNIT SIX: Tracheostomy Care 910
Assisting with Tracheostomy Intubation 911
Performing Tracheostomy Suctioning 912
Inflating a Tracheal Tube Cuff 914
Cleaning the Inner Cannula and Ostomy 914
Changing Tracheostomy Tube Ties 916
for Twill Tape Ties 916
Capping with a Passey–Muir Valve 917
DOCUMENTATION 918
CRITICAL THINKING APPLICATION 919

UNIT SEVEN: Chest Drainage Systems 921
Maintaining a Two-Bottle Drainage/Suction System 922
for Gravity Drainage 922
for Suction 922
Setting Up and Maintaining a Disposable Water Seal Chest Drainage System 923
Administering Autotransfusion Using Pleur-Evac ATS 925
Assisting with Removal of Chest Tube 926
DOCUMENTATION 927
CRITICAL THINKING APPLICATION 928
GERONTOLOGIC CONSIDERATIONS 929
MANAGEMENT GUIDELINES 929
CRITICAL THINKING STRATEGIES 931

CHAPTER 27
Circulatory Maintenance 932

Learning Objectives 933
Terminology 933
THEORETICAL CONCEPTS
The Circulatory System 934
Electrical Conduction 935
Pacemakers 936
ECG 936
Alterations in Circulation 936
Hemorrhage 937
Shock 937
Heart Failure 937
Ischemia 938
Thrombosis and Embolism 938
Altered Circulation 938
Assessment 938
Emergency Life Support Measures 938
Early Defibrilation Programs in Hospitals 939
Planning and Intervention 939
Fetal Monitoring 939
NURSING DIAGNOSES 941

UNIT ONE: Control of Bleeding 942
Using Digital Pressure 943
Using Pressure Dressing 943
DOCUMENTATION 944
CRITICAL THINKING APPLICATION 944

UNIT TWO: Circulatory Maintenance 945
Applying Graduated Compression Stockings (Elastic Hosiery) 946
Applying Pneumatic Compression Devices 947
DOCUMENTATION 950
CRITICAL THINKING APPLICATION 951

UNIT THREE: Electrocardiogram (ECG) Monitoring 952
Monitoring the ECG 953
Interpreting an ECG Strip 955
Recording a 12-Lead ECG 957
Monitoring Clients on Telemetry 959
DOCUMENTATION 961
CRITICAL THINKING APPLICATION 961

UNIT FOUR: Emergency Life Support Measures 963
Administering Basic Life Support to an Adult 964
for Unresponsiveness 964
for Airway 964
for Rescue Breathing 966
for Circulation 966
for Continuing CPR 967
Placing Victim in Recovery Position 968
Administering CPR to a Child 968
Providing Bag–Valve–Mask Ventilation 969
Using an Automated External Defibrillator (AED) 970
Administering the Heimlich Maneuver for Conscious Client 971
Administering the Heimlich Maneuver for Unresponsive Client 972
Calling a Code 973
Maintaining the Emergency "Crash" Cart 975

Performing Defibrillation 975
Providing Care Following Code 975
DOCUMENTATION 975
CRITICAL THINKING APPLICATION 976

UNIT FIVE: Pacemaker Management 977
Assisting with Pacemaker Insertion 978
Maintaining Pacemaker Function 979
Providing Client Teaching 980
DOCUMENTATION 981
CRITICAL THINKING APPLICATION 981

UNIT SIX: Fetal Monitoring 983
Auscultating Fetal Heart Tones 984
Applying External Electronic Fetal Monitoring 984
Interpreting Electronic Fetal Monitoring Tracings 985
Assessing Periodic Fetal Heart Changes 986
DOCUMENTATION 989
CRITICAL THINKING APPLICATION 989
GERONTOLOGIC CONSIDERATIONS 990
MANAGEMENT GUIDELINES 991
CRITICAL THINKING STRATEGIES 992
Cross reference: Chapter 33, Advanced Nursing Skills

CHAPTER 28
Intravenous Therapy 993
Learning Objectives 994
Terminology 994
THEORETICAL CONCEPTS
Fluid and Electrolyte Balance 995
  Fluids 995
  Electrolytes 996
Fluid and Electrolyte Imbalance 996
IV Administration 997
NURSING DIAGNOSES 997

UNIT ONE: Initiating Intravenous Therapy 998
Preparing the Infusion System 999
Adding Extension Tubing 1001
Preparing the Venipuncture Site 1002
Inserting a Winged Needle 1003
Inserting an Over-the-Needle Catheter 1006
DOCUMENTATION 1009
CRITICAL THINKING APPLICATION 1009

UNIT TWO: Intravenous Management 1010
Regulating Infusion Flow Rate 1011
Using an Electronic Flow-Control Device 1012
Using a Syringe Pump 1013
Managing the IV Site 1014
  for IV Administration Sets 1014
  for Converting from Continuous IV to a "Lock" 1015
  for Applying a Transparent Dressing 1015
Converting IV to Saline Lock 1016
Changing Gown for Client with IV 1017
Discontinuing an IV 1018
DOCUMENTATION 1019
CRITICAL THINKING APPLICATION 1020

UNIT THREE: Intake and Output 1021
Monitoring Intake and Output 1022
Monitoring IV Intake 1024
DOCUMENTATION 1024
CRITICAL THINKING APPLICATION 1025

UNIT FOUR: IV Medication Administration 1026
Adding Medication to IV Solution 1027
Using a Secondary ("Piggyback") Bag 1027
Using a Volume Control Set 1029
Using a Peripheral Saline Lock 1030
Administering Medications by Peripheral IV Line Injection "Push" 1031
DOCUMENTATION 1032
CRITICAL THINKING APPLICATION 1032

UNIT FIVE: Blood Transfusions 1033
Administering Blood through a Y-Set 1034
Administering Blood through a Straight Line 1036
Administering Blood Components 1037
Monitoring for Potential Complications 1037
DOCUMENTATION 1040
CRITICAL THINKING APPLICATION 1040
GERONTOLOGIC CONSIDERATIONS 1041
MANAGEMENT GUIDELINES 1041
CRITICAL THINKING STRATEGIES 1043

CHAPTER 29

Central Vascular Access Devices 1044

Learning Objectives 1045
Terminology 1045
THEORETICAL CONCEPTS
Central Vascular Access Devices 1046
Peripheral Catheter 1046
Midline Catheter 1046
Central Vascular Access Devices 1046
Client Selection for CVADs 1047
Subcutaneously Implanted Ports 1047
Peripheral Insertion of a Central Catheter (PICC) 1047
Total Parenteral Nutrition 1047
NURSING DIAGNOSES 1048

UNIT ONE: Percutaneous Central Vascular Catheters 1049
Assisting with Percutaneous Central Vascular Catheterization 1050
Changing a Central Line Catheter Dressing 1051
Infusing IV Fluids Through a Central Line 1053
Drawing Blood from Central Line Catheter 1055
Applying a BIOPATCH 1057
Changing an Access Cap 1058
Measuring and Monitoring Central Venous Pressure (CVP) 1059
DOCUMENTATION 1061
CRITICAL THINKING APPLICATION 1061

UNIT TWO: Total Parenteral Nutrition/Total Nutrient Admixture 1063
Assisting with Catheter Insertion 1064
Maintaining Hyperalimentation Infusions (TPN) 1066
Changing Hyperalimentation (TPN) Dressing and Tubing 1067
Maintaining Hyperalimentation for Children 1068
DOCUMENTATION 1068
CRITICAL THINKING APPLICATION 1069

UNIT THREE: Lipid Emulsion Therapy 1070
Infusing IV Lipids 1071
DOCUMENTATION 1072
CRITICAL THINKING APPLICATION 1073

UNIT FOUR: Tunneled Central Vascular Access Devices (CVADs) 1074
Maintaining the Hickman or Broviac CV Catheter 1075
Changing the Hickman or Broviac CV Catheter Dressing 1076
Maintaining the CV Catheter with Groshong Valve 1076
for 10- or 20-mL Irrigation 1077
Drawing Blood from the CV Catheter with Groshong Valve 1078
DOCUMENTATION 1078
CRITICAL THINKING APPLICATION 1079

UNIT FIVE: Implanted Subcutaneous Port 1080
Accessing and Flushing an Implanted Port Using a Huber Needle 1081
Administering Drugs via a Subcutaneous Implanted Port 1082
Administering Infusions via a Subcutaneous Port 1083
Drawing Blood from an Implanted Subcutaneous Port 1084
DOCUMENTATION 1085
CRITICAL THINKING APPLICATION 1085

UNIT SIX: Peripherally Inserted Central Catheter (PICC) 1086
Maintaining the PICC 1087
Changing the PICC Dressing 1088
Drawing Blood from the PICC 1090
Removing the PICC 1090
DOCUMENTATION 1091
CRITICAL THINKING APPLICATION 1091
GERONTOLOGIC CONSIDERATIONS 1092
MANAGEMENT GUIDELINES 1092
CRITICAL THINKING STRATEGIES 1094

CHAPTER 30

Orthopedic Interventions 1095

Learning Objectives 1096
Terminology 1096
THEORETICAL CONCEPTS
Restoring Function 1097
Fractures 1097
Casts 1098

Traction 1098
Acute Compartment Syndrome 1099
Joint Replacement (Arthroplasty) 1099
Hip Fracture 1100
Amputation 1100
Orthopedic Assessment 1101
NURSING DIAGNOSES 1101

UNIT ONE: Application of Immobilizing Devices 1102
Applying a Sling 1103
Applying Spiral Bandage 1104
Applying a Figure-Eight Bandage 1104
Applying a Splint 1105
Applying a Cervical Collar 1106
Applying a Jewett–Taylor Back Brace 1106
DOCUMENTATION 1107
CRITICAL THINKING APPLICATION 1107

UNIT TWO: Cast Care 1109
Caring for a Wet Cast 1110
Assessing a Casted Extremity 1111
Instructing Client in Self Care 1112
DOCUMENTATION 1113
CRITICAL THINKING APPLICATION 1113

UNIT THREE: Traction 1114
Maintaining Skin Traction 1115
Maintaining Skeletal Traction 1117
Maintaining an External Fixator Device 1119
Maintaining Halo Traction 1120
DOCUMENTATION 1121
CRITICAL THINKING APPLICATION 1121

UNIT FOUR: Clients with an Amputation 1123
Positioning and Exercising the Stump 1124
Shrinking/Molding the Stump 1125
DOCUMENTATION 1126
CRITICAL THINKING APPLICATION 1126

UNIT FIVE: Client with Joint Replacement 1127
Caring for a Client with Hip Arthroplasty 1128
for Bed Positioning 1128
for Strengthening Exercises 1128
for Mobility and Dislocation Prevention 1129
for Assistive Devices and Adaptive Aids 1129
Caring for a Client with Knee Arthroplasty 1130
for Bed Positioning 1130
for Strengthening Exercises 1130
for Getting Out of Bed 1131
DOCUMENTATION 1131
CRITICAL THINKING APPLICATION 1131

UNIT SIX: Stryker Frame 1132
Using a Stryker Wedge Turning Frame 1133
Turning from Supine to Prone 1133
Using a Stryker Parallel Frame 1133
Assisting Client with Bedpan 1134
DOCUMENTATION 1134
CRITICAL THINKING APPLICATION 1134
GERONTOLOGIC CONSIDERATIONS 1135
MANAGEMENT GUIDELINES 1135
CRITICAL THINKING STRATEGIES 1137

CHAPTER 31
Perioperative Care 1138

Learning Objectives 1139
Terminology 1139
THEORETICAL CONCEPTS
The Surgical Experience 1140
Perioperative Care 1140
Intraoperative Stage 1142
NURSING DIAGNOSES 1144

UNIT ONE: Stress in Preoperative Clients 1145
Preventing Anxiety and Stress 1146
Reducing Anxiety and Stress 1146
Assisting the Client Who Uses Denial 1147
DOCUMENTATION 1147
CRITICAL THINKING APPLICATION 1147

UNIT TWO: Preoperative Teaching 1148
Providing Surgical Information 1149
for the Preoperative Client in the Hospital 1149
for the Preoperative Client in an Outpatient Setting 1149
for the Intraoperative Client 1149
for the Postoperative Client 1150

Providing Client Teaching 1150
Providing Family Teaching 1150
Teaching for Laser Therapy 1151
Teaching for Lithotripsy 1152
Teaching for Diagnostic Laparoscopy 1153
Teaching for Arthroscopy 1154
Instructing in Deep Breathing Exercises 1155
Instructing in Coughing Exercises 1155
Providing Instruction to Turn in Bed 1156
Instructing in Leg Exercises 1156
DOCUMENTATION 1156
CRITICAL THINKING APPLICATION 1156

UNIT THREE: Preoperative Care 1158
Obtaining Baseline Data 1159
Preparing the Surgical Site 1159
Preparing the Client for Surgery 1161
Administering Preoperative Medications 1164
DOCUMENTATION 1164
CRITICAL THINKING APPLICATION 1165

UNIT FOUR: Conscious Sedation 1166
Preparing Client for Conscious Sedation 1167
Monitoring Client During Procedure 1168
Caring for Client Following Conscious Sedation 1169
DOCUMENTATION 1169
CRITICAL THINKING APPLICATION 1170

UNIT FIVE: Postanesthesia Care Unit (PACU) and Discharge 1171
Providing Postanesthesia Care 1172
Discharging Client from Postanesthesia Unit to Nursing Unit 1172
Discharging Client from Phase II Unit to Home 1174
DOCUMENTATION 1174
CRITICAL THINKING APPLICATION 1175

UNIT SIX: Postoperative Care 1176
Providing Postanesthesia Care 1177
Administering Postanesthesia Medications 1177
DOCUMENTATION 1178
CRITICAL THINKING APPLICATION 1178
GERONTOLOGIC CONSIDERATIONS 1179
MANAGEMENT GUIDELINES 1180
CRITICAL THINKING STRATEGIES 1182
Cross reference: Chapter 16, Pain Management

CHAPTER 32
End-of-Life Care 1183

Learning Objectives 1184
Terminology 1184
THEORETICAL CONCEPTS
Loss and Grieving 1184
  Stages of Grief 1185
Stages of Dying 1185
Core Principles for End of Life Care 1186
Managing Pain 1186
The Hospice Option 1187
NURSING DIAGNOSES 1188

UNIT ONE: The Grief Process 1189
Understanding Grief 1190
Assisting with Grief 1190
DOCUMENTATION 1191
CRITICAL THINKING APPLICATION 1191

UNIT TWO: The Dying Client 1192
Supporting the Client Near the End of Life 1193
Providing Pain Management at the End of Life 1195
Assisting the Dying Client 1196
Supporting the Family or Caregiver 1198
DOCUMENTATION 1199
CRITICAL THINKING APPLICATION 1199

UNIT THREE: Postmortem Care 1200
Providing Postmortem Care 1201
CRITICAL THINKING APPLICATION 1202
GERONTOLOGIC CONSIDERATIONS 1203
MANAGEMENT GUIDELINES 1203
CRITICAL THINKING STRATEGIES 1204

CHAPTER 33
Advanced Nursing Skills 1205

Learning Objectives 1206
Terminology 1206

THEORETICAL CONCEPTS
Advanced Skills in Nursing Practice 1207

UNIT ONE: Pulmonary Artery Pressure (Hemodynamic) Monitoring 1209
Leveling and Zeroing the Monitor System 1211
Assisting Physician with Catheter Insertion 1212
Obtaining Pressure Readings 1214
Measuring Cardiac Output 1215
DOCUMENTATION 1215
CRITICAL THINKING APPLICATION 1216

UNIT TWO: Arterial Blood Pressure Monitoring 1217
Performing the Allen's Test 1218
Assisting with Arterial Line Insertion 1219
Monitoring Arterial Blood Pressure 1219
Withdrawing Arterial Blood Samples 1221
Removing Arterial Catheter 1222
DOCUMENTATION 1223
CRITICAL THINKING APPLICATION 1223

UNIT THREE: Cardiac Emergencies 1225
Maintaining the Emergency Cart 1226
Checking Contents of the Emergency Cart 1227
Calling a Code 1228
Performing Defibrillation 1228
Administering Advanced Life-Support Medications 1230
Assisting with Elective Synchronized Cardioversion 1231
DOCUMENTATION 1233
CRITICAL THINKING 1233

UNIT FOUR: Mechanical Ventilation 1235
Alterations of Ventilation and Gas Exchange 1236
Caring for Clients on Ventilators 1236
Weaning the Mechanically Ventilated Client 1239
DOCUMENTATION 1240
CRITICAL THINKING APPLICATION 1240
GERONTOLOGIC CONSIDERATIONS 1242
MANAGEMENT GUIDELINES 1242
CRITICAL THINKING STRATEGIES 1244
Cross reference: Chapter 27, Circulatory Maintenance

CHAPTER 34
Community-Based Nursing 1245
Learning Objectives 1246
THEORETICAL CONCEPTS
Introduction 1246
- Legal Issues in Home Care 1247
- Home Care Definition 1248
- Home Health Team 1248
- Referral to Home Care 1248
- Transition from Hospital to Home 1249
- Client Teaching 1249
- Adapting Care to the Home Setting 1249
- Plan of Treatment 1249
- Documentation 1249

NURSING DIAGNOSES 1251

UNIT ONE: Admission to Home Care 1252
Identifying Eligibility for Medicare Reimbursement 1254
Completing Admission Documentation 1255
Maintaining Nurse's Safety 1255
Assessing Home for Safe Environment 1256
Evaluating Client's Safety 1257
Assessing Caregiver's Safety 1257
Assessing for Elder Abuse 1258

UNIT TWO: Infection Control 1259
NURSING DIAGNOSES 1260
Preparing for Client Care 1261
Disposing of Waste Material in the Home Setting 1261
Cleansing Thermometers 1262
Caring for an AIDS or HIV Client in the Home 1262
Cleansing Equipment in the Home Setting 1263
Teaching Preventive Measures in the Home 1263
Teaching Safer Practices to IV Drug Users 1264

UNIT THREE: Body Mechanics 1265
NURSING DIAGNOSIS 1266
Positioning Nonhospital Bed for Client Care 1267
Moving a Helpless Client Up in Bed Without Assistance 1267

UNIT FOUR: Hygienic Care 1268
Bathing 1269

Skin Care 1269
Pressure Ulcer Care 1269
Hair Care 1269
NURSING DIAGNOSES 1270
Bathing Client in the Home 1270
Transferring Client to Tub or Shower 1270
Adapting Bedmaking to the Home 1271
Providing Pressure Ulcer Care 1271
Preparing Normal Saline 1271
Removing Lice 1272

UNIT FIVE: Medications 1273
NURSING DIAGNOSES 1274
Administering Medications 1274
Sterilizing Nondisposable Medication Equipment 1275

UNIT SIX: Total Nutrient Admixture 1276
Total Nutrient Admixture (TNA) 1277
NURSING DIAGNOSES 1278
Administering Total Nutritional Admixture (TNA) in the Home 1278
Monitoring Client on TNA 1279
Discontinuing TNA Infusion 1279

UNIT SEVEN: Elimination 1281
Urinary Elimination 1282
Bowel Elimination 1282
NURSING DIAGNOSES 1283
Using Clean Technique for Intermittent Self-Catheterization 1283
for Female Client 1283
for Male Client 1284
Providing Suprapubic Catheter Care 1284
Administering Continuous Ambulatory Peritoneal Dialysis (CAPD) 1285
for Draining Fluid 1285
for Infusing Dialysate 1286
Changing Dressing for CAPD Client 1286
Instructing Client in Colostomy Irrigation 1286

UNIT EIGHT: Respiratory Care 1288
NURSING DIAGNOSES 1289
Caring for Oxygen Equipment 1290
Teaching Safety Measures for Oxygen Use 1290
Managing Ventilator Equipment 1290
Providing Catheter Care for Transtracheal Catheter 1291
for Heimlich Micro-Trach 1291
for SCOOP Catheter Cleaning in Place 1291
for SCOOP Catheter Cleaning After Removal 1292
Teaching the Client Catheter Care 1293
Teaching Tracheostomy Suction 1293
Cleaning Suction Equipment 1293
Teaching Tracheostomy Care 1294

UNIT NINE: Circulatory Care 1295
NURSING DIAGNOSES 1296
Monitoring Pacemaker at Home 1297
Checking with Pacemaker Clinic via Telephone 1297
Instructing in Use of Holter Monitor 1298
Teaching Care of Implantable Cardioverter–Defibrillator 1298

Bibliography 1300

Index 1308

GUIDE TO

CLINICAL NURSING SKILLS

SIXTH EDITION

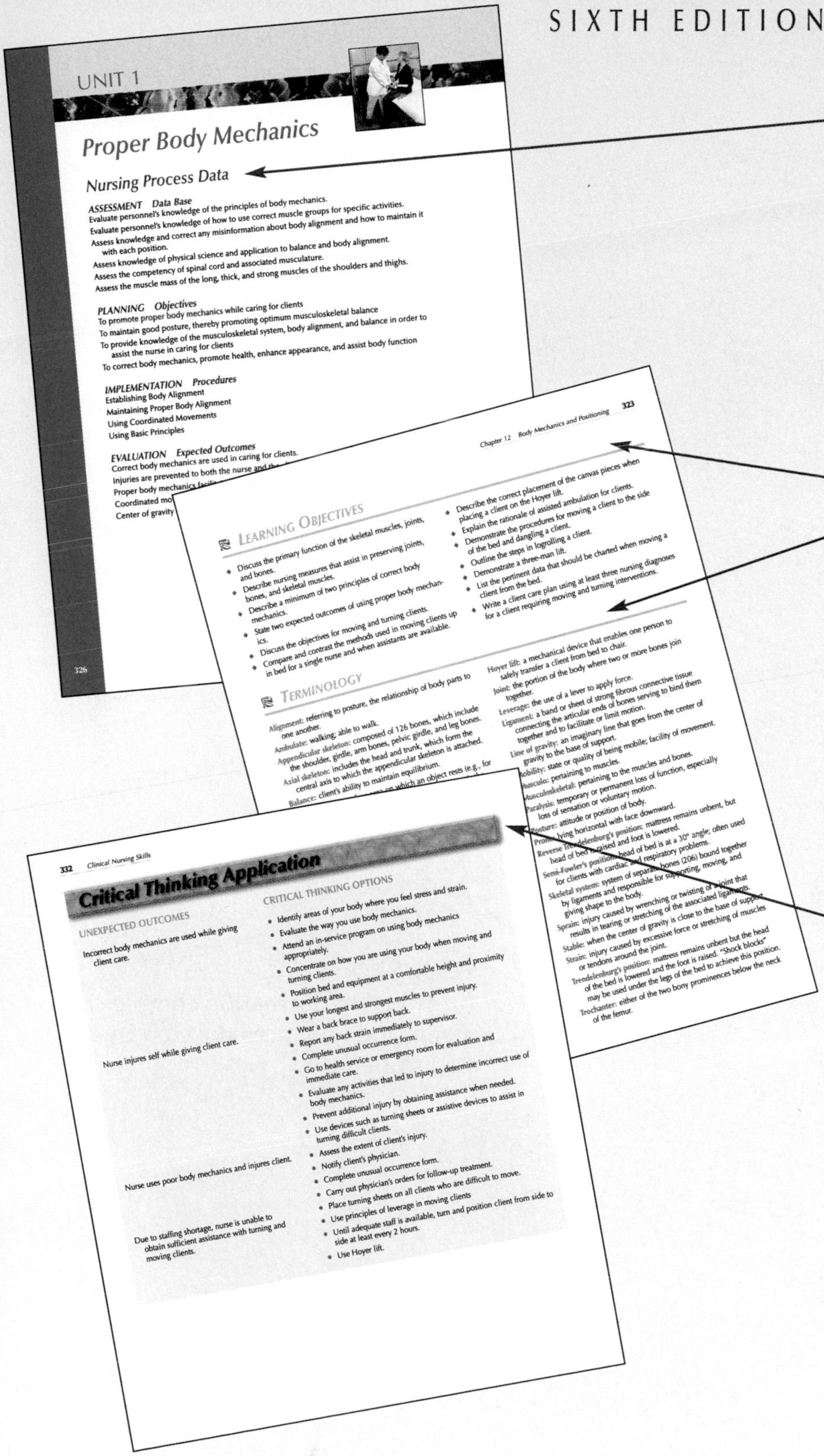

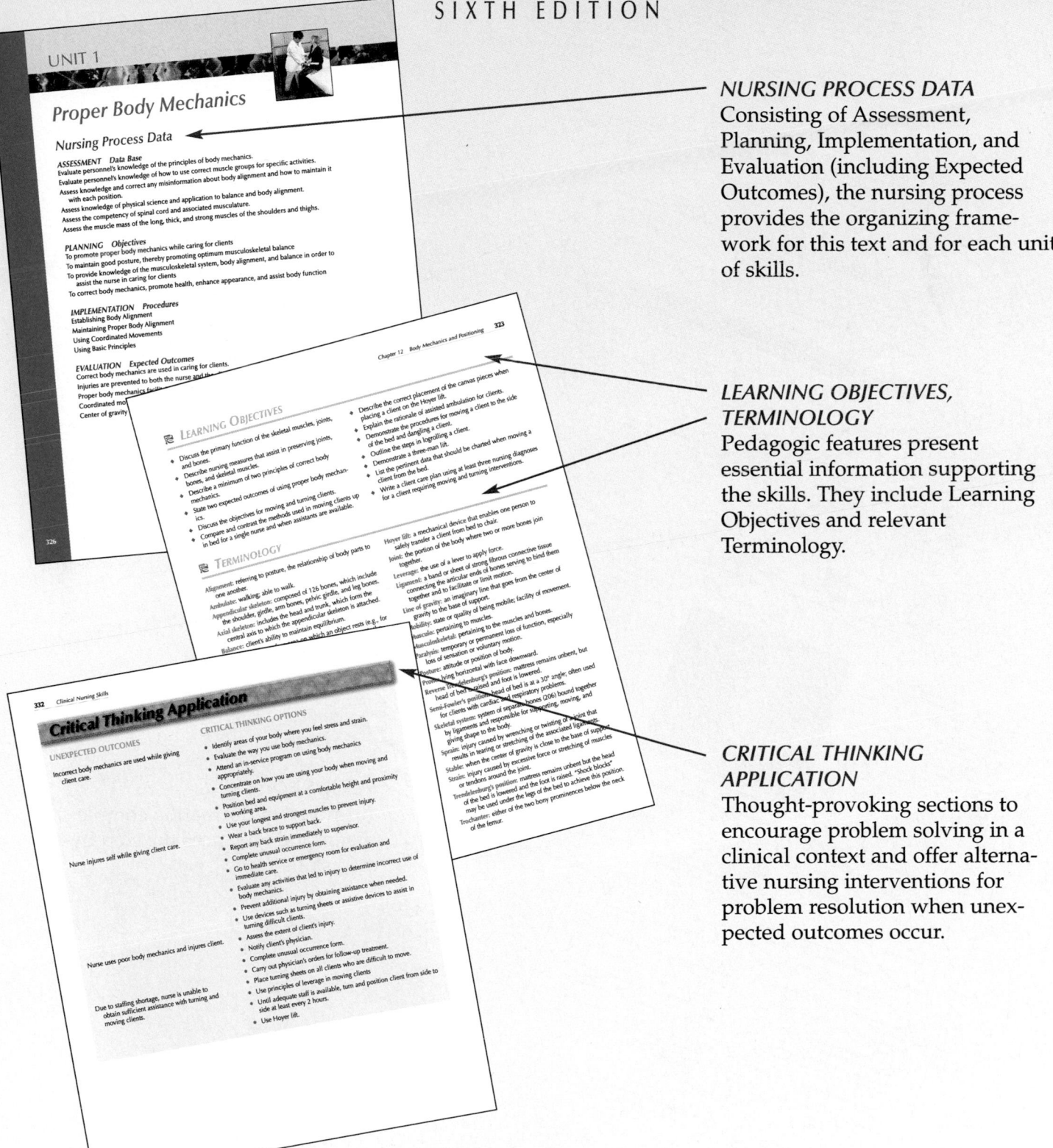

NURSING PROCESS DATA
Consisting of Assessment, Planning, Implementation, and Evaluation (including Expected Outcomes), the nursing process provides the organizing framework for this text and for each unit of skills.

LEARNING OBJECTIVES, TERMINOLOGY
Pedagogic features present essential information supporting the skills. They include Learning Objectives and relevant Terminology.

CRITICAL THINKING APPLICATION
Thought-provoking sections to encourage problem solving in a clinical context and offer alternative nursing interventions for problem resolution when unexpected outcomes occur.

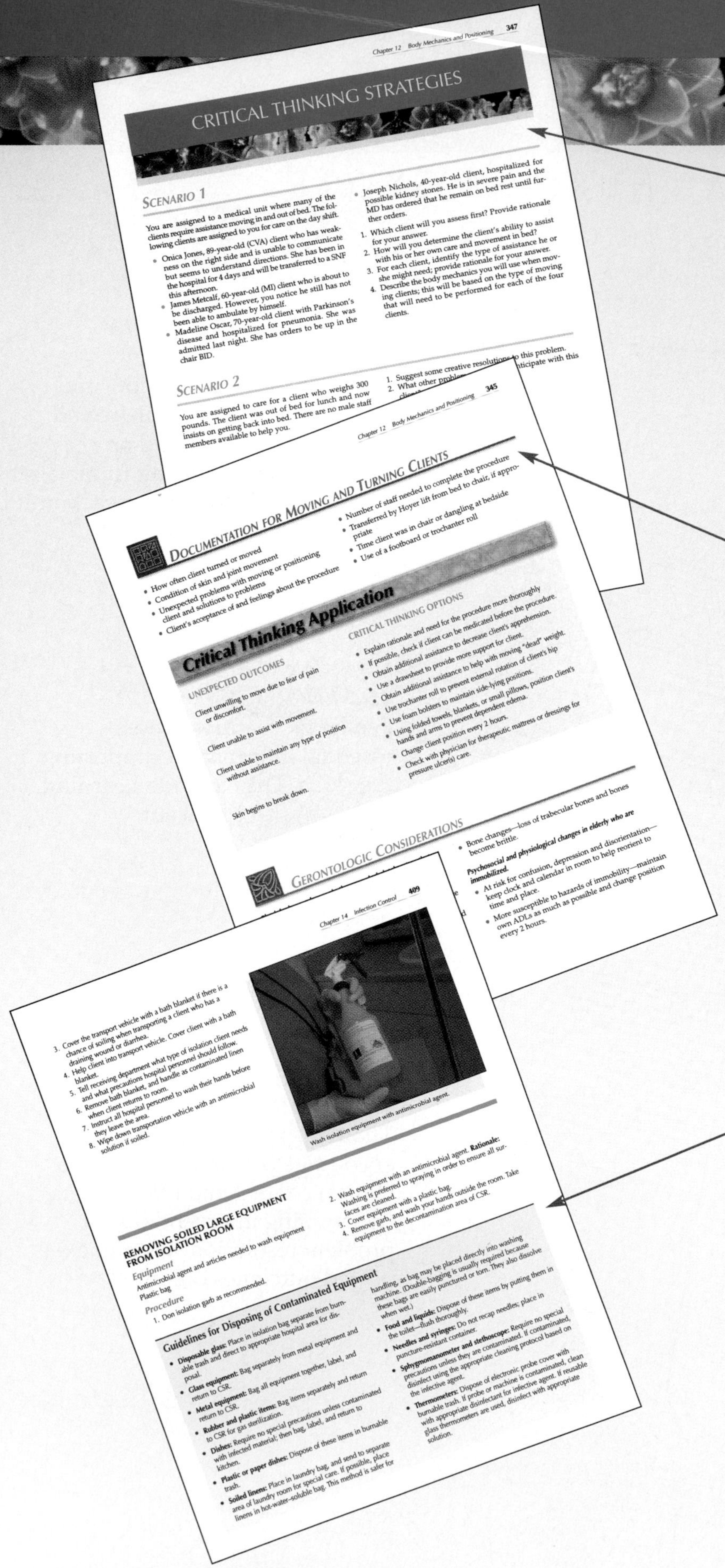

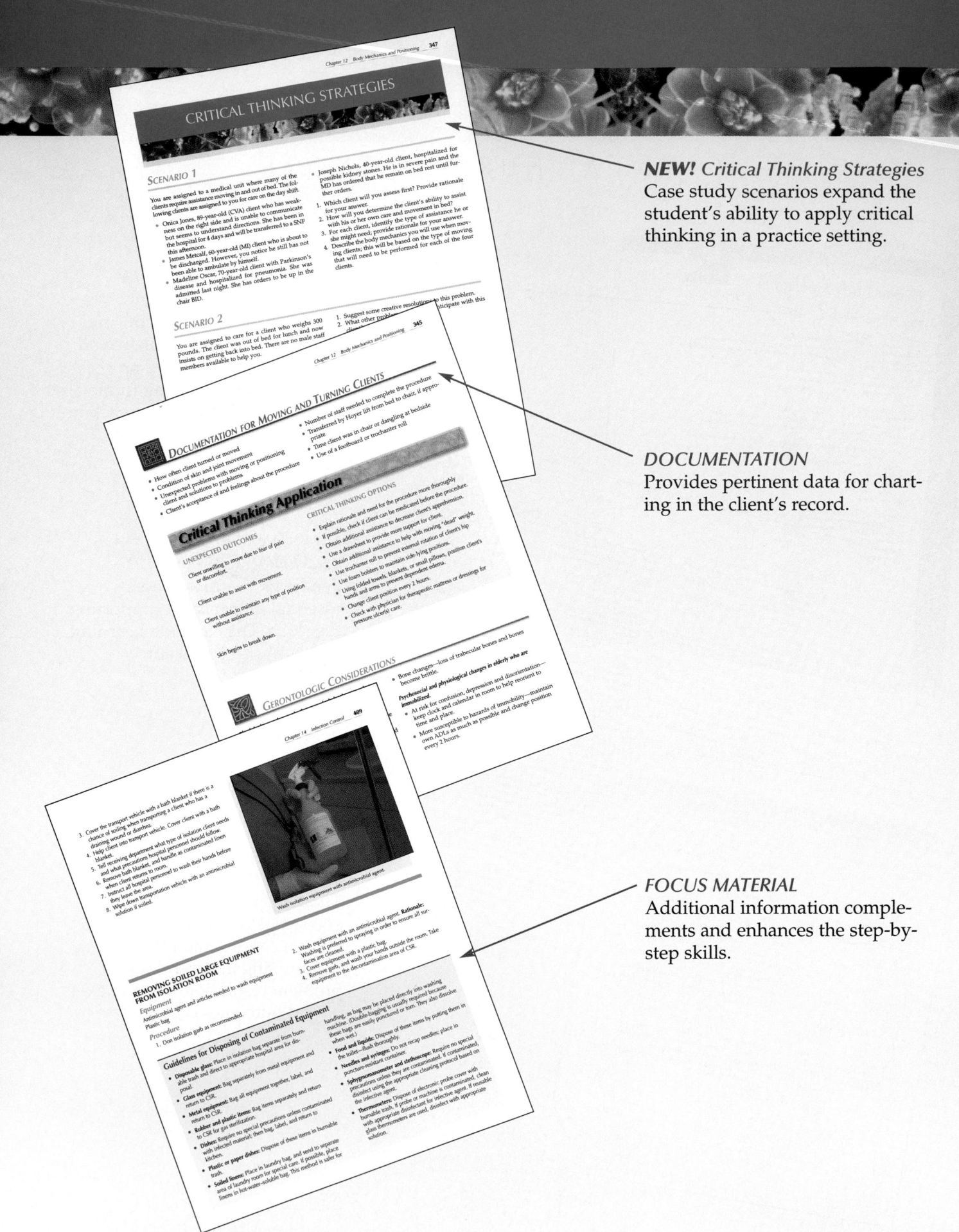

***NEW!** Critical Thinking Strategies*
Case study scenarios expand the student's ability to apply critical thinking in a practice setting.

DOCUMENTATION
Provides pertinent data for charting in the client's record.

FOCUS MATERIAL
Additional information complements and enhances the step-by-step skills.

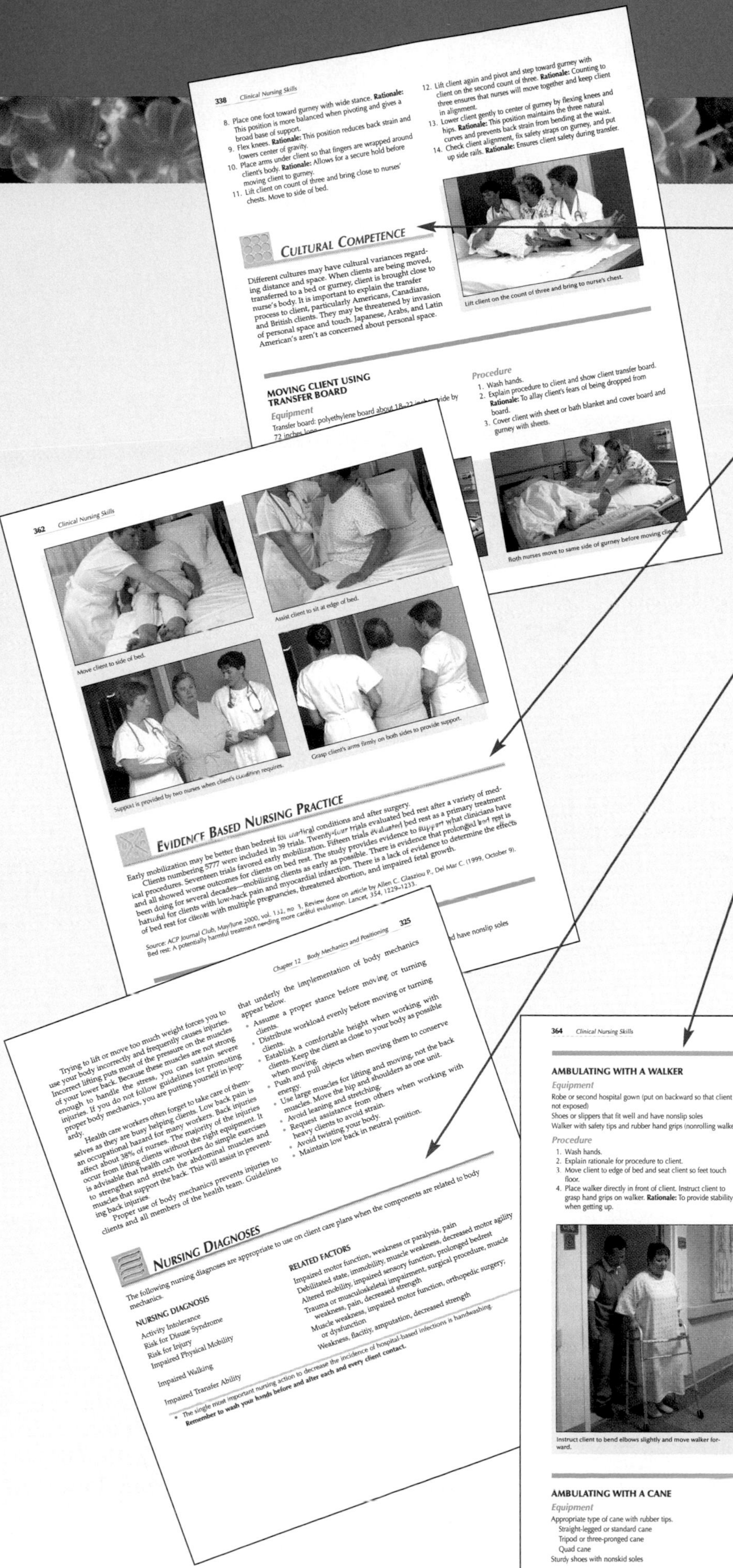

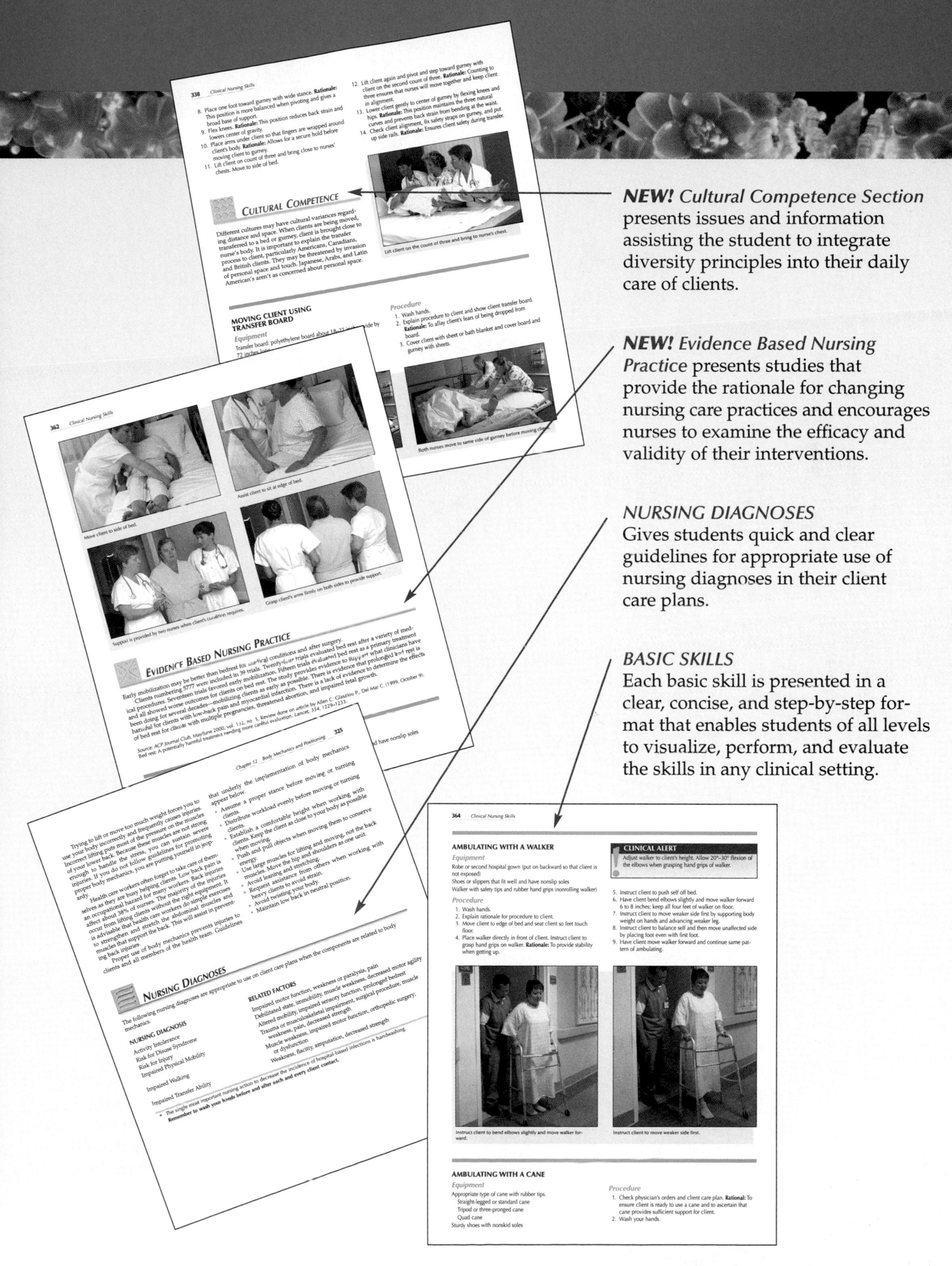

NEW! Cultural Competence Section presents issues and information assisting the student to integrate diversity principles into their daily care of clients.

***NEW!** Evidence Based Nursing Practice* presents studies that provide the rationale for changing nursing care practices and encourages nurses to examine the efficacy and validity of their interventions.

NURSING DIAGNOSES
Gives students quick and clear guidelines for appropriate use of nursing diagnoses in their client care plans.

BASIC SKILLS
Each basic skill is presented in a clear, concise, and step-by-step format that enables students of all levels to visualize, perform, and evaluate the skills in any clinical setting.

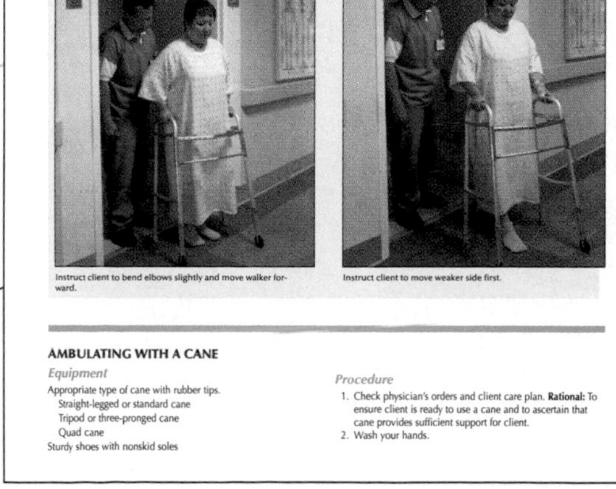

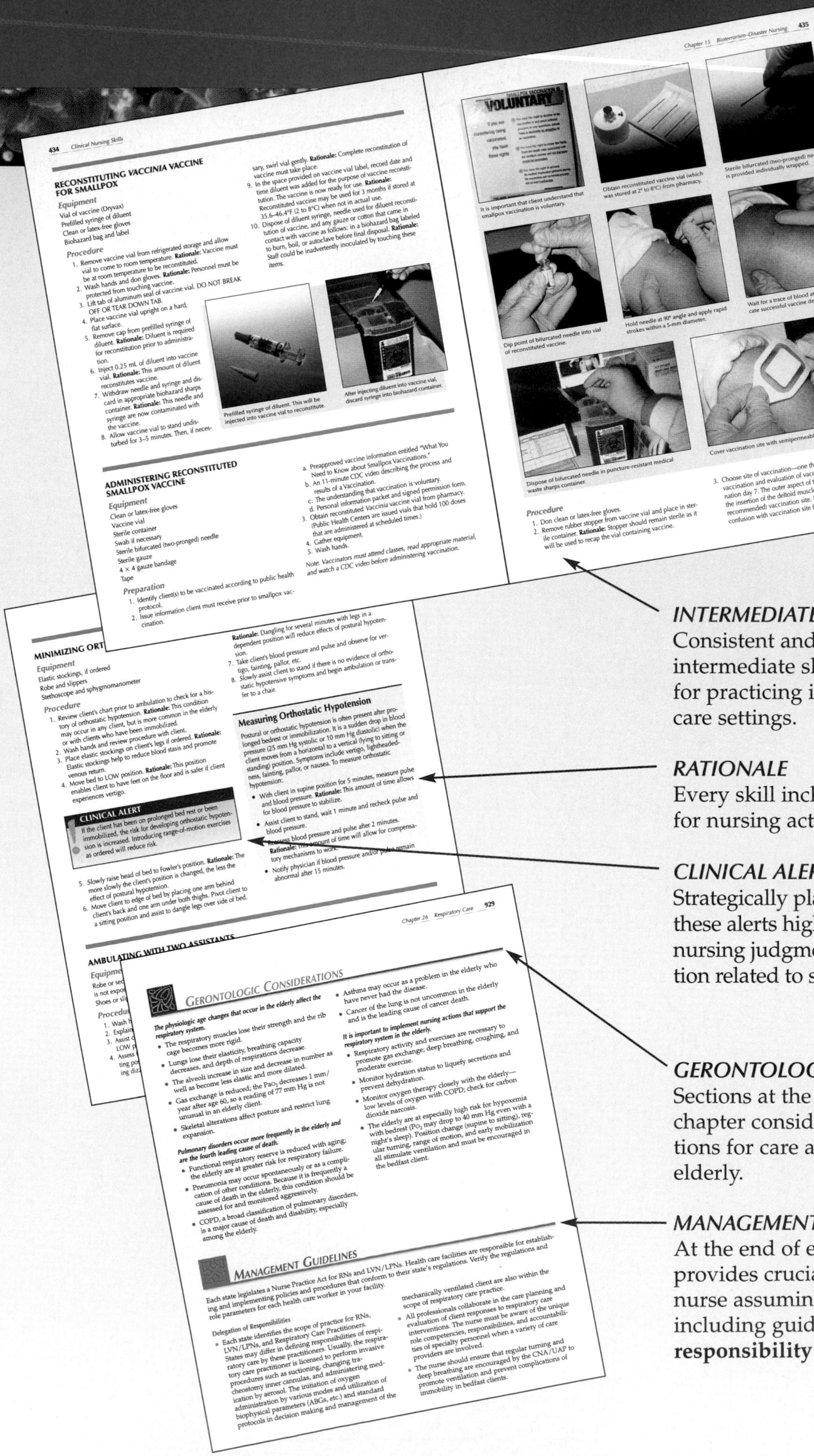

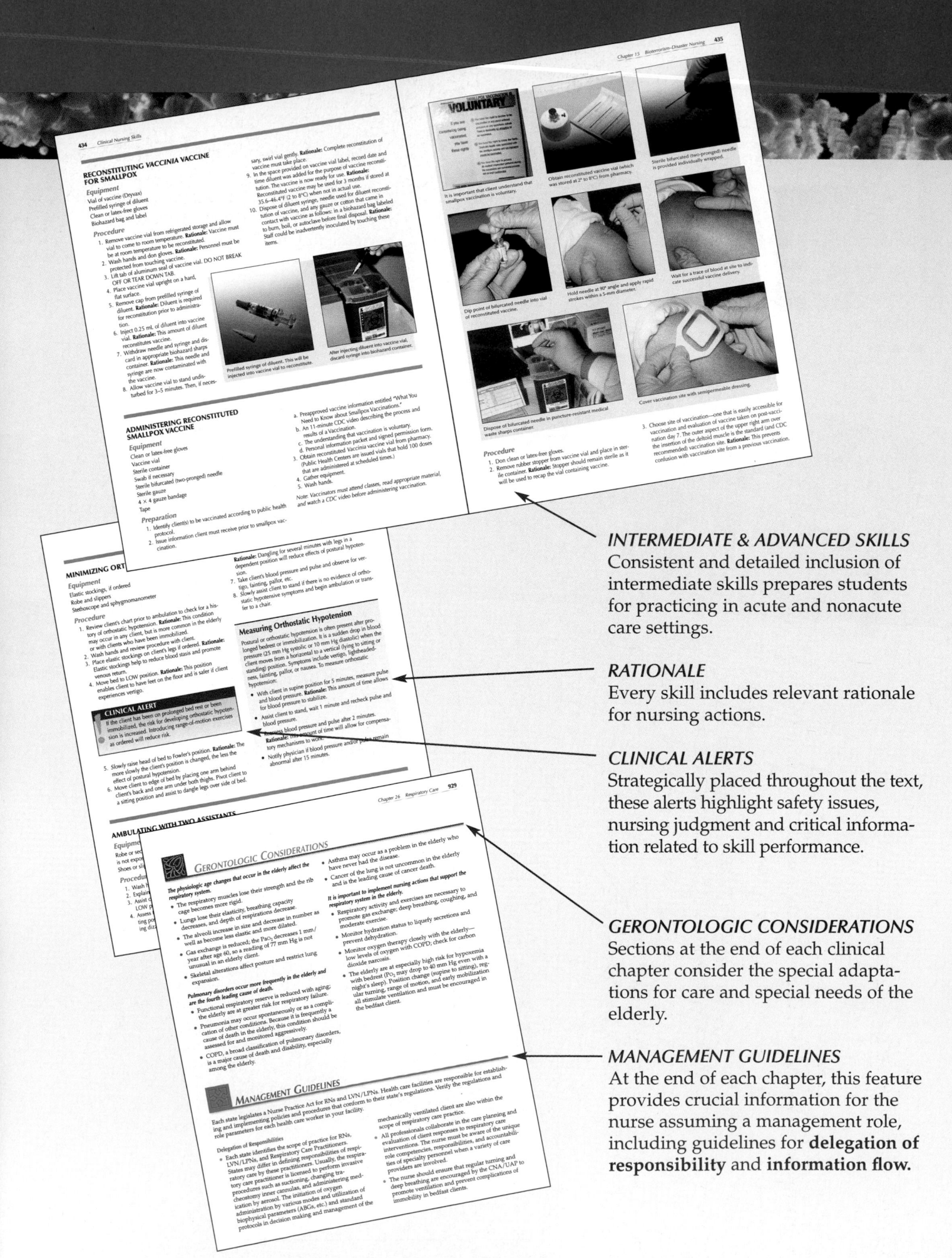

INTERMEDIATE & ADVANCED SKILLS

Consistent and detailed inclusion of intermediate skills prepares students for practicing in acute and nonacute care settings.

RATIONALE

Every skill includes relevant rationale for nursing actions.

CLINICAL ALERTS

Strategically placed throughout the text, these alerts highlight safety issues, nursing judgment and critical information related to skill performance.

GERONTOLOGIC CONSIDERATIONS

Sections at the end of each clinical chapter consider the special adaptations for care and special needs of the elderly.

MANAGEMENT GUIDELINES

At the end of each chapter, this feature provides crucial information for the nurse assuming a management role, including guidelines for **delegation of responsibility** and **information flow.**

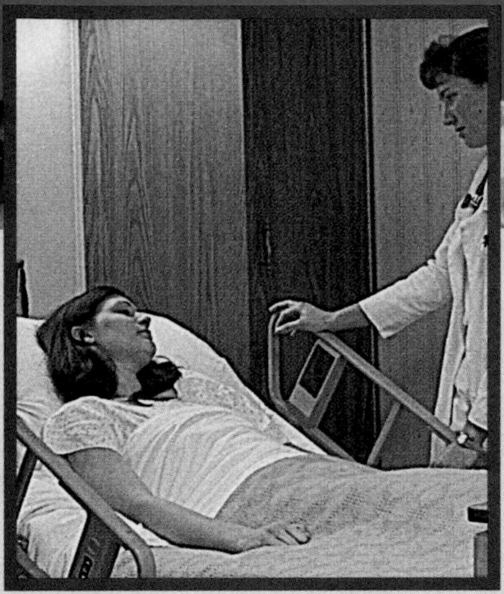

CHAPTER 1

Professional Nursing

Professional Role 2
Standards and Statutes 4
Clients' Rights 7
Clinical Practice 10
Medical Asepsis Principles 14
Protocol for Procedures 18

MANAGEMENT GUIDELINES 19

CRITICAL THINKING STRATEGIES 20

LEARNING OBJECTIVES

- Discuss what is meant by the concept "professional role of the nurse."
- Define the purpose of "A Code for Nursing Students."
- Define the term *accountable.*
- List three ways you can assist the client to assume and adapt to the client role.
- Identify the guidelines that will assist you to convey nursing competence to your clients.
- Describe the Nurse Practice Act.
- Define the term *nurse licensure.*
- State four functions of the Board of Registered Nursing.
- Discuss four grounds for licensure revocation for professional misconduct.
- Explain the legal issues of drug administration.
- Describe what is meant by "clients' rights."
- List four actions or guidelines that you need to complete to prepare for daily client care.
- Describe the steps of planning for client care.
- Explain what is meant by "Advance Directives."

PROFESSIONAL ROLE

As you enter the profession of nursing, you will experience some of the most frustrating and some of the most rewarding situations of your life. To decrease the frustrations and increase the positive experiences, this chapter introduces you to the role of the nurse. Emphasis is placed on those procedures that will assist you to become a functioning member of the health team, even with limited experience.

The information in this chapter will help you through the first few critical days of your clinical experience. In addition, legal aspects of the nursing profession are discussed to help you become aware of the far-reaching consequences of nursing actions. Clients' rights and the Nurse Practice Act (also called the Nursing Practice Act in some states) are also presented for your information.

As a nurse you will be held accountable and responsible for your actions. What does all this mean? To be accountable means that you must answer for all your activities surrounding client care. Accountability can be observed and measured by a variety of factors. It is reflected in the nurse's ethical integrity. Nursing actions are evaluated against a set of standards, frequently referred to as standards of professional performance. In this evaluation the nurse is judged according to predetermined factors in which all nurses should be competent.

Responsibility means that the nurse is conscientious and honest in all professional activities. A good example of responsibility deals with not betraying confidential information concerning clients in the hospital. In addition, a responsible nurse respects clients' rights and abides by the Patient's Bill of Rights.

Nurses must function within the Nurses' Code of Ethics. The Code of Ethics is a set of formal guidelines for governing professional action. It assists the nurse in problem solving where judgment is required. More emphasis is now being placed on the professional organizations to uphold the Code of Ethics and to admonish those nurses who violate the code. The Code of Ethics was revised in June 2001 by the American Nurses Association. The Code should be reviewed as you progress in the program. The National Student Nurses Association, Inc., also developed the Code of Academic and Clinical Conduct in April 2001. The Code provides guidance for nursing students in the personal development of an ethical foundation as both a nurse and human being.

Assuming the Nursing Role

Your actions, both verbal and nonverbal, influence the client's feelings and ideas regarding your level of competence, the role of nursing in administering care, and the client's overall adaptation to health care facilities. Assuming a professional role means that you behave as a professional person. Following the guidelines below will assist you to convey nursing competence, not only to clients but also to your peers and other nursing staff.

- Always dress neatly in appropriate, clean attire, and follow the dress code of your school or facility.
- Keep hair off collar and fingernails cut short. Wear clear nail polish, not colored polish. Synthetic nails are not allowed as they harbor bacteria.
- Speak in correct English without slang or inappropriate language.
- Relate to the clients as worthwhile individuals who deserve respect and consideration. Call the client by his or her surname, and use the appropriate honorific (Mr., Ms., Miss, Mrs.). Do not use nicknames or first names.
- Do not "talk down" to or patronize the client. Remember that the client knows more about his or her own body, symptoms, feelings, and responses than anyone else. Listen and pay attention to what the client says about himself or herself or the underlying feelings that are not expressed.
- Remain in a professional role at all times. Do not socialize with the clients. Clients should view you as a

A Code for Nursing Students

As students are involved in the clinical and academic environments, we believe that ethical principles are a necessary guide to professional development. Therefore, within these environments we:

1. Advocate for the rights of all clients.
2. Maintain client confidentiality.
3. Take appropriate action to ensure the safety of clients, self, and others.
4. Provide care for the client in a timely, compassionate and professional manner.
5. Communicate client care in a truthful, timely, and accurate manner.
6. Actively promote the highest level of moral and ethical principles and accept responsibility for our actions.
7. Promote excellence in nursing by encouraging lifelong learning and professional development.
8. Treat others with respect and promote an environment that respects human rights, values, and choice of cultural and spiritual beliefs.
9. Collaborate in every reasonable manner with the academic faculty and clinical staff to ensure the highest quality of client care.
10. Use every opportunity to improve faculty and clinical staff understanding of the learning needs of nursing students.
11. Encourage faculty, clinical staff, and peers to mentor nursing students.
12. Refrain from performing any technique or procedure for which the student has not been adequately trained.
13. Refrain from any deliberate action or omission of care in the academic or clinical setting that creates unnecessary risk of injury to the client, self, or others.
14. Assist the staff nurse or preceptor in ensuring that there is full disclosure and that proper authorizations are obtained from clients regarding any form of treatment or research.
15. Abstain from the use of alcoholic beverages or any substances in the academic and clinical setting that impair judgment.
16. Strive to achieve and maintain an optimal level of personal health.
17. Support access to treatment and rehabilitation for students who are experiencing impairments related to substance abuse and mental or physical health issues.
18. Uphold school policies and regulations related to academic and clinical performance, reserving the right to challenge and critique rules and regulations as per school grievance policy.

Source: National Student Nurses' Association, Inc. April 6, 2001.

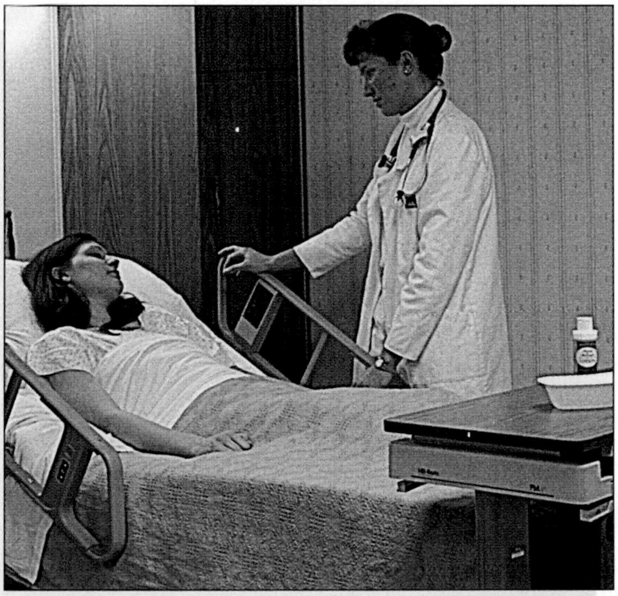

Relate to clients as worthwhile individuals who deserve respect and consideration.

knowledgeable professional who brings healing, caring, and teaching roles to the relationship.

- Use yourself as a therapeutic tool to convey caring and healing. Use body language to reinforce honest and direct verbalization, not to contradict it.
- Be accountable and answerable for your behavior and nursing actions and the nursing care you are expected to provide. If you do not understand what is expected, seek assistance from a staff member. Your responsibility is to remain reliable, honest, and trust-worthy in administering nursing care.
- Maintain client confidentiality. Do not talk about clients in public areas. Follow HIPAA standards.

The Client Role

Assisting the client to adapt to hospitalization is one of the primary functions of the nurse. The less resistive the client is to receiving treatment during hospitalization, the more open he or she is to curative methods. The nurse can assist in adaptation by understanding that all clients have individual needs, concerns, and perceptions that require discussion and planning as they take on the role of client in the health care setting. You must accept the client's perceptions of his or her new surroundings. If possible, try to accommodate client's wishes, assess previous concepts of illness and hospitalization, and discuss previous experiences. Be aware that anxiety is a natural reaction to an unfamiliar setting, to new procedures, and to new people. If, for example, a client is extremely fatigued or overwhelmed by traveling to the hospital and the admission procedure, you can help him or her adapt to the surroundings, regain a sense of control and identity, and accept the changed circumstances.

Another way to assist the client to retain his or her identity and uniqueness is to communicate with the client as an individual. Ask questions and observe verbal responses as well as nonverbal cues. Provide ways to care for a client's personal possessions, clothing, and physical comfort so that the client adapts more easily to the change in environment and feels more secure and in control.

Be aware that the medical condition is only one part of the client's life and that the changes that have led up to admission affect other areas of his or her well-being. Clients may have concerns about new routines, financial matters, their families, or their future. By responding to clients' total needs at the time of admission, you can help them establish a positive attitude toward their total care.

Acknowledge and accept any statements or behavior the client uses to adapt to his or her new surroundings. Even though various cultures and groups differ in their response to illness and some responses may differ from your personal beliefs, acknowledge the client's individuality. Cultural groups often utilize traditional health care providers, identified and respected by the specific cultural group. Concepts of illness, wellness, and health are part of the client's total belief system and must be recognized by the nurse as part of what makes the client an individual. Support the client's beliefs and behavior as long as they do not increase the risk of injury or illness. Be sensitive to any past health care experiences that may influence the client's feelings at the time of admission. A prior experience in the hospital may determine how a client responds to the current environment and how he or she accepts treatment.

STANDARDS AND STATUTES

Legal issues and regulations play a dominant role in nursing practice today. The law provides a framework for establishing nursing actions in the care of clients. Laws determine and set boundaries and maintain a standard of nursing practice.

The Nurse Practice Act defines professional nursing and recommends those actions that the nurse can practice independently and those actions that require a physician's order before completion.

Each state has the authority to regulate and they administrate health care professionals. Although the provisions of Nurse Practice Acts are quite similar from state to state, it is imperative that the nurse know the licensing requirements and the grounds for license revocation defined by the state in which he or she works.

Legal and ethical standards for nurses are complicated by a myriad of federal and state statutes and the continually changing interpretation of them by the courts of law. Nurses are faced today with the threat of legal action based on negligence, malpractice, invasion of privacy, and other grounds. This chapter covers the basic legal issues and topics, from clients' rights and nurses' liability in the administration of drugs and grounds for proceedings to address professional misconduct.

The Nurse Practice Act

The Nurse Practice Act is a series of statutes enacted by a state to regulate the practice of nursing in that state. Subjects covered by Nurse Practice Acts include definition of the scope of practice, education, licensure, and grounds for disciplinary actions. Nurse Practice Acts are quite similar throughout the United States, but the professional nurse is held legally responsible for the specific requirements for licensure and regulations of practice as defined by the state in which she or he works.

The responsibilities of the professional nurse involve a level of performance for a defined range of health care services. These services include assessment, planning, implementation, and evaluation of nursing action, as well as teaching and related services, such as counseling. Skills and functions that professional nurses perform in daily practice include:

- Provide direct and indirect client care services
- Perform and deliver basic health care services
- Implement testing and prevention procedures
- Observe signs and symptoms of illness
- Administer treatments per physician's order
- Observe treatment reactions and responses
- Administer medications per physician's order
- Observe medication responses and any side effects
- Observe general physical and mental conditions of individual clients
- Provide client and family teaching
- Act as a client advocate when needed
- Document nursing care
- Supervise allied nursing personnel
- Coordinate members of the health care team

Nurse Licensure

The authorization to practice nursing is defined legally as the right to practice nursing by an individual who holds an active license issued by the state in which she or he intends to work. The licensing process is administered by the Board of Registered Nursing, frequently called the BRN (or BON). This board may also grant endorsement or reciprocity to an applicant who holds a current license in another state. The applicant for RN licensure must have attended an accredited school of nursing, be a qualified nursing professional or paraprofessional, or have met specific prerequisites if licensed in a foreign country.

Board of Registered Nursing Functions

- Establishes and oversees educational standards
- Establishes professional standards
- Monitors examinations for licensure (NCLEX)
- Registers and renews nurses' licenses
- Conducts investigations of violations of the statutes and regulations
- Issues citations
- Holds disciplinary hearings for possible suspension or revocation of the license
- Imposes penalties following disciplinary hearings
- Establishes and oversees diversion programs in some states

Standards of Clinical Nursing Practice

The American Nurses Association first published these standards in 1973. The standards were revised in 1991 and updated in 1998. The standards apply to all registered nurses working in clinical practice regardless of clinical specialty, practice setting, or educational preparation. These standards have shaped nursing practice and have helped both nurses and others understand what nursing is and does.

The standards describe a competent level of professional nursing care and professional performance common to all nurses engaged in clinical practice. This includes descriptions of the responsibility and accountability of the professional.

The standards of practice consists of two segments: Standards of Care which describe the six standards of care using the nursing process; and the eight Standards of Professional Performance. These standards describe a competent level of behavior in the professional role.

Nurses in specialty nursing practice, such as critical care nursing or neonatal nursing, practice under standards that further define the responsibilities in these settings. The nursing specialties and appropriate groups, with the American Nurses Association, determine these standards.

Nurses practicing at an advanced level are accountable for meeting and maintaining the basic standards of clinical nursing practice in addition to the Scope and Standards of Advanced Practice Registered Nursing.

Standards of Clinical Nursing Practice

Standards of Care

- Assessment
- Diagnosis
- Outcome Identification
- Planning
- Implementation
- Evaluation

Standards of Professional Performance

- Quality of Care
- Performance Appraisal
- Education
- Collegiality
- Ethics
- Collaboration
- Research
- Resource Utilization

Liability and Legal Issues

Each state defines and regulates the grounds for professional misconduct. Even though many states have similar standards the practicing nurse must know how his or her state defines professional misconduct. The penalties for professional misconduct include probation, censure and reprimand, suspension of license, or revocation of license. The state's Board of Registered Nursing (BRN) has the authority to impose any of these penalties for

American Nurses Association Standards of Professional Performance

I. Quality of Care: The nurse systematically evaluates the quality and effectiveness of nursing practice.

II. Performance Appraisal: The nurse evaluates one's own nursing practice in relation to professional practice standards and relevant statutes and regulations.

III. Education: The nurse acquires and maintains current knowledge and competence in nursing practice.

IV. Collegiality: The nurse interacts with, and contributes to the professional development of, peers and other health care providers as colleagues.

V. Ethics: The nurse's decisions and actions on behalf of patients are determined in an ethical manner.

VI. Collaboration: The nurse collaborates with the patient, family, and other health care providers in providing patient care.

VII. Research: The nurse uses research findings in practice.

VIII. Resource Utilization: The nurse considers factors related to safety, effectiveness, and cost in planning and delivering patient care.

Source: American Nurses Association. (1998). *Standards of Clinical Nursing Practice* (2nd ed.). Washington, DC: Author.

Standards of Care (Example)

Standard II. Diagnosis

The nurse analyzes the assessment data in determining diagnoses.

Measurement Criteria

1. Diagnoses are derived from the assessment data.
2. Diagnoses are validated with the patient, family, and other health care providers, when possible and appropriate.
3. Diagnoses are documented in a manner that facilitates the determination of expected outcomes and plan of care.

professional misconduct. Any one of the following actions would be considered professional misconduct.

- Obtaining an RN license through misrepresentation or fraudulent methods
- Giving false information on application for license
- Practicing in an incompetent or gross negligent manner
- Practicing when ability to practice is severely impaired
- Being habitually drunk or dependent on drugs
- Furnishing controlled substances to himself or herself or to another person
- Impersonating another certified or licensed practitioner or allowing another person to use his or her license for the purpose of nursing
- Being convicted of or committing an act constituting a crime under federal or state law
- Refusing to provide health care services on the grounds of race, color, creed, or national origin
- Permitting or aiding an unlicensed person to perform activities requiring a license
- Practicing nursing while license is suspended
- Practicing medicine without a license
- Procuring, aiding, or offering to assist at a criminal abortion
- Holding oneself out to the public as a "nurse practitioner" without being certified by the BRN as a nurse practitioner (in some states)

Drugs and the Nurse

In their daily work, most nurses handle a wide variety of drugs. Failure to give the correct medication or improper handling of drugs may result in serious problems for the nurse due to strict federal and state statutes relating to drugs. The Comprehensive Drug Abuse Prevention Act of 1970 provides the fundamental federal regulations for compounding, selling, and dispensing narcotics, stimulants, depressants, and other controlled items. Each state has a similar set of regulations for the same purpose.

Noncompliance with federal or state drug regulations can result in liability. Violation of the state drug regulations or licensing laws are grounds for the Board of Registered Nursing to initiate disciplinary action.

Negligence/Malpractice

The doctrine of negligence rests on the duty of every person to exercise due care in his or her conduct toward others from which injury may result. To find liability there must be a duty of care on the part of the nurse and a causal relationship between damage or harm to the client as well as an act or an omission to act by the nurse.

Gross negligence is the intentional failure to perform a duty in reckless disregard of the consequences affecting the client. It is viewed as a gross lack of care to such a level as to be considered willful and wanton. Gross negligence can be due to improper use of restraints, client falls, or medication errors that lead to a client injury.

Criminal negligence also consists of a duty on the part of the nurse and an act that is the proximate cause of the injury or death of a client. This type of negligence is usually defined by statute and as such is punishable as a crime. The act being punished would be a flagrant and reckless disregard of the safety of others and/or a willful disregard to the injury liable to follow so as to convert the act into a crime when it results in personal injury or death.

Guidelines for Drug Administration

- Nurses must not administer a specific drug unless allowed to do so by the particular state's Nurse Practice Act.
- Nurses must not administer any drug without a specific physician order.
- Nurses are to take every safety precaution in whatever they are doing.
- Nurses are to be certain that employer's policy allows them to administer a specific drug.
- Nurses must not administer a controlled substance if the physician's order is outdated.
- A drug may not lawfully be administered unless all the above items are in effect.
- Nurses are not permitted to fill prescriptions and in most states cannot write prescriptions.
- General rules for drug dispensing:
  - Never leave prepared medicines unattended.
  - Always report errors immediately.
  - Send labeled bottles or packages that are unintelligible back to pharmacist for relabeling.
  - Store internal and external medicines separately if possible.

One is not "negligent" unless he or she fails to exercise the degree of reasonable care that would be exercised by a person of ordinary prudence under all the existing circumstances in view of probable danger of injury. The death or serious injury of a client following a medication or IV error can result in criminal negligence.

Malpractice is any professional misconduct that is an unreasonable lack of skill or fidelity in professional duties. In a more specific sense it means bad, wrong, or injurious treatment of a client resulting in injury, unnecessary suffering, or death to a client proceeding from ignorance, carelessness, lack of professional skill, disregard of established rules, protocols, principles or procedures, neglect, or a malicious or criminal intent.

Civil Law	Criminal Law
Contract	Assault
Unintentional tort	Battery
Intentional tort	Murder
Negligence	Manslaughter

It is the nurse's legal duty to provide competent, reasonable care to clients. To ensure that this occurs the nurse must know the standards of care, develop consistent patterns of practice that meet the standards, and reflect his or her action in accurate and complete documentation. Legal action against nurses has been increasing over the last decade. Nursing actions which constitute a breach of a standard of care that can lead to injury of a client include such actions as not inserting a Foley catheter correctly; not taking appropriate steps to decrease a client's temperature; not reporting unusual or worsening condition of the client to his or her physician; and not preventing falls. All of these situations can lead to malpractice suits.

Legal doctrine holds that an employer may also be liable for negligent acts of employees in the course and scope of employment. Physicians, hospitals, clinics, and other employers may be held liable for negligent acts of their employees. This doctrine does not support acts of gross negligence or acts that are outside the scope of employment.

CLIENTS' RIGHTS

State and federal regulations governing health care facilities mandate that certain rights be afforded clients receiving health care. Hospitals and health care facilities must have established policies that discuss client rights and how staff are to adhere to them.

Because clients' rights may conflict with nursing functions, you should be familiar with the key elements of these rights. It is important to remember that within a health care system, all clients retain their basic constitutional rights, such as freedom of expression, due process of law, freedom from cruel and inhumane punishment, equal protection, and so forth. Clients also have the right to know the identity of all health care providers and others involved in their care, which includes student nurses. All health care workers must wear a name badge indicating their title (e.g., Jane Doe, Student Nurse). The name of the nursing program is also included on the name badge. Most badges include a photo ID in addition to the name.

The first Patient's Bill of Rights was adopted by the American Hospital Association in 1973, and a revision was approved in 1992. The President introduced a new Patient's Bill of Rights in 2002 with stipulations that provide uninsured workers credits to purchase health care coverage, to increase spending for veterans' health, and to provide Medicare recipients coverage for prescription drugs. At the time of this writing, the bill has yet to pass Congress. Legislation is pending.

Under the Patient's Bill of Rights, hospitals must provide a foundation for understanding and respecting the rights and responsibilities of clients, their families, physicians, and other caregivers. The hospital must ensure and respect the role of clients in decision making about treatment choices and other aspects of their care. There must be a sensitivity to cultural, racial, linguistic, religious, age, and gender differences. In addition, the needs of persons with disabilities must be considered when providing health care services. Each hospital is encouraged to tailor its bill of rights to its particular community and client population. Individualization to the community ensures that the families and their specific rights are considered when the bill of rights is written.

The following is a summary of the rights that can be exercised on the client's behalf by a designated surrogate or by the client him- or herself. It is the nurse's responsibility to know what the document states in each facility and how the information is provided to the client.

HIPAA

The Health Insurance Portability and Accountability Act (HIPAA), enacted into law in 1996 and phased in gradually, requires the Secretary of Health and Human Services (HHS) to devise standards to improve Medicare and Medicaid programs and the efficiency and effectiveness of the health care system. It ensures continuing health care insurance if the client has had existing group insurance, proposes standards for electronic transactions and security signatures, and ensures privacy of individual health information. The privacy rule component went into effect on April 14, 2003. It requires health care providers to take reasonable measures to protect against unauthorized disclosures of personal medical information. This law also requires client consent before any information is given to employers, lenders, or any other health care agencies.

Consent to Receive Health Services

There are two major forms of consent signed by clients in a health care facility. The first consent is completed at the

The Client's Bill of Rights

1. The client has the right to considerate and respectful care.
2. The client has the right to and is encouraged to obtain from physicians and other direct caregivers relevant, current, and understandable information concerning diagnosis, treatment, and prognosis. In emergencies, the client is entitled to the opportunity to discuss and request information related to specific procedures and/or treatments, the risk involved, and the financial implications of the treatment choices, etc. Clients also have the right to know the identity of health care professionals caring for them.
3. The client has the right to make decisions about the plan of care prior to and during the course of treatment and to refuse a recommended treatment or plan of care to the extent permitted by law and hospital policy and be informed of medical consequences of this action.
4. The client has the right to have an advance directive and have the hospital honor the intent of the directive to the extent permitted by law and hospital policy. The institution must advise clients of their rights under state law and hospital policy to make informed medical choices. Hospitals must identify if a client has an advance directive and place it in the client records.
5. The client has the right to every consideration of privacy including examination, treatment, consultation, and case discussion.
6. The client has the right to expect all communications and records pertaining to his/her care be treated as confidential by the hospital, except in cases as suspected abuse and public health hazards.
7. The client has the right to review the records pertaining to his/her medical care and have the information explained or interpreted as necessary, except when restricted by law.
8. The client has the right to expect that, within its capacity and policies, a hospital will make reasonable response to the request of a client for appropriate and medically indicated care and services.
9. The client has the right to ask and be informed of the existence of business relationships among the hospital, educational institutions, other health care providers, or payers that may influence the client's treatment and care.
10. The client has the right to consent to or decline to participate in proposed research studies or human experimentation affecting care and treatment or requiring direct client involvement, and to have those studies fully explained prior to consent.
11. The client has the right to expect reasonable continuity of care when appropriate and to be informed by physician and other caregivers of available and realistic client care options when hospital care is no longer appropriate.
12. The client has the right to be informed of hospital policies and practices that relate to client care, treatment, and responsibilities, including grievances and conflicts.

Figure 1-1 *Source:* American Hospital Association, revision October 21, 1992. New revision pending, 2003.

time of admission; the client signs the form in the admissions office or in the emergency department, wherever the admission is initiated. This agreement usually indicates that the client has agreed to such things as medical treatment, x-ray examinations, blood transfusions, and injections. The second type of consent is for invasive testing procedures, such as a liver biopsy, surgery, special studies involving dye injection, or other treatments in which there are risks associated with the procedure.

Consent is the client's approval to have his or her body touched by specific individuals, such as doctors, nurses, and laboratory technicians. Informed consent refers to the process of informing the client prior to granting a consent regarding treatment, such as tests and surgery, and must be understood by the client in terms of the intended outcome and the potential harmful results. The client may rescind a prior consent verbally or in writing.

The authority to sign a consent must be given by a mentally competent adult. Court-authorized persons may give consent for mentally incompetent adults. In emergency situations, if the client is in immediate danger of serious harm or death, action may be taken to preserve life without the client's consent.

The nurse's liability in terms of consent is to ensure that the client is fully informed before being asked to sign a consent form. The physician, nurse, or other health personnel must inform the client of any potentially harmful effects of the treatment. If this is not done, it may result in the nurse's being held personally liable. The nurse must respect the right of a mentally competent adult client to refuse healthcare; however, a life-threatening situation may alter the client's right to refuse treatment.

Nurses' Responsibilities

Clients are protected by law (invasion of privacy) against unauthorized release of personal clinical data, such as symptoms, diagnoses, and treatments. Nurses, as well as other health care personnel, may be held personally liable for invasion of privacy, should litigation arise from the unauthorized release of client data. Advances in technology, including computerized medical databases, the internet, and telehealth, pose potential (unintentional) breaches of confidentiality and privacy. Changes in technology have changed not only the delivery of health care, but the system used to record and retrieve health information.

The computer, fax machine, and the phone calls between facilities and agencies leave the client at risk for information dissemination to unintended sources. Information is readily available to anyone walking by a fax machine or a computer. Confidential information, however, may be released with the client's consent. Information release is mandatory when ordered by a court or when state statutes require reporting child abuse, communicable diseases, or other incidents. Nurses have a legal and ethical responsibility to become familiar with their employer's policies and procedures regarding protection of clients' information.

Medical records are the key written account of such client information as signs and symptoms, diagnosis, treatment, and responses to treatment. Not only do these records document care given to clients, but they also provide effective means of communication among health care personnel. These records contain important data for insurance and other expense claims and are used in court in the event of litigation.

Health care professionals are becoming more aware of the implications of clients' rights as society in general becomes more aware of every human being's basic rights. Although there are still gaps in the legal process, many states are beginning to grapple with the status of laws applicable to clients who are hospitalized. It is essential that nurses be aware of the particular state's laws and statutes affecting clients and themselves. Nurses as well as physicians are accountable for their actions, and the threat of civil and criminal prosecution is becoming more prevalent. The American Nurses Association has developed a position statement supporting the principles of client privacy and confidentiality as a commitment to client advocacy.

Patient Self-Determination Act

Patient Self-Determination Act of 1991 (PSDA) is a federal law that applies to all health care institutions receiving Medicaid funds. It imposes on the state and providers of health care such as hospitals, nursing homes, hospices, home health agencies, and prepaid health care organizations, certain requirements concerning advance directives and an individual's rights under state law to make decisions concerning medical care; this includes the right to accept or refuse medical or surgical care. The PSDA defines an "advance directive" as a written instruction, such as a living will or durable power of attorney for health care. A competent adult can communicate preferences about future medical treatment through the advance directives. Clients must be provided written documentation regarding their rights to formulate advance directives, such as living wills and durable power of attorney for health care. Clients must be made aware of their rights to make decisions about these issues on admission to all health care facilities and health maintenance organizations (HMOs); however, they are not required to sign an advance directive if they do not choose to do so. The directives allow clients to control their own healthcare decisions, even if they become incapacitated in the future.

Classifications of Law Related to Nursing

Classification	Example
Constitutional	Clients' rights to equal treatment
Administrative	Licensure and the state BRN
Labor relations	Union negotiations
Contract	Relationship with employer
Criminal	Handling of narcotics
Tort	
Medical malpractice	Reasonable and prudent client care
Product liability	Warranty on medical equipment

Advance Medical Directives

Advance medical directives are of two types: treatment directives, such as living wills, and appointment directives, such as durable power of attorney for health care. An advance medical directive is a document that allows clients to make legal decisions about how they wish to receive future medical treatment. It is written and signed before any such care becomes necessary. Within this document, the client may indicate the person or persons he or

Advance Directives

An advance directive allows the client to participate in the following decisions:

- Choosing health care providers such as physicians and nurses.
- Deciding who may have access to medical records.
- Choosing the type of medical treatments the client desires.
- Consenting to or refusing certain types of medical treatments.
- Choosing the agent who will make decisions about the client's health care when the client is unable to do so.

she wishes to make medical decisions in situations in which the client is unable to do so. The document needs to be signed and witnessed, and copies should be kept on file in the physician's office and the hospital. The witness to this document should not be a hospital employee, relative, or heir to the estate. Advance directives vary among states and therefore the nurse must be knowledgeable about the use and type of directives in the state in which he or she practices. An advance directive does not need to be written, reviewed, or signed by an attorney. It must, however, be witnessed by two individuals.

Living Will A living will is a type of advance directive, indicating the client's wishes regarding prolonging life using life support measures, refusing or stopping medical interventions, or making decisions about his or her medical care when the client is diagnosed as having a terminal or permanent unconscious condition. It does not apply to any other health care decisions. Living wills are executed while the client is competent and able to make sound decisions. As conditions change, a living will needs to be evaluated for relevance. (States differ in their acceptance of living wills as legal documents.)

Durable Power of Attorney for Health Care This legal document must be prepared and signed while the client is competent. The document gives power to make health care decisions to a designated individual (agent) in the event the client is unable to make competent decisions for him or herself. The designated person is obligated to follow the directives outlined in the document. The document gives the client's agent specific health care decisions or the authority to make any and all health care decisions the client would make if able. Decisions regarding withdrawing or using life support, organ donation, or consent to treatment or procedures are included in the directives. As long as the client is competent, the agent does not have the authority to make treatment decisions.

The major difference between living wills and the durable power of attorney is that the durable power of attorney is more flexible. A living will is used only if the client's condition is terminal or they are in a permanently unconscious state. A living will only allows the client to direct that life-sustaining treatments be withheld or withdrawn. The durable power of attorney is not limited to terminal or permanent unconscious conditions. It also addresses all types of health care decisions, including life-sustaining treatments.

Clients should be encouraged to carry a card in their wallet indicating they have a living will and/or durable power of attorney on file. The name of their agent should be listed.

Do Not Resuscitate

A "Do Not Resuscitate" (DNR) or sometimes called "Do Not Attempt to Resuscitate" (DNAR) order is another type of advance directive. A DNR is a request to not have cardiopulmonary resuscitation (CPR) if the client ceases to breathe or is unable to sustain a heartbeat. An advance directive form can be signed at any time before or during hospitalization. When signed, the physician places a DNR notation in the client's medical chart. (*See* Chapter 32.)

CLINICAL PRACTICE

Before your first clinical experience, you should review the most essential components of client care to enable you to practice safe and efficient nursing care. Guidelines for clinical practice, the parts of a client chart, communication techniques, principles of medical asepsis, a basic nursing assessment, and protocols for nursing care procedures are presented to give you confidence and background information in providing nursing care.

Guidelines for Clinical Practice

Before attempting to provide client care, you need to familiarize yourself with all aspects of the care the client requires. The following guidelines will assist you in this preparation. Usually, the preparation is completed the night before you go to the clinical setting. If this is not possible, you need to identify those aspects of preparation that will render you a safe practitioner.

- Obtain the clinical assignment in sufficient time to be able to prepare for safe practice.
- Read client's chart or computer data and obtain information necessary to assist you in client care. This usually encompasses the following items: history and physical, physician's progress notes, graphic sheet, medication record, laboratory findings, nurses' notes or flow sheets or both, admissions data base, client care plan, Kardex card, and physician's orders. Each of these documents is illustrated later in this chapter.
- Review all procedures that you will provide for the client. Use your skills and fundamentals books for your review.
- Research the diagnosis so that you are more aware of signs and symptoms the client may exhibit. Identify alterations from normal such as altered laboratory values, vital signs, and so forth.
- Research all medications you will administer to the client. Many instructors require that medication cards be completed on all medications prior to administration.
- Plan your day's schedule by developing a time management plan to help keep you organized and to enable you to complete client care in a timely manner.
- Practice charting the procedures you will be administering so that you can identify appropriate vocabulary and include necessary information. Pertinent charting

24-HOUR CLOCK

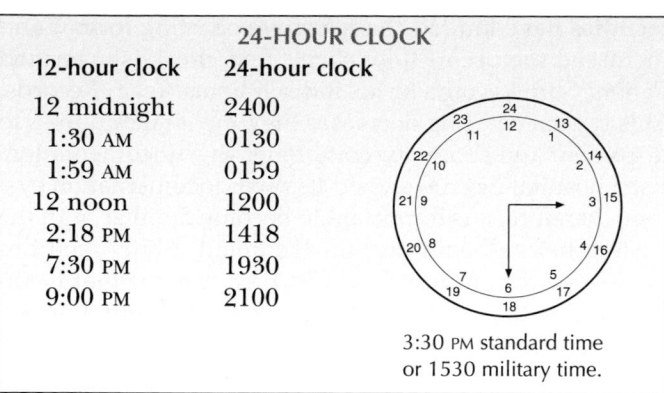

12-hour clock	24-hour clock
12 midnight	2400
1:30 AM	0130
1:59 AM	0159
12 noon	1200
2:18 PM	1418
7:30 PM	1930
9:00 PM	2100

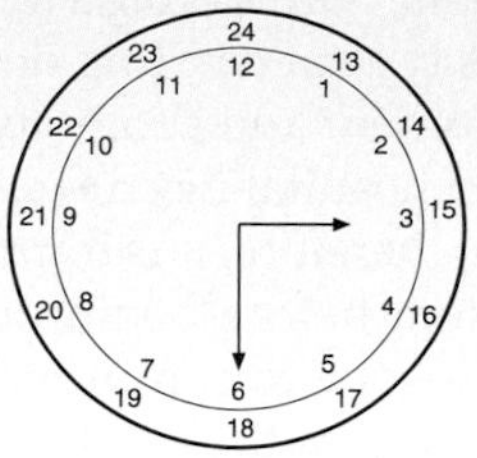

3:30 PM standard time or 1530 military time.

Figure 1-2

information is included with each procedure described in this text.

- Complete a clinical prep sheet as required by the instructor. The sheet usually has a section for all pertinent data.

Military Time The use of "military time" is becoming more common in health care facilities today. One advantage of using this time frame is that the confusion of whether something is ordered or documented in the A.M. or P.M. is avoided. "Military time" describes time as a 24-hour clock rather than the standard 12-hour clock like your watch. Midnight is identified as 24:00, 1:00 A.M. is 01:00, 3:00 P.M. is 15:00, etc. Review both the 24-hour clock and the chart above to acquaint yourself with this method of keeping time.

Providing Client Care

You have prepared for this clinical practice before coming to the nursing unit. Now you receive an update on the client's condition, and a team leader or nurse preceptor goes over nursing procedures you will be completing. This is accomplished during a report period. Each hospital has a method for presenting the report. Some facilities tape a report from the off-going shift that is listened to by the on-coming staff. Other nursing units give a verbal report in which they review the information obtained by the previous shift. Facilities where primary nursing is practiced have a one-to-one report between the on-coming nurse and the off-going nurse for a specific group of clients. At this time a work sheet is completed that lists times for treatments and medications. Following the report, the team leader or your preceptor nurse goes over all aspects of the care you will deliver for the client. This is the time to ask any questions you may have regarding policy or procedure for the nursing unit or the client. Your medications are checked at this time to ensure that you have all necessary medications and equipment to prepare and administer the drugs.

The following outline of client care will assist you in planning your nursing care for the day.

1. Wash your hands.
2. Gather equipment, such as a stethoscope, sphygmomanometer, thermometer, and linen.
3. Check the client's identaband. Introduce yourself to the client and explain the nursing care you will be giving.
4. Check if the client has any preference for the order in which the care is to be given.
5. Complete a nursing assessment. You may use the basic nursing assessment outlined in this chapter as a guide if your instructor does not have one she or he prefers you to use.
6. Document your findings as you are completing the physical assessment, and enter it in the nurses' notes section of the chart or on the flow sheet.
7. Take vital signs if it is the policy of the unit.
8. Don gloves (if appropriate) and complete all nursing interventions, and document the findings immediately after completion.
9. Administer all medications. Document medication administration in the appropriate place, and observe for signs of side effects or unusual findings.
10. During your nursing care, practice good communication techniques.
11. Complete all charting.
12. Terminate the relationship with the client.
13. Report off to the appropriate person.
14. Wash your hands after providing nursing care and before leaving the nursing unit.

Client's Records

Become familiar with each form, its placement in the chart, and the information that it contains. Brief examples of some of these forms are included in this chapter and examples of these forms are included in Chapter 3.

Kardex The Kardex card represents the "hub" for all client activities. Physician's orders are transcribed on the card. Laboratory tests, medications, and activity levels are just a few items documented in designated areas of the Kardex.

Computerized client information is replacing the Kardex card in many facilities today. The same information is contained on the electronic version, but in many cases, the information is more up to date.

Care Plan Client care plans vary among health care facilities. The more common individualized handwritten care plan is being replaced by preprinted standardized care plans, computerized care plans, or critical pathways. Regardless of the type of care plan used, the purpose does not change. Care plans are written guidelines for client care that all health care workers use to deliver individualized care. Most care plans today are termed Multidisciplinary Care Plans as all health team providers document treatments and observations on one form. Pertinent data regarding client care needs can be communicated to all providers using the multidisciplinary care plan. Client teaching is frequently detailed on the same form.

Critical or Clinical Pathway You may see either of these terms used to describe an approach to deliver collaborative, outcome-driven health care to clients. These documents are another approach to providing individualized care to clients. Interventions and outcomes are progressively outlined within the pathway as illustrated.

Client's Chart

The chart itself contains several forms that are important to your preparation and administration of nursing care. Be sure to familiarize yourself with the specific forms in the health care facility where you have your clinical experience. The following forms are intended to be just examples.

Nurses' Notes Nurses' notes are documents that contain clinical observations and nursing interventions. Many facilities have limited the narrative charting format and increased the use of flow sheets and checklists, termed Patient Care Records or Multidisciplinary Team Records. This type of charting decreases the time it takes nurses to document and promotes comprehensive documentation. Each hospital has developed its own documentation system; therefore, it is important to become familiar with the system before beginning to document. Many facilities have gone to computerized charting systems that facilitate a more thorough mechanism for data input. In-service education programs on use of the computer for charting and data retrieval needs to be completed before clinical experience is begun to ensure that you can obtain all the necessary information to provide safe care for the client.

Medication Records Medication records are usually similar to those illustrated (Chapter 18). All medications should be documented on a medication record. Some facilities chart routine medications on one medication sheet and prn and one-time only medications on another sheet. Check the institution's policy for each record's use.

Graphic Records Vital signs are recorded on the graphic sheet, including blood pressure, pulse, respirations, tem-

COMMUNITY HOSPITAL

CLIENT CARE PLAN

Client Information

Discharge Criteria
1) Lungs clear to auscultation.
2) Voiding qs and continent of urine.
3) Verbalizes an understanding of discharge instructions and medications.
4)

Admitting Diagnosis

Relevant Info:

Date	Problem/Need	Expected Outcome/Goal	CP	DL	Nursing Interventions	Update / DC	Initial
3/22/04	(1.) Ineffective Breathing Pattern related to pain.	Absence of respiratory complications.	q2h x24h then q4h x48h then q8h q3-4 h	POD 3 3/25 3 pm	1a. Encourage turning, coughing and deep breathing exercises (TCDB) q2h. b. Teach client to splint incision when coughing. c. Instruct in use of breathing device, if ordered. d. Place in semi-Fowler's position. e. Assess need for pain med. f. Medicate for pain 1/2hr. before TCDB. g. Auscultate breath sounds.		
	2. Altered Urinary Elimination related to incontinence.	Continent of urine. Absence of urinary tract infection (UTI).	q4h	cath. out	2a. Check urinary output for signs and symptoms of UTI, ie. color, odor, consistency. b. Provide catheter care according to protocol. c. Force fluids to 2500mL. d. Give cranberry juice, 240mL q shift.		
3/22/04	(3.) Knowledge Deficit related to administration of discharge meds.	Verbalizes understanding of discharge meds, including listing signs and symptoms of side effects.	q24h	prior to disch	3a. Instruct in action of Maxaquin b. Review side effects with client and/or family. c. Have client state signs and symptoms of side effects prior to discharge. d. Provide Take Home Medication pamphlet.		

Figure 1-3 Standardized care plan.

COMMUNITY HOSPITAL

CLIENT CARE PLAN
Individualized

Client Information

Discharge Criteria
1) *Wound healing progressing satisfactorily*
2) *Verbalizes ability to care for wound at home*
3) *Verbalizes understanding of discharge instructions*
4)

Admitting Diagnosis

Relevant Info:

Date	Problem/Need	Expected Outcome/Goal	CP	DL	Nursing Interventions	Update/DC	Initial
3/22/04	*Impaired skin integrity*	*Wound healing s̄*	*q̄4h*	*Prior*	*4a. Place on Lt side c̄ chux under hips & abd.*		
	related to prolonged	*s̄ complications*		*to dis-*	*Gently move into this position. Do not rush c̄ move.*		
	immobility			*charge*	*b. Note drainage location, quantity color & odor.*		
					c. Irrig. wound c̄ 50 ml. saline solution. Use		
					asepto syringe. Catch solution in emesis basin.		
					d. Cover wound with ABD dressings. Use		
					Montgomery straps.		

Figure 1-4 Individualized client care plan.

perature and pain level. Most facilities have included the pain scale on the graphic record as it is referred to as the fifth vital sign. Weight is also included on this form. Intake and output results may be recorded on this record or on a separate form depending on the facility.

Physician's Orders Physician's orders may be written on forms with carbon copies attached, are preprinted, or are computerized, depending on the facility. If the orders are carbon copied, copies can be sent to the pharmacy and to the lab, with the original retained in the client's chart. Computerized orders can be easily utilized by all hospital departments.

Physician's Progress Notes Physician's progress notes (Fig. 1-11) contain daily observations and thoughts regarding treatments, signs, and symptoms experienced by the client, operative risks explained to the client, and the client's responses to therapy.

History and Physical The physician's report of his assessment is written on a special form (Fig. 1-12). Most hospitals type the history and physical from notes dictated by the physician. When this occurs, it may be several days before this information is available.

Laboratory Forms Laboratory results are sent back to the unit on the original laboratory order form (Figs. 1-13, 1-14). The information from each form may be transcribed to a laboratory data flow sheet. This sheet provides a valuable overview of all laboratory results. Computerized reports of laboratory findings may be used in some facilities.

Basic Nursing Assessment

Each nurse develops her or his own routine for completing a basic nursing assessment. There is no right or wrong way, although it should be consistent and complete. The following outline for basic assessment is a simple approach to the assessment and one you may wish to adopt until you have established a good system for yourself.

The basic assessment is completed at the beginning of each shift. The assessment should take no longer than 5 to 10 minutes to complete. You should focus on the specific physiologic system that correlates with the client's diagnosis. For a more in-depth discussion of each system in the assessment, see Chapter 11 on physical assessment.

The following outline will assist you in completing a basic physical assessment.

1. Vital signs:
   a. Temperature (method dictated by condition)
   b. Radial pulse: rate, volume, and rhythm
   c. Respirations: rate, depth, and rhythm
   d. Blood pressure: Korotkoff's sounds
   e. Pain: location and intensity of pain; use pain scale to determine pain level.
2. Response to medications if given
3. Emotional responses: client behavior, reactions, and demeanor; general mood (crying, depression)
4. Skin, hair, and nails: Skin: presence or absence of abrasions, contusions, tears, erythema, pressure ulcers, incision line, color, turgor, temperature, edema. Inspect hair distribution, thickness or thin-

ness, texture, and amount. Inspect nails for curvature and angle, texture, color and surrounding tissue.

5. Musculoskeletal: activity level, general mobility, gait, range of motion
6. Neurological: pupils (size, response, equality); hand grips; strength and sensation of all extremities; ability to follow commands; level of consciousness
7. Respiratory: breath sounds; sputum color and consistency; cough (productive or nonproductive)
8. Cardiovascular: heart sounds; presence of pulses; edema; presence of hair on extremities
9. Gastrointestinal: bowel pattern and sounds; presence of nausea or vomiting; abdominal distention; consumption of diet
10. Genitourinary: voiding; color, odor, and consistency of urine; dysuria; vaginal drainage or discomfort; penile discharge

If any unusual findings are assessed, complete a more in-depth assessment of the particular system affected. Throughout the day, continue to assess changes in the client's condition by paying particular attention to the alterations from normal that you identified in the initial assessment. At the end of the shift, make a notation of any changes in the client's condition.

MEDICAL ASEPSIS PRINCIPLES

Microorganisms are found everywhere in nature. Pathogenic microorganisms, or pathogens, cause disease; nonpathogenic microorganisms, or nonpathogens, do not cause disease. Some microorganisms are nonpathogens in their normal body environment. An example of this is *Escherichia coli*, which is normally present in the intestinal tract and does not cause a problem until it inhabits another environment such as the urinary tract.

The spread of microorganisms is prevented by the use of two forms of asepsis: medical asepsis and surgical asepsis. Medical asepsis occurs when there is an absence of pathogens. Surgical asepsis occurs when there is an absence of all organisms. Medical asepsis is often referred to as "clean technique," whereas surgical asepsis is termed "sterile technique." A discussion of surgical asepsis can be found later in this book. This chapter discusses medical asepsis as it affects nursing care.

Principles of medical asepsis are used in all aspects of client care. In fact, the use of medical asepsis begins before you report to the nursing unit. To ensure protection for the client, you begin practicing medical asepsis by limiting jewelry to only a wedding band and perhaps small earrings for pierced ears when administering client care. Fingernails are short and in good repair. Your hair is off your collar and under control to prevent contaminating sterile fields and falling into client's food or wounds.

While providing client care, the following principles should be kept in mind:

- Linen rooms or carts are considered clean; therefore linen not used for client care cannot be returned.

Day 3 **POD 2**	**Day 4** **POD 3**	**Day 5** **POD 4**
• **q 8 hr.** ✓ Basic assessment, CMS, Drsg, I&O, SPO_2, VS, IV site, skin assessment. • ✓ Homan sign. HV dc'd. • Oxygen protocol.	• **q 8 hr.** ✓ Basic assessment, CMS, Drsg, I&O, past or present IV site healing, skin assessment, Homan sign. • Oxygen protocol.	• **q 8 hr.** ✓ Basic assessment, skin, assessment, CMS, Drsg, I&O, Homan sign. • Oxygen protocol. • ✓ past or present IV site healing.
• ↑ gait training. • Ambulate BID if able.	• Ambulate BID. • PT/Nursing.	• Ambulate BID. • PT/Nursing.
• TED/SCD, I.S., TCDB. Foley remains if needed or until Epidural dc'd. • *Hip Precaution for hemiathroplasty only*	• TED/SCD • DC Foley. • TCDB, especially prior to SpO_2✓. • *Hip Precaution for hemiathroplasty only*	• TED/SCD. • TCDB. • *Hip Precaution for hemiathroplasty only*
• Stool softener, Iron supp. BID (hold if GI upset). Cathartic if no BM. • Anticoagulant.	• Stool softener, Iron supp. BID (hold if GI upset). • Anticoagulant.	• Stool softener, Iron supp. BID (hold if GI upset). • Anticoagulant.
• IV TKO, IVL, or DC if not needed (leave IVL until Epidural dc'd).	• IV dc'd.	
• Diet as tolerated.	• DAT.	• DAT.
• If PCA or Epidural taper dose & give PO pain meds.	• Taper and DC PCA; give PO pain meds. ✓ $SpO_2 \times 1$. SpO_2 reading.	• PO pain meds, reassessing pain level.
• Analgesia method.	• Analgesia method, Pharmaceutical & non-pharmaceutical pain control. • Discharge plan reinforced.	• Understands Ortho inst, risk of DVT/PE, Hip precautions. • Reinforce any instruction given. • Answer any questions patient may have.
• BCP CN or RN to notify MD if platelet count shows 100,000 drop in past 24 hr.	• BCP CN or RN notify MD if platelet count shows 100,000 drop in past 24 hr.	• As indicated.
• PT BID. • Chaplain Services & Dietary consult PRN.	• PT. Chaplain Services & Dietary consult PRN.	• PT. Chaplain Services & Dietary consult PRN.
• SS assess if needed for SNF transfer (notify SS if min. assist needed).	• Discharge decision, S.S. assess if needed and not done.	• Arrange equipment needed for home. • Complete transfer sheet or discharge instructions.
Shift: 7-3 / 3-11 / 11-7 — Circle Yes (Y) or No (N) Y N / Y N / Y N Ambulation started (PT).	Shift: 7-3 / 3-11 / 11-7 — Circle Yes (Y) or No (N) Y N / Y N / Y N Voiding without Foley. Y N / Y N / Y N SS note re. discharge plan (SS).* Y N / Y N / Y N BM passed (RN). Y N / Y N / Y N Pain managed with PO medicine (RN).*	Shift: 7-3 / 3-11 / 11-7 — Circle Yes (Y) or No (N) Y N / Y N / Y N Discharge plan reinforced (RN). Y N / Y N / Y N Discharged to appropriate care level (RN).

11-7	11-7	11-7
11-7	11-7	11-7
7-3	7-3	7-3
7-3	7-3	7-3
7-3	7-3	7-3
3-11	3-11	3-11
3-11	3-11	3-11
3-11	3-11	3-11

Figure 1-5 Clinical pathway.

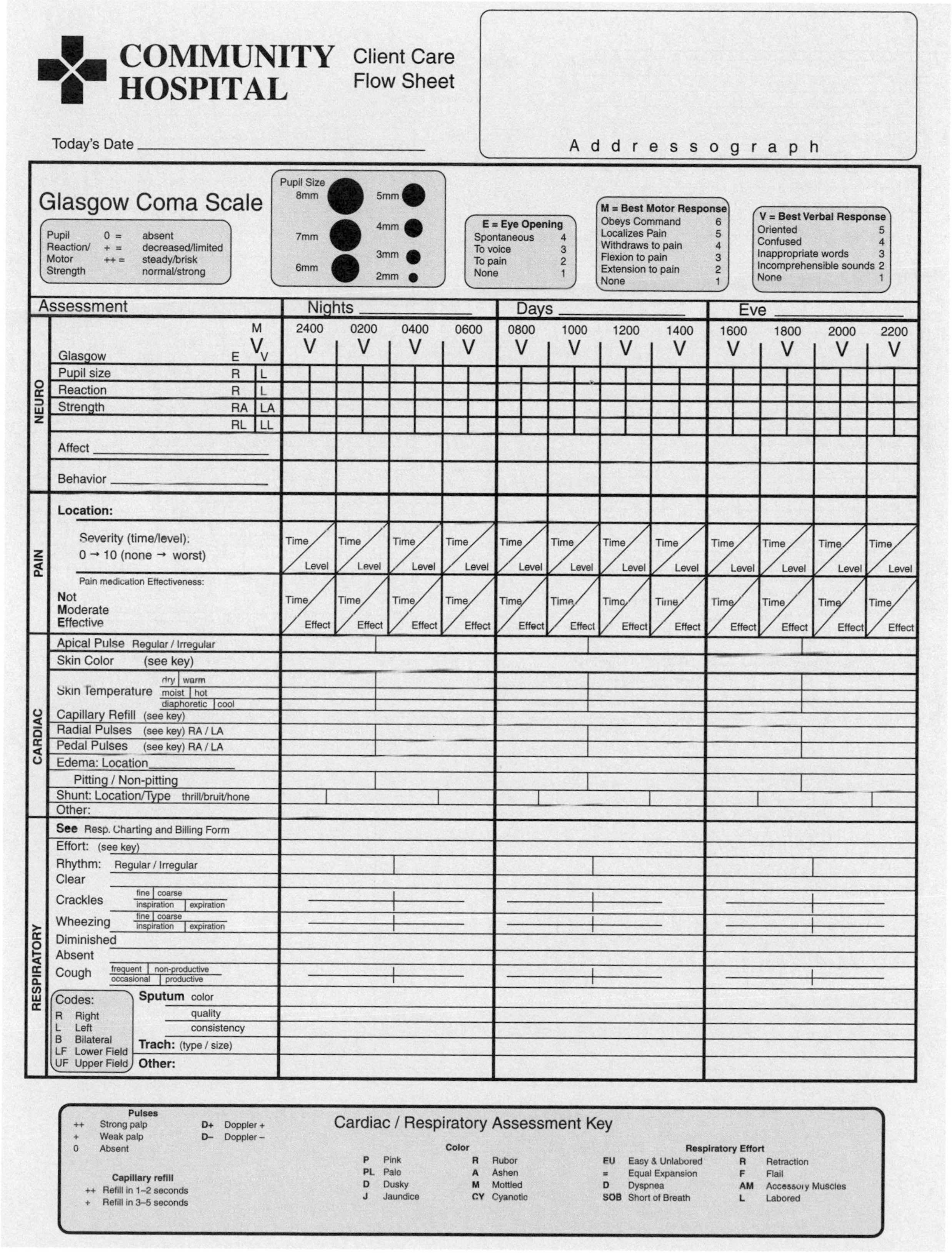

COMMUNITY HOSPITAL

Client Care Flow Sheet

Today's Date ____________

Addressograph

Glasgow Coma Scale

Pupil Reaction/ Motor Strength		
0 =	absent	
+ =	decreased/limited	
++ =	steady/brisk	normal/strong

Pupil Size: 8mm, 7mm, 6mm, 5mm, 4mm, 3mm, 2mm

E = Eye Opening	
Spontaneous	4
To voice	3
To pain	2
None	1

M = Best Motor Response	
Obeys Command	6
Localizes Pain	5
Withdraws to pain	4
Flexion to pain	3
Extension to pain	2
None	1

V = Best Verbal Response	
Oriented	5
Confused	4
Inappropriate words	3
Incomprehensible sounds	2
None	1

Assessment	Nights ____				Days ____				Eve ____			
	2400	0200	0400	0600	0800	1000	1200	1400	1600	1800	2000	2200
NEURO: Glasgow E M V	V	V	V	V	V	V	V	V	V	V	V	V
Pupil size R L												
Reaction R L												
Strength RA LA												
RL LL												
Affect ____												
Behavior ____												
PAIN: Location:												
Severity (time/level): 0 → 10 (none → worst)	Time / Level	Time / Level	Time / Level	Time / Level	Time / Level	Time / Level	Time / Level	Time / Level	Time / Level	Time / Level	Time / Level	Time / Level
Pain medication Effectiveness: Not Moderate Effective	Time / Effect	Time / Effect	Time / Effect	Time / Effect	Time / Effect	Time / Effect	Time / Effect	Time / Effect	Time / Effect	Time / Effect	Time / Effect	Time / Effect
CARDIAC: Apical Pulse Regular / Irregular												
Skin Color (see key)												
Skin Temperature dry / warm; moist / hot; diaphoretic / cool												
Capillary Refill (see key)												
Radial Pulses (see key) RA / LA												
Pedal Pulses (see key) RA / LA												
Edema: Location____												
Pitting / Non-pitting												
Shunt: Location/Type thrill/bruit/hone												
Other:												
RESPIRATORY: See Resp. Charting and Billing Form												
Effort: (see key)												
Rhythm: Regular / Irregular												
Clear												
Crackles fine / coarse; inspiration / expiration												
Wheezing fine / coarse; inspiration / expiration												
Diminished												
Absent												
Cough frequent / non-productive; occasional / productive												
Sputum color												
quality												
consistency												
Trach: (type / size)												
Other:												

Codes:
R Right
L Left
B Bilateral
LF Lower Field
UF Upper Field

Cardiac / Respiratory Assessment Key

Pulses
++ Strong palp
+ Weak palp
0 Absent
D+ Doppler +
D– Doppler –

Capillary refill
++ Refill in 1–2 seconds
+ Refill in 3–5 seconds

Color
P Pink
PL Pale
D Dusky
J Jaundice
R Rubor
A Ashen
M Mottled
CY Cyanotic

Respiratory Effort
EU Easy & Unlabored
= Equal Expansion
D Dyspnea
SOB Short of Breath
R Retraction
F Flail
AM Accessory Muscles
L Labored

Figure 1-6 Flow sheet.

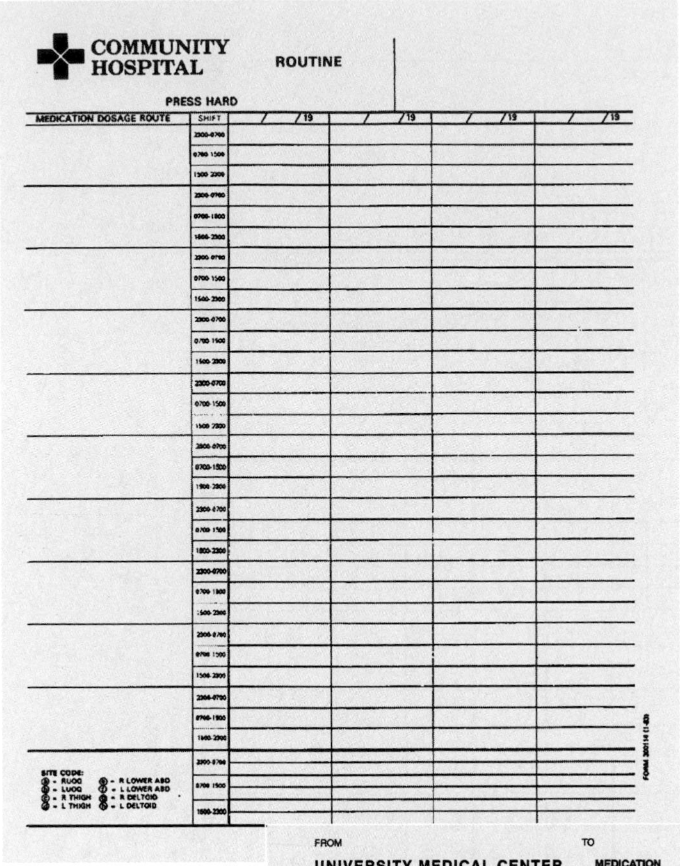

Figure 1-7 Medication record.

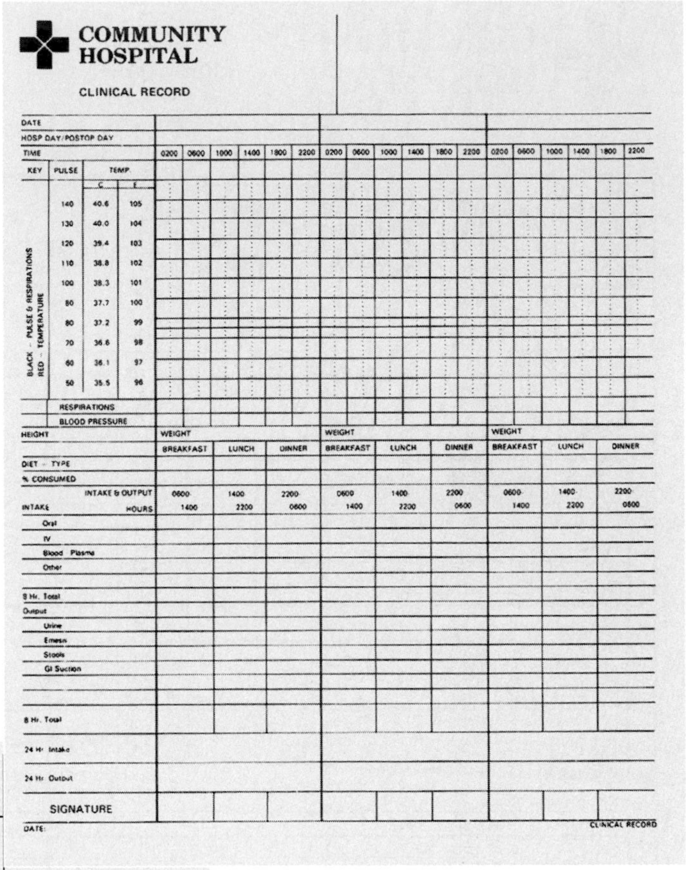

Figure 1-9 Graphic record.

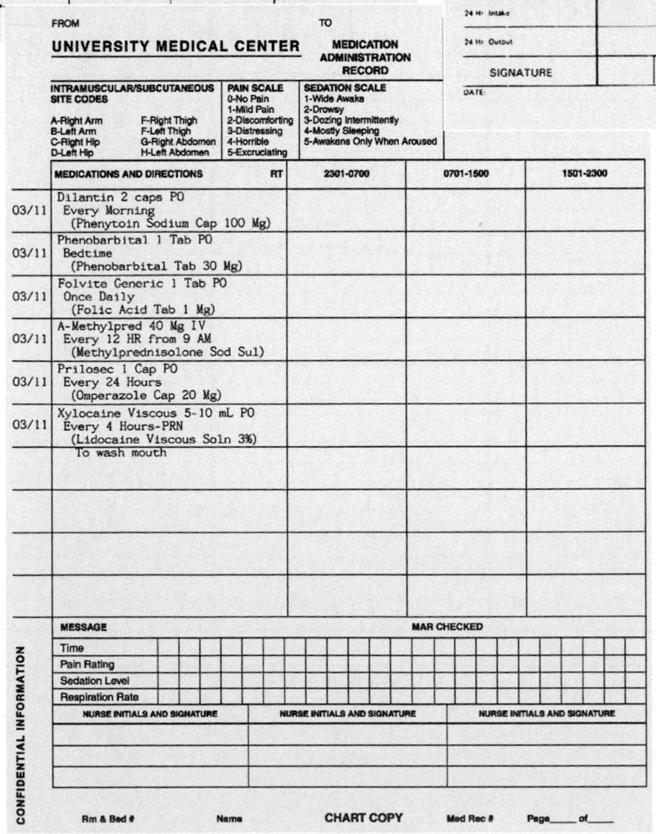

Figure 1-8 Medical administration record (MAR).

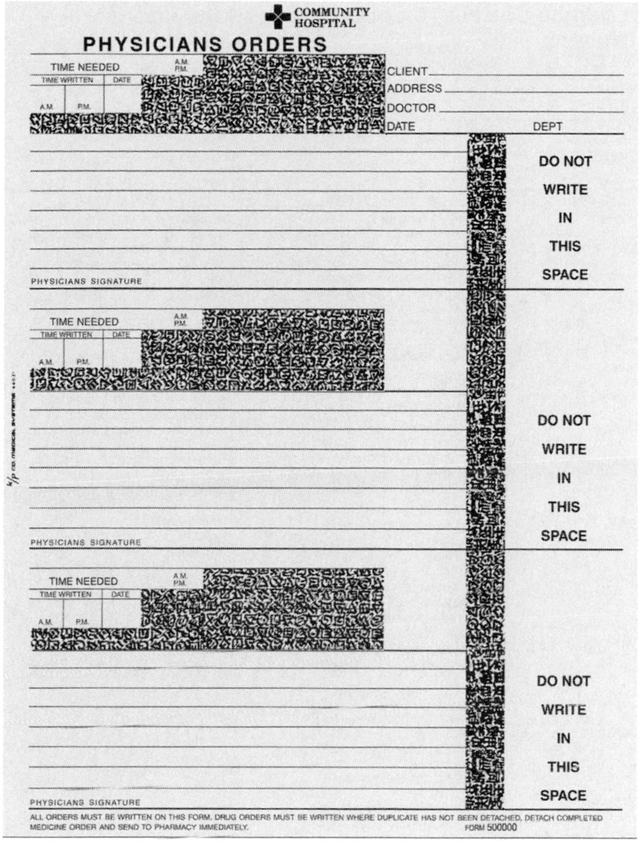
COMMUNITY HOSPITAL

PHYSICIANS ORDERS

TIME NEEDED A.M. P.M.
TIME WRITTEN DATE
A.M. P.M.
CLIENT
ADDRESS
DOCTOR
DATE DEPT

DO NOT WRITE IN THIS SPACE

PHYSICIANS SIGNATURE

TIME NEEDED A.M. P.M.
TIME WRITTEN DATE
A.M. P.M.

DO NOT WRITE IN THIS SPACE

PHYSICIANS SIGNATURE

TIME NEEDED A.M. P.M.
TIME WRITTEN DATE
A.M. P.M.

DO NOT WRITE IN THIS SPACE

PHYSICIANS SIGNATURE

ALL ORDERS MUST BE WRITTEN ON THIS FORM. DRUG ORDERS MUST BE WRITTEN WHERE DUPLICATE HAS NOT BEEN DETACHED. DETACH COMPLETED MEDICINE ORDER AND SEND TO PHARMACY IMMEDIATELY. FORM 500000

Figure 1-10 Physician's order sheet.

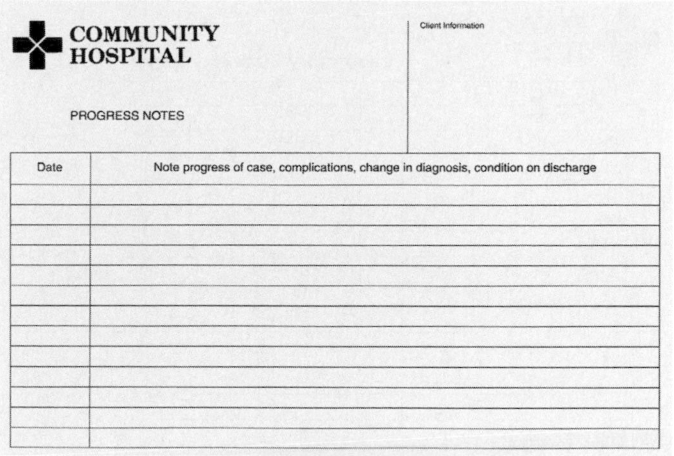
COMMUNITY HOSPITAL

PROGRESS NOTES

Client Information

Date	Note progress of case, complications, change in diagnosis, condition on discharge

Figure 1-11 Physician's progress notes.

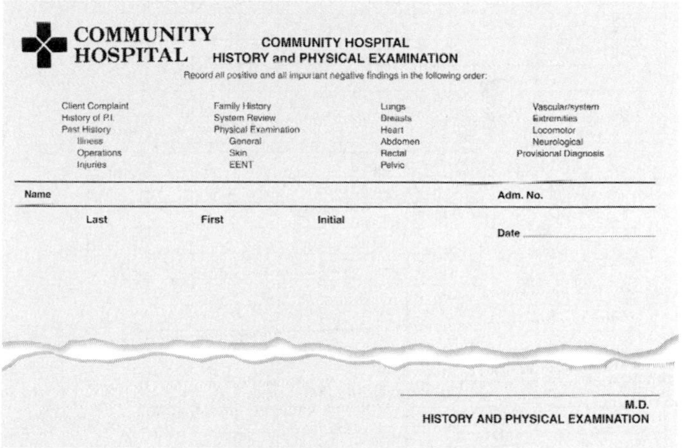
COMMUNITY HOSPITAL

COMMUNITY HOSPITAL
HISTORY and PHYSICAL EXAMINATION

Record all positive and all important negative findings in the following order:

Client Complaint, History of P.I., Past History, Illness, Operations, Injuries; Family History, System Review, Physical Examination, General, Skin, EENT; Lungs, Breasts, Heart, Abdomen, Rectal, Pelvic; Vascular system, Extremities, Locomotor, Neurological, Provisional Diagnosis

Name Adm. No.
Last First Initial
Date

M.D.
HISTORY AND PHYSICAL EXAMINATION

Figure 1-12 Physician's history and physical record.

- Utility rooms are designated as areas for clean and dirty supplies. Cross-contamination must be avoided by not placing articles in the wrong area.
- Linen and articles are carried away from your uniform and are not held close to your body.
- Articles dropped on the floor are considered contaminated and must be discarded appropriately. If linen is accidentally dropped on the floor, it is placed in a soiled linen hamper.
- Clients are to wear slippers or shoes when out of bed.
- Each client has his or her own supplies and equipment, which are not used by other clients. Sterilization or disinfection of equipment is carried out between use.
- If you are not feeling well, you should not report for clinical experience. If you are running a temperature or have a cold and a runny nose, call the appropriate person and report that you are ill.
- Paper tissue is used for removing client's secretions. Discard the tissue in the trash basket.
- Equipment is cleaned and rinsed with cold water to remove secretions or substances before being returned to the central supply area. Heat coagulates the substances and makes it more difficult to remove.
- Soap and water are considered the best cleansers because they help break down soil so it can be more readily removed. Detergents may be more effective in hard or cold water; however, tissue damage can result from their use. Germicides may be added to soap or detergent and increase the effectiveness of the cleansing agent.
- Friction is used to facilitate soil removal. A brush, sponge, or cloth may be used to produce the friction.
- When aseptic technique is used, cleaning is conducted from the cleanest to the least clean area. For example, always clean the incision area from the center of the incision to the periphery of the skin.

Handwashing

The single most effective medical aseptic practice is handwashing. When you first arrive at the nursing unit and before beginning nursing practice, you should complete a medical handwashing procedure. The important concept to remember is that you soap and rinse your hands twice before providing any nursing care to the client. Hands are

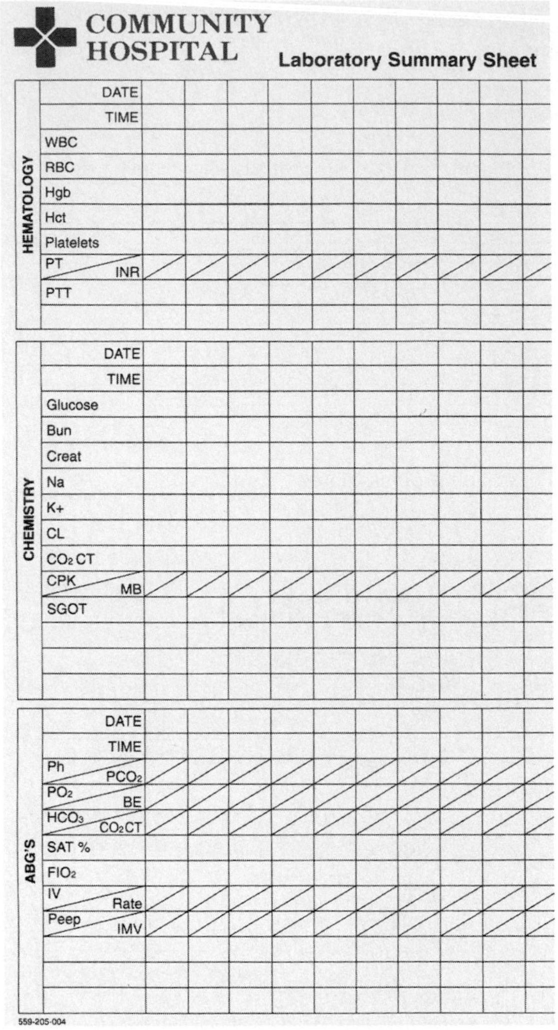

COMMUNITY HOSPITAL
Laboratory Summary Sheet

HEMATOLOGY
DATE
TIME
WBC
RBC
Hgb
Hct
Platelets
PT / INR
PTT

CHEMISTRY
DATE
TIME
Glucose
Bun
Creat
Na
K+
CL
CO_2 CT
CPK / MB
SGOT

ABG'S
DATE
TIME
Ph / PCO_2
PO_2 / BE
HCO_3 / CO_2CT
SAT %
FIO_2
IV / Rate
Peep / IMV

559-205-004

Figure 1-13 Laboratory results flow sheet.

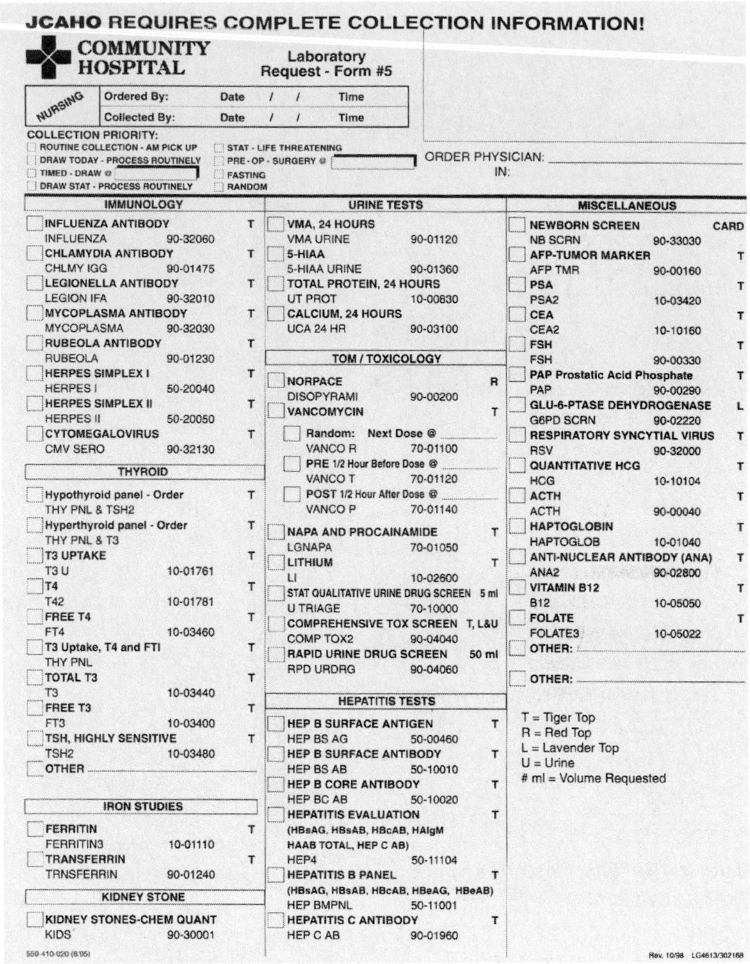

JCAHO REQUIRES COMPLETE COLLECTION INFORMATION!

COMMUNITY HOSPITAL
Laboratory Request - Form #5

NURSING
Ordered By: Date / / Time
Collected By: Date / / Time

COLLECTION PRIORITY:
ROUTINE COLLECTION - AM PICK UP
DRAW TODAY - PROCESS ROUTINELY
TIMED - DRAW @
DRAW STAT - PROCESS ROUTINELY
STAT - LIFE THREATENING
PRE-OP - SURGERY @
FASTING
RANDOM

ORDER PHYSICIAN:
IN:

IMMUNOLOGY
INFLUENZA ANTIBODY T
INFLUENZA 90-32060
CHLAMYDIA ANTIBODY T
CHLMY IGG 90-01475
LEGIONELLA ANTIBODY T
LEGION IFA 90-32010
MYCOPLASMA ANTIBODY T
MYCOPLASMA 90-32030
RUBEOLA ANTIBODY T
RUBEOLA 90-01230
HERPES SIMPLEX I T
HERPES I 50-20040
HERPES SIMPLEX II T
HERPES II 50-20050
CYTOMEGALOVIRUS T
CMV SERO 90-32130

THYROID
Hypothyroid panel - Order T
THY PNL & TSH2
Hyperthyroid panel - Order T
THY PNL & T3
T3 UPTAKE T
T3 U 10-01761
T4 T
T42 10-01781
FREE T4 T
FT4 10-03460
T3 Uptake, T4 and FTI T
THY PNL
TOTAL T3 T
T3 10-03440
FREE T3 T
FT3 10-03400
TSH, HIGHLY SENSITIVE T
TSH2 10-03480
OTHER

IRON STUDIES
FERRITIN T
FERRITIN3 10-01110
TRANSFERRIN T
TRNSFERRIN 90-01240

KIDNEY STONE
KIDNEY STONES-CHEM QUANT
KIDS 90-30001

URINE TESTS
VMA, 24 HOURS
VMA URINE 90-01120
5-HIAA
5-HIAA URINE 90-01360
TOTAL PROTEIN, 24 HOURS
UT PROT 10-00830
CALCIUM, 24 HOURS
UCA 24 HR 90-03100

TOM / TOXICOLOGY
NORPACE R
DISOPYRAMI 90-00200
VANCOMYCIN T
Random: Next Dose @
VANCO R 70-01100
PRE 1/2 Hour Before Dose @
VANCO T 70-01120
POST 1/2 Hour After Dose @
VANCO P 70-01140
NAPA AND PROCAINAMIDE T
LGNAPA 70-01050
LITHIUM T
LI 10-02600
STAT QUALITATIVE URINE DRUG SCREEN 5 ml
U TRIAGE 70-10000
COMPREHENSIVE TOX SCREEN T, L&U
COMP TOX2 90-04040
RAPID URINE DRUG SCREEN 50 ml
RPD URDRG 90-04060

HEPATITIS TESTS
HEP B SURFACE ANTIGEN T
HEP BS AG 50-00460
HEP B SURFACE ANTIBODY T
HEP BS AB 50-10010
HEP B CORE ANTIBODY T
HEP BC AB 50-10020
HEPATITIS EVALUATION T
(HBsAG, HBsAB, HBcAB, HAIgM HAAB TOTAL, HEP C AB)
HEP4 50-11104
HEPATITIS B PANEL T
(HBsAG, HBsAB, HBcAB, HBeAG, HBeAB)
HEP BMPNL 50-11001
HEPATITIS C ANTIBODY T
HEP C AB 90-01960

MISCELLANEOUS
NEWBORN SCREEN CARD
NB SCRN 90-33030
AFP-TUMOR MARKER T
AFP TMR 90-00160
PSA T
PSA2 10-03420
CEA T
CEA2 10-10160
FSH T
FSH 90-00330
PAP Prostatic Acid Phosphate T
PAP 90-00290
GLU-6-PTASE DEHYDROGENASE L
G6PD SCRN 90-02220
RESPIRATORY SYNCYTIAL VIRUS T
RSV 90-32000
QUANTITATIVE HCG T
HCG 10-10104
ACTH T
ACTH 90-00040
HAPTOGLOBIN T
HAPTOGLOB 10-01040
ANTI-NUCLEAR ANTIBODY (ANA) T
ANA2 90-02800
VITAMIN B12 T
B12 10-05050
FOLATE T
FOLATE3 10-05022
OTHER:
OTHER:

T = Tiger Top
R = Red Top
L = Lavender Top
U = Urine
# ml = Volume Requested

559-410-020 (8/95)
Rev. 10/98 LG4613/302168

Figure 1-14 Laboratory order forms.

washed before all procedures and in between clients. Antibacterial gels are used between clients if hands are not dirty. The specific step-by-step handwashing procedure is covered in Chapter 14, Infection Control.

Clean, nonsterile gloves are worn when touching blood, body fluids, secretions, excretions, and contaminated items. Gloves are discarded immediately after use in an appropriate container. Gloving decreases the risk of cross-contamination between clients and between clients and health care workers. Handwashing is completed following removal of gloves.

PROTOCOL FOR PROCEDURES

Each procedure in this textbook follows a basic protocol. To save space and prevent repetition, all steps in the protocol are frequently not outlined in detail for each procedure. Remember, however, that these steps are important and must be followed if complete and responsible nursing care is to be delivered to the patient.

- Check physician's orders.
- Check client care plan, clinical pathway, or Kardex.
- Identify client.
- Introduce yourself to the client.
- Explain procedure to be done.
- Answer client's questions and reinforce teaching.
- Wash your hands.
- Gather equipment and fill out charge slips.
- Take all of the required equipment to the room.
- Provide privacy for the client by drawing curtain or screen around bed.
- Raise bed to HIGH position.
- Lower side rail nearest you.
- Drape client (if appropriate).
- Don gloves (if appropriate).
- Perform procedure according to protocol.
- Clean client as necessary.
- Remove drape and position client for comfort.
- Remove gloves.

- Raise side rail to UP position.
- Lower bed.
- Replace call bell.
- Pull back curtain or remove screen.
- Remove equipment and clean, dispose, and disperse used equipment.
- Wash hands.
- Document or chart findings.

MANAGEMENT GUIDELINES

Each state legislates a Nurse Practice Act for RNs and LVN/LPNs. Health care facilities are responsible for establishing and implementing policies and procedures that conform to their state's regulations. Verify the regulations and role parameters for each health care worker in your facility.

Delegation of Responsibilities

- As an RN you will be held accountable and responsible for your actions. You must know the health care worker's level of client care tasks that can be assigned. The Nurse Practice Act for both RN and Vocational/Practical Nurse must be adhered to when assigning client care. The skill level and scope of practice of unassisted licensed personnel must be evaluated before assigning client care.
- The RN must abide by and function within the American Nurses Association Code for nurses. The RN is responsible for the appropriate delegation of nursing tasks to others in order to provide safe, competent client care.
- Legal issues and regulations must be followed in order to establish appropriate client care standards when delegating to other health care workers. The RN has a responsibility for a level of performance which must be carried out and cannot be delegated, including health care teaching, initial assessment, and the administration of IV medications.
- The signing of a consent form for surgery or an invasive procedure may be delegated to the LVN/LPN, and in some facilities a ward clerk may obtain the consent. Informed consent is the responsibility of the physician; however, most facilities allow nurses and other health care workers to witness the client's signature on the consent form after an explanation has been provided by the physician. Some facilities require that a physician obtain the signed consent form. The signature of the witness indicates only that he or she obtained the client's signature on the form. The RN is still responsible for ensuring that the client understands what the procedure is, including potential complications. If the client is unsure of the procedure, the physician needs to be notified to reexplain the procedure until the client understands.

Information Flow

- Each member of the nursing unit should be given appropriate directions on the tasks to be completed, keeping in mind the legal issues surrounding delegation. Assign only those tasks the health care worker is legally responsible to carry out.
- The RN must ensure that proper consent forms are signed by the client prior to invasive procedures or surgery. Even when the task of witnessing a consent form signing is delegated, the RN is responsible for ensuring it is completed and placed in the client's chart. Ask the delegee to inform you when all paperwork is completed for the procedure in order for you to check the forms.
- Ensure that all health care workers are aware of DNR orders. Make sure the Kardex or plan of care adequately states the DNR order, and provide that information during report.
- Give specific directions to health care workers regarding the client information you wish reported and how you wish to receive it (i.e., written or verbal).
- Provide current information to health care workers in a timely manner as it impacts their care of the client (i.e., changes in activity or diet orders).

CRITICAL THINKING STRATEGIES

SCENARIO 1

As a new student you are going into the hospital to prepare for the clinical experience tomorrow morning. There are two stages of preparation. The first stage is obtaining all the necessary information you will need to provide safe care. The second stage is reviewing your textbooks and lecture notes to gain an understanding of the client's diagnosis, medications, lab values, and diagnostic tests that will be done during his/her hospitalization.

1. If you have only a limited time to review the client's chart, what sections of the chart will provide you with sufficient information to render you safe to care for the client?
2. In preparing for clinical practice, what information is essential to review in addition to the data you have obtained from the clinical record? Where is the most appropriate place to find this information?
3. List the priority interventions you will carry out within the first hour of the clinical experience. Explain the rationale for your answers.

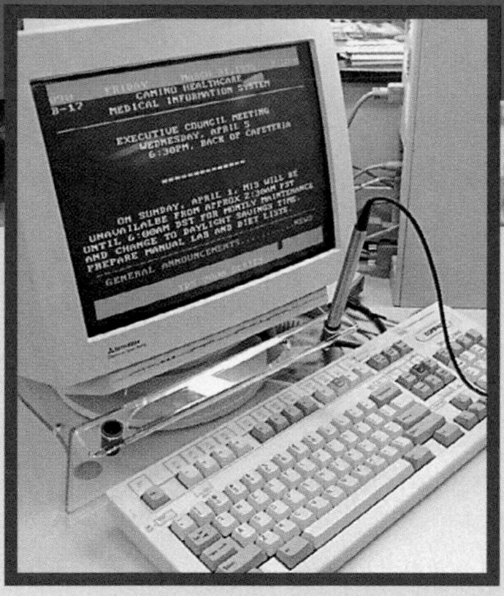

CHAPTER 2

Nursing Process and Critical Thinking

Nursing Process 22
Critical Thinking 24
Nurses Are Critical Thinkers 25
Nursing Diagnosis 27
Evidence Based Nursing Practice 30

MANAGEMENT GUIDELINES 31

CRITICAL THINKING STRATEGIES 32

LEARNING OBJECTIVES

- Define the term *critical thinking.*
- Explain how critical thinking is used in each step of the nursing process.
- Define the term *nursing process.*
- Describe how the nursing process relates to nursing.
- Discuss the term *assessment,* and describe how it influences the nursing process.
- List the components of the assessment step.
- Describe the primary purpose of the analysis phase of the nursing process.
- Define outcome identification and planning, and give an example of this step in the nursing process.
- Define what is meant by the implementation phase of the nursing process.
- Explain evaluation and include your understanding of why it is an important step in the nursing process.
- Define the term *nursing diagnosis.*
- Differentiate nursing diagnosis from medical diagnosis.
- Compare and contrast the two-part and three-part Nursing Diagnosis Statement.
- Define evidence based nursing practice.
- State two examples of nursing diagnoses.

NURSING PROCESS

Nursing process is a familiar term in nursing and is used as a way of organizing nursing actions in health care delivery. It is a systematic, problem-solving approach to client care. It is considered a critical thinking competency that assists the nurse to intervene in client care. The nurse's actions are based on reasoning and scientific knowledge. By definition, the term *process* refers to a series of actions that lead toward a particular result. When attached to nursing, the term *nursing process* becomes a general description of nursing: assessment, analysis/nursing diagnosis, planning, implementation, and evaluation. The nursing process is used to diagnose and treat human responses to health and illness (American Nurses Association, 1980). The nursing process provides an organized structure and framework for the delivery of nursing care in all settings. It provides the basis for critical thinking in nursing. Although the five steps can be described separately and in logical order, in practice the steps overlap and events may not always occur in the order listed here. For purposes of understanding this process, however, it is appropriate to work through each phase in logical progression.

The five steps of the nursing process are presented, defined, and illustrated to assist you in understanding the importance of integrating this framework in your beginning mastery of nursing content. A model of each step will enable you to visualize how the individual components can be translated into direct nursing actions or behaviors.

Assessment

Assessment, the first step in the nursing process, refers to the establishment of a data base for a specific client. Assessment requires skilled observation, reasoning, and a theoretical knowledge base to gather and differentiate, verify and organize data, and document the findings. The nurse gathers information relevant to the client from a variety of sources and then assigns meaning to this data. Assessment is a critical phase because all the other steps in

Assessment

Gather data
  Objective data
  Subjective data
Verify data
Confirm observations
Organize data
Make inferences from data
Communicate data

Observe—Interview—Examine

Identify client needs
Be aware of staff reactions to client
Assess sources of data
  Client history
  Data from family
  Client status—physical/emotional
  Signs and symptoms
  Test results and findings
Recall stored knowledge

the process depend on the accuracy and reliability of the assessment. Assessment is based on concepts of physiology, pathophysiology, psychology, and social adjustment.

Nursing Diagnosis

Nursing diagnosis is an integral component of the nursing process. Following the assessment step of the nursing process, the formulation of a nursing diagnosis is made. Nursing diagnosis is the statement of a client problem derived from the systematic collection of data and its analysis. It is a clinical judgment about a designated client, family, or community that provides the basis for completion of the nursing process. Nursing diagnosis includes the etiology, when known, and relates directly to the defining characteristics, both major and minor. Nursing diagnosis provides the foundation for each individual client's therapeutic plan of care, and once it is established, the nurse is accountable for actions that occur within the scope of this nursing diagnosis framework.

Nursing diagnosis is a clinical judgment about individual, family, or community responses to actual or potential health problems/life processes. Nursing diagnoses provide the basis for selection of nursing interventions to achieve outcomes for which the nurse is accountable (North American Nursing Diagnosis Association, 1997). The nurse must use critical thinking and decision-making skills when determining nursing diagnoses.

Nursing Diagnosis

Analyze and synthesize collected data

Examine defining characteristics, both major and minor

Determine clusters of clues

Identify related factors

Identify potential nursing diagnoses

Develop nursing diagnosis appropriate to client problem

Outcome Identification and Planning

This phase refers to the identification of nursing actions that are strategies for achieving the goals or the desired outcome of nursing care. The planning and outcome phase should be directly related to solving or alleviating the problems identified in the nursing diagnosis. It includes a plan, short- and long-term client-centered goals, strategies for goal outcome, and nursing measures for the delivery of care. During this phase, the nursing diagnoses are prioritized to meet the client's immediate needs.

Clients should be involved in the planning phase to ensure that the client's and the health care team members' goals are congruent. If they are not, goal achievement can be impaired. Planning focuses on the development of a plan of care individualized for a specific client.

Planning

Identify short- and long-term goals and outcomes

Prioritize nursing diagnoses

Develop a plan based on goals and outcomes, including a teaching plan

Anticipate needs of client and family based on priorities

Select nursing behaviors needed to accomplish goals

Specify deadlines for completion of plan

Coordinate care and community resources

Consider contingencies for modifying plan

Record relevant information

Planning is based on the client's health care needs, selected goals, and strategies directed toward goal achievement. It is a plan of care in which the appropriate nursing actions and the client's desires are considered and chosen to achieve a goal.

Implementation

The fourth phase in the nursing process is the implementation, or intervention, phase. This phase refers to the priority nursing actions or interventions performed to accomplish a specified goal. It explicitly describes the action component of the nursing process. This phase involves initiating and completing those nursing actions

Implementation

Implement client care plan by giving direct care based on goals and outcomes

Perform actions and procedures in accordance with client needs

Counsel and teach client or family or both

Use preventive, palliative, or emergency measures for client's welfare

Encourage independence and self-care

Motivate and maintain optimum wellness

Communicate to client's family and allied staff

Supervise work of staff for whom nurse is responsible

Record data

Continue assessment process

necessary to accomplish the identified client goals and outcomes. Nursing actions must be appropriate, individualized for the client, and based on safe nursing practice; they should be formulated on scientific principles and derived from the problem-solving process. Finally, the interventions must be congruent with the total medical as well as nursing treatment plan. Implementation of the plan involves giving direct care to the client to accomplish the specified goal.

Implementation is based on accurate and complete assessment, interpretation of data, identified client needs, goals and outcomes, analysis, nursing diagnosis, and strategies to achieve goals.

Evaluation

The final phase of the nursing process is evaluation. Evaluation is the examination of the outcome of nursing actions or the extent to which the expected outcomes or goals were achieved. Was the goal achieved? What parts of the goal were not achieved? Was client behavior modified? Evaluation is a necessary phase to complete the nursing process. It allows the nurse to continue to identify goals in the overall treatment plan and to alter the current plan to the client's needs.

Evaluation is based on the previous phases of the nursing process (assessment, analysis, outcomes and planning, and implementation). The evaluation phase completes the process and examines the outcome.

The nursing process has provided the framework for the immense amount of nursing content that is contained in this textbook. The rationale for choosing this framework is that it provides a way to organize and present nursing knowledge as well as being an essential component of providing quality client care.

Evaluation

Determine effects of nursing actions

Determine extent to which goals and outcomes were achieved

Examine appropriateness of nursing actions

Investigate effect and degree of compliance for client and family

Reassess care plan—judge if goal modification is necessary

Consider alternative nursing actions

Record client responses

CRITICAL THINKING

All nurses are required to use critical thinking skills as they provide nursing care for clients. The National League for Nursing even requires that graduates of all types of nursing programs demonstrate critical thinking skills upon graduation. Nurses are expected to not only master nursing content in all disciplines, but to think creatively, solve problems, communicate, and use reflective judgment in the practice of nursing. Critical thinking involves problem solving and decision-making processes, but it is a more complex process. Critical thinkers look at a particular problem and then reflect back on previous nursing or life experiences as they clearly define the problem, analyze the data, and determine appropriate interventions to solve the problem.

There is no single accepted definition, but many authors have defined critical thinking in terms that are relevant to nursing. Critical thinking can be defined by looking first at what *critical* means. It comes from the Greek word *kritikos*, meaning "critic." To be critical means to ask questions, to analyze, to examine your own thinking and the thinking of others (Chaffee, 1994). Critical thinking focuses on judgment, and nurses in particular must use reflective judgment because each clinical situation they encounter is different and unique. Effective critical thinking and problem solving actually depend on relevant knowledge and previous experience (Facione 1998; McKeachie, 1999). The definition of critical thinking by Scriven and Paul (1996) for the National Council for Excellence in Critical Thinking Instruction is widely accepted today by many in the field of education. "Critical thinking is an intellectually disciplined process of actively and skillfully conceptualizing, applying, analyzing, synthesizing, and/or evaluating information gathered from, or generated by observation, experience, reflection, reasoning, or communication, as a guide to belief and action." To expand on this statement further, critical thinking requires cognitive skills, the ability to ask pertinent questions, knowledge, and the ability to think clearly. As stated, an important aspect of critical thinking is also the ability to use reflection and language properly. Reflection is the ability of thinking back or recalling an earlier clinical situation, remembering nursing actions which worked, and determining if this information is helpful in the current situation. The ability to use language is associated with the ability to think meaningfully. Thinking and language are closely related processes (Miller & Babcock, 1996). To become a critical thinker the nurse must use language accurately. If nurses are unable to use appropriate terminology, communication with the client and other health care workers may be impaired. In addition to these skills, nurses need to be creative thinkers in order to develop appropriate plans of care for clients.

Critical thinking competencies are the cognitive processes a nurse uses to make judgments. Specific critical thinking competencies in clinical situations include: diagnostic reasoning, clinical inferences, and clinical decision making. These competencies are used by many health care professionals. The nursing process is considered the specific critical thinking competency in nursing. Diagnostic reasoning is a series of clinical judgments made during and after data collection, resulting in an informal judgment or formal diagnosis (Carnevali & Thomas, 1993). This process assists in making clinical inferences or judgments about a client's plan of care. The clinical decision-making process uses reasoning to ensure that after evaluating all options available the best options are chosen to improve the client's health status.

Critical thinking skills assist the nurse to look at all aspects of a situation and then arrive at a conclusion. Critical thinkers identify and question assumptions, determine what is important in each situation, and examine each alternative before making an informed decision. When critical thinking is employed in a clinical situation you would expect that one would examine ideas, beliefs, principles, assumptions, conclusions, statements, and inferences before coming to a conclusion and then making a decision. The conclusions and decisions made by nurses affect clients' lives; therefore they must be guided by precise, disciplined thinking which leads to accurate and complete data collection. While examining the situation, using these concepts, the nurse would also be using scientific reasoning, the nursing process, and decision-making processes.

NURSES ARE CRITICAL THINKERS

Nurses are required to be problem solvers and decision makers, to acquire nursing judgment skills, and to think critically in order to practice in today's nursing climate. Decision-making and problem-solving skills are necessary for managing and delivering client care. Both of these skills require critical thinking.

Watson and Glaser have described critical thinking as a process that defines a problem, selects pertinent information for a solution, recognizes stated and unstated assumptions, formulates and selects relevant hypotheses, draws conclusions, and judges the validity of inferences. The outcome of critical thinking is forming a conclusion and stating the justification for that conclusion. This is what differentiates critical thinking from usual thinking.

Nurses who are considered critical thinkers are those who use logic, creativity, and good communication, and are flexible and competent in delivery of client care. Additional attitudes attributed to nurses who are considered critical thinkers include: open-minded, empathetic, realistic, and team players.

Nurses use critical thinking skills as they relate theory to practice, apply the nursing process in client care, and make critical clinical decisions. The ability to use critical thinking skills assists the nurse to recognize and analyze problems and to solve them using a systematic approach.

To acquire critical thinking skills, the nurse must first develop a sound theoretical knowledge base. This means studying the concepts appropriate to each clinical discipline (i.e., disease state and client problem in each area of nursing practice) and transferring that knowledge to clinical situations in order to provide safe client care and make independent judgments. In addition to reflecting on previous knowledge, the nurse gains immeasurable experience in the identification of clients' problems with each clinical experience. Over time, the nurse is able to select the best solution for assisting clients to resume a healthy state.

Critical thinking is a process as well as a cognitive skill that is used to identify and define problems, assess clients, and evaluate their responses to treatment and care. Nurses select and classify data and organize it into clusters or patterns to formulate nursing diagnoses. Critical thinking is used when alternative nursing actions are evaluated and the most appropriate action is selected for each client problem. After the client intervention is carried out, the effectiveness of the intervention and client outcome is evaluated using critical thinking. It is easy to see from this statement that critical thinking is used throughout the steps of the nursing process.

Problem-solving methodologies have been used throughout your educational process as you faced everyday situations. The nursing process provides the basis for critical thinking in nursing when problem-solving is required in client care. The following examples demonstrate how critical thinking is used throughout the five steps of the nursing process. When the steps are followed consistently and accuracy of the data is maintained, you will develop habits that promote critical thinking in nursing.

Assessment in Critical Thinking

Identifying essential assessment data and where the data can be found requires critical thinking. Obtaining, classifying, and organizing data is a principal function of critical thinking.

One of the leading causes of errors in making clinical judgments or decisions is the collection of inaccurate or incomplete data during the assessment phase. The data collection or assessment step of the nursing process assists the nurse to predict, detect, prevent, and control client problems. A nurse with good critical thinking skills develops a systematic approach to obtaining and validatory data. This includes identifying all aspects of data collection, i.e., review the client's chart, ask pertinent questions, and complete the assessment in a systematic manner. If an assessment tool is used, ensure that thought goes into the way the data is recorded; don't just write information down in a rote manner. Review the assessment form to determine if additional or more in-depth information is required based on the initial findings—this action involves critical thinking. Ask yourself, "is this information relevant?" and "do I need to assess anything else?" Listen to the client. Clients provide important subjective data to add to objective information. Once all of the data is collected, it should be validated to ensure that data is not missing and that it is correct. It needs to be organized or categorized in a usable system. Clustering of similar information assists the nurse in forming a picture of the client's problems and strengths. Critical thinking is necessary to determine the significance of reported data, and clustering identifies if patterns of behavior or responses exist. Clustering data helps determine relevant from irrelevant data as well as gaps in information. It also pinpoints cause-and-effect relationships. Once the clustering is completed; inferences may be formulated.

Nursing Diagnosis in Critical Thinking

A nursing diagnosis is the identification of a client problem. Before a nursing diagnosis is made, the nurse has critically analyzed synthesized, clustered, and interpreted all the collected data. Use of critical thinking skills is essential in this step of the nursing process. As you cluster data, you are applying the scientific principle of classifying information in order to determine if relationships exist among the data and whether data is relevant or irrelevant in this situation. As information is clustered, inconsistencies among the collected data may prompt the nurse to look for additional assessment findings. Determining when additional information is needed for an accurate diagnosis prevents the nurse from making a very common critical thinking error—making a judgment based on incomplete information. After the data is clustered, the nurse begins to look at patterns of functioning (NANDA Nursing Diagnoses categorization). This is a major step toward identifying the client's problems. The identification of this information assists the nurse in determining the appropriate nursing diagnosis. Identifying patterns requires the critical thinking skills associated with a sound scientific knowledge base. The nurse must differentiate the normal from the abnormal findings, as well as the risk factors for abnormal patterns of functioning. Using a nursing diagnosis reference book will assist the nurse in clarifying data relevant to defining characteristics or risk factors related to the client's clinical manifestations.

During this step of the nursing process, actual client problems are identified, potential problems are predicted, and priorities are established. Establishing nursing diagnoses is an important independent action of the nurse; however, medical diagnoses must be considered as well. Nursing diagnoses cannot be treated in isolation. Collaborative problem identification and treatment with other health care workers form the basis of client care. Priorities of care are determined by the severity of the client's problems. These priorities are identified within the planning and intervention steps of the nursing process.

Planning in Critical Thinking and Outcome Identification

Client's long- and short-term goals are formulated after deliberating with the client, family, and other health care team members. Defining realistic goals that are acceptable to the client requires critical thinking. A prioritized plan of care is developed during this phase of the nursing process that includes client outcomes.

Determining client outcomes, as stated, is the foundation of this step in the nursing process. Determining outcomes (goals) and interventions are paramount to providing effective client care. Outcomes are time specific. Long-term outcomes or goals are usually based on what is expected by the time of discharge from a nursing unit or a facility. Short-term outcomes are based on time frames as short as by the end of the shift, within twenty-four hours, etc. The long-term goal or discharge expected outcome should be determined before other outcomes and interventions can be initiated. When setting priorities for client problems, keep in mind that treating these problems must be addressed on the plan of care in order to achieve the client's discharge goal or outcome. There are two critical thinking skills inherent in this step. One is listing the client problems and determining whether there are relationships between the problems; and two, assigning the problems by highest priority. These critical thinking skills require sound scientific principles and scientific method, clinical judgment, reasoning skills, and goal-directed thinking.

When listing the actual and potential problems identified by the assessment data, identify which problems need immediate intervention and those which are underlying causes of the problems. Those situations identified as causing the problem must be assigned the highest priority, as they need to be resolved in order for the client to resume a healthy lifestyle. After listing the problems, determine if there are relationships among the problems. If relationships exist, the problems contributing to the effects of other problems should receive a high priority. Using Maslow's Hierarchy of Human Needs is a method employed by many nurses to determine prioritization of problems. Maslow lists problems with survival needs (food, fluids, oxygen) as the highest priority. These needs must be addressed first in the plan of care for the client's well-being.

To write specific, realistic, client-centered outcomes, the problems must be stated clearly. Outcomes are derived directly from the problem statement, and the subject of the problem statement is the client. An example of a clear, client-centered outcome is "The client will ambulate the length of the hall before discharge." Remember, problem statements are written as nursing diagnoses as well as client problems. An example of a client outcome utilizing a nursing diagnosis example is "The client will demonstrate accurate administration of insulin according to the guidelines established by the diabetic educator within 24 hours of admission." This outcome is directly related to a "Knowledge deficit: Insulin Administration" nursing diagnosis. You will also notice there is a time-specific statement included within the outcome statement. This time frame assists the nurse to evaluate outcome achievement or reevaluate the plan of care.

Implementation in Critical Thinking

Nursing interventions are specific strategies developed to achieve positive client outcomes. These interventions are determined by using the critical thinking skills of generalizing, explaining, and predicting outcomes. After consideration of all identified possible actions, nursing interventions are implemented.

Identifying appropriate nursing actions is critical to the outcome of client care. Determining these actions requires critical thinking skills. These skills include the ability to identify specific actions, predict and monitor the client's response to the actions, and weigh risks and consequences of each action. Examining the risks and consequences of an action, a nurse is determining the most beneficial and least harmful approach to client care. When interventions are clearly delineated on the plan of care, the likelihood of the actions being carried out is enhanced. The more specific the intervention, the greater chance of success for the intervention. If increasing fluid intake is the intervention, specifics as to fluid likes and dislikes of the client should be addressed. For example, "Client prefers noncarbonated beverages at room temperature." Another example of a specific intervention is "Ambulate the client after his bath, before lunch, and before dinner." This would be appropriate for the goal to ambulate the length of the hall by discharge. Putting times for interventions or distances for ambulation increases the likelihood of compliance with the intervention by all health care workers.

Evaluation in Critical Thinking

During the final phase of the nursing process, the nurse critically analyzes each of the client outcomes. If the client need was not satisfied, the plan is revised. Clearly documenting a comprehensive plan provides the basis for evaluation. Evaluating progress toward outcome achievement assists the nurse in evaluating the effectiveness of the plan. A critical thinking question during this phase of the nursing process is "How well did the client accomplish the goal?" The nurse might also ask "What could have been done differently?"

In addition to using critical thinking skills when providing client care, nurse managers use these skills in assigning client care and delegating activities, an example of which is the assignment of client care to a nursing assistant. The nurse manager must determine the skill level of the nursing assistant and the critical nature of the client, as well as other staffing assignments before the assignment is completed.

NURSING DIAGNOSIS

An important implication of nursing diagnosis is that it refers to a health problem or condition that nurses are legally licensed to treat. The establishment and acceptance of this diagnostic category demonstrates recognition and legal sanction of nursing as a profession with its own body of knowledge, education, and experience.

The term *nursing diagnosis* is not comparable to or the same as a medical diagnosis. The major differences in medical and nursing diagnoses is the focus on illness, injury, or disease by the physician. The nursing diagnosis focuses on the response to actual or potential health problems or life processes. Medical diagnoses do not vary until treatment is completed, whereas the nursing diagnosis is fluid and changes as the client's condition or response to treatment changes. Nursing diagnosis is derived from the assessment phase of the nursing process and is based on both subjective and objective data. As the data base evolves, patterns of health problems emerge, and alterations from normal health states are identified. A nursing diagnosis is a statement of an actual health problem or a risk or wellness statement within the client's biologic, social, or personal system. The specific problem identified implies that the nurse is qualified and prepared to intervene and treat that condition. The nurse is not legally able to intervene and treat a medical diagnosis without specific physician's orders. Thus, the nurse is not able to intervene if the client has a diagnosis of, for example, *potential atelectasis* or *pneumonia*. This is a medical diagnosis, whereas *ineffective breathing pattern* is a nursing diagnosis and nursing interventions can be instituted to assist the client.

Comparison of Diagnoses

Medical	Nursing
Cancer of Liver	Acute pain
Congestive Heart Failure	Excess fluid volume
Chronic Obstructive Pulmonary Disease	Ineffective breathing patterns

TABLE 2–1 Nursing Diagnosis: Risk for Impaired Skin Integrity

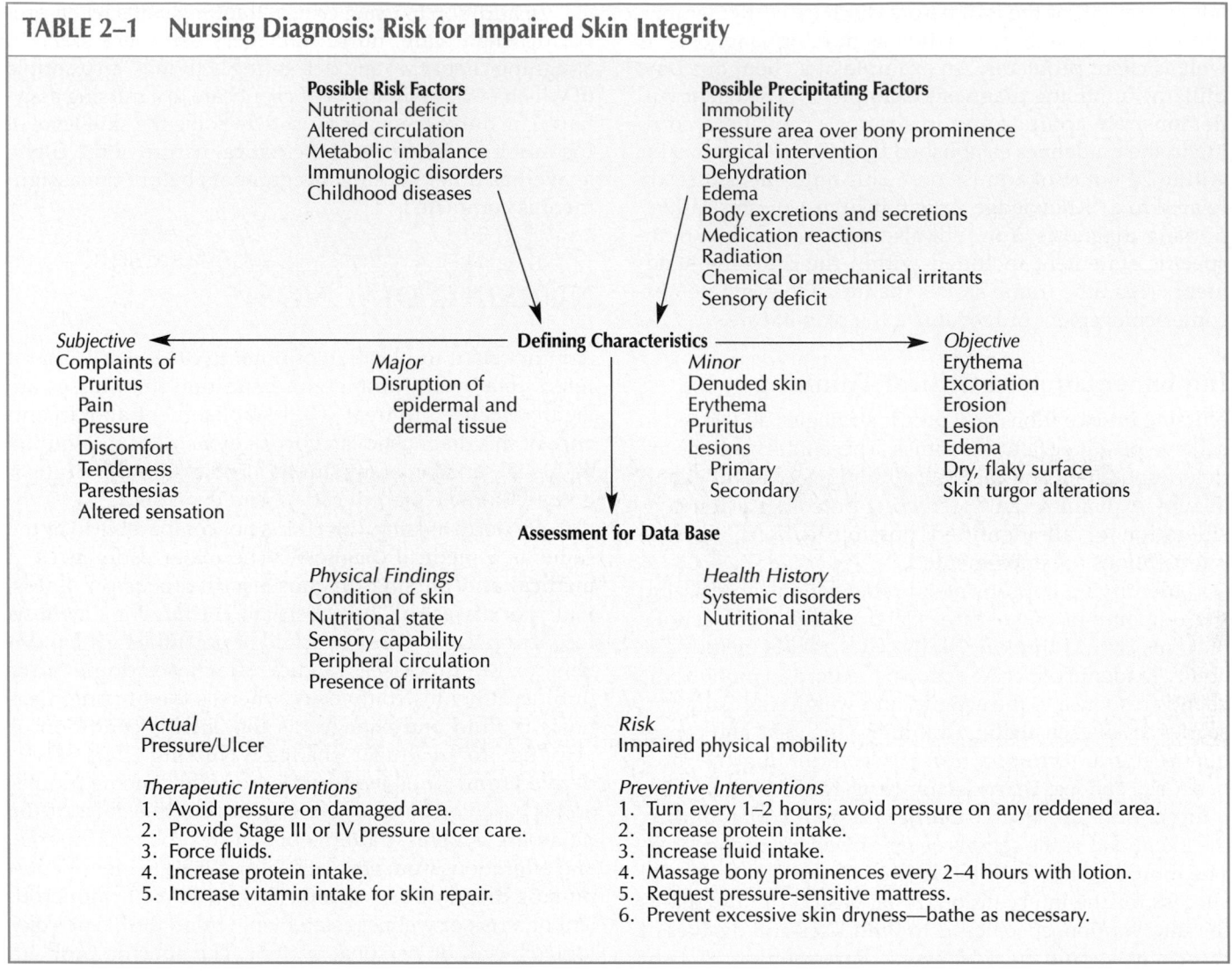

Possible Risk Factors
Nutritional deficit
Altered circulation
Metabolic imbalance
Immunologic disorders
Childhood diseases

Possible Precipitating Factors
Immobility
Pressure area over bony prominence
Surgical intervention
Dehydration
Edema
Body excretions and secretions
Medication reactions
Radiation
Chemical or mechanical irritants
Sensory deficit

Defining Characteristics

Subjective
Complaints of
- Pruritus
- Pain
- Pressure
- Discomfort
- Tenderness
- Paresthesias
- Altered sensation

Major
Disruption of epidermal and dermal tissue

Minor
Denuded skin
Erythema
Pruritus
Lesions
- Primary
- Secondary

Objective
Erythema
Excoriation
Erosion
Lesion
Edema
Dry, flaky surface
Skin turgor alterations

Assessment for Data Base

Physical Findings
Condition of skin
Nutritional state
Sensory capability
Peripheral circulation
Presence of irritants

Health History
Systemic disorders
Nutritional intake

Actual
Pressure/Ulcer

Therapeutic Interventions
1. Avoid pressure on damaged area.
2. Provide Stage III or IV pressure ulcer care.
3. Force fluids.
4. Increase protein intake.
5. Increase vitamin intake for skin repair.

Risk
Impaired physical mobility

Preventive Interventions
1. Turn every 1–2 hours; avoid pressure on any reddened area.
2. Increase protein intake.
3. Increase fluid intake.
4. Massage bony prominences every 2–4 hours with lotion.
5. Request pressure-sensitive mattress.
6. Prevent excessive skin dryness—bathe as necessary.

Nursing diagnoses provide a written communication to all health care workers regarding the client's status. The use of nursing diagnoses provides a vocabulary that is used to describe specific nursing practice, research, and education. It provides a method to synthesize and communicate nurses' observations and judgments to all members of the health care team. Nursing diagnoses are being used to form a basis for the development of nursing theory.

Types of Nursing Diagnoses

According to Carpenito and the North American Diagnosis Association, a nursing diagnosis can be written as an actual, risk, or a wellness or syndrome type of statement.

Actual: The nurse has validated an actual nursing diagnosis using clinical judgment, and the client has presented with a major defining characteristic.

Risk: Based on clinical judgment, the client is more vulnerable to develop the problem than others in similar circumstances. This may also be referred to as a "potential problem."

Wellness: Based on clinical judgment, the client is in transition from a specific level of wellness to a higher level of wellness.

Syndrome: A syndrome diagnosis comprises a cluster of actual or risk nursing diagnoses that are predicted to present in a certain situation or event.

The term *possible diagnosis* is not considered a type of diagnosis. It is an option indicating some data are present to confirm the diagnosis but the data is incomplete or insufficient. Writing a nursing diagnosis as "possible" alerts other nurses of your concern that there is insufficient data to support your concern but you have a hunch that a problem exists. Further data collection is needed to confirm or deny the diagnosis.

Diagnostic Statement

The diagnostic statement describes the health status of the client and the factors that have contributed to the status. These statements have been developed through research by the North American Nursing Diagnosis Association (NANDA) and are termed Nursing Diagnoses. NANDA approved the new Taxonomy II Nursing Diagnosis in April 2000 at the 14th biennial conference. The Taxonomy II format allows more flexibility of the nomenclature and it makes it easier to make changes when new additions and modifications are made.

The Taxonomy of Nursing Diagnosis is a classification in which the diagnostic labels are grouped in nine patterns of human responses. Each diagnosis is grouped in one of these human responses:

- Exchanging
- Communicating
- Relating
- Valuing
- Choosing
- Moving
- Perceiving
- Knowing
- Feeling

Components of Nursing Diagnosis

There are basically two formats used to devise the Nursing Diagnosis. The two-part statement and the three-part statement.

A two-part statement is the most common type of format used in practice. The first component is the *Diagnostic Label* or problem statement. This describes the client's response to an actual, possible, or risk health problem or a wellness condition. The second component, *Etiology*, is the cause or contributing factor to the problem. The two components are linked by the *"related to(r/t)"* term.

A three-part statement includes the *Diagnostic Label*, *Etiology*, and the *Defining Characteristics*. *Defining Characteristics* are defined as signs and symptoms or clinical manifestations and subjective and objective data. The characteristics are linked to the other two components by the term *"as evidenced by"* statement. Defining characteristics are divided into major and minor categories. To state an *Actual* nursing diagnosis, the client must exhibit at least one or more major defining characteristics. Minor defining characteristics may or may not be present.

A one-part statement is used infrequently with a Wellness or Syndrome diagnosis. Related factors are not present with Wellness or Syndrome diagnosis. The diagnostic statement would indicate only "Potential for enhanced well-being."

The following are examples of nursing diagnoses written in a two-part and three-part statement.

An *Actual Nursing Diagnosis*, written as a three-part statement:

DIAGNOSTIC LABEL (Problem)	Impaired transfer ability
CONTRIBUTING FACTORS (Etiology or Cause)	Related to inability to move left side
CLINICAL MANIFESTATIONS (Defining Characteristics)	Evidenced by flaccid paralysis of left side

A *Risk or Possible Diagnosis*, written as a two-part statement, when there are no defining characteristics:

DIAGNOSTIC LABEL (Problem)	Impaired walking
RISK FACTORS	Related to long leg cast secondary to fractured femur

Nursing diagnoses provide the basis for selection of nursing interventions to achieve outcomes for which the nurse is accountable. In 1987, the Center for Nursing Classification at the University of Iowa College of Nursing introduced the Nursing Interventions Classification (NIC) system and in 1991 the Nursing Outcomes Classification (NOC) system. These classifications were developed for use with NANDA and other diagnostic systems. The NIC includes physiological and psychosocial interventions to treat and prevent illness and promote health for clients, families, and the community. NOC has developed standardized outcomes to measure the effects of nursing interventions. These outcomes can be used in all settings and with all client populations. NIC and NOC have not been accepted and implemented to the extent of NANDA.

The PES framework is a commonly used approach or organizing framework developed by Marjory Gordon that uses the three-part diagnostic statement.

P refers to the *problem*, or state of health, of the individual, family, or community. This problem is expressed as clearly as possible, for example, Impaired Skin Integrity.

E describes the *etiology*, or probable cause, of the health problem. This may refer to many factors that include client behaviors, environmental components, or the interaction of both. The etiology is combined with the problem statement by using the words "related to," for example, prolonged bed rest.

S signifies the relevant *signs and symptoms*—usually a summary of the objective assessment findings (signs) and subjective data reported by the client (symptoms). The phrase that connects this part of the statement is "as evidenced by," for example, Impaired Skin Integrity, "related to" prolonged bed rest, as evidenced by a 2 × 2 cm circular red lesion or erythematous macules with moderate serosanguinous drainage.

Although there are several approaches to formulating a statement of Nursing Diagnosis, the PES system is used by many schools of nursing throughout the United States. The Nursing Diagnoses are continually changing as the NANDA research continues. New diagnoses are introduced at the biennial meeting.

EVIDENCE BASED NURSING PRACTICE

This term is relatively new to the practice of nursing, even though nursing has recognized the importance of research as an essential basis for its development. Other health-related disciplines have long relied on this type of empirical data when making clinical decisions.

Taylor-Piliac define evidence based nursing practice as the application of the best available empirical evidence that applies recent research findings to clinical practice in order to aid clinical decision making.

The levels of evidence vary among researchers. Some researchers believe that the synthesis and use of scientific information comes from randomized clinical trials. Others look at the process more broadly and include information gleaned from case reports and expert opinion to guide health care decisions.

The University of Minnesota Evidence-Based Health Care Project concludes that evidence based practice solves problems by carrying out four steps:

1. Identify issues or problems based on analysis of current nursing knowledge and practice.
2. Identify relevant research through literature search.
3. Evaluate research by using criteria that has scientific merit.
4. Interventions are selected by using the most valid evidence.

Evidence based nursing, on the other hand, is the process by which nurses make clinical decisions using research evidence, clinical practice experience, and client preferences.

Nurses must recognize the importance of using research findings in clinical practice. It is paramount that nurses begin to not just read research articles but critically examine the content of the article. Once research data is available, the nurse must be allowed to make changes in clinical practice based on the findings. In many facilities this involves research teams that review current literature and then make appropriate recommendations for clinical practice. Unfortunately, very little is known about the best methods for implementing research evidence into nursing practice. Evidence based nursing will strengthen client outcomes, improve client safety, provide effective nursing practice, and increase nursing's credibility among other health care professionals and the general public. This should be considered another step in developing nursing's theory base.

One note of caution when you are reading about evidence based practice: Do not confuse it with best practices. These terms are sometimes used interchangeably, but they do not mean the same thing. *Best practices* is a term used to describe nursing interventions that have proven effective in promoting positive client outcomes or in reducing overall costs to the client or facility. Best practices are not necessarily based on research findings.

Evidence Based Research Project

When completing an evidence based research project you need to complete the following steps:

STEP 1 State the question you wish to study. It may be a simple question related to a standard nursing procedure that has been done a certain way for many years, or it may be a totally new way of completing a procedure.

STEP 2 Gather the evidence (information). Do a literature search, use the Internet, review medical and nursing studies reported in journals that relate to your subject of interest.

STEP 3 Analyze and assess the evidence. Did it come from a valid source? Who did the study, and how was the study actually conducted?

STEP 4 Based on research findings, conduct a pilot study to validate your hypothesis. Individuals can make changes in a pilot study, but for an institution to make changes a plan must be developed, it must be based on research findings, and it must be formally implemented.

STEP 5 Obtain feedback from individuals involved in the research. Monitor the research and identify the specific response(s) and alterations that have occurred in the practice setting as a result of the research findings.

STEP 6 Analyze and report the outcome resulting from the research project. Reporting a change in practice that improves nursing procedures will encourage others to make changes in practice settings as well.

Source: Cathryn Domrose, *NurseWeek*, November 19, 2001. Information based on interviews with nurse researchers and clinicians including: Lisa Sams, Carolyn K. Davis, Kathleen Stevens, Brigitte Failner.

Evidence based practice highlights can be found throughout the book. It will provide you with a framework for determining the effectiveness of selected nursing skills and practice issues. As you proceed through your nursing program, you will be exposed to additional evidence based practice research and its effect on clinical practice.

MANAGEMENT GUIDELINES

Each state legislates a Nurse Practice Act for RNs, LVN/LPNs, and advanced nursing practioners. Health care facilities are responsible for establishing and implementing policies and procedures that conform to their state's regulations. Verify the regulations and role parameters for each health care worker in your facility.

Delegation of Responsibilities

- The RN's responsibility when delegating client care tasks is to ensure that the care plan is followed for each client. Information contained on the care plan is reported to each health care worker assigned to client care.
- The RN is responsible for implementing the nursing process in all aspects of client care. LVN/LPNs may be assigned to carry out tasks within the nursing process, such as assessing clients after the initial assessment and executing interventions based on the client care plan. The RN, however, is ultimately responsible for client care, developing the plan of care, and ensuring that the plan is followed.
- The LVN/LPN may assist the RN in planning and updating the plan of care, but may not be responsible for this action.
- Assistive personnel, such as unlicensed assistive personnel (UAP) and CNAs, are delegated client tasks, but do participate in the actual development of the plan of care. Their input is valuable and should be considered when changes in the plan of care is necessary.
- Critical thinking processes are used by all health care workers as they provide client care. The RN has a more expanded scientific knowledge base and experience in utilizing these skills to provide the leadership necessary for effective and safe client care.

Information Flow

- The RN synthesizes client data and determines the most appropriate health care worker to provide care to each client in her/his assignment.
- Each health care worker is given a report on activities to be completed during the shift.
- Dissemination of client care information is based on the client's plan of care.
- Directions are given to all health care workers indicating the type of client information the nurse needs immediately and information that can be given during report times. For example, if a client has a fever, the RN may want to know the temperature as soon as it is obtained.

CRITICAL THINKING STRATEGIES

SCENARIO 1

You have been assigned to care for Mr. Peters, a 76-year-old widower who was admitted with the diagnosis of congestive heart failure. He has lived alone for the last 2 years since his wife died. His children live about 1 hour away and visit him once a month. The children ordered Meals on Wheels for him, but he refused to eat the food that was delivered. "I can do my own cooking, I am not an invalid," was the answer when the nurse asked why he didn't like the Meals on Wheels program. He had not seen the physician for at least 2 years. At the last visit, the physician prescribed a moderately low-sodium diet, Lasix 40 mg daily, Calan, and multiple vitamins. His admitting vital signs were BP 180/90, P 98, R 22. His weight indicated a gain of 10 pounds since the last visit. His physical assessment indicated rales in the lung bases, 3+ edema of the ankles, and difficulty breathing in the supine position.

1. How will you use the nursing process to determine an accurate assessment data base?
2. What information is missing that might be important to the nurse to assist in planning care for this client? What is the best approach for obtaining the information?
3. Identify at least four nursing diagnoses that are relevant for this client's plan of care. Write a two-part and a three-part diagnostic statement for each nursing diagnosis.
4. Using a nursing diagnosis book, list the major and minor defining characteristics for the four nursing diagnosis listed in question 3.
5. Identify the priority nursing diagnosis, and provide the rationale for your decision.
6. Develop a very brief nursing care plan using the nursing process format as outlined in the text.

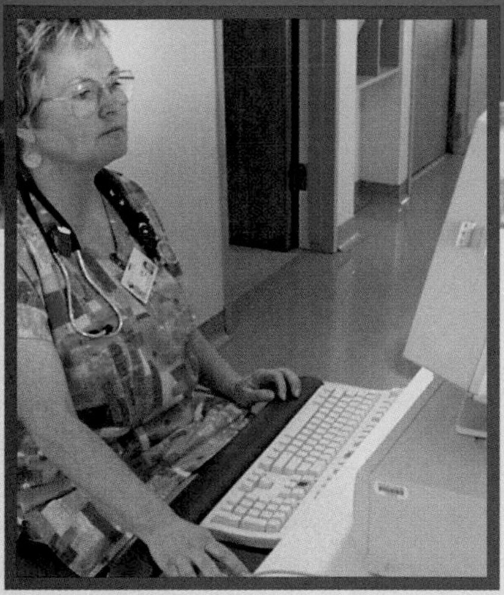

CHAPTER 3

Managing Client Care: Documentation and Delegation

Client Care Plans 35
- Types of Plans 35
- Components of a Care Plan 35
- Critical Paths or Clinical Pathways 38

Charting 40
- Charting—A Method of Communication 40
- Charting Format 41
- Charting for Potential Legal Problems 41
- Forensic Charting 41
- Charting and the Nursing Process 42
- Charting Systems 42

Legal Forms of Documentation 53
- Unusual Occurrence, Variance, or Incident Report 53
- Consent Forms 54

Reporting 56

Delegating Client Care 56
- Client Acuity Systems 57
- RN Delegation 57
- Parameters of Delegation 58

Student Clinical Planning 59
- Time Management 59

Word Roots, Prefixes and Suffixes 59

MANAGEMENT GUIDELINES 61

CRITICAL THINKING STRATEGIES 63

LEARNING OBJECTIVES

- Describe the components of the client care plan.
- State the two types of client care plan.
- Explain the method for individualizing the care plan when a standard care plan is used.
- Define the term "client problem or need."
- State the most important reason for using nursing diagnosis in care planning.
- Define the use of deadlines and checkpoints in the client care plan.
- State how the client care plan and nurses' notes relate to each other.
- Compare and contrast a clinical pathway and a client care plan.
- Explain at least three purposes of charting.
- Describe at least three major components of accurate charting.
- Differentiate between the advantages and disadvantages of the three charting systems: source-oriented, problem-oriented, and computer-assisted charting.
- Complete a charting exercise in all three charting systems using a simulated situation.
- List the four items that should be charted for every client.
- Discuss the relationship between the nursing assessment data base, nursing problem list, and problem-oriented medical records.
- Define the terms "subjective" and "objective data," "assessment," and "plan" when referring to SOAP notes.
- Describe the legal ramifications for completing unusual occurrence reports.
- Discuss specific client activities requiring consent forms.
- Discuss the legal risks of computer charting.
- Discuss the RN's role in delegating client care.
- Complete a data collection tool based on a clinical situation.
- Develop a time-management work sheet for client care.

TERMINOLOGY

Acuity system: a method for determining staffing requirements based on the assessment of client needs.

Care Plan, Client: a plan of care, usually written, that meets the special needs of each client.

Charting: process of recording information about a client concerning the progress of his or her disease and treatment.

Charting by exception: documenting only exceptions to predetermined nursing standards in a narrative format.

Clinical pathways: interdisciplinary client care plans using specific assessments, interventions, and outcomes for specified health-related conditions.

Computer-assisted charting: client information is entered into the computer for storage and retrieval at a later time.

Delegation: transferring to a competent individual the authority to perform a selected task in a selected situation.

Flow sheets: client data are recorded or graphed to show patterns or alterations in findings.

Focus charting: charting on one "focus" area. Using DAR format (data, action, response).

Kardex: a convenient and readily accessible file of cards containing current client information.

Nursing process: a set of actions that includes assessment, planning, intervention, and evaluation.

Problem-oriented medical record (POMR): a client record that is organized according to the person's specific health problems.

Report: to give an account of something that has been seen, heard, done, or considered.

SOAP notes: nursing notes organized consistently by what the client feels "subjectively"; what the nurse observes "objectively"; how the nurse "assesses" the situation; and what the nurse "plans."

SOAPIE: nursing notes similar to SOAP with additional data; implementation (i) and evaluation (e).

Source-oriented charting: information in the chart is organized according to its source, for example, physician's progress notes, nurses' notes.

Systems charting: charting or documentation relative to the assessment data obtained during the physical assessment of the client.

Unusual Occurrence: recording of an unusual happening or event that could affect client or staff safety; also commonly referred to as variance or incident report.

CLIENT CARE PLANS

Documentation is a major component of the nurse's role. Importance is based on several factors: evaluation of planned client care, communication to other health care professionals, Joint Commission on Accreditation of Healthcare Organizations (JCAHO) and client safety regulations, reimbursement from the federal government, and legal implications. If a treatment, medication, or activity has not been documented in the chart, legally it is very difficult to prove that the client actually received the care. Contact with the client and care delivered to the client must be documented. One of the most useful tools to provide this care is the client care plan.

Client care plans are an integral part of providing nursing care. Without them, quality and consistency of client care may not be obtained. Client care plans provide a means of communication among nurses and other health care providers. The plan should serve as a focal point for client care assignments and reporting.

In earlier years the JCAHO required an individualized care plan be developed for each client (Long, 1994). According to the guidelines from JCAHO, the client or family must be involved in the development of the care plan and it must be interdisciplinary. One reason the critical or clinical pathway is becoming more popular is the interdisciplinary approach involved in this system. Some facilities still use the standardized or individualized care plan. The only modification they need to make is to ensure that multidisciplinary planning and intervention are included in the care of each client. Documentation of client care must also be interdisciplinary.

Regardless of the type of care plan used, the following information should be included: client's needs or problems both actual and potential, stated as nursing diagnoses; expected outcomes or short-term goals; nursing interventions or actions; and discharge criteria or long-term goals.

Once the goals of client care are established, they are included in a multidisciplinary care plan. Each step in meeting these goals is detailed, including specific observations and how often the observations are made. Step-by-step directions are included for difficult problems, such as lengthy and involved dressing changes. Individualized client teaching programs are described on the care plan. As is evident, all of this information is essential in providing continuity of client care.

Types of Plans

Client care plans consist of two types: an individualized care plan, completely written by the nurse and other health team members for each specific client, and a standard client care plan. Because of the time required to write individualized care plans, hospital nursing departments are developing preprinted standard care plans based on the most frequent hospital admission diagnoses for the hospital. The standard care plan, based on the facility's standards of nursing practice, are guidelines that outline the usual problems or needs that occur with a specific diagnosis. It contains a list of usual nursing actions or interventions and the standard expected outcomes for each problem. Advantages for using standard care plans include: standards of care are established for diagnoses which result in effective care for each client; continuity of care is established; all nurses provide the same level of care; documentation time is decreased; and documentation is more accurate. The major disadvantage is the risk that individualized client care may not be provided. The care plan becomes a part of the permanent client record.

Components of a Care Plan

Individualizing Care Plans All clients must have an individualized plan of care even though the standard care plan is used. To individualize the care plan, space is generally provided at the end of the preprinted form to allow the nurse to identify unusual problems or needs. Standard care plans are individualized by activating only those problems that pertain to a particular client. The nurse may add another problem to the bottom of the form to further individualize the care plan.

Initiating the Plan The client care plan is formulated after the assessment phase of the nursing process. The nurse, after completing the nursing history and assessment, determines if a standard care plan is available for the client's medical diagnosis or if an individualized care plan must be written. If a standard care plan is available, the nurse need only circle, date, and initial the needs that are relevant for that client. When an individualized care plan is being written, the nurse translates the client's needs or problems into nursing diagnoses and writes them on the care plan. Nursing diagnoses are the acceptable terminology for use on client care plans throughout the country. The terminology was established by the National Conference on Classification of Nursing Diagnosis, published for the first time in 1973.

Identifying Client Problems or Needs A client problem or need is a condition that requires assistance or intervention from a health care team member to return the client to a healthy state. The client problem is identified as any unmet need. It can be as basic as the need for adequate comfort or nourishment to the more complex psychosocial needs.

On many care plans, problems are identified as either actual or potential. An actual problem is one that exists at that time. Interventions are planned to resolve or alter

COMMUNITY HOSPITAL

CLIENT CARE PLAN

Client Information

Discharge Criteria
1) Lungs clear to auscultation.
2) Voiding qs and continent of urine.
3) Verbalizes an understanding of discharge instructions and medications.
4)

Admitting Diagnosis

Relevant Info:

Date	Problem/Need	Expected Outcome/Goal	CP	DL	Nursing Interventions	Update / DC	Initial
3/22/04	(1.) Ineffective Breathing Pattern related to pain.	Absence of respiratory complications.	q2h x24h then q4h x48h then q8h q3-4 h	POD 3 3/25 3 pm	1a. Encourage turning, coughing and deep breathing exercises (TCDB) q2h. b. Teach client to splint incision when coughing. c. Instruct in use of breathing device, if ordered. d. Place in semi-Fowler's position. e. Assess need for pain med. f. Medicate for pain 1/2hr. before TCDB. g. Auscultate breath sounds.		
	2. Impaired Urinary Elimination related to incontinence.	Continent of urine. Absence of urinary tract infection (UTI).	q4h	cath. out	2a. Check urinary output for signs and symptoms of UTI, i.e. color, odor, consistency. b. Provide catheter care according to protocol. c. Force fluids to 2500mL. d. Give cranberry juice, 240mL q shift.		
3/22/04	(3.) Deficient Knowledge related to administration of discharge meds.	Verbalizes understanding of discharge meds, including listing signs and symptoms of side effects.	q24h	prior to disch	3a. Instruct in action of Maxaquin b. Review side effects with client and/or family. c. Have client state signs and symptoms of side effects prior to discharge. d. Provide Take Home Medication pamphlet.		
	4. Impaired Skin Integrity related to prolonged immobility.	Skin clean and intact.	q4h q2h	prior to disch	4a. Provide skin care. Use lotion. b. Turn side to side. c. Keep linens dry and wrinkle free.		

*You may use approved abbreviations from the facility when writing care plans.

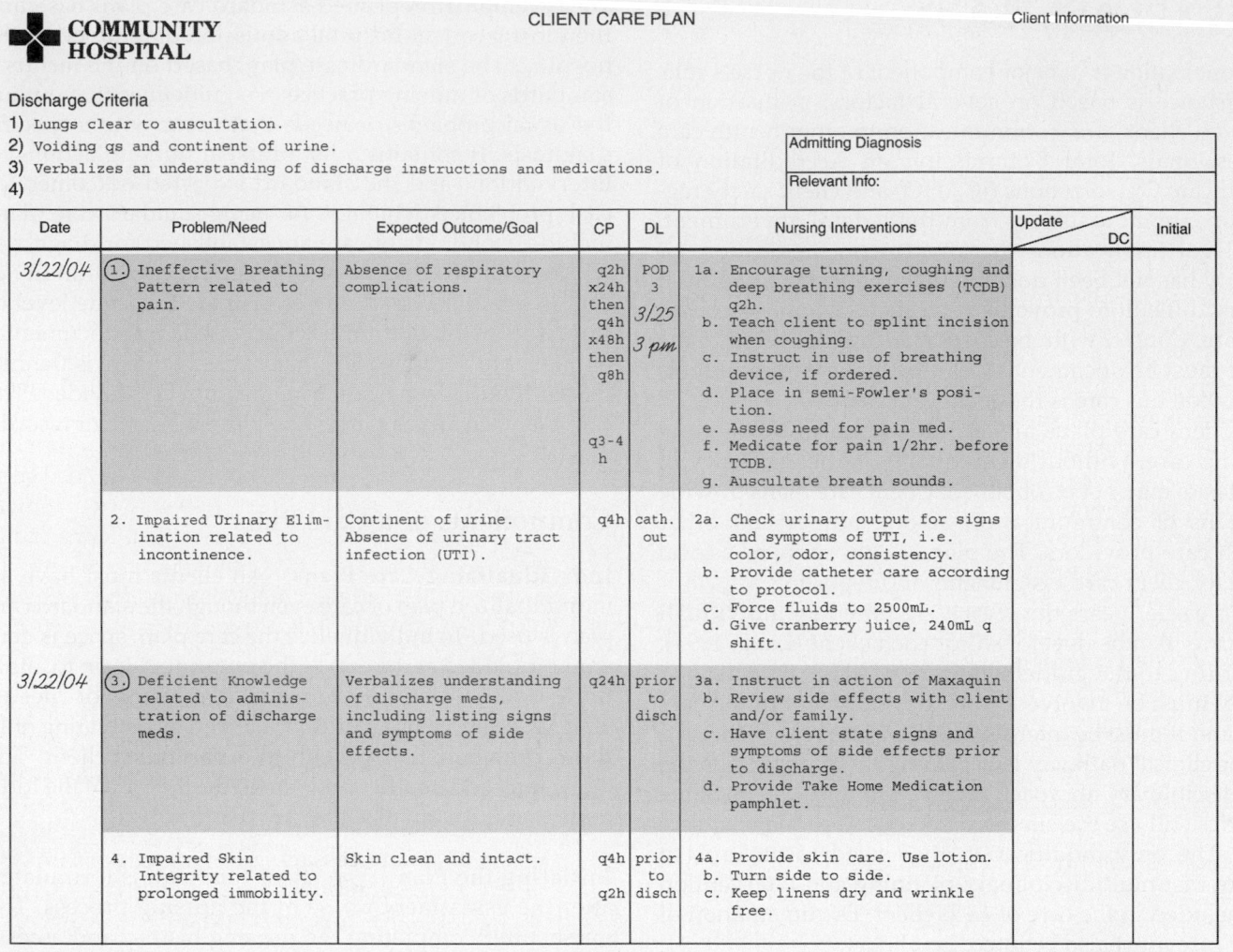

Preprinted standardized client care plan using Nursing Diagnosis format.

the problem. A potential problem describes a condition that frequently occurs with the client's diagnosis or health problem. An actual problem, for example, is a reddened coccyx related to urinary incontinence. Interventions are developed to treat the reddened area to prevent further breakdown or pressure ulcer formation. A potential problem, such as "Ineffective Breathing Patterns *related* to acute pain" following gallbladder surgery, could affect any client with that condition. Interventions are planned to prevent the problem. Some potential problems are identified to assess more carefully for them. For example, a debilitated client with poor nutrition is assessed for possible wound infection.

Formulating Nursing Diagnoses Using a nursing diagnosis to state the client's real or potential problems takes the problem out of the realm of medical diagnosis. Nursing diagnosis does not focus on a problem or disease state but rather on a physical, psychological, or behavioral response. Nursing diagnosis can change frequently as the client's health status changes and potential health problems become actual health problems. The nursing diagnosis approach, unlike the medical model or systems approach to care planning, allows for this flexibility in focus.

The use of nursing diagnosis in care planning is a universal method of communication to all health team members. When the diagnosis "Impaired Skin Integrity" is written, the entire health team knows that the client has a broken area on the skin with destruction of skin layers. The relationship of skin impairment to cause is usually stated as "Impaired Skin Integrity, *related to* prolonged immobility."

Expected Outcomes or Goals After the problems have been identified, the nurse sets goals or expected outcomes for client care that are congruent with the goals of the client or significant other. Client-centered goals should be clear, concise, realistic, and should identify specific observable and measurable behaviors. Expected outcomes or goals should indicate what is to be expected when the goal is achieved, by whom, when, to what degree of accuracy, and should be time-limited. The Client Care Plan on page 36, shows several examples of a client-centered goal and the nursing interventions necessary to attain each goal.

Client care plans must include both short- and long-term goals. Long-term goals are frequently stated as discharge criteria and as such should be met prior to discharge, if possible. Short-term goals usually appear in the form of expected outcomes for each problem.

They are designed as stepping stones to assist the client to meet discharge criteria or long-term goals. Some hospitals, particularly rehabilitation facilities, use short-term goals differently. They frequently set weekly steps or phases in the rehabilitative process that clients meet before the final expected outcome is achieved. For example, to meet the long-term goal of ambulation without use of devices, a short-term goal is to ambulate with a walker without assistance. These types of goals are prioritized and updated regularly.

Interventions After problems and expected outcomes are written on the care plan, the nurse determines appropriate nursing interventions that meet the goals of care. Interventions, if written properly, specify the exact nursing actions to be carried out or provide explicit instructions on how care is to be delivered. Time and frequency of the intervention should also be provided.

Checkpoints and Deadlines The standard care plan illustrated in this text includes checkpoint (CP) and deadline (DL) columns. The checkpoint indicates how often the action or intervention should be checked, observed, or carried out and therefore how often it should be charted. The deadline column indicates the time when the goal should be met or the action is no longer necessary. It is important to document the exact time and date when the nursing action should be completed to communicate this information to the entire nursing staff. On the sample Client Care Plan on page 36, notice that item 1—Ineffective Breathing Pattern—should be alleviated by the third postoperative day, in this case, March 25 at 3:00 P.M. The checkpoints are listed in sequence to meet the goal. For the first 24 hours the nursing interventions (la through 1d) should be completed every 2 hours and then advanced to every 4 hours for the next 48 hours.

Updating Care Plans To ensure that client care plans are current and relevant, they should be reviewed on a daily basis and updated at least every 24 to 48 hours. There are several ways to update a care plan. Some facilities have spaces designated on the nursing Kardex or nurses' notes. In the figure, the update column is used when the original deadline is reached but the problem persists. A new deadline must then be established. If the ineffective breathing pattern exists beyond the third postoperative day, a new time frame for goal achievement is determined and documented in the update column.

Activating Care Plans When standard care plans are used, a systematic approach to activation and deactivation must be understood by all nursing personnel. As already stated, a common approach is to circle, date, and initial problems that are relevant for the individual client. Any problem that is not circled remains inactivated and should not be assessed, treated, or documented. From the example, you can see that the client has two of the problems listed, an ineffective breathing pattern and a knowledge deficit regarding discharge medication. Items 1 and 3 are circled. In the date column, date, time, and initials of the nurse activating the problem are entered. The second problem is not activated; therefore a circle is not placed around the number.

Inactivating Care Plans To inactivate the problem, a single line through the problem or intervention with a black pen can be made. In the update/DC column the date, time, and nurse's initials should be placed next to the crossed out, inactivated information. If only one of the interventions is not necessary, a line is drawn through that intervention and initials placed next to it in the initial column. The other interventions are left current and active.

Evaluating Care Plans The evaluation of how well the client care plan was individualized to meet the needs of the client is tested at discharge. If the care plan was appropriate, the discharge criteria are met. The nursing interventions and problems are then inactivated or discontinued. Frequently, there are clients who, on discharge, have not met the discharge criteria for various reasons. The documentation in the chart should reflect those problems that still exist, the extent to which the problem is being resolved, and additional information to indicate which plans were formulated for goal achievement.

Changing Care Plan Formats As computers are being used more commonly to document nursing care and workplace redesign is transforming how we deliver nursing care, the type and method of using the nursing care plan is changing. JCAHO's requirements are becoming more flexible and are allowing new ways to document client care. Critical paths, protocols, and standardized nursing care plans are used with or are replacing the more traditional care plans.

Computerized Client Care Plans The format used in computer software packages individualizes client care plans according to each health care facility's specifications. This type of format is very popular now that computerized documentation systems have been implemented in many facilities. Preparation time for writing individualized care plans is decreased and standardized plans are developed and written by clinical experts. One disadvantage of this software is that nurses must carefully determine the relevance and appropriateness of the care plan for each individual client. The care plan for each client is generated by the computer each shift. Changes must be entered into the computer frequently to ensure the accuracy of the plan.

Critical Paths or Clinical Pathways

This type of documentation is used primarily with managed care delivery systems. In this system, traditional nursing care plans do not exist. A critical path or clinical pathway is a standardized multidisciplinary plan of care developed for clients with common or prevalent conditions. It is a tool developed collaboratively by all health team members to facilitate achievement of client outcomes in a predictable and established time frame. The clinical pathways are used on each shift to direct and monitor client care. The plan indicates the actions and interventions achieved at designated times in order to meet the criteria for reimbursable length of stay. For example, a client with a total hip replacement has a critical path that states time frames for out of bed, gait training, and ambulation listed under the physical activity section of the form. On the second postoperative day the client should move from bed to chair with assistance. Nursing diagnoses are not always incorporated in the critical path. Documentation of nursing activities completed in response to the critical path varies according to facility policies and guidelines. Some facilities initial each

CLINICAL PATHWAY FOR OPERATIVE HIP

Use Ortho **Admit Orders**	**Day 1** **Admit/ to OR in 24–36 hrs.** **Date** ____________	**Day 2** **Post Operative Day (POD) 1**
Assessment A *If mechanical fall with no medical hx of problems, then surgery immediately. If hx of medical problems eval. suggested.*	• **Adm. assessment, q 8 hr.** ✓ Basic assessment, CMS, HV Drsg, I&O, IV, skin assess, B/S, flatus. **q 4 hr. Post-op** ✓ VS, O_2 protocol. SpO_2 reading (see graphic)	• **q 8 hr.** ✓ Basic assessment, CMS, HV Drsg, I&O, SpO_2, VS, IV site, skin assess. sign. • BID ✓ Homan sign. Oxygen protocol.
Physical Activity P • Ambulate BID if able.	• Bedrest, move in bed with assistance. • Pre admit activity level:	• OOB chair. • Commode with help. • Transfer & gait training.
Treatment T *Hip Precautions for hemiarthroplasty only*	• Incentive Spirometry (IS), TCDB, TED/ Sequential Compression Device (SCD). • Foley cath. insert	• TED/SCD, I.S., TCDB. • Foley cath. remains if needed. • *Hip Precaution for hemiathroplasty only*
Medications IV, PO, IM, SQ, etc. M	• Ancef pre operative. • Ancef 8 hr. × 24 hr. (after Surgery). Antiemetic PRN, Anticoagulant.	• Stool softener • Iron supp. BID (hold if GI upset). • Anticoagulant.
IV Fluids/Blood Products I	• Transfuse blood if needed. • IV at 75–100cc till tol. P.O. then switch to IVL.	• IV at TKO or IVL.
Nutrition N	• Advance diet as tolerated.	• Diet as tolerated.
Comfort/Pain C	• PCA or other pain medication as ordered by Surgeon or Anesthesia.	• PCA or other pain medication as ordered by Surgeon or Anesthesia.
Education E	• Pre & Post op. Patient Clinical pathway, TED/SCD, Analgesia method. • Discharge plan reinforced.	• Reinforce Post op. & Clinical pathway, TED/SCD, Analgesia method.

Clinical Pathway for Operative Hip Care.

MULTIDISCIPLINARY PROBLEM RECORD

When a particular problem no longer exists the caregiver should yellow out the problem and date when it was resolved. • Review and update problem list q shift. •

Date/Time		Problem #	PROBLEM State the problem with description of findings	INTERVENTION Refer to Pathways, Flow Sheets, Standards of Care as appropriate	EVALUATION Reassessment of problem or results of interventions	Initial

A form used in Variance Charting.

day's completed tasks on the critical path document, whereas others use flow charts and narrative charting.

If the client does not achieve the expected outcome in the specified time, a "variance" occurs, and an individual plan of care is developed that may then incorporate nursing diagnosis. For example, if a client is unable to ambulate by day three, a nursing diagnosis can be used to individualize the client's variance from the critical path expectations. An individualized care plan is initiated, and charting continues on the variance until it is resolved. The individualized section of the care path is usually found on the back of the form. In the sample "Clinical Pathway for Operative Hip" the form used to chart the variance is termed "Multidisciplinary Problem Record". The problem is identified and listed as problem 1. In the space provided for the PROBLEM—a nursing diagnosis is used or a client problem is listed. Interventions are developed and an evaluating section is added. All other documentation continues on the care path.

In addition to the pathway and multidisciplinary problem record, the more sophisticated clinical pathways also include an admitting assessment, nursing history including risk factors for falls and skin, nutrition risk evaluation and social or cultural variables. An ongoing admission data base is included in the packet. Also, this section contains a discharge planning risk assessment and multidisciplinary team conference section. Routine Assessment and Care Record frequently are included in this system of documentation.

There are several advantages for using critical or clinical pathways including continuity of care among all health care workers—discharge planning is begun on admission, and teaching plans are initiated early in the hospitalization. Clinical or critical pathways have been proven to reduce length of hospital stay, complications, and costs. Client satisfaction has also increased with the use of pathways.

Not all clients can be placed on pathways. For more complex clients, those requiring specialized care or clients experiencing complications, individualized care plans are more appropriate.

Protocols There are several uses for protocols within the various health care settings. Protocols can be used when specific equipment, such as a Roto Bed, is used in client care. They are also useful for specific nursing interventions such as administration of IV antifibrinolytic agents. In both of these situations, specific actions must be taken to ensure accurate and safe care of clients requiring these treatments. Using protocols in these situations promotes safety.

Protocols can be used in conjunction with standard care plans, individualized care plans, and critical paths. The use of protocols decreases the amount of documentation required on the care plan as actions and interventions are described in detail on the protocol.

In some areas of the hospital, protocols are used in place of care plans. This is particularly true in emergency departments, outpatient surgery, labor and delivery, postanesthesia departments, and operating rooms. Protocols for client care in each of these areas are practical because clients have common needs. For example, clients in the postanesthesia area must have their respiratory status monitored, fluid balance maintained, and level of consciousness assessed. These clients must also meet certain criteria for discharge from the unit. There is no real requirement for an individualized plan of care for the clients in these settings. The time spent in these specialty areas is usually very limited and the service very specific.

CHARTING

Next to direct client care, charting is one of the nurse's most important functions. Charting, the process of recording vital information, serves many important purposes:

- Charting communicates information, such as facts, figures, and observations, to other members of the client's health care team.
- Charting assists supervisory personnel to evaluate the staff's performance on a day-by-day basis for specific clients.
- Charting provides a permanent record for future reference that may become a legal document in the event of litigation or prosecution.

Charting—A Method of Communication

Complete and accurate charting is essential to protect both the client and the nurse. In communicating your observations and actions, charting helps to ensure both quality and continuity of health care for your clients. Information recorded by you becomes a valuable data base for nurses on subsequent shifts. Then, when you reassume responsibility for the client, you can determine what events occurred during prior time periods. Frequently, a client's reaction time is nearly as important as the reaction itself; therefore accuracy of time observations becomes an integral part of the charting process. In addition to the client's attending physician, other personnel interested in the chart may include the infection control nurse, discharge coordinator, utilization review personnel, or other hospital staff specialists who are checking on the client's progress or lack of positive reaction to treatment.

The client, as an individual, should receive individualized attention that focuses on his or her specific needs. As these needs are identified by each member of the health care team, they can be communicated to the others. Since nurses have the greatest amount of direct client contact, it is appropriate for the nurse to coordinate the important function of charting.

Charting provides one means for assessing the quality and effectiveness of nursing care. Nurse managers, team leaders, and supervisors use nurses' notes as a basis for staff evaluations. Because charts are documented descriptions of nursing actions, the quality of nursing care may be evaluated on the basis of the quality of charting notes.

Since charting describes nursing interventions and their outcomes, other healthcare personnel can determine if subsequent treatment should be changed.

A client's record includes all charting and becomes part of a legal document. Should a client's hospital record be introduced in court, the notes become a legal record of the care provided by each health care provider. Legally, care that is not recorded is considered to be care that was not provided. It is necessary therefore to chart all care that you *do* provide, as well as any care that you *do not* provide.

The legal requirement for charting is found in state laws and professional requirements. For example, Title 22 of the California Code of Regulation states

> Nurses' notes which shall include but not be limited to the following: concise and accurate record of nursing care administered; record of pertinent observations including psychosocial and physical manifestations as well as incidents and unusual occurrences, and relevant nursing interpretation of such observations; name, dosage and time of administration of medications and treatment. Route of administration and site of injection shall be recorded if other than by oral administration; record of type of restraint and time of application and removal. The time of application and removal shall not be required for soft tie restraints used for support and protection of the patient.

In addition to the nurses' notes, Title 22 requires that a written client care plan must be a permanent part of the medical record.

> There shall be a written patient care plan developed for each patient in coordination with the total health team. This plan shall include goals, problems/needs, and approach and shall be available to all members of the health team.

The JCAHO also states its requirements for documentation in its nursing care standards. Examples of the documentation standards include: an admission assessment performed and documented by a registered nurse that includes consideration of biophysical, psychosocial, environmental, self-care, educational, and discharge planning; nursing care based on identified nursing diagnoses or client care needs and client care standards; needs that are consistent with the therapies of other disciplines;

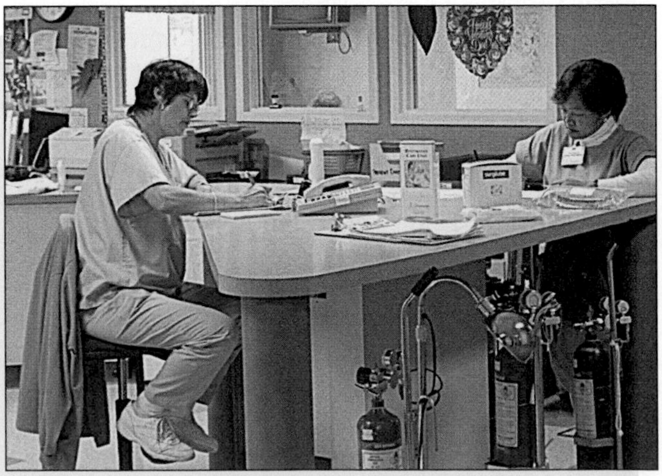

Charting is completed immediately following client care.

interventions identified to meet the client's needs; the actual client care provided while hospitalized; educational information provided; and the ability of the client or family to manage the continuing care on discharge.

Charting Format

The format of the chart varies from hospital to hospital. Most important is the content of the notes. First, your notes should describe the assessment that you completed at the beginning of your shift. This information provides a baseline for changes that may occur later in the client's condition. If there are no such changes, this fact should be entered as the final note. Some hospitals require that all parts of the assessment be documented; others require that only abnormalities be documented.

As your shift progresses, you should always include certain items in your notes, including changes in the client's medical, mental, or emotional condition. Nurses are well attuned to medical changes, such as shock, hemorrhage, or a change in level of consciousness; however, the nurse may overlook subtle emotional changes. Anger, depression, or joy should also be documented because these emotions often are indications of the client's response to the illness. Recording these changes is absolutely necessary if other nurses are to act appropriately during subsequent shifts. You should also chart if *no* changes occurred in the client's condition so that treatments can be modified as necessary. Normal aspects of the client's condition should be noted also.

Reactions to any unscheduled or prn medications must be recorded. Because each medication is given to meet a specified need, the client's response or lack of response must be recorded to document whether the need was met. To complete this part of the entry, note the time the medication was given, the problem for which the medication was given, and the expected solution. For example: "7 A.M. c/o moderate RUOQ abdominal incisional pain, '7' on pain scale. Roxanol, 30 mg, PO for pain." When the effects of the medication are known, write another note: "8 A.M. States pain relieved."

Finally, it is important to record the client's response to teaching. These notes may describe return demonstrations, verbalization of learning, or resistance to instruction. Because most teaching takes place over a period of days, record both what you taught and how the client responded. Then other nurses will know whether to repeat the previous instructions, reinforce them, or start a new topic.

Frequently, repetitive aspects of nursing care, such as vital signs and intake and output, are recorded on flow sheets. If flow sheets are used, you need not repeat the same information in your notes. An exception is an abnormal measurement that is a part of a larger assessment. For example: "c/o sharp abd. pain. BP 78/50. P 136. Skin cold & diaphoretic. NG tube draining bright red bloody fluid with small clots. Reported to Dr. Jones."

Charting for Potential Legal Problems

- Use facts. If you chart "physician notified," include time called, facts you gave, and his or her response.
- Do not use pat phrases. Be specific and use individual assessment parameters. Do not chart global assessments such as "IV running."
- Be professional when you chart. Do not make interpretations; state what happened, for instance, "suggested to physician that client requires heart monitor" and physician responded "case does not warrant a monitor." If this client were later to be involved in a lawsuit, these notes indicate that the nurse was observant, alert, and aware that the client might be in danger.
- Do not use words such as *mistake* or *accident*; write specifically what incident occurred and what actions were taken.
- Do not use tentative or vague statements such as *appears* or *apparently*.
- Use correct language and medical terms. Do not use slang, pat phrases, or abbreviations that are not generally accepted.
- Use correct grammar and spelling.
- Do not chart for someone else.
- Do not chart ahead of time. Chart after the care is complete, but do not wait until the end of the shift.
- Do not alter a medical record. Draw a single line through an incorrect entry and initial and date the error.
- Write in late entries when you think about them; do not try to go back into earlier charting and insert the information. Label the information as "late entry" and put the time it actually happened in the entry.
- Countersign care given by assistive staff only if the facility allows you to countersign, and then do so only after you review the entry and are familiar with the care provided to the client.
- Chart potentially serious situations; include observations, reports to the physician and supervisor, and whether any action was taken. Be precise; add quotes or specific communication. This is the only kind of charting that holds up in court.
- Report problems to appropriate authorities, such as suspected child abuse to social services.
- Provide the best care you are capable of giving; then precisely chart your observations, interventions, and communications; this is the best deterrent to later legal problems.

Forensic Charting

The content of nurse's notes may affect the outcome of criminal investigations; when charting, especially in the

ER, OR, or suspected assault cases, nurses must document exactly and carefully. Forensics is not only linked to criminal investigations; it is the connection between medical data and the legal process. Nurses must be aware that their documentation may be involved in a future legal case.

Charting and the Nursing Process

The nursing process provides the framework for decision making throughout all phases of nursing care. The components of the nursing process are assessment, planning, implementation (or intervention), and evaluation. This cycle is applied by the nurse both to routine situations and critical care emergencies.

It is important to relate the nursing process to charting because for experienced nurses, the process may become only a mental exercise. The nurse "thinks through" the situation, makes decisions, takes action, and then observes the results. Unless the entire process is recorded on the client care plan and documented in the chart, the next nurse who encounters a similar situation with the same client is deprived of important and potentially valuable background data. The second nurse, without knowing the full background, may repeat the entire process, resulting in a loss of valuable time and an increase in client discomfort. When similar nursing interventions completed by different nurses have the same positive results, the client experiences a feeling of reassurance that may not be achieved if each nurse attempts a totally different set of interventions to reach the same objective.

The client, in a strange environment with unknown people doing unfamiliar and often uncomfortable things, often tries to find reassurance in any type of routine. The client soon expects a certain procedure to be done by the same person in the same way and at a predictable hour. Changes in the procedure are often upsetting to the client. It is imperative that the steps of any procedure, especially those that are complicated or personalized to the client, be documented in detail on the client care plan so that each nurse does it the same way. The detailed description of how to perform a dressing change, however, is written in the client's care plan, not in the nurses' notes.

The nurses' notes describe the amount, color, consistency, and odor of the drainage. In addition, the amount and type of irrigating solution and type of abdominal dressing are noted. It is important to add a statement as to the client's tolerance of the procedure.

Charting Systems

The three main charting systems are *source-oriented*, *problem-oriented*, and *computer-assisted* charting. Two additional systems used are *focus charting* and *charting by exception*. The most common system is the *source-oriented chart*, so named because the information is organized and presented according to its source. For example, there are separate sections for doctors' progress notes, nurses' notes, and respiratory therapy notes. To obtain a complete "picture" of the client, one must read through all sections and piece together the separate bits of data. This may be a time-consuming process, and the result may not produce an accurate or complete assessment of the client. Narrative charting is found within this charting system.

A second system for chart organization is the *problem-oriented medical record*. In this system the chart is based on the problem list—all problems, present or potential, identified with that client. Using the problems as reference points, each person giving care charts progress notes on the same sheets. In this way assessment of a specific incident by everyone concerned (e.g., physician, RN, dietitian, enterostomal therapist) is in the same location, and the client's overall picture can be easily seen.

The third method of organizing data is *computer-assisted charting*. This type of charting constantly updates information from many sources. For example, physiologic measurements are recorded and updated on the computer terminal at least hourly. The information is easily retrievable by the nursing personnel as questions arise. Reference material for common nursing problems ensures quick reference and easily retrieved information to provide safe nursing care.

Focus charting. As the name implies, it makes client needs or problems the focus of care in the progress notes. This method moves away from labeling client status a problem because it includes the client's condition, nursing diagnosis, signs or symptoms, or a significant client event or change in status (need for surgical intervention). Focus charting is similar to SOAP (subjective, objective, assessment, plan) charting except it uses the term *focus* in place of *problem*, which eliminates the negative connotation of the word *problem*. The focus is not necessarily written as a nursing diagnosis. The progress notes are organized using the DAR format: data, action, and response. Data includes the information that supports the focus; action is the nursing intervention used to treat the problem; and response is how the client responds to the intervention and the outcome. The following is an example:

D: Client found grimacing, hands clenched, and body rigid. Verbalized pain at 9 on pain scale.

A: Administered 15 mg MS IV push. Called physician to request PCA for client.

R: Pain moderately relieved after 35 minutes. Able to understand instruction in use of PCA.

Charting by exception. (CBE) is a system that focuses on significant findings or deviations from the norm. It reduces time spent documenting and reduces multiple data entries in the record. It uses flow sheets, protocols and standards of practice, nursing diagnosis, care plans, SOAP progress notes, and a nursing database. A nursing and physician order flow sheet is used to document physical assessments and implementation of physician and nursing orders as well as completion of nursing and physician orders. The form also contains the teaching record and discharge notes. Only changes or findings significantly different from the norm are documented. Nurses chart only when the client does not meet the predetermined standard or norm. All exceptions to the standards must be documented narratively. When nurses see entries in the chart, it alerts them that something unusual has occurred with the client. An additional advantage in CBE charting is that all flow sheets are kept at the bedside, which eliminates the need to transcribe information from a work sheet to the permanent record.

Some legal or reimbursement issues, such as admissibility in court, may be related to charting by exception. At this time the rule "if it wasn't charted, it wasn't done" is still the prevailing attitude in legal issues.

Source-Oriented Systems Charting Systems charting is a common and efficient way of organizing client information in source-oriented nurses' notes. An outline of the systems to be reviewed, and sometimes specific subheadings for each, is established. Medical units may use one type of systems nurses' notes, and critical care may use another.

At the beginning of the shift, the nurse performs a physical assessment on each client to determine that client's current status. This information becomes the initial systems charting. When changes occur, they are noted with the time under the appropriate system. If no changes occur during the shift, no other charting of this type may be necessary.

To record all pertinent client information, several flow sheets are commonly used in conjunction with the systems form. One flow sheet is the vital signs sheet, which contains information, such as temperature, pulse, blood pressure, respiration, urine output, hemodynamic monitoring values, infusion rates of vasoactive drugs, and daily weights. Other flow sheets may include a medication and an intake and output record. Special sheets, such as neurologic monitoring sheets and diabetic sheets, are used as necessary. Flow sheets eliminate the need to write excessive notes and avoid duplication of information. Flow sheets do not negate the need for narrative descriptions.

Refer back to the client care plan to ensure that all problems have been assessed and documentation completed. It is a good idea to check the care plan several times a day.

Source-Oriented Narrative Charting Narrative charting is based on chronology rather than systems. Information is charted in chronologic order, regardless of the subject of the note. For example, the nurses' notes for a client could appear as follows:

0730	Blood glucose 240 mg/dL
0745	5 units Reg. Insulin administered Rt. Abd.
0815	Assessment completed.

The primary deficiency of narrative charting is that it is very easy to chart without specifying why the client is in the hospital or what the client's overall condition is. Note the example illustrated above. Why is the client in the hospital? What is the client's general condition? How is the client progressing?

COMMUNITY HOSPITAL

ICU NEURO/SPINAL FLOW CHART

Date: 3/22/04			Time:	8 am		
Pupils			Right: size	4 mm		
			Reaction	S		
			Left: Size	4 mm		
			Reaction	S		
			Visual Acuity	C		
Mental Status						
COMA SCALE	Eyes Open		Spontaneously			
			To Speech			
			To Pain	+		
			Never			
	Verbal Response		Clear			
			Confused			
			Inappropriate	+		
			Incomprehensible			
			None			
MOVEMENT	Arms		Normal Power			
			Weakness	+		
			Flexion			
			Extension			
			No Response			
	Legs		Normal Power			
			Weakness	+		
			Flexion			
			Extension			
			No Response			
Reflexes			Gag/Cough	0		
			Corneal	+		
			Babinski R/L	+/+		
			Oculocephalic	0		
Respiratory			Pattern	Reg.		
			Rate	28		
Seizures			Type	0		
			Duration			
			Fluid Drainage from Ears or	0		
			Nose	0		

Signature D. Jones RN

Neurologic flow sheet.

When using narrative charting, an assessment should be performed at the beginning of the shift and as needed thereafter. When assessment is the initial entry in narrative charting, subsequent entries are more relevant and understandable. This combination of assessment and narrative charting is the best technique to ensure that adequate information about the client is recorded for all personnel who use nurses' notes.

There is a tendency for hospitals to move away from traditional narrative charting to focus on charting by exception charting. Because the client's chart is considered a legal document, it is important that nurses chart relevant, accurate, and appropriate information in a timely manner. The following rules for charting narrative notes will assist you in maintaining an acceptable chart.

1. Use black ink, not felt pen or pencil. Black ink microfilms best.
2. Correct errors by drawing a single line through the error, write the words *mistaken entry* (ME) above it, and then initial the error. The error must be readable. Ink eradication, erasures, or use of occlusive materials is not acceptable. The word *error* is no longer advised because juries tend to associate the word *error* with an actual nursing care mistake.
3. Sign each entry with your first initial, last name, and status; for example, SN for student nurse, LVN for licensed vocational nurse, or RN for registered nurse. Script, not printing, is used for the signature. Each signature should appear at the righthand margin of the nurses' notes.

Narrative Charting

Advantages

- Can be used in conjunction with flow sheets and other documentation systems
- Quick method of charting chronologic data
- Familiar method of charting
- Easy to use
- Used in all types of clinical settings

Disadvantages

- Lack of systematic structure leading to difficulty in determining data relationships
- Time consuming
- Frequently lacks information on client care outcomes
- Difficult to monitor data for quality assurance
- Relevant information found in several areas in chart

4. Notes should appear on each succeeding line. Lines should not be omitted in the nurses' notes. A horizontal line is drawn to "fill up" a partial line. Continuous charting is done for each entry unless a time change occurs. You may or may not need a new line for each new idea or statement, depending on agency protocol.
5. Entries should be concise. Complete sentences are not required. Start each entry with a capital letter, and end the entry with a period even if the entry is a single word or phrase.
6. The date is entered in the data column on the first line of every page of nurses' notes and whenever the date changes.
7. Time is entered in the time column whenever a new time entry occurs. Do not put time changes in the text of the nurses' notes. If only one time is entered for block charting, enter the last time you were with the client.
8. Chart objective facts, not your interpretations. For example, chart "ate 100%," not "good appetite." If the client complains, place the complaint in quotation marks to indicate that it is his or her statement. For example, "c/o chest pain radiating down left arm."
9. Objective data is to be charted as well. In addition to the statement offered by the client, the nurse should chart his or her observations: "Skin cold and clammy. Diaphoretic. Vital signs stable."
10. Refusal of medications and treatments must be documented. A circle is placed around the time the medication or treatment is to be given in the appropriate area of the chart. An explanation as to the reason the medication was not given is entered in the nurses' notes.
11. Sign each entry before it is replaced in the chart rack. An entry is not to be left unsigned. If all the charting is completed for the shift at one time, a single signature is placed at the end of the charting.
12. Accuracy is important. Describe behaviors rather than feelings. This allows other health team members to determine the client's actual problems.
13. Chart only those abbreviations and symbols approved by the facility. Information can be misinterpreted or misleading when unfamiliar abbreviations are used. (See the listing at the end of the chapter for examples of commonly used abbreviations.)
14. Spell correctly, using proper terminology and grammar.
15. Write legibly. If your writing is not legible, then print.
16. Only chart what you personally have done or observed. An exception to this rule is when you are responsible for charting for nonprofessional personnel.
17. Do not use the word "client" in the chart. The chart belongs to that client.

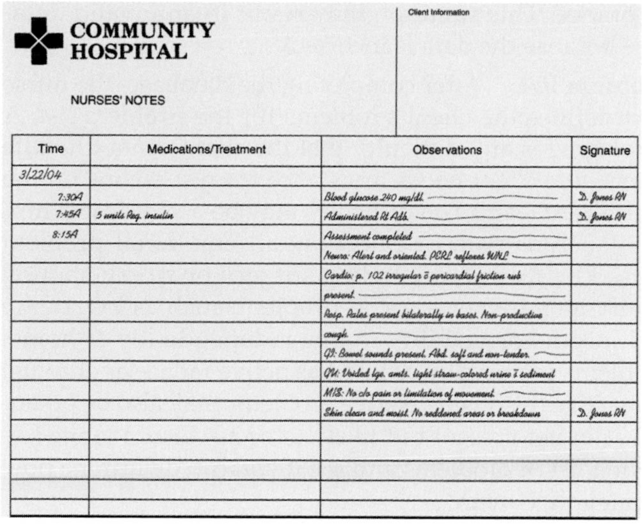
COMMUNITY HOSPITAL

NURSES' NOTES

Client Information

Time	Medications/Treatment	Observations	Signature
3/22/04			
7:30A		Blood glucose 240 mg/dl.	D. Jones RN
7:45A	5 units Reg. insulin	Administered Rt Adb.	D. Jones RN
8:15A		Assessment completed	
		Neuro: Alert and oriented. PERL reflexes WNL	
		Cardio: p. 102 irregular c̄ pericardial friction rub	
		present.	
		Resp. Rales present bilaterally in bases. Non-productive	
		cough.	
		GI: Bowel sounds present. Abd. soft and non-tender.	
		GU: Voided lge. amts. light straw-colored urine c̄ sediment	
		M/S: No c/o pain or limitation of movement.	
		Skin clean and moist. No reddened areas or breakdown	D. Jones RN

Source-oriented narrative charting using systems charting format.

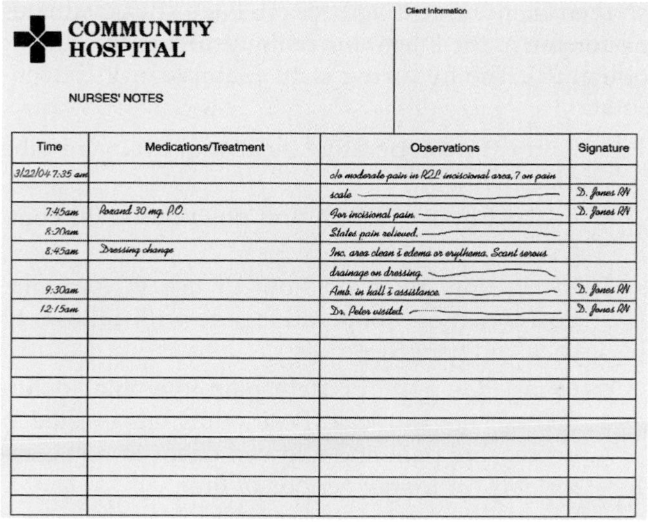
COMMUNITY HOSPITAL

NURSES' NOTES

Client Information

Time	Medications/Treatment	Observations	Signature
3/22/04 7:35 am		c/o moderate pain in RLL incisional area, 7 on pain	
		scale	D. Jones RN
7:45am	Roxand 30 mg. P.O.	For incisional pain.	D. Jones RN
8:20am		States pain relieved.	
8:45am	Dressing change	Inc. area clean c̄ edema or erythema. Scant serous	
		drainage on dressing.	
9:30am		Amb. in hall c̄ assistance.	D. Jones RN
12:15am		Dr. Peter visited.	D. Jones RN

Nurses' notes in narrative charting.

18. Do not double chart. If something appears on a flow sheet, it does not need to appear on the nurses' narrative record unless there is an alteration from normal.
19. Do not squeeze information into a space because you forgot to chart it earlier. Add the information on the first available line. Write in the time the event occurred, not the time you entered the information the words *late entry* can be inserted before the charting.
20. The following information should be charted.
    a. Physician's visits.
    b. Times the client leaves and returns to the unit, mode of transportation, and destination.
    c. Medications (chart immediately after given). Include dosage, route of administration (if parenteral, where given), whether pain was relieved (if pain medication), and side effects.
    d. Treatments (chart immediately after given).

A new form of narrative charting, assessment–intervention–response (AIR), has been introduced that presents a more efficient and effective method of organizing and simplifying this type of charting. In the assessment (A) section of the chart, the nurse summarizes data and impressions of problems found via assessment. The intervention (I) section is for summaries about interventions based on assessment findings. The summary may include a condensed nursing care plan or plans for additional monitoring. The response (R) section focuses on the client's response to nursing interventions. Each assessment and intervention is labeled so that other nurses can chart pertinent responses. With appropriate flowsheets and the AIR method of narrative charting, client care is more clearly and concisely documented.

The AIR Format

A Respirations 30 and labored. Rales bilateral in the bases.
I Deep breathing and coughing, incentive spirometer with Mucomyst. Up in chair.
R Respiration 24, decreased intensity of rales but still present.

Problem-Oriented Medical Records and PIE The second major type of charting is the problem-oriented medical records, or POMR. This system focuses on a specific problem or complaint; it differs from source-oriented narrative charting, not only in format but in philosophy. Problem-oriented medical records focus on the client's status rather than on the source of the information, such as department or member of the health care team who is originating the information. Narrative charting typically consists of doctors' progress notes, physical therapy progress notes, nurses' notes, and respiratory therapy progress notes. With POMR, only one set of progress notes is used, and all personnel caring for the client record their data on this set.

The PIE charting format, which stands for problem-identification, intervention, and evaluation, is a newer, condensed version of the problem-oriented charting system. This type of charting uses the nursing process and nursing diagnosis while incorporating the plan of care into the nurses' progress notes. The PIE charting system does not use the traditional nursing care plan. Client problems, teaching needs, and discharge planning needs are identified during the initial client assessment, the P of the PIE format. Based on the assessment, nursing diagnoses are identified and numbered on a problem list. Interventions that are carried out are documented for each specific nursing diagnosis (I). Each shift evaluates the outcome of the interventions in resolving the client's problem (E). The following is an example of PIE documentation:

P#1: Pain r/t postoperative incisional drainage tube placement.

P: Instruct in use of PCA and positioning for comfort.

I: Instruction given on how to use PCA pump. Positioned on unoperative side with pillows to back and between knees.

E: Using PCA appropriately, pain tolerable, identified as 3 on pain scale. Positioning has assisted in decreasing pain and allowed client to rest comfortably for longer periods of time.

In its purest form, a POMR consists of five distinct parts: the data base (initial assessment), problem list, initial plan, progress notes, and discharge summary. The data base is made up of information from and about the client that is used to develop the problem list. Because the POMR system is systematic and well defined, the data base consists of specific types of data, including the chief complaint (why the client came to the hospital), personal and family medical history, allergies and reactions, medications taken at home, physical assessment, mental and emotional assessment, and lifestyle.

Database. Development of a complete data base requires skill and practice. Basic features of client interviewing and physical assessment are covered in other sections of this text, but a few tips and reminders may help to sharpen your skills. First, select a time mutually acceptable to you and the client. Know how much time you have for the interview and whether the client has scheduled appointments or tests. Be aware of the client's physical and emotional comfort, the physical environment of the interview location, and pending mealtimes. Second, consider how your questions might affect the client. Phrase questions that require the client to explain and answer—a "yes" or "no" is not sufficiently informative. Do not make the client defensive by being judgmental about his or her actions. Clients who believe you do not approve of their actions often withhold potentially important information. Third, avoid leading statements. Many clients try to respond in an agreeable manner. For example, "You don't . . ." statements may be answered by "No, of course not." Also, avoid using medical jargon unfamiliar to the client. Some words you use daily may be unknown to your client. The client answers what he or she thinks you asked to avoid showing ignorance. This situation may result in an invalid database because the data is incorrect.

Problem list. After completing the database, the nurse next defines the client problems for the problem list. A "problem" is any difficulty that the client cannot handle alone—the client needs assistance from someone on the health care team. The difficulty may be a physical symptom, such as pain or infection; an emotional problem caused by fear of impending surgery or worry about a family member; or a social problem, such as loss of job and income or inability to live independently at home. Problems are usually defined as active (acute or chronic) or inactive (resolved). Active problems may also be potential—not yet present but likely to occur. Examine the following list of problems and see if you can determine how to categorize them.

Medical diagnoses are included on the problem list if they are definite. If they are only tentative, the client's symptoms should be put on the list until the actual diagnosis is made. Of course, many of the symptoms may qualify as part of the nursing diagnosis. For example, anxiety related to one's medical diagnosis is a nursing diagnosis.

Upper GI bleeding, 3 days' duration	Active
Children, 2 and 5 years old, at home with father	Active
Possible skin breakdown	Active—Potential
Appendectomy 1954	Resolved
Asthma since childhood	Active—Chronic

The categories of the POMR closely approximate the steps in the nursing process. The database and problem list equate to assessment; the initial plan equates to plan-

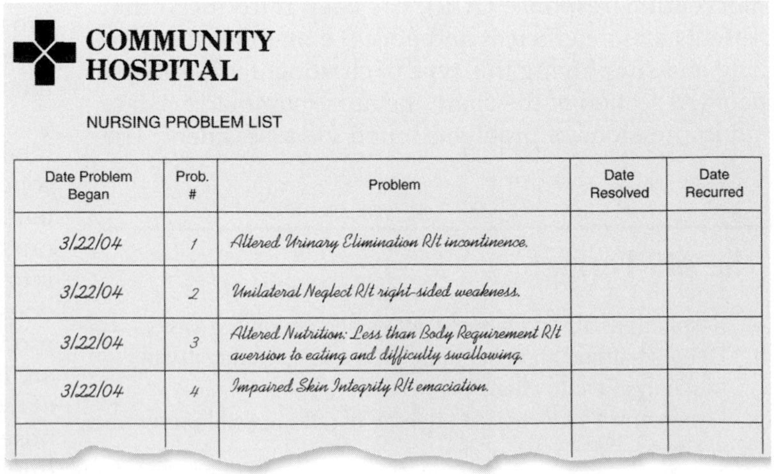
COMMUNITY HOSPITAL

NURSING PROBLEM LIST

Date Problem Began	Prob. #	Problem	Date Resolved	Date Recurred
3/22/04	1	Altered Urinary Elimination R/t incontinence.		
3/22/04	2	Unilateral Neglect R/t right-sided weakness.		
3/22/04	3	Altered Nutrition: Less than Body Requirement R/t aversion to eating and difficulty swallowing.		
3/22/04	4	Impaired Skin Integrity R/t emaciation.		

POMR: Problem list.

ning; the progress notes discuss intervention; and the discharge summary is an evaluation.

Initial plan. After you complete the database and start the problem list, you then formulate the client care plan (CCP). For each major problem or group of problems, the CCP should include the following information: date, problem, expected outcome, check point, deadline, and nursing actions.

Progress notes. In the POMR system, one set of progress notes is used by everyone. This means that all members of the health care team write their observations on the same part of the chart. The entries on the problem list are always numbered, so when the nurse, physician, and the respiratory therapist all refer to problem 3 in their progress notes, everyone knows that they are referring to "Ineffective airway clearance, *related* to pain."

Within the well-organized POMR system, progress notes have a specific format, usually called SOAP or SOAPIE. These acronyms translate as:

Subjective: Client's symptoms and own description of problem.

Objective: Clinical findings; include observations and factual data; for instance, intake and output, vital signs, drainage, presence of rash.

Assessment: Statements about the problem based on subjective and objective data. Nursing diagnoses may be written here.

Plan: What you decide to do about the problem.

Implementation: Your nursing interventions.

Evaluation: How the implementation worked.

When writing progress notes, remember that a separate SOAP or SOAPIE note is needed for each problem. You should not combine problems. It is not always necessary to include the I, E, portions of the note; however, always include the S, O, A, and P parts, even if the client does not supply subjective statements.

Discharge summary. The discharge summary, the final step in the POMR system as well as all forms of charting, includes both a summary of the client's hospitalization and documentation of client teaching. SOAPIE notes are again used as the charting format, and a summary should be written for each problem on the problem list. If the problem is fully resolved during hospitalization, that fact and the date it occurred (from the progress notes) are all that is necessary. The discharge summary is not a day-by-day account of the client's stay but a short review. It is beneficial to

SOAP and SOAPIE Charting

Problem 1

Fluid Volume, Excess, *related to* poor compliance to medication administration.

- S "My rings are tight and my shoes don't fit."
- O Fingers are edematous. 3+ pitting edema of both ankles.
- A Fluid overload as a result of refusing diuretics.
- P Elevate feet. Explain necessity for diuretics. Administer drug, obtain order for IM med if nec. Observe dietary intake of Na^+ to determine if compliant to diet.

- I Client education completed regarding use of LASIX.
- E Could state signs and symptoms of low potassium.

Problem 2

Ineffective Airway Clearance, *related to* pain.

- S "I'm having difficulty bringing up mucus."
- O Lungs sound congested, rales present bilaterally in lower bases.
- A Unable to deep breathe and cough due to high abdominal incision.
- P Elevate HOB 45 degrees. Enc. coughing and deep breathing. Medicate for pain q3h. Splint inc. when coughing.

- I Expectorating large amounts of clear mucus.

COMMUNITY HOSPITAL

Client Information

PROGRESS NOTES

Date	Note progress of case, complications, change in diagnosis, condition on discharge
3/22/04	Problem #3
	S Refuses to eat. States "I'm afraid to swallow because I choke sometimes and don't like the food."
	O Has difficulty swallowing fluids. Chokes if not sitting upright.
	A Swallowing difficulty—probably related to CVA.
	P Contact dietician to see client re: food preferences.
	Place in high-Fowler's position when feeding.
	Feed slowly and reassure client often.

POMR: Progress notes using SOAP charting.

COMMUNITY HOSPITAL

PROGRESS NOTES

Client Information

Date	Note progress of case, complications, change in diagnosis, condition on discharge
3/22/04	Mr. Rappaport was admitted to the restorative care unit on 3/15/00 with right-side weakness, difficulty swallowing,
	inability to perform ADL's, 10# weight loss, and coccyx area reddened with Stage 1 pressure ulcer. Laboratory values WNL,
	except for a urinary tract infection 1 week prior to admission which has been resolved with P.O. Gantrisin (Problem #1)
	Continues to exhibit right-sided weakness. Unable to perform ADL's right handed (Problem #2) O.T. working on alternative
	ways to become independent in ADL's. Instructions given to client to swallow on left side. Weight loss has stabilized, dietition
	working with client to determine food preferences. Hi-protein, hi-calorie liquids between meals started 4/10/00. (Problem #3)
	Skin care with transparent dressings continues. Area remains unchanged. (Problem #4) Plan is to begin preparation for
	discharge. Instructions on dietary needs and skin care given to wife and daughter. O.T. will continue at home to work on
	ADL's. D. Jones RN

POMR: Discharge summary.

include specific highlights such as the highest serum glucose level or the highest temperature, but all the values need not be included. Remember, a separate SOAPIE note should be written for each problem that is not fully resolved at the time of the discharge.

All invasive procedures, surgical interventions, and major diagnostic tests should be listed and the results outlined. Braces, equipment, and supplies (e.g., for dressing changes, catheterizations) should be included in the summary. If the equipment or braces are difficult to use or apply, it is helpful if pictures or diagrams are included. Completed client teaching, discharge medications, and specific teaching regarding the medications should also be documented.

Referrals to other health care services should be identified with the name of the agency and the contact person listed on the chart. If clients are being discharged to other health care facilities or to a visiting nurse, it is helpful if they receive not only a copy of the discharge summary but a copy of the last client care plan. This provides for a smooth transition of care from one health care setting to another.

Because of the many changes necessary when implementing POMR, hospitals often use only part of it or are changing to it in stages; therefore it is common to find situations in which parts of several systems are in use. For example, SOAP nursing notes may be used and the remainder of the chart is source oriented, or doctors may use the problem list and SOAP progress notes and nurses use systems charting for nurses' notes. Although progress is rather slow, it appears that many more hospitals are adopting the POMR system, not only for its format and ease of use, but also for its completeness on documenting client care.

Computer-Assisted Charting

Computer-assisted charting can be implemented by itself or as in most cases, it is a component of a facility medical information system. There are so many constraints on time and resources that this type of system is becoming a necessity for health care agencies today. Inaccurate documentation has a significant impact on quality of client care, costs, and revenues. Redundant information input wastes valuable nursing time. Missing or incomplete documentation is costly and frustrating. If supplies or treatments are not documented, payment cannot be obtained.

Nursing information systems can manage clinical data in a variety of health care settings. These systems allow nurses to provide and access accurate and timely information. This type of charting allows the nurse to select content phrases on a screen that automatically builds a comprehensive record without inputting all the individual pieces of information.

Computer-assisted charting can be accomplished in a nurses' station or at the bedside. Most of the necessary documentation can be done at the bedside if the equipment is available. This includes vital signs, admission assessment, nursing assessment, intake and output records, client education records, and client care plans. Once the information is entered into the computer, it can be disseminated to different reports without the nurse's

Problem-Oriented Charting

Advantages

- Focuses on client problem
- Implements problem-solving approach
- Ease in retrieving information about each problem
- Problem resolution is clearly documented
- Problem list assists in identifying priority needs of client
- May be used effectively in acute or long-term care settings
- Consistency in documentation format
- Effectively uses nursing process in documentation
- Readily used in conjunction with standard nursing care plan
- Integrated documentation system promotes collaboration among all health care providers
- PIE charting uses flow sheet, which decreases documentation time and redundancy

Disadvantages

- Difficult to obtain agreement on what should be included in record
- Physicians vary in their acceptance of all disciplines using same list
- Duplication of information necessary on several forms
- Need for constant updating of problem list and determining whose responsibility it is to do so
- Format is frequently not used in pure form, making it difficult to use effectively
- Not efficient because each problem requires a separate POMR entry
- PIE charting incorporates use of care planning, which is responsibility of RN; therefore it is difficult to use LVNs in documentation system

intervention. Some of the documentation systems offer packages, such as customized flow sheets for each nursing unit in the hospital, and individualized critical pathways for each service area in the facility. Laboratory results, respiratory therapy notes and client care documentation are fully integrated into the electronic chart. Management reports can also be generated through this type of system. Shift reports, client acuity, and client care plan variance can be generated in some systems.

Computer systems record, store, and retrieve many pieces of data about the client that must be communicated

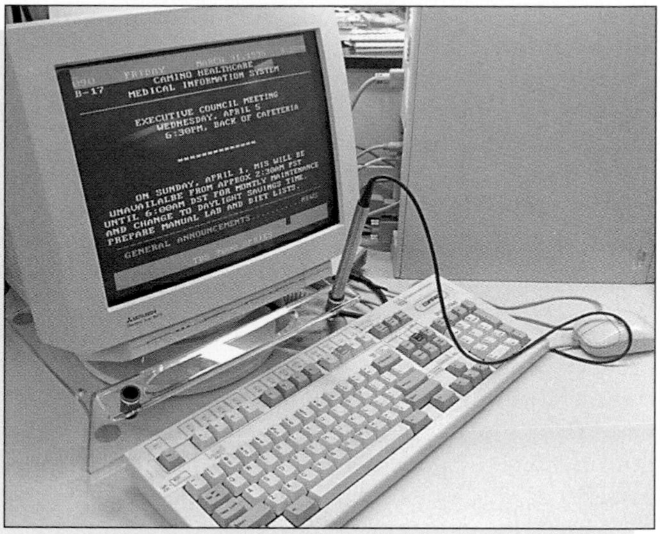

Light pen is used to record information into computer terminal.

throughout the hospital for the client to receive optimal care. For example, when a client is admitted and the physician enters orders into the computer, many things automatically happen. The dietary department is notified of the diet needs, pharmacy is notified of medications and IVs that are ordered, CSR is notified of special equipment needs, and the laboratory is notified of required tests. It is no longer necessary for the nurse to make out and deliver requests to all these departments and then arrange for delivery or pick up of the desired items. Each nursing unit has several computer terminals, or the terminals may be at the bedside. Before accessing the terminal, the sign-on code must be entered. Each person accessing information must have their own sign-on code. This prevents unauthorized persons from accessing confidential infor-

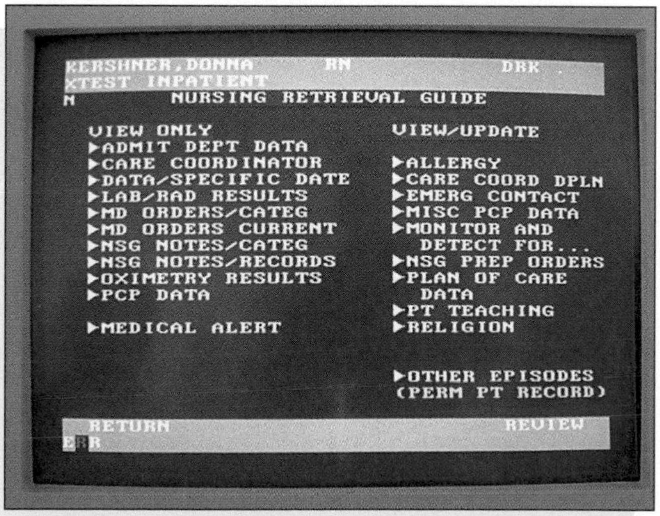

Nurses choose specific category of data from screen.

mation. After sending the code by pressing a SEND button, the nurse can select the section of the record needed. The lightpen is pointed at the data category and after pressing the button on the pen, the selection comes up on the screen. The most common category selections are nurses' notes, physician orders, laboratory or x-ray reports, and client care plans.

Hospitals usually have programs that contain special matrices of "Nursing Retrieval Guide(s)." Once the retrieval guide appears on the screen, the nurse can choose the specific category of data needed. Much of the routine ordering and care a nurse gives can be charted rapidly and completely in a matter of seconds using this system.

When the nurse has completed the charting, the information is displayed. At this time the nurse can make corrections, additions, or deletions. If the data displayed are correct, the nurse enters the data and it becomes a permanent part of the computer record for that client, and a hard copy is printed out to be put in the chart.

When the client is to be discharged, the nursing discharge summary is completed. This shows not only the client's physical condition but also the status of client teaching and follow-up plans. Again, it is simply punched or tapped on the terminal and the data are displayed. This information and the client instruction sheet generated by the computer are sent home with the client.

Computer-Assisted Charting

Advantages

- Quick communication between departments
- Quick access to information
- Increases accuracy and speed of documentation
- Improves documentation and meets JCAHO standards
- Tracks client outcomes
- Increases speed and completeness of reimbursement through accurate documentation
- Information is legible

Disadvantages

- Computer system is expensive to purchase and update
- "Downtime" can create problems of not receiving information or it is not charted on time
- Computer may increase charting time if number of terminals is insufficient
- Nurses rely on computers and don't question information when it may be wrong

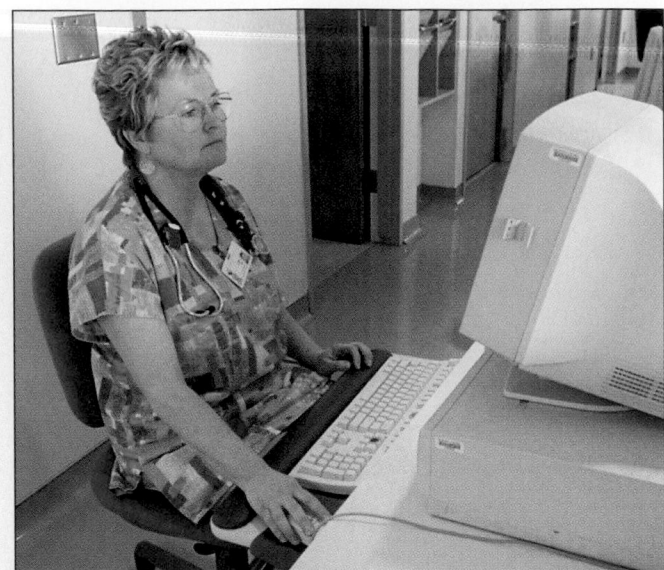

Each nursing unit has several computer terminals for documentation.

In addition to making the charting of client care and the communication between departments much simpler and less time-consuming, the computer provides reference material for common nursing problems. For example, a matrix may show the signs and symptoms associated with diabetes mellitus. If the nurse is unsure of the signs and symptoms of the different forms of this disease, he or she can easily find them in the computer, and, if needed, this information can be printed out and put in the chart. In this way the nurse can be quickly updated about the client's condition and thereby provide optimal care.

As in many professions, use of the computer in nursing and medicine has become more common and its pos-

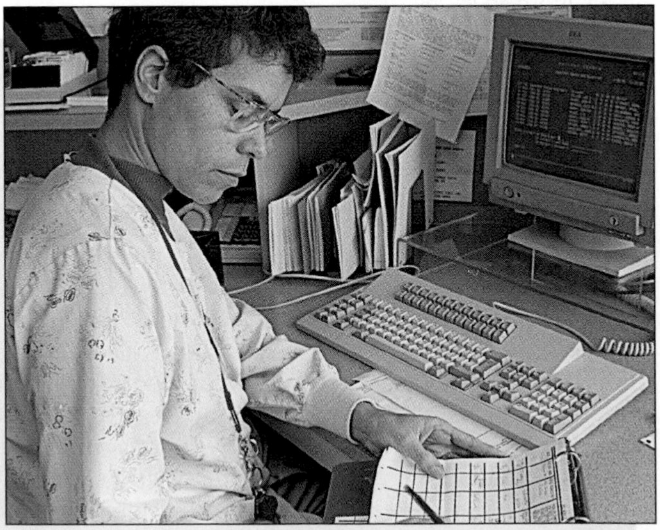

Entry data becomes part of permanent record.

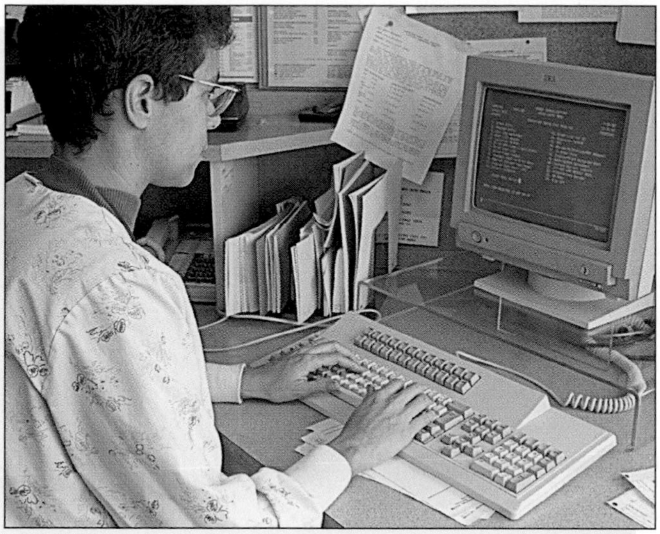

Client data is entered into computer at nurse's station.

sible uses are rapidly expanding. In the very near future, automated speech recognition will allow nurses to document into the computer by just speaking. Also, handwriting recognition programs are being tested and will soon be available. This will allow nurses to write, rather than type, information into a book-sized computer. If learning the skills of computer use is viewed as a challenge and the reward is more efficient nursing care and less time spent on paperwork, the learning time will have been well spent.

Bedside E-documentation. Electronic charting is becoming more familiar in hospitals and clinics. Portable bedside and handheld computers have the following advantages:

- Data is entered into the client's chart immediately.
- This method saves nurses' time.

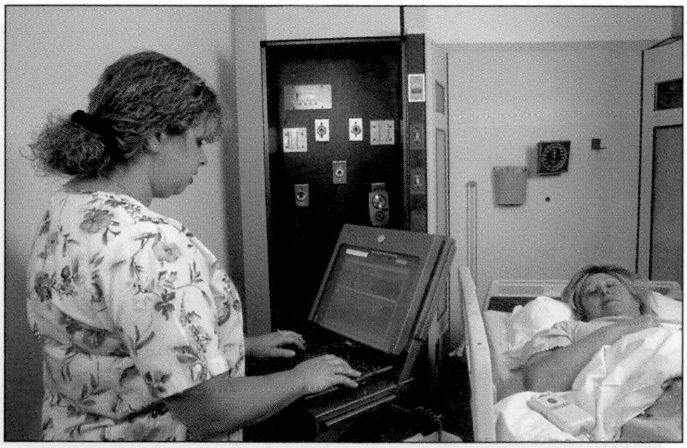

Portable bedside computer unit facilitates client charting.

- Entry may be more accurate, because it is entered immediately after the intervention.
- Charges to the client are automatic.

There are disadvantages to using E-documentation. The computer may not be equipped for narrative charting, and if there is a central data bank, a computer problem could effect obtaining important client information.

At this time there are many issues with E-documentation, but for expediency (especially with the shortage of nurses), it will probably become a primary mode of client charting.

Minimizing Legal Risks of Computer Charting

The American Nurses' Association, the American Medical Record Association, and the Canadian Nurses' Association offer guidelines and strategies for computer safety in charting.

- Your personal password or computer signature should not be given to anyone: neither another nurse on the unit, a float nurse, nor a physician. The hospital issues a short-term password with access to certain records for infrequent users.
- Do not leave a computer terminal unattended after you have logged on. Most computers do have a timing device that shuts down a terminal when it has not been used for a certain time.
- Computer entries are part of the client's permanent record and, as such, cannot be deleted. It is possible, however, to correct an error before the material has been stored. If the entry has already been moved to storage, handle the error by marking the entry "mistaken entry," add correct information, and date and initial the entry. If you record information in the wrong chart, write "mistaken entry," add "wrong chart," and sign off.
- Once information about a client is stored, it is difficult to delete accidentally. Do check that stored records have back-up files. This is an important safety check. If you inadvertently delete a part of the permanent record (this is difficult to do, since the computer always asks if you are sure), type an explanation into the computer file with date, time, and your initials. Submit an explanation in writing to your supervisor.
- Do not leave computer information about a client displayed on a monitor where others have access to it. Also, do not leave printed files unattended. Keep a log that accounts for every copy of a computerized file that you have generated from the system.
- A positive diagnosis of human immunodeficiency virus (HIV) or hepatitis B virus (HBV) is part of the client's confidential record. Disclosure of this information to

```
CCU-9061
01/04/04   12:49 PM     QAZ$$P     PAGE 001                     MEDICAL CARE PLAN
BRAUN, SALLY                                          F  65  CC13  SERV    MED
ADM:  01/01/04   MURPHY, PAUL MD                            07:00 AM 01/04/04
CARE COORINDATOR: JANE DAYTON, RN
==============================================================================
ADVANCE DIRECTIVE: N                ACCOM CODE:   **/STD ACCOM-CRIT CARE
DIAGNOSIS:
  DIVERTICULITIS OF COLON 56211
  CLINICAL PATH: EMERGENT COLORECTAL SURGERY
  01-03-04: PERFORATED CECUM; FECAL PERITONITIS; ILEOCOLECTOMY

VITAL SIGNS:
  01/03  VITAL SIGNS, T-P-R/BP, Q2H, (CCAC)

DIET AND FLUID BALANCE;
  01/03  DIET: NPO-EXC-ICE, (CCAC)
  01/03  IV LINE-START D5/.45% NACL, 1000ML W, KCL 20MEQ, CONT TIL DC'D,
         125ML/HR (31/125GTT) *CONT TIL DC'D*, <01/03/99-..>, (CCAC)
  01/03  CONNECT NG TUBE, SUCTION LOW CONTINUOUS, (CCAC)
  01/03  IRRIGATE/INSTILL, NG TUBE, WITH NORM SALINE, 20ML, Q4H, OR PRN,
         <01/03/99-..>, (CCAC)
  01/03  RECORD I 7 O, (CCAC)
  01/03  FOLEY CATH TO GRAVITY DRAINAGE, (CCAC)
  01/04    #2 197 IV LINE- D5/.45% NACL, 1000ML W, KCL 20MEQ, 125ML/HR
           (31/125GTT) *CONT TIL DC'D*, SCHED FOR APPROX 01:10 AM

HYGIENE/ACTIVITY/SAFETY:
  01/03  ACTIVITY, AMBULATE WITH ASSIST, (CCAC)
  01/03  POSTIONING: ELEVATE HD OF BED 30DEG, (CCAC)
  01/04  ACTIVITY, UP IN CHAIR-WITH ASSISTANCE--WHEN EXTUBATED, (CCAC)
OTHER CATEGORIES INCLUDED ARE:
PROCEDURES
MISCELLANEOUS ORDERS
ALLERGIES
```

Client care plan.

```
CCU     -9065
01/04/04        12:50 PM
                NURSING DATA         **PRINT**      3
BED 404B
MATSON, EDWARD
                         01/04/04
09:30AM  RESPIRATORY ASSESSMENT. . . . LUNG
SOUNDS: CLEAR BILAT POST--DENIES
SHORTNESS OF BREATH ON ROOM AIR. (LCC )
09:30AM  MUSCULOSKELETAL ASSSESSMENT. . . .
CIRCULATION: PEDAL PULSE PRESENT
BILATERAL. . . . CIRCULATION: --1+ PEDAL
EDEMA BILATERALLY. (LCC )
09:30AM  CARDIOVASCULAR ASSESSMENT --NO
SALINE LOCK. (LCC )
09:30AM  ABDOMINAL ASSESSMENT. . . .
ABDOMEN: SOFT. . . . BOWEL SOUNDS: PRESENT
         (LCC )
```

Example of nurses' notes documented in computer.

COMMUNITY HOSPITAL

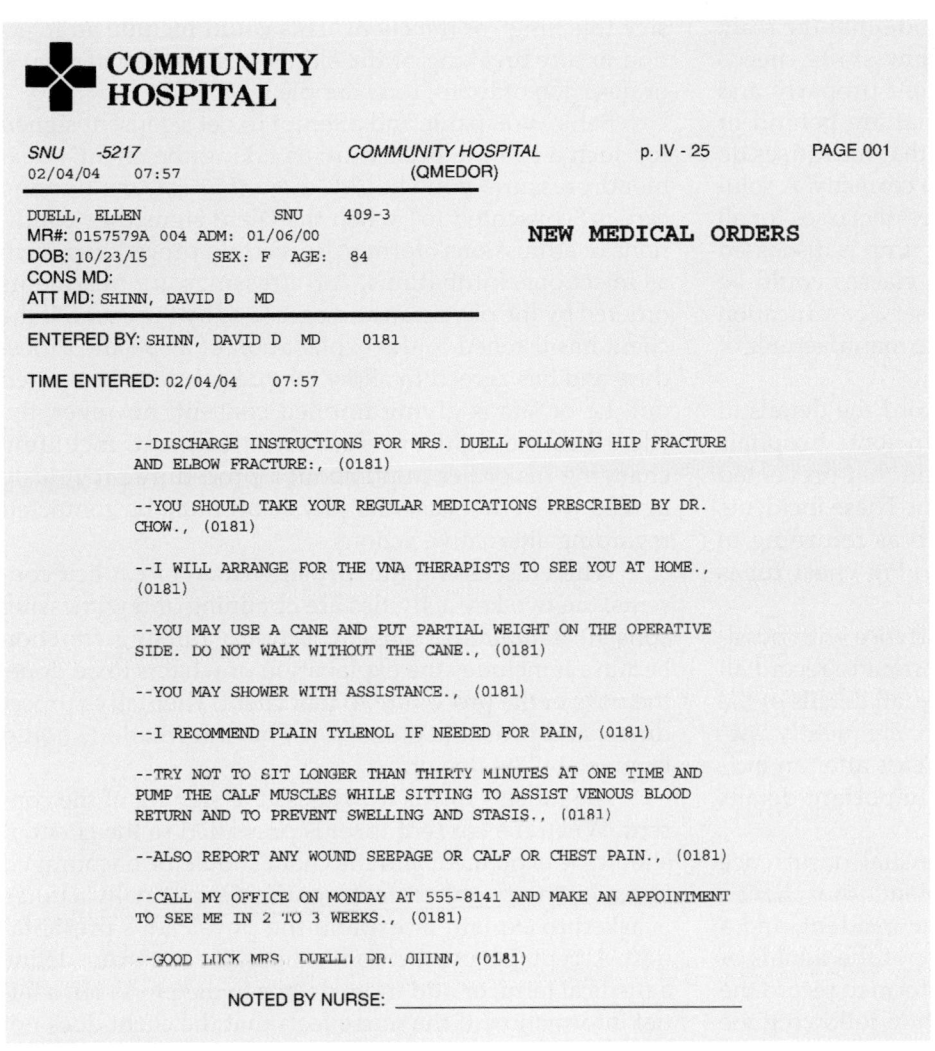

SNU -5217 COMMUNITY HOSPITAL (QMEDOR) p. IV - 25 PAGE 001
02/04/04 07:57

DUELL, ELLEN SNU 409-3
MR#: 0157579A 004 ADM: 01/06/00
DOB: 10/23/15 SEX: F AGE: 84
CONS MD:
ATT MD: SHINN, DAVID D MD

NEW MEDICAL ORDERS

ENTERED BY: SHINN, DAVID D MD 0181

TIME ENTERED: 02/04/04 07:57

--DISCHARGE INSTRUCTIONS FOR MRS. DUELL FOLLOWING HIP FRACTURE AND ELBOW FRACTURE:, (0181)

--YOU SHOULD TAKE YOUR REGULAR MEDICATIONS PRESCRIBED BY DR. CHOW., (0181)

--I WILL ARRANGE FOR THE VNA THERAPISTS TO SEE YOU AT HOME., (0181)

--YOU MAY USE A CANE AND PUT PARTIAL WEIGHT ON THE OPERATIVE SIDE. DO NOT WALK WITHOUT THE CANE., (0181)

--YOU MAY SHOWER WITH ASSISTANCE., (0181)

--I RECOMMEND PLAIN TYLENOL IF NEEDED FOR PAIN, (0181)

--TRY NOT TO SIT LONGER THAN THIRTY MINUTES AT ONE TIME AND PUMP THE CALF MUSCLES WHILE SITTING TO ASSIST VENOUS BLOOD RETURN AND TO PREVENT SWELLING AND STASIS., (0181)

--ALSO REPORT ANY WOUND SEEPAGE OR CALF OR CHEST PAIN., (0181)

--CALL MY OFFICE ON MONDAY AT 555-8141 AND MAKE AN APPOINTMENT TO SEE ME IN 2 TO 3 WEEKS., (0181)

--GOOD LUCK MRS. DUELL! DR. SHINN, (0181)

NOTED BY NURSE: ______________________

Computerized medical orders.

unauthorized people may have legal implications. If the diagnosis is entered as any other diagnosis, take steps to follow your hospital's confidentiality procedures. Check your state's special protocols for treatment of a client's HBV or HIV status.

LEGAL FORMS OF DOCUMENTATION

Unusual Occurrence, Variance, or Incident Report

Unusual occurrence, also called incident report (IR), or unexpected occurrence serves three main purposes: to help document quality of care, to identify areas where in-service education is needed, and to record the details of an incident for possible legal reference.

With some staff nurses, unusual occurrence forms have a poor reputation and, perhaps, with some justification. When something goes wrong and a nurse is told to "make out a report," it is interpreted as a form of punishment.

Although this form should be completed regularly with any unusual occurrence and may, on occasion, be used as a form of reprimand, they are no more nor less than what their title suggests: a report of an incident.

As a tool for documenting quality of care, unusual occurrences inform the quality assurance coordinator and the head nurse of areas of practice on the unit that need improvement. For example, there may be an increase in the number of clients who fell out of bed. Further research may show that because the census is up, the staff is very busy and is forgetting to reposition clients' overbed tables. In their attempts to get water or tissues, for example, more clients are falling out of bed. The solution to the problem may be to speak with the staff regarding the consequences of this action, and as a group find a mutually acceptable way of preventing this type of incident from recurring.

Unusual occurrences also suggest and document the need for in-service education. For example, when an unusual number is written regarding a new piece of equipment, the head nurse may conclude that the staff, especially those on evening and night shifts, needs instruction on operating this equipment properly and effectively. Another example is IVs that are behind or ahead of schedule. This might indicate that the nurses do not know how to regulate the IV pump correctly. A solution to this problem is to conduct a series of classes for all shifts in which the operation of the IV pump is discussed and hands-on practice is given. Such classes could be given by someone in the hospital's in-service education department or by a representative of the manufacturer of the IV pumps.

Unusual occurrences may also record the details of an occurrence for possible legal use. In some hospitals unusual occurrences cover any situation that prevented the client from having a normal recovery. These incidents could include nonnursing actions such as returning to surgery for control of bleeding or having chest tubes inserted for a pneumothorax.

When completing an unusual occurrence with possible legal implications, it is doubly important to record all details of the incident. It is not easy to recall details of the care you gave a client 1 or 2 months ago. Frequently lawsuits are not filed for months or even years after an incident, so it is essential that you record important details promptly.

Information to record on the unusual occurrence includes general details of the incident, the client's response, your action or reaction to the incident, and a list of other personnel who were aware of the details of the incident. Often there is space on the form to record the physician's report of the client's condition following the incident. To fill in the section regarding the physician's report, the nurse later copies the doctor's progress notes from the chart onto the form. At no time is the unusual occurrences given to the physician. This is a written document between the hospital and its insurance carrier, not the physician.

On completion, unusual occurrences are forwarded to the unit manager or head nurse and then to nursing administration. Information from the report of interest to in-service education or quality assurance departments can be obtained at this time. Ultimately, the unusual occurrence is passed along to the hospital's legal department to be retained indefinitely in the event that legal action is later initiated on behalf of the client.

Consent Forms

When an individual enters a hospital, some of his or her basic legal rights are affected. So that these rights are not violated, the client must give permission (consent) for all treatment. If consent is not obtained, the hospital, physician, or nurse may be charged with committing "battery" against the client. Battery, as defined by law, is an "offensive touching" of the client. This could include an injection or any breaking of the skin's surface, use of x-rays, or insertion of tubes, for example.

Before you panic and attempt to get a consent signed for such a routine procedure as taking the client's next blood pressure, you should know that routine nursing care is "consented to" when the client signs the "conditions of admissions" form. Also, certain procedures, such as injections, intubations, and dressings are treatments ordered by the physician and agreed to by the client. If the client has listened to the explanation of a specific procedure and has agreed to allow the procedure to be carried out, he or she is giving implied consent; however, the client has the right to refuse any treatment, including changing his or her mind about a procedure previously agreed to. In that case the physician must be contacted regarding alternative actions.

When discussing the formal written or explicit consents, the two key activities are obtaining and witnessing consent. Obtaining consent is not a nursing function because it includes the explanation of what is to be done, the risks of the procedure to that client, alternative procedures, and probable outcomes. This information should be given by the doctor.

The nurse's role is to witness the signing of the consent. When the consent form is presented to the client, it should be explained, and the client should be encouraged to read it thoroughly before signing. Occasionally a nurse is asked to explain or expand the physician's presentation. Acceptable practice is for the nurse to clarify, define a medical term, or add more details to the physician's initial information. If the nurse feels that the client does not really understand what is going to occur, it is the nurse's responsibility to notify the doctor to give further explanation before the client signs the consent. An easy way to determine what the client understands is to ask him or her to repeat the physician's explanation. Under ordinary circumstances, only one witness to signing the consent is necessary. The witness does not have to be an RN, just someone over the age of 18 years.

There are many rules and regulations governing consents. If you have questions about them, consult the consent manual for your hospital, or a supervisory person. There are several important situations in which more information may be needed. One relates to the client's mental competency. Generally, the client must sign personally, and spouses are unable to sign for the client. Permanent incompetence usually involves legal action to assign someone else as conservator. Temporary incompetence may be the result of hospital treatments, such as drugs or anesthetics. When a narcotic or sedative has been given, at least 4 hours lapsed time is recommended before the client is considered competent to sign a consent. A second situation concerns the client who is a minor. The age of consent varies by state and also according to specific

Unusual occurrence, variance or incident report.

UNUSUAL OCCURRENCE

COMPLETE IMMEDIATELY FOR EVERY INCIDENT AND SEND TO ADMINISTRATOR

HOSPITAL NAME ____________

ADMINISTRATOR:
Please forward to Hospital Attorney

CITY ____________

FOR ADDRESSOGRAPH PLATE ____________

CONFIDENTIAL REPORT OF INCIDENT (NOT A PART OF MEDICAL RECORD)

CLIENT ____________ (LAST NAME) (FIRST NAME) AGE ____ SEX ____ (M OR F) ROOM ____

ADMITTING DIAGNOSIS ____________ DATE OF ADMISSION ____________

ATTENDING PHYSICIAN ____________ DATE OF INCIDENT ____________ TIME ____ M

WERE BED RAILS UP? ____________ WAS SAFETY BELT IN USE? ____________

WAS CLIENT RATIONAL? ____________ HI LO BED POSITION ____________

SEDATIVES ____________ DOSE ____________ TIME ____________

NARCOTICS ____________ DOSE ____________ TIME ____________

GIVEN WITHIN 12 HOURS PREVIOUS TO INCIDENT

TIME DOCTOR WAS CALLED ____ A.M. ____ P.M. TIME RESPONDED ____ A.M. ____ P.M.

(I.E., HOUSE PHYSICIAN-RESIDENT-INTERN-ETC.)

I NOTIFIED DR. ____________ TIME ____ M BY ____________

NURSE'S ACCOUNT OF THE INCIDENT (INCLUDE EXACT LOCATION)

LIST PERSONS FAMILIAR WITH DETAILS OF INCIDENT - AND OTHER CLIENTS IN THE SAME ROOM

NAME ____________ ADDRESS ____________

NAME ____________ ADDRESS ____________

NAME ____________ ADDRESS ____________

HISTORY OF INCIDENT AS RELATED BY CLIENT ____________

DATE OF REPORT ____________

COMMUNITY HOSPITAL

Client Information

AUTHORIZATION FOR AND CONSENT TO SURGERY, ADMINISTRATION OF ANESTHETICS, SPECIAL DIAGNOSTIC OR THERAPEUTIC PROCEDURES

Date ____________ Time ____________

Your admitting physician is ____________, M.D.

Your surgeon is ____________, M.D.

1. The hospital staff and facilities assist your physicians and surgeons in the performance of various surgical operations and other diagnostic and therapeutic procedures. These surgical operations and special diagnostic or therapeutic procedures all may involve calculated risks of complications, injury or even death, from both known and unknown causes and no warranty or guarantee has been made as to result or cure. Except in a case of emergency or exceptional circumstances, these operations and procedures are not performed upon clients unless and until the client has had an opportunity to discuss them with his/her physician. Each client has the right to consent to or to refuse any proposed operation or special procedure (based upon the description or explanation received).
2. Your physicians and surgeons have determined that the operations or special procedures listed below may be beneficial in the diagnosis or treatment of your condition. Upon your authorization and consent, the operations or special procedures will be performed by your physicians and surgeons and their staff. The persons in attendance for the purpose of administering anesthesia or performing other specialized professional services, such as radiology, pathology and the like, are not the agents, servants or employees of the hospital or your physician or surgeon, but are independent contractors performing specialized services on your behalf and, as such, are your agents, servants, or employees. Any tissue or member severed in any operation will be disposed of in the discretion of the pathologist, except ____________ and those body parts specified as donor organs.
3. Your signature opposite the operations or special procedures listed below constitutes your acknowledgement (a) that you have read and agreed to the foregoing, (b) that the operations or special procedures have been adequately explained to you by your attending physicians or surgeons and that you have all of the information that you desire, and (c) that you authorize and consent to the performance of the operations or special procedures.

Operation or Procedure

Signature ____________ Client

Signature ____________ Witness

(If client is a minor or unable to sign, complete the following): Client is a minor, is unable to sign because

Father ____________ Guardian ____________

Mother ____________ Other person and relationship ____________

Consent form.

situations, such as emancipation (being away from the family and self-supporting) and the type of medical problem (reportable diseases or pregnancy). An associated problem may arise when deciding who can legally sign for a minor.

REPORTING

A shift-to-shift report should be given not only from the Kardex but from the client care plan. There is no need to review particular procedures for such activities as dressing changes, when they are outlined on the care plan. A simple statement to the effect that the procedure is listed on the care plan is all that is necessary. This decreases both time and repetition of information.

To avoid confusion from shift to shift, specific times for treatments and for activities of daily living (ADLs) are indicated. For example, it is noted on the care plan that the client prefers his bath before 8 A.M. to avoid having to ask him every day when he wants his bath. This consistency promotes a feeling of confidence in the nursing staff and alleviates fear.

Intrashift Reports Reporting your observations and interventions to other health team members is as essential as documenting them on the client's chart. Intrashift reports are usually verbal reports relayed to team members, team leaders, or charge nurses to keep them informed of changes in the client's conditions. Examples of findings that need to be communicated to other health team members include significant changes in vital signs, unusual responses to treatments, medications, or changes in the client's physical or emotional condition.

Intershift Reports Intershift reports disseminate client information between shifts. It may be accomplished through a verbal report or by tape recording the information. The intershift report should include the following data: client's name, room number, physician's name, diagnosis, and date of surgery when appropriate. In addition, report unusual findings based on the nursing assessment, response to treatments or medications, unusual occurrences, laboratory results, laboratory studies, tests to be completed on the next shift, and any physical or psychosocial problems that exist.

Physician Notification Physicians should be notified whenever treatment or nursing care parameters are exceeded, significant alterations occur in physical assessment findings, or abnormal laboratory findings and test results are obtained.

Before calling the physician, have all data available to allow you to answer questions: current vital signs, laboratory results, when medications were given last, and so on. It is a good idea to have the entire chart with you.

When calling the physician, identify yourself by name, your status (RN or SN), nursing unit, and the client's name. State the exact reason you are calling. Give pertinent and succinct information.

Nurse Manager Written or verbal reports are given to nurse managers, nursing supervisors, or clinical coordinators during each shift. The report includes information on all critically ill clients, those with unusual occurrences or complications, and clients with conditions that are difficult to manage. It is also a good idea to alert the supervisor to problems with families, physicians, or other health disciplines so she or he can assist you in the problem solving.

Client Care Conferences Client care conferences and care plans play an integral role in planning and delivering health care for difficult or unusual problems. The client care conference can focus on developing the care plan or on identifying difficult problems. A conference can be scheduled to plan appropriate interventions and to inform all health team members of the goals for that client's care.

DELEGATING CLIENT CARE

Client care assignments should be based on careful analysis of each client's needs and goals of care. The care plan may be consulted for an effective use of health care team members to their best advantage as well as for the client's welfare. A client requiring extensive sterile dressing changes, frequent assessments, and IV medications is more appropriately assigned to a professional nurse. A client who is convalescing following a stroke and requires mainly bathing and ambulation assistance can usually be assigned to another member of the health team such as a nursing assistant.

In most health care facilities, delegating client care to health care workers has become a financially driven reality. RNs have less responsibility for actual direct care activities such as hygienic care, ambulation, and feeding. However, delegation of these tasks is under the jurisdiction of the RN. To delegate appropriate tasks, the nurse must be familiar with the Nurse Practice Act for RNs and Licensed Vocational Nurses (LVNs) in their state and with the hospital's job descriptions for each level of health care worker. More unlicensed assistive personnel (UAP) are being employed by facilities as a method of cost containment. The goal is still to deliver service to the clients. This classification of health care worker includes many titles, such as patient focused care technician, patient care technician, UAP, and nurse assistant. This level of health care worker provides basic care functions and can be a help to the overburdened nurse. UAPs must receive training in the skills they are to perform before client care is assigned.

The usual tasks assigned to these workers are similar to CNAs with added responsibilities such as changing clean dressings or suctioning long-standing tracheostomies using clean technique. The RN is still responsible for the care that is provided by this category of health care worker. Because of this, many state boards of nursing have developed position statements and guidelines to help RNs delegate activities safely. Guidelines vary among states, so you need to check your state's guidelines. Also, there are general guidelines that should be followed regardless of the state in which you practice. According to the National Council of State Boards of Nursing (NCSBN), tasks that involve nursing judgment and the need to assess the client's responses to the care plan must not be delegated to any other level of worker than an RN. Any nursing intervention that requires independent, specialized nursing knowledge, skill, or judgment can only be delegated to an RN, according to the American Nurses Association. The hospital cannot expand the duties of health care workers beyond those legally allowed by the state. The hospital may, however, decrease their task levels and require certification or credentials for some tasks.

Client Acuity Systems

State law, such as Title 22 of the California Code of Regulation, provides information on how staffing is determined in hospitals within that state. Title 22 states the following regulations regarding staffing.

> There shall be a method for determining staffing requirements based on assessment of client needs. This assessment shall take into consideration at least the following:
>
> 1. The ability of the client to do self-care
> 2. Degree of illness
> 3. Requirements for special nursing activities
> 4. Skill level of personnel required in delivery care
> 5. Placement of the client in the nursing unit
>
> There shall be documentation of the methodology used in making staffing determinations. Such documentation shall be part of the records of the nursing service and be available for review.

Various systems to determine staffing patterns have been used for many years. With the advent of diagnosis-related groups (DRGs), acuity systems for planning staffing needs are being used in many hospitals. This system forms the basis for client care delivery. Categories of nursing care are identified, and a numerical value is assigned to each category. These categories of care include areas such as ADLs, ambulation, client teaching, and medication administration. The numerical values assigned to each category are based on a point scale. For example, using a scale of 1 to 5, a score of 1 indicates the client can function independently in certain tasks; a score of 5 indicates complete dependency on a caregiver for that category.

The scores from all categories are totaled; this score is divided by the number of categories in the acuity system. The final score is designated as the client's acuity level, which is determined for each 8-hour shift. Every nursing unit has a predetermined number of client care hours assigned for each acuity level. For example, a client acuity level of 4.0 on the day shift is allotted 2.8 hours of nursing care for that shift.

After all clients in the nursing unit are assigned an acuity level, the total client care acuity number is used to determine the number of nursing staff required for the next shift. Then, the acuity level of individual clients is used to plan care assignments for the staff. A nurse may be able to safely care for a total acuity of 16. This method seems equitable, since each staff member is assigned to clients based on acuity. Thus, instead of assigning the nursing staff to clients based on room location or number of clients, the acuity level is used to allocate staff resources. Staffing patterns based on the acuity system have been found to be the most practical, equitable, and manageable.

RN Delegation

Delegation is defined as "transferring to a competent individual the authority to perform a selected nursing task in a selected situation." (Source: National Council of State Boards of Nursing). State licensing laws designate that nurses are legally accountable for quality of care and for direct client care. For example,

- RNs decide which tasks to delegate and under what circumstances.
- RNs must know what is safe delegation of nursing care tasks.
- RNs must supervise (monitor and evaluate) outcomes for all delegated tasks.

RNs must know the legal scope of practice of other licensed providers. They must also know competency of licensed and unlicensed personnel as well as the tasks which may be delegated.

- Some states identify tasks that may *not ever* be delegated (such as a sterile dressing to unlicensed personnel).
- RNs may *not* delegate assessment, evaluation, or nursing judgment functions.

RNs and LVNs must check with their own states' laws and regulations to determine which activities may *not* be performed by unlicensed personnel (UAPs).

RN Responsibilities That Cannot Be Delegated

- Data entry into client's charts for all unlicensed personnel to whom tasks are delegated.
- Initial health assessments (only by RN).
- Care plan objectives—checked by RN if completed by LVN.

- Review data obtained by other health care workers.
- Complete referral form for additional client services.
- Receive reports of client conditions and any unexpected findings from delegated activities.
- Identify parameters for which worker is to notify nurse.
- Carry out pain management activities (epidural narcotic analgesia done only by RN).
- Check advanced directives in client's chart.
- Organ donation—RN or LVN responsible for carrying out hospital policies.
- Complete discharge teaching plan.

Parameters of Delegation

Many state boards of nursing have identified the parameters of delegation. Examples of these "Rights of Delegation" are:

Right Task—a task that can be legally delegated to an LVN/LPN, PCT, or UAP. Check the state nurse practice act to determine if the caregiver is trained to perform the task. Judge if the UAP or LVN is competent to perform the task.

Right Circumstances—the LVN, PCT, or UAP understands the elements of the procedure and the RN is assured that the UAP can perform the procedure safely in an appropriate setting. Caregiver is able to collect the right supplies to perform the procedure.

Right Person—the right person (RN or LVN) delegates the right task (legally can be delegated to a UAP) to the right person (legally can perform the task) on the right client (stable with predictable outcomes).

Right Communication—person delegating the task (RN or LVN) has described the task clearly including directions, special steps of the task, and the expected outcomes.

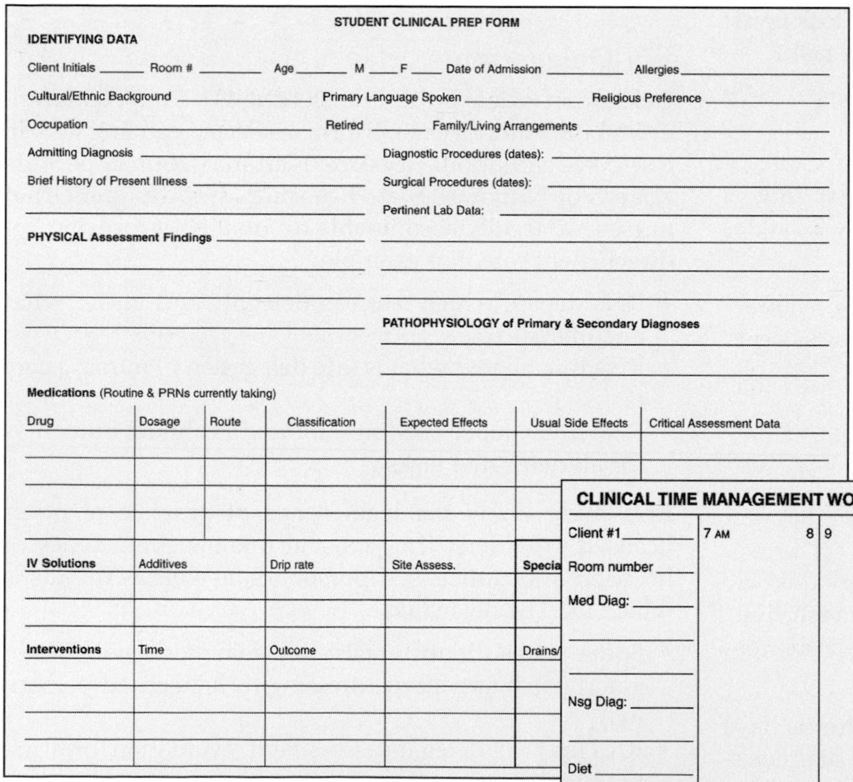

STUDENT CLINICAL PREP FORM

IDENTIFYING DATA

Client Initials ______ Room # ________ Age ________ M ____ F ____ Date of Admission __________ Allergies ____________

Cultural/Ethnic Background ____________ Primary Language Spoken ____________ Religious Preference ____________

Occupation ____________ Retired ________ Family/Living Arrangements ____________

Admitting Diagnosis ____________ Diagnostic Procedures (dates): ____________

Brief History of Present Illness ____________ Surgical Procedures (dates): ____________

Pertinent Lab Data: ____________

PHYSICAL Assessment Findings ____________

PATHOPHYSIOLOGY of Primary & Secondary Diagnoses ____________

Medications (Routine & PRNs currently taking)

Drug	Dosage	Route	Classification	Expected Effects	Usual Side Effects	Critical Assessment Data

IV Solutions	Additives	Drip rate	Site Assess.	Specia[l]

Interventions	Time	Outcome		Drains/

Clinical Prep Form.

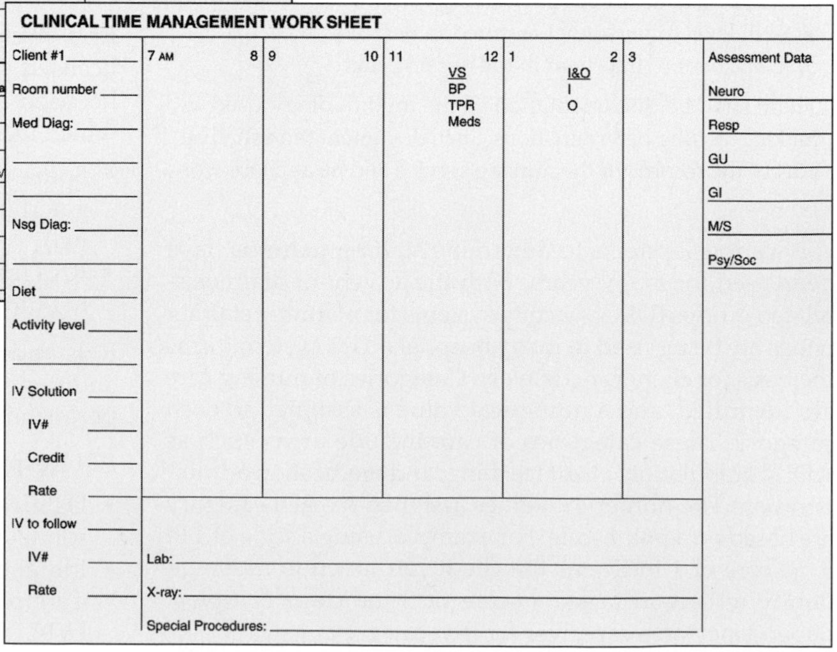

CLINICAL TIME MANAGEMENT WORK SHEET

Client #1 ______	7 AM 8	9 10	11 12	1 2	3	Assessment Data
Room number ______			VS BP TPR Meds	I&O I O		Neuro
Med Diag: ______						Resp
						GU
						GI
Nsg Diag: ______						M/S
						Psy/Soc
Diet ______						
Activity level ______						
IV Solution ______						
IV# ______						
Credit ______						
Rate ______						
IV to follow ______						
IV# ______	Lab: ____________					
Rate ______	X-ray: ____________					
	Special Procedures: ____________					

Time Management Work Sheet.

Right Supervisor—the RN or LVN delegating the activity answers the UAP's questions and

Source: Smith, S. F. (2001). *Sandra Smith's Review of Nursing for NCLEX-RN.* Englewood Cliffs, NJ: Prentice Hall Health.

STUDENT CLINICAL PLANNING

Preclinical Planning To assist students with client care planning prior to clinical experience, many nursing programs have developed a Student Clinical Prep Form. This form helps focus the student's attention on the information necessary to ensure safe nursing practice. Most forms of this type, such as the example provided, include information related to the client's biographical data, history and physical assessment findings, medical diagnosis, nursing diagnosis, medications including IVs, and nursing interventions.

Time Management

Implementing time management techniques during your student clinical experience will assist you not only in organizing client care management but also in completing your assignment efficiently. Some techniques you may find helpful are listed below.

- Design a time management work sheet you can follow.
- Collect the appropriate information you will require to identify client care tasks (e.g., RN report, care plan, Kardex, medication record).
- Identify specific tasks of client care and the time frame needed for completion.
- Prioritize tasks included in the client care plan.
- Make an initial visit to assess your client's status.
- Revise priorities based on your assessment.
- Plan nursing interventions in sequence.
- Group and sequence client care activities for completion in the same time frame. Allocate sufficient time to complete client assignment.
- Consider client's wishes for completing nonpriority tasks, such as bathing and grooming.
- Identify tasks for which you will require assistance.
- Notify the appropriate colleague to assist you (e.g., ambulating your client).
- Identify and collect necessary equipment for task completion.
- Complete client care, implementing the prioritized plan of action (POA) using your time management work sheet.
- Allocate appropriate time to interact with your client.
- Mark off tasks on the time management sheet as you complete them, leaving a record for giving verbal report to the nurse when leaving the unit.
- Document client care as soon as feasible, or at least every 2 hours, on the appropriate records.

Word Roots, Prefixes and Suffixes

a, an: without, not
ab: away from
abd: abdominal
ac: before meals
acro: extreme, top, extremity
acu: sharp
ad, al: to, toward
adeno: gland
adip: fat
ad lib: freely, as desired
-aemia: blood
aero: air, gas
-aesthesia: sensation
-al: action, process
alg: pain
-algesia, algia: suffering pain
amb: ambulatory, walking
amput: cut away, cut off
amt: amount
ante: before
anti: against, opposed to
ap, apo: away from
arteri: artery
arthro: joint
-ase: enzyme
aur: ear
auto: self
bacill: rod
bacter: rod
bi: double, two
bid: twice each day
bile: bile
bio: life
blephar: eyelid
BM: bowel movement
brachi: arm
brady: slow
BRP: bathroom privileges
bucc: check
c̄: with
cale: stone
capit: head
cardi, cardio: heart
cathart: cleansing
caud: tail
cav: hollow
cec: blind
cent: hundred

(continues)

Word Roots, Prefixes and Suffixes *(continued)*

-chem, -chemo: chemical
chole: bile
chron: time
cid: kill
-cide: causing death
cili: eyelid
circum: ring, circle
C/O: complains of
cogni: know
colo: colon
com, con: with, together
crani: skull
cry: cold
cut: skin
cyan: blue
cyst: bladder
cyt: cell
-cyte: cell
DC: discontinue
demi: half
dent: tooth
derm: skin
di, dis: double, separation, reversal
dors: back
dur: hard
dy: two
-dynia: pain
dys: abnormal, different
e, ec: out from
-ectomy: cutting out
em, en: in, within
embol: inserted a wedge
-emesis: vomiting
-emia: blood
emulsi: milk out, exhaust
endo: within
entero: intestinal
epi: upon
erythro: red
eso: inside
-esthesia: sensation
et: and
eu: normal
ex: out of
exo: the outside, beyond
fore: before, in front of
gastro: stomach
genito: genital
-gens, -gent: clan, tribe
glosso: relating to the tongue
glyco: sugar
-gram: tracing, a mark
-graphy: a writing, a record
grav: heavy
gyn: woman
H_2O: water
hemi: half
hemo: blood
hepar, hepatio: liver
hisc: open
homeo: same, similar
homo: same, similar
HS: bedtime
hydro: related to water
hyper: above, beyond
hypo: under, below
I&O: intake and output
-iasis: condition, pathologic state
ile, ilo: intestine
in: not, within, into
in: inch
incont: incontinent
infra: below
inter: between
intra: inside
is: equal
isch, ischo: hold, suppress
-ism: condition, theory
itis: inflammation
juxta: next to
latero: side
lb or #: pound
leuko: white
lip: fat
lith: stone
ly: loose, dissolve
-lysis: dissolving, decomposition
macro: large, big
mal: bad, poor
mamm: breast
man: hand
mani: mental alterations
megaly: large
meta: beyond
metra, metro: uterus
micro: small
ne: young, new
nebul: cloud, mist
necr, necro: dead
neo: new
neuro: nerve
noct: night
-nos, -noso: disease
npo: nothing by mouth
nucleo: nucleus
nutri: nourish
ob: against
oc: occlude
olig: few, small
oob: out of bed
opisth: backward
-opsy: examination
opthalm: eye
-orrhaphy: repair of
ortho: straight, normal
-osis: process, condition
oss, ost: bone

-ostomy: creation of an opening
-otomy: opening into
palp: touch, feel
pan: all, entire
para: beside, beyond
paten, patent: spreading open
path: disease, sickness
pc: after meals
ped, pedi, pedo: foot
ped, pedo: child
pen: lack of
per: by, through
peri: around
pet: tend toward
pha: speak
phag: eat
phleb: vein
phon: sound
phot: light
phthi: waste away
-phylaxis: protection
-plasm: to mold
-plasty: formed or repaired by plastic surgery
platy: broad, flat
-plegia: paralysis
pleur: rib
plur: more
pne: breathing
-pnea: respiration, respiratory condition
pneumo: air, gas, lung
post: after, behind
pre: before
prn: whenever necessary
pro: before
pruri: itch
pseud, pseudo: false
psych: the soul, mind
-ptosis: a lowered position of an organ
pulmo: lung
pur: pus
pyo: pus
pyro: fire
qd: every day
qh: every hour
qid: four times each day
qs: as much as required
q2h: every 2 hours
q3h: every 3 hours
q4h: every 4 hours
ren: kidneys
retro: backwards
-rhage, -rhagia: hemorrhage, excessive flow or discharge
s̄: without
-sclerosis: dryness, hardness
-scopy: to see
sedat: soothed, calm
semi: half
sens: sense
sept: wall off
socio: social
som: sleep
spiro: breathe
stasis: stoppage, slowing
stat: immediately
steat: fat
sub, sup: under, below
super: over, above, higher
syn: with, together
tach: fast
therapeu: serve, treatment
therm: heat
thromb: clot
tid: three times each day
-tomy: cut
top: place
toxic: poisonous
troch: wheel
trop: turn, change
-trophy: nutrition, nourishment
ultra: beyond, excessively
un: one
-uria: a specific condition of, or related to urine
vaso: vessel
veno: vein
ventro: abdomen
°: degree

MANAGEMENT GUIDELINES

Each state legislates a Nurse Practice Act for RNs and LVN/LPNs. Health care facilities are responsible for establishing and implementing policies and procedures that conform to their state's regulations. Verify the regulations and role parameters for each health care worker in your facility.

Delegation of Responsibilities

- The RN must complete the initial assessment, develop the client care plan, and develop the teaching plan. These activities cannot be delegated to any other health care team worker.
- Tasks which require judgment or the need to assess outcomes of the task may not be delegated to other health care team workers.
- Before delegating any client care to an LVN/LPN, review the Nurse Practice Act and the facility policies to determine which tasks may be delegated and which may not be delegated.
- Before delegating client care to Unlicensed Assistive Personnel (UAP), review the board of nursing (BRN) guidelines in your state as well as the facility policy governing their skill level. Remember the facility may decrease the level of responsibility for health care workers, but they cannot exceed the skill level outlined in Practice Acts or the BRN guidelines.
- When delegating client care, refer to the Kardex as well as the client care plan or critical pathway to determine the level of care required in order to appropriately assign the health care workers. Assign clients according to care needs, not location of rooms.
- Charting basic care modalities such as hygienic care can be assigned to CNAs and UAPs when flow sheets are used. These caregivers cannot be assigned to complete narrative charting.
- LVNs/LPNs are responsible for charting using all formats: narrative, flow sheets, problem-oriented, and computer-assisted charting.
- RNs are responsible for the data entry in charts for all unlicensed health care workers.

Information Flow

- Information relative to client care is provided both in written and verbal communication. Written information is found on the Kardex card, client care plan or critical pathway. Verbal communication consists of the shift and team report and directions provided to the workers throughout the shift. When assigning client care to health care workers, the RN uses both communication processes. When directions are given to health care workers, the Kardex card and care plan or pathway is the foundation for client information. This information is provided in a verbal report at the beginning of the shift. Two-way communication is encouraged throughout the shift, as client's needs change or new orders are written for client care.
- Verbal reports can be given individually or to a group of health care workers. It depends on the type of health care delivery system that is employed in the facility.
- Specific information regarding client care must be provided to each health care worker. This information includes: activity level, vital sign times, diet, ability to perform ADLs, procedures or treatments that will be conducted during the shift and the approximate time this will occur, specimens needing collection, as well as any safety precautions necessary, visual and hearing deficits, dentures, and specific tasks to be completed by the health care worker.
- Communicate with all members of the health care team through the multidisciplinary care plan. Ensure they follow the plan of care and document to the care plan.
- After receiving report from unlicensed health care workers, the RN must complete the charting except where flow sheets are used.
- The RN is responsible for the accuracy of all documentation, including information contained in the flow sheet; therefore, it should be checked each shift.
- Licensed nursing staff should review the documentation for the past 24 hours before beginning nursing care. The chart will provide details on the client's status including assessment findings, response to pain medication, and client's response to treatments. Continuity of care can be provided when client information is known.
- The RN should review necessary data, obtained by reading the chart, with the unlicensed personnel to provide for continuity of care.
- RNs should review principles of charting with personnel if guidelines for charting are not being followed. The records are permanent and reflect the care provided the client while hospitalized. The chart can be subpoenaed if a lawsuit is filed.

CRITICAL THINKING STRATEGIES

SCENARIO 1

Determine appropriate delegation of client activities for a staff team on a unit. This scenario does not take into consideration the acuity of the client, only the nursing tasks needed for the day shift. Each facility and state have differing policies regarding personnel; therefore, these policies need to be reviewed before this activity is completed.

The team consists of 1 RN, 1 LVN/LPN and 1 UAP. There are 10 clients and 2 unoccupied beds. There is a charge nurse and ward clerk assigned to the nursing unit. There are two other teams and these three teams make up the medical–surgical nursing unit.

RM 601A	Mr. Rodrigues, 98, admitted 24 hours earlier Diagnosis: congestive heart failure Bed rest, bed bath and assistance with oral hygiene, daily weight, I&O Vital signs q 4 hrs., low sodium diet, restricted fluids to 1500mL IV #2 1000mL D5/.2NS with 20mEq KCL at 50mL/hr—800mL remaining IV medications: Lasix 40mEq BID Oral medications: Digoxin 0.25mg daily, vitamin supplement
RM 601B	Mr. Jamisen, 69, admitted this A.M. Diagnosis: coronary artery disease Surgery at 10 A.M.: triple by-pass—will go to ICU following surgery Preop checklist and client teaching has been completed Preop meds on call to OR IV medications IV #1 1000mL D5/.2NS at 75mL/hr
RM 602A	Mrs. Jones, 59, admitted 2 days ago Diagnosis: cholelithiasis Surgery 2 days ago: Laparoscopic cholecystectomy Ambulate ad lib, self care Oral medications for pain IV discontinued at 8 A.M. To be discharged today with discharge teaching
RM 602B	Not occupied
RM 603A	Mrs. Henderson, 38, admitted yesterday Diagnosis: metastatic cancer to the brain CAT scan scheduled for 12 noon IV #2 1000mL D5W with 20 mEq KCL at 50mL/hr Assist with ADLs Vital signs and neuro checks q 4 hrs, I&O Oral medications for pain
RM 603B	Miss Johnson, 70, admitted 3 days ago Diagnosis: pancreatic cancer with metastasis to the lungs Chair TID, and ambulate to bathroom Vital signs q 4 hrs Spirometry q 4 hrs with RT Deep breathing and coughing exercises q 4 hrs Nasotracheal suction PRN IV #5 1000mL D5W at 50 mL/hr PCA pump for pain medication Chemotherapy IV daily
RM 604A	Mr. Scott, 64, admitted this AM Diagnosis: benign prostatic hypertrophy Surgery for TURP at 1 P.M.—to return to the nursing unit Needs preop teaching and a surgical checklist completed
RM 604B	Mr. Jackson, 37, admitted last night Diagnosis: torn ACL Surgery this A.M. at 7:30—will return to unit by 10:30 A.M. CPM ordered postop
RM 605A	Mrs. Price, 89, admitted 1 week ago Diagnosis: terminal heart failure, semi-comatose Complete ADLs, keep comfortable, turn q 2 hrs Vital signs q 8 hrs, I&O Foley catheter to drainage IV #8 D5/.45 NS with 40mEq KCL at KO rate
RM 605B	Not occupied

RM 606A Mrs. Fellipe, 28, admitted last evening
Diagnosis: gastroenteritis for past 4 days
Ambulate to bathroom, chair as tolerated
Independent in ADLs
Vital signs q 4 hrs, NPO, I&O
IV #3 1000mL NS with 40mEq KCL at 125mL/hr

RM 606B Mrs. Blake, 48, admitted yesterday
Diagnosis: sickle cell crisis
Bed rest until pain subsides
Vital signs q 4 hrs, I&O, diet as tolerated
Oral medications: folic acid, nonsteroidal antiinflammatory drug
Narcotic analgesic medication for pain
IV #3 1000mL D5/.2NS with 40mEq KCL at 125mL/hr

1. Determine the appropriate staff assignment for this client roster. What information do you need to complete this assignment?
2. How would you as team leader make client assignments for each individual staff member?
3. How do the theory of delegation and the facility/state policies of delegation impact on your assignment?
4. What additional factors would you need to consider in making these assignments?

SCENARIO 2

You are assigned to provide nursing care for Mr. Fred Smith, 39 years of age. He is admitted to the hospital for severe dehydration due to the effects of chemotherapy. On your initial rounds at 7:30 A.M., you find him sleeping. His respirations are labored and stertorous. His color is ashen, eyes sunken, and skin dry. At 8 A.M. you enter the room and find him awake. He complains of being very thirsty and wants a glass of water. He cannot tolerate oral fluids and is receiving IV fluids with KCl added because of his nausea and vomiting on admission the day before. After taking his vital signs (T: 100.6; P: 100; R: 32) you give him his bath and make his bed. You notice he has reddened areas over his coccyx and on his elbows and heels, each area about the size of a quarter. His skin is dry and peeling. Drainage from his Foley catheter is a dark amber color with a very strong odor. You measure the urine at 8 A.M. The total is 75 mL. The last output was measured at 6 A.M.

1. How would you chart the information obtained from the simulated situation? What would be appropriate forms to use?
2. What assessment information (that you just charted) would require nursing interventions?
3. If you were assigning this client to a team member, who would be most appropriate—RN, LVN/LPN, or CNA?

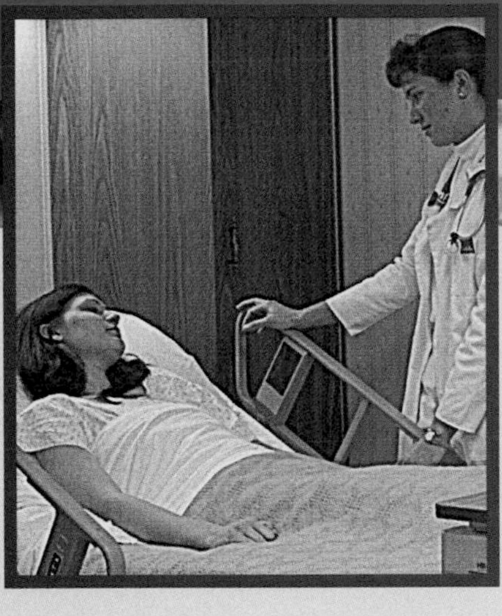

Communication and Nurse–Client Relationship

THEORETICAL CONCEPTS

UNIT ONE: **Therapeutic Communication** 74
- Introducing Yourself to a Client 75
- Beginning a Client Interaction 75
- Assessing Cultural Preferences 75
- Assessing Spiritual Issues 76
- Assisting a Client to Describe Personal Experiences 76
- Encouraging a Client to Express Needs, Feelings, and Thoughts 77
- Using Communication to Increase a Client's Sense of Self-Worth 77

UNIT TWO: **Nurse–Client Relationship** 79
- Initiating a Nurse–Client Relationship 80
- Facilitating a Nurse–Client Relationship 80
- Terminating a Nurse–Client Relationship 80

GERONTOLOGIC CONSIDERATIONS 81

MANAGEMENT GUIDELINES 82

CRITICAL THINKING STRATEGIES 83

LEARNING OBJECTIVES

- Define the term *communication.*
- Explain why communication is an important concept in nursing.
- Describe what is meant by the communication process.
- Discuss four factors that affect communication.
- List five examples of therapeutic communication.
- List five examples of blocks to communication.
- Explain why multicultural health care is important and discuss the term *cultural diversity.*
- List three components of a cultural sensitivity assessment.
- List two questions that would elicit information about the client's spiritual issues.
- Demonstrate the steps for beginning a client interaction.
- Explain why it is therapeutic to encourage the client to express feelings and thoughts.
- State two nursing diagnoses that relate to communication with clients.
- Describe the phases of a nurse–client relationship.
- List three components for maintaining a nurse–client relationship.
- Describe the rationale for discussing termination at the beginning of the relationship.

TERMINOLOGY

Acceptance: favorable reception; basic acknowledgment.

Agitation: excessive restlessness and increased mental and especially physical activity.

Anxiety: a state of uneasiness and distress; diffuse apprehension.

Apprehension: a fearful or uneasy anticipation of the future; dread.

Assistance: aiding, helping, or giving support.

Attitude: a state of mind or feeling with regard to some matter; disposition.

Behavior: the actions or reactions of persons under specified circumstances.

Clarify: to make clear or easier to understand.

Cliché: stereotyped response; a trite or overused expression or idea.

Cognition: the mental process or faculty by which knowledge is acquired.

Communication: the exchange of thoughts, information, or messages.

Confusion: disorder; jumble; distraction; bewilderment.

Congruence: agreement; conformity.

Consent: to agree; to be of the same mind.

Convey: to communicate or make known; to impart.

Coping mechanism: a means by which to adjust or adapt to disequilibrium; defense mechanism against anxiety.

Counseling: to give support or to provide guidance.

Cultural diversity: differences among people with respect to their values, beliefs, language, customs and general patterns of behavior.

Cultural sensitivity: being aware of and accepting diversity among people.

Depression: a mental state characterized by dejection, lack of hope, and absence of cheerfulness.

Emotion: any strong feeling, as of joy, hate, sorrow, love.

Empathy: ability to readily comprehend the feelings, thoughts, and motives of another person.

Esteem: to consider as of a certain value; regard; respect.

Ethnocentrism: belief in the superiority of one's own ethnic group.

Evaluate: to examine and judge; appraise.

Expression: to manifest or communicate; make known.

Feedback: the return of information to the place of origin.

Helping relationship: an interaction of individuals that sets the climate for movement of the participants toward common goals.

Maladaptive: inability to, or faulty adjustment or adaptation.

Multicultural health care: a consideration of client's varying cultures (including beliefs, values, customs, traditions, language, etc.) when delivering health care.

Noncompliance: failure or refusal to go along with a plan or program.

Nonverbal communication: aspects of communication that are not content (such as body language or gestures) but still convey meaning.

Overdependence: the state of needing or relying on someone or something too much.

Perception: the process of receiving and interrupting sensory impressions.

Rapport: a feeling of mutual trust experienced by persons in a satisfactory relationship.

Refer: to send or direct someone for action or help.

Relationship: an interaction of individuals over a period of time.

Self-esteem: a sense of pride in oneself; self-love.

Social: involvement with communities and other persons.

Spiritual assessment: assessing a client's religious or spiritual beliefs and values.

Support: to lend strength or give assistance to.

Termination: the end of something; a limit or boundary; conclusion or cessation.

Therapeutic: having medicinal or healing properties; a healing agent.

Understanding: to perceive and comprehend the nature and significance of; to know.

Validate: to substantiate or verify.

Verbal communication: the words, content, or information conveyed in the message.

COMMUNICATION

Communication is the process of sending and receiving messages by means of symbols, words, signs, gestures, or other actions. It is a multilevel process consisting of the content, or information, part of the message and the part that defines the meaning of the message. Messages sent and received define the relationship between people. From the point of view of a learned skill, communication is intended to accomplish a defined goal. It is the transmission of facts, feelings, and meaning through the communication process.

The communication process forms one of the primary bases for administering all skills. Without clear communication the nurse cannot assess, administer, or evaluate his or her actions in performing the skill. The principles of therapeutic communication also form a basis for interviewing and counseling skills.

Communication is a vital element in nursing. Everything that occurs within the nurse–client interaction involves some form or mode of communication, whether it includes listening to an upset family member, assisting a client in health teaching, or performing a nursing procedure. Without communication the nurse could not give nursing care.

The communication process includes both verbal and nonverbal expressions and is affected by the intrapersonal framework of the person, the relationship between the participants, and the purpose of the sender. The content of the message and the context also influence the communication process. The manner in which the message is sent and the effect on the receiver also play a role in the eventual outcome of the communication process. As you can see, the communication process can be very complex. As a beginning practitioner, however, the most important factor to remember is that *what* you say and *how* you say it has a very great influence on your client.

One of the most important skills you must master is to be able to talk therapeutically to clients and to be able to listen to them. Nurse–client communication is an intimate process of providing nursing care. In fact, the initial step in the nursing process—assessment—comprises observation, interview, and examination. The interview involves talking and listening to the client. Initially, it may be difficult for you to concentrate on both talking and listening, since you have not yet mastered the basic skills, such as a bed bath or taking vital signs. As you gain experience, however, these skills will become more familiar and you can focus on the communication-interaction process with the client.

Guidelines That Influence Effective Communication

- A person cannot *not* communicate. This idea is basic to communication. We have an inherent need to communicate, whether it be verbal or nonverbal. Even silence is a form of communication.
- There is a content, or informational, value to messages sent and received that explains what the message is about and expresses how the sender regards the receiver.
- The message sent is not necessarily the meaning received.
- Messages contain overt and covert meanings. The sender is aware of the overt, or direct, meaning and may or may not be aware of the hidden, or covert, meaning.
- Communication becomes dysfunctional when a person does not assume responsibility for his or her communication. Dysfunctional communications result from failing to learn to communicate properly and leaving the responsibility for communicating to others.

Learning to talk with clients and listening to them is the beginning of a nurse–client relationship. Some of you come to nursing with many of these basic communication skills already mastered. Others experience shyness, hesitancy, and awkwardness in relating to clients. Try to keep in mind that you are being educated to be a professional person—a nurse—and as such you have a great deal to give to your clients. They will learn to respect your skill, value your presence, and depend on you when they are ill. One of the most rewarding aspects to nursing is experiencing a communication between you and your client. If you do feel shy or hesitant, remember that communication skills can be learned. Begin by practicing or role playing with your classmates until you feel comfortable in the initial phases of a relationship.

All communication between nurse and client should be therapeutic, whether it involves obtaining information for an assessment, interacting with the client during a bed bath, or doing client teaching. The difference between therapeutic communication and a therapeutic relationship is that a relationship has a beginning, middle, and end with specified goals for each phase. Therapeutic communication techniques should be used in all forms of communication.

Guidelines for Communicating with Clients

In establishing nurse–client communication, some basic guidelines should be remembered.

- Accept the client as a valued and worthwhile individual, for this acceptance is a prerequisite for a nurse–client relationship.
- Be aware of the total client, not just his or her physical needs. The client's social, emotional, and spiritual needs are also important.
- Understand your own needs, feelings, and reactions so that they do not interfere with the therapeutic process with the client.
- Be prepared to feel some degree of emotional involvement with your client, evidencing caring and concern for his or her welfare. At the same time, however, it is necessary to maintain objectivity.
- Remember that the nurse–client interaction is a professional one. As such, you as the nurse possess the skills, abilities, and resources to relieve the other person's pain and discomfort and your client seeks comfort and assistance for alleviation of some existing problem.
- A nurse–client relationship does not require a long-term agreement or formal meetings between nurse and client to be effective. You may still meet the objectives of such a relationship in a short clinical experience.
- Take an active role and guide the conversation if the client is overly hesitant. For example, "I'm here to listen to any concerns you might have, Mr. Smith. You were mentioning having trouble understanding. . . ."
- Give broad opening statements and ask open-ended questions to help the client describe what is happening to him or her. Pick up cues and follow through with the subject that the client introduces to provide continuity.
- Use body language to convey empathy, interest, and encouragement to facilitate communication.
- Use silence as a therapeutic tool, as it allows the client to pace and direct his or her own communications. Long periods of silence, however, may increase the client's anxiety level, so use this technique wisely.

THERAPEUTIC COMMUNICATION TECHNIQUES

Communication includes the totality of the human person and reflects what is happening within and outside of us. Body sensations, thoughts, feelings, emotions, ideas, perceptions, judgments, previous experiences, and memories are all part of how and what we communicate. Effective, functional communication only occurs when what is happening within is congruent with what we share with the outside. It is important to be a therapeutic as well as a functional communicator and not to disturb the communication process by using nontherapeutic techniques or blocks to communication.

Therapeutic communication techniques assist the flow of communication and always focus on the client. Nontherapeutic communication techniques block or hinder communication and generally focus on the nurse and meet the nurse's needs. The major therapeutic and nontherapeutic techniques are listed below.

Acknowledgment. Acknowledging the client without inserting your own values or judgments. Acknowledgment may be simple and with or without understanding, verbal or nonverbal.

Example: In the response "I hear what you're saying," the nurse acknowledges a statement without agreeing with it.

Example: "Yes, go on." "Uh huh."

Clarification. Clarifying the client's message. Check out or make clear either the intent or hidden meaning of the message, or determine if the message sent was the message received.

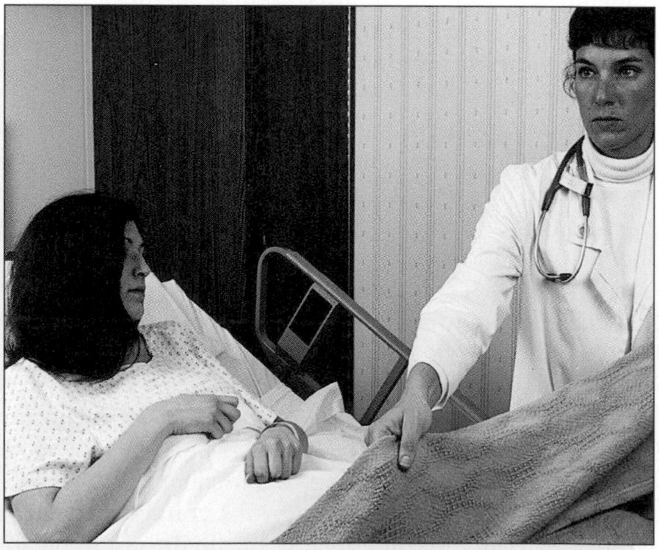

Therapeutic communication implies the nurse is focusing on the client. Here we see an example of nontherapeutic communication.

Example: "I don't understand. Can you say it in a different way."

Example: "Are you saying . . ." (Repeat meaning of client's message.)

Feedback. Using feedback to relay to the client the effect of his or her words. This method helps keep the client on course or alters the course. It involves acknowledging, validating, clarifying, extending, and altering.

Example: "You changed the bag on your colostomy very well."

Example: "When you say that, it makes me feel uncomfortable." (If the client is making personal comments about the nurse.)

Focus. Focusing or refocusing on the client's statement. Pick up on central topics or "cues" given by the client.

Example: "You were telling me how hard it is to talk to your doctor."

Example: "You said the Doppler test tomorrow is frightening."

Incomplete Sentences. Encouraging the client to continue.

Example: "Then your life is . . ."

Listening. Consciously receiving the client's message.

Example: Listening eagerly, actively, responsively, and seriously.

Minimum Verbal Activity. Keeping your own verbalization minimal and letting the client lead the conversation.

Example: "You feel . . .?"
"Go on."

Mutual Fit or Congruence. Creating harmony of verbal and nonverbal messages.

Example: A client is crying, and the nurse says, "I'll sit with you awhile," and puts his or her hand on the client's shoulder.

Example: A client tells the nurse he or she feels fine, but the client's body language indicates that he or she is in pain. "You say you feel fine, but you look like you are in pain."

Nonverbal Encouragement. Using body language to communicate interest, attention, understanding, support, caring, and listening to promote data gathering.

Example: The nurse nods appropriately as the client talks.

Example: The nurse leans forward.

Open-Ended Questions. Asking questions that cannot be answered with a simple "yes" or "no" or "maybe." Generally ask questions requiring an answer of several words to broaden conversational opportunities and to help the client communicate.

Example: "How is your PCA working?" rather than "Is the pain gone?"

Reflection. Identifying and sending back a message acknowledging the feeling or repeating the last few words the client said. (Conveys acceptance and great understanding.)

Example: ". . . distrust your diagnosis?"

Restatement. Repeating the client's statement as encouragement for him or her to continue.

Example: "You said that you can't bear to look at your stoma."

Validation. Verifying the accuracy of the sender's message.

Example: "Yes, it is confusing when so many staff are in the room."

BLOCKS TO COMMUNICATION

Changing the Subject. Introducing new topics inappropriately, a pattern that may indicate anxiety.

Example: The client is crying and discussing his or her fear of surgery when the nurse asks, "How many children do you have?"

False Reassurance. Using clichés, pat answers, "cheery" words, advice, and "comforting" statements in an attempt to reassure the client. Most of what is called "reassurance" is really false reassurance.

Example: "It's going to be all right."

Example: "Don't worry. This pain medication always works."

Giving Advice. Telling the client what to do. Giving your opinion or making decisions for the client implies he or she cannot handle his or her own life decisions and that you are accepting responsibility for him or her.

Example: "If I were you. . . ."

Example: "You should try some alternative treatments."

Incongruence. Sending verbal and nonverbal messages that contradict one another; two or more messages, sent via different levels, seriously contradicting one another. The contradiction may be between the verbal/nonverbal content or time/space content.

Example: "I'd like to talk to you" (but I'm just too busy), said while nurse is turning away from the client.

Assumptions. Making an assumption about the meaning of someone else's behavior that is not validated by the other person.

Example: The nurse finds the suicidal patient smiling and tells the staff he's in a cheerful mood and much better.

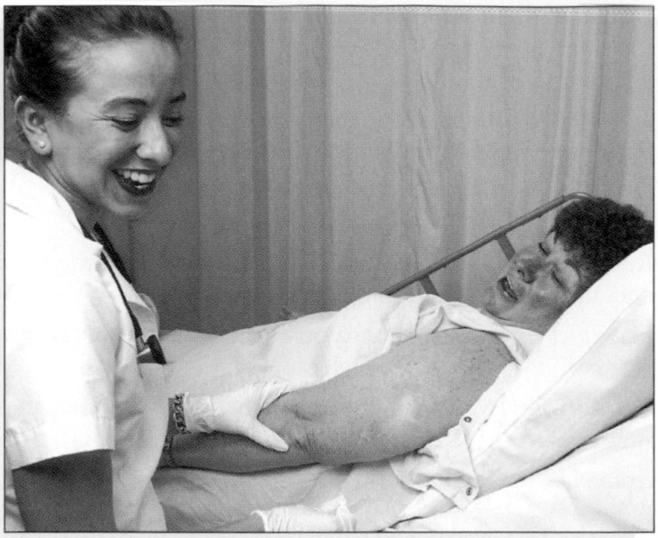

Within the interpersonal framework, nurses share part of who they are with the client.

Invalidation. Ignoring or denying another person's presence, thoughts, or feelings.

Example: Client: "Hi, how are you?" Nurse: "I can't talk now, I'm on my way to lunch."

Overloading. Talking rapidly, changing subjects, and giving more information than can be absorbed at one time.

Example: "I see you're 48 years old and were admitted yesterday. Have you had a physical assessment? Where do you come from?"

Social Response. Responding in a way that focuses attention on the nurse instead of the client.

Example: "This sunshine is good for my roses. I have a beautiful rose garden."

Underloading. Remaining silent and unresponsive, not picking up cues, and failing to give feedback.

Example: Nurse asking, "I hope your pain is better" as he or she smiles and walks away.

Value Judgments. Giving one's own opinion, moralizing or implying one's own values by using words such as *nice*, *good*, *bad*, *right*, *wrong*, *should*, and *ought*.

Example: "I think he's a very good doctor."

Example: "I think it's good that you decided to have the blood transfusion."

MULTICULTURAL HEALTH CARE

As we move into the 21st century, there are demographic shifts occurring that will change the direction of health care. The last census showed that almost 29% of the population is comprised of people of color, and over 12% are of Hispanic or Spanish origin. The total foreign-born population in 1990 was almost 20 million, or 8% of the total population, and 14 million Americans did not speak English. This trend can be expected to increase as the new census statistics are tallied. In fact, those groups that were minority may now be classified as majority.

Because of this change in the United States population demographics, there are emerging barriers to health care for many groups of people. Perhaps the greatest barrier is language and, since communication is an essential component of providing nursing care, it is important to consider under the topic of communication. Other barriers may be living in urban, poor neighborhoods, poor prevention practices such as poor nutrition, as well as beliefs that affect how certain cultural groups understand illness and respond to treatment. Perhaps the greatest barrier for many of these ethnic groups is poverty. Those in the lower socio-economic group have reduced access to health care, including health insurance, availability and location of health facilities, transportation, and so on.

Cultural Competence

It is important for nurses to understand the impact of various cultures on the health care practices if they are to become culturally competent. As more and more people are immigrating to this country, nurses will be faced with cultural diversity problems in administering health care. Cultural diversity implies the range of differences in values, beliefs, customs, folklore, traditions, language, and patterns of behavior for the various cultural groups. For example, people from different cultures define personal space differently. Some may prefer closer personal contact, while others are offended by a person moving into their personal space. The nurse needs to be aware that personal space is related to culture, gender, and group behavior. Because all of these aspects potentially affect how an individual experiences, copes with, and responds to illness, nurses must be aware of these cultural differences.

Cultural Sensitivity

Nurses must become sensitive to people from cultures other than their own, if they are to meet the needs of their clients. People from different cultures may have different beliefs and values about illness and treatment, and different health practices and patterns of behavior. In order to treat the client holistically, the nurses should be aware of these differences and be able to incorporate them into the individual client's plan of care. For example, if a Native American is a client and this person believes in and values shamanic healers, the nurse could formulate a plan that includes a healer visiting the client. This addition to the care plan could occur without interfering with the Western approach in which the primary provider would be a physician.

Cultural Assessment

When completing a total assessment on a client, the individual cultural components that would be important to include are:

- Cultural background and orientation
- Communication patterns (based on culture)
- Nutritional practices
- Family relationships
- Beliefs and perceptions relating to health, illness and treatment modalities
- Values relating to health practices
- Education
- Issues affecting the delivery of health care

Spiritual Assessment

When you are completing a total client assessment, it is important to include a spiritual assessment. This need not be invasive or intrusive. The purpose of such an assessment is to open the channels of communication so that the client will feel comfortable in discussing spiritual issues. If the client experiences no opening from the nurse, he or she may conclude that the nurse does not wish to discuss spirituality; therefore, just asking a few pertinent questions during a general assessment may accomplish the goal of opening communication.

RELATIONSHIP THERAPY

Nurses are given the unique opportunity to share part of who they are with others who have asked directly or indirectly for assistance. It is within this interpersonal framework that the nurse–client relationship begins to develop and take on its individual characteristics.

Both individuals bring into the relationship their thoughts, feelings, sense of self or self-worth, behavior patterns, abilities to adapt and cope, belief systems, and points of view about life and how they interact with it. Within all these complex variables, there is a commonly shared point at which the nurse–client relationship begins.

This relationship may be defined as the interaction between the nurse and a client with shared therapeutic goals and objectives. Characteristics of the relationship include acceptance, honesty, understanding, and empathy of the nurse toward the client who is willingly or unwillingly seeking help. Generally, it is important for the nurse to view the client as a unique individual who is responsible for his or her own feelings, actions, and behaviors and who is an active participant in a health care program. The relationship is more effective if the client shows a willingness to accept responsibility and actively participates in the therapeutic relationship. This is not always possible and the nurse must begin the relationship by accepting the level at which the client is able to participate. This, at times, is a difficult and frustrating process. The goal of relationship therapy is to assist the client to identify and meet his or her own needs. The nurse may assist the client in reaching the goals by demonstrating acceptance so that the client may experience the feeling of being accepted as an individual; by developing mutual trust through consistent, congruent nursing behaviors; by providing corrective emotional experiences to increase self-esteem; and finally by creating a safe, supportive environment. Some degree of emotional involvement and honest, open communication is essential throughout the relationship. The nurse must encourage the client to express his or her feelings, concerns, expectations, fears, and the like within safe limits.

Relationship Principles

Principles underlying a helping relationship include:

- Awareness of the total client, including emotional and physical needs, cultural and spiritual needs.
- Some degree of emotional involvement while maintaining objectivity.
- The setting of appropriate limits and consistency in behavior while caring for the client.
- Open, honest, clear communication.
- Encouragement of the expression of feelings.
- Focus on "here and now."

Dangers to the relationship include overemotional involvement and judgmental attitudes on the part of the nurse and the staff.

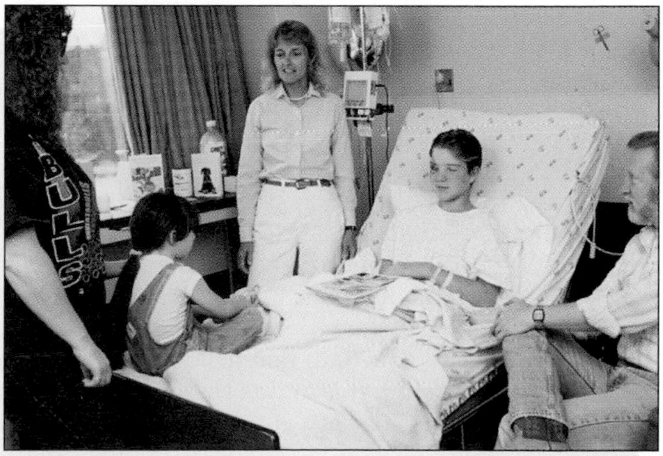

Relationship therapy includes bringing the family together to discuss client care needs.

TABLE 4–1 Religious Diversity Considerations for Client Care

Religious Orientation	Baptism	Death Rituals	Health Crisis	Diet
Adventist	Opposed to infant baptism	No last rites	Communion or baptism may be desirable	No alcohol, coffee, tea, or any narcotic
Baptist	Opposed to infant baptism	Clergy supports and counsels	Some believe in healing and laying on of hands Some sects resist medical help	Condemn alcohol Some do not allow coffee and tea
Islam	No baptism	Prescribed procedures by family for washing body and shrouding after death	No faith healing Ritual washing after prayers every day	Prohibit alcohol and pork
Buddhist	Rites are given after child is mature	Send for Buddhist priest Last rite chanting	Family should request priest to be notified	Alcohol and drugs discouraged; some are vegetarian
Christian Scientist	No baptism	No last rites No autopsy	Deny the existence of health crises Many refuse all medical help, blood transfusions, or drugs	Alcohol, coffee, and tobacco viewed as drugs and not allowed
Episcopalian	Infant baptism mandatory	Last rites not essential for all members	Medical treatment acceptable	Some do not eat meat on Fridays
Jehovah's Witness	No infant baptism	No last rites	Opposed to blood transfusions	Do not eat anything to which blood has been added
Judaism	No baptism but ritual circumcision on eighth day after birth	Ritual washing of body after death	All ill people seek medical care Treatment supersedes dietary restrictions	Orthodox observe kosher dietary laws, which prohibit pork, shellfish, and the eating of meat and milk products at the same time
Methodist	Baptism encouraged	No last rites	Medical treatment acceptable	No restrictions
Mormon	Baptism eight years or older	Baptism for the dead can be done by proxy	Do not prohibit medical treatment, although they believe in divine healing	Do not allow alcohol, caffeine, tobacco, tea, and coffee
Roman Catholic	Infant baptism mandatory	Last rites required	Sacrament of the sick	Most ill people are exempt from fasting

Note: There may exist circumstances that require a court order to supervene religious practices (e.g., a blood transfusion to save the life of a child).

Phases in Nurse–Client Relationship Therapy

There are three phases in a traditional nurse–client relationship.

Initiation, or Orientation, Phase In the initial interaction with the client, you introduce yourself and establish the boundaries of the relationship. It is also the phase in which you identify problems, expectations, and relevant issues (cultural and spiritual) that need to be addressed during the relationship. It is at this stage in the relationship that you would identify any impairments such as hearing, speaking, developmental, or psychological, that must be taken into account so that adjustments in the relationship may be made.

Continuation, or Active Working, Phase This is the phase in which you would develop a working relationship, and in conjunction with meeting the client's needs, begin resolving the client's problems: for example, working with the client to handle his pain; teaching the client to care for a new device, such as a colostomy; or implementing a plan to increase the client's independent functioning.

Termination Phase At this final phase, when the client is soon to be discharged; you would follow the plan that you began when the client was admitted: for example, anticipate problems the client will face when he goes home; complete discharge planning and teaching; deal with client's fears about being on his own after leaving the hospital.

NURSING DIAGNOSES

The following nursing diagnoses may be appropriate to include in a client care plan when the components are related to establishing and maintaining a nurse–client relationship.

NURSING DIAGNOSIS	RELATED FACTORS
Impaired Verbal Communication	Psychologic barrier, inability to speak dominant language, impaired cognitive function, lack of privacy
Powerlessness	Perceived lack of control resulting in dissatisfaction
Impaired Social Interactions	Lack of motivation, anxiety, depression, lack of self-esteem, disorganized thinking, delusions, hallucinations
Social Isolation	Hospitalization, terminal illness
Disturbed Thought Processes	Depression, anxiety, fear of unknown, emotional trauma, unclear communication, negative response from others

- The single most important nursing action to decrease the incidence of hospital-based infections is handwashing. **Remember to wash your hands or use antibacterial gel before and after each and every client contact.**

UNIT 1

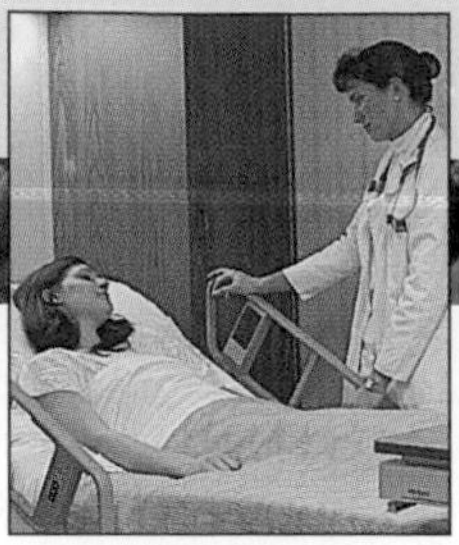

Therapeutic Communication

Nursing Process Data

ASSESSMENT **Data Base**

Determine client's ability to process information at the cognitive level.

Evaluate mental status data to establish baseline for intervention.

Evaluate client's ability to communicate on a verbal level.

Observe what is happening with the client here and now.

Identify client's developmental level so interaction expectations will be realistic.

Assess client's anxiety level because anxiety interferes with communication.

Assess client's cultural background.

PLANNING **Objectives**

To assist client to meet his or her own needs

To assist client to experience the feeling of being accepted

To increase client's self-esteem

To provide a supportive environment for change

To institute therapeutic rather than casual or nongoal-oriented communication

To affect or influence the client's physical, emotional, and social environment

To be sensitive to client's cultural orientation

IMPLEMENTATION **Procedures**

Introducing Yourself to a Client

Beginning a Client Interaction

Assessing Cultural Preferences

Assessing Spiritual Issues

Assisting a Client to Describe Personal Experiences

Encouraging a Client to Express Needs, Feelings, and Thoughts

Using Communication to Increase a Client's Sense of Self-Worth

EVALUATION **Expected Outcomes**

Client develops the ability to assess and meet his or her own needs.

Communication becomes clearer, more explicit, and centered on problem areas.

A supportive environment is created so that the client can reduce the level of anxiety and experience change.

Cultural diversity is accepted by the health care team.

INTRODUCING YOURSELF TO A CLIENT

Procedure

1. Obtain client assignment.
2. Read chart and review physician's orders.
3. Check client care plan.
4. Clarify any questions about client assignment.
5. Proceed to client's room and check room number.
6. Introduce yourself to the client. (Example: "Good morning, Mr. Jones. My name is Miss Barnes. I am a student nurse from the Bellington School of Nursing, and I will be caring for you today.")
7. If the client is blind, introduce yourself as you come into the room: tell exactly what you are doing and when you are leaving. **Rationale:** Blind clients become anxious when they hear someone enter the room who does not speak.
8. Begin to establish a nurse–client relationship using clear, open communication.

BEGINNING A CLIENT INTERACTION

Procedure

1. Following introduction (at which time you call the client by name and tell the client your name), relate purpose of interaction.
2. Tell client specifically what you will be doing in terms of his or her care.
3. Ask if the client understands or has any questions.
4. Encourage client to describe how he or she is feeling at the time (especially focusing on the pain level).
5. Encourage client to participate in his or her care—both verbally and nonverbally.
6. Pay attention to communication as well as the procedure you are administering. **Rationale:** Often, your best database is drawn from observation.
7. Assess nonverbal behavior and determine if it fits (is congruent) with verbal communication, especially when you are evaluating pain level.
8. Complete communication by asking client for feedback.

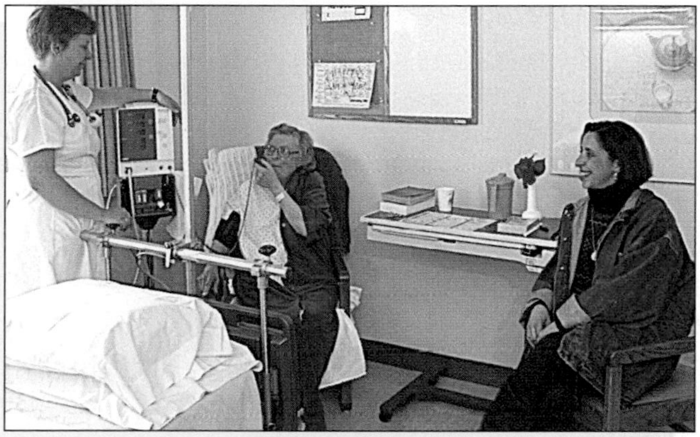

When interacting with a client, the nurse includes friends as an important element in client's support system.

9. Complete interaction by telling client when you will return.
10. Follow through on agreed-upon meeting time to build client trust.

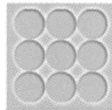

CULTURAL COMPETENCE

One way to become culturally competent is to learn the language that a majority of your clients speak—this will give you insight into the culture and help you recognize individual cultural impediments to the client's receiving health care.

Source: Gaskill, M. (May 6, 2002). Just say the words. *NurseWeek:* Santa Clara, CA.

ASSESSING CULTURAL PREFERENCES

Procedure

1. Review client history related to cultural orientation to determine if adequate information pertaining to cultural preferences is included. **Rationale:** A complete history will detail cultural diversity patterns.
   a. Ethnic heritage and language.

b. Family organization and role of members.
c. Dietary practices and knowledge about nutrition.
d. Education, formal and informal.
e. Health care practices and beliefs.

2. Determine client's perception of illness based on cultural beliefs.
3. Validate verbal and nonverbal communication from client based on cultural understanding. **Rationale:** When the client's cultural background is different from the nurse's, communication problems may result.
4. Consider using an interpreter if communication seems unclear. **Rationale:** An interpreter will facilitate communication and reduce stress on the client.
5. Examine expectations of health care based on the client's cultural influences. **Rationale:** Health care should be congruent with the client's expectations or a positive outcome of treatment may be in jeopardy.

ASSESSING SPIRITUAL ISSUES

Procedure

1. Ask the client relevant questions concerning spiritual issues. **Rationale:** If the nurse never opens this subject, the client will not feel free to discuss spiritual issues.
   a. Do you have a spiritual component in your life?
   b. If so, how will this help you during your illness?
   c. Is there any particular person or spiritual advisor that you would like me to contact for you?
   d. Is there anything that I (as your nurse) can do to support your spiritual beliefs?
2. Are there any spiritual issues that you would like to discuss? If so, let's arrange a time to talk about these issues. **Rationale:** this approach will open communication and notify the client that you are willing to discuss these issues.

EVIDENCE BASED NURSING PRACTICE

Religion Makes a Difference

A nationwide study of 21,000 people from 1987 to 1995 found a seven-year difference in life expectancy between those who never attended religious spiritual services and those who attended more than once a week.

Source: Sullivan, M, MD. (October 1, 2001). *Integrative medicine.* Boulder, CO: Bottom Line Personal.

ASSISTING A CLIENT TO DESCRIBE PERSONAL EXPERIENCES

Procedure

1. Encourage client to describe his or her perceptions and feelings.
2. Focus on communication as well as body reactions.
3. Don't dominate the conversation. **Rationale:** The less you say, the more you encourage spontaneity and verbalization from the client.
4. Assist client to clarify feelings.
5. Maintain an accepting, nonjudgmental attitude. **Rationale:** Making value judgments, even nonverbal ones, negatively affects the nurse–client relationship.
6. Give broad opening statements, and ask open-ended questions. **Rationale:** This open approach enables the client to describe what is happening.

Communicating with the Hearing Impaired

If your client is hearing impaired, it is very important to establish a method of communication (pen and pencil, sign language, speaking loudly and clearly). Other factors to take into consideration when communicating with the hearing impaired are to pay attention to the client's nonverbal cues, decrease background noise such as television, and always face the client when speaking. It is also important to check with the family as to how they communicate with the client. Finally, it may be necessary to contact the appropriate department resource person for this type of disability.

ENCOURAGING A CLIENT TO EXPRESS NEEDS, FEELINGS, AND THOUGHTS

Procedure

1. Focus on feelings rather than superficial topics during interactions.
2. Assist client to identify thoughts and feelings.
3. Pick up on verbal cues, leads, and signals from the client.
4. Convey attitude of acceptance and empathy toward the client. **Rationale:** Being aware of your own feelings and attitudes and separating them from the client's contributes to acceptance.
5. Note what is said as well as what is not said.
6. Assist the client to become aware of differences between behavior, feelings, and thoughts.
7. Give honest, nonjudgmental feedback to the client.

USING COMMUNICATION TO INCREASE A CLIENT'S SENSE OF SELF-WORTH

Procedure

1. Use body language as well as verbal communication to convey empathy. **Rationale:** Sitting down at the client's bedside or not acting as if you are in a hurry encourages communication.
2. Respect the client's need for emotional privacy, but be available to client.
3. Encourage the client to apply the problem-solving approach to different situations.
4. Be nonjudgmental (see example of making judgmental responses.)
5. Mutually identify goals to meet the client's individual needs.
6. Keep all agreements with the client.
7. Become the client's advocate.
8. Give client positive feedback when appropriate.

DOCUMENTATION FOR THERAPEUTIC COMMUNICATION

- Identification of client needs
- Explicit goals of interaction
- Communication patterns of client
- Emotional state of client
- Expressed feelings and thoughts if relevant
- Cultural issues if relevant
- Spiritual issues if relevant

Critical Thinking Application

UNEXPECTED OUTCOMES	CRITICAL THINKING OPTIONS
Therapeutic communication is not achieved.	• Eliminate blocks to communication from interaction style. If a block does occur, recognize it. Move to correct communication by using therapeutic modes of communication. • Evaluate your own process of communication during and after interaction. • If client needs to verbalize and you cannot help him or her do so, contact another nurse or the social worker.
Client's demanding behavior interferes with the therapeutic communication process.	• Do not ignore demands; they will only increase in intensity. • Attempt to determine causal factors of behavior, such as high anxiety level. • Set limits to response patterns when client is demanding. Control own feelings of anger and irritation. • Teach alternative means to getting needs met.
Cultural preferences/issues were not recognized, so communication was hindered.	• Complete a cultural assessment before revising a plan of care. • Bring in a translator to converse with the client to establish baseline communication. • Evaluate values, beliefs, preferences, and expectations related to health care.
Spiritual issues were not discussed until the client asked for a priest or minister.	• At this time, assess the client's spiritual beliefs and ask if there is any way you can assist him/her in this area.

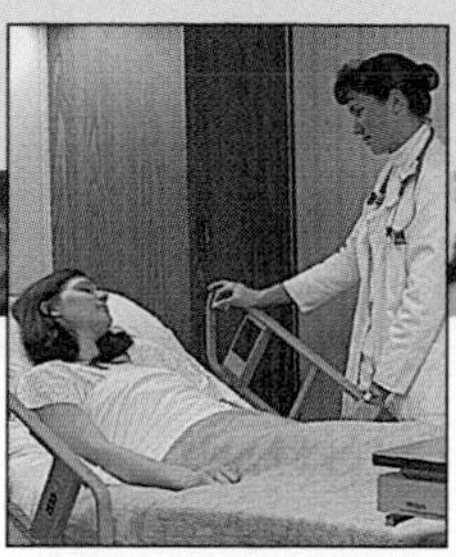

Nurse–Client Relationship

Nursing Process Data

ASSESSMENT *Data Base*

Determine the purpose of establishing a nurse–client relationship.

Consider the overall condition of client to determine if he or she can benefit from a nurse–client relationship.

A specific relationship could feed into secondary gains of anxiety.

An individual with chronic organic brain disorder cannot benefit from a relationship per se.

Identify client expectations of a therapeutic relationship to determine if you can meet these needs.

Examine your own feelings and expectations to evaluate potential effect on such a relationship.

PLANNING *Objectives*

To provide an environment in which client can feel secure enough to alter behavior patterns

To allow a client to experience a positive, satisfying relationship

To enable client to test more adaptive ways to handle anxiety

To provide a climate conducive to raising the client's self-esteem

To allocate enough time to complete planned process of interaction

To terminate relationship successfully

IMPLEMENTATION *Procedures*

Initiating a Nurse–Client Relationship

Facilitating a Nurse–Client Relationship

Terminating a Nurse–Client Relationship

EVALUATION *Expected Outcomes*

Principles of therapeutic communication are used.

Boundaries of professional relationship are maintained.

The appropriate environment for interaction is established.

Termination of the relationship is completed successfully.

INITIATING A NURSE–CLIENT RELATIONSHIP

Procedure

1. Assess client's symptoms and problems, and communicate a willingness to help alleviate these discomforts.
2. Establish a beginning relationship. **Rationale:** Open, honest, congruent communication and consistent behavior help lay the groundwork for trust in a relationship.
3. Establish mutual goals as a basis for the relationship. **Rationale:** Goals mutually set and agreed on are more easily accepted by both parties in the relationship.
4. Be consistent in your behavior; do what you say you will do, and only make promises you are willing to keep. **Rationale:** The most important element is the beginning of trust. Without trust the nurse–client relationship is ineffective.
5. Encourage client's participation in his or her care. **Rationale:** This focus enhances compliance to treatment.

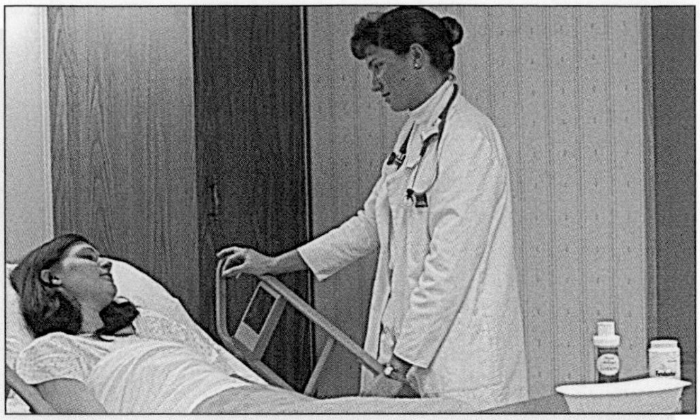

Initiating a relationship is an important component of client care.

6. Approach client in a warm, accepting manner. **Rationale:** The client may interpret a cool, aloof manner as lack of interest.

FACILITATING A NURSE–CLIENT RELATIONSHIP

Procedure

1. Assume the role of facilitator in the relationship.
2. Accept client as having value and worth as an individual. **Rationale:** Basic acceptance is a fundamental prerequisite of a relationship.
3. Provide a safe environment conducive to client's willingness to share.
4. Maintain the relationship on a professional level. **Rationale:** Responding on a professional rather than a social level defines the relationship.
5. Keep interaction reality oriented, that is, in the here and now. **Rationale:** Discussion of past or future experiences does not contribute to a change in behavior now.
6. Listen actively; that is, responding to the client's cues.
7. Use nonverbal communication to support and encourage client.
   a. Recognize meaning and purpose of nonverbal communication, especially in assessing pain.
   b. Keep verbal and nonverbal communication congruent.
8. Focus content and direction of conversation on client's cues, not on social or superficial topics.
9. Interact on client's intellectual, developmental, and emotional level.
10. Focus on "how," "what," "when," "where," and "who" rather than "why." **Rationale:** Asking "why" places the client on the defensive because it requires justification of behavior.
11. Teach client problem solving to correct maladaptive patterns.
12. Assist client to identify, express, and cope with feelings.
13. Help client develop alternative coping mechanisms that are more adaptive.
14. Recognize a high level of anxiety, and assist client to deal with it.

TERMINATING A NURSE–CLIENT RELATIONSHIP

Procedure

1. Work closely with the client in discharge planning and in planning the termination of the relationship from its beginning. **Rationale:** This approach promotes the client's independence and increases his or her sense of self-esteem.
2. Anticipate problems of termination and plan for their resolution. **Rationale:** Saying goodbye is often uncomfortable and difficult for both the client and the nurse.
3. Be aware that the client's behavior may reflect fear that he or she can't cope at home, overdependence, depression, and withdrawal. **Rationale:** Allowing this behavior to be expressed helps the client to work it through.
4. Do not terminate the relationship too abruptly or allow it to persist beyond the client's needs.
5. Complete a satisfactory termination of the relationship. **Rationale:** This enables the client to move on.

DOCUMENTATION FOR NURSE–CLIENT RELATIONSHIP

- Primary goals of nurse–client relationship and identified client needs
- Ongoing process of relationship therapy, including client's expressed feelings, thoughts, and so forth
- Client's behavior and changes in behavior, both positive and negative
- Cues to other team members on how best to relate to this particular client
- Elements of discharge planning

Critical Thinking Application

UNEXPECTED OUTCOMES	CRITICAL THINKING OPTIONS
Client refuses to participate in a nurse–client relationship.	• Comply with client's request, and do not force or impose relationship therapy. • Continue to offer relationship therapy at intervals. • Suggest that another team member attempt to establish a relationship.
Nurse–client relationship frequently degenerates into a social conversation.	• Reevaluate the goals for the relationship, and remind client of terms originally established. • Set firm limits, and continually reexamine progress.
Termination of the nurse–client relationship is not successful.	• Reexamine the process of termination (termination should begin at the beginning of the relationship). • Devote more interaction time to this aspect of the relationship. • Attempt to elicit feelings about termination from the client as well as examining your own feelings.
Nurse–client relationship cannot be established due to cultural differences.	• Allow the client's behavior to be expressed without making value judgments, and assist the client to discuss his or her feelings. • The nurse may make a special effort to understand the cultural preferences of the client. • Consider finding another nurse to establish the relationship—one with a similiar background.

GERONTOLOGIC CONSIDERATIONS

Physical changes that affect communication

- Hearing changes (e.g., presbycusis, tympanic membrane atrophy, and distorted sounds) may make communication difficult. The nurse must speak clearly, loudly, and in view of the client. Use simple sentences, request feedback to validate understanding.
- Visual changes, such as presbyopia, and pupil, cornea, and lens impairment may diminish visualization. The nurse should be aware of eye changes and check that client sees clearly enough to perform required activities.

Psychosocial changes that affect communication

- Relationships change with age. There is a loss of nurturing functions within the family. The nurse may need to perform this function with the elderly.
- Role changes within and outside the family occur—loss of spouse and loss of support systems. Elderly may require more support from caregivers.
- Elderly have fears of physical dependency, chronic illness, and loneliness. Caregiver may need to address these fears and work with client through communication and relationship to reduce them.

MANAGEMENT GUIDELINES

Each state legislates a Nurse Practice Act for RNs and LVN/LPNs. Health care facilities are responsible for establishing and implementing policies and procedures that conform to their state's regulations. Verify the regulations and role parameters for each health care worker in your facility.

Delegation of Responsibilities

- Evaluation of cultural diversity and spiritual issues should be completed by either the RN or LVN, not by a nursing assistant (NA).
- A full history completed by the RN or LVN.
- Care plan objectives relating to communication, spiritual issues and cultural differences completed by the RN or checked by the RN if completed by the LVN.

Information Flow

- All staff caring for the client from a different cultural heritage should be informed of special needs of the client based on cultural diversity theory.
- The unit manager should include special needs of the client based on communication patterns and cultural background when making staff assignments. (For example, is there a nurse from the same cultural background or who speaks the same language as the client who can be assigned to that client's care.)
- Assign a nurse that is comfortable dealing with spiritual issues if the initial assessment indicates the client wishes to discuss these issues.

CRITICAL THINKING STRATEGIES

SCENARIO 1

A 25-year-old male comes to the emergency department. He has a bleeding wound on his arm, and he refuses surgical intervention when told he must remove his clothes and jewelry.

1. What effect would this client response have on the initial nursing plan of care?
2. What is your understanding of this client response? What are some questions you might ask the client?
3. Describe the strategies and goals you would devise to solve this problem.
4. Describe the measures you would implement to resolve this situation.

SCENARIO 2

A client has just been admitted with a diagnosis of rectal cancer. He is scheduled for surgery the next day. When you are completing an assessment and you ask about spiritual beliefs, the client says, "I'm a washed-out Catholic and I don't think I'm going to live, so what's the sense in talking about it?"

1. What would be the consequence of not responding to the client's comments about spiritual beliefs?
2. How would the goals of establishing a nurse–client relationship and assessing spiritual beliefs overlap in this situation?
3. Describe the actions you would take to engage this client in a discussion about these issues.

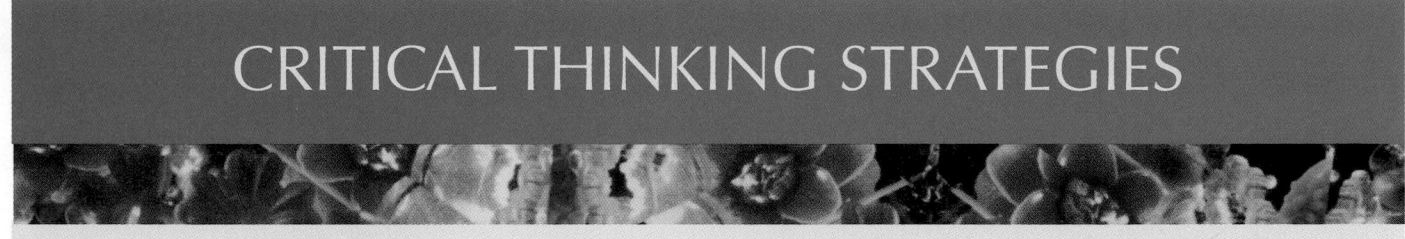

CHAPTER 5

Admission and Discharge

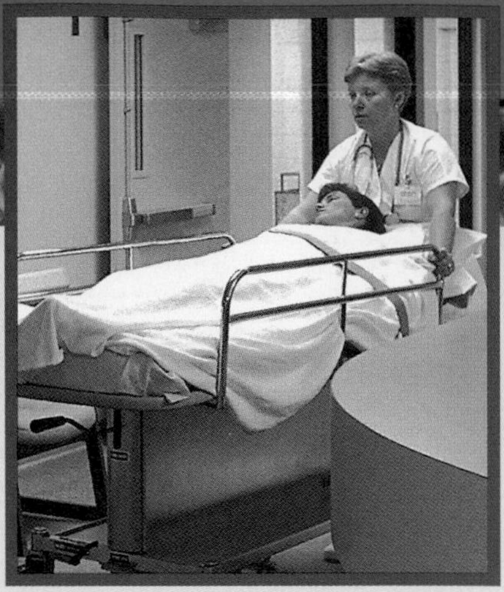

THEORETICAL CONCEPTS

UNIT ONE: **Admission and Transfer** **90**
Admitting a Client 91
Transferring a Client 93

UNIT TWO: **Height and Weight** **95**
Measuring Height and Weight 96

UNIT THREE: **Discharge** **99**
Discharging a Client 100
Discharging a Client Against Medical Advice (AMA) 101

GERONTOLOGIC CONSIDERATIONS 102

MANAGEMENT GUIDELINES 103

CRITICAL THINKING STRATEGIES 104

LEARNING OBJECTIVES

- Explain the steps of admitting a client to a health care unit.
- Describe the client assessment that is completed at the time of admission.
- List the data that are included in charting when admitting a client to the health care environment.
- Describe the disposition process for client's valuables when hospitalized.
- Outline the steps in transferring a client within the hospital environment.
- Describe two suggested solutions for clients who are unable to adapt to the hospital environment.
- Discuss the discharge procedures when a client leaves the health care unit.
- Identify three suggested solutions for a client leaving the hospital against medical advice.
- Describe the expected outcomes for clients being discharged from the hospital, including meeting the criteria in the initial plan of care.
- Complete discharge charting on a client record using specific criteria.
- State what is meant by advanced directives.
- List documents that may be included in the admission record (Patient's Bill of Rights, Advance Directives, DNAR, etc.).

TERMINOLOGY

Adaptation: ability to adjust to a change in environment.
Admit: the process of signing a client into the hospital.
Ambulatory: able to walk, or not confined to bed.
Assessment: critical evaluation of information; the first step in the nursing process.
Behavior: a person's total activity—actions or reactions; especially, conduct that can be observed.
Caring: thoughtful attentiveness accompanied by responsibility.
Client Care Plan: a plan for care of a specific client or one designed especially for one client.
Comfort: to ease physically; relieve, as of pain.
Communication: to convey or transmit knowledge, information, or messages to another person.
Diagnostic test: a test used to determine a diagnosis or to determine the cause and nature of a pathological condition.
Disability: a disabled state or condition; incapacity.
Discharge: to let go, as in discharging a client from the hospital.
Empathy: the vicarious experience of another's situation.
Home care assistance: nursing care given in the client's home.
Identaband: a band, usually worn on a client's wrist, with the client's name and medical record number.
Limitation: the state of being limited or restricted.
Maladaptation: inability to adjust to a change in environment.
Potential: possible but not yet realized.
Procedure: a particular way of accomplishing a desired result.
Stress: a state of agitation that renders the body out of balance.
Supervise: to direct or inspect performance; to oversee.
Termination: the spatial or temporal end of something; a limit or boundary.
Therapeutic: having healing or curative powers.
Transfer: to convey or shift from one person or place to another.
Transition: the process or an instance of changing from one form, state, activity, or place to another.
Verbalize: to express in words (written or spoken).
Volunteer: a person who performs or gives his or her services of his or her own free will.

ADMISSION, TRANSFER, AND DISCHARGE

The admission procedure for clients can be a negative experience if it is impersonal, mechanized, or impolite. It can be a positive step in health care if handled with attention and care. The impressions formed by the clients during the admission process strongly affects their attitude toward their total care. Because the admission procedure can be the initial introduction into the health care system, the nurses should consider this process a key step in client care.

Admission to the Hospital

The process of admitting a client to a health care facility varies in institutions, such as nursing homes, clinics, and hospitals. Regardless of the size or type of facility, the admission process is vitally important to provide safe, adequate care. Because the nurse–client relationship begins with admission, the nurse should have a thorough understanding of the standard admission process.

If a client enters the hospital in an emergency situation, he or she may feel insecure or fearful because he or she has had little time to make plans concerning family, travel, finances, or employment. When a client enters the hospital for elective treatment or surgery, the nurse has a little more time to orient and prepare the client for a hospital stay.

When the client arrives at the hospital, the first contact is usually with the admitting receptionist, who assigns a hospital number and interviews the client. If preadmission material was mailed to the client, it is verified by the receptionist at this time; otherwise, the client must answer questions about age, address, financial or insurance status, next of kin, religion, employment, and consent for treatment. If the client cannot answer these questions due to age or condition, a relative usually gives the information. A parent or guardian must do this for a child.

During admission, clients should be requested to send valuables home with their family. There may be a safe available in the hospital but it is preferable not to leave the valuables in the hospital. Clients also receive identification bracelets or identabands at this time.

If the client brings home medications or herbal supplements to the hospital, they should be placed in the client's medication drawer, or sent home (according to agency policy). No medication is to be kept at the client's bedside unless there is a specific physician's order that it be placed there.

In some circumstances, upon a physician's order, a client's labeled home medication may be stored in the client's medication drawer, and then administered by nursing staff in lieu of a hospital-dispensed preparation. In this case, the medication administration record (MAR) reflects that the client supplies the particular medication and the agency does not charge for dispensing it.

Prehospital laboratory procedures and x-rays should be done before admission for elective procedures. If not, the client should have them done immediately before being taken to his or her room or shortly after admission. These procedures may take several hours. Delays in completing them may result in physical and emotional strain for the client. Delays may also occur in the treatment of the client.

The client is directed or escorted to the clinical laboratory for baseline values on hemoglobin, hematocrit, complete blood count, differential, and serologic screening for sexually transmitted diseases. Depending on the policy of the facility, the client may then proceed to the electrocardiographic laboratory and to radiology to obtain a chest x-ray.

Clients admitted under emergency situations will have their laboratory studies and x-rays completed in the emergency department or after they are admitted to the nursing unit. The same panel of routine admission studies are usually ordered for these clients.

Admission to the Nursing Unit

When admission to the hospital is complete, the client is either directed to the nursing unit or escorted by a volunteer. The client may be met by a staff nurse assigned to admissions for that day or by the nurse who will be working with the client during the client's stay in the hospital. It is at this time that the nurse must begin to assess the client's needs and to plan care. The registered nurse is required to prioritize the client's needs and to initiate the nursing care plan or clinical pathway.

In 1992, the Joint Commission on Accreditation of Healthcare Organizations (JCAHO) required every person admitted to the hospital to have an admission assessment completed or directed by a registered nurse within a specified time frame.

When you meet a client, introduce yourself and any other personnel who will provide care, including the ward clerk. Explain your role and functions to the client. Your initial contact leaves a lasting impression, so try to present information in an uninterrupted, organized, and friendly manner. If other clients are in the room, introduce them to the new client.

Tell the client about mealtimes, visiting hours, telephone use, requests for clergy, recreational and lounge use, physicians' visits, and other schedules. Drugs may *not* be kept at the bedside without a physician's order. Some hospitals have printed booklets describing this information. The more information your client receives, the more control he or she has over the environment.

Help the client become familiar with his or her immediate physical space by showing the location and the operation of the intercom system or call bell, the location of the bathroom, and the operation of the call system inside the bathroom. If electric beds are used, show the client how to operate bed controls. You may also want to show the client how to operate the television and the radio set.

Because clients may not be sure of their role while in the hospital, many hospitals have adopted versions of the American Hospital Association's *Patient's Bill of Rights* (see

Admission Protocol

- Advance directives are made available to clients.
- The client's bill of rights is presented to each client.
- The admission assessment is completed by a registered nurse within a specified time after admission.
- All clients must be clearly identified by a legible identification band.
- When consent forms are required (for surgical procedures), they must be signed by an adult or guardian who is mentally competent. The adult must give voluntary consent, understand the risks and benefits of the treatment, and have the opportunity to ask questions.

Bill of Rights, Chapter 1, pg. 8.). This bill includes the following rights: to obtain information about the client's illness or injury, to refuse medication or treatment, to participate in his or her own care, to know the rationale and risks of the treatment, and to receive courteous care. Make sure your clients understand their rights. Clear, uncomplicated explanations help them adapt to their new environment.

Effective December 1991, *The Patient Self-Determination Act* was implemented. This act requires all Medicare and Medicaid recipient hospitals to provide clients with information regarding their rights to reject medical treatment and write advance directives. The facilities must also provide education to the staff and the community on the law and policies governing these issues.

Once you have completed introductions and the environmental orientation, you may begin the nursing history and assessment to establish baseline data about the client's general condition (see Chapter 11, Physical Assessment).

Client Transfer

Clients are frequently transferred from one unit to another as their condition fluctuates. When a client is moved, all of the records, charts, medications, MAR, belongings, and personal hygiene and special equipment are transferred with him or her. After accompanying the client to a new unit, introduce him or her to new roommates, the charge nurse, and the nurse who will be responsible for his or her care. Assist him or her to get settled in the new room. Make a complete report to the nursing staff using the client care plan or clinical pathway.

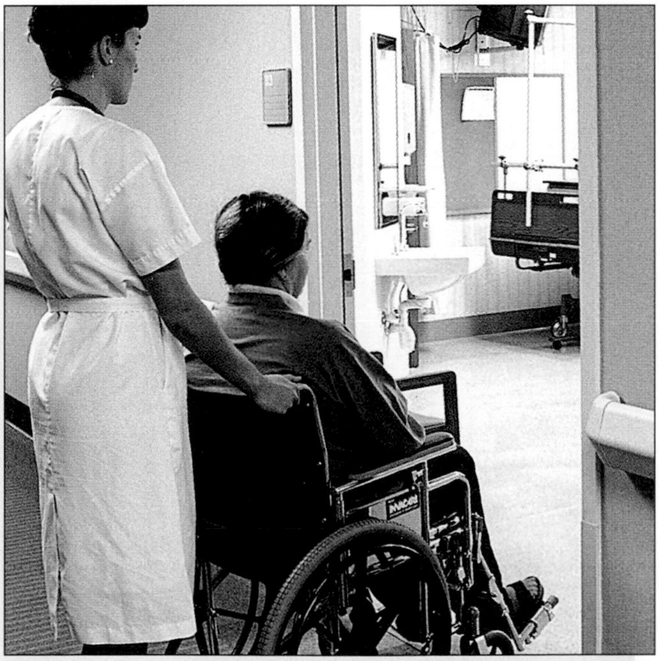

Client may be admitted to the hospital in a wheelchair.

The new unit's receiving nurse has an obligation to *validate* all information relayed about the client, to perform an independent client history and physical assessment and to handle the client's transfer as a "new admission" to the receiving unit. The client also has a right to receive an orientation to the new setting just as that provided in the previous setting.

Sometimes clients are transferred within the same unit (e.g., from a semiprivate to a private room or vice versa) for various reasons. Clients may also be transferred from one unit to *another unit in the agency* as their condition fluctuates. While these transfers are readily accomplished within a short time-frame, communication about such transactions may be delayed and confusion about a client's identification or location may result in the client's injury.

Always ensure that the client's chart reflects the client's *current room number* and that *all* departments participating in the client's care are informed about the client's transfer to a new room number.

A client's transfer to another facility, and sometimes to another unit within the same facility, *closes* the current hospital record just as if it were a "discharge." A new record is established when the client arrives at the new receiving unit (equivalent to a new hospital admission). In these circumstances, a copy of the client's records may or may *not* accompany the client, therefore, a thorough report of the client's pretransfer hospital course and current health status *must* be thoroughly communicated to receiving personnel in order to facilitate continuity of care.

Discharge from the Agency

When a client is discharged from a health care unit, preparations must be made to help the client transfer

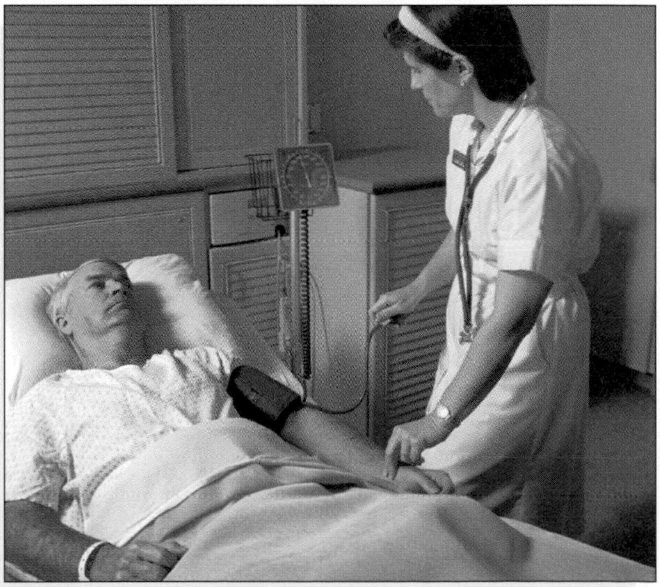

Vital signs are obtained during the admission procedure.

COMMUNITY HOSPITAL

ADMISSION QUESTIONNAIRE

Addressograph Plate

Please answer the following questions so that we may plan your nursing care more efficiently and your discharge when it occurs. If you do not understand a question, please ask for help.

1. What health problem was responsible for admission to the Hospital at this time? ______
2. How long have you had this problem? ______
3. Briefly state what your understanding is of your present problem. ______
4. If known, what are your doctor's plans for you? ______
5. How long do you expect to be in the Hospital? ______
6. List any other health problems you are aware of besides the one hospitalized for: ______
7. List any major health problems, illnesses, surgeries, or hospitalizations you have had in the past, including the date of each:
   ______ (Date)
   ______ (Date)
8. Do you have any food allergies or restrictions?
   If yes, explain ______

Sample of Admission Questionnaire.

COMMUNITY HOSPITAL

BELONGINGS LIST

Patient's Name ______ Date ______

Male ❑ Female ❑

Admitting Unit ______

❑ Discharged

❑ Deceased

❑ Transferred

Unit and Rm # From ______

Unit and Rm # To ______

CLOTHING LIST				MISCELLANEOUS	
PLEASE DESCRIBE	NUMBER	PLEASE DESCRIBE	NUMBER	PLEASE DESCRIBE	NUMBER
Bathrobe		Shoes		Cane	
Belt		Slacks/Shorts		Crutches	
Blouse		Slippers		Dentures ❑ Upper ❑ Lower ❑ Partial	
Coat		Skirts			
Dress		Sweater		Flowers or Plants	
Gloves		Tie		Glasses or Contact Lenses	
Gown		Underclothes		Jewelry Remaining with Pt.	
Hat					
Helmet					
Hose/Socks/Pantihose				Luggage	
Jacket				Radio	
Pajamas				Wallet/Purse	
Shirt				Watch	
				Wig	

Signature of Person Listing ______

Signature of Personnel Handling Belongings ______

Signature of Receiving Personnel or Relative ______

If Relative: Address ______ Phone ______

Belongings List may be completed by nursing staff or security staff.

from a dependent role to a more independent role. Discharge from the hospital can be a welcome relief for the client, but it can also be a time of anxiety and fear. During this transition, the nursing staff can facilitate the process by being aware of individual client needs.

During the discharge process, you must take into consideration the physical, emotional, and psychosocial needs of the client and family. Sometimes hospitalization introduces the client to a lifelong need to chronically adapt to declining physical health and to chronically affiliate with the health care system. The nurse must be empathetic to the client's response at "discharge" and approach the client with all possible options for continued care, educational and financial resources, and any other services to assist the client to adapt to a chronic situation. Your responsibilities for the discharge process include assessing the client's posthospitalization needs and planning with the client and family to meet discharge needs. It is also important to communicate with appropriate health care team members and community agencies. The final responsibilities of the discharge process are to terminate the nurse–client relationship and evaluate the discharge process.

See Chapters 6 (Client Education and Discharge Planning) and 34 (Home Care Management) for further information on discharging clients to home or another health care facility.

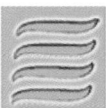

NURSING DIAGNOSES

The following nursing diagnoses may be appropriate to include in a client care plan when the components are related to admission, transfer, and discharge of a client.

NURSING DIAGNOSIS	RELATED FACTORS
Impaired Adjustment	Change in self concept, loss of function, dependence
Anxiety	Actual or perceived threat to self-concept, threat to biologic integrity, unfamiliar environment and treatments, change in socioeconomic status
Anticipatory Grieving	Loss of function, change in lifestyle, lack of social support system, change in social role or economic status
Ineffective Health Maintenance	System impairment, surgery, musculoskeletal impairment, visual disorders, external devices
Social Isolation	Hospitalization, chemical dependency, altered appearance
Fear	Unknown outcome of hospitalization, medical or surgical treatments
Powerlessness	Actual or perceived lack of control over situation, not participant in decision-making regarding treatment, lack of privacy

- The single most important nursing action to decrease the incidence of hospital-based infections is handwashing. **Remember to wash your hands or use antibacterial gel before and after each and every client contact.**

UNIT 1

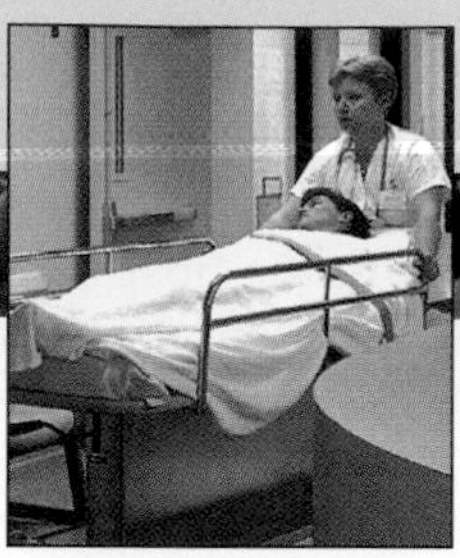

Admission and Transfer

Nursing Process Data

ASSESSMENT *Data Base*

Observe and record client's physical, emotional, and intellectual status.

Observe and record client's ability to adapt to the environment of a hospital unit. Observe for disabilities or limitations.

Identify medications client is currently taking.

Assess the client's level of comfort or discomfort.

Determine client's understanding of his or her disease and its limitations.

Assess condition prior to transfer.

Obtain a thorough report of client's progress and status when receiving from another unit.

PLANNING *Objectives*

To assist client to adapt to hospital environment with minimal distress

To encourage the client to participate in his or her own plan of care

To provide a comfortable and aesthetically pleasing environment for the client

To provide the client with some control over his or her immediate environment

To provide the client with an opportunity to verbalize his or her feelings about hospitalization

To facilitate transfer if required

To facilitate safe and individualized continuity of care

IMPLEMENTATION *Procedures*

Admitting a Client

Transferring a Client

EVALUATION *Expected Outcomes*

Client adapts to hospital environment.

Client participates in his or her own plan of care.

Client exercises some degree of control over his or her environment.

Client accepts transfer to new unit.

Clients individual needs are accommodated.

ADMITTING A CLIENT

Equipment

Admission kit for personal hygiene or individual hygiene articles; hospital gown

Thermometer

Blood pressure cuff and stethoscope

Urine container, if specimen needed

Kardex card, client care plan, or clinical pathway

Client's chart

Addressograph labeled containers for client's dentures, etc.

Agency nursing history and assessment form

Procedure

1. Introduce yourself to the client and family and begin to establish a therapeutic nurse–patient relationship.
2. Orient client to hospital room and introduce the client and family to staff and to roommate if present. **Rationale:** Reduces anxiety about hospital stay.
3. Check physician's orders for treatments to be instituted immediately. **Rationale:** This prevents delay of treatments that could affect client's condition.
4. Explain equipment and hospital routines. Check that identa-band is placed on client's wrist. Place allergy band on wrist as needed.
5. Assist client to don hospital gown.
6. Complete a general nursing assessment.
7. Obtain client's health history and physical assessment. **Rationale:** Complete history provides total picture of client's condition and problems.

Obtaining a Nursing History

- Past medical history or health problems, including those for which client was not hospitalized
- Signs and symptoms of current problems according to client's perceptions
- Assessment of health status (include lifestyle, habits)
- Diet and nutrition, hydration status, elimination, exercise, habits (i.e., smoking, drinking), sleep patterns, cognitive function
- Relationships and social support systems; emergency contacts
- Values, beliefs, religious or spiritual practices
- History of allergies, (drugs and foods) and restrictions
- Medication history—use and allergies
- Risk factors for health—weight, smoking habit, age, general health, and so on
- Client's knowledge of illness (understanding of present illness) and expectations of care
- Risk analysis for discharge (ability to manage self-care at home)
- Special data base for elderly client: level of independence, ability to complete activities of daily living (ADLs), side effects of medications, history of recent loss of loved one, management of chronic conditions

8. Obtain the client's weight and height.
9. Obtain urine specimen if needed and take vital signs.
10. Inform laboratory that client is available for chest x-ray and routine blood work if not obtained earlier.
11. Initiate client's care plan or clinical pathway; Identify client's problem areas and needs. Identify clients at risk for falls and post a head-of-bed (HOB) alert for any identified risk.
12. Notify physician that the client has been admitted, and obtain orders if policy permits.
13. Reassess client's level of comfort and ability to adapt to hospitalization.
14. Complete client teaching for all unfamiliar procedures or interventions.
15. Fill out Kardex card and client care plan.
16. Document information on appropriate forms in chart.

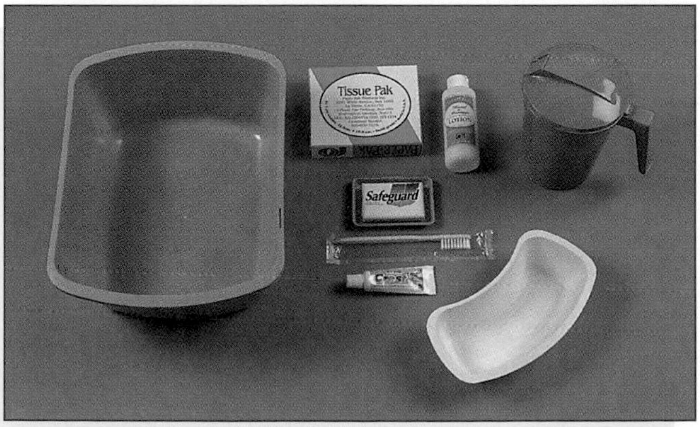

The admission kit usually contains basic personal hygiene items.

COMMUNITY HOSPITAL

NURSING HISTORY / ASSESSMENT

White areas may be completed by patient / family.
Shaded areas must be completed by nurse / N.A.

CONFIDENTIAL INFORMATION

PATIENT'S NAME

INFORMATION PROVIDED BY ☐ Patient ☐ Family ☐ Friend ☐ Unable to Obtain

DATE OF ADMISSION | TIME OF ADMISSION

ROUTE OF ADMISSION ☐ Ambulatory ☐ Wheelchair ☐ Stretcher

ORIENTATION TO UNIT ☐ Floor Brochure ☐ Channel 50 / 52 ☐ Call Light ☐ Bed Control ☐ Emergency Light ☐ Telephone ☐ Visiting hr ☐ Mealtime

HEALTH PERCEPTION / HEALTH MANAGEMENT PATTERN

DESCRIBE YOUR USUAL STATE OF HEALTH ☐ Excellent ☐ Good ☐ Fair ☐ Poor

WHY ARE YOU BEING ADMITTED TO THE HOSPITAL?

Please list any medical problems or previous surgeries below. Include pacemakers, artificial joints, or diabetes.

PROBLEM / SURGERY	DATE

IMMUNIZATIONS ☐ Influenza ☐ Pneumonia

☐ Pacemaker ☐ Artificial Joint ☐ Diabetes

MEDICATIONS – List medications, including aspirin, laxatives, birth control pills, cough medicines, vitamins, herbal supplements, non-prescriptions, all prescriptions.

NAME	DOSE	FREQUENCY	LAST DOSE

DISBURSEMENT OF VALUABLES ☐ Patient ☐ Home ☐ Security

VALUABLES KEPT BY PATIENT

VITAL SIGNS

STATED WEIGHT Kg	ACTUAL WEIGHT Kg	STATED HEIGHT cm	ACTUAL HEIGHT cm
BP	Temp. °C	PULSE	RESPIRATION

ADVANCE DIRECTIVE INFORMATION

Do you have an Advance Directive? (Also may be called a Living Will) ☐ Yes ☐ No

If so, is it on file at this facility. ☐ Yes ☐ No

If not, will you bring / send a copy? ☐ Yes ☐ No

If you do not have an Advance Directive, do you want one? ☐ Yes ☐ No ☐ Not Sure

Do you want help with this? ☐ Yes ☐ No

☐ See Progress Note for additional comments. Date & Time:

Are you an Organ Donor? ☐ Yes ☐ No

If necessary, would you consent to a blood transfusion? ☐ Yes ☐ No

ALLERGIES

NAME (Drug or Other)	DESCRIBE REACTION

Latex Rubber ☐ Yes ☐ No ☐ Unknown

Shellfish ☐ Yes ☐ No ☐ Unknown

X-Ray Dye ☐ Yes ☐ No ☐ Unknown

EDUCATIC

WHAT DO YOU KNOW ABOUT

DO YOU WANT INFORMATION ILLNESS, TREATMENT, OR ME

WHAT INFORMATION WOULD

DO YOU UNDERSTAND WHAT BEEN TOLD SO FAR?

IS THERE A CULTURAL OR LA ☐ No ☐ Yes Exp

Interpreter Name

Phone #

CONFIDENTIAL INFORMATION

DISCHARGE PLANNING NEEDS

COMMUNITY AGENCIES CURRENTLY USED ☐ Home Health ☐ Meals on Wheels ☐ Assistance Program ☐ Other

WHO IS AVAILABLE TO HELP YOU WHEN YOU RETURN HOME?

DO YOU ANTICIPATE ANY PROBLEM CARING FOR YOURSELF WHEN YOU RETURN HOME? ☐ No ☐ Yes Explain:

EMERGENCY CONTACTS

NAME	RELATIONSHIP	TELEPHONE #

Areas within BOLD lines may contain information written elsewhere on the chart. If that is i... please indicate where the information may be found (Example: "See ODSU Form")

1229-1 (1/01)

Nursing History/Assessment Form (a)

COMMUNITY HOSPITAL

NURSING HISTORY / ASSESSMENT

White areas may be completed by patient / family.
Shaded areas must be completed by nurse / N.A.

CONFIDENTIAL INFORMATION

ACTIVITY / EXERCISE PATTERN

PHYSICAL LIMITATIONS

Hearing	☐ Yes	☐ No
Sight	☐ Yes	☐ No
Speech	☐ Yes	☐ No
Mobility	☐ Yes	☐ No

FUNCTIONAL ABILITY LEVEL
0 = Self Care
1 = Requires equipment
2 = Requires supervision or assistance
3 = Requires equipment & supervision / assistance
4 = Total care required

___ Feeding ___ Dressing
___ Bathing ___ Bed Mobility
___ Ambulating ___ Toileting

PHYSICAL AIDS	HOSPITAL	HOME	N/A
Glasses	☐	☐	☐
Contacts	☐	☐	☐
Hearing Aid	☐	☐	☐
Dentures	☐	☐	☐
Partial	☐	☐	☐
Complete	☐	☐	☐
Cane	☐	☐	☐
Walker	☐	☐	☐
Wheelchair	☐	☐	☐
Prosthesis	☐	☐	☐
______	☐	☐	☐
______	☐	☐	☐

GENERAL SAFETY
High Risk for Fall (HRFF)
Any one indicator checked indicates HRFF

History of Falls	☐
Impaired Mobility	☐
Impaired Cognition	☐
Sensory Deficit	☐
Incontinence or Urgency	☐
Age over 75	☐
Any other reason for which the health card team judges the patient to be at risk	☐

Central Line ☐ Yes ☐ No Type ______ Dialysis Access ______

PAIN MANAGEMENT (Cognitive—Perceptual Pattern)

Have you experienced any discomfort / pain in the past 24 hours? ☐ Yes ☐ No
If yes, how did you treat this pain? ______

Was the treatment of pain / discomfort effective? ☐ Yes ☐ No

ELIMINATION PATTERN

Last Bowel Movement ______
Normal Bowel Pattern ☐ Yes ☐ No ______
Regular ☐ Yes ☐ No ______
Laxatives / Enemas ☐ Yes ☐ No ______
Problems Urinating ☐ Yes ☐ No ______

ROLE / RELATIONSHIP-SEXUALITY / REPRODUCTIVE PATTERN

Do you have any emotional, family, or home concerns that need to be addressed during this hospitalization? ☐ Yes ☐ No

Possibly pregnant? ☐ Yes ☐ No Last Period ______ Do you feel safe in home? ☐ Yes ☐ No

Comments:

VALUE / BELIEF PATTERN

Do you have any special request with regard to your religious beliefs while you are in the hospital? ☐ Yes ☐ No

Comments:

NUTRITION / METABOLIC PATTERN

Special Diet at Home ☐ Yes ☐ No Specify ______

Food Allergies ☐ Yes ☐ No Specify ______

NUTRITION SCREEN

READ THE QUESTIONS BELOW. CIRCLE THE NUMBER IN THE YES COLUMN FOR THOSE THAT APPLY TO YOU.	NO	YES
Without wanting to, have you lost 10 pounds or more within the last 6 months?	0	1
Do you have a pressure sore or non-healing / infected wound?	0	1
Have you had daily nausea, vomiting, or diarrhea lasting more than 5 days?	0	1
Has your food intake declined within the past 3 months due to chewing / swallowing problems?	0	1
Have you been hospitalized for an illness or a surgery for more than 7 consecutive days within the past 3 months?	0	1
Total the nutritional score (all "yes" answers) and enter in the computer. **At nutrition risk** = any "yes" answer. (Score 1–5)	TOTAL:	

Do you have any concerns that have not been discussed? ☐ No ☐ Yes Please explain below:

RN SIGNATURE	DATE	TIME

1229-2 (1/01)

CONFIDENTIAL INFORMATION

Nursing History/Assessment Form (b)

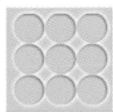

CULTURAL COMPETENCE

The American health care system emphasizes medical science and care, informed consent, self-care, advance directives, and risk management. In contrast, clients of other cultures may prefer to rely on faith in God, beliefs, hope, and acceptance of fate as their primary coping mechanisms. A medical interpreter's assistance may be sought to help bridge these two sets of values and to help the client understand the hospitalization experience. The nurse should be aware of different cultural responses to Western protocols. For example: Chinese-Americans believe the number 4 is unlucky because it sounds like the Chinese word for death; if possible, do not assign 4 as a room number.

TRANSFERRING A CLIENT

Equipment

Wheelchair or gurney
Warm covering for gurney
Client's records, chart, and client care plan
Medications and MAR
Personal hygiene equipment
Special equipment (e.g., sheepskin)
Personal belongings
Valuables receipt

Procedure

1. Obtain physician's order if needed. **Rationale:** Physicians order client transfers from and to critical care unit. They do not always order transfers within departments.
2. Contact admitting office to arrange for transfer.
3. Communicate with transfer unit to determine the best time for moving the client.
4. Inform and talk to client of impending transfer. **Rationale:** Discussing the rationale for transfer and eliciting the client's feelings facilitate adjustment to the transfer unit.
5. Gather equipment, belongings, and records.
6. Wash hands. **Rationale:** This prevents transfer of microorganisms to new unit.
7. Obtain necessary staff assistance for smooth transfer.
8. Transfer client to wheelchair or gurney unless client is remaining in bed for the transfer. Use protective belts, if necessary.
9. Cover client to provide warmth and to avoid exposure during transfer.
10. Notify head nurse when you arrive on the new unit.
11. Introduce and acquaint client with new roommates.
12. Introduce client to new staff, especially the nurse who will be caring for the client that day.
13. Give a complete report to staff, using the client care plan or clinical pathway and Kardex. Give information concerning individualized care needs, client problems, progress, when next medications or treatments are due. If necessary, give phone report to receiving nurse. **Rationale:** Complete communication maintains continuity of care after transfer.
14. Notify physician when client's transfer is completed.
15. Notify the switchboard and admitting office when transfer is completed. A written transfer slip must be sent to the appropriate departments.
16. Notify dietary department, x-ray, and the laboratory if tests were scheduled or results pending.
17. Determine that valuables receipt is either with client or on chart.

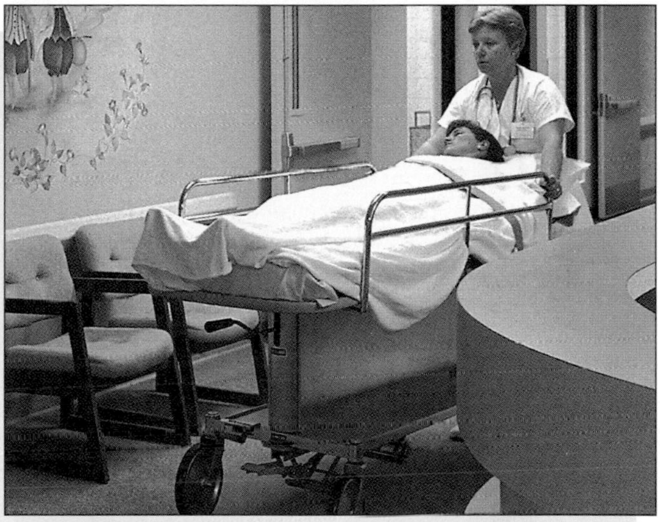

Clients may be admitted or transferred on a gurney

CLINICAL ALERT

When a client is moved to another bed or room *within the same unit,* make certain the room/bed number is changed on the client's chart, MAR, and all other documents at the time the client is transferred.

DOCUMENTATION FOR ADMITTING AND TRANSFERRING

- Admission procedures
- Adaptation to hospitalization
- Client history and admission assessment data: height, weight, vital signs, physical assessment findings
- Laboratory specimens obtained and sent
- Types of x-rays
- Transfer, time of arrival to new unit, method of transfer, and condition of the client
- Posted alerts regarding client's special needs (e.g., risk for falls)
- Inventory of client's valuables and home medications

Critical Thinking Application

UNEXPECTED OUTCOMES	CRITICAL THINKING OPTIONS
Client is unable to adapt to hospital environment.	• Assess physiologic and emotional basis for maladaptation. Request consultation with nurse manager, client advocate, physician.
Client resists transfer; appears anxious.	• Allow client an opportunity to ventilate feelings. • If possible, allow some choice (room, bed, number of roommates) in new unit.
Following transfer, client's personal belongings are lost.	• Return to previous unit and check with staff. • Ascertain that belongings were in fact at the hospital. • Check the clothing list for actual articles brought to hospital.

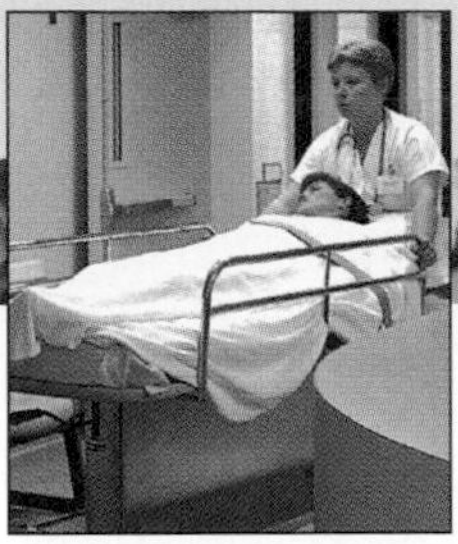

UNIT 2

Height and Weight

Nursing Process Data

ASSESSMENT Data Base
Check the need for daily or weekly body weight measurements.

Determine appropriate method for obtaining client's weight (bedside scale, bed scale).

Determine ability to stand for height measurement.

PLANNING Objectives
To establish baseline data to check against total body fluid balance

To identify excess or deficits of fluid balance

To establish baseline data for diagnostic tests that involve dye and radioactive material injections

To determine drug dosage

To determine nutritional status in relation to body requirements (see Chapter 19)

IMPLEMENTATION Procedures
Measuring Height and Weight

EVALUATION Expected Outcomes
Client's weight, depending on status, disease state and therapy, shows expected losses, gains, or stabilization.

Weight is obtained and recorded as ordered by the physician.

Height is obtained and recorded on admission form.

MEASURING HEIGHT AND WEIGHT

Equipment

Balance beam scale (for clients who are able to stand without assistance)

Bed scale (for clients who are confined to bed or who are unable to stand) or

Bed scale (built into the bed)

Floor scale (for clients in wheelchairs) with height bar

Paper towel

Preparation

1. Weigh client in the morning before breakfast.
2. Ask client to void before weighing.
3. Use the same scale each time you weigh the client. **Rationale:** For consistency in weight from day to day, keep variables the same as possible.
4. Make sure the client wears the same type of clothing (e.g., gown or robe) for each weighing.
5. If the client is bedridden, weigh linens used for covering the client each time the client is weighed.
6. Change wet gowns or heavily saturated dressings before weighing the client.

Procedure

1. Transport client to scale or bring scale to bedside.
2. Balance scale so that weight is accurate (See Table 5–1 for desirable weight based on sex and height.)
3. Place a clean paper towel on scale and ask client to remove shoes.
4. Assist client to stand on scale.
5. Move weights until the weight bar is level or balanced.
6. Record weight on appropriate record.
7. Ask client to face front so back is toward scale's balancing bar.
8. Instruct client to stand erect.
9. Place L-shaped sliding height bar on top of client's head.

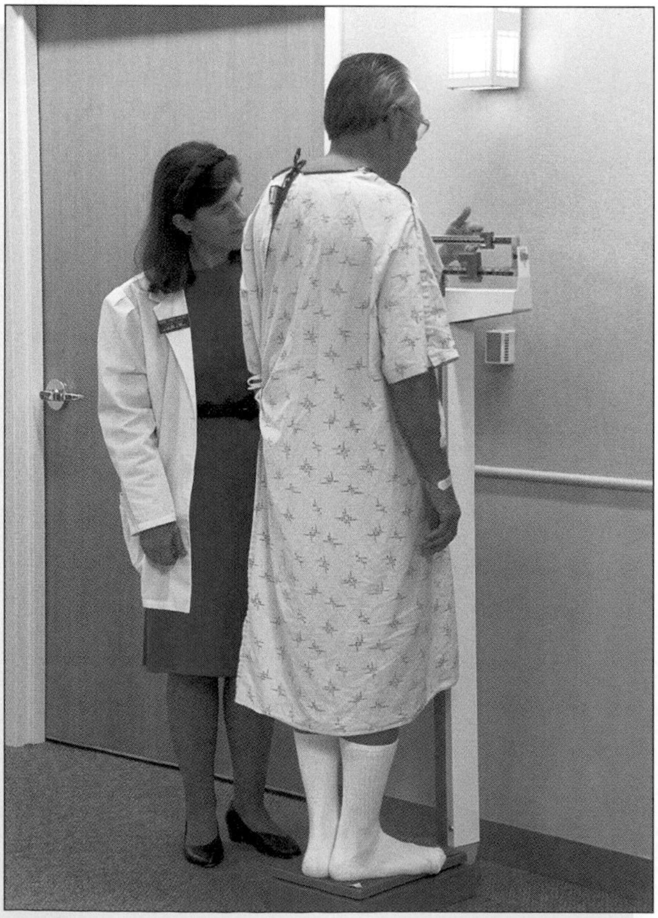

Weigh client in the morning, before eating or drinking, using the same scale each time.

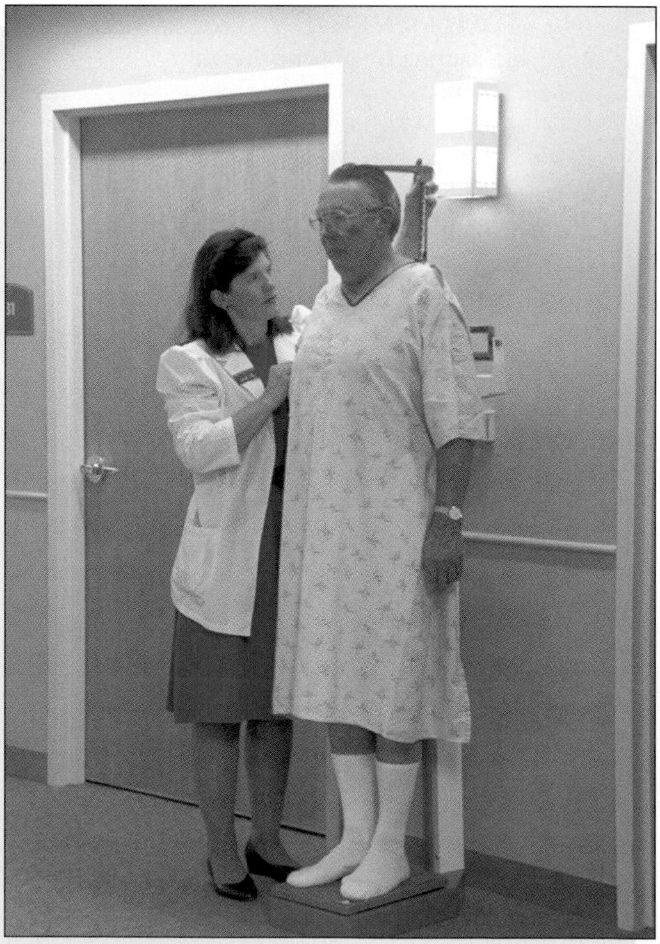

Instruct client to stand erect to measure height.

TABLE 5–1 Weight Chart (Desirable Weights in Pounds, According to Frame—in Indoor Clothing)

WOMEN Height Feet	Inches	Small Frame Pounds	Medium Frame Pounds	Large Frame Pounds	MEN Height Feet	Inches	Small Frame Pounds	Medium Frame Pounds	Large Frame Pounds
4	10	92–98	96–107	104–119	N/A		N/A	N/A	N/A
4	11	94–101	98–110	106–122	N/A		N/A	N/A	N/A
5	0	96–104	101–113	109–125	N/A		N/A	N/A	N/A
5	1	99–107	104–116	112–128	N/A		N/A	N/A	N/A
5	2	102–110	107–119	115–131	5	2	112–120	118–129	124–141
5	3	105–113	110–122	118–134	5	3	115–123	121–133	129–144
5	4	108–116	113–126	121–138	5	4	118–126	124–136	132–148
5	5	111–119	116–130	125–142	5	5	121–129	127–139	135–142
5	6	114–123	120–135	129–146	5	6	124–133	130–143	138–156
5	7	118–127	124–139	133–150	5	7	128–137	134–147	142–161
5	8	122–131	128–143	137–154	5	8	132–141	138–152	147–162
5	9	126–135	132–147	141–158	5	9	136–145	142–156	151–170
5	10	130–140	136–151	145–163	5	10	140–150	146–160	155–174
5	11	134–144	140–155	149–168	5	11	144–154	150–165	159–179
6	0	138–148	144–159	153–173	6	0	148–158	154–170	164–184
6	1	N/A	N/A	N/A	6	1	152–162	158–175	168–189
6	2	N/A	N/A	N/A	6	2	156–167	162–180	173–194
6	3	N/A	N/A	N/A	6	3	160–171	167–185	178–199
6	4	N/A	N/A	N/A	6	4	164–175	172–190	182–204

Height is in feet and inches, including shoes. Weight is in pounds, including indoor clothing. Assumption: Male indoor clothing with shoes weighed seven pounds. Female clothing with shoes weighed four pounds. Identify clothes client wore for accurate weight.

For girls between 18 and 25, subtract 1 pound for each year under 25.

Source: Blue Cross/Blue Shield of Delaware, 1997; American Heart Association.

10. Read client's height as measured.
11. Record height on appropriate record.
12. Throw away paper towel (if used) and assist client back to room.

DOCUMENTATION FOR HEIGHT AND WEIGHT

- Time height and weight measured
- Client's height and weight measurement recorded on graphic sheet and MAR (if indicated)
- Type and identifying number of scale used for weighing
- Weight of any attached equipment shoes or clothing that adds to client's actual weight

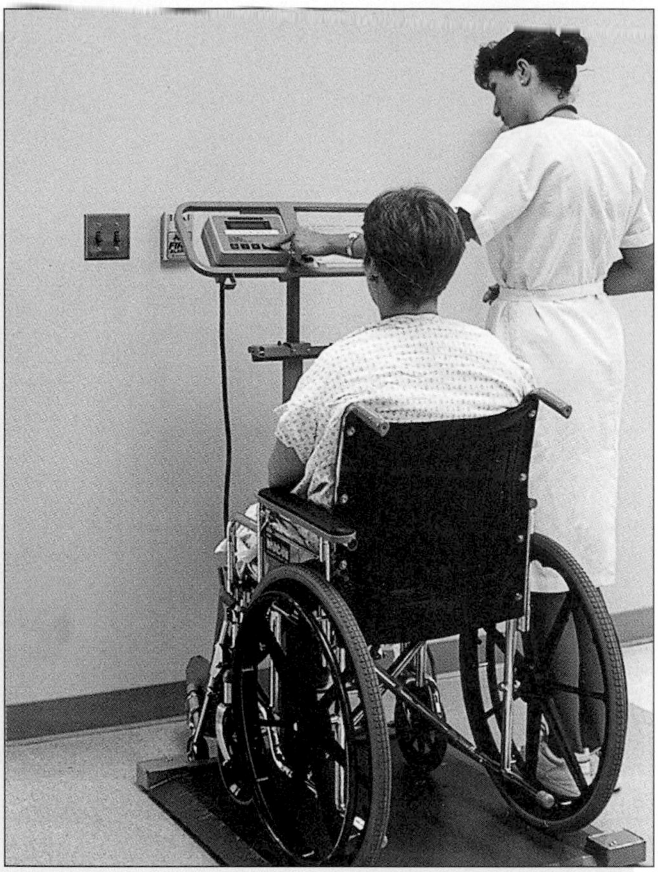

Scales accommodate wheelchairs for daily weighing of client.

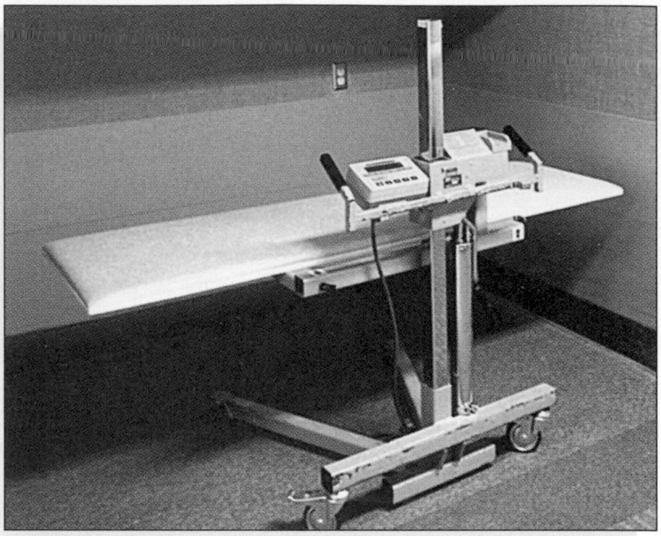

Bed scale is used to weigh clients who are on complete bed rest.

Critical Thinking Application

UNEXPECTED OUTCOMES	CRITICAL THINKING OPTIONS
Weight varies excessively from one day to the next.	• Check if same scale was used for both weighings. • Check what clothing or linen was on the client when he or she was weighed on both days. • Check that scale was balanced appropriately. • Reweigh the client to determine if an error was made in the weight.
Client is too critically ill to be weighed accurately because of mechanical devices used to sustain life.	• Estimate weight loss and gain by assessing other factors, such as skin turgor, output, presence of edema. • Weigh the client on a bed scale and note equipment used.

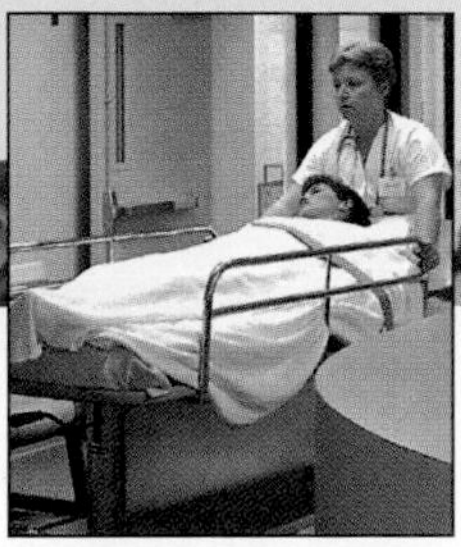

Discharge

Nursing Process Data

***ASSESSMENT* Data Base**

Verify order for client's discharge.

Identify discharge destination (home, rehabilitation unit, extended care setting, etc.)

Assess client's feelings about discharge.

Review care plan or clinical path to determine client's progress toward goal achievement during hospitalization.

Identify client's teaching needs for discharge.

Assess need for health care assistance in the home.

Determine that discharge needs have been addressed by dietitian (OT) (PT), social worker, or other specialist.

Verify that client is ready for discharge.

Try to determine reason for client's intent to leave the hospital against medical advice.

***PLANNING* Objectives**

To prepare the client for discharge and complete discharge planning

To assist in the transfer of a client whose condition necessitates care at another facility

To allow the client to verbalize his or her feelings about discharge and to identify the client's strengths and weaknesses

To help the client become aware of potential changes in environment and lifestyle due to his or her disability or limitation

To provide client with instructions for self-care and follow-up care

***IMPLEMENTATION* Procedures**

Discharging a Client

Discharging a Client Against Medical Advice (AMA)

***EVALUATION* Expected Outcomes**

Client verbalizes his or her feelings about being discharged and identifies strengths and weaknesses.

Client is aware of potential changes in environment and lifestyle due to his or her disability or limitations.

Client and family discuss how they can work together to help the client maximize his or her potential.

Client knowledgeably discusses all points included in the nurse–client teaching, including medication and self-care.

Home care assistance is arranged when needed.

DISCHARGING A CLIENT

Equipment

Agency's discharge instructions form

Educational pamphlets

Telephone numbers and information regarding clinic appointments or special groups

Specific equipment, such as wheelchair or commode, needed on discharge

Medications

Materials for dressing changes (if indicated) or anti-embolic stockings and any additional items dispensed to client transport vehicle for discharge

Preparation

1. Determine that physician's discharge orders have been written.
2. Notify family or significant other to arrange transportation. If unavailable, notify discharge coordinator for arrangements.
3. Notify all hospital departments: admitting, cashier, dietary.
4. Ensure that all laboratory work, x-rays, treatments, and procedures are completed prior to discharge.
5. Obtain adaptive aids or other supplies client may need.
6. Provide opportunities for client to discuss impending discharge.
7. Complete client teaching if applicable. (See Chapter 6, Client Education and Discharge Planning.)

Procedure

1. Review details of discharge with client (See Discharge Planning unit in Chapter 6).
2. Complete written instructions on Discharge Instructions form using lay terminology that client can understand.
3. Review any teaching and answer questions about medications, diet, bathing, any activity restrictions (e.g., lifting, sexual activity, driving) physical/wound care, use of special equipment or supplies and follow-up appointments.
4. Explain how to recognize complications and what to do if they occur.
5. Have client sign discharge form and provide the client with a copy.
6. Place agency copy of client's signed discharge instructions form on client's chart.
7. Assist client to retrieve safeguarded valuables per agency policy.
8. Terminate relationship with client. **Rationale:** Providing an opportunity for the client to express

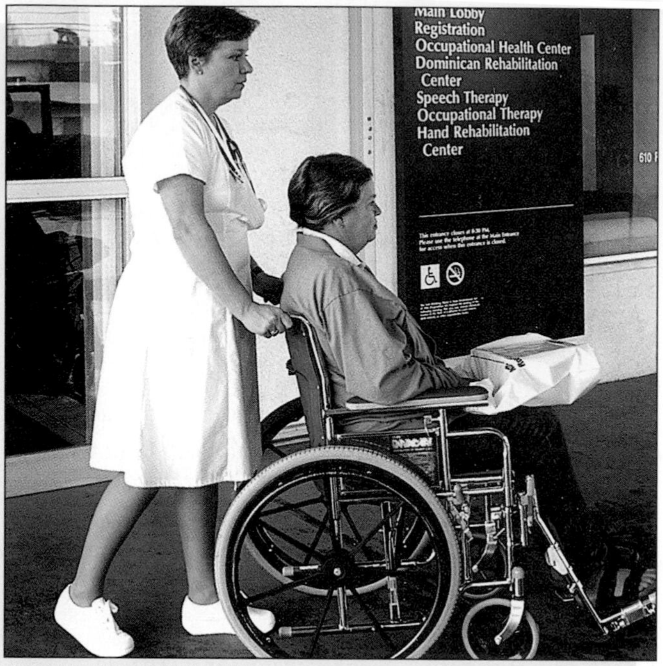

Clients are discharged in a wheelchair for their safety.

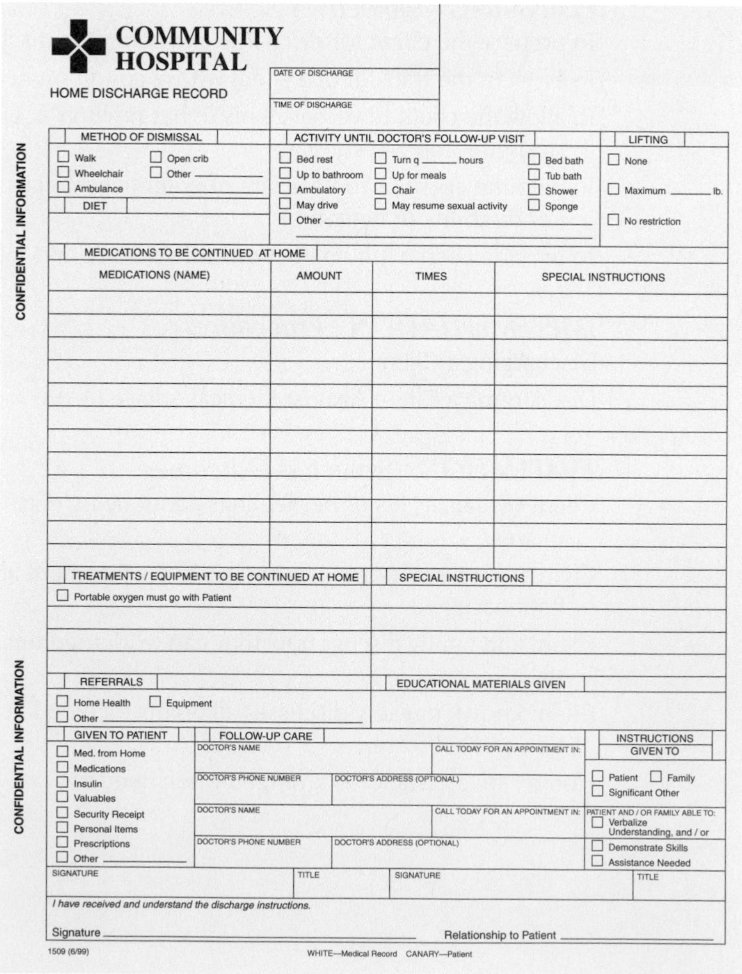

COMMUNITY HOSPITAL

HOME DISCHARGE RECORD

DATE OF DISCHARGE

TIME OF DISCHARGE

CONFIDENTIAL INFORMATION

METHOD OF DISMISSAL
☐ Walk ☐ Open crib
☐ Wheelchair ☐ Other ____
☐ Ambulance

DIET

ACTIVITY UNTIL DOCTOR'S FOLLOW-UP VISIT
☐ Bed rest ☐ Turn q ____ hours ☐ Bed bath
☐ Up to bathroom ☐ Up for meals ☐ Tub bath
☐ Ambulatory ☐ Chair ☐ Shower
☐ May drive ☐ May resume sexual activity ☐ Sponge
☐ Other ____

LIFTING
☐ None
☐ Maximum ____ lb.
☐ No restriction

MEDICATIONS TO BE CONTINUED AT HOME

MEDICATIONS (NAME)	AMOUNT	TIMES	SPECIAL INSTRUCTIONS

TREATMENTS / EQUIPMENT TO BE CONTINUED AT HOME
☐ Portable oxygen must go with Patient

SPECIAL INSTRUCTIONS

CONFIDENTIAL INFORMATION

REFERRALS
☐ Home Health ☐ Equipment
☐ Other ____

EDUCATIONAL MATERIALS GIVEN

GIVEN TO PATIENT
☐ Med. from Home
☐ Medications
☐ Insulin
☐ Valuables
☐ Security Receipt
☐ Personal Items
☐ Prescriptions
☐ Other ____

FOLLOW-UP CARE
DOCTOR'S NAME | CALL TODAY FOR AN APPOINTMENT IN:
DOCTOR'S PHONE NUMBER | DOCTOR'S ADDRESS (OPTIONAL)
DOCTOR'S NAME | CALL TODAY FOR AN APPOINTMENT IN:
DOCTOR'S PHONE NUMBER | DOCTOR'S ADDRESS (OPTIONAL)

INSTRUCTIONS GIVEN TO
☐ Patient ☐ Family
☐ Significant Other
PATIENT AND / OR FAMILY ABLE TO:
☐ Verbalize Understanding, and / or
☐ Demonstrate Skills
☐ Assistance Needed

SIGNATURE | TITLE | SIGNATURE | TITLE

I have received and understand the discharge instructions.

Signature ____ Relationship to Patient ____

1509 (6/99) WHITE—Medical Record CANARY—Patient

Home Discharge Record.

feelings and impressions contributes to a positive termination.

9. Follow agency's procedure for client discharge, including time and method of leaving hospital unit.
10. Document time and method of client's discharge, destination, individual accompanying, and any supplies, prescriptions, sent with client.
11. Notify appropriate departments of client's discharge.

DISCHARGING A CLIENT AGAINST MEDICAL ADVICE (AMA)

Equipment

Client's record

Form for discharge against medical advice (AMA)

Procedure

1. If client insists on leaving the hospital, notify physician immediately.
2. Ascertain from the client exactly why he or she wants to leave the hospital.
3. Explain and validate the physician's reasons that continued hospital care is necessary.
4. Explain risks of leaving hospital (AMA). **Rationale:** Some insurance companies may not pay for hospitalization if the client leaves AMA.
5. If client still insists on leaving, offer him or her the appropriate form and request him or her to sign it. The nurse cosigns the document. **Rationale:** This form states that the hospital is relieved from responsibility for the client's condition.

> **CLINICAL ALERT**
>
> Refer to agency SOPs (Standard Operating Procedures) for specific instructions related to client admission, transfer, or discharge.

6. If the client refuses to sign the form, note this fact on the form and have it witnessed. **Rationale:** This fulfills legal requirements if the client insists on discharge AMA without signing form.
7. Put the copy of the form on the client's chart.
8. Document verbatim statement in nurses' notes indicating reason for leaving.
9. Offer teaching and prepared materials to client.
10. Notify the appropriate people—the physician, the nursing supervisor, administration—when the client leaves.
11. Escort the client to the door as you would any discharged client. If client refuses assistance, document on nurses' notes. **Rationale:** The hospital is still responsible for the client while he or she is on hospital property.
12. Notify relatives if you are concerned for client's safety.

DOCUMENTATION FOR DISCHARGING A CLIENT

- Day-to-day preparatory activities, such as teaching, return demonstrations, discussion with dietitian
- If specific discharge forms or client teaching sheets are used, record data using these forms
- Discharge data, such as time, how discharged (ambulatory, wheelchair, ambulance), if accompanied by relative or nurse, and client's physical and psychosocial condition
- Discharge medications, special equipment, and materials taken home by client
- Discharge criteria that was not met and reason criteria was not met as identified on client care plan
- Client's signed Release from Responsibility for Discharge (AMA) form
- Individuals notified of client's discharge AMA

Critical Thinking Application

UNEXPECTED OUTCOMES	CRITICAL THINKING OPTIONS
Client is discharged to an extended care facility (ECF).	• Reinforce physician's explanation as to why client needs to go to an ECF. • Provide time for client and family to deal with the loss of the client's independence and his or her previous role in the home setting.
Client does not understand the discharge process.	• Repeat information as needed to help clarify unfamiliar terms or statements. • Explain to the client's relative the necessary care that will be required on discharge.
Client wants to leave the hospital AMA.	• Attempt to identify client's reasons for wanting to leave AMA. • In case of a minor or mentally incompetent client, contact agency's attorney ASAP. • Provide alternatives to leaving the hospital. • Do not force the adult client to remain in the hospital, but do encourage discussion about the situation. • Notify the charge nurse or supervisor that he or she should contact the client advocate, a social worker, or the clergy to discuss the situation with the client. • If possible, consult your hospital's policies and procedures regarding AMA before releasing client. • Have client sign AMA form, if possible. • If client will not sign AMA form, have another nurse witness refusal, and chart details of discharge.

GERONTOLOGIC CONSIDERATIONS

U.S. demographics affect hospital admissions.

- Estimated in 2001, more than 33 million persons (12.4% of the U.S. population) are over age 65—U.S. Census Bureau.
- Average life expectancy has increased to 75 years.
- Health care services are used more by the aged than any other group.
- The older the age of the person, the longer stay in the hospital.
- Three out of four elderly people die of heart disease, cancer, or stroke.

Elderly clients admitted to the hospital require special consideration.

- Level of fatigue and pain may be pronounced; thus, admission procedure may need to be altered to meet client's needs.
- May require special, repeated orientation due to confusion, impairment in hearing, visualization, mobilization, and so forth.
- Special attention may need to be oriented to family of the elderly client.
- Special problems associated with age need to be anticipated and nursing care planned to intervene appropriately.
- Discharge planning needs to take into account client's age and handicaps.

MANAGEMENT GUIDELINES

Each state legislates a Nurse Practice Act for RNs and LVN/LPNs. Health care facilities are responsible for establishing and implementing policies and procedures that conform to their state's regulations. Verify the regulations and role parameters for each health care worker in your facility.

Delegation of Responsibilities

- Delegation tasks for the admission of a new client may be divided into three task areas:

  A CNA may assist the client into bed, place their personal items in a designated area, describe the room environment including the use of the call bell, telephone, television, visiting hours, mealtimes, and other hospital services. The CNA may also take vital signs, obtain height and weight measurements.

  The LVN/LPN may complete a health history form, obtain admission data required by the hospital, witness consent forms, and complete the same tasks identified above.

  The RN is responsible for the initial health assessment, reviewing the data obtained by other health care workers, initiating the client care plan or clinical pathway, developing the teaching plan that is required, and beginning the discharge plan. The health assessment must be completed in a specified time frame according to JCAHO guidelines.
- An RN must complete a referral form for additional client services when needed. An LVN/LPN may complete discharge teaching following the established discharge teaching plan.
- Escorting a client out of the hospital can be delegated to a volunteer, CNA, or LVN/LPN. Many facilities have escort services which utilize volunteers.

Information Flow

- It is important to remember that clients being admitted to the hospital is usually frightened and unsure of the events that will take place. It is important to communicate their needs to all staff members assigned to provide care. This will provide for consistency in care and make them feel more at ease.
- A complete report on the newly admitted client must be given to all team members. If an LVN/LPN or CNA assisted in the admission process, they must provide immediate feedback to the RN manager regarding their findings.
- The client Kardex and MAR must be completed in a timely manner to facilitate safe and effective care for the client. It is often the responsibility of the unit secretary to initiate the documentation; however, it is the responsibility of the RN to check the documents for accuracy and completeness.
- A client care plan or clinical pathway must be established within a designated time frame. The time is determined by the facility.
- Shift report must contain a brief history and overview of the client's assessment, reason for admission, specific treatments, procedures, and anything pertinent to their needs.

CRITICAL THINKING STRATEGIES

SCENARIO 1

Mr. Moore has been told by his cardiologist that his coronary arteriogram indicates he has three-vessel disease and he is a candidate for coronary bypass surgery. The surgery is scheduled and Mr. Moore is directed to the facility's preadmission testing unit 1 week before admission for preliminary blood work and preoperative instructions. At this time he receives a packet of information ("Open Heart Surgery Patient Instructions"). One week later he is admitted to the hospital.

1. What is the advantage of providing the client with information this far in advance of surgery?
2. Which member of the team is most appropriate to complete this admission?
3. Based on this admission data, who would be the team member to initiate a clinical path?
4. How does the clinical path facilitate the client's admission, transfer, and discharge processes? Are there drawbacks?

SCENARIO 2

A female client has been admitted to the nursing unit with the diagnosis of acute abdominal pain. You are assigned to admit her to room 113. The chart only contains the following demographic data: lives locally, is 28 years old, recently married. Her husband is at the bedside and is very concerned with his wife's pain. As you walk in the room to complete the admission process, she is writhing in pain and crying loudly.

1. To prepare for the admission interview, what will you do first? Why?
2. State how you will ask the client to describe her pain.
3. What questions might be appropriate to ask regarding the abdominal pain?
4. What assessment data is priority for this client?
5. How is this information utilized in the development of a client plan of care?

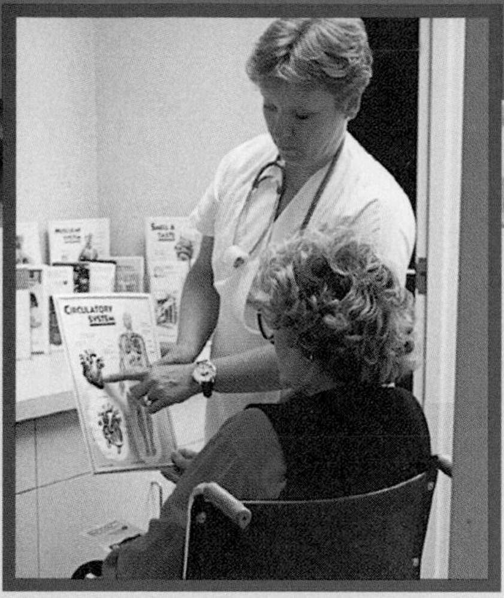

CHAPTER 6

Client Education and Discharge Planning

THEORETICAL CONCEPTS

UNIT ONE: **Client Education** 113
- Collecting Data and Establishing Rapport 114
- Determining Readiness to Learn 115
- Assessing Learning Needs 115
- Determining Appropriate Teaching Strategy 117
- Selecting the Educational Setting 118
- Implementing the Teaching Strategy 119
- Evaluating Teaching and Learning 120

UNIT TWO: **Discharge Planning** 122
- Preparing a Client for Discharge 123
- Completing a Discharge Summary 124

GERONTOLOGIC CONSIDERATIONS 125

MANAGEMENT GUIDELINES 126

CRITICAL THINKING STRATEGIES 127

Learning Objectives

- Define the process of client education.
- Discuss the meaning of the term *learning theory*.
- Outline the process of collecting client data.
- Describe the relationship of the nursing process to client education.
- Explain how the nursing process relates to client education.
- List two factors to consider when you are determining the appropriate teaching strategy.
- Define cultural competence.
- Identify one strategy to determine readability level of written material.
- List and describe two specific teaching strategies appropriate for clients and families.
- Describe how to develop an evaluation tool.
- Discuss the meaning of the term *discharge planning*.
- List three risk factors that require discharge planning.
- Identify the steps necessary to complete a discharge summary.

Terminology

Assessment: the first step in identifying client's knowledge base is to set meaningful learning goals and strategies.

Client education: the process of influencing behavior and teaching the client self-care techniques so that he or she can resume responsibility for certain aspects of health care following discharge from the health facility.

Compliance: follow-through on advice and direction by medical personnel to promote wellness and rehabilitation.

Comprehensive health care: a total system of health care that takes the whole person into account.

Counseling: to give support or to provide guidance.

Culture: a way of living, thinking, and behaving. It is learned within the family and guides the way we solve problems in our daily lives.

Cultural competence: a set of congruent behaviors, attitudes, and policies that enables nurses and other health care workers to work effectively in a cross-cultural situation.

Diagnosis-related groups (DRGs): categorization of disease diagnoses that standardizes the reimbursement of government funds for number of days in the hospital.

Discharge: to let go, as in discharging a client from the hospital; the flowing away of a secretion or excretion of pus, feces, urine.

Discharge planning: systematic process of planning for client care following discharge; includes client needs, goals of care, and strategies for implementation.

Evaluation tool: a test, questionnaire, or direct observation that evaluates the effectiveness of the teaching.

Helping relationship: an interaction of individuals that sets the climate for movement of the participants toward common goals.

Home care assistance: nursing care provided by licensed and unlicensed personnel in the client's home setting.

Learning: The process of conceptual change, within the framework of the client's perceptions, that leads to modifications in behavior.

Maladaptive: inability to, or faulty adjustment or adaptation.

Readiness to learn: a component of the learning process; referring to the psychologic state of being open and accepting of new information and the learning process.

Relationship: an interaction of individuals over time.

Resistance: inability to listen and participate in discussion of health behavioral changes.

Support: to lend strength or give assistance to.

Termination: the end of something; a limit or boundary; conclusion or cessation.

Therapeutic: having medicinal or healing properties; a healing agent.

Transfer: to convey or shift from one person or place to another.

Transition: the process or an instance of changing from one form, state, activity, or place to another.

Transitional care: the process of facilitating the transition or move between hospital and home to maintain continuity of health care.

Understanding: to perceive and comprehend the nature and significance of, to know.

Validate: to substantiate or verify.

CLIENT EDUCATION

Client education is one of the most important responsibilities of the professional nurse. With advancing medical science and an increasing number of clients with long-term degenerative illnesses, client teaching/learning can impact the client's health and how he/she adapts to the illness. The emergence of consumer involvement in health care, recognition of cost benefits, shorter hospital stays, and clients being discharged while still requiring care all contribute to the need for client education. Research has documented the benefits of client education and the reasons it is essential to make client teaching a nursing priority. The Joint Commission on Accreditation of Healthcare Organizations (JCAHO) has devised Patient and Family Education (PF) Standards for agencies accredited by them. JCAHO looks for evidence of three major processes involved in client education: the hospital's internal focus on education, direct education of the client and family, and evaluation of how well the education program achieves the identified goals.

Client education must be relevant and sensitive to the client's perceptions and family structure, especially cultural beliefs and practices. For example, if a nurse wants to teach a Chinese diabetic client about diet, the nurse should make suggestions that include foods the patient likes to eat (rice, stir-fry vegetables) and avoid foods with hidden sugars (sweetened soy milk). Diet may also be closely tied to a client's perception of social values. Eating may not be merely for nutrients, but also a gesture of politeness and social interaction.

Because clients have a right to know about their illness and any procedures being performed, client education is an expected standard for nursing practice (see JCAHO Standards). The education plan must take into account the client's cultural beliefs, literacy level, and be age appropriate. Clients have the right to maintain and honor their cultural beliefs, values, and practices while hospitalized. One in every three Americans represents an ethnically diverse culture. Because of these statistics, it is important that nurses gain a greater awareness of the various cultures in order to provide culturally competent care.

JCAHO stresses the need for multidisciplinary care planning and client education. With several health care team members employed in client teaching, it is essential that good communication among the disciplines be maintained. This will prevent repetition of teaching by different disciplines, and thus prevent confusion on the part of the client and the family. A documented teaching plan assists in identifying the content to be covered and the discipline responsible for each section of the teaching plan.

The goal of client and family education is to promote optimal health of the client. To achieve this goal, clients and families must learn in a way that is meaningful and acceptable to their concept of self and in relationship to the illness. Thus, learning is a process of conceptual change within the framework of the client's perceptions that leads to behavioral change. To be effective, the nurse must utilize excellent listening and communication skills to establish rapport, facilitating the teaching/learning process. The nurse must also teach the information in a way that the client and family can understand and in which they can actively participate.

Once a client has received a new diagnosis or new information about his/her condition, the nurse needs to start with what the client knows and believes about the disease. Often, when the nurse talks with the client about his/her condition, it helps the client recognize and ponder what he/she knows and expects may happen as a result of the condition. Clients need to be able to identify and understand what the illness is, effects of the treatment, whether it is acute or chronic, the short- and long-term outcomes, and whether it is controllable or curable.

Discussing possible effects of the illness will help the client accept the condition, be open for new ideas or teaching, and be motivated to learn and change. The client must recognize his/her gaps in knowledge and misconceptions, and then assimilate and act on new information. When the client and the family assist in goal setting and the information is presented based on their preferences, learning becomes more meaningful. Thus, the client will be able to apply the information and change specific behaviors as needed.

Once the client is motivated to learn, the nurse must be sure that the information is correct, consistent, and concise. The information should be presented utilizing proven teaching/learning principles. These principles include interactive learning; providing a conducive environment; utilizing client's learning style; appropriate method of information delivery; content taught in a simple to complex format; family involvement; use of simple understandable terms; use of an interpreter when necessary; and having written material in the client's predominant language. Follow-up phone calls or home/office visits are an excellent way to reinforce and evaluate the effectiveness of the teaching/learning.

The client education plan is a component of the total nursing care plan, which is part of the nursing process. Thus, the same principles of the nursing process are an integral part of client education. Because nurses are the principal providers of care, they usually provide the leadership role in directing the education plan for the client and family. Nurses provide the communication link between all members of the team to ensure the client's teaching goals are met in a timely manner.

Client education, when viewed as a process rather than the simple action of imparting information, assists the client to actively participate in his or her health plan for wellness. Individualized to the client and included as part of a total care plan, client education contributes to continuity of care following discharge. Another advantage of using this approach is that all nursing personnel may participate in a coordinated effort to implement teaching and evaluation of care can be accomplished.

Readiness to Learn

Readiness to learn is an essential component of the learning process. One of the principles of client education and adult learning is that the goals are constructed mutually with the nurse, the client, and the family. When goals are arrived at as a consensus between nurse and client, the readiness to learn is enhanced. Desired outcomes of client education are formulated as goals. Objectives can be stated as specific statements related to a goal. The more clearly stated the goals and objectives, the more directed the planned interventions. Written as behavioral objectives, evaluating the outcome is easier.

Most nurses recognize that the client may resist learning and cannot be forced to learn; the nurse can only assist the client, encourage him or her, and facilitate learning. To master information, the client must have internalized some form of motivation to learn; for example, the client realizes that to adequately control diabetes and feel better, he or she must understand the relationship of insulin and food to body needs.

Resistance to Change

Many clients appear to resist change, even when changing would result in a positive outcome. When this occurs, the process of learning is blocked. As a nurse educator, you are functioning as an agent of change and dealing with resistance to change is a necessary task. There are several reasons underlying resistance; one of the most common is that change is frightening, even when a person consciously wishes to alter his or her behavior. Also, if a person perceives change as a possible threat, he or she may resist. Another cause of resistance is inaccurately perceiving the reason for or effect of change. Other sources of resistance include psychologic inflexibility, cultural practices, inability to tolerate change, and not believing that change will have a positive effect.

The nurse is both an educator and an agent of change. If the client resists change (the teaching process) attempting to identify the reason for that resistance and altering the teaching approach accordingly may assist the nurse to accomplish the goals of client education.

Barriers to Change	Nursing Approaches
Perceived threat or fear of change	Identify specific fears or threats and impart accurate information that may reduce fears. Focus on the positive outcome of change.
Inaccurate perceptions of effect of change	Clarify client perceptions. Impart accurate information, and discuss results of behavior change.
Disagreement that change is positive	Work to agree on mutual goals and demonstrate positive outcomes so client views change as positive rather than negative.
Psychologic resistance or perceived loss of freedoms or behaviors	Focus on discussion of client's perceived loss of freedom and demonstrate willingness to alter plan or adapt to client's needs.
Inability to tolerate change	Recognize that low tolerance is often caused by fear—allaying fear through developing trust, being supportive when client attempts to change, and giving positive feedback decreases fear of change.

Malcolm Knowles, author of *The Modern Practice of Adult Education*, discusses strategies for adult learning. He suggests that adult learning and readiness to learn are influenced by developmental tasks. It may be useful for the nurse to review Erik Erikson's eight stages of human development and the tasks associated with each stage when determining the client's readiness to learn.

Client education is more than imparting information to a client; it is the process of influencing behavior. As such, it needs to be directed towards the client's thinking to be able to make meaningful behavioral changes. When goals are mutually agreed on and clearly stated, the learner understands what is expected, the nurse understands his or her role and can evaluate it, and the results can more easily be measured.

Tips to Facilitate Client-Focused Education

- Get to know the client, his/her knowledge level, perception, current practices, and preferences.
- Determine client's goals and readiness to learn, and individualize ways to achieve goals.
- Take into account client's goals, learning style, special skills, cultural beliefs, and developmental level.
- Utilize simple language and interact at client's level with empathy and concern.
- Utilize a variety of materials and methods that encourage active learning and participation.
- Plan for right time and right place to maximize client and family learning.
- Follow-up at another time to clarify information and reassess learning.

Student Nurse's Role in Client Education

As we discussed in the beginning of the chapter, the nurse's role has changed during the last 30 years. Now, a major constituent of the nurse's responsibility is to follow through on client care and implement discharge planning. Client education is an important component of the planning, especially since the majority of clients require assistance to maintain their health status when they leave the hospital. Learning new skills and understanding the disease process, medications, and treatments provide the self-care tools to return to a wellness state. Nursing students are learning to be practitioners; their learning takes place in a curriculum that is based on the nursing process. Since client education is considered a part of total client care within this framework, student nurses should understand the principles of client education and learn to include this process as part of the nursing care they administer to their clients.

DISCHARGE PLANNING

Recent changes in health care delivery systems, as an attempt to contain rapidly rising costs, has altered client care. The number of hospital days for clients in acute care hospitals has decreased; frequently, these clients are discharged still needing care; and this care is frequently delivered in the home setting. Most clients, especially those who are high risk, benefit from the process of discharge planning. Discharge planning is defined as the systematic process of planning for client care after discharge from the hospital. The emphasis and goal of discharge planning is to meet client needs through continuity of care—from an acute care setting to a discharge facility.

When the client is admitted and the care plan formulated, discharge planning should be initiated. The process includes an assessment of the client and family needs; the physical, emotional, and psychosocial status; home environment, and family and community resources.

Discharge planning involves multidisciplinary action with participation by all members of the health care team including the client and family. Many of the larger hospitals have discharge planners or coordinators. These staff are considered part of the health care team; they orchestrate the discharge planning. This is especially important when the client is considered high risk. More often, however, the staff or head nurse is responsible for discharge planning. With the assistance of social workers or community-based nurses, the staff identifies and anticipates client needs and formulates a plan for meeting these needs after discharge from the hospital.

JCAHO Standards for Client Education

- Hospital plans for and supports the provision and coordination of client education activities.
- Hospital identifies and provides the resources necessary for achieving educational objectives.
- Education process is coordinated among appropriate staff or disciplines who are providing care or services.
- Client receives education and training specific to the client's assessed needs, abilities, learning preferences, and readiness to learn as appropriate to the care and services provided by the hospital.
- Client is educated, based on assessed needs, about how to safely and effectively use medications, according to law and regulation, and the hospital's scope of services, as appropriate.
- Client is educated about nutrition interventions, modified diets, or oral health, when applicable.
- Hospital ensures client is educated about how to safely and effectively use medical equipment or supplies, as appropriate.
- Client is educated about pain and managing pain as part of treatment, as appropriate.
- Client is educated about habilitation or rehabilitation techniques to help him or her be more functionally independent, as appropriate.
- Client is educated about other available resources, and when necessary, how to obtain further care, services, or treatment to meet his or her identified needs.
- Education includes information about client's responsibilities in his or her care.
- Education includes self-care activities, as appropriate.
- Discharge instructions are given to client and those responsible for providing continuing care.

Note: Academic education is provided for a hospitalized child or adolescent, either directly by the hospital or through other arrangements, when appropriate.

Source: Adapted from Joint Commission on Accreditation of Healthcare Organizations (JCAHO). *Comprehensive Accreditation Manual for Hospital: The Official Handbook.* JCAHO Patient and Family Education (PFE 2000) Standards. Oakbrook Terrace, IL.

Risk Factors for Discharge Planning

- Elderly age group
- Multisystem disease process
- Major surgical procedure
- Chronic or terminal illness
- Emotional or mental instability
- Inadequate or inappropriate living arrangement
- Lack of transportation
- Financial insecurity
- Unsafe features in the home

Successful discharge planning includes

1. A total plan of care from the acute care setting to recovery at home or another healthcare facility.
2. Appropriate teaching for family and client in self-care.
3. Knowledge of the necessary procedures for self-care, as well as emergency procedures.
4. Appropriate agencies involved in transition to the home care setting.

A new approach to discharge planning is transitional care using transition specialists. This category of practitioner was implemented to facilitate the transition from hospital (where discharge planning is initiated) to recovery (in the home). The transition specialist meets with the family and client in the acute setting, begins discharge planning, and usually makes a home visit before the client is discharged. Following discharge to the home, this specialist is available to the client and family. This type of transitional care and coordination has proven to be cost-effective and has improved the quality of client care.

Federal Requirements for Discharge Planning Process

- Hospitals must identify at an early stage of hospitalization all Medicare clients who are likely to suffer adverse health consequences on discharge if there is no planning.
- The hospital must provide a discharge planning evaluation.
- A registered nurse, social worker, or other qualified person must develop or supervise development of the evaluation.
- Discharge planning must include an evaluation of the likelihood of needing posthospital services and of the availability of the services.
- The evaluation must include the client's capacity for self-care or the possibility of the client being cared for in the environment from which the client entered the hospital.
- The evaluation must be completed on a timely basis so that appropriate arrangements for posthospital care are made before discharge.
- The discharge planning evaluation must be in the client's medical record.

Communication between the client, family, and health care agencies is essential for effective discharge planning. The nurse establishes a dialogue between these various people and coordinates the discharge plan before the client leaves the hospital. When referrals to other agencies are necessary, these are initiated before the client is discharged. The nurse, if there is no discharge planner available, is responsible for coordinating such referrals—including signed physician's orders for specific care, treat-

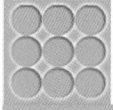

Cultural Competence

It is essential to remember that all client teaching plans and strategies must consider cultural aspects in the planning phase. Cultural differences affect client's open-mindedness to client education and their willingness to listen to the teaching and then being compliant with the changes that need to occur. Cultural differences affect client's attitudes about illness, health care workers and treatment modalities. JCAHO has mandated that there must be greater awareness of diversity, attention to the needs of special populations, and staff training to meet their needs.

All cultures have health beliefs about illness; what causes it and what cures it, as well as who they will allow to treat them. It is important for nurses to understand each culture's differences, as it will impact the client teaching process. The following table summarizes cultural beliefs that may have an affect on health care and client teaching.

TABLE 6–1 Cultural Beliefs Affecting Client Teaching

Ethnic Group	Cultural Beliefs
Asian/Pacific Islander	Extended family has large influence on client.
	Older family members are honored and respected, and their authority is unquestioned.
	Oldest male is decision maker and spokesman.
	Strong emphasis on avoiding conflict and direct confrontation.
	Respect authority and do not disagree with health care recommendations—but; they may not follow recommendations.
Chinese	Chinese clients will not discuss symptoms of mental illness or depression because they believe this behavior reflects on family; therefore, it may produce shame and guilt.
	Use herbalists, spiritual healers, and physicians for care.
Japanese	Believe physical contact with blood, skin diseases, and corpses will cause illness.
	They also believe improper care of the body, including poor diet and lack of sleep, causes illness.
	They believe in healers, herbalists and physicians for healing, and energy can be restored with acupuncture, and acupressure.
	They use group decision making for health concerns.
Hindu and Muslim	Indians and Pakistanis do not acknowledge a diagnosis of severe emotional illness or mental retardation because it reduces the chance of other family members getting married.
Vietnamese	Vietnamese accept mental health counseling and interventions particularly when they have established trust with the health care worker.
Hispanic	Older family members are consulted on issues involving health and illness.
	Patriarchal family—men make decisions for family.
	Illness is viewed as God's will or divine punishment resulting from sinful behavior.
	Prefer to use home remedies and consult folk healers known as curanderos rather than traditional Western health care providers.
African-American	Family and church oriented.
	Extensive extended family bonds.
	Key family member is consulted for important health-related decisions.
	Illness is a punishment from God for wrongdoing, or is due to voodoo, spirits, or demons.
	Health prevention is through good diet, herbs, rest, cleanliness, and laxatives to clean the system.
	Wear copper and silver bracelets to prevent illness.
Native American	Oriented to the present.
	Value cooperation.
	Value family and spiritual beliefs.
	Strong ties to family and tribe.
	Believe state of health exists when client lives in total harmony with nature.
	Illness is viewed as an imbalance between the ill person and natural or supernatural forces.
	Use medicine man or woman known as a shaman.
	Illness is prevented through elaborate religious rituals.

ments, or medications, so that the client can be reimbursed by third-party payment.

Included in the discharge plan is a discharge summary. This summary includes an overall review of hospitalization activities and the client's learning needs. There is a statement indicating how well the learning needs have been met, the client teaching completed, short- and long-term goals of care, referrals made, and coordinated care plan to be implemented after discharge.

Since 1988, hospitals have been mandated by federal requirements to provide a discharge planning process for all Medicare clients. These same requirements now apply to all clients within hospitals in the United States.

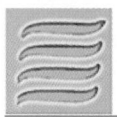

NURSING DIAGNOSES

The following nursing diagnoses are appropriate to include in a client care plan when the components are related to establishing and maintaining client teaching and discharge planning.

NURSING DIAGNOSIS	RELATED FACTORS
Impaired Verbal Communication	Cognitive impairment, auditory impairment, language barrier
Ineffective Health Maintenance	Cultural and religious beliefs, information misinterpretation, lack of education, lack of motivation, inadequate health care services
Knowledge Deficit	Inadequate understanding of condition, misinformation, language differences
Noncompliance	Impaired ability to perform tasks, poor self-esteem, lack of motivation
Relocation Stress Syndrome	Changes associated with transfer between facilities or facility and home, effects of losses associated with moving, stress in family members
Ineffective Role Performance	Change in self-perception of role; change in others' perception of role as a result of an altered health status which leads to denial of learning need
Ineffective Denial	Attempt to disavow need to alter lifestyle by avoiding client teaching

- The single most important nursing action to decrease the incidence of hospital-based infections is handwashing. **Remember to wash your hands or use antibacterial gel before and after each and every client contact.**

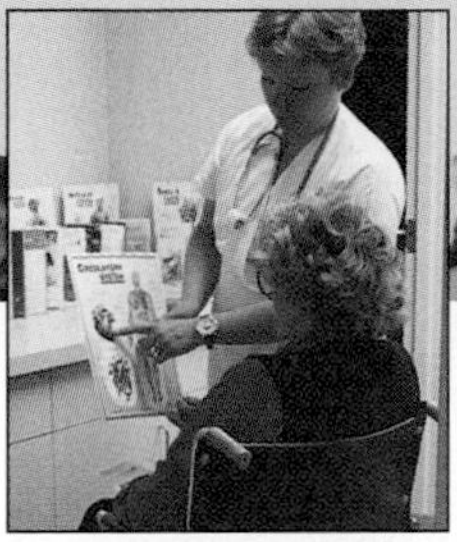

Client Education

Nursing Process Data

ASSESSMENT Data Base

Assess high-risk criteria for client education.
Determine the need for client teaching program.
Identify client learning style and preferences.
Assess knowledge and skill level of client.
Assess motivation to learn.
Assess readiness and openness to learning.
Identify health beliefs and practices.
Assess developmental and educational level of client.
Determine appropriate methodology for client teaching sessions.
Identify appropriate adjunctive materials, such as audiovisual aids, to enhance learning process.
Assess appropriate setting for the individual client.

PLANNING Objectives

To develop a plan in the nursing process framework
To determine teaching priorities and establish learning objectives
To select appropriate teaching strategies
To increase client's knowledge so as to positively affect health status
To increase client's self-esteem by encouraging participation in goal selection and implementation program
To encourage client to acknowledge individual responsibility for health behaviors and health status
To improve client's ability to make informed decisions affecting health status
To facilitate behavioral changes that are conducive to optimum health status
To provide continuity of care when the client is moving from one health care setting to another

IMPLEMENTATION Procedures

Collecting Data and Establishing Rapport
Determining Readiness to Learn
Assessing Learning Needs
Determining Appropriate Teaching Strategy
Selecting the Educational Setting
Implementing the Teaching Strategy
Evaluating Teaching and Learning

EVALUATION Expected Outcomes

Client's knowledge regarding his or her health status has increased.

Client's ability to make informed and effective health-related decisions, based on accurate information and awareness of self, has improved.

Effective use of the health care delivery system has been promoted.

Continuity of care and information exchange has occurred between health agencies or between the hospital and client's home and family.

The nurse has evaluated his or her teaching effectiveness and revised the plan, teaching style, and content as necessary.

Increased compliance to medical regimen as demonstrated by client's ability to manage condition/disease process.

COLLECTING DATA AND ESTABLISHING RAPPORT

Equipment

Nursing care plan in the nursing process

Room or suitable setting to complete assessment

Adjunct materials, such as audiovisual equipment, charts, and illustrations

Written materials, such as outlines or other handouts

Equipment for demonstration and return demonstration

Documentation forms: Kardex, client's chart

Preparation

1. Develop a nursing care plan in the nursing process format.
2. Use communication and relationship skills. **Rationale:** These skills encourage client's participation in the plan.
3. Avoid a judgmental attitude to prevent client telling the nurse what client thinks the nurse wants to hear. **Rationale:** An open nonjudgmental attitude assists client to be honest with feelings.
   a. Use "how" questions to facilitate communication. **Rationale:** "How" is more effective than "why" in a question, as "why" tends to set up a defensive reaction to the question.
   b. Use verbal and nonverbal behavior and congruence of both to build relationship with the client.
4. Use assessment (observation) skills. **Rationale:** This establishes a database.
5. Request demonstration of a skill previously learned or currently used (e.g., giving self an insulin injection). **Rationale:** Client's ability to demonstrate skill assists you to evaluate ability to perform, as well as mastery of previous teaching principles.

Procedure

1. Identify personal characteristics.
   a. Age and sex.
   b. Educational level.

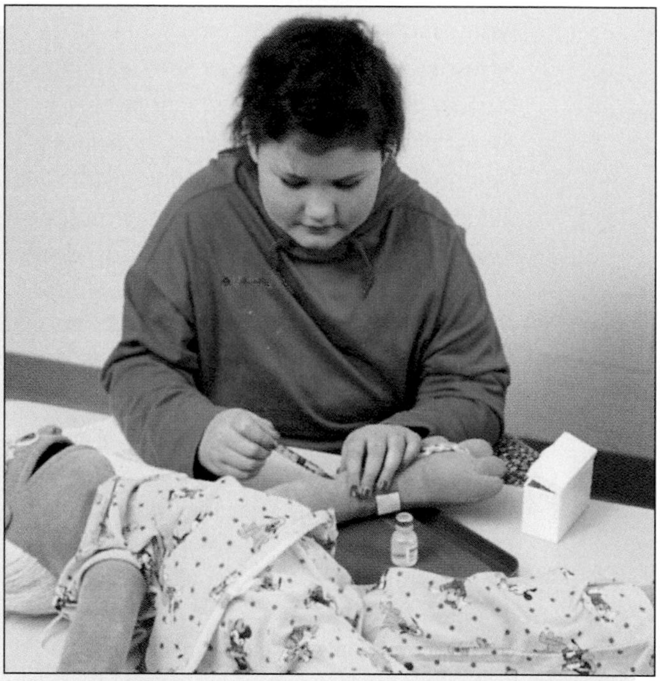

When collecting data to determine learning needs and strategies, use age-appropriate materials.

   c. Marital status.
   d. Family composition and living situation.
   e. Ethnic group and cultural practices pertinent to language skill & preference.
   f. Learning style preference.
2. Identify support systems available; both personal and community.
3. Identify values and attitudes toward self and others having his or her particular disease or condition.
4. Assess knowledge base—anatomy and physiology (normal and disease-related) and the disease process—by asking specific questions.

5. Evaluate capacity and ability to perform specific skills, including those previously learned.
6. Assess knowledge of rationale behind specific skills.
7. Evaluate patterns of coping.
   a. Past experiences of self and others in relation to the disease.
   b. Perception by client of how ill he or she is at this time.
   c. Reactions to stress and ways of managing anxiety.
   d. Current level of self-management.
   e. Willingness of client to change behavior.

DETERMINING READINESS TO LEARN

Procedure

1. Determine client's physiologic readiness.
   a. Degree of physical comfort of client (level of pain), level of alertness, ability to concentrate, degree of interest.
   b. Acuteness of the illness and its influence on client's ability to learn.
   c. Environmental factors that may affect client's degree of readiness.
   d. Safety issues and need for supervision.
2. Evaluate client's psychologic readiness.
   a. State of client's feelings and their influence on receptivity to learning. **Rationale:** An angry and hostile client is not going to absorb information until his or her anger is acknowledged or worked through.
   b. Psychologic barriers (for example, the presence of denial) and their influence on the learning process.
   c. Client's intellectual capacity and level of comprehension.
3. Assess client's willingness to make changes and be compliant with the teaching plan.
4. Assess families ability and willingness to participate in teaching.
   a. Determine willingness to participate in actual hospital instruction.
   b. Determine cognitive ability to understand instruction.
   c. Evaluate the extent of time and active participation of the family during instruction.
   d. Assess the interaction of the client and family during client teaching. **Rationale:** This will provide data on potential compliance and noncompliance issues related to the teaching plan.
5. Assess the extent of support and actual care the family members will provide for the client at home. **Rationale:** This will determine the extent of the instruction necessary for the family.

> **CLINICAL ALERT**
>
> JCAHO Standards for Patient and Family Education require that client's learning needs, preferred learning styles, literacy level, educational level, language spoken and understood, and learning readiness are assessed.

ASSESSING LEARNING NEEDS

Procedure

1. Assess if client has learning needs related to diagnosis, hospitalization, surgical procedures, or treatments.
   a. Ask specific questions related to what physician has told client related to specific learning need(s).
   b. Ask client what he/she is most interested in learning about specific learning need(s).
   c. Ask client to tell you in his/her own words what they know about specific learning need(s).
2. Interview client to determine what his/her daily life is like. **Rationale:** The information will assist you in determining impact of changes in client's lifestyle brought on by illness or condition. This will help you determine how to approach the teaching plan.
   a. Ask client to describe his/her usual daily routine.
   b. Determine if anything has changed with this pattern since illness.
   c. Describe hobbies or sports activities in which client participates.
   d. Describe normal workday and what activities are involved with employment, if still working.
   e. Discuss usual family responsibilities. Will the family be involved with his/her care?
3. Determine client's age and developmental level. **Rationale:** Knowing client's developmental level is necessary to provide the most effective teaching strategies.
4. Determine clients learning style. **Rationale:** This will assist in matching the most appropriate teaching strategy for client education.
   a. Ask questions related to what time of day he/she learns best.

Family Assessment should be an integral part of planning an effective teaching plan if family members will be affected by, or part of, the care of the client. Include the following information in the assessment.

- Which family members will be involved with care of client?
- Can family members provide care necessary or will additional support be necessary?
- Does home environment support client's care at home?
- Are any changes to home necessary to provide a safe environment?
- Do family members speak English and have basic literacy skills?
- Are there any cultural belief conflicts that could inhibit adequate care in home?
- Do family members interact in a supportive manner with the client?
- What do family members know about the client's condition? Do they need additional teaching?

b. Determine if he/she learns best by reading, listening, hands-on learning, or a combination of styles.
c. Use a commercial learning style inventory, if available.

5. Complete a cultural assessment. **Rationale:** To develop a culturally responsive teaching plan based on client's beliefs.
   a. Determine client's belief about illness.
   b. Determine how strong the client's belief system is relative to his/her traditional culture.
   c. Determine whether he/she uses folk medicine practices and uses a traditional healer. Clients from Asia, Africa, and South America are more likely to maintain this cultural component of their former country.
   d. Identify if traditional dietary habits are practiced in the home. If so, these should be included in the teaching plan, particularly nutritional counseling.
6. Determine client's educational and literacy levels. **Rationale:** Client's may seem disinterested in learning when, in fact, they do not understand what is being said and are embarrassed to ask. This can lead to missed physician appointments, noncompliance with treatment or medication usage, and even disability.
   a. Determine client's reading level by measuring his/her reading and comprehension skills.

CLINICAL ALERT

Agencies contract with telephone language lines to provide interpreter services. These services are available through AT&T Language Line Services and Pacific Interpreters Inc. on a 24-hour basis and in over 140 languages.

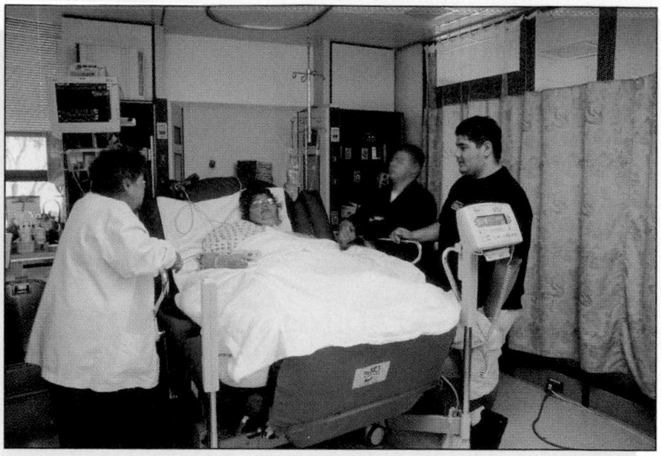

Include family in teaching, particularly if they will play a role in caring for client.

   b. Use a test of reading and comprehension to obtain a client profile before beginning teaching process. **Rationale:** To determine most appropriate written material for client.
7. Assess client's ability to speak and read English.
   a. Determine if client requires an interpreter during assessment of learning needs and teaching process.
   b. Ensure that words you use in client's language are correct for the situation.
   c. Do not use slang that could be misunderstood.
   d. Use simple words and phrases to allow interpreter to relate the intent of your statement.
8. Use assessment data and assessment instrument to jointly determine client's learning needs: educational, physical, psychosocial, and financial needs.
9. Formulate needs as goals.
10. Prioritize learning needs or goals.
11. Review with client alternative resources available to accomplish goals.
12. Determine ability of facility, family, staff, or multidisciplinary team to meet goals or learning needs.
13. Identify potential barriers to learning.

CLINICAL ALERT

The Rapid Estimation of Adult Literacy in Medicine (REALM) reading test can be easily administered in a few minutes. This test provides the reading grade level for clients who read below ninth-grade level. Words the client reads are all common health terms. The client reads as many words as he/she can correctly pronounce. A chart is used to convert raw scores obtained from word reading into a reading grade estimate.

Source: REALM, Department of Internal Medicine, Louisiana State University (MC-S), P.O. BOX 33932,

a. Physical: visual or auditory, pain level, literacy level, reading level.
b. Emotional barriers: stress or anxiety, inability to focus on information.
c. Language or culture: ability to understand and speak English, beliefs about health, folk practices or communication style differences.

14. Obtain verbal or written contract with client for educational program.
15. Refer client to other resources or agencies when appropriate.

DETERMINING APPROPRIATE TEACHING STRATEGY

Procedure

1. Consider the following factors when determining appropriate strategy:
   a. Input from client about how he or she learns best.
   b. Specific task or nature of the content to be transmitted and how it is best learned.
   c. Client attention span and retention ability.
   d. Reading level of client.
   e. Teaching materials and resources available.
   f. Time, availability, skills, and abilities of staff; appropriate use of paraprofessional and professional staff.
   g. Participation by members of other health care disciplines as part of a team.
   h. Determination of most appropriate time for teaching.
2. Use appropriate reading material for individual client.
   a. Determine reading level of written material.
   b. Use a readability formula to determine most appropriate written information for client.
   c. Use brochures, handout and written material written at a sixth grade level if client has low literacy skills. **Rationale:** Seventy-five percent of the adults in the United States should be able to read the material.
   d. Use short, common words in written material. **Rationale:** Medical terminology may be misunderstood.
   e. Make sentences 10 words or less and written in active voice.
   f. Make paragraphs short with one focus.
   g. Use large type (fonts) and lowercase letters. **Rationale:** Large font size is easier for clients with visual impairments or elderly clients, and lowercase letters are easier to read.
   h. Use diagrams and photos when ever possible to make a point.
   i. Set realistic goals and only one or two objectives for each teaching session. **Rationale:** Overloading client with information will not allow him/her to master information necessary for compliance.
   j. Ensure client completes a return demonstration, if appropriate. **Rationale:** This assists you to determine the extent to which client understands information presented. The greater the understanding and ability to perform a particular skill, the greater the compliance to treatment.
3. Determine which type of teaching strategy will be effective in a given situation.
   a. Group process: use of principles from group dynamics, mental health, or other related fields to enhance learning or behavior changes in a small group setting.
   b. Lecture–discussion: presentation of content in a didactic fashion with opportunity for questions and interaction during or at the conclusion of the presentation.
   c. Demonstration–return demonstration: demonstration (videotape) by the instructor with practice by the learner and return demonstration of mastery of the skill.
   d. Role playing: assumption of roles by various participants or learners for the purpose of clarifying various aspects of a situation.

CLINICAL ALERT

Readability Formulas

The Fry Formula assesses three samples of 100 words from different parts of a written handout and is useful to determine client's reading grade level. The Simplified Measure of Gobbledygook (SMOG) formula is very similar. The Fry Formula plots the average number of syllables and average number of sentences on a graph that then shows grade level. The SMOG formula also measures the number of syllables in a particular sample of written material which is then converted by a chart that determines reading grade level.

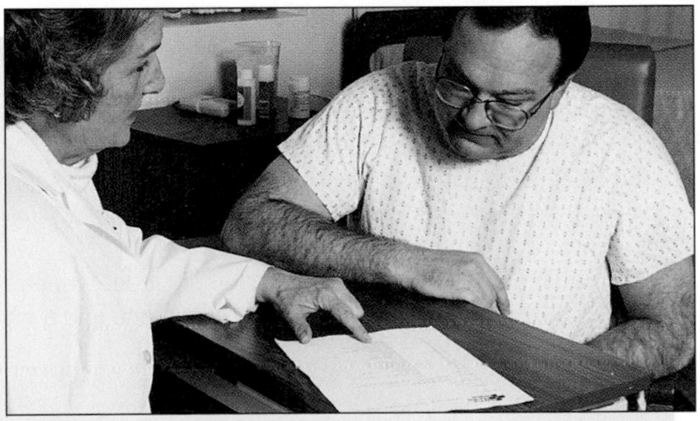

Determine which teaching strategy will be most effective for client.

   e. Games: structured game situation with rules designed for the learner to accomplish specific educational objectives.
4. Select appropriate teaching adjuncts based on developmental level, learning style, and reading literacy.
   a. Videotape or videocassette programs.
   b. Films; slide and tape presentations.
   c. Diagrams, charts, and illustrations.
   d. Programmed instruction materials.
   e. Books.
   f. Pamphlets and other written handouts.
5. Provide language-specific material for non–English-speaking clients.
   a. Photos.
   b. Models of specific body parts.
   c. Audio tapes in specific language.

EVIDENCE BASED NURSING PRACTICE

Silent Clients

A qualitative study in Finland (N = 38 patients, N = 19 nurses) found that 18 clients who were identified as aloof or silent spoke little about themselves and followed the lead of the nurse. The nurse often used communication techniques that did not facilitate communication and were nontherapeutic. The study concluded that client's quietness or silence in client education settings "was complex, supported by the hospital's institutional standard, nurses' lack of expertise, and client's restrictive and face-saving speech". This underscores the necessity that client education be client focused, based on client's knowledge, experience, and preferences, rather than comply to a preset standardized, structured format.

Source: Kettunen, T., Poshiparta, M., Limatainen, L., et al. (2001). Taciturn patients in health counseling at a hospital: passive recipients or active participators? *Qualitative Health Research*, May (11), 399–422. From *Evidence-Based Nursing, 5*(1), January 2002, p. 30.

SELECTING THE EDUCATIONAL SETTING

Procedure

1. Choose an appropriate setting based on selected teaching strategy and available facility space.
2. Evaluate types of setting most appropriate to individual client and client's learning needs.
3. Consider an informal setting.
   a. Spontaneous teaching interactions between nurse and client can occur at any time in any setting.
   b. Usually no formal plan or evaluation tool is used.
4. Consider a formal setting.
   a. Teaching is carried out in a specified area of the facility such as an in-service classroom.
   b. Teaching can occur independently, such as with audiovisual programmed instruction modules or in a group setting.
   c. Formal plan for the teaching program includes written goals, objectives, teaching strategies, content, and evaluation method.

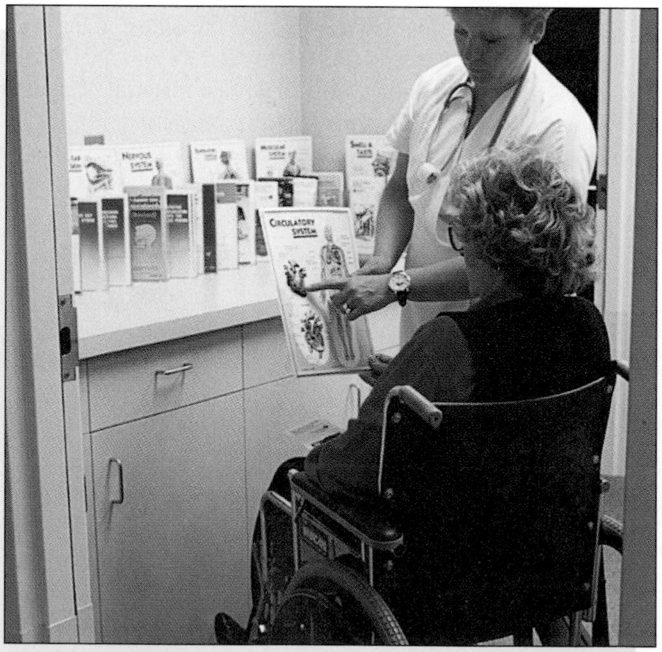

After selecting the appropriate setting, choose the teaching adjuncts.

IMPLEMENTING THE TEACHING STRATEGY

Procedure

1. Gather teaching materials appropriate for client's learning needs and teaching strategy.
2. Sit with client in designated setting, and establish a warm and accepting relationship. **Rationale:** This is conducive to teaching and assists client in learning.
3. Specify previously established mutual goals and behavioral objectives of the program. **Rationale:** Mutually agreed-on goals promote acceptance of teaching strategy by the client.
4. Clarify or reclarify contract, agreements, or expected outcomes with individual or group. **Rationale:** Beginning at the level of understanding of person or group facilitates the process.
5. Assess teaching situation for any modifications needed and adjust plans accordingly.
6. Teach content or components of the plan to client. **Rationale:** Sticking to the plan and not deviating or going off on a tangent reinforces your commitment to help client master the content.
7. Use appropriate communication skills throughout session. **Rationale:** Therapeutic communication techniques enhance learning environment.
8. Request feedback (evaluation interchange) during teaching process. **Rationale:** Feedback lets you know how client is understanding content and allows for modification as indicated.
9. Plan for short teaching sessions on a frequent basis.
10. Adhere to agreed-on starting and ending times; negotiate any changes. **Rationale:** This encourages client to trust you.
11. Provide closure to teaching situation by summarizing and reiterating agreements made, actions to be taken, or subsequent events to follow.
12. Provide positive reinforcement if not done previously. **Rationale:** This approach increases self-esteem and encourages learning in client.
13. Terminate teaching session by establishing time for next client contact.
14. Do postassessment of your own participation, and plan for corrections and improvements in presentation. **Rationale:** Ongoing evaluation assists in final step of nursing process evaluation.
15. Reinforce teaching throughout hospitalization.
    a. Use return demonstration of skills frequently throughout hospital stay.
    b. Review teaching content through use of video-tapes and reading material.
    c. Provide positive reinforcement for changes in behavior.
    d. Discuss teaching content and written information by asking pertinent questions and providing answers to client's questions.

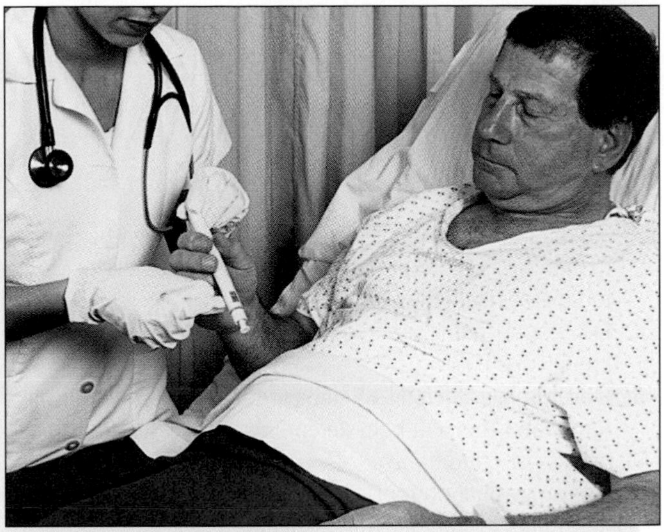

Demonstration is an important component of teaching strategy.

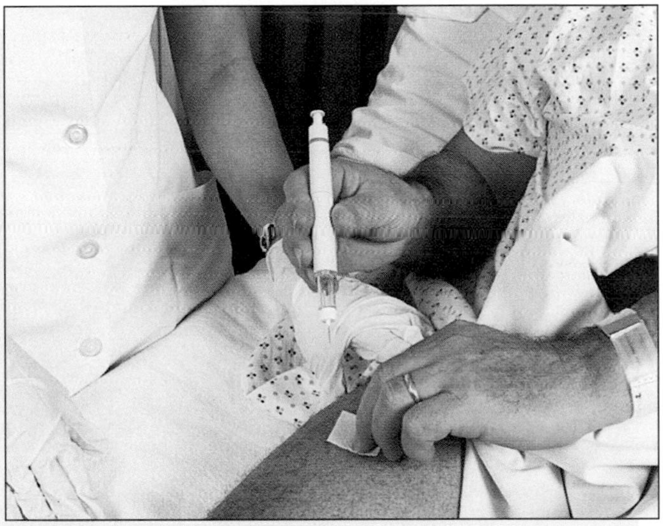

Request a return demonstration to evaluate client understanding.

16. Send teaching plan and written materials home with client and family.
17. Place copy of written instructions in chart for documentation. Instructions must be signed by client. This stays in chart.
18. Provide copy of teaching plan and written material to home health agency if referral has been made for visiting nurse. **Rationale:** This promotes consistency in information dissemination and reinforces teaching provided to client while hospitalized.

EVALUATING TEACHING AND LEARNING

Procedure

1. After demonstrating skill(s), ask client to complete a return demonstration. Evaluate client's ability to perform tasks.
2. Ask client and/or family to explain demonstration using own words.
3. Ask client and/or family specific questions regarding information provided. **Rationale:** To determine necessity of reinforcing or reteaching information.
4. Develop a simple pre and post test to determine client's knowledge base.
5. Develop hypothetical situations for client to problem solve. **Rationale:** This will help determine client's understanding of disease or condition.
6. Use an evaluation tool, if appropriate. **Rationale:** Evaluating with a specific tool focuses the evaluation phase better.
   a. Evaluate forms, format, and types of tools available for evaluation.
      (1) Pretest–posttest: measures changes in (e.g., knowledge level, attitudes, values).
      (2) Questionnaire: completed by client to report attitudes, certain behaviors, and, most frequently, level of satisfaction with the teaching program.
      (3) Physiologic tracers: determined prior to teaching episode to be the criterion of measurement of success (e.g., changes in blood pressure values after teaching program for hypertensive clients).
      (4) Direct observation of behavior changes: report of level of performance during return demonstrations.
   b. Choose an evaluative tool based on goals and objectives of the teaching program. **Rationale:** The purpose is to achieve goals, thus evaluative tool should be based on goals.

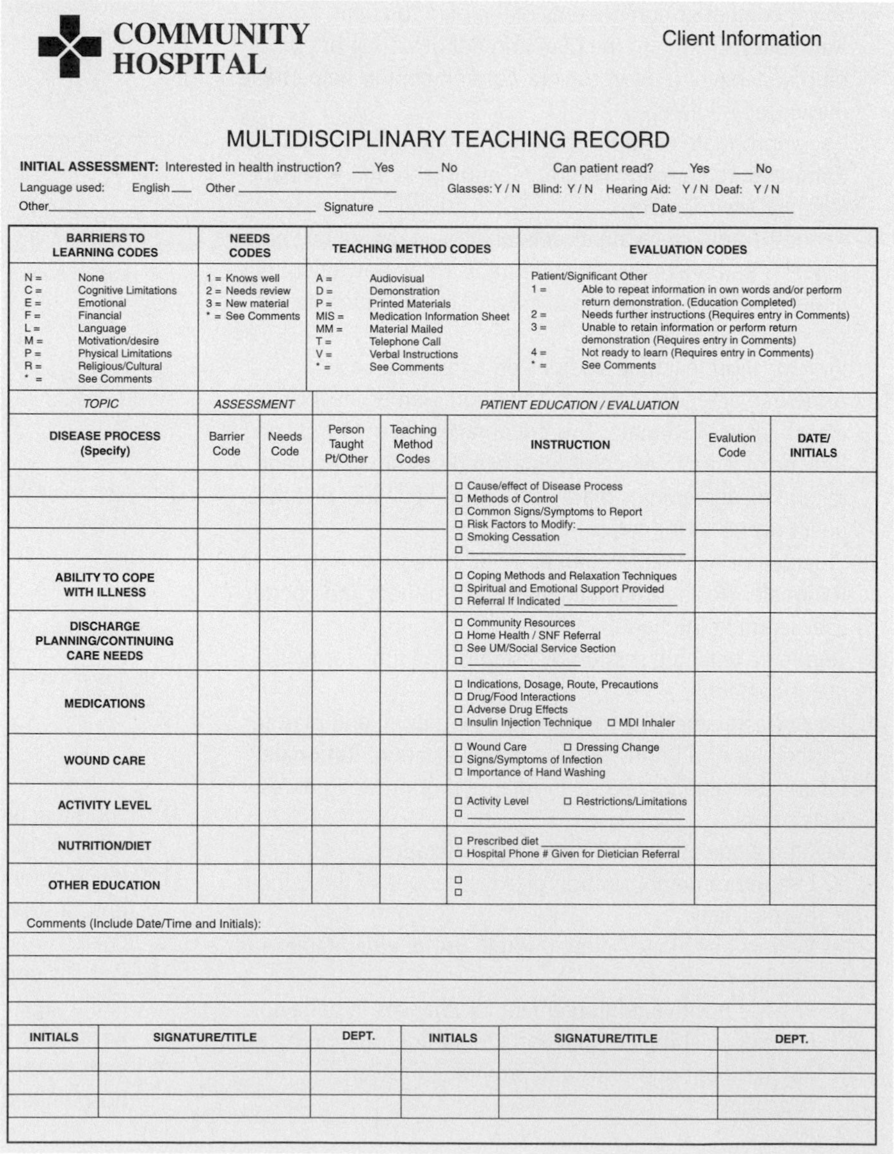

COMMUNITY HOSPITAL

Client Information

MULTIDISCIPLINARY TEACHING RECORD

INITIAL ASSESSMENT: Interested in health instruction? ___Yes ___No Can patient read? ___Yes ___No

Language used: English___ Other ______________ Glasses: Y / N Blind: Y / N Hearing Aid: Y / N Deaf: Y / N

Other______________ Signature ______________ Date ______________

BARRIERS TO LEARNING CODES	NEEDS CODES	TEACHING METHOD CODES	EVALUATION CODES
N = None C = Cognitive Limitations E = Emotional F = Financial L = Language M = Motivation/desire P = Physical Limitations R = Religious/Cultural * = See Comments	1 = Knows well 2 = Needs review 3 = New material * = See Comments	A = Audiovisual D = Demonstration P = Printed Materials MIS = Medication Information Sheet MM = Material Mailed T = Telephone Call V = Verbal Instructions * = See Comments	Patient/Significant Other 1 = Able to repeat information in own words and/or perform return demonstration. (Education Completed) 2 = Needs further instructions (Requires entry in Comments) 3 = Unable to retain information or perform return demonstration (Requires entry in Comments) 4 = Not ready to learn (Requires entry in Comments) * = See Comments

TOPIC	*ASSESSMENT*		*PATIENT EDUCATION / EVALUATION*				
DISEASE PROCESS (Specify)	Barrier Code	Needs Code	Person Taught Pt/Other	Teaching Method Codes	**INSTRUCTION**	Evalution Code	**DATE/ INITIALS**
					☐ Cause/effect of Disease Process ☐ Methods of Control ☐ Common Signs/Symptoms to Report ☐ Risk Factors to Modify: ______ ☐ Smoking Cessation ☐ ______		
ABILITY TO COPE WITH ILLNESS					☐ Coping Methods and Relaxation Techniques ☐ Spiritual and Emotional Support Provided ☐ Referral If Indicated ______		
DISCHARGE PLANNING/CONTINUING CARE NEEDS					☐ Community Resources ☐ Home Health / SNF Referral ☐ See UM/Social Service Section ☐ ______		
MEDICATIONS					☐ Indications, Dosage, Route, Precautions ☐ Drug/Food Interactions ☐ Adverse Drug Effects ☐ Insulin Injection Technique ☐ MDI Inhaler		
WOUND CARE					☐ Wound Care ☐ Dressing Change ☐ Signs/Symptoms of Infection ☐ Importance of Hand Washing		
ACTIVITY LEVEL					☐ Activity Level ☐ Restrictions/Limitations ☐ ______		
NUTRITION/DIET					☐ Prescribed diet ______ ☐ Hospital Phone # Given for Dietician Referral		
OTHER EDUCATION					☐ ☐		

Comments (Include Date/Time and Initials):

INITIALS	SIGNATURE/TITLE	DEPT.	INITIALS	SIGNATURE/TITLE	DEPT.

Multidisciplinary Teaching Record.

DOCUMENTATION FOR CLIENT EDUCATION

- Client's learning needs
- Client's learning objectives and goals set by client and staff
- Topics or subjects covered as a part of client education process, such as medications, procedures, dietary plan, activity restrictions, or follow-up care
- Teaching strategies used
- Degree of client's participation in the teaching activity
- Client's reading level
- Client's learning style preference
- Progress in meeting the expected outcomes of teaching
- Client's emotional response to the learning process
- Information or equipment sent home with client
- Client's developmental level

Critical Thinking Application

UNEXPECTED OUTCOMES	CRITICAL THINKING OPTIONS
Client's health status or treatment compliance has not improved as a result of the teaching program.	• Reevaluate nursing care plan according to the nursing process. • Reassess client for barriers to learning. • Assess client's reading and developmental levels. • Reevaluate testing tool. • Review client's learning style preference. • Determine readability level of written material. • Problem solve with client as to next step to take. • Request assistance from in-service consultant for determining which aspects of the teaching program were not successful and why. • Assist in revising parts of the program and restructure for individual client needs.
Client is hostile to teaching program.	• Attempt to determine underlying reason for hostility. • Terminate this session of teaching program, but tell client you will return tomorrow or at a later time. • Bring another nurse along to assist you in teaching as well as to help you evaluate reason for hostility.
Client's ability to make informed and effective health-related decisions, based on accurate information and awareness of self, has not improved.	• Assist client to take realistic responsibility for ineffective decisions without guilt and shame attached. • Assist client to identify those areas in which he or she is willing to make changes and support development of a plan of action. • Refer to other resources such as groups with like conditions (e.g., cancer, diabetes).
Client is unable to understand client teaching due to language barrier.	• Identify a volunteer or family member who can be used as an interpreter. • Use the AT&T Information line. • Obtain teaching material in client's native language. • Use photos or models, or make drawings that depict task to be performed.

UNIT 2

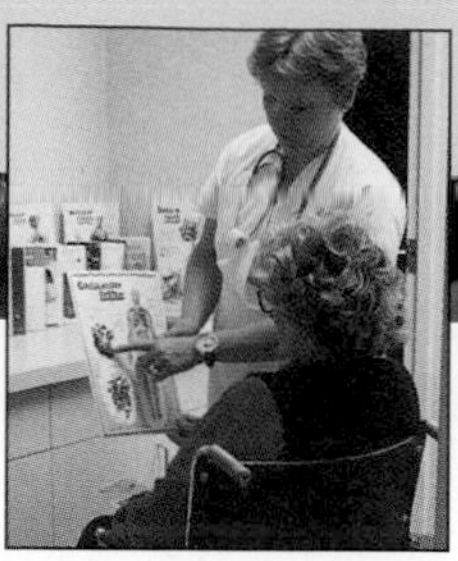

Discharge Planning

Nursing Process Data

ASSESSMENT ***Data Base***

Determine if client requires discharge planning.

Determine if client is in a high-risk category.

Assess special needs of client for individualized planning.

Assess need for multidisciplinary health care workers.

Determine information needed for compiling discharge summary.

PLANNING ***Objectives***

To complete a discharge risk factor assessment when admitting a client

To determine health care workers needed for discharge planning

To make appropriate referrals for client discharge

To complete discharge teaching

To develop a discharge plan

To complete a discharge summary

IMPLEMENTATION ***Procedures***

Preparing a Client for Discharge

Completing a Discharge Summary

EVALUATION ***Expected Outcomes***

Discharge teaching is completed.

Discharge planning is effective.

Discharge summary is completed.

PREPARING A CLIENT FOR DISCHARGE

Procedure

1. Obtain admission history, physical, and hospital progress notes.
2. Determine risk factors for discharge planning.
3. Refer high-risk clients to discharge coordinator or social service department, if appropriate.
4. Develop discharge plan (if not already completed) including short- and long-term goals in conjunction with physician and client.
5. Evaluate degree to which client education plan was implemented; reinforce aspects that were incomplete or refer to home agency.
6. Identify need for follow-up care after discharge in conjunction with physician.
7. Make appropriate agency referrals.
8. Complete a discharge referral form, and communicate directly with referral agency about client. (*Note: Health care agency may prefer their own discharge form to be completed rather than documentation in the nurses' notes.*)
9. Develop written discharge instructions for client and family, including medication administration times, dose, and side effects; treatments to be carried out at home for in a facility); potential side effects or complications from treatments or surgery; when to notify physician regarding symptoms; etc.
10. Update client care plan, and send copy to referral agency.
11. Send client teaching plan and materials to referral agency. **Rationale:** To maintain consistency in client teaching.
12. Document discharge summary.

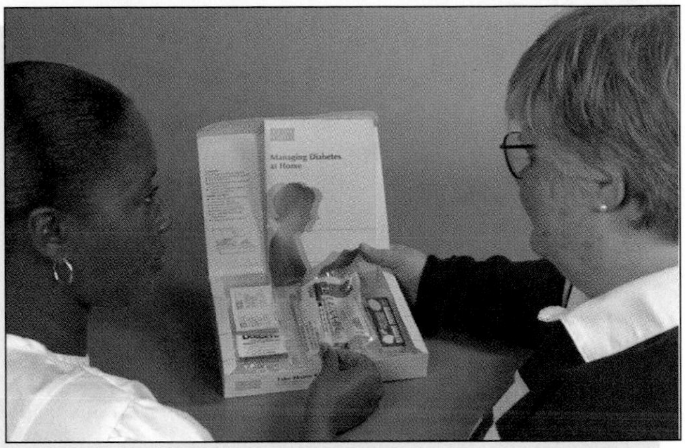

Discharge teaching is an important component of the discharge plan.

DISCHARGE PLAN

Medicare No. ____________
MediCal No. ____________

Name ____________
Admission Date ____________ Discharge Date ____________

1. Living arrangement: Alone ____________ With ____________
2. Residence after discharge: ____________
   Name and address of nearest relative or friend: ____________
3. Financial situation: Needs assistance ____________ Covered ____________
4. Agency Referrals: Discharge Coordinator ____________
   Home Health: ____________

DISCHARGE INSTRUCTIONS

Medications

Name/Dose	Time	Special Instructions

Potential Side Effects ____________

Nutrition
Special Diet ____________
Restrictions ____________

Treatments
Special Equipment Resources and Instructions ____________

Discharge Nursing Evaluation

	Independent	Needs Assistance	Dependent	Plan
Personal Needs (ADLs)				
Dressing self				
Bathing				
Skin condition				
Mobility				
Walking				
Bed rest				
Sensory capability				
Glasses				
Hearing aid				
Mental State				
Confused				
Alert				
Oriented				

SUMMARY OF CARE PLAN

Follow-up Care: Call Dr. ____________ for appointment in ______ weeks
Telephone No.: ____________

Other relevant information

❒ Pain rating @ discharge ___/10
❒ Pain Pamphlet given
❒ Prescription given **–or–**
❒ No medication given
❒ Additional instructions given

Sample Discharge Plan form.

COMPLETING A DISCHARGE SUMMARY

Procedure

1. Document a complete physical and psychosocial assessment at time of discharge.
2. Review vital sign ranges, and state latest vital signs.
3. Identify activity level of client.
4. Describe use of adaptive devices or equipment needs.
5. Review client teaching plan. Provide explanation of areas where teaching was adequate and where additional reinforcement is required.
6. Identify prescribed medications, dosage, and administration times. Provide information on client's knowledge of medication.
7. Describe goal achievement based on client care plan. Describe action taken if goal not achieved.
8. Identify referral agencies contacted.
9. Provide information regarding instructions on physician office visits, appointments to health care agencies, or support services.
10. Describe client's condition at time of discharge.
11. Document discharge instructions provided to client and family.
12. Describe method of discharge (e.g., wheelchair) and person accompanying client at discharge.
13. State means of discharge transportation (e.g., private car, ambulance).
14. Specify discharge facility where client is going.

DOCUMENTATION FOR DISCHARGE PLANNING

- Discharge teaching completed
- Discharge plan completed including risk factors, short- and long-term goals, and degree to which plan was implemented
- Need for follow-up after discharge
- Referral agencies contacted
- Discharge summary form completed; discharge instructions including medications, treatments, etc.

Critical Thinking Application

UNEXPECTED OUTCOME	CRITICAL THINKING OPTIONS
Client is discharged before discharge plan is completed.	• Continue to complete discharge plan, and send to referral agency. • Verbally communicate to referral agency and discuss discharge needs of client.
Discharge plan does not contain adequate data.	• Reassess parameters of a discharge plan, and revise accordingly. • Elicit assistance from another nurse or supervisor to revise discharge plan.
Goals of discharge plan were not accomplished.	• Attempt to assess reason goals were not met. • Reformulate or revise goals so that they are mutually agreed on and more realistic. • Request assistance from expert health care workers or in-service consultant.
Discharge referral plan is not implemented and client receives no referral notice before discharge.	• Attempt to contact other referral agencies to provide continuity of care for client. • Notify physician and discharge coordinator (if available) of necessity of providing follow-through care after discharge.

GERONTOLOGIC CONSIDERATIONS

Teaching Strategies

Memory changes occur with the elderly population.

- There is better short-term memory with auditory rather than visual presentation of information.
- Structure should be brief and simple.
- Repetition is important.
- Older clients learn better by doing, using multiple senses, than by reading instructions.
- Memory is better for things considered important.
- Clients remember best what is told *first*.
- Declining mentation is not inevitable with aging, but some memory loss is usual.

Retention facts that underlie teaching strategies. People remember

- 5–10% of what they read.
- 10–20% of what they hear.
- 30–50% of what they hear and verbalize.
- 70% of what they verbalize and write.
- 90% of what they say as they perform a task.

Interventions for teaching the elderly

- Speak distinctly and sit close to learner.
- Face the learner so that lip reading can supplement hearing.
- Use visual aids and verbal teaching.
- Decrease extraneous noise.
- Use printed materials with large type and high contrast.
- Limit use of blue, green, and violet illustrations. Use red.
- Avoid totally dark room for audiovisual presentations.
- Increase time allowed for psychomotor skills, and allow time for repetition.
- Slow the pace of presentation.
- Give small amounts of information at one time.
- Use analogies and examples to explain information. Mnemonic devices are helpful to compensate for imperfect memory.
- Establish attainable short-term goals.
- Encourage participation in goal setting and planning.
- Integrate new behaviors with previously learned ones.
- Focus on problem solving, not just delivery of facts.
- Apply teaching to present situation.
- Bolster self-esteem and self-confidence in self-care.
- Stress the "why" of what is presented.
- Recognize that the elderly client may prefer to be alone when learning.
- Make follow-up phone calls, if indicated, to check on the client, reinforce teaching, or to clarify any misunderstanding.

Discharge Planning

A discharge plan for the elderly contains some of the same components as a plan for a younger adult; at every step in the plan, however, the coordinator must remember that this is an elderly person and he or she must be evaluated for the ability and resources to manage at home. This is especially so if the elderly person lives alone or with another elderly person. Following are several issues that the discharge planner must consider when formulating the plan:

- Was the person functioning independently at home before hospitalization, and is it realistic to expect him/her to do so again?
- Does this person have capable family or friend resources to assist with functioning in the home (in addition to the necessary professional resources)?
- What is the baseline health status of the person (assuming he/she recovers from the current hospitalization), and does this status allow for independent functioning following hospitalization?
- What are the long-term financial resources of the elderly person and do special measures need to be initiated for coverage?
- If the elderly person cannot return to the facility he or she was in prior to hospitalization, what special arrangements need to be made?
- Special considerations the discharge planner must take into account when coordinating a plan for an elderly individual. For example:
  1. Does the person have a hearing or visual impairment that interferes with learning?
  2. Does the teaching need to be done in written form (not just verbal)?

3. Would a return demonstration of care procedures by the home health nurse be beneficial after the client has returned home?
4. Will the anxiety level of the client to be discharged interfere with understanding and learning?
5. Is the health status of the client a way of gaining attention? If so, this need should be separated from the needs of self-care following discharge. It is important to convey this need to the follow-up caregiver.

MANAGEMENT GUIDELINES

Each state legislates a Nurse Practice Act for RNs and LVN/LPNs. Health care facilities are responsible for establishing and implementing policies and procedures that conform to their state's regulations. Verify the regulations and role parameters for each health care worker in your facility.

Delegation of Responsibilities

- RNs must develop the teaching and discharge plans based on the assessment of client needs. The Nurse Practice Act sets the standards for who assesses and plans client care. Multidisciplinary team input is critical and a major component of both plans. The nurse is usually the coordinator of most client care plans and teaching plans.
- Once the teaching and discharge plans have been developed, other members of the health care team may participate in implementing them.
- LVN/LPNs follow the guidelines established in the teaching plans. They can assist with the discharge plans; however, an RN must write the discharge referral summary and communicate with the referring agency.

Information Flow

- The teaching plan should be developed in concert with the client and family. Mutually acceptable goals should be established with realistic time frames.
- The teaching plan is initiated early in the hospitalization. It must be written because it is a permanent part of the client record. It is updated as goals are achieved.
- Team members are kept apprised of the progress toward meeting the teaching goals by updates during shift report.
- Client information is disseminated between referral agencies and the hospital through a written discharge summary and/or referral sheet. The data in the summary includes pertinent information on the hospitalization and the condition at discharge, the medications and treatments the client is to continue to take, and specific equipment required for client care.

CRITICAL THINKING STRATEGIES

SCENARIO 1

Mr. John Johanson, age 58, was admitted to the medical unit with a diagnosis of congestive heart failure. He is African-American, 5′7″, and weighs 260 pounds. He is a cross-country truck driver. He lives alone when not working. He usually watches TV and eats fast foods or frozen dinners. This is his second hospital admission in the last month. His vital signs are: BP 230/108, P 108 and irregular, R 36. He has bibasilar rales, and a 3+ pitting edema of the lower extremities. His point of maximal impulse (PMI) is at the sixth intercostal space (ICS), midaxillary line. He states he is short of breath and has had difficulty ambulating the last few days. He states he has tried to lose weight but even after dieting he gains more weight back. When asked about his smoking habits, he states he knows he is not supposed to smoke and he has tried to stop, but with his work it is too difficult because he is alone so much. He states he is on blood pressure drugs, but unsure of the name.

1. Identify the current nursing diagnoses by priority and provide rationale for answers.
2. From this data, what would you conclude are the teaching needs by priority and develop a teaching plan for Mr. Johanson.
3. Are there any cultural considerations that need to be taken into account when considering his teaching plan? If so, identify actions you will take relative to the cultural considerations.
4. Briefly outline how you will determine when it is appropriate to initiate the teaching plan.
5. Describe the discharge plan you might develop for Mr. Johanson.

CHAPTER 7

Safe Client Environment and Restraints

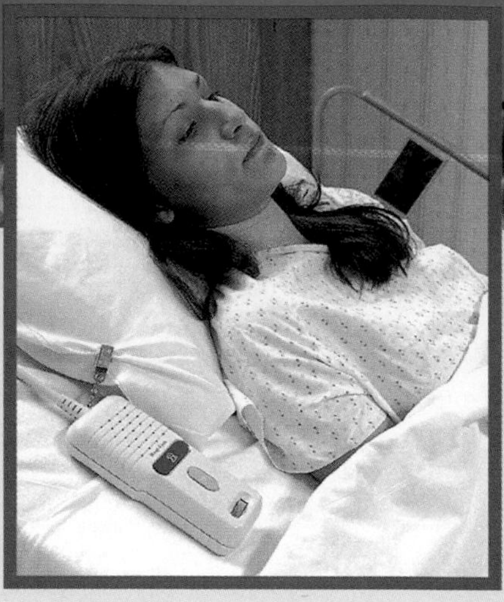

THEORETICAL CONCEPTS

UNIT ONE: A Safe Environment 140
- Preventing Client Falls 141
- Preventing Thermal/Electrical Injuries 142
- Providing Safety for Clients During a Fire 143
- Providing Safety for Clients Receiving Radioactive Materials 144

UNIT TWO: Restraints 146
- Managing Clients in Restraints 147
- Applying Torso/Belt Restraint 148
- Using Wrist Restraints 149
- Using Mitt Restraints 150
- Using Elbow Restraints 151
- Applying a Vest Restraint 152
  - *for Client in Bed* 152
  - *for Client in Wheelchair* 153
- Applying Mummy Restraints 154

GERONTOLOGIC CONSIDERATIONS 157

MANAGEMENT GUIDELINES 157

CRITICAL THINKING STRATEGIES 158

LEARNING OBJECTIVES

- Define the term *adaptation.*
- Describe three characteristics that influence adaptation.
- Outline four sociocultural dimensions of environmental adaptation.
- State two nursing diagnoses relevant to maintaining a safe environment.
- Outline the objectives for providing a safe environment.
- Identify clients who are at high risk for falls.
- List and briefly describe at least four guidelines for using restraints to prevent mechanical injuries.
- Explain four methods of preventing drug injuries.
- List the guidelines for providing safety when clients are receiving radioactive materials.
- Demonstrate two methods of client evacuation when a fire occurs in a nursing unit.
- Demonstrate the application of wrist restraints.
- Demonstrate the application of a torso/belt restraint.
- Identify at least five actions to maintain a safe environment for infants.
- List the components that should be included when charting for application of restraints.

TERMINOLOGY

Adaptation: ability of an organism to adjust to a change in environment.

Ambiance: the pervading atmosphere of the surrounding environment.

Ambulation: to move from place to place by walking.

Aseptic: sterile; a condition free from bacteria and infection.

Assessment: critical evaluation of information; the first step in the nursing process.

Behavior: a person's total activity—actions or reactions; especially conduct that can be observed.

Chemical restraint: use of a sedating psychotropic drug to manage or control behavior.

Comprehensive healthcare: a total system of healthcare that takes the whole person into account.

Contaminated waste: radioactive waste, which, if improperly disposed of, may be harmful or cause a radiation hazard.

Decibel: a unit for measuring difference in acoustic signals; a unit of intensity and volume of sound.

Ecosystem: the biologic and physical dimensions of the environment that refers to all living and nonliving elements.

Epidemiologist: one who studies the causes, distribution, and frequency of disease outbreaks in a human community.

Homeostasis: a state of equilibrium of the internal environment.

Hygiene: pertinent to a state of health and its preservation.

Limitation: the state of being limited or restricted.

Licensed independent practitioner (LIP): an individual licensed by the state or institution who is permitted to provide and monitor conscious sedation to clients, and order restraints or seclusion. This practitioner is either a physician, dentist, advanced nurse practitioner, or physician's assistant.

Maladaptation: inability of an organism to adjust to a change in environment.

Mechanical restraint: containment of a person in a chair or bed to provide safety.

Nosocomial: infection or disease originating in a hospital.

Physical restraint: any manual method or physical or mechanical device that restricts freedom of movement, or normal access to one's body, material, or equipment, attached to or adjacent to the client's body that he/she cannot easily remove. Holding a client in a manner that restricts his/her movement.

Physiologic: in accord with or characteristic of the normal functioning of a living organism.

Psycho: prefix referring to the mind or mental processes of an individual.

Psychosocial: a term that refers both to psychologic and social factors.

Restraint: any involuntary method (chemical or physical) of restricting an individual's freedom or movement, physical activity, or normal access to the body.

Seclusion: the involuntary confinement of a person in a locked room.

Sentinel event: any unexpected occurrence involving death or serious physical or psychological injury, or the risk thereof.

Sociocultural: a term that refers both to society and culture.

Stress: pressure, strain, or force sufficient to throw an individual out of balance.

Supervise: to direct or inspect performance; to oversee.

Therapeutic: having healing or curative powers.

Thermal: pertaining to using, producing, or caused by heat.

ORIENTATION TO THE CLIENT ENVIRONMENT

Maintaining Homeostasis

As a nurse, one of your primary responsibilities is to make sure your clients have a safe and comfortable health care environment. It is your responsibility to help clients adapt to this environment as well as to their health care in general.

From a holistic view, the term *environment* can generally be explained as the total of all conditions and influences, both external and internal, that affect the life and development of an organism. As human beings we are constantly exposed to changing physical, biologic, and social conditions. To survive, we continually assess our relationship to our changing surroundings. We also learn how to make adjustments that help us control and improve our environment. This complex process is called *adaptation.*

Adaptation includes psychologic and physiologic adjustments. People in most situations are able to control or adapt to their immediate surroundings. Although no two people respond to the environment in exactly the same way, common principles related to adaptation can be found in all human beings:

- All adaptations are attempts to maintain optimum physical and chemical states, or homeostasis.
- Individuals retain their own identity and uniqueness regardless of the degree of adaptation required.
- Adaptation affects all aspects of human existence.
- Human beings have limits in the process and degree of their adaptation.
- Adaptation is measured in relationship to time.
- Adaptive responses to the environment may or may not be adequate or appropriate.
- Adaptive attempts may be stressful.
- The degree and process of adaptation varies from individual to individual.
- Adaptation is an ongoing process about which the individual may be consciously or unconsciously aware.

Each of us adjusts to our immediate environment in a way that is unique to us. When this environment changes suddenly, for instance when we are hospitalized, we may not be able to adapt independently to our immediate surroundings safely and comfortably. It is at this point that assistance must be provided.

CHARACTERISTICS THAT INFLUENCE ADAPTATION

The characteristics that make all people unique also provide information about the process of adaptation to the environment. These factors must be considered when assessing clients' needs and abilities to safely adjust to their immediate surroundings.

Age

A client's age is a critical factor in the assessment process. Because terms such as *elderly* and *young* can be interpreted in many different ways, the nurse may need to look at the client's developmental stage (physical and mental growth) rather than at the client's chronologic age.

As people develop, sensory receptors help process day-to-day events. Human beings learn how to protect themselves and how to adjust to changing needs through experiencing these events. During the learning process, young children may require entirely different protection than teenagers. Even a 30-year-old man who has learned through experience how to protect himself in a routine environment may not have adequate skills in an unfamiliar atmosphere.

The older adult often requires special assistance. Sensory and motor changes, such as slowness of movement, postural instability, decreased vision or hearing, and even diminished acuity for taste and touch, are not uncommon. These changes can result in an altered ability to sense and adapt to harmful environmental stimuli. The older person may not see or hear an approaching car, detect the taste of spoiling food, or move quickly enough to avoid falling.

Mental Status

The ability to perceive and react to environmental stimuli is closely related to mental status. Adapting to a new or different environment requires learning through experience and possessing a cognitive awareness of the immediate surroundings. Making adjustments to the environment requires stimuli to travel over the sensory pathways of nerves to the central nervous system. To respond to stimuli, such as avoiding a burn from a hot object, motor neurons carry impulses to muscles to cause an involuntary reflex action, such as withdrawing the hand from hot water. Sensory impulses traveling to the cerebral cortex of the brain inform the person that this stimulus is potentially harmful. Voluntary movement then provides additional adaptation.

Consciousness is the state in which individuals are aware of themselves and their relationship to their surroundings. Unconsciousness indicates a lack of awareness and inability to cognitively respond to the environment. Levels of consciousness range from fully conscious to nonresponsive. Difficulty in adapting to the immediate environment due to alterations in mental status can manifest itself in a variety of ways:

- Confused clients often view their environment in a distorted way. This condition can lead to extreme behavioral changes, injury, or combativeness.
- Neurologically injured clients may have decreased perception of stimuli such as heat, cold, pain, or friction. In extreme cases, they may have no perception of any stimuli.
- Paralysis inhibits movement and is accompanied by a loss of position sense (dangling limbs or poor body alignment).
- Alterations in communication, sight, or hearing are barriers to identifying hazards and sharing fears or concerns with others.
- Fluctuating levels of consciousness create difficulty in promoting self-care and self-image.

Continuous assessment of changes in the client's ability to relate and adapt to the environment is essential. Ability to adapt influences the type and amount of assistance the client needs, especially while in less than familiar surroundings.

States of Illness

Illness or injury causes a person to focus more intensely on him or herself. The very nature of disease or trauma requires the individual to use physical and mental energy to adapt to the situation and to become more egocentric. A client often cannot perform even the simplest daily activity. Fatigue or pain may render clients helpless. Assistance with activities, such as bathing, eating, skin care, and elimination, may be necessary.

Some medications produce such side effects as drowsiness, which prevent the individual from adequately assessing the environment. Perceptions may be distorted, and the client is more vulnerable to hazards.

Emotional stress and anxiety can occur in mild to acute degrees. Although mild anxiety very often increases perceptual awareness, acute anxiety reduces perceptual awareness.

Because an individual is able to focus only on a specific amount of stimuli at one time, additional stimuli that may be equally important are not perceived. Potential environmental dangers are not processed. The client whose energy is focused on pain may not even hear instructions from the nurse. Depressed clients also require assistance. Depression often results in slower than normal responses to stimuli. Alcohol, a central nervous system depressant, also causes dull, slow reactions to stimuli.

When pain, anxiety, illness, injury, weakness, medications, or even lack of sleep cause a decrease in sensory acuity, awareness of potential hazards is altered. The client may not be able to make the necessary biologic, physical, or emotional adjustments to adapt to the immediate environment. Any of these conditions necessitates immediate assessment and action.

PHYSICAL AND BIOLOGICAL DIMENSIONS

The influences that make up an environment include the basic categories of biological and physical conditions. The biological dimensions of our environment covered in this section include all living things, such as plants, animals, and microorganisms. Water, oxygen, sunlight, organic compounds, and other components in which living things exist and develop make up the physical dimensions of an environment.

As you become more aware of the factors that affect environmental adaptation, providing a safe and comfortable atmosphere for your clients becomes a greater challenge. As you assess your clients and help them adapt to the environment of a health care facility, you should consider the following essential elements: space, lighting, humidity, temperature, ventilation, sound levels, surfaces and equipment, safety, food and water, and waste disposal.

Adequate Space

Everyone needs space in which to grow and develop. This space may consist of a room or an area as small as a shelf or corner. No matter what form space takes, individuals need to feel they have control over it—that they can arrange it or decorate it to their liking.

Providing space for clients encourages stimulation and experimentation. Toddlers need the space of an area like a recreation room for discovery and motor skills, since playtime is their primary source of development. Adults often enjoy the social activities of a lounge but may also require well-defined personal areas even if these areas are as simple as a bedside table or a bulletin board.

Natural and Artificial Light

Light, like space, is necessary for growth and development. The production of vitamin D, a critical component of bone metabolism, occurs from ultraviolet radiation on the skin. Natural light also helps wounds heal. In a hospital setting, natural light can be used to decrease feelings of isolation and to encourage clients to continue their normal routine.

Whether natural or artificial, adequate light is essential for the preservation of sight, for safety, and for accurate assessments and nursing care. Because eye strain, as well as nervousness and fatigue, can result from improper lighting, care should be taken to avoid glare, sharp contrast, and flickering lights. Night lights promote safety and orientation for the elderly.

Humidity and Temperature

The ability to adapt to changes in humidity or temperature is directly related to comfort. Most people in this country are comfortable at a room temperature of between 18.3° and 25°C (65°–77°F) with the humidity at 30% to 60%. People in other cultures function equally well at lower or higher readings.

Conditions that may inhibit a person's ability to adjust to high temperatures include excessive physical work, dehydration, extremes in age (the very young and very old), decreased physical fitness, and inappropriate clothing. An individual who has difficulty adapting to high temperatures may experience a rapid rise in pulse rate, cramps, nausea, and vomiting. Severe inability to adapt to heat can result in heat stroke and death.

An individual who has difficulty adapting to lower temperatures may experience a change in behavior, depressed vital signs, and eventual unconsciousness. Hypothermia, or abnormally low body temperature, occurs when there is an imbalance between heat loss and heat production.

Extremes of heat or cold increase the incidence of infection and add to discomfort. Temperatures in health-care institutions can be regulated with air conditioners and dehumidifiers, although care should be taken to avoid drafts and excessive dryness.

Ventilation

Particular attention should be given to assessing the movement of air within a client's immediate environment. An adequately ventilated room should contain a comfortable amount of moisture; be free of irritating pollutants, odors, or noxious fumes; and be at a tolerable temperature.

Adequate ventilation is especially important when more than one client is in a room. Other areas requiring optimum ventilation are operating rooms, delivery rooms, nurseries, isolation rooms, and sterile supply rooms.

A properly functioning ventilation system reduces airborne contaminants by regulating the amount of air movement within an enclosed area. When ventilation cannot be maintained by using doors and windows, mechanical devices, such as fans or air conditioners, may be used.

Clients requiring airborne isolation are placed in private rooms where the ventilation system is a directional air flow negative-pressure ventilation system. Six to twelve air exchanges per hour occur with this system.

Comfortable Sound Levels

Noise can be defined as any undesirable sound. The intensity and kind of noise that is comfortable is highly individual and related to past experiences. A businessman who lives on a busy street in a city may not adjust well to the absolute quiet he may experience at night in a hospital room. On the other hand, a farmer from a rural community may be disturbed by the slightest sound. Infants often sleep peacefully in an atmosphere of loud noise and activity.

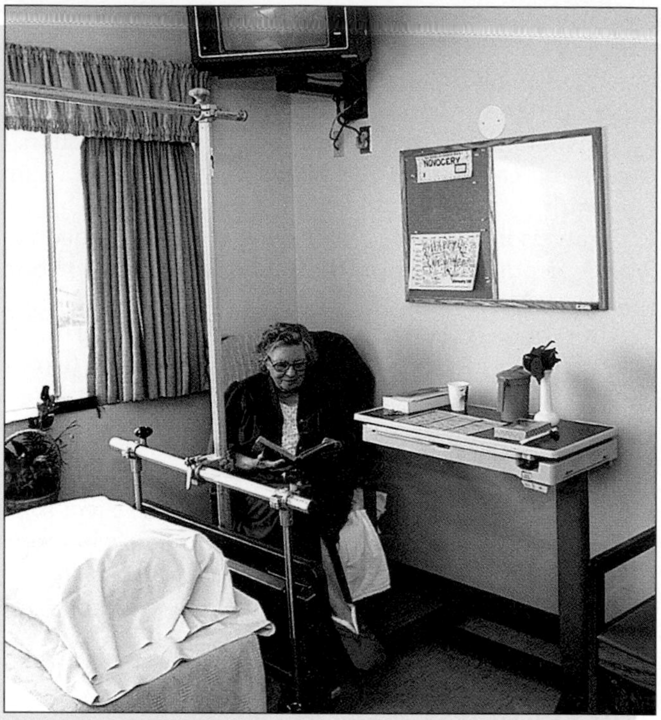

Provide a comfortable environment with space for personal effects.

Decibel is the unit for measuring the intensity of noise. At close range noise produced from heavy traffic, for example, has a decibel measure of 90, whereas a whisper at 3 feet has an intensity of 20 decibels.

At certain levels noise is considered hazardous. Temporary or permanent hearing loss or damage can occur when noise is present for a prolonged time at intensities over 90 decibels. Other effects of sustained loud noise are muscle tension, increased blood pressure, blood vessel constriction, pallor, increased secretion of the adrenal hormone, and nervous tension.

The pitch, quality, and duration of noise may also affect the client's environment. Unwanted sounds produced by sirens, traffic, and aircraft are often beyond the control of the nurse. But noise within a hospital setting, such as television, call systems, careless handling of dishes and other equipment, visitors, excessive conversation at the nurses' station, and some care-related sounds (e.g., beeping monitors) can be controlled.

Nursing personnel should always be aware of the noise level and its effects on the clients' well-being. Very ill individuals are often more sensitive to excessive or meaningless stimuli. Certain sounds can be reassuring because they represent activity or assistance to the client.

Furniture: Bed Safety

Today, most health care facilities are designed to be attractive, orderly, efficient, and clean. Since a person's outlook is strongly influenced by the surroundings, careful attention to appearance and cleanliness can assist with adjustment to the health care environment. Although it is essential to assess the routines and standards of cleanliness of each client, the nurse may also have to teach the client how to organize and clean up. In some cases, instruction to the client may be critical to maintaining or improving a health care condition.

The standards and routine cleaning procedures of the hospital are generally not a nursing function now because hospital housekeeping has become a specialized occupation. Maintaining an organized, clean environment, however, requires coordination by all health care providers.

Furnishings should be arranged to be physically safe, comfortable, aesthetically appealing for the client, and easily cleaned. Adequate cleaning of the room should be done at a time of day that is coordinated with the client's needs so that the resulting sense of security adds to the client's ability to adapt adequately to the surroundings. The ambiance of the room and a sense of order contribute to the client's sense of well-being.

Hospital beds are usually adjustable in height from the floor; when the bed is in LOW position, the client can more easily and safely get in or out of it; when it is in HIGH position, the nursing staff can more efficiently render care. The head and sometimes the knee areas of the bed can be elevated; this is accomplished by electric controls or infrequently by hand cranks. The cranks, if used, are at the foot of the bed, with the "head" crank on the left and the "knee" crank on the right. Remember to replace the cranks under the bed when not in use. This placement prevents the hospital staff from running into them. The electric controls are found on the foot, the side of the bed, or on the side rails. When placed at the side, the client can more easily control bed positions. Bed wheels should be equipped with locks and kept in locked position.

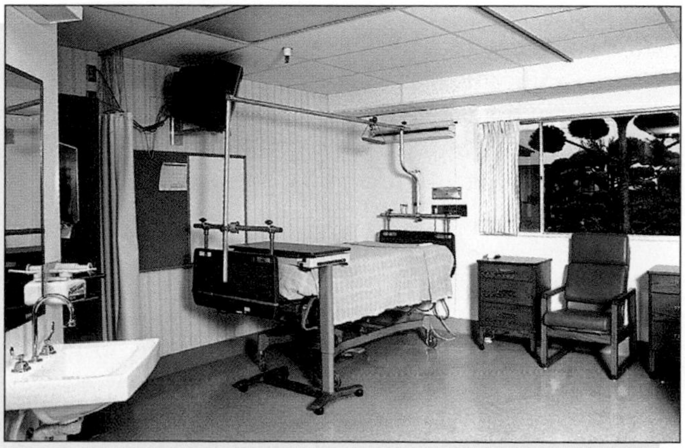

A pleasant environment promotes a sense of well-being.

For many years, side rails have provided what everyone thought was safe nursing care, protecting clients from injury as a result of falling out of bed. Changes are now occurring in both long-term care and acute care settings regarding the use of side rails. The Health Care Financing Administration (HFCA) and the Food and Drug Administration (FDA) have established new guidelines that decrease the routine use of side rails. There is still controversy over the safety of side rails. HCFA believes that regardless of whether side rails are used as restrictive or assistive devices, risk of client entrapment in the side rails overshadows the potential benefit. Elderly clients and those with altered mental status are at high risk for injury when side rails are routinely used.

HCFA has stated that a half- or quarter-length upper side rail is not considered a restraint if the client uses it as an aid for moving in and out of bed. A full-length or four half-length rails are not considered restraints if the client requests them in order to feel more secure, and if he is able to lower them by himself before getting into or out of bed.

Nurses must assess appropriateness for side rail use for each client and inform both client and family of benefits and risks for their use. These assessments must be completed according to hospital policies and procedures to ensure that client is not at risk for injury if they are in use.

The overbed table is adjustable in height and slides over the bed to provide space for self-care activities or additional working surface for the nurse. The overbed table may also be used when the client sits in a chair. Small bed trays are sometimes convenient when the overbed table cannot be used.

The bedside table, similar to a nightstand, holds the client's personal possessions in drawers. A cabinet section in the table can be used to store bathing or toiletry equipment, and the top provides space for the client's familiar items, such as pictures or books.

A chair with firm back and arm supports should always be a part of the client's furnishings. Chairs should be made of durable, easily cleanable materials, such as plastic or Naugahyde. The client should be instructed to avoid contact between skin surfaces and the chair when sitting in a chair. A small towel or blanket can be placed under the client for this purpose.

A signaling system is also essential for the client to call for assistance. A signaling system may be an intercom, buzzer, electric light, or handbell. Whatever device is available must be within the client's reach and ability to use.

Food and Water

Fresh, nourishing food and clean water are vital to recovering and maintaining health and must be planned for and ensured in appropriate amounts in health care facilities. A client's well-being can be positively affected by the ingestion of the correct number of calories, fat, proteins, carbohydrates, minerals, vitamins, and water, but it is well known that many people have nutritional habits that can negatively affect their well-being. A careful nutritional assessment is a critical step in helping the client adjust to the environment.

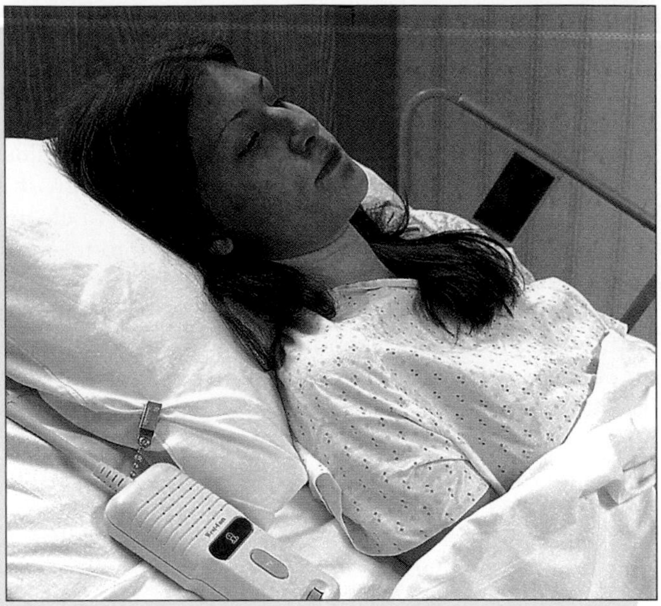

Ensure that call light or other summoning device is within easy reach of client to provide access to nursing staff.

Hazardous Products and Waste Management

All waste products, whether contaminated equipment, blood or body fluid, waste, garbage, soiled dressings, refuse, or hazardous products, must be handled and disposed of in a way that prevents risk for injury or illness.

Nurses must be aware of potential dangers to themselves as well as to their clients when handling and disposing of hazardous materials. Just a few of the hazardous chemicals that nurses and other health care workers may be exposed to include: disinfectants such as isopropyl alcohol and iodine; sterilizing agents such as formaldehyde and ethylene oxide; and anesthetic waste gases such as nitrous oxide and Fluothane. Antineoplastic agents used in cancer treatment may also pose a hazard even when proper prevention policies and procedures are in place. All health care agencies have specific-guidelines regarding the handling and disposal of such materials. For example, unit Material Safety Data Sheets provide information about area-specific chemical hazards and precautionary measures. Each toxic agent sheet (Material Safety Data Sheet) in the facility details information on the chemical's makeup, its health effects, exposure information, and emergency care procedures. These are available and accessible to the staff.

The U.S. Public Health Service Centers for Disease Control and Prevention, the Environmental Protection Agency, the Occupational Health and Safety Administration (OSHA), the American Hospital Association, and state departments of health are some of the agencies that prepare guidelines for the handling and disposal of biohazards and dangerous products. Familiarity with general and unit-specific hazards and adherence to recommended standards for their control is essential for safe nursing practice. OSHA requires hospitals to educate employees about chemical hazards and to train them in safety precautions before they work in an area where toxic agents are used. Most hospitals require annual hazardous chemical training as part of their required staff development and training updates. (Refer to Chapter 14, Infection Control, for more details in handling hazardous material.)

In some health care facilities, a position of infection control nurse has been created to gather data on the type and frequency of various infections found in the hospital. These data help the infection control nurse to locate the source of the problem, predict its spread, and identify the best method of preventing its recurrence. Many of the nosocomial (hospital-originated) diseases can be traced to inadvertent transmission by care providers. Each nurse plays a significant role in establishing a safe environment for the client by using standard precautions in client care and by handling and disposing of biohazards appropriately (see Chapter 14, Infection Control).

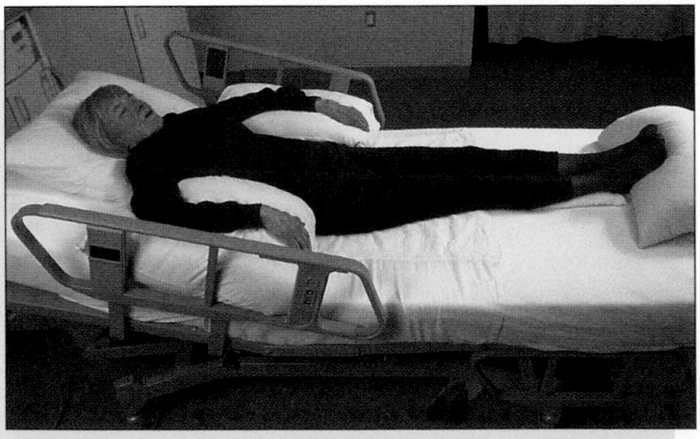

Half-length side rails can be requested by clients to use as an assistive device.

SOCIOCULTURAL DIMENSIONS

The first two dimensions of the environment, the biologic and physical, or ecosystem, refer to all living and nonliving elements. The third dimension of an environment is sociocultural, which includes both past and present influences from the people and the culture surrounding the individual. Customs, religious and legal systems, and economic and political beliefs are all part of this environment. This dimension also involves responses and adjustments to the ideals, concepts, beliefs, activities, and pressure of various groups, such as social clubs, peer groups, or colleagues.

Organization of Time

How clients perceive and deal with time and the passing of time depends on their age, immediate situation, culture, and past experiences as well as their present physical and emotional condition. To a mother waiting for her child to return from surgery, hours seem like days. Small children generally do not have a well-developed sense of time. A 3-year-old may act out feelings of abandonment when separated from a parent for just a few minutes. In an intensive care unit, time can be severely disrupted, since health care activities continue around the clock. The ability to organize time is a critical element in adaptation. Helping clients assess and plan their time is one of the most important ways you can help them cope with their new surroundings.

Privacy

Many people who enter a health care facility fear exposure and loss of identity. Providing privacy for a client is more than a luxury or a mere courtesy. It is necessary and vitally important to the individual's attitude toward health care.

Clients should be given as much privacy as possible. Most individuals give clues to the nurse about the degree of privacy they need. The client's culture, past experience, values, and age should all be considered when planning for privacy.

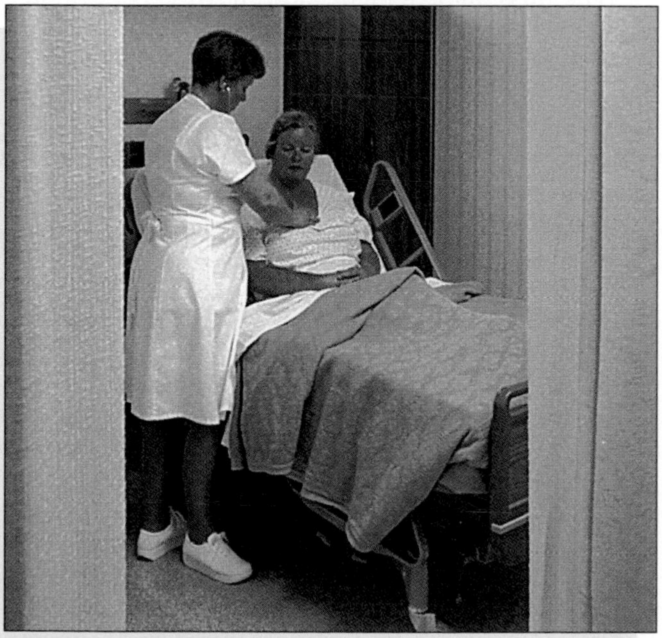

Clients should be given as much privacy as possible by drawing curtains or using screens.

Hospital routines should be planned to promote privacy. If an embarrassing or upsetting situation occurs, the feelings of the client must be protected. People require time and space to think, organize, and reflect. Privacy is necessary for human development even at home. In the hospital, privacy is critical to the client's attitude and well-being.

Privacy can be promoted by drawing curtains or screens. Doors and window shades may also be used. Signs stating "Do Not Enter without checking at desk," posted on room entrances give the client a sense of security from disturbances. This is especially important during physical examinations, personal care, or emotional upset. Knocking or asking for permission to enter the client's room or area promotes mutual respect and enhances a sense of emotional space.

Privacy also extends beyond the physical need of the individual. Health status, conversation, and records are privileged information. A more trusting, therapeutic relationship evolves if the client understands that confidences shared with nurses are used appropriately.

Individualized Care

Providing an environment that is comfortable, safe, and individualized to meet the specific needs of a client is a challenging task. The client's ability to adapt to the immediate environment can either improve or interfere with his or her well-being. To assist the client in adjusting to the environment, a careful assessment of the situation should always include the person's usual routines, self-care abilities, cultural beliefs, current perceptions, and past experiences. To promote the best adaptation to a different environment, encourage as much independence as possible with each client. You may be required to use your resourcefulness, imagination, and ingenuity to assist the client through difficult periods. Ongoing assessment and open communication between client and staff is essential if positive adaptation is to occur.

Hospitalized clients also need emotional space. This form of space is that psychological area where the person can experience a sense of self. This is particularly difficult to achieve in a hospital setting when caretakers exercise control over many of the activities of daily living. It is important that the staff be aware of this psychological need so that they can provide adequate privacy, quiet, and freedom of choice over all of the areas that the client can control. The staff must also be aware that the client rarely needs to relinquish total responsibility for his or her care.

Information and Teaching

The amount of information the client has about the environment and immediate situation directly affects his or

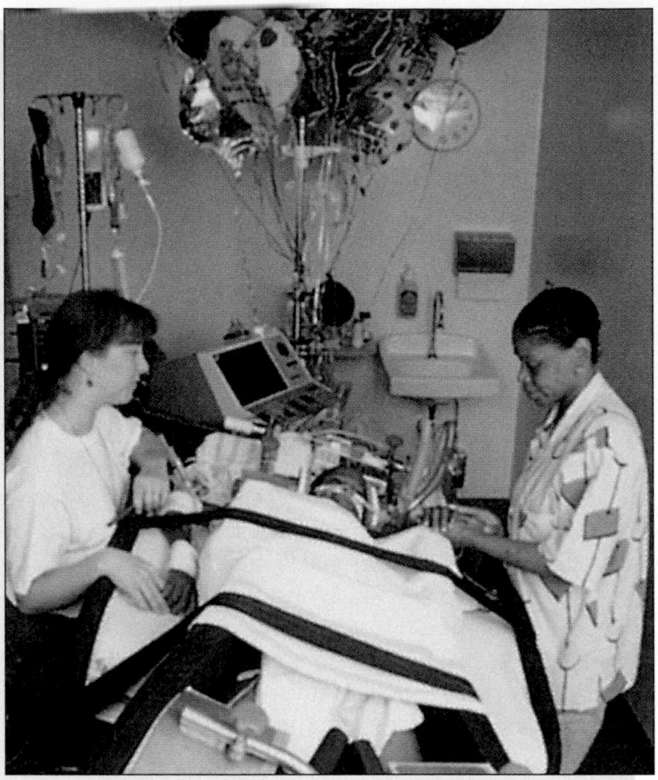

Providing an environment that is both safe and individualized is a challenging task for the nursing staff.

her ability to adjust safely and comfortably. When the individual is given information and explanation about strange equipment, diagnostic procedures, or unfamiliar health care personnel, fears and feelings of helplessness can be reduced and a shared sense of responsibility

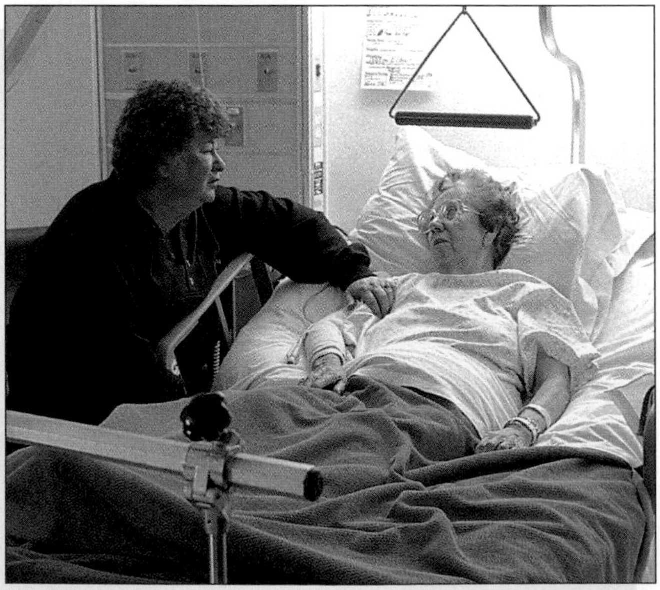

Providing a safe environment involves instructing the client, family, and visitors in safety measures.

enhanced. The client becomes more capable of asking questions and expressing concerns if prepared for unfamiliar occurrences.

Providing the client and his or her family, if appropriate, with information about the client's environment is the responsibility of the nurse. As more people assume the role of consumers of health care, there is more demand for knowledge about aspects of healthcare. Including the client in planning and caring for himself or herself promotes a sense of responsibility, independence, and self-respect.

Teaching the client about various aspects of health care is one method of information sharing. Over the years, the focus has changed from the professional staff doing everything for the client to helping the client be more independent. This change enables the client to adapt to the environment with guided assistance from nurses. As the client learns about his or her own healthcare and becomes involved in meeting his or her particular needs, a sense of trust, responsibility, and usefulness develops.

A SAFE ENVIRONMENT

JCAHO is committed to improving safety for clients and residents in health care organizations. About 50% of the JCAHO standards are directly related to safety. JCAHO has standards that address restraints and seclusion, environment of care (fire drills, medical equipment monitoring), physical environment, and infection control policies, to name only a few.

The mission statement indicates it is continuously trying to improve the safety and quality of care provided to the public through its accreditation standards. In July 2001, additional client safety standards went into effect for hospitals. These standards address a number of significant client safety issues including the requirement that hospitals have the responsibility to inform a client if he or she has been harmed by the care provided.

One of the policies implemented by JCAHO in 1996 addresses sentinel events. This policy ensures that health care organizations identify sentinel events and take action to prevent their recurrence. These events include an unexpected death or serious physical or psychological injury. Serious injuries such as the loss of limb or function are also included in this policy. All sentinel events are documented, and this documentation is forwarded to JCAHO.

JCAHO released the study on the top 10 Sentinel Events from January 1995 to June 2002. The list at the top of the facing page is a part of the 1,747 events that occurred during that time.

Providing a safe environment involves a number of people, including the client, visitors, and health care providers. Providing protection from hazardous situa-

Top Ten Sentinel Events

Event	Number of occurrences
Client suicide	289
Operative/postoperative complications	215
Medication error	199
Wrong-site surgery	197
Delay in treatment	97
Client fall	83
Death or injury to client who was physically restrained	83
Assault/rape/homicide	72
Transfusion error	48
Perinatal death/loss of function	44

Source: Joint Commission on Accreditation of Healthcare Organizations, June 26, 2002. Sentinel Event Statistics, Oakbrook Terrace, Il.

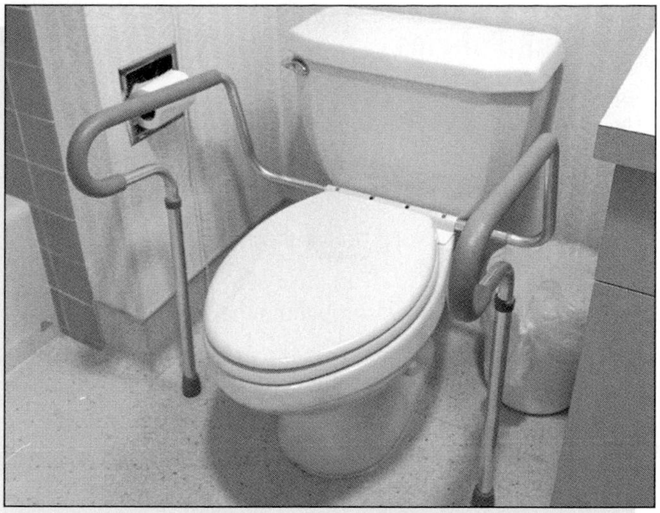
Rails next to the toilet assist in preventing client falls.

tions and education about safety precautions is one of your most important responsibilities as a nurse.

Clients who are moved from their usual environment into one that is unfamiliar and often frightening may act in ways that are very different from their usual behavior. A threatening situation can interfere with the individual's adaptation to the immediate surroundings.

The design and decor of the client's room must satisfy two needs: comfort and safety. Tasteful, unobtrusive colors help to normalize the hospital room. Interesting color combinations and patterns generally appeal more to the senses than do the traditional white or green choices. Pictures, flowers, cards, colorful linens, and curtains can add variety and familiarity to a room.

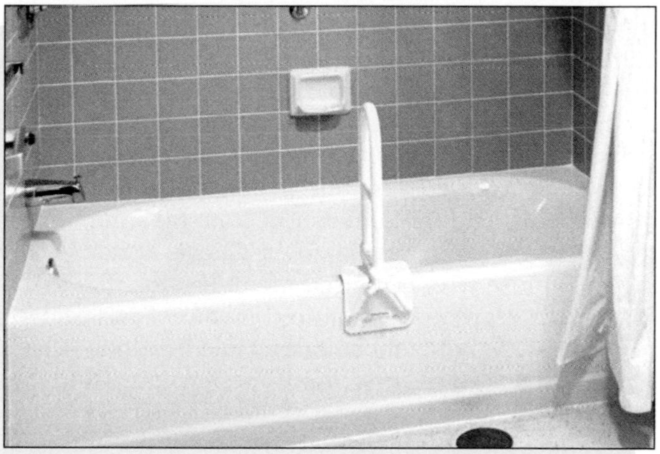
Safety features such as handrails assist in preventing client falls.

Safety Precautions

The client's age and health status influence the specific safety precautions that need to be taken to provide a safe environment. For example, infants require constant supervision, since they may attempt to put anything in their mouths or noses.

Preschool-aged children can be taught more detailed aspects of safety. Fire precautions and guidelines for bathing should be stressed.

Elementary school-aged children can usually protect themselves from hazards. They do, however, require instruction on how to operate mechanical equipment as well as information about fires and emergency exits.

All hospitals in the United States are required to be smoke-free facilities. Teenagers, adolescents, and adults should be given instruction about nonsmoking, the use of special equipment, and emergency exits. In addition, general information regarding their safety during hospitalization should be explained.

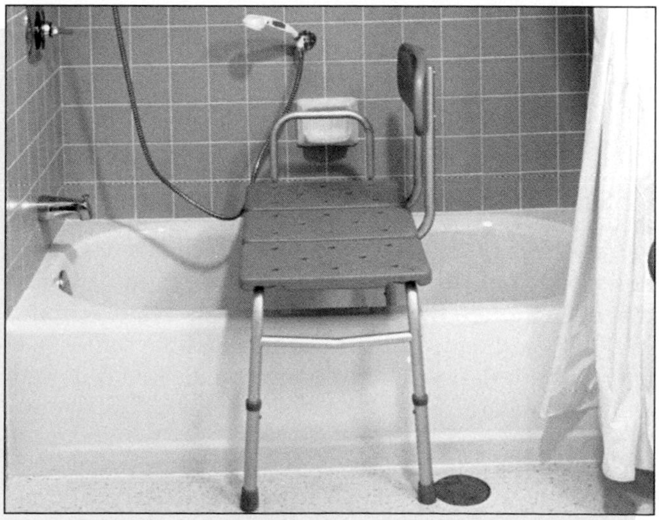
Shower chairs provide for client safety.

Smoking Policies

Joint Commission for Accreditation of Health Care Organizations (JCAHO) standards require hospital smoking policies be disseminated and enforced throughout hospital buildings.

- Directives on smoking policy should be conveyed to each client on admission.
- Smoking is prohibited throughout the hospital.
- A physician may write orders for an exception to this policy for an individual client.
- A designated smoking area may be made available for family or visitors. (See Chapter 26 for safety measures for clients receiving oxygen therapy.)

Client Falls

It is estimated that one third of individuals over 65 years, and over half of individuals over 80 will fall at least one time per year. It has been shown that most of the falls in the hospital have occurred from or near the client's bed. Other common areas where falls occur include the bathroom and corridor. Even though much research has been done on falls and fall prevention, it is still a major problem for health care organizations. Clients at risk for falls include: those with impaired mental status due to confusion, disorientation, impaired memory, and inability to understand, and those taking medications such as sedatives, tranquilizers, antihypertensives, and beta blockers.

A fall risk assessment is now part of the admission assessment of all clients. If the client is at high risk for falling, appropriate interventions are implemented immediately.

Evidence Based Nursing Practice

Do Side Rails Prevent Falls?

A New Zealand study of almost 2,000 clients tested a new policy of restricting side rails. The results revealed that even though the use of side rails decreased (from 29% to 7%), the mean fall rate remained the same (36.6 falls/100 admissions). However, the falls that did occur were less severe.

Source: Hanger, H. C., et. al. (July 1999). "An analysis of falls in the hospital: Can we do without bedrails?" *Journal of the American Geriatric Society, 47*(5):529; *RN, 62* (7.1).

Elderly adults are especially at risk for injury from falls. Decreased sensory acuity, decreased balance and postural instability, acute confusion or chronic physical problems such as arthritis contribute to the high risk for falls among the elderly. Specialized safety equipment, such as toilet and bathtub railing and modified seats, are often used in geriatric units to decrease risk of injury during bathroom use.

It is sometimes difficult to balance the need for client safety with that for autonomy. Surveillance by agency personnel or family members, use of alarm systems or special monitoring devices provide alternatives to use of restraints in promoting client safety.

Guidelines for the Use of Restraints

For many years, it was believed that restraining a client or placing a client in seclusion was considered a method to protect the client or the staff from injury. After much research into the subject, it has been determined that use of restraints is very problematic and actually leads to severe client injury and even death.

Because of client injury or potential injury from use of restraints or seclusion, both JCAHO and the Health Care Financing Administration (HCFA) have developed regulations regarding use of restraints in acute care, long-term care, and psychiatric settings. The standards require that the facility exhaust all reasonable alternatives before a client is placed in restraints or seclusion. HCFA standards used in long-term and psychiatric settings are more stringent than JCAHO. A licensed independent practitioner (LIP) is permitted by the state and hospital to order a restraint or seclusion. HCFA requires that restraints can only be implemented with an order from a physician or LIP. An LIP must evaluate the client in person within one hour of implementation of restraints. Orders for restraints can be written for up to 4 hours for an adult. The order can be renewed every 4 hours, up to a total of 24 hours. JCAHO allows that following an assessment by an RN, restraints may be implemented and then the physician must be contacted within a specified time frame. Each facility determines the time frame for rewriting restraint orders. Restraints must be evaluated every 8 hours for clients over 18 years of age, every 2 hours for clients 9–17, and 1 hour for children under 9 years. Facilities may choose to be more restrictive, but they cannot be less restrictive in the time frame for renewal of orders.

Documentation of the client's symptoms that lead to the implementation of restraints must be both subjective and objective and derived from a clinical evaluation. All less restrictive interventions utilized must be documented as well.

When restraints are employed, they must be an appropriate method of restraint and be used in the least restrictive manner. The family, significant other, or guardian must be informed immediately when restraints are required. Many hospitals use "sitters" in place of restraints for clients whenever possible. Family members may be called on to sit with the client as well.

Devices and immobilization that are considered protective interventions but not "restraint" interventions include arm boards for IV stabilization, procedural immobilization such as the temporary use of soft restraints to prevent a client from interfering with a related treatment, or soft restraints and tabletop chairs that are used as a temporary preventative measure.

Restraint Guidelines

- Review hospital policy for the use of restraints.
- Requires a physician's order.
- Use restraints for the client's protection and to prevent injury only if all other less restrictive measures are not effective.
- Use the least amount of restraint possible. A torso belt is least restrictive, limb restraint is more restrictive, and chemical (medication) is *most* restrictive.
- Allow clients as much freedom of movement as possible. Use slip knots for quick release. Do not use square knots or bows.
- Always explain the purpose of the restraint to the client and family. Afford as much dignity to the client as possible.
- Remember that restraints can cause emotional, mental, and physical deterioration and increase the risk of injury if falls occur.
- Remember that circulation and skin integrity can be affected by restraints.
- Special precautions should be taken for adult females in restraints to protect breast tissue.
- Clients must be observed every 15 minutes.
- Release restraints every 2 hours for at least 5 minutes, to inspect tissues and provide joint range of motion and position change to prevent circulatory impairment. When a client is combative, release only one restraint at a time.
- Assess and provide for client's fluid and elimination needs, pain management, and position change every 2 hours.
- Pad bony prominences, such as wrist and ankles, beneath a restraint.
- Attempt to make restraints as inconspicuous as possible for the sake of the client's relatives and friends, who may be upset by seeing restraints.
- Clearly document rationale and precautions taken for client safety.
- Notify family, significant other, or guardian if restraints are necessary.
- Enlist support of family members or significant other to sit with client rather than implement restraints.

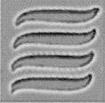

Nursing Diagnoses

The following nursing diagnoses may be appropriate to include in a client care plan when the components are related to maintaining a safe environment.

NURSING DIAGNOSIS	RELATED FACTORS/RISK FACTORS
Risk for Injury	Motor, sensory, or cognitive alterations; elimination urgency; bleeding tendency; physiologic instability due to medications, aging, illness, environmental hazards.
Disturbed Sensory Perception	Medications, decreased sensory acuity, altered level of consciousness, mental status changes, environmental conditions.
Impaired Tissue Integrity	Chemical, thermal, or mechanical factors, decreased mobility, nutritional deficiency.
Self-Mutilation	Labile behavior, depression, guilt, inadequate coping.

- The single most important nursing action to decrease the incidence of hospital-based infections is handwashing. **Remember to wash your hands or use antibacterial gel before and after each and every client contact.**

UNIT 1

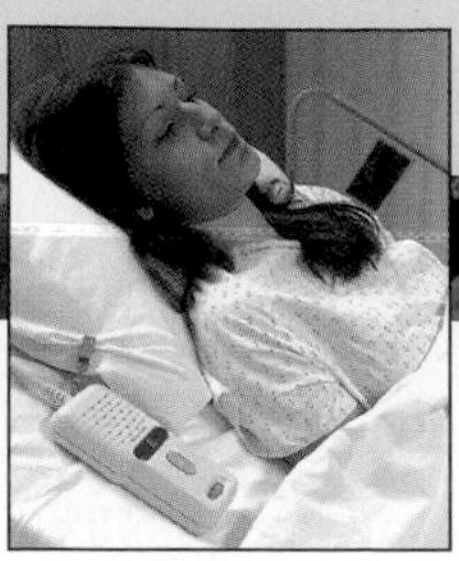

A Safe Environment

Nursing Process Data

ASSESSMENT *Data Base*

Identify client's age, previous or chronic sensory impairments, previous level of mobility, ambulatory aids used, and general health history.

Assess the client's reliability as an accurate health historian.

Identify any alteration of sensory or motor abilities or emotional adaptation due to illness, injury, or hospitalization.

Observe and record client's present level of consciousness, orientation, mobility, and any sensory or motor restrictions.

Evaluate client's ability to comprehend instruction about how to use potentially dangerous equipment.

Evaluate client's ability to make judgments.

Assess need for specific precautions to promote a safe environment.

Assess type of fire extinguisher needed for specific types of fires or use ABC extinguisher.

Assess the need for protection while administering care to clients with radioactive implant.

PLANNING *Objectives*

To provide protection when states of illness decrease the individual's ability to receive and interpret environmental stimuli

To assist client to interpret environmental stimuli relevant to his or her safety

To determine safety equipment necessary to promote a safe environment

To place all personal articles and call light within easy reach of client

To enhance degrees of mobility in a safe environment

To determine that all electrical equipment is intact and operated safely

To determine the protective devices needed when caring for clients receiving radioactive material

IMPLEMENTATION *Procedures*

Preventing Client Falls

Preventing Thermal/Electrical Injuries

Providing Safety for Clients During a Fire

Providing Safety for Clients Receiving Radioactive Materials

EVALUATION *Expected Outcomes*

Client's immediate environment is safe from potential mechanical, chemical, and thermal or electrical hazards.

All personal articles and call light are within easy reach of the client.

Client receives information regarding mechanical, chemical, and thermal safety precautions appropriate to his or her needs.

All electrical equipment is intact and operated safely.

If oxygen is used, appropriate safety measures are in effect.

Personnel are protected from radioactive material.

PREVENTING CLIENT FALLS

Equipment

Side rails, handrails

Alarm systems

Restraints

Locks for movable equipment, such as beds, wheelchairs and gurneys

Procedure

1. Assess all clients for risk factors for falls.
2. Orient new clients to their surroundings, including use of call light.
3. Instruct ambulatory client in use of toilet and shower controls and emergency signals in bathroom.
4. Place bed in low position when you are not providing direct client care.
5. Determine appropriateness for side rail use.
6. Keep half side rails up for all heavily sedated, elderly, confused, and immediate post-surgical clients according to hospital policy.
7. Place articles, such as call light, cups, and water within the client's reach.
8. Pad bed rails for client with high risk for seizures.
9. Remind client and hospital personnel to lock beds, wheelchairs and gurneys and to release the lock only after client is secure for transport.
10. Tell clients who are weak, sedated, in pain, or who have had surgery to ask for assistance before getting out of bed.

> **CLINICAL ALERT**
>
> To prevent at-risk clients from falling out of bed, consider using one of the following interventions:
>
> - Use a mattress with raised edges; use body-length pillows, rolled blankets, or "swimming noodles" (foam flotation aids) under mattress edges.
> - Place mat on floor next to bed.
> - Place client in a very low to ground bed (7 to 13 inches above floor).
> - Use bed alert alarms.
> - Use half or three-fourth length side rails.

EVIDENCE BASED NURSING PRACTICE

Falls in Hospitals

Rigorous research methods were rarely used for falls research, and as a result potential biases and errors threaten their findings. Because of these limitations, the following summary of research findings are considered opinions of respected authorities, based on clinical experience, descriptive studies, or reports of expert committees. Additional research using controlled, randomized trials should be implemented to substantiate the following outcomes of studies conducted by various individuals and groups.

Some studies suggest that clients at risk for falls include those with increased age, those taking certain medications, decreased mental status, impaired mobility, and those with special toileting needs. Other research suggests that age does not play a role in increased falls.

Clients with a history of falls are also at greater risk for additional falls. One study identified that between 16% and 52% of clients may experience more than one fall during their hospitalization.

Impaired mental status was the most commonly identified factor in hospitalized clients who fell. It has not been substantiated as to what constitutes impaired mental status that leads to falls.

Source: Best Practice; Evidence Based Practice Information Sheets for Health Professionals, "Falls in Hospitals," Vol. 2, Issue 2, 1998, ISSN 1329-1874.

CLINICAL ALERT

Multiple intervention fall prevention programs should be implemented in all health care facilities to decrease or prevent falls. Fall prevention interventions should include the following:

- Client risk assessment
- Identify high-risk clients and implement a plan of action to prevent falls
- Educate staff in fall prevention programs
- Decrease environmental risks, obstacles, and clutter
- Implement grab bars in bathroom, and stabilize beds
- Support client's elimination needs
- Monitor client's reaction to medications
- Assist clients with mobility
- Monitor client's mental status
- Institute interventions to prevent falls from bed
- Use safety straps or seat belts when in wheelchairs or geri-chairs
- Involve family members in client prevention program

11. Use two staff to transport client on gurney or wheelchair when nonattached equipment, such as chest-tube system or IV poles, must accompany client in transport.
12. Respond to client's summons as soon as possible.
13. Make sure floors are free of debris that might cause clients to slip and fall. Spilled liquids should be wiped up immediately. Encourage housekeepers to use signs for slippery areas.
14. Check to see that client's unit and hallway are neat and free of hazardous obstacles, such as foot stools, electrical cords, or shoes.

CLINICAL ALERT

There is a tendency for multiple fallers to repeat the type and location of the fall on successive falls (e.g., use of commode). Studies have identified a variety of fall risk factors and have led to the development of a number of fall risk assessment tools. Clients at high risk for fall GENERALLY demonstrate more than one of the following:

- History of falls
- Advanced age
- Sensory or motor impairment
- Urgent need for elimination
- Postural blood pressure instability

for the High-Risk Client

15. Attend to acute changes in client's behavior (e.g., hallucinations, abrupt disorientation or altered responses or cognitive impairment). Monitor client frequently.
16. Continuously orient the disoriented client.
17. Assess and respond to fluid and elimination needs every two hours.
18. Employ bed, chair, and wander alarms.
19. Assign aides or elicit the assistance of sitters or family to monitor the high-risk client; make certain they inform you when they leave the client's side.
20. Relocate high-risk client to room near nurses' station.
21. Utilize a recliner chair for client safety.
22. Keep intercom open between client's room and nurses' station.
23. Secure physician's specific orders if restraints are deemed absolutely necessary.

PREVENTING THERMAL/ELECTRICAL INJURIES

Equipment

Fire extinguishers

Covers for heat and cold application devices

Procedure

1. Make sure that all electrical apparatuses are routinely checked and maintained. Look for safety inspection expiration dates on biomedical equipment.
2. Have all electrical appliances brought to the hospital by client (radios, electric razors, hair dryers, etc.) inspected by hospital maintenance staff. It is best to discourage use of nonhospital equipment.
3. Make sure water in the tub or shower is not more than 110°F (95°F for those with circulatory insufficiency).
4. When heating pads, sitz bath, or hot compresses are used, check the client frequently for redness. Maximum temperature should not exceed 105°F (95°F for those with circulatory insufficiency).
5. Hospitals do not allow smoking in the facility. There may be designated smoking areas outside the building. Inform clients and visitors about the hospital's smoking regulations. Do not allow confused, sedated, or severely incapacitated clients to smoke without direct supervision.
6. Store all combustible materials securely to prevent spontaneous combustion.
7. Make sure that all staff and employees participate in and understand fire safety measures, such as extinguishing fires and plan for evacuating clients.
8. Report and do not use any apparatus that produces a shock, has a broken plug or ground pin, or has a frayed cord.
9. Never apply direct heat (e.g., heating pad) to ischemic tissue—doing so increases the tissue's need for oxygen.

> **CLINICAL ALERT**
>
> The elderly, diabetic, or comatose client is especially vulnerable to thermal injuries.

10. Turn equipment off before unplugging it. **Rationale:** This prevents sparks that can cause a fire.
11. Plug devices that require a high current (i.e., ventilators or radiant warmers) into separate outlets. **Rationale:** This prevents overloading the circuit that could lead to a fire.
12. Use only three-pronged grounded plugs.

PROVIDING SAFETY FOR CLIENTS DURING A FIRE

Equipment

Appropriate extinguisher for fire:
- Water type
- Soda-acid type
- Foam type
- Dry chemical type
- Carbon dioxide type
- ABC extinguisher

Procedure

1. Follow hospital policy and procedure for type of fire safety program and for ringing the fire alarm to summon help.
2. Secure the burning area by closing all doors and windows.
3. Shut off all possible oxygen sources and electrical appliances in the fire area.
4. Remove all clients from the immediate area to a safe place. Be familiar with fire exits and agency evacuation plan.
5. To remove a client safely from the fire, use carrying method that is most comfortable for you and safe for client.
   a. Place blanket (or bedspread) on floor. Lower client onto blanket. Lift up head end of blanket and drag client out of danger.
   b. Use two-person swing method. Place client in sitting position. Form a seat by having two people clasp forearms or shoulders. Lift client into "seat" and carry out of danger.
   c. Carry client using "back-strap" carry method. Step in front of client. Place client's arms around your neck. Grasp client's wrists and hold tight against your chest. Pull client onto your back and carry to safety.
6. If possible, employ the appropriate extinguishing method without endangering yourself. Fire extinguishers should not be used directly on a person.
7. Be familiar with the different types of fire extinguishers and their location.

Class A

a. Water-under-pressure type or soda-acid type.
b. Use on cloth, wood, paper, plastic, rubber, or leather.
c. Never use on electrical or chemical fires due to danger of shock.

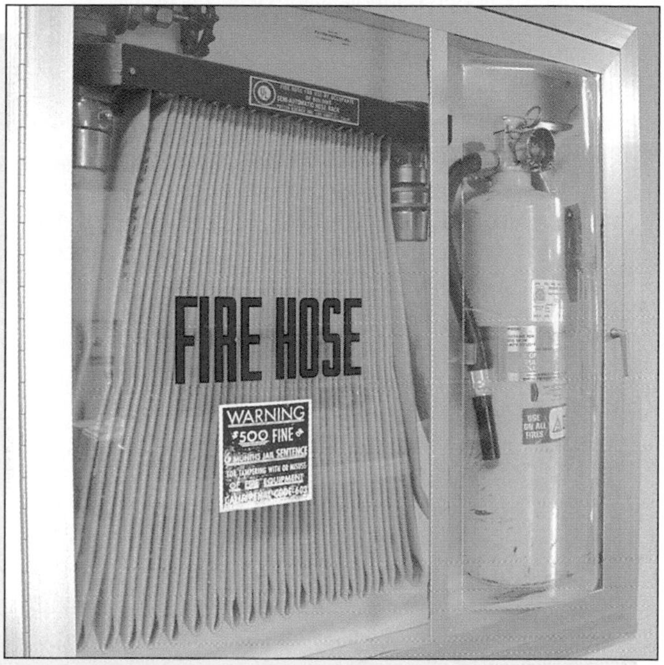

Become familiar with the location and use of fire extinguishers in the hospital.

Class B

a. Foam, dry chemical, carbon dioxide types.
b. Use on fires such as gasoline, alcohol, acetone, oil, grease, or paint thinner and remover.
c. Class A extinguisher is never used on class B fires.

Class C

a. Dry chemical or carbon dioxide types.
b. Use on electrical wiring, electrical equipment, or motors.
c. Class A or class B extinguishers are never used on class C fires.

Class ABC combination

a. Contains graphite.
b. Use on any type of fire.
c. Most common extinguisher in use.

8. Keep fire exits clear at all times.

PROVIDING SAFETY FOR CLIENTS RECEIVING RADIOACTIVE MATERIALS

Equipment

Protective shields for x-ray
Lead-shielded container if required
Film badge if required
Sign for client's door: "Caution, Radioactive Material"

Procedure

1. Review these guidelines:
   a. Determine the type and amount of radiation used and its side effects and hazards.
   b. Increased time in the presence of a radioactive source increases exposure to radiation. Rotate care providers.
   c. Shields, such as lead walls or lead aprons, are used as protection from radioactive source.
   d. Exposure is greater the closer the person is to the radioactive source.
   e. When not in use, radioactive material must be stored in lead-shielded containers.
2. If nurse or family member is assisting with a radioactive procedure, they must put on a shield.
3. If a radioactive implant is used in a client, all nurses and visitors must be protected with a shield. Limit exposure with the client.
4. Keep track of how much time is spent in the presence of radioactive material. Request film badge if in area where ionizing radiation is used frequently.
5. Constantly assess and support clients who are undergoing radiation therapy. Bed rest, isolation, and unpleasant side effects are sometimes common.
6. Follow guidelines for working with clients with unsealed sources of Iodine-131.

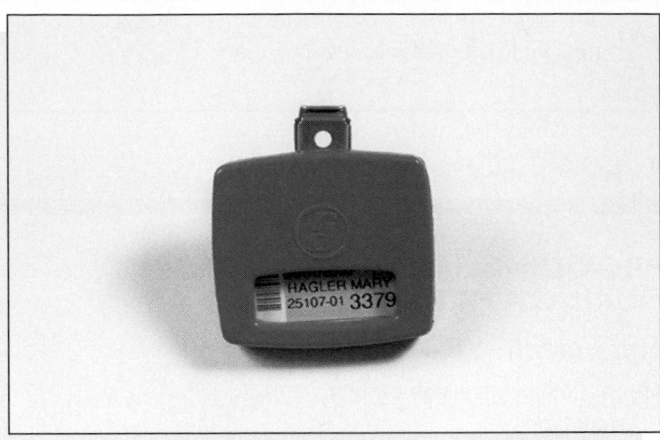

Wear film badge when client has radioactive material in place.

   a. Wear rubber gloves at all times when providing care.
   b. Wash gloves before removing, and place in designated waste container.
   c. Wash hands with soap and water after removing gloves.
   d. Dispose of all bed linen in contaminated linen bag.
   e. Wrap all nondisposable items that have come in contact with client's blood, saliva, or gastric juices in plastic bag. Send to appropriate hospital department for decontamination (usually nuclear medicine department).
   f. Notify radiation safety officer (usually in radiology department) if clothes or shoes have been contaminated.

CLINICAL ALERT

Pregnant nurses should check hospital policy regarding working with clients receiving radioactive materials.

General Guidelines for Radiation Precautions*

Radioactive Implant

Care time not to exceed 15 minutes per employee per day.

No pregnant woman or anyone under age 18 should enter room.

No special handling of excreta other than universal precautions.

Bath usually omitted, client movement restricted.

Visitors limited to 1 hour/day, keeping distance from client.

All linens, gloves, trash, dressings, and so on kept in room until cleared by radiation safety officer.

Systemic Radioactive Material

No lab specimens to be taken without consent of radiation safety officer.

Use disposable dietary tray.

Handle all excreta and secretions with gloves.

Have client use toilet—flushing twice.

Shielding not needed.

No visitors without special instructions.

Keep gloves, dressings, linens, and trash in contaminated container.

*Note: See Institutional Policy for Specifics.

DOCUMENTATION FOR PROVIDING A SAFE ENVIRONMENT

- Assessment notes
- Actual incidents involving mechanical, chemical, or thermal trauma
- Client education given
- Safety devices used

Critical Thinking Application

UNEXPECTED OUTCOMES	CRITICAL THINKING OPTIONS
The client, nurse, or visitor experiences an accident or injury related to mechanical, chemical, or thermal trauma.	• Provide immediate first aid or care • Assess vital signs, and notify physician. • Report the incident according to hospital procedure. Unusual occurrence forms are used to protect the injured individual, the nurse, and the hospital. • Review safety procedures to ensure a safe environment. • Report all malfunctioning equipment immediately to the proper department.
Unfamiliarity with hospital fire and disaster protocol results in poor performance.	• Review protocols frequently to update knowledge base. • Participate in fire and disaster drills to become familiar with protocols.
Radium implant becomes dislodged and falls out.	• Put on lead gloves, pick up radium with forceps and place in lead-shielded container in client's room. • Notify physician and hospital radiation safety officer immediately. • Never touch radioactive source directly.
Spillage of excreta from client with systemic radioactive therapy.	• Cover spillage with absorbent material and notify radiation safety officer. • Wash with soap and water if skin contaminated. Notify radiation safety officer.

UNIT 2

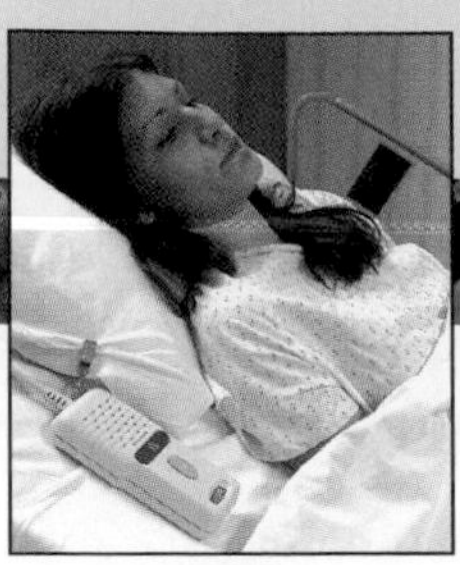

Restraints

Nursing Process Data

ASSESSMENT **Data Base**

Assess client's risk for falls on an ongoing basis.

Assess need for fall prevention measures.

Identify least restrictive type of restraint, if needed.

Assess area under and surrounding a restraint to ensure it is not restrictive.

Evaluate client's response to restraint use.

PLANNING **Objectives**

To identify clients who are at risk for injury

To prevent a client from injuring himself (herself) or others

To employ fall prevention measures

To obtain physician's order for restraints if deemed absolutely necessary

To apply restraints safely and effectively

To restrain a child's elbow to prevent the child from reaching an incision

To promote client safety when ambulating or sitting in a chair

IMPLEMENTATION **Procedures**

Managing Clients in Restraints

Applying Torso/Belt Restraint

Using Wrist Restraints

Using Mitt Restraints

Using Elbow Restraints

Applying a Vest Restraint

for Client in Bed

for Client in Wheelchair

Applying Mummy Restraints

EVALUATION **Expected Outcomes**

Client is prevented from injuring himself (herself) or others.

Restraints are applied appropriately.

Client does not develop complications due to restraint use (e.g., agitation, pressure sores, circulatory disturbance).

Child is prevented from reaching the incision site.

MANAGING CLIENTS IN RESTRAINTS

Equipment

Appropriate restraint, limb, torso, and vest

Preparation

1. Identify and evaluate if all less restrictive measures have been explored before the client is placed in restraints.
2. Call physician or LIP for restraint order before applying restraints. If restraints must be placed before the order is obtained, ensure the order is obtained within one hour for either a nonbehavioral health client or a behavioral health client.

NOTE: Follow guidelines for obtaining restraint orders and updating orders according to hospital policy.

3. Ensure that a face-to-face assessment is completed on the client within 8 hours for a nonbehavioral health client, and 1 hour for a behavioral (psychiatric) health client.
4. Ensure that restraint orders are renewed every 24 hours or sooner according to facility policy for nonbehavioral health clients, or every 4 hours for behavioral health clients. Children from 12 to 17 must have orders renewed every 2 hours, for a maximum of 24 hours.
5. Establish and implement a plan of care for the client to eliminate the need for restraints.
6. Discuss the use of restraints with the client and family members. If possible, elicit the support of the family or use sitters to stay with the client rather than place the client in restraints.

Procedure

1. Gather appropriate restraint.
2. Seek the client's cooperation with restraint procedure, if possible.

There are three types of restraints used in clinical practice:

1. *Chemical:* Sedating psychotropic drugs to manage or control behavior. Psychoactive medication used in this manner is an inappropriate use of medication.
2. *Physical:* Direct application of physical force to a client, without the client's permission, to restrict his or her freedom of movement.
3. *Seclusion:* Involuntary confinement of a client in a locked room.

Physical force may be applied by individuals, mechanical devices, or a combination of any of them.

Source: JCAHO, 2000.

CLINICAL ALERT

Restraints are indicated only if there is no other viable option available to protect the client; and then they are implemented only when the client is assessed and evaluated by an appropriate licensed independent practitioner.

3. Apply restraint according to specific directions.
4. Monitor and assess the client every 15 minutes.
5. Release restraint at least every two orders and provide:
   a. Toileting.
   b. Fluids and food.
   c. Hygiene care such as brushing teeth or washing face and hands.
   d. Check circulation and skin, provide skin care.
   e. Check for body alignment.
   f. Provide range of motion to all joints, particularly those in restraints.
6. Avoid application of force on long bone joints when applying or repositioning a restraint.
7. Take vital signs every 8 hours unless indicated more frequently.
8. Bathe client every 24 hours.
9. Do not interrupt the client's sleep unless indicated by his/her medical condition.
10. Ensure that a new order and the physician or LIP completes a medical assessment every 24 hours.
11. Obtain a physician's order and discontinue restraints as soon as it is clinically indicated.
12. Document all assessments and findings on appropriate forms.

CLINICAL ALERT

In acute medical and post-surgical care, a restraint may be necessary to ensure that an IV or tube feeding is not removed, or the client cannot be allowed out of bed following surgery. This type of medical restraint may be used temporarily to limit mobility or prevent injury to the client. This is not considered a restraint as discussed above.

Additional types of activities that may constitute a restraint include:

- Tucking a client's sheet so tight that he/she cannot move.
- Using a side rail to prevent a client from voluntarily getting out of bed.
- Placing the client in a geri-chair with a table.
- Placing a wheel-chair bound client so close to the wall that it prevents them from moving.

TABLE 7–1 Methods to Decrease Use of Physical or Chemical Restraints

Environmental Alterations	Physiological Approaches
• Use alternatives such as wedge or roll cushions for positional support • Adjust lighting at night to decrease fear of unknown and facilitate vision of where bed is in room • Use rolled edge mattresses • Use low level beds (7–13 in. from floor) • Place mats on floor in case of client fall • Use special beds • Place in special unit where client can be watched more carefully • Use sitters or family members • Use upper side rails only for aid in turning and moving	• Potential complication assessment; i.e., increased temperature or hypoxia • Pain relief • Comfort measures • Physical therapy/exercises **Psychosocial Interventions** • Identify and alter factors that are causing client anxiety, if possible • Talk with client • Involve client in activities that take his or her mind off what is happening • Encourage interaction with family members by phone if necessary

APPLYING TORSO/BELT RESTRAINT

Equipment

Safety belt restraint (usually 2 inch soft webbing material) with waist and side belts (for bed)

Procedure

1. Check physician's order and client care plan for torso/belt restraint.
2. Obtain belt. (Belts usually have a key locked buckle to prevent slipping and to provide a snug fit.)
3. Explain necessity for safety belt to client and family.
4. Apply torso restraint as follows:
   a. Slip waist belt through flat buckle, adjusting to client's size.
   b. Snap hinged plate shut by hooking plain end of key over cross bar and lifting upward.
   c. Attach side belts to bed frame in similar manner.
   d. Release restraint by hooking green end of key over cross bar from below and pulling downward.
5. Document time, rationale, and type of safety belt used in nurses' notes, along with client monitoring, client response, frequency of care measures, and time and rationale for discontinuing restraint. Documentation must be done every 15 minutes.

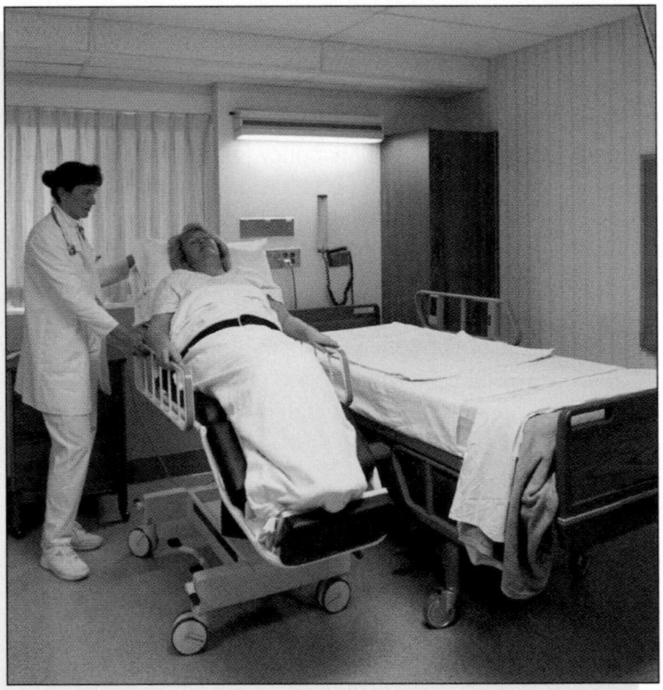

Some belts have a key-locked buckle to prevent slipping and to provide a snug fit.

EVIDENCE BASED NURSING PRACTICE

Deaths Due to Use of Physical Restraint or Seclusion

A 50-state survey by the *Hartford Courant* in 1998 identified at least 142 deaths related to the use of physical restraint or seclusion since 1988. The true number of deaths is much higher since data regarding this type of information is not public information. According to statistical projections commissioned by the *Courant* and conducted by the Harvard Center for Risk Analysis, between 50 and 150 deaths occur every year across the country due to improper restraint procedures. Based on this data, it was felt there is a critical need for mandated monitoring of the use of restraints and seclusion.

Source: Position Statements: Reduction of Patient Restraint and Seclusion in Health Care Settings, www://ana.org/readroom/position/ethics.

USING WRIST RESTRAINTS

Equipment

Commercial cloth restraints with flannel padding
Ace bandages of appropriate size for area to be immobilized
Call bell for communication

Procedure

1. Attempt all other methods of client protection or less restrictive measures before applying restraints.
2. Check physician's order for wrist or ankle soft restraint. If necessary, place restraint on client, then phone physician or LIP for orders within one hour of application of restraint.
3. Obtain soft restraints.
4. When applying restraint, place padded section over the wrist or ankle.
5. Secure restraint by pinching long-pronged adapter and inserting into buckle end of restraint, or follow manufacturer's directions.

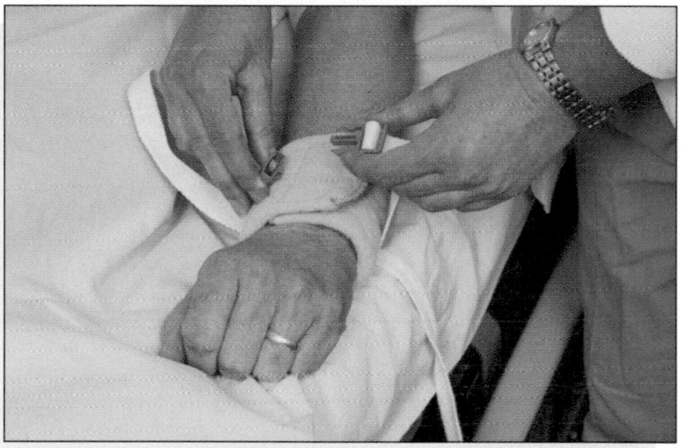

Secure restraint by pinching long-pronged adapter and inserting into buckle end of restraint.

6. Attach other end of restraint under movable portion of bed frame by using a half-bow knot. **Rationale:** This is a quick release knot and will untie quickly in an emergency.

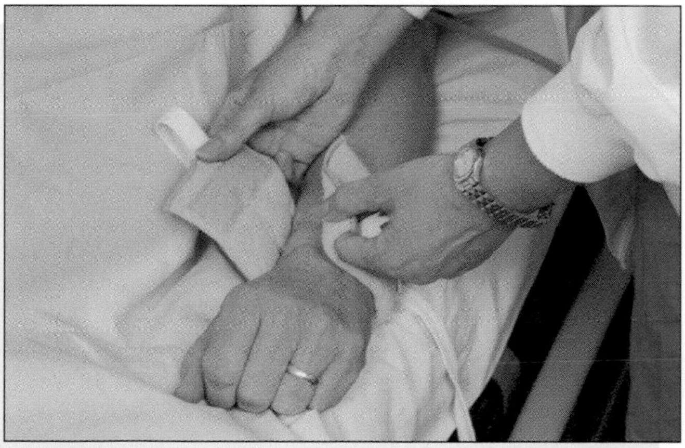

First, apply padded portion of restraint around wrist or ankle.

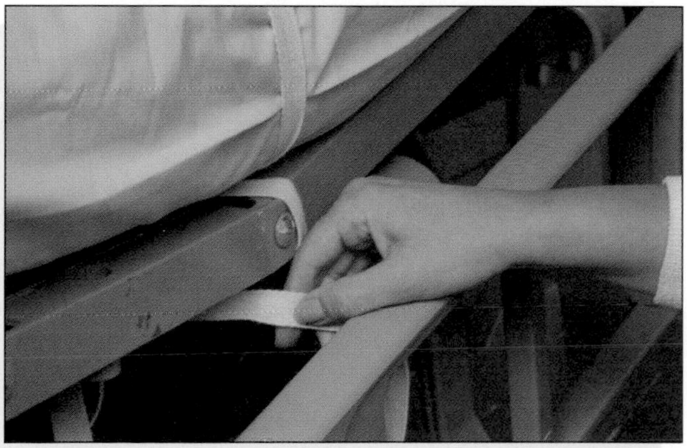

Secure restraint under moveable part of bed, using slipknot.

CLINICAL ALERT

Always keep scissors in easy access to facilitate cutting restraints in case of an emergency.

7. Release restraints every 2 hours to:
   a. Check limb circulation and skin condition.
   b. Provide extremity range of motion.
   c. Change client's position.
   d. Attend to elimination, fluid, or other needs.
8. Document use of and rationale for wrist restraints in nurses' notes. Identify all less restrictive actions tried before restraints.
9. Monitor client every 15 minutes.

CLINICAL ALERT

Limb, vest, and mitt restraints are considered a Type II restraint. A Type I restraint is a four-point locked restraint. Type I restraints are used primarily in psychiatric or emergency room settings.

If using *any* locked restraint, keep the key in client's room taped to the top of bed or near "stat" call button. It must be in sight and easily accessible in case of emergency.

Alternate Type of Soft Restraint

- Slide strap through slit in restraint.
- Tighten strap, leaving fingerbreadth space between restraint and client's limb.

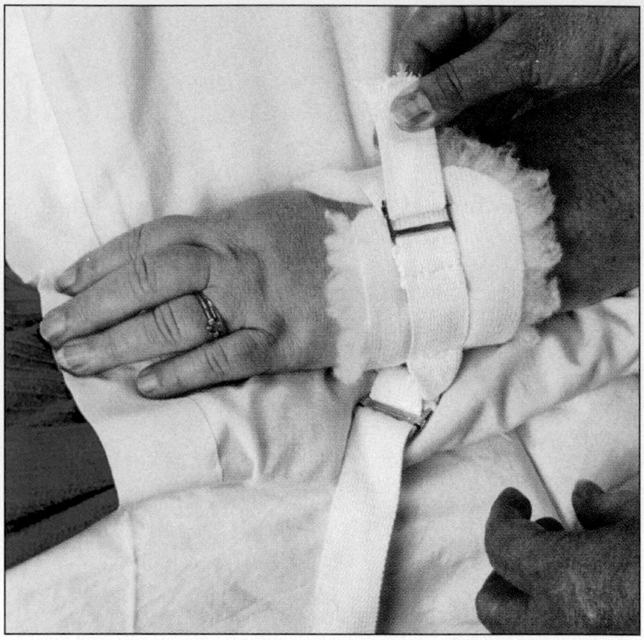

Precautions for Using Restraints

- Try restraint-free alternatives before restraints.
- Use correct size and apply according to manufacturer instructions.
- Follow facility's written policy on restraint use.
- Tie restraints only to bedsprings or frame.
- Supervise client closely and relieve restraints every two hours.
- Ensure that physician or LIP sees client within 8 hours if client is in medical surgical section of facility, or 1 hour if client is in mental health section.

USING MITT RESTRAINTS

Equipment

Mitt restraint
Gauze padding
Call bell for communication

Procedure

1. Check physician's order, or after placing mitt restraint, phone physician or LIP for orders.
2. Determine if less restrictive actions could be used.
3. Wash hands.
4. Obtain appropriate size mitt restraint and gauze padding, if needed.
5. Identify the client by checking identaband.
6. Explain steps and purpose of procedure to family and client (to gain his or her cooperation) if client is able to understand.
7. Raise bed to high position.
8. Lower side rail.

9. Check condition of skin and circulation in involved extremity.
10. Wrap fingers with gauze to absorb moisture and prevent abrasion, if necessary.
11. Apply mitt; secure wrist ties snugly, but maintain circulation by assuring that 2 fingers can be slipped under the restraint.
12. For hand control, use slip knot to tie restraints to immovable part of bed frame, not to side rail.
13. Place call bell within access and monitor client every 15 minutes.
14. Remove mitt every 2 hours to:
    a. Check adequacy of circulation and skin condition.
    b. Provide extremity range of motion.
    c. Change client's position.
    d. Provide for fluid, elimination, or other needs.
15. Reapply mitt.
16. Raise bedrail and lower bed, according to facility policy.
17. Wash hands.
18. Chart on nurses' notes: client behavior necessitating restraint; all less restrictive actions taken, condition of skin, adequacy of circulation of involved extremity; time of mitt application; times of release and observed responses, and care needs met. Documentation must be done every 15 minutes.

CLINICAL ALERT

Restraints are never used as a substitute for surveillance. *Note: In confused ambulatory clients, restraint use has been associated with increased falls.*

USING ELBOW RESTRAINTS

Equipment

Elbow restraint
Soft padding

Procedure

1. Check physician's order. This type of restraint, if used for medical procedures or to protect IVs, does not require specific restraint orders.
2. Obtain elbow restraints (many types are available).
3. Explain necessity of restraints to child's parents.
4. Place restraints over elbow of both arms. You may need to insert tongue blades into pockets of restraint.
5. Wrap restraints snugly around the arm. Secure by tying the restraints at the top. Many restraints have ties long enough to cross under the child's back and tie under the opposite arm.
6. For small infants and children, tie or pin restraints to their shirts.
7. Release the restraints every 2 hours to allow joint mobility.
8. Assess position of restraints, circulation, skin condition, and sensation every hour.
9. Provide diversionary activity for small child.
10. Encourage parents or hospital personnel to hold child to promote a feeling of security.
11. Document use of restraints in nurses' notes. Document release of restraints, skin, and circulatory condition. Documentation must be done every 15 minutes.

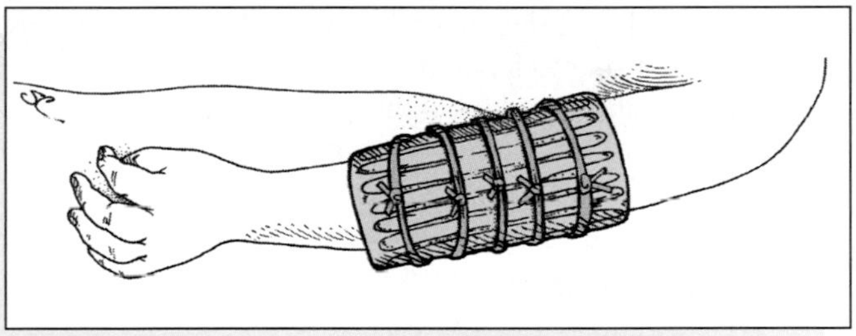

Elbow restraints prevent children from reaching equipment.

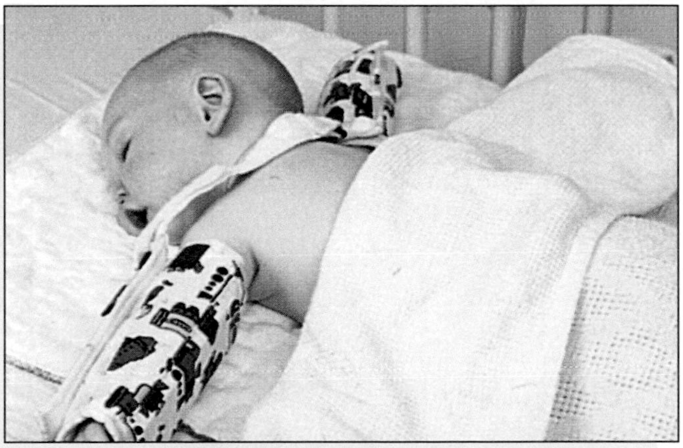

Elbow restraints may be used to prevent child from reaching his or her face or head.

APPLYING A VEST RESTRAINT

Equipment

Safety vest
Call bell for communication

Procedure

for Client in Bed

1. Check physician's order or apply vest and call physician or LIP within 1 hour for order.
2. Determine if less restrictive actions could be used.
3. Explain necessity for jacket or vest restraint to client and family.
4. Place vest over gown.
5. Place safety vest on client so that closed side of vest is in back and front side of vest crosses over chest or according to manufacturer's directions. **Rationale:** This prevents choking if client slumps forward.
6. Bring strap through slit in front of the vest. **Rationale:** Criss-crossing vest in the back may cause serious injury.
7. Tie straps to nonmovable upper section of bed frame using slipknot. **Rationale:** This position minimizes risk of inadvertent release, which may cause subsequent injury.

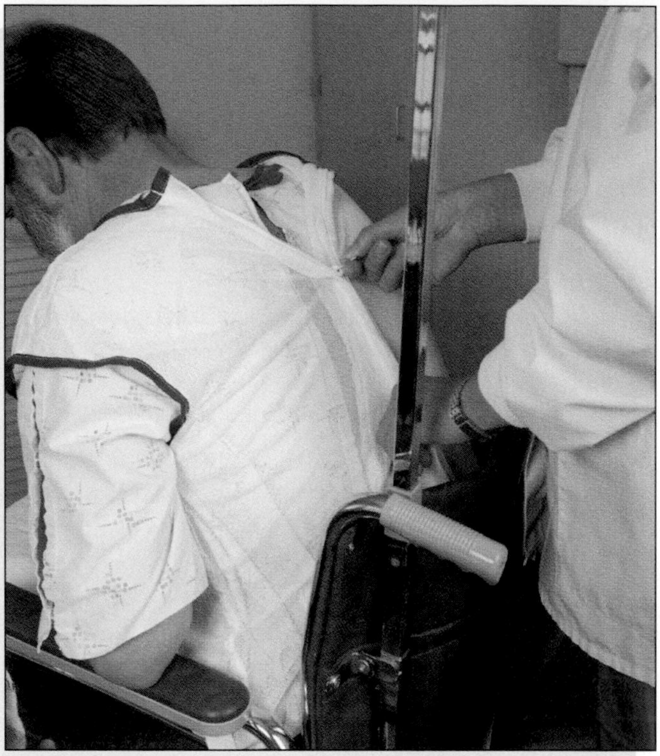
Zip vest from bottom to top at client's back.

CLINICAL ALERT

The use of vest restraint has been associated with serious injury, including client suffocation.

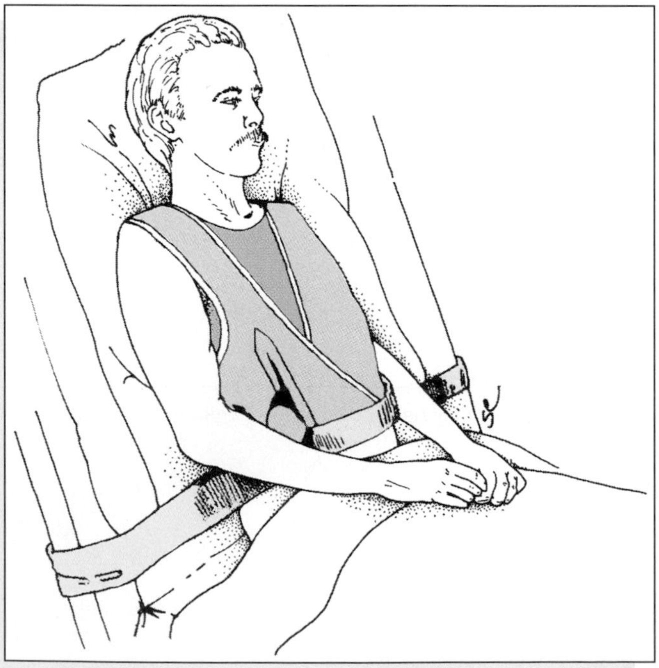
Vest restraint can be used for client on bed rest.

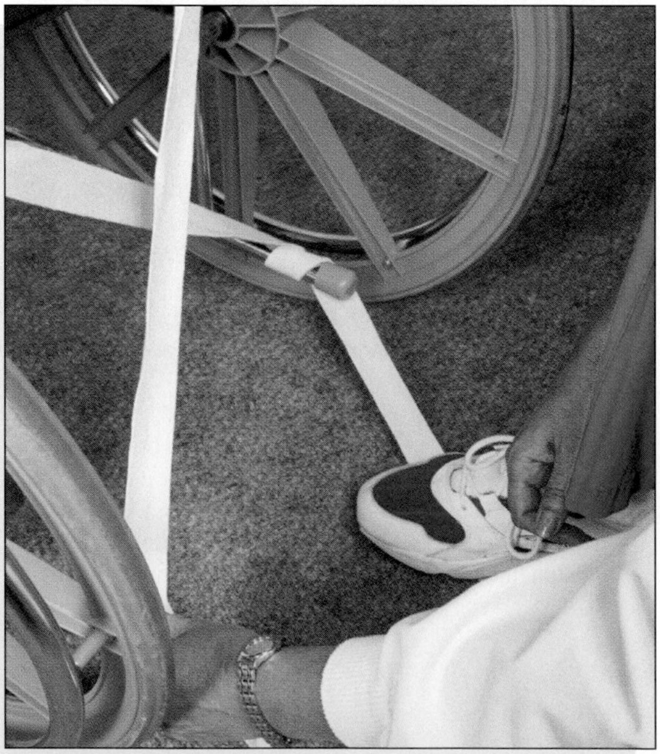
Pull vest tails under armrests and cross tails in back of chair. Wrap tails around immovable kickspur.

8. Observe client every 15 minutes to ensure proper fit of jacket.
9. Release vest restraint every 2 hours. Follow interventions for releasing restraints of all types.
10. Document use and rationale for restraint in nurses' notes every 15 minutes.
11. Document client assessment and attendance to fluid and elimination needs regularly.

for Client in Wheelchair

1. Place client in wheelchair with buttocks against chair back.
2. Place vest on client, zipper vest is best. Zip vest from bottom to top. Ensure that there is adequate space between vest and client. **Rationale:** To prevent constriction from vest that is too tight.
3. Pull straps at 45-degree angle to rear of seat and pull vest tails under armrests and cross tails in back of chair. **Rationale:** Tying vest tails in back of chair prevents client from reaching the tails and untying the vest.
4. Wrap tails around immovable kickspur. **Rationale:** This anchors the tails and prevents client from slipping out of restraints.
5. Tie each tail to kickspur using half-bow knot. **Rationale:** This type of knot is used because it can be quickly released if necessary.
6. Check client every 15 minutes to ensure vest is on correctly and client is not in compromising situation.
7. Document every 15 minutes according to policy.

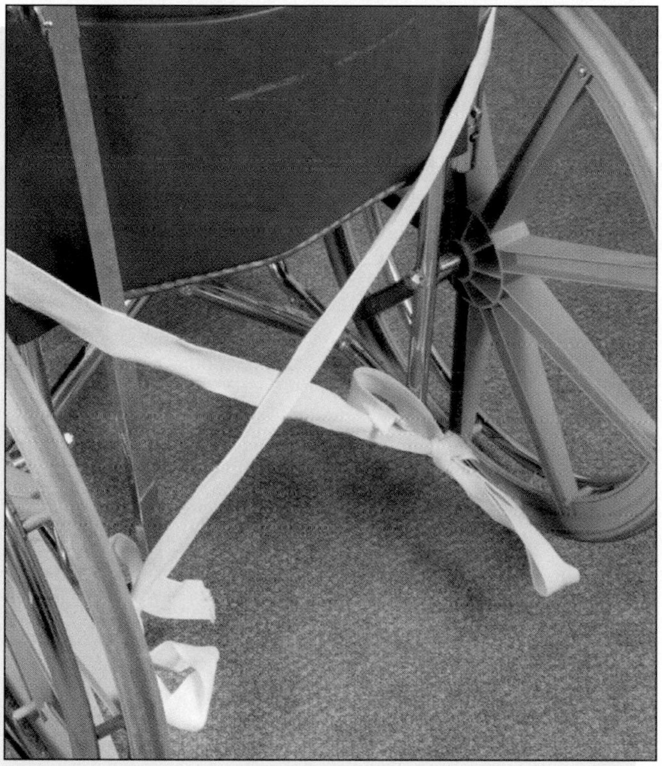

Tie each tail to kickspur using half-bow knot.

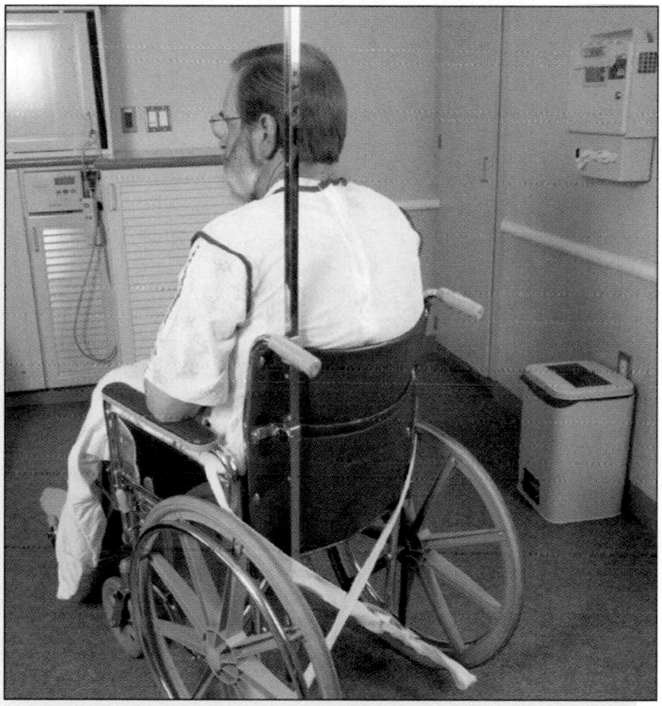

Check client every 15 minutes while in restraint.

Tying a Half-Bow Knot

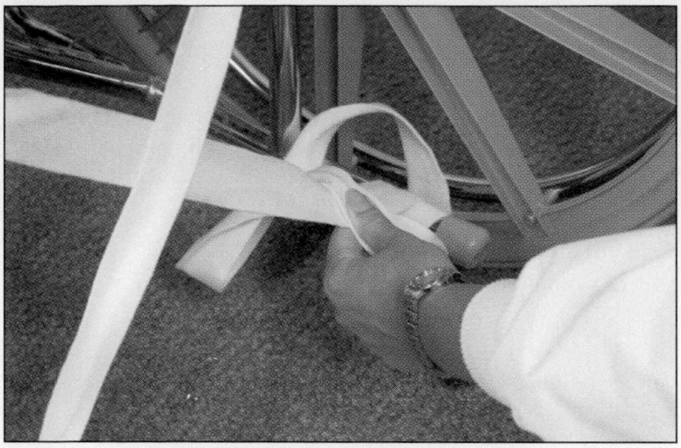

Place restraint tie around wheelchair kickspur. Bring free end up, around, under, and over attached end of tie and pull tight.

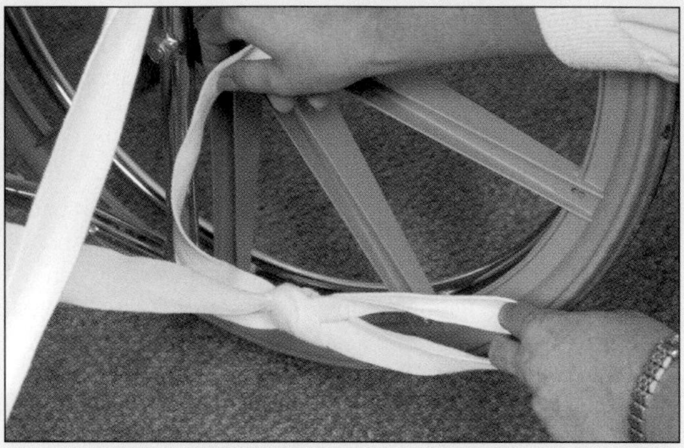

Tighten free end of tie and bow until knot is secure.

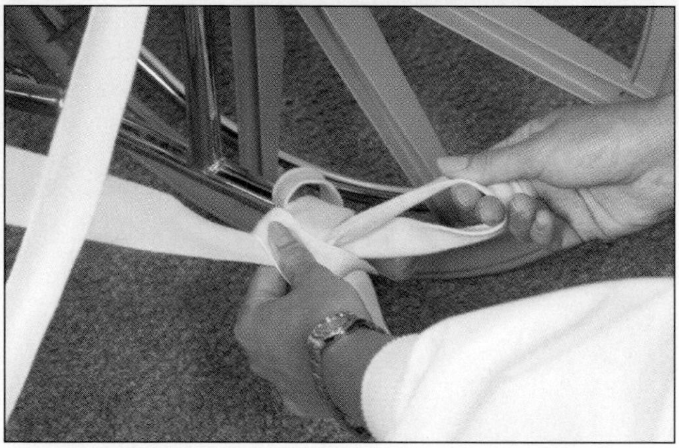

Take free end over and under attached end of tie, but this time make half-bow loop.

CLINICAL ALERT

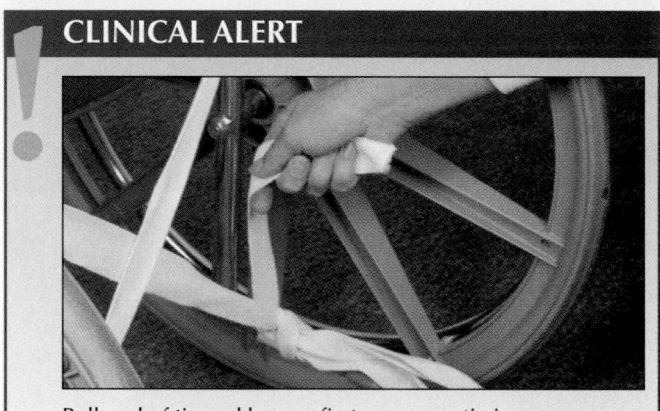

Pull end of tie and loosen first crossover tie in an emergency.

APPLYING MUMMY RESTRAINTS

Equipment

Blanket large enough to fit child

Procedure

1. Place the blanket on a secure surface.
2. Fold down one corner of the blanket until the tip reaches the middle of the blanket.
3. Place the baby in a diagonal position with the head halfway off the folded edge of the blanket.
4. Bring one side of the blanket over the infant's arm and trunk, and tuck it under the other arm and around the back.

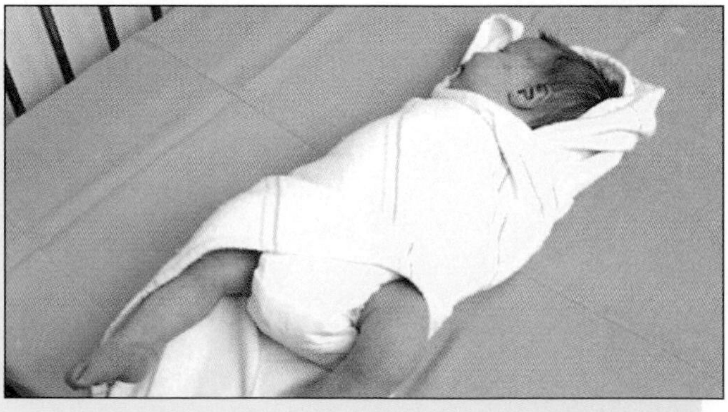

A mummy restraint is used when certain procedures are to be done.

5. Tuck the bottom part of the blanket up onto the infant's abdomen.
6. Fold the second side over the infant, and tuck it snugly around the body.
7. Use the restraint only until procedure is completed.

Mummy boards with Velcro straps are used more often in the hospital setting. A diaper or Chux is placed on the board, the infant is placed on the board and secured with the Velcro straps.

CLINICAL ALERT

Generally, restraint policies do not apply to:

- Restriction for security purposes.
- Procedure-related immobilization (e.g., for medical, surgical, or diagnostic procedure).
- Use of adaptive support devices (e.g., brace, orthopedic appliances).
- Use of medical protective devices (e.g., tabletop chairs, bed rails).
- Voluntary restraint (client consent).

DOCUMENTATION FOR APPLYING RESTRAINTS

- Description of specific behaviors leading to restraint.
- Note all less restrictive techniques used. If less restrictive techniques were not used, provide rationale.
- Extent to which client is able to cooperate with restraint procedure.
- Any injury to client or others.
- All observation data for entire length of restraints. Usually, a form is completed.
- Justification and reassessment for continued use of restraints.
- Document review of care plan for effectiveness or rationale for ineffectiveness of care plan.

DATE: ____________ UNIT: ____________ REASON FOR RESTRAINT: ____________

SUGGESTED ALTERNATIVES TO RESTRAINT USE CONSIDERED DURING THE RE-ASSESSMENT PROCESS:

TIME

___ ___ ___ Met patient s comfort needs
___ ___ ___ Changed or elimin ated bothersome treatments
___ ___ ___ Modified the environment
___ ___ ___ Reality orientation and psychosocial interventions
___ ___ ___ Provided companionship and supervision
___ ___ ___ Offered diversion and physical activities
___ ___ ___ Designed creative alternatives

CODES:

DESCRIPTION
2P = 2 POINT 3P = 3 POINT
4P = 4 POINT G = GERICHAIR
M = MITTENS 4S = 4 SIDERAILS WITH PROTECTIVE PADS

LEVEL OF CONSCIOUSNESS
A = ALERT
D = DROWSY
C = CONFUSED

RESPONSE
C = CALM
A = AGITATED
S = SLEEPING

RESTRAINT RESOLUTION
A = APPLIED
R = RELEASED
A/R = APPLIED & RELEASED

EFFECT
A = ADEQUATE
I = INADEQUATE

SIGN/CIRCULATION
I = INTACT R = BROKEN
R = REDDENED M = MOTTLED
P = PULSES PALPABLE

RANGE OF MOTION
Y = YES
N = NO
S = SLEEPING

POSITION
R = RIGHT SIDE
L = LEFT SIDE
S = SUPINE
P = PRONE

FLUIDS/NOURISHMENT/TOILETING
Y = YES
N = NO
R = REFUSED
*SEE OBSERVATIONS

TIME	0800	1000	1200	1400	1600	1800	2000	2200	2400	0200	0400	0600
NOTE: PATIENT IS MONITORED EVERY 15 MINUTES. DOCUMENT EVERY 2 HOURS.												
DESCRIPTION												
LEVEL OF CONSCIOUSNESS												
RESPONSE to RESTRAINT												
RESTRAINT RESOLUTION												
EFFECT of RESTRAINT												
SKIN/CIRCULATION												
NOTE: PATIENT IS MONITORED AND DOCUMENTED ON EVERY 2 HOURS.												
RANGE OF MOTION												
POSITION												
FLUIDS/ NOURISHMENT												
TOILETING												
INITIALS												

SIGNATURE/TITLE	INITIALS	SIGNATURE/TITLE	INITIALS	SIGNATURE/TITLE	INITIALS
SIGNATURE/TITLE	INITIALS	SIGNATURE/TITLE	INITIALS	SIGNATURE/TITLE	INITIALS
SIGNATURE/TITLE	INITIALS	SIGNATURE/TITLE	INITIALS	SIGNATURE/TITLE	INITIALS

COMMUNITY HOSPITAL

PATIENT I.D. #
NAME
SEX AGE SS #
BIRTH DATE MED. REC. # FIN. CLASS
DOCTOR ADMIT. DATE

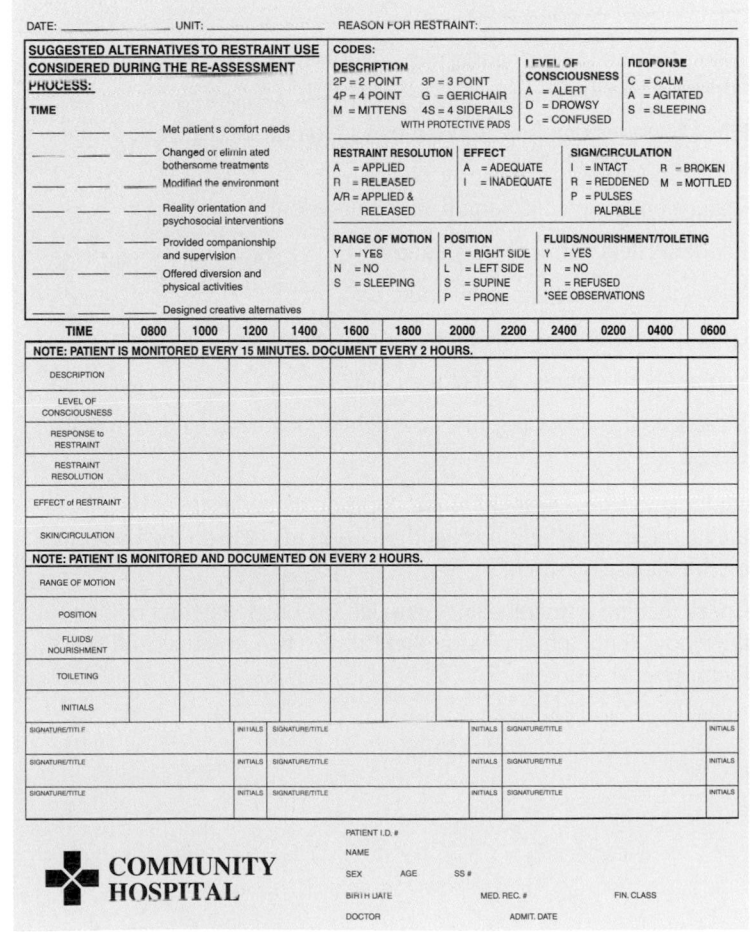

Restraint/Seclusion Flow Sheet.

Critical Thinking Application

UNEXPECTED OUTCOMES	CRITICAL THINKING OPTIONS
Skin abrasion, maceration, or rash occurs following application of restraints.	• Reassess absolute need for restraint. • Reassess application method. • Increase padding of soft restraints before application. • Keep restraints off as much as possible and have staff or family member stay with client.
Impaired circulation or edema evidenced by change in color, sensation, movement, and blanching of nail beds.	• On observation of signs of neurovascular changes, immediately release restraints. • Massage area gently to increase circulation. • If extremity is edematous, elevate extremity above level of heart. Encourage range of motion. • Request order for different type of restraint.
Client unties restraints.	• Camouflage restraint to decrease client's awareness. • Reassess need for restraint. • Exhaust alternative measures to promote safety. • Anticipate and attend to client's needs.
Client with history of falling has developed acute cognitive changes.	• Alert all personnel that client is high risk for fall. • Review medication regimen (e.g., Demerol and psychoactive drugs can cause acute confusion). • Assess for physiologic causes (e.g., hypoxemia, infection, pain) and address alterations. • Place bedside commode and remove obstacles; provide good lighting as well as night light. • Reduce environmental stimuli (e.g., television). • Reorient client with each encounter. • Move client for better surveillance. • Employ monitoring alarm/device or engage family attendance. • Request floor mattress or recliner chair.
Child is able to reach incision site even with elbow restraints in place.	• Make sure the elbow restraints are tight enough and extend over the elbow. • Tie the one elbow restraint to the opposite elbow restraint by placing the tie under the child's back and securing the tie with the upper tie on the opposite restraint. • Check that the restraint is large enough to completely immobilize the elbow. If not, obtain a larger size or use two restraints and tie them together securely.

GERONTOLOGIC CONSIDERATIONS

Safety precautions for the elderly

- Assure sensory adaptive devices are used (glasses, hearing aid).
- Use one-half to three-quarter rails rather than full rails.
- Provide adequate lighting.
- Provide and encourage use of call bell/summons device.
- Assess fluid and elimination needs regularly.
- Promote ADLs and exercise to maintain muscle strength and flexibility.
- Heed client's summons promptly.
- Put necessary articles for personal hygiene and activities of daily living within easy reach.
- Provide nonslip mats and grab bars in bath tubs, showers, and near toilets.
- Use shower chair.
- Mop up spills promptly.
- Keep hallways clear of obstacles.
- Lock all equipment when not moving client.
- Provide handrails in hallways.
- Maintain a consistent environment: keep furniture in established places.

Preventing thermal injury

- Skin is fragile and prone to injury as client's age increases. Use thermal treatments with caution. Do not apply *direct* heat to areas with ischemic tissue.
- Check skin frequently when any type of heat therapy (e.g., Aqua K pad) is used.
- Check water temperature before placing client in bathtub (95°F for the elderly and those with peripheral circulation impairment).

Wandering-client management plan

- Clients who are identified as potential wanderers from a facility or at risk for falls should wear a monitor device.
- Monitors come in various models, each one designed to identify clients who move away from a designated monitor zone.
- Clients need to be checked regularly to ensure the monitor is appropriately positioned and the alarm functions properly.

MANAGEMENT GUIDELINES

Each state legislates a Nurse Practice Act for RNs and LVN/LPNs. Health care facilities are responsible for establishing and implementing policies and procedures that conform to their state's regulations. Verify the regulations and role parameters for each health care worker in your facility.

Delegation of Responsibilities

- Before nursing staff is assigned to care for clients requiring restraints, the team leader and/or charge nurse must ensure they have been properly educated in the legal requirements as well as in the application of restraints.
- All personnel must be aware of environmental and client risks for injury. Remind staff to notify RN of risks.
- Nurses must help identify clients at high risk for injury and must be familiar with agency plan/protocol for the prevention of injury.
- Nurses must individualize restraint implementation.

Information Flow

- Clients at high risk for injury: Report client risk behaviors, attempts to determine underlying cause, attempted alternative protective measures, and rationale for choice of restraint.
- Document type and time restraint initiated, regular monitoring, and client response. According to the FDA, approximately 20 clients die every year from protective restraints. It is critical to instruct all personnel (including CNAs and UAPs who may not administer the restraints, but give client care and therefore, observe restraint use) in the proper use of restraints.

CRITICAL THINKING STRATEGIES

Scenario 1

As you enter Mrs. Lake's room, you find her with one leg over the side rail, making attempts to get out of bed unassisted. Mrs. Lake is an 82-year-old client with a history of congestive heart failure (CHF). When you question what she is doing, she tells you, "I need to go to the bathroom." She also tells you she is sure her dog needs to be let out because she hasn't been able to get out of the bed all morning. This is your second day caring for Mrs. Lake. Your initial assessment on admission 2 days ago included her being oriented to person, place, time, and thing. The night shift reported off saying she was disoriented all night.

1. What is your first nursing action? Provide rationale for your response.
2. What additional priority nursing actions are justified for Mrs. Lake?
3. What additional information do you need to gather to determine the next step in her plan of care?
4. If, in the assessment completed by the RN it is determined she needs to be closely monitored for possible falls, what interventions, by priority, will you implement?
5. Identify the legal requirements that must be implemented when a client is placed in restraints.
6. What documentation must be provided when a client is placed in restraints?

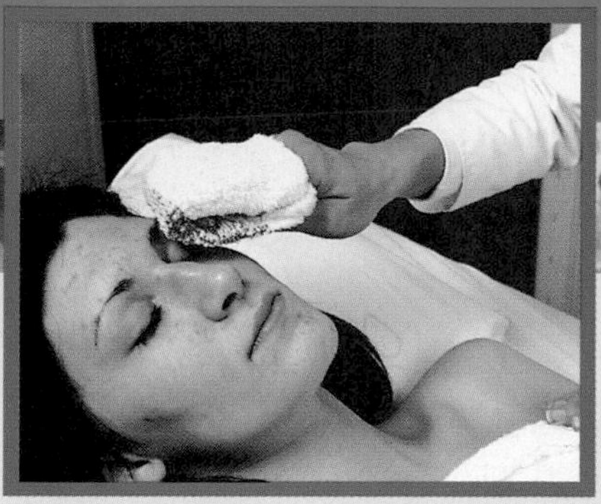

CHAPTER 8

Bathing, Bedmaking, and Maintaining Skin-Integrity

THEORETICAL CONCEPTS

UNIT ONE: Bedmaking 165
- Folding a Mitered Corner 166
- Changing a Pillowcase 166
- Making an Unoccupied Bed 166
- Making a Surgical Bed 169
- Changing an Occupied Bed 169

UNIT TWO: Bath Care 172
- Folding a Washcloth Mitt 173
- Providing Morning Care 173
- Bathing an Adult Client 174
- Bathing Using Disposable System 176
- Bathing an Infant 177
- Bathing in a Hydraulic Bathtub Chair 178

UNIT THREE: Skin Integrity 180
- Monitoring Skin Condition 181
- Preventing Skin Breakdown 182
- Preventing Skin Tears 183
- Managing Skin Tears 184

UNIT FOUR: Evening Care 188
- Providing Evening Care 189
- Providing Back Care 189

GERONTOLOGIC CONSIDERATIONS 191

MANAGEMENT GUIDELINES 192

CRITICAL THINKING STRATEGIES 193

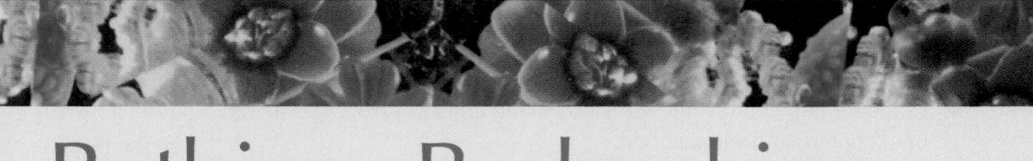

Learning Objectives

- Compare and contrast the steps in making an occupied, unoccupied, and surgical bed.
- Demonstrate the skill of folding a mitered corner.
- Outline the steps in bathing a bedridden adult client.
- Differentiate between bathing a bedridden client and a critically ill client.
- Compare and contrast the differences in bathing an infant and an adult client.
- State the advantages of using a commercial bathing system.
- Describe the assessment modalities completed while bathing a client.
- Outline the steps in providing morning care.
- Describe the skin assessment steps that must be completed on a daily basis.
- Describe the changes in skin that occur with aging and appropriate nursing interventions to prevent a skin tear.
- Describe briefly the components of evening care.
- Define the three back care strokes and their use in back care.
- Complete client charting for evening care on nurses' notes.
- Write three nursing diagnoses appropriate for providing basic hygienic care to clients.

Terminology

Bedmaking

Anesthesia (surgical, recovery) bed: a bed made in a specific manner for the client who is returning to the bed after having anesthesia or surgery.

Closed bed: a bed not being used by a client; the linens are left to cover the bed.

Occupied bed: the client remains in the bed while it is being made.

Open bed: a bed being used by a client; the linens are folded down.

Unoccupied bed: the client is out of the bed while it is being made.

Equipment Used with Beds

Aside from the standard types of equipment used on the basic hospital bed, specialized equipment can be added to meet the client's healthcare needs.

Balkan overbed frame: an overhead bar used to support a trapeze, or a series of pulleys and weights used for traction equipment.

Footboard: usually a solid support placed on the bed where the soles of the feet touch. It is secured to the mattress or bed frame. Footboards are used to prevent permanent plantar flexion (footdrop) and to exercise leg muscles. The footboard may also have side supports to help maintain proper alignment of feet.

Sheets for Bedmaking

Contour sheets: sheets that have elastic at each corner; fitted sheets.

Drawsheets: sheets made of fabric or waterproof material that are placed across the shoulder-to-knee area of the bed and tucked in on the sides.

Full sheets: regular full-length flat sheets that can be used as the top and bottom sheet.

Incontinent pads: large, disposable pads that can be placed under the buttocks area, head, drains, or any place where excess moisture or fluid may collect on the bed.

Pull sheets: sheets placed across the shoulder-to-knee area of the bed. The sides are not tucked under the mattress. The sheet is kept wrinkle-free and folded under the client. Pull sheets are used to lift the client in the bed.

Levels of Personal Care

Complete care: the client requires total assistance from the nurse because he or she is able to do little or nothing for him or herself. Complete bathing, skin care, oral care, nail and hair care, care of the feet, eyes, ears, and nose, and a total bed linen change are usually provided.

Early morning care: this type of care may or may not be a routine in some hospitals. If early morning care is provided, it is usually given by the night shift nurses. It may include bathing the hands and face, use of the bedpan or urinal, oral care, and other preparations before breakfast.

Evening care (H.S. care, hour of sleep care): evening care is usually provided to prepare the client for a relaxing, uninterrupted period of sleep. Activities include oral care, partial bathing, skin care and a soothing back massage, straightening or changing the bed linen, and offering the bedpan or urinal. The client should also be assessed for the need of food, drink, or medication before sleep.

OR care: clients who will be undergoing surgery or diagnostic tests may be required to bathe the evening before. Partial bathing is sometimes allowed in the morning if time permits. If the client is not allowed to have anything by mouth, care must be taken not to allow swallowing of water or dentifrice while providing oral care. The client is usually given a clean gown. All dentures, hairpins, makeup, nail polish, contact lenses, and jewelry are removed. Valuables are locked up. The client is encouraged to void before leaving for the operating room.

Partial care: the client performs as much of his or her own care as possible. The nurse completes the remaining care.

Skin Care

Acne: skin condition due to irritation and infection of the sebaceous glands.

Bedsore: a synonym for decubitus or pressure ulcer—area of cellular necrosis due to decreased circulation.

Blanching: a whitish hue to an area of the skin when pressure is applied.

Ecchymosis: collection of blood underneath skin surface; bruise.

Emollient: soothing, softening agent applied to body surfaces.

Epidermis: superficial, or top, layer of skin.

Erythema: redness of skin associated with rashes, infections, and allergic responses.

Hyperemia: influx of blood into an area causing redness to the skin.

Ischemia: decreased, insufficient blood supply to body area.

Lesion: an area of broken skin as a result of trauma or a pathologic interruption of tissue.

Necrosis: cellular death resulting from decreased blood flow to tissue.

Pediculosis: infestation of lice.

Pediculus capitis: head lice.

Pediculus corporis: body lice.

Pediculus pubis: crab lice.

Petechiae: pinpoint reddish spots.

Pressure ulcer: a synonym for bedsore or pressure sore area of cellular necrosis due to decreased circulation.

Purpura: reddish purple area.

Shearing force: layers of skin moving on each other.

Skin tear: Traumatic wound resulting from separation of the epidermis from the dermis.

Turgor: the degree of elasticity of the skin.

Back Care

Effleurage: long stroking motions of the hands up and down the back. Hands do not leave the skin surface. Pressure is light.

Petrissage: pinching of the skin, subcutaneous tissue, and muscle as you move up and down the client's back.

Tapotement: alternate striking of fleshy part of hands on client's back as you move up and down the back.

GENERAL TERMINOLOGY

Assessment: the collection, verification, organization, interpretation, and documentation of client data; the first step in the nursing process.

Complete bath: all areas of the body are bathed. This bath can be done completely by the nurse or by the client.

Cyanosis: blueness of the skin related to decreased oxygenation of the blood.

Dermis: layer of skin below the epidermis containing blood and lymphatic vessels, nerves, nerve endings, glands, and hair follicles.

Epidermis: superficial, avascular layer of skin primarily used for protection.

Erythema: a redness of the skin due to congestion of the capillaries.

Excreta: waste matter; materials cast out by the body.

Fissure: a groove, slit, or natural division; ulcer or crack-like sore.

Flush: a redness of the face and neck.

Hypoallergenic: against allergy, as hypoallergenic tape.

Incurvate: curved, especially inward.

Inflammation: swelling, pain, heat, and redness of tissue.

Intervention: the act of coming between, so as to hinder or modify.

Jaundice: yellowish appearance caused by deposition of bile pigment in the skin.

Mucosa: mucous membrane lining passages and cavities communicating with the air.

Pallor: paleness; absence of skin coloration.

Partial bath: certain parts of the body are bathed such as the face, hands, under arms, back, and perineal area. Another definition of a partial bath is a bath that occurs when the nurse bathes areas which the client cannot reach and the client washes all other areas.

Pigment: any normal or abnormal coloring of the skin.

Plaque: a patch on the skin or on a mucous surface; a blood platelet.

Pressure point: area for exerting pressure to control bleeding; an area of skin that can become irritated with pressure, especially over bony prominences.

Sensory deprivation: enforced absence of usual and accustomed sensory stimuli.

Sensory overload: too much stimuli for the senses to adjust to at once.

Therapeutic bath: these baths require a physician's order and are used for specific conditions. The order should include type of bath, water temperature, and solution to be used.

Ulcer: an open sore or lesion of the skin or mucous membrane of the body.

BASIC HEALTH CARE

Clients enter the hospital environment because of an accident or acute illness requiring immediate care, or because the physician has recommended diagnostic procedures or surgery. The latter is commonly referred to as an "elective admission." Whatever the reason, the client must rapidly alter everyday routines and activities of daily living. The client may be concerned about his or her health and well-being and may experience varying degrees of anxiety as a reaction to unfamiliar procedures, hospital personnel, and the hospital environment.

After the client has been admitted to the health care unit, many independent actions, such as bathing, personal hygiene, and general care, may be curtailed by the nature of the illness and confinement. The client may require assistance with even the simplest of actions. Without therapeutic intervention, the total adaptation process may be put in jeopardy as additional physical problems occur.

Knowing when and how to intervene and performing such skills as bedmaking, bathing, and personal hygiene facilitate the client's process of adapting to the health care.

When the client is confined to bed even for a short time, comfort is essential in order to promote rest and sleep. Beds must be kept clean, free of debris and wrinkles, to prevent skin irritation and breakdown. The bed needs to be straightened frequently during the day to accomplish this. If the client is to remain in bed for an extended time, all care and daily routines are directed from bed. It becomes the center of activity.

There are many different types of beds and related equipment available to meet the special health care needs of individual clients.

Types of Beds

The hospital bed is a standard twin-size bed in a frame that allows for different positions to facilitate care and comfort for the client. The height, head, and foot positions in most beds are electrically operated to assist both the client and the nursing staff. The nurse instructs the client in the proper use of bed controls and in bed positions that could be dangerous for the client.

Support Surfaces

Support surfaces such as mattress overlays filled with foam, gel, or water are commonly used as the first line of defense against skin breakdown. These surfaces prevent pressure on bony prominences, thus reducing pressure ulcer incidence. They are cost-effective surfaces that prevent pressure ulcers in clients who are classified as low risk (class I and II pressure ulcers). These surfaces can also be used to treat those clients who already have pressure ulcers.

Foam overlay (Bio-Gard, Geo-Matt) support surfaces are used for prevention in low-risk clients. The foam pads are ventilated for moisture control and have an anti-shearing surface. Foam mattresses (Comfortline Ultimate, basic PRIMA, and SimpliMATT) can be placed on top of existing mattresses. DUO DETEQ, an alternating therapy system mattress, is used as a replacement for the mattress. A third type of support system, the continuous airflow system (ACUCAIR), is also placed over an existing mattress. It keeps skin dry with the continuous airflow and moisture control feature. It also reduces friction and shear. This system is portable and easily transported and placed on the existing mattress.

Specialty Beds

New types of specialty beds are used to provide care to clients at risk for developing pressure ulcers. Clients requiring the specialty beds are those at high risk for skin breakdown or pressure ulcers. Clients most susceptible to these conditions (where a specialty bed is critical), include spinal cord injury clients or those who need frequent turning and are difficult to move.

Specialty beds replace the entire hospital bed and are classified as high air-loss (Clinitron Elexis, Rite Hite, Fluid Air ELITE), low air-pressure (Flexicare and Kin Air IV), and air-filled (Pressure Guard CFT, Fluid Air, Clinitron). High-air loss beds are used for clients with stage III and IV pressure ulcers. These beds have anti-friction/shear surfaces and built-in scales. Low-air loss beds are used for clients who are difficult to reposition or when moving is contraindicated. Air-filled beds are used for clients who require minimal movement. It makes turning easy and facilitates drainage.

There are two additional types of beds used as preventative or treatment measures for very difficult clients. The first type, the kinetic beds (TotalCare, SpO_2RT, and RotoRest) is used to provide continuous passive motion or oscillation for clients with unstable spines. The second type of bed, the bariatric bed (Magnum, Burke, BariKare), is used with obese clients. These beds have a special feature that not only allows clients to be weighed in the bed, but it converts into a chair.

Bathing

Routine bathing is an essential component of daily care. It is essential to prevent body odor, because excessive perspiration interacts with bacteria to cause odor. Dead skin cells can lead to infection if impaired skin integrity occurs. Excessive bathing, on the other hand, can be dangerous to elderly clients. In the aged, the skin may become dry and cracked, which can also lead to infection.

There are several types of commercial body cleansing systems currently used in hospitals and other health care facilities. The systems are a body bath, shampoo, and a perineal care package. The bath system uses disposable washcloths to cleanse the client. This type of system cleans, moisturizes, conditions, and protects the skin; therefore, it is a good alternative for elderly clients or clients with sensitive skin. The system provides ingredients that are hypoallergenic and bactericidal.

Bathing promotes a feeling of self-worth by improving the person's appearance. Relaxation and improved circulation are benefits of bathing and play a therapeutic role in the care of clients on bedrest. The apocrine glands, found in the axillae and pubic areas, produce sweat, which leads to odor. Therefore, special bathing considerations should be given to these areas.

In addition to the therapeutic effects, the bath affords the nurse time to spend in communication and assessment. Assessment of skin conditions, mobility, and self-care deficits can be detected while bathing the client.

Bathing is accomplished in a variety of ways, according to the client's needs, condition, and personal habits. Bathing is necessary to cleanse the skin and to promote circulation. Baths may also be used as a treatment to promote healing for a client with burns. Various types of bathing include:

- Complete bed bath: The client, who is usually totally dependent, is bathed by the nurse due to physical or mental incapacity. The client is encouraged to complete as much of his or her bath as possible.
- Partial bath: Face, axilla, hands, back, and genital area are bathed. Partial bath may be completed by client or nurse.
- Therapeutic bath: This bath is used as part of a treatment regimen for specific conditions, such as skin disorders, burns, high body temperature, and muscular injuries. Medicinal substances, such as oatmeal, Aveeno, and cornstarch, may be included in the bath water.
- Shower: Preferred method of bathing if client is ambulatory or can be transported to use a shower chair.
- Tub bath: Used by ambulatory clients as well as those who must be assisted by a device such as the Hoyer lift.
- Cooling bath: the client is placed in a tub of tepid water to reduce body temperature.

Skin Conditions

The skin is the largest organ of the body and is frequently not assessed, or even thought of, as far as nursing interventions are concerned. Skin is exposed to environmental risks, physical, and mechanical injury. Skin is composed of the epidermis (outer layer) and the dermis (inner layer). The skin provides protection, thermoregulation, excretion, metabolism, sensation, and communication for the body.

Skin types, colors, textures, and condition are as different and unique as each person. The condition of a client's skin is determined by his or her health status, age, activity level, and environmental exposure. For example, the skin of an infant is often more sensitive and delicate than that of an adult because it has not been exposed to many environmental elements. Most infants cannot tolerate strong soaps and lotions, and must be handled gently to avoid trauma. Adolescents are affected by acne and have areas of increased oil secretion. Adults may have drier skin, especially as they age. Older adults cannot always tolerate harsh soaps because their skin is more delicate. They require less frequent bathing and more lubrication with oil-rich creams and lotions.

According to Payne and Martin skin tears or a traumatic wound usually occurs on the extremities of elderly clients as a result of friction, or shearing and friction forces, which result in separation of the epidermis from the dermis. This occurs more frequently with elderly clients as a result of changes in their skin. The epidermis gradually thins, as a result of loss in dermal thickness, and becomes more susceptible to mild mechanical trauma. In addition, the skin loses its elasticity as elastin fibers decrease. This leads to a less effective barrier against fluid loss, bruising, and infection. Impaired thermoregulation leads to decreased tactile sensitivity and pain perception. Blood vessels become thin and fragile, which presents as purpura or the appearance of little hemorrhages under the skin. Skin tears seem to appear at the site where purpura is present. Skin tears are more prevalent on the arms and hands, but can occur anywhere on the body. A skin tear on the back or buttocks is often mistaken for a pressure ulcer; however, the etiology of a skin tear is different.

Maintaining skin integrity is an integral part of providing nursing care; being aware of the client's skin condition and alterations in the integrity is a critical aspect of providing total client care.

NURSING DIAGNOSES

The following nursing diagnoses may be appropriate to include in a client care plan when the components are related to basic care of the client.

NURSING DIAGNOSIS	RELATED FACTORS
Activity Intolerance	Prolonged bed rest, surgery, pain, treatment schedule, weakness, fatigue
Ineffective Health Maintenance	Ineffective coping, lack of motivation, motor impairment, lack of financial resources
Bathing/Hygiene Self-Care Deficit	Lack of coordination, motor impairment, visual disorders, surgery, muscle weakness, pain
Impaired Skin Integrity	Surgery, immobility, prolonged bed rest, mechanical factors (shearing force, pressure)

- The single most important nursing action to decrease the incidence of hospital-based infections is handwashing. **Remember to wash your hands or use antibacterial gel before and after each and every client contact.**

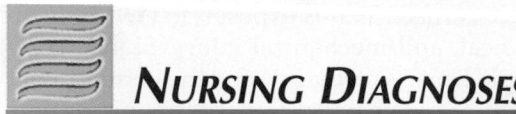

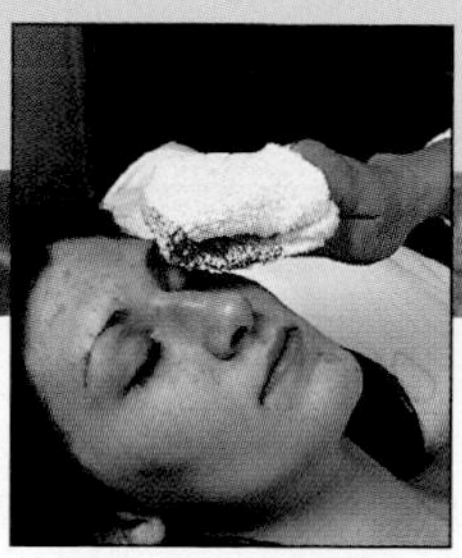

Bedmaking

Nursing Process Data

ASSESSMENT Data Base

Assess the client's need to have linen changed.

Determine if the client's present condition permits a change of bed linen.

Determine how many and what type of linens are required.

Check client's unit for available linens.

Determine client's prescribed level of activity and any special precautions in movement.

Assess client's ability to get out of bed during linen change.

PLANNING Objectives

To provide a clean, comfortable sleeping and resting environment for the client

To eliminate irritants to skin by providing wrinkle-free sheets and blankets

To avoid client exertion by making bed while occupied (Do not move client more than necessary)

To enhance client's self-image by providing a clean, neat, and comfortable bed

To properly dispose of soiled linens and prevent cross-contamination

To correctly align clients to assist in promoting a physically and emotionally safe and comfortable position

To prevent stress to the nurse's back or limbs during procedure

IMPLEMENTATION Procedures

Folding a Mitered Corner

Changing a Pillowcase

Making an Unoccupied Bed

Making a Surgical Bed

Changing an Occupied Bed

EVALUATION Expected Outcomes

Client states he or she is rested during and after bedmaking procedure.

Bed remains clean, dry, free of wrinkles or other skin irritants, and at a comfortable temperature.

Skin remains free of irritation caused by contact with linens.

The nurse feels no stress to back or limbs during the procedure.

FOLDING A MITERED CORNER

Equipment

Same as for an unoccupied bed

Procedure

1. Tuck sheet tightly and smoothly under mattress at top or bottom of the bed depending on where mitered corner is needed.
2. Grasp edge of sheet with hand and bring sheet onto mattress so that edge forms a right angle.
3. Tuck lower edge of sheet under mattress.
4. Place finger on sheet where it meets mattress and lower top of sheet over finger. **Rationale:** This action makes the mitered corner neat and tight.
5. Remove finger without disturbing folds.
6. Tuck sheet securely under mattress.

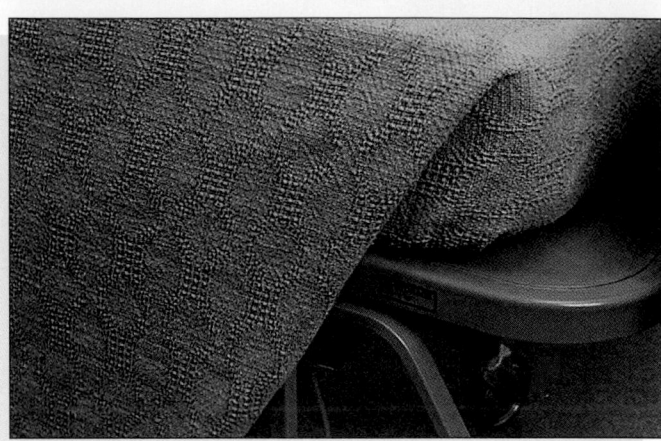

Mitered corners keep bed linens tight and wrinkle-free.

CHANGING A PILLOWCASE

Equipment

Clean pillowcase

Procedure

1. Wash your hands.
2. Pick up center of closed end of pillowcase.
3. Continue to firmly grip end of pillowcase; then with other hand gather pillowcase from open end and fold back (inside-out) over closed end.
4. Pick up center of one end of pillow with the hand holding the gathered pillowcase.
5. Pull pillowcase over pillow with other hand. Do not place pillow or case under arm, chin, or in teeth. **Rationale:** Contamination occurs from using these methods.
6. Adjust pillow corners in pillowcase by placing hand between case and pillow.

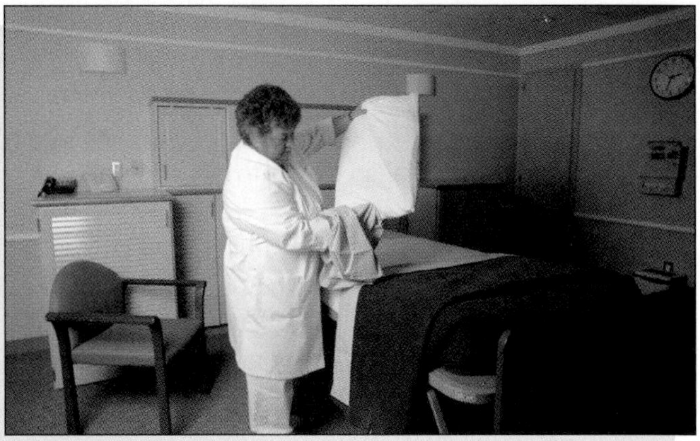

Pick up center of one end of pillow with the hand holding the gathered pillowcase and pull case over pillow with other hand.

MAKING AN UNOCCUPIED BED

Equipment

Chair or table
Linen hamper
Linens (in order of use):
- Bath blanket
- Mattress pad, optional
- Bottom sheet
- Drawsheet
- Incontinent pad, if needed
- Top sheet
- Blanket
- Bedspread
- Pillowcase
- Clean gloves, as needed

Preparation

1. Gather linen and hamper and bring to room.
2. Explain need for client to be out of bed during procedure.

3. Wash your hands. Don gloves if needed
4. Assist client out of bed and into chair.
5. Arrange second chair and hamper conveniently for use.
6. Place linen on chair; ensure chair is clean. **Rationale:** This action provides a clean surface and promotes infection control.
7. Place linen on chair in order of use; pillow case at bottom.
8. Remove call signal from linen.
9. Adjust bed to a comfortable working height.

Procedure

1. Lower both side rails and place bed in flat position.
2. Loosen linen on all sides, including head and foot of the bed.
3. Remove spread and blanket. If they are to be reused, fold them and place on the chair.
4. Remove top, draw, and bottom sheet, and place in linen hamper. **Rationale:** Never place dirty linen on the floor as cross-contamination occurs from this action.
5. Push mattress to head of bed. Center the mattress if necessary.
6. If mattress pad is not changed, smooth out wrinkles and recenter pad on the bed surface. **Rationale:** Wrinkles can cause skin abrasions if skin is compromised by age, disease, or malnutrition.
7. Make up one side of the bed, then move to the other side of bed and make it. **Rationale:** This step saves time and energy.
8. Place contour bottom sheet on mattress, and continue making bed at Step 13. If using a flat bottom sheet, place the center fold of the sheet in the middle of the mattress with the end of the sheet even with the end of the mattress.
9. Unfold the bottom sheet, and cover the mattress.
10. Tuck the top of the sheet under the head of the bed.
11. Miter the corner of the bottom sheet at the head of the bed. (See procedure for mitered corner.) **Rationale:** A mitered corner is tighter and less likely to come apart.
12. Tuck the remaining side of the bottom sheet well under the mattress.
13. If the client needs a drawsheet, center the drawsheet on the bed and open drawsheet top to opposite side. Tuck the sheet under the mattress. Smooth out wrinkles.
    a. If a pull sheet is needed, fold drawsheet in half or quarters. Position sheet in middle of bed. **Rationale:** Pull sheets are used with heavy or difficult-to-move clients.
    b. If absorbent pad is needed, center it on bed over draw or pull sheet.

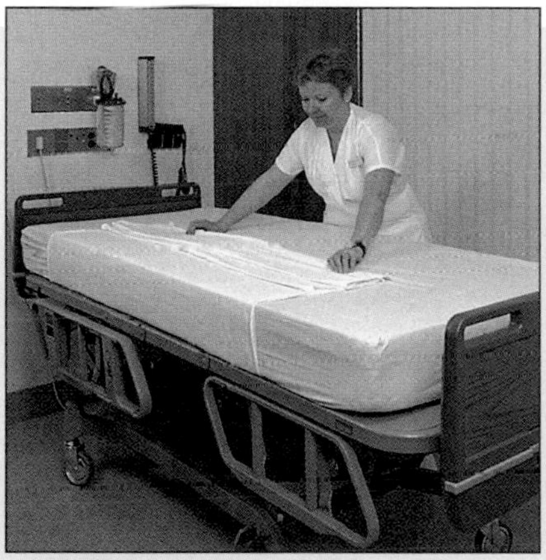

Tuck drawsheet in tightly.

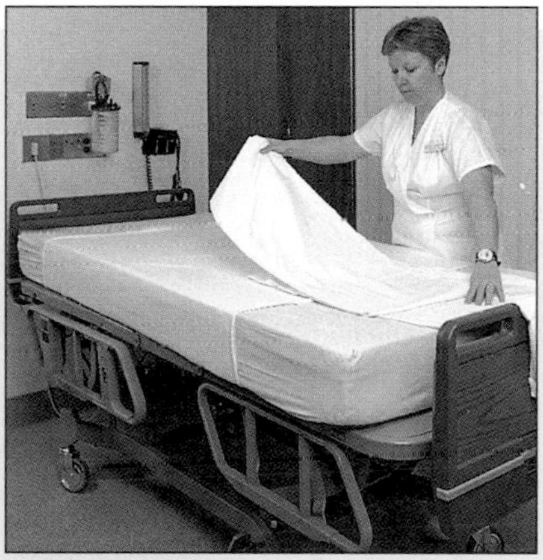

Unfold bottom sheet to cover mattress.

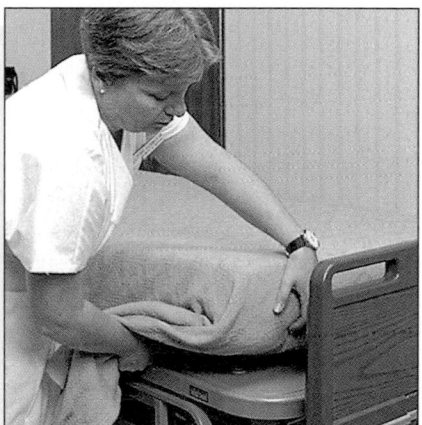

Smooth linen before mitering corners.

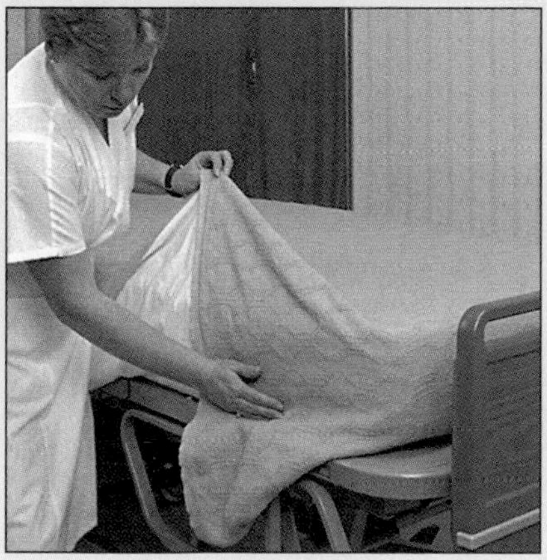

Form triangle and tuck in linen.

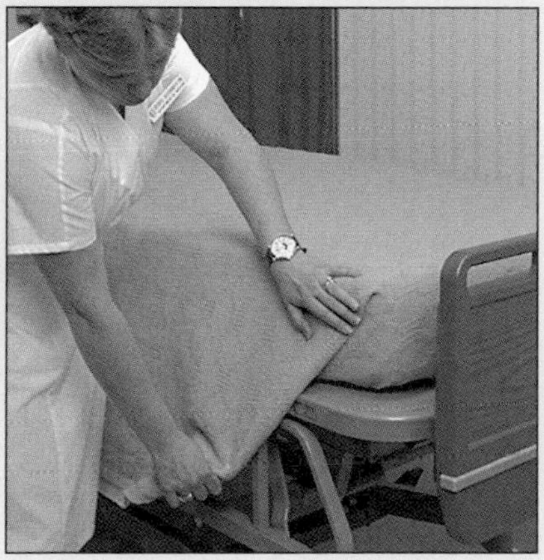

Pull down top linen while holding corner.

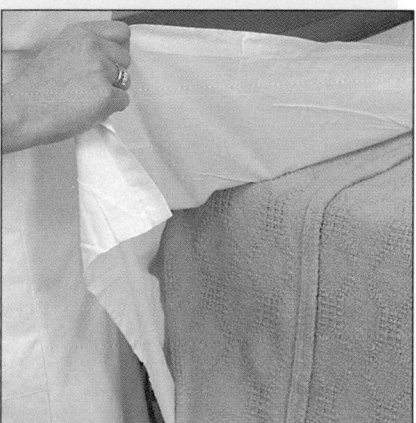

Fold cuff of sheet over spread.

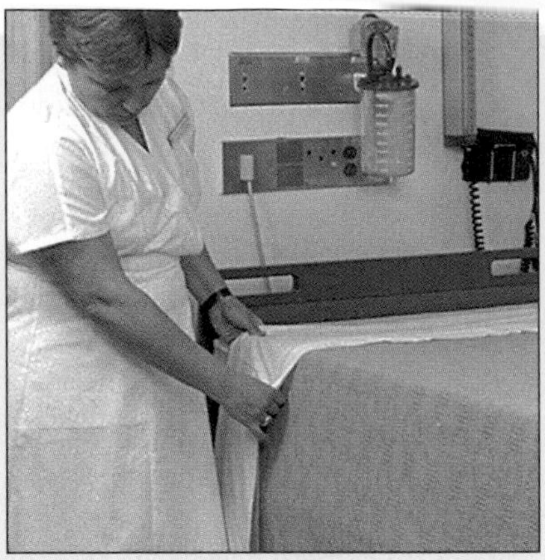

Fold sheet over spread and leave cuff.

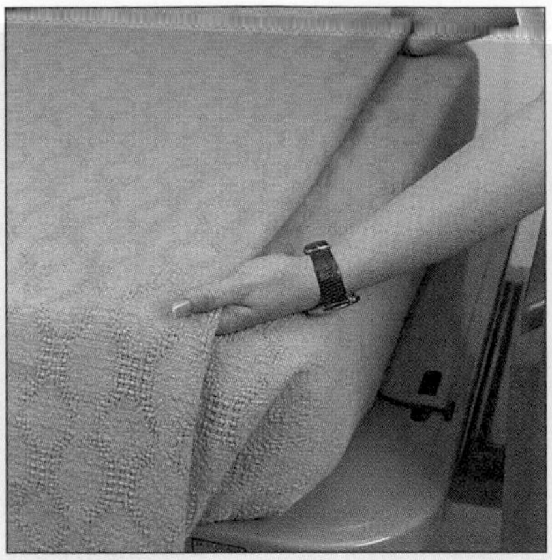

Pleat top linen to allow space for feet.

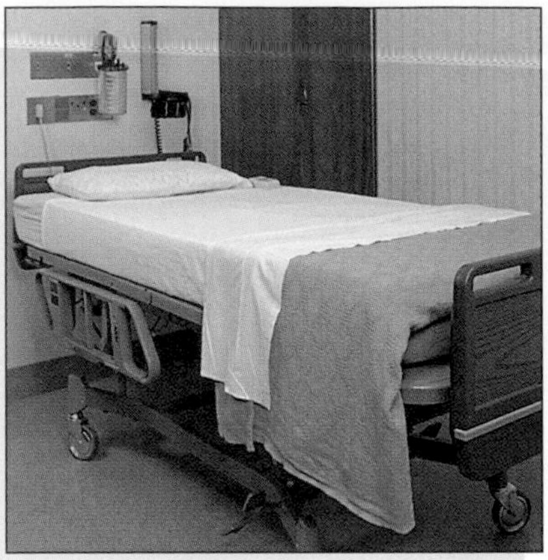

Fanfold linen to foot of bed.

14. Move to the other side of the bed. Pull linen toward you and straighten out linen.
15. Tuck the top of the sheet under the head of the bed if using a flat sheet.
16. Miter the corner of the bottom sheet at the head of the bed if not using a contour sheet.
17. Tuck remaining bottom sheet well under the mattress. Gather sheet into your hand, lean away from the bed, and pull sheet downward. Tuck sheet under mattress.
18. If drawsheet is used, tighten and tuck the same as bottom sheet.
19. Straighten out absorbent pad and pull sheet if used.
20. Place top sheet, blanket, and spread full length on top of bed.
21. Leave a cuff of top sheet and spread at the head of the bed. **Rationale:** This prevents client's face from rubbing against blanket.
22. Tuck sheet, spread, and blanket well under foot of mattress, one side at a time.
23. Miter corners at the foot of the bed, one side at a time.
24. Make a small pleat or slightly loosen linen to allow room for client's feet.
25. Fanfold linen to foot of bed.
26. Change pillowcase. See skill "Changing a Pillowcase."
27. Return bed to lowest position. Reattach call signal to linens.
28. Pull side rail up on side furthest from client.
29. If the unit is unassigned, leave top linen pulled up, covering the bed.
30. Dispose of soiled laundry.

Principles of Medical Asepsis

- Place dirty linen in hamper.
- Do not place dirty linen on floor.
- Discard all unused linen from client area.
- Do not transfer linen from one client area to another.
- Do not allow dirty linen to touch uniform.

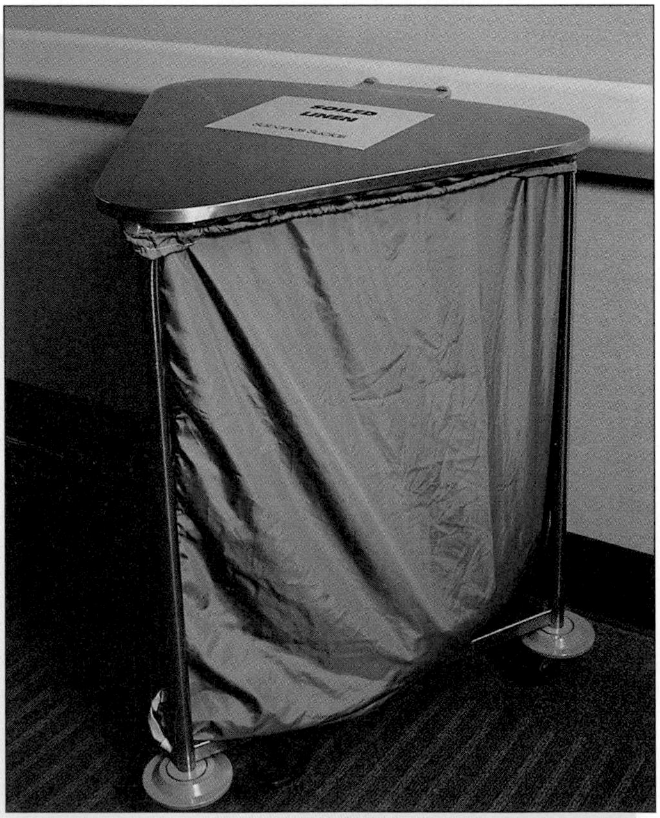

Keep linen hamper covered to prevent spread of microorganisms. Hamper can be taken into the client's room.

MAKING A SURGICAL BED

Equipment

Same as for an unoccupied bed.

Procedure

1. Wash your hands.
2. Bring linens to the room.
3. Arrange chair and linen hamper conveniently for use.
4. Place linen on chair. Ensure that chair is clean.
5. Raise bed to highest position.
6. Place the bottom sheet on the bed, using the same method as for making an unoccupied bed.
7. Place a drawsheet and absorbent pad on the bed.
8. Lay top sheet, blanket, and bedspread over top of bed.
9. Fold up linen from foot, head, and one side of the bed toward center of the bed.
10. Fold bottom and top edges nearest you to the opposite side, forming a triangle. Pick up center point of triangle.
11. Fanfold linen to side of bed. **Rationale:** Folding linen at side of the bed facilitates moving surgical clients into the bed.
12. Leave bed in HIGH position to facilitate easy transfer of surgical client from gurney to bed.
13. Change pillowcase and leave on chair or at foot of bed.
14. Move all objects away from bedside area. **Rationale:** This allows surgical gurney to be placed close to bed for client transfer.
15. Wash your hands.

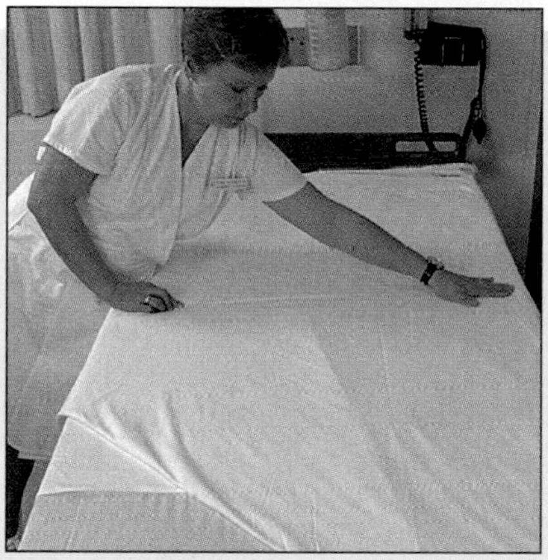
Place draw sheet and absorbent pad on bottom sheet.

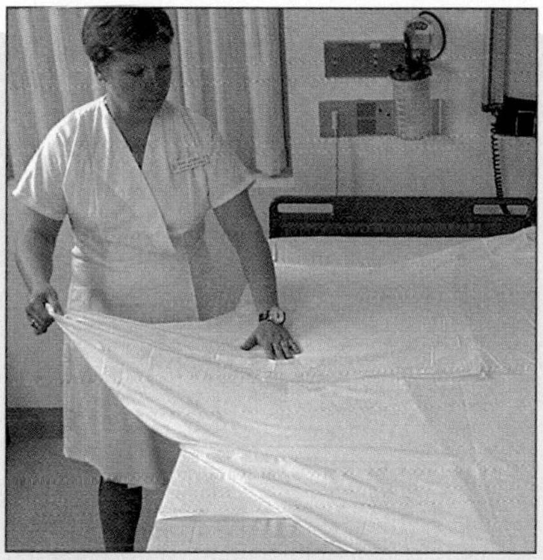
Fold bottom and top edges to opposite side forming a triangle.

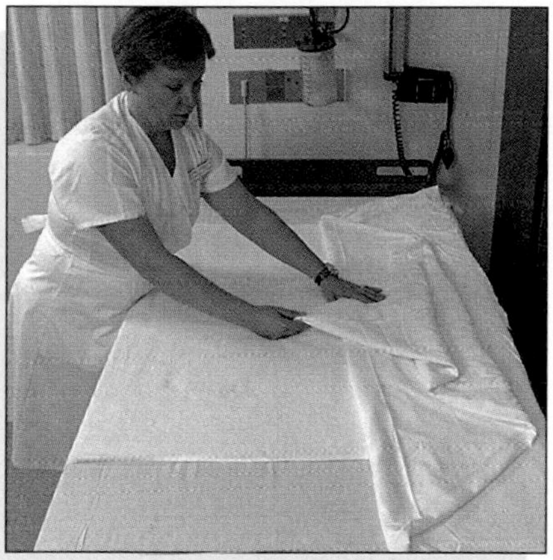
Fanfold linen to opposite side of bed for transferring client.

CHANGING AN OCCUPIED BED

Equipment

Chair or table
Linen hamper
Linens (in order of use):
- Bath blanket
- Mattress pad, optional
- Bottom sheet
- Cloth drawsheet
- Incontinent pad, if needed
- Top sheet
- Blanket
- Bedspread
- Pillowcase

Clean gloves, if indicated

Preparation

1. Talk with the client and explain how he or she can be involved in the procedure.
2. Explain the sequence for the procedure.
3. Arrange furniture and equipment (e.g., linen hamper and chair) for convenience of use.
4. Wash your hands and collect the linen.
5. Place linen on chair; ensure that chair is clean.
6. Remove call signal from linens.
7. Pull curtain closed. **Rationale:** This provides privacy for the client.
8. Adjust the bed to a comfortable working height with side rails up. Help client into a supine position.
9. Don gloves if bed linen is soiled with body fluids.

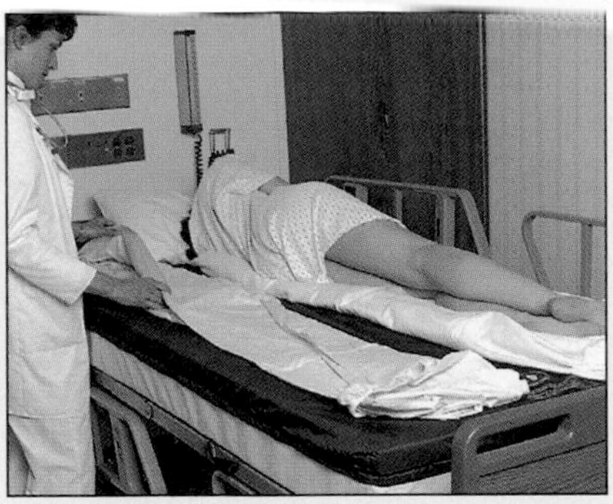

Place center of sheet in middle of bed.

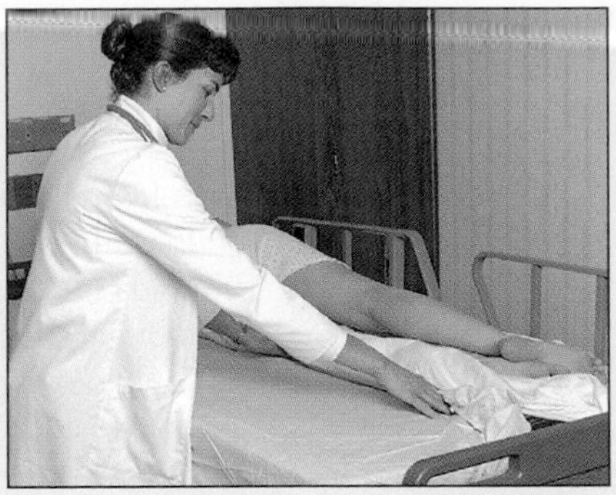

Tighten bottom sheet under mattress.

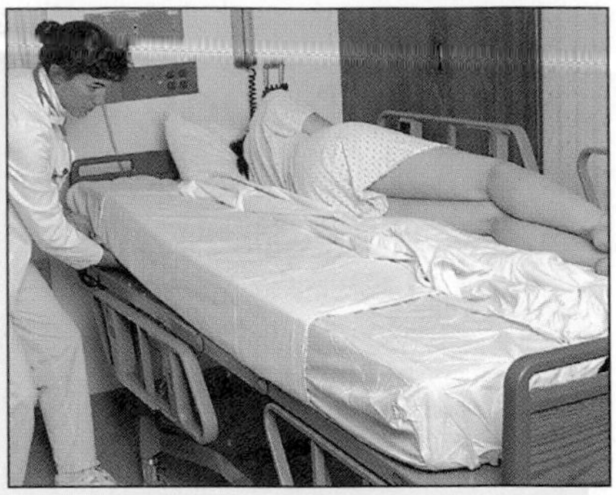

Place drawsheet in middle of bed.

Procedure

1. Lower side rail on your side of the bed, but make sure side rail on opposite side is in UP position. **Rationale:** This ensures client safety as client rolls to edge of bed.
2. Loosen top linens.
3. Remove spread, sheet, and blanket at the same time the bath blanket is pulled over client. **Rationale:** Blanket keeps client warm during bed change. If they are to be reused, fold them and place on the chair.
4. Place top sheet in linen hamper.
5. Push mattress to head of bed. Center the mattress if necessary.
6. Assist client to the side of the bed, place in side-lying position facing away from you as near the far side rail as possible.
7. Loosen bottom linens on your side of the bed.
8. Push dirty linen under or as close as possible to client.
9. Smooth out wrinkles and recenter pad on the bed surface if mattress pad is used but not changed. **Rationale:** Wrinkles may cause skin irritation.
10. Place clean bottom sheet on mattress with client on the opposite side of the bed. Place the center fold of the sheet in the middle of the mattress with the end of the sheet even with the end of the mattress.
11. Unfold the bottom sheet and cover the mattress. Make sure the clean bottom sheet is underneath any used linen. **Rationale:** This keeps the clean linen uncontaminated.
12. Tuck the top of the sheet under the head of the bed, or position contour sheet around corner of mattress.
13. Miter the corner of the bottom sheet at the head of the bed if flat sheet is used.
14. Tuck the remaining bottom sheet well under the mattress from head to foot.
15. Center drawsheet on the bed, if the client requires a drawsheet, and fanfold half of the sheet under the client. Tuck side of the sheet under the mattress. Smooth out wrinkles.
    a. Fold drawsheet in half or quarters if a pull sheet is needed. Position sheet in middle of bed. Fanfold half of the pull sheet under client.
    b. Fanfold absorbent pad and center it on bed under client's buttocks. Place the pad, absorbent side up and plastic side down, close to the client. **Rationale:** This position makes it easy to pull through to the other side of the bed.
16. Help the client roll over to the other side of the bed.
17. Tell the client why there is a hump of linen in the center of the bed. Make the client comfortable.
18. Raise the side rail. Move to other side of bed.

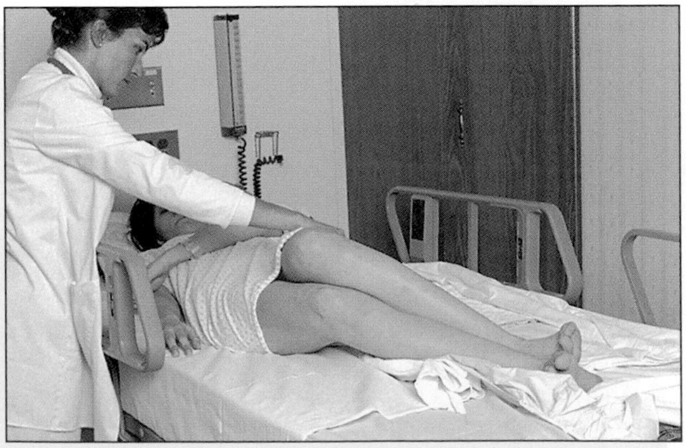

Assist client to roll over to other side of bed.

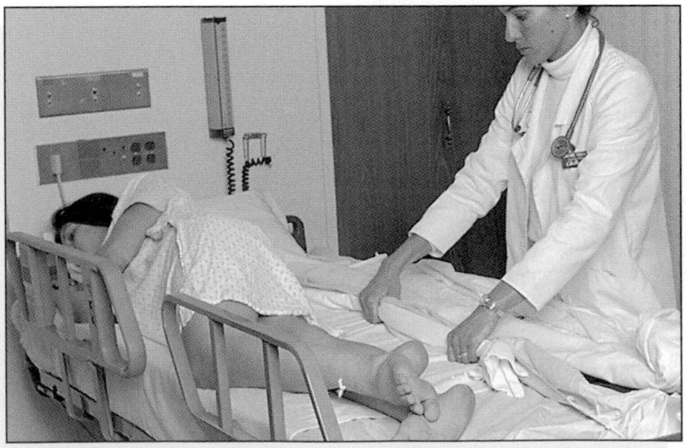

After raising side rail, pull linen toward you.

19. Move linens to the other side of the bed, by gently pulling linens toward you.
20. Lower side rail, and loosen bottom sheets.
21. Pull dirty linen to side of bed and roll into a bundle at the foot of the bed or place linen in linen hamper. **Rationale:** This reduces the spread of microorganisms.
22. Never place dirty linen on the floor. **Rationale:** Cross-contamination occurs from this action.
23. Pull clean linen across mattress and straighten under client.
24. Miter the top corner of the flat bottom sheet or tuck contour sheet over mattress edge.
25. Gather bottom sheet into your hand, lean away from the bed, and pull linens downward at an angle. Tuck remaining bottom sheet well under the mattress. If drawsheet is used, tighten and tuck it in the same way.
26. Help the client into a supine position and adjust the pillow.
27. Place top sheet, blanket, and spread over the client. Leave at least a 6-inch cuff of top sheet at the head of the bed.
28. Remove bath blanket, and straighten top sheet and blanket.
29. Miter corners at foot of bed.
30. Pull up all layers of linen at client's toes. Make a small pleat. **Rationale:** This allows room for client's feet and prevents sheets from rubbing on client's toes.
31. Raise side rail.
32. Remove pillow from bed, and change pillowcase.
33. Return bed to lowest position. Reattach call signal to linens.
34. Position client for comfort.
35. Dispose of soiled laundry.
36. Remove gloves if used and wash your hands.

DOCUMENTATION FOR BEDMAKING

- Specific linens or equipment that cause discomfort for the client
- Special requirements for linens (e.g., certain detergents or elimination of starch)
- Use of pull sheets, incontinent pads, or specified ways to keep bed dry

Critical Thinking Application

UNEXPECTED OUTCOMES	CRITICAL THINKING OPTIONS
Client refuses to have bed made.	• Assess reason for refusal. Client may be in pain or does not want to be disturbed. • Offer to make the bed at a later time. • Change only the pillowcase and drawsheet, if client allows. • Beds do not need to be changed unless soiled or damp so allow client's independence if possible.
Cross-contamination occurs from improper linen disposal.	• Provide adequate linen hampers for the nursing personnel. • Attend in-service education programs on infection control.
Client's skin becomes irritated from linen or begins to break down.	• Obtain hypoallergenic linen. • Place special mattress under client. • Provide skin care with lotion.
The nurse feels stress on back during bedmaking.	• Make sure bed is positioned for comfort of the nurse. High position is generally used. • If client is heavy, ask for assistance with bedmaking, especially in moving side to side. • Use full sheet or Booster Lift for turning. • Attend in-service classes on preventing back strain.

UNIT 2

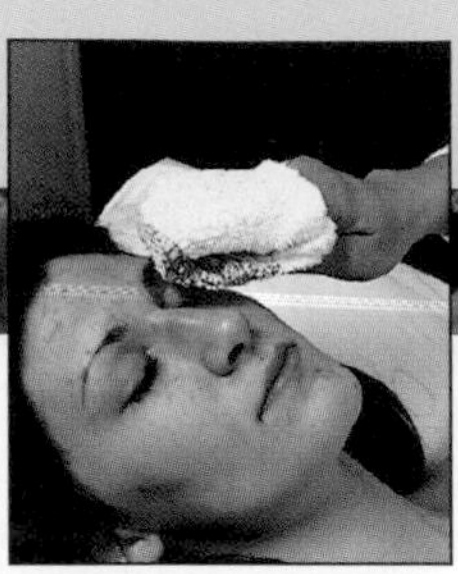

Bath Care

Nursing Process Data

ASSESSMENT Data Base

Assess client's need for bathing and other personal hygiene activities.

Check client's activity order. Note special precautions related to movement or exercise.

Assess client's ability to perform his or her own care and determine how much assistance he or she needs.

Discuss client's preferences for the bathing procedure, bath, and personal articles.

Check client's room for availability of bathing articles and linens.

Assess client's skin (see Unit 3 on Skin Integrity).

PLANNING Objectives

To decrease the possibility of infection by removing excessive debris, secretions, and perspiration from the skin

To promote circulation

To maintain muscle tone through active or passive movement during bathing

To alternate points of pressure on the body by changing client's position during the bath

To provide comfort for the client

To assess the client's overall status, skin condition, level of mobility, comfort

IMPLEMENTATION Procedures

Folding a Washcloth Mitt

Providing Morning Care

Bathing an Adult Client

Bathing an Infant

Bathing in a Hydraulic Bathtub Chair

Bathing the Critically Ill

EVALUATION Expected Outcomes

Client's skin is free of excessive perspiration, debris, secretions, and offensive odors.

Body positions have been changed and muscles and joints have been exercised actively or passively during the bath.

Client feels comfortable and does not complain of pain, fatigue, or itching, irritated or excessively dry skin.

Client participates in bath procedure to the best of his or her ability.

The nurse has assessed the integrity and condition of the client's skin and the level of mobility, comfort, or pain.

FOLDING A WASHCLOTH MITT

Procedure

1. Unfold the washcloth.
2. Place one corner of cloth in the palm of your hand, just above your fingers.
3. Wrap one edge of the cloth around the palm and fingers.
4. Anchor cloth with your thumb.
5. Bring far edge of cloth up and tuck under edge in palm of hand.
6. If washcloth is too small to fold, make into a square. **Rationale:** This prevents water from dripping onto client or bed.

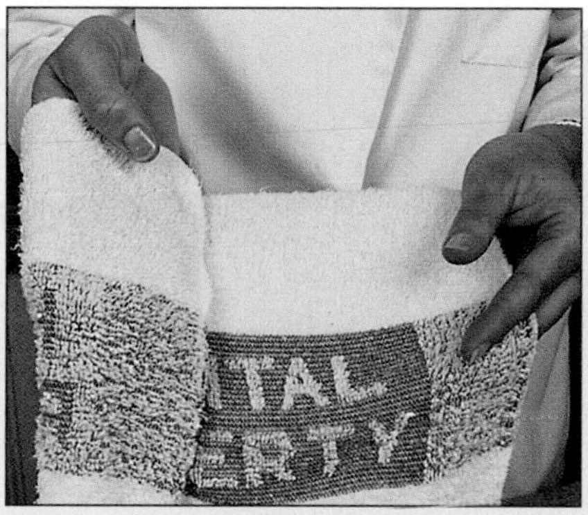

Wrap one edge of cloth around palm and fingers.

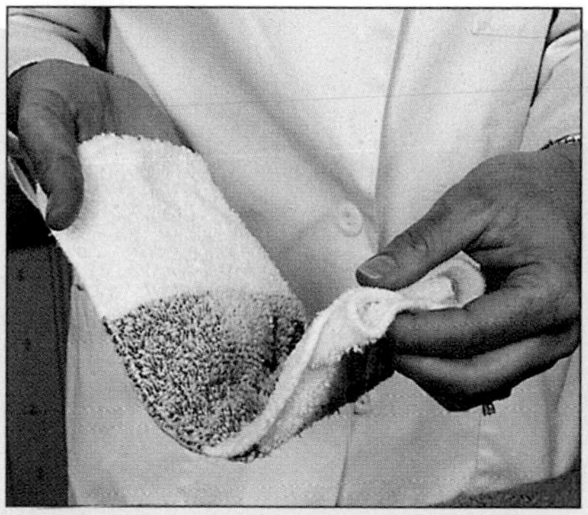

Wrap cloth around hand and anchor with thumb.

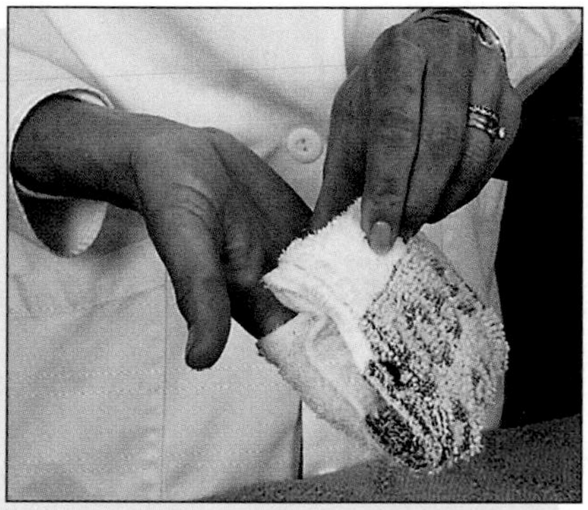

Tuck far edge of cloth under edge in palm of hand.

PROVIDING MORNING CARE

Equipment

Basin of warm water
Soap
Towel and washcloth
Emesis basin
Toothbrush and paste
Bedpan or urinal
Toilet tissue
Clean gloves

Preparation

1. Determine if client wishes morning care. **Rationale:** Morning care is provided to "freshen" the client in preparation for breakfast, physicians' visits, and procedures occurring prior to bathing.
2. Wash your hands. **Rationale:** When providing morning care to several clients, it is important to wash your hands between clients so that microorganisms are not transmitted from one client to another.
3. Gather equipment and take it to client's room.
4. Explain that early morning care is available while client remains in bed. If client is able, assist him or her to the bathrooms.
5. Provide privacy.

Procedure

1. Wash your hands.
2. Offer bedpan or urinal and assist client as needed. Don gloves when giving client bedpan or urinal.
3. Move bed to comfortable working height, and lower side rail.
4. Put equipment on over-bed table within reach.
5. Wash client's face and hands or assist as needed. Dry face and hands.
6. Offer oral hygiene. Assist as needed. Gloves should be worn if client needs assistance with oral hygiene.
7. Hold emesis basin so client can rinse after brushing teeth.
8. Assist client to comfortable position.
9. Reposition bed, and replace side rails.
10. Remove equipment and draw curtains.
11. Remove gloves, if used.
12. Wash hands.

BATHING AN ADULT CLIENT

Equipment

Basin or sink with warm water (110°–115°F)
Soap and soap dish
Personal articles (i.e., deodorant, powder, lotions)
Laundry hamper
Two to three towels and washcloth
Gloves if appropriate
Bath blanket
Clean pajamas or hospital gown
Table for bathing equipment
Shaving equipment for male patients

Preparation

1. Provide a comfortable room environment (i.e., comfortable temperature, lighting).
2. Talk with client about plan for bathing to meet personal care needs.
3. Encourage client to bathe him or herself. **Rationale:** To increase independence, promote exercise and a sense of self-worth.
4. Explain any unfamiliar methods or procedures regarding bathing.
5. Wash your hands.
6. Collect necessary equipment, and place articles within reach on over-bed table.
7. Ask the client if he or she needs to void or defecate before starting the bath. **Rationale:** Warm water of the bath and movement can stimulate the client to void.
8. Position the bed at a comfortable working height.
9. Ensure privacy.

Procedure

1. Place bath blanket over client and over top linen. Loosen top linen at edges and foot of bed.
   a. Remove dirty top linen from under bath blanket, starting at client's shoulders and rolling linen down toward the client's feet.
   b. Ask client to grasp and hold top edge of bath blanket to keep it in place while you pull linen to foot of bed.
   c. Place dirty linen in laundry hamper.
2. Help client to the side of the bed closest to you. Keep the side rail on the far side of the bed in the UP position.
3. Remove client's gown. Keep client covered with bath blanket. Place gown in laundry bag. **Rationale:** To protect client's modesty and keep client warm during bathing.
4. Remove pillow if client can tolerate.
5. Place towel under client's head.
6. Don clean gloves if risk of exposure to body fluids when bathing client. **Rationale:** To maintain Standard Precautions.
7. Make a mitt with a washcloth. Fold washcloth around your hand as illustrated previously. **Rationale:** This prevents wet ends of cloth from annoying client.
8. Bathe client's face. **Rationale:** Begin bath at cleanest area and work downward toward feet.
   a. Wash around client's eyes, using clear water. With one edge of washcloth, wipe from the inner canthus toward the outer canthus. **Rationale:** This prevents secretions from entering lacrimal duct. Using a different section of the washcloth, repeat procedure on other eye. Dry thoroughly.
   b. Wash, rinse, and dry client's forehead, cheeks, nose, and area around lips. Use soap with client's permission.
   c. Wash, rinse, and dry area behind and around the client's ears.
   d. Wash, rinse, and dry client's neck.
9. Remove towel from under client's head.
10. Bathe client's upper body and extremities. Place towel under area to be bathed.
    a. Wash both arms by elevating client's arm and holding client's wrist. Use gentle strokes from the wrist toward the shoulder, including the axillary area. **Rationale:** This helps promote circulation.
    b. Wash, rinse, and dry client's axillae. Apply deodorant and powder if desired.
    c. Wash client's hands by soaking them in the basin or with a washcloth. Nails can be cleaned now or after the bath.
    d. Keeping chest covered with the towel, wash, rinse, and thoroughly dry client's chest, especially under breasts. (Apply powder or cornstarch under breasts if desired).
11. Bathe client's abdomen. Using a towel over chest area and bath blanket, cover areas you are not bathing. Wash, rinse, and dry abdomen and umbilicus. Replace bath blanket over client's upper body and abdomen.
12. Bathe client's legs and feet. Place towel under leg to be bathed. Drape other leg, hip, and genital area with the bath blanket.
    a. Carefully place bath basin on the towel near the client's foot.
    b. With one arm under the client's leg, grasp the client's foot and bend knee. Place foot in basin of water.
    c. Bathe client's leg, moving toward hip. Rinse and dry client's leg. **Rationale:** This promotes circulation.
    d. Wash client's foot with washcloth. Rinse and dry foot and area between toes thoroughly.
    e. Carefully move basin to other side of bed, and repeat procedure for client's other leg and foot.

CLINICAL ALERT

Bathe lower extremities gently if client is at high risk for deep vein thrombosis. DO NOT rub legs. This action could dislodge a clot.

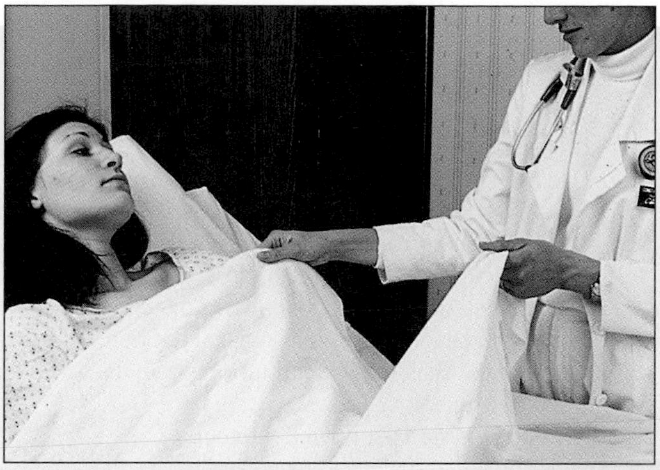

Remove top linen and replace with bath blanket.

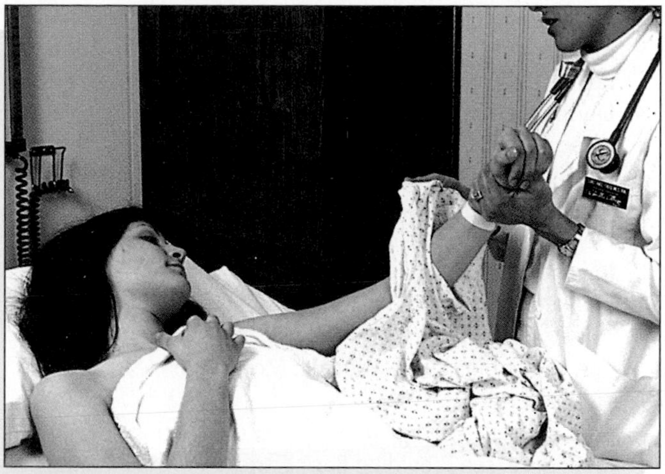

Remove gown while covering client with bath blanket.

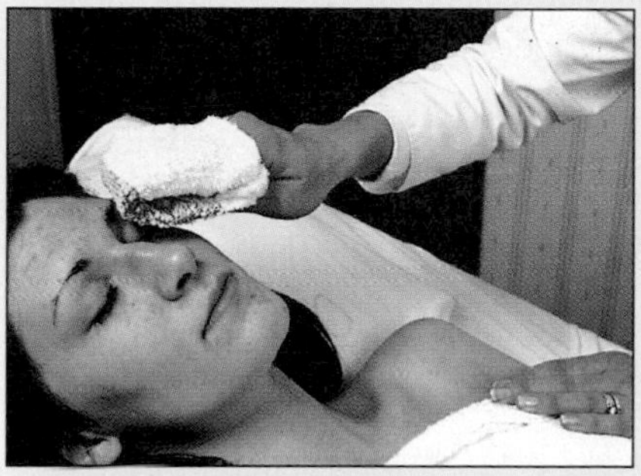

Wash eyes first, from inner to outer canthus.

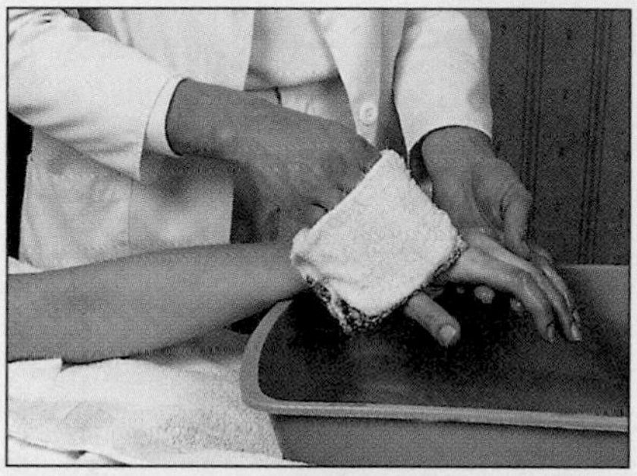

Wash hands by soaking them in a basin.

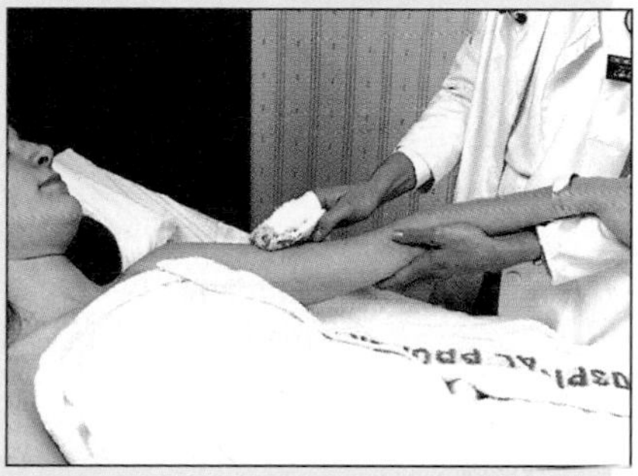

Support wrist when washing client's arm.

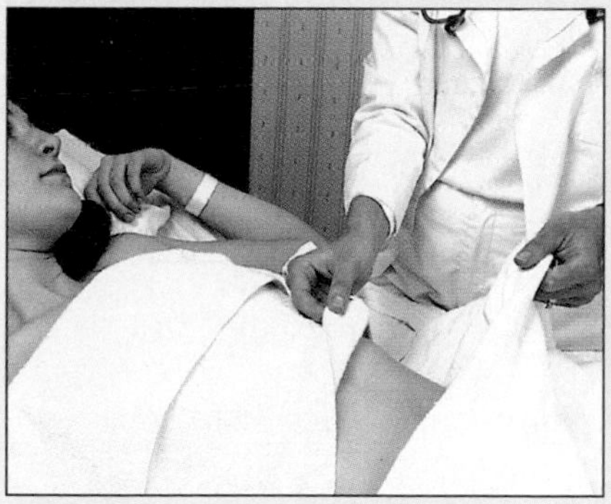

Keep client covered with towel during bath.

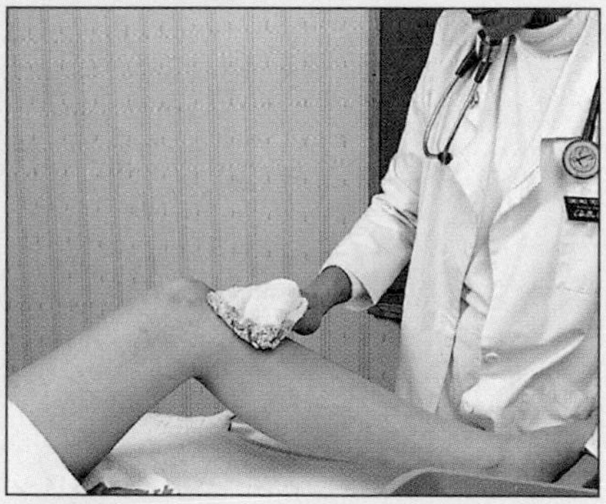

Wash client's legs and feet for a total bed bath.

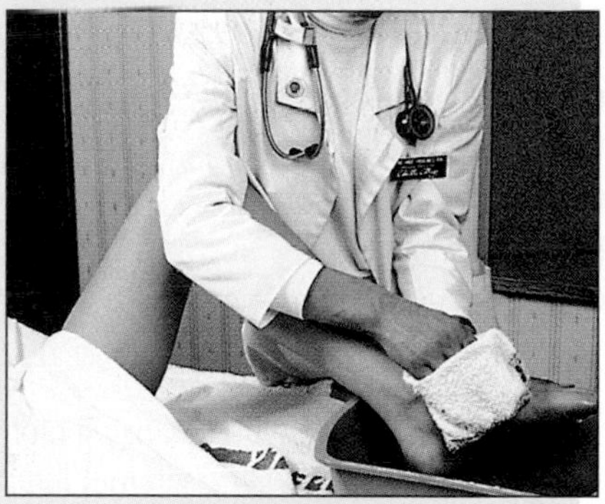

Place client's feet in basin while bathing.

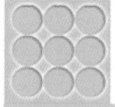

CULTURAL CONSIDERATIONS

When providing hygienic care for clients, the nurse needs to assess the client's usual pattern of bathing, hygienic products usually used, and cultural rituals and beliefs.

Modesty and bathing rituals and beliefs must be considered in caring for clients. For example, some cultures and religions do not allow members of the opposite sex to see them from the waist to the knees (Gypsy culture, Southeast Asian cultures). Hispanic women have a strong sense of modesty and do not want health care workers to see them unclothed.

13. Change bath water. Raise side rails when refilling basin. **Rationale:** This ensures client safety. Check the water temperature before continuing with the bath.
14. During the bath, continuously assess the client's skin and musculoskeletal system. Careful attention should be paid to the verbal statements and nonverbal expressions. **Rationale:** This data yields information about client's overall condition.
15. Help client turn to a side-lying or prone position. Place towel under area to be bathed. Cover client with a bath blanket.
16. Wash, rinse, and dry client's back, moving from the shoulders to the buttocks. **Rationale**: Move from clean to dirty area on body.
17. Provide back massage now or after completion of bath. (For procedure, see Providing Back Care.)
18. Bathe client's genital area. Cover all body parts except area to be bathed. Place towel under client's hips.

for Female Client

a. Bathe perineum from pubis to rectum. **Rationale:** This prevents contamination from the rectal area.
b. Use separate areas of the washcloth for each stroke.
c. Discard soiled washcloths as needed.
d. Clean the labia majora by separating the labia and clean between the majora and labia minora.
e. Wash, rinse, and dry the clitoris, urethral meatus, and vaginal orifice.
f. Ensure all folds of skin are thoroughly dry.

for a Male Client

a. Place a towel under the penis.
b. Hold the penis by the shaft. If the client is uncircumcised, retract the foreskin before washing. **Rationale:** This prevents the formation of phimosis.
c. Using a circular motion, wash, rinse, and dry the meatus of the penis and glans in an outward direction.
d. Gently replace foreskin to its original position.
e. Cleanse the shaft of the penis moving from the tip to the base of the penis.
f. Wash, rinse, and pat dry the scrotum.

19. Remove gloves and place in receptacle.
20. Assist client to dress in a clean hospital gown or pajamas.
21. Clean and store bath equipment. Dispose of dirty linen.
22. Proceed with any other personal hygiene activities as needed.
23. Replace call light, lower bed, and place side rails in UP position before leaving client.
24. Remove gloves, if used, and wash your hands.

BATHING USING DISPOSABLE SYSTEM

Equipment

Commercial cleansing system
Bath blanket
Clean gown
Disposable bag
Clean gloves, if appropriate

Preparation

1. Obtain package with cleansing cloths. Cloths are premoistened with an aloe and vitamin E formula.
2. Heat package in microwave for no more than 45 seconds. **Rationale:** Increased time could lead to excessive heat and burning of the skin. The commercial system can be used at room temperature.
3. Explain procedure to client. **Rationale:** This procedure may be new to the client and an explanation is needed to ensure client understands the difference between a bed bath and a bath using a cleansing system. The client may not think he has had a complete bath but only "a sponge bath."
4. Wash your hands.
5. Don gloves if there is a risk of contact with body secretions.
6. Replace top linen and gown with bath blanket.

Procedure

1. Open package and remove one cloth at a time.
2. Remove bath blanket at each site when cleansing with cloth.

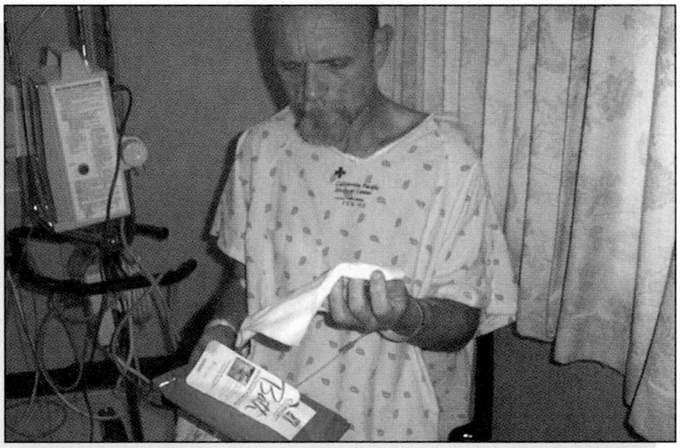

Each towel is used once and discarded.

3. Replace bath blanket when cloth removed. **Rationale:** To prevent client chilling.
4. Use a new cloth for each section of the body as follows:
   a. Face, neck, and chest
   b. Right arm and axilla
   c. Left arm and axilla
   d. Perineum
   e. Right leg
   f. Left leg
   g. Back
   h. Buttocks

5. Discard cloth after cleansing each area. Rinsing is not required with this system. Replace bath blanket over each part of the body after it has been cleaned. **Rationale:** To prevent the client from becoming chilled.
6. Place clean gown on client.
7. Place client in comfortable position.
8. Discard cloths in appropriate receptacle in dirty utility room.
9. Wash your hands.
10. Document bath on flow sheet or nurses' notes.

BATHING AN INFANT

Equipment

Tub or basin filled with warm water (100°F)
Two towels
Washcloth
Suction bulb
Mild soap
Cotton balls
Blanket
Clean clothing
Clean gloves, if indicated

Preparation

1. Provide a comfortable room environment (i.e., comfortable temperature, lighting.)
2. Wash your hands.
3. Collect necessary equipment, and place articles within reach.
4. Position the bed at a comfortable working height.
5. Place towel, laid out in diamond fashion, on bed next to basin.
6. Don gloves if there is a risk of exposure to body secretions.

Procedure

1. Test water temperature with your wrist or elbow.
2. Lift infant using football hold.
3. Remove all clothing except shirt and diaper.
4. Cover infant with towel or blanket. Never let go of the infant during the bath. **Rationale:** This is a safety intervention.
5. Clean infant's eyes, using a cotton ball moistened with water. Wipe from inner to outer canthus, using a new cotton ball for each eye. **Rationale:** This procedure prevents water and particles from entering the lacrimal duct.

CLINICAL ALERT

Discharge is present for 2 to 3 days due to prophylactic eyedrops administered at birth.

6. Make a mitt with the washcloth.
7. Wash infant's face with water.

Some facilities use disposable cleansing systems to bathe neonates and infants. There are four infant-size washcloths for infants up to 25 pounds. The bathing procedure is the same for infants and adults.

8. Suction nose, if necessary, by compressing suction bulb prior to placing it in nostril. **Rationale:** This prevents aspiration of moisture. Release bulb after it is placed in nostril.
9. Wash infant's ears and neck, paying attention to folds; dry all areas thoroughly.
10. Remove shirt or gown.
11. Remove diaper by picking up infant's ankles in your hand.
12. Pick up infant and place feet first into basin or tub. Immerse infant in tub of water only after umbilical cord has healed. Pick up infant by placing your hand and arm around infant, cradling the infant's head and neck in your elbow. Grasp the infant's thigh with your hand. **Rationale:** The umbilical cord is kept dry to prevent infection and encourage it to "fall off."
13. Wash and rinse the infant's body, especially the skin folds.
14. Wash infant's genitalia.
    a. For a female infant: Separate labia and with a cotton ball moistened with soap and water, cleanse downward once on each side. Use a new piece of cotton on each side.
    b. For an uncircumcised male infant: Do not force foreskin back. Gently cleanse the exposed surface with a cotton ball moistened with soap and water.
    c. For a circumcised male infant: Gently cleanse with plain water.
15. Wrap the infant in a towel and use a football hold when washing an infant's head. Soap your own hands and wash infant's hair and scalp, using a circular motion. Rinse hair and scalp thoroughly. **Rationale:** Football hold is the most secure for active infants.
16. Place infant on a clean, dry towel with head facing the top corner and wrap infant.
17. Use the corner of the towel to dry infant's head with gentle, yet firm, circular movements.
18. Replace infant's diaper and redress in a new gown or shirt.
19. Provide comfort by holding the infant for a time following the bath procedure.
20. Wash your hands.

BATHING IN A HYDRAULIC BATHTUB CHAIR

Equipment

Two towels and washcloth
Soap
Clean gown, robe, and slippers

Procedure

1. Bring client to tub room in wheelchair.
2. Fill tub with water and check temperature. **Rationale:** Temperature must not be over 105°F or client may burn skin.
3. Release chair to lowest point beside tub, and place towel on floor under chair.
4. Move client into bathtub chair, and attach seat belt.
5. Swing chair into position over tub.
6. Direct client to move legs down, then lower chair into low position in the tub filled with water.
7. When client is finished bathing, reverse chair out of tub.

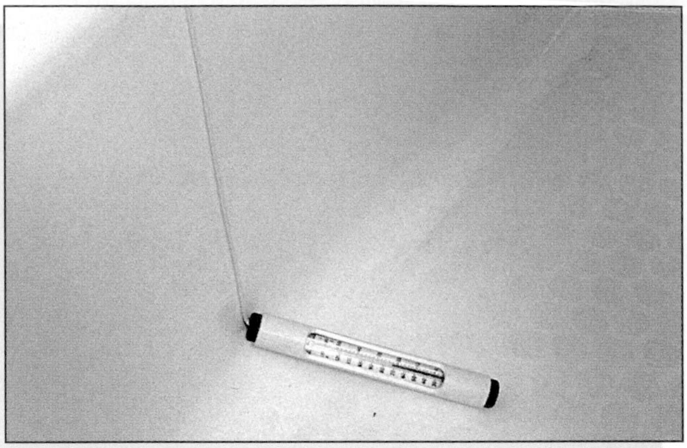

Check that water temperature is not above 105°F for safety.

8. Assist client to towel dry.
9. Put clean gown, robe, and slippers on client and transport to room.

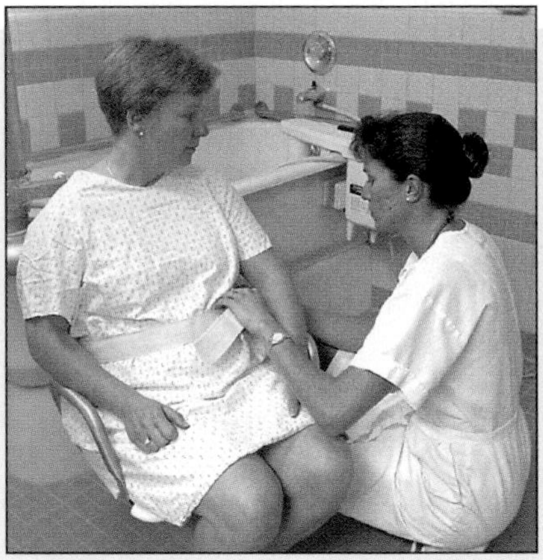

Attach seat belt before swinging chair over the tub.

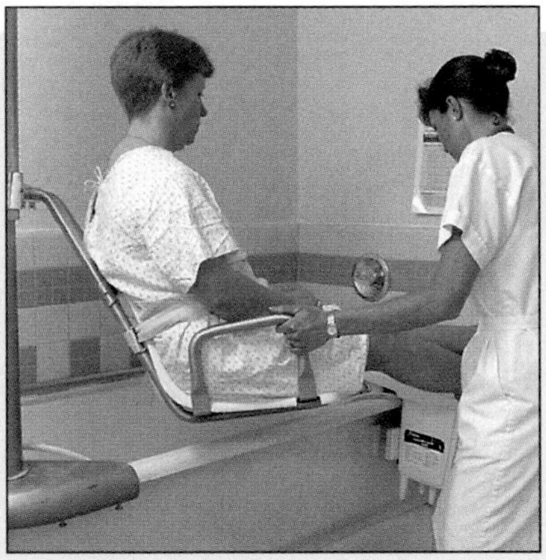

Support client in chair as chair is swung over tub.

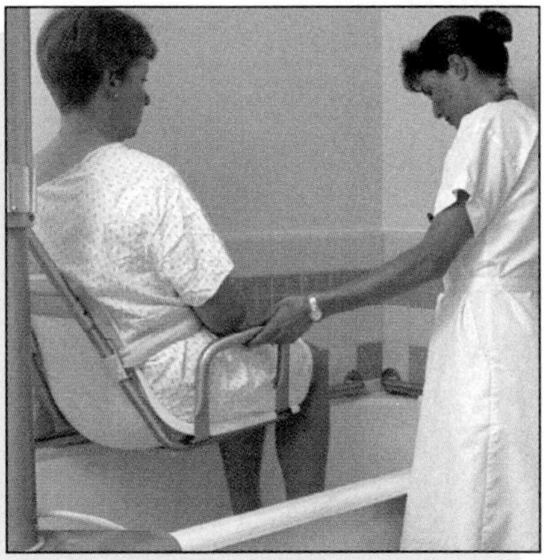

Lower chair into tub filled with water.

DOCUMENTATION FOR BATH CARE

- Client's overall ability to participate in own care
- Type of bath given (i.e., complete or partial) and by whom (e.g., client, nurse, family member)
- Condition of client's skin and any interventions provided for the skin (e.g., lotion, massage)
- Client's educational needs regarding hygienic care
- Information shared with client or family
- Infant bath demonstration to parents with return demonstration

Critical Thinking Application

UNEXPECTED OUTCOMES	CRITICAL THINKING OPTIONS
Client is unwilling to accept a complete bed bath.	• Respect client's wishes and take other opportunities for assessment. • Have client wash hands, face, and genitals. You should wash back and give back care. Reexplain the purpose of the bath to the client and request client participation.
Client is too shy to allow bath.	• Respect client's privacy and only wash areas client wishes you to do. • Give assistance so client can bathe him or herself. • Allow spouse or parent to give bath if this is more acceptable to client.
Client complains of dry, itching skin following the bath.	• Assess for cause of itching. • Ask physician for an order for special lotion. • Do not use soap for the bath.

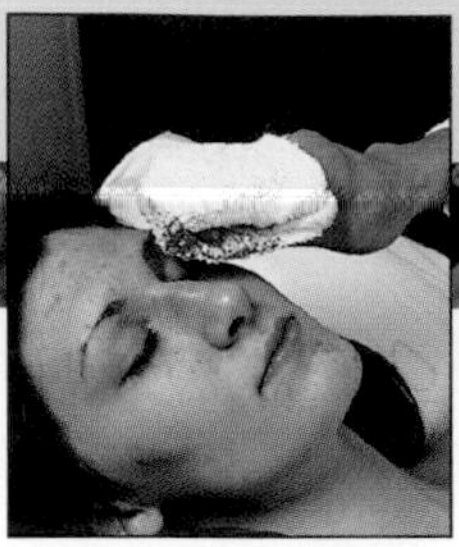

Skin Integrity

Nursing Process Data

ASSESSMENT Data Base

Assess for signs of skin breakdown or the eruption of lesions.
Assess color of skin.
Assess color of mucous membranes.
Check for alterations in skin turgor.
Evaluate for complaints of itching, tingling, or numbness.
Evaluate texture of skin.
Assess general hygienic state.
Observe skin for increased or decreased pigmentation and discoloration.
Evaluate client's condition to determine appropriate support surface or specialty bed.

PLANNING Objectives

To maintain intact skin without signs of ischemia, hyperemia, or necrosis
To recognize a break in skin integrity
To avoid introduction of pathogens through break in skin
To prevent skin breakdown from pressure points or strain
To prevent excessive dryness, flaking, itching, or burning
To use heat support surface or specialty bed to prevent or treat altered skin integrity.

IMPLEMENTATION Procedures

Monitoring Skin Condition
Preventing Skin Breakdown
Managing Skin Tears

EVALUATION Expected Outcomes

Client's skin remains intact without signs of ischemia, hyperemia, or necrosis.
Client is able to change position without evidence of pressure areas.
Client's skin does not show signs of dryness, flaking, itching, or burning.
Client does not complain of pain.

MONITORING SKIN CONDITION

Equipment

Artificial light for observation if natural light is not available
Bath blanket
Gown
Clean gloves, if indicated

Procedure

1. Explain monitoring process to client.
2. Provide privacy for client, and wash your hands.
3. Remove linens and gown if necessary. Cover client with bath blanket.
4. Compare color of client's skin with normal range of color within the individual's race. Observe for pallor (white color), flushing (red color), jaundice (yellow color), ashen (gray color), or cyanosis (blue color).
5. Place the back of your fingers or hand on client's skin to check temperature. *Consider the temperature of the room and of your hands.* **Rationale:** The back of the hand is more sensitive to changes in temperature than the palm.
6. Correlate abnormalities in skin color with changes in skin temperature. **Rationale:** Skin temperature reflects blood circulation in the dermis layer.
7. Observe for areas of excessive dryness, moisture, wrinkling, flaking, and general texture of skin.
8. Gently pick up a small section of the skin with your thumb and finger. Observe for ease of movement and speed of return to original position to check for skin turgor. **Rationale:** Degree of hydration is reflected in the skin turgor or elasticity of the skin.
9. Press your finger firmly against client's skin for several seconds (especially ankle area). After removing your finger, observe for lasting impression or indentation. **Rationale:** This identifies the degree of edema based on the level of indentation. 1+ to 5+ indicates edema of 1 cm to 5 cm.

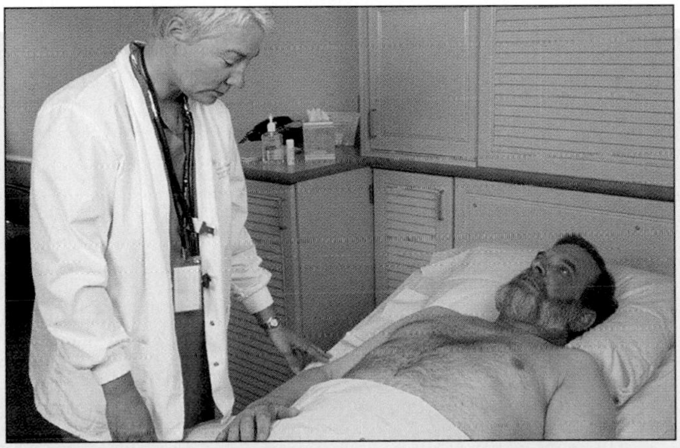

Compare color of client's skin with normal range of color within the individual's race.

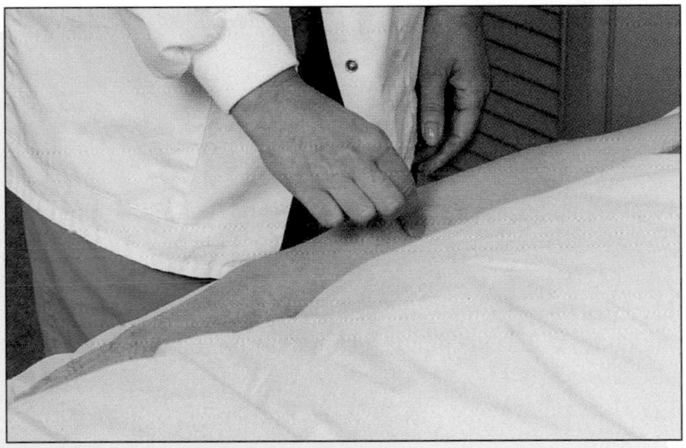

Gently pick up a small section of skin with your thumb and finger to check for skin turgor.

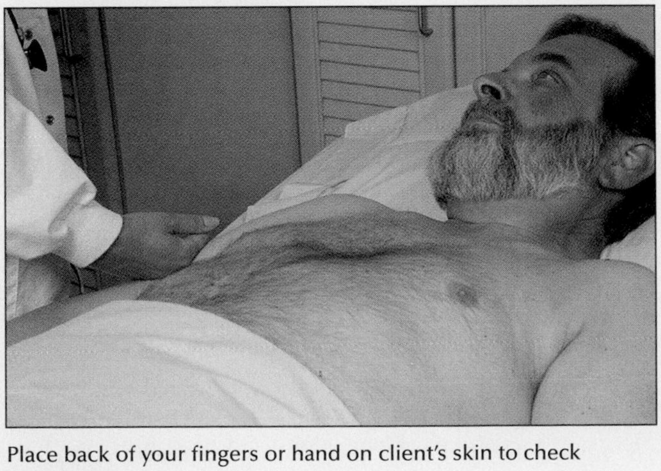

Place back of your fingers or hand on client's skin to check temperature.

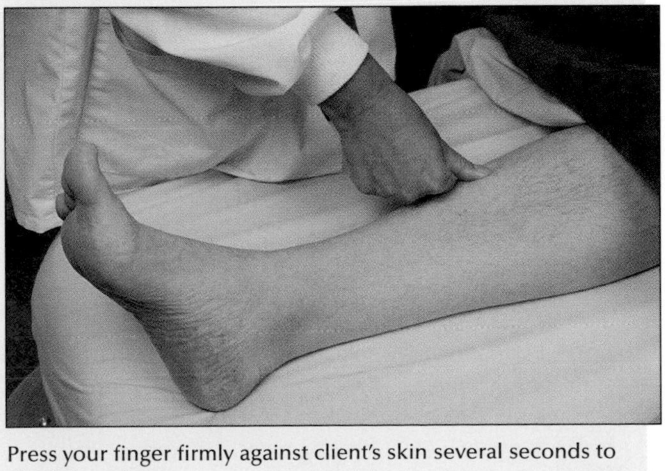

Press your finger firmly against client's skin several seconds to check for edema.

TABLE 8–1 Potential Skin Problems

Skin Condition	Problem	Nursing Responsibility
Xeroderma, or dry skin	If skin is extremely dry, it could crack and become infected May cause pruritus	Maintain skin integrity Bathe less frequently Use superfatted soap Use tepid, not hot, water and rinse well after bathing Relieve discomfort Use emollient or moisturizing lotion after bathing Encourage nutritious diet Increase fluid intake Maintain cool, humid environment
Skin rash or contact dermatitis. May be allergic or nonallergic reaction	Erythema, flat or raised eruptions and inflammation Could cause pruritus, discomfort, and infection if scratched	Avoid soap and heat, and rubbing area Bathe area: may use antiseptic soap with orders Apply ordered lotion or spray (steroids) to prevent itching Use cool, wet dressing
Abrasions	Break in skin integrity could result in infection Healing may be prolonged due to age (poor circulation, etc.)	Wash abrasions with soap and water Apply lotion as ordered
Fungal skin infection	Fungal skin infection: common in diabetics, those on antibiotics or immunosuppressive therapy, those who are incontinent	Apply topical antifungal medication as ordered Dry skin folds well before applying antifungal medication Apply medication sparingly to prevent skin from becoming too moist Keep incontinent clients dry and provide good perineal care Avoid using plastic pants or liners next to client's skin Use nonocclusive dressings if needed

10. When checking skin temperature and texture of skin, note the client's response to heat, cold, gentle touch, and pressure.
11. Observe the amount of oil, moisture, and dirt on the skin surface. **Rationale:** Degree of moisture or dryness indicates disease states or hydration status.
12. Note presence of strong body odor or odor in the skin folds.
13. Use a disposable blunt-ended probe such as a comb to detect small moving white specks. **Rationale:** Lice or white specks may be present on head as well as in pubic area when body lice are present.
14. Observe for areas of broken skin (lesions) or ulcers. If present, wear gloves. Check if lesions are present over entire body or if they are localized to a specific area.
15. Check for skin discolorations (e.g., ecchymosis, petechiae, purpura, erythema, and altered pigmentation). **Rationale:** These signs are indications of generalized disease states, such as leukemia, vitamin deficiency, or hemophilia.

PREVENTING SKIN BREAKDOWN

Equipment

Skin lotion
Pressure-relieving mattress
Clean gloves if open lesions are present

Procedure

1. Inspect skin daily; observe the client's most vulnerable body surfaces for ischemia, hyperemia, or broken areas.
2. Change the client's body position at least once every 2 hours to rotate weight-bearing areas. Use turning techniques. **Rationale:** To minimize skin injury caused by friction and shear forces. Observe all vulnerable areas at this time. Include right and left lateral, prone, supine, and swimming-type positioning if possible.
3. Massage client's skin and pressure-prone areas, if skin is not reddened, when client changes position. **Rationale:** Massage increases risk of breakdown in clients with reddened areas over bony prominences.
4. Lubricate dry, unbroken skin to prevent breakdown. Use cornstarch and creams or protective barriers such as skin sealants.
5. Apply lotion to bedridden client's sacrum, elbows, and heels several times during the day.

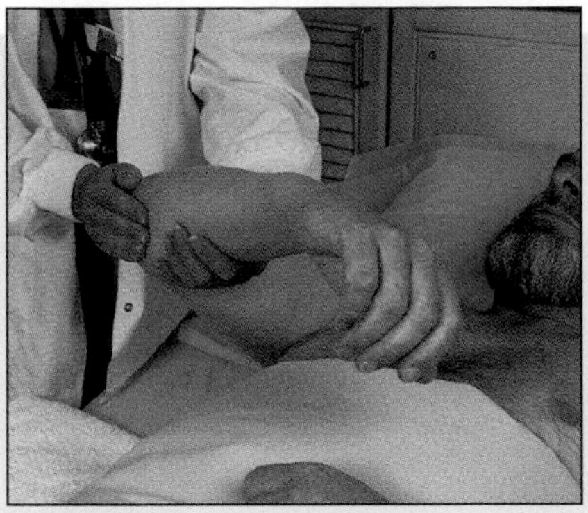
Observe client's most vulnerable body surfaces for ischemia, hyperemia, or broken skin.

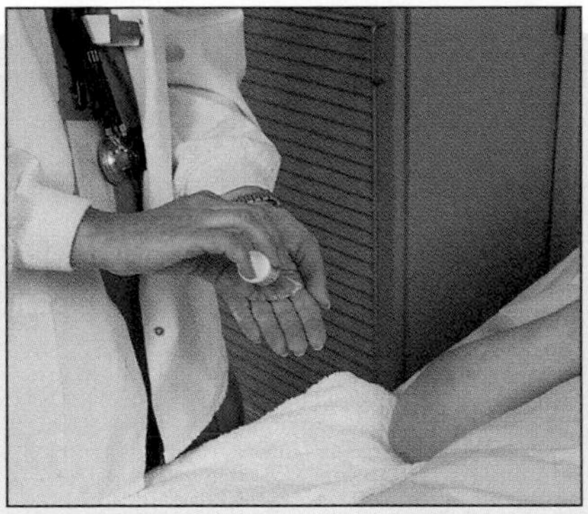
Lubricate dry, unbroken skin to prevent breakdown.

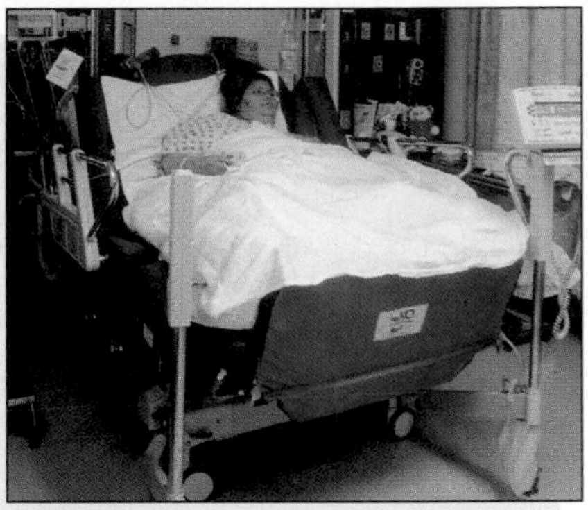
High-risk, obese clients should be placed on BariKare beds.

6. Cleanse skin with warm water and a mild pH-balanced cleansing agent, then apply moisturizers and a barrier cream as ordered.
7. Protect healthy skin from drainage secretions.
8. Use protective padding on heels and elbows if needed.
9. Keep linens clean, dry, and wrinkle-free.
10. Encourage active exercise or range-of-motion exercise.
11. Encourage client to eat a well-balanced diet with protein-rich foods and adequate fluids.
12. Teach client and family how to prevent pressure areas and pressure ulcer formation.

Products used to prevent skin breakdown and treat impaired skin integrity are selected based on client's skin type, product application, cost, and desired outcome.

CLINICAL ALERT

New guidelines from the U.S. Department of Health and Human Services advocate no skin massage on reddened skin or skin that has a potential for breakdown because massage causes friction and shearing.

PREVENTING SKIN TEARS

Equipment

Lift or turning sheet
Padding for bedrails, or other equipment
Pillows and blankets
Paper tape
Moisturizing agent for skin
Clean gloves as needed

Preparation

1. Identify clients at risk for developing skin tears. **Rationale:** Clients at risk are those on bedrest, those with purpura or ecchymosis, paper-thin skin, poor vision resulting in accidental bumping into objects.
2. Identify the category of skin tear, if present. **Rationale:** To determine correct nursing action to be completed.
3. Wash hands before providing client care.

Procedure

1. Use lift sheet or The Booster lift device when moving clients at risk for developing skin tears. **Rationale:** This will assist in preventing tears resulting from friction or shearing.

Payne–Martin Classification System for Skin Tears

Category I: skin tears without tissue loss

Linear type: epidermis and dermis pulled apart

Flap type: epidermal flap completely covers dermis to within 1 mm of the wound margin

Category II: skin tears with partial tissue loss

Scant tissue loss type: 25% or less of epidermal flap lost

Moderate to large tissue loss type: more than 25% epidermal flap lost

Category III: skin tears with complete tissue loss, no epidermal flap

Source: Payne, R. L. and Martin, M. L. (1998). *Ostomy Wound Management, Classification System for Skin Tears, 39,* 16–26.

2. Remove tape from dressings carefully; use only paper or nonadherent dressing for at-risk clients, if possible.
3. Assist clients with ambulation if unsteady gait. Remove objects in pathway. **Rationale:** To prevent client from bumping into objects and causing bruises and cuts or from falling.
4. Ensure clients use glasses, if necessary, when ambulating or transferring into chair. **Rationale:** To prevent falling or unsteady gait due to impaired vision.
5. Place padding on beds, wheelchairs, or equipment. **Rationale:** To prevent client from rubbing on hard surfaces and causing bruising.
6. Don gloves and apply moisturizing agent to dry skin to keep moist.
7. Remove gloves and place in appropriate receptacle.
8. Wash hands.
9. Document findings in chart.

CLINICAL ALERT

Ensure that all health care workers are aware of proper handling of elderly clients with fragile skin. Slight friction and shearing can create a skin tear when turning or lifting these clients.

MANAGING SKIN TEARS

Equipment

Saline
Nontoxic wound cleanser
Moist wound dressing (e.g., Hydrogel, foam, petrolatum ointment)
Nonadherent dressings
Steri-strips
Gauze
Clean gloves

Procedure

1. Wash hands and don clean gloves.
2. Remove old dressing being careful to not cause additional skin damage. Moisten dressing with saline before removing if dressing sticks to skin.
3. Assess for signs of infection.
4. Cleanse skin tear with saline or nontoxic wound cleanser. Be careful not to put pressure on skin as you are cleaning. **Rationale:** To prevent additional trauma to skin.
5. Place steri-strips over edges of skin flap to approximate edges of tear and surrounding tissue. **Rationale:** To promote healing.
6. Apply moist wound dressing over tear site.
7. Secure nonadherent dressing with gauze.
8. Change dressings according to hospital policy.
9. Remove gloves and place in appropriate receptacle.
10. Wash hands.
11. Document findings in chart.

SUPPORT SURFACES AND SPECIALTY BEDS

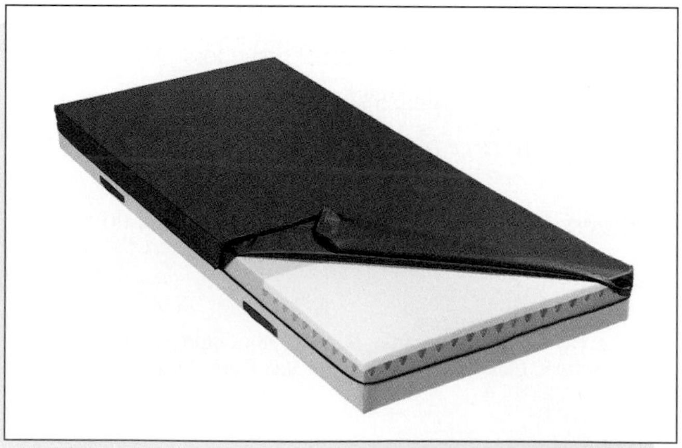

FirstStep Select, an overlay mattress from KCI.

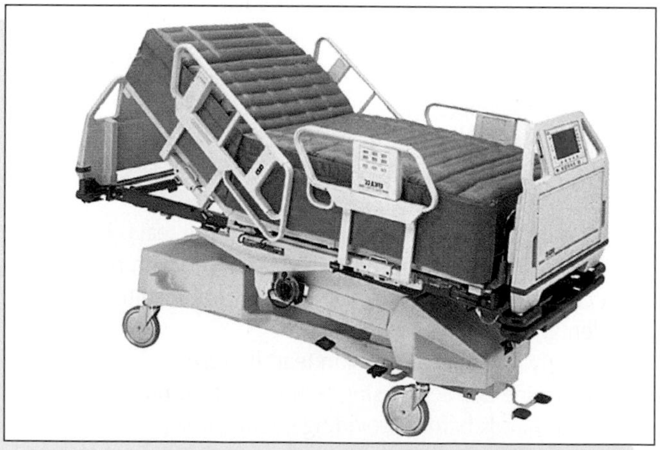

Active low-air-loss beds gently pulsate or rotate from side to side. The EFICA-CC (illustrated courtesy of Hill-Rom) offers automatic pressure adjustment. Other brands include Biodyne, Restcue, and Pulmonair 40.

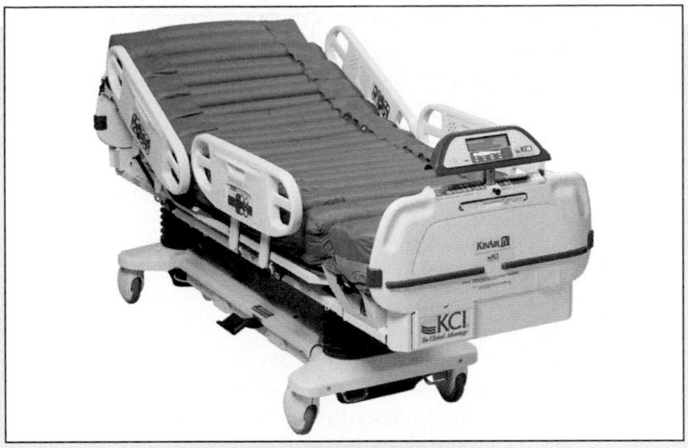

KinAir IV, a low-air-pressure bed from KCI.

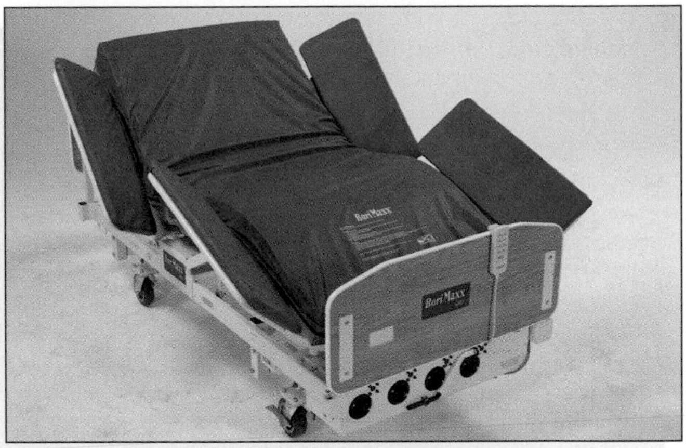

BariKare, a bariatric pressure bed from KCI.

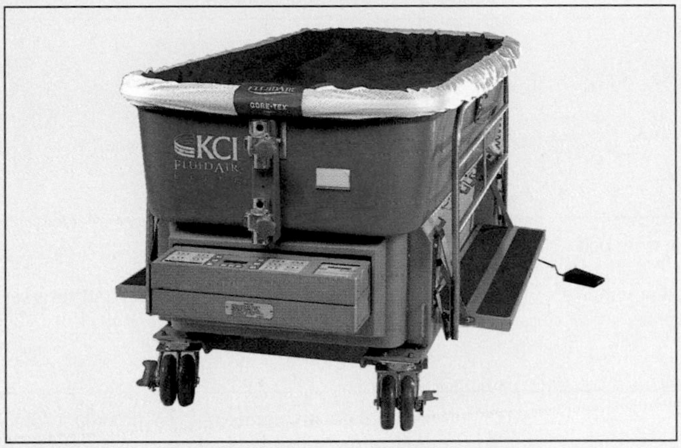

FluidAir Elite, a high-air-pressure bed from KCI.

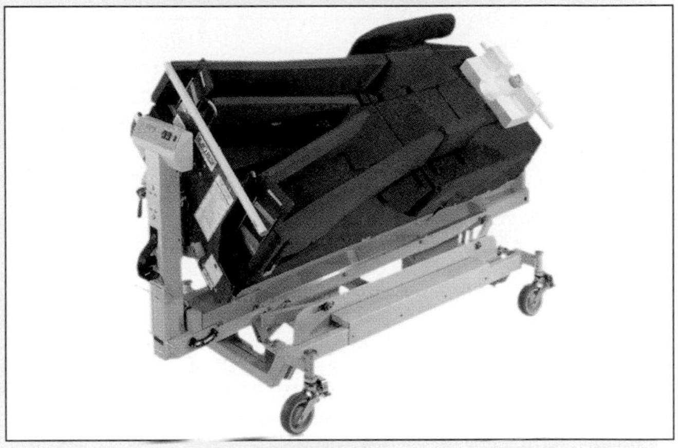

RotoRest Delta, a kinetic bed from KCI.

DOCUMENTATION FOR SKIN INTEGRITY

- Client's skin condition: odor, temperature, turgor, sensation, cleanliness, integrity
- Client's mobility
- Turning frequency and client positioning
- Type of care given (e.g., massage, bathing)
- Client's complaints about skin or pressure ulcer
- Time and method used to obtain wound specimen
- Type of lesion, location, size, shape, color
- Alterations in sensation in skin lesion area
- Skin or body odor
- Presence of skin tear and assessment findings
- Treatment given for skin tear

TABLE 8–2 Therapeutic Beds

Type of Bed	Bed Features and Benefits	Client Recommendations
Low-air-loss Flexicair (MC3) KinAir (KCI) Mediscus SMI 3000	Segmented cushions minimize shear and friction Automatic pressure adjustment Air flows through mattress and sheets to client's skin, which aids evaporation of moisture and reduces temperature Quick adjustment for CPR Built-in scale Bed-exit alarm Extended safety sides U-shaped cushions provide relief for head, sacral area, and heels	Clients at high risk for skin breakdown Clients with pulmonary problems—reduces risk of airborne contamination Clients with external fixators, heavy casts, or who are obese Clients with skin grafts, flaps, and all four stages of pressure ulcers
Air fluidized or high-air-loss Rite Hite, Clinitron II Skytron Fluid Air (KCI) SMI 5000	Fluid-like movement places minimum pressure on bony prominences Drying effect of beads prevents skin breakdown Offers softer surface than any other bed	Severe skin disorders Pressure ulcers Burns Generalized massive edema Poor wound healing Geriatric or orthopedic clients
Active low-air-loss EFICA-CC (illustrated) Biodyne Restcue Pulmonair 40	Built-in scale CPR deflation control Automatic pressure adjustment Gently pulsates or rotates side to side Protects skin integrity Promotes removal of pulmonary secretions Stimulates capillary blood flow	Massive edema Congestive heart failure Sepsis Critical care clients Pneumonia or other pulmonary problems with compromised skin integrity
Bariatric Patient Care Systems MAGNUM II (Hill-Rom) BariKare (KCI)	Chair position allows sitting up without transferring from bed Control lower extremity edema Upper body x-rays can be easily obtained while client remains in bed Low air loss Percussion and palpation easily done	Obese clients up to 850 lbs. Difficult clients to move in or out of bed Client's requiring Trendelenburg's position and reverse Trendelenburg's position
Kinetic SpO_2RT Dynamic Air Therapy RotoRest	Continuous lateral rotation 20–40 degrees Enhanced surface system Increased client comfort Easy for one care giver to provide care Less need for client transfer Decreases length of time on ventilators Decreases length of hospital stays Built-in bed scales on some models	Clients with pulmonary conditions; pneumonia, COPD Skin complications related to bed rest Spinal cord–injured clients

Critical Thinking Application

UNEXPECTED OUTCOMES	CRITICAL THINKING OPTIONS
Skin is erythematous but remains intact.	• Monitor fluid balance and nutritional status. • Obtain pressure-relieving mattress. • Turn client every 2 hours.
Client cannot be positioned in a manner to avoid erythematous areas entirely.	• Turn at least every hour. • Do not turn on erythematous site. • Use protocol for stage 1 ulcer treatment on affected area.
Skin integrity is interrupted, even with skin care.	• Use aseptic technique in treating area to prevent spread of bacteria and promote wound healing. • Use appropriate skin care products.
Skin tear occurs.	• If skin is sensitive and breakdown occurs over large area, the use of a Clinitron unit or fluid bed might be indicated (Table 8-2).

UNIT 4

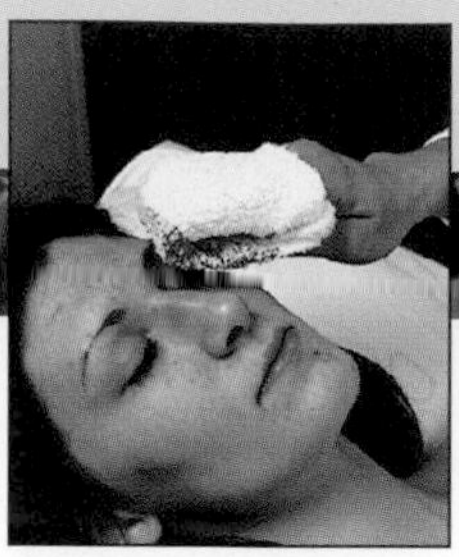

Evening Care

Nursing Process Data

ASSESSMENT Data Base

Review client's usual routines prior to sleep:
- Usual time of sleep and length of sleeping period
- Personal hygiene routines
- Temperature of room and number of blankets
- Anticipated elimination needs
- Religious or meditation needs

Evaluate client's understanding and acceptance of safety precautions, such as use of side rails.

Assess client's needs for comfort and security.
- Dressings
- Medication
- Linen change or adjustment
- Positioning
- Television, radio, light
- Communication needs

Assess physical and emotional status during evening care.

Assess condition of back, especially bony prominences.

PLANNING Objectives

To encourage a period of comfortable, uninterrupted rest

To evaluate the client's present health status

To make observations about the client's physical and emotional status

To provide time for the client and nurse to review the day's events

To provide time for the client to communicate needs and questions regarding health care

To provide the client with a clean, secure environment in which to sleep

IMPLEMENTATION Procedures

Providing Evening Care

Providing Back Care

EVALUATION Expected Outcomes

Client states he or she is comfortable and ready for sleep in a safe, clean environment.

Client has the time to talk about concerns or ask questions.

The nurse is able to evaluate the client's health care status.

PROVIDING EVENING CARE

Equipment

Towels, washcloth
Clean linens if needed
Basin of warm water, soap
Dental items (i.e., toothbrush, dentifrice, denture cup)
Emesis basin, cup
Fresh pitcher of water if allowed
Skin care lotion and powder if desired
Personal care items (e.g., deodorant, skin moisturizers)
Bedpan, urinal, toilet paper
Miscellaneous supplies as needed (e.g., dressing, special equipment)
Clean gloves, if indicated

Preparation

1. Explain the needs and benefits of evening care; discuss how the client can be involved.
2. Collect and arrange equipment.
3. Adjust the bed to a comfortable working height, and assist the client into a comfortable position.
4. Ensure privacy.
5. Wash your hands.
6. Don gloves if indicated.

Procedure

1. Offer bedpan or urinal if client is unable to use bathroom. Assist with handwashing.
2. If client needs or requests a bath, provide assistance as needed.
3. Assist with mouth and dental care as needed.
4. Remove equipment, extra linens, and pillows if possible. Remove stockings, ace wraps, and binders.
5. Change dressings. Perform any required procedural techniques.
6. Wash face, hands, and back. Provide back massage.
7. Assist with combing or brushing hair if desired.
8. Replace antiembolic (elastic) stockings and binders.
9. Replace soiled linen, or straighten and tuck remaining linen. Fluff pillow and turn cool side next to client.
10. Straighten top linens. Provide additional blankets if desired.
11. Remove any additional equipment. Place call signal and water (if allowed) within client's reach.
12. Administer sleeping medication if ordered and client requests.
13. Assess for pain.
14. Assist client into a comfortable position.
15. Ensure that the client's environment is safe and comfortable.
16. Raise side rails, place bed in LOW position, and turn lighting to low.

Note: Side rails are now considered restraints. Check with your facility about agency policies on use of side rails. See Chapter 7, page 133.

17. Remove gloves, if used.
18. Wash your hands.

PROVIDING BACK CARE

Equipment

Basin of warm water
Washcloth
Towel
Soap
Skin care lotion

Procedure

1. Check skin for reddened areas before beginning back rub.
2. Explain the purpose of a back rub, and ask client if he or she would like one.
3. Provide privacy.
4. Wash your hands with warm water.
5. Warm lotion by holding bottle under water.
6. Raise bed to comfortable height for you, and assist the client into a comfortable prone or semiprone position. Keep farthest side rail in UP position.
7. Drape bed clothes for warmth, and untie the client's gown. Wash back with warm water and soap if necessary.
8. Place lotion on your hands.
9. Once you place your hands on a client's back to begin a back rub, your hands should remain in constant skin contact with the client until back rub is complete. **Rationale:** To prevent "tickling" sensation.
10. Repeatedly move your hands up on either side of the client's spine, across shoulders, and down the lateral aspects of the back using the effleurage stroke, applying firm and steady pressure.
11. Then rub your hands over the scapular area, extending over the upper shoulders, using a circular motion.
12. Move your hands down the center of the client's back to sacral area.
13. Massage with a figure-eight motion from the sacrum out over each buttock.

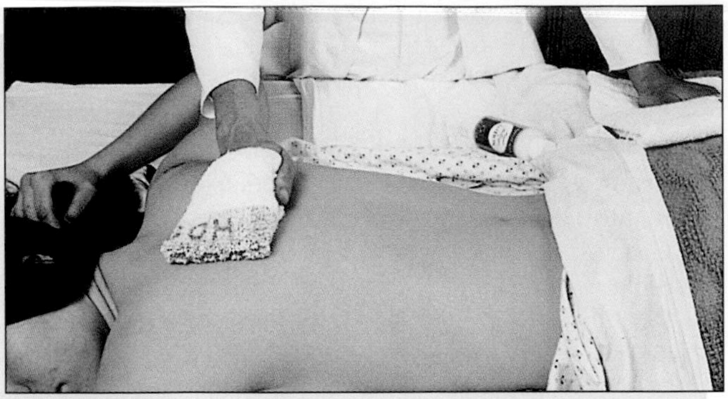

Wash back with soap and water, then dry thoroughly before beginning back rub.

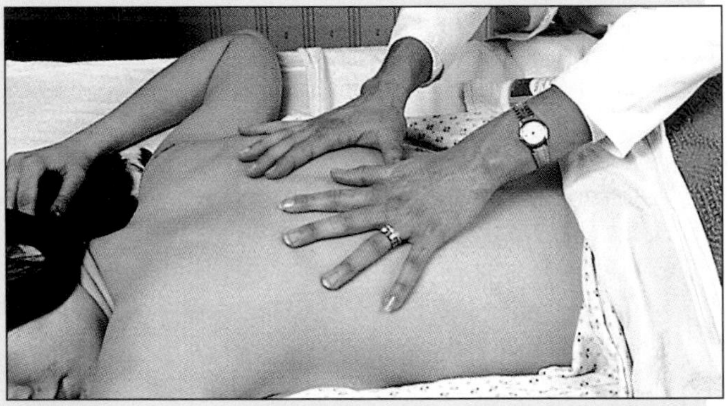

Without lifting hands from skin surface, massage in continuous motion.

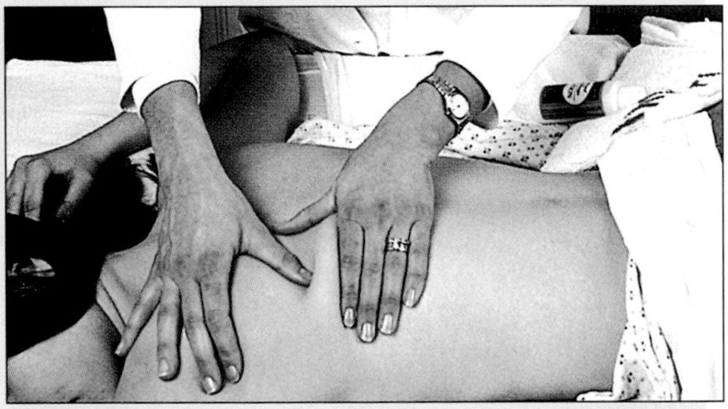

The petrissage, or kneading stroke, is used over the shoulders and along back.

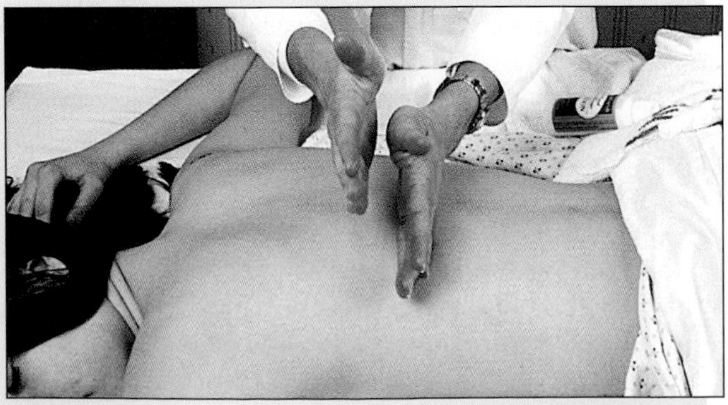

The tapotement stroke stimulates the skin as the hands move up and down the back.

14. Finally, rub lightly up and down the back a few strokes before lifting hands from client's back.
15. Assess skin for color, turgor, skin breakdown.
16. When stimulation is desired, the back and buttocks can be lightly struck with the fleshy sides of your hands, called tapotement. Using an alternating rhythm, move up and down the back several times. In addition, kneading can be accomplished by picking up the skin between the thumb and fingers as you move up the back. This movement is called petrissage.
17. Close client's gown, pull up bedcovers, and assist client to change position if desired. Place side rails in UP position. Place bed in LOW position.
18. Return lotion to the proper area.
19. Wash your hands.

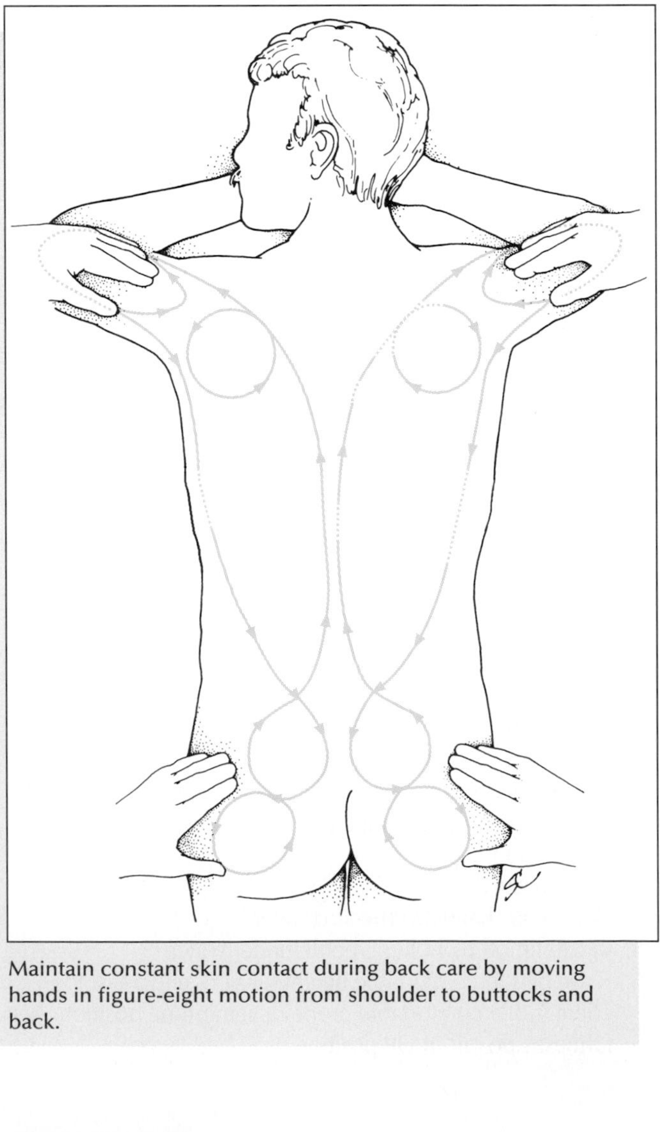

Maintain constant skin contact during back care by moving hands in figure-eight motion from shoulder to buttocks and back.

DOCUMENTATION FOR EVENING CARE

- Client's level of comfort or discomfort
- Type of care given (i.e., back care, evening care)
- Any significant complaints
- Nature of client teaching if done
- Medication required for discomfort or sleep
- Client's physical and emotional status after evening care completed

Critical Thinking Application

UNEXPECTED OUTCOMES	CRITICAL THINKING OPTIONS
Client misinterprets back care from nurse and makes sexual advances.	• Set firm limits by explaining therapeutic purpose of back care. • Tell client that if he or she cannot accept back care as part of the therapeutic regimen, you will stop.
Client refuses back care because he or she thinks you are too busy or disinterested.	• Make sure you offer the back care in an unhurried and meaningful manner. Do not allow the client to misinterpret your offer for care. • Return to client and offer back care later in the evening.
Client is unable to sleep even after evening care is given.	• Encourage verbalization of fears. • Check to see if sleeping medication can be given. • Provide additional back care.

GERONTOLOGIC CONSIDERATIONS

Factors that can increase risk of skin breakdown and delay wound healing.

- Inadequate nutritional intake.
- Compromised immune system.
- Compromised circulatory and respiratory systems.
- Poor hydration.
- Decreased mobility and activity.

Skin changes with age.

- Delayed cellular migration and proliferation.
- Skin is less effective as barrier and slow to heal.
- There is increased vulnerability to trauma.
- There is less ability to retain water.
- Geriatric skin is dry (osteotosis) due to decreased endocrine secretion and loss of elastin. This can cause pruritus, which could lead to skin ulceration.
- Increased skin susceptibility to shearing stress leading to blister formation and skin tears.
- There is increased vascular fragility.

The skin of the elderly should be assessed.

- Decreased temperature, degree of moisture, dryness resulting from decreased dermal vascularity.
- Skin not intact, open lesions, tears, pressure ulcers as a result of increased skin fragility.
- Decreased turgor, dehydration as a result of decreased oil and sweat glands.
- Pigmentation alterations, potential cancer.
- Pruritus—dry skin most common cause because of decreased oil and sweat glands.
- Bruises, scars from increased skin fragility.

Bathing may minimize dryness.

- Have client take complete bath only twice a week.
- Use superfatted or mild soap or lotions to aid in moisturizing.
- Use tepid, not hot, water.
- Apply emollient (lanolin) to skin after bathing.

MANAGEMENT GUIDELINES

Each state legislates a Nurse Practice Act for RNs and LVN/LPNs. Health care facilities are responsible for establishing and implementing policies and procedures that conform to their state's regulations. Verify the regulations and role parameters for each health care worker in your facility.

Delegation of Responsibilities

- All personnel interacting with clients must report any client risk behaviors or signs or symptoms that are unusual or new. Since activities of bathing or bedmaking have predictable outcomes and do not require nursing judgment, they are usually delegated to CNAs or UAPs. When these activities of daily living are delegated to a CNA or unlicensed personnel, the professional nurse remains responsible for total client care and should receive a complete report from the staff member assigned to the client.
- Even though unlicensed personnel are qualified to complete many tasks that involve activities of daily living, if the client is critically ill or unstable, the RN or LVN/LPN should be assigned to such a client. The professional nurse may observe the client's total condition, thereby avoiding complications caused by missed assessment parameters.

Information Flow

- CNAs and UAPs must report any unusual or unanticipated signs or symptoms or risk behaviors to the RN or LVN/LPN responsible for the client's care. This report should include mental status as well as previously unreported physical signs and symptoms observed during the interaction period.
- Clients with skin tears may be referred to the wound care specialist if the facility has one on staff. This would be especially beneficial if the tear is a category II or III.

CRITICAL THINKING STRATEGIES

SCENARIO 1

An 89-year-old male was admitted earlier today and you were assigned to admit him and provide nursing care for the remainder of the shift (4 hours). His admitting diagnosis is dehydration due to prolonged nausea and vomiting. He lives with his 88-year-old wife. They have some home health care twice a week, and a nursing assistant assists them with bathing and personal hygienic care. He is usually very active, walking, gardening, and attending church every week.

Your nursing history indicates he has not been out of bed for three days. He was unable to get to the bathroom and used a urinal, which proved to be difficult for him to manage and he spilled some urine each time he used it. He has not had a bath for 4 days and has not brushed or cleaned his dentures.

1. Considering the client's issues related to bathing and bedmaking, what is your priority assessment when completing the initial assessment? Provide the rationale for your answer.
2. What information would you place on his care plan to prevent skin breakdown? List the risk factors the client probably exhibited.
3. Outline the nursing interventions that will be incorporated in his plan of care for the pressure ulcer?
4. What would you consider priority for his bathing needs? Provide the rationale for your answer.
5. Identify the major preventative measures to prevent skin breakdown or tears that will need to be discussed with the nursing assistant who will continue to care for him when he returns home.

SCENARIO 2

The client develops a skin tear on the greater trochanter the second day after admission.

Refer to Scenario 1.

1. Identify risk factors for developing a skin tear.
2. Describe the nursing interventions that will treat the skin tear.
3. Are there any bathing changes that will need to be carried out during the time the treatment for the skin tear is being done?

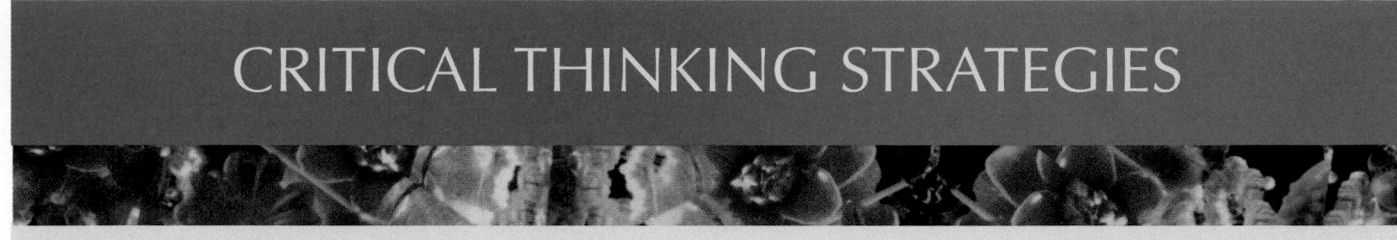

CHAPTER 9

Personal Hygiene

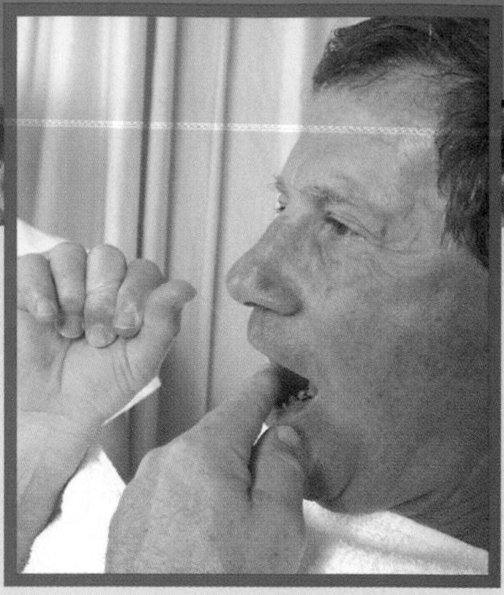

THEORETICAL CONCEPTS

UNIT ONE: **Oral Hygiene** **198**
- Providing Oral Hygiene 199
- Flossing Client's Teeth 200
- Providing Denture Care 201
- Providing Oral Care for Unconscious Clients 202

UNIT TWO: **Hair Care** **204**
- Providing Hair Care 205
  - *for Routine Hair Care 205*
  - *for Tangled Hair 205*
  - *for Coarse or Curly Hair 205*
- Shampooing Hair 205
  - *for Client in a Chair 206*
  - *for Client on a Gurney 206*
  - *for Client on Bed Rest 206*
  - *for Client Using Disposable System 206*
- Shaving a Client 207

UNIT THREE: **Pediculosis** **209**
- Removing Lice and Scabies 210

UNIT FOUR: **Foot Care** **213**
- Providing Foot Care 214
- Providing Nail Care 214

UNIT FIVE: **Bedpan, Urinal, and Commode** **216**
- Using a Bedpan and Urinal 217
- Assisting Client to Commode 218

UNIT SIX: **Perineal and Genital Care** **220**
- Draping a Female Client 221
- Providing Female Perineal Care 221
- Providing Incontinence Care 222
- Providing Male Perineal Care 223

UNIT SEVEN: **Eye and Ear Care** **225**
- Providing Routine Eye Care 226
- Providing Eye Care for Comatose Client 226
- Providing Postoperative Socket Care 226
- Removing and Cleaning an Artificial Eye 227
  - *for Heavy Mucus Deposit 228*
- Removing and Cleaning Contact Lenses 228
- Cleaning and Checking a Hearing Aid 229

GERONTOLOGIC CONSIDERATIONS 231

MANAGEMENT GUIDELINES 231

CRITICAL THINKING STRATEGIES 232

LEARNING OBJECTIVES

- Discuss oral hygiene needs of clients.
- Outline the procedure for flossing teeth.
- Compare and contrast oral hygiene for clients with natural teeth and dentures.
- Demonstrate safety awareness when providing oral care for unconscious clients.
- Identify the appropriate method of hair care according to client's condition.
- Outline the steps for shaving a male client.
- State the rationale for preventing prolonged scalp contact with solutions used to treat pediculosis.
- Discuss rationale for cutting nails straight across.
- Demonstrate proper draping technique for female clients.
- Demonstrate the skill of placing a bedpan for a bedridden client.
- Describe the steps in providing perineal care for male and female clients.
- Describe nursing actions necessary to care for clients with a prosthetic eye or contact lenses.
- State two suggested solutions when hearing is not improved after cleaning a hearing aid.
- Demonstrate the procedure for replacing an artificial eye.
- State at least two nursing diagnoses pertinent to clients requiring assistance with personal hygiene.

TERMINOLOGY

Abrasion: the scraping away of a portion of skin or of a mucous membrane as a result of injury.

Adaptation: an alteration or adjustment by which an individual can improve his or her relationship to the environment.

Antibacterial: any substance that fights against or suppresses bacteria.

Anticoagulant: any substance that suppresses or counteracts coagulation of blood.

Aspiration: to withdraw fluid that has abnormally collected in an area to obtain a specimen.

b.i.d.: two times daily.

Canthus: the angle at either end of the slit between the eyelids.

Capillary: minute blood vessel joining arterioles and venules; carries blood, forming the capillary system.

Congenital: present at birth, as a congenital anomaly or defect.

Cornea: the clear, transparent anterior portion of the fibrous coat of the eye.

Debilitated: to become feeble; tired; loss of strength.

Decalcification: the act of removing calcium, the basic component of bones and teeth.

Decubitus: old term for pressure ulcer.

Dental plaque: a thin film on the teeth made up of mucin and colloidal material found in saliva.

Edema: a local or generalized condition in which there is excess fluid in the tissues.

Emesis: vomiting.

Epidermis: the outer layer of skin.

Eversion: a turning outwards.

Excoriation: the abrasion of the epidermis or of the coating of any organ of the body.

Expectoration: expulsion of mucus or phlegm from the throat or lungs.

Fissure: a groove, slit, or natural division; ulcer or crack-like sore.

Floss: a waxed or unwaxed tape or thread used to clean between teeth.

Fungus: a vegetable cellular organism that subsists on organic matter.

Genitals: organs of generation; reproductive organs.

Hemorrhage: abnormal internal or external discharge of blood.

Holistic: the philosophy that an individual must be looked at as a whole rather than a sum of the parts.

Hygiene: the study and observance of health rules.

Hypoallergenic: against allergy, as hypoallergenic tape.

Impetigo: inflammatory skin disease marked by isolated pustules that become crusted and rupture.

Incontinent: inability to retain urine or feces through loss of sphincter control.

Incurvate: curved, especially inward.

Intervention: the act of coming between, so as to hinder or modify.

Irritation: a source of annoyance; incipient inflammation, soreness or roughness, or irritability of a body part.

Labia: the lips of the vulva.

Lesion: an injury or wound; a single infected patch in a skin disease.

Metabolism: the sum of all physical and chemical changes that take place within an organism; all energy and material transformations that occur within living cells.

Microorganism: a minute living body such as a bacterium or protozoon not perceptible to the naked eye.

Mucosa: mucous membrane lining passages and cavities communicating with the air.

Nasolacrimal: pertinent to the nose and lacrimal apparatus.

Ophthalmic solution: solution designed especially for the eyes.

Oral: concerning the mouth.

Palate: the roof of the mouth.

Parotid gland: either of the largest of the paired salivary glands, located below and in front of each ear.

Pediculosis: infestation with lice.

Perineum: the external region between the vulva and anus in a female or between the scrotum and anus in a male.

Plaque: a patch on the skin or on a mucous surface; a blood platelet.

Pressure point: area for exerting pressure to control bleeding; an area of skin that can become irritated with pressure, especially over bony prominences.

Sclera: the tough, white, fibrous outer envelope of tissue covering all of the eyeball except the cornea.

Semi-Fowler's position: semisitting position.

Systemic: pertinent to the whole body rather than to one of its parts.

Thrush: fungus infection of mouth or throat, especially in infants and young children and in clients with AIDS.

Ulcer: an open sore or lesion of the skin or mucous membrane of the body.

Urethra: canal for the discharge of urine extending from the bladder to the outside.

Vascular: pertinent to or composed of blood vessels.

HYGIENIC CARE

Unfamiliar or life-threatening conditions affect the client's adaptation to the health care system. A holistic approach on the part of the nurse provides individualized care and assists the client to adapt. Basic hygiene care is an integral part of the total treatment program. Together with its role in enhancing the client's adaptation to the hospital environment and sense of self-worth, it provides an opportunity to do a total assessment and evaluation. This time also allows for establishing a working relationship with the client and offers an opportunity to reduce stress by discussing fears and concerns about being in the hospital or the care being received.

The manner in which hygienic care is provided by nursing staff influences the client's perception of the staff. If care is administered in a professional and efficient manner, the client's confidence in the health care system is increased. The need to provide personal hygiene depends on each client's physical state and ability to care effectively for him or herself. Your first responsibility is to assess the client's level of ability. After gathering this data, you should assist the client as necessary, providing any assistance or teaching he or she may require.

Oral Hygiene

The condition of the oral cavity has a direct influence on an individual's overall state of health. Dental diseases require a "host" (the tooth and gum), an "agent" (plaque), and an "environment" (e.g., the presence of saliva and food). When plaque comes in contact with bacterial enzymes, carbohydrates, and acids, cavitation begins as the enamel of the tooth is decalcified. As long as food and plaque remain in the oral cavity, the possibility of dental decay increases. In the hospital the incidence of caries (cavities) can be decreased by using a dentifrice containing fluoride, proper brushing and flossing, and adequate nutrition. Clients at risk for poor oral hygiene include those who are NPO, mouth breathers, and those with oral surgery.

Hair Care

The appearance and condition of a client's hair may reflect his or her general physical and emotional status, individuality and feelings of worth, and the ability to care for him or herself. When complex medical care is required during illness or trauma, hair care is often neglected.

Hair care is an important aspect of regular hygiene. To prevent damage to the hair, scalp, and surrounding skin, and to promote the client's sense of well-being, you should assess the condition of a client's hair. Based on the assessment, provide hair and scalp care, shampooing, and shaving, and intervene to correct special problems.

Foot Care

The feet are especially susceptible to discomfort, trauma, and infection due to the amount of stress they must endure as well as to their distance from main blood supplies. Many conditions can be avoided if proper foot care is taken. The more common foot problems include

- *Incurvated or ingrown toenails:* The corners of the nail tend to press into skin, causing pain, ulceration, and infection.
- *Cracks and fissures between toes:* This problem often occurs as a result of excessively dry skin.
- *Athlete's foot:* Irritation characterized by itching, burning skin; caused by an easily transmitted fungus.
- *Corns:* High calluses caused by pressure on toes, joints, or bony prominences.

- *Plantar warts:* A virus manifested as a deep, often painful wart on the soles of the feet.
- *Calluses:* Thickened epidermis over areas of pressure.
- *Decreased circulation to the feet:* A problem that is often caused by diabetes, vascular diseases, or the constriction of major vessels to the lower extremities.

Perineal and Genital Care

The perineum consists of the area between the thighs and from the anterior pelvis to the anus. This area contains organs and structures related to sexual functioning, reproduction, and elimination.

Hygienic care involves cleaning the perineum and genitalia to prevent bacterial growth, which can rapidly increase in this warm, dark, moist environment. Perineal care is often provided as a routine part of bathing but may be required more frequently to prevent skin irritation, infection, discomfort, or odor.

All clients are susceptible to perineal irritation or infection. Clients who are especially vulnerable are those who are immobilized, incontinent, debilitated, postsurgical, or comatose; those who have indwelling catheters; those who have metabolic and fluid balance disorders; or those who require systemic medications.

Eye Care

The usual eye care provided for hospitalized clients is for the comatose client and the client with contact lenses. Fortunately, not too many clients require enucleation of the eye and the need for an artificial eye.

Several types of contact lenses are used by clients. The older, hard lenses were the first on the market and were made of solid plastic. They were easy to keep clean because they did not absorb proteins from the eye. They do inhibit oxygenation of the cornea; therefore, they must not be worn for long periods of time.

Soft lenses, the most popular of the lenses, allow more oxygenation of the cornea, but require care because they are less durable and carry a risk of contamination from collection of bacteria, dirt, and chemicals. Extended-wear lenses, another type of soft contact lenses, are worn for a number of days (usually up to 7) without being removed. The Food and Drug Administration (FDA) has just approved the use of continuous 30-day lenses. It is recommended that the lenses be removed every 30 days, cleaned, disinfected, and replaced or discarded. Lenses should not be replaced for 24 hours to allow the eye to rest. There are reported side effects with these lenses, including conjunctivitis, dry eyes, and mild burning or stinging. Some clients use disposable extended-wear lenses. These are considered one-time-only contacts and are discarded, not cleaned, after they are removed.

Individuals who wear contact lenses must be aware of environmental contaminants such as dust, smoke, and sprays because they can irritate the eyes. Certain drugs cause a decrease in the eye fluid on which the contact lens floats and can lead to irritation of the eye. Common drugs that can lead to this problem include antihistamines, birth control pills, and alcohol. Clients who use eye cosmetics must apply the makeup before they insert the contact lenses so makeup doesn't get on the lenses.

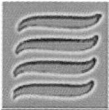

NURSING DIAGNOSES

The following nursing diagnoses may be appropriate to include in a client care plan when a client is admitted and requires basic hygiene care.

NURSING DIAGNOSIS	RELATED FACTORS
Deficient Knowledge	Misinformation or lack of information, impaired cognitive function, lack of motivation
Impaired Oral Mucous Membrane	Inadequate oral hygiene, chemotherapy, malnutrition, dehydration, infection, mechanical trauma
Noncompliance	Inability to perform tasks, disability, impaired memory
Bathing/Hygiene Self-care Deficit	Impaired motor or cognitive function, pain, disease condition, surgery
Situational Low Self-esteem	Impaired motor or cognitive function, chronic illness, chronic pain

- The single most important nursing action to decrease the incidence of hospital-based infections is handwashing. **Remember to wash your hands or use antibacterial gel before and after each and every client contact.**

UNIT 1

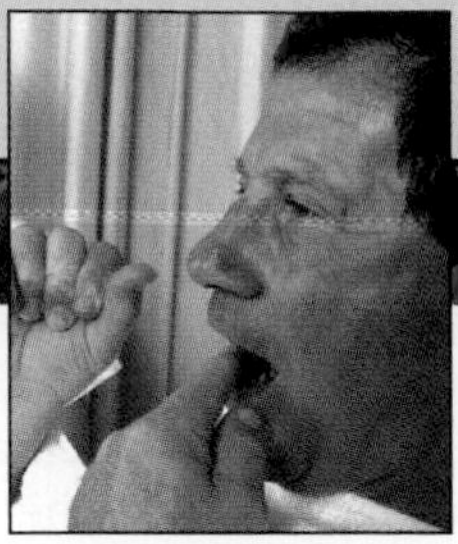

Oral Hygiene

Nursing Process Data

ASSESSMENT *Data Base*

Assess whether client wears dentures.

Evaluate client's knowledge of oral hygiene techniques.

Assess condition of client's oral cavity, teeth, gums, and mouth.

Assess for color, lesions, tenderness, inflammation, intactness of teeth, and degree of moisture or dryness of the oral cavity.

Observe external and internal lips.

Assess palate (roof and floor of mouth), and inspect under tongue.

Assess entire oral mucosa, noting inside of the cheek.

Observe tongue. Note tip, sides, back position, and underside.

Evaluate condition of gums and teeth.

Assess condition of throat as client says "Ah."

If dentures or orthodontic appliances are used, observe relationship of the appliances to client's oral cavity (i.e., fit, irritation, condition of dentures).

PLANNING *Objectives*

To remove plaque and bacteria-producing agents from oral cavity

To allow nurse to assess client's oral health status, knowledge, and routines of oral care

To decrease possibility of irritation or infection of oral cavity

To remove unpleasant tastes and odors from oral cavity

To provide comfort for client

To provide client teaching when appropriate

IMPLEMENTATION *Procedures*

Providing Oral Hygiene

Flossing Client's Teeth

Providing Denture Care

Providing Oral Care for Unconscious Clients

EVALUATION *Expected Outcomes*

The oral health status of client has been assessed and documented by nurse.

Oral hygiene care is provided without complications.

Plaque and bacteria-producing agents are removed.

PROVIDING ORAL HYGIENE

Equipment

Toothbrush: small enough to reach back teeth; soft and rounded with nonfrayed rows of nylon bristles
Dentifrice: client's choice, preferably one containing fluoride; special paste for dentures
Cup of water
Emesis basin or sink
Dental floss: regular or fine, waxed or unwaxed, depending on client's needs
Tissues or towel
Mouthwash if desired
Clean gloves

Preparation

1. Wash your hands.
2. Collect necessary equipment. Assist client with the arrangement of equipment if necessary.
3. Assist client to sink or provide privacy if care is to be given in bed.
4. Help client into a comfortable semi-Fowler's position or a sitting position.
5. Don clean gloves, if dentures are present, and help client remove them if necessary. Place dentures in denture cup.
6. Inspect surface of mouth for any abnormalities.
   a. Inspect surface of mouth, especially buccal mucosa (it should be pink, smooth, and moist), for any abnormalities. **Rationale:** Alterations from normal may indicate presence of disease states such as measles, mumps, or Addison's disease.
   b. Examine condition of teeth and gums. Be alert to changes in gums. **Rationale:** Gingival hypertrophy, crevices between teeth and gums, pockets of debris, and bleeding with slight pressure are indicative of gingivitis.
   c. Ask client about usual oral care routines.
7. Elicit any concerns, comments, or questions client may have about his or her oral health status.
8. Determine oral hygiene needs based on findings.
9. Assess client's need for teaching. Consider educational level, physical, emotional and mental state, previous experiences, and cultural differences.
10. Assess client's physical condition. Consider diagnoses, treatments, fluid status, drugs, diet, and level of comfort or pain.
11. Assess client's ability to care for him or herself.

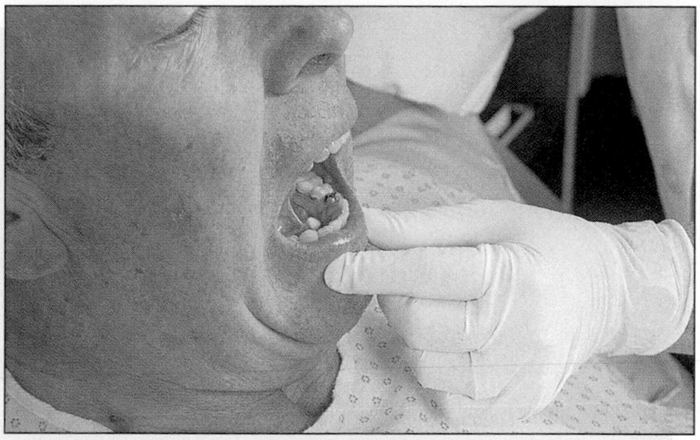

Inspect surface of mouth for abnormalities.

Procedure

1. Wash your hands and don clean gloves.
2. Request that client open mouth wide and hold emesis basin under chin.
3. Instruct client to complete following steps or provide the care yourself. Direct the bristles of the toothbrush toward the gum line for all areas to be brushed. **Rationale:** Action removes food particles from gum line and stimulates the gums.
4. Keep the brush positioned over only two or three teeth at a time. Use small rotating movements to cover the outside surfaces of all teeth.
5. Clean the inner surfaces of all back teeth, using the brushing method described above.
6. Use a firm back-and-forth motion, to clean the flat chewing surfaces.
7. Use the bristles on the end of the toothbrush and rotate the brush back and forth across the teeth to clean the inner surfaces of the front teeth.

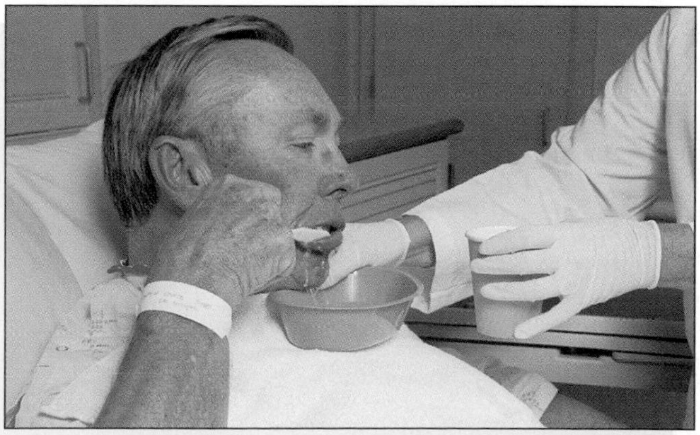

Providing oral hygiene is an essential component of client care.

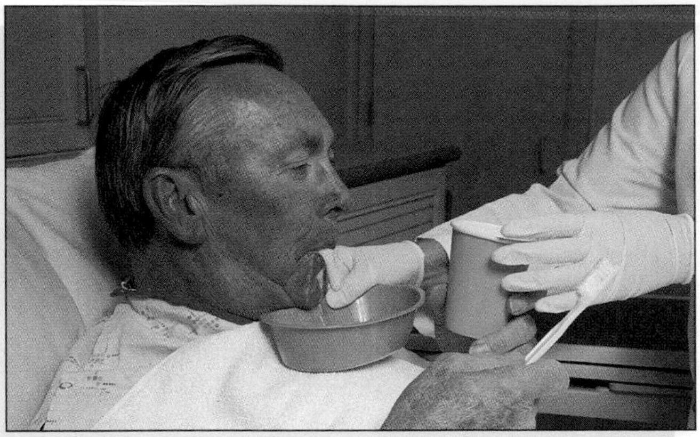

Assist client to rinse mouth with water.

8. Lightly brush all areas of the tongue—this improves the breath. Be careful not to stimulate gag reflex.
9. Rinse the client's mouth thoroughly with water.
10. Inspect oral cavity, and repeat brushing if necessary.

Sonic Toothbrush

Many dentists and dental hygienist's recommend the use of a sonic toothbrush, especially for clients with plaque formation, stains, and periodontal pockets. The usual recommended time for brushing is two minutes twice a day. The toothbrush is charged by plugging the charger into the electrical outlet; therefore, electrical safety procedures must be followed. Do not store or place the charger where it can come in contact with water. Client instructions for using the toothbrush are printed on the owner's manual and must be clearly understood before attempting to use the toothbrush. ***NOTE:*** *If the client brings the toothbrush to the hospital, it is not necessary to charge it if hospitalization is less than two weeks. If hospitalization is beyond two weeks or the toothbrush needs charging, instruct the client's relatives to take the brush home and charge it. It is required by most hospitals that any electrical appliance brought into the hospital must be checked for safety by the hospital engineering department.*

Client Teaching

Begin teaching client about oral care during your initial assessment. Focus teaching on oral health needs and care. You may want to incorporate the following techniques:

- A demonstration and return demonstration to illustrate correct dental care techniques.
- Disclosure tablets or solution that temporarily stains dental plaque pink. This technique helps the client to see where plaque appears on the teeth. After applying tablets or solution, ask the client to brush and floss until plaque is removed.

11. Floss thoroughly, using approximately 12–15 inches of floss loosely wrapped around one finger of each of your hands. Flossing removes plaque from between teeth.
12. Floss between each tooth by looping floss around each edge of the tooth and sliding floss down to the gum line.
13. Rinse client's mouth thoroughly with water.
14. Wipe off client's mouth and chin.
15. Wash client's toothbrush, rinse, and put it and paste away and return additional equipment.
16. Remove gloves and place in appropriate receptacle.
17. Wash your hands.
18. Check to see that client is comfortable.

FLOSSING CLIENT'S TEETH

Equipment

Dental floss 12–15 inches long—two pieces
Cup of water
Emesis basin
Towel
Clean gloves

Preparation

1. Discuss with client when he or she would prefer flossing teeth, after brushing or after morning care is completed.
2. Instruct client in procedure if he or she is able to floss; otherwise, you carry out procedure.
3. Gather necessary equipment.
4. Wash your hands and don gloves. **Rationale:** This is an important step, as gloves prevent the transmission of microorganisms to the client's mouth and to the nurse.

Procedure

1. Place client in sitting position and move bed to HIGH position.
2. Place towel under client's chin and emesis basin within reach.

3. Cut dental floss into two 12- to 18-inch lengths.
4. Instruct or assist client to complete the following steps.
   a. Wrap one length of floss loosely around index fingers of both hands.
   b. Hold floss taut between two hands, and gently pull back and forth between each tooth.
   c. Move floss up and down sides of teeth to clean plaque. Go as near gum line as possible without injury to gum. Pull floss back and forth gently, working back toward the biting surface of each tooth. Repeat other edge of each tooth, using a new section of floss. **Rationale:** Overly vigorous flossing can damage gums.
   d. Floss each tooth several times until all particles of food are removed.
5. Assist client to rinse mouth and expectorate into emesis basin.
6. Remove basin and wipe client's mouth with towel.
7. Remove gloves and wash hands.
8. Lower bed and return client to comfortable position.

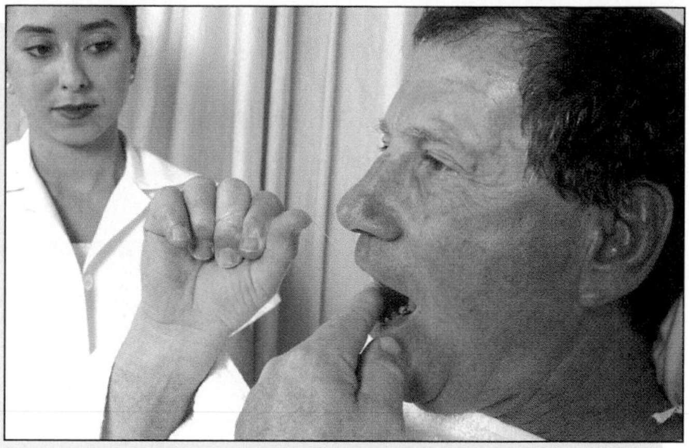

Instruct client to floss to prevent build-up of plaque and food particles between the teeth.

PROVIDING DENTURE CARE

Equipment

Denture toothbrush
Denture cup
Cleanser or effervescent tablets for dentures
Clean gloves
Mouthwash, if desired

Procedure

1. Encourage client to use dentures. **Rationale:** Dentures improve speech, make eating easier, and improve the shape of the mouth, appearance, and self-image.
2. Wash your hands and don gloves.
3. Help client remove dentures. If client is unable to do this, carefully place your finger on the edge of the upper denture. **Rationale:** This action breaks the seal at the roof of the mouth and allows the denture to easily slide out. Lower denture generally lifts out easily.
4. If client is unable to clean own dentures, place them in an unbreakable container. Either wash dentures over a basin or carry them to the sink. Place a paper towel or washcloth on the bottom of the sink. **Rationale:** To cushion the surface in case you accidentally drop a denture.
5. Hold one denture in your hand. With your other hand, use a toothbrush or special denture brush and a cleaning agent, such as a commercially prepared paste or solution, to brush the denture. Use the same brushing motion as with natural teeth.
6. Rinse denture thoroughly in cold water. **Rationale:** Hot water can damage dentures.

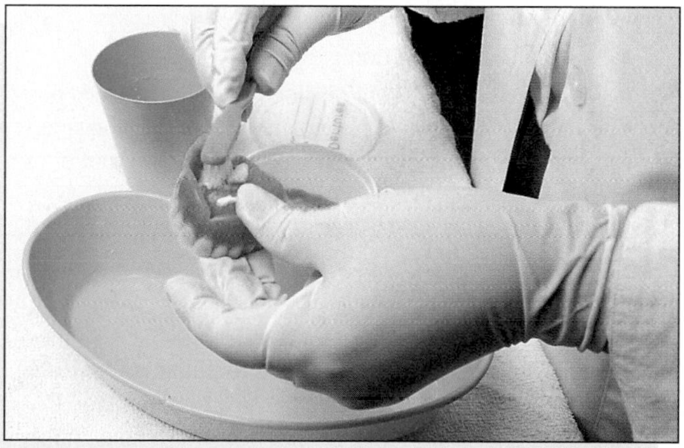

Hold dentures securely while brushing.

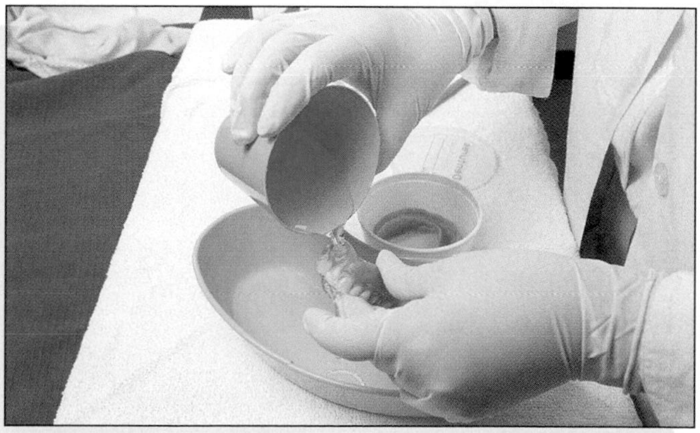

Rinse dentures in cold water.

7. If dentures are to remain out of the mouth for a period of time, as at night, store them in a clearly labeled, unbreakable container of cold water.
8. If dentures are to be worn immediately, help client to rinse oral cavity with warm water or mouthwash.
9. You may also gently brush client's gums and tongue. **Rationale:** To remove bacteria and freshen breath.
10. Help client replace dentures.
11. Remove gloves, and place in appropriate receptacle.
12. Wash your hands.

PROVIDING ORAL CARE FOR UNCONSCIOUS CLIENTS

Equipment

Mouth swabs (lemon-glycerin type)
Lubricant for lips
Waterpik devices or brush
Bulb syringe
Tongue blades
Clean gloves

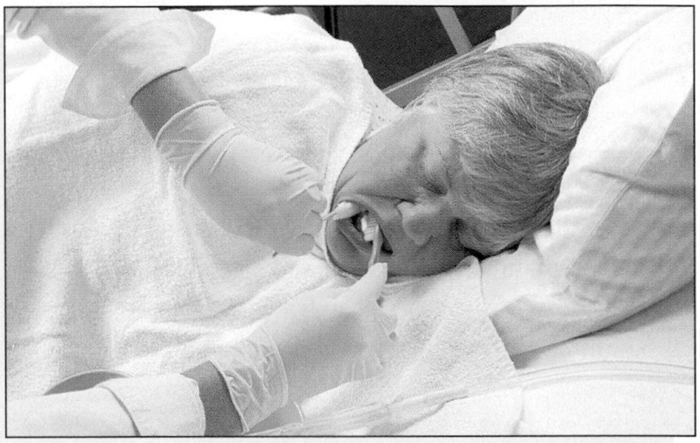

Use padded tongue blade when brushing teeth.

Procedure

1. Gather equipment.
2. Wash your hands and don gloves.
3. If possible, position client on side in a semi-Fowler's position. If this is not possible, turn client's head to the side. **Rationale:** Allows fluid to drain or be suctioned out of mouth and thus prevents aspiration.
4. Place a bulb syringe or suctioning equipment nearby. **Rationale:** Safety precaution to use for suctioning oral cavity as needed.
5. Place a small amount of toothpaste on brush. Brush the external surfaces of the teeth in the routine manner, using less water on the brush. You may use a tongue blade to move the cheeks and lips. Do not put your fingers in the client's mouth. **Rationale:** This prevents accidental closing down on toothbrush and biting your finger.
6. To clean the inner surfaces of the teeth, use a padded tongue blade to separate the upper and lower sets of teeth. Brush the teeth and tongue in the usual manner.
7. Rinse the client's mouth carefully, using very small amounts of water that can be suctioned.
8. Lubricate client's lips with petroleum jelly.
9. Provide oral care frequently—as often as every 2 hours if necessary. **Rationale:** Oral care maintains adequate oral health.
10. Remove gloves, and place in appropriate receptacle.
11. Wash your hands.

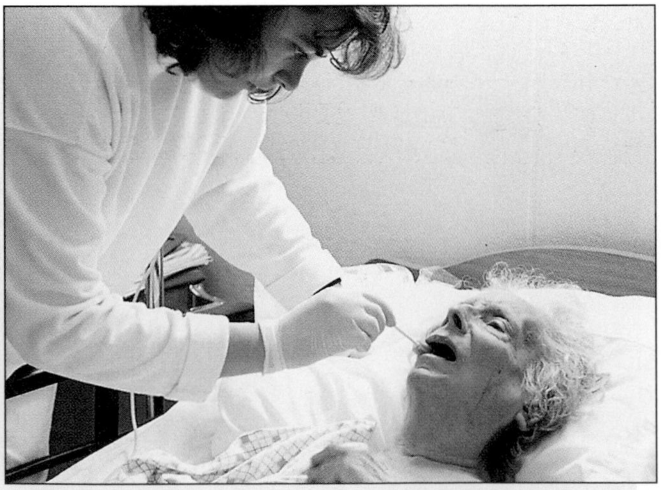

Check facility policy for use of mouth swabs.

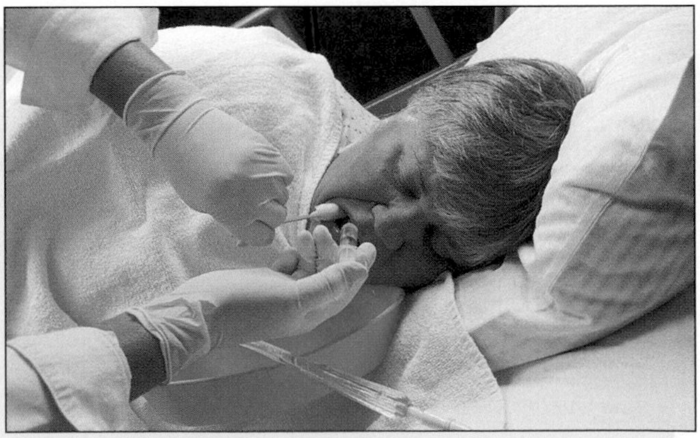

Rinse mouth using water-filled syringe.

DOCUMENTATION FOR ORAL HYGIENE

- Findings of assessment of mouth; condition of gums, mucous membranes, and teeth
- Assessment of client's oral hygiene needs
- Planning steps taken to meet client's oral hygiene needs
- Oral care provided or observed
- Effectiveness of oral care on client's teeth, gums, mucosa
- Client's reaction and level of comfort
- Client's level of participation in oral care
- Client's participation in nurse–client teaching

Critical Thinking Application

UNEXPECTED OUTCOMES	CRITICAL THINKING OPTIONS
Even with increased oral hygiene, client still has odorous breath.	• Use antiseptic mouthwash between oral hygiene care. • Notify the physician, as this could be a symptom of systemic disease. • Obtain dental consultation to check for presence of dental caries or gum disease. • Examine client's nutritional intake. Absent nutrients or imbalanced intake of fats, protein, or carbohydrates can result in bad breath.
Client complains of extreme oral mucosal irritation or sensitivity.	• Request physician's order for one of the following solutions: Saline solutions: for soothing, cleansing rinses Anesthetic solutions: to dull extreme pain in the oral cavity Effervescent solutions (e.g., hydrogen peroxide or ginger ale) to loosen and remove debris from the mouth Coating solutions (e.g., Maalox) to protect irritated surfaces Antibacterial—antifungal rinses (e.g., nystatin [mycostatin]) to prevent the spread of organisms that cause thrush
Vigorous flossing results in bleeding and sore gums.	• Give client warm antiseptic mouthwash to relieve soreness. • Investigate gum condition and refer for consultation.
Client needs care after oral surgery or oral trauma.	• Oral care following surgery or trauma is always ordered by physician. No oral hygiene care should be attempted until physician has clearly defined the specific care. • Suctioning equipment should always be present. • Assessment of client's head, face, neck, and general status is critical at this time.
Normal stimulation and cleaning is not sufficient to remove debris and plaque for the unconscious client.	• Try flossing teeth to dislodge debris. • Provide mouth care with toothbrush and dentifrice at least b.i.d. • Check with physician and order sonic toothbrush.
Parotid gland inflammation can occur with improper oral hygiene.	• Rinse mouth with mouthwash. • Use swab to reach back in oral cavity along mandible to temporomandibular area. • Floss teeth at least daily.

UNIT 2

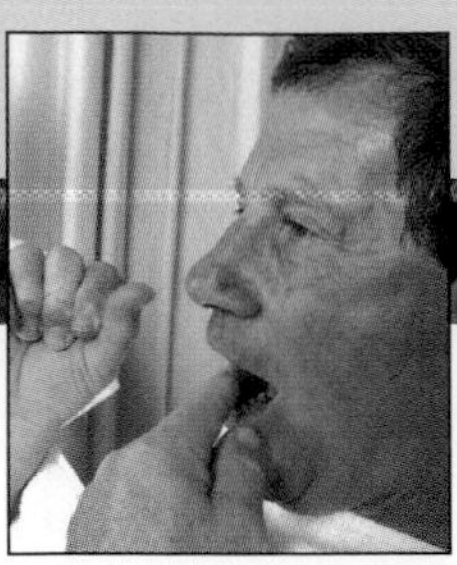

Hair Care

Nursing Process Data

ASSESSMENT *Data Base*
Review general physical assessment findings.
Elicit information regarding loss of hair, tenderness of scalp, or itching.
Determine client's ability to perform own hair care.
If unable to care for own hair find out who usually assists client.
Observe client's hair and scalp, noting the following:
- Texture
- Color
- Degree of thickness and hair distribution
- Degree of gloss or shine
- Dryness or oiliness
- Areas of irritation, rash, or scaliness on the scalp or surrounding skin
- Matting or snarls
- Pediculosis (lice)

Assess usual hair care routines, products, and appliances.
Assess method for providing hair care (e.g., in bed, on gurney, in wheelchair).
Determine client teaching needs regarding hair care.

PLANNING *Objectives*
To prevent irritation to the scalp and damage to the hair
To help maintain or improve client's existing condition of hair and scalp
To promote circulation to the hair follicle and growth of new hair
To distribute oils along the hair shaft
To promote self-esteem

IMPLEMENTATION *Procedures*
Providing Hair Care
- *for Routine Hair Care*
- *for Tangled Hair*
- *for Coarse or Curly Hair*

Shampooing Hair
- *for Client in a Chair*
- *for Client on a Gurney*
- *for Client on Bedrest*
- *for Client Using a Disposable System*

Shaving a Client

EVALUATION Expected Outcomes

Hair and scalp assessment are performed without complications.
Client's hair and scalp are clean, comfortable, and styled according to client's preference.
Client is comfortable and rested following shampooing.
Shaving is accomplished without discomfort.

PROVIDING HAIR CARE

Equipment

Blunt-ended comb or pick
Brush
Towel
Mirror
Hair care products and ornaments

Preparation

1. Determine client's hair care needs.
2. Wash your hands.
3. Help client into a comfortable position to perform hair care.
4. Collect and assemble equipment.

Procedure

for Routine Hair Care

1. Place all hair care items within reach.
2. Place towel over client's shoulders.
3. Brush or comb client's hair from scalp to hair ends, using gentle, even strokes.
4. Style hair in a manner suitable to client.
5. Replace hair care items in appropriate place, and clean items as needed.
6. Wash your hands.

for Tangled Hair

1. Hold client's hair above the tangle to prevent discomfort.
2. Using a wide-toothed comb, gently comb tangle. Use short, gentle strokes. Work out the tangle from the end of hair shafts toward the scalp. Work on small amount of tangle at one time. **Rationale:** Working on large tangles results in broken ends and damaged hair shafts.
3. You may also apply small amounts of vinegar or conditioner or alcohol to client's hair to make combing the tangle easier.
4. Style the client's hair in a manner that prevents further tangling (e.g., a loose braid placed in an area that does not put pressure on the head).

for Coarse or Curly Hair

1. Comb hair in small sections to remove tangles.
2. Use a comb or pick to comb hair in small sections.
3. Apply a small amount of oil to dry or flaking areas of the scalp.
4. Using a wide-toothed comb or pick, gently lift hair and smooth out evenly.
5. If corn-rowing is desired, make small rows of braids close to the scalp in the client's choice of design. (This type of braid is left in the hair for a longer time.)

SHAMPOOING HAIR

Equipment

Two bath towels
Washcloth
Shampoo
Conditioner, if desired
Shampoo board for clients confined to bed
Hair dryer, if allowed in hospital

for Disposable System

Package containing shampoo cap
Face or bath towel
Hair care products, as requested by client
Comb and/or brush

Note: Ensure that electrical equipment is checked by maintenance department before using. ***Rationale:*** *This confirms that equipment is grounded and mechanically safe.*

Preparation

1. Determine client's hair care needs.
2. Wash your hands.
3. Collect and assemble equipment.
4. Help client into a comfortable position to perform hair care.
5. Shampooing the hair can be accomplished in a variety of ways depending on the client's usual routine and physical condition. In many institutions, a physician's order is necessary before shampooing a client's hair.
6. If possible, the easiest way to shampoo is to assist the client while he or she is in the shower. Caution should be taken to prevent the client from becoming overly tired or weak while in the shower.

Procedure

for Client in a Chair

1. Have shampoo items readily available.
2. Drape one towel over client's shoulders and around neck. Place another towel within reach.
3. Face client away from sink. Lock wheels of wheelchair.
4. Pad the edge of the sink with a towel or bath blanket.
5. Ask client to lean head and neck against sink.
6. Using a washcloth to protect client's eyes, wet hair, and gently make a lather with shampoo.
7. Rinse thoroughly, and repeat if necessary.
8. Towel dry, add conditioner if desired, and rinse again.
9. Using a dry towel, pat hair dry, and wrap turban style to transport back to bed.
10. Use hair dryer if available.
11. Style as desired.
12. Replace equipment.

for Client on a Gurney

1. Have shampoo items readily available.
2. Position gurney with head end at sink.
3. Lock wheels on gurney. **Rationale:** This prevents the gurney from moving away from the sink.
4. Pad the edge of the sink with a towel or bath blanket.
5. Move the client's head just beyond the edge of the gurney to allow water to run off more easily.
6. Put a pillow or a rolled blanket under the client's shoulders to help elevate and extend the head.

> **CLINICAL ALERT**
>
> If the client is elderly, do not press the neck down on the edge of the sink—this position can diminish circulation to the brain and has been reported to be a possible cause of strokes.

7. Drape one towel over client's shoulders and around neck. Place another towel within reach.
8. Use a washcloth to protect client's eyes. Wet hair and gently make a lather with shampoo.
9. Rinse thoroughly and repeat if necessary.
10. Towel dry, add conditioner if desired, and rinse again.
11. Using a dry towel, pat hair dry, and wrap turban style to transport back to room.
12. Use hair dryer if available.
13. Style as desired.
14. Replace equipment.

for Client on Bed Rest

1. Place shampoo board, if available, under the client's head. This allows water and soap to run off into a basin at the side of the bed.
2. Drape one towel over client's shoulders and around neck. Place another towel within reach.
3. Place client's head on shampoo board.
4. Using a washcloth to protect client's eyes, wet hair, and gently make a lather with shampoo.
5. Rinse thoroughly, and repeat if necessary.
6. Towel dry, add conditioner if desired, and rinse again.
7. Using a dry towel, pat hair dry, and wrap turban style.
8. Remove equipment from bed.
9. Change gown and linen if wet.
10. Use hair dryer if available.
11. Style as desired.
12. Replace all equipment.
13. Wash your hands.

for Client Using Disposable System

1. Heat shampoo package in microwave for no more than 30 seconds.

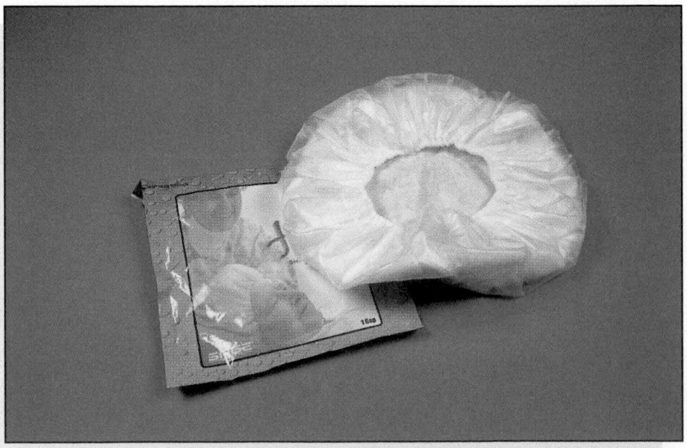

Shampoo system activated by microwave.

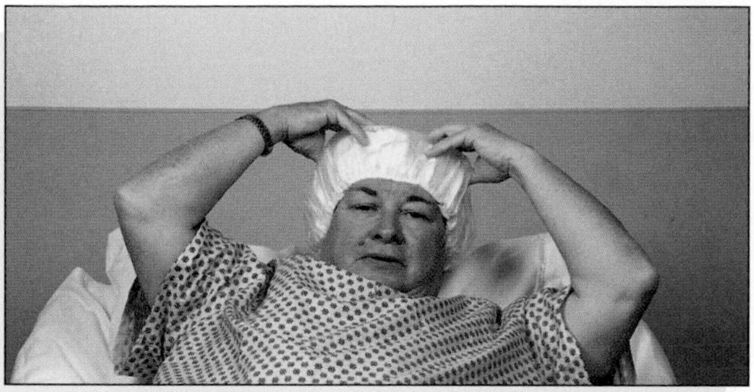

Disposable shampoo cap can be used for clients on bed rest.

2. Open package and check if cap is too warm. **Rationale:** Clients react to heat at different temperatures; therefore, check the cap temperature with client before placing on client's head.
3. Place cap on head. Ensure that all hair is contained within the cap. For longer hair, place cap on top of head and then tuck all hair up inside cap.

CLINICAL ALERT

If hair is tangled, the cap may need to stay on for longer period of time in order to saturate hair. If blood or other secretions are present on hair, they may need to be removed using the washcloths from the disposable bath system before attempting to shampoo the hair.

4. Gently massage cap with hands, 1–2 minutes for short hair and 2–3 minutes for longer hair. **Rationale:** This will assist in saturating the hair with the solution.
5. Remove cap and place in appropriate receptacle.
6. Towel dry hair.
7. Complete hair care according to client's needs and desires.

Note: Disposable hair care systems provide a quick and easy way to freshen client's hair with minimal client movement.

SHAVING A CLIENT

Equipment

Safety or electric razor, specific to client's needs or wishes
Shaving cream
Aftershave lotion (optional)
Two towels
Basin of warm water

Preparation

1. Place client in sitting position.
2. Place towel over chest and under chin.
3. Put up mirror on overbed table.
4. Determine how the client usually shaves (i.e., use of safety edge or electric razor; special products).
5. Check to see if the client has excessive bleeding tendencies due to pathologic conditions (hemophilia) or the use of specific medications (anticoagulants or large doses of aspirin). **Rationale:** If client is accidentally cut, it could lead to some loss of blood.

Procedure

1. If using a safety edge razor:
   a. Don gloves and apply a warm, moist towel to soften the hair.
   b. Apply a thick layer of soap or shaving cream to the shaving area.
   c. Holding skin taut, use firm but small strokes in the direction of hair growth.
   d. Gently remove soap or lather with a warm, damp towel. Inspect for areas you may have missed.
2. If using electric razor:
   a. Use rotating motion of razor and start from lateral aspect of face and move toward chin and upper lip area.
   b. Clean razor with brush or remove head and clean facial hair from head of razor.
3. Apply aftershave lotion or powder as desired.
4. Reposition client for comfort if needed.
5. Remove gloves and replace equipment.

CLINICAL ALERT

According to the hospital policy, be sure to have the electric razor checked for safety aspects. Some hospitals do not allow clients to use their own electric razors.

Documentation for Hair Care

- Documentation of hair care assessment and needs
- Shampooing method, outcomes, problems encountered
- Client's tolerance to hair care
- Shaving done
- Unusual bleeding from shaving

Critical Thinking Application

UNEXPECTED OUTCOMES	CRITICAL THINKING OPTIONS
Extreme matting, snarling, blood, or nonremovable substances appear in client's hair.	• Never cut a client's hair unless it is absolutely necessary. Check hospital policy regarding hair cutting. • Apply alcohol to tangled hair or blood-soaked hair. Keep in place 5 minutes. Wash hair with shampoo to remove alcohol and blood. • Secure permission of family or physician.
Client is cut during shaving procedure.	• Assess extent of cut, and place a clean towel on the area with pressure to stop bleeding. • If cut appears to be more than a nick, report to physician, and fill out unusual occurrence report.
Shaving is difficult and painful for the client.	• Place warm towels on area to be shaved for 15 minutes. • Apply more shaving cream. • Ensure that razor is sharp.

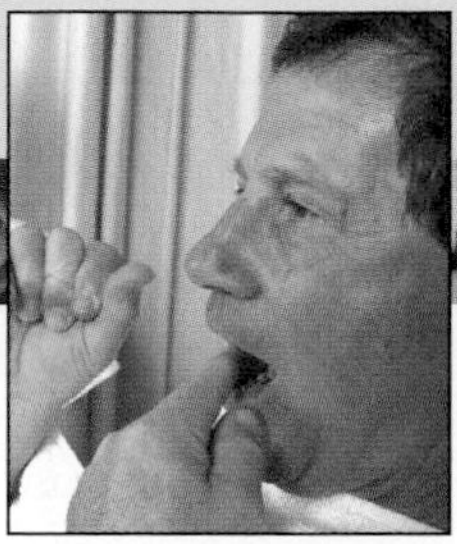

Pediculosis

Nursing Process Data

ASSESSMENT ***Data Base***

Observe head (scalp), body (beard, eyebrows, arms, legs), and pubic areas for the following signs:

- Small, hemorrhagic areas on the skin
- Scratches on the skin
- Habitual itching and scratching
- Insect-type bites or pustular eruptions behind the ears or hairline
- Small, white dandruff-like particles

Assess client's personal hygiene, living conditions, contact or exposure to others with lice (e.g., school-aged children, sexual partners, siblings).

PLANNING ***Objectives***

To remove lice from client's hair and prevent further skin problems such as impetigo or infection

To remove cause of itching and intense need to scratch scalp

To control spread to others

IMPLEMENTATION ***Procedures***

Removing Lice and Scabies

EVALUATION ***Expected Outcomes***

Lice removed following treatment.

Client verbalizes cause of problem and preventive measures.

REMOVING LICE AND SCABIES

Equipment

Isolation bags (optional)
Lindane: Gammabenzene, Kwell, or Scabene
1% permethrin cream rinse (NIX)
Trimethoprim sulfamethoxazole (Bactrim); oral antibiotic
Clean linen
Fine-tooth "nit" comb
Disinfectant for comb
Clean gloves
Towels

Procedure

1. Don clean gloves. Gloves are used even when completing treatment at home.
2. Remove and bag client's clothing and linens. Client's clothes do not need to be bagged separately and placed in isolation bags if standard precautions are used.
3. Notify physician and other health care providers of lice or scabies infestation.
4. Begin treatment as ordered by physician.

for Using Lindane Lotion for Scabies

a. Remove all oil-based hair dressings and skin lotions or creams; dry skin and cool before applying Lindane.
b. Shake lotion container well. Apply thin film of lotion over entire body, excluding face and urethral meatus. Ensure all body creases and folds have adequate lotion applied.
c. Rub in thoroughly; allow skin to dry and cool after application. Leave on skin for 8–12 hours.
d. Shower or bathe to remove lotion.

for Using Lindane Shampoo for Lice

a. Shampoo hair by wetting hair and then applying shampoo. Work drug into hair thoroughly and allow to remain on hair for 4 minutes. Before rinsing hair add small amount of water to form a thick lather, then rinse hair thoroughly.
b. Use "nit comb" or tweezers to remove remaining nit shells.

CLINICAL ALERT

Product can be poisonous if misused. Convulsions have been reported in connection with Lindane shampoo therapy, especially with accidental oral ingestion.

CLINICAL ALERT

Permethrin stays on the hair shaft for up to 14 days; therefore, recurrence of lice infestations rarely happens.

c. Monitor body and hair for signs of lice. If living lice are present after 7 days, repeat shampoo.
d. Instruct client or family to monitor for side effect; eczematous eruptions. Inhalation adverse effects include; headache, nausea, vomiting, irritation of the ear, nose, and throat.

for Using Permethrin(Nix) for Lice or Scabies

a. Shampoo hair with regular shampoo, rinse, and towel dry.
b. Shake lotion well before applying. Nix is only used on hair, not on skin.
c. Saturate damp hair with lotion and keep in place for 10 minutes.
d. Rinse hair thoroughly and dry with clean towel.
e. Inspect hair shafts daily for at least 7 days.
f. Regular shampooing may be initiated within a day. **Rationale:** Residual deposits of the drug on the hair shaft is not reduced with regular shampooing.
g. Instruct client or family to monitor for side effects of drug: pruritus, transient tingling, burning, stinging, numbness, erythema, edema, rash.

5. Disinfect combs and brushes with the shampoo.
6. Remove gloves.
7. Wash hands.

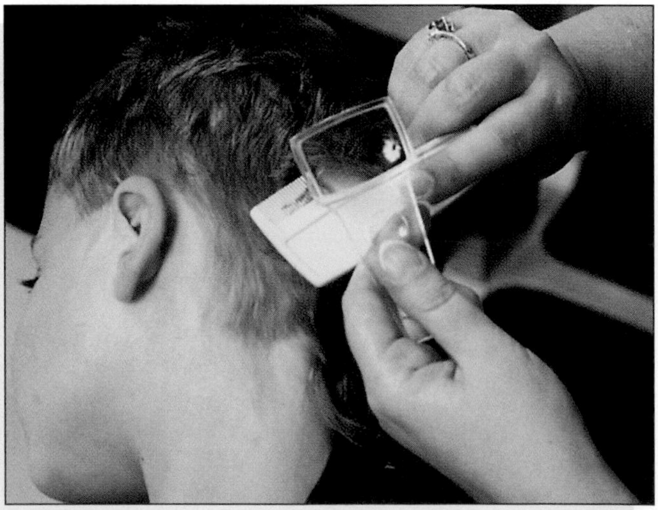

Use magnifying glass when inspecting for head lice.

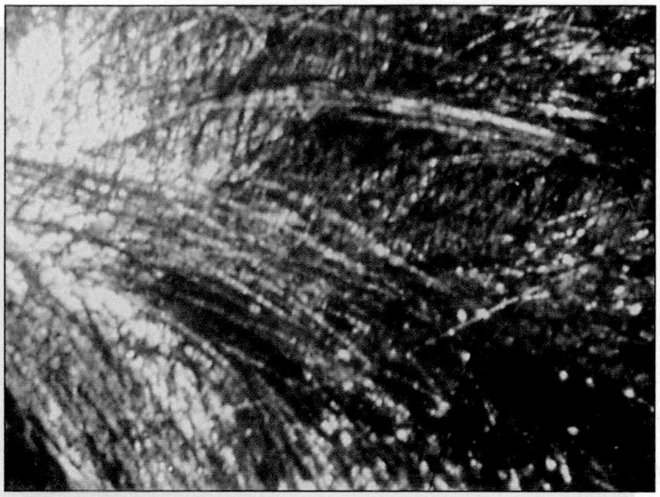

Examine hair closely for white nits on hair shaft.

8. Instruct client or parent to check hair and use "nit comb" every 2 to 3 days until lice are gone and to check skin for removal of scabies. (Pruritus may last for 2 weeks following treatment.)
9. Wash clothes and linens in hot water (130°) or dry them using high heat.
10. Place stuffed toys in hot dryer.
11. Instruct client or family to vacuum furniture and floors to rid house of lice. **Rationale:** Head lice need a human host and therefore do not survive long after falling off head.
12. Administer Bactrim if ordered. **Rationale:** It destroys lice.
13. Discuss the cause, treatment, and preventive measures regarding lice infestation with client and family.

Evidenced Based Nursing Practice

Head Lice Infestation

In a randomly assigned study, 115 children, age 2–13 (mostly girls), were assigned to three groups. One group received only cream rinse (Nix), one group only the oral antibiotic (Bactrim), and one group received the combination of the oral antibiotic and the cream rinse. At both 2 and 4 week follow-up appointments, more than 90% of the children receiving the combination therapy were lice free compared to 80% or less in the other two groups. No major side effects were noted in any of the 3 groups of children.

Source: Head lice infestation: single drug versus combination therapy with one percent permethrin and trimethoprim/sulfamethoxazole. *Pediatrics 2001,* March (107) E30. Authors: Hipolito, R. B., Mallorca, F. G., Zuniga-Macaraig, Z. O., et.al.

Documentation for Removing Lice and Scabies

- Location of lice infestation
- Notification of physician and health care providers
- Nursing interventions and the results obtained
- Client teaching activities

Critical Thinking Application

UNEXPECTED OUTCOMES	CRITICAL THINKING OPTIONS
Special shampoo is left on hair/scalp too long.	• Observe for irritation or burning after rinsing out the shampoo. • If scalp is burned, notify physician for a medication order. • Do not repeat treatment unless specifically ordered by physician.
Other clients or staff become infested with lice.	• Isolate the client's linen and personal hair grooming equipment to prevent spread of lice. • Instruct client or staff on use of medicated lotion, shampoo, or combination therapy.
Lice are not eliminated with treatment.	• Repeat treatment using combination therapy as ordered by physician. • Do not repeat treatment for 7 days.

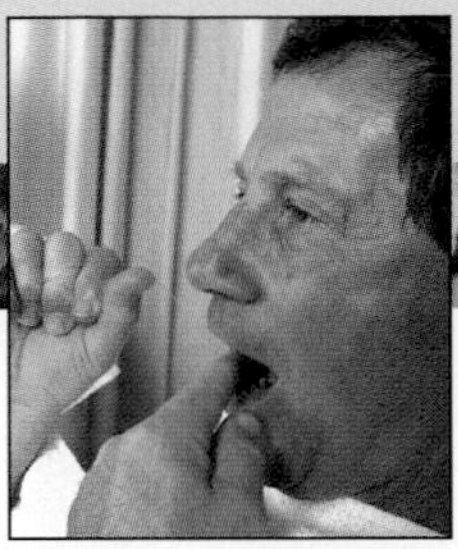

Foot Care

Nursing Process Data

ASSESSMENT Data Base

Review data from general physical assessment.

Observe the color of the client's feet and lower extremities.

Assess temperature of each foot.

Note color, shape, condition, contour, and length of toenails.

Assess speed of color return when nailbed is depressed (capillary refill).

Inspect skin of entire foot (including corner of toes, between toes, and heels) for irritation, cracking, lesions, corns, calluses, deformities, and edema.

Assess mobility of ankle and toes. (Footdrop or plantar flexion and eversion of feet can occur during prolonged bed rest.)

Assess cleanliness of feet.

Inspect client's shoes for excessive wear and proper fit.

During assessment, gather data from the client about level of comfort, pain, or tenderness.

PLANNING Objectives

To provide for specific foot care needs

To encourage self-care and prevention of future problems

To prevent infection, discomfort, deformities, circulatory problems, and odor

IMPLEMENTATION Procedures

Providing Foot Care

Providing Nail Care

EVALUATION Expected Outcomes

Foot care provided without complications.

Client's feet are clean and appear free of complicating conditions, such as excessive moisture, calluses, corns, blisters, abrasions, or infection.

Client and family understand the importance and techniques for proper foot care.

PROVIDING FOOT CARE

Equipment

Basin of warm water
Soap or emollient agent
Washcloth
Two towels
Toenail clippers
Nail file, emery board, pick, or orangewood stick
Skin care lotion or lanolin
Clean gloves (use if risk of contacting body fluids)

Preparation

1. Determine foot care needs based on client's condition and assessment data.
2. Check physician's orders and client care plans.
3. Collect necessary equipment.
4. Help client into a chair in a comfortable sitting position if possible.
5. Discuss procedure with client.
6. Wash your hands.

Procedure

1. Place towel or bath mat on floor in front of client.
2. Place basin of warm water on towel.
3. Help client place feet in basin.
4. Add emollient agent to water, if desired.
5. Assist client with other personal hygiene activities while feet are soaking. Let feet soak for 10 minutes.
6. Using a washcloth, gently wash client's feet with soap and water.
7. Dry each foot thoroughly with a second towel. Dry between each toe.

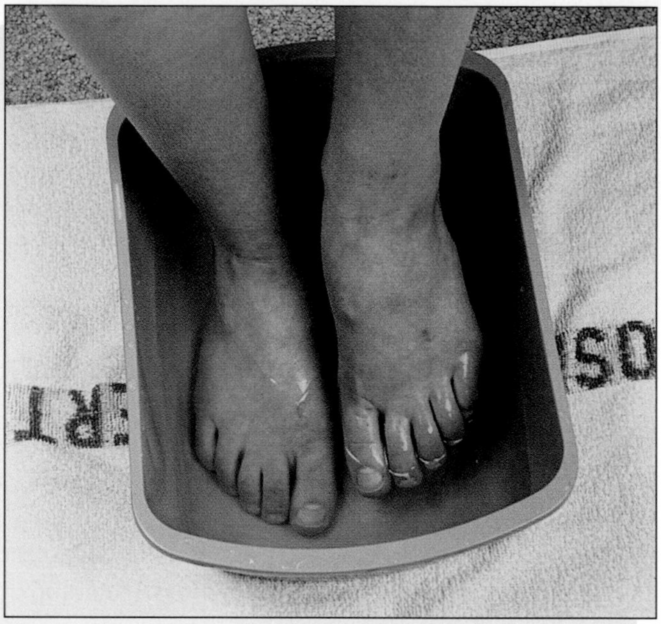

Place towel on floor in front of client and place feet in basin for soaking.

8. Using nail clippers, cut straight across the nails. **Rationale:** Prevents trauma to surrounding tissue.
9. Clean underneath and on sides of nails using a file or orangewood stick.
10. If necessary, push back cuticles using an orangewood stick. Smooth rough edges with an emery board.
11. Apply lotion to entire foot focusing on callused or dry areas. If client's feet are cracking or excessively dry, instruct client to use a deep-penetrating moisturizer like shea butter.
12. Assist client in putting on clean socks and shoes or slippers.
13. Replace equipment.
14. Assist client to bed or position for comfort in chair.
15. Wash your hands.

PROVIDING NAIL CARE

Equipment

Basin of warm water
Towel
Scissors or nail clippers
File or emery board
Orangewood stick
Clean gloves

Procedure

1. Check hospital policy on nail cutting. Some institutions do not allow nurses to cut client's nails if the client has diabetes mellitus, peripheral vascular disease, or a localized condition such as a fungus infection. Thick, mycotic, or ingrown toenails should not be cut by the nurse. Request that a podiatrist see the client.
2. Wash your hands and don clean gloves.

3. Position client for comfort.
4. Expose one extremity at a time.
5. Soak nails if softening is needed. Dry nails.
6. Cut toenails straight across with scissors or clippers. **Rationale:** Rounding off toenails may break the skin or cause ingrown toenails.
7. Smooth cut edges with file or emery board. Be careful to not injure surrounding skin.
8. Clean under nail with orangewood stick.
9. Reposition client.
10. Remove and clean equipment.
11. Remove gloves and wash your hands.

CLINICAL ALERT

Check policy of hospital regarding cutting of nails. Some healthcare facilities require that only a podiatrist cut nails.

DOCUMENTATION FOR FOOT AND NAIL CARE

- Initial assessment findings and overall status of client's feet
- Foot and nail care needs and plans
- Care given and results of care
- Any abnormalities
- Involvement in client or family teaching
- Referral to podiatrist if necessary

Critical Thinking Application

UNEXPECTED OUTCOMES	CRITICAL THINKING OPTIONS
Client has excessively dry, scaly skin, even after routine foot care.	• Apply alkali solutions as ordered, such as Epsom salts or bicarbonate of soda, to soften skin and remaining scales. Repeated soakings are usually necessary. • Apply lanolin or shea butter moisturizer.
Client's feet are excessively moist.	• Give foot care twice a day. • Use moisture-absorbing powder.
Client has large calluses on feet.	• After soaking, obtain an order to rub a pumice stone or an abrasive material on the callused area. Calluses are never cut from the skin due to possible scarring to the epidermis. • For diabetic clients, obtain services of a podiatrist.
Client has mycotic nails.	• Report to physician so podiatrist can be consulted.

UNIT 5

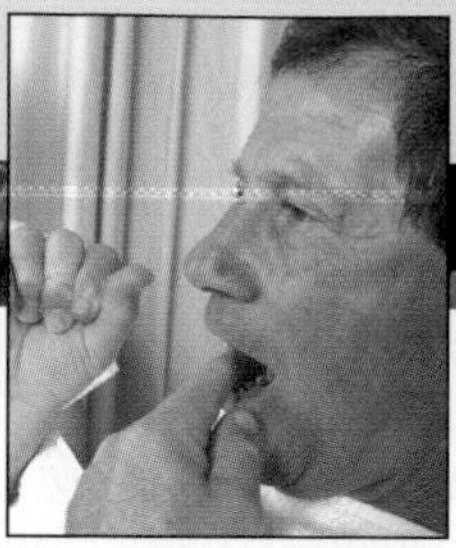

Bedpan, Urinal, and Commode

Nursing Process Data

ASSESSMENT Data Base

Determine client's usual voiding pattern.

Assess client's ability to assist with the procedure.

PLANNING Objectives

To assist the client to void when on bed rest or unable to urinate

To help client void 200–500 mL of urine without discomfort or difficulty

IMPLEMENTATION Procedures

Using a Bedpan and Urinal

Assisting Client to Commode

EVALUATION Expected Outcomes

Client voids 200–500 mL of urine without discomfort or difficulty.

Bladder does not become distended.

Genitourinary system is free of infection.

USING A BEDPAN AND URINAL

Equipment

Bedpan or urinal
Toilet tissues
Absorbent pad, if needed
Clean gloves

Procedure

1. Wash your hands and don gloves.
2. Obtain bedpan or urinal and warm pan or urinal by running warm water around the edges of the receptacle if cold.
3. Provide privacy.
4. Elevate the head of the bed.
5. Place client in a supine position, if possible, or position on edge of bed or in a chair.
6. Instruct the client to sit on bedpan or urinal. If the client needs assistance, follow these steps:

for Using a Bedpan

a. Place absorbent pad under hips, if needed.
b. Raise the client's hips and slip your arm under the client or turn the client on his or her side. Roll the client onto the pan.
c. Place a rolled towel or blanket under the client's sacrum. **Rationale:** This provides comfort by padding the bony area.

for Using a Urinal

a. Place the base of the urinal flat on the bed between the client's thighs.
b. Position the client's penis over the urinal.

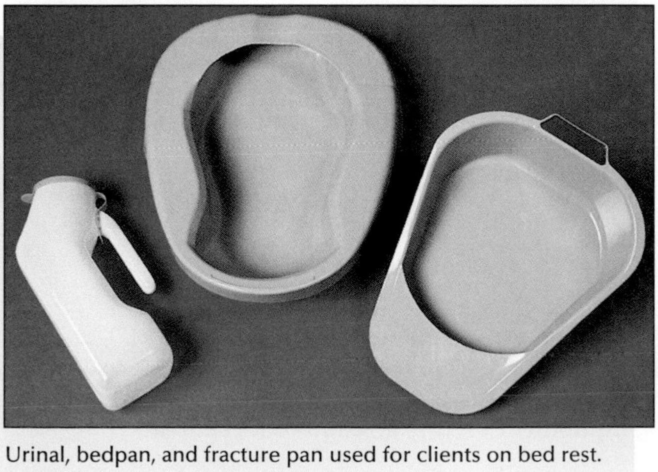

Urinal, bedpan, and fracture pan used for clients on bed rest.

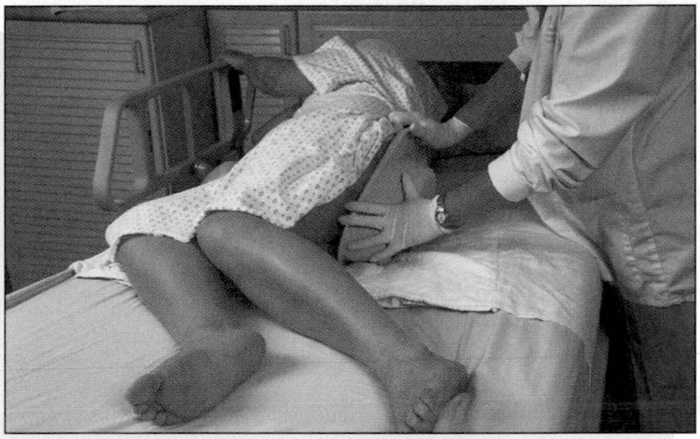

Turn client to side to position on bedpan.

Note: It may be easier for clients to use a urinal if they sit on the edge of the bed.

7. Place the signal light or call bell and toilet tissue within easy reach.
8. When the client has voided, remove the bedpan or urinal and assist with wiping as necessary.
9. Provide an opportunity for the client to wash his or her hands.
10. Reposition the client for comfort, pull back curtains.
11. Measure intake and output if required.
12. Empty bedpan or urinal, clean equipment, and return to proper area in client's room.
13. Remove gloves and wash your hands.

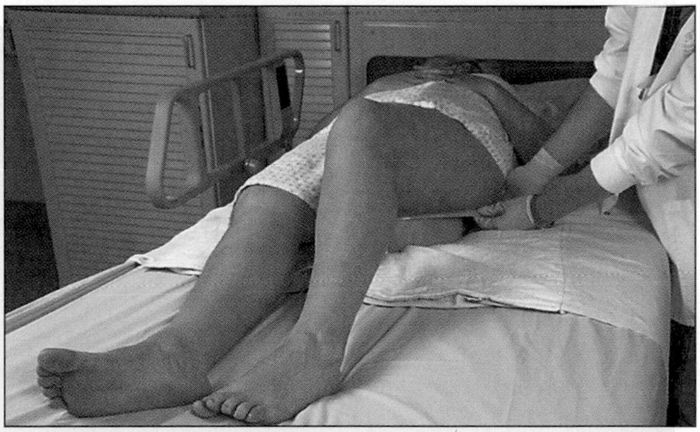

Roll client onto pan and make comfortable.

ASSISTING CLIENT TO COMMODE

Equipment

Commode with locking wheels or rubber-tipped legs
Toilet tissue
Nurse's call bell
Slippers
Bath blanket

Procedure

1. Place commode at foot of bed. Be sure to lock wheels on commode if needed.
2. Place slippers on client.
3. Move client to edge of bed and assist to a sitting position at edge of bed.
4. Instruct client to grasp your shoulders.
5. Place your hands securely around client. **Rationale:** To stabilize client for transfer.
6. Pivot client in front of commode.
7. Lower client onto commode, using correct body mechanics; ensure client is securely positioned on commode.
8. Place toilet tissue within easy reach.
9. Cover client with bath blanket for warmth and privacy.
10. Place call bell within easy access of client.
11. Provide privacy by closing curtains and shutting door.

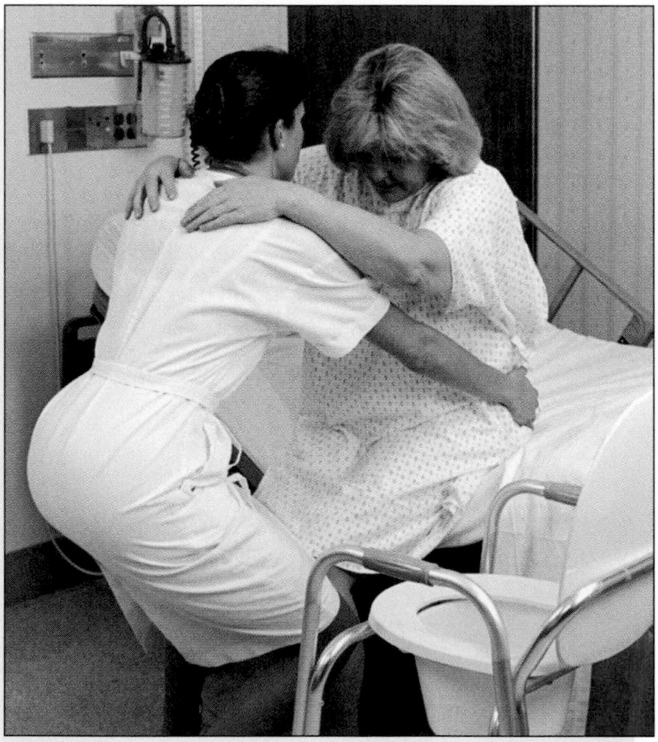

Use correct body mechanics when guiding client to commode.

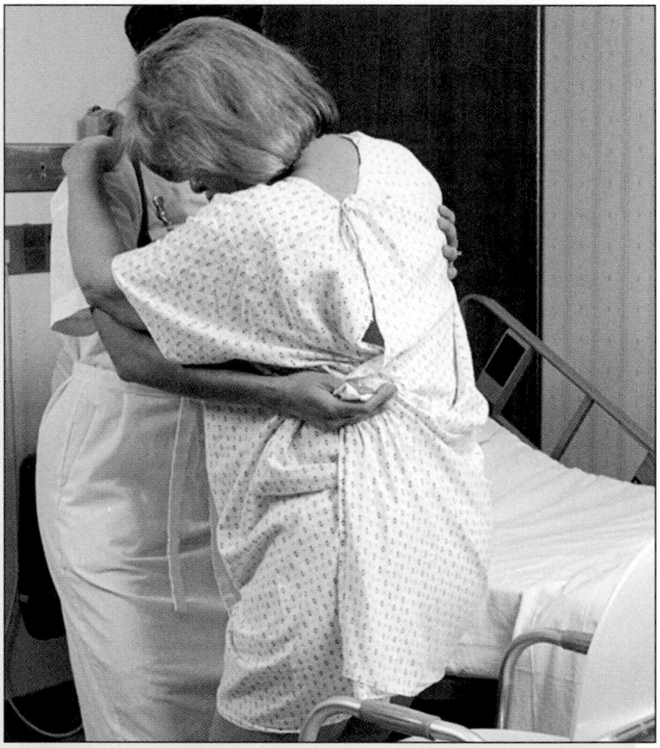

Pivot with client and bend knees when seating client.

DOCUMENTATION FOR BEDPAN, URINAL, AND COMMODE

- Amount, color, appearance, and odor of urine
- Techniques effective in stimulating voiding
- Equipment used (e.g., commode, bedpan)

Critical Thinking Application

UNEXPECTED OUTCOMES	CRITICAL THINKING OPTIONS
Client is unable to turn and has difficulty raising hips.	• Use a fracture pan rather than a bedpan. Powder the fracture pan. • Insert the fracture pan with the flat side toward the head, under the client's thighs.
Client is unable to void on bedpan.	• Assess reason. • Maintain complete privacy. • Run water in sink. • Massage the lower abdomen. • Place a hot washcloth on the abdomen. • Pour warm water over the perineum with client positioned on toilet or bedpan. • Give client a sitz bath after obtaining an order.

UNIT 6

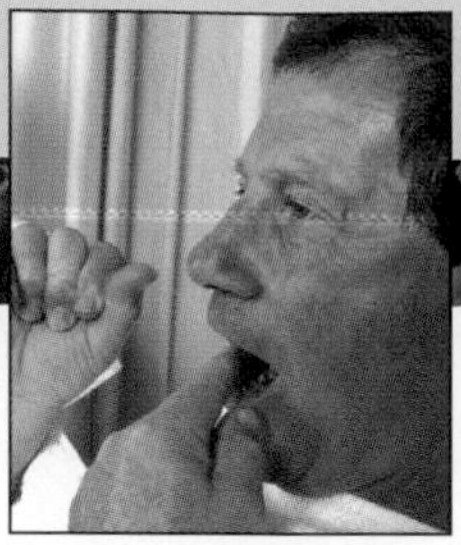

Perineal and Genital Care

Nursing Process Data

ASSESSMENT ***Data Base***

Review general assessment data about client.

Observe for signs of perineal itching, burning on urination, or skin irritation. Ask client if he or she experiences any of these problems.

Assess client's ability to bathe him or herself and to perform perineal care.

While providing privacy, assess the perineal–genital area for abnormal secretions, ulcerations, skin excoriations and sensitivity, drainage (amount, consistency, odor, color), swelling, enlarged lymph glands, catheter patency, and comfort.

Assess client's learning needs related to perineal and genital care.

PLANNING ***Objectives***

To decrease the growth of bacteria

To remove excessive secretions

To promote healing after surgery and vaginal deliveries

To prevent the spread of microorganisms for clients with indwelling catheters

To increase client comfort

IMPLEMENTATION ***Procedures***

Draping a Female Client

Providing Female Perineal Care

Providing Incontinence Care

Providing Male Perineal Care

EVALUATION ***Expected Outcomes***

Perineal care has been comfortably and effectively provided.

Perineal area is clean, odor-free, and without irritation or discharge.

DRAPING A FEMALE CLIENT

Equipment

Bath blanket

Procedure

1. Bring bath blanket to bedside.
2. Identify client and explain procedure.
3. Provide privacy.
4. Wash your hands.
5. Place bed in HIGH position, and lower side rail nearest you.
6. Place bath blanket over client's top linen so that one corner of the blanket is pointed toward the client's head to form a diamond shape over the client.
7. Instruct client to hold onto bath blanket. Fanfold linen to foot of bed.
8. Request that client flex knees and keep them apart with feet firmly on bed.

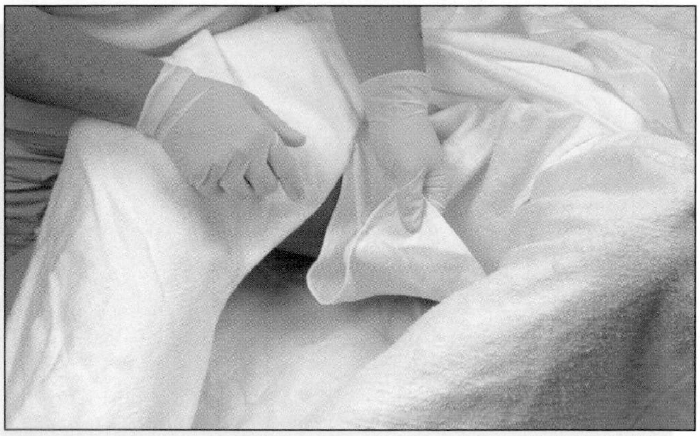

Draping protects client's privacy when performing perineal care.

9. Wrap lateral corners of bath blanket around feet in a spiral fashion until they are completely covered.
10. The corner of the blanket between knees and extending over perineum can later be folded back over the abdomen.

PROVIDING FEMALE PERINEAL CARE

Equipment

Bath blanket or sheet
Two bath towels
Protective pad
Washcloths
Clean gloves

Preparation

1. Check to see if specific physician orders are to be followed.
2. Talk with client about how she can perform care or assist with procedure. **Rationale:** This gives client a sense of control.
3. Collect and arrange necessary equipment.
4. Provide privacy by closing door and pulling drapes.
5. Wash your hands.
6. Position client in a comfortable position in bed. Head of bed can be elevated to low-Fowler's position. Drape according to procedure described above.
7. If possible, encourage the client to bend her knees and separate her legs. **Rationale:** The perineal area can be cleansed more efficiently in this position.

Procedure

1. Place a protective pad or towel under the client's hips. **Rationale:** Keeps the linen clean and dry.
2. Don gloves.
3. Lift corner of drape away from perineal area.
4. Place washcloth into basin. Rub cloth with soap, wring out excess water.
5. Fold washcloth into mitt or gather into palm of hand. (Refer to Folding a Mitt in Chapter 8).

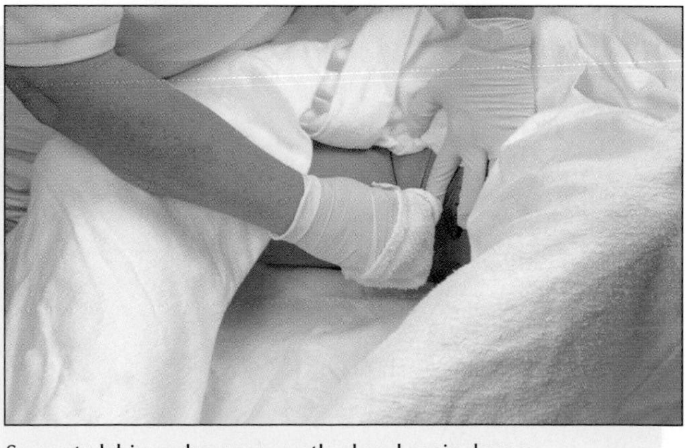

Separate labia and expose urethral and vaginal areas.

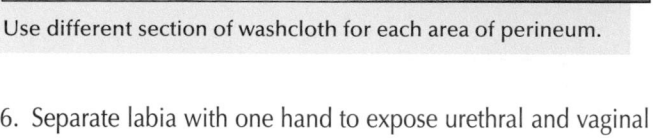

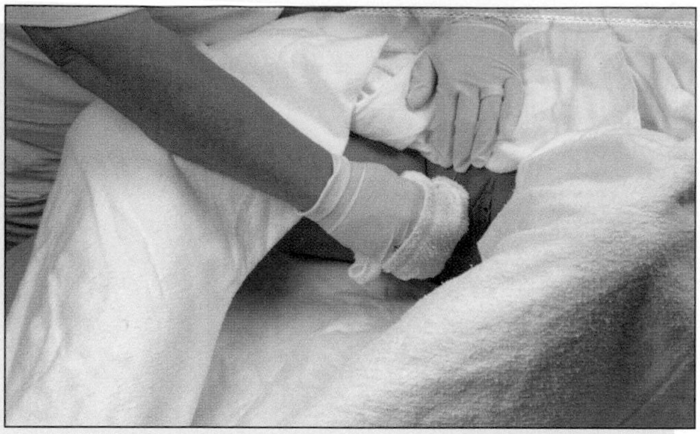
Use different section of washcloth for each area of perineum.

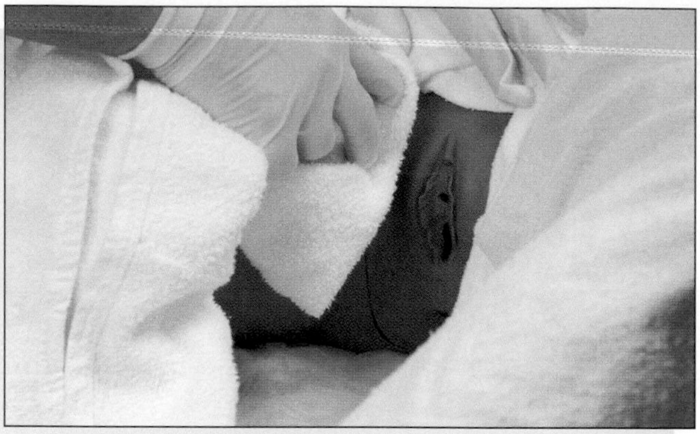
Thoroughly pat dry perineal area.

6. Separate labia with one hand to expose urethral and vaginal openings.
7. Wash labia minora, from front to back, in a downward motion on one side. **Rationale:** This promotes the principle of washing from a clean to a dirty area.
8. Change washcloth area or obtain new washcloth if first one is soiled. Repeat cleansing stroke on opposite side. **Rationale:** This prevents cross-contamination between areas.
9. Place washcloth in water, resoap, wring dry, and form a mitt, using new section of washcloth to continue washing perineal area.
10. Wash external labia (labia majora) and perineal area from front to back.
11. Change area of washcloth and cleanse opposite side of external labia and perineal area.
12. Thoroughly pat dry perineal area. **Rationale:** Prevents moisture accumulation and potential fungal infections.
13. Change washcloth area and clean around anal area. **Rationale:** Anal area is last to be washed to prevent cross-contamination.
14. Discard washcloths and package in appropriate receptacle.
15. Remove gloves.
16. Position client for comfort.
17. Wash your hands.

CULTURAL COMPETENCE

Cultures define cleanliness in different ways. Western cultures, because of the abundance of detergents and washing machines, value clean clothes. Parts of India, Thailand, and Africa have only river water available for washing clothes, therefore do not place importance on clean clothes.

Anglo-Americans are fastidious about body cleanliness and the absence of body odor. The use of perfumes, deodorants, and aftershave lotions is a major part of their hygienic care. In European cultures, natural body odor is thought to have sex appeal.

PROVIDING INCONTINENCE CARE

Equipment

Package with premoistened perineal washcloths
Clean linen, gown as needed
Clean gloves

Preparation

1. Provide privacy for client and explain what you will be doing.
2. Obtain package of three washcloths premoistened with 3% dimethicone, a transparent barrier that remains on the skin

to protect it. **Rationale:** This protective barrier is less messy than zinc oxide or other petroleum-based barriers and it seals out wetness on the perineum.

3. Place in microwave for 12 seconds. **Rationale:** Warming for a longer time can potentially burn the client's perineum. Washcloths may be used at room temperature.
4. Take warmed package to room.
5. Don clean gloves.

Procedure

1. Remove soiled gown and place in linen hamper.
2. Open package.
3. Clean soiled area by cleansing from front to back, using a different cloth for each area of the perineum. The cloths provide moisturizing, deodorizing, and a barrier protection. Discard soiled washcloths and package in appropriate receptacle.
4. Place new gown on client and change linen as needed.
5. Place client in position of comfort.
6. Remove gloves and place in appropriate receptacle.
7. Wash hands.

PROVIDING MALE PERINEAL CARE

Equipment

Bath blanket or sheet
Two bath towels
Protective pad or plastic sheet
Washcloth
Basin of warm water
Clean gloves

Preparation

1. Collect and arrange necessary equipment.
2. Talk with client about how he can perform care or assist with procedure.
3. Ask client to attempt to empty bladder.
4. Provide privacy by closing door and pulling drapes.
5. Wash your hands and don gloves.
6. Cover client with bath blanket or towel over abdomen and cover client's legs with sheet or towel, exposing genital area as little as possible. **Rationale:** This contributes to client's comfort and privacy.

Procedure

1. Place washcloth in basin. Apply soap to washcloth.
2. Wring washcloth out to remove excess water. **Rationale:** This will prevent the protective pad from getting too wet.
3. If the client has not been circumcised, retract his foreskin carefully to expose the glans penis.
4. Gently but securely hold the shaft of the penis in one hand.
5. Using a circular motion, start at the tip of the penis and wash downwards toward the shaft with soap and water. Do not repeat washing over an area without using a clean area of the washcloth. **Rationale:** This procedure prevents cross-contamination.

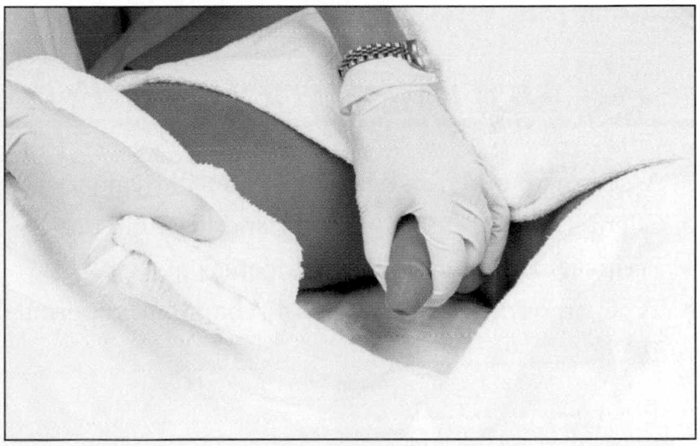

Hold shaft of penis in one hand.

6. Rinse out washcloth and rinse area thoroughly.
7. Replace the foreskin over the glans penis.
8. Wash around the scrotum using a new washcloth.
9. Rinse out washcloth and then rinse area thoroughly.
10. Wash the anus last.

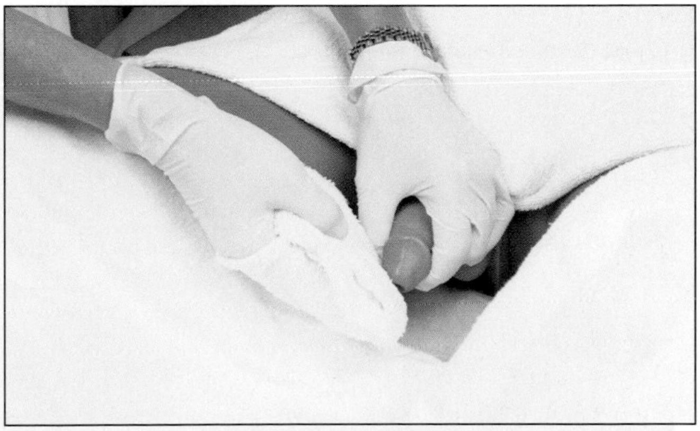

Use circular motion, starting at tip of penis and wash toward shaft.

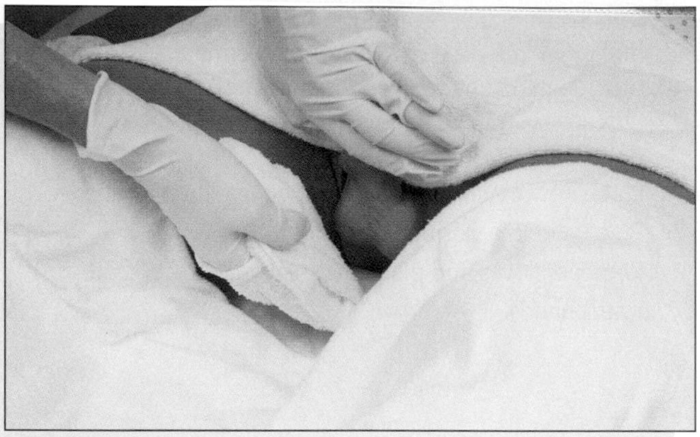

Wash around scrotum using new washcloth.

11. Rinse out washcloth and rinse anal area.
12. Dry all areas.
13. Remove articles and cover client.
14. Reposition client for comfort.
15. Remove gloves, and place in appropriate receptacle.
16. Wash your hands.

Documentation for Perineal and Genital Care

- Assessment and care needs for perineal hygiene
- Client's level of understanding and teaching needs
- Perineal care provided and outcomes of care
- Type, amount, consistency of discharge from perineal area
- Response of client to procedure
- Incontinence, number of times, and interventions attempted to control incontinence

Critical Thinking Application

UNEXPECTED OUTCOMES	CRITICAL THINKING OPTIONS
Client has foul odor even after perineal care.	• Obtain order for sitz bath. • Request order for medicated solution. • Request culture of discharge so the appropriate treatment can be instituted.
Client develops urinary tract infection.	• Instruct client on proper technique for perineal care. • Instruct female clients to wash from anterior to posterior aspects of perineum, using different sections of cloth for each wipe. • Instruct male clients to wash from urethral opening down the shaft of the penis.

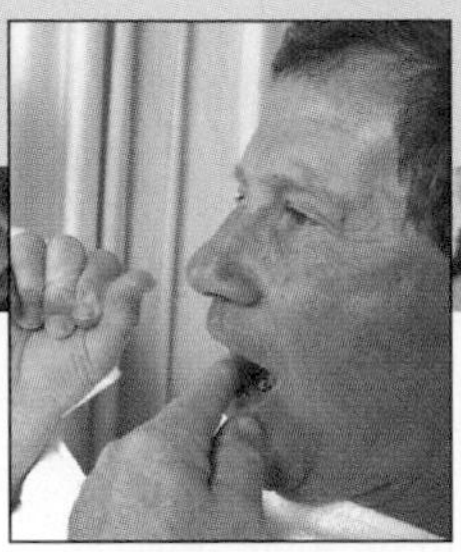

UNIT 7

Eye and Ear Care

Nursing Process Data

ASSESSMENT *Data Base*

Assess if client is using eyeglasses or contact lenses, has an artificial eye, or is experiencing any eye problems.

Observe client's eyes for symmetry and clarity.

Assess skin surrounding client's eyes for excessive dryness, scaling, and irritation.

Assess eyes for discomfort, irritation, edema, crustation, sties, and lesions.

Assess eye socket for potential complications.

Assess artificial eye for signs of tearing or itching.

Assess client's knowledge related to care of contact lenses.

Observe client's tear ducts and sclera for inflammation and excessive tearing.

Assess client's pupils for response to light.

Observe client's eye movements or muscle action.

Evaluate ability to hear and usefulness of hearing aid.

PLANNING *Objectives*

To ensure that eyes and surrounding skin areas are clear, comfortable, and free of crustation

To improve or maintain the client's vision

To prevent irritation and infection

To maintain or improve the client's appearance and self-esteem

To increase ability to hear

IMPLEMENTATION *Procedures*

Providing Routine Eye Care

Providing Eye Care for Comatose Client

Providing Postoperative Socket Care

Removing and Cleaning an Artificial Eye

for Heavy Mucus Deposit

Removing and Cleaning Contact Lenses

Cleaning and Checking a Hearing Aid

EVALUATION *Expected Outcomes*

Eyes and surrounding area are clear and free of crustation.

Eye socket remains free of infection.

Vision is maintained or improved.

Hearing is improved.

PROVIDING ROUTINE EYE CARE

Equipment

Small basin
Water or normal saline solution
Washcloth or cotton balls
Clean gloves

Preparation

1. Determine client's eye care needs, and obtain physician's order if needed.
2. Explain necessity for and method of eye care to client. Discuss how client can assist you.
3. Collect necessary equipment.
4. Wash your hands and don gloves.

Procedure

1. Use water or saline at room temperature.
2. Using the washcloth or cotton balls dampened in water or saline, gently wipe each eye from the inner to outer canthus. Use separate cotton ball or corner of washcloth for each eye. **Rationale:** To prevent cross-contamination from one eye to the other.
3. If crusting is present, gently place a warm, wet compress over eye(s) until crusting is loosened.

PROVIDING EYE CARE FOR COMATOSE CLIENT

Equipment

Water or normal saline solution
Washcloth, cotton balls, tissues
Sterile lubricant or eye preparations if ordered by the physician
Eye dropper or asepto bulb syringe
Eye pads or patches
Clean gloves

Procedure

1. Wash your hands and don clean gloves.
2. Cleanse the eyes using a dampened washcloth or cotton balls dampened in water or saline. Gently wipe each eye from inner to outer canthus. Use separate cotton ball or corner of washcloth for each eye. **Rationale:** Wiping from inner canthus to outer prevents particles and fluid from entering nasolacrimal duct.
3. Use a dropper to instill a sterile ophthalmic solution (liquid tears, saline, methylcellulose) every 3 to 4 hours as ordered by physician. (See procedure for *Instilling Eyedrops* in Chapter 18.) **Rationale:** To prevent corneal drying and ulceration.
4. Keep client's eyes closed if blink reflex is absent. If eye pads or patches are used, explain their purpose to client's family. Do not tape eyes shut. **Rationale:** Corneal abrasions and drying occur when eyes lose blink reflex.
5. Remove gloves and wash hands.
6. Remove patch and evaluate condition of eye every 4 hours.

PROVIDING POSTOPERATIVE SOCKET CARE

Equipment

Conformer (plastic or silicone)
Facial tissue
Washcloth
Baby shampoo
Cotton-tipped applicator sticks
Opticlude eye patch

Procedure

1. Explain procedure to client.
2. Provide privacy.
3. Place client in a semi to high Fowler's position
4. Instruct client to not rub his/her eyelids from nose toward side of face. This is a down and outward motion. **Rationale:** The conformer can become dislodged.

5. Instruct client to close his/her eyes before wiping eye toward nose in a horizontal direction.
6. Wipe lids toward the nose with a facial tissue or warm washcloth to remove secretions and tears.
7. Clean dried secretions from lid margins with a cotton-tipped applicator soaked in baby shampoo.
8. Instruct client to take any medications that are prescribed. **Rationale:** Antibiotic ointment or drops can get into socket through holes in conformer.
9. Apply Opticlude patch if desired. Usually, a few days postop client does not need to wear a dressing, but may wish to keep socket covered.

CLINICAL ALERT

A conformer made of plastic or silicone is placed in socket following removal of an eye. The conformer is used to maintain orbit volume and to form lid pockets that will eventually hold artificial eye in place. The conformer is not to be removed, as it is used to maintain necessary space for artificial eye.

10. Instruct client on how to replace conformer if it should fall out.
    a. Wash his/her hands.
    b. Lift upper lid with thumb or forefinger of one hand.
    c. Slide conformer under upper lid.
    d. Hold conformer in place and pull down on lower lid. **Rationale:** This assists conformer to slip back into socket.

CLINICAL ALERT

Check with ophthalmologist regarding frequency of cleansing artificial eyes. Physicians are not in agreement with this procedure. Some recommend removing eye at regular intervals, while others recommend handling prosthesis only when necessary in order to prevent infection of the socket. Some clients are instructed to not remove the prosthesis between their yearly visit to the ocularist who cleans and polishes the eye. The yearly cleaning and polishing extends life of the prosthesis and returns luster to eye.

REMOVING AND CLEANING AN ARTIFICIAL EYE

Equipment

Suction cup (optional)
Water or hard contact lens solution
Mild soap (Ivory)
Facial tissue
Washcloth
Towel
Clean gloves
3% hydrogen peroxide, if needed
Small container
Baking soda

Preparation

1. If possible, encourage client or family member to care for client's artificial eye.
2. If assisting with artificial eye care, assess client's usual method for cleansing.
3. Gather equipment.
4. Wash your hands and don gloves.

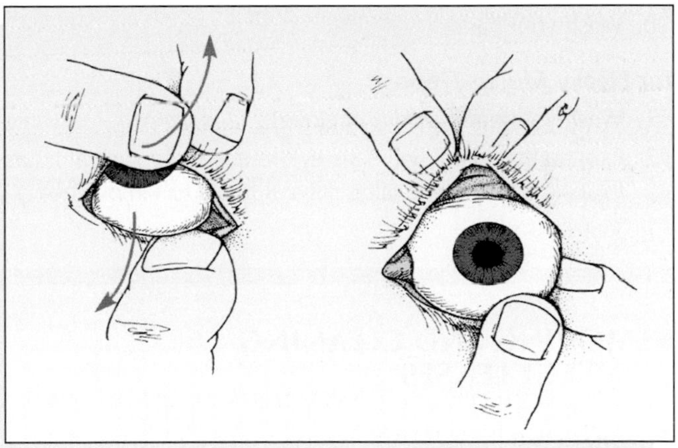

Removal of eye prosthesis.

Procedure

1. Place towel on overbed table. Remove eye while working over table. **Rationale:** In case the eye should come loose when using suction cup or you accidently drop it.
2. Hold the palm of your nondominant hand below artificial eye.
3. Remove prothesis using your hand or a suction cup.
    a. When using your hands to remove prosthesis, depress lower lid and pull down and outward away from nose with index finger of dominant hand so bottom edge of

prosthesis slides out of socket and into your nondominant hand.

b. When using a suction cup, lift upper eyelid with your index finger to keep eyelashes out of the way. Moisten tip of suction cup with water, squeeze suction cup and gently place tip on middle of prosthesis while releasing pressure to create suction. While pulling gently on suction cup and prosthesis, depress lower lid downward and pinch it inward slightly toward socket. Prosthesis should come out easily. Keep your nondominant hand below socket. **Rationale:** To prevent dropping of eye if it comes loose from suction cup.

4. Wash prosthesis in water and a mild soap like Ivory liquid. A "hard contact" lens cleaning solution can be substituted for soap and water. **Rationale:** This removes most of surface accumulations and reduces irritation to eyelids.
5. Moisten a facial tissue and rub prosthetic eye to remove surface secretions. Rinse thoroughly with water before reinserting eye.
6. Inspect tissue in and around eye for swelling or drainage.
7. Wash eyelid and dry, wiping from inner to outer canthus. **Rationale:** Direction is more sanitary because it prevents contaminating tear duct.
8. Moisten prosthesis, lift upper eyelid and slide into place.
9. Remove gloves and dispose of supplies.
10. Wash your hands.

for Heavy Mucus Deposit

1. Wash your hands and don gloves.
2. Explain that client will have eye removed for several hours to soak. **Rationale:** It takes several hours to remove heavy mucus deposits. Instruct client on procedure so he/she can complete it at home if necessary.
3. Remove artificial eye using steps outlined in above skill.
4. Place artificial eye in container with 3% hydrogen peroxide. Use sufficient quantities of hydrogen peroxide to completely cover eye.
5. Soak prosthesis several hours or overnight in hydrogen peroxide solution if there is a heavy mucus deposit that is not removed with usual washing procedure.
6. Rinse prosthesis thoroughly and place in a container with ½ tsp. baking soda and cold water. Soak for 30 minutes. **Rationale:** This neutralizes hydrogen peroxide.
7. Wipe surface of prosthesis with a damp facial tissue to remove any residual protein deposits.
8. Rinse well using water or soft contact lens saline solution.
9. Reinsert eye into socket.
10. Remove gloves and wash hands.

CLINICAL ALERT

Do not clean prosthesis with abrasives or sterilizing agents, because they will attack the acrylic that encompasses artificial eye.

REMOVING AND CLEANING CONTACT LENSES

Equipment

Towel
Contact lens container
Commercially prepared cleaning solution
Commercially prepared disinfecting solution
Commercially prepared rinsing and storing solution
Enzymatic agent (protein remover)
Clean gloves

Procedure

1. Place client in supine position, and place a towel under the client's chin.
2. Wash hands and don gloves.
3. Place the tip of your thumb across the lower lid below its margin.
4. Place the top of the forefinger of the same hand on the upper lid above its margin.
5. Spread eyelids apart as wide as possible and locate outer edges of soft lens which should appear as a rim around outer edge of iris.
6. Place thumb and forefinger directly on soft lens.

CLINICAL ALERT

Extended-wear (overnight) contacts, rigid or soft, increase the risk of corneal ulcers, infection-caused eruptions on the cornea that can lead to blindness. Symptoms include visual changes, eye redness, eye discomfort or pain, and excessive tearing.

7. Gently remove lens from surface of eyeball by squeezing lens between thumbs and fingertip. **Rationale:** Cornea is avascular and use of contact lenses interrupts flow of oxygen into cornea. Removing lenses for a period of time allows oxygen to reach cornea and thus prevent corneal complications.
8. Release eyelids.
9. Place lens in palm of hand or place disposable lenses in trash. Disposable lenses are not to be cleaned or reused. There is not a lens cleaner available for these lenses.
10. Place 2–3 drops of cleaning solution on lens.
11. Clean lens thoroughly by rubbing between fingertip and palm of hand for 20–30 seconds.
12. Rinse lens thoroughly with sterile saline solution or rinsing solution. Use only lens cleaning system recommended by ophthalmologist. Do not interchange cleaning solution systems.
13. Place lens in disinfecting solution according to physician directions. Time varies from hours to one full day. **Rationale:** This destroys microorganisms on lenses.

CLINICAL ALERT

Clean, rinse, and disinfect reusable lenses each time they are removed regardless of number of times each day. Always store lenses in storage solution, not water. Microorganisms from water can feed on corneal tissue.

Client Teaching

Instruct the client in the following safety issues:

- Notify physician immediately if eyes are red, not comfortable, or you can't see clearly.
- Use only rinsing solution, not saliva, to wet lenses.
- Use only commercially prepared saline solution or rinsing solution to cleanse lenses.
- Do not interchange types of lens cleaning systems.
- Maintain lens-care regimen prescribed by physician.
- Put on makeup before inserting lenses.
- Use appropriate type of lenses for their intended use. Do not use daily-wear lenses at night or disposable lenses more than once.

14. Rinse lens thoroughly with rinsing solution.
15. Repeat procedure on second lens.
16. Use enzyme tablet or solution according to physician orders, usually weekly. **Rationale:** This removes stubborn protein and lipids.
17. Clean lens container daily and leave open to dry. Replace as directed by physician, either weekly or monthly.

CLEANING AND CHECKING A HEARING AID

Equipment

Soap
Water
Petroleum jelly
Pipe cleaner
Cotton-tipped applicator
Hearing aid batteries
Clean gloves

Procedure

1. Determine ability of client to perform all or part of cleaning procedure, and teach procedure when necessary. Have client remove hearing aid if able to do so.
2. Wash hands and don gloves.
3. Wipe casing with dry cloth.
4. Check batteries if hearing aid has not been functioning. Insert new batteries, matching positive (+) and negative (−) signs.
5. Examine cord for breaks; replace as necessary.
6. Before inserting ear mold, cleanse outer ear gently with cotton-tipped applicator.
7. Turn receiver switch to ON. Assist client to adjust volume control to desired level. If whistling or feedback noises occur, check for tightness of fit as ear mold probably has not been inserted properly.
8. Place hearing aid in container when not in use, and place in bedside stand.
9. Remove gloves.
10. Wash your hands.

DOCUMENTATION FOR EYE AND EAR CARE

- Documentation of eye assessment and eye care needs
- Method and outcome of eye care provided
- Condition of eye and surrounding structure
- Condition of eye socket
- Client's response to client teaching regarding contact lenses
- Response to using hearing aid
- Improved hearing after cleaning
- Client's ability to insert, remove, and clean hearing aid

Critical Thinking Application

UNEXPECTED OUTCOMES	CRITICAL THINKING OPTIONS
Eyelids become crusted from exudate.	• Place warm, moist washcloth across eyes and leave in place for several minutes. • Moisten cotton applicator stick with sterile saline, and gently twist the applicator stick over crusted surface to assist in removing crust.
You are unable to replace the artificial eye or contact lens.	• If client is unable to assist, ask relatives for help. • Do not use force. Leave lens or eye out until someone who is able to replace it is available.
Artificial eye itches	• Usually due to protein accumulation (from tear layer) on front surface of eye causing an allergic reaction. • Clean artificial eye. • Apply eye drops prescribed by physician.
Artificial eye tears	• Caused by more fluid-producing tissues in an ophthalmic socket than in a normal eye. • With an artificial eye there is an increase in tears, mucus, and oil from tear layer leading to increased tearing. • Insert eyedrops prescribed by physician, particularly in locals with dry heat.
Wrong solution used on contact lens causes excessive tearing and burning sensation when lens is placed in eye.	• Immediately remove lens from eye, and place in proper storage container. • Immediately rinse client's eye with copious amounts of sterile water. • Have client checked immediately by ophthalmologist for emergency care of potentially burned cornea.
Hearing did not improve with cleaning of hearing aid.	• Check if receiver switch is ON. • Check if batteries are properly in place and that the poles match: positive (+) and negative (−). • Recheck hearing aid with expert.

GERONTOLOGIC CONSIDERATIONS

Clients with dentures require special nursing care

- Check for proper fit when replacing dentures. Ill-fitting dentures interfere with chewing and can lead to altered nutrition. Loss of teeth may limit meal planning and the nurse should assist the client to choose a balanced diet taking into account tooth loss.
- Monitor denture cleaning to ensure client has fresh-tasting mouth to encourage eating. Elderly clients have decreased sensitivity to sweet, sour, salty, and bitter tastes; thus, they may compensate by using extra salt. The nurse can counsel the client on alternative seasonings and request dietary consultation.

Nails and hair change with age

- As client's age increases, nails become soft, fragile, and lusterless. Diabetic clients require a physician's order to cut nails.
- Nails should be kept trimmed (straight across with no jagged edges) so skin that is at risk is not scratched and opened.

A positive body image is enhanced with good personal hygiene. Nursing care should focus on assisting the client to maintain good personal hygiene.

MANAGEMENT GUIDELINES

Each state legislates a Nurse Practice Act for RNs and LVN/LPNs. Health care facilities are responsible for establishing and implementing policies and procedures that conform to their state's regulations. Verify the regulations and role parameters for each health care worker in your facility.

Delegation of Responsibilities

- The staffing patterns today often require that Certified Nursing Assistants (CNAs) or Unlicensed Assistive Personnel (UAPs) complete personal hygiene activities for most clients because these activities have a predictable outcome and do not require nursing judgment. However, performing these tasks for the client provides an excellent forum for client assessment. When the tasks are delegated to other personnel, the RN and LPNs responsible for client care must receive specific reports of the client's condition and any unexpected findings. The CNAs and UAPs should receive specific instructions regarding the condition of each client and what to observe for.
- The team member delegating staff assignments should try to implement a staffing pattern that allows professional nurses to be assigned to complete general care, including personal hygiene activities, at least every other day so that important assessment parameters are not missed.
- Check facilities procedure manual for appropriate health care worker to remove and replace eye prosthesis and contact lenses.

Information Flow

- CNAs and UAPs should be educated, encouraged, and rewarded with positive feedback when they give excellent reports on the client for whom they have performed the tasks of personal hygiene. When the unit is extremely busy, this may be the major source of information the professional nurse receives about the client for whom he or she is legally responsible.

CRITICAL THINKING STRATEGIES

SCENARIO 1

You have been assigned to two clients for the 7 A.M. to 12 noon clinical experience.

Client 1: A 68-year-old female with a total hip replacement 2 days ago. Her past history indicates she had a cataract removed 2 months ago and had a lens fitted a week ago. She has developed a very uncomfortable incision site. It is red and tender to touch. Her dressings are somewhat moist without observable drainage on the dressings. Her vital signs indicate a temperature of 101°F, P 90, R 28 and unlabored. She tells you she doesn't feel like doing anything today.

Client 2: An 80-year-old female with a fractured hip, unrepaired, admitted this morning from a local long-term care facility. She is in severe pain and requires pain medications every 4 hours. She is unable to use the patient-controlled analgesia (PCA) because she forgets how it works. Her physical assessment indicates her skin is reddened around the coccyx and very dry. She appears to be unkempt, and her hair is matted.

1. Based on the scenario what is your first action after you hear report? Provide rationale for your answer.
2. Identify the assessment you will complete on each client. What information will you be gathering in order to make a decision on nursing care for the shift?
3. List, in priority, the nursing care you will provide for each client and provide rationale for your decision.
4. Which client will you assess first and why?
5. Which of the personal hygiene skills will you administer to each client? Will any adjustments need to be made in the skill in order to provide care for the client? Please state the changes that will need to be made.

CHAPTER 10

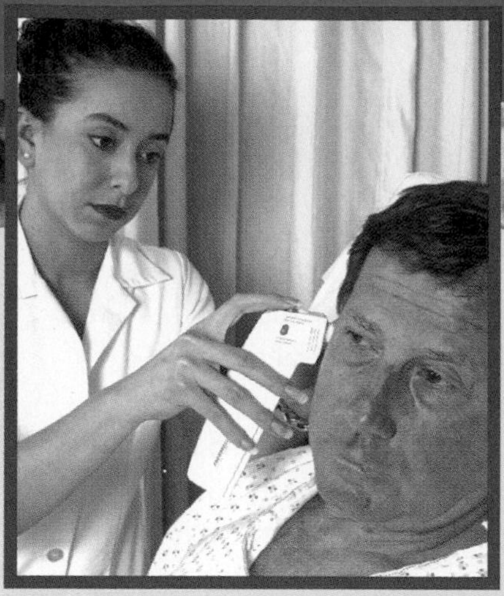

Vital Signs

THEORETICAL CONCEPTS

UNIT ONE: **Temperature 243**
- Using a Digital Thermometer 244
  - *for Oral Temperature 244*
  - *for Axillary Temperature 245*
- Using an Electronic Thermometer 245
  - *for Oral Temperature 245*
  - *for Rectal Temperature 246*
- Measuring an Infant or Child's Temperature 246
  - *for Oral Route 247*
  - *for Rectal Route 247*
  - *for Axillary Route 247*
- Using an Infrared Thermometer for Tympanic Temperature 247
- Using a Heat-Sensitive Wearable Thermometer 248

UNIT TWO: **Pulse Rate 250**
- Determining a Radial Pulse 251
- Taking an Apical Pulse 252
- Taking an Apical–Radial Pulse 253
- Palpating a Peripheral Pulse 254
- Monitoring Peripheral Pulses with Doppler Ultrasound Stethoscope 255

UNIT THREE: **Respirations 258**
- Obtaining the Respiratory Rate 259

UNIT FOUR: **Blood Pressure 261**
- Measuring a Blood Pressure 262
- Palpating Systolic Arterial Blood Pressure 265
- Measuring Lower-Extremity Blood Pressure 265
- Measuring Blood Pressure by Flush Method in Small Infant 266
- Using a Continuous Noninvasive Monitoring Device 267

GERONTOLOGIC CONSIDERATIONS 269

MANAGEMENT GUIDELINES 270

CRITICAL THINKING STRATEGIES 271

Cross Reference, Assessing Pain—Pain Management, Chapter 16

Learning Objectives

- Identify the cardinal signs that reflect the body's physiologic status.
- List three mechanisms that increase heat production.
- Explain how disease alters the "set point" of the temperature-regulating center.
- Define hypothermia and list the symptoms of this condition.
- Differentiate between the oral, rectal, axillary, and tympanic methods of taking temperature.
- Describe two nursing actions that can be performed when temperature is not within normal range.
- Describe at least three different types of pulses.
- Discuss the pulse, and indicate how it is an index of heart rate and rhythm.
- Compare normal heart rate range for adults and children.
- Identify the characteristics of peripheral pulses.
- Define the term "respiration."
- List the normal respiratory rate for adults and children.
- Explain four types of abnormal respiratory patterns.
- Identify four factors that affect blood pressure.
- Demonstrate the method of palpating systolic arterial blood pressure.

Terminology

General Terminology

Antipyretic: an agent that reduces febrile temperatures.

Apex: the pointed end of a cone-shaped part or organ (e.g., lower heart, upper lung).

Arteriosclerosis: an arterial disease characterized by inelasticity and thickening of the vessel walls with lessened blood flow.

Atherosclerosis: a form of arteriosclerosis in which there are localized accumulations of lipid-containing material within the internal surfaces of blood vessels.

Atrial: pertaining to the atrium, the upper cardiac chamber that receives blood from the lungs and systemic circulation.

Autoregulation: the intrinsic ability of an organ or tissue to maintain blood flow despite changes in arterial pressure.

Axilla: armpit.

Cardiac output: the amount of blood ejected by the heart or the stroke volume (SV) times the heart rate (CO = SV × HR).

Cardio: pertaining to the heart.

Cardiogenic: having origin in the heart itself.

Chemoreceptor: a sense organ or sensory nerve ending that is stimulated by and reacts to chemical stimuli.

Contractility: having the ability to contract or shorten muscle tissue or cells.

Core temperature: the body's interior deep tissue temperature (e.g., the abdominal cavity).

Diastole: the period in which the heart dilates and fills with blood; the period of relaxation.

Doppler: a type of ultrasound stethoscope or probe that uses an ultrasound beam to detect blood flow.

Febrile: feverish, increased body temperature.

Fibrillation: quivering, involuntary contraction of individual muscle fibers.

Hypertension: blood pressure that is considered to be higher than the normal range.

Hyperthermia: unusually high body temperature.

Hypervolemia: abnormal increase in the volume of circulating body fluid.

Hypotension: blood pressure that is lower than the normal range.

Hypothalamus: the part of the brain that lies below the thalamus; it maintains or regulates body temperature, certain metabolic processes, and other autonomic activities.

Hypothermia: a body temperature below the average normal range.

Hypovolemia: diminished blood volume.

Infarction: an area of tissue in an organ or part that undergoes necrosis following cessation of blood supply.

Ischemia: local and temporary hypoxia due to obstruction of the circulation to a part.

Korotkoff's sounds: low-frequency sounds that are regarded by the American Heart Association as the best index of blood pressure in an adult—sounds are produced as a result of changes in blood flow through a compressed artery.

Myocardium: the middle muscle layer of the walls of the heart.

Palpate: to examine by touch; feel.

Peripheral: pertinent to the periphery, away from the central structure.

Peripheral vascular disease: indicates diseases of the arteries and veins of the extremities, especially those conditions that interfere with adequate flow of blood.

Piloerection: hair standing on end when heat production is stimulated through vasoconstriction.

Pyrogen: any substance that produces fever.

Set point: the constant temperature that the hypothalamus (the body's thermostat) strives to maintain.

Shock: state of inadequate tissue perfusion resulting from circulatory failure, precipitated by many factors and identified by various signs and symptoms.

Sphygmomanometer: instrument for indirectly determining arterial blood pressure.

Thermoregulation: the body's physiological function of heat regulation to maintain a constant internal body temperature.

Valsalva's maneuver: attempt to forcibly exhale with the glottis, nose, and mouth closed, producing an increased intrathoracic pressure.

Vasoconstriction: constriction of the blood vessels and stimulation of heat production.

Vasodilation: dilation of blood vessels, and the inhibition of heat production.

Pulse Terminology

Atrial fibrillation: atrial arrhythmia characterized by rapid, random contractions of the atrial myocardium causing a rapid, irregular ventricular rate.

Bigeminal pulse: a regularly irregular pulse where every second beat has a decreased amplitude.

Bradycardia: a pulse rate below 60 BPM.

Bounding pulse: pulse pressure is increased. It is felt as a slapping against the fingers because of the rapid upstroke and quick downstroke. It is seen in conditions of increased cardiac output, such as exercise, anxiety, alcoholic intake, and pregnancy. It is also noted in pathology with fever, anemia, hyperthyroidism, liver failure, complete heart block with bradycardia, and hypertension.

Normal pulse: pulse is smooth and rounded and is felt as a sharp upstroke and gradual downstroke. Provides information about cardiac status and blood volume. Correlates with cardiac contraction.

PMI: apical pulse or point of maximum impulse; palpated at 5th intercostal space, left midclavicular line. Pulses occurs with contraction of left ventricle.

Premature beats: a pacemaker outside the sinus node fires earlier than the sinus node, the normal pacemaker of the heart. Since the beat is early, the stroke volume is less because the ventricles do not have time to fill. This condition causes a pause in rhythm, which may result in a pulse deficit.

Pulse deficit: occurs when the heart rate counted at the apex by auscultation is greater than the heart rate counted by palpation of the radial pulse. The pulse wave is not transmitted to the periphery to produce a palpable radial pulse.

Pulsus alternans: rhythm is regular but the amplitude alternates from beat to beat. May be related to left ventricular failure.

Pulsus paradoxus: detected by blood pressure measurement. The disappearance of Korotkoff's sounds during inspiration phase of breathing, with sounds appearing throughout the respiratory cycle (during inspiration and exhalation) at a pressure 10 mm Hg lower than heard during exhalation alone. This phenomenon occurs in COPD and with cardiac tamponade and should be further evaluated.

Pulse pressure: the difference between systolic and diastolic pressure (about 30 to 40 points).

Sinus arrhythmia: common in children and young adults. The rate accelerates with inspiration and slows with expiration.

Tachycardia: heart rate greater than 100 BPM.

Weak or thready pulse: pulse pressure is diminished. It is smooth and rounded, but is felt as a gradual upstroke and prolonged downstroke. It is commonly seen in conditions resulting in decreased cardiac output, such as heart failure and shock, and with obstruction to left ventricular ejection, such as aortic stenosis.

Respiratory Terminology

Apnea: absence of breathing.

Biot's respirations: abrupt interruptions between a faster, deeper respiratory rate.

Bradypnea: slow, regular respirations. Rate is below 10 per minute.

Cheyne–Stokes: periods of apnea appear throughout cycle. Respirations become deeper and faster than normal followed by a slower rate and progressing to periods of apnea lasting from 15 to 60 seconds.

Hyperpnea: abnormal increase in depth and rate.

Kussmaul's respirations: deep, gasping breathing. Attempt to blow off carbon dioxide as respiratory compensation for metabolic acidosis (e.g., diabetic ketoacidosis).

Sonorous: loud breathing.

Stertorous: loud, noisy breathing.

Tachypnea: respiratory rate increased above 24 breaths per minute. Rate remains regular but shallow in pattern.

VITAL SIGNS

Vital signs, also termed cardinal signs, reflect the body's physiologic status and provide information critical to evaluating homeostatic balance. Vital signs include four critical assessment areas: temperature, pulse, respiration, and blood pressure. The term "vital" is used because the information gathered is the clearest indicator of overall health status. These four signs form baseline assessment data necessary for an ongoing evaluation of a client's condition. If the nurse has established the normal range for a client, deviations can be more easily recognized. Although not a cardinal sign, pain is now considered the 5th vital sign and must be assessed at the same time.

Routine vital signs (including pain assessment) are important to assess on every client. These parameters should be assessed by a staff member who is familiar with the client's health history so results can be evaluated against previous data. Vital signs should be taken at regular intervals and serial readings are important with all vital signs. In fact, trends yield more information than singular readings. The more critical the client's condition, the more often these signs need to be taken and evaluated. They are not only indicators of a client's present condition but also cues to a positive or negative change in status.

Obtaining the total picture of a client's health status is a major objective of client care. Although vital signs yield important information in themselves, they gain even more relevance when compared with the client's diagnosis, laboratory tests, history, and records. The five vital signs are as follows:

1. *Temperature* represents the balance between heat gain and heat loss and is regulated in the hypothalamus of the brain. Variations in temperature indicate the health status of the body; thermostatic function may be altered by pyrogens, nervous system disease, or injury.
2. The *pulse* is an index of the heart's action; by evaluating its rate, rhythm, and volume, one can gain an overall impression of the heart's action.
3. *Respiration*, the act of bringing oxygen into the body and removing carbon dioxide, yields data on the client's entire breathing process. When the pattern of respiration is altered, ongoing evaluation yields important cues to a client's changing condition.
4. *Blood pressure* readings provide information about the condition of the heart, the arteries and arterioles, vessel resistance, and the cardiac output. Serial readings provide the best indication of a client's cardiovascular status.
5. *Pain assessment* that is ongoing and constant is essential to maintain the client's homeostasis and quality of life. Pain assessment provides information on location, quality, and intensity, as well as outcomes of relief measures. (See Vital Sign Assessment record.)

Factors Influencing Vital Signs

Factors that cause alterations in vital signs include age, gender, race, heredity, medications, lifestyle, environment, pain, exercise, anxiety, stress, metabolism, circadian rhythms, and hormones. The normal variations in vital signs may be caused by age, disease, trauma, etc. The most common alterations are listed below.

Age Age influences body temperature. Body temperature varies from 96.0°–99.5°F in newborns and 96.8°–98.3°F in elderly clients due to thermoregulation deficiencies in both age groups. Newborns have an immature thermoregulation mechanism that causes temperature fluctuations in response to the environment. Elderly clients have an ineffective thermoregulating system due to physiological changes of aging. These changes are related to loss of subcutaneous fat, decreased sweat glands, reduced metabolism, and poor vasomotor control. Environmental conditions may also play a role in an elderly person's ability to effectively adapt body heat and cooling to changes

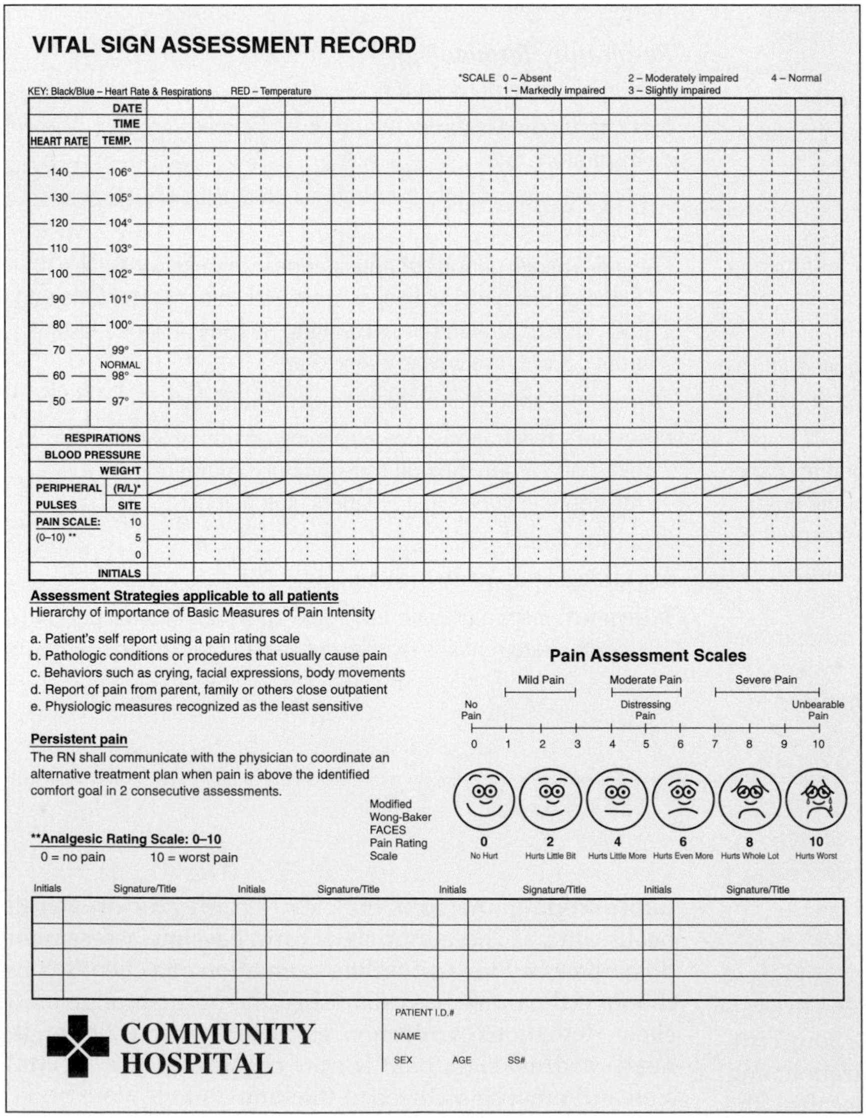
VITAL SIGN ASSESSMENT RECORD

KEY: Black/Blue – Heart Rate & Respirations RED – Temperature

*SCALE 0 – Absent 1 – Markedly impaired 2 – Moderately impaired 3 – Slightly impaired 4 – Normal

	DATE
	TIME
HEART RATE	TEMP.
140	106°
130	105°
120	104°
110	103°
100	102°
90	101°
80	100°
70	99°
60	NORMAL 98°
50	97°
	RESPIRATIONS
	BLOOD PRESSURE
	WEIGHT
PERIPHERAL	(R/L)*
PULSES	SITE
PAIN SCALE: (0–10) **	10
	5
	0
	INITIALS

Assessment Strategies applicable to all patients
Hierarchy of importance of Basic Measures of Pain Intensity

a. Patient's self report using a pain rating scale
b. Pathologic conditions or procedures that usually cause pain
c. Behaviors such as crying, facial expressions, body movements
d. Report of pain from parent, family or others close outpatient
e. Physiologic measures recognized as the least sensitive

Persistent pain
The RN shall communicate with the physician to coordinate an alternative treatment plan when pain is above the identified comfort goal in 2 consecutive assessments.

****Analgesic Rating Scale: 0–10**
0 = no pain 10 = worst pain

Initials	Signature/Title	Initials	Signature/Title	Initials	Signature/Title	Initials	Signature/Title

COMMUNITY HOSPITAL

PATIENT I.D.#
NAME
SEX AGE SS#

Vital Sign Assessment Record.

in external temperature. Respirations vary according to age as well. Newborns have a respiratory range of 30–80 breaths/minute with an average rate of 32 breaths/minute. As age increases, respirations decrease; adults average 16 breaths/minute. The pulse rate also decreases with age. Newborns average 140 beats/minute and adults average 80 beats/minute. On the other hand, blood pressure may increase with age. The newborn's mean blood pressure is 65/42 while the normal adult client's blood pressure ranges from 120/80 to 100/60.

Gender Women experience greater temperature fluctuations than men, probably due to hormonal changes. Temperature variations occur during the menstrual cycle. During menopause, the instability of the vasomotor controls leads to periods of intense body heat and sweating.

Race and Heredity Studies have been mostly inconclusive as to race and heredity being related factors in vital signs alteration. Blood pressure alterations appear to be the main difference in vital signs, usually as a result of particular groups being more susceptible to hemodynamic alterations. African Americans are more prone to high blood pressure resulting from increased salt sensitivity or increased blood cholesterol levels.

Medications Some medications can directly or indirectly alter temperature, pulse, respirations, and blood pressure. For example, narcotic analgesics can depress the rate and depth of respirations and lower blood pressure.

Pain Acute pain leads to sympathetic stimulation which in turn increases the heart rate, respiratory rate, and blood pressure. Chronic pain decreases the pulse rate as a response to parasympathetic stimulation, and may decrease heart rate and respirations.

Circadian Rhythms Biologic rhythms, or biorhythms, control certain physiological patterns in conjunction with environmental factors. The most familiar biorhythm is the circadian rhythm that controls sleep patterns. These rhythms influence blood pressure (pressure is lowest in the morning and peaks in late afternoon and evening) and temperature (highest in the evening—8 P.M. to 12 midnight—and lowest in the early morning—4 to 6 A.M.).

TEMPERATURE

Temperature control of the body is a homeostatic function, regulated by a complex mechanism involving the hypothalamus. The temperature of the body's interior (core temperature) is maintained within ±1°F except in the case of febrile illness. The surface temperature of the skin and tissues immediately underlying the skin rises and falls with a change in temperature of the surrounding environment. Core temperature is maintained when heat production equals heat loss. The temperature regulating center in the hypothalamus keeps the core temperature constant. Temperature receptors, which determine if the body is too hot or too cold, relay signals to the hypothalamus.

Regulatory Mechanisms

When the body becomes overheated, heat-sensitive neurons stimulate sweat glands to secrete fluid. This enhances heat loss through evaporation. The vasoconstrictor mechanism of the skin vessels is reduced, thereby conducting heat from the core of the body to the body surface. Heat loss occurs through radiation, evaporation, and conduction.

When the body core is cooled below 98.6°F (37°C), heat conservation is affected. Intense vasoconstriction of the skin vessels results. There is also piloerection and a decrease in sweating to conserve heat. Heat production is stimulated by shivering and increased cellular metabolism.

The "set point" is the critical temperature level to which the regulatory mechanisms attempt to maintain the body's core temperature. Above the "set point," heat-losing mechanisms are brought into play, and below that level heat-conserving and heat-producing mechanisms are set into action.

Disease can alter the "set point" of the temperature-regulating center to cause fever, a body temperature above normal. Inflammation, brain lesions, pyrogens from bacteria or viruses, or degenerating tissue (i.e., gangrenous areas or myocardial infarction) also increase the "set point." Dehydration can cause fever due to lack of available fluid for perspiration and by increasing the "set point," which brings more heat-conserving and heat-producing mechanisms into play. When the "thermostat" is suddenly set higher, the client complains of feeling cold, has cool extremities, shivers, and has piloerection. Hypoxia can occur due to increased oxygen use with the increased metabolism of heat production. When the "thermostat" returns to normal, heat-losing mechanisms again are activated. The client feels hot and starts perspiring. Other symptoms of fever the client may experience are perspiration over the body surface; body warm to touch; flushed face; feeling cold alternately with feeling hot; increased pulse and respirations; malaise and fatigue; parched lips and dry skin; and convulsions, especially with rapid temperature rise in children.

When the body temperature falls below the normal range, the client experiences hypothermia and complains of being cold, shivers, and has cool extremities. Hypothermia may be caused by accidental cold exposure, frostbite, or GI hemorrhage. Medically induced hypothermia is used for some cardiovascular and neurosurgical interventions. The ability of the hypothalamus to regulate body temperature is greatly impaired when the body temperature falls below 94°F (34.4°C) and is lost below 85°F (29.4°C). Cellular metabolism and heat production are also depressed by a low temperature.

Measuring Body Temperature

Oral or rectal temperatures reflect the body's core temperature. Tympanic and axillary temperatures are somewhat variable but are clinically acceptable for tracking important changes. The normal range of an oral temperature is 97°–99.5°F, or 36°–37.5°C. Rectal temperatures are approximately 1°F higher, ear canal 0.5° higher, and axillary temperatures are 1°F lower than oral readings. Body temperature may vary according to age (lower for the aged), time of day (lower in the morning and higher in the afternoon and evening), amount of exercise, or extremes in the environmental temperature.

The thermometer is the instrument used to measure body heat. Oral and rectal (also used for axillary temperature) thermometers in hospitals are commonly, as of 2002, digital and disposable. Prior to 1998, when the American Hospital Association agreed to eliminate mercury from the health care environment, mercury thermometers were used in hospitals. The thermometer is marked in degrees and tenths of degrees with either a Fahrenheit or Celsius (centigrade) scale and a range of 93°–108°F (34°–42.2°C).

Electronic thermometers are also now widely used in hospitals. They have disposable covers, which promote infection control, and therefore should always be used. The electronic thermometer plugs into a receptacle and has a heat sensor that records the client's core temperature in seconds. The ear canal provides another noninvasive site for temperature measurement using infrared thermometers.

Heat-sensitive tapes are also used to record temperature. A chemical strip tape is applied to the skin, and color changes indicate the temperature level. A continuous-reading wearable tape can be used for 2 days; the temperature is also read by a change in color. These tapes are both disposable and nonbreakable. They are most appropriate for use with small children, and in situations when proper cleaning of the thermometer is difficult.

Fever Signs

Fever is considered to be any abnormal elevation of body temperature (over 100.8°F). The most common signs and symptoms are:

- Perspiration over the body surface
- Body warm to the touch
- Chills and shivers
- Flushed face
- Client complaints of feeling alternately cold and hot
- Increased pulse and respirations
- Complaints of malaise and fatigue
- Parched lips and dry skin
- Convulsions, especially in children

PULSE

The pulse is an index of the heart's rate and rhythm. The apical pulse rate is the number of heart beats per minute. With each beat, the heart's left ventricle contracts and forces blood into the aorta. Closure of the heart valves creates the sounds heard. The forceful ejection of blood by the left ventricle produces a wave that is transmitted through the arteries to the periphery of the body. The pulse is a transient expansion of peripheral arteries resulting from internal pressure changes. If cardiac output is reduced (such as with a premature or irregular heart beat) the peripheral pulse is weak, if felt, or skipped so that the radial pulse rate is less than the apical rate; the difference is called a "pulse deficit." The pulse wave is influenced by the elasticity of the larger vessels, blood volume, blood viscosity, arteriolar and capillary resistance.

Circulatory System Control

The circulatory system is under the dual control of the autonomic nervous system and autoregulation (at the microcirculation level). This dual control allows the circulatory system to vary blood flow to meet the body's requirements. Local control of blood flow is called autoregulation. Blood flow is adjusted according to oxygen need based on changing metabolic activity of different tissues.

The autonomic nervous system regulates circulation through the vasomotor center in the medulla oblongata. Stimulation of the sympathetic nervous system causes vasoconstriction, increased heart rate and cardiac contractility, and a resulting increase in blood pressure. On the other hand, sympathetic inhibition causes vasodilation, reduced heart rate, and a reduction in blood pressure.

Pressure receptors, called baroreceptors, located in the walls of the carotid sinus and arch of the aorta also influence the vasomotor center. Decreased circulating volume (as in hemorrhage) stimulates these receptors, which then transmit signals to the vasomotor center to stimulate the sympathetic nervous system. Resulting cardiovascular responses divert blood flow to vital organs.

Heart Rate and Rhythm

A normal adult heart rate is from 60 to 100 beats per minute (BPM), the average rate is 72 BPM. Rates are slightly faster in women, and more rapid in children and infants (90–140 BPM: Table 10–1). The resting heart rate usually does not change with age. Tachycardia is a pulse rate over 100 BPM. Bradycardia is a pulse rate below 60 BPM.

When taking a client's pulse, be aware that many pathologic conditions produce bradycardia. Among the most common causes are decreased thyroid activity, hyperkalemia, cardiac conduction blocks, and increased intracranial pressure.

Tachycardia is associated with stressful conditions, hypoxia, exercise, and fever. Client conditions, such as congestive heart failure, hemorrhage and shock, dehydration, and anemia produce tachycardia as a compensatory response to poor tissue oxygenation.

Heart rhythm is the time interval between each heartbeat. Normally, the heart rhythm is regular, although slight irregularities do not necessarily indicate cardiac malfunction. An irregular cardiac rhythm, especially if sustained, requires cardiac evaluation because it may be indicative of cardiac disease.

Variance in heart rate, either increased or decreased, may be attributed to many factors, such as drug intake, lack of oxygen, loss of blood, exercise, and body temperature. When evaluating a pulse rate, it is important to ascertain the normal baseline for each client and then to determine variances from the normal for that particular client. The heart normally pumps about 5 L of blood through the body each minute. This cardiac output is calculated by multiplying the heart rate per minute by the stroke volume, the amount of blood ejected with one contraction. Increasing the heart rate is one of the first compensatory mechanisms the body employs to maintain cardiac output.

Evaluating Pulse Quality

The quality of the pulse is determined by the amount of blood pumped through the peripheral arteries. Normally, the amount of pumped blood remains fairly constant; when it varies, it is also indicative of cardiac malfunction. A so-called bounding pulse occurs when the nurse is able to feel the pulse by exerting only a slight pressure over the artery. If, by exerting pressure, the nurse cannot clearly determine the flow, the pulse is called weak or thready.

The arterial pulse can be felt over arteries that lie close to the body surface and over a bone or firm surface that can support the artery when pressure is applied. The radial artery is palpated most frequently because it is the most accessible. The femoral and carotid arteries are used in cases of cardiac arrest to determine the adequacy of perfusion.

Peripheral pulses may be absent or weak. The amplitude of a pulse depends on the degree of filling in the artery during systole (ventricular contraction) and emptying during diastole (ventricular relaxation). It is important to note characteristics of peripheral pulses: 0 = absent; 1+ = weak; 2+ = diminished; 3+ = strong; and 4+ = full and bounding. (Use the system described in your hospital procedure manual.)

When peripheral pulses cannot be palpated, a Doppler ultrasound stethoscope is used by the nurse to confirm the presence or absence of the pulse. Remember, the pulse is not always an accurate indication of the force of cardiac contractions. If cardiac contractions are weak or ventricular filling is incomplete, the pulse is weak; however, in the case of aortic stenosis, the pulse may be weak in spite of forceful cardiac contraction.

The pulse should be taken frequently (every 15 minutes to 1–2 hours) on an acutely ill hospitalized client and less frequently (every 4–8 hours) on more stable hospitalized clients. Once a week or even once a month is adequate for clients in long-term care facilities. Do not wait

TABLE 10–1 Vital Sign Chart for Children

Age	Normal Pulse Range	Normal Pulse Average	Blood Pressure Average	Respiration Average
Newborn	110–180	140	90/55	30–50
1 year	80–150	120	90/60	20–40
2 years	80–130	110	95/60	20–30
4 years	80–120	100	99/65	20–25
6 years	75–115	100	100/56	20–25
8 years	70–110	90	105/56	15–20
10 years	70–110	90	110/58	15–20

until the next routinely scheduled time if the client develops unexpected symptoms or has experienced trauma.

RESPIRATION

Respiration is the process of bringing oxygen to body tissues and removing carbon dioxide. The lungs play a major role in this process. Another respiratory function is to maintain arterial blood homeostasis by maintaining the pH of the blood. The lungs accomplish this by the process of breathing.

Breathing consists of two phases, inspiration and expiration. Inspiration is an active process in which the diaphragm descends, the external intercostal muscles contract, and the chest expands to allow air to move into the tracheobronchial tree. Expiration is a passive process in which air flows out of the respiratory tree.

The respiratory center in the medulla of the brain and the level of carbon dioxide in the blood both control the rate and depth of breathing. Peripheral receptors in the carotid body and the aortic arch also respond to the level of oxygen in the blood. To some extent, respiration can be voluntarily controlled by holding the breath and hyperventilation. Talking, laughing, and crying also affect respiration.

The diaphragm and the intercostal muscles are the main muscles used for breathing. Other accessory muscles, such as the abdominal muscles, the sternocleidomastoid, the trapezius, and the scalene, can be used to assist with respiration if necessary.

Evaluating Respirations

The quality of breathing is important baseline information. Normal breathing, termed eupnea, is almost invisible, effortless, quiet, automatic, and regular. When the breathing pattern varies from normal, it needs to be evaluated thoroughly. For example, bronchial sounds heard over the large airways are fairly loud. There is normally a pause between inspiration and expiration. Softer sounds are heard over peripheral lung areas, and there are no pauses between inspiration, which is a long sound, and expiration, which is a short sound. If breathing is noisy, labored, or strained, an obstruction may be affecting the breathing pattern that could lead to major alterations in homeostasis.

In addition to evaluating the breathing pattern, it is also necessary to evaluate the rate and depth of breathing. The normal rate for a resting adult is 12–18 breaths per minute. A rate of 24 or above is considered tachypnea, and a rate of 10 or less is considered bradypnea. The rate for infants ranges from 20–30 breaths per minute and is often irregular. Older children average about 20–26. The ratio of pulse to breathing is usually 5:1 and remains fairly constant.

The depth of a person's breathing (tidal volume) is the amount of air that moves in and out with each breath. The tidal volume is 500 mL in the healthy adult. Alveolar air is only partially replenished by atmospheric air with each inspiratory phase. Approximately 350 mL (tidal volume minus dead space) of new air is exchanged with the functional residual capacity volume during each respiratory cycle. Accurate tidal volume can be measured by a spirometer, but an experienced nurse can judge the approximate depth by placing the back of the hand next to the client's nose and mouth and feeling the expired air. Another method of estimating volume capacity is to observe chest expansion and to check both sides of the thorax for symmetrical movement.

After assessing the pattern, rate, and depth of breathing, it is important to observe the physical characteristics of chest expansion. The chest normally expands symmetrically without rib flaring or retractions. In addition, observation of chest deformities should also be made, as all of these signs yield information about the respiratory process and overall health status of the client.

BLOOD PRESSURE

The heart generates pressure during the cardiac cycle to perfuse the organs of the body with blood. Blood flows from the heart to the arteries, into the capillaries and veins, and then flows back to the heart. Blood pressure in the arterial system varies with the cardiac cycle, reaching the highest level at the peak of systole and the lowest level at the end of diastole. The difference between the systolic and diastolic blood pressure is the pulse pressure, which is normally 30–50 points (mm Hg).

There are seven major factors that affect blood pressure.

Cardiac Output The force of heart contractions (the amount of blood ejected by the heart) influences blood pressure, especially systolic pressure.

Peripheral Vascular Resistance Resistance to the flow of blood is due to resistant vessels under the influence of the autonomic nervous system. Peripheral vascular resistance is the most important determinant of diastolic pressure.

Elasticity and Distensibility of Arteries Elasticity refers to the action of the blood vessel walls to spring back after blood is ejected into them. When blood is ejected into the aorta and large arteries, the arterial vessel walls distend. Recoil during diastole propels blood through the arterial tree and maintains diastolic pressure. Both elasticity and distensibility decrease with age, resulting in increased systolic pressure and slightly increased diastolic pressure.

Blood Volume Increased blood volume causes an increase in both systolic and diastolic blood pressure, whereas decreased blood volume causes the reverse effect. Hemorrhage decreases blood pressure whereas overhydration from excessive blood transfusions may cause an increase in blood pressure.

Blood Viscosity Blood viscosity (thickness) influences blood flow velocity through the arterial tree. For example, increased viscosity, which occurs with polycythemia, increases resistance to blood flow, whereas decreased viscosity, resulting from anemia, decreases resistance.

Hormones and Enzymes These substances have an important influence on blood pressure. For example, epinephrine and norepinephrine produce a profound vasoconstrictor effect on peripheral blood vessels (mediators of the sympathetic nervous system). Aldosterone (released by the adrenal cortex), renin (released by the juxtaglomerular apparatus of the kidney), and angiotensin (activated by the renin response) also produce effects that raise blood pressure. Histamine and acetylcholine (a parasympathetic mediator) cause vasodilation, therefore lowering blood pressure.

Chemoreceptors Chemoreceptors in the aortic arch and carotid sinus also exert control over the blood pressure. They are sensitive to changes in PaO_2, $PaCO_2$, and pH. Decreased PaO_2 stimulates the chemoreceptors, which stimulate the vasomotor center. Increased $PaCO_2$ and decreased pH directly stimulate the vasomotor center, causing increased peripheral vascular resistance.

Measuring Blood Pressure

Measuring arterial blood pressure provides important information about the overall health status of the client. For example, the systolic pressure provides a data base about the condition of the heart and great arteries. The diastolic pressure indicates arteriolar or peripheral vascular resistance. The pulse pressure, or difference between the systolic and diastolic pressure, provides information about cardiac function and blood volume. A single blood pressure reading, however, does not provide adequate data from which conclusions can be drawn about all of these factors. Rather, a series of blood pressure readings should be taken to establish a baseline for further evaluation.

The *indirect method* of taking a blood pressure using a recently calibrated anaeroid manometer and a stethoscope is accurate for most clients. New electronic blood pressure devices constantly monitor systolic, diastolic, and mean readings at preset time intervals and are helpful to measure blood pressure trends in clients who are at risk for hyper- or hypotension. These devices also provide a printout if needed for documentation. If a stethoscope is unavailable or the brachial artery amplitude is decreased, the brachial or radial artery can be palpated as the blood pressure cuff is inflated to determine the systolic blood pressure (palpated pulse disappears at this point). Alternatively, an inflated blood pressure cuff may be slowly deflated and the point at which distal pulsation is first palpated reflects systolic blood pressure. Those who are severely hypotensive or hypertensive (hemodynamically unstable), have low blood volume, or are on rapid-acting IV vasoconstricting or vasodilating drugs should have blood pressure measured by direct (intraarterial) method. The *direct method* is continuous and measures mean arterial pressures. A needle or catheter is inserted into the brachial, radial, or femoral artery. An oscilloscope displays arterial pressure waveforms.

Normal blood pressure in an adult varies between 100 and 120 systolic and 60 and 80 diastolic (See box on page 267). As blood moves toward smaller arteries and into arterioles, where it enters the capillaries, pressure falls to 35. It continues to fall as blood goes through the capillaries, where the flow is steady and not pulsatile. As blood moves into the venous system, pressure falls until it is the lowest in the venae cavae.

Blood pressures vary widely. A blood pressure of 100/60 may be normal for one person but may be hypotensive for another. Hypotension (90–100 systolic) in a healthy adult without other clinical symptoms is little reason for concern.

Blood pressure readings are recorded in association with Korotkoff's sounds. These sounds are described as "K" phases. The systolic, or first, pressure reading occurs with the advent of the first Korotkoff's sound. The systolic reading represents the maximal pressure in the aorta following contraction of the left ventricle and is heard as a faint tapping sound.

Korotkoff's Sound Phases

Phase I: The pressure level at which the first faint, clear tapping sounds are heard. The sounds gradually increase in intensity as the cuff is deflated. This phase coincides with the reappearance of a palpable pulse (systolic sound).

Phase II: That time during cuff deflation when a murmur or swishing sounds are heard.

Phase III: The period during which sounds are crisper and increases in intensity.

Phase IV: That time when a distinct, abrupt, muffling of sound (usually of a soft, blowing quality) is heard (diastolic sound in children or physically active adults).

Phase V: That pressure level when the last sound is heard and after which all sound disappears (second diastolic sound).

Source: American Heart Association, 1996.

According to American Heart Association standards, the diastolic, or second, reading should be taken at the time of the last Korotkoff's sound (phase V) for adults. The diastolic reading represents the minimal pressure exerted against the arterial walls at all times. In children under age 13, pregnant women, and clients with high cardiac output or peripheral vasodilation, sounds are often heard to a level far below muffling and sometimes to levels near 0. In these individuals, muffling (phase IV) should be used to indicate diastolic pressure, but both muffling (phase IV) and disappearance (phase V) should be recorded (e.g., 110/80/20).

Frequency of blood pressure assessment should be individualized or as ordered. Blood pressure for an acutely ill client should be taken every 15 minutes to 1–2 hours and the blood pressure of more stabilized clients should be taken every 4–8 hours to once a day. Clients with severe hypotension or hypertension, with low blood volume, or those on vasoconstrictor or vasodilator drugs require checking every 5–15 minutes.

PAIN

According to JCAHO, pain should be considered the fifth vital sign. Pain must be evaluated every time vital signs are taken, and it should be documented on the vital sign record. Refer to Chapter 16, Pain Management, for a more in-depth explanation of pain and the options available for pain management.

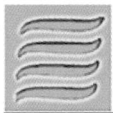

NURSING DIAGNOSES

The following nursing diagnoses are appropriate to use on client care plans when the components are related to vital signs.

NURSING DIAGNOSIS	RELATED FACTORS
Cardiac Output, Decreased	Hypovolemia, rapid pulse, changes in breathing patterns, alteration in heart rhythm or rate, or vascular tone
Fluid Volume Deficit	Excessive urinary output, abnormal fluid loss, infection, fever
Fluid Volume Excess	Decreased cardiac output, fluid retention, inflammatory process, low protein diet, increased fluid intake
Tissue Perfusion, Altered (Cardiopulmonary)	Vascular disorders, hypovolemia, medications, hypoxemia
Airway Clearance, Ineffective	Obstruction of airway, increased secretions, fatigue
Ventilation, Inability to Sustain Spontaneous	Metabolic factors; respiratory muscle fatigue
Breathing Pattern, Ineffective	Change in rate, depth or pattern of breathing that alters normal gas exchange
Thermoregulation, Ineffective	Disease, infection, drug reactions, or damage to the hypothalamic temperature-regulating center; possibly dehydration
Pain, Chronic Pain	Chronic disease conditions, tissue trauma, injury

- The single most important nursing action to decrease the incidence of hospital-based infections is handwashing. **Remember to wash your hands or use antibacterial gel before and after each and every client contact.**

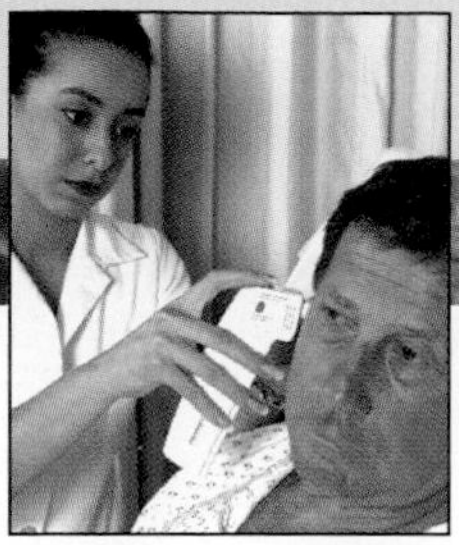

Temperature

Nursing Process Data

ASSESSMENT Data Base

Determine number of times temperature needs to be taken daily.

Assess temperature in relationship to time of day and age of client.

Compare temperature with other vital signs to establish baseline data.

Determine the method most appropriate for obtaining temperature.

Oral Method

Accurate method of determining body temperature

Used only for alert and cooperative clients; not unconscious clients

Not appropriate for use with tachypneic or mouth-breathing clients

Not appropriate for clients with oral inflammatory processes

Delivery of oxygen by nasal cannula does not affect oral temperature readings

Determine client has not taken hot or cold liquids or smoked for 15 to 30 minutes prior to taking temperature orally

Rectal Method

Appropriate for tachypneic, uncooperative, confused, or comatose clients or for clients on seizure precautions

Used for clients with open-mouth breathing, such as those with nasal or oral intubation

Appropriate for clients with wired jaws, facial fractures, or other abnormalities, or for clients with nasogastric tubes who cannot breathe easily with mouth closed

Contraindicated for infants or clients who have had surgery involving the rectum

Axillary Method

Least accurate, but safe

Often used for infants and young children

Used in recovery rooms to avoid turning clients

Time consuming

Electronic Thermometer

Accurate for oral or rectal temperature measurement, but inaccurate for axillary temperature measurement

Prevents infection between clients

Time efficient and easy to read

Infrared Ear Thermometer

Measures body heat radiating from the tympanic membrane

Noninvasive, safe, efficient

Less sensitive in detecting fever in the very young child and infant

Heat Sensitive Tape

Disposable and nonbreakable

Appropriate for children and when proper cleaning of thermometer is difficult

PLANNING Objectives

To determine if core temperature is within normal range

To provide baseline data for further evaluation

To determine alterations in disease conditions

IMPLEMENTATION Procedures

Using a Digital Thermometer

for Oral Temperature

for Axillary Temperature

Using an Electronic Thermometer

for Oral Temperature

for Rectal Temperature

Measuring an Infant or Child's Temperature

for Oral Route

for Rectal Route

for Axillary Route

Using an Infrared Thermometer for Tympanic Temperature

Using a Heat-Sensitive Wearable Thermometer

EVALUATION Expected Outcomes

Temperature is within normal range.

Temperature readings are compared with age, time of day, and previous readings.

Alterations in temperature are detected early and treatment begun.

Appropriate method of temperature taking is determined for each client.

Correct length of time is used for thermometer insertion to obtain an accurate reading.

USING A DIGITAL THERMOMETER

Equipment

Client's individual digital thermometer

Gloves, if necessary

Procedure

1. Wash hands.
2. Don gloves if risk of contact with saliva.

for Oral Temperature

a. Wait 20–30 minutes to take oral temperature if client has been eating, drinking, chewing gum, smoking, or exercising. **Rationale:** These activities may alter core temperature.
b. Place thermometer in client's mouth under front of tongue, and along gum line. **Rationale:** Location ensures contact with large vessels under tongue.

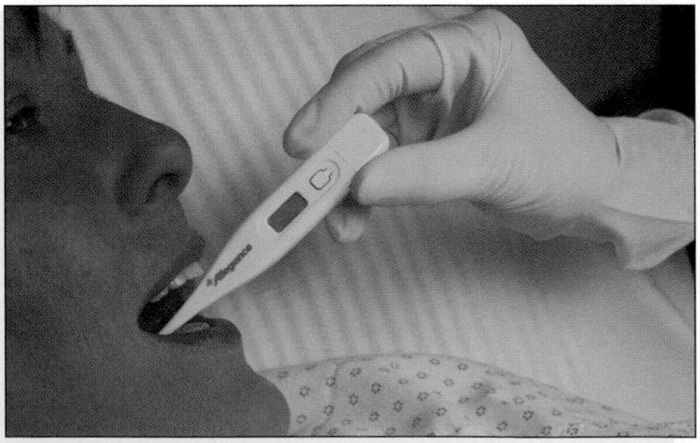

Place thermometer in client's mouth under tongue.

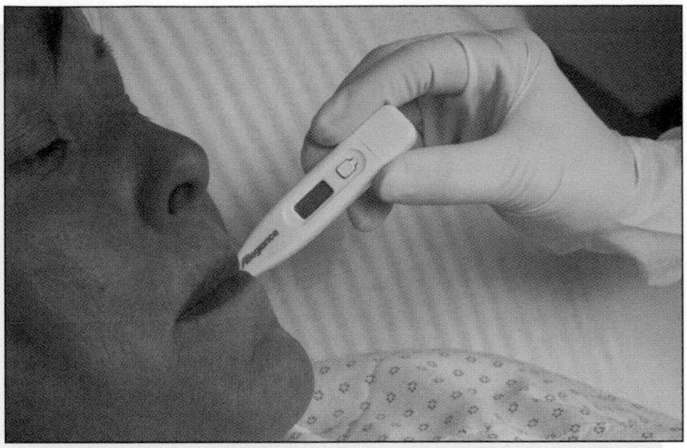

Ask client to hold lips closed and leave thermometer in place 45–90 seconds.

c. Have client hold lips closed and leave thermometer in place 45–90 seconds. **Rationale:** Open-mouth breathing produces abnormally low readings.
d. Remove thermometer and read temperature displayed in digital window.

for Axillary Temperature

a. Assist client to comfortable position and expose axilla area.
b. Dry axilla if necessary. **Rationale:** A false low reading may result if axilla is moist.

Mercury Thermometers

Mercury thermometers are no longer used in hospitals. In 2001, a U.S. senator introduced a comprehensive bill to totally eliminate and retire mercury because of its toxic effects on people and the environment. This bill will allow consumers to trade in thermometers for mercury-free ones, prohibit the sale of mercury-containing items, and generally eliminate the use of mercury in the United States.

TABLE 10–2 Comparing Centigrade and Fahrenheit Temperatures

Centigrade (C)	Fahrenheit (F)
36.0	96.8
36.5	97.7
37.0	**98.6**
37.5	99.5
38.0	100.4
38.3	101.0
39.0	102.2
39.5	103.1
40.0	104.0

To convert degrees F to degrees C, subtract 32, then multiply by 1.8.
To convert degrees C to degrees F, multiply by 1.8, then add 32.

c. Place thermometer in center of axilla and lower arm down across chest. **Rationale:** This position allows thermometer to be in contact with large vessels.
d. Leave in place 1–2 minutes. **Rationale:** Axilla temperature recordings take a longer time to register.

3. Record temperature noting route and return thermometer to its case at client's bedside stand.
4. Wash hands.

CLINICAL ALERT

Temperature varies with time of day: It is highest between 5 and 7 P.M. and lowest between 2 and 6 A.M. This variation is termed circadian thermal rhythm. A consistent method of body temperature measurement should be used so that readings are comparable.

USING AN ELECTRONIC THERMOMETER

Equipment

Electronic thermometer unit with digital readout and probe
Disposable cover for thermometer
Lubricant on tissue (for rectal temperature)
Clean gloves

Procedure

1. Wash your hands and don gloves, if necessary.
2. Remove thermometer from charger unit.
3. Place carrying strap around your neck.
4. Grasp probe at top of stem using your thumb and forefinger. **Rationale:** Pressure on top releases the ejection button.
5. Firmly insert probe in disposable probe cover.
6. Provide privacy for rectal temperature.

for Oral Temperature

a. Instruct client to open mouth. Slide probe under front of client's tongue and along the gum line in the sublingual pocket. **Rationale:** The larger blood vessels in the pocket more accurately reflect the core temperature.

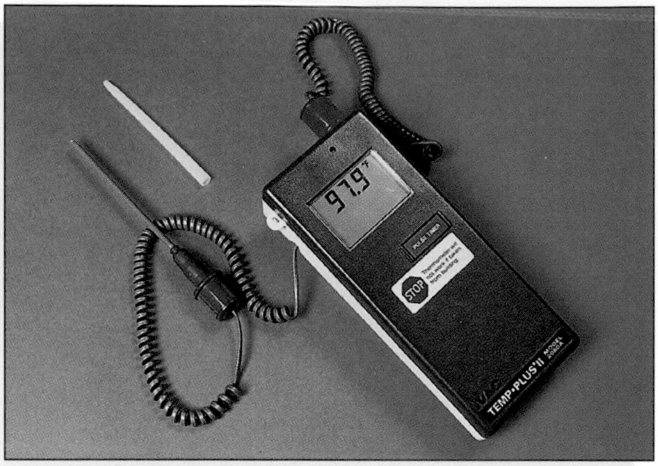

Electronic thermometer unit with digital probe.

b. Instruct client to close lips (not teeth). Lips should close at the ridge on the probe cover.

for Rectal Temperature

a. Don clean gloves. **Rationale:** Prevents exposure to feces.
b. Position client on side facing away from you, separate buttocks, instruct client to take in a deep breath, and insert covered and lubricated probe ¼ to 1½ inches (depending on client's age) through anal sphincter.

CLINICAL ALERT

The temperature of an unconscious client is never taken by mouth. The rectal or tympanic method is preferred.

Rationale: Taking in a deep breath relaxes the sphincter and the lubrication prevents tissue trauma.
c. Position probe to side of rectum to ensure contact with tissue wall. **Rationale:** This ensures probe is in contact with large vessels of rectal wall.

7. Remove probe when audible signal occurs. Client's temperature is now registered on the dial.
8. Discard oral probe cover into trash by pushing ejection button.
   a. Discard rectal probe cover, tissue, and gloves. **Rationale:** Proper disposal prevents transmission of microorganisms.
   b. Wipe anal area to remove lubricant and stool.
9. Assist client to comfortable position.
10. Wash your hands.
11. Record temperature, and then return probe to storage well. **Rationale:** This ensures that system is ready for next use.
12. Return thermometer unit to charging base. Ensure charging base is plugged into electric outlet.

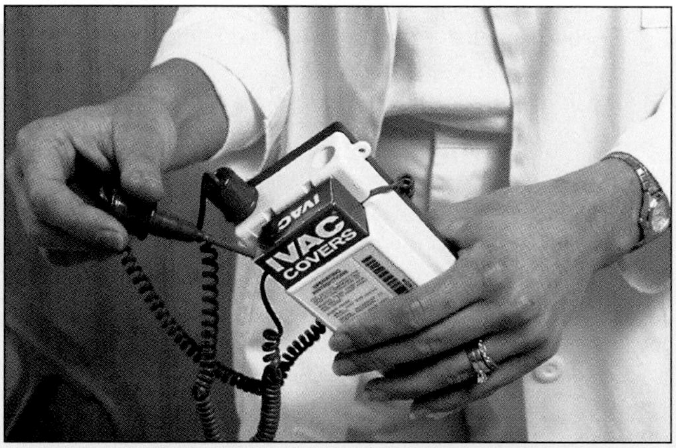

Cover probe of thermometer before taking temperature.

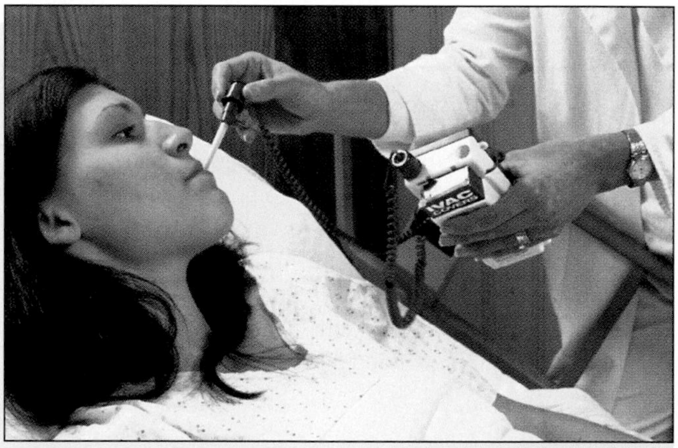
Slide probe under front of tongue to sublingual pocket.

MEASURING AN INFANT OR CHILD'S TEMPERATURE

Equipment

Digital or electronic thermometer with disposable probe cover
Water-soluble lubricant
Gloves, if necessary

Procedure

1. Determine appropriate thermometer and route for child. **Rationale:** Oral route is appropriate for child over 3 years of age and electronic, nonbreakable thermometer is preferred.
2. Wash hands.

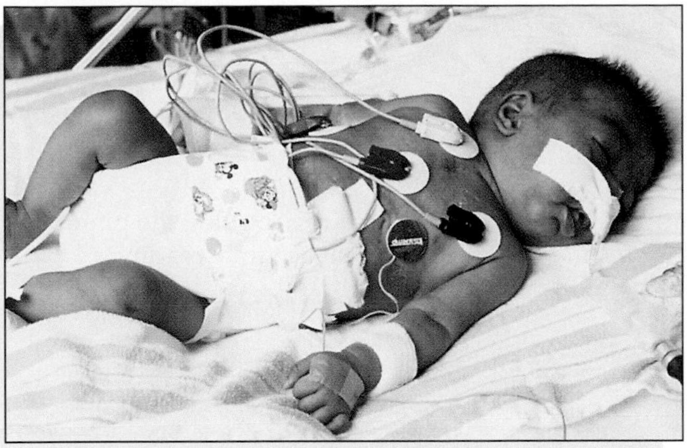

The axillary method is often used for children who are unconscious, have seizures, or have a structural abnormality.

3. Explain procedure at child's level of understanding.
4. Remove probe from cover or attach probe tip to electronic thermometer.

for Oral Route (only for child 3 years or older)

a. Place probe under child's tongue, one side or the other.
b. Have child close mouth and either hold thermometer in place or monitor while taking temperature.
c. Leave digital thermometer in place 45–90 seconds or remove electronic thermometer when audible signal occurs.

for Rectal Route

a. Place infant or child in prone or side-lying position.
b. Lubricate probe.
c. Insert thermometer ¼ to ½ inch into rectum for infant—½ to 1 inch for child, and hold in place.
d. Turn on scanner and follow directions.
e. Remove probe when tone or beep is heard.

for Axillary Route

a. Assist infant or child to a comfortable position and expose axilla.
b. Dry axilla if necessary. **Rationale:** A moist axillary area can produce a false low reading.
c. Place thermometer in center of axilla. Lower child's arm down and across the chest. **Rationale:** This position ensures that thermometer remains in contact with large vessels of axilla.
d. Leave in place 1–2 minutes or until tone is heard. **Rationale:** Axillary temperature recordings take longer to register than oral or rectal.

5. Read and record temperature, indicate method.
6. Discard probe cover into trash by pushing ejection button, or return digital thermometer into its case.

USING AN INFRARED THERMOMETER FOR TYMPANIC TEMPERATURE

Equipment

Infrared thermometer unit
Disposable probe cover

Procedure

1. Wash hands.
2. Attach disposable cover centering probe on film and press firmly until backing frame of probe cover engages base of probe. **Rationale:** Cover protects client from transmission of microorganisms.
3. Turn the client's head to one side and stabilize the client's head.
4. Pull pinna upward and backward for an adult or down and backward for a child. **Rationale:** This procedure provides better access to the ear canal.
5. Center probe and gently advance into ear canal to make a firm seal, directing probe toward tympanic membrane. **Rationale:** Pressure close to the tympanic membrane seals ear canal and allows for accurate reading.
6. Press and hold temperature switch until green light flashes and temperature reading displays (approximately 3 seconds). **Rationale:** Method records core body temperature.
7. Remove thermometer. Discard probe cover.
8. Return thermometer to home base or storage unit for recharge.

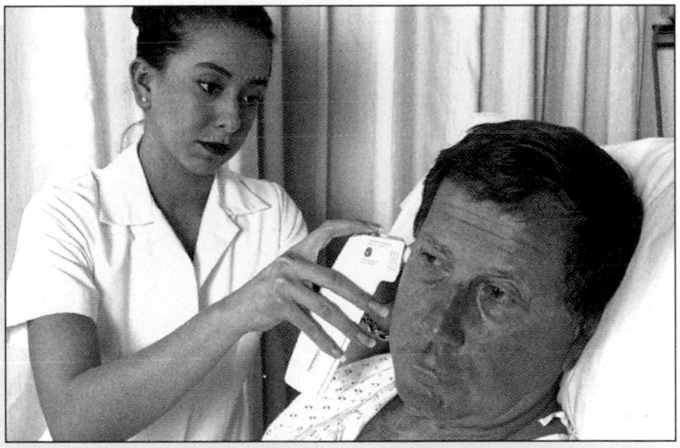

The tympanic route for taking a temperature is advised for clients over 3 months of age.

9. Keep lens clean using lint-free wipe or alcohol swab, then wipe dry. Do not use povidone-iodine (Betadine).
10. Wash hands.

CLINICAL ALERT

Do not use ear thermometer in infected or draining ear, or if adjacent lesion or incision exists.

Evidence Based Nursing Practice

Correct Technique for Taking a Tympanic Temperature

Studies on the correct technique for taking a tympanic temperature indicated that the ear tug (pulling the pinna upward and backward for an adult and down and backward for a child) is essential for an accurate reading. Eliminating this step will not allow the thermometer to be directly at the tympanic membrane.

Source: Best Practice, Vital Signs (1999), vol. 3, no. 3, p. 5. http://www.joannabriggs.edu.au.

USING A HEAT-SENSITIVE WEARABLE THERMOMETER

Equipment

Wearable thermometer (TraxIt), chemical strip tape or liquid crystal thermometer

Procedure

1. Check orders for continuous-reading thermometer.
2. Dry forehead or axilla area, if necessary.
3. Place strip on forehead or deep in client's axilla—may stay in place for 2 days.
4. Read correct temperature by checking color changes or dots that turn from green to black.
5. Record temperature on appropriate form or record.

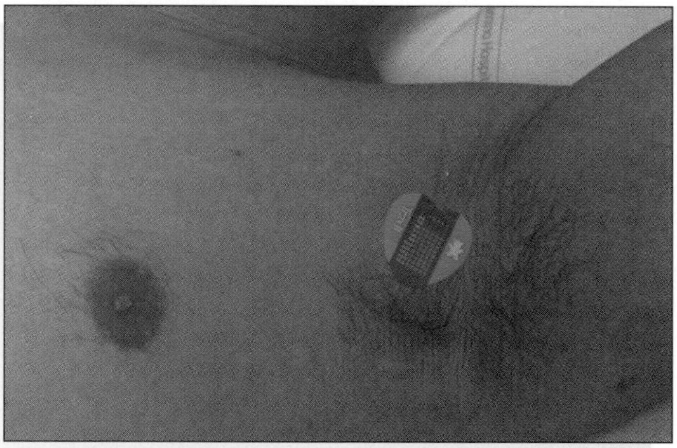

Place TraxIt®, a continuous-reading wearable thermometer, deep in client's axilla.

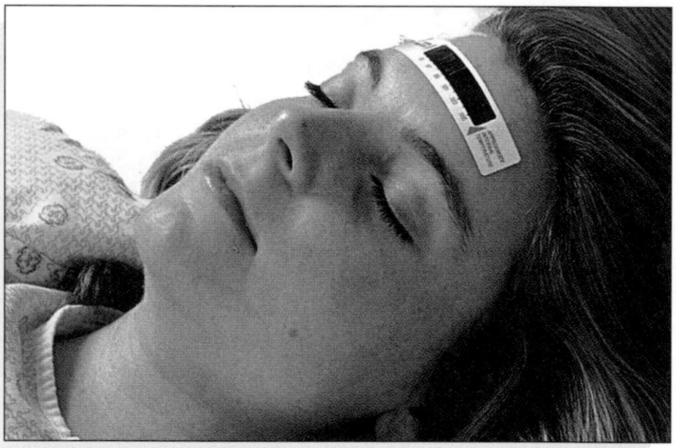

Liquid crystal thermometer is placed against lower forehead for 15 seconds.

Documentation for Temperature

- Site designated: "O" (oral), "R" (rectal), "A" (axillary), or "T" (tympanic)
- Temperature recorded on temp sheet and graph
- Nursing interventions used for alterations in temperature
- Condition of skin related to alterations from normothermia (e.g., diaphoresis)
- Signs and symptoms associated with alterations in temperature (e.g., shivering, dehydration)

Critical Thinking Application

UNEXPECTED OUTCOMES	CRITICAL THINKING OPTIONS
Fever develops.	• Check possible sources of infection, and take preventative measures. • Notify physician. • Employ cooling methods if temperature is dangerously high, such as tepid sponge bath, cool oral fluids, ice packs, or antipyretic drugs. • Assess all vital signs.
Despite initial cooling measure, temperature remains elevated due to hypothalamus damage from brain disease or injury.	• Notify physician, and request cooling blanket. • Monitor temperature every 15–30 minutes and record. • Continue to administer antipyretic drugs as ordered.
Temperature remains elevated because of bacterial-produced pyrogens.	• Check for order to obtain culture of possible sources of infection • Give antipyretic drugs as ordered. • Decrease room temperature and remove excess covers. • Give tepid sponge bath.
Temperature remains subnormal.	• Extreme low temperature can cause vasoconstriction; assess for blood clots. • Institute measures to promote vasodilation (application of warmth). • If extremity is ischemic, monitor that heat source does not exceed body temperature.

UNIT 2

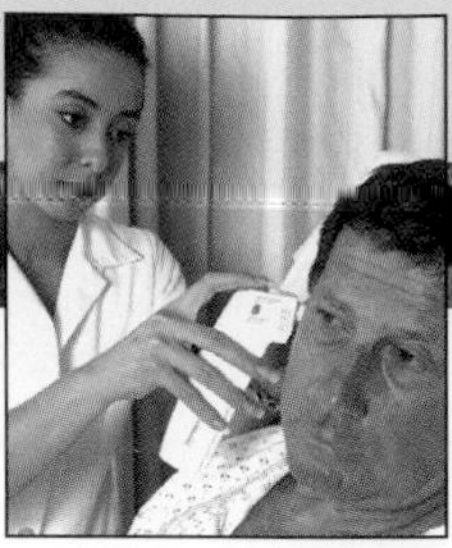

Pulse Rate

Nursing Process Data

ASSESSMENT Data Base

Assess appropriate site to obtain pulse.

Check pulse with health status changes, as ordered by physician, or before administering certain medications.

Assess for rate, rhythm, volume, and quality.

Assess an apical pulse on clients with irregular rhythms or those on cardiac medications.

Obtain baseline peripheral pulses with initial assessment or in any client going for cardiac or vascular surgery. Also obtain pulse for medical clients with diabetes, arterial occlusive diseases, atherosclerosis, or aneurysm, or any color or temperature changes in the periphery.

Obtain an apical–radial pulse when deficits occur between apical and radial measurements.

Assess the need to monitor pulses with an ultrasound or electronic device.

PLANNING Objectives

To determine if the pulse rate is within normal range and if the rhythm is regular

To evaluate the quality (amount of blood pumped through peripheral arteries) of arterial pulses

To determine if peripheral pulses are equal in amplitude when compared to corresponding pulses

To determine presence of peripheral pulses with ultrasound device when palpation is ineffective

To monitor and evaluate changes in the client's health status

To determine apical pulse rate before heart medications are administered

IMPLEMENTATION Procedures

Determining a Radial Pulse

Taking an Apical Pulse

Taking an Apical–Radial Pulse

Palpating a Peripheral Pulse

Monitoring Peripheral Pulses with Doppler Ultrasound Stethoscope

EVALUATION Expected Outcomes

Pulse is palpated without difficulty.

Pulse rate is within normal range and rhythm is regular.

All peripheral pulses are equal in amplitude when compared to the corresponding pulse on the other side and when compared to the next proximal site.

Apical pulse is easily detected and counted.

DETERMINING A RADIAL PULSE

Equipment

Watch with sweep second hand or digital watch

Procedure

1. Wash your hands.
2. Check client identaband and place client in comfortable position.
3. Ask about activity level within last 15 minutes. **Rationale:** Pulse rate increases with activity, then returns to preactivity rate.
4. Palpate arteries by using pads of the middle three fingers of your hand. **Rationale:** The nurse may feel own pulse if palpating with the thumb.
   a. Radial artery is usually used because it lies close to the skin surface and is easily accessible at the wrist.
   b. Press the artery against the bone or underlying firm surface to occlude vessel, and then gradually release pressure. **Rationale:** Too much pressure obliterates the pulse.
   c. Note quality (strength) of pulse. **Rationale:** Strength of the pulse is an indication of stroke volume.
   d. If pulse is difficult to palpate, try exerting more pressure on the most distal palpating finger. **Rationale:** This amplifies the pulse wave against the two more proximal palpating fingers.
5. Count pulse for 30 seconds, and multiply by two to obtain pulse rate. **Rationale:** This is sufficient time for rate determination if pulse rhythm is regular.
6. Count radial pulse for at least 1 minute if rhythm is irregular or difficult to count. **Rationale:** It may take a minute or so to detect the irregularity. This method assists you to count the pulse more accurately.
7. Check to see that client is comfortable.
8. Wash your hands.
9. Record pulse rate, rhythm, and strength (volume).

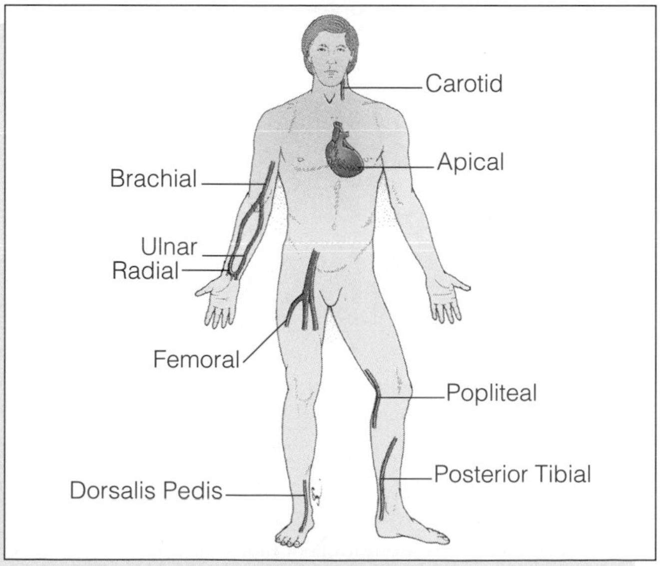

Radial artery is the most commonly used site for determining pulse rate.

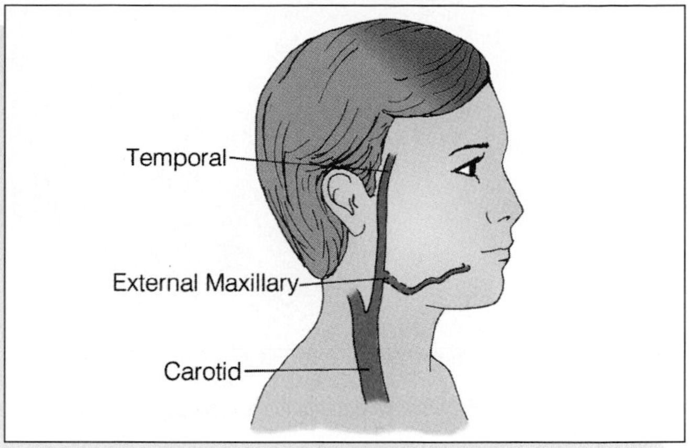

Carotid artery is used when other sites are inaccessible.

TABLE 10–3 Pulse Quality
Pulse quality is determined by the amount of blood pumped through the peripheral arteries. The amount of pumped blood usually remains fairly constant; when it varies, it is also indicative of cardiac malfunction.
• **Bounding pulse:** Occurs when the nurse is able to feel the pulse by exerting only a slight pressure over the artery. May occur with increased stroke volume.
• **Weak or thready pulse:** Occurs if, by exerting firm pressure, the nurse cannot clearly determine the flow. May be associated with decreased stroke volume.
• **Pulsus alternans:** A regular pulse that the nurse feels as strong alternating with weak beats. May be related to left ventricular failure.
• **Bigeminal pulse:** Every second beat has a decreased amplitude. May be due to premature contractions.

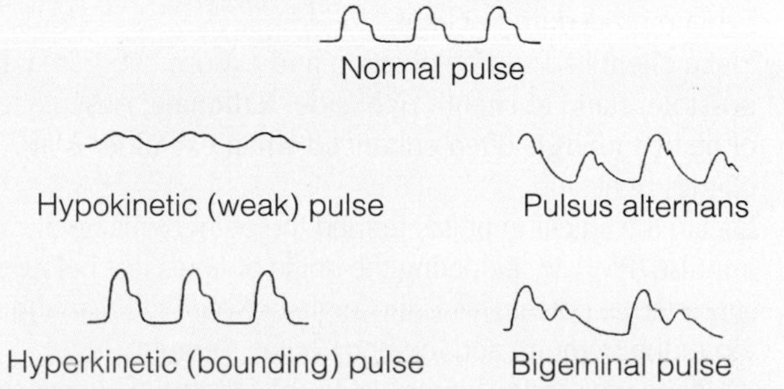

Source: LeMone, P., and Burke, K. M. *Medical–Surgical Nursing: Critical Thinking in Clinical Care* (2nd ed.). Upper Saddle River, NJ: Prentice Hall Health, 2000, p. 1186.

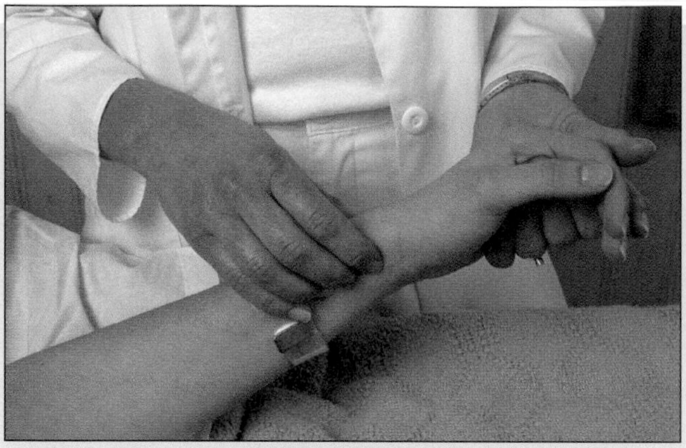

Palpate radial pulse by using pads of middle three fingers, not thumb, for accurate results.

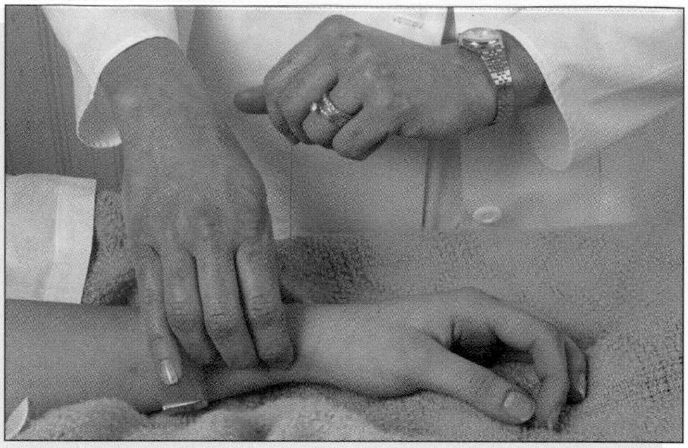

Count pulse for at least 30 seconds and multiply by two to obtain pulse rate.

EVIDENCE BASED NURSING PRACTICE

Pulse Rate Measurement

Studies have indicated that the accuracy of pulse rate measurement is influenced by the number of counted seconds (counting the pulse for 60 seconds is more accurate than 15 or 30 seconds). However, clinical significance of the result is not clear, so length of count period may be of limited significance.

Source: Best Practice, Vital Signs (1999), vol. 3, no. 3, p. 2. http://www.joanna-briggs.edu.au.

TAKING AN APICAL PULSE

Equipment

Watch with sweep second hand
Stethoscope

Procedure

1. Gather equipment.
2. Wash your hands.
3. Check client's identaband. Provide privacy.
4. Explain procedure to client.
5. Place client in a supine position and expose chest area. If possible, stand at client's right side. **Rationale:** Ausculation of heart sounds is often enhanced when examiner is at client's right side.
6. Locate the apical impulse, termed the point of maximal impulse (PMI), by palpating the angle of Louis just below the suprasternal notch. This is the angle between the manubrium, top of the sternum, and the body of the sternum.
   a. Place your index finger just to the left of the client's sternum, and palpate the second intercostal space.
   b. Place your middle finger in the third intercostal space, and continue palpating downward until you locate the apical impulse at the fifth intercostal space.

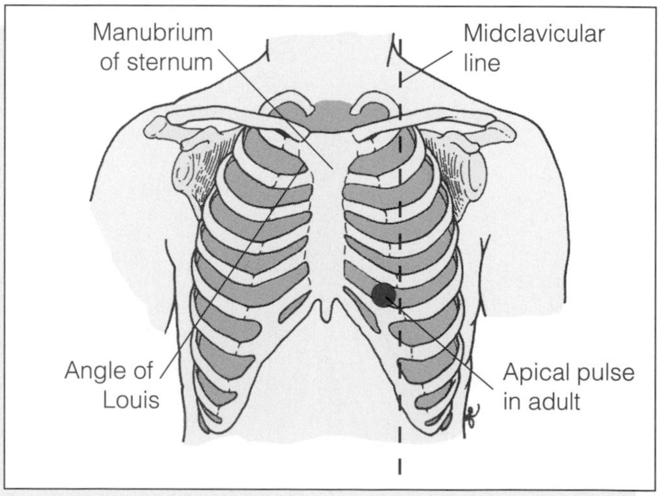

Apical pulse site in adult.

   c. Move your index finger laterally along the fifth intercostal space to the midclavicular line (MCL).
7. Warm the stethoscope in the palm of your hand for 5–10 seconds. **Rationale:** Warming the stethoscope prevents startling the client.

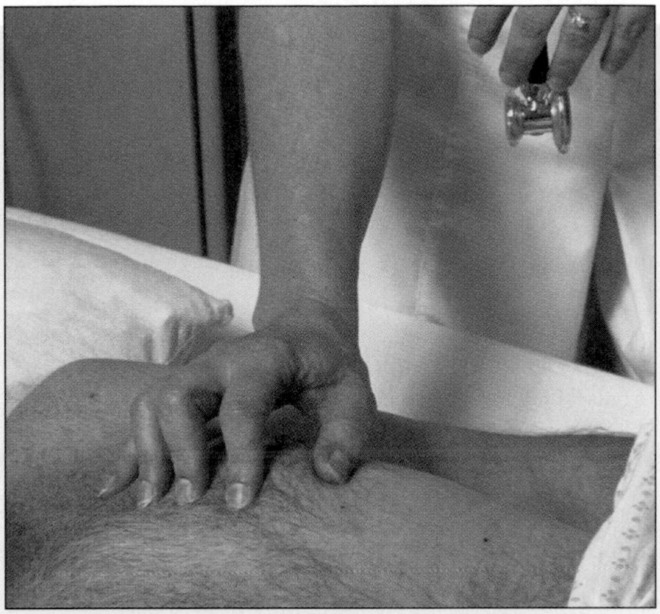

Place middle finger in third intercostal space and continue to move downward to fifth intercostal space.

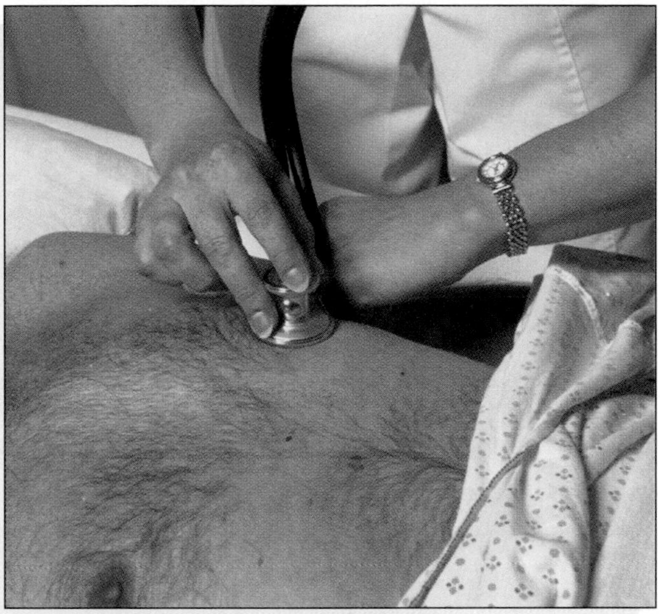

Accurate apical pulse is found in fifth intercostal space, left of sternum at midclavicular line, or at Erb's point.

8. Count client's apical pulse.
   a. Place diaphragm of stethoscope firmly over apical impulse site. **Rationale:** Heart sounds are high pitched and most clearly heard with diaphragm of stethoscope.
   b. Count the rate for 1 minute when taking an apical pulse. Count lub-dub sound as one beat. **Rationale:** More accurate readings are obtained over 1 minute, especially if pulse is irregular.
   c. Determine if there is a regular pattern to any irregularity or if it is chaotically irregular. **Rationale:** This finding helps describe the rhythm disturbance.
9. Check to see that client is comfortable.
10. Wash your hands and clean stethoscope, if necessary.
11. Record apical pulse rate, rhythm, and intensity.

TAKING AN APICAL–RADIAL PULSE

Equipment

Watch with sweep secondhand
Stethoscope
Another nurse to assist with procedure

Note: An experienced nurse may be able to assess apical and radial rates simultaneously without an assistant.

Procedure

1. Gather equipment.
2. Wash your hands.
3. Check client's identaband.
4. Provide privacy.
5. Explain procedure to client especially if two nurses are taking the pulse. **Rationale:** Clients may be apprehensive when two nurses are at the bedside, so a full explanation helps allay fears.
6. Assist client to a supine position and expose chest area.
7. Place watch where clearly visible to both nurses. **Rationale:** Both nurses count pulse rates within the same time span, preferably using one watch.
8. Warm stethoscope in palm of your hand. **Rationale:** Prevents startling the client with cold stethoscope.
9. Locate radial pulse. The second nurse locates apical pulse at the fifth intercostal space left of sternum at the midclavicular line, and firmly places diaphragm of stethoscope on the site. **Rationale:** Firm application helps transmit high-pitched heart sounds.
10. With assistant, select number on watch to start counting pulse (e.g., 12:00).
11. Signal to the other nurse with your hand when to start taking the pulse and when to stop. Both nurses simultaneously count pulse for 1 full minute.
12. Auscultate the apical pulse and palpate the radial pulse simultaneously (preferably using two nurses, one at each site).

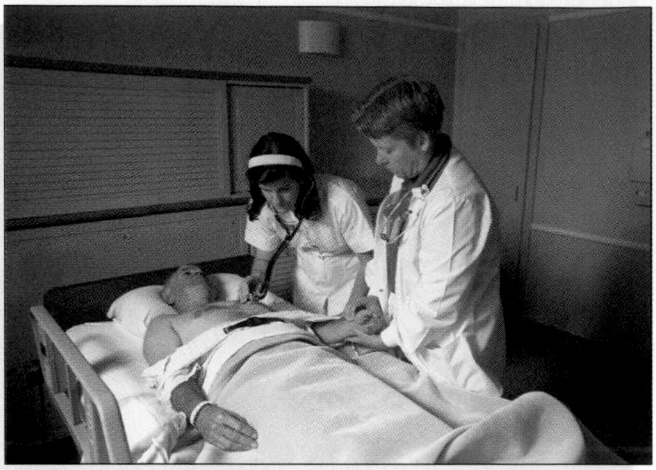

Second-nurse locates apical pulse at the fifth intercostal space and midclavicular line.

a. Note a pulse deficit when rhythm is irregular. **Rationale:** Atrial dysrhythmias and premature ventricular beats generally produce pulse deficits (apical greater than radial rate). A pulse deficit results from the ejection of a volume of blood that is too small to initiate a peripheral pulse wave.
b. If a significant pulse depicit is found, assess for other abnormal signs (BP).
c. Assess pulse volume by feeling the pressure of the beat. The quality is described as normal, weak, strong, or bounding.

13. Subtract radial rate from apical rate to obtain pulse deficit. **Rationale:** The pulse deficit represents the number of ineffective or nonperfused heartbeats.
14. Position client for comfort.
15. Wash your hands.
16. Chart apical and radial rate and pulse deficit.

PALPATING A PERIPHERAL PULSE

Equipment

Felt-tipped pen
Watch with second hand

Procedure

1. Gather equipment.
2. Wash your hands.
3. Check client's identaband.
4. Provide privacy. Explain procedure.
5. Place client in a supine position with relaxed legs.
6. Palpate peripheral pulses: radial, carotid (when other sites are inaccessible), brachial, femoral, popliteal, dorsalis pedis, posterior tibial. (For special cases, after carotid surgery, palpate temporal pulse also.)
7. Compare pulse sites bilaterally by palpating with pads of the middle three fingers of your hand.
8. Press artery against the bone or underlying firm structure to occlude vessel and then gradually release pressure.
9. Palpate weak pulses gently. **Rationale:** Too much pressure obliterates a weak pulse.

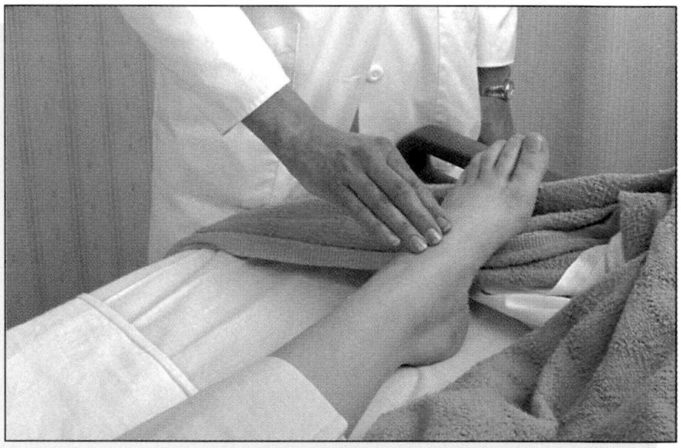

Apply firm pressure against underlying structure, then release to find peripheral pulse.

10. Assess if bilateral pulses are equal in amplitude (strength).
    a. If pulse is not immediately palpable, examine adjacent area. **Rationale:** This action identifies where interruption or alteration in circulation occurs in an extremity.
    b. Since pulse locations differ, mark pulse locations with felt-tipped pen, especially when they are difficult to palpate. **Rationale:** Marking site allows the next nurse to find location without spending extra time.

Characteristics of Peripheral Pulses

0 = Absent
1+ = Weak
2+ = Diminished
3+ = Strong
4+ = Full and bounding

CLINICAL ALERT

If palpating the carotid pulse, avoid pressing on the carotid sinus in the upper neck area near the jaw. *Do not* palpate both carotids simultaneously because this decreases blood flow to the brain.

c. Compare presence and characteristic of peripheral pulses with previous findings. **Rationale:** This action allows early identification of alterations in peripheral circulation.

11. Check to see that client is comfortable.
12. Wash your hands.
13. Record pulse rate, rhythm, pattern, and volume.

MONITORING PERIPHERAL PULSES WITH DOPPLER ULTRASOUND STETHOSCOPE

Equipment

Doppler ultrasound stethoscope or probe
Conductive jelly (not K-Y)

Procedure

1. Gather equipment.
2. Wash your hands.
3. Check client's identaband and explain procedure to client.
4. Provide privacy.
5. Uncover extremity to be assessed.
6. Place extremity in a comfortable position.
7. Plug headset (stethoscope) into one of the two outlet jacks located next to the volume control. If not using stethoscope, plug probe into monitor.
8. Apply conductive gel to client's skin. **Rationale:** The ultrasound beam travels best through gel and requires an airtight seal between the probe and the skin.
9. Hold probe (at tapered end of plastic core) against skin at a 90° angle to the blood vessel being examined.
10. Turn on Doppler by pressing down the "ON."
11. Move probe over site if pulse is not detected. Keep it in direct contact with skin, and adjust volume to detect blood

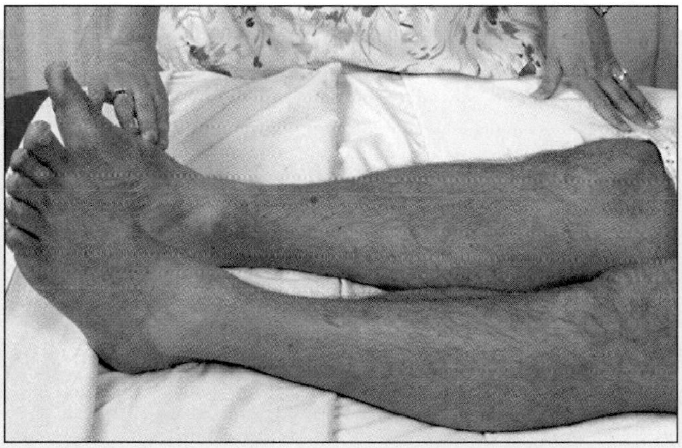

Try to find peripheral pulse with fingers before applying gel.

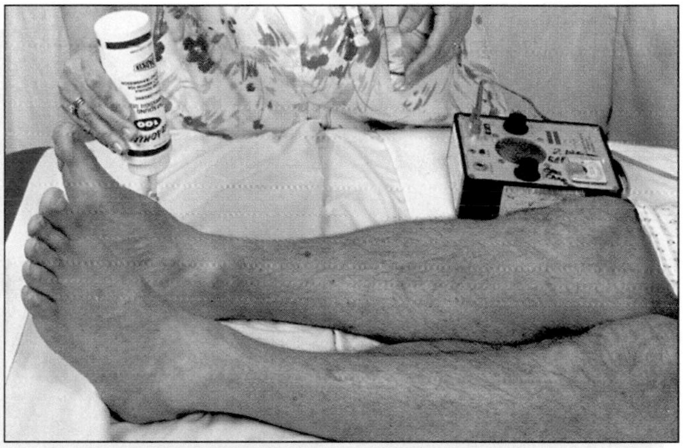

Apply gel to skin to facilitate beam transmission.

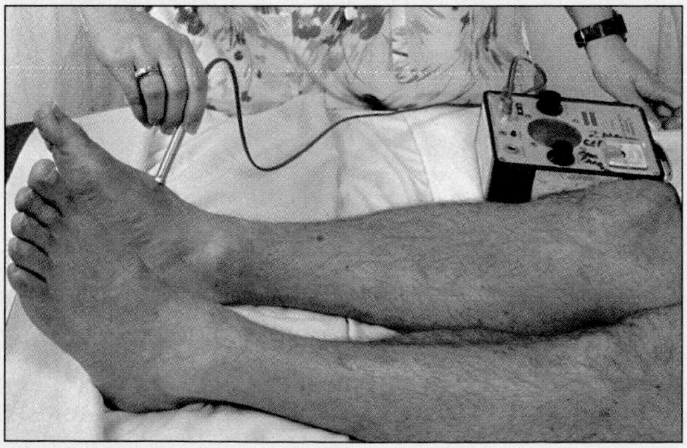

Hold probe against skin at 90° angle.

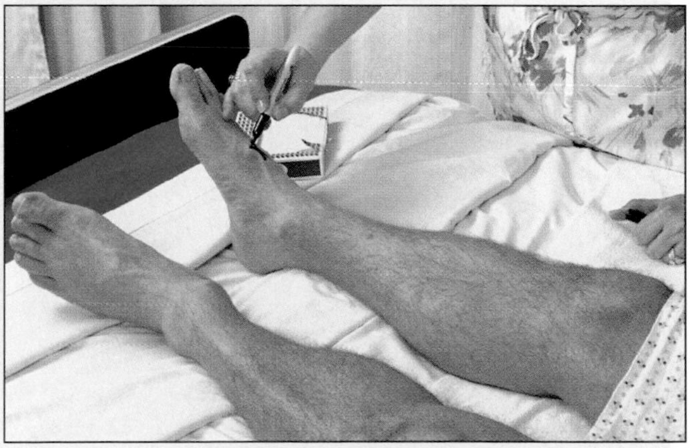

Mark site where pulsations were heard.

flow. **Rationale:** This action should facilitate detection of whooshing pulse sounds.
12. Reapply new gel if pulse is still not detected and, with light pressure, place probe over site and turn switch ON. Increase volume control, or check if batteries are weak.
13. Mark site where pulsations were heard. **Rationale:** This facilitates future assessments.
14. Clean gel from skin and Doppler probe. Replace cover over extremity.
15. Position client for comfort.
16. Replace Doppler equipment to appropriate location.
17. Wash your hands.

Documentation for Taking a Pulse

- Type of pulse taken
- Rate, rhythm, intensity, and quality of pulse
- Pulse deficit if any present
- Characteristics of all peripheral pulses—use rating scale
- Use of Doppler stethoscope if needed
- Effects of nursing or medical treatments on abnormal pulse rates or rhythms

Critical Thinking Application

UNEXPECTED OUTCOMES	CRITICAL THINKING OPTIONS
Apical, femoral, and carotid pulse is absent.	• *Note:* For all unexpected outcomes assess all vital signs and status of the client. • Immediately call a Code. • Initiate CPR immediately, and continue to assess the femoral or carotid pulse during resuscitation. • For absent femoral pulse, assess for systemic circulation and presence of disorders affecting circulation to extremities. • Use Doppler stethoscope to assess for presence of pulse.
Abnormal heart beats are present.	• Relieve anxiety, fear, or stress through communication and pertinent information. • If client has pain, relieve with change of position, back rub, and analgesic.
Tachycardia (pulse rate over 100 BPM in adults or 140 in children):	• Decrease heart rate by reducing an elevated temperature to normal. • Take vital signs every 15 minutes to 2 hours until condition stabilizes and pulse rate is within normal limits. • Determine significance of pulse rate as it affects blood pressure, sensorium, and client comfort. • Notify physician if persistent tachycardia continues or if there is a change in blood pressure. • Determine if tachycardia is normal for this client.

UNEXPECTED OUTCOMES	CRITICAL THINKING OPTIONS
Bradycardia (pulse rate less than 60 in adults or less than 70 in children):	• Notify physician for electrocardiogram request to determine if heart block is present. • If client is on digitalis, hold the drug, or on beta blockers or other medications, notify physician. • Have atropine and temporary pacemaker available for physician if pulse is consistently slow (less than 50) and client is not an athelete (who may well have a pulse less than 50). • Continue monitoring pulse rate every 15 minutes to 2 hours until pulse is within normal limits.
Ectopic Beats (premature ventricular or atrial contractions)	• Relieve pain if irregularity is due to premature beats associated with pain. • Administer oxygen if client has an order to do so. • If associated with stimuli from noise, visitors, caffeinated beverages, or smoking, eliminate the cause of the stimulation. • Notify physician to request a medical order for an electrocardiogram since premature beats in a client with myocardial infarction may be potentially harmful. • Obtain order from physician to draw serum electrolytes, especially magnesium or potassium. Low levels can cause ectopic beats. • Continue monitoring pulse rate every 15 minutes to 2 hours until irregularity is controlled.
Peripheral pulse is absent.	• Assess for other signs and symptoms of circulatory impairment.
Loss of peripheral pulse.	• Use a Doppler ultrasound and stethoscope to find pulse and report to physician.
Doppler stethoscope unable to detect sounds.	• Check that conductive jelly is used because salt from K-Y Jelly can damage the probe. • Check that batteries are less than 6 months old. The date should be indicated on all batteries. • Use alkaline batteries; they last longer. • Check that abnormal pressure is not applied, as this obliterates pulse.
Client is in isolation and requires vascular assessment.	• Clean with gas sterilization after discontinuing use of Doppler stethoscope. • Do not clean with alcohol or autoclave.

UNIT 3

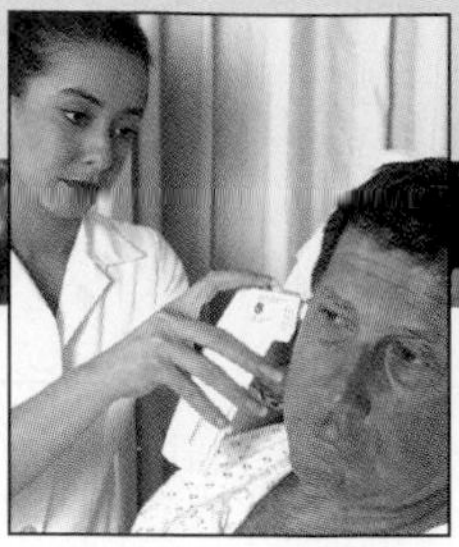

Respirations

Nursing Process Data

ASSESSMENT ***Data Base***

Assess client's respiratory rate, depth, and rhythm.

Evaluate any abnormalities noted during inspection and palpation or by percussion and auscultation.

Assess presence of dyspnea or cyanosis.

Assess for presence of abnormal sounds, such as stertorous or sonorous breathing.

Assess if accessory muscles are used for breathing.

PLANNING ***Objectives***

To note respiratory rate, rhythm, and depth

To establish baseline information on admission to the unit

To note labored, difficult, or noisy respirations or cyanosis

To identify alterations in respiratory pattern resulting from disease condition

To compare if respiratory rate is within normal range with pulse and blood pressure readings

IMPLEMENTATION ***Procedures***

Obtaining the Respiratory Rate

EVALUATION ***Expected Outcomes***

Regular rate of breathing and symmetrical respiratory excursion is established.

Client exhibits quiet, effortless breathing.

OBTAINING THE RESPIRATORY RATE

Equipment

Watch with a second hand

Procedure

1. Wash your hands.
2. Check clients identaband and explain procedure to client.
3. Check lighting to ensure it is adequate for procedure.
4. Maintain client's privacy.
5. Place hand on chest or observe chest rise and fall and count respirations.
6. Note relationship of inspiration to expiration. Note also depth and effort of breathing.

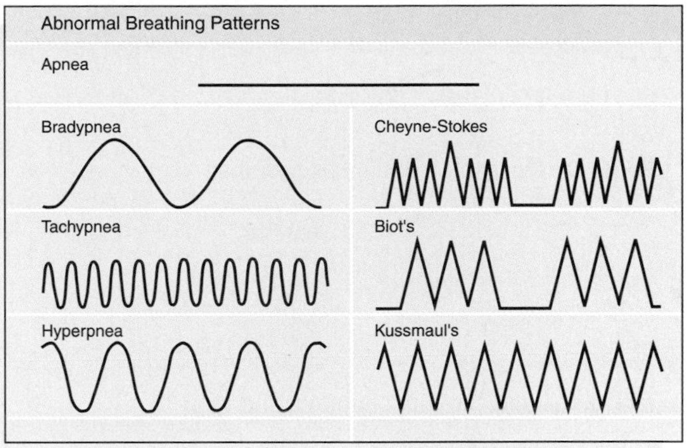

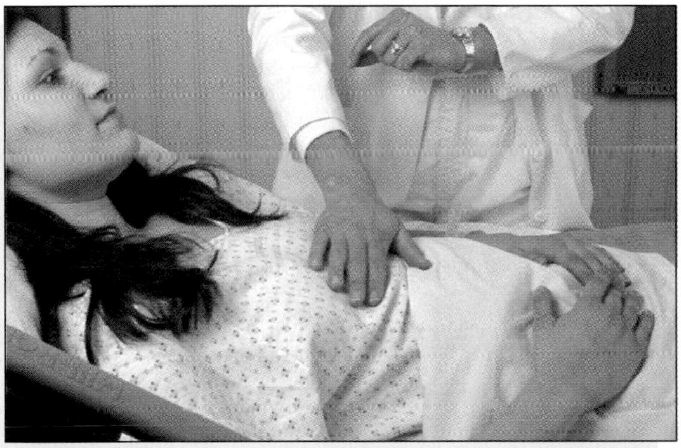
Place hand on chest when respirations are difficult to count.

7. Count respirations for preferably one minute, or for 30 seconds and multiply by 2. **Rationale:** One full minute is more accurate for abnormal breathing patterns.
8. Wash your hands.
9. Compare respiratory rate with previous recordings.
10. Record respiratory rate. Record if rhythm or depth altered from normal.

Normal Respiratory Rate

Adults: 12–20 per minute

Young children: 20–25 per minute

Infants: Up to 40 per minute

EVIDENCE BASED NURSING PRACTICE

Accuracy in Counting Respirations

One study found that counting respirations for 15 seconds versus a full minute produced a significant difference in the rate; thus, the conclusion is that respirations should be counted for a full minute.

Source: *Best Practice*, Vital Signs (1999), vol. 3, no. 3, p. 2. http://joannabriggs.edu.au.

DOCUMENTATION FOR RESPIRATION

- Rate, depth, and rhythm of respirations
- Abnormal sounds associated with breathing
- Effectiveness of therapy if needed to correct respiratory problems
- Ratio of inspiration and expiration
- Alterations from baseline respiratory patterns

Critical Thinking Application

UNEXPECTED OUTCOMES	CRITICAL THINKING OPTIONS
Apnea (absence of breathing) occurs, may be intermittent.	• *Note:* For all unexpected outcomes, assess client for all vital signs and comfort/condition. • Begin artificial ventilation by mouth-to-mask, mouth-to-nose, or other airway adjunct method at the rate of 12 per minute for an adult or 20 per minute for a child. • Summon help immediately; call a Code.
Tachypnea (rate faster than normal and more shallow >24) occurs.	• Relieve anxiety, fear, and stress through communication and pertinent information. • Relieve fever if that is the cause. • Correct respiratory insufficiency with low-flow oxygen administration, good pulmonary toilet, and deep breathing and coughing exercises.
Bradypnea (rate slower than normal <10) occurs.	• If due to respiratory depressant drugs, such as opiates, barbiturates, and tranquilizers, be prepared to assist respirations or administer mouth-to-mask resuscitation. • Administer oxygen at 4–6 L/min via nasal cannulae as ordered. If client has COPD use 2 L/min. • Stimulate client to take breaths at least 10 times per minute.
Hyperpnea (increased depth of respiration) occurs.	• Rest after period of exertion. • Relieve fear, anxiety, or stress. • May be indicative of respiratory compensation for metabolic acidotic state (Kussmaul pattern).
Cheyne–Stokes respirations (respiratory cycle in which respirations increase in rate and depth, then decrease, followed by a period of apnea) occur.	• Follow physician's orders to treat underlying disease state (e.g., heart failure, increased intracranial pressure). • Monitor respirations every 15 minutes to hourly, depending on client's status. • Be prepared to administer CPR if apnea occurs. • Evaluate cause—one of the indicators that death is approaching.
Biot's (irregular pattern—slow and deep or rapid and shallow, followed by apnea) respirations occur.	• Assess for central nervous system (CNS) abnormalities (increased intracranial pressure, meningitis).
Kussmaul's (deep and gasping breaths—more than 20 breaths/minute) respirations occur.	• Follow orders to treat for renal failure, septic shock, or diabetic ketoacidosis.

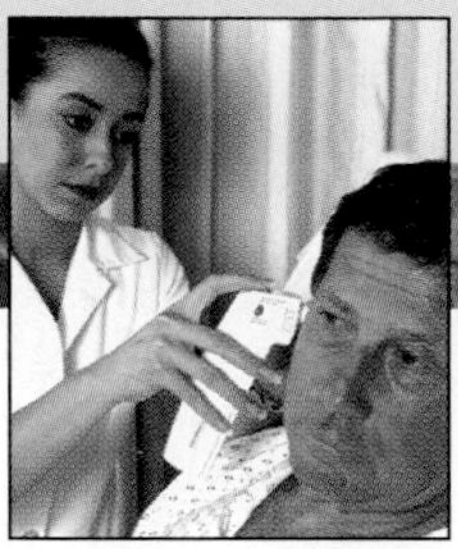

Blood Pressure

Nursing Process Data

ASSESSMENT ***Data Base***

Assess blood pressure initially and whenever client's status changes.

Assess size of cuff needed for accurate reading.

Assess the beginning and disappearance of Korotkoff's sounds during a blood pressure reading.

Assess presence of factors that can alter blood pressure readings.

Note any changes from prior assessments.

PLANNING ***Objectives***

To determine if arterial blood pressure reading is within normal range for the individual client

To assess condition of heart, arteries, blood vessel resistance, and stroke volume

To establish a baseline for further evaluation

To identify alterations in blood pressure resulting from a change in disease condition

To correlate blood pressure readings with pulse and respirations

IMPLEMENTATION ***Procedures***

Measuring a Blood Pressure

Palpating Systolic Arterial Blood Pressure

Measuring Lower Extremity Blood Pressure

Measuring Blood Pressure by Flush Method in Small Infant

Using a Continuous Noninvasive Monitoring Device

EVALUATION ***Expected Outcomes***

Blood pressure is within normal to high normal range (systolic: 100–140; diastolic: 60–85 mmHg).

Alterations in blood pressure are identified early and appropriate treatment initiated.

Severely altered blood pressure readings are rechecked with different equipment or validated by another nurse.

Unstable blood pressure readings are monitored frequently for trend recognition.

MEASURING A BLOOD PRESSURE

Equipment

Sphygmomanometer with proper size cuff
Stethoscope

Procedure

1. Gather equipment. Clean stethoscope prior to use. Be sure the cuff is an appropriate size for the client. **Rationale:** A cuff that is too narrow results in erroneously high readings; a cuff too large may result in false low readings.
2. Provide quiet environment.
3. Wash your hands.
4. Check client's identaband.
5. Explain procedure to client. If client is a child, take blood pressure after the other vital signs. **Rationale:** This intervention may upset the child and affect pulse and respirations.
6. Place client in relaxed reclining or sitting position. **Rationale:** Blood pressure should be the same in either position.
7. Prepare client for blood pressure reading.
   a. Assess if client has smoked or exercised within last 15 minutes. Prepare client for blood pressure reading.
   b. Allow client to rest several minutes before beginning a reading.
   c. Client should be instructed not to cross legs or talk during the procedure. **Rationale:** Client activities and a slouched position yield false high readings.
8. Expose upper part of client's arm and position it with palm upward, arm slightly flexed with the whole arm supported at heart level. **Rationale:** If arm is below level of heart, the blood pressure reading is higher than normal, and if above the heart, is lower than normal.
9. Choose appropriate size cuff and wrap totally deflated cuff snugly and smoothly around upper part of arm (lower border of cuff 1 inch above antecubital space) with center of cuff bladder over brachial artery (pressure dial at zero).
10. Locate and palpate brachial artery with fingertips (medial aspect of antecubital fossa).
11. Position stethoscope ear pieces in ears. The ear pieces should tilt slightly forward. **Rationale:** Sounds are heard more clearly.
12. Ensure stethoscope hangs freely from ears. **Rationale:** Rubbing of stethoscope against an object can cause artifact and inaccurate readings.
13. Close valve on sphygmomanometer pump.
14. Inflate cuff rapidly (while palpating radial artery) to a level 30 points mm Hg above level at which radial pulsations are no longer felt. **Rationale:** This level ensures that cuff is inflated to a pressure exceeding the client's systolic pressure. Slow inflation can yield gaps in pressure readings.
15. Note level and rapidly deflate, waiting 60 seconds. **Rationale:** This is enough time for venous congestion to decrease.
16. Place bell (or diaphragm) of stethoscope lightly on the medial antecubital fossa where brachial artery pulsations are located and rapidly inflate cuff to 30 points/mm Hg above point where radial pulse disappeared. **Rationale:** This pressure ensures that cuff is inflated to exceed client's systolic pressure.
17. Deflate cuff gradually at a constant rate by opening valve on pump (2–4 points mm Hg/second) until the first Korotkoff's sound is heard. This is the systolic pressure, or phase I, of Korotkoff's sounds. **Rationale:** Slower or faster deflation yields false readings.

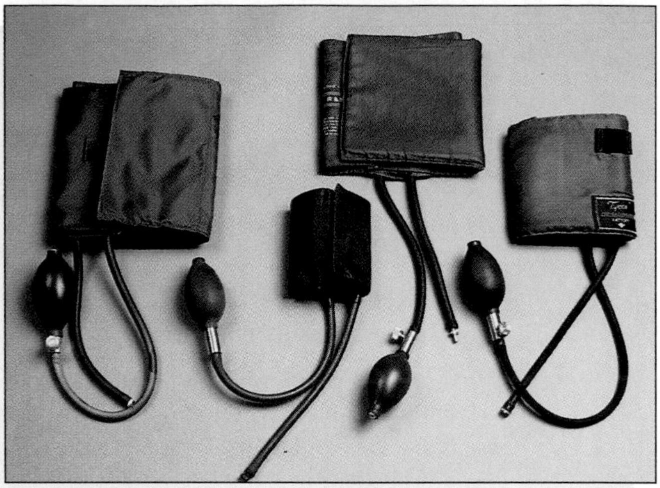
Blood pressure cuffs are available in various sizes.

Blood Pressure Cuff Sizes

- Standard (12–14 cm wide) for the average adult arm.
- Narrower cuff for infant, child, or adult with thin arms.
- For children (younger than 13 years) the bladder should be large enough to encircle the arm completely (100%).
- Wider cuff (18–22 cm) for client with obese arms or thigh pressure readings.

The cuff's inflatable bladder width should be 40% of the circumference of the limb on which it is used. The length of the bladder should be twice its width.

CLINICAL ALERT

When a client moves from recumbent to standing position, systolic pressure can fall 10–15 points mm Hg and diastolic may rise by 5 points mm Hg.

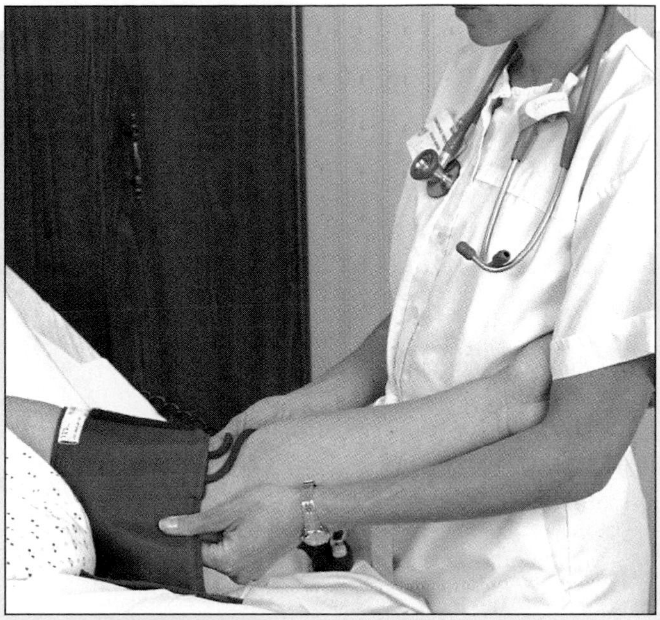
Wrap blood pressure cuff snugly around upper arm.

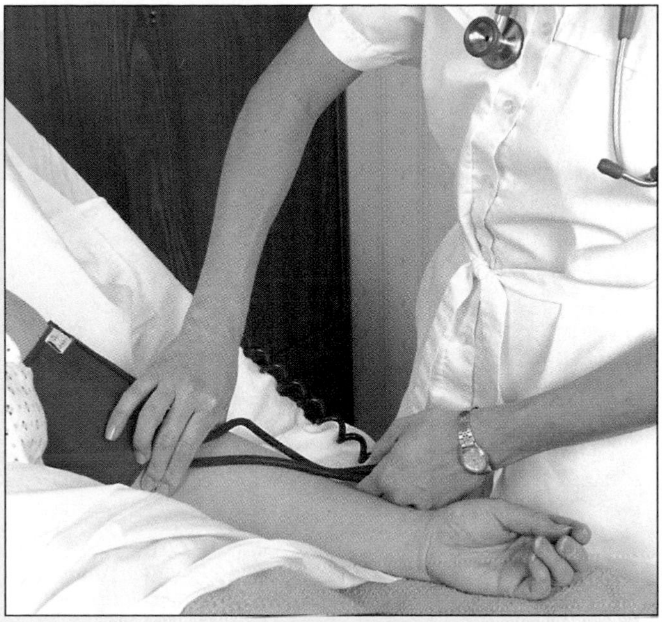
Palpate brachial artery on medial antecubital fossa.

18. Read pressure on manometer at eye level. **Rationale:** This ensures accurate reading.

CLINICAL ALERT

The American Heart Association recommends routine use of the *bell* of the stethoscope for blood pressure (Korotkoff's sounds) auscultation.

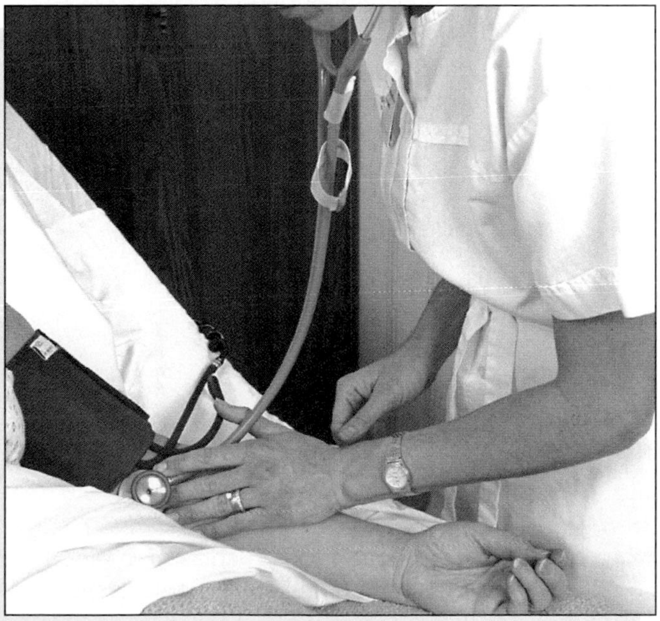
Place stethoscope on medial antecubital fossa.

19. Continue to deflate cuff at a rate of 2–4 points mm Hg/second. Do not reinflate without letting cuff totally deflate. **Rationale:** Reinflating cuff results in erroneously high readings.
20. Note point at which Korotkoff's sounds begin (phase I), and when they disappear completely (phase V). Disappearance of sounds (phase V) is regarded by the American Heart Association as the best index of diastolic blood pressure in individuals over age 13. If the child is younger than 12 years, the best indication of diastolic pressure is the distinct muffling of sounds at phase IV.

Note: Some facilities require that all five phases be recorded.

21. Do not leave cuff inflated for a prolonged period. **Rationale:** Leaving cuff inflated produces client discomfort.
22. Deflate cuff completely and wait at least 1–2 minutes before rechecking the blood pressure. **Rationale:** This allows time for blood vessels to return to normal.

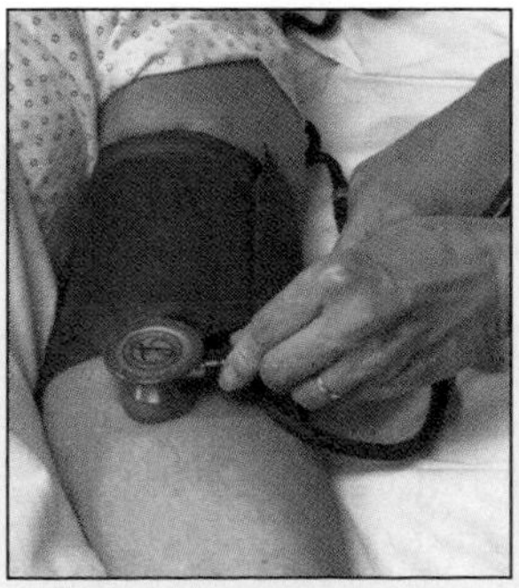
Bell of stethoscope.

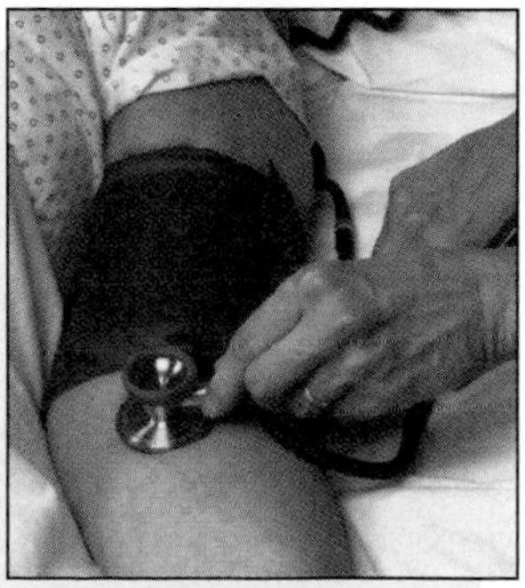
Diaphragm of stethoscope

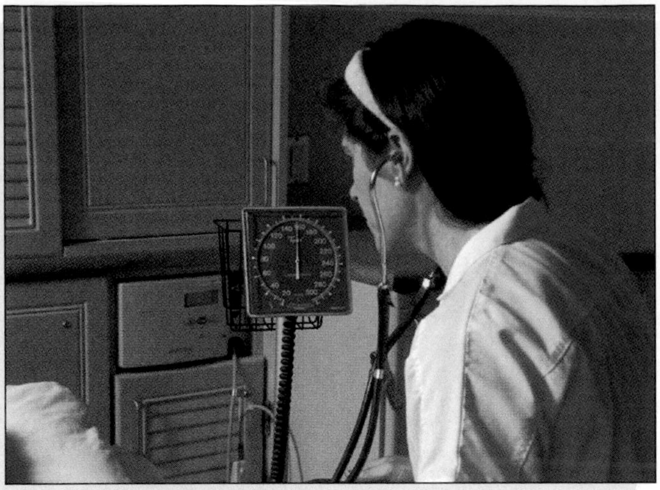
Read manometer at eye level.

Note: Check level of comfort of client and level of consciousness (as well as other vital signs) when evaluating blood pressure reading. If all signs and symptoms don't correlate, reevaluate blood pressure.

CLINICAL ALERT

Routinely, blood pressure for an acutely ill client should be taken every 1–2 hours and blood pressure for more stabilized clients should be taken every 4–8 hours. Clients with severe hypotension or hypertension, with low blood volume, or on vasoconstrictor or vasodilator drugs may require checking every 15 minutes.

23. Remove cuff from client's arm.
24. Check that client is comfortable.
25. Compare blood pressure reading with previous recordings.
26. Wash your hands.
27. Record blood pressure readings using two phases: 120/80 where 120 is the systolic (phase I) and 80 is the diastolic (phase V) pressure; or three phases: 130/110/80 where 130 is the systolic (phase I), 110 is the first diastolic (phase IV), and 80 is the second diastolic (phase V) pressure.
28. Repeat this procedure on the opposite arm if this is an initial reading.

EVIDENCE BASED NURSING PRACTICE

Stethoscope Accuracy in Measuring Blood Pressure

Studies indicate that when measuring the blood pressure, accuracy is much higher when using the bell (rather than the diaphragm) of the stethoscope.

Source: Best Practice, Vital Signs (1999), vol. 3, no. 3, p. 3. http://www.joannabriggs.edu.au.

EVIDENCE BASED NURSING PRACTICE

Body Position Influence on Blood Pressure

When the client's arm was placed above or below the level of the heart, BP changed by as much as 20 points mm Hg. Therefore, it is recommended that clients sit with their arm supported horizontally at heart level.

Studies showed that when hypertensive clients crossed their legs while having their BP taken, the systolic readings rose by 9.45 points mm Hg and the diastolic rose by 3.7 points mm Hg. Clients should have their feet on the floor during a BP measurement.

Sources: Best Practice, Vital Signs (1999), vol. 3, no. 3, p. 3. http://www.joannabriggs.edu.au. Fitzpatrick, F., Ortiz, L., et al. (1999). *Nursing Research 48* (2), 105.

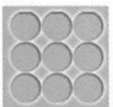

CULTURAL COMPETENCE

Many cultures believe that certain substances protect one's health. For example, Italians, Greeks, and Native Americans believe that garlic or onions eaten raw or worn on the body will prevent an illness such as high blood pressure. If a client wishes to include these items in his or her diet or wear them, the nursing staff should respect this practice, since it is an important cultural tradition for many groups.

PALPATING SYSTOLIC ARTERIAL BLOOD PRESSURE

Equipment

Sphygmomanometer with proper size cuff

Procedure

1. Gather equipment. Check that cuff is appropriate size for client. **Rationale:** A cuff that is too narrow results in erroneously high readings.
2. Wash your hands.
3. Check client's identaband.
4. Explain procedure to client.

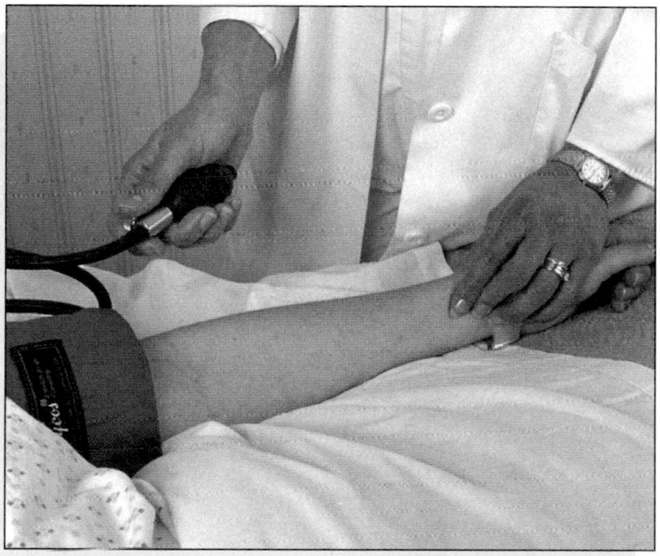

Palpate radial artery while inflating cuff and releasing pressure.

5. Place client in relaxed position, and support arm at heart level.
6. Wrap cuff snugly and smoothly around the upper part of the arm (1 inch above antecubital space) with center of bladder over brachial artery.
7. Keep pressure level in cuff at zero.
8. Locate radial artery pulsations on cuffed arm.
9. Inflate cuff rapidly (while palpating radial artery), to a level 30 points mm Hg above level at which radial artery pulsations are no longer felt. **Rationale:** This level ensures that cuff is inflated to a pressure exceeding client's systolic pressure.
10. Continue to palpate artery and release pressure from cuff slowly (2–3 points mm Hg/second). The first palpated beat is the systolic pressure. This should be the same point at which the last pulsation was felt during inflation of cuff.
11. Remove cuff and return equipment.
12. Wash your hands.
13. Record systolic blood pressure reading as "palpated systolic pressure."

CLINICAL ALERT

- Avoid measuring blood pressure in an arm with extensive axillary node dissection (e.g., radical mastectomy) or an arteriovenous fistula (e.g., for dialysis).
- Ultrasound techniques such as using a Doppler stethoscope can be used to measure systolic blood pressure when auscultatory sounds are too faint to be heard.

MEASURING LOWER-EXTREMITY BLOOD PRESSURE

Equipment

Stethoscope

Sphygmomanometer with standard or large-size cuff

Procedure

1. Gather equipment.
2. Wash your hands.
3. Check client's identaband.
4. Explain procedure to client.
5. Wrap cuff snugly and smoothly around lower leg with cuff's distal edge at the malleolus.
6. Locate either the dorsalis pedis or posterior tibial artery pulsations.
7. Inflate cuff rapidly while palpating foot artery, to a level 30 points mm Hg above level at which artery pulsations are no longer felt.
8. Place bell (or diaphragm) of stethoscope quickly on pulse site.
9. Deflate cuff slowly (2–4 points mm Hg/second) while auscultating sounds over the selected artery.
10. Remove cuff and return equipment.
11. Check to see that client is comfortable.
12. Record readings for first (systolic) and last (diastolic) sounds, noting site and client position.

for Alternative Methods

13. Measure blood pressure in thigh by using a large cuff with bladder placed over posterior mid thigh and bottom edge

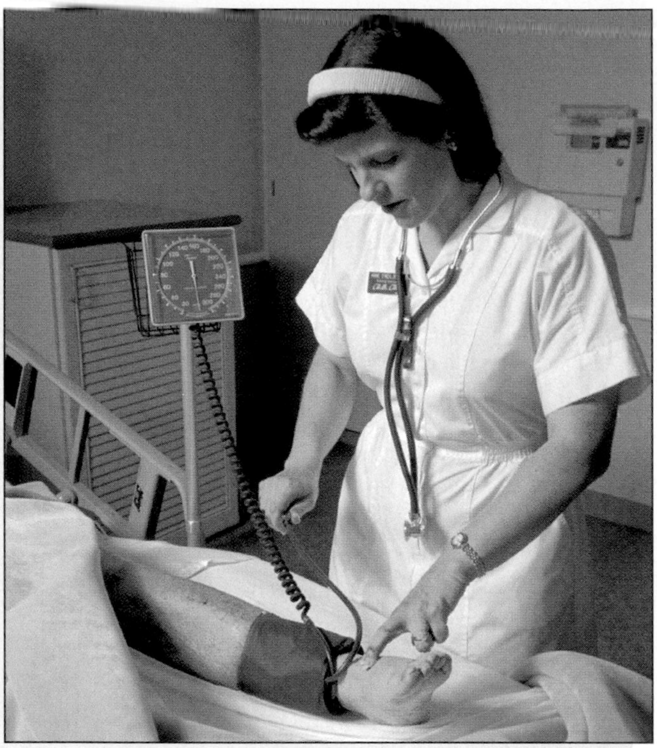
Wrap cuff snugly around lower leg and locate dorsalis pedis.

above knee. **Rationale:** The cuff bladder must be directly over the posterior popliteal artery for accurate reading. Listen with stethoscope at popliteal fossa with client in prone position, or supine with knee flexed enough for stethoscope placement.

Note: The systolic pressure is 20 to 30 points mm Hg higher than in the brachial artery. The diastolic pressure is the same.

14. Measure blood pressure in forearm by placing appropriate size cuff around forearm 13 cm from elbow; listen for Korotkoff's sounds over radial artery at wrist.
15. Compare blood pressures measured indirectly in the arm, leg, and thigh to reveal similar values. Measurements may be difficult to obtain in clients with peripheral vascular disease.

CLINICAL ALERT

Traditionally, vital signs provided the basis for assessing the need for and adequacy of sedation in critically ill clients. If the client is on drug therapy, vital signs may not always be a reliable indicator of sedation, because they do not directly reflect the level of consciousness.

MEASURING BLOOD PRESSURE BY FLUSH METHOD IN SMALL INFANT

Equipment

Sphygmomanometer with appropriate cuff
Elastic bandage
Assistant for observing flush
Well-lighted room

Procedure

1. Gather equipment.
2. Wash your hands.
3. Check client's identaband.
4. Wrap blood pressure cuff snuggly and smoothly just above wrist or ankle.
5. Elevate extremity above heart level.
6. Wrap elastic bandage firmly around exposed hand or foot. **Rationale:** Bandage compression empties the veins.
7. Lower extremity to heart level when compression is complete.
8. Inflate cuff rapidly to 200 points mm Hg.
9. Remove elastic bandage.
10. Deflate cuff slowly (not exceeding 5 points mm Hg/second).
11. Instruct assistant to watch for appearance of flush in the extremity distal to cuff. **Rationale:** An assistant is necessary so that pressure at which flush appears can be precisely noted. This reading more clearly reflects the *mean* blood pressure than the systolic pressure.
12. Document that blood pressure was taken by flush method.

CLINICAL ALERT

Flush pressures are taken on small infants or on adults when unable to auscultate or palpate blood pressure readings.

USING A CONTINUOUS NONINVASIVE MONITORING DEVICE

Equipment

Blood pressure cuff
Display monitor
Readout paper for monitor

Procedure

1. Check clients identaband and wash hands.
2. Gather equipment. Select proper size blood pressure cuff. Attach the cuff to the air hose by firmly pushing the valve from the cuff into the air hose and twisting to secure fit.
3. Squeeze the air from the cuff.
4. Wrap the cuff securely around the extremity (usually the arm).
5. Turn power switch ON.
6. Position the extremity at the level of the heart. **Rationale:** If arm is below heart level, reading will be higher than normal.
7. Set arterial pressure alarm limits by pushing *Alarm* to ON and set both HIGH and LOW parameters by depressing the *Alarm* button until the parameters read out on the digital display. **Rationale:** The alarm parameters provide a safety factor by alerting the nurse when the readings exceed the parameters.
8. Test time cycles by turning wheel (found above alarm button) to 1 minute and check for cycling effects. Then, to set automatic cycle time, move the wheel to desired time increments.
9. Press *Start* button for approximately 4 seconds to activate printer for readout of blood pressure; press again to begin reading. Systolic, diastolic, mean arterial pressures, and heart rates can be monitored with this system.
10. Alternate extremities if device is used for a prolonged period of time.
11. Check position of cuff and skin under cuff frequently. **Rationale:** It is important to note bruises or skin trauma, and to check if position of cuff has changed.

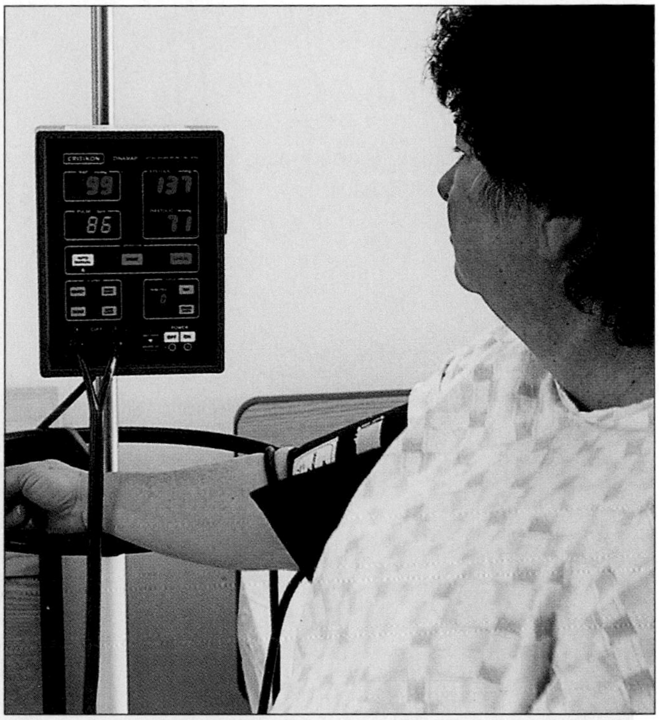

Continuous monitoring of blood pressure is done by attaching cuff to display monitor.

Blood Pressure Classification

Blood Pressure	Systolic	Diastolic
Normal	<120	<80
Pre HBP	120 to 139	80 to 89
Stage I HBP	140 to 159	90 to 99
Stage II HBP	160 and higher	100 and higher

Source: National Heart, Lung and Blood Institute, 2003, May.

DOCUMENTATION FOR BLOOD PRESSURE

- Two phases of Korotkoff's sounds (e.g., 120/80) and site
- Three phases of Korotkoff's sounds (e.g., 130/110/80) and site
- Response to alternative nursing actions
- Response to position changes

Critical Thinking Application

UNEXPECTED OUTCOMES	CRITICAL THINKING OPTIONS
Blood pressure reading is abnormally high without apparent physiologic cause.	• Check if arm was unsupported • Check if cuff was too narrow. • Check if cuff was not snug. • Check if cuff was deflated too slowly or reinflated during deflation causing venous engorgement and abnormally high diastolic readings. • Ask if client has pain, was anxious (white coat syndrome), or had just exercised, eaten, or smoked. Recheck pressure as indicated. • Check blood pressure on both arms. The normal difference from arm to arm is usually no more than 5 points mm Hg. • Check if insufficient rest before assessment.
Blood pressure reading is very low and there are no significant clinical indicators.	• Assess if cuff is too wide. • Check if client's arm was above heart level. • Check if inflation was too slow. This reduces intensity of Korotkoff's sounds. • Assess if Korotkoff's sounds were barely audible. Raise client's arm, and then recheck. Sounds should be louder. • Identify if stethoscope was misplaced and was not on brachial artery. • Take blood pressure 3 minutes after client rises from supine to standing if postural hypotension is suspected.
Hypotension (systolic pressure less than 90 mm Hg) develops.	• Take all vital signs more frequently (every 15 minutes to 2 hours) until condition has stabilized. • Place client in supine position with lower extremities elevated 45° and head on pillow. • Assess cause of hypotension, and notify physician. • Increase or administer fluids as ordered by physician. • Observe postoperative clients for signs of bleeding. • Administer oxygen.
Blood pressure cannot be measured on upper extremity due to casts or other causes of inaccessibility.	• Use lower extremity to obtain blood pressures. Systolic pressure in thigh is usually 20–30 points mm Hg higher than in arms, but diastolic pressure is equivalent to arm readings.
Korotkoff's sounds cannot be heard due to hypotension.	• Use the palpation method or ultrasound technique. Client may be candidate for intraarterial (direct method) pressure monitoring.
Hypertension (blood pressure consistently over 140/90, mm Hg) develops.	• For clients with severe, acute hypertension, take vital signs more frequently (every 15 minutes to 2 hours) until condition has stabilized. • Notify physician • If client is anxious or excited, institute relaxation techniques to lower blood pressure. • Allow client to rest after strenuous exercise.

UNEXPECTED OUTCOMES	CRITICAL THINKING OPTIONS
	• Relieve pain with reassurance, change of position, and analgesia as ordered by physician. • For clients with essential hypertension, administer antihypertensive and diuretic drugs as ordered by the physician. Evaluate response by checking blood pressure in reclining, sitting, and standing position. Instruct client in diet therapy, such as low salt, low fat, and inclusion of vitamins and garlic.
Continuous BP monitoring system displays 00 instead of blood pressure reading. (00 indicates the unit is unable to determine parameters.)	• Check cuff placement and size to determine if appropriately placed.

GERONTOLOGIC CONSIDERATIONS

Cardiac status—changes

- Changes in cardiovascular status with aging are often insidious and may become apparent when system is stressed and there is increased demand for cardiac output (which may occur with illness and hospitalization). Nursing care assessment should focus on client's cardiovascular status, even when diagnosis does not include a cardiac condition.
- Blood pressure measurement should take age into account. If client has severe joint stiffness, pseudohypertension may be present. If this is suspected, raise the cuff pressure above the systolic blood pressure and, if the radial pulse remains palpable, the reading may show 10 to 15 points mm Hg in error.
- Postural hypotension is common in the elderly (positional drop of less than 20 points mm Hg); nurses should take note when helping a client out of bed. Hypertension is also common in this age group.
- A rise in blood pressure may be associated with reduced cardiac output, vasoconstriction, increased blood volume, or fluid overload.
- Pulse changes, particularly an irregular pulse, can be related to hypoxia, airway obstruction, or electrolyte imbalance.
- The arteries in elderly clients may feel stiff and knotty due to decreased elasticity. Excessive pressure to site when taking pulse may obliterate it. The normal rate is 60–90 beats per minute.
- If pulses are not palpated, the Doppler may need to be used.

Respiratory status—changes

- Changes in the respiratory system may be subtle and gradual with the elderly: oxygen saturation is decreased to 93%–94%; there is often poor cough response and incomplete lung expansion—all of which leads to increased risk of pulmonary infection when the elderly client is hospitalized.
- Slightly irregular breathing patterns are not unusual in the elderly.

Temperature—changes

- With the elderly, temperature may be as low as 95°F. Because they may be easily dehydrated with increased temperature, nursing assessment should include baseline temperature at admission and continued monitoring during hospitalization.
- Elderly who have acute infections may have a subnormal temperature.
- Increased temperatures can lead to increased metabolism, thus increasing the body's demand for oxygen. This causes the heart to work harder.
- Oral temperatures are the preferred method for obtaining the elderly client's temperature.

MANAGEMENT GUIDELINES

Each state legislates a Nurse Practice Act for RNs and LVN/LPNs. Health care facilities are responsible for establishing and implementing policies and procedures that conform to their state's regulations. Verify the regulations and role parameters for each health care worker in your facility.

Delegation of Responsibilities

- Taking vital signs for clients may be assigned to any health care worker provided they have been assessed for competency in the procedure. This includes LVN/LPN, CNA, UAP, and EMT.
- The registered nurse must identify parameters for which the health care worker is to notify the nurse; i.e., blood pressure above or below a certain reading, pulse rate, or irregular pulse.
- The nurse must provide detailed explanations and/or demonstrate alterations in the procedure or specific methods of obtaining the vital signs to CNA, UAP or EMTs.
- Obtaining peripheral pulses by use of the Doppler is the responsibility of the RN or LVN. A CNA or UAP is not responsible for using the Doppler.
- The CNA or UAP may monitor the blood pressure using the noninvasive monitoring device; however, the CNA or UAP is not responsible for initiating the procedure or setting the alarms.

Information Flow

- Directions must be given to health care workers on documentation procedures. Do they complete the graphic record, write the findings on a vital sign sheet at the nurses' desk, or give the results to the nurse?
- The registered nurse must evaluate all abnormal or changed vital signs identified by the health care workers. The nurse maintains total responsibility for client care even though someone else performs the task of taking the vital signs.
- The registered nurse must ensure that the health care workers know the parameters for reporting unusual vital signs. Periodic checks with the workers may be necessary.

CRITICAL THINKING STRATEGIES

SCENARIO 1

Mr. Trager (age 92) has been admitted to your unit with a temperature of 103°F, BP 140/90, P 114, and R 30 and labored. He reports a history of 3 days of diarrhea and fever, and asks you for something to drink.

1. From your analysis of the admission data, determine the following:
   a. Appropriate nursing diagnosis in priority for this client.
   b. The metabolic effects of fever on pulse and respiration.
   c. Age factors that contribute to the existing problem.
2. What are the other assessment findings indicative of the diagnosis established from primary admitting data?
3. Develop a plan of care for this client.
4. Describe the evaluative outcomes for problem resolution.

SCENARIO 2

Mr. Sondheim is admitted to the hospital with unstable hypertension for evaluation. He has a family history of hypertension and heart disease. The nurse will complete a physical exam and a history.

1. What information is missing in the family history that the nurse will want to elicit from the client?
2. Which questions regarding lifestyle would be appropriate to ask?
3. Which aspects of client teaching would the nurse want to cover before Mr. Sondheim is discharged?

CHAPTER 11

Physical Assessment

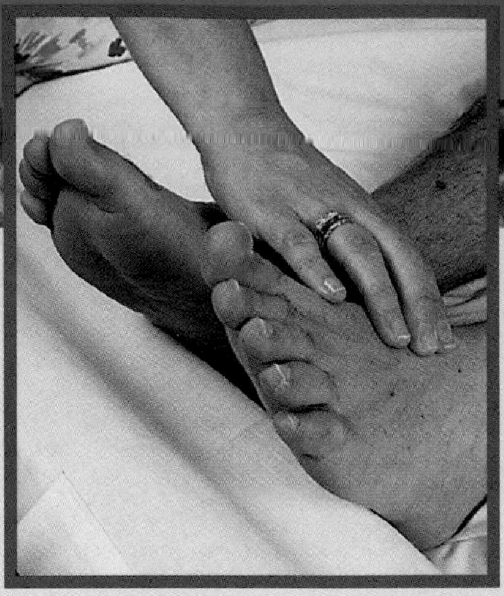

THEORETICAL CONCEPTS

Examination Techniques 274
Focus Assessment 275
Physical Assessment 276
Neurologic Assessment 276
Assessment of the Head and Neck 282
Assessment of the Skin 286
Assessment of the Chest: Lungs, Breasts, and Heart 288
Assessment of the Abdomen, Liver, and Genitourinary Tract 295
Mental Health Assessment 299
Mental Status Assessment 299

OBSTETRICAL ASSESSMENT 302

NEWBORN ASSESSMENT 308
Apgar Scoring 311

PEDIATRIC ASSESSMENT 311

GERONTOLOGIC CONSIDERATIONS 317

MANAGEMENT GUIDELINES 320

CRITICAL THINKING STRATEGIES 321

LEARNING OBJECTIVES

- Outline the essential elements obtained from a health history.
- List the four techniques of physical assessment.
- Demonstrate six steps of the focus assessment.
- Describe the abnormal manifestations associated with each specific body system for one client with whom you are familiar.
- List four normal responses that determine the client's level of consciousness.
- Describe four abnormal responses in pupil assessment.
- State three assessment components of the skin.
- Describe normal and abnormal lung sounds.
- Outline the steps of breast assessment.
- Identify the four areas for heart sound auscultation.
- List at least five essential elements included in a mental status assessment.
- Compare and contrast three elements of the antepartum obstetrical assessment.
- Relate the elements of a "9" score on the Apgar test.
- Describe basic components of a pediatric physical assessment.

ASSESSMENT

Basic assessment discussed in this chapter can be performed in less than 10 minutes using a stethoscope, penlight, reflex hammer, your hands, and observational skills. Although you may not be able to perform assessment rapidly at first, you will have many opportunities to practice your skills, because every client should be assessed at least once a shift.

While interviewing the client, note such characteristics as hair, skin, posture, facial expression, and body language—in other words, the general appearance of the client. Then proceed with a head-to-toe systems assessment using the four techniques of assessment: inspection, palpation, percussion, and auscultation. This IPPA sequence is used for all systems except for the abdominal assessment, which requires auscultation *before* palpation and percussion. Palpation and percussion are performed using fingers and hands to assess abnormalities of sound, such as vocal fremitus, enlarged organs, organ displacement, and chest expansion. Auscultation is accomplished by using a stethoscope to listen to breath, heart, and bowel sounds. Observe the client's response as each system is assessed.

Equipment

The stethoscope is the primary instrument used for assessment. Remember that any movement of the tubing or chest piece by clothing or hands can cause extraneous noise that obliterates the sounds you want to hear. The diaphragm piece should be applied firmly to the skin. It enhances high-pitched sounds (breath sounds, normal heart sounds, bowel sounds). The bell piece should be placed very lightly to pick up low-pitched sounds, such as vascular sounds and abnormal heart sounds. If the bell is pressed firmly, it stretches the skin and acts as a diaphragm. Other instruments used include the penlight, reflex hammer, ophthalmoscope, otoscope, and tuning fork.

HEALTH HISTORY

A total client assessment begins with a nursing health history. Using open-ended questions such as "tell me about . . .," collect data about past health conditions, current problems, and present needs. The information is obtained through objective (observed) and subjective (stated by client) data collection.

Information obtained from the interview and the physical assessment constitutes the basis for identifying nursing diagnoses and establishing the individualized client care plan. A complete health history includes the following elements:

- *Biographic information:* age, sex, educational level, marital status, living arrangements.
- *Chief complaint:* condition that brought client to health care facility; reason for visit; any recent changes.
- *Present health status or illness:* onset of the problem; clinical manifestations, including severity of symptoms; pain characteristics if present.
- *Health history:* general state of health, past illnesses, surgeries, hospitalizations, allergies, otc's, herbal supplements, current medications, and general habits such as smoking, alcohol consumption, or recreational drug use.
- *Family history:* age and health status of parents, siblings, and children; cause of death for immediate family members.
- *Psychosocial factors, lifestyles:* cultural beliefs that influence health management; religious or spiritual beliefs.
- *Nutrition:* dietary habits, preferences, or restrictions.
- *Domestic violence:* (JCAHO requirement).

NURSES' ROLE

The nurse's role in assessing the client and obtaining a health history has expanded dramatically over the last 40 years. Today nurses must be adequately instructed to perform a total assessment, as well as a focus assessment, including the use of instruments, formerly the domain of physicians only. The skill of performing a physical assessment must be practiced repeatedly to acquire expertise.

EXAMINATION TECHNIQUES

Inspection

Observe the client while facing him or her in the bed or chair. Observe the client's skin color and texture; check for lesions and hair distribution. Look at overall body structure. If the client can be out of bed, observe gate and stance. Note all parts of the body as the examination proceeds. Inspection also evaluates verbal and behavioral responses and mental status.

Palpation

Obtain information by using the hands and fingers to palpate. A light or deep palpation depends on the area being palpated. The palmer surface of fingers and finger pads are used to determine position of the organs, size and consistency, fluid accumulation, pain, and masses. The ulnar surface of the hand is used to distinguish vibration and temperature. The moisture and warmth of the skin can also be determined during palpation.

Percussion

Produces sound waves by using the fingers as a hammer. Place the interphalangeal joint of the middle finger on the skin surface of the nondominant hand. Using the tip of the middle finger of the dominant hand, strike the placed finger. Vibration is produced by the impact of the fingers striking against underlying tissue. Sound or tone of the vibration is determined by body area or organ percussed. Normal lung areas produce a resonance sound; liver sounds are dull and a flat sound is heard over muscle.

Auscultation

Place the stethoscope on the client's bare skin to listen for the presence and characteristics of sound waves. The bell of the stethoscope is used to detect low-pitched sounds; the diaphragm detects high-pitched sounds. Note variations in intensity, pitch, duration, and quality.

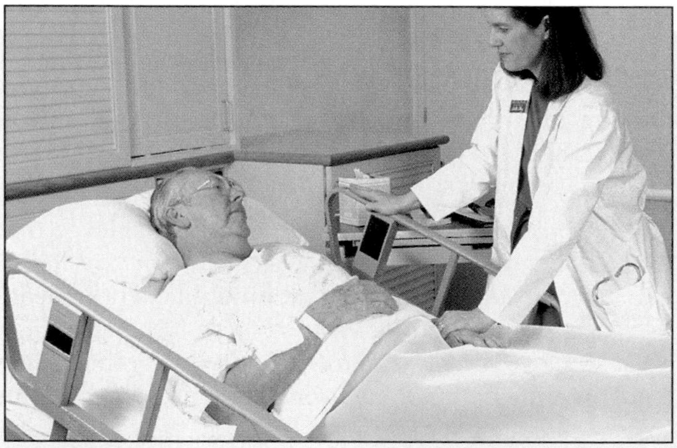

1 Inspection.

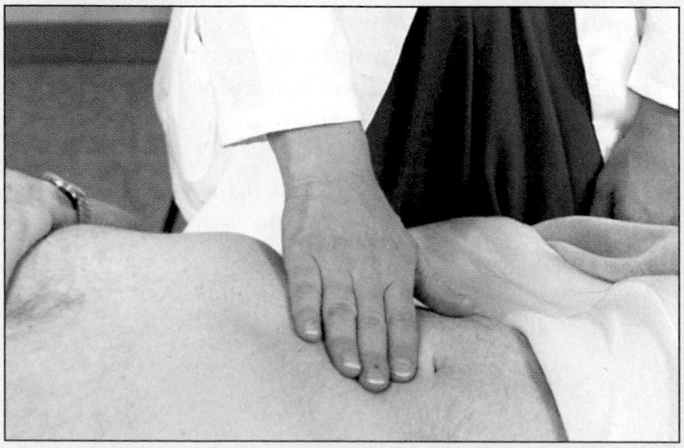

2 Palpation.

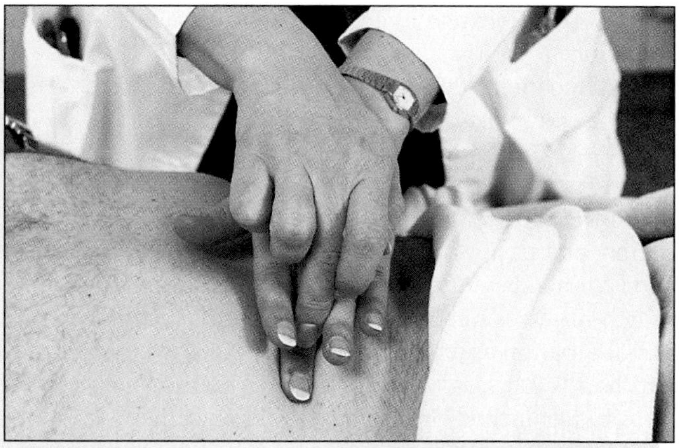

3 Percussion.

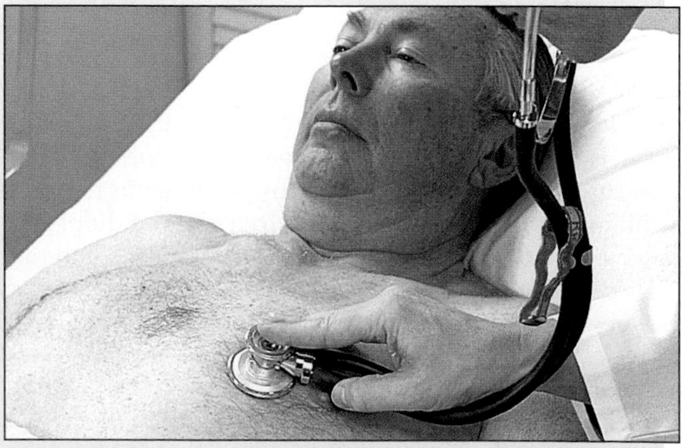

4 Auscultation.

FOCUS ASSESSMENT

A full physical assessment is completed upon admission. A focus assessment, also called a bedside or shift assessment, is performed at the beginning and ending of the shift and concentrates on the vital assessment parameters; tracks changes from shift to shift and should take no more than 5 minutes to complete. Several activities in the assessment can be completed at the same time. Usually, it is individualized to fit the client's condition, diagnosis, and level of acuity.

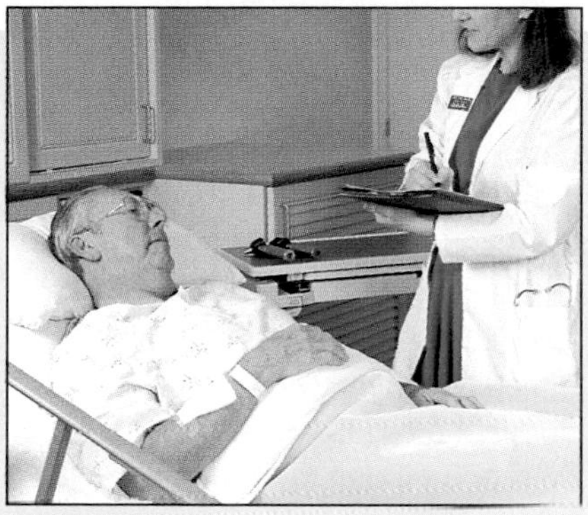

Step 1.

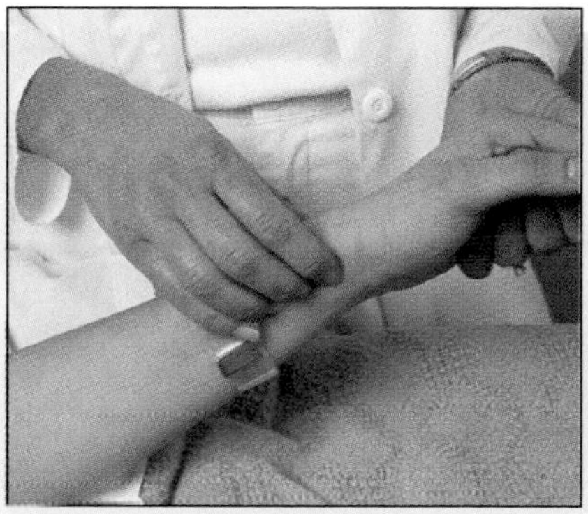

Step 2.

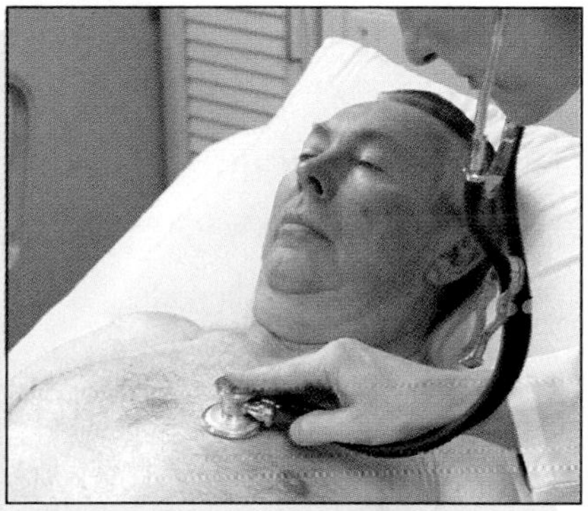

Step 3.

Step 1

Evaluate the client's level of consciousness, eye contact and responsiveness, color and texture of the skin, any IVs, dressings or tubes visible. Ask appropriate questions to determine orientation to time and place. Establish the nurse–client relationship at this time.

Step 2

Assess vital signs. While taking the client's pulse, feel skin temperature and moisture. Check bilateral radial pulses. Observe for edema in face or neck. Individualize the assessment; for example, with a neurological condition, check pupils.

Step 3

Remove client's gown or raise gown. Use stethoscope to listen to heart sounds, apical pulse and breath sounds bilaterally. Observe breathing patterns, symmetry of chest movement, shape of chest, and depth of respirations. Check for skin turgor.

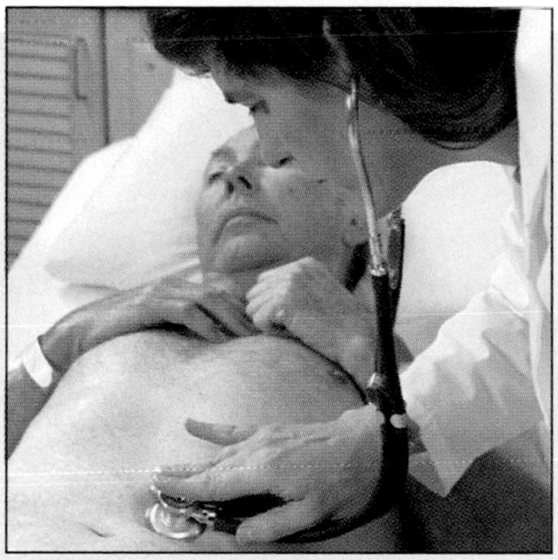

Step 4.

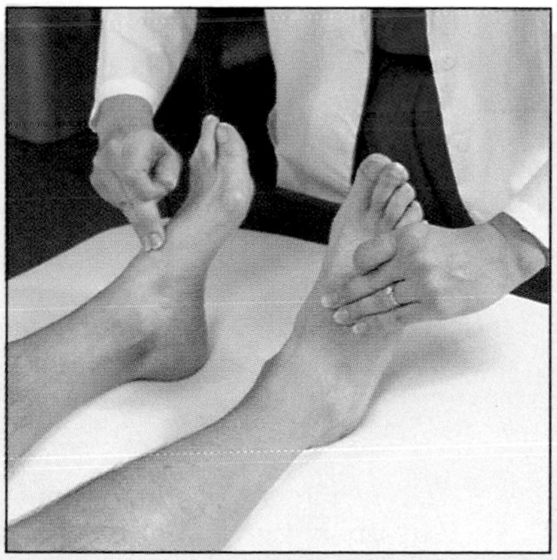

Step 5.

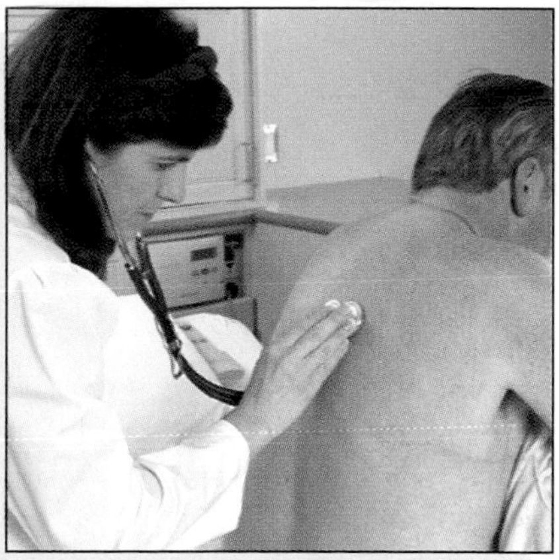

Step 6.

Step 4

Auscultate abdomen for bowel sounds. Use palpation and percussion techniques only if appropriate to diagnosis. Palpate bladder if necessary (based on output). If catheter is in place, observe urinary output for color, odor, consistency, and amount.

Step 5

Assess lower extremities for warmth, color, moisture, presence of pedal or popliteal pulses, muscle tone and sensation. Assess for pedal edema or general edema in the lower extremities. Check traction or casted areas for skin breakdown, alignment and placement.

Step 6

Have client turn onto side or sit at edge of bed. Assess posterior lung fields and symmetry of chest movement with inspiration. Assess skin for pressure areas, particularly coccyx and heels when client returns to side-lying position. Evaluate client's ability to move in bed.

PHYSICAL ASSESSMENT

Neurologic Assessment

The neurologic examination begins with the initial contact with the client. Evaluation of verbal responses, movement, and sensation is carried out throughout the examination. In addition, functions of the cerebrum, cerebellum, cranial nerves, spinal cord, and peripheral nerves are assessed. The level of consciousness is the most sensitive and reliable index of cerebral function.

Assessment	*Normal*	*Abnormal*
Level of Consciousness		
Evaluate **verbal responses** If client seems awake and alert but does not respond properly, check to see if client is blind, deaf, or speaks another language	Alert Mood appropriate to situation Responds to verbal command Answers questions appropriately Speaks clearly Oriented to time, person, place, and purpose Recent and remote memory intact	Drowsy Difficult to awaken Unable to give date, month, place Irritable Memory defect Difficulty finding words Does not recognize family Does not respond to own name
Observe and test symmetry of **motor responses** on both sides of body	Eyes open Follows command to stick out tongue, squeeze fingers, move extremities	Eyes closed Does not follow directions to stick out tongue, squeeze fingers, or move extremities
Exert pressure on nailbed with pen Apply pressure to supraorbital ridge Pinch Achilles tendon Test each side independently	Responds to painful stimuli by reaching out or trying to stop pressure	Does not localize or withdraw from painful stimuli or withdraws abnormally Assumes *decorticate posturing* (legs extended; feet extended with plantar flexion; arms internally rotated and flexed on chest): may be due to lesion of corticospinal tract near cerebral hemisphere Assumes *decerebrate posturing* (arms stiffly extended and hands turned outward and flexed; legs extended with plantar flexion): may be due to lesion in diencephalon, pons, or midbrain Assumes *flaccid posturing* (no motor response): may be due to extreme brain injury to motor area of brain *Involuntary movements* *Choreiform* (jerky and quick): present in Sydenham's chorea *Athetoid* (twisting and slow): present in cerebral palsy *Tremors:* hyperthyroidism, cerebellar ataxia, parkinsonism *Spasms:* cord-injured clients *Seizures:* brain injury, heat stroke, electrolyte imbalance *Asterixis:* metabolic encephalopathy due to liver or kidney failure

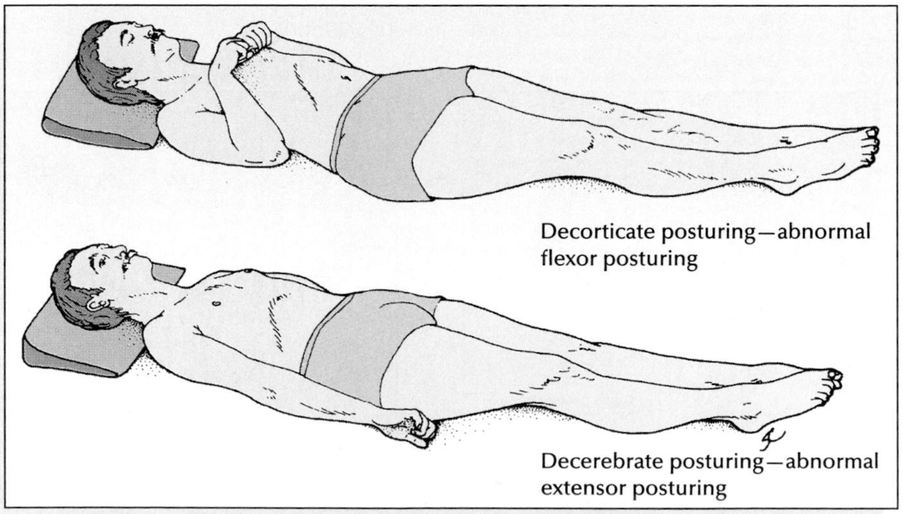

Assessment	*Normal*	*Abnormal*
Pupil Assessment		
Observe **appearance of pupils** by holding eyelids open and checking for:		
Size of pupils	Diameter: 1.5–6 mm	Unilateral dilation: sign of third cranial nerve involvement Bilateral dilation: sign of upper brain stem damage Unilateral dilation and nonreactive: sign of increased intracranial pressure (ICP) or ipsilateral oculomotor nerve (III) compression from tumor or injury
Shape of pupils	Round and midposition	Midposition and fixed: sign of midbrain involvement Pinpoint and fixed: sign of pontine involvement or opiate effect
Equality of pupils	Equal	Unequal: sign that parasympathetic and sympathetic nervous systems are not in synchronization
Observe **reaction to light** by using penlight in darkened room Open eyelid being tested; cover opposite eye	Pupil constricts promptly	Sluggish reaction: early warning of deteriorating condition Light reflex is the most important sign differentiating structural (cranial involvement) from metabolic coma due to extracranial cause (e.g., diabetic coma), which does not alter light reflex

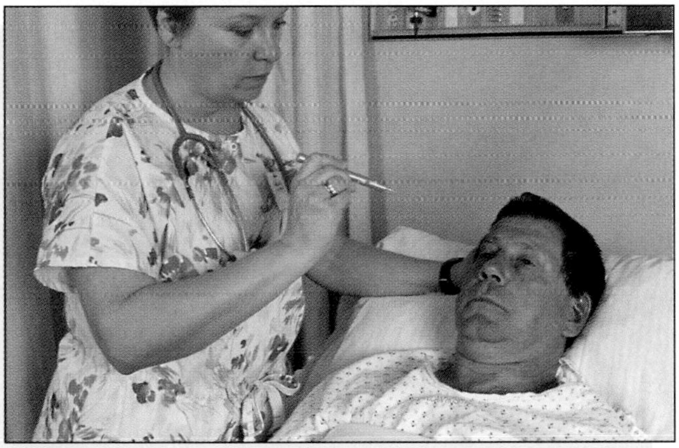

Move light toward client's eye from side position.

Observe consensual **light reflex** Hold both eyelids open Shine light into one eye only Observe opposite eye	Both pupils constrict	Pupil does not constrict: sign that connection between brain stem and pupils is not intact
Check **accommodation** (ability of lens to adjust to objects at varying distances)	Lens can adjust	When the lens thickens (often in the fifth decade of life) accommodation can be limited

PHYSICAL ASSESSMENT *(continued)*

Assessment	*Normal*	*Abnormal*
Motor Function Assessment		
Assess bilateral **muscle strength** Test hand grip by asking client to squeeze your fingers	Muscle strength is equal bilaterally	Absent or weak muscle function on one side may be sign of hemiplegia (paralysis of one side of the body); or hemiparesis (weakness on one side); paraplegia (paralysis of the legs or lower part of the body); tetraplegia or quadriplegia (paralysis of arms and legs)
Test arm strength by asking client to close eyes and hold arms out in front with palms up	Maintains position for 20–30 seconds	Cannot maintain position—downdrifts one extremity

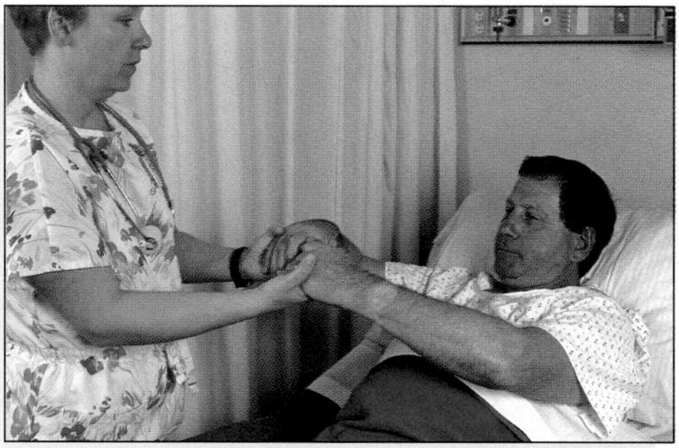

Test client's hand grip.

Assessment	*Normal*	*Abnormal*
Assess **flexion** and **extension** strength in extremities		
Stand in front of client, place your hand in front of client, and ask client to push your hand away Place your hand on client's forearm and ask client to pull arm upward	Equal response in both arms	Unequal response in arms Asymmetrical response Inability to perform movements
Position client's leg with knee flexed and foot resting on bed; as you try to extend leg, ask client to keep foot down Place one hand on client's knee and one hand on client's ankle; ask client to straighten leg as you apply resistant force to knee and ankle	Equal response in both legs	Unequal response in legs
Assess **muscle tone** Flex and extend client's upper extremities to assess how well client resists your movements	Client resistance is apparent	Increased resistance: sign of increased muscle tone from muscle rigidity or spasticity in upper motor neuron (UMN) lesions, such as with CVA and parkinsonism Decreased resistance to leg extension and arm flexion in UMN lesion (CVA)
Flex and extend client's lower extremities to assess resistance		Weakness in lower motor neuron (LMN) and cerebellar lesion

Assessment	Normal	Abnormal
Assess **coordination**	Client able to perform coordinated movements on request: hand, foot, hand and leg positioning	Uncoordinated movements: may be due to cerebellum or basal ganglia involvement
Hand coordination Ask client to pat both thighs as rapidly as possible Ask client to turn hands over and back in quick succession		
Ask client to touch thumb with each finger in rapid succession—repeat with other hand		Clumsy movement with cerebellar involvement
Foot coordination Place your hands close to client's feet Ask client to tap your hands alternately with the balls of feet		
Hand positioning coordination With client's eyes open, extend your hand in front of client's face		
Ask client to touch nose with index finger several times in rapid succession		Tremor as nose is approached indicates cerebellar involvement
Repeat test with client's eyes closed		Inability to perform task with eyes closed: may be due to loss of positioning sense
Leg positioning coordination Ask client to put heel on opposite knee and to slide heel down leg to foot		
Assess **reflexes**		
Blink reflex Hold client's eyelid open Approach client's eye unexpectedly from side of head Complete corneal touch	Eyes close immediately	Absence of blink response; eyelid continuously in open position: due to fifth or seventh cranial nerve (pons) involvement; blindness
Gag and swallow reflex Open client's mouth and hold tongue down with tongue blade Touch back of pharynx on each side with applicator stick	Gag and swallow reflex present	Absence of gag and swallow reflex; inability to swallow food or liquid: due to ninth or tenth cranial nerve (medulla) involvement
Plantar reflex Run top of pen along outer lateral aspect from heel to little toe of client's foot Continue tracing a line across ball of foot toward great toe	Toes are pointed down	Babinski response: great toe dorsiflexes; other toes fan on foot of paralyzed side in CVA, and bilaterally in spinal cord injury (SCI)

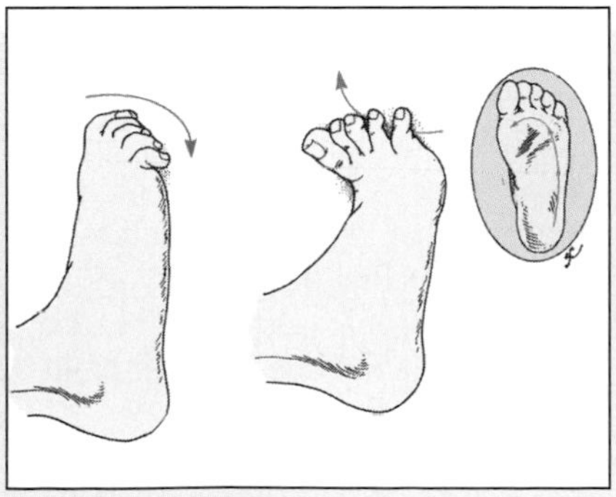

Testing plantar reflex.

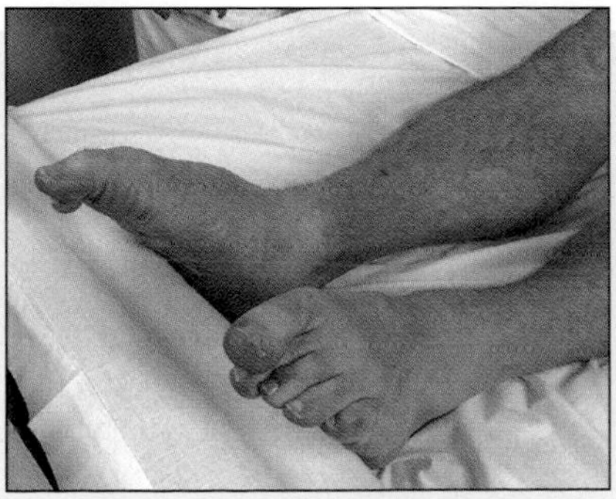

Negative Babinski.

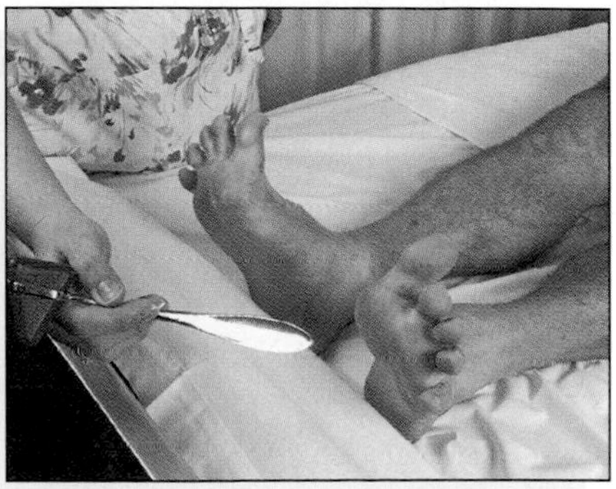

Positive Babinski.

PHYSICAL ASSESSMENT (*continued*)

Assessment	*Normal*	*Abnormal*
Deep tendon reflex		
Ask client to relax Position limb to be assessed so that muscle is somewhat stretched Using reflex hammer, strike tendon quickly Assess according to scale	Biceps reflex: flexion at elbow and contracting of biceps muscle Triceps reflex: extension at elbow and contraction of triceps muscle Patellar reflex: extension of knee and contraction of quadriceps	Absent or diminished: sign of cervical cord (C–5 or C–6) involvement Absent or diminished: C–7 or C–8 cord involvement Absent or diminished: L2–3 or L3–4 cord involvement
Grading Scale 4+ Hyperactive or exaggerated 3+ More brisk than usual but not indicative of disease state 2+ Average or normal 1+ Slightly diminished, low normal 0 No response		Indicates upper motor neuron (UMN) lesion or SCI Seen with lower motor neuron (LMN) lesion
Sensory Function Assess **superficial sensations**		
Pain Ask client to close eyes Stroke or touch skin with safety pin, alternating blunt end and sharp end of pin Ask client to distinguish sharp and dull pain	Ability to distinguish between sharp and dull sensations	Alterations in pain or temperature sensations: indicate lesion in posterior horn of spinal cord or spinothalamic tract of cord
Temperature Fill two test tubes with water, one hot, one cold Ask client to close eyes and touch client's skin with test tubes	Ability to distinguish between hot and cold	
Touch Ask client to close eyes Stroke cotton wisp over client's skin	Ability to identify light touch—equal bilaterally	Anesthesia = loss of light touch Analgesia = absence of sense of pain Hypalgesia = decreased pain sensation Hyperalgesia = exaggerated sensitivity to pin prick (pain)
Positioning Ask client to close eyes Grasp client's finger with your thumb and index finger Move client's finger up and down Ask client to identify direction finger is moving Repeat with great toe	Ability to identify position or mimic position with other hand	Inability to determine direction of movement: may be due to posterior column or peripheral nerve disease
Vital Signs		
Assess **respiration** Assess rate and pattern of breathing	Regular rate: 12–20 breaths per minute	Cheyne–Stokes (rhythmic increase in depth of breathing followed by period of apnea) may be due to deep cerebral or cerebellar lesion or condition altering cerebral perfusion Central neurogenic (sustained) hyperventilation due to upper brain stem involvement Ataxic (Biot's) breathing unpredictably irregular, due to lower brain stem involvement

Assessment	*Normal*	*Abnormal*
Monitor arterial blood gases if signs of respiratory imbalances occur	pH: 7.35–7.45 P_{CO_2}: 35–45 mm Hg HCO_3: 22–26 mEq/L	Alterations in pH and P_{CO_2} values indicate respiratory imbalances: pH below 7.35 and P_{CO_2} above 45: sign of respiratory acidosis (hypoventilation) pH above 7.45 and P_{CO_2} below 35: sign of respiratory alkalosis (hyperventilation) HCO_3 above 26 indicates metabolic compensation for chronic respiratory acidosis (hypoventilation)
Assess **temperature** If client is semiresponsive or nonresponsive, take rectal or tympanic temperature If rectal temperature is contraindicated or there are signs of increased ICP, use alternate method.	Ability to maintain normal body temperature (approximately 98.6°F, or 37°C)	Inability to maintain normal temperature: may be due to damage to hypothalamus No sweating below level of injury; due to spinal cord injury Hypothermia
Assess **apical** and **radial pulses** Note character of pulses Count heart rate Count radial pulse rate	Regular rhythm Rate 60–100 BPM Apical and radial rates are equal	Fast heart rate due to decreased blood volume, arrhythmia, heart failure, fever, medulla dysfunction Irregular rhythm with premature beats due to hypoxia, cardiac irritability, or electrolyte imbalance Pulse deficit due to premature beats or ineffectual cardiac contraction.
Assess **blood pressure** Position neurologic clients in low- to semi-Fowler's position	Normal pressure (range 120/80–140/90)	Systolic blood pressure rises with diastolic pressure remaining same (widening pulse pressure): sign of increased intracranial pressure Blood pressure over 140/85 is a sign of hypertension Blood pressure below 90/60 is a sign of hypotension

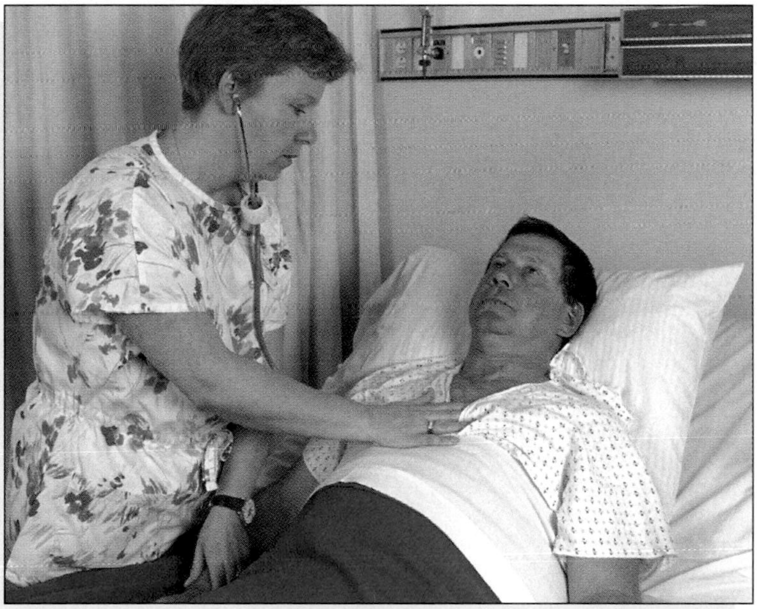

Assess client's apical pulse.

ASSESSMENT OF THE HEAD AND NECK

The names of the regions of the head are derived from the bones that form the skull. Knowing the names of the bones and regions of the skull can assist in describing the location of the physical findings.

An understanding of the function of each lobe of the brain allows the nurse to be able to identify potential client problems when an injury occurs to that portion of the brain.

The brain comprises three segments: the brain stem, cerebrum, and the cerebellum. There are 12 cranial nerves, which are discussed later in this chapter, and 31 pairs of spinal nerves with dorsal and ventral roots.

The brain stem is divided into four sections: The *diencephalon* comprises the thalamus, which screens and relays sensory impulses to the cortex, and the hypothalamus, which regulates the autonomic nervous system, stress response, sleep, appetite, body temperature, water balance, and emotions. The *midbrain* is responsible for motor coordination and conjugate eye movements. The *pons* controls involuntary respiratory reflexes and contains projection tracts between the spinal cord, medulla, and brain. The *medulla* contains cardiac, respiratory, vomiting, and vasomotor centers. In addition, all afferent and efferent nerve tracts must pass between the spinal cord and brain through the medulla.

The cerebral hemispheres have an outer layer formed by cellular gray matter, called the cerebral cortex. The two cerebral hemispheres are divided into four major lobes. The frontal lobe controls emotions, judgments, motor function, and the motor speech area. The parietal lobe integrates general sensations; interprets pain, touch, and temperature; and governs discrimination. The temporal lobe contains the auditory center and sensory speech center. The occipital lobe controls the visual area. The cerebellum coordinates muscle movement, posture, equilibrium, and muscle tone.

The 12 cranial nerves are summarized in Table 11–1. The 2nd through 12th nerves arise from the brain stem. The cranial nerves are 12 pairs of parasympathetic nerves with their nuclei along the brain stem.

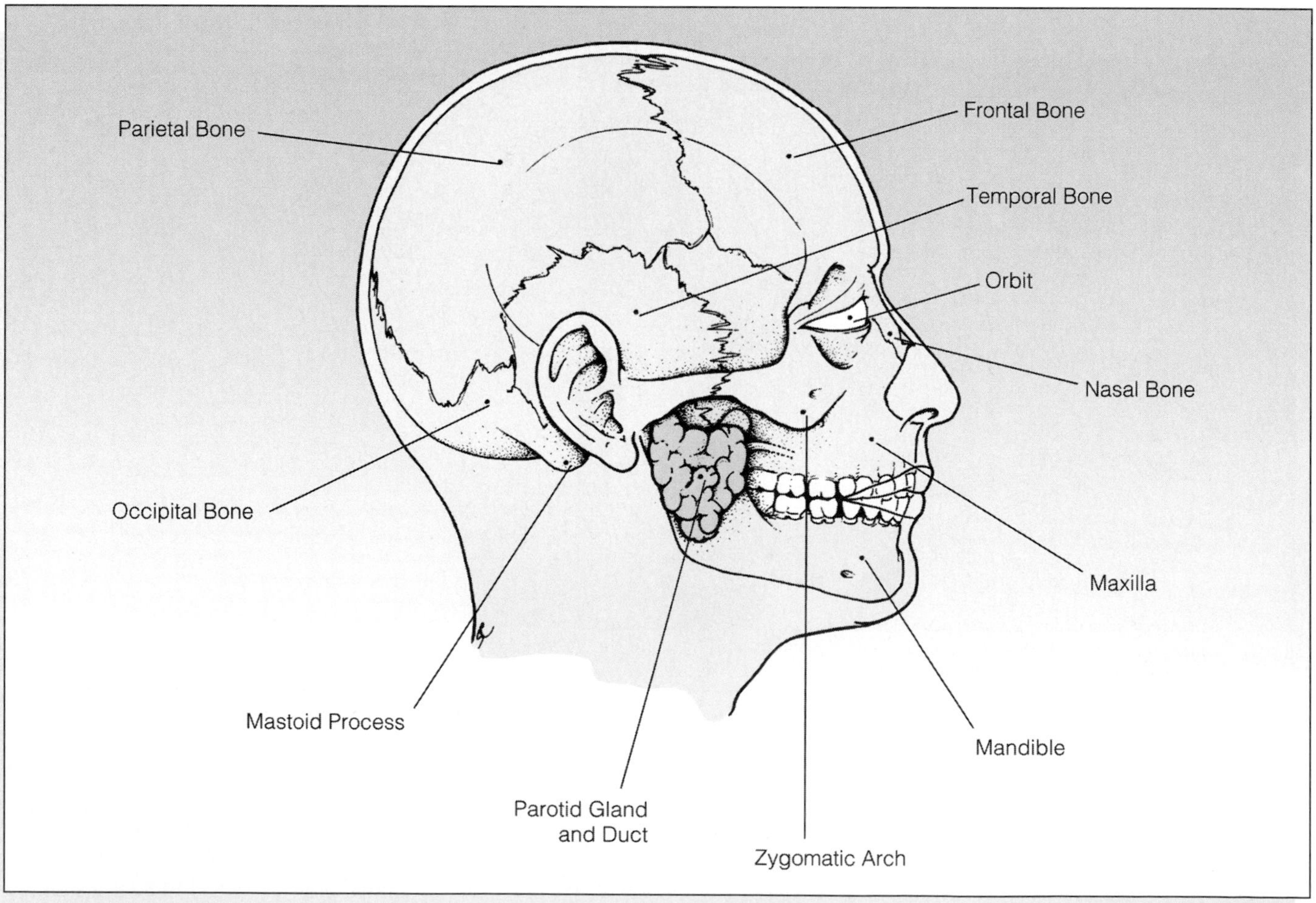

Bones that form the skull.

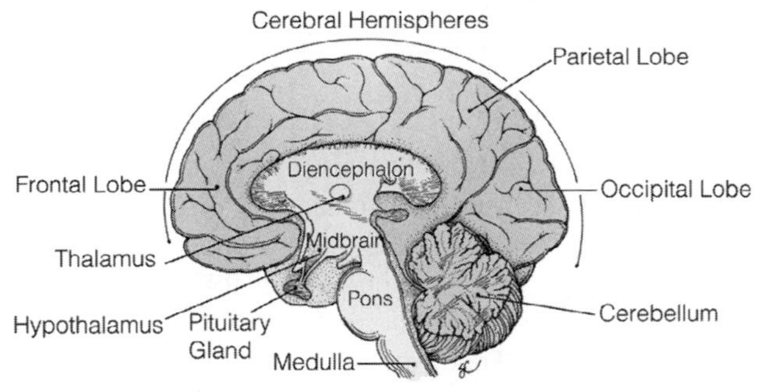

Lobes of the brain.

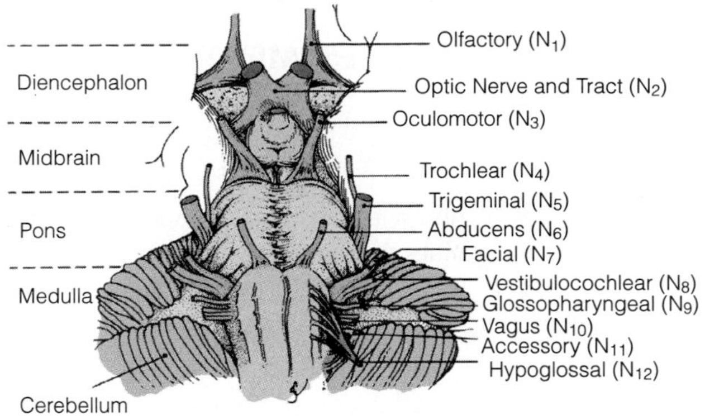

Brain segments and cranial nerves.

TABLE 11–1 Cranial Nerves and Their Function

Cranial Nerve	Function	Testing Cranial Nerves
I Olfactory	Sensory nerve	Recognizes odor in each nostril separately (e.g., coffee)
II Optic	Sensory nerve: conducts sensory information from the retina	Demonstrates visual acuity: can read newsprint
III Oculomotor	Motor nerve: controls four of the six extraocular muscles; raises eyelid and controls the constrictor pupillae and ciliary muscles of the eyeball	Responds to light: pupils constrict; moves eyes medially; elevates upper eyelid
IV Trochlear	Motor nerve: controls the superior oblique eye muscle	Move eyes to the right, up then down, and to the left.
V Trigeminal	Mixed nerve with three sensory branches and one motor branch: the ophthalmic branch supplies the corneal reflex	Demonstrates normal facial sensation; clenches teeth with no lateral jaw deviation; blinks as wisp touched to cornea
VI Abducens	Motor nerve: controls the lateral rectus muscle of the eye	Moves eyes laterally
VII Facial	Mixed nerve: anterior tongue receives sensory supply, motor supply to glands of nose, palate lacrimal submaxillary, and sublingual; motor branch supplies hyoid elevators and muscles of expression and closes eyelid	Elevates eyebrows; puffs cheeks; recognizes tastes (sugar, salt)
VIII Acoustic	Sensory nerve with two divisions: hearing and semicircular canals	Hears whisper with each ear separately
IX Glossopharyngeal	Mixed nerve: motor innervates parotid gland; sensory innervates auditory tube and posterior portion of taste buds	Demonstrates gag reflex to tongue blade when touched to back of tongue
X Vagus	Mixed nerve: motor branches to the pharyngeal and laryngeal muscles and to the viscera of the thorax and abdomen; sensory portion supplies the pinna of the ear, thoracic, and abdominal viscera	Same as IX
XI Accessory	Motor nerve: innervates the sternocleidomastoid and trapezius muscles	Shrugs shoulders
XII Hypoglossal	Motor nerve: controls tongue muscles	Sticks tongue out in midline without deviation

HEAD AND NECK ASSESSMENT

Assessment	*Normal*	*Abnormal*
Eye Assessment		
Note **visual acuity** by observing client performance of activities of daily living	Adequate performance of activities of daily living	Age related macular degeneration (AMD) Hyperopia (farsightedness) Myopia (nearsightedness)
Factors influencing visual acuity include client's previous status and age	Appropriate responses to environment	Cataract (opacification of the lens) Enucleation (loss of an eye): may have prosthesis in place
Note exact location, size, and color of any **external lesions** Palpate for mobility and firmness	No external lesions	Circumocular ecchymosis: may be sign of basal skull fracture Xanthelasma (small, yellowish, well-circumscribed plaques): may appear on eyelids of clients with lipid disorders. *Example:* atherosclerosis

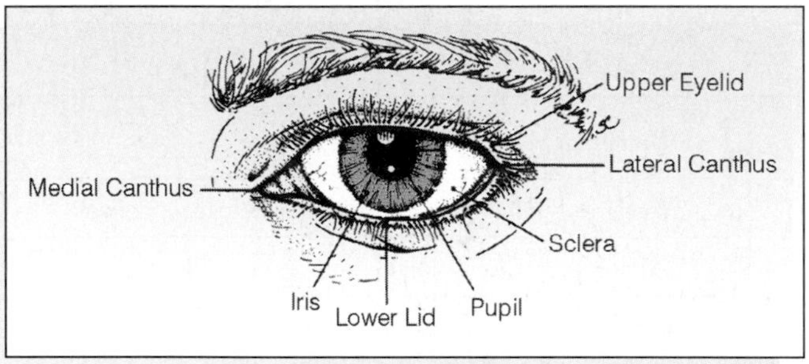

Anatomy of the eye.

Assessment	*Normal*	*Abnormal*
Note **equality of eyelid movement**	Eyelids are equal in movement	Ptosis (paralytic drooping of the upper eyelid)
Note color, consistency, amount, and origin of **discharge** from eyes	No discharge	Sty or hordeolum Thick white discharge; may be due to conjunctivitis
Note **internal lesions**	No internal lesions	Conjunctival or ciliary injection (dilatation of the blood vessels)
Assess differences between **pupil size and reaction** Note presence of hemorrhage	Both pupils are the same size	Anisocoria (indicates unequal pupil size): may be indicative of neurologic trauma or deficit Corneal edema (very soft, movable mass that looks like raw egg white): frequently occurs in clients who have increased intracranial pressure Arcus senilis (partial or complete whitish circle near the outer edge of the cornea); usually due to aging; does not affect vision

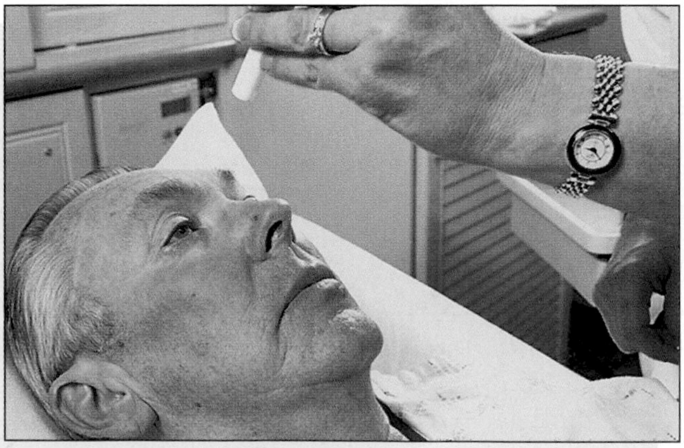

Assess pupil size and reaction.

Assessment	Normal	Abnormal
Ear Assessment		
Note **auditory acuity** by asking client to indicate if he or she hears normal sounds as you make them	Adequate responses to normal sounds Auditory changes due to aging	Deafness or impaired hearing; excess cerumen in auditory canal Abnormal sounds in the ears (ringing or buzzing) may be caused by ototoxic drugs

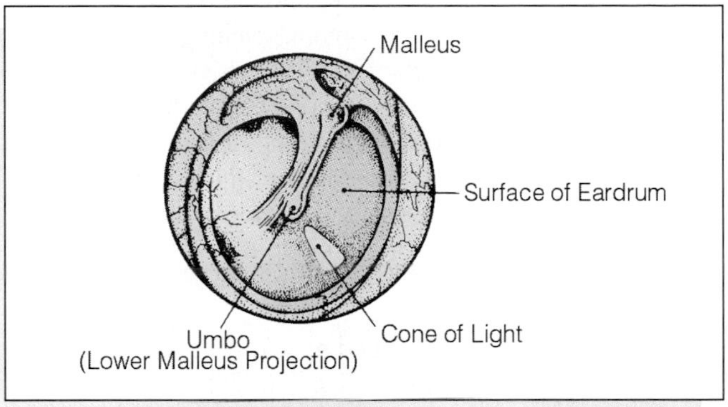

Anatomy of the tympanic membrane (ear drum).

Assessment	Normal	Abnormal
Note exact size, color, and location of any **external** lesions Palpate lesions for mobility and firmness	No external lesions	Battle's sign (ecchymosis behind the ear). may be sign of basilar skull fracture

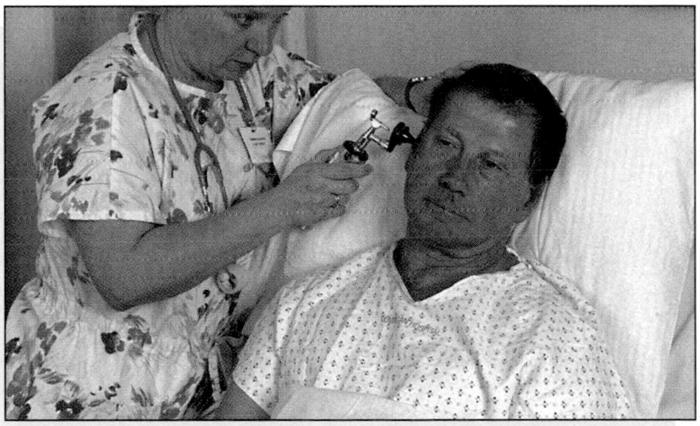
Position otoscope in ear before viewing.

Assessment	Normal	Abnormal
Note color, quantity, and consistency of any **discharge** from the ears Test clear fluid for glucose using a Labstix	No discharge Wax buildup Glucose test negative	Redness, swelling, and pain may be signs of otitis externa Cerebrospinal fluid leak: may be due to head injury. If drainage is blood and CSF, it will develop a "halo" with a reddish area in the center surrounded by a whitish circle if placed on white material Perforation of tympanic membrane: serosanguineous or purulent drainage Glucose test of clear drainage is positive if CSF

HEAD AND NECK ASSESSMENT (*continued*)

Assessment	*Normal*	*Abnormal*
Nose Assessment		
Note any **structural changes** in the nose by observing client breathe	Regular breathing with mouth closed	Breathing through the mouth only: furuncles may occlude breathing
Gently occlude one nostril at a time; ask client to breathe through the nonoccluded nostril	Breathing through nonoccluded nostril	Obstruction in the nose due to deviated nasal septum, swelling of the nasal turbinates, or excessive mucus secretions
Note color, quantity, and consistency of any **discharge** from the nose	Minimal discharge	Cerebrospinal fluid leak (fluid tests positive for glucose with Labstix) Copious, watery-to-thick, mucopurulent discharge: may be due to acute rhinitis Excessive buildup of mucous secretions
Mouth and Lip Assessment		
Note size, color, and location of any **external lesions** Palpate for mobility and firmness	No external lesions	Dehydrated mouth or lips Fissures Pressure sores Necrosis
Note size, color, and location of any **internal lesions** Palpate for mobility and firmness	No internal lesions	Candidiasis (a fungal infection indicated by adherent, white patches)
Neck Assessment		
Note any **lesion or swelling** in the neck	Occasional small, mobile, discrete, nontender lymph nodes	Enlarged tender immobile nodes
Ask client to relax and flex neck slightly Palpate the neck, using the pads of your fingers to move the skin and underlying tissues		

ASSESSMENT OF THE SKIN

The skin is the body's first line of defense against disease and injury. It is made up of three layers: the epidermis, the dermis, and the subcutaneous tissues.

The epidermis is divided into two avascular, or bloodless, layers: an outer layer that consists of dead keratinized cells and an inner layer that consists of live cells where keratin and melanin are formed. The dermis contains blood vessels, connective tissue, sebaceous glands, and some of the hair follicles. The subcutaneous tissues contain the remainder of the hair follicles, fat, and the sweat glands.

Hair, nails, sweat glands, and sebaceous glands are appendages of the skin. There are two types of sweat glands: eccrine and apocrine. Eccrine glands are distributed over most of the body except for the palms and soles. These glands help control body temperature through their sweat production. The apocrine glands are found mainly in the axillary and genital areas and are stimulated by emotional stress. Bacterial decomposition by aprocrine sweat glands causes adult body odor.

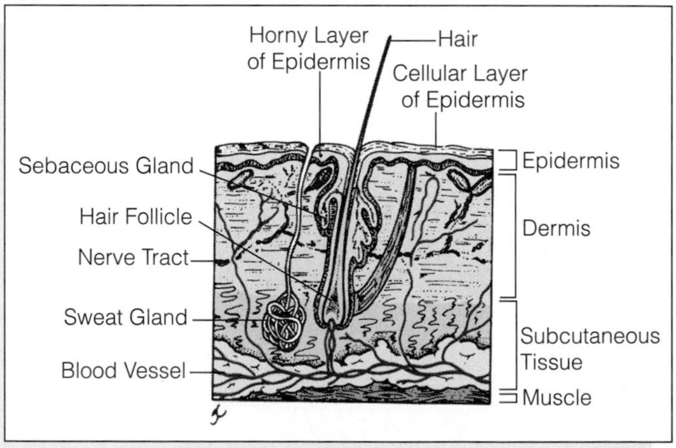

Anatomy of the skin.

SKIN ASSESSMENT

Assessment	*Normal*	*Abnormal*
Note **color** of the skin by assessing the oral mucous membranes, the conjunctiva, and the nailbeds	Pink, tan, or brown, depending on the client's basic skin color	Pallor (decrease in color) *Example:* anemia from acute blood loss (hemorrhage), renal failure, dietary deficiencies, or arterial insufficiency Jaundice (icterus): due to the presence of conjugated or unconjugated bilirubin in the blood and tissues; appears most frequently in the face and sclerae; seen best under natural light *Example:* liver disease Cyanosis (blue, bluegray, or purple discoloration of the skin and mucous membranes): caused by hypoxia, a result of an increased amount of reduced hemoglobin Peripheral: seen in nailbeds and earlobes *Example:* vasoconstriction, venous insufficiency Central: seen in nailbeds, lips (circumoral), and oral mucosa Erythema (redness of the skin): caused by capillary congestion; occurs with inflammation or infection; usually a local finding

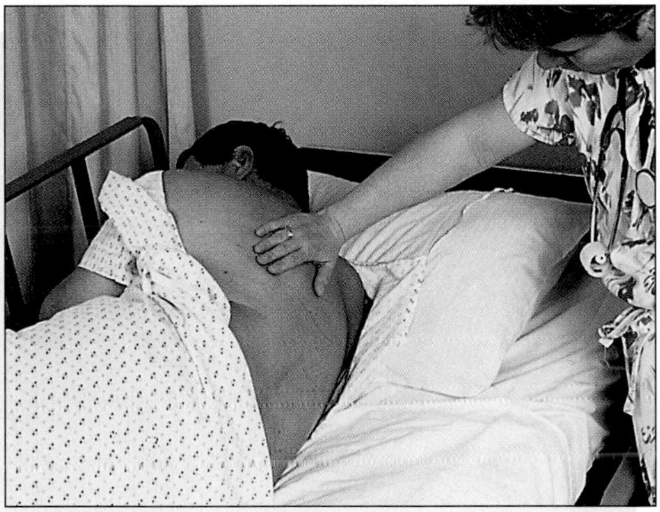

Check quality of the skin.

Assessment	*Normal*	*Abnormal*
Note **pigmentation**	Discolored spots may be due to normal aging	Hyperpigmentation (especially in skin creases) *Example:* use of oral contraceptives, pregnancy, Addison's disease, and hyperthyroidism
Note **turgor** and **mobility**	Smooth and elastic	Tight or stretched and difficult to move: due to local or generalized edema Wrinkled: due to dehydration or caused by rapid weight loss
Pinch skin over the sternum If the fold persists, skin turgor is poor	Resilient and supple	Thin and translucent (parchment) *Example:* chronic steroid use Thin, shiny, and smooth with alopecia on lower extremities *Example:* chronic arterial insufficiency
Assess for **edema** Press finger firmly for 5 seconds into skin on top of foot or inner ankle bone	Resilient and no depression remains after pressure released	Pitting edema: excess interstitial fluid *Example:* congestive heart failure, renal failure, cirrhosis of the liver, venous stasis

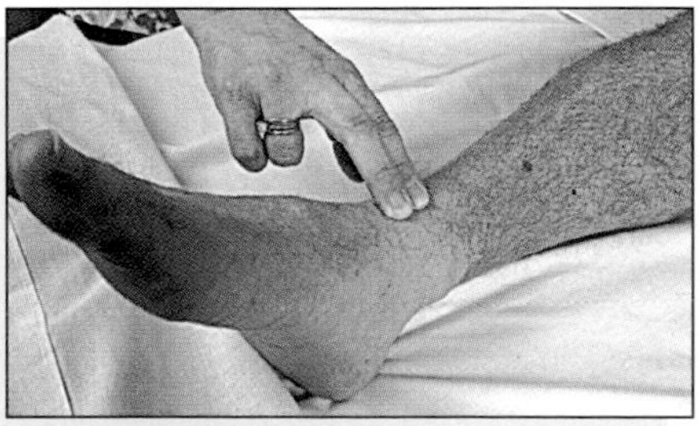

Check client for edema.

Assessment	*Normal*	*Abnormal*
Note **moistness** and **temperature** of the skin	Warm and dry	Warm (hot) and moist due to temperature elevation

SKIN ASSESSMENT (*continued*)

Assessment	*Normal*	*Abnormal*
		Cool and moist (cold and clammy): may be due to shock states Abnormally dry: may be due to dehydration, decreased sebaceous gland secretions, or the excessive use of soap
Assess for **sensation**—response to external stimuli	Feels touch, sensitive to heat and cold and pressure	Absence of touch or pain sensation *Example:* spinal cord injury or nerve damage Diminished heat and cold sensation *Example:* peripheral vascular disease Itching and tingling *Example:* peripheral vascular disease, peripheral neuropathy, allergy
Note **lesions** on the skin Physical characteristics include color, elevation, shape, mobility, and contents	No lesions present	Macules (flat localized changes in color) *Example:* petechiae, first-degree burns, purpura Papules, plaques, nodules (solid, elevated, varying in size) *Example:* psoriasis, xanthomas Cancerous lesions *Examples:* Basal cell epithelioma—small, smooth papule with atrophic center Melanoma—pigmented tumor; may arise from a blue-black mole Squamous cell—macules with indistinct margins; surface may be crusted Wheals (elevated, circumscribed, transient) *Example:* urticaria, insect bites Vesicles and bullae (clear, fluid-filled pockets between skin layers) *Example:* second-degree burns Pustules (vesicles or bullae filled with purulent exudate) *Example:* furuncles, acne

ASSESSMENT OF THE CHEST: LUNGS, BREASTS, AND HEART

The chest, or thorax area, extends from the base of the neck to the diaphragm. The overall shape of the thorax should be elliptical, although deformities such as barrel chest, pigeon chest, or funnel chest do occur. Total assessment includes the external aspect: the nurse should observe for movement, posture, shape, and symmetry, especially of the breast and axilla area, and the internal components of the lungs and the heart.

The lungs anteriorly extend from 2 to 4 cm above the inner third of the clavicle to the eighth rib at the midaxillary line and the sixth rib at the midclavicular line.

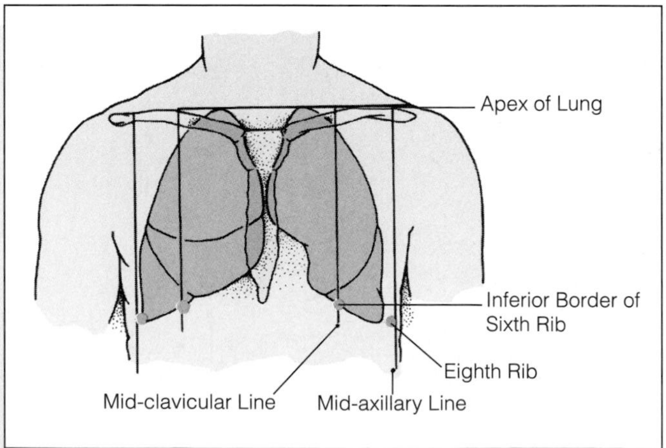

Anterior anatomical relationship of lungs to skeletal structure.

Posteriorly the lungs extend from the third thoracic spinous process and descend to the tenth process or, on deep inspiration, to the twelfth process.

Chest assessment begins with inspection, proceeds to palpation, and then to auscultation. Breath sounds of clients differ due to the depth of breathing, underlying disease, or obesity. Because of these differences, it is difficult to compare the breath sounds of one client with another. The basic principle to remember when auscultating the lungs is to do a comparison between the right and left lung. To make these comparisons, begin auscultating at the apices of one lung, alternating sides as you work down through both lungs. By comparing similar areas in both lungs, you can note changes and determine causes for these changes more easily.

Examination of the chest usually proceeds from posterior to anterior. For posterior assessment of the lungs, place the client in an upright sitting position with shoulders pulled forward. For anterior assessment, the client can be sitting or supine (especially if female). If the client is lying on his or her side, the lung closest to the bed is mechanically compressed, and true lung sounds cannot be heard.

Ask the client to breathe a little deeper than usual through the mouth. Breathing through the nose produces extra sounds that mask true lung sounds.

The heart is located directly behind the sternum, with the left ventricle projecting into the left chest. The heart is usually thought to be in the left chest for two reasons: the left ventricle produces the most movement (ventricular contraction), and three of the valve sound areas are located to the left of the sternum.

The action of the heart should be assessed both proximally and distally. Proximal assessment involves evaluating heart sounds, heart rate, and rhythm to obtain information about the mechanical activity of the heart. Distal assessment involves evaluating the peripheral pulses to obtain information about the effectiveness of the heart's pumping action.

One method for assessing heart sounds is to start at the aortic area, moving slowly across to the pulmonic area, down to the tricuspid area, and over to the mitral area. This same general progression can also be used in reverse, starting at the mitral area and progressing up to the aortic area. Most clinicians begin the assessment at the mitral area, which is the point of maximum impulse and where the apical pulse is the loudest.

The most important point to remember in heart assessment is to use the same method every time, repeating the same steps in the same sequence. By using one systematic approach, you learn how to compare the different sounds more easily and not neglect to listen to all areas on the chest.

Breast assessment should include observing for lumps, drainage, dimpling of breast tissue, and presence of asymmetry. The client should also be asked if she has noted any recent changes.

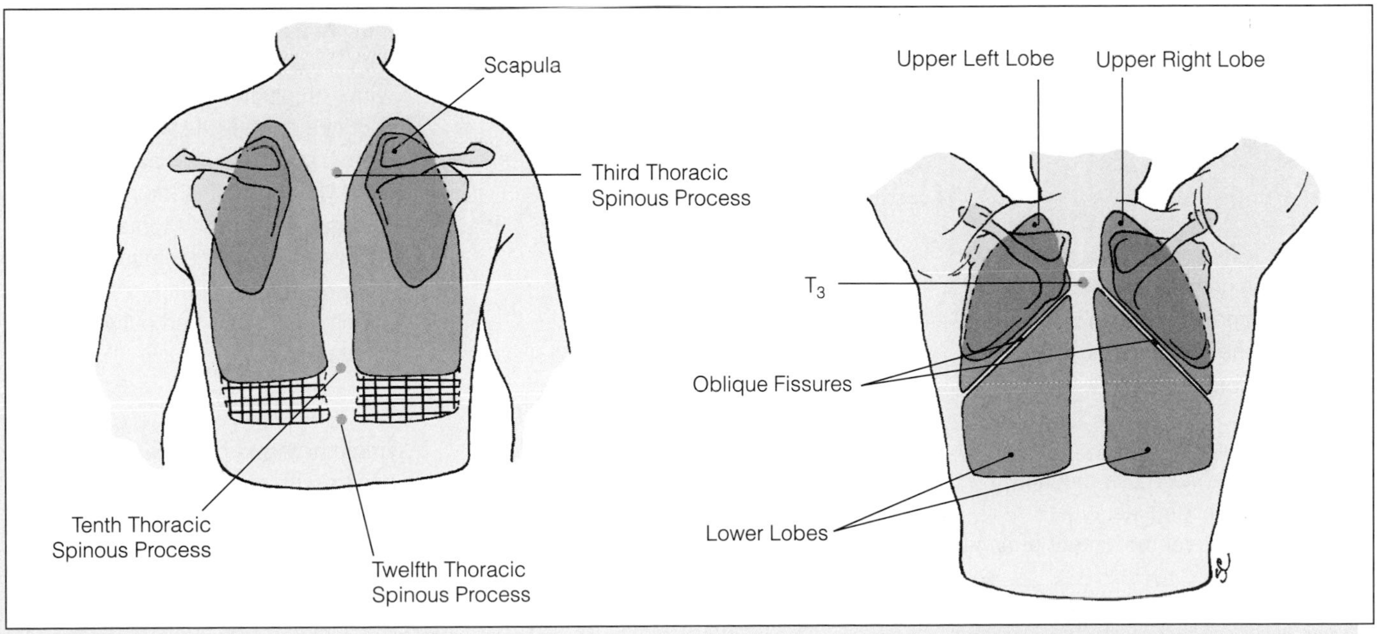

Posterior relationship of lung lobes to skeletal structures.

CHEST ASSESSMENT

Assessment	*Normal*	*Abnormal*
Chest Assessment		
Note respiratory rate—increase may be due to fever, pain, anxiety	A normal or increased rate does not assume a normal tidal volume	Clients may have an increased rate to compensate for decreased tidal volume, but the resultant minute volume is still not sufficient. (Normal minute volume is 6–8 L/minute.) Increased depth: due to neurologic disease, intracranial pressure (ICP) from trauma, drug overdose, exertion, fear, or anxiety Decreased depth: due to neurologic disease, ICP from trauma, drug overdose, respiratory disease, pneumothorax, or pain
Note the **general appearance** of the chest and movement when client breathes	Straight spine, level shoulders	Breathes sitting forward with arms on pillows or overbed table (present with emphysema)
	Relaxed breathing; rib cage moves symmetrically with respirations	Uses accessory muscles (i.e., scalene, trapezius, sternocleidomastoid, pectoralis, or intercostal)
Note **shape of chest**	Anterior–posterior dimension is half of lateral dimension	Anterior–posterior dimension increased in emphysema (barrel chest) Deformities such as scoliosis (lateral curvature), kyphosis (forward curvature), or kyphoscoliosis
Note **position of ribs**	Slant downward	Horizontal is common in COPD Bulging of interspaces during exhalation with retraction on inhalation (present with asthma and emphysema) Chest tilted to one side when client sits or stands: may be due to pain in ribs or chest wall or trauma (i.e., fractured ribs or surgery such as a thoracotomy)
Measure **chest excursion** for range and symmetry: place hands parallel to 10th rib (under scapulae) with thumbs beside spine. Bunch up fold of skin pushing thumbs medially. Ask client to inhale	On inhalation, the thumbs move equidistant away from midline indicating equal expansion	Flail chest: occurs when four or more ribs are broken; area collapses inward during inhalations and outward on exhalation
For anterior assessment, place hands over lower thorax, push medially, then have client inhale. Note equidistant lateral movement of hands		Asymmetrical (unequal) chest expansion occurs with pneumothorax, fractured ribs, atelectasis, or when client's chest splints due to pain

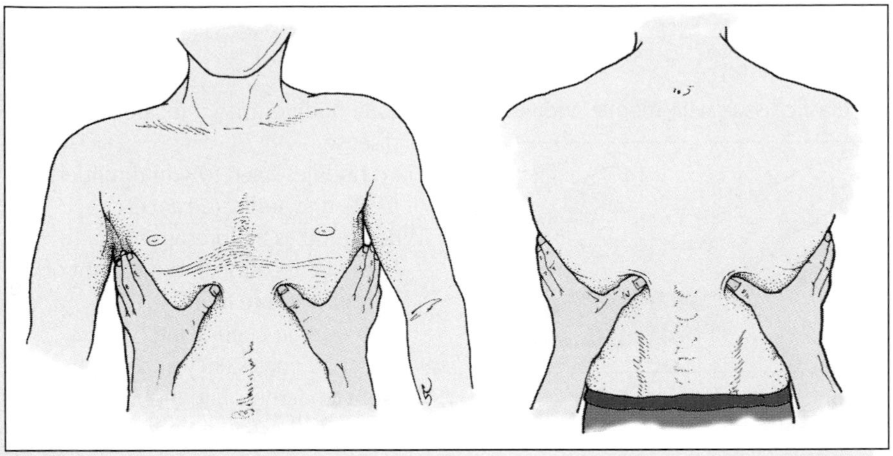

Measure chest excursion while client takes deep breath.

Assessment	Normal	Abnormal
Tactile and Vocal Fremitus		
Tactile fremitus (vibrations felt on surface of chest as sound passes through tissue) Palpate upper thorax and ask client to say "ninety-nine"; vibrations detected as hands move down thorax	Varied because it depends on thickness of chest wall	Decreased sounds: obesity, emphysema, pneumothorax, and possible asthma Increased sounds: heard when lung is filled with fluid-consolidation (pneumonia) or tumors Absent sounds: atelectasis or pleural effusion Asymmetric sounds: abnormal Normal sounds: found with bronchitis or pulmonary edema
Breast Assessment		
Inspect **size, symmetry,** and **contour** of breasts, comparing one side with the other Place client in sitting position Have client remove clothing from waist up Have client raise arms over her head	Size varies with each client Breasts should be fairly equal in size and contour and symmetric in position	Masses, skin thickening, dimpling, or flattened areas: indicate possible cancer
Color, edema, and **venous pattern of skin**	Normal skin color with darker area surrounding nipples No edema or prominent vessels	Erythema: indicates infection or inflammatory carcinoma Edema or increased venous prominence: indicates carcinoma
Inspect **size and shape of nipples** Note direction in which they point, and any **rashes** or **discharge** To palpate breasts, position client supine or on side	Simple inversion of nipples is common	Flattening, nipple retraction, or axis deviation of nipple points: may be due to fibrosis associated with cancer Ulcerations of nipples and areola: may be due to Paget's disease Discharge: may not be malignant but should be observed closely

CHEST ASSESSMENT (*continued*)

Assessment	*Normal*	*Abnormal*
Place a pillow under the shoulder of the side being examined Using three fingers in a circular motion, compress breast tissue gently against chest wall Systematically examine entire breast, top to bottom, moving medially to laterally into the axilla	Soft, elastic tissue with mobile nodules	Mobile nodules may indicate cystic disease Hard nodules fixed to skin or underlying tissue may indicate cancer When nodules are present Describe location and quadrant of breast where found Note size in centimeters Describe consistency and shape Note tenderness and mobility of nodule in relationship to underlying tissue

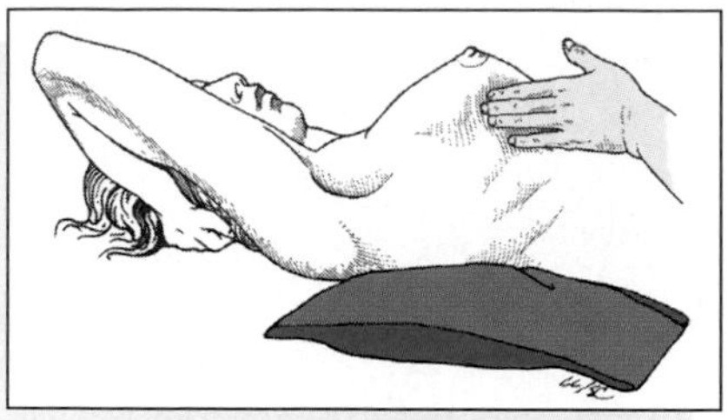

Examine breast tissue in circular movement.

Assessment	*Normal*	*Abnormal*
Palpate nipples		
Compress nipple and areola between thumb and index finger to inspect for discharge	No discharge or small amount of milky discharge in previously nursing mother	Bloody discharge: may indicate papilloma
Note **elasticity**	Elastic, no retraction of nipple	Loss of elasticity: indicates possible cancer
Observe for erection of nipple with palpation		Inversion, flattening, or retraction: may indicate cancer
Lung/Respiratory Assessment		
Complete a **general assessment** of the lungs		
Respiratory rate	12–20 respirations/minute	Increased respiratory rate: may be due to increased metabolic needs (fever), mechanical injury, surgery, or trauma to chest wall
Respiratory depth or volume	Normal depth is equal to about 500 mL	
Auscultation: note location and quality of **lung sounds**		
Note presence of *adventitious (extra) sounds*, such as crackles, wheezes, and rhonchi, or pleural friction rub	No extra sounds heard—symmetrical areas should be the same in quality and intensity	*Discontinuous Sounds:* *Crackles* (rales) are due to sudden opening of closed airways, indicating hypoventilation; usually heard as soft, high-pitched scratching sounds, like hair strands rubbing together at end of inspiration Heard in dependent areas of bedridden clients or in early CHF. Simulate by rubbing hair together in front of your ear *Continuous Sounds:* *Wheezes* are produced by air passing through airways narrowed by edema, spasm or mucus; may be heard on inspiration but more often louder on expiration; high-pitched and musical *Rhonchi* are low-pitched rumbling, coarse; sounds heard on inhalation and exhalation. May be cleared with coughing. *Sibilant wheezes* are high-pitched, musical sounds; may be caused by asthma, increased secretions, or edema

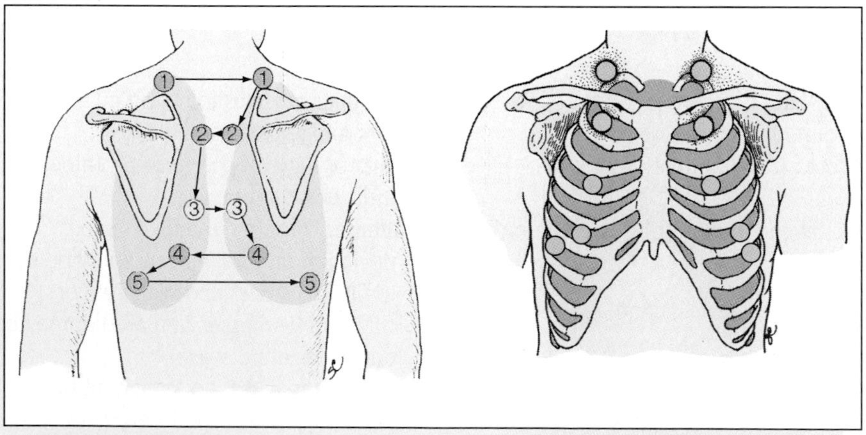

Stethoscope placement sites for posterior (left) and anterior (right) auscultation of breath sounds. Follow arrows for sequence of examination.

Assessment	Normal	Abnormal
		Pleural friction rub is produced when inflamed pleurae rub together in the absence of normal pleural fluid; localized, high-pitched, harsh, and scratchy; frequently transient; may be heard on inspiration and expiration *Stridor* is an inspiratory wheeze heard in the neck due to partial obstruction at the tracheal or laryngeal level

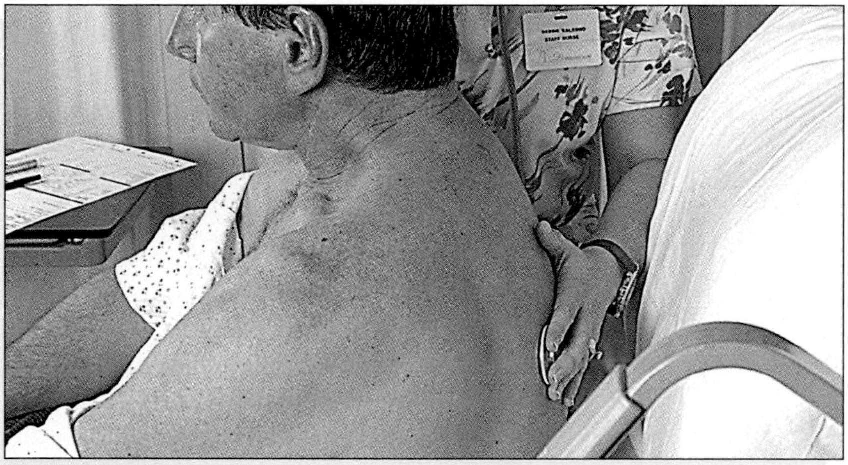

Listen to posterior breath sounds.

Assessment	Normal	Abnormal
Evaluate *breath sounds*		
Bronchovesicular breath sounds Heard over the mainstem bronchi below the clavicles and adjacent to the sternum, between scapulae	Moderate to high pitch, with moderate amplitude Hollow, muffled quality Inspiration and expiration equal in duration	Bronchial or bronchovesicular sounds heard in the perimeter where vesicular sounds are expected indicate consolidation such as pneumonia. The client's spoken and whispered words are also clearly heard by the examiner over consolidated lung areas
Vesicular (normal) breath sounds Heard over lung parenchyma (heart will mask breath sounds on the left side)	Low to medium pitch, with low amplitude Soft, whooshing quality	Breath sounds may be absent over areas of atelectasis, pneumothorax, or pleural effusion
Lungs extend anteriorly to the sixth intercostal space	Inspiration two to three times longer than expiration	
Bronchial breath sounds Heard over the trachea above the sternal notch	High pitch and amplitude Harsh, loud, tubular quality Expiration longer than inspiration	
Lungs extend posteriorly to T10 on expiration, to T12 on deep inspiration		Breath sounds are decreased (faint) with hypoventilation, early atelectasis, and COPD
Heart Assessment		
Evaluate **atrioventricular heart sounds** (S_1 heart sound). Use diaphragm of stethoscope—best for picking up high-pitched sounds	S_1 (the first heart sound, a combination of the mitral and tricuspid closure) heard best over the mitral and tricuspid areas. S_1 louder than S_2 in this area	Heart sounds not heard in the area prescribed (e.g., with left ventricular hypertrophy, mitral sound moves laterally)
Mitral value sounds Heard best at left, fifth intercostal space at, or medial to, the midclavicular line		
Tricuspid valve sounds Heard best at fifth intercostal space, left sternal border	S_1 also heard at this area and is louder than S_2	

CHEST ASSESSMENT (*continued*)

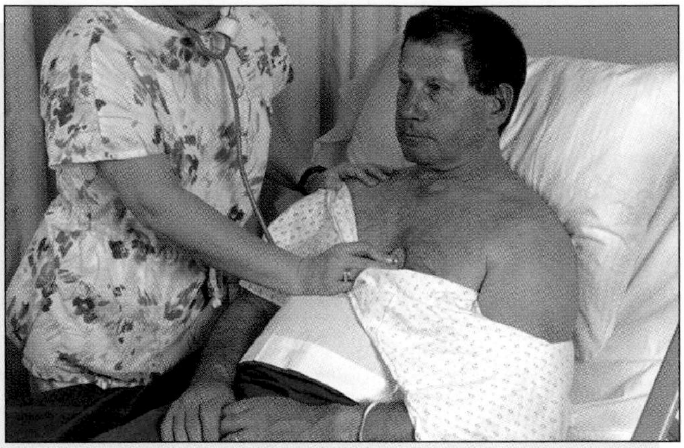

Auscultate heart sounds.

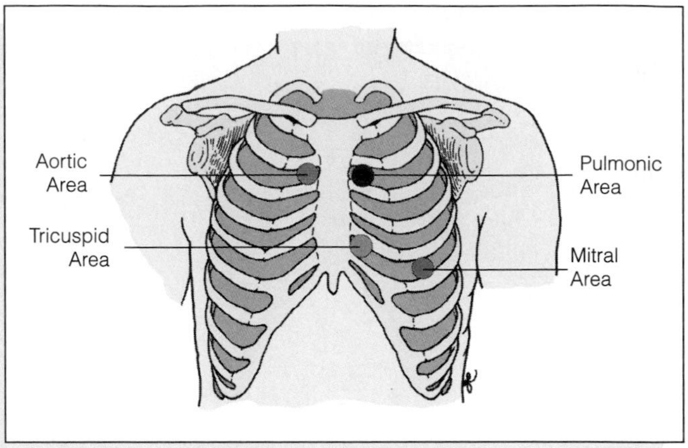

S_1 heard best over mitral and tricuspid areas.
S_2 heard best over aortic and pulmonic areas.

Assessment	*Normal*	*Abnormal*
Evaluate **semilunar heart sounds** (S_2 heart sounds)	S_2 (the second heart sound, a combination of the aortic and pulmonic closure): heard best over the aortic and pulmonic areas	Sounds altered with aortic stenosis (thrill) and hypertension (accentuated sound)
Aortic valve sounds Heard best at second intercostal space, right sternal border		
Pulmonic valve sounds Heard best at second intercostal space, left sternal border	Part of S_2 is louder than S_1 in this area. May be heard separately from aortic closure if client inhales deeply	Accentuated with pulmonary hypertension
Evaluate presence of **diastolic heart sounds**		
Use bell of stethoscope—best for picking up low-pitched sounds Place lightly on chest with client in left side lying position	Quiet and low-pitched	
S_3 (ventricular gallop) Heard just after S_2, at the apex or at lower, left sternal border	May be a physiologic finding in children and young adults Abnormal finding in older clients	Almost always signifies heart failure in client over age 40
S_4 (atrial gallop) Heard just before S_1, at the apex or at lower, left sternal border; occurs when blood flow from atrial contraction meets increased resistance in ventricle	Normal finding in elderly	Heard in older individual with hypertension
Assess for **heart murmurs,** heard between heart sounds Produced by atypical flow of blood through the heart (e.g., irregularity or partial obstruction, increased flow in normal area, flow into dilated chamber, flow through abnormal passage); regurgitant flow Occurs during systole (between S_1 and S_2) or during diastole (between S_2 and S_1)	Faint sound More common during systole Often found in children and young adults	Faint or loud enough to be heard without a stethoscope Occurs during systole or diastole (diastolic murmurs are almost always pathologic)—found in older clients with heart disease or infants and children with congenital heart defects

Assessment	*Normal*	*Abnormal*
Evaluate the **apical pulse** when assessing for general heart rate and rhythm of contractions	Regular rhythm Heart rate: 60–100 beats/minute	Irregular rhythm (dysrhythmia) may be regularly irregular or irregularly irregular (i.e., atrial fibrillation)
Auscultate at the apex of the heart (left, fifth intercostal space at the midclavicular line)	Moderate bradycardia common in well-trained athletes	Bradycardia (less than 60 beats/minute)
Palpate and view pulse on chest wall if client's chest wall is thin enough	Mild tachycardia possible with stress, infection, or fever	Tachycardia (more than 100 beats/minute)
Assess for **irregular apical pulse** With another nurse, take apical and radial pulses *simultaneously*		
Compare beats per minute for both pulses	Equal apical and radial pulses = no pulse deficit	Fewer beats at the radial area may indicate an irregular apical pulse, producing ineffective pumping
Palpate **peripheral pulses:** radial, brachial, femoral, popliteal, dorsalis pedis, posterior tibial (For special cases, after carotid surgery, palpate temporal pulse also)	Easily palpated Equally strong on both sides Posterior tibial pulse usually weaker than femoral	Difficult to palpate Unequal pulses Weak pulse Absent pulses
Guidelines for palpating peripheral pulses: If pulse is not immediately palpable, examine adjacent area—pulse locations differ with clients		
Palpate weak pulses gently so that you do not obliterate pulse with too much pressure		
If you cannot differentiate your pulse from client's pulse, check your radial or carotid pulse, or observe monitor pattern		
When peripheral pulses cannot be palpated, use a Doppler ultrasound stethoscope and grade according to scale		

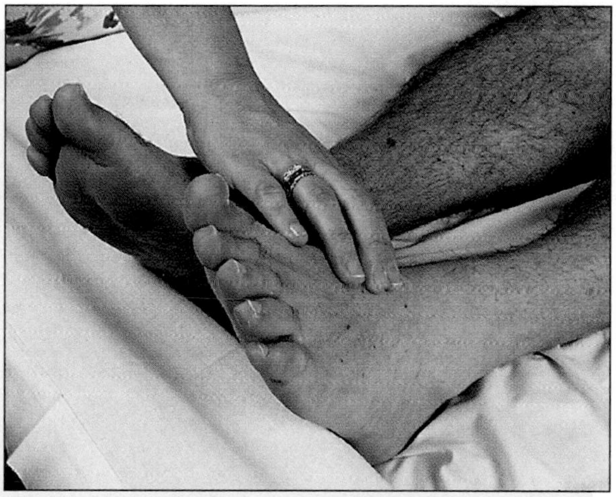
Palpate peripheral pulse, dorsalis pedis.

ASSESSMENT OF THE ABDOMEN, LIVER, AND GENITOURINARY TRACT

The abdomen extends from the diaphragm to the pelvis. Generally speaking, there are two body systems present in this area: the gastrointestinal system and the genitourinary system.

The gastrointestinal system begins at the mouth and consists of the esophagus, stomach, the small and large intestines, and associated organs that include the liver, pancreas, and spleen.

The urinary tract consists of the kidneys, ureters, bladder, and the urethra. The urinary tract should be assessed frequently and accurately because changes in urine production reflect changes in other body systems.

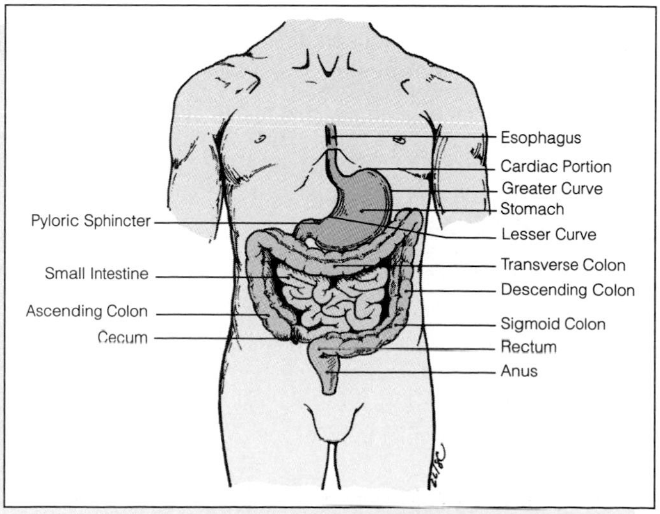

Assessment requires knowledge of abdominal organ anatomy.

The most common way to assess the urinary tract is to note the quantity and quality of the urinary output. Some medications or foods produce unusual odors and colors in urine (e.g., sulfasalazine [Azulfidine] turns urine a yellow-orange color; asparagus gives urine a musty odor).

External male genitalia include the penis, the scrotum, and the testicles. External female genitalia include the vulva, the urethral orifice, and the vagina.

ASSESSMENT OF THE ABDOMEN, LIVER, AND GENITOURINARY TRACT

Assessment	*Normal*	*Abnormal*
Abdomen		
Have client lie flat in bed At the client's abdominal level, inspect the **general contour** of the abdomen	Abdomen flat from chest to pubis with concave indentation at umbilicus	Scaphoid (concave) abdominal contour: due to inadequate nutritional intake to meet caloric need or inadequate food absorption Distended abdomen: caused by gas and fluid accumulation due to lack of peristalsis, hemorrhage, or intestinal leakage after trauma (e.g., auto accident or surgery), or ascitic fluid (e.g., liver or cardiac failure)
Inspect for bruising around umbilicus and over planks	No change of skin color around umbilicus or flanks	Acute abdomen
Observe for scars, stretch marks, dilated veins, presence of hernia	Correlate with health history	Dilated veins caused by liver disease Bulge seen with defect in abdominal wall
Assess **circumference** for intraabdominal hemorrhage or ascites by placing a tape measure around the largest circumference of the abdomen and drawing two lines around client's entire abdomen, one line at the top of the tape measure, one line at the bottom of the tape measure; perform measurement when client exhales	No increase in abdominal circumference	Abdominal circumference increases steadily within 1–2 hours
Auscultate abdomen to assess presence and quality of **bowel sounds**		
Place diaphragm of stethoscope firmly on right lower quadrant and count sounds for 1 minute	Bowel sounds gurgle, about 5–30 per minute	Increased bowel sounds: due to blood in GI tract, diarrhea, or to partial bowel obstruction (sounds become high-pitched and tinkling or come in "rushes," followed by silence as obstruction progresses)
Listen at all quadrants, near the center, for several minutes if sounds not heard initially	Varying frequency of sounds with clients and time of day (i.e., more sounds right before and after eating)	
	Decreased or absent bowel sounds after surgery After general anesthesia, normal sounds in 1–2 days	Bowel sounds hypoactive, quiet, and infrequent: may be due to peritonitis, paralytic ileus, or no obvious cause
	After abdominal surgery, normal sounds in 3–5 days	Absent bowel sounds: may be due to complete bowel obstruction or systemic illness

Assessment	*Normal*	*Abnormal*
Palpate abdomen to determine condition of **abdominal muscles** and organs beneath muscles Assist client to relax, lie flat in bed, and flex knees. Have client mouth-breathe	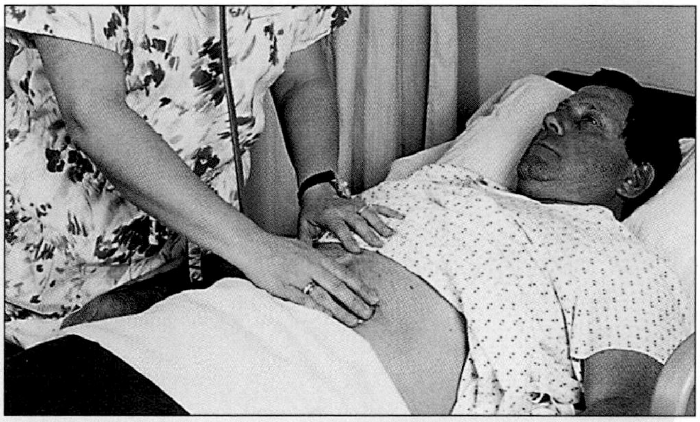 Palpate client's abdomen.	
Place your hand flat on client's abdomen, holding your four fingers together and depressing ½ inch	Soft, pliant musculature when relaxed	Rigid, tender muscles/pain produced with cough: may be due to presence of muscle spasm, inflammation or infection (peritonitis)
Have client cough to determine any areas of abdominal tenderness	Cough does not produce pain in abdomen	
Begin palpation at the pubis, moving upward. Palpate any problem areas last to minimize effects of discomfort Palpate all quadrants of abdomen to assess organs contained in each quadrant Superficial palpation: use slight pressure only	No bulges felt No masses felt	Pain or tenderness with quick release of pressure indicates rebound tenderness suggesting peritoneal inflammation If hernia is suspected, have client raise head and shoulders and observe for abdominal bulge
Deep palpation: indent the abdominal wall 4–5 cm—may use one hand over the other to apply pressure	No masses felt	Masses felt with colon disease, vascular aneurysm, dilated bowel, distended bladder, or cancer
Palpate **liver** by placing left hand behind 11th and 12th ribs with right hand on right abdomen lateral to rectus muscle	Normal liver (difficult to palpate) may feel like sharp ridge with smooth surface	Tenderness may be due to inflammation (hepatitis) Enlarged liver with nontender edge may be due to cirrhosis
Urinary Tract Assessment		
Assess the **external urethra**	Orifice is pink and moist; clear, minimal discharge	Burning or pain at urethral orifice: may indicate urinary infection
Assess the quantity, color, odor, specific gravity, and pH of **urine output**	Output: 1200–1500 mL/24 hours, or 30–50 mL/hour—should equal oral and IV intake	Increased output: may indicate increased intake, diuresis, potential diabetes mellitus, or inappropriate antidiuretic hormone (ADH) response (e.g., diabetes insipidus) Frequent small amounts of urine output indicate urinary retention or urinary tract infection Decreased output: may indicate dehydration, acute nephritis, cardiac disease, renal failure, or excess ADH response (e.g., head injury)

ASSESSMENT OF THE ABDOMEN, LIVER, AND GENITOURINARY TRACT (*continued*)

Assessment	*Normal*	*Abnormal*
	Clear, yellow-amber color (vegetarians may have slightly cloudy urine)	Cloudy (turbid): may indicate possible urinary tract infection Dark amber: may indicate very concentrated urine due to dehydration Dark amber to green: may indicate hepatitis or obstructive jaundice
	Slight odor (ammonia-like odor indicates that specimen has been sitting for some time)	Foul-smelling: may indicate urinary tract infection, drug or specific food ingestion (e.g., asparagus) Sweet odor: may indicate acetone from ketoacidosis (i.e., diabetes mellitus)
	Specific gravity: 1.003–1.030	Specific gravity of more than 1.030: indicates dehydration Constant specific gravity of 1.010, regardless of fluid intake: indicates renal failure
	pH range from 4.5–7.5; average is 6–7	Acidic pH—when below 6.0 may indicate starvation or acidosis Alkaline pH greater than 7.0: indicates metabolic alkalosis or alkaline ash diet (e.g., vegetarian)
Assess for **blood** in urine using Hemastix or Labstix	No blood present	Smokey to mildly pink-tinged to grossly red-colored urine: indicates blood in urine
Palpate for **bladder distention**	Not normally palpated	Distended bladder (firm, round mass) accompanied by discomfort and urge to void: indicates urine retention (common following surgery, where catheter is not used)
Assess for **pain**	No pain	Severe pain in the flank region (below rib cage posteriorly and lateral to spine): indicates kidney infection or stones
Genital Assessment		
Visually examine the **male genitalia** Retract the foreskin of the uncircumcised penis to note cleanliness, any **lesions,** and **discharge**	Clean No odor No lesions	Unclean Odor Lesions and discharge may indicate venereal disease or cancer
Lift scrotum to inspect for rash	No discharge Size of penis and scrotum vary	Oval and round, dark erosion: may indicate syphilitic chancre
Noting groin area, ask client to strain down	Urethra opens midline of the tip of the glans No bulges in groin area	Hypospadias: due to congenital displacement of the urethral meatus Bulge on straining seen with hernias Indurated nodule or ulcer: may indicate carcinoma
Using thumb and first two fingers, gently palpate each testicle for size, shape, and consistency	Two testicles in the scrotum No nodules felt, no swelling or tenderness	Mass in scrotum: indicates possible hernia, hydrocele, testicular tumor, or cyst Pain indicates inflammatory disease
Visually examine **female genitalia**	Clean No odor	Unclean Odor (musty with bacterial infection)
Assess for signs of sexual abuse	No signs	Bruises, welts, burns, unusual swelling

Assessment	*Normal*	*Abnormal*
Assess for **lesions** or **discharge** or complaints of itching	Minimal, clear discharge Menstrual flow Lochia (normal discharge after delivery) No lesions No pruritus	Thick; thin, white, yellowish, or green discharge: may indicate trichomoniasis Thick, white, and curdy discharge with pruritus may indicate candidiasis Lesions: could indicate syphilitic chancre, herpes infection, venereal wart, or carcinoma of vulva

MENTAL HEALTH ASSESSMENT

The mental assessment is completed throughout the physical assessment during the history taking. It is not generally considered a separate entity. Mood, memory, orientation, and thought processes can be evaluated while obtaining the health history. Nutritional preferences and restrictions can be determined as a part of a client care plan and may or may not be included in the general client assessment.

A spiritual assessment can be obtained as a part of the health history, although specific sociocultural beliefs may need to be ascertained separately. The purpose of a spiritual assessment is to facilitate the client adapting to the hospital environment and to help the staff understand stressors the client may be experiencing as a result of belief systems.*

The purpose of a mental status assessment is to evaluate the present state of psychologic functioning and to monitor safety needs of the client. It is not designed to make a diagnosis; rather it should yield data that contribute to the total picture of the client as he or she is functioning at the time the assessment is made.

The specific rationale for completing a mental status assessment is:

- To collect baseline data to aid in establishing the cause, diagnosis, and prognosis
- To evaluate the present state of psychologic functioning
- To evaluate changes in the individual's emotional, intellectual, motor, and perceptual responses
- To determine the client's ability to cope with the present situation
- To assess the need and availability of support systems
- To ascertain if some seemingly psychopathologic response is, in fact, a disorder of a sensory organ (i.e., a deaf person appearing hostile, depressed, or suspicious)
- To determine the guidelines of the treatment plan
- To document altered mental status for legal records

The initial factors that the nurse must consider in completing a mental status assessment are to correctly identify the client, the reason for admission, record of previous mental illness, present complaint, any personal history that is relevant (living arrangements, role in family, interactional experience, history of alcoholism, domestic violence), family history if appropriate, significant others and available support systems, assets, and interests.

The actual assessment process begins with an initial evaluation of the appropriateness of the client's behavior and orientation to reality. The assessment continues by noting any abnormal behavior and ascertaining the client's chief verbalized complaint. Finally, the evaluation determines if the client is in contact with reality enough to answer particular questions that further assess the client's condition.

**Note:* For more information on a spiritual–religious assessment, see Chapter 4.

MENTAL STATUS

Assessment	*Normal*	*Abnormal*
General Appearance, Manner, and Attitude		
Assess **physical appearance**	General body characteristics, energy level	Inappropriate physical appearance, high or low extremes of energy
Note **grooming,** mode of dress, and **personal hygiene**	Grooming and dress appropriate to situation, client's age, and social circumstance Clean	Poor grooming Inappropriate or bizarre dress or combination of clothes Unclean

MENTAL STATUS (*continued*)

Assessment	*Normal*	*Abnormal*
Note **posture**	Upright, straight, and appropriate	Slumped, tipped, or stooped
Note speed, pressure, pace, quantity, volume, and diction of **speech**	Moderated speed, volume, and quantity Appropriate diction	Tremors Accelerated or retarded speech and high quantity Poor or inappropriate diction
Note relevance, content, and organization of **responses**	Questions answered directly, accurately, and with relevance	Inappropriate responses, unorganized pattern of speech Tangential, circumstantial, or out-of-context replies
Expressive Aspects of Behavior		
Note **general motor activity**	Calm, ordered movement appropriate to situation	Overactive (e.g., restless, agitated, impulsive) Underactive (e.g., slow to initiate or execute actions)
Assess **purposeful movements and gestures** Assess style of **gait**	Reasonably responsive with purposeful movements, appropriate gestures	Repetitious activities (e.g., rituals or compulsions) Command automation Parkinsonian movements Ataxic, shuffling, off-balance gait
Consciousness		
Assess **level of consciousness**	Alert, attentive, and responsive Knowledgeable about time, place, and person	Disordered attention; distracted, cloudy consciousness Delirious Stuporous
Thought Processes and Perception		
Assess **coherency, logic,** and **relevance** of thought processes by asking questions about personal history (e.g., "Where were you born?" "What kind of work do you do?")	Clear, understandable responses to questions Attentiveness	Disoriented in time, place, person Disordered thought forms Autistic or dereistic (absorbed with self and withdrawn); abstract (absent-mindedness); concrete thinking (dogmatic, preaching)
Assess **reality orientation:** time, place, and person awareness	Orderly progression of thoughts based in reality Awareness of time, place, and person	Disorders of progression of thought; looseness, circumstantial, incoherent, irrelevant conversation, blocking Delusions of grandeur or persecution: neologisms, use of words whose meaning is known only to the client Echolalia (automatic repeating of questions) No awareness of day, time, place, or person
Assess **perceptions** and reactions to personal experiences by asking questions, such as "How do you see yourself now that you are in the hospital?" "What do you think about when you're in a situation like this?"	Thoughtful, clear responses expressed with understanding of self	Altered, narrowed, or expanded perception illusions Depersonalization

Assessment	Normal	Abnormal
Thought Content and Mental Trend		
Assess degree of anxiety Ask questions to determine general themes that identify **degree of anxiety** (e.g., "How are you feeling right now?" "What kinds of things make you afraid?")	Mild or 1+ level of anxiety in which individual is alert, motivated, and attentive	Moderate to severe (2+ to 4+) levels of anxiety
Assess **ideation** and **concentration**	Ideas based in reality Able to concentrate	Ideas of reference Hypochondria (abnormal concerns about health) Obsessional Phobias (irrational fears) Poor or shortened concentration
Mood or Affect		
Assess prevailing or **variability in mood** by observing behavior and asking questions, such as "How are you feeling right now?" Check for presence of abnormal **euphoria**	Appropriate, even mood without wide variations high to low	Cyclothymic mood swings; euphoria, elation, ecstasy, depressed, withdrawn
If you suspect **depression,** continue questioning to determine depth and significance of mood (e.g., "How badly do you feel?" "Have you ever thought of suicide?")	May be sad or grieving but mood does not persist indefinitely	Flat or dampened responses Inappropriate responses Ambivalence
Memory		
Assess **past and present memory** and **retention** (ability to listen and respond with understanding or knowledge); ask client to repeat a phrase (e.g., an address)	Alert, accurate responses Able to complete digit span Past and present memory appropriate	Hyperamnesia (excessive loss of memory); amnesia; paramnesia (belief in events that never occurred) Preoccupied Unable to follow directions
Assess **recall** (recent and remote) by asking questions, such as "When is your birthday?" "What year were you born?" "How old are you?" "Who is the president of the United States now?"	Good recall of immediate and past events	Poor recall of immediate or past events
Judgment		
Assess **judgment, decision-making ability,** and **interpretations** by asking questions, such as "What should you do if you hear a siren while you're driving?" "If you lost a library book, what would you do?"	Ability to make accurate decisions Realistic interpretation of events	Poor judgment, poor decision-making ability, poor choice Inappropriate interpretation of events or situations
Awareness		
Assess **insight,** the ability to understand the inner nature of events or problems, by asking questions, such as "If you saw someone dressed in a fur coat on a hot day, what would you think?"	Thoughtful responses indicating an understanding of the inner nature of an event or problem	Lack of insight or understanding of problems or situations Distorted view of situation

MENTAL STATUS (*continued*)

Assessment	*Normal*	*Abnormal*
Intelligence		
Assess **intelligence** by asking client to define or use words in sentences (e.g., recede, join, plural)	Correct responses to majority of questions	Incorrect responses to majority of questions indicate possible severe psychiatric disorders
Assess **fund of information** by asking questions, such as "Who is president of the United States?" "Who was the president before him?" "When is Memorial Day?" "What is a thermometer?" (Consider client's cultural and educational background and his or her grasp of English)	Correct responses to majority of questions	Deteriorated or impaired cognitive processes
Sensory Ability		
Assess the **five senses** (i.e., vision, hearing, taste, feeling, and smell)	Able to perceive, hear, feel, touch appropriate to stimulus	Lack of response Suspicious, hostile, depressed Kinesthetic imbalance
Developmental Level		
Assess **developmental level** compared with normal	Behavior and thought processes appropriate to age level	Wide span between chronologic and developmental age Mentally retarded
Lifestyle Patterns		
Identify **addictive patterns** and effect on individual's overall healthy	Normal amount of alcohol ingested Smoking habits, number of years Prescriptive medications Adequate food intake for physical characteristics	High quantity of alcohol taken frequently Heavy smoker Addicted to illegal drugs Habituative medication; user of over-the-counter or legal medications Anorexic eating patterns Obese or overindulgence of food
Coping Devices		
Identify **defense-coping mechanisms** and their effect on individual	Conscious coping mechanisms used appropriately, such as compensation, fantasy, rationalization, suppression, sublimation, or displacement Mechanisms effective, appropriate, and useful	Unconscious mechanisms used frequently, such as repression, regression, projection, reaction formation, insulation, or denial Mechanisms inappropriate, ineffective, and not useful

OBSTETRICAL ASSESSMENT

Assessment	*Normal*	*Abnormal*
Baseline Data		
Assess **breasts** and **nipples**		
Contour and size		
Presence of lumps	No lumps	Lumps
Secretions	Colostrum secretions in late first trimester or early second trimester	Secretions, other than colostrum

Assessment	Normal	Abnormal
Assess **abdomen**		
Contour and size		
Changes in skin color	*Linea nigra* (black line of pregnancy along midline of abdomen) Primiparas: coincidentally with growth of fundus Multiparas: after 13–15 weeks' gestation	
Striae (reddish-purple lines)	On breasts, hips, and thighs during pregnancy After pregnancy, faint silvery-gray	
Scar, rashes, or other skin disturbances	Usually none present	
Fundal height in centimeters (fingerbreadths less accurate): measure from symphysis pubis to top of fundus	Fundus palpable just above symphysis at 8–10 weeks Halfway between symphysis and umbilicus at 16 weeks Umbilicus at 20–22 weeks	Large measurements: EDC is incorrect; tumor; ascites; multiple pregnancy; polyhydramnios, hydatidiform mole Less than normal enlargement: fetal abnormality, oligohydramnios, placental dysmaturity, missed abortion, fetal death
Perineum: assess for scars, lesions, or discharge	None present	Rash, warts, discharge
Evaluate **weight**		
Take **vital signs, blood pressure** (BP), **temperature, pulse,** and **respiration** (TPR)		
Evaluate **lab findings**		
Urine: sugar, protein, albumin	Negative for sugar, protein, and albumin throughout pregnancy	Positive for sugar, protein, and/or albumin
Hematocrit (HCT)	38%–47%	
Hemoglobin (Hgb)	12–16 gm/dL	
Blood type and Rh factor		If Rh negative, father's blood should be typed If Rh positive, titers should be followed; possible RhoGAM at termination of pregnancy
Pap smear		
VD smears and screening		
Antepartum Assessment		
Evaluate **weight** to assess maternal health and nutritional status and growth of fetus	First trimester: 3–4 lbs Second trimester: 12–14 lbs Third trimester: 8–10 lbs Minimum weight gain during pregnancy: 24 lbs	Inadequate weight gain; possible maternal malnutrition Excessive weight gain: if sudden at onset, may indicate preeclampsia; if gradual and continual may indicate overeating
Evaluate **blood pressure**	Fairly constant with baseline data throughout pregnancy	Increased: possible anxiety (client should rest 20 to 30 minutes before you take BP again) Rise of 30/15 above baseline data: sign of preeclampsia Decreased: sign of supine hypotensive syndrome. If lying on back, turn client on left side and take BP again

OBSTETRICAL ASSESSMENT (*continued*)

Assessment	*Normal*	*Abnormal*
Evaluate **fundal height**	Drop around 38th week: sign of fetus engaging in birth canal Primipara: sudden drop Multipara: slower, sometimes not until onset of labor	Large fundal growth: may indicate wrong dates, multiple pregnancy, hydatidiform mole, polyhydramnios, tumors Small fundal growth: may indicate fetal demise, fetal anomaly, retarded fetal growth, abnormal presentation or lie, decreased amniotic fluid
Determine **fetal position,** using **Leopold's maneuvers.** Complete external palpations of the abdomen to determine fetal position, lie, presentation, and engagement		
First maneuver: to determine part of fetus presenting into pelvis	Vertex presentation	Breech presentation or transverse lie
Second maneuver: to locate the back, arms, and legs: fetal heart heard best over fetal back		
Third maneuver: to determine part of fetus in fundus		
Fourth maneuver: to determine degree of cephalic flexion and engagement		

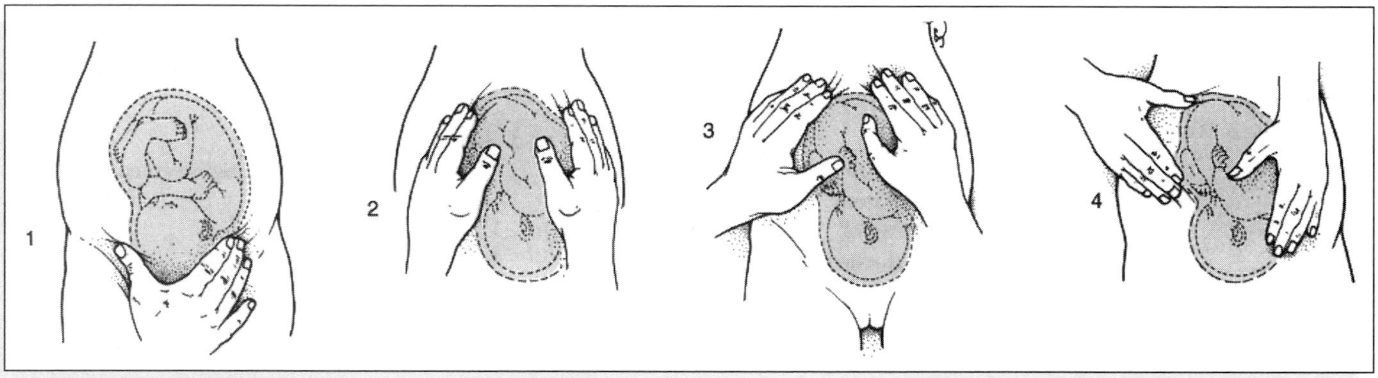

Steps of Leopold's maneuvers.

Assessment	*Normal*	*Abnormal*
Evaluate **fetal heart rate** by quadrant, location, and rate	120–160 beats/min	>160 or <120: may indicate fetal distress *Notify physician*
Check for presence of **edema**	In lower extremities toward end of pregnancy	In upper extremities and face: may indicate preeclampsia
Evaluate **urine** (clean catch midstream)	Negative for sugar, protein, and albumin	Positive for sugar: may indicate subclinical or gestational diabetes Positive for protein and/or albumin: may indicate preeclampsia
Evaluate **levels of discomfort**		
Intrapartum Assessment		
Assess for **lightening** and **dropping** (the descent of the presenting part into the pelvis)	Several days to 2 weeks before onset of labor Multipara: may not occur until onset of labor Relief of shortness of breath and increase in urinary frequency	No lightening or dropping: may indicate disproportion between fetal presenting part and maternal pelvis

Assessment	*Normal*	*Abnormal*
Check if **mucous plug** has been expelled from cervix	Usually expelled from cervix prior to onset of labor	
Assess for **"bloody show"**	Clear, pinkish, or blood-tinged vaginal discharge that occurs as cervix begins to dilate and efface	
Assess for **ruptured membranes**		
Time water breaks	Before, during, or after onset of labor	Breech presentation: frank meconium or meconium staining
Color of **amniotic fluid**	Clear, straw color	Greenish-brown: indicates meconium has passed from fetus, possible fetal distress Yellow-stained: fetal hypoxia 36 hours or more prior to rupture of membrane or hemolytic disease
Quantity of amniotic fluid	Normal is 500 to 1000 mL of amniotic fluid, rarely expelled at one time	**Polyhydramnios**—excessive amniotic fluid over 2000 mL Observe newborn for congenital anomalies: craniospinal malformation, orogastrointestinal anomalies. Down's syndrome, and congenital heart defects **Oligohydramnios**—minimal amniotic fluid, less than 500 mL Observe newborn for malformation of ear, genitourinary tract anomalies, and renal agenesis
Odor of fluid	No odor	Odor may indicate infection; deliver within 24 hours
Fetal heart rate	120–160 beats/min Regular rhythm	Decreased: indicates fetal distress with possible cord prolapse or cord compression Accelerated: initial sign of fetal hypoxia Absent: may indicate fetal demise
Labor and Delivery Assessment		
Evaluate Contractions		
Frequency: from start of one contraction to start of next	3–5 minutes between contractions	Irregular contractions with long intervals between: indicates false labor
Duration: from beginning of contraction to time uterus begins to relax	50–90 seconds	>90 seconds: uterine tetany; stop oxytocin if running
Intensity (strength of contraction): measured with monitoring device	Peak 25 mm Hg End of labor may reach 50–75 mm Hg	>75 mm Hg: uterine tetany or uterine rupture
First-Stage		
Latent phase (0–4 cm dilation)	0–3 to 4 cm; average 6.4 hrs	Prolonged time in any phase: may indicate poor fetal position, incomplete fetal flexion, cephalopelvic disproportion, or poor uterine contractions
Active phase (4–8 cm)		
Transitional phase (8–10 cm)	Length of time varies—may be 1–2 hours	If total labor <3 hours: indicates precipitous labor, increasing risk of fetal complications, or maternal lacerations and tears
Assess for **bloody show**		
Observe for presence of **nausea or vomiting**		
Assess **perineum**	Beginning to bulge	

OBSTETRICAL ASSESSMENT (*continued*)

Assessment	*Normal*	*Abnormal*
Evaluate **urge to bear down**		Often uncontrolled Multipara: can cause precipitous delivery "Panting" (can be controlled until safe delivery area established)
Second stage (10 cm to delivery)	Primipara: up to 2 hours Multipara: several minutes to 2 hours	>2 hours: increased risk of fetal brain damage and maternal exhaustion
Assess for **presenting part**	Vertex with ROA or LOA presentation	Occiput posterior, breech, face, or transverse lie
Assess **caput** (infant head) Multipara: move to delivery room when caput size of dime Primipara: move to delivery room when caput size of half dollar	Visible when bearing down during contraction	"Crowns" in room other than delivery room: delivery imminent (do not move client)
Assess **fetal heart rate** Bradycardia, drop of 20 beats/min below base line (↓120 beats/min) Tachycardia, increase in FHR over 160 beats/min for 10 min	120–160/min	Decreased: may indicate supine hypotensive syndrome (turn client on side and take again) Hemorrhage (check for other signs of bleeding: notify physician) Increased or decreased: may indicate fetal distress secondary to cord progression or compression (place client in Trendelenburg's or knee–chest position; give oxygen if necessary; inform physician)
Evaluate **fetal heart rate tracing**	Short-term variability is present Long-term variability ranges from 3–5 cycles/min	Absence of variability (no short term or long term present) Severe variable decelerations (fetal heart rate <70 for longer than 30–45 seconds with decreasing variability)
Deceleration	Early deceleration (10–20 beat drop) Recovery when acme contraction passes—often not serious	Monitor closely—distinguish from late deceleration (10–20 beat decrease with hypertonic contraction); leads to fetal distress
Variable deceleration; decrease in FHR, below 120/min	Mild; may be within normal parameters—continue to monitor	Cord compression—may result in fetal difficulty
Loss of beat-to-beat variation	If continues less than 15 minutes, no problem apparent	Late deceleration pattern occurs—monitor for hypertonic contraction; leads to fetal distress
Evaluate **breathing**	Controlled with contractions	Heavy or excessive: may lead to hyperventilation and/or dehydration
Evaluate **pain** and **anxiety**	Medication required after dilated 4–5 cm unless using natural childbirth methods	Severe pain early in first stage of labor: inadequate prenatal teaching, backache due to position in bed, uterine tetany
Third stage (from delivery of baby to delivery of placenta)	Placental separation occurs within 30 minutes (usually 3–5 min)	Failure of placental separation Abnormality of uterus or cervix, weak, ineffectual uterine contraction, tetanic contractions causing closure of cervix >3 hours: indicates retained placenta
Fourth stage (first hour postpartum)		Mother in unstable condition (hemorrhage usual cause)

Assessment	Normal	Abnormal
		Highest risk of hemorrhage in first postpartum hour
Temperature	36.5°C–37.5°C	>37.5°C: may indicate infection Slight elevation: due to dehydration from mouth breathing and NPO
Pulse	Pulse: 60–100	Increased: may indicate pain or hemorrhage
Respiration	Respirations: 12–22	
Blood pressure	Blood pressure: 140–120/80	Increased: may indicate anxiety, pain, or posteclamptic condition Decreased: hemorrhage
Postpartum Assessment		
Assess **vital signs** every 15 minutes for 1 hour, every 30 minutes for 1 hour, every hour for 4 hours, every 8 hours, and as needed	Pulse may be 45–60/min in stage 4 Pulse to normal range about third day	Decreased BP and increased pulse: probably postpartum hemorrhage Elevated temperature >38°C indicates possible infection Temperature elevates when lactation occurs
Assess **fundus** every 15 minutes for 1 hour, every 8 hours for 48 hours, then daily	Firm (like a grapefruit) in midline and at or slightly above umbilicus Return to prepregnant size in 6 weeks: descending at rate of 1 fingerbreadth/day	Boggy fundus: immediately massage gently until firm; report to physician and observe closely; empty bladder; medicate with oxytocin if ordered Fundus misplaced 1–2 fingerbreadths from midline: indicates full bladder (client must void or be catheterized)
Assess **lochia** every 15 minutes for 1 hour, every 8 hours for 48 hours, then daily		
Color	3 days postpartum: dark red (rubra) 4–10 days postpartum: clear pink (serosa) 10–21 days postpartum: white, yellow brown (alba)	Heavy, bright-red: indicates hemorrhage (massage fundus, give medication on order, notify physician) Spurts: may indicate cervical tear No lochia: may indicate clot occluding cervical opening (support fundus; express clot)
Quantity	Moderate amount, steadily decreases	Foul: may indicate infection
Odor	Minimal	
Assess **breasts** and **nipples** daily	Days 1–2: soft, intact, secreting colostrum Days 2–3: engorged, tender, full, tight, painful Day 3+: secreting milk Increased pains as baby sucks: common in multiparas	Sore or cracked (clean and dry nipples; decrease breast-feeding time; apply breast shield between feeding) Milk does not "let down": help client relax and decrease anxiety; give glass of wine or beer if not culturally, religiously, or otherwise contraindicated
Assess **perineum** daily	Episiotomy intact, no swelling, no discoloration	Swelling or bruising: may indicate hematoma
Assess **bladder** every 4 hours	Voiding regularly with no pain	Not voiding: bladder may be full and displaced to one side, leading to increased lochia (catheterization may be necessary)
Assess **bowels**	Spontaneous bowel movement 2–3 days after delivery	Fear associated with pain from hemorrhoids

OBSTETRICAL ASSESSMENT (*continued*)

Assessment	*Normal*	*Abnormal*
Assess mother–infant **bonding**	Touching infant, talking to infant, talking about infant	Refuses to touch or hold infant
Evaluate **Rh-negative status**	Client does not require RhoGAM	RhoGAM administered
Maternal History: Definition of Terms		
Abortion: pregnancy loss before fetus is viable (usually <20 weeks or 500 g) *Gravida:* any pregnancy, including present one	*Multigravida:* refers to second or any subsequent pregnancy *Para:* past pregnancies that continued to viable age (20 weeks); infants may be alive or dead at birth	*Nullipara:* refers to female who has never carried pregnancy to viable age for fetus *Multipara:* refers to female who has given birth to two or more viable infants; either alive or dead
Primigravida: refers to first-time pregnancy	*Primipara:* refers to female who has delivered first viable infant; born either alive or dead	

NEWBORN ASSESSMENT

Assessment	*Normal*	*Abnormal*
Skin Assessment		
Note skin **color** and **lesions**	Pink Mongolian spots Capillary hemangiomas on face or neck Localized edema in presenting part Cheesy white vernix Desquamation (peeling off) Milia (small white pustules over nose and chin) Jaundice after 24 hours; gone by second week	Cyanosis, pallor, beefy red Petechiae, ecchymoses, or purpuric spots: signs of possible hematologic disorder Café au lait spots (patches of brown discoloration): possible sign of congenital neurological disorder Raised capillary hemangiomas on areas other than face or neck Edema of peritoneal wall Poor skin turgor: indicates dehydration Yellow discolored vernix (meconium stained) Impetigo neonatorum (small pustules with surrounding red areas) Jaundice at birth or within 12 hours Dermal sinuses (opening to brain) Holes along spinal column Low hairline posteriorly: possible chromosomal abnormality Sparse or spotty hair: congenital goiter or chromosomal abnormality
Note color of **nails**	Pink	Yellowing of nail beds (meconium stained)
Note **skin tone**	Strong, tremulous	Flaccid, convulsions Muscular twitching, hypertonicity
Head and Neck Assessment		
Note **shape of head**	Fontanels: anterior open until 18 months; posterior closed shortly after birth	Depressed, fontanels indicate dehydration; closed or bulging indicate congenital anomalies; full or bulging indicate edema Cephalohematoma that crosses the midline Microcephaly and macrocephaly

Assessment	Normal	Abnormal
Assess **eyes**	Slight edema of lids	Purulent discharge Lateral upward slope of eye with an inner epicanthal fold in infants not of Asian descent Exophthalmos (bulging of eyeball): may be congenital anomaly, sign of congenital glaucoma or thyroid abnormality Enophthalmos (recession of eyeball): may indicate damage to brain or cervical spine
	Pupils equal and reactive to light by 3 weeks of age Intermittent strabismus (occasional crossing of eyes)	Constricted pupil, unilateral dilated fixed pupil, nystagmus (rhythmic nonpurposeful movement of eyeball): continuous strabismus
	Conjunctival or scleral hemorrhages	Haziness of cornea
	Symmetrical light reflex (light reflects off each eye in the same quadrant): sign of conjugate gaze	Absence of red reflex; asymmetrical light reflex
Note **placement of ears,** shape and position		Low-set ears: may indicate chromosomal or renal system abnormality
Assess **nose**	Discharge, sneezing	Thick, bloody nasal discharge
Assess **mouth**	Sucking, rooting reflexes	Cleft lip, palate
	Retention cysts	Flat, white nonremovable spots (thrush)
	Occasional vomiting	Frequent vomiting: may indicate pyloric stenosis Vomitus with bile: fecal vomiting Profuse salivation: may indicate tracheoesophageal fistula
Assess **neck**	Tonic neck reflex (Fencer's position)	Distended neck veins Fractured clavicle Unusually short neck Excess posterior cervical skin Resistance to neck flexion
Assess **cry**	Lusty cry	Weak, groaning cry: possible neurological abnormality High-pitched cry: newborn drug withdrawal; hoarse or crowing inspirations; catlike cry: possible neurological or chromosomal abnormality
Chest and Lung Assessment		
Assess **chest**	Circular Enlargement of breasts Milky discharge from breasts	Depressed sternum Retractions, asymmetry of chest movements: indicates respiratory distress and possible pneumothorax
Assess **respirations/lungs**	Abdominal respirations	Thoracic breathing, unequal motion of chest, rapid grasping or grunting respirations, flaring nares
	Respiration rate: 30 to 50	Deep sighing respirations
	Respiration movement irregular in rate and depth	Grunt on expiration: possible respiratory distress
	Resonant chest (hollow sound on percussion)	Hyper-resonance of chest or decreased resonance

NEWBORN ASSESSMENT (*continued*)

Assessment	Normal	Abnormal
Heart Assessment		
Assess the **rate, rhythm,** and **murmurs** of the heart	Rate: 100–160 at birth; stabilizes at 120–140	Heart rate >200 or <100
	Regular rhythm	Irregular rhythm
	Murmurs: significance cannot usually be determined in newborn	Dextrocardia, enlarged heart
Abdomen and Gastrointestinal Tract Assessment		
Assess the **abdomen**	Prominent	Distention of abdominal veins: possible portal vein obstruction
Assess the **gastrointestinal tract**	Bowel sounds present	Visible peristaltic waves Increased pitch or frequency: intestinal obstruction Decreased sounds: paralytic ileus Distention of abdomen
	Liver 2 to 3 cm below right costal margin	Enlarged liver or spleen
	Spleen tip palpable	Midline suprapubic mass: may indicate Hirschsprung's disease
	Umbilical cord with one vein and two arteries	One artery present in umbilical cord: may indicate other anomalies
	Soft granulation tissue at umbilicus	Wet umbilical stump or fetid odor from stump
Genitourinary Tract Assessment		
Assess **kidneys and bladder**	May be able to palpate kidneys	Enlarged kidney
	Bladder percussed 1 to 4 cm above symphysis pubis	Distended bladder; presence of any masses
Assess the **genitalia**	Edema and bruising after delivery	Inguinal hernia
	Unusually large clitoris in females a short time after birth	Ambiguous genitalia (chromosomal abnormality)
	Vaginal mucoid or bloody discharge may be present in the first week	
Urethral orifice	Urethra opens on ventral surface of penile shaft	Hypospadias (urethra opens on the inferior surface of the penis) Epispadias (urethra opens on the dorsal surface of the penis) Ulceration of urethral orifice
Testes	Testes in scrotal sac or inguinal canal	Hydroceles in males
Spine and Extremities Assessment		
Assess the **spine**	Straight spine	Spina bifida, pilonidal sinus; scoliosis
Assess **extremities**		Asymmetry of movement
	Soft click with thigh rotation	Sharp click with thigh rotation: indicates possible congenital hip Uneven major gluteal folds: indicates possible congenital hip Polydactyly (extra digits on a hand or foot); syndactyly (webbing or fusion of fingers or toes)
Assess **anus and rectum**	Patent anus	Closed anus: no meconium

TABLE 11–2 Apgar Scoring

Sign	0	1	2
Heart rate	Absent	Slow (less than 100)	Over 100
Respiratory effort	Absent	Slow, irregular	Good, crying
Muscle tone	Flaccid	Some flexion of extremities	Active motion
Reflex irritability	No response	Cry	Vigorous cry
Color	Blue, pale	Body pink, extremities blue	Completely pink

Apgar scoring system is a method of evaluating a newborn's condition at 1 and 5 minutes after birth.

- Newborns who score 7–10 are considered free of immediate danger.
- Newborns who score 4–6 are moderately depressed.
- Newborns who score 0–3 are severely depressed.

Scores less than 7 at 5 minutes, repeat every 5 minutes for 20 minutes. Infant may be intubated unless 2 successive scores of 7 or more occur.

PEDIATRIC ASSESSMENT

Assessment	*Normal*	*Abnormal*
Measurements		
Measure **height** and **weight** and plot on a standardized growth chart	Height/weight proportional Sequential measurements: pattern follows normal growth curves	Height/weight below fifth percentile Sudden drop in percentile range of height and/or weight: possible sign of disease process or congenital problem Sudden and persistent increase (above 95th percentile)
Assess **temperature** (axillary or tympanic until 6 years of age)	Axillary 36.5°–37.5°C (97.7°F) Elevations following eating or playing not unusual Rectal 36.6°–37.2°C (97.8°F)	Temperature of 104°–105°F: corresponds roughly with 101°–102°F in an adult Large daily temperature variations Hypothermia: usually result of chilling
Measure **circumference of head and chest** Examine or check circumferences when child is less than 2 years old Compare measurements with standardized charts	Head at birth: about 2 cm greater than chest During first year: equalization of head and chest After 2 years: rapid growth of chest; slight increase in size of head	Increase in head circumference greater than 2.5 cm per month: sign of hydrocephalus
Assess **pulse** apically	Birth–1 year: 100–180 1 year: 80–150 2 years: 80–130 3 years: 80–120 Over 3 years: 70–110	Pulse over 180 *at rest* after first month of life: cardiac or respiratory condition Inability to palpate or very weak femoral and pedal pulses: possible coarctation of the aorta

PEDIATRIC ASSESSMENT (*continued*)

Assessment	*Normal*	*Abnormal*
Assess **respirations**	Birth: 30–50 6 years: 20–25 Puberty: 14–16 (Young children have abnormally high respiration rate with even slight excitement)	Consistent tachypnea: usually a sign of respiratory distress Respiratory rate over 100; lower respiratory tract obstruction Slow rate: may be sign of CNS depression
Assess **blood pressure**	Birth: 55–60/80–90 1 year: 90–60 Rise in both pressures: 2–3 points per year of age Adult level reached at puberty	Elevated blood pressure in upper extremities *and* decrease in lower extremities: coarctation of aorta Narrowed pulse pressure (normal or elevated diastolic with lowered systolic; less than 30 points difference between systolic and diastolic readings): possible sign of aortic or subaortic stenosis or hypothyroidism Widened pulse pressure: possible sign of hyperthyroidism
Appearance		
Observe **general appearance**	Alert, well-nourished, comfortable, responsive	Lethargic, uncomfortable, malnourished, gross anomalies, dull
Listen to **voice and cry**	Strong, lusty cry	Weak cry, low- or high-pitched cry: may indicate neurological problem or chromosomal abnormality Stridor: possible upper airway edema or obstruction or hoarse cry
	Facial expression animated No indications of pain	Expressionless, unresponsive Doubling over, rubbing a body part, general fretfulness, irritability
Assess presence of **odor**	No odor	Musty odor: sign of phenylketonuria, diphtheria Odor of maple syrup: may be maple syrup urine disease Odor of sweaty feet: one type of acidemia Fishy odor: may be metabolic disorder Acetone odor: acidosis, particularly diabetic ketoacidosis
Skin Assessment		
Assess **pigmentation**	Usually even Pigmented nevi common Large, flat, black and blue areas over sacrum, buttocks (mongolian spots)	Multiple cafe au lait spots: possible neurofibromatosis Cyanosis Jaundice Pallor
Assess **lesions**	Usually none Adolescence: acne	Erythematous lesions Multiple macules, papules, or vesicles Petechiae and ecchymoses: may indicate coagulation disorder
Assess **signs/symptoms of abuse**	None present	Hives (allergy) Subcutaneous nodules: may indicate juvenile rheumatoid arthritis Any unexplained bruises, welts, scars, burn marks, rope marks, failure to thrive, x-ray findings of multiple bone injuries, passive, noncommunicating child

Assessment	*Normal*	*Abnormal*
Note **consistency of skin**	Good turgor Smooth and firm Check fontanel in infant	Poor turgor Dryness Edema Lack or excess of subcutaneous fat: sign of malnutrition or excess nutrition (obesity)
Assess **nails**	Nailbeds: normally pigmented Good nail growth	Cyanosis Pallor Capillary pulsations Pitting of the nails: possible sign of fungal disease or psoriasis Broad nailbeds: possible sign of Down's syndrome or other chromosomal abnormality
Assess **hair** (consistency appropriate to ethnic group)	No excessive breaking Consistent growth pattern	Dry, coarse, brittle hair: possible sign of hypothyroidism Alopecia (loss of hair): may be psychosomatic or due to drug therapy Unusual hairiness in places other than scalp, eyebrows, and lashes: may indicate hypothyroidism, vitamin A poisoning, chronic infections, reaction to Dilantin therapy Tufts of hair over spine or sacrum: may indicate site of spina bifida occulta or spina bifida Absence of the start of pubic hair during adolescence: possible hypothyroidism, hypopituitarism, gonadal deficiency, or Addison's disease
Assess **lymph nodes**	Nontender, movable, discrete nodes up to 3 mm in diameter in occipital, postauricular, parotid, sub-maxillary, sublingual, axillary, and epitrochlear nodes Up to 1 mm in diameter inguinal and cervical nodes	Tender or enlarged nodes: may be sign of systemic infection
Head and Neck Assessment		
Assess **scalp**	Usually without lesions	Ringworm, lice
Assess frontal and maxillary **sinuses**	Nontender	Tenderness: indicative of inflammatory process Seborrheic dermatitis
Assess **face**	Symmetrical movement	Asymmetry: signs of facial paralysis Twitching: could be due to psychosomatic causes; vitamin/mineral deficiency
Evaluate the eyes Gross screening of vision Snellen chart	With younger child, ability to focus and follow movement and to see objects placed a few feet away	Inability to follow movement or to see objects placed a few feet away
Sclerae	Completely white	Yellow sclera: sign of jaundice Blue sclera: may be normal or indicative of osteogenesis imperfecta

PEDIATRIC ASSESSMENT (*continued*)

Assessment	*Normal*	*Abnormal*
Placement in eye socket	Normally placed	Exophthalmos (protrusion of eyeball) Enophthalmos (deeply placed eyeball)
Iris	At rest: upper and lower margins of iris visible between the lids	Setting sun sign (iris appears to be beneath lower lid): if marked, may be sign of increased intracranial pressure or hydrocephalus
Movement	In newborn, intermittent strabismus or nystagmus	Fixed strabismus or intermittent strabismus continuing after 6 months of age: indication of muscle paralysis or weakness Involuntary, repetitive oscillations of one or both eyes: normal with *extreme* lateral gaze Nystagmus: may be cerebellar dysfunction indicative of use of certain drugs (anticonvulsants, barbiturates, alcohol)
Eyelids	Fully covers eye Fully raised on opening	Ptosis of eyelid: may be an early sign of a neurological disorder Sty
Conjunctiva	Clear	Inflammation (conjunctivitis) Hemorrhage Stimson's lines (small red transverse lines on conjunctiva)
Cornea	Clear	Opacity: sign of ulceration Inflammation Redness
Discharge	Tears	Purulent discharges: note amount, color, consistency (bacterial conjunctivitis)
Pupils	Round, regular Clear, equal Brisk reaction to light Accommodation reflex (ability of lens to adjust to objects at different distances)	Sluggish or asymmetrical reaction to light: indicates intracranial disease Lack of accommodation reflex
Lens	Clear	Opacities (cataracts)
Evaluate the **ears**		
Sinuses	No abnormality	Small holes or pits anterior to ear: may be superficial but could indicate the presence of a sinus leading into brain
Position	Top of ear above level of eye	Top of ear below level of eye: associated with some congenital defects
Discharge	None	Discharge: note color, odor, consistency, and amount
Hearing	In infant: turning to sound In older child: responds to whispered command	Diminished hearing in one or both ears
Assess the **nose**	No secretions	Secretions: note characteristics Any unusual shape or flaring of nostrils
	Breathing through nose	Breathing through mouth
Assess the **mouth**		Circumoral pallor: possible sign of cyanotic heart disease, scarlet fever, rheumatic fever, hypoglycemia; also seen in other febrile diseases

Assessment	Normal	Abnormal
		Asymmetry of lips: seen in nerve paralysis
	Intact palate	Cleft palate
	Teeth in good condition	Delayed appearance of deciduous teeth: may indicate cretinism, rickets, congenital syphilis, or Down's syndrome; may also be normal
	In older child presence of permanent teeth	Poor tooth formation: may be seen with systemic diseases
		Green or black teeth: seen after iron ingestion or death of tooth
		Stained teeth: may be seen after prolonged use of tetracyclines
Assess the **gums**	Retention cysts in newborn	Inflammation, abnormal color, drooling, pus, tenderness
		Black line along gums: may indicate lead poisoning
Assess the **tongue**	Moves freely	Tremors on protrusion: may indicate chorea, hypothyroidism, cerebral palsy
		Protruding tongue—Down's syndrome
		White spots (thrush)
		Tongue-tie (frenulum)
	Pink, with conical, filiform nontender papillae	Strawberry tongue (scarlet fever)
Assess the **throat**	Tonsils normally enlarged in childhood	White membrane over tonsils (diphtheria)
		White pus on sacs, erythema (bacterial pharyngitis), tender: vitamin deficiencies, anemia
Assess the **larynx**	Normal vocal tones	Hoarseness or stridor: possible upper respiratory tract obstruction
Assess the **neck**	Short in infancy	
	Lengthens at 2–3 years	
	Trachea slightly right of midline	Trachea deviated to left or right: may indicate shift with atelectasis
Thyroid	Not enlarged	Enlarged: may be due to hyperactive thyroid, malignancy, goiter
Movement	Full lateral and upward/downward motion	Limited movement with pain: may indicate meningeal irritation, lymph node enlargement, rheumatoid arthritis, or other diseases
Lungs and Thorax Assessment		
Assess the **lungs**	Normally clear and equal breath sounds bilaterally	Presence of rhonchi, crackles, or wheezes
		Diminished breath sounds heard over parts of lung
	No retractions	Mild to severe intercostal or sternal retractions indicative of respiratory distress
	Symmetry of diaphragmatic movement	Asymmetry of movement (phrenic nerve damage)
Assess the **sputum**	None or small amount of clear sputum in morning	Thick, tenacious sputum with foul odor
		Blood-tinged or green sputum
Assess the **breasts**	Slightly enlarged in infancy	Discharge or growth in male
	Generally slightly asymmetrical at puberty	Masses (especially solid, fixed nonmobile) in older adolescent

PEDIATRIC ASSESSMENT (continued)

Assessment	Normal	Abnormal
Heart Assessment		
Assess **heart sounds**	S_1, S_2, S_3	S_4 indicates congestive heart failure
Assess **femoral pulses**	Strong	Weak
Note **edema**	None present	Edema—note location (initially periorbital) and duration, bulging fontanelles
Note **clubbing** of fingers	None present	Clubbing—congenital cyanotic heart defects; note location and duration
Note **murmurs**		Murmur grade three or higher is always abnormal No change in quality with positional changes
Note **cyanosis**	None normally present	Circumoral or peripheral cyanosis: indicates respiratory or cardiac disease (hypoxemia); congenital heart defects
Abdomen Assessment		
Assess **skin condition**	Soft	Hard, rigid, tender
Assess for **peristaltic motion**	Not visible	Visible peristalsis—may indicate pyloric stenosis (olive-shaped mass, palpable, in area of pyloris)
Assess **shape**	"Pot-bellied" toddlers Slightly protuberant in standing adolescent	Large protruding abdomen: may indicate pancreatic fibrosis, hypokalemia, rickets, hypothyroidism, bowel obstruction, constipation, inguinal hernias, unilateral or bilateral: observe for reducibility
	Umbilical protrusion	Umbilical hernia
Genitourinary Tract Assessment		
Assess **female genitalia**		
Discharge	Mucoid, no odor	Foul or copious discharge; any bleeding prior to puberty
Assess **male genitalia**	Orifice on distal end of penis	Hypospadias or epispadias (urethral orifice along inferior or dorsal surface)
Presence of urethral orifice		
Urethral opening	Normal size	Stenosis of urethral opening
Foreskin	Covers glans completely	Foreskin incompletely formed ventrally when hypospadias present
Placement of testes	Descended testes	Undescended testes Enlarged scrotum
Signs of abuse	No signs	Bruises, welts, swelling
Assess **urine output**	Full, steady stream of urine	Urine with pus, blood, or odor (infection) Excessive urination or nocturia: possible sign of diabetes
Check **anus and rectum**	No masses or fissures present	Hemorrhoids, fissures, prolapse, pinworms Dark ring around rectal mucosa: may be sign of lead poisoning
Musculoskeletal Assessment		
Assess **extremities**	Coloration of fingers and toes consistent with rest of body	Cyanosis—indicates respiratory or cardiac disease, or hypothermia in newborn Clubbing of fingers and toes indicates cardiac or respiratory disease

Assessment	Normal	Abnormal
	Quick capillary refill on blanching	Sluggish blood return on blanching indicates poor circulation
	Temperature same as rest of body	Temperature variation between extremities and rest of body indicates neurological or vascular anomalies
	Presence of pedal pulses	Absence of pedal pulses indicates circulatory difficulties
	No pain or tenderness	Presence of localized or generalized pain
	Straight legs after 2 years of age	Any bowing after 2 years of age may be hereditary or indicate rickets
	Broad-based gait until 4 years of age; feet straight ahead afterwards	Scissoring gait indicates spastic cerebral palsy Persistence of broad-based gait after 4 years of age indicates possible abnormalities of legs and feet or balance disturbance Any limp or ataxia
Assess **spine**	No dimples	Presence of dimple or tufts of hair indicates possible spina bifida
	Flexible	Limited flexion indicates central nervous system infections Hyperextension (opisthotonos) indicates brain stem irritation, hemorrhage, or intracranial infection
Have child bend forward at waist and check level of scapulae (scoliosis screening)	No lateral curvature or excessive anterior posterior curvature Scapulae at same height	Presence of lordosis (after age 2 years), kyphosis, or scoliosis
Assess **hips**		Asymmetrical thigh folds, clicks on adduction—hip dysplasia
Assess **joints**	Full range of motion without pain, edema, or tenderness	Pain, edema, or tenderness indicates tissue injury
Assess **muscles**	Good tone and purposeful movement	Decreased or increased tone
	Ability to perform motor skills approximate to development level	Spasm or tremors may indicate cerebral palsy Atrophy or contractures

Gerontologic Considerations

Head and Neck and Neurologic System

Physiologic Changes with Age

- Decreased speed of nerve conduction and delay in response and reaction time, especially with stress.
- Diminution of sensory faculties; decreased vision, loss of hearing, diminished sense of smell and taste, greater sensitivity to temperature changes with low tolerance to cold.
- Tooth loss.
- Poor dentition, inadequate chewing, poor swallowing reflex.
- Condition of teeth, gums, buccal cavity.
- Periodontal disease.

Taste sensation decreases.

- Chronic irritation of mucous membranes.
- Atrophy of up to 80% of taste buds.
- Loss of sensitivity of those on tip of tongue first: sweet and salt.
- Loss of sensitivity of those on sides later: salt, sour, bitter.

Assessment

- Facial symmetry.
- Poor reflex reactions.
- Level of alertness—presence of organic brain changes: memory impairment.
- Motor function—strength.

Skin

Physiologic Changes with Age

Skin less effective as barrier.

- Decreased protection from trauma.
- Less ability to retain water.
- Decreased temperature regulation.

Skin composition changes.

- Dryness (osteotosis) due to decreased endocrine secretion.
- Loss of elastin.
- Increased vascular fragility.
- Thicker and more wrinkled on sun-exposed areas.
- Melanocyte cluster pigmentation.

Sweat glands.

- Decreased number and size.
- Decreased function of sebaceous glands.

Hair

- General hair loss.
- Decreased melanin production.
- Facial hair increases in women.

Nails more brittle and thick.

Assessment

Skin.

- Temperature, degree of moisture, dryness.
- Intactness, open lesions, tears, decubiti.
- Turgor, dehydration.
- Pigmentation alterations, potential cancer.
- Pruritus—dry skin most common cause.

Bruises, scars.

Condition of nails (hard and brittle).

- Presence of fungus.
- Overgrown or horny toenails, ingrown.

Condition of hair.

Infestations (scabies, lice).

Chest

Physiologic Changes with Age

Respiratory muscles lose strength and become rigid.

Ciliary activity decreases.

Lungs lose elasticity.

- Residual capacity increases.
- Larger on inspiration.
- Maximum breathing capacity decreases; depth of respirations decreases.

Alveoli increase in size, reduce in number.

- Fewer capillaries at alveoli.
- Dilated and less elastic alveoli.

Gas exchange is reduced.

- Arterial blood oxygen Pa_{O_2} decreases to 75 mm Hg at age 70.
- Arterial blood carbon dioxide Pa_{CO_2} unchanged.

Coughing ability is reduced—less sensitive mechanism.

More dependent on the diaphragm for breathing.

System less responsive to hypoxia and hypercardia.

Assessment

- Shape of chest excursion.
- Lung and breath sounds.
- Quality of cough, if present; sputum.

Rib cage deformity.

Dyspnea, hypoxia, and hypercarbia.

Breast—size, symmetry, contour.

- Presence of lumps.
- Size and shape of nipples.

Heart

Physiologic Changes with Age

Mitral and aortic valves thicken and become rigid.

Cardiac output decreases 1% per year after age 20 due to decreased heart rate and stroke volume.

Vessels lose elasticity.

- Less effective peripheral oxygenation.
- Position change from lying-to-sitting or sitting-to-standing can cause blood pressure to drop as much as 65 mm Hg.

Increased peripheral vessel resistance.

- Blood pressure increases: systolic may normally be 170 mm Hg, diastolic may normally be 95 mm Hg.

- Smooth muscle in arteries is less responsive.

Blood clotting increases.

Assessment

Heart sounds—murmurs.

Peripheral circulation, color, warmth.

- Apical pulse.
- Jugular vein distention.

Orthostatic hypotension.

- Dizziness.
- Fainting.

Edema.

Activity intolerance.

Dyspnea.

Transient ischemic attacks (TIAs).

Abdomen

Physiologic Changes with Age

Esophagus dilates, decreased motility.

Stomach.

- Hunger sensations decrease.
- Secretion of hydrochloric acid decreases.
- Emptying time decreases.

Peristalsis decreases and constipation is common.

Absorption function is impaired.

- Body absorbs less nutrients due to reduced intestinal blood flow and atrophy of cells on absorbing surfaces.
- Decrease in gastric enzymes affects absorption.

Hiatal hernia common (40–60% of elderly).

Diverticulitis common (40% over age 70).

Liver.

- Fewer cells, with decreased storage capacity.
- Decreased blood flow.
- Enzymes decrease.
- Increased risk for drug toxicity.

Impaired pancreatic reserve.

Decreased glucose tolerance.

Assessment

- Indications of possible hiatal hernia.
- Bowel distention.
- Bowel sounds.

Genitourinary Tract

Physiologic Changes with Age

Kidneys.

- Smaller due to nephron atrophy.
- Renal blood flow decreases 50%.
- Glomerular filtration rate decreases 50%.
- Tubular function diminishes: less able to concentrate urine; lower specific gravity; proteinuria 1+ is common; blood urea nitrogen (BUN) increases 21 mg%.

Renal threshold for glucose increases.

Bladder.

- Muscle weakens.
- Capacity decreases to 200 mL or less, causing frequency.
- Emptying is more difficult, causing increased retention.
- Increased risk of incontinence.

Prostate enlarges to some degree in 75% of men over age 65; hypertrophy.

Menopause occurs by mean age of 50.

Perineal muscle weakens.

Vulva atrophies.

Vagina.

- Mucous membrane becomes dryer.
- Elasticity of tissue decreases, so surface is smooth.
- Secretions become reduced, more alkaline.
- Flora changes.

Sexuality.

- Older people continue to be sexual beings with sexual needs.
- No particular age at which a person's sexual functioning ceases.
- Frequency of genital sexual behavior (intercourse) may tend to decline gradually in later years, but capacity for expression and enjoyment continue far into old age.

Assessment

- Condition of skin—dehydration.
- Urinary output; blood in urine; color; specific gravity; prothrombin time (PT).
- Incontinence.
- Bladder distention.
- Genital assessment.

Musculoskeletal System

Physiologic Changes with Age

Contractures.

- Muscles atrophy, regenerate slowly, strength diminishes.
- Tendons shrink and sclerose.

Range of motion of joints decreases.

- Lack of adequate joint motion, ankylosis.
- Slight flexion of joints.

Assessment

Mobility level.

- Ambulate with more difficulty.
- Limitation to movement.
- Muscle strength cramps.
- Gait becomes unsteady.

Presence of kyphosis.

Pain in joints.

MANAGEMENT GUIDELINES

Each state legislates a Nurse Practice Act for RNs and LVN/LPNs. Health care facilities are responsible for establishing and implementing policies and procedures that conform to their state's regulations. Verify the regulations and role parameters for each health care worker in your facility.

Delegation of Responsibilities

- RNs must complete the admission assessment and document the findings. They cannot delegate this activity to anyone else on the team.
- LVN/LPNs may complete focus assessments each shift; however, any changes in assessment findings must be reported and verified with the RN.
- Unlicensed assistive-personnel may not perform assessments on clients.
- LVN/LPNs delegated the responsibility to complete focus assessments on clients must have clear direction on what is essential information to report back. Remind the LVN/LPN they must verify with the RN any changes identified in the assessment.
- Remind LVN/LPNs that if there are any questions on the client status as a result of their assessment, they must notify the RN immediately.

Information Flow

- Changes in assessment data identified in report or in the client's chart must be reported to the appropriate nurse assigned to complete the focus assessment.

CRITICAL THINKING STRATEGIES

SCENARIO 1

Mrs. Smiley has had a history of hypertension for several years. She has recently experienced an inability to use her right arm and leg and has lost ability to express herself. She has been admitted to your unit with the diagnosis of R/O left CVA (stroke) and has been placed on a continuous heparin IV drip.

1. Based on admitting data, make a judgment about what deviations from normal you would find in the physical examination.
2. List appropriate nursing diagnoses based on her physical state and immobility status (this affects virtually all systems).
3. In view of all these existing and potential problems, identify *priority* concerns (all are important concerns) for this client.
4. Develop a plan of care addressing these priority concerns.

SCENARIO 2

You are caring for a woman in labor and monitoring the fetal heart rate. You note that early deceleration has occured (a 10- to 20-beat drop in the fetal heart rate)

1. From these symptoms, indicate your priority intervention.
2. What would you conclude about the viability of the fetus?
3. What does this change in condition of the fetus imply?

CHAPTER 12

Body Mechanics and Positioning

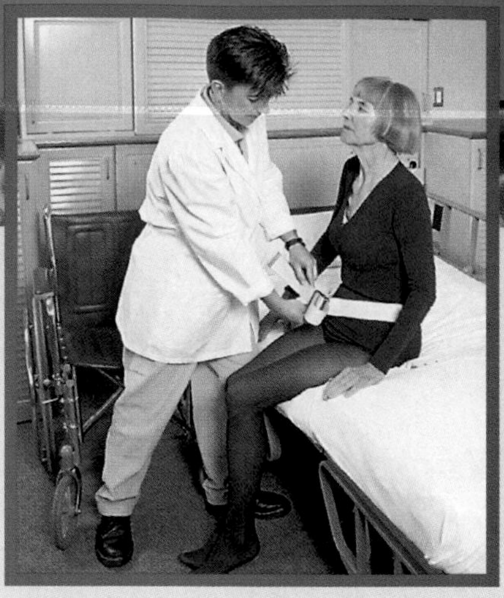

THEORETICAL CONCEPTS

UNIT ONE: **Proper Body Mechanics** **326**

Establishing Body Alignment 327
Maintaining Proper Body Alignment 328
Using Coordinated Movements 329
Using Basic Principles 329

UNIT TWO: **Moving and Turning Clients** **333**

Turning to Lateral Position 335
Turning to a Prone Position 335
Moving Client Up in Bed 336
Moving Client with Assistance 337
Transferring Client from Bed to Gurney 337
Moving Client Using Transfer Board 338
Dangling at the Bedside 339
Moving from Bed to Chair 340
Using a Hoyer (Sling) Lift 342
Logrolling the Client 343
Using a Footboard 344
Placing a Trochanter Roll 344

GERONTOLOGIC CONSIDERATIONS 345

MANAGEMENT GUIDELINES 346

CRITICAL THINKING STRATEGIES 347

Learning Objectives

- Discuss the primary function of the skeletal muscles, joints, and bones.
- Describe nursing measures that assist in preserving joints, bones, and skeletal muscles.
- Describe a minimum of two principles of correct body mechanics.
- State two expected outcomes of using proper body mechanics.
- Discuss the objectives for moving and turning clients.
- Compare and contrast the methods used in moving clients up in bed for a single nurse and when assistants are available.
- Describe the correct placement of the canvas pieces when placing a client on the Hoyer lift.
- Explain the rationale of assisted ambulation for clients.
- Demonstrate the procedures for moving a client to the side of the bed and dangling a client.
- Outline the steps in logrolling a client.
- Demonstrate a three-man lift.
- List the pertinent data that should be charted when moving a client from the bed.
- Write a client care plan using at least three nursing diagnoses for a client requiring moving and turning interventions.

Terminology

Alignment: referring to posture, the relationship of body parts to one another.

Ambulate: walking; able to walk.

Appendicular skeleton: composed of 126 bones, which include the shoulder girdle, arm bones, pelvic girdle, and leg bones.

Axial skeleton: includes the head and trunk, which form the central axis to which the appendicular skeleton is attached.

Balance: client's ability to maintain equilibrium.

Base of support: surface area on which an object rests (e.g., for a client lying in prone position, the base of support is the entire undersurface of the body).

Body mechanics: movement of the body in a coordinated and efficient way so that proper balance, alignment, and conservation of energy is maintained.

Brachial plexus: network of spinal nerves supplying arm, forearm, and hand.

Cartilage: bone-like tissue of the very young that is replaced by bone tissue through the process of ossification. In adults cartilage is found in such areas as the nose, ears, and knees.

Center of gravity: midpoint or center of the body weight. In an adult it is the midpelvic cavity between the symphysis pubis and umbilicus.

Dangle: to have a client sit on the edge of the bed with feet in a dependent position, flat on floor, if possible.

Dorsiflexion: flexion of the foot at the ankle joint; the act of turning the foot and toes upward, as in standing on the heel.

Flexion: the act or condition of being bent.

Footdrop: a falling or dragging of the foot from paralysis of the flexors of the ankle.

Fowler's position: head of bed is at a 45° angle; client's knees may or may not be flexed.

Gravity: the force that pulls objects toward the earth's surface.

High-Fowler's position: head of bed is at a 60° angle; often used to achieve maximum chest expansion.

Hoyer lift: a mechanical device that enables one person to safely transfer a client from bed to chair.

Joint: the portion of the body where two or more bones join together.

Leverage: the use of a lever to apply force.

Ligament: a band or sheet of strong fibrous connective tissue connecting the articular ends of bones serving to bind them together and to facilitate or limit motion.

Line of gravity: an imaginary line that goes from the center of gravity to the base of support.

Mobility: state or quality of being mobile; facility of movement.

Musculo: pertaining to muscles.

Musculoskeletal: pertaining to the muscles and bones.

Paralysis: temporary or permanent loss of function, especially loss of sensation or voluntary motion.

Posture: attitude or position of body.

Prone: lying horizontal with face downward.

Reverse Trendelenburg's position: mattress remains unbent, but head of bed is raised and foot is lowered.

Semi-Fowler's position: head of bed is at a 30° angle; often used for clients with cardiac and respiratory problems.

Skeletal system: system of separate bones (206) bound together by ligaments and responsible for supporting, moving, and giving shape to the body.

Sprain: injury caused by wrenching or twisting of a joint that results in tearing or stretching of the associated ligaments.

Stable: when the center of gravity is close to the base of support.

Strain: injury caused by excessive force or stretching of muscles or tendons around the joint.

Trendelenburg's position: mattress remains unbent but the head of the bed is lowered and the foot is raised. "Shock blocks" may be used under the legs of the bed to achieve this position.

Trochanter: either of the two bony prominences below the neck of the femur.

MUSCULOSKELETAL SYSTEM

The musculoskeletal system protects the body, provides a structural framework, and allows the body to move. The primary structures in this system are muscles, bones, and joints.

Skeletal Muscles

Skeletal muscles move the bones around the joints by contracting and relaxing so that movement can take place. Each muscle consists of a body, or belly, and tendons, which connect the muscle to another muscle or to bone.

When skeletal muscles contract, they cause two bones to move around the joint between them. One of these bones tends to remain stationary while the other bone moves. The end of the muscle that attaches to the stationary bone is called the origin. The end of the muscle that attaches to the movable bone is called the insertion.

Muscles are designated flexors or extensors according to whether they flex the joint (decrease the angle between the bones) or extend the joint (increase the angle between the bones). For example, when the deltoid muscle contracts, it abducts the arm and raises it laterally to the horizontal position. The anterior fibers aid in flexion of the arm, and the posterior fibers aid in extension of the arm.

Joints

Joints are the places where bones meet. Their primary function is to provide motion and flexibility. Although the internal structure of joints varies, most joints are composed of ligaments, which bind the bones together, and cartilage, or tissue, which covers and cushions the ends of the bones.

Bones

Bones provide the major support for all the body organs. Bone is composed of an organic matrix, deposits of calcium salts, and bone cells. The organic matrix provides the framework and tensile strength for the bone. The calcium salts, which are about 75% of the bone, provide compressional strength by filling in the matrix. As a result, it is very difficult to damage a bone by twisting it or by applying direct pressure.

Bone cells include osteoblasts, osteocytes, and osteoclasts. Osteoblasts deposit the organic matrix; osteocytes and osteoclasts reabsorb this matrix. Because this process is usually in equilibrium, bone is deposited where it is needed in the skeletal system. If increased stress is placed on a bone, such as the stress of continued athletic activity, more bone is deposited. If there is no stress on a bone, as is often the case with clients on prolonged bedrest, part of the bone mass is reabsorbed, or lost.

SYSTEM ALTERATIONS

Alterations in mobility can result from problems in the musculoskeletal system, the nervous system, and the skin. A primary cause for alterations in muscles is inactivity. With forceful activity muscles increase in size. With inactivity muscles decrease in size and strength. When clients are in casts or in traction, on prolonged bedrest, or unable to exercise, their muscles become weak and atrophied.

Alterations in joints result when mobility is limited by changes in the adjacent tissues. When muscle movement decreases, the connective tissue in the joints, tendons, and ligaments becomes thickened and fibrotic.

Chronic flexion and hyperextension can also cause alterations in the joints. Chronic flexion can cause joints to become contracted in one position so that they are unmovable. Hyperextension occurs when joints are extended beyond their normal limits, which is usually 180°. The results of hyperextension are pain and discomfort to the client and abnormal stress on the ligaments and tendons of the joints.

Alterations in bone are caused by disease processes, decalcification and breaks caused by trauma, or twisting. Encouraging clients to stand and to walk is important because the body functions best when it is in a vertical position. Physical activity forces muscles to move and increases blood flow, which improves metabolism and facilitates such body functions as gastrointestinal peristalsis.

Nursing Measures

Nursing care measures to preserve the joints, bones, and skeletal muscles should be carried out for all clients who require bedrest. Positions in which clients are placed, methods of moving, and turning should all be based on the principles of maintaining the musculoskeletal system in proper alignment. The nurse must also use good body mechanics when moving and turning clients to preserve her or his own musculoskeletal system from injury.

BODY MECHANICS

Knowledge of a client's body and how it moves is important. Knowledge of your own body and what happens to it when you care for clients with altered mobility is also important. Before you lift or move a client, determine the causes and consequences of the client's illness. This knowledge enables you to move the client without causing additional discomfort. Before you begin, thoroughly explain the procedures you will be completing so that you obtain the client's cooperation.

Trying to lift or move too much weight forces you to use your body incorrectly and frequently causes injuries. Incorrect lifting puts most of the pressure on the muscles of your lower back. Because these muscles are not strong enough to handle the stress, you can sustain severe injuries. If you do not follow guidelines for promoting proper body mechanics, you are putting yourself in jeopardy.

Health care workers often forget to take care of themselves as they are busy helping clients. Low back pain is an occupational hazard for many workers. Back injuries affect about 38% of nurses. The majority of the injuries occur from lifting clients without the right equipment. It is advisable that health care workers do simple exercises to strengthen and stretch the abdominal muscles and muscles that support the back. This will assist in preventing back injuries.

Proper use of body mechanics prevents injuries to clients and all members of the health team. Guidelines that underly the implementation of body mechanics appear below.

- Assume a proper stance before moving or turning clients.
- Distribute workload evenly before moving or turning clients.
- Establish a comfortable height when working with clients. Keep the client as close to your body as possible when moving.
- Push and pull objects when moving them to conserve energy.
- Use large muscles for lifting and moving, not the back muscles. Move the hip and shoulders as one unit.
- Avoid leaning and stretching.
- Request assistance from others when working with heavy clients to avoid strain.
- Avoid twisting your body.
- Maintain low back in neutral position.

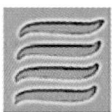

NURSING DIAGNOSES

The following nursing diagnoses are appropriate to use on client care plans when the components are related to body mechanics.

NURSING DIAGNOSIS	RELATED FACTORS
Activity Intolerance	Impaired motor function, weakness or paralysis, pain
Risk for Disuse Syndrome	Debilitated state, immobility, muscle weakness, decreased motor agility
Risk for Injury	Altered mobility, impaired sensory function, prolonged bedrest
Impaired Physical Mobility	Trauma or musculoskeletal impairment, surgical procedure, muscle weakness, pain, decreased strength
Impaired Walking	Muscle weakness, impaired motor function, orthopedic surgery; or dysfunction
Impaired Transfer Ability	Weakness, flacidity, amputation, decreased strength

- The single most important nursing action to decrease the incidence of hospital-based infections is handwashing. **Remember to wash your hands or use antibacterial gel before and after each and every client contact.**

UNIT 1

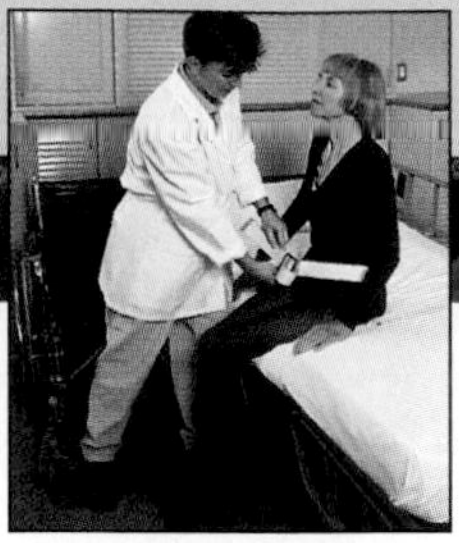

Proper Body Mechanics

Nursing Process Data

ASSESSMENT ***Data Base***
Evaluate personnel's knowledge of the principles of body mechanics.

Evaluate personnel's knowledge of how to use correct muscle groups for specific activities.

Assess knowledge and correct any misinformation about body alignment and how to maintain it with each position.

Assess knowledge of physical science and application to balance and body alignment.

Assess the competency of spinal cord and associated musculature.

Assess the muscle mass of the long, thick, and strong muscles of the shoulders and thighs.

PLANNING ***Objectives***
To promote proper body mechanics while caring for clients

To maintain good posture, thereby promoting optimum musculoskeletal balance

To provide knowledge of the musculoskeletal system, body alignment, and balance in order to assist the nurse in caring for clients

To correct body mechanics, promote health, enhance appearance, and assist body function

IMPLEMENTATION ***Procedures***
Establishing Body Alignment

Maintaining Proper Body Alignment

Using Coordinated Movements

Using Basic Principles

EVALUATION ***Expected Outcomes***
Correct body mechanics are used in caring for clients.

Injuries are prevented to both the nurse and the client.

Proper body mechanics facilitate client care.

Coordinated movements prevent client discomfort.

Center of gravity is maintained when lifting objects.

ESTABLISHING BODY ALIGNMENT

Procedure

1. Determine need for assistance in moving or turning a client. **Rationale:** Half of all back pain is associated with lifting or turning clients. The most common back injury is strain on the lumbar muscle group.
2. Establish a firm base of support by placing both feet flat on the floor, with one foot slightly in front of the other.
3. Distribute weight evenly on both feet.
4. Slightly bend both knees. **Rationale:** Allows strong muscles of legs to do the lifting.
5. Hold abdomen firm and tuck buttocks in so that spine is in alignment. **Rationale:** This position protects the back.
6. Hold head erect, and secure firm stance.
7. Use this stance as the basis for all actions in moving, turning, and lifting clients.
8. Maintain weight to be lifted as close to your body as possible. **Rationale:** This position maintains the center of gravity and provides leverage that reduces lower back strain.
9. Align the three natural curves in your back (cervical, thoracic, and lumbar). **Rationale:** Weight of client is evenly distributed throughout spine, lowering risk of back injury.

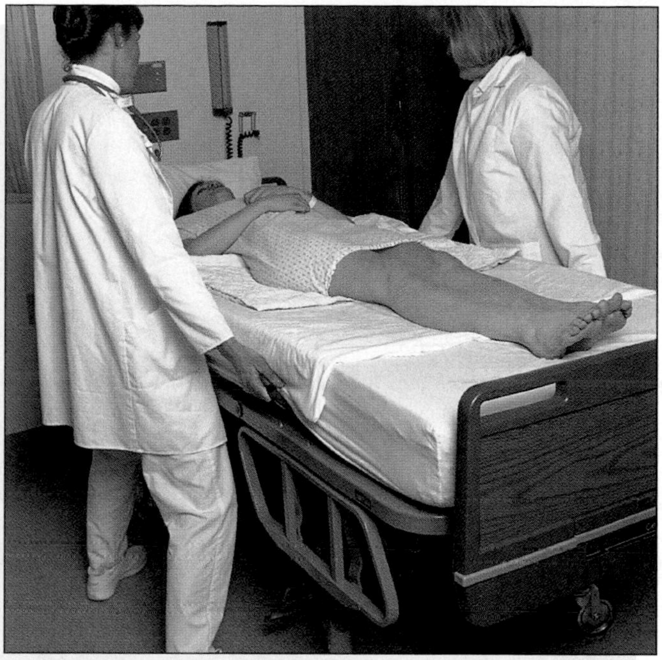

Determine need for assistance with moving client.

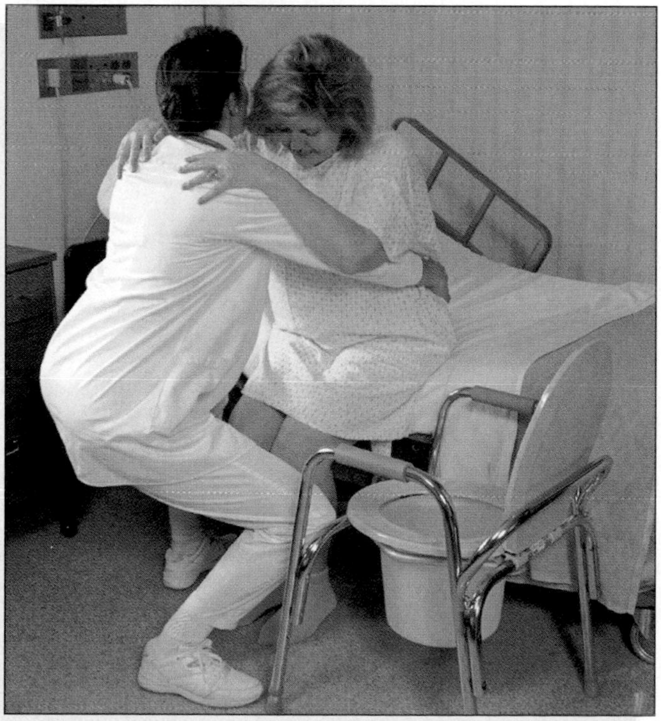

Hold head erect and secure firm stance to work without causing injury.

10. Wear a back brace for moving, lifting, or turning. **Rationale:** Brace protects and supports back and keeps body in alignment.
11. Prevent twisting your body when moving the client. **Rationale:** This prevents injury to the back.

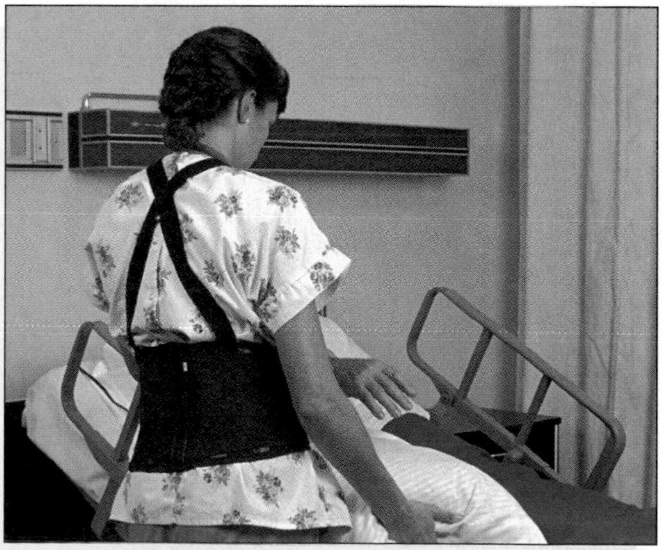

Wear a back brace to support back and keep body in alignment. Back brace benefit is controversial.

MAINTAINING PROPER BODY ALIGNMENT

Procedure

1. Begin with the proper stance established in the previous intervention.
2. Evaluate working height necessary to achieve objective.
   a. Test parameters of possible heights (i.e., bed moves within an approximate range of 18 inches from floor).
   b. Establish a comfortable height in which to work; usual height is between waist and lower level of hip joint.
3. Test that this level minimizes muscle strain by extending your arms and checking that your body maintains proper alignment.
4. If you need to work at a lower level, flex your knees. **Rationale:** Bending over at the waist results in back strain.
5. Make accommodations for working at high surface levels. **Rationale:** Reaching up may result in injury to the back through hyperextension of muscles.
6. Work close to your body so that your center of gravity is not misaligned and your muscles are not hyperextended. **Rationale:** This prevents back strain.
7. Use your longest and strongest muscles (biceps, quadriceps, and gluteal) when moving and turning clients.
8. Whenever possible, roll, push, and pull objects instead of lifting.

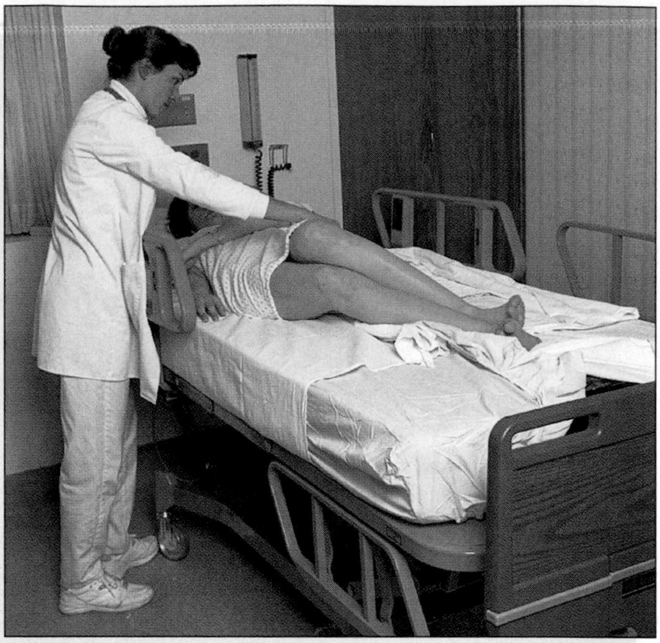

Ensure that height of bed allows you to work without causing injury.

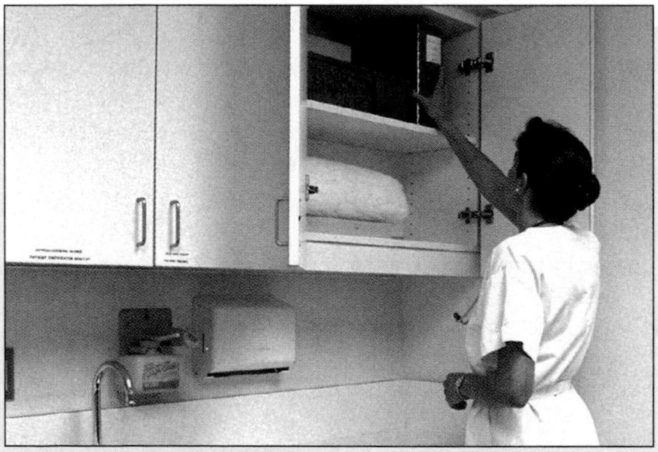

Correct: Keep body in correct alignment when turning and reaching for objects to prevent muscle strain or back injury.

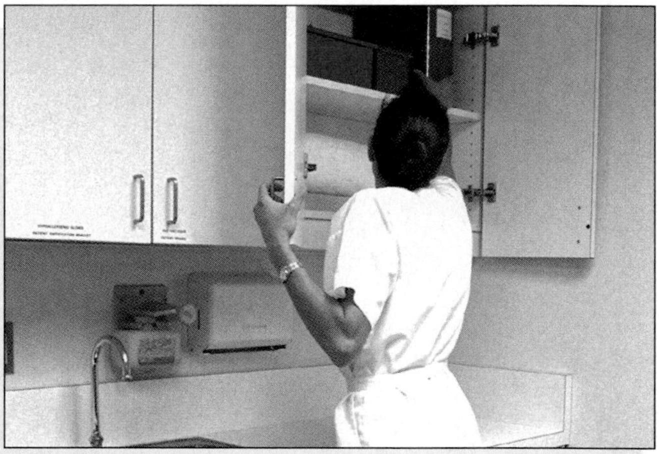

Incorrect: Do not use stretching or twisting movements when you reach for objects out of close proximity to your body.

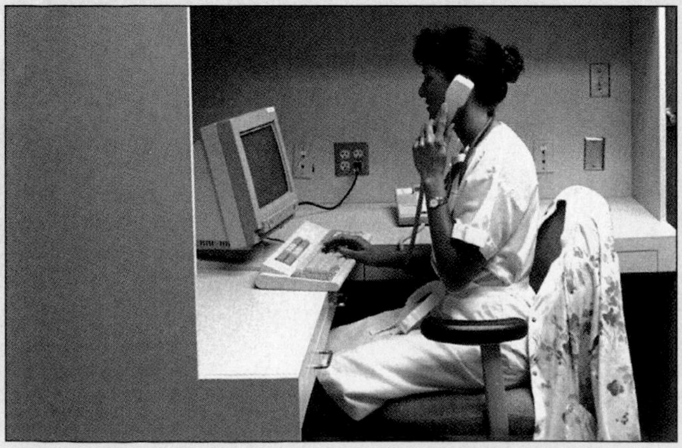

Correct: Work close to the body so that center of gravity is not misaligned.

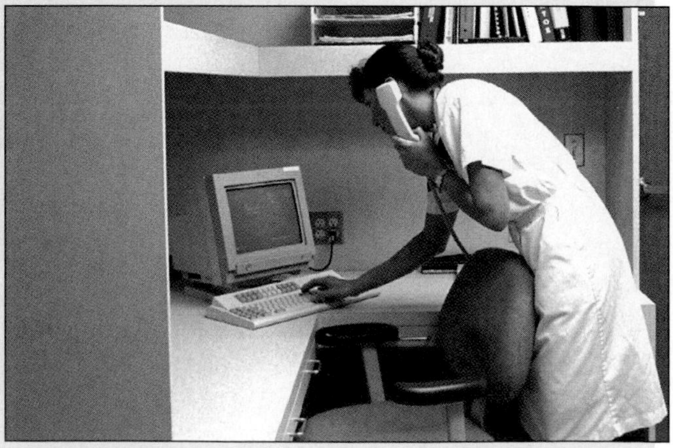

Incorrect: Bending over incorrectly could injure back muscles and cause undue strain.

USING COORDINATED MOVEMENTS

Procedure

1. Plan muscle movements to distribute workload before you actually begin turning, moving, or lifting clients.
   a. Establish a clear plan of action before you begin to move.
   b. Take a deep breath so oxygen is available for energy expenditure.
   c. Tense antagonistic muscles (abdomen) to those you will be using (diaphragm) in preparation for the movement.
   d. Release breath and mobilize major muscle groups (abdominal and gluteal) to do the work.
2. Move muscles in a smooth, coordinated manner. **Rationale:** This avoids putting strain on one muscle and is more efficient.
3. Do not make jerky, uncoordinated movements. **Rationale:** This may cause injury or frighten the client.
4. When you are working with another staff member, coordinate plans and movements before implementing them.

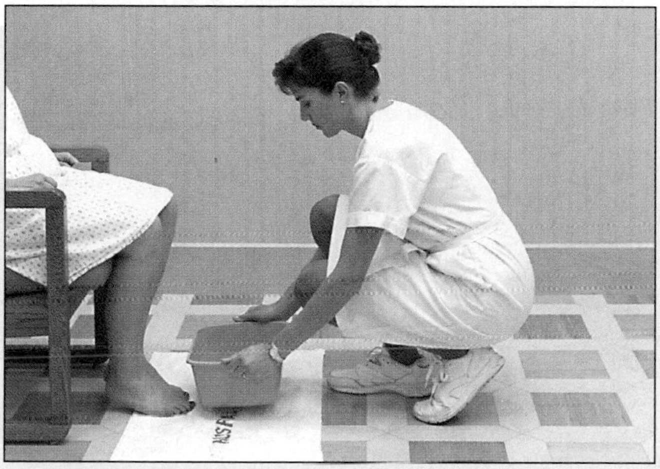

Correct: Move muscles as a unit and in alignment rather than twisting.

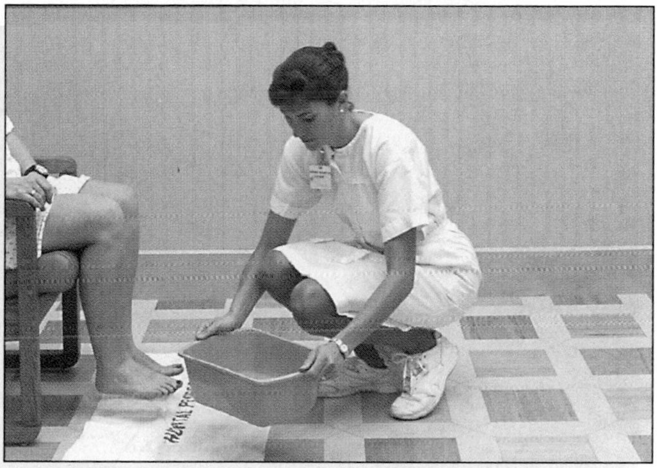

Incorrect: Do not twist or rotate upper body when working at lower surface levels.

USING BASIC PRINCIPLES

Procedure

1. Move an object by pushing and pulling to expend minimal energy.
   a. Stand close to the object.
   b. Place yourself in proper body alignment stance.
   c. Tense muscles, and prepare for movement.
   d. Pull toward you by leaning away from the object and letting arms, hips, and thighs (*not back*) do the work.

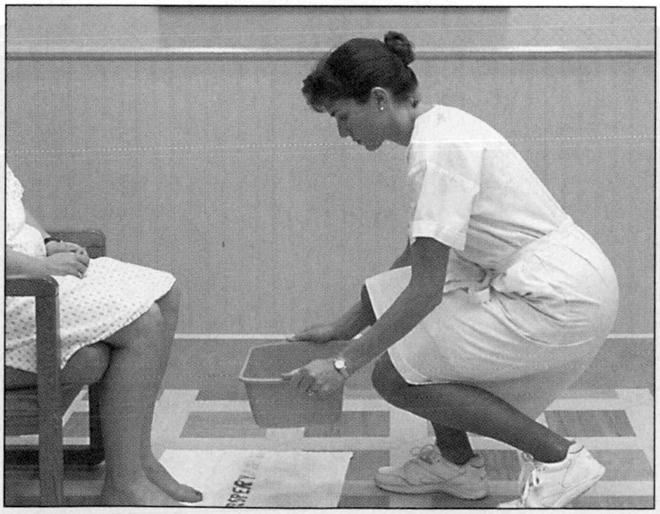

Correct: Keep body in proper alignment by bending knees and keeping back straight when lifting objects.

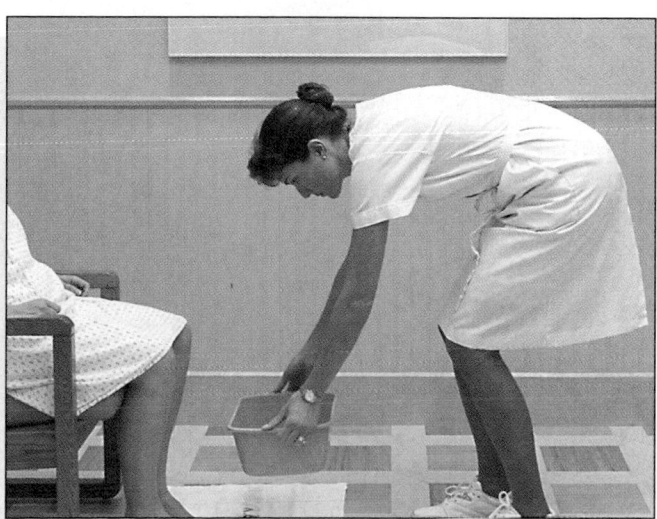

Incorrect: Prevent injury to back muscles; for proper alignment, bend at knees and use leg muscles.

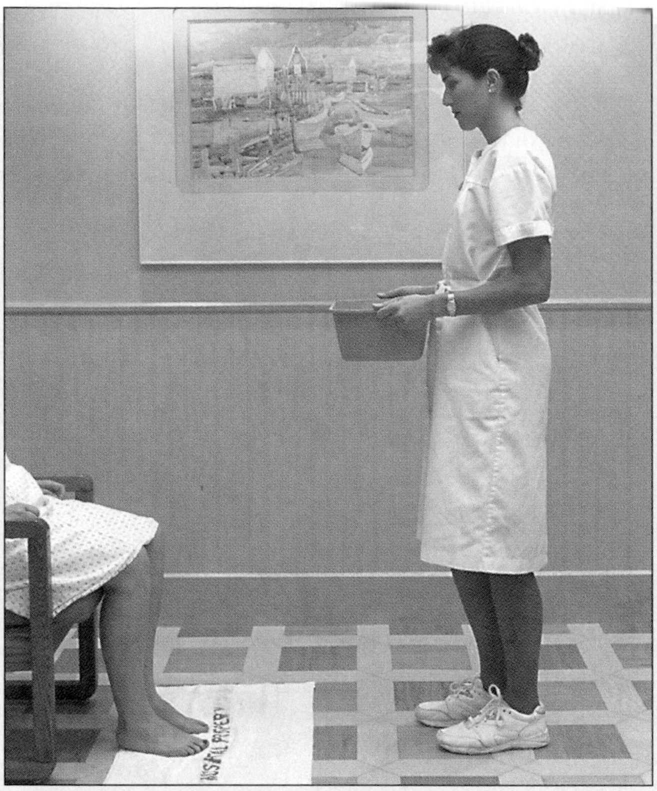

Correct: Hold objects close to the body to prevent muscle strain and possible back injury.

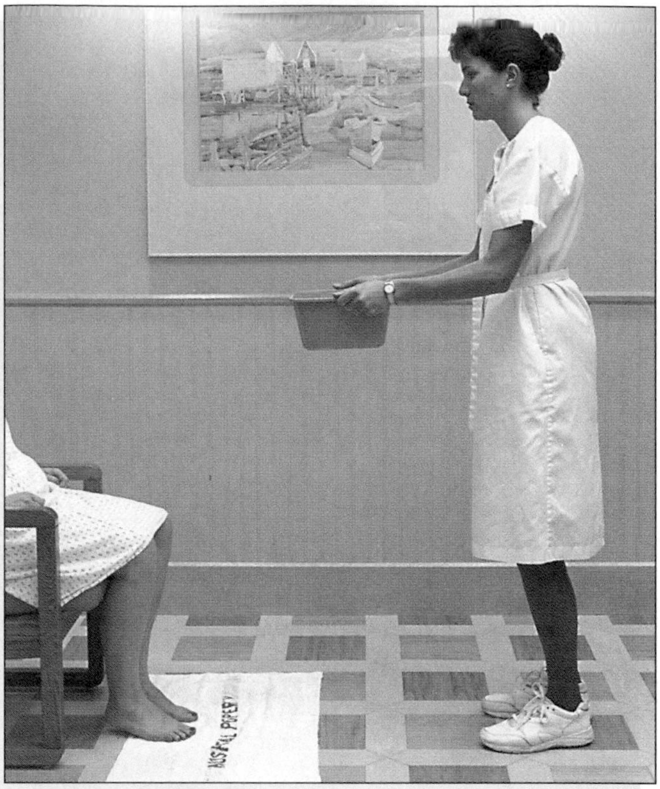

Incorrect: Holding objects away from the body may cause back strain or injury.

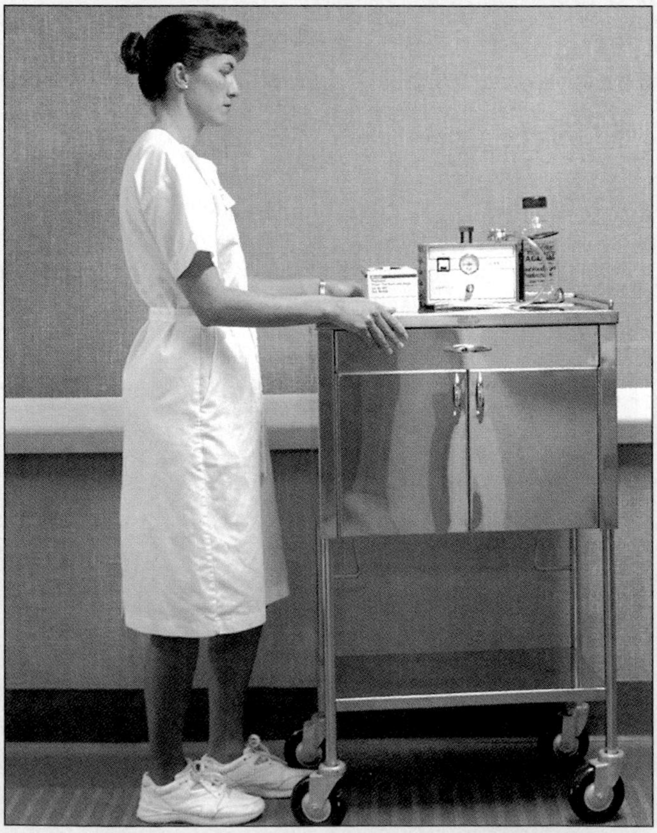

Correct: When pushing an object, place yourself in proper body alignment.

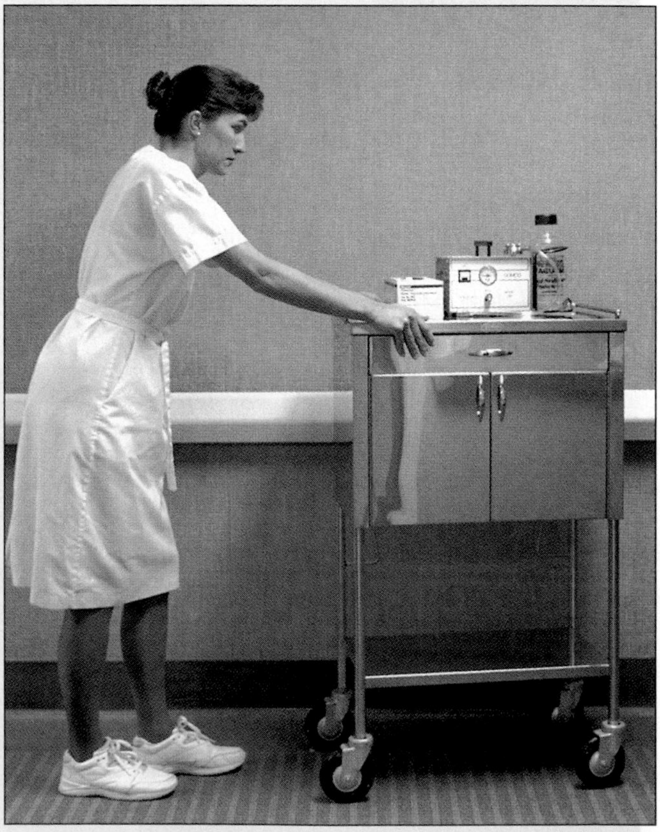

Incorrect: Standing away from object puts body out of proper alignment.

   e. Push away from you by leaning toward object, using body weight to add force.
2. When changing direction, use pivotal movement—moving muscles as a unit and in alignment, rather than rotating or twisting upper part of body.
3. When working at lower surface levels, do not stoop by bending over. Flex body at knees and, keeping back straight, use thigh and gluteal muscles to accomplish task.
4. Use muscles of arms and upper torso in an extended, coordinated movement parallel to body stance when reaching to prevent twisting or hyperextension of muscles.
5. Lift or carry clients or objects with the maximum use of these body alignment principles:
   a. Determine that the movement is within your capability to perform without injury.
   b. Place yourself in proper body alignment stance.
   c. Stand close to and grasp the object or person near the center of gravity.
   d. Prepare muscles by taking a deep breath, and set muscles.
   e. Lift object with arms or by stooping and using leg and thigh muscles.
   f. Carry object or person close to your body to prevent strain on your back.
   g. Take frequent rest periods to prevent additional strain.

Documentation for Body Mechanics

- Injury to client resulting from poor body mechanics
- Devices needed for turning and moving
- Number of personnel required for turning and moving
- Ways in which client assists in moving
- Special requirements of client for proper body alignment, such as support pillows

Critical Thinking Application

UNEXPECTED OUTCOMES	CRITICAL THINKING OPTIONS
Incorrect body mechanics are used while giving client care.	• Identify areas of your body where you feel stress and strain. • Evaluate the way you use body mechanics. • Attend an in-service program on using body mechanics appropriately. • Concentrate on how you are using your body when moving and turning clients. • Position bed and equipment at a comfortable height and proximity to working area. • Use your longest and strongest muscles to prevent injury.
Nurse injures self while giving client care.	• Wear a back brace to support back. • Report any back strain immediately to supervisor. • Complete unusual occurrence form. • Go to health service or emergency room for evaluation and immediate care. • Evaluate any activities that led to injury to determine incorrect use of body mechanics. • Prevent additional injury by obtaining assistance when needed. • Use devices such as turning sheets or assistive devices to assist in turning difficult clients.
Nurse uses poor body mechanics and injures client.	• Assess the extent of client's injury. • Notify client's physician. • Complete unusual occurrence form. • Carry out physician's orders for follow-up treatment.
Due to staffing shortage, nurse is unable to obtain sufficient assistance with turning and moving clients.	• Place turning sheets on bed for all clients who are difficult to move. • Use principles of leverage in moving clients. • Until adequate staff is available, turn and position client from side to side at least every 2 hours. • Use Hoyer lift.

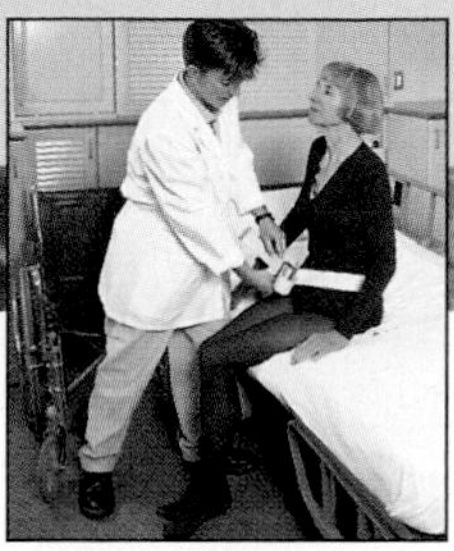

Moving and Turning Clients

Nursing Process Data

ASSESSMENT *Database*
Observe the client and identify ways to improve the client's position and alignment.
Determine the client's physical ability to assist you with positioning.
Note the presence of tubes and incisions that alter the positioning and alignment procedures.
Assess joint mobility.
Assess skin condition with each turn.

PLANNING *Objectives*
To provide increased comfort
To provide optimal lung excursion and ventilation
To prevent contractures due to constant joint flexion
To promote optimal joint movement
To help maintain intact skin
To prevent injury due to improper movement

IMPLEMENTATION *Procedures*
Turning to Lateral Position
Turning to a Prone Position
Moving Client Up in Bed
Moving Client with Assistance
Transferring Client from Bed to Gurney
Moving Client Using Transfer Board
Dangling at the Bedside
Moving from Bed to Chair
Using a Hoyer (Sling) Lift
Logrolling the Client
Using a Footboard
Placing a Trochanter Roll

EVALUATION *Expected Outcomes*
Client's comfort is increased.
Skin remains intact without evidence of breakdown.
Breathing is adequate and unlabored.
Joint movement is maintained.
Footdrop is prevented.
Body alignment is maintained.

TABLE 12–1 Bed Positions for Client Care

Positions	Placement	Use
High-Fowler's	Head of bed 60° angle	Thoracic surgery, severe respiratory conditions
Fowler's	Head of bed 45°–60° angle; hips may or may not be flexed	Postoperative, gastrointestinal conditions, promotes lung expansion
Semi-Fowler's	Head of bed 30° angle	Cardiac, respiratory, neurosurgical conditions
Low-Fowler's	Head of bed 15° angle	Necessary degree elevation for ease of breathing, promotes skin integrity, client comfort
Knee-Gatch	Lower section of bed (under knees) slightly bent	For client comfort; contraindicated for vascular disorders
Trendelenburg's	Head of bed lowered and foot raised	Percussion, vibration, and drainage (PVD) procedure; promotes venous return
Reverse Trendelenburg's	Bed frame is tilted up with foot of bed down	Gastric conditions, prevents esophageal reflux

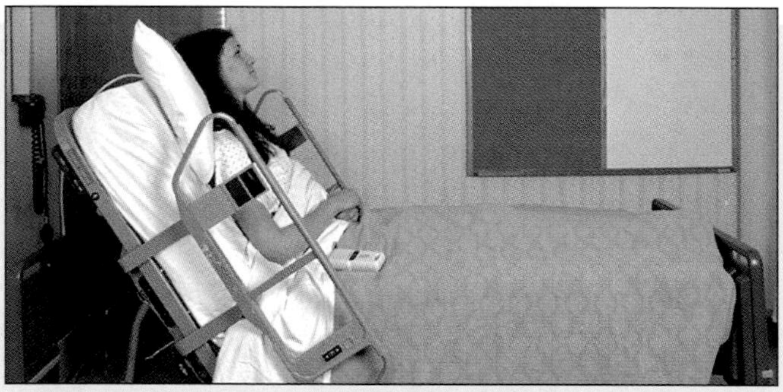

High-Fowler's position at 60° angle.

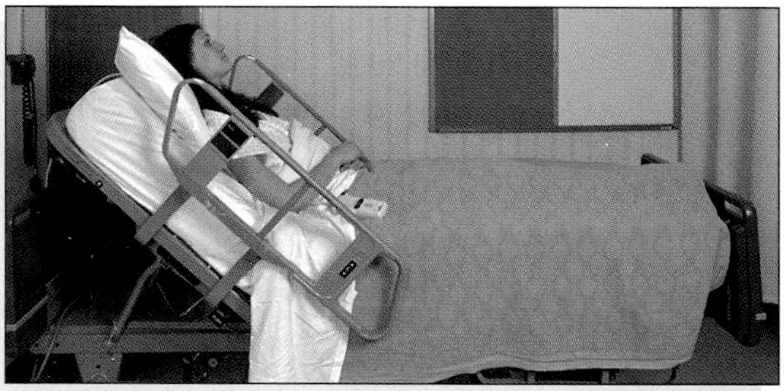

Fowler's position at 45°–60° angle.

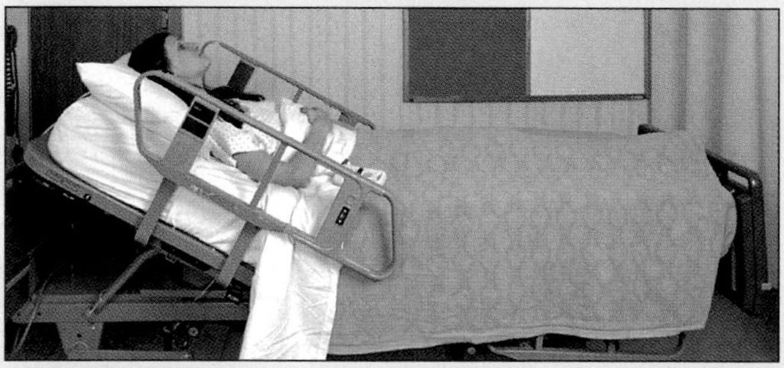

Semi-Fowler's position at 30° angle.

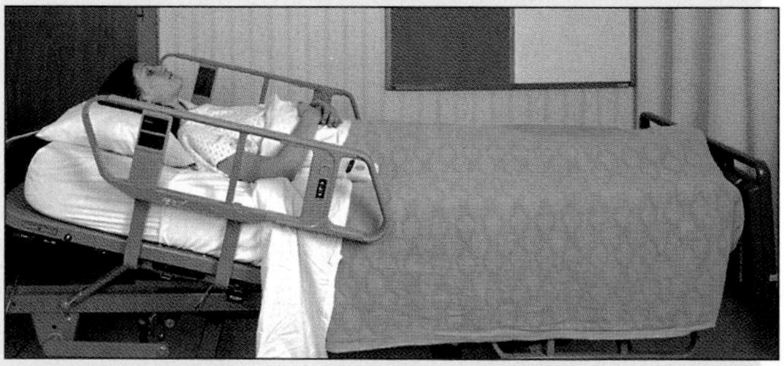

Low-Fowler's position at 15° angle.

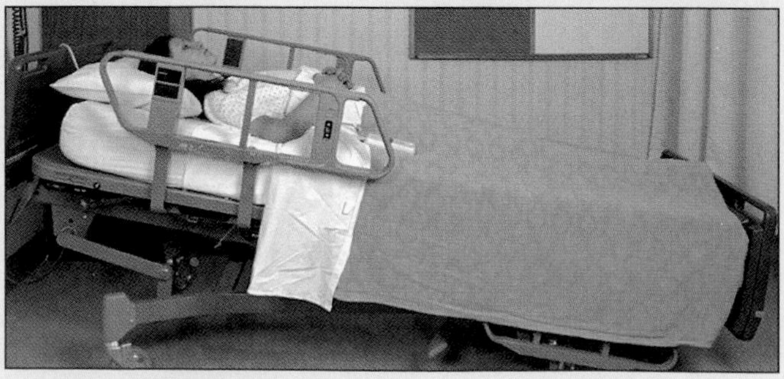

Reverse Trendelenburg's position.

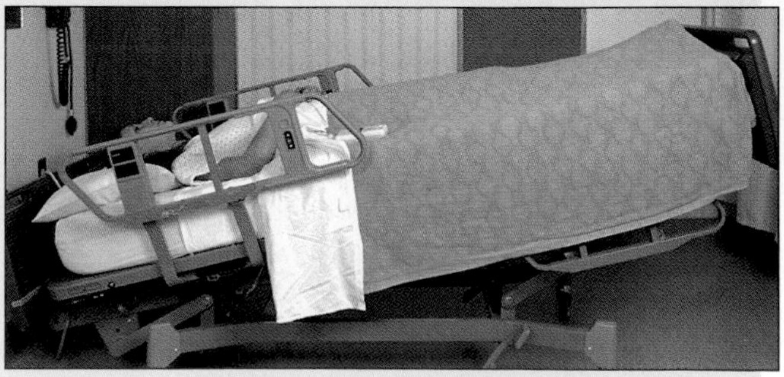

Trendelenburg's position.

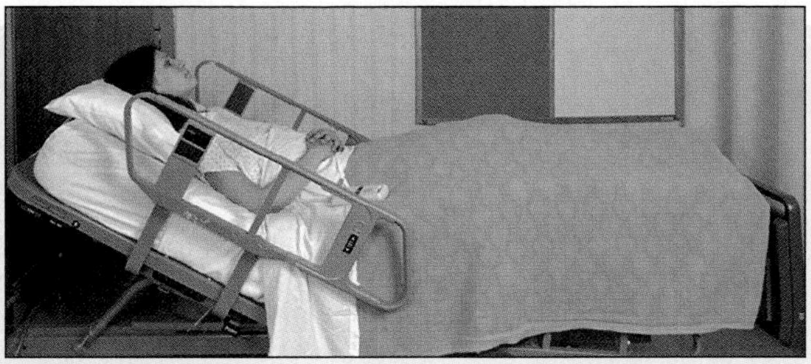

Elevated knee gatch.

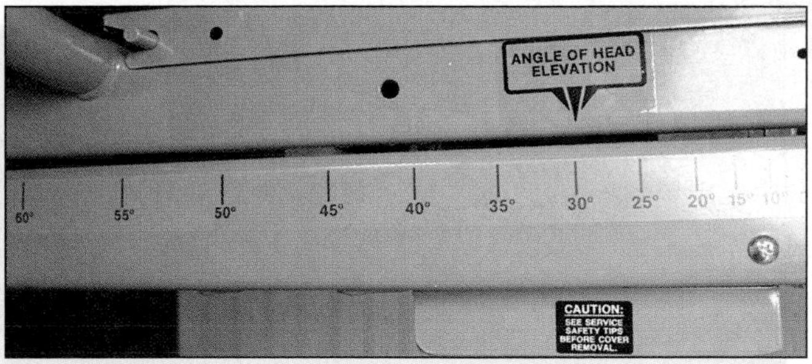

Angle gauge on bed.

TURNING TO LATERAL POSITION

Equipment

Pillows for positioning
Turning sheet
Drawsheet for trochanter roll

Procedure

1. Identify client and wash hands.
2. Explain rationale for procedure to client.
3. Lower head of the bed completely or to a position as low as client can tolerate.
4. Elevate bed to a comfortable working height.
5. Move client to your side of bed. Put side rails up, and move to other side of bed.
6. Flex client's knees.
7. Place one hand on client's hip and one hand on client's shoulder; roll onto side.
8. Position pillow to maintain proper alignment.
9. Be sure to position client's arms so they are not under the body.

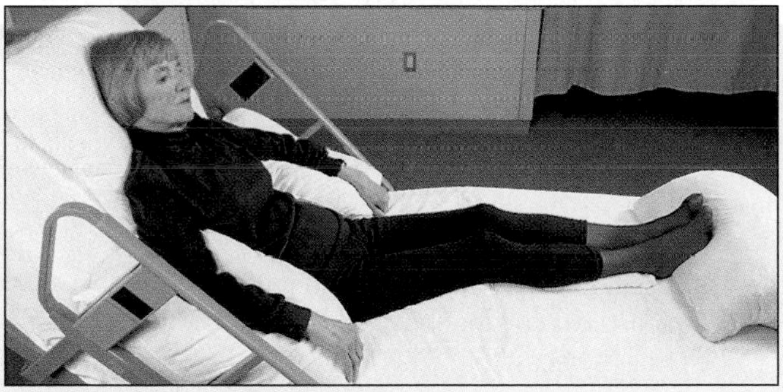

Use pillows to support proper alignment.

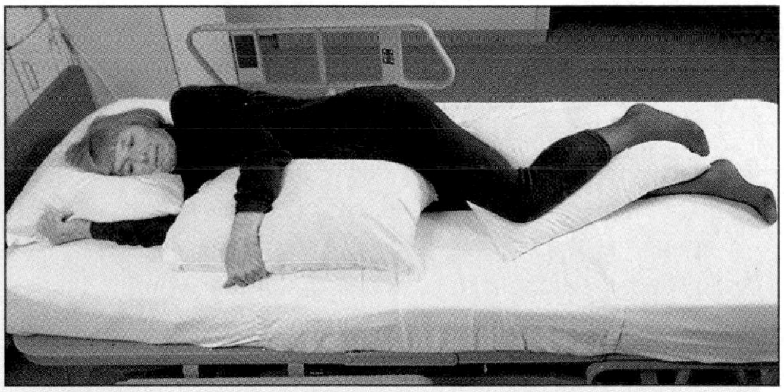

Lateral (side-lying) position.

TURNING TO A PRONE POSITION

Equipment

Pillows for positioning
Turning sheet

Procedure

1. Identify client and wash hands.
2. Explain rationale for procedure to client.
3. Lower head of bed completely or to a position that is as low as client can tolerate.
4. Elevate bed to a comfortable working height.
5. Move client to side of bed away from side where he or she will finally be positioned.
6. Position pillows on side of bed for client's head, thorax, and feet.
7. Roll client onto pillows, making sure that client's arms are not under his or her body.
8. Reposition pillows as necessary for client's comfort.

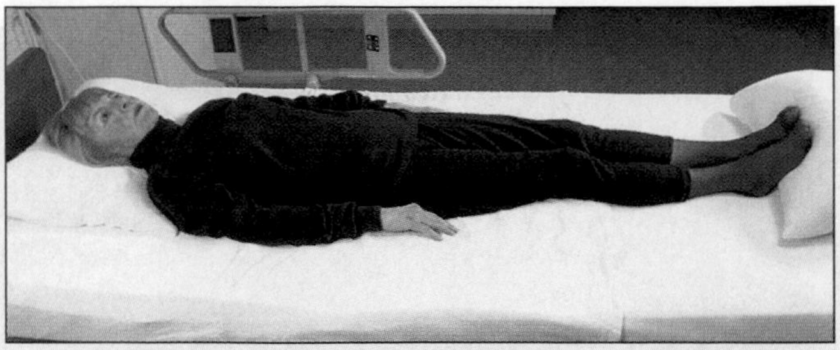
Supine position.

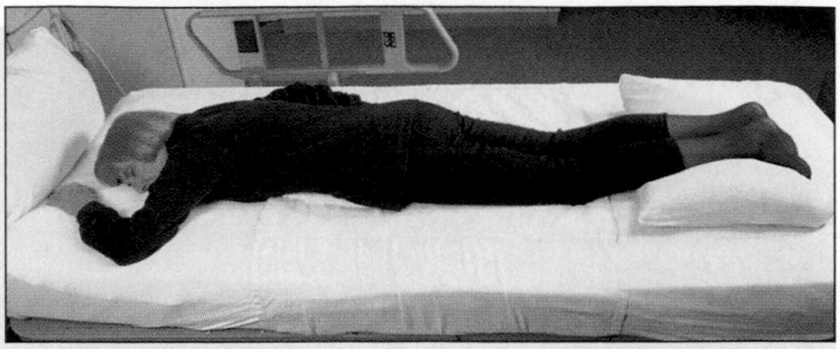
Prone position.

MOVING CLIENT UP IN BED

Equipment

Trapeze (optional)
Turning sheet

Procedure

1. Identify client and wash hands.
2. Explain rationale for procedure to client.
3. Lower head of bed so that it is flat or as low as client can tolerate.
4. Raise bed to a comfortable working height. **Rationale:** Allows nurse's center of gravity to assist in turning.
5. Remove pillow and place it at head of bed. **Rationale:** This prevents striking client's head against bed.
6. Place one arm under client's shoulders and other arm under client's thighs.
7. Flex your knees and hips. Move feet close to bed.
8. Place your weight on your back foot.
9. Instruct client to put arms across chest, bend legs, and put feet flat on the bed.
10. Shift your weight from back to front foot as you lift client up in bed. **Rationale:** Shifting weight reduces force needed to move client up in bed.

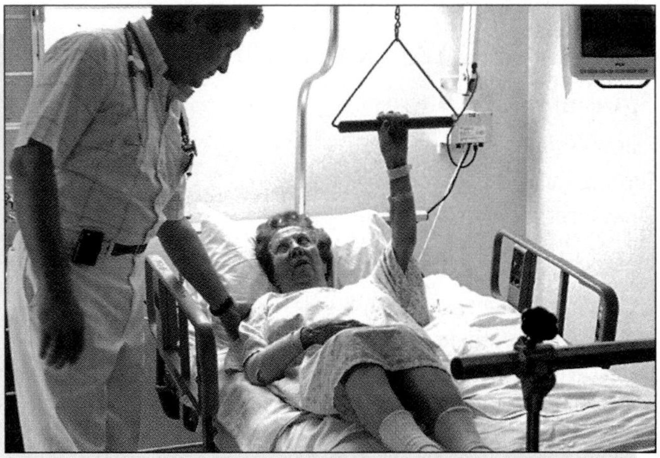
Encourage client to help when moving up in bed.

Note: There are several other methods of moving a client up in bed—including using client's elbows, lifting under the back, and having client use the trapeze.

11. Ask client to push with feet as you move him/her.
12. Position client comfortably, replacing pillow and arranging bedding as necessary.

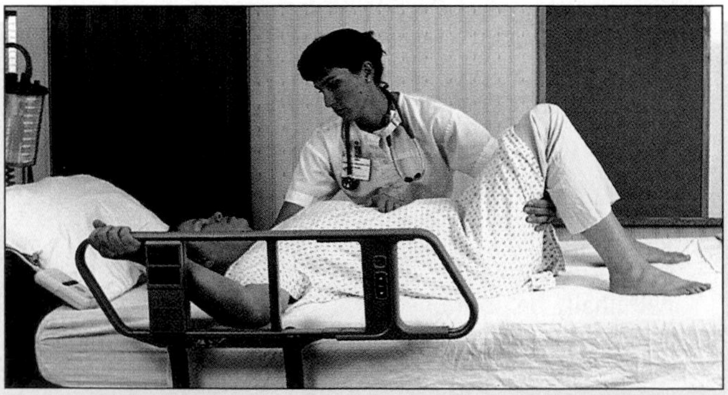
Place one arm under shoulders and other under thighs.

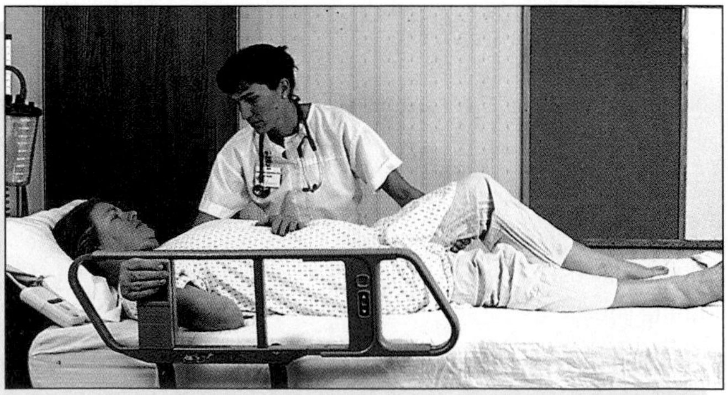
Maintain proper body alignment when moving client up in bed.

MOVING CLIENT WITH ASSISTANCE

Equipment

Drawsheet folded to use as lift sheet

Procedure

1. Identify client and wash hands.
2. Explain rationale for procedure to client.
3. Lower head of bed so that it is flat or as low as client can tolerate.
4. Raise bed to a comfortable working height.
5. Remove pillow, and place it at head of bed. **Rationale:** To prevent head being bumped when moved.
6. Coordinate the movements of all nurses. **Rationale:** One nurse is responsible for stating when to move client, "on count of three."
7. Position client with two nurses or staff members.
   a. First position: Position one nurse on each side of client. Assume broad base of support; position front foot facing head of bed, body slightly turned toward head of bed. Each nurse should have one arm under client's shoulders and one arm under the client's thighs. Ask client to bend knees.
   b. Alternate position: Position one nurse at client's upper body. Nurse's arm nearest head of the bed should be under client's head and opposite shoulder. Nurse's other arm should be under client's closest arm and shoulder. Position other nurse at client's lower torso. Nurse's arms should be under client's lower back and thighs.
   c. Second alternate position—Using pull sheet: Place folded drawsheet under client's body extending from shoulder line to just below buttocks. Position one nurse on each side of bed. Roll up sides of lift sheet as close as possible to sides of client. Assist client to flex knees, if possible. Each nurse firmly grasps sheet at level of client's upper back with one hand and at level of buttocks with other hand. Each nurse places weight on back foot. Then with one firm, coordinated, rocking movement (shifting weight from back to front foot), lift client toward head of bed.
   d. Place client in a comfortable position.

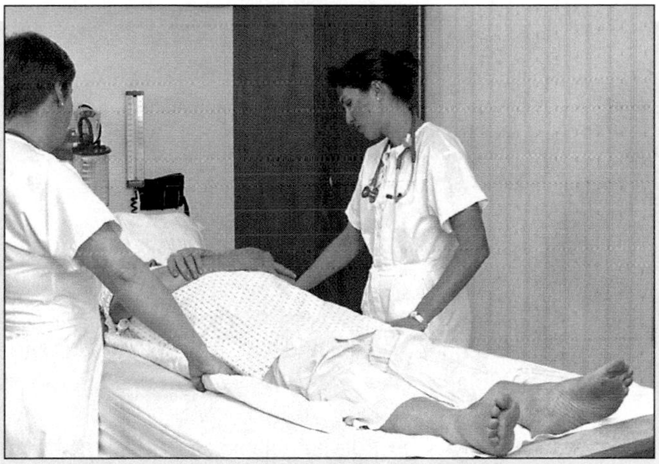

Hold drawsheet firmly and close to client for proper support.

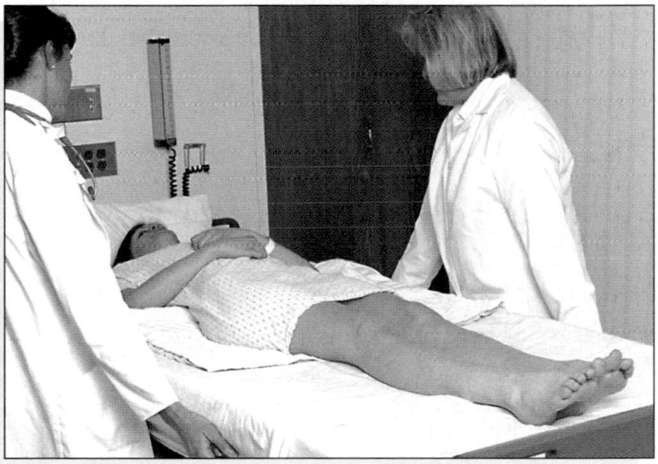

Shift weight from back to front leg when moving client up.

TRANSFERRING CLIENT FROM BED TO GURNEY

Procedure

1. Wash hands.
2. Position gurney at right angle (90°) to bed and lock brakes.
3. Elevate bed to height of gurney and lock wheels. **Rationale:** When two beds are the same height it is easier and safer to transfer client.
4. Place bed in flat position and lower side rails on side nearest nurses.
5. Position two to three nurses on side toward which client will move.
6. Place one nurse at head and shoulders, one at hips, and third nurse at thighs and ankles of client. If two nurses are used, place one nurse at head and shoulders and second nurse at waist and thighs. **Rationale:** These positions will distribute client's weight evenly.
7. Place client's arms across chest.

8. Place one foot toward gurney with wide stance. **Rationale:** This position is more balanced when pivoting and gives a broad base of support.
9. Flex knees. **Rationale:** This position reduces back strain and lowers center of gravity.
10. Place arms under client so that fingers are wrapped around client's body. **Rationale:** Allows for a secure hold before moving client to gurney.
11. Lift client on count of three and bring close to nurses' chests. Move to side of bed.
12. Lift client again and pivot and step toward gurney with client on the second count of three. **Rationale:** Counting to three ensures that nurses will move together and keep client in alignment.
13. Lower client gently to center of gurney by flexing knees and hips. **Rationale:** This position maintains the three natural curves and prevents back strain from bending at the waist.
14. Check client alignment, fix safety straps on gurney, and put up side rails. **Rationale:** Ensures client safety during transfer.

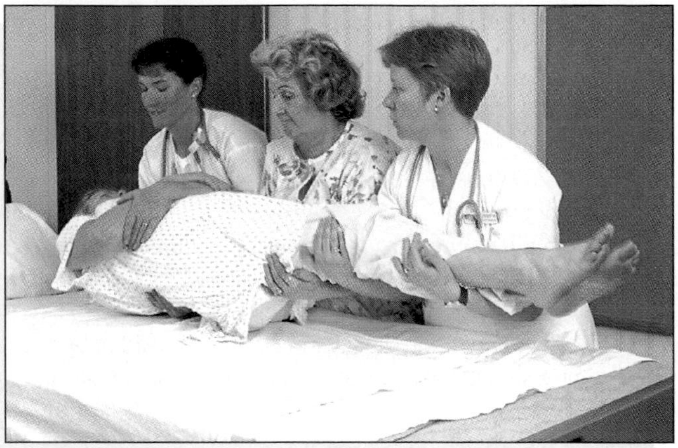
Lift client on the count of three and bring to nurse's chest.

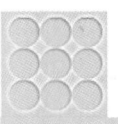

CULTURAL COMPETENCE

Different cultures may have cultural variances regarding distance and space. When clients are being moved, transferred to a bed or gurney, client is brought close to nurse's body. It is important to explain the transfer process to client, particularly Americans, Canadians, and British clients. They may be threatened by invasion of personal space and touch. Japanese, Arabs, and Latin American's aren't as concerned about personal space.

MOVING CLIENT USING TRANSFER BOARD

Equipment

Transfer board: polyethylene board about 18–22 inches wide by 72 inches long
Sheets to cover board, gurney, and client
Bath blanket (optional)
Gurney, bed, or CT table

Procedure

1. Wash hands.
2. Explain procedure to client and show client transfer board. **Rationale:** To allay client's fears of being dropped from board.
3. Cover client with sheet or bath blanket and cover board and gurney with sheets.

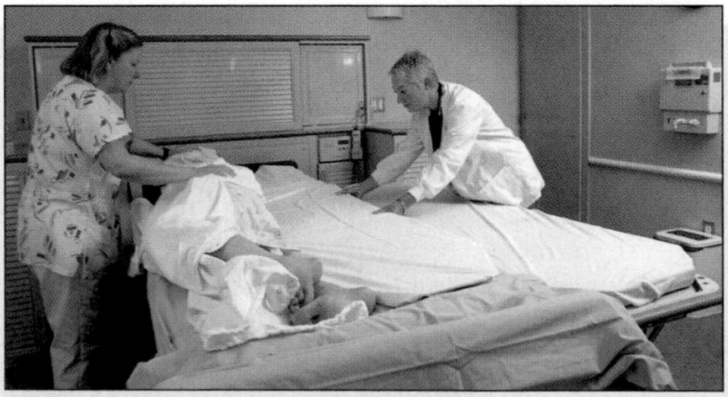
Move client to side of bed in lateral position.

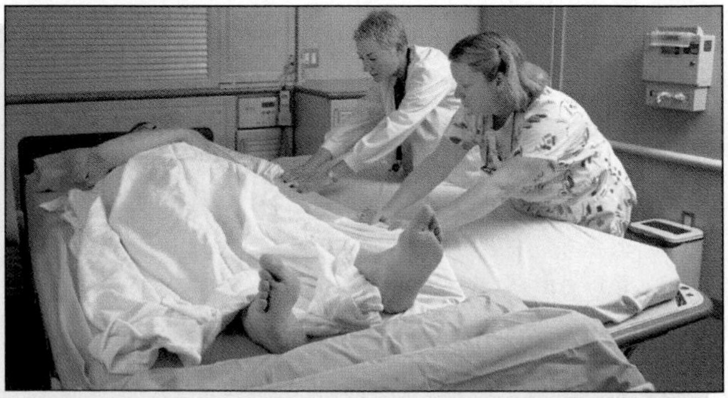
Both nurses move to same side of gurney before moving client.

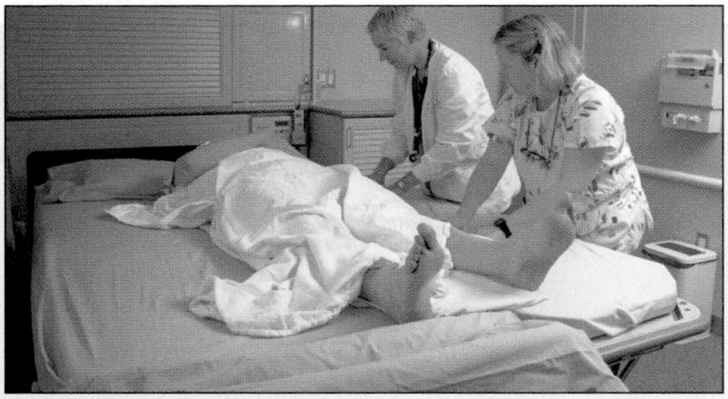

Use handholds on board to move client to gurney; maintain proper body mechanics.

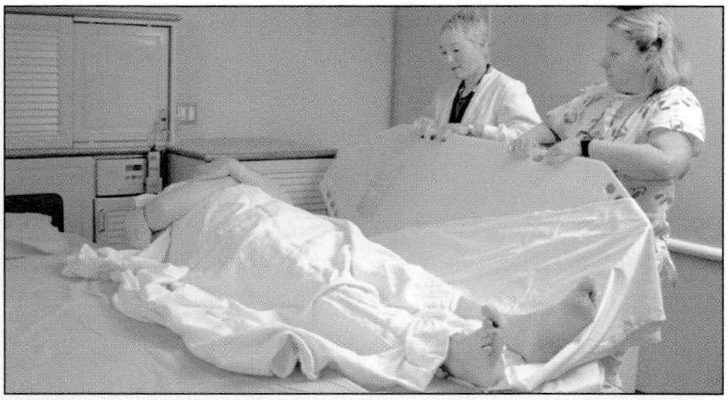

Remove transfer board after centering client on gurney.

4. Position client on side of bed away from gurney in lateral position.
5. First nurse supports client while second nurse places board as close to client as possible. **Rationale:** This allows client to be positioned on entire board after turn.
6. Instruct client to turn onto back, directly onto board. Client may need assistance to turn.
7. Place both nurses on side of gurney or bed toward which client will be turned.
8. Assume appropriate body mechanics (broad base of support, one foot in front of the other, knees and hips flexed). Place weight on front foot.
9. Transfer weight on count of three from front to back foot as you lift board and pull it toward you.
10. Center client on gurney or bed and remove board by pulling board out and up using handholds along edge of board and using good body mechanics.
11. Place side rails in UP position, or according to facility policy.

DANGLING AT THE BEDSIDE

Procedure

1. Wash hands.
2. Explain procedure to client.
3. Lower bed to lowest position.
4. Move client to edge of bed and instruct client to bend knees. **Rationale:** This allows client to easily move legs and feet over side of bed onto floor.
5. Turn client onto side, keeping knees flexed, or place bed in Fowler's position (head elevated at 45° angle). **Rationale:** This position is sometimes preferred; it may be easier for nurse to pivot client to sitting position.
6. Stand at client's hip level. Assume broad base of support with forward foot closest to client. Flex your knees, hips, and ankles.

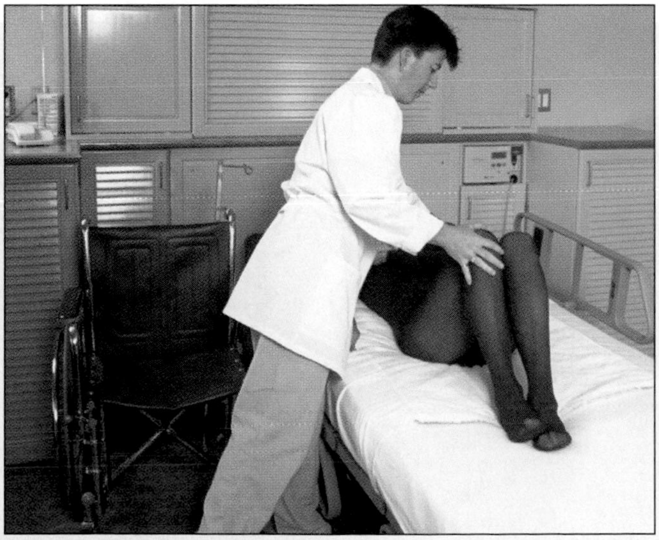

Move client to side of bed and instruct to flex knees.

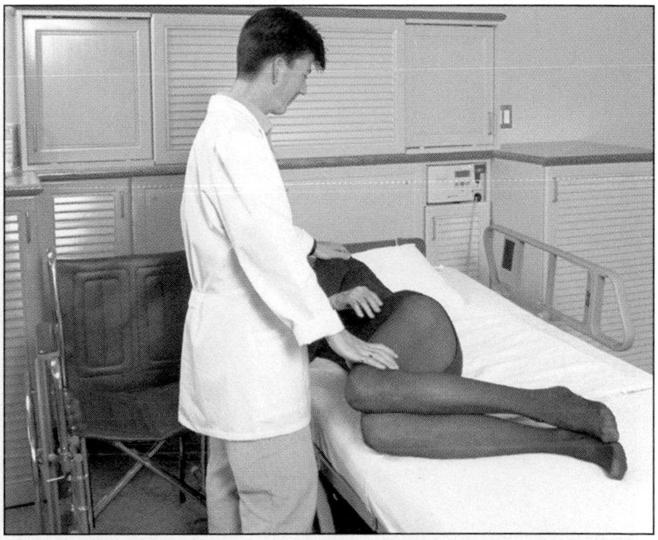

Turn client onto side, maintaining knees in flexed position.

7. Place one of your arms under client's shoulders and other arm beneath client's thighs near knees. **Rationale:** This prevents client falling backward onto bed.
8. Lift client's thighs slightly and pivot on balls of your feet as you move client into sitting position. Use gluteal, abdominal, leg, and arm muscles to move client.
9. Stand in front of client until client is stable in upright position. **Rationale:** Client may experience orthostatic hypotension if he/she has been on bed rest for a period of time.
10. Take vital signs especially if this is first time client is dangled. **Rationale:** To determine if orthostatic hypotension is present.
11. Dangle client with feet flat on the floor for a few minutes before transferring to chair or ambulating. **Rationale:** When feet are on floor, it helps to prevent clot formation.

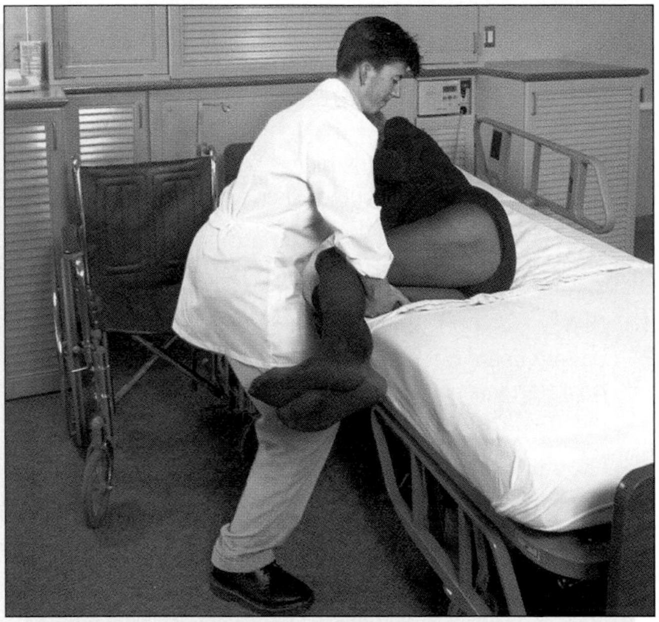
Maintain broad base of support as you pivot client to sitting position.

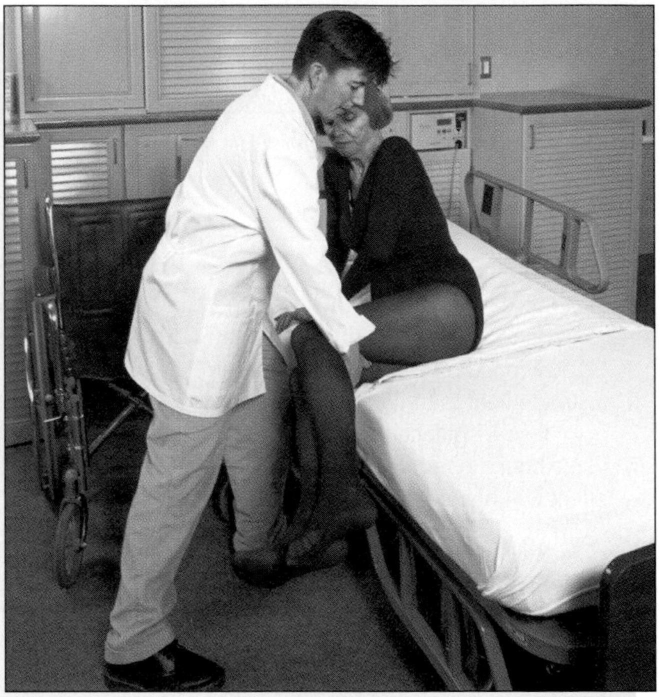
Dangle client with feet flat on floor for several minutes before transferring to chair or ambulating.

MOVING FROM BED TO CHAIR

Equipment

Chair
Bath blanket

Procedure

1. Identify the client and wash hands.
2. Lock bed in place.

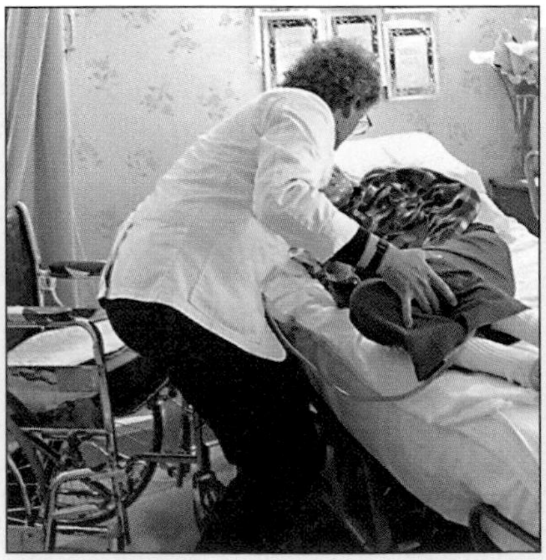
Move client to the side of bed before positioning.

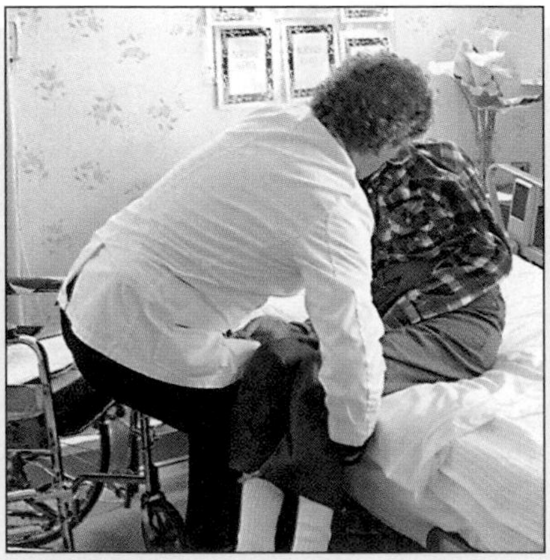
Pivot client and dangle feet before placing feet flat on floor.

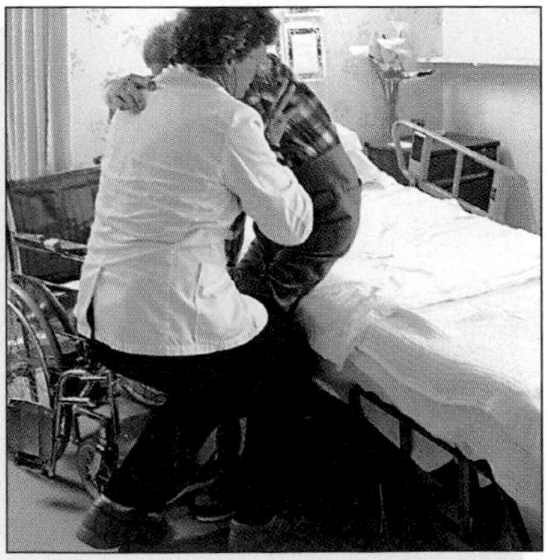
Have client reach arm across shoulder for balance.

3. Place chair at head of bed. Be sure to lock chair wheels or have someone hold chair as you move client.
4. Follow steps 4–6 in skill *Dangling at the Bedside.*
5. Dangle client until he or she is stable.
6. Give client nonslip shoes or slippers.
7. Have client reach across chair and grasp chair arm, if possible. **Rationale:** Helps stabilize client to prevent falls during transfer to chair.
8. Place your hands under client's axilla or around client's back.
9. Place your feet slightly to side and in front of client.
10. Rock client and, on count of three, pivot client into chair.
11. Position client in chair to prevent pressure areas. If client has circulatory impairment, elevate legs while out of bed. **Rationale:** This promotes venous return.

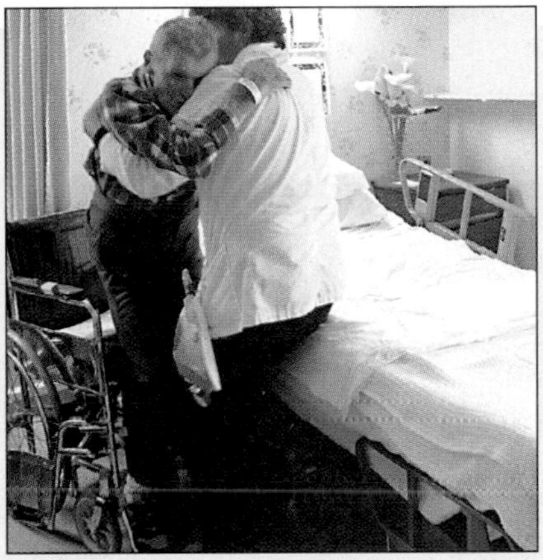

Stabilize client by positioning nurse's foot at the outside edge of client's foot.

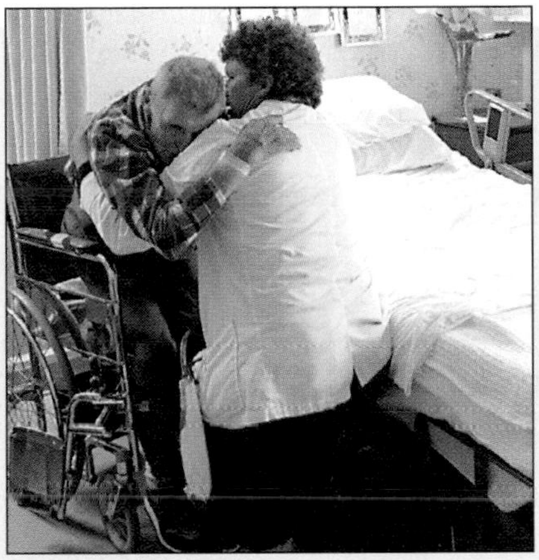

Pivot client into chair using leg muscles instead of back muscles.

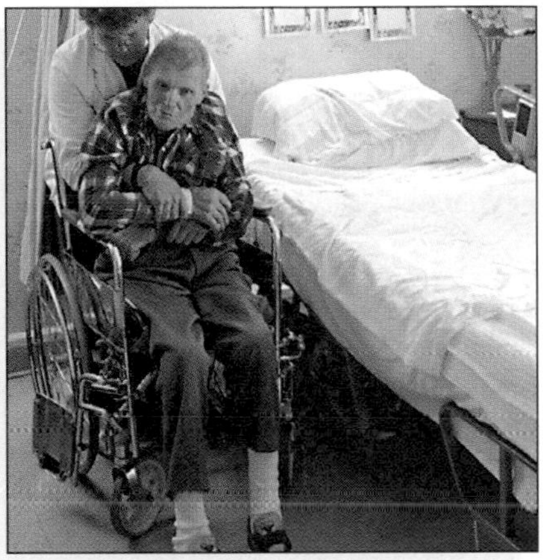

Pull client back and up in wheelchair for better posture.

Use of Safety Belt in Transferring Client from Bed to Chair

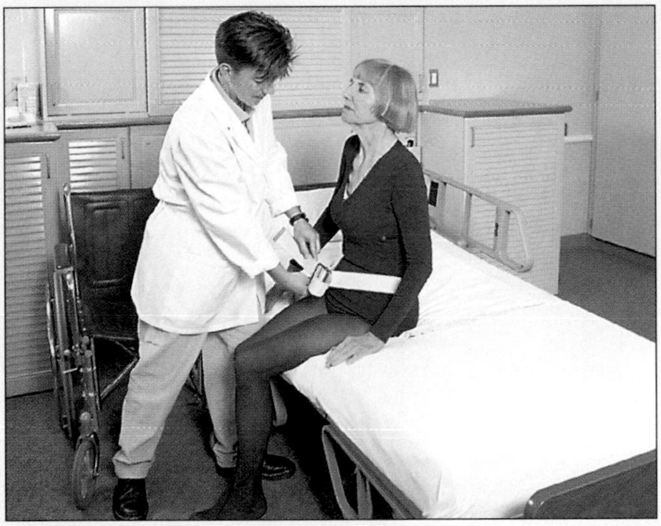

1. Place safety belt around client's waist while client is in sitting position on the edge of the bed (dangling).

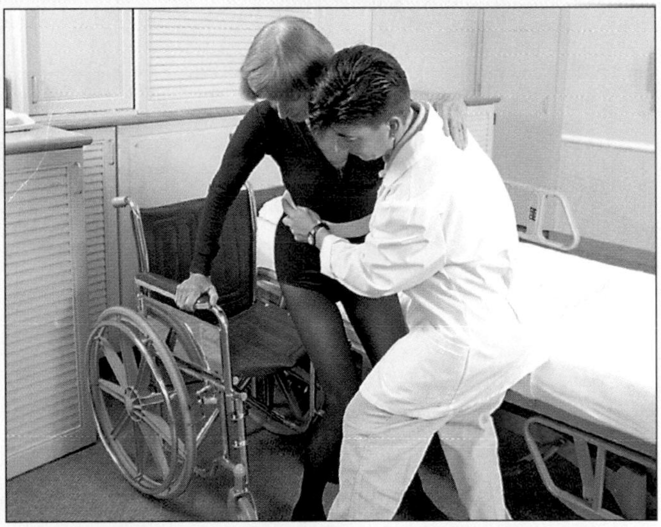

2. Grasp safety or transfer belt with left hand. Place right hand around client's waist and guide into chair.

Client Lifts and Transfer Devices

There are four different types of client lift and transfer devices: sliding boards, for transferring a client from a bed to a gurney, portable sling lifts for lifting clients out of bed and moving to another location; standing aids for helping a client stand on his own for transport, and ceiling lifts used to raise and briefly suspend client above the bed.

USING A HOYER (SLING) LIFT

Equipment

Hoyer lift base
2 canvas pieces: 1 large, 1 small
2 sets of canvas straps

Procedure

1. Check orders and client care plan. Determine that lift can safely move the weight of the client.
2. Explain procedure to client. **Rationale:** Clients may be frightened by use of a mechanical device.
3. Wash your hands.
4. Bring Hoyer frame to bedside.
5. Provide privacy for client.
6. Lock wheels of bed.
7. Place client's chair by the bed. Allow adequate space to maneuver the lift.
8. Raise bed to HIGH position and adjust head and knee gatch so that mattress is flat.
9. Keep side rail on opposite side in UP position.
10. Roll client away from you.
11. Place lower edge of wide canvas piece under client's knees.
12. Place upper edge of narrow canvas piece under client's shoulders.
13. Raise side rail on your side of bed.
14. Move to opposite side of bed, and lower side rail.
15. Roll client away from you to opposite side, and straighten out canvas pieces. Turn client to supine position.
16. Place U base of frame under bed on side where chair is positioned.
17. Lock wheels of frame. Lower side rail.
18. Attach canvas straps from swivel bar to each canvas piece using hooks.
19. Place straps evenly on canvas pieces. Sling extends from shoulders to knees. **Rationale:** This supports client's weight equally.
20. Elevate head of bed.
21. Raise client by turning release knob clockwise to close pressure valve.
22. Pump lift handle until client is lifted clear of the bed.
23. Maneuver client over the chair.
24. Lower client by turning release knob *slowly* counterclockwise.
25. Guide client into chair.
26. Align client into chair.
27. Remove straps from bar, and move lift out of the way.
28. Check for client's comfort in chair; place call bell close at hand.
29. Wash your hands.
30. Return client to bed using reverse method.

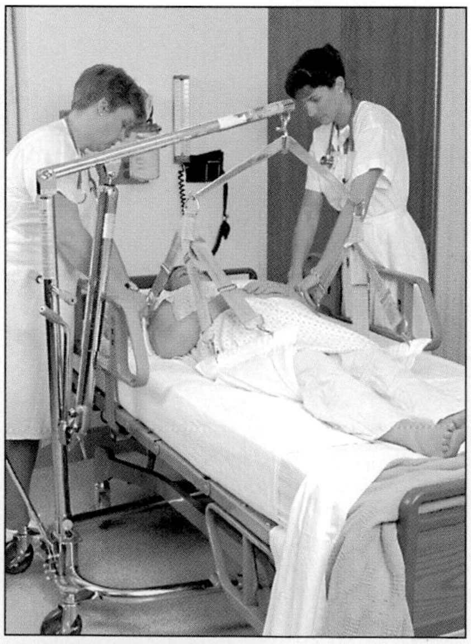

Place canvas piece under client from knees to shoulders.

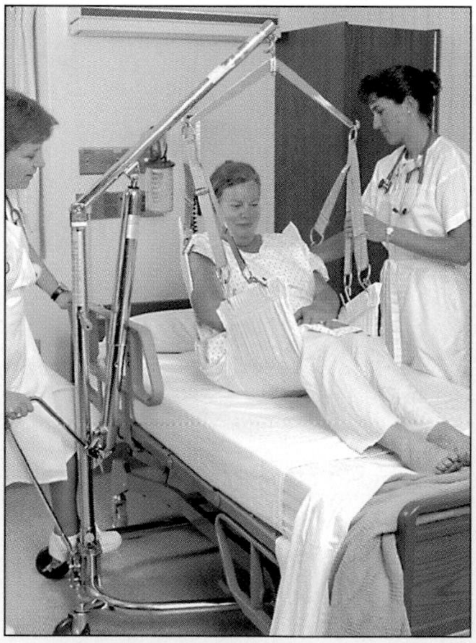

Raise client off bed by turning release knob clockwise.

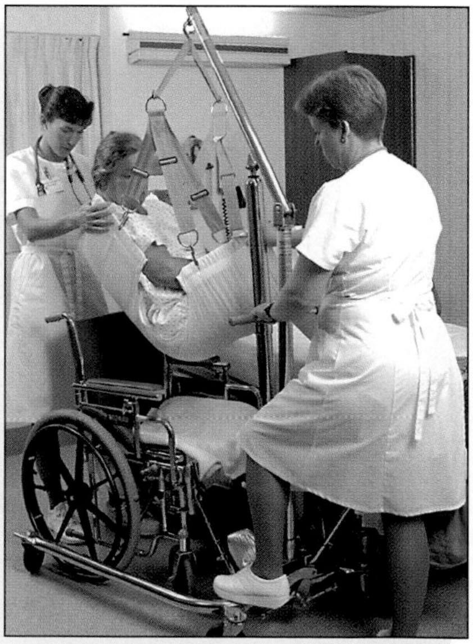

Use one nurse to stabilize client as second nurse guides client into chair.

LOGROLLING THE CLIENT

Equipment

Pillows, towels, blankets for positioning
Turning sheet

Procedure

1. Check order for logrolling client and client care plan as to exactly why client needs to be logrolled.
2. Wash your hands.
3. Obtain sufficient assistance to complete procedure with ease. Three nurses are preferable.
4. Place a pillow between the client's knees before moving the client. **Rationale:** To prevent adduction of hip. This will prevent spinal torque.
5. Position two nurses on side of bed to which client will be turned. Position third nurse on other side of bed.
6. Designate person at head of bed to be in charge of coordinating move.
7. Assume correct position for client move;
   a. Nurse at head: one arm supports client's head, second arm supports shoulders and neck.
   b. Second nurse: one hand grasps client's other shoulder, the other hand and arm around knee.
   c. Third nurse: on the opposite side of the bed, nurse holds drawsheet firmly to support torso. **Rationale:** This maintains the body in alignment.
8. Instruct client to place arms across chest to keep body straight.
9. Assume broad stance with one foot ahead of the other and knees flexed.
10. Rock onto back foot, and use leg and arm muscles to move client in one coordinated movement when nurse at head of bed signals. **Rationale:** To maintain proper alignment, all of the body parts must be moved at the same time. If not, injury to client's neck and spinal column may occur.
11. Maintain client's position in alignment with pillows, towels, or folded blankets.
12. Change client's position frequently (minimum 2 hours) according to physician's orders.

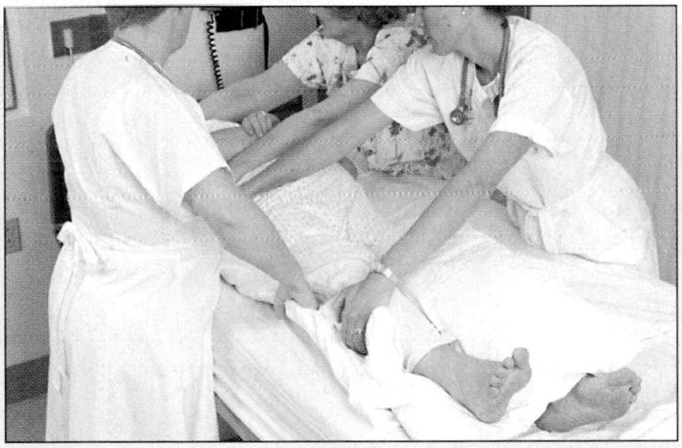

1. Position nurses on each side of client

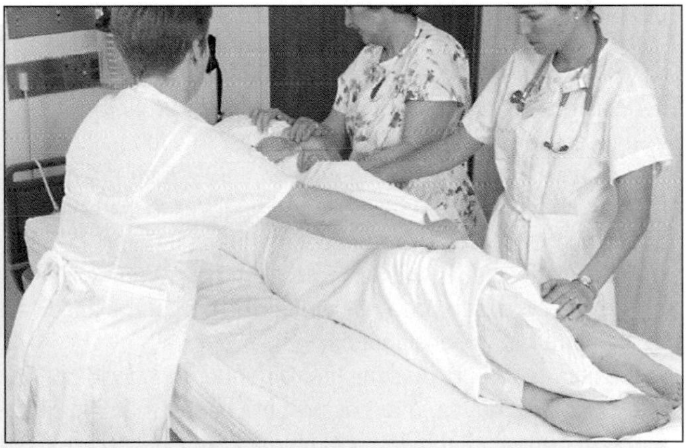

2. Maintain proper alignment while turning client.

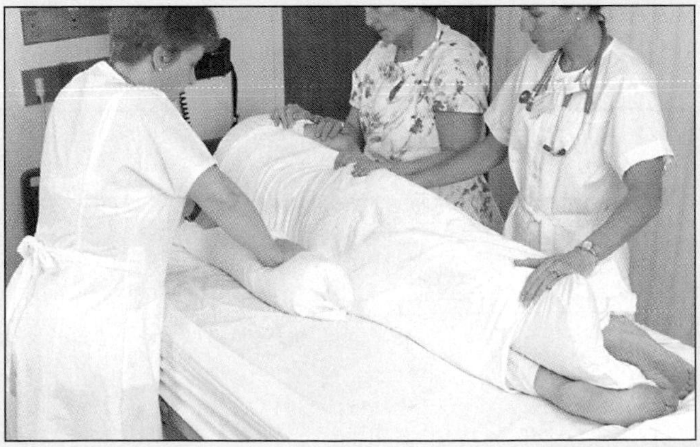

3. Maintain client's position with pillow support under client's back.

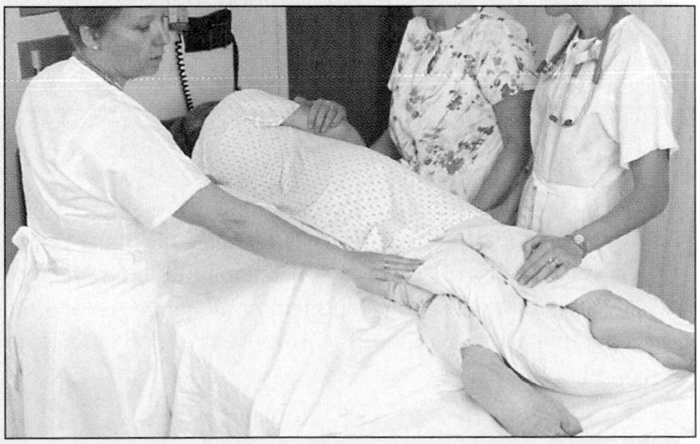

4. After positioning pillow, allow client to lean back for support.

USING A FOOTBOARD

Equipment

Footboard

Procedure

1. Provide a footboard if client is unable to place feet in dorsal flexion or plantar flexion is continuous.
2. Cover footboard with a bath blanket to protect feet from rough surfaces.
3. Place footboard on bed in a place where client's feet can firmly rest on it without sliding down in bed.
4. Observe legs to ensure that they are not in a flexed position when feet are against the board.
5. Tuck top linen under mattress at foot of bed, and bring linen up over the footboard to the top of the bed. Do not drape top linen over footboard as it can easily be pulled off the bed.

> **CLINICAL ALERT**
>
> Footboards are used to prevent plantar flexion. Extended periods of plantar flexion can lead to footdrop.

Note: Clients are encouraged to wear high-top sneakers while on bedrest, along with the footboard. **Rationale:** *Aids in preventing footdrop.*

6. Put feet and ankles through range-of-motion exercises every 4 hours for clients on prolonged bedrest.
7. Observe heels and ankles frequently for signs of breakdown.
8. Place pillow under client's calves (not under heels) allowing heels to be off mattress if skin breakdown is assessed.

PLACING A TROCHANTER ROLL

Equipment

Bath blanket

Procedure

1. Wash hands and place client in supine or prone position.
2. Place folded bath blanket on bed next to client.
3. Extend blanket from greater trochanter to thigh or knee.
4. Place blanket edge under leg and buttocks to anchor.
5. Roll bath blanket toward client by rolling it under.
6. Rotate affected leg to slight internal hip rotation. **Rationale:** The purpose is to prevent external rotation of the head of the femur in the acetabulum.
7. Tighten the roll by tucking the roll under the hip joint.
8. Allow affected leg to rest against trochanter roll. Hip should be in normal alignment, not internally or externally rotated. Patella should be facing upward if client in supine position. **Rationale:** This is used most commonly for clients who have a muscle weakness or paralysis of that side of the body.

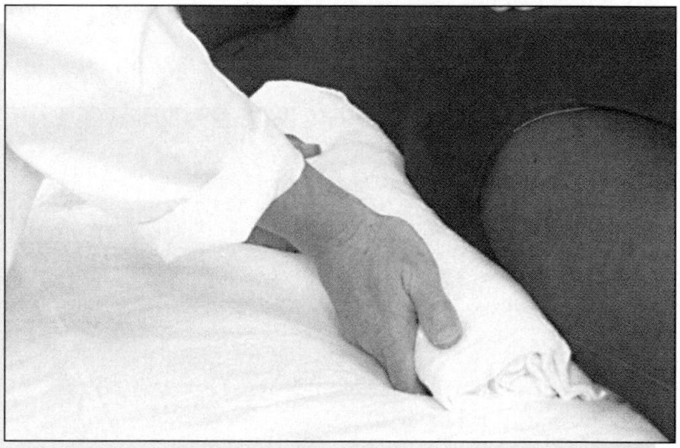

Use trochanter rolls made from bath blankets to align client's hips.

Handroll Positioning

When positioning clients who are on long-term bed rest, all areas of the body must be considered. Handrolls made from folded washcloths rolled into a cone shape (or commercially available) may be used to position and maintain wrist and fingers in a functional position. The purpose is to prevent deformity and contractures.

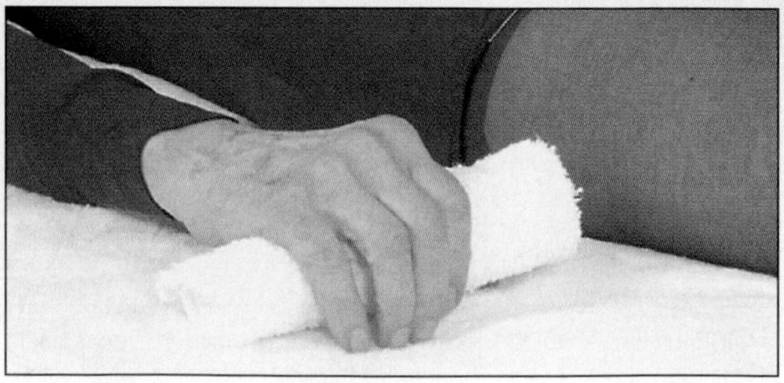

DOCUMENTATION FOR MOVING AND TURNING CLIENTS

- How often client turned or moved
- Condition of skin and joint movement
- Unexpected problems with moving or positioning client and solutions to problems
- Client's acceptance of and feelings about the procedure
- Number of staff needed to complete the procedure
- Transferred by Hoyer lift from bed to chair, if appropriate
- Time client was in chair or dangling at bedside
- Use of a footboard or trochanter roll

Critical Thinking Application

UNEXPECTED OUTCOMES	CRITICAL THINKING OPTIONS
Client unwilling to move due to fear of pain or discomfort.	• Explain rationale and need for the procedure more thoroughly • If possible, check if client can be medicated before the procedure. • Obtain additional assistance to decrease client's apprehension.
Client unable to assist with movement.	• Use a drawsheet to provide more support for client. • Obtain additional assistance to help with moving "dead" weight.
Client unable to maintain any type of position without assistance.	• Use trochanter roll to prevent external rotation of client's hip • Use foam bolsters to maintain side-lying positions. • Using folded towels, blankets, or small pillows, position client's hands and arms to prevent dependent edema.
Skin begins to break down.	• Change client position every 2 hours. • Check with physician for therapeutic mattress or dressings for pressure ulcer(s) care.

GERONTOLOGIC CONSIDERATIONS

Physiologic age changes in the musculoskeletal system that affect nursing care of the elderly.

- Contractures—muscles atrophy, regenerate slowly; tendons shrink and sclerose.
- Range of motion of joints decreases—lack of adequate joint motion, ankylosis.
- Mobility level is limited—muscle strength lessens and gait may be unsteady.
- Kyphosis occurs—cervical vertebrae may be flexed; intervertebral discs narrow.
- Bone changes—loss of trabecular bones and bones become brittle.

Psychosocial and physiological changes in elderly who are immobilized.

- At risk for confusion, depression and disorientation—keep clock and calendar in room to help reorient to time and place.
- More susceptible to hazards of immobility—maintain own ADLs as much as possible and change position every 2 hours.

Nursing care for positioning elderly clients.

- Ambulate within limitations of age.
- Alter position every 2 hours; align correctly.
- Prevent osteoporosis of long bones by providing exercises against resistance as ordered.
- Provide active and passive exercises—rest periods necessary and exercise paced throughout the day for the elderly.
- Provide range-of-motion exercises to all joints three times a day.
- Educate family that allowing the client to be sedentary is not helpful.
- Encourage walking, which is best single exercise for the elderly.

Management Guidelines

Each state legislates a Nurse Practice Act for RNs and LVN/LPNs. Health care facilities are responsible for establishing and implementing policies and procedures that conform to their state's regulations. Verify the regulations and role parameters for each health care worker in your facility.

Delegation of Responsibilities

- All levels of health care workers can be assigned to move and turn clients, and provide assistance with transfers.
- Positioning clients in bed can be assigned to all levels of health care workers.
- Frequently, the physical therapist is assigned to work with postoperative clients or clients requiring special transfer techniques or ambulation until clients are released to nursing.
- Before assigning staff to logroll a client or use the Hoyer lift for moving a client out of bed, ensure they have been properly instructed in the procedures and safety issues associated with these activities.

Information Flow

- The RN must give specific directions to the health care workers on appropriate positions for clients on bed rest or specifics on how to transfer clients to a chair or gurney.
- Before physical therapy releases clients to nursing for transfer or ambulation activities, the RN must obtain explicit information on the procedures to be used. This information must be written on the Kardex, as well as reviewed with all staff assigned to the client.
- A team conference may be necessary if special equipment or specific activities are required by a client. This conference ensures all staff will be given a demonstration and provided information necessary for safe client care.
- The RN must ensure that all new personnel are proficient in transfers, logrolling and use of the Hoyer lift before assigning them to care for clients requiring these skills.
- It is crucial for safe client care that the RN monitors health care workers when they perform logrolling or use the Hoyer lift after the initial demonstration.

CRITICAL THINKING STRATEGIES

SCENARIO 1

You are assigned to a medical unit where many of the clients require assistance moving in and out of bed. The following clients are assigned to you for care on the day shift.

- Onica Jones, 89-year-old (CVA) client who has weakness on the right side and is unable to communicate but seems to understand directions. She has been in the hospital for 4 days and will be transferred to a SNF this afternoon.
- James Metcalf, 60-year-old (MI) client who is about to be discharged. However, you notice he still has not been able to ambulate by himself.
- Madeline Oscar, 70-year-old client with Parkinson's disease and hospitalized for pneumonia. She was admitted last night. She has orders to be up in the chair BID.
- Joseph Nichols, 40-year-old client, hospitalized for possible kidney stones. He is in severe pain and the MD has ordered that he remain on bed rest until further orders.

1. Which client will you assess first? Provide rationale for your answer.
2. How will you determine the client's ability to assist with his or her own care and movement in bed?
3. For each client, identify the type of assistance he or she might need; provide rationale for your answer.
4. Describe the body mechanics you will use when moving clients; this will be based on the type of moving that will need to be performed for each of the four clients.

SCENARIO 2

You are assigned to care for a client who weighs 300 pounds. The client was out of bed for lunch and now insists on getting back into bed. There are no male staff members available to help you.

1. Suggest some creative resolutions to this problem.
2. What other problems would you anticipate with this client?

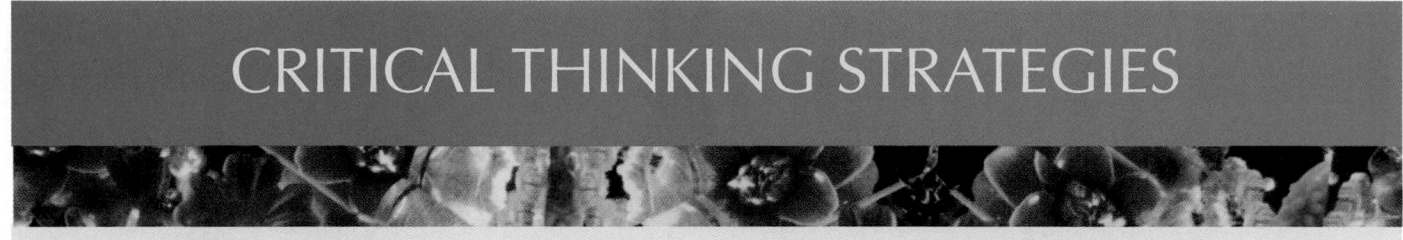

CHAPTER 13

Exercise and Ambulation

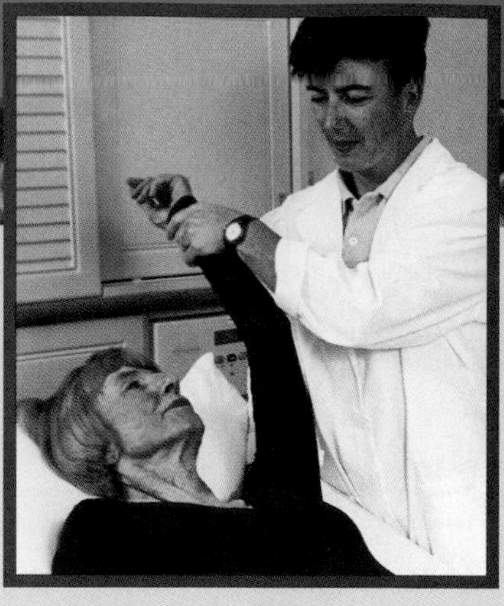

THEORETICAL CONCEPTS

UNIT ONE: **Range of Motion** 354
- Performing Passive Range of Motion 355
- Teaching Active Range of Motion 359

UNIT TWO: **Ambulation** 360
- Minimizing Orthostatic Hypotension 361
- Ambulating with Two Assistants 361
- Ambulating with One Assistant 362
- Ambulating with a Walker 364
- Ambulating with a Cane 364

UNIT THREE: **Crutch Walking** 367
- Teaching Muscle-Strengthening Exercises 368
- Measuring Client for Crutches 368
- Teaching Crutch Walking: Four-Point Gait 369
- Teaching Crutch Walking: Three-Point Gait 369
- Teaching Crutch Walking: Two-Point Gait 370
- Teaching Swing-To Gait and Swing-Through Gait 370
- Teaching Upstairs and Downstairs Ambulation with Crutches 371
- Teaching Moving In and Out of Chair with Crutches 372

GERONTOLOGIC CONSIDERATIONS 373

MANAGEMENT GUIDELINES 374

CRITICAL THINKING STRATEGIES 375

Cross reference: Continuous Passive Motion Machine, Chapter 30

Learning Objectives

- Define rehabilitative nursing.
- Compare and contrast preservative and restorative methods of care.
- Identify the joints and the type of movement they allow.
- Compare and contrast passive and active range of motion.
- Demonstrate passive range-of-motion exercises using all muscle groups.
- Explain the rationale of assisted ambulation for clients.
- Complete a client-teaching guide for clients requiring muscle-strengthening exercises.
- Demonstrate the proper method for measuring crutches.
- Name and discuss four crutch-walking gaits.
- Demonstrate four crutch-walking gaits.
- List the components of crutch walking that require documentation.
- Write three nursing diagnoses that are appropriate for clients requiring exercise and ambulation activities.

Terminology

Abduction: movement of a bone away from the midline of the body or body part, as in raising the arm or spreading the fingers.

Adduction: movement of a bone toward the midline of the body or part

Alignment: arranged in a straight line; position of body parts in relation to each other.

Ambulate: walking; able to walk.

Antagonists: muscles that exert an action opposing that of prime mover.

Atrophy: a wasting of any organ or body part due to lack of nutrients or oxygen.

Base of support: foundation on which a person's body weight is supported.

Balance: a result of body alignment that maintains equilibrium.

Cardiovascular: pertaining to heart and blood vessels.

Circumduction: movement of a bone in a circular direction so that the distal end scribes a circle while the proximal end remains stationary, as in "winding up" to throw a ball.

Contractility: ability of muscle to shorten, tighten, and contract.

Dorsiflexion: flexion of the foot at the ankle joint; the act of turning the foot and toes upward, as in standing on the heel.

Elasticity: ability of strained muscle to regain original size and shape when applied force is removed.

Eversion: turning outward; movement of the foot at the ankle joint so that the sole faces outward.

Excitability: capacity of muscle to respond to stimulus without intervention of motor nerves.

Extensibility: ability of muscle to stretch in response to applied force.

Extension: a movement that increases the angle between two bones, straightening a joint.

Fibrotic: pertinent to fibrosis, the formation of fibrous material.

Flaccidity: decrease in muscle tone.

Flexion: a movement that decreases the angle between two bones; the act of bending a joint.

Fracture: any break or crack in a bone

Hyperextension: continuation of extension beyond the anatomic position, as in bending the head backward.

Hypertrophy: increased muscle fiber leading to increased muscle shape and size.

Inversion: turning inward; movement of the foot at the ankle joint so that the sole faces inward.

Ligament: a band or sheet of strong fibrous connective tissue connecting the articular ends of bones serving to bind them together and to facilitate or limit motion.

Mobility: state or quality of being mobile; facility of movement.

Musculoskeletal: pertaining to the muscles and bones.

Paralysis: temporary or permanent loss of function, especially loss of sensation or voluntary motion.

Plantar flexion: extension of the foot at the ankle joint; the foot and toes are turned downward toward the sole of the foot, as in standing on tiptoe.

Posture: attitude or position of body.

Prime movers: muscles responsible for the primary movement of contraction.

Pronation: rotation of the forearm so that the palm faces backward or downward; movement of the whole body so that the face and abdomen are downward.

Prone: lying horizontal with face downward.

Protraction: movement of the clavicle (collar bone) or mandible (lower jaw) forward on a plane parallel to the ground.

Proximal: nearest the point of attachment or reference point.

Range-of-motion: extent to which a joint can move through active or passive exercises.

Retraction: movement of the clavicle or mandible backward on a plane parallel to the ground.

Rotation: movement of a bone around its own axis, as in moving the head to indicate "no" or turning the palm of the hand up and then down.

Spasticity: increase in muscle tension.

Sprain: injury caused by wrenching or twisting of a joint that results in tearing or stretching of the associated ligaments.

Strain: injury caused by excessive force or stretching of muscles or tendons around the joint.

Supination: rotation of forearm so that the palm faces forward or upward; movement of the whole body so that the face and abdomen are upward.

Synergists: muscles that enhance action of prime mover.

Tendons: fibrous connective tissue serving for the attachment of muscles to bones and other parts.

Tonicity: ability of muscle to maintain steady contraction, which determines its firmness.

Ulcer: an open area of the skin or mucous membrane.

REHABILITATION CONCEPTS

Rehabilitative nursing involves the prevention and correction of alterations in the musculoskeletal system. In fact, the definition of rehabilitative nursing is the process of restoring a person's ability to live and work in as normal a manner as possible. To assist clients to achieve and maintain optimal mobility, both preservative and restorative methods are used.

Preservative methods, such as exercises and assisted ambulation, include those interventions that are needed to help clients maintain their normal mobility. Because the changes that occur in the human body when a person is hospitalized are varied and subtle, preservative methods are used with every client. Restorative methods, such as crutch walking and splinting, are used with clients who have decreased mobility caused by such factors as debilitating illness or major surgery. The purpose for applying restorative methods is to assist the client in achieving the level of mobility he or she enjoyed before becoming ill.

The general goals for using these methods are to assist the client to strive for optimal function, to prevent further injury, and to restore normal function. To achieve these goals of care, it is important for the nurse to accept the philosophy underlying rehabilitative nursing: that every illness is accompanied by the intrinsic threat of disability and that this part of total client care must begin with the initial client contact. Finally, it is important to accept that the principles of rehabilitation are basic to the care of all clients and that rehabilitation must be begun early in the client's hospitalization.

Being hospitalized and immobile seriously affects a person's body image, behavior, and overall adaptation and adjustment. The greater the disability, the more these aspects of a person's life are affected. The nurse's responsibility in providing total client care is to be aware of these responses and to take them into account when developing a client care plan.

MUSCULOSKELETAL SYSTEM

The musculoskeletal system is comprised of bones, muscles, joints, cartilage, bursa, tendons, and ligaments. The bones form the infrastructure of the system. The ability of bones to provide weight bearing and mobility is in direct relationship to the size and shape of the bones.

Joints, in conjunction with muscles, provide motion and flexibility. Skeletal muscles are under voluntary control as a result of being innervated by somatic nerves. Muscles, through their ability to contract, convert energy into mechanical work, maintain body alignment, and cause movement.

The muscular system is a system of more than six hundred fibers that are attached to bones. The system allows for body movement under the control of the voluntary nervous system. Muscles provide for body movement or locomotion, support the body, and perform several body functions, such as the partial production of heat. The fibers of the voluntary muscles are grouped together in a sheath of connective tissue. Each bundled group of muscle fibers is surrounded by a connective tissue sheath. The sheath tissue may be continuous with fibrous tissue that extends from the muscle as a tendon.

There are several properties of muscle fibers. The first is excitability, or the capacity of a muscle to respond to stimulus without intervention of the motor nerves. Another property is contractility, the ability of a muscle to shorten, tighten, or contract. Muscles are also able to maintain steady contraction (tonicity), stretch in response to applied force (extensibility), and regain their original size and shape when applied force is removed (elasticity).

Muscle Function

Skeletal muscles produce body movements by pulling on the bones. Bones serve as levers, and joints serve as fulcrums of these levers. Each muscle has a point of origin and a point of insertion that are usually attached to the bone. Muscles that move a body part usually do not extend over that part. These muscles usually perform with group action; some contract, and others relax. Prime movers are muscles responsible for the primary movement of contraction. Antagonists are muscles that exert an action opposing that of the prime movers. Synergists are muscles that enhance action of the prime mover. The accessory parts to muscles are the ligaments and the tendons.

JOINTS

A joint of the body is the point at which two or more bones join together. The function of a joint is skeletal flexibility and motion. Joints are classified according to structural variations that allow for different kinds of movements. There are three main types of classification: synarthrotic, amphiarthrotic, and diarthrotic joints.

Synarthrotic joints are immovable and include those areas where tissue grows between articulating surfaces, such as the suture lines of the skull. Amphiarthrotic joints have limited movement. Diarthrotic joints have two freely movable parts. This type of joint is a cavity enclosed by a capsule lined with synovial membrane, which secretes a lubricant. The following types of joint movement allow for structural variations.

- Hinge type allows single directional movement (elbow).
- Ball-and-socket type allows bending (hip).
- Saddle type allows multidirectional shifting (thumb).
- Pivot type allows rotary movement (neck, cervical spine).
- Gliding type allows limited sliding of bones against each other (wrist, ankle, invertebral joints).

Each of these types of joints have specific kinds of movements they can perform. These movements can be described in relationship to the three body planes: sagittal, transverse, and coronal. The sagittal plane divides the body into two portions with a straight vertical line between the two parts. The transverse plane divides the body into upper–lower portions with a horizontal line. The coronal plane divides the body into anterior–posterior portions at right angles to the sagittal plane. The joints accomplish a variety of movements that range from flexion–extension to rotation and circumduction. For definitions of joint movements through the planes of the body, refer to the following.

Joint Movements

Abduction: Movement of a bone away from the midline of the body or body part, as in raising the arm or spreading the fingers.

Eversion: Turning outward; movement of the foot at the ankle joint so that the sole faces outward.

Flexion: A movement that decreases the angle between two bones; the act of bending a joint.

Protraction: Movement of the clavicle (collar bone) or mandible (lower jaw) forward on a plane parallel to the ground.

Pronation: Rotation of the forearm so that the palm faces backward or downward; movement of the whole body so that the face and abdomen are downward.

Circumduction: Movement of a bone in a circular direction so that the distal end scribes a circle while the proximal end remains stationary, as in "winding up" to throw a ball.

Adduction: Movement of a bone toward the midline of the body or part.

Inversion: Turning inward; movement of the foot at the ankle joint so that the sole faces inward.

Extension: A movement that increases the angle between two bones, straightening a joint.

Hyperextension: Continuation of extension beyond the anatomic position, as in bending the head backward.

Retraction: Movement of the clavicle or mandible backward on a plane parallel to the ground.

Supination: Rotation of forearm so that the palm faces forward or upward; movement of the whole body so that the face and abdomen are upward.

Rotation: Movement of a bone around its own axis, as in moving the head to indicate "no" or turning the palm of the hand up and then down.

EXERCISE

Muscles that are not used become weak and shortened. During prolonged bed rest, strength and endurance decrease rapidly. Clients can regain muscle strength and mobility by practicing specific groups of exercises daily. Promoting exercise, both passive and active, is one of the most important nursing functions. The purpose of exercises is to promote proper alignment, prevent contractures, stimulate circulation, and prevent thrombophlebitis and pressure ulcers. Exercise reduces joint pain and stiffness and increases flexibility and endurance. Exercise also prevents edema of the extremities and promotes lung expansion.

The nurse both performs and teaches several types of exercises as a component of providing total client care. Passive exercises are carried out by the therapist or nurse without assistance from the client. These exercises enable the client to retain as much joint range of motion as possible, as well as stimulating circulation. Active exercises, although supervised by the nurse, are performed by the client. These exercises increase muscle strength when the client is partially immobile.

Resistive exercises, another rehabilitative measure, provide resistance in order to increase muscle power. These active exercises are performed by the individual working against resistance. Isometric or muscle-setting activities are similar to resistive exercises. These exercises maintain strength in a muscle when the joint is immobilized. They are performed by the individual without assistance.

Range-of-motion (ROM) exercises are the most common form of exercises for maintaining joint mobility and increasing maximal motion of a joint when the client is totally or partially immobilized. These exercises are completed by the nurse or physical therapist. The therapist puts an extremity through its full range so that the joint is moved through all the appropriate planes. Before beginning these exercises, it is important that the nurse assess the client's condition and the baseline ROM capabilities, establish the extent of ROM to be carried out, and ensure that the client is comfortable. Be aware that clients might be fearful of this type of exercise and that a full explanation of what you are going to do is helpful to allay fears. Enlist the cooperation of the client for maximum benefit. Discontinue all range-of-motion exercises if the client complains of pain, for it is at this point that the exercises become counterproductive.

AMBULATION

Ambulation, or walking, is an important function that most of us accomplish automatically; that is, without thinking or conscious effort. When a person has been immobilized, confined to bed following surgery or an injury, or unable to ambulate, this seemingly simple activity can become a major hurdle to overcome. The longer a person is immobilized, the more difficult it is to regain ambulatory ability; likewise, the sooner a person begins to ambulate after being bedridden, the more easily he or she will regain preimmobilization status. Early ambulation decreases hospitalization time and prevents complications, such as paralytic ileus or thrombophlebitis.

The human body functions best when it is frequently placed in a vertical position. Ambulation improves physical and mental well-being. Ambulation increases muscle strength and joint mobility. It also increases respiratory exchange, gastrointestinal muscle tone, and circulation. Without stress on bones, calcium deposits occur and renal problems increase from calcium-based calculi.

Balance, coordination, and good body alignment are aspects important to walking. One must be able to move forward and maintain an upright balance; use muscles, bones, and joints correctly for coordination; and keep the head erect and vertebral column fairly straight with feet and knee caps pointed forward in order to maintain good body alignment.

The major muscle groups used for walking are the thigh and leg muscles. If these muscles have not been used or exercised because the client has been in bed for a long time, ambulation must be accomplished step by step. Weak muscles cannot support a human frame for the mechanics of walking. It is important, then, to begin the process of ambulation by administering muscle-strengthening exercises. Several different types of exercises were described previously; however, the most important preambulatory preparation is quadriceps-setting and gluteal-setting exercises. Carried out several times a day, these exercises restore muscle strength and prepare the legs for weight bearing.

Before actually assisting the client to walk, explain exactly what you are going to do, and prepare the client by doing the ambulatory procedure in stages. For example, begin with the muscle-strengthening exercises. Then assist the client to sit up in bed to determine if he or she is experiencing vertigo. Have the client move to the side of the bed with legs down, and only when he or she is ready and feels comfortable in doing so, assist the client to stand beside the bed. You may decide to take the client's vital signs after dangling to determine if they are stable. Allow the client to remain there with the bed as support until he or she feels totally secure. Finally, and with the assistance of one or two nurses (depending on the assessment of the client's ability and readiness to ambulate), have the client walk by taking short steps and walking only as long as he or she can tolerate. Do this several times a day, and it will not be long before the client's legs are strengthened, and he or she can graduate to one assistant, a walker, or cane. Throughout this procedure, do not allow the client to lose confidence in the ability to walk or your ability to support and assist while regaining his or her independence of action.

A variety of assistive devices are available to give the client support when ambulating. Such devices may give the client confidence (especially important with the elderly), stability, support for a weak limb, or reduce the pressure on a limb. These devices may include canes (standard cane, T-handled cane, tripod cane, and quad cane) and walkers (standard, with wheels, or a hemi-walker). Other assistive devices include crutches, used to lessen or remove weight from one or both legs.

CRUTCHES

Crutches are an aid to walking by providing support during ambulating when the lower extremities are unable to support the body weight. It is hoped that this situation is temporary, but even if it is permanent, crutches do allow independence of movement that otherwise could not occur.

There are three main types of crutches: the axillary (most common for short-term use), the Lofstrand, or Canadian (a forearm crutch with a metal band and handle), and the platform, for clients who are unable to use their wrists to bear weight.

Several safety factors should be taken into account before assisting the client to use crutches. The measurement should be 5 cm (2 inches) from the axillary fold to the crutch bar. The handpiece should be adjusted to allow 20° to 30° elbow flexion, and rubber suction tips should be placed on the bottom of the crutches. Finally, the client should be informed that while using crutches, one needs well-fitting shoes with nonslip soles.

The type of crutch used by the client depends on the ability to ambulate, the muscle strength needed for support, and the individual needs of the client.

NURSING DIAGNOSES

The following nursing diagnoses are appropriate to use on client care plans when the components are related to exercise and ambulation needs of clients.

NURSING DIAGNOSIS	RELATED FACTORS
Activity Intolerance	Nutritional disorders, surgery, disease states, impaired motor function, pain
Impaired Home Maintenance Management	Chronic debilitating disease, injury, surgery, lack of knowledge, insufficient funds, lack of support or community resources
Acute Pain	Altered body function (muscle spasms or rigidity), musculoskeletal disorders, inflammation, immobility
Impaired Physical Mobility	Neuromuscular impairment, musculoskeletal impairment, surgical procedure, trauma
Self-Care Deficit (specify)	Neuromuscular impairment, surgery, musculoskeletal impairment, visual disorders, external devices, decreased strength and endurance

- The single most important nursing action to decrease the incidence of hospital-based infections is handwashing. **Remember to wash your hands or use antibacterial gel before and after each and every client contact.**

UNIT 1

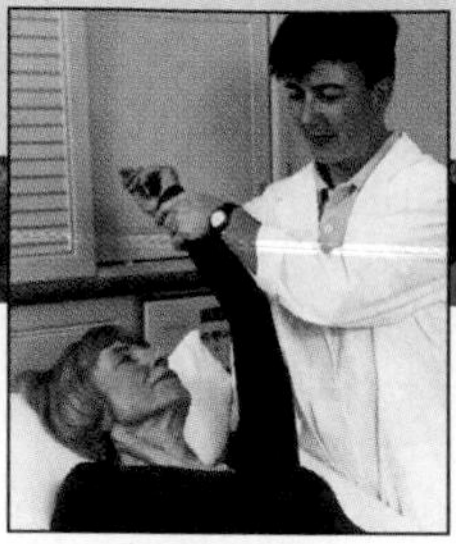

Range of Motion

Nursing Process Data

ASSESSMENT *Database*

Determine client's physical ability to perform exercises (i.e., level of consciousness, presence of casts, traction).

Ascertain client's baseline level of joint movement and muscle strength.

Note amount of spontaneous movement shown by the client.

Assess client's understanding of ROM exercises.

PLANNING *Objectives*

To improve or maintain joint function

To improve or maintain muscle tone and strength

To counteract effects of prolonged bed rest or immobilization

To prevent contractures

To increase client comfort

To prepare the client for ambulation

IMPLEMENTATION *Procedures*

Performing Passive Range of Motion

Teaching Active Range of Motion

EVALUATION *Expected Outcomes*

Client experiences improved range of motion and muscle tone.

Client is comfortable following range-of-motion exercises.

Client is able to ambulate without difficulty following a period of bed rest.

PERFORMING PASSIVE RANGE OF MOTION

Equipment

Hospital bed

Procedure

1. Wash hands.
2. Explain rationale for procedure to client.
3. Position client on his or her back with bed as flat as possible. Place bed in high position.
4. Expose limb to be exercised.
5. Put all joints through range of motion slowly and gently (Tables 13–1 and 13–2). Start at head.
6. Protect against gravity and detrimental movement when performing range-of-motion exercises.
7. Provide support above and below joint using a cradling support while performing the exercises.
8. Follow sequence of exercises for upper and lower body according to chart.

TABLE 13–1 Range of Motion: Upper Body

	Neck	Shoulder	Elbow	Forearm	Wrist	Finger and Thumb
Flexion	Move head forward 90° with chin on chest	Raise arm 180° from side to above head	Bend elbow so arm moves up toward shoulder		Bend hand 90° toward inner arm	Make a fist so fingers are all bent inward
Extension	Move head up from chest 90° to erect position	Move arm to side of body	Straighten elbow and return to position		Move hand straight pointed out	Move fingers 90° to straight position
Hyperextension	Move head backwards 90°	Move arm to back of body at 50° angle			Bend hand up and back 90° toward arm	Move fingers up toward back of hand
Abduction		Hold arm away from side 180° to above head			Bend wrist out away from arm	Spread fingers as much as possible
Adduction		Move arm from side across chest			Bend wrist inward toward radius	Move fingers and thumb together
External Rotation		Hold arm out to side with elbow bent 45°; move forward so palm faces forward				
Internal Rotation		Move arm to side at shoulder level with elbow bent 45°. Lower arm so palm faces back				
Rotation	Move head in circular motion—90° left, then 90° right					
Circumduction		Move arm in full circle				
Supination				Rotate forearm 90° so palm is up		
Pronation				Rotate forearm 90° so palm is down		

TABLE 13–2 Range of Motion: Lower Body

	Trunk	Hip	Knee	Ankle	Toes
Flexion	Bend forward 90°	Move leg forward and up 90°	Bend knee 90°; foot moves back and up		Point down 90°
Extension	Stand in straight position	Move leg in straight alignment with trunk	Move foot 90° with knee straight and leg in line with body		Straight out from foot
Hyperextension	Bend backward 30°	Move leg backward 50°			Point up 45°
Lateral Flexion	Bend to both sides 45°				
Internal Rotation		Turn leg and foot inward 90°			
External Rotation		Turn leg and foot outward 90°			
Circumduction		Move leg in circle 360°			
Abduction		Move leg away from body 45°			Spread apart 15°
Adduction		Move leg toward body 45°			Bring together in normal position
Rotation	Move in circle 360° from waist				
Plantar Flexion				Point toes downward	
Dorsiflexion				Point toes upward	
Eversion				Move sole of foot lateral to outside	
Inversion				Move sole of foot medial to inside	

9. All joints should be put through five full-range-of-motion exercises to each joint at least twice daily.
10. Encourage client to do active exercises as soon as possible. **Rationale**: Passive exercises only help prevent contractures, but do not maintain muscle.
11. Discontinue exercises if client complains of pain or discomfort.
12. Reassess client's ability to perform ROM exercises and adjust schedule accordingly.

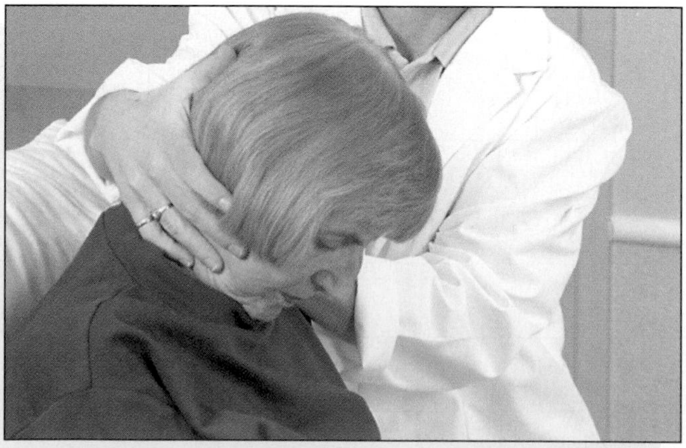
Flexion of neck—Move head forward 90° with chin on chest.

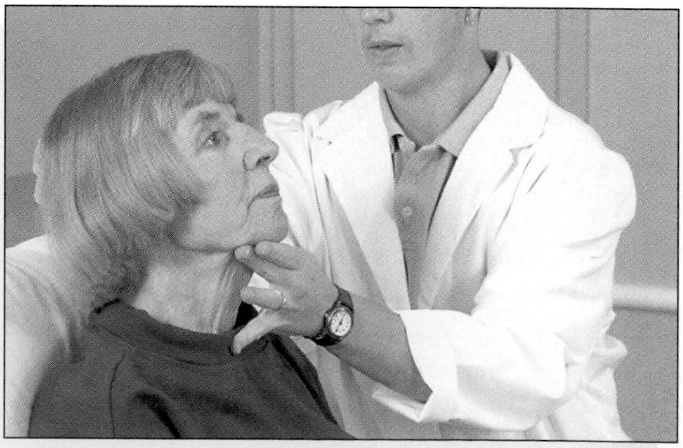
Extension of neck—Move head up from chest 90°.

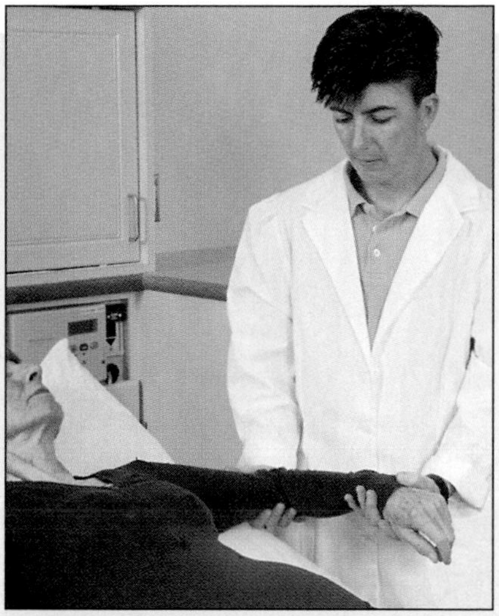
Internal rotation of shoulder.

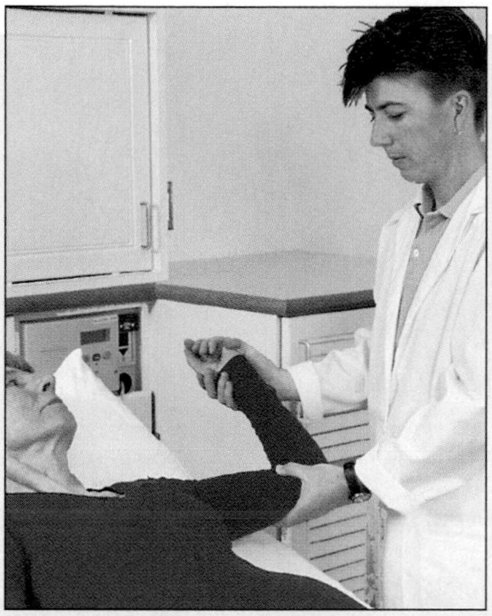
External rotation of shoulder.

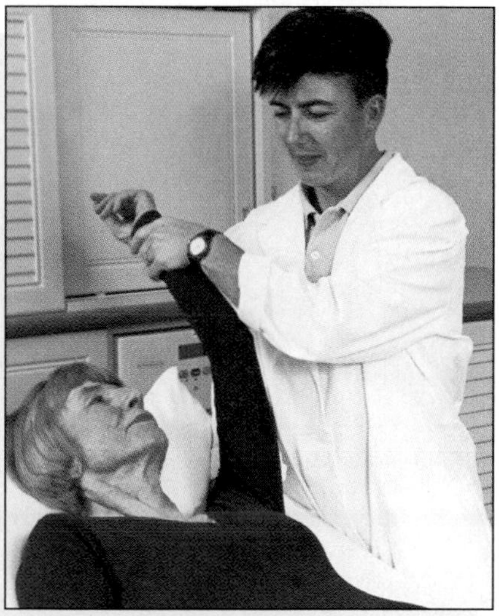
Abduction of shoulder.

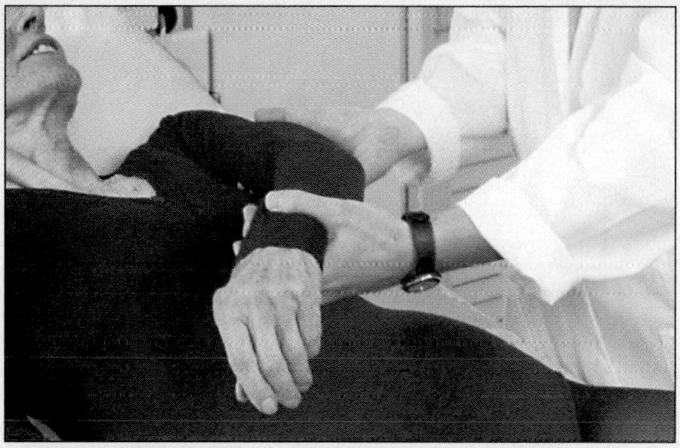
Adduction of shoulder.

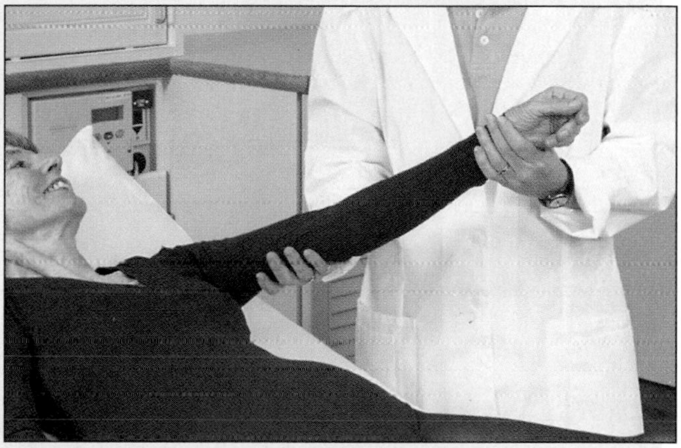
Extension of elbow.

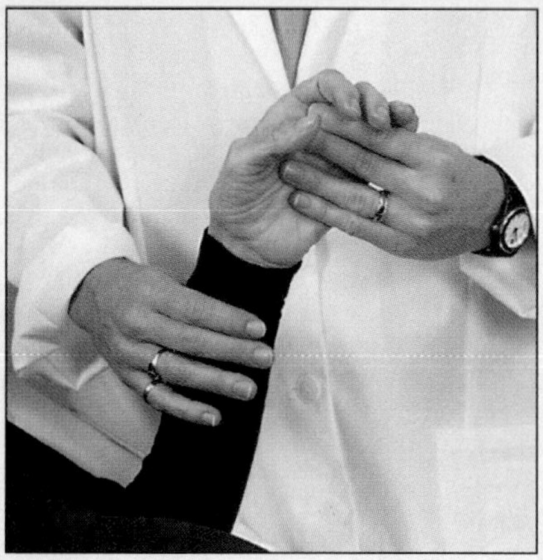
Rotation of the wrist.

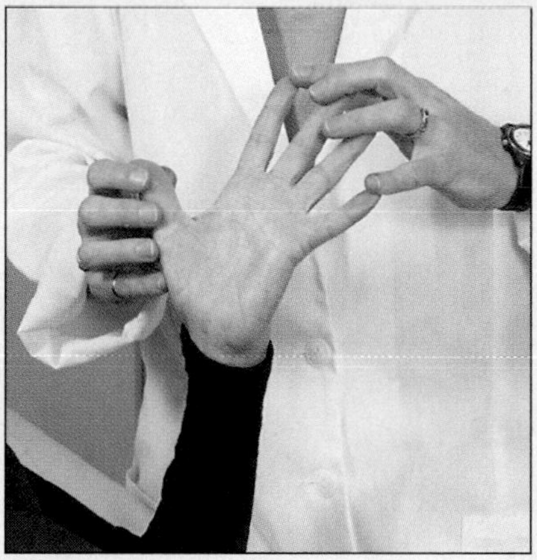
Extension of finger joints.

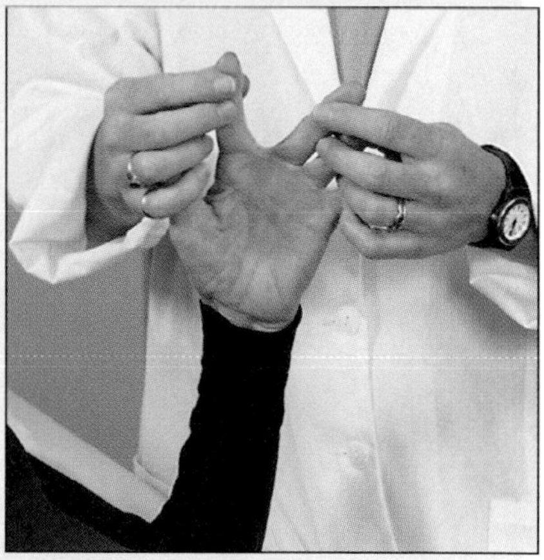
Adduction–abduction finger exercises.

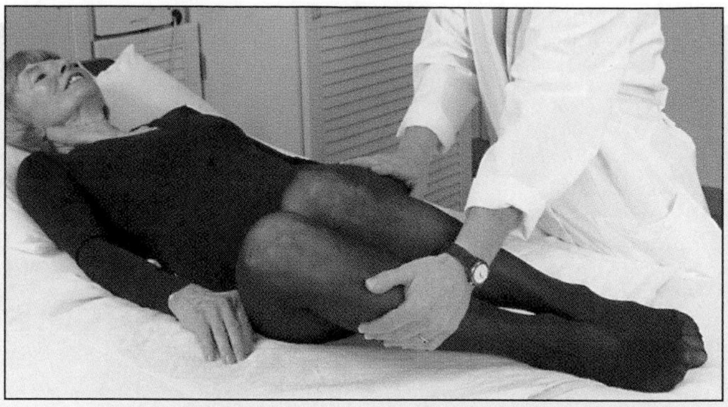

Rotate lower trunk outward 90°.

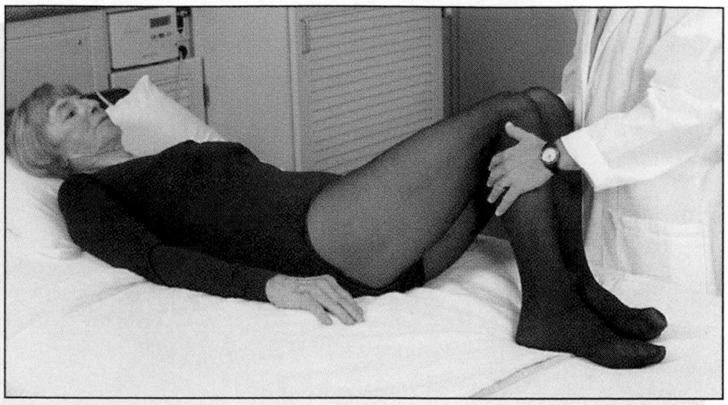

Rotate lower trunk to other side 90°.

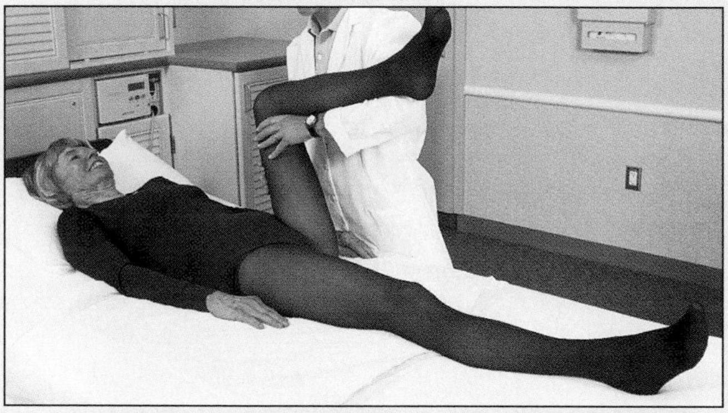

Flex hip and knee.

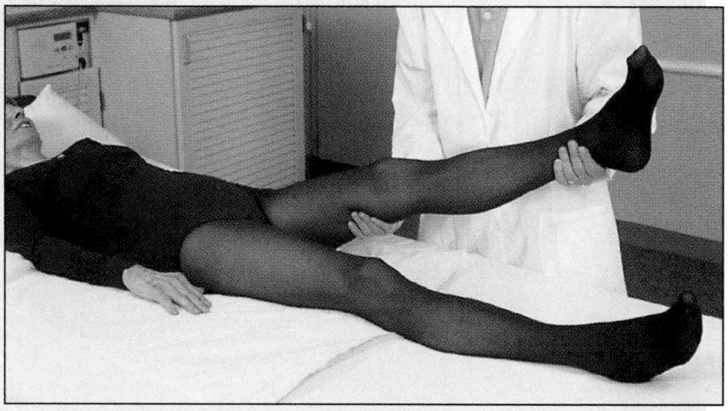

Straight leg raise.

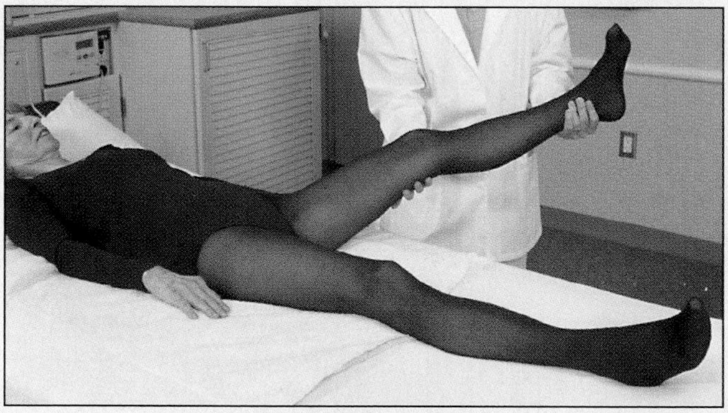

Abduction—Move leg away from the body.

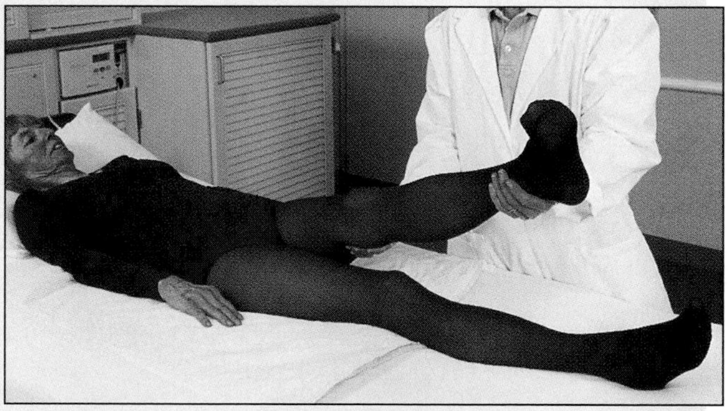

Adduction—Move leg toward midline of body.

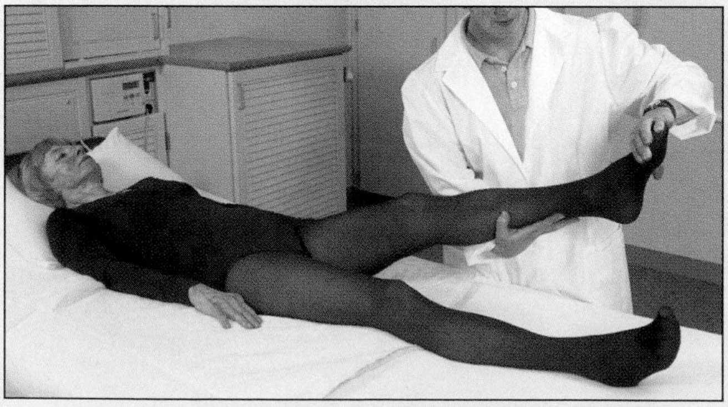

Plantar flexion—Move foot down and away from leg.

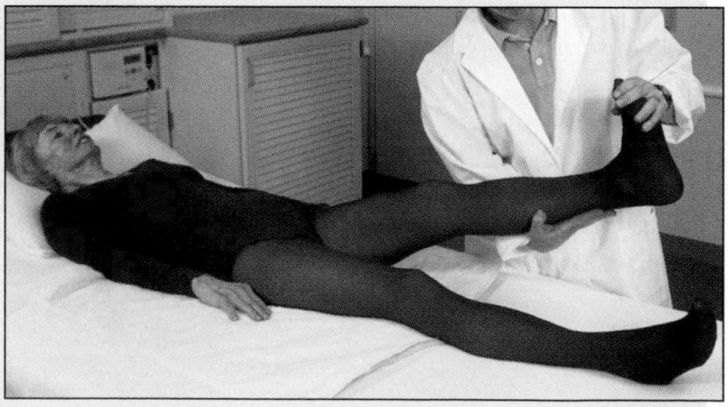

Dorsiflexion—Move foot up and toward leg.

TEACHING ACTIVE RANGE OF MOTION

Equipment

Hospital bed
Sturdy nonslip shoes or slippers

Procedure

1. Explain the rationale for the procedure to the client.
2. Demonstrate the exercises that the client should perform.
3. Watch as the client does the exercises.
4. Assist with the exercises as needed.
5. Correct any problems you notice in the client's performance.
6. Encourage client to perform as much of the exercises as possible.
7. Instruct client to do range-of-motion exercises every 4 hours, exercising all joints.

DOCUMENTATION FOR RANGE OF MOTION

ROM Exercises

- Amount of time needed to complete exercises
- Any changes in condition of joint or joint mobility
- Movements that caused unusual pain or discomfort
- Amount of client participation
- Specific joints put through range of motion
- Alterations in usual procedure

Critical Thinking Application

UNEXPECTED OUTCOMES	CRITICAL THINKING OPTIONS
Client continues to lose mobility and strength despite nursing intervention.	• Discuss the need for additional measures to improve joint range with the health team. • Assess client for the need to use splints and braces to maintain the best physiologic position between exercise periods, and discuss your findings with the physician.
Client experiences pain and discomfort during range-of-motion exercises.	• Assess amount and type of pain and report findings to physician. • Reevaluate your technique to ensure you are performing the exercises correctly. • Start exercises with less stress on joints. Do exercises for a shorter period of time and gradually increase time and range of joint mobility.

UNIT 2

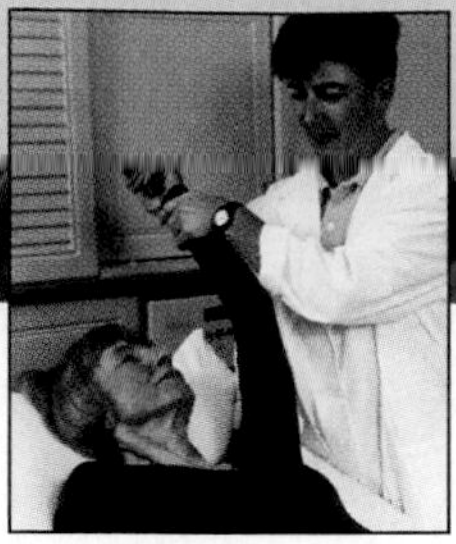

Ambulation

Nursing Process Data

ASSESSMENT *Database*

Assess client's previous activity level.

Check physician's orders for activity.

Assess vital signs and physical ability to ambulate.

Assess need for safety belt.

Assess client for dizziness when moved into an upright sitting position.

Determine if client feels pain from operative site.

Observe client's balance.

Assess any sensory deficits (visual, perceptual).

PLANNING *Objectives*

To promote increased feelings of physical and mental well-being

To develop increased tolerance for exercise

To decrease hospitalization time

To regain independence of action by regaining ability to walk

To prevent paralytic ileus by increasing abdominal wall and gastrointestinal tract muscle tone

To prevent thrombophlebitis by increasing circulation in the legs

To promote healing by increasing circulation and muscle contraction

IMPLEMENTATION *Procedures*

Minimizing Orthostatic Hypotension

Ambulating with Two Assistants

Ambulating with One Assistant

Ambulating with a Walker

Ambulating with a Cane

EVALUATION *Expected Outcomes*

Feelings of physical and mental well-being increased.

Balance and muscle tone improve.

Client progresses from needing assistance with ambulation to becoming independent in ambulation.

Complications of immobility are prevented with ambulation.

MINIMIZING ORTHOSTATIC HYPOTENSION

Equipment

Elastic stockings, if ordered
Robe and slippers
Stethoscope and sphygmomanometer

Procedure

1. Review client's chart prior to ambulation to check for a history of orthostatic hypotension. **Rationale:** This condition may occur in any client, but is more common in the elderly or with clients who have been immobilized.
2. Wash hands and review procedure with client.
3. Place elastic stockings on client's legs if ordered. **Rationale:** Elastic stockings help to reduce blood stasis and promote venous return.
4. Move bed to LOW position. **Rationale:** This position enables client to have feet on the floor and is safer if client experiences vertigo.

CLINICAL ALERT

If the client has been on prolonged bed rest or been immobilized, the risk of orthostatic hypotension is increased. Raising and lowering HOB several times to stimulate baroreceptors will help to prevent this condition.

5. *Slowly* raise head of bed to Fowler's position. **Rationale:** The more slowly the client's position is changed, the less the effect of postural hypotension.
6. Move client to edge of bed by placing one arm behind client's back and one arm under both thighs. Pivot client to a sitting position and assist to dangle legs over side of bed. **Rationale:** Dangling with feet flat on floor for several minutes with legs in a dependent position will reduce effects of postural hypotension.
7. Take client's blood pressure and pulse and observe for vertigo, fainting, pallor, etc.
8. *Slowly* assist client to stand if there is no evidence of orthostatic hypotensive symptoms and begin ambulation or transfer to a chair.

Measuring Orthostatic Hypotension

Postural or orthostatic hypotension is often present after prolonged bedrest or immobilization. It is a sudden drop in blood pressure (25 mm Hg systolic or 10 mm Hg diastolic) when the client moves from a horizontal to a vertical (lying to sitting or standing) position. Symptoms include dizziness, lightheadedness, fainting, pallor, or nausea. To measure orthostatic hypotension:

- With client in supine position for 5 minutes, measure pulse and blood pressure. **Rationale:** This amount of time allows for blood pressure to stabilize.
- Assist client to stand, wait 1 minute and recheck pulse and blood pressure.
- Reassess blood pressure and pulse after 2 minutes. **Rationale:** This amount of time will allow for compensatory mechanisms to work.
- Notify physician if blood pressure and/or pulse remain abnormal after 15 minutes.

AMBULATING WITH TWO ASSISTANTS

Equipment

Robe or second hospital gown (put on backwards so that client is not exposed)
Shoes or slippers that fit well and have nonslip soles

Procedure

1. Wash hands.
2. Explain the rationale for the procedure to the client.
3. Move client to side of bed and assist client to sit on the edge after placing bed in LOW position.
4. Assess the client for dizziness or faintness. Keep client in sitting position until he or she is able to stand without becoming dizzy. **Rationale:** Orthostatic hypotension can occur with prolonged bedrest (See skill *Minimizing Orthostatic Hypotension*).
5. Position one nurse on each side of the client and have each nurse grasp the client's upper arm with the hand that is closest to the client.
6. Have each nurse grasp the client's hand with the other hand.
7. Encourage the client to maintain erect posture and look straight ahead, not down.
8. Ask the client to lift each foot to take a step. The client should not shuffle.
9. Walk the client only as far as he or she is capable of walking and returning without exhaustion.

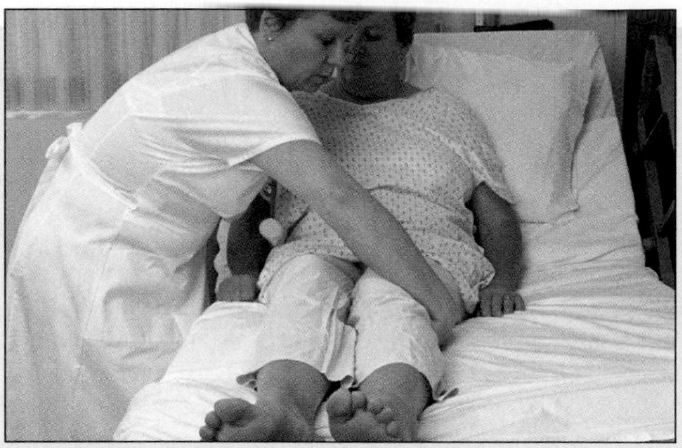

Move client to side of bed.

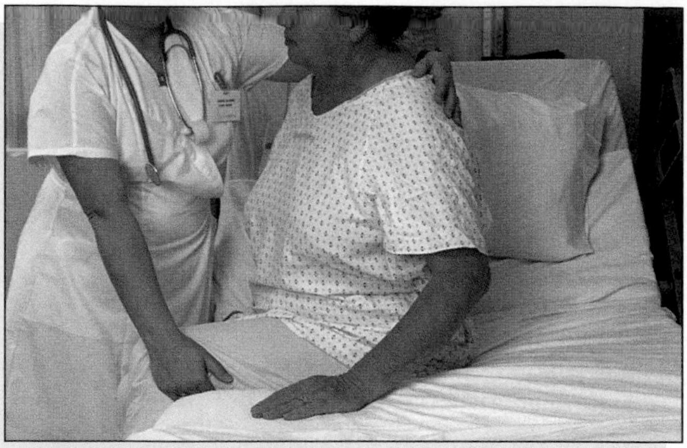

Assist client to sit at edge of bed.

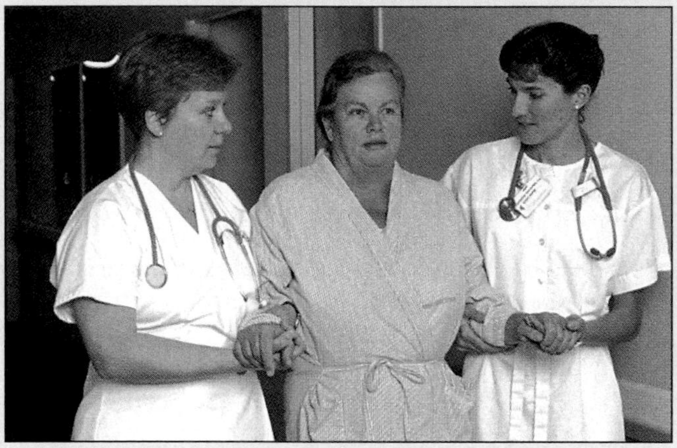

Support is provided by two nurses when client's condition requires.

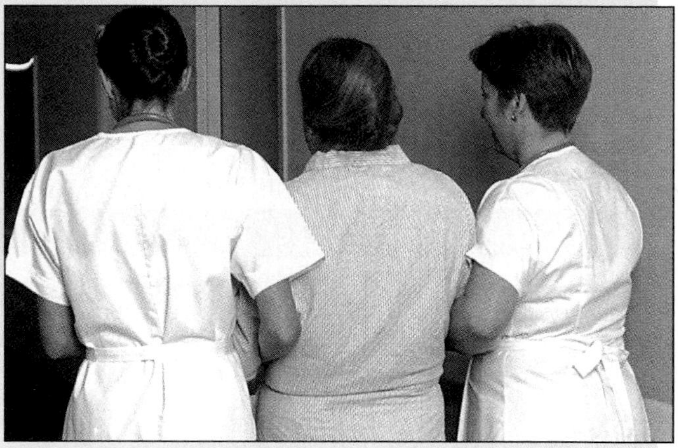

Grasp client's arms firmly on both sides to provide support.

EVIDENCE BASED NURSING PRACTICE

Early Mobilization Promotes Better Outcomes

Clients numbering 5777 were included in 39 trials. Twenty-four trials evaluated bed rest after a variety of medical procedures. Seventeen trials favored early mobilization. Fifteen trials evaluated bed rest as a primary treatment and all showed worse outcomes for clients on bed rest. The study provides evidence to support what clinicians have been doing for several decades—mobilizing clients as early as possible. There is evidence that prolonged bed rest is harmful for clients with low-back pain and myocardial infarction. There is a lack of evidence to determine the effects of bed rest for clients with multiple pregnancies, threatened abortion, and impaired fetal growth.

Source: ACP Journal Club, May/June 2000, vol. 132, no. 3. Review done on article by Allen, C., Glasziou, P., Del Mar, C. (1999, October 9). Bed rest: A potentially harmful treatment needing more careful evaluation. *Lancet, 354*, 1229–1233.

AMBULATING WITH ONE ASSISTANT

Equipment

Robe or second hospital gown (put on backward so that client is not exposed)

Shoes or slippers that fit well and have nonslip soles

Safety belt if indicated

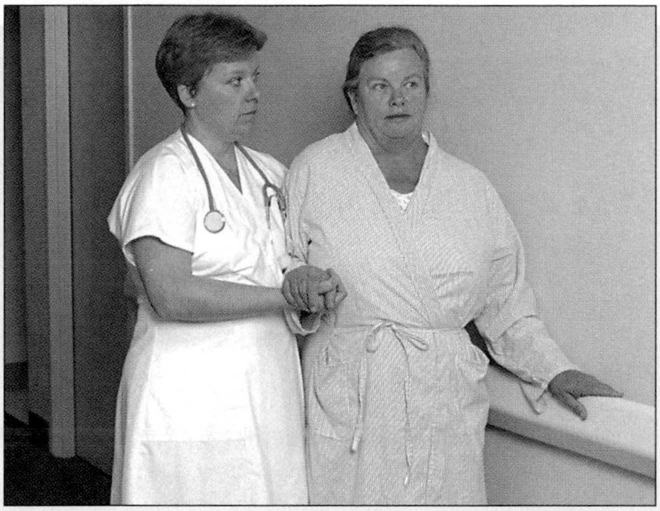

Grasp client around waist and stabilize, holding other arm.

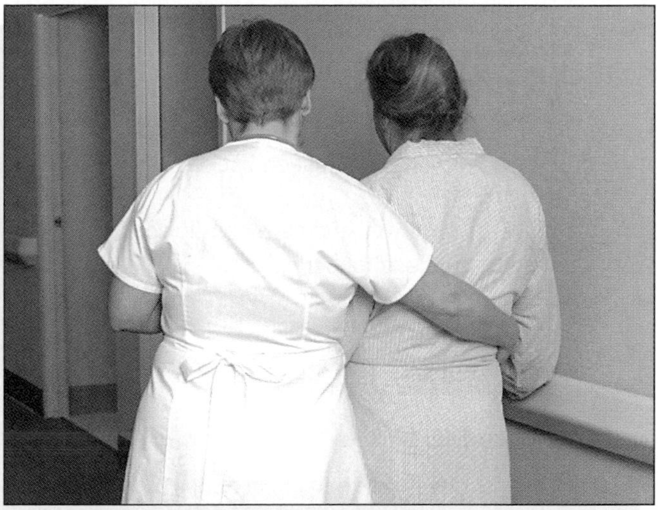

Use wall rail if available to support client.

Procedure

1. Check client's chart for ambulation problems, orthostatic hypotension, or any specific physician's orders.
2. Wash hands.
3. Explain the rationale for the procedure to the client.
4. Help the client sit on the side of the bed after placing bed in LOW position.
5. Assess the client for vertigo or faintness. **Rationale:** Keeping client in this position until he or she is able to stand without becoming dizzy will prevent falling.
6. Apply safety belt if client is unsteady. **Rationale:** Provides support if client is weak and prevents injury.
7. Help the client to stand and observe his/her balance.
8. Grasp client around waist to stabilize, and grasp arm with other hand to guide client.
9. Stand on weaker side, when client is moderately weak; for cerebrovascular accident (CVA) client—stand on unaffected side. **Rationale:** Flaccid muscles on affected side do not provide sufficient muscle strength for you to grasp and support client.
10. Encourage client to maintain good posture and to look straight ahead. **Rationale:** Tendency is for client to look down, which may increase vertigo.
11. Instruct client to lift each foot to take a step, not to shuffle.
12. Walk client as far as he or she is capable of walking without becoming exhausted. Remember client must walk back to room, so take this into consideration when walking. A wheelchair or walker can be pushed behind client so if he becomes tired he can sit down.

CLINICAL ALERT

If the client is collapsing, try to break the fall with your body and guide client to the floor. If the client is unsteady or appears to be falling, support his or her body, especially the head and trunk, maintaining your body in good alignment with line of gravity within your base of support. This alignment prevents injury to yourself, while giving the client adequate support. If necessary, guide the client all the way to the floor.

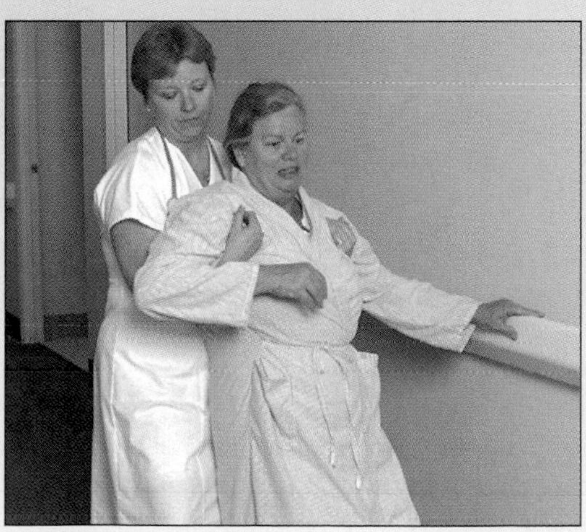

Grasp client under both arms if she begins to fall.

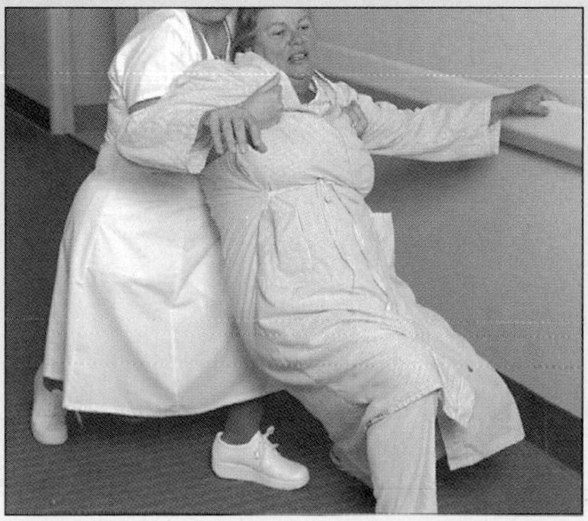

Break client's fall using your body to prevent injury.

AMBULATING WITH A WALKER

Equipment

Robe or second hospital gown (put on backward so that client is not exposed)

Shoes or slippers that fit well and have nonslip soles

Walker with safety tips and rubber hand grips (nonrolling walker)

Procedure

1. Wash hands.
2. Explain rationale for procedure to client.
3. Move client to edge of bed and seat client so feet touch floor.
4. Place walker directly in front of client. Instruct client to grasp hand grips on walker. **Rationale:** To provide stability when getting up.

> **CLINICAL ALERT**
>
> Adjust walker to client's height. Allow 20°–30° flexion of the elbows when grasping hand grips of walker.

5. Instruct client to push self off bed.
6. Have client bend elbows slightly and move walker forward 6 to 8 inches; keep all four feet of walker on floor.
7. Instruct client to move weaker side first by supporting body weight on hands and advancing weaker leg.
8. Instruct client to balance self and then move unaffected side by placing foot even with first foot.
9. Have client move walker forward and continue same pattern of ambulating.

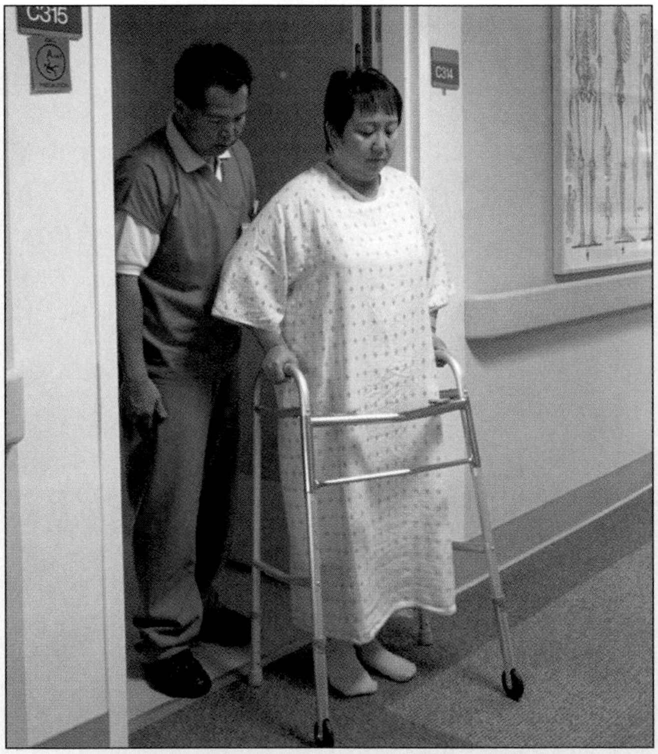

Instruct client to bend elbows slightly and move walker forward.

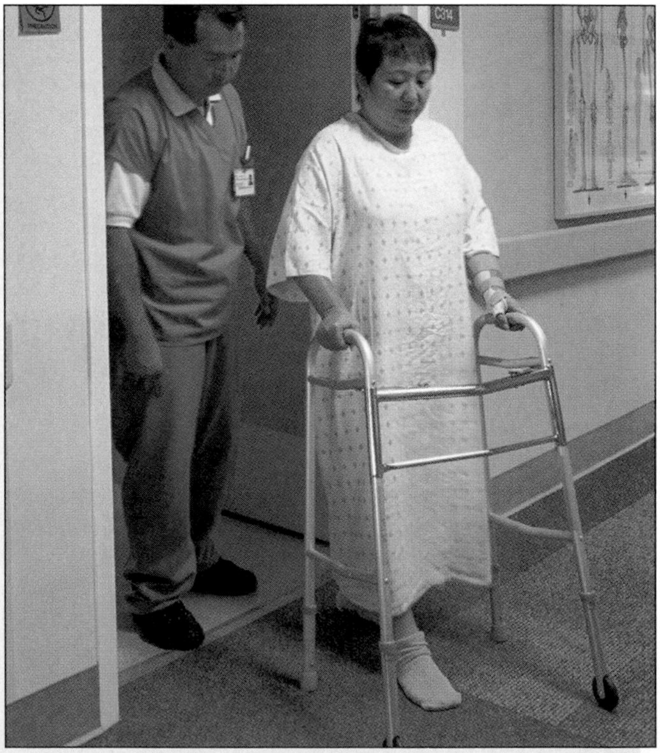

Instruct client to move weaker side first.

AMBULATING WITH A CANE

Equipment

Appropriate type of cane with rubber tips.

- Straight-legged or standard cane
- Tripod or three-pronged cane
- Quad cane

Sturdy shoes with nonskid soles

Procedure

1. Check physician's orders and client care plan. **Rational:** To ensure client is ready to use a cane and to ascertain that cane provides sufficient support for client.
2. Wash your hands.

3. Explain the purpose of using a cane for ambulation, and answer client questions.
4. Demonstrate use of cane if client is unfamiliar with its use.
5. Assist client to put on appropriate shoes and socks for walking.
6. Assist client to standing position with feet firmly on the floor.
7. Instruct client to hold cane on the stronger side of the body. **Rationale:** This offers the most support.
8. Check that cane extends from greater trochanter to floor with 20°–30° for elbow flexion. **Rationale:** If cane is too long or too short, client may injure back.
9. Place cane about 12 inches in front of the foot and slightly to the outside. **Rationale:** This position provides the best balance, because the client's center of gravity is within the base of support.
10. Determine that client can maintain balance and does not experience dizziness before taking the first step.
11. Move cane 4 inches (10 cm) in front of client and then move affected leg forward, even with the cane.
12. Instruct client to shift his or her weight to affected leg and cane. Then move unaffected leg forward, ahead of cane.
13. Move cane forward, then bring affected leg forward until it is even with cane. Repeat these steps when walking with the cane.
14. Accompany client by walking beside him or her on the unaffected side. **Rationale:** If the client loses his or her balance, supporting client on unaffected side is most effective. Simply insert your hand and arm underneath the client's axilla and support his or her arm with your other hand.
15. Evaluate client's ability to use the cane, and instruct about its use as needed.
16. Reinforce the client's achievement to assist him or her to gain confidence in ambulating.
17. Continue to accompany client until the time for walking is completed.
18. Assist client to return to the room and to bed if indicated.
19. Position client for comfort.
20. Assess client's response to ambulation.
21. Wash hands.
22. Chart client's progress, and evaluate plan for increased periods of ambulation in terms of client's capability.

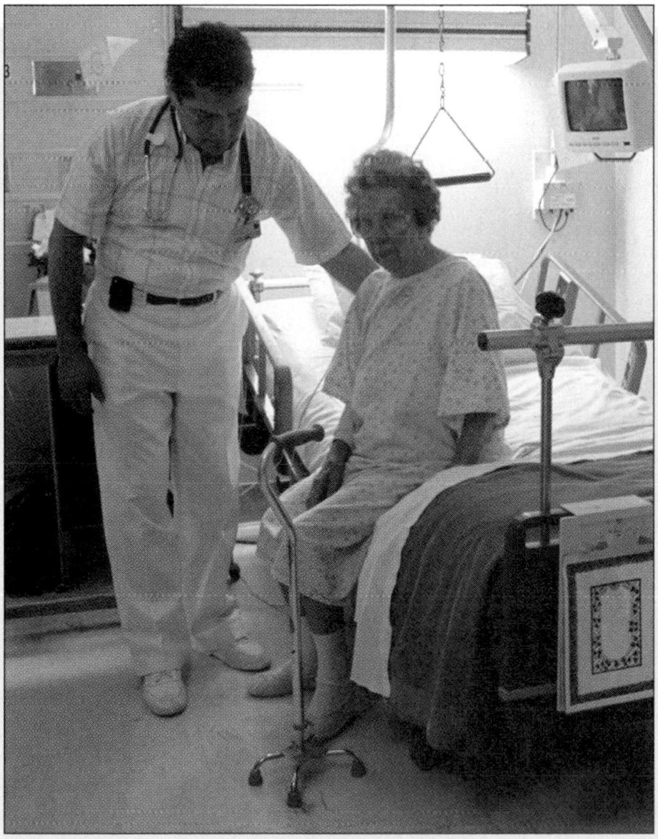

Direct client to hold cane on stronger side of body.

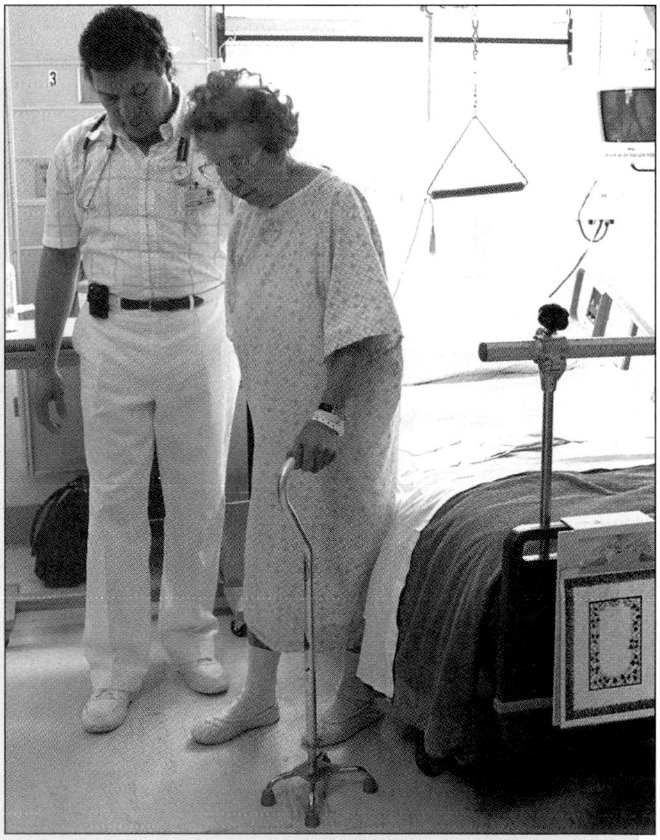

Instruct client to move affected leg forward first, even with cane.

DOCUMENTATION FOR AMBULATION

- Client's ability to balance
- Time and distance of ambulation
- Strength and/or weakness of lower extremities
- Use of correct procedure for walker or cane
- Client's perceptions of ambulation

Critical Thinking Application

UNEXPECTED OUTCOMES	CRITICAL THINKING OPTIONS
Client experiences vertigo or feels faint.	• If in the client's room, help the client return to the chair or bed. • If in the hall, ease the client down the wall to the floor. Do not attempt to hold the client. • Summon help if possible.
Client is too weak to ambulate.	• Provide active and passive ROM. • Begin ambulation protocol as soon as possible.
Client is heavy or has poor balance.	• Ask other nurses or staff to help you ambulate the client until able to walk on his or her own. • If necessary, enlist the aid of a stronger assistant whose presence may give the client additional psychologic as well as physical support. • Gradually increase ambulation as muscle tone improves and balance improves.
Client feels unsafe to ambulate.	• Ambulate more frequently for shorter periods and with more assistance to increase confidence. • Medicate at least 1 hour before ambulation to decrease pain. • With abdominal surgery, check with physician for an order for a binder to decrease fear of dehiscence and pain. • Establish rapport with the client so you can discuss fears about ambulation.

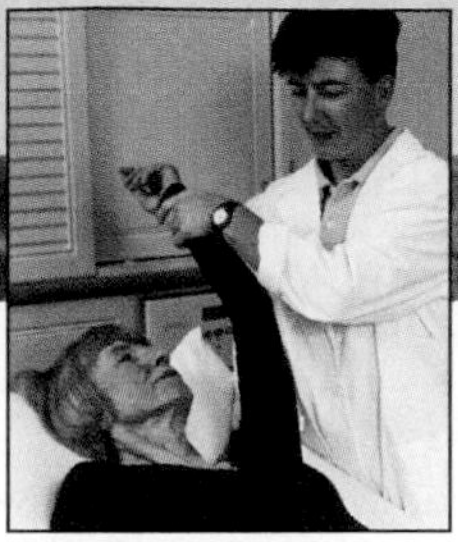

UNIT 3

Crutch Walking

Nursing Process Data

ASSESSMENT Database

Assess physical ability to use crutches and strength of the client's arm, back, and leg muscles.

Observe client's ability to balance self.

Note any unilateral or unusual weakness or vertigo.

Assess which gait is appropriate for client.

Assess client's understanding of crutch-walking technique.

PLANNING Objectives

To improve client's ability to ambulate when he or she has lower extremity injury

To increase muscle strength, especially in the arms and legs

To increase feeling of well-being when client can ambulate

To promote joint mobility

IMPLEMENTATION Procedures

Teaching Muscle-Strengthening Exercises

Measuring Client for Crutches

Teaching Crutch Walking: Four-Point Gait

Teaching Crutch Walking: Three-Point Gait

Teaching Crutch Walking: Two-Point Gait

Teaching Swing-To Gait and Swing-Through Gait

Teaching Upstairs and Downstairs Ambulation with Crutches

Teaching Moving In and Out of Chair with Crutches

EVALUATION Expected Outcomes

Client's ability to ambulate is improved.

Muscle strength of client's arms and legs is improved.

Client experiences a feeling of well-being.

TEACHING MUSCLE-STRENGTHENING EXERCISES

Equipment

Books, boards, or other firm surface for each hand

Procedure

1. Explain the rationale for the exercises to the client.
2. Check the client care plan for orders.
3. Demonstrate the exercises that client will practice.

for Quadriceps-Setting Exercises

a. Try to hyperextend the client's leg by pushing the popliteal area (the area behind knee) into the bed and lifting heel off the bed.
b. Instruct client to contract muscle for a count of 5, then relax for a count of 5.
c. Have client repeat exercise 2–3 times, gradually working up to 10–15 times an hour.

for Gluteal-Setting Exercises

a. Tell client to pinch his or her buttocks together for a count of 5 and then to relax for a count of 5.
b. Have client repeat exercise 10–15 times an hour.

for Pushups in Sitting Position

a. Tell client to sit up in bed with arms at sides.
b. Put books, boards, or something firm under the client's hands and have the client push down, raising hips off the bed. (This exercise may also be practiced while sitting in a chair.)
c. Have client repeat exercise until he or she can do 10–15 pushups an hour.

for Pushups in Prone Position

a. Tell client to lie prone in bed.
b. Ask client to place hands on the bed, close to the shoulders.
c. Tell client to extend arms and to push the upper part of the body into an upright position.
d. Have client repeat exercise until he or she can do 10–15 pushups an hour.

4. Monitor as the client performs the exercises, and correct any problems that may occur.
5. Assess the client for increasing strength as he or she continues to practice the exercises.

MEASURING CLIENT FOR CRUTCHES

Equipment

Measuring tape
Hard-soled street shoes

Procedure

1. Explain the rationale for the procedure to the client.
2. Tell client to put on the shoes she or he will be wearing when using the crutches.
3. Ask client to lie flat in bed with arms at sides.
4. Measure the distance from the client's axilla (armpit) to a point 15 to 20 cm (6–8 inches) out from heel.
5. Adjust hand bars on the crutches so that the client's elbows are always slightly flexed.
6. Tell the client to stand with the crutches under the arms.
7. Measure the distance between the client's axilla and the arm pieces on the crutches. You should be able to put two of your fingers in the space between the axilla and the crutch bar. **Rationale:** Crutches that do not fit the client correctly or crutches that are used incorrectly can damage the brachial plexus and cause paralysis of the arms.

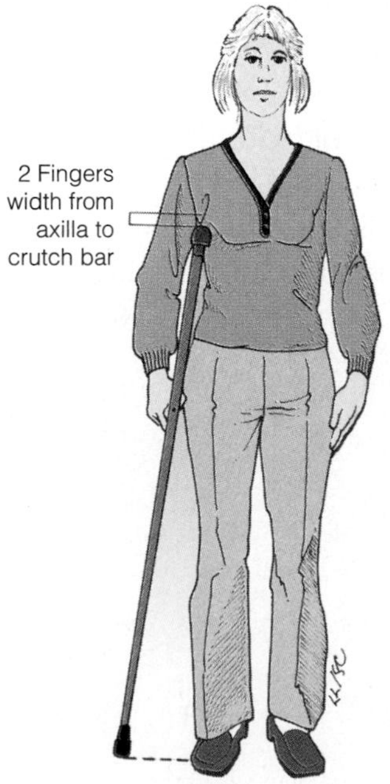

Measure from axilla to heel for crutch height.

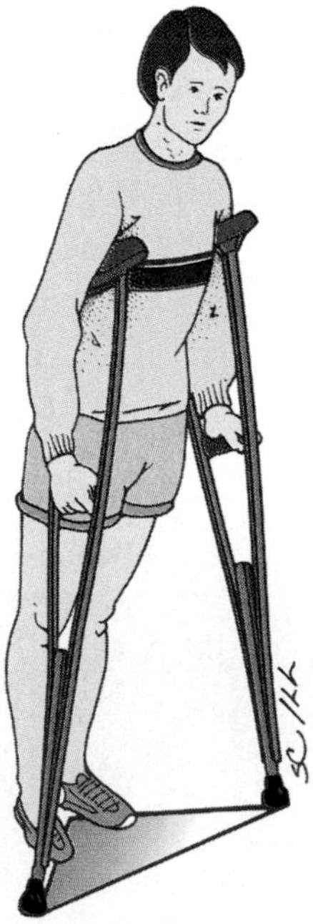

Tripod crutch stance for balance in crutch walking.

TEACHING CRUTCH WALKING: FOUR-POINT GAIT

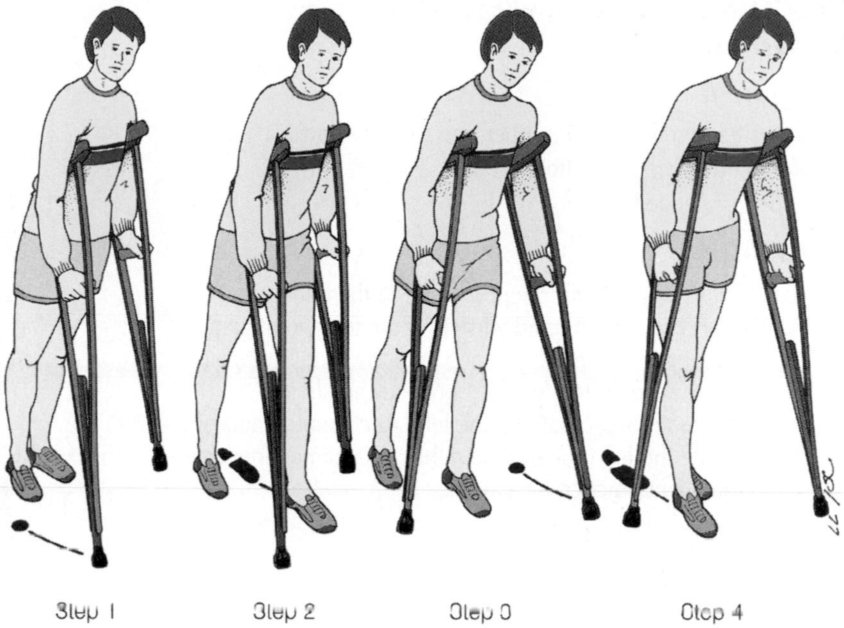

Four-point gait.

Equipment

Properly fitted crutches with rubber tips and arm pads
Regular, hard-soled street shoes
Safety belt, if needed

Procedure

1. Explain the rationale for the procedure to the client.
   a. The gait is rather slow but very stable.
   b. The gait can be performed when the client can move and bear weight on each leg.
2. Demonstrate the crutch-foot sequence to the client.
   a. Move the right crutch.
   b. Move the left foot.
   c. Move the left crutch.
   d. Move the right foot.
3. Help the client practice the gait. Be ready to help with balance if necessary.
4. Assess client's progress, and correct mistakes as they occur.

TEACHING CRUTCH WALKING: THREE-POINT GAIT

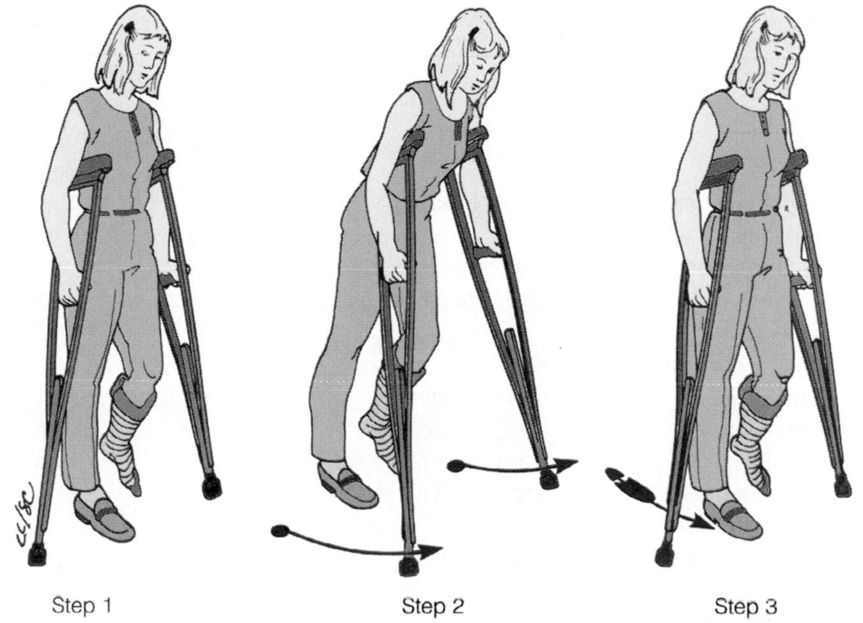

Three-point gait.

Equipment

Properly fitted crutches with rubber tips and arm pads
Regular, hard-soled street shoes
Safety belt, if needed

Procedure

1. Explain the rationale for the procedure to the client.
   a. The gait can be performed when the client can bear little or no weight on one leg or when the client has only one leg.
   b. This gait is fairly rapid and requires strong upper extremities and good balance.
2. Demonstrate the crutch-foot sequence to the client.
   a. Two crutches support the weaker extremity.
   b. Balance weight on the crutches.
   c. Move both crutches and affected leg forward.
   d. Move unaffected leg forward.
3. Assess the client's progress, and correct any mistakes as they occur.
4. Remain with client until crutch safety is ensured.

TEACHING CRUTCH WALKING: TWO-POINT GAIT

Equipment

Properly fitted crutches with rubber tips and arm pads
Regular, hard-soled street shoes
Safety belt, if needed

Procedure

1. Explain the rationale for the procedure to the client.
   a. This procedure is a rapid version of the four-point gait.
   b. This gait requires more balance than the four-point gait.
2. Demonstrate the crutch-foot sequence to the client.
   a. Advance the right foot and the left crutch simultaneously.
   b. Advance the left foot and the right crutch simultaneously.
3. Help the client practice the gait.
4. Assess the client's progress, and correct any mistakes as they occur.

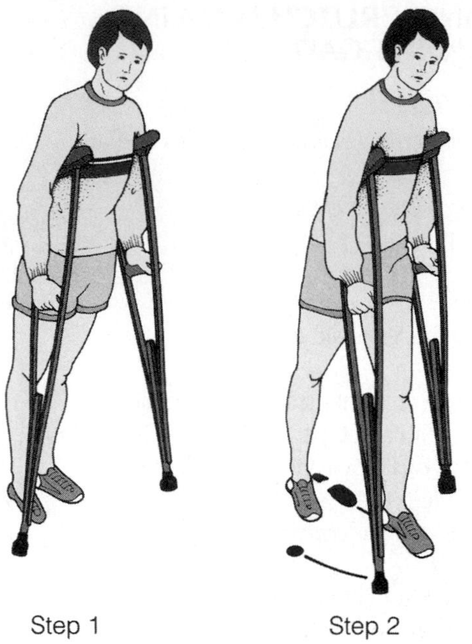

Two-point gait.

TEACHING SWING-TO GAIT AND SWING-THROUGH GAIT

Equipment

Properly fitted crutches with rubber tips and arm pads
Regular, hard-soled street shoes
Safety belt, if needed

Procedure

1. Explain the rationale for the procedure to the client.
   a. These gaits are usually performed when the client's lower extremities are paralyzed.
   b. The client may use braces.
2. Demonstrate the crutch-foot sequence to the client.
   a. Move both crutches forward.
   b. Swing-to gait: Lift and swing the body to the crutches.
   c. Swing-through gait: Lift and swing the body past the crutches.
   d. Bring crutches in front of the body and repeat.
3. Help the client practice the gaits.
4. Assess the client's progress, and correct any mistakes as they occur.

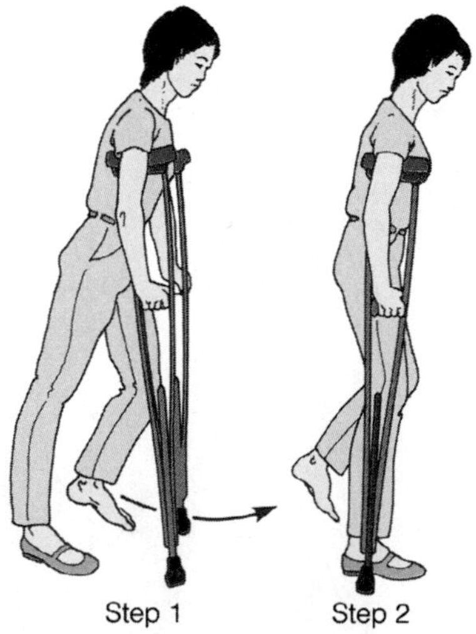

Swing-to-gait.

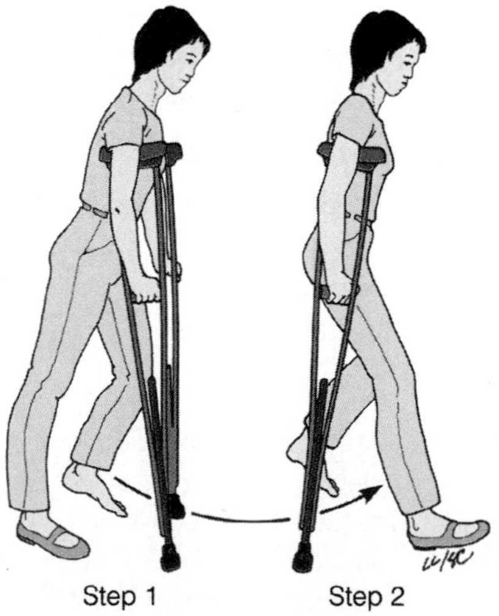

Swing-through-gait.

TEACHING UPSTAIRS AND DOWNSTAIRS AMBULATION WITH CRUTCHES

Equipment

Properly fitted crutches with rubber tips and arm pads
Regular, hard-soled street shoes
Safety belt, if needed

Procedure

1. Explain rationale for the procedure to the client.
2. Apply safety belt if client is unsteady or requires support.
3. Demonstrate procedure using a three-point gait.

for Going Downstairs

a. Start with weight on the uninjured leg and crutches on the same level.
b. Put crutches on the first step.
c. Put weight on the crutch handles and transfer unaffected extremity to the step where crutches are placed.
d. Repeat until client understands the procedure.

for Going Upstairs

a. Start with the crutches and unaffected extremity on the same level.
b. Put weight on the crutch handles and lift the unaffected extremity onto the first step of the stairs.
c. Put weight on the unaffected extremity and lift other extremity and the crutches to the step.
d. Repeat until client understands the procedure.

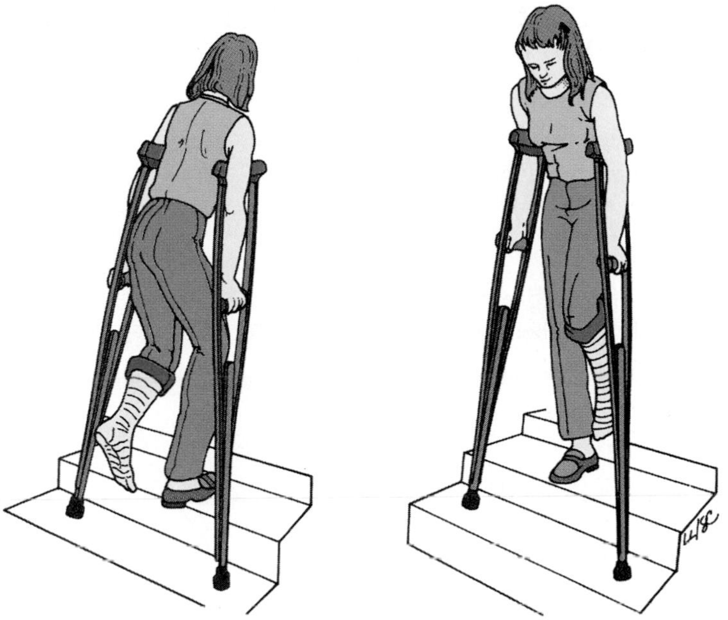

4. Help the client practice.
5. Make sure that the client has adequate balance. Be ready to assist if necessary.
6. Assess the client's progress, and correct any mistakes as they occur.

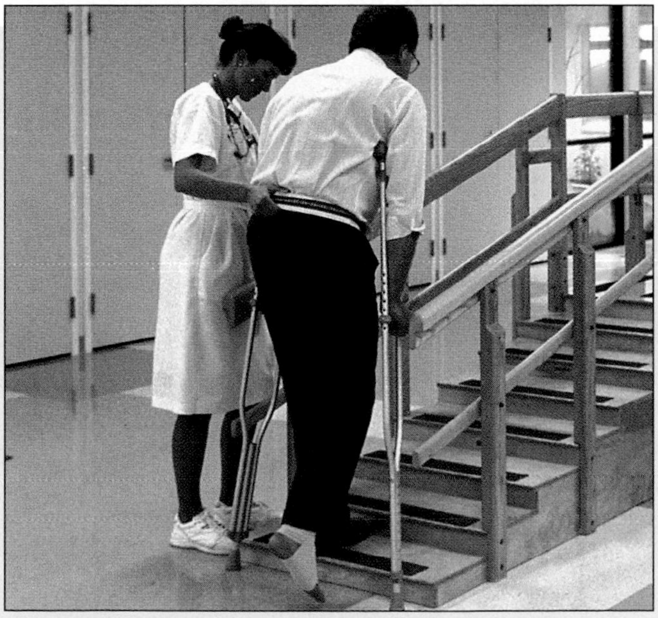

Use safety belt when client is first learning to manipulate stairs.

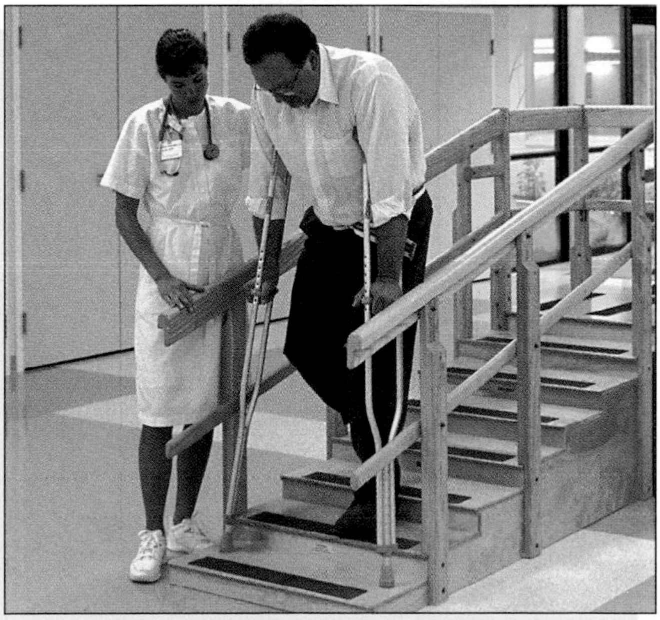

Demonstrate going up or down stairs using a three-point gait.

TEACHING MOVING IN AND OUT OF CHAIR WITH CRUTCHES

Equipment

Properly fitted crutches with rubber tips and arm pads
Regular, hard-soled shoes
Safety belt, if needed

Procedure

1. Explain procedure to client.
2. Apply safety belt if client is unsteady with crutches.
3. Instruct client to follow these steps.

for Moving into Chair

a. Stand in front of the chair, facing forward.
b. Place both crutches in hand on affected side.
c. Hold onto chair arm on unaffected side.
d. Lower self into chair by bending knees and hips.

for Moving out of Chair

a. Move forward in chair by using unaffected side to slide body to edge of chair.
b. Hold onto chair arm on unaffected side.
c. Place both crutches in hand on affected side.
d. Lift self out of chair by grasping the chair arm and supporting self with crutches.
e. Place crutches in front and slightly to side of body and begin crutch walking.

DOCUMENTATION FOR CRUTCH WALKING

- Time and distance of ambulation on crutches
- Balance
- Problems noted with technique
- Remedial teaching
- Client's perceptions of ambulation with crutches
- Ability to move in and out of chair

Critical Thinking Application

UNEXPECTED OUTCOMES	CRITICAL THINKING OPTIONS
Client states he or she is frightened of the crutches.	• Observe as the client practices the procedures to make sure that he or she is completing the steps correctly for each gait. • Explain that it takes time to become proficient. • Reassure the client that he or she will improve with continued practice. • Assess the client's ability to use the crutches and evaluate level of confidence. • Check with physician about obtaining an order for a walker until the client feels more confident.
Client fears falling while dependent on crutches.	• Slow down crutch protocol until client gains confidence at every level of mastery (e.g., four-point gait to two-point gait). • Remain with client and give verbal reassurance and feedback for improvement.
Shoulder girdle is too weak to bear client's weight for crutch support.	• Increase exercise of shoulder (biceps and triceps setting) to gain strength. • Request physician to write an order for overhead frame with trapeze for shoulder exercise sets.

UNEXPECTED OUTCOMES	CRITICAL THINKING OPTIONS
Slipping occurs with crutch walking.	• Check crutch tips to ensure they cover all metal or wood. • Observe the client's stance or gait to determine if it is too broad. • Be sure that floor surface is dry and free of scatter rugs.
Client complains of numbness and tingling in fingers when crutch walking.	• Remeasure distance between axilla and crutch bars to determine if two finger breadths can be inserted. • Observe client's gait to determine if he or she is leaning on crutch inappropriately.

GERONTOLOGIC CONSIDERATIONS

The elderly can suffer impaired mobility and disability due to decreased physical function or accidents.

- Nearly 23% of older people living in the community have some degree of disability.
- Persons 85 and older constitute 27% of those who have impaired mobility.
- Impaired mobility can lead to many subsequent problems, including depression, negative self-image, dependent behavior, and loss of independence.
- Effects of disability can influence the individual's body image, physical appearance, and bodily sensations.
- Posture becomes more flexed and center of gravity shifts.

Special assessment parameters are important for the elderly.

- Specific source of disability or impaired mobility
- Presence of accompanying disease state: arthritis, stroke, dementia, diabetes, CHF, COPD
- Presence of pain
- Condition of skin
- Drug effects: sedation, incontinence, orthostatic hypotension
- Motivation for rehabilitation
- Nutritional status
- Best assistive aid for client
- Be aware of any vision problems your client may have, especially cataracts, glaucoma, or macular degeneration. Note poorly lighted areas in the home or dark areas in the corridors, throw rugs, uneven or uncarpeted areas adjoining carpeted areas, etc. which may cause the client to stumble or fall.
- Check your client's ability to be mobile—their gait, balance, posture, and whether the client shuffles or is able to pick up his or her feet. Check if the client leans forward and is therefore off balance. Poor or unsteady mobility is often a direct cause of falling.
- Assess the client's degree of muscle strength and/or loss of flexibility because as age increases, strength declines, resulting in a fall. Even a poor hand grip can be dangerous if the client is walking downstairs. If leg muscles are weak, it may be difficult to get off a bed or up from a chair and the client may lose his or her balance.
- Assess for certain medications the client is taking which may cause vertigo, poor balance, blurred vision, weakness, or even drowsiness. Review the medications for elderly clients, keeping in mind the fact that they may require only half the normal dose due to their age and inability to metabolize drugs. The use of alcohol may contribute to falls in the home environment, so if the client uses alcohol there should be client teaching that focuses on the potential danger.
- Chronic diseases such as osteoarthritis, Parkinson's, Alzheimer's, and diabetes with peripheral neuropathy can all contribute to falls. Clients who have these diseases may require special assessment and interventions to prevent falls.
- Most elderly clients are aware of the danger of falling and breaking a hip or a leg, so fear is usually present when they are moving or walking. Proper intervention and instructions with an assistive device (canes, walkers, wheelchairs, etc.) will help to allay these fears which may become so overpowering that they cause immobilization and depression. Even fear itself, with its concomitant caution, may result in a fall; if

the nurse can work with the client to discuss fears about falling and specific behaviors to prevent falling, it would be very therapeutic.

Develop nursing care plan to meet elderly client's needs.

- Focus on disability or impaired mobility.
- Establish supportive relationship.
- Teach activities of daily living. Determine activities that must be accomplished each day for individual to care for own needs and be as independent as possible.
- Increase activities as individual progresses and is able to assume activity.
- Give positive reinforcement for all effort expended.

MANAGEMENT GUIDELINES

Each state legislates a Nurse Practice Act for RNs and LVN/LPNs. Health care facilities are responsible for establishing and implementing policies and procedures that conform to their state's regulations. Verify the regulations and role parameters for each health care worker in your facility.

Delegation of Responsibilities

- Range of motion is usually performed by a licensed physical therapist. If this staff member is not available, the nurse or health care worker must understand the principles of the skill before performing it on the client. Range of motion is important for the client who is immobilized or on long-term bedrest, so if the skill is ordered more than once per day, it will probably be delegated to a nurse, CNA, or UAP. This staff member should be assigned to observe and be checked by personnel who understand the skill.
- Ambulation may be done by any health care worker and is often assigned to a CNA or UAP. However, the first time a client is ambulated, an assessment is very important for safety reasons and this should be performed by an RN or LVN/LPN. In some medical–surgical settings, a physical therapist may ambulate specific high-risk clients for the first time. A licensed nurse performing this task will minimize the possibility of orthostatic hypotension occurring, because assessment and vital signs are an important part of the skill.
- Crutch walking is a skill often performed initially with specialized personnel such as the physical therapist. However, the nurse should understand the principles of crutch walking so that he or she may reinforce the correct steps of the procedure whether the client is in the hospital or in the home setting.

Information Flow

- Range-of-motion and muscle-strengthening exercises, ambulation, and crutch walking should all be included in the verbal report at change of shift to all personnel and charted in the client's record.
- Any problems that occur with the exercises or ambulation should also be noted and, if present, the task should be reassigned to licensed personnel. It is especially important to note occurrence of orthostatic hypotension and what actions were effective to minimize the effects on the client.

CRITICAL THINKING STRATEGIES

SCENARIO 1

You are assigned to care for two clients during the day shift.

Client A: A 65-year-old obese client who had a hysterectomy yesterday. Her orders include ambulation and up-in-chair TID on the first postop day.

Client B: A 70-year-old female client who is to be discharged today after having an inguinal hernia repair yesterday.

1. What is your priority of care for these two clients?
2. What assessment will you focus on for both clients and which assessment will be your priority?
3. Briefly describe the discharge teaching that will be done for Client B.

When you approach Client B and tell her you would like to do her discharge teaching, she informs you, "Oh at my age, I can be a couch potato so I don't need you to tell me anything."

4. What is your best response?
5. Based on the information provided, what generalizations can you make about the general health and projected health of this client?
6. What is the primary danger to the health of this client? Describe how you will explain this to the client.
7. What plan (part of discharge teaching) can you devise to positively affect this situation?

You have elicited the help of a nursing assistant to help you ambulate Client A. As you are ambulating the client, she begins to fall.

8. What steps should both you and the nursing assistant take to prevent client injury?
9. After your initial intervention, what other actions should be taken for this client?
10. What preliminary actions should have been taken to prevent this from happening?

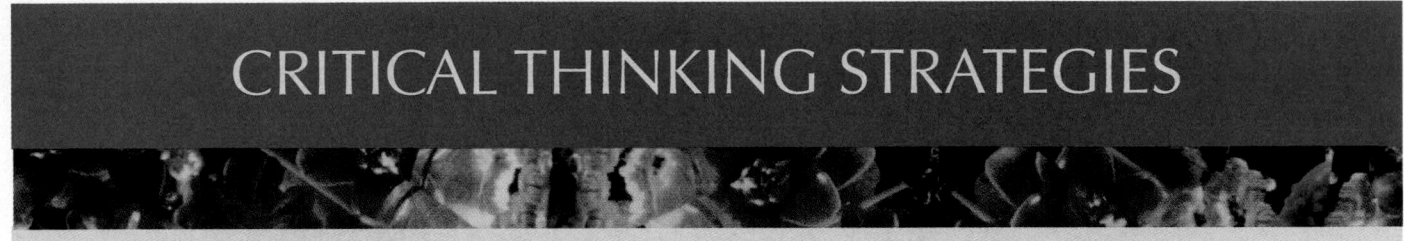

CHAPTER 14

Infection Control

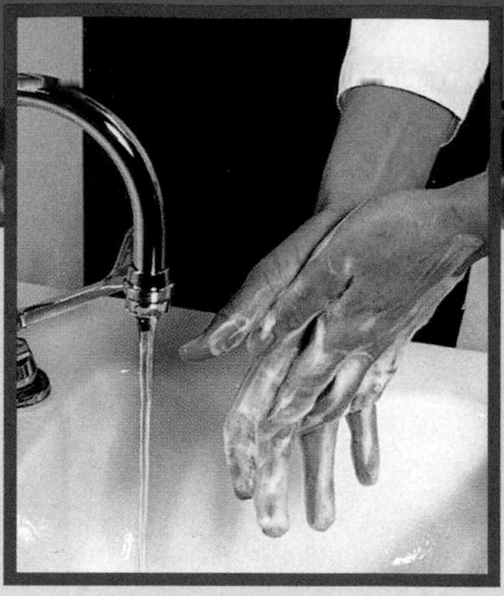

THEORETICAL CONCEPTS

UNIT ONE: **Basic Medical Asepsis** **390**

Handwashing (Medical Asepsis) 391

for Using Waterless Antiseptic Agents 393

Cleaning Washable Articles 393

Donning and Removing Clean Gloves 393

Managing Latex Allergies 395

UNIT TWO: **Standard Precautions (Tier One)** **397**

Donning Protective Gear Utilizing Standard Precautions 398

Exiting a Client's Room Utilizing Standard Precautions 399

UNIT THREE: **Isolation** **402**

Preparing for Isolation 403

Donning and Removing Isolation Attire 403

Using a Mask 405

Assessing Vital Signs 406

Removing Items from Isolation Room 406

Utilizing Double-Bagging for Isolation 406

Removing a Specimen from Isolation Room 408

Transporting Isolation Client Outside the Room 408

Removing Soiled Large Equipment from Isolation Room 409

GERONTOLOGIC CONSIDERATIONS 410

MANAGEMENT GUIDELINES 411

CRITICAL THINKING STRATEGIES 412

LEARNING OBJECTIVES

- Describe and draw the six steps in the chain of infection.
- Explain what is meant by the body's natural defenses.
- List and describe eight conditions that predispose clients to infection.
- Describe what is meant by the term *nosocomial infection* and discuss one intervention that will help to prevent it.
- List the major organisms responsible for nosocomial infections.
- State the main purpose of handwashing.
- Demonstrate donning and removing a gown.
- Define the terms *surgical asepsis* and *medical asepsis.*
- Outline the steps in donning isolation clothing before entering an isolation room.
- Outline the steps in removing isolation clothing before leaving the room.
- State the isolation procedure for removing specimens and equipment from an isolation room.
- Describe the modes of transmission of HIV.
- List three precaution principles and explain their main purpose.
- List blood and body fluid protection protocol.
- Describe the difference between the first and second tier of precautions.

TERMINOLOGY

AIDS: acquired immunodeficiency syndrome—a serious condition characterized by a defect in natural immunity against disease. When the immune system is suppressed, the individual is vulnerable to a host of opportunistic infections.

Antibody: protein substance developed by the body to fight disease organisms. Not effective against a virus that is inside the cells.

Antimicrobial: an agent that prevents the development or pathogenic action of microbes.

Antiseptics: agents that are applied to body tissues, such as skin or mucous membrane, to destroy or retard the growth of microorganisms.

Asepsis: the absence of disease-producing microorganisms.

Aseptic technique: a method to eliminate contamination, germs, or infection.

Autoinfections: infections that arise from an individual's own body flora.

AZT: an antiviral drug currently being used as an effective drug against HIV.

Bacteriostatic: a substance that prevents the growth or multiplication of bacteria.

Barrier nursing: any technique that reduces the risk of cross-contamination.

Biohazard waste: any solid or liquid waste that may present a threat of infection.

Carrier: a person or animal without signs of illness but who carries pathogens on or within his or her body that can be transferred to others.

Cell-mediated immunity: reactions to antigens by cells rather than antibody molecules present in body fluids.

Chemotaxis: attraction and repulsion of living protoplasm to a chemical stimulus.

Cofactors: existing characteristics in the individual which may make them more susceptible to the AIDS virus.

Colonization: organisms present in body tissue but not multiplying or invading the tissue.

Contagious disease: a disease conveyed easily to others.

Contamination: introduction of disease, germs, or infectious materials into or on normally sterile objects.

Detergent: compounds (surfactants) that possess a cleaning action, often referred to as soaps. They are composed of a hydrophilic and a lipophilic substance.

Disinfectants: chemical agents that are used to destroy or reduce microorganisms on inanimate surfaces and objects.

Disinfection: a process that employs physical and chemical means to remove, control, or destroy most of the organisms that may be present on equipment or materials.

Duration of the infectious challenge: sustained exposure to even a relatively small number of organisms that poses a significant risk to the client (e.g., intravenous catheters become colonized with microorganisms).

Endogenous: organisms natural to an individual's own body.

Enteric precautions: isolation practices designed to prevent transmission of pathogens through contact with fecal matter and vomitus.

Exogenous: organisms external to an individual's own body.

False negative: a negative test in someone who in fact has been infected by a microorganism but for some reason has not developed antibodies.

False positive: a positive test for an antibody. Usually the result of an artifact of the laboratory test; the person has not in fact been exposed to the microorganism. All persons who test positive should have the test repeated.

Granulation: formation of granules (roughened prominences). Each granulation represents an outgrowth of new capillaries and enriched blood supply.

Host: an animal or person on which or within which microorganisms live.

Humoral immunity: acquired immunity in which the circulating antibody is predominant.

Hygiene: study of health and observance of rules pertinent to health.

Incubation period: the time between infection from a microorganism and the onset of symptoms. Seems to range from 6 months to 7 years for AIDS. Not everyone who is exposed to the virus develops the disease.

Infection: establishment of a disease process that involves invasion of the body tissue by microorganisms and the reaction of the tissues to their presence and to the toxins generated by them.

Isolation technique: practices designed to prevent the transmission of communicable diseases.

Kaposi's sarcoma: a type of cancer usually occurring on the surface of the skin or in the mouth. Kaposi's sarcoma may also spread to internal organs of the body and may be responsible for death.

Latex: natural rubber used in many gloves and medical equipment. Latex proteins can enter the body and cause latex allergy.

MDR-TB: multidrug-resistant tuberculosis is an in vitro resistant strain of TB to antituberculosis drugs.

Medical asepsis: all practices that limit the number and growth of microorganisms and their transmission.

Microorganism: minute living body, such as a bacterium, protozoan, or virus, not perceptible to the naked eye.

Nosocomial infection: an infection acquired while in the hospital that was not present or incubating at the time of admission.

Opportunistic infections: illness or diseases that would not be a threat to anyone whose immune system is functioning normally, but in a person with AIDS may be responsible for death.

Opsonin: a substance in blood serum that acts on microorganisms and other cells and facilitates phagocytosis.

Outbreak: a critical incident in which infections occur above an established level and are caused by the same infective agent.

Pathogen: a microorganism that can cause infectious disease in the human body.

PEP: postexposure prophylaxis; recommendations from the CDC on how to treat a health care worker's exposure to HIV.

Pneumocystis carinii pneumonia: PCP is a parasitic infection of the lungs. This is one of the two rare diseases that affect 85% of AIDS clients. PCP has symptoms similar to other severe forms of pneumonia.

Primary immune response: response that occurs when the B cell recognizes an antigen, becomes activated, and divides into more memory cells.

Protective isolation: practices designed to protect a highly susceptible person from contagious diseases, reverse isolation.

Protocol: description of steps taken in exact order—may be legally binding.

Resident (normal) flora: organisms natural to an individual's own body. Organisms multiply in the environment, not merely survive there.

Retrovirus: a virus with a life cycle in which the genetic information is in reverse of that in an ordinary virus: the RNA code is transcribed backward into DNA.

Sepsis: condition resulting from the presence of pathogenic bacteria and their products.

Sterile: free from any living microorganisms.

Subungual: an area beneath a fingernail or toenail.

Surgical asepsis: practices which will maintain area free from microorganisms, as by a surgical scrub, or sterile technique.

Susceptible sites: an area that is sensitive to or can be invaded by a bacterium or other infectious agent.

Virulence: recognized pathogenic organisms designated because of their ability to invade and propagate in normal, intact, uncompromised individuals. Some organisms that are avirulent for normal individuals become pathogenic when defense mechanisms are impaired.

Virus: minute, parasitic organism that depends on nutrients inside cells for its metabolic and reproductive needs. These organisms cause a variety of infectious diseases and stimulate host antibodies. Unlike a bacteria, viruses are unable to survive long on their own and are not affected by antibodies.

Waterless antiseptic agent: an antiseptic agent that does not require use of exogenous water. Agent dries automatically after applying to hands and rubbing hands together.

CHAIN OF INFECTION

For an infection to occur a chain of events must take place. If the chain is broken through the implementation of infection control measures, the infection is less likely to occur. The chain of infection involves six steps.

Infectious Agent (Microorganism) The first step in the chain involves the presence of an infectious agent, or microorganism. Whether the microorganism is capable of producing an infection depends on a number of circumstances: the virulence and number of organisms present, the susceptibility of the host, the existence of a portal of entry, and the affinity of the host to harbor the microorganism.

Reservoir A reservoir must provide a favorable environment for growth and multiplication of the microorganism. These reservoirs include the respiratory, gastrointestinal, reproductive and urinary tract, and blood.

Portal of Exit The third link in the chain must be a portal of exit, which allows the microorganism to move from the reservoir to the host. Without a portal of exit an infection cannot occur. The portal of exit is directly associated with the reservoir. For example, if the reservoir is the respiratory tract, the portal of exit is through sneezing, coughing, breathing, or talking. If the reservoir is blood, the portal of exit is through an open wound, needle puncture site, or nonintact skin surface.

Mode of Transmission. The fourth step is transmission of microorganisms. There are five routes of transmission; the three primary routes are contact, droplet, and airborne. Two lesser routes are common vehicle (transmission by contaminated items such as food, water, devices, or equipment) and vector borne (transmission by vectors such as mosquitoes fleas, rats, etc.). This last mode of transmission is more significant in other parts of the world than in the United States.

Contact transmission, the most frequent source of nosocomial infection, is transmitted via two modes—direct and indirect contact. Direct contact involves a direct transmission, body-to-body, and the physical transfer of microorganisms from one infected person to another, for example, through sexual contact, kissing, or even touch. It also may occur when a health care worker touches a client, gives a client a bath, or performs other care activities. Indirect transmission involves contact with a contaminated intermediate object such as a needle, instrument, or dressing. This also occurs when contaminated hands are not washed and gloves are not changed between clients.

Droplet transmission is a form of contact transmission, but the mechanism of pathogen transfer is so different that it is considered a separate route of transmission. It occurs when droplets from the infected source person are projected a short distance to the host's nasal mucosa, mouth, or conjunctiva. These droplets are not suspended in the air, so it is not considered airborne transmission.

Airborne transmission occurs by dissemination of either small particle nuclei of evaporated droplets or dust particles containing the infectious agent. These agents can be dispersed widely by air currents, as with Legionnaire's disease, and may be inhaled by a susceptible host. These microorganisms include *Mycobacterium tuberculosis*, rubeola, and varicella viruses.

Portal of Entry The most effective barrier to transmission of microorganisms is an intact skin. For an infection to occur it must have a means of entering the body. A disruption in the integrity of the skin provides such a portal of entry for microorganisms. Microorganisms also enter the body the same way they leave the body. The respiratory system provides a viable portal of both exit and entry.

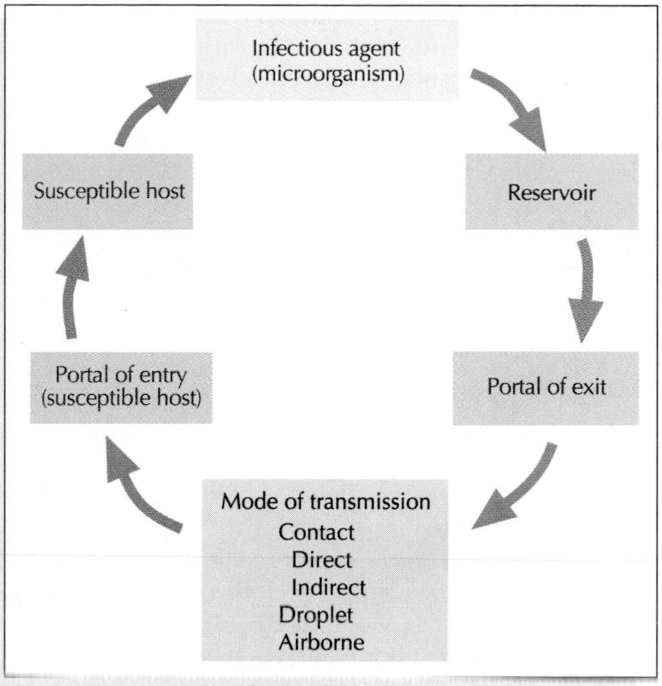

Six steps in the chain of infection.

Susceptible Host For an infection to occur a susceptible host is needed—someone who is "at risk." This includes clients who are immunosuppressed, fatigued, stressed, anemic, not immunized, poorly nourished, or those who have underlying diseases. Hospitalized clients with wounds, catheters, and IVs are at high risk for developing infections. Clients who require invasive procedures, blood specimen collections, and surgery are also in the high-risk category.

BARRIERS TO INFECTION

An individual's ability to resist infection is determined by the status of the body's defense mechanisms and by the person's general health. Factors that contribute to susceptibility to infection include altered nutritional status, stress, fatigue, disease, drugs, metabolic functions, and age. Clients with severe underlying diseases are most likely to develop nosocomial infections. The body is protected against infection by immunities, by the inflammatory process, and by anatomic barriers that include the skin and mucous membranes.

When the integrity of the skin or mucous membrane is broken, both resident and transient flora or bacteria have a direct route to the internal tissues of the body. To prevent the spread of infection, the body's internal defense mechanisms mobilize and begin clearing and repairing the damaged site. How quickly a wound heals depends on the degree of vascularization in the injured area, the location and cleanliness of the wound, and the degree of tissue damage.

The second way the body resists infections is through immunity, antitoxins, and vaccines. Natural immunity is inherited. Acquired immunity occurs after an individual has been exposed to a disease or infection or has been vaccinated.

The third way the body resists infection is through the inflammatory process. Inflammation involves use of metabolic energy, increased blood flow to the inflamed area, and, in many cases, drainage of inflammatory debris to the external environment.

When an area becomes inflamed, cells at the site activate the plasmin system, the clotting system, and the kinin system. The result of the activation of these systems is the release of histamine, which creates increased vascular permeability around the injured site, and the release of chemotoxic agents, which summon phagocytes into the vascular and tissue spaces. Phagocytes are white blood cells that combat and prevent infection by ingesting harmful microorganisms.

The Body's Natural Defenses

Any alteration in the body's natural defenses increases the probability that an infection will occur. Almost any organism can be the cause of a significant nosocomial infection, given the proper circumstances. Some of the variables that help determine which organism emerges as the pathogen are the virulence and number of organisms, the exposure and attachment of the organism to a susceptible site, and the duration of the client's exposure to the infectious challenge. The following formula illustrates these variables.

$$\frac{\text{Dose} \times \text{Virulence}}{\text{Host Resistance}} = \text{Infection}$$

Using this formula, the client's risk factors can be evaluated. The inherent health and immunologic status of the client are also major factors in determining whether an infection occurs.

Alterations in the skin barrier include any physiologic break in the integrity of the skin. Intentional breaks are caused by the use of percutaneous catheters and needles and by surgical procedures. Unintentional causes of skin breakdown include the development of pressure ulcers and traumatic wounds.

CONDITIONS PREDISPOSING TO INFECTION

Certain conditions and invasive techniques predispose clients to infection because the integrity of the skin is broken or the illness itself establishes a climate favorable for the infectious process to occur. Among the most common are surgical wounds, changes in the antibacterial immune system, or alterations in the respiratory tract or genitourinary tract. Implants such as heart valves, prosthetic grafts, or vascular grafts can lead to nosocomial septicemias. The extensive use of IV therapy in clients has increased infections dramatically.

Surgical Wounds

It has been documented that the longer a person is hospitalized prior to the surgical procedure the greater the risk of postsurgical infection. Other factors that influence infection rates are duration of time in the operating room, time surgery is done (between midnight and 8:00 A.M. is period of greatest risk), whether the client has postsurgical drains in place, and if the surgery enters a colonized or infected part of the body.

It is useful for the nurse to be aware of conditions that increase the risk of postoperative infection. Risk reduction measures include preoperative showering with an antiseptic solution; the use of depilatory creams or the clipping of hair in lieu of shaving the surgical site, and keeping the incision site covered with a dry sterile dressing. A wet dressing, through osmosis and diffusion, pulls organisms down into the wound from the surface. This is particularly important during the first 45 hours before the wound becomes "watertight." Research shows that preoperative shaving results in disruption of normal flora on the surface of the skin.

Antibacterial Immune Mechanisms

There are three categories of abnormalities in antibacterial immune mechanisms: those affecting inflammatory responses, those affecting phagocytic functions, and those affecting opsonins (humoral immunity).

Anything that interferes with the migration of phagocytic cells to the area of contamination or with the physical contact of phagocytes and bacteria enhances the development of an infection. Examples of such interferences include deficient blood supplies, the presence of ischemic or dead tissue, sutured material, foreign bodies, and hematomas. Vasopressor agents, radiation injury, uremia, severe nutritional deficiencies, and steroid therapy inhibit the synthesis of antibodies and other essential proteins.

Clients with severe thermal injuries and severe nutritional deficiencies have abnormalities involving the number of neutrophils collected at the site of an inflammatory response and defects of bactericidal chemotoxic capacity. Clients with Hodgkin's disease have a specific defect in cell-mediated immunity.

Genetic inabilities to synthesize complement components or specific antibodies can cause abnormalities in opsonins. Burn clients may have complement inactivated by a circulating substance released by the damaged tissue. Without complement, lysis of cells and destruction of bacteria cannot take place.

Respiratory Tract

Common alterations in the respiratory tract that facilitate the development of an infection include endotracheal intubation, tracheostomy, bronchotracheal suctioning, and stasis due to poor respiratory excursion for clients on bed rest.

The bronchi and trachea are so sensitive to foreign matter that they initiate the cough reflex whenever irritation occurs. Ciliated, mucus-coated epithelium lining the trachea and lungs aids in clearing the respiratory tract of bacteria and mucus by the beating motion of the cilia. Intubation bypasses the cough reflex and compromises the effectiveness of this action. Although the trachea is usually considered sterile, it does not remain sterile after 48–72 hours of intubation. Infections associated with endotracheal intubation include pneumonia, tracheitis, and purulent bronchitis.

Catheters placed directly in the trachea can force pathogenic microorganisms into the respiratory system. In addition, catheters may damage the mucous lining of the respiratory tract, further compromising the effectiveness of its clearing mechanisms.

Genitourinary Tract

Instrumentation, including catheterization of the bladder, and complicated obstetric delivery after prolonged confinement in bed are two procedures that introduce potentially pathogenic bacteria into the genitourinary tract. Acute urinary tract infection and pyelonephritis often occur after the use of a catheter or cystoscope.

The most common alteration is the placement of an indwelling urinary catheter. Research has demonstrated that significant bacteriuria develop in only 2% of the clients who have a single "straight" catheterization (in and out) to empty a distended bladder. Although bacteriuria may be considered benign and usually resolves after removal of the catheter, bacteriuria following catheterization may result in symptomatic cystitis and, occasionally, in acute pyelonephritis, chronic pyelonephritis, and persistent asymptomatic bacteriuria. Lack of adequate fluid intake, improper positioning of the catheter and bag, use of an open versus a closed drainage system, and inadequate emptying of the bladder all serve to increase the risk of infection in the catheterized client.

Invasive Devices

Most nosocomial septicemias occur as a result of significant alterations in normal host defenses. These infections may be primary (caused by direct introduction of microorganisms into the bloodstream) or secondary (arising from an infection at another site such as the urinary tract). In fact, the most common site for a nosocomial infection is the urinary tract.

The use of IV therapy greatly increases the risk of introducing harmful microorganisms. The incidence of septicemia in clients receiving IV therapy varies from 0 to 8%.

Septicemia may also be caused by the introduction of microorganisms from contaminated fluids, infected venipuncture sites, or foci of septic thrombophlebitis as a complication of using an indwelling IV catheter.

Infusion-related sepsis is associated with contaminated infusion fluid, which may be contaminated either during manufacturing (intrinsic contamination) or during hospital use (extrinsic contamination).

Venipuncture Sites

The wounds made by a percutaneous stick at the venipuncture site may become colonized or infected. This opening provides a reservoir for bacteria that could move along the catheter into the bloodstream.

Organisms that travel down the catheter ultimately reside in the thrombus, which is usually present on the catheter tip. Around the thrombus, bacteria are shielded from the immune response and antibiotics. When these microorganisms attain a critical level, they seed the bloodstream and cause bacteremia. Site infections can be reduced by several methods: selecting a catheter appropriate to the size of the vein; avoiding sites near joints; the performance of proper site preparation; maintaining a regimen for site care; and changing the site every 48–72 hours as well as maintaining a closed system of therapy. Discontinuing IVs started in emergency situations like codes or "field starts" in which proper site hygiene wasn't carried out also reduces IV-related infections.

Total Parenteral Nutrition Therapy

Total parenteral nutrition therapy (TPN) is a means of achieving an anabolic state in clients who would otherwise be unable to maintain normal nitrogen balance. Problems with IV-related sepsis in TPN are the same as those seen in conventional IV therapy, only greatly magnified. The hypertonic solution used with these clients supports the growth of a wide variety of organisms, especially fungus, to a greater extent than conventional IV solutions. Clients on TPN are critically ill and malnourished. Peripheral inserted central catheter (PICC) lines are usually inserted for TPN infusions. These lines may not be changed for months. Infection control is of critical importance with TPN. Meticulous site care must be done at least every 3 days to preserve the site, and aseptic technique used when changing solution, tubing, dressings, and filters.

Implanted Prosthetic Devices

Commonly used implanted devices include artificial cardiac valves, synthetic vascular grafts, orthopedic prosthetic joints, neurosurgical shunts, and cerebrospinal fluid pressure monitoring devices. Most infections associated with prosthetic devices require long-term IV antibiotic therapy. If the infection is not controlled, removal and replacement of the prosthesis is indicated.

NOSOCOMIAL INFECTIONS

Nosocomial infections are infections that are acquired while the client is in the hospital—infections that were not present or incubating at the time of admission. The morbidity is high; this condition affects more than 2 million people and, in 2000, it was estimated to cause or contribute to 103,000 deaths in the United States. It has an economic toll of more than $ 4.5 billion annually. Many of these infections are caused by pathogens transmitted from one client to another by health care workers. Nosocomial infections are usually caused by poor handwashing technique or no handwashing between clients. Handwashing is the single most important intervention to prevent these infections; various studies have shown that there is very poor compliance with handwashing techniques by health care workers. Other interventions important to the prevention of nosocomial infections are the use of sterile technique when indicated, keeping the environment as free as possible of pathogens, and identifying and protecting at-risk clients. The CDC has studied rates of the four "hot spots"—infections of surgical sites, the bloodstream and urinary tract, and ventilator–associated pneumonia in intensive care units.

There are three major organisms responsible for the majority of nosocomial infections: *Clostridium difficile*, methicillin-resistant *Staphylococcus aureus* (MRSA), and vancomycin-resistant enterococcus (VRE). The most common organism, *C. difficile* is an anaerobic, gram-positive, spore-forming bacillus associated with infectious diarrhea (CDAD). Twenty to forty percent of hospitalized clients become colonized within a few days of entering the hospital. Because it is often resistant to antimicrobial therapy, it is able to proliferate in the hospital setting.

The second most common infection, affecting 40% of all critically ill or immunosuppressed clients, is nosocomial pneumonia. The leading cause of this condition is gram-positive *Staphylococcus* that is methicillin resistant. This condition often occurs in clients who have invasive procedures such as intravenous or respiratory therapy treatments or surgical procedures. Health care personnel easily transmit MRSA to clients because it frequently colonizes skin. Vancomycin, the drug of choice to treat MRSA, is losing its effectiveness as a treatment.

VRE is a gram-positive bacterium normally found in flora of the gastrointestinal tract. When this bacterium mutated and became resistant to common antimicrobial therapies, it became a major cause of nosocomial infections in the hospital setting.

For the last 4 years there has been a new type of antibiotic available to fight resistant infections. An example of this drug (the first entirely new type of antibiotic in 35 years) is Zyvox. This drug and others of its genre are the drugs of choice for VRE and MRSA.

STANDARD PRECAUTIONS

In 1985, universal precautions were instituted as a result of the human immunodeficiency virus (HIV) epidemic in the United States. Blood and body fluid precautions were practiced on all clients regardless of their potential infectious state.

In 1987, body substance isolation (BSI) was proposed. The intent of this isolation system was to isolate all moist and potentially infectious body substances (blood, feces, urine, sputum, saliva, wound drainage, and other body fluids) from all clients, regardless of their infectious status, primarily through the use of gloves.

In the late fall of 1994, the CDC drafted new guidelines. The revised guidelines contain two tiers of precautions. The first tier, **standard precautions,** blends the major features of universal precautions (blood and body fluids precautions) and body substance isolation into a single set of precautions to be used for the care of all clients in hospitals, regardless of their diagnosis or presumed infection status. The new standard precautions apply to blood, all body fluids, secretions, and excretions, whether or not they contain visible blood; nonintact skin; and mucous membranes. These precautions are designed to reduce the risk of transmission of both recognized and unrecognized sources of infection in hospitals. As a result of the new category of standard precautions, clients with diseases or conditions that previously required category-specific or disease-specific precautions are now covered under this category and do not require additional precautions.

The second tier, **transmission-based precautions,** is designed only for the care of specified clients. This tier reduces the disease-specific precautions into three sets of precautions based on routes of transmission. These categories are designed for clients documented or suspected to be infected or colonized with highly transmissible or epidemiologically important pathogens for which additional precaution must be used to interrupt transmission

Handwashing, Hand Antisepsis, and Gloving CDC Recommendations

- Hands must be washed with antiseptic soap and water or alcohol-based handrub:
  1. Before and after client contact and between clients.
  2. After contact with a source of microorganisms.
  3. After removing gloves. Before donning gloves.
  4. After touching equipment or surfaces that may be contaminated.
- Gloves should be used as an adjunct to, not a substitute for, handwashing.
  1. Remove gloves and wash hands after any hand contaminating activity.
  2. Change gloves between clients.
  3. Change gloves during care of a single client when moving from one procedure to another. (This is critical when moving from a contaminated to a clean body site.)
  4. Use disposable gloves only once.
  5. Do not touch any body surface that is moist without gloves. (Moisture can be considered potentially contaminated.)
  6. Have latex-free gloves available for personnel with an allergy or sensitivity to latex.
  7. Decontaminate hands before donning sterile gloves.

to others in the hospital. The three types of transmission-based precautions include airborne, droplet, and contact precautions. Airborne precautions reduce the risk of airborne transmission of infectious agents, such as measles, varicella, and tuberculosis. Droplet precautions are used to prevent the transmission of diseases, such as meningitis, pneumonia, scarlet fever, diphtheria, rubella, and pertussis. Contact precautions are used for clients known or suspected to have serious illnesses easily transmitted by direct contact, such as herpes simplex, staphylococcal infections, hepatitis A, respiratory syncytial virus, and wound or skin infections.

All three types of precautions may be used at one time when multiple routes of transmission are suspected in a client. These precautions are always used in conjunction with standard precautions. Table 14–1 outlines recommendations for transmission-based precautions.

Fundamental Principles Certain fundamental principles should be applied to all clients. The first is handwashing. Handwashing is the single most important means of preventing the spread of infection. (People carry between 10,000 and 10 million bacteria on each hand.) A second fundamental principle involves the use of gloves. Gloves are worn to provide a protective barrier, prevent gross contamination of the hands when touching body substances or blood, and reduce the risk of exposure to blood pathogens. Gloves also prevent the spread of microorganisms to other clients and to health care personnel.

The third fundamental principle is the proper placement of clients in the hospital to prevent the spread of microorganisms to others or to the client. Clients may not always be placed in private rooms when they are infected. They can be placed in a room where the second client has the same infectious process.

The fourth fundamental principle is the appropriate use of isolation equipment to prevent the spread of microorganisms to health care workers and other clients. The equipment required is based on the specific transmission route of the microorganism. Specific handling of client care items needs to be considered in preventing the spread of infection.

Handwashing Wash hands with nonantimicrobial soap or use waterless antiseptic agent for routine handwashing and after removing gloves. An antimicrobial or antiseptic agent should be used for control of specific outbreaks of infection.

Gloves Clean, nonsterile gloves (or latex-free gloves if latex allergy is present) are worn when touching blood, body fluids, secretions, excretions, and contaminated items. Put gloves on just before touching mucous membranes and nonintact skin. Remove gloves immediately after use, and wash hands before touching noncontaminated items and environmental surfaces or giving care to another client. Gloves should be discarded immediately and not reused.

Mask, Eye Protection, Face Shield Wear mask and eye protection during procedures in which splashes or sprays could come in contact with eyes and mucous membranes.

Principles of Handwashing

- Wash hands thoroughly at the beginning of the shift before providing client care.
- Wash hands for 10–15 seconds before and after providing client care.
- Wash hands before and after preparing medications.
- Wash hands after handling soiled linen, equipment, or supplies.
- Wash hands between contact with different clients.
- Wash hands after removing gloves.
- Wash hands after you have sneezed or coughed.
- Wash hands before and after eating.
- Wash hands just before leaving the nursing unit.

TABLE 14–1 HICPAC* Recommendations for Transmission-Based Precautions

	Contact	Droplet	Airborne
Purpose	Prevent transmission of known or suspected infected or colonized microorganisms by direct hand or skin-to-skin contact that occurs when providing direct client care. Conditions in which contact precautions are required: diphtheria, herpes simplex, scabies, *Staphyloccus* infection, hepatitis A, and respiratory syncytial virus wound or skin infection	Prevent transmission of large-particle droplets, larger than 5 microns (μm) (i.e., diphtheria, pertussis, streptococcal pharyngitis, pneumonia, scarlet fever, meningitis, rubella)	Prevent transmission of small-particle residue of 5 microns (μm) or smaller droplets (i.e., measles, varicella, tuberculosis)
Client Placement	• Private room • Can be placed in room of client with same microorganism	• Private room • Can be placed in room of client with same diagnosis	• Private room • Can be placed in room of client with same diagnosis • Monitor negative air pressure • Keep door closed • Keep client in room
Respiratory Protection	• Mask not necessary	• Use mask when working within 3 feet of client	• Respiratory protective equipment • Do not enter room of clients with rubeola or varicella if susceptible to these infections
Gloves and Gown	• Wear gloves when entering room • Change gloves after contact with infective material, such as wound drainage or fecal material • Wash hands immediately after removing gloves • Wear gown when working with clients with diarrhea, ostomies, or wound drainage not contained in dressing • Wear gown if contact with client or environment will occur	• Follow standard precautions	• Follow standard precautions
Client Transport	• Transport only if essential • Ensure precautions are maintained to minimize risk of transmission	• Transport only if essential • Place mask on client when outside room	• Transport only if essential • Place mask on client when outside room
Client Care Items	• Client care items and environmental surfaces are cleaned daily • Dedicate equipment to single client use (i.e., stethoscope, thermometer)		

*Hospital Infection Control Practices Advisory Committee.

Source: Adapted from Department of Health and Human Services: CDC, *Federal Register,* "Recommendations for Isolation Precautions in Hospitals" (1997).

Face shields protect the mucous membranes of the eyes, nose, and mouth from splashes of blood, body fluids, secretions, and excretions. Suctioning clients and assisting physicians in insertion of hemodynamic monitoring lines are examples of situations in which this type of protection is required.

Gown Nonsterile disposable gowns are used to protect the skin and clothing from contamination while providing client care. Gowns should be worn whenever there is a risk of contamination from blood, body fluids, secretions, or excretions. Soiled gowns should be removed immediately and hands washed to prevent the spread of microorganisms.

Linen Transport soiled linens in a manner that prevents skin and mucous membrane exposure, contamination of clothing, and transfer of microorganisms to other clients and environments. This is usually accomplished through double-bagging linen before taking it to the laundry facility.

Occupational Health and Blood-borne Pathogens Take precautions to prevent injuries caused by needles, scalpels, or other sharp instruments or devices. Only use safety needles. Never recap used needles, purposely bend or break needles by hand, remove needles from disposable syringes, or otherwise handle needles directly. All such instruments should be placed in puncture-resistant containers for disposal. The use of needleless systems for IV management has dramatically decreased needle stick injuries.

Mouth pieces, resuscitation bags, or other ventilation devices should be used as an alternative to mouth-to-mouth resuscitation.

Client Placement Clients who are at risk for contaminating the environment or who are unable to maintain appropriate hygiene or environmental control should be placed in a private room. If this is not possible, other arrangements need to be made in consultation with the hospital's infection control department.

In addition to health care workers following standard precautions, the following guidelines should be considered when providing client care:

- Health care workers who have open lesions, upper respiratory infections, or weeping dermatitis should refrain from all direct client contact and from handling client care equipment.
- Because of the risk of transmission of HIV and hepatitis B virus (HBV) from mother to fetus, pregnant health workers should be especially familiar with, and strictly adhere to, precautions to minimize risk of these viruses. Currently, pregnant health care workers are not known to be at greater risk of contracting HIV or HBV than other workers.

Health Care Worker Protection Act In 1997 the "Health Care Worker Protection Act" was passed to assist in the reduction of health care workers who are accidentally exposed to potentially contaminated, infected blood via a needle stick. This act makes the use of safe needle devices a requirement if the facility receives Medicare funding. The impetus for the bill was a direct result of statistics from the Centers for Disease Control and Prevention (CDC) indicating that more than 800,000 needle sticks and sharps injuries were being reported yearly. This is the most common cause of health care worker-related exposure to blood-borne pathogens. Needle stick injuries caused by hollow-bore needles accounted for 86% of all reported occupational HIV exposures. Nurses make up 24% of all the cases of HIV infection among health care workers known or thought to have been infected on the job. For more information, refer to the PEP protocol (PEP) described later in this chapter.

More than 20 pathogens can be transmitted through small amounts of blood. In addition to HIV and Hepatitis B, syphilis, varicella-zoster, and Hepatitis C can be transmitted via this route. Hepatitis B is the most common infectious disease transmitted through work-related exposure to blood. About 5,100 health care workers become infected with Hepatitis B each year.

ACQUIRED IMMUNODEFICIENCY SYNDROME

Epidemiology and Modes of Transmission

The incidence of acquired immunodeficiency syndrome (AIDS) has grown exponentially since it was first recorded in 1981. The statistics are chilling: The U.S. cumulative number of AIDS cases reported to the CDC as of June 2001 is 793,026; 649,186 cases are males, 134,845 are females, and 8,994 are children under age 13. Estimates are that there will be 75 million HIV cases in the top five industrial nations by 2010. AIDS has become the second leading killer of young men 24–44 years old and the fifth leading killer of U.S. women. AIDS will be the third most common cause of death in the United States. Cases have been reported from all 50 states and three U.S. territories. AIDS is perhaps the most serious epidemic facing the modern world, making knowledge about it and techniques for caring for the AIDS client mandatory learning for all nurses. No one is immune to AIDS.

The two major risk groups continue to be homosexual or bisexual men and IV drug abusers, which make up over two-thirds of all AIDS cases. AIDS incidence increased most dramatically among women, African-Americans, and people infected heterosexually. Prior to the introduction of combination therapies for HIV, AIDS incidence was increasing each year. The epidemic has slowed significantly from the early years when increases were 65–95% each year. In 1996, the estimated AIDS incidence dropped for the first time, decreasing by 6%. Deaths from the disease also decreased by 25%. The decrease is thought to be related partially as a result of prevention efforts targeted at high-risk populations. In addition, the new therapies have extended the life span of individuals with AIDS.

African-Americans and Hispanics have been disproportionately affected by the HIV epidemic over the last decade. Homosexual sex and IV drug abuse evenly resulted in AIDS cases among the African-American men. Heterosexual contact cases increased slightly over the same time frame. The incidence of female African-American cases increased significantly among infected heterosexuals (about 11%).

Definitions

Acquired Immunodeficiency Syndrome AIDS is the most severe form of a continuum of illnesses associated with HIV infection. AIDS is defined by the CDC as an HIV infection in a person with a CD4+ T-lymphocyte count of less than 200 cells/microliter (μL) of blood or a CD4+ percentage of less than 14. Twenty-six clinical conditions are listed in the CDC AIDS surveillance case definition in category C. Once clients have a condition listed in category C, they remain in that surveillance category. Among those 26 conditions listed in the category are cytomegalovirus (CMV) retinitis; Kaposi's sarcoma; *Mycobacterium avium* complex (MAC) (which includes the *M. avium* and *M. intracellulare* organisms) or *M. kansasii*; *Mycobacterium tuberculosis*, any site; *Pneumocystis carinii*; and recurrent pneumonia.

Proper Handling of Biohazard Waste

Speaking for the Florida Department of Health and Rehabilitation Services, an epidemiologist stated that there was an 80% reduction in exposure to biohazard material in seven Florida hospitals following the enactment of the Florida Administrative Code. This code is an example of the principles that additional states are beginning to enact.

What Is Biohazard Waste?

Any solid or liquid waste that may present a threat of infection is considered "biohazard." This could include laboratory waste, blood or blood products, body fluids, absorbent material saturated with blood or body fluids (either wet or dry), discarded sharps, and nonabsorbent disposable devices (such as drains, excretions, gloves, urine specimens, etc.).

Why Separate Biohazard from Other Medical Waste?

It is critical that the biohazard waste be separated at the point of origin or before it leaves the client's room. This reduces the risk of exposure considerably. The principles of separation are:

- Use an impermeable red plastic bag labeled "biohazard"; close bag securely while inside the client's room.
- Use a second red-labeled bag outside the room and place the inside bag in it so that the waste is "double-bagged."
- Do not place red-labeled bag with other waste material, because it could contaminate all waste.
- Sharps should be separated from all other waste and placed in a leak and puncture proof container with a biohazard symbol on the outside.
- Fiberboard waste containers should NOT contain scalpels.
- Do not overfill sharps containers, because items could fall out.

Storage of Biohazard Material

Biohazard waste must be appropriately sealed. It may be stored for 30 days; time starts when material is placed in the sharps container or biohazard bag. All biohazard waste must be restricted, locked up, or placed in a separate storage area. Biohazard waste must be in a room with *no* carpeting. Sealed cement is necessary so that a spill can be cleaned up. Biohazard material must be labeled correctly so that there is a tracking method for each bag, container, etc. Labels should say "medical waste" and "biohazard" and be dated when the bag was first placed in the area.

Transporting Biohazard Waste

When transporting biohazard waste within the facility, containers must remain intact. Trash chutes must *not* be used. Outdoor containers should be secured against vandalism and marked or labeled.

A contingency plan for spilled material:

- Spilled or leaked biohazard material must be cleaned with industrial strength detergent, and then disinfected.
- Onsite treatment and disposal of waste must be steamed, incinerated, or cleaned with an alternative method (chemical, dry heat, etc.).
- Each facility must post a "Spill Contingency Plan" which includes which substance to be used to disinfect.

If each facility has an administrative code that includes a total plan, policies, and procedures for dealing with biohazard waste, as well as a training program for all employees in how to handle biohazard waste, the incidence of exposure could be dramatically decreased.

Source: Florida Department of Health and Rehabilitation and Services.

Human Immunodeficiency Virus HIV is a blood-borne infective retrovirus that invades the CD4+ T-lymphocyte (immunity) cell, renders it useless, and then duplicates itself by means of that cell. With loss of the client's immune function, the disease becomes clinically manifested. Infection with HIV progresses to AIDS in at least 35% of those infected. Once a client has been diagnosed with HIV, the usual approach to care includes evaluation of the immune system and classification by CDC grouping, (A) asymptomatic, (B) acute symptomatic, and (C) AIDS-indicator conditions. Identification and treatment of infectious and neoplastic complications, initiation of approved antiretroviral therapy, and consideration of experimental measures are also included in the evaluation.

HIV is transmitted through high-risk behaviors or other contact with the virus, including

- Sexual contact with HIV-infected individuals
- Sharing needles with HIV-infected individuals
- Transfusions of blood or blood products from infected individuals (not common today, but new cases are still reported)
- Babies who become infected from the mother before or during birth, or through breast-feeding
- Contact with contaminated needles, blood, secretions, or excretions from an HIV-infected client

Health Care Workers' Exposure to HIV

Prospective studies of health care workers have estimated that the average risk for HIV transmission after a percutaneous exposure to HIV-infected blood is approximately 0.3% and after a mucous membrane exposure is 0.09%. Risk factors for transmission by skin exposure and fluid or tissue exposure has not been quantified. The CDC states that 600,000 to 800,000 needle stick injuries occur each year with potential risk of HIV exposure (CDC statistics, 2002). Considerations that influence the use of postexposure prophylaxis (PEP) include the timing of the PEP—how soon after exposure PEP was begun—and the belief that the infection can be prevented or improved by the use of the antiretroviral drugs.

In 1997, the Public Health Service updated recommendations for management of health care worker exposure to HIV and recommendations for PEP. The decision to recommend HIV PEP takes into account the nature of the exposure, needle stick or mucous membrane contact, and the amount of blood or body fluid involved in the exposure. Other considerations include exposure to a virus known or suspected to be resistant to antiretroviral drugs. Pregnancy is also a consideration. Risk factor assessments are key determinants of PEP. Health care facilities should have the protocols available, and prompt reporting and postexposure care should be considered a health care emergency and treated as such. This includes access to clinicians who can provide postexposure care during all working hours and the antiretroviral agents for PEP immediately available. Health care workers must be educated to report occupational exposures immediately after they occur because PEP is most likely to be effective if implemented as soon after the exposure as possible. Not all exposures with HIV-infected blood or body fluids will result in the need for PEP.

An exposure is defined as a percutaneous injury, contact of mucous membrane or nonintact skin, or contact with intact skin when the duration of contact is prolonged or involves an extensive area, with blood, tissue, or other body fluids. Body fluids include semen, vaginal secretions, or other body fluids contaminated with visible blood (cerebrospinal, synovial, pleural, amniotic fluids, peritoneal, pericardial). There is no evidence that tears, sweat, nonbloody urine or feces transmit HIV.

A risk assessment is performed on all health care workers who have been exposed to potentially HIV-infected blood or body fluids. The Public Health Service has devised a two-step algorithm to determine the risk of transmission for the worker. If it is determined that a high risk of transmission has occurred, the health care worker would be started on a PEP regimen.

Recommendations for PEP include a basic 4-week regimen of two drugs (zidovudine and lamivudine) for most HIV exposures. An expanded regimen that includes the addition of a protease inhibitor (indinavir or nelfinavir) is recommended for HIV exposures that pose an increased risk of transmission or when there is a known or suspected resistance to one or more of the antiretroviral agents recommended for PEP.

OTHER INFECTIOUS DISEASES

Tuberculosis

Tuberculosis is an infectious disease caused by the tubercle bacillus *Mycobacterium tuberculosis*. The main reservoir for the organism is the human respiratory tract, and transmission occurs between individuals through respiratory contact. The tubercle bacillus enters the respiratory tract on droplets transmitted through productive coughing from the infected individual. Symptoms may occur in 4–12 weeks after exposure or may go unnoticed for many years. Active pulmonary tuberculosis has a slow, insidious onset. The progression of the active disease and symptoms of cough, weight loss, and fever usually occur within the first two years after the infection. Latent infections which are asymptomatic are not infectious and may last a lifetime. Without treatment tuberculosis progresses to other body sites. Disseminated tuberculosis occurs in many of the body areas, not just the lungs. The incidence of tuberculosis cases in this country has increased greatly, due in large part to the AIDS epidemic. Immunosuppressed hosts are very vulnerable to the bacillus. In addition to immunosuppressed individuals, others considered at high risk for infection include alcoholics; IV drug abusers; individuals who share a closed environment with the infected individual; residents of institutions such as long-term care and correctional facilities; foreign-born individuals from countries with a high prevalence of tuberculosis, such as Asia, Latin America, Africa, Mexico, and the former Soviet Union; low-income populations who are medically underserved; and clients who are noncompliant and do not complete the appropriate drug therapy. Health care workers who come in contact with any of the high-risk populations are at risk for infection.

A growing number of clients develop MDR-TB, multidrug-resistant tuberculosis. This type of tuberculosis is invitro resistance of a strain of TBC to antituberculosis drugs. The disease can progress from diagnosis to death in as short a period as 4–16 weeks. The increasing incidence of MDR-TB can be attributed to delays in treatment, inadequate isolation and infection control practices, and lack of follow-through after hospital discharge. Clients develop resistance to the standard drug regimen as a result of noncompliance and/or inappropriate drug therapy. MDR-TB is also caused by person-to-person contact through sneezing or coughing, or from a person with primary drug resistance.

Early recognition and treatment of tuberculosis must be initiated promptly and isolation measures instituted to prevent the spread of the disease. The CDC describes effective tuberculosis control requirements as early identification, isolation, and treatment of persons with active tuberculosis. The purified protein derivative (PPD) skin test is used to quickly identify the infection in the absence of clinical symptoms. Sputum specimens for AFB and culture and sensitivity and chest x-rays are also ordered to rule out TB. A PPD skin test is read 48–72 hours after the injection. A positive skin test is indicated by an induration of 5–10 mm at the site of the injection. A two-step method is now being used, particularly with health care workers. This procedure involves the first PPD injection to be given and read within 48–72 hours. If the PPD is negative or doubtful the PPD is repeated in one week. If the client has a positive reaction, he or she is started on a prophylaxis regimen. A client who is known to be HIV-positive with a 5 mm or larger induration at the site of the PPD injection should be considered positive for tuberculosis.

The CDC recommendation for tuberculosis isolation includes a directional air-flow, negative-pressure ventilation system in the room of tuberculosis clients. Negative-pressure ventilation pulls air away from hallways and exhausts it out of the room to areas away from air intake vents. Six air changes each hour is required to provide microbial dilution within the room. Ultraviolet irradiation lamps can be used to supplement ventilation systems when the risk of tuberculosis transmission is high.

Anyone entering the client's room should wear a mask that forms a tight-fitting seal against particulates 1–5 microns (μ). Two examples of tuberculosis masks are the high-efficiency particulate air (HEPA) mask used for suspected or confirmed multidrug-resistant (MDR) tuberculosis and the disposable submicron mask used for confirmed tuberculosis. Disposable particulate respirators are suggested by the CDC when adequate ventilation is not available in the room. All treatments and procedures should be performed in the client's room if at all possible. If the client must leave the room, a valveless particulate respirator must be used.

Viral Hepatitis

There are six forms of hepatitis. Each form differs in regard to incubation period, route of transmission, antigenic properties, and progression to chronicity. All forms of hepatitis produce an inflammatory response to the liver which is characterized by liver cell necrosis, inflammation, and cell regeneration. The three major forms of hepatitis are Hepatitis A Virus (HAV), Hepatitis B Virus (HBV), and Hepatitis C Virus (HCV). Hepatitis D Virus (HDV) is not as common and Hepatitis E Virus (HEV) is rare in the United States. Hepatitis G Virus (HGV) is a recently isolated blood-borne infectious agent transmitted by needle-sticks and blood transfusions.

Hepatitis A (HAV) is spread via the fecal–oral route and sexual transmission. Poor sanitation and handwashing is a major source of infection. Approximately 152,000 infections occur in the United States each year. Ninety-nine percent of those infected recover without any serious problems. HAVRIX vaccine is available to prevent HAV. Once exposed to the infection or as a preventative therapy, immune serum globulin is administered intramuscularly.

Hepatitis B (HBV) is spread through infected blood or body fluids and through two nonparenteral routes, sexual contact and perinatal transmission. Contaminated needles, syringes, and blood products are the most common mode of transmission, although about 30% of the cases are spread through sexual contact. An estimated 140,000 individuals are infected yearly in the United States. Two to ten percent of adults become chronically infected with HBV following an infection. HBV is 100 times more infectious than HIV. HBV vaccine provides active immunity in over 95% of recipients. The two common vaccines are Engerix-B and Recombivax HB. Hepatitis B immune globulin provides passive immunity to individuals who have had contact with HBV-contaminated material.

Hepatitis C (HCV) is transmitted primarily by contact with contaminated blood and blood products. Eighty-five percent of those infected with HCV will remain chronically infected. Chronic HCV infection is the main causal factor for nearly one third of all liver transplants. There are three types of interferon used to treat HCV.

The CDC recommends the use of standard precautions with clients known to have hepatitis. The precautions should be maintained for one week after the onset of symptoms.

Severe Acute Respiratory Syndrome (SARS)

In 2003, there was a multi-country outbreak of a virus suspected to be a mutated form of the corona-virus (the common cold). The specific SARS pathogen is not known. There is speculation that this new virus has jumped from animal to human, setting up the possibility for a worldwide pandemic like the 1918 swine or Spanish flu that infected millions of people around the world and killed more than 20 million. Jumping species, from animal to human and being able to transmit person-to-person, is the worst possible combination of events because it can cause havoc in a non-immune population. Because of this potential for disaster, the World Health Organization issued a global alert when this corona virus rapidly spread to 26 countries. At this initial juncture, it was critical to employ stringent infection control protocols because both the exact pathogen, as well as the transmission mode, continued to elude scientists.

The primary symptoms of SARS are malaise, aching muscles, a persistent fever >38°C or 100.4°F, dry cough, shortness of breath or breathing difficulties, and an almost normal white blood count. People with these symptoms, who have recently traveled to or been in the far East, are advised to see a doctor immediately. The unusual and discriminating characteristic of this illness is that while it appears to be a flu-like illness, the symptoms persist and simply do not go away. Administering anti-viral drugs (i.e., ribovirin, a drug also used to treat hepatitis C) does not appear to be effective. At this point, there is only supportive treatment including oxygen and ventilatory assistance when necessary.

Total infection control precautions are essential to prevent transmission. These would include goggles or glasses to protect mucous membranes of the eyes, N95 mask, gown, and gloves. In addition, washing hands carefully is essential. Utilizing all of these protective measures has been shown to protect health care workers as long as they are careful not to touch contaminated surfaces or clothing after removing isolation gear. In the initial stages, SARS was transmitted to health care personnel because they did not adhere to precise precautions while caring for SARS clients. Also, it was discovered that this particular virus can live for 24 hours or longer on various surfaces, making it even more dangerous.

At the time of this publication, SARS has not been contained, additional cases are developing and the death rate is rising, even though it is only about 9% for those who contract the virus and are under 50 years old. For those over 50, the death rate is much higher. Even if this particular condition is eliminated, new viruses and bacteria will appear on the world stage and many of them could be mutated forms, not responsive to current antibiotics. Our transient and mobile global society makes it imperative that intervention and containment occur rapidly to prevent a worldwide pandemic when a new or mutated pathogen appears. The other imperative is that health care workers protect themselves using infection control protocols so that the spread of a new pathogen is contained in health care settings.

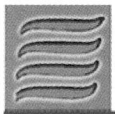

NURSING DIAGNOSES

The following nursing diagnoses may be appropriate to use on client care plans when the components are related to clients requiring isolation protocol or sterile procedures.

NURSING DIAGNOSIS	RELATED FACTORS
Altered Health Maintenance	Participation in high-risk activities, substance abuse, infectious states, religious or cultural beliefs detrimental to health
Risk for Infection	Immunosuppressed hospitalized clients, HIV/AIDS clients, invasive procedures, lack of immunization
	Inadequate defenses (loss of skin integrity, leukopenia, low hemoglobin)
Ineffective Therapeutic Regimen Management	Choices of daily living precludes maintaining treatment modalities, e.g., drug therapy, handwashing
Ineffective Community Coping	Deficits in social support, disease follow-up protocols, inadequate resources for disease prevention
Deficient Knowledge	Lack of access to health care facilities, lack of education, cognitive limitation
Noncompliance	Lack of motivation, education or readiness, information misinterpretation, cultural or religious beliefs
	Medical condition (communicable disease, HIV-positive), hospitalization, terminal illness
Latex Allergy Response	Allergies to certain foods, allergy to latex, lack of safety procedures for latex allergy
Ineffective Protection	Poor compliance to protocols, lack of knowledge, lack of resources

- The single most important nursing action to decrease the incidence of hospital-based infections is handwashing. **Remember to wash your hands or use antibacterial gel before and after each and every client contact.**

UNIT 1

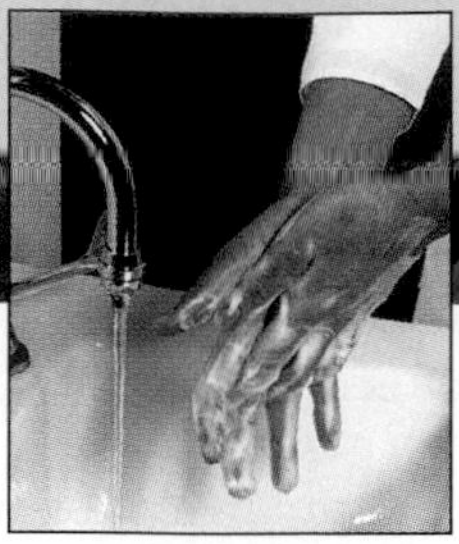

Basic Medical Asepsis

Nursing Process Data

ASSESSMENT *Data Base*

Assess method of handwashing that is most appropriate for assigned task.

Identify clients at risk for infection.

Assess availability of equipment for frequent handwashing (soap and water or antiseptic cleansing agent).

Evaluate health status of the nurse.

Check agency policy for handwashing protocol.

Assess need for use of unsterile gloves.

Assess nurses and clients for latex allergies.

Assess need for latex-free equipment and/or environment.

PLANNING *Objectives*

To deliver client care with pathogen-free hands

To prevent pathogenic microorganisms from spreading client to client, environment or health care personnel to client

To protect clients from cross-contamination

To protect health care workers

IMPLEMENTATION *Procedures*

Handwashing (Medical Asepsis)

For Using Waterless Antiseptic Agents

Cleaning Washable Articles

Donning and Removing Clean Gloves

Managing Latex Allergies

EVALUATION *Expected Outcomes*

Infection is prevented from spreading.

Cross-contamination is prevented.

Health care workers are protected from infection.

HANDWASHING (MEDICAL ASEPSIS)

Equipment

Nonantimicrobial soap* for routine handwashing
Orangewood stick for cleaning nails, if available
Running warm water
Paper towels
Trash basket

*According to 1997 HICPAC recommendations.

> **CLINICAL ALERT**
> Nurses must wash hands for 10–15 seconds before and after each direct contact with a client or each use of client care items to prevent spread of infection.

Compliance Studies for Handwashing

- A study of 2,800 opportunities for handwashing showed only a 48% compliance.
- Another study showed hands were washed only 8.5–9.5 seconds; a minimum of 10–15 seconds is necessary to prevent spread of infection.
- Compliance with handwashing technique is higher among nurses than physicians and other health care personnel; however, it is estimated to be only 30–50%.

Source: Centers for Disease Control and Prevention.

Procedure

1. Stand in front of but away from sink. **Rationale:** Uniform should not touch sink to avoid contamination.
2. Ensure that paper towel is hanging down from dispenser.
3. Turn on water using foot pedal or faucet so that flow is adequate, but not splashing.
4. Adjust temperature to warm. **Rationale:** Cold does not facilitate sudsing and cleaning; hot is damaging to skin.

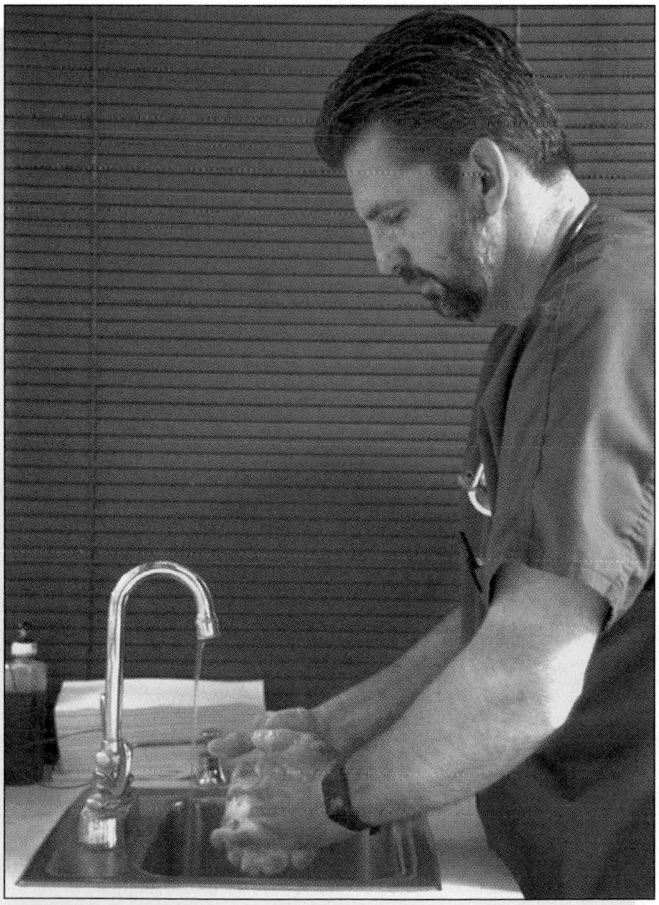

The single most important nursing action to decrease the incidence of hospital-based infection is washing your hands.

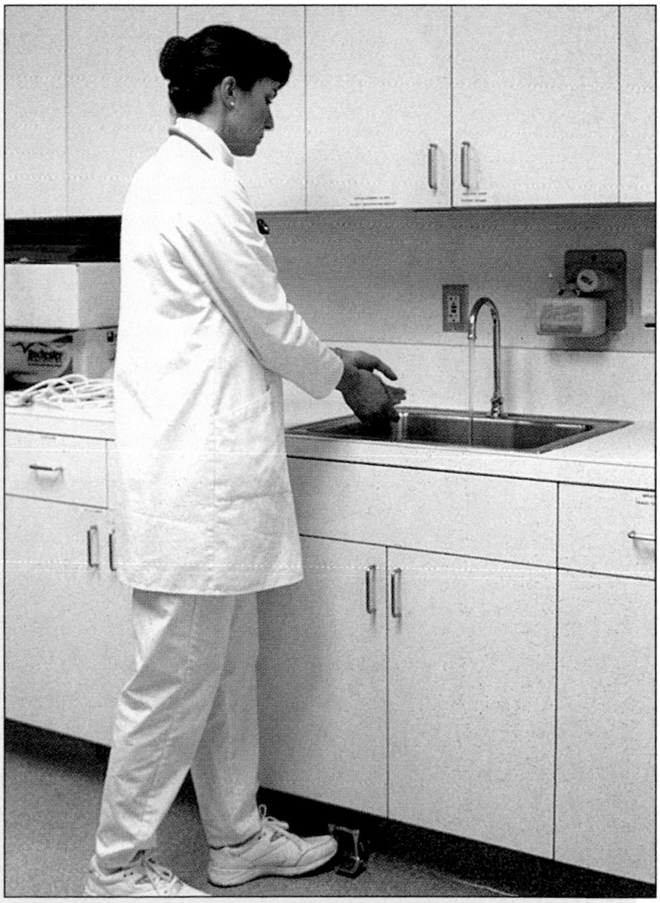

Use foot pedals when available to prevent contamination of hands.

5. Wet hands under running water. **Rationale:** Wet hands facilitate distribution of soap over entire skin surface.
6. Place a small amount, one to two teaspoons (3–5 mL) of liquid soap on hands. Thoroughly distribute over hands. Soap should come from a dispenser, not bar soap. **Rationale:** This prevents spread of microorganisms.
7. Rub vigorously, using a firm, circular motion, while keeping your fingers pointed down, lower than wrists. Start with each finger, then between fingers, then palm and back of hand. **Rationale:** This creates friction on all surfaces.
8. Wash your hands for at least 10–15 seconds. **Rationale:** Duration of washing is important to produce mechanical action and to allow antimicrobial products time to achieve desired effect.
9. Clean under your fingernails with an orangewood stick. (This should be done at least at start of day and if hands are heavily contaminated.)

CLINICAL ALERT

CDC Alert: The CDC has stated that health care workers in contact with clients must remove all fake fingernails to maintain infection control principles.

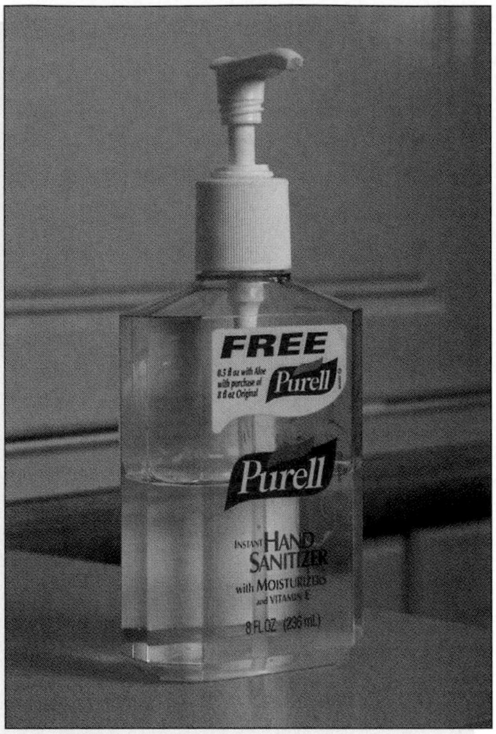

Waterless hand sanitizer kills 99.9% of the most common germs in 15 seconds.

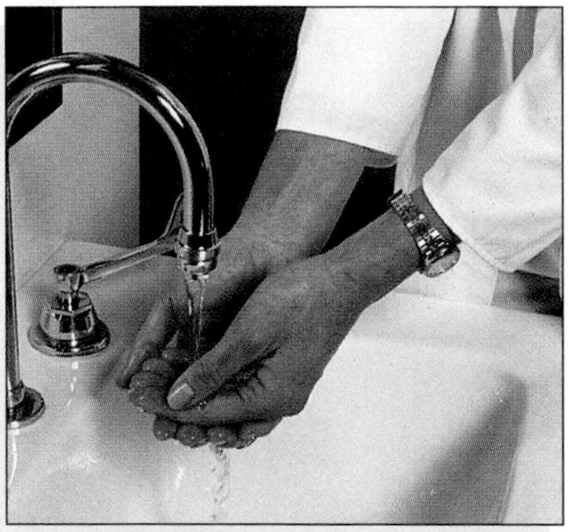
Wet hands thoroughly before applying soap to facilitate removal of pathogens.

10. Rinse your hands under running water, keeping fingers pointed downward. **Rationale:** This position prevents contamination of arms.
11. Resoap your hands, rewash, and rerinse if heavily contaminated.
12. Dry hands thoroughly with a paper towel, while keeping hands positioned with fingers pointing up. **Rationale:** Moist hands tend to gather more microorganisms from the environment.
13. Turn off water faucet with dry paper towel, if not using foot pedal. **Rationale:** to avoid recontaminating the hands.

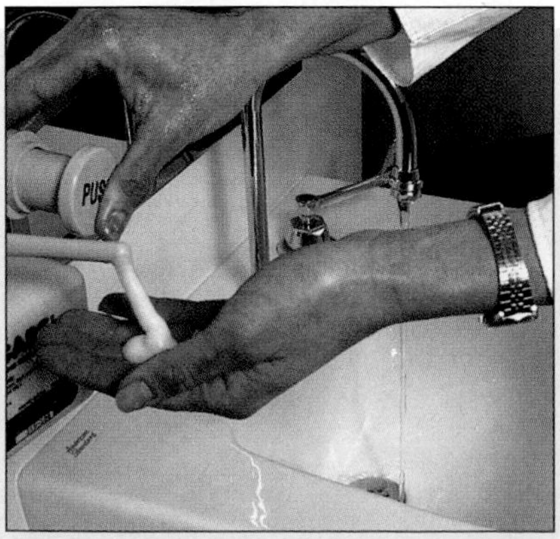
Use a generous amount of soap and friction during handwashing procedure.

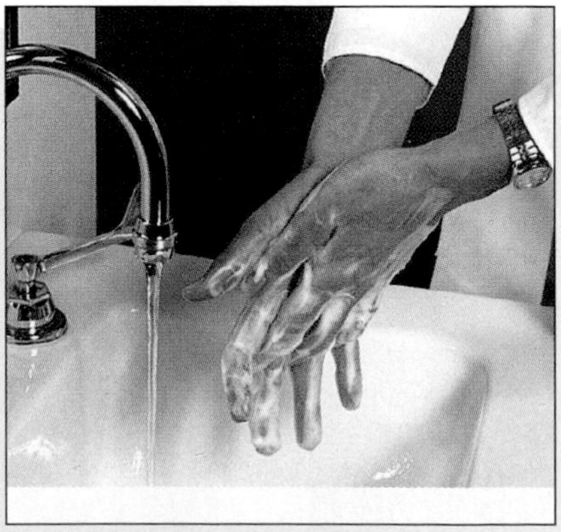
Keep fingers pointed down during handwashing to prevent contaminating arms.

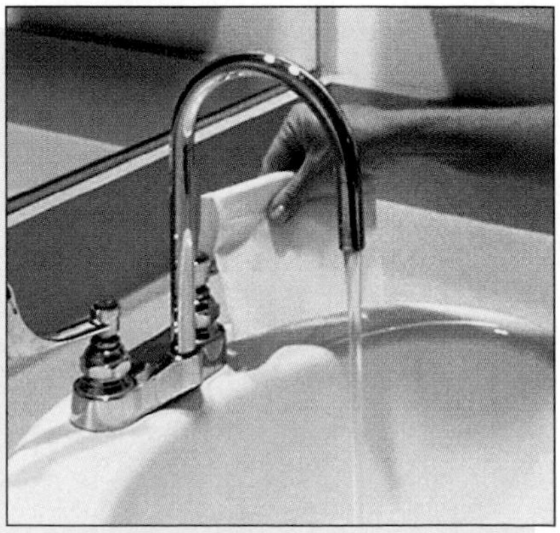
If foot pedal is not available, turn water faucet off using paper towel.

14. Restart procedure at step 5 if your hands touch the sink anytime between steps 5 and 13.

for Using Waterless Antiseptic Agents

1. Check dirt on hands and use waterless agent only if hands are clean.
2. Apply small amount of alcohol-based rub (3–5 mL) on palm of hand.
3. Rub hands together vigorously, covering all surfaces, sides of hands and fingers. **Rationale:** Failure to cover all surfaces can leave contaminated areas on the hands.
4. Rub hands until dry—waterless agent will dry quickly and automatically without using a towel.

CLINICAL ALERT

Antimicrobial soap or waterless agent should be used when there is identified resistant bacteria, colonization outbreaks, or hyperendemic infections.

CLINICAL ALERT

Hands soiled with dirt or organic matter require soap or detergents that contain antiseptic and water to effectively clean.

Evidence Based Nursing Practice

Improving Hand Hygiene

The leading cause of health care–acquired infections and spread of multiorganisms is inappropriate or inadequate hand hygiene. Nine studies (between 1977 and 2000) demonstrated the impact of hand hygiene on the risk of acquiring infections. One of these studies showed that endemic MRSA was eliminated in 7 months in a neonatal ICU following the introduction of a new hand antiseptic.

Source: Webster, J., Faoagil, J., Cartwright, D. (1994). Elimination of MRSA from a neonatal ICU after hand washing with Triclosan. *Journal of Pediatric Child Health, 30,* 59–64.

CLEANING WASHABLE ARTICLES

Equipment

Article to be washed
Antiseptic solution (according to hospital policy)
Running warm water
Paper towels
Trash basket
Clean gloves

Procedure

1. Wash your hands and don clean gloves.
2. Rinse under cold running water. **Rationale:** Cold water removes organic material. Hot water coagulates protein of organic material (pus, blood) and it adheres to a surface.
3. Wash with warm, soapy water using friction or follow hospital protocol for cleaning equipment.
4. Rinse well with clear, hot water.
5. Dry thoroughly.
6. Return to proper place or prepare for sterilization or disinfection if indicated.
7. Remove gloves and wash your hands.

DONNING AND REMOVING CLEAN GLOVES

Equipment

Clean gloves
Trash receptacle

Procedure

1. Wash your hands. **Rationale:** Donning gloves with unclean hands can transfer microorganisms outside gloves.
2. Remove glove from glove receptacle.

3. Hold glove at wrist edge and slip fingers into openings. Pull glove up to wrist.
4. Place gloved hand under wrist edge of second glove and slip fingers into opening.
5. Remove glove by pulling off, touching only outside of glove at cuff, so that glove turns inside out.
6. Place rolled-up glove in palm of second hand.
7. Remove second glove by slipping one finger under glove edge and pulling down and off so that glove turns inside out. Both gloves are removed as a unit.
8. Dispose of gloves in proper container, not at bedside.
9. Wash your hands.

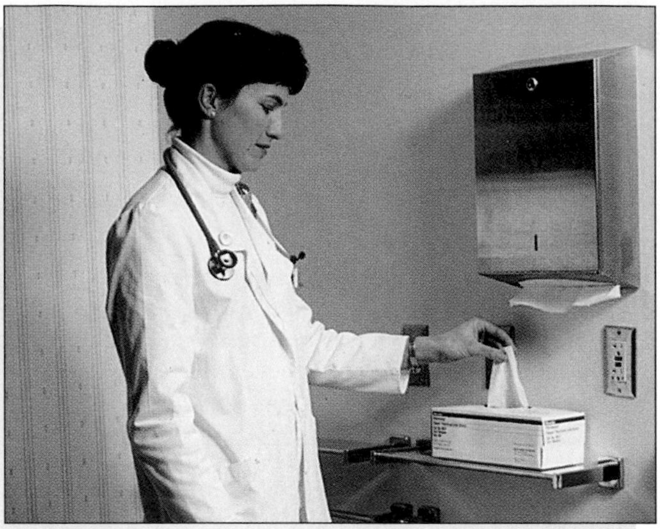

Clean gloves need to be easily accessible for health care workers.

CLINICAL ALERT

Latex allergy or hypersensitivity can be life-threatening, so recognize the primary symptoms in both clients and staff.

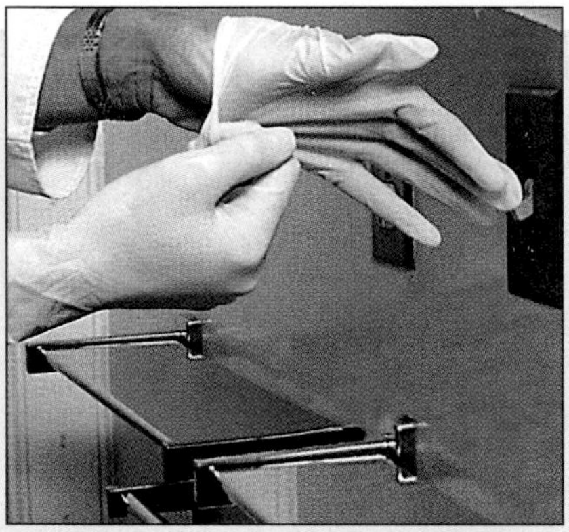

Pick up glove at wrist edge and slip fingers into openings.

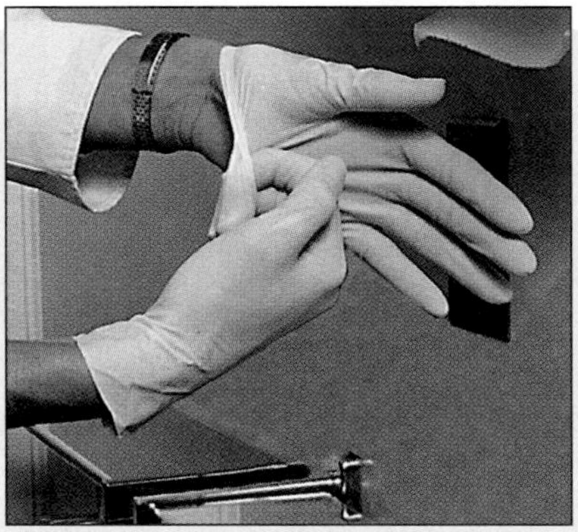

Remove glove by pulling off without touching hand with soiled glove.

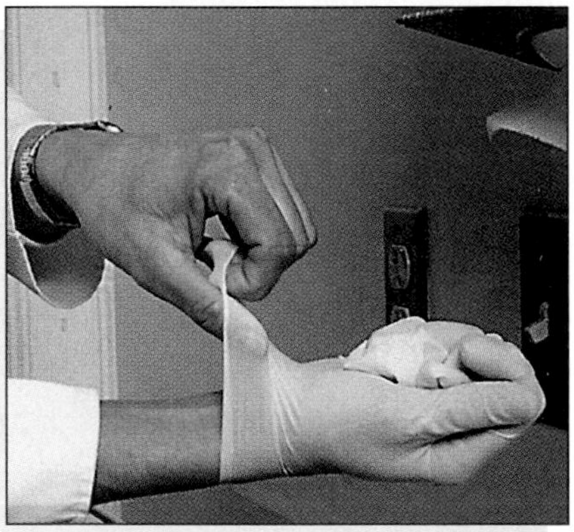

Place rolled up glove in palm of second hand and then remove glove.

EVIDENCE BASED NURSING PRACTICE

The Effectiveness of Gloves

Numerous studies have proven the effectiveness of gloves in preventing contamination of health care worker's hands. One study found that those who wore gloves during client contact had contaminated hands with an average bacterial count of 3/minute of client care compared to a count of 6/minute for those not wearing gloves.

Source: Pitlet, D., et al. (1999). Bacterial contamination of the hands of hospital staff during routine client care. *Archives of Internal Medicine, 159,* 821–826.

Glove Selection

- Use sterile gloves for procedures involving contact with normally sterile areas of the body.
- Use examination gloves for procedures involving contact with mucous membranes, unless otherwise indicated, and for client care or procedures that do not require use of sterile gloves.
- Change gloves between clients.
- Do not wash, disinfect, or reuse surgical or examination gloves.
- Use general purpose utility gloves (rubber household gloves) for housekeeping tasks that involve potential blood contact and for instrument cleaning and decontamination procedures.

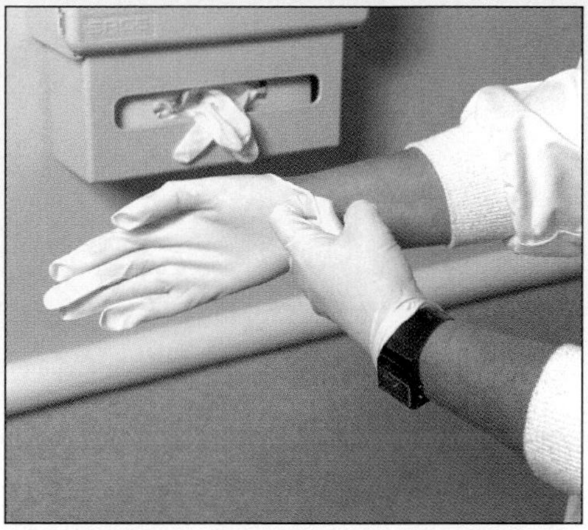

EVIDENCE BASED NURSING PRACTICE

The Importance of Wearing Gloves in Client Care

This study demonstrated that nurses doing "clean" activities such as lifting clients; taking blood pressure, pulse, or oral temperatures; or even touching a client could contaminate their hands with a bacterial count of 100 to 1,000 CFU of *Klebsiella* during such a procedure.

Source: Caswell, M., Phillips, I. (1997). Hands as route of transmission for *Klebsiella* species. *British Medical Journal, 2,* 1315–1317.

MANAGING LATEX ALLERGIES

Equipment

Latex-free gloves
Latex-free syringes
Latex-free IV tubing and bags of solution
Latex-free cart with supplies for client with latex allergy

Procedure

1. Assess clients at high risk or suspected sensitivity to latex (high latex exposure, congenital defects, indwelling catheters, etc.).
2. Assess clients and staff with allergies to avocados, bananas, kiwi, or chestnuts. **Rationale:** They may have cross-sensitivity to latex.
3. Recognize symptoms of latex allergy.
   a. Contact dermatitis.
   b. Type IV: facial swelling, itching, hives, rhinitis, eye symptoms.
   c. Type I: potentially dangerous bronchospasms, generalized edema, difficulty breathing, cardiac arrest.

Provide a latex-free cart—supplies for staff and clients with latex allergy.

4. Replace latex-containing products (especially gloves) with nonlatex alternatives.
5. Obtain a latex-free cart when a client is identified as having a latex allergy.
   a. Place cart inside client's room.
   b. Check that cart is supplied with latex-free gloves, syringes, IV tubes, suction catheters, etc.
6. Ensure that anaphylaxis medication is available for both clients and staff if latex allergy is suspected. **Rationale**: If there is a severe reaction, this medication may be lifesaving.

DOCUMENTATION FOR BASIC MEDICAL ASEPSIS

- Infection control measures used
- Clean gloves used for procedure
- Latex allergy identified
- Use of latex-free gloves

Critical Thinking Application

UNEXPECTED OUTCOMES	CRITICAL THINKING OPTIONS
Infection occurs in client.	• Assess mode of transmission of microorganism. • Administer antibiotics specific to microorganism as ordered. • Review handwashing technique. • Attend in-service program on infection control procedures. • Notify nurse manager of allergy.
Latex allergy identified in health care worker or client.	• Institute latex safety procedures for staff and client (if identified). • Educate staff about latex allergy. • Replace latex-containing objects (particularly gloves) with nonlatex alternatives. • Create a latex-free environment in which those who are allergic can work safely.

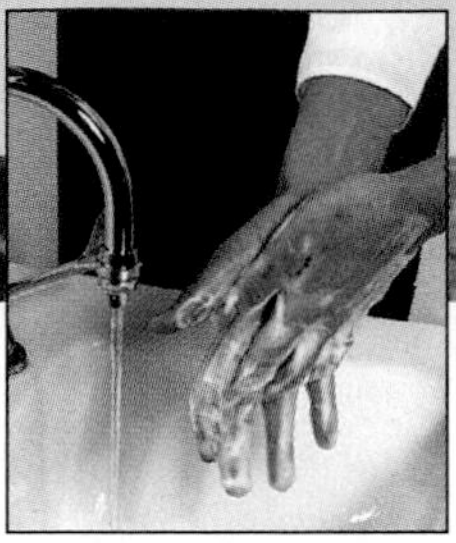

Standard Precautions (Tier One)

Nursing Process Data

ASSESSMENT Data Base

Assess for skin integrity.

Assess for presence of drainage from lesions or body cavity.

Assess for ability to deal with oral secretions.

Assess for compliance to hygiene measures (i.e., covering mouth when coughing, ability to control body fluids).

Assess ability to carry out activities of daily living (ADLs).

Assess extent of barrier techniques needed (i.e., gloves, gown, mask, protective eyewear).

Assess need for special equipment (i.e., hazardous waste bags, plastic bags for specimens).

PLANNING Objectives

To prevent the spread of the microorganism to health professionals

To reduce potential for the transmission of microorganisms

To protect hospital personnel and others from contamination

To provide appropriate equipment and techniques for preventive measures

To prevent clients (especially compromised clients) from acquiring nosocomial infections.

IMPLEMENTATION Procedures

Donning Protective Gear Utilizing Standard Precautions

Exiting a Client's Room Utilizing Standard Precautions

EVALUATION Expected Outcomes

The microorganism is not transmitted to other individuals.

The health care worker is protected from the microorganism.

Appropriate nursing interventions are carried out for the client.

STANDARD PRECAUTIONS
For all patient care

PROCEDURE					
Talking to patient					
Adjusting IV fluid rate or non-invasive equipment					
Examining patient *without* touching blood, body fluids, mucous membranes	X				
Examining patient *including* contact with blood, body fluids, mucous membranes	X	X			
Drawing blood	X	X			
Inserting venous access	X	X			
Suctioning	X	X	*Use gown, mask, eyewear if bloody body fluid splattering is likely*		
Inserting body or face catheters	X	X	*Use gown, mask, eyewear if bloody body fluid splattering is likely*		
Handling soiled waste, linen, other materials	X	X	*Use gown, mask, eyewear only if waste or linen are extensively contaminated and splattering is likely*		
Intubation	X	X	X	X	X
Inserting arterial access	X	X	X	X	X
Endoscopy	X	X	X	X	X
Operative and other procedures which produce extensive splattering of blood or body fluids.	X	X	X	X	X

DONNING PROTECTIVE GEAR UTILIZING STANDARD PRECAUTIONS

Equipment

Disposable gloves
Gown
Mask
Protective eyewear

Procedure

1. Wash hands using nonantimicrobial soap and dry.
2. Put on gown by placing one arm at a time through sleeves. Wrap gown around body so it covers clothing completely. **Rationale:** Gowns are worn when it is likely that personal clothing will come in contact with blood, body fluids, secretions, and excretions.
3. Bring waist ties from back to front of gown or tie in back, according to hospital policy. **Rationale:** This will ensure that entire clothing is covered by the gown preventing accidental contamination.
4. Tie gown at neck or adhere Velcro strap to gown.
5. Don mask. **Rationale:** Masks are worn when there is an anticipated contact with respiratory droplet secretions (e.g., client with suspected or known tuberculosis), the client has a persistent cough and does not cover mouth, or when suction will be performed.
6. Don protective eyewear such as face shield. **Rationale:** Face shields will protect the nurse from splashing of blood or body fluids while caring for clients.
7. Don disposable gloves. **Rationale:** Gloves will prevent contamination of hands when there is contact with blood, body fluids, secretions, or excretions.

Standard Precaution Guidelines

The following standard precautions are recommended for use with clients to prevent transmission of infectious agents. Please follow these guidelines when caring for clients.

- Wash hands thoroughly after removing gloves and before and after all client contact.
- Wear gloves when there is direct contact with blood, body fluids, secretions, excretions, and contaminated items. This includes a neonate before first bath. Wash as soon as possible if unanticipated contact with these body substances occurs.
- Protect clothing with gowns or plastic aprons if there is a possibility of being splashed or direct contact with contaminated material.
- Wear masks, goggles, or face shield to avoid being splashed; includes during suctioning, irrigations, and deliveries.
- Do not break or recap needles, discard them intact into puncture-resistant containers.
- Place all contaminated articles and trash in leakproof bags. Check hospital policy regarding double-bagging.
- Clean spills quickly with a 1:10 solution of bleach, or according to facility policy, or EPA approved germicide if spill occurs in an HIV/AIDS client's room.
- Place clients at risk for contaminating the environment in a private room with separate bathroom facilities, or with another client with same infectious organism.
- Transport infected clients using appropriate barriers, i.e., mask and gown.

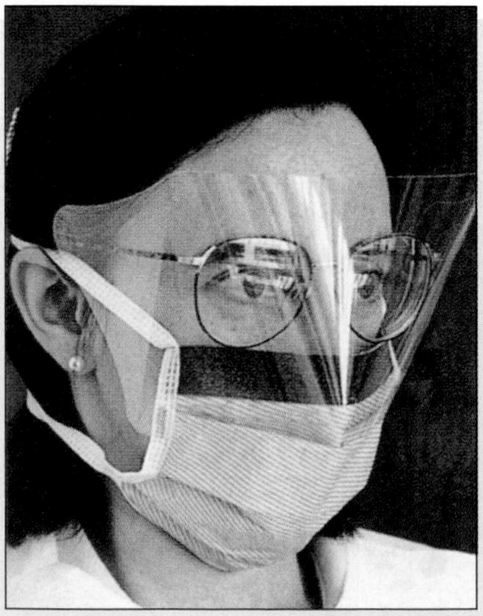

Face shield should be used when there is a risk of splashing from body fluids or blood.

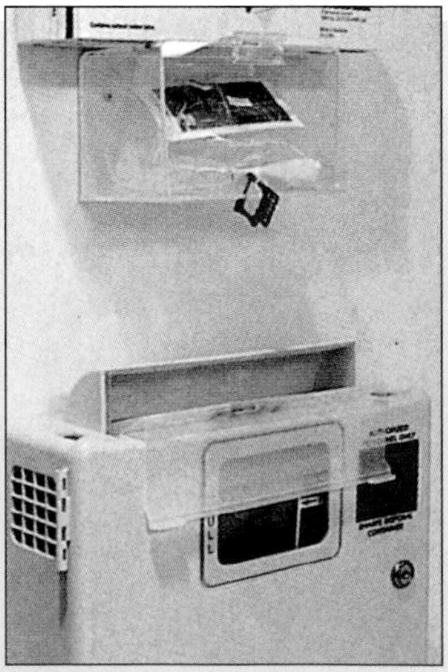

Place sharps container in area for easy access.

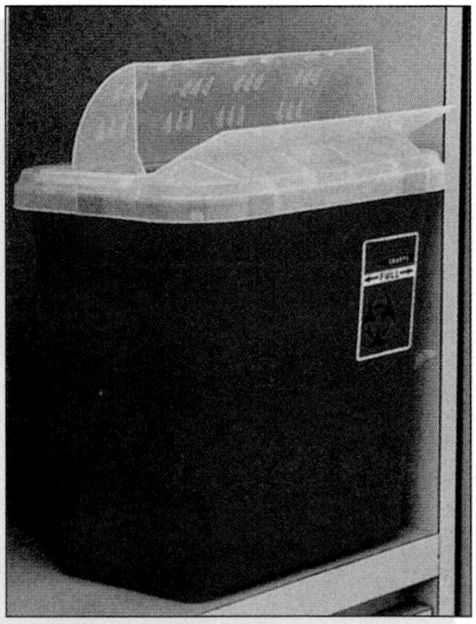

Larger sharps containers are available for areas where usage is greater.

EXITING A CLIENT'S ROOM UTILIZING STANDARD PRECAUTIONS

Equipment

Linen hamper
Garbage bag

Procedure

1. Untie string of gown at waist. **Rationale:** Any surface below waist level is considered contaminated, therefore the strings at the waist are untied before removing gloves.
2. Remove first glove by turning it inside out, place rolled-up glove in second hand, remove second glove by slipping one finger under glove edge and pulling glove off. Dispose of them in garbage bag.
3. Untie gown at neck. **Rationale:** The back of the neck is considered clean and the tie should not be touched with contaminated gloves.
4. Take off gown by pulling down from shoulders, turn gown inside out, and pull arms out of gown. **Rationale:** The inside of the gown is not considered contaminated and therefore, if it accidently touches your uniform, it will not be contaminated.
5. Dispose of gown in linen hamper. If disposable, place in garbage bag.
6. Remove protective eyewear.
7. Remove mask and place in garbage bag.
8. Wash hands in room.
9. Exit room and wash hands at nearest sink. **Rationale:** To prevent spread of microorganisms.
10. Dispose of all double-bagged equipment by taking to "dirty" utility room. Send specimens to laboratory and deposit linen in appropriate linen hamper.
11. Wash hands.

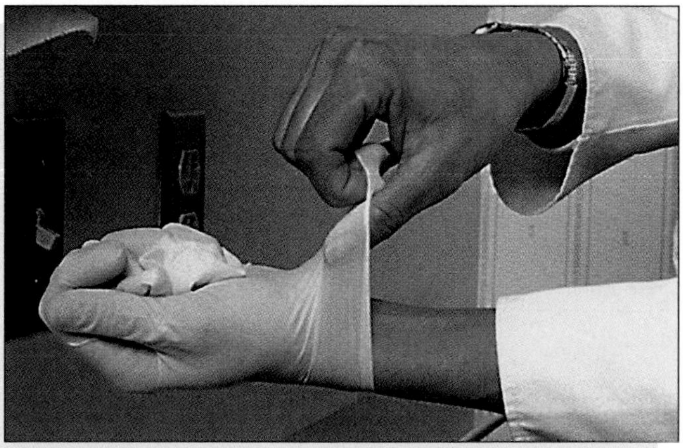

Place rolled-up glove in palm of second hand. Remove second glove by slipping one finger under edge and pulling down and off so that glove turns inside out. Both gloves are removed as a unit.

CLINICAL ALERT

Disposal Precautions

Secretion: Client should be instructed to expectorate into tissue held close to mouth. Suction catheters and gloves should be disposed of in impervious, sealed bags.
Excretion: Excrement should be disposed of by flushing into sewage system. Strict attention should be paid to careful handwashing; disease can be spread by oral–fecal route.
Blood: Needles and syringe should be disposable. Used needles should not be recapped. They should be placed in a puncture-resistant container that is prominently labeled "isolation." Specimens should be labeled "blood precaution."

HIV–HBV CLINICAL ALERT

Sample protocol for accidental contact with blood or body fluids.

1. Any percutaneous or mucocutaneous exposure should receive immediate first aid.
   a. Percutaneous exposure—a break in the skin caused by contaminated needle or sharp instrument, broken glass container holding blood or body fluids, or human bite.
   b. Mucocutaneous exposure—body fluid contact to open wounds, nonintact skin (eczema), or body fluid splash to mucous membranes (mouth, eyes).
2. Apply immediate first aid to site.
   a. Needle stick or puncture wound: Scrub area vigorously with soap and water for 5 minutes.
   b. Oral mucous membrane exposure: Rinse area several times with water.
   c. Ocular exposure: Irrigate immediately with water or normal saline solution.
   d. Human bite: Cleanse wound with povidone–iodine (Betadine) and sterile water.
3. Report unusual occurrence to the charge nurse or supervisor. (*See* explanation of form and sample in Chapter 3.)
4. Complete an unusual occurrence form and follow reporting requirements mandated by OSHA.
5. Follow facility protocol for emergency care. If risk assessment indicates, follow PEP protocol.
6. Document circumstances of exposure, postexposure management, counseling, and follow-up procedures in health care worker's confidential medical file.

Note: Use of antiseptics is not contraindicated; however, they have not been proven effective in postexposure care.

DOCUMENTATION FOR STANDARD PRECAUTIONS

- Standard precautions maintained
- Client's response to care and protocol used
- Specimens sent to laboratory if appropriate
- Disposal precautions utilized if appropriate

Critical Thinking Application

UNEXPECTED OUTCOMES	CRITICAL THINKING OPTIONS
Contaminated blood or body fluid comes in contact with your skin or mucous membranes.	• Report incident, and complete unusual occurrence report. (Very important for follow-up legal and medical implications.) • Follow hospital guidelines (they may differ per facility) for postexposure prophylaxis (PEP). • HIV exposure should be immediately reported, as most hospitals offer AZT preventive therapy. This therapy should be administered within 1 hour, not more than 24 hours after exposure. • Obtain AIDS antibody test in ensuing months. • Continue to monitor own health status and carry out specific activities to build immune system. Do not smoke or drink excessively. Eat well-balanced meals with reduced fat intake. Take vitamin supplements designed to boost immune system (vitamin C, beta-carotene, vitamin A, Coenzyme Q 10, zinc). Check with nutritionist or holistic physician for complete protocol. Exercise frequently. Obtain adequate sleep and rest. Learn and practice stress reduction activities (stress is known to lessen effectiveness of immune system).
Working with AIDS clients becomes extremely stressful, and you experience burn-out.	• Request consultation therapy to handle feelings and learn new methods of coping with stress. • Leave this type of work temporarily. • Change other aspects of your life to reduce stress. • Follow above-mentioned regimen to enhance immune system.

TABLE 14–2 Basic and Expanded HIV Postexposure Prophylaxis Regimens

Regimen Category	Application	Drug Regimen
Basic	Occupational HIV exposures for which there is a recognized transmission risk	4 weeks (28 days) of both zidovudine 600 mg every day in 2 or 3 divided doses **and** lamivudine 150 mg twice a day. Now available combined as combivar, single tablet given 2x daily.
Expanded	Occupational HIV exposures that pose an increased risk for transmission (e.g., larger volume of blood and/or higher virus titer in blood)	Basic regimen plus **either** indinavir 800 mg every 8 hours on an empty stomach **or** nelfinavir 750 mg three times a day with meals or snacks.

Recommendations for the Selection of Drugs for PEP

The selection of a drug regimen for HIV PEP must strive to balance the risk for infection against the potential toxicity of the agent(s) used. Because PEP is potentially toxic, its use is not justified for exposures that pose a negligible risk for transmission. Also, there is insufficient evidence to recommend a highly active regimen for all HIV exposures. Therefore, two regimens for PEP are provided: a "basic" two-drug regimen that should be appropriate for most HIV exposures and an "expanded" three-drug regimen that should be used for exposures that pose an increased risk for transmission or where resistance to one or more antiretroviral agents is known or suspected. When possible, the regimens should be implemented in consultation with persons having expertise in antiretroviral treatment and HIV transmission.

Source: CDC (2001) Morbidity and Mortality Weekly Report (MMWR). cdc.gov/mmwr/preview/mmwrhtml/rr5011a4.htm.

*Indinavir should be taken on an empty stomach (i.e., without food or with a light meal) and with increased fluid consumption (i.e., drinking six 8-oz glasses of water throughout the day); nelfinavir should be taken with meals.

UNIT 3

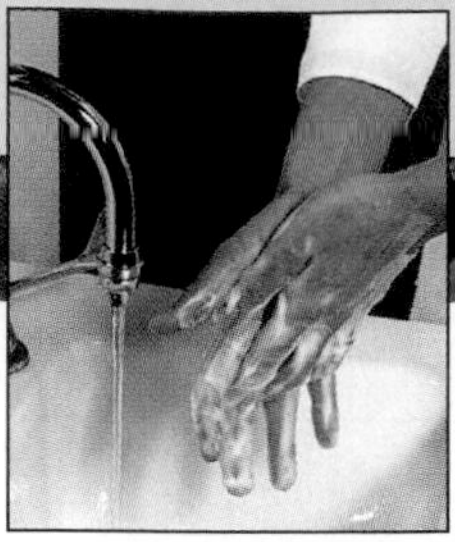

Isolation

Nursing Process Data

ASSESSMENT Data Base
Identify appropriate times for handwashing.
Identify type of protective clothing required for barrier nursing.
Identify epidemiology of the disease to determine how to prevent infection from spreading.
Identify equipment needed to prevent spread of organisms.
Assess method of terminal cleaning and disposing of equipment.

PLANNING Objectives
To prevent the spread of endogenous and exogenous flora to other clients
To reduce potential for transferring organisms from the hospital environment to the client
To protect hospital personnel from becoming infected
To prevent immunosuppressed clients from acquiring nosocomial infections

IMPLEMENTATION Procedures
Preparing for Isolation
Donning and Removing Isolation Attire
Using a Mask
Assessing Vital Signs
Removing Items from Isolation Room
Utilizing Double-Bagging for Isolation
Removing a Specimen from Isolation Room
Transporting Isolation Client Outside the Room
Removing Soiled Large Equipment from Isolation Room

EVALUATION Expected Outcomes
Isolation environment is maintained to prevent contamination of surrounding area.
Personnel working with isolation clients remain free of infection.

PREPARING FOR ISOLATION

Equipment

Specific equipment depends on isolation precaution system used
Soap* and running water
Isolation cart containing masks, gowns, gloves, plastic bags, isolation tape
Linen hamper and trash can, when needed
Paper towels
Door card indicating precautions

Procedure

1. Check physician's order for isolation.
2. Obtain isolation cart from central supply, if needed.
3. Check that all necessary equipment to carry out the isolation order is available.

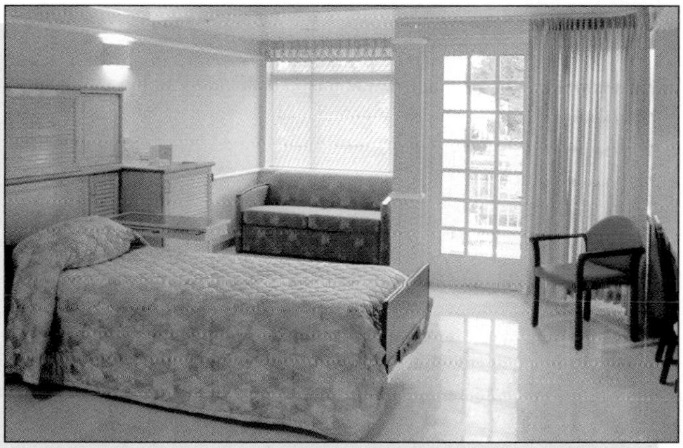

Client's isolation room with directional air-flow negative pressure ventilation system.

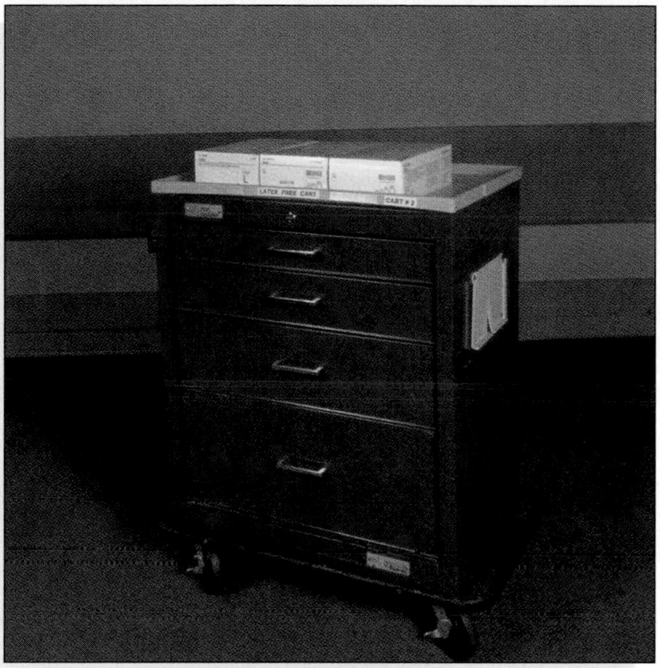

Place isolation cart outside client's door when cart is required.

4. Place isolation card on the client's door.
5. Ensure that linen hamper and trash cans are available, if needed.
6. Explain purpose of isolation to client and family.
7. Instruct family in procedures required.
8. Wash hands with antimicrobial soap† before and after entering isolation room.

*Type of antimicrobial soap or agent depends on infectious agent and client condition.

DONNING AND REMOVING ISOLATION ATTIRE

Equipment

Gown
Clean gloves

Procedure

for Donning Attire

1. Wash and dry hands.
2. Take gown from isolation cart or cupboard. Put on a new gown each time you enter an isolation room.
3. Hold gown so that opening is in back when you are wearing the gown.
4. Put gown on by placing one arm at a time through sleeves. Pull gown up and over your shoulders.
5. Wrap gown around your back, tying strings at your neck.
6. Wrap gown around your waist, making sure your back is completely covered. Tie strings around your waist.
7. Don eye shield and/or mask, if indicated. **Rationale:** Mask is required if there is a risk of splashing fluids.

Hospital policy in the United States may require staff to use plastic aprons instead of long-sleeved gowns for isolation protocol. This alternative is acceptable for infection control as long as gloves are worn, skin on arms is intact, and rigorous handwashing includes the arms.

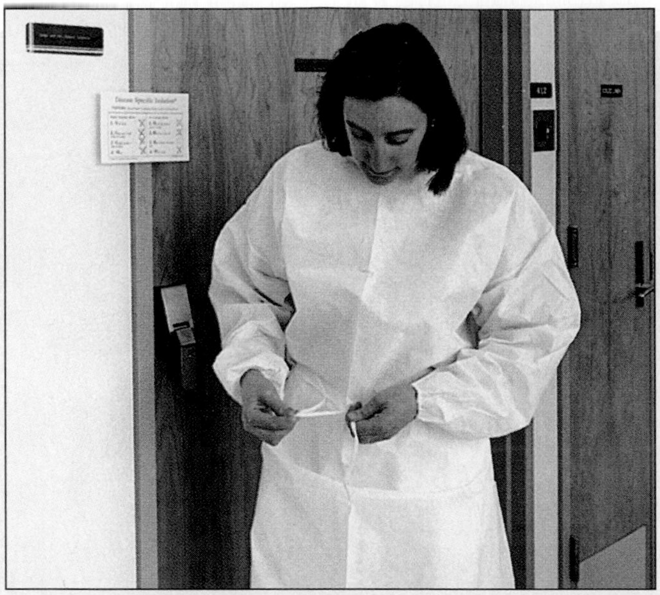

Isolation gown is put on before mask, eye shield, or gloves.

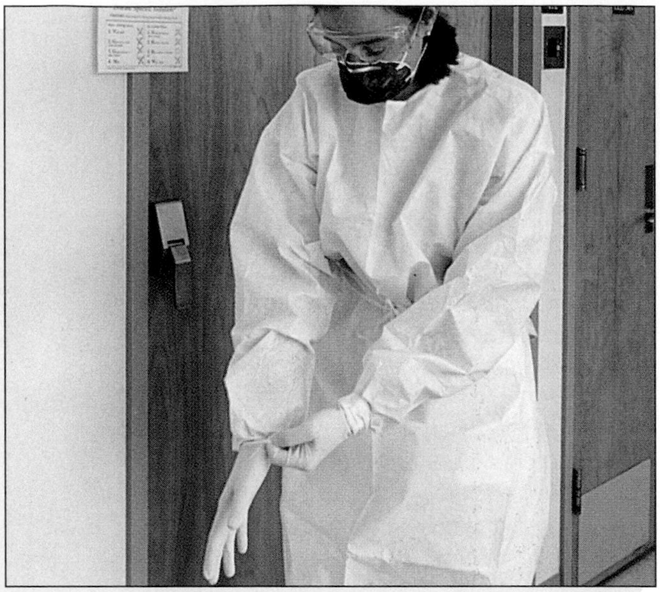

Cover wristlets completely to prevent contamination of exposed skin.

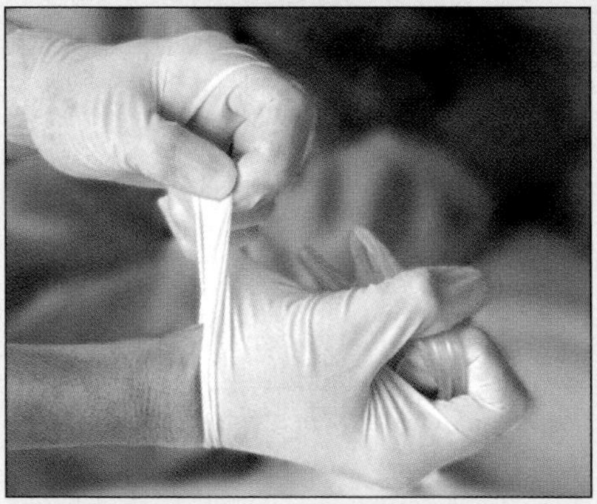

Remove gloves before gown, mask, or eye shield.

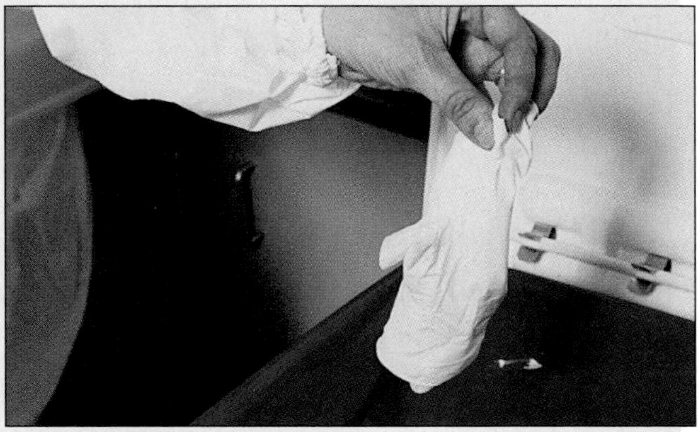

Dispose of gloves in appropriate receptacle.

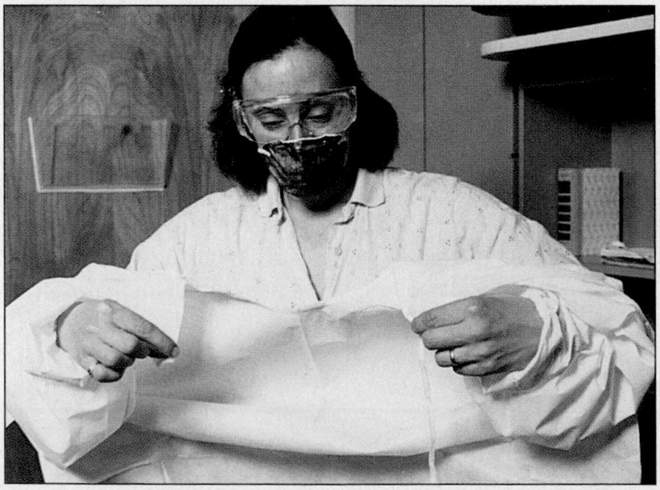

Pull gown off shoulders, then down over arms.

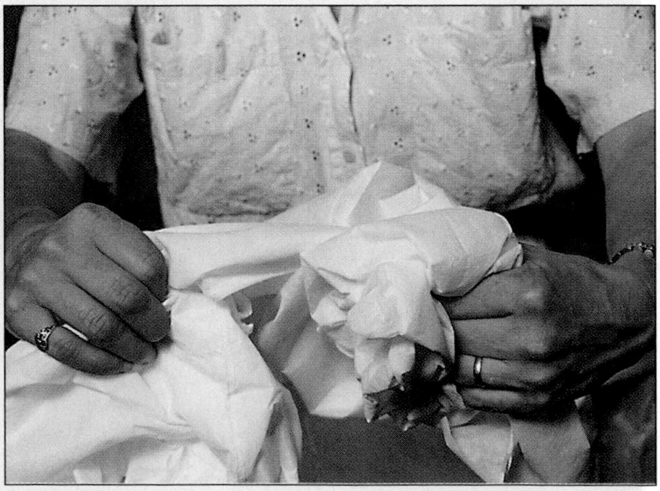

Hold gown away from body when rolling inside out.

8. Don clean gloves and pull gloves over gown wristlets. **Rationale:** Prevents contamination of exposed skin.

for Removing Attire

1. Untie gown waist strings.
2. Remove gloves and dispose of them in garbage bag.
3. Next, untie neck strings, bringing them around your shoulders so that gown is partially off your shoulders.
4. Using your dominant hand and grasping clean part of wristlet, pull sleeve wristlet over your nondominant hand. Use your nondominant hand to pull sleeve wristlet over your dominant hand.
5. Grasp outside of gown through the sleeves at shoulders. Pull gown down over your arms.
6. Hold both gown shoulders in one hand. Carefully draw your other hand out of gown, turning arm of gown inside out. Repeat this procedure with your other arm.
7. Hold gown away from your body. Fold gown up inside out.
8. Discard gown in appropriate place.
9. Remove eye shield and/or mask and place in receptacle.
10. Wash your hands. **Rationale:** This prevents cross-infection to other clients.

CLINICAL ALERT

Some isolation gowns do not tie at the neck, they slip over the head. When removing these gowns, pull shoulders forward to loosen the Velcro at the neck area. Remove gown in the same manner as you would if tied at the neck.

USING A MASK

Equipment

Clean mask

Procedure

1. Obtain mask from box.
2. Position mask to cover your nose and mouth.
3. Bend nose bar so that it conforms over bridge of your nose.
4. If you are using a mask with string ties, tie top strings on top of your head to prevent slipping. If you are using a cone-shaped mask, tie top strings over your ears.
5. Tie bottom strings around your neck to secure mask over your mouth. There should be no gaps between the mask and your face.
6. *Important:* Change mask every 30 minutes or sooner if it becomes damp. **Rationale:** Effectiveness is greatly reduced after 30 minutes or if mask is moist.
7. Wash your hands before removing mask.

CLINICAL ALERT

Respiratory N95 or HEPA (high-efficiency particulate air) masks are recommended for suspected or confirmed multidrug-resistant tuberculosis.

- Masks are fitted to worker.
- Wear mask until it becomes difficult to breathe. This indicates mask is clogged.
- When not in use, store mask in zip-lock bag in safe area.
- Masks are expensive and can be used repeatedly until it is difficult to breathe through them.

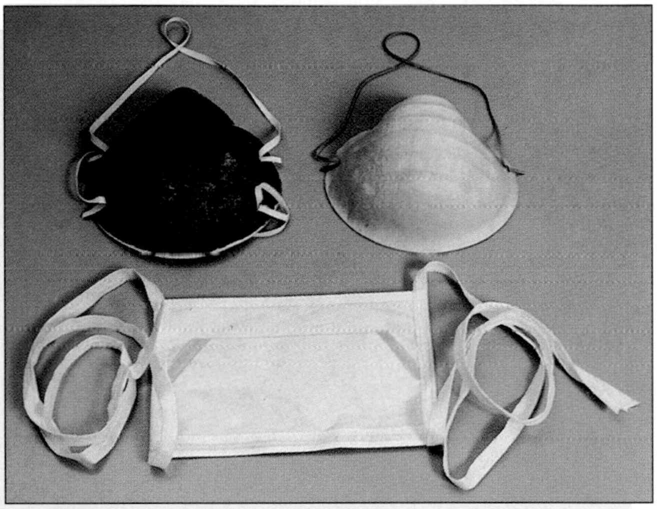

Sample masks used for isolation protocol.

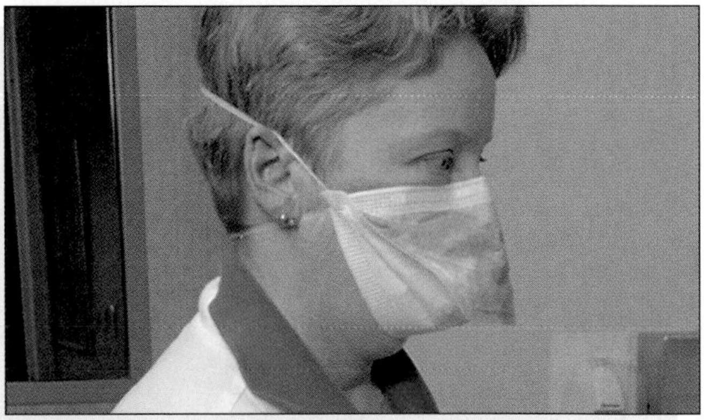

Particulate filter respirator mask must be airtight.

8. To remove mask, untie lower strings first, or slip elastic band off without touching mask. **Rationale:** Only strings are considered clean.
9. Discard mask in a trash container.
10. Wash your hands.

> **CLINICAL ALERT**
> Protective eyewear such as goggles and face shield are worn when there is a risk of splashes or sprays from blood, secretions, excretions, or body fluids. Eyewear is removed before taking off mask.

ASSESSING VITAL SIGNS

Equipment

Thermometer
Stethoscope
Blood pressure cuff and sphygmomanometer
Thermometer stand
Watch with sweep second hand
Isolation clothing

Procedure

1. Wash your hands.
2. Don isolation clothing as required by type of isolation.
3. Proceed to take vital signs as you would for any client.
4. Place equipment in appropriate area if it is to be left in room. Follow appropriate protocol to remove equipment from isolation room.
5. Remove isolation clothing according to protocol.
6. Wash hands.
7. Wipe watch if accidentally contaminated. Use appropriate solution.

REMOVING ITEMS FROM ISOLATION ROOM

Equipment

Large red isolation bags
Specimen container
Plastic bag with biohazard label
Laundry bag
Red plastic container for sharps
Cleaning articles

Procedure

1. Place laboratory specimen in plastic bag. Affix biohazard label to plastic bag.
2. Dispose of all sharps in appropriate red plastic container in room.
3. Place all linen in linen bag.
4. Place reusable equipment such as procedure trays in plastic bags. **Rationale:** Appropriate separation of equipment from isolation room alerts central supply staff that it is contaminated and special handling needs to be carried out.
5. Dispose of all garbage in plastic bags.
6. Double bag all material from isolation room. Follow procedure for *Utilizing Double-Bagging for Isolation.* **Rationale:** All material removed from an isolation room is potentially contaminated. This will prevent spread of microorganisms.
7. Replace all bags, such as linen bag and garbage bag, in appropriate container in room.
8. Clean client's room as necessary, using germicidal solution, according to facility protocol.
9. Prepare to leave the client's room.

UTILIZING DOUBLE-BAGGING FOR ISOLATION

Equipment

2 isolation bags
Items to be removed from room
Gloves

Procedure

1. Follow dress protocol for entering isolation room, or, if you are already in the isolation room, continue with Step 2.
2. Close isolation bag when it is one-half to three-fourths full. Close bag inside the isolation room.

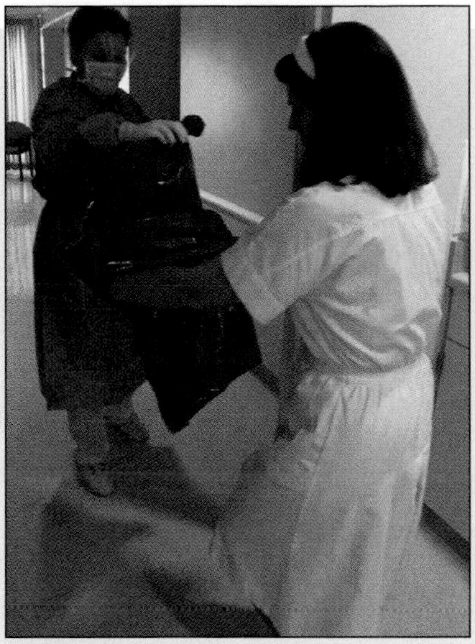

Place bag from inside room into bag held open from outside room.

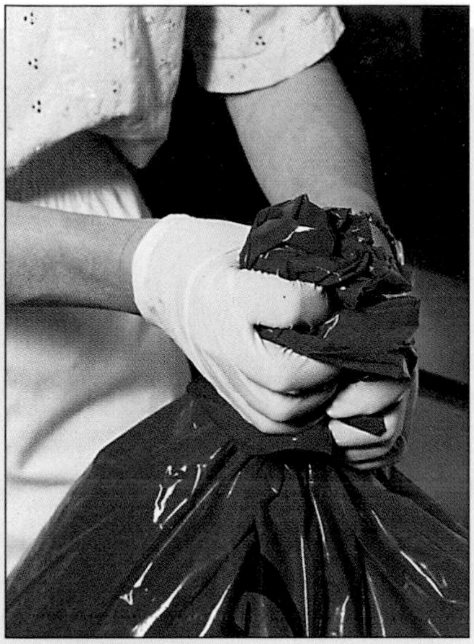

Close bag securely and label contents, if necessary.

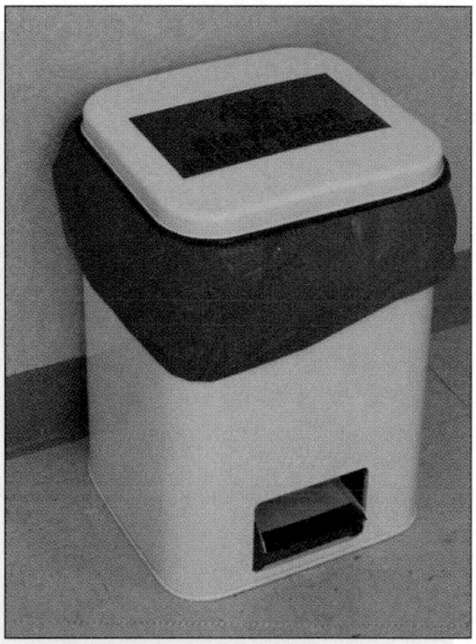

Set up new biohazard bag for continued use in client's room.

CLINICAL ALERT

Linen and burnable trash are disposed of in same manner. Ensure that when placing bags in containers in "dirty" utility room you place in correct container according to bag contents.

3. Double bag for safety if outside of bag is contaminated, if the bag could be easily penetrated, or if contaminated material in the bag is heavy and could break bag.
4. Set up a new bag for continued use inside room. Bag is usually red with the word "Biohazard" written on outside of bag.
5. Place bag from inside room into a bag held open by a second health care worker outside room if double-bagging is required. Second health care worker makes a cuff with the top of the bag and places hands under cuff. **Rationale:** This prevents hands from becoming contaminated.
6. Place bag into second bag without contaminating outside of the bag. Secure top of bag by tying a knot in top of bag.
7. Take bag to designated area where biohazard material is collected, usually "dirty" utility room.
8. Remove gloves and wash hands.

Three Requirements for Double-Bagging

Outside of bag is contaminated.

Bag could easily be penetrated.

Contaminated material is heavy and could break bag.

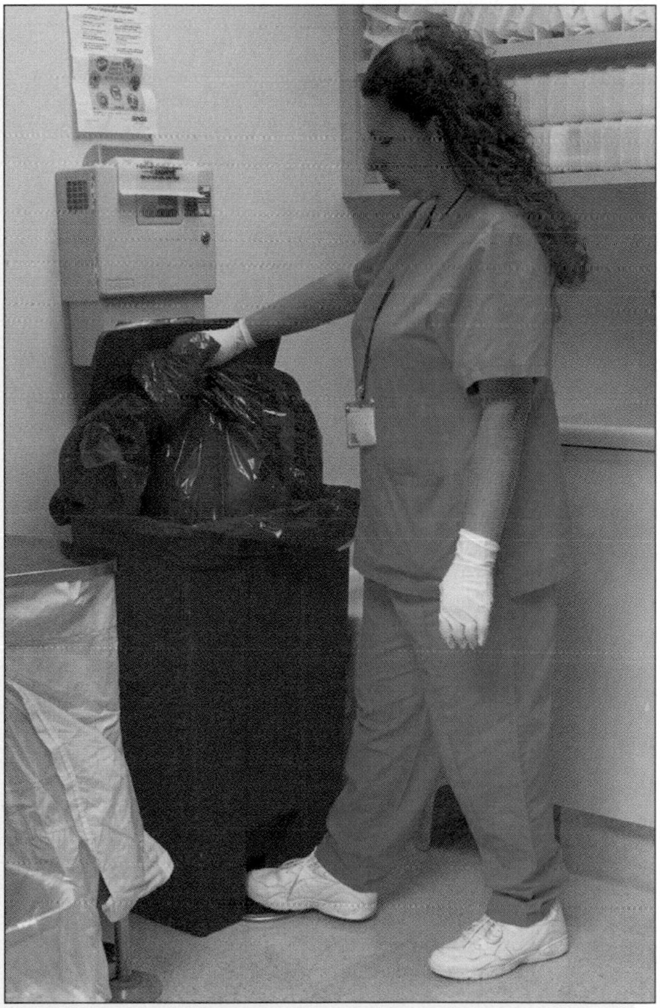

Place red biohazard bag in specified area for disposal.

REMOVING A SPECIMEN FROM ISOLATION ROOM

Equipment

Specimen container
Clean biohazard bag

Procedure

1. Follow dress protocol for entering isolation room, or, if you are already in the isolation room, continue with Step 2.
2. Mark a specimen container with the client's name, type of specimen, and the word "isolation" before entering an isolation room.
3. Collect specimen, and place container in a clean plastic biohazard bag outside the room. **Rationale:** Use clear bags so that laboratory personnel can see the specimen easily.
4. Wash your hands.
5. Send specimen to laboratory with appropriate laboratory request form.

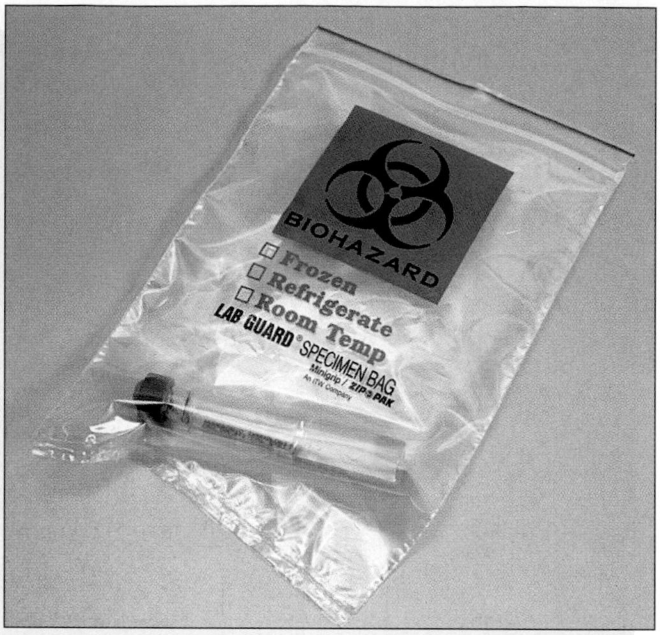

Biohazard bag for transportation of specimens from isolation room.

TRANSPORTING ISOLATION CLIENT OUTSIDE THE ROOM

Equipment

Transport vehicle
Bath blanket
Mask for client if needed

Procedure

1. Explain procedure to client.
2. If client is being transported from a respiratory isolation room, instruct him or her to wear a mask for the entire time out of isolation. **Rationale:** This prevents the spread of airborne microbes.
3. Cover the transport vehicle with a bath blanket if there is a chance of soiling when transporting a client who has a draining wound or diarrhea.
4. Help client into transport vehicle. Cover client with a bath blanket.
5. Tell receiving department what type of isolation client needs and what precautions hospital personnel should follow.
6. Remove bath blanket, and handle as contaminated linen when client returns to room.
7. Instruct all hospital personnel to wash their hands before they leave the area.
8. Wipe down transportation vehicle with an antimicrobial solution if soiled.

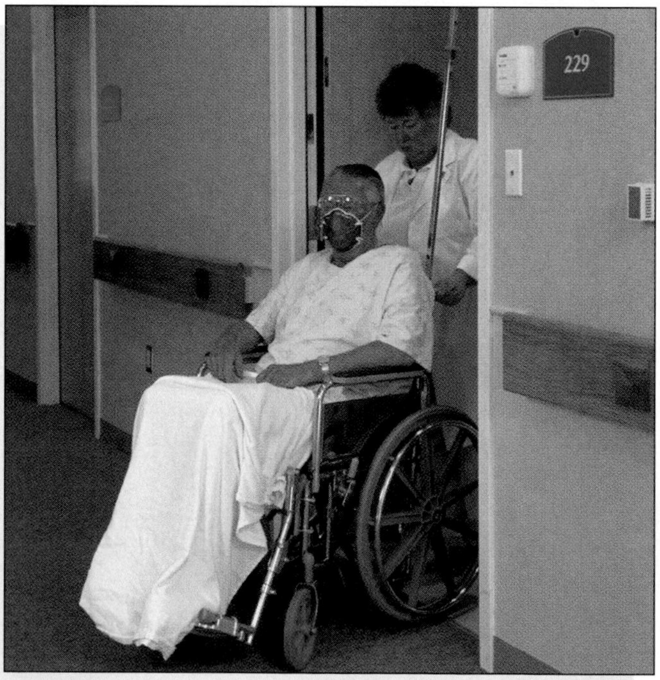

Place surgical mask on client if he needs to be transported outside room.

REMOVING SOILED LARGE EQUIPMENT FROM ISOLATION ROOM

Equipment

Antimicrobial agent and articles needed to wash equipment
Plastic bag

Procedure

1. Don isolation garb as recommended.
2. Wash equipment with an antimicrobial agent. **Rationale:** Washing is preferred to spraying in order to ensure all surfaces are cleaned.
3. Cover equipment with a plastic bag.
4. Remove garb, and wash your hands outside the room. Take equipment to the decontamination area of CSR.

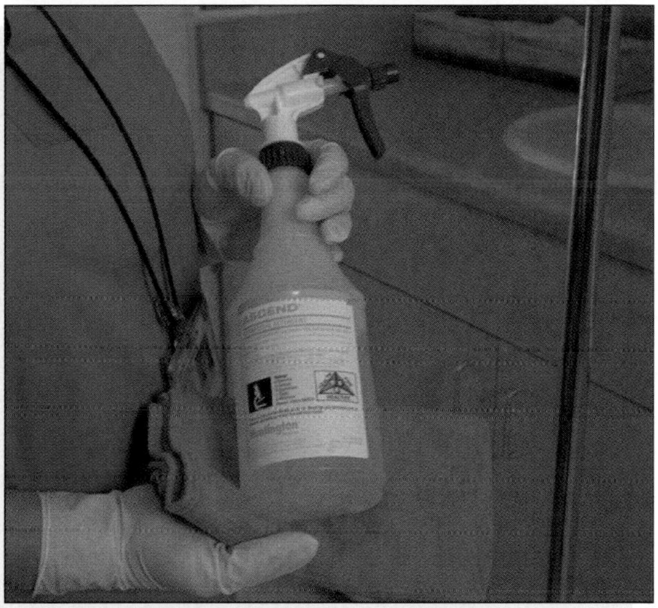

Wash isolation equipment with antimicrobial agent.

Protocol for Leaving Isolation Room

Untie gown at waist.

Take off gloves.

Untie gown at neck.

Pull gown off and place in laundry hamper.

Take off goggles or face shield.

Take off mask.

Wash hands.

Guidelines for Disposing of Contaminated Equipment

- **Disposable glass:** Place in isolation bag separate from burnable trash and direct to appropriate hospital area for disposal.
- **Glass equipment:** Bag separately from metal equipment and return to CSR.
- **Metal equipment:** Bag all equipment together, label, and return to CSR.
- **Rubber and plastic items:** Bag items separately and return to CSR for gas sterilization.
- **Dishes:** Require no special precautions unless contaminated with infected material; then bag, label, and return to kitchen.
- **Plastic or paper dishes:** Dispose of these items in burnable trash.
- **Soiled linens:** Place in laundry bag, and send to separate area of laundry room for special care. If possible, place linens in hot-water–soluble bag. This method is safer for handling, as bag may be placed directly into washing machine. (Double-bagging is usually required because these bags are easily punctured or torn. They also dissolve when wet.)
- **Food and liquids:** Dispose of these items by putting them in the toilet—flush thoroughly.
- **Needles and syringes:** Do not recap needles; place in puncture-resistant container.
- **Sphygmomanometer and stethoscope:** Require no special precautions unless they are contaminated. If contaminated, disinfect using the appropriate cleaning protocol based on the infective agent.
- **Thermometers:** Dispose of electronic probe cover with burnable trash. If probe or machine is contaminated, clean with appropriate disinfectant for infective agent. If reusable thermometers are used, disinfect with appropriate solution.

Documentation for Isolation

- Type of isolation protocol being practiced
- Client's reactions to sensory deprivation
- Specimens sent to laboratory
- Vital signs if appropriate

Critical Thinking Application

UNEXPECTED OUTCOMES	CRITICAL THINKING OPTIONS
Outbreak of disease occurs in isolation environment.	• Identify cause of outbreak, and contact the infection control practitioner for consultation. • Examine handwashing and infection control practices among staff. • Attend in-service education program on isolation techniques to increase your awareness of appropriate procedures.

Gerontologic Considerations

- Social isolation resulting from infection control requirements is more intense with the elderly. They need frequent contact with health care workers. Sometimes being ill is the only attention they receive.
- Elderly clients can become confused in the hospital and when placed in isolation, there is an even greater risk. Frequent monitoring for safety issues is necessary.
- Frequent explanations of why isolation is necessary is important for the elderly. They may have a lapse of memory and forget earlier discussion about isolation.
- Ensure that call lights are easily accessible and the client understands how to call for assistance. They may have impaired hearing and sight, which can interfere with communications.

MANAGEMENT GUIDELINES

Each state legislates a Nurse Practice Act for RNs and LVN/LPNs. Health care facilities are responsible for establishing and implementing policies and procedures that conform to their state's regulations. Verify the regulations and role parameters for each health care worker in your facility.

Delegation of Responsibilities

- LVN/LPNs and CNAs may be assigned to clients requiring infection control precautions and barriers. Ensure that all health care workers have been properly educated in infection control procedures before assigning them to clients requiring these measures.
- It is the RN's responsibility to make assignments that take into account the type of isolation precautions and potential cross-contamination of other clients in the care of the health care worker. For example, the same health care worker should not take care of a client in contact isolation and an immunosuppressed client.

Information Flow

- Ensure that appropriate designations are posted on the door of the room indicating the type of isolation precautions necessary for the client.
- Indicate the type of isolation precautions on the Kardex card.
- During shift report and team report, review the type of isolation precautions being maintained for the client.
- Inform and instruct all visitors on the isolation precautions.
- Monitor that all hospital staff practice good handwashing technique. Review appropriate technique with those who do not practice these techniques.
- Review isolation precautions, particularly standard precautions, with all new personnel and on a regular basis with all personnel to ensure compliance with hospital policy.
- Monitor health care workers for appropriate use of gloves, masks, and gowns when caring for clients in isolation. Instruct health care workers in proper use of these items when providing client care.

CRITICAL THINKING STRATEGIES

SCENARIO 1

You are assigned to care for two clients. One client has just returned from surgery for an abdominal resection. The second client is hospitalized with an acute case of tuberculosis.

1. Is this assignment appropriate, considering the two diagnoses? Provide a rationale for the answer.
2. What special precautions will you take when providing care for these two clients?
3. CDC guidelines are specific for clients with tuberculosis. Identify the differences in providing care for this client versus other clients requiring barrier nursing.
4. Describe the procedure for leaving the tuberculosis client's room. Provide a rationale for the prioritized steps.

SCENARIO 2

You are assigned to take two clients' vital signs, complete a focus assessment, provide hygienic care, monitor IVs, and complete a dressing change for a client with an abdominal resection.

1. What task will have priority with this assignment?
2. Develop a time management plan and provide a rationale for the time frames and activities.

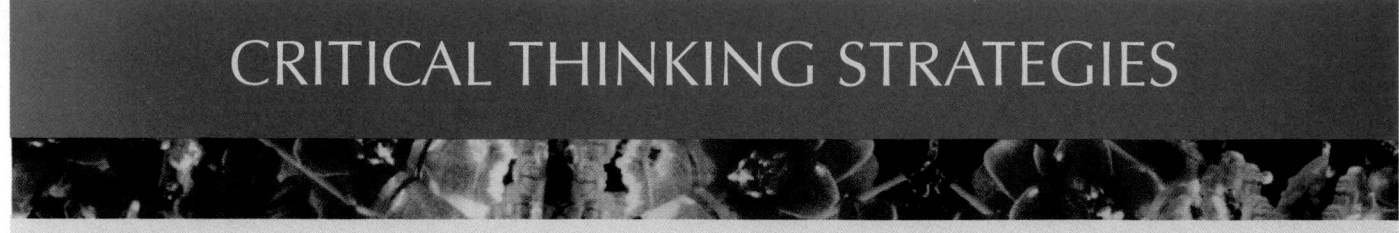

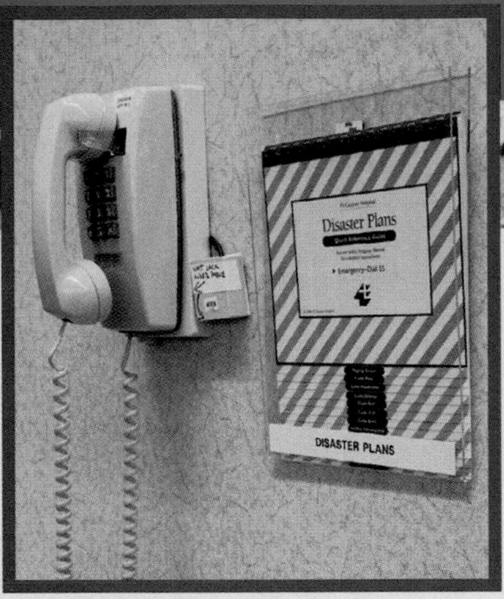

CHAPTER 15

Bioterrorism–Disaster Nursing

THEORETICAL CONCEPTS

UNIT ONE: Bioterrorism Agents, Antidotes, and Vaccinations 427

Identifying Agents of Biological Terrorism 428
Prioritizing High-Risk Groups for Smallpox Vaccination 433
Reconstituting *Vaccinia* Vaccine for Smallpox 434
Administering Reconstituted Smallpox Vaccine 434
Understanding Post-Vaccination Reactions 436
Instructing Client in Post-Vaccination Evaluation 437
Identifying Indications for *Vaccinia* Immune Globulin (VIG) Administration 438
Collecting and Transporting Specimens 438
Identifying Chemical Agent Exposure 439
Triaging for Chemical Agent Exposure 440
Managing Care After Chemical Agent Exposure 441
Identifying Acute Radiation Syndrome 441

UNIT TWO: Personal Protective Equipment and Decontamination 444

Implementing Hospital Infection Control Protocol 445
Decontaminating via Triage 447
Choosing Protective Equipment for Biological Exposure 448
Choosing Protective Equipment for Chemical Exposure 450
Choosing Protective Equipment for Radiological Attack 450
Decontaminating Victims Following a Biological Terrorist Event 451
Decontaminating Victims Following a Chemical Terrorist Event 451
Decontaminating Victims Following Radiation Exposure 452
Controlling Radiation Contamination 453

UNIT THREE: Triage and a Communication Matrix 455

Establishing Triage Treatment Areas 456
Establishing Public Health Parameters 456
Developing a Communication Network 457
Establishing Viable Communication 458
Treating Life-Threatening Conditions 458
Assessing Victims Post-Triage 459
Caring for Those Who Died 460
Caring for Clients with Psychological Reactions 461
Identifying Post-Traumatic Stress Disorder 461

GERONTOLOGIC CONSIDERATIONS 463

MANAGEMENT GUIDELINES 463

CRITICAL THINKING STRATEGIES 464

LEARNING OBJECTIVES

- Discuss the concept of preparedness for a terrorism attack.
- List the effects on infrastructure that may result from a mass casualty incident.
- Describe the communication network necessary to ensure delivery and transmission of accurate information during or following a disaster.
- Compare and contrast external and internal communication systems.
- State the chain of command and reporting requirements when a mass casualty incident occurs.
- Explain the term *triage* and outline at least one strategy for implementing triage.
- Differentiate between a chemical and a biological attack.
- Participate in bioterrorism-related education and training for health care professionals.
- Discuss diversity considerations when health care workers are responding to a terrorist event.
- List at least two ethical issues you might encounter during a mass casualty event.
- Define the terms *disaster, terrorism, weapons of mass destruction*, and *mass casualty incident.*
- List signs and symptoms of various biological agents and describe how to distinguish between them.
- Discuss the clinical features of smallpox.
- Identify the high-risk groups for smallpox vaccination.
- Demonstrate the procedure for smallpox vaccination (include reconstituting *vaccinia* vaccine).
- State the primary reaction stages of smallpox vaccination.
- Describe the steps of collecting and transporting a potentially contaminated clinical specimen.
- Describe the major agents of a chemical attack.
- Outline the ways that chemical agents can be disseminated (including pulmonary, cyanide, vesicant, and nerve agents).
- List the primary interventions necessary to care for clients following chemical exposure.
- Describe how to measure external radiation levels.
- Define *acute radiation syndrome.*
- Review the equipment included in Standard Precautions.
- List the steps of decontamination via triage.
- Explain the protective equipment necessary for biological exposure (individualize for anthrax, plague, botulism, and smallpox).
- Differentiate decontaminating victims following a biological and chemical attack.
- List the equipment necessary for decontamination following radiation exposure.
- Demonstrate decontamination procedures for victims of a radiological attack.
- Discuss establishing public health parameters for triage.
- List the steps of triage.
- Explain collaborative communication.
- Demonstrate the steps of treating life-threatening conditions.
- Describe psychological reactions to a bioterrorism attack.
- Discuss post-traumatic stress disorder.

TERMINOLOGY

Aerosol: very fine liquid or solid particles suspended in air—small particles in a gaseous medium.

Airborne: microorganisms spread by droplets dispersed in the air; a deliberate release of pathogens; could be carried out by using an aerosol delivery system.

Antimicrobial: an agent that prevents the development or pathogenic action of microbes.

Antidote: a substance that neutralizes a poison or the effects of a poison.

Bioterrorism: the planned, deliberate use of a chemical or biological agent (bacteria, virus, fungi, or toxin) with the intent to harm or kill people. Bioterrorism is a general term used to encompass all forms of terrorism.

Centers for Disease Control and Prevention (CDC): a U.S. government agency with the stated purpose of preventing the transmission of communicable diseases. This agency is responsible for identifying and disseminating standards and guidelines for isolation precautions.

Chemical terrorism: use of a chemical agent (nerve, blood, blister, volatile) with intent to harm or kill people.

Communicable disease: a disease that can be transmitted person-to-person.

Community disaster plan: a document that specifies who is in charge, lines of communication, and agencies and resources that will be involved.

Contamination: introduction of disease, germs, or infectious materials into or onto normally sterile objects.

Decontamination: process of removing contamination from people, equipment, or environment—usually done through a physical (i.e., shower) or chemical process.

Disaster: an event of such magnitude that essential services are disrupted and current resources are overwhelmed.

Emergency: any event or situation that occurs as an unexpected and sudden incident, demanding immediate action.

Equivalent dose: a measure of the effect that radiation has on humans—takes into account the type and absorbed dose of radiation.

Exposure: inhalation or contamination by a substance that contains a biological, chemical, or radioactive agent.

Federal Bureau of Investigative (FBI): investigate agency of United States Department of Justice; it has authority and responsibility to investigate specific crimes, such as a bioterrorism event.

Federal Emergency Management Agency (FEMA): primary or lead federal agency that responds to a disaster, such as a terrorism incident.

First responder: first trained personnel to arrive at an emergency.

Hazardous material: any substance that is potentially toxic to a biological system.

HAZMAT model: hazardous materials; this model is used for situations involving certain toxic or chemical exposures.

Homeland Security: the Dept. of Homeland Security (DHS) coordinates all activities related to a terrorist attack.

Immunization: process of rendering a person immune, usually done through vaccination.

Incident Command System (ICS): local and national command structure that organizes emergency responses.

Incubation period: time between infection from a microorganism and onset of symptoms.

Infection: establishment of a disease process that involves invasion of body tissue by microorganisms, reaction of tissues to their presence, and to toxins generated by them.

Inhalation: exposure to a substance through the respiratory tract.

Isolation: practices or actions designed to prevent transmission of communicable diseases.

Ionizing radiation: radiation that has the energy to cause atoms to lose electrons and become ions—alpha, beta, gamma, and x-rays are examples.

Isotopes: elements that have neutrons (they have neither a positive nor negative charge). Not all isotopes are radioactive; those that are, are called radionuclides. Cobalt-69 is an example of a radioactive isotope.

Mass casualty incident (MCI): an incident or emergency event associated with many casualties (airplane crash, terrorism, chemical spill) that has a negative impact on emergency resources.

Microorganism: a minute living body, such as a bacterium, protozoan, or virus, not perceptible to the naked eye.

NBC: military acronym for nuclear, biological, and chemical weapons.

Nerve agent: chemical agent that acts on the body by disrupting normal function of the nervous system.

Occupational Safety and Health Administration (OSHA): section of the Department of Labor that develops and implements regulations requiring employers to have safety policies and to provide training and personal protective equipment to employees who may be exposed to toxic substances.

Outbreak: critical incident in which infections occur above an established level and are caused by the same infective agent.

Pandemic: denotes a disease that affects the population of a large region, country, or continent.

Pathogen: microorganism that can cause disease; may be bacteria, fungi, parasites, or viruses.

Percutaneous agent: substance that can be absorbed through the skin.

Personal protective equipment (PPE): equipment for protection of emergency personnel; includes gloves, masks, gowns, eye shields, biohazard bags, and in some cases, head and shoe covers.

Poison: any substance that enters the body by absorption, ingestion, inhalation or infection, and interferes with normal physiological functions.

RAD: radiation absorbed dose—the unit of measure for radiation exposure.

Radiation: energy in the form of waves or particles that is emitted from radioactive material or equipment.

Radioactive contamination: radioactive material distributed over some area, equipment, or person; must be decontaminated.

Radiation dose: quantity of radiation energy deposited in a material by the radiation to which victim is exposed.

REM: roentgen equivalent man—the unit of dose or measure—takes into account type of radiation producing the exposure.

Sodium hypochlorite: 0.5% diluted bleach is the active ingredient used for decontamination.

START: acronym that stands for "simple treatment and rapid triage" an initial triage system used for triaging large numbers of victims.

Standard (Universal) Precautions: a system of disease control; assumes that direct contact with body fluids is infectious and recommends a series of procedures to protect the staff.

Threat assessment: an assessment of a community's vulnerability and risk potential.

Toxin: poisonous substance produced by a living organism.

Trauma: multisystem condition or injury that is potentially life threatening to the individual.

Vaccine: preparation of a killed or weakened microorganism used to induce immunity against disease.

Vesicles: blisters on the skin.

Virulence: the power of a microorganism to cause disease in a given host.

Virus: an infectious microorganism that normally lives within other living cells and cannot reproduce outside the cell.

Weapons of mass destruction (WMD): nuclear, biological, chemical, incendiary, or conventional explosive agents that pose a threat to health, safety, food supply, property, or the environment.

INTRODUCTION

America's world changed on September 11, 2001. From this time, our greatest challenge became to adopt the awareness that we are no longer invulnerable; that biological, chemical, and nuclear terrorism is a future reality; and that we must change our perspective of how to function in the world. Senator Bill Frist stated it clearly, "The United States faces a grave and growing threat from bioterrorism."

Four years ago, this chapter would never have been written. Today, a page in history has been turned, and the medical community—indeed the world—must face terrorism and the probability of disasters caused by terrorism. We cannot predict—we can prepare. In order to steer a course toward a viable future, we must be prepared to cope with such a disaster.

Preparedness for a terrorist-caused disaster is critical for containment and protection of the population. There must be coordinated emergency preparedness plans in place in order that a prompt and effective response to a biological, chemical, or radiation attack is initiated. Nurses are an important part of this response.

The Centers for Disease Control and Prevention (CDC) has developed a strategic plan based on five focus areas, the first of which is preparedness.

- Preparedness and prevention
- Detection and surveillance
- Diagnosis and characterization of biological and chemical agents
- Response
- Communication

Meeting this new challenge will require preparedness in all communities, cities, and states in the United States of America.

Disaster Defined

Disaster is defined as an event of such magnitude that essential services are disrupted and current resources are overwhelmed. Disasters may be natural (caused by an earthquake, hurricane, tornado, blizzard, flood, etc.) or caused by human actions such as civil disturbance, a hazardous material incident, or act of terrorism.

Whatever the cause, disasters have several characteristics in common: They are unexpected and there has been little or no warning; lives, public health, and the environment are endangered; emergency services and personnel must be called to action if not available during the initial stages of the disaster. The terrorist attack that occurred in Washington, D.C., and New York on September 11, 2001, was just such an event. It was an event that carried an unforeseen and immediate threat to public health and required the intervention of others to provide outside resources.

PUBLIC POLICY

Mass Casualty Characteristics

- Mass casualty incidents are community-wide incidents—not confined to individual hospitals.
- Event occurs in local community.
- Local government provides "first responders."
- State and federal government will be involved if incident is large enough.
- Hospitals are last link in community response to mass casualty incident.
- Hospitals will receive most seriously injured and ill casualties.

Hospitals are the most comprehensive community health resource. As the last link in the community chain of readiness, the hospital is the organization that will have to, by default, make up for the inadequacies in community preparedness.

Hospitals must follow federal legislation known as EMTALA (the Emergency Medical Treatment and Labor Act), which governs what a hospital must do when clients present themselves. If the emergency department is closed because of client overload or to protect the health of current clients, by federal law the hospital is not allowed to turn away clients. EMTALA ensures that all individuals who appear at an emergency department must be screened, evaluated, and stabilized before being transferred. Triage is not equivalent to medical screening, so a hospital could easily be overwhelmed in a disaster, even when victims are processed in the field via triage.

Also, this legislation is still in place even if the community designates some hospitals to receive victims of a disaster and others to remain open to clients not exposed to the contaminant. Authorities are suggesting that an open dialogue with the federal government (officials of the Department of Health and Human Services [HHS]) to revise provisions of EMTALA is necessary, now that the potential for mass casualty disaster is present.

Bioterrorism Response Act

The Public Health Security and Bioterrorism Response Act of 2002, signed into law in June 2002, authorized $4.3 billion to combat terrorism. The federal government has focused on three components: detection, treatment, and containment.

One aspect of the law will be to allocate funds for the training of health care workers, including nurses. The ANA, together with HHS, has established the National Nurses Response Team (NNRT). This team, made up of a large number of nurses, is poised to respond to any major disaster, such as an anthrax or smallpox attack.

These nurses, as well as other health care professionals, will be "federalized," thus receiving umbrella coverage for licensure, liability, and expenses. Deployments will be limited to 2 weeks. In the law-signing ceremony, President Bush pointed out that biological attacks could occur covertly, and health care professionals may well be the first to recognize such an attack. He went on to say, "The speed with which they detect and respond to a threat to public health will make the difference between containment and catastrophe."

Disaster Impact on the Infrastructure

When a disaster occurs, the impact on the infrastructure may be severe. Services and delivery systems, transportation, utilities, fuel, food, water supplies, and communication systems may be affected. Disaster experts point out that when one of the support systems breaks down, it has a domino effect and all elements of the infrastructure could be affected. According to Community Emergency Response Team (CERT)* information, some of the ways in which the infrastructure can be affected following a disaster are shown below.

Service	Effect
Transportation	Inability to get emergency service personnel into the affected area.
	Inability to transport victims away from the area.
Electrical	Increased risk of fire and electrical shock.
	Possible disruption to transportation system if downed lines are across roads.
Telephone	Lost contact between victims, service providers, and family members.
	System overload due to calls from/to friends or relatives.
Water	Disruption of service to homes, businesses, and medical providers.
	Inadequate water supply for firefighting.
	Increased risk to public health if there is extensive damage to the water supply or if it becomes contaminated.
Fuel Supplies	Increased risk of fire or explosion from ruptured fuel lines.
	Risk of asphyxiation from natural gas leaks in confined areas.

*The Community Emergency Response Team (CERT) concept was originally developed and implemented by the City of Los Angeles Fire Department following the 1987 Whittier Narrows earthquake. They realized that citizens would likely be on their own at least during the early stages of a catastrophic disaster, and thus, there was a need for a Disaster Preparedness program. So far, thousands of people and hundreds of teams have been trained.

Disaster Mitigation

When examining how to mitigate the effects of a disaster, safety precautions and preparation must be considered first, that is, personal safety, home preparation, and community preparation. Individual safety and home preparation need to be dealt with on a personal level. Focusing on both natural disasters, such as earthquakes and floods, and man-made disasters, each family or community should develop a Preparedness Plan. In addition, each health care facility must have their own Preparedness Plan, developed enough to implement under the chaotic circumstances of a disaster.

The purpose of this chapter is to focus on man-made disasters, such as a terrorism event, and how the medical community, specifically nurses, could develop their own Preparedness Plan to cope with a mass casualty disaster.

Community Response Plan

Apart from personal safety and home preparation prior to a disaster, a planned community response is a critical element. A CERT that is trained and prepared to intervene will do more to mitigate disaster outcomes than any other planned approach. A CERT organizational structure would look like this:

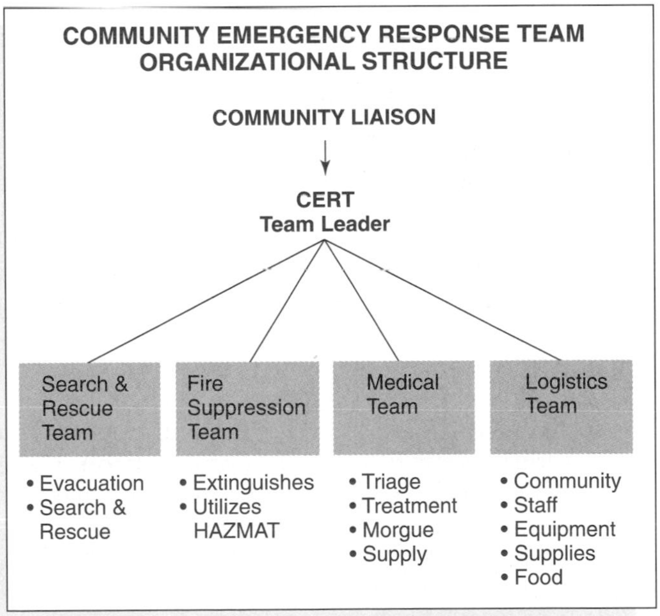

Strategic Plan for Responding to Biological or Chemical Terrorism

The CDC has formulated a Strategic Planning Workgroup to combat the deliberate dissemination of biological or chemical agents. The plan encompasses detection and surveillance, laboratory analysis, emergency response, and communication systems. Success of the plan hinges

Bioterrorism Emergency Questionnaire

A 42-item questionnaire was developed for health care facilities to assess their preparedness and capacity to respond to and treat victims of a biological incident. This document should be completed and the results evaluated by any facility that has not developed a plan for preparedness.

Source: Bioterrorism Questionnaire: Bioterrorism Emergency Planning and Preparedness Questionnaire for Healthcare Facilities. http:www.ahrq.gov/news/press/pr2002/ (may be reproduced without permission) bioterrpr.htm (PDF file 135KB; text version).

on the relationship between medical and public health professionals working together for emergency management.

Five Focus Areas in the CDC's Strategic Plan

- *Preparedness and Prevention:* Emergency coordinated preparedness teams are to be developed in all cities and states in order to respond effectively. The CDC will assist in developing tools and strategies to prevent and mitigate illness and injury.
- *Detection and Surveillance:* Early detection is critical for prompt responding. The CDC will develop disease surveillance systems, as well as mechanisms for detecting, evaluating, and reporting suspicious events. This will be done in partnership with front-line medical–hospital emergency professionals. Reporting of unexplained injuries and illnesses will be part of routine surveillance systems.
- *Diagnosis and Characterization of Biological–Chemical Agents:* The CDC and its partners will create a multilevel laboratory response network to analyze biological agents. Diagnostic technology will be disseminated to state laboratories for diagnostic confirmation and reference support for terrorism response teams.
- *Response:* The CDC will develop a comprehensive public health response to a terrorist event that will encompass investigation, medical treatment, prophylaxis for infected persons and disease prevention and decontamination measures.
- *Communication Systems:* The ability of the United States to be prepared and intervene effectively when a terrorist event has been identified is dependent on well-trained health care and public health professionals having access to emergency information via state-of-the-art communication systems. Effective communication with the public is also essential. Through this sophisticated communication network, the CDC will disperse information regarding disease outbreaks, dissemination of diagnostic results, and emergency health information.

JCAHO Standards

The Joint Commission on Accreditation of Healthcare Organizations (JCAHO) has focused on security management and has developed a plan that describes how the organization will establish and maintain a security program to protect those involved. The plan provides for designation of personnel who will report and investigate security incidents, provide identification for participants, and control access and egress to sensitive areas. In addition, JCAHO will provide an education program and performance standards for a mass casualty event.

A COMMUNICATION NETWORK FOR DISASTER MANAGEMENT

Everyday communication systems are likely to be overwhelmed in a disaster. Preparing for this eventuality by establishing backup and redundant communication systems is essential.

First responders will be local. They will work in conjunction with the state and federal organizations, and therefore, there must be an integrated system of in-hospital and out-of-hospital team members with state and federal agencies.

Local systems, both in and out of the hospital, will comprise the critical human infrastructure for responding to weapons of mass destruction (WMD) incidents. Communication coordination will be an essential component in this infrastructure system. One measure is to include a 24-hour wireless radio dedicated communication system to communicate with other health care facilities if telephone lines and the Internet do not function.

Communication among the triage team (out-of-hospital) establishing victim care priorities, the hospital or treatment staff (in-hospital), and state and federal agencies' forensic investigation needs must also be established as a cooperative effort. Training through drills and scenarios would provide practice so that these vital communication functions would be implemented instantly if there were to be a WMD incident.

Following from the local communication structure, where there should be one single community-identified person or small group in command acting as liaison agent, the state and federal response teams will be integrated into the communication system. An example of a local system used nationally might be the Incident Command System (ICS), commonly used among EMS personnel. It is a logical management command and control structure that should be part of hospital planning. Specific roles and positions carry specific duties and responsibilities. Each position has a prioritized list of tasks that are checked off as they are completed. When an emergency occurs, the "incident commanders" take command. They can, in turn, appoint liaison or safety officers or any other position to communicate back to any local or regional ICS, according to the needs created by the emergency. This system organizes emergency responses in five categories: command, planning, operations, logistics, and administration.

Internal (or In-Hospital) Communication

Hospitals will have to expand their sphere of influence to include community-level teams. They must have an ongoing, open channel of communication with emergency response teams, who will have been notified first of a mass casualty incident. A community-wide network, all using the same channel of communication, is necessary.

Family and friends, calling to learn about their loved ones following the arrival of casualties, will rapidly overload the system and isolate the hospital. To cope with this eventuality, a single communication site for obtaining victim and locator information should be established. The Red Cross or comparable organization could serve as this third-party, off-site source of information.

A clear and open information system, using both telecommunications and a position-to-position cascade in the event of the primary system being overloaded, is nec-

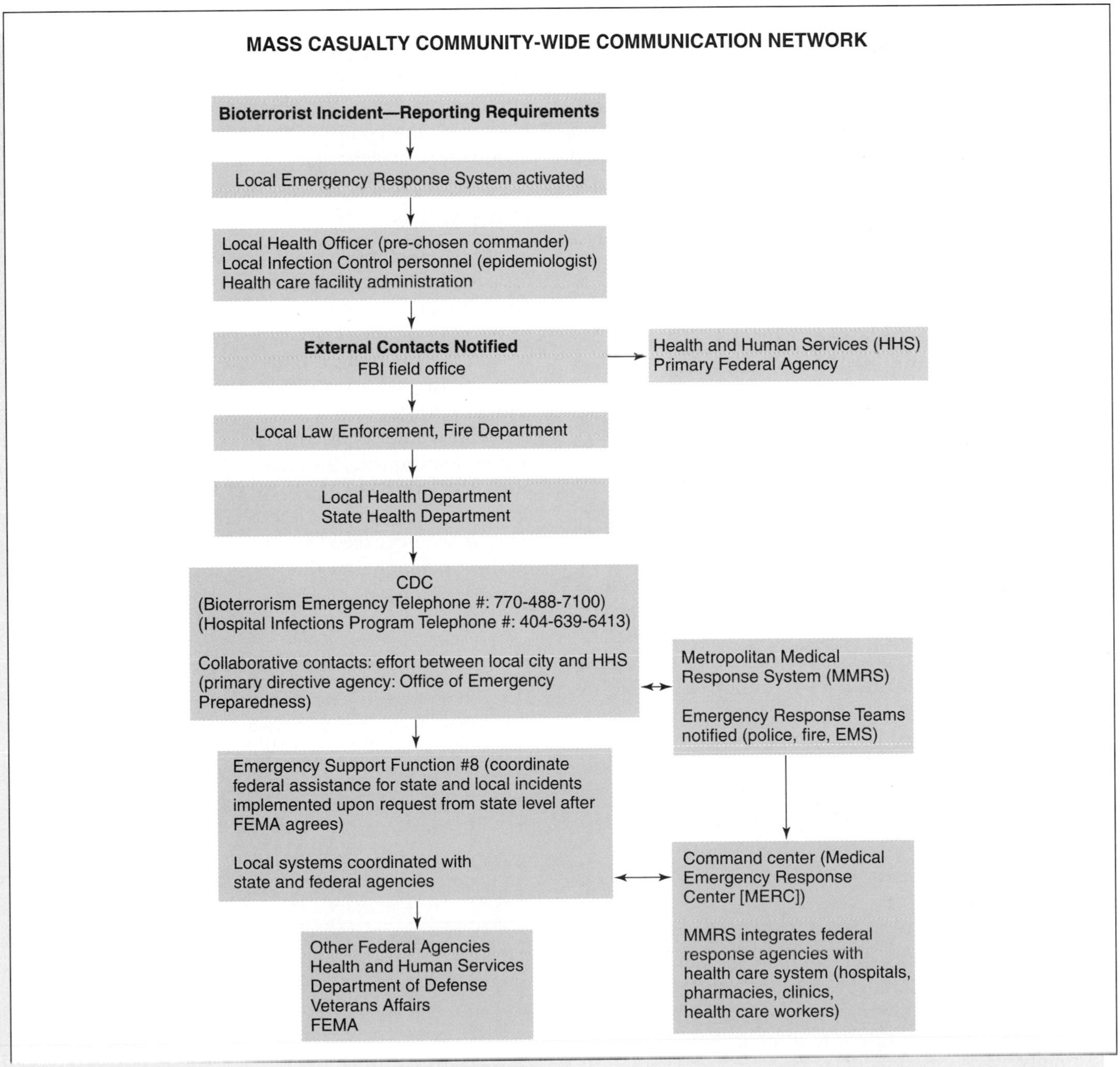

essary. This cascade should be designated by position (e.g., emergency room supervisor), not person, due to turnover, multiple shifts, and personnel reassignment during a disaster. One hospital instituted a text message alert system by pager that could be sent to many personnel at one time. In addition to a communication system being established, adequate equipment, such as cell phones, walkie-talkies, even runners, must be available because current phone land lines may be totally overwhelmed.

TRIAGE

Triage is from a French word (*trier*) meaning to sort. It is a medical process of prioritizing treatment urgency. One example of a triage system is START, an acronym for "simple triage and rapid treatment." This is a standardized system that provides a framework for triage decisions, especially useful for triaging large numbers of victims at an emergency incident. START was developed in the 1980s in California as a way of preparing for a disaster.

Emergency department personnel use the triage system to quickly assess large numbers of people with multiple problems. Rapid identification in the hospital is important to determine which clients require immediate treatment and which can safely wait.

There are varying methods of categorizing triage. One option is as follows:

1. **Emergent** triage refers to a life-threatening or potentially life-threatening condition that requires immediate treatment. These conditions could include multisystem failure, cardiopulmonary arrest, bleeding, airway loss, multiple trauma, severe shock, cervical spine injury, and so on.
2. **Immediate** or Urgent triage is not life-threatening or acute, but refers to clients who need treatment as soon as possible (within 2 hours). These clients have stable vital signs and there is no immediate crisis. This category would include fever, minor burns, lacerations, significant pain, and fractures.
3. The third category is **Nonemergent** or Nonurgent, including clients who have a condition that would not be affected by a delay in treatment. These are clients with chronic or minor injuries, strains, rash, back pain, and so on.

A second way of implementing the strategy of triage is as follows:

1. **Immediate (I)**—the victim has a life-threatening injury (airway, bleeding or shock) that demands immediate attention (the same as Emergent);
2. **Delayed (D)**—an injury that does not jeopardize the victim's life if definitive treatment is delayed; and finally,
3. **Dead (DEAD)**—no respiration after two attempts to open airway. (CPR is not performed in a disaster environment because it demands extensive resources, including personnel time.)

The above strategy will probably be the one used if there is a mass casualty disaster, because **the goal of triage is to do the greatest good for the greatest number**. Triage must occur as quickly as possible after victims are located.

Triage Victim Flow

From triage, victims are taken to a designated medical treatment area (Immediate Care, Delayed Care, or Morgue), and from there, transported out of the disaster area (see flow chart below). There are various methods of implementing triage that include minimal to massive numbers of victims. Whichever triage method or strategy is chosen, the community or identified team must be aware of the specific categories.

Field Triage

Rapid assessment remains essential. During a disaster, instead of a finite number of victims coming to emergency departments that are able to utilize all of the hospital's resources, victims arrive in huge numbers and overwhelm the emergency department; or, there are actually so many injured, triage must occur in the field. Thus, the term *field triage*.

This would be used in case of a major disaster—either natural (earthquake, tornado, hurricane), or one caused by man, including events such as a chemical spill, plane crash, explosion, fire, or a terrorist event. The numbers of injured would exceed the resources of any emergency medical personnel at the scene. Thus, decisions will be

TRIAGE VICTIM FLOW CHART*

Incident Location	Triage	Medical Treatment	Transportation
		Delayed Care Area	Air Transportation
Search and Rescue	Triage Team	Immediate Care Area	Transportation Manager
		Morgue	Ground Transportation

*CERT Training: Participant Handbook.

triage driven, not treatment driven. These victims would be classified according to a color coding tag system.

Colored Tags		*Classification*
Red	=	Emergent
Yellow	=	Immediate
Green	=	Urgent
Blue	=	Psychological Support or First-Aid level
Black	=	Dead or Imminently Terminal

Catastrophic Triage

When events are cascading out of control or disaster has wiped out primary treatment resources, the choice of triage system will be limited. Basically, there are two options. One option is to follow first and second steps and the other is severely limited to those who have the potential to survive—they will be Red Tagged. Thus, triage categories change during a disaster. The primary assessment is one of acuity, but the victim must have the ability to survive. Making these decisions will be terribly difficult, but this system seems to be the only realistic method of categorizing victims of a deadly disaster.

First Step The most direct and expedient method of field triage would be to evaluate victims according to these categories:

I = Immediate
D = Delayed
Dead = Dead

Everyone must be tagged.

Second Step Treat victims immediately.

Check airway and breathing rate	▶	Initiate airway management
Check circulation	▶	Initiate bleeding control
Check mental status	▶	Treat for shock

Document Results

Necessary for effective deployment of resources

Information on location of victims

Quick record of number of casualties by degree of severity

Triage and Decontamination

While triage is an essential component of disaster management, decontamination prioritization is also critical. This is a process to determine the need for and order of victim decontamination. Both processes may be implemented simultaneously. The same triage rule of thumb applies; namely, **providing the greatest benefit for the greatest number**.

If there are mass casualty victims inside a "hot zone," the Incident Commander may assign personnel to manage both medical triage and decontamination. The first step may be to group victims into ambulatory and nonambulatory categories. Prioritization of these victims may be done using the medical triage system, START.

The highest priority for Ambulatory decontamination (classified as *Immediate*) casualties includes:

- Victims closest to the point of release
- Those who report exposure to aerosol
- Victims with evidence of liquid deposits on skin or clothing

Triage Categories

Field Triage

Red	=	Emergent (hyperacute—1st priority)
Yellow	=	Immediate (serious—2nd priority)
Green	=	Urgent (injured—3rd priority)
Blue	=	First aid
Black	=	Dead or dying

Catastrophic Triage (First Option)

I	=	Immediate (life threatening)
D	=	Delayed (may delay treatment without death)
Dead	=	Dead

Catastrophic Triage (Second Option)

Red Tag = Potential to survive
No other victims tagged.

START Categories

Color Tag			**Decontamination Priority**
Red Tag	=	Immediate	1. Serious signs/symptoms Known agent contamination
Yellow Tag	=	Delayed	2. Moderate-to-minimal signs/symptoms Known agent or aerosol contamination Close to point of release
Green Tag	=	Minor	3. Minimal signs/symptoms No known exposure to agent
Black Tag	=	Deceased/ Expectant	4. Very serious signs/ symptoms Grossly contaminated Unresponsive

- Those who are clinically symptomatic (i.e., shortness of breath) but were not as close to point of release
- Victims evidencing conventional injuries, such as open wounds

Nonambulatory casualties includes:

- Victims who are unconscious or unresponsive and will remain in place while further prioritization for decontamination occurs
- Those triaged as *Delayed* (casualties who may have serious injuries, but can wait without compromising the outcome)

Highest priority for overall decontamination includes casualties:

- Who are medically triaged as *Immediate*
- In need of lifesaving medical procedures that can be performed on the spot
- Who have been exposed to nerve agents—decontamination as soon as possible may be lifesaving

Post-Triage Organization

Following evaluation and prioritizing victims into treatment groups and providing immediate lifesaving measures, clients will be transported to three locations: Immediate Treatment, Delayed Treatment, and the Morgue.

Treatment area personnel will then:

1. Perform additional *triage* as needed.
2. Complete *physical assessment* (head-to-toe) to determine extent of injuries.
3. Render *first aid* if needed.

Following this post-triage assessment, personnel will provide immediate treatment for burns, open wounds, fractures, sprains, hypothermia, frostbite, and so on. Following triage and post-triage assessment, it is essential to document the number of victims in each category (Immediate, Delayed), as well as the Dead victims. See Unit 3 for skills in Post-Triage.

The number of victims may exceed local capacity for treatment. Survivors will assist others, but it cannot be assumed they will know how to give lifesaving aid or post-disaster survival techniques. Therefore, outside resources will be requested. For example, the U.S. government has an action plan in place.

This federal response plan includes a stockpile of specialized medical supplies assembled in eight guarded secret warehouses nationwide. More than 100 air-cargo containers (each one fills a Boeing 747) are ready to be sent to any city in the United States within 12 hours. State and local officials will be able to track the cargo sent by ground transport to a final, local destination.

When the CDC, in consult with local officials, agrees that an attack has occurred and the local system is insufficient to cope, a container of supplies will be dispersed, as well as physicians and health personnel, if needed.

WEAPONS OF MASS DESTRUCTION

Biological Agents

Biological terrorism is the use of specific agents to cause harm or kill people, and includes the use of organisms such as bacteria, viruses, and toxins. The use of biological agents as weapons poses a difficult problem for public health officials because these agents present with an insidious onset and mimic natural epidemics of influenza. Symptoms may take days to develop before victims seek medical care.

These agents are classified as a threat to national security because they possess unique characteristics:

- Agents that are easily disseminated or transmitted person to person and could be dispersed over a wide geographical area
- Agents that cause high mortality with the potential for major public health impact
- Agents that require specific actions in order that public health preparedness is secured

Biological weapons have a history that goes back as far as the sixth century. Recent history reveals the fact that many nations have biowarfare capability with agents such as anthrax, plague, and smallpox. In spite of the fact that the Geneva convention prohibited use of biological and chemical warfare, and in 1972 many nations agreed to stop research, the United States remains vulnerable to a biowarfare attack.

A biological agent cannot be detected directly. The way it will be identified is when victims arrive at clinics and hospitals and, either through the awareness and perception of professionals who correlate the unusual influx of victims with similar symptoms, or through a retrospective of "putting the pieces together," the biological cause will be identified.

To accomplish the goal of identifying a biological attack, several steps need to be taken.

1. Set up bioterrorism education programs and training for health care professionals who must be able to recognize signs and symptoms of a biological attack.
2. Prepare and distribute educational materials that will inform and remind health care professionals of the signs and symptoms of various biological weapons.
3. Establish communication systems to ensure that accurate information is delivered.
4. Recognize the signs and symptoms of major high-priority agents. For example,
    - *Variola major* (smallpox)

- *Bacillus anthracus* (anthrax)
- *Trancisella tularensis* (tularemia)
- *Yersinia pestis* (plague)
- *Clostridium botulinum* toxin (botulism)

Chemical Agents

Chemical terrorism is the deployment of chemical weapons with the intention of causing havoc, harm, and death to the recipients. The release of these weapons will quickly cause death, especially if released in an enclosed space. The U.S. Army Medical Research Institute of Chemical Defense has classified these agents as potential weapons. These chemical weapons can be pulmonary agents (phosgene, chlorine), cyanide agents (hydrogen cyanide), vesicant agents (mustard, oxime), nerve agents (tabun, sarin, VX), or incapacitating agents (agent 15, BZ). These weapons will inflict painful external and internal injuries, psychological devastation, and death. An act of chemical terrorism is likely to be overt because the effects of these agents on people are immediate and obvious; the agents are absorbed through the skin, mucous membranes, or pulmonary system.

Perhaps the most dangerous of these agents are nerve gases (sarin, tabun, VX), which are extremely toxic and easy to disseminate in the air. These nerve agents are designed to kill people by binding up a compound known as acetylcholinesterase, which is the body's "off" switch. When acetylcholinesterase is significantly decreased or absent in the body, the glands and voluntary muscles continue to be stimulated, eventually wear out, and the body can no longer sustain healthy function.

Decontamination of some chemical agents is time and labor intensive and requires tremendous resources. However, if chemical agents are widely dispersed, every one of thousands of persons affected cannot be individually decontaminated. Also, decontamination may not be required for certain chemical incidents. The triage team may remove victims to an uncontaminated area and/or send victims home to shower.

Radiation

The threat of terrorists using nuclear or radioactive materials in the United States is considered to be real. While we cannot predict which form this terrorist event might take, we can prepare to cope with the situation should it arise.

Radiation presents unique characteristics, in that exposure may occur without individuals coming in direct contact with the source of radiation. With other bioterrorism agents, the victim must be in contact with the material, either through inhalation, ingestion, or through the skin.

Radioactive substances emit radiation in the form of rays (waves) or extremely small particles. *Waveforms* are x-ray and gamma rays; *particle forms* are alpha, beta, and neutron. Ionizing radiation is radiation that has enough energy to cause atoms to lose electrons and become ions. Charged particles are emitted from ionizing radiation. These particles (alpha and beta) are the most likely to be dispersed following a terrorist attack. They may adhere to airborne dust particles or attach to clothing, and could be inhaled, causing internal contamination. Beta rays are found in "fallout" and alpha particles are emitted from plutonium. Gamma rays, also an example of ionizing radiation, are emitted in a nuclear blast and have high penetration potential, causing severe damage to the individual, but do not require decontamination. In the event of a nuclear attack, both rays and particle forms are likely to be dispersed.

A cell that has been exposed to any type of radiation is damaged and may die. If a terrorist event causes radiation to be released, it could result in either external or internal hazards that could be major or insignificant.

Internal–External Exposure Exposure to radiation from a source outside the body is external exposure; exposure from inside the body is internal. Internal exposure occurs when radioactive material is assimilated into body tissues. This occurs from inhalation, ingestion, or insertion, such as a radioactive implant of iodine-131. A critical point of discrimination is whether the victim was exposed to or contaminated by radiation. If exposed, the victim is *not* a hazard to others. The radiation is absorbed by or passes through the body, but does not result in radioactive contamination.

Radioactive contamination as radioactive particulate material is a major cause for concern. The source of contamination, resulting from spillage, leakage, deliberate dispersal, or attached to dust particles in the air, can be passed on to health care workers. If this were to occur, it could become an internal exposure hazard as it is incorporated into the body, as well as an external exposure.

Measuring Radiation The term *RAD* (radiation absorbed dose) is a unit of measure for radiation exposure; 1 RAD results in absorption of 100 ergs of energy/gram of tissue exposed. The international system now measures the unit of exposure by Gray (Gy); thus, the amount of absorbed radiation is more commonly

---

A possible terrorism event involving radiation dispersal could be:

- An attack on a nuclear facility or detonated nuclear weapon
- A radiation dispersal device: "dirty bomb" (embedding radioactive material in a conventional explosive)
- Radioactive material dispersal

Bioterrorism Agents

Disease	Signs & Symptoms	Incubation Period	Person-to-Person Transmission
Anthrax (Inhalational)	Nonspecific flulike, with fever, malaise, fatigue, cough. Delayed symptoms—severe respiratory distress.	1–7 days (usually 48 hours). Can be 6 weeks.	No.
Botulism (Inhalational)	Increasing muscle weakness, drooping eyelids, blurred vision, difficulty speaking and swallowing; progresses down body to paralysis.	12–36 hours after exposure.	No.
Pneumonic Plague	Sudden onset of high fever, chills, chest pain, headache, and cough with bloody sputum. Possibly vomiting and diarrhea. Advanced: skin lesions, respiratory failure.	2–3 days (1–6 days after exposure).	Yes, through droplet, aerosol.
Smallpox	Sudden onset of high fever, headache, and backache. Then, painful rash of small, red spots starts on face and spreads over entire skin surface. Progresses from macules to papules.	7–17 days after exposure (average is 12 days).	Yes, airborne, droplet or direct contact with skin lesions (until scabs fall off—3–4 weeks).
Typhoid Tularemia	Sudden onset of high fever, weakness, weight loss, chest pain, and cough.	3–5 days after exposure.	No.
Viral Hemorrhagic Fevers (Filoviruses, such as Ebola and Marburg, and arenaviruses, such as Lassa and Junin)	Sudden onset of fever, muscle aches, and profound weakness, followed by circulatory compromise.	2–21 days after exposure.	Yes, risk higher during late stages of disease.

measured by the Gray, rather than RAD (1 Gy equals 100 RADs).

Radiation dose is a specific calculated measurement of the amount of energy deposited in the body. The unit of dose is called REM, which takes into account the type of radiation. It is not necessary for the reader to understand the technical specifics of exposure and dose. It is important to know how to measure external radiation levels and to understand the dangers of exposure.

A survey instrument measures radiation levels. The readout is in units of R (which can be either RAD or REM), which is exposure or dose. An instrument reading of 50R/hr tells the health care worker that if he stays in the exposed area for 1 hour, he will receive a 50-RAD exposure. Some instruments measure dose over time, called radiation dosimeters; these instruments should be worn by personnel working in a contaminated area. A radiation detection device (film badge) should be worn by personnel who come in contact with the exposed area or victims. Both survey instruments and dosimeters have limitations. In the case of survey instruments, they need to be recalculated at regular intervals and, because they use batteries, should be checked and replaced periodically. Dosimeters also must be zeroed and checked at regular intervals.

Health Effects of Radiation A victim contaminated by radiation is at risk—how much risk is dependent on how much radiation is absorbed. Victims who absorb less than 0.75 Gy will not experience symptoms of exposure. Those who absorb 8 Gy could die. Between 0.75 and 8 Gy, the victim could develop acute radiation syndrome (ARS). See box on page 442.

Low exposures do not cause major damage, such as bone marrow damage or birth defects. High exposure may kill cells and significantly increases the incidence of cancer. Regardless of the type of exposure, triage must focus on life-threatening injury before radiological injury.

Background Radiation We are all exposed to a certain amount of radiation from our daily environment. This is known as background radiation and is derived from natural sources such as radiation from outer space; industrial, academic, or military uses of radiation; and radiation used in medicine. All these sources combine to give us a background radiation dose of 0.360 REM per person per year.

ETHICAL CONSIDERATIONS

When we consider the profession of nursing, a central theme must be the ethical considerations of the practice of nursing. Under the chaotic and challenging conditions of a terrorist event, ethics may seem unimportant; while they

Treatment	Death Rate if Untreated	Death Rate if Treated	Isolation Precautions/ Standard Precautions
Antibiotics, including ciprofloxacin 500 mg PO q12 hrs. Doxycycline 100 mg PO q12 hrs; also, combined IV and PO.	High	Improved chances for survival. Once symptoms appear, treatment is less effective.	Standard Precautions.
Antitoxin—requires skin testing. Supportive care and ventilate until victim can breathe on his own.	High.	Low, if breathing can be supported for duration of illness (weeks to months, in some cases).	Standard Precautions.
Antibiotics, including ciprofloxacin 400 mg IV q12 hrs. Doxycycline 200 mg PO, then 100 mg PO q12 hs.	Almost always fatal.	Treatment is highly effective if taken within 24 hours of first symptoms.	Bubonic form: Standard Precautions Pneumonic form: Standard Precautions plus Droplet Precautions until 48–72 hours after antibiotic treatment.
Vaccination is effective if given within 3–4 days of exposure; passive immunization with VIG if 3 days post-exposure.	3–30%.	If vaccinated, less than 1%.	Strict Isolation Precautions: Airborne (includes N95 mask) and Contact, in addition to Standard Precautions.
Antibiotics, including doxycycline and ciprofloxacin.	33%.	1–3% if treated within 24 hours of exposure.	Standard Precautions.
Little is known. Antiviral agents, such as ribavirin, may be useful.	15–90%.	Unknown.	Strict Isolation Precautions, including negative-pressure room with anteroom.

may not be addressed overtly during a disaster, ethical considerations form the bedrock of nursing interventions.

In the midst of a crisis, when resources are limited or unavailable, and the emergency medical and nursing staff do not have the capability of handling the disaster, decision making, nursing judgments, indeed, even functioning ability will rest on one's code of ethics. To review the Nurses Code of Ethics, see Chapter 1, page 3.

DIVERSITY CONSIDERATIONS

If a mass casualty terrorist event were to occur in the United States, many citizens could potentially be harmed. Because approximately 30% of our population is nonwhite, it is important for nurses to be aware of the impact of culture, beliefs, and values on responses to a disaster. Simply being aware of diversity within populations will assist the emergency team to recognize different responses to a mass casualty incident and to relate in a sensitive, appropriate manner.

During the initial assessment following a disaster, the nurse should be aware of the following cultural components:

- Language—(non–English-speaking) communication
- Cultural background and beliefs
- Values, patterns relating to health practices
- Religious practices—limitations
- Nutritional parameters

SUMMARY

In November 2001, 800 public health and military professionals participated at a joint conference. They identified the chief challenge in formulating a strategic plan for preparedness response as "lack of training among front-line responders—physicians and nurses—and inadequate planning at the local, state, and federal levels." Combining these deficit areas—lack of planning, identified skills, and training—helps us to design a framework for nurses to acquire the knowledge necessary for strategic planning and preparedness. Nurses are a vital part, along with physicians and other health care professionals, of preparedness programs throughout the country. Nurses must identify their own skill level and the skills necessary to participate as members of the medical response team.

The term *skill* may be applied to performance. A complex series of actions to accomplish a task may be called skilled performance. A skill can be learned, but it takes experience in performing step-by-step actions before a well-defined response pattern is accomplished. In addition, the change from hesitant responses in the middle of performing a skill to a competent, automatic response takes place only with practice. Thus, the skills necessary to participate in a medical response system when there has been a disaster caused by a WMD must be identified, practiced, and mastered.

This chapter will identify certain skills, drawn from performance-based learning objectives, that nurses must acquire to become high-level task performers on a disaster response team.

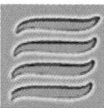

NURSING DIAGNOSES

The following nursing diagnoses are appropriate to use on client care plans when the components relate to a client who requires treatment related to a disaster.

NURSING DIAGNOSIS	RELATED FACTORS
Ineffective Community Coping	Disaster-overwhelmed community resources Lack of access to health care facilities Infrastructure (services) not functioning at 100% Deficits in social support
Ineffective Protection	First responders' and health care personnel protection not appropriate for identified bioterrorism agent
Deficient Knowledge	Lack of information about bioterrorism agent, triage, decontamination methods, treatment
Ineffective Role Performance	First responders and health care personnel unclear about or unable to function in designated roles
Ineffective Community Therapeutic Regimen Management	First responders and health care personnel unclear about or unable to function in designated roles Communication network inadequate for crisis
Effective Therapeutic Regimen Management	Community and health care facilities have Preparedness Plan in place Educational materials, training, and practice have prepared team to function effectively in a disaster

Note To Readers

The skills in this chapter have been formulated according to the latest information and protocols available at the time of publication. Because this topic is new and in transition with new information integrated as events change, please check periodically with the appropriate government sources (i.e., CDC, DHS, NIOSHA, AHA, APIC, JCAHO, FEMA, etc.) for the latest information and updates on procedures and protocols.

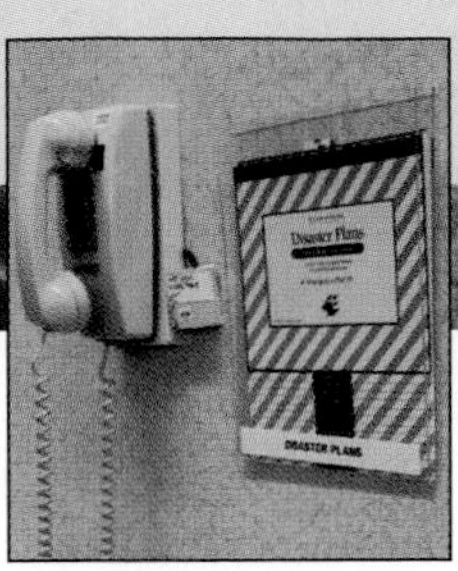

Bioterrorism Agents, Antidotes, and Vaccinations

Nursing Process Data

ASSESSMENT *Data Base*

Identify epidemiologic features

- Rapidly increasing incidence of specific signs and symptoms
- Unusual number of clients seeking care, especially with flulike symptoms, fever, respiratory complaints
- An endemic disease that rapidly emerges
- Clusters of clients from one area
- Large numbers of fatalities

Identify mode of dissemination and incubation period.

Assess the appropriate therapy/antidotes necessary to treat victims of a bioterrorist attack.

Determine clients who could be in a high-risk group for smallpox vaccination.

Assess need for smallpox vaccination.

Observe post-vaccination reactions and compare with adverse reactions.

Assess client's understanding of post-vaccination evaluation.

Assess need for collecting a clinical specimen to identify a specific bioterrorism agent.

Identify acute radiation syndrome.

Assess radiation dose exposure of client.

PLANNING *Objectives*

To recognize a possible terrorist attack

To provide clinical knowledge to recognize features of a biological–chemical–nuclear attack

To enhance ability to detect a biological attack by distinguishing signs and symptoms of various agents

To participate in an effective medical response to a terrorist attack

To provide focused educational content for health care professionals as knowledge base

To possess the skills to initiate an effective response to a terrorist event

To identify the steps of reconstituting smallpox vaccine

To be able to recognize post-vaccination reactions (expected and adverse) and instruct clients in these reactions

To identify need for *vaccinia* immune globulin (VIG)

To know how to collect and transport a clinical specimen

IMPLEMENTATION *Procedures*

Identifying Agents of Biological Terrorism

Prioritizing High-Risk Groups for Smallpox Vaccination

Reconstituting *Vaccinia* Vaccine for Smallpox

Administering Reconstituted Smallpox Vaccine

Understanding Post-Vaccination Reactions

Instructing Client in Post-Vaccination Evaluation

Identifying Indications for *Vaccinia* Immune Globulin (VIG) Administration
Collecting and Transporting Specimens
Identifying Chemical Agent Exposure
Triaging for Chemical Agent Exposure
Managing Care after Chemical Agent Exposure
Identifying Acute Radiation Syndrome

EVALUATION Expected Outcomes

Bioterrorism agent is identified by recognizing specific epidemiological features.
Clients exposed to biological–chemical–radiological agents are identified.
Victims of bioterrorism attack are treated successfully.
Health care workers and clients receive smallpox vaccinations as needed.
High-risk persons for receiving smallpox vaccinations are identified.
Post-vaccination reactions are expected and normal, not adverse.
Appropriate clinical specimens are collected.
Radiation dose of health care workers remains at safe level.

IDENTIFYING AGENTS OF BIOLOGICAL TERRORISM

ANTHRAX

Definition: An acute infectious disease caused by *Bacillus anthracis*, a spore-forming gram-positive bacillus. Human anthrax occurs in three forms: inhalation (the form most dangerous), cutaneous, or gastrointestinal.

Procedure

1. Recognize clinical features.
   a. Inhalation or pulmonary form.
      1. Early signs and symptoms: developing within days, nonspecific flulike illness with malaise, dry cough, mild fever, and headache.
      2. Delayed signs and symptoms: severe respiratory distress, hemodynamic collapse—victim may die, even with antibiotic treatment.
   b. Cutaneous form.
      (1) Early signs and symptoms: local skin involvement with intense itching; painless, papular lesions (commonly seen on head, forearms, or hands).
      (2) Delayed signs and symptoms: papular lesion turned vesicular, developing into black eschar with edema.
   c. Gastrointestinal form (from contaminated meat).
      (1) Early signs and symptoms: abdominal pain, nausea and vomiting, severe diarrhea.
      (2) Delayed signs and symptoms: gastrointestinal bleeding and fever; usually fatal after progression to toxemia and sepsis.
2. Know mode of dissemination and incubation period.
   a. Inhalation of spores: aerosol—no person-to-person transmission. Incubation: 2–60 days (usually 48 hours).
   b. Cutaneous: direct contact with skin lesions.
   c. Gastrointestinal ingestion of contaminated food: no person-to-person transmission; incubation: 1–7 days.

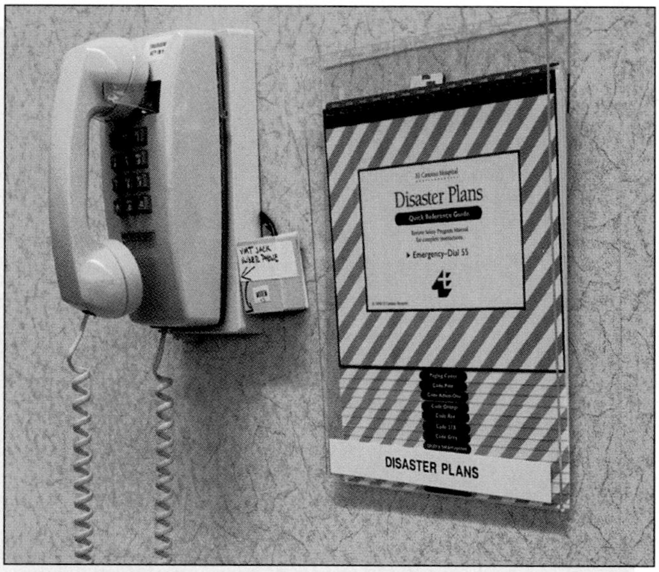

Be familiar with disaster and preparedness plan in the hospital. Perform mock disaster scenarios to maintain skill level and knowledge of procedures if disaster occurs.

3. Manage decontamination.
   a. Remove contaminated clothing.
   b. Instruct clients to shower thoroughly with soap and water.
   c. Instruct personnel to use Standard Precautions.*
   d. Decontaminate environment with 0.5% diluted bleach (1 part to 9 parts water), or EPA-approved germicidal agent.
4. Institute isolation precautions.
   a. Inhalation—Standard Precautions,* wash victim thoroughly (use 0.5% diluted bleach for visible contamination); store clothing in sealed plastic bag with biohazard label.

Understand the Danger of Biologically Toxic Agents

1. Biological incidents will be the most difficult of all attacks for the community to recognize and effectively coordinate a response.
2. Most viruses are useful as bioterror agents—they cause unique signs and symptoms that require intervention and isolation of the victims to prevent spread.
3. Specific incapacitating viral or bacterial agents slowly produce signs and symptoms.
   a. Signs and symptoms are nonspecific and difficult to recognize; onset of incident may remain unknown for days before symptoms appear.
   b. It may be necessary to identify "clusters" of illness—many victims in one location become sick within a short period of time.
4. If agents are detected early, most can be treated with antibiotics or antivirals.
5. The most common form of agents that could be used in a bioterror attack are bacteria.

   b. Cutaneous—contact precautions (gown and gloves).
   c. Gastrointestinal—Standard Precautions.*
5. Assign client placement.
   a. Private room placement *not* necessary.
   b. Airborne transmission does *not* occur.
   c. Skin lesions may be transmitted by direct skin contact only.
6. Implement therapy for anthrax infection.
   a. Ciprofloxacin 400 mg IV q8–12 hrs; 500 mg PO q12 hrs; doxycycline 200 mg IV (1 dose); 100 mg IV q8–12 hrs; or 100 mg PO q12 hrs, or amoxicillin may also be ordered.
   b. Continue treatment for 60 days.
   c. Mass casualty—oral therapy with standard doses.

**Standard Precautions: See Chapter 14, pg. 382.*

PLAGUE

Definition: Acute, severe bacterial infection, caused by gram-negative bacillus. Seen in bubonic or pneumonic form; caused by bacillus *Yersinia pestis.* A bioterrorism outbreak could be airborne, causing pneumonic plague.

Procedure

1. Recognize clinical features.
   a. Bubonic form.
      (1) Swollen, tender lymph nodes (femoral or inguinal commonly most involved).
      (2) High temp 103.1–105.8°F (39.5 to 41°C), chills.
      (3) Pulse rapid, hypotension.
      (4) Extreme exhaustion.
   b. Pneumonic form.
      (1) High fever, chills, tachycardia, headache.
      (2) Cough with foamy hemoptysis.
      (3) Tachypnea and dyspnea.
2. Know mode of dissemination and incubation period.
   a. Transmitted from rodents to humans by infected fleas; incubation 2–8 days.
   b. Human-to-human transmission occurs by inhaling droplets through cough.
   c. Bioterrorism-related through dispersion of aerosol; incubation: 1–3 days.
3. Manage decontamination—procedure should be done in a room designed for this purpose or at a special site outside the hospital.
   a. Instruct clients to remove clothing and store in closed plastic biohazard bags.
   b. Instruct clients to shower thoroughly with soap and water—include all crevices.
   c. Home decontamination: employ Standard Precautions (gloves, gown, face shield, when necessary).
   d. Use 0.5% diluted bleach or EPA-approved germicidal agent.
4. Institute isolation precautions.
   a. Bubonic form—routine aseptic (Standard) Precautions.

A Holistic Approach to Coping with Plague

Athens, 200 B.C.: Hippocrates uses precious oils to protect and treat his patients. It is known that essential oils, volatile molecules, float in the air and enter the olfactory system where the limbic system is stimulated to release chemical messages that activate a physical response. Oils have the ability to oxygenate, transport nutrients, and heal. One particular oil blend, "Thieves," was created from research looking back to the fifteenth century when four thieves used clove, rosemary, lemon, cinnamon, and eucalyptus to protect themselves while robbing plague victims in England. The thieves did not die from plague, while hundreds of thousands did. These oils may be used today to protect oneself from certain diseases.

Source: Young, D., Gary, N.D. (2002). *An introduction to young living essential oils* (10th ed.), Payson, UT: Young Living.

   b. Pneumonic form—add droplet precautions to Standard Precautions (eye protection and surgical mask when within 3 feet of client) until 72 hours of antimicrobial therapy.
5. Assign client placement.
   a. Bubonic form—private isolation room or cohort with clients with similar symptoms.
   b. Maintain at least 3 feet between clients when cohorting is not possible.
   c. Do not place client with immunosuppressed client.
6. Implement therapy.
   a. Doxycycline 100 mg 2 × daily.
   b. Ciprofloxacin 500 mg 2 × daily.

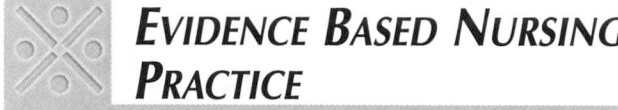

EVIDENCE BASED NURSING PRACTICE

Lessons Learned from a Full-Scale Bioterrorism Exercise

In May 2000, three hospitals in metropolitan Denver and officials from local, state, and federal agencies participated in a simulated bioterrorism attack exercise involving the simulated release of *Yersinia pestis* aerosol that infected 2,000 people. During the attack, decision making became inefficient and many problems were identified. The single most important lesson learned from this experience was that three aspects must receive equal effort: controlling the spread of disease, triage, and treatment of ill persons.

In May, 2003, additional full-scale bioterrorism exercises were conducted in three cities—Miami, Seattle, and Chicago. The results are not available at this time, but questions asked included how fast were victims treated, and how to prevent rescuers from becoming victims. It is hoped that while practice may improve proficiency, lessons learned will never have to be implemented.

Source: Hoffman, R., & Norton. J. (2000 Dec.). Colorado Dept. of Public Health and Environment. *Emerging Infectious Diseases, 6*(6), 652–653.

BOTULISM

Definition: A muscle-paralyzing disease caused by an anaerobic gram-positive bacillus that produces a potent neurotoxin. Food-borne botulism is the most common form; inhalational botulism is most likely to occur through a bioterrorist release of aerosol.

Procedure

1. Recognize clinical features.
   a. Food-borne botulism.
      (1) Gastrointestinal symptoms: nausea, vomiting, diarrhea.
      (2) Leads to symptoms of inhalational botulism.
   b. Inhalational botulism.
      (1) No fever—client is responsive.
      (2) Symmetric cranial nerve paralysis: drooping eyelids, blurred vision, diplopia, difficulty swallowing, dry mouth.
      (3) Symptoms progress to paralysis of arms, respiratory muscles, and legs.
      (4) Symptoms may be confused with Guillain-Barré syndrome or myasthenia gravis.
2. Know mode of dissemination and incubation period.
   a. Food-borne botulism: generally transmitted through toxin-contaminated food; incubation is 12–36 hours after ingestion.
   b. Inhalational botulism: transmitted through aerosolization of the toxin. Incubation is 24–72 hours postexposure.
3. Manage decontamination.
   a. Client does not require decontamination.
   b. Contaminated clothing washed with commercial soap
4. Institute isolation precautions.
   a. No evidence of person-to-person transmission.
   b. Standard Precautions for clients.
5. Assign client placement: client room selection and care according to facility policy. Client-to-client transmission does not occur.
6. Implement therapy.
   a. Early recognition of botulism important for administration of antitoxin that may stop or reduce paralysis.
   b. Administer trivalent botulinum antitoxin (per CDC orders); requires skin testing due to 95% hypersensitivity reactions.
   c. Monitor client for respiratory failure and provide supportive care.

TYPHOIDAL TULAREMIA

Definition: A disease caused by *Francisella tularensis* bacterium. It is extremely infectious and can be transmitted via aerosol or contaminated water or food.

Procedure

1. Recognize clinical features.
   a. Early symptoms: headache, cough, fever, and chills, malaise.
   b. Delayed symptoms: pharyngeal ulcers, pleuritic chest pain, pneumonia, pericarditis—may progress to respiratory failure.
2. Know mode of dissemination and incubation period.
   a. Bioterrorism mode is aerosol.
   b. This disease may not be recognized unless a bioterrorism attack is suspected.
   c. Incubation period: 2–12 days (average 3–5 days) after exposure.
3. Manage decontamination: general decontamination measures for clothing of infected person—shower with soap or

use 0.5% diluted bleach. Because there is no person-to-person transmission, no other measures are necessary.
4. Institute isolation precautions.
   a. This disease is not transmitted person to person, so isolation measures are not required.
   b. Standard Precautions recommended.
5. Assign client placement: cohort clients and do not place with immunosuppressed clients.
6. Implement therapy: ciprofloxacin 250 mg. PO q12 hrs × 14 days, streptomycin 15 mg/Kg BID IM × 10–14 days or gentamicin 1.5 mg/Kg q8 hrs IV × 10–14 days.

EVIDENCE BASED NURSING PRACTICE

Nurse Hotlines—A Source for Identifying Epidemics

In this study, the nurse hot line showed a 17% increase in calls when the 1993 Milwaukee cryptosporidium outbreak occurred. The conclusion is that nurse hot line calls are a potential source of public surveillance for identifying epidemics of emerging infectious diseases or bioterrorism attacks.

Source: Rodman, J., Frost, F., & Jakubaoski, W. (1998). *Using hot line calls for disease surveillance.* Southwest Center for Managed Care Research and EPA.

VIRAL HEMORRHAGIC FEVER (VHF)

Definition: An infection caused by agents such as Ebola, Marburg, Larsa, Argentine, yellow and dengue fevers. These viruses could be life-threatening (moderately high lethality) and could be delivered by aerosol in a biological attack.

Procedure

1. Recognize clinical features.
   a. Each illness has unique clinical manifestations; however, some features are similar.
   b. Characterized by abrupt onset of fever, myalgia, headache, prostration.
   c. Other signs and symptoms are nausea and vomiting, diarrhea, pain in abdomen and chest, cough, and pharyngitis.
   d. A maculopapular rash, prominent on the trunk, develops in most clients 5 days after onset of illness.
   e. Bleeding manifestations may occur as the disease progresses. Even though it is rare for this life-threatening condition to occur, bleeding (intracranial hemorrhage) could result; hence, the term, hemorrhagic fever.
2. Know mode of dissemination and incubation period.
   a. Viruses are zoonotic (animal-borne), but can be spread person-to-person.
   b. All viruses (except dengue fever) could be spread by aerosol in a biological attack.
   c. Incubation period: usually 5–10 days, with a range of 2–21 days.
3. Manage decontamination: the virus is transmitted person-to-person; decontamination with overt attack: victim undresses, showers with soap or 0.5% diluted bleach.
4. Institute isolation procedures.
   a. Communicable person-to-person; risk is highest after infection has progressed. Isolation precautions (including airborne and contact), including respirators, face shields, gowns, gloves, shoe and head covers.
   b. Negative-pressure ventilated rooms with an anteroom.
5. Assign client placement.
   a. Clients should be under strict isolation precautions, including a negative-pressure room with anteroom.
   b. Only clients with the same form of hemorrhagic infection should be cohorted.
6. Implement therapy.
   a. Primarily supportive.
   b. Ribavirin, 30 mg/Kg IV × 1 dose; 15 mg/Kg IV q6 hrs × 4 days.

Q FEVER

Definition: A rickettsial organism (*Coxiella burnetii*), naturally found in sheep, cattle, and goats. Bioterrorism mode of dissemination will be aerosol or food supply sabotage.

Procedure

1. Recognize clinical features.
   a. Early signs and symptoms: headache, fever, chills, malaise, diaphoresis, anorexia; insidious onset with nonspecific flulike symptoms.
   b. Delayed signs and symptoms: double vision, sore throat, cough, chest pain, nuchal rigidity, encephalitis, hallucinations, weight loss.
   c. Differential diagnosis: atypical pneumonias.
2. Know mode of dissemination and incubation period.
   a. Aerosol or food supply.
   b. Incubation period: 10–40 days (average 10–14 days).
3. Manage decontamination.
   a. Have victim undress and shower thoroughly with soap. May use 0.5% diluted bleach.
   b. Clean environment with 0.5% diluted bleach.
4. Institute isolation precautions: none required. Rarely transmitted person to person. Use Standard Precautions.
5. Assign client placement: transmissibility rare, so clients can be cohorted.
6. Implement therapy.
   a. Tetracycline 500 mg PO q6 hrs × 5–7 days; doxycycline 100 mg PO q12 hrs × 5–7 days.
   b. Continue treatment for 2 days post-febrile condition.

RICIN TOXIN

Definition: Produced from the castor bean plant and secreted in castor seeds; *Ricinus communis* is a cytotoxin that blocks protein synthesis, killing the cell.

Procedure

1. Recognize clinical features.
   a. Signs and symptoms depend on route of exposure. Diagnosis is difficult. ELISA test of blood will identify ricin.
      (1) Ingestion: nausea, vomiting, diarrhea, and severe abdominal cramps occur before vascular collapse (GI bleeding), leading to death on 3rd day.
      (2) Aerosol—inhalation: cough, fever, hypothermia, and hypotension (usually nonspecific symptoms); cardiovascular collapse leads to death in 36–48 hours.
   b. This biotoxin has been used by assassins; causes death within minutes when placed on the skin. In 2003, ricin was found in a terrorist cell in England—potential use unknown.
2. Know mode of dissemination and incubation period.
   a. Ricin will be delivered via the castor bean through a chemical process (ingested) or through inhalation method.
   b. Incubation period is within hours to days (ingestion: 3 days; inhalation 3–4 days).
3. Manage decontamination.
   a. Ingested biotoxin does not require decontamination.
   b. Aerosol exposure—victim should shower with soap or use 0.5% diluted bleach.
4. Institute isolation precautions. This toxin is not transmitted to others, but Standard Precautions should be implemented.
5. Assign client placement. There is no communicability person to person or transport through the skin, so placement is planned to protect client's immune system.
6. Implement therapy. There is no approved antitoxin treatment or prophylaxis (vaccination) at this time.
   a. Therapy is supportive; give oxygen and hydration.
   b. If there is ingestion, GI decontamination would be implemented.

SMALLPOX

Definition: An acute viral disease caused by the *variola virus*. It was eradicated worldwide in 1977, and in the early 1980s routine vaccinations were discontinued. Because there is a large nonimmune population, authorities fear it could be a bioterrorism weapon, transmitted via the airborne route as aerosol or by infected human vectors.

Procedure

1. Recognize clinical features.
   a. Initially, symptoms resemble an acute viral illness like influenza with high fever, myalgia, headache, and backache.
   b. Rash appears (when smallpox becomes most contagious), progressing from macules to papules (in 1 week) to vesicles, and scabs over in 1–2 weeks.
   c. Distinguishing rash from varicella (chickenpox): smallpox has a synchronous onset on face and extremities, rather than arising in 'bunches,' starting on the trunk.
2. Know mode of dissemination and incubation period.
   a. Smallpox is transmitted by large and small respiratory droplets; thus, both respiratory and oral secretions spread the disease, as well as lesion drainage and contaminated objects such as bed linens.
   b. Clients are considered more infectious if they are coughing or have a hemorrhagic form of the disease.
   c. Vaccination effective if given within 3–4 days.
   d. Incubation: 7–17 days; average is 12 days.
3. Manage decontamination.
   a. Decontamination of clients is not indicated with smallpox.
   b. Careful management using contact precautions of potentially contaminated equipment and environmental surfaces—clean, disinfect, and sterilize when possible.
   c. Dedicated or disposable equipment for each client should be used.
4. Institute strict isolation precautions *immediately*.
   a. Airborne and contact precautions in addition to Standard Precautions; includes gloves, gown, eye shields, shoe covers, and correctly fitted masks (very important).
   b. Airborne precautions: Microrganisms transmitted by airborne droplet nuclei (particles 5 microns or smaller).
      (1) Respiratory protection when entering client's room (particulate respirators, N95); must meet National

Dangers of Smallpox Vaccination: The Debate Continues

Smallpox vaccination results in 2–4 deaths per million—as many as 1,000 deaths could occur if everyone in the United States were to be vaccinated. In 2003, there are 300 million doses of vaccine available, enough to vaccinate everyone in the United States. Live virus is dangerous, especially to those who have a compromised immune system, those with cardiovascular conditions, and those with skin diseases, such as eczema and psoriasis. Those who were already vaccinated 30 years ago have been tested and some have been found to have what appears to be a significant level of immunity; but, is it enough? Others who received vaccinations in the 1970s and earlier are believed to have no useful immunity. There is still a debate: Should the vaccinations be voluntary? Should only first responders and emergency personnel receive vaccinations? Should only those who were never vaccinated receive vaccination?

Institute for Occupational Safety and Health (NIOSH) standards for particulate respirators.
   (2) Isolate in room under negative pressure with high-efficiency particle air filtration.
- c. Contact precautions: Clients known to be infected or colonized with organisms that can be transmitted by direct contact or indirect contact with contaminated surfaces.
   (1) Wash hands using antimicrobial agent when entering and leaving room.
   (2) Don gloves when entering room.
   (3) Wear gown for all client contact or contact with client's environment.
   (4) Wear gown when entering room and remove before leaving isolation area.

5. Assign client placement.
   a. Rooms must meet ventilation and engineering requirements for airborne precautions.
      (1) Monitored negative air pressure with 6–12 air exchanges/hr.
      (2) Appropriate discharge of air to outdoors, or high-efficiency filtration of air.
   b. Door to room must remain closed; private room is preferred. Clients with same diagnosis may be cohorted.
   c. Limit transport of clients; use appropriate mask if unavoidable.
6. Implement therapy.
   a. Post-exposure immunization (*vaccinia* virus) is available.
      (1) Vaccination alone if given within 3–4 days of exposure.
      (2) Passive immunization (VIG) if greater than 3 days post-exposure.
      (3) VIG given at 0.6 mL/kg IM. See administration skill, pg. 435. Check with CDC for up-to-date recommendations.
   b. Prophylactic care with precautions.

PRIORITIZING HIGH-RISK GROUPS FOR SMALLPOX VACCINATION

Procedure

1. Identify health care workers. **Rationale:** All persons potentially exposed to the virus must be evaluated for possible vaccination.
   a. Personnel involved in evaluation, care, or transportation of confirmed, probable, or suspected smallpox clients.
   b. Laboratory personnel involved in collection or processing of clinical specimens.
   c. Other persons with increased likelihood of contact with infectious materials from a smallpox client (laundry or medical waste handlers).
   d. Other persons or staff who have a reasonable probability of contact with smallpox clients or infectious materials (e.g., selected law enforcement, emergency response, or military personnel).
   e. Because of potential for greater spread of smallpox in a hospital setting due to aerosolization of the virus from a severely ill client, all individuals in the hospital may be vaccinated.
2. Identify clients exposed to the smallpox virus. **Rationale:** The sooner clients are identified, the earlier they can receive smallpox vaccination, which must be given within 4 days to be effective.
   a. Persons who were exposed to initial release of the virus.
   b. Persons who had face-to-face, household, or close-proximity contact (<2 meters = 6.5 feet) with a confirmed or suspected smallpox client after client developed fever and until all scabs have separated (no longer infectious).
3. Determine contraindications for vaccination of noncontacts. **Rationale:** Persons with certain medical conditions are known to have a higher risk of developing severe complications following vaccination with *Vaccinia* vaccine.
   a. Persons with diseases or conditions which cause immunodeficiency, such as HIV, AIDS, leukemia, lymphoma, persons with cardiac conditions, therapy with alkylating agents, antimetabolites, radiation, or large doses of corticosteroids.
   b. Persons with serious, life-threatening allergies to the antibiotics: polymyxin B, streptomycin, tetracycline, or neomycin. **Rationale:** Dryvax contains trace amounts of these antibiotics.
   c. Persons who have ever been diagnosed with eczema, even if the condition is mild or not presently active.

> **CLINICAL ALERT**
>
> A household member who has eczema or a history of eczema who has been exposed to a recently vaccinated household member is at higher risk for developing a post-vaccine complication from the vaccination site of the vaccinated person.

   d. Women who are pregnant.
   e. Persons with other acute or chronic skin conditions such as atopic dermatitis, burns, impetigo, or varicella zoster (shingles). These persons should not be vaccinated until the condition resolves.

RECONSTITUTING *VACCINIA* VACCINE FOR SMALLPOX

Equipment

Vial of vaccine (Dryvax)
Prefilled syringe of diluent
Clean or latex-free gloves
Biohazard bag and label

Procedure

1. Remove vaccine vial from refrigerated storage and allow vial to come to room temperature. **Rationale:** Vaccine must be at room temperature to be reconstituted.
2. Wash hands and don gloves. **Rationale:** Personnel must be protected from touching vaccine.
3. Lift tab of aluminum seal of vaccine vial. DO NOT BREAK OFF OR TEAR DOWN TAB.
4. Place vaccine vial upright on a hard, flat surface.
5. Remove cap from prefilled syringe of diluent. **Rationale:** Diluent is required for reconstitution prior to administration.
6. Inject 0.25 mL of diluent into vaccine vial. **Rationale:** This amount of diluent reconstitutes vaccine.
7. Withdraw needle and syringe and discard in appropriate biohazard sharps container. **Rationale:** This needle and syringe are now contaminated with the vaccine.
8. Allow vaccine vial to stand undisturbed for 3–5 minutes. Then, if necessary, swirl vial gently. **Rationale:** Complete reconstitution of vaccine must take place.
9. In the space provided on vaccine vial label, record date and time diluent was added. The vaccine is now ready for use. **Rationale:** Use reconstituted vaccine for time period recommended by manufacturer if stored at 35.6–46.4°F (2 to 8°C) when not in actual use.
10. Dispose of diluent syringe, needle used for diluent reconstitution of vaccine, and any gauze or cotton that came in contact with vaccine as follows: in a biohazard bag labeled to burn, boil, or autoclave before final disposal. **Rationale:** Staff could be inadvertently inoculated by touching these items.

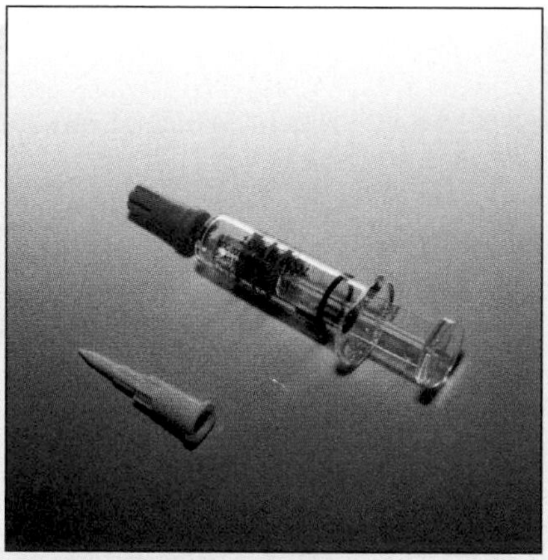
Prefilled syringe of diluent. This will be injected into vaccine vial to reconstitute.

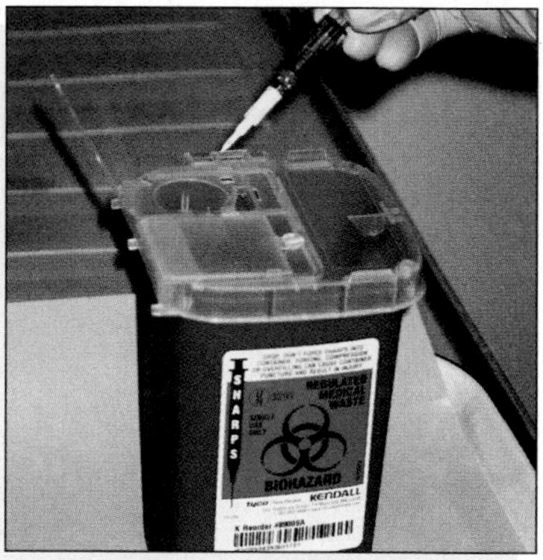

After injecting diluent into vaccine vial, discard syringe into biohazard container.

ADMINISTERING RECONSTITUTED SMALLPOX VACCINE

Equipment

Clean or latex-free gloves
Vaccine vial
Sterile container
Swab if necessary
Sterile bifurcated (two-pronged) needle
Sterile gauze
4 × 4 gauze bandage
Tape

Preparation

1. Identify client(s) to be vaccinated according to public health protocol.
2. Issue information client must receive prior to smallpox vaccination.
   a. Preapproved vaccine information entitled "What You Need to Know about Smallpox Vaccinations."
   b. An 11-minute CDC video describing the process and results of a Vaccination.
   c. The understanding that vaccination is voluntary.
   d. Personal information packet and signed permission form.
3. Obtain reconstituted *Vaccinia* vaccine vial from pharmacy. (Public Health Centers are issued vials that hold 100 doses that are administered at scheduled times.)
4. Inspect vaccine for particulate matter or discoloration; if present, do not use.
5. Gather equipment.
6. Wash hands.

Note: Vaccinators must attend classes, read appropriate material, and watch a CDC video before administering vaccination.

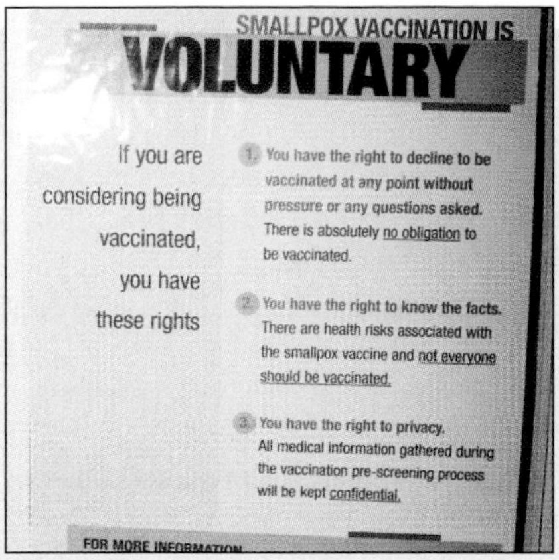

It is important that client understand that smallpox vaccination is voluntary.

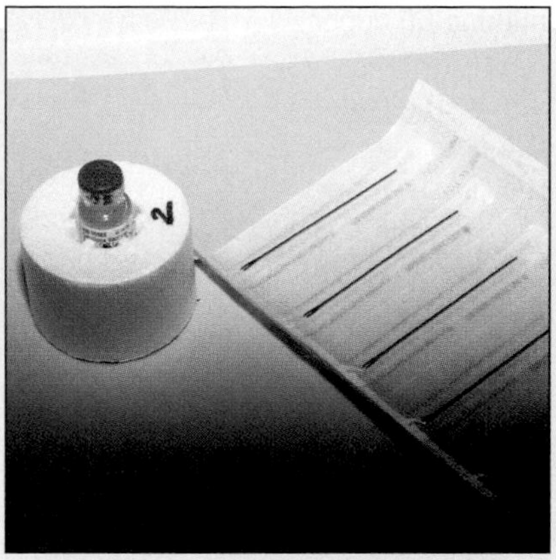
Obtain reconstituted vaccine vial (which was stored at 2° to 8°C) from pharmacy.

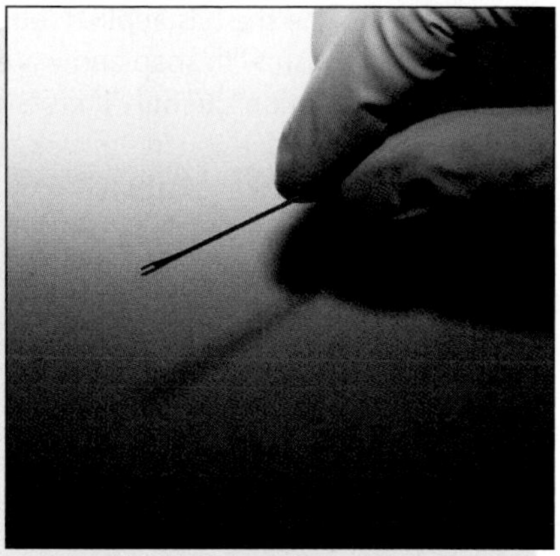
Sterile bifurcated (two-pronged) needle is provided individually wrapped.

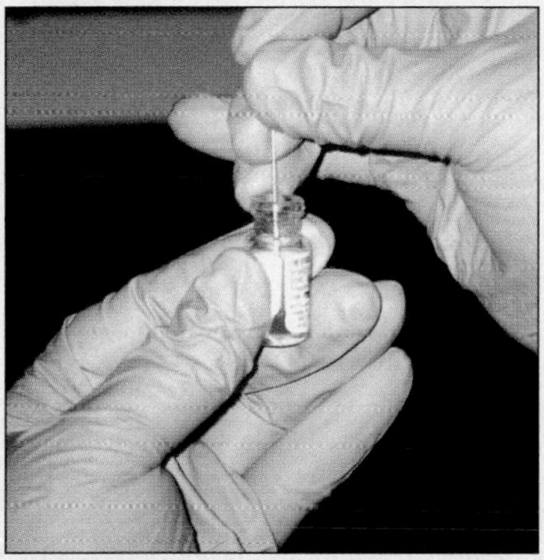
Dip point of bifurcated needle into vial of reconstituted vaccine.

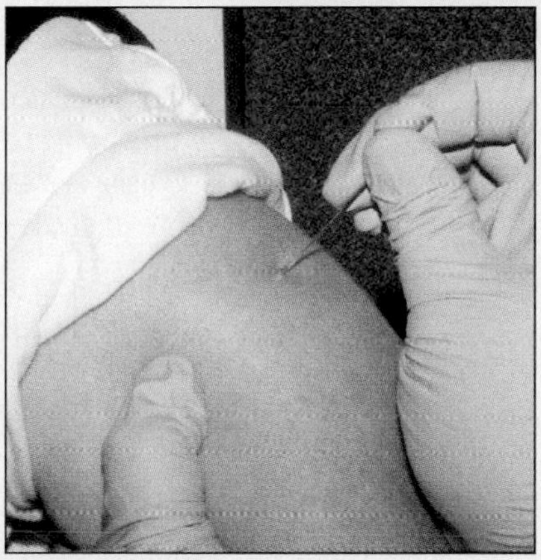
Hold needle at 90° angle and apply rapid strokes within a 5-mm diameter.

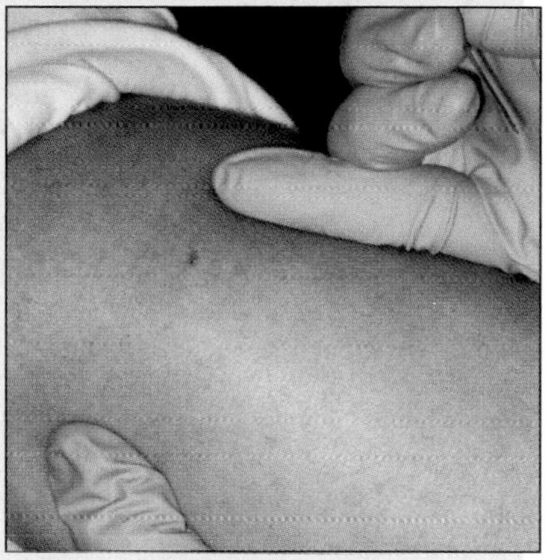
Wait for a trace of blood at site to indicate successful vaccine delivery.

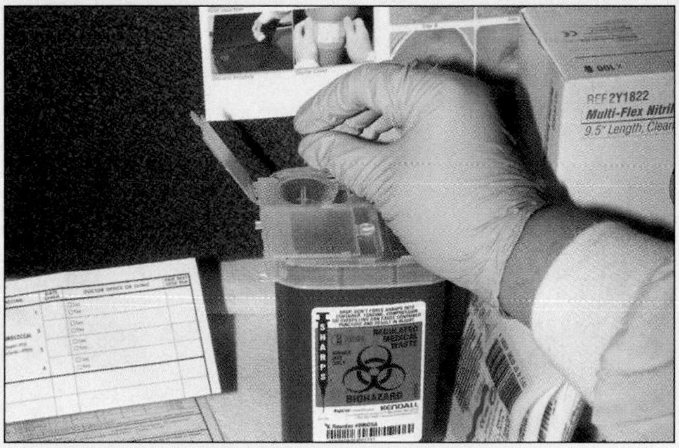
Dispose of bifurcated needle in puncture-resistant medical waste sharps container.

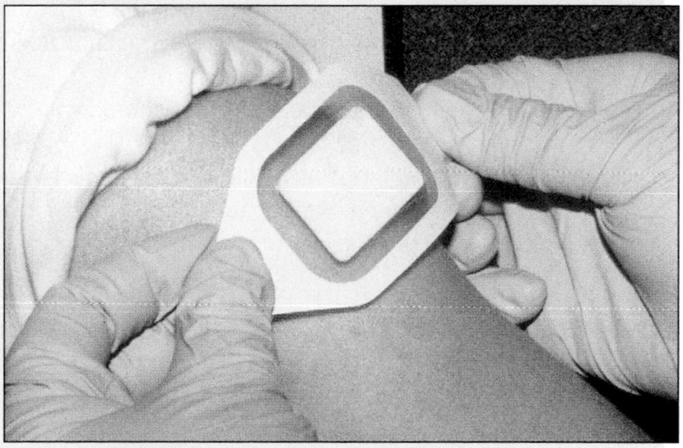
Cover vaccination site with semipermeable dressing.

Procedure

1. Don clean or latex-free gloves.
2. Remove rubber stopper from vaccine vial and place in sterile container. **Rationale:** Stopper should remain sterile as it will be used to recap the vial containing vaccine.
3. Choose site of vaccination—one that is easily accessible for vaccination and evaluation of vaccine taken on post-vaccination day 7. The outer aspect of the upper right arm over the insertion of the deltoid muscle is the standard (and CDC recommended) vaccination site. **Rationale:** This prevents confusion with vaccination site from a previous vaccination.

4. Ask client if he/she has applied lotion or anything on upper arm. If so, wash with soap and water.
5. Clean vaccination site only if grossly contaminated. Let dry thoroughly. Under no circumstances apply alcohol to the skin (per CDC 2002). **Rationale:** Alcohol will inactivate vaccine deposited on skin.
6. Dip point of a sterile bifurcated needle into vial of reconstituted vaccine and withdraw needle perpendicular to the floor.

Note: Needles are designed to hold designated dose of vaccine (2.5 μL) between needle prongs to allow delivery to skin surface.

CLINICAL ALERT

Do not redip needle into vaccine vial if needle has touched skin. This contaminates the vial.

7. Hold skin of upper arm taut and place wrist firmly on the arm.
8. Hold needle at a 90° angle (perpendicular) to skin and apply up-and-down (perpendicular) strokes rapidly within a 5-mm diameter area.
   a. First-time smallpox vaccination recipients: Deliver 3 strokes with a bifurcated needle. Observe for blood appearing within 15–30 seconds. If blood does not appear, deliver 3 additional punctures with the *same* needle *without* reinserting needle into the vaccine vial. **Rationale:** New guidelines from the Advisory Committee on Immunization Practices (APIC) were announced February, 2003, to change the number of strokes from 15 to 3 for first-time recipients to conform to the FDA approved package insert from Wyeth, the manufacturer of the Dryvax vaccine.
   b. Revaccination recipients: Deliver 15 up-and-down strokes with a bifurcated needle.
9. Examine for a trace of blood at vaccination site, which usually takes 15 to 30 seconds to appear. **Rationale:** This indicates successful vaccine delivery.

CLINICAL ALERT

When administering smallpox vaccination, strokes should be made rapidly and be sufficiently vigorous to elicit a trace of blood at vaccination site. If trace of blood does not appear, strokes have not been sufficiently vigorous and procedure should be repeated.

10. Cover vaccination site with gauze bandage and tape or semipermeable dressing. **Rationale:** This prevents contact transmission of virus to unvaccinated persons (people with contraindications to vaccination) or inadvertent inoculation of another body site.
    a. Keep vaccination covered until scab separates.
    b. Change dressing if exudate builds up. The CDC recommends changing dressing daily, or every 3 days.

Note: The CDC recommends using a semipermeable dressing (Tegaderm) when at a work site, in public, or for showering. When site is totally blocked from air, skin at site might soften and wear away.

11. Dispose of bifurcated needle in a puncture-resistant medical waste sharps container. **Rationale:** Bifurcated needle is for single usage only.
12. Instruct client to keep site dry and not to rub or scratch vaccination site.

Note: Vaccinia virus may be recovered from vaccination site, beginning at the time of development of a papule (2 to 5 days post-vaccination) until scab separates from skin (14–21 days post-vaccination) and underlying skin has healed.

13. Recap vial with sterile rubber stopper and store capped vial at 35.6–46.4°F (2 to 8°C.) Note number of doses left in vial. **Rationale:** This temperature will allow vaccine to be saved for subsequent use.
14. Remove gloves, discard in appropriate hazardous waste receptacle, and wash hands thoroughly.

UNDERSTANDING POST-VACCINATION REACTIONS

Procedure

1. Identify persons who should be revaccinated. **Rationale:** If the vaccination did not take, the individual will remain vulnerable to the smallpox virus.
   a. They will have delayed type of skin sensitivity consisting of *erythema only* within 24–48 hours.
   b. This represents a response to inert protein in a previously sensitized person and can occur in a highly immunized person or in individuals with little or no immunity; it is indistinguishable from the immediate or immune reaction.
2. Confirm successful vaccination and enter results in client's record. **Rationale:** So that the client will not have to be revaccinated.
   a. Presence of a pustular lesion in previously unvaccinated persons.

b. Pustular lesion or an area of definite induration or congestion surrounding a central lesion 7 days following revaccination in a previously vaccinated person.
c. Vaccinees who do not exhibit a "major" reaction at vaccination site on day 7 should be revaccinated.

3. Recognize adverse reactions. **Rationale:** Identifying an adverse reaction is important so that VIG may be administered.
   a. The overall risk of serious complications following vaccination with *vaccinia* vaccine appears to be low.
   b. Complications occur more frequently in persons receiving their first dose of vaccine, and among young children (<5 years of age).
   c. The *most frequent* complications of vaccination are inadvertent inoculation, generalized vaccinia, eczema vaccination, progressive vaccinia, and post-vaccination encephalitis.
   d. Unexpected cardiovascular complications resulted in reevaluation of the vaccination program in 2003.
4. Document results on vaccination record in client's chart.

INSTRUCTING CLIENT IN POST-VACCINATION EVALUATION

Procedure

1. Tell client that successful vaccination is normally associated with tenderness, redness, swelling, and a lesion at the vaccination site.
2. Instruct client that vaccination may also be associated with fever for a few days, malaise, and enlarged, tender lymph nodes in the axilla of the vaccinated arm.

Note: These symptoms are more common in older children and clients receiving their first dose of vaccine [15–20%] than in persons being revaccinated [0–10%].

3. Check for inoculation site becoming reddened and pruritic 3–4 days after vaccination and every 3 days following; place results in the record. **Rationale:** This is a primary reaction following vaccination.
   a. A vesicle surrounded by a red areola, enlarges, becomes umbilicated, and then pustular by the 7th to 11th day after vaccination.
   b. The pustule begins to dry, redness subsides, and lesion becomes crusted between 2nd and 3rd week.
4. Inform client that by the end of the 3rd week, scab falls off, leaving a permanent scar that at first is pink in color, but eventually becomes flesh-colored.
5. Instruct person who has been previously vaccinated (a partially immune person) that an attenuated primary vaccine site reaction will occur with the following characteristics.
   a. Absence of fever or constitutional symptoms.
   b. Papule by 3rd day that becomes vesicular by 5th to 7th day, and dries shortly thereafter.
   c. A relatively small vesicle and areola.
   d. Scar, if present, is usually insignificant and disappears within 1–2 years.

> **CLINICAL ALERT**
> Instruct client to wash hands thoroughly after touching vaccination site to prevent inadvertent inoculation at another site.

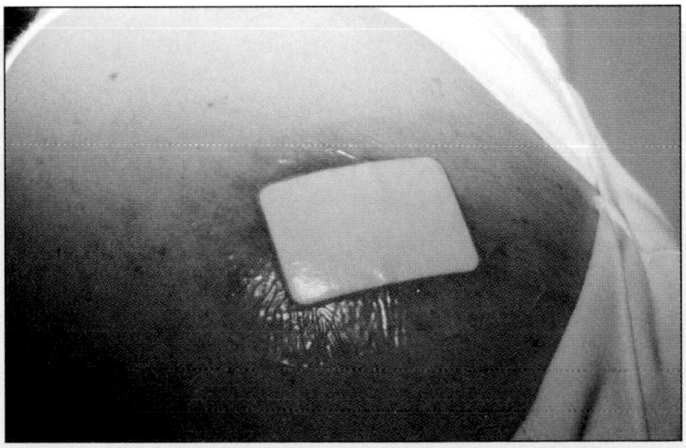

Example of semi-permeable dressing covering site at eighth day postvaccination.

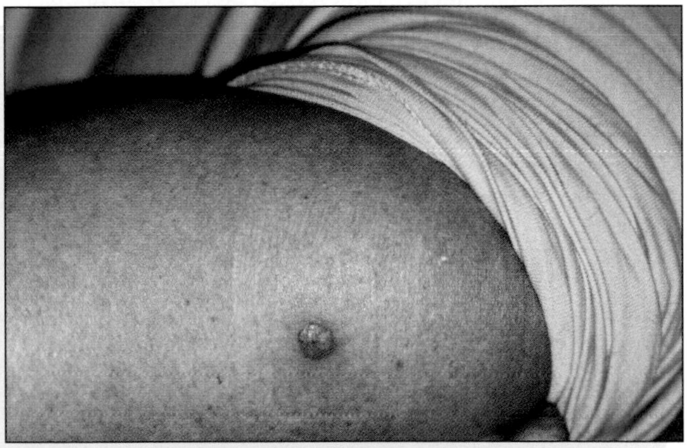

Example of pustular lesion 8 days following revaccination in a previously vaccinated person.

Evidence Based Nursing Practice

Complications from Inadvertent Inoculation

Inadvertent smallpox inoculation at other sites accounts for about 50% of all complications following primary and revaccination. This complication of vaccinia vaccination occurs at a rate of about 1 in 2000 primary vaccinations and usually results from auto-inoculation when virus is transferred by hand from the site of vaccination to other areas. The most common sites involved are the face, eyelid, nose, mouth, genitalia, and rectum. Most lesions will heal without specific therapy.

Source: Vaccination guidelines for state and local health agencies (2002). Centers for Disease Control, U.S. Department of Health and Human Services.

IDENTIFYING INDICATIONS FOR *VACCINIA* IMMUNE GLOBULIN (VIG) ADMINISTRATION

Procedure

1. Identify post-vaccination complications for which VIG may be indicated. **Rationale:** VIG is indicated for some complications, but not others.
   a. Eczema vaccinatum.
   b. Progressive *vaccinia* (*vaccinia* necrosum).
   c. Severe generalized *vaccinia* if client has a toxic condition or serious underlying illness.
   d. Inadvertent inoculation of eye or eyelid without vaccinial keratitis.
2. Check physician's orders for VIG treatment of complications due to *vaccinia* vaccination.
3. Administer VIG intramuscularly (IM) as early as possible after onset of symptoms.
4. Give VIG in divided doses over a 24–36-hour period. Doses may be repeated at 2–3-day intervals until no new lesions appear. **Rationale:** Because the therapeutic dose of VIG may be large (e.g., 0.6 mL/Kg body weight), it is given in divided doses.
5. Instruct staff VIG is not indicated for treatment of post-vaccination encephalitis and is contraindicated for vaccinial keratitis.

Possible Adverse Reactions to Smallpox Vaccination

- *Inadvertent Inoculation at Another Site:* Virus is transferred by hand from vaccination site to another body area. Most lesions heal without therapy.
- *Generalized Vaccinia:* Bloodborne dissemination of vaccinia virus resulting in vesicular rash of varying extent (occurs 1 in 5000 vaccinations). Usually self-limiting.
- *Eczema Vaccinatum:* Skin lesions that cover area affected by eczema or a chronic skin condition. Illness (fever, lymphadenopathy) is usually mild, but can be fatal (occurs 1 in 26,000 primary vaccinations).
- *Progressive Vaccinia:* Severe and potentially fatal; occurs in persons with immune deficiencies. Characterized by failure of lesion to heal with progressive necrosis. VIG is used to treat condition.
- *Post-Vaccination Encephalitis:* All symptoms of encephalitis occur between 8–15 days post-vaccination. Incidence is 1 in 300,000 vaccinations, and there is no cure.
- *Cardiac complications:* Heart inflammation (myocarditis, pericarditis), angina and a few heart attacks have occurred. Incidence is 1 in 20,000 individuals vaccinated for the first time. Experts are evaluating the connection.

COLLECTING AND TRANSPORTING SPECIMENS

Equipment

Disposable gown
1 N95 mask
Eye shield
Shoe covers
2 pair gloves
2 zip-closure plastic bags
2 biohazard bags
Label for specimen and chain of custody form

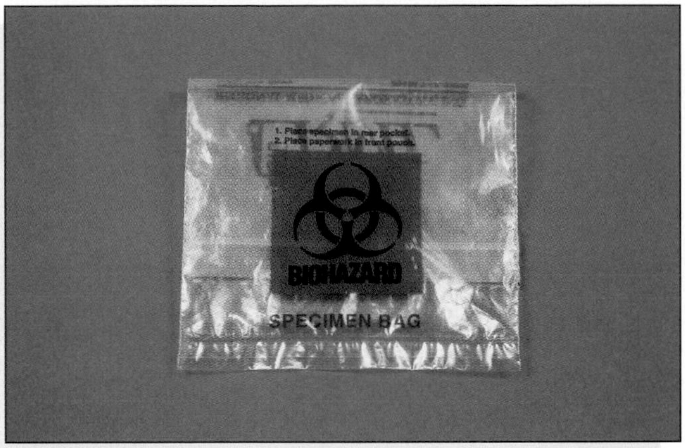

Procedure

1. Acquire and follow specific recommendations for diagnostic sampling of the specific agent.
   a. Perform all sampling according to Standard Precautions. **Rationale:** For protection of health care workers.
   b. Check that laboratory has capacity and equipment to handle specific sample. There are 4 laboratory levels.

Note: Proposed laboratory levels (A through D): local clinical labs for minimal identification of an agent; county or state labs; state and other large labs with advanced capacity for testing; and level D, CDC, or select Department of Defense labs with Bio Safety Level (BSL) testing capacity.

2. Wear protective gear when entering environment where potential for exposure exists. **Rationale:** It is important to safeguard health and safety of persons collecting specimen.
   a. Disposable gown.
   b. Properly fitted N-95 mask. *Note: Mask will not protect males with beards.*
   c. Gloves.
   d. Eye shield.
   e. Shoe covers if indicated.
3. Choose gown with sleeve cuffs that can be covered by stretching gloves up and over cuff. **Rationale:** No skin should be exposed.
4. Collect specimen and place in appropriate container (zip-closure plastic bag, sealed).
5. Remove original gloves handling specimen, and place in biohazard container. **Rationale:** These gloves may have been contaminated.
6. Don new pair of gloves.
7. Place specimen bag in second zip-closure bag and seal, or if specimen is large, in trash bag.
8. Remove protective gear and place in biohazard bag. **Rationale:** Protective equipment may be contaminated.

> **CLINICAL ALERT**
> Be careful not to contaminate outside of either disposal bag during handling.

9. Label specimen on outside of bag with appropriate label: date, person collecting specimen, location, and contact person.
10. Wash hands.
11. Document specimen collection in duplicate, fill out worksheet, "Possible Biological Agent Exposure Contact." **Rationale:** This will warn staff who transport specimen to protect themselves.
12. Give to person designated for this location.
13. Collect an acute phase serum sample, as well as a later convalescent serum sample. **Rationale:** The two samples will be compared as follow-up study.
14. Transport specimens by coordinating with local, state health departments, and the FBI.
    a. Include a chain of custody form with specimen information from moment of collection, completed each time specimen is transferred to another party.
    b. Plan ahead for care of specimens by having appropriate packaging materials and transport media available.

IDENTIFYING CHEMICAL AGENT EXPOSURE

Procedure

Note: Chemical agents may be solid, liquid, or gas; there are numerous ways of disseminating the agent.

1. **Pulmonary agents:** such as chlorine, chloropicrin or phosgene, when inhaled produce pulmonary edema with little damage to other pulmonary tissues (with resulting hypoxemia) and hypovolemia.
   a. Immediate symptoms are irritation of eyes, nose, and upper airways—often not distinctive enough to be recognized as chemical agent exposure.
   b. Two to 24 hours later, victim develops chest tightness, shortness of breath with exertion (later, at rest).
   c. Cough produces clear, frothy sputum, fluid that leaked into lungs.
   d. If symptoms begin soon after exposure, death may occur within hours.

> **CLINICAL ALERT**
> Suspect a chemical agent exposure if health care facility is presented with several nontrauma clients with similar symptoms.

2. **Cyanide agents:** may be gases or solids, such as hydrogen cyanide or cyanogens chloride; with high concentrations death occurs in 6 to 8 minutes.
   a. Initial symptoms are burning irritation of eyes, nose, and airways, and smell of bitter almonds.
   b. Victim's skin may be acyanotic, cherry-red (oxygenated venous blood), or normal.
   c. Large amount of gas inhaled: hyperventilation, convulsions, cessation of breathing (3 to 5 minutes), and no heartbeat (6 to 10 minutes).
3. **Vesicant agents:** cause vesicles or blisters. Common agents are sulfur mustard and lewisite. More lethal than pulmonary agents and cyanide.
   a. Mustard—initial symptoms not observable. Effects begin hours after exposure: erythema, burning and itching with blisters; burning of eyes; airway pain, sore throat, nonproductive cough.
   b. Lewisite—oily liquid that results in topical damage. Vapor causes immediate pain, burning and irritation of eyes, skin and upper airways.

   Note: This is distinguishing feature of lewisite versus mustard when initial symptoms are not observable.

   Cellular damage occurs that can result in hypovolemic shock.
4. **Nerve agents:** liquids or vapors that are the most toxic of all chemical agents. Common agents are Sarin, tabon, Soman, GF, and VX.
   a. Nerve agents block the enzyme acetylcholinesterase, so activity in organs, glands, muscles, smooth muscles, and central nervous system cannot turn off; body systems wear out.
   b. Effects of nerve agent depends on route (vapor or droplet) of exposure and amount; it is felt within seconds.
      (1) Felt first on face: eyes, nose, mouth, and lower airways—watery eyes, runny nose, increased salivation, and constriction of airways, shortness of breath.

CLINICAL ALERT

The most common sign of nerve vapor exposure is constricted pupils (miosis) with reddened, watery eyes.

      (2) Large concentration of vapor: loss of consciousness, convulsions, no breathing.

TRIAGING FOR CHEMICAL AGENT EXPOSURE

Procedure

1. **Pulmonary agents.**
   a. Victim complaining of dyspnea within 6 hours of exposure requires immediate intervention—bed rest (no exertion) and oxygen.
   b. Continued care.
      (1) Continue airway support with oxygen.
      (2) Monitor for hypovolemia and correct acidosis.
      (3) If symptoms are not present within 12 hours, and x-ray, physical exam, and ABGs normal, client may be discharged.
2. **Cyanide agents.**
   a. Antidotes should be administered within minutes of inhalation if client has seizures or respiratory symptoms.
   b. Mild symptoms: give supportive care and monitor.
3. **Vesicant agents.**
   a. Almost all victims will have delayed treatment for skin, eyes, and airway injuries.
   b. Clients with severe airway injury (dyspnea) require intensive pulmonary care.
4. **Nerve agents.**
   a. Victims exposed to liquid nerve agent who show signs of nerve exposure must be decontaminated immediately.

   Rationale: Rapid decontamination will decrease reaction, but not prevent it.
   b. Administer antidotes immediately according to symptoms—multiorgan involvement, respiratory difficulty, convulsions.
   c. Victims suspected of exposure, but who present with no symptoms may have delayed treatment.

Triage in the Hot Zone Following a Chemical Agent Terrorist Attack

- First responders will probably not be able to identify the exact agent.
- Early intervention is critical for nerve agents and cyanide.
- Pulmonary agent exposure will be treated later.
- Intervention in the hot zone generally has to do with airway, breathing, and circulation (ABCs); add antidotes for nerve agents.

MANAGING CARE AFTER CHEMICAL AGENT EXPOSURE

Procedure

1. **Pulmonary agents:** Client with pulmonary edema must be on immediate bed rest with no exertion and receive oxygen.
2. **Cyanide agents:** Administer antidotes.
   a. Client inhales amyl nitrite, or is given sodium nitrite IV (10 mL; 300 mg); frees bound cyanide from hemoglobin to allow O_2 transport.
   b. Sulflur thiosulfate IV (50 mL; 12.5 gm); sulfur converts cyanide to form a nontoxic substance.
   c. Give antidotes sequentially and slowly, titrated to monitor effects; ventilate with oxygen, and correct acidosis.
3. **Vesicant agents.**
   a. Mustard: Immediate decontamination (within 1 minute) will minimize damage; longer will be too late. Irrigate affected skin areas and eyes frequently and apply antibiotics to skin 3 to 4 times/day.
   b. Lewisite: Similar to mustard. Immediate decontamination is important. An antidote for systemic lewisite is British anti-Lewisite (BAL), a drug given IV for heavy metal poisoning.
4. **Nerve agents.**
   a. Personal protection equipment is necessary when decontaminating victims. Decontamination must take place first, before management begins.
   b. Antidotes:
      (1) *Atropine* 2 to 6 mg (average dose 2 to 4 mg) IM. 2 mg more may be administered in 5 to 10 minutes if no improvement. A high initial dose is necessary to block excess neurotransmitter, especially if victim is unconscious.
      (2) *Protopam*, an oxime, 600 mg given slowly IV to counteract nerve agent by removing agent from the enzyme.
      (3) *Valium* might be used for prolonged convulsions.
   c. The military has a device (Mark I Auto-Injection Kit) that holds 2 spring-powered injectors containing two antidotes, Atropine and Protopam, that can be used effectively and quickly to administer antidotes.

IDENTIFYING ACUTE RADIATION SYNDROME

Procedure

1. Assess for an acute illness characterized by manifestations of cellular deficiencies. **Rationale:** Early recognition of the body's reaction to ionizing radiation is important.
   a. Prodromal period: loss of appetite, nausea, vomiting, fatigue, and diarrhea.
   b. Latent period: symptoms disappear for a period of time.
   c. Overt illness follows the latent period—infection, electrolyte imbalance, diarrhea, bleeding.
   d. The final phase is a period of recovery or death.
2. Determine the radiation dose, if possible.

> **CLINICAL ALERT**
> The higher the radiation dose, the greater the severity of early effects and possibility of late effects.

3. Attempt to identify dose exposure of client. **Rationale:** Treatment is according to dose exposure.
   a. Dose less than 2 Gy (200 RADS) is usually not severe; nausea and vomiting seldom experienced at 0.75–1 Gy (75–100 RADS) of penetrating gamma rays.
      (1) Hospitalization unnecessary at less than 2 Gy, thus outpatient care indicated.

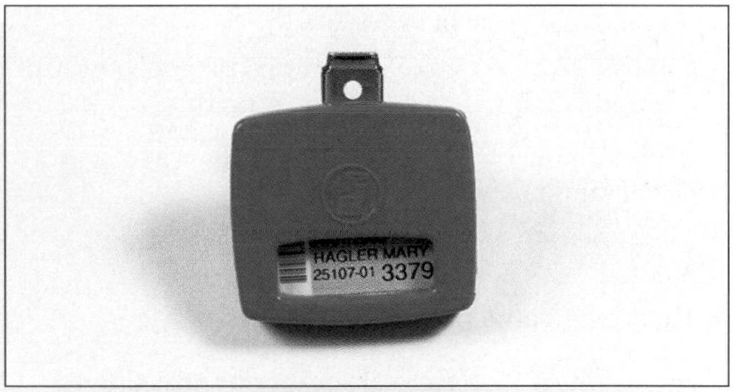

Wear film badge when likely to be exposed to radioactive material.

      (2) Closely monitor and administer frequent CBC with differential blood tests.
   b. Dose greater than 2 Gy (200 RADS).
      (1) Signs and symptoms become increasingly severe with increased dose.
      (2) See box on page 442 for description of four syndromes.
   c. Give supportive care—treat gastric distress with H_2 receptor antagonists (Tagamet, Pepcid, etc.).
   d. Prevent and treat infections—monitor viral prophylaxis.
   e. Consult with hematologist and radiation experts.
   f. Observe for erythema, hair loss, skin injury, mucositis, weight loss, and fever.

4. Identify if radiation dose includes radioactive iodine. **Rationale:** Uptake of this isotope could destroy thyroid tissue.

5. Administer potassium iodide before exposure, if possible, or as soon as available (within 4 hours). **Rationale:** Blocks uptake of specific damaging isotope which protects thyroid tissue.

Acute Radiation Syndromes

- *Hematopoietic syndrome:* Characterized by deficiencies of red blood cells, lymphocytes and platelets, with immunodeficiency; increased infectious complications, including bleeding, anemia, and impaired wound healing.
- *Gastrointestinal syndrome:* Characterized by loss of cells lining intestinal crypts and loss of mucosal barrier with alterations in intestinal motility; fluid and electrolyte loss with vomiting and diarrhea; loss of normal intestinal bacteria, sepsis, and damage to the intestinal microcirculation, along with the hematopoietic syndrome.
- *Cerebrovascular–central nervous system syndrome:* Primarily associated with effects on the vasculature and resultant fluid shifts. Signs and symptoms include vomiting and diarrhea within minutes of exposure; confusion, disorientation, cerebral edema, hypotension, and hyperpyrexia. Fatal in short time.
- *Skin syndrome:* Can occur with other syndromes; characterized by loss of epidermis (and possibly dermis) with "radiation burns."

Source: Oak Ridge Institute for Science and Education (2002). Guidance for Radiation Accident Management, "Managing Radiation Emergencies." www.orau.gov/reacts/syndrome.htm.02/21/02.

Documentation for Bioterrorism Agents, Antidotes, and Vaccinations

Agents of Bioterrorism Identified

- Clinical features of agent (anthrax, plague, botulism, typhoid, VHF, Q fever, smallpox, ricin)
- Incubation period
- Decontamination, if necessary
- Client placement and isolation precautions implemented
- Therapy–treatment implemented

Clients to Whom *Vaccinia* Smallpox Vaccine Administered

- Post-vaccination reactions noted
- Adverse reactions of smallpox vaccination assessed
- Client to whom *vaccinia* immune globulin (VIG) administered
- Specimens collected and destination of transport (Lab)

Chemical Agents Identified (Pulmonary, Cyanide, Vesicant, Nerve)

- Triaging, if necessary, for chemical exposure
- Treatment administered to chemically exposed client

Acute Radiation Syndrome Identified

Critical Thinking Application

UNEXPECTED OUTCOMES	CRITICAL THINKING OPTIONS
Epidemiologic features of disease cannot be identified.	• Examine clusters or unusual numbers of clients with similar signs and symptoms by communicating with other hospitals in the community. • Gather specimens and send them to the appropriate laboratory. • Institute Standard Precautions plus airborne and contact precautions until specific agent is identified.
An effective community response to a terrorist attack is unlikely (hospital does not have a Preparedness Plan in place).	• Form a hospital committee to prepare a Preparedness Plan. • Collect educational materials to fill in areas of content the response team requires to function effectively in the event of a disaster. • Set up practice sessions with post evaluation to increase response effectiveness. • Establish a communication network, so it is already in place in the event of a terrorist attack; assign roles and a command center spokesman.
The U.S. government orders your hospital staff to vaccinate a targeted population for smallpox.	• Collect the necessary material to identify high-risk clients and have the knowledge base to perform the skill of administering smallpox vaccinations. • Practice administering smallpox vaccinations without using the actual vaccine until staff is proficient in the skill.
Client receives smallpox vaccination and inadvertently inoculates eye.	• Request orders to administer VIG IM for complications, if client is appropriate. • Assess that no new lesions appear after VIG doses given over 24–36 hours.

UNIT 2

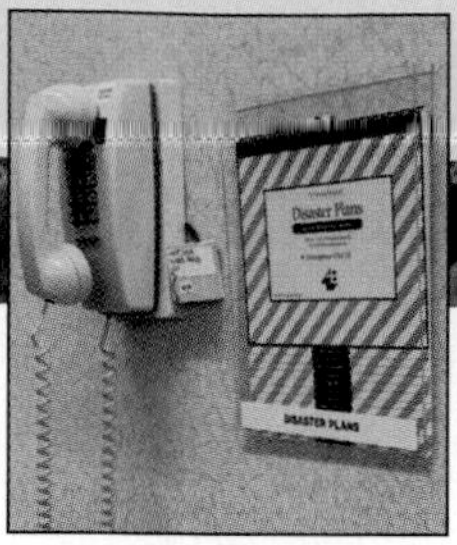

Personal Protective Equipment and Decontamination

Nursing Process Data

ASSESSMENT Data Base

Identify clients who present risk to health care professionals.

Assess need for special equipment (biohazard bags, specimen bags, etc.).

Determine type of protection equipment required according to an identified biohazard (biological, chemical, or radiological).

Assess need for decontaminating victims prior to triage.

Assess strategy for decontamination at site of incident.

Assess need for mass casualty decontamination.

PLANNING Objectives

To select and utilize appropriate personal protection equipment

To demonstrate Standard Precaution techniques

To demonstrate behaviors that help to ensure personal safety

To understand containment principles to avoid spreading contamination

To prevent further spread of biological–chemical–radiological agents with appropriate decontamination procedures

To understand principles of decontaminating via triage

To prevent spread of bioterrorism agents by following guidelines of mass casualty decontamination

IMPLEMENTATION Procedures

Implementing Hospital Infection Control Protocol

Decontaminating via Triage

Choosing Protective Equipment for Biological Exposure

Choosing Protective Equipment for Chemical Exposure

Choosing Protective Equipment for Radiological Attack

Decontaminating Victims Following a Biological Terrorist Event

Decontaminating Victims Following a Chemical Terrorist Event

Decontaminating Victims Following Radiation Exposure

Controlling Radiation Contamination

EVALUATION Expected Outcomes

Appropriate infection control protocols (Standard Precautions) are instituted.

Special equipment is available following a hazardous event.

Appropriate protective equipment is used for the particular biohazard agent present.

Decontamination procedures via triage are implemented appropriately.

Decontamination procedures are implemented according to particular biological–chemical–radiological agent present.

Mass casualty decontamination via triage is carried out effectively.

Radiation exposure is controlled.

IMPLEMENTING HOSPITAL INFECTION CONTROL PROTOCOL

Equipment

Handwashing material
Gloves
Masks (HEPA or N95 for respiratory problems, pneumonia, plague, smallpox, etc.)
Eye shields or face shields
Gowns
Disinfecting material

Procedure

1. Utilize Standard Precautions for all clients admitted to or arriving at the hospital. For specific protocols and skills, see Chapter 14, Infection Control. **Rationale:** Agents of bioterrorism are generally not transmitted person to person.
2. Follow routine client placement for normal number of admissions.
   a. Isolate suspicious cases.
   b. Group similar cases.
3. Utilize alternative placement for large numbers of clients.
   a. Co-group clients with similar syndromes in a designated area.
   b. Establish designated unit, floor, or area in advance.
   c. Place clients based on patterns of airflow and ventilation with respirator problems, smallpox, or plague. **Rationale:** Transmission is through droplets (touching).
   d. Place clients after consultation with engineering staff. **Rationale:** Adequate plumbing and waste disposal must be available.
4. Control entry to client designated areas. **Rationale:** Minimizes possibility of transmission to other clients and staff.
5. Transport bioterrorism clients as little as possible—limit to essential movement. **Rationale:** This practice will reduce opportunity for microorganism transmission within facility.
6. Clean, disinfect, and sterilize equipment according to principles of Standard Precautions.
   a. Use procedures facility has in place for routine cleaning and disinfection.
   b. Have available approved germicidal cleaning solutions.
   c. Contaminated waste should be sorted and disposed of in accordance with biohazard waste regulations. See Handling Biohazard Waste in Chapter 14, page 386.
   d. For clients with bioterrorism-related infections, use Standard Precautions for cleaning unless infecting organism indicates special cleaning.

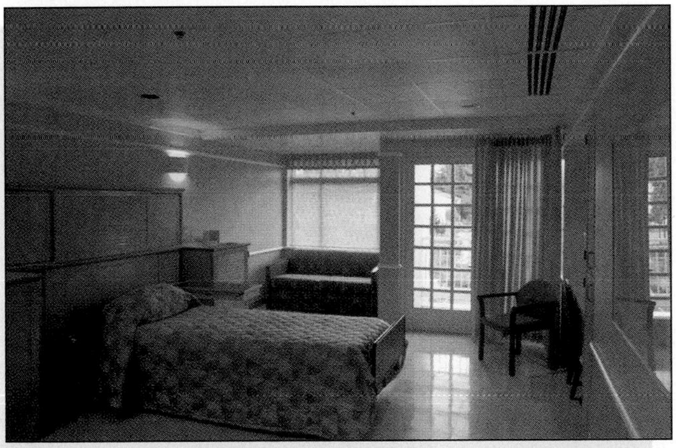

Clients who are placed in isolation require a room with a directional air flow, negative-pressure ventilation system with minimum of 6 to 12 air exchanges per hour.

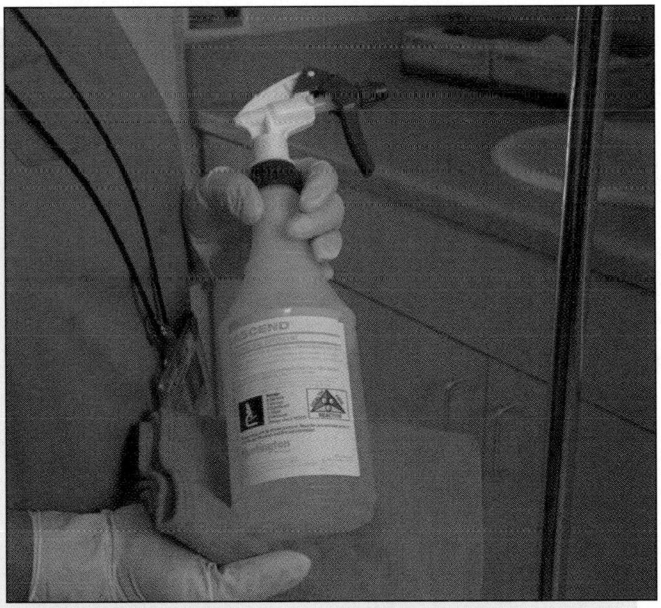

Clean all reusable large equipment thoroughly with antimicrobial or antiseptic agent as required by hospital policy.

Standard Precautions

Washing hands	Use antimicrobial soap or waterless antiseptic agent to clean hands.
Donning gloves	Wear clean nonsterile gloves—to protect health care personnel from touching blood, body fluids, secretions, excretions, and contaminated items.
Donning a gown	A clean, nonsterile gown will protect skin and prevent soiling of clothes.
Wearing a mask	Wear a mask to protect mucous membranes of nose and mouth for workers and victims.
Wearing special masks: HEPA or particulate filter respiratory mask	When bioterrorism agent is suspected and is transmitted via aerosol or airborne, special masks are indicated.
Wearing eye or face shield	Shield will protect mucous membranes of eyes from splash or spray of victim's body fluids.

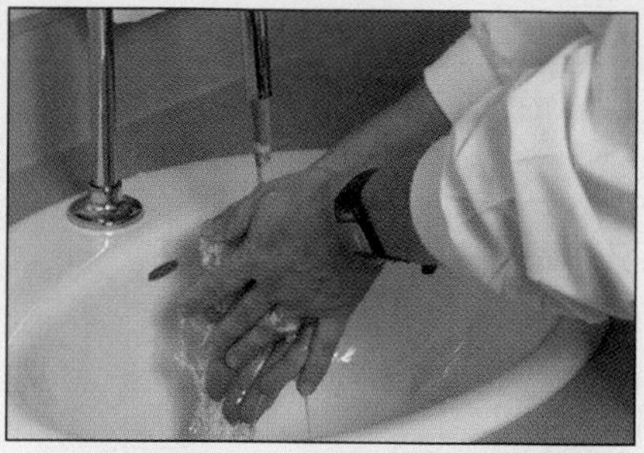

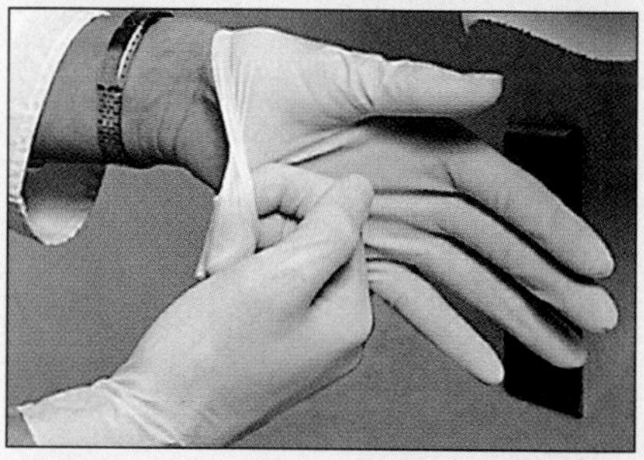

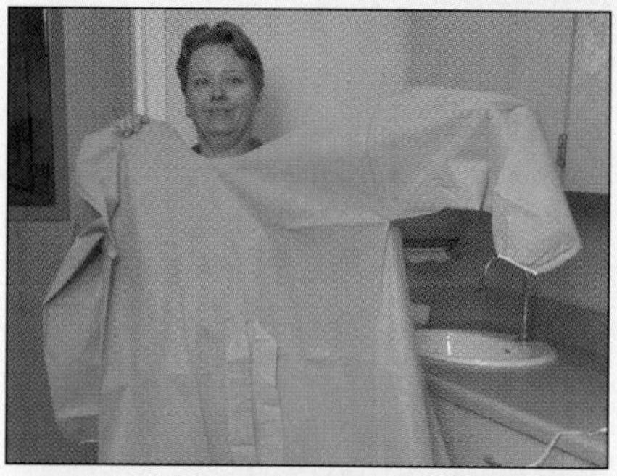

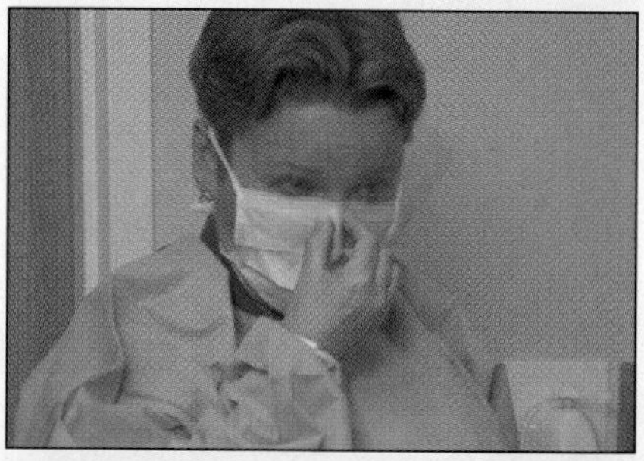

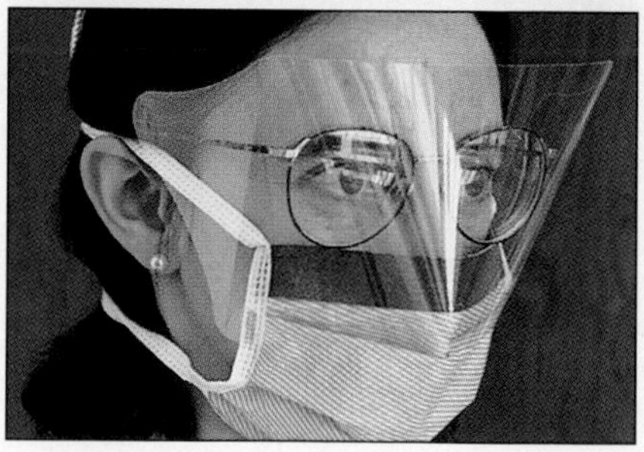

See more complete explanation of Standard Precautions in Chapter 14, Infection Control.

Glove Protection from Toxic Chemicals

- OSHA's new PPE standard requires companies to perform a hazard assessment to determine the need for protective clothing.
- Wide variations in chemical resistance of gloves and protective clothing make equipment selection difficult.
- Many factors affect the performance of gloves during actual use. Toxic chemicals such as pesticides, aromatic amines, and isocyanates can permeate gloves and protective clothing. In addition, flexing, stretching, pressure, and abrasion are physical factors that can cause premature breakthrough.
- A new generation of products produce a color change when permeation occurs, thus providing a method for field validation of the efficacy of protective clothing.
- PERMEA-TEC™ sensors are an example—they are attached to hands before gloving. The detector is placed on thumb, middle finger, and palm, as these areas represent the highest area of contact and abrasion.
- Sensors should be checked hourly to determine when breakthrough occurs, indicating gloves must be changed.

Source: Colormetric Laboratories Inc. (© 1999—modified April 8, 2002). www.clilabs@clilabs.com.

DECONTAMINATING VIA TRIAGE

Equipment

Personal protection equipment including clothing
Water source
Soap
0.5% sodium hypochlorite (HTH chlorine or diluted bleach) cleaning solution
Towels
Waste container for contaminated clothes
Masking tape, 2 inches wide
Body bags
Film badge or chemical agent detector

Procedure

1. Decontaminate at scene of incident (hot zone). **Rationale:** Prevents hospital system from absorbing contaminated victims and protects health care providers and uncontaminated casualties.
2. Familiarize emergency personnel with stages of decontamination. **Rationale:** Effective decontamination is essential for victim and staff protection.
   a. Gross decontamination.
      (1) Decontaminate those who require assistance.
      (2) Remove and dispose of exposed victim's clothing. **Rationale:** This will remove 70–80% of contaminant.
      (3) Perform a thorough head-to-toe tepid water rinse. **Rationale:** Cold water can cause hypothermia and hot water can result in vasodilation, speeding distribution of the contaminants.
   b. Secondary decontamination.
      (1) Perform a full-body rinse with clean tepid water. **Rationale:** Water is an effective decontaminant because of rapidity of application.
      (2) Wash rapidly from head to toe with cleaning solution (HTH chlorine is effective) and rinse with water. **Rationale:** HTH chlorine can decontaminate both chemical and biological contaminants.

Note: Undiluted household bleach is 5.0% sodium hypochlorite.

   c. Definitive decontamination.
      (1) Perform thorough head-to-toe wash and rinse.
      (2) Dry victim and don clean clothes.
3. Initial decontamination may be accomplished by the fire department with hoses spraying water at reduced pressure. **Rationale:** This will remove a high percentage of contaminant at an early stage.
4. Decontaminate salvageable clients first. **Rationale:** This allows those in need of medical intervention to be treated.
   a. Nonsymptomatic and ambulatory victims have lowest priority for decontamination. **Rationale:** The goal is to decontaminate victims who have been exposed, yet are salvageable.
   b. Clients who are dead or unsalvageable have lowest priority for decontamination.
5. Reduce extent of contamination in facility by decontaminating clients prior to receiving in health care facility. **Rationale:** Necessary to ensure safety of clients and staff.
   a. Establish decontamination site outside facility using a decontamination tent prior to needing it. **Rationale:** To protect clients and staff inside facility.
   b. Set up procedures for decontamination, depending on infectious agent.
6. Implement procedure for decontaminating client.
   a. Don appropriate personal protective gear before assisting clients to decontaminate.

b. Remove contaminated clothing and place in appropriate double biohazard bags.
c. Instruct or assist client to shower with soap and water. **Rationale:** Bathing clients in bleach may be potentially harmful. For specific infections, diluted bleach 0.5% is indicated.
d. Use clean water, normal saline, or ophthalmic solution for rinsing eyes.

Guidelines for Setting Up Site for Decontamination

- Establish upwind from contamination area.
- Set up site on a downhill slope, if possible, or on flat ground (so that runoff can be captured).
- Have water source available and, if possible, decontamination solution.
- Have decontamination equipment available, if possible.
- Supply personal protection equipment for health care personnel.
- Notify health care facilities nearby to be available, if possible.
- Maintain security and privacy for site.
- Institute post-decontamination monitoring and checks.

Source: Maniscalco, P., Christen, H. (2002). *Understanding terrorism and managing the consequences,* Brady-Prentice Hall, Upper Saddle River, NJ: Pearson Education.

CHOOSING PROTECTIVE EQUIPMENT FOR BIOLOGICAL EXPOSURE

Equipment

Listed below in procedure

Procedure

1. Plan for protection from biological hazards.
   a. First responders to a biological hazard may be exposed to bacteria, viruses or toxins via inhalation (through respiratory tract) or ingestion (contact with mucous membranes of eyes, nasal tissues, or open cuts).
   b. Biological weapons are particles and will not penetrate proper protective equipment.
   c. Respirators—type selected according to hazard identified and its airborne concentration.
      (1) High level of protection: Self-contained breathing apparatus (SCBA) with full facepiece. Provides highest level of protection against airborne hazards when used correctly. **Rationale:** Reduces exposure to hazard by a factor of 10,000.
      (2) Minimal level of protection: Half-mask or full facepiece air-purifying respirator with particulate filters like N95 (used for TB) or P100 (used for hantavirus).
      (3) Full facepiece respirator (P100 or HEPA filters) used if agent was *not* aerosoled or dissemination was by letter or package that could be bagged.
   d. Protective clothing includes gloves and shoe covers—necessary for full protection. **Rationale:** Prevents skin exposure and/or contamination of other clothing.
      (1) Level A Protective Suit used when a suspected biological incident occurs and type, dissemination method, and concentration is unknown.
      (2) Level B Protective Suit used when biological aerosol is no longer present.

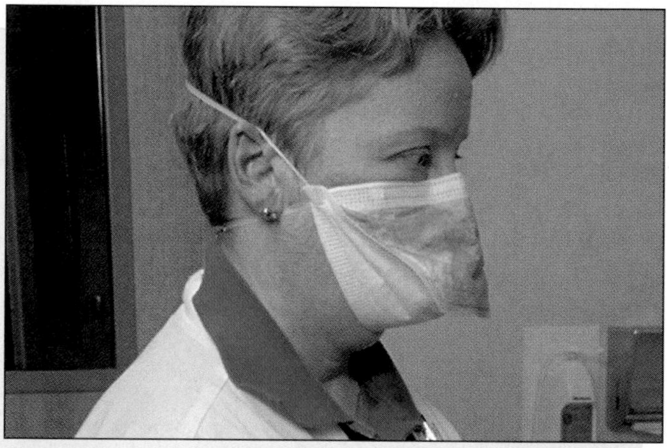

For minimal protection, use particulate filter N95 or HEPA filter respirator when you may be exposed to an unknown biological hazard.

   e. If possible, have biological detection equipment in place—SMART tickets are a handheld point detection system developed by the Navy Medical Institute. Instrument captures antigen and changes color according to 8 different biological agents detected.
2. Identify *anthrax* precautions.
   a. Implement and maintain Standard Precautions (gowns, gloves, and mask). Use Contact Precautions for cutaneous anthrax.

b. Isolation or decontamination is not implemented. **Rationale:** Anthrax is not transmitted by person-to-person contact.
c. If client has been exposed and clothing may be contaminated, decontamination is advised.

3. Identify *plague* precautions.
   a. In a bioterrorism attack, bacterium (*Yersinia pestis*) may be spread by inhalation of droplets, aerosols, or disseminated via infected fleas or other biting insects. **Rationale:** Droplet precautions are used until client has been treated for 2–3 days (gown, gloves, and mask).
   b. Strict isolation until client has been treated for 2–3 days. **Rationale:** So that airborne contaminants do not spread throughout the hospital or community.
   c. Decontamination precautions: soap/shower; 0.5% diluted bleach for visible contamination.
   d. Disinfect environment: 0.5% diluted bleach or EPA approved detergent.
4. Identify *botulism* precautions.
   a. A bioterror attack could disseminate an aerosol of the bacterium or purified neurotoxins. Therefore, use Standard Precautions. **Rationale:** If toxin is used, there is no danger of person-to-person transmission.
   b. Decontamination procedures: toxin may be removed from skin by soap and water.
   c. Place contaminated clothes in sealed plastic bag for biohazard disposal.
   d. Other precautions:
      (1) Environment: diluted bleach 0.5%, 15–20 seconds, or EPA-approved germicidal detergent.
      (2) Boil water for 15 minutes.
      (3) Cook food at 176°F for 30 minutes.
5. Identify *smallpox (variola)* virus.
   a. Spread through airborne or direct contact with skin lesions or secretions. Use Standard Precautions with airborne (respiratory isolation; N95 or P100 mask) and contact precautions (gown and gloves). **Rationale:** Virus is spread through droplet or contact; therefore, isolation decontamination precautions are used.
   b. Isolate and quarantine victim immediately and place in negative pressure room with HEPA filtration or direct exhaust to the outside.
   c. All direct contacts are quarantined for at least 17 days. **Rationale:** Incubation period is 7–17 days.
   d. Cleanse with soap/shower; use 0.5% diluted bleach for gross or visible contamination.
   e. Place mask on victim, if not in isolation. **Rationale:** Virus is spread through airborne method so mask will protect others.
   f. Health care workers maintain standard/airborne/contact precautions for minimum 17 days (until all scabs separate). **Rationale:** When scabs separate, client is no longer contagious.
   g. All bedding and clothing must be autoclaved or laundered in hot water and bleach.
6. Identify *brucellosis* precautions.
   a. Bioterrorism mode of dissemination could be aerosol or food supply sabotage. Standard Precautions indicated. If lesions are draining, use contact precautions.
   b. Decontamination—victim should undress and use soap/shower.
   c. Environment: 0.5% bleach.
7. Identify *typhoidal tularemia* precautions.
   a. Bioterrorism mode of dissemination would probably be aerosol with nontransmission. Use Standard Precautions.
   b. Isolation/decontamination precautions. Victim should undress, use soap and shower. For visible contamination, use 0.5% bleach.
   c. Environment: 0.5% bleach.
8. *Viral encephalitides* precautions.
   a. Bioterrorism mode of dissemination is aerosol. Use Standard Precautions.
   b. Isolation/decontamination precautions. Victim should undress, use shower with soap and large quantity of water.
   c. Mosquito control × 72 hours.
   d. Environment: 0.5% bleach.

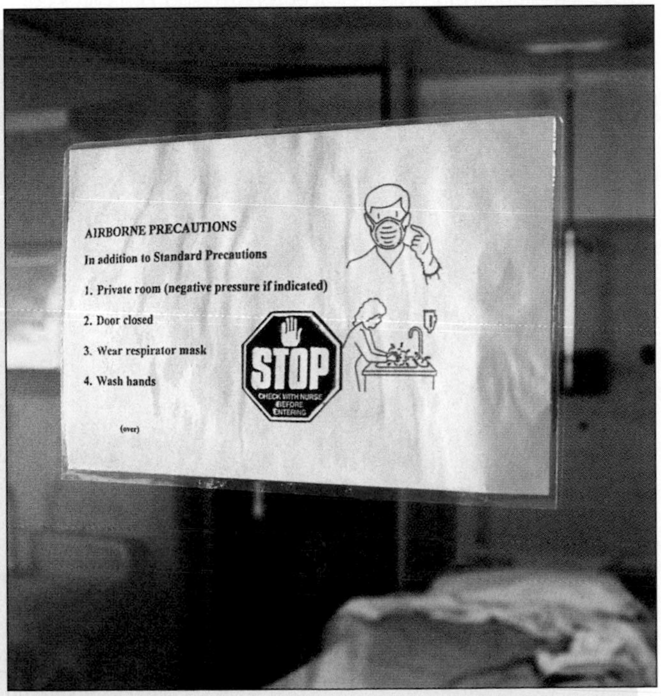
AIRBORNE PRECAUTIONS
In addition to Standard Precautions
1. Private room (negative pressure if indicated)
2. Door closed
3. Wear respirator mask
4. Wash hands
STOP
CHECK WITH NURSE BEFORE ENTERING
(over)

Institute airborne precautions when certain bioterrorism agents such as plague and smallpox are suspected.

The U.S. Government is now launching an early warning system that detects bioterrorism agents released into the air. Adapting 3000 existing monitors that now are used for air pollution, this system could detect biological agents, such as smallpox or anthrax. Results of early warnings could be confirmed at a network of laboratories within 24 hours using DNA analysis.

CHOOSING PROTECTIVE EQUIPMENT FOR CHEMICAL EXPOSURE

Equipment

Listed below in procedure.

Procedure

1. Identify victims who were exposed to chemical substance. **Rationale:** Early identification is essential to save lives, especially from nerve agents or cyanide.
2. Cover all skin surfaces with protective clothing impervious to chemicals. **Rationale:** Necessary for protection until exact chemical agent is identified.
   a. Use Mission Oriented Protective Posture (MOPP) suit, if available (chemical protection suit).
   b. Use fire department chemical suits as alternative.
3. Don masks with filtered respirator. (HEPA filter respirator—P100 with full facepiece—and fit-tested N95 meet CDC performance criteria for chemical exposure.) **Rationale:** Chemicals can be inhaled.
4. Wear boots or boot covers. **Rationale:** Feet should be covered to prevent tracking contaminant.
5. Initiate decontamination procedures with trained personnel.
   a. Decontaminate at site, if possible.
   b. Otherwise, decontaminate outside of facility.
6. Use chemical detection devices, if available. **Rationale:** Devices would validate presence or absence of agent.
   a. M8 Paper: Sheet of chemically treated paper—if colored spots appear within 20 seconds, chemical agent is present.
   b. M9 Tape: Affix adhesive backed paper to equipment or protective clothing—color changes when exposed to chemical agent.
   c. M2S6A1 Chemical Agent Detector Kit: Can detect nerve, blister or blood agent vapors; a glass ampule contains substance that, when placed on test spot, changes color.
   d. Chemical Agent Monitors (CAMs): Contain a microprocessor chip that identifies presence of certain nerve and blister agents.

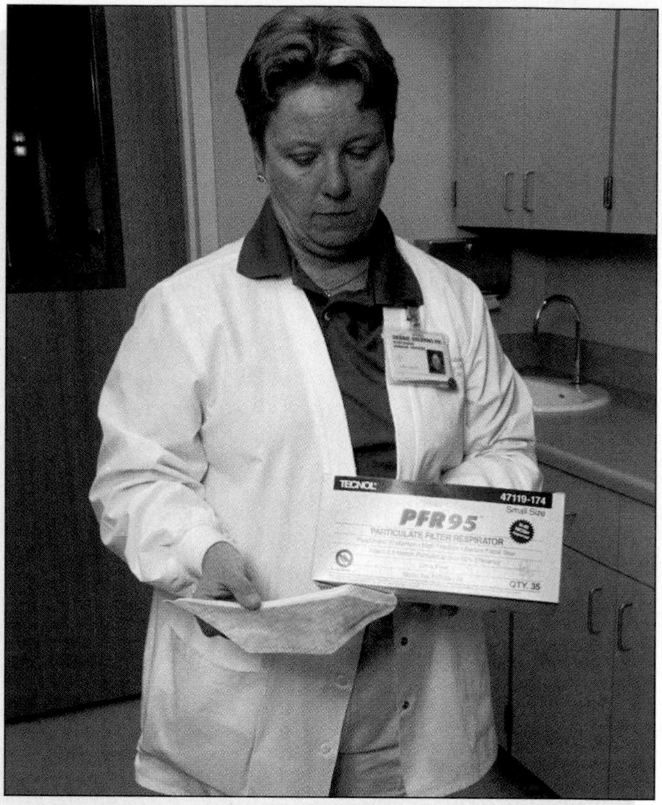

For chemical or certain biological exposure, masks with HEPA filtered respirator or N95 should be used.

CHOOSING PROTECTIVE EQUIPMENT FOR A RADIOLOGICAL ATTACK

Equipment

Listed below in procedure.

Procedure

1. Identify victims contaminated by radiation. **Rationale:** If victim is contaminated, clothes, skin, etc., can transmit contamination to others.
   a. If victim was exposed to ionizing radiation (most common are alpha, beta particles, and gamma rays), contamination occurred.
   b. The higher the dose of radiation, the greater the severity of contamination.
2. Don protective clothing: basic gear will stop alpha and some beta particles, not gamma rays. **Rationale:** Necessary to protect responders from exposure and to prevent cross-contamination, exposing other clients.
   a. Scrub suit.
   b. Gown and cap.
   c. Mask.
   d. Eye shield.
   e. Double gloves—one pair under cuff of gown and taped to close all entry; second pair can be removed and/or replaced.
   f. Masking tape, 2 inches wide.
   g. Shoe cover with all seams taped.
   h. Radiation detection device: able to detect energy emitted from a radiation source. Several detectors available: Geiger counters, dosimeters, etc.
   i. Film badge.

3. Transport victim to facility.
   a. If victim is not decontaminated at site, set up portable decontamination unit prior to entering facility.
   b. Double-bag all victim's clothing in sealed biohazard plastic bags marked "Radioactive."
4. Institute decontamination procedures.
   a. Open wounds or nonintact skin: irrigate with sterile water or normal saline (NS); cover with dry, sterile dressing.
   b. Eyes: irrigate with sterile water of NS according to skill, "Irrigating the Eyes," Chapter 18.
   c. Intact skin: wash skin with soap and warm water. Bleach, 0.5%, may also be used.
   d. Radiation burns: treat as other burns are treated.
5. Recheck radiation levels at each stage of treatment until reduced to background levels.
6. Dispose of used protective gear appropriately. **Rationale:** This gear is radiologically contaminated waste, and to prevent cross-contamination it must be treated as such.

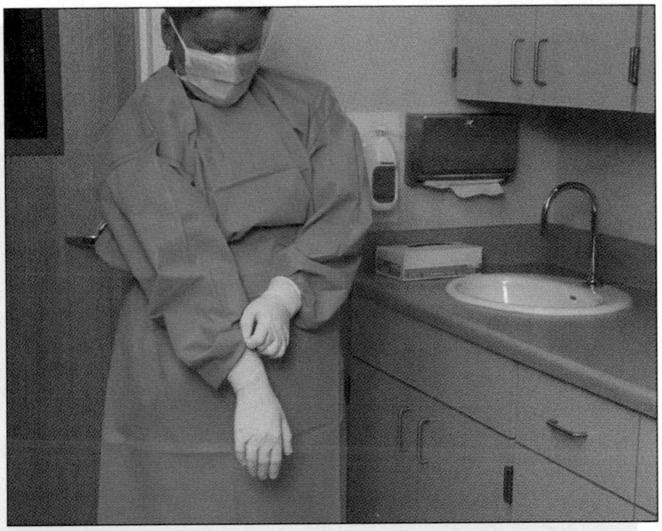

When exposed to radiological material, double gloves that cover all skin exposure should be worn.

DECONTAMINATING VICTIMS FOLLOWING A BIOLOGICAL TERRORIST EVENT

Equipment

Protective clothing for health care worker
Biohazard bags
Soap and water; diluted sodium hypochlorite (bleach)

Procedure

1. Don protective clothing and adhere strictly to Standard Precautions for emergency personnel. **Rationale:** This will prevent secondary contamination of personnel.
2. Identify dermal exposure, if possible. **Rationale:** Biological agents are difficult to detect.
3. Remove victim's clothing as soon as possible and place in biohazard bags. **Rationale:** If victim was exposed, clothing is contaminated.
4. Cleanse exposed areas using soap and tepid water (large amounts) or diluted sodium hypochlorite (0.5%).
5. Send victims home, if possible, to continue decontamination procedure by washing thoroughly with soap and water.
   a. Instruct victims to monitor for signs and symptoms of agent.
   b. Inform victim of results of lab analysis as soon as possible.

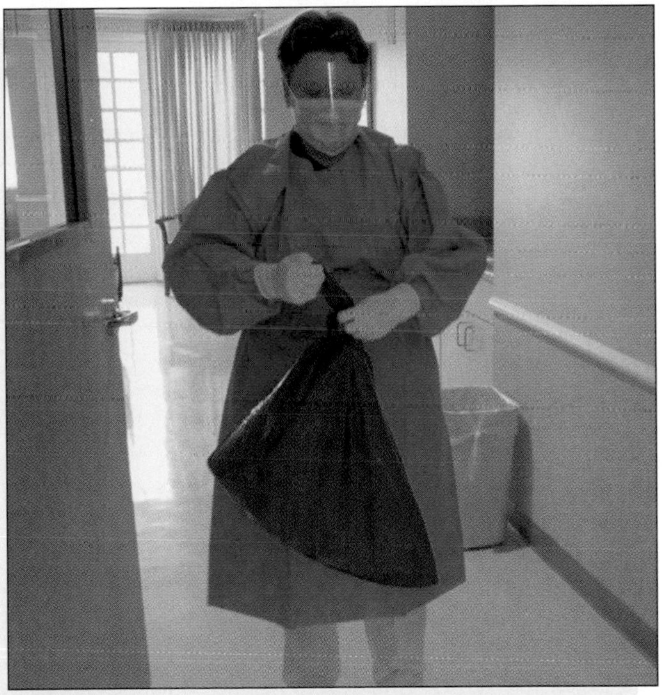

Dispose of all contaminated clothing in appropriate biohazard bags.

DECONTAMINATING VICTIMS FOLLOWING A CHEMICAL TERRORIST EVENT

Equipment

Protective equipment for health care workers
Biohazard bags
Soap and water; diluted sodium hypochlorite (bleach)
Saline or isotonic bicarbonate
Chemical agent monitor or M8 paper

Procedure

1. Know general principles to guide actions following a chemical agent incident.*
   a. Expect a 5:1 ratio of unaffected:affected casualties.
   b. Decontaminate immediately (ASAP).
   c. Disrobing is decontamination, head to toe; the more removal, the better.
   d. Large volume water flush is best decontamination method.
   e. Following exposure, first-responders must decontaminate immediately to avoid serious effects.
2. Practice triage guidelines for Mass Casualty Decontamination.* **Rationale:** Chemical exposure can be deadly, so early decontamination is critical. Decontaminate according to:
   a. Casualties closest to point of release.
   b. Casualties reporting exposure to vapor or aerosol.
   c. Casualties with liquid deposits on clothing or skin.
   d. Casualties with serious medical conditions.
   e. Casualties with conventional injuries.
3. Decontaminate victims as early as possible. **Rationale:** Requirements differ according to type of chemical agent used: sarin dissipates quickly in the air; VX remains lethal for hours.
   a. Nerve agents may be absorbed on all body surfaces—must be removed quickly to be effective.
   b. Vesicant (blister) agents are not always identified due to latent effects.
4. Treat eyes and mucous membranes with special protocol.
   a. Flush with copious amounts of water. **Rationale:** Eyes and mucous membranes are too sensitive to use other skin decontaminant solutions.
   b. If available, isotonic bicarbonate (1.26%) or saline (0.9%) may be used as a flushing agent.
5. Monitor victim for remains of agent or contaminant using chemical agent monitor (CAM) or M8 paper for chemical agents. **Rationale:** To validate removal of contaminant.

Note: Skin decontamination kits are (M258A1) available designed for chemical decontamination. They hold wipes that contain a solution that neutralizes most nerve and blister agents.

**Source:* Guidelines for Mass Decontamination During a Terrorist Chemical Agent Incident. U.S. Army Soldier and Biological Chemical Command, Jan. 2000. (Download at http://www2.sbccom.army.mil/hld.)

DECONTAMINATING VICTIMS FOLLOWING RADIATION EXPOSURE

Equipment

Personal protection equipment including self-contained breathing equipment and flash suits, if indicated
Surgical attire or disposable garments, shoe covers, eye shield, gloves, and masks with respirators
Water source and container to catch runoff
Bins for contaminated clothing
Biohazard bags
Vacuum cleaner with HEPA filter
Radiation dose meter

Procedure

1. Determine cause of incident to identify radiation exposure or contamination. **Rationale:** Exposure does not necessarily indicate need for decontamination.
   a. First responders may be told by those requesting assistance that there has been a radiation-exposure event.
   b. First responders may recognize radiation exposure from observation at incident site.
2. Understand difference between exposure and contamination.
   a. Exposed victim: presents no hazard, requires no special handling, and presents no radiological threat to personnel. **Rationale:** This is no different from client who has had diagnostic x-rays.
   b. Externally contaminated victim: may mean individual has come in contact with unconfined radioactive material. **Rationale:** Any person or object contaminated by radioactivity must be considered contaminated. Steps should be taken to minimize contamination.
   c. Internal contamination: occurs by inhalation or ingestion (airborne radioactive particles) or through an open wound. *Usually* this form of contamination is not a hazard to others.
3. Use appropriate personnel protection equipment (PPE). **Rationale:** This will protect personnel who may come in contact with contaminated victim.
   a. If radiation incident is suspected, self-contained breathing apparatus (SCBA) and flash suits are indicated. **Rationale:** This will reduce potential exposure of health-care providers. Inhalation of radioactive particles is cross-contamination hazard.
   b. If SCBA suits not available:
      (1) Use surgical attire or disposable garments (such as those made of Tyvek).
      (2) Use eye protection and double gloves.
      (3) Use masks with respirators. **Rationale:** These will protect health care workers from inhaling radioactive particles leading to internal contamination.
   c. It is important to recognize that external radiation (such as penetration by gamma rays) is *not* dangerous to emergency personnel—the only exception to this rule is a rare

neutron radiation exposure. **Rationale:** Gamma ray radiation is absorbed by or passes through the body, but does not leave radioactive contamination.
   d. If monitoring for radiation is not available, consider all clients contaminated.
   e. Personnel should minimize time in radiation zone. **Rationale:** Radiation exposure depends on time, distance, and shielding.
4. Triage client's medical condition first, regardless of radiation exposure. **Rationale:** First priority is delivery of emergency medical services, including transport.
   a. Administer emergency medical treatment to radiation-exposed clients.
   b. Decontaminate clients who have been contaminated on the scene before transport.
5. Complete decontamination of victims. **Rationale:** Until decontamination is complete, victims are an exposure risk to selves, staff, and others.
   a. Remove client's clothing and have client do a total body wash, scrubbing skin with soap and soft brush. **Rationale:** Removal of victim's clothing will reduce 80% of the contamination.
   b. Place contaminated clothing in bins or biohazard bag labeled "Radioactive."
   c. Capture runoff of water; contain and label "Radioactive."
   d. Wash area down between washing victims. **Rationale:** This will prevent transfer of contaminated material.
   e. Capture material with vacuum cleaner with HEPA filter, if appropriate. **Rationale:** This prevents release of radioactive material into the air.
   f. Monitor client with radiation meter to measure radiation.
6. Implement isolation techniques for contaminated victims. **Rationale:** To confine contamination and protect personnel.

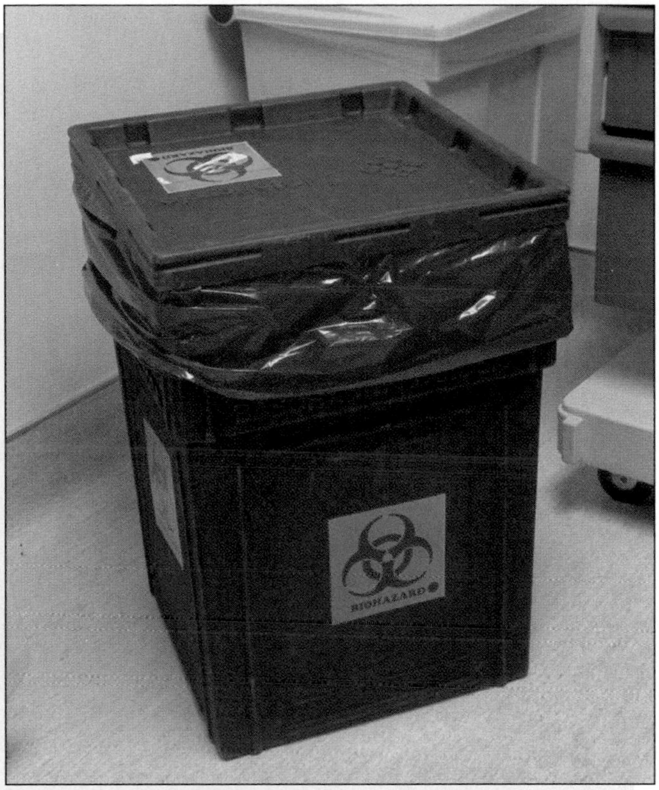

Place contaminated clothing in bins or biohazard bag labeled "RADIOACTIVE" if that is source of contamination.

7. Determine source of radiation, type of radioactive material, length of time of exposure, if possible. **Rationale:** This is valuable data for long-term interventions, but does not alter immediate handling and transport of victim.

CONTROLLING RADIATION CONTAMINATION

Equipment

Soap and water
Disposable client equipment
Biohazard bags
Wide tape
White tape
Heavy, wide paper
Plastic-lined containers
Radiation meter

Procedure

1. Decontaminate all victims; remove all clothing and complete a full body wash. **Rationale:** This will reduce most of the contamination.
2. Institute isolation techniques. **Rationale:** This will confine contamination and protect others.
3. Decontaminate equipment touched by client.
   a. Gurney used to transfer client.
   b. Equipment used in client care (BP cuff, stethoscope, etc.)
   c. Ambulance.
4. Decontaminate care providers who touched or moved client. **Rationale:** Protective clothing may be contaminated.
5. Examine surrounding area (walls, floor that client may have touched).
6. Control entry and exit of victims. **Rationale:** Radioactive particles adhere to dust, may become airborne, and can contaminate other clients and personnel.
   a. Mark entry area with white tape to differentiate areas.
   b. Restrict access to controlled area.

c. Monitor everyone leaving controlled area—have persons cleared by radiation safety officer.
7. Cover floor areas with rolls of heavy, wide paper and tape securely to floor. **Rationale:** To prevent tracking of contaminants.
8. Control waste by using large plastic-lined containers for contaminated articles.
9. Monitor radiation by using meter.

DOCUMENTATION FOR PERSONAL PROTECTIVE EQUIPMENT AND DECONTAMINATION

- Specific infection control protocols implemented (i.e., Standard or Airborne Precautions)
- Personal protection gear and equipment used
- Decontamination site established
- Decontamination procedure used for biological or chemical event
- Radiation exposure decontamination procedure

Critical Thinking Application

UNEXPECTED OUTCOMES	CRITICAL THINKING OPTIONS
Mass casualty disaster occurs with hundreds of victims affected in one area.	• Don protective gear before approaching WMD site. • Identify weapon or agent used to create disaster, if possible. • Institute field triage (triage first done at site before victims sent to community health care facilities). • Decontaminate victims at site before transporting to treatment facility.
Type of personal protection equipment is unknown for agent exposure.	• It is critical that response team be fully protected; thus, choose highest level of equipment; that is, assume you need: (1) airborne protection with respirators—self-contained breathing apparatus (SCBA) with full face piece. (2) full Level A protective suit. (3) shoe covers and double gloves. (4) biological detection device, if available.
Clients are admitted with potential radiation exposure.	• Determine if radiation is exposure or contamination; if the latter, use protective gear and radiation dose meter. • Decontaminate clients by removing all clothing and giving a full body wash—institute isolation techniques. • Decontaminate all equipment, surfaces, and personnel that came in contact with client. • Administer treatment according to dose exposure: supportive care, frequent blood tests (CBC and differential), and prevent infection.

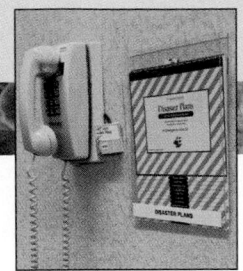

Triage and a Communication Matrix

Nursing Process Data

ASSESSMENT *Data Base*

Assess the need to establish triage treatment areas.
Validate that public health parameters are established.
Observe that the steps of triage are followed.
Assess that victim is not in immediate danger or, conversely, requires immediate intervention.
Assess vital signs of victims.
Assess the treatment steps necessary to treat life-threatening conditions.
- Observe for signs of respiratory distress.
- Assess need for establishing an airway.
- Observe for amount and source of bleeding and need for intervention.
- Recognize shock state and need for intervention.

Assess victims post-triage and observe for any signs or symptoms that indicate major injury.
Identify victims having a severe psychological reaction to bioterrorism event.
Assess possibility of post-traumatic stress syndrome developing.
Assess that lines of communication are established and activated.
Assess that Federal Response Plan is activated.
Assess that external, internal, and collaborative communication networks are in place.

PLANNING *Objectives*

To establish a triage site taking into account public health parameters
To establish triage treatment areas appropriate to number and injuries of victims
To follow steps of triage
To observe for any signs/symptoms that indicate major injury
To treat life-threatening conditions
To care for clients with major psychological reactions to bioterrorism event
To prevent post-terrorism trauma
To develop a communication network including external, internal, and collaborative

IMPLEMENTATION *Procedures*

Establishing Triage Treatment Areas
Establishing Public Health Parameters
Developing a Communication Network
Establishing Viable Communication
Treating Life-Threatening Conditions
Assessing Victims Post-Triage
Caring for Those Who Died
Caring for Clients with Psychological Reactions
Identifying Post-Traumatic Stress Disorder

EVALUATION Expected Outcomes

Appropriate triage site is established.
Steps of triage evaluation are followed.
Assessment is completed before treatment is begun.
Appropriate intervention is implemented for life-threatening conditions.
Victims are assessed post-triage.
Severe psychological reactions are recognized and plan for intervention instituted.
Lines of communication are established.
Federal Response Plan is activated, if needed.

ESTABLISHING TRIAGE TREATMENT AREAS

Procedure

1. Assign roles to personnel in treatment areas.
2. Select a site as soon as possible—advance planning is essential.
   a. Select safe area, free of hazards and debris.
   b. Position site upwind of hazard zone.
   c. Determine whether site is accessible to transportation vehicles (ambulances, trucks, helicopters).
   d. Be sure site is able to expand.

> **CLINICAL ALERT**
> Survey entire scene, including area above you, for threats to your safety before beginning triage or team work.

3. Protect treatment area and delineate area using tarps, etc. If possible, do not contaminate a crime scene.
4. Set up signs to identify subdivisions of area.
   a. I = Immediate care.
   b. D = Delayed care.
   c. Dead = Dead for morgue.
5. Establish I and D areas close together. **Rationale:** Facilitates verbal communication between workers who can also share medical supplies and transfer victims quickly when status changes.
6. Position victims in head-to-toe configuration, with 2–3 feet between victims. **Rationale:** This system will effectively use space and personnel.
7. Establish morgue site secure and away (and not visible) from medical treatment areas.

ESTABLISHING PUBLIC HEALTH PARAMETERS

Equipment

Soap and water; antibacterial gel
Gloves
Mask and goggles
Biohazard waste disposal containers
Plastic bags
Water purification equipment
Search and rescue equipment

Procedure

1. Assign personnel to monitor public health concerns where disaster victims are sheltered. **Rationale:** To avoid or minimize spread of disease.
2. Have available search and rescue safety equipment.
   a. Helmet or hardhat.
   b. Goggles.
   c. Sturdy work gloves and shoes.
   d. Clothing appropriate for weather conditions.
   e. Dust mask or appropriate filtered mask (see Protection section).
   f. Rescue whistle.
3. Maintain proper hygiene by washing hands and using gloves.
   a. Wash hands with soap and water if dirty or antibacterial gel between victims.
   b. Wear gloves at all times.
   c. Change gloves between victims if possible. If not, clean them between victims in a bleach and water solution (1 part bleach to 9 parts water).
4. Wear a mask and goggles.
5. Avoid direct contact with body fluids.
6. Maintain sanitation.
   a. Mark and have available specific biohazard waste disposal containers where bacterial sources (gloves, dressings, etc.) are discarded.
   b. Place waste products in plastic bags and bury them in designated area.
   c. Bury human waste.

7. Purify water for drinking, cooking, medical use, if potable water is not available.
   a. Boil water at rolling boil for 10 minutes.
   b. Use water purification tablets.
   c. Use unscented liquid bleach (16 drops per gallon of water or 1 teaspoon per 5 gallons; mix and let stand for 30 minutes).

ORGANIZATION OF MEDICAL OPERATIONS FOLLOWING A DISASTER*

TRIAGE	TRANSPORT	TREATMENT	MORGUE	SUPPLY
• Triager • Transcriber • Back-up	• Litter Bearers • Back-up	• Immediate - TX Leader • Delayed - TX Leader	• Security • Identification • Location • Disposition	• Procurement • Distribution

* CERT Training: Participant Handbook

Steps of Triage

1. Don protective gear for own safety.
2. Evaluate disaster scene: stop, look, listen, check safety.
3. Perform voice triage—tell victims who you are and ask them to walk (if possible) to your team.
4. Conduct triage: **I (Immediate), D (Delayed) and Dead.** All victims must be tagged.
5. Treat **I** (Immediate) victims (airway, bleeding, shock).
6. Document results.

DEVELOPING A COMMUNICATION NETWORK

Procedure

1. Understand lines of communication. **Rationale:** When lines of communication are compromised, effective triage and intervention cannot take place.
   a. Mass casualty incident occurs.
   b. Local public health official notifies FBI—lead agency for crisis plan.
   c. FBI notifies DHS, HHS, CDC, and FEMA.
   d. State health agency requests CDC to deploy response teams if needed.
2. Understand the network of communication that will be activated in response to a suspected or actual bioterrorism event.
   a. Emergency response team:
      Local and state public health officials.
      Infection control personnel in notified facilities.
      FBI field offices (Dept. of Homeland Security).
      CDC.
      Local emergency medical services (EMS).
      Local police and fire departments.
   b. In turn, the Federal Response Plan will be activated.
3. Activate Federal Response Plan. **Rationale:** When the local area cannot cope with the disaster, federal assistance is available.
   a. Department of Health and Human Services (HHS) is primary agency.
   b. Office of Emergency Preparedness is action agency.
   c. Emergency Support Function N8 coordinates federal assistance to supplement state and local resources (directed by HHS).
   d. Implemented when state requests assistance and FEMA agrees.

EVIDENCE BASED NURSING PRACTICE

Who Can You Count On?

Research has repeatedly shown that disasters result in increased pro-social behavior, where cooperation and consensus are present during the emergency response phase, and self-interested activity is set aside.

Source: Tierney, K., Lindell, M., Perry, R. (2001). *Facing the unexpected: Disaster preparedness and response in the US.* Joseph Henry Press.

ESTABLISHING VIABLE COMMUNICATION

Procedure

1. Set up **external communication** system designated spokesperson.
   a. A viable system will minimize disruption.
   b. All communication goes through designated spokesperson—no staff will communicate with the public, press, or outside persons.
2. Report to appointed community-wide regional spokesperson or small group designated as being in command throughout the incident. Spokesperson will be in charge of coordination of all media relations. **Rationale:** One person or small group in charge will minimize confusion.
3. Set up a single community site for family and friends to obtain victim-locator information. **Rationale:** More than one site will lead to mass confusion.
   a. Provide clear, consistent, and verifiable information to clients and general public.
   b. Plan in advance methods and channels of communication to be used to inform the public.
4. Establish **internal communication.**
   a. Determine position (not person) that will be in charge (i.e., emergency department supervisor, called "incident commander"). **Rationale:** Position, rather than person, will negate confusion when there is staff turnover, multiple shifts, or reassignment of staff.
   b. Communicate only through established lines of communication with designated commander or liaisons.
5. Establish a **collaborative communication system.**
   a. Establish ongoing, open channels of communication with emergency response teams. **Rationale:** Response teams may have first awareness of the disaster and will need to communicate with the hospital.
   b. Appoint person (reporting to spokesperson) to collaborate with response team and link to community representative.
   c. Develop a community-wide communications network. **Rationale:** If different organizations cannot communicate with each other, precious time will be lost.

Note: Local areas are beginning to establish their own interconnected networks to facilitate communication. For example, all of New York City's hospitals are connected via the Internet, so if victims begin to funnel into several facilities, their symptoms can be quickly correlated to establish a diagnosis.

   d. Test the communications network so overload does not occur in the event of a mass casualty incident.
6. Develop clear communication systems that have access to telecommunications as well as a person-to-person communication system. **Rationale:** This position-to-position or person-to-person system is necessary if telecommunications are overwhelmed or unavailable.
   a. Use pagers, walkie-talkies, and the Internet via e-mail as substitutes for communication network during a disaster.
   b. Develop horizontal and vertical relationships between organizations, governmental and private, that will have to work together in a mass casualty event.

CLINICAL ALERT

The goal of disaster medical interventions is to do the greatest good for the greatest number of victims.

TREATING LIFE-THREATENING CONDITIONS

Equipment

Protective gear
Dressings/Bandages
Tourniquets
Stethoscope
Tongue blades
Automated external defibrillator (AED), if available

Procedure

1. Implement Simple Triage and Rapid Treatment (START). **Rationale:** This is the first step for treating multiple casualties in a disaster.
2. **Check breathing immediately.**
   a. Open airway. **Rationale:** If airway is obstructed, victim cannot get oxygen.
   b. Move fast—time is critical. **Rationale:** Heart function will be affected within minutes, and brain damage is possible after 4 minutes.
   c. Check if tongue is obstructing airway. **Rationale:** This is the most common airway obstruction (especially when victim is positioned on back).
3. Use head-tilt/chin-lift method if victim is not breathing and airway is not obstructed.
   a. Touch victim and shout, "CAN YOU HEAR ME?" **Rationale:** To ensure victim has not fainted.
   b. If victim does not respond, place one hand on forehead, two fingers of other hand under chin, and tilt jaw

upward and head back slightly. **Rationale:** This position opens airway.
c. Look for chest to rise, listen for air exchange, and feel for abdominal movement. **Rationale:** Reliable indicator of open airway is feeling or hearing air movement.
d. If no response (victim does not start breathing), repeat procedure. (If AED is available, may apply to victim.)
e. If victim does not respond after second attempt, move on to next victim. **Rationale:** Goal of disaster intervention is to do the greatest good for the greatest number of victims.
f. If the victim begins breathing, maintain airway (hopefully with a volunteer holding airway open) or place soft object under victim's shoulders to elevate them, keeping airway open.

4. **Control bleeding. Rationale:** If bleeding is not controlled within a short period of time, victim will go into shock. Loss of 1 liter of blood—out of a total of 5 in the human body—will present risk of death.
5. Identify type of bleeding.
   a. Arterial bleeding (spurting blood)
   b. Venous bleeding (flowing blood)
   c. Capillary bleeding (oozing blood)
6. Choose appropriate method to control bleeding.
   a. Direct local pressure—place direct pressure over wound (using clean or sterile pad) and press firmly. **Rationale:** 95% of bleeding can be controlled by direct pressure with elevation.
   b. Maintain compression by wrapping wound firmly with pressure bandage.
   c. Elevate wound above level of heart.
   d. Use pressure point to slow blood flow to wound, brachial point for arm, femoral point for leg. **Rationale:** Using pressure on a pulse point on a major artery will slow blood flow.
7. Use tourniquet if bleeding cannot be controlled by other methods (consider this a last resort). **Rationale:** Tourniquets can pose serious risks to affected limbs.
   a. Incorrect material or application can cause more damage and bleeding; if too tight, nerves, blood vessels, or muscles may be damaged.
   b. If tourniquet is left in place too long, limb may be lost.
   c. If tourniquet is applied, leave in plain sight and affix label to victim's forehead, stating time tourniquet was applied.
   d. Notify physician to remove tourniquet.
8. **Recognize and treat shock. Rationale:** If the victim remains in shock, it will lead to death of cells, tissue, and organs.
   a. Body will initially compensate for blood loss, so signs of shock may not be observable.
   b. Continually evaluate victim's condition.
9. Observe for signs/symptoms of shock.
   a. Rapid, shallow breathing (<30/min).
   b. Cold, pale skin (capillary refill <2/sec).
   c. Failure to respond to simple commands.
10. Administer treatment for shock.
    a. Position victim supine with feet elevated 6–10 inches.
    b. Maintain open airway.
    c. Maintain body temperature (cover ground and victim).
    d. Avoid rough or excessive handling, and do not allow victim to eat or drink.

Steps of Trauma Assessment Applied to Triage

1. Perform a rapid systematic assessment. **Rationale:** Trauma is a multisystem condition so all systems must be assessed.
2. Complete a primary trauma assessment. **Rationale:** To identify victim's primary and critical problem.
   a. Airway.
   b. Breathing capability.
   c. Shock—circulation and bleeding.
   d. Neurological—level of consciousness, mental status.
   e. Exposure to contaminate.
   f. Disability.
   g. Evacuation necessity.
3. Complete a secondary assessment (post-triage) that includes a focus assessment.

CLINICAL ALERT

Experts agree that 49% of disaster victims could be saved by providing simple medical care for life-threatening conditions: airway obstruction, bleeding, and shock.

ASSESSING VICTIMS POST-TRIAGE

Procedure

1. Perform head-to-toe assessment, always in the same order. **Rationale:** Performing assessment in same way every time will enable you to complete it more quickly and accurately.
   a. Head
   b. Neck
   c. Shoulders
   d. Chest
   e. Arms
   f. Abdomen
   g. Pelvis

h. Legs
i. Back

2. Complete assessment before beginning any treatment. **Rationale:** In order to prioritize treatment interventions, a complete assessment must be done.
3. Observe for any sign/symptom that indicates major injury.
   a. Assess how person received injury (mechanism of injury)
   b. Airway obstruction
   c. Signs of shock
   d. Labored or difficult breathing
   e. Excessive bleeding
   f. Swelling/bruising
   g. Severe pain
4. Provide immediate treatment. During treatment, reclassify victim, if necessary.
5. Assess that victim is not in immediate danger. If available staff, continue to assess for signs of head, neck, and spinal injury.
   a. Change in level of consciousness (unconscious, confused)
   b. Unable to move body part
   c. Severe pain in head, neck, back
   d. Tingling or numbness in extremities
   e. Difficulty breathing or seeing
   f. Heavy bleeding/blood in eyes or nose
   g. Seizures
   h. Nausea, vomiting
   i. Possible closed compression injury (e.g., victim found under collapsed structure)
6. Immobilize head, neck, or spine by keeping spine in straight line, putting cervical collar on neck, or placing victim on board—if equipment is available.
7. Document who person is and relevant medical information.
   a. Available identifying data
   b. Description, clothing
   c. Injuries
   d. Treatment
   e. Transfer location

Phases of Death Due to Trauma

Phase 1	Death within minutes due to overwhelming and irreversible damage to vital organs.
Phase 2	Death within several hours due to excessive bleeding.
Phase 3	Death within several days or weeks due to infection or multiple system failure (not from injury per se).

Experts agree that over 40% of disaster victims in Phases 2 and 3 of death could be saved by providing basic medical care.

Source: American College of Surgeons.

CULTURAL COMPETENCE

During a disaster, it remains a priority for staff to address ethnic, religious, and cultural customs of diet, death, and burial.

CARING FOR THOSE WHO DIED

Procedure

1. Tag victims pronounced DOA (dead on arrival).
   a. Add special tag "not to remove personal effects."
   b. Incorporate special instructions for people performing autopsies, preparing bodies for burial or transportation.
2. Place bodies in cordoned off area for field triage. **Rationale:** Decontamination may have to be completed before transport.
3. Notify those performing post-mortem care of victim's diagnosis. **Rationale:** For protection of staff handling post-mortem care.
   a. Autopsies performed carefully using all personal protective equipment and Standard Precautions, including use of masks and eye protection.
   b. Incorporate any special instructions about biological–chemical–radiological agent present.
4. Complete a record for all bodies including identification, name of person declaring death, diagnosis, if known, name of agency removing body, etc.

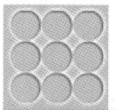

CARING FOR CLIENTS WITH PSYCHOLOGICAL REACTIONS

Procedure

1. Expect major psychological reactions of fear, panic, anger, horror, paranoia, etc., following a bioterrorism event.
2. Plan prior to such an event for professional and educated volunteers to be on site.
3. Minimize fear and panic in staff.
   a. Provide educational materials that include risks to health care workers, accurate information of bioterrorism facts, plans for protecting workers, and how to use personal protection equipment.
   b. Encourage team participation in disaster drills. **Rationale:** Experience in handling a disaster will build confidence and allay anxiety.
4. Cope with psychological reactions of fear and anxiety.
   a. Minimize panic by clearly explaining care given with explanations.
   b. Offer rapid evaluation and treatment and avoid isolation, if possible. **Rationale:** Waiting for evaluation and treatment (as well as isolation) will cause anxiety.
5. Treat major anxiety reactions in unexposed persons with factual information, reassurance, and medication, if indicated. **Rationale:** Anxiety is communicable; prompt intervention will allay group anxiety. ("Worried well" persons could overwhelm hospitals if they leave disaster area and go to closest health care facility.)
6. Prevent post-terrorism trauma. **Rationale:** Early intervention may reduce stress disorder.
   a. Gather victims into a group with a skilled therapist soon after event (within 24 hours) to prevent a major post-trauma reaction.
      (1) Early opportunity for catharsis will help prevent suppression of traumatic event emotions.
      (2) Group victims according to age and experience.
   b. Follow initial group meeting with subsequent meeting within one week to discuss feelings about event. **Rationale:** Research has found that group meetings following traumatic event has eliminated 80% post-traumatic stress disorder.

EVIDENCE BASED NURSING PRACTICE

Studies on mass casualty incidents have reported enormous stress and pressure faced by health workers. Effective response to the crises requires considerable support services for themselves.

Source: Caro, D. (1999). Towards integrated crisis support of regional emergency networks. *Health Care Management Review, 24*(4), 7–19.

CLINICAL ALERT

If a disaster occurs, be alert to signs of disaster trauma in yourself and/or coworkers, and take steps to alleviate stress before it becomes incapacitating.

IDENTIFYING POST-TRAUMATIC STRESS DISORDER

Procedure

1. Recognize possibility of existing condition.
   a. Traumatic event occurs and is reexperienced as flashbacks, dreams, or memory state.
   b. Abreaction occurs: vivid recall of painful experience with original emotions.
   c. Individual cannot adjust to event.
2. Assess signs and symptoms of anxiety and depression. **Rationale:** Early recognition will assist in therapeutic intervention.
   a. Emotional instability, withdrawal, and isolation
   b. Nightmares, difficulty sleeping
   c. Feelings of detachment or guilt
3. Assess aggressive or acting-out behavior; may be explosive or impulsive behavior.
4. Assist client to go through recovery process. **Rationale:** Client may have to be assisted through recovery steps to reach adjustment.
   a. Recovery—reassure client that he is safe following experience of the traumatic event.
   b. Avoidance—client will avoid thinking about traumatic event; support client.
   c. Reconsideration—client deals with event by confronting it, talking about it, and working through feelings.
   d. Adjustment—client rehabilitates and adjusts to environment following event; client functions well and is able to view future positively.

Documentation for Triage and Communication Matrix

- Triage treatment areas established—note site and subdivisions
- Triage format for assessing victims
- Public health parameters followed
  - Protection equipment used for site selection and maintenance
  - Sanitation procedures
  - Purified water procedure
  - Search and rescue procedures
- Protection gear and equipment used for triaging victims
- Procedures implemented for individual life-threatening conditions
- Post-triage assessment of victim
- Assessment of psychological reactions
- Interventions for identifying post-traumatic stress disorder
- Communication network established
  - Internal communication lines
  - External communication lines
  - Collaborative communication lines

Critical Thinking Application

UNEXPECTED OUTCOMES	CRITICAL THINKING OPTIONS
Triage site does not conform to public health requirements.	• Assign additional personnel to monitor for public health concerns (in addition to triage and treatment). • Collect waste in disposable containers for human waste or place in plastic bags and bury. • Boil water or use water purifying tablets if potable water is not available. • Use diluted bleach (0.5%) to decontaminate surfaces.
Multiple casualties exhibit life-threatening conditions	• Implement triage principles—simple triage and rapid treatment (START)—check breathing, control bleeding, and treat shock. • Assess and treat victims post-triage and post-initial interventions, then refer to community facility.
Large group of victims are experiencing major psychological reactions of fear, panic, and horror.	• Assign personnel and/or volunteers to separate and group victims according to age and degree of reaction. • Assign skilled therapist to work with group at least 15–30 minutes, allowing them to talk about their fears and feelings. • Refer victims to post-trauma group to prevent post-traumatic stress disorder.

GERONTOLOGIC CONSIDERATIONS

Under the circumstances of a bioterrorism event, all victims will be triaged and treated according to the system established. The elderly will be included in general triage decisions according to their injuries, not age, so this chapter does not include gerontologic considerations.

MANAGEMENT GUIDELINES

Delegation of Responsibilities

- Pre-emergency/disaster planning and coordination will have (should have) occurred prior to the terrorist event.
- Personnel roles and lines of authority will have been previously delineated so health care workers will refer to the Preparedness Plan posted in each facility and report to the designated superior or Incident Command Center.
- Each member of the responder team should have an identified role, have practiced actions necessary to perform in this role, studied the educational materials, and demonstrated knowledge necessary to perform in this designated role.
- Role responsibilities must be decided before a disaster occurs. For example, in one disaster scenario, the nursing supervisor is responsible for setting up the command center, the administrator will be in contact with outside resource organizations, and the director of nursing will do the administrator's functions.
- Because emergency response teams must work together as a team, be flexible and adapt to the requirements of a changing situation, team response must have practice sessions.
- Duties of command center designated person:

  Find adequate nursing personnel and assign roles and responsibilities

  Assign responsible person to switchboard

  Limit all routine nonemergency admissions

  Refer all public information calls and media to designated place

Information Flow

Once a disaster has been declared, the information flow is delineated in the Preparedness Plan.

- Reporting of the incident takes place (see Reporting Requirements on page 419).
- The community liaison notifies ▶ Community Emergency Response Team (CERT) team leader (out-of-hospital staff), who notifies ▶ medical–nursing group (in-hospital staff).
- Federal agencies notified.
- A community-wide network is established—all using the same channels of communication.
- Position-to-position (not person) cascade of communication (community liaison ▶ command center person ▶ team leader) is established.
- A single off-site communication center for family and friends of victims must be established to avoid overloading system.

CRITICAL THINKING STRATEGIES

SCENARIO 1

Your hospital has not developed a total Preparedness Plan, including specific recommendations and strategies.

1. What are the implications of this situation under disaster conditions? Include a list of several consequences.
2. What strategies would you suggest to increase hospital administration awareness?
3. Describe the steps you would suggest to alter this situation so that a viable Preparedness Plan is in place.

SCENARIO 2

A Russian organized crime syndicate has stolen radioactive isotopes from an unprotected nuclear research facility and sold the material to an al Qaeda group. This terrorist group smuggled the material into the United States via Canada. At a professional football game, this group detonates the weapon, creating a small explosion that rapidly spreads radiological material. The firefighters and police who rushed to the site had no radiation detectors, so they were exposed to radiological fallout. HAZMAT teams were sent to the area, detected radiation, and set up decontamination equipment.

You are part of the Preparedness Plan team for the local hospital in charge of the command center. Upon being notified of the disaster:

1. What additional information does your team need to make decisions about coping with this disaster?
2. What are the priority actions you would take?
3. What further assessment of contamination is necessary?
4. Describe the special protective equipment your team would require.

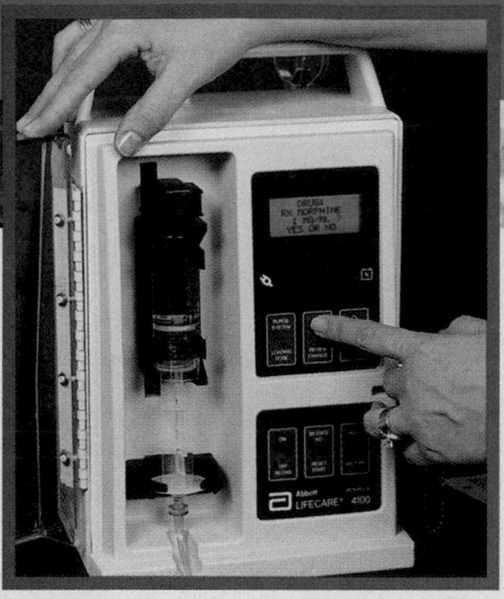

CHAPTER 16

Pain Management

THEORETICAL CONCEPTS

UNIT ONE: **Nonpharmacological Pain Relief** 477
- Alleviating Pain Through Touch (Massage) 478
- Using Relaxation Techniques 478

UNIT TWO: **Pharmacological Pain Management** 480
- Administering Pain Medications 481
- Administering Epidural Narcotic Analgesia 481
  - *for Bolus Injection* 483
  - *for Continuous Infusion* 483
- Qualifying the Client for PCA 483
- Administering PCA 484
- Terminating a PCA Infusion 487
- Teaching PCA to a Client 487

GERONTOLOGIC CONSIDERATIONS 491

MANAGEMENT GUIDELINES 492

CRITICAL THINKING STRATEGIES 493

Cross Reference: End-of-Life Care, Chapter 32

LEARNING OBJECTIVES

- Discuss what is meant by the experience of pain.
- Explain the use of endorphins for pain control.
- Describe the body's physiologic response to pain.
- Identify the most important information elicited from the client regarding pain.
- Discuss what it means for the nurse to be the client's advocate in relation to pain control.
- Discuss the main components of JCAHO's Standards for Pain Management.
- Discuss the gate control theory.
- Outline the main points of one nonpharmacological method of relieving pain.
- Describe two different pain scales.
- Discuss two advantages of epidural narcotic analgesia.
- List three criteria for client selection for PCA.
- Explain what is meant by establishing the client control mode.
- Describe the steps of teaching PCA to a client.
- Discuss two components of pain management.

TERMINOLOGY

Acupressure: Chinese method of treatment that involves compression of certain areas of the body by following a system of meridians or energy flow.

Adaptive reaction: a response by which the person attempts to improve or alter his or her condition in relation to the environment.

Alleviate: to make more bearable; reduce (pain, grief, or suffering).

Angina: a sense of suffocation with symptoms of severe, steady pain and feeling of pressure in region of the heart.

Arrhythmia: irregular rhythm.

Arthritis: inflammation of a joint, usually accompanied by pain and frequently, deformity.

ATC: around-the-clock medication for persistent pain.

Autogenic training: a method of deep muscle relaxation that enables one to reduce the stress response, regain homeostasis, and prepare to handle additional stress.

Autoimmunization: immunity produced by an attack of the disease or by processes occurring within the body.

Autonomic nervous system: the part of the nervous system that regulates the functioning of internal organs and glands; it controls such functions as digestion, respiration, and cardiovascular activity.

Behavior: the manner in which one acts.

Biofeedback: a training technique that uses monitoring instruments to assist people to control stress-related disorders through self-regulation of internal functions.

Booster dose: an additional dose given to a client on a prn basis. Ordered by physician, administered by RN.

Brady: prefix indicating slow.

Bradycardia: slowed heart action, below 60 BPM.

Cardiovascular: pertaining to the heart and blood vessels.

Cerebral cortex: the extensive outer layer of gray tissue of the cerebral hemispheres (brain), responsible for higher nervous functions.

Coping mechanisms: means by which an individual adjusts or adapts to a threat or a challenge; actions that assist in maintaining homeostasis.

Diaphoresis: profuse sweating.

Dynamics of homeostasis: danger or its symbols, whether internal or external, resulting in the activation of the sympathetic nervous system and the adrenal medulla. The organism prepares for fight or flight.

Emotional: affected by strong feelings, as of joy and sorrow.

Endorphins: a naturally occurring body chemical similar to morphine but many times stronger.

Fight or flight: one's immediate response to stress that is, although archaic and often inappropriate, part of our central nervous system biologic heritage.

Four (4)-hour limit (mL): the maximum amount of drug that can be administered to client during a 4-hour period.

Gastrointestinal: pertaining to the stomach and the intestine.

General adaptation syndrome: a general theory of stress response formulated by Dr. Hans Selye; describes the action of stress response in three stages: the alarm reaction, the stage of resistance, and the stage of exhaustion.

Health: the state of physical, psychologic, and sociologic well-being.

Hypertension: a condition in which the client has a higher blood pressure than judged to be normal.

Illness: a state characterized by the malfunction of the biopsychosocial organism.

Insomnia: inability to sleep.

Ischemic: local and temporary anemia due to obstruction of the circulation to a part.

JCAHO: Joint Commission on Accreditation of Healthcare Organizations—sets standards of care and accredits health care facilities.

Loading dose (optional): initial dose given to client as ordered by physician.

Lockout interval: period during which the PCA cannot be activated and no analgesic can be delivered by client. (A booster dose can be given during lockout interval if ordered.)

Meditation: the act of reflecting on or pondering; contemplation.

Musculoskeletal: pertaining to the muscles and the skeleton.

Nausea: inclination to vomit, usually preceding emesis.

Opioid (narcotic) addiction: pattern of compulsive drug use characterized by continued craving for the narcotic—creates both a psychological and physiological dependence.

Pain: a sensation in which a person experiences discomfort, distress, or suffering. There are three main types of pain: acute, chronic, and malignant.

Parasympathetic nervous system: a division of the autonomic nervous system that regulates acetylcholine and conserves energy expenditure; it slows down the system.

PCA—Patient-controlled analgesia: a method of delivering pain medication via IV pump. Within physician-ordered parameters, the client can control the medication amount necessary to manage his or her pain level.

Physiologic: concerning body function.

Psychogenic: of mental origin.

Referred pain: pain felt in a part removed from its point of origin.

Regression: a turning back or return to a former state.

Relaxation: a lessening of tension or activity in a part.

Resistance: opposition to or the ability to oppose.

Stamina: constitutional energy; strength; endurance.

Stress: a nonspecific response of the body to any internal or external event or change that impinges on a person's system and creates a demand.

Stressor: a specific demand that gives rise to a coping response.

Sympathetic nervous system: a division of the autonomic nervous system that controls energy expenditure and mobilizes for action when confronted with a threat.

Tachy: prefix meaning fast.

Tachycardia: abnormal rapidity of heart action; above 100 BPM.

TENS—Transcutaneous electrical nerve stimulation: a noninvasive method to relieve pain that involves stimulation to the skin via a mild electric current.

Tolerance: a larger and larger dose of an opioid is required to have the same effect.

Touch: a tactile sense.

Visceral: pertaining to internal organs.

Wellness: a state of physical, psychologic, and sociologic well-being of a whole person.

COPING WITH PAIN

Pain is now considered the fifth vital sign and, according to JCAHO Standards for Pain Management, is essential to regularly assess and manage in order to maintain the client's homeostasis and quality of life.

The experience of pain is direct and personal. In this culture we tend to view pain as a negative condition and often go to any lengths to avoid the sensation. The positive aspect of pain is that it is an early warning system; its presence triggers an awareness that something is wrong in the body. Without the sensation of pain we could not survive, because pain provides the cues that allow us to modify our reactions and direct our behavior. One perspective of pain is that it is a message to our conscious self to check out any pain sensation before it gets worse, for that is the nature of pain. Without intervention the condition may well get worse.

Margo McCaffery, a nurse–author who writes about caring for the client in pain, defines pain as "whatever the patient experiencing pain says it is, existing whenever he says it does." The nurse is totally dependent on the client to describe the sensation of pain, identify the location, and tell about what kind of pain is being experienced.

The most important information in pain assessment, then, is the client's report. The pain experience is totally subjective. The onset of acute pain stimulates the sympathetic nervous system "fight or flight" response that results in certain signs or symptoms. While observation of these symptoms provides objective data, it cannot be considered conclusive evidence to the identification of pain—that must come from the client.

The sensation of physical pain arouses some specific responses in the client. The sympathetic nervous system

Types of Pain

Acute pain	Pain that occurs only in a defined period of time (6 months or less), and is caused by specific stimuli that damages the tissue. Usually of recent onset and varies in intensity.
Chronic pain	Prolonged, persistent nonmalignant pain that occurs over a 6 month period or longer. Pain varies in intensity and may serve no useful function.
Malignant pain	Recurrent, acute episodes of pain, which may also include chronic pain. This pain may vary in intensity and have rapid or slow onset. It may last longer than 6 months and be intractable.

response is usually stimulated by superficial pain, and the parasympathetic nervous system response is usually stimulated by deeper pain and results in the slowing down of all the systems to conserve energy.

Theories of Pain

The neurophysiologic basis of pain can be explained by several theories, none of which is mutually exclusive nor totally comprehensive.

Specificity Theory This theory suggests that certain pain receptors are stimulated by a specific type of sensory stimuli that sends impulses to the brain. This theory dealt with the physiologic basis for pain but did not take into account the psychologic components of pain, nor the degree of pain tolerance.

Pattern Theory This theory attempts to include factors that were not adequately explained by the specificity theory. This theory suggests that pain originates in the dorsal horn of the spinal cord. A certain pattern of nerve impulses is produced and results in intense receptor stimulation that is coded in the central nervous system (CNS) and signifies pain. Like the specificity theory, the pattern theory does not explain the psychologic factors of pain.

Gate Control Theory One of the most popular and credible concepts is the gate control theory. The first premise of the gate control theory is that the actual existence and intensity of the pain experience depends on the particular transmission of neurologic impulses. Secondly, gate mechanisms along the nervous system control the transmission of pain. Finally, if the gate is open, the impulses that result in the sensation of pain are able to reach the conscious level. If the gate is closed, the impulses do not reach the level of consciousness and the sensation of pain is not experienced.

Three primary types of neurologic involvement affect whether the gate is open or closed. The first type involves activity in the large and small nerve fibers that affect the sensation of pain. Pain impulses travel along small-diameter fibers. The large-diameter nerve fibers close the gate to the impulses that travel along the small fibers. The technique of using cutaneous stimulation on the skin, which has many large-diameter fibers, may help to close the gate to the transmission of painful impulses, thereby relieving the sensation of pain. Interventions that apply this theory to practice include massage, hot and cold applications, touch, acupressure, and transcutaneous electric nerve stimulation. These interventions are described in detail later in this chapter.

The second form of neurologic involvement is the impulses from the brain stem that affect the sensation of pain. The reticular formation monitors in the brain stem regulate sensory input. If the person receives adequate or excessive amounts of sensory stimulation, the brain stem transmits impulses that close the gate and inhibit pain impulses from being transmitted. If on the other hand, the client experiences a lack of sensory input, the brain stem

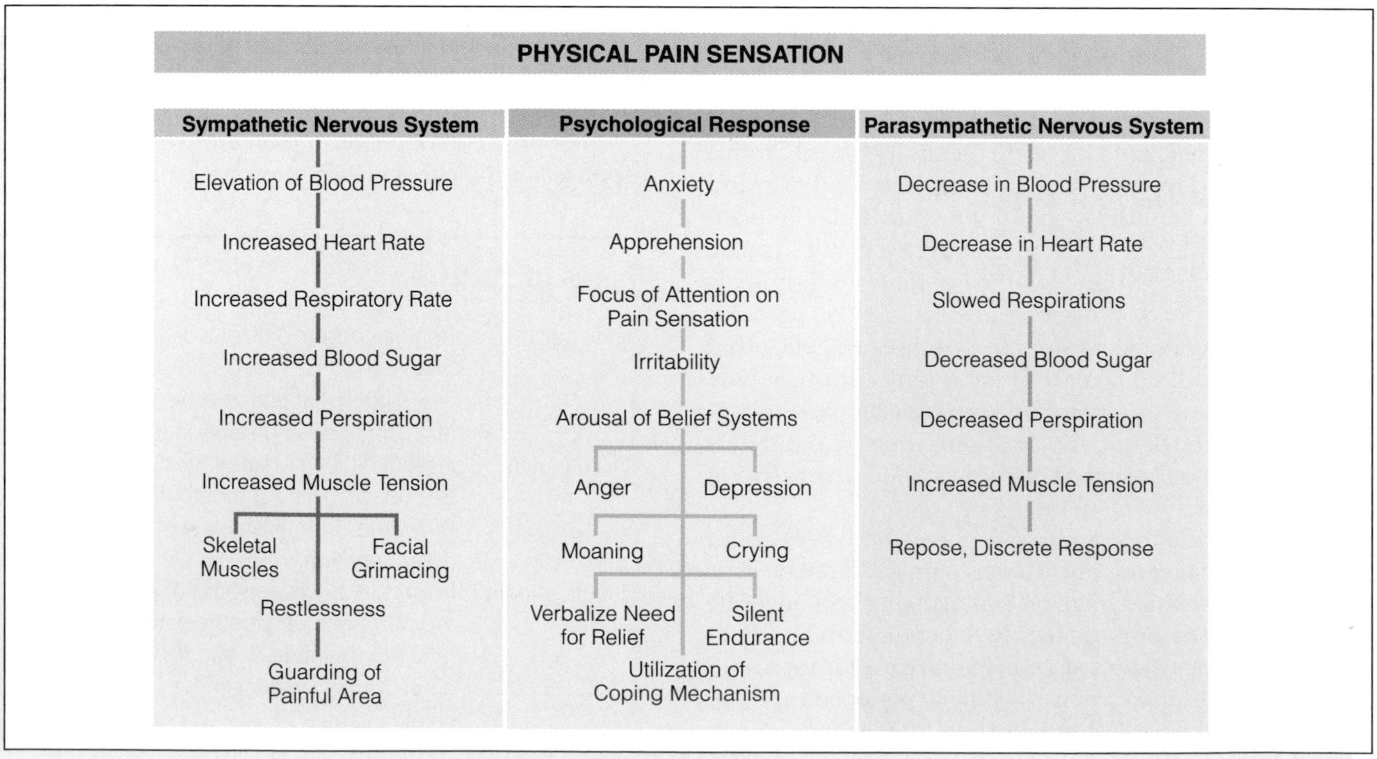

does not inhibit the pain impulses, the gate is open, and the pain impulses are transmitted. Interventions that apply to this part of the gate control theory are those related in some way to sensory input, such as techniques of distraction, guided imagery, and visualization.

The third type of neurologic involvement is the neurologic activities or impulses in the cerebral cortex and thalamus. A person's thoughts, emotions, and memories may activate certain impulses in the cortex that trigger pain impulses, which are transmitted to the conscious level. Past experiences relating to pain affect how the client responds to current pain. For this reason, it is important to explore the client's previous experiences and teach the client what to expect from the present situation. Interventions that apply to this part of the gate control theory include using and teaching various relaxation techniques, teaching the client about what expectations to have about pain as related to a specific illness, allowing the client to feel he or she has some control over the taking of medication for pain relief, and giving medications properly (i.e., preventively, before the pain is so severe that the client fears he or she will receive no relief).

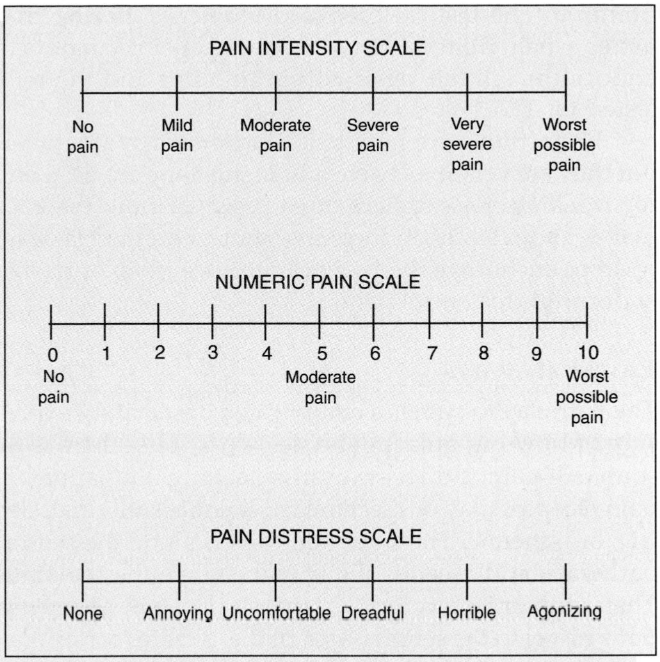

Acute Pain Management: Operative or medical procedures and trauma. Source: U.S. Department of Health and Human Services, Public Health Service.

The Discovery of Endorphins

A relatively recent theory of pain relief was developed when Avron Goldstein, looking for morphine and heroin receptors, discovered that receptors in the brain fit only morphine or morphine-like molecules. He asked himself why these receptors were located in the brain, when opiates are not naturally found in this area. The answer, learned through diligent research, is that the brain produces natural brain opiates. These substances are hormones, chemicals produced by different parts of the body to regulate certain biologic processes. At present, five of these natural opiates have been found. Three are called endorphins, one dynorphin, and one enkephalin. Endorphins fit into special cells, called receptors, and thereby activate their regulating powers. In addition to endorphin "keys" and receptor "locks," researchers have found antilocks, called antagonists, that keep endorphins from working. Endorphin receptors and antilocks have been found throughout the body—in the stomach, intestines, pancreas, spinal cord, and bloodstream, as well as the brain.

A beta-endorphin is 50 times stronger than morphine, and a dynorphin is 190 times stronger than mor-

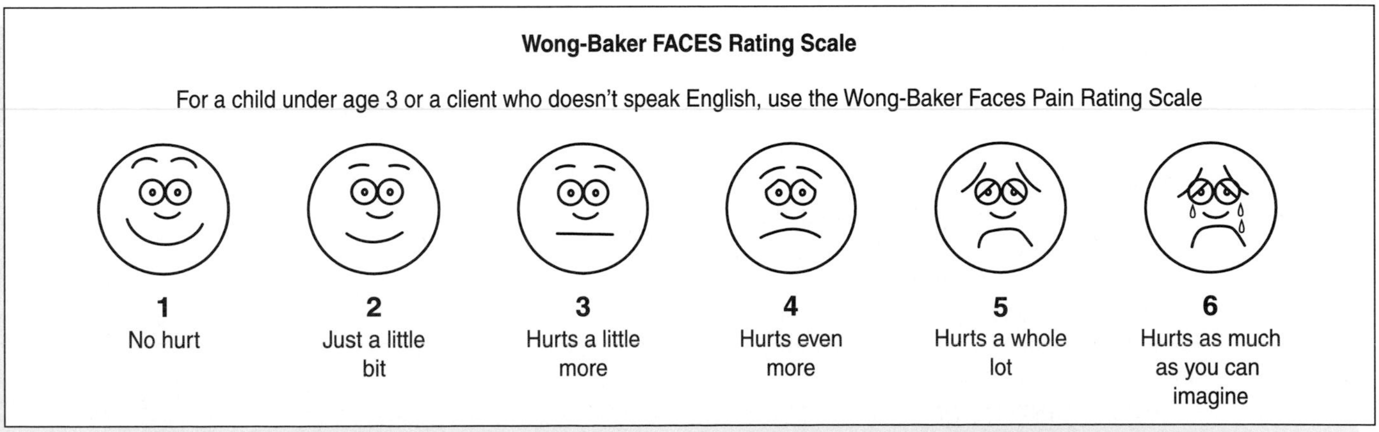

Ask the client to choose the face that best describes how he or she feels pain. Try to be specific about which pain (injection or incision), where it hurts, and what time (now, earlier, after lunch, etc.). *Source:* Wong-Baker FACES Pain Rating Scale (from Wong, D. L., et al., 1999. *Nursing Care of Infants and Children* [6th ed.] St. Louis, Mosby.)

phine. In one test, 14 men and women suffering from extreme pain from cancer were given tiny injections of an endorphin. All felt relief within minutes and the relief lasted for 1 to 3 days.

Endorphins are now being produced synthetically, but they are very expensive and at this time are used only for research. Researchers must discover how the body makes and releases endorphins before a method is developed to encourage the body to produce more of its own endorphins to control pain.

Pain Pathways

The pathway to pain is a complicated, fascinating expression of how our amazing bodies work. First there is the source of pain, a direct causative factor. Stimulation of a pain receptor may be mechanical, chemical, thermal, electric, or ischemic. The sensation travels along the sensory pathways and ascends the spinal cord to the thalamus. The autonomic nervous system is activated, and sensations travel to the sensory area of the cerebral cortex. Pain reception occurs in the thalamus, where awareness and integration take place, and pain interpretation occurs in the cerebral cortex. Once awareness of pain takes place and it has been interpreted by the cerebral cortex, the person becomes aware and the response patterns are activated.

The Pain Experience

The pain experience is a mixture of physical sensations, physiologic changes, and psychosocial (including psychological, sociocultural, and environmental) factors. The client's interpretation of the physical sensation is influenced by the client's culture, previous experiences with and without pain, beliefs about self, interpretation of the future, present environment, and the persons in that environment. The intensity of pain is influenced by what the sensation means to the client, the client's level of anxiety, degree of fatigue, and the number of stressors in the client's environment.

There are several methods of assessing the degree or level of pain a client may be experiencing. Note the examples of pain scales you may use to assess your client's pain. After explaining the scale you are using, ask your client what level of pain he or she is experiencing at the moment. You may use a numeric scale of 1 to 10, an intensity scale with 3 or more categories to rate client pain, a pain distress scale, or the Wong–Baker FACES scale. Note the photo in which the nurse is wearing a FACES scale badge. The FACES pain scale is very important for pediatric clients, since children may have difficulty verbalizing the degree of pain they are experiencing. The different faces help them relate to pain by how sad the face appears, thus identifying for the nurse the level of pain they are feeling. Whichever scale is chosen, maintain its use throughout the course of pain control.

Assessing Pain in a Cognitively Impaired or Nonverbal Client

Many clients who have diminished cognitive function (for example, Alzheimer's, psychosis, dementia, senility) can

How to Measure Pain

Location	Ask the client to locate pain on or within the body—exactly where is the pain felt?
Intensity	Determine strength, power, or force of the pain the client is experiencing. Use numeric or verbal scales or the faces pictures.
Quality	Determine the features or characteristics that distinguish this pain, such as searing, dull, throbbing, sharp, burning, etc.
Pattern	Ask client how pain changes and timing of the pain, such as is it continuous, steady, intermittent, transient?

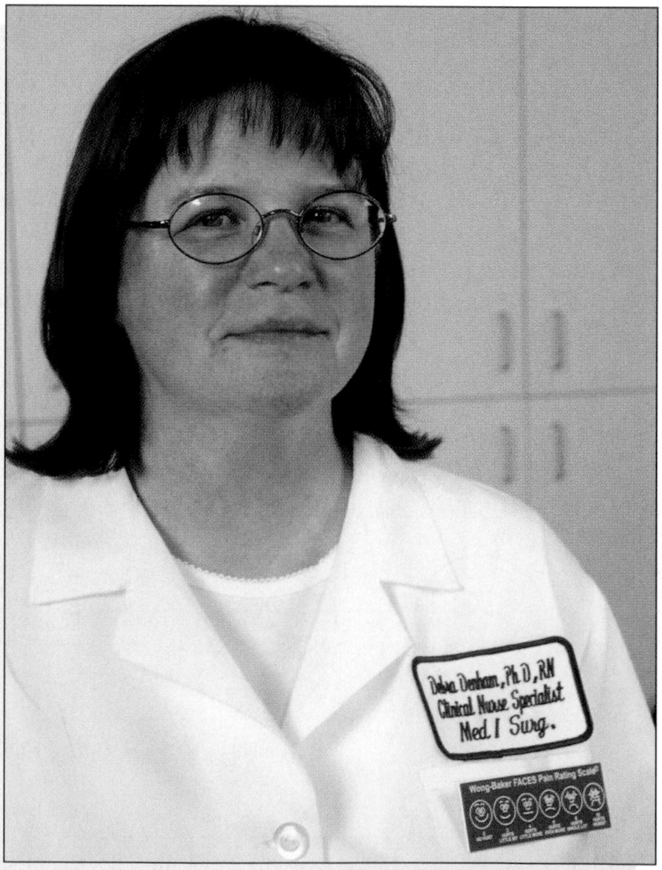

Nurse's badge with Wong-Baker FACES Pain Rating Scale reminds both nurse and client to pay attention to pain level.

still respond appropriately when asked about the level of pain they are experiencing.

If you cannot elicit a response or if the client cannot respond verbally, then nonverbal cues must be assessed: facial expression, behavior, unusual movements, vocal sounds (moaning), or muscle contractions, especially around the eyes.

After establishing a baseline pain level and medicating, evaluate changes in the client. From this outcome, the nurse should be able to build a plan for future pain management.

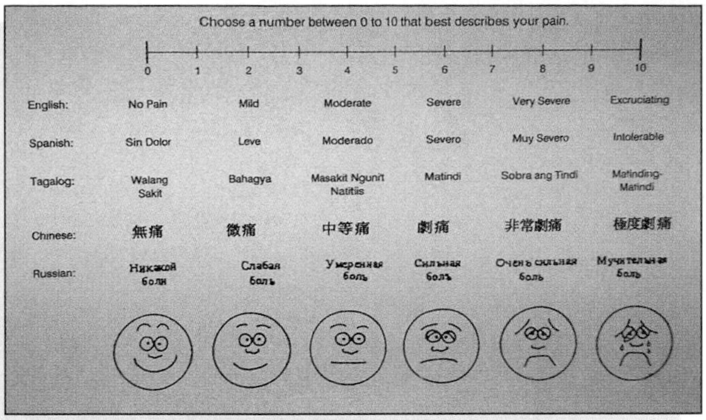

A multilanguage pain chart facilitates an accurate description of pain.

JCAHO Standards for Pain Management

In 2000, JCAHO described the appropriate standards for pain management for all health care facilities. The standards below were adapted from the comprehensive accreditation manual for hospitals.

- *Recognize that clients have the right to appropriate assessment and management of pain.* Pain assessment is to be considered a priority; in fact, it is now considered by many facilities and several states, to be the fifth vital sign. This will enable the client's pain level to be assessed as frequently as vital signs.
- The facility must provide appropriate pain assessment tools (see pain scales and faces), and *pain levels should be recorded so that regular reassessment and follow-up can be done.*
- *Policies will be in place so that clients will be treated for pain, and adequate doses of opioids to relieve pain without unacceptable side effects will be given. Clients will be involved in their own pain management.*
  - *If a facility, such as a long-term home care facility, cannot treat the client adequately for pain, the client should be referred to an appropriate facility.*
  - *Facilities should collect data to monitor the effectiveness of pain management.*
  - *Facility staff should receive education so they are competent in pain assessment and management.*
  - *Clients and their families should be informed about pain management and client's needs for symptom control, and these should be included in discharge planning.*

Again, in 2001, JCAHO released revised standards for the assessment and management of pain. They stated that all health care facilities are expected to comply with these standards and that accreditation will be granted only on this basis. Margo McCaffery, an expert on pain management, believes that JCAHO's revised standards may do more to improve pain management than any other development in managing pain.

NONINVASIVE PAIN RELIEF

When a method to relieve pain is noninvasive, it is safer and results in less potential side effects for the client. Such measures are becoming the pain control choice of the future.

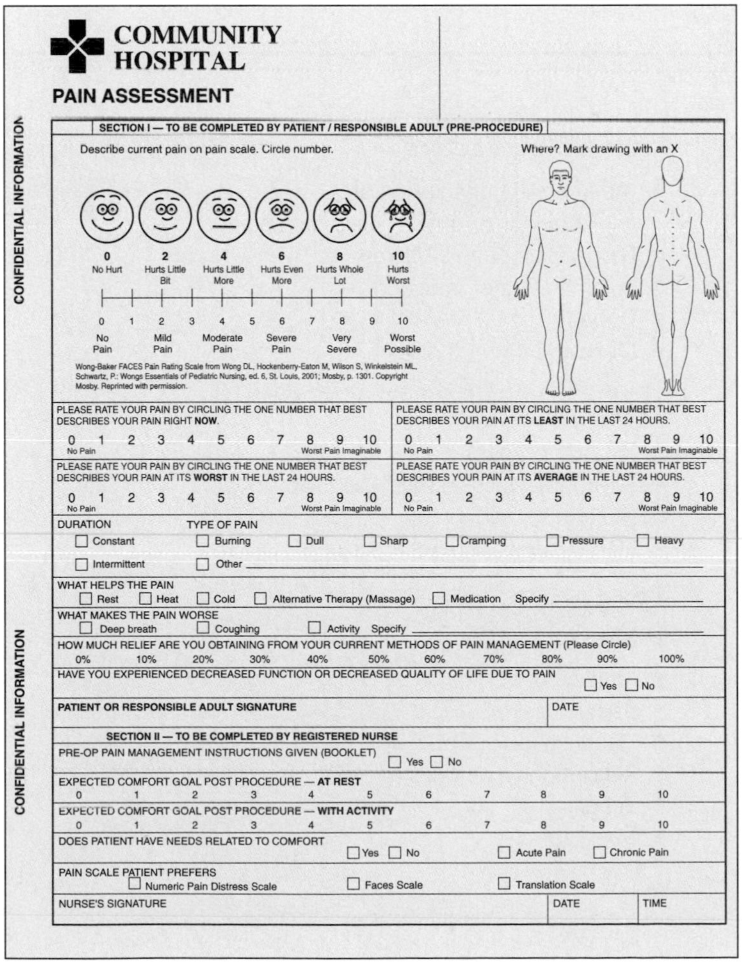

COMMUNITY HOSPITAL

PAIN ASSESSMENT

CONFIDENTIAL INFORMATION

SECTION I — TO BE COMPLETED BY PATIENT / RESPONSIBLE ADULT (PRE-PROCEDURE)

Describe current pain on pain scale. Circle number.

0 No Hurt · 2 Hurts Little Bit · 4 Hurts Little More · 6 Hurts Even More · 8 Hurts Whole Lot · 10 Hurts Worst

0 1 2 3 4 5 6 7 8 9 10

No Pain · Mild Pain · Moderate Pain · Severe Pain · Very Severe · Worst Possible

Wong-Baker FACES Pain Rating Scale from Wong DL, Hockenberry-Eaton M, Wilson S, Winkelstein ML, Schwartz, P.: Wongs Essentials of Pediatric Nursing, ed. 6, St. Louis, 2001; Mosby, p. 1301. Copyright Mosby. Reprinted with permission.

Where? Mark drawing with an X

PLEASE RATE YOUR PAIN BY CIRCLING THE ONE NUMBER THAT BEST DESCRIBES YOUR PAIN RIGHT **NOW**. 0 1 2 3 4 5 6 7 8 9 10 No Pain — Worst Pain Imaginable	PLEASE RATE YOUR PAIN BY CIRCLING THE ONE NUMBER THAT BEST DESCRIBES YOUR PAIN AT ITS **LEAST** IN THE LAST 24 HOURS. 0 1 2 3 4 5 6 7 8 9 10 No Pain — Worst Pain Imaginable
PLEASE RATE YOUR PAIN BY CIRCLING THE ONE NUMBER THAT BEST DESCRIBES YOUR PAIN AT ITS **WORST** IN THE LAST 24 HOURS. 0 1 2 3 4 5 6 7 8 9 10 No Pain — Worst Pain Imaginable	PLEASE RATE YOUR PAIN BY CIRCLING THE ONE NUMBER THAT BEST DESCRIBES YOUR PAIN AT ITS **AVERAGE** IN THE LAST 24 HOURS. 0 1 2 3 4 5 6 7 8 9 10 No Pain — Worst Pain Imaginable

DURATION: ☐ Constant ☐ Intermittent

TYPE OF PAIN: ☐ Burning ☐ Dull ☐ Sharp ☐ Cramping ☐ Pressure ☐ Heavy ☐ Other ______

WHAT HELPS THE PAIN: ☐ Rest ☐ Heat ☐ Cold ☐ Alternative Therapy (Massage) ☐ Medication Specify ______

WHAT MAKES THE PAIN WORSE: ☐ Deep breath ☐ Coughing ☐ Activity Specify ______

HOW MUCH RELIEF ARE YOU OBTAINING FROM YOUR CURRENT METHODS OF PAIN MANAGEMENT (Please Circle)
0% 10% 20% 30% 40% 50% 60% 70% 80% 90% 100%

HAVE YOU EXPERIENCED DECREASED FUNCTION OR DECREASED QUALITY OF LIFE DUE TO PAIN ☐ Yes ☐ No

PATIENT OR RESPONSIBLE ADULT SIGNATURE ______ DATE ______

SECTION II — TO BE COMPLETED BY REGISTERED NURSE

PRE-OP PAIN MANAGEMENT INSTRUCTIONS GIVEN (BOOKLET) ☐ Yes ☐ No

EXPECTED COMFORT GOAL POST PROCEDURE — **AT REST**
0 1 2 3 4 5 6 7 8 9 10

EXPECTED COMFORT GOAL POST PROCEDURE — **WITH ACTIVITY**
0 1 2 3 4 5 6 7 8 9 10

DOES PATIENT HAVE NEEDS RELATED TO COMFORT ☐ Yes ☐ No ☐ Acute Pain ☐ Chronic Pain

PAIN SCALE PATIENT PREFERS ☐ Numeric Pain Distress Scale ☐ Faces Scale ☐ Translation Scale

NURSE'S SIGNATURE ______ DATE ______ TIME ______

CONFIDENTIAL INFORMATION

Pain assessment form.

Pain Management Guidelines

The University of Iowa has developed guidelines for acute pain management, including a set of major recommendations. The main topics covered are:

- Complete a baseline pain assessment including pain level.
- Educate client and family about pain management.
- Monitor the acute pain the client is experiencing, including intensity, duration, and effect of pain.
- Follow guidelines of pharmacological management.
- Implement nonpharmacological management.
- Assess the effectiveness of pain management.

Current practice for controlling pain is to use both drugs and nondrug options because both, separately or combined, meet the objectives of relieving pain and making the client more comfortable.

Nondrug options may include the use of specific cognitive–behavioral techniques—deep breathing, visualization, imagery; physical agents—electric stimulators, massage–vibration, and biofeedback systems; and various adjunct therapies—cold therapy, heat therapy, or counterirritants.

The nonpharmacological approach (Table 16–2) is appropriate for clients who are receptive to alternative methods; who have a high level of anxiety around the issue of pain; who would benefit from reducing dependence on drug therapy; who anticipate long-term or have chronic pain; or who receive inadequate pain relief from pharmacological interventions.

The Nurse's Role

Pain reduction methods include a wide range of techniques and medications. Rarely is pain relief successfully achieved with only one method. Even massive doses of narcotics do not always control pain effectively—especially when it has been allowed to escalate.

One of the most important influences on pain relief is the relationship that exists between nurse and client. With most methods (the exception is PCA), the nurse has the power to relieve pain or to withhold pain relief. This knowledge creates anticipatory anxiety for the client. The client may request less medication when the nurse is supportive, caring, and assists with pain management.

The single most critical factor in achieving pain relief

Characteristics of Pain

Location

- Area of the body
- Diffuse or localized
- Radiates and area involved

Quality

- Stabbing, knife-like
- Throbbing
- Cramping
- Vise-like, suffocating
- Searing, burning
- Superficial, deep

Intensity

- Rate on scale: 0–10 (0 = no pain,10 = most pain ever experienced)

Factors Associated with Pain

- Nausea
- Vomiting
- Bradycardia, tachycardia
- Hypotension, hypertension
- Profuse perspiration
- Apprehension or anxiety

Precipitating Factors

- Motion affecting incision area (e.g., coughing, turning, deep breathing)
- Fear and emotional distress
- Inflammation or infection
- Trauma
- Disease state

Aggravating Factors

- Position changes
- Environmental stressors
- Fatigue
- Inadequate pain relief measures

Alleviating Factors

- Position change
- Medications
- Biofeedback
- Visualization
- Relaxation techniques
- TENS
- Massage

TABLE 16–1 Pain Management

Effective Pain Management	Barriers to Effective Pain Control
• Listens to and believes clients when they describe the level of pain they are experiencing.	Insensitive response or not believing the client's subjective experience of pain.
• Intervenes or administers the pain medication when it is needed.	Nurse wants reassurance the pain really necessitates medication—does not just respond to the client's request.
• Does not allow the pain to escalate but anticipates when pain medication is needed.	Believes drug tolerance will make the medication less effective, so the less medication given, the better.
• Works with the client to control the pain and requests different medications or dosages from the physician when needed.	Believes the physician knows best about the amount of pain medication for the client.
• Is not concerned about addiction when administering pain medication. (The incidence of opioid addiction in hospitalized clients is less than 1%.)	Concerned about drug dependence or addiction—believes it is more important than effective pain management.
• Understands the various actions of drugs and their role in pain control.	Inadequate knowledge about pain medications, so dosage, duration of action, or synergistic drug interactions are miscalculated.

is for the nurse to be the client's advocate. The comfort of the client is the nurse's primary concern.

Nursing interventions that provide effective pain relief, in addition to pain medication, are those that encourage behaviors that assist the client not to focus on pain. For example, when the client is talking about something of great interest or pleasure, he or she is not thinking about pain. Teaching the client techniques, such as deep, slow breathing and relaxation, lessens pain, whereas muscle tension and anxiety increase it. If the nurse teaches pain relief techniques before surgery, the client can more easily implement them when the pain is intense. The nurse may also encourage the client to use techniques that he or she has already found effective, no matter how "unscientific" they may be. Whatever method or technique the nurse uses to assist the client with relieving pain, the single most critical intervention is a caring and supportive attitude.

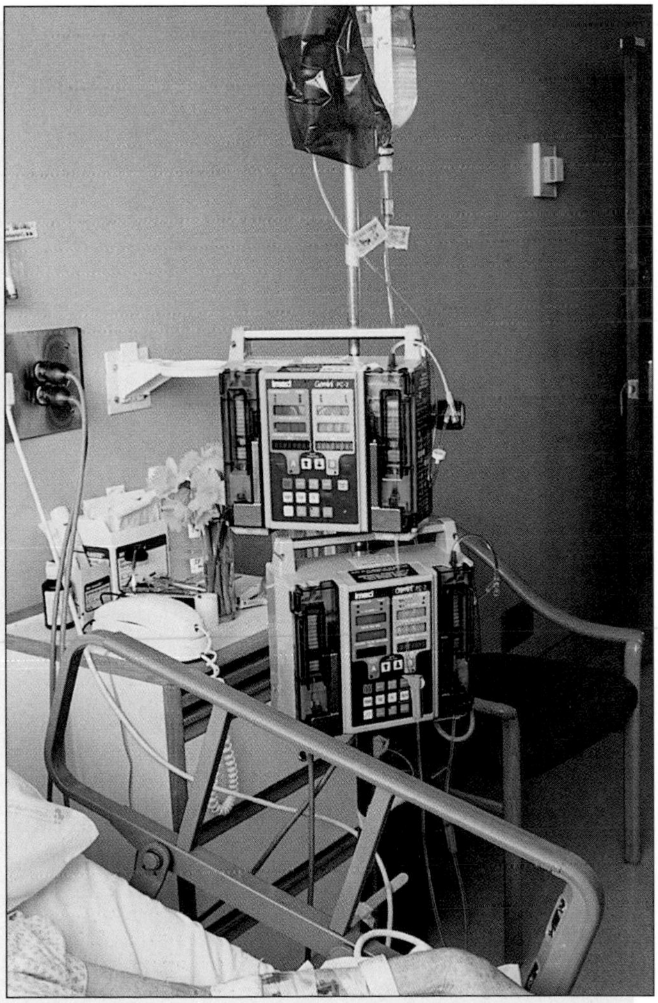

Continuous IV narcotic drip for pain control.

TECHNIQUES FOR PAIN CONTROL

Patient-Controlled Analgesia (PCA)

One of the most successful methods of pain relief to be introduced in the last few years is patient-controlled

Pain—the Fifth Vital Sign

California has passed into law the requirement that pain be considered the fifth vital sign. It must assessed and documented at the time other vital signs are taken. The Veterans Administration, as well as many other states and facilities, has incorporated pain on their vital signs graphic record.

TABLE 16–2 Nonpharmacological Approaches to Pain

Physical Methods	Advantages
TENS—stimulating skin with mild electric current—provides pain relief by blocking pain impulses to the brain (*See Community Based Nursing*, Chapter 34)	Noninvasive method Higher level of activity Studies show more effective for postoperative pain Gives staff confidence they can assist client with pain Choice for chronic pain
Acupuncture—ancient Chinese form of treating diseases through insertion and manipulation of needles at specific points on the body	Insertion of thin needles is not painful to the client Pain relieving capacity extends beyond actual procedure Method may provide relief when no other method works
Biofeedback—electric monitoring device that feeds back effect of behavior so client can control internal processes (e.g., heartbeat)	Noninvasive method Completely controlled by client Promotes stress reduction as well as pain relief After mastery, instruments are not needed to achieve result
Vibration or massage—hands-on manipulation of muscles or electrical form of massage (vibration)	Noninvasive method—electrically alleviates pain by numbness or paresthesia or through touch Increases circulation and endorphins to area Relaxes muscles and reduces tension on nerves and promotes relaxation Useful only for light to moderate pain
Cold therapy—cold wraps, gel packs, cold therapy, ice massage; do not use on irradiated tissue or when clients have peripheral vascular disease	Relieves pain faster than heat therapy Numbs nerves and decreases inflammation and spasms Effective for nerve, abdominal, and lower back pain Alters pain threshold Decreases tissue injury response
Heat therapy—hot wraps, dry heat, moist heat; do not use on irradiated tissue or tumors	Noninvasive method Decreases pain by reducing inflammation Promotes relaxation of muscles Increases vasodilation and blood flow to area Facilitates clearance of tissue toxins and fluids
Counterirritants—mentholated ointments or lotions (Ben-Gay or Icy Hot)	May contain salicylates (reduces inflammation) but dangerous if client has potential bleeding problems May be irritating to the skin—potential skin breakdown
Acupressure application—based on the ancient Chinese method of acupuncture, this method involves using specific points located on meridians at various places on the body	Noninvasive method Redirection of energy flow through pressure on meridian points Reduces pain and increases endorphins
Cognitive–Behavioral Methods	**Advantages**
Relaxation—body relaxation of muscles used with imagery, therapist instruction	Relaxes tense muscles and reduces stress Effective in reducing pain Easy to learn and implement techniques for self-mastery Reduces fear and anxiety connected to pain
Imagery—visualization technique of forming sensory images, or seeing in the "mind's eye" an image that distracts from the sensation of pain	Effective in reducing pain Client can control use and timing of technique Reduces high-level anxiety connected to pain
Deep breathing—techniques using breath to control pain	Effective in reinforcing body relaxation and visualization Reduces pain through breath control; increases oxygen utilization
Hypnosis—creating a state of altered consciousness so that client is susceptible to instruction	Effective with a client who is suggestive and who experiences tension and anxiety accompanying pain

analgesia (PCA). The primary purpose of PCA is to allow the client to self-administer an analgesic dose of medication predetermined by the physician. PCA enables the client to assess and control his or her own pain level. This method of pain control has been found to be very efficacious because the client feels in more control of his or her life situation, there is no significant difference in the amount of analgesic medication used (if anything, it is usually less), and this method of pain control is less time-consuming for the nurse.

Epidural Pain Control

An effective technique for controlling pain is the use of an epidural catheter. The advantage of epidural pain control is that the narcotic moves directly from the epidural space into the spinal fluid and binds with opiate receptors in the spinal cord, blocking reception of pain. Administered by this method, the required drug dose is considerably lower because it is not metabolized in the liver.

Direct IV Pain Control

In addition to the new methods of pain control, a client may receive a continuous infusion via direct IV. The dosage may be titrated to achieve pain relief with the lowest dose (10 mg or ⅙ gr of morphine sulfate). The dose is individualized according to the client's needs, tolerance, and response. When pain relief is not achieved, increments of at least 25% of the previous dose should be implemented. When morphine is administered IV, a dark bag should be placed over the narcotic bag because the medication is light-sensitive.

Breakthrough Pain Control

There are two major types of pain—continuous and breakthrough. Many clients with cancer experience long periods of persistent pain and may also experience severe flare-ups that occur even when the client is on around-the-clock (ATC) medication. Studies suggest that nearly 70 percent of cancer clients experience breakthrough pain. These episodes typically last about 30 minutes, but tend to totally decimate the client.

Generally, breakthrough pain occurs as two types:

- Incident pain—caused by movement or activity (for example, sitting up, walking, or coughing).
- Spontaneous pain—does not seem to be linked to any specific source, but occurs with no warning or relation to activity or movement.

Breakthrough pain can be managed by different protocols, some of which are listed below.

- Increasing the dose of ATC so that breakthrough pain is eliminated—this method is not always advisable because sedation and other side effects of the drug may occur.
- Changing the ATC so that relatively constant analgesia occurs (use long-acting oral opioids or fentanyl patches).
- Prescribing a supplemental dose of a short-acting morphine-like drug so that it is taken 30 minutes before incident pain when this type of pain is predictable.
- When spontaneous pain occurs, instruct the client to take the dose as soon as possible after onset. At this point in pain control, this is the best plan, even though there may be a "pain gap." New drugs, currently being researched in clinical trials, may solve this problem.
- A new delivery method, oral transmucosal, delivers fentanyl citrate via a sucker. An example of this drug is Actiq, 1,600 µg/sucker. This has the advantage of being quickly absorbed through the mucous membrane of the mouth and working rapidly to control breakthrough pain. This medication should be taken only by clients already taking prescription opioid (narcotic) drugs on a regular schedule.

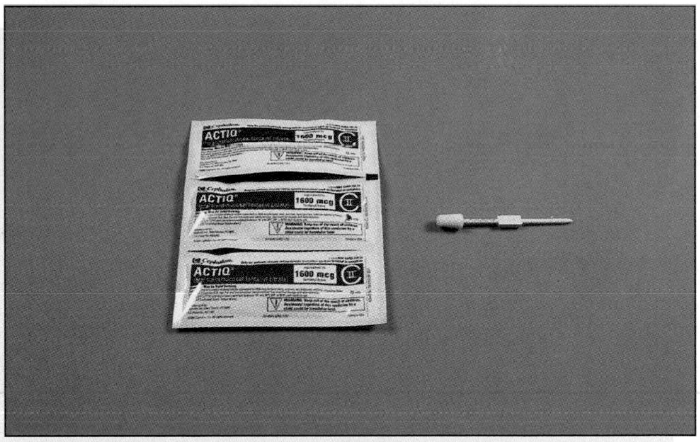

A new method for managing breakthrough pain is oral transmucosal, delivering medication via a sucker.

NURSING DIAGNOSES

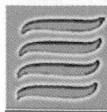

The following nursing diagnoses may be appropriate to include on client care plans when the components are related to alleviating pain in a client.

NURSING DIAGNOSIS	RELATED FACTORS
Anxiety	Anticipation of discomfort, fear, helplessness, inability to relax
Fear	Long-term disability, terminal disease, hospitalization, invasive procedures, lack of knowledge, surgery and its outcome
Pain (acute, chronic)	Trauma, immobility, surgery, chronic illness
Ineffective Coping	Poor adjustment to pain/illness, fear

- The single most important nursing action to decrease the incidence of hospital-based infections is handwashing. **Remember to wash your hands or use antibacterial gel before and after each and every client contact.**

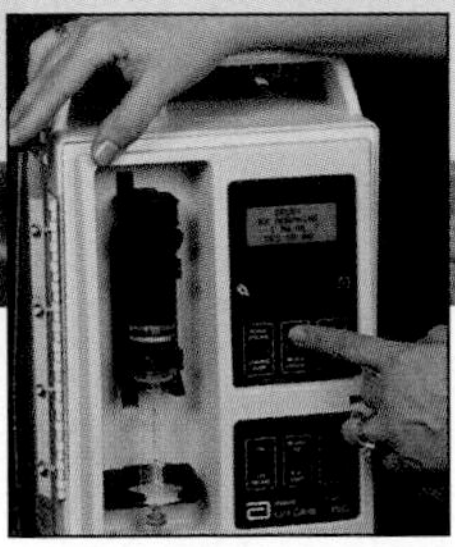

UNIT 1

Nonpharmacological Pain Relief

Nursing Process Data

ASSESSMENT Data Base

Assess type of pain.

- Acute pain: short duration of a few seconds to 6 months
- Chronic pain: longer duration of 6 months to years
- Malignant pain: severe and constant and resistant to relief measures

Choose a pain intensity scale and identify the level or degree of pain the client is experiencing.

Assess nonverbal indications of pain.

Assess client's behavioral responses to pain.

- Depression, withdrawal, or crying
- Stoicism or expressive

Assess location, quality, intensity, onset, duration, pattern, aggravating factors, associated factors, and relief or alleviating factors. (See *Physical Pain Sensation* chart p. 468.)

PLANNING Objectives

To relieve pain or prevent pain from escalating by relaxing muscles; muscle tension increases the pain

To decrease client's anxiety that present and future pain relief will not be achieved

To bring pain relief to a level acceptable to the client

To educate clients to communicate their pain level

IMPLEMENTATION Procedures

Alleviating Pain through Touch (Massage)

Using Relaxation Techniques

EVALUATION Expected Outcomes

Pain is controlled to the client's satisfaction.

Pain is relieved and does not interfere with ambulation or sitting in a chair.

Client experiences pain relief from relaxed muscles.

Client's anxiety level is low as related to pain.

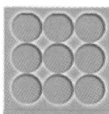

CULTURAL COMPETENCE

Health care personnel working in a variety of settings maintain that pain is a culturally influenced phenomenon. How pain is experienced and expressed varies by cultural group. For example, some cultures (such as the Italians and Jewish people) encourage open expression of feelings like pain, while others (the stoic English, Irish, and Chinese) believe that pain is something to be ignored or endured in silence. This was demonstrated by Zborowski's study done as early as the 1950s. While these general conclusions may lead to stereotyping, it is important to consider the impact of the individual's culture in the assessment of pain level.

Source: Spector, R. (2001). *Cultural Diversity in Health and Illness.* (5th ed.) Upper Saddle River, NJ: Prentice Hall Health.

ALLEVIATING PAIN THROUGH TOUCH (MASSAGE)

Equipment

Cream
Massage oil

Procedure

1. Determine whether client achieves more relief from pain with massage over painful area, near painful area, or from foot rub, back rub, or hand rub.
2. Warm your hands by rubbing them together or rinsing in warm water.
3. Warm lotion to be used by holding closed bottle under warm running water.
4. Massage area of client's choice with slow and steady motion.
5. Use deep pressure or light stroking motion, whichever is more comfortable for the client. **Rationale:** Relaxed muscles result in a decreased pain level.

USING RELAXATION TECHNIQUES

Equipment

A printed relaxation technique (the nurse can read slowly until client learns technique)
A cassette recorder and tape

Procedure

1. Help client assume a comfortable position.
   a. If lying, place support under knees, lower legs, and under head. Be sure body is in good alignment.
   b. If sitting, sit comfortably positioned with both feet on the floor, hands on knees, back straight, and head balanced comfortably straight.
2. Instruct client to inhale deeply, hold breath for a moment, then exhale deeply. Repeat several times.
3. Give the following instructions to client, using a slow, soothing voice.
   a. Continue to breathe in and out slowly. Concentrate on my voice and follow my words.
   b. Find a point of tension in your body.
   c. As you identify the tension, tense the area up even more.
   d. Then relax the area, letting all the tension drain out.
4. Continue with these instructions until the client has had time to relax all points of tension.
5. To end the process, instruct the client to open eyes slowly and say, "I feel relaxed and awake."

DOCUMENTATION FOR NONPHARMACOLOGICAL PAIN RELIEF

- Describe the client's pain, including onset, pattern, location, quality, intensity, precipitating factors, associated factors, and aggravating factors.
- Describe alleviating factors, including what the client does to relieve pain as well as nursing assistance
- Describe behavioral changes due to pain relief or the absence of objective changes in response to nursing interventions
- If there is a poor response to therapy, state what other measures will be attempted, and chart results
- Continue to document attempts to relieve pain until relief occurs and the client is satisfied

Critical Thinking Application

UNEXPECTED OUTCOMES	CRITICAL THINKING OPTIONS
Client achieves no relief from massage.	• Try combining method with use of medications (i.e., while waiting for the medication to take effect). • Client has to trust the technique before it can be effective. Have client talk to another person who has found technique helpful.
Client cannot focus on relaxation technique.	• Start with very simple breathing techniques and progress slowly to relaxation and visualization.

UNIT 2

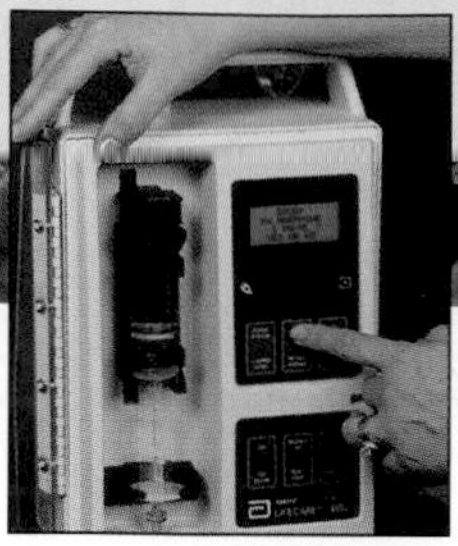

Pharmacological Pain Management

Nursing Process Data

ASSESSMENT Database

Assess client's type, description, rating (use a pain intensity scale), and level of pain.
Assess vital signs for baseline comparison.
Assess allergy to pain medication—morphine.
Assess patency of IV lines.
Assess sedation level of client on epidural analgesia.
Assess insertion site for drainage, inflammation, etc.
Assess potential use of PCA as method of pain control.
Assess reliability of candidate—ability to self-administer PCA.
Assess client throughout PCA therapy (every 2 hours during first 24 hours, then every 4 hours).

PLANNING Objectives

To prevent pain from retarding recovery
To prevent pain from causing nausea and vomiting, a decrease in fluid intake which results in fluid and electrolyte imbalance
To prevent pain from causing undue fatigue
To prevent pain from inhibiting moving, ambulating, turning, and coughing; pain increases the possibilities of secondary problems from inactivity (e.g., pneumonia, emboli)
To provide a consistent level of pain control without unacceptable side effects
To enable the client to feel in control of his or her pain management
To decrease the client's anxiety around the pain control issue
To allow the client, according to needs for pain control, to self-administer pain medication via PCA

IMPLEMENTATION Procedures

Administering Pain Medications
Administering Epidural Narcotic Analgesia
  for Bolus Injection
  for Continuous Infusion
Qualifying the Client for PCA
Administering PCA
Terminating a PCA Infusion
Teaching PCA to a Client

EVALUATION Expected Outcomes

Client feels competent to self-administer pain medication via PCA.
PCA infuser works efficiently to administer medication.
IV site used to administer PCA remains free of complications.
Pain is controlled to client's satisfaction.
Client's anxiety level remains low or manageable around issue of pain control.

ADMINISTERING PAIN MEDICATIONS

Equipment

Pain Assessment Scale
Appropriate pain medication

Procedure

1. Assess pain intensity by selecting a pain tool based on client's preference.
   a. Verbal description scale.
   b. Numeric rating scale.
   c. FACES pain scale.
2. Check physician's orders for changes in pain medication.
3. Administer pain medication or request change in dosing schedule of infusion, PCA, etc.
4. Record results and set schedule for follow-up reassessment.

EVIDENCE BASED NURSING PRACTICE

Pain in the Cognitively Impaired

In a study of 217 cognitively impaired nursing home clients, 62% reported pain when asked directly. The pain scale most easily understood was a 0 to 5 scale using words from "no pain" to "worst pain."

Source: McCaffery, M. (July 1999). Assessing pain in a confused or nonverbal patient. *Nursing 99, 29*(7), 18.

Pain Management Options

Prior Treatments

IM injections of morphine (or Demerol)

Intermittent IV dosing

New Standards of Pain Care

Continuous IV infusion of pain medication

PCA—combination of continuous infusion with client-controlled bolus dosing for breakthrough pain

Epidural analgesia (continuous infusion or PCA analgesia)

Adjunctive medications, i.e., anti-inflammatory, antiemetics to enhance effects of opioids

Transition to long-acting oral meds before discontinuing IV analgesics

ADMINISTERING EPIDURAL NARCOTIC ANALGESIA

Note: Many hospitals require specific certification before the RN can administer narcotics via an indwelling epidural catheter. A student nurse should not administer solutions via epidural catheter unless there is specific agency protocol that allows it.

Equipment

Labels for safety precautions:
  At head of bed: "Epidural Protocol Client"
  At end of catheter: "Epidural Catheter"
3-mL syringe and ampule of naloxone hydrochloride (Narcan: 0.4 mg) as ordered at bedside
Ambu bag at bedside
Respiratory record, apnea monitor, or pulse oximeter
Sterile gloves
Tape

for Bolus Injection
Prediluted preservative-free narcotic as ordered
12-mL safety syringe with filter needle
20-gauge 1-inch needle
Antimicrobial swabs (no alcohol)
Sterile 2 × 2 gauze

for Continuous Infusion
Infusion pump
IV tubing
Prediluted preservative-free narcotic container

Preparation

1. Check physician's orders for epidural narcotic indicating minimum and maximum dosage.
   a. Preservative-free narcotic and dose; preservative-free saline and amount ordered.
   b. Interval between doses.
   c. Infusion rate and concentration, if appropriate.
2. Check that safety sign is over bed: "Epidural Protocol Client."
   Rationale: Identifies client to all staff as having epidural tubing.
3. Check that catheter is labeled "Epidural catheter."
   Rationale: Identifies catheter and avoids confusing epidural catheter with IV tubing.

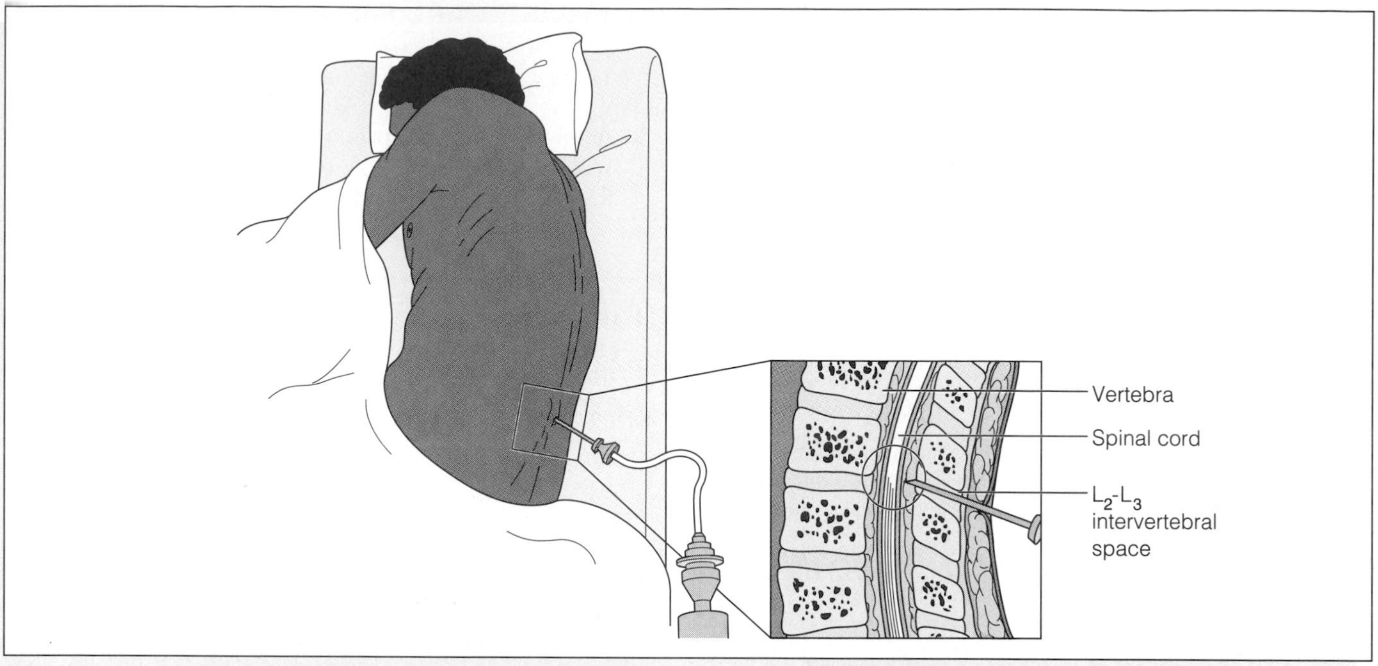

Placement of indwelling catheter in the epidural space.

CLINICAL ALERT

Place IV line as far as possible from an epidural catheter and label epidural catheter to avoid mistaking it for IV catheter—this could be a *fatal* mistake. Some catheters are specifically labeled. For example, the DuPen permanent epidural catheter has a yellow band near the Luer-Lok tip that has a sign "Epidural catheter—not an IV access."

4. Check that a Narcan ampule and 3-mL syringe are at bedside. **Rationale:** Respiratory depression can be treated with IV Narcan, a narcotic antagonist.
5. Check that there is IV access for administration of Narcan. **Rationale:** It may be necessary to quickly administer a narcotic antagonist if respiratory depression occurs.

Note: IV should be accessed with needleless syringe. If a needle must be used for injection into an IV system, use one no longer than 1 inch and no smaller than 25 gauge.

6. Check that Ambu bag is available on unit. **Rationale:** Necessary for complication of respiratory depression.
7. Check if an apnea monitor or pulse oximeter is ordered. **Rationale:** It is important that clients are monitored closely (at least for the first 12 hours) because of dangerous side effects, especially respiratory depression.
8. Assemble equipment.
9. Wash your hands, and maintain strict aseptic technique. **Rationale:** Maintaining sterility of insertion site, administered solutions, and infusion lines decreases potential for complications.
10. Check client's identaband.

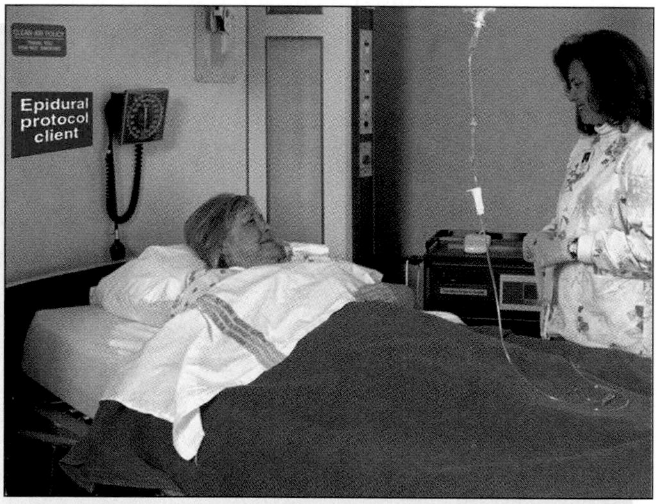

When a client is receiving epidural analgesia, there should be a sign over the bed stating "Epidural Protocol Client."

Narcotic Administration

Narcotics Commonly Administered Via Epidural Continuous Infusion

- Hydromorphone hydrochloride (Dilaudid: 0.05–0.3 mg/hr)
- Fentanyl (50–150 μg/hr)
- Morphine sulfate (Duramorph: 0.2–1.0 mg/hr)

Procedure

for Bolus Injection

1. Put on sterile gloves and maintain sterile technique.
2. Wipe narcotic vial with antiseptic swab.
3. Draw up ordered dose of prediluted preservative-free narcotic in 12-mL syringe with filter needle.
4. Change filter needle to needleless cannula.
5. Expel air from syringe.
6. Verify narcotic with a second nurse before administering. **Rationale:** It is important to take every precaution to prevent inadvertent administration of a drug that could cause spinal cord damage.
7. Disinfect catheter injection port (Luer-Lok port or the injection cap) with nonalcohol antimicrobial wipe. **Rationale:** Alcohol must *never* be used because it is extremely toxic to the spinal cord.

CLINICAL ALERT

If more than 1 mL of fluid or blood is returned during aspiration of the catheter, the procedure *must be terminated* (because the catheter may have migrated) and physician notified.

8. Dry injection cap or port with sterile 2 × 2 gauze.
9. Insert cannula into injection cap or port, and attempt to aspirate for 30 seconds. **Rationale:** See Clinical Alert above.

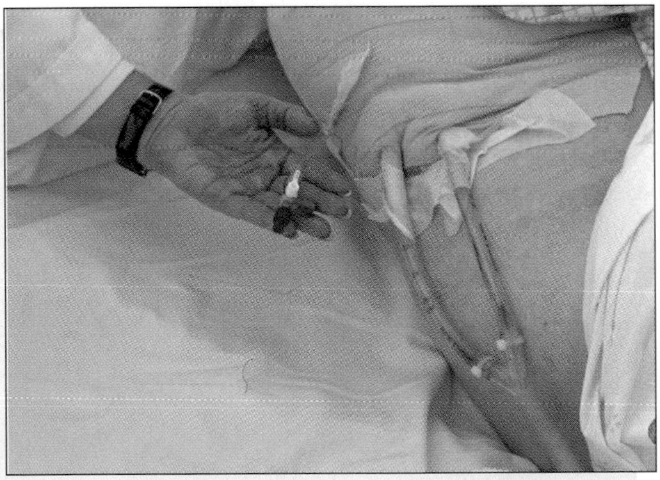

Intrapleural catheter may be used for pain medication instillation.

10. Inject medication slowly.
11. Remove cannula from injection cap or port.
12. Dispose of syringe in appropriate container.
13. Check that a sterile, occlusive dressing is over insertion site. Dressing is changed every 72 hours (certified RN or MD to change dressing) or when wet.
14. Tape all injection ports on epidural line if there is no continuous infusion. **Rationale:** This will prevent injecting a solution meant for the IV line into the epidural line.
15. Closely monitor respirations every 1 hour for 24 hours or use apnea monitor or pulse oximeter. **Rationale:** Due to risk of respiratory depression, close monitoring after administration of an epidural narcotic is essential.
16. Monitor vital signs: BP and pulse every 30 minutes for 1 hour after initial epidural dose, then every 8 hours.
17. Monitor for possible side effects of narcotic administration: respiratory depression, urinary retention, nausea and vomiting, and pruritus.
18. Document dose and client status.

CLINICAL ALERT

Low molecular weight heparin (LMWH) should NOT be used with epidural or spinal analgesia.

for Continuous infusion

1. Check physician's orders for epidural narcotic.
2. Check that safety signs are near bed and label is on catheter.
3. Wash hands and don gloves.
4. Attach container of narcotic to infusion pump tubing.
5. Prime tubing (see Chapter 28 for step-by-step instruction).
6. Attach proximal end of tubing to pump and distal end to epidural catheter.
7. Tape all connections securely.
8. Set infusion pump to ordered calibration.
9. Observe for side effects of narcotic or client response and pain level.
10. Dispose of gloves and wash hands.
11. Chart pump reading every hour for 12–24 hours or as dictated by institutional policy.
12. Record narcotic on appropriate sign-out sheet.

QUALIFYING THE CLIENT FOR PCA

Procedure

1. Determine whether physician wishes to use PCA for pain control.
2. Determine if client is a candidate for PCA.
   a. Check criteria for client selection.
   b. After explaining PCA, determine if client wishes to use this method of pain control.

CLINICAL ALERT

Determine if client is allergic to pain medication prescribed—usually morphine or meperidine.

3. Determine which type—electronic or mechanical—PCA unit is appropriate.
   a. A mechanical device is fed by gravity rather than electricity; it is simple, inexpensive, disposable, and does not interfere with the client's mobility.
   b. A pump or electronic device has a computer for dosage monitoring, is more flexible, and can be reset as necessary.
4. Assess any allergy to prescribed pain medication.
5. Perform basic physical assessment before initiating PCA.
   a. Establish baseline vital sign chart.
   b. Specifically assess client's respiratory system for ongoing evaluation during PCA therapy.

Criteria for Client Selection for PCA

- Clients requiring parenteral analgesic treatment.
- Clients requiring postoperative pain relief.
- Trauma clients who have clear sensorium.
- Clients suffering from chronic pain (terminal cancer).
- Clients who are mentally alert and able to understand and comply with procedure instructions.
- Clients without a handicap that impairs ability to use PCA.
- Clients with no prior addiction to drugs or alcohol.
- Eighteen years of age is the usual minimum age for PCA use, but it has been used in children as young as 7 years of age.

ADMINISTERING PCA

Equipment

Note: This skill applies to the Abbott Lifecare PCA Plus II pump. Specific steps of administering PCA vary with different manufacturers' equipment.

Specific physician's orders for PCA
Gloves
PCA infuser pump
PCA administration tubing
IV start kit, tubing, catheter, and ordered fluid
Extension set with Luer-Lok adapter
Analgesic medication cartridge and injector (vial injector)
PCA administration record
PCA booklet for client

Preparation

1. Check that physician's orders, including medication orders for PCA, are complete.

Note: Morphine is available in 30-mL vial injectors (concentration of 1 mg/mL or 5 mg/mL).

2. Check client's identaband.
3. Assemble IV administration set (refer to Chapter 28, *Preparing the Infusion System*).
   a. Wash your hands and don gloves.
   b. Start IV line. **Rationale:** This establishes venous access for PCA.
4. Assemble PCA vial injector following manufacturer's instructions.
   a. Snap caps from injector (plunger) and vial.
   b. Connect plunger to vial by twisting them together.
   c. Prime unit by pushing down on injector to release air.
   d. Connect PCA tubing to injector.
5. Prime PCA tubing only to the "Y," then clamp tubing. **Rationale:** Clamping above the Y prevents the narcotic going into the primary line.
6. Attach maintenance IV to unprimed portion of the Y. **Rationale:** To establish primary infusion.
7. Tape maintenance IV securely to Y of PCA tubing. **Rationale:** This is necessary if there is no Luer-Lok on PCA tubing (Abbott).

EVIDENCE BASED NURSING PRACTICE

Client Satisfaction with Pain Assessment

A nationwide database of more than 400 hospitals demonstrated that client satisfaction with pain control rose from 678 to 898 when the hospitals changed their pain assessment format to include more frequent pain assessment, greater use of PCA, and reduced use of IM pain medication. Nurses' attitude about medicating for pain also changed during the study.

Source: (Dec., 1999), Improved Satisfaction Through Better Pain Control, *RN, 29*(12), 30-0-P.

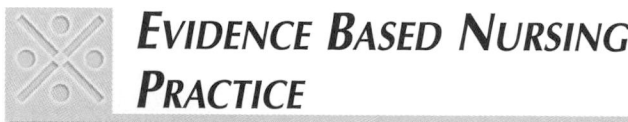

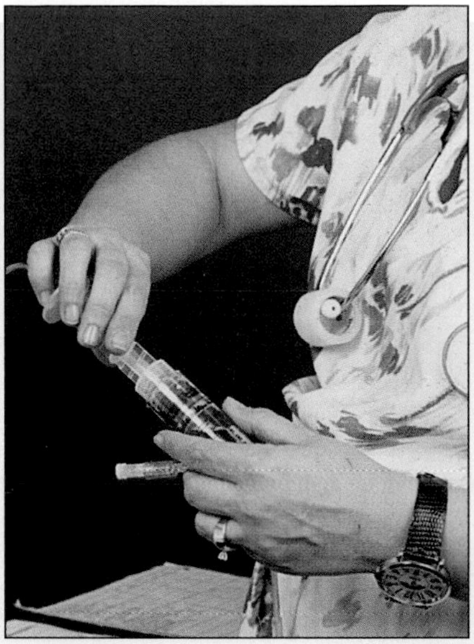
Connect plunger to vial.

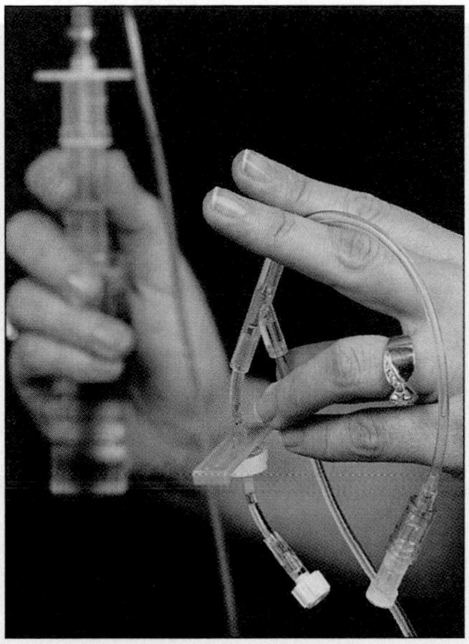
Prime PCA tubing to Y connector.

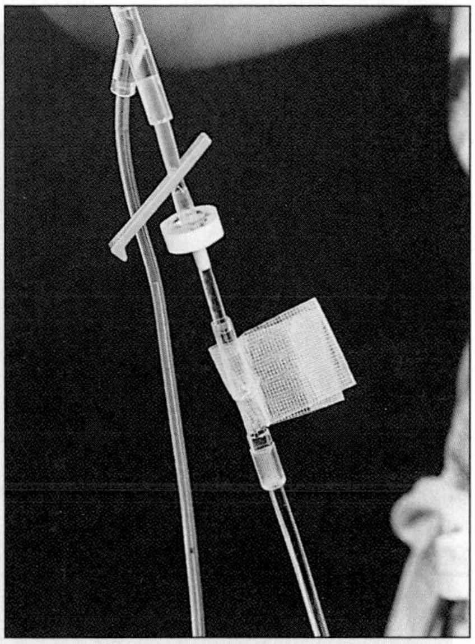
Tape maintenance IV securely.

8. Prime lower tubing of PCA set with IV solution from the gravity administration set. **Rationale:** This clears air from tubing.
9. Close slide clamp on PCA tubing. **Rationale:** Closing slide clamp maintains prime and prevents air entry.
10. Open flow control clamp on IV. **Rationale:** This clears medication already primed with maintenance IV.
11. Explain ongoing procedure to client. (You have already completed client teaching regarding pain management with use of PCA infuser.)
12. Leave PCA booklet with client for referral during pain control time.

CLINIC AL ALERT

To administer blood or any other medication incompatible with pain medication, you must establish a second IV site.

PCA Infuser Pump

PCA infuser pumps are made for home or hospital use. These special pumps allow the client to control three parameters of medication delivery:

- Stopping and starting a continuous infusion.
- Titrating the hourly dose within a preset range of milligrams per hour.
- Administering a bolus dose within preset parameters.

Procedure

1. Unlock by turning key, and open door of infuser.
2. Activate drive release mechanism by pinching spring-loaded lever, and move drive assembly to uppermost position.
3. Load vial injector into vial injector holder by moving drive assembly downward. (Be sure calibrations are visible.)
4. Clamp securely, and listen for "click" sound. **Rationale:** Click lets you know vial injector is properly inserted and locked into position.
5. Rotate vial injector in holder, and inspect for leakage or cracks. **Rationale:** Improper loading may cause vial injector to crack. Vial injector may not leak until delivery pressure is applied. Cracked vial injector may cause overdelivery of medication to client.

CLINICAL ALERT

If vial injector is cracked and unusable, discard contents in presence of another licensed RN and sign off on narcotic record or follow hospital protocol for disposal of narcotic. Replace with new vial injector.

6. Validate drug dose as you continue to activate PCA by responding to screen (e.g., drug—morphine 1 mg, yes or no?).
7. Set PCA parameters for infusion according to manufacturer's instructions.
   a. Press on–off button to turn on infuser. **Rationale:** When machine is turned on, DOOR OPEN and VOLUME DELIVERED messages appear.
   b. Use dose volume control to set DOSE VOLUME to be delivered. **Rationale:** Limits the total amount of drug the client can receive/dose.

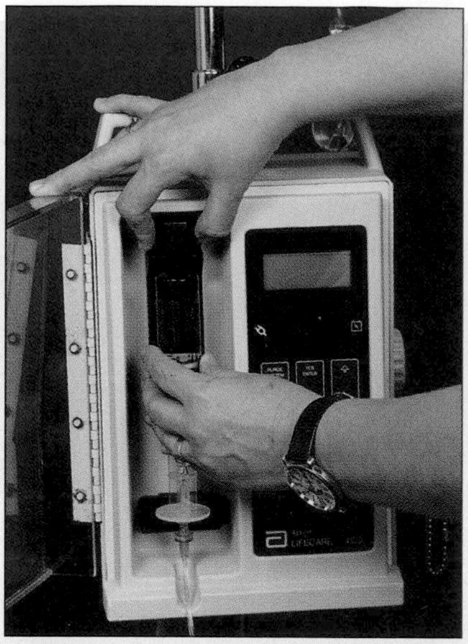
Load vial injector into holder

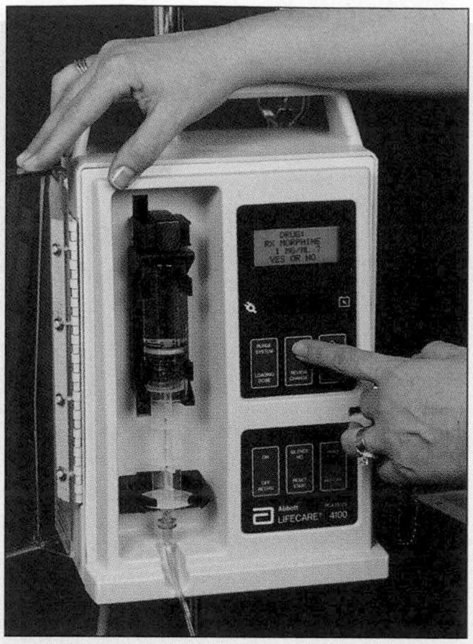
Validate drug dose on screen

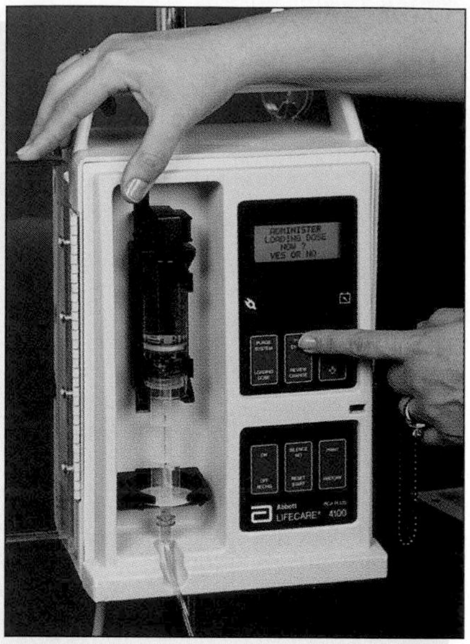
Administer loading dose

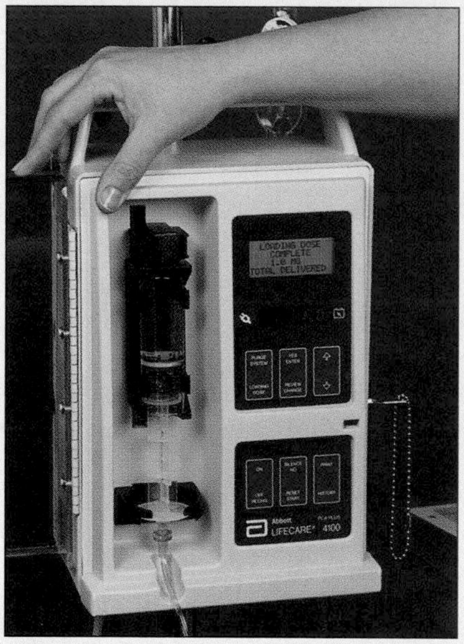
Read screen for loading dose complete.

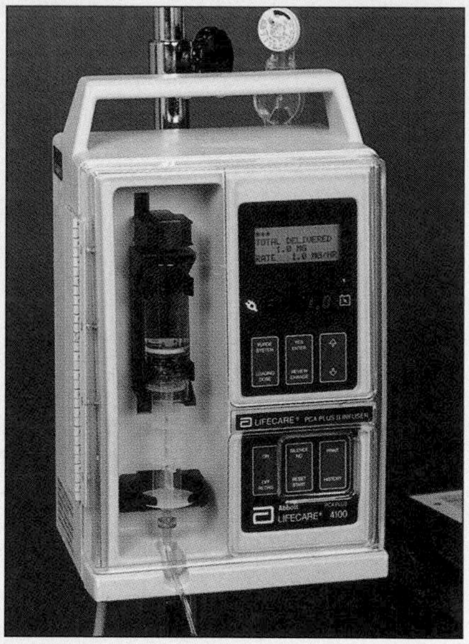
Read screen for total delivered dose.

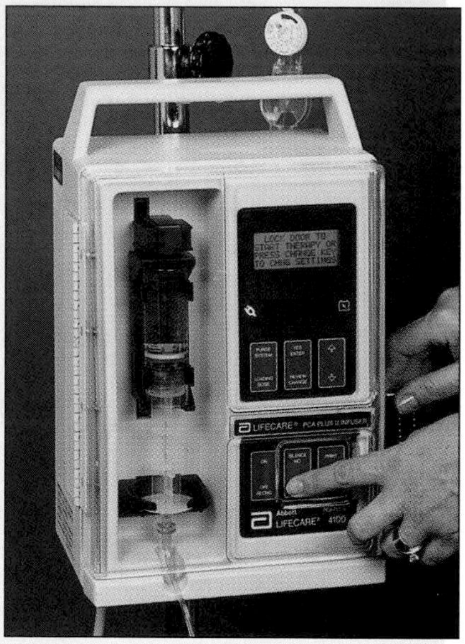
Lock door to begin therapy.

   c. Set LOCKOUT INTERVAL (generally between 5 and 10 minutes). **Rationale:** Period during which PCA cannot be activated.
   d. Check that slide clamps on PCA infuser are open.
8. Calculate for loading dose the number of milliliters needed for correct milligram dose.
   a. Press and release LOADING DOSE.
   b. Check that display screen shows volume delivered.
   c. Monitor respirations every 15 minutes after loading dose until stable.
9. Set 4-HOUR LIMIT by calculating maximum dose client may receive in a 4-hour period. Control ranges from 5 to 30 mL in 5-mL increments. **Rationale:** This allows 30 mL to be the maximum amount that can be delivered in 4 hours.

Dose Calculation

- The PCA infuser delivers in milliliters. The nurse must calculate the number of milliliters needed for the correct milligram dose. Examples: 10 mg (1 mL) every 10 minutes; 40 mg (4 mL) every 10 minutes.
- The maximum rate of administration is 20 mL/hour.

10. Close and lock security door to initiate client control. Remove key and place with narcotic keys or follow hospital protocol. **Rationale:** Door must be locked to read READY message. This indicates infuser is now in client control mode and that first dose is available to client.
11. Hand control button to client.
12. Review client instructions.
13. Monitor client status every 2 hours for 24 hours and revise parameters with physician, if necessary.

PRN Booster Dose via PCA

If physician so orders, a booster dose may be given to a client on a PRN basis. All booster doses must be administered by an RN.

- Open door.
- Set DOSE VOLUME to dose ordered.
- Set LOCKOUT INTERVAL to 00.
- Administer dose.
- Set dose back to original order.
- Set LOCKOUT INTERVAL to original order.
- Close and lock door.

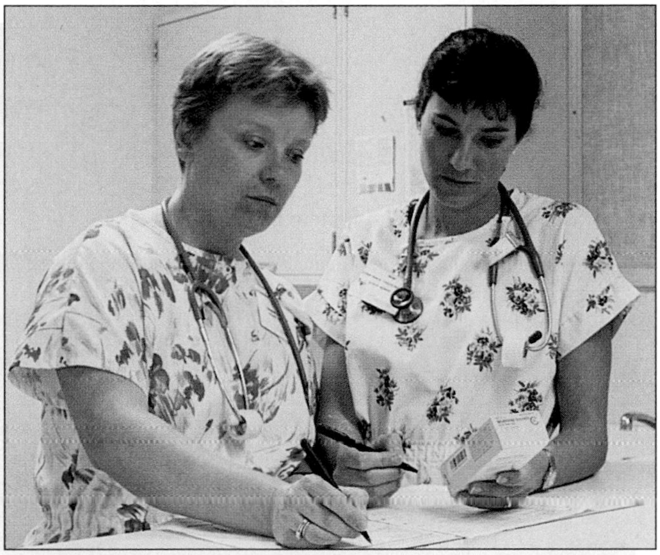

Check narcotic dose with a second nurse.

TERMINATING A PCA INFUSION

Procedure

1. Close manual slide clamp proximal to Luer-Lok connector on vial injector.
2. Unlock and open security door.
3. Remove vial injector from PCA infuser, and disconnect from set.
4. Press OFF button to turn off PCA infuser.
5. Continue or discontinue IV as required.
6. Record and dispose of PCA narcotic vial injector per hospital policy for disposal of narcotic drugs.
7. Dispose of narcotic that remains in vial injector per protocol. **Rationale:** Narcotics must be accounted for by cosignature on controlled narcotic record or per individual hospital protocol.

TEACHING PCA TO A CLIENT

Preparation

1. Determine if client is a candidate for PCA (see skill in this chapter *Qualifying the Client for PCA*).
2. Allow client to directly handle equipment and practice using a "dummy" PCA button. **Rationale:** This reduces fear of technology and teaches basic steps of PCA.

Procedure

1. Demonstrate how PCA device works.
   a. Set the pump's controls to deliver pain medication.
   b. Instruct client that if amount of medication is not sufficient to control pain, he or she may press a button to deliver an additional bolus.
   c. Tell client that after each bolus, client must wait a minimum amount of time (usually 5–10 minutes) before delivering another dose. **Rationale:** This protects client from receiving too much medication.
   d. Dose may be adjusted to maintain pain control. **Rationale:** When clients control their own medication dose, studies indicate usage is not excessive.
   e. Have client explain and demonstrate PCA use before initiating therapy.
2. Clarify with client how he or she administers medication dose when pain is felt. **Rationale:** Self-control of pain medication has been found to be very successful with clients

and less time-consuming for the nurse. There is no significant difference in amount of medication used.

3. Program PCA infuser for continuous infusion plus a bolus dose.
   a. Establish amount of narcotic needed to control client's pain (i.e., give 1–5 mg morphine every 10 minutes until pain is relieved).
   b. Set pump's hourly infusion rate to equal total milligrams per hour needed to control pain.
4. Reassure client that PCA will control, but not totally abolish, pain. **Rationale:** Continuous infusion supplemented by small boluses provides steady relief (more so than IM injections) but does not eliminate pain.
5. Teach client how to evaluate pain level on a five-point scale. If client's pain is not sufficiently relieved, medication dose is increased. **Rationale:** When clients know they can control their pain level, they feel less helpless and more empowered.
   1 = Pain relieved
   2 = Occasional discomfort
   3 = Decreased pain intensity, e.g., able to walk, cough
   4 = Minimal pain relief
   5 = No pain relief
6. Evaluate client's response to medication schedule. **Rationale:** It is important to check for adverse effects of sedation to avoid complications or necessity of revising dose parameters.
7. Reassess client's ability to control pain level and effectiveness of medication dosage to control pain.
8. Teach client importance of not letting family member (or anyone other than client) activate PCA pump.

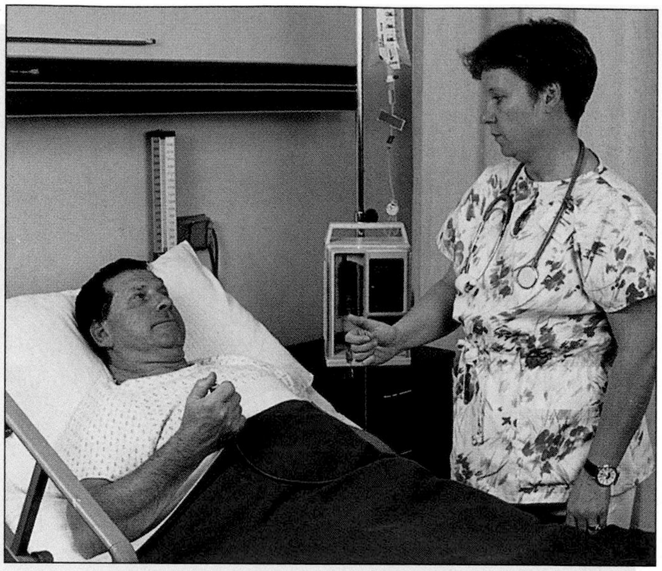

Teach PCA procedure to client.

9. Teach client potential adverse effects (sedation, respiratory depression) if anyone other than client activates pump.
10. Instruct client to notify staff if machine malfunctions (alarm sounds or message display indicates a problem), pain is not controlled or changes in severity, or if he or she has any questions.

PATIENT CONTROLLED ANALGESIA (PCA)—USING THE PCA INFUSION PUMP

DATE:	TIME:	DRUG ALLERGIES:

A. DRUG/CONCENTRATION: Check One
Morphine = 1 mg/mL .... ☐
Meperidine = 10 mg/mL .... ☐
Other ________ ________ = mg/mL .... ☐

B. PCA/BASAL (Patient Controlled with Background Continuous Infusion)
Please specify doses in mL rather than mg when ordering.

1. Specify DOSE (patient controlled): ________ mL
   Pump range is 0.1–9.9 mL
   Suggested dose: Morphine 0.5–1.5 mL (0.5–1.5 mg)
   Meperidine 0.5–1.0mL (5-10mg)

2. Specify DELAY (PCA dose lockout interval): ________ min
   Pump range is 3–60 min
   Suggested interval: 10–15 min

3. Specify BASAL RATE (continuous infusion): ________ mL/hr
   Pump range is 0.0–10.0 mL/hr
   Suggested continuous rate: Morphine 1.0–2.5 mL/hr (1.0–2.5 mg/hr)
   Meperidine 1.0–1.5 mL/hr (10–15 mg/hr)

4. Specify 1 HOUR LIMIT (maximum combined PCA + basal rate): ________ mL
   Pump range is 1.0–30 mL
   Suggested limit: Morphine 5–10 mL/hr (5–10 mg)
   Meperidine 4.0–5.5 mL/hr (40–50 mg)

5. Specify BOLUS dose (initial loading dose) if desired: ________ mL
   Specify if bolus dose may be repeated and frequency/interval:
   ____
   Pump range is 0.0–9.9 mL
   Suggested bolus dose: Morphine 3–5 mL (3–5 mg)
   Meperidine 2.0–2.5 mL (20–25 mg)

C. Additional PCA orders: ________

D. If patient persistently complains of inadequate analgesia, notify Physician.

Physician's Signature: ________

PCA Administration Record.

DOCUMENTATION FOR PHARMACOLOGICAL PAIN RELIEF

- Pain onset, pattern, description, location, intensity
- Amount and type of pain medication administered
- Sedation level of client
- Interventions, level of pain relief
- Side effects—pruritus, nausea, and vomiting
- Vital signs

for Epidural Analgesia

- Pain relief from medication
- Side effects—pruritus, nausea and vomiting
- Condition of insertion site
- Vital signs

for PCA

- Assess and chart on client using PCA infuser every 4 hours (after initial 24 hours), unless otherwise ordered.
- Describe respirations every 2 hours, and compare to baseline assessment sheet.
- Record sedation and pain legend every 4 hours. Include degree of pain relief obtained from PCA.
  1 = Wide awake
  2 = Drowsy
  3 = Dosing intermittently
  4 = Mostly sleeping
  5 = Only awakens when disturbed
- Initiate new PCA administration record for each narcotic vial injector used.

for PCA Record

- Chart appropriate entries throughout your shift. To determine amount of medication administered, press TOTAL DOSES and multiply by number of milliliters prescribed.
- Chart LOADING DOSE and time administered separately on medication record.
- Chart wasted narcotic—cosigned per hospital policy.
- Verify and document that calculated volume remaining and actual volume remaining in syringe are the same. Report any discrepancy and follow hospital procedure for incorrect narcotic count.

Critical Thinking Application

UNEXPECTED OUTCOMES	CRITICAL THINKING OPTIONS
for Administering Pain Medication	
Client says that pain medication is not helping the pain.	• Reassess tolerance level of client (check if client has previously been on high doses of a narcotic, thus developing a high tolerance level). • Check that pain dose is adequate for pain management. • Request consultation with physician to increase or change pain medication (remember, the nurse is the client's advocate).
Client appears overly sedated.	• Hold the next pain medication until client can be evaluated—notify the physician. • Check other drugs client is taking—there may be a synergistic effect.
for Epidural Analgesia	
Client develops constipation from regularly administered narcotic preparations.	• Obtain order for and administer stool softener and peristaltic stimulant. • Encourage intake of high-fiber diet, if not contraindicated. • Encourage adequate fluid intake.

UNEXPECTED OUTCOMES	CRITICAL THINKING OPTIONS
Client develops respiratory depression and appears to be sedated.	• Check sedation level (drug may have been absorbed by systemic vasculature and epidural veins and ended up in high concentrations in the brain). • Reduce rate of epidural and notify physician. • Check on other drugs the client is taking—there may be a synergistic effect. • Nursing assessment: respirations, ability to cough and deep breathe, auscultate chest, arterial blood gases. • Check that Narcan is at the bedside—may be ordered if respirations are too slow (this drug reverses analgesia so monitor for high pain level returning).
Client develops nausea and vomits.	• Assess cause of problem—consider pain, ileus, as well as reaction to drug. • Administer antiemetics as ordered, and protect client from aspiration. • Keep client NPO until cause of problem is discovered.
Client complains of numbness in legs and motor weakness but has no pain.	• Turn epidural infusion off until normal sensations return, then restart infusion at 2 to 4 mL/hr lower than original rate. • Monitor for pain relief. • Chart nursing actions and client response.
Catheter insertion site is red and warm to touch, and drainage is noted.	• Check temperature and vital signs and notify physician.
for PCA	
Vial injector is incorrectly positioned or empty.	• Close slide clamp. • Press SILENCE. • Check vial injector for contents and position. Properly install it or replace with new vial injector. • Open slide clamp.
Alarm signal flashes.	• Press SILENCE to mute alarm temporarily.
Security door is closed and locked and a. Dose volume and lockout interval controls combined allow more than 20 mL/hr, *or* b. Dose volume is greater than 5 mL or at 0.0 mL/hr, *or* c. Lockout interval is less than 5 minutes.	• Unlock and open security door. • Reset DOSE VOLUME and/or LOCKOUT INTERVAL to proper values. • Close and lock security door and remove key. • READY message appears.
Alarm signal flashes and fluid delivery stops. Audible alarm sounds.	• Close slide clamp. • Press SILENCE (mutes alarm for 1–5 minutes). • Plug into AC outlet as soon as possible to recharge battery. (With a discharged battery, there is a blank message panel, loss of cumulative volume and total dose information, and nonoperation of PCA infuser.)
Alarm bar flashes because door has been open 10 minutes.	• Press SILENCE to mute for an additional 10 minutes, *or* • Close and lock security door.

UNEXPECTED OUTCOMES	CRITICAL THINKING OPTIONS
Client exhibits bradypnea, hypotension, nausea, vomiting, or dizziness.	• Monitor sedation level—remember the goal of PCA is to control pain without sedation. • Report to physician that medication parameters are resulting in oversedation.
Client experiences breakthrough pain.	• Readjust the medication or dosage level or bolus level (according to orders) so that breakthrough pain does not occur.
Client is insecure and anxious about using PCA mode of pain control.	• Determine which steps client feels insecure about completing, and reteach procedure while demonstrating steps.
Medication, either type or dose, is not sufficiently controlling client's level of pain.	• Reevaluate medication and dose parameters with physician.

GERONTOLOGIC CONSIDERATIONS

The incidence of pain in the elderly has not been well studied and this population presents several pain management problems.

- Elderly people often suffer acute and chronic painful diseases or have multiple diseases, thus they often have more than one source of pain.
- Elderly are at increased risk for drug–drug as well as drug–disease interactions.
- Studies show the incidence of pain is twofold higher in those over 60. Acutely painful conditions affect the elderly disproportionately (herpes zoster, arthritis, polymyalgia rheumatica, peripheral vascular disease).
- Elderly may have impaired senses (vision, hearing) and an impaired ability to express themselves.

Pain assessment is more complex and difficult with the elderly.

- The elderly may report pain differently (not as clearly) as younger clients due to physiologic, psychologic, and cultural changes associated with aging.
- Clinicians often hold the mistaken belief that the elderly have increased pain thresholds; they may be more stoic about experiencing, thus reporting pain.
- Cognitive impairment (which may occur in as many as 50% of the institutionalized elderly) may interfere greatly with the assessment of pain. Even though behavior may be assessed (restlessness, groaning, agitation) it is nonspecific and subject to interpretation.
- See Gerontologic Considerations for Medications in Chapter 18 for specific guidelines for drug use with the elderly.

Traditional approaches to pain control may not work with the elderly.

- Universal use of pain series may not be possible with visual, hearing, and motor impairments.
- Clients may report pain initially, but recall (due to cognitive impairment) may not be possible.
- Pain assessment may require frequent monitoring. Monitoring may have major implications for quality of care and quality of life, so facilities with limited staff may result in poor pain control in the elderly.
- The elderly are at risk for over- and undertreatment. Adverse drug reactions are more prevalent with the elderly.
- Attitudes among healthcare professionals may also impede appropriate care (partially due to belief that acute and chronic pain are a normal component of aging).

MANAGEMENT GUIDELINES

Each state legislates a Nurse Practice Act for RNs and LVN/LPNs. Health care facilities are responsible for establishing and implementing policies and procedures that conform to their state's regulations. Verify the regulations and role parameters for each health care worker in your facility.

Delegation of Responsibilities

- Noninvasive pain management techniques can be delegated to any staff member who feels comfortable performing and/or has experience in using touch (massage) or relaxation techniques. If TENS is used for pain control, the nurse must understand the basic principles of how this method works.
- The nurse, RN or LVN/LPN, is the primary individual who is responsible for pain management. He or she does this through the nurse–client relationship by becoming the client's advocate. Therefore, a professional nurse must manage the client's pain in order to identify the intensity, codify the degree, and evaluate the response to pain medication, and intervene as necessary with the physician to change the medication protocol.
- Administration of Epidural Narcotic Analgesia *must* be done by an RN and, in many hospitals, the nurse must have special certification. This skill may *not* be delegated to a nonprofessional staff member.
- Initial administration of PCA must be done by an RN or experienced LVN/PN. It may not be delegated to a UAP, nor may the UAP administer a booster dose.
- PCA may be managed and taught to the client by an RN or LVN/LPN *if* two parameters exist: (1) The Nurse Practice Act and agency protocol in the state allows it, and (2) The nurse has the information and experience to qualify the client and teach the procedure (under physician's orders). Nonprofessional staff may *not* perform this skill.

Information Flow

- It is critically important that the RN inform all staff where epidural narcotic analgesia is being used.
- Safety precautions (written labels) *must* be placed in the appropriate places, such as "Epidural Protocol Client" at the head of the bed, and the catheter labeled "Epidural Catheter" to avoid injuring the client.
- It is also imperative that the RN communicate to other nurses through the client's written records, labeling the IV line, and verbally through report that the client is receiving epidural anesthesia, and that the IV line be placed as far as possible from the epidural catheter. If an epidural catheter is mistaken for an IV line, it could be a *fatal* mistake.
- Because the nurse is the client's advocate in pain control, he or she must receive adequate feedback from all staff who interact with the client so that a viable pain management program can be implemented. It is the nurse's responsibility to inform the auxillary staff caring for the client to report how the client is managing pain.

CRITICAL THINKING STRATEGIES

SCENARIO 1

The client assigned to you has a diagnosis of advanced Alzheimer's disease and cancer with bone metastases. He is a 65-year-old man recently hospitalized. You know he is in pain, but he is unable to relate the degree of pain clearly to the staff or his family.

1. What is the most appropriate method of assessing pain in this client?
2. When considering this client, what is unique about the pain assessment in this situation?
3. What are some possible plans/goals to deal with this client's pain?
4. What are some of the risks in implementing the plan?

SCENARIO 2

The client has a PCA in place but constantly complains that the pain medication is not working. When asked if he uses the bolus dose, he says that he is constantly "locked out."

1. What further assessment, if any, is necessary with this client?
2. Describe the goals and strategies you would devise to handle this situation.
3. What are the best actions you can carry out to meet these goals?

CHAPTER 17

Alternative Therapies and Stress Management

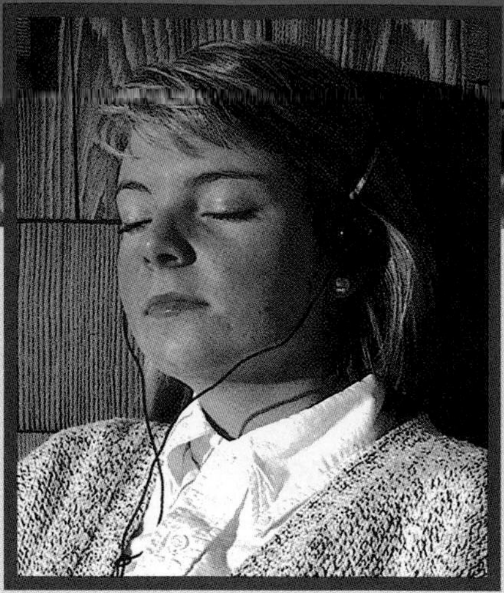

THEORETICAL CONCEPTS

UNIT ONE: **Stress and Adaptation** **507**
- Determining the Effect of Stress 508
- Determining Response Patterns 508
- Managing Stress 509
- Manipulating the Environment to Reduce Stress 509
- Teaching Coping Strategies 509
- Managing Stress Using a Holistic Model 510
- Teaching Controlled Breathing 510
- Teaching Body Relaxation 511
- Using Meditation as an Alternative Therapy 512

GERONTOLOGIC CONSIDERATIONS 513

MANAGEMENT GUIDELINES 513

CRITICAL THINKING STRATEGIES 514

LEARNING OBJECTIVES

- Define the term *stress* according to Hans Selye.
- Discuss the psychologic effect of stress on the body.
- Describe the body's physiologic response to stress, and include at least two body systems.
- List at least three different categories of stressors.
- Identify at least five danger signals of stress.
- Discuss a specific alternative method used to control stress.
- Discuss complementary and alternative medicine (CAM) and how it can be applied to nursing.
- Choose two alternative therapies, discuss the major components and relate how you use them with clients.
- Practice breathing techniques and discuss how you would teach this to a client.

TERMINOLOGY

Adaptive reaction: a response by which the person attempts to improve or alter his or her condition in relation to the environment.

Alleviate: to make more bearable; reduce (pain, grief, or suffering).

Anxiety: a state of uneasiness and distress; diffuse apprehension.

Apathy: indifference; insensibility; without emotion; sluggish.

Apprehension: a fearful or uneasy anticipation of the future; dread.

Ataraxia: the absence of all anxiety.

Autonomic nervous system: the part of the nervous system that regulates the functioning of internal organs and glands; it controls such functions as digestion, respiration, and cardiovascular activity.

Cerebral cortex: the extensive outer layer of grey tissue of the cerebral hemispheres (brain), responsible for higher nervous functions.

Complementary/alternative medicine (CAM): a set of practices that encompass many treatments and ideologies outside of mainstream medicine.

Coping mechanisms: means by which an individual adjusts or adapts to a threat or a challenge; actions that assist in maintaining homeostasis.

Defense mechanisms: conscious or unconscious processes used to protect oneself from threats or to alleviate anxiety.

Dynamics of homeostasis: danger or its symbols, whether internal or external, resulting in the activation of the sympathetic nervous system and the adrenal medulla. The organism prepares for fight or flight.

Emotional: strong feelings, as of joy and sorrow.

Fight or flight: one's immediate response to stress that is, although archaic and often inappropriate, part of our central nervous system's biologic heritage.

General adaptation syndrome: a general theory of stress response formulated by Dr. Hans Selye; describes the action of stress response in three stages: the alarm reaction, the stage of resistance, and the stage of exhaustion.

Hallucination: false perception having no relation to reality and not accounted for by external stimuli.

Health: the state of physical, psychologic, and sociologic well-being.

Holistic: a way of looking at individuals and organisms as a whole rather than a sum of the parts.

Homeostasis: the maintenance of a constant state in the internal environment through self-regulatory techniques that preserve an organism's ability to adapt to stress.

Hypertension: a condition in which the client has a higher blood pressure than judged to be normal.

Illness: a state characterized by the malfunction of the biopsychosocial organism.

Insomnia: inability to sleep.

Lifestyle: the manner in which one is accustomed to living.

Meditation: the act of reflecting on or pondering; contemplation.

Musculoskeletal: pertaining to the muscles and the skeleton.

Pain: a sensation in which a person experiences discomfort, distress, or suffering.

Parasympathetic nervous system: a division of the autonomic nervous system that regulates acetylcholine and conserves energy expenditure; it slows down the system.

Perspective: subjective evaluation of relative significance; a view.

Psychogenic: of mental origin.

Relaxation: a lessening of tension or activity in a part.

Stamina: constitutional energy; strength; endurance.

Stress: a nonspecific response of the body to any internal or external event or change that impinges on a person's system and creates a demand.

Stressor: a specific demand that gives rise to a coping response.

Sympathetic nervous system: a division of the autonomic nervous system that controls energy expenditure and mobilizes for action when confronted with a threat.

Tachycardia: abnormally rapid heart action; above 100 beats per minute.

Tranquilizer: a drug that acts to reduce tension and anxiety without interfering with normal mental activity.

Wellness: a state of physical, psychological, and sociologic well-being of a whole person. Synonym for health.

STRESS

Stress is a universal phenomenon; all human beings in all cultures experience it as a part of their everyday existence. Although stress is a natural component of life, it can sap energy and contribute to the presence of disease. The concept of stress has been with us since the beginning of time, but it was not until William Osler and Walter Cannon began their investigations in the early 1900s that stress was actually linked to illness. By 1950, Hans Selye, a Canadian endocrinologist and biologist, scientifically demonstrated that stress plays a major role in certain diseases, such as gastric ulcers and high blood pressure. Since Selye's early research, authorities from medicine as well as all areas of science have studied and written thousands of articles on this subject. With the undeniable fact that stress affects an individual's total life, nurses should have a basic understanding of this phenomenon, its effect on humans, how humans cope and adapt to stress, and how the nurse can deal with his or her own stress and help clients deal with theirs. To examine stress and its influence on human beings in this culture, we have to examine the total scope of life experience. The stress of life is life itself according to Dr. Barbara Brown, a nurse–author.

Western medicine is entering an era of transformation. The whole context of the medical profession is changing. Clients and professionals alike are examining alternatives to traditional patterns of treatment and are devising new modes of health care delivery. These changes are occurring at a time when the health care system in this country, and indeed the world, desperately needs a new structure to deal with health and illness.

Perhaps the greatest impetus for these changes has developed in response to new knowledge about the role of stress in our lives. Selye, the acknowledged expert on stress, believed that efforts to manage and find cures for diseases is ineffective as an approach to wellness. He and other prominent scientists think that a viable answer is to examine our ability to cope and adapt to stress. Arnold Fox, MD, stated that stress is either the main cause or a strong contributing factor in all diseases of humankind. In fact, most scientists now attribute 70–80% of all diseases to stress and lifestyle.

The view that disease is caused by invading microorganisms, or that ill people are merely victims, or even that all disease can be cured by modern science is misleading and limiting. New definitions of existing problems necessitate finding new solutions. The current emphasis on stress is relevant to our times, and nurses need to recognize and understand stress and its influence on individuals, on the profession, and, most particularly, on clients.

Stress is a difficult term to define precisely, for it does not have a single specific source or one definite response. Selye stated that stress may be viewed as the common denominator of all the body's adaptive reactions. Stress may be grief as well as joy, pleasure as well as unhappiness, cold as well as heat, fear as well as elation. In fact, stress covers the total range of mental, emotional, and physical demands on the body, and responds with predictable biochemical and general adaptation changes. If the body is in a state of balance and the whole organism functions in harmony, the body is healthy. Stress can be defined as a state of arousal or agitation that throws the body out of balance. Although a certain amount of stress is necessary for survival, when it becomes prolonged and intense, our adaptive responses weary, and the negative aspects begin to take their toll on our bodies and our minds. When this occurs, it can be said that disease or dis-ease has overtaken the body and an unhealthy state exists.

The Effect of Stress

Physiologically, stress may be viewed as the experience an individual has when the demands placed on the body exceed the ability to cope, and the body is thrown out of balance. Chemically, stress initiates certain bodily processes, such as the "fight-or-flight" mechanism, which result in a threat to homeostasis. Early in the 1900s Walter Cannon, a Harvard physiologist, coined the term *homeostasis*. As a result of his work, certain adjustment mechanisms of the body, such as blood sugar level, temperature, and hydration, were identified. According to Cannon, the stress response resulted in these mechanisms being activated, which in turn threw the body out of balance.

Rather than a specific response, Hans Selye focused on a general adaptation process as a response to stress. This process is the body's attempt to adapt and maintain homeostasis. Selye further defined stress as the rate of wear and tear on the body and stated that the only freedom from stress is death.

Selye's *general adaptation syndrome* occurs in three stages. The first stage, the *alarm stage*, occurs when the generalized response throughout the body responds to stressors, such as trauma, infection, pain, cold, heat, and fear. The purpose of the alarm reaction is to mobilize the body's defenses to meet the stressor. Biochemically, during the alarm stage, the adrenal cortex produces the anti-inflammatory hormones, the adrenocorticotropin hormones (cortisone and cortisol), and the proinflammatory hormones (aldosterone and desoxycorticosterone). This is called the shock phase because it is when the autonomic nervous system comes into full play.

The second stage, *resistance*, occurs when the body's defenses are mobilized to produce hormones to cope with the alarm stage. The body chemistry either repels or adapts to the stressor. During this phase the organism may be successful in adapting to the stressor, and, if so,

TABLE 17–1 Selye's Stress Adaptation Syndrome

Stage	General Function	Interpersonal	Behavioral	Affective	Cognitive	Physiological
1 Alarm reaction	Mobilization of body defenses	Interpersonal communication effectiveness decreases	Task oriented Increased restlessness Apathy, regression Crying	Feelings of anger, suspiciousness, helplessness Anxiety level increases	Alert Thinking becomes narrow and concrete Symptoms of thought blocking, forgetfulness, and decreased productivity	Muscle tension Increase in epinephrine and cortisone Stimulation of adrenal cortex and lymph glands Increase in blood pressure, pulse, blood glucose
2 Stage of resistance	Adaptation to stresses Resistance increases	Interpersonal communication self-oriented Uses interpersonal relationships to meet own needs	Automatic behaviors Self-oriented behaviors Fight or flight behavior apparent	Increased use of defense mechanisms Emotional responses may be automatic or exaggerated	Thought processes more habitual than problem-solving oriented	Hormonal levels return to prealarm stage if adaptation occurs Physiological responses return to normal or are channeled into psychosomatic symptoms
3 Stage of exhaustion	Depletion or exhaustion of organs and resources Loss of ability to resist stress	Disintegration of personal interactions Communication skills ineffective and disorganized Self-oriented	Restless, withdrawn, agitated; may become violent or self-destructive Diminished productivity	Depressed, flat or inappropriate affect Exaggerated or inappropriate use of defense mechanisms Decreased ability to cope	Thought disorganization, hallucinations, preoccupation Reduced intellectual processes	Exhaustion, with increased demands on organism Adrenal cortex hormone depletion Death, if stress is continuous and excessive

the biochemical changes resulting from the alarm phase return to the prealarm stage. Any life change causes alarm and resistance, and the stress accrued through life reduces the body's adaptive abilities.

The *final stage* occurs when the stress is prolonged and the body can no longer cope effectively. The result is exhaustion and the body may become ill with disease. The organism's adaptive abilities are depleted, and the organism loses its ability to deal with the stress. The organism goes into shock, and, if the stress is not alleviated, the result may be death of the organism. The general adaptation syndrome varies widely in intensity. Reaction to positive stimuli, such as getting married or a job promotion, also activates a stress response. The response may, however, result in less damage than a negative stressor, even though it does temporarily throw the body out of balance. Furthermore, a person does not respond with the same intensity to all negative stressors. For example, one doesn't respond with the same degree of intensity to jumping in a cold pool as to turning a corner and seeing a man with a gun.

The *local adaptive syndrome* is the manifestation of stress in a limited part of the body. The body responds locally to the stressor, such as a burn or cut to a finger. The local response may also trigger a general response if the ability of the body to respond to the specific area is greatly affected by the condition of the whole organism. An upper respiratory infection causes a much different response within a healthy child than in a child with cystic fibrosis. The better the organism as a whole adapts to stress, the more effective the local adaptive response.

Individual Responses to Stress

Responses to stress, then, can be categorized into several different patterns: the *physiologic response,* in which there is loss or gain in weight over time, hormone levels increase, blood pressure increases, or possibly a somatoform (psychosomatic) symptom appears; the *psychologic response,* which may also result in a psychosomatic illness or psychiatric manifestations, such as depression, mania, withdrawal from reality, or anxiety; and, the *behavioral response,* in which one hits out, becomes aggressive (fights), or withdraws; one may also become immobilized, or turn inward (physical or emotional flight). The *interpersonal mode* can reflect stress when communication

Signals of Stress

Physiologic	
Fatigue, lethargy	Pain—backache, teeth grinding
Muscle tension—neck, back, legs, and so forth	Excessive sweating
Frequent headaches—tension, migraine	Heart problems—palpitations, racing, variable heartbeat, chest pain
Shaking, trembling, spasms	Breathing complications—hyperventilation
Cold extremities, poor circulation	High blood pressure
Digestion disturbances—acid, nausea, gas, cramps, colitis	Skin eruptions—rash, hives, itching, eczema, acne
Eating disorders—compulsive eating, loss of appetite	Sexual difficulties—impotence, low libido (desire), nonorgasmic, vaginitis
Elimination disorders—diarrhea, constipation	Amenorrhea (absence of menstrual period)
Sleep problems—insomnia, nightmares, excessive sleep, early awakenings	
Psychologic	
Anxiety	Confusion
Panic disorder	Helplessness
Depression	Apathy
Pessimism	Alienation
Melancholy	Isolation
Impatience	Numbness
Anger	Self-consciousness
Irritability	Purposelessness
Boredom	
Behavioral Indicators	
Restlessness	Indecisiveness
Loss of memory, poor concentration	Tardiness
Nervous mannerisms—tics, grimaces, finger tapping, hair twisting	Inflexibility
Speech difficulties—stuttering, stammering	Nonproductivity
Hyperactivity	Poor problem solving
Disorganization	Alcohol and drug abuse
Passivity	Phobic responses
Aggressiveness	Overeating

effectiveness decreases, relationships deteriorate, trust in others diminishes, and the ability to form and maintain close, intimate, loving ties with another person decreases. Finally, the affective response may be present when one's emotions are affected so that anxiety is high and emotions are unstable, labile, unpredictable, and inappropriate to the situation. All of the above-mentioned modes of response relate to the negative elements of response patterns. Of course, these modes can be used in a positive way so that stress becomes nondetrimental. There is no way to eliminate stress completely, but individuals can learn to minimize the harmful effects and use their response modes in a positive way.

Stressors may be chemical, physical, developmental, and emotional. Graduating from nursing school, being promoted, failing to be promoted, having arguments, and playing a tough game of racquetball are all stressful events and require adaptation and change at some level. By understanding stress, we can more easily identify stress factors and their effects on clients who need or seek health care. Whether a client is having a baby, undergoing open-heart surgery, or seeking counseling for emotional problems, each of these individuals is experiencing stress in his or her own particular manner. How the individual adapts or fails to adapt depends on several factors: personality and emotional makeup and past experiences in dealing with stress (response repertoire).

People are able to create many different forms of disease as well as emotional and spiritual scars. And the more we use up our reserves of adaptation energy, the more likely we are to age and hasten our death. In fact, Selye warned that there is no evidence that the basic reserves of energy for adaptation can be restored. These may be genetically programmed. The more reserves we use handling everyday stress, the less we have for major crises or for growing older. The latest research indicates that there is a direct relationship between the amount of stress encountered in everyday life and aging.

Danger Signals of Stress

- Depression, lack of interest in life
- Uncontrolled hyperactive behavior
- Lack of concentration, inability to focus
- Feelings of unreality
- Loss of control, emotional instability
- Pervasive high anxiety level
- Physical manifestations
  Irregular heartbeats
  Tremors, tics
  Gastrointestinal disturbance
  Skin disturbance
  Changes in respiratory patterns
- Insomnia
- Disease
- Increased dependence on alcohol, drugs

Stress and Disease

Stress and an individual's method of handling it have been associated with the risk of developing heart disease, cancer, and other illnesses. Although stress is an inevitable part of life, excessive amounts of it can contribute to poor health. When one goes through a very stressful period, it is important to work through that stress, rather than ignore it.

The mechanisms by which stress leads to disease may differ for heart disease and cancer. Perceived stress leads to a release of adrenaline, cortisol, and other hormones within the body. These substances, in turn, increase the heart rate, blood pressure, cholesterol level, and platelet stickiness. When stress becomes chronic, these physiologic changes can accelerate atherosclerosis, the process that causes coronary heart disease.

Individuals with Type A behavior are known to be at increased risk of heart disease. Type A behavior is defined as having a constant sense of time urgency and a feeling of free-floating anger at the world in general. These behavior patterns can be seen as a maladaptive way of dealing with chronic stress. The famous study of the causative factors in heart disease, the Framingham study, examined many aspects of heart disease. Results revealed that males who were classified as Type A developed chest pains three times as often as their more peaceful Type B counterparts. Another fascinating conclusion was that those who remained calm and serene (Type B personalities) rarely developed high cholesterol levels regardless of their diet.

Chronic stress causes changes in the immune system that can interfere with its ability to recognize and destroy cancerous cells. Several researchers have shown that cancer clients have a characteristic personality pattern years before the cancers are diagnosed. Part of this personality pattern involves difficulty dealing with stress and turning conflict inward instead of confronting it directly.

It is important to remember that the stress syndrome can be both positive and negative. Any change or alteration in the balance of life can create stress. The Holmes and Rahe stress scale is an excellent example of the varying conditions in life that result in stress. We are all unique individuals, and we respond differently to various stressors. Thus, it does not matter whether the stress is positive or negative, light or severe. What matters is how we develop adaptive mechanisms to cope with these stressors. The ability to cope or solve a problem can be translated as the ability to withstand stress and create life experiences that do not work against us. The implications of stress theory—that by being able to withstand stress, by coping with it, diluting it when it occurs, or eliminating it we can actually affect our life—are tremendously exciting. It means that we are not doomed to inevitable illness later in life, nor are we preprogrammed for premature aging. In fact every individual controls his or her own health. To quote the *Journal of American Medical Association*, "Nature did not intend us to grow old and ill; we were designed to die young in old age but free of disease." In other words, even when we are old we should feel "young" (healthy) and be free of disease.

Along with coping with one's own stress, it is the responsibility of the nurse to be aware that clients suffer from stress phenomena and that part of the nurse's role is to assist clients to adapt and cope with stress.

Guidelines for Implementing Stress Objectives in Nursing

The nurse must have an understanding of the role of stress.

- Understand and accept the theory of stress—what it is and what effect it has on the body.
- Be aware of how stress manifests: tiredness, apathy, frequent illness, lack of interest or liveliness, unwillingness to seek out new challenges, inability to cope with change, and many other symptoms.
- Recognize the factors that increase stress, both positive and negative (illness, hospitalization, pain, marriage, family pressures, etc.).
- Assist in making a plan and implementing it, designing specific actions to reduce stress, such as relaxation methods, meditation, exercise.
- Work out a plan with the individual about how to control, alter, or change stressors in his or her life.

Stress and a Satisfying Life

Understanding stress teaches you critical principles for creating a healthy and satisfying life. Consider the following principles, and reflect on how you can use stress in your life to positive advantage.

- **Stress does not come from the outside; you generate it totally within yourself.** In Hans Selye's definition, stress is the nonspecific reaction to any demand. An upcoming exam may be a stressor; your reaction may or may not be stress. A specific response to the exam (assuming you want to get a good grade in the course) is to study extra hard. But nonspecific reactions, which do not serve specifically to resolve the imbalance of having an upcoming exam and wanting to do well, may also include a certain amount of fear, even panic. You might eat more, smoke cigarettes, pace the floor, or have difficulty sleeping. You yourself, not the exam, have generated these reactions—they are the symptoms of stress.
- **You cannot see stress directly; you can only experience its symptoms.** No one can see love, but we all know its symptoms: the fluttering heart, butterflies in the stomach, inability to concentrate on other things, tendency to think about a loved one all the time. You must discover your personal characteristic symptoms of stress. You might overeat or get headaches or skin rashes. You might become short-tempered. Learn to recognize your symptoms as not actual problems but bodily warning lights signalling an imbalance. Merely seeking immediate relief from the symptoms through drugs, sex, or other distractions is like painting over the warning light to keep it from bothering you. You must look deeper within your system to discover and correct the imbalance.
- **Your attitude plays a significant role in illness and wellness.** While working at the University of Chicago with professionals who experienced constant pressure, researcher Susanne Kobasa demonstrated that the primary difference between those who became ill and those who stayed well was attitude. Those who stayed well tended to be committed to their jobs, viewed problems as challenges not obstacles, and felt a sense of control—they believed their actions and presence actually made a difference. Your attitude, beliefs, and conceptualization of what is happening to you determine your internal reaction to those events and, therefore, determine your stress level.

  The challenge is to shift your attitudes so that you look for the positive side of events—not a phoney positive attitude that turns one into a "Pollyanna" who fails to recognize painful situations or major problems, but a "can do" attitude.
- **Stress is essential to everything you enjoy.** We all love the feeling of victory, and this feeling of achievement is proportional to the challenge. Think about what makes you feel happiest, most excited and enthusiastic. Having your team win a football game in the final two minutes is more exciting and memorable than when the team wins by a large margin over a poor team. When you have learned a subject well, how much better it feels to handle successfully a challenging set of final exam problems rather than a bunch of boring multiple-choice questions that test only a small part of what you've learned in the course.

  Coping with stress requires exploring the inner you, utilizing and reinforcing your creativity, skill, and strength. Stressful events and periods in our lives can help us grow to be better able to make the most of our lives. Learning to truly celebrate your successes will increase your joy, personal satisfaction, and enthusiasm.
- **A healthy life is a balance of stress and relaxation.** In nature, stress and tension alternate with relaxation. Your heart contracts and relaxes to keep your blood flowing. Your breath enters and leaves. Your busy, complex world provides plenty of stress; most of us must work diligently to find relaxation techniques and time to balance this stress. Few aspects of our culture really encourage us to acknowledge the importance of relaxation. Can you imagine one of your professors, as the assignment is being collected, asking if you made sure to do your 20-minute meditation last night?
- **You must take responsibility for your own life, including its stress.** Only you can really make your life better. No one else can feel or deal with your symptoms of stress. Take responsibility for dealing effectively with stressors. Focus on wellness, not illness. Practice self-awareness, self-education, and self-responsibility. Create a stress management program, motivate yourself to follow it, and update it regularly until it becomes an automatic part of your life.

Emmett E. Miller, MD

Emmett E. Miller, MD, is a leading practitioner of psychophysiological medicine, which relates mental processes to physical health and optimal performance. Dr. Miller has developed a unique series of self-improvement audio tapes and experiential videotapes relating to stress management, self-improvement, and health and wellness. He is a frequent guest speaker at health conferences and workshops. Dr. Miller maintains a private practice in hypnotherapy, preventive medicine, and psychotherapy in Los Altos, California.

The nurse may carry out specific behaviors in the hospital setting to reduce stress.

- Identify the stressors affecting the client now.
- Counsel the client and family on the theory of stress; together, examine how the client's particular stressors affect his or her lifestyle.
- Reinforce the client's adaptive process by meeting his or her needs, listening to concerns, administering care, and providing emotional support.
- Assist the client to alter adaptive behaviors to cope more effectively with stress.
- Remember that laughter decreases stress, so maintain a light rather than a depressed or morbid attitude.

A NEW PARADIGM FOR HEALTH

The way the Western world views health is undergoing a change. Even the terms we use to describe health are changing; new terms, like *holistic health* and *alternative, unconventional*, or *complementary medicine* are being heard more frequently in both medical and nonmedical circles. In the past, good health meant the absence of disease. The new definition of health goes beyond physical health to encompass the health of the whole person, including mental, emotional, and spiritual health. The World Health Organization (WHO) formulated a new definition of health in 1970 that has significantly influenced the medical model of health care. WHO described health as "a state of complete physical, mental, and social well-being, not merely the absence of disease or infirmity." What made this definition innovative is that it took into account the mind as well as the body. In fact, this new interpretation of health almost enters the spiritual dimension. Though critics have pointed out that by this definition no one is truly healthy, it is the beginning of a view of health as an open system in a holistic framework. A holistic redefinition of health emphasizes high-level wellness or going beyond the absence of disease toward one's maximum health potential. This section focuses on the connection among mind, body, spirit, and environment and discusses how one can use this connection to reach the possible highest level of health and wellness.

A Holistic Approach to Health

From the 1990s into the new century, we are witnessing a significant growth in many dimensions of health. As shown in a recent Gallup survey completed for *American Health Magazine*, many people in society now include a very broad range of issues in the concept of personal health. Certainly their top health concern is still oriented toward personal health—"staying free of disease." The third-highest priority, however—"living in an environment with clean air and water"—expresses a much more global health perspective. Many of their top concerns show not only physical status but also mental and emotional status as important components of personal health. Today's significant health goals may even include having a positive outlook on life and sharing love with friends and family. Wellness can be thought of as a state of being; holistic health is the means of achieving it.

The term *holistic* implies wholeness; a harmonious individual that integrates mind, body, and spirit into a functioning unit. A holistic stress model implies modifying all parts of one's life so that stress is both encountered and alleviated from an integrated perspective.

In the modern era, holistic medicine postulates a constant interchange between mind and body, psyche and soul. Carl Jung was one of the first physicians and therapists to discuss the prevention of illness in terms of using one's inner resources. He discussed the inner self and themes of self-renewal in relation to growth, spirituality, and health. As our body of research knowledge grows, more and more physicians are employing spiritual growth techniques as a health tool. For example, Dr. Carl Simonton has been using meditation and imagery as adjunct therapy for clients with cancer and has shown that clients recover faster and have less pain when guided imagery is used. He has also demonstrated that cancer clients showed a heightened immune response. Dr. Joan Borysenko at the Harvard Mind–Body Clinic is also using meditation as a medical tool; Dr. Norman Shealy, founder of the American Holistic Medical Association and the Shealy Institute for Comprehensive Pain and Healthcare, has used alternative methods of health care for many years. The current literature, much of it authored by prominent physicians, exemplifies today's trend toward the holistic, or alternative, model.

The holistic paradigm suggests that the body, psyche, and environment are one and interact as an open system. This idea can assist us to view our client's health as well as our personal health from a new dimension. In the holistic view, health care includes three types of actions: disease and injury prevention, treatment, and health promotion.

Alternative treatments may include treatments that require involvement on the client's part, such as changes in eating patterns and other lifestyle behaviors; or physical treatments, such as acupuncture or vitamin therapy. The client is counseled to take the initiative and assume responsibility for his or her own health, and the role of the nurse and physician is to guide clients to various health care options. Truly holistic treatment involves an integrated assessment of all aspects of health.

More and more university medical centers are opening a hospital-based alternative department and consider it an integral component of a new health care model.

Integrated programs that are customized to meet the unique needs of the organization and the community appear to be the direction of health care in the United States.

COMPLEMENTARY AND ALTERNATIVE MEDICINE (CAM)

Alternative, or complementary, medicine is not nearly as unknown, untried, or unaccepted as traditional physicians believed. For the first time, in 1993, physicians learned, through the *New England Journal of Medicine*, that Americans made 425 million visits to alternative providers, compared with 388 million visits to all other mainstream primary care physicians. Many physicians, on learning the results of this survey, were stunned because they had no idea Americans were seeking alternative therapies in such numbers. Now it is estimated that 627 million Americans use alternative therapies while only 386 million visit conventional practitioners. Visits to alternative therapists have increased from 33% of the population to 69%. Another startling fact was that 72% of those using alternative therapies did not tell their primary care physician. In the late 1990s, over $27 billion per year is spent on alternative medicine, an out-of-pocket cost to the consumer.

The National Institutes of Health, a conservative, scientifically based organization, is now dispensing 150 million (still a fraction of its $10.3 billion annual budget) to the Office of Alternative Medicine. This office was founded because of congressional pressure to investigate new approaches to the degenerative diseases killing Americans.

In 1997, several national insurance companies elected to begin reimbursing their clients for selected alternative treatments. Among the companies are Blue Cross–Blue Shield, Alliance for Alternatives in Health Care, Inc., Oxford Health Plan, and Aetna US Life. Alternative treatments reimbursed include acupuncture, massage therapy, and body therapies such as Rolfing, chiropractic, stress reduction, and homeopathic therapy.

Legal Implications of Alternative Therapy

There are currently several bills pending in the U.S. House of Representatives and the Senate that will allow authorized health care providers to give alternative treatments, provided the client is fully informed about the type of treatment, the risks and benefits, and conventional therapy that is available. Written consent is necessary only if the therapy is invasive (acupuncture) or can cause the client harm.

If the client does request information about alternative approaches to illness, the nurse should discuss this request with the client's physician and unit manager or supervisor. The nurse may even contact the client advocate or ombudsman and ask them to talk with the client and honor the request. In many states, there are staff personnel and physicians who are open to alternative therapy and even encourage in the client's right to take responsibility for their own health. In such a situation, the personnel may work as a team in conjunction with the client to explore all of the available treatment options, including alternative therapy.

Alternative Treatment Methods

A new direction in alternative medicine is called *integrative medicine*, a blending of the best of conventional methods with high-tech and alternative therapies. This method combines drugs, surgery, high-tech treatments and mind–body practices as well as alternative treatments. It remains client-centered.

Following is a short sampling of the more than 200 alternative treatment methods that may be used alone or in tandem with conventional medical treatments. Alternative methods may be classified as lifestyle (holistic medicine; nutrition), botanical (homeopathy, herbal, aromatherapy), manipulative (chiropractic, acupressure and acupuncture, reflexology, massage), and mind–body (meditation, guided imagery, biofeedback, color healing, and hypnotherapy).

Acupuncture An ancient Chinese method of relieving pain and treating disease, acupuncture is based on the belief that energy, or *qi*, flows along 12 lines or meridians in the body creating a balance between two principles of nature called yin and yang. Each meridian is connected to a particular organ or system. It is believed that lack of energy flow or blocked energy along the meridians leads to illness or disease. Acupuncture treatment involves inserting sharp needles under the skin along the meridian lines, thereby unblocking energy, stimulating flow, and restoring balance and health of internal organs. Since the 1960s in the United States, Chinese doctors, as well as some U.S. physicians, have performed major surgery with acupuncture as the only anesthetic.

Applied Kinesiology Applied kinesiology is a form of evaluation based on the theory that the condition of a person's muscles reflects certain internal disorders or problems. Body imbalances or disorders are identified when certain muscle groups are tested and appear weak. Certain foods, medications, or herbs are held in a person's hand or placed next to their skin. If the substance is not appropriate for the body, the muscles respond to testing by appearing weak. When the substance is removed, the muscles regain their strength. Based on identifying weak muscles, various treatments, such as vitamins, herbs, diet therapy, acupressure, or chiropractic, are suggested.

Aromatherapy Essential oils are the aromatic liquids extracted from herbs, plants, and flowers. These oils have been used to treat various conditions and have been an important part of medical lore for thousands of years. For example, there are 188 references to essential oils in the Bible. Modern aromatherapy became known in the 1930s, but it was not until the 1990s that aromatherapy emerged as a major mode of alternative treatment.

Essential oils can be included in the genre of vibrational therapy because specific oils have their own vibrational level or life force and, as such, work differently in the body. Dr. Robert Becker, in his book *The Body Electric*, discusses the fact that the human body has an average electrical frequency and the health of a person depends on their particular body frequency. Research at the State University in Cheny, Washington, determined that the average body frequency is 62–68 Hertz (Hz). When the frequency drops, the immune system is compromised and various illnesses may ensue. Based on this research, scientists found that pollutants lower the body frequency. For example, canned or processed foods have a frequency of zero, fresh produce 15 Hz, and essential oils start at 52 Hz and go as high as 320 Hz (which is organic, pure rose oil). Essential oils have the ability to penetrate the human body through either the skin or olfactory receptors. Supporters of this form of alternative therapy believe that essential oils are a most effective healing agent and they are noninvasive. Examples of commonly used oils are lemon and thyme oil, used to kill strep, staph, and TB; lavender, used as a relaxing or sleep enhancing oil; and peppermint, used to aid digestion. This mode of treatment would be used to supplement, not replace, other treatment methods.

Ayurveda A form of medicine that originated in India, ayurveda, meaning the science of life, has been practiced in India for over 5000 years and has just recently become known in the West. This system is based on the concept of three metabolic body types: slim, athletic, and heavy. Each body type utilizes food and herbs in a different way, thus treatment includes dietary changes, herbs, and exercise, as well as specific practices, such as yoga, meditation, massage with herbal remedies, and medicated inhalations. This form of medicine has recently gained popularity in the West after several Indian physicians opened clinics based on this system of treatment. Notable among them is Dr. Deepak Chopra, an endocrinologist, who has written many popular books on the subject.

Biofeedback This technique employs an instrument to monitor physiologic processes of the body and to "feed back" measurements to the individual being monitored. A scale, thermometer, and pulse monitor are common feedback devices, as are more technically sophisticated machines having electronic sensors and digital readouts. Recent research has confirmed that many people can influence or control their autonomic processes (heart rate, blood pressure, temperature, digestive functions, etc.). As the client becomes more adept at controlling body responses, the need to use monitoring devices decreases—and the mental skills can be used independently.

Chiropractic Originating in ancient Greece and literally meaning "done by the hands," chiropractic suggests that one cause of disease and dysfunction in the body is a misalignment of the spinal column that interferes with proper nerve function. These conditions cause or contribute to some diseases and lower the body's resistance to others. Spinal adjustments and manipulation restore structural integrity, thus enabling the body to heal itself. Studies have shown that chiropractic can relieve pain and structural disorders in the joints and muscles. The focus of treatment is general and includes correction of such disorders as headaches; allergies; pain in the back, hip, or spinal column; or gastrointestinal problems.

Energy Medicine This contemporary aspect of health views the human body as comprised of electronic vibrations. Interventions involving the energy field will interface with environmental, spiritual, and vibrational aspects of healing. Special high and low frequencies of sound and light are already being used for healing. For example, sound therapy is used to speed healing through a cast; full-spectrum light frequencies are being used to affect moods such as seasonal affective disorder (SAD). Other examples of energy/vibrational/frequency healing are Reike healing, in which the healer has progressed through two or three extensive education levels of mastery; therapeutic touch, which also entails learning the techniques via a seminar or educational program; and energy healing, which is simply the transmission of the healer's energy into the client's body. Documented studies have shown that certain individuals have this ability to transmit healing energy to others. In fact, a special photographic process called Kirlian photography has shown the energy moving from healer to client.

Herbal Medicine All cultures from ancient times onward have used herbs to cure illness. Indeed, many drugs commonly used today are derived from herbs. Nearly one-fourth of all medications have at least one ingredient that is plant based. The World Health Organization (WHO) estimates that 80% of the world population includes herbal medicines as part of their health practices.

Other countries are far ahead of the United States in integrating herbal products into mainstream medicine. WHO's *Guidelines for the Assessment of Herbal Medicine* state that historical use is a valid way to document safety and efficacy in the absence of scientific evidence to the contrary. European herbs are among the world's best-studied medicines. Some are even prescribed by physicians in Europe because they are so effective in treating diseases. In the United States, more and more holistic physicians are incorporating herbs into their medical practice, both because they are effective and because they have far fewer side effects than drugs.

Homeopathy Based on the work of the German physician Dr. Samuel Hahnemann in the early 1800s, homeopathy is a system of treatment that rests on the theory that extremely minute doses of certain substances, usually herbal or chemical, cause a response in a person that mimics a particular disease. These substances, or homeopathic remedies, are administered to a person with a disease exhibiting a similar symptom pattern, stimulating the body's natural healing response. This is called "treatment by similars, or like cures like." The practice of homeopathy is becoming more popular; there is even a software package designed to assist physicians in the homeopathic diagnosis and treatment of disease.

Massage Of all the alternative treatments, massage may be the oldest form of medicine known to man. Historical records indicate that the Chinese, in 3000 B.C., wrote about massage, and both the Greeks and Romans considered massage a therapy. Massage was introduced to the United States in 1877 by Dr. S. Mitchell, and schools of massage proliferated in both the United States and Britain.

With the introduction of electrical treatments, the application of massage began to diminish as a part of recommended physiotherapy. However, today, the application of touch to the skin to relieve tension in muscles, ligaments, tendons, and joints is an accepted nonpharmacological approach to decrease pain.

Naturopathy Founded almost 100 years ago, this form of medicine includes natural therapeutics such as nutrition, herbs, homeopathy, massage, exercise, and even acupuncture. Drugs are not in this repertoire. Naturopathy school of thought believes that diseases are the body's attempt to heal itself through release of impurities. Treatments are designed to increase the client's "vital force" by eliminating toxins, thus allowing the body to heal.

Nutrition The holistic approach dictates that an individual pay close attention to nutritional status as a critical component of wellness. Research strongly points to diet as a major contributor to health or disease. This is especially so when a person has a diet of high saturated fat, refined sugars, additives, preservatives, or junk food. It is also current thinking that a high-carbohydrate diet contributes to obesity. Nutrition can also play a major role in prevention of disease; more and more emphasis is currently being placed on the role of antioxidants (vitamins C, E, beta-carotene, pycnogenol, etc.) in preventing such diseases as cancer and heart disease.

There is much controversy today over whether the average American consumes a diet that provides enough of the essential nutrients to prevent disease and aging. The pro argument group says that if you follow the USDA Pyramid Food Guide, you do not need to supplement your diet. The opposing argument says that the quality of food today (unless you are eating a majority of organic/natural foods) is so deficient in nutrients that you cannot sustain a healthy diet.

To follow preventive guidelines for better health, most alternative physicians and health care workers advocate supplementing diet with a broad-based multiple vitamin/mineral capsule daily, preferably with natural, food-based (not synthetic) nutrients. This prescription would include basic vitamins, all the minerals (including trace minerals), antioxidants, essential fatty acids (Omega 3 and 6), the carotinoids, coenzyme Q10, nutrients for the eyes such as lycopene and lutein, and bioflaonoids.

Reflexology Also called "zone therapy," reflexology is a method of treatment that proposes that diseases and organ dysfunction can be both diagnosed and treated by pressing on certain areas of the hands or feet. Each area of the body is represented by a corresponding area on the feet or hands; pressing on specific points is said to stimulate blood, nutrient, and energy flow to the diseased area of the body.

Relaxation and Visualization Stress experts have carefully studied the effects of deep relaxation on the mind and body. They found that individuals who regularly practice relaxation exercises experience less stress than people who don't. The relaxation response is actually the physiologic opposite of the stress response. People adept at invoking the relaxation response use their minds to control their autonomic nervous system—oxygen consumption, respiratory rate, heart rate, blood pressure, and muscle tension. Their alpha brain waves, the waves associated with feelings of well-being, increase. Effective body relaxation techniques have existed for centuries. Several have gained significant popularity in recent years. The following short descriptions should familiarize you with the leading techniques.

1. *Deep Breathing:* Emphasized by virtually all relaxation exercises, deep breathing is a key to reducing stress. When you are tense, your breathing becomes rapid, irregular, and shallow. Healthy deep breathing increases the amount of oxygen in your blood, cleanses your system of carbon dioxide and other waste chemicals, relaxes your muscles, and encourages your heart rate to return to normal. Learning to take deep, slow, full breaths and exhale completely effects mastery of this key relaxation technique. B. K. S. Iyengar, a world-

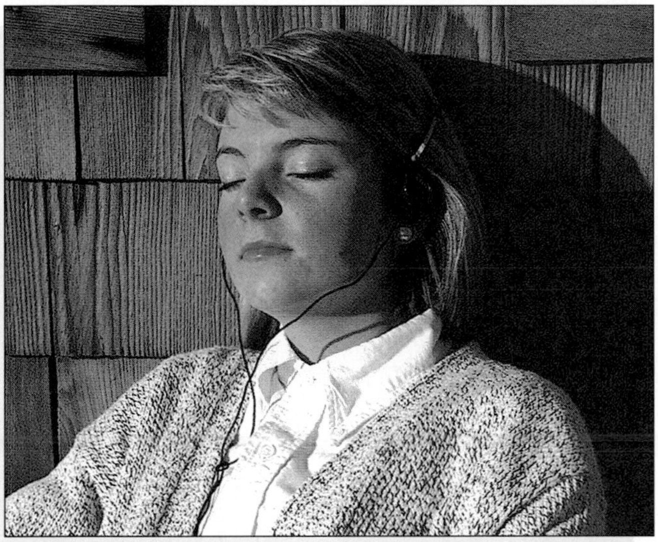

Sound and visualization are alternative treatment methods.

class yoga teacher, suggests a breathing technique for stress reduction. Try it and instruct your clients in this technique.

- Inhale as you normally do.
- Exhale as you normally do.
- Pause as long as comfortable.
- Repeat the first three steps.

Simple? Yes. Effective? Yes. This technique allows lungs to empty more completely, continuing the normal exhalation process. Why is this simple exercise effective? Because the completed exhalation enables the mind to quiet—a rest from the jumble of one thought upon another. Iyengar says that if you learn this "secret," you can control stress. It also provides the foundation for meditation.

2. *Autogenic Training:* In this form of relaxation, warmth and heaviness are visualized: two physical sensations associated with the relaxed state. The warmth represents increased blood flow throughout the body, and heaviness is perceived as relaxation of the skeletal muscles. During progressive relaxation, specific muscles or groups of muscles are tensed and released throughout the body. This technique is especially effective for clients who are fearful and stressed.
3. *Meditation:* Originating thousands of years ago, meditation is based on Eastern cultures and religions. The effects of meditation are similar to those associated with deep relaxation. Meditation is the process of bringing the mind to stillness. It sounds easy, but if you have tried meditation, you know from experience how difficult and frustrating this process can be. There are many methods of meditation, from the traditional transcendental meditation (TM) and Zen meditation to the repetition of a word such as "one," advocated by Dr. Herbert Benson of Harvard University. TM is a structured form of meditation popularized in the United States in the 1960s by Maharishi Mahesh Yogi. In TM, a mantra is selected (a word or sound) that is repeated mentally while the person is seated quietly in a tranquil place.

   Perhaps the easiest meditation technique is to sit in a comfortable position with the spine straight (the lotus position is perfect if the legs can stand it), eyes closed, and to relax. While meditating, one concentrates on relaxing the muscles and organs throughout the body, then focuses on breathing. One is to inhale fully, then exhale, watching the breath come out "in one's mind's eye." If a thought comes in, it should be made to slip away and one should continue inhaling and exhaling. No thoughts should be allowed to rush in to break the concentration.
4. *Visualization:* Visualization is a proven technique for healing, stress management, and positive goal attainment. When a mental picture is created, the body responds as if it were a real experience. Visualization can assist a client to feel more confident in circumstances filled with uncertainties. It can also assist with reducing pain. Teach the client to first relax (through one of the techniques mentioned in this chapter), then deep breathe, and finally to see the pain in the mind's eye becoming less and less severe.

T'ai Chi Ch'uan This slow, graceful Chinese technique for relaxation is actually a system to both stimulate and balance subtle life energies. Thirty minutes a day devoted to the gentle, flowing movements of t'ai chi is relaxing, centering, and invigorating—a great way to relax and an interesting alternative to energetic Western exercise.

Yoga Yoga is an ancient Indian discipline that begins with postures, or asanas, that stretch and strengthen muscles. It progresses to meditative relaxation or breathing techniques. Yoga is not sport or exercise as such; nor does it have to be a religion. The system is devised completely for health and well-being. The best way to begin yoga is to find an experienced teacher who can correct postures and guide the individual through the breathing and relaxation exercises.

NURSING DIAGNOSES

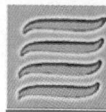

The following nursing diagnoses may be appropriate to include in a client care plan when the components are related to decreasing stress and promoting adaptation.

NURSING DIAGNOSIS	RELATED FACTORS
Anxiety	Increased stress, for instance, illness, trauma, loss
Ineffective Individual Coping	High stress on person, for example, individual inability to adapt, length and duration of stressor
Defensive Coping	Denial of problem, rationalization of failure, such as increased demands on individual
Disturbed Energy Field	Decreased immune response, increased stress level, poor integration of mind–body energy.
Altered Health Maintenance	High stress level, from illness, abuse, or psychologic factors
Social Isolation	Maladaptive coping to stressor, such as long-term or high level of stress
Post-trauma Syndrome	Reexperiencing a traumatic event, exhibiting altered lifestyle, psychic numbness
Pain (acute, chronic)	Trauma, immobility, illness, or disease

- The single most important nursing action to decrease the incidence of hospital-based infections is handwashing. **Remember to wash your hands or use antibacterial gel before and after each and every client contact.**

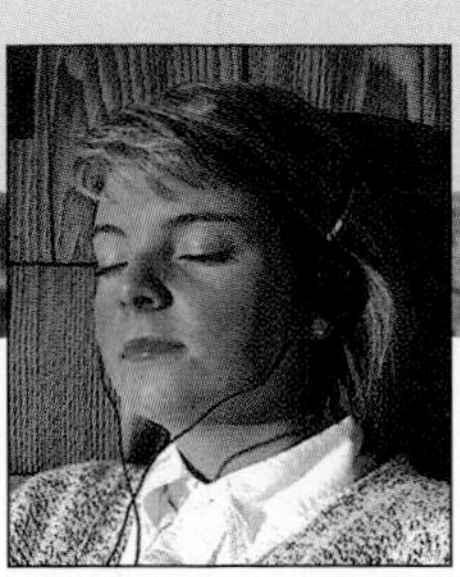

UNIT 1

Stress and Adaptation

Nursing Process Data

ASSESSMENT *Data Base*

Identify the client who demonstrates stressed behavior.

Evaluate, with the client, the past and present stressors that the client has experienced.

Evaluate the stressors' effect on the client's body and signs of distress in the body.

Examples of physiological stress effects:

- *Cardiovascular system:* increased pulse and blood pressure, evidence of angina, arrhythmias, migraine headaches, disturbance of heat and cold mechanisms
- *Gastrointestinal system:* ulcers, ulcerative colitis, constipation or diarrhea, imbalance in sugar absorption
- *Musculoskeletal system:* backache, tension headaches, arthritis, proneness to accidents
- *Autoimmune system:* infections, flu, allergies, rheumatoid arthritis, cancer

Assess client's level of energy and the degree to which it is depleted.

Evaluate client's awareness of thoughts, attitudes, values, and beliefs that influence stress response and adaptation.

Assess present level of distress in the client's body.

Assess possible causes of stress that are affecting client:

- *Environmental stressors:* input overload, such as sights, sounds, smells; actions and demands of others in the environment; or monotony
- *Physical stressors:* hunger, heat or cold, dangerous environment, injury, or pain
- *Emotional stressors:* loss of something of value, frustrations of needs and drives, threats to self-concept
- *Psychosocial stressors:* Conflicting cultural values (e.g., the American values of competition and assertiveness vs. the need to be dependent)
- *Future shock:* physiologic and psychological stress resulting from an overload of the organism's adaptive systems and decision-making processes brought about by too rapidly changing values and technology
- *Cultural shock:* stress developing in response to the transition from a familiar environment to unfamiliar one; involves unfamiliarity with communication, technology, customs, attitudes, and beliefs (e.g., immigrating, being confined in a hospital or prison); crowding, and urban life
- *Job choice and the work environment* (About 80% of the workers in our country are estimated to be unhappy in their jobs.)

Assess the factors that influence how the client responds to stress:

- *Characteristics of the stressful event:* magnitude, intensity, duration
- *Client's biologic and psychologic inclinations*
- *Appropriateness of support system*

Life changes according to a stress scale (Holmes & Rahe 1967)

PLANNING *Objectives*

To identify presence of stress in client

To identify how stress affects the body

To identify the current sources that result in stressed behavior

To determine the client's response to stress

To evaluate stress interventions that have a positive effect on stressed client

IMPLEMENTATION *Procedures*

Determining the Effect of Stress
Determining Response Patterns
Managing Stress
Manipulating the Environment to Reduce Stress
Teaching Coping Strategies
Managing Stress Using a Holistic Model
Teaching Controlled Breathing
Teaching Body Relaxation
Using Meditation as an Alternative Therapy

EVALUATION *Expected Outcomes*

Client is able to evaluate the general stressors and identify sources of stress in his or her life.
Client is aware of response patterns to stress and is able to alter patterns appropriately.
Client is aware of body–mind stress and its influence on his or her body.
Client is able to reduce environmental stressors.
Client is able to identify and alleviate stress caused by mental concerns.

DETERMINING THE EFFECT OF STRESS

Procedure

1. Identify client's stress tolerance level.
   a. Recognize the body's alarm signals (see major signals in assessment).
   b. Assess signal correctly as signifying high level of stress.
2. Discuss the concept of stress to elicit understanding of the effect on client's body.
   a. Stress may be physical, chemical, or emotional and may cause bodily or mental tension that may be a factor in disease causation.
   b. Stress tends to alter existing equilibrium.
3. Encourage client to feel free to discuss life patterns that relate to stress.
4. Discuss the effect of stress. **Rationale:** Directing the conversation to the emotional, mental, and social sources of stress assist the client in examining its total effect.
5. Assist the client in formulating a plan to reduce or eliminate at least some sources of stress.

Hans Selye's Definition of Stress

- Stress is a specific syndrome that consists of all nonspecifically induced changes within the biologic system.
- The body is the common denominator of all adaptive responses.
- Stress is manifested by measurable changes in the body.
- Stress causes a multiplicity of changes in the body.

DETERMINING RESPONSE PATTERNS

Procedure

1. Evaluate adaptation factors that influence stress management.
   a. *Age:* adaptation is greatest in youth and young middle life and least at the extremes of life.
   b. *Environment:* does environment support managing stress?
   c. *Time:* the client can more easily adapt to stress over a period of time than suddenly.
   d. *Flexibility:* degree of flexibility of the individual influences survival.
   e. *Expenditure of energy:* the individual usually uses the adaptation mechanism that is most economic in terms of energy.
   f. *Presence of illness:* disease decreases the person's capacity to adapt to stress.

2. Assess the effects of stress on the client.
   a. Increased anxiety, anger, helplessness, hopelessness, guilt, shame, disgust, fear, frustration, or depression.
   b. Behaviors resulting from stress:
      (1) Apathy, regression, withdrawal.
      (2) Crying, demanding.
      (3) Physical illness.
      (4) Hostility, manipulation.
      (5) Senseless violence, lashing out.

EVIDENCE BASED NURSING PRACTICE

The Opposite of a Stress Response

In many studies, Herbert Benson, MD, of "The Relaxation Response" fame found that the opposite of a stress response (physiological response) can be achieved by completing only two steps: repeating a prayer, word, sound, phrase, or movement, and disregarding all other thoughts (as in meditation, yoga, etc.).

Source: Benson, H. (1984). *The relaxation response.* New York: Times Books.

MANAGING STRESS

Procedure

1. Discuss the client's body response to stress.
   a. The body's response to stress is a self-preservation mechanism that automatically and immediately becomes activated in times of danger.
   b. Assist client to understand response patterns.
2. Teach client to be aware of stress sensations in his or her body—recognize physical symptoms.
3. Suggest that client frequently monitor thought patterns to identify those thoughts that cause automatic tensing responses (tight muscles, increase in heartbeat, butterflies in stomach.)
4. Assist client to decide whether these thoughts are essential to survival or if they can be changed, eliminated, or replaced.
5. Assist client in planning to set aside periods each day for self stress evaluation.
6. Provide problem-solving assistance so the client can examine new, more appropriate response patterns.
7. Refer client to resources (therapy classes, books, relaxation tapes) that will assist in developing new responses.

MANIPULATING THE ENVIRONMENT TO REDUCE STRESS

Procedure

1. Modify client's external environment so that adaptation responses are within his or her capacity.
2. Support the efforts of the client to adapt or to respond.
3. Provide client with the materials required to maintain constancy of his or her environment.
4. Understand the body's mechanisms for accommodating stress.
5. Prevent additional stress.
6. Reduce external stimuli and input through senses.
7. Reduce or increase physical activity depending on the cause of and response to stress.

TEACHING COPING STRATEGIES

Procedure

1. Analyze client's stress status.
   a. Estimate total amount of stress client is experiencing—too high a level of stress indicates need for intervention.
   b. Recognize where in body or mind the stress is manifesting.
2. Discuss various options for reducing stress—which alternatives fit with client.

3. Suggest client use diversion methods of coping.
   a. *Physical diversion*: jogging, swimming, cooking, cleaning.
   b. *Mental diversion*: reading, painting, going to a movie, or simply thinking about a pleasant memory.
4. Plan with client how to use rest as a way to cope with stress.
   a. Vacation, leave of absence from job, frequent naps.
   b. Eliminate or decrease major stressors so result is rest from stress input.
   c. Plan with client how to manage time so that input can be reduced and goals limited.
5. Teach client how to use concentration, body relaxation, breathing, or meditation techniques to relieve mind stress.
6. Remind client that laughter is a great tranquilizer and healer as well as a stress reducer, and assist client to plan how to use this method.

Suggestions for Coping with Stress

- Rank tasks to be completed, and identify activities that need to be accomplished.
- Forget unimportant details; do not try to remember too many things. Concentrate on the essential issues and details.
- Eliminate past unpleasant events from the mind and focus on the present.
- Do not cling to unpleasant experiences and emotions that impair emotional ability to respond to here and now.
- Discard habit of anticipating negative outcomes, which is often worse than the actual event.
- Do not yearn for things relating to the past or the future; focus attention on present desires.

MANAGING STRESS USING A HOLISTIC MODEL

Procedure

1. Manage stress through exercise.
   a. Poor physical condition becomes a stressor—this state contributes to lethargy, a constant fatigue level, low resistance for illness, and lessens adaptive responses.
   b. Good physical condition results in stamina, reserves necessary to withstand stress, and protection against unpredictable stress periods.
   c. Exercise prepares the body physically for stress caused by environmental conditions.
   d. Consistent exercise prepares body to handle stress emotionally.
2. Manage stress through diet.
   a. Certain foods and drug substances (caffeine, alcohol, sugar, junk foods, preservatives, tobacco) are potent stressors to our bodies.
   b. Consuming high-stress foods results in negative body changes, such as hypertension, high cholesterol, labile blood sugar levels, and a rapid, bounding pulse rate.
   c. Consuming a low-stress diet results in more energy and stamina to cope with stress.
   d. Teach client that a low-stress diet includes reducing saturated fat, and limiting protein intake to 10–15% of consumed calories. Remainder of intake should be raw or barely cooked vegetables, fruits, whole grains, nuts, low-fat dairy products, and plenty of liquids. Eliminate sodas, caffeine products, and most alcohol. Exclude refined sugars and carbohydrates and convenience or processed foods.
   e. Encourage the use of vitamin supplements: vitamin C, B-complex, mineral supplements. Assist client to examine diet and experiment with different vitamin-mineral supplements.
3. Manage stress by altering lifestyle patterns.
   a. Counsel clients to eliminate unnecessary stressors in their life—change parts of life that are particularly stressful.
   b. Assist client to develop personal methods for coping with stress: walking in the woods, painting, listening to music, reading, or practicing yoga.
   c. Encourage client to assess lifestyle periodically and alter habits as necessary to reduce stress.

TEACHING CONTROLLED BREATHING

Procedure

1. Instruct client to sit so that his or her back is well supported, with spine straight but not rigid.
2. Have client place feet flat on floor and place hands on legs.
3. If client is lying down, have him or her place hands at side.
4. Suggest client find a comfortable position, close eyes, and take a deep, slow breath through nostrils.

5. Continue giving the client the following instructions.
   a. Extend your abdominal muscles.
   b. Hold your breath for the count of four. Then very slowly release the air through slightly parted lips, making a whoosh sound.
   c. When you think that all the air is out, hold your stomach in to push out even more air.
   d. Repeat this breathing pattern several times so that your body relaxes.

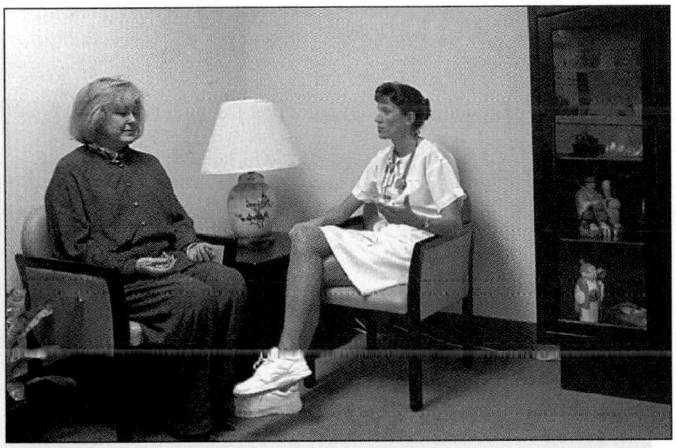
Find a quiet room to teach relaxation process.

   e. Breathe in through your nostrils to the count of four—1-2-3-4. Hold it—1-2-3-4—and expel the breath all the way out slowly, slowly releasing the air through your mouth.
   f. As the air goes out, feel all of the tension drain out with it.
   g. Now double the count, and breathe in slowly, filling your lungs all the way to the top to the count of eight. 1-2-3-4-5-6-7-8. Hold it—1-2-3-4—and now slowly release the breath—5-6-7-8.
   h. Again breathe in slowly to the count of 10 and count for the client—1-2-3-4-5-6-7-8-9-10. Hold it to the count of eight—1-2-3-4-5-6-7-8—and slowly release the air through your mouth to the count of 10—1-2-3-4-5-6-7-8-9-10. Pause.
   i. Continue with your regular breathing pattern, letting the air breathe for you.
6. Stop the process by having the client open his or her eyes.

If you are motivated to learn CAM techniques, there are numerous classes available. In fact, to implement certain CAM therapies such as Reike, therapeutic touch, acupressure, or acupuncture, you will need specialized classes/training.

TEACHING BODY RELAXATION

Procedure

1. Place client in a comfortable position.
   a. Have client sit so that back is well supported and spine is straight. Have client put both feet on the floor and hold hands comfortably in lap.
   b. If sitting is uncomfortable, have client lie on a bed and support areas of the body so that he or she is comfortable.
2. Instruct client to concentrate on each key muscle of the body, tensing and relaxing each muscle until it is totally relaxed.
3. Ask client to tense and release the muscles in the left toes, left foot, left calf, left thigh, and left leg.
4. Now have the client continue the process on the right leg, trunk, upper torso, arms, shoulders, neck, and face. Then have the client check to see that every muscle is relaxed.
5. Ask the client to check for tight areas, any tension, any uncomfortable areas or sensations and then to let it all go. Ask the client if he or she is willing to let all of the tension go.
6. Ask client to practice being totally relaxed.

CULTURAL COMPETENCE

Allowing for a religious or spiritual component in the care plan will enhance the client's ability to cope. Benson (1997) found that when religious beliefs were added to relaxation response procedures, worries and fears improved greatly.

Source: Fontaine, K. (2000). *Healing practices.* Upper Saddle River, NJ: Prentice Hall.

USING MEDITATION AS AN ALTERNATIVE THERAPY

Procedure

1. Meditation is the process of relaxing the body and focusing and quieting the mind. The essence of this method depends on the ability to concentrate on an object, a word, or nothing at all.
2. The process of meditation begins with slow, quiet breathing and deep muscle relaxation. (See Alleviating Stress Using Controlled Breathing and Body Relaxation.)
3. Instruct the client in meditation techniques—suggest books or tapes that focus on meditation.
4. Encourage the client to begin meditation—suggest positive outcomes.
   a. During meditation, there is a decrease in oxygen consumption, blood pressure, pulse rate, respiration, brain wave activity, and blood lactate level (high in anxious people).
   b. Research indicates that meditation has a measurable effect on stress-related conditions.

DOCUMENTATION FOR STRESS AND ADAPTATION

- Identification of stressed behavior observed in client
- Separation of physical from emotional and environmental stressors
- How client is responding to stress
- Pertinent verbalizations of client related to stress
- Nursing interventions related to stress reduction

Critical Thinking Application

UNEXPECTED OUTCOMES	CRITICAL THINKING OPTIONS
Client moves into the stage of exhaustion, and stress becomes dangerous to health.	• Immediately take measures to remove stressors through medication, complete rest, and so forth. • Implement specific stress-reducing measures, such as relaxation processes, visualization, and biofeedback.
Client refuses to acknowledge that stress is affecting his or her life.	• Attempt to elicit feelings of client before giving information about the role of stress and effect on one's body. • Refer client to resources, articles, and knowledgeable persons who can discuss the effect of stress and the importance of eliminating stressors.

Gerontologic Considerations

The influence of stress on aging is significant and affects response and coping ability.

- Nearly 23% of older people living in the community have some degree of disability.
- Elderly have less resistance to stressors: mental, emotional, environmental, and physical.
- Homeostatic imbalance is more common in the elderly and causes additional stress on the body.
- Adaptation to stress lessens with age (depends in part on genetic makeup and personal learning to deal with life crises).
- Nursing care should focus on adaptive responses to stress—assist client to develop mechanisms to deal with the stress of illness and hospitalization.

Management Guidelines

Each state legislates a Nurse Practice Act for RNs and LVN/LPNs. Health care facilities are responsible for establishing and implementing policies and procedures that conform to their state's regulations. Verify the regulations and role parameters for each health care worker in your facility.

Delegation of Responsibilities

- Stress assessment should be assigned to an RN or LVN with experience evaluating stress in clients and one who understands Selye's model of stress.
- An LVN assigned to a client who needs coping strategies for stress should check the care plan with an RN or team leader.
- Teaching a client body relaxation, controlled breathing, or meditation should be done by an experienced nurse—RN or LVN.

Information Flow

- Integrating stress reduction and coping strategies into a client's care plan should be shared by the total staff interacting with the client to maintain a consistent approach.
- The staff approach should have outcome behaviors designated so that the strategies can be evaluated as to effectiveness and efficacy for the client.

CRITICAL THINKING STRATEGIES

SCENARIO 1

Robert Warren is 40 years old and works as an administrative assistant for a senator in Washington, D.C. Before his admission to the hospital, he had no history of heart trouble and had no other major health problems. He is overweight by 30 pounds, complains of difficulty sleeping for several years, and has admitted to several brief depressive episodes that he has handled by either working longer hours or becoming intoxicated with alcohol. He does admit to overuse of alcohol on a daily basis.

Robert complains of burnout related to his work. Although he admires and supports his boss, he also competes with him and secretly believes he would make a better senator. Another area of concern is his marriage, which he says is dull except for an explosive argument every few weeks. Robert has been having affairs with other women regularly for the past few years. He and his wife have no children. Robert's admission diagnosis is acute myocardial infarction.

1. What are the consequences of Robert's adhering to this life-style behavior?
2. Which assessment parameters for stress are important for this client? Be specific about the areas of stress in the assessment.
3. In what ways can you assist this client to improve his coping with stress? (Robert's nutrition and exercise plans are deferred because he is currently in a cardiac rehabilitation program which daily monitors his diet and exercise.)
4. How might you test the result of stress reduction behaviors?

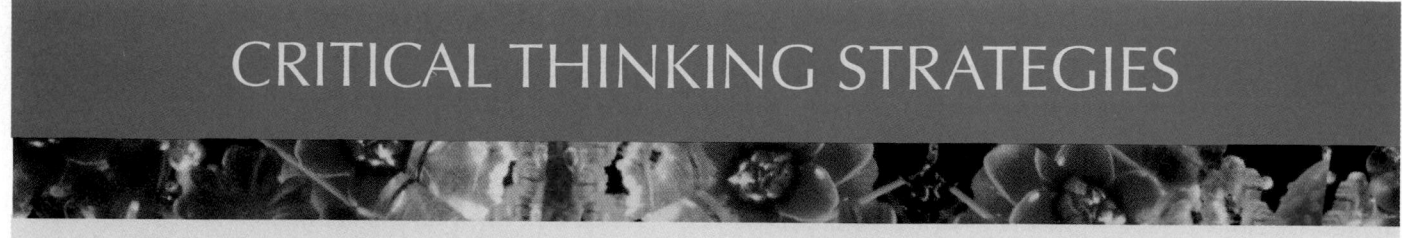

CHAPTER 18

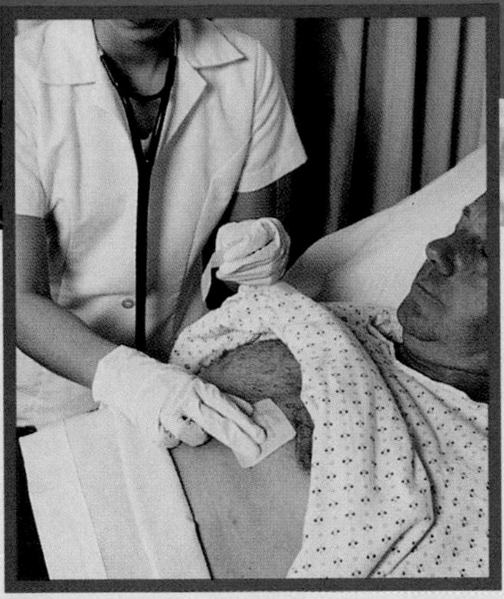

Medication Administration

THEORETICAL CONCEPTS

UNIT ONE: **Medication Preparation** 520
- Preparing Medications 521
- Converting Dosage Systems 523
- Calculating Dosages 523
- Using the Narcotic Control System 524
- Using an Automated Dispensing System 524
- Administering Medication Protocol 526

UNIT TWO: **Oral Medications** 528
- Preparing Oral Medications 529
  - *for Liquid Medications* 529
  - *for Crushing or Altering Medications* 529
- Administering Oral Medications to Adults 531
- Administering Medications per NG or Enteral Tube 531
- Administering Oral Medications to Children 532
  - *for Liquid Medication* 532

UNIT THREE: **Topical Medications** 534
- Applying Topical Medications 535
- Applying Cream to Lesions 535
- Applying Transdermal Medications 536
- Instilling Ophthalmic Drops 537
- Administering Ophthalmic Ointment 537
- Irrigating the Eye 538
  - *for Bilateral Irrigation* 538
- Adminstering Otic Medications 539
- Irrigating the Ear Canal 539

UNIT FOUR: **Mucous Membrane Medications** 542
- Administering Sublingual Medications 543
- Instilling Nose Drops 543
- Administering Metered-Dose Inhaled (MDI) Medications 544
- Using MDI with Spacer 545
- Administering Inhaled Medication by Non-pressurized (Nebulized) Aerosol (NPA) 546
- Administering Rectal Suppositories 546
- Administering Vaginal Suppositories 547

UNIT FIVE: **Parenteral Administration** 549
- Preparing Injections 550
- Administering Intradermal Injections 554
- Administering Subcutaneous (Sub Q) Injections 555
- Preparing Insulin Injections 556
- Teaching Use of Insulin Pump 560
- Administering Subcutaneous (Sub Q) Heparin/LMWH 562
- Administering Intramuscular (IM) Injections 563
- Using Z-Track Method 567

GERONTOLOGIC CONSIDERATIONS 570

MANAGEMENT GUIDELINES 571

CRITICAL THINKING STRATEGIES 572

Learning Objectives

- Explain the concepts of drug absorption, distribution, biotransformation, and excretion.
- List the seven parts of a medication order.
- State the "five rights" for administering medications.
- Describe the medication cart and its purpose.
- Identify three nursing actions to prevent medication errors.
- Outline steps for applying a transdermal medication.
- List factors to assess before applying medications to the skin or mucous membranes.
- Describe steps for instilling eyedrops.
- Outline the process of eye and ear irrigations.
- Contrast the procedure for instilling ear medication in adults and children.
- Outline steps used when preparing parenteral medications.
- Demonstrate correct calculation and preparation of a complex medication order.
- Compare insulin types, their onset, peak, and duration of action.
- List four important factors to assess when administering parenteral medications.
- State four techniques to alleviate pain with parenteral injections.
- Describe the injection technique using the Z-track method.
- List steps for inserting a rectal or vaginal suppository.
- List factors to include in charting medications.

Terminology

Absorption: the passage of a substance from administration site into the bloodstream.

Addictive: causing enslavement to some habit.

Allergy: an antigen–antibody reaction or sensitivity to a substance.

Anaphylaxis: a shock state due to an antigen/antibody reaction to a foreign substance (e.g., medication).

Anesthesia: partial or complete loss of sensation with or without loss of consciousness as a result of injury, disease, or administration of a drug.

Aseptic: sterile; condition free from germs and infection.

Aspirate: to remove by suction.

Biotransformation: metabolic conversion of a drug into inactive metabolites that are readily excreted from the body.

Bronchodilatation: dilatation of the airways.

Cerumen: protective secretion produced by the outer ear canal.

Circulation: movement of blood in a circular course, exiting through the aorta and coming back into the heart via the venae cavae.

Compatible: able to mix with another substance without destructive changes.

Congestion: the presence of an excessive amount of blood or fluid in an organ or in tissue.

Contaminate: to soil, stain, or pollute; to render impure.

Contraindication: any circumstance indicating the inappropriateness of a form of treatment otherwise advisable.

Dosage: the amount of medicine to be administered to a client at one time.

Drug: any substance that when taken into the living organism may modify one or more of its functions.

Dyspnea: a subjective feeling of difficulty in breathing.

Ecchymosis: irregularly formed hemorrhagic area of the skin; a bruise.

Generic: common or general name for a drug as opposed to a brand name.

Instillation: slowly pouring or dropping a liquid into a cavity or onto a surface.

Intradermal: within the dermal layer of the skin; injection here used for testing allergies, immune responses.

Intramuscular: within a muscle; injected medication is rapidly absorbed due to rich vascular supply.

Intravenous: administration into a vein for immediate drug action.

MAR: medication administration record.

Medicine: a drug or remedy.

Metabolism: the biological process of changing a substance so that it (a) is less active, and (b) can be excreted.

Narcotic: a controlled substance that depresses the central nervous system, thus relieving pain and producing sedation.

Nebulizer: a device for breaking a drug into small particles to produce a mist or fog for inhalation.

Ophthalmic: topical route for administering eye medications.

Otic: topical route for administering ear medications.

Parenteral: absorption route for administering medications other than the GI tract requiring medicated injection.

Peristalsis: a progressive, wavelike movement that occurs involuntarily in the intestines of the body.

Subcutaneous: third layer of skin which contains fat, with few blood and lymph vessels; route for injected medication. Results in slower absorption.

Sublingual: under the tongue.

Systemic: pertinent to the whole body rather than one specific area.

Therapeutic: having medicinal or healing properties.

Tonicity: state of normal tension (e.g., muscular) or normal osmolality (body fluid).

PHARMACOLOGIC AGENTS

The term *medication* refers to approved therapeutic (pharmacologic) agents applied to or introduced into the body to produce specific local or systemic physiologic effects. The term *medication* usually refers to a chemical compound that is produced in a pharmaceutical laboratory and is prescribed by a physician to be administered to a client to prevent, treat, or cure illness. These agents should be differentiated from over-the-counter products such as vitamins, minerals, nutritional supplements, and botanical agents (herbs, phytomedicines) which also affect the body. While such agents are available to the public and commonly used for self-treatment, they are not officially regulated or monitored in the United States. It is important to assess the client's use of pharmaceutical agents as well as over-the-counter products or supplements, since there is potential for dangerous interactive effects.

Pharmacologic agents have a generic (patented official) name (e.g., acetaminophen), and a trade or brand name (created by the particular manufacturer) which is capitalized (e.g., Tylenol). Generic formulations are usually less expensive than brand name products.

BIOLOGIC EFFECTS OF DRUGS

The ultimate effect of a drug is influenced by four biologic processes: absorption, distribution, metabolism (biotransformation), and excretion. These processes determine the onset, duration, and intensity of a drug's action.

Absorption This process refers to the movement of the drug from the administration site into the bloodstream. The route of administration determines whether or not a drug is confined to one area of the body to exert a *local effect*, or is absorbed by the vascular system and distributed to body tissues for a *systemic effect*. The oral route (PO) is most frequently used for drug administration. Drugs may be given PO to exert a local effect (e.g., cough medicine, antacid), but more commonly the drug dissolves and is absorbed by the GI tract to exert a systemic effect. Liquid forms are absorbed more quickly. Most drugs are absorbed in the small intestine via the large vascular mucosal surface. The alkaline environment of the intestines enhances this absorption process. GI absorption is influenced by the pH, the presence or absence of food, concomitant ingestion of other drugs, solubility of the drug, and blood flow to the absorption site. In general, bioavailability of oral drugs is decreased because after absorption, the drug is circulated to the liver (first pass) and metabolized before reaching the circulation.

Medications applied "topically" to the skin (dermal) or eye (ophthalmic) or into the ear canal (otic) are often administered for local action. The skin is also used for transdermal (percutaneous) absorption of drugs via patches, which release a medication continuously for a systemic effect.

Mucous membranes provide a variety of convenient sites for drug administration to achieve a local or systemic effect by absorption. Sites include sublingual and buccal areas, the nose or respiratory tract (by inhalation), the eye, vagina, and rectum.

The parenteral route (by injection) provides the most direct, reliable, rapid drug absorption. Methods of parenteral administration include intradermal, subcutaneous (Sub Q), intramuscular (IM), and intravenous (IV). Site selection depends on the drug, its action, and client factors. For example, a client with a severe allergic reaction receives epinephrine IV (directly into the bloodstream) because this route bypasses the process of absorption and provides immediate distribution and drug action in an emergency situation.

Distribution Distribution refers to the process by which a drug is transported by the blood to the site of action. This process requires adequate cardiac output and tissue perfusion. Some of the drug binds to plasma protein and may compete with other drugs for this storage site. The rest is transported in "free" form through the circulation. It is the "free" form that is pharmacologically active. The "free" drug crosses cell membranes and as it is metabolized and excreted, the protein-bound drug is freed for action. Lipid-soluble drugs are distributed to and stored in fat and then released slowly into the bloodstream when drug administration is discontinued. The distribution process requires adequate cardiac output and tissue perfusion, while the rate of diffusion is influenced by the drug's protein-binding capacity, its solubility, the amount of drug in the plasma and the presence of physiologic barriers such as the blood–brain and placental barriers.

Metabolism Metabolism or biotransformation refers to the enzymatic process by which a "free" drug is converted to an inactive and harmless form that can be excreted. Most drugs are metabolized in the liver where some drugs are converted into metabolites that are more pharmacologically effective than their "parent" form. Some drugs given orally are significantly inactivated by "first passing" through the liver before entering the general circulation to be transported to the site of action. Oral doses of these drugs must be higher than parenteral doses, and some drugs totally inactivated by "first pass" must be given parenterally. Other sites of drug metabolism include the lungs, kidney, plasma, and intestinal mucosa.

Excretion This is the final process by which the drug is eliminated from the body. The kidneys are the most important route of excretion because they eliminate both the pure drug as well as metabolites of the parent drug. During excretion, substances are filtered through the glomeruli, secreted by the tubules, and then either reabsorbed by the tubules or directly excreted and eliminated through urine. Other routes of excretion include the lungs (by exhalation), GI tract, saliva, sweat, and breast milk.

Medication biodynamic processes and the individual client's response to drug therapy are influenced by many factors including a client's body weight, body mass index, age, sex, acid–base and fluid and electrolyte balance, biorhythms, and general health and nutritional status. In addition, ethnic origin and genetic and immunologic factors affect biodynamics, as do psychological, emotional, and environmental influences. The term *drug polymorphism* is applied to these variations in clients' response to medications.

ADMINISTERING MEDICATIONS SAFELY

A medication must have physician's order or prescription before it can be legally administered to a client. If a written order is illegible or is questionable for any reason, the physician must be notified for clarification. In many agencies it is the pharmacist's responsibility to contact the prescriber to clarify unclear or questionable orders. If a medication order is spoken aloud or over the phone ("verbal" or oral order), there is greater risk of error. Some agencies restrict verbal orders to emergencies only. Always repeat the verbal order to avoid misinterpretation, have the prescriber spell out the name of the medication and dosage, and have another person listen to the order as well. Get the prescriber's phone number, then record the order onto the client's chart directly (rather than transcribing from scrap paper). This order must be signed by the prescriber within 24 hours.

Verbal orders should not be taken if the prescriber is present and the chart is available, nor are they appropriate for complex therapeutic protocols (e.g., chemotherapy). To avoid error, it is better to have the prescriber e-mail or fax the medication order.

Seven Parts of Medication Orders

- Client's name
- Date medication was ordered
- Name of medication
- Medication dosage
- Route of administration and any special instruction for administration
- Time and frequency medication is to be given
- Signature of individual ordering the drug

Common communication breakdowns leading to medication errors include:

- Unapproved or unclear abbreviations (e.g., use "mcg" rather than μg and use "units" rather than U)
- Illegible writing
- Misplaced or unnoticed decimals (e.g., .2 rather than 0.2)
- Verbal orders
- Incomplete orders

Source: Institute for Safe Medication Practices (2001).

Medication orders may be *routine* (administered as ordered until discontinued by the prescriber), *one-time-only*, *"stat"* (immediately), or PRN (administered when the client needs the medication within the specified time interval, e.g., q4h). The continued validity of any medication order should be evaluated since prescribers sometimes forget to discontinue medications no longer appropriate for the client's condition.

While the physician prescribes the medication and the pharmacist dispenses it, the nurse is responsible for validating, preparing, and administering medications safely and in accordance with agency policies and procedures. The nurse who prepares the medication must also give it to the client, then document the medication, time, dosage, and route on the client's record. In addition, the nurse assesses and documents the client's response to the drug administered. If the client is allergic to a medication, an anaphylactic reaction may occur. This is an immediate, life-threatening reaction which means that the client is hypersensitive to the drug. Prompt assessment and immediate intervention with epinephrine (Adrenalin) is indicated. If a medication is refused by the client, record it, and report to physician via a note on the chart.

Safe administration requires adherence to the "Six Rights" (originally five) each time a medication is given in order to decrease the risk of a medication error.

Safety Precautions

When you administer drugs, you must follow certain safety rules, also known as "The Six Rights." These rules are to be carried out each time you give a drug to a client.

The Six Rights

- Right medication. Compare drug container label to the medication sheet (MAR) three times. Note expiration date. Know action, dosage, and method of administration. Know side effects of the drug.

- Right client. Check the room and bed number and client's identaband; have client state name.
- Right time. Medication given 30 minutes before or after time ordered is acceptable.
- Right method or route of administration. If a change in route is indicated, request new orders from physician.
- Right dose. Validate calculations of divided doses with another nurse. Check heparin, insulin, and digitalis doses with another nurse. Know the usual dose and question any dose outside safe range.
- Documentation is now considered to be the sixth client right; the nurse should document the name of the drug, the dose and route, and time administered. Also, the client's reaction to the medication is important to include.

Two new rights are under consideration:

- Right to know—client has the right to know about drug he or she is taking.
- Right to refuse—client has the right to refuse to take a medication.

In the event of a medication error, the physician must be notified immediately so that potential danger to the client is minimized. Follow your agency's unusual occurrence or variance reporting procedure to facilitate audits that help identify and rectify sources of medication errors.

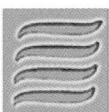

NURSING DIAGNOSES

The following nursing diagnoses are appropriate to use on client care plans when the components relate to a client who requires treatment with medications.

NURSING DIAGNOSIS	RELATED FACTORS
Altered Health Maintenance	Lack of education or readiness to learn, cognitive impairment, lack of equipment, inadequate support systems, inadequate financial resources, religious beliefs, cultural beliefs/values
Deficient Knowledge Regarding Medications	Inadequate understanding of condition, treatment, or self-care needs
Noncompliance to Medication Regimen	Impaired ability to perform tasks, side effects of therapy, nontherapeutic environment, denial of condition, lack of information, poor self-esteem, nonsupportive family

- The single most important nursing action to decrease the incidence of hospital-based infections is handwashing. **Remember to wash your hands or use antibacterial gel before and after each and every client contact.**

UNIT 1

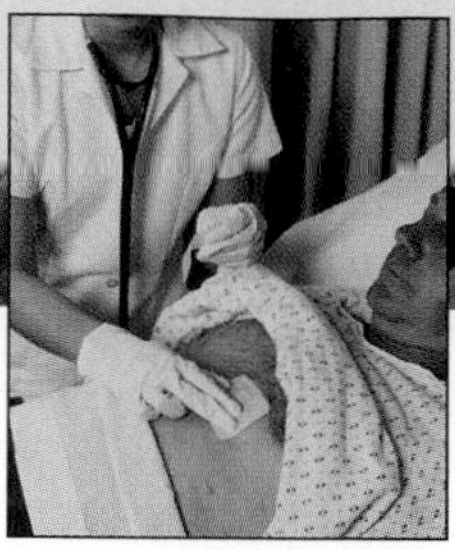

Medication Preparation

Nursing Process Data

ASSESSMENT *Data Base*

Validate medication to be given with physician's order and client's MAR.

Know desired therapeutic action of the drug, side effects, and adverse reactions.

Assess for potential drug interaction with client's other medications or contraindication to administration (allergy, lab data, vital signs, unsafe dose).

Identify route for drug administration.

Recognize need to calculate drug dosage and seek verification of calculation by another nurse.

Validate drug and dosage of certain critical drugs with another nurse.

PLANNING *Objectives*

To understand the drug's action and rationale for administration to the client (desired therapeutic effect)

To prepare the appropriate medication to be given by the correct route

To have another nurse double check dosage calculations and preparation of certain critical drugs

To anticipate potential side effects or adverse client reactions and be prepared to take corrective actions

IMPLEMENTATION *Procedures*

Preparing Medications

Converting Dosage Systems

Calculating Dosages

Using the Narcotic Control System

Using an Automated Dispensing System

Administering Medication Protocol

EVALUATION *Expected Outcomes*

Rationale for medication administration is clear and therapeutic effect is anticipated.

Medication is withheld if administration is contraindicated by assessment findings.

Dosage calculations are accurate and validated.

Medication is prepared appropriately according to procedure for route of delivery.

Medication is administered according to the "six rights."

PREPARING MEDICATIONS

Equipment

Reference resource (e.g., PDR, pharmacology textbook, drug handbook)
Calculator (if indicated)
Medication administration record sheet (MAR)
Client's chart

Procedure

1. Check physician's orders and client's MAR for medications client is to receive (drug, dosage, route of administration, time intervals).
2. Identify any unfamiliar drugs.

> **CLINICAL ALERT**
>
> Individual drugs are designed to be administered by specific route—be sure to check drug labels for appropriate route of administration.

3. Research unfamiliar drugs using appropriate reference.
   a. Generic and trade name.
   b. Drug classification and major uses.
   c. Pharmacologic actions.
   d. Safe dosage, route, and time of administration.
   e. Side effects; adverse reactions.
   f. Nursing implications.
   g. Complete client teaching as needed.
4. Review client's record for allergies, lab data, any factor (e.g., NPO status, planned procedures) that contraindicates administration of ordered medications.
5. Check client's MAR with previous day's MAR every 24 hours for each drug's dosage, route, and time to be given. **Rationale:** Any new medication, discontinued medications, or altered dosages must be identified before continuing with medication preparation.

Note: The pharmacy monitors the client's ordered medications and produces the MAR sheet each day.

6. Validate carefully that MAR is consistent with physician's most recent order for each medication.

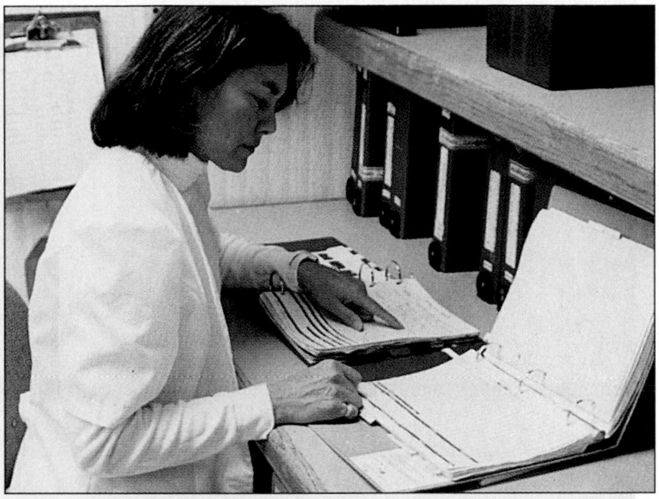

Check physician's order against medication record sheet.

Rationale: Some medication dosages are adjusted on a daily basis.

7. Wash your hands.
8. Take medication cart, if facility uses this system, to client's room.

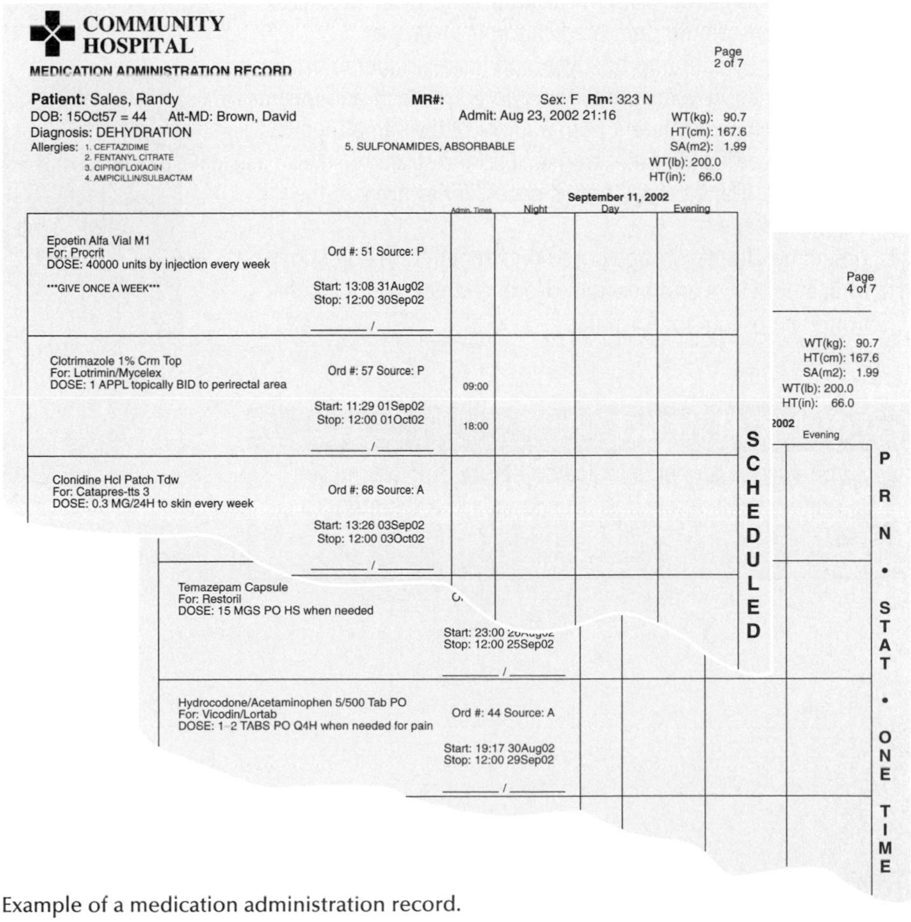

COMMUNITY HOSPITAL
MEDICATION ADMINISTRATION RECORD
Page 2 of 7
Patient: Sales, Randy MR#: Sex: F Rm: 323 N
DOB: 15Oct57 = 44 Att-MD: Brown, David Admit: Aug 23, 2002 21:16
Diagnosis: DEHYDRATION
Allergies: 1. CEFTAZIDIME 2. FENTANYL CITRATE 3. CIPROFLOXACIN 4. AMPICILLIN/SULBACTAM 5. SULFONAMIDES, ABSORBABLE
WT(kg): 90.7 HT(cm): 167.6 SA(m2): 1.99 WT(lb): 200.0 HT(in): 66.0
September 11, 2002
Admin. Times | Night | Day | Evening

Epoetin Alfa Vial M1
For: Procrit
DOSE: 40000 units by injection every week
GIVE ONCE A WEEK
Ord #: 51 Source: P
Start: 13:08 31Aug02
Stop: 12:00 30Sep02

Clotrimazole 1% Crm Top
For: Lotrimin/Mycelex
DOSE: 1 APPL topically BID to perirectal area
Ord #: 57 Source: P
Start: 11:29 01Sep02
Stop: 12:00 01Oct02
09:00
18:00

Clonidine Hcl Patch Tdw
For: Catapres-tts 3
DOSE: 0.3 MG/24H to skin every week
Ord #: 68 Source: A
Start: 13:26 03Sep02
Stop: 12:00 03Oct02

SCHEDULED

Page 4 of 7
WT(kg): 90.7 HT(cm): 167.6 SA(m2): 1.99 WT(lb): 200.0 HT(in): 66.0
Evening

Temazepam Capsule
For: Restoril
DOSE: 15 MGS PO HS when needed
Stop: 12:00 25Sep02

Hydrocodone/Acetaminophen 5/500 Tab PO
For: Vicodin/Lortab
DOSE: 1–2 TABS PO Q4H when needed for pain
Ord #: 44 Source: A
Start: 19:17 30Aug02
Stop: 12:00 29Sep02

PRN • STAT • ONE TIME

Example of a medication administration record.

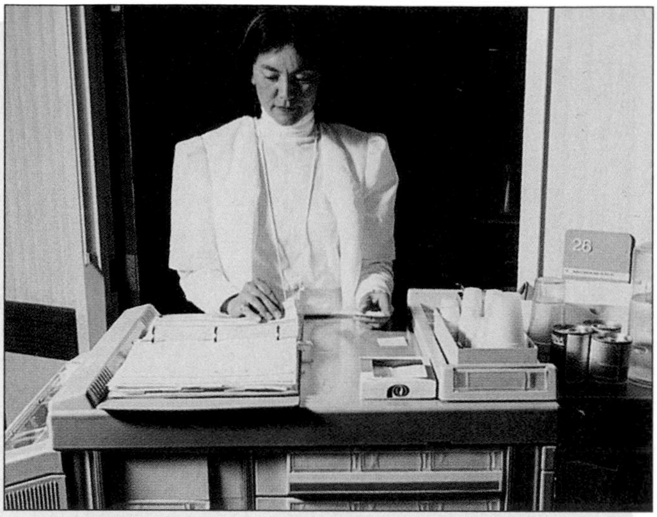

Take medication cart to client's room.

9. Open medication cart; take out client's medication drawer.
10. Starting at the top of the medication record check each medication in order against the medication packages in the drawer. Ensure that all doses for your shift are there. Pharmacy restocks cart every 24 hours. **Rationale:** If a dose is missing, or too many doses remain, check medication record for possible error in administration.
11. Compare drug label with MAR. **Rationale:** This is a safety check to ensure the right medication is given.
12. Retrieve medication to be given and inspect label to assure that medication is indicated for ordered route of administration. **Rationale:** Different preparations of the same medication are used for different routes of administration.
13. Determine if any calculation is necessary to prepare the correct dosage.
14. Calculate client's dosage based on strength of medication, if indicated. Have another nurse double check your calculation. (See p. 523 for formulas.)

> **CLINICAL ALERT**
>
> If client assessment is indicated before drug administration (e.g., BP), leave dose in wrapper as a reminder to do so.

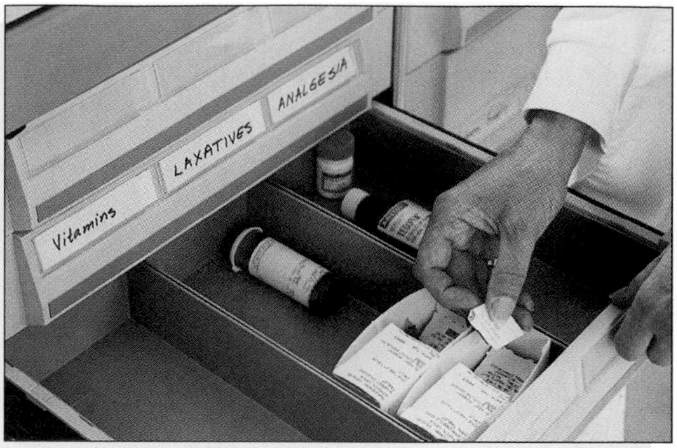

Locate medications in client's drawer. Retrieve medication to be given and inspect label.

15. Prepare medication as indicated for nonparenteral or parenteral route, checking drug label before, during, and after preparation.

> **CLINICAL ALERT**
>
> Check medication label three times:
> - When retrieving the medication from storage area.
> - When preparing the medication.
> - When returning the medication to storage area.

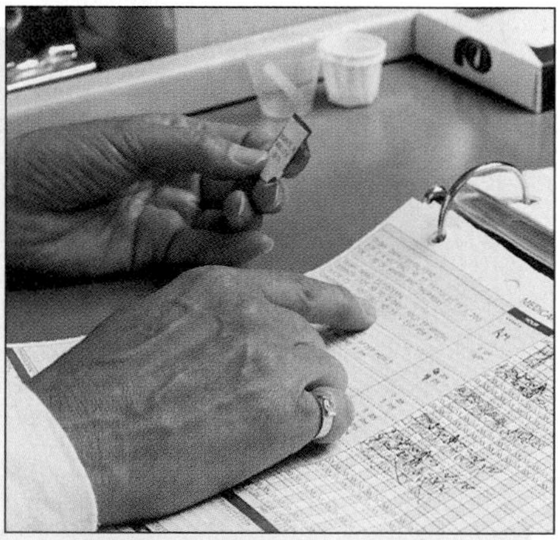

Check individually wrapped medication against client's MAR.

CONVERTING DOSAGE SYSTEMS

Procedure

1. To make conversions from the metric to apothecaries' or household systems, it is necessary to memorize or refer to equivalency tables.
2. To convert milligrams to grains, use the following formula:

$$\frac{1 \text{ gr}}{\text{milligrams per grain}} = \frac{\text{Dose desired}}{\text{Dose on hand}}$$

$$\frac{1}{60} = \frac{X}{180}$$

$$60x = 180$$

$$X = 3 \text{ gr}$$

3. You may also use ratio and proportion to calculate dosage:

   1 gr:60 mg: :X gr:180 mg

   $60X = 180$

   $X = 3$ gr
4. To convert milligrams to milliliters, you can set up a direct proportion and, following the algebraic principle, cross multiply.
5. Check Conversion Tables in the Drug Supplement at the end of the chapter.

CALCULATING DOSAGES

Equipment

Orders for dosage of medication needed
Dosage of medication on hand

Procedure

1. To calculate oral dosages, use the following formula. (D and H must be in same unit of measure.)

$$\frac{D}{H} = X$$

   where D = dose desired; H = dose on hand; and X = dose to be administered.

   Example: Give 500 mg of ampicillin sodium when the dose on hand is in capsules containing 250 mg.

$$\frac{500 \text{ mg}}{250 \text{ mg}} = 2 \text{ capsules}$$

2. To calculate dose when in liquid form, use the following formula

$$\frac{D}{H} \times Q = X$$

   where D = dose desired; H = dose on hand; Q = quantity; and X = amount to be administered

   Example: Give 375 mg of ampicillin when it is supplied as 250 mg/5 mL.

$$\frac{375 \text{ mg}}{250 \text{ mg}} \times 5$$

$$1.5 \times 5 = 7.5 \text{ mL}$$

3. To calculate parenteral dosages, use the following formula:

$$\frac{D}{H} \times Q = X$$

   Example: Give client 40 mg gentamicin C complex sulfate. On hand is a multidose vial with a strength of 80 mg/2 mL.

$$\frac{40}{80} \times 2 = 1 \text{ mL}$$

4. To calculate dosages for infants and children using BSA:

$$\frac{\text{BSA*}}{1.7} \times \text{adult dose} = \text{pediatric dose}$$

   * BSA = body surface area.

   See *Pediatric Nursing,* 3rd., by Jane Ball and Ruth Bindler, 2003, Prentice Hall, for complete discription of method to determine Body Surface Area.
5. To calculate dosages for infants and children using Clark's weight rule:

$$\text{Child's dose} = \frac{\text{Child's wt. in lbs.}}{150} \times \text{Adult dose}$$

6. Check your calculations before drawing up the medications.

Note: Calculation of Solutions is in the drug supplement section at the end of the chapter.

USING THE NARCOTIC CONTROL SYSTEM

Equipment

Medication record sheet
Narcotic sign-out sheet
Medication

Procedure

for Client Administration

1. Check client's medication sheet for narcotic order.
2. Check dose and time last narcotic was administered.
3. Unlock and open narcotic drawer, and find appropriate narcotic container.
4. Count the number of pills, ampules, or prefilled cartridges in container.
5. Check the narcotic sign-out sheet, and check that the number of narcotics in drawer matches the number on specific narcotic sign-out sheet. **Rationale:** Laws on controlled substances require careful monitoring of narcotics.
6. Correct any discrepancy before proceeding with narcotic administration.
7. Sign out for the narcotic on the narcotic sheet after taking narcotic out of drawer.
8. Lock drawer after dispensing medication.
9. Administer medication according to specific oral or parenteral procedure.

CLINICAL ALERT

A licensed person must sign for each narcotic dispensed from the medication drawer.

10. Document narcotic on client's medication record according to usual procedure. Include client's pain rating (e.g., 8/10) and sedation level before and after narcotic administration according to agency policy.

for Unit Narcotic Stock

11. Check narcotic counts every 8 hours. One off-going and one on-coming *licensed* nurse must check the narcotics together. The number on each narcotic sign-out sheet must match the number of that particular narcotic remaining in the drawer.
12. Explore any discrepancy in stock and recorded dispensed narcotic numbers. **Rationale:** Counts must balance. It is the nurse's responsibility to account for all controlled substances dispensed.
13. Licensed nurses cosign the narcotic record if the count is accurate.

CLINICAL ALERT

If the narcotic depresses breathing, note client's level of sedation and respiratory rate before administering, and document assessment according to agency policy.

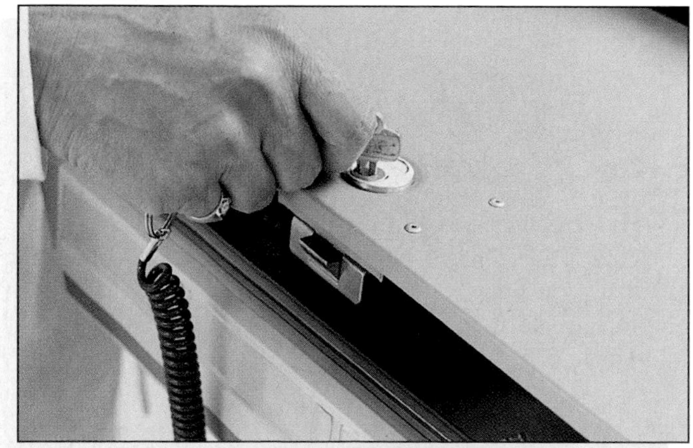

Lock narcotic drawer after removing medication. Keep key with you at all times.

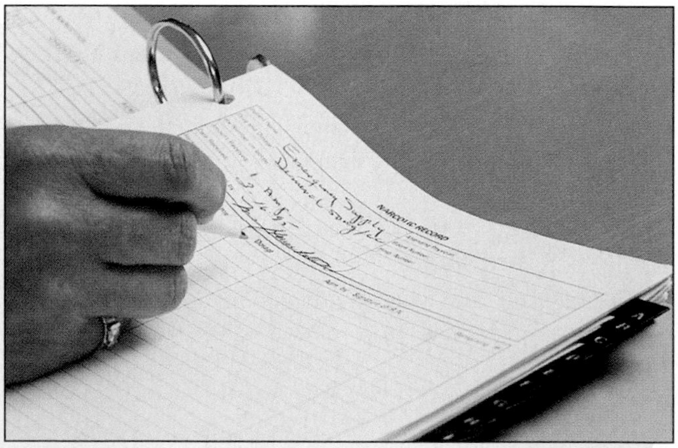

Sign on specific narcotic sign-out sheet after taking narcotic out of drawer.

USING AN AUTOMATED DISPENSING SYSTEM

Equipment

Automated dispensing system (e.g., PYXIS)
Client's medication record

Preparation

See *Preparing Medications.*

Procedure

1. Enter your user ID code number and user password or scanned fingerprint. **Rationale:** This process controls access to medication/narcotics.
2. Select desired client from list to access client's file.
3. Validate with client's medication record, select desired medication and dose on monitor screen. **Rationale:** Client is directly billed for medication.
4. Enter a witness ID/scan (by another nurse) to validate wasted medication, if partial dose is needed.
5. Remove the appropriate medication when drawer opens.
6. Close drawer and exit system.
7. Prepare medication and administer according to route.

> **CLINICAL ALERT**
>
> The usual checks and balances between nurses and pharmacists may be bypassed with automated dispensing systems, increasing the risk for medication errors.

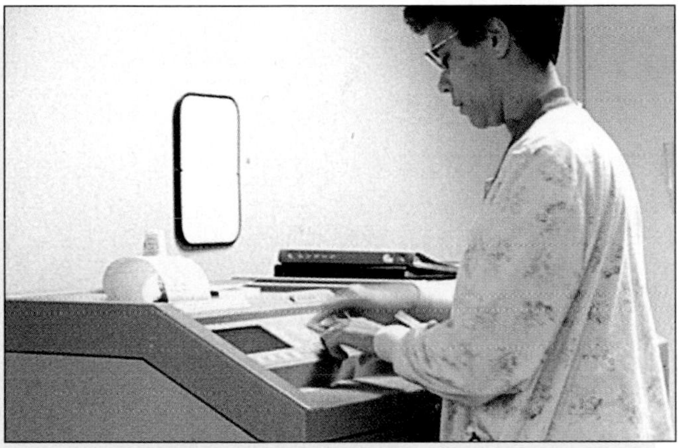

Obtain code number (user ID) from the pharmacy.

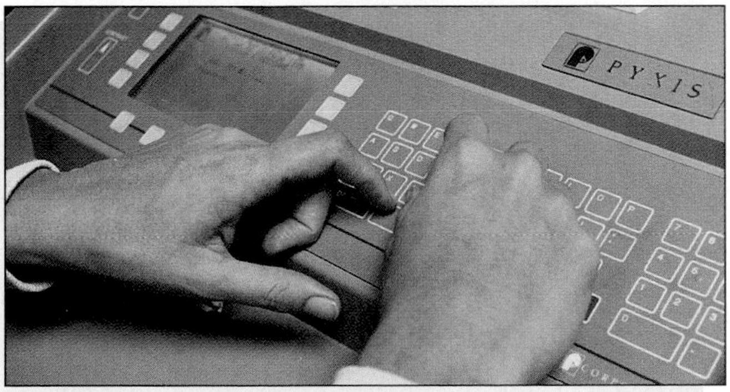

Enter code to open specific drawer for client's drug.

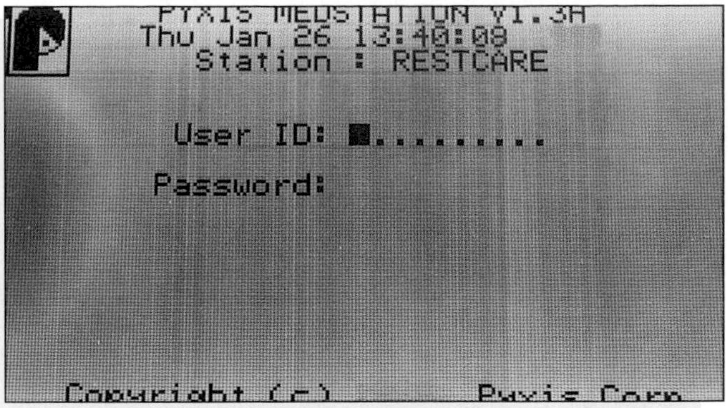

Enter user ID number and user password.

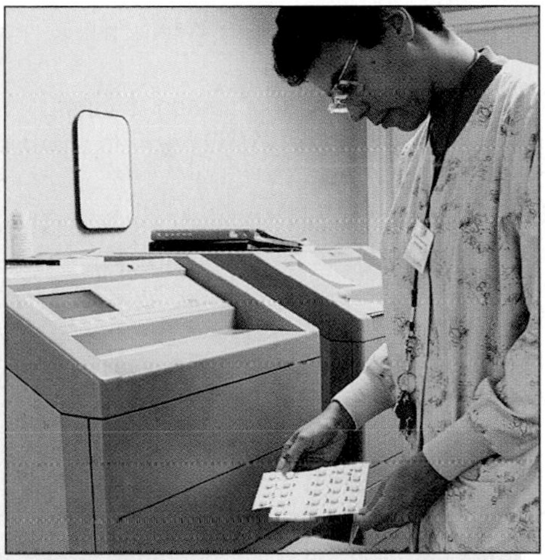

Check number of drugs remaining.

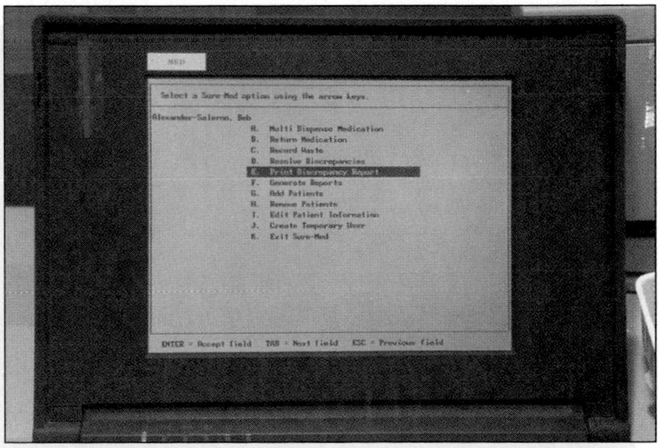

If there is a discrepancy, print report.

ADMINISTERING MEDICATION PROTOCOL

Equipment

Prepared medication
Gloves (if indicated)
Stethoscope

Preparation

See *Preparing Medications.*

Procedure

1. Check client's room number against the medication record and lock the medication cart before entering client's room, if cart is used. **Rationale:** Locking cart is a safety measure.
2. Check client's identaband and ask client to state name.
3. Provide privacy.
4. Explain procedure and purpose of medication to client.
5. Assist client to appropriate position for medication administration.
6. Check client's vital signs if indicated before administering medication. **Rationale:** Medication's effects may cause hemodynamic instability if client's vital signs are at the high or low extreme of normal.
7. Wash hands and don gloves if indicated. **Rationale:** Parenteral and enteral medication administration require the use of gloves.
8. Administer medication according to route procedure and adhering to the "Six Rights" of medication administration.
9. Dispose of equipment appropriately; then remove gloves, if used, and wash your hands.
10. Record administered medications in client's record; the time, medication given, dosage, route (including site of injection), and any relevant assessment findings.

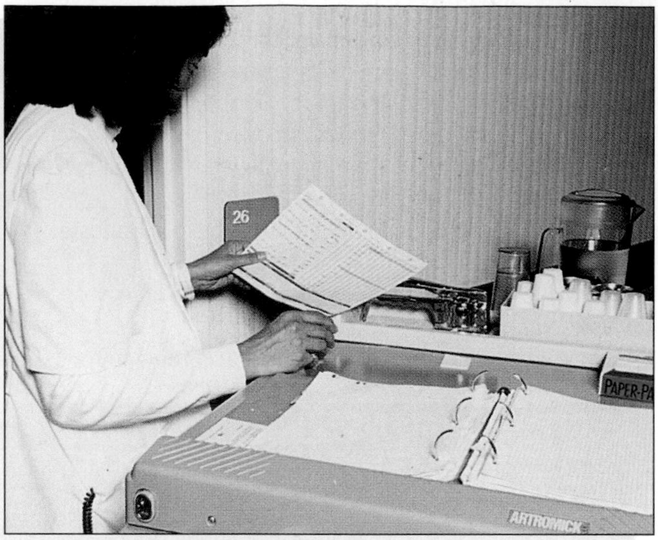

Check room number against medication record.

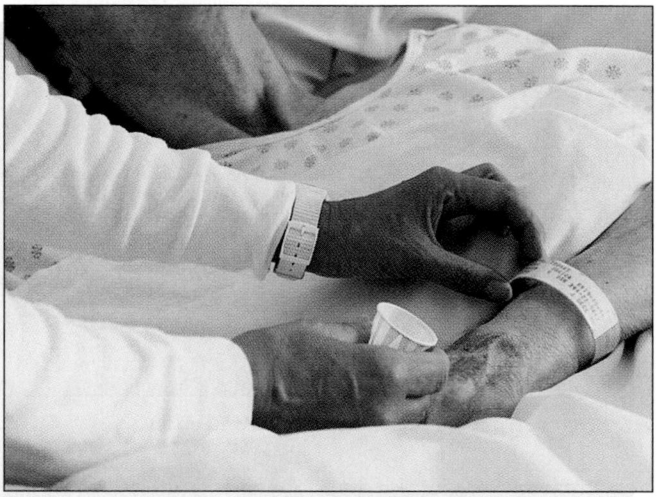

Check client's identaband and ask client to state name.

CLINICAL ALERT

Checking client's identity includes checking name and hospital number on identaband against the MAR. This is a new JCAHO requirement.

Abbreviations *frequently misinterpreted* include:

- AU (each ear) misinterpreted as OU (each eye). Do not use AU.
- Per os (orally) misinterpreted as OS (left eye). Use "PO."
- qd (each day) misinterpreted as qid (four times a day). Use "daily."
- qhs (at bedtime) misinterpreted as qh (every hour). Use "nightly."

EVIDENCE BASED NURSING PRACTICE

Medication Errors—A Growing Problem

One study of 5000 medication errors found that the most common errors resulting in client death were wrong dose (40.9%), wrong drug (16%), and wrong route (9.5%). In 2001, more than 100,000 medication errors were reported. Of these, 2539 resulted in injury, including 14 deaths.

Source: Carroll, P. (2003, January). Medication errors. *RN,* 66(1), 52–57.

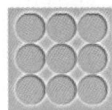

CULTURAL COMPETENCE

One genetic factor noted to differ among ethnic groups is variation in metabolic pathways which may accelerate or decelerate drug metabolism. It is also thought that the pathophysiology of various disease states may differ among populations based on genetic determination. For example, Black clients respond differently to different antihypertensives than whites do. Blacks respond better to diuretics than they do to beta blockers and angiotensin-converting enzyme (ACE) inhibitors for hypertension.

Some agents within drug classes are more effective than others for different populations. Asians metabolize psychotropic agents slower than other ethnic groups, so lower doses may be indicated.

The nurse should obtain a list of each client's current medications as well as any alternative therapies used so that possible untoward interactions can be prevented.

Medication Safety Measures

- Keep all medicines in locked carts or cabinets.
- Do not store dangerous drugs (e.g., concentrated KCl, NaCl, magnesium sulfate) in locked carts.
- Avoid the use of stock or "borrowed" medications.
- Keep narcotics in double-locked cabinets or PYXIS. Count all narcotics with oncoming staff at the end of each shift.
- Clearly label and separate topical medicines from parenteral or oral medicines.
- Check with another nurse (1) mathematical calculations for dosages and (2) dispensed/prepared "high alert" drugs and those for high risk clients (e.g., insulins, heparin, digoxin, and hemodynamic agents if not premixed).
- Do not leave any medication at client's bedside unless there is a specific physician's order to do so.
- Report any errors in drug administration to charge nurse and client's physician immediately. Monitor the client closely for adverse effects. Document the drug given, and complete a written variance report.
- Provide complete instruction to clients regarding medication to be used at home.
- Make sure every physician involved with the client is aware of medications the client is taking at home.

Critical Thinking Application

UNEXPECTED OUTCOMES	CRITICAL THINKING OPTIONS
Nurse is unsure of correct dosage when calculating client's drug order.	• Use a calculator. Request that another nurse check calculation or conversion. Seek agency pharmacist's assistance.
Client returns from surgery and medication orders are unclear.	• Clarify with physician which medications are to be discontinued or renewed postoperatively. (All medications given before surgery are automatically cancelled postoperatively.)
Narcotic count and sign-out narcotics sheets do not agree.	• Check medications sheets for narcotics signed out to specific clients. • Check with other nurses who may have administered narcotics. • Submit report if sign-out sheets cannot be verified.

UNIT 2

Oral Medications

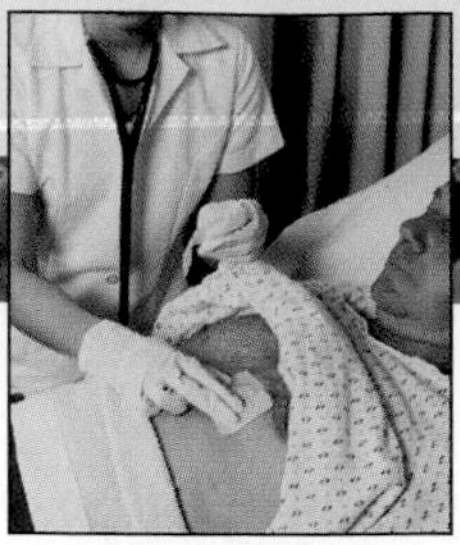

Nursing Process Data

ASSESSMENT *Data Base*

Check that medication is to be given by oral route.

Determine that client is not NPO.

Determine that client is able to take medication orally.

- Client is alert.
- Swallow/gag reflex is present.
- No risk of aspiration exists.
- Client is not nauseated/vomiting.

Determine that medication can be safely altered if necessary for administration.

PLANNING *Objectives*

To provide an easy, inexpensive, and convenient route for administering medications

To ensure that client is able to take oral medication

To safely administer an altered oral medication

To facilitate administration of oral medication to the client with swallowing difficulty (dysphagia)

To administer oral medication to an adult or child

IMPLEMENTATION *Procedures*

Preparing Oral Medications

- *for Liquid Medications*
- *for Crushing or Altering Medications*

Administering Oral Medications to Adults

Administering Medications per NG or Enteral Tube

Administering Oral Medications to Children

- *for Liquid Medication*

EVALUATION *Expected Outcomes*

Medication is given according to the "Five Rights" of safe administration.

Client takes medication orally without difficulty.

Client experiences intended therapeutic drug effect.

Client demonstrates knowledge about oral medications.

PREPARING ORAL MEDICATIONS

Equipment

Oral medication: tablet, capsule, or liquid from bottle or unit dose.

Client's preference of water, juice, milk, or other vehicle (e.g., jelly, yogurt, pudding) to assist swallowing (if not contraindicated for drug absorption)

Mortar and pestle to crush or pill cutter to divide medication if necessary

Measuring spoon, calibrated dropper, syringe or medicine cup, straw as indicated for particular client's need

Preparation

1. Follow all steps for Medication Administration.
2. Wash hands.

Procedure

for Liquid Medications

1. Remove bottle lid and place topside down to avoid contamination.
2. Hold bottle with label facing up to avoid dripping medication onto label.
3. Set medication cup on firm surface and pour liquid medication; read fluid dispensed at eye level, *read at lowest point of meniscus.* **Rationale:** This reading ensures accurate dose of medication.
4. Wipe bottle lip before replacing cap. Check medication label again. **Rationale:** This safety check ensures correct drug and dosage.
5. Return multidose bottle to storage area. Sign out for any narcotic dispensed on narcotic sheet with date, client's name, room number, physician's name, dosage, your signature, and any wasted narcotic (co-signed by another nurse).
6. Remember to check the label three times:
   a. When taking the medication container from storage place.
   b. When placing medication into medicine cup.
   c. When returning medication container to storage place.

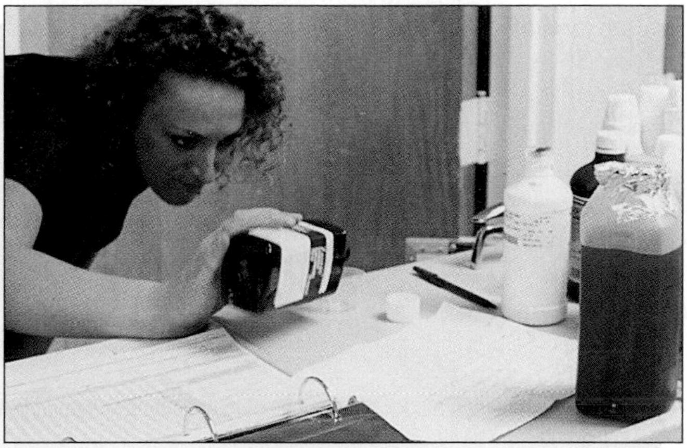
Pour liquid at eye level to read dose correctly.

for Crushing or Altering Medications

1. Leave pill in unit dose packaging and place on firm surface. **Rationale:** Labeled packaging maintains identity and prevents loss of medication. If client does not take medication, it can be returned to drawer.
2. Pound pill with pestle or other tool to crush, pulverizing thoroughly or place pill between two soufflé cups before crushing. **Rationale:** The cups confine the medication.
3. Remove any uncrushed pill coating if medication is to be given per feeding tube. **Rationale:** To prevent tube clogging.
4. Check orders for partial dose medication. Place tablet in pill cutter if scored. **Rationale:** Unscored tablets should *not* be cut. Send to pharmacy for appropriate dose.
5. If giving orally, mix pulverized medication (or powder from opened capsule) carefully in small amount of soft food (pudding, jelly, applesauce). **Rationale:** For many clients with swallowing difficulty, soft food is easier to swallow than liquid.

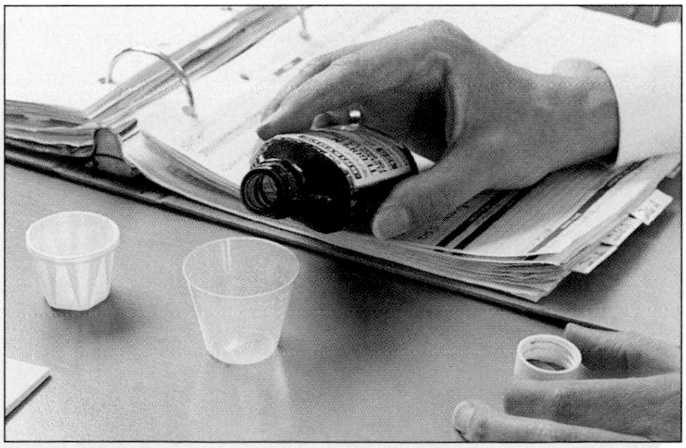
Pour liquid while holding bottle with label up.

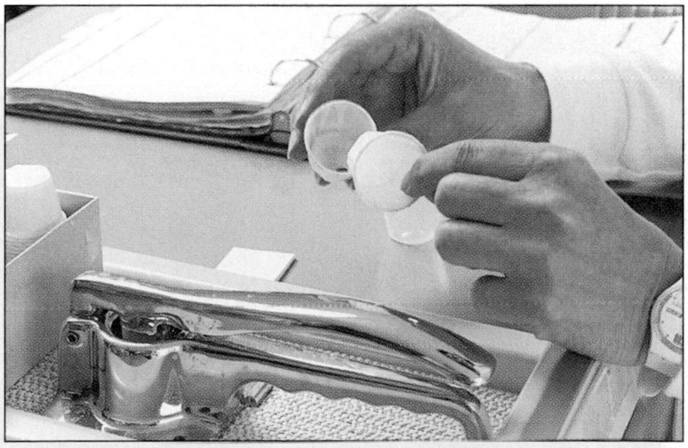
Place tablet in cup and put second cup on top.

6. Open capsule and sprinkle "beads" over soft food to administer. Warn client not to chew the "beads." **Rationale:** Beads are formulated for a sustained timed release therapeutic effect.
7. Ensure client has received all of medication.
8. Offer liquid or food to cleanse palate.

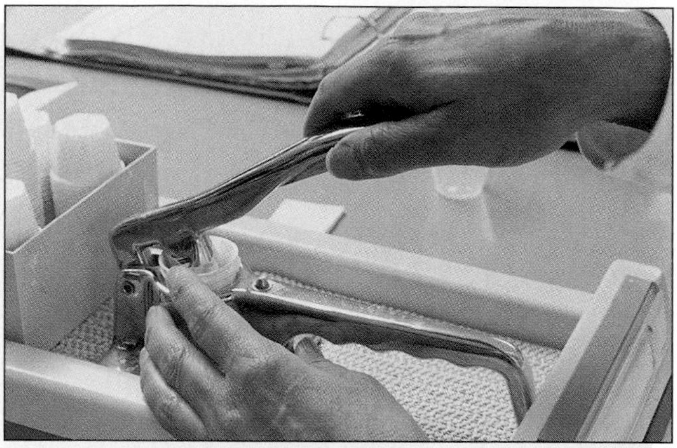

Place pill in crusher to crush tablet.

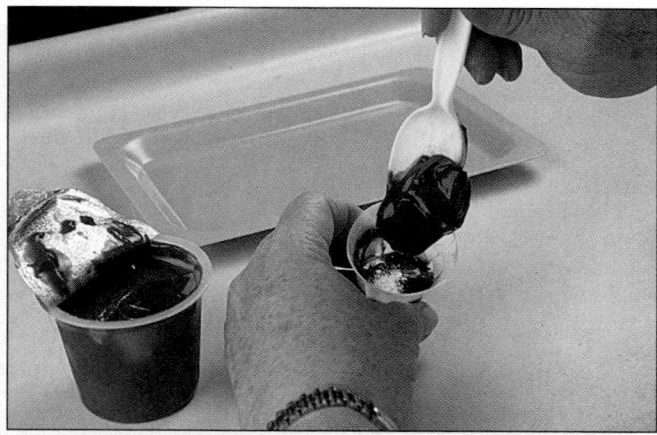

Mix pulverized medication for powder medication (for powder from opened capsule) carefully in small amount of soft food (pudding, jelly, applesauce).

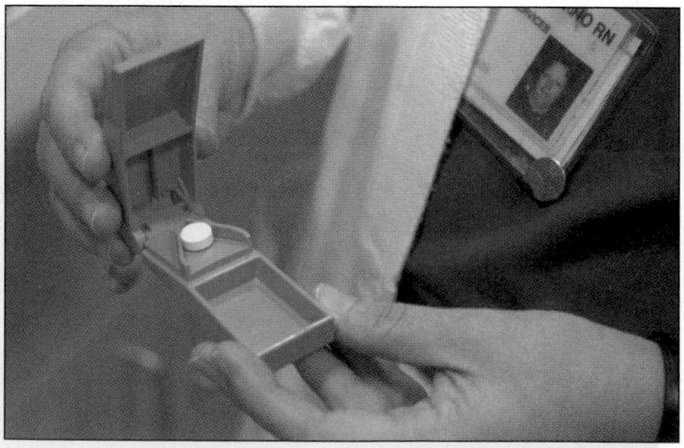

If partial dose is ordered and tablet is scored, place tablet in pill cutter to be cut.

General Precautions for Altering Oral Medications

Unsafe Actions

- *Do not* crush enteric coated or gel-coated tablets. **Rationale:** Coatings allow intestinal absorption of the drug, protect the medication from stomach acid, or protect the stomach from the medication.
- *Do not* crush long-acting tablets. **Rationale:** Sustained action over hours is the advantage of extended release versions of drugs. Crushing could yield a toxic dose and eliminate the sustained action needed through the day.
- *Do not* try to open sealed capsules.
- *Do not* crush contents of capsules (e.g., spansule) with beads or pellets. **Rationale:** These are intended for sustained release action.
- *Do not* give sublingual formulations orally. **Rationale:** Ingredients may be inactivated by stomach acid.
- *Do not* crush sublingual formulations.
- *Do not* give oral medications sublingually. **Rationale:** This could yield a toxic dose since the medication would be absorbed directly into the bloodstream and skip intended pass through the liver for early metabolism before entering the bloodstream.

Safe Actions

- Scored tablets may be split. If a tablet is not scored, return to pharmacy for right dose.
- Chewable medications *can be* crushed safely.
- If a capsule opens easily, powder from the capsules *can be* mixed with food or liquid.
- Liquid-filled capsule contents *can be* (a) squeezed out through a hole punched with a large gauge needle, or (b) aspirated, then mixed with food or liquid. Liquid-filled capsules should not be administered sublingually.
- Beads from opened capsules *can be* sprinkled over soft food to administer, but should not be chewed.
- A sublingual formulation still *can be* given sublingually if the client is NPO.

ADMINISTERING ORAL MEDICATIONS TO ADULTS

Equipment

See Equipment for Dispensing Oral Medications.

Preparation

1. Follow steps for Administering Medication Protocol, Unit 1.
2. Follow procedure for Preparing Oral Medications.
3. Wash hands.

Procedure

1. Take medication tray/cart to client's room; check room and bed number against medication record.
2. Check client's identaband and ask client to state name so you are sure you have correct client.
3. Place client in sitting position
4. Explain what type of medication you are giving and its purpose.
5. Determine if bedside assessment is indicated before administering medication (e.g., vital signs) and assess client.
6. Remove medication from packet and place into medication cup.
7. Hand medication cup to client if assessment findings do not contraindicate administration.
8. Offer glass of water or other liquid. **Rationale:** Aids swallowing dilution and absorption of medication.
9. Make sure client swallows medication.
10. Discard used medicine cup.
11. Record medication on client's record, including assessment findings, if indicated.
12. Assess client for therapeutic drug action and possible side effects or adverse reactions.

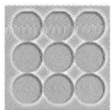

CULTURAL COMPETENCE

Cultural and genetic factors affect how a client reacts to medications. Physiologic rhythms, cultural acceptance, use of alcohol, and stress may either inhibit or accelerate drug biodynamics.

Cultural factors include values and beliefs, educational level, previous experiences, family influence, and physician/client relationship. The use of "natural" remedies can also alter the client's response to drug therapy.

ADMINISTERING MEDICATIONS PER NG OR ENTERAL TUBE

Equipment

See Equipment for Preparing Oral Medications.
Water for diluting and flushing
50-mL irrigating piston syringe
Clean gloves

CLINICAL ALERT

Consult with pharmacist before deciding to alter the form of *any* medication. Have pharmacist substitute liquid form of medication if available, or substitute a short-acting formulation that can be safely crushed for administration. Contact the physician for a substitute medication if formulation alternatives are unavailable.

Preparation

1. Follow steps for Medication Administration, Unit 1.
2. Follow procedure for Preparing Oral Medications.
3. Wash hands.

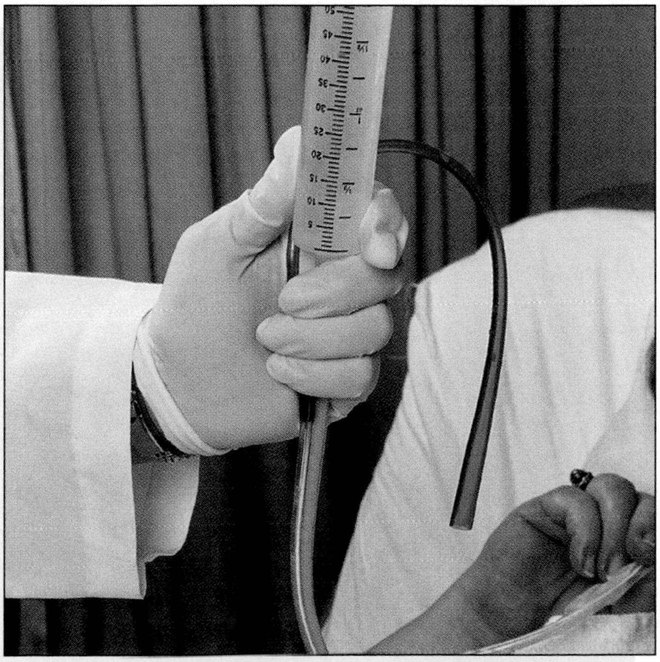

Administer each medication separately, allowing to flow through NG tube by gravity.

Procedure

1. Stop any continuous tube feeding for 30 minutes if medication is to be given on empty stomach.
2. Dilute crushed tablet or powder from capsule in 30 mL warm water.
3. Don gloves.
4. Disconnect NG tube from feeding system.
5. Insert 50 mL syringe into NG tube and aspirate to check residual volume. Return residual and flush NG tube. **Rationale:** To validate gastric capacity for receiving medication and flush solution.
6. Administer each medication separately, allowing to flow through tube by gravity.
7. Flush tube with 15–30 mL water after each medication, monitoring amount of flush to record on I&O sheet. **Rationale:** Flushing reduces risk of tube clogging.
8. Restart tube feeding at appropriate time.

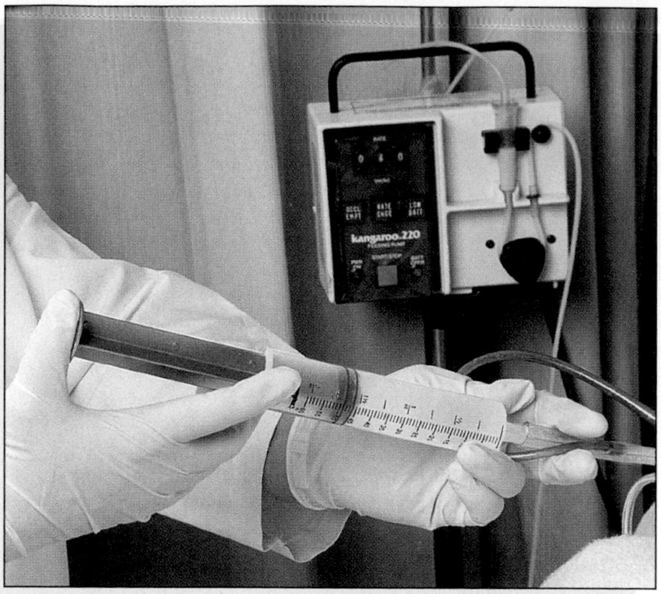

Flush tube (not blue pigtail) with 15–30 mL water after each medication (monitor amount) record on I&O sheet.

ADMINISTERING ORAL MEDICATIONS TO CHILDREN

Equipment

See Equipment for Preparing Oral Medications.

Preparation

1. Follow procedure for Preparing Oral Medications
2. Wash hands.

Procedure

1. Check child's identaband and have child state name.
2. Tell the child it is time to take medicine and explain rationale for medication to family. **Rationale:** Teaching needs may be met at this time.
3. Assess any indicated assessment findings before medication administration.
4. Allow the child to select which medication to take first. **Rationale:** Child exercises some control if allowed to make choices.
5. If indicated, tell the child that the medication is mixed with food/liquid and doesn't taste like the food or liquid without medication.
6. Ask family about best way to administer medication. **Rationale:** Consideration of preference makes administration easier.
7. Administer medication (or medication/food mixture) considering child's developmental level.
8. Follow with fluids of child's choice.
9. Confirm that medication has been swallowed.
10. Offer praise to the child for taking medication.

for Liquid Medication

1. Place dropper or syringe in buccal area of child's mouth, aiming toward cheek.
2. Allow child to suck or squeeze medication slowly into mouth—or allow infant to suck medication from nipple.

DOCUMENTATION FOR ORAL MEDICATIONS

Client's Medication Record

- Name of medication
- Dosage
- Route
- Time administered
- Initials of nurse administering medication
- Signature of nurse identifying initials

Nurses' Notes

- Client's assessment parameters
- Record PRN, STAT, and one-time-only medications
- Name of medication, dosage, route, time administered
- Client's response
- Signature of nurse

Critical Thinking Application

UNEXPECTED OUTCOMES	CRITICAL THINKING OPTIONS
Client has an allergic or anaphylactic response to medication.	• Immediately stop or hold medication. • Notify physician at once; prepare to administer epinephrine to dilate bronchi and support blood pressure. • If reaction is severe: Keep client flat in bed with head elevated. Take vital signs every 10–15 minutes; stay with client. Assess for hypotension or respiratory distress. Establish airway, if necessary. Have emergency equipment available. Provide psychologic support to client to alleviate fears. Record type and progression of reactions.
Client has difficulty swallowing tablets or capsules.	• Use mortar and pestle to crush medications if appropriate and administer to client mixed with juice or a food, such as applesauce or jelly. • If totally unable to swallow medications, do not attempt administering by mouth. Ask physician to order same or comparable medication by a more appropriate route (e.g., parenteral, rectal).
Client is nauseated and oral medications have not been taken.	• Hold medication. Notify physician for antiemetic medication order and alternate route for administering necessary medications. • Administer antiemetic if ordered, then administer medication when client's nausea is relieved.

UNIT 3

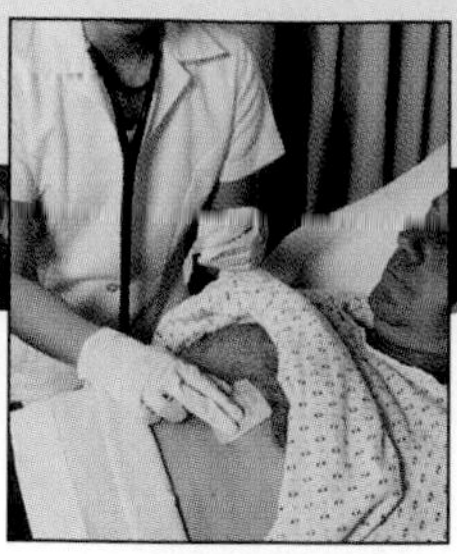

Topical Medications

Nursing Process Data

ASSESSMENT Data Base

Assess for proper route of medication administration.

Observe skin for open lesions, rash, or redness.

Determine drug manufacturer's recommended site for transdermal application.

Assess that area for transdermal application is dry, hairless, intact.

Assess for allergies as reported by client or noted in client's chart.

Assess condition of ear or eye and surrounding area.

Determine purpose for eye or ear irrigation.

Assess client's ability to cooperate with eye/ear medication administration or irrigation.

PLANNING Objectives

To provide local anesthetic, anti-inflammatory or anti-infective effect to a specified part of the body

To provide slow continuous transdermal absorption of medication

To decrease intraocular pressure

To prevent unwanted systemic effect of topically applied eye medication

To provide pupil dilation to facilitate eye examination or therapeutic procedure

To remove debris or neutralize chemical action and minimize eye injury

To soften and remove cerumen (ear wax)

IMPLEMENTATION Procedures

Applying Topical Medications

Applying Creams to Lesions

Applying Transdermal Medications

Instilling Ophthalmic Drops

Administering Ophthalmic Ointment

Irrigating the Eye

for Bilateral Irrigation

Administering Otic Medications

Irrigating the Ear Canal

EVALUATION Expected Outcomes

Client's discomfort (itching, pain) is minimized

Infection is controlled/prevented

Undesired systemic effects of topically applied medication do not occur

Eye examination is successfully completed

Intraocular pressure is reduced

Hazardous chemical action is neutralized and injury is minimized

Client's hearing is improved

APPLYING TOPICAL MEDICATIONS

Equipment

Medication container (tube or jar)
Soap and water to cleanse skin
Clean gloves
Tongue blade
Gauze or transparent dressing (as indicated)
Tape
Pen (to label dressing, if indicated)

Preparation

See Preparing Medications.

Procedure

1. Take medication container and dressing supplies to client's room.
2. Check room and bed number against client's record and check client's identaband, asking client to state name.
3. Provide privacy.
4. Explain procedure and purpose to client.
5. Wash hands and don clean gloves.
6. Cleanse skin site with soap and water and dry thoroughly.
7. Squeeze medication from tube or use a tongue blade to take cream/ointment from medication container.
8. Spread small quantity of medication smoothly and evenly with gloved hand over client's skin following direction of hair follicles. **Rationale:** Gloves facilitate smooth application of ointment.

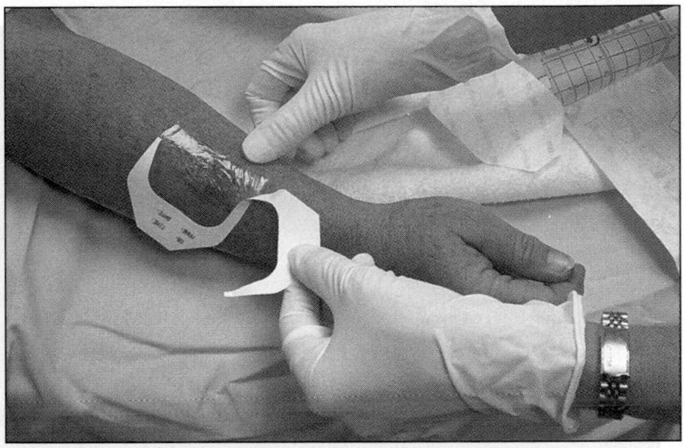

Apply dressing; then label with date, time, and initials.

9. Apply dressing if indicated. **Rationale:** Dressing may ensure that medication is not rubbed off.
10. Label dressing with date, time, and your initials.
11. Remove gloves and wash your hands.
12. Check that client is comfortable.
13. Return medication container to storage area.

> **CLINICAL ALERT**
>
> Systemic absorption of topical medication from open lesions can result in toxic reactions.

APPLYING CREAM TO LESIONS

Equipment

Medication container (tube or jar)
Sterile normal saline for cleansing
Sterile gauze pads for cleansing site
Sterile tongue blade
Mask (see agency policy)
Sterile gloves
Sterile gauze or transparent dressing (or commercially prepared burn dressing)
Kerlix gauze wrap or stretch body net to secure dressing
Pen for labeling dressing

Preparation

See Applying Topical Medications.

Procedure

1. Take medication to client's room; check room and bed number against medication record.
2. Check client's identaband and ask client to state name.
3. Provide privacy.
4. Wash your hands, don mask and clean gloves.
5. Remove previous dressing if present.
6. Note characteristics of site and cleanse area as ordered with sterile gauze pads and saline. Remove gloves.
7. Open medication container.
8. Don sterile gloves.
9. If no dressing is ordered, use gloved hand to apply medication directly to lesion; apply medication sparingly to 1/16-inch thickness. **Rationale:** To provide an occlusive effect.
10. If dressing is ordered, apply thin layer of medication to sterile gauze, then apply dressing to lesion area.
11. Secure dressing with Kerlix wrap or body net if large area is involved.
12. Label dressing with date, time, and your initials.
13. Check to assure that client is comfortable following procedure.
14. Remove gloves and wash your hands.
15. Return medication container to appropriate storage area.

APPLYING TRANSDERMAL MEDICATIONS

Equipment

Medication patch or tube
Gloves
Premeasured medication administration paper
Soap and water
Clear plastic wrap (optional)
Tape and pen for labeling dressing

Preparation

See Preparing Medications.

1. Obtain transdermal patch or premeasured paper that accompanies medication tube.
2. Carefully read the manufacturer's directions for application. **Rationale:** Directions as well as application areas of the body differ.

Procedure

1. Take medication to client's room, check room and bed number against medication record.
2. Check identaband, and ask client to state name.
3. Provide privacy.
4. Wash your hands.
5. Don gloves. **Rationale:** Gloves prevent you from absorbing medication through fingertips.
6. Alternate areas with each dose of medication to prevent skin irritation. Remove and discard previous medicated paper/patch and cleanse area prior to applying new dose. Observe for any skin reaction.
7. Place prescribed medication directly on paper (usually ½–1-inch strip).
8. Apply medicated paper to clean, dry, hairless, intact skin.
9. Use paper to spread medication paste over a 2-inch area. Secure paper with tape or cover medicated area with plastic wrap and tape.
10. For patch, remove protective covering and immediately apply patch to clean, dry, hairless, intact skin.
11. Remove gloves and wash your hands.
12. Label patch or paper with date, time, and your initials.
13. Return medication to appropriate storage area.

Manufacturers' directions for application of transdermal agents differ significantly. Body temperature and blood flow to different regions influence the suggested application site. Always adhere to the manufacturer's specific guidelines and precautions when administering these systems.

CLINICAL ALERT

Dispose of used transdermal patch in biohazard box to protect others from exposure to medication.

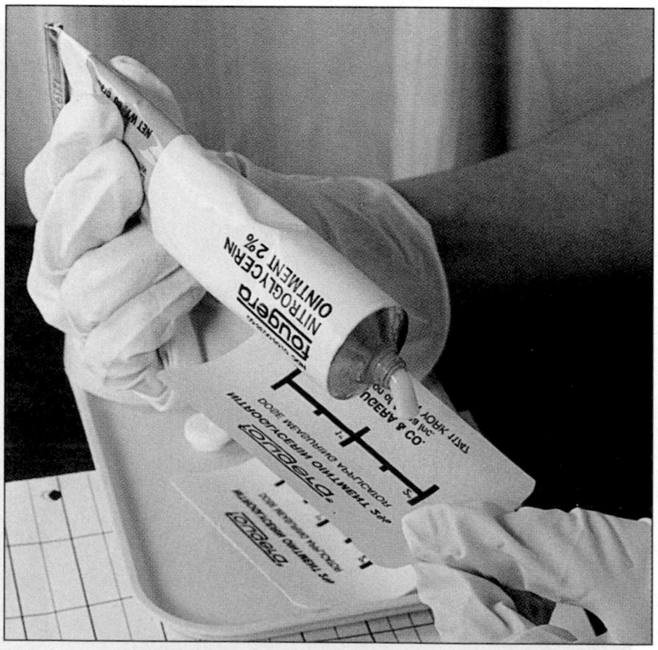

Use premeasured paper to measure medication dosage.

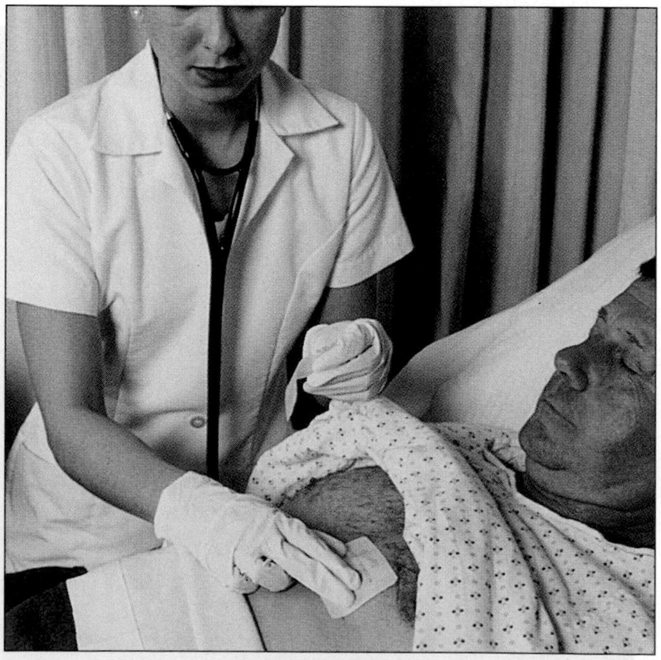

Wear gloves to prevent drug absorption through fingertips.

INSTILLING OPHTHALMIC DROPS

Equipment

Eye medication in ocumeter container
Gloves
Tissues

Preparation

1. Compare the medication record with physician's order.
2. Gather necessary equipment.
3. Remove the medication from the medication cart.
4. Compare the label on the medication container to the medication record. **Rationale:** This is a safety check to ensure that medication is for ophthalmic instillation.

Procedure

1. Take medication to client's room; check room and bed number against medication record.
2. Check identaband, and ask client to state name.
3. Wash your hands and don gloves.
4. Explain procedure and purpose of medication to client.
5. Tilt client's head slightly backward and ask client to look up. **Rationale:** The cornea is protected as client looks up.
6. Uncap ocumeter, placing cap on its side.
7. Give tissue to client for wiping off excess medication.
8. Place ocumeter ½–¾ inch above eyeball with dominant hand. **Rationale:** This position reduces risk of dropper touching eyeball and causing injury.
9. Place nondominant hand on cheekbone and hand holding dropper on top.
10. Expose lower conjunctival sac by pulling down on cheek, creating a "cup."

CLINICAL ALERT

Apply pressure to inner canthus for 2 minutes to prevent rapid drug absorption if eyedrops have potential systemic effects (e.g., bradycardia due to timolol maleate [Timoptic] drops for glaucoma).

Abbreviations for Eye Medication Administration

OS = Left eye
OD = Right eye
OU = Both eyes

11. Drop prescribed number of drops into center of conjunctival sac. **Rationale:** Placing medication directly on cornea could cause injury to cornea.
12. Apply pressure to inner canthus, if indicated.
13. Ask client to gently close eyelids and move eyes. **Rationale:** This distributes solution over conjunctival surface.
14. Very gently massage closed lid for client who cannot cooperate (e.g., comatose client).
15. Remove excess medication with tissue.
16. Remove gloves and wash your hands.
17. Replace medication in appropriate place.

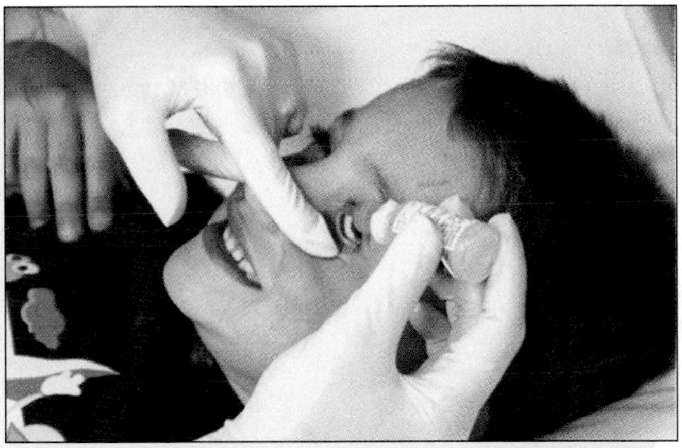

Use nondominant hand to pull lower lid down. Drop eye medication in the center of lower conjunctival sac.

ADMINISTERING OPHTHALMIC OINTMENT

Equipment

Eye ointment in tube
Tissues
Gloves

Preparation

See Instilling Ophthalmic Drops.

Procedure

1. Take medication to client's room, check room and bed number against medication record.
2. Check identaband and ask client to state name.
3. Explain procedure and purpose to client.
4. Wash hands and don gloves.

5. Take protective guard off medication tube and lay on its side.
6. Expose lower conjunctival sac by pulling down on cheek or grasping lower lid below client's eye lashes to form a trough.
7. Instruct client to look upward. **Rationale:** To keep cornea out of way of medication administration area.
8. Place medication tube tip ½–¾ inch above exposed conjunctival sac.
9. Squeeze ribbon of ointment along middle third of inside edge of lower lid.
10. Ask client to close eyelids and move eyes, or gently massage closed lid to distribute medication.
11. Remove excess medication from client's eye area with tissue.
12. Caution client that ointment will cause vision to be temporarily blurred.
13. Recap and replace medication.
14. Remove gloves and wash your hands.

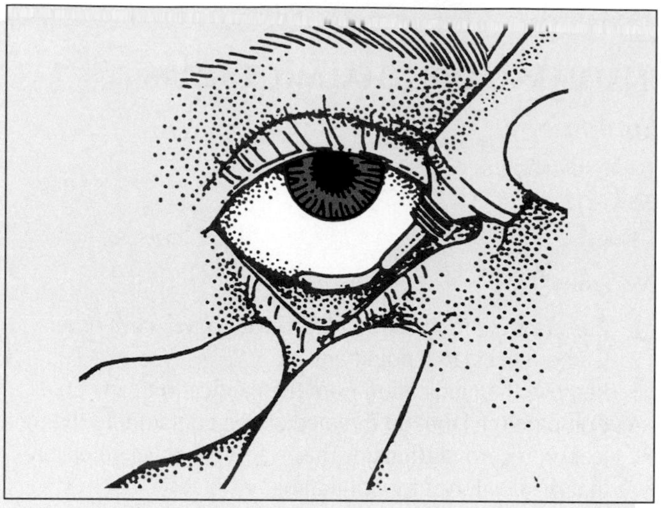

Squeeze ointment along middle third of inside edge of lower lid and ask client to close eyes.

IRRIGATING THE EYE

Equipment

500 mL bag of sterile normal (isotonic) saline *or* bottle of sterile pH-balanced commercial eye irrigating solution (e.g., Dacriose)
IV administration tubing
IV fluid pole for elevation
Nasal cannula (as for oxygen delivery)
Tape
Sterile gauze pads
Absorbent pad or towel
Clean gloves

Preparation

1. Check physician's order for irrigation.
2. Wash hands.
3. Gather equipment.
4. Warm irrigating solution to body temperature by placing container in dry heating pad.

Procedure

1. Take equipment to client's room, check room and bed number against medication record.
2. Check client's identaband and ask client to state name.
3. Provide privacy.
4. Explain procedure and purpose to client.
5. Place client in semi-Fowler's position, turned to side of client's affected eye.
6. Have client hold curved basin on cheek under affected eye.
7. Don gloves.
8. Using your thumb and forefinger, open client's eye to expose lower conjunctival sac by pulling the sac down toward cheek.
9. Place eye irrigation bottle spout tip ¾ inch above client's inner canthus, pointing downward toward the outer canthus.
10. Squeeze bottle, allowing irrigating solution to flow into client's conjunctival sac to remove debris.
11. Continue irrigating for 10 minutes or until eye is cleansed completely.
12. Note results of debris returned with irrigation.
13. Wipe client's eyelid with gauze, wiping from inner to outer canthus.
14. Dispose of equipment in appropriate area.
15. Remove gloves and wash hands.
16. Assist client to comfortable position.
17. Document irrigation and results.

for Bilateral Irrigation

1. Spike saline bag with IV tubing and hang bag on pole.
2. Affix end of IV tubing to nasal cannula, then fit cannula around client's head (or around ears as for oxygen administration) securing prongs at bridge of client's nose with tape.
3. Start flow of saline solution from IV bag and allow to flush client's eyes to neutralize a chemical exposure.
4. Increase flow rate, then continue wide open irrigation until 500 mL has been used over a ten minute period.
5. Follow steps 12–17 above.

ADMINISTERING OTIC MEDICATIONS

Equipment

Prescribed ear medication
Dropper for Instilling medication
Gloves

Preparation

1. Compare the medication record with the most *recent* physician's order.
2. Gather necessary equipment.
3. Remove the medication from the medication cart.
4. Compare the label on the medication bottle to the medication record. **Rationale:** Safety check.
5. Before preparing medication for administration, warm medication bottle to body temperature. **Rationale:** Instillation of cold medication can cause vertigo.

Procedure

1. Take medication to client's room, and check room number against medication card or sheet.
2. Check identaband, and ask client to state name.
3. Explain procedure and purpose to client.
4. Wash your hands.
5. Don gloves.
6. Position client on side, with ear to be treated in the uppermost position. **Rationale:** This position allows medication to enter external ear canal by gravity.
7. Fill medication dropper with prescribed amount of medication.

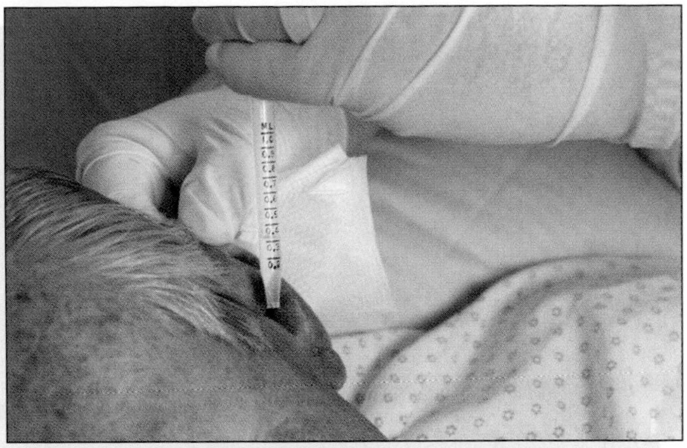

Lift pinna upward and backward to instill eardrops in an adult.

8. Prepare client for instillation of ear medication as follows:
   a. *Infant.* Draw the pinna gently downward and backward. **Rationale:** This separates the drum membrane from the floor of the cartilaginous canal.
   b. *Adult.* Lift pinna upward and backward. **Rationale:** This position straightens the ear canal.
9. Instill medication drops, holding dropper slightly above ear. **Rationale:** This position protests dropper from contamination.
10. Instruct client to remain on side for 5–10 minutes following instillation. **Rationale:** Prevents medication from escaping and facilitates distribution.
11. Dispose of gloves and wash hands.

IRRIGATING THE EAR CANAL

Equipment

Asepto or irrigating syringe
Prescribed irrigating solution or tap water
2 basins: round basin, curved basin
Absorbent pad or towel
Cotton ball

Preparation

(Client may have instilled wax-softening eardrops several hours prior to irrigation.)

1. Check physician's order for irrigation.
2. Wash hands.
3. Gather equipment.
4. Warm irrigating solution to body temperature. **Rationale:** Cold solution can precipitate nausea and vertigo.

Procedure

1. Take equipment to client's room, check room and bed number against medication record.
2. Check client's identaband and ask client to state name.
3. Provide privacy.
4. Explain procedure and purpose to client.
5. Don clean gloves.
6. Place client in Fowler's position and place absorbent towel over client's chest and shoulders.
7. Pour irrigating solution into round basin.
8. Place curved basin under ear to catch irrigating solution.
9. Fill syringe with irrigating solution.
10. Open and straighten client's ear canal by pulling the pinna up and backward for adult or down for an infant or child. **Rationale:** This action allows the solution to flow into ear canal.
11. Hold irrigating syringe at entrance to ear canal without occluding meatus. **Rationale:** Entering ear canal can cause impaction.
12. Push plunger, directing flow of solution toward the top of the canal. **Rationale:** This action allows the flow to reach the entire length of canal.

13. Note return flow throughout procedure.
14. After solution has ceased to flow, dry outside of ear.
15. Return client to comfortable position and place cotton ball in ear canal to absorb excess fluid. **Rationale:** This reduces risk of external otitis.
16. Return used equipment to appropriate area.
17. Remove gloves and wash your hands.
18. Document irrigation and results.

CLINICAL ALERT

Ensure that client's tympanic membrane is intact before irrigating the ear. Water should not be used to irrigate the ear to remove an organic foreign body (e.g., insect or bean) since water may cause the object to swell.

DOCUMENTATION FOR TOPICAL MEDICATIONS

Client's Medication Record

- Time administered
- Name of medication
- Dosage
- Route
- Site of application
- Initials of nurse administering medication
- Signature by nurse which identifies initials

Nurses' Notes

- Record PRN, STAT, and one-time-only medications
- Time administered, name of medication, dosage, route, site
- Client's response to application
- Condition of area treated
- Signature of nurse

Critical Thinking Application

UNEXPECTED OUTCOMES	CRITICAL THINKING OPTIONS
Client develops skin irritation due to medication.	• Notify the physician so that medication may be discontinued.
Client has allergic response (rash or itching).	• Hold medication; notify physician. • Obtain order for antihistamine or topical anti-inflammatory agent if necessary. • Continue to monitor client.
Transdermal patch does not stay on skin.	• Cover with plastic wrap and/or tape in place.
Risk for eye infection because of break in aseptic technique.	• Medication dropper is contaminated. Discard dropper and obtain new one. • Review the recommended procedures for administering the medication, and have another nurse observe until skill of administering eye medications is perfected.
Irritation of eye occurs.	• Notify physician for new orders. • Obtain orders for sterile soaks to ease pain and discomfort.
Blink response (corneal protection) lost due to neurologic condition.	• Obtain order for artificial tears to protect cornea. Keep eyelid closed with tape.
While administering ear drops, client moves unexpectedly, causing medication to run down client's neck.	• Repeat explanation of procedure to client. • Readminister medication while holding client in the correct position. Keep client positioned on side for 15 minutes after instillation.

UNEXPECTED OUTCOMES	CRITICAL THINKING OPTIONS
Client complains ear medication is too warm.	• Check to ensure medication is heated only to 98.6°F. • Observe client for any untoward effects.
Client complains of nausea or vertigo following ear medication instillation.	• Warm medication to body temperature. Cold medication may cause these effects.
Client's earwax does not clear with ear irrigation.	• Inform client that ear impaction is usually self-induced by cleaning the ear improperly. • Teach client to clean only external opening of the ear with washcloth over index finger, and not to enter ear canal. • Consult with physician to order wax-softening eardrops to instill the night before irrigation.

UNIT 4

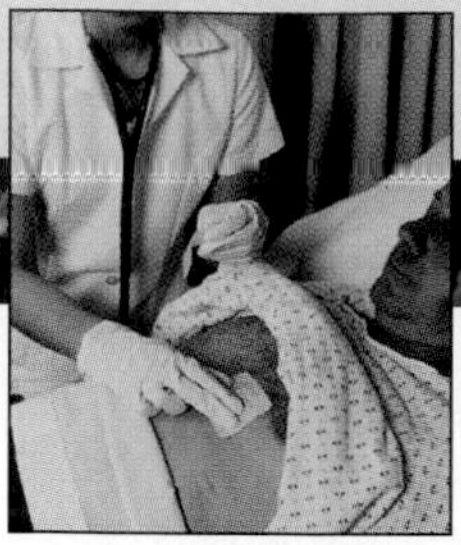

Mucous Membrane Medications

Nursing Process Data

ASSESSMENT Data Base

Assess that drug can be administered sublingually.

Assess client's ability to understand and follow directions.

Assess vital signs, SpO_2, relevant to medication action.

Assess for dyspnea, labored breathing, wheezing.

Determine possible undesired systemic effects of inhaled agents (tremor, nausea, tachycardia).

Review physician's orders for medication and diluent to be administered, and frequency of treatments.

Observe amount and character of expectorated sputum.

Determine need for other respiratory techniques.

Assess client's breath sounds before and after each treatment.

Assess client's bowel elimination pattern.

PLANNING Objectives

To provide appropriate surface for rapid absorption of medication for systemic effect

To confine drug action to a local area

To facilitate ease and consistency of self-administration of medication

To decrease client's work of breathing

To provide alternate route of medication administration when client is NPO/nauseated

To promote bowel elimination

To combat infection

To deliver aerosolized medications

To temporarily decrease the work of breathing

To promote better ventilation

To loosen secretions

IMPLEMENTATION Procedures

Administering Sublingual Medications

Instilling Nose Drops

Administering Metered-Dose Inhaled (MDI) Medications

Using MDI with Spacer

Administering Medication by Nonpressurized (Nebulized) Aerosol (NPA)

Administering Rectal Suppositories

Administering Vaginal Suppositories

EVALUATION Expected Outcomes

Chest pain is relieved due to rapid systemic response to sublingual medication administration.

Desired local effect of medication is achieved without undesired systemic effects.

Client's wheezing, shortness of breath, and work of breathing are reduced with inhaled medication.

Client's nausea/discomfort is relieved with suppository administration.
Nebulized medication delivered to small airways.
Client is able to expectorate secretions.
Client's breathing is eased and exercise capacity increased.
Breath sounds are improved.
Spirometry and SpO_2 are improved.

ADMINISTERING SUBLINGUAL MEDICATIONS

Equipment

Sublingual medication (e.g., nitroglycerin tablets in a dark bottle). *Tablets lose potency when exposed to light; opened bottle should be replaced in 3 months.*
or
Nitrolingual aerosol spray in canister

Preparation

1. *See* Preparing Medications, Unit 1.
2. Assess vital signs if administering sublingual nitroglycerine. (*Systolic BP should not be lower than 90 mm Hg*).
3. Place client in a sitting position.

Procedure

1. Follow steps for preparing and administering oral medications, *except:*
   a. Explain that client must not swallow drug or eat, smoke, or drink until medication is completely absorbed.
   b. Ask client to place tablet under the tongue or to hold tongue up so tablet can be placed under tongue. **Rationale:** Absorption is rapid and complete due to the vast network of capillaries in this area.
   c. Alternate: hold nitrolingual canister vertically with spray opening as close to mouth as possible. Deliver 1 or 2 metered sprays onto or under tongue, then have client close mouth immediately. Tell client not to inhale medication.
2. Evaluate client for drug action and possible side effects (e.g., headache).

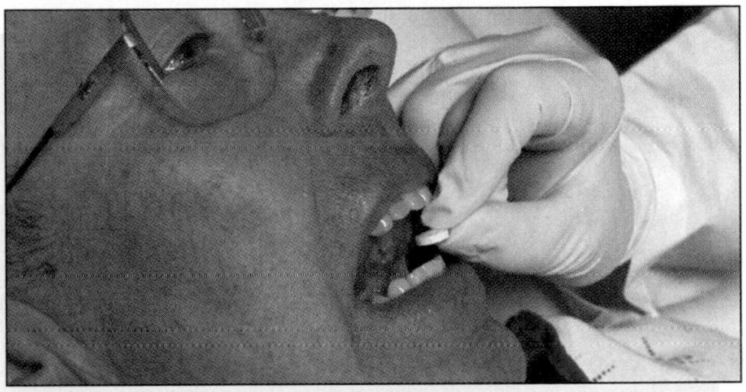
Sublingual medication is placed under client's tongue for rapid absorption.

CLINICAL ALERT

When administering rapid-acting (sublingual) nitroglycerin, monitor client's response closely and record. If chest discomfort is not relieved in 5 minutes, a repeat dose is indicated and physician should be notified. No more than 3 doses should be administered in a 15-minute period. Monitor client's BP for potential hypotensive effect and hold dose if systolic BP is less than 90 mm Hg.

INSTILLING NOSE DROPS

Equipment

Medication bottle
Dropper
Tissues

Preparation

1. *See* Preparing Medications, Unit 1.
2. Wash hands.

Procedure

1. Take equipment to client's room; check room and bed number against medication record.
2. Check client identaband and have client state name.
3. Place client in sitting position with head tilted back or in supine position with head tilted back over pillow.
4. Fill dropper with prescribed amount of medication.
5. Place dropper just inside the nares and instill correct medication dosage. Repeat procedure in other nares.
6. Wipe away any excess medication with tissue.
7. Instruct client not to sneeze or blow nose and to keep head tilted back for 5 minutes to prevent medication from escaping.
8. Check to see that client is comfortable before leaving room.
9. Wash hands.
10. Return medication to appropriate storage area.

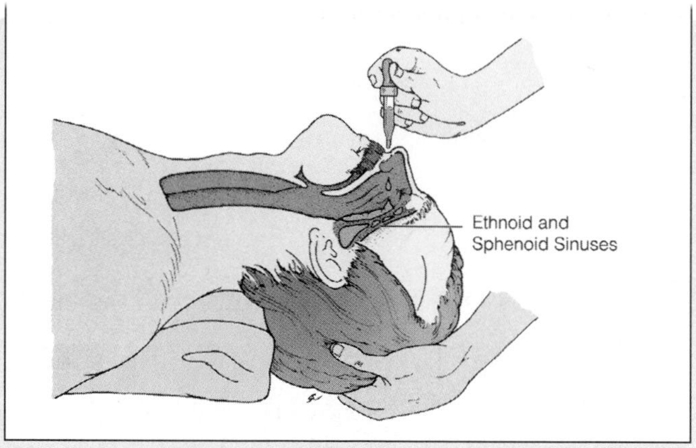

Instruct client to tilt head backwards and place dropper inside nares when instilling nose drops.

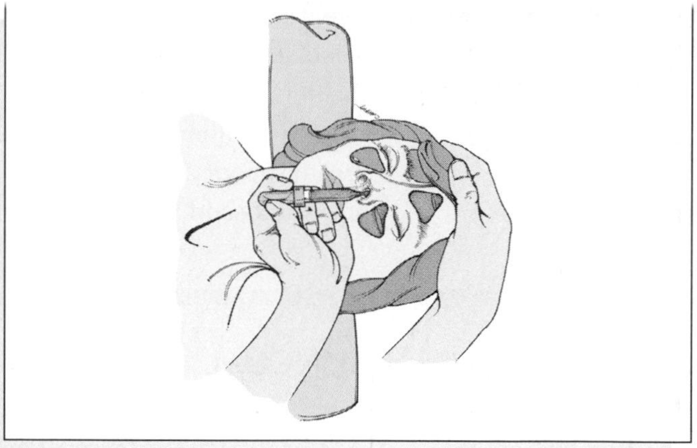

Tilt client's head back for nose drops to reach maxillary and frontal sinuses.

ADMINISTERING METERED-DOSE INHALED (MDI) MEDICATIONS

Equipment

Prescribed medication canister
Metered-dose inhaler (MDI) dispenser (actuator or holder)
Spacer or holding chamber (if ordered)
Tissues

Preparation

1. Compare medication record with physician's order.
2. Wash your hands.
3. Gather equipment.
4. Compare label of drug canister to client's medication record.

Procedure

1. Take medication canister and MDI dispenser to client's room.
2. Check client's identaband and have client state name.
3. Provide privacy.
4. Explain procedure and purpose to client.
5. Assist client to standing or sitting position.
6. Insert canister (stem down) into longer part of metered-dose dispenser. (For new canister, test spray [prime] MDI into air one or two times. **Rationale:** This is done *only* with new canister to ensure patency of unit.)
7. Shake MDI with canister to mix medication and propellant. (*Shake canister before each MDI puff*). **Rationale:** Without shaking propellant, little or no medication will be delivered.
8. Instruct client to remove mouthpiece and hold inhaler 2 inches away from mouth (following manufacturer's instructions). Mist is to be *inhaled* into airways. **Alternately,** place mouthpiece in mouth, holding cannister upright.

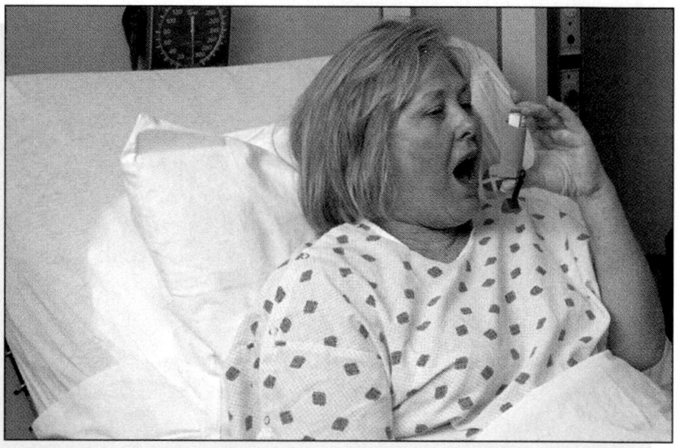

Depress inhalation device while inhaling slowly (3–5 seconds) and deeply through mouth.

9. Instruct client to exhale through pursed lips. **Rationale:** Exhaling through pursed lips increases exhaled volume, allowing room for a greater *inspiratory* volume.
10. Instruct client to depress inhalation device, releasing a puff of medication while inhaling slowly and deeply (3–5 seconds). **Rationale:** With slow deep inhalation, medication goes to lower respiratory tract.
11. Tell client to hold breath for 10 seconds, then remove unit and slowly exhale though pursed lips. **Rationale:** Holding the breath allows time for the medication to be absorbed.
12. Assess client's breathing and reaction to medication. **Rationale:** With certain drugs, heart rate may increase.
13. Provide tissues. **Rationale:** Inhaled medication may stimulate coughing.
14. Instruct client to wait one or two minutes between inhalations and to shake canister before each puff. **Rationale:** Waiting between doses helps prevent paroxysmal bronchospasm.

15. Have client replace mouthpiece cap.
16. Caution client not to increase dose without physician's order. **Rationale:** Potential side effects of an increased dose could be serious.
17. Have client rinse mouth after using MDI that contains steroids.
18. Teach client to remove canister and to clean mouthpiece *daily*, washing with soap and water and allowing to air dry. **Rationale:** These devices are sites for microbial growth.
19. Instruct client to rinse mouth after use and to not swallow the water.
20. Review medication side effects with client. **Rationale:** Client continues home therapy and should be aware of self-monitoring needs.
21. Wash hands.
22. Document procedure and results.

Inhaled Medications

- Inhaled medications provide relief for bronchospasm, wheezing, asthma, or allergic reactions.
- Medications include bronchodilators, steroids, and antimediators.
- Common systemic side effects include tremors, nausea, tachycardia, palpitations, nervousness, and dysrhythmias.

Client Teaching

- Canister must be shaken before each puff so that propellant and medication are adequately combined. Priming sprays are performed only with a new canister (canister volume allows for this).
- Prime new MDI by spraying into the air 4 times. Prime inhaler that has not been used for 4 weeks by spraying once into the air.
- Tell client to keep track of number of puffs used in order to plan for refill of prescription.

USING MDI WITH SPACER

Equipment

See Administering MDI Medications.

Preparation

1. *See* Administering MDI Medications.
2. Wash hands.

Procedure

1. Assemble medication canister in MDI.
2. Insert MDI mouthpiece into spacer. **Rationale:** Research indicates a MDI inhaler fitted into a spacer improves airway delivery of medication because large drops do not fall into the mouth.
3. Remove mouthpiece cover from spacer.
4. Hold upright and shake MDI with spacer to mix medication and propellant.
5. Instruct client to exhale slowly through pursed lips.
6. Instruct client to close lips around spacer mouthpiece. **Rationale:** Spacer eliminates need for simultaneous hand action and mouth inspiration coordination.
7. Activate MDI canister, pressing down with fingers, pushing it further into plastic adapter. **Rationale:** This releases metered dose of medication into spacer.

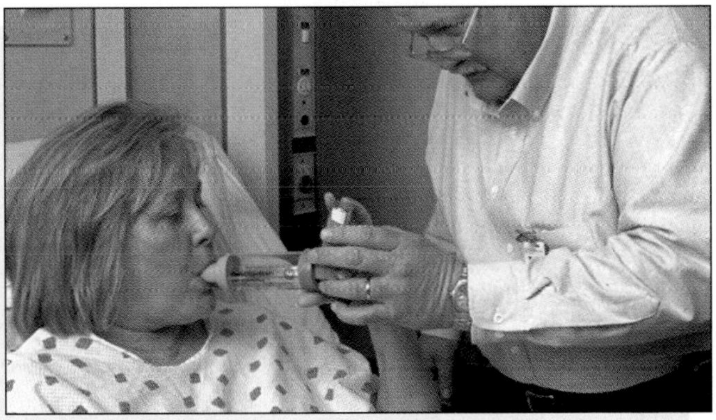

Hold canister upright when using MDI with spacer.

8. After activation, instruct client to inhale slowly and deeply through mouth and hold breath for 10 seconds.
9. Instruct client to exhale and relax.
10. Provide water mouth rinse following inhaled corticosteroids. **Rationale:** To prevent oral candidiasis.
11. Remove drug canister and clean mouthpiece and spacer daily, washing with soap and water.

CLINICAL ALERT

If several types of medications are used, follow this sequence: Quick-acting bronchodilator (e.g., albuterol sulfate); slower-acting bronchodilator (e.g., ipratropium bromide [Atro-vent]); antimediators (e.g., steroids).

CLINICAL ALERT

Several medications are available as *dry powder inhalers* (DPIs). These contain no propellant, and spacers are not used. DPIs are administered with the client's neck hyperextended. The client's lips are placed around the mouthpiece of the dispenser, and inspiration is quick and deep. Dry powder delivery is actuated by a *fast inhalation.*

EVIDENCE BASED NURSING PRACTICE

Why Use a Spacer with MDI?

Only 10–15% of inhaled (MDI) medications reach the small airways, but use of a spacer can increase this by about 12%.

Source: Togger, D., & Brenner, P. (2001). Metered dose inhalers. *American Journal of Nursing, 101*(10), 29.

ADMINISTERING MEDICATION BY NONPRESSURIZED (NEBULIZED) AEROSOL (NPA)

Equipment

Nebulizer medication chamber
T-piece, mouthpiece or mask
Corrugated tubing
Air flow tubing
Prescribed medication (e.g., bronchodilator)
Prescribed diluent (normal saline)
Wall source (or other source) for compressed air, or oxygen with flowmeter

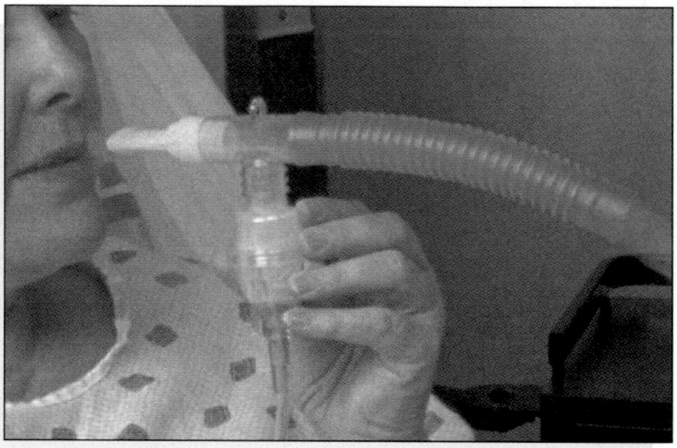

Nonpressurized aerosol (NPA) treatment in progress.

Preparation

1. Wash hands.
2. Dilute medication as ordered and place in nebulizer chamber.
3. Attach one end of tubing to compressed air source.
4. Attach other end of tubing to nozzle at side or bottom of nebulizer.
5. Keep nebulizer chamber vertical, and connect top of chamber to mask or T-piece sidearm.
6. Hold mouthpiece in its protective cover, and attach to one end of T-piece.
7. Attach corrugated tubing to other end of T-piece.

Procedure

1. Turn on air or oxygen (8 L/min) source, and observe for mist flow.
   a. If the client is receiving 3 L/min or less of oxygen therapy, deliver aerosolized medications with compressed air (yellow wall outlet).
   b. If the client is receiving 4 L/min or more of oxygen therapy, deliver the aerosol medication with the oxygen flowmeter (green wall outlet) set at 8 L/min.
2. Have client place mouthpiece in mouth and close lips.
3. Instruct client to breathe normally in and out of mouthpiece or mask.
4. Have client take a deep breath and hold for several seconds, then exhale slowly every 3–5 breaths. (Treatment is complete when all medication is used and no mist is seen.)
5. Turn power (air or O_2 flow) off, and unplug compressor (if used), or reset prescribed O_2 flow rate.
6. Clean mouthpiece, and place equipment in plastic bag at bedside. (Dispose of and replace components according to agency policy.)

ADMINISTERING RECTAL SUPPOSITORIES

Equipment

Suppository as ordered from refrigerator
Clean gloves
Water-soluble Lubricant (K-Y jelly)
Paper towel

Preparation

1. *See* Preparing Medications, Unit 1.
2. Compare the medication record with the most recent physician's order.

3. Wash your hands.
4. Gather necessary equipment.
5. Retrieve medication from refrigerator.
6. Compare the medication label with client's MAR.
7. Place suppository, lubricant, and paper towel on a tray if not using medication cart.
8. Check drug information to determine side effects to observe for following insertion.

Procedure

1. Take equipment to client's room.
2. Check room number against client's MAR.
3. Check client's identaband and have client state name.
4. Explain procedure and purpose to client.
5. Provide privacy.
6. Place client in Sims' (left lateral) position.
7. Squeeze dollop of lubricant onto paper towel.
8. Remove foil wrapper from the suppository.
9. Moisten suppository tip with warm water or lubricant to facilitate insertion.
10. Don clean gloves and inspect anal area for hemorrhoids.
11. Instruct client to bear down to identify anal opening and insert the suppository about 1½ inches into the rectal canal beyond the anal sphincter. **Rationale:** Prevents suppository from slipping out.

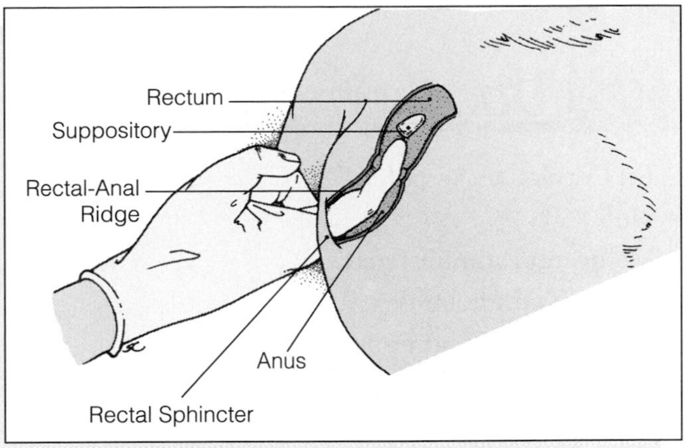

Insert rectal suppository beyond the anal–rectal ridge to ensure it is retained.

12. Instruct client to lie quietly for 15 minutes while medicine is absorbed, and that suppository may take up to one hour to be effective.
13. Dispose of equipment and gloves and wash your hands.
14. Return after 15 minutes to ensure client is comfortable.
15. Chart medication and results obtained.

ADMINISTERING VAGINAL SUPPOSITORIES

Equipment

Prescribed vaginal suppository
Client's applicator (should be kept in client's room)
Clean gloves

Preparation

1. *See* Preparing Medications, Unit 1.
2. Compare the medication record with the most recent physician's order.
3. Wash your hands.
4. Gather necessary equipment.
5. Remove the medication from medication cart.
6. Compare the medication label to the client's MAR.

Procedure

1. Take equipment to client's room, and check room number against client's MAR.
2. Check client's identaband and ask client to state name.
3. Provide privacy.
4. Explain procedure and purpose to client.
5. Don gloves.
6. Place client in dorsal recumbent or Sims' position.
7. Remove foil wrapper from suppository. Insert into applicator.
8. Don clean gloves.

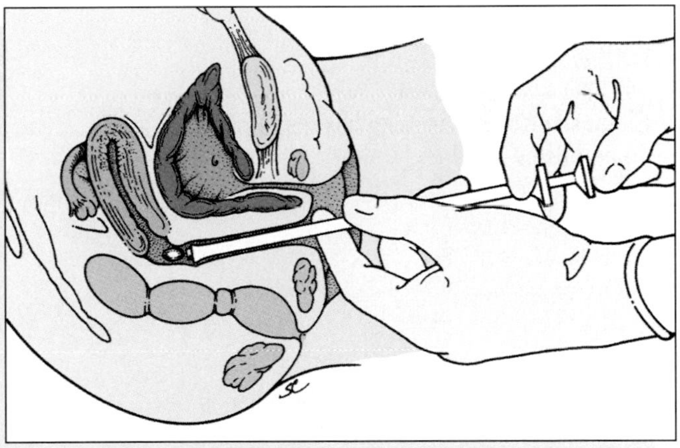
Insert vaginal suppository at least two inches into vaginal canal using applicator as shown.

9. Insert applicator with suppository into the vaginal canal at least 2 inches. **Rationale:** Prevents suppository from slipping out.
10. Instruct client to lie quietly for 15 minutes until the suppository is absorbed.
11. Discard equipment, wash applicator, and return to appropriate place in client's room.
12. Remove gloves and wash your hands.
13. Chart medication and assessment findings (e.g., discharge, odor).

DOCUMENTATION FOR MUCOUS MEMBRANE MEDICATIONS

Client's Medication Record

- Time
- Medication administered
- Route of administration
- Initials of nurse administering medication
- Signature of nurse identifying initials

Nurses' Notes

- Time
- Name of medication, dosage, route pre *and* post administration assessment findings (chest discomfort, vital signs, SpO_2, breath sounds)
- Physician notification, if done
- Results of suppository action

Critical Thinking Application

UNEXPECTED OUTCOMES	CRITICAL THINKING OPTIONS
Client's discomfort is not relieved with sublingual nitroglycerin.	• Check bottle for expiration date—potency is lost 3 months after opening bottle. • Administer second tablet in 5 minutes—if discomfort continues, notify physician and obtain stat ECG. • Administer no more than 3 tablets/sprays in a 15 minute period. • Monitor for blood pressure effect—hold medication if systolic BP is less than 90 mm Hg. • Consult with physician for blood test for possible myocardial injury and need for continuous cardiac monitoring.
Client states that breathing has not improved after using inhaler.	• Place client in Fowler's position. Validate that MDI/spacer/NPA device is functioning properly (e.g., canister shaken before use). • Check number of doses left in MDI canister (*see box*). • Validate that client's lips have tight fit around MDI mouthpiece so mist is inhaled. • Instruct client to hold breath 10 seconds after MDI use and to wait 2 minutes between puffs.
Client using MDI reports painful white patches in mouth.	• Instruct client to use spacer with MDI steroid medication. • Instruct client to rinse mouth with water and expectorate after administering MDI steroid. • Notify physician of findings.
Client fails to have BM post laxative suppository administration.	• Reassess abdomen and check client for rectal fecal impaction. • Consult with physician to order oil-retention enema or cleansing enema. • Teach client ways to prevent constipation.
Client is unable to retain vaginal suppository.	• Administer vaginal suppository at bedtime to prevent medication leakage.

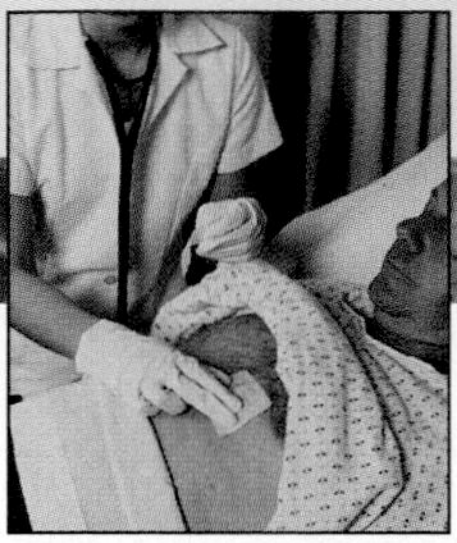

UNIT 5

Parenteral Administration

Nursing Process Data

ASSESSMENT *Data Base*

Check that appropriate method for administration of drug was ordered.

Assess condition of administration site for presence of lesions, rash, inflammation, lipid dystrophy, ecchymosis.

Assess client's understanding of medication action.

Check client's written history and ask for oral history for past allergic reactions. (Do not rely solely on client's chart.)

Review client's chart noting previous injection sites, especially insulin and heparin administration sites.

PLANNING *Objectives*

To ensure proper route of drug administration

To protect self from harm when administering parenteral injections

To administer medication parenterally according to the "Five Rights"

To reduce discomfort with medication injection

To alternate injection sites for consistent absorption of medication

To observe and report side effects/adverse effects of drug administration

IMPLEMENTATION *Procedures*

Preparing Injections

for Withdrawing Medication from a Vial

Administering Intradermal Injections

Administering Subcutaneous (Sub Q) Injections

Preparing Insulin Injections

for One Insulin Solution

for Two Insulin Solutions

Teaching Use of Insulin Pump

Administering Subcutaneous (Sub Q) Heparin/LMWH

Administering Intramuscular (IM) Injections

Using Z-Track Method

EVALUATION *Expected Outcomes*

Injection is completed without technical complications.

Needlestick injury does not occur.

Injection is as painless as possible.

Medication therapeutic effect is achieved.

Injection sites remain without lesions.

PREPARING INJECTIONS

Equipment

Medication in vial or ampule
Vial of compatible diluent (if necessary)
Syringe of closest capacity to hold medication with appropriate-size needle and integrated safety feature
Antimicrobial wipes

Procedure

1. Wash your hands.
2. Obtain equipment for injections.
3. Select the appropriate size needle, considering route, desired site, client's size and viscosity of medication. **Rationale:** The larger the gauge number, the *smaller* the needle lumen. Larger gauges produce less tissue trauma and are used for aqueous solutions. Smaller gauges are required for viscous solutions such as hormones.
4. Assemble the syringe and needle, maintaining sterility.
5. Fill syringe with medication or proceed to subsequent skills.

CLINICAL ALERT

Federal needlestick safety legislation **requires** health care facilities to implement devices that protect against accidental needlesticks.

for Withdrawing Medication from a Vial

1. Remove the vial cap.
2. Open antimicrobial wipe, and cleanse the rubber top of the vial. **Rationale:** Manufacturer does not guarantee sterility of rubber top.
3. Tighten needle to syringe. Remove needle guard.
4. Pull back on plunger to fill syringe with an amount of air equal to amount of solution to be withdrawn. **Rationale:** The displacement of solution with air is necessary to prevent the formation of a vacuum in the sealed vial.

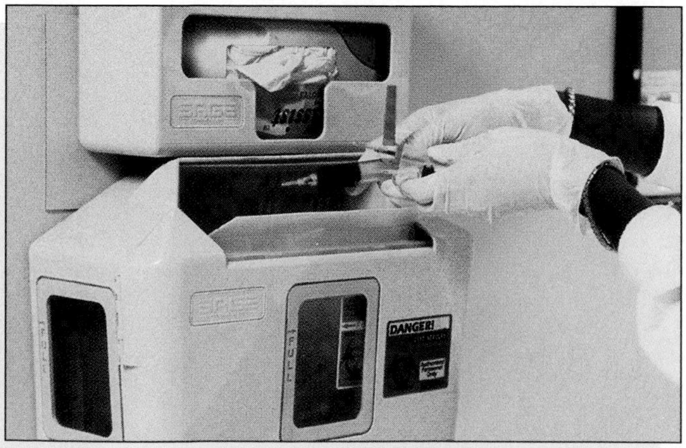

Discard syringe following injection in biohazard container.

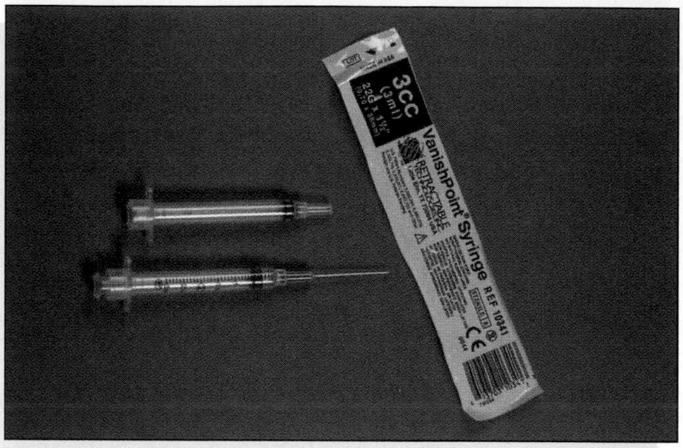

Health care facilities must use safety needles to conform to needlestick safety legislation.

EVIDENCE BASED NURSING PRACTICE

Needlestick Injuries

Six percent of needlestick injuries involve safety devices with shielding, retracting, or blunting safety features. Most injuries occur after use and before disposal. In some cases, the protective features are not activated. Puncture-proof sharps disposal containers continue to play an important role in preventing injury.

Source: Jagger, J., Perry, J. (2002). Realistic Expectations for Safety Devices, *Nursing 2002, 32*(3), 72.

CLINICAL ALERT

When injecting a medication that is irritating to the tissues (e.g., Vistaril), change needle before administering intramuscular injection to the client.

Selecting the Appropriate-Size Needle

- *Intradermal injections:* 1 mL tuberculin syringe with short bevel, 25–27 gauge, $\frac{3}{8}$–$\frac{1}{2}$ inch needle.
- *Subcutaneous injections:* 0.5–3 mL syringe with 25–29 gauge, $\frac{3}{8}$–$\frac{5}{8}$ inch needle.
- *Intramuscular injections:* 1–5 mL syringe with needle gauge and length appropriate for muscle site; deltoid muscle requires 23–25 gauge, $\frac{5}{8}$–1 inch needle; needle sizes for the vastus lateralis and gluteus muscles vary from 18 to 23 gauge, needle lengths, 1–1$\frac{1}{2}$ inch.

Types of Injections

Intradermal Injections

- Injection sites: inner aspect of forearm or scapular area of back; upper chest, medial thigh.
- Purpose: to test for antigens (tubercle bacillus, allergens).
- Amount injected: ranges from 0.01 to 0.1 mL.
- Absorption rate: slow.

Subcutaneous Injections

- Injection sites: fatty tissue of abdomen, lateral and posterior aspects of upper arm or thigh, scapular area of back, upper ventrodorsal gluteal areas.
- Purpose: for medications that are absorbed slowly.
- Amount injected: variable—small amount of fluid, no more than 2 mL. If repeated doses are necessary, alter site accordingly.

Intramuscular Injections

- Purpose: to promote rapid absorption of the drug; to provide an alternate route when drug is irritating to subcutaneous tissues.
- Amount injected: variable—may be large amount of fluid. If more than 5 mL for adult or 3 mL for child and 1 mL for infant, divide dose into two syringes.
- Absorption rate: depends on circulatory state of client.
- Injection sites:

Ventrogluteal Injection Site (preferred site for IM injection)

Place client in side-lying position.

Use right hand for left anterior hip, or left hand for right anterior hip.

Identify greater trochanter and place palm at site.

Keep palm on greater trochanter and point index finger toward client's anterior superior iliac spine and fan out other 3 fingers.

Form "V" area with index finger separated from other 3 fingers.

Inject medication at 90° angle within "V" area.

Dorsogluteal Injection Site (least desirable for IM injection)

Place client in prone position.

Identify greater trochanter by placing hand on site.

Identify postero-superior spine (prominence) of iliac crest.

Draw imaginary line between trochanter and posterior superior iliac spine.

Locate injection site above imaginary line drawn between these 2 boney landmarks (this site will help to prevent injury to sciatic nerve).

Inject medication with long needle into dorsogluteal site at 90° angle.

Vastus Lateralis Injection Site

Place client in supine position with thigh available.

Identify greater trochanter and lateral femoral condyle.

Using middle third and anterior lateral aspect of thigh, select site.

Inject medication directly into muscle at 90° angle.

Deltoid Injection Site (solution must be nonirritating)

Expose client's upper arm.

Deltoid site is two fingerbreadths below acromion process.

Place left hand on acromion process and right index finger two fingerbreadths below.

Inject limited medication volume (0.5 to 1 mL) in deltoid IM site at 90° angle.

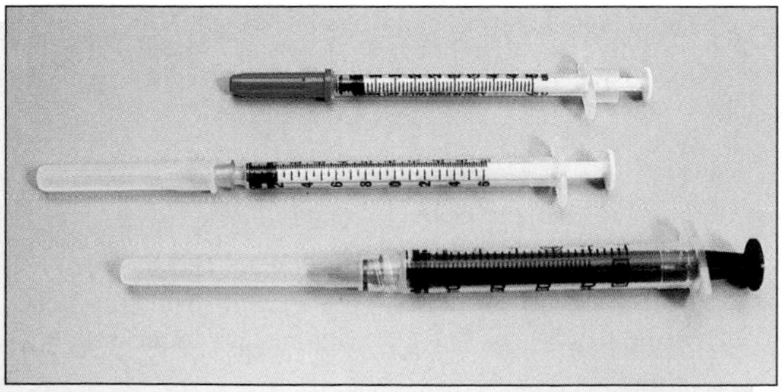

Three types of syringes: tuberculin, insulin, and 3-mL.

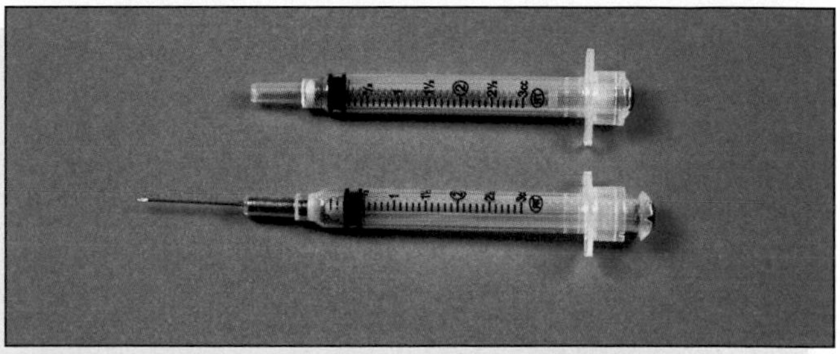

Safety syringe with retractable needle (below) and needle retracted into barrel (above).

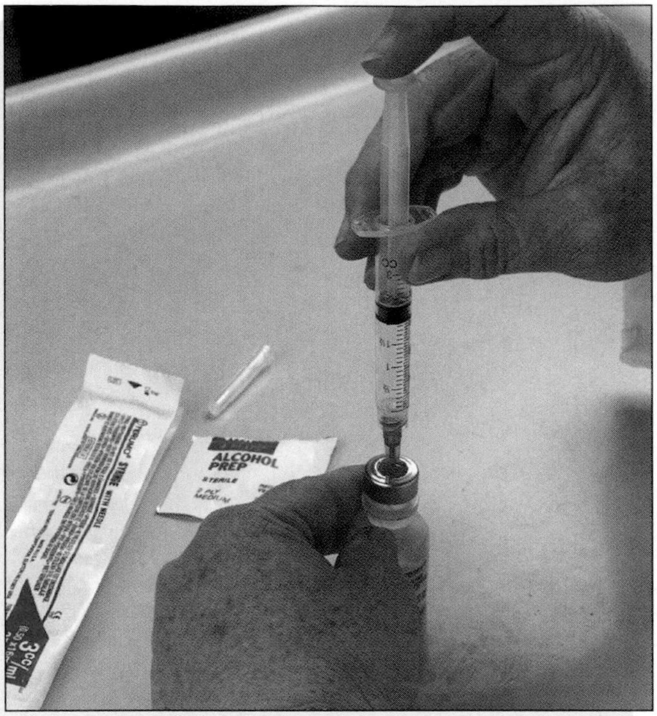

Insert needle into upright vial and inject air into vacant area, keeping needle above surface of medication.

5. Insert needle into upright vial. Inject air into vacant area of vial keeping needle bevel above surface of medication. **Rationale:** Air creates positive pressure within vial allowing accurate withdrawal of medication.
6. Invert vial, and pull plunger to extract desired amount of medication. Touch only syringe barrel and plunger tip. **Rationale:** This prevents contamination of the plunger, inside of barrel, and medication.
7. Expel any air bubbles from syringe at this time by tapping the side of syringe sharply with your finger or pen below the air bubble. **Rationale:** Air bubbles form in syringe due to dead air space in needle hub. Removing air bubbles while needle remains within the inverted vial avoids accidental contamination of needle and facilitates easy removal of air and accurate withdrawal of solution.

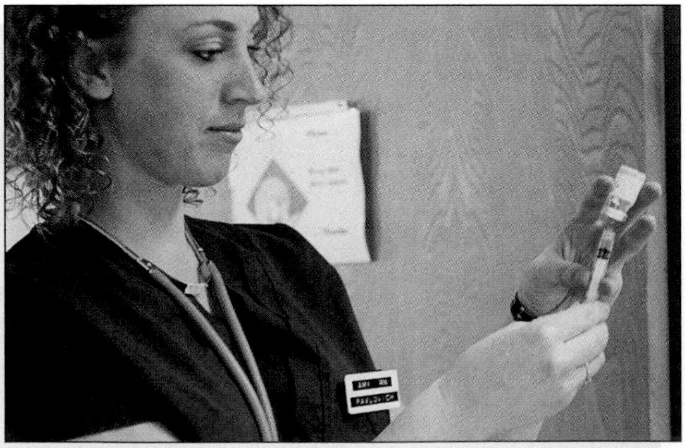

Invert vial to extract desired amount of medication.

CLINICAL ALERT

If multiple-use vials are opened, they should be marked with the date and time the container is entered and nurse's initials. Consult the product label or package insert to determine if refrigeration is necessary. Unless contamination is suspected, the Centers for Disease Control and Prevention (CDC) recommends that the vial be discarded either when empty or on the expiration date set by the manufacturer.

8. Recheck amount of medication in syringe.
9. Turn vial to upright position and remove needle. **Rationale:** Removing needle from inverted vial may cause leaking of medication from needle insertion site.
10. Replace needle guard using scoop method.
11. Recheck medication label and dosage against medication record and any dosage calculation. **Rationale:** This is a second safety check.
12. Replace or dispose of medication vial, checking label once again. **Rationale:** This is a third safety check.

for Combining Medications in One Syringe Using Two Vials

1. Prepare both vials by removing caps and cleansing tops with separate antimicrobial wipes.

CLINICAL ALERT

Check appropriate text or consult agency pharmacist to ensure compatibility of medications before combining in a syringe for injection.

2. Draw air into syringe equal to amount of solution to be removed from *second* vial. Inject air into *second* vial. Do not withdraw medication at this time. **Rationale:** Air creates positive pressure within the vial allowing withdrawal of solution.

Reconstituting Powdered Medication

- Insert needle into upright powdered medication vial.
- Remove the amount of air equal to desired quantity of diluent; this provides space for the diluent.
- Inject diluent into upright powdered medication vial.
- Remove needle and cover with guard.
- Rotate powdered medication vial with diluent between palms. Do not shake vial because shaking creates air bubbles and may cause difficulty withdrawing medication dose.
- Withdraw medication from vial.

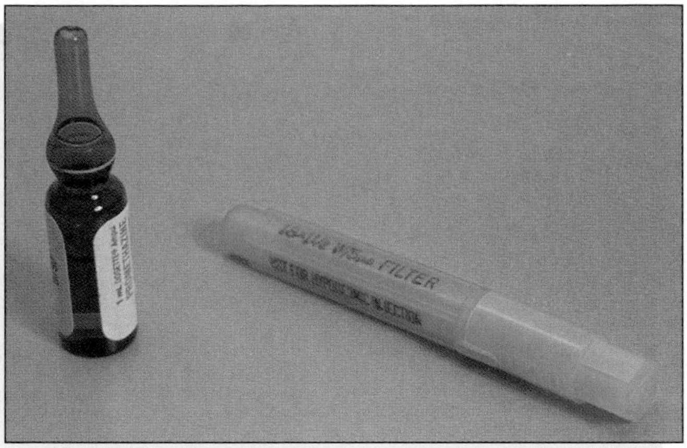

A special filler needle may be used to prevent aspirating glass when withdrawing solution from an ampule.

3. Draw air into syringe equal to amount of solution to be removed from *first* vial and inject it into *first* vial.
4. Invert first vial and withdraw ordered amount of medication without removing syringe.
5. Expel all air bubbles from syringe.
6. Recheck amount of solution and remove syringe from vial.
7. Insert needle into *second* vial, invert, and carefully withdraw exact amount of solution ordered. **Rationale:** Withdrawing excess solution from second vial results in an inaccurate dosage of medication. If this occurs, syringe must be discarded and procedure begun again.

for Withdrawing Medication from an Ampule

1. Move solution from neck to body of ampule by tapping stem sharply or holding neck of ampule between thumb and forefinger and flicking wrist.

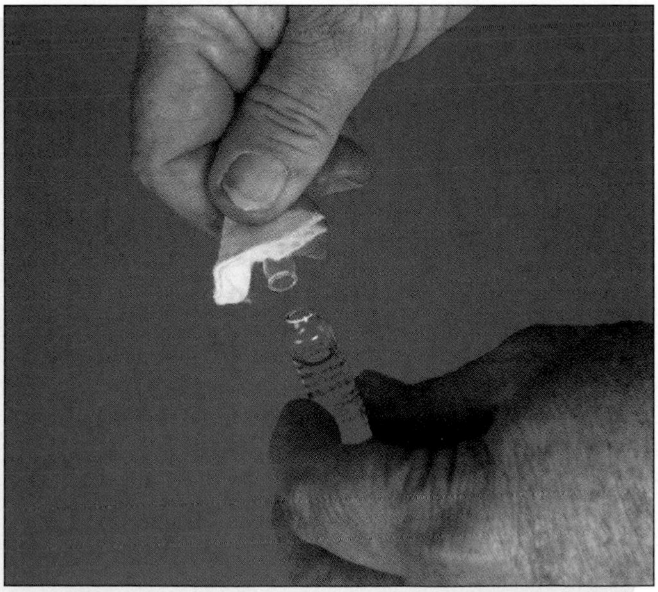

Using alcohol swab or dry gauze square, grasp and snap off stem of ampule, breaking away from you.

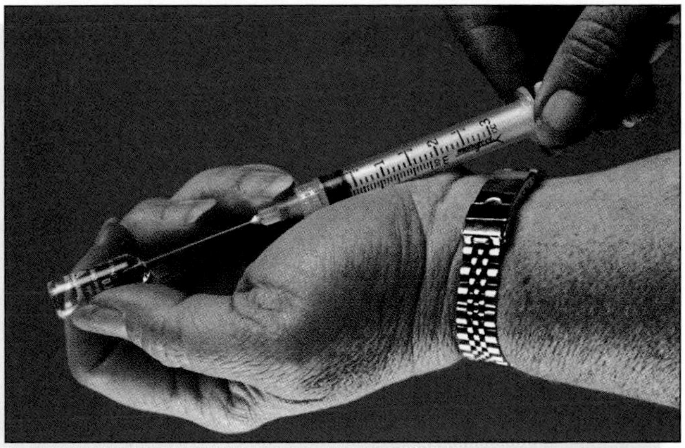

Tilt or invert ampule to withdraw appropriate amount of medication.

2. Grasp top (stem) of ampule between thumb and forefinger of one hand and grasp body of ampule with other hand. Using a pad, break stem away from you. (If ampule is not scored, partially file neck of ampule). **Rationale.** Gauze pad protects hands and breaking away from you prevents injury from glass fragments.
3. Set the ampule upright. It is not necessary to add air prior to withdrawing the medication.
4. Use a special filter needle to withdraw solution, if indicated. **Rationale:** Filter needle prevents aspiration of glass when withdrawing solution from ampule.
5. Remove needle guard and insert needle into ampule without touching sides of ampule. If needle is sufficiently long, medication may be withdrawn with ampule in upright position. When a short needle is used, invert ampule and withdraw appropriate amount of medication. **Rationale:** Surface tension prevents solution from leaking out of inverted ampule.
6. Return ampule to upright position and withdraw needle.
7. Tap syringe barrel below bubbles to dislodge air bubbles to hub of syringe.
8. Eject air with syringe in an upright position. If amount of solution is overdrawn, invert syringe and remove excess solution into a nearby receptacle.
9. Cover needle with guard, using scoop method.

for Combining Medications Using Alternative Method

1. Draw up ordered dose from each vial or ampule into two separate syringes. First syringe must be able to hold entire volume of combined medications.
2. Remove needle from first syringe.
3. Pull back plunger of first syringe to allow space for volume of second medication to be added.
4. Insert needle of second syringe into hub of first syringe.
5. Slowly inject medication of second syringe into first syringe hub, then withdraw needle.
6. Attach new needle to first syringe.
7. Discard needles and second syringe.

for Preparing Prefilled Medication Cartridge Syringe

1. Hold barrel of cartridge syringe (e.g., Tubex) in one hand and pull back on plunger with other hand.
2. Insert prefilled medication cartridge, needle first, into cartridge barrel.
3. Twist cartridge syringe flange clockwise until it is secure.
4. Screw plunger rod onto screw at bottom of medication cartridge until it fits firmly and tightly into rubber stopper.
5. Remove needle guard and any air bubbles.
6. Determine if dosage in cartridge is greater than required amount. If so, invert Tubex and gently expel excess medication, being careful to maintain sterility of needle. **Rationale:** If permanent needle is contaminated, the cartridge becomes contaminated and must be discarded.
7. Replace needle guard, using scoop method.

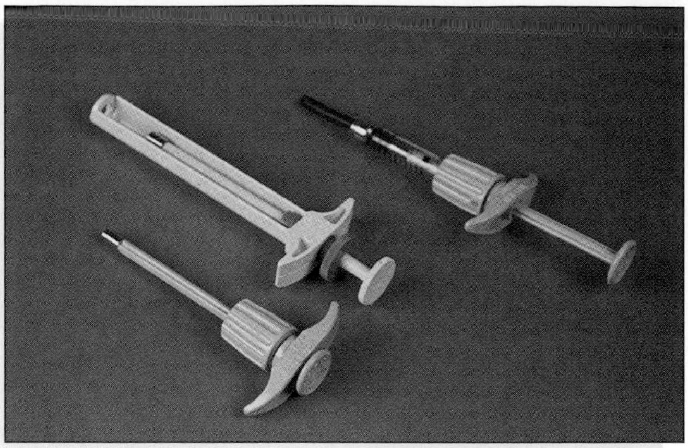

Prefilled medication cartridge and cartridge syringes.

ADMINISTERING INTRADERMAL INJECTIONS

Equipment

Medication (e.g., 0.1 mL Purified Protein Derivative Antigen for tuberculin testing)

Unit dose (1 mL) tuberculin syringe with ¼–⅜″ 27-gauge needle

Antimicrobial wipes

Gauze pads

Clean gloves

Pen to mark injection site

Preparation

Follow steps for Preparing Injections.

Procedure

1. Take prepared injection to client's room, checking room and bed number against client's medication record.
2. Check client's identaband and ask client to state name.
3. Explain procedure and purpose to client.
4. Wash hands and don gloves.
5. Select lesion-free injection site on undersurface, upper third of forearm for skin testing.
6. Cleanse area with antimicrobial wipe, using circular motion outward from site and allow to dry.
7. Remove needle guard.
8. Grasp the client's dorsal forearm to gently pull the skin taut on ventral forearm.
9. Holding syringe almost parallel to skin, insert needle at a 10°–15° angle with bevel facing up, about 1/8 inch. Needle point should be visible under skin. DO NOT ASPIRATE.
10. Inject medication slowly, observing for a wheal (blister) formation and blanching at the site. **Rationale:** This indicates that the medication was injected within the dermis. If no wheal develops, injection was given too deeply.
11. Withdraw needle at same angle as inserted. Pat area gently with dry gauze pad but DO NOT MASSAGE. **Rationale:** Massaging could disperse medication.
12. Activate needle safety feature and discard syringe unit in puncture proof container.
13. Mark injection site with pen for future assessment.
14. Return client to comfortable position.
15. Dispose of gloves and wash hands.
16. Record site and antigen in client's record.

CLINICAL ALERT

For tuberculin testing, instruct client to return and have the site checked by the health care provider in 48 to 72 hours.

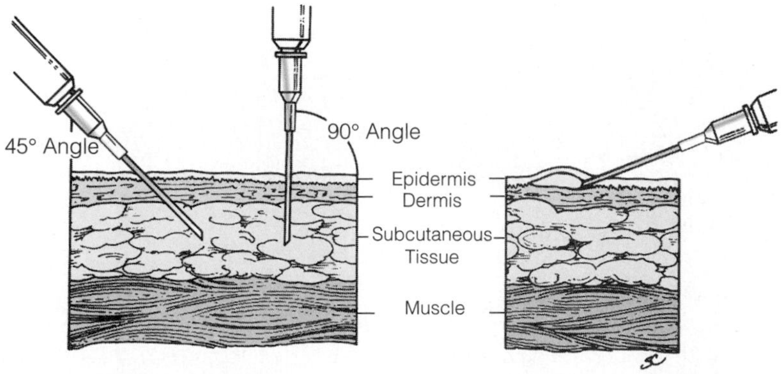

Insert needle at 45° or 90° angle into tissue for subcutaneous injection.

Insert needle at 15° angle just under the epidermis for intradermal injection.

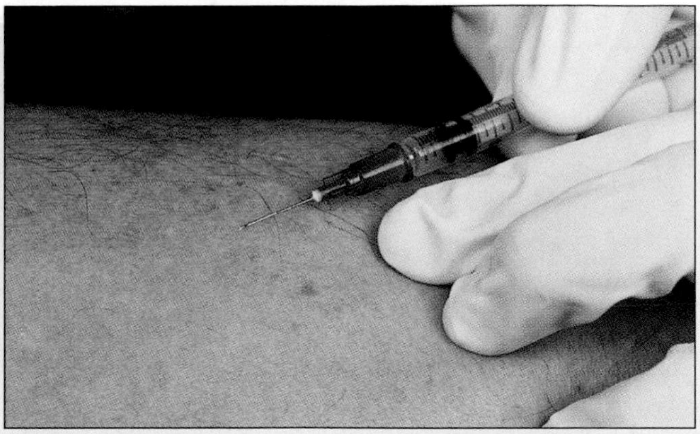

Insert needle with bevel up for intradermal injection.

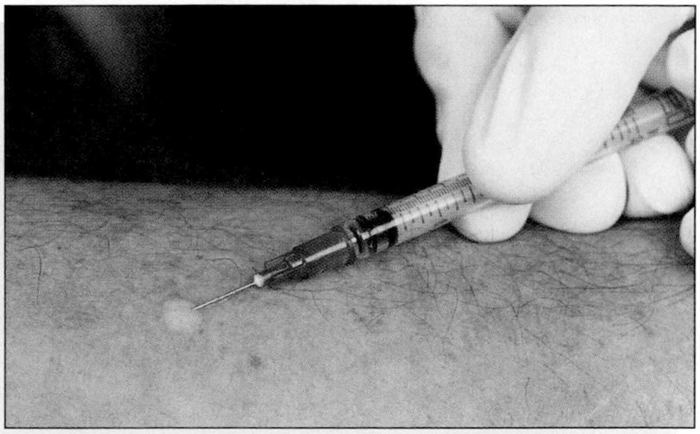

Inject solution to form wheal on skin.

ADMINISTERING SUBCUTANEOUS (SUB Q) INJECTIONS

Equipment

Nonirritating medication
3-mL syringe with 5/8-inch needle (usual 25–27 gauge)
Antimicrobial wipes
Clean gloves

CLINICAL ALERT

Irritating medications such as Vistaril must not be administered subcutaneously, as a sterile abscess or tissue necrosis may result. Such medications should be administered by another route.

Preparation

See steps for Preparing Injections.

Procedure

1. Take prepared injection to client's room, checking room and bed number against client's medication record.
2. Check client's identaband and ask client to state name.
3. Explain procedure and purpose to client.
4. Wash hands and don gloves.
5. Select fatty site for injection (e.g., abdomen, avoiding 2 inch radius around umbilicus, alternating sites for each injection. **Rationale:** This prevents repeated trauma to tissue.
6. Cleanse area with antimicrobial wipe, using circular motion from inside outward. **Rationale:** This action supports the principle of moving from clean to dirty area.
7. Remove needle guard.
8. Use thumb and forefinger and gently grasp loose area ("pinch an inch") of fatty tissue on appropriate site (e.g., posterior-lateral aspect, middle third of arm.) **Rationale:** This ensures insertion of medication within subcutaneous tissue, not muscle.

   Note: Spreading the skin is acceptable when there is substantial fatty tissue.

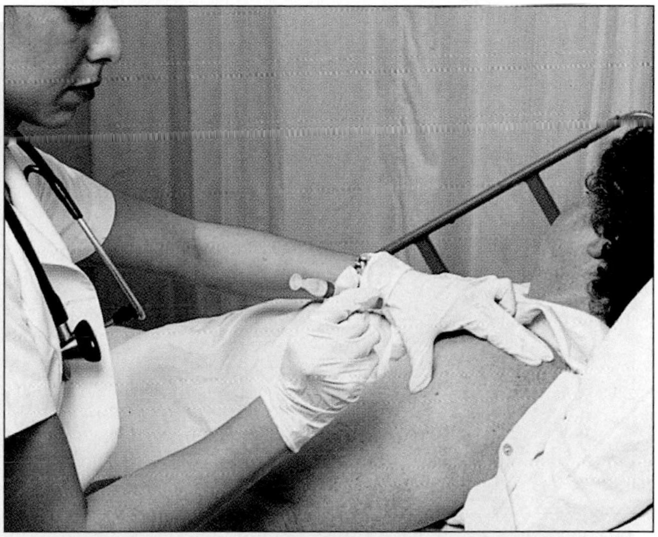

The upper arm can be used for both IM and Sub Q injections.

9. Hold syringe like a dart between the thumb and forefinger.
10. Insert needle at a 45° or 90° angle. A 90° angle is used more commonly due to short needles on prepackaged syringes. **Rationale:** Angle varies with the amount of subcutaneous tissue, selected site and needle length.
11. Continue to hold tissue and aspirate by pulling back on plunger with thumb of dominant hand. If no blood appears, administer injection. If blood appears, withdraw needle, activate safety feature and discard, then prepare a new injection. **Rationale:** Blood indicates needle has entered a blood vessel. Injecting the drug IV may be dangerous.
12. Inject medication slowly.
13. Wait 10 seconds, then withdraw needle quickly and activate needle safety feature.
14. Release tissue and massage area with swab (if indicated). **Rationale:** Massaging area aids absorption.
15. Discard needle/syringe unit in puncture-proof container.
16. Return client to position of comfort.
17. Discard gloves and wash your hands.
18. Record medication and site used.

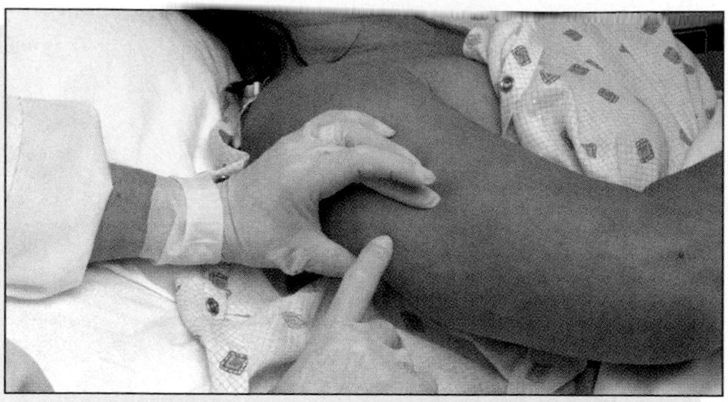

Select site on lateral aspect of mid-upper arm.

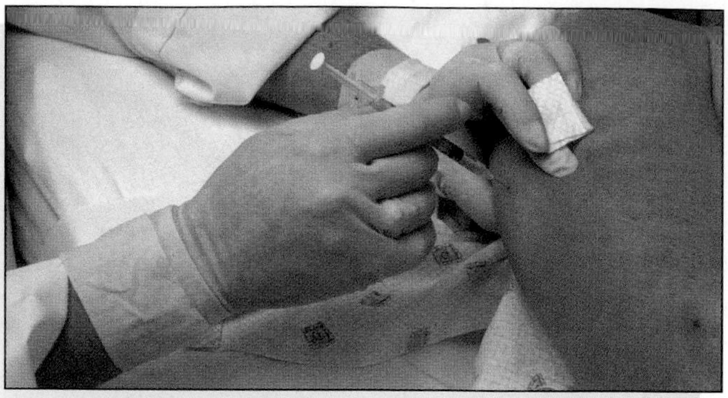

Insert needle at 45 or 90° angle, using short needle for Sub Q.

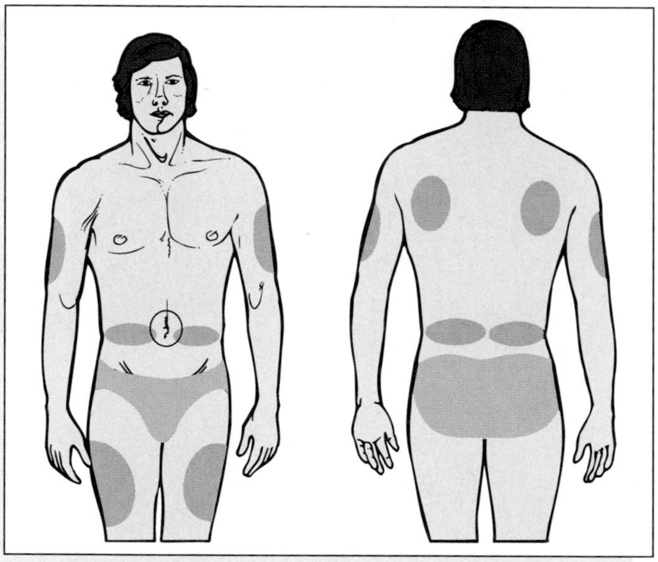

Sites for subcutaneous injections given routinely. (Avoid umbilicus area.) Abdomen site preferred.

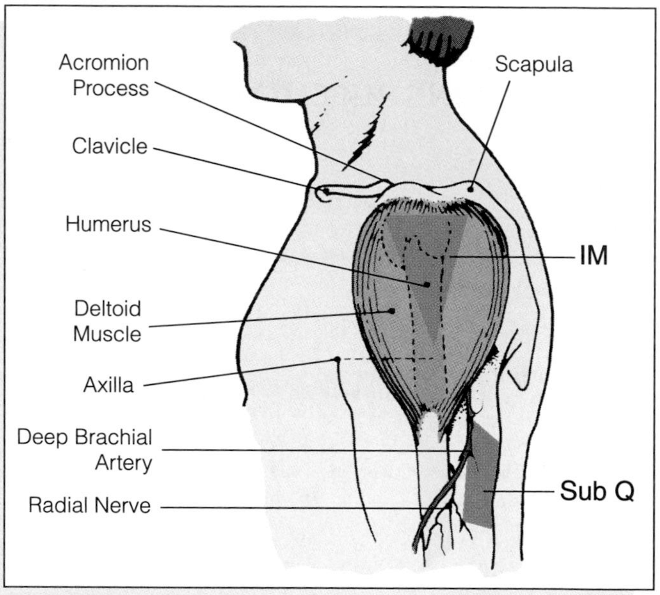

IM injection in upper arm. Lower shaded area for Sub Q injection.

PREPARING INSULIN INJECTIONS

Equipment

Insulin(s) vials

Unopened vials of insulin should be stored in refrigerator unless it is Lantus, or completely used in 28 days.

Opened vial of insulin should be kept at room temperature and should be discarded after 28 days

Temperature extremes will cause loss of potency

Do not use insulin that has clumping, frosting, or precipitation

Insulin syringe: 100 units (100)/1 mL, U30 and U50 syringes are available with 27–29-gauge needle

Antimicrobial swabs

Clean gloves

Preparation

1. *Follow steps for Preparing Injections.*
2. Obtain client's blood glucose level *prior to preparation* to determine appropriate administration of insulin. *See* Chapter 20 (Specimen Collection) for finger stick blood.

for Newly Diagnosed Diabetic Client

a. Explain to client that the dose of insulin must be adjusted according to blood glucose test results.
b. Explain that there is a variation in levels—the lowest blood glucose level is before meals and highest 1–2 hours after meals.
c. Goal of treatment is to eliminate wide swings in glucose levels.

CLINICAL ALERT

Hypoglycemia (blood sugar <70) is the most common adverse effect of insulins. Client should wear Med-Alert bracelet/ID to alert others. The client should be instructed to carry at least 15 g fast-acting sugar (e.g., glucose tablet, 1 T sugar, jelly, honey, or canned cake frosting) to be taken in the event of a hypoglycemic reaction.

3. Check latest insulin order and rotation chart for injection sites.

Procedure

1. Wash your hands.
2. Rotate intermediate or long-acting (cloudy) insulin vial gently in your hands. **Rationale:** This brings cloudy insulin solution into suspension. Clear insulins do not require this.
3. Wipe top of insulin bottle with antimicrobial swab.
4. Remove needle guard and place on tray.
5. Pull plunger of syringe down to desired amount of medication (e.g., 12 units). Inject amount of air into air space, not into insulin solution. **Rationale:** Injecting air directly into insulin solution causes bubbles and makes medication withdrawal difficult to control.

CLINICAL ALERT

Long-acting insulin, LANTUS (glargine) is a clear solution. It is *not* to be mixed with any other type of insulin or solution. It is given subcutaneously and is not intended for IV use. It must be refrigerated but dose is given at room temperature.

6. Withdraw ordered amount of insulin into syringe.
7. Validate medication record, insulin bottle, and prepared syringe with an RN for accuracy. **Rationale:** Double checking insulin helps safeguard against errors.
8. Remove needle from vial and expel air from syringe.
9. Replace needle guard.
10. Take medication to client's room.
11. Follow steps for administration of medications by subcutaneous injection.

CLINICAL ALERT

Do not massage site following injection of certain drugs such as insulin or heparin because this hastens absorption and drug action and may cause tissue irritation. Hold wipe over injection site for several seconds.

TABLE 18–1 Insulin Types and Therapeutic Action (in minutes/hours*)

Types	Onset	Peak	Duration
Rapid-acting (clear solution)			
Humalog® (Lispro) NovoLog® (Aspart)	5–15 min	60–90 min	3–5 hrs
Short-acting (clear solution)			
Novolin R Humulin R Velosulin BR (buffered insulin for insulin pumps)	0.5–1 hr	2–4 hrs	5–7 hrs
Intermediate-acting (cloudy solution)			
Humulin N (NPH) Novolin N (NPH)	1–2 hrs	6–12 hrs	16–24 hrs
Humulin L Novolin L	2 hrs	6–8 hrs	16–22 hrs
Mixtures (cloudy solution)			
Humulin 70/30 (70% NPH, 30% Regular) Novolin 70/30 (70% NPH, 30% Regular) Humulin 50/50 (50% NPH, 50% Regular)	30 min	2–12 hrs	24 hrs
Humalog 75/25 (75% lispro protamine suspension, 25% lispro)	15 min	1 hr	24 hrs
Long-acting			
Humulin Ultralente *(cloudy solution)* Lantus (glargine) *(clear solution)*	4–6 hrs	16–20 hrs	28 hrs

*The time of insulin action may vary significantly in different clients, and in the same client at different times.

Insulin is biologically engineered through the process of recombinant-DNA technology. Insulin is produced by different companies who use different names for short, intermediate, or long acting forms of insulin or their mixtures.

NPH = neutral protamine Hagedorn

Premixing Types of Insulin

- Mixing NPH and Lente insulin is not recommended. **Rationale:** NPH is phosphate buffered and will combine with zinc in Lente insulin. This will result in a precipitate of zinc phosphate and conversion of long-acting properties of Lente into an unpredictable form of short-acting insulin.
- Mixtures of rapid acting (Humalog) and intermediate or long acting insulin should be administered within 15 minutes before a meal.
- Mixtures of NPH and regular (short acting) insulins can be used immediately, or stored (in upright needle-up position) for use within 30 days.
- Do not reuse syringe if mixing insulins. (Instruct client to follow this guideline at home.)

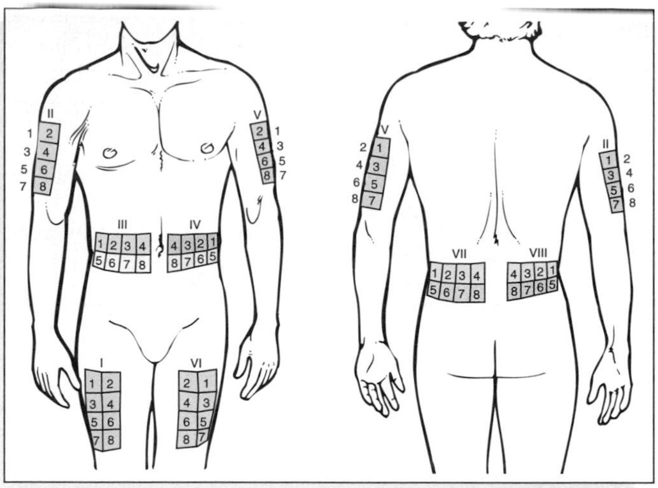

Instruct the client to inject into sites on the abdomen (where absorption rate is faster) and, only if necessary, rotate to other sites systematically. Injecting within an anatomic area prevents localized changes in fatty tissue and promotes stable insulin absorption rates. Injections should be ½ to 1 inch apart.

Evidence Based Nursing Practice

Using an Insulin Pen Accurately

In a recent study, 9% of 109 clients who used intermediate acting insulin failed to properly mix (roll) their insulin pens resulting in erratic insulin delivery (5% to 214% intended dose).

Source: Cohen, M. (2000). Medication errors. *Nursing 2000, 30*(3), 18.

Teaching Clients How to Use an Insulin Pen

1. Check for diamond symbol (◆) in window to indicate pen has been primed.
2. Turn dose knob clockwise until arrow (→) is viewed in window.
3. Pull dose knob out in direction of arrow until a "0" appears in the dose window. (A dose cannot be dialed until the dose knob is pulled out.)
4. Turn dose knob clockwise until correct dose appears in window.
5. Turn pen up and down to create suspension.
6. Place needle immediately before injection, and remove immediately after injection.

   Note: If insulin pen has short (3/16 inch) needle, do not pinch up before injection; inject insulin over 6 to 7 seconds.
7. Follow manufacturer's instructions carefully regarding pen system use.

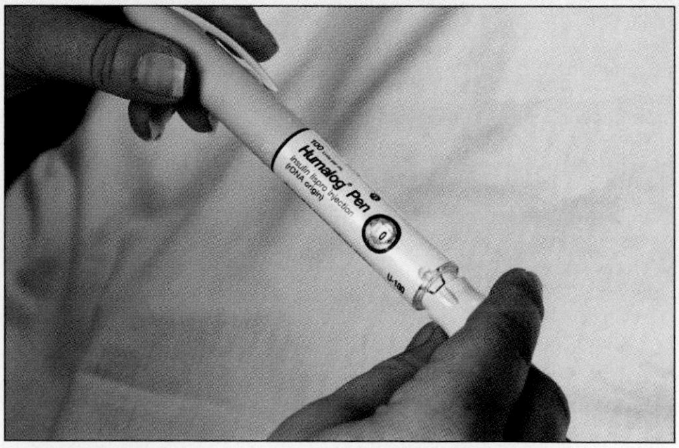

Pull dose knob until "0" appears before turning knob to correct dose.

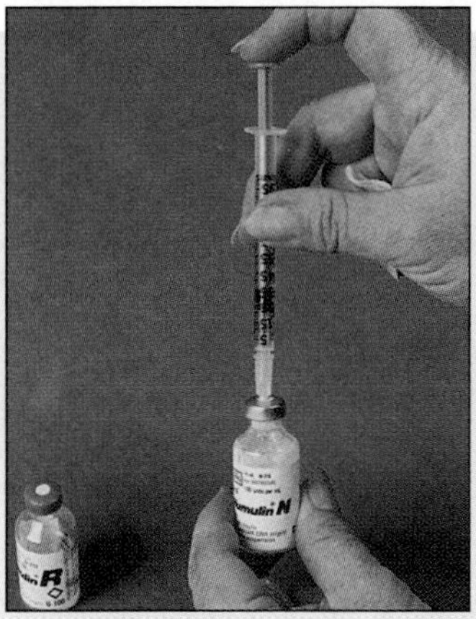

Step 1: Inject prescribed amount of air into intermediate-acting (cloudy) insulin vial without needle touching solution.

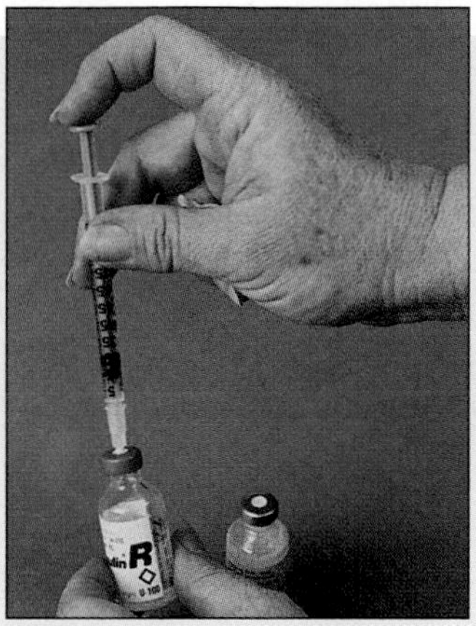

Step 2: Inject prescribed amount of air into rapid- or short-acting (clear) insulin vial. Do not withdraw needle.

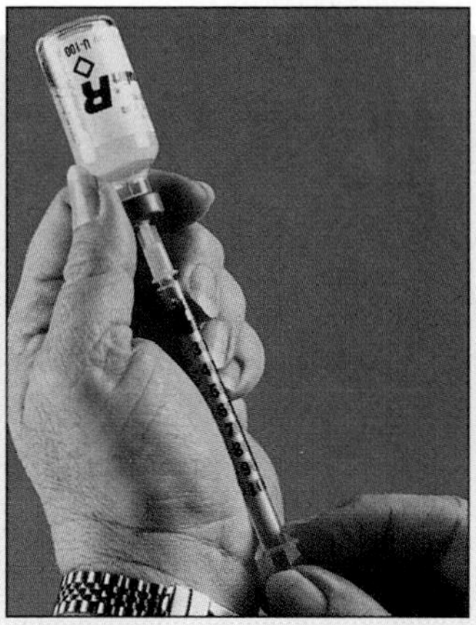

Step 3: Invert vial of rapid or short acting insulin, withdraw prescribed amount of medication, and withdraw needle from vial.

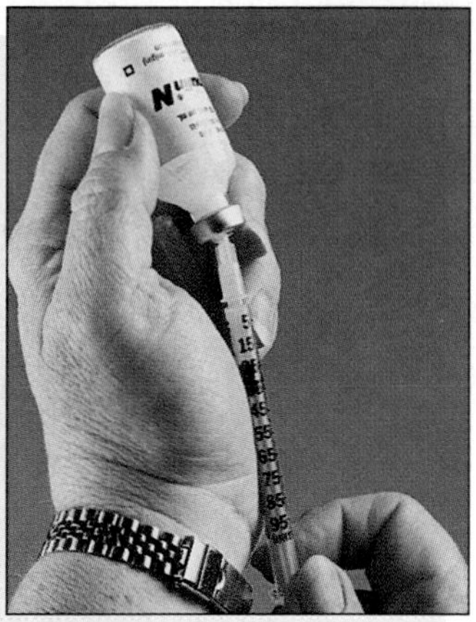

Step 4: Invert intermediate-acting insulin vial and withdraw exact amount without injecting insulin into bottle.

Note: Some clients prefer to reuse syringes until needle becomes dull. This is practical and safe if the needle is recapped after each use. Clients should consult their physician before initiating syringe reuse.

for Two Insulin Solutions

1. Check medication orders and rotation chart for injection sites.
2. Wash your hands.
3. Follow steps for combining medications in one syringe using two vials.
4. Rotate cloudy intermediate or long-acting insulin **Bottle (A)** between hands. **Rationale:** This brings cloudy solution into suspension.
5. Wipe top of both insulin bottles with alcohol.
6. Take needle guard off and place on tray.
7. Pull plunger of syringe down to *desired total units* of insulin.
8. Insert needle and inject prescribed amount of air into **Bottle A** *(cloudy)* insulin. Do not touch insulin solution with the needle. **Rationale:** This prevents contamination of the second bottle B *(clear rapid or short-acting insulin).*
9. Inject air into insulin **Bottle B** and withdraw medication. **Rationale:** Withdrawing *clear* insulin first prevents inadvertent injection of intermediate-acting insulin into rapid or short acting insulin bottle which would inactivate its rapid action.
10. Check dose with another nurse and both sign MAR. **Rationale:** Double checking helps ensure accurate dosage.
11. Withdraw needle from bottle and expel all air bubbles.
12. Invert **Bottle A** and insert needle. Take care not to inject any rapid, short-acting *(clear)* insulin into intermediate-acting (cloudy) insulin bottle. This can be avoided by holding steady pressure on plunger when inserting needle into bottle.
13. Pull back on plunger to obtain exact prescribed amount of intermediate or long-acting insulin. The total insulin dose now includes both the clear insulin, previously drawn up into syringe, and the intermediate or long-acting cloudy insulin you have just drawn up.

CLINICAL ALERT

Insulin type and brand should remain consistent for an individual client.

14. Withdraw needle from bottle and replace needle guard.
15. Follow protocol for administration of medications by subcutaneous injections.

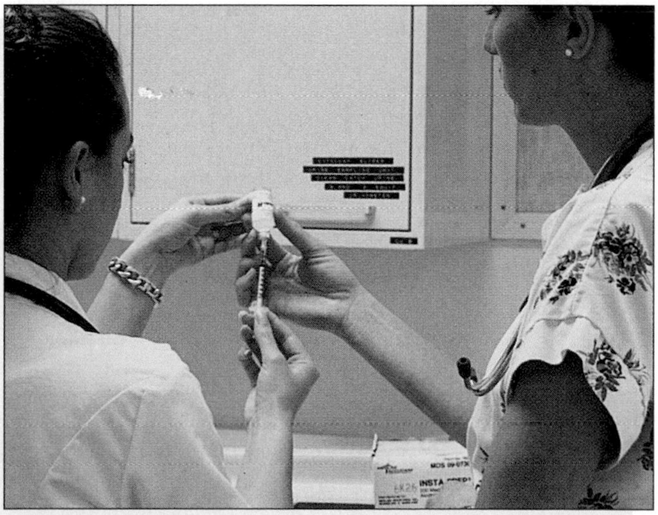

Double check insulin dose with a second nurse to help prevent errors in preparation.

EVIDENCE BASED NURSING PRACTICE

The Importance of Double Checking Drug Dose

- Double checks have revealed that up to 4.2% of *prescriptions* are filled erroneously.
- Double checks help the nurse identify mistakes which are difficult for one's self alone to recognize.
- Double checks work best when each nurse calculates desired dosages *independently* rather than having another nurse "*verify*" what has been prepared.

Source: Cohen, M. (2002). Double checking for errors. *Nursing 2002, 32*(3), 18.

TEACHING USE OF INSULIN PUMP

Equipment

Insulin pump (MiniMed or Disetronic)
Insulin syringe
Infusion sets (e.g., Sof-Set catheter, bent and straight needles with 24–42-inch plastic tubing)
Batteries (MiniMed: 3 standard Everready 357 1.5v batteries, 8 wks average life; Disetronic battery available through Disetronic)
Insertion device (e.g., Sof-Serter)
Skin prep (alcohol, Betadine, or Hibiclens)
Adhesive (Polyskin, Opsite, or Tegaderm dressing)
Velosulin BR (Regular short-acting buffered insulin)
Humulin R or Novolin R

Note: There are two rapid-acting human insulin analogs: Humalog® (Lispro) and NovoLog® (Aspart). The timing of these insulins more closely resembles the way the body makes insulin when food is ingested. This type of insulin works faster and has a shorter duration of action.

Procedure

1. Inform client of advantages of using Continuous Subcutaneous Insulin Infusion (CSII) with an insulin pump. **Rationale:** In teaching a new method, this enhances acceptance.
   a. CSII is a form of intensive insulin therapy used to optimize glycemic control and prevent or slow the progression of long-term complications of diabetes.
   b. CSII more closely mimics release of insulin by pancreas with basal and bolus insulin infusion.

CLINICAL ALERT

Insulin pump management and education should be done by a registered nurse certified in insulin pump therapy in collaboration with a physician.

- Basal: amount of insulin delivered hourly in attempt to maintain blood glucose.
- Bolus: amount of insulin delivered immediately prior to meals or for episodes of hyperglycemia.

   c. Lifestyle advantages: flexibility; client does not have to strictly adjust meal time, exercise, or sleep schedules to coincide with peak action time of an intermediate insulin, since only *Regular* (short-acting) insulin is used.
   d. Less risk of severe hypoglycemia compared with multiple daily injections.
   e. Children as young as 8 years are now using the insulin pump.

Note: Continuous Subcutaneous Insulin Infusion (CSII) is a form of intensive insulin therapy utilized as an alternative to multiple daily injection for some individuals in an attempt to achieve optimal glycemic control. Insulin pumps are manufactured by two companies that provide 24-hour emergency and technical information: MiniMed Technologies, Sylmar, CA (1-800-826-2099), and Disetronic Medical Systems, Minneapolis, MN (1-800-280-7801). All models are battery-powered and deliver basal and bolus doses.

2. Client selection criteria.
   a. Requires conscientious client or child committed to perform multiple daily blood glucose monitoring.
   b. Requires motivated client or child to accept greater levels of responsibility for self-care and problem-solving with CSII.
   c. Availability of supportive health care team or family with expertise in CSII therapy.
3. Teach client and/or family how to operate insulin pump.
   a. Provide instructional materials on insulin pump operation (literature and video tape tutorials available through manufacturer).
   b. Instruct client on basic modalities of pump operation and programming steps (varies with model of pump).

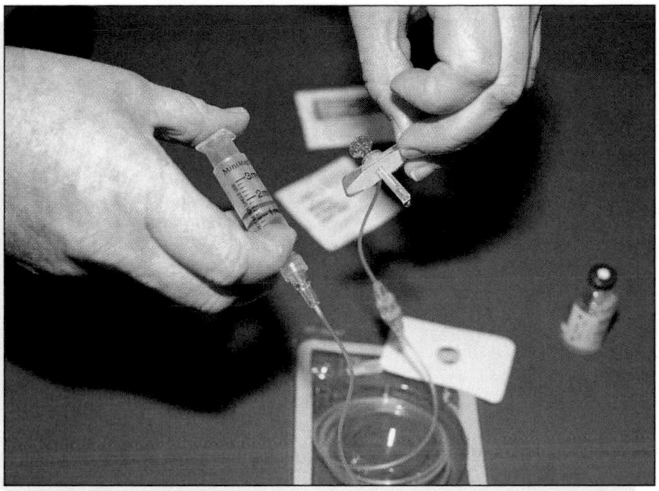

Infusion set is primed with regular short-acting insulin.

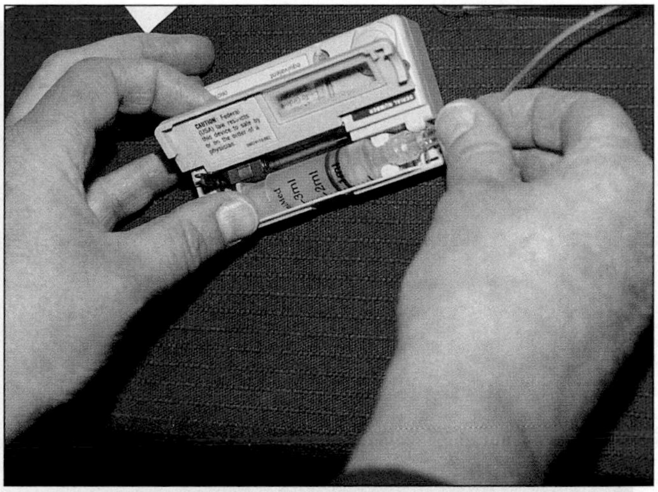

Position syringe securely in pump.

c. Basal rate can be set for lower at night and higher 3–4 hours before breakfast, then intermediate for the rest of the day.
d. Bolus doses can be given before meals.
e. Alarms notify client if reservoir is empty, catheter obstructed, battery "Low," or pump malfunctioning.
f. Review necessity of self-monitoring blood glucose before meals, bedtime, and at 0300. Additional testing is necessary for insulin dose adjustments, illness, and physical exercise. **Rationale:** Frequent monitoring assists proper dosage of bolus and basal rates.

4. Instruct client on preparation of insulin infusion set.
   a. Filling of reservoir/cartridge (every 24 hours at same time every day) and proper priming and placement into pump. **Rationale:** Changing at the same time every day establishes a routine.
   b. Selection and preparation of infusion site (abdomen is preferred site for insertion as insulin absorption is faster and more predictable due to less physical movement).

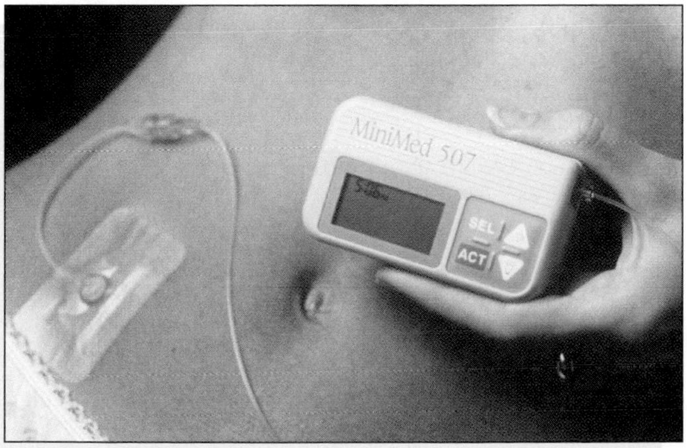

MiniMed 507 Insulin Pump attached to fusion set. Abdominal site is preferred because insulin absorption is faster and most predictable.

CLINICAL ALERT

If insulin must be discontinued, the tube cannot be clamped. The tubing or needle must be removed or the pump must be turned off, because the pump is a pressure pump.

Avoid areas around waistline and pantline and 1 inch from umbilicus. New insertion site should be 1–2 inches away from previous site.
   c. Proper insertion of catheter-over-needle or needle.
   d. Application of sterile dressing.
   e. Rotation of sites and changing of catheter or needle every 48 hours. Instruct client to observe for signs of redness, tenderness, and drainage on daily basis. Reinforce to change site with new infusion set, to alternate site, and to report problems promptly to health care provider. **Rationale:** To prevent site problem and to ensure uniform insulin absorption.
   f. Reinforce monitoring blood glucose 3 hours after insertion and/or removal of catheter/needle. **Rationale:** Suspect improper insertion of catheter/needle, or accidental removal if blood glucose is 240 mg/dL with 2 sequential testings.

5. Instruct client in self-management skills for episodes of acute complications of diabetes.
   a. HYPOGLYCEMIA (e.g., due to physical exercise or a missed meal) = temporary stopping of insulin infusion and changes in basal/bolus rates. (See Alert).

CLINICAL ALERT

Ketoacidosis can occur if insulin delivery is interrupted.

b. HYPERGLYCEMIA (e.g., due to sick day) = increases of basal/bolus rates.
c. Fasting states (e.g., surgery, diagnostic testing) = adjustments in basal/bolus rates as needed.
d. Instruct client to carry backup batteries, insulin, infusion sets and insulin syringes, and at least 15g carbohydrate to be taken in event of hypoglycemic reaction.
e. Instruct client to be familiar with pump alarms and interventions for troubleshooting.
f. Instruct client to wear Med-Alert bracelet and carry medical identification, emergency phone number of healthcare professionals, and 24-hour emergency hotline phone number of pump manufacturer for technical support.
g. Inform client to remove pump before exposure to x rays, MRIs, and CAT scans and have hospital personnel place pump in alternative room.
h. Advise client to avoid submersion of insulin pump in water (e.g., swimming, showering). **Rationale:** Not all models of insulin pumps are waterproof.

6. Instruct client on cleaning and maintenance of pump and how to order additional supplies.
7. Provide resources for client: community insulin pump support groups, educational literature, Internet information provided online by manufacturer.

ADMINISTERING SUBCUTANEOUS (SUB Q) HEPARIN

Equipment

Heparin in vial (*carefully note units per mL*)
1 mL tuberculin syringe or unit dose syringe with small (25–29) gauge needle
or
Low-molecular-weight heparin in prefilled syringe
Antimicrobial swabs
Gloves

> **CLINICAL ALERT**
> Heparin is available in a variety of strengths (e.g., 1,000 units/mL or 5,000 units/mL vials). *Carefully* check vial units per mL before drawing into syringe and have another nurse double-check your prepared injection.

> **CLINICAL ALERT**
> Subcutaneous injection of low-molecular-weight (LMW) heparin involves *low doses* that help prevent clot formation but do not alter blood coagulation studies. LMW administration is less time–consuming and does not require as much monitoring as conventional heparin.

Preparation

1. *See* Preparing Injections.
2. Double check heparin prepared dose with another nurse.
3. Place client in supine position.
4. Wash hands.

Note: Some facilities advocate adding air to syringe to create air lock. ***Rationale:*** *Prevents tracking of medication on skin and decreases bruising. (To avoid loss of drug, do not clear needle of air before injecting 30 to 40 mg of LMWH).*

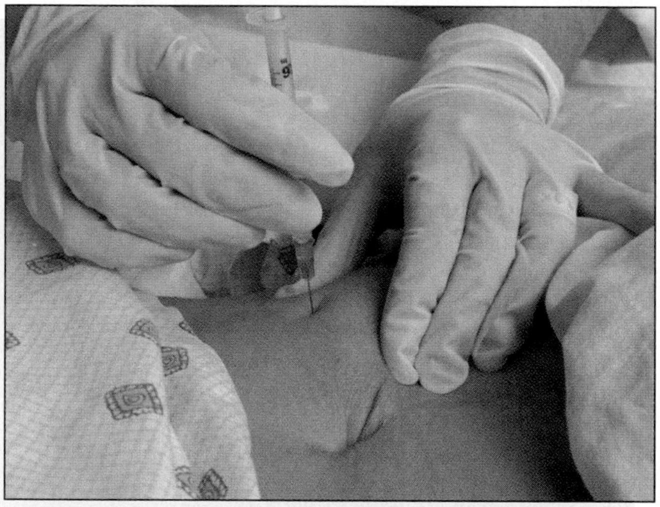

Select site at least two finger breadths from umbilicus.

Procedure

1. Take prepared injection to client's room, check room and bed number against client's MAR.
2. Check client's identaband, and ask client to state name.
3. Provide privacy.
4. Explain procedure and purpose to client.
5. Don gloves.
6. Select site on client's lower abdomen (at least two fingerbreadths from umbilicus) or select area of fatty tissue above iliac crest. **Rationale:** Heparin should not be administered IM or in the extremities.
7. Avoid ecchymotic area or lesions.
8. Cleanse site gently with antimicrobial swab, using circular motion from inside outward.
9. Gently pinch an inch of subcutaneous tissue (fat roll) between thumb and forefinger of nondominant hand and hold fat pad throughout injection.

10. Hold syringe between thumb and forefinger of dominant hand and insert full length of needle into skinfold at a 90° angle.
11. Inject medication slowly *without* aspirating first. **Rationale:** Aspiration can rupture small vessels and increase risk of bleeding into tissue.
12. Wait 10 seconds before gently withdrawing needle at same angle in which it entered skin. **Rationale:** This allows heparin to absorb into tissue and minimizes bruising.
13. Press and hold swab over injection site. **Rationale:** This prevents back-tracking of medication.
14. Do not massage area. **Rationale:** This may cause bruising.
15. Activate needle safety feature and discard syringe in puncture-proof container.

CLINICAL ALERT

To prevent tissue damage and bruising, do not aspirate or massage heparin injections.

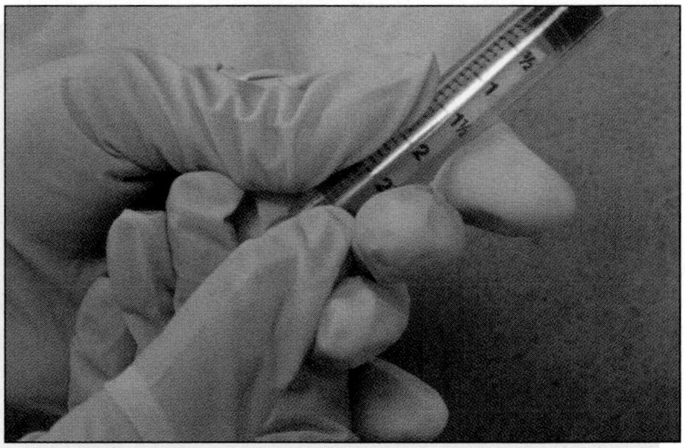

Activate needle safety feature; then, dispose of syringe in sharps container.

16. Return client to position of comfort.
17. Remove gloves and wash hands.
18. Document injection.

ADMINISTERING INTRAMUSCULAR (IM) INJECTIONS

Equipment

Medication vial or ampule
3-mL syringe with 1–1½ inch needle (21–23 gauge)
2 antimicrobial swabs
Gloves

Preparation

See Preparing injections.

CLINICAL ALERT

Ventrogluteal site is safer and preferred over dorsogluteal whenever possible, because dorsogluteal area is especially vulnerable to nerve and vascular injury.

Procedure

1. Take prepared injection to client's room. Check room number against client's MAR.
2. Check client's identaband, and have client state name.
3. Explain procedure to client.
4. Provide privacy for client.
5. Wash hands and don gloves.
6. Select injection site, identifying landmarks. Consider client's size, amount and viscosity of medications being injected. Alternate sites each time injections are given.
7. Cleanse area with antimicrobial swab, using circular motion from inside outward.

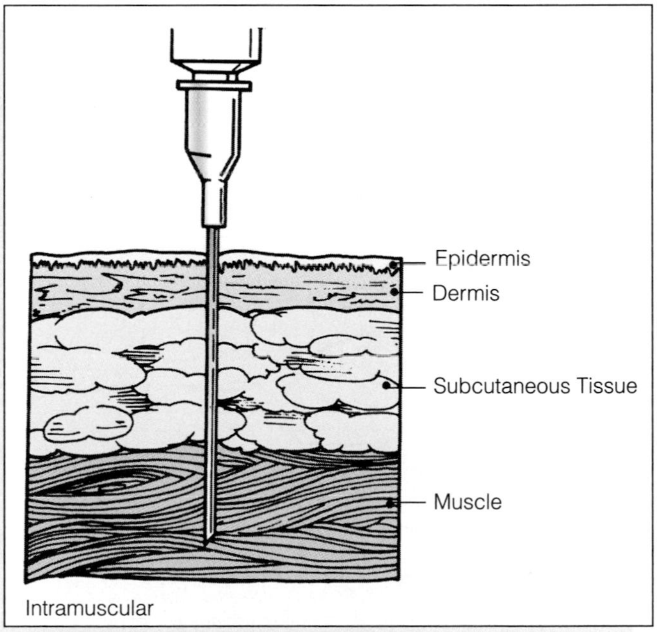

Insert needle at 90° angle for IM injections into muscle.

8. Do not add air to syringe. If tracking medication is a potential problem, use Z-track method.
9. Spread skin taut between thumb and forefinger (grasping muscle is acceptable in pediatric and geriatric clients with less fatty tissue) to ensure needle placement in muscle belly.
10. Insert needle at a 90° angle to the muscle, using a quick, darting motion. **Rationale:** This angle facilitates medication reaching muscle.

11. Pull back on plunger; if blood returns, discard and prepare a new injection. **Rationale:** The appearance of blood indicates needle has entered a blood vessel, and medication injected directly into bloodstream may be dangerous.
12. Inject medication slowly. **Rationale:** This allows time for medication to disperse through tissue.
13. Withdraw needle quickly, and massage area with antimicrobial swab.
14. Activate needle safety feature.
15. Dispose of syringe/needle unit in puncture-proof container.
16. Return client to comfortable position.
17. Discard gloves and wash hands.
18. Chart medication and site of injection.

Techniques for Minimizing Pain During IM Injections

- Encourage client to relax.
- If medication is irritating, use a new needle for injection.
- Place client on side with upper knee flexed for ventrogluteal, or flat on abdomen with toes turned inward for dorsogluteal injection.
- Avoid injecting into sensitive or hardened tissue.
- Compress tissue at injection site.
- Ensure that needle length reaches muscle for IM injection.
- Prevent antiseptic from clinging to needle during insertion by waiting until skin prep is dry.
- Reduce puncture pain by "darting" needle quickly into muscle.
- Use as small a gauge needle as possible.
- Inject medication slowly.
- Maintain grasp on syringe; do not move needle once inserted.
- Withdraw needle quickly after injection.
- Use Z-track technique.
- EMLA cream may be applied 30 to 40 minutes prior to injection.

VENTROGLUTEAL INJECTION SITE

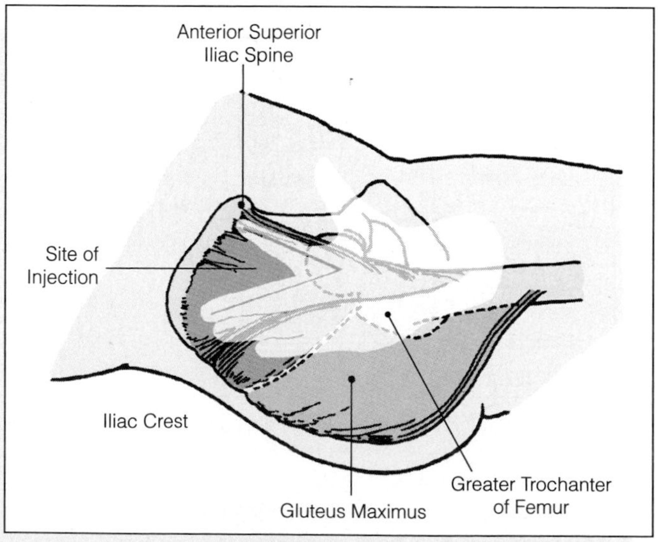

Overlay of hand shows area of injection into ventrogluteal site for IM injections (client's right side)

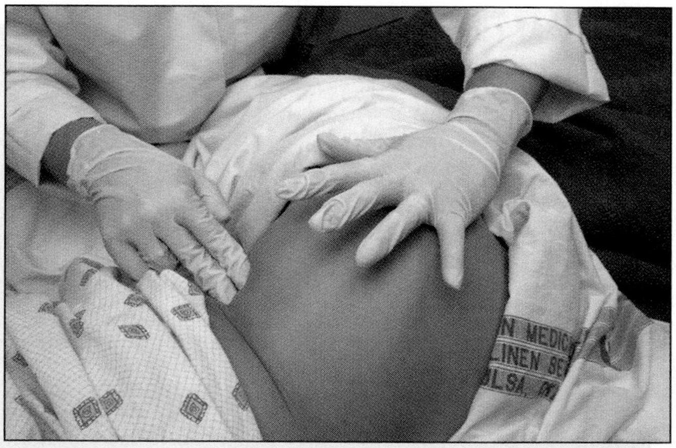

With client left side-lying, identify right greater trochanter; place palm at site.

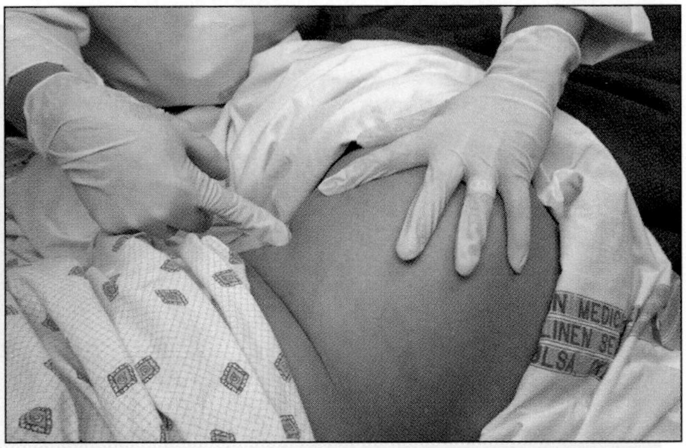

Place palm on greater trochanter and point to anterior iliac spine.

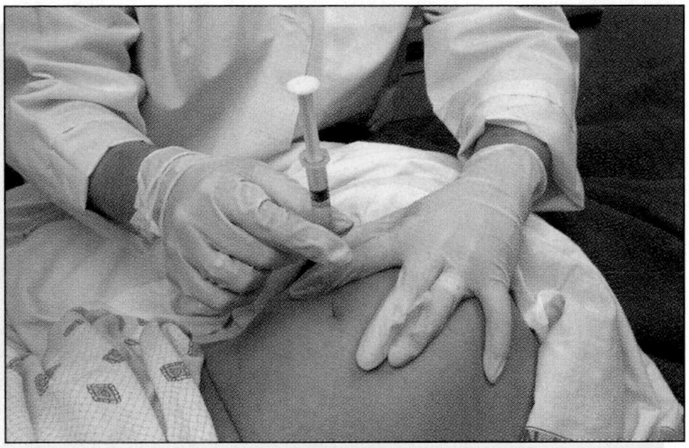

Inject medication at 90° angle within "V" area.

DORSOGLUTEAL INJECTION SITE

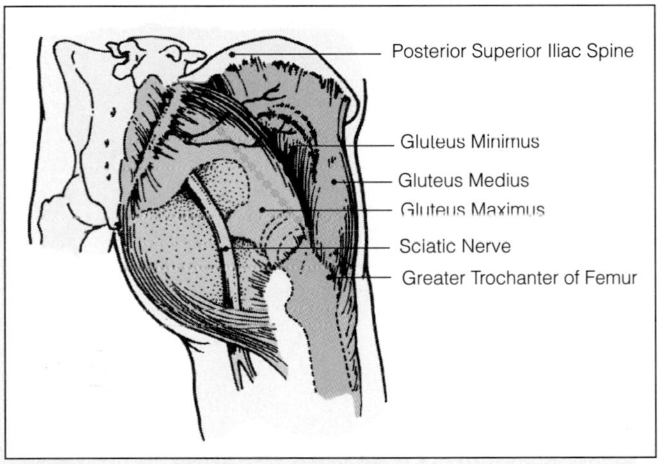

Place injection above and outside diagonal line for dorsogluteal injection.

CLINICAL ALERT

Do not use the upper outer quadrant of the buttocks to identify the dorsogluteal injection site. The buttocks include fat tissue that extends well below the gluteal muscle and varies significantly among individuals. Intersecting vertical and horizontal lines on the buttocks can easily include the sciatic nerve and major blood vessels in the upper outer quadrant, possibly exposing them to serious and permanent injury if an injection is placed there.

CLINICAL ALERT

Chemical injury to the sciatic nerve can occur even with injection of irritating medications *near* the nerve. To avoid sciatic nerve injury, locate dorsogluteal injection site above imaginary line drawn between two boney landmarks.

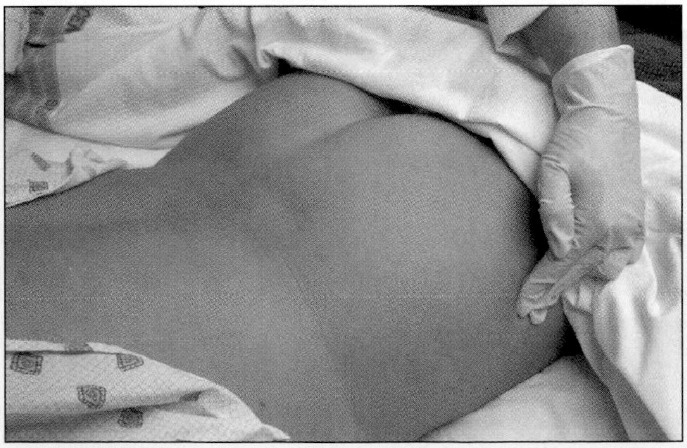

Locate greater trochanter to identify dorsogluteal site.

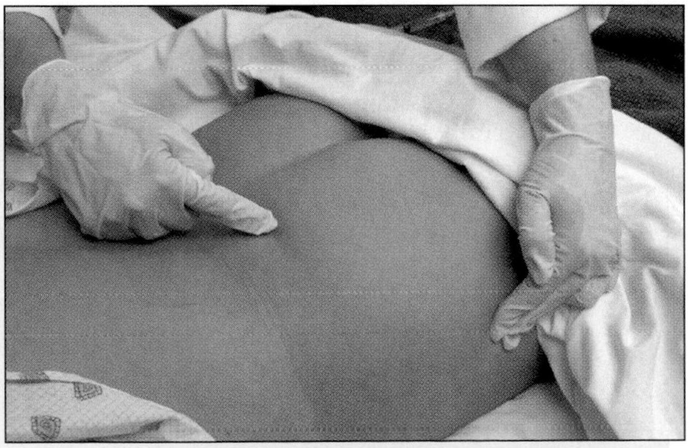

Locate posterosuperior spine of iliac crest.

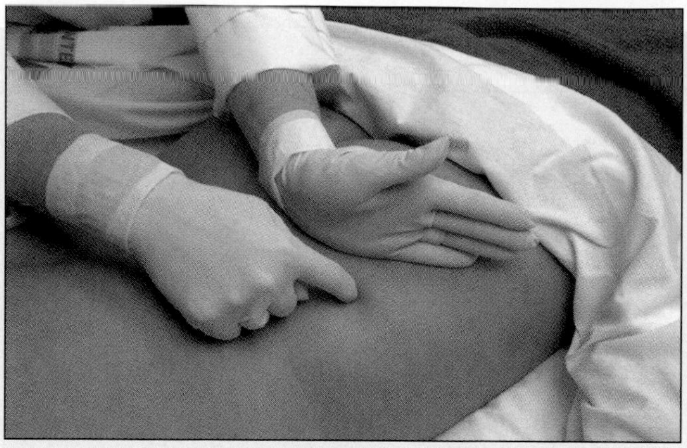

Draw imaginary line between trochanter and iliac spine.

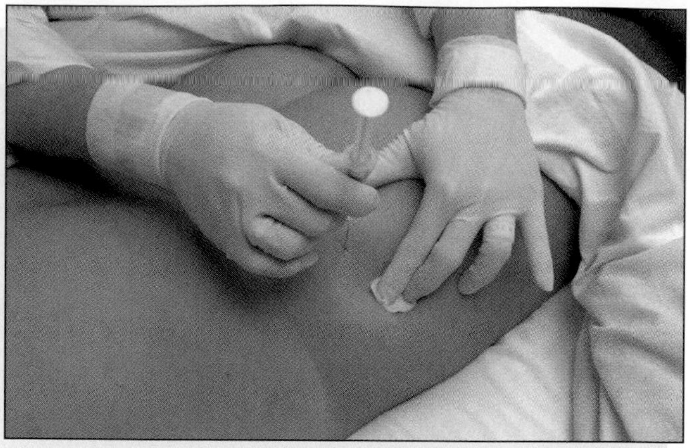

Inject medication directly into dorsogluteal site at 90° angle.

VASTUS LATERALIS INJECTION SITE

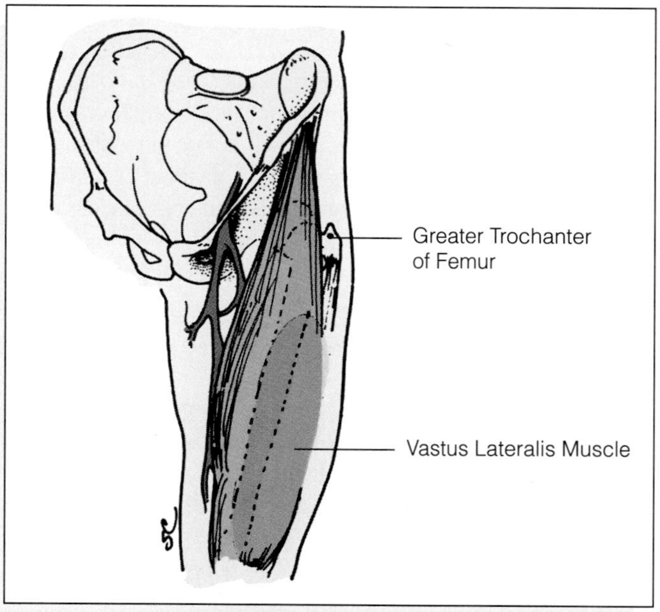

Shaded area indicates site location for vastus lateralis injection.

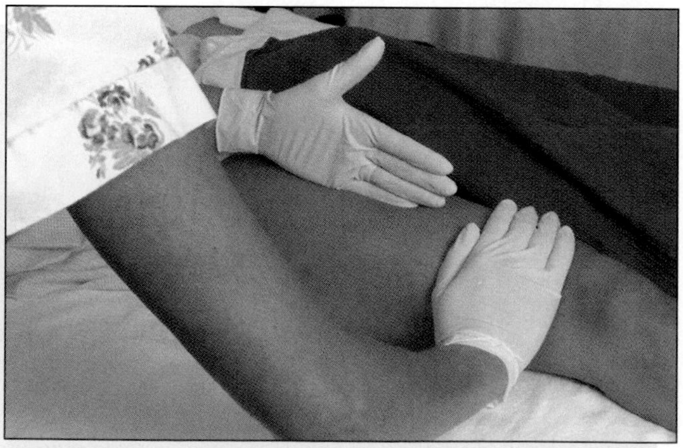

Select site using middle third and anterior lateral aspect of thigh.

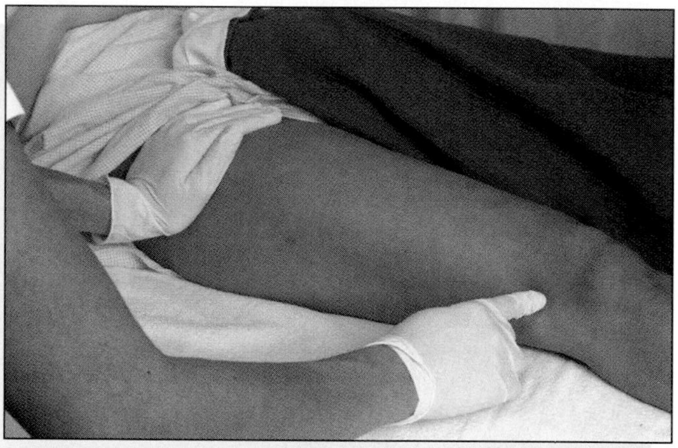

Vastus lateralis: identify greater trochanter and lateral femoral condyle.

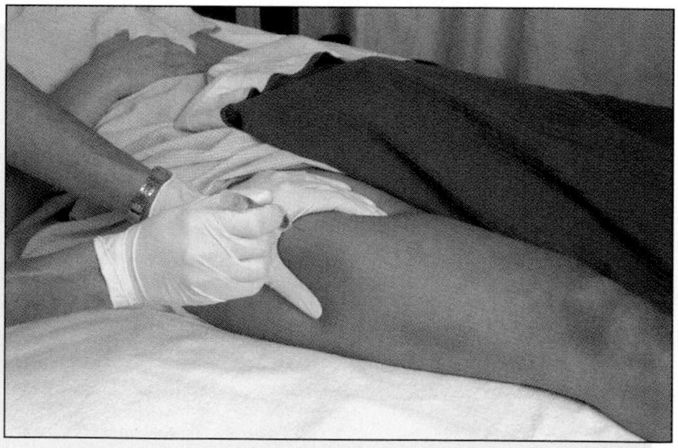

Inject medication at 90° angle directly into muscle.

DELTOID INJECTION SITE

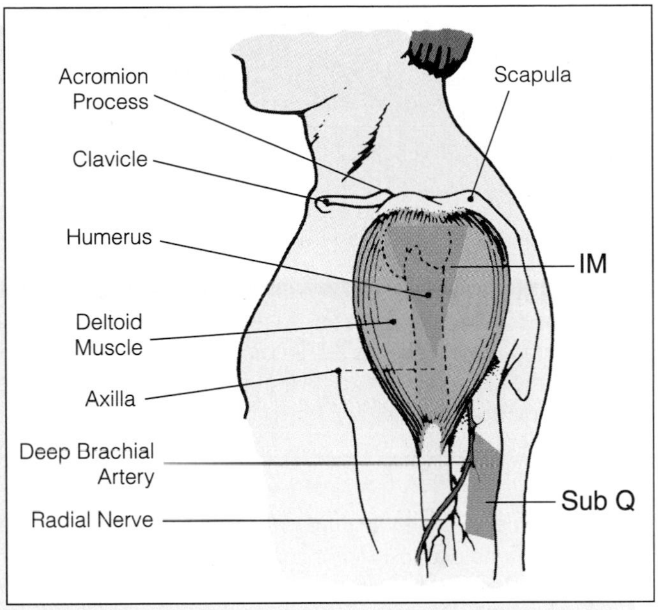

Locate deltoid site on outer lateral aspect of upper arm.

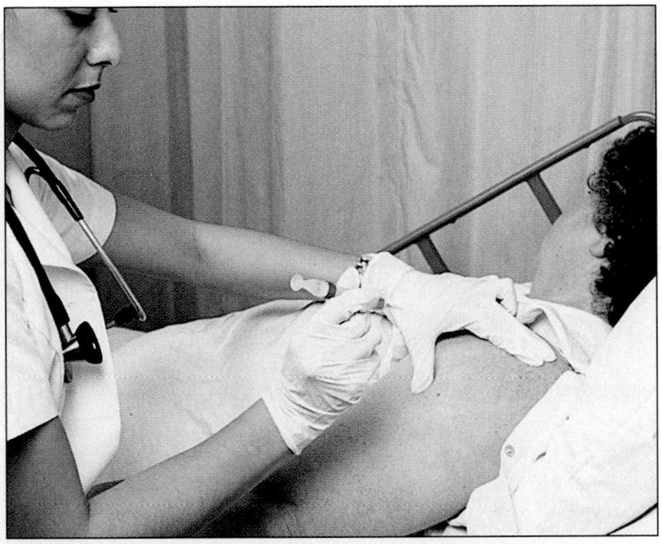

Inject medication (0.5 1 mL) within area two fingerbreadths below lower edge of acromion for top boundary, opposite axilla for bottom boundary.

EVIDENCE BASED NURSING PRACTICE

Choose the Right Needle Size

A 5/8-inch needle won't reach deltoid muscle in 17% of men and 50% of women. A 1-inch needle is better for men (130–260 lb) and women (132–198 lb).

Source: Zucherman, J. (2000, November 18). The importance of injecting vaccines into muscle. *British Medical Journal.*

USING Z-TRACK METHOD

Equipment

Syringe
2 needles (one 2-inch needle)
Medication
Antimicrobial swabs
Gloves

Preparation

See Preparing Injections.

Procedure

1. Gather equipment.
2. Draw up prescribed medication into syringe.
3. Do not add air to syringe for Z-track method. **Rationale:** A seal is provided by pulling skin to the side, then releasing after injecting medication.

> **CLINICAL ALERT**
>
> The Z-track method prevents "tracking" and is used for administering medications that are especially irritating to subcutaneous and nerve tissue (e.g., imferon or Vistaril).

4. Attach new 2-inch sterile needle to syringe. **Rationale:** A new needle prevents introducing medication that could be

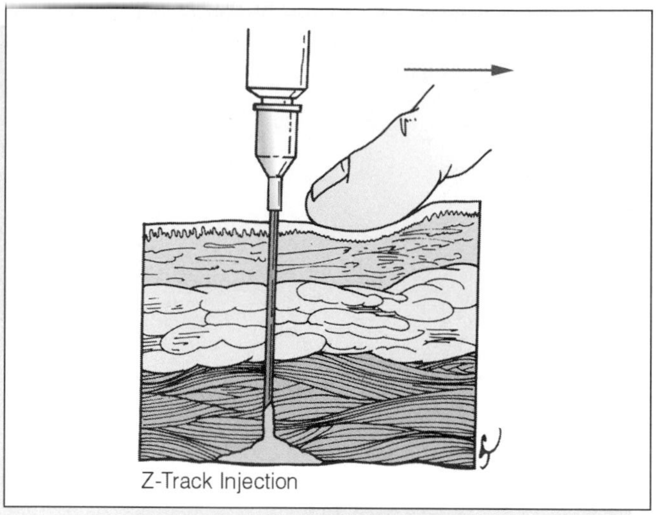

Z-Track Injection

irritating to tissue. A long needle allows medication to go deep into the muscle.

5. Take medication to client's room; check room number against MAR.
6. Check identaband, and ask client to state name.
7. Provide privacy.
8. Explain procedure and purpose to client.
9. Wash hands and don gloves.
10. Place client in prone position, if possible. **Rationale:** This position provides the best perspective for identifying dorsogluteal landmarks: posterosuperior iliac crest and greater trochanter.
11. Cleanse site with antimicrobial wipe.
12. Pull skin 1–1½ inch laterally away from injection site. **Rationale:** This tissue displacement creates a track that keeps medication from seeping into subcutaneous tissue.
13. Maintain displacement and insert needle at a 90° angle. Aspirate by pulling back on plunger to see if needle is in blood vessel. If so, discard and prepare new injection.
14. Inject medication slowly and wait 10 seconds keeping skin taut. **Rationale:** Permits muscle relaxation and absorption of medication.
15. Withdraw needle and release retracted skin. **Rationale:** Lateral tissue displacement interrupts needle track and seals medication in the muscle when the tissue is released.
16. Apply light pressure with swab. Do not massage. **Rationale:** Massage may disperse medication into subcutaneous tissue and cause tissue irritation.

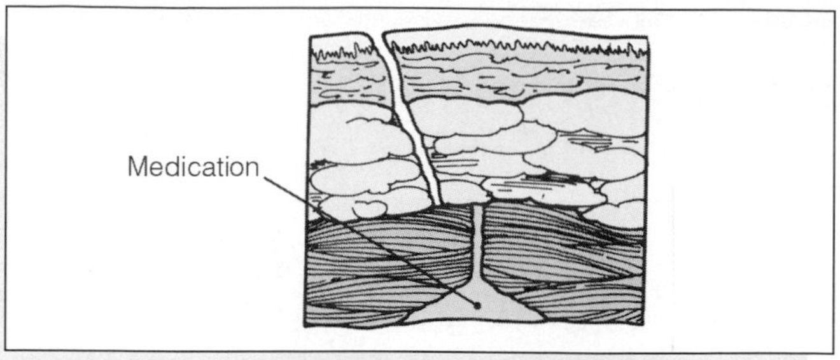

Z-track is used to prevent backflow of medications into Sub Q tissue.

CLINICAL ALERT

If client is obese, use a 2–3-inch needle so that medication is absorbed into muscle (not fat) tissue and blood level of drug is achieved.

17. Activate needle safety feature.
18. Return client to a position of comfort and safety.
19. Discard gloves and equipment in appropriate area.
20. Wash your hands.
21. Document administration of medications in the medication record.

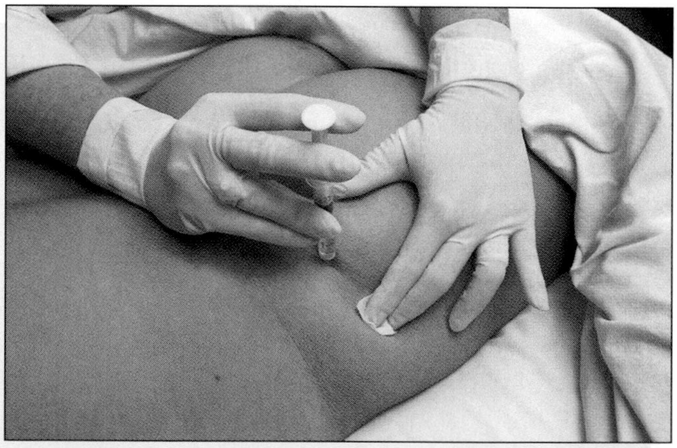

Maintaining displacement, insert needle at 90° angle. Aspirate by pulling back on plunger, checking to see if needle is in blood vessel. If blood is aspirated, discard and prepare new injection.

CHARTING FOR PARENTERAL MEDICATIONS

Client's Medication Record

- Time administered
- Name of medication
- Dosage
- Route
- Injection site
- Initials of nurse administering medication
- Signature by nurse (to identify initials)

Nurses' Notes

- Record PRN, STAT, intradermal, and one time only medications
- Name of medication, dosage, route, site, time administered
- Client's pre- and postinjection assessment findings (pain rating, sedation, and relevant laboratory)
- Signature of nurse

Critical Thinking Application

UNEXPECTED OUTCOMES	CRITICAL THINKING OPTIONS
Client complains of pain when injection is administered at dorsogluteal IM site.	• Assess site of injection, neurovascular status of extremity. Document findings. • Notify physician. • Obtain order for warm, moist packs. • Fill out unusual occurrence form. • Take greater care to identify anatomic landmarks. Place client prone (on abdomen). Use dorsogluteal site ONLY when necessary. • Locate a line from posterosuperior iliac spine to the greater trochanter of the femur; inject lateral and slightly superior to midpoint of line. Use Z-track technique. Inject into muscle at a 90° angle.
Medication is administered using wrong parenteral route.	• Notify physician, and complete unusual occurrence form. • Medications may need to be administered to reverse the action of the medication. • Monitor client's response closely and report adverse findings immediately. • Medication administered IM or IV rather than sub Q leads to faster absorption rates; therefore an assessment needs to be done to determine effects. (IV administration has immediate action.)
Ecchymosis occurs following heparin injection.	• Rotate injection site. Do not inject medication into ecchymotic area. • Do not aspirate before injection or massage site following needle withdrawal. • When forming fat pad in preparation for injection site, do not pinch tightly. • Apply ice to area before injecting heparin.

UNEXPECTED OUTCOMES	CRITICAL THINKING OPTIONS
Client has an anaphylactic allergic reaction to medication.	• Maintain patent airway. • Position client for optimal cerebral perfusion—trunk horizontal, legs elevated. Stay with client. • Notify physician immediately. • Be prepared to carry out the following actions following physician's orders. Administer oxygen 6 L/minute via nasal cannula. Insert IV line for fluid resuscitation and drug delivery. Administer epinephrine for bronchodilitation. Monitor client for response to treatment. Monitor vital signs frequently until the client's status is stabilized. • Record incident and place allergy alert bracelet on client. • Fill out unusual occurrence form.

GERONTOLOGIC CONSIDERATIONS

Twenty percent of the 32 million elderly Americans not living in nursing homes are prescribed at least one medication considered potentially harmful.

Major problems with prescriptive drugs in the elderly.

- Drug interactions—many seniors use multiple physicians and pharmacies, creating risk of drugs that interact thereby causing adverse reactions.
- Medication errors—the more medications a person takes the greater risk of medication error (people over age 75 take an average of 17 prescriptions annually).
- Noncompliance—not taking right dose at right time or discontinuing drug without consultation; common due to lack of understanding about reason to take drug and general knowledge base of drug action.
- Unpredictable drug action—physiologic changes in the elderly associated with age and disease may alter effects of the drugs.
- Drug side effects not recognized—elderly not aware or do not understand potential dangerous side effects of drugs.
- Inadequate monitoring—elderly often alone or not monitored consistently, so drug problems are not identified.
- Cost of drugs—multiple medications are costly for many elderly, so they may reduce the frequency of dosing or stop taking a drug.

The elderly are at risk for drug toxicity.

- Altered liver function, slows medication metabolism.
- Altered renal excretion, slows drug excretion.
- Reduced protein level (increased ratio of fat to muscle) decreases medication binding and increases free circulating drug levels.
- Increased CNS sensitivity to drugs that interfere with neurotransmitters that regulate brain function.

Drugs the elderly should avoid.

- Sedatives/hypnotics
- Tranquilizers (antianxiety medications)
- Anticholinergics (belladonna alkaloids, antispasmodics)

MANAGEMENT GUIDELINES

Each state legislates a Nurse Practice Act for RNs and LVN/LPNs. Health care facilities are responsible for establishing and implementing policies and procedures that conform to their state's regulations. Verify the regulations and role parameters for each health care worker in your facility.

Delegation of Responsibilities

- Registered and licensed vocational nurses are responsible for administering oral and parenteral medications to client. In some non-acute facilities, such as residential homes, geriatric technicians may administer medications following standard procedures.
- Individuals administering medications must be knowledgeable about the RATIONALE for their use. This insight cues the need for specific pre- and post-administration individual client assessment (responses such as vital signs, lab values, adverse reactions) as an integral part of this deceptively simple skill.
- Unlicensed assistive personnel are not trained (or expected) to obtain and interpret essential client data necessary for decision making when administering medications. However, if they are assigned to administer daily care, they should be informed what to observe for and report to the RN or LVN.

Information Flow

- *Immediately report to physician:*
  All errors in medication administration (and complete agency variance report)
  Ineffective client responses to medication including adverse responses (vital signs, rash, paradoxical reaction, etc.)
  Reports of abnormal relevant lab data (e.g., toxic drug levels)
- *Report to relief staff:*
  All of the above PLUS:
  Any new or discontinued medication orders
  PRN, STAT, and one-time-only medications given
  Effectiveness of medication therapy

CRITICAL THINKING STRATEGIES

SCENARIO 1

Your client has recently suffered a "brain attack" (stroke), which has caused him to have difficulty swallowing (dysphagia) and places him at risk for aspiration. When the previous shift nurse attempted to have him take his oral medications with water, he coughed and choked violently, so the nurse discontinued efforts to complete his medication administration. One of this client's most important medications is Inderal LA 80 mg, a timed-release capsule that is given once a day. This long-acting capsule cannot be opened and its contents emptied for convenient administration without interfering with the timed-release property of its formulation.

1. What types of consult would provide assistance in decision making about this client's swallowing problem and medication administration?
2. What actions would facilitate this client's swallowing and decrease the risk of aspiration?
3. What alternative method is there for administering the Inderal LA?
4. How will the nurse communicate adjustments in administration to the other staff members?

SCENARIO 2

This is Nancy Drew's third hospitalization for diabetic ketoacidosis this year. She has been an insulin-dependent diabetic for 5 years (since age 9). For several years, Nancy has controlled the condition using two daily insulin injections, a combination of regular and NPH (intermediate-acting) before breakfast and dinner.

This year Nancy made the cheerleading A squad—quite an achievement and an honor—requiring practice before and after school, enrollment in gymnastics class, and participation at evening and weekend games, some of which were out of town. In addition, Nancy must attend cheerleading camp this summer and is preparing for all-state competition trials.

Nancy's condition is stabilized during hospitalization, and shortly before discharge she confides in you that she hates needles, that "the shots really hurt," and, in fact, she prepares the syringes and sometimes just throws them away. In addition, she has experienced low blood sugar on occasion while cheerleading and knows that something happens with her insulin "overreacting" at these times; it makes her uncoordinated and "confused," but she just can't take time out to ingest sugar. She is afraid of losing her position on the A squad—she worked so hard to get there.

1. Based on this data, identify Nancy's psychosocial needs and developmental tasks at age 14.
2. What are the implications of insulin absorption and action as influenced by exercise and site of administration?
3. Describe actions that can decrease pain associated with medications.
4. Suggest an alternative way for Nancy to maintain her insulin coverage without discomfort and erratic absorption rates.

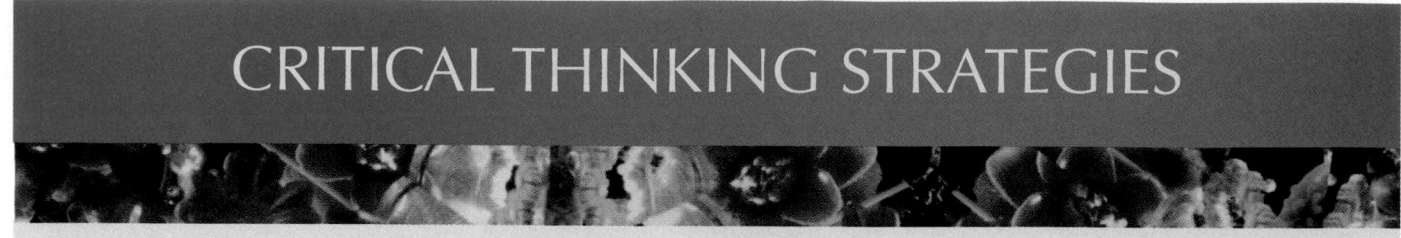

DRUG SUPPLEMENT

CALCULATIONS OF SOLUTIONS

Types of Solutions

1. Volume to volume (vol/vol): a given volume of solute is added to a given volume of solvent.
2. Weight to weight (wt/wt): a stated weight of solute is dissolved in a stated weight of solvent.
3. Weight to volume (wt/vol): a given weight of solute is dissolved in a given volume of solvent, which results in the proper amount of solution.

Preparing Solutions

Solutions of Varying Strengths

Determine the strength of the solution, the strength of the drug on hand, and the quantity of solution required.

Use this formula for preparing solutions:

$$\frac{D}{H} \times Q = X$$

where D = desired strength; H = strength on hand; Q = quantity of solution desired; and X = amount of solute.

Example: You have a 100% solution of hydrogen peroxide on hand. You need a liter of 50% solution.

$$\frac{50}{100} \times 1{,}000 \text{ mL} = 500 \text{ mL (solute)}$$

If the strength desired and strength on hand are not in like terms, you need to change one of the terms.

Example: You have 1 L of 50% solution on hand. You need a liter of 1:10 solution. 1:10 solution is the same as 10%.

$$\frac{10\%}{50\%} \times 1{,}000 \text{ mL} = 200 \text{ mL (solute)}$$

Add 200 mL of the drug to 800 mL of the solvent to make a liter of 10% solution.

Volume to Volume Solutions

Use the formula:

$$\frac{D}{H} \times Q = X$$

Example: Prepare a liter of 5% solution from a stock solution of 50%.

$$\frac{5\%}{50\%} \times 1{,}000 \text{ mL} = 100 \text{ mL}$$

Add 100 mL to 900 mL of diluent to make 1 L of 5% solution.

Solutions from Tablets

Use the formula:

$$\frac{D}{H} \times Q = X$$

where X = amount per number of tablets used.

Example: Prepare 1 L of a 1:1000 solution, using 10-gr tablets.

$$\frac{1/1000}{10 \text{ gr}} \times 1{,}000 \text{ mL} = X$$

First convert 10 gr to grams so the numerator and denominator are in the same unit of measure. 1 g = 15 gr; therefore 10 gr = 2/3g. Now substitute the new numbers in the formula and solve for X.

$$\frac{1/1000}{2/3} \times \frac{1000}{1} \text{ mL} = X$$

$$\frac{3}{2000} \times \frac{1000}{1} = X$$

$$X = 2/3 \text{ or } 1\tfrac{1}{2} \text{ tablets}$$

Place 1½ tablets into the liter of solution and dissolve.

ABBREVIATIONS AND SYMBOLS

aa	of each
a.c.	before meals
ad lib.	freely, as desired
b.i.d.	twice each day
c̄	with
cc	cubic centimeter
C	carbon
Ca	calcium
Cl	chlorine
dr *or* ʒ	dram
et	and
GI	gastrointestinal
gt *or* gtt	drop(s)
H_2O	water
H_2O_2	hydrogen peroxide
IM	intramuscular
in.	inch
K	potassium
lb *or* #	pound
m	minimum (a minimum)

Mg	magnesium	q4h	every 4 hours
mL	milliliter	R_x	treatment, "take thou"
N	nitrogen, normal	s̄	without
Na	sodium	s̄s̄	one-half
NPO	nothing by mouth	STAT	immediately
oob	out of bed	t.i.d.	three times each day
os	mouth	tsp	teaspoon
oz *or* ℥	ounce	WBC	white blood count
p.c.	after meals	°	degree
per	by, through	–	minus, negative, alkaline reaction
prn, or PRN	whenever necessary		
q.d.	every day	+	plus, positive, acid reaction
q.h.	every hour	%	percent
q.i.d.	four times each day	v	Roman numeral 5
q.s.	as much as required, quantity sufficient	vii	Roman numeral 7
		ix	Roman numeral 9
q2h	every 2 hours	xiii	Roman numeral 13
q3h	every 3 hours		

CONVERSION TABLES

Household Equivalents (Volume)

Metric	Apothecary	Household
0.06 mL	1 minim	1 drop
5(4) mL	1 fluid dram	1 teaspoonful
15 mL	4 fluid drams	1 tablespoonful
30 mL	1 fluid ounce	2 tablespoonfuls
180 mL	6 fluid ounces	1 teacupful
240 mL	8 fluid ounces	1 glassful

Apothecary Equivalents (Volume)

Metric		Apothecary
1 mL	=	15 minims
1 cc	=	15 minims
0.06 mL	=	1 minim
4 mL	=	1 fluid dram
30 mL	=	1 fluid ounce
500 mL	=	1 pint
1,000 mL (1 L)	=	1 quart

Apothecary Equivalents (Weight)

Metric		Apothecary		
1.0 g	*or*	1,000 mg	=	gr xv
0.6 g	*or*	600 mg	=	gr x
0.5 g	*or*	500 mg	=	gr viiss
0.3 g	*or*	300 mg	=	gr v
0.2 g	*or*	200 mg	=	gr iii
0.1 g	*or*	100 mg	=	gr 1½
0.06 g	*or*	60 mg	=	gr 1
0.05 g	*or*	50 mg	=	gr ¾
0.03 g	*or*	30 mg	=	gr ½
0.015 g	*or*	15 mg	=	gr ¼
0.010 g	*or*	10 mg	=	gr ⅙
0.008 g	*or*	8 mg	=	gr ⅛
4 g			=	1 dr
30 g			=	1 oz
1 kg			=	2.2 lbs

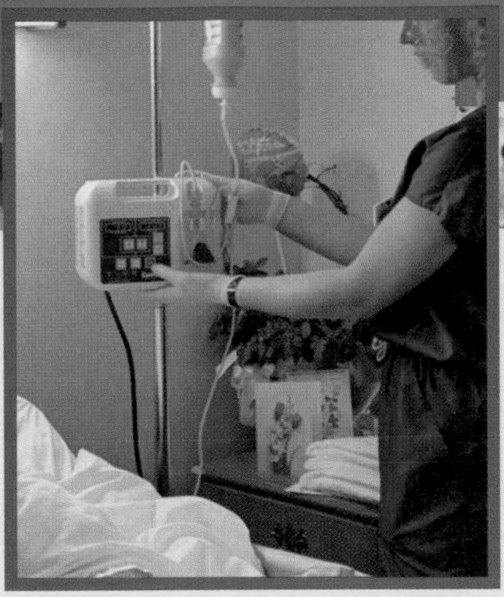

CHAPTER 19

Nutritional Management and NG Intubation

THEORETICAL CONCEPTS

UNIT ONE: **Modified Therapeutic Diets** 588

Restricting Dietary Carbohydrates 589
Restricting Dietary Protein 589
Restricting Dietary Fat 589
Restricting Mineral Nutrients 590
Providing Nutrient Enhanced Diets 590
Providing Modified Diets 591
for Dietary Fiber 591
for Postoperative Diet Progression 591
Providing Consistency Diets 592
for Bland Diet 592
for Mechanical Soft Diet 592
for Pureed Diet 593

UNIT TWO: **Nutrition Maintenance** 595

Serving a Food Tray 596
Assisting the Visually Impaired Client to Eat 596
Assisting the Dysphagic Client to Eat 597

UNIT THREE: **Gastrointestinal Intubation** 599

Inserting a Large-Bore Nasogastric (NG) Tube 600
for Testing Blood in Gastric Specimen 601
for Decompressing the GI Tract 603
Irrigating/Maintaining a Nasogastric (NG) Tube 605
Performing Gastric Lavage 606
Administering Poison Control Agents 607
Removing an NG or Nasointestinal Tube 607

UNIT FOUR: **Enteral Tube Feedings** 610

Giving an Intermittent Feeding via Large-Bore Nasogastric Tube 611
for Intermittent Feeding via Gastrostomy Tube 613
Dressing the Gastrostomy Tube Site 614
Inserting a Small-Bore Feeding Tube 615
Providing Continuous Feeding via Small-Bore Nasointestinal/Jejunostomy Tube 616

GERONTOLOGIC CONSIDERATIONS 619

MANAGEMENT GUIDELINES 621

CRITICAL THINKING STRATEGIES 623

Cross Reference: Hyperalimentation (TPN) and Lipids (Chapter 29)

LEARNING OBJECTIVES

- List the essential nutrients necessary to sustain life.
- Outline the primary differences between vitamins and minerals.
- Describe the primary functions of the gastrointestinal system and accessory organs.
- Discuss precautions used for dysphagic clients.
- Identify the assessment categories important for a total nutritional assessment.
- Describe a sodium-restricted diet and list at least three foods high in sodium.
- Explain what is meant by a postoperative diet protocol.
- Outline the steps for inserting a nasogastric tube.
- Identify the primary steps of administering a tube feeding.
- Discuss at least two potential problems that may occur with a tube feeding and the suggested solutions.
- Outline emergency management to decontaminate the GI tract of toxins/poisons.
- Contrast aspects of gastric vs intestinal tube feedings.
- Discuss potential problems that may occur with tube feedings and possible solutions.

TERMINOLOGY

Alimentary: of or pertaining to nutrition.

Anabolism: reaction in which small molecules are put together to form larger ones—repairing or building up cells.

Anorexia: loss of appetite for food.

Aspirate: to remove fluids or gases by suction.

Aspiration: accidental inspiration of fluid or a foreign body into the airway.

Calorie: the amount of heat necessary to raise the temperature of 1 kilogram of water 1°C. This is the "small" calorie. The dietary, or large, Calorie represents 1000 of these calories, or 1 kilocalorie.

Carbohydrates: a group of chemical substances, including sugars, glycogen, starches, dextrins, and celluloses, that contain only carbon, oxygen, and hydrogen.

Cardio: prefix pertaining to the heart.

Carina: point at which the trachea divides into the right and left bronchi.

Cardiovascular: term that pertains to the heart and blood vessels as cardiovascular system.

Catabolism: reaction in which large molecules are broken down into smaller ones—process of breaking down cells.

Diabetic: one who has inadequate production and/or use of insulin.

Diet: liquid and solid food substances regularly consumed.

Digestion: the process by which food is broken down mechanically and chemically in the gastrointestinal tract.

Diverticulosis: diverticula of the colon without inflammation or symptoms.

Dumping syndrome: symptoms that develop due to rapid entry of undigested food into the jejunum.

Dysphagia: difficulty swallowing.

Emaciation: a condition characterized by extreme leanness or thinness.

Emesis: the act of vomiting.

Enteral nutrition: provision of nutrients via the gastrointestinal tract (includes oral feedings).

Enterostomy: opening into the stomach or jejunum through which a feeding tube can be inserted.

Fat: substance made up of carbon, hydrogen, and oxygen, occurring naturally in most foods but especially in meat and dairy products.

Food supplement: a preparation added to the regular diet that aids nourishment.

Gavage: introduction of nourishment into the GI tract by mechanical means.

Gastrointestinal: term that pertains to the stomach and intestines.

Hematemesis: vomitus containing blood.

Hydrogenation: a chemical process by which hydrogens are added to monounsaturated or polyunsaturated fats, making the fats more saturated.

Hyperalimentation: the process of nourishing the body through parenteral means.

Hyperglycemia: condition characterized by an increase in blood sugar.

Hypertonic: solution having a higher osmotic pressure or tonicity than a solution to which it is compared.

Hypoglycemia: condition characterized by a deficiency of sugar or glucose in the blood.

Ileus: obstruction of the intestine caused by paralysis of the intestinal muscles.

Ingest: the process of taking material into the gastrointestinal tract.

Jejunostomy: surgical creation of a permanent opening into the jejunum.

Kwashiorkor: a state of extreme malnutrition due to severe protein insufficiency.

Lavage: to wash.

Lumen: the inner open space of a tube.

Malnutrition: a condition characterized by a lack of necessary food substances or improper absorption and distribution of food substances in the body.

Minerals: inorganic elements or compounds.

Nasogastric tube: a tube that is passed through the nose and into the stomach.

Nasointestinal tube: small bore flexible tube passed through the nose and advanced to the proximal intestine to be used for short-term feeding.

Nausea: a feeling of sickness accompanied with the urge to vomit.

Nutrient: nourishing; food item that supplies the body with necessary elements.

Obstruction: blocking of a structure that prevents it from functioning normally; obstacle.

Parenteral nutrition: process of providing nutrition via a route other than the alimentary canal, such as intravenous.

PEG: percutaneous endoscopic gastrostomy.

Polyunsaturated: term usually referring to a fat, indicating that the carbon chain has more than one double bond. These fats tend to have higher densities (HDL) than saturated fats.

Projectile vomiting: the expulsion of vomitus with great force.

Proteins: substances that contain amino acids essential for growth and repair of tissues.

Renal: term that pertains to the kidney.

Saturated fatty acid: fatty acid carrying the maximum possible number of hydrogen atoms.

Sepsis: pathologic state usually febrile, resulting from the presence of microorganisms or their poisonous products in the bloodstream.

Trans-fatty acid: a partially hydrogenated mono- or polyunsaturated fat.

Trauma: an injury or wound.

Unsaturated fatty acid: fatty acid that lacks hydrogen atoms and has at least one double bond between carbons (includes polyunsaturated and monounsaturated fatty acids).

Uremia: toxic condition associated with end-stage renal disease and the retention of nitrogenous substances in the blood.

Vitamins: a group of organic substances essential for life.

NUTRITIONAL MANAGEMENT

Nutrition is comprised of essential nutrients—carbohydrates, fats, proteins, vitamins, minerals, and water—all of which are necessary for growth and development through the life cycle. When these are supplied to the body in proper balance, the body uses them for energy, growth and development, tissue repair, and regulation and maintenance of body processes.

Food is undeniably necessary for maintenance of life, and is, as a symbol, equally important to man's psychological health. Food has powerful social meaning as it promotes hospitality, companionship, and kinship, and perpetuates ethnic heritage and traditional customs. While these emotional and social aspects are influential in food choices, they are not necessarily based on an awareness of the importance of nutrition in health.

Proper balanced nutrition helps to promote health and prevent illness, and is essential to maintain normal metabolic processes of growth, development, and healing. The recommended dietary allowance (RDA), designed by the U.S. Department of Agriculture is a widely accepted standard for levels of nutrient sufficiency to meet the needs of *healthy* persons. As with any balance, excesses or deficiencies of these RDA goals can have general and long-lasting adverse effects on health.

ESSENTIAL NUTRIENTS

Essential nutrients cannot be synthesized by the body, but healthy individuals can *satisfy* essential nutrient (RDA) recommendations by following food group intake guidelines illustrated in the "Food Guide Pyramid" published by the U.S. Department of Agriculture. ("Food Guide Pyramids" have also been developed for the elderly, children, vegetarians, and for various ethnic groups [Mediterranean, Asian, and Latin American] to promote healthful nutrition.) This pyramid depicts a *hierarchy* that encourages intake from all food groups but emphasizes *greater* consumption of foods at the big *base*, and lesser consumption of foods at the smaller *apex*. These foods provide the following *essential* nutrients (**macronutrients** include carbohydrates, fats, and proteins; **micronutrients** include vitamins and minerals).

The food guide recommendations are easy to follow because one can select from a variety of foods *within* each major food group. Selections should be relatively low in fat (particularly saturated, hydrogenated and trans-fatty acids, and cholesterol), salt, and simple or refined sugars. It is also important to understand what constitutes a single food group "serving"; one 6-ounce pretzel eaten at the fair would satisfy all the bread group recommendation for one day. Seldom referred to, the "Food Guide

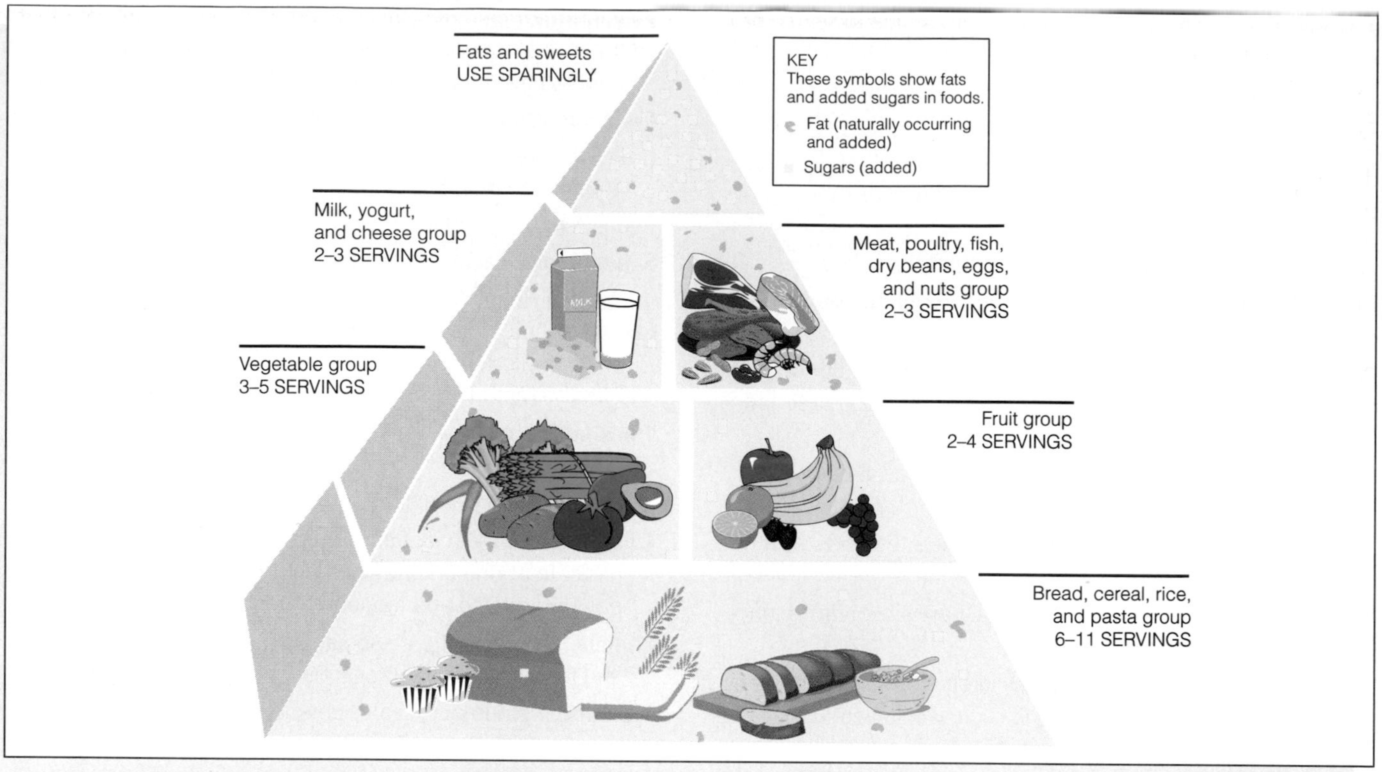

USDA Food Guide Pyramid (U.S. Department of Agriculture, U.S. Department of Health and Human Services, Washington, D.C., 2002).

Pyramid" also lists the amount of food that counts as one serving.

In addition to following recommendations in these guides, food intake should be balanced with regular physical activity in order to maintain ideal body weight and avoid obesity (excess amount of body fat), which is the greatest form of malnutrition in the United States. Obesity is associated with increased morbidity and mortality. It is recommended that body mass index (weight in kilograms divided by height in meters squared) should be kept within the range of 20–26.

TABLE 19–1 Food Guide Pyramid: Serving Size

What Counts as One Serving?		
Milk, yogurt, and cheese		
1 cup milk or yogurt	1.5 oz natural cheese	2 oz processed cheese
Meat, poultry, fish, dry beans, eggs, and nuts		
2–3 oz cooked lean meat, poultry, or fish		½ cup cooked dry beans, 1 egg, or 2 tbsp peanut butter, (counts as 1 oz of meat)
Vegetables		
1 cup raw, leafy vegetables	½ cup other vegetable, cooked or chopped, raw	¾ cup vegetable juice
Fruits		
1 med apple, banana, orange	½ cup chopped, cooked, or canned fruit	¾ cup fruit juice
Bread, cereal, rice, and pasta		
1 slice bread	1 oz ready to eat cereal	½ cup cooked cereal, rice, or pasta

MACRONUTRIENTS

Carbohydrates

Carbohydrates are the chief source of energy and contain carbon, hydrogen, and oxygen. Carbohydrates include sugars, starches, and cellulose. Simple sugars, such as fruit sugar, are easily digested. Starches, which are more complex, require more sophisticated enzyme processes to be reduced to glucose, the end product of carbohydrate metabolism. Glucose, which is converted sugars and starches, appears in the body as blood sugar and is "burned" as fuel by the tissues. Some glucose is processed by the liver, converted to glycogen, and stored by the liver for later use.

Ingesting too many carbohydrates crowds out other important foods and prevents the body from receiving the necessary nutrients for healthy maintenance. Too few carbohydrates may lead to loss of energy, depression, ketosis, and a breakdown of body protein. Although differences in individual body structure, energy expenditure, basal metabolism, and general health status determine the amount and kind of carbohydrates that should be consumed for optimal health, there are general guidelines. While the average American diet provides 45% of calories from carbohydrate, it is recommended that simple (refined) sugars be limited to 10% of total calories since they contain no nutrients. The Select Committee on Nutrition and Human Needs of the U.S. Senate recommends 55–60% of calories come from complex carbohydrates.

Fats

Fats or lipids are the second important group of nutrients. Fats also provide energy. In fact, when oxidized, they are the most concentrated sources of energy and, as such, furnish the calories necessary for survival. Fats also act as carriers for the fat-soluble vitamins, A, D, E, and K. Consuming too much fat can lead to weight problems and poor metabolism of food products. The optimal percentage of fat in the diet is 25–30% of our daily caloric intake, but the average American diet provides 35–40% of calories from fat. High-fat diets increase the risk of developing atherosclerotic cardiovascular disease and cancer.

Fatty acids are the basic components of fat and comprise two main groups. Saturated fatty acids usually come from animal sources. It is recommended that we *decrease* total fat intake and *substitute* saturated (hydrogenated) fats with polyunsaturated and monounsaturated fats. Saturated fats are solid at room temperature and should not exceed 10% of calories; cholesterol intake should be limited to less than 300 mg daily. Unsaturated fatty acids primarily come from vegetables, nuts, or seed sources. In the unsaturated group are three essential fatty acids. These acids are called "essential" because they are necessary to ensure health and growth and the body cannot manufacture them. They must therefore be obtained from the diet. These three acids are linoleic acid, arachidonic acid, and linolenic acid. They are necessary for healthy blood, arteries, nerves, and skin. A deficiency in this group leads to skin problems and illness.

Essential Body Nutrients

- Carbohydrates
  - Monosaccharides
    - Glucose, fructose, galactose
  - Disaccharides
    - Sucrose, lactose, maltose
  - Polysaccharides
    - Starch, dextrin, glycogen, cellulose, hemicellulose
- Fats
  - Linoleic acid, linolenic acid, arachidonic acid
- Proteins
  - Amino acids
    - Phenylalanine, lysine, isoleucine, leucine, methionine, valine, tryptophan, threonine, and histidine (required by infants, not adults)
- Vitamins
  - Fat-soluble
    - Vitamins A, D, E, and K
  - Water soluble
    - Vitamins B_1, B_2, B_6, B_{12}, niacin, pantothenic acid, folacin, biotin, choline, *meso*-inositol, *para*-aminobenzoic acid, and vitamin C
- Minerals
  - Major elements
    - Calcium, chloride, iron, magnesium, phosphorous, potassium, sodium, sulfur
- Water
  - Trace elements

Proteins

Proteins, the third essential group of nutrients, are complex organic compounds that contain amino acids. Proteins are critical to all aspects of growth and development of body tissues. They are necessary for the building of muscles, blood, skin, internal organs, hormones, and enzymes and are also a source of energy when there is insufficient carbohydrate or fat in the diet. When protein is spared, it is either used for tissue repair and maintenance or converted by the liver and stored as fat.

When digested and broken down, proteins form 20 amino acids. (Some nutritional experts maintain that there are 22 essential amino acids.) These amino acids are then absorbed from the intestine into the bloodstream and carried to the liver for synthesis into the tissues and organs of the body. They are the chemical basis for life, and if just one is missing, protein synthesis decreases or even stops. All but nine of the amino acids can be produced by the body. These nine must be obtained from the diet. Eight essential amino acids are required by all humans. Infants require one more, histidine. If all are present in a particular food, the food is a "complete protein." Foods that lack one or more of these essential amino acids are called "incomplete proteins." Most meat and dairy products are complete proteins, and most vegetables and fruits are incomplete. When several incomplete proteins form the major portion of a person's diet, they should be combined carefully so that the result is a balance yielding complete protein. For example, the combination of beans and rice is perfectly balanced to give a complete protein food.

It is difficult to determine the exact amount of protein needed to supply all of the essential amino acids because there are many variables. Height and weight, level of activity, and nutritional and health status all influence the amount of protein necessary for a healthy body. The National Research Council recommends that 0.42 gram (g) of protein be consumed per day per pound of body weight or 56 g/day for men and 45 g/day for women. The optimal healthy diet should be 10 to 12% protein, rather than the 17% that most Americans consume as part of their total calorie intake. It appears that as long as the essential amino acids are included in the diet, the total grams of protein can be reduced.

Protein deficiency can affect the entire body—organs, tissues, skin, and muscles—as well as certain body processes. If a child is deficient in protein, he or she may suffer from kwashiorkor, a disease resulting in physical and mental impairment and, if severe enough, death. If an adult is deficient in protein, his or her stamina, mental state, and ability to withstand stress and infection is affected. Protein deficiency also interferes with recovery from diseases or surgery.

Protein is very plentiful in the body. It is an integral part of all cells and essential for growth and development. Just like fats and carbohydrates, adequate protein must be consumed in balance with other nutrients for human survival.

Water

Although not specifically a nutrient, water is essential for survival. Water is involved in every body process from digestion and absorption to excretion. It is a major portion of circulation and is the transporter of nutrients throughout the body.

Body water performs three major functions: it gives form to the body, constituting 50–75% of the body mass; it provides the necessary environment for cell metabolism; and it maintains a stable body temperature.

Almost all foods contain water that is absorbed by the body. The average adult body contains about 53 liters of water and loses 2.8 liters a day. If a person suffers severe water depletion, dehydration can result and can eventually lead to death. A person can survive several weeks without food but only days without water. In order to prevent dehydration (water loss exceeding water intake), a general requirement is to drink 2–3 liters of water daily, or 1 mL/kcal expenditure. Measures of intake and output assist the health care team in identifying and correcting body water imbalances.

MICRONUTRIENTS

Vitamins

Vitamins are organic food substances and are essential in small amounts for growth, maintenance, and the functioning of body processes. Vitamins are found only in living things—plants and animals—and usually cannot be synthesized by the human body.

Vitamins can be grouped according to the substance in which they are soluble. The fat-soluble group includes vitamins A, D, E, and K. These vitamins are measured in international units. Each unit generally refers to the amount of the vitamin needed to produce a change in the nutritional health of a laboratory animal. The water-soluble vitamins include eight B complex vitamins, vitamin C, and the bioflavonoids. These are usually measured in milligrams.

Vitamins have no calorie value, but they are as necessary to the body as any other basic nutrient. Currently, there are about 20 substances identified as vitamins, but recent research is concerned with identifying even more of these substances since they are so essential to survival.

For many years research groups have attempted to determine basic vitamin requirements for various age groups. The most commonly used are the listings of the Recommended Dietary Allowances (RDA) and Adequate Intakes (2001), based on standards established by the National Academy of Sciences.

Minerals

Minerals are inorganic substances, widely prevalent in nature, and essential for metabolic processes. Minerals are grouped according to the amount found in the body. *Major minerals* include calcium, magnesium, sodium, potassium, phosphorus, sulfur, and chlorine, all of which have a known function in the body. Major minerals are measured in milligrams. A second group—*trace minerals*—are iron, copper, iodine, manganese, cobalt, zinc, fluorine, selenium, and molybdenum. These minerals are measured in micrograms, and their function in the body remains unclear. There remains another group of trace minerals (such as boron, silica, nickel, vanadium, etc.) found in scanty amounts in the body and whose function is also unclear. Minerals form 60–90% of all inorganic material in the body and are found in bones, teeth, soft tissue, muscle, blood, and nerve cells.

Vitamins for Everyone

In fact, a recent article in the *Journal of the American Medical Association* advocated that everyone, young and old, should take a basic multivitamin and mineral daily supplement.

Source: See Journal of the American Medical Association, p. 596.

Minerals act on organs and in metabolic processes. They act as catalysts for many reactions, such as controlling muscle responses, maintaining the nervous system and acid–base balance, transmitting messages, maintaining cardiac stability, and regulating the metabolism and absorption of other nutrients. Even though they are considered separately, all minerals work synergistically with other minerals, and their actions are interrelated. A deficiency in one mineral, therefore, affects the action of others in the body. It is essential that adequate minerals be ingested because a mineral deficiency can result in severe illness. Likewise, excessive amounts of minerals can throw the body out of balance and may be toxic to the body. This is especially so of certain trace minerals.

Sufficient minerals can be supplied by adequate diet. Even though RDAs have not been established on all minerals, a diet that contains all the other nutrients usually supplies the necessary amount of minerals for the body. Many nutritionists and biochemists, however, recommend a daily basic vitamin–mineral supplement to ensure adequate levels.

RDAs AND DRIs

The **RDAs** for essential nutrients judged to be adequate for a healthy person provides most fat-soluble and water-soluble vitamins and minerals. These needs are met by ingesting a variety of common foods. Excessive levels of dietary supplements in excess of the RDAs (e.g., use of multivitamins) may have toxic systemic effects.

In addition to the RDAs for essential *macronutrients,* **DRIs** (dietary reference intakes) recognize the health benefits of other dietary (*micronutrient*) components in the prevention of chronic diseases. Recommendations for micronutrients are evolving. DRIs include a set of values called **Upper Intake levels.** These values represent the maximum amount of a nutrient that is safe for most people on a daily basis. These values may be found at the National Academy of Sciences, courtesy of the National Academy Press, Washington, D.C.

- **In 1997,** the DRI recommended intake of *five nutrients for bone health*: calcium, phosphorus, magnesium, vitamin D, and fluoride.
- **In 1998,** recommendations were expanded to include the *eight B vitamins* and choline.
- **In 2000,** the focus relates to *beta carotene and antioxidant nutrients* (vitamins C and E and selenium).
- **In 2001,** recommendations included fat-soluble vitamins A and K and a dozen minerals.

As new knowledge surfaces about the importance of nutrients for basic health, the recommended intake reflects this increased awareness. The box, left column, shows an example of the changes in recommended nutrients over the previous 5 years.

NUTRITIONAL ASSESSMENT

No single parameter is sufficient to determine a client's nutritional status. Initial screening of the hospitalized client is performed by the professional nurse on admission.

In general, the nurse asks the client about a recent change in body weight of 10 pounds or more in the last 6 months, nausea, vomiting, diarrhea lasting more than 5 days, any declining food intake, difficulty chewing or swallowing, and time/duration of recent hospitalizations. Results of this screening may classify the client at "nutrition risk" (need for dietitian consult). Unfortunately, many clients are unable to provide the essential subjective information.

Objective measures of nutritional status include weight in relation to height, monitoring dietary intakes with calorie counts, examination for signs of micronutrient deficiencies, and laboratory tests such as serum albumin, transferrin, and prealbumin; tests of cellular immunity; and total lymphocyte count. Other measures include evaluation of body composition by visual inspection or anthropometric measurements (triceps skin fold, mid-arm muscle circumference). *See* Nutritional Assessment Parameters, Table 19–2.

ASSIMILATION OF NUTRIENTS

Following the discussion of the essential body nutrients, it is now important to identify how these elements are broken down, absorbed, and used in the body. Nutrients, in most cases, are ingested through the mouth, and must be broken down by the body. This process is called digestion. It starts in the mouth, and continues in the stomach and the small and large intestines.

The total daily energy requirement of an individual is the number of calories needed to replace the energy loss from the metabolic rate, plus loss from a person's physical, emotional, and mental output. The number of calories ingested should be directly related to maintaining an adequate energy level and supporting the body's metabolic processes.

Gastrointestinal Tract

The main functions of the gastrointestinal system are the secretion of enzymes and electrolytes to break down raw materials that are ingested; the movement of the ingested products through the system; the complete digestion of

TABLE 19–2 Nutritional Assessment Parameters

Clinical Assessment	Normal	Abnormal
Dietary Data		
Appetite	Remains unchanged	Increased or decreased recently Particular cravings
Nutritional intake	Adequate foods and fluids to supply body nutrients Nonallergic response to major food groups	Elimination of certain food categories that results in limited nutrients Emphasis on some food groups (sugar) to the exclusion of others (vegetables) Allergic response to certain foods
Caloric intake	Average 28 KcaL/Kg/day	Constant use of fad diets to lose weight Use of drugs or chemicals that interfere with appetite or nutrient assimilation
Meal patterns	3–6 home-prepared meals/day Adequate time and calm atmosphere for meals	Fast-food or packaged foods Missed meals, constant snacking, or overeating Eating "on the run" or hurried
General Appearance	Alert, responsive healthy appearing eyes and skin	Listless, dull, nonresponsive Skin and eyes appear unhealthy
Physical factors	Adequate chewing and swallowing capability Mouth and gums healthy so food can be ingested Physical exercise adequate for calorie intake	Teeth or gums in poor condition or ill-fitting dentures Swallowing impairs ingestion Inadequate physical exercise to burn calories
Presence of disease	No disease process that interferes with nutrient assimilation No congenital condition or postsurgery condition that interferes with nutrient assimilation	Disease present that interferes with ingestion, digestion, assimilation, or excretion Congenital condition, rehabilitation phase, or postsurgery that interferes with food assimilation
Elimination schedule	Regular, adequate elimination of foods Absence of constant flatus, discharge, or mucus	Irregular or painful elimination Presence of constant flatus Presence of discharge, blood, or mucus
Anthropometric Measurements		
Height	For bedridden clients, measure arm span—fully extend arms 90° angle to body and measure from tip of one middle finger to the tip of other middle finger for estimated height	Loss of 2–3 inches in height may indicate osteoporosis
Weight—compared to ideal and usual body weight	Ideal body weight 100 lbs (female); 106 lbs (male) for 5 feet height + 5 lbs for each 1 inch over 5 feet (female) and 6 lbs for each 1 inch over 5 feet (male). Small frame minus 10% Large frame plus 10%	Changed—markedly increased or decreased recently: important indicator of changed nutritional status Loss of more than 10% weight for prior 6 months should be clinically evaluated.
Body Mass Index Ratio of weight in kilograms and height in meters.	18.5–24.9	Less than 18.5—underweight 25–29—overweight 30–39—obese
Triceps skinfold measurement (mm)	Standard values—male to female 12.5–16.5	If values change over months, may indicate a chronic condition
Circumference of upper arm (cm)	29.3–28.5	
Midarm muscle circumference (cm)	25.3–23.2	Hydration status may influence results

TABLE 19–2 Nutritional Assessment Parameters *(continued)*

Clinical Assessment	Normal	Abnormal
Biochemical Assessments*		Examples of possible disease conditions:
Serum albumin	3.5–5.0 g/dL	Decrease signifies lowered nutritional status—protein deficient
Serum transferrin binds iron to plasma and transports to bone marrow	200–430 mg/dL	Reduced levels may indicate chronic diseases and protein deficiency Elevated levels—anemias, liver damage, lead toxicity
Hemoglobin	Male—13.5–17 g/dL Female—12–15 g/dL	Decreased related to iron deficiency (anemias and leukemia)
Prealbumin (PA) serum	20–50 mg/dL	Decreased—protein wasting diseases, malnutrition (< 10.7 indicates severe nutritional deficiency) Elevated—Hodgkin's disease
Blood urea nitrogen/creatinine	10:1–20:1	Nitrogen imbalance, inadequate renal functioning
24-hour urinary nitrogen	Positive balance	Inadequate protein intake
Sociocultural Data		
Cultural–religious factors	Ability to afford adequate foods in all food categories Cultural beliefs that do not eliminate whole food groups Religious beliefs that do not eliminate whole food groups	Economic position that precludes purchase of adequate food Religious or cultural beliefs that interfere with receiving balanced diet (macrobiotic diets) Inadequate knowledge, experience, or intelligence to prepare healthy meals
Ethnicity	Traditional foods that do not eliminate whole food groups	Beliefs and ethnic preference that eliminate major nutrients from the diet
Lifestyle	Well-balanced meals that include all nutrients Food does not lose all nutrient value in preparation	Fast-paced stressful lifestyle that incorporates fastfood or convenience foods deficient in nutrients or imbalanced (high-fat)

*Laboratory test parameters differ among laboratories. Check the reference range for the specific lab where the client's blood or urine was tested.

nutrients and their absorption into the blood; and the storage or excretion of the end products of digestion.

Chewing food is the first stage of breaking down food. When nutrients reach the stomach, both mechanical and chemical digestive processes occur.

The average meal remains in the stomach for 3 hours where digestion continues. The stomach's secretion of hydrochloric acid and pepsin break down proteins, while the *acid pH* environment helps protect against ingested pathogens. Vomiting or suction removal of *acid* gastric contents (primarily HCl, Na, and K) can lead to fluid and electrolyte imbalance with metabolic *alkalosis* (high bicarbonate and elevated pH on arterial blood gases [ABGs]). H_2 receptor antagonists (e.g., cimetidine) make gastric secretions less acid, so their administration reduces the risk of metabolic alkalosis and electrolyte disturbance in clients who require gastric secretion suction (decompression).

The stomach's mechanical processes occur with intervals of peristalsis and relaxation of the pyloric sphincter as gastric content (chyme) moves into the small intestine (duodenum). Digestive processes continue within the small intestine (duodenum, jejunum, ileum) as enzymes break down protein to amino acids, fats to glycerol and fatty acids, and carbohydrates to monosaccharides. Here, most nutrients and water are absorbed into the circulation. While 7–10 liters of electrolyte-rich secretions mix with the chyme, only 600–800 mL enter the large intestine. Small intestine secretions have an *alkaline pH*, making this environment more vulnerable to bacterial invasion. *Alkaline* intestinal fluid loss (e.g., due to diarrhea, intestinal decompression), can lead to fluid and electrolyte imbalance with metabolic *acidosis* (low bicarbonate and low pH on ABGs).

The ileocecal valve separates the small intestine from the large intestine. In the large intestine, fluids and electrolytes continue to be absorbed to solidify the stool, and mucus is secreted to lubricate waste as it moves toward the rectum for storage and final elimination of stool which contains approximately 200 mL water.

The Accessory Organs

The accessory organs of the gastrointestinal tract also play an important role in the use of nutrients. These organs include the tongue, salivary glands, teeth, liver, gallbladder, and pancreas.

The liver is especially important because it has a major role in the metabolism of carbohydrates, fats, and proteins. In carbohydrate metabolism, the liver converts glucose to glycogen and stores it. The liver then can reconvert glycogen to glucose when the body requires higher blood sugar. The process of releasing carbohydrates (end products) into the bloodstream is called glycogenolysis.

The liver metabolizes fats through the process of oxidation of fatty acids and the formation of acetoacetic acid. Also, the liver forms lipoproteins, cholesterol, and phospholipids and converts carbohydrates and protein to fats.

Proteins are metabolized in the liver, where deamination of amino acids takes place. Also in this process, the formation of urea and plasma proteins is completed. Finally, the interconversion of amino acids and other compounds occurs in the liver.

The gallbladder's primary function is to act as a reservoir for bile. When fatty materials are in the duodenum, liberation of cholecystokinin is stimulated and the gallbladder contracts, causing the relaxation of the sphincter of Oddi. Bile emulsifies fats through constant secretion (500–1000 mL in 24 hours).

The pancreas secretes pancreatic juices that contain enzymes for the digestion of carbohydrates, fats, and proteins. Enzymes are secreted as inactive precursors that do not become active until secreted into the small intestine. In the intestine, the enzyme trypsin acts on proteins to produce peptones, peptides, and amino acids; pancreatic amylase acts on carbohydrates to produce disaccharides; and pancreatic lipase acts on fats to produce glycerol and fatty acids.

In summary, the alimentary tract's primary function is to provide the body with a continuous supply of nutrients by ingestion and moving food and fluids, secreting digestive juices for breaking down the food, and absorbing the resulting nutrients, water, and electrolytes. Nutrients are essential for life, but their simple ingestion into the body is not sufficient for survival. They must be broken down, absorbed, and used efficiently if the body is to remain in proper balance or homeostasis.

GASTROINTESTINAL DYSFUNCTIONS

Dysphagia

Dysphagia (difficulty swallowing) may be due to dysfunction of neurologic pathways or from dysfunction of muscles of the swallowing tract. It occurs in as many as 60% of stroke clients and 50% of those with Parkinson's disease. Others who experience *dysphagia* are those with esophageal reflux, cerebral palsy, multiple sclerosis, polio, amyotrophic lateral sclerosis and myasthenia gravis. The most serious complication of dysphagia is aspiration of liquid or food into the lungs, creating an environment conducive to bacterial growth. A protective cough normally prevents aspiration, but 50% of clients who aspirate do so *without* coughing, so aspiration goes undetected until pneumonia develops. A complex disorder, dysphagia requires an individualized diagnosis and management by collaborative experts: radiologist, occupational therapist, speech pathologist, and dietitian.

GI Hemorrhage

The gastric blood from GI hemorrhage is an irritant that usually triggers vomiting, which may aggravate the bleeding. Clients with impaired liver function are an example of those most likely to experience a gastric bleed, but these clients are also unable to process the protein load created by digestion and absorption of blood. The digestion of blood can cause a precipitous rise in serum ammonia, which can lead to altered neurologic function (somnolence, loss of coordination, coma). Lavage (washing) per gastric intubation removes blood to prevent this "metabolic encephalopathy," and also allows estimation of the client's acute blood loss. This same lavage process may be used to remove ingested poisonous substances in order to prevent their digestion and absorption.

Intestinal Obstruction

When gastrointestinal processes are disrupted, intestinal "obstruction" develops. Cessation of peristalsis (ileus) due to neurogenic impairment (traumatic stress), abdominal pathology, electrolyte imbalance (hypokalemia), or bowel manipulation (as in surgery) results in altered GI movement and absorption, allowing secretions and gas to accumulate. Temporary decompression to remove fluids and gas may be necessary in some instances because progressive accumulation of gases and fluid distends the bowel, compresses bowel wall capillaries, and can lead to septic shock, as well as hypovolemic shock. Decompression may also alleviate pain, nausea and vomiting, and reduce the possibility of aspiration.

Decompression Decompression requires the insertion of a nasogastric tube, which is connected to continuous or intermittent negative pressure suction while the client is kept NPO and given IV fluids. Since gastrointestinal secretions are isotonic with extracellular fluid, a guideline for fluid replacement is to administer a volume of normal saline (or one-half normal saline with KCl) equivalent to the previous day's drained secretions. It is important to check client's voiding record before adding KCl to IV fluids. A unique feature of the GI tract is that its nutrition is derived directly (rather than from the bloodstream), so early ambulation, termination of decompression, and resumption of PO intake are recommended. The return of bowel sounds and passage of flatus are indicators that GI function has returned and is able to accommodate PO intake.

NORMAL AND THERAPEUTIC NUTRITION

Normal nutrition is based on recommended daily dietary allowances. These standards are scientifically designed for the maintenance of nearly all healthy people in the United States.

Therapeutic nutrition is a modification of nutritional needs based on the disease condition or the excess or deficit of a nutrition state. Combination diets, which include alterations in minerals, vitamins, proteins, carbohydrates, fats, as well as fluid and texture, are prescribed.

Whether a normal or a therapeutic diet is being considered, a person's cultural, socioeconomic, and psychologic influences, as well as the physiologic requirements, must be taken into account for effective nutrition; thus, in any given situation, the nutritional requirements must be considered within the context of the total needs of an individual.

Diet Related to Risk for Heart Disease

Since the 1950s, when the lipid hypothesis was introduced, the amount of saturated fat and cholesterol in the diet was implicated as a risk for coronary artery disease. Anyone who had a cholesterol level over 200 was told they were in jeopardy; later, research showed that it was not just the total cholesterol level, but the ratio of "good" cholesterol or high-density lipoproteins (HDLs) to "bad" cholesterol or low-density lipoproteins (LDLs).

New theories of risk continue to emerge. One that is supported by hundreds of clinical studies is that a high concentration of homocysteine in the blood is a serious risk factor for heart disease. For example, two major studies published in the *Annals of Internal Medicine* as early as September 7, 1999, showed that even mildly elevated levels of homocysteine were associated with an increased risk of death from cardiovascular disease. A more current analysis of observational studies suggests that elevated homocysteine may be a modest predictor of ischemic heart disease and stroke risk in healthy populations (*JAMA*, October 2002). How is this related to diet? Supplements of folic acid, vitamin B_6, and vitamin B_{12} lower homocysteine levels.

Homocysteine is an amino acid that is formed when there is a high consumption of methionine in the diet; methionine is found in meats and dairy products. Homocysteine is a chemical that, when circulating in excess levels in the bloodstream, can damage artery walls, causing the vessel to trap circulating cholesterol. Current thinking is that the trigger that starts this process is not simply cholesterol or fat, but a high level of homocysteine. A healthy level of homocysteine is 8.72 µmol/L for men and 7.52 µmol/L for women. The *New England Journal of Medicine* recently published a study that showed elevated homocysteine is a risk factor 14.4 times greater than high cholesterol for cardiovascular disease. Increasing daily intake of the major B vitamins (folic acid, pyridoxinen, and vitamin B_{12}) may reduce homocysteine levels.

Nutritional Problems in the Hospital

In a hospital, nutrition is frequently neglected as a vital component of client care. Clients may become more malnourished the longer they remain in a hospital.

For clients who seem to be stable on admission and give no history of nutritionally related food problems, the usual hospital diet is adequate; however, all clients must be reassessed periodically to prevent nutritional problems from developing. A periodic assessment is especially important for clients hospitalized for a long time. In many long-term care facilities, clients are weighed monthly.

For clients identified as having a nutritional problem, a nursing care plan must be developed. To treat these clients correctly, the cause of depletion must first be determined. Research indicates that poor food intake is the leading cause of malnutrition. Reasons for poor food intake include fear, anxiety, or depression prior to or during hospitalization. Some clients may not be capable of feeding themselves or may have poorly fitting dentures. Treatment and therapy may limit a client's ability to eat or interfere with his or her appetite. Also, some clients may have the desire to eat and have a good appetite, but shortly after eating a certain food, experience cramps, pain, gas, or diarrhea or feel nauseous or vomit. This eventually leads to less food intake. Whatever the source, the cause of depletion must be determined to prevent further malnutrition.

ENTERAL FEEDING FOR NUTRITIONAL SUPPORT

Well-nourished clients can tolerate a short period of *caloric balance deficit* such as that occurring with a brief illness or surgery, because the body's fat stores provide calories during such periods. Nutrient guidelines for healthy persons, however, are not meant to meet the needs of clients whose nutritional status is altered by illness that affects oral intake and nutrient digestion, its absorption or utilization. Studies indicate that malnutrition (protein and calorie deficiency) is present in as many as 50% of hospitalized clients, and that clients become more malnourished the longer the hospital stay. Clients with negative nitrogen balance (reduced serum albumin, reduced prealbumin) have already lost structural and functional proteins, have poor surgical outcomes, increased infection rates and prolonged hospital stays. Enteral nutrition may be prescribed for these clients, those unable or unwilling to eat, or those who need a supplement to ingested food, as well as for clients in catabolic states with intensive caloric requirement (e.g., burn, trauma client).

Enteral feeding is preferred over parenteral (intravenous) nutrition because it is safer, less expensive, and associated with fewer complications. It helps to maintain GI function and speeds regeneration of the small intestine, which receives its nutrition from food directly rather than from the bloodstream. Enteral nutrition preserves production of humoral antibodies, reduces gut bacterial overgrowth, and, by helping to maintain the gut's protective mucosal barrier, reduces risk of sepsis. Since the intestine is less prone to ileus than the stomach and large intestine, postoperative feeding into the small intestine is feasible even though the client is "NPO."

Enteral formulas come in powder form to reconstitute, or as ready-to-use liquids. They contain all or just one of the following: protein, carbohydrates, fat, electrolytes, and vitamins and minerals, depending on the client's needs. Isotonic formulas provide 1 cal/mL and are most commonly used. Modified formulas are available for clients with specific nutritional requirements: lactose-free or lactose-containing, fiber-containing, elemental (predigested), or modular formulations that provide additional macronutrient components (lipid, carbohydrate, or protein). Specialized formulas are also available for trauma clients or those with pulmonary disease (low-carbohydrate formula), renal failure, diabetes, liver failure, or immune deficiency.

Many types of nasogastric/nasointestinal tubes are available for enteral feeding. Large-bore nasogastric tubes are inserted for short-term (one week) intermittent feedings which are delivered by gravity through a syringe or in an infusion pump 4–6 times daily. If nutritional support is indicated for an extended period (6 weeks), a long, soft, flexible, small-bore tube made of silastic or polyurethane is placed nasointestinally (advanced beyond the pylorus). Small-bore tubes are more comfortable for the client, and feeding may be continuous infusion using a pump. The client's position must be kept with head of bed elevated 30°. Feeding into the small intestine is associated with greater risk of infection due to the intestine's alkaline (less protected) environment.

For clients with a history of gastric reflux or tube feeding–related aspiration pneumonia, a small-bore jejunostomy tube may be placed surgically or by laparoscopy. Special "dual-purpose tubes" (e.g., Moss) can be placed at the time of surgery to provide gastric decompression and simultaneous (early postoperative) feeding into a functional small intestine while the client is NPO (e.g., Moss tube).

For *extended nutritional support*, (feeding over 6 weeks), tubes are placed surgically through the abdominal wall, directly into the stomach (gastrostomy, percutaneous endoscopic gastrostomy [PEG] or small intestine (jejunostomy). These directly placed tubes are secured by stabilizing bars (bumpers), a large mushroom tip, or a balloon inflated with water (similar to a Foley retention catheter).

Therapeutic Management

After determining the cause and the extent of depletion, the next step is to institute therapeutic procedures that meet the needs of the client. In selecting nutrients, the dietitian will evaluate the status of the client's gastrointestinal tract to determine if modifications in nutrients are necessary. For example, can the client split intact protein into the peptides and amino acids needed for absorption? Can the client tolerate the osmotic load of monosaccharides or disaccharides? Is the client fat intolerant, or does he or she need special fat? Is the client lactose intolerant? Can the client eat normally?

Most of us consider that eating and mealtime is a social time. Frequently, however, nurses place clients in uncomfortable and even unsocial positions so that eating is not a pleasure. In preparing the client's environment for eating, try to make him or her as comfortable as possible. For example, it is important to plan painful or uncomfortable procedures so that they are not immediately before or after meals. Position the client as near to normal as possible; that is, sitting in a chair, dangling on the side of the bed, or with the bed elevated 90°. Provide a bright, nonodorous environment. If possible, position roommates so they can converse while eating if they so desire. Check the client care plan for client preferences: cultural or religious limitations as well as allergies and personal likes or dislikes. Food trays should be checked for compliance with orders and client preferences. If the client is NPO, be sure that a sign is posted on the unit door and that the client does *not* receive a tray.

When you are preparing to assist the client to eat, lower the side rail and place the tray table over the client's lap low enough so that he or she can see what is on it. If the tray is not neatly arranged, rearrange it. Food appearance and presentation influence appetite. Assist the client with whatever is needed, such as cutting meat. If the client is unable to drink from a glass, provide a straw or special cup.

Be sensitive to the client's response to food, and continually attempt to orient feeding to meet the client's needs. If the client has diminished sight or is blind but able to feed him or herself, tell the client what is on the tray and the position of each item. Often, it is clearer to describe position of foods by a clock; for example, chicken at 12, green beans at 3 o'clock.

After therapeutic diets have been ordered, it is critical that the nurse be aware of compliance by the client. The nurse is most closely involved with the client and is the one who can best determine the client's actual intake. The nurse should ensure that the client is not receiving inappropriate foods from other sources and that the client is actually eating the foods prescribed. If the prescribed diet is not meeting the client's needs, an alternative method of feeding might be considered. For example, if oral feedings prove inadequate, then alternative methods, such as feeding by nasogastric, nasoduodenal, or nasojejunal tube, should be considered. A variety of delivery systems and methods of enteral feeding are now available for adequate care of the client. The particular choice should be based on the individual client's needs and requirements.

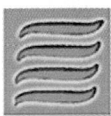

NURSING DIAGNOSES

The following nursing diagnoses are appropriate to use on client care plans when the components are related to nutritional problems or nutritional health maintenance.

NURSING DIAGNOSIS	RELATED FACTORS
Deficient Knowledge	Lack of appropriate dietary information, misinterpretation of information, cognitive limitation, inadequate motivation
Noncompliance to Diet	Chronic illness, disease-related symptoms, side effects of therapy, financial status, cultural practices
Imbalanced Nutrition: Less than Body Requirements	Impaired swallowing, faulty metabolism, dysphagia, altered level of consciousness, inadequate absorption, eating disorders
Imbalanced Nutrition: More than Body Requirements	Lack of basic nutritional knowledge, excessive intake in relation to metabolic requirements, decreased activity patterns, decreased metabolic needs, eating disorders

- The single most important nursing action to decrease the incidence of hospital-based infections is handwashing. **Remember to wash your hands or use antibacterial gel before and after each and every client contact**.

UNIT 1

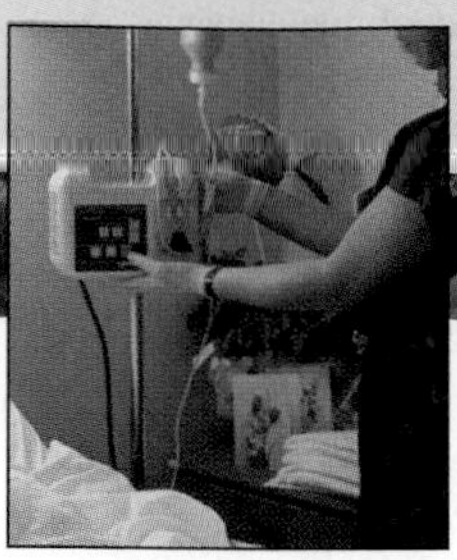

Modified Therapeutic Diets

Nursing Process Data

ASSESSMENT Data Base

Assess total health status of client—physical, emotional, and mental status.

Determine appropriateness of prescribed therapeutic diet as related to altered state of health.

Evaluate ability of client to tolerate diet.

Assess client's acceptance of diet regimen.

Refer to general assessment steps in maintaining normal nutritional status.

Assess client's dietary preferences.

PLANNING Objectives

To maintain balanced health status

To meet nutritional needs based on alterations in client's health status

To allow client to tolerate foods and nutrients more efficiently

To design a therapeutic diet with which client will comply

To identify client who requires specialized dietary consultation

IMPLEMENTATION Procedures

Restricting Dietary Carbohydrates

Restricting Dietary Protein

Restricting Dietary Fat

Restricting Mineral Nutrients

Providing Nutrient Enhanced Diets

Providing Modified Diets

Providing Consistency Diets

EVALUATION Expected Outcomes

Client complies with prescribed therapeutic diet.

Client tolerates diet well, and diet meets nutritional and health status requirements.

Therapeutic diet assists in management of client's health problem.

Client verbalizes knowledge of therapeutic diet.

Therapeutic diet conforms to ethnic preferences and cultural orientation.

Therapeutic diet can be implemented in home setting.

RESTRICTING DIETARY CARBOHYDRATES

1. Reactive hypoglycemia occurs when most of the glucose moves from blood into cells and results in abnormally low blood glucose levels (<70 mg/dL).
   a. Foods prescribed are high in protein and a variety of complex carbohydrates, consumed in 5 or 6 small meals per day.
   b. Foods restricted are simple carbohydrates; for example, sugar, syrup, candy.
2. Nutrition is one of the cornerstones of treatment for diabetes.
   a. Foods included on the diet are balanced and provide protein, fat, and carbohydrates in relation to an individual's needs.
   b. Foods limited are refined or simple sugars.
   c. Counting grams of carbohydrates and using the glycemic index (describes how much blood glucose level rises with a specific food when compared with an equivalent amount of glucose) are nutritional tools for managing diabetes.

RESTRICTING DIETARY PROTEIN

1. A **restricted protein diet** is used for renal impairment (uremia), hepatic coma, and cirrhosis (according to individual requirements).
   a. Control end products of protein (nitrogenous waste) metabolism by limiting protein intake.
   b. Protein allowance is decreased to 0.8mg/kg/day.
   c. Limits high-protein foods, such as eggs, meat, milk, and milk products.
2. A **PKU diet** is an amino acid metabolism abnormality diet used for phenylketonuria (PKU), galactosemia, and lactose intolerance.
   a. Reduce or eliminate the offending enzyme in the food intake of protein, and use substitute nutrient foods.
   b. Avoid milk and milk products as they constitute the main source of enzymes for the three diseases.
   c. Employ substitutes to meet daily allowances.

RESTRICTING DIETARY FAT

1. A **restricted fat diet** is used to manage cardiovascular diseases, diabetes mellitus, and high serum cholesterol levels.
   a. Focuses on restriction of saturated (hydrogenated) fats and cholesterol to treat dyslipidemia and reduce risk for coronary artery disease. These fats are solid or semi-solid at room temperature.
   b. Lipid levels goals = total cholesterol <200 mg/dL, LDL-C <130 mg/dL, HDL-C > 45 males and 55 females mg/dL and triglycerides < 150 mg/dL.
   c. Restrict total fat to 30% (or less) of calories, achieve normal body weight by reducing calorie intake; restrict saturated fat to 10% (or less) of calories and reduce cholesterol to 300 mg per day.
   d. Substitute saturated and trans-fats with monosaturated fats found primarily in plant products, use low-fat or nonfat products; increase intake of fruits and vegetables and essential fatty acids.
   e. Limit high-cholesterol foods found in animal products, such as egg yolk, red meat, shellfish, organ meats, bacon, and pork.
2. A **modified-fat diet** is used according to individual tolerance in malabsorption syndromes, (cystic fibrosis, gallbladder disease, obstructive jaundice, and liver disease).
   a. Attempt to lower fat content in diet when there is inadequate absorption of fat.
   b. Avoid such foods as gravies, fatty meat and fish, cream,

CULTURAL COMPETENCE

When a special diet is prescribed, it should be consistent with the client's cultural background, income, physical needs, and religious practices. For example, Jewish people do not combine certain foods on the same tray. So, to comply with Kosher laws, do not combine meat and dairy products.

fried foods, rich pastries, whole-milk products, cream soups, salad and cooking oils, nuts, and chocolate. Allow eggs (3–5 per week), lean meat, and small amount of butter or butter substitute.

3. Increase unsaturated fats and decrease saturated fats and trans fats, found in fast and fried foods. (These are fats that result from hydrogenation.)
   a. There are two kinds of unsaturated fats.
   b. Polyunsaturated fats: diet is used to manage and decrease risk of cardiovascular diseases.
   c. Monounsaturated fats (olive oil, canola oil, avocados, pecans, almonds): reduce risk of some diseases such as diabetes and cardiovascular disease.

RESTRICTING MINERAL NUTRIENTS

1. A **restricted sodium diet** is used to manage hypertension, hepatitis, congestive heart failure (edema), renal insufficiency, cirrhosis of the liver, and adrenal cortical treatment.
   a. Correct or control the retention of sodium and water in the body by limiting sodium intake. May be done by restriction of salt in the diet or in combination with medications.
   b. Restrict salt in cooking or at the table. In clients requiring dietary modification in salt intake, any product containing sodium, such as soda bicarbonate, may be prohibited (typical diet provides 4–6 g of sodium/day).
   c. Explain sodium restrictions in diet.
      Mild: 2–3 g sodium (no added salt provides 3 g of sodium/day)
      Moderate: 1,000–1,500 mg sodium
      Strict: 500 mg sodium
      Be aware of sodium content of some medications (e.g., antacids).
2. A **low-calcium diet** may be used to prevent formation of calcium oxalate stones.

Foods High in Sodium and Potassium

Foods High in Sodium

- Table salt and all prepared salts, such as celery salt
- Smoked meats and salted meats
- Most frozen vegetables or canned vegetables with added salt
- Butter, margarines, and cheese
- Quick-cooking cereals
- Shellfish and frozen or salted fish
- Seasonings and sauces
- Canned soups
- Chocolates and cocoa
- Beets, celery, and selected greens (spinach)
- Anything with salt added, such as potato chips, popcorn

Foods High in Potassium

- Fruit juices, such as orange, grapefruit, banana, raw apple
- Instant, dry coffee powder
- Egg, legumes, whole grains
- Fish, fresh halibut, codfish
- Pork, beef, lamb, veal, chicken
- Milk, skim and whole
- Dried dates, prunes
- Bouillon and meat broths

PROVIDING NUTRIENT ENHANCED DIETS

1. An **increased potassium diet** is used to manage diabetic acidosis, extended use of certain diuretics or steroids, burns (after first 48 hours), vomiting, fevers, COPD, and may have an antihypertensive effect.
   a. Replace potassium loss from the body with specific foods high in potassium or a potassium supplement. (Severe loss is managed with intravenous therapy.)
   b. Avoid no specific foods unless there is a sodium restriction because some foods high in potassium are also high in sodium.

2. A **high-iron diet** is used to manage anemias (blood loss, nutritional), and malabsorption syndrome.
   a. Replace a deficit of iron caused by inadequate intake or chronic blood loss.
   b. Include foods high in iron content, such as organ meats (especially liver), meat, egg yolks, whole-wheat products, seafood, leafy vegetables, nuts, dried fruit, and legumes.
3. A **high-calcium diet** is used to prevent osteoporosis, prevent and treat hypertension.
   a. Increases normal adult intake of 1 g/day to 1.5 g/day for postmenopausal female.
   b. Recommends use of *fortified* low-fat and nonfat products.
   c. Clients who are lactose intolerant should use leafy green vegetables and nonliquid dairy products (cheese, yogurt).

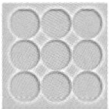

Cultural Competence

Food is one of the most interesting aspects about any culture.

- American acculturation tends to *replace* traditional habits, tastes, and preferences with a detrimental *switch* to highly processed foods.
- This may account for increased rates of illness and death from heart disease and cancer in some populations.
- While not all cultural food habits are healthy, they are *usually* higher in fiber and vitamins than the typical American diet, and should be encouraged.

General recommendations:

- Food preferences should be maintained.
- Focus education on food practices and preparation, possible health hazards, and importance of role modeling for children.

PROVIDING MODIFIED DIETS

for Dietary Fiber

1. There are two types of fiber: insoluble fibers found in the cell walls of plants do not dissolve in water, so they speed up elimination of waste products; soluble fibers (oat bran) dissolve in water. They decrease blood cholesterol levels and slow absorption of glucose, so blood sugar levels are reduced in diabetes.
2. A **high fiber diet** is prescribed to treat constipation and diverticulosis.
   a. Suggest foods high in fiber or residue, such as any beans, fruits, vegetables, whole grain breads and cereals, and especially unrefined bran.
   b. Instruct client that foods low in carbohydrates are usually high in residue.
3. A **low fiber diet** is used to manage ulcerative colitis, postoperative colon and rectal surgery, diverticulitis (when inflammation decreases, diet may revert to high residue), diarrhea, and enteritis.
   a. Inform client that low-residue foods are ground meat, fish, broiled chicken without skin, creamed cheeses, limited fat, warm drinks, refined strained cereals, and white bread.
   b. Instruct client that foods high in carbohydrates are usually low in fiber or residue.

for Postoperative Diet Progression

1. A **special postoperative surgical diet** is necessary to promote wound healing, avoid shock from decreased plasma proteins and circulating red blood cells, prevent edema, and promote bone healing.
   a. Provide 2,800 total calories for tissue repair and even greater calories for extensive repair.
   b. Fluid intake is 2,000–3,000 mL/day for uncomplicated surgery and 3,000–4,000 mL/day for sepsis or renal damage. Seriously ill clients with drainage can require more.
2. **Diet progression protocol** progresses from nothing by mouth the day of surgery to a general diet within a few days following surgery. Check facility diet manual for progression of diet. Foods allowed in each phase of the progressive diet may include those listed here. In addition, the following diets, mechanical soft and pureed, may be included in the diet progression.
   a. A *clear-liquid diet* is 1,000–1,500 mL/day and comprises water, tea, broth, gelatin, and juices (apple, cranberry), or clear carbonated beverages. Avoid juices with pulp.
   b. A *full-liquid diet* lacks many nutrients, so it is used temporarily. Includes any food that is liquid at room temperature—clear liquids, milk and milk products, custard,

puddings, creamed soups, sherbet, ice cream, and any fruit juice.

c. A *surgical soft diet* is full liquid and pureed vegetables, eggs (not fried), milk, cheese, fish, fowl, tender beef, veal, potatoes, and cooked fruit. Include foods that are easy to chew and digest and limited in fiber; do not include gas-formers.

d. General diet: Take into consideration specific alterations necessary for client's health status.

Bland Diet Allowances

Foods Allowed

- Milk, butter, eggs (not fried), custard, vanilla ice cream, cottage cheese
- Cooked refined or strained cereal, enriched white bread
- Gelatin; homemade creamed, pureed soups
- Baked or broiled potatoes

Examples of Foods That Are Eliminated

- Spicy and highly seasoned foods
- Raw foods
- Very hot and very cold foods
- Gas-forming foods (varies with individuals)
- Coffee, alcoholic beverages, carbonated drinks
- High fat contents (some butter and margarine allowed)

PROVIDING CONSISTENCY DIETS

for Bland Diet

1. A bland diet is used to promote the healing of the gastric mucosa by eliminating food sources that are chemically and mechanically irritating. Bland diets may be used to manage duodenal ulcers, gastric ulcers, and postoperative stomach surgery.
   a. Instruct client that bland diets are presented in stages with the gradual addition of certain foods.
   b. Provide frequent, small feedings during active stress periods.
2. Establish regular meals and food patterns when condition permits.

for Mechanical Soft Diet

1. A mechanical soft diet is used when clients
   a. Are edentulous.
   b. Have poorly fitted dentures.
   c. Have difficulty chewing.
   d. Do not chew food thoroughly.

Nutrient Requirements for Healing*

- Total calories per day:
  2,800 for tissue repair
  6,000 for extensive repair
- Protein:
  40–50 g/day average person
  50–75 g/day early in postoperative period
  100–200 g/day if needed for new tissue synthesis
- Carbohydrates:
  55–60% of calories—sufficient in quantity to meet calorie needs and allow protein to be used for tissue repair
- Fat:
  25–30%—not excessive as it leads to poor tissue healing and susceptibility to infection
- Vitamins:
  Vitamin C—up to 1 g/day for tissue repair
  Vitamin B—increased above normal for stress management
  Vitamin A—adjuncts autoimmune system
  Vitamin E—increases O_2 to tissues
- Minerals:
  Zinc—tissue repair
  Selenium—cell repair
  Calcium/magnesium—relaxes nerves and maintains electric stimulation

**This is an example of nutrients necessary for healing. Each diet should be individualized and a consult is required.*

2. Any food that can be easily broken down can be included in this diet. It allows clients variations in tastes that are not allowed on a soft diet (chili beans).

for Pureed Diet

1. A pureed diet provides food that has been blenderized to a smooth consistency.
   a. Mainly used for clients with dysphagia or those who are unable to chew.
   b. Often used with small babies.
   c. Some hospitals provide this type of diet for gastrostomy feedings.
2. When assisting clients with this type of diet, talk with them about the meal, describing the different foods. When the texture is all the same, distinguishing between foods is difficult.
3. Do not mix all pureed food together or feed out of one bowl or dish. Try to keep foods separate and feed alternately, with dessert last.

DOCUMENTATION FOR MODIFIED THERAPEUTIC DIETS

- Type of diet provided
- Client's daily weight
- Intake and output
- Client's understanding of dietary restriction
- Any client or family teaching provided
- Nutritional consult requested
- Client's tolerance of diet progression
- Community agency referral offered

Critical Thinking Application

UNEXPECTED OUTCOMES	CRITICAL THINKING OPTIONS
Client is noncompliant to diet.	• Elicit client's feelings to determine exactly what is behind the noncompliance. • Check method of diet preparation and administration to see if it is attractive and appealing. • Ensure that environment is conducive to eating. • Notify dietitian to discuss diet with client.
Client with sodium-restricted diet states that food has no taste.	• Recommend use of lemon, herbs, and spices to add flavor to foods. • Encourage client to avoid processed foods, frozen entrees, salty snacks. • Inform client that salt craving decreases over time with change in diet. • Consult physician for recommendation of potassium-containing salt substitute.
Client on a fat-restricted diet asks what foods to eat/avoid.	• Suggest client remove all visible fat from and limit intake of red meats. • Encourage to substitute poultry (skin removed) and fish for red meat. • Limit intake of butter, salad dressings, trans-fatty (partially hydrogenated) products. • Use low-fat or nonfat products. • Increase intake of fruits, vegetables, and legumes.

UNEXPECTED OUTCOMES	CRITICAL THINKING OPTIONS
Postmenopausal client has lactose intolerance but is concerned about need for increased calcium to prevent osteoporosis.	• Consult with registered dietitian. • Encourage intake of nonliquid dairy products (yogurt, cheese). • Suggest intake of leafy vegetables, canned fishes. • Calcium carbonate supplements are best absorbed. • Recommend calcium carbonate supplement in low dose (500 mg or less), several times/day for better absorption and efficacy.

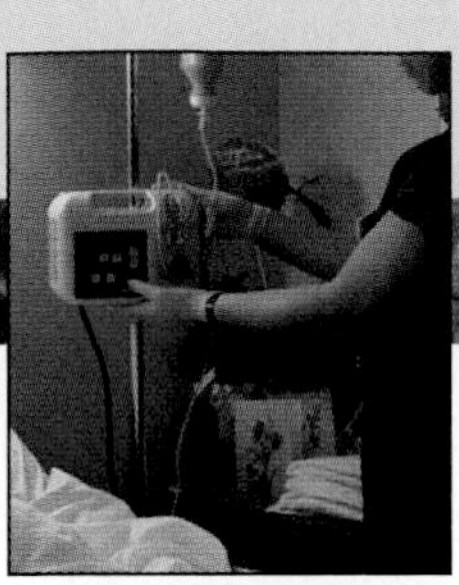

UNIT 2

Nutrition Maintenance

Nursing Process Data

ASSESSMENT *Data Base*

Check appropriate dietary order.

Assess client's nutritional needs.

Determine client's sociocultural orientation.

Obtain client's diet history, and determine eating habits and food preferences.

Assess client's ability to comply with diet regimen.

Assess client's fluid intake needs.

Check recommended daily dietary allowances and essential body nutrients.

Evaluate results of the following data:

- Analysis of appropriate diagnostic tests.
- Alterations in health status that indicate need for therapeutic vs. regular diet.

Assess client's risk for aspiration.

Check for specific instructions for positioning and feeding technique for the dysphagic client.

PLANNING *Objectives*

To provide a nutritional diet based on individual needs

To identify the client who exhibits nutritional deficits and to determine an appropriate diet

To provide nutritional requirements for clients unable to consume oral feedings

To provide a diet that is tolerated physiologically and emotionally by the client

To assist the visually impaired client to self-feed.

To utilize techniques that minimize risk for aspiration in the dysphagic client.

IMPLEMENTATION *Procedures*

Serving a Food Tray

Assisting the Visually Impaired Client to Eat

Assisting the Dysphagic Client to Eat

EVALUATION *Expected Outcomes*

Appropriate consultation assists in individualizing nutritional plan of care.

Client receives a balanced diet that meets nutritional requirements.

Diet is acceptable to client's taste and cultural orientation.

Visually impaired client is able to self-feed.

Dysphagic client is able to eat using adaptations to prevent aspiration.

SERVING A FOOD TRAY

Equipment

Diet slip completed
Diet tray
Over-bed table
Utensils
Protective covering

Preparation

1. Obtain dietary consult, if necessary, to meet client's needs.
2. Elicit food preferences of the client.
3. Send request to the diet kitchen for the specific diet.
4. Check client care plan for changes in diet.
5. Check all diet trays before serving to ensure the diet provided is the one ordered.
6. Ensure that hot food is hot and cold food is cold.
7. Keep food trays attractive. Avoid spilling liquids on tray.
8. Assist client to empty bladder if needed and wash hands.
9. Remove unpleasant objects from area.

Procedure

1. Wash your hands and assist client to wash hands.
2. Raise bed to HIGH position, and lower side rail.
3. Assist client to sitting position if possible.
4. Place protective covering over gown.
5. Place tray on tray table. Position table so client can see food.
6. Assist client as needed (e.g., cut meat, open milk carton). Always leave call bell within reach.
7. Check on client during meal to determine if assistance is necessary.
8. Reposition tray table at bedside when completed.
9. Provide hand cleaning and oral care.
10. Offer bedpan or assistance to commode or bathroom.
11. Raise side rail.
12. Position bed for comfort.
13. Note amount of food eaten.
14. Remove food tray from room.
15. Wash your hands.
16. Chart amount eaten. If necessary, record liquid intake.

> **CLINICAL ALERT**
>
> Clients sensitive to latex have potential for serious allergic reactions to some plant proteins. Cross-reactivity to latex has been shown with foods such as avocado, banana, papaya, chestnuts, kiwi, potatoes, and tomatoes. Clients with allergy to these foods may have latex allergy and vice versa.

EVIDENCE BASED NURSING PRACTICE

Doctors Recommend Vitamins

A physician from Harvard Medical School and his colleagues reviewed studies published between 1966 and 2002 that suggested a link between diseases such as cancer and heart disease and vitamin intake. These researchers concluded that everybody, regardless of age or health status, should take a daily multivitamin–mineral supplement.

Source: Fairfield, K., & Fletcher, R. (2002, June). Vitamins for chronic disease prevention in adults. *Journal of the American Medical Association, 19,* 3116–3126.

ASSISTING THE VISUALLY IMPAIRED CLIENT TO EAT

Procedure

1. Check client care plan for current changes in diet.
2. Check room number, client's identaband and allergy band, and have client state name.
3. Wash your hands.
4. Raise head of bed to HIGH position, and lower side rail.
5. Assist client to wash hands and face.
6. Place client in sitting position if possible.
7. Place protective covering over gown.
8. Place tray on tray table. Position table so client can see food.
9. Stand or sit facing client. (Bed is in low position if you are sitting.)
10. Assist client by using the following technique:
    a. Use the clock system by describing food arrangement on the plate.

b. Tell the client the time on the clock at which food is placed; for example, "The corn is at 4 o'clock and the chicken is at 8 o'clock."
c. Encourage the client to feed him or herself, but remain with client if possible.
11. Encourage the client to hold glass, bread, finger foods.
12. Allow client time to chew and swallow.
13. Provide fluids throughout meal.
14. Alternate foods; don't feed all meat then all vegetable.
15. Allow client to rest at intervals during the feeding.
16. Talk with client during meal. **Rationale:** Talking with the client makes mealtime more pleasant and encourages client not to hurry.
17. Reposition tray table at bedside when completed.
18. Provide hand cleaning and oral care if desired.
19. Raise side rail.
20. Position bed for comfort. Lower bed if it is raised.
21. Note amount of food eaten.
22. Remove food tray from room.
23. Wash your hands.
24. Chart amount eaten. If necessary, record I&O.
25. Place call bell within client's reach.

ASSISTING THE DYSPHAGIC CLIENT TO EAT

Equipment

Protective covering
Provision for oral care and hand washing
Towel
Penlight to inspect oral cavity
Oral suction catheter connected to suction source

Preparation

1. Note specific instructions for feeding technique (diet and positioning) prescribed by speech or swallowing specialist; for example, cornstarch, Thickit, or rice cereal to thicken food, as prescribed. **Rationale:** clients with swallowing problems find it easier to swallow full liquids.
2. Check if client is receiving oral and enteral feeding; stop the enteral solution about one hour before oral feeding.
3. Eliminate environmental distractors such as television, radio.
4. Ensure that temperature of food is appropriate.

Procedure

1. Wash your hands.
2. Check client's identaband and allergy bracelet and have client state name.
3. Provide client privacy.
4. Maintain bed in LOW position and lower side rail.
5. Assist client to sit upright, hips flexed slightly greater than 90° with shoulders and face slightly forward, and chin parallel to the floor or slightly tucked. **Rationale:** Gravity assists proper bolus movement to the stomach.

Note: Prescribed position is different for specific dysphagias. Some types of dysphagia necessitate client positioning to one side, or with head rotated toward the stronger or weaker side, or even side-lying. Instructions should be placed in client's record, care plan, and posted at client's head of bed.

6. Assist client to wash hands before eating.
7. Place protective covering over client's gown.
8. Place tray on table and towel under plate. **Rationale:** This stabilizes plate while feeding.
9. Suction oral secretions before feeding, if necessary.
10. Sit at client's side, or sit facing client.
11. Encourage self-feeding.
12. Instruct client to take (or offer) small portions of food at first (0.5 to 1 tsp at a time), bites manageable in size but large enough to require chewing.
13. Instruct client to eat food first, without accompanying liquid, reserving *all* liquid intake until after finishing food. **Rationale:** Using liquids to wash down boluses of food pushes the food down too rapidly.
14. Instruct client to perform an exaggerated sucking motion at the beginning of each swallow with chin tucked slightly. **Rationale:** Decreases risk of aspiration.
15. Allow client to concentrate on swallowing *without* distractions such as conversation or television. **Rationale:** For the dysphagic client, swallowing takes concentration; talking increases risk for aspiration.
16. Make sure client is swallowing every mouthful. **Rationale:** Buildup may occur on weak side of mouth or pharynx.
17. Observe client closely for evidence of aspiration (e.g., cough), and suction oropharynx if indicated.
18. Help with feeding only if client shows signs of weakness, fatigue.
19. Provide positive reinforcement for accomplishment.
20. Assist with oral care and handwashing following meal.
21. Remove food tray and raise side rails as indicated.
22. Place call bell in reach.
23. Record percentage of food eaten and amount of liquid intake (if indicated).
24. Maintain client's sitting position for 30 minutes after eating.
25. Carefully observe client with impaired communication for 30 minutes after the first few servings.

> **CLINICAL ALERT**
>
> The use of a straw increases risk of aspiration because the dysphagic client has less control over the amount of fluid intake. Similarly, the dysphagic client should not be fed with a syringe.

DOCUMENTATION FOR NUTRITION MAINTENANCE

- Appetite
- Food intake (percentage eaten)
- Tolerance to diet
- Weight
- Liquid intake
- Feeding techniques for the dysphagic client

Critical Thinking Application

UNEXPECTED OUTCOMES	CRITICAL THINKING OPTIONS
Client is unable to assimilate foods metabolically.	• Document on client care plan, and make staff report of abnormal results of diagnostic tests which identify assimilation problems. Assist the physician in altering the method of feeding (enteral or parenteral).
Client vomits or has diarrhea.	• Evaluate allergic responses to food. Review history and physical to determine any existing food allergies. • Obtain order for clear liquid diet, gradually progressing back to regular diet. • Assess overall health status (e.g., temperature, obstruction).
Cultural preferences or psychosocial behavior interferes with eating.	• Modify diet to conform to client's desires. • Request consultation with dietician.
Client appears to be aspirating food (coughing, hoarseness, noisy breathing).	• Instruct client to cough to determine if airway is clear. Assess lungs thoroughly. • Suction if necessary. • Instruct client not to talk when eating to concentrate on swallowing. • Obtain speech therapy consult for swallow evaluation.

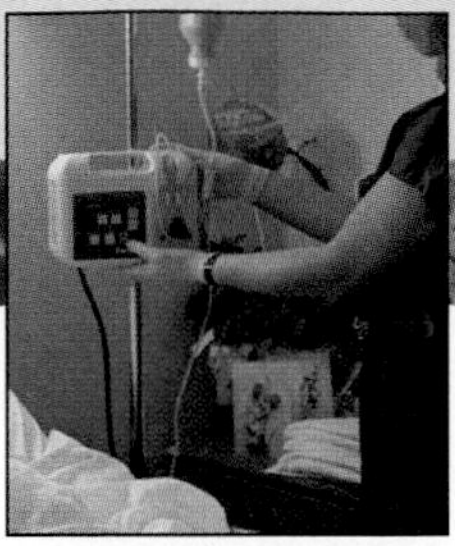

Gastrointestinal Intubation

Nursing Process Data

ASSESSMENT *Data Base*

Evaluate oral intake and diet history.

Assess nutritional requirements. Does the client have special needs?

Assess overall status necessitating GI decompression (gastric surgery, intestinal obstruction)

Assess other medically related nutritional problems.

Assess status of GI tract; bowel sounds.

Assess capacity to chew and swallow, presence of gag reflex.

Assess patency of nares.

Check for vomiting, diarrhea, or abdominal distention.

Assess risk for aspiration.

PLANNING *Objectives*

To provide alternative means of providing nutrients for clients with functional gastrointestinal tract

To provide means of nutrition if there is an inability to swallow or an existing obstruction in upper alimentary canal

To provide increased nutrient requirements above oral consumption

To maintain fluid and electrolyte balance

To perform gastric lavage to remove blood, fluid or particles, or to prevent digestion and absorption of poison

To absorb and remove ingested toxins

To provide nasal/oral hygiene for the client who is NPO

To maintain decompression tube patency

IMPLEMENTATION *Procedures*

Inserting a Large-Bore Nasogastric (NG) Tube

for Testing Blood in Gastric Specimen

for Decompressing the GI Tract

Irrigating/Maintaining a Nasogastric (NG) Tube

Performing Gastric Lavage

Administering Poison Control Agents

Removing an NG or Nasointestinal Tube

EVALUATION *Expected Outcomes*

NG tube is inserted into stomach.

NG tube placement is validated.

Appropriate residual is obtained from aspiration of stomach contents.

Client complies with feeding procedure.

Intake and output balance is maintained.
Nasogastric tube functions efficiently and remains patent.
Electrolyte imbalance does not occur.
Client does not develop parotiditis or nasal irritation.
Client does not develop respiratory complications.
Blood/toxic substance is removed by lavage and not digested and absorbed.
Client's gastrointestinal function returns to normal.

INSERTING A LARGE-BORE NASOGASTRIC (NG) TUBE

Equipment

Plug with tubing or suction source
Single-lumen Levin tube or double-lumen Salem sump tube and antireflux valve
Water-soluble lubricant
Hypoallergenic tape (2.5 cm or 1 inch) or commercial tube-holder
pH chemstrip or Gastroccult testcard and developer
Towel
Emesis basin
Tissues
Safety pin with rubber band
Stethoscope
Tongue blade
Glass of water with straw
50 mL catheter-tip syringe
Clean gloves
Indelible pen or piece of tape for marking tube
Spindle adapter

Preparation

1. Check physician's order and client care plan for inserting an NG tube.
2. Determine size of catheter based on length of time it will remain in place, client size, and viscosity of feeding solution as ordered. Check tube for defects and flush with water to check for patency.
3. Check client's identaband and have client state name.
4. Discuss procedure with client. **Rationale:** Demonstration and display of items to be used helps to allay client's fear and to gain cooperation.
5. Provide privacy.
6. Gather equipment.

Procedure

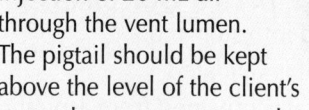

1. Wash hands. Don clean gloves.
2. Position client at 45° angle or higher with head of bed elevated.
3. Examine nostrils, and select the most patent nostril by having client breathe through each one. **Rationale:** The nostril with greater airflow should be chosen for insertion.
4. Place a towel over client's chest and an emesis basin within reach; establish a cueing signal for client to use to stop you momentarily. **Rationale:** Client may experience discomfort or gag during tube insertion.
5. Measure from tip of nose to earlobe to xiphoid (NEX) process of sternum to determine appropriate length for tube insertion.

CLINICAL ALERT

- Nurses never insert or withdraw an NG tube for clients recovering from gastric surgery. The suture line could easily be interrupted, and hemorrhage could occur.
- Never insert an NG tube in a client after nasal, craniofacial, or hypophysectomy surgery.

Gastric (Salem) Sump Tube

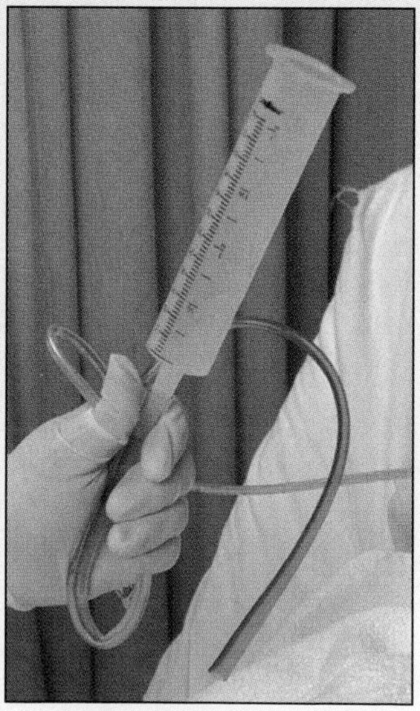

This gastric tube is a double lumen radiopaque plastic tube with a blue pigtail at the outer end. The pigtail provides an air vent to keep pressure from building in the stomach when the salem tube is attached to suction. It is NOT used for irrigation, obtaining a specimen, etc. However, if pigtail is blocked and requires irrigation, following irrigation, the pigtail should be cleared with an injection of 20 mL air through the vent lumen. The pigtail should be kept above the level of the client's stomach to prevent stomach contents from leaking out.

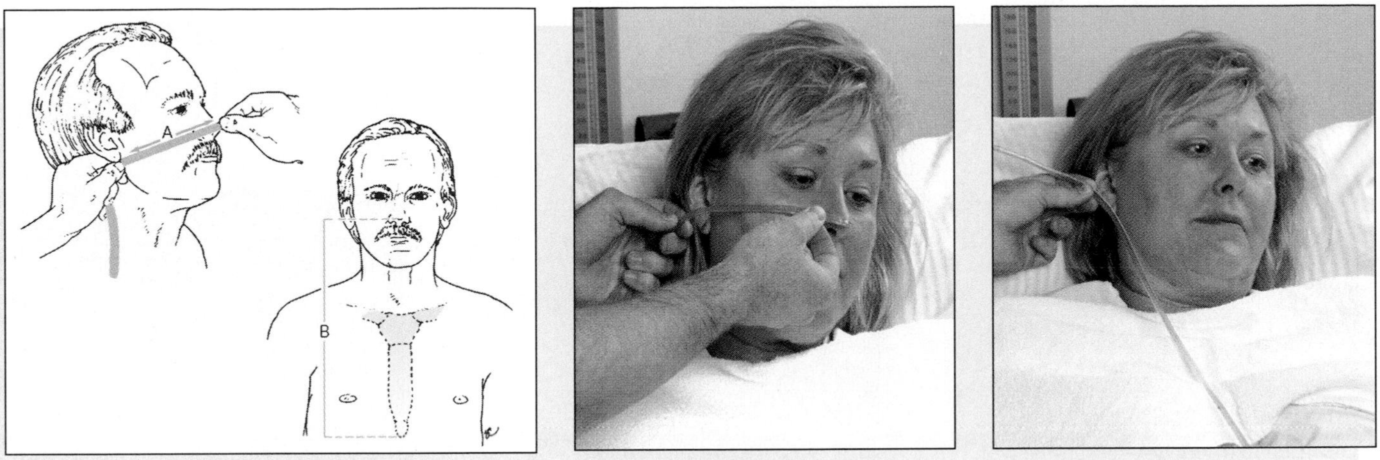

For inserting a nasogastric tube, measure from tip of nose to earlobe to xiphoid process of sternum to determine length for tube insertion.

6. Coil end of tube over fingers. **Rationale:** This softens tube and facilitates insertion.
7. Lubricate first 4 inches of tube with water-soluble lubricant. **Rationale:** Oil-based lubricant could cause respiratory complications.
8. Insert tube through nostril to back of throat. Aim the tube toward back of throat and down. Suggest client swallow sips of water to assist tube insertion. **Rationale:** Sips of water through a straw may aid in advancing tube.

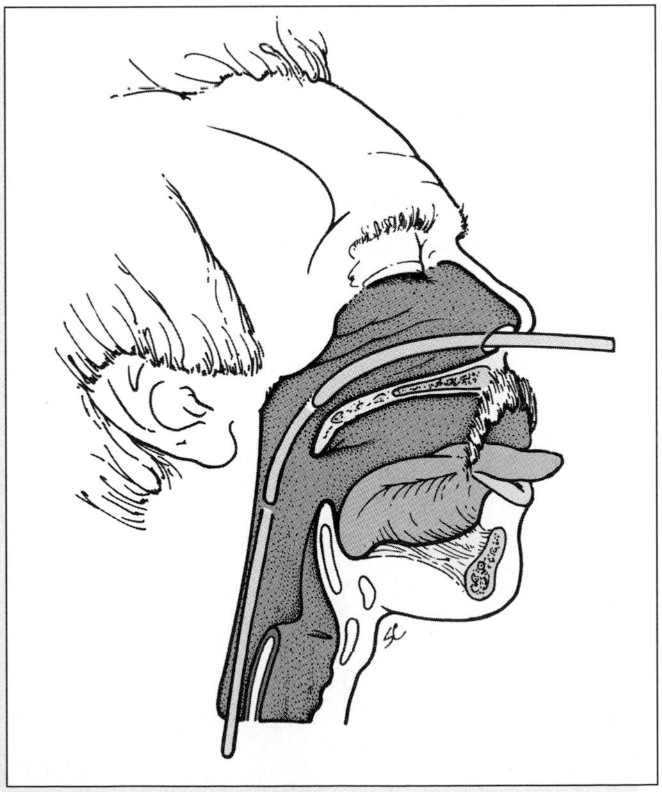
NG tube inserted through naris to stomach.

CLINICAL ALERT

Coughing and choking are normal responses for some clients; however, choking and coughing plus *cyanosis* or inability to speak indicate that the tube may be in the airway.

9. Instruct client to flex head forward. **Rationale:** This position assists in tube insertion after tube has passed through nasopharynx and reduces risk of tube entering trachea.
10. Listen for air exchange at 25-cm (carina) level; if no sound is heard, advance tube. **Rationale:** If sound is heard, tube may be advancing into airway and should be removed.
11. Continue advancing tube, having client dry swallow or giving client sips of water, until mark is reached.
12. Attach syringe to free end of NG tube to check position of tube.
13. Inject 10–15 mL of air through NG tube, and listen with the stethoscope over stomach for a rush of air or "whoosh" sound. **Rationale:** This is one method of checking that tube has reached client's stomach.

Note: This method cannot be used alone to determine placement.

14. Aspirate gastric contents with 50-mL syringe and check pH. See p. 604, *Method of Determining Gastric pH*; if it is 0–4, tube is in stomach. (Intestinal sites and the pulmonary tree indicate a pH range of 6–7.) **Rationale:** This is essential for determining tube position.

for Testing Blood in Gastric Specimen

a. Note *color* of secretions. **Rationale:** Coffee ground appearance may represent digested blood, while bright red color may indicate active bleeding or ingestion of red food.
b. Place one drop of aspirate onto Gastroccult test area. (*See* photo in Determining Gastric pH.)
c. Apply two drops of Gastroccult developer directly over the sample in the Gastroccult test area.

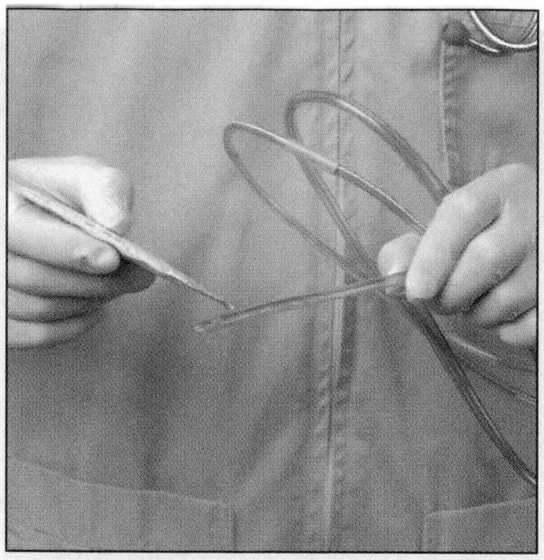

Lubricate first 4 inches of NG tube with water-soluble lubricant.

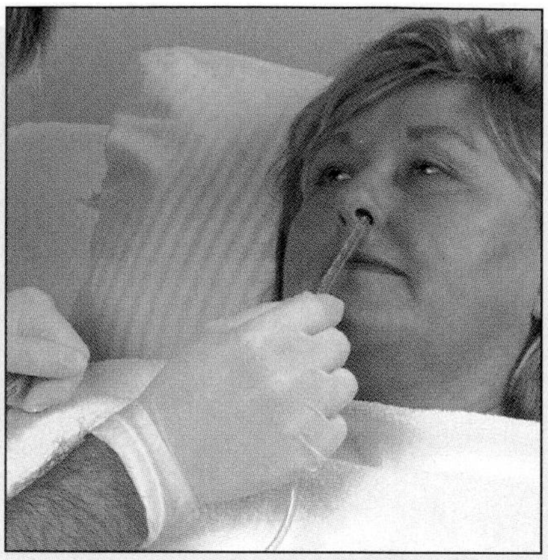

Insert NG tube through client's more patent nostril.

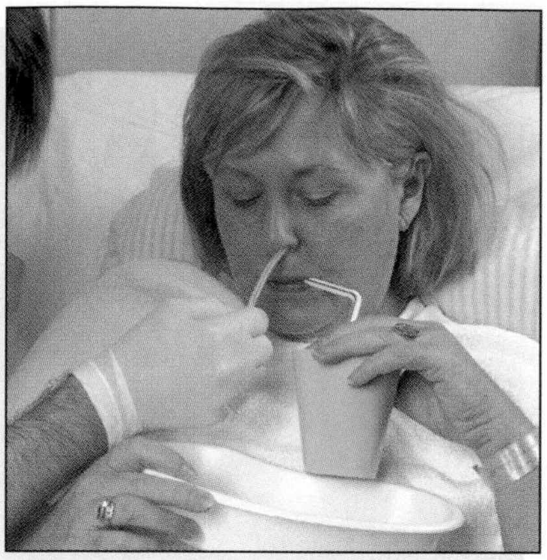

Instruct client to flex head forward and take sips of water.

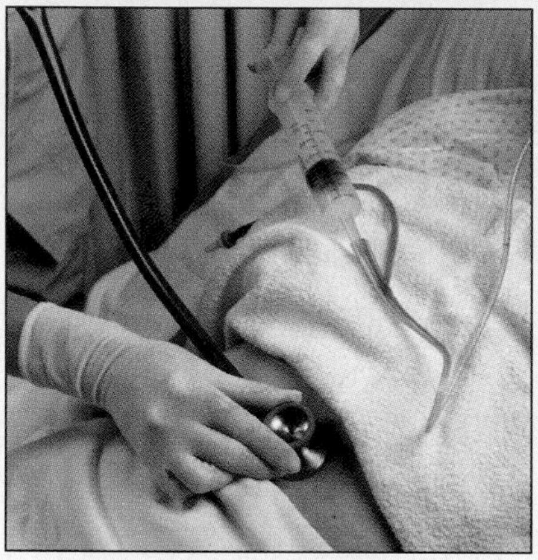

Place stethoscope over client's epigastric region, then inject air and listen for whooshing sound.

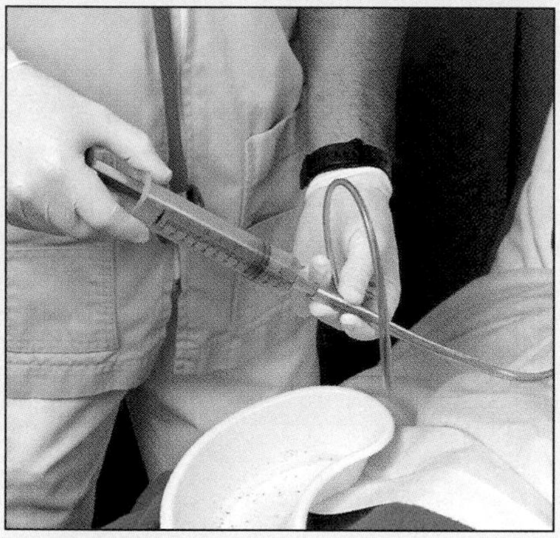

Aspirate gastric contents to check color and pH.

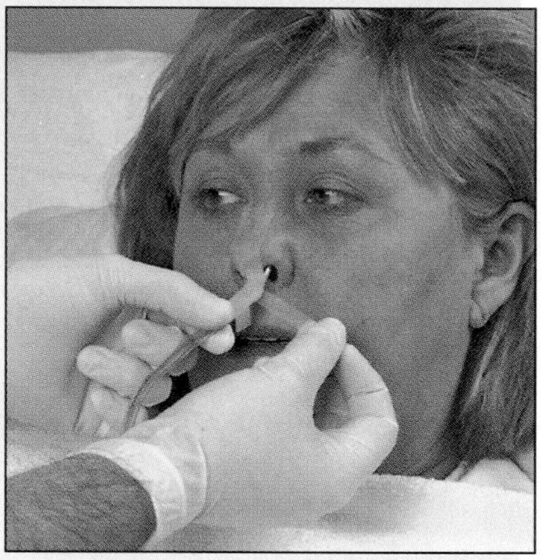

Tape tube securely to client's nose to prevent tube migration.

d. Read occult blood results within 60 seconds; any blue color indicates presence of blood.

Note: to determine if reagents in developer are functioning properly, add one drop of developer between positive and negative areas. The positive Performance Monitor area should turn blue within 10 seconds and the negative area should not turn blue.

15. Tape tube securely to nose or use an attachment device. (StatLock-NG Securement Device is flexible, yet resistant to tearing and adheres strongly to skin.) **Rationale:** When tube

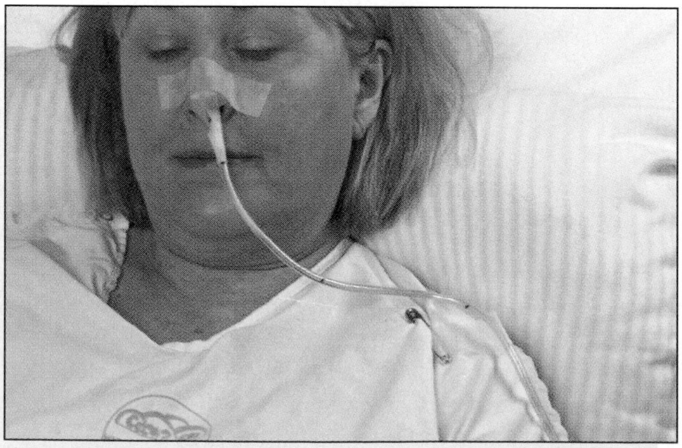

Secure tube by pinning to client's gown or bed linen, above level of stomach.

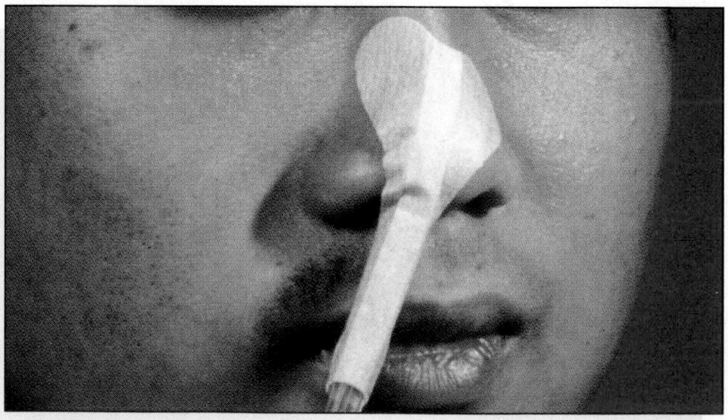

StatLock-NG Securement Device prevents tissue trauma.

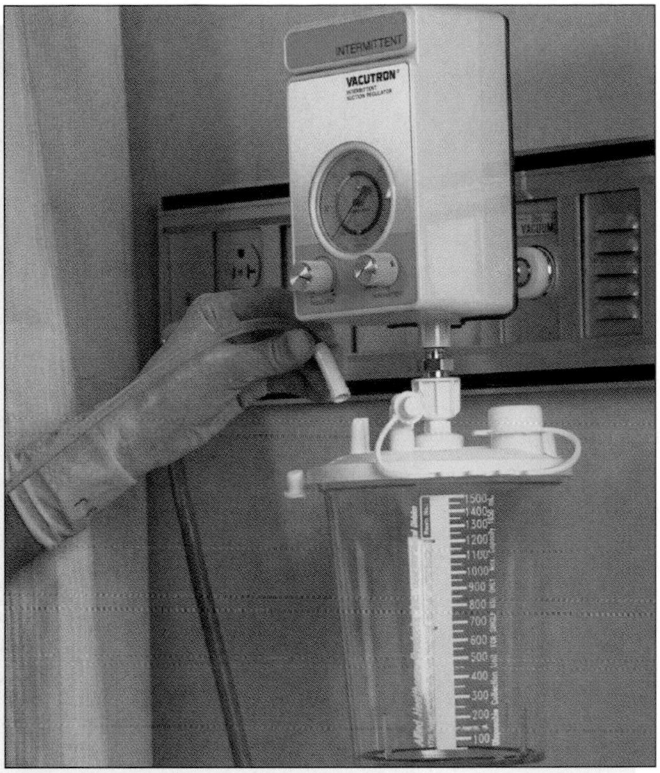

Connect suction tubing to suction source.

is taped securely, tissue trauma caused by pull on sides of nostril will be minimized.

a. Cut tape about 3 inches long.
b. Split ½ of tape lengthwise.
c. Place unsplit end of tape over bridge of nose, with bifurcated ends hanging free.

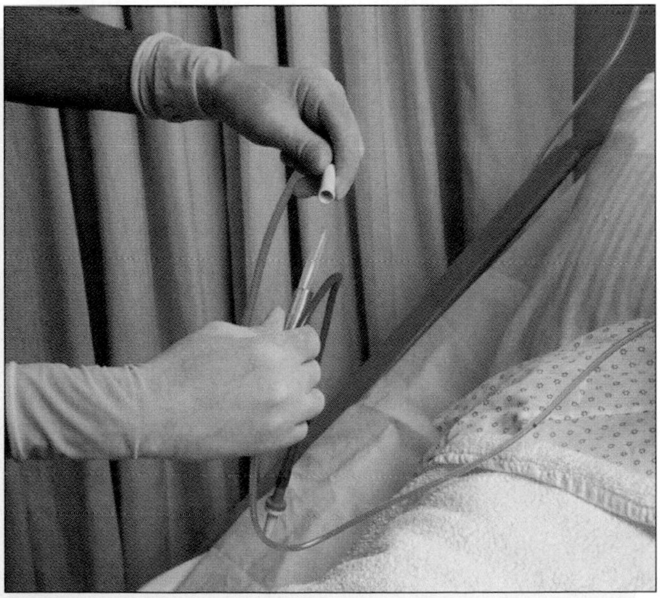
Tapered adapter is inserted to connect NG tube to suction tubing.

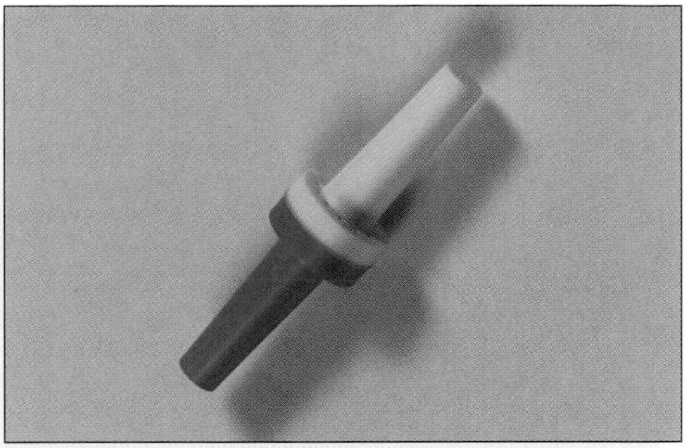
Insert blue side of antireflux valve into Salem sump tube blue pigtail.

d. Wrap each end of tape around the tube where it exits from the nose.

16. Plug end of tube or connect it to suction machine.

for Decompressing the GI Tract

a. Connect suction tubing to suction source.
b. Connect tapered adapter between suction tubing and Levin (single-lumen) NG tube and set suction on *intermittent low* (40 mm Hg) for decompression.

Clients who are unable to ingest food or take fluids by mouth should receive regular oral and nasal hygiene to keep mucous membranes moist and to help prevent infection of the parotid glands. Oral hygiene also reduces the risk of aspiration pneumonia, as it decreases the number of pathogens in oropharyngeal secretions. Chewing gum or sucking on sugar-free candy also helps stimulate salivation, but excessive use can stimulate gastric secretions and electrolyte imbalance.

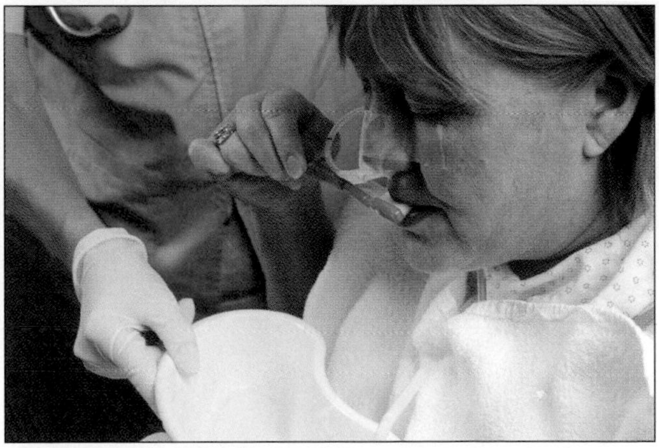
Provide regular nasal and oral hygiene to keep mucous membranes moist and help prevent parotiditis.

Rationale: Intermittent suction allows gastric tube suction force to be intermittently released, thereby reducing risk of mucosal erosion.
Or

c. Connect larger lumen of Salem sump tube to *continuous low* suction (30–40 mm Hg) or to *intermittent high* suction (120 mm Hg). **Rationale:** Continuous suction can be used because air vent lumen prevents excessive pressures from developing in stomach.

17. Secure tube with tape/rubber band pinned to client's gown or bed linen, leaving some degree of slack for head movement.
18. Implement procedure below when double-lumen (Salem sump) tube is used.
    a. Stabilize blue pigtail above level of stomach. **Rationale:** Helps to prevent siphoning into sump (pigtail) tubing.
    b. Insert antireflux valve (blue tip) into blue pigtail of Salem tube. **Rationale:** Antireflux valve allows air to enter tube, yet prevents leakage of gastric secretions.
19. Provide oral and nasal hygiene.
20. Remove gloves and wash hands.
21. Position client for comfort.

Method of Determining Gastric pH

Gastric pH is used to help determine NG tube placement, to assess gastric contents and to evaluate and treat certain disease conditions.

Procedure

- Complete initial steps as for any procedure: gather equipment, explain procedure to client, wash hands and don gloves. *Note: When testing for pH wait at least 1 hour after medication or an NG feeding.*
- Attach a 50 mL syringe with catheter tip to the NG tube and flush with 20 mL of air.
- Aspirate 5–10 mL of gastric secretions.
- Note color of secretions—gastric secretions are greenish to tan or off-white; respiratory secretions are clear to light yellow with mucus; duodenal samples are usually deep yellow. *Color of secretions does not guarantee correct placement.*
- Place 5 mL into a small cup or emesis basin and dip test paper into the cup, place a sample on the pH test paper, or using applicator, apply one drop of gastric sample to pH test area on gastroccult card.
- Read chemstrip pH within 30 seconds by comparing the color of the paper with the pH color guide.
- Gastric contents are usually 0–4.0. If the NG tube is in the pulmonary tree, it will be 6 or more. If the NG tube has passed into the intestines, the pH is more than 6 and could be 7.0–8.0.
- If clients are receiving medications that raise gastric pH, or have gastric bleeding or esophageal reflux, pH measurement may be unreliable.
- Document result of gastric pH specimen.

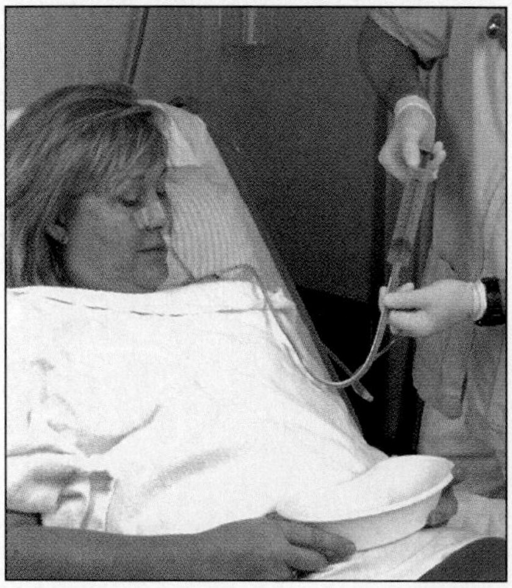
Aspirate 5–10 mL of gastric secretions to test pH.

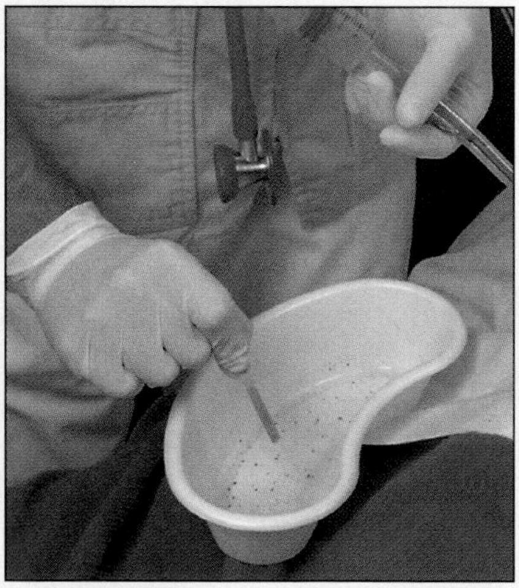
Dip test paper into gastric secretion to test pH.

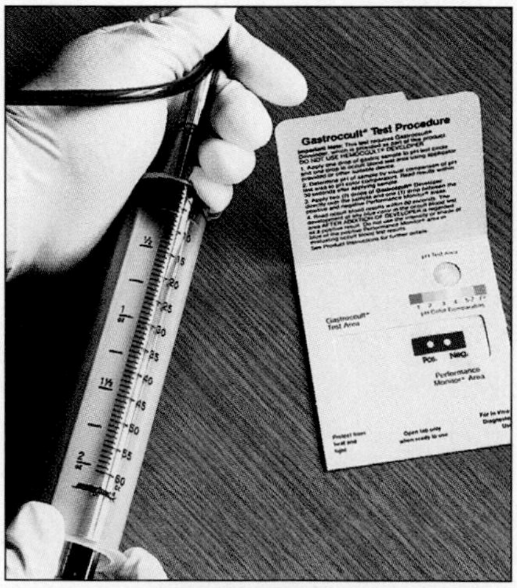

Place small drop on card to check pH.

IRRIGATING/MAINTAINING A NASOGASTRIC (NG) TUBE

Equipment

Disposable irrigation set
Emesis basin
Towel
50-mL syringe with catheter tip
Normal saline irrigation solution and container
I&O record sheet
Clean gloves

Preparation

1. Check orders and client care plan.
2. Wash hands.
3. Check client's identaband and provide privacy.
4. Explain procedure to client.
5. Place client in semi-Fowler's position.

Procedure

1. Don clean gloves.
2. Disconnect NG tube from suction source if necessary.
3. Place towel under NG tube to protect sheets and place emesis basin nearby.
4. Check for NG tube placement by following steps 12 through 14 in previous skill. **Rationale:** Solution could be instilled in lungs if NG tube is not in the stomach.
5. Draw up 20–30 mL normal saline into irrigating syringe (amount varies with physician's orders).
6. Gently instill normal saline into NG tube or remove syringe plunger, pour NS into syringe barrel, and allow solution to flow in by gravity. Do not force the solution.
7. Repeat procedure if necessary.

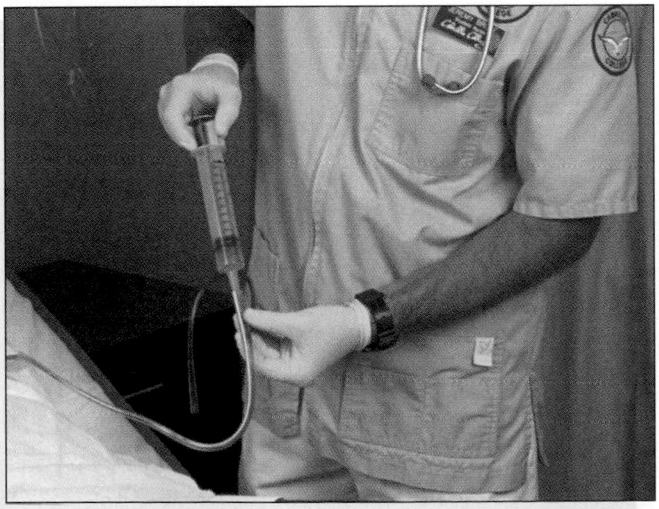

Aspirate secretions to check tube placement before instilling saline solution.

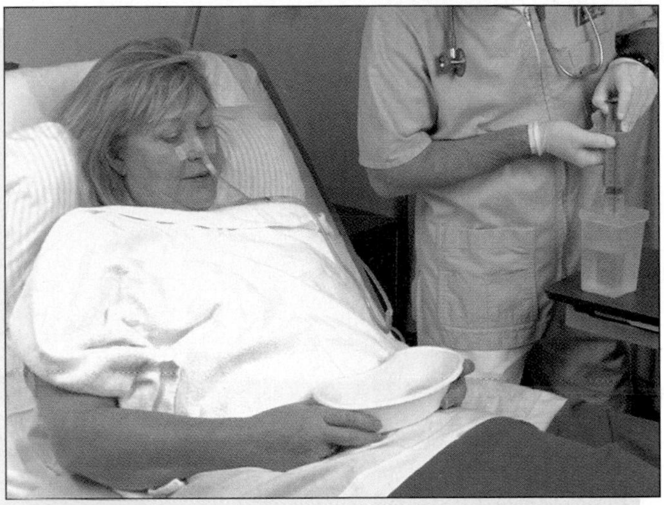

For irrigating NG tube, draw up 20–30 mL normal saline into irrigating syringe.

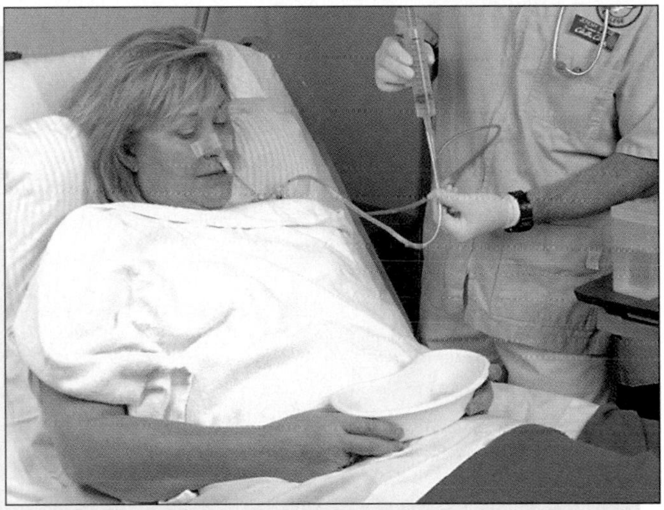

Gently instill normal saline into NG tube or allow solution to flow by gravity.

- If water rather than normal saline is used to irrigate enteral decompression tubes, the production of gastric secretions will increase and increasing amounts of electrolytes will be washed out. Similarly, if the client is NPO but ingests ice chips ad lib, electrolyte imbalance due to washout can occur, causing metabolic alkalosis.
- Limit the use of ice chips by substituting chips made from an electrolyte solution, and provide oral hygiene to keep the client's mucous membranes moist for comfort.
- If the client is receiving adequate parenteral hydration (IV fluids), excessive thirst should not be experienced.

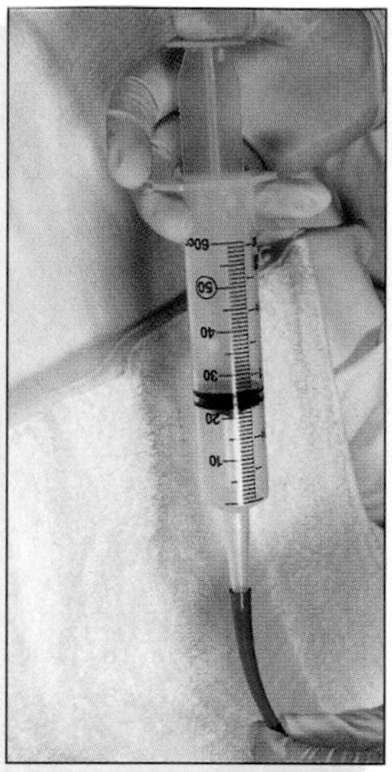

Follow Salem tube irrigation with injection of air into pigtail to clear, then reinsert antireflux valve.

8. Reconnect to suction or plug tube.
9. Record on I&O sheet the irrigation solution.
10. Remove gloves and wash your hands.
11. Reposition client for comfort.

CLINICAL ALERT

If NG tube is connected to suction, disconnect tube from suction before beginning irrigation procedure, then reconnect to suction following irrigation.

PERFORMING GASTRIC LAVAGE

Equipment

Large-bore (37–40 Fr) Ewald or orogastric tube (client may have endotracheal tube in place if comatose)
Large irrigating syringe with adapter
Container for aspirate
Lavage fluid, normal saline, or water
Container for specimen
Water-soluble lubricant
Standby suction available
Towel
Pen and tape
Gloves

Preparation

1. Check physician's orders for gastric lavage and solution to be used.
2. Determine if client is alert or comatose.
3. Gather equipment.
4. Wash hands and don gloves.

Procedure

1. Measure for tube insertion using the following guidelines.
   a. Measure distance from bridge of nose to earlobe to xiphoid process.
   b. Mark with pen or tape.
2. Place client at 45° with head of bed elevated.
3. Lubricate tube with water-soluble lubricant.
4. Insert tube orogastrically (about 50 cm or 20 inches).
5. Auscultate stomach during an injection of air with a syringe to confirm location of tube.
6. Aspirate gastric contents with syringe before instilling solution. Save specimen for analysis.
7. Repeatedly instill 50–100 mL normal saline or water and aspirate contents.
8. Monitor carefully volume instilled and character and volume of aspirated contents. **Rationale:** This will assist in determining net volume if there is blood loss.
9. Continue repeating process until gastric return is clear, or as ordered.
10. Complete procedure. Stomach will be left empty. Activated charcoal will be instilled (as ordered) or a saline cathartic will be given.
11. Pinch tube for removal, wrap in towel, and dispose of equipment.
12. Remove and dispose of gloves and wash hands.
13. Record vital signs frequently and monitor client's response closely.

Gastric lavage is used to remove unabsorbed poisons from the stomach or to diagnose gastric hemorrhage. It also assists in arresting hemorrhage and removing liquid from the stomach.

CLINICAL ALERT

Some authorities recommend water to lavage the stomach of blood since it breaks up clots more easily than saline solution, is less expensive, and is readily available.

ADMINISTERING POISON CONTROL AGENTS

Equipment

Large (37–40 Fr NG tube)
Activated charcoal or prescribed antidote
Equipment for inserting a nasogastric tube
50–100 g activated charcoal or prepackaged charcoal/sorbitol product mixed with water to consistency to administer through tube
Or
Balanced propethylene glycol–electrolyte solution (e.g., GoLYTELY) for bowel irrigation

Preparation

See Preparation for Inserting a Nasogastric Tube

Note: Client may have an endotracheal tube in place.

Procedure

1. Ensure that client has bowel sounds present.
2. Insert large bore (37–40 Fr) flexible tube nasogastrically or orogastrically.
3. Place comatose *intubated* client in a head-down, left side-lying position or place cooperative alert client on commode.
4. Aspirate gastric contents and save.
5. Administer activated charcoal slurry and repeat if ordered or, for cooperative client, administer balanced electrolyte solution per NG tube at a rate of 1–2 L/hr until rectal runout is clear.

Activated Charcoal for Ingested Poisons

Activated charcoal adsorbs significant amounts of certain poisons, especially when a person overdoses. The earlier charcoal is given, the more effective it is. The amount given is 5–10 times that of the suspected poison or, if the poison is unknown, 50–100 g for adults.

CLINICAL ALERT

Studies indicate that activated charcoal alone adsorbs most drugs and poisons in the GI tract, and has some ability to draw certain toxins out of circulation and back into the gut where they are bound and then excreted. Since activated charcoal is thought to be as effective as administration of ipecac to induce vomiting, ipecac use is now limited to the home for immediate use in the alert client after known ingestion of a poison.

REMOVING AN NG OR NASOINTESTINAL TUBE

Equipment

Towel, paper towel
Stethoscope
Container of sterile normal saline solution
50-mL syringe with catheter tip
Tissues
Gloves
Tube plug

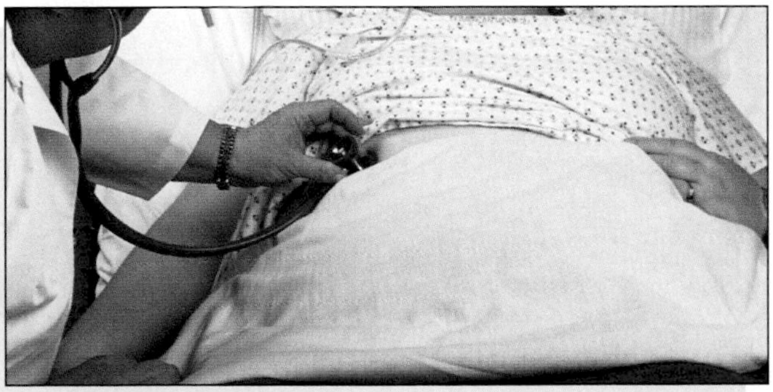

Assess client for return of bowel sounds before removing NG tube.

Preparation

1. Check physician's orders for NG tube removal.
2. Assess client to determine that bowel sounds have returned; auscultate to right of umbilicus as alternative to all four sites.

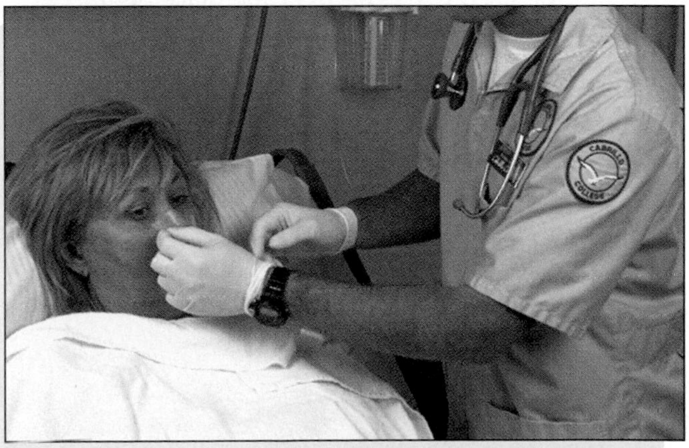

Clamp tube, unpin tube, and loosen tape on nose securing NG tube.

3. Prepare client for tube removal by explaining that it may cause some nasal discomfort, coughing, sneezing, or gagging.
4. Wash hands and don gloves.

Procedure

1. Provide tissues and place towel over client's chest.
2. Flush NG/NI tube with 20 mL normal saline. **Rationale:** To clear tube so that GI contents do not inadvertently drain into esophagus on tube removal.
3. Follow saline flush with a bolus of air. **Rationale:** To free tube from stomach/intestinal lining.
4. Unpin tube from client's gown and loosen tape that secures tube to client's nose.
5. Turn off suction and disconnect NG tube.
6. Plug tube or clamp it by folding it over in your gloved hand.
7. Pinch tube close to client's naris, have client take a deep breath and hold it while you withdraw the tube. **Rationale:** Holding breath closes glottis and helps prevent aspiration.
8. Wrap tube in paper towel to remove from client's view.
9. Offer oral and nasal hygiene.
10. Empty and record amount and character of drainage.
11. Discard disposable equipment and return reusable equipment to appropriate area.
12. Remove and dispose of gloves and wash hands.

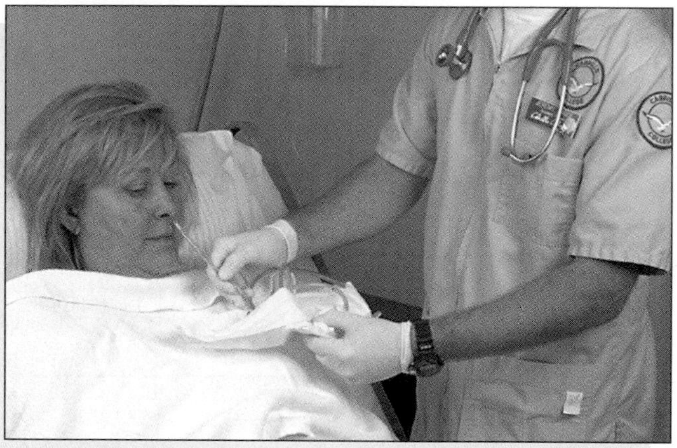

Have client hold breath and remove NG tube with continuous steady pull.

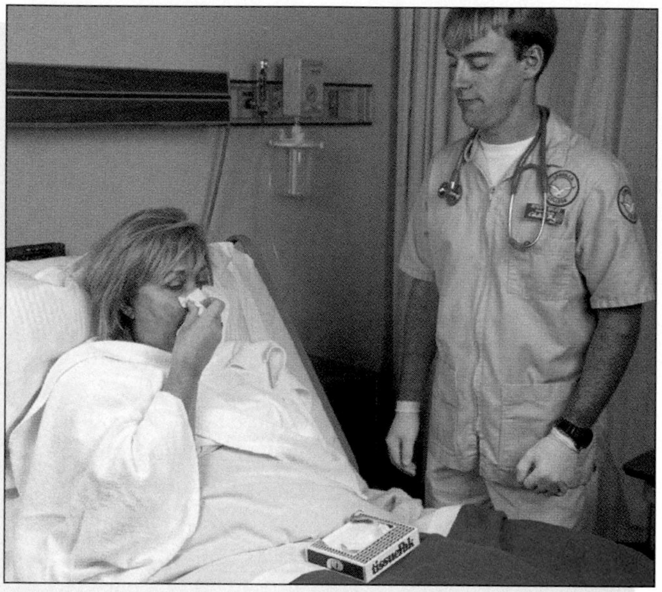

Offer oral and nasal hygiene after removing tube.

Documentation for Gastrointestinal Intubation

- Type of tube inserted
- Technique used to assess NG tube placement
- Character and amount of drainage
- Type of suction and pressure setting used
- Frequency and solution used for irrigations
- Abdominal and elimination assessment findings (return of bowel sounds, passage of flatus)
- Net return for lavaged client (amount of irrigant instilled subtracted from amount of aspirated return).
- Frequent vital signs (if indicated)
- Nasal and oral hygiene measures
- Client's tolerance of decompression
- Results of gastric specimen testing (blood, pH)
- Decontaminating agents used for detox

Critical Thinking Application

UNEXPECTED OUTCOMES	CRITICAL THINKING OPTIONS
NG tube is difficult to advance.	• Select more patent nostril: Have client compress each nostril and breathe in to determine which is more patent. • Rotate tube or withdraw slightly, then try to advance, but do not force. • Relubricate tube and try again. • Stiffen tube by cooling in iced water. • Have client hold ice chips in mouth for a few minutes to numb nasal passage and suppress gag reflex.
Client coughs, is unable to speak and becomes *cyanotic* during tube insertion.	• Remove tube immediately as these indicate that tube is being advanced into client's airway.
Salem sump pigtail leaks gastric contents.	• Flush with normal saline, then with air to clear. • Keep blue pigtail at level above client's stomach. • Insert antireflux valve plug (blue side into blue pigtail lumen).

UNIT 4

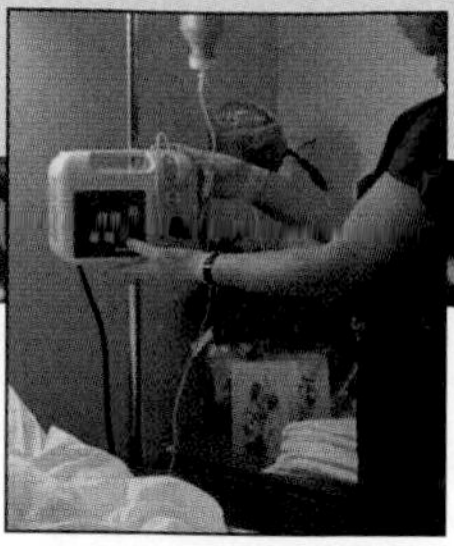

Enteral Tube Feedings

Nursing Process Data

ASSESSMENT Data Base

Assess client's nutritional status.

Physician's order for enteral feeding.

Determine rationale for prescribed enteral feeding.

Ensure appropriate placement of NG/NI tube using a variety of means.

Perform abdominal assessment (assure presence of bowel sounds unless feeding is given into small intestine).

Assess client's elimination pattern and characteristics.

PLANNING Objectives

To provide nutrients to the client who is unable to ingest normally

To correct nutritional deficiency in selected clients

To prevent respiratory complications

To prevent fluid and electrolyte imbalance

To promote healing of enterocutaneous fistula by direct mucosal feeding

PROCEDURES Interventions

Giving an Intermittent Feeding via Large-Bore Nasogastric Tube

for Intermittent Feeding via Gastrostomy Tube

Dressing the Gastrostomy Tube Site

Inserting a Small-Bore Feeding Tube

Providing Continuous Feeding via Small-Bore Nasointestinal/Jejunostomy Tube

EVALUATION Expected Outcomes

Validation measures indicate feeding tube is appropriately placed.

Aspirated residual volumes indicate adequate gastric emptying.

Client's nutritional needs are met.

Respiratory complications do not occur.

Fluid and electrolyte imbalance does not occur.

Gastrostomy/Jejunostomy tube site remains free of irritation or leakage.

GIVING AN INTERMITTENT FEEDING VIA LARGE-BORE NASOGASTRIC TUBE

Equipment

Antimicrobial swabs
Pen to mark date and time on equipment
Prescribed nutritional formula/product
Calibrated container for measuring formula
Irrigating syringe (50 mL) with catheter tip
pH indicator strip
Normal saline for flushing
Stethoscope
Towel
Gloves
Clean dressing for gastrostomy site, if needed

Preparation

1. Check physician's order for type, amount and frequency of feeding.
2. Swab unopened formula container top with alcohol.
3. Pour prescribed amount of formula into container (if refrigerated, warm formula by placing container in hot water; do not use microwave to warm formula).
4. Date and refrigerate opened formula can (discard in 24 hours).
5. Wash hands.
6. Maintain artificial airway cuff inflation during feeding (if indicated).

Procedure

1. Check client's identaband and have client state name.
2. Provide privacy and explain procedure and purpose to client.
3. Assess client's abdomen to verify presence of bowel sounds. **Rationale:** Absence of bowel sounds indicates lack of peristalsis, and gastric feeding should not be given.
4. Check mark on tube at exit site. **Rationale:** To check for possible migration of tube.
5. Don gloves.
6. Elevate client's head of bed 30°–45° angle or high Fowler's.
7. Place towel under work area.
8. Remove white tip of antireflux valve from NG tube.
9. Insert syringe into NG tube to validate gastric placement. **Rationale:** Tube could have migrated between feedings.
   a. Auscultate "whoosh" of injected air.
   b. Check color and test pH of aspirate (once every 8 hours after first 24 hours of tube placement).
   c. Aspirate gastric contents to determine residual volume. **Rationale:** Feeding should be withheld if residual volume is greater than one-half the amount of previously delivered feeding.
   d. Return aspirated contents to stomach. **Rationale:** This helps prevent electrolyte imbalance.

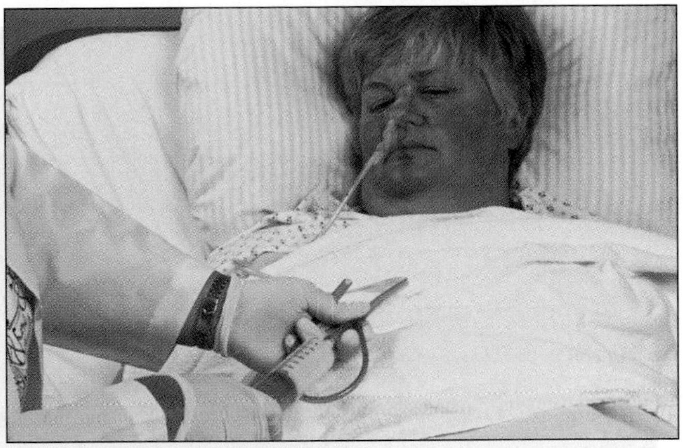
Aspirate gastric contents to determine residual volume; then return contents to stomach to prevent electrolyte imbalance.

10. Preflush prior to feeding, if necessary.
11. Pinch tubing. **Rationale:** This procedure prevents air from entering stomach.
12. Remove plunger from barrel of syringe, and attach barrel to NG tube.
13. Fill syringe with formula. (If using feeding bag, adjust drip rate to infuse over 30 minutes. Usually drop factor on feeding bags is 20 drops/mL.)

CLINICAL ALERT

Gastric ileus or delayed emptying may result in retention of forced feedings and impose a serious risk of aspiration and death, especially when feedings are continuous. To reduce the risk of aspiration:

- Aspirate gastric contents (NG tube) to determine retention before administering any intermittent feeding.
- For intermittent feedings, the residual volume should not be greater than one-half the amount of the previously delivered feeding.
- Regularly analyze residuals with continuously infused feeding to evaluate whether retained amount is significant. For instance, if the formula is infusing at 100 mL/hr and aspirated volume is greater than 100 mL, the stomach is not emptying as fast as the feeding is being infused.
- Keep the head of bed elevated at all times for *continuous* feeding, and for 1 to 2 hours following an intermittent (bolus) feeding.
- Report delayed gastric emptying to the physician for possible pharmacologic management.
- Check placement of NG tube prior to administering medications and every 8 hours for continuous feeding.

TABLE 19–3 Comparison of Enteral Tube Feeding Methods

	Advantages	Disadvantages
Nasogastric	• Easily placed. • Intermittent feeding is possible, so client is less confined. • Large-volume feeding may be delivered less often. • Tube placement does not require x-ray confirmation. • Acid environment may reduce infection. • Less risk of dumping syndrome. • Uses normal gastric emptying, preventing intestinal overload. • Less expensive; no feeding pump required.	• Limited to 1 wk use. • Gastric retention, reflux, and aspiration are possible. • Large tube is uncomfortable and visible to others. • Naris ulceration may occur. • Allows regurgitation by interfering with normal upper and lower esophageal sphincter function. • Gastric ulceration or fistulae may occur.
Gastrostomy or PEG	• Long-term use is possible. • Allows intermittent feeding. • Normal gastric emptying occurs. • Tube is not visible to others. • Medication administration is easier. • Less risk of infection. • Client can ambulate. • Esophageal irritation is avoided.	• Requires surgical placement with sedation or local anesthetic. • Requires local skin care. • May ulcerate gastric mucosa.
Nasointestinal	• Smaller tube is more comfortable. • Less risk of reflux and aspiration.	• Requires x-ray confirmation. • Tube is more difficult to place. • Client is still at risk for aspirating nasopharyngeal and gastric contents. • Elevated position must be maintained. • Constant infusion used; intermittent feeding not recommended because of osmotic response of small intestine. • Cramping, vomiting, distention, and diarrhea more common. • Requires pump; more expensive. • Tube can displace back into stomach (with constant infusion, this increases risk of aspiration). • Medication administration is difficult (liquid form preferred). • Greater risk of infection due to alkaline environment. • Limited to 4 wk use.
Jejunostomy	• Tube position is guaranteed. • Tube is not visible. • Possibly less risk of reflux and aspiration.	• Requires general anesthesia for placement. • Continuous infusion is required. • Local skin care is required. • Cramping, vomiting, distention, and diarrhea are more common. • Other disadvantages associated with nasointestinal feeding.

14. Hold container no more than 18 inches above client's stomach. **Rationale:** Holding container too high increases flow rate; rapid infusion can cause diarrhea.
15. Allow formula to infuse slowly (between 20 and 35 minutes) through the tubing. Clamp tubing or continue to fill syringe before syringe empties; do not allow syringe to "run dry." **Rationale:** If syringe runs dry before the addition of more formula, air enters stomach.
16. Follow tube feeding with water flush in amount ordered (usually 30–60 mL). **Rationale:** Water cleans tube and prevents obstruction with formula.
17. Reinsert antireflux valve.
18. Maintain head of bed elevation at least 1 to 2 hours.
19. Wash, rinse, and dry equipment after each feeding. Markdate and change syringe daily.
20. Return equipment to client's bedside.
21. Give prescribed amount of water between feedings, PO or per tube, if tube feeding is sole source of nutrition.
22. Provide oral hygiene.
23. Remove gloves and wash hands.

CLINICAL ALERT

Instances of death have been associated with systemic *absorption* of blue dye, which has been added to enteral formula (client's skin and internal organs become blue). It is thought that dye translocates by inhibiting the normal protective barrier processes of the gastrointestinal tract. Large containers of blue dye have been found to be contaminated. Dye is added to formula only on a physician's prescription and a single dose (blue dye: FD&C#1, FDA approved) unit should be used. Do *not* open any closed system (e.g., ready-to-hang formula container) to add dye.

EVIDENCE BASED NURSING PRACTICE

Adding Blue Dye to Enteral Feedings

A research study of patients receiving oral or enteral feedings with blue dye added has demonstrated that clinically significant aspiration occurred in 33% of the enterally fed patients. Positive glucose oxidase strip readings were present in 87% of patients with positive aspiration while blue discoloration was detected in only 27% of patients. This research does not support the use of blue coloring for identification of aspiration. Furthermore, multiple-dose blue dye containers may be a source of respiratory infections.

Source: Fellows, et al. (2000). Evidence-based practice for enteral feedings: Aspiration prevention strategies, bedside detection and practice change. *Medsurg Nursing, 9*(1), 27–31.

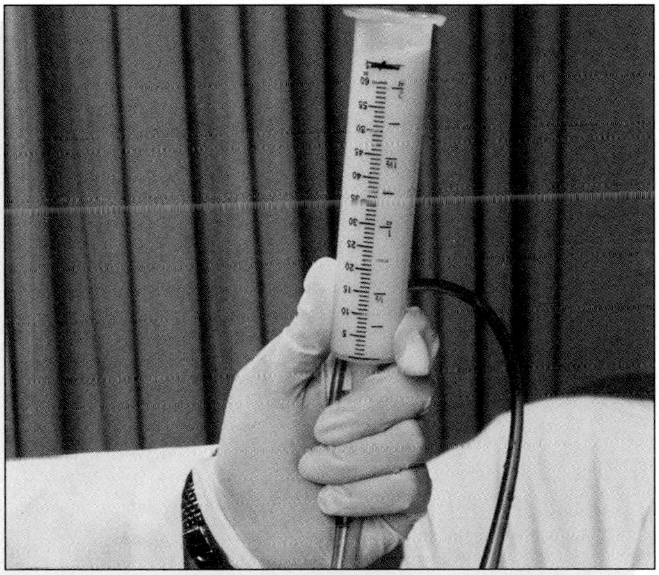

Allow feeding to flow by gravity and clamp tubing before syringe empties, or continuously fill syringe before it completely empties.

for Intermittent Feeding via Gastrostomy Tube

1. Check length of exposed tubing.
2. Aspirate to check residual volume. **Rationale:** Increased residuals may indicate delayed gastric emptying or that gastrostomy tube's internal stabilizer has migrated and is obstructing pyloric outlet.
3. Hold syringe no higher than 18 inches above client's stomach and administer 30 mL of water to flush and test patency of tubing. Clamp tubing by folding before syringe empties. **Rationale:** To prevent administering air into client's stomach.

CLINICAL ALERT

If gastrostomy tube residual is unobtainable, the tube may be displaced between client's stomach and abdominal wall, in which case administration of feeding could result in peritonitis.

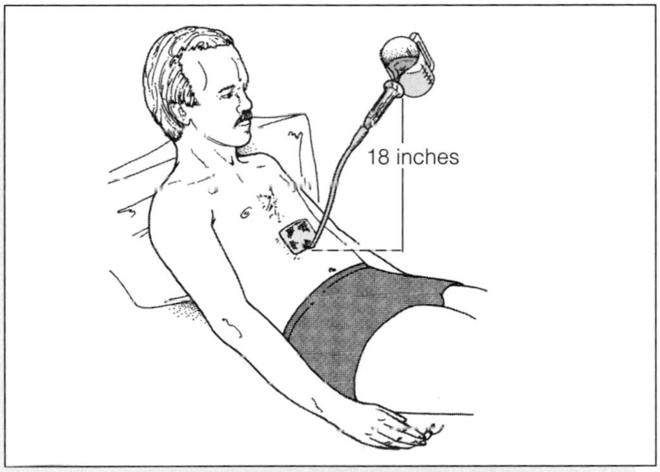

Allow feeding to flow by gravity through gastrostomy tube.

4. Insert empty syringe into gastrostomy tube opening and administer feeding, no higher than 18 inches above client's stomach, allowing formula to flow by gravity.
5. Proceed as in previous skill with flushing, then reinsert tube plug.

CLINICAL ALERT

Vomiting and pulmonary aspiration are more likely to occur in any client with delayed gastric emptying. Stop feedings if the client experiences abdominal distention, GI distress, or increasing residuals.

Note: Gastrostomy site may be left open to Air.

6. Remove dressing (if dressing is used,) around gastrostomy site.
7. Wash, rinse, and dry skin. Assess skin condition.
8. Apply clean dressing. (*See* Skill "Dressing the Gastrostomy Tube Site.")
9. Maintain head of bed elevation 30–60 minutes.

EVIDENCE BASED NURSING PRACTICE

PEG Tube Feedings Influence on Health Status

In a study of 150 patients (mean age of 78.9), 70% of those receiving PEG tube feedings had no significant improvement in functional, nutritional or overall health status.

Source: Callahan, C., et al. (2000). Outcomes of percutaneous endoscopic gastrostomy among older adults in a community setting. *Journal of American Geriatric Society, 48*(9), 1054.

DRESSING THE GASTROSTOMY TUBE SITE

Equipment

Normal saline; dated and initialed container left at client's bedside.
4 × 4 gauze squares or swabs and dilute peroxide
Protective skin barrier paste (if indicated)
Prepared split gauze dressing (occlusive dressing encourages fungal growth)
Gloves
Tape
Pen to label dressing

Preparation

1. Gather equipment.
2. Wash hands.

Procedure

1. Check client's room number and identaband and have client state name.
2. Provide privacy and explain procedure and purpose to client.
3. Don gloves.
4. Remove old dressing and discard.
5. Inspect exit site for signs of irritation or leakage.
6. Open packet of gauze squares and saturate with dilute peroxide.
7. Cleanse around exit site, then rotate external bumper 90°.
8. Dry site.
9. Apply thin layer of protective skin barrier paste to site (if excoriated). **Rationale:** To protect the skin from leakage; physician should be notified.
10. Place split dressing over (not under) external bar. **Rationale:** Dressing placed under the external bar can cause erosion of gastric tissue or abscess of the abdominal wall due to pressure on the internal bar within the stomach.
11. Secure dressing with tape (if necessary) and if external tube is long, secure it to dressing with tape. **Rationale:** To prevent inadvertent pulling and dislodgement of tube.

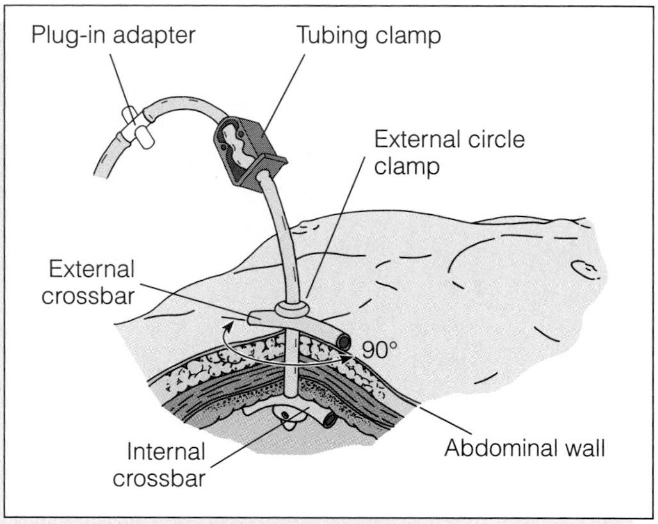

Change tube dressing when wet, or daily, placing dressing *over* external crossbar.

12. Mark dressing with your initials, date and time.
13. Remove gloves and wash hands.
14. After one week, cleanse site with soap and water and leave open to air, according to physician's orders.

Clients requiring *sustained* enteral feeding, may prefer a low profile gastrostomy tube. These tubes are inserted several (3+) months after the gastrostomy tract (stoma) has healed. They fit close to the skin, so are less apt to be pulled out or get in the way of daily activities. In addition, some incorporate a one-way antireflux valve which opens for feedings and also prevents backflow of gastric contents.

Since products differ, refer to the manufacturer's instructions for the specific tube your client has had inserted.

INSERTING A SMALL-BORE FEEDING TUBE

Equipment

Feeding tube package, small-bore (8–12 Fr) radiopaque nasointestinal feeding tube (43–60 inch) with stylet and weighted tip
Administration set with pump or controller
50 mL syringe, normal saline solution
Clean gloves
Water-soluble lubricant (if needed)
Micropore or adhesive tape
Glass with water and straw, if appropriate
Stethoscope
Towel and tissues
Safety pin or clip
Emesis basin
pH chemstrip
Pen for marking tube

Preparation

1. Validate physician's orders.
2. Gather equipment.
3. Check client's room number and identaband.
4. Provide privacy.

Procedure

1. Wash hands.
2. Explain procedure to client.
3. Elevate head of bed at least 45°. Place towel over chest, provide tissues and emesis basin.
4. Determine length of tube for insertion into stomach. Use distal end of feeding tube, and measure from tip of nose to earlobe to xiphoid process and add 10 inches. Place tape on tube to mark position.
5. Check that guidewire does not protrude through holes in feeding tube. Reposition guidewire as necessary. **Rationale:** This will prevent trauma or damage to the mucosa.
6. Don gloves.
7. Lubricate tip of feeding tube with water-soluble lubricant. Tubes with surface lubricant need to have tip of tube moistened in water to activate lubricant.
8. Assess nares to determine patency. **Rationale:** The appropriate nostril to use for tube insertion is the more patent one.

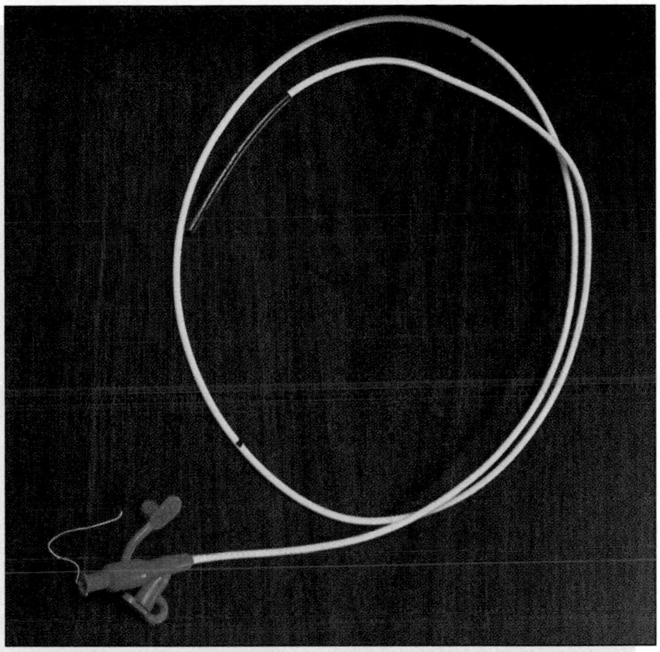

Check that guidewire (stylet) does not protrude through holes in feeding tube. Reposition guide if necessary.

9. Instruct client to hyperextend neck.
10. Insert feeding tube through patent nostril and gently advance tube.
11. Ask client to flex head forward and swallow when tube reaches pharynx. (Stimulation of gag reflex is normal with tube insertion.) **Rationale:** This will assist tube to move into esophagus. Hyperextension at this stage may open airway and tube could move into trachea.
12. Pull back on tube if client begins to cough or show signs of respiratory distress. **Rationale:** Tube has entered trachea not esophagus.
13. Wait several seconds, then advance tube asking client to swallow when tube reaches pharynx.
14. Advance tube to premeasured position; stop and listen at tube tip for breathing sounds. **Rationale:** If you can hear air exchange, tube could be in respiratory tract.
15. Tape tube in place.

EVIDENCE BASED NURSING PRACTICE

In a study comparing the use of water versus cranberry juice as a irrigant to maintain patency of small-bore feeding tubes, tubes irrigated with water were found to have significantly lower incidence of occlusion than those irrigated with cranberry juice.

Source: Frankel, E., et al. (1998). Methods of restoring patency to occluded feeding tubes. *Nutrition in Clinical Practice, 13,* 120–131.

16. Flush tube (side port) with 30–60 mL air, then attempt to aspirate contents; reposition client and repeat aspiration if necessary to obtain a specimen.
17. Test aspirated secretions for color and pH. **Rationale:** As tube advances into small intestine, pH becomes higher (>5).
18. Do not remove guidewire. **Rationale:** Once guidewire is removed it cannot be reinserted to manipulate tube placement.
19. Turn client to right side-lying. **Rationale:** To allow natural digestive reflexes to expel tube from stomach and into small intestine. Most tubes migrate into small intestine in 24 hours.
20. Obtain x-ray to determine feeding tube placement. DO NOT INITIATE FEEDING until desired placement is confirmed, and guidewire is removed.
21. Once position is validated, connect feeding tube to feeding administration set.
22. Flush feeding tube with water (using at least a 30-mL syringe, as a smaller syringe could cause too much pressure in the tube) every 4 hours as ordered, or following administration of formula or medication. **Rationale:** This maintains patency of tube; small-bore tubes may become obstructed.
23. Check tape daily that secures tube to nostril. Keep nares clean. Secure tube by pinning or clipping to gown.
24. Replace small-bore tube every 3–4 weeks or as ordered. **Rationale:** Small-bore tubes can become contaminated or obstructed.
25. Administer daily mouth care to client.
26. Remove gloves, wash hands, and make client comfortable.

Safety Concerns: Small-bore Feeding Tubes

- Do not allow formula to hang for over 4 hours.
- Change formula bag/reservoir and administration set daily.
- Discard closed formula system after 24 hours.
- If small bore nasointestinal feeding tube fails to migrate into the small intestine, consult physician to prescribe a prokinetic medication (e.g., metoclopramide) to induce transpyloric passage of the tube.

PROVIDING CONTINUOUS FEEDING VIA SMALL-BORE NASOINTESTINAL/ JEJUNOSTOMY TUBE

Equipment

Prescribed formula in closed ready to infuse system (preferred)
Formula reservoir or bag (if necessary for open system)
Infusion pump (not to exceed 40 psi)
Administration tubing compatible with pump
Label or pen
60 mL sterile syringe
Sterile normal saline solution or warm water
Gloves, if indicated

Preparation

1. Check physician's order for feeding formula (type and volume to administer).
2. Check x-ray report. **Rationale:** Validates that tube has advanced beyond client's pyloric valve or to proximal jejunum.
3. Wash hands.
4. Gather equipment.
5. Mark date on formula, reservoir, administration tubing (to be changed daily).
6. Don gloves for inspection of jejunostomy site.

Procedure

1. Fill with enough formula to limit hang time to 4 hours if using reservoir or bag for continuous intestinal feeding.

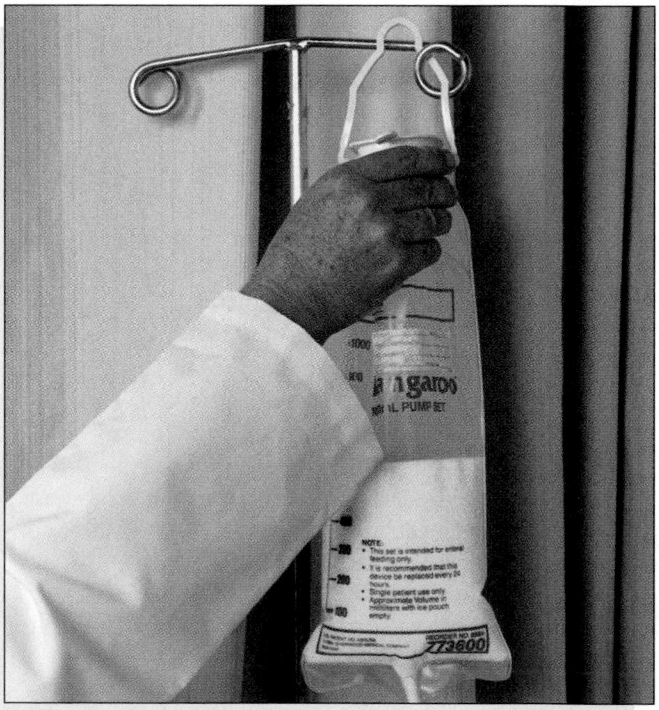

If using open system reservoir or bag for continuous feeding, fill with enough formula to limit hang time to 4 hours.

Rationale: To reduce risk of infection since intestine is a less protected (alkaline) environment.
2. Connect administration tubing to formula reservoir (con-

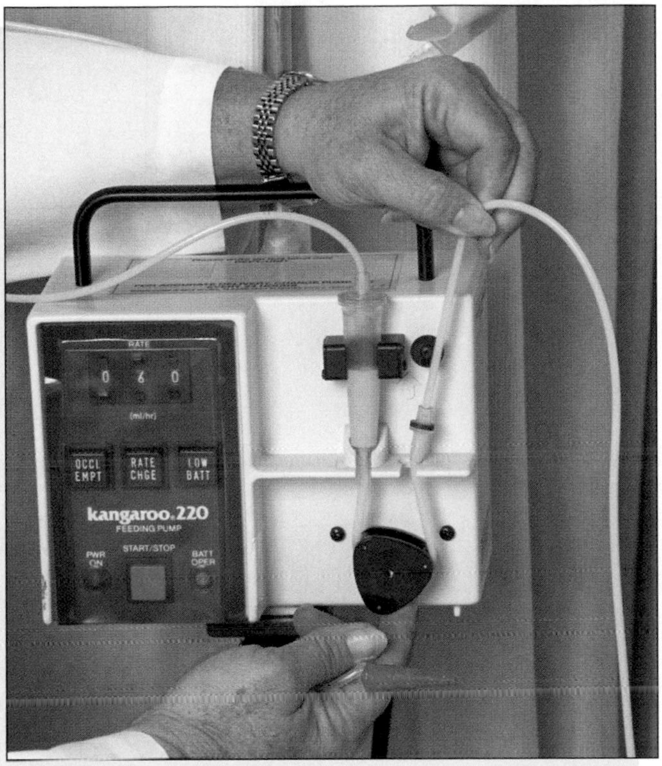

Thread tubing through pump per manufacturer's instructions. Pump must not exceed 40 psi.

tainer or bag) and prime tubing per manufacturer's instructions.

3. Thread tubing through pump per manufacturer's instructions.
4. Note mark on client's feeding tube to determine if migration has occurred.
5. Connect primed formula tubing to client's small-bore nasointestinal tube. Initiate feeding with isotonic (300 mOsml) or slightly hypotonic formula. **Rationale:** To prevent dumping syndrome (cramping and diarrhea).

Note: Alternate method is to connect formula tubing to client's surgically established jejunostomy feeding tube.

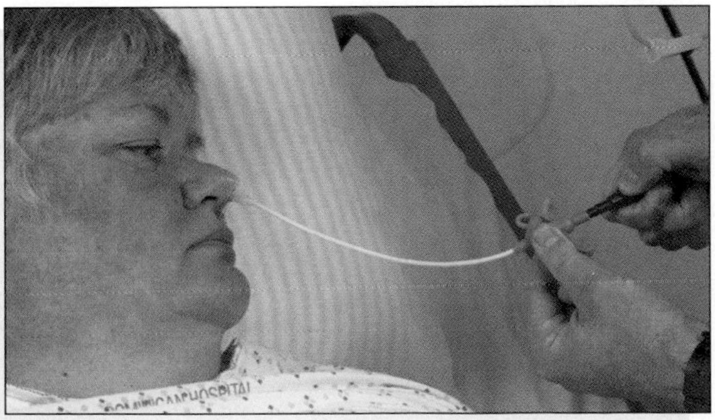
Connect feeding tube to client's small-bore nasointestinal tube.

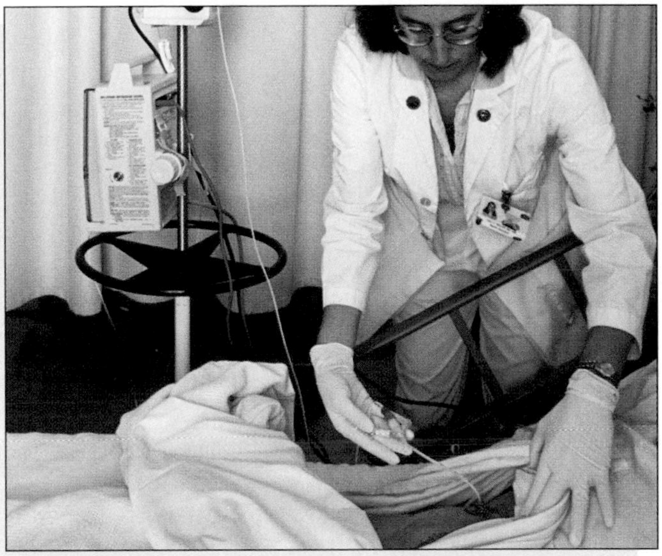
Connect continuous feeding system to client's surgically placed jejunostomy tube.

6. Start feeding at slow constant infusion rate (25–50 mL/hr). **Rationale:** Slow increase in feeding volume is better tolerated. (Maximum rate is 100–150 mL/hr).
7. If client tolerates feeding, increase rate in 8–24 hours (increase by 25–50 mL/hr to prescribed rate).
8. Keep client's head of bed elevated at 30°–45° angle *at all times* if infusion is continuous. **Rationale:** To reduce risk of aspiration.
9. Using side-port, flush small-bore continuous feeding tube every 4–6 hours, and before and after medication, with 30 mL of warm water. **Rationale:** To prevent tube clogging.
10. Obtain a new sterile syringe each time closed system side-port is used for flushing.
11. Rinse open system reservoir thoroughly before adding additional formula.

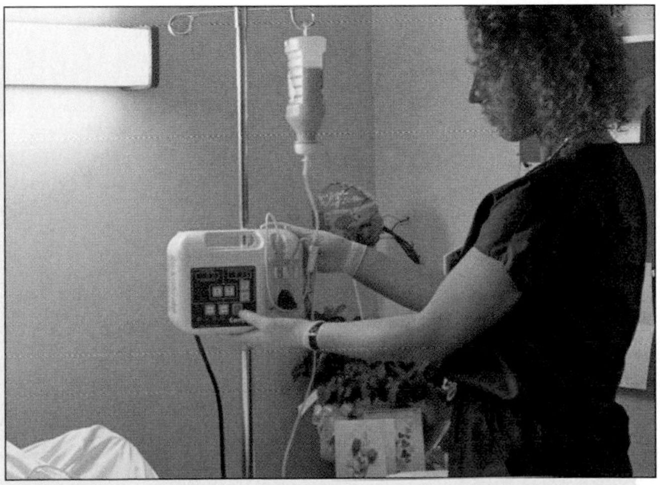
Start continuous feeding at slow rate (25–50 mL/hr).

CLINICAL ALERT

The pH method for determining tube placement may not be useful during *continuous* NG/NI feeding because the infused formula raises gastric pH and lowers intestinal pH. The continuous-feeding aspirate will look like formula, may be curdled or bile stained. A sudden increase in residual volume may indicate that a nasointestinal tube has become displaced upward into the stomach.

CLINICAL ALERT

If client is receiving continuous feeding, maintain HOB elevation at 30°–45° at all times.

Turn off feeding 1 hour before client must be repositioned at less than 30° for any procedure or transport.

DOCUMENTATION FOR ENTERAL TUBE FEEDINGS

- Date and time of procedure
- Placement of nasointestinal tube and x-ray validation of proper placement
- External length of exposed tubing
- Methods of validating tube placement
- Quantity and character of aspirated residuals (color, pH, other tests)
- Amount and type of formula/decontaminant given
- Frequent vital signs (if indicated)
- Head of bed elevation during and following feeding
- Frequency of tube irrigation and type of irrigant used
- Abdominal assessment findings (distention, nausea, vomiting, bowel sounds)
- Daily weight
- Intake and output
- Tube exit site assessment
- Application of dressing to exit site
- Oral hygiene provided
- Bowel elimination pattern and characteristics

Critical Thinking Application

UNEXPECTED OUTCOMES	CRITICAL THINKING OPTIONS
PEG external bar cannot be rotated.	• If PEG tube is immobile, notify physician immediately.
X-ray shows nasointestinal tube remains in stomach.	• Position client on right side to promote tube movement to distal antrum. • Report to physician and request order for medication to facilitate tube movement. (metoclopramide). • Delay any feeding until x-ray confirms that tube is in small intestine.
Feeding tube cannot be aspirated or flushed and formula is leaking from insertion site; occlusion alarm sounds continuously.	• Try flushing tube with warm water and small-volume (5 mL) luer lock syringe. • Use push and pull technique. • *Do not* use carbonated beverage or juice for irrigation • *Do not* use stylet (guidewire) to unclog tube. • Use declogging system suggested by tube manufacturer—if not successful, notify physician.

UNEXPECTED OUTCOMES	CRITICAL THINKING OPTIONS
Client develops diarrhea when feeding is started.	• Consult dietitian about osmolarity of formula (hyperosmolar formula causes diarrhea) • Decrease formula feeding and/or bolus feeding rate. • Do not add blue dye to formula.
Client develops diarrhea due to system contamination.	• Use careful handwashing when setting up or opening system. • Check expiration date on formula container. • Change formula reservoir, administration set or delivery syringe daily, maintain asepsís. • Do not add blue due to formula. • Use side port stopcock rather than disconnecting tube system to aspirate or deliver fluid.
Gastric residual is greater than 50% of amount administered in previous feeding.	• Withhold feeding temporarily and recheck. • Consult dietician for more isotonic formula. • Assess bowel sounds and report increasing residuals to physician.

GERONTOLOGIC CONSIDERATIONS

Dietary needs of the elderly include

Energy (caloric) requirement: 2,000–2,400 kcal/day (may adjust to energy expenditure and physical activity).

Protein: 10% of energy requirement, increases to 20% of energy requirement during periods of stress (surgery, infection, burn).

Fiber: 20–35 g/day of fiber (five servings of fruit per day).

Fluids: 1,500–2,000 mL of water/day or 30 mL/kg body weight.

Vitamins: same as for younger adult except for vitamins D, B_6, and B_{12}. *Significant deficiencies in* serum *levels of vitamins and minerals are rare in healthy older adults.*

Vitamin D requirement is 10 mg/day for adults 51–70 and 15 mg/day for those over age 70.

Vitamin B_6 intake should be 1.7 mg/day for men and 1.5 mg/day for women over age 51 (25% of elderly are deficient in vitamin B_6).

Vitamin B_{12} intake should be 2.4 mg for all adults over age 51 (about 15% of elderly are deficient in vitamin B_{12}).

Minerals: increased need only if for 10 ng/day of iron.

The elderly are at high risk for malnutrition due to age-related physiologic changes, health care status, and lifestyle factors.

Physiologic changes associated with aging.

- Between ages 25 and 70, percentage of body fat doubles and lean body mass decreases by about one third.
- Metabolic rate decreases 20% in men and 13% in elderly women; energy requirements decrease, there is reduced hunger and increased satiety due to increased levels of cholecystokinin, so food intake decreases.
- Esophageal and intestinal motility decrease.
- Saliva production decreases.
- Gastric secretions decline by 30% in adults over age 65, increasing risk for malabsorption of vitamin B_{12}, calcium, iron, folate, and possibly zinc.
- Lactose intolerance (more prevalent in elderly than younger adults) increases risk for calcium and vitamin D deficiency.
- Gastric emptying is slowed.
- Protein reserves may be inadequate for periods of stress, sepsis, or injury leading to protein—calorie malnutrition.

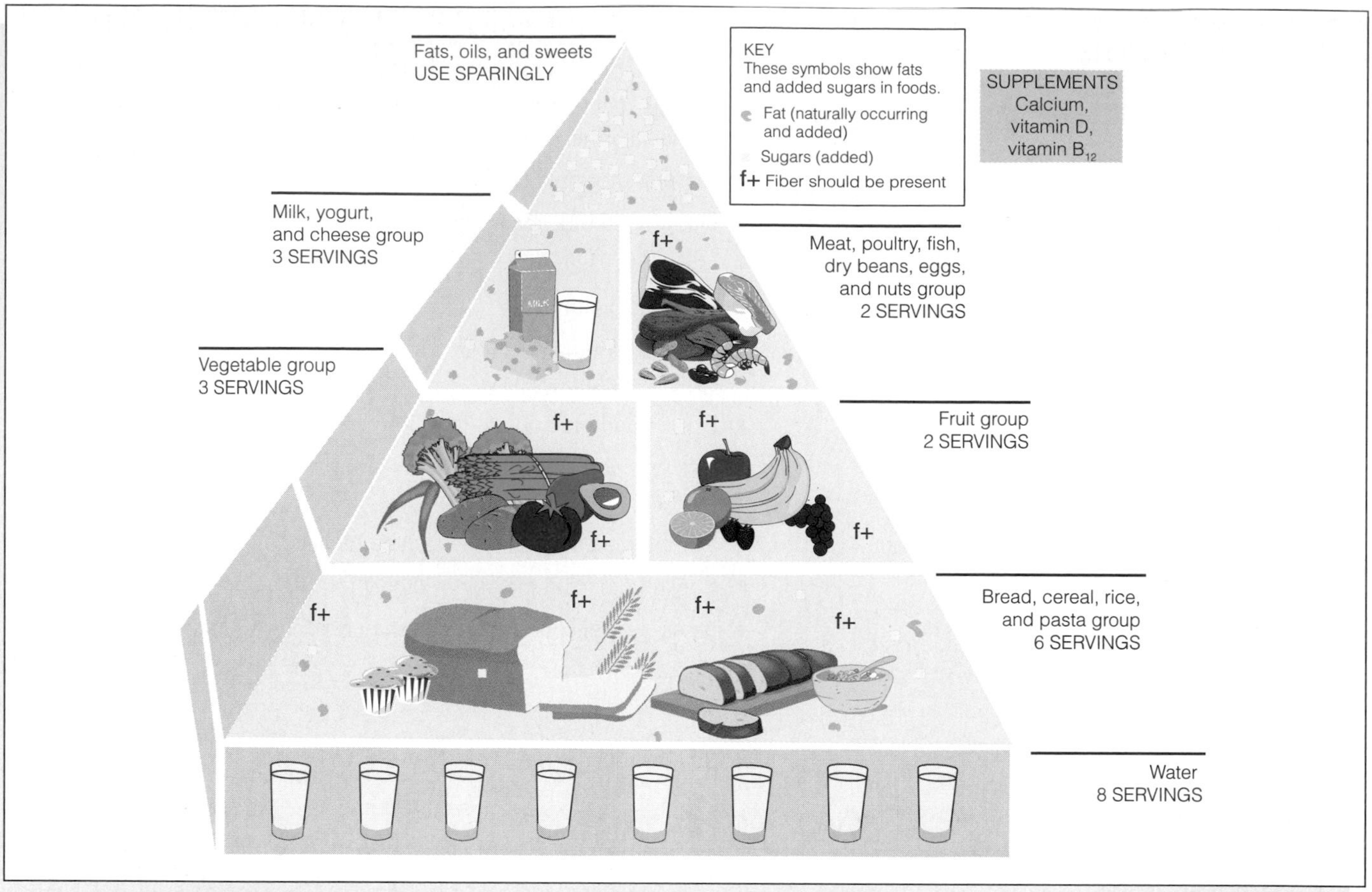

Revised Food Guide Pyramid for the Elderly*

The U.S. Government has revised the food pyramid to meet the needs of the healthy elderly over age 70. It differs from the standard pyramid by including eight 8-ounce glasses of pure water, needed by the aging body to prevent dehydration and constipation, and nutrient supplements of calcium, vitamins D and B_{12} which many elderly lack. Also different from the standard pyramid, this one does not set a limit on food servings but does encourage the elderly to limit intake of fats, oils and sweets.

*US Dept. of Agriculture Human Nutrition Research Center on Aging, Tults University, Boston, MS.

- Loss of sense of smell (in over 50% of those age 65–80 and 75% in those over age 80).
- Decline in thirst drive (risk for dehydration).

Health status factors.

- Poor dentition (up to 37% of elderly are edentulous). Loss of dentition is not due to the normal aging process but to improper oral hygiene and or inadequate nutrition beginning at an earlier age.
- Ill-fitting dentures causing pain limiting variety and quantity of intake.
- Swallowing or self-care deficit disorders (e.g., neuromuscular disorders, Parkinson's, Alzheimer's).
- Psychological changes (depression, cognitive impairment).
- Effect of medications (altered metabolism, anorexia, nausea, diarrhea, cognitive disturbance).
- Inappropriate diet prescription (low-salt, low-cholesterol or low-calorie diet).
- Medical conditions (e.g., COPD, heart failure, cancer resulting)

Lifestyle factors.

- Alcoholism
- Inadequate income
- Decreased physical activity, lack of transport, isolation
- Cultural values
- Lack of monitoring/caregiving

Assessment parameters for nutritional status of the elderly client in addition to the above risk factors include:

- Anthropometric values:

Body weight = men should weigh 106 lb for 5 feet plus 6 lb for each additional inch in height. Women should weigh 100 lb for 5 feet plus 5 pounds for each additional inch in height. Significant weight loss is more than 10% of body weight over the last 6 months or more than 7.5% over the last 3 months or more than 5% over the last month.

Body mass index risk for malnutrition:

Mild = BMI is 17.0–18.4

Moderate = 16.0–16.9

Severe = less than 16.0

- Biochemical indicators of *malnutrition* include:

  Serum albumin below 3.5 mg/L (increased risk for infection, pressure ulcers, prolonged hospitalization)

  Low serum cholesterol
- Serum creatinine (reflects muscle mass)

  Moderate deficit if 60–79% of predicted

  Severe deficit if less than 60% of predicted

MANAGEMENT GUIDELINES

Each state legislates a Nurse Practice Act for RNs and LVN/LPNs. Health care facilities are responsible for establishing and implementing policies and procedures that conform to their state's regulations. Verify the regulations and role parameters for each health care worker in your facility.

Delegation of Responsibilities

- The professional nurse is responsible for the client's basic nutritional assessment (an evaluation tool) if a dietician is not available. A nonprofessional (CNA or UAP) is not trained to assess this information. A periodic nutritional assessment should be completed for any client who is hospitalized for a long period of time.
- The UAP (unless specifically trained by a swallowing specialist) should not be allowed to feed or assist in feeding the dysphagic client. The licensed professional should monitor and evaluate the UAP's adherence to client-specific feeding instructions.
- Generally, serving a food tray or feeding a client is assigned to the nonprofessional staff. These staff should be reminded to report any unusual complaints or poor intake of food based on the client's care plan.
- Insertion of NG tubes is performed by a physician, an RN, or an LVN/LPN. A CNA or UAP may measure and record drainage from an NG tube and provide oral hygiene.
- Enteral feedings should be given by professional nurses, but some facilities do allow trained nonprofessionals to administer the feedings.
- If medication is administered through a (double lumen) tube, refer to agency protocol to determine who may administer the medication. According to some facilities, it is only an RN or LVN/LPN who may administer medication.

Information Flow

- Changes in GI therapy or nutritional support orders as well as significant changes in client data regarding tolerance of nutritional therapies (including laboratory data and client's elimination pattern) should be communicated to all staff.
- NPO or positioning requirements should be posted at the client's head of bed (HOB) and communicated to all attending staff (orally and by written plan of care).
- Specific instructions and special techniques for feeding the dysphagic client should be posted at the client's HOB.
- The UAP should report to the nurse when a feeding pump alarm sounds, or when additional formula is needed.
- The UAP should report to the nurse if a client's NG tube is leaking or if the client becomes nauseated or vomits.
- Clients who are taking enteral feedings should be working with a Nutrition Support Team (NST) in accordance with the American Society for Parenteral and Enteral Nutrition. The nursing staff should work with and communicate through this team, because they are trained to follow this aspect of the care plan.
- The nurse assigned to the client is the essential link between the client and the team, thus both verbal and written reports are important for continuity of care and assessment of the nutritional status of the client.

- It is also important for the nurse to teach the client and his or her family about the need for and routine of nutritional support through enteral feedings.
- Following initial nutrition screening by the admitting nurse, the physician, or other appropriate member of client's care team (e.g., speech or occupational therapist), the Nutrition Support Team for individualized assessment of clients should be contacted. Areas for assessment are:

Nutrition risk on screening
Extended ICU stay
Any type of nutrition support (tube feeding, TPN)
Latex allergy
75 years and older and having surgery
Liquid diet or NPO for more than 3 days
Pregnant or lactating but not admitted for delivery

CRITICAL THINKING STRATEGIES

SCENARIO 1

Mrs. Ramsey, age 62, has been admitted to the hospital with complaints of painful abdominal distention and signs of dehydration after 2 days of vomiting. She is diagnosed with small bowel obstruction due to adhesions (scar tissue) from a remote abdominal hysterectomy.

1. What are the pathophysiologic effects of intestinal obstruction?
2. What potential fluid and electrolyte problems occur with small bowel obstruction?
3. How does the loss of gastric secretions differ from the loss of intestinal secretions?
4. What are the body's normal compensatory mechanisms for acid–base imbalances due to loss of gastrointestinal fluids?
5. What interventions help to correct these imbalances?

SCENARIO 2

An elderly client (age 64) is admitted to the hospital for a hip replacement. When you are taking a history, you note that she appears to be malnourished.

1. What additional dietary information would be important to include in the database for this client?
2. Evaluate the assessment parameters in terms of the nutritional needs of the elderly and examine how this client fits into the model.
3. Identify the primary parameters to be included in the discharge plan for this client.

SCENARIO 3

Mr. Bradley has been diagnosed with cancer of the liver and is admitted to the hospital with brain metastases. He complains of no appetite, refuses most meals, and is becoming significantly malnourished with drastic weight loss. Impairment of his hepatic and neurologic status has caused intermittent periods of nonresponsiveness and inability to eat.

Mr. Bradley's family is asking about alternative nutrition options and the physician is requesting that they make decisions about the treatment options.

1. If nutritional support is indicated, what are the processes normally followed?
2. Who has the primary decision making power about medical treatments such as nutritional support?
3. Do health care providers have an obligation to provide extraordinary care?
4. Once initiated, can health care providers discontinue artificial feeding?
5. In what ways can health care providers provide symbolically significant care?

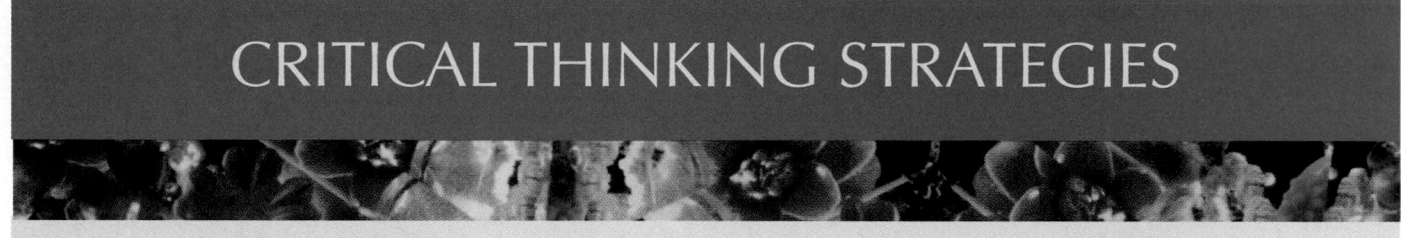

CHAPTER 20

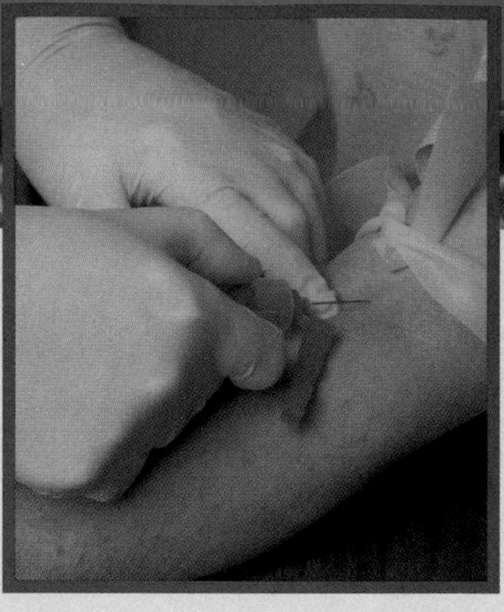

Specimen Collection

THEORETICAL CONCEPTS

UNIT ONE: **Urine Specimens** **629**

Collecting Midstream Urine 630

Collecting 24-Hour Urine Specimen 631

UNIT TWO: **Infant Urine Specimen** **633**

Collecting a Specimen from an Infant 634

UNIT THREE: **Stool Specimens** **635**

Collecting Adult Stool Specimen 636

Collecting Stool for Ova and Parasites 636

Collecting Infant Stool Specimen 637

Testing for Occult Blood 637

for gamma Fe-Cult Plus 637

for Hemoccult 638

for Gastroccult 638

Collecting Stool for Bacterial Culture 638

Teaching Parents to Test for Pinworms 638

UNIT FOUR: **Blood Specimens** **640**

Withdrawing Venous Blood (Phlebotomy) 641

Using Vacutainer System 641

Withdrawing Arterial Blood 643

Collecting a Specimen for Culture 644

Obtaining Blood Specimen for Glucose Testing (Capillary Puncture) 645

Measuring Blood Glucose Using Chemstrip 645

Measuring Blood Glucose Using Glucometer 646

Monitoring Glucose: Sure Step FLEXX 646

for Quality Control 646

for Measuring Blood Glucose 647

Measuring Blood Glucose Using Lifescan One-Touch II 647

UNIT FIVE: **Sputum Collection** **650**

Obtaining Sputum Specimen 651

Using Suction Trap 652

Collecting Specimen by Transtracheal Aspiration 652

UNIT SIX: **Throat and Wound Specimens for Culture** **654**

Obtaining a Throat Specimen 655

Obtaining Wound Specimen for Aerobic Culture 655

Obtaining Wound Specimen for Anaerobic Culture 656

GERONTOLOGIC CONSIDERATIONS 657

MANAGEMENT GUIDELINES 658

CRITICAL THINKING STRATEGIES 659

LEARNING OBJECTIVES

- Discuss the nursing responsibilities for reporting abnormal laboratory values.
- Describe the major client instructions that ensure an uncontaminated midstream urine specimen.
- State two objectives for obtaining a stool specimen.
- List four precautions that must be carried out when obtaining a stool specimen for parasite identification.
- Demonstrate the procedure for testing for occult blood.
- State necessary documentation when collecting a stool specimen.
- Explain the objectives for collecting a sputum specimen.
- Outline the steps of collecting a sputum specimen from a suction trap.
- Compare and contrast obtaining an aerobic and anaerobic culture.
- State the purpose for using an autolet.
- Demonstrate the use of the autolet to obtain a capillary blood specimen.
- Write two nursing diagnoses which are relevant for specimen collection.
- Demonstrate the removal of blood using a vacutainer.
- List specimen collections requiring specific consent forms.
- State two critical-thinking solutions for the problem of blood not flowing into the syringe when withdrawing blood.
- State the nursing action when a hematoma occurs at the puncture site.

TERMINOLOGY

Aerobe: a microorganism that lives and grows in the presence of free oxygen.

Albuminuria: the presence of albumin in the urine.

Anaerobe: an organism that lives and grows in the absence of molecular oxygen.

Antimicrobial: an agent that prevents the multiplication of microorganisms.

Antimicrobic: preventing the development or pathogenic action of microbes.

Asepsis: prevention of contact with microorganisms.

Aspiration: the removal of fluids or gases from a cavity by the application of suction.

Autolet: a small instrument with lancet used to obtain a capillary blood specimen; usually used to measure blood glucose level.

Bacteria: unicellular plant-like microorganisms lacking chlorophyll.

Cannula: a tube for insertion into a duct or cavity.

Culture: to grow microorganisms or living tissue cells in a special medium.

Dermis: synonym for corium; the skin layer beneath the epidermis; contains vascular connective tissue.

Excoriation: a breakdown of the epidermis.

Expectorant: an agent that facilitates the removal of the secretions of the bronchopulmonary mucous membrane.

Exudate: material obtained from a wound as the result of the inflammatory process.

Genitourinary: pertaining to the genital and urinary systems.

Glucose: a monosaccharide, the end product of carbohydrate metabolism; also known as dextrose; found in the normal blood.

Glycosuria: the presence of sugar in the urine.

Granulocytes: a granular leukocyte.

Hematuria: blood in the urine.

Hypovolemia: diminished circulating fluid volume.

Inflammatory process: localized response when injury or destruction of tissue has occurred; destroys, wards off, or dilutes the causative agent or the injured tissue.

Intracellular: inside the cell.

Micturition: the process of emptying the urinary bladder; voiding.

Occult blood: blood in minute quantities, can be recognized only by microscopic examination or by chemical means.

Parasite: an organism that lives within, on, or at the expense of another organism, known as the host.

Patency: the state of being freely open.

Pathogen: disease-producing organism.

Pinworm: oxyurid parasite of the intestine, usually *Enterobrus vermicularis.* Commonly found in children. Piperazine is drug of choice.

Polyuria: the excessive production and elimination of urine.

Purulent: containing pus, or caused by pus.

Pus: an inflammation product containing leukocytes and exudate.

Septic: pertinent to pathologic organisms or their toxins.

Septicemia: presence of pathologic bacteria in the blood.

Skin turgor: the tension or fullness of the cells.

Specific gravity: weight of a substance compared with an equal volume of water. Water is 1.000.

Specimen: a sample taken to show or to determine the character of the whole, as a specimen of urine.

Sputum: substance expelled by coughing or clearing the throat.

Stool: waste matter discharged from the bowels.

Transtracheal: passage of a tube or needle through the wall of the trachea.

Urinary tract infection (UTI): an infection of the urinary tract, including all or part of the organs and ducts participating in the secretion and elimination of urine.

Vacutainer: a plastic adapter that fits onto a double-ended needle for obtaining a venous blood sample.

Venipuncture: puncture of a vein with a needle or catheter.

Venous: pertaining to the veins; unoxygenated blood.

Viscosity: resistance offered by a fluid; property of a substance that is dependent on the friction of its component molecules as they slide by each other.

LABORATORY TESTS

Laboratory tests are an adjunct for diagnosing health care problems and assessing the health status of clients. Test findings can reveal occult problems, determine the stage of disease, estimate the activity of the disease process, and measure the effect of therapy. Multiple laboratory tests are usually ordered not only to assist in diagnosing problems but also to rule out certain disease states.

Laboratory tests can be analyzed individually or as a part of a screening panel. For example, a routine urinalysis screens for the chemical makeup of the urine as well as color, clarity, and presence of abnormal cells. Blood chemistry components can be tested individually as well as in combination through a multiparameter test. These tests provide data on 8, 12, or 16 different elements of blood, depending on the laboratory equipment. It is more cost-effective when all the tests are run simultaneously with one blood specimen. For example, a "panel 12" analyzes the following tests: total protein, albumin, calcium, inorganic phosphorous, cholesterol, glucose, BUN, uric acid, creatinine, total bilirubin, alkaline phosphatase, and SGOT.

Every laboratory establishes its own normal values for each test. The normal values are generally printed on each laboratory slip to facilitate comparisons with the client's findings. Healthy clients do not always fall within the calculated laboratory norms. The physician, considering other variables, must judge the value and diagnostic implications of these tests.

Nursing Responsibility

Nursing responsibilities associated with the collection of specimens range from client education to reporting abnormal laboratory findings to the appropriate health team member. When specimens are ordered, it is essential that the client understands the full importance of "how" and "why" the specimen is to be obtained. If sterile or clean technique is required, client teaching can provide an understanding of the process. If the client is involved with obtaining the specimen, precise instructions should be given.

To prevent unnecessary lost time and cost to the client, the nurse must be well informed of the correct procedure for obtaining, handling, and processing each specimen. If the nurse is unfamiliar with the procedure, he or she should refer to the nursing procedure or laboratory manual for the health care facility. Specific directions are written for most tests performed by the laboratory. If there is any question about the procedure, the laboratory should be called for directions before obtaining the specimen.

The physician should be notified immediately of any abnormal laboratory findings which could be potentially life-threatening. Verbal communication is the most appropriate and efficacious method. When the nurse leaves written messages on the chart, several hours may elapse before the physician sees the findings.

The nurse should also document when abnormal results are reported to the physician. Documentation should include date, time, tests, and the orders taken. If results were left with another person such as office personnel, the name of the person receiving results should be documented.

All clients admitted to a healthcare facility have at least one laboratory specimen collected during their hospitalization. The most frequent laboratory tests ordered are those involving the urine and blood.

It is the nurse's responsibility to be aware of any and all legal implications of specimen collection. Reporting certain tests, such as HIV testing, requires a specific consent; likewise, certain test results are required to be reported to ensure public safety. It is important to remember that all client information, including laboratory results, is confidential.

Urine Tests

Nursing responsibilities include collecting, temporarily storing, and performing tests on the urine specimen. Timed urine specimens are usually left in the nursing unit until completion of the test. When urine specimens are retained in the nursing unit, the nurse must take special care in the storing and handling of the specimen to ensure reliable results. Generally, urine specimens collected over a period of hours must be refrigerated or have preservatives added to the specimen to ensure accurate results.

Preservatives, such as hydrochloric acid or thymol, prevent deterioration of the specimen.

Most urine specimens are collected as clean-catch, or midstream, specimens and sent directly to the laboratory. Single urine specimens are obtained through random sampling. It is best to obtain the first voided specimen in the morning for routine urine tests. This specimen is more concentrated, and the pH is more acidic. The midstream method of urine collection necessitates that proper instructions be given to the client in cleansing the genitalia and obtaining the specimen.

When timed specimens are ordered, the nursing role encompasses not only the handling of the urine specimen but also precise instructions to the client for collecting the specimen. The collection of urine needs to start and finish at the designated time. Timed tests vary from 2 hours to 24 hours. Assessment for amylase and bilirubin can be done on a 2-hour collection. Creatinine clearance and estriol determination require a 24-hour specimen. A 24-hour urine specimen that is started at 9 A.M. must be finished at 9 A.M. the next day in order to obtain accurate results. Instructions to the client include voiding at 9 A.M., discarding that urine specimen, and collecting the rest of the urine at 9 A.M. the next morning.

Clinitest, Acetest, and the test for specific gravity are usually performed by the nurse and are not done by the laboratory. Nurses should follow the specific procedures for each test to obtain accurate results.

Blood Tests

Even though blood studies are carried out on venous, capillary, or arterial blood, the usual sample is obtained from venous blood. Capillary blood specimens are usually used to obtain specimens from infants and neonates. In adult clients blood glucose and hemoglobin levels can be determined from capillary blood. Arterial samples are obtained for blood gas determination and cultures.

Venipunctures must be carried out keeping in mind that hemoconcentration and hemolysis can occur if the procedure is done improperly. Hemoconcentration results from prolonged use of a tourniquet. Hemolysis may occur from using a small bore needle for the venipuncture of rapidly infusing blood into the specimen tubes. Using a larger bore needle for performing the venipuncture and taking the cap off the specimen tubes is recommended to prevent hemolysis.

If a needle and syringe are used for drawing blood, the top should be removed from the blood tube. After removing the top, slowly inject the blood into the test tube. When blood is ejected through both the needle and the rubber stopper, hemolysis occurs and the specimen is destroyed.

Blood specimens are placed in specific blood tubes according to the type of test ordered and sent to the laboratory for analysis. Each health care facility has a list of blood tests that are analyzed from blood in a specific color-top test tube. The colored top on the test tube indicates whether or not the tube contains a preservative. When whole blood is required for the test, an anticoagulant, such as heparin or trisodium citrate, is placed in the test tube to keep the blood from clotting. When serum is needed for the laboratory test, no preservative is added to the blood as the clot is used for the test. If the test tube contains a preservative, the tube should be gently rotated back and forth with palms of hands to prevent the blood from clotting.

Some blood tests require that the client fast for several hours prior to obtaining the specimens. Other blood tests have no special requirements for collection. Blood studies requiring a fasting specimen for accuracy include fasting blood sugar, lipid panels, glucose tolerance tests, and insulin levels.

Test Tube Types for Specimen Collection

This list is an example of color-identified test tubes for blood draw. Each color indicates the specific test ordered and contains the appropriate additive/preservative.

Clotted Blood/Serum

Gray and Red (polymer barrier)
Yellow and Red (polymer barrier)
Red
Gold
Orange
Brown
Yellow and Green
Royal Blue—no additive
Brown—no additive

Whole Blood

Lavender (Purple)
Green
Black
Yellow

Whole Blood/Plasma

Green and Brown
Green (Yellow top)
Light Green
Light Blue
Lavender (Purple) (same as above for EDTA)
Gray
Green
Royal Blue

Cultures

Specimens from the throat, eyes, nose, vagina, wounds, sputum, stool, urine, and blood are often ordered to be cultured for pathogens. Special tubes or containers with culture media are used for organism growth. The culture is prepared in the laboratory according to the type of test ordered. It is essential that the proper technique be used to place the specimen in the appropriate container to ensure accurate results. Specimens obtained for culture and sensitivity require immediate processing and must be sent directly to the laboratory after they are obtained. If a time lapse occurs, the specimen may need to be discarded and a new one obtained. If the specimen is allowed to dry before the examination, the organism cannot be transferred to the slide and, thus, to the culture medium.

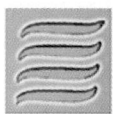

NURSING DIAGNOSES

The following nursing diagnoses may be appropriate to include in a client care plan when the components are related to collecting specimens.

NURSING DIAGNOSIS	RELATED FACTORS
Anxiety	Dread of unknown outcome, results of specimen tests
Ineffective Coping	Fear, external stress, situational crisis
Deficient Knowledge	Inaccurate collection of specimen (e.g., instruction not clear, unable to hear or see well enough to complete collection)
Noncompliance to Test Requirements	Inadequate understanding of the purpose or value of diagnostic test (e.g., language and cultural barriers)
Acute Pain	Invasive procedure, altered body function, recent surgery
Risk for Infection	Invasive procedure, contamination from poor technique of specimen collection

- The single most important nursing action to decrease the incidence of hospital-based infections is handwashing. **Remember to wash your hands or use antibacterial gel before and after each and every client contact.**

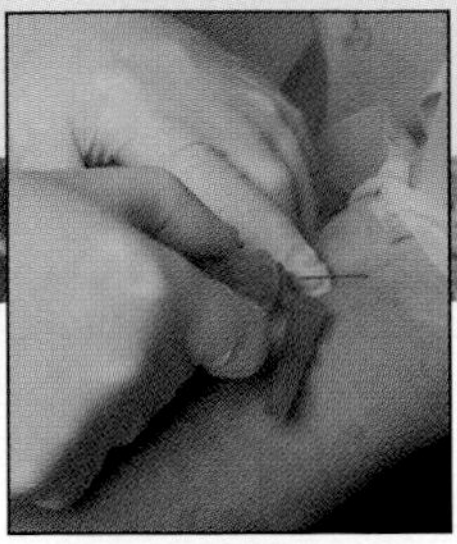

UNIT 1

Urine Specimens

Nursing Process Data

ASSESSMENT Data Base

Assess client's ability to understand instructions and to obtain specimens properly.

Identify if signs and symptoms of urinary tract infections are present: frequency, urgency, dysuria, hematuria, flank pain, fever, and cloudy urine with sediment.

PLANNING Objectives

To instruct the client in the method for obtaining a specimen

To obtain an uncontaminated urine specimen for culture and sensitivity

To maintain the collection of urine for 24 hours

IMPLEMENTATION Procedures

Collecting Midstream Urine

Collecting 24-Hour Urine Specimen

EVALUATION Expected Outcomes

Client is able to obtain urine specimen.

Uncontaminated urine specimen is obtained.

24-hour urine specimen is completed appropriately.

COLLECTING MIDSTREAM URINE

Equipment

Soap and water
Cleaning swab or bactericidal soap
Sterile specimen container
Label for container
Clean gloves

Procedure

1. Gather equipment.
2. Wash your hands.
3. Identify client by checking identaband.
4. Explain procedure to client.
5. Don clean gloves and provide perineal care as needed.
6. Instruct client to collect specimen in bathroom or place on bedpan.

> **CLINICAL ALERT**
>
> Do not use alcohol-containing wipes for cleansing before collecting urine for suspected drug abuse.

7. Instruct client to clean the urinary meatus and obtain urine specimen.

for a Male

a. Don clean gloves and open container.
b. Cleanse end of penis with cleansing swab using circular motion and moving from middle toward outside. **Rationale:** Always swab from clean to dirty area to decrease bacteria levels.
c. Ask client to initiate urine stream.
d. After single stream achieved, pass specimen bottle into stream and obtain urine sample. At least 30 mL must be obtained for adequate specimen. **Rationale:** The microorganisms which accumulate at the urinary meatus have been flushed out with the original stream of urine and are not collected in the specimen.

for a Female

a. Don clean gloves and open container.
b. Spread labia minora with nondominant hand.
c. Cleanse area with disinfectant swab, beginning above the urethral orifice and moving posteriorly.

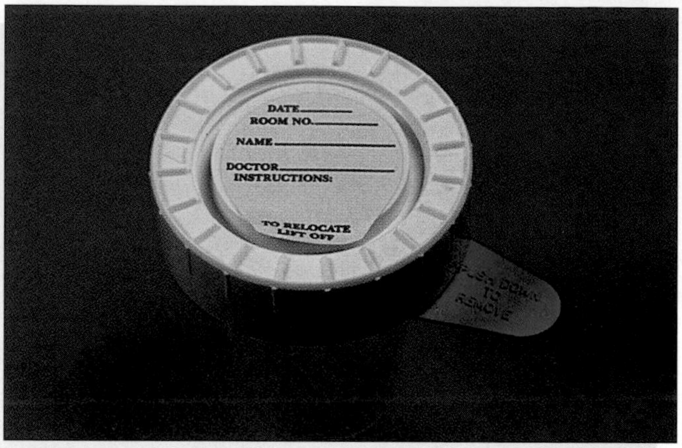

Sterile urine specimen container.

d. Ask client to initiate urine stream. Hold labia open throughout the voiding process.
e. After single stream achieved, pass specimen bottle into the stream and obtain sample of 50 ml (½ full).

8. To prevent contamination of specimen with skin flora, instruct the client to remove the bottle before the flow of urine stops and before releasing the labia or penis.
9. Instruct client to completely empty bladder.
10. Wipe off outside of container after replacing cap.
11. Remove gloves and wash your hands.
12. Label the specimen (as appropriate) with client's name, room number, medical record number, date, time, and physician's name.
13. Take it specimen to laboratory within 15 minutes. If this is not possible, refrigerate specimen. **Rationale:** Delays in testing may decrease glucose ketone, bilirubin, and urobilinogen values. Falsely elevated bacteria counts can also occur if specimen is not refrigerated.

> **CLINICAL ALERT**
>
> A contaminated specimen is the single most common reason for inaccurate reporting on urinary cultures and sensitivities. To prevent contamination, place cap of container with sterile side up while collecting specimen and do not touch inside of container.

COLLECTING 24-HOUR URINE SPECIMEN

Equipment

Urine specimen container
Preservative, if required
Requisition slip
Label for specimen
Sign that urine collection is in progress
Container with ice, if needed

Note: 24-hour urine specimens must be collected for the entire time ordered. To obtain accurate finding, the laboratory needs the entire urine specimen. The start and stop dates and times should be reported at change of shift.

> **CLINICAL ALERT**
>
> Note any dietary restriction or medication precautions in preparation for 24-hour urine collection.

Procedure

1. Explain procedure to client. Stress the importance of saving all urine for 24 hours.
2. Place sign in client's bathroom stating that 24-hour urine specimen is in progress with start and stop date and time.
3. Collect urine specimen and discard it. **Rationale:** The first specimen is considered "old urine" or urine in the bladder before test began. Test begins with an empty bladder.
4. Record date and time of first specimen on label, and place bottle in appropriate area. Depending on hospital protocol, specimens may be refrigerated, placed on ice, or left in the client's bathroom.
5. Add preservative, if required.
6. Post sign in appropriate place, if other than client's bathroom.
7. Place all urine voided in specimen container. Instruct client *not* to urinate directly into the large collection container.
8. Request client to void exactly 24 hours after first specimen was obtained. Place voided urine in container.
9. After the last voided specimen is placed in the container, cover and send entire specimen to the lab with the proper requisition.
10. Remove sign, and remind client that the test is completed.
11. If a specimen is accidentally discarded, obtain a new container, note the new date and time, and restart the procedure.
12. For creatinine clearance test: Instruct client to avoid caffeine-containing drinks including coffee, tea, and most soft drinks. Drink plenty of water before and during 24-hour collection.

DOCUMENTATION FOR URINE SPECIMENS

- Method used to obtain specimen
- Color, consistency, and odor of urine
- Amount of urine obtained (record this amount on the intake and output record also)
- Time specimen sent to laboratory
- Refrigeration, if required
- Exact time for 24-hour specimen

Critical Thinking Application

UNEXPECTED OUTCOMES	CRITICAL THINKING OPTIONS
Client is unable to assist with obtaining a sterile specimen.	• Place female client in bed and, after cleaning perineum thoroughly, place on sterile or clean bedpan. Cleanse perineal area with swab and obtain specimen according to procedure. • Assist client into bathroom. Assist client to cleanse perineum, instruct to start urine stream, and place the sterile specimen container under the stream to collect specimen. • For male clients, cleanse the penis, and place a sterile or clean urinal under the client. Instruct to start stream of urine and then place sterile container under stream. • Notify physician. Consider catheterization.
Urine specimen contaminated with feces or toilet paper.	• Instruct client on need for accuracy and compliance to urine collection.
Client cannot void on command at completion of test.	• Instruct client to void as close to time as possible. • Chart exact time when last specimen collected on both urine bottle and lab slip. Notify lab of findings.
Urine specimen discarded before 24-hour sample collected.	• If time period is close to 24 hours, call laboratory to determine if test can be completed on sample collected. • If 24-hour sample must be started again, instruct client of necessity to save all urine. • Place signs indicating 24-hour test collection in progress on bathroom door and client's bedside stand. • Mark in bold or underlined print in Kardex indicating 24-hour urine collection in progress.

UNIT 2

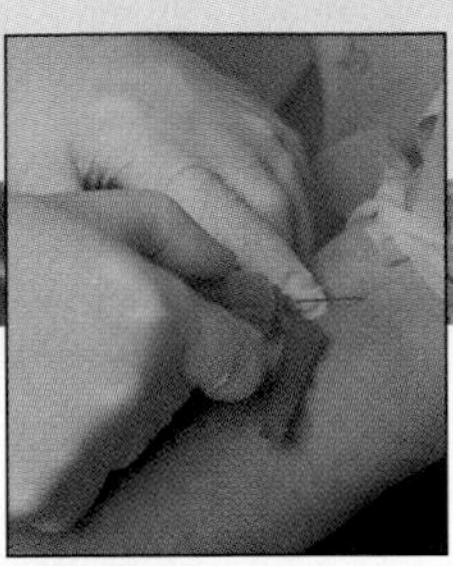

Infant Urine Specimen

Nursing Process Data

ASSESSMENT *Data Base*
Determine the purpose for which the specimen is being obtained.

Determine how the collection is to be obtained.

Assess parents' understanding of the purpose for the procedure.

PLANNING *Objectives*
To obtain a clean urine specimen for urinary system diagnosis tests

To obtain urine specimen for routine hospital admission or as a preoperative urine sample

To provide a method for ensuring collection of all urine when a 24-hour urine collection is ordered

IMPLEMENTATION *Procedures*
Collecting a Specimen from an Infant

EVALUATION *Expected Outcomes*
An uncontaminated urine specimen is obtained.

Family is able to assist in collecting urine from small children.

COLLECTING A SPECIMEN FROM AN INFANT

Equipment

Cleansing solution
Towel
Pediatric urine collector
Diapers
Appropriate specimen containers
Clean gloves (2 pair)
Clean specimen container
Label for specimen

Procedure

1. Gather equipment.
2. Wash your hands. Don clean gloves.
3. Identify correct child by checking identaband.
4. Cleanse and dry child's perineum.
5. Remove paper backing from the adhesive on the urine collector.
6. Apply urine collector to child's perineum, avoiding extension over anus to prevent contamination.
   a. *Male:* Place child's penis through the opening of the collector.
   b. *Female:* Place the opening of the collection bag over the child's urinary meatus.
7. Remove gloves.
8. Place a diaper on the child to help hold the collector in place.

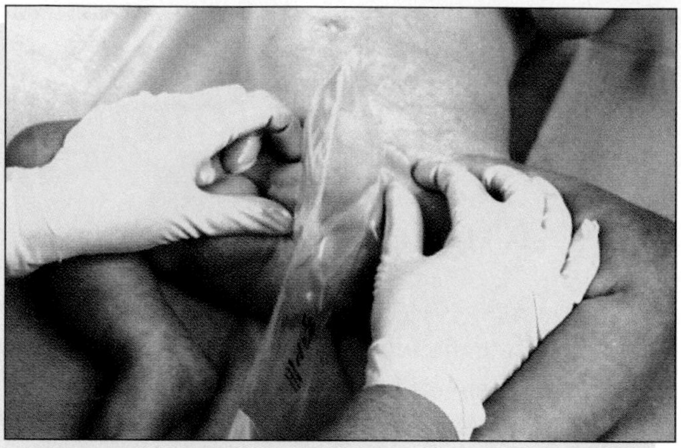

Remove adhesive backing from urine collection bag and place securely over penis.

9. Wash your hands.
10. Check the collector every 15 minutes until a specimen is obtained.
11. Don clean gloves.
12. Remove the collector and place in a urine specimen container.
13. Place clean diaper on child.
14. Remove gloves and wash your hands.
15. Send the urine specimen to the lab either by placing the urine collection bag in a urine container or pouring urine from collection bag into the urine container.
16. Label the container with the child's name, date and time of collection, and the initials of the nurse doing the collection.

DOCUMENTATION FOR COLLECTING A SPECIMEN FROM AN INFANT

- Amount, color, character, and odor of urine
- Time specimen obtained and sent to laboratory
- Condition of perineum

Critical Thinking Application

UNEXPECTED OUTCOMES	CRITICAL THINKING OPTIONS
Specimen is lost because collector does not adhere.	• Obtain a new collection bag, and repeat the procedure. • Tape bag in place with nonallergenic paper tape if necessary.
Specimen is lost because collection bag is the wrong size.	• Obtain appropriate size bag, and repeat the procedure.
Specimen cannot be obtained with a collection bag.	• Notify the physician that you are unable to obtain urine specimen. • If possible keep diapers off and observe when infant urinates; attempt to obtain specimen.

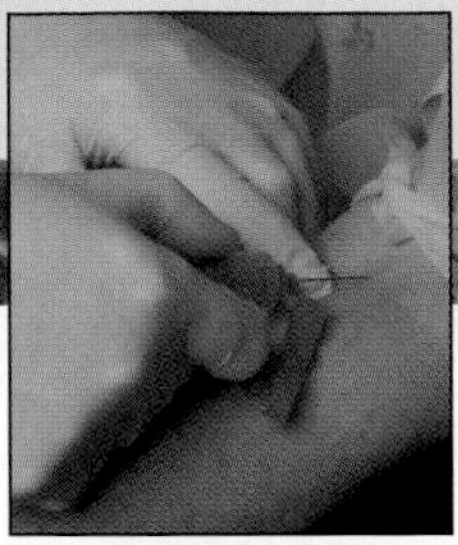

UNIT 3

Stool Specimens

Nursing Process Data

ASSESSMENT *Data Base*
Determine the purpose for the test.
Check whether the specimen must be sent to the laboratory immediately.
Determine the eliminatory status of the client (i.e., liquid vs. formed stools).
Assess gastrointestinal tract dysfunction.

PLANNING *Objectives*
To obtain stool specimens for diagnosing dysfunction in bowel elimination
To assess for perforation or bleeding from a gastric ulcer
To detect presence of ova and parasites
To determine presence of pinworms

IMPLEMENTATION *Procedures*
Collecting Adult Stool Specimen
Collecting Stool for Ova and Parasites
Collecting Infant Stool Specimen
Testing for Occult Blood
for gamma Fe-Cult Plus
for Hemoccult
for Gastroccult
Collecting Stool for Bacterial Culture
Teaching Parents to Test for Pinworms

EVALUATION *Expected Outcomes*
Specimen meets laboratory requirements for diagnostic testing.
Client does not experience undue discomfort or embarrassment during procedure.
Cellophane tape test completed.

COLLECTING ADULT STOOL SPECIMEN

Equipment

Waxed cardboard or plastic container with cover
Tongue blade
Label for container
Clean bedpan or bedside commode
Clean gloves

Procedure

1. Check the client's identaband, and explain the procedure to the client.
2. Determine if dietary restrictions are required prior to specimen collection.
3. Before collecting stool specimen, ask the client to void. Tell client not to void on the specimen. **Rationale:** This prevents contamination of specimen with urine, which could result in inaccurate test results.
4. Don gloves.
5. Clean out all urine from the bedpan or bedside commode.
6. Raise the head of the bed so that client can assume a squatting position on the bedpan, or help client sit on the bedside commode.

> **CLINICAL ALERT**
> Do not allow urine or water to come in contact with the stool specimen.

7. Provide privacy until client has passed a stool.
8. Remove the bedpan or bedside commode. If necessary, help the client clean perineum.
9. Use tongue blade to obtain and place a small portion (2 teaspoons) of the formed stool in a waxed cardboard or plastic container. (For some tests you may need to collect the entire specimen.) Do not contaminate inside of container.
10. Discard remaining stool, and clean bedpan or bedside commode.
11. Remove gloves, and wash your hands.
12. Label container with client's name.
13. Fill out laboratory request for appropriate test.
14. Take specimen to laboratory immediately. **Rationale:** Specimen may need to be refrigerated or examined immediately after collection.

COLLECTING STOOL FOR OVA AND PARASITES

Equipment

Waxed cardboard or plastic container with cover
Tongue blade
Label for container
Clean bedpan or bedside commode
Clean gloves

Procedure

1. Follow the steps for *Collecting Adult Stool Specimen.* Don clean gloves to collect stool specimen.
2. Collect exudate, mucus, and blood with all specimens.
   a. Place stool into container (with a preservative fluid).
   b. Mash the specimen in the container until mixed well with preservative. **Rationale:** Parasites thrive in this type of medium.
3. Replace and tighten cup. Shake the contents until mixed well.
4. Keep specimens at body temperature to be examined within 30 minutes. **Rationale:** Organisms must be seen in their active stages, as loose, fluid stools are likely to contain trophozoites or intestinal amoebas and flagellates.
5. There is usually no need to maintain well-formed or semiformed stool specimens at body temperature or to examine them quickly even though they may contain ova or cystic form of parasites.

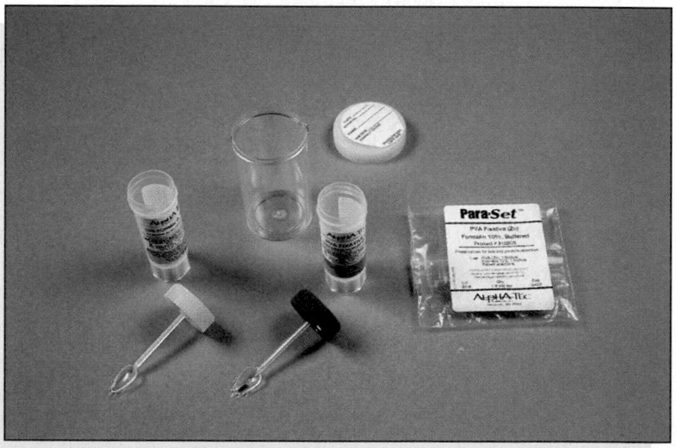

Equipment necessary for collecting ova and/or parasite specimen.

6. Collect complete stools after purgative medications are administered.
7. When the presence of tapeworms is suspected, all stools must be examined in their entirety in order to find the head of the parasite.
8. Do not give barium, oil, and laxatives containing heavy metals that interfere with the extraction process for 7 days prior to stool examination. **Rationale:** Ova or cysts are not revealed.

9. Use only normal saline solution or tap water if an enema must be administered to collect specimens. Do not use soap suds or other substances.
10. Do not contaminate the specimen with urine as it kills amoeba.
11. Collect three random, normally passed stool specimens to ensure accurate test results.
12. Provide air freshener, if needed.

COLLECTING INFANT STOOL SPECIMEN

Equipment

Diaper
Plastic diaper liner
Waxed cardboard or plastic container with cover
Cotton swabs
Label for container
Clean gloves

Procedure

1. Place a clean, disposable diaper on the child or infant.
2. Check diaper frequently so that you obtain a specimen that is not contaminated with urine.
3. If child is passing liquid stools, place a plastic liner inside the diaper.
4. Don clean gloves before taking diaper off child and collecting specimen.
5. Use cotton swabs to procure the specimen.
6. Place specimen in stool container.
7. Remove gloves, wash hands, label, and send to lab immediately with client's name and medical record number.

TESTING FOR OCCULT BLOOD

Equipment

Clean bedpan or bedside commode
Tongue blade
Guaiac test (Hemoccult) or gamma Fe-Cult packet
Guaiac solution
Glacial acetic acid
Hydrogen peroxide
Clean gloves

Procedure

1. Explain need for stool specimen to client.
2. Provide privacy.
3. Position client on bedpan or commode.
4. Don clean gloves.
5. Take stool specimen to bathroom or utility room.
6. Prepare slide for testing according to packet instructions:

for gamma Fe-Cult Plus

a. Smear thin layer of stool on panel number 1.
b. Obtain second specimen from a different part of stool specimen and smear thin layer on panel number 2.
c. Turn packet over, and remove perforated flap (marked Not to Be Opened by Patient).
d. Add 2 drops of Fe-Cult developing solution to test area over smear of stool.
e. Read and record test results within 30 seconds. **Rationale:** Color reaction fades within 2–3 minutes.

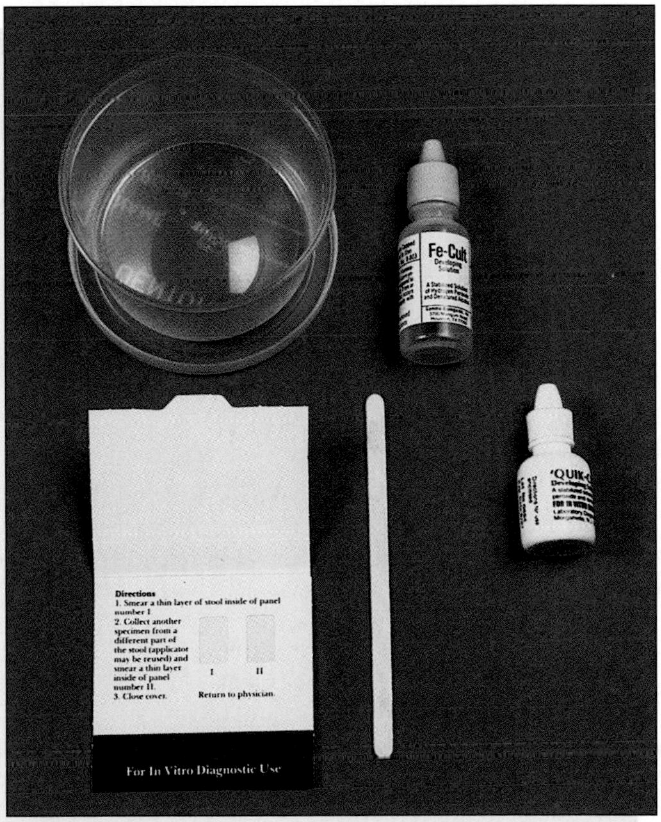

Supplies needed for testing stool for occult blood.

Any trace of blue indicates a positive result. No trace of blue indicates a negative result.

for Hemoccult

a. Follow steps a and b for Fe-Cult Plus test.
b. Wait 3–5 minutes before processing test.
c. Turn packet over, and lift flap.
d. Apply 2 drops of Hemoccult developer over each smear.
e. Read and record test results within 60 seconds.

CLINICAL ALERT

Overt bleeding from hemorrhoids or menstrual bleeding renders the test inaccurate.

f. Apply 1 drop of Hemoccult developer between the + and – quality monitor test strip (orange section at bottom of packet).

CLINICAL ALERT

A hemoccult processing test cannot be used for gastric contents. A gastroccult test must be used.

g. Interpret results within 10 seconds. If the positive side turns blue, the test slide is accurate.

7. Discard filter paper or packet.
8. Remove gloves and wash your hands.
9. Check facility policy for testing. Some laboratories conduct studies.
10. Document stool smear results and confirm quality monitor test.

for Gastroccult

Note: See procedure in *Chapter 19, Nutrition Maintenance and NG Intubation*, p. 601.

COLLECTING STOOL FOR BACTERIAL CULTURE

Equipment

Waxed cardboard container with cover
Tongue blade
Label for container
Clean bedpan or bedside commode
Clean gloves

Procedure

1. Follow steps for *Collecting Adult Stool Specimen.* Don clean gloves before collecting stool specimen.
2. Collect exudate, mucus, and blood with all specimens.
3. Place a small amount of feces in a waxed cardboard container (if entire specimen is not needed).
4. Remove gloves, wash hands, and send entire specimen to the laboratory immediately after collection. If there is any delay, the specimen must be iced.
5. Report and calculate on the basis of daily output any stool specimens that are to undergo chemical analysis.

TEACHING PARENTS TO TEST FOR PINWORMS

Equipment

Specimen container with paddle
Clean gloves

Procedure

1. Explain procedure to child and parent.

Note: This test is rarely done or seen in hospital settings, so if pinworms are suspected, the parents can be taught how to obtain specimen at home.

2. Parents may choose to wear clean gloves.
3. Instruct parents to make collection upon arising in the morning before bathing, cleansing, or passing a bowel movement.

Note: For very active children, specimens may be collected a few hours after going to bed, while the child is sleepy and more cooperative. **Rationale:** Pinworms, when present, migrate out of the anus to lay eggs during sleep.

4. Remove cap in which is inserted a plastic paddle with one side coated with a nontoxic, adhesive material. This side is

CLINICAL ALERT

After treatment (drug of choice is mebendazole) and to prevent reinfection, use meticulous cleaning practices and teach parents of child to do the same.

marked "sticky side." Do not touch this side with fingers.

5. Separate buttocks and press the sticky side against several areas around anus using moderate pressure.
6. Replace the paddle in tube. Be sure there is no stool on paddle.
7. Label container with your full name, medical record number, and date.
8. Keep specimen at room temperature until all specimens are collected (on consecutive days). Return all tubes to the doctor.

Documentation for Stool Specimens

- Date and time specimens collected
- Date and time specimens sent to laboratory
- Number of specimens sent to laboratory
- Description of stool: color, amount, odor, and any purulent patches or blood noted
- Dietary restrictions imposed
- Condition of perianal skin, if client is having diarrhea
- If serial stool specimens are needed, record each specimen on the Kardex card as well as the chart

Critical Thinking Application

UNEXPECTED OUTCOMES	CRITICAL THINKING OPTIONS
Client is embarrassed by having to give stool specimen.	• Place a bedpan or other collection device under the toilet seat in bathroom to obtain specimen. • If client is confined to bed, pull sheets over client's legs and draw curtains around the bed until procedure is completed. • If odor occurs from passage of stool, spray room with air freshener.
Client is unable to pass adequate stool for specimen collection.	• Notify physician to obtain order to give a normal saline or tap water enema.
Client passes liquid stools.	• Determine if part or entire specimen is required for test. • Obtain a plastic container with a cover and several large cotton swabs. Dip cotton swabs into the liquid stool. Place swabs in plastic container. After procedure, pay close attention to skin care. A protective ointment may be necessary to protect skin from liquid stools.

UNIT 4

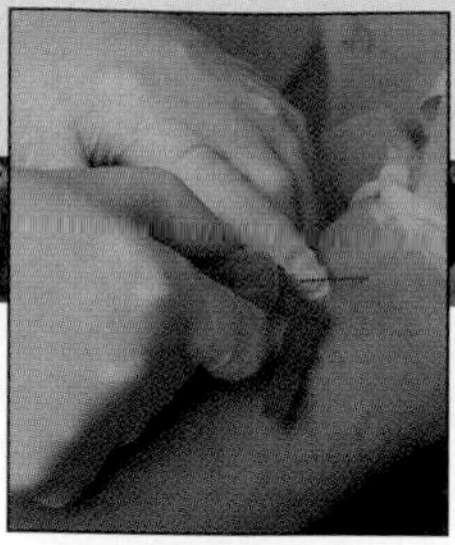

Blood Specimens

Nursing Process Data

ASSESSMENT **Data Base**

Check order for blood withdrawal in client's chart.

Note specific requirements for the test (e.g., fasting or administration of medications prior to the test).

Check to see if the test is routine or urgent.

Assess veins for venipuncture site.

PLANNING **Objectives**

To obtain an uncontaminated blood specimen

To obtain a blood sample without complications, such as hematoma formation or excessive oozing at the site

To obtain specimens of blood that can be used to diagnose the client's illness

To obtain and transfer specimens without destroying red blood cells

To ensure accurate test results by making sure the client follows all requirements for the test (e.g., fasting)

To ensure accurate test results by selecting the right tube for the right test

To ensure that uncontaminated blood specimen for culture is obtained

To obtain an accurate blood glucose level

IMPLEMENTATION **Procedures**

Withdrawing Venous Blood (Phlebotomy)

Using Vacutainer System

Withdrawing Arterial Blood

Collecting a Specimen for Culture

Obtaining Blood Specimen for Glucose Testing (Capillary Puncture)

Measuring Blood Glucose Using Chemstrip

Measuring Blood Glucose Using Glucometer

Monitoring Glucose: Sure Step FLEXX

for Quality Control

for Measuring Blood Glucose

Measuring Blood Glucose Using Lifescan One-Touch II

EVALUATION **Expected Outcomes**

Blood sample is obtained without complications, such as hematoma formation or excessive oozing at the site.

Uncontaminated blood specimen is obtained.

Blood samples are sent to the laboratory in the proper tubes.

Blood glucose level obtained.

WITHDRAWING VENOUS BLOOD (PHLEBOTOMY)

Equipment

5-mL or 10-mL safety syringe
20-gauge 1-inch needle(s)
Antimicrobial wipe (with blood alcohol specimen, use nonalcohol solution)
Appropriate plastic laboratory tubes
Dry, sterile sponges
Tourniquet
Absorbent pad or towel
Clean gloves
Laboratory slip

Preparation

1. Check physician's orders for tests to be obtained.
2. Wash your hands.
3. Gather equipment.
4. Open sterile packages.

Procedure

1. Identify client by checking identaband; introduce yourself and explain the procedure.
2. Don clean gloves.
3. Place extremity straight and in dependent position, if possible.
4. Place absorbent pad or towel under arm. **Rationale:** This prevents soiling the linen with blood.
5. Place equipment close to work area.
6. Place a tourniquet 4–6 inches above the client's elbow. (If client has an IV or fistula in place, place the tourniquet *on the other arm.*) Tighten the tourniquet and tell the client to open and close fist. **Rationale:** Muscle contraction increases blood flow to arm.
7. Cleanse antecubital fossa (inner aspect of elbow) with antimicrobial wipe starting at vein site and moving in a circular motion about 2 inches away from vein. **Rationale:** A larger vessel is more appropriate than a smaller vessel for blood draw.
8. Let site dry. **Rationale:** This reduces bacteria on skin surface when dry.
9. Hold skin taut with nondominant hand. Perform a venipuncture with bevel of needle pointed up at a 30° angle.
10. Lower needle toward skin after needle has entered vein. **Rationale:** This decreases risk of accidentally penetrating the other side of vein.
11. Thread needle along path of vein. Watch for backflow of blood in syringe.
12. Pull syringe plunger back gently, and check for placement of the needle in the vein. If placement is correct, release tourniquet, wait a few seconds to allow fresh blood to flow into the vein, and then pull back gently on the plunger.
13. Fill syringe to desired amount.
14. Remove needle from vein, cover venipuncture site with a sterile sponge, and press the sponge firmly on the site for 2–3 minutes. (Client may be able to hold sponge in place.)
15. Do not remove top from laboratory tube. Place needle straight through top.
16. Gently eject blood down the side of the tube. Do not allow blood to foam or splash. **Rationale:** Red blood cells can be destroyed if the blood sample is not handled carefully.
17. Replace tube top, and rotate blood gently to mix blood with tube contents. *Alternative method:* Needle can be inserted through rubber stopper of test tube if 20-gauge needle is used. Inject blood slowly into test tube to prevent hemolysis of cells.
18. Label tube promptly. Write client's name, date, and time. You may also need to write initials of the person who drew the specimen if this information is required by hospital policy.
19. Check client's venipuncture site for oozing. Continue to press sponge firmly over site if clots have not begun to form at site.
20. Dispose of shielded needle and syringe in biohazard receptacle.
21. Remove gloves, wash hands.
22. Take blood specimens to a designated station or laboratory according to hospital procedure.

USING VACUTAINER SYSTEM

Equipment

Vacutainer assembly with shielded or blunting needle
Antimicrobial wipe (with blood alcohol specimen, use nonalcohol solution)
Plastic vacuum blood collection tubes, placed in order of collection
Dry, sterile sponges
Double-ended needle that screws into the adapter
Clean gloves
Tourniquet
Tape
Laboratory slip

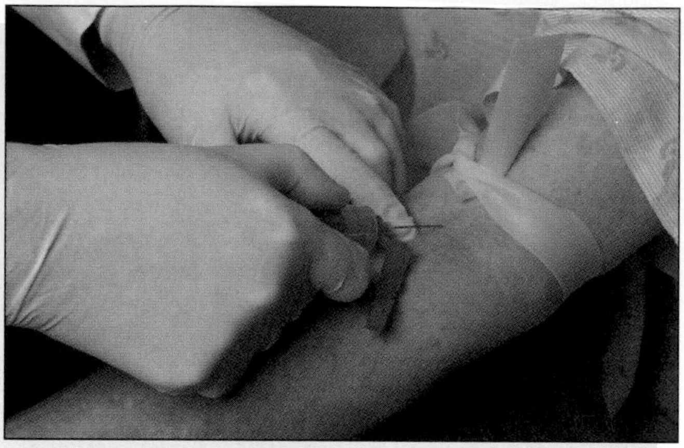
Clamp vein down by placing forefinger below puncture site and insert needle at 15–30° angle.

Preparation

1. Check physician's orders for tests to be obtained.
2. Wash your hands.
3. Obtain plastic adapter, double-ended needle that screws into the adapter, and appropriate vacuum specimen tubes.
4. Screw the double-ended needle into the plastic adapter, with the shorter needle facing the plastic adapter.
5. Explain procedure to client.
6. Don clean gloves.

Procedure

1. Follow steps 1–12 in *Withdrawing Venous Blood.*
2. Once the needle is positioned inside vein and blood return is visualized, insert blood collection tube into plastic holder while holding the plastic adapter steady. Press the vacuum tube firmly into the short needle so that it pierces the top of the tube. Blood should begin to spurt quickly into the tube until the tube is filled or vacuum is used.
3. Instruct client to relax fist and release tourniquet. **Rationale:** Hemolysis occurs with prolonged tourniquet use.
4. Release the tube, and set it aside. Attach another tube to Vacutainer, or prepare to remove needle.
5. Place sponge over needle site, and remove needle while applying gentle pressure to site.
6. Hold sponge on site for 2–3 minutes. Do not have client bend elbow. **Rationale:** Bending the elbow can facilitate formation of a hematoma.
7. Place Vacutainer with needle in biohazard container.
8. Check if tube contains additive, gently invert to mix and label specimen tubes.
9. Remove gloves, and wash your hands.
10. Complete laboratory slip, and take specimen to designated station or laboratory.

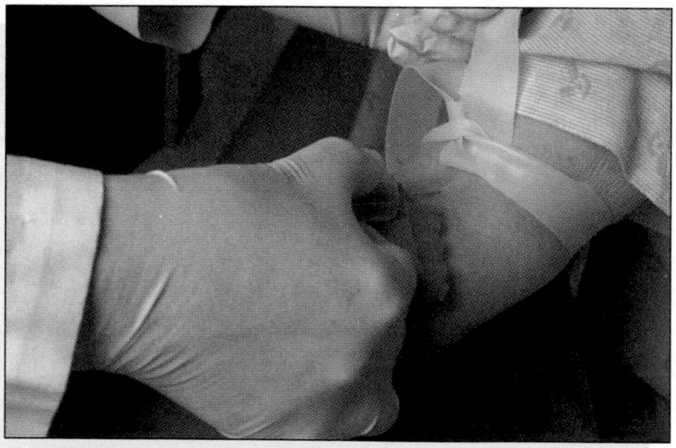
When blood begins to fill tube, tell client to relax fist and release tourniquet.

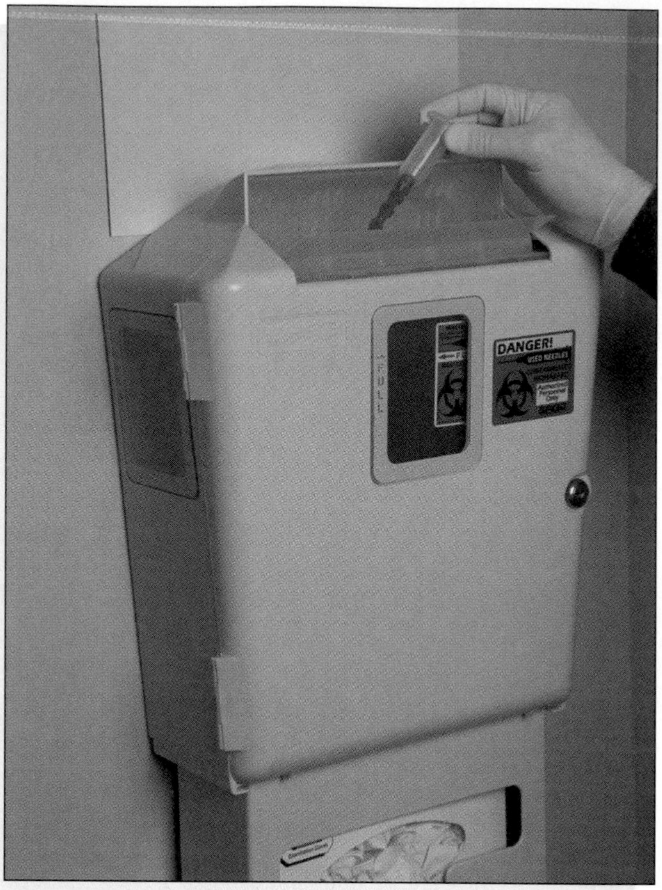

Place vacutainer with safety needle attached into biohazard container.

WITHDRAWING ARTERIAL BLOOD

Equipment

3-mL syringe with 22-gauge 1-inch needle with safety guard
Syringe cap/stopper
1:1000 solution heparin
Antimicrobial swabs (2)
2 × 2 gauze pad
Nonallergenic tape
Plastic bag filled with crushed ice
Clean gloves
Goggles and mask
Laboratory requisition
Label for syringe

Preparation

1. Check physician's orders for test to be performed. (Usual test is arterial blood gases.)
2. Assemble equipment.
3. Wash hands.
4. Wipe top of heparin bottle with antimicrobial swab.
5. Uncap needle and insert into heparin bottle.
6. Withdraw ½ to 1 mL of heparin solution into syringe.
7. Prepare syringe by pulling plunger back entire length of syringe, rotate syringe to allow heparin to coat syringe sides.
8. Express excess Heparin into sink.
9. Call laboratory to apprise them of specimen being sent for ABGs according to hospital policy.

Procedure

1. Take equipment into room and place on overbed table.
2. Check identaband.
3. Explain procedure and purpose of test.
4. Don clean gloves, goggles, and mask.
5. Palpate selected radial site with fingertips. **Rationale:** To determine best site for puncture. Allen's test should precede an arterial puncture if there is a question of poor collateral circulation.
6. Hyperextend wrist slightly. **Rationale:** This position will stabilize radial artery.
7. Cleanse puncture site with antimicrobial swab using a circular motion beginning over the artery site. Place swab on inside of packet and in close proximity to site.
8. Keep fingertip of nondominant hand over puncture site. **Rationale:** To maintain puncture site location.
9. Pick up syringe and hold needle bevel in uppermost position and insert needle into artery at a 45° angle.
10. Do not advance needle once blood is observed flowing into syringe.
11. Hold needle steady and allow blood to fill syringe. Pulsations from artery will assist in filling syringe. Do not draw back on syringe. **Rationale:** Drawing back on syringe can cause air bubbles to fill syringe and inaccurate ABGs results will occur.
12. Place 2 × 2 inch gauze next to needle site and withdraw needle when syringe is filled.
13. Immediately apply pressure over site with gauze. Maintain pressure for 5–10 minutes. **Rationale:** Prolonged pressure over arterial puncture site will prevent bleeding.
14. Monitor puncture site for signs of oozing. When bleeding has stopped, place 2 × 2 gauze over site and apply tape as you would for a pressure dressing.
15. Expel any air bubbles from syringe. Activate needle guard.
16. Label syringe.
17. Place syringe in plastic bag filled with ice. Close plastic bag.
18. Remove gloves and wash hands.
19. Complete laboratory requisition slip. Indicate client's temperature and oxygen percentage as necessary.
20. Take specimen to laboratory immediately.

Allen's Test

Allen's test is performed to determine adequacy of collateral perfusion before arterial blood stick.

- Ask client to rest hands facing upward.
- Observe color changes in palm.
- Ask client to make a tight fist (to force blood from hand).
- Compress the radial and ulnar arteries by applying direct pressure using index and middle fingers (obstructs blood flow to hand).
- Ask client to clench and unclench fist several times.
- Ask client to relax hand in a slightly flexed position. Hand should appear blanched due to absence of blood flow.
- Release pressure on ulnar artery and note if fingers and palm flush within 5 minutes. This is a positive test for patency.
- If fingers and palm remain pale, do not use this site for arterial puncture; test other extremity.

COLLECTING A SPECIMEN FOR CULTURE

Equipment

2 sets of paired culture media bottles (aerobic and anaerobic)
Blood withdrawal equipment (e.g., 2 needles and syringe with attached needle)
Povidone–iodine (Betadine) swab
2 antimicrobial swabs
Additional needles
Clean gloves

Preparation

1. Check physician's orders.
2. Wash your hands.
3. Gather equipment.
4. Don clean gloves.
5. Explain procedure to client.

Procedure

1. Cleanse skin with antimicrobial wipe. Allow skin to dry.
2. Prepare skin with povidone–iodine. Cleanse starting at vein site and moving in circular motion outward 2 inches.

> **CLINICAL ALERT**
>
> Check with physician—blood culture may be ordered prior to client beginning antibiotic therapy.

3. Allow skin to dry.
4. Remove povidone–iodine with antimicrobial wipe.
5. Perform venipuncture.
6. Withdraw 20 mL of blood from vein without IV. Do not draw specimen through catheter. **Rationale:** Fluid from IV alters results.
7. Remove needle used for venipuncture and replace with new sterile needle. **Rationale:** Contamination may result if needle used to puncture skin is reused.
8. Swab top of paired blood culture bottles with povidone–iodine swab and then antimicrobial swab, and inject 8–10 mL blood into each bottle according to hospital policy. Gently rotate bottle to mix well. Change needle each time so new sterile needle is used for each bottle.
9. Draw a second sample of blood after 15 minutes or according to hospital policy. Use percutaneous stick if required by hospital policy. (Prepare skin with povidone–iodine solution again.)

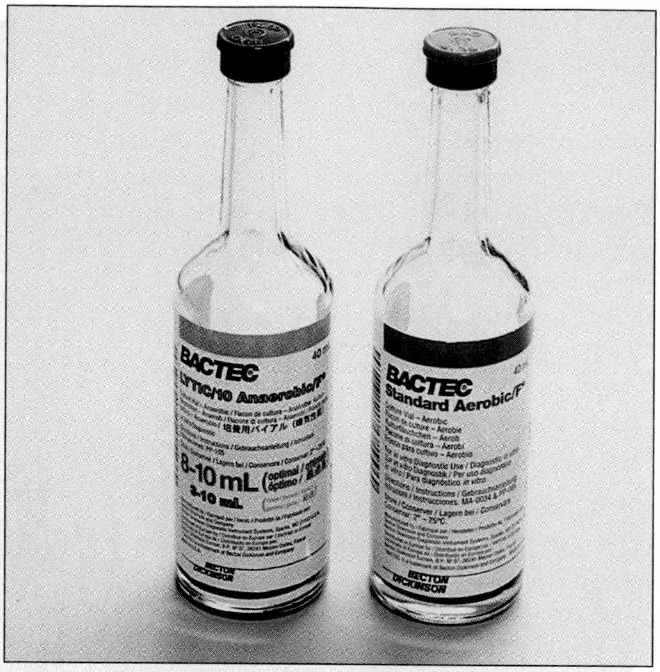

Inject blood into both aerobic and anaerobic culture bottles.

10. Place in second set of paired blood culture bottles, using single sterile needle technique.
11. Remove gloves and wash hands.
12. Label bottles, and transport to lab immediately. Include site where blood specimens were obtained.

Principles of Measuring Blood Glucose

- Bedside glucose testing is used only to monitor progress of treatment and not to establish a diagnosis of diabetes.
- Specimens used for glucose testing must be whole blood (capillary, arterial, or venous).
- Appropriate nursing actions need to be taken whenever client results exceed critical lab values (check facility policies).
- For a critical value, the FIRST action is to repeat the test.
- Test strip bottle should be dated when opened and recapped firmly between uses to protect strips.

OBTAINING BLOOD SPECIMEN FOR GLUCOSE TESTING (CAPILLARY PUNCTURE)

Equipment

Automatic lancet (i.e., Autolet or Glucolet)
Penlet
Soap and water
Cotton ball, sterile sponges
Clean gloves

Preparation

1. Gather equipment—automatic lancet or Autolet wallet—and take to bedside.
2. Wash your hands.
3. Don gloves.

Procedure

1. Wash client's fingertip (especially side of finger where lancet will puncture, or heel for infant), with soap and water. **Rationale:** Use soap and water if repeated sticks are to be done, as alcohol toughens skin and may change reading.
2. Gently manipulate finger or heel to determine if good blood supply is available.
3. Take cover off Penlet or Lancet (disposable).
4. Place lancet in Penlet, push and twist in place.
5. Twist cover of lancet pen to remove.
6. Replace cover of Penlet.
7. Cock Penlet to pull lancet back into Penlet.
8. Place tip of sampling pen against side of finger or heel.
9. Activate to force the lancet downward by pressing gently on the activating button. The lancet punctures the skin immediately.
10. Gently massage the base of the finger, stroking toward the puncture site. Do not squeeze or apply pressure to site. **Rationale:** Massaging increases blood flow to the fingertip.

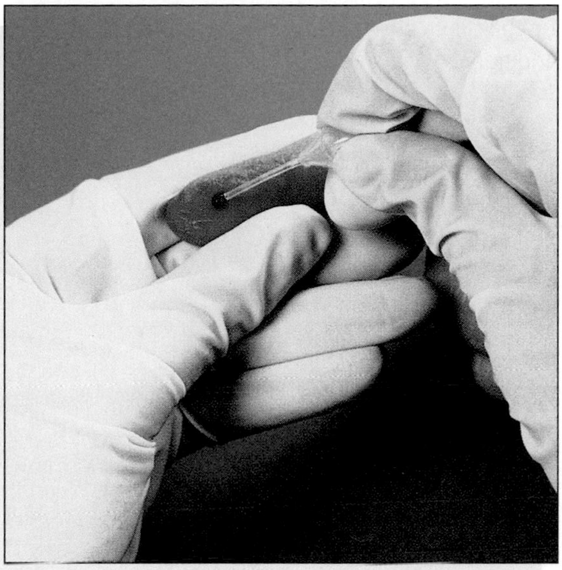

Fill tubing of capillary bulb when obtaining blood specimen.

11. Wait a few seconds to allow blood to collect at puncture site.
12. Place a large drop of blood onto both zones of the reagent area on Chemstrip. May use capillary suction bulb to obtain blood specimen. Place tip of capillary bulb at base of blood drop. *Do not* fill bulb with blood. Fill only tubing with blood.
13. Rotate finger tips when doing capillary punctures.
14. Wipe puncture site with cotton ball to seal.
15. Discard used equipment.
16. Remove gloves and wash hands.
17. Document results.

MEASURING BLOOD GLUCOSE USING CHEMSTRIP

Equipment

Reagent strips (Chemstrips)
Color chart
Blood specimen
Cotton ball
Clean gloves

Procedure

1. Follow steps in *Obtaining Blood Specimen for Glucose Testing.*
2. Place blood specimen on reagent area of Chemstrip.
3. Start the timer simultaneously with dropping blood on strip.
4. Wait 60 seconds, wipe blood from Chemstrip using dry cotton ball.

AtLast Blood Glucose System

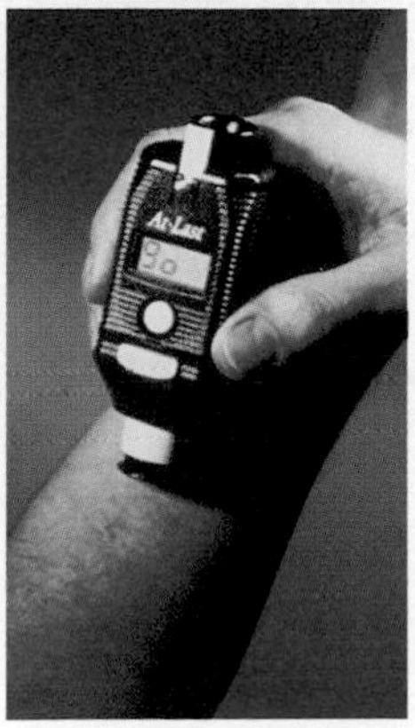

This device allows the client to use alternative sites, such as forearms, upper arms, and thighs, to obtain blood specimens. These sites are less sensitive than the fingertips, thus decreasing the discomfort of the frequent "sticks" for blood glucose monitoring. This new system functions the same as other monitors. It should increase compliance and improve diabetic control, particularly for clients who have been monitoring their glucose for a long time.

5. Wait additional 60 seconds and match color chart for results.
6. If color chart indicates reading is darker than 240 mg/dL, wait additional 60 seconds and compare Chemstrip with color scale.
7. Check Kardex or physician's orders for insulin, and administer prescribed dose.
8. Remove gloves and wash hands.
9. Document results of blood glucose and insulin dosage on diabetic record and medication sheet.

MEASURING BLOOD GLUCOSE USING A GLUCOMETER

Equipment

Glucometer blood glucose monitor
Chemstrips including calibration strip
Dry cotton ball
Clean gloves

Preparation

1. Remove calibration strip from bottle of Chemstrips.
2. Compare lot numbers on calibration strip to lot number on side of Chemstrip bottle. These must match.
3. Place calibration strip in meter by opening door and inserting top of strip into slot on right side of meter.
4. Insert strip until you hear a "click."
5. Close door.
6. Push ON/OFF button. Numbers 888 should appear on screen.
7. Open door of monitor.
8. Push black button on the left side of door, and slide Chemstrip under strip guide with test pads facing up.
9. Close door quickly. Numbers 000 should be displayed on screen indicator. If not, open and close door again.
10. Open door and remove strip. Leave door open.
11. Don clean gloves.

Procedure

1. Obtain blood specimen according to steps 1 through 11 in skill *Obtaining Blood Specimen for Glucose Testing.*
2. Insert Dextrose Stix into Glucometer according to manufacturer's instructions.
3. Wait 30 seconds or time noted by manufacturer. **Rationale:** Time necessary for blood to penetrate Dextrose Stix.
4. Start timer.
5. Read digital display when alarm sounds. **Rationale:** Alarm indicates glucose reading is ready.
6. Dispose of Dextrose Stix.
7. Turn off Glucometer.
8. Remove gloves and wash hands.
9. Document findings on appropriate record.

Note: Many hospitals have changed to glucometers that can "download" results, such as the Sure Step Flexx BG meter.

MONITORING GLUCOSE: SURE STEP FLEXX

Equipment

Sure Step Flexx blood glucose monitor
Blood glucose test strips
High and low control solutions
Single use blood-letting device
Antimicrobial skin preparation pad
Lint free cloth, such as 2 × 2 gauze
Prepackaged disinfectant towelette, moistened with 1:10 dilution of 5.25% sodium hypochlorite, i.e., "Gluco-Chlor" towelette
Clean gloves

Procedure

for Quality Control

1. Turn on the meter.
2. Check the battery status to ensure adequate power.
3. Press continue.
4. Select Quality Control (QC) Test from main menu by touching appropriate area on the screen.

CLINICAL ALERT

Quality control for the Flexx (with documentation) is required on a regular basis to verify test results when client data is entered.

5. Select Control Test by touching "HIGH" or "LOW" area on the screen to indicate which control test is to be done.
6. Enter operator ID assigned by specific facility.
7. Select Control Solution Lot Number from list displayed, or enter it manually. Verify lot number on control solutions.
8. Select Test Strip Lot number (and code) from this list displayed, or enter in manually. Verify lot number (and code) on test strips.
9. Shake Control Solution vial gently. Check confirmation dot on back of test strip to ensure it is completely blue.
10. Apply one drop of Control Solution to pink test square on test strip.

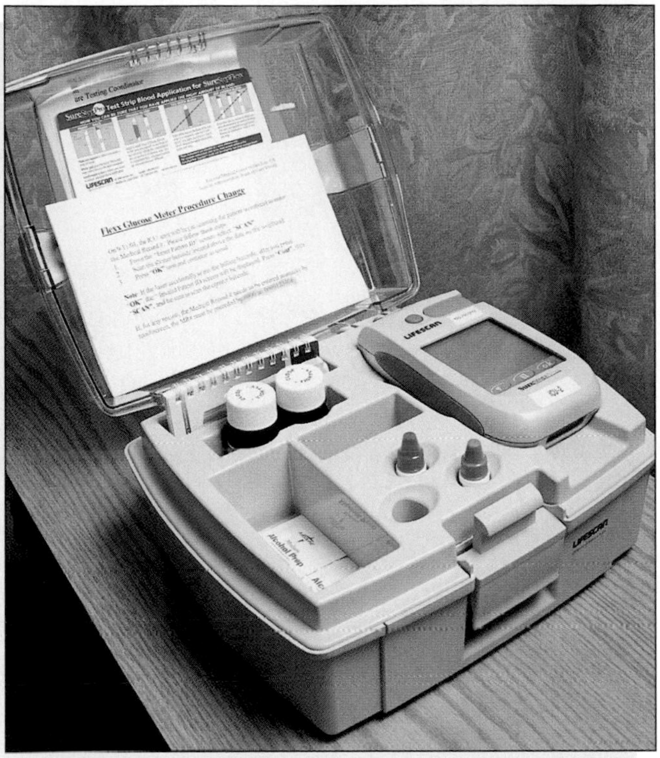

Sure Step Flexx blood glucose monitoring equipment.

11. Insert test strip into test holder within 2 minutes of applying Control Solutions. The white side of test strip tip should be facing up. Firmly push strip into meter.

CLINICAL ALERT

The test strip must be *completely* inserted to receive accurate results.

12. Check result which appears in approximately 30 seconds. Control Solution test results should fall within expected ranges printed on test strip bottle. If Control Solution test results fall outside expected control range, "ENTER NOTE" and follow recommendations.
13. Remove test strip and dispose of it according to facility policy and procedure.
14. Quality Control test must be completed for both "HIGH" and "LOW" controls.

for Monitoring Blood Glucose

1. Wash hands and don gloves.
2. Press power button to turn on meter.
3. Check battery status as status screen appears.
4. Press "CONTINUE." Select "PATIENT TEST" from Main Menu.
5. Enter operator ID and press "OK."
6. Check to ensure Code Number displayed on meter matches code number on test strip bottle.
7. Enter client's ID (medical record number), and press "OK."
8. Select Test Strip Lot Number (and code) from list displayed, or enter in manually. Verify lot number (and code) displayed on screen.
9. Follow steps in *Obtaining Blood Specimen for Glucose Testing.*
10. Apply drop of blood to test strip by carefully touching pink test square on test strip. Check "Confirmation Dot" on back of test strip to verify that it has turned completely blue.
11. Use 2 × 2 gauze pad and apply direct pressure to puncture site to control bleeding.
12. Insert test strip into test strip holder within 2 minutes of applying blood.

CLINICAL ALERT

The test strip must be *completely* inserted to receive accurate results.

13. Check results which appear in approximately 30 seconds.
14. Evaluate client results that fall above or below the Critical Lab Values limit.
    a. Press "Enter Note" and choose one to three comments, if indicated, that correspond to client's current situation.
    b. Follow appropriate nursing actions as determined by facility policy and procedure.
15. Press "OK" and remove test strip from meter.
16. Remove gloves and dispose of gloves and test strip according to facility policy.

MEASURING BLOOD GLUCOSE USING LIFESCAN ONE-TOUCH II

Equipment

Penlet II
Sterile lancet
One-Touch II meter
Test strip
Soap and water
Clean gloves
Tissue or sterile gauze squares

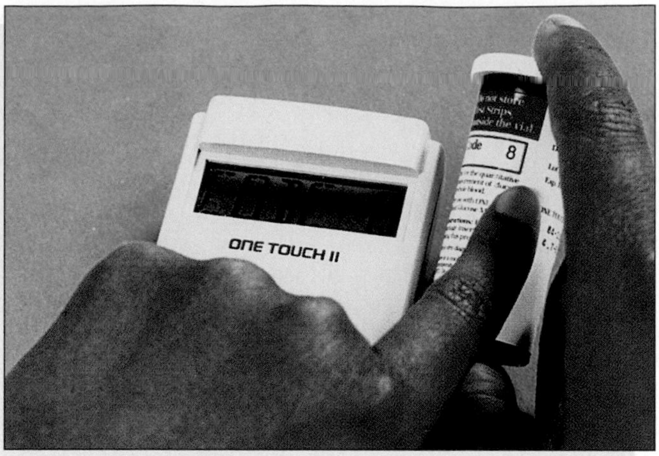

Ensure code number on test strip matches code number on meter.

Preparation

1. Check physician's orders for specific times.
2. Wash your hands.
3. Gather equipment.
4. Check that code number on test strip matches code number on meter. **Rationale:** If code number is not the same, incorrect blood glucose readings occur. Turn meter to ON. The word "Code" and the number appear on the display for several seconds. Code numbers range from 1 to 16.
5. Explain procedure to client.
6. Don clean gloves.

Procedure

1. Instruct client to wash hands with soap and warm water. **Rationale:** Warm water stimulates the flow of blood to the fingers.
2. Instruct client to place arm at side of body for 10–15 seconds. **Rationale:** Blood is brought to fingertips for ease in obtaining sample.

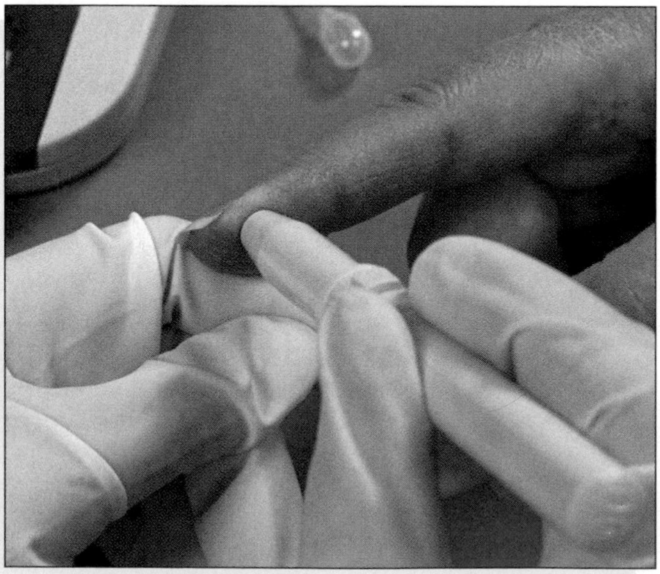

Place tip of pen against side of fingertip.

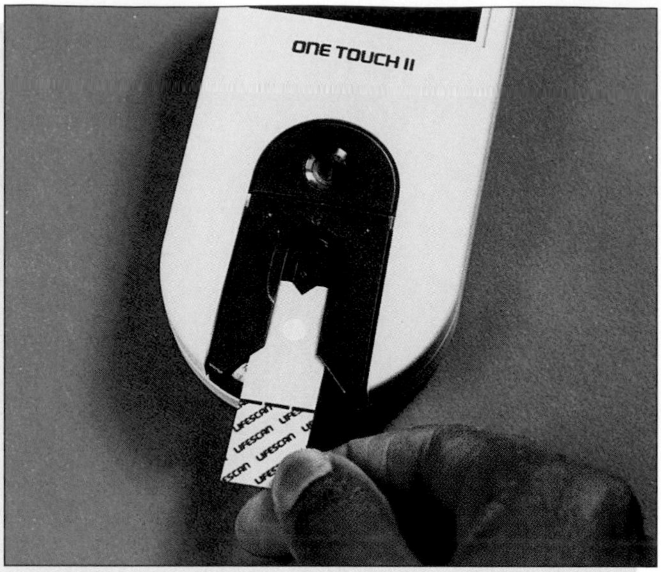

Insert strip, test spot up, into meter until it stops.

3. Remove Penlet II cap by pulling it straight out.
4. Insert sterile lancet into lancet holder twisting into place. Do not line up ridges on the lancet with the slots in the lancet holder.
5. Replace Penlet II cap and cock Penlet to pull lancet back into Penlet.
6. Choose a lateral surface of a fingertip. Rotate sites for sticks. **Rationale:** Rotating sites decrease callous formation and bruising of fingertips.
7. Hold Penlet II firmly against side of finger and press release button.
8. Squeeze finger gently to obtain drop of blood.
9. Place tip of capillary bulb at base of blood drop and fill tubing with blood.

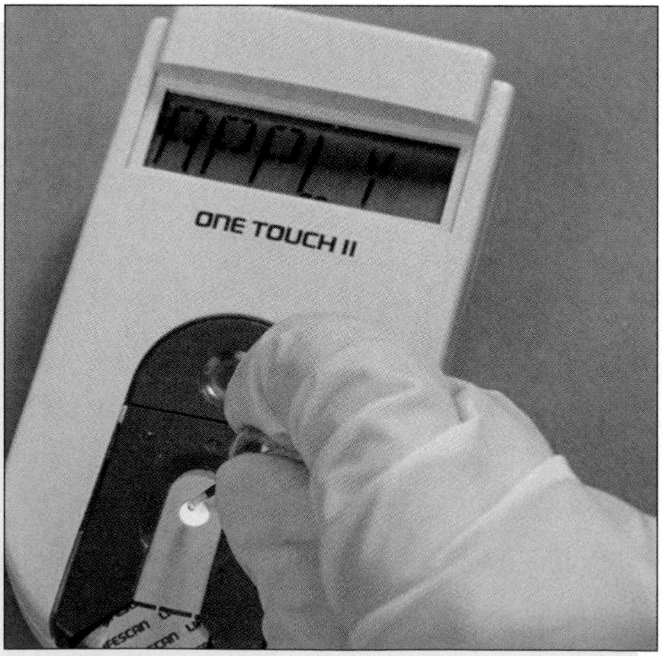

Place large drop of blood on test strip.

10. Turn meter ON.
11. Remove test strip from bottle and insert test strip into meter until it stops, notched end first and test spot side up.
12. Place large drop of blood on test strip. Do not smear blood on test spot or add additional blood after test begins.
13. Wait for the beeping sound (45 seconds) to obtain reading.
14. Use tissue or gauze to apply firm pressure over puncture site.
15. Remove lancet by removing Penlet II cap. Pull back on dark gray sliding barrel until lancet drops out into biohazard container.
16. Clean Penlet II sampler and cap with soap and water.
17. Remove test strip, and place in disposal bag.
18. Remove gloves and wash your hands.
19. Document findings, and administer insulin as needed.

Documentation for Blood Specimens

- Date and time of blood withdrawal
- Date and name(s) of test(s) for which blood was drawn
- Any unusual conditions in either the client or specimen
- Site where blood cultures were obtained for capillary specimen
- Results of blood glucose reading
- Insulin administered: type, amount, location of injection
- Notification of physician of critical lab values, orders or interventions

Critical Thinking Application

UNEXPECTED OUTCOMES	CRITICAL THINKING OPTIONS
Veins roll away from needle when performing a venipuncture.	• Stabilize vein by applying traction to skin below needle insertion site. • Common occurrence in elderly. Use a 5°–15° angle when inserting needle into vein as elderly client's veins are superficial.
Blood does not flow into the syringe.	• Check the position of the needle in the vein. • Pull needle back slightly away from the wall of the vein. Rotate needle gently. Do not pull excessively on the plunger, especially if the vein is small, since this movement may cause the vein to collapse.
Blood does not flow into the vacuum tube.	• Check the position of the needle in the vein. If vacuum in the tube is lost or if the vein is not large enough, discard the tube and get another. • If there is pressure on the vein for vacuum pull, select a larger vein or use a syringe and needle instead of the Vacutainer method.
Unable to get blood sample with Autolet.	• Check that fingertip or heel is not toughened with overuse of alcohol sponges. Should use soap and water to clean area. • Choose an alternative site and repeat the stick. • Stroke gently from base of finger toward the tip. Do not apply firm massage as it can interfere with blood flow.
Meter shows not enough blood.	• Remove test strip, and insert new strip. • Obtain new blood drop. • Ensure blood drop is sufficient to form a round, shiny drop that covers entire strip. • Complete procedure.

UNIT 5

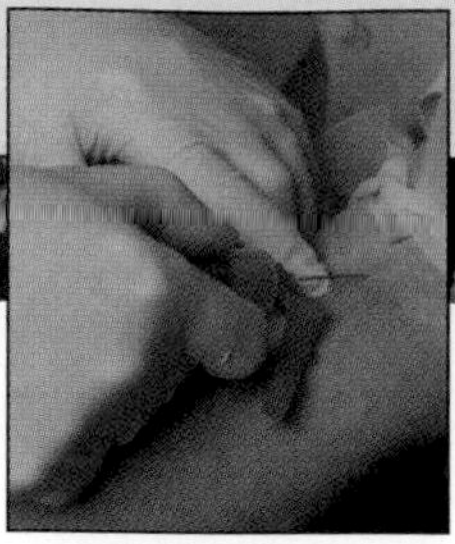

Sputum Collection

Nursing Process Data

ASSESSMENT *Data Base*

Check diagnosis for indication of need for specimen.

Observe client's ability to cough up specimen. You may need to assist the client while obtaining a specimen, or suction equipment may be necessary.

Determine the degree of pain the client can tolerate.

Check client's understanding of procedure so sputum and not saliva is obtained.

PLANNING *Objectives*

To obtain adequate sputum specimen for laboratory examination

To identify predominant organisms, if respiratory disease is present

To maintain client's respiratory status during and after procedure

IMPLEMENTATION *Procedures*

Obtaining Sputum Specimen

Using Suction Trap

Collecting Specimen by Transtracheal Aspiration

EVALUATION *Expected Outcomes*

Adequate sputum specimen is obtained for laboratory examination.

Client's respiratory status is maintained during and after procedure.

OBTAINING SPUTUM SPECIMEN

Equipment

Sputum specimen container and label
Biohazard bag for delivery of specimen to laboratory
Tissues
Laboratory requisition slip
Clean gloves
Gown, mask (HEPA or N95 if client has TB), goggles, if needed

Preparation

1. Check orders and client care plan.
2. Gather equipment.
3. Wash your hands.
4. Provide privacy.
5. Place client in sitting position.

> **CLINICAL ALERT**
>
> *Note:* A first specimen obtained in the early morning before eating or drinking provides the best sputum sample. Chest physiotherapy may be helpful in mobilizing secretions just prior to sputum collection.

Procedure

1. Explain procedure and rationale to client.
2. Have client rinse mouth before coughing to remove any oral contaminants.
3. Don clean gloves. Don mask, gown, goggles if client requires assistance with procedure.
4. Instruct client to breathe in and out deeply 2 to 4 times. Then give a series of low, deep coughs to raise sputum from the lungs. **Rationale:** Deep coughs produce sputum rather than saliva.
5. Obtain 1–2 teaspoons of sputum in container; close and seal lid.
6. Follow directions on specimen container to complete closing system.
7. Label specimen tube directly and place in biohazard transport bag.
8. If client is unable to produce sputum specimen, assist client by placing palms of your hands or a rolled pillow around incision area if client is inhibited by pain. **Rationale:** Wrapping a sheet around chest or abdomen also provides support for body walls during coughing.
9. Remove gloves, gown, mask, and goggles and wash hands.
10. Evaluate client's status after procedure.
11. Deliver sputum to the laboratory within 30 minutes after collection. Obtain specimen during treatment if client is receiving IPPB or PVD.

> **CLINICAL ALERT**
>
> Know what test the sputum is being collected for:
> - Routine culture—sterile container
> - Acid-fast bacilli (AFB)—sterile container
> - Cytology—container contains a preservative warning: preservative is poisonous

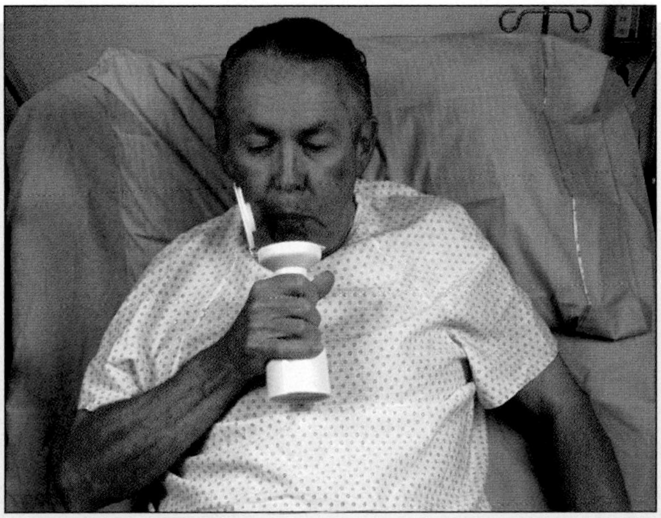

Instruct client to lift hinged lid of sputum collection system, and expectorate directly into sterile container.

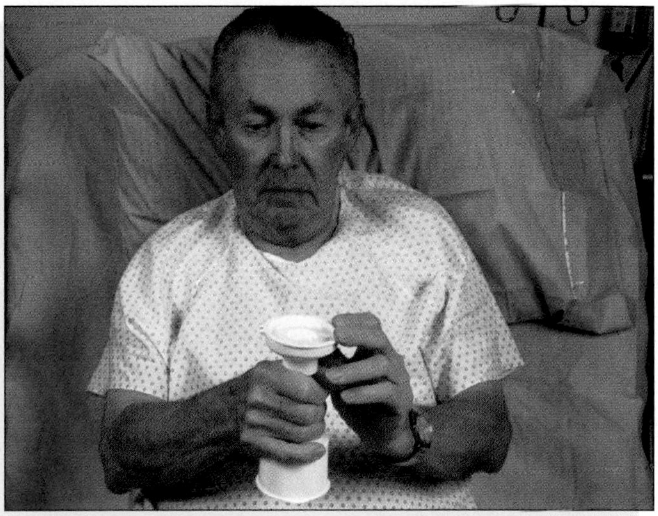

Instruct client to obtain 1–2 teaspoons of sputum, close and seal lid of container.

USING SUCTION TRAP

Equipment

Suction machine
Sterile catheter and glove
Sterile saline
Sterile sputum trap
Culture tube
Biohazard disposal bag
Clean gloves
Gown, mask, goggles

Preparation

1. Check physician's orders and client care plan for type of equipment needed.
2. Wash your hands.
3. Gather equipment.
4. Explain procedure to client.
5. Provide privacy.
6. Don clean gloves, goggles, gown, and mask as appropriate.

Procedure

1. Set up suction equipment.
2. Attach sputum trap between suction catheter and tubing. Maintain trap in upright position throughout procedure.
3. Complete suctioning as for nasooropharyngeal suctioning using sterile technique.
4. Place your thumb on top of sputum trap to monitor; remove your thumb and provide intermittent suction, lifting thumb at intervals until 3–5 mL specimen is collected.
5. Suction no more than 10 seconds at a time. **Rationale:** This prevents removal of too much oxygen.

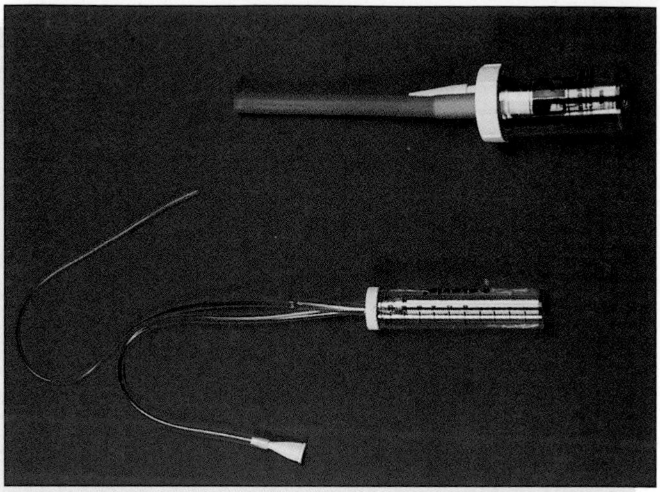

Two common types of suction traps used in client care.

6. Turn off wall suction.
7. Label specimen container: client's name, date, time, and physician.
8. Cap suction trap and place it in biohazard bag. Follow agency protocol for double-bagging specimens before transporting to laboratory.
9. Remove gloves and other equipment (mask, gown, and goggles if used) and dispose of in appropriate receptacle.
10. Send specimen that was collected in trap to laboratory. (In many hospitals suction tube is also sent to the lab with specimen.)
11. Place client in a comfortable position.
12. Wash your hands.

COLLECTING SPECIMEN BY TRANSTRACHEAL ASPIRATION

Equipment

No. 14 needle with polyethylene tubing or small intracatheter (IV catheter)
Sterile saline and 3–5 mL syringe
Skin-cleansing solution dictated by hospital policy
Xylocaine injection
Clean gloves

Procedure

1. Explain procedure to client.
2. Collect equipment.
3. Provide privacy for client.
4. Wash your hands and don gloves.
5. Position client by hyperextending client's neck and placing a pillow under shoulders.
6. Cleanse cricothyroid area of neck with antimicrobial solution.
7. Physician will anesthetize area with Xylocaine.
8. Physician will insert 14-gauge needle into cricothyroid area, thread polyethylene tubing through needle, withdraw needle, and leave tubing in place.
9. Attach syringe (3–5 mL) with 1–2 mL sterile saline into polyethylene tubing.
10. Inject saline into polyethylene tubing to initiate coughing response.
11. To obtain specimen, immediately pull back on barrel of syringe.
12. Withdraw catheter and apply pressure over puncture site.
13. Place sputum secretions in sterile container, label container, and send it to laboratory.
14. Remove gloves and wash your hands.
15. Position client for comfort.

Documentation for Sputum Collection

- Date and time of collection
- Amount, color, and consistency of sputum
- Mechanical sputum trap used for collection
- Client's tolerance of procedure

Critical Thinking Application

UNEXPECTED OUTCOMES	CRITICAL THINKING OPTIONS
Pain inhibits client from coughing.	• If diagnosis permits, support painful area with rolled pillows or tight sheets so that external pressure equals internal pressure, thus minimizing pain and discomfort. • Before beginning procedure, ask client to take several deep breaths. These breaths may trigger the cough reflex and aerate the lungs. • Give client pain medication as ordered 15–30 minutes before obtaining the specimen.
Client develops coughing spasms during procedure.	• Press your third finger lightly over the client's trachea in the cricoid hollow. This pressure releases the nerve that innervates the coughing reflex. • Report to physician to obtain an order for nebulization.
Unable to obtain sputum specimen.	• Notify physician for orders: bronchodilator drugs, nebulization treatment. • Perform chest physiotherapy to mobilize secretions for expectoration before obtaining sputum specimen. • Attempt procedure early in the morning when mucus has collected during the night and is more easily expectorated. • Obtain order for aerosol therapy.

UNIT 6

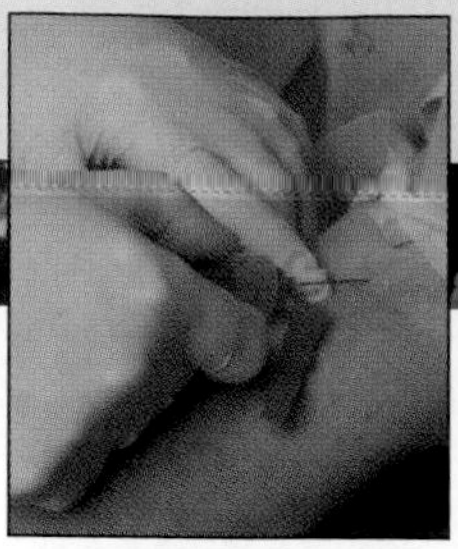

Throat and Wound Specimens for Culture

Nursing Process Data

ASSESSMENT ***Data Base***

Identify appropriate container for specimen swabs or material.
Determine time frame for expediting specimen to lab.
Assess exact area for specimen.
Assess client's ability to cooperate with procedure.
Assess wound and drainage.

PLANNING ***Objectives***

To obtain an uncontaminated specimen for study
To place specimen swab or material in container using appropriate techniques
To send specimen to laboratory within specified time frame

IMPLEMENTATION ***Procedures***

Obtaining a Throat Specimen
Obtaining Wound Specimen for Aerobic Culture
Obtaining Wound Specimen for Anaerobic Culture

EVALUATION ***Expected Outcomes***

Uncontaminated specimens obtained.
Specimens placed in appropriate culture medium container.
Specimens sent to laboratory in timely manner.

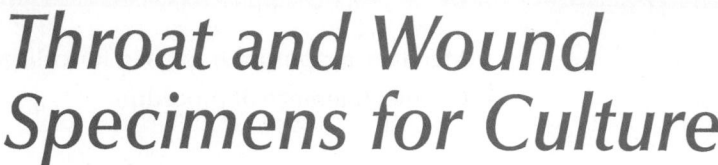

OBTAINING A THROAT SPECIMEN

Equipment

Tongue depressor
Culture tube with applicator stick
Light source
Clean gloves

Preparation

1. Check physician's orders.
2. Gather equipment.
3. Explain procedure to client.
4. Position client in Fowler's position.
5. Place treatment light or face client toward natural light source to provide good lighting.
6. Wash your hands and don clean gloves.

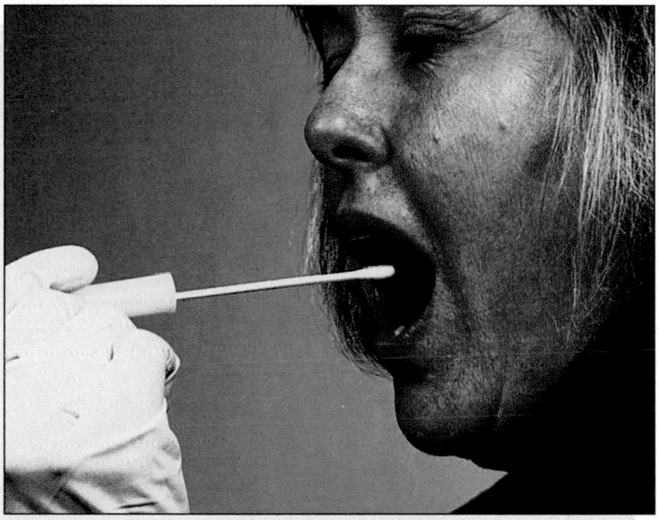

After swabbing throat, remove applicator stick being careful not to touch any part of the mouth.

Procedure

1. Remove the sterile applicator from the culture tube by rotating cap to break seal.
2. Ask the client to tilt head back and open mouth.
3. Use tongue depressor if desired to depress tongue. **Rationale:** Prevents tongue from contaminating the swab.
4. Swab the back of the throat along the tonsillar area from left to right. **Rationale:** Swab only one side of the throat. A second specimen of the other side may be taken; check hospital protocol.
5. Remove the applicator stick, and place in the specimen tube.
6. Push the stick into the tube until the swab is saturated with culture medium and cap reaches black dot. **Rationale:** This places the applicator tip into the culture medium to preserve bacteria until laboratory can complete test.
7. Position client for comfort.
8. Remove gloves and wash your hands.
9. Label specimen tube, and send to laboratory immediately. **Rationale:** To ensure accurate identification of microorganisms.

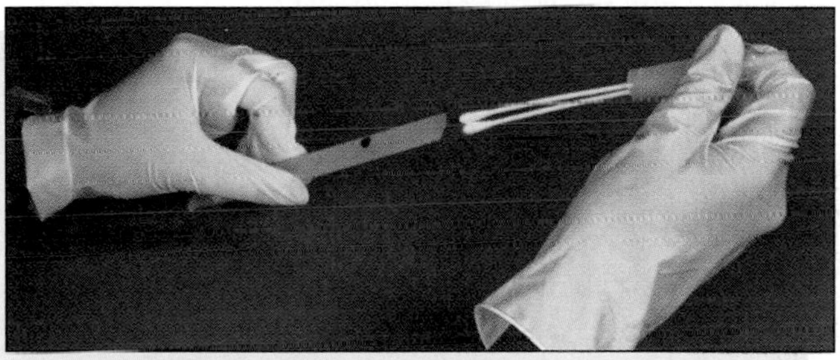

Push applicator stick into specimen tube, being careful not to contaminate stick.

OBTAINING WOUND SPECIMEN FOR AEROBIC CULTURE

Equipment

Culture transport swab with transport medium
Laboratory slip
Clean gloves, 2 pair
Sterile gloves
Dressing material
Disposal bag
Biohazard bag

Preparation

1. Check physician's orders and client care plan.
2. Wash your hands.

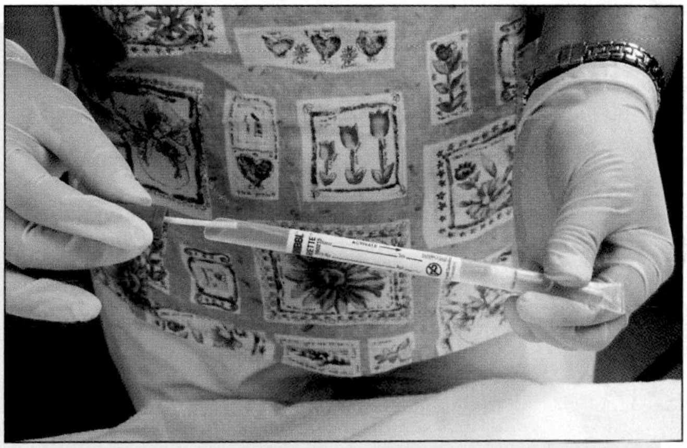

Push tip of swab into liquid culture medium.

> **CLINICAL ALERT**
> Large wounds should have separate cultures taken from different areas of the wound.

3. Gather equipment.
4. Explain procedure to client.
5. Open all sterile dressing material, and arrange for easy access during dressing change.

Procedure

1. Don clean gloves.
2. Remove and discard soiled dressing from wound into disposal bag.
3. Remove gloves, discard into disposal bag, and don clean gloves.
4. Remove swab, and wipe swab in wound. Obtain culture from active drainage area.
5. Avoid touching skin edges or other surfaces that will contaminate swab.
6. Return swab to container.
7. Crush transport medium vial, and push swab tip into contact with transport medium.
8. Close container.
9. Place specimen in sealed biohazard bag.
10. Write any recent antibiotic or antifungal therapy on laboratory requisitions. **Rationale:** These drugs may lead to false-negative results from the culture.
11. Remove clean gloves, wash hands.
12. Don sterile gloves, and replace dressing.
13. Remove gloves, discard, and wash your hands.
14. Transport specimen to laboratory within 30 minutes. Do not refrigerate. **Rationale:** This ensures organisms are still viable.

OBTAINING WOUND SPECIMEN FOR ANAEROBIC CULTURE

Equipment

Anaerobic transport medium kit with swab
Laboratory slip
Clean gloves
Sterile gloves
Dressing material
Disposal bag
Plastic bag

Preparation

1. Check physician's orders and client care plan.
2. Wash your hands.
3. Gather equipment.
4. Explain procedure to client.
5. Open all sterile dressing material, and arrange for easy access during dressing change.

Procedure

1. Don clean gloves.
2. Take off dressing from wound, and discard in disposal bag.
3. Remove gloves and don clean gloves.
4. Remove specimen swab, and wipe in wound as you did with aerobic culturing. Be sure you do not tip anaerobic transport medium tube because it contains carbon dioxide. **Rationale:** Tipping "spills" the gas out, making it useless to transport anaerobic organisms.

> **CLINICAL ALERT**
> Obtain wound specimen for both aerobic and anaerobic organisms during scheduled dressing change before any medication or antimicrobial agents have been applied.

5. Return swab to container. *Do not* touch sides of container with applicator.
6. Fill out or affix label to specimen and place specimen in sealed plastic bag.
7. Write any recent antibiotic or antifungal therapy on laboratory requisition. **Rationale:** These drugs can lead to false-negative results.
8. Transport specimen to laboratory *immediately*. Do not refrigerate specimen.
9. Alternative method:
   a. Draw up exudate in syringe with all air expelled or have a physician aspirate the wound.
   b. Inject drainage into anaerobic culture tube.
   c. Transport specimens to laboratory *immediately*. **Rationale:** Anaerobic organisms may appear on gram stain even though they are not grown in the culture.
10. Remove clean gloves, wash hands, don sterile gloves.
11. Replace sterile dressing following protocol.
12. Remove sterile gloves.
13. Wash your hands.

DOCUMENTATION FOR OBTAINING SPECIMEN FOR CULTURE

- Assessment of wound and drainage
- Date and time specimen collected
- Type of culture obtained (aerobic or anaerobic)
- Site where culture obtained
- For wound specimens, document an assessment of wound and drainage
- Time specimen sent to lab

Critical Thinking Application

UNEXPECTED OUTCOMES	CRITICAL THINKING OPTIONS
Inner surface of collection container contaminated while inserting swab into the culture medium container.	• Obtain new specimen and send to laboratory
Anaerobic specimen not sent to laboratory immediately.	• Obtain new specimen and send to laboratory.
Anaerobic specimen not sent in appropriate container with hydrogen gas.	• Obtain appropriate container and send new specimen to laboratory.
Wound culture produces false-negative results.	• Check if antibiotics or antifungal medications had been administered. If so, notify laboratory and provide specific drugs administered.

GERONTOLOGIC CONSIDERATIONS

- Elderly clients may not clearly hear and understand the directions given regarding specimen collection. Ask specific questions to ensure compliance.
- Determine client's ability to follow directions for obtaining specimens such as urine and stool. Hearing and vision may be impaired, thereby interfering with their ability to follow through on specimen collection.
- Assess client's ability to accurately use blood glucose–monitoring equipment. Finger dexterity may be altered due to stroke, arthritis, or other chronic conditions, thus preventing them from being able to use the equipment or obtain the blood specimen.
- Residual urine may increase as a result of changes in the bladder tone, leading to urinary stasis and potential bacterial proliferation. This leads to bladder infections, necessitating accurate identification of bacteria. This is accomplished through analysis of urine obtained from specimens free of contamination. Ensure client understands the procedure for obtaining an uncontaminated urine specimen. The nurse may need to obtain the specimen if the client is unable to do so without contaminating it.
- Avoid obtaining blood specimens from client's arm if neurological or vascular alterations are present.
- Client's receiving anticoagulant/antiplatlet therapy require a longer pressure time over the venipuncture site to prevent bleeding.
- Elderly clients have large rolling veins that make it appear easier to perform a venipuncture. In fact, they tend to collapse and rupture quite easily. They may not require a tourniquet for venipuncture.
- Minimize the amount of tape used over IV site to prevent skin breakdown.

MANAGEMENT GUIDELINES

Each state legislates a Nurse Practice Act for RNs and LVN/LPNs. Health care facilities are responsible for establishing and implementing policies and procedures that conform to their state's regulations. Verify the regulations and role parameters for each health care worker in your facility.

Delegation of Responsibilities

- CNAs can be assigned to obtain specimens that are nonsterile and noninvasive. Examples of these specimens include urine and stool collections.
- Unlicensed Assistive Personnel (UAP) and CNAs have been instructed in some areas to take blood measurements using the Accu-Chek and Glucometer machines. You will need to check with the facility policy and procedure manual for directions. Most states consider this an invasive technique and do not allow this level of health care worker to perform the task.
- LVN/LPNs can obtain most specimen collections except withdrawing blood. This task requires that they have additional education and be IV certified in order to obtain the blood specimens.

Information Flow

- It is very important that all staff members are aware of clients needing specimen collection. Many of the specimens, particularly blood specimens, require fasting. Shift and team reports should identify those clients with special needs relative to obtaining all specimens.
- When 24-hour specimens are being collected ensure that signs are posted in the client's room to remind all health care workers to save the specimens. This is usually for a 24-hour urine specimen collection.
- Remind LVN/LPN to notify the RN of blood glucose findings, even if they are administering the insulin. It is the RN's responsibility to know these facts.
- Remind all health care workers to notify the nurse manager when any specimen has been collected. Follow the procedure for the facility for sending the specimen to the laboratory. Some facilities have personnel who pick up specimens from the nursing unit; others require the unit staff to take the specimen to the laboratory.
- Inform the health care workers about specimens that must be taken to the laboratory immediately after collection.

CRITICAL THINKING STRATEGIES

SCENARIO 1

You have been assigned to collect specific specimens on several clients. Ms. Saunders is scheduled to have a 24-hour urine specimen collected.

1. When will you start collecting the specimen? List parameters necessary for accurate collection.
2. If the 24-hour urine specimen becomes contaminated with stool, what nursing action is indicated?

SCENARIO 2

Mrs. Block has orders for a stool specimen to be collected for presence of amoeba. When you collect the specimen from her, urine is mixed with the stool.

1. What is the nursing action?

SCENARIO 3

Mr. Jarvis has recently been diagnosed with diabetes, and you are assigned to collect a blood specimen for glucose testing.

1. Describe the activities you would perform to complete this assignment.
2. If the results exceed critical lab values, what is the implication of this result?
3. What actions will you take?

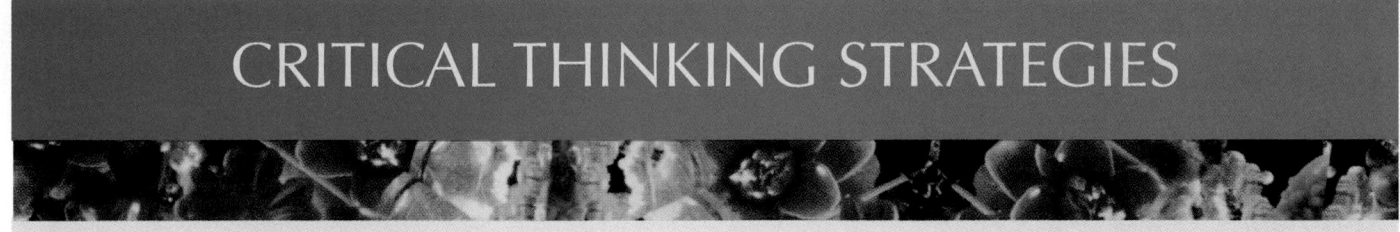

CHAPTER 21

Diagnostic Procedures

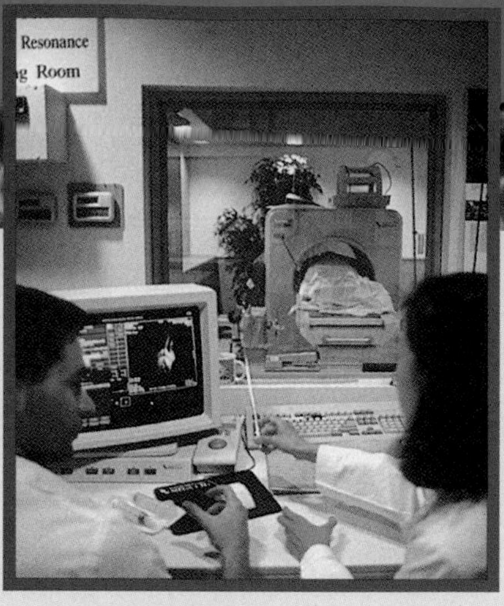

THEORETICAL CONCEPTS

UNIT ONE: **X-Ray Studies** **666**

Preparing for X-ray Studies 667

for Oral Cholecystography 667

for Intravenous Pyelography (IVP) 668

for Myelography 668

for Arteriography 669

for Computed Tomography (CT Scan) 669

for Cardiac Catheterization 670

for Bone Densitometry 670

for Magnetic Resonance Imaging (MRI) 671

for Mammography 672

UNIT TWO: **Nuclear Scanning** **674**

Preparing for Nuclear Scans 675

for Bone Scan 675

for Lung Scan 675

for PET Scan 676

for Nuclear Cardiography 676

for Thyroid Scan 677

Teaching for Nuclear Scan 677

UNIT THREE: **Barium Studies** **679**

Preparing for Barium Studies 680

for Barium Enema 680

for Barium Swallow Study 680

for Small Bowel Follow-Through 681

UNIT FOUR: **Endoscopic Studies** **682**

Preparing for Endoscopic Studies 683

for Arthroscopy 683

for Bronchoscopy 683

for Colonoscopy 684

for Cystoscopy 684

for Gastrointestinal Tract Endoscopy 685

for Laparoscopy 685

for Sigmoidoscopy 685

UNIT FIVE: **Fluid Analysis and Microscopic Studies** **688**

Assisting with Lumbar Puncture 689

Assisting with Liver Biopsy 690

Assisting with Thoracentesis 691

Assisting with Paracentesis 692

Assisting with Bone Marrow Aspiration 693

Assisting with Vaginal Examination and Papanicolaou (Pap) Smear 693

Assisting with Amniocentesis 694

GERONTOLOGIC CONSIDERATIONS 695

MANAGEMENT GUIDELINES 696

CRITICAL THINKING STRATEGIES 697

LEARNING OBJECTIVES

- Describe the major components of client teaching for diagnostic studies.
- List at least three preparatory functions for clients undergoing diagnostic studies.
- Explain the importance of determining allergic responses to shellfish before clients undergo contrast media studies.
- List the signs and symptoms that occur when the client experiences an allergic reaction.
- Explain the reason for giving blocking agents before administering radioisotopes to clients.
- Outline the nursing care responsibilities when a client returns from myelography
- Discuss the nursing care responsibilities when a client returns from arteriography
- Describe the care necessary after cardiac catheterization care to prevent postprocedure complications.
- Explain the steps you would take if a client is given medication prior to a GI series.
- Describe client positions for at least four diagnostic procedures commonly performed at the bedside.
- Compare and contrast postprocedure nursing observations for clients undergoing liver biopsy, paracentesis, and thoracentesis.
- Explain the nurse's role during procedures that use fiberoptic scopes.
- Describe how ultrasonography is used for diagnostic studies.
- Describe the data that should be included in the charting for clients undergoing diagnostic procedures.

TERMINOLOGY

Abscess: a localized collection of pus in any part of the body.

Allergy: an altered reaction of body tissues to a specific substance; essentially an antibody—antigen reaction and may be due to the release of histamine.

Amniocentesis: puncturing the amniotic sac, usually by using a needle and syringe, to remove amniotic fluid for assessment of fetal maturity.

Antiemetic: an agent that prevents or arrests vomiting.

Arteriography: study using radiopaque dye injected into an artery to assess arteries.

Barium: a radiopaque compound used in roentgenography of the gastrointestinal tract.

Bone Densitometry: Test used to determine bone mineral content and density; used to diagnose osteoporosis.

Bronchoscopy: a visualization of the larynx, trachea, and bronchi through a flexible scope.

Catheterization: use or passage of a catheter, a tube for evacuating or injecting fluids.

Centesis: perforation or puncture through the skin to obtain fluid.

Cholangiography: x-ray examination of the bile ducts.

Cholecystogram: x-ray picture of the gallbladder.

Computed Tomography (CT Scan): a scanning technique that provides a series of detailed visualizations.

Contrast medium: a radiopaque substance used during x-ray examination to provide a contrast in density between the tissue being filmed and the medium.

Contusion: an injury in which the skin is not broken.

Craniotomy: incision involving the skull.

Crepitus: a crackling breath sound.

Diagnosis: method or art of identifying the disease or condition a person has or is believed to have.

Diaphoresis: profuse sweating.

Dissipate: to scatter, disperse, dispel, disintegrate.

Dyspnea: shortness of breath.

Endoscopy: visualization of body organs and cavities using an endoscope (tubular instrument with light source and viewing lens).

Enema: introduction of a solution through a tube into the rectum or colon.

Fiberoptic scope: flexible scope that uses fiberoptic materials for visualization. These materials transmit light along its course by reflecting it from the side or wall of the fiber. Devices using fiberoptic materials are used in endoscopic examinations.

Fluoroscopy: type of examination using a screen to view shadows with the aid of x-rays.

Lithotomy: incision into the bladder for removing a stone.

Lumbar: pertaining to the loins and lower vertebrae in the back.

Magnetic Resonance Imaging (MRI): is a nonivasive test that uses a magnetic field with radio frequency waves to produce cross-sectional images of the body.

Mammography: x-ray examination of breast used to detect breast cancer.

Myelography: x-ray inspection of the spinal cord by the use of radiopaque medium.

Neoplasm: a new and abnormal formation of tissue, as a tumor or growth.

npo: nothing by mouth.

Oliguria: diminished amount of urine formation.

Paracentesis: puncture of the abdominal cavity for the removal of fluid.

Peripheral: outer part or surface of a body.

PET Scan: imaging technique used to scan entire body or its various regions.

Pyelo: pertaining to the pelvis of the kidney.

Pyelography: x-ray study of the renal pelvis and ureter.

Scintillation: the emissions from radiographic substances; a subjective sensation of seeing sparks.

Septicemia: blood poisoning; septic products in blood and tissue.

Tachycardia: fast pulse above 100 BPM.

Thoracentesis: surgical puncture of the chest wall for the removal of fluid.

Tumor: uncontrolled new growth or tissue forming an abnormal mass that performs no physiologic function.

Urticaria: a vascular reaction of the skin characterized by the eruption of pale elevated wheals, which are associated with severe itching.

Ventro: denoting the abdomen or ventral (anterior) surface of the body.

Vertigo: sensation of moving or having objects move when they are actually still.

TEST PREPARATION

Diagnostic tests play a major role in the diagnosis and care of clients. Diagnostic testing is as important as a thorough history and physical examination. The results from diagnostic tests can confirm or eliminate client diagnosis. In addition to assisting with the identification of disease states, diagnostic tests assist with monitoring diseases as interventions and treatments are established. With cost containment a major issue in health care today it is imperative that tests are scheduled appropriately, the client is prepared for the tests, and specimens, if any, are collected and disseminated efficiently. Many tests are completed on an outpatient basis; therefore, very explicit information must be provided to the client. Many procedures begin the preparation 1 or 2 days in advance of the actual test. Clients must thoroughly understand this and be able to comply with the instructions in order to obtain an accurate result.

Nurses play a major role in client preparation for diagnostic tests. Client education is one of the most important means to promote an accurate test result. The educational process begins with a discussion of the test itself, the preparation necessary for an accurate result, and the posttest interventions if any.

Many types of diagnostic tests are being utilized in the health care industry today. This chapter contains only a few of the most common tests. There is a brief overview of pretest preparation and any posttest interventions commonly done following the test. As client education is a major role of the nurse, it is highlighted throughout the chapter.

The responsibility of the nurse begins with the initial scheduling of the test and continues after the results of the test are explained to the client. The physician explains the results of the test, but the nurse answers questions, interprets terminology, and listens to the client express his or her feelings or apprehensions.

The preparation of clients for diagnostic tests must be done on an individual basis. Some clients are well informed about the test they are scheduled to take. They know about diet and fluid restrictions, what to expect during the procedure, whether or not there is any discomfort with the test, and how long the procedure takes. Others need a great deal of explanation. Also, some clients prefer not to be given any explanation about the test. Nurses need to respect the client's preferences and provide only information requested, unless it in some way is a danger to the client.

Undergoing diagnostic tests can be frightening for clients; they are often unaware of what the procedure involves and worry about the outcome. Communication involves an active, verbal interchange of ideas as well as an astute observation of the client's nonverbal cues, and can be hindered by this fear. One effective way to allow clients time to think about questions is to provide a printed form explaining the diagnostic test. The form may cover such information as how long a test takes, equipment used for the test, and any sensations experienced during the test. Leaving the form at the bedside can stimulate interest and prompt the shy, reserved client to ask questions when you return later.

Most diagnostic procedures are done on an outpatient basis. This makes it imperative that the nurse provides the necessary information about the procedure. Instructions are sent home with the client that include preprocedural preparation. When the client arrives for the diagnostic test, time should be allotted to answer questions, reassure the client, and determine if the preprocedure preparation was followed.

Another important aspect of teaching involves the way in which the nurse approaches the client. The nurse should avoid giving the impression that she/he is in a hurry and that she/he has no time to answer any questions. On the other hand, be aware of the client's ability to pay attention to what you have to say. If the client seems distracted, he or she may be worried about finances, about who is watching the children, or whether or not their job will be waiting after discharge from the hospital. This preoccupation may prevent assimilation of knowledge and the client may be unprepared for the events that follow.

Remember, the client probably does not know medical jargon; therefore, explain procedures in terms the client can understand. If the client looks puzzled and does not ask any questions, evaluate how you presented the information.

Feedback is the only way in which you can evaluate the learner's knowledge. Feedback can be in the form of direct questioning about certain aspects of the test. Feedback can also be determined through direct observation of facial expressions, posturing, and activities.

Instituting Standard Precautions

Standard precautions must be instituted whenever there is a risk of exposure to body fluids for the healthcare worker. Protective barriers, gloves, and gown must be used whenever an invasive procedure is performed. A mask and/or goggles are worn if there is a risk of splashing blood or body fluids during the procedure. Gloves must be worn by healthcare providers when handling specimens such as blood or cerebrospinal fluid.

X-ray Studies

Many x-rays use the normal contrasts of the body, such as air, water in soft tissues, and bone; however, for some tests a contrast medium is required. Plain radiology is performed without contrast material. These include x-rays of chest, skull, abdomen, and bones. Several types of contrast media are used routinely, including barium sulfate, helium, carbon dioxide, iodized oils, and organic iodides.

One of the major problems with the use of some contrast media is the adverse reaction or sensitivity that can occur. This is more common when iodine preparations are used. The degree of reaction varies from mild (such as nausea) to severe (such as cardiovascular collapse). The usual symptoms include urticaria, hives, dyspnea, nausea, vomiting, and decreased blood pressure.

Clients allergic to food, especially shellfish, or drugs are often allergic to some dyes used in diagnostic studies, particularly those that are iodine-based. Following injections of iodine dye, many tests are abnormal for varying lengths of time. Urine sodium, specific gravity, protein, and osmolality are abnormal for 16 hours. Urine catecholamines are also abnormal for 16 hours.

Barium can cause some uncomfortable feelings and problems with the gastrointestinal tract, but with proper postprocedure care this condition can be greatly reduced.

Fluoroscopy, x-rays that pass through the body to a fluorescent viewing screen, and the less often used tomography (replaced by the CT scan), a sequence of x-ray films each representing a section of tissue at different levels, have been very important in diagnosing and confirming clients' conditions. Two very common uses of fluoroscopy are upper GI barium swallow studies and angiography procedures to guide catheters to predetermined positions, such as in cardiac catheterization. The Computed Tomography (CT) scan passes x-rays through the body organs at many angles.

Ultrasound Studies

Ultrasonography can be done alone or with other procedures. Sound waves produced by ultrasound differentiate normal from diseased tissue. The sound waves are transmitted through fluid, but not bone, air, or contrast material. It is usually performed in physicians' offices or outpatient settings. Ultrasound is painless, requiring only that the client lie quietly during the 15–30-minute procedure. There is no risk to the procedure; therefore, it can be repeated frequently without side effects. This procedure needs to precede barium studies because barium impedes transmission of sound waves. It requires that a gel be placed over the site of the organ to be tested. This provides an air-free barrier between the probe (which holds the transducer) and the skin. The probe is passed over the specific body area, and ultrasonic waves are transmitted through the tissue. The transducer converts the echoes to electric impulses and transforms them into visual images. There is no preprocedural or postprocedural care for the client because it is a noninvasive procedure, except for an ultrasound of pelvic organs. The client needs to drink four glasses of water to promote a full bladder. The full bladder enhances transmission of sound waves and thus improves visualization of organs.

Echocardiography is a procedure similar to ultrasound. It is a painless, noninvasive technique that uses transducers and oscilloscopes similar to those in ultrasound procedures. The echocardiogram records heart motion, not heart outline. There is no preparation or postprocedure alteration in activity for this procedure.

Doppler ultrasonography is used to evaluate blood flow through carotid arteries or peripheral blood vessels. Deep vein thrombosis and peripheral vascular disease are diagnosed using this diagnostic test. A handheld transducer transmits high-frequency sound waves to an artery or vein. The sound waves strike the moving RBCs and are reflected back to the transducer, which amplifies the sound and produces a graphic recording.

Nuclear Scanning

Radioisotopes distribute uniformly through normal tissue, but unevenly in pathologically involved or diseased tissue. The radionuclide atom emits radioactive particles (photons in the gamma radiation range) which have short half lives. The most commonly used are gallium, thallium, and iodine. A scanning procedure involves less radiation exposure than a chest x-ray.

Radioisotopes tend to concentrate in specific organ tissues and thus are more effective when administered for scanning a particular organ. For example, technetium-99m is specifically used for thyroid scanning while thallium-201 (^{201}TI) is used to evaluate blood flow through vessels that are too small to visualize with a cardiac catheterization procedure. This is often termed a *myocardial perfusion scan*. Technetium-99m is also used for cardiac scanning. The newer thallium imagery is three-dimensional; the camera moves around the client in a 180°–360° arc. The three-dimensional view is more precise in identifying abnormalities. Scanning allows visualization of organs that are unobservable by x-ray alone. Tumors present as areas of reduced radioisotopic activity. Radioisotope studies are contraindicated with pregnancy, breast-feeding mothers, or persons who are allergic to the radioisotopes.

The radioactive isotopes are administered intravenously or orally to the client. A specified time elapses before the scanning is done. This allows time for the radioactive material to reach the specific tissue under study. Then, a scanning device is used to record the concentration of radiation that emerges from the radioisotope.

Some clients are given blocking agents before the administration of the radioisotope. This prevents the radioactive material from entering organs other than those being studied. A common blocking agent is Lugol's solution, which is given to a client who is having a study done on an organ other than the thyroid gland.

Microscopic Studies

Microscopic studies are necessary for diagnosis and treatment of many diseases and infectious processes. Specimens are collected from tissues, blood, organ biopsies, and secretions, in addition to other sources such as blood and urine.

Biopsies involve the physician's taking a piece of tissue from the designated area to be used for microscopic evaluation. Biopsies can be done on endometrial tissue, the lung and liver, and bone marrow aspiration, to name a few areas. Information obtained from the biopsy can indicate pathologic conditions, diseases, and treatment for infections.

Endoscopic Studies

An endoscopy refers to inspection of an internal body organ and cavities by introducing an instrument called an endoscope. Biopsies of suspicious tissue, removal of abnormal growths, injection of blood vessels, dilation and stent procedures, and surgical procedures can all be accomplished through the endoscope.

Endoscopes are either rigid or flexible and have a light source and viewing lens that allows the physician to observe the specified area. Scopes can be inserted through body orifices or through small incisions. Rigid scopes are used mostly for operative laparoscopic procedures. Flexible fiberoptic scopes are used in pulmonary and GI endoscopy. Because the scope is flexible, light can be transmitted around corners and thus provide a view of body structures not visible by older rigid scopes.

Fluid Analysis Studies

Normal body fluids can provide information concerning the client's health status. Body fluids frequently studied include CSF analysis, and condition of the fetus and its environment. Abnormal accumulation of fluids within the body can be analyzed by aspirating the fluid and sending it to the laboratory for studies. The most common areas where fluid needs to be removed include the abdomen and pleural space. Most often, the fluid is removed for therapeutic purposes, although it may be removed for diagnostic purposes. Once fluid is removed, it is measured and samples are sent to the laboratory for analysis.

Magnetic Resonance Imaging (MRI)

The MRI procedure has revolutionized diagnostic medicine. The procedure identifies the distribution of hydrogen molecules in the body using a three-dimensional process. The images are translated by computer and differentiate normal from abnormal tissue structure and blood flow. It uses a strong magnetic field in conjunction with radio frequency waves to transmit signals from body cells to the computer. The computer produces cross-sectional images of the body. The procedure is noninvasive and does not involve harmful exposure to radiation. The MRI detects and describes soft tissue abnormalities and yields information about the chemical nature of the cells. Gray and white brain matter can be differentiated and brain tumors and vascular abnormalities identified.

The MRI is the diagnostic procedure of choice for detecting most brain abnormalities, abnormal blood flow through coronary arteries, assessing kidney flow, heart defects, and a myriad of other abnormalities and defects. This procedure has replaced the need for arthrography and myelography. It has been used as a diagnostic tool in the diagnosis of multiple sclerosis; however, it has limited ability to detect plaque as the client ages. The procedure is noninvasive and does not involve harmful exposure to radiation.

Assisting the Physician during Tests

Nurses are frequently called on to assist the physician with procedures at the bedside as well as in the treatment room. The procedures presented in this chapter are the most common ones performed in the hospital unit. It is important that the nurse be aware of the correct client positioning in order to facilitate the procedure, decrease complications, and decrease the time it takes to complete the procedure.

Some diagnostic tests frequently used in the past are used less frequently today. One such procedure is the lumbar puncture. Removal of fluid from the spinal tract may cause the brain, because of edema, to herniate down through the tentorium. Because of this complication, a lumbar puncture is not done on a client with head trauma or potential increased intracranial pressure. The CT scan is now frequently used to determine intracranial bleeding.

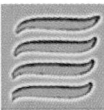

NURSING DIAGNOSES

The following nursing diagnoses may be appropriate to include in a client care plan when the components are related to clients undergoing diagnostic procedures.

NURSING DIAGNOSIS	RELATED FACTORS
Anxiety	Apprehension regarding test or procedure outcome
Fear	Results of diagnostic test, change in health status, threat to self-concept
Risk for Deficient Fluid Volume	Reaction to contrast media, NPO status, side effects of medication
Deficient Knowledge	Misunderstanding of instructions or information, inadequate data or explanation of procedure (maintaining position after spinal tap, liver biopsy)
Noncompliance	Inability to follow directions as a result of poor health status, cultural influences or patient's value system

- The single most important nursing action to decrease the incidence of hospital-based infections is handwashing. **Remember to wash your hands or use antibacterial gel before and after each and every client contact.**

UNIT 1

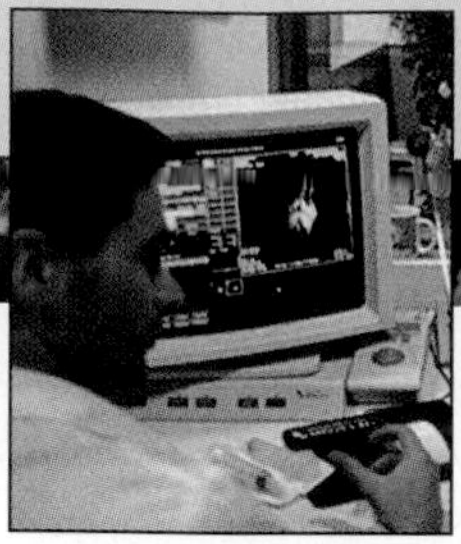

X-Ray Studies

Nursing Process Data

ASSESSMENT ***Data Base***

Assess client's knowledge of procedure to be done.

Identify any history of drug or food allergies.

Evaluate client's ability to follow directions before and during the test.

Assess vital signs and document for baseline data.

PLANNING ***Objectives***

To determine if the client is physically prepared for the test

To determine if the client is psychologically prepared for the test

To determine if the client is at risk for an allergic reaction

To determine if the client is able to cooperate with the preparation and completion of the test.

IMPLEMENTATION ***Procedures***

Preparing for X-Ray Studies

- *for Oral Cholecystography*
- *for Intravenous Pyelography (IVP)*
- *for Myelography*
- *for Arteriography*
- *for Computed Tomography (CT) Scan*
- *for Cardiac Catheterization*
- *for Bone Densitometry*
- *for Magnetic Resonance Imaging (MRI)*
- *for Mammography*

EVALUATION ***Expected Outcomes***

Client is able to complete the test without untoward effects.

Client understands procedure and has anxiety level under control.

Client is properly prepared for diagnostic test.

PREPARING FOR X-RAY STUDIES

Equipment

Signed consent form
Pajama bottoms and hospital gown
Allergy identaband, if needed
Wheelchair

> **CLINICAL ALERT**
>
> Ensure that female client is not pregnant nor is there a chance of being pregnant before performing any diagnostic tests using x-rays.

Procedure

for All X-Ray Studies

1. Identify the specific diagnostic test to be performed (Table 21–1).
2. Determine if any tests must precede others in order to schedule test appropriately.
3. Obtain client's history to determine allergies to food or drugs, and note these on the chart. Notify physician of findings.
4. Identify specific preparations that need to be carried out before the studies.
5. Monitor food and fluid restrictions that need to be altered for the studies.
6. Obtain special consent forms for all invasive diagnostic studies after the physician has explained the study to the client.
7. Provide client teaching regarding the purpose of the study, including any special preparation required and restrictions imposed by the study.
8. Provide psychological support and reassurance to the client.
9. Obtain orders regarding medications or nutrition for clients with special problems, such as diabetes or seizure disorders.
10. Carry out safety precautions immediately prior to the study:
    a. Check identaband for accuracy.
    b. Have client void if necessary.
    c. Remove client's hairpins, jewelry, and dentures if necessary.
    d. Chart premedication given.
    e. Monitor safe transfer from the bed to gurney or wheelchair.
    f. Accompany client to x-ray department if needed. (Usually, nurses accompany critically ill clients.)

for Oral Cholecystography

1. Explain purpose for procedure to client—x-ray provides visualization of gallbladder.
2. Identify allergies to shellfish or iodine. Notify physician if allergy is noted.
3. Obtain consent form.

> **CLINICAL ALERT**
>
> Symptoms of contrast media reactions:
> - Urticaria, hives
> - Nausea, vomiting
> - Respiratory distress
> - Decreased blood pressure
>
> Clients allergic to food or drugs may also be allergic to contrast media used for diagnostic studies.

TABLE 21–1 X-Ray Studies

Diagnostic Test	Rationale
Oral Cholecystography	To visualize shape and position of the gallbladder and to identify the presence of stones
Intravenous Pyelography	To visualize structures of the urinary tract
Myelography	To visualize the subarachnoid space to identify abnormalities
Arteriography	To visualize abnormalities or obstructions to specific blood vessels
Computed Tomography	To visualize a cross-section of the brain to precisely localize intracranial lesions
Cardiac Catheterization	To measure oxygen concentration, provide blood samples, determine cardiac output, and visualize coronary arteries
Bone Densitometry	To determine bone mineral density and strength of bone
Magnetic Resonance Imaging	To visualize inner structures of body
Mammography	To determine presence of breast pathology

4. Instruct client to eat low-fat meal evening before test.
5. Administer iodine radiopaque medication 2 hours after dinner. Drug: iopanoic acid (Telepaque).
   a. Number of tablets administered is based on client's weight.
   b. Tablets are given 5 minutes apart with 8 oz. of water for each tablet. Usually 6 tablets are given.
   c. Inform client that diarrhea is a common side effect.
6. Keep client NPO after administration of contrast medium. **Rationale:** This prevents contraction of gallbladder and expulsion of radiopaque dye.

CLINICAL ALERT

Do not schedule test after barium study because it precludes visualization of gallbladder.

CLINICAL ALERT

Ultrasound has replaced the oral cholecystogram test in most cases. It may still be used, however, if ultrasound results are inconclusive.

7. Take client to x-ray department.
8. Explain details of procedure to client.
   a. X-ray client in standing and lying positions for good visualization of gallbladder and common bile duct. Test takes about 1 hour.
   b. Feed client a fatty meal to test ability of the gallbladder to contract.
   c. If visualization does not occur, additional medications may be given and the test repeated the following day, or an IV cholangiogram may be done.
9. Explain postprocedure care to client.
   a. Mild dysuria can occur. **Rationale:** Dye is excreted through the kidneys.
   b. Observe for allergy symptoms from dye.

for Intravenous Pyelography (IVP)

1. Follow steps as appropriate in *Preparing for X-Ray Studies.*
   a. Give client clear liquid diet the evening before the IVP and maintain NPO status after 12 midnight. Some facilities allow clear liquid diet in morning.
   b. Give laxative or cathartic as ordered, usually 24 hours before test. **Rationale:** To eliminate feces and gas to provide better contrast.
   c. Identify allergies to shellfish or iodine. **Rationale:** Other contrast material will be used in place of iodine contrast media.
   d. Obtain consent.
   e. Take client to x-ray department when notified.
2. Explain details of procedure to client.
   a. Client is positioned in supine position.
   b. Flat plate of abdomen taken. **Rationale:** Ensure no residual stool which could interfere with visualization of renal system.
   c. Test dose of contrast medium may be injected intradermally for clients with a history of allergies. The contrast material is administered if there is no reaction within 15 minutes of test dose.
   d. IV is inserted and contrast medium injected as a large single dose.
   e. X-rays are taken over period of 30 minutes to 1 hour to determine extent to which dye is filtered through the kidneys.
3. Warn client that contrast medium can cause feelings of nausea, shortness of breath, and a hot, flushed effect.
4. Return client to room and resume ordered activity level.
5. Encourage fluids, and resume usual diet. Fluids should include at least 24 ounces of water. **Rationale:** Increasing fluid intake prevents osmotic diuresis from contrast medium.
6. Monitor client for at least 24 hours for signs and symptoms of reactions to contrast medium such as oliguria, nausea, and vomiting.

for Myelography

1. Follow steps as appropriate in *Preparing for X-Ray Studies.*
   a. Explain procedure to client—test identifies abnormalities of spine and subarachnoid space.
   b. Identify allergies to shellfish, iodine, or other contrast media.
   c. Keep client NPO for 3–4 hours before test.
   d. Obtain baseline levels of motor and sensory function and vital signs.
   e. Assess for signs of ICP. **Rationale:** This test is contraindicated for clients with ICP. Brain herniation can occur.
   f. Obtain consent form.
   g. Medicate with sedative if ordered. **Rationale:** This provides client comfort.
   h. Take client on gurney to x-ray department.
2. Explain details of procedure to client.
   a. Client is placed either in prone position with pillow under abdomen or side-lying with knees drawn up to abdomen and chin on chest. **Rationale:** This position allows physician to visualize ruptured disc or neoplasms.
   b. A lumbar puncture needle is inserted between the vertebrae into the subarachnoid space.
   c. A small amount of cerebrospinal fluid is sent to lab for study.
   d. Contrast medium is injected, and client is tilted on table to allow flow of dye to designated areas of spine to visualize it by x-rays.
   e. Oil-based contrast medium, Pantopaque, is removed through aspiration. Explain to client that sudden sharp pain in legs may occur.
   f. Water-based contrast medium, metrizamide, is absorbed and excreted through kidneys. It is not removed by

aspiration. Most facilities now use Omnipaque because it has far fewer side effects.
   g. Procedure lasts about 1 hour.
   h. Client is returned on gurney to room.
3. After the test.
   a. Keep client in prone position or supine position for 8 hours for water-based or 12 hours for oil-based contrast. May turn side to side. **Rationale:** This position prevents a headache and CSF leaks.
   b. Keep head of bed elevated 30°–50°. If procedure has included water-soluble dye medium, client may be on bedrest for up to 24 hours. **Rationale:** This position reduces rate of upward displacement of dye.
4. Observe for seizure activity if metrizamide used for procedure. It can precipitate seizures. Do not give medications that can decrease seizure threshold.
5. Monitor vital signs and motor and sensory function.
   a. Cervical myelogram: Check upper and lower extremities and bladder function.
   b. Lumbar myelogram: Check lower extremities and bladder function.
6. Medicate for pain as ordered, usually with a mild sedative.
7. Increase fluids to at least 2,500 mL each day for 2 days. **Rationale:** Fluids rehydrate and replace cerebrospinal fluid and may prevent headache following procedure. Offer diet.
8. Monitor output, and observe for distention.
9. Observe puncture site for 24 hours for bleeding, hematoma, or edema.
10. Observe for complication of chemical or bacterial meningitis: fever, stiff neck, photophobia or delayed reaction to dye.
11. Use comfort measures and relaxation techniques when needed.

CLINICAL ALERT

A myelogram is performed less frequently today because of the wide use of the MRI and CT scanning. The MRI is more accurate for viewing spinal cord and surrounding structures.

for Arteriography

1. Follow steps as appropriate in *Preparing for X-Ray Studies.*
2. Explain purpose of procedure to client—examination of arteries to determine abnormalities in blood flow.
3. Identify allergies to shellfish, iodine, or any contrast media. Ask client if taking anticoagulants.
4. Obtain baseline CBC, PT/PTT, and APTT.
5. Obtain consent form.
6. Keep client NPO for 2–8 hours or as ordered.
7. Shave and scrub puncture site when ordered.
8. Have client void before procedure.
9. Obtain vital signs and check peripheral pulses. **Rationale:** To provide comparison data following procedure.
10. Administer preprocedure medications if ordered, and transport client to x-ray department.
11. Explain details of procedure to client.
    a. Client is positioned supine on x-ray table.
    b. Puncture site will be scrubbed and a local anesthetic administered. Catheter is inserted into brachial or femoral artery.
    c. Contrast medium will be injected to visualize abnormalities or obstruction to specific vessels. Inform client that warm flush may be felt when dye injected.
    d. Client may be instructed to hold breath for x-rays. Procedure takes about 1 hour if an automatic film changer is used.
    e. Catheter is removed and pressure dressing applied over site.
12. Client is returned on gurney to room and instructed to remain in bed for 2 hours.
13. Monitor vital signs, pulses, and puncture site, as with surgical clients. **Rationale:** To identify potential complications.
14. Observe for signs of shock and presence of pain, which indicate hemorrhage or thrombosis.
15. Observe for symptoms of delayed allergic reaction to dye, such as nausea, vomiting, tachycardia, and sweating. **Rationale:** Delayed reactions can occur up to several hours following the procedure.
16. Notify physician immediately if unusual symptoms are present. **Rationale:** Immediate medical intervention is necessary to prevent anaphylaxis.
17. Apply ice pack or pressure dressing to puncture site if ordered. Do not flex the involved extremity.
18. Maintain bed rest with head elevated slightly for at least 8 hours. Check hospital policy for time.
19. Offer fluids and diet as ordered and tolerated.
20. Provide comfort measures as needed.

for Computed Tomography (CT Scan)

1. Explain purpose of procedure to client—CT scans give outlines of bone tissue and fluid structures due to tumors and hematomas. Tomography can be performed on abdomen, brain, or chest.

Xenon Computed Tomography

This test is relatively new and is used to evaluate cerebral blood flow. The new technique precisely measures blood flow to various areas of the brain. It can define the degree and extent of ischemia in acute neurologic conditions such as stroke. This technology detects changes hours to days before changes can be seen on the MRI or CT. The client inhales a xenon/oxygen gas mixture for approximately 4–5 minutes, during which time CT data is obtained. The xenon gas travels to regions of the brain where it is distributed to tissue in proportion to blood flow and lipid content (xenon is fat soluble). A computer actually calculates blood flow to many different areas of the brain and within minutes the computer provides precise measurements of cerebral blood flow.

2. Identify allergies to shellfish or iodine if contrast medium is used.
3. Obtain consent if contrast medium is used or facility requires.
4. Place client on NPO for 4 hours if contrast medium is used. **Rationale:** Dye can cause nausea; NPO prevents emesis and potential aspiration.
5. Administer preprocedure medication if ordered.
6. Remove all metal objects, such as hair clips, necklace, and jewelry. **Rationale:** Metal objects block bony structures on the film.
7. Take client on gurney to x-ray department.
8. Explain equipment and procedure to client.
9. Explain client will have IV injection of contrast material if enhanced study is to be done. Explain that a warm, flushed feeling or nausea can occur.
10. Explain that client will be placed in an encircling body scanner.
11. Instruct client to lie very still during the procedure and to not touch area to be scanned. **Rationale:** Movement causes artifact on the image.
12. Return client to room.
13. Provide diet and encourage fluids to 3000 mL or as ordered. **Rationale:** Increasing fluids assists in eliminating the contrast medium more quickly.
14. Observe for signs of delayed allergic reaction if contrast study is done.

for Cardiac Catheterization

1. Explain purpose for procedure to client—to visualize heart structures and coronary blood flow and measure oxygen saturation, cardiac output and heart pressures. Used most often to determine the cause of chest pain in adult clients. Procedure takes about one hour.
2. Obtain consent form.
3. Identify allergies to drugs, iodine, shellfish, or any other contrast media.
4. Check if client is on anticoagulants. Contact physician for instructions related to drug administration.
5. Complete prep and shave of groin or brachial area (or both). Mark peripheral pulses for past catheterization assessment.
6. Establish baseline data for vital signs, peripheral pulses, coagulation studies (PTT, PT), ACT and ECG pattern.
7. Place client on NPO 4–6 hours before test.
8. Before procedure, obtain vital signs, take weight, and have the client void.
9. Administer preprocedure medication, usually Valium and atropine.
10. Take client on gurney to cardiac catheterization lab.
11. Explain equipment and details of procedure to client.
    a. Client is strapped onto a table. ECG leads and blood pressure equipment are applied.
    b. Groin or brachial area is scrubbed and injected with Xylocaine.
    c. Catheter is placed in femoral artery and advanced to cardiac chambers.
    d. When contrast medium is injected for coronary artery visualization, explain to client that a warm, flushed feeling, shortness of breath, or nausea can occur.
    e. Instruct client to report any chest pain immediately.
    f. Client is asked to hold breath about 10 seconds during contrast medium injection.
    g. Reinforce that client will not fall off table as he or she may be turned on side for cineangiography. Total procedure takes 1–1½ hours.
    h. Following catheterization, pressure is applied to puncture site for 10–15 minutes.
12. Transport client on gurney to room.
13. Provide postcardiac catheterization care.
    a. Monitor vital signs, puncture site, heart and lung sounds, and peripheral pulses as with a surgical client.
    b. Elevate extremity used for catheterization site. Keep extremity extended. **Rationale:** Position promotes blood supply back to heart and prevents thrombus formation.
    c. Apply pressure dressing to puncture site if bleeding continues.
    d. Encourage fluids and diet when vital signs are stable and no evidence of nausea or drowsiness is present.
    e. Monitor for signs and symptoms of allergic response.
    f. Monitor for signs of clot induced stroke or myocardial infarction.
14. Position client for comfort. Place on back for several hours after the procedure, then turn from side to side.

for Bone Densitometry

1. Discuss procedure with client prior to scheduled test and ask pertinent questions for the record.
    a. Determine if barium studies have been done within last 10 days. **Rationale:** Barium may falsely increase bone density of lumbar spine.

Procedures Done During Cardiac Catheterization

Transluminal Coronary Angioplasty: Specially designed catheter is introduced into the coronary arteries and placed across the stenotic area of the artery. The artery is then dilated by controlled inflation of the balloon for a few seconds. Coronary stents can be placed at the site of the stenosis after angioplasty. The stent is used to keep the coronary artery patent.

Laser Arterectomy: Permanent procedure to open coronary arteries that have plaque deposits using laser therapy.

Angioplasty: Catheter is placed in a stenotic area and a balloon is inflated and forcefully dilates the stenotic area. The client is monitored during the procedure using ECG tracings. If myocardial ischemia is present during the procedure, the balloon is removed.

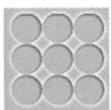

CULTURAL COMPETENCE

A cross-culture assessment questionnaire should be offered to clients who may have differences in understanding or following directions in preparation for diagnostic procedures. In some cultures, it is difficult for clients to admit they do not understand what is being said to them. Westerners are bold and direct when asking questions so we expect the same from clients of different cultures.

With the "push" to get clients in and out of procedure rooms, communication and understanding can be compromised. However, while preparing for the procedure, talking with the client can provide the comforting measures necessary to allow them to participate appropriately during the procedure. Ask clients which family member should be included in the discussion and client teaching regarding the diagnostic procedure. Pay close attention to what family members say. They can provide valuable information regarding the client's understanding or fear of the procedure. In some cultures words such as cancer, surgery, or death are not used. In many Middle Eastern cultures you do not speak of death, it is viewed as a breach in the nurse–client relationship. Modesty is an issue with some cultures. This varies greatly among cultures and individuals within those cultures. Be sensitive to this issue and allow the client to undress in private if at all possible.

Source: Heinekine, J., & McCoy, N. (2000, January). Establishing a bond with clients of different cultures. *Home Healthcare Nurse, 18*, (1), 45.

   b. Instruct client that no specific pretest fasting, blood work, or sedation needs to be done.
   c. Instruct client to go to outpatient x-ray or hospital facility according to instructions (there are no preparations for study, so it is usually not important to come early for test).
   d. Instruct client not to wear jewelry, belt buckles, or zippers to x-ray department and to remove coins and keys from pocket; clothing need not be removed for test.
   e. Determine if client has had previous bone density tests or fractures. Document findings for physician.
2. Explain that there is no pain or discomfort associated with test.
3. Explain that false positive results can include previous fractures and previous bone scans.
4. Explain procedure to client.
   a. Client will be placed on an imaging table with legs supported on padded box. **Rationale:** Position flattens pelvis and lumbar spine.
   b. Images of lumbar and hip bones are projected on a computer monitor.
   c. Each machine scans the bones of the finger, heel, and forearm differently, so specific instructions will be given according to machine descriptions.
   d. After computer screen calculates bone mineral density, it is compared with existing data from healthy 25–35-year-old women and a T score is determined. The T score indicates the strength of the bone. The positive T score indicates a bone that is stronger than normal. A negative T score indicates the bone is weaker than normal. Z scores are also obtained. These scores compare clients matched for age, sex, race, height, and weight.
5. Instruct client that no specific postprocedural care is required. There are no side effects or complications associated with the test.

for Magnetic Resonance Imaging (MRI)

1. Evaluate client for following conditions. **Rationale:** These conditions exempt clients from having MRI because the magnet can move and displace metal, such as clips and staples, or cause a malfunction.
   a. Clients with pacemakers, insulin pumps, or other implanted electrical devices.
   b. Clients with hip prostheses, cardiac surgery, or metal implants.
   c. Clients with vascular clips and staples from recent surgery.
   d. Pregnant clients should not be scanned even though there is no definitive evidence of harm to fetus.
   e. Clients with cardiac or respiratory complications may be excluded.
2. Check for allergies if contrast medium is to be used. Two common contrast mediums are gadodiamide and gadopentatediameglumine.
3. Instruct client to remove all metal or magnetically sensitive objects: jewelry, watches, hair clips, credit cards.

CLINICAL ALERT

Clients who are extremely claustrophobic may require conscious sedation or may be moved to a nonenclosed MRI. If sedated, client must be monitored for at least 1 hour before discharge.

4. Describe MRI machine and procedure to client—it provides a clear picture of the inner structures of the extremities, brain, and spinal cord, and it clearly reproduces soft tissue, ligaments, and nerves; often used for determining response to radiotherapy and chemotherapy.
   a. Client needs to lie flat, still, and relax inside the tube magnet. **Rationale:** Movement can produce artifact on image.
   b. Procedure lasts 20–60 minutes. During time client is in the machine he/she can talk to and hear staff. Prism glasses may be worn so client can see outside scanner.
   c. Entire body is encased in machine.
   d. Inform client he or she will feel nothing but may hear noises represented by a grating or loud buzzing sound, lasting 5 minutes. **Rationale:** Noises are caused by changing magnetic fields.
   e. Inform client he or she will have ear plugs in place but will be able to communicate with MRI staff through microphone. **Rationale:** This allays feelings of claustrophobia.
   f. Instruct client in relaxation techniques.
5. Instruct client to void before procedure. **Rationale:** This prevents the need for client to void while undergoing procedure.

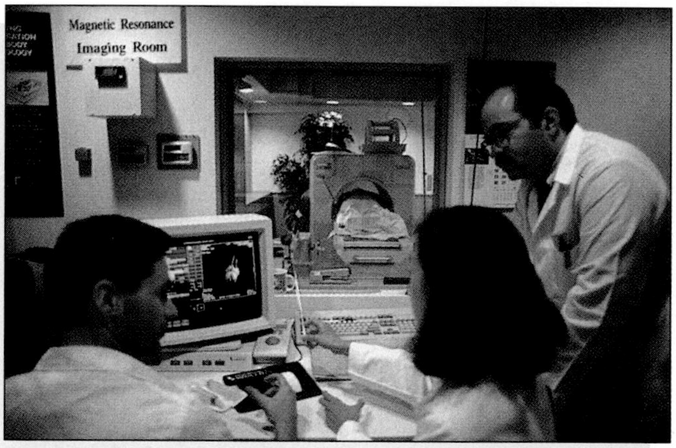

Magnetic resonance imaging (MRI) machine.

6. Administer premedication as ordered, usually Valium.
7. Place client in a comfortable position on table.
8. Instruct client on feelings of warmth or shortness of breath if contrast medium is used during procedure.
9. Transport client to room following procedure.
10. Observe for symptoms of delayed reaction to contrast material if used during procedure.

for Mammography

1. Instruct client to not wear deodorant or talcum powder. **Rationale:** It can interfere with the reading of the mammogram.
2. Instruct client not to wear jewelry around neck.
3. Review client's history regarding breast implants or previous breast surgery, lumps or unusual findings on monthly examinations. **Rationale:** Included on health record so radiologist has an accurate assessment of mammogram findings.
4. Explain procedure to client—may cause some momentary discomfort when x-ray cone compresses breast tissue; discomfort does not last after release of cone. **Rationale:** Compression of breast provides better visualization of breast tissue.
5. Explain that there is minimal radiation exposure from this procedure.
6. Instruct client to take off clothing above waist, including bra, and put x-ray gown on so it ties in front.
   a. One breast is placed on x-ray plate and the cone is brought down on breast to compress it.
   b. The breast will be placed in different positions to view the entire breast tissue.
   c. The second breast is done in same manner.
7. Instruct client to wait when mammography is finished until films are processed. **Rationale:** Sometimes additional films will need to be taken; this prevents client from having to return to the department.
8. Instruct client in self breast examination, if necessary, and answer questions before client leaves.
   a. Test results are usually mailed to client.
   b. If the mammography is being done for diagnostic purposes, the mammogram may be read and results are immediately available for client.

DOCUMENTATION FOR X-RAY STUDIES

- Preparation completed (e.g., NPO, clear liquid dinner)
- Client teaching completed
- Medication administered Allergies noted
- Unusual anxiety or fears of client
- How client transported to test
- Time sent and returned from test
- Postprocedure care
- Appearance of dressing or puncture sites

Critical Thinking Application

UNEXPECTED OUTCOMES	CRITICAL THINKING OPTIONS
Client has allergic reaction.	• Follow protocol or standing orders for allergic reactions. • Start O_2 at 6 L/min unless otherwise contraindicated. Use nasal cannula. • Place in semi- or high-Fowler's position if not contraindicated. • Administer medications as outlined in protocol or according to physician's orders. • Provide reassurance and encouragement. • Have client take slow, deep breaths. • If nausea or vomiting occur, obtain an order for an antiemetic from the physician.
Client is given meal when on NPO status.	• Call x-ray and change time of test. If possible, arrange for test to be done later in the day to avoid additional hospitalization. • Instruct client on what NPO means.
Client very apprehensive and refuses test at last minute.	• Identify reasons for anxiety and attempt to allay fears. • Notify physician and ask if he or she wants to cancel or postpone test to later time. Do not attempt to "talk client into it."
Bleeding or hemorrhage occurs from arteriogram puncture site.	• Notify physician. • Apply direct pressure until pressure dressing can be applied. • Monitor amount of blood loss and possible signs and symptoms of shock. • Elevate and keep extremity in extension position.
Client develops irregular pulse following cardiac catheterization.	• Notify physician immediately • Prepare for possible code and IV administration of medication. • Monitor vital signs frequently.
Bleeding occurs at catheter insertion site following cardiac catheterization.	• Apply pressure dressing. • Elevate extremity. • Monitor peripheral pulse and vital signs. • If bleeding does not subside, notify physician.

UNIT 2

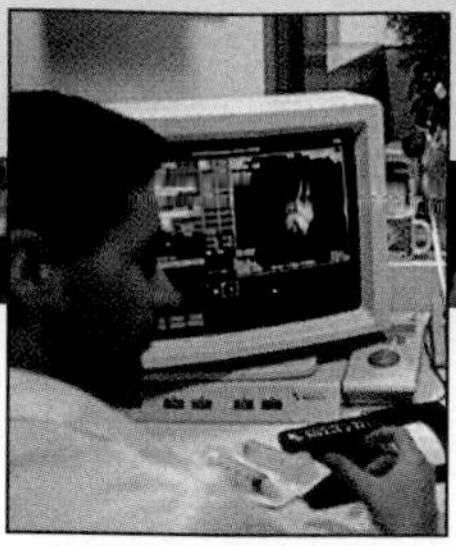

Nuclear Scanning

Nursing Process Data

ASSESSMENT *Data Base*

Assess client's understanding of nuclear imaging and the specific diagnostic test he or she is to receive.

Assess client's ability to tolerate procedure (e.g., swallowing iodine solution, fasting).

Determine client's psychologic needs in relation to the nuclear scan.

Identify any allergies the client may have to radioactive materials.

Assess need to remain with client during procedure.

Assess vital signs and document for baseline data.

PLANNING *Objectives*

To diagnose tumors, metastatic disease, abnormal conditions, cardiac and other organ abnormalities via noninvasive method

To prepare the client physically for the nuclear diagnostic test

To prepare the client psychologically to prevent undue stress

To complete client teaching to ensure the client understands the procedure

IMPLEMENTATION *Procedures*

Preparing for Nuclear Scans

- *for Bone Scan*
- *for Lung Scan*
- *for PET Scan*
- *for Nuclear Cardiography*
- *for Thyroid Scan*

Teaching for Nuclear Scan

EVALUATION *Expected Outcomes*

Client is physically prepared for the diagnostic study.

Client is psychologically prepared for the diagnostic study.

Client discusses rationale for the diagnostic test.

PREPARING FOR NUCLEAR SCANS

Equipment

Signed consent form
IV equipment (for most scans)
Hospital gown and pajama bottoms

Preparation

1. Identify the specific diagnostic test that is to be performed (Table 21–2).
2. Determine if any tests must precede others in order to schedule test appropriately.

Note: Technetium-99m, gallium, thallium, and iodine are used commonly for scanning. Technetium-99m is used extensively because it has a 6 hour half-life and emits low levels of gamma rays.

3. Identify specific preparations that need to be carried out before the studies. Check for recent exposure to radionuclids. **Rationale:** May interfere with current study.
4. Monitor fluid alterations that need to precede the studies.
5. Obtain special consent forms if required by facility after the physician has explained the study to the client.
6. Provide client teaching regarding the study, including any special preparation required for the study.
7. Provide psychologic support and reassurance to the client.
8. Explain that radiation exposure is minimal and limited.
9. Record client's height and weight.
10. Carry out safety precautions immediately prior to the study:
    a. Check identaband for accuracy.
    b. Check for allergies.
    c. Chart premedication if given.
    d. Monitor safe transfer from the bed to gurney or wheelchair.
    e. Accompany client to nuclear medicine department if needed. (Usually, nurses accompany critically ill clients.)

for Bone Scan

1. Follow steps as appropriate in *Preparing for Nuclear Scans.*
    a. Explain purpose for procedure to client—usually done to detect metastatic cancer. If client is of child-bearing age, determine whether she is pregnant. If so, test cannot be done.
    b. No fasting or sedation is required.
    c. Have client ready for injection of radionuclide material, probably Technetium-99m, 1–3 hours before scan.
    d. Force fluids between injection of isotope and scan.
    e. Have client void before going to x-ray.
    f. Take client to nuclear medicine department.
2. Explain procedure.
    a. Client is positioned supine under scintillation camera (camera records radiation emitted by skeleton).
    b. Instruct client to remain very still for 20 minutes to ensure observation of bone abnormalities.
    c. Client will be repositioned to prone and lateral positions during scan.
    d. Return client to room.
3. Instruct client to resume activities and diet. **Rationale:** There is no problem with radiation exposure because only tracer doses of radioisotopes are used.
4. Force fluids for 2–3 hours after scan. **Rationale:** To promote renal filtering of excess tracer. Trace elements are excreted in 6–24 hours.

for Lung Scan

1. Follow steps as appropriate in *Preparing for Nuclear Scans.*
    a. Explain purpose for procedure—used to detect pulmonary embolism.
    b. Obtain consent if required.
    c. Obtain chest x-ray 24–48 hours before scan.
    d. Transport client to nuclear medicine department.
    e. Ensure all jewelry is removed.
2. Explain details of procedure.
    a. Explain equipment to client.
    Closed-breathing system is used when ventilation scan is done.
    Scintillation camera.

TABLE 21–2 Nuclear Studies

Diagnostic Test	Rationale
Bone Scan	To diagnose metastatic bone disease, osteomyelitis, or fractures
Lung Scan	To diagnose pulmonary embolism, pneumothorax, or assess pulmonary status before lung surgery
PET Scan	To scan whole body or its various areas; used in diagnosis; especially useful in diagnosing epilepsy
Cardiology Scan	To diagnose coronary artery disease, cardiomyopathy, valvular heart disease, or to assess cardiac status and analyze ventricular function
Thyroid Scan	To diagnose thyroid nodules, abnormal function, or thyroid cancer

b. Client is injected intravenously with a tracer amount of radioactive material—usually, radionuclide-tagged MAA (macroaggregated albumin with Technetium) is used.
c. Client is positioned in several ways to obtain clear images.
d. Client is instructed to breathe through a closed system until all radioactive gas is cleared from the system.
e. Instruct in use of mouthpiece or nose clips if used.
f. Client is instructed to lie quietly for 30 minutes as radiography is completed—Gamma ray detector is passed over client, records radionuclide uptake on film.

3. Transport client on gurney to room.
4. Instruct client to resume prestudy activities.

for PET Scans

1. Follow steps as appropriate in *Preparing for Nuclear Scans.*
2. Explain that purpose of test is to scan the whole body or its various regions. It aids in determining focal area for seizure activity and is used to help diagnose epilepsy. It is also useful in determining brain region for surgical removal of affected area when medication resistance is present.
3. Assess client and take complete history to determine if client is pregnant. Determine if client is claustrophobic or anxious. **Rationale:** Test cannot be performed if client is pregnant. Client must be able to lie still during the entire process, including a minimum of 45 minutes with his or her head inside scanner.
4. Premedicate with nonaspirin analgesia if client has arthritis or lower back pain that could prevent client from lying still for prescribed time. **Rationale:** Sedatives are avoided if at all possible because they alter metabolism. If necessary, chloral hydrate could be used; it has fewest adverse effects.
5. Instruct client to stay NPO for 6–8 hours, if glucose metabolism is measured.
6. Instruct client to avoid caffeine, alcohol, and nicotine on day of test.
7. Explain procedure:
   a. Reassure client that there is no discomfort except lying on a hard surface for up to three hours.
   b. Ensure client has not taken aspirin or other anticoagulants for several days prior to scan.
   c. Explain that an arterial line with be inserted to obtain blood samples.
   d. Explain that a peripheral intravenous catheter will be inserted to inject radioisotope.
   e. Instruct client to lie quietly for 45 minutes. Lights will be dim. **Rationale:** This is time for radioisotope uptake to occur, as isotopes are circulating to the brain.
   f. Monitor vital signs as indicated.
   g. Explain that actual scan time is about 45 minutes. He or she must remain quiet with head in scanner during this entire time. **Rationale:** Any motion, moving, or talking can detract from the quality of image.
   h. Explain that arterial blood samples may be drawn from arterial line during scan.
8. Provide postprocedural instructions.
   a. After scan, IV and arterial lines will be discontinued.
   b. Client can resume normal activities and meals.
   c. Monitor for signs of seizure activity or adverse effects if seizure did occur during scan.
   d. If sedative was given, do not allow client to drive or engage in any hazardous activities until sedative has worn off. Instruct client to have someone drive him/her home.

for Nuclear Cardiography

1. Follow steps as appropriate in *Preparing for Nuclear Scans.*
2. Instruct client that radioactive tracer substances are used to detect and evaluate cardiovascular abnormalities. Alterations of left ventricular muscle function and coronary blood flow are evaluated.
3. Instruct client in specific activities related to the test (i.e., exercise on a treadmill, holding certain medications, fasting). See step 2 for specific cardiology test.
4. Explain that short fasting time may be necessary.
5. Following isotope injection, 15 minutes to 4 hours later scan will be performed.
6. Instruct client in nuclear medicine department.
   a. Gamma ray detector is placed over heart.
   b. Placed in several positions during scan.
   c. Scan records images of heart.

Common Tests in Nuclear Cardiology

Technetium pyrophosphate scan. This binds with calcium and creates an area of increased radionuclide uptake. The client receives an injection into the antecubital vein. He or she then waits 2 hours while the renal system clears the drug. A special camera scans the heart to identify areas of increased uptake of the radioisotope. The radioisotope accumulates in damaged areas of the heart and shows any evidence of a recent MI. Scan also called a myocardial Infusion Scan.

Thallium scan. A medication (^{201}Tl) is injected into the antecubital vein and scanning is done within 4–10 minutes. Necrotic or ischemic tissue does not reflect the radioisotope as tissue with normal blood supply and healthy cells does. To detect myocardial scarring and perfusion, an acute or chronic MI, or the evaluation of prior cardiac surgery are the primary purposes for this test.

Thallium scan with exercise. When this test involves exercise, it takes 1 hour and 15 minutes; 3 hours later, a 30-minute resting scan is performed. Imaging with exercise may demonstrate perfusion problems not apparent when the client is at rest.

Gated cardiac blood pool scan. The client receives an intravenous injection of a red blood cell tagging agent and ECG leads are positioned on him or her. The computer is then synchronized with the ECG reading. This test evaluates left ventricular function.

7. Evaluate client's status following the scan.
   a. Encourage fluids to excrete isotopes.
   b. Apply pressure over venipuncture site if necessary.

for Thyroid Scan

1. Follow steps as appropriate in *Preparing for Nuclear Scans.*
2. Purpose of scan is to diagnose thyroid nodules, abnormal thyroid function, or thyroid cancer.
3. Explain procedure to client.
   a. Instruct client not to consume any iodine compounds (vitamin or mineral supplements that may contain iodine or iodized table salt) or eat any foods that contain iodine—especially seafood, which has a high iodine content. **Rationale:** Consuming iodine products interferes with the test.
   b. Instruct client not to take thyroid or antithyroid drugs or x-ray contrast medium before the test, usually 6 weeks before test. **Rationale:** These materials interfere with the thyroid scan.
   c. Tell client that after the initial oral radioactive Technetium he or she must return to the lab 24 hours later. Some labs do scanning after 2 hours of injestion of Technetium.
   d. Instruct client that no isolation is needed following scan.

TEACHING FOR NUCLEAR SCANS

Procedure

1. Inform client that test is to be performed in the nuclear medicine department.
   a. The department name alone may be frightening to the client.
   b. Taking the client to the department ahead of time may help to decrease anxiety.
2. Explain to the client that he or she will be receiving an injection of a radioisotope through a vein. The exceptions to this procedure are a lung scan in which the isotope is administered through an oxygen mask and a gastric-emptying scan in which the isotope is given orally with food.
   a. Inform client that this isotope emits a harmless amount of radiation.
   b. Also inform client that the camera used for scanning does not emit radiation. The camera detects a small and harmless amount of radiation from the isotope as it is lodged in the part of the body being imaged.
3. Explain to the client that he or she will be lying on a table (he or she will not be confined in an enclosed space) while the camera is positioned above or below the table.
4. Assure the client that someone will be with him or her throughout the test, contrasting this procedure with x-rays for which the technician must leave the room or with the MRI for which the client enters a tube-like structure.
5. Tell the client that if he or she is in pain, he or she may receive an analgesic during the procedure, as he or she must remain still while the camera is scanning the body.

DOCUMENTATION FOR NUCLEAR SCANNING

- Client teaching completed
- Client's emotional state
- Any radioisotopes given on the unit
- Preprocedural preparation completed (i.e., enema or laxative)
- Means by which client transported to nuclear medicine department
- Time client sent to and returned from scan

Critical Thinking Application

UNEXPECTED OUTCOMES	CRITICAL THINKING OPTIONS
Client appears not to understand purpose of diagnostic test.	• Observe for nonverbal cues or misunderstandings in order to clarify • Provide alternative teaching aids. • Show client the equipment if necessary. • Ask client to repeat explanation to you.
Client is unable to cooperate during the procedure.	• If not contraindicated by condition, ask physician for sedation order. • Nursing staff members may be asked to help client remain quiet. If so, wear lead apron shield.
Client is uncomfortable during procedure.	• Reposition client for comfort if possible. (It may not be possible depending on area of body to be scanned.) • Provide support by propping client in position needed for scanning. • Assist client to focus on other things (e.g., the ball game, weather, or something pleasant).

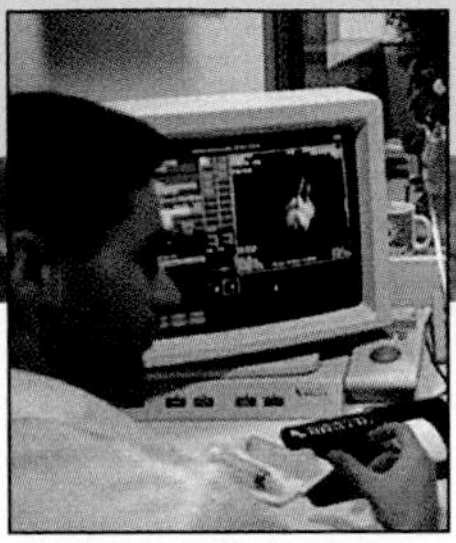

UNIT 3

Barium Studies

Nursing Process Data

ASSESSMENT *Data Base*

Assess results of laxative and enema administration to ensure a clean colon for the study. Notify physician if client is unable to "hold" enema solution.

Evaluate client's ability to cooperate with test.

Evaluate client's knowledge of test.

PLANNING *Objectives*

To determine the client's ability to understand the preparatory process

To clean out colon in order to ensure visualization of colon

To prepare the client psychologically for the test

IMPLEMENTATION *Procedures*

Preparing for Barium Studies

for Lower GI or Barium Enema

for Upper GI or Barium Swallow Study

for Small Bowel Follow-Through

EVALUATION *Expected Outcomes*

Client is able to cooperate with test.

Client's colon is clear of stool.

Barium is expelled following test.

PREPARING FOR BARIUM STUDIES

Equipment

Signed consent if agency requires
Enema tube and bag
Ordered solution for enema
Laxative
Wheelchair

Procedure

1. Identify the specific diagnostic test that will be performed (Table 21–3).
2. Explain purpose for procedure to client.
3. Obtain consent for specific test to be performed.
4. Instruct client to prepare for test.
   a. Stay on low-residue diet 1 to 2 days before test, and a clear liquid diet from lunch the day before test. No dairy products.
   b. Take one glass of water or clear fluid every hour for 8–10 hours.
   c. Administer one full bottle (10 oz) of magnesium citrate or X-prep at 2 P.M. day before test.
   d. Administer three 5-mg Dulcolax tablets at 7 P.M., evening before test.
   e. Keep NPO after Dulcolax tablets.
   f. Administer a suppository or a cleansing enema (or both if necessary) in early morning on day of test. Ensure bowel is clear; liquid return should be clear. If not, notify x-ray department.

> **CLINICAL ALERT**
> If client has suspected bowel obstruction, no cathartics are given.

5. Carry out safety precautions immediately prior to the procedure:
   a. Check identaband for accuracy.
   b. Monitor safe transfer from bed to gurney or wheelchair.

for Barium Enema

1. Transport client to radiology department usually via wheelchair.
2. Explain details of procedure to client.
   a. A balloon rectal tube is inserted and balloon is tightly inflated against anal sphincter. **Rationale:** To keep barium in rectum during study.
   b. Client is turned side to side while dripping barium into rectum using gravity flow for infusion.
   c. Barium flow is monitored by fluoroscopy continuously and colon is examined as barium goes through colon.
   d. Barium is drained out and an x-ray is taken to determine if barium has been expelled.
   e. Entire procedure takes 15 minutes to 1 hour.

TABLE 21–3 Barium Studies

Diagnostic Test	Rationale
Lower GI Studies	
Barium Enema	To visualize the lower GI tract for contour, patency, position and mucosal pattern of colon
Upper GI Studies	To visualize the upper GI tract; pharynx, esophagus and stomach
Barium Swallow	To visualize the esophagus
Small Bowel Follow-Through	To visualize the duodenum, jejunum, and ileum

> **CLINICAL ALERT**
> Barium studies should follow IVPs, ultrasound examinations, and arteriograms because barium interferes with visualization of other structures. Barium enema should precede barium swallow.

3. Transport client to room.
4. Force fluids with electrolytes unless contraindicated.
5. Administer laxative or enema as ordered. **Rationale:** To facilitate bowel evacuation.
6. Ensure client has bowel movement within 2–3 days.

for Barium Swallow Study

1. Explain purpose of procedure to client.
2. Instruct client to stay on low residue diet 1–3 days before procedure, if ordered and to stay NPO for 8 hours before test.
3. Administer laxative or enema evening before procedure, particularly if this test follows barium enema study.

Small Bowel Enema

Barium is injected into a tube placed in the small bowel. This procedure provides better visualization of the entire small bowel because the barium solution is not diluted by juices from the GI tract. This test is used when bowel obstruction is suspected.

> **CLINICAL ALERT**
> Gastrografin, a water soluble contrast material, should be used if there is a risk for leakage of contrast material through a perforation of the GI tract.

4. Instruct client not to smoke. **Rationale:** Smoking causes an increase in flow of digestive juices.
5. Transport to radiology department.
6. Explain details of procedure to client.
   a. Client is instructed to drink a cup of flavored barium, usually in milkshake-like form, under fluoroscopic exam.
   b. Client is instructed to turn to several positions while x-rays are obtained.
   c. X-rays are taken every 30 minutes as barium advances.

for Small Bowel Follow-Through

   a. Barium swallow may be extended to examine duodenum and small bowel.
   b. Films can be taken as long as 24 hours later.

7. Transport client to room.
8. Force fluids unless contraindicated.
9. Administer cathartic.
10. Ensure bowel movement within 2–3 days. Enema may need to be administered.

> **CLINICAL ALERT**
> Obtain specific orders for enemas when client has severe abdominal pain, ulcerative colitis, or history of megacolon. Do not follow general preprocedural orders.

DOCUMENTATION FOR BARIUM STUDIES

- Laxative administered
- Type, amount of fluid, number of enemas administered
- Enema result, consistency of stool, color of returning enema solution
- Unusual symptoms such as pain, bleeding, or nausea associated with enemas
- Color of stool following test

Critical Thinking Application

UNEXPECTED OUTCOMES	CRITICAL THINKING OPTIONS
Barium is unable to be expelled even following administration of laxatives and enemas.	• Obtain order for and administer oil-retention enema • Administer tap water enema following oil-retention enema. • Continue to administer laxatives until barium is expelled.
Laxatives or enemas (or both) are ordered for clients with ulcerative colitis or severe abdominal pain.	• Do not administer either the laxative or enema without checking with the physician. • If physician confirms order, carefully administer small amount of enema fluid, and observe and document effects on client. • Chart the type of pain, if any characteristics of stool, and any symptoms noted while enema is administered. • If client complains of excruciating pain, stop procedure and notify the physician.
Client's medications are administered in error.	• Notify x-ray department, and ask for specific orders as to what action needs to be taken regarding the test. • Inform physician, complete a medication error form and send to nursing office. An incident form may need to be completed as well. • If this is a frequent problem on the unit or in the hospital, an in-service education program should be given that includes a discussion of when medications should be given and when held.

UNIT 4

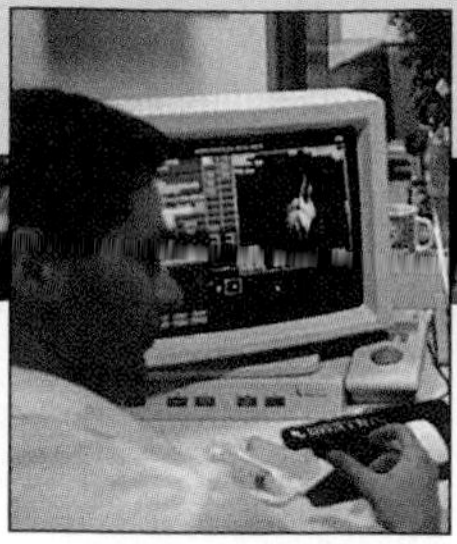

Endoscopic Studies

Nursing Process Data

ASSESSMENT Data Base

Assess vital signs prior to and during studies, if indicated. Some studies require general anesthesia or conscious sedation, and scope is used that could result in perforation and bleeding.

Assess client's knowledge of procedure to be done.

Evaluate baseline laboratory tests, particularly those for potential bleeding problems, if biopsy is to be done.

Evaluate if client is at risk for complications, especially infection (antibiotics may need to be ordered).

Assess biopsy site for indications of bleeding.

Evaluate for signs of infection following procedure.

PLANNING Objectives

To provide information regarding procedure to decrease client's anxiety

To determine if previous studies were completed using barium

To evaluate potential for complications following procedure

To position client on table correctly to facilitate optimal visual outcome and aid in diagnosing condition

IMPLEMENTATION Procedures

Preparing for Endoscopic Studies

for Arthroscopy

for Bronchoscopy

for Colonoscopy

for Cystoscopy

for Gastrointestinal Tract Endoscopy

for Laparoscopy

for Sigmoidoscopy

EVALUATION Expected Outcomes

Client is prepared psychologically and physically for endoscopic procedure.

Diagnostic procedure performed with minimal discomfort.

Direct observation and endoscopy provides for biopsy, removal of abnormal tissue, and minor surgical procedures.

Endoscopy allows for observation of body structures through use of video camera.

TABLE 21–4 Endoscopic Procedures

Diagnostic Test	Rationale
Arthroscopy	To evaluate meniscus cartilage or ligament injury; to differentiate arthritic inflammation from injury
Bronchoscopy	To visualize larynx, trachea, bronchi, and alveoli; to diagnose bleeding sites and obtain sputum specimens
Colonoscopy	To visualize rectum and colon; to obtain tissue biopsy and remove polyps
Cystoscopy	To visualize urethra, bladder, ureters, prostate; to place stents
Gastrointestinal tract endoscopy (EGD)	To visualize esophagus, stomach, and duodenum; to obtain specimen for cell studies
Laparoscopy	To visualize abdominal cavity; to perform surgical interventions
Sigmoidoscopy	To visualize anus, rectum, sigmoid colon; to remove polyps, obliterate hemorrhoids

PREPARING FOR ENDOSCOPIC STUDIES

Procedure

1. Explain test to client.
2. Obtain signed consent form.
3. Complete preparation according to endoscopic test being performed.
4. Place on NPO status for 8–12 hours for gastroscopy and as directed for other procedures.
5. Remove dentures for bronchoscopy, gastroscopy procedures.
6. Provide bowel prep for laparoscopy, sigmoidoscopy or colonoscopy to cleanse all fecal material from colon. **Rationale:** Allows adequate visualization of mucosa.
7. Obtain lab results for bleeding and clotting factors, Hgb, Hct, electrolytes if potential bleeding could occur or possible biopsy will be done with endoscopy.
8. Complete physical assessment to determine risk factors for possible complications and allergies.
9. Notify special procedure room staff and physician of potential problems with client's condition that could interfere with procedure.

for Arthroscopy

1. Follow steps in *Preparing for Endoscopic Studies* as it applies to this procedure.
2. Explain that arthroscopy allows direct visualization of specific anatomic site (i.e., knee joint). Small trocars are placed into joint and surgical procedure is completed with direct vision of a camera attached to arthroscope.
3. Explain that client usually receives local anesthesia and procedure takes 30 minutes to 2 hours.
4. Instruct client to remain NPO from midnight if general anesthesia is to be given.
5. Instruct client in use of crutches, if necessary.
6. Shave hair 6 inches above and below involved joint, if ordered.
7. Explain procedure to client.
   a. Anesthesia is given, either local or general.
   b. Leg is scrubbed, elevated, and wrapped in elastic bandage from toes to lower thigh. **Rationale:** Reduce blood flow from lower extremity.
   c. Physician places tourniquet or instills saline solution in client's knee before insertion of scope. **Rationale:** To reduce bleeding.
   d. Knee is placed at 45° angle.
   e. Small incision is made in skin around knee and scope is inserted into joint space.
   f. Procedure is completed, joint is irrigated, medication to decrease inflammation is injected into knee.
   g. Sutures or butterfly tapes are placed on skin with pressure dressing applied over site.
8. Assess client's neurovascular status immediately after procedure.
9. Assess vital signs and observe site for potential complications (i.e., bleeding, edema, or excessive drainage).
10. Provide discharge teaching.
    a. Elevate knee at all times when sitting, minimize use of joint for several days.
    b. Apply ice packs according to physician's orders.
    c. Instruct client to observe for potential complications: fever, redness around site, excess drainage, or alteration in color of drainage, pain, increased edema.
    d. Ambulation with crutches is usually allowed on same day as surgery.
    e. Remind client to make postop physician appointment according to orders.

for Bronchoscopy

1. Follow steps for *Preparing for Endoscopic Studies* as it applies to this procedure.
2. Explain purpose of procedure to client.

3. Explain that test provides endoscopic visualization of larynx, trachea, and bronchi through insertion of flexible fiberoptic bronchoscope. Biopsies may be taken and cultures obtained during procedure.
4. Place client on NPO for 6–8 hours before procedure. **Rationale:** This decreases risk of aspiration while gag reflex is blocked during the procedure.
5. Instruct client to practice good oral hygiene.
6. Obtain baseline data: vital signs and respiratory assessment. **Rationale:** This provides comparison data after procedure.
7. Remove dentures. **Rationale:** This prevents damage or lodging of dentures in the throat during procedure.
8. Premedicate client with sedative and atropine if ordered. **Rationale:** These medications inhibit vagal stimulation, suppress gag reflex, and decrease the client's anxiety.
9. Client is placed in sitting or supine position in operating room or special procedure room.
10. Explain procedure to client.
    a. Physician sprays nasopharynx and oropharynx with topical anesthetic. **Rationale:** This prevents laryngospasm, depresses gag reflex, and prevents discomfort when scope is inserted.
    b. Client is instructed to avoid swallowing anesthetic agent. Instruct client to expectorate into emesis basin.
    c. Bronchoscope is inserted into mouth and advanced to trachea and bronchi.
    d. Tissue specimens or secretions are collected and sent to laboratory for study.
    e. Bronchoscope is removed.
11. Cleanse client's nose of lubricant following removal of scope.
12. Provide postprocedures care.
    a. Monitor vital signs and respiratory status as with a surgical client. **Rationale:** This determines possible complications, such as bleeding or hypoxia.
    b. Monitor for bloody sputum. **Rationale:** Bleeding can occur as a result of the bronchoscopy. Notify physician immediately if this occurs.
    c. Instruct client not to eat or drink until gag reflex returns, usually 1–2 hours. **Rationale:** Aspiration can occur when gag reflex is absent.

for Colonoscopy

1. Follow steps in *Preparing for Endoscopic Studies* as it applies to this procedure.
2. Explain that procedure visualizes rectum, colon, and small bowel to detect pathologic conditions.
3. Place client on liquid diet and Dulcolax tabs 2 days before procedure, if ordered. May use just one day prep with Colyte.
4. Instruct client to drink electrolyte laxative solution (Golytely or Colyte) the day before procedure. Take according to directions, usually 8 ounces every 15 minutes until 1 gallon taken. Entire gallon should be taken in 4 hours. Solution should be chilled (more palatable) and swallowed quickly. **Rationale:** This osmotic solution works quickly and produces a clear colon in about 4 hours if directions are followed accurately. Watery diarrhea usually begins 30–60 minutes after first glass taken.
5. Explain side effects of nausea and fluid and electrolyte imbalance to client, especially elderly clients.
6. Instruct client to not take any routine or pm medications when drinking electrolyte solution. **Rationale:** The medications will not be digested.
7. Obtain baseline vital signs.
8. Start peripheral IV and medicate client with a narcotic analgesic (usually Versed) as ordered.
9. Take client to special procedure room.
10. Explain procedure to client.
    a. Position client on left side with legs drawn up.
    b. Scope is inserted through rectum and advanced through the sigmoid, descending, transverse, and ascending colon.
    c. Client may experience discomfort when air is instilled into colon to open colon and advance scope.
    d. Valium may be administered if client is anxious.
    e. Biopsy forceps or brush is inserted through scope to obtain specimens for study.
    f. Tissue or secretions obtained are placed in specimen container.
    g. Scope is removed, and rectal area cleaned and dried.
11. Instruct client in discharge teaching: to report any rectal bleeding, abdominal pain, distention, or purulent rectal drainage. **Rationale:** These symptoms indicate possible bowel perforation or hemorrhage.
    a. Instruct client to resume normal diet and force fluids after test.
    b. Instruct client that he or she may experience flatulence from air instillation.
12. Monitor vital signs as with any client. **Rationale:** Vital sign changes indicate complications, especially increased temperature and pulse and decreased blood pressure.

for Cystoscopy

1. Follow steps in *Preparing for Endoscopic Studies* as it applies to procedure.
2. Explain that cystoscopy is used to evaluate conditions associated with urinary tract: urethra, bladder, lower ureters. It is used for both diagnostic and therapeutic procedures.
3. Instruct in bowel prep, if ordered.
4. Keep client NPO if general anesthesia is given.
5. Administer preprocedural medications one hour before test.
6. Place client in lithotomy position. Provide covering to preserve modesty and prevent chilling.
7. Prepare external genitalia with antimicrobial swabs.
8. Explain procedure to client.
    a. Local anesthetic may be instilled into urethra before scope is inserted if under local anesthesia.
    b. Cystoscope is inserted through the urethra to inspect bladder and urethral wall and facilitate a biopsy.

c. Bladder is filled with sterile irrigating solution to assist in distending the bladder and irrigating bladder of clots. **Rationale:** Irrigation allows for better visualization of bladder.
d. Biopsy forcep may be passed through cystoscope to obtain tissue.
e. Bladder is emptied, and scope removed.

9. Provide post test instructions. Instruct client to:
   a. Observe closely for signs of septicemia (i.e., chills, fever, flushed feeling).
   b. Force fluids unless contraindicated.
   c. Monitor urine for persistent bright red color.
   d. Assess for severe pain (colicky pain is normal with urethral catheterization), continual burning, and frequency.
10. Monitor vital signs.
11. Palpate client for bladder distention and ensure client voids before discharge. **Rationale:** Urinary retention can be caused by edema from instrumentation.

for Gastrointestinal Tract Endoscopy

1. Follow steps in *Preparing for Endoscopic Studies* as it applies to this procedure.
2. Explain that this procedure is used to visualize upper GI tract by inserting flexible fiber-optic–lighted scope.
3. Keep NPO for 6–12 hours.
4. Remove dentures.
5. Explain procedure to client.
   a. Client taken to special procedure room.
   b. Client is awake during procedure, usually takes 20–30 minutes.
   c. Cardiac monitoring and pulse oximetry are done.
   d. Throat is anesthetized by swabbing with local anesthetic, usually Xylocaine. **Rationale:** To decrease gag reflex.
   e. Client is sedated with intravenous medication (usually Valium or Versed). Atropine may be administered to decrease secretions.
   f. Client is placed in left lateral recumbent position.
   g. Endoscope passed through esophagus to the duodenum. Can evaluate all structures as scope goes through the GI tract (termed EGD).
   h. Air is introduced through scope to distend upper GI tract. **Rationale:** To maximize visualization.
   i. Specimens may be taken and sent to lab.

EGD and ERCP

The esophagogastroduodenoscopy (EGD) can be used therapeutically for cautery and injection of sclerosing agents on bleeding varices.

Endoscopic retrograde cholangiopancreatography (ERCP) provides visualization of the bile and pancreatic ducts. Stones can be removed and stents placed in the bile ducts to drain bile.

6. Provide postprocedure care.
   a. Monitor vital signs as for surgical client.
   b. Check for signs and symptoms of bleeding or perforation. **Rationale:** Sharp, intense pain in stomach or chest and cool, pale skin indicate perforation.
   c. Check gag reflex. **Rationale:** May take 2–3 hours before gag reflex returns.
   d. Keep side rails up until effects of medications have subsided.
   e. Provide ice chips or throat lozenges for sore throat.

for Laparoscopy

1. Follow steps in Preparing for Endoscopic studies as it applies to this procedure.
2. Explain that scope is inserted through abdominal wall and into peritoneum to visualize abdominal and pelvic organs—used to assist in diagnosing pathologic conditions of pelvic and abdominal area.
3. Complete bowel prep as ordered.
4. Instruct in NPO status after midnight. Client receives general anesthesia.
5. Shave and prep abdomen as ordered.
6. Start a peripheral IV as ordered.
7. Have client void just before surgery. **Rationale:** To prevent accidental penetration of distended bladder during procedure.
8. Insert Foley catheter and NG tube before or after anesthesia administration, according to facility policy. **Rationale:** To prevent complications associated with penetration of distended stomach or bladder with needle placement.
9. Explain procedure to client.
   a. Client is placed in supine position on operating room table.
   b. Skin preparation is completed using antimicrobial swabs.
   c. Blunt-tipped needle is inserted through small incision in periumbilical area and into peritoneal cavity.
   d. Peritoneal cavity is filled with CO_2. **Rationale:** Separates abdominal wall from intra-abdominal viscera to allow better visualization of pelvic and abdominal structures.
   e. Scope is inserted through trocar and procedure completed.
   f. Scope is removed and CO_2 is allowed to escape.
   g. Incision is closed with butterfly tape, spray tape, or sutures and covered with transparent dressing.
10. Provide general postop care.
11. Instruct client in discharge teaching.
    a. Observe site for signs of infection, bleeding, increased pulse rate or fever. Notify physician immediately if these signs occur.
    b. Instruct client that he or she will have shoulder or subcostal discomfort for 24 hours. Medicate for pain as needed.

for Sigmoidoscopy

1. Follow steps in *Preparing for Endoscopic Studies.*
2. Explain that test allows for visualization of rectum and sigmoid colon.

3. Administer tap water or disposable (e.g., Fleets) enema as ordered the evening before the procedure. Clients with ulcerative colitis will not have enema ordered. Oral cathartic may also be given.
4. Allow clear, light breakfast on day of test.
5. Have client void before procedure.
6. Explain procedure to client.
   a. Client is placed on special table in special procedure room or in physician's examining room.
   b. Position in a knee–chest position if using examination table and rigid scope. Place on left side with right leg bent and placed over left leg if using flexible scope.
   c. Drape client to provide for modesty and warmth.
   d. Physician examines the rectum digitally first.
   e. Lubricated scope is advanced through anus into the rectum to visualize any abnormality of rectum, sigmoid colon, and large bowel.
   f. Client may feel pressure and need to have a bowel movement. Assure client this is usual feeling.
   g. Air may be introduced to increase visualization of bowel wall.
   h. Suction equipment passed through the scope may be used to remove secretions for better visualization of colon.
   i. Biopsy may be obtained by passing a snare through scope.
   j. Scope is removed, and client's rectal area is cleaned and dried.
   k. Gloves are applied if nurse is assisting with cleaning. Remove gloves and wash hands.
   l. Have client remain flat for 10–15 minutes before leaving room.
7. Instruct client in discharge teaching.
   a. Resume preexamination activities.
   b. Monitor stools for bleeding. Bloody stools are normal first 1–2 days after test.
   c. Instruct client to avoid enema or barium studies for at least 1 week.
   d. Observe for signs of increased abdominal distention, increased tenderness, or rectal bleeding.

DOCUMENTATION FOR ENDOSCOPIC STUDIES

- Test preparation completed
- Client teaching completed and client's ability to understand procedure evaluated
- Client's tolerance of procedure
- Preprocedure and postprocedure vital signs, if required
- Record type of specimen taken and sent to lab
- Specific postprocedure care given and client's response to treatment
- Specific signs and symptoms indicating potential complications

Critical Thinking Application

UNEXPECTED OUTCOMES	CRITICAL THINKING OPTIONS
Lower gastrointestinal tract not clear and sigmoidoscopy not completed.	• Repeat laxative and enemas per physician orders. • Observe results of enema; if solution not clear, notify physician.
Vertigo occurs while maintaining knee–chest position during sigmoidoscopy.	• Have client lie in supine position for few minutes. • Have client assume standing position slowly.
Upper gastrointestinal bleeding begins when scope inserted.	• Insert nasogastric tube, and apply suction. • Monitor vital signs for evidence of shock.
Potential colon perforation following endoscopic procedure.	• Assess for abdominal distention, tenderness, and pain. • Notify physician immediately. • Ensure client has a patent IV line, if not, insert peripheral line.
Potential infection following cystoscopy.	• Instruct client to force fluids to maintain constant flow of urine and prevent accumulation of bacteria in bladder. • Instruct client on signs and symptoms of sepsis; fever, flushing, chills, increased pulse rate, and feeling faint. Instruct client to notify physician immediately if any of these occur. • If client has been given prophylactic antibiotics, instruct in taking them as ordered. Do not stop taking the medication; take entire prescription.

UNIT 5

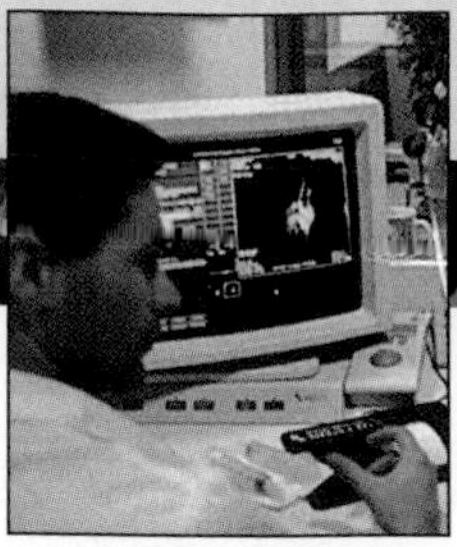

Fluid Analysis and Microscopic Studies

Nursing Process Data

ASSESSMENT *Data Base*

Assess vital signs prior to, during, and following the procedure.

Assess client's ability to maintain position necessary for procedure.

Assess client's knowledge of the procedure to be performed.

Review pertinent laboratory tests prior to procedure.

Evaluate signs and symptoms that indicate a potential problem could exist if test performed.

PLANNING *Objectives*

To provide reassurance for clients undergoing diagnostic tests

To position the client in a manner that facilitates the introduction of a needle through the skin surface to obtain a fluid or tissue sample

To obtain tissue or fluid to determine presence of infection or diseases

To obtain body fluids for specific disease analysis

To aspirate fluid to relieve pressure on body organs

IMPLEMENTATION *Procedures*

Assisting with Lumbar Puncture

Assisting with Liver Biopsy

Assisting with Thoracentesis

Assisting with Paracentesis

Assisting with Bone Marrow Aspiration

Assisting with Vaginal Examination and Papanicolaou (Pap) Smear

Assisting with Amniocentesis

EVALUATION *Expected Outcomes*

Client is prepared psychologically and physically for procedure.

Diagnostic tests performed with minimal discomfort.

Vital signs remain within normal range.

Specimens sent to lab in appropriate container and in a timely manner.

TABLE 21–5 Diagnostic Procedures

Diagnostic Test	Rationale
Lumbar Puncture	To obtain a cerebrospinal fluid specimen to determine presence of microorganisms, RBCs, or WBCs
Liver Biopsy	To obtain a specimen to determine presence of tumor or disease
Thoracentesis	To remove fluid from the thoracic cavity; to obtain a specimen cell study
Paracentesis	To remove fluid from the abdominal cavity; to obtain a specimen for cell study
Bone Marrow Aspiration	To study cells obtained from the specimen
Vaginal Examination and Papanicolaou Smear	To determine cell changes through a smear; to obtain a specimen for venereal disease identification
Amniocentesis	To remove amniotic fluid for studies of fetal maturity and genetic abnormalities

ASSISTING WITH LUMBAR PUNCTURE

Equipment

Diagnostic tray or equipment specific for procedure
Bath blanket
Sterile collection bottles or test tubes if indicated and not on tray
Sterile gloves
Xylocaine injection or EMLA cream if not on tray
Examining light
Clean gloves

Procedure

1. Explain that an LP is used for diagnosis of tumors, hemorrhage, infection, and autoimmune diseases involving CNS.
2. Explain procedure—a hollow core needle is placed in the subarachnoid space at L3–4 or L4–5 to facilitate measuring CSF pressure and obtaining fluid for testing.
3. Obtain consent.
4. Instruct client to empty bowel and bladder.
5. Wash your hands.
6. Obtain tray and any additional equipment needed, such as sterile gloves, bath blanket.

CLINICAL ALERT

This procedure is contraindicated in clients with increased intracranial pressure. A reduction in pressure may cause a herniation of the brain stem.

7. Position client in lateral recumbent position with back at the edge of the examining table. Cover with bath blanket, exposing only client's back.
8. Open sterile tray if requested by physician. Pour antiseptic solution into sterile medicine cup if needed.
9. Pull client's knees up to abdomen and flex chin on chest. **Rationale:** This position widens the space between the spinous processes of the lower lumbar vertebrae for ease of needle insertion.
10. Place pillows between knees. **Rationale:** This prevents upper legs from sliding off lower legs.
11. Assist client in relaxation exercises or instruct in deep, slow breathing through the mouth.
12. Use xylocaine or EMLA cream around site before needle insertion by physician.
13. Explain that he or she must remain still without movement during test.
14. Assist physician with the Queckenstedt's test when requested. After opening pressure is obtained, apply compression to neck veins with your fingers.
15. Don clean gloves and assist physician as directed.

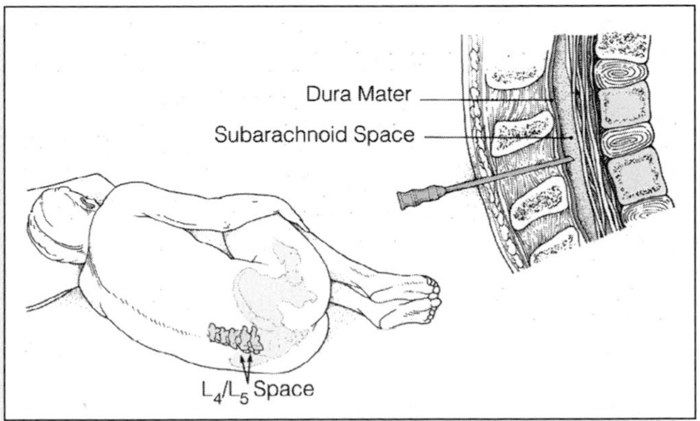

Place client in Sims' position to facilitate needle insertion for lumbar puncture.

16. Label cerebrospinal fluid samples with number on each specimen container.
17. After removal of needle, apply Band-Aid to puncture site.
18. Remove gloves and wash hands.
19. Fill out lab slips for appropriate test (i.e., cell count, serology).
20. Instruct client to lie flat for 4–24 hours, depending on hospital policy. Head is to remain flat and even with position of body. **Rationale:** To reduce CSF leakage.
21. Encourage fluids if not contraindicated by client's condition. **Rationale:** To reduce chance of headache.

CLINICAL ALERT

Queckenstedt's test is used to identify blockage of CSF flow in the spinal subarachnoid space. Generally when neck pressure is applied, there is a rapid rise in pressure level on the manometer with a return to normal within seconds when pressure is released.

22. Observe for spinal fluid leak from puncture site.
23. Check for headaches or alterations in neurologic status.

ASSISTING WITH LIVER BIOPSY

Equipment

Same as for *Assisting with Lumbar Puncture*

Preparation

1. Obtain lab values, such as prothrombin time, bleeding time, and platelet count if ordered.
2. Determine if a blood typing and crossmatching is needed.
3. Determine if client is to be NPO.
4. Explain that tissue will be removed after special needle is inserted into liver. Tissue will be studied to determine presence of disease.
5. Obtain consent.
6. Assess if client has any allergies to topical anesthetic agents.

Procedure

1. Wash your hands.
2. Take vital signs. **Rationale:** This provides baseline data to compare with postprocedure data.
3. Administer sedative as ordered.
4. Obtain tray and any additional equipment needed, such as sterile gloves, sandbag, bath blanket.

CLINICAL ALERT

A liver biopsy is contraindicated in clients with platelet counts below 50,000/mm or prolonged prothrombin time. Bleeding can occur following the procedure.

5. Place client in supine position at the right edge of the bed. Raise right arm and extend it over the left shoulder behind the head. If possible, turn head to left side. **Rationale:** This position provides maximal exposure of right intercostal space.

Note: Left lateral position can be used for biopsy.

6. Open sterile tray if requested by physician.
7. Local anesthesia is used around puncture site.
8. Instruct client to inhale and exhale deeply several times and then exhale and hold breath while physician inserts the biopsy needle. **Rationale:** Holding the breath prevents the needle from tearing the diaphragm or lacerating the liver as it descends during exhalation.

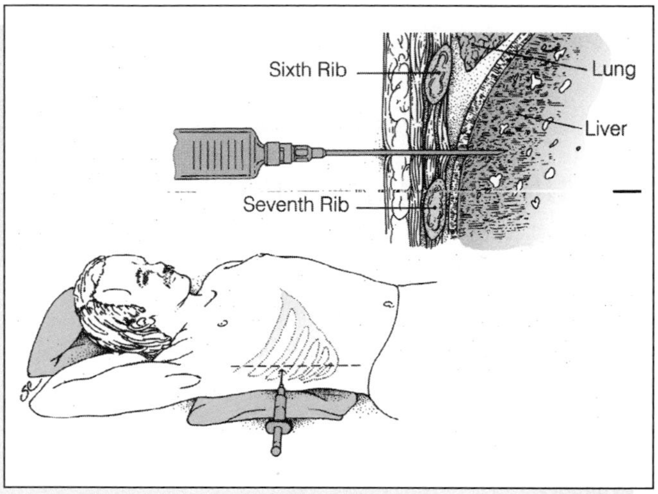

Instruct client to raise arm over head to facilitate needle insertion for liver biopsy.

9. Instruct the client to breathe normally after the physician removes the needle.
10. Don clean gloves and place Band-Aid over puncture site.
11. Position client on right side for 2–4 hours. A folded blanket may be placed under client's right side to provide hemostasis. **Rationale:** This position compresses the liver against the chest wall, thereby decreasing risk of hemorrhage.
12. Remove gloves and wash your hands.
13. Instruct client to remain on bed rest for 24 hours.
14. Assess for signs of hemorrhage at least every hour for 12 hours.
15. Monitor vital signs as you would for a surgical client (e.g., every 15 minutes for 1 hour).
16. Assess rate, rhythm, and depth of respirations.
17. Assess breath sounds and check for signs of dyspnea and restlessness. **Rationale:** Lung may be punctured during biopsy.
18. Send specimen to lab.

ASSISTING WITH THORACENTESIS

Equipment

Same as for *Assisting with Lumbar Puncture*

Preparation

1. Explain purpose of procedure to client.
2. Explain that needle is inserted into pleural space for removal of fluid for either diagnostic tests or to relieve pleural pressure.
3. Obtain consent.
4. Ensure chest x-ray film has been taken. **Rationale:** This film is used to compare with the film taken after the procedure.
5. Assess if client has any allergies to topical anesthetic agents.
6. Explain that movement or coughing must not be done during procedure; to prevent lung or pleural damage.

Procedure

1. Wash your hands.
2. Take vital signs, and complete a respiratory assessment. **Rationale:** This information provides postprocedure comparisons and early identification of potential complications.
3. Administer sedative as ordered.
4. Position client on edge of bed with arms crossed and resting on the overbed table. **Rationale:** This position provides good access to the intercostal spaces and facilitates fluid removal.

Note: Client can be placed in side-lying position on unaffected side if unable to sit up.

5. Provide adequate warmth and covering for client using bath blanket.
6. Place unwrapped sterile tray on bedside stand.
7. Open sterile gloves as indicated. Maintain sterile technique throughout procedure.
8. Assist physician as needed with skin prep.
9. Don clean gloves. Instruct client not to cough, take a deep breath, or move during placement of needle by the physician.
10. Following insertion of needle into pleural space observe client for pallor, dyspnea, tachycardia, chest pain, or vertigo. Report these findings immediately to the physician. **Rationale:** These symptoms occur with a pneumothorax.

Note: Blunt-tip, soft catheter-over-needle is used more often than a needle to prevent pneumothorax.

11. Apply pressure dressing (as determined by policy) after fluid and needle are removed. Remove gloves and wash hands.

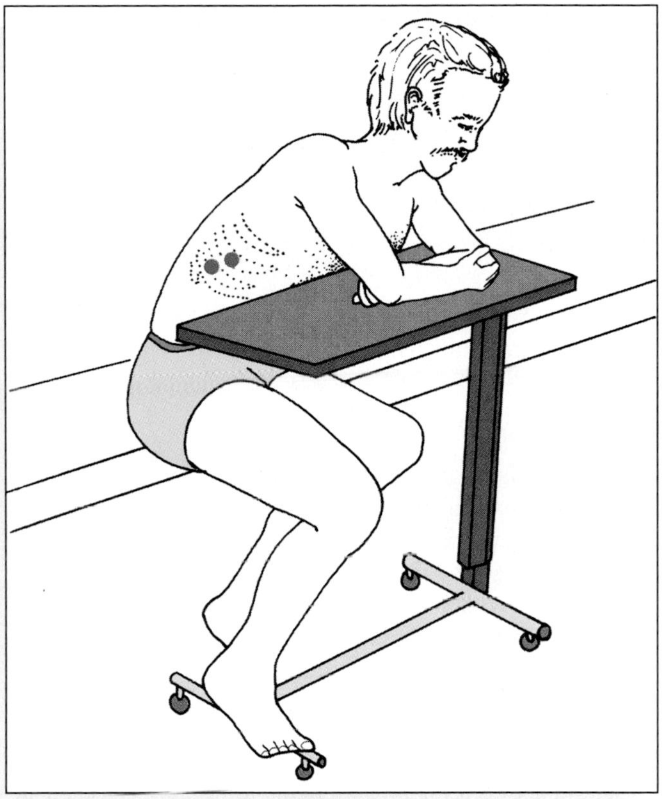

Place client in a leaning forward position to expose intercostal space for thoracentesis.

12. Observe client every 5 minutes for ½ hour for pulmonary edema (blood-tinged sputum), crepitus, cardiac distress (changes in respirations, pulse, or color), or a shift in the mediastinum.
13. Place client on unaffected side with head elevated 30° for at least 1 hour.
14. Monitor vital signs and breath sounds as with postoperative clients for 2 hours.
15. Observe dressing, change as needed. **Rationale:** Drainage is a common occurrence following a tap.
16. Obtain chest x-ray following procedure to check for pneumothorax.
17. Record color, amount, consistency, and samples of fluid obtained.
18. Complete lab slips, and send specimen to lab.

ASSISTING WITH PARACENTESIS

Equipment

Same as for *Assisting with Lumbar Puncture*
- Chair
- Drape
- Sterile tray
- Sterile gloves
- Bucket

Dressing—elastic adhesive patch
Blood pressure equipment
Clean gloves

Preparation

1. Explain purpose of procedure to client.
2. Explain that needle is inserted into peritoneal cavity and fluid removed for fluid analysis or to remove fluid from cavity to promote comfort and increase respiratory status.
3. Obtain consent.
4. Assess if client has any allergies to topical anesthetic agents.
5. Assess if client has coagulation abnormalities or bleeding tendencies. Procedure is contraindicated in these clients.
6. Wash your hands.
7. Assess client's abdominal girth and bowel sounds. **Rationale:** This information provides postprocedure comparisons and early identification of potential complications.
8. Weigh client. **Rationale:** This information can be used to assess fluid loss following the procedure.
9. Have client empty bladder. **Rationale:** This prevents accidental puncture of the bladder during the procedure.

Procedure

1. Place client in Fowler's position on chair or on edge of bed with legs spread apart.
2. Drape client, and provide adequate warmth and covering with a bath blanket.
3. Obtain vital signs, and observe client for pallor and vertigo during procedure. **Rationale:** These symptoms are indicative of shock.
4. Position and open tray on over-bed table.
5. Open sterile gloves if needed.
6. Assist physician in preparing skin with antiseptic solution and topical anesthesia or as needed.
7. Don clean gloves.
8. Physician inserts trocar needle, or cannula through small incision. Plastic tubing is attached to cannula to facilitate fluid removal.
9. Observe total amount of fluid aspirated. Usually no more than 1000 mL is removed at one time. **Rationale:** Removing larger amounts of fluid can lead to hypotension and hyponatremia.
10. Apply pressure dressing following removal of needle. **Rationale:** This prevents bleeding from puncture site.
11. Remove gloves, and place in appropriate receptacle.
12. Wash your hands.
13. Return client to bed and place in semi- to high-Fowler's position. **Rationale:** These positions usually are most comfortable for client and promote lung expansion.
14. Observe for leakage at puncture site or scrotal edema in male client.
15. Monitor vital signs and observe closely for signs of hypotension. Monitor urine output and color, and dressing every 15 minutes for at least 2 hours; every hour for 4 hours; every 4 hours for 24 hours.
16. Assess bowel sounds, and measure abdominal girth. **Rationale:** To monitor for signs of perforated bowel or peritonitis.
17. Weigh client when vital signs are stable. **Rationale:** This prevents hypotension.
18. Reinforce or change dressings as needed.
19. Monitor serum protein and electrolytes, particularly sodium. **Rationale:** Fluid contains high levels of protein that is removed with this procedure.
20. Record color, amount, consistency, and samples obtained from paracentesis, and send to laboratory.

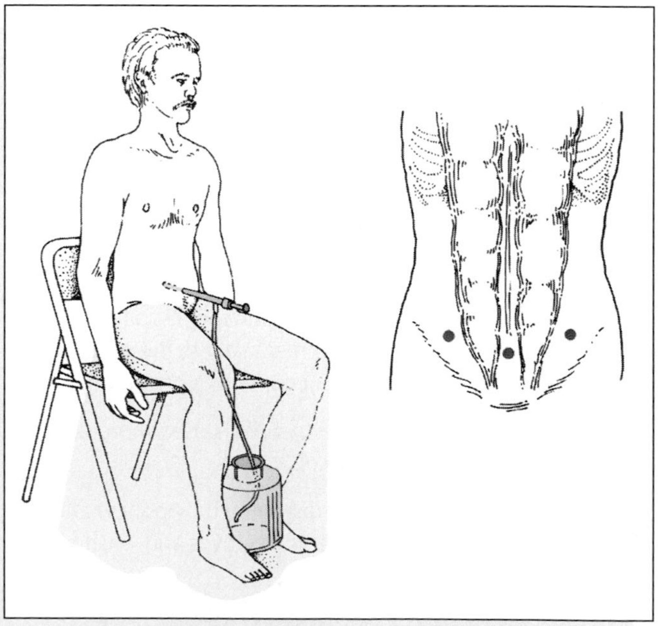

Position client in chair to facilitate trocar insertion and drainage for paracentesis.

ASSISTING WITH BONE MARROW ASPIRATION

Equipment

Same as for *Assisting with Lumbar Puncture*
2 slides
Preservative spray

Procedure

1. Explain purpose of procedure.
2. Explain procedure.
3. Explain that client will experience discomfort or pressure when needle is inserted.
4. Obtain consent.
5. Obtain tray and provide any additional equipment needed, such as specimen container or gloves.
6. Assess coagulation studies and report unusual findings to physician.
7. Premedicate with prescribed drugs.
8. Position client in supine position if sternum or anterior iliac crest is the biopsy site, or prone if posterior iliac crest is the biopsy site. Place a sandbag under iliac crest area if physician requires.
9. Open tray on over-bed table.
10. Assist physician as needed.

Note: A large-bore needle containing a stylus is inserted into bone. Stylus is removed and ½ to 2 mL bone marrow removed as specimen, spread on slides, and sprayed with preservative.

11. Don sterile gloves.
12. Apply direct pressure for 5–15 minutes following removal of needle. **Rationale:** To prevent bleeding.
13. Cover puncture site with sterile pressure dressing. Ice pack may be applied to help control bleeding:
14. Remove gloves and wash hands.
15. Monitor vital signs, and observe puncture site for drainage, edema, or pain, as with surgical client. **Rationale:** To monitor for signs of infection. Call physician for temperature above 101°F.
16. Position the client for comfort.
17. Properly label specimens, and send to laboratory.
18. Evaluate client for signs of shock or infection.

ASSISTING WITH VAGINAL EXAMINATION AND PAPANICOLAOU (PAP) SMEAR

Equipment

Two slides
Cytology container
Fixative agent
Vaginal speculum, several sizes
Gloves
Water-soluble lubricant jelly
Examining light

Preparation

1. Explain purpose of procedure.
2. Explain that test is performed to detect neoplastic cells in cervical and vaginal secretions.
3. Instruct client not to douche for 18–72 hours before exam.
4. Instruct client that test should be done 2 weeks after start of last menses.

Procedure

1. Instruct client to empty bladder.
2. Assist client to examination room.
3. Instruct client to remove clothing below the waist, including underwear, and don gown.
4. Position client on examining table in lithotomy position using stirrups.
5. Provide adequate coverings to preserve modesty and prevent chilling.
6. Open speculum package, gloves, and lubricant. Place on tray. Place cytology slides and container on tray.
7. Label two slides with client's name and area from where specimen is obtained.
8. Position light for good exposure.
9. Stay with client if she is a child or physician is a male.
10. Assist physician as needed.
11. Place slides in cytology container, and send to the lab. Complete all cytology forms. Client's medical history and reason for examination is written on request form.
12. Assist client in perineal care.
13. Assist client to dress if necessary.

ASSISTING WITH AMNIOCENTESIS

Procedure

1. Explain purpose for procedure to client. *Note: Test is to withdraw fluid for analysis to check fetal maturity status, sex of fetus, genetic or chromosomal abnormalities, hereditary metabolic disorders, anatomical abnormalities or fetal distress.*
2. Obtain consent, both mother and father.
3. Have client void prior to test. **Rationale:** This prevents injury to the bladder.
4. Transport client to treatment room.
5. Instruct client to lie quietly in supine position for 30 minutes.
6. Obtain fetal heart tones, and mothers blood pressure.
7. Open amniocentesis tray and gloves. Place Xylocaine nearby if not included on tray. **Rationale:** Procedure is performed under sterile conditions to prevent infection.
8. Explain details of procedure to client.
   a. Physician prepares abdomen with povidone–iodine (Betadine) or alcohol.
   b. Xylocaine injection provides local anesthesia for needle insertion area.
   c. Needle is inserted, and amniotic fluid is withdrawn.
   d. Amniotic fluid is placed in light resistant specimen container and labeled with client's name. Appropriate lab slips are completed. **Rationale:** To prevent breakdown of bilirubin.
   e. Procedure takes about 10 minutes.
9. Don sterile gloves and place small dressing or Band-Aid over needle site.
10. Remove gloves and wash hands.
11. Monitor fetal heart tones, and observe for signs of labor.
12. Instruct client to notify physician of any unusual occurrences, signs of labor, or signs of infection.
13. Give RhoGam if woman is Rh-negative. **Rationale:** There is a risk of immunization against fetal blood (hemolytic disease).

DOCUMENTATION FOR FLUID ANALYSIS AND MICROSCOPIC STUDIES

- Preparation completed for test
- Client teaching completed and client's ability to understand procedure evaluated
- Consent form signed
- Client's tolerance of procedure
- Fluid or specimens sent to laboratory for analysis
- Preprocedure and postprocedure vital signs if required
- Record color and amount of fluid withdrawn from paracentesis, thoracentesis, or lumbar puncture
- Type of dressing applied
- Specific position assumed after procedure as indicated
- Abnormal findings following procedure indicating potential complications

Critical Thinking Application

UNEXPECTED OUTCOMES	CRITICAL THINKING OPTIONS
Client has spinal fluid leak following lumbar puncture.	• Keep client in supine position. • Notify physician. • Keep sterile dressing over puncture site. Do not allow dressing to become wet. • If leak persists, physician may place client in Trendelenburg's position to prevent headache. This position is contraindicated in clients with increased intracranial pressure or following a craniotomy.
Client complains of shortness of breath or expectorates blood-tinged sputum following a thoracentesis.	• Place client in Fowler's position. • Assess vital signs. • Administer oxygen. • Monitor breath sounds. • Notify physician and check on order for chest x-ray. • Have chest tube insertion tray available. • Allay client's fears, and provide emotional support.
Urine output is blood-tinged following paracentesis or amniocentesis.	• Notify physician at once; bladder may have been punctured during procedure. • Monitor vital signs for shock. • Maintain client on bed rest. • Observe for urine output.

Gerontologic Considerations

Elderly clients requiring diagnostic tests are at risk for the following problems:

- Dehydration can result from fluid restriction, use of contrast agents for the tests, and bowel preparation using enemas. Osmolar imbalances and hypovolemia can result from the dehydration.
- Extracellular fluid volume excess can occur if large volumes of fluid are required for the test. Renal studies, which usually require the use of large volumes of fluid, should not be considered if the client is at risk for circulatory overload. Elderly clients may have a compromised cardiorespiratory status. A secondary choice of tests may need to be considered such as a CT scan.
- Renal dysfunction resulting from multiple tests using contrast agents should be avoided. Acute renal failure can result from multiple tests with contrast agents in elderly clients who already have a compromised renal system. Spacing tests over time helps prevent this problem.

Nursing responsibilities for elderly clients requiring diagnostic tests should include the following:

- Carefully monitor fluid and electrolyte balance.
- Adequately hydrate client prior to and following tests unless contraindicated.
- Monitor laboratory tests, such as electrolytes and osmolarity.
- Monitor intake and output frequently.
- Monitor vital signs.
- Weigh clients who are at risk for fluid volume disturbances.
- Complete physical assessment, including mental status, each shift, and report unusual findings to physician.

MANAGEMENT GUIDELINES

Each state legislates a Nurse Practice Act for RNs and LVN/LPNs. Health care facilities are responsible for establishing and implementing policies and procedures that conform to their state's regulations. Verify the regulations and role parameters for each health care worker in your facility.

Delegation of Responsibilities

- LVNs/LPNs and RNs may both be assigned to care for clients undergoing diagnostic tests. Nurses are frequently working in X-ray and Diagnostic Procedure Laboratories today and assisting physicians with invasive procedures. Technicians are also educated to work in areas such as cardiac catheterization labs. These technicians are not nursing personnel. In most cases, radiologic technologists assist with the various procedures within the X-ray and Diagnostic Procedure Labs.
- When invasive procedures such as liver biopsy and paracentesis are performed on the nursing unit, either an LVN/LPN or RN is assigned to assist the physician.
- Preprocedure and postprocedure interventions are assigned to the LVN/LPN or RN for direct responsibility. A CNA may assist the nurse by taking vital signs.
- Only RNs can transport clients who have received conscious sedation for a procedure.

Information Flow

- All staff members must be aware of clients undergoing diagnostic tests. This information is disseminated through shift and team reports. It is also written on the Kardex card or is on the client's information sheet on the computer. If premedication is required, this information is found on the Medication Administration Record as well. If the client is NPO for the test, a sign must be placed in the client's room indicating this status.
- Specific directions must be given to the staff member assigned to the client to inform them of their client care responsibilities both pre- and postprocedure.
- The RN must assess the knowledge base of the staff member assigned to assist the physician with any procedure being performed on the unit. This is to ensure safety for the client.
- The RN collaborates with the physician to identify any specific equipment or needs he or she may have for the procedure being performed on the unit.

CRITICAL THINKING STRATEGIES

SCENARIO 1

Mr. Michael Spicer, a 72-year-old retired fireman, is scheduled for the following diagnostic procedures as an outpatient. He has started his testing with a barium enema. You have been asked to call him and instruct him about the procedures.

Diagnostic Tests to be Completed

- IV pyelography
- Bone scan
- Sigmoidoscopy

1. What is the priority question you should ask? Provide rationale for your answer.
2. When beginning the discussion about the IVP, what is your priority question? Provide rationale for your answer.
3. Identify the most important postprocedure client education regarding the IVP. Provide rationale for your answer.
4. The client asks you if he will be radioactive and a risk to his family following the bone scan. What is your best response?
5. Briefly explain the preprocedure prep for the sigmoidoscopy.

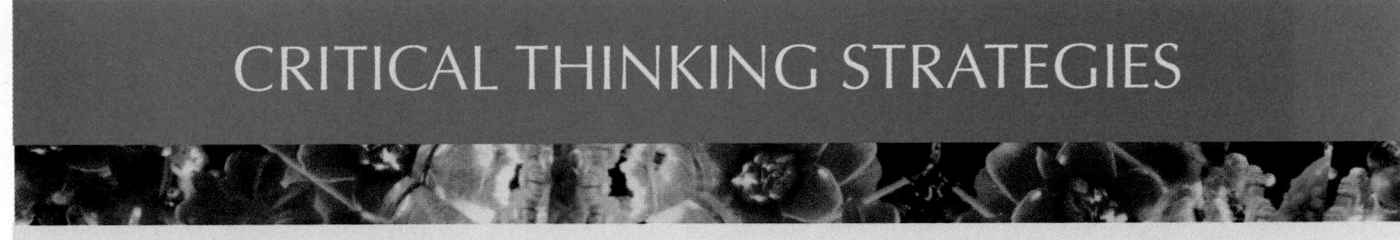

CHAPTER 22

Urinary Elimination

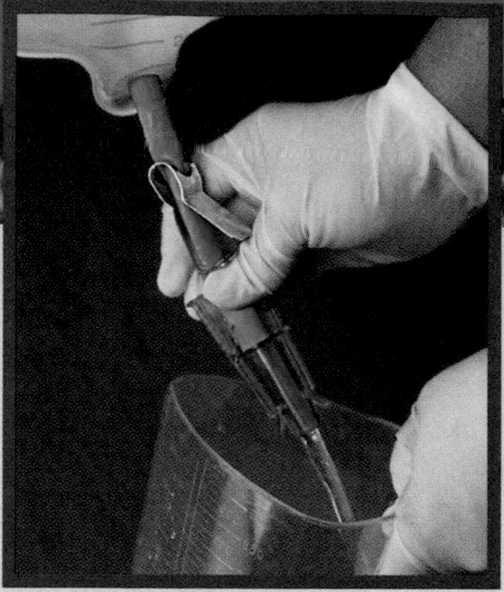

THEORETICAL CONCEPTS

UNIT ONE: **Intake and Output** **704**
- Measuring Intake and Output 705

UNIT TWO: **External Catheter System** **708**
- Applying a Condom Catheter 709
- Attaching Catheter to Leg Bag 709

UNIT THREE: **Catheterization** **712**
- Draping a Female Client 713
- Using a Bladder Scanner 713
- Inserting a Straight Catheter (Female) 714
- Inserting a Straight Catheter (Male) 716
- Inserting a Retention Catheter (Female) 717
- Inserting a Retention Catheter (Male) 721
- Providing Catheter Care 722
- Removing a Retention Catheter 723

UNIT FOUR: **Bladder Irrigation** **726**
- Irrigating by Opening a Closed System 727
- Irrigating a Closed System 728
- Maintaining Continuous Bladder Irrigation 729

UNIT FIVE: **Suprapubic Catheter Care** **732**
- Providing Suprapubic Catheter Care 733

UNIT SIX: **Specimens from Closed Systems** **735**
- Collecting Specimen from a Closed System 736

UNIT SEVEN: **Urinary Diversion** **738**
- Applying a Urinary Diversion Pouch 739
- Obtaining Specimen from an Ileal Conduit 742
- Catheterizing Continent Urinary Reservoir 742

UNIT EIGHT: **Hemodialysis (Renal Replacement Therapy)** **745**
- Providing Hemodialysis 746
- Ongoing Care of Hemodialysis Client 748
- Terminating Hemodialysis 748
- Maintaining Central Venous Dual-Lumen Catheter (DLC) 749

GERONTOLOGIC CONSIDERATIONS 752

MANAGEMENT GUIDELINES 752

CRITICAL THINKING STRATEGIES 754

Cross reference: Urine Studies in Chapter 20
Peritoneal Dialysis (CAPD) in Chapter 34
Self-Catheterization (Male and Female) in Chapter 34
Suprapubic Catheter Care at Home in Chapter 34.

LEARNING OBJECTIVES

- Describe the process of urine production.
- List four alterations that result in urinary elimination problems.
- State two nursing diagnoses that relate to urine elimination.
- Complete an intake and output bedside record.
- Compare and contrast the steps for inserting a straight catheter in a male and female client.
- Describe the major parameters needed to preserve a sterile environment when inserting a catheter.
- Demonstrate the clamping protocol used for clients with suprapubic catheters.
- Explain how a catheter is attached to a leg bag.
- Identify the most important advantages of a suprapubic catheter.
- List the major steps of irrigating by opening a closed urinary system.
- Outline the steps necessary to obtain a urine specimen from a closed urinary drainage system.
- Outline the steps for applying a urinary diversion pouch.
- Describe rationale for renal replacement therapy.
- List safety precautions for maintaining a fistula or graft for vascular access for hemodialysis.

TERMINOLOGY

Albuminuria: the presence of albumin in the urine.

Anemia: a condition in which the number of circulating red blood cells, or hemoglobin, is reduced.

Antibiotic: a substance that inhibits or destroys other organisms, especially bacteria.

Antidiuretic: Pituitary hormone that causes water reabsorption by the distal tubule of the nephron.

Anuria: a total suppression or lack of production of urine (less than 100 mL/day).

Arteriovenous: extracorporeal circuit created with arterial to venous blood flow. The client's blood pressure forces blood through a hemofilter and back to a venous return access.

A-V fistula: anastomosis of a vein with an artery as an access site for hemodialysis.

Azotemia: increased levels of BUN and creatinine in the blood.

Bactericidal: able to destroy bacteria.

Calyx: any cuplike division of the kidney pelvis.

CAPD: continuous ambulatory peritoneal dialysis.

Catheterization: a sterile tube insertion for the injection of or removal of fluids from a vessel or body cavity.

CCPD: continuous-cycle peritoneal dialysis.

CVVH: continuous venovenous hemofiltration.

Dehydration: the process of losing water as in depriving the body tissues of water.

Dialyzer: artificial kidney.

Distention: stretching out or inflating of an organ such as the bladder.

Diuresis: the excessive production of urine.

Dorsal: pertaining to the back.

Dysuria: difficult or painful urination.

Edema: a condition in which body tissues contain an excessive amount of fluid.

Electrolyte: composed of acids, bases, and salts; a compound that develops an electrical charge when dissolved in water.

End-stage renal disease: the loss of 80% of kidney nephrons resulting in accumulation of nitrogenous wastes in the blood and uremia.

Excoriation: a breakdown of the epidermis.

Foley catheter: a type of indwelling tube that is inserted through the urethra into the bladder to provide continuous urinary drainage.

Genitourinary: pertaining to the genital and urinary systems.

Hemodialysis: provides an artificial kidney function through use of a shunt pumping blood to a machine for blood purification.

Hydrostatic pressure: pumping force created by the mean arterial blood pressure, or a pump.

Incontinence: inability to retain urine.

Indwelling urethral catheter: a retention, or Foley, catheter.

Infection: condition in which the body or a part is invaded by a pathogenic agent.

Irrigation: the flushing of a tube, canal, or area with solution.

Malpighian corpuscle: a spheric body consisting of a glomerulus and Bowman's capsule found in the cortex of a kidney.

Micturition: the process of emptying the urinary bladder; voiding.

Nocturia: excessive urination during the night.

Oliguria: diminished production of urine (<400 mL/day).

Patency: the state of being freely open.

Peri: prefix meaning around or about.

Peristalsis: a progressive wavelike movement that occurs involuntarily in hollow tubes in the body, especially the alimentary tract.

Polyuria: the excessive production and elimination of urine (output > 2 liters/day).

Pyuria: the presence of pus in the urine.

Renal: pertaining to the kidney.

Sediment: a substance settling at the bottom of a liquid.

Septic: pertinent to pathogens or their toxins.

Septicemia: presence of pathogens in the blood.

Shock: a state of inadequate tissue perfusion.

Specific gravity: weight of a substance compared with an equal volume of water. Water is 1.000.

Stoma: surgically created opening.

Ultrafiltrate: fluid collection from the blood which is isotonic and devoid of red blood cells or protein.

Urethra: a canal for the discharge of urine from the bladder to the outside.

Urinary diversion: an alternate route for urine elimination.

Urinary tract infection (UTI): an infection of the urinary tract, including all or part of the organs and ducts.

Venovenous: extracorporeal circuit created using a dual-lumen hemodilaysis catheter inserted into a central vein. Blood flow through the dialysis circuit is pump controlled.

URINARY SYSTEM

The primary structures of the urinary system are the kidneys, ureters, bladder, and urethra. Each kidney produces urine, which is carried to the bladder by a ureter that is about 25 cm (10 inches) long and 0.6 cm in diameter. Peristaltic waves, pressure, and gravity propel urine through the ureters so that it can be discharged into the bladder.

The bladder serves as a reservoir for urine until voiding takes place. When micturition, or urination, occurs, urine passes through two sphincters and is transported from the bladder to the external environment through the urethra. The kidneys are essential to life, but the collection system is not.

The anatomic position of the bladder and the structure of the urethra differ in males and females. The bladder is posterior to the symphysis pubis. In a female the bladder is anterior to the vagina and the neck of the uterus. In a male the bladder is anterior to the rectum. The urethra of the female is about 4 cm (1.5 inches) long, and the male urethra is 20 cm (8 inches) long.

The urethra, bladder, ureters, and kidney pelves are lined with a continuous layer of mucous membrane. Because there is continuity of the lining, bacteria introduced into the normally sterile system can spread throughout the tract. When the bladder is empty, the lining falls into folds that provide pockets where bacteria can multiply. Since the membrane is highly vascular, bacteria can easily enter the bloodstream and septicemia can result.

Urine Production

Nephrons, the functional units of the kidneys, produce urine. Each nephron consists of a renal corpuscle and a renal tubule, which is surrounded by a capillary bed. Each kidney has approximately a million nephrons.

Urine formed in the renal tubule enters a collecting duct. The collecting ducts from a number of nephrons attach to a single, larger collecting duct, which empties urine into the kidney calyx. The urine collects in the renal pelvis until enough accumulates to flow to the bladder. If movement of urine from the pelvis is interrupted, infection, hydronephrosis, or formation of calculi may occur.

Blood is circulated to kidneys by way of the renal artery. This artery branches into arterioles, which supply a capillary tuft (glomerulus) filter. Under the influence of blood pressure, plasma is forced through the glomerulus and enters renal tubules. Filtered blood then passes from the glomerulus through an efferent arteriole and finally a capillary system that surrounds the renal tubules (peritubular capillaries). Kidneys filter approximately 140 liters of blood each day, but only 1500 mL of urine is produced. As blood pressure falls, urine production decreases.

The plasma that is filtered into the renal tubule contains water, glucose, electrolytes, and nitrogenous wastes. This "filtrate" is then modified as it moves through the tubular system. Substances such as medications are secreted from the peritubular capillaries and into the filtrate for elimination. Most of the plasma fluid is reabsorbed into the bloodstream by way of peritubular capillaries, and excess fluid is removed along with acid waste products (urea, creatinine, hydrogen ion) in the form of urine. Through this process, kidneys maintain fluid and electrolyte and acid–base balance. In addition to urine production, kidneys play an important role in maintenance of blood pressure by secreting renin, activation of vitamin D to facilitate calcium absorption, and stimulation of red blood cell production by erythropoietin. It is easy to appreciate that loss of kidney function has a profound and widespread effect on homeostasis since it influences elimination of waste products, bone metabolism, blood pressure, tissue oxygenation (RBC production), acid–base balance, and fluid and electrolyte balance.

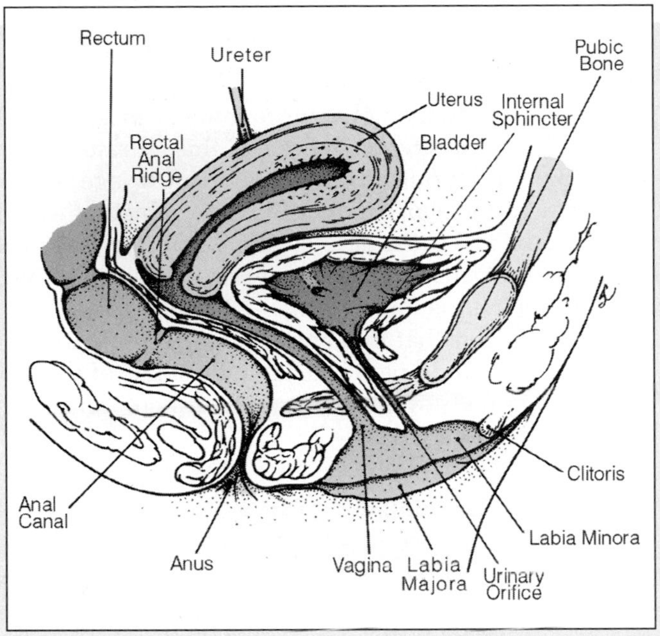

Female genitourinary system.

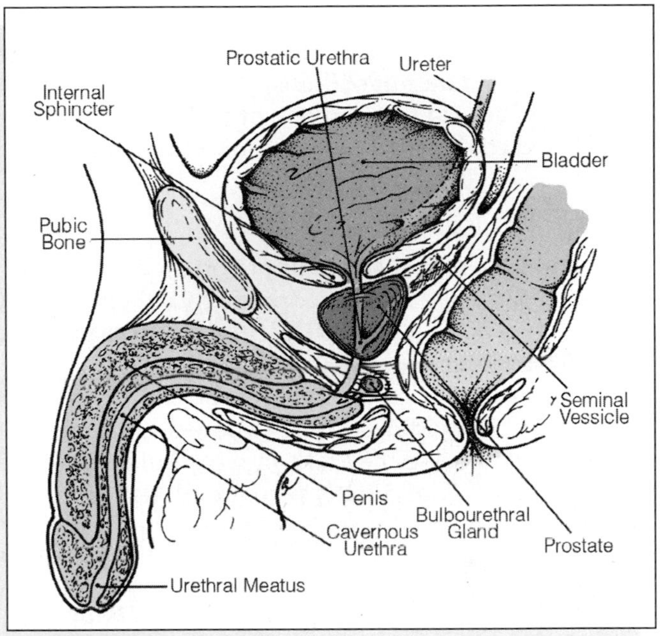

Male genitourinary system.

Micturition

Micturition (urination) is a voluntary response to pressure changes within the bladder. When urine begins to collect, the muscular walls of the bladder are relaxed, with little change in pressure. After about 300 mL of urine accumulates, the bladder walls tighten, and pressure increases. This rising pressure stimulates receptors in the bladder wall, which send impulses to the spinal cord. After 400–500 mL of urine is collected, the bladder walls contract and the internal sphincter relaxes, causing a sense of urgency to void. When urine enters the urethra, the external sphincter relaxes and voiding occurs.

Micturition can occur sooner if the tone of the bladder is increased because of such factors as emotional stress or infection. Micturition can be delayed by voluntary contraction of the external sphincter or practicing pelvic floor exercises. Once the volume of urine reaches about 700 mL, however, most individuals lose their ability to delay micturition.

If an individual is unable to void, as much as 1000 mL of urine can accumulate in the bladder. When a large volume of urine is retained, the bladder's lining and blood vessels can be damaged by the increased stretching and pressure. When this happens, an individual experiences pain, restlessness, chilling, flushing, headache, diaphoresis, and a rise in blood pressure.

TABLE 22–1 Tubular Alterations of Filtrate

Proximal tubule and descending limb	Obligatory water reabsorption, which accounts for about 80% of the absorption of water, occurs in the proximal tube and descending limb. Glucose, amino acids, vitamins, and sodium are actively reabsorbed. Chloride, sulfate, phosphate ions, and urea are passively reabsorbed. Bicarbonate is actively reabsorbed in relation to systemic pH. Water is reabsorbed with these substances, leaving the filtrate osmotic pressure unchanged.
Loop of Henle	Sodium is actively transported from the filtrate in the ascending limb into the medullary interstitial fluid, thus raising its osmotic pressure. This rising pressure causes more water to be reabsorbed from the descending limb and the collecting duct and results in the concentration of the urine.
Distal tubule and collecting ducts	Facultative or optional reabsorption of water, which accounts for about 10%–15% of the absorption of water, occurs in the distal tubule and collecting ducts. Sodium is actively reabsorbed in exchange for secreted potassium or hydrogen. As water continues to be reabsorbed, the filtrate becomes more concentrated and its volume is greatly reduced.

ALTERATIONS IN URINARY ELIMINATION

Alterations in urinary elimination can result from changes in the intake and output of fluids, obstructions to the flow of urine, changes in the secretion of antidiuretic hormone (ADH), and changes in blood volume or blood pressure.

Alterations Related to Fluids

The average person takes in approximately 2600 mL of fluid each day: 1200 mL from drinking, 1100 mL from the water content of food, and 300 mL from changes in metabolism. An increase or decrease in fluid intake results in a parallel increase or decrease in urine output.

Healthy individuals rarely experience decreases in urine output because they take in more fluids whenever they are thirsty. Individuals who are ill, however, may experience decreases in urine output because they are unable to respond to the thirst response, their intake is limited due to testing that requires NPO preparations, or their IV fluid intake is insufficient to balance fluid losses.

Fluid is lost from the body not only from urine, but also through respiration, perspiration, and feces. On a daily basis, most individuals lose approximately 2400 mL of fluid: 1500 mL through urine output, 200 mL through respiration, 600 mL through perspiration, and 100 mL through the elimination of feces. Individuals who are ill may also lose fluids through vomiting, bleeding, wound drainage, and suctioning/decompression.

Alterations Related to Obstructions

A decrease in the output of urine may also be caused by an obstruction (tumor, clot, tissue hypertrophy) to the flow of urine from the bladder. If the obstruction is large enough, the bladder does not empty completely. Instead, it retains fluid and, over time, becomes distended. Individuals who have obstructions in the urinary tract experience the need to void more frequently. When they do void, however, they eliminate only very small amounts of urine.

Alterations Related to Aldosterone and Antidiuretic Hormone

Changes in the secretion of ADH and aldosterone also alter urine output since these hormones control the amount of water that is reabsorbed in the distal renal tubules and collecting ducts. Common factors that increase the secretion of ADH and aldosterone and reduce urine output include emotional stress, accidental or surgical trauma, pain, hemorrhage, decreased cardiac output, anesthesia, and drugs, such as morphine and barbiturates. Factors that reduce the secretion of ADH and thus increase urine output include alcohol, caffeine, cold, and disease states and medications such as diuretics

Alterations Related to Changes in Blood Volume

Because the production of urine is influenced by the volume of blood filtrate, decreases in this filtrate lead to reductions in the output of urine. Hemorrhage, severe dehydration, and shock reduce the flow of blood through the glomeruli and cause decreases in the filtrate. If the volume of the filtrate is reduced substantially, severe oliguria, or even anuria, may occur.

Other factors that may increase or decrease the output of urine include pathophysiologic states of the kidneys or other body systems, drugs, treatment modalities, diet, and metabolic rate.

Alterations in Disease States

Urinary diversion is required when the bladder is obstructed or has been removed due to disease or trauma. Diversion can be created anywhere along the urinary pathway, and is named for the structure involved in the diversion. The most common urinary diversion is the ileal conduit, named because it uses the ileum of the bowel to form the conduit. A segment of the ileum close to the ileocecal valve is resected with its mesentery intact to create the conduit. The proximal end of this segment is closed and the distal segment is brought out through the lower quadrant of the abdominal wall to form the stoma. The ureters are anastomosed to the ileal segment at the proximal end or side of the conduit.

This type of diversion is an incontinent urinary diversion. Another example of an incontinent urinary diversion is a ureterostomy, which diverts urine directly through a ureteral stoma on the abdomen. Clients with incontinent diversions must wear an appliance for urine collection.

Ileal *reservoirs* are continent diversions that do not require the use of a collection device. The ileal pouch is created with valves that allow it to function as a "bladder," which is regularly emptied by client self-catheterization through the abdominal stoma.

TABLE 22–2 Urine Exam: What To Look For
Urine color
Clarity and odor
Urine pH
Urine specific gravity
Protein, glucose, and ketone bodies
Urine sediment: red and white blood cells, casts, crystals, and bacteria

The "neo bladder" is created by connecting the ureters to a segment of ileum that is connected to the urethra. The client has no stoma; therefore, no collection device is required. The "bladder" is emptied by timed voiding or urethral self-catheterization.

Alterations Related to End-Stage Renal Disease

Loss of nephron function is irreversible in chronic renal disease. The glomerular filtration rate slows, and the functioning nephrons cannot eliminate creatinine, urea, and nitrogen in sufficient amounts to maintain homeostasis. The client proceeds through three phases, reduced renal reserve, renal insufficiency, and then the final phase, end-stage renal disease. During the first phase, the client is usually asymptomatic with intact excretory and regulatory renal functions, even though there is a 40% to 75% loss of nephrons. In the second phase the client becomes "azotemic" (the BUN and serum creatinine levels rise), as 80% of the nephron function is lost. Reabsorption of electrolytes by the renal tubules decreases and the kidneys lose their ability to concentrate urine. In the final stage, 10% of normal kidney function remains. Excretory, regulatory, and hormonal renal functions are impaired and the kidneys are no longer able to maintain homeostasis. Usually during the later segment of the second stage of renal failure, the client and family determine the most appropriate long-term treatment for the client. Renal replacement therapies include hemodialysis; continuous ambulatory peritoneal dialysis (CAPD); continuous-cycle peritoneal dialysis (CCPD); or renal transplant.

NURSING INTERVENTIONS

The primary purpose for performing nursing interventions associated with urinary elimination is to maintain the integrity of the urinary system, which allows the body to eliminate excess fluid and wastes, and thereby promote homeostasis.

Aseptic technique is essential whenever performing procedures that could introduce bacteria into the urinary tract. Handwashing, using sterile gloves, and maintaining a closed urinary collection system decrease the incidence of ascending bladder contamination and subsequent urinary tract infection. Securing catheters to the skin minimizes to-and-fro motion, thus reducing infections of the urinary tract. Maintaining aseptic technique throughout dialysis procedures is necessary to prevent infection in grafts, fistulae, and catheters.

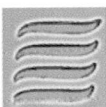

NURSING DIAGNOSES

The following nursing diagnoses may be appropriate to use on client care plans when the components are related to promoting urine elimination.

NURSING DIAGNOSIS	RELATED FACTORS
Impaired Urinary Elimination	Incontinence, lack of muscle tone, urinary tract infection, motor or sensory impairment, abdominal surgery
Body Image Disturbance	Alteration in body appearance, urinary diversion stoma, use of appliance, catheter presence
Fluid Volume Excess	Decreased urine output, renal system dysfunction, decreased cardiac output
Ineffective Individual Coping	Poor adjustment to illness or treatment, chronic disease state
Noncompliance	Inadequate knowledge base, denial of health status, cultural or spiritual beliefs
Urinary Retention	Inability to void, bladder distention or atony, surgical repair
Incontinence (stress, reflex urge, punctional, total)	Inability to retain urine related to stress, surgery, anatomical or functional problems, infection, motor or sensory impairment
Risk for Infection	Vascular access site, altered immunity, urine retention, presence of catheter, malnutrition

- The single most important nursing action to decrease the incidence of hospital-based infections is handwashing. **Remember to wash your hands or use antibacterial gel before and after each and every client contact.**

UNIT 1

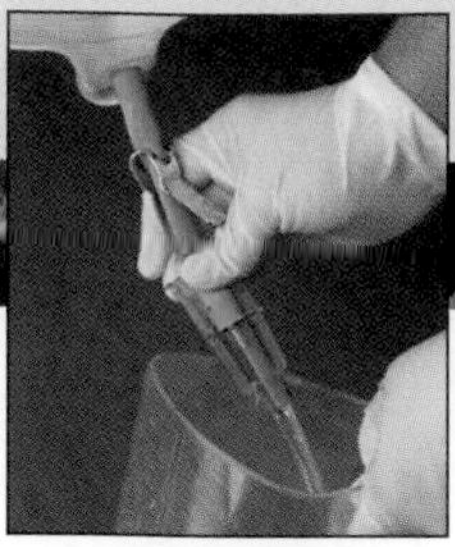

Intake and Output

Nursing Process Data

ASSESSMENT ***Data Base***

Assess if strict measurement of intake and output is ordered.

Assess client's ability to assist in keeping intake and output record.

Assess all potential sources of intake (e.g., IVs, oral fluids) and output (e.g., urine, drainage from tubes).

Observe color, clarity, and odor of urine.

Determine all forms where documentation of intake and output must occur.

Assess for signs of dehydration.

Evaluate weight changes (most accurate assessment of fluid balance).

PLANNING ***Objectives***

To accurately measure all sources of fluid intake

To accurately measure all sources of fluid output

To identify alterations in fluid balance based on urine and weight assessment

To record data on appropriate records

IMPLEMENTATION ***Procedures***

Measuring Intake and Output

EVALUATION ***Expected Outcomes***

All sources of intake and output are identified.

Intake and output measurements are accurately maintained.

Signs of fluid imbalance are identified.

Intake and output records are current and accurate.

MEASURING INTAKE AND OUTPUT

Equipment

I&O bedside form with fluid conversions
I&O chart record
Client's own graduated container
Bedpan or urinal
Clean gloves
Antimicrobial swab

Preparation

1. Explain purpose of keeping I&O record to client.
2. Instruct client to keep record of all fluids taken orally. Keep an I&O record at the bedside for the client to document intake.
3. Instruct client to void into bedpan or urinal, not into toilet.
4. Instruct client not to place toilet tissue in bedpan or defecate in bedpan.

Procedure

Oral Intake

1. Measure all fluid intake (including oral, IV, fluid medications, and tube feedings) according to hospital values (e.g., cup = 150 mL, glass = 240 mL).
2. Record time and amount of fluids in the appropriate space on bedside form.
3. Check hospital procedure manual or the bedside I&O record for approximate amounts of fluid containers.
4. Transfer 8-hour total fluid intake from bedside I&O record to graphic sheet for 24-hour I&O record on chart.
5. Record all forms of fluid intake in the total amount column of the 24-hour record (IVs and oral fluid).
6. Complete 24-hour intake record by adding together all three 8-hour totals.

Output

1. Don clean gloves to measure output from all sources.
2. Empty urinal, bedpan, or drainage bag into graduated container. **Rationale:** Measurement is only approximate from drainage bag or "hat." (Include other sources of output such

BEDSIDE INTAKE AND OUTPUT RECORD

Name ____________ Date ________

Room # ________

	Intake			Output		
	Oral	IV		Urine	Emesis	Drainage
7 am – 3 pm			7 am – 3 pm			
Total			Total			
3 pm – 11 pm			3 pm – 11 pm			
Total			Total			
11 pm – 7 am			11 pm – 7 am			
Total			Total			
24hr Total			24hr Total			

Measurements

Glass 240cc
Cup 150cc
Bowl 150cc
Juice Glass 100cc
Coffee Pot 240cc

Ice Cream 100cc
Jello 100cc
Ice Chips 5cc/Cube

Beside Intake and Output Record.

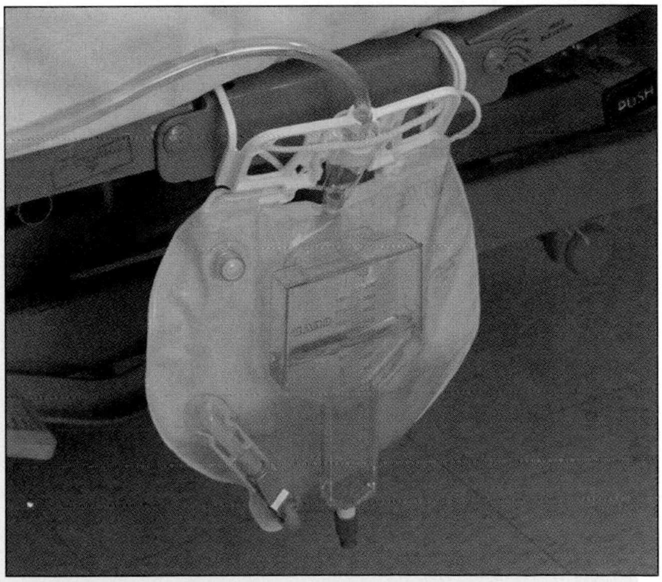

Close monitoring of urine output is accomplished when calibrated drainage bag has a urimeter.

Methods to Stimulate Voiding

- Run water in sink.
- Massage the lower abdomen.
- Place a hot washcloth on the abdomen.
- Pour warm water over the perineum with client positioned on toilet or bedpan.
- Obtain order for sitz bath.
- Put oil of wintergreen on a cotton ball in the bedpan or urinal.

as drainage, diarrheal stools, draining wounds or emesis on output record.)

3. To drain urine collection bag:
   a. Slip spigot from bag sleeve.
   b. Use client's individual (labeled) graduated receptacle.
   c. Unclamp spigot and drain bag—do not allow spigot to touch sides of receptacle.
   d. Swab end of spigot with antimicrobial swab before replacing into bag sleeve.
4. Remove gloves, and wash hands.
5. Record time and amount of output on bedside I&O record.
6. Complete 24-hour output record by adding together all three output totals, and place total on graphic sheet.
7. Notify physician of any significant imbalance; more intensive monitoring may be indicated. **Rationale:** Hourly urine output less than 25–30 mL/hour for two consecutive hours or 24-hour urine output less than 500 mL can indicate dehydration or internal bleeding and can result in acute renal failure.

CLINICAL ALERT

Use client's own graduated receptacle when measuring output. Change gloves and wash hands between each client.

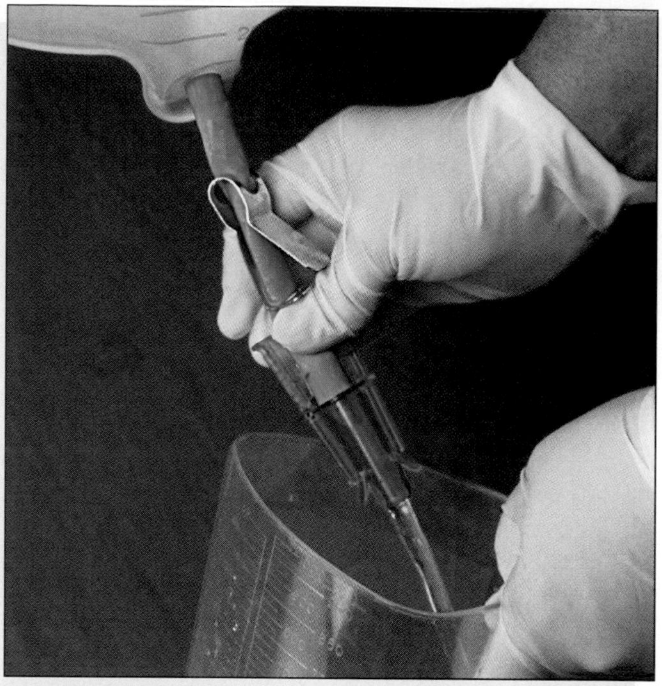

Empty urinal, bedpan, or Foley drainage bag into client's individual (labeled) graduate or commode "hat" and note amount of urine.

Documentation for Intake and Output

- Time and amount of all oral fluid intake
- 8-hour totals of all IV and enteral fluids
- 24-hour total of all fluid intake
- Time and amount of all urinary output
- Time and amount of all drainage (e.g., NG)
- 8-hour total of all fluid output
- 24-hour total of all fluid output

Critical Thinking Application

UNEXPECTED OUTCOMES	CRITICAL THINKING OPTIONS
Fluid balance is not correct as stated on I&O record.	• Recheck addition, then report to charge nurse so he or she can determine if all nurses are keeping accurate records. • Check if client or family can help with keeping the I&O record. • Check the addition on the I&O record to see if an error was made.
Client unable to maintain an intake of at least 1,500 mL.	• Ensure that fluid restriction is not ordered. • Check if the client is able to drink fluids independently or if assistance is needed. • Ensure that adequate fluids are available for the client. • Offer fluids regularly.
Client voids in toilet when on I&O monitoring.	• Document on I&O sheet, "voided in toilet." • Provide additional verbal instructions indicating all urine must be measured and recorded. • Place sign above toilet indicating "All urine must be measured and recorded."

UNIT 2

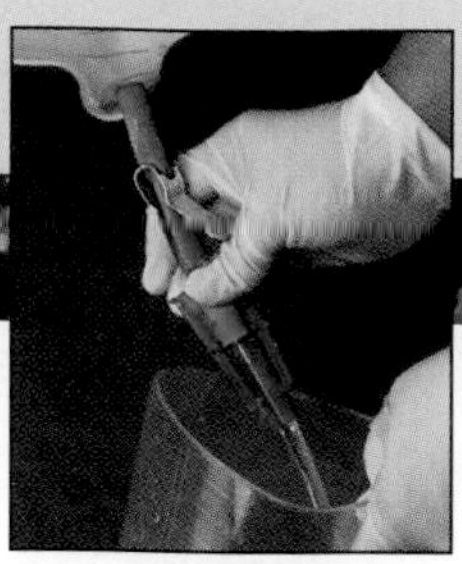

External Catheter System

Nursing Process Data

ASSESSMENT *Data Base*

Assess that client is able to empty bladder completely and spontaneously.

Assess the genital area for signs of irritation and edema during the use of condom catheter.

Assess activity level of client to determine when a leg bag or a continuous drainage system is necessary.

PLANNING *Objectives*

To provide a means for managing incontinence

To provide a means of collecting urine in a system that allows client ambulation

To prevent skin breakdown due to incontinence of urine

To prevent urinary tract infections in clients who are at risk and require a method of urine collection

IMPLEMENTATION *Procedures*

Applying a Condom Catheter

Attaching Catheter to Leg Bag

EVALUATION *Expected Outcomes*

Urine collection enhances client's lifestyle.

Client remains dry.

Genital area remains free of skin breakdown due to incontinence.

Client is able to ambulate with inconspicuous urine collection system.

APPLYING A CONDOM CATHETER

Equipment

Soap, water, towel, washcloth
Commercial condom catheter; select appropriate size
Leg bag or bedside drainage system
Skin barrier prep
Clean gloves
Drape
Scissors

Preparation

1. Check physician's orders and client care plan.
2. Gather equipment.
3. Identify client and explain procedure.
4. Wash your hands and provide privacy.
5. Raise bed and lower side rail on working side of bed. Place client flat supine.
6. Don clean gloves.
7. Drape for privacy.
8. Wash genital area with soap and water, and dry area thoroughly.
9. Clip hair from base of penis if necessary. **Rationale:** To avoid catching in adhesive strip.

Procedure

1. When commercial condom catheters are used, apply protective coating to skin on penile shaft and allow to dry completely (60 seconds).
2. Peel off paper from both sides of the adhesive liner according to product instructions.
3. Spirally wrap the adhesive liner around the penile shaft behind the glans.

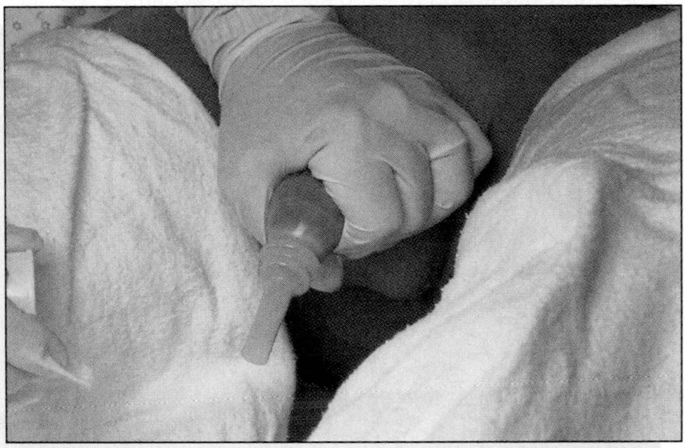

After unrolling condom onto penis, apply pressure to ensure smooth fit.

4. Take the condom catheter and place the prerolled sheath so funnel is against the glans, but *not* rubbing it.
5. Unroll the condom up the penis until it is completely over the adhesive liner.
6. Gently squeeze condom against liner to seal it after sheath is completely rolled over the penis. Do not wrinkle as wrinkles cause urine to leak through catheter.
7. Attach condom to a drainage system. The drainage system can be a leg bag or a bedside drainage system depending on activity level and condition of client.
8. Lower bed, and raise side rail or assist client out of bed if he is to be ambulated.
9. Remove gloves, and wash your hands.
10. Assess penis 30 minutes after condom applied to check for edema, discoloration, and urine flow. **Rationale:** This detects complication with application.

ATTACHING CATHETER TO LEG BAG

Equipment

Leg bag
Antimicrobial swabs
Clean gloves

Procedure

1. Obtain order for leg bag from physician.
2. Gather leg bag and alcohol wipe.
3. Identify client and explain procedure.
4. Provide privacy.
5. Raise bed, and lower side rail on working side of bed.
6. Wash hands and don clean gloves.
7. Disconnect drainage tubing from indwelling or condom catheter.

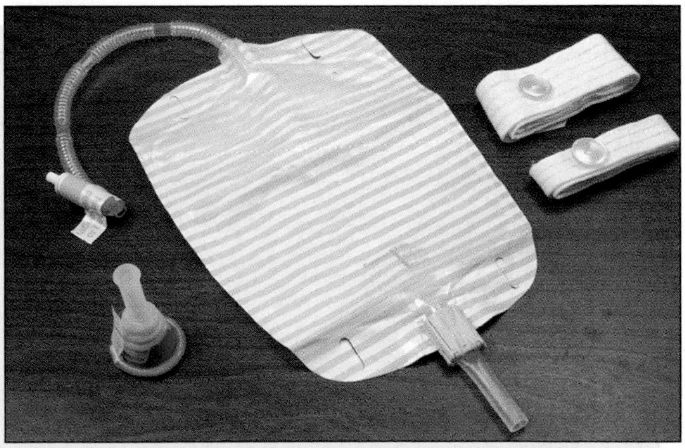

Leg bag uses Velcro strap to secure to leg.

8. Cap bedside drainage tubing end with protective cap from leg bag. **Rationale:** To maintain sterility of connecting parts.
9. Wipe leg bag and catheter connectors with swab.
10. Connect tip of leg bag into catheter.
11. Place cap from leg bag tip on collection tubing.
12. Secure leg bag to thigh by placing Velcro strap through bag and around leg.
13. When removing leg bag, disconnect catheter from leg bag and wipe each connection end with alcohol wipes.
14. Take leg bag cap off drainage tubing and replace it on leg bag.
15. Connect catheter to drainage tubing.
16. Lower bed and raise side rail.
17. Rinse leg bag in warm soap and water, and place in bath room to dry.
18. Remove gloves and wash your hands.

CLINICAL ALERT

Use of an external urine collection system is recommended for incontinent men without urine retention. These devices are comfortable, and there is less bacteriuria than with indwelling catheters.

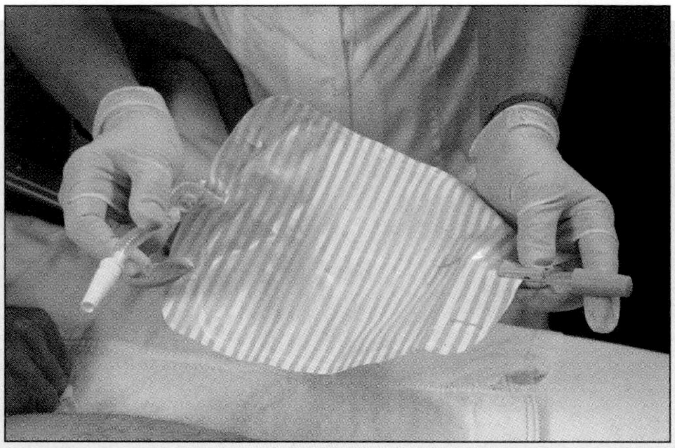

Connect longer tube from leg bag to catheter.

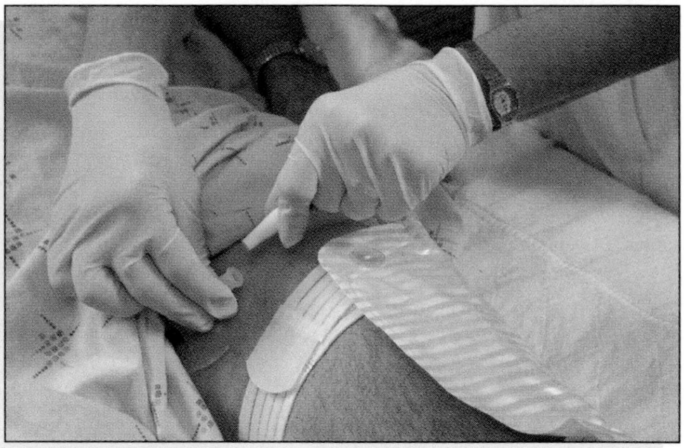

Maintain sterility when placing the tip of leg bag into catheter.

Documentation for External Catheter

- Type of condom catheter applied
- Size of catheter used
- Condition of genital area
- Protective coating (prep) applied to skin
- Type of drainage collection device attached
- Amount, color, and odor of urine obtained
- Client's tolerance of procedure and ability to perform self-care

Critical Thinking Application

UNEXPECTED OUTCOMES	CRITICAL THINKING OPTIONS
Incontinence continues with use of condom catheter.	• Use smaller condom to provide wrinkle-free application. • Replace adhesive strips for better condom adherence. • Make sure penis is dry before applying condom system.
Penis becomes reddened and excoriated.	• Remove condom catheter • Notify physician for topical medication order. • Apply adult briefs, and change frequently. Keep condom off penis until area is healed. • Wash perineal area frequently. • Ensure drainage collection system is dependent of condom tubing to promote gravity flow.

UNIT 3

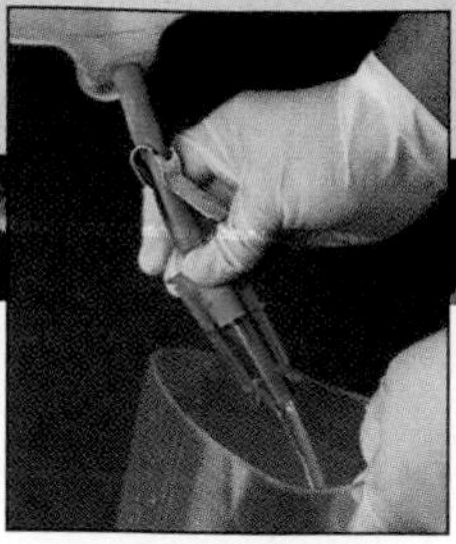

Catheterization

Nursing Process Data

ASSESSMENT ***Data Base***

Assess the client's bladder for distention.

Assess purpose of catheterization or urine output monitoring.

Check physician's orders for method of catheterization to be done.

Assess urinary meatus for exudate or inflammation.

Assess character and amount of urine.

Note client's I&O balance.

PLANNING ***Objectives***

To prevent or relieve discomfort due to bladder distention

To promote urinary elimination

To obtain a sterile urine specimen

To provide continuous urinary bladder drainage

To provide bladder irrigation

To measure the amount of residual urine (post void)

To monitor the output of a critically ill client

IMPLEMENTATION ***Procedures***

Draping a Female Client

Using a Bladder Scanner

Inserting a Straight Catheter (Female)

Inserting a Straight Catheter (Male)

Inserting a Retention Catheter (Female)

Inserting a Retention Catheter (Male)

Providing Catheter Care

Removing a Retention Catheter

EVALUATION ***Expected Outcomes***

Residual urine measured.

Bladder is decompressed, relieving discomfort.

Sterile urine specimen obtained.

Catheterization performed using sterile technique.

Retention catheter inserted without difficulty.

Catheter is removed as soon as possible.

DRAPING A FEMALE CLIENT

Equipment

Bath blanket

Procedure

1. Bring bath blanket to bedside.
2. Identify client, and explain procedure.
3. Provide privacy.
4. Wash your hands.
5. Place bed in HIGH position, and lower side rail nearest you.
6. Place bath blanket over client's top linen so that one corner of the blanket is pointed toward the client's head to form a diamond shape over the client.
7. Instruct client to hold onto bath blanket. Fanfold linen to foot of bed and place on chair.
8. Request that client flex knees and keep them apart with feet firmly on bed.
9. Wrap lateral corners of bath blanket around feet in a spiral fashion until they are completely covered.
10. The corner of the blanket between knees and extending over perineum can later be folded back over the abdomen. **Rationale:** Draping provides for warmth and unnecessary exposure of genital area until procedure is performed.

Note: Draping is not always done, but may be appropriate for certain cultures for the modest females.

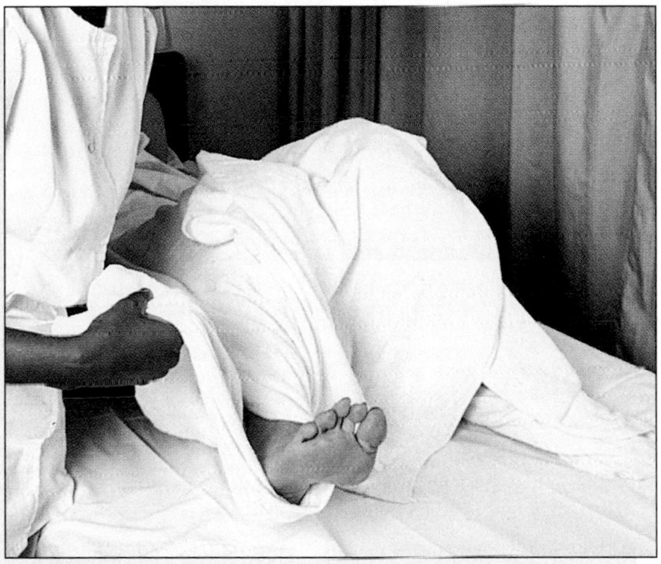

Use bath blanket to drape client before catheterization.

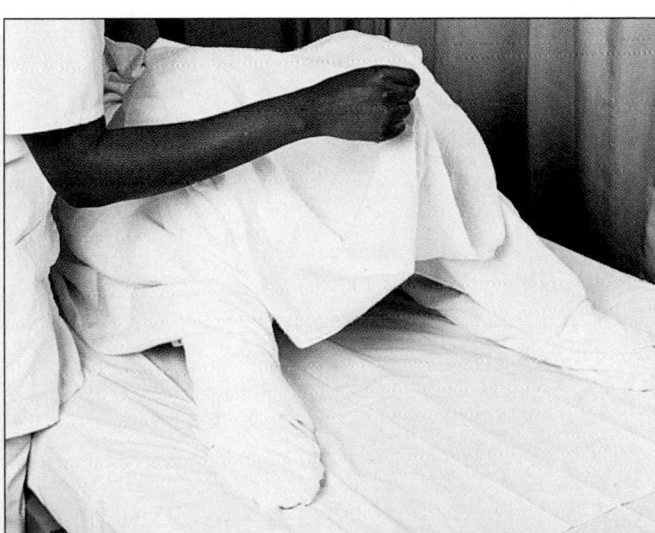

Corner of blanket is folded back over abdomen to expose perineum.

USING A BLADDER SCANNER

Equipment

Ultrasound BladderScan device
Ultrasound conducting gel
Tissues

Preparation

1. Check physician's order to evaluate client's bladder.
2. Identify client and explain procedure and purpose.
3. Ask client if she has had hysterectomy or is pregnant. **Rationale:** Scanner is not indicated for pregnant clients.
4. Provide privacy.
5. Determine time and amount of last void or assist client to empty bladder if residual volume is to be evaluated.
6. Determine that client does not have an indwelling catheter. **Rationale:** Scanner reflects off the catheter bulb giving an echo reading.
7. Wash hands.
8. Place client flat supine and palpate client's bladder to locate.

Procedure

1. Turn the device on and press "SCAN."
2. Apply conducting gel to scanner head.
3. Select MALE or FEMALE mode on scan unit. Select *MALE MODE* if female client has had a hysterectomy.
4. Fanfold linens to expose client's suprapubic area.

5. Place head of scanner 3 cm above client's symphysis pubis and align the icon.
6. Press scanhead button and hold scanner until a beep is heard.
7. Scan until bladder image is lined up on crosshairs.
8. Take several scans at different angles and press DONE when finished.
9. Press PRINT for a printout of client's bladder volume in milliliters.
10. Wipe gel from client's skin.
11. Reposition client for comfort.

INSERTING A STRAIGHT CATHETER (FEMALE)

Equipment

Disposable catheterization tray with straight catheter (14 Fr), and specimen cup
Bath blanket or turn sheet
Additional light source, if needed
If necessary for cleansing, towel, washcloth, basin with warm water and soap
Clean gloves

Note: This skill may be indicated after client voids to determine residual volume.

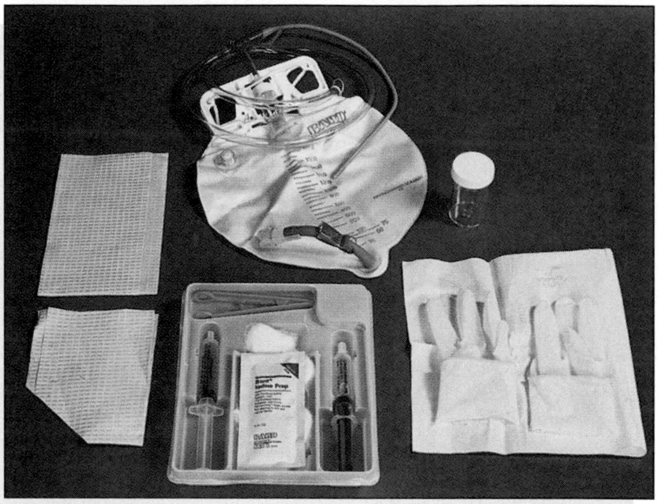

Disposable kit includes equipment necessary for performing a catheterization. (Retention catheter/Foley is shown above).

Preparation

1. Bring equipment to client's room.
2. Check lighting source.
3. Identify client, and explain procedure and need for client to keep knees positioned during procedure.
4. Provide privacy.
5. Wash your hands.
6. Place bed in HIGH position, and lower side rail on working side.
7. Fold linens to foot of bed and cover client's lower body with bath blanket.
8. Provide perineal care, if necessary, with soap and water using clean gloves. Dry perineum thoroughly.
9. Discard towels, water, and replace basin.
10. Dispose of gloves, and wash your hands.
11. Drape the client (see *Draping a Female Client*).
12. Have client bring knees up and out. May need assistance to keep knees in this position. **Rationale:** This position provides for good visualization of urinary meatus.
13. Adjust light source to ensure that meatus is adequately exposed.
14. Fold up bath blanket corner to expose perineum.

EVIDENCE BASED NURSING PRACTICE

Regaining Voiding Ability

In hip surgery patients, those receiving intermittent catheterization regained satisfactory voiding quicker than those with an indwelling catheter.

Source: Cravens, D., & Zweig, S. (2000). Urinary catheter management. *American Family Physician, 61*(2), 369–375.

Estimating Bladder Fullness

- The bladder is not normally palpable until it contains over 150 mL of urine.
- Normally, suprapubic percussion produces a hollow sound. A dull or flat sound indicates bladder distention.
- A bulge may be noted in the suprapubic area when the bladder contains 500 mL.
- Pain may not be felt until the bladder has distended to the umbilicus (1400–1900 mL).
- Subjective symptoms are not reliable indicators of bladder fullness.

Procedure

1. Open sterile package by tearing the package on the lined edge of plastic wrap. Place plastic wrap at foot of bed for waste disposal.
2. Place cath tray on bed between client's legs.
3. Fold back drape to expose perineum.
4. Open white outer wrap away from sterile package with last turn toward client.
5. Remove sterile absorbent pad, and position plastic side down under client's buttocks. Have client lift buttocks if able. Position pad by holding corners of pad only. **Rationale:** Pad creates a sterile field.
6. Put on sterile gloves.
7. Remove sterile articles from tray, and arrange conveniently on sterile field or place tray onto field.
8. Open package, and pour antiseptic solution over cotton balls.
9. Uncap syringe filled with lubricant, or tear open lubricant package, pick up catheter tip, and lubricate the tip of the catheter generously. Place catheter back on tray. May place lubricant on sterile field and put catheter tip on lubricant and leave in place. **Rationale:** Removing catheter from sterile container (tray) increases risk of contamination.
10. If specimen is required, uncap sterile specimen container.
11. Move catheter tray close to client.
12. Place sterile fenestrated drape over perineum exposing meatus (optional).
13. Prep client's meatus:
    a. Separate the client's labia minora with your nondominant hand (maintain separation throughout prep).
    b. With your dominant hand, *use forceps* to pick up an absorbent ball that has been saturated with antiseptic solution. (If Betadine swabs are used, pick up one swab.)
    c. Cleanse client's meatus with one downward stroke of forceps or swab. **Rationale:** Using a downward stroke cleans from least contaminated to most contaminated area.
    d. Discard absorbent ball or swab in the plastic cover at foot of bed. **Rationale:** Using a new cotton ball or swab with each downward stroke prevents transfer of microorganisms.
    e. Repeat step c at least three to four times.
    f. Continue to hold client's labia apart until you insert catheter. **Rationale:** This prevents contamination of urinary meatus.
14. Discard preps in plastic bag at the foot of the bed as appropriate. Using sterile gloved hand, pick up lubricated catheter keeping drainage end in collection container, and insert 2 inches or until urine begins to flow.
15. Move nondominant hand from holding labia open to hold catheter in place.
16. Place sterile specimen container under drainage end of catheter if specimen is needed, and fill container with approximately 30 mL of urine.
17. Replace catheter drainage end into collection container, and allow urine to flow until it ceases.
18. Pinch catheter closed when urine ceases to flow, and remove gently and slowly.
19. Remove drapes and dry the perineum.
20. Position client for comfort, put the bed in LOW position with the side rails up.
21. Measure and record urine output on the I&O bedside record.
22. Discard gloves and equipment appropriately.
23. Wash your hands.
24. Send specimen to lab if indicated and document findings.

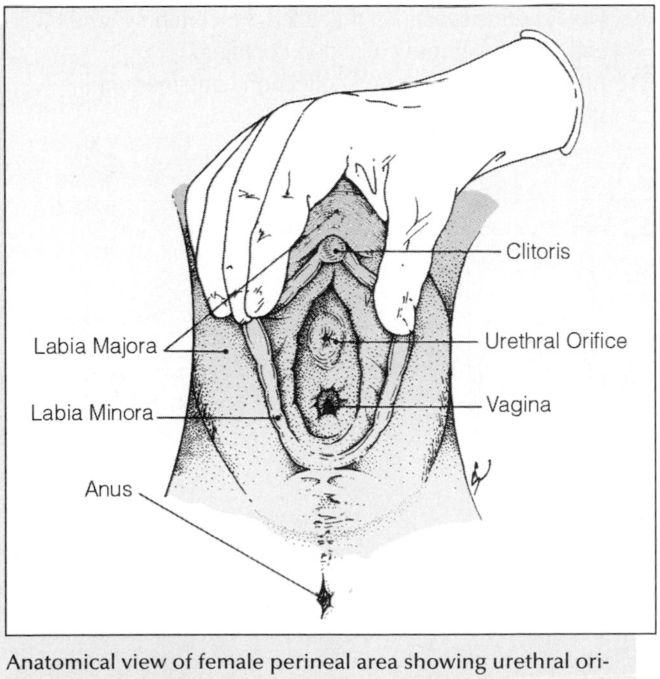

Anatomical view of female perineal area showing urethral orifice.

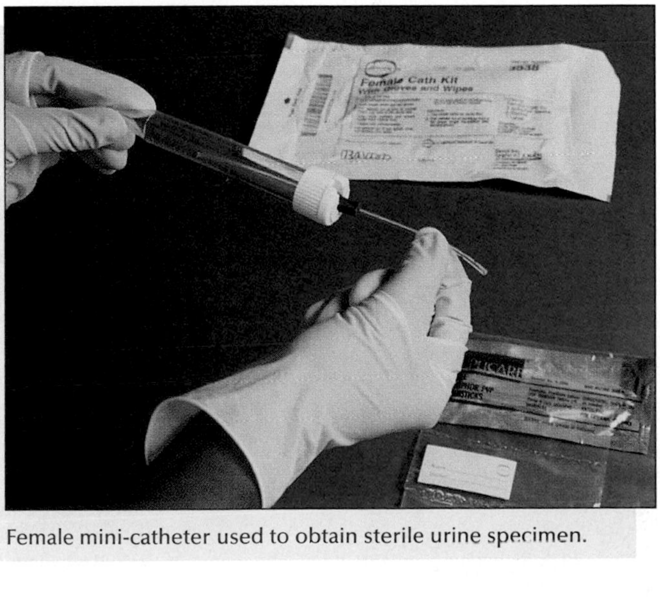

Female mini-catheter used to obtain sterile urine specimen.

INSERTING A STRAIGHT CATHETER (MALE)

Equipment

Same as for *Inserting a Straight Catheter (Female)*
2% lidocaine gel for lubricant, if ordered

Preparation

1. Follow steps 1 through 6 in *Inserting a Straight Catheter (Female).*
2. Place client in a supine position with knees slightly apart. **Rationale:** This position relaxes abdominal and perineal muscles.
3. Drape client by placing a bath blanket or draw sheet over chest area and fanfold top linen down to cover lower extremities, exposing only genital area.
4. Don clean gloves, and wash genital area if necessary.
5. Remove gloves, and prepare for catheterization.

Procedure

1. Open sterile package by tearing the package on the lined edge of plastic wrap. Place plastic wrap at foot of bed for waste disposal.
2. Place sterile kit at client's side near thigh.
3. Open outer wrap away from sterile package with last turn toward penis.
4. Don sterile gloves.
5. Place first drape over thighs and under penis.
6. Place fenestrated drape over penis.
7. Open antiseptic package and pour solution over cotton balls. Open lubricant packet syringe—eject from syringe onto sterile field.
8. Hold penis upright with your nondominant hand.
9. With your dominant hand, use forceps to pick up cotton ball saturated with antiseptic solution or pick up Betadine swab.
10. Cleanse meatus with circular stroke using cotton ball or swab. Discard cotton ball or swab into plastic bag at foot of bed.
11. Repeat circular cleansing motion prep around tip of penis. Cleanse three times using a new cotton ball or swab each time.
12. Continue to hold penis with your nondominant hand.
13. Discard forceps into plastic bag.
14. Lubricate catheter about 3–4 inches using generous amount of lubricant.
15. *Alternate Method:* Insert tip of lubricant syringe at urethral opening and instill lubricant (or 2% lidocaine, if ordered) directly into urethra. (If cath tray does not have syringe, place sterile syringe on tray before gloving.) **Rationale:** This facilitates catheter placement by expanding and anesthetizing urethra, especially for the client with enlarged prostate.
16. Pick up catheter with sterile gloved hand about 8–10 cm (3–4 inches) from tip of catheter.
17. Lift penis to a 90° angle (perpendicular to body) and exert slight traction by pulling upward. **Rationale:** This movement straightens the urethra for easier insertion of catheter.
18. Insert catheter about 20 cm (8 inches) until urine begins to flow.
19. If catheter meets resistance decrease angle of penis to 45°, twist catheter and ask client to take a deep breath. **Rationale:** Taking a deep breath helps relax external sphincter. If persistent resistance is felt and catheter cannot be inserted without difficulty, remove catheter and notify physician.
20. Obtain urine specimen if needed. Pinch tubing, and transfer end of catheter into collection container.
21. Allow urine to drain into collection container until flow stops.

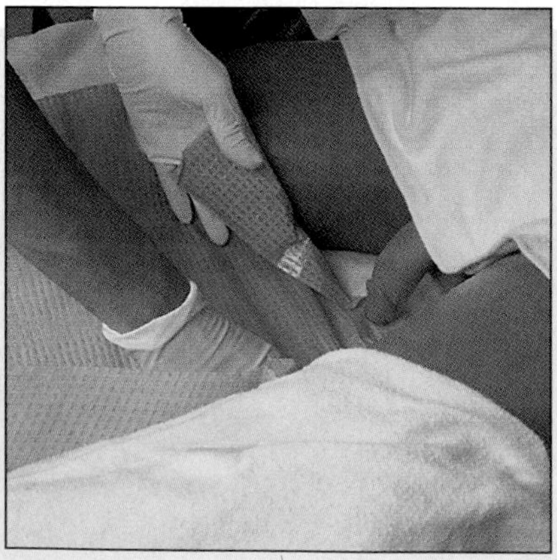

Place absorbent pad, with plastic side down, under penis to establish sterile field.

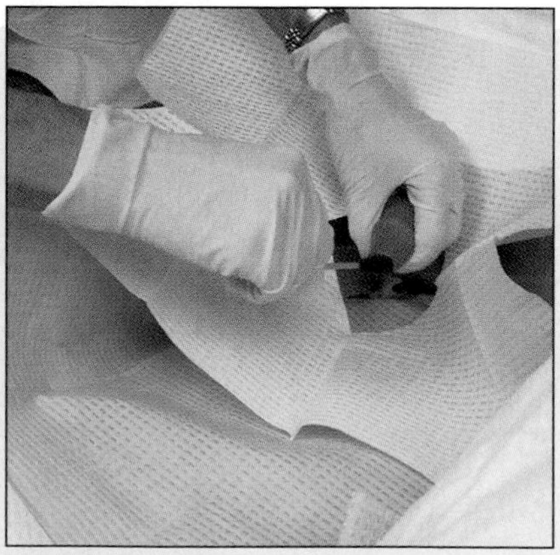

Prep head of penis, starting at meatus and cleansing outward in a circular motion.

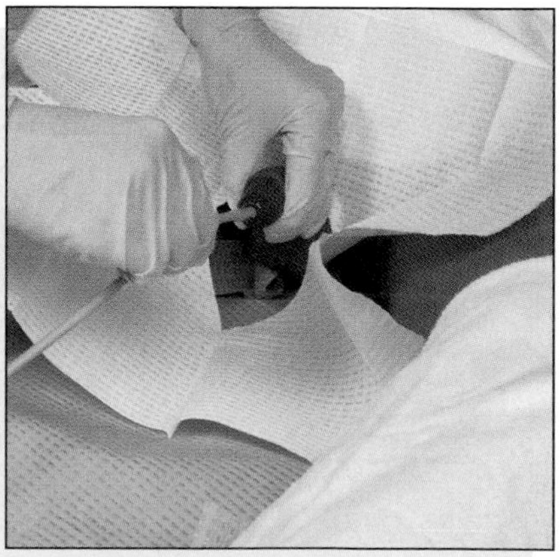

Insert amply lubricated catheter until urine flows.

22. Remove catheter, place lid on specimen bottle.
23. Dry penis and remove drapes.
24. Make client comfortable. Place bed in LOW position with side rails up.
25. Discard equipment in appropriate container.
26. Remove gloves and wash hands.
27. Send specimen to lab and document findings.

INSERTING A RETENTION CATHETER (FEMALE)

Equipment

Disposable retention catheter kit with appropriate size catheter (size 14–16 for adult female, and size 16–18 for adult male)
Closed drainage set, if not included in kit
Additional lighting, if needed
Bath blanket
Towels, washcloth
Clean gloves
Basin with warm water
Soap
Tape or commercial catheter holder

Preparation

Same as for *Inserting a Straight Catheter (Female)*.

Procedure

1. Don clean gloves, complete perineal care, and remove gloves.
2. Open sterile package by tearing the package on the lined edge of plastic wrap. Place plastic wrap at foot of bed for waste disposal.
3. Place catheter and bag on bed between client's legs.
4. Fold back corner of bath blanket to expose perineum.
5. Open white outer wrap away from package with last turn toward client.
6. Remove sterile absorbent pad, and position under client's buttocks plastic side down. Have client lift buttocks if able. Position pad by holding corners of pad only. **Rationale:** Holding onto the edges keeps the center sterile.
7. Put on sterile gloves, and separate the two containers. Place container with cotton balls, antiseptic solution packet, and lubricant toward client. Place container with catheter and bag toward foot of bed (next to first container).
8. Open package, and pour antiseptic solution over cotton balls.
9. To test catheter balloon.
   a. Remove rubber protector and insert tip of the prefilled syringe into catheter side arm to inflate balloon.
   b. Ensure that at least 10 mL sterile water is in syringe as the balloon usually holds more than 5 mL of water. **Rationale:** The catheter can fall out if not secured with appropriately inflated balloon. Standard catheters have 5-mL balloons.
   c. If balloon malfunctions after testing, replace it before continuing with procedure.

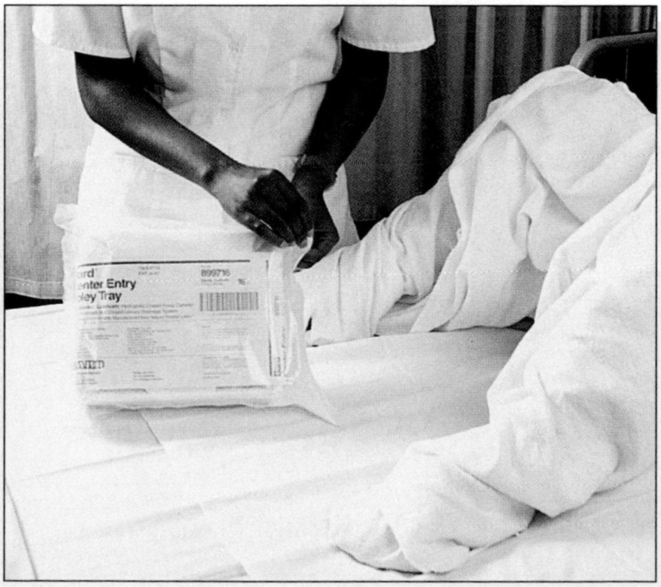

Open sterile package by tearing it along lined edge of plastic wrap.

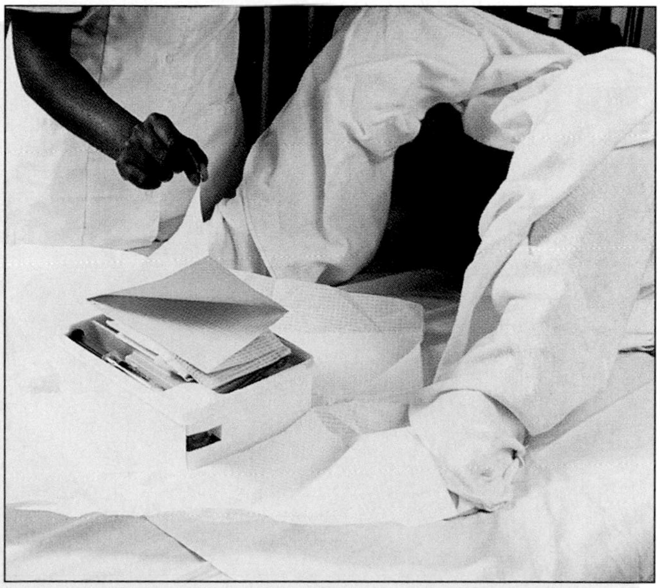

Remove sterile absorbent pad and place it under client's buttocks.

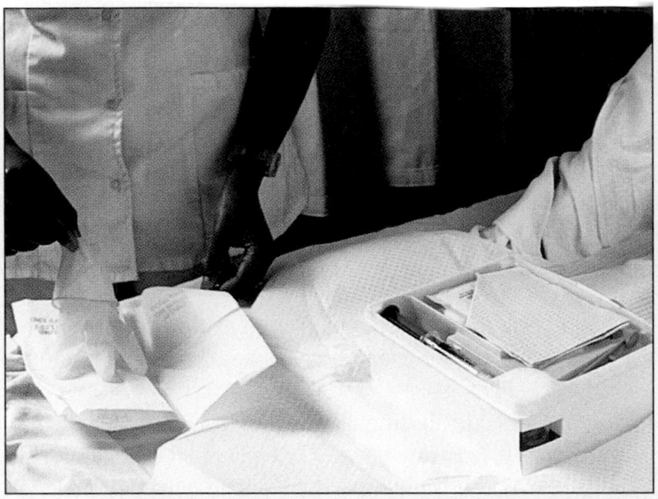

Put on sterile gloves, being careful not to contaminate sterile field.

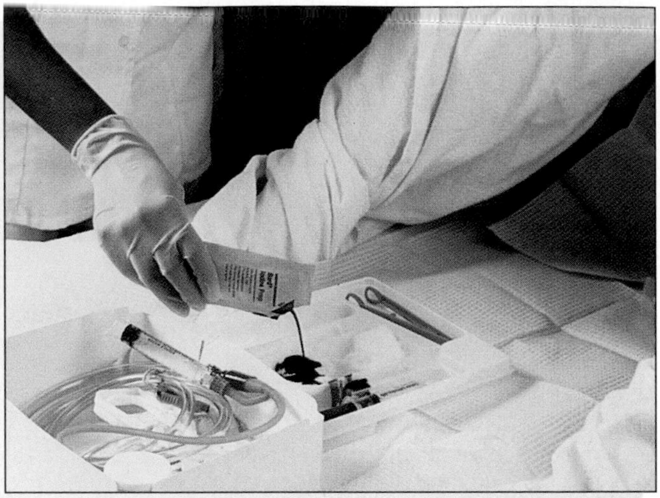

Pour antiseptic solution completely over cotton balls.

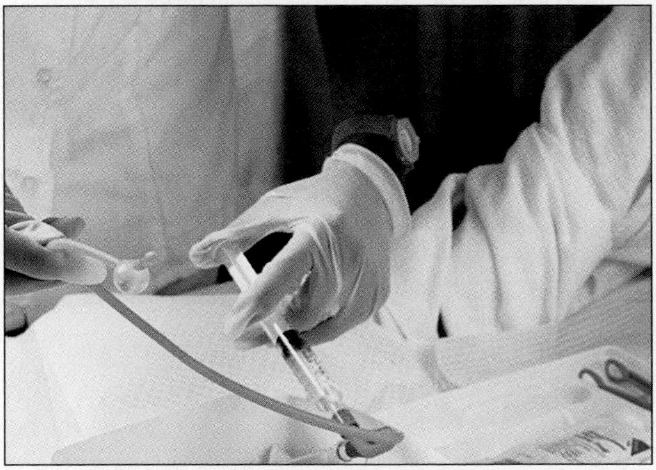

Test catheter balloon by inserting prefilled syringe into catheter.

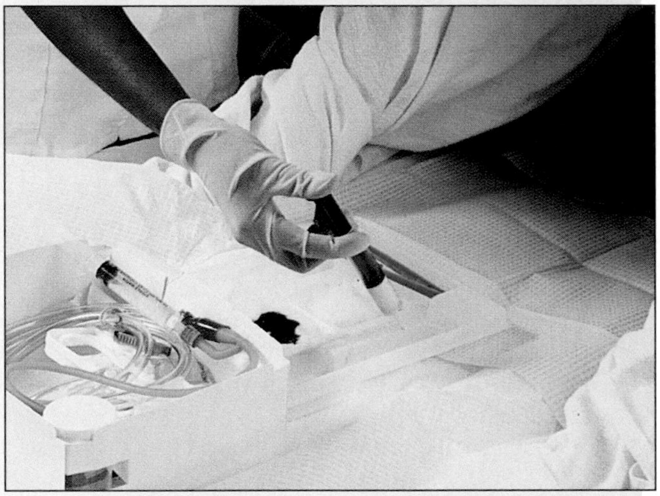

Uncap lubricant syringe and squeeze lubricant onto tray.

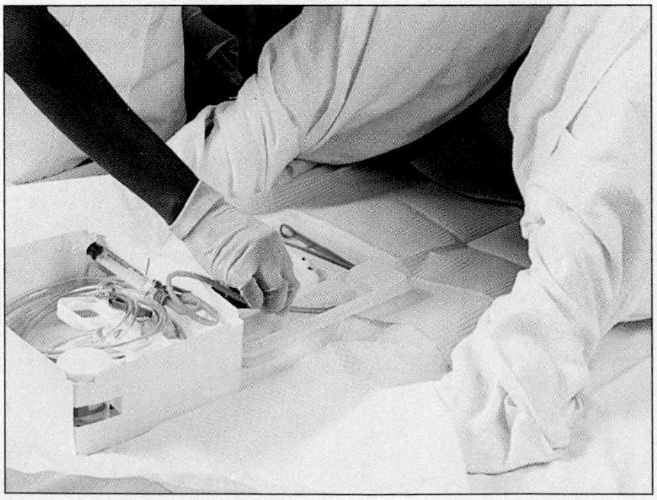

Lubricate tip of catheter to facilitate insertion without trauma.

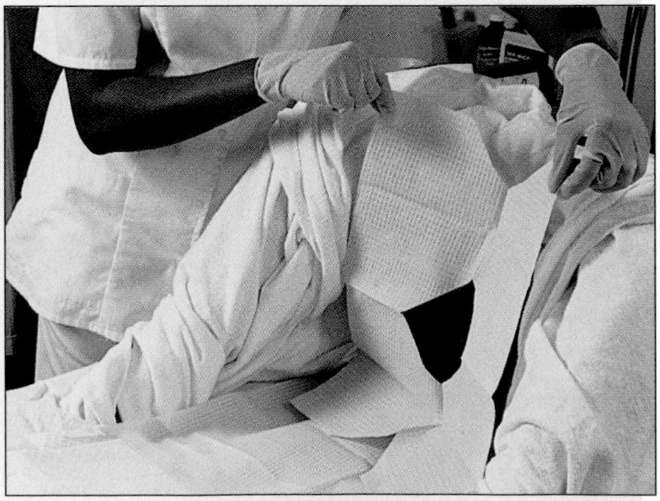

Position sterile fenestrated drape over client to expose genitalia.

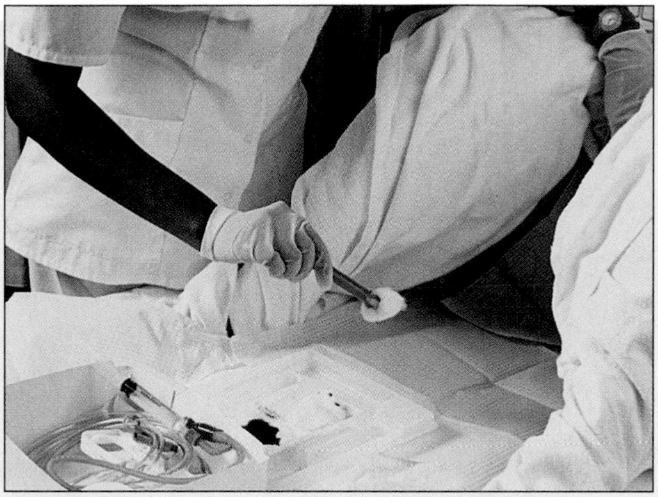

Cleanse meatus by using downward strokes with cotton balls.

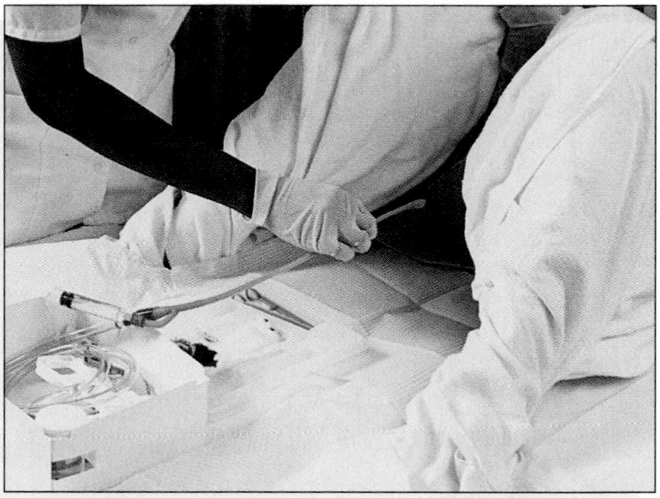

Insert catheter while holding labia apart to prevent contamination.

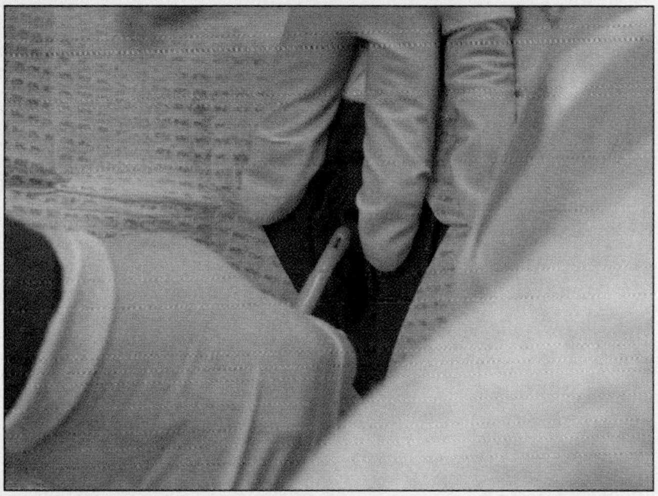

Insert catheter into meatus 1½ to 2 inches until urine begins to flow.

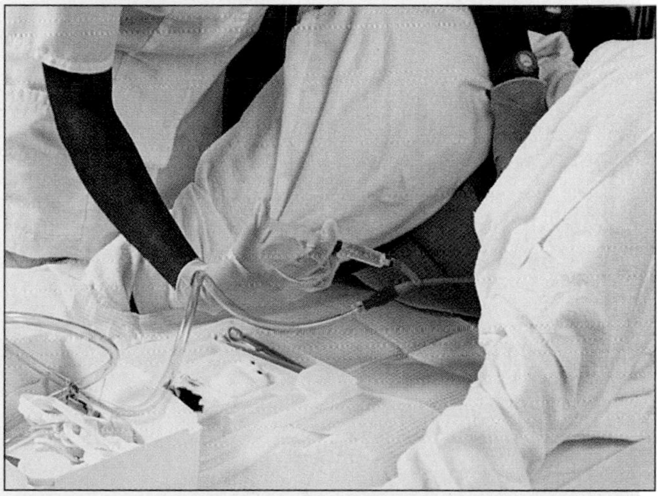

Inject water from prefilled syringe into catheter balloon after inserting catheter.

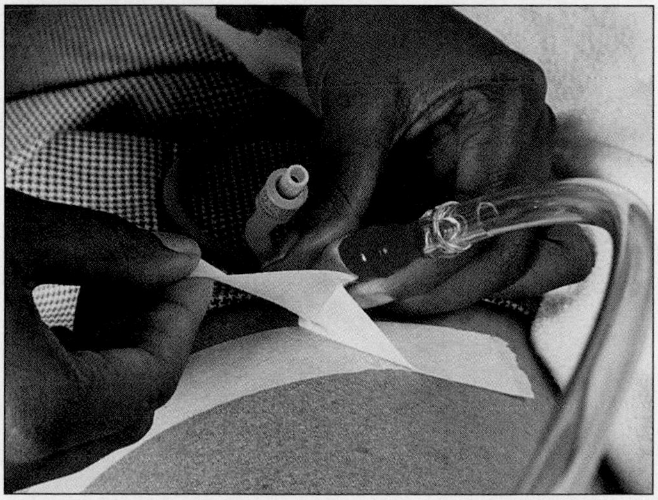

Tape catheter to side of client's thigh using nonallergenic tape.

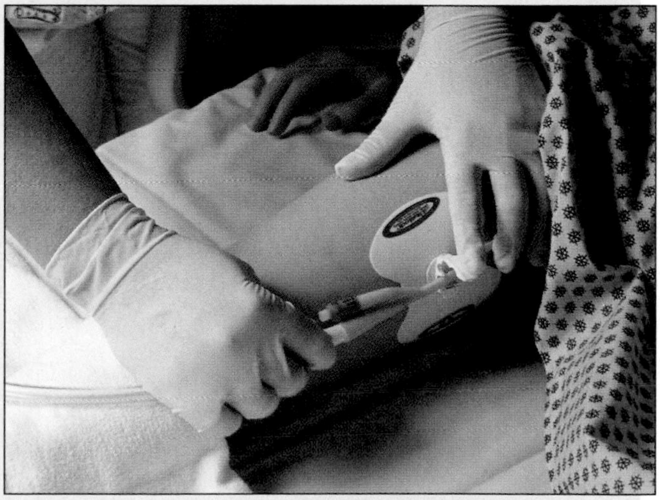

Commercial holder (StatLock Foley) stabilizes catheter to minimize urethral trauma.

10. After testing balloon, pull back on syringe to remove fluid and deflate balloon. **Rationale:** Testing is done to ensure that balloon inflates without leaking.
11. Uncap syringe filled with lubricant or open package, and generously lubricate tip in lubricant. Keep catheter on tray. **Rationale:** Lubricating the catheter prevents friction and trauma to the meatus and urethra.
12. Position fenestrated drape over the client to expose the genitalia (optional).
13. Prep client's meatus:
    a. Separate client's labia minora with your nondominant hand.
    b. With your dominant hand, *use forceps* to pick up an absorbent cotton ball that has been saturated with antiseptic solution.
    c. Cleanse client's meatus with one downward stroke of forceps or swab. Discard absorbent cotton ball or swab in plastic bag at foot of bed.
    d. Repeat step c at least three to four times.
    e. Continue to hold the client's labia apart until you insert the catheter.
14. Discard forceps in plastic bag at foot of bed.
15. With uncontaminated hand, take catheter from tray, and insert gently into meatus 2 inches or until urine starts to flow.
16. Guide the catheter gently just beyond the point at which urine begins to flow. **Rationale:** Inserting catheter further into bladder ensures it is beyond neck of the bladder.

CLINICAL ALERT

Chronic irritation and inflammation of bladder mucosa due to long-term (over 8 months) presence of an indwelling catheter (urethral or suprapubic) is associated with an increased risk for bladder cancer.

17. Inject entire contents of prefilled (9 mL sterile water) syringe into the side arm of the catheter used for balloon inflation. **Rationale:** Injection fills catheter lumen as well as inflation balloon.
18. If client complains of pain on balloon inflation, immediately aspirate the sterile water. **Rationale:** The catheter may be in the urethra rather than the bladder.
19. Retract the catheter until you feel resistance. **Rationale:** This indicates the correct position.

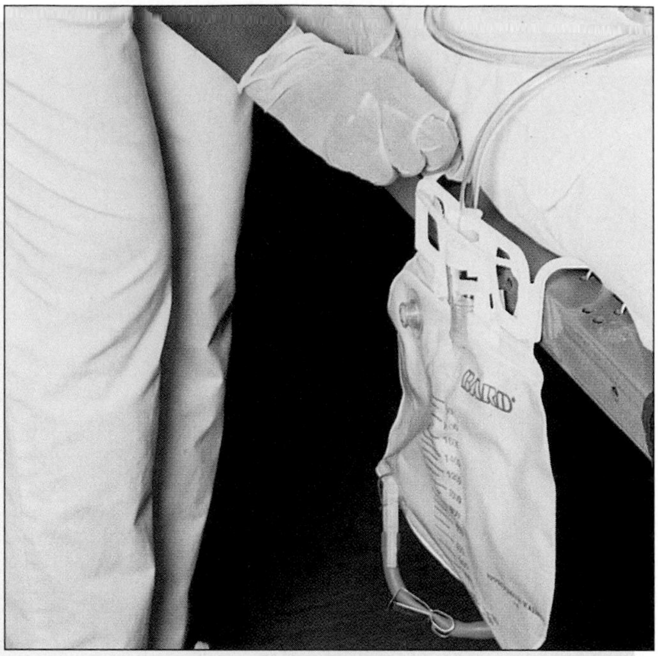

Attach drainage bag to bed frame to promote gravity drainage of urine—always keep bag below level of client's bladder.

20. Apply catheter holder or tape catheter to client's thigh. Place one piece of tape on leg. Take second piece of tape and encircle catheter leaving two "tails" on tape. Secure "tails" from tape on catheter to tape on leg. **Rationale:** To stabilize catheter and minimize urethral trauma.
21. Attach drainage bag to bed frame (not side rails); coil tubing to allow free gravity flow of urine.
22. Cleanse client's perineum of antiseptic solution. Remove drapes.
23. Reposition client for comfort; put bed in LOW position with side rails up.
24. Remove all equipment, including gloves, and discard disposable trash in appropriate container.
25. Measure and record urine output on I&O.
26. Wash your hands.

CLINICAL ALERT

Never obtain a urine specimen from the catheter drainage bag. Pathogens in drainage bag urine do not necessarily represent those present in lower urinary tract.

INSERTING A RETENTION CATHETER (MALE)

Equipment

Same as for *Inserting a Retention Catheter (Female)*

Preparation

1. Follow steps 1 through 6 in *Inserting a Straight Catheter (Female).*
2. Place client in a supine position with knees slightly apart. **Rationale:** This position relaxes abdominal and perineal muscles.
3. Drape client by placing a bath blanket over chest area and fanfold top linen down to cover lower extremities, exposing only perineal area.
4. Don clean gloves and wash client's perineal area if necessary.
5. Remove gloves and prepare for catheterization.

Procedure

1. Open sterile package by tearing package on lined edge of plastic wrap. Place plastic wrap at foot of bed for waste disposal.
2. Place sterile kit on client's thighs if client is cooperative, or at client's side near thigh.
3. Open outer white wrap away from sterile package with last turn toward penis.
4. Place sterile drape over thighs and under penis.
5. Don sterile gloves.
6. Place container with cotton balls or swabs and lubricant toward client. Place container with catheter and bag toward foot of bed (next to first container).
7. Open package and pour antiseptic over cotton balls or open Betadine swab package.
8. To test catheter retention balloon, remove rubber protector, and insert tip of the prefilled syringe into catheter side arm to inflate balloon.
9. After testing balloon, pull back on syringe to remove fluid. **Rationale:** Testing is done to ensure that balloon inflates without leaking.
10. Lubricate catheter generously about 3–4 inches or, if using alternate method, insert lubricant directly into the urethra using a prefilled syringe.
11. Position fenestrated drape over the penis.
12. Hold penis upright with your nondominant hand. Hold sides of penis to prevent closing of urethra.
13. With your dominant hand, use forceps to pick up cotton ball saturated with antiseptic solution or pick up swab.
14. Cleanse meatus first with one circular stroke using the forceps or Betadine swab.
15. Discard swab into plastic wrap at foot of bed.
16. Repeat circular prep around head of penis. Cleanse three times using a new cotton ball or Betadine swab each time. **Rationale:** Using a circular motion around head of penis prevents bacteria from entering urinary meatus.
17. Continue to hold penis with your nondominant hand.
18. Discard forceps into plastic bag as appropriate.

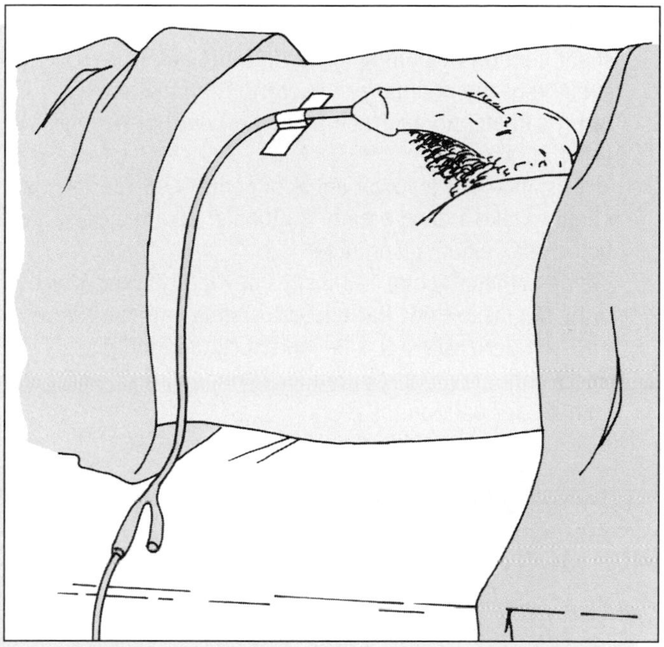
Tape catheter to abdomen to prevent pressure on penoscrotal angle.

EVIDENCE BASED NURSING PRACTICE

Risks for Urinary Retention

In this study, risks for urinary retention was greater in elderly patients receiving over 4000 mL of IV fluids perioperatively in a 24-hour period, and on prolonged bedrest (over 24 hours). Length of anesthesia time, history of urinary problems, and type of analgesic did not correlate with incidence of urinary retention.

Source: Wynd, C., et al. (1996). Factors influencing postoperative urinary retention following orthopaedic surgical procedures. *Orthopaedic Nursing, 15*(1), 43–49.

19. Pick up catheter with sterile hand about 8–10 cm (3–4 inches) from tip of catheter.
20. Lift penis to a 90° angle (perpendicular to body) and exert slight traction by pulling upward. **Rationale:** This movement straightens the urethra for easier insertion of catheter.
21. Insert catheter about 20 cm (8 inches) until urine begins to flow.
22. If resistance is met lower angle of penis to 45° and ask client to take a deep breath. **Rationale:** Taking a deep breath helps relax external sphincter.
23. Guide catheter gently 1–2 inches beyond point at which urine begins to flow. **Rationale:** Inserting catheter further into bladder ensures it is beyond neck of bladder.
24. Inject entire contents of prefilled syringe into side arm of catheter for balloon inflation.
25. Retract catheter until you feel resistance.
26. Tape catheter to abdomen with 1-inch tape. Alternative taping to upper thigh. **Rationale:** This prevents pressure on the penoscrotal angle.
27. Attach drainage bag to bed frame (not side rails).
28. Reposition client for comfort; put bed in LOW position with side rails up.
29. Remove all equipment, including gloves, and discard disposable trash in the appropriate container.
30. Measure and record urine output in I&O bedside record.
31. Wash your hands.
32. Document findings.

PROVIDING CATHETER CARE

Equipment

Commercially prepared kit *or* periwipes or antiseptic solution
Cleansing swabs or sterile cotton balls
Clean gloves
Bowl
Paper bag
Soap and water
Two washcloths
Towel

Preparation

1. Check physician's orders and client care plan.
2. Gather equipment.
3. Identify client by checking identaband.
4. Provide privacy.
5. Wash hands.
6. Explain procedure to client.
7. Raise bed, and lower side rail on working side.

Procedure

1. Place client in supine position, and expose perineal area to easily visualize the meatus.
2. Open catheter care kit or assemble equipment on over-bed table within easy reach.
3. Pour antiseptic solution over cotton balls or open package of cleansing swabs.
4. Place paper bag near working area, if used.
5. Remove tape.
6. Put on clean gloves.

for Female

a. Cleanse urinary meatus using circular motion moving from middle toward outside with washcloth, soap and water, antiseptic soaked cotton ball, or swab.
b. Dispose of cotton ball into paper bag. **Rationale:** This motion prevents bacteria from entering the urinary meatus.
c. Gently pull catheter taut and cleanse with new washcloth, swab, or cotton ball from catheter insertion site down catheter tubing approximately 4–5 inches toward drainage bag.
d. Dispose of cotton ball into paper bag.

for Circumcised Male

a. With mitten washcloth, soap, and water, cleanse around urinary meatus.
b. Dry area with towel.

Complications Associated with Long-Term Indwelling Catheter Placement

- Urinary tract infections
- Catheter leaks
- Bladder spasms
- Urethral erosion
- Urethritis
- Epididymitis
- Prostatitis
- Scrotal abscess
- Prostatic abscess
- Urinary stones
- Urethral sphincter damage
- Bladder cancer

c. Using separate washcloth, clean area between scrotum and rectal area, then dry.
d. Place soiled linen in hamper.

for Uncircumcized Male

a. Retract foreskin back away from catheter.
b. With mitten washcloth, soap, and water, cleanse around urinary meatus.
c. Dry penis with towel.
d. After drying, pull foreskin back around the catheter.
e. Place soiled linen in hamper.

7. Remove gloves and discard. Retape catheter.
8. Position client for comfort.
9. Lower bed, and raise side rail.
10. Discard equipment.
11. Wash hands.

REMOVING A RETENTION CATHETER

Equipment

10-mL syringe without needle
Paper towel
Soap, water, towel
Clean gloves
Client's calibrated graduate

Preparation

1. Check physician's orders for removing catheter.
2. Wash your hands.
3. Gather equipment.
4. Explain procedure to client.
5. Provide privacy.
6. Don clean gloves.

> **CLINICAL ALERT**
> Do not aspirate balloon vigorously. Doing so may collapse inflation lumen and prevent balloon deflation.

Procedure

1. Remove tape attaching catheter to client.
2. Insert syringe hub into balloon port of catheter. Do not cut port with scissors. **Rationale:** Balloon may not totally deflate if port is cut.
3. Withdraw fluid from balloon (usually 5–10 mL water in balloon).
4. Pull gently on catheter to ensure balloon is deflated before attempting to remove. **Rationale:** Damage to urethra can occur if balloon is not totally deflated.
5. Hold a paper towel under catheter with your nondominant hand.
6. If resistance is not met, slowly withdraw catheter allowing it to fall into paper towel.
7. Disconnect catheter bag from bed frame.
8. Empty catheter drainage bag into graduate and measure.
9. Record output on I&O bedside record.
10. Dispose of catheter in appropriate receptacle.
11. Wash perineum with soap and water. Dry thoroughly. Remove gloves.

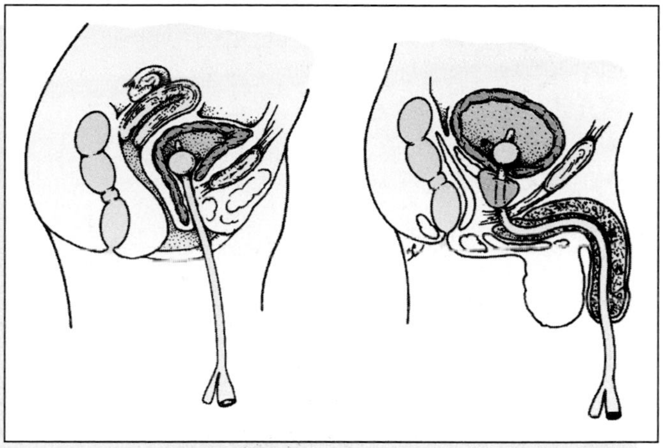

Balloon must be deflated before removing to prevent damage to urethra.

12. Position client for comfort.
13. Wash your hands.
14. Instruct client to drink oral fluids as tolerated and observe for signs and symptoms of urinary tract infections (burning, frequency, urgency).
15. Offer bedpan or urinal after removing catheter, until voiding occurs. Keep accurate I&O record.
16. Report to physician if client has not urinated in 8 hours.

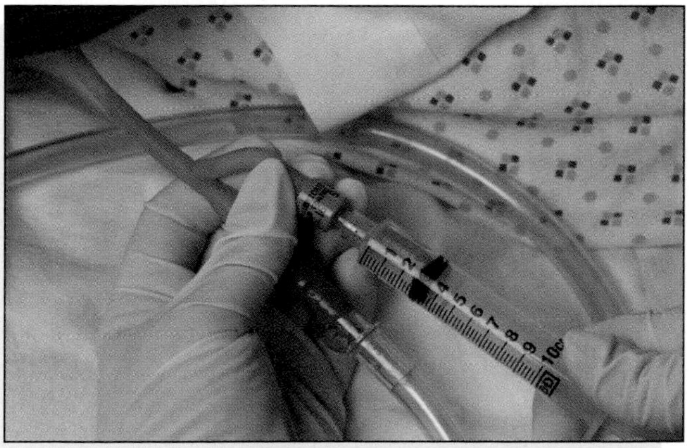

Insert syringe hub into balloon port and withdraw fluid (size of balloon is specified in print).

DOCUMENTATION FOR CATHETERIZATION

- Time and purpose
- Type and size of catheter
- Amount, color, and odor of urine obtained
- Client's tolerance of procedure
- Specimen sent to lab (if ordered)
- Catheter care provided
- Condition of urinary meatus
- Catheter removed
- Voiding: time and amount after catheter removal
- Intake and output
- Residual volume amount and time since last void

Critical Thinking Application

UNEXPECTED OUTCOMES	CRITICAL THINKING OPTIONS
Bladder scan gives no reading	• Make certain that adequate conducting gel has been used. • Have obese client bend knees so that feet are flat on the bed. • Have thin client partially sit up to compress abdomen. • Apply more pressure with scanhead, depressing 1–2 inches into client's abdomen.
Catheter is inserted in the vagina of a female client.	• Leave the catheter in place and follow these actions: a. Have someone obtain a new catheter and new gloves. You may need a whole new kit if contamination of the sterile field has occurred. b. Reposition your fingers to assist in visualizing the urethral meatus. c. Locate the client's urinary meatus before inserting the catheter and repeat procedure.
Catheter is contaminated when attempting to insert.	• Obtain a new catheter and repeat the catheterization. • If the sterile field has been contaminated, obtain a new catheter kit. Repeat the procedure.
Unable to insert catheter into a male client.	• Obtain a new catheter kit and follow these actions. a. Hold penis vertical to client's body. b. Insert catheter while applying slight traction by gently pulling upward on the shaft of the penis. c. If you encounter resistance, rotate the catheter, increase the traction, and lower the angle of the penis slightly.
Urine leaks around catheter.	• Catheter may not be inserted above sphincter, but rather in the urethral channel. It may be necessary to insert a new catheter. • Check amount of fluid in catheter balloon. If balloon is underinflated, leakage may occur. • Fill balloon to 10 mL with sterile water to provide sufficient volume to fill catheter inflation lumen as well. Bacteriostatic water and sodium chloride contain substances which affect the integrity of the balloon.

UNEXPECTED OUTCOMES	CRITICAL THINKING OPTIONS
Urine exceeds 500 mL with catheterization.	• Clamp catheter for 10 minutes and then unclamp. • If bladder appears to be grossly distended when palpated, insert Foley catheter instead of straight catheter. a. If urine exceeds 500 mL, inflate balloon and clamp for 10 minutes. b. Open clamp and drain remaining urine. c. Monitor client's vital signs; watch for hypotension, pallor, diaphoresis.

UNIT 4

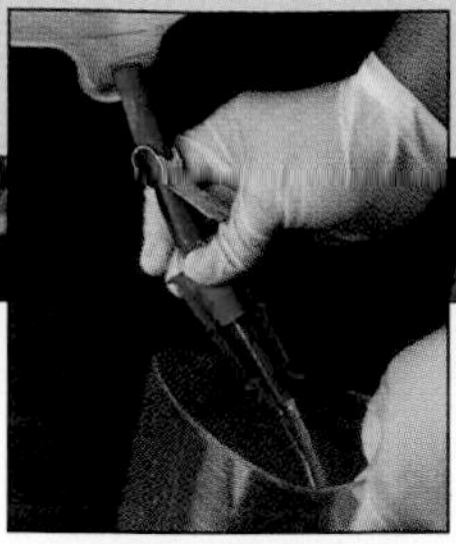

Bladder Irrigation

Nursing Process Data

ASSESSMENT ***Data Base***

Determine rationale for irrigation.

Note rate of urine flow from bladder, color of urine, presence of clots or debris.

Assess for distended bladder.

Assess for bladder discomfort.

Note client's I&O balance.

PLANNING ***Objectives***

To remove blood clots from client's bladder

To ensure patency of drainage system

To relieve bladder spasms

IMPLEMENTATION ***Procedures***

Irrigating by Opening a Closed System

Irrigating a Closed System

Maintaining Continuous Bladder Irrigation

EVALUATION ***Expected Outcomes***

Blood clots are removed from client's bladder.

Continuous flow of solution is maintained to evacuate clots and prevent catheter obstruction.

Catheter remains patent and unobstructed by clots or sediment.

Net urine output is determined.

IRRIGATING BY OPENING A CLOSED SYSTEM

Equipment

Sterile irrigation set with catheter tip syringe (new set for each irrigation)
Clean gloves,
Sterile normal saline irrigant (or solution as ordered)
Catch basin
Antiseptic swab
Absorbent pad
Sterile protective cap for tubing
Pain or antispasmodic medication

Preparation

1. Check physician's order for system irrigation and client care plan.
2. Gather equipment.
3. Check client's identaband.
4. Explain procedure and rationale to client.
5. Wash your hands.
6. Premedicate client as indicated. **Rationale:** Manual irrigation causes painful bladder spasms.
7. Provide privacy, and place client in a comfortable position. The dorsal-recumbent position is most convenient if client can tolerate this position. Raise bed, and lower side rails if needed.

Procedure

1. Fanfold linen to expose catheter.
2. Palpate client's bladder to check for distention.
3. Open sterile container on bed or on over-bed table. Maintain sterility of inside of the container.
4. Don clean gloves.

CLINICAL ALERT

Opening a closed urinary drainage system is indicated as a last resort to reestablish catheter patency. Manual irrigation should NOT be performed with transurethral resection of a bladder tumor due to risk of bladder rupture.

5. Place an absorbent pad under connection of tubing and catheter. **Rationale:** This will form a working field for irrigating catheter.
6. Pour irrigant into solution container.
7. Place syringe in container. Do not contaminate syringe tip.
8. Place catch basin on pad to form working field. (Always keep syringe tip and irrigant uncontaminated.)
9. Disconnect catheter from drainage tube. Place sterile protective cap over the end of the drainage tube. **Rationale:** This will prevent contaminating tip of tubing.
10. Coil tubing on bed.
11. Place catheter over edge of catch basin. **Rationale:** If end of catheter touches covers, underpad, exposed skin surfaces, or drainage tube, it will be contaminated.
12. Insert irrigating syringe into catheter and attempt to aspirate any obstructing debris. **Rationale:** If irrigation is performed without removing debris, it can be forced into bladder and result in infection.
13. Withdraw irrigating solution into syringe.
14. Instill 30–50 mL of irrigant into catheter with a gentle but firm pressure.
    a. Remove syringe and allow solution to drain.
    b. Lower catch basin to facilitate solution return via gravity or aspirate instilled solution.

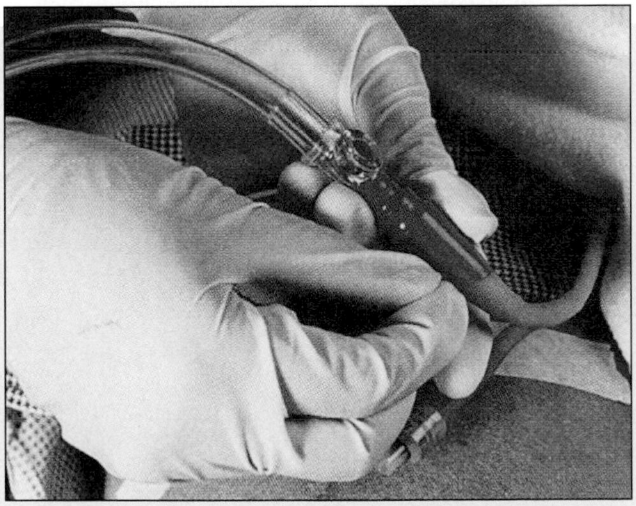

Carefully remove sealing tape to access catheter.

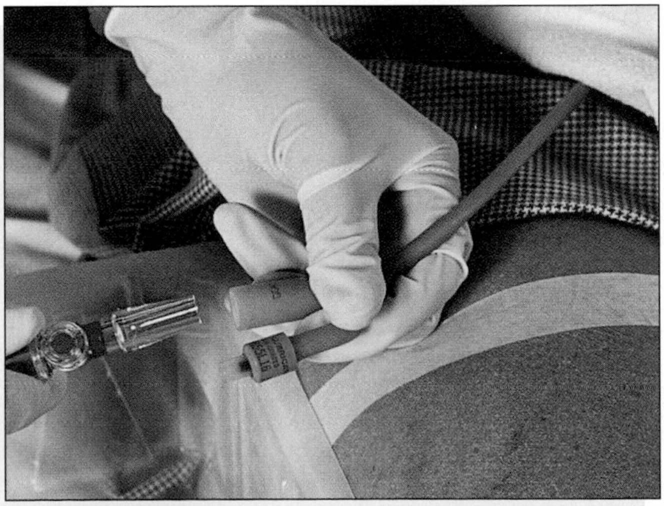

Disconnect catheter from drainage tubing; cover tubing end with sterile cap.

c. Continue to irrigate client's bladder with 30–50 mL of irrigant until fluid returns are clear or clots removed.
15. Remove the protective cap from drainage tube and wipe it with an antiseptic swab.
16. Wipe end of catheter with an antiseptic sponge, and connect the catheter to the drainage tube.
17. Ensure straight line from tubing to drainage bag. Curl excess tubing loosely on bed and secure tubing to linen.
18. Tape catheter to inner thigh for a female and to abdomen for a male.
19. Lower bed and raise side rails.
20. Discard equipment and remove gloves.
21. Make sure client is clean and comfortable. Place call light within easy reach.
22. Wash your hands.
23. Measure amount of return. Subtract any irrigating solution used to irrigate from the client's I&O record.

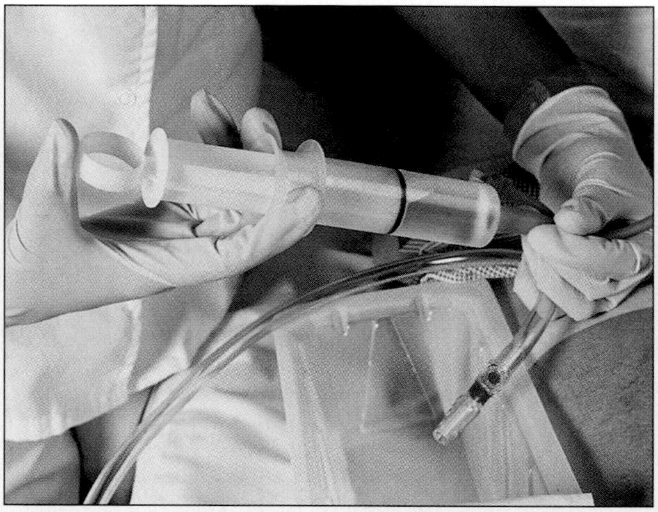

Instill 30–50 mL of irrigant into catheter to irrigate an open system.

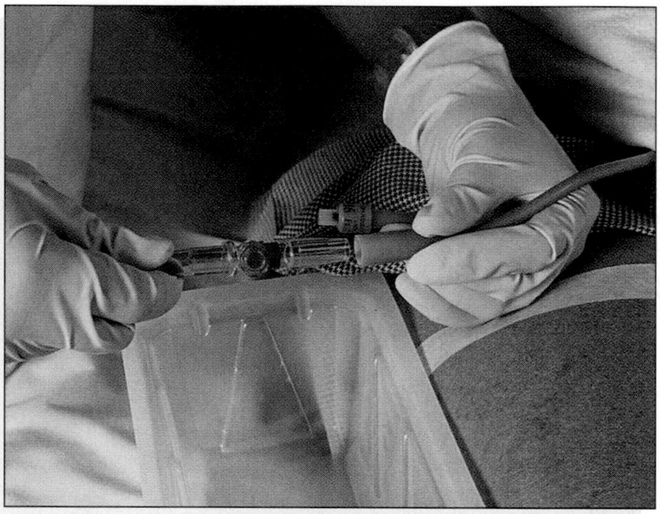

Reconnect catheter to drainage tubing using aseptic technique.

IRRIGATING A CLOSED SYSTEM

Equipment

Irrigation set
30-mL syringe with needleless cannula
Alcohol or povidone–iodine (Betadine) swab
Ordered irrigating solution (normal saline)
Clamp for drainage tubing
Clean gloves
Prepared pain medication, if ordered

Preparation

1. Check physician's order and client care plan.
2. Gather equipment.
3. Check client's identaband. Explain procedure and rationale to client.
4. Wash hands.
5. Provide privacy, and place client in dorsal-recumbent position, if tolerated.
6. Raise bed, and lower side rail on working side of bed.
7. Don clean gloves.
8. Premedicate client if ordered.
9. Empty client's urinary drainage bag and record amount.

Procedure

1. Open sterile container. Maintain sterility on inside of the container.
2. Place absorbent pad under end of catheter to form a working field.
3. Pour irrigant into solution container.
4. Clamp tubing just distal to injection port.

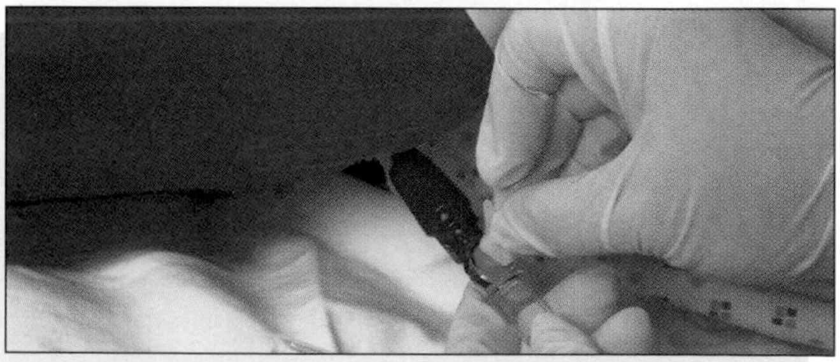

Prep injection port on catheter drainage tubing before inserting needleless cannula.

5. Swab tubing injection port with alcohol or Betadine solution.
6. Insert the needleless cannula into tubing injection port.
7. Attempt to aspirate obstructing clot or debris. **Rationale:** Irrigation without first attempting removal of debris can force it into bladder, resulting in infection.
8. Withdraw irrigating solution into syringe.
9. Swab injection port again.
10. Inject solution slowly into port. **Rationale:** To prevent back pressure in urinary drainage system.
11. Remove syringe from injection port.
12. Unclamp drainage tube, and lower catheter. **Rationale:** This facilitates drainage.
13. Repeat irrigation steps until return is free of clots and debris.
14. Lower bed and raise side rail.
15. Dispose of equipment and remove gloves.
16. Wash your hands.
17. Measure amount of return. Subtract the irrigating solution from the client's I&O record.

MAINTAINING CONTINUOUS BLADDER IRRIGATION

Equipment

Irrigating solution (2,000 mL sterile normal saline) as prescribed
IV tubing with roller clamp
IV pole
Alcohol or povidone–iodine (Betadine) swab
Clean gloves

Procedure

1. Check physician's orders and client care plan.
2. Note if client has triple lumen indwelling catheter and drainage bag.
3. Place label on irrigating bag. Include client's name, date, room number, type of solution, and additives.
4. Check client's identaband.
5. Explain procedure to client and provide privacy.
6. Wash your hands and don clean gloves.
7. Remove protective covering from spike on tubing, and insert spike into insertion port of solution container. Use aseptic technique.
8. Hang irrigating solution container on IV pole and prime tubing. Height of pole is usually 24–36 inches above bladder.
   a. Remove protective cover from end of tubing using aseptic technique.
   b. Open roller clamp, and allow irrigating solution to run through tubing until all air is expelled. **Rationale:** This prevents air from entering bladder and causing discomfort.
   c. Close roller clamp.
9. Connect tubing to catheter irrigating (indwell) lumen using aseptic technique.
10. Remove gloves.
11. Adjust drip rate of irrigating solution by adjusting the clamp on the tubing to increase or decrease based on urine outflow color.

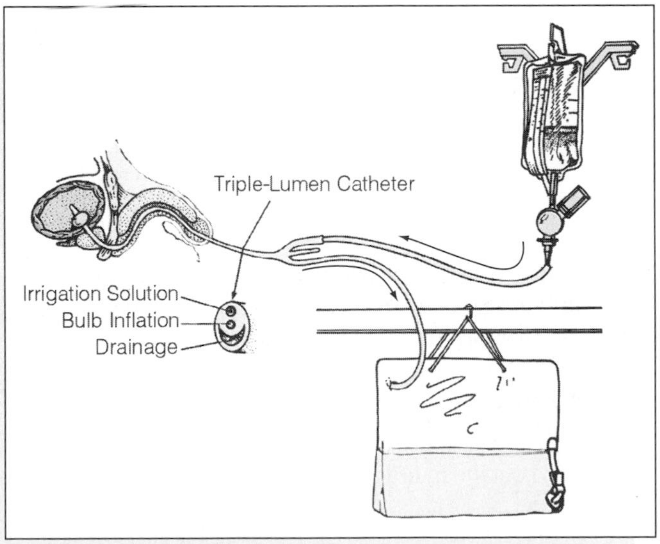

Maintain continuous bladder irrigation by using a triple-lumen catheter for procedure.

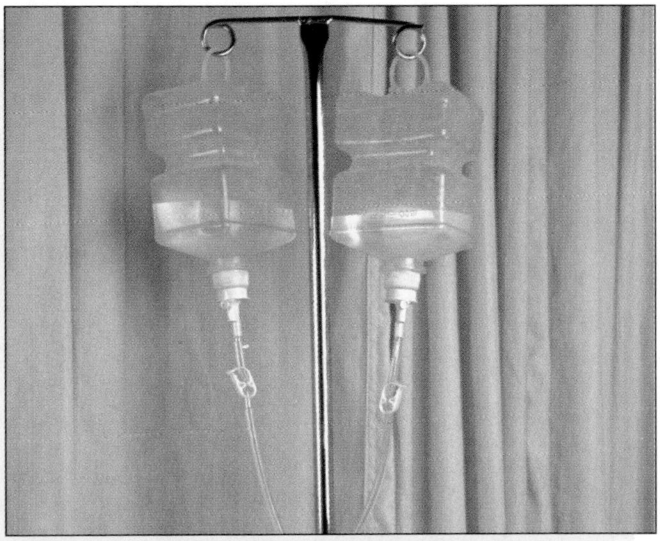
Hang irrigating solution on IV pole at height of 24–36 inches above bladder.

a. Infuse continuously to keep urine drainage pink to clear.
b. When drainage is dark red or contains blood clots, increase drip rate. **Rationale:** Increased drip rate will clear the drainage and flush out clots.
c. Change irrigation solution bottle using aseptic technique.

12. Check for bladder distention or abdominal pain; note urine color.
13. Monitor urine output at least every hour to observe patency of system.
14. Empty drainage bag as needed. Subtract amount of irrigant infused from total output to obtain urine output and record.
15. Maintain catheter traction if taped to thigh. **Rationale:** This promotes venous hemostasis.
16. Remove gloves and wash hands.

Note: Procedure is done to flush clots and debris from bladder following prostatic surgery, and to prevent catheter obstruction and promote patency.

DOCUMENTATION FOR BLADDER IRRIGATION

- Type and amount of solution administered for irrigation
- Rate of administration of irrigating solution
- Description of urinary output, including color and presence of clots or debris
- Any signs of discomfort or cramping
- Medication given for pain.
- Amount of actual urine output (total urine output minus amount of irrigant instilled)

Critical Thinking Application

UNEXPECTED OUTCOMES	CRITICAL THINKING OPTIONS
Irrigation flow is not infusing at prescribed rate.	• May need to raise or lower IV standard with attached irrigation bag to assist in regulating flow using gravity. • Move the flow adjuster clamp to a new site on the tubing if flow is slower than ordered. Tubing may be collapsed due to constant pressure from clamp. • If infusion rate slows, may indicate clots are blocking flow. Irrigate catheter following physician's orders.
Irrigation solution is not returned because of an obstruction in the system.	• Follow these steps to obtain irrigation solution: a. Check tubing for kinks. b. Have client change position. c. Aspirate the solution from the catheter, using moderate "pull back" pressure. d. If the irrigant does not return, palpate the client's bladder and instill 30–50 mL of irrigating solution to agitate and clear any clots. e. If irrigant does not return, reconnect urinary system and observe for 30 minutes. Bladder spasms can block the flow of urine through the system. f. If irrigant still does not return after performing the above procedures, notify physician for further orders.
Client experiences excessive bladder spasms.	• Notify physician to obtain an order for urinary antispasmodic. • Assist client to change position.

UNEXPECTED OUTCOMES	CRITICAL THINKING OPTIONS
Bright red drainage continues even when solution flow rate is increased.	• Notify physician immediately. • Obtain vital signs and continuously monitor. • Continue to infuse solution at a rapid rate to flush client's bladder until you obtain physician's orders. • Do not allow client to cough. • Keep client's catheter-taped leg straight to maintain traction on catheter inflation bulb.

UNIT 5

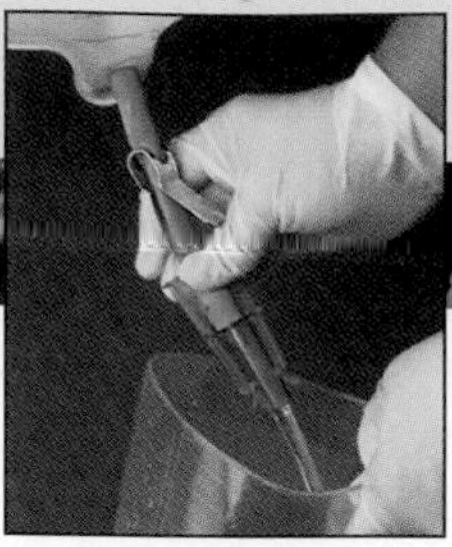

Suprapubic Catheter Care

Nursing Process Data

ASSESSMENT Data Base

Observe for urine flow through catheter.

Observe for excessive bleeding through catheter or at insertion site.

Check that suture site is clean, dry, and intact.

Check that straight drainage is maintained.

Assess that fluid intake is at least 2,000 mL daily.

Assess client for pain, bladder distention, or spasms.

Assess client's ability to assist with clamping procedure.

Assess client's ability to tolerate catheter being clamped.

PLANNING Objectives

To prevent urinary tract infection when a suprapubic catheter is inserted

To maintain a patent suprapubic catheter

To monitor the catheter clamping procedure

To prevent infection at catheter insertion site

To provide discharge teaching if catheter is to remain in place when client is discharged

IMPLEMENTATION Procedures

Providing Suprapubic Catheter Care

EVALUATION Expected Outcomes

Catheter remains patent; bladder drains completely.

Client voids spontaneously after routine clamping.

Client remains free of urinary tract infections.

Insertion site is clean and dry.

PROVIDING SUPRAPUBIC CATHETER CARE

Equipment

Closed drainage system, including Foley catheter tubing and bag
Catheter clamp and plug
Dry sterile dressing and tape if ordered
Cleansing solution
Clean gloves
Sterile gloves

Preparation

1. Check physician's orders and client care plan.
2. Explain purpose of catheter.
3. Describe procedure for monitoring and clamping suprapubic catheter.
4. Wash your hands.
5. Provide privacy.

Procedure

1. Observe catheter for patency. **Rationale:** The most common problem with suprapubic catheters is occlusion with sediment or clots.
   a. First 24 hours: check the catheter every hour to detect possible obstruction. Urine output should be in excess of 30 mL/hour.
   b. Second day: check the catheter every 8 hours.
   c. Third day: check the catheter when the catheter is unclamped.
2. Maintain a closed drainage system. Do not open system to irrigate or obtain urine sample.
3. Observe for signs and symptoms of urinary tract infection (color, odor, presence of sediment).
4. Keep the dressing dry around site of insertion. Apply a new dressing, maintaining sterile technique, every morning and as necessary at other times.
   a. Wash hands and don clean gloves.
   b. Remove old dressing and discard in appropriate container.
   c. Wash hands and open sterile supplies.
   d. Open cleansing solution and pour over sterile gauze.
   e. Don sterile gloves.
   f. Assess skin surrounding suprapubic catheter.
   g. Cleanse area with cleansing solution. Allow to dry.
   h. Apply sterile dressing and secure with tape.
   i. Remove gloves and supplies and discard in appropriate container.
   j. Wash hands.
5. Perform clamping protocol according to physician orders. Use this protocol or clamp according to facility policies and procedures.
   a. Explain the clamping procedure and ask client to help you monitor the clamping.
   b. Instruct client to notify you if he or she feels fullness in the bladder during clamping.
   c. Don clean gloves.
   d. Clamp the catheter.
6. Empty the drainage bag or remove drainage tubing from catheter, maintaining aseptic technique.
   a. Place drainage tubing in sterile package to maintain sterility.
   b. Place catheter plug in catheter end.
   c. Remove gloves.
   d. Record urine output on I&O bedside record.
   e. Leave the catheter clamped or plugged for 3–4 hours depending on client's level of comfort and physician's orders.
7. At 3- to 4-hour intervals, or when client feels fullness in bladder, ask client to void normally. Don clean gloves to measure the urine and record output on I&O bedside record.
8. Immediately after client voids, unclamp catheter and leave unclamped for 5 minutes, collecting the residual urine.
   a. Don clean gloves to measure the residual urine following unclamping of the catheter.
   b. Reclamp catheter.
   c. Send a urine specimen to laboratory after the first clamping. **Rationale:** This checks for the presence of microorganisms.
9. Repeat clamping protocol every 3–4 hours according to physician orders. The catheter may be open to drainage from bedtime until 6 in the morning.
10. When the client is voiding normally, clamp the catheter throughout the night in preparation for its removal.
11. When the client's residual urine output is less than 100 mL or retains less than 20% of residual urine on two successive checks, notify the physician for removal of the catheter.

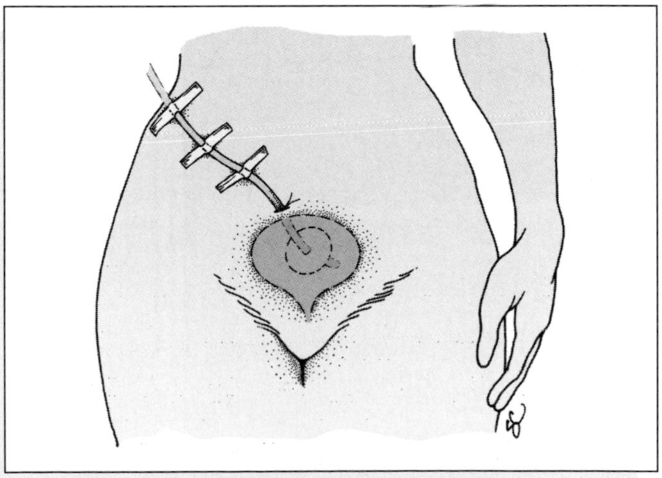

Tape catheter and connect to a closed system.

12. Apply a Band-Aid or small 2 × 2 sterile dressing over the insertion site.
13. Dispose of the catheter in biohazard bag.
14. If the client is discharged from the hospital with the catheter, provide the following teaching for home care:
    a. Instruct the client to drink one glass of fluid every hour while awake.
    b. Instruct client to follow clamping procedure when awake or as instructed by physician.
    c. Instruct the client to leave the catheter open to the drainage system at night. (Drainage system may be urinary tubing and bag or leg bag.)
    d. Tell client to notify physician if dysuria occurs when voiding or if urine becomes cloudy, odorous, or full of sediment.

DOCUMENTATION FOR SUPRAPUBIC CATHETER CARE

- Time catheter clamped
- Length of time clamped
- Client's ability to void spontaneously
- Client's feelings of fullness
- Time specimen sent to laboratory
- Color, amount, and odor of urine obtained
- Color, amount, and odor of residual urine

Critical Thinking Application

UNEXPECTED OUTCOMES	CRITICAL THINKING OPTIONS
Suprapubic catheter was not sutured in place and becomes dislodged.	• Place sterile dressing over puncture site. Do not attempt to replace the catheter. • Notify physician immediately. • Have new suprapubic catheter ready for insertion by physician.
Client develops urinary tract infection.	• Observe client for signs and symptoms of urinary tract infection: temperature; cloudy, foul-smelling urine with sediment present; bladder spasms. • Inform physician of possible urinary tract infection and obtain order for urinary antibiotic. • Force fluids to at least 2000 mL per day unless contraindicated by diagnosis. Give cranberry juice or fluids that acidify urine. • Clarify physician's order for protocol regarding clamping catheter or keeping the catheter open to straight drainage while evidence of infection is present.
Client unable to void spontaneously through urethra.	• Notify physician for orders.

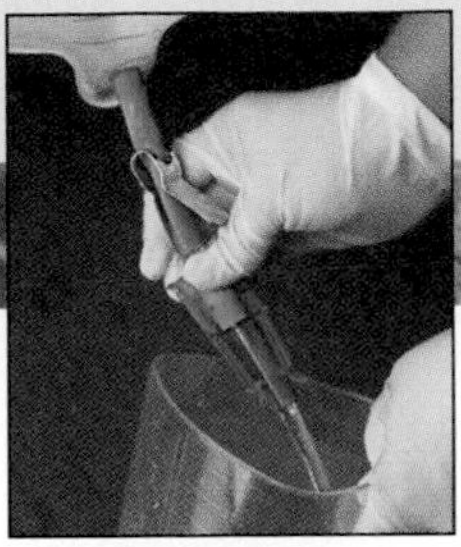

Specimens from Closed Systems

Nursing Process Data

ASSESSMENT *Data Base*

Assess the type of specimen needed: Sterile specimens for culture and sensitivity tests; clean specimens for urinalysis.

Check to see if the closed urinary system has a port for obtaining a specimen or catheter is made of self-sealing material (not silastic or silicone).

Identify amount of urine needed for specimen.

PLANNING *Objectives*

To prevent urinary infection by obtaining a urine specimen without interrupting a closed urinary drainage system

To determine the specific microorganism causing a urinary tract infection

To obtain a urine specimen for use in a diagnostic urinary workup

IMPLEMENTATION *Procedures*

Collecting Specimen from a Closed System

EVALUATION *Expected Outcomes*

Noncontaminated urine specimen is obtained from the closed urinary drainage system.

Catheter does not develop a leak from improper puncture for urine specimen.

COLLECTING SPECIMEN FROM A CLOSED SYSTEM

Equipment

Catheter tubing clamp
Syringe with needleless cannula
Sterile specimen container and label
Antimicrobial or alcohol swab
Clean gloves

Procedure

1. Gather equipment.
2. Identify client by checking identaband.
3. Explain the procedure and rationale to the client. Clamp drainage tubing for 15 minutes. **Rationale:** This ensures urine specimen is adequate.
4. Wash your hands and don gloves.
5. Wipe the aspiration port of the drainage tubing with the antimicrobial or alcohol swab.
6. Insert needleless cannula at a 30°–45° angle into aspiration port. Allow urine to accumulate in tubing. (2 mL urine is sufficient for a specimen.)
7. Aspirate the urine sample by gently pulling back on syringe plunger, and then remove syringe.
8. Wipe aspiration port with antimicrobial swab. Remove clamp.
9. Empty syringe into sterile urine container. (Sometimes urine is sent to the laboratory in special collection syringe.)
10. Remove and discard gloves.
11. Wash your hands.
12. Label container, and take it to the laboratory within 15 minutes. If this is not possible, refrigerate specimen.

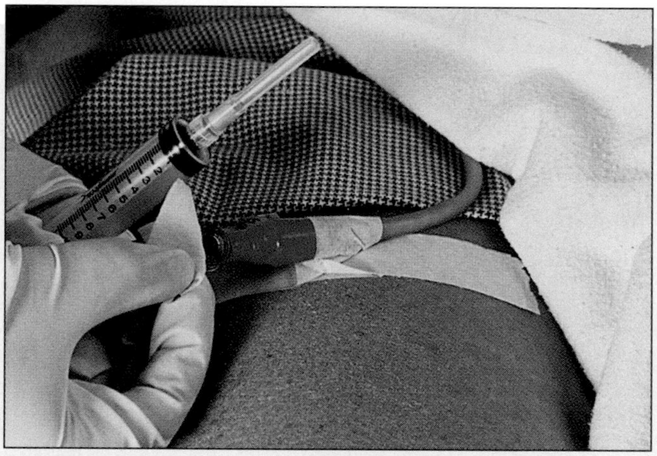

Wipe aspiration port before inserting sterile syringe and needle or syringe with needleless cannula.

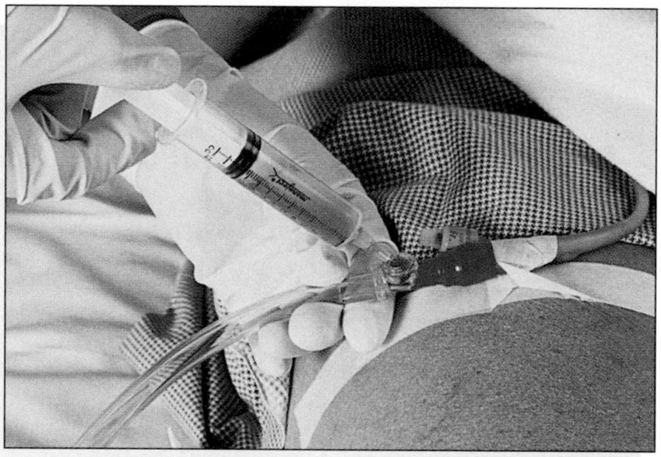

Insert needle or needleless cannula at 30°–45° angle into aspiration port and gently pull back on barrel of syringe.

DOCUMENTATION FOR SPECIMENS FROM CLOSED SYSTEMS

- Type of specimen obtained
- Mode of obtaining specimen from port
- Color, consistency, and odor of urine
- Time of urine collection
- Time specimen sent to laboratory

Critical Thinking Application

UNEXPECTED OUTCOMES	CRITICAL THINKING OPTIONS
Insufficient amount of urine available when specimen collection is attempted.	• Clamp catheter tubing for 30 minutes. • Reposition client. • Check for kinking of catheter.
Signs and symptoms of urinary tract infection occur.	• Notify the physician of client's signs and symptoms. • Make sure there are no kinks in urinary system tubing or that the system is not clamped off. This ensures that the urine drains into the catheter bag and does not stagnate in bladder. • Give ordered antibiotics on correct time schedule. • Do not interrupt the closed urinary drainage system.
Bacteremia develops secondary to urinary tract infection.	• Administer antibiotics as ordered. • Encourage client to force fluids to flush out bladder. • Use cranberry juice or other acid-producing (noncitric) juices. • Obtain frequent vital signs and assessment data. • Observe color and clarity of urine for further infectious problems.

UNIT 7

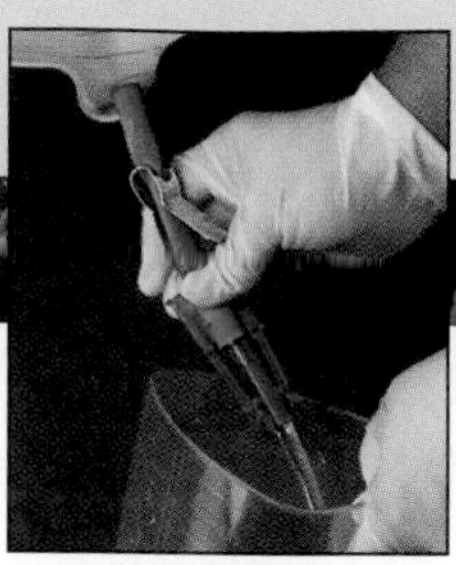

Urinary Diversion

Nursing Process Data

ASSESSMENT *Data Base*

Assess location of stoma on client's abdomen. (Depends on type of diversion.)

Determine type of urinary diversion.

Observe stoma color (same color as mucous membrane lining the mouth).

Assess skin for erythema and excoriation.

Assess presence of ureteral stents for new ureterostomy.

Assess most appropriate pouching system for client. (System depends on client's age, manual dexterity, and size of stoma.)

Assess client's ability to manage self-care.

Assess urine output (amount and character).

PLANNING *Objectives*

To provide a pouching system that prevents skin irritation

To instruct the client in self-care

To monitor stoma for viability

To obtain a sterile urine specimen

IMPLEMENTATION *Procedures*

Applying a Urinary Diversion Pouch

Obtaining Specimen from an Ileal Conduit

Catheterizing Continent Urinary Reservoir

EVALUATION *Expected Outcomes*

Client demonstrates self-care skills.

Pouching system fits tightly, and skin remains free of irritation.

Sterile urine specimen is obtained.

Stoma remains viable.

Urine output balances intake

APPLYING A URINARY DIVERSION POUCH

Equipment

One- or two-piece urinary pouch with skin barrier, flange, and spigot at bottom of pouch to empty urine
Items to clean stoma (e.g., soft cloth or gauze sponges) and warm water
Plastic bag for disposal of used equipment
Tissue for drying skin
Tissue or tampon for wicking stoma
Underpad to protect bedding
Scissors if indicated
Protective barriers such as skin prep, skin gel, or protective barrier film
Stoma measuring guide
Clean gloves

Preparation

1. Check physician's order and client care plan. Pouch should be changed every 3–7 days.
2. Gather equipment.
3. Wash your hands.
4. Identify client and explain procedure.
5. Provide privacy.
6. Place client in supine position or in a position that promotes self-care.
7. Place bath blanket over client's chest and position top covers over lower abdomen.
8. Place protective pad under client.

Procedure

1. Don clean gloves.
2. Prepare new urinary pouch. First measure stoma site with measuring guide, unless pouch has pre-cut opening.
3. Trace size of stoma on wafer and cut 1/16–1/8 inch larger than size. **Rationale:** This small opening prevents leakage of effluent onto skin; however, the size is large enough to prevent pressure on the stoma from the wafer rubbing on skin.

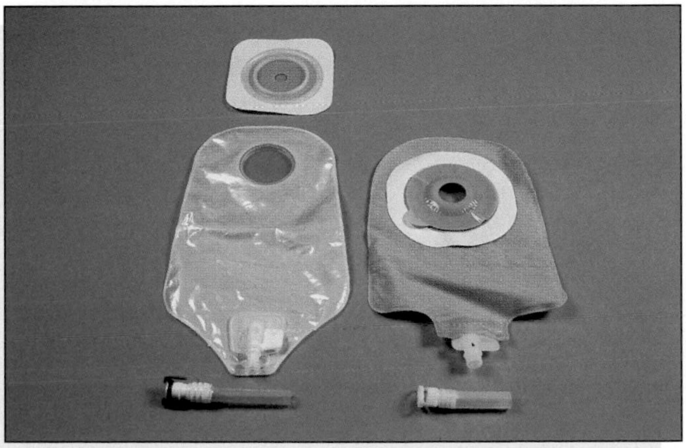

One-piece and two-piece urinary diversion appliances.

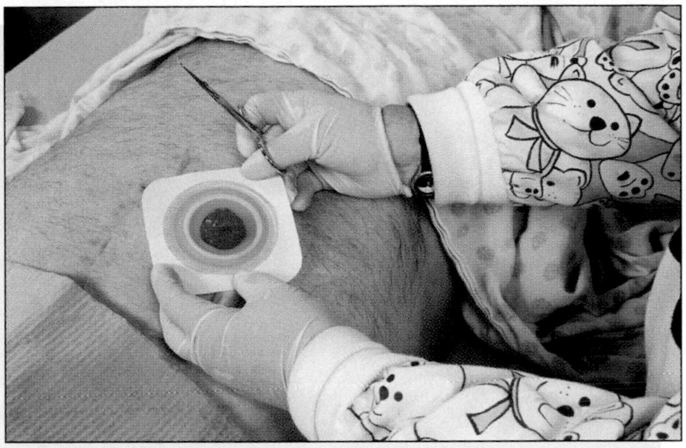

Cut wafer opening slightly larger than stoma.

4. Snap pouch onto flange.
5. Empty, then remove old pouch, and discard in plastic bag. Remove wafer slowly beginning at top and use gauze to press skin away as wafer is peeled off.
6. Wash skin with warm water and dry thoroughly. **Rationale:** Chemical or perfumed wipes can irritate delicate skin so should not be used to clean around stoma.

Note: Stoma may bleed slightly when wiped.

7. Check stoma for healing; it should be bright red and moist, round and raised 1/2–1 inch above skin surface (or may be flush).

Note: This may be an appropriate time to teach client to check status of stoma and skin around stoma.

8. Wick stoma with tissue or tampon. **Rationale:** To keep urine from contact with skin during pouch change.
9. Check skin surrounding stoma to ensure effluent hasn't been draining under wafer causing skin irritation.
10. Apply protective barrier to healthy skin surrounding stoma or to wafer if indicated. **Rationale:** Protective barriers contain alcohol and cause burning and pain, and may interfere with seal.

CLINICAL ALERT

Thin plastic tubes (stents) may be placed in each ureter during surgery. These exit stoma and remain in place for up to 10 days. They serve to maintain patency until swelling has subsided at ureteroileal anastamosis site (6–10 days). Their presence and length of exposure should be documented. The surgeon should be notified when they wash out into collection appliance.

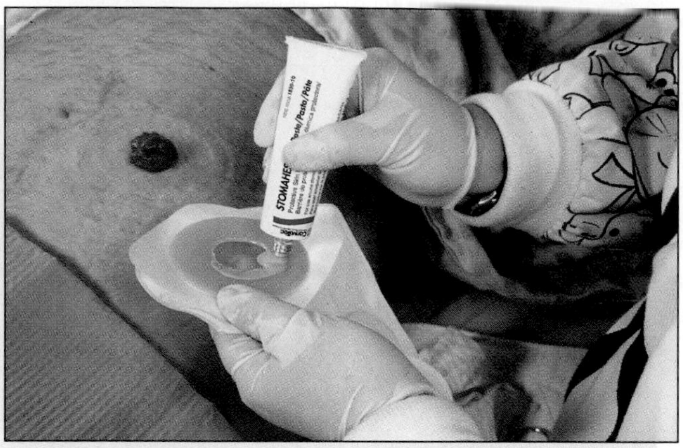

Apply protective barrier paste to wafer, if indicated.

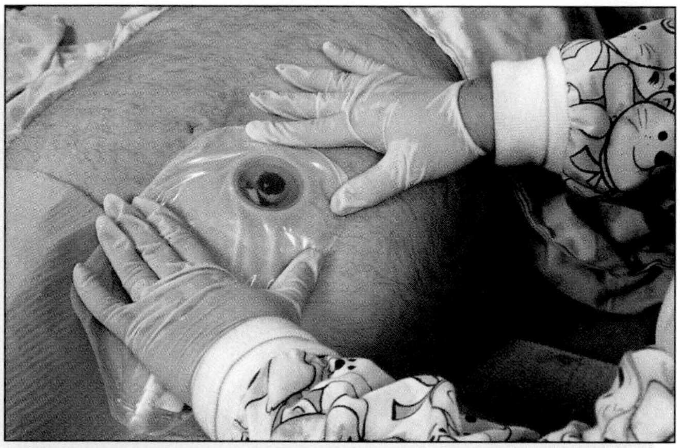

Apply pouch and press firmly to facilitate seal.

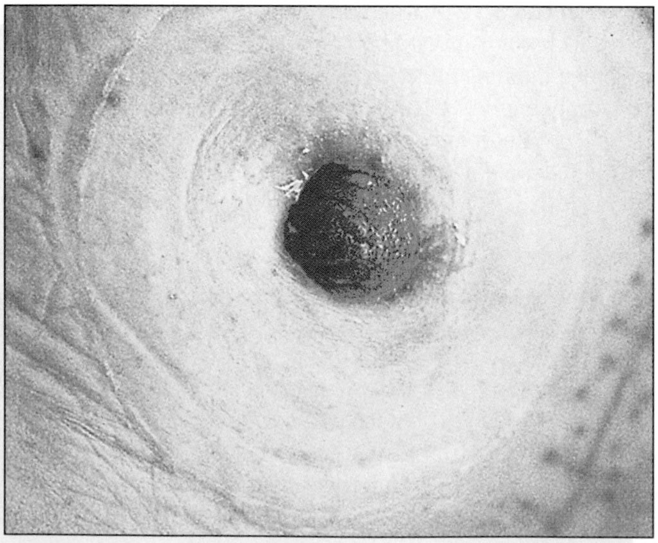

Well-healed urinary diversion stoma.

Client Teaching for Emptying Appliance

Instruct client to

- Empty appliance when 1/3 full.
- Use bathroom if possible.
- Place distal end of pouch between thighs into toilet.
- Open drainage port to allow urine to drain.
- Clean drain port with soapy warm water.
- Close drainage port.
- Wash hands.

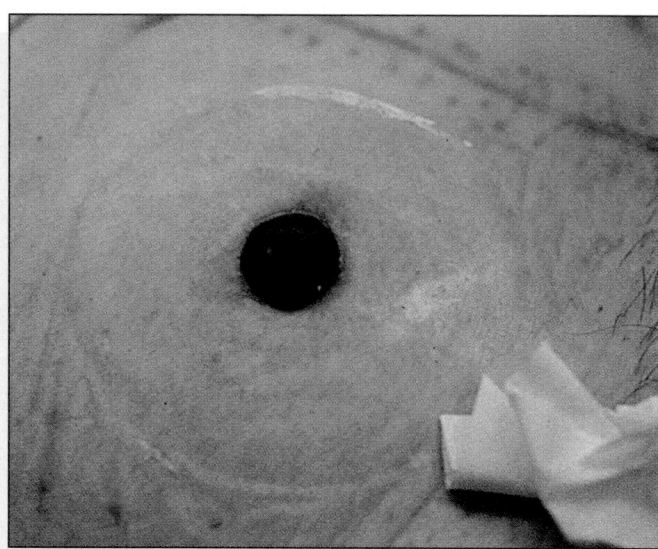

Ileal conduit stoma.

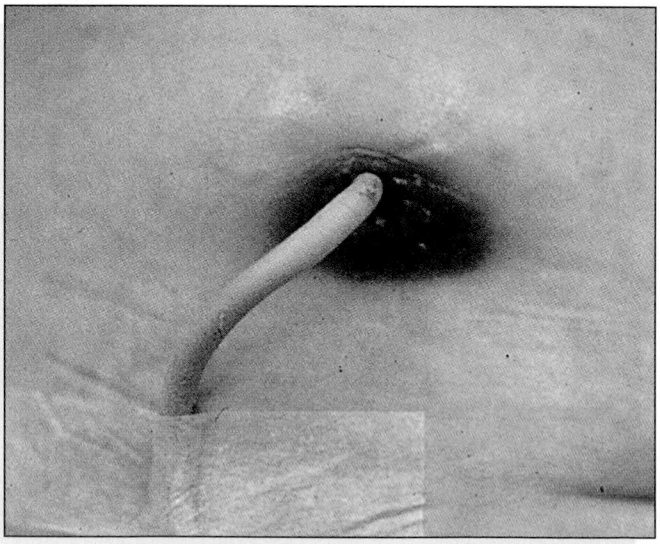

Ureterostomy with catheter.

Four Types of Urinary Diversion	Nursing Considerations
Ileal or Colonic Conduit	
• Urostomy constructed from portion of bowel—ileum is resected and an internal pouch formed and attached to abdominal wall. • Ureters are connected to internal pouch. • An external appliance collects urine output. • Stoma is larger than ureterostomy.	• Care of urinary appliance. • Monitor periostomal skin for breakdown. • Monitor stoma.
Continent Urostomy (Kock's Reservoir)	
• Reservoir is constructed from ileum and ascending colon. Two nipple valves are created by pulling ileum back onto itself. • Ureters are implanted near internal nipple valve (valve prevents reflux). • Outlet valve is attached to abdominal wall and stoma. • Catheters are inserted to drain urine.	• Instruct in clean intermittent self-catheterization every 2–4 hours.
Indiana Pouch	
• Internal pouch is created from the ascending colon and terminal ileum. • Pouch is larger than Kock's reservoir. • Catheters are inserted into internal pouch to drain urine.	• Instruct in clean intermittent self-catheterization every 2–4 hours. • Monitor for electrolyte imbalance; reservoir may absorb urea and electrolytes.
Neo Bladder	
• Created from cecum or ileum with ureters attached. • Has no stoma. • Requires no external appliance. • Preserves normal body image.	• Client may eliminate with timed voiding. • May require self urethral catheterization.

11. Let dry thoroughly.
12. Remove paper from adhesive on wafer or one-piece appliance.
13. Remove wick and center wafer or pouch over stoma; apply to dry skin, starting at bottom, and working up around stoma.
14. Attach pouch to gravity drainage bag only while client is in bed. Pouch has a spout at end to drain urine. Empty pouch when one-third full.
15. Discard equipment in appropriate receptacle.
16. Remove gloves and wash hands.

OBTAINING SPECIMEN FROM AN ILEAL CONDUIT

Equipment

Sterile catheter kit
Prep solution
Sterile saline or water
Underpad
New urinary pouch
Supplies to apply new pouch
Bath blanket, towels
Clean gloves
Soap and water

Preparation

1. Check physician's orders and client care plan.
2. Gather equipment.
3. Wash your hands.
4. Explain procedure to client.
5. Provide privacy.
6. Place bath blanket over client's chest and position top covers over lower abdomen.
7. Place towels around stoma. **Rationale:** Urine will leak around catheter.
8. Don gloves.

Procedure

1. Open sterile packages.
2. Remove pouch. *Note:* Do not use pouch contents to obtain urine specimen. Remove gloves.
3. Put on sterile gloves.
4. Place sterile drape over stoma.
5. Remove top from specimen container, and place end of catheter into container.
6. Apply lubricant to catheter.
7. Use forceps to pick up cotton ball and prep stoma with solution and rinse with sterile saline or water.
8. Insert tip of catheter into stoma. When abdominal musculature relaxes, slide catheter into conduit, approximately 1½ inches.
9. When urine specimen is obtained (usually not more than 5–25 mL), clamp catheter with fingers and remove.
10. Return lid to specimen container and apply label.
11. Remove completely any residual prep solution and lubricant; wash and dry peristomal area.
12. Replace pouch, or apply new pouch.
13. Remove gloves and wash hands.
14. Send specimen to lab immediately or refrigerate.

CATHETERIZING CONTINENT URINARY RESERVOIR

Equipment

Clean catheter
Water-soluble lubricant
Clean gloves
Bedpan (if client unable to use toilet)
Plastic bag
Warm water and soap
Washcloth, towel

Preparation

1. Check physician's orders and client care plan.
2. Gather equipment.
3. Identify client and explain procedure.
4. Wash hands and don gloves.
5. Provide privacy.
6. Position client on chair facing toilet or place bedpan next to client if on bedrest.

Procedure

1. Remove appliance or dressing if present.
2. Remove clean catheter from plastic bag.
3. Lubricate tip of catheter.
4. Insert catheter 1½–2 inches into stoma. Place distal end of catheter into toilet or bedpan.
5. Instruct client to take deep breath as you gently insert catheter through nipple valve until urine returns. **Rationale:** When the abdominal muscles are relaxed it is easier to advance catheter through nipple valve.
6. Leave catheter in place until urine stops draining.
7. Pinch catheter, and remove gently.
8. Wash and dry peristomal area with soap and water.
9. Replace pouch or dressing if needed. Assist client back to bed, or position for comfort.
10. Clean catheter with warm soap and water, allow to dry, and place in clean plastic bag. Return to storage area in client's bathroom.
11. Remove gloves and wash hands.

Documentation for Urinary Diversion

- Color and amount of urine obtained from catheterizing continent reservoir
- Catheter size used for catheterization
- Status of ureteral stents, if present
- Peristomal skin and stoma condition
- Client's acceptance of stoma, participation in self-care
- Type and method of drainage pouch applied
- Specimen sent to lab

Critical Thinking Application

UNEXPECTED OUTCOMES	CRITICAL THINKING OPTIONS
Appliance does not keep client dry.	• Check area for crease or dip in skin which allows urine to pool and leak out. • Fill in area with skin barrier to prevent pooling. • Belt may be applied to minimize leak if it appears on one side only. • Try applying another type of appliance. • If leak due to dissolving of skin barrier, change more frequently or change to different barrier. • Advise client to avoid using soaps or wipes to clean the area because they interfere with pouch adhesions.
Client unable to manage own urinary diversion.	• Simplify pouch procedure if possible. Provide detailed instruction in a more simplified manner if possible. • Include family in teaching to enable them to support and assist the client. • May need referral to home health care facility for follow-up care.
Unable to insert catheter into conduit.	• Insert catheter into stoma but do not force it. Wait for a few seconds to see if abdominal muscles relax enough to allow catheter to slide in. If not, notify physician. • Have client take in a deep breath to relax abdominal muscles.
No urine obtained from conduit.	• Rotate catheter, or position client on side to allow urine to flow into catheter. As little as 1–3 mL is needed for culture and sensitivity.
Odor in appliance.	• Odor usually due to alkaline urine in pouch turning to ammonia. Keep urine acidic by taking vitamin C, 500 mg b.i.d. to t.i.d., and drinking cranberry juice. Other citrus juices should be avoided because they form an alkaline ash. • Wash urinary equipment with mild soap and water and rinse in vinegar weekly. • Inform client that certain foods and drugs, such as asparagus and vitamin B complex, give an odor to the urine. The pouch should be emptied frequently if these substances are ingested. • Cloudy and strong odor to urine may be due to urinary tract infection. Advise physician, and collect sterile urine specimen.

UNEXPECTED OUTCOMES	CRITICAL THINKING OPTIONS
Unable to insert catheter into continent reservoir.	• Instruct client to take in deep breath as you gently push catheter into nipple valve. • Notify physician if catheterization unsuccessful; nipple valve may be malfunctioning.
Erythematous vesicular rash appears on periostomal skin.	• A possible allergic reaction. Even though the pouch material is hypoallergenic, this can appear. • Avoid use of chemical wipes and perfumed soaps.

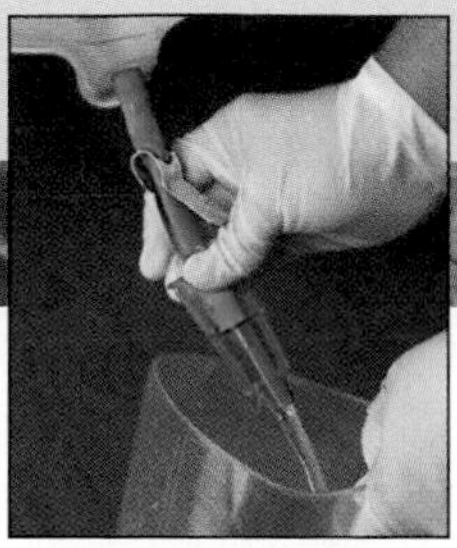

Hemodialysis (Renal Replacement Therapy)

Nursing Process Data

ASSESSMENT **Data Base**

Review dialysis orders.

Assess patency of vascular access.

Femoral vein catheter: dual-lumen vascular device used for immediate vascular access in life-threatening situations.

Central venous dual-lumen catheter (DLC): vascular device placed in internal jugular vein used for temporary access for acute hemodialysis clients.

Permanent dual-lumen catheter (PDLC): vascular device inserted through internal jugular vein and advanced to SVC.

Arteriovenous fistula: surgically created internal anastomosis between an artery and vein; used for clients undergoing chronic hemodialysis.

Arteriovenous graft: surgically implanted synthetic material (Gortex) or biologic material (human umbilical vein) used for anastomosis between an artery and vein for clients undergoing chronic hemodialysis.

Review chart and laboratory reports for factors that may alter management of dialysis (especially potassium, sodium, calcium and phosphorus levels, albumin, hemoglobin, hematocrit levels, BUN, and creatinine).

Assess vital signs.

Assess causes of hypotension: fluid loss; hypoalbuminemia; large interdialytic weight gain.

Check serum electrolytes, BUN, and creatinine before and after dialysis according to physician orders.

Weigh client before and after dialysis to determine fluid loss.

PLANNING **Objectives**

To remove end-products of protein metabolism: urea, creatinine, and uric acid

To remove excess fluid, thereby reestablishing fluid balance

To maintain or restore normal level of electrolytes in the body

To maintain a patent access site for hemodialysis

To maintain patent catheters centrally placed

To instruct the client in self-care

IMPLEMENTATION **Procedures**

Providing Hemodialysis

Providing Ongoing Care of Hemodialysis Client

Terminating Hemodialysis

Maintaining Central Venous Dual-Lumen Dialysis Catheter (DLC)

*(See Chapter 34 for CAPD Skill)

EVALUATION Expected Outcomes

Asepsis is maintained throughout the procedure.

Creatinine and BUN levels are reduced, and electrolyte balance remains in a satisfactory state.

Excess fluid is reduced.

Toxic substances are removed.

Access site remains patent.

Client is able to care for self following client teaching.

PROVIDING HEMODIALYSIS

Equipment

Dialyzer (types are hollow fiber or cellulose acetate)
1000-mL bag of 0.9% normal saline IV solution
Machine blood lines
Fistula needles, 15/16 gauge, 1–1½ inches in length
Sterile gauze pads, alcohol swabs, and povidone–iodine swabs
Two 3-mL syringes
Two 20-mL syringes
Drape
Client mask
Hemostats, cannula clamps
Tape
Sterile gloves and clean gloves
Gown
Protective goggles and face mask or visor shield
12-mL syringe
Heparin solution 1000 U/mL
Hemastix

Preparation

1. Obtain dialysate bath composition as ordered.
2. Set up 1000-mL IV of normal saline using IV tubing in blood line set.
3. Load heparin pump (e.g., 8 mL heparin) per manufacturer's instructions. **Rationale:** Heparin is added to system just before blood enters dialyzer to prevent clotting. The clotting mechanism is activated when blood moves outside body and is in contact with foreign substances.
4. Check location of nearest emergency power outlet. **Rationale:** To maintain electric current if routine power fails.
5. Test dialysis machine for presence of bleach with Hemastix. **Rationale:** This detects presence of caustic agents that could result in client complications.
6. Prime dialyzer and arterial and venous blood lines with saline.
7. Hang additional IV solution of saline. **Rationale:** Saline infusions must be available immediately for rapid reversal of hypotension or discontinuation of dialysis.
8. Connect pressure monitor lines to both arterial and venous drip chambers. **Rationale:** This monitors the amount of hydrostatic pressure exerted on blood in the ultrafiltration process used to extract fluid throughout dialysis treatment.
9. Set the alarm pressures—high and low.
10. Connect air leak detector to venous drip chamber.
11. Test all machine alarms—venous and arterial pressure, air detector, and blood leak detector.
12. Connect arterial and venous lines for recirculation with adapter, and turn blood pump to 200 mL/min.
13. Document alarm checks in dialysis log.

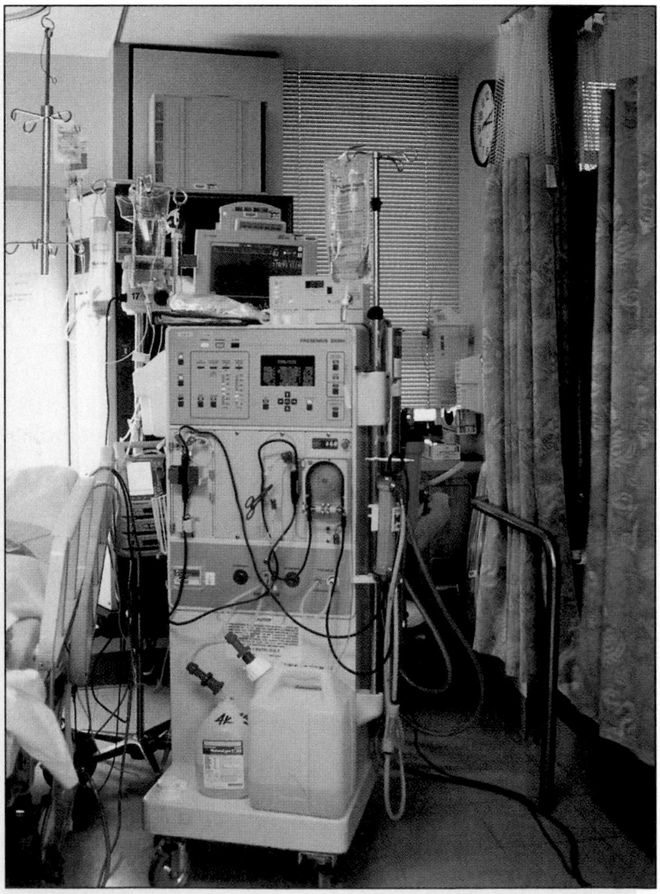

Hemodialysis unit used to treat renal failure clients.

The Hemodialysis Process

Hemodialysis works by removing blood from the client's arterial access site (graft, fistula, or catheter) circulating it through a tubing system to a dialyzer. In the dialyzer, which acts like a semipermeable membrane, fluid, electrolytes, and toxins are removed from the blood through a process of convection, osmosis, and diffusion. The blood then flows from the dialyzer through a tubing system to the client's venous access site. Fluid is removed through the use of hydrostatic pressure applied to the blood and a negative hydrostatic pressure applied to the dialysate bath. The difference between these two pressures is termed transmembrane pressure and this results in the process of ultrafiltration.

CLINICAL ALERT

When a hemodialysis client is hospitalized:

1. Place an identifying bracelet on access arm.
2. Post safety precautions at head of bed.
3. Notify dialysis specialty nurse of client's admission to hospital.

Procedure

for AV Fistula or Graft

1. Place blood line at the same level as the bed.
2. Don mask and gown. Put on goggles, and wash hands.
3. Don clean gloves, and remove dressing, if used. Remove and discard gloves.
4. Don sterile gloves.
5. Clean access site using alcohol swab, then povidone–iodine swab. Using a circular motion, cleanse from needle insertion site outward. Allow to dry. **Rationale:** Cleansing occurs from cleanest to dirtiest area preventing contamination of the site.
6. Insert needles into fistula or graft. Tape securely to extremity.
7. Obtain blood for predialysis blood samples as ordered by the physician. (Usually electrolytes, hematocrit, clotting time, etc.)
8. After blood is drawn for lab work, heparin bolus should be given to client according to physician's order—start heparin pump at ordered rate.
9. Prime the extracorporeal circuit with blood.
   a. Connect arterial tubing of the blood line to client's arterial site.
   b. Connect venous tubing.
   c. Unclamp venous blood line.
   d. Unclamp arterial blood line.
   e. Clamp saline infusion line.
10. Note time of dialysis initiation.

Blood Flow for Dialysis

An adequate vascular access should permit blood flow to the dialyzer of 200–450 mL/min. Optimal blood access and blood flow to the dialyzer influences dialysis efficiency.

11. Tape all connections securely; secure blood tubing to client's extremity.
12. Set alarm pressures—high and low.
13. Establish blood flow rate (usually 300–450 mL/min).
14. Ensure that access connections are visible.
15. Check client's blood pressure and pulse once dialysis has been initiated, then every 30 minutes unless otherwise indicated.
16. Assess client at least every 30 minutes for vital signs and potential complications.
17. Administer any ordered medication through the venous line. **Rationale:** Medication infuses into client, not machine.
18. Turn heparin infusion off last 30–60 minutes or as ordered.

Safety Precautions for Fistula or Graft

- Feel for vibration (thrill) over access site regularly.
- Do not measure blood pressure on extremity.
- Do not perform venipuncture in extremity.
- Counsel client not to wear constrictive clothing on extremity.
- Counsel client to avoid lying on extremity.
- Avoid carrying heavy loads with access extremity.
- Immediately report swelling, discoloration, drainage, or coldness, numbness, or weakness of hand.

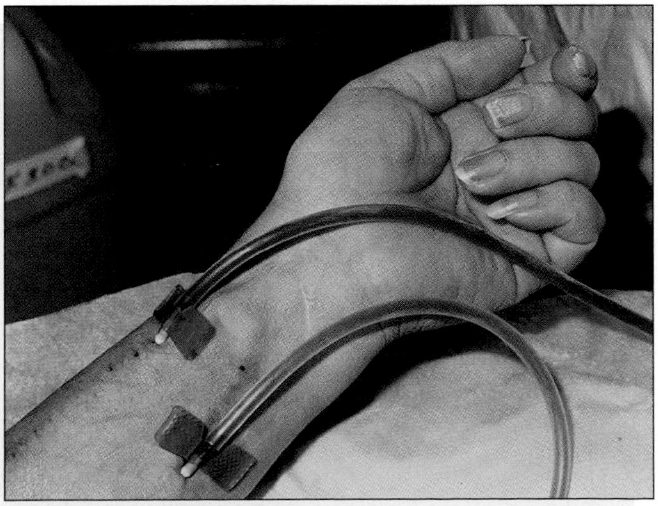

Arterial and venous needles placed in graft for hemodialysis.

Assessing Arteriovenous Fistula

- Wash your hands.
- Position client's arm so fistula is easily accessed.
- Palpate the area to feel for thrill (vibration). This indicates arterial to venous blood flow and fistula patency.
- Auscultate with a stethoscope to detect a bruit (swishing noise). This indicates a patent fistula.
- Palpate pulses distal to fistula to check circulation.
- Observe capillary refill in extremity digits.
- Assess for numbness, tingling, coldness, pallor, or alteration in sensation in digits of fistula extremity.
- Assess for signs and symptoms of infection: redness, edema, soreness, warmth, or increased temperature.

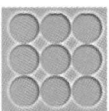

CULTURAL COMPETENCE

- African-Americans have a more rapid decline in glomerular filtration rate than do Caucasians.
- Hypertensive African-Americans have decreased renal excretion of sodium, making sodium restriction an important factor in treatment.
- Hypertension, diabetes, and ESRD are 3–4 times more common in African-Americans and American Indians than in Caucasians.

PROVIDING ONGOING CARE OF HEMODIALYSIS CLIENT

Procedure

1. Limit fluid intake to prescribed amount (e.g., 1,500 mL/day).
2. Maintain diet as prescribed: high-quality protein 1 g/kg ideal body wt/day; sodium 2–3 g/day; potassium, average 1.5–2.5 g/day.
3. Check BP for hypertension/hypotension; check temperature for possible infection.
4. Auscultate heart and lung sounds for signs of fluid overload (pulmonary edema and pericarditis).
5. Provide access site care.
6. Observe mental status—indicative of fluid and electrolyte imbalance or thrombus.
7. Administer Epogen, if ordered, to improve hemoglobin level (given at time of dialysis).
8. Encourage regular rest periods.
9. Weigh daily to assess fluid accumulation.
10. Use antibacterial soap and lotion to bathe. **Rationale:** This decreases risk of staphylococcal infections.
11. Determine that client understands when and how to take medications (e.g., Tums with meals).
12. Provide continued emotional support.
    a. Allow for expression of feelings about change in body image and role performance.
    b. Encourage expression of fears.
    c. Encourage family support.
    d. Give support for required change in lifestyle.

Note: Dialysis adequacy is improved with increased prescription, conversion of catheters to grafts or fistulas, and by not shortening treatments.

TERMINATING HEMODIALYSIS

Equipment

Clean gloves
Gown
Goggles
Mask
Nonsterile pads
Tubing clamps

EVIDENCE BASED NURSING PRACTICE

Survival Rate in Hemodialysis Clients

This study revealed that elderly ESRD clients receiving hemodialysis during morning hours have a higher survival rate than those undergoing dialysis in the afternoon. Previously identified risk factors for this study did not account for these differences.

Source: Bliwise, D. et al (2001). Survival by time of day of hemodialysis in an elderly cohort. *JAMA, 286*(21), 2690–2694.

Procedure

1. Don gloves, gown, goggles, and protective mask.
2. Remove tape and dressing to visualize needle insertion site.
3. Place pads under connectors.
4. Open IV of normal saline to return blood on the arterial side of tubing.
5. Start blood pump at 200 mL/min.
6. Return venous blood.
7. Clamp lines.
8. Remove needles according to unit protocol.
9. Measure and record postdialysis vital signs and weight.

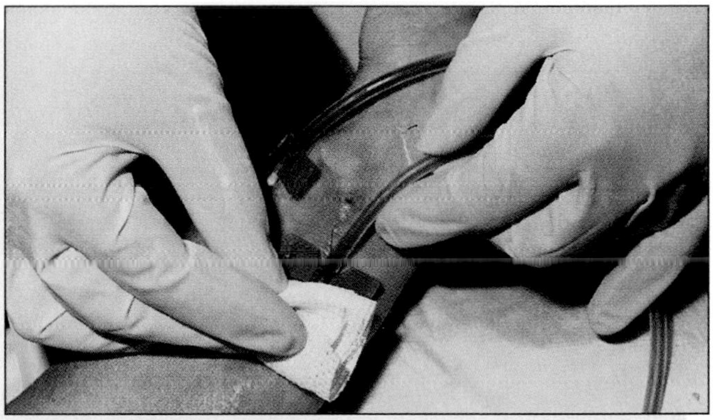

Remove arterial and venous needles, using needle safety shields.

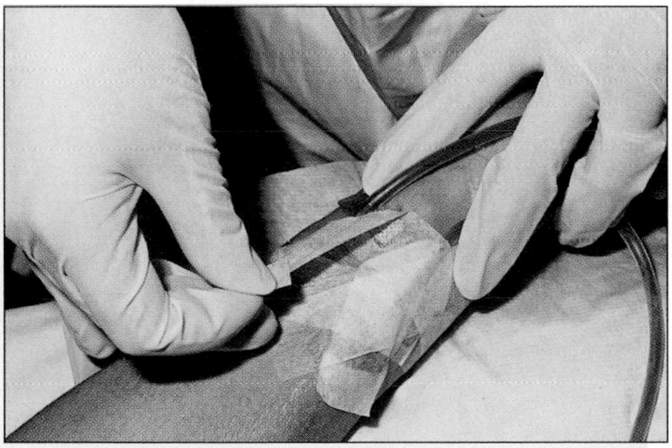

Carefully remove tape from needle sites.

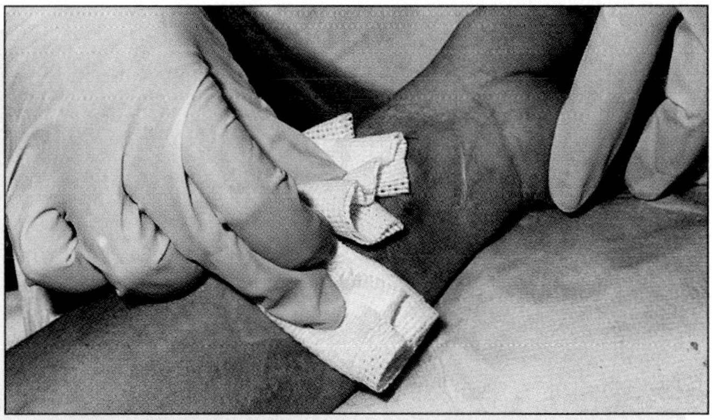

Apply pressure over needle site for 5 to 10 minutes.

MAINTAINING CENTRAL VENOUS DUAL-LUMEN DIALYSIS CATHETER (DLC)

Equipment

Heparin 1000 U/mL
Sterile normal saline
Povidone–iodine swabs, Betadine spray
Sterile 4 × 4 gauze pads
Sterile transparent occlusive dressings
Tape
Luer-Lok catheter caps
Nonsterile drape
Two 3-mL syringes
Two 20-mL syringes
Clean gloves
Two masks
Sterile gloves

Preparation

1. Wash your hands.
2. Fill two 20-mL syringes with 20 mL each of normal saline, and two 3-mL syringes with 3 mL of 1000 μ/mL heparin.
3. Mask client and self, and don clean gloves.
4. Place drape under catheter lumens.
5. Remove gauze wrap from lumens, if present, and discard in appropriate receptacle.
6. Remove gloves.

> **CLINICAL ALERT**
>
> Femoral dialysis DLCs are changed every 3 days. The client is not allowed to flex leg or ambulate.

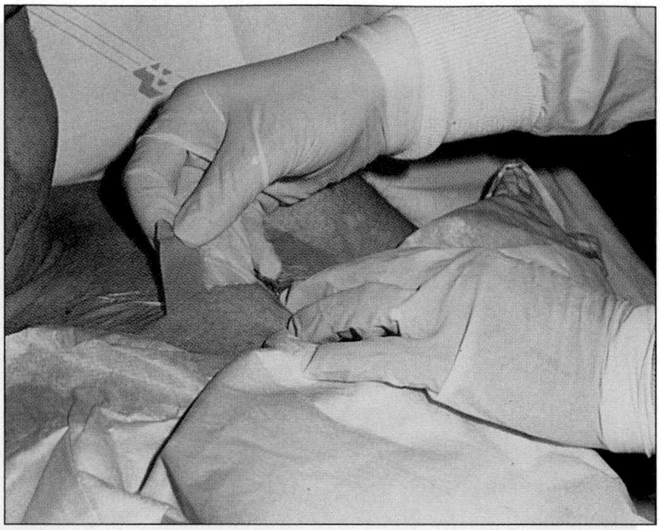

Maintain sterility while carefully removing dressing from dual-lumen catheter.

Procedure

1. Open sterile supplies.
2. Holding corner of 4 × 4, place under catheter lumens.
3. Spray lumens with Betadine and allow to dry.
4. Don sterile gloves.
5. Remove old lumen caps.
6. Use 4 × 4 gauze to pick up new caps and place on lumens.
7. Unclamp and inject 20 mL saline solution into each lumen using positive pressure technique.
8. Inject 3 mL heparin into each catheter using positive pressure technique.
9. Reclamp lumens.
10. Remove old dressing, and discard in biohazard receptacle.
11. Cleanse area surrounding catheter with povidone–iodine swabs using circular motion. Begin at catheter insertion site and work outward.
12. Place sterile transparent dressing over catheter insertion site.

Note: Provide catheter site care after each dialysis. Dressing is not required after permanent catheter site epithelializes around catheter (about 2 weeks).

13. If desired, wrap lumens in gauze and tape. **Rationale:** To prevent skin irritation from lumen clamps.
14. Dispose of equipment in biohazard receptacle.
15. Remove gloves and mask, and discard.
16. Wash hands.
17. Monitor daily for signs of infection, bleeding, or displacement of catheters.

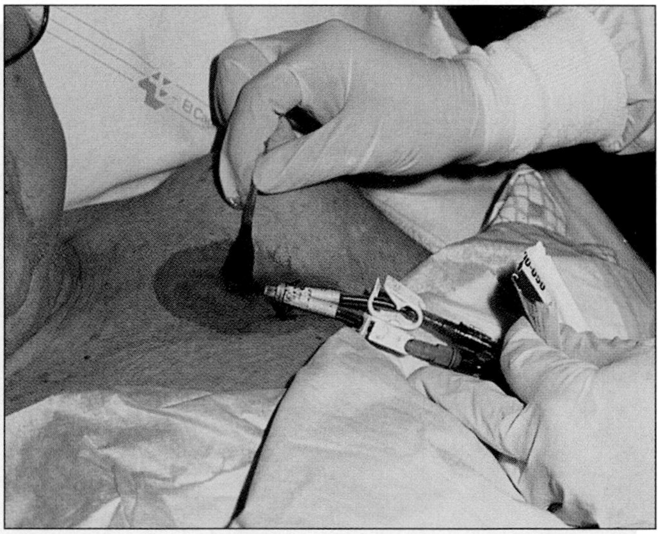

Cleanse catheter insertion site with povidone–iodine swabs using circular motion.

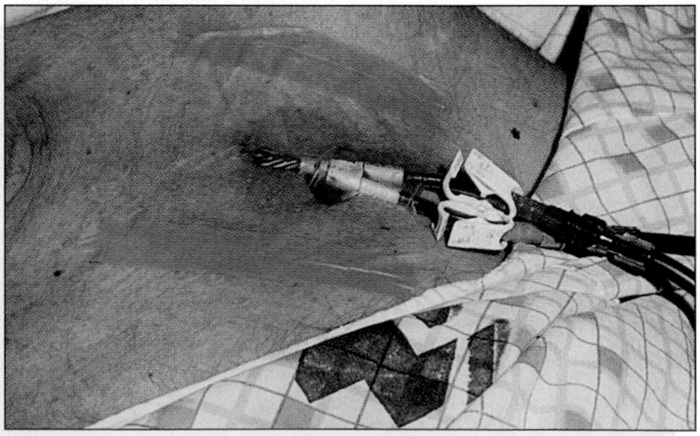

Monitor frequently for signs of infection, bleeding, or catheter displacement.

> **CLINICAL ALERT**
>
> Central venous dual-lumen dialysis catheter (DLC) maintenance (heparin "pack" and site dressing) is performed *only* by the nephrology nurse following a dialysis treatment. These catheters are not maintained the way CVADs are. Instead, they are "packed" with *undiluted* heparin following dialysis, then "unpacked" (3 mL blood withdrawn from catheter) prior to the next dialysis treatment.

Documentation for Hemodialysis

- Predialysis assessment, subjective and objective data
- Status of fistula or graft access site and distal circulation
- Time dialysis initiated and terminated
- Dialyzer type and dialysate used
- Volume of blood processed
- Any complications during procedure and actions taken
- Client symptoms at 30 minute intervals
- Vital signs every 30 minutes
- Postdialysis assessment

Critical Thinking Application

UNEXPECTED OUTCOMES	CRITICAL THINKING OPTIONS
Decreased peripheral pulse, thrill, or bruit in fistula or graft.	• Notify physician promptly of potential access clotting. (Success of declotting depends on speed with which it is instituted.) • Client may be sent to radiology for vascular procedure.
Hypotension occurs during dialysis.	• After careful assessment administer normal saline or concentrated saline bolus into the extracorporeal circuit. • If hypotension is severe, place client in Trendelenburg's position if tolerated; consult physician about administration of mannitol (plasma expander), blood, or vasopressors. • Before future dialyses, consult with physician about using smaller volume dialyzer, less ultrafiltration, or intermittent normal saline doses to maintain blood pressure.
Bleeding occurs during dialysis.	• If blood leak alarm sounds, observe dialysate. If no blood is apparent, check dialysate with Hemastix since air bubbles can cause false alarms. • If bleeding or blood leak is present, discontinue dialysis without returning client's blood.
Alarms sound during dialysis.	• Before dialysis, thoroughly familiarize yourself with alarm sounds, functions, and trouble-shooting maneuvers. • When alarms sound, quickly check for possible causes, such as obstructions or separations of tubing. • In an emergency, such as clots, air emboli in venous line, or failure of bypass mode, clamp venous blood line tubing immediately, and place client in Trendelenburg's position on left side.
Near the end of or following dialysis, the client develops restlessness, confusion, seizures, headache, nausea, vomiting, or hypertension.	• Suspect dialysis disequilibrium if client develops these symptoms. • Consult physician, and implement orders to slow blood flow rate or discontinue dialysis. • Administer medications as ordered (hypertonic saline or mannitol) to control symptoms. • For future dialyses, consult with physician about possible orders regarding prevention, such as earlier dialysis before BUN rises excessively or shorter dialysis treatment.
Hypervolemia occurs; PAP, PWP, CVP increases.	• Clamp replacement port to stop fluid infusion. • Notify physician immediately.

GERONTOLOGIC CONSIDERATIONS

Some changes in the urinary system that occur naturally with aging may be difficult to differentiate from pathologic processes.

Changes seen with aging include:

- Reduced activation of vitamin D results in decreased absorption of calcium from the gut.
- Reduction in glomerular filtration rate and decrease of renal nephrons (reduced by 30–50% by age 75).
- Medications eliminated by the kidneys may require dosage modification; the elderly client should be monitored closely for signs of drug toxicity.
- Lower specific gravity of urine occurs due to decreased ability to concentrate urine; may cause nocturia.
- Any acute fluid loss may cause renal insufficiency.
- The bladder has reduced holding capacity, weaker smooth muscle contractility and decreased sphincter tone, but lack of bladder control is *not* a normal part of aging.
- Urgency as well as urge incontinence and nocturia are common among all elderly clients due to decreased bladder capacity.
- In the elderly, postvoiding residual volume increases, but remains within the normal range, usually no more than 50 mL.
- Prostatic enlargement in men causes obstruction with resultant urinary retention and UTIs.
- Reduced estrogen levels in women lead to atrophy of tissues that line and surround the urethra, bladder outlet, and vagina, contributing to urinary incontinence.
- Many elderly have coexistent urge and stress incontinence.
- Women may experience weakening of pelvic muscles, causing urethral shortening and urinary retention.

MANAGEMENT GUIDELINES

Each state legislates a Nurse Practice Act for RNs and LVN/LPNs. Health care facilities are responsible for establishing and implementing policies and procedures that conform to their state's regulations. Verify the regulations and role parameters for each health care worker in your facility.

Delegation of Responsibilities

- CNAs may document intake and output findings on bedside records. Some facilities allow CNAs to chart these findings on flow sheets. Please check the facility policies and procedures regarding this.
- UAPs may apply condom catheters, and provide catheter care.
- Unlicensed Assistive Personnel (UAPs) may perform the same tasks as the CNA. In addition, many states are allowing "clean" catheterization on clients requiring long-term procedures. It is advisable to check the policy and procedure manual to determine the tasks UAPs may perform.
- Technicians may be trained to perform certain tasks in hemodialysis units. They may initiate the dialysis treatment and monitor clients while they are on dialysis but may not give medications or make nursing judgments.
- LVN/LPNs are assigned to care for clients requiring catheterization, and instillation of medication into the bladder and irrigating a closed urinary system with a physician's order.
- LVN/LPNs may be assigned to clients with urinary diversion. They may change pouches and empty continent ileostomies.
- Most LVN/LPNs do not work with hemodialysis clients. They can work in a hemodialysis unit with additional training, much like the technician. They are not assigned to maintain central venous dual-lumen catheters or to work with clients requiring venovenous hemofiltration.

Information Flow

- It is very important that all staff be informed about which clients require intake and output recordings. I&O records should be at the bedside to remind everyone to record the findings.

- Hemodialysis grafts/fistulas and distal circulation of the involved extremity must be assessed frequently after the initial placement, and regularly thereafter.
- Health care team members should report any complaints of pain or discomfort from the client, as well as unusual odor, color, or abnormal findings from urinary catheter drainage systems.
- Urinary diversion pouches should be emptied when ⅓ full. If the facility policy does not allow ancillary personnel to complete this task, the nurse will instruct them to observe the amount of urine in the pouch and report when it needs to be emptied.
- Hemodialysis technicians must be instructed on client's parameters while on dialysis. They should be instructed to immediately report deviations from the norm to the RN. The RN is ultimately responsible for the care of all clients, regardless of who is assigned to monitor the dialysis treatment.

CRITICAL THINKING STRATEGIES

SCENARIO 1

Your 55-years old neighbor confides in you that every time she coughs or sneezes she loses urine. She asks if this is normal since so many of her friends have the same problem.

1. Describe various types and causes of urinary incontinence.
2. What lifestyle changes help to correct stress incontinence?
3. What noninvasive measures help to correct stress incontinence?

SCENARIO 2

Mrs. Christofferson, a 64-year-old female client, is a first-day postoperative client. She had a bowel resection yesterday. The physician ordered her Foley catheter discontinued at 8 A.M. this morning. His additional order is to check for residual urine after her first voiding.

1. The client has not voided since the Foley catheter was removed 2 hours earlier. What is your priority nursing intervention?
2. The client voids 600 mL of urine 6 hours after the Foley catheter was removed. What further actions should the nurse take at this time?
3. Checking for residual urine, you obtain 120 mL of urine. What is your next intervention? What alternative action might you take if you suspect the client may exceed the normal amount of residual urine?

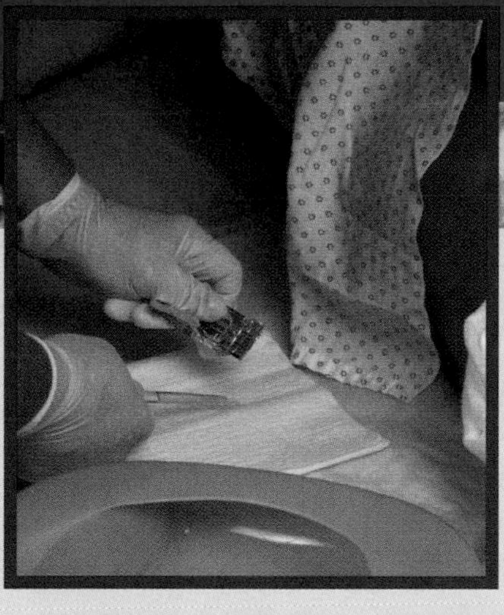

CHAPTER 23

Bowel Elimination

THEORETICAL CONCEPTS

UNIT ONE: **Bowel Evacuation** 763
- Removing a Fecal Impaction 764
- Providing Digital Stimulation 764
- Developing a Regular Bowel Routine 765
- Administering a Suppository 766

UNIT TWO: **Enema Administration** 768
- Administering a Large-Volume Enema 769
- Administering an Enema to a Child 771
- Administering a Small-Volume Enema 772
- Administering a Retention Enema 772
- Administering a Return Flow Enema 773

UNIT THREE: **Fecal Ostomy Pouch Application** 775
- Applying a Fecal Ostomy Pouch 776

GERONTOLOGIC CONSIDERATIONS 782

MANAGEMENT GUIDELINES 782

CRITICAL THINKING STRATEGIES 784

Cross Reference: Colostomy Irrigation (See Home Care, Chapter 34); Bedpan (See Personal Hygiene, Chapter 9).

LEARNING OBJECTIVES

- Explain both the mechanical and chemical aspects of digestion.
- Compare and contrast hypermotility with hypomotility.
- Discuss what is meant by obstruction of the bowel.
- Describe the anatomic locations for an ileostomy, cecostomy, or colostomy.
- List the components of a good bowel training program.
- Outline the essential steps in administering a tap water or saline enema to an adult client.
- Describe the precautions necessary when performing digital stimulation to remove a fecal impaction.
- Compare and contrast stoma care of an ileostomy and a colostomy.
- Outline the steps for developing a regular bowel routine.
- Describe at least three interventions used when skin is denuded from leakage.
- Describe at least three precautions necessary when applying a fecal ostomy pouch.
- Discuss the corking and intubation procedure for client with a continent ileostomy.

TERMINOLOGY

Anal fissure: a small linear ulcerated area in the anal area.

Bacteria: unicellular plantlike microorganisms lacking chlorophyll.

Bowel: the intestine.

Bowel movement: the emptying of the intestinal tract.

Carminative: an agent that removes gases from the gastrointestinal tract.

Cathartic: a drug to induce emptying of the intestinal tract; a laxative.

Chyme: the viscous, semifluid contents of the stomach present during digestion of a meal. Chyme then passes through the pylorus into the duodenum, where further digestion occurs.

Colitis: inflammation of the colon.

Colon: the large intestine, which extends from the cecum to the anus.

Colostomy: an artificially created opening from the colon to the abdominal surface for the elimination of waste.

Constipation: difficulty or straining in defecation and infrequent bowel movements over an extended period of time.

Defecation: emptying of the intestinal tract; bowel movement.

Diarrhea: the passage of unformed liquid stools.

Digestion: the process by which food is broken down, mechanically and chemically, in the gastrointestinal tract.

Diverticulitis: inflammation of diverticuli in the intestinal tract causing stagnation of feces in the small distended sacs (diverticula).

Diverticulum: an outpouching of the mucous membrane of the intestine.

Emulsification: the breaking down of large fat globules in the intestine to smaller, uniformly distributed particles.

Enema: the introduction of fluid through a tube into the lower intestinal tract.

Feces: intestinal waste products consisting of bacteria and secretions of the liver, in addition to a small amount of food residue.

Fistula: an abnormal tubelike passage from a normal cavity or tube to a free surface or another cavity.

Flaccid: relaxed, flabby; having defective or absent muscle tone.

Flatulence: excessive gas in the stomach and intestines.

Gastrointestinal: having to do with the stomach and intestines.

Hemorrhoids: abnormally distended rectal veins due to a constant increase in venous pressure.

Hypermotility: unusually quick motility in the gastrointestinal tract.

Hyperreflexia: increased action of reflexes.

Hypertonic: having a higher osmotic pressure than normal body fluid.

Hypomotility: unusually slow motility of the gastrointestinal tract.

Ileostomy: an artificially created opening from the ileum to the abdominal surface for the elimination of wastes.

Impaction: condition of being tightly wedged into a place, as of feces in the bowel.

Integumentary: relative to a covering, as the skin.

Laxative: a mild-acting drug to induce emptying of the intestinal tract.

Mucosa: mucous membrane.

Necrosis: death of areas of tissue or bone caused by enzymatic action or lack of circulation.

Obstipation: the act or condition of obstructing; extreme constipation due to obstruction.

Occlude: to block off, obstruct.

Occult blood: blood in such minute quantities that it can only be detected by a microscope or chemical means.

Ostomy: a surgically formed artificial opening that serves as an exit site for the bowel or intestine.

Parasite: an organism that lives within, on, or at the expense of another organism, known as the host.

Perforation: the act or process of making a hole, such as that caused by an ulcer.

Peristalsis: a progressive wave-like movement that occurs involuntarily as in the gastrointestinal tract.

Reflux: a return of or backward flow.

Sphincter: circular band of muscle fiber constricting a natural orifice.

Stoma: an artificially created opening between two passages or between a passage and the body surface.

Stool: waste matter discharged from the bowels.

Suppositories: semisolid substances for introduction into the rectum, vagina, or urethra where they dissolve; serves as a vehicle for medicines to be absorbed.

Villi: short filamentous processes found on certain membraneous surfaces.

ANATOMY AND PHYSIOLOGY

The gastrointestinal system converts food into products that can be used as nutrients on the cellular level and disposes of wastes incurred in the process. The primary structures in this system include the mouth, esophagus, stomach, small intestine, and large intestine.

The mouth, esophagus, and stomach are the structures of the upper gastrointestinal tract, where the process of digestion begins. The small intestine, where digestion is completed and most absorption takes place, is a 12-foot tube composed of the duodenum, jejunum, and ileum. The large intestine is made up of the cecum, colon, and rectum. The cecum contains the ileocecal valve and the appendix. The colon is divided into the ascending, transverse, descending, and sigmoid colon. The rectum extends from the sigmoid colon to the anus. The terminal end of the rectum is called the anal canal and is guarded by the internal and external sphincter muscles. The chief functions of the colon are to reabsorb water and sodium and to store wastes.

Digestion is accomplished mechanically and chemically. Food is mechanically churned through the intestinal tract by sharp contractions, or peristaltic waves, of the circular and longitudinal muscles of the intestinal wall. Muscular sphincters and valves are located at strategic points throughout the intestinal tract. These structures help propel the food bolus or feces at appropriately timed intervals in a process called rhythmic segmentation. The sphincters and valves, when functioning properly, prevent reflux of contents. Peristaltic waves, coupled with rhythmic segmentation, allow maximal contact between food and the bowel wall so that chemical reactions can accomplish digestion and absorption can take place.

The chemical aspects of digestion in the small intestine begin in the duodenum with the introduction of pancreatic juices and bile. Pancreatic juices are rich in enzymes, which work to break down proteins and fats and to complete the transformation of starch to sugar. Bile, secreted by the liver, aids in the emulsification and absorption of fats. These substances work in an alkaline medium that combines with the acidity of chyme to provide a neutral pH in the duodenum, thereby protecting the duodenal mucosa.

In the 20 feet of jejunum and ileum, approximately 3,000 mL of digestive enzymes are secreted. These enzymes, which are secreted by the mucus glands of the intestines, complete the digestive processing of food prior to absorption. Again, the alkaline nature of these secretions works to protect the mucous membrane of the intestinal tract.

The peristaltic activity of the gastrointestinal tract, as well as its secretory functions, is governed, to a large degree, by parasympathetic and sympathetic nerve fibers.

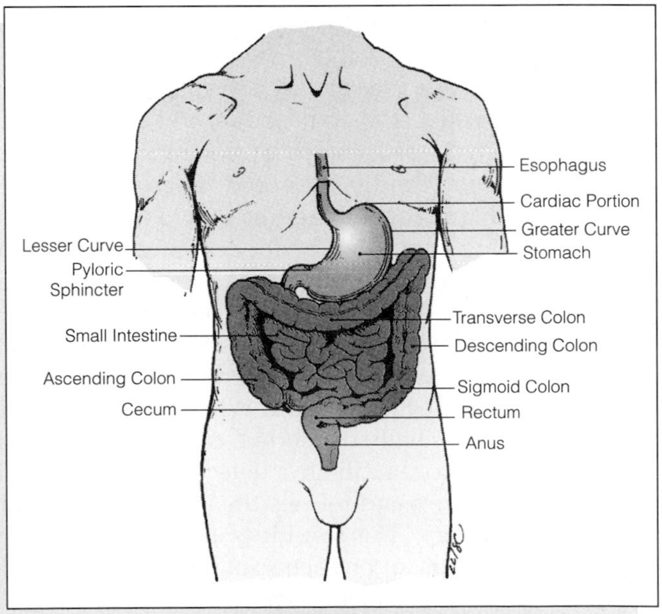

Anatomy of the gastrointestinal tract.

Stimulation of the parasympathetic system increases the activity of the intestinal tract, while stimulation of the sympathetic nervous system inhibits activity in the tract. The internal anal sphincter, however, is activated by sympathetic stimulation, whereas the external anal sphincter is under voluntary control.

Absorption, another primary function of the small bowel, is the passage of prepared materials from the gastrointestinal lumen to the blood and cells. Most absorption in the small intestine results from the churning action of the bowel. Chyme is continually exposed to the circular folds of the mucosal surface, which is lined with thread-like projections called villi. Villi serve as the sites of absorption of fluid and nutrients. The duration of contact between chyme and the mucosal surface of the bowel is very important in absorption. Hypermotility in the small intestine can result in decreased contact with the mucosal wall and deficient absorption; hypomotility can result in increased absorption of fluids as well as problems with elimination.

The circulatory system delivers nutrients to tissue cells and transports the waste products of metabolism. The small bowel and colon are supplied by the superior and inferior mesenteric arteries. Blood that contains absorbed nutrients is carried from the gastrointestinal tract by the superior and inferior mesenteric veins, which become a part of the portal system delivering blood to the liver. Each villus on the intestinal wall contains a network of small capillaries, which absorb sugar and amino acids, and a central lymph channel, which absorbs fatty acids and glycerol. When circulation is compromised, absorption is decreased and cells are lost.

By the time chyme reaches the ileocecal valve—the junction between the small and large intestines—most nutrients have been absorbed. Whereas 3 L of fluid pass through the small bowel, only 500 mL actually pass through the ileocecal valve. The semiliquid material received by the large intestine consists of living and dead bacteria, undigested food and residue, and cell debris. As residue is slowly passed along the colon by peristaltic-like mass movements, fluid is absorbed. These movements occur relatively infrequently (perhaps two or three times per day) and are stimulated by the entrance of food into the stomach by the gastrocolic reflex.

Absorption of fluid in the colon takes place primarily in the ascending and transverse colon. Fecal masses are stored in the sigmoid colon and move into the rectum with mass peristaltic movement. When the rectum fills and becomes sufficiently distended, centers in the sacral area of the spinal cord facilitate a defecation reflex, which contracts the rectum and relaxes the internal and external anal sphincters. The resulting urge, facilitated by higher centers, leads to contraction of the abdominal, perineal, and diaphragmatic muscles. Willful defecation is a coordinated, learned habit. Voluntary inhibition of the act returns the stool to the sigmoid colon.

DEFECATION

Defecation is defined as evacuation of the bowel. The pattern of defecation varies with each individual. It can occur from several times each day to two to three times each week. The type and amount of stool evacuated is also individualized. It is determined by such factors as diet and normal changes in the intestinal flora. Additional factors that influence bowel patterns include age, fluid intake, exercise, psychologic factors, alterations in lifestyle, and medications.

For healthy bowel elimination, the client needs to have sufficient bulk (cellulose and fiber) to produce adequate fecal volume. Food intake at specified times and food that does not produce flatulence are also important for healthy elimination. Daily fluid intake of 2000 to 3000 mL is essential to promote adequate urine output, as well as maintain a soft stool for easy elimination. Daily exercise stimulates peristaltic activity, facilitating bowel movements.

Normal feces are composed of about 75% water and 25% solid material. The stool is soft, but formed, and the color ranges from light to dark brown. The color of the stool is due to the presence of stercobilin and urobilin, derived from bilirubin. In the absence of bile pigment the stool takes on a characteristically clay-colored or white appearance. The action of bacteria in the colon plays a role in the color of the stool. Ingestion of certain foods, drugs, and vitamins can alter the color and consistency of the stool. The nurse must complete an accurate bowel history to determine normal or abnormal findings. Conclusions should not be made on observation alone. Iron supplements, vitamins with iron, beets, red peppers, licorice, grape juice, and spinach affect the color of the stool, which could lead to an incorrect conclusion of blood in the stool. Feces that are red or black in color can be a direct result of ingestion of these foods. Medications can also affect the color and consistency of the stool. General anesthetics block parasympathetic stimulation to the colon, leading to potential constipation. In addition to consistency and distinct color of the feces there is an odor associated with the feces. The odor is a result of the action of microorganisms on the chyme.

Abnormal characteristics of the feces include the presence of exudate, parasites, fat, and large amounts of mucus. Large amounts of mucus are generally associated with an inflammatory process of the bowel. The stool appears slimy in this condition. Diseases, such as ulcerative colitis or Crohn's disease, produce a stool with large amounts of pus when inflammation is present. Stools with abnormally high fat content are foul-smelling and float to the top of the water. Children with cystic fibrosis commonly produce this type of stool.

Constipation

Because many factors influence the development of constipation, the management of it is also individualized according to each client's need. There is acute and chronic constipation, each a result of certain problems and each requiring their own form of management.

Acute constipation is usually managed with suppositories, enemas, or osmotic laxatives to clear the rectum. A bowel program is usually indicated following the initial treatment. Usually, there is a modification of the diet and fluid intake in addition to education about bowel habits.

Chronic constipation requires the use of bulk forming agents if the client has a low dietary fiber and no specific underlying cause for the constipation. Osmotic agents may be effective for immediate results but the goal of the bowel management program is to establish regular bowel habits, using only small doses of laxatives.

ALTERATIONS IN ELIMINATION

By-products of digestion must be continually eliminated to maintain normal body function. Alterations in normal elimination can result from changes in motility, obstruction of the lumen of the bowel, circulatory deficiencies, disease process, and surgically induced alterations to the structures of the intestinal tract.

Changes in Motility

Motility in the gastrointestinal system is the ability to move spontaneously. Normal motility of the bowel provides peristaltic activity that pushes and churns food and chyme through the upper tract and feces through the lower tract at timed intervals.

Hypermotility may be caused by direct stimulation or irritation of the autonomic nervous system, as well as by inflammatory processes in the gastrointestinal tract. Stimulation of parasympathetic nerves promotes peristalsis and increases bowel muscle tone. Increased peristalsis speeds the propulsion of chyme through the upper tract, resulting in deficient absorption of nutrients. When increased peristalsis speeds the propulsion of feces through the lower tract, diarrhea occurs.

Stimulation of the autonomic nervous system may be psychic in origin. Anxiety, for example, may be mediated through either parasympathetic nerves, with resultant diarrhea, or through sympathetic nerves, with resultant constipation. The action on the parasympathetic nervous system of certain drugs may also cause hypermotility of the intestine. Antihypertensive drugs, such as reserpine, and cholinergic drugs can cause diarrhea by their stimulation of parasympathetic nerves.

Hypermotility caused by the stimulating effect of an irritant on intestinal peristalsis may arise from infectious agents, chemical agents, or inflammatory disease processes. The most common intestinal irritants are the products of certain bacteria that release toxins in the digestive tract. Chemical agents that irritate the intestinal mucosa include cytotoxic drugs, castor oil, and quinidine. Ulcerative and inflammatory disease processes include diverticulitis, tuberculous lesions, ulcerative colitis, and Crohn's disease.

Hypomotility may be caused by direct stimulation or blockage of the autonomic nervous system, intestinal muscle weakness, and chemical agents that inhibit peristalsis and induce flaccidity in the intestinal tract. Decreased peristalsis causes chyme to move sluggishly through the upper tract so that fluids are overabsorbed. Decreased peristalsis also slows the propulsion of feces through the lower tract and causes constipation, fecal impaction, and obstruction.

Stimulation or blockage of the autonomic nervous system may be congenital in origin, as is the case in Hirschsprung's disease, where the absence of parasympathetic nerve ganglia results in failure of peristalsis of the affected portion of the bowel. The effects of trauma or toxins on autonomic innervation of the intestine, which occur with paralytic (adynamic) ileus, inhibit motility to the point of obstruction.

Intestinal muscle weakness that results from disease processes, old age, or a lack of essential vitamins (notably the B group) or electrolytes (particularly potassium) may all contribute to hypomotility. Certain drugs, such as codeine and morphine, can also cause hypomotility by relaxing the smooth muscles of the digestive tract and by increasing spasms of the intestinal sphincters.

Obstruction of the Lumen of the Bowel

Obstruction of the lumen of the bowel may be partial or complete. The severity of the obstruction depends on the region of the bowel that is affected, the degree to which the lumen is occluded, and the degree to which the circulation in the bowel wall is disturbed.

A small-bowel obstruction that occurs as a consequence of persistent vomiting (reverse peristalsis) can cause severe disturbances in the electrolyte balance of the body. Large-bowel obstructions, even if complete, are not as dramatic, provided that the blood supply to the colon is not disturbed.

The causes of intestinal obstruction are varied. In rare instances, obstruction may result when a foreign body, such as a large fruit stone or a mass of parasitic worms, becomes lodged in the bowel. More frequently, intestinal obstructions are caused by strictures, adhesions, hernia, volvulus, intussusception, polyps, neoplasms, and fecal impactions.

The physiology of an obstruction in the lumen of the bowel is generally the same, regardless of cause. As the lumen of the bowel is blocked, the body attempts to overcome the obstruction by increasing peristalsis. During this process, liquid feces move past the site of obstruction and

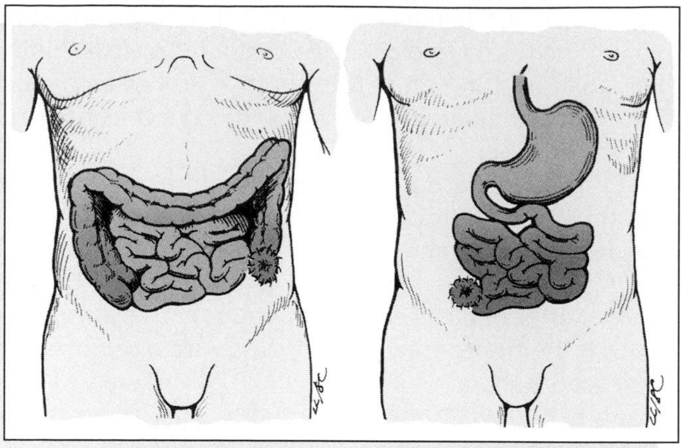

A sigmoid colostomy. An ileostomy.

Potential Postoperative Complications

- Hemorrhage
- Shock
- Thrombophlebitis
- Pulmonary embolism
- Sepsis
- Paralytic ileus
- Intestinal obstruction
- Impaired intestinal absorptive capability
- Leaky anastomosis
- Stoma necrosis

cause diarrhea and increased obstruction, which leads to constipation. Within several hours peristalsis is reduced, and the bowel becomes flaccid. As intraluminal pressure builds up, fluid is retained and absorption decreases. The increased intraluminal pressure then leads to the compression of the bowel wall and its capillaries, which causes necrosis of the bowel wall.

Circulatory Deficiencies

An adequate circulatory flow is essential for maintaining the structure of the bowel and for carrying on cellular nutrition. Any interruption of the arterial blood supply inhibits the bowel function. An occlusion of the circulatory flow, also called an intestinal infarction, results in gangrene of the bowel unless surgical intervention is carried out. A partial occlusion of the mesenteric arteries due to atherosclerosis can cause intestinal angina, a condition that occurs when the blood supply is increasingly interrupted.

Surgically Induced Alterations in Bowel

When alterations in bowel elimination become life threatening and medical management fails, surgical intervention becomes necessary. Diversionary surgical procedures of the bowel include cecostomy, ileostomy, and colostomy.

An ostomy may be temporary or permanent, depending on the etiology. The most common indication for a permanent ostomy is low cancer of the rectum or advanced metastic cancer involving the colon. A temporary ostomy may be performed because a bowel prep could not be done due to obstruction and/or perforation, or to protect a distal surgery of the colon. Ileostomy and colostomy are the most frequent type of fecal diversion. Children with certain congenital intestinal disorders may require an ostomy. These are usually temporary and reversed once the child reaches a certain weight.

A cecostomy is a surgically created opening from the cecum through the abdominal wall. This procedure is a quick and temporary method to decompress the right side of the colon. This is usually done with the insertion of a catheter into the colon. This catheter requires frequent irrigation to ensure patency. If stool leaks around the site, a pouch should be applied to collect the output.

An ileostomy is a surgically created opening from the terminal ileum through the abdominal wall. The entire large intestine is bypassed or removed. Permanent ileostomies are usually performed on clients with Crohn's disease of the entire large intestine and those clients with a weakened rectal sphincter, which would leak stool if a pull-through procedure was performed.

In recent years, new surgical procedures have eliminated many permanent ileostomies. Clients with polyposis or ulcerative colitis may choose to have a Kock Continent Ileostomy or an internal reservoir of the ileum constructed at the rectum. The Kock reservoir consists of an internal pouch with two limbs of the ileum, one forming an internal valve. Continence occurs as a result of the stool collecting in the internal pouch. The pouch must be intubated four to six times a day to evacuate the stool. The rectal reservoir is created by joining the ileum to the anus after the colon is removed. The client will have four to ten stools a day and must have good sphincter control. Any of the surgeries that remove or bypass the large intestine produce a soft-to-watery effluent that contains water and many digestive enzymes that have not yet been absorbed by intestinal villi. The daily output varies from 500 to 2000 mL.

A colostomy is a surgically created opening from the colon through the abdominal wall and can be created using any segment of the large intestine. With a colostomy, the diseased portion of the colon is bypassed or removed and a portion of healthy colon is brought to the outside of the abdomen to form a stoma. The type of stoma is named after the segment of bowel used to form the stoma. The farther to the right side of the colon the stoma is placed will determine the type of output from the stoma.

TABLE 23–1 Comparison Chart for Ostomies

Colostomy	Ileostomy
Etiologic Factors	
Cancer of colon Traumatic or congenital disruption of intestinal tract Diverticulitis	Ulcerative colitis Crohn's disease (regional ileitis) Birth defects Trauma Protect distal surgery Distal obstruction
Surgical Procedure	
Portion of colon brought through abdominal wall	Portion of ileum brought through abdominal wall
Bowel Control	
Sigmoid—Sometimes Ascending—No	None
Stool Consistency	
Sigmoid—Formed Ascending—Semiformed	Liquid to semisoft
Irrigation for Bowel Control	
Sigmoid	No
Use of Appliance	
Yes, use nondrainable	Yes
Nursing Care Priorities	
Maintain skin integrity a. Keep skin clean and dry b. Provide skin barrier c. Ensure proper fit of appliance	Same as colostomy
Fluid Requirement	
Sigmoid—Normal intake Transverse—8–10 glasses per day	8–10 glasses per day
Diet Control	
Avoid gas-forming foods, Eat in moderation odor-forming foods Chew food well	Same as colostomy
Medications	
Sigmoid—none Transverse—Avoid enteric coated meds May need Na replacement Vitamins, especially K minerals	Same as colostomy B_{12}
Psychosocial	
Promote self-image Refer to Ostomy Club	Same as colostomy

The most common surgery performed for cancer of the colon is a low anterior resection. In this procedure a wide excision of the tumor and surrounding lymph nodes is made and the remaining colon is reconnected. The client may have a diverting ostomy proximal to the resected area to protect the surgical site from leakage.

Abdominal–perineal resections with permanent sigmoid colostomy are usually done only when the tumor is located too low in the rectum for the client to maintain continence. Output from colostomies on the left side of the intestine will eventually become formed and firm, since most of the water has been absorbed by the time the feces reaches these portions of the colon.

A descending colostomy is usually temporary. It is seen frequently in children with congenital disorders. Adults may have a descending colostomy following trauma or severe diverticulitis when perforation is present.

A transverse colostomy can be located anywhere along the transverse colon. It is also usually temporary and is done for either a bowel obstruction or perforation.

Colostomies can also be named for the way they are constructed. A loop colostomy is a very quick surgical procedure to exteriorize the bowel. A loop of intestine is brought out to the surface of the abdomen and some type of plastic bridge is placed under the loop to prevent it from falling back inside the abdomen. This bridge is left in place for 7–14 days until the abdominal wall has sealed. In any of the surgeries in which the rectum is left the client can expect to pass any old stool remaining from before surgery, plus mucus produced by the lining of the intestine on an ongoing basis. A double-barrel colostomy is one that has two stomas. One is the proximal or functional stoma. The second is the distal stoma that connects the remaining stoma and rectum. This stoma is often referred to as a mucus fistula. It may put out mucus or old stool from before surgery, especially if the client is totally obstructed distal to the stoma.

An end colostomy has only one stoma, which originates from the proximal portion of the bowel. The distal end of the colon is either resected or is closed off with sutures and remains in the abdomen. This can also be called a Hartman's procedure. All of these ostomies can be reversed once the distal site is healed and an adequate bowel prep can be done.

Colostomy irrigations are not commonly used today to establish regularity of bowel elimination. Clients usually reestablish bowel habits similar to those prior to the surgery. There may still be some clients who do perform daily irrigations; however, there are situations when irrigations must not be done. Irrigations are always contraindicated in clients with unstable fluid and electrolyte balance and in those clients in whom vagal stimulation is dangerous. Irrigations are also contraindicated when clients are receiving radiation therapy or are experiencing chemotherapy-induced diarrhea.

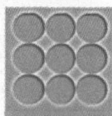

CULTURAL COMPETENCE

When providing nursing care for clients requiring an intervention for bowel elimination, remember that many cultures are very modest and do not like to talk about elimination issues. Respectful approaches and providing privacy during the procedure are critical for all clients but especially for some cultures, in order for them to feel comfortable with the task that needs to be completed. This is especially true for Chinese-Americans, who may request to use the toilet and not a bedpan. Arab-Americans prefer to wash rather than use toilet paper after every urination and bowel movement. They may insist on using a bidet to wash up. Muslims may require additional bathing rituals.

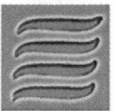

NURSING DIAGNOSES

The following nursing diagnoses may be appropriate to use on client care plans when the components are related to alterations in bowel elimination.

NURSING DIAGNOSIS	RELATED FACTORS
Body Image Disturbed	Presence of stoma, fear of rejection, psychosocial factors
Risk for Constipation	Inadequate intake of fluid or bulk, decreased exercise, disease states, medication, personal habits
Diarrhea	Nutritional intake, medication, disease state
Anticipatory Grieving	Loss of body contiguity, operative procedure (colostomy, ileostomy)
Health Maintenance, Ineffective	Cognitive impairment, depression, immobility, cultural beliefs, lack of social support
Skin Integrity Impaired	Skin irritation or breakdown, poor pouching techniques, incontinence or diarrhea, poor-fitting equipment, economic situation
Noncompliance	Inability to manage equipment, impaired manual dexterity, poor vision
Fluid Volume Deficient	Effluent from ileostomy is watery to semisoft; excessive use of enemas or laxatives
Knowledge Deficient	Inability to manage ostomy, constipation

- The single most important nursing action to decrease the incidence of hospital-based infections is handwashing. **Remember to wash your hands or use antibacterial gel before and after each and every client contact.**

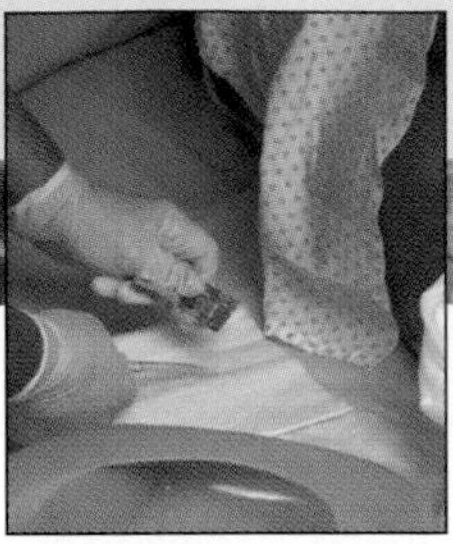

UNIT 1

Bowel Evacuation

Nursing Process Data

ASSESSMENT ***Data Base***

Assess for symptoms indicating presence of impaction: nausea; headache; abdominal pain; malaise, or abdominal distention.

Evaluate client's diet.

- Amount of high-bulk foods.
- Amount of fluid intake daily.

Evaluate client's physical status.

- Extent of physical exercise performed daily.
- Ability to ambulate (i.e., spinal cord injury, CVA).
- Ability to perform bed exercises, abdominal exercises.
- Extent of disease process.
- Medications routinely taken.

Assess effectiveness of drugs, such as stool softeners, bulk formers, suppositories.

Assess time of day client usually evacuates bowels, any changes in normal routine.

Identify client's ability to adapt and psychologic readiness for the above program.

Identify position most effective for bowel evacuation.

Assess consistency and amount of stool for abnormal findings (diarrhea or fecal impaction).

Assess when client had last bowel movement.

Assess for abdominal distention and bloating.

Assess perianal area for tears, ulcerations, or excoriation.

Assess for post-operative constipation.

PLANNING ***Objectives***

To promote regular bowel evacuation

To prevent constipation

To remove a fecal impaction

To establish a bowel program to which the client can easily adapt

To develop a bowel program that the client can perform him or herself

To relieve pain and discomfort

IMPLEMENTATION ***Procedures***

Removing a Fecal Impaction

Providing Digital Stimulation

Developing a Regular Bowel Routine

Administering a Suppository

EVALUATION ***Expected Outcomes***

Client establishes regular bowel evacuation program.

Constipation is prevented.

Fecal impaction is removed.

Client is able to evacuate bowel at a convenient and consistent time.

Client is free of pain, flatus, and discomfort.

REMOVING A FECAL IMPACTION

Equipment

Clean gloves, 2 or 3 pair
Water-soluble lubricant
Absorbent pad
Washcloth and towel
Bath blanket
Bedpan
Basin of warm water

Preparation

1. Check physician's order for impaction removal if the client is at risk for possible complications from vagal stimulation (i.e., cardiac or spinal cord injured client). **Rationale:** Vagal stimulation can result from manual removal of feces. It should be used only as a last resort and with specific physician's order. It causes a decreased pulse rate by decreasing conductivity at the sinoatrial (S-A) node and decreasing the rate of impulse firing at the node.
2. Gather equipment.
3. Identify the correct client, and explain procedure.
4. Provide privacy.
5. Wash your hands.

Procedure

1. Obtain baseline pulse and blood pressure.
2. Place client on left side with knees flexed.
3. Place absorbent pad on bed. Cover with bath blanket.
4. Place bedpan next to client's buttocks.

CLINICAL ALERT

Stimulation of rectum could result in excessive vagal nerve stimulation with subsequent cardiac arrhythmias.

5. Don gloves, and lubricate fingers of dominant hand. You may want to double-glove dominant hand to prevent contamination if glove tears.
6. Ask client to take a deep breath and exhale slowly through the mouth as your index finger is gently inserted into rectum. **Rationale:** Encouraging breathing assists in relaxing the sphincter.
7. Gently remove the hardened stool by working the forefinger into and around the mass to break it up.
8. Allow client to rest between digital removal if any untoward effects, such as palpitations or faintness, are exhibited.
9. Obtain vital signs if client complains of any discomfort.
10. Provide hygienic care, as needed.
11. When stool is removed, change gloves; wash and dry buttocks thoroughly.
12. Dispose of stool in toilet or send stool specimen to laboratory.
13. Clean bedpan, and replace in appropriate area.
14. Remove gloves and wash your hands.
15. Position client for comfort.
16. Wash your hands.
17. Follow physician's orders for administering a cleansing enema or inserting a suppository. **Rationale:** These procedures will assist in the removal of any remaining feces.

Note: An oil retention enema may be used prior to removing the impaction.

PROVIDING DIGITAL STIMULATION

Equipment

Bath blanket (optional)
Clean gloves, 1 or 2 pair
Lubricant
Bedpan or commode
Absorbent pad
Washcloth and towel
Medication if ordered
Toilet tissue

Procedure

1. Check physician's orders and client care plan. Determine client's usual bowel habits and time of evacuation.
2. Wash hands.

3. Gather equipment.
4. Identify the correct client, and explain procedure.
5. Provide privacy and place absorbent pad on bed as necessary.
6. Place client in position in the bed for bowel evacuation (bedpan in place). Place client in either left or right lateral position—if on right side, sigmoid is uppermost and assists with feces removal.
7. Place bath blanket over client if appropriate.
8. Don gloves, and lubricate fingers of nondominant hand. You may want to double-glove to prevent contamination if gloves tear. **Rationale:** Lubrication reduces resistance by fingers moving through anal sphincter.
9. Insert finger into rectum 1½–2 inches.
10. Move your finger from side to side in a circular motion to slightly stretch the rectal wall. Move toward the spine and not the bladder to prevent injury to the bladder.
11. Instruct client to take slow, deep breaths during procedure.
12. Continue stretching the rectal wall for 1–3 minutes until the internal sphincter muscle relaxes.
13. Work with client to discover an associated stimulus to help establish a good bowel routine. **Rationale:** Abdominal massage, coughing, deep inhalations, and tightening of abdominal muscles, in conjunction with digital stimulation, assist in bowel evacuation.
14. Repeat digital stimulation for 1–3 minutes at 5-minute intervals up to 20 minutes if a bowel movement does not occur.
15. Place stool in bedpan as it is removed.
16. Use two fingers if necessary to break up hard stool for evacuation to occur.
17. Assess vital signs if prolonged digital removal is required. **Rationale:** Vagal nerve stimulation can occur.
18. Assess for bleeding.
19. After bowel evacuation occurs, assist the client with cleaning and drying perineum.
20. Remove equipment from room.
21. Wash equipment, and return to storage area.
22. Discard gloves and wash hands.
23. Position the client for comfort.

> **CLINICAL ALERT**
>
> A daily routine should be set up for at least 2–3 weeks to establish a pattern.

DEVELOPING A REGULAR BOWEL ROUTINE

Equipment

Clean gloves, 1 or 2 pair
Lubricant
Bedpan or commode
Absorbent pad
Specific enema if ordered
Washcloth and towel

Preparation

1. Check physician's orders and client care plan.
2. Identify the correct client, and explain procedure.
3. Identify time of day client usually evacuates bowels.
4. Evaluate diet, exercise, former use of medications for bowel evacuation.
5. Administer the following drugs as ordered:
   a. Stool softener (Colace, Dialose, DCS, coloxyl) daily.
   b. Bulk former (Metamucil or FiberCon)—q.d. to t.i.d.
   c. Mild laxative (Senokot, Doxidan, Dulcolax) 8 hours before program.
   d. Suppository (glycerin or Dulcolax) just before digital stimulation.
6. Wash your hands.

Procedure

1. Don gloves. You may want to double-glove to prevent contamination if glove tears.
2. Perform digital stimulation ½ hour after dinner or breakfast or according to client's time schedule for evacuation (see previous intervention).
3. Place client on toilet or commode. (Use bedpan if client is on bed rest.)
4. Remove gloves.
5. Wash your hands.
6. Provide privacy and sufficient time for evacuation.
7. Don gloves.
8. Wash and dry perineal area if client is unable to do so.
9. Remove gloves.
10. Place client in wheelchair or bed and position for comfort.
11. Wash your hands.
12. Wean client away from suppositories and laxatives when spontaneous bowel movements occur with digital stimulation.

Bowel Training

Good bowel training programs include

- Initiation of defecation on demand with digital stimulation and abdominal massage
- Evacuation at same time each day
- Proper diet, increased fiber and fluids
- Daily physical exercise regimen
- Client and family education

EVIDENCE BASED NURSING PRACTICE

Management of Constipation in Older Adults

Studies conducted in Britain and the United States indicate that between 10% and 18% of otherwise healthy adults have frequent straining on defecation. Constipation appears to be more common in women than men, and about 20% of the elderly identify the problem. Constipation may occur secondary to other conditions such as colorectal cancer or strictures. It is also associated with contributing factors such as inadequate fluid intake, absence of dietary fiber, caloric intake, and lack of exercise. In addition to these factors, clients in the hospital may have a lack of privacy and inconvenience or lack of toilet facilities, which can lead to constipation.

A variety of products have been studied to determine if any of them prevent constipation. Some studies support the effectiveness of supplementing the diet with bran but its effectiveness has not been supported by randomized controlled trials.

Other studies suggest that fiber may be effective in improving bowel movement frequency in the ambulatory client, while stimulant and osmotic laxatives may be more effective than bulk-forming agents for the immobilized client.

Source: Management of constipation in older adults, *Best Practice, 3*(1), 1999.

ADMINISTERING A SUPPOSITORY

Equipment

Clean gloves
Lubricant
Bedpan or commode
Absorbent pad (optional)
Suppository as ordered
Washcloth and towel
Paper towel

Procedure

1. Check physician's orders and client care plan.
2. Wash your hands.
3. Gather equipment.
4. Identify the correct client, and explain procedure.
5. Provide privacy. Place client in Sims' position.
6. Place bed protector on bed if necessary.
7. Don gloves, lubricate fingers of nondominant hand.
8. Place small amount of lubricant on paper towel.
9. Open suppository foil; lubricate tip of suppository. **Rationale:** This prevents tissue damage and promotes easy insertion of suppository.
10. Instruct client to breathe through mouth. **Rationale:** This relaxes anal sphincter.
11. Insert suppository (usually glycerin) with pointed end first, and place high in rectum beyond external and internal sphincters, approximately 3–4 inches (approximately 10 cm). **Rationale:** This prevents expulsion of suppository.
12. Push the suppository against the side of the rectal wall. Ensure it is not placed into fecal mass. **Rationale:** It is ineffective if placed in feces as it cannot be absorbed.

CLINICAL ALERT

If client has a spinal cord injury, observe for signs of autonomic hyperreflexia (goose pimples, pounding headache, hypertension, perspiration above level of spinal cord injury).

If signs and symptoms of autonomic hyperreflexia occur, discontinue digital stimulation, apply Nupercainal and Xylocaine ointment around anus and rectum as ordered. This anesthetizes the area and decreases the stimulation that caused the response. Wait 10 minutes for symptoms to decrease, and then gently remove the feces.

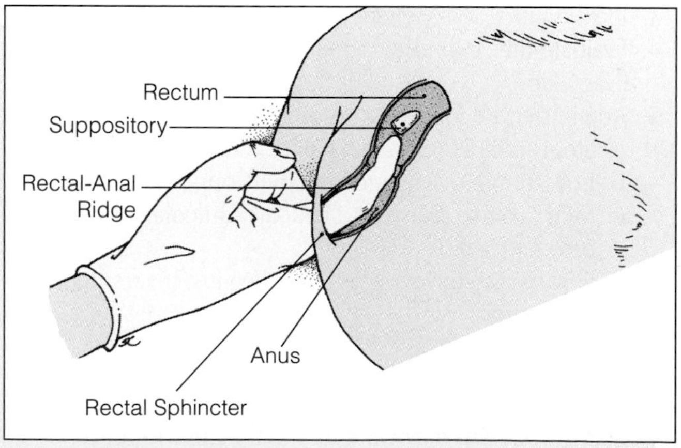

Insert rectal suppositories beyond the rectal–anal ridge for retention.

13. Instruct client to stay in Sims' position for at least 5 minutes. **Rationale:** This position helps retain the suppository.
14. Place client on toilet or commode. If bowel movement does not occur in 30 minutes, perform digital stimulation. A suppository is usually effective within 30 minutes.
15. Repeat with stronger suppository if ordered (Dulcolax) after 30 minutes if there are no results.
16. Allow client to retain Dulcolax suppository for 30 minutes. If no results, do digital stimulation again.
17. Following bowel evacuation, cleanse and dry perineal area.
18. Remove gloves, and wash your hands.
19. Position client in wheelchair or bed.

DOCUMENTATION FOR BOWEL EVACUATION

- Type and number of suppositories used
- Digital stimulation used
- Approximate time used for digital stimulation
- Amount, consistency, characteristics of stool
- Protocol for bowel evacuation for client
- Untoward complications of bowel training program
- Nursing interventions needed to correct complications

Critical Thinking Application

UNEXPECTED OUTCOMES	CRITICAL THINKING OPTIONS
When digital stimulation is performed, client exhibits reflex spasm that prevents stool expulsion.	• Apply local anesthetic around rectum and anus, if ordered. • Wait for spasm to relax, and then proceed with stimulation.
Client develops diarrhea.	• Identify possible cause of diarrhea. • Observe dietary intake for possible cause. Provide for bulk. • Hold the laxatives and stool softeners temporarily. • Instruct client to eat yogurt and drink milk if not contraindicated by condition. • Inform physician of diarrhea and obtain orders for Kaopectate. Administer 2 teaspoons after each loose stool for 24 hours. • Check with physician if medications should be readjusted for bowel training as needed.
Client exhibits signs and symptoms of vagal response during removal of fecal impaction.	• Immediately discontinue procedure. • Place client in shock position. • Monitor vital signs every 5–15 minutes until condition is stable. • Notify physician of findings and request medication order for antispasmodic such as atropine. • Be prepared for "Code" situation, even though it is not likely to occur.
Effective bowel evacuation program is not established.	• Ask dietitian for altered diet (including more fruits and vegetables). • Check if contraindication exists for increasing fluids to 3000 mL daily. • Obtain order from the physician to administer a different stool softener and bulk former or increase dosage. • Have client increase physical activity, especially exercise of the abdominal muscles if not contraindicated by condition. • Ensure that client begins bowel training program ½ hour after a meal.

UNIT 2

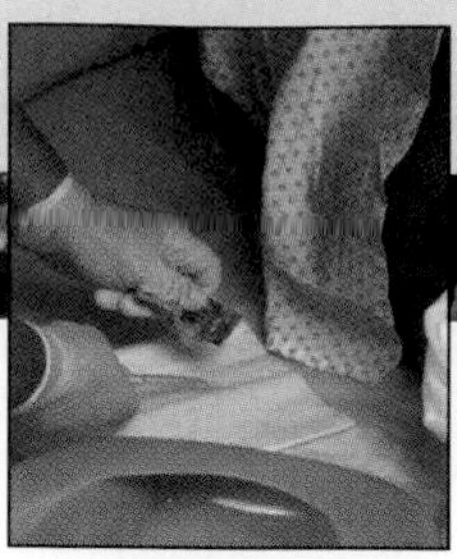

Enema Administration

Nursing Process Data

ASSESSMENT ***Data Base***

Review client's present and past eliminatory status.
Assess the need for an enema.
Evaluate amount of solution a client can tolerate.
Assess if fecal impaction is present.
Assess the degree of abdominal distention.
Assess degree of sphincter control.
Assess current medical regimen.
Assess dietary history.
Assess vital signs before and after procedure, as necessary.

PLANNING ***Objectives***

To relieve constipation
To relieve fecal impactions
To cleanse the bowel prior to surgery, or diagnostic examination
To evacuate the bowel in clients with neurologic dysfunction
To provide nutrients
To introduce an exchange resin
To relieve abdominal distention
To stimulate peristalsis

IMPLEMENTATION ***Procedures***

Administering a Large Volume Enema
Administering an Enema to a Child
Administering a Small Volume Enema
Administering a Retention Enema
Administering a Return Flow Enema

EVALUATION ***Expected Outcomes***

Client experiences increased comfort and relief from abdominal distention.
Returns are clear if preparing client for diagnostic examination or surgery.
Relief obtained from fecal impaction.
Return of solution plus formed, soft feces is complete.

ADMINISTERING A LARGE-VOLUME ENEMA

Equipment

Fluid container with attached rectal tube (size 22–30, straight, or French, for adults)
Normal saline, tap water, soap 750–1000 mL of solution
Water-soluble lubricant
Bath blanket
IV pole
Clean bedpan, commode, or toilet
Bed protector pad
Skin care items (e.g., soap, water, towels)
Two pair of clean gloves
Toilet tissue

Preparation

1. Check physician's orders and client care plan.
2. Gather equipment.
3. Identify correct client and explain the procedure. Explain the benefits of relaxing and taking periodic deep breaths.
4. Provide privacy.
5. Wash your hands.

Procedure

1. Fill water container with 750–1000 mL of lukewarm solution, 105°–110°F. **Rationale:** Solutions that are too hot or too cold or solutions that are instilled too quickly can cause cramping, damage to rectal tissues, and extreme shock.
2. Allow solution to run through tubing until air is removed. Clamp tube. **Rationale:** If air is instilled during procedure, client experiences discomfort as a result of distension of the colon.
3. Hang container on IV pole next to bed.
4. Raise bed to HIGH position, and lower side rails on side where you will be working.
5. Don gloves.
6. Place bed protector under client.
7. Place bedpan within easy reach, or place commode near bed.
8. Place client on left side in Sims' position. **Rationale:** To facilitate flow of solution using contour of bowel.
9. Provide privacy, and drape client with bath blanket.
10. Lubricate tip of tubing with generous amount of water-soluble lubricant.
11. Gently spread buttocks, instruct client to take a slow breath, and insert tubing 3–4 inches.
12. Raise the solution container to a maximum height of 18 inches when giving a high enema and 12–18 inches when giving a low enema. **Rationale:** To assist in fluid movement, turn client to supine position midway through procedure, then to right side.
13. Open regulating clamp and allow solution to flow slowly. **Rationale:** If the flow is slow, client experiences fewer cramps. The client will also be able to tolerate and retain a greater volume of solution.
14. Hold tubing in place in client's rectum at all times. Keep a bedpan nearby.

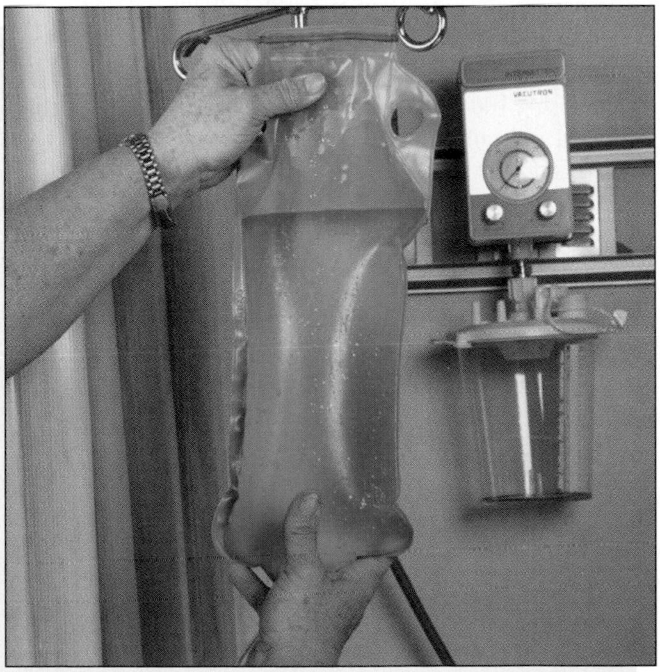

Fill bag to 750 or 1000 mL with tepid solution.

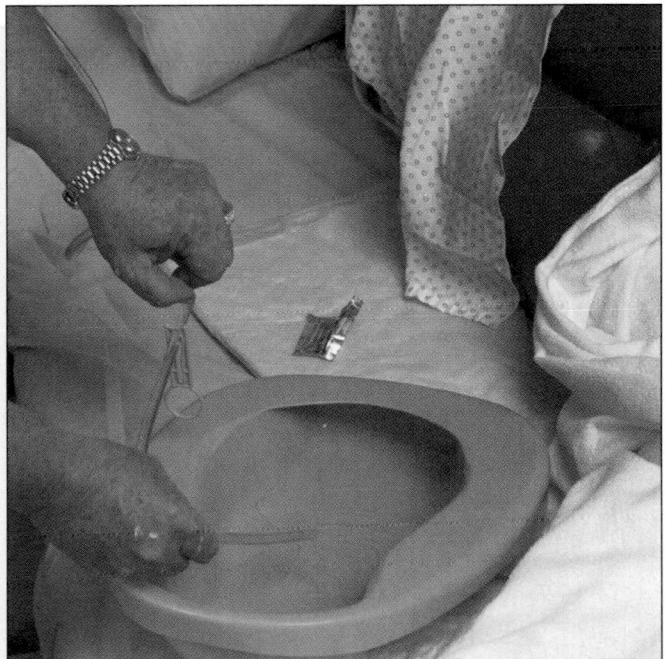

Allow solution to run through tubing to expel air.

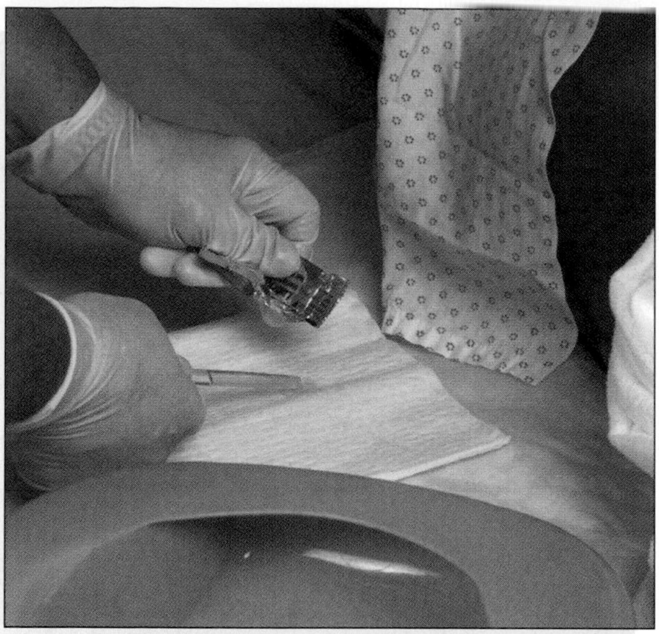

Lubricate tip of tubing to prevent rectal injury.

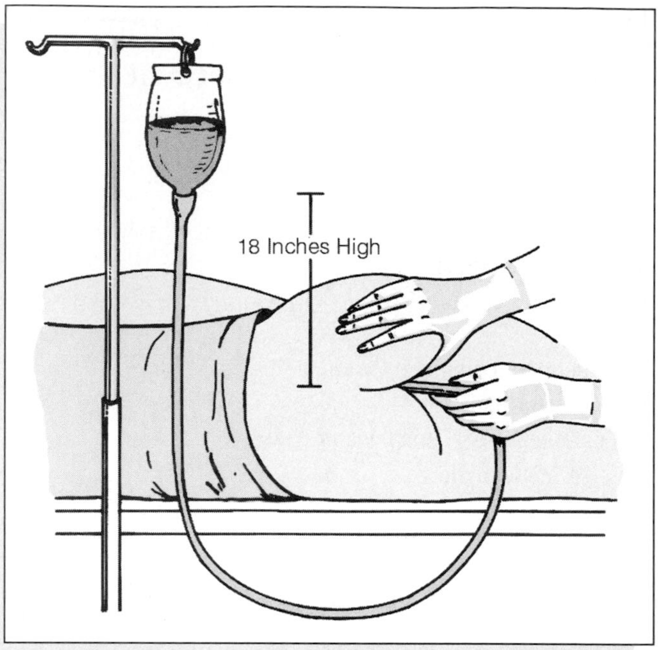

Place enema solution container no more than 18 inches above rectum for safety.

Types of Enemas

Cleansing

- Stimulates peristalsis through irritation of colon and rectum and by distention. Agents: Soap suds, tap water, and saline.
- *Soap suds:* Mild soap solutions stimulate and irritate intestinal mucosa. Strong soap solutions can cause severe irritation of the mucous membrane of the colon. Dilute 3–5 mL mild soap in 1000 mL of water.
- *Tap water:* Give with caution to infants or to adults with altered cardiac and renal reserve. Tap water is a hypotonic solution.
- *Saline:* For normal saline enemas, use a smaller volume of solution. Hypertonic solutions draw fluid into the colon from the body tissues. These solutions are mildly irritating to the mucous membrane of the colon.

Retention

- Solution or nutrient is retained for specified time. Agents: mineral oil, olive oil, cottonseed oil, liquid petrolatum. Nutrient agent: dextrose solution.
- *Emollient (Oil):* Lubricates the rectum and colon protecting the intestinal mucous membrane. Feces absorb oil and become softer and easier to expel. Client retains enema for prescribed time, usually 30–60 minutes.
- *Nutritive:* Provides nourishment in temporary or emergency situations. Enema is retained.

Distention Reduction

- Provides relief from flatus causing distention. It improves ability to expel flatus. Types: carminative and return flow.
- *Carminative:* Two common types include: 1-2-3 enema (30 g of magnesium sulfate, 60 g of glycerin, and 90 mL warm water) and milk and molasses (180–240 mL of equal amounts).
- *Return flow:* Harris flush most common. Mild colonic irrigation using 100–200 mL of enema solution. After instillation, enema container is lowered and solution siphoned back into container.

Medicated

- Enemas containing drugs used for reducing bacteria or removing potassium. Agents: Kayexalate and neomycin.
- *Kayexalate:* A resin is introduced into the large intestine removing the excess potassium by exchanging it for sodium ions.
- *Neomycin:* Antibiotic solution used to reduce bacteria prior to bowel surgery.

15. Lower solution container or momentarily clamp tubing if client experiences cramping, is unable to retain solution, or exhibits anxiety. Resume infusion of solution after a few minutes.
16. After you have instilled the solution, gently remove the tubing. Instruct client to hold solution for 10–15 minutes or as long as tolerated. **Rationale:** The longer the solution is retained the more effective the results.
17. Clean and dispose of equipment.
18. Place client on bedpan, elevate the head of the bed so that client can assume a squatting position on bedpan, or assist to commode.
19. Remove gloves, and wash hands.
20. Provide privacy until client has expelled total volume of instilled solution.
21. Don clean gloves before removing bedpan, or assist client to bed.
22. Remove bedpan when client is ready, and immediately empty, clean, and replace to proper storage area.

TABLE 23–2 Fluid Volume for Enema Administration

Infant	50–150 mL
Toddler	250–350 mL
Child	300–500 mL
Adolescent	500–750 mL
Adult	750–1000 mL

23. Assist client with perineal care, and help client to assume a comfortable position.
24. Lower bed and raise side rails.
25. If client is on strict I&O, measure returns. **Rationale:** To make sure total volume of the solution is expelled.
26. Remove gloves and wash your hands.

ADMINISTERING AN ENEMA TO A CHILD

Equipment

Water container with attached rectal tube (size 14–18 straight [French] for children, and size 10–12 French or infant enema syringe with bulb for infants)
Normal saline, tap water, soap solution
Water-soluble lubricant
Clean potty chair for children
Bed protector
Skin care items (e.g., soap, water, towels)
Clean gloves

Preparation

1. Check physician's orders and client care plan.
2. Gather equipment.
3. Provide privacy for child.
4. Wash your hands.
5. Identify correct client, and explain procedure to child or family. Take time to calm a frightened child and to answer the child's questions.

Procedure

1. Fill water container with 100°F solution (500 mL or less for child, 150 mL or less for an infant).
2. Open clamp and allow solution to run through the tubing so that air is removed.
3. Clamp tube and hang solution container on IV pole.
4. Place bed protector under child.
5. Place child on left side or in knee–chest position. **Rationale:** To facilitate flow of solution using contour of bowel.
6. Don clean gloves.
7. Lubricate tip of tubing or infant enema syringe with bulb.
8. Gently separate buttocks and insert catheter or syringe into child's rectum (1–1½ inches for infants, 2–3 inches for children).
9. Elevate solution container no more than 12–18 inches. **Rationale:** Height increases pressure of solution entering colon—too much pressure may damage colon.
10. Open clamp and allow solution to flow slowly for 10–15 minutes.
11. After you have instilled the solution, close clamp and gently remove the tubing or syringe.
12. Hold child's buttocks together or tape them with hypoallergenic paper tape. If child is toilet trained, place a potty chair nearby.
13. Retain solution 10–15 minutes for cleansing enemas.
14. Place the child on a potty chair or bedpan to expel solution.
15. If there are no contraindications, you may gently massage child's abdomen to help child expel returns.
16. If the child wants to be left alone while expelling returns, provide privacy. Child should expel the total volume of the instilled solution.
17. Remove the potty chair or bedpan.
18. Clean the child's perineal area, and help child assume a comfortable position.
19. Estimate returns of solution. **Rationale:** To determine that the child expelled the total volume of the solution.
20. Clean all equipment, and replace in appropriate area.
21. Remove gloves and wash your hands.

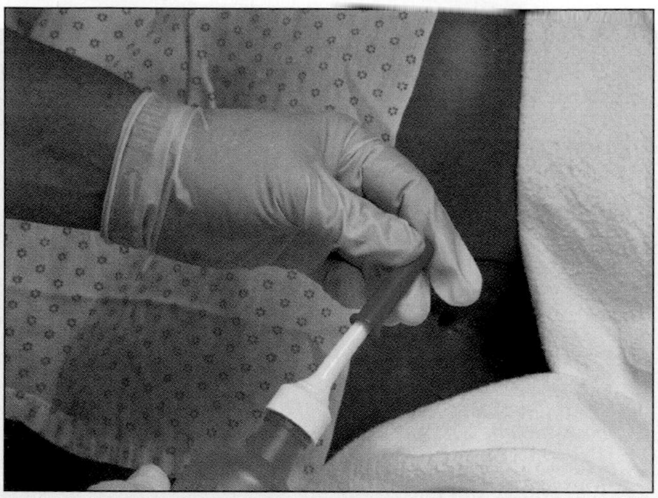
Remove cap from container and ensure that it is lubricated.

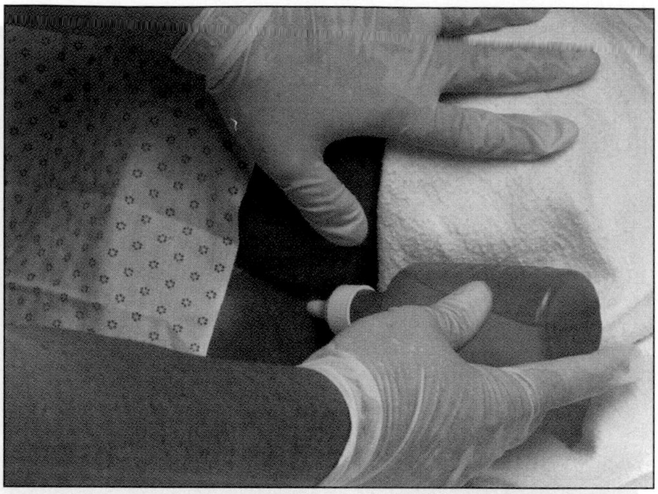
Insert tip of container gently into rectum and expel all fluid.

ADMINISTERING A SMALL-VOLUME ENEMA

Equipment

Commercially prepared enema
Water-soluble lubricant
Bedpan, commode, toilet
Two pair of clean gloves
Bed protector
Skin care items (e.g., soap, water, towels)

Preparation

1. Check physician's orders and client care plan.
2. Gather equipment.
3. Wash your hands.
4. Identify correct client and explain the procedure. Explain the benefits of relaxing and taking periodic deep breaths.
5. Place bed protector under client.
6. Place client on left side in a Sims' position.
7. Provide privacy.
8. Don clean gloves.

Procedure

1. Read directions on enema container.
2. Lubricate with water-soluble lubricant if necessary. (Usually rectal tube is self-lubricated.)
3. Expose the anal opening to assist you in inserting the tube without traumatizing the tissue.
4. After inserting rectal tube, gently squeeze the container, and empty entire 120 mL of hypertonic solution.
5. Keep pressure on container while removing from rectum. **Rationale:** To prevent solution from being drawn back into container.
6. Instruct client to hold solution 5–7 minutes.
7. When ready to expel solution elevate the head of the bed so that the client can assume a squatting position on the bedpan. If able, client may expel solution in toilet.
8. Remove and dispose of gloves.
9. Provide privacy until the client has expelled the total volume of the instilled solution.
10. Don gloves and remove bedpan if client using bedpan.
11. Assist client with perineal care, and help client to assume a comfortable position.
12. Measure returns if on strict I&O.
13. Dispose of equipment, and remove gloves.
14. Wash your hands.

ADMINISTERING A RETENTION ENEMA

Equipment

Commercially prepared disposable oil retention enema
Oil: Adult 150–200 mL, child 75–100 mL, 91°F
Water-soluble lubricant
Bedpan or commode
Bed protector
Skin care items (e.g., soap, water, towels)
Clean gloves

Preparation

1. Identify and prepare client as for any enema.
2. Provide privacy.
3. Gather equipment—disposable oil retention enema is administered like a small enema. Read directions on enema container.
4. Wash hands and don clean gloves.

Procedure

1. Explain steps of procedure to client.
2. Raise bed to HIGH position.
3. Place bed protector on bed.
4. Expose anal opening, and gently insert rectal tube tip of container 3–4 inches. Commercially prepared enemas are prelubricated.
5. Squeeze contents slowly, and empty entire amount into rectum.
6. Keep container compressed and remove rectal tube gently. **Rationale:** To prevent solution from being drawn back into container.
7. Lower bed.
8. Discard equipment and gloves, following Standard Precautions. Wash hands.
9. Explain to client that oil should be retained for 30–60 minutes before it is expelled. **Rationale:** Purpose of enema is to soften stool.
10. A cleansing enema may need to be given to remove oil and stimulate defecation.

ADMINISTERING A RETURN FLOW ENEMA

Equipment

Fluid container with attached rectal tube
Normal saline or tap water at 105°–110°F
Water-soluble lubricant
Clean bedpan
Bed protector
Skin care items (e.g., soap, water, towels)
Clean gloves

Preparation

1. Check physician's orders and client care plan.
2. Gather equipment.
3. Provide privacy.
4. Wash your hands.
5. Check identaband.
6. Fill fluid container with 100–200 mL of ordered solution; check that temperature is between 105°–110°F.
7. Allow solution to run through tubing so that air is removed. **Rationale:** If air is instilled during procedure, client experiences discomfort.
8. Hang container on IV pole.

Procedure

1. Explain procedure to client. Explain the benefits of relaxing and taking periodic deep breaths during procedure.
2. Raise bed to HIGH position, and lower side rails.
3. Don gloves.
4. Place bed protector under client.
5. Place client on left side in Sims' position. **Rationale:** This position facilitates instillation of fluid.
6. Lubricate tip of tubing with water-soluble lubricant.
7. Gently spread buttocks, and insert tubing 3–4 inches into client's rectum, past external and internal sphincters. Avoid traumatizing hemorrhoids during insertion. **Rationale:** Vagal nerve stimulation from enemas may cause cardiac arrhythmias.
8. Raise water container to a maximum height of 18 inches above bed.
9. Open clamp and allow solution to flow slowly into rectum and sigmoid colon. If cramping occurs, clamp tube for a few minutes and then continue infusion.
10. Lower solution container below level of rectum and allow all fluid to flow back into container.
11. Raise container 18 inches above rectum and allow solution to flow back into rectum.
12. Repeat inflow–outflow process 5–6 times, changing solution when it becomes thick with feces. **Rationale:** This assists in stimulating intestinal peristalsis with expulsion of flatus.
13. Provide privacy until client has expelled total volume of instilled solution following last inflow–outflow series.
14. Assist client with perineal care, and help client assume a comfortable position.
15. If client is on strict I&O, measure returns to make sure total volume of solution is expelled.
16. Clean all equipment, and replace in bathroom or appropriate location.
17. Remove gloves and wash your hands.
18. Lower bed and raise side rails.

Documentation for Enema Administration

- Purpose of enema
- Time enema given
- Volume and type of solution used
- Results obtained: amount, consistency, and color
- Any unexpected outcomes and measures taken to remedy problems
- Client's reactions to procedure
- Relief of flatus

Critical Thinking Application

UNEXPECTED OUTCOMES	CRITICAL THINKING OPTIONS
Client expels solution prematurely.	• Calm and ease client's distress by reassuring him or her as you clean the equipment. • Place bedpan under client. Place client in semi-Fowler's position with knees flexed. • Hold the rectal tube in client's rectum between thighs. Slow the water flow, and continue with the enema.
Client complains of severe and sudden abdominal pain, nausea, and distention.	• Remove tubing, and notify physician immediately of possible perforation. (This is an uncommon complication.) • Assess vital signs. If you suspect cardiac dysrhythmias, remove bedpan and notify physician immediately. • Be prepared to administer emergency drugs, such as atropine. • If an IV is not in place, start an IV of 5% dextrose in water (D_5W) using a large-bore needle for emergency use.
The flow of water is impeded or an obstruction is felt.	• Open clamp on tubing. Allow a small amount of solution to flow. (The warm solution may help relax the internal sphincter.) • Withdraw tube slightly, and reinsert. • Gently perform a digital examination for the possibility of fecal impaction. Break up impaction if present. Ask physician for order to give a retention enema, followed by a cleansing enema 2–3 hours later.
Client cannot return enema solution.	• Gently massage client's abdomen if not contraindicated. • Replace rectal tube. Lower the enema bag below the level of the bed. • If client is not uncomfortable, do nothing. If client complains of discomfort or pain, notify physician.
Enema returns are not clear prior to surgery or diagnostic testing.	• Repeat enema. If, after three enemas, returns are still not clear, notify physician of findings. • May need to give an enema with a stronger solution. • Physician may need to order magnesium citrate or electrolyte solution (i.e., GoLYTELY).
Fecal impaction is not relieved.	• Check orders for oil retention enema. • Check catheter size needed. • Obtain order for and use digital stimulation and manual extraction of feces if not contraindicated by diagnosis of cardiac or neurologic involvement.

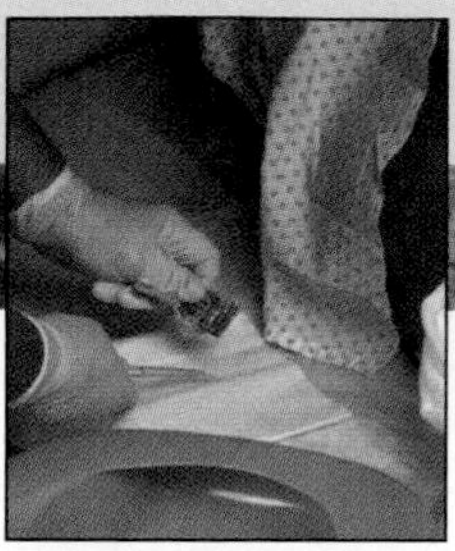

UNIT 3

Fecal Ostomy Pouch Application

Nursing Process Data

ASSESSMENT *Data Base*

Assess type and location of stoma (section of bowel used to create stoma).

Observe stoma color, which should be beefy red and moist.

Inspect client's abdomen for creasing, firmness, softness, contour, scars, folds, and incisions.

Inspect client's periostomal skin for signs of erythema, excoriation, ulceration, and fistula formation.

Assess how far stoma protrudes above skin surface; it should be ½–1 inch.

Assess size of stoma.

Assess output of effluent including amount, consistency, odor.

Assess client's learning abilities, age, manual dexterity, and visual acuity.

PLANNING *Objectives*

To collect effluent for accurate assessment of output in the hospital

To collect effluent for the comfort of the client

To contain drainage and odors so that the client feels that he or she is socially acceptable

To protect peristomal skin from erythema, excoriation, and infection

To protect the client's clothing

IMPLEMENTATION *Procedures*

Applying a Fecal Ostomy Pouch

EVALUATION *Expected Outcomes*

Pouch remains intact without leakage for 3–5 days.

Pouching system provides maximal skin protection.

Pouching system remains odorproof for 3–5 days.

Client gradually assumes an active role in applying the pouch.

Client's skin remains free of erythema or excoriation.

APPLYING A FECAL OSTOMY POUCH

Equipment

1 or 2 piece transparent ostomy pouch with attached skin barrier
Warm water
Soft cloths
Bath blanket
Plastic bag for pouch disposal
Tail closure or night adaptor for pouch
Clean gloves
Measuring guide
Tissues
Scissors

Preparation

1. Check client care plan.
2. Determine exact supplies client uses.
3. Gather equipment.
4. Explain procedure to client.
5. Provide privacy.
6. Raise bed to high position.
7. Wash hands and don gloves.

Procedure

1. Place bath blanket over client. Place absorbent pad or towels under client. **Rationale:** To protect bed from spillage.
2. Observe placement of stoma. **Rationale:** To determine normal amount of output and consistency. (Immediately after surgery, all stomas will have very liquid stool and high flatus output.)
3. Empty old pouch into bedpan or toilet.
4. Remove old pouch by pushing against skin as you pull backing from skin and discard in plastic bag. Save tail closure on bottom of pouch.
5. Measure output, if ordered.
6. Clean skin and stoma gently with warm water and soft cloth. **Rationale:** Oily substances can interfere with pouch adhesive.

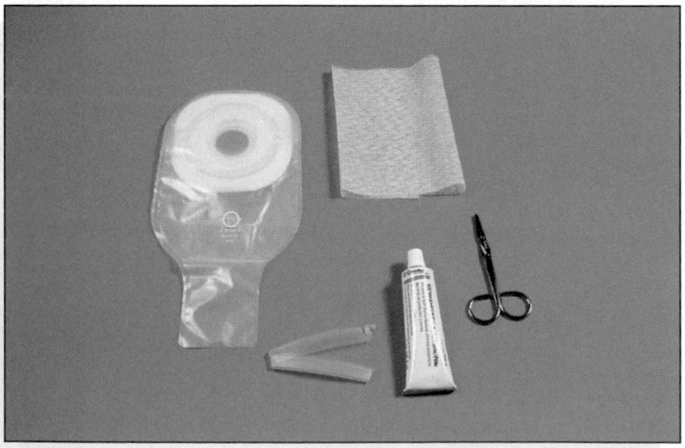

Supplies needed to change one-piece pouches.

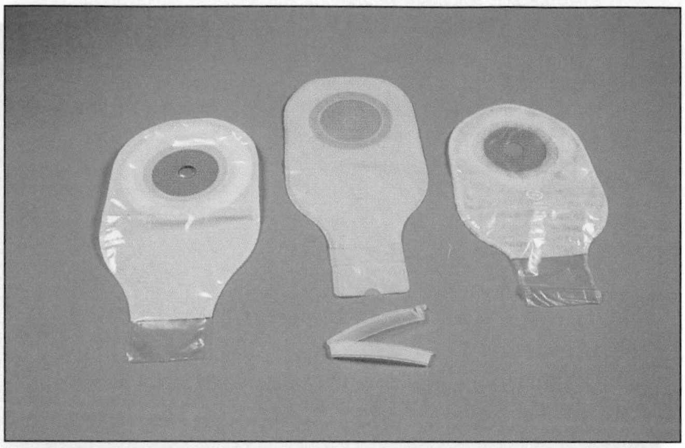

One-piece pouches.

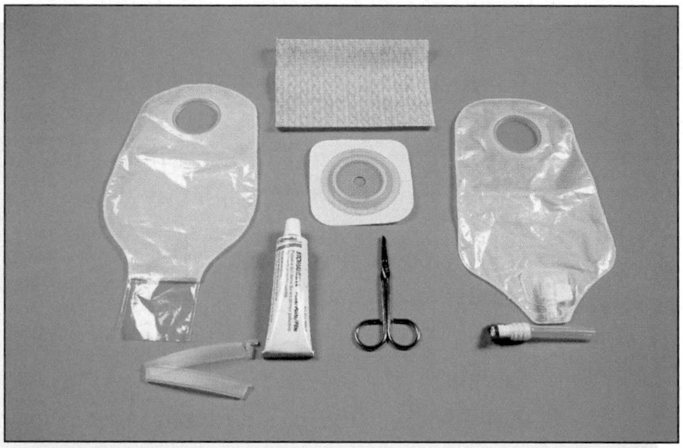

Supplies needed to change two-piece pouches.

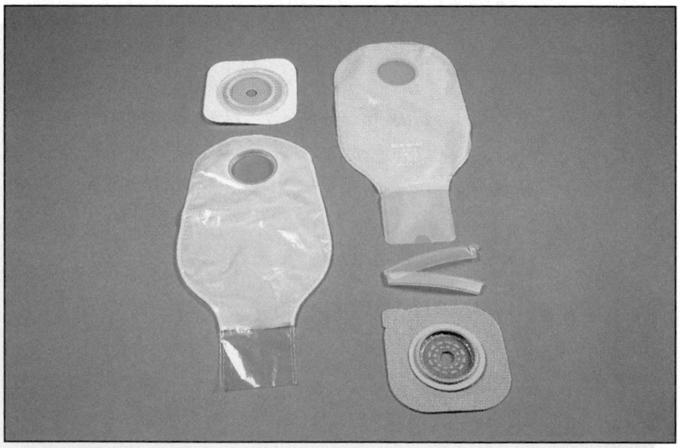

Two-piece fecal pouches.

CLINICAL ALERT

To promote the client's self-esteem and body image, be aware of your own body language. Even subtle changes in the way you look at the stoma could indicate disgust or disapproval and an altered self-esteem could result.

7. Dry skin well with soft cloth. Keep tissues available if stoma functions while pouch is off.
8. Observe skin and stoma for changes in size, ulceration, and color (stoma should be a beefy red).
9. Measure stoma with measuring guide.
10. Trace measured pattern on pouch.
11. Cut pouch to pattern, making sure opening is large enough to encircle stoma without pushing on edges. **Rationale:** No skin should appear between the pouch edge and the stoma.
12. If using a two-piece pouch, snap the wafer and pouch together: (*See* photo sequence for alternate method of using two-piece pouch.)
13. Remove paper from skin barrier on pouch and save it. **Rationale:** This may be used as a pattern for next pouch change.
14. Apply a ring of skin barrier paste to opening on pouch.
15. Remove paper from outer ring.
16. Center and apply pouch to clean and dry skin. Smooth edges of adhesive to skin. **Rationale:** If adhesive is wrinkled, it may result in leakage from pouch.
17. Pouches can be applied over an incision. **Rationale:** Incisions are sealed within 24 hours of surgery.
18. Close and secure end of pouch with tail closure.
    a. Ensure bowed end is next to body. **Rationale:** This provides a better fit to body, and prevents outpouching of clamp through clothing.
    b. Lay hook on top of bag and fold bag 1 inch over end of pouch.
    c. Squeeze clamp together to close.
19. Remove soiled pouch and tissues from bedside.
20. Remove gloves and wash hands.
21. Position client for comfort. Return bed to low position.
22. Put away supplies and reorder as necessary.

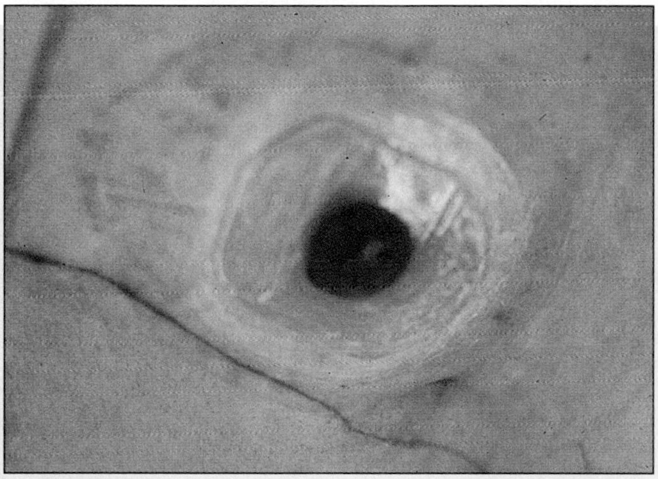
Viable stoma.

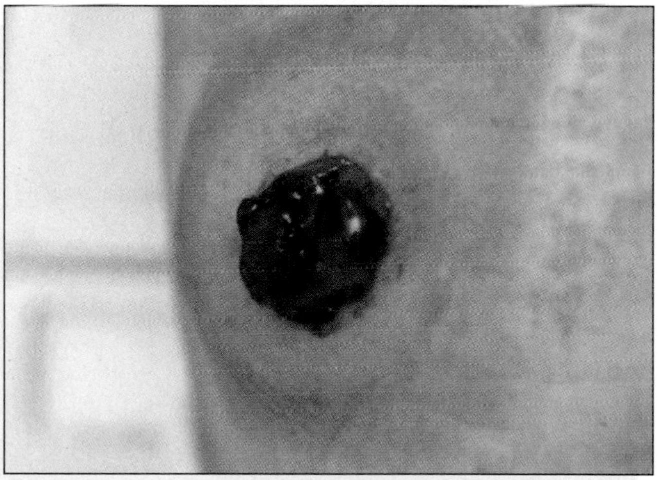
Nonviable stoma.

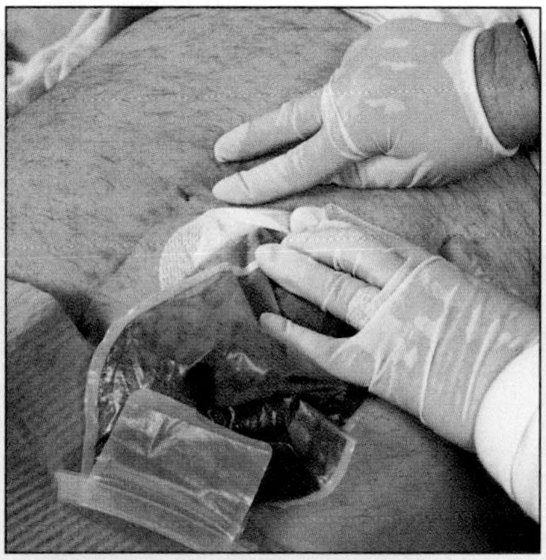
Starting at upper corner, remove old pouch.

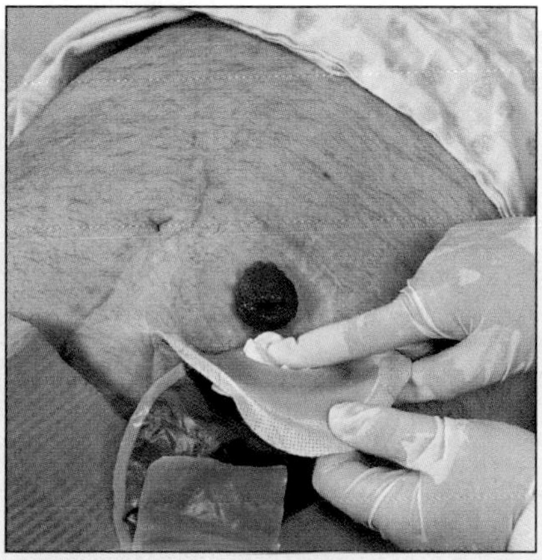
As you remove old pouch, push against skin while pulling on pouch.

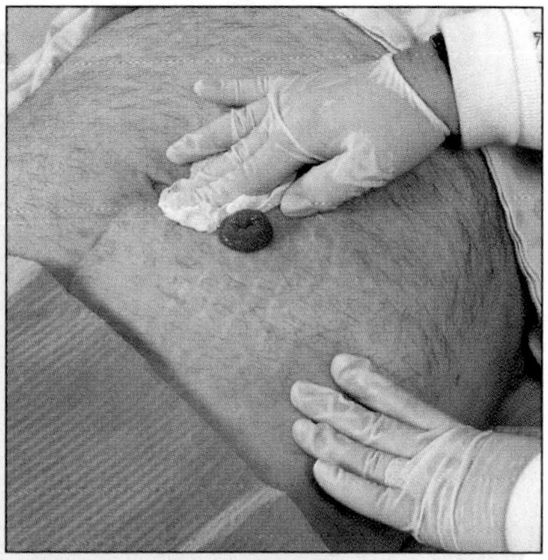
Clean skin with warm water; dry well.

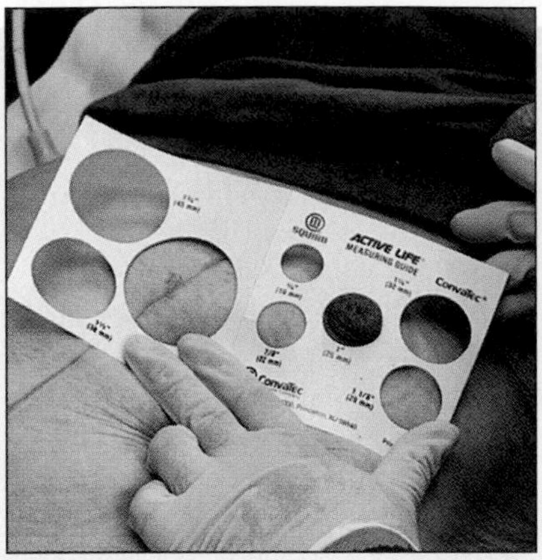

Measure stoma size.

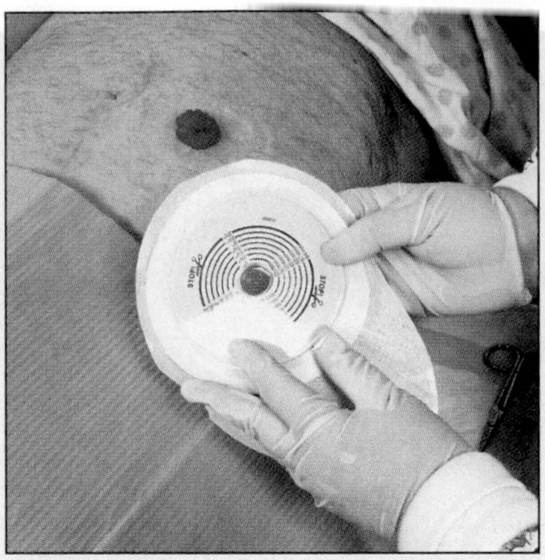

Remove plastic covering from one-piece pouch.

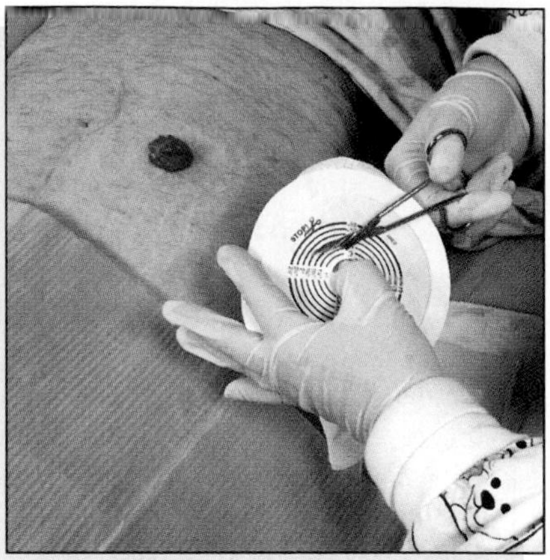

Cut pouch opening to exact size of stoma.

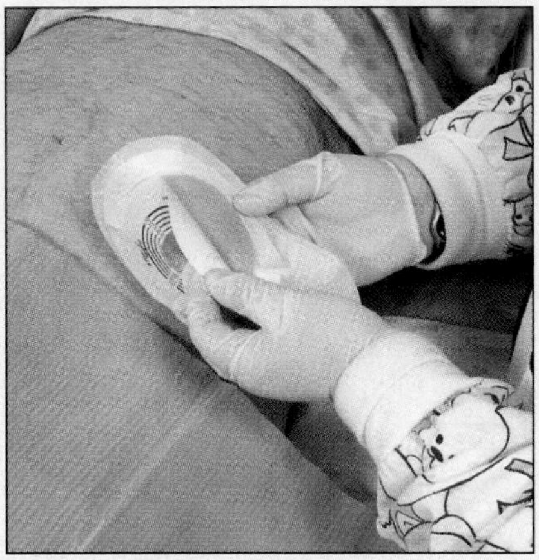

Remove paper from inner wafer. Save pattern for future pouch changes.

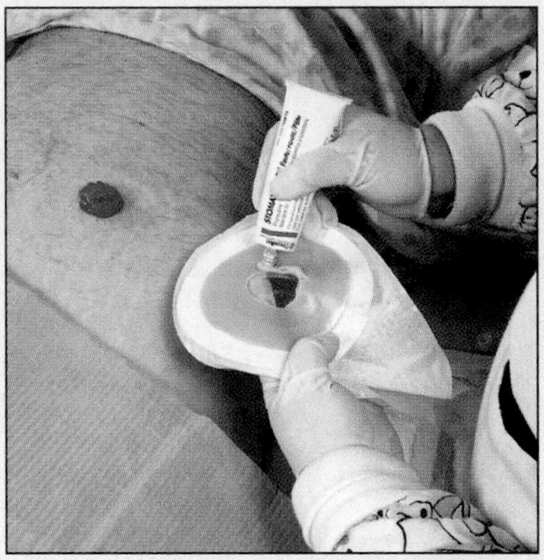

Apply ring of paste to opening on pouch.

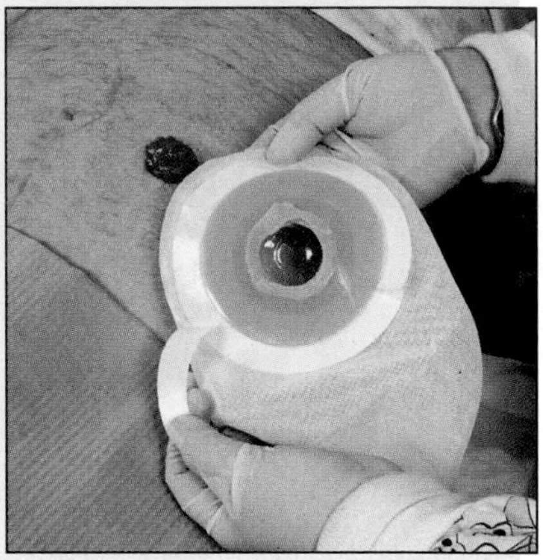

Remove paper from outer adhesive ring of pouch.

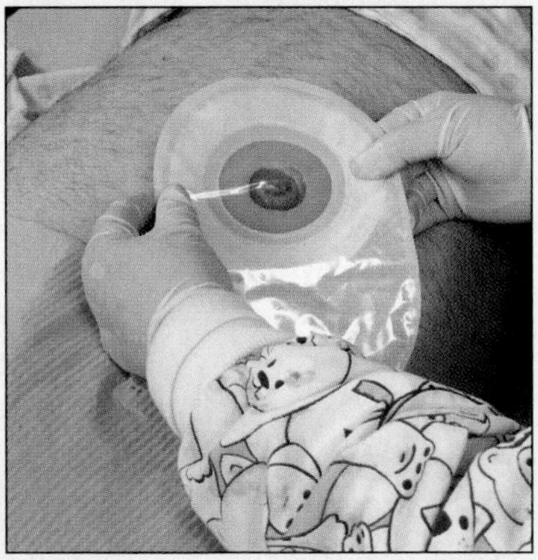

Center and apply pouch to clean, dry skin.

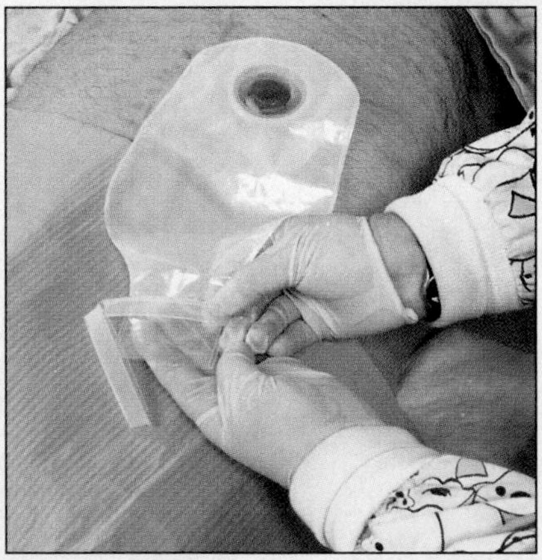

After applying one-piece pouch, clamp bottom of pouch.

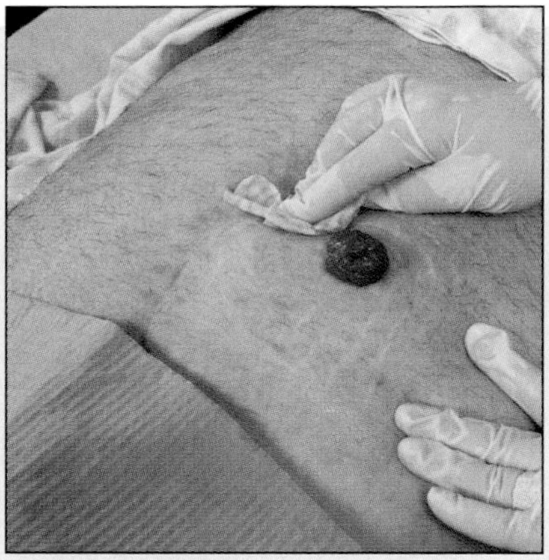
Clean and dry skin thoroughly before applying two-piece pouch.

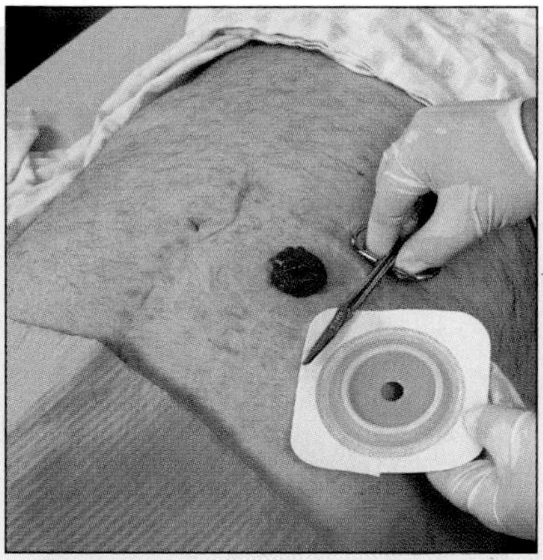
Cut opening of a two-piece pouch to exact size of stoma.

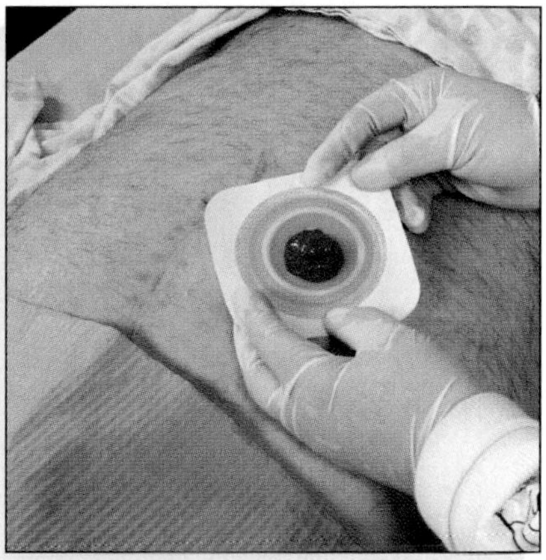
Check size of opening to ensure proper fit.

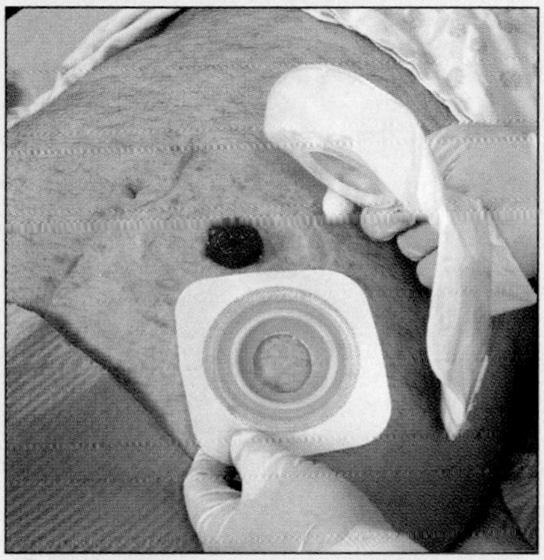
Snap pouch onto wafer when using a two-piece pouch.

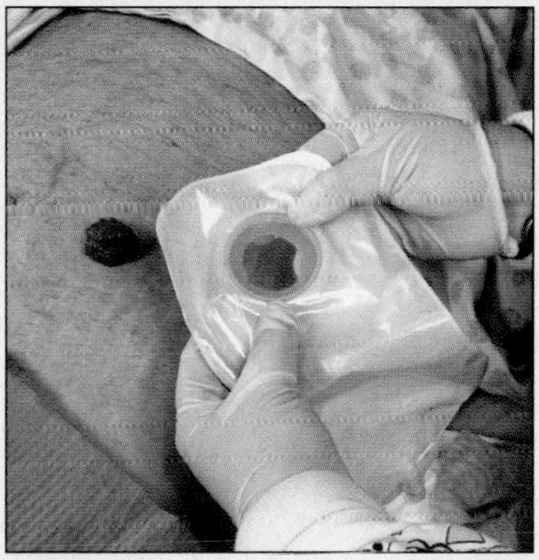
Check for secure fit by tugging at bottom of pouch.

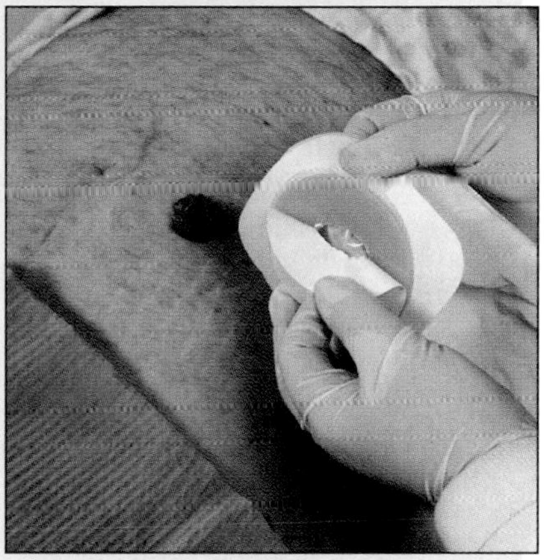
Remove paper from inner barrier.

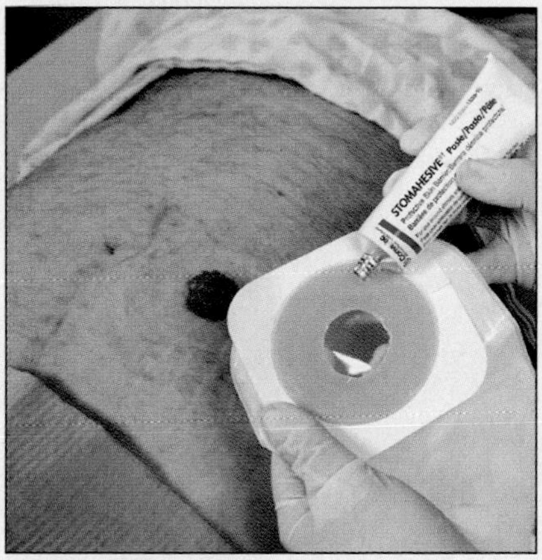

Apply paste to inner circle of wafer.

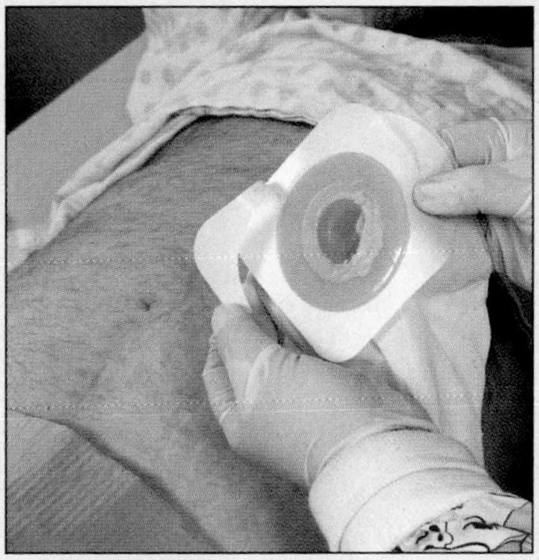
Remove paper from outer adhesive ring.

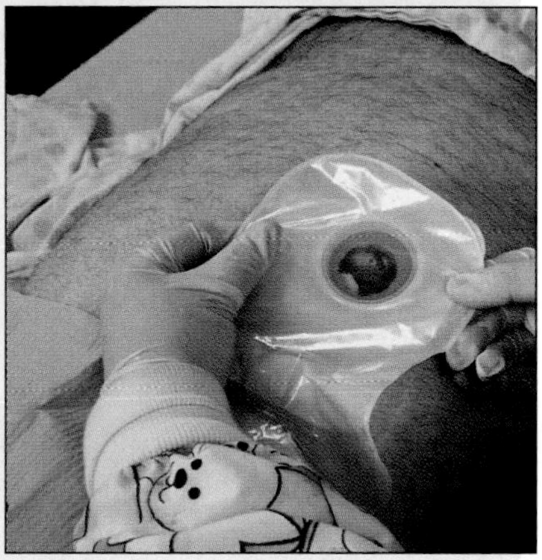
Center pouch over stoma and press onto skin.

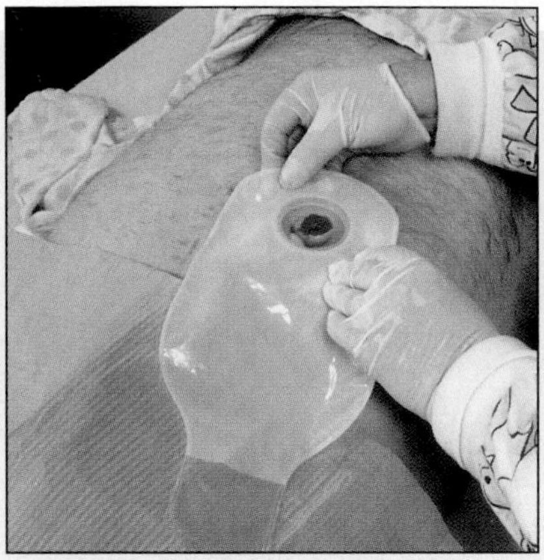

Secure adhesive to skin.

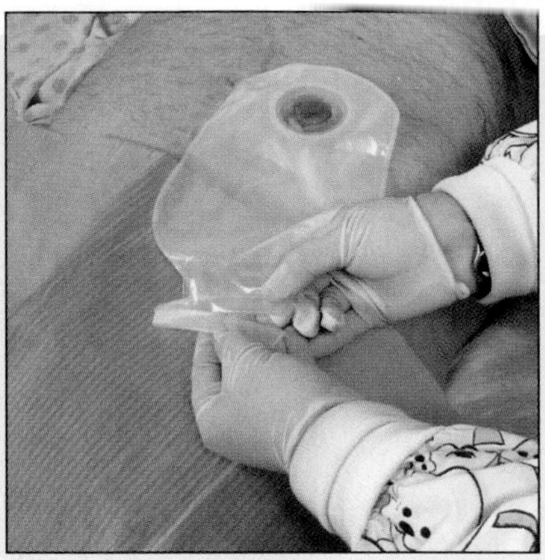

Clamp bottom of pouch.

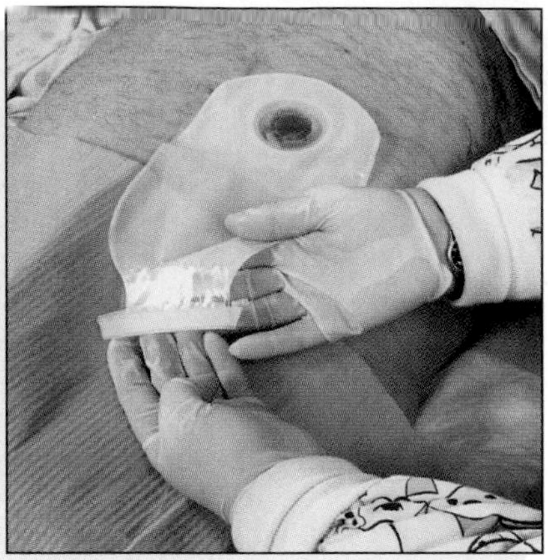

Check that pouch clamp is secure.

Client Teaching

- Empty pouch when one-third full of stool or flatus.
  a. Empty into toilet.
  b. Pouch should last for 3–4 days.
- Empty each morning and last thing at night even if not one-third full.
- Check seal on daily basis for tight fit, change if needed.
- Instruct client to always carry a supply of ostomy equipment for emergency use.
- Instruct client on emptying and cleaning pouch, opening and closing clamp, observing and cleaning periostomal area, and changing pouch.
- Have client return demonstration until able to perform activities correctly.

Loop Colostomy with Rod

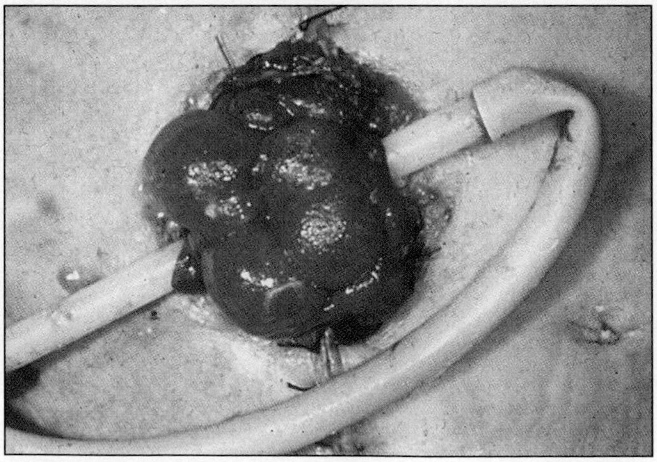

A loop of bowel is brought onto abdomen and is supported by a plastic rod.

Loop Colostomy with Rod Removed

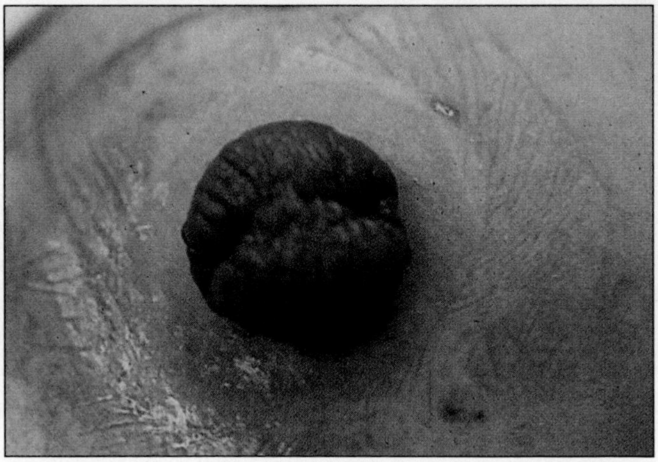

Two openings are made in colostomy.

Proximal loop is functional and discharges fecal material.

Distal end is nonfunctional and discharges only mucus.

DOCUMENTATION FOR FECAL OSTOMY POUCH APPLICATION

- Type of pouch and skin barrier used
- Time pouch applied
- Time pouch emptied
- Amount, color, and consistency of stool emptied from pouch
- Presence or absence of flatus through the stoma
- Location of stoma
- Client participation in and toleration of pouch application
- Condition of peristomal skin and stoma, including color and size
- Condition of incision line (i.e., any redness or swelling)
- Condition of abdomen (e.g., distention)
- Client teaching, which has been completed

Critical Thinking Application

UNEXPECTED OUTCOMES	CRITICAL THINKING OPTIONS
Stoma appears dark, dusky-colored, or black.	• Notify physician of findings, and document in chart. (Usually indicates stoma is ischemic.)
Stoma becomes ulcerated or cut.	• Examine pouching system to see if opening of pouch may be cutting into stoma. • Recut opening to exact size of stoma.
Stoma remains a persistent pale pink.	• Request physician to order Hgb, Hct (usually the result of low Hgb). • Instruct client to monitor effluent for constipation if iron preparation ordered.
Bleeding occurs when stoma is touched.	• Observe and note—usual occurrence postoperatively.
Erythematous rash at site of pouch.	• Assess for allergic reaction to product being used. • May need to change to different type of adhesive on pouch or change to a pouch with no adhesive.
Papular rash appears on peristomal skin.	• Assess for possible yeast sensitivity. • Be sure skin is clean and dry before applying pouch. • Do not rinse pouch with water because this traps water under wafer. • May need to use antifungal powder on skin with each pouch change until skin clears.
Skin is denuded from leakage.	• Evaluate cause of leakage. • Be sure pouch is cut to correct size. • May need to fill any creases around stoma with skin barrier paste. • May need to use secondary skin barrier like Eakin seal. • May need to attach belt to minimize lateral leakage. • Change to a product like durahesive that swells around stoma preventing leakage and holds up well to liquid output.

UNEXPECTED OUTCOMES	CRITICAL THINKING OPTIONS
	• Be sure pouch is emptied before it is over ⅓ full of stool or flatus, since an overfull pouch can break seal of pouch.
	• Pouches should not be changed more than once daily.
Client experiences itching or burning under appliance.	• May be a sign that stool is undermining seal of pouch.
Client not coping with altered body image.	• Refer to United Ostomy Association, the Crohn's and Colitis Foundation of America, American Cancer Society or the local Enterostomal Therapy nurse.

GERONTOLOGIC CONSIDERATIONS

- Elderly clients frequently have concomitant cardiac problems, which can be affected by vagal stimulation during fecal removal or enema administration. Check with the physician before these skills are performed on elderly clients. Monitor the pulse carefully during the procedure.
- Fecal impaction is not uncommon with elderly clients due to decreased mobility and exercise, dietary habits, and tendency to overuse enemas and laxatives.
- Encourage clients to decrease use of laxatives and enemas, increase fluid intake and fiber in diet, and increase exercise. Dehydration resulting from inadequate fluid intake leads to constipation and fecal impaction.
- To select the proper ostomy appliance for an elderly client, the nurse must determine if the client has any physical limitations that could influence the type of appliance needed. These limitations include poor vision, use of only one hand, arthritis, and inability to perform cleaning and pouching procedure.

MANAGEMENT GUIDELINES

Each state legislates a Nurse Practice Act for RNs and LVN/LPNs. Health care facilities are responsible for establishing and implementing policies and procedures that conform to their state's regulations. Verify the regulations and role parameters for each health care worker in your facility.

Delegation of Responsibilities

- A CNA or unlicensed assistive personnel (UAP) may be assigned to administer a disposable enema or tap water enema in most facilities. This information is presented in the CNA curriculum. These personnel are not allowed to administer enemas with medications or a Harris flush.
- An LVN/LPN may be assigned to insert a rectal tube, administer enemas, and perform colostomy care.
- In some rehabilitation settings, aides may be instructed to administer glycerine suppositories. This requires additional training. Check facility policy and procedure manuals to determine which health care worker may be assigned to this task.
- A CNA cannot be assigned to perform a fecal impaction removal because of the risk of a vagal response during the procedure.

Information Flow

- Information relative to bowel elimination is provided both through report and written information on the Kardex card.
- Before delegating any of the tasks associated with bowel elimination to a CNA or UAP, determine their knowledge base to perform the task. Ask them to explain the procedure if you are unsure of their ability to perform the task.

- When an LVN/LPN or RN is assigned to perform colostomy care or assist a physician with an intestinal tube insertion, ensure he or she is familiar with the procedure. Review the procedure as needed.
- Clients who require a bowel program need instruction on the process so they may become independent in the skill. If someone else will be assisting them with this procedure, they should be included in the teaching process. The RN is responsible for establishing the teaching program. An LVN/LPN may assist in carrying out the plan.
- When special steps or supplies are needed to perform a task (i.e., colostomy care), information should be written on the client care plan or clinical pathway. This allows all staff to perform the procedure the same way. Clients feel more secure when procedures are completed in a uniform method.

CRITICAL THINKING STRATEGIES

SCENARIO 1

You are assigned to a 74-year-old man who had a transverse colostomy for cancer 4 days ago. During the night report, you heard the night nurse say his pouch is leaking and he is very angry with the staff for causing the mess. As you prepare to enter his room, you decide how to approach him.

1. Determine the most appropriate communication technique to use with the client. Provide rationale for your response.
2. As you observe the stoma and pouch, you determine the leak is at the bottom of pouch.
   a. State two reasons the pouch may be leaking.
   b. Describe your initial nursing action after you assess the leaking pouch.
   c. What steps do you take to ensure the new pouch will not leak?
3. After removing the first pouch, you assess the skin and determine the periostomal skin to be erythematous and the stoma reddened and slightly edematous.
   a. What is your priority nursing intervention? Provide the rationale for your response.
   b. After completing the priority intervention, what is your next action?
4. Following the application of the new pouch, you determine that a teaching plan needs to be developed for the client.
   a. Describe the method of developing a teaching plan for this client.
   b. After developing a plan, indicate the first step the nurse should incorporate to implement the plan.
   c. Describe your rationale for the first step of the teaching plan.
   d. List at least three nursing diagnoses that are appropriate for this client's care plan.
   e. Identify at least one community resource that is appropriate for a referral.

SCENARIO 2

You assess Mrs. Jacob, a 65-year-old who had a colostomy performed 6 days ago, for cancer of the descending colon. When you tell her you will be instructing her on how to apply a new pouch, she starts to cry and says, "No, I don't want to know how because all it does is leak everywhere."

1. Identify the initial nursing intervention and discuss additional actions you would take to resolve this problem.
2. Describe the assessment database that should be completed before a plan can be implemented.
3. Outline the steps in designing a client teaching plan for a client with an ostomy.

CHAPTER 24

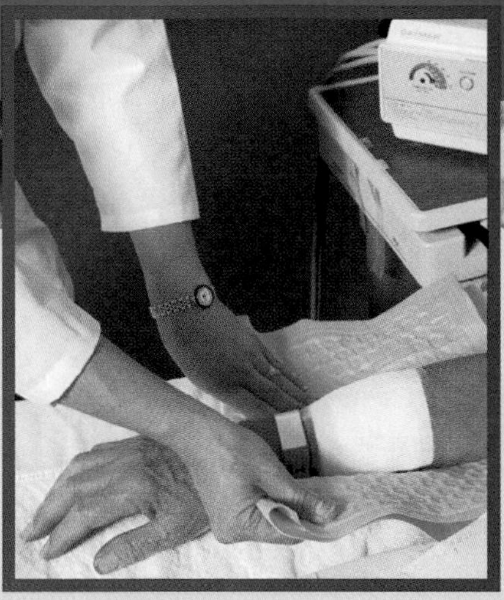

Heat and Cold Therapies

THEORETICAL CONCEPTS

UNIT ONE: **Heat Therapies** **792**

Applying a Commercial Heat Pack 793

Monitoring an Infant Radiant Warmer 793

Applying an Aquathermic Pad 794

Applying a Hot Moist Pack 795

Assisting with a Sitz Bath 796

UNIT TWO: **Cold Therapies** **798**

Applying an Ice Pack/Commercial Cold Pack 799

Applying a Disposable Instant (Chemical) Cold Pack 800

UNIT THREE: **Systemic Cooling Therapies** **802**

Providing a Tepid Bath 803

Using a Cooling Blanket 804

GERONTOLOGIC CONSIDERATIONS **808**

MANAGEMENT GUIDELINES **809**

CRITICAL THINKING STRATEGIES **810**

LEARNING OBJECTIVES

- Describe the mechanisms responsible for the body's heat loss and heat production.
- Discuss the role of the hypothalamus in the body.
- List at least three adaptive processes that maintain the body temperature within a normal range.
- Discuss how heat transmission occurs.
- Describe the physiologic effects of heat applications.
- Describe the physiologic effects of cold applications.
- Differentiate local vs systemic thermal therapies.
- Identify various modes of heat therapy (local and systemic).
- Identify various modes of cold therapy (local and systemic).
- Identify indications and contraindications for various heat and cold therapies.
- List four safety factors to consider when applying heat and cold treatments.
- List two safety factors used to prevent skin irritation for infants in a radiant warmer.
- Demonstrate preparation of the infant radiant warmer.
- Describe major nursing interventions performed for clients requiring a cooling blanket.
- State two nursing diagnoses related to thermal treatments.
- Predict the type of thermal agent that would be most therapeutic for a particular client's condition.

TERMINOLOGY

Ambient temperature: temperature of the air surrounding a person.

Antipyretic: an agent that reduces febrile temperatures.

Compress: a pad of cloth applied firmly to a part of the body; compress may be dry or wet, cold or warm.

Conduction: heat transfer between materials of different temperatures that are in direct contact with each other (e.g., hot or cold pack).

Convection: heat transfer by circulation of a medium of a different temperature (e.g., whirlpool, blood circulation).

Cryotherapy: transfer of heat from the client by use of a cooling agent.

Cyanosis: bluish coloring of the skin and the mucous membrane due to decreased oxygenation.

Erythema: increased reddish color of the skin due to vasodilatation of capillaries.

Evaporation: absorption of heat (energy) as a result of conversion of a material from a liquid to a vapor state (e.g., sweating, spraying).

Fever: regulated rise in body temperature to a new hypothalamic "set point"; usually mediated by internal stimuli (e.g., pyrogenic cytokines).

Hyperemia: increased blood supply to an area.

Hyperthermia: nonregulated rise in core body temperature exceeding 41.5°C; usually due to external stimuli that cause excessive endogenous heat production or reduced capacity to lose heat (e.g., environmental exposure, CNS injury, medications).

Hypothermia: a reduction in core body temperature below 35°C due to exposure to cool or cold temperatures (e.g., environment, infusions). Mild = 34°C, moderate = 30°C, severe = less than 30°C.

Insulator: substance that is a poor conductor or a nonconductor of heat; a substance that helps prevent the escape or entrance of heat.

Mottling: blue-gray to purplish blotches seen usually peripherally; it is usually the result of peripheral vasoconstriction.

Pallor: loss of reddish hue due to superficial vasoconstriction produced by sympathetic stimulation.

Radiation: exchange of heat directly without an intervening medium (e.g., heat lamp).

Shivering thermogenesis: production of body heat by shivering or muscle contraction (tremors).

Suppuration: the process of pus formation.

Thermogenesis: heat production by the body.

Thermotherapy: transfer of heat to a client by use of a heating agent.

Vasoconstriction: a narrowing of blood vessels.

Vasodilation: expansion of blood vessels.

Vasomotor: pertaining to nerves having muscular control of the blood vessel walls.

TEMPERATURE CONTROL

The temperature of the human body is regulated and maintained by a group of interrelated feedback systems. When these homeostatic mechanisms are altered by disease or environmental conditions, the body may need assistance to regain its normal temperature.

Temperature control of the body is a homeostatic function that balances heat production and loss to maintain body temperature within a fairly constant range. The body uses neuronal pathways to collect, organize, and transmit temperature information. These pathways also transmit physiologic responses to produce temperature adjustments. The main integrative function is carried out by the hypothalamus.

The hypothalamus is the body's thermostat, and it functions to maintain the body as close as possible to a constant, or "set point," temperature. Information reaches the hypothalamus by indirect and direct means: indirectly through receptors and directly by circulating blood. The hypothalamus triggers body response in the tissues and vasomotor tone in the organs to produce shivering, sweating, and changes in conduction, convection, evaporation, and radiation. The body uses these physiologic processes to alter temperature.

The body continuously strives to maintain a constant optimal temperature. As heat is gained through metabolism, exercise, or environmental factors, the body throws off excess warmth through convection, conduction, or evaporation. In contrast, on sensing a loss of heat (cold), the body triggers one or more processes to produce heat (thermogenesis), conserve it, or dissipate it. Although these dynamic processes cannot be observed, their resulting effects, such as violent shivering, are readily evident. The hypothalamus continuously makes adjustments, varying in intensity, to maintain the core body temperature.

Our body works to maintain a neutral thermal environment. We consciously and unconsciously alter levels of activity in response to the physiologic stimulus from the body's thermostat, the hypothalamus. When we sense cold, we huddle or curl up to decrease heat lost from the body surface. When warm, we extend our bodies and separate our limbs. There are sensors in the hypothalamus and in the dermis that are distributed widely over the body surface. These sensors react to changes in temperature. In fact, the hypothalamus is sensitive to very minute changes, as slight as 0.01°C in the circulating blood.

Adjustment Processes

An important adjustment process is heat conservation. When the body perceives a cooling sensation, heat-conserving and heat-producing mechanisms are activated. Vessel constriction, a heat-conserving mechanism, removes warmed blood from the surface area of the skin. This reduces heat loss to the cooler exterior through conduction. Sweating removes heat from the body through the process of evaporation. The piloerector muscles contract, raising all the body hairs, to create an insulating (nonconductive) layer of air around the body. The latter reaction produces "goose flesh" and may lead to the behavioral response of huddling, curling up, or adding clothing to modify the microenvironment.

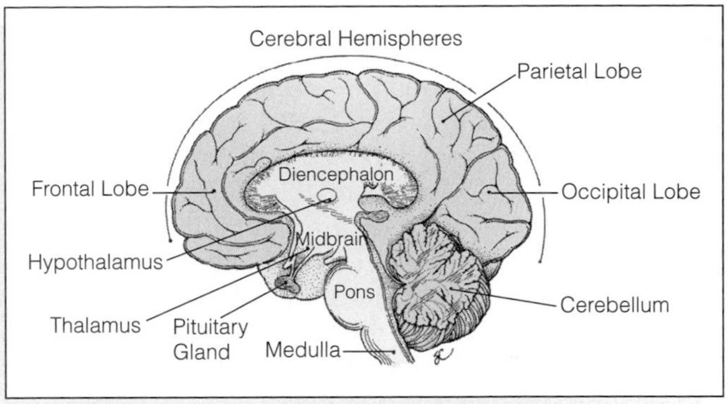

The hypothalamus is located in the diencephalon portion of the brain. It controls the body's thermostat.

An emotional reaction can also produce a vasomotor response. Psychologic perception of danger triggers the body's alarm system causing epinephrine to be released. This results in vasoconstriction on the periphery of the body, piloerection, and increased respiratory rate.

Heat production, or thermogenesis, is a progressive adaptive process. A mild cold stimulus causes an increase in respiratory rate. This is the result of the increased oxidative process going on in muscles as they are tensing. More oxygen is consumed, shivering begins as muscle tension increases, and heat is produced. This process continues until the temperature, as sensed by the thermostat hypothalamus, is high enough or has reached the "set point."

A second kind of thermogenesis, nonshivering thermogenesis, also activates metabolic processes. Production of norepinephrine, mediated through neuroendocrine control, stimulates the metabolism of brown fat. Oxygen consumption is raised during this process, heat is produced, and body temperature increases. Brown adipose tissue has a special kind of cell structure and is normally present in newborns. Newborns, incapable of shivering, still are able to produce body heat through metabolic processes. Brown adipose tissue reserves are felt to decrease with age, which perhaps explains why we feel extremes of cold more severely as we grow older.

In contrast, when the body perceives excess heat, opposite measures are activated. Sources of excess body heat may be internal (excessive muscle activity) or external (a very warm environment). The adaptability of the multiple systems to maintain temperature within the critical range is again demonstrated when mechanisms are activated to dissipate heat. The thermostat of the hypothalamus and the peripherally situated warmth receptors provide neurologic information to set the cooling mechanisms in motion. Peripheral vasodilatation occurs, and warmed blood is brought to the surface of the body. Surface vessels dilate, promoting radiation of heat away from the body. Behavioral responses are to remove insulative layers and to extend our body to increase the surface area for greater heat conduction. Heat conservation mechanisms are reduced, muscle activity is decreased, and heat production is minimized.

All thermoregulatory activities require functional pathways for receptors and effectors. Physiologic systems must be healthy and intact to respond to the constant adjustments. The behavioral–intellectual systems must also function effectively to be able to manipulate the immediate environment to maintain body temperature. Our ability to adapt to alterations in temperature is affected by many external factors, such as pathogens; medications; physical disorders; and general health conditions related to age, circulation, physical fitness, and nutrition.

Heat and cold therapies utilize physical principles/processes of *conduction, convection, evaporation*, and *radiation* to manipulate heat *transfer*. The body uses these same *processes of heat transfer* to retain heat (when the body is too cold) or to release heat (when the body is too hot) in an attempt to normalize body temperature.

Processes of Heat Transfer

Conduction is heat transfer through *direct* contact with a cooler object. The greater the temperature difference, the faster heat will transfer; very hot or very cold applications can cause tissue injury.

Different objects have different heat conductivity: the body's superficial tissues transfer (conduct) heat readily, but cooling or warming the surface has little impact on changing the temperature of deeper tissues. Metal conducts heat readily, but air has low conductivity. Therefore, metal objects should be removed from the treated area, and a towel may be placed under a hot or cold pack to trap air (insulate) and limit heat transfer in order to prevent tissue injury.

Convection is heat transfer by direct contact with a *circulating medium* (agent in motion) and another material of a different temperature. Therapeutic examples include whirlpool, aquathermic pad, cooling blanket, irrigations or infusions. Heat transfer by convection is more rapid than heat transfer by conduction, and convection modalities that circulate fluid are more effective than those that circulate air. The body utilizes convection by circulating warm blood away from and cooler blood into an area to stabilize tissue temperature.

Evaporation is heat transfer by conversion of a liquid to a *vapor*. Heat transfer by evaporation is more effective than heat transfer by air current (radiation). Evaporation of sweat serves to cool the body as long as the humidity of the environment is low enough to support evaporation. Another example is a moist open body cavity that loses heat to the cooler environment of the surgical suite. Therapeutic examples of evaporation include tepid sponging, or cold spraying.

Radiation is heat transfer through the air (no intervening medium) from a *warmer* to a *cooler* area. Since the exposed head is responsible for 65% of our body heat loss, a head covering will help prevent radiant heat loss. An example is putting a cap on a newborn's head.

THE INFLAMMATORY PROCESS

Almost all types of injury, arising from both external and internal sources, may cause an inflammatory response. Common causes of this process are trauma, surgery, extremes of heat and cold, damage to the body tissues, and chemicals. Inflammation may be acute, subacute, or chronic.

When acute inflammation occurs, you will recognize the common symptoms of redness, swelling, heat and

TABLE 24–1 Physiologic Effects of Heat and Cold Therapies

Thermotherapy	Cryotherapy
Increases superficial temperature Increases local metabolic rate Dilates arterioles and capillaries Enhances blood flow to area (including nutrients and phagocytic WBCs) Increases capillary permeability Improves lymphatic and venous drainage of fluid and metabolites. Promotes inflammation Enhances flexibility of muscles, ligaments Provides *analgesia* via gating mechanism Reduces edema *not* associated with acute inflammation	Reduces local tissue temperature Decreases cellular metabolism Constricts arterioles, capillaries and decreases blood flow, venous and lymphatic drainage. Reduces capillary permeability Reduces delivery of phagocytes Slows nerve conduction Reduces edema formation and accumulation Has extreme *anesthetic* effect via gating mechanism Decreases muscle spasticity

pain, or loss of function. When an individual experiences acute inflammation, it may manifest in two ways: as a vascular or cellular blood cell response. When a vascular response occurs, vasoconstriction is followed by vasodilation (warmth and redness are the characteristics). Then, swelling occurs, caused by an increase in capillary permeability, which results in fluid escaping into the tissues. The seriousness of the injury dictates the degree of response. For example, it may be an immediate or transient response or a sustained reaction that continues for several days and results in actual damage; or it could be a delayed response, which could occur with a sunburn or radiation injury. A cellular blood response to acute inflammation occurs when leukocytes move into the area of injury.

The signs and symptoms of inflammation are actually produced by chemical mediators, such as histamine (the first mediator in the inflammatory response), plasma proteases (kinins such as bradykinin), and prostaglandins, which contribute to vasodilation, capillary permeability, pain and fever, and leukotrienes. Cytokines are also mediators of inflammation and participate in a variety of cellular responses. Finally, inflammatory exudates are produced in this process, which include serous, fibrinous, and other forms of exudates. Healing occurs after the inflammatory process has resolved and regeneration or cell replacement takes place.

Heat and cold therapy has been used for many years as treatment for the symptoms of inflammation. Heat and cold therapies are commonly applied superficially to inhibit or enhance the inflammation that accompanies acute tissue injury (e.g., musculoskeletal sprain, strain, fracture, or surgery). Cold (cryo) therapies reduce inflammation; heat (thermo) therapies enhance inflammation. For each degree centigrade increase or decrease in the injured site's temperature, the tissue metabolic rate is increased or decreased by 13%. The magnitude of this response is influenced by the temperature of the modality, duration of therapy, and surface area exposed to the treatment.

Conditions That Affect Adaptive Processes

Pathogens in the form of viruses and bacteria can trigger fever, generally a temperature of over 38.3°C, or 101°F. Fever caused by a pathogenic process is a thermoregulation disorder in which the "set point" is displaced upward. In response, the body perceives it is cold and seeks to conserve heat (i.e., shivering). Age, the duration and amount of temperature increase, and the overall disease condition are variables influencing the body's reaction.

Fever makes clients feel uncomfortable, so antipyretic agents are frequently used. In fact, many studies substantiate that fever as a natural defense correlates positively with a quicker recovery and improved survival rates. While antipyretic agents do reduce fever, their benefit has not been established beyond that of making clients feel more comfortable. In contrast, *external* cooling measures (tepid sponging and the use of cooling blankets) are *ineffective antipyretics* because they only lower skin temperature. If the hypothalamic set point is high, external cooling will induce adverse counteractive mechanisms (shivering). Shivering imposes a tremendous metabolic burden by increasing metabolic rate and oxygen demand four to fivefold.

Medications can alter the "set point" of the hypothalamus as well as affect one's ability to shiver or to exert vasomotor control. Drugs such as Thorazine or Phenergan may suppress the brain's temperature regulatory center.

Disorders of or damage to a major adaptive system can make it more difficult for the body to cope with even small changes. For example, the skin is a major organ in the cooling and heating of the body. A severe inflammation or skin infection may render this system unresponsive to temperature fluctuations.

Other health conditions that affect the adaptive processes are poor circulation to the skin, which makes heat dissipation difficult; dermatitis, which decreases the ability of temperature sensors and circulation to respond; and an insufficient amount of muscle mass, which decreases thermogenesis.

Hyperthermia (Body Temperature Exceeding 41.1°C)

Hyperthermia is a *heat-related* emergency that can cause irreversible brain damage. It differs from fever because it is not mediated by pyrogenic cytokines but develops when the body's metabolic heat production or environmental heat load exceeds the body's ability to lose heat. The body's core temperature may exceed 41.1°C even though the hypothalamic temperature set point is *normal*. Vasodilation and sweating attempt to lower body temperature and no diurnal temperature variation or shivering is observed. Hyperthermia may be caused by strenuous exercise, environmental exposure (heat stroke) or CNS injury.

In contrast to fever, antipyretic agents are contraindicated, and hyperthermia responds to external cooling measures that combine evaporation and convection such as water spraying and warm air fanning. More aggressive cooling measures (cold immersion, cooling blanket) *may* induce shivering by creating a skin to core temperature gradient. The cool skin will initiate shivering before the brain temperature cools.

Hypothermia (Body Temperature of 35°C)

Hypothermia may be due to environmental exposure to cold with insufficient protection, loss of thermoregulation secondary to CNS pathology/injury or multiple trauma, The skin is colder than core tissues, creating a skin to core temperature gradient that results in vasoconstriction and shivering. Active external rewarming of the hypothermic client should be avoided because it can result in metabolic acidosis when peripheral vessels dilate and accumulated tissue acids enter the circulation. As cold blood returns to the warmer core *further* core cooling "afterdrop" occurs and arrhythmias may result. Passive measures such as a warm environment and simple blanket are preferred in management of the hypothermic client. Clients who are hypothermic due to head injury have better outcomes if maintained hypothermic with no attempts at rewarming.

In certain situations, hypothermia may be therapeutically *induced* to protect vital organs because it provides metabolic quiescence. Studies indicate that hypothermia induced by surface cooling is not helpful in head-injured clients, but may improve neurologic outcomes in survivors of cardiac arrest, and may be beneficial in the early treatment of stroke clients undergoing reperfusion therapy. Since surface applications make skin colder than core tissues, they will cause shivering, which must be prevented by medical management.

Central (internal) cooling, during cardiac or neurosurgery is another manipulation that creates a core to skin temperature gradient that can induce postoperative shivering. Rewarming the blood before terminating surgery helps to warm core tissues, but peripheral vasculature remains constricted for some time, unable to receive the warmed blood. Later, as peripheral vessels open, cool blood from the periphery moves to mix with warmer blood in the core and central temperature drops 2°–5°C ("afterdrop"). A warming blanket may be used to help prevent heat loss. Even a combination of measures fails to promote homogeneous body rewarming, therefore, pharmacologic agents that blunt hypothalamic responses and dilate vascular beds are necessary adjuncts to suppress shivering in the centrally cooled client postoperatively.

Alterations in body temperature are influenced by the body systems' integrity, age, particular disease process, and temperature stresses that a healthy person in a moderately neutral environment may experience. Many of these alterations may have temporary as well as chronic qualities. Persons may need assistance for a relatively short time or for the rest of their lives. It is apparent that assistance is often needed to maintain body temperature. Nursing attention and action can make a difference in many situations vital to the client's comfort, healing, and coping.

COLD THERAPIES (CRYOTHERAPIES)

Cold therapies facilitate heat transfer *from* the body, and are the treatment of choice immediately following local tissue injury, and throughout the acute inflammatory phase. Cold applications are usually accompanied by compression and elevation of the affected area (see *Orthopedic Measures,* Chapter 30). Intermittent cold therapy is beneficial as long as the temperature of the injured area continues to be elevated. Once the local temperature returns to normal, acute inflammation has probably resolved and cryotherapy can be discontinued.

TABLE 24–2 Indications for Cold Therapies

Indications	Contraindications
Acute inflammation, acute or chronic pain	Impaired circulation (peripheral vascular disease)
Acute swelling or bleeding	Raynaud's disease/phenomenon
Muscle spasm	Hypersensitivity to cold
Strain, sprain, or contusion	Decreased sensation

Cryotherapy's primary benefit is the inhibition of local enzymatic/metabolic activity, limiting further tissue injury. Cold constricts vessels (controls bleeding), reduces edema formation, decreases nerve conduction velocity, increases the pain threshold, and decreases muscle spasticity. Paradoxical cold induced vasodilation may occur when applications to *distal* extremities (fingers, toes) exceed 15 minutes at temperatures below 1°C. The amount of vasodilation is usually small, but should be avoided in certain situations and therapy time should be limited to 15 minutes or less when treating *distal extremities*. Longer treatment durations may be used for other areas of the body. With cold therapy, the area temperature remains lower than normal for 1 or 2 hours *after* removal of the cooling modality, so applications are usually repeated every 1–2 hours.

HEAT THERAPIES (THERMOTHERAPIES)

The physiologic effects of heat are generally opposite to those of cold. Heat applications are *inappropriate* during the acute inflammatory phase of musculoskeletal injury (with the exception of neck or back muscle strain), but are beneficial for subacute and chronic inflammation. Heat promotes *analgesia* and sedation by stimulating nerve endings and blocking pain transmission by the gate control theory of pain modulation. The benefits of heat therapy last only as long as the heat stimulus is applied. When removed, effects quickly disappear.

Heat facilitates soft tissue *repair* by increasing delivery of nutrients and oxygen and removal of cellular debris. Heat relaxes skeletal muscles, increases elasticity, and decreases viscosity of connective tissue and thereby facilitates other treatments by producing relaxation.

TABLE 24–3 Indications for Heat Therapies

Indications	Contraindications
Subacute or chronic inflammation	Acute musculoskeletal injury
Subacute or chronic pain	Impaired circulation (peripheral vascular disease)
Subacute edema	Sensory impairment
Muscle soreness	Bruising or bleeding
Infection (supports suppuration)	Open wound
Consensual vasodilation	

Although tissue conduction of heat is limited to a depth of about 2 cm, burns can occur if heat application is too hot or prolonged, or if the tissue is unable to mount the increased metabolic demand imposed. The body tends to acclimate to (annihilate) heat therapies; therefore, insulation is recommended with heat applications. Superficial heating therapies that get *cooler* during application (e.g., moist packs) are safer than therapies with a constant maintained temperature (e.g., heating pad).

A unique benefit of heat is its ability to inhibit sympathetic nervous system outflow. Heat promotes vasodilation both at the site of application *and* in distal cutaneous vessels ("consensual vasodilation"). By way of this spinal cord reflex, heat may be applied proximally (e.g., to low back) to increase *peripheral* circulation and facilitate healing in an area that lacks sufficient circulation or sensation to tolerate the *direct* application of heat.

The following considerations for client safety are important when applying heat and cold treatments.

- In most hospitals, the water temperature is controlled at a temperature not to exceed 110°F (43.3°C) to prevent client injury.
- A protective layer of petroleum jelly may be used to prevent tissue damage when hot packs are applied.
- Place hot pack on client's skin for a few seconds, then remove and check condition of skin before leaving pack on the prescribed length of time.
- Monitor vital signs frequently when systemic cold is applied.
- When using hypothermia blanket, use towels to wrap hands and feet to protect skin from injury.
- Observe skin for purplish color, and check client for numb feeling after cold applications are removed.

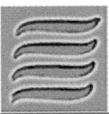

NURSING DIAGNOSES

The following nursing diagnoses are appropriate to use on client care plans when the components are related to thermic treatments.

NURSING DIAGNOSIS	RELATED FACTORS
Ineffective thermoregulation	Anesthesia, medications, alcoholism, infection, CNS injury, environmental exposure
Deficient knowledge	*Lack of understanding* about inflammatory process; rationale and hazards of heat/cold therapies
Risk for peripheral neurovascular dysfunction	Prolonged application of heat or cold therapy to joints or areas with impaired circulation
Hyperthermia	CNS injury, strenuous exercise, environmental exposure, medications
Hypothermia	CNS injury, environmental exposure, major trauma, surgery, alcoholism, medications
Risk for impaired Skin Integrity	Prolonged use of cold or heat therapy, excessive temperature of therapy, impaired sensation, impaired circulation.

- The single most important nursing action to decrease the incidence of hospital-based infection is handwashing. **Remember to wash your hands or use antibacterial gel before and after each and every client contact.**

UNIT 1

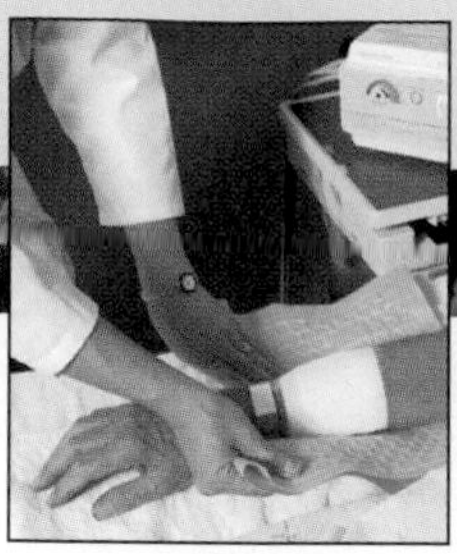

Heat Therapies

Nursing Process Data

ASSESSMENT *Data Base*

Review client's history for possible circulatory problems (peripheral vascular disease, diabetes).

Determine site and type and duration of therapy to be applied.

Determine rationale for heat therapy.

Assess area to be treated.

Determine client's ability to sense temperature at site.

Assess skin condition before and after therapy.

PLANNING *Objectives*

To increase circulation to area.

To provide analgesia

To promote suppuration/inflammatory process

To facilitate mobilization of interstitial fluid

IMPLEMENTATION *Procedures*

Applying a Commercial Heat Pack

Monitoring an Infant Radiant Warmer

Applying an Aquathermic Pad

Applying a Hot Moist Pack

Assisting with a Sitz Bath

EVALUATION *Expected Outcomes*

Circulation is increased to area.

Local pain is reduced.

Inflammation/suppuration is enhanced.

Tissue fluid is mobilized/edema reduced.

APPLYING A COMMERCIAL HEAT PACK

Equipment

Prepackaged heat pack
Tape

Procedure

1. Check physician's orders for type and duration of heat treatment.
2. Wash your hands.
3. Gather equipment.
4. Explain procedure to client.
5. Provide privacy.
6. Remove heat pack from outer wrapper.
7. Break inner seal by holding pack tightly in the center and in an upright position.
8. Squeeze firmly to break seal. **Rationale:** Breaking the seal activates the chemical ingredients and produces the heat.
9. Check for leakage from pack. Remove pack immediately if leakage occurs. **Rationale:** Chemicals from the pack may burn the skin.
10. Gently shake the pack, then apply to treatment area.
11. Remove pack after 5 minutes, and assess skin for erythema.
12. Replace pack and secure with tape. Keep in place 15–30 minutes or as ordered by physician.
13. Place call bell in clients' reach.
14. Remove pack, and discard in appropriate container.
15. Wash your hands.

MONITORING THE INFANT RADIANT WARMER

Equipment

Radiant warmer with skin or rectal probe
Bedding appropriate for warmer

Preparation

1. Several different radiant warmers, or infant care centers, are available. Follow the manufacturer's operating instructions for safety and to determine if a manual or proportional controller is used. (General operating instructions and protocols are presented here.)
2. Check caster locks to make certain that each caster is in locked position.
3. Adjust procedure table to desired position.
4. Plug line cord into a three-wire receptacle.
5. Turn power switch ON; the red pilot light and the alarm indicator should glow. Turn alarm switch ON to test alarm system.
6. Turn manual knob to automatic.
7. Install skin or rectal probe in controller and set switch to either rectal or skin, depending on which probe is being used.
8. Warm unit for 7 minutes.
9. Adjust temperature to degree ordered; temperature is dialed on digital temperature set switch.
10. Wash your hands.

Procedure

1. Place infant in warmer.
2. Attach skin probe.
   a. Place 1-cm skin probe with polished surface touching skin to left of the umbilicus.
   b. Use a rectal probe if hospital protocol permits.

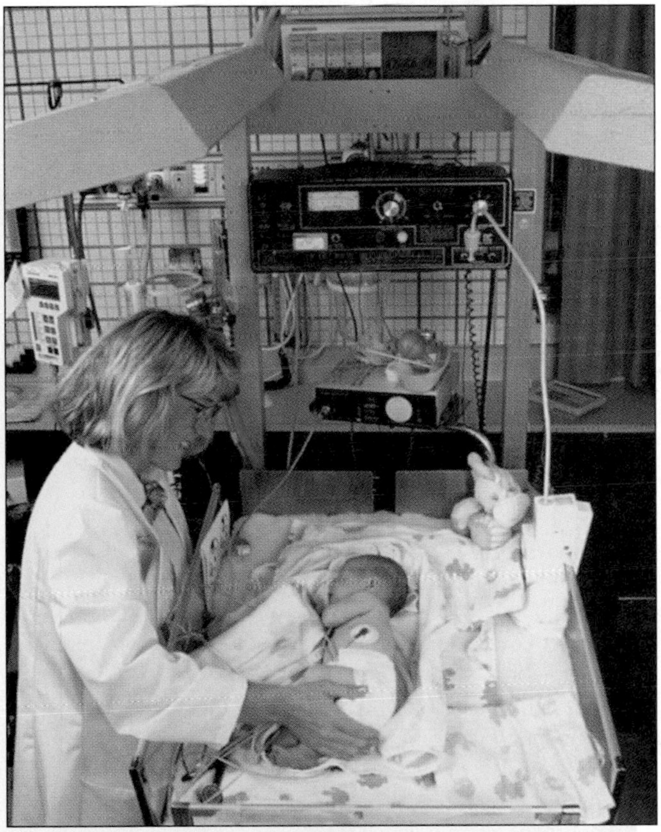

Type 1: Infant overhead warmer used to maintain body temperature.

3. Monitor placement of skin probe.
   a. Inspect infant's skin under probe at regular intervals. **Rationale:** Infant's skin is delicate and irritates easily.
   b. Change the probe location if irritation begins to appear.

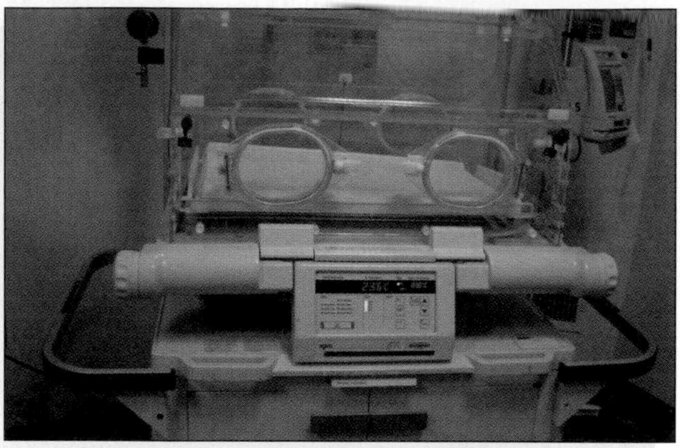

Type 2: Infant radiant warmer used to maintain body temperature—used without clothes on infant.

c. Do not use adhesive tape or pads. **Rationale:** These may cause skin irritation or allergic reactions. Infant's skin is very thin and fragile.

4. Allow 3–5 minutes for probe to reach infant's temperature.
5. Activate audible alarm by setting switch to ON. **Rationale:** If the infant's temperature exceeds 102°F (38.8°C), the audible alarm sounds and the visible alarm light flashes.
6. Wash your hands.

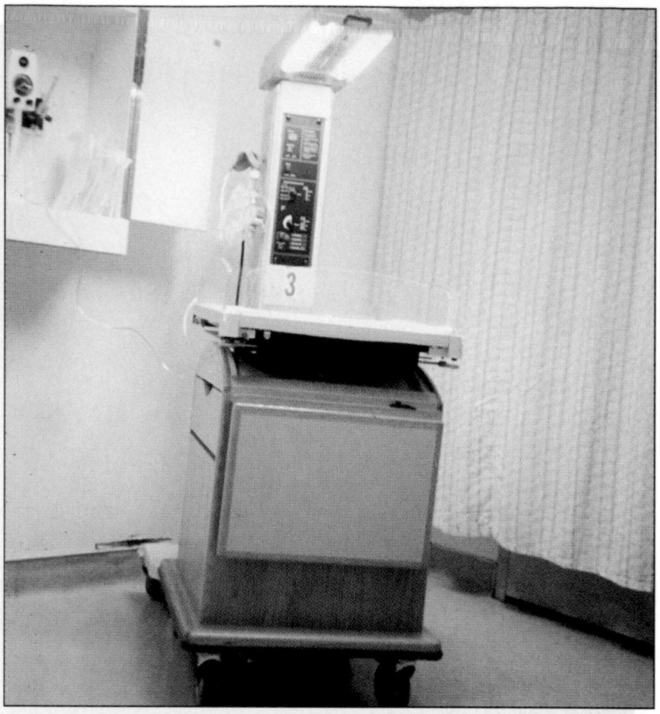

Type 3: Infant warmer most often used in birthing room to maintain body heat while examining newborn.

APPLYING AN AQUATHERMIC PAD

Equipment

Aquathermic reservoir container with pump
Aquathermic pad (disposable)
Distilled water
Tape

Preparation

1. Review physician's orders to determine treatment area, type of application, and temperature of treatment.
2. Wash hands.
3. Gather equipment, and check it for safety factors (e.g., frayed cords, water leaks).
4. Take equipment to client's room and identify client.
5. Connect aquathermic pad to pump hoses (male and female fittings).
6. Snap locking rings into place to ensure hose fittings are snug, then open hose clamps.
7. Fill reservoir ⅔ full with *room temperature* distilled water.
8. Place pump on bedside stand or other surface at or *above* level of the pad. **Rationale:** If pump is placed below pad level, water will drain back into pump when it is shut off.
9. Use plastic key to set reservoir temperature as ordered, then remove key. **Rationale:** Temperature range is 30–42°C. Removing key prevents tampering.
10. Plug pump into grounded wall outlet.

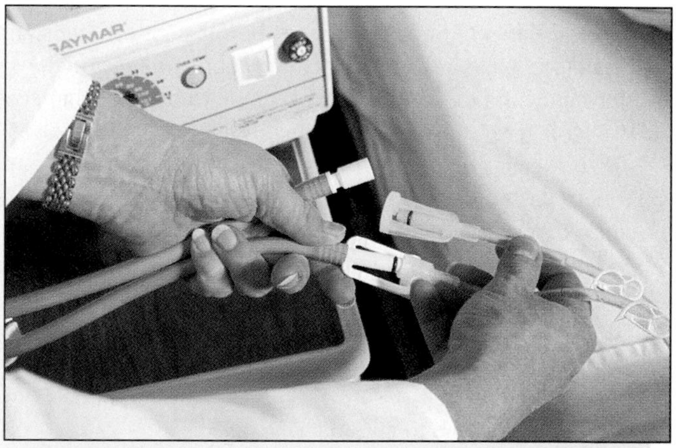

Connect Aqua-K pad to pump hoses.

11. Turn pump power switch "ON." Set temperature is reached in about 20 minutes.

CLINICAL ALERT

Do not allow the client to lie on a "constant heat source" such as a heating pad or aquathermic pad.

CLINICAL ALERT

Contraindications to heat therapies include acute injury or inflammation, recent or potential hemorrhage, deep-vein thrombophlebitis, impaired circulation, impaired sensation, and impaired mentation.

When treating an area where skin is not intact, cover lesion with sterile gauze and insulating barrier before applying heat (see *Wound Care,* Chapter 25).

Procedure

1. Explain procedure to client and provide privacy.
2. Apply aquathermic pad with its *coiled surface* against client's extremity or over moist pack that has been placed on area to be treated.
3. Secure pad with tape if necessary; *do not use safety pins.* **Rationale:** Pins can pierce coils in pad.
4. Check client's skin after 2–3 minutes. **Rationale:** This is to assess for possible skin reaction caused by a hot pad.
5. Instruct client to notify you if the pad seems too warm. **Rationale:** This prevents burning of skin.
6. Remove pad after 15–20 minutes. Observe area for redness, pain, or any untoward reaction.
7. When pad is used to keep dressings or soaks warm, continue treatment longer than 20 minutes if ordered. Treatment may be continuous when used for clients with back pain.

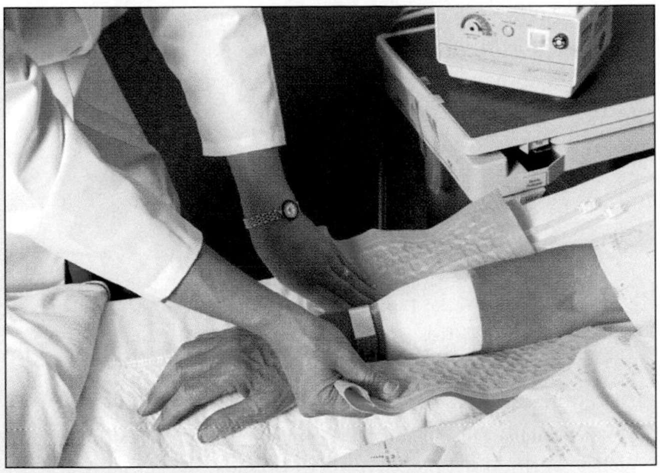

Aquathermic pad is a form of heat therapy.

8. Turn pump "OFF." Close hose clamps; hold hose with connectors above pump and pad. **Rationale:** Prevents water spillage.
9. Remove aquathermic pad and join male and female connectors.
10. Place pad on bedside stand until next treatment or place in appropriate disposal area.
11. Reposition client for comfort.
12. Wash your hands.

APPLYING A HOT MOIST PACK

Equipment

Box of 4 × 4 gauze sponges or other absorbent material necessary for size of area to be treated
Hot tap water or ordered solution and container
Plastic moisture barrier (plastic bag)
Or
Aquathermic pad (optional)
Tape
Bath thermometer
Gloves

CLINICAL ALERT

Do not apply heat to an edematous area until the reason for edema has been determined.

Preparation

1. Check orders for type of hot moist treatment ordered, length of treatment, and time interval between treatments.
2. Gather specific equipment for type of hot moist pack ordered.
3. Place material in a warming solution (usually water).
4. Determine amount of time elapsed since last application.
5. Considering age of client, body part involved, and type of treatment, determine safe temperature of application to prevent burning. **Rationale:** Water temperature in hospitals is usually controlled at 43.3°C/110°F, but the individual client may require altered temperature.
6. Identify correct client and explain treatment.
7. Wash hands.

Procedure

1. Position client appropriately to expose and assess area to be treated. **Rationale:** Open wounds are generally *not* treated with heat application because heat increases the area's need for oxygen and may injure granulation tissue. Heat therapy to a recent bruise can restart bleeding.
2. Assess client's ability to sense touch and heat/cold at site to be treated. **Rationale:** Impaired skin sensation may contraindicate therapy.

3. Remove any jewelry from area to be treated. **Rationale:** Decreases risk of burn due to conductive potential of metal.
4. Open container of gauze sponges. Open ABD outer wrap if used.
5. Don gloves.
6. Saturate gauze sponges (or other selected material) with warm water (no greater than 43.3°C). *Note: Water in hospitals is usually controlled at 43.3°C.*
7. Pick up soaked sponges and wring out excess solution.
8. Place warm moist pack over area to be treated.
9. Use plastic barrier or aquathermic pad to mold and secure pack to site. **Rationale:** Barrier helps maintain heat by preventing evaporative cooling.
10. Set aquathermic pad temperature at 41°C. **Rationale:** While the warm moist pack will cool quickly, the aquathermic pad maintains heat—*this also increases the risk of burns.*
11. Use tape to secure the barrier. Do not allow client to lie on pack or pad.
12. Assure that nurse call system is in client's reach. **Rationale:** Client should summon nurse if discomfort is felt.
13. Assess area in 5 minutes for signs of redness, mottling, or blistering. **Rationale:** These may be signs of burning. Thermotherapy should be discontinued and a cool pack should be applied.
14. Remove and dispose of pack after 20 minutes or as prescribed.
15. Assess and dry the treated area. **Rationale:** Slight redness and warmth are expected responses.
16. Document procedure and client's response to treatment.
17. Discard gloves and wash your hands.

ASSISTING WITH A SITZ BATH

Equipment

Disposable sitz bath with tubing and bag
Warm water (40°–43°C) *Note: Cold temperature may be indicated for client's situation.*
Towels for drying
Thermometer
Clean gloves, if needed

Preparation

1. Verify physician's order for sitz bath, duration and frequency of treatments
2. Raise toilet seat and place sitz bath basin with "FRONT" facing the front of the toilet bowl.
3. Fill basin with warm water (40°–43°C) ½ to ⅔ full
4. Close flow tubing clamp.
5. Open top of plastic bag and fill with hot water (40°–43°C).
6. Hang bag at a level higher than the sitz basin so that fluid will flow by gravity.
7. Insert tubing through front or rear entry hole in sitz bath, then snap or secure tubing into channel or "eye" in bottom of basin.
8. Wash hands.

Procedure

1. Identify client by checking identaband and asking client to state name.
2. Explain procedure and rationale for sitz bath.
3. Assist client to treatment area with *accessible call bell.*
4. Provide privacy by placing sign on door.
5. Check to assure that temperature of thermotherapy water is 40.5°–43.3°C *Note: Most hospitals control water temperature so that it will not exceed 110°F* or 43.3°C.
6. Assist client to sit in sitz bath for 15–20 minutes.
7. Maintain water temperature by continually adding water of appropriate temperature to bag. **Rationale:** Overflow will drain into toilet through openings in back of basin.

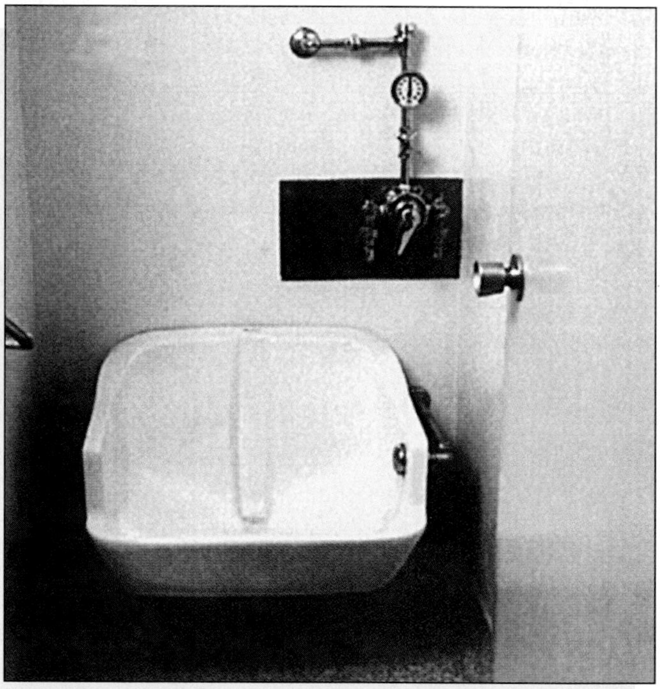

While some facilities still use a permanent sitz bath, most offer clients a disposable unit due to infection control practices.

8. Upon completion, assist client to dry area and allow client to sit briefly to allow normalization of blood pressure and to prevent hypotension upon standing. **Rationale:** Orthostatic hypotension may occur with rapid position change following warm sitz bath due to vasodilation.
9. Empty and rinse client's sitz basin and store in convenient location for future use. If drainage present, don clean gloves.
10. Discard soiled linen.
11. Wash your hands.

Documentation for Heat Therapies

- Time of application
- Type of heat therapy applied
- Area of body treated
- Status of area pre- and post-treatment
- Positioning of area treated
- Duration of treatment
- Client's response to treatment

Critical Thinking Application

UNEXPECTED OUTCOMES	CRITICAL THINKING OPTIONS
Client reports that heat therapy is ineffective.	• Inform client that accommodation to heat reduces awareness but that therapeutic effect continues and increasing heat can cause burning.
Swelling is not reduced with heat therapy.	• Reinforce importance of resting area until swelling is reduced. • Consult with physician regarding discontinuing therapy after a 2-day trial and the need for anti-inflammatory medication or reevaluation.
Client experiences pain, asks about alternative measures for relief	• Try local heat for analgesia at site free of malignancy, infection, or circulatory insufficiency. • Cold therapy may be an option, or heat/cold alternating therapy—as counterirritants, these therapies alter nerve transmission.
Pain in affected area is increased.	• Assess if application is too hot. • Ensure that temperature is not over 110°F (43.3°C) if a heating pad is used. • Observe surrounding skin for erythema or burning.
Client refuses to keep application intact.	• Elicit reason for uncooperative behavior. Determine if client is uncomfortable. • Explain rationale for treatment.
Pack is difficult to secure due to affected area or activity of client.	• Use a roll of Kerlix (wide gauze) to wrap and mold the pack to the body. • Use a small sheet to wrap around the trunk. • Have a person (parent for child) hold the pack in place only if absolutely necessary.
Elderly client is confused and does not follow treatment.	• Assign health care team member to stay with client during treatment, or schedule treatment when client can be checked on frequently.
Aquathermic pump signals "Over Temp."	• Check reservoir water level; it may be low or empty. • Be sure to use room temperature (not hot) distilled water in reservoir. Check that hoses are not kinked or hose clamps closed.

UNIT 2

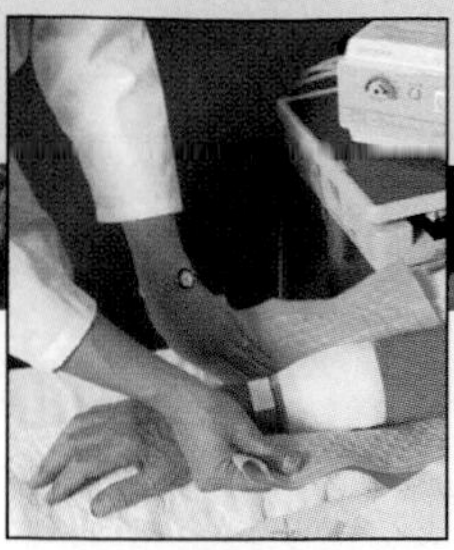

Cold Therapies

Nursing Process Data

ASSESSMENT Data Base
Review client's history for possible circulatory problems (Raynaud's, diabetes, cold sensitivities)
Determine purpose for cryotherapy
Assess site to be treated
Determine client's ability to sense temperature at site.
Assess skin condition before and after therapy

PLANNING Objectives
To reduce metabolic process
To promote vasoconstriction
To decrease edema
To achieve an anesthetic effect
To reduce muscle spasticity and promote motion

IMPLEMENTATION Procedures
Applying an Ice Pack/Commercial Cold Pack
Applying a Disposable Instant (Chemical) Cold Pack

EVALUATION Expected Outcomes
Inflammatory response is controlled
Bleeding is reduced/controlled
Anesthetic response is achieved
Spasticity is reduced
Motion is facilitated

APPLYING AN ICE PACK/COMMERCIAL COLD PACK

Equipment

Small plastic bag, ice bag, or glove (consider size to be treated and necessity to mold)
Flaked or crushed ice
Salt
Or
Reusable silicone gel cold pack that has been in freezer (−5°C) for at least 1.5 hours before initial use
Moist cloth or towel
Elastic bandage or towel
Tape (*do not use pins*)
Pillows

Preparation

1. Verify physician's order for type of cold pack, duration and frequency of therapy.
2. Fill ice bag ½ to ⅔ full. **Rationale**: Space allows bag to conform to treatment area.
3. Remove excess air from bag. **Rationale**: Facilitates molding to treatment area.
4. Add salt to ice if a colder slush mixture is needed.
5. Take equipment to client's room.
6. Wash hands.

> **CLINICAL ALERT**
> - Gel packs provide more aggressive cooling than ice bags, so deserve greater caution.
> - During cold therapy, erythema will occur.
> - The client will experience four stages of cold progression: cold/stinging/burning/numbness.
> - Discontinue therapy upon numbness.

Procedure

1. Validate client by checking identaband and having client state name.
2. Provide privacy.
3. Explain procedure and rationale to client. Discuss sensory experiences to expect with cold therapy.
4. Position client to expose area to be treated and remove any jewelry if present.
5. Assess client's ability to sense touch and heat/cold at site to be treated. **Rationale:** Impaired skin sensation may contraindicate therapy.
6. Use pillows or other item to elevate area to be treated. **Rationale:** Elevation promotes venous return, reduces swelling and pain.
7. Place moist towels directly onto skin area. **Rationale:** A moist towel facilitates tissue cooling. A dry towel can be used for less intense cooling.

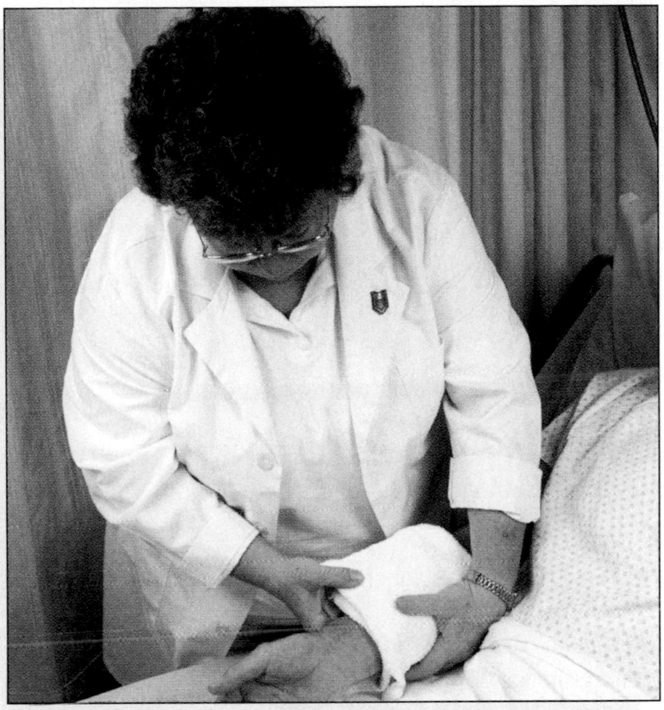

Wrap and tape towel around pack to secure.

8. Place ice/cold pack atop moist towel and mold it to fit the treatment area. **Rationale:** Manufacturer's instructions vary among products and must be followed for safe use.
9. Secure pack in place with toweling or elastic wrap using tape. **Rationale:** Outer wrap decreases warming effect of environmental air.
10. Place call bell within client's reach.
11. Assess client and treatment site in 5 minutes. **Rationale:** If mottling or blisters occur, or client reports numbness, discontinue pack immediately.
12. Limit treatment time to 10–15 minutes or as prescribed. **Rationale:** A reusable cold pack usually loses its effectiveness after 15 minutes. Application time can be increased if cold is applied over bandages or against a cast.
13. Assess treatment area for adverse signs (wheals, cyanosis, pallor, pain, or tingling/numbness *distal* to treatment over a superficial nerve such as the radial nerve at the lateral elbow).
14. Discard used towels in linen hamper.
15. Return reusable ice bag or cold pack to freezer for at least 30 minutes before reusing.

> **CLINICAL ALERT**
> Never apply a fully cooled *reusable cold pack* directly to the skin; also, do not overinsulate the area.
>
> Bony areas (knee, ankle, elbow) usually require half the treatment time as fatty areas. Superficial nerves at these joint sites are especially vulnerable to cold-induced neuropathy, especially if cold is combined with compression.

Evidence Based Nursing Practice

Postoperative Cold Therapy

While several studies have demonstrated that the use of cold over compression reduces bleeding and swelling and improves return to motion, this research study concludes that compression is just as effective as cold post total knee surgery, and is more cost effective.

Source: Smith, J. et al (2002). A randomized, controlled trial comparing compression bandaging and cold therapy in postoperative total knee replacement surgery. *Orthopaedic Nursing, 21*(2), 61–66.

APPLYING A DISPOSABLE INSTANT (CHEMICAL) COLD PACK

Equipment

One time only use instant chemical cold pack (kept at room temperature)
Moist cloth or towel (if indicated on pack instructions)
Elastic bandage or towel
Tape
Pillows

Preparation

1. Review orders, and check length of treatment.
2. Gather equipment.
3. Wash your hands.
4. Identify client by checking identaband.
5. Explain procedure.
6. Provide privacy and position client.

> **CLINICAL ALERT**
>
> Do *not* apply an instant chemical pack to the *face* and never use pins to secure pack. Leakage of chemical contents can cause serious injury. If contents are exposed to skin, immediately flush with copious amounts of water and notify physician.

Procedure

1. Grasp top of cold pack, and shake contents to bottom of bag.
2. Hold package in the middle with both hands, or follow manufacturer's directions on package.

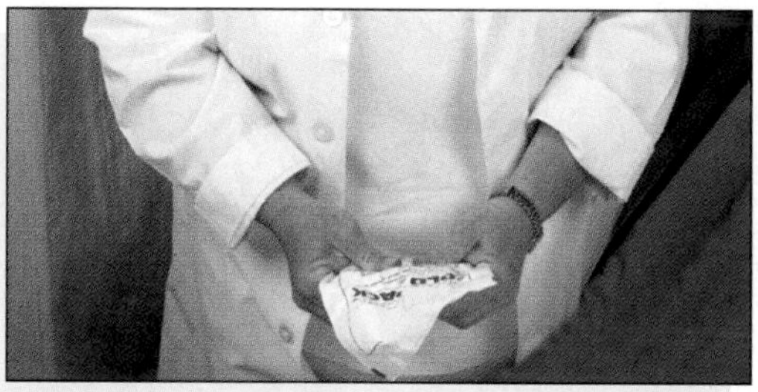

Follow manufacturer's instructions to activate chemical cold pack.

3. Locate inner pouch and squeeze the package firmly to break the inner pouch.
4. Shake the package gently to mix the chemicals together.
5. Check that package is not punctured or opened. **Rationale:** If solution touches the skin, the chemicals can burn the skin.
6. Use pillows or other item to elevate area to be treated. **Rationale:** Elevation promotes venous return, reduces swelling and pain.
7. Apply pack *directly* to skin, *or* place disposable cold pack atop towel (according to instructions). **Rationale:** The degree of cold is *not* great with a chemical cold pack.
8. Mold pack to fit area and secure in place with toweling or elastic wrap and tape. **Rationale:** Outer wrap decreases warming effect of environmental air.
9. Place call bell within client's reach.
10. Assess client and treatment site in 5 minutes. **Rationale:** If mottling or blisters occur, or client reports numbness, discontinue pack immediately.
11. Limit treatment time to 30 minutes or as prescribed.
12. Dispose of "one time only use" pack. **Rationale:** Product cannot be reused by freezing as frostbite may result.
13. Wash your hands.

DOCUMENTATION FOR COLD THERAPIES

- Specific cold application used
- Time of treatment
- Area of body treated
- Status of area pre- and post-treatment
- Positioning of area treated
- Duration of treatment
- Effectiveness of treatment
- Client's response to procedure

Critical Thinking Application

UNEXPECTED OUTCOMES	CRITICAL THINKING OPTIONS
Local edema is not reduced.	• Elevate extremity above level of heart. • Ensure that body surface is sufficiently covered with cold application to cause vasoconstriction. • Apply cold treatment for first 24 hours until edema has dissipated, as ordered.
Bleeding continues even with cold applications.	• Reassess area for possible "bleeders," which may require cautery or ligation by the physician. • Apply pressure to site to stop bleeding.
Area to be treated is near superficial nerve.	• Use caution: reduce time and duration of cold application. • Ask client to report any itching or tingling and discontinue therapy if these occur.
Hand develops waxy white sheen, mottling, and blisters during local ice therapy.	• Immerse part in moving water at 40°–42°C until area flushes (about 30 minutes). • Do not apply dry heat, keep area uncovered at room temperature. • Do not rub part; keep part elevated.

UNIT 3

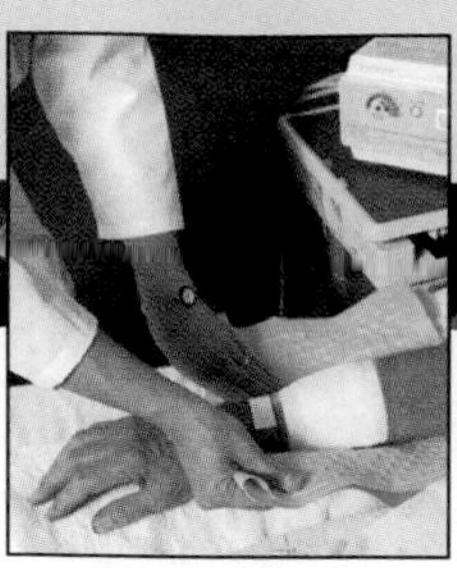

Systemic Cooling Therapies

Nursing Process Data

ASSESSMENT *Data Base*

Determine if client's temperature can be reduced by less intensive measures.

Assess skin condition, especially of nose, ears, hands, and feet, before, during, and following treatment.

Determine client's ability to tolerate treatment.

Assess baseline data (i.e., vital signs, neurologic signs, mental status, peripheral circulation).

Assess that the cooling blanket and machine are functioning properly.

Evaluate ECG findings throughout treatment, if client is monitored.

Assess fluid and electrolyte balance (especially potassium level).

Evaluate fluid intake and output throughout treatment.

Assess for early indicators of shivering.

Assess if medications have been administered.

PLANNING *Objectives*

To protect the skin from injury during use of the cooling blanket

To prevent shivering during cold applications

To ensure that the cooling blanket functions properly

To reduce body's internal (core) temperature

To decrease metabolic processes, thereby preventing irreversible states

IMPLEMENTATION *Procedures*

Providing a Tepid Bath

Using a Cooling Blanket

EVALUATION *Expected Outcomes*

Skin remains free of injury during use of the cooling blanket.

Cooling blanket functions properly.

Client's internal temperature is reduced without any untoward effects.

Shivering is avoided during use of the cooling blanket.

PROVIDING A TEPID BATH

Equipment

Water or other coolant at prescribed temperature
Basin or tub
Washcloth and towels
Thermometer
Bath blanket
Electric fan

Preparation

1. Review order for bath.
2. Note temperature of solution ordered and length of time of application.
3. Gather equipment, and bring to client's room. Identify client.
4. Provide privacy, and explain procedure.
5. Wash your hands.
6. Obtain vital signs for baseline data.

Procedure

1. Remove client's clothing to allow for cooling and observation. Use bath blanket for privacy.
2. Observe skin surface before applying cold wrap or sponging.
3. Monitor skin color and vital signs every 15–30 minutes during cooling.
4. Immerse washcloths or material for sponging in ordered solution, generally 70°–80°F (21°–27°C).
5. Wring out excess solution, and place cloths on forehead, back of neck, axilla, groin, and wrists. **Rationale:** The vascularity of these areas promotes cooling.
6. Depending on type of bath, change wraps or soaks every 5 minutes. **Rationale:** This prevents wraps from holding body heat.

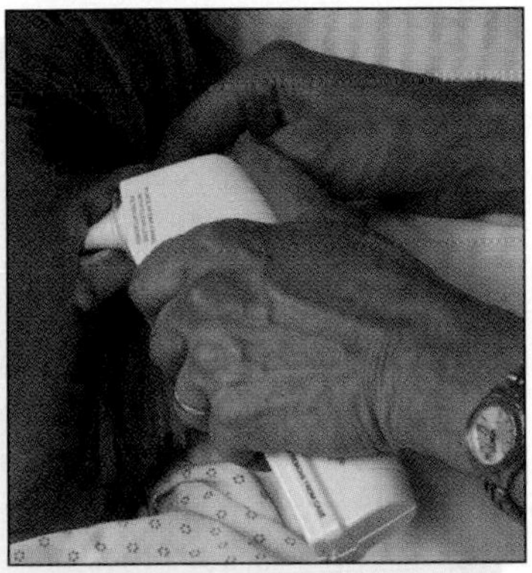

Monitor client's temperature before, and every 25 minutes during sponging.

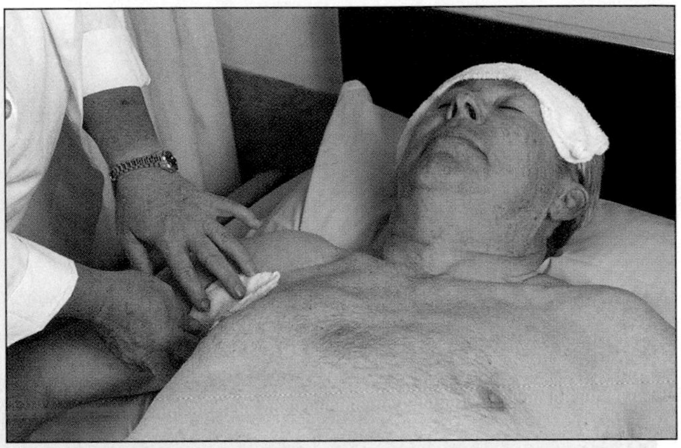

Place tepid cloths to vascular areas of body to promote conduction of client's body heat.

7. Stop the treatment if shivering occurs. **Rationale:** If the body senses a loss of heat, it attempts to produce it by thermogenesis, conserve it, or dissipate it.
8. Cool the air to 68°–72°F (20.0°–22.2°C). **Rationale:** Enhances therapy by convection and evaporation.
9. Promote movement of air (fanning) if possible.
10. Take temperature every 15 minutes. When temperature has decreased to desired level, dry skin and replace light covering over client and reposition for comfort. **Rationale:** A thin client will cool faster than one with more subcutaneous fat.

> **CLINICAL ALERT**
>
> Tympanic temperature readings best reflect core temperature, since the tympanic membrane and hypothalamus have a common blood supply. Prevent false low readings by positioning the probe snugly to seal the ear canal from ambient air.

11. Continue to take vital signs every 1–2 hours until temperature is stabilized.
12. Provide high-calorie diet. **Rationale:** Increased temperatures cause an increased metabolic rate. Carbohydrates, proteins, and 2500–3000 mL fluid intake is essential for maintaining homeostasis.
13. Place cloths in linen hamper and return equipment to utility or storage area.
14. Wash your hands.

EVIDENCE BASED NURSING PRACTICE

Effective Ways to Reduce Fever

There is no statistical difference in fever reduction between use of cooling blanket vs. tepid water sponge bathing; however, cooling blankets are associated with significantly *more* shivering. Cooling blankets do appear to reduce fever effectively in heavily sedated or paralyzed critically ill clients.

Source: Manthous, (1995). *American Journal of Respiratory Critical Care Medicine, 151,* 10–14.

USING A COOLING BLANKET

Equipment

Thermal (heating/cooling) unit
Distilled water
Rectal thermometer probe and lubricant
Disposable thermal (cooling) blanket
1 sheet or thin blanket
Covering for client
4 towels
Tape
Lower extremity (or foot) compression wraps
Tympanic thermometer
Sphygmomanometer
Stethoscope
Continuous ECG monitoring (if indicated)
Supplemental oxygen therapy equipment

Preparation

1. Check physician's orders for desired client temperature.
2. Identify medications client has received (antipyretic, narcotic, sedative, or paralytic agents).
3. Gather equipment and take to client's room.
4. Connect power card to grounded outlet.
5. Ensure that reservoir (distilled water) level is adequate.
6. Wash your hands.
7. Identify client and explain procedure.
8. Provide privacy.
9. Obtain baseline vital signs.

CLINICAL ALERT

Paralytic agents prevent *shivering* but have no effect on wakefulness or sensory perception, including perception of pain. With compete paralysis, pain might be manifested as increased heart rate, increased blood pressure, or sweating. Never assume that a client receiving a paralytic agent is asleep. Continually inform client about care, offer reassurance, and provide pain relief while the paralyzing effect of the drug persists.

EVIDENCE BASED NURSING PRACTICE

Hypothermia Improves Stroke Outcome

A study of stroke patients indicates that induced hypothermia to 32°C for a 3-hour period with cooling blankets and ice water/alcohol bath *improved* outcomes. Hypothermia reduces ischemic damage and reperfusion injury following thrombolysis, and reduces bleeding risk associated with administration of tPA. It may also help prevent hyperthemia associated with shift of the third ventricle during an intracerebral hemorrhage.

Source: Mitka, M. (2001). Playing it cool in stroke research. *Journal of the American Medical Association, 285*(10), 1282.

Procedure

1. Place the cooling blanket on bed, and connect it to the machine.
   a. Push the tab. Insert male tubing connector of the cooling pad into inlet opening. Release the tab.
   b. Repeat connection using the outlet opening.
   c. Turn the unit ON by pushing power switch.
2. Place a sheet or a thin bath blanket over the cooling blanket. **Rationale:** A cover over pad reduces risk of client injury.
3. Place client on the cooling blanket. Wrap client's legs and feet in compression wraps. **Rationale:** This helps to prevent thrombus formation and reduces edema.
4. Wrap client's lower arms and hands and lower legs and feet (and scrotum if indicated) in towels and tape to secure. **Rationale:** This provides insulation to prevent tissue injury and prevents stimulation of skin thermoreceptors that initiate *shivering* before brain temperature cools.
5. Set the master temperature control to either automatic or manual operation. **Rationale:** There are two separate temperature controls, one for automatic and one for manual operation.

for Automatic Control

a. Insert lubricated probe into client's rectum 2 inches.
b. Set temperature control at the desired temperature (fluid temperature set point).
c. Turn automatic mode light on and press "START". **Rationale:** The pad fluid temperature will adjust automatically to bring client's temperature to a selected set point.
d. Check that the pad temperature limits are set at desired safety limits.
e. Remove and clean rectal probe every 4 hours.

for Manual Control

a. Insert lubricated probe into client's rectum 2 inches.
b. Observe that the manual mode light is on.
c. Monitor the fluid set point, which indicates temperature of pad. **Rationale:** This ensures pad temperature is maintained at desired level.

6. Set the temperature control to 37°C, and begin lowering temperature 1°C every 15 minutes until 33° or 34°C is reached (or set temperature as ordered). **Rationale:** Thermal blanket will cool client at this temperature independent of client's temperature.
7. Monitor client's tympanic temperature every 15 minutes. **Rationale:** This measurement reflects core temperature since the hypothalamus and tympanic membrane share a common blood supply.
8. Observe client for signs predicting onset of shivering: ECG muscle tremor artifact, visible facial muscle twitchings, hyperventilation, and verbalized sensations.
9. If manifestations of shivering occur notify physician and obtain order for IV medications, usually chlorpromazine.
10. While client undergoes hypothermia, monitor vital signs every 15–30 minutes during reduction of temperature control and then every 2 hours. **Rationale:** Monitoring allows for continual evaluation of client response.
11. Monitor ECG if the client has cardiac disease (possible arrhythmias) or hypokalemia. **Rationale:** Serum potassium levels fluctuate with induced hypothermia.
12. Observe obese clients for fluid balance alterations.
13. Monitor client's serum glucose. **Rationale:** Insulin levels are decreased with induced hypothermia. Glucose levels may rise with shivering.
14. Remove and clean rectal probe every 4 hours.
15. Check physician's order for and apply thigh-high support stockings or compression wraps. **Rationale:** Stockings prevent venous stasis.
16. Turn, cough, and deep-breathe client every 30 minutes.
17. Monitor client's skin condition and bony prominences every 2 hours. **Rationale:** Client is at risk for pressure ulcers when skin temperature is lowered and there is moisture present.

CLINICAL ALERT

Remove any jewelry and select gowns without metal snaps to prevent excess conduction. Keep the client and blanket covering dry to prevent frostbite.

18. Turn off unit when client's temperature is 1°–3°C above desired temperature. **Rationale:** Cooling will continue upon discontinuation of therapy.
19. Monitor vital signs every 15 minutes during warming.
20. Observe for edema. **Rationale:** This is caused by increased cell permeability, acidosis due to shivering, fluid imbalance, and hypothermia.
21. Clean and return equipment to central supply following use. Dispose of blanket.
22. Monitor client's vital signs frequently after discontinuation of treatment.
23. Make client comfortable.
24. Wash your hands.

Classification of Hypothermia

Mild	32°–37°C	89.6°–98.6°F
Moderate	28°–32°C	82.4°–89.6°F
Severe	20°–28°C	68.0°–82.4°F

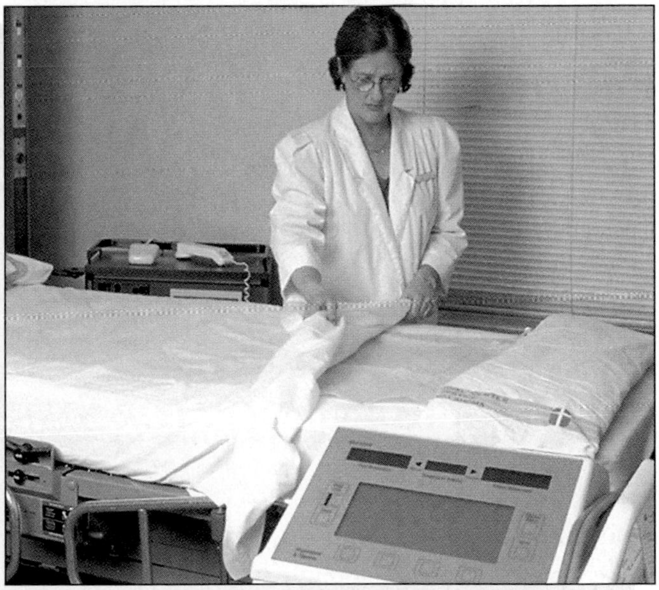

Disposable cooling blanket is covered by sheet to protect client's skin.

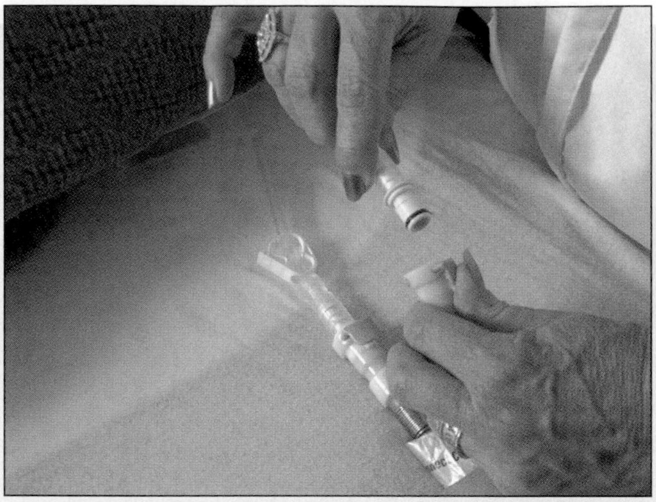

Connect two ends of tubing—one from blanket, the other from machine.

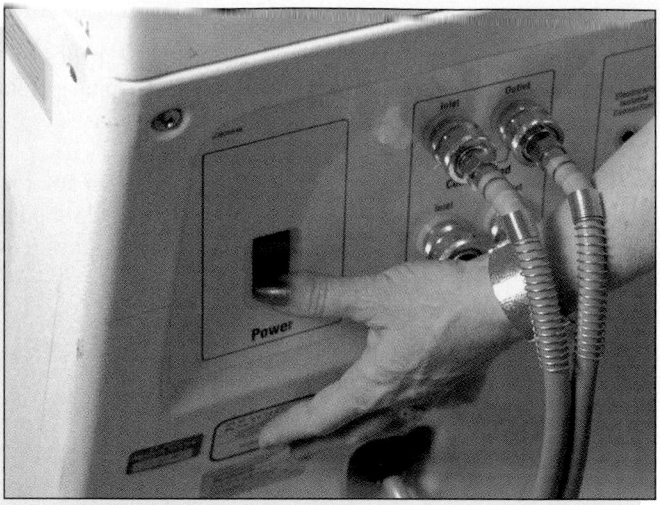

After machine is powered and connected to blanket, push unit ON button.

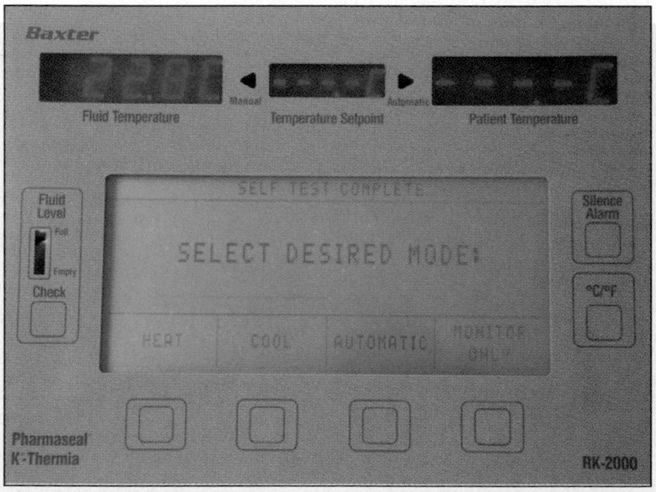

After checking fluid level, select desired mode: heat, cool, automatic or monitor.

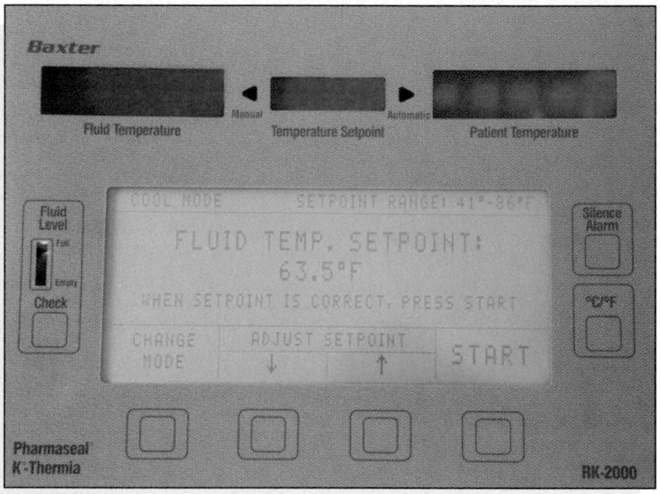

Set fluid temperature to ordered set point, and press START.

DOCUMENTATION FOR SYSTEMIC COOLING THERAPIES

- Baseline vital signs
- Assessment for early signs of shivering
- Type and duration of sponging
- Application of compression wraps
- Cooling blanket "mode" and temperature settings
- Application of insulating covers to extremities and scrotum
- Client's temperature and other vital sign trends and methods of measuring
- Client's monitored cardiac rhythm
- Serum glucose monitoring
- Client's response to cooling therapy and any adverse effects
- Physician notification of client's response (if indicated)
- Medications administered

Critical Thinking Application

UNEXPECTED OUTCOMES	CRITICAL THINKING OPTIONS
Client's core temperature decreases rapidly to desired level.	• Turn off cooling blanket. • Take top blanket off if you are using one.
Client begins to shiver.	• Stop the procedure or warm the solution a few degrees (or both). • Monitor temperature because shivering causes an increase in the metabolic rate leading to an increase in heat production. • Monitor temperature every 15 minutes to detect additional temperature decrease. • If temperature continues to drop, the blanket can be turned on to the warming control and the client can be warmed. • Contact physician for medication order (narcotic or sedative agent). • Provide supplemental oxygen therapy.
The rectal temperature probe does not seem to be accurate, or differs from tympanic measurement.	• Assess client's skin condition for cold, presence of peripheral pulses, and ability to feel pressure; check rectum for presence of stool. • Continue taking client's temperature every 2 hours with tympanic thermometer. • Calibrate the thermistor to ensure that the temperature reading of the thermistor is accurate.
Client's core temperature is not reduced.	• Check the master temperature control to see what limits are set. May need to decrease lower limit. Check with physician. • Contact physician for additional cooling blanket and place a top cooling pad on client to provide a greater body surface area in contact with pads. • Place a blanket over the top pad to insulate and provide a more effective and rapid control of temperature. • Attach small cooling pads to the extra connections on the machine to provide cold areas to body where the arteries are close to the surface, such as groin, axilla, and neck. • Discuss need for cold water spray and warm air fan to reduce client's temperature. • Consider that cutaneous vasoconstriction due to external cooling may be conserving core body heat. • Discuss need for more aggressive internal cooling measures (e.g., cold peritoneal lavage).
Skin is injured during use of the cooling blanket.	• Make sure client is turned every 30 minutes. • Lubricate skin with petroleum jelly to provide protection. • Wrap client's hands and feet securely to prevent frostbite. • Check bony prominences at least every hour. • Ensure that the master control temperature is not set too low. • Chart changes in skin condition.

UNEXPECTED OUTCOMES	CRITICAL THINKING OPTIONS
Cooling blanket does not function properly.	• Check that plug is connected to the outlet. • Check that the fluid level is sufficient and that unit freezing has not occurred. • Check that the thermistor probe is properly connected. • Check that the cool limit on the pad is not set too high. • Check that there is no constriction through pads or tubing.

GERONTOLOGIC CONSIDERATIONS

Elderly clients are more susceptible to injury from heat and cold therapy as a result of physiologic changes or medical conditions.

- There is increased epidermal replacement time and cells are replaced more slowly in the elderly.
- Skin in the elderly is thin and contains less moisture.
- The elderly have a reduced sensitivity to pain, and therefore may not feel untoward effects of heat and cold treatment.
- Temperature needs to be decreased when using heat therapy because the elderly client's skin burns more easily.

Vital signs and frequent assessment may need to be carried out during heat and cold therapy as vasodilation from heat or vasoconstriction from cold can cause changes in cardiac function and blood pressure.

- Peripheral circulation may be compromised due to atherosclerosis or microvascular disease.
- Sensation in distal extremities may be impaired in elderly clients with neuropathy due to diabetes.
- The elderly may take medications that decrease sweating (anticholinergics for Parkinson's) or increase heat production (CNS stimulants or lithium).
- Temperature threshold for sweating is higher in the elder client and ability to mount a metabolic response to temperature loss is limited.
- Living conditions and financial limitations may not afford adequate environmental control.
- Hemodynamic responses to heat/cold therapies may be more unpredictable.

MANAGEMENT GUIDELINES

Each state legislates a Nurse Practice Act for RNs and LVN/LPNs. Health care facilities are responsible for establishing and implementing policies and procedures that conform to their state's regulations. Verify the regulations and role parameters for each health care worker in your facility.

Delegation of Responsibilities

- RNs may assign LPN/LVNs to perform any of the skills covered in this chapter. For example, they may set up a sterile field for a dressing change, apply heat or ice to an extremity, set up a hypothermia blanket or give a sitz bath.
- Assessment before delegation and evaluation of the client's response during and following therapy is required of licensed delegate.
- Systemic cooling or heating therapies are indicated for critically ill clients in special care settings who may be sedated or pharmacologically paralyzed. These clients are generally monitored and cared for exclusively by licensed personnel.
- CNAs and UAPs may be assigned to do many of the skills with supervision. They are not trained to do sterile dressings and should not be assigned to use infant radiant warmers or hypothermia blankets without special guidance and supervision.

Information Flow

- Because many of the procedures in this chapter are performed by unlicensed personnel, there must be excellent reporting to the nurse responsible for client care. The treatment effect of these measures will influence client health, so outcomes of the procedures must be charted as well as verbally reported to the nurse.
- Any adverse responses (local or systemic) should be reported to prescribing physician so that corrective measures can be provided.

CRITICAL THINKING STRATEGIES

SCENARIO 1

Mrs. Moore is a 52-year-old client who has been admitted to your unit following a laparoscopic cholecystectomy. She has a peripheral IV infusion of 5% dextrose in 0.45% NS infusing at 120 mL/hr in the cephalic vein at the left wrist. She receives intermittent antibiotic therapy by IV piggyback. The infusion also facilitates PCA Morphine for client-controlled pain management.

One hour after the evening IV antibiotic administration, she calls the nurse and reports a discomfort in her left arm. Assessment findings include discomfort in the area, slight pallor, swelling (lower arm circumference 1.5 inches greater than contralateral arm), and coolness to touch.

1. Based on assessment findings, what is the probable complication and what are possible causes?
2. What should the nurse's first action be?
3. How should the area be treated?
4. When are heat or cold therapies indicated to manage IV complications?

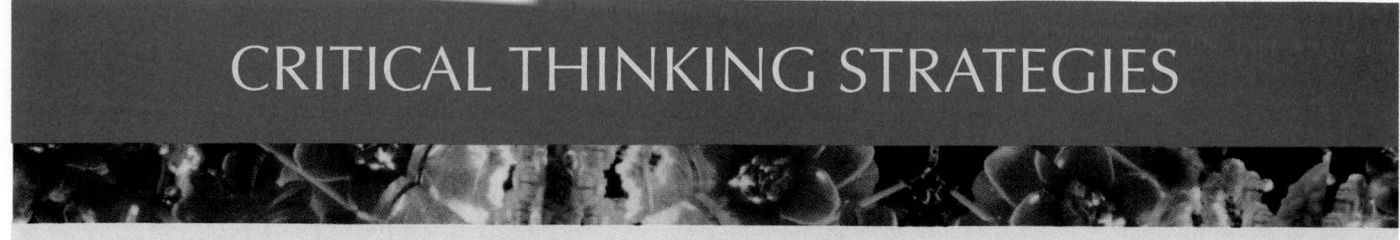

CHAPTER 25

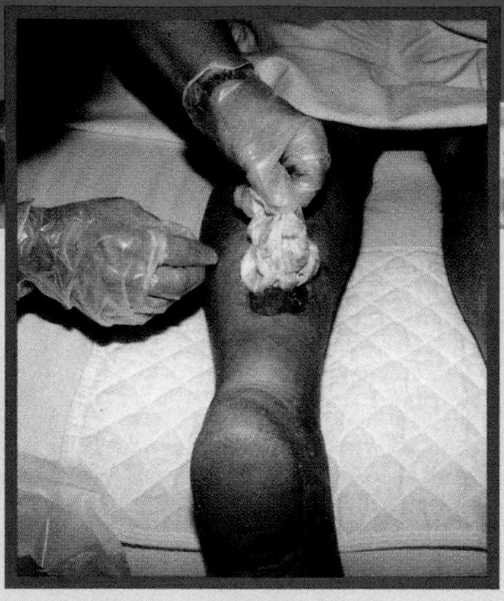

Wound Care and Dressings

THEORETICAL CONCEPTS

UNIT ONE: **Measures to Prevent Infection 819**

Completing a Surgical Hand Scrub 820
Donning Sterile Gloves 820
Pouring from a Sterile Container 822
Preparing a Sterile Field 822
Preparing a Sterile Field Using Prepackaged Supplies 824
Preparing for Dressing Change with Individual Supplies 824

UNIT TWO: **Dressing Change 826**

Changing a Dry Sterile Dressing 827
Removing Sutures 828
Removing Staples 829

UNIT THREE: **Wound Care 831**

Assessing a Wound 832
Changing a Wound Dressing 834
Packing a Wound 836
Changing a Dressing for a Venous Ulcer 837
Assessing Ankle–Brachial Index (ABI) 840
Caring for a Wound with a Drain 840
Applying an Abdominal Binder 842
Maintaining Wound Drainage System 842
Irrigating Wounds 844

UNIT FOUR: **Wet-to-Moist Dressings 847**

Applying Wet-to-Moist Dressings 848

UNIT FIVE: **Pressure Ulcers 850**

Preventing Pressure Ulcers 853
Applying Transparent Adhesive Film Dressing 854
Using Hydrocolloid Dressing 857

UNIT SIX: **Adjunctive Wound Care Therapy 861**

Using Electrical Stimulation 862
Using Noncontact Normothermic Wound Therapy 863
for Using Warm-Up® Therapy System 863
for Changing Wound Cover 864
for Charging Batteries 864
Using Vacuum-Assisted Closure 865
for Removing Dressing 866
for Disconnecting V.A.C.® Unit 866
for Reconnecting V.A.C.® Unit 866
for Changing Canister 866

GERONTOLOGIC CONSIDERATIONS 867

MANAGEMENT GUIDELINES 868

CRITICAL THINKING STRATEGIES 869

Cross reference: Chapter 8 for Special Beds

LEARNING OBJECTIVES

- Describe the three phases of wound healing.
- Define the three types of wound healing.
- Discuss three factors that affect wound healing.
- State three complications associated with wound healing.
- State criteria used to assess a wound.
- Compare and contrast the four stages of pressure ulcers.
- Write three nursing diagnoses for a client requiring wound care.
- State three goals of wound care.
- Discuss the effect of topical agents in wound healing.
- Differentiate between clean, contaminated, and infected wounds.
- Compare and contrast clean and sterile technique.
- Explain appropriate use of dressings: gauze, adhesive clear film, hydrocolloid, and hydrogel.
- Outline the steps in irrigating a wound.
- List steps to obtain a wound specimen for culture.
- Perform the steps of a surgical hand scrub.
- Prepare a sterile field for a dressing change.
- Demonstrate the steps of putting on sterile gloves.
- Describe the procedure for cleaning around a drain site.
- List steps used to maintain a Hemovac or Jackson–Pratt suction drain.
- Demonstrate changing a sterile dressing.
- Outline the steps for removal of staples and sutures.
- Outline the procedure for changing a wet-to-moist dressing.
- Compare and contrast the three adjunctive wound care therapies.
- Complete charting on a wound assessment and wound care.

TERMINOLOGY

Adhesions: formation of fibrous scar tissue around the incision as a result of surgical intervention. Adhesions can cause obstruction or malfunction by distorting the organ.

Adjunctive wound care therapy: wound treatments other than dressings and cleansing agents.

Aerobe: a microorganism that lives and grows in the presence of free oxygen.

Anaerobe: an organism that lives and grows in the absence of molecular oxygen.

Antimicrobial: an agent that prevents the multiplication of microorganisms.

Asepsis: prevention of contact with microorganisms.

Collagen formation: formation of the protein substance of the white fibers of skin, bone, and cartilage.

Debris: remains of damaged or broken-down tissue or cells.

Decubitus ulcer: see pressure ulcer.

Dehiscence: a bursting open, as a graafian follicle or wound, especially abdominal wounds.

Dermis: synonym for corium; the skin layer beneath the epidermis; contains vascular connective tissues.

Edematous: the presence of abnormally large amounts of fluid in the intercellular tissue spaces of the body.

Electrical stimulation of wound: transfer of electrical current through contact with moist wound bed.

Epidemiology: division of medical science concerned with defining and explaining the interrelationships of the host, agent, and environment in causing disease.

Epithelium: outer covering of the body; top layer of skin.

Erythema: redness of the skin due to congestion of capillaries.

Evisceration: protrusion of the viscera; removal of the viscera.

Exudate: material obtained from a wound as the result of the inflammatory process.

Gangrene: death and putrefaction of body tissue precipitated by poor or absent blood supply to the tissue. Occurs as a result of infection, injury, or disease processes.

Granulation: formation of granules; fleshy projections formed on the surface of a gaping wound that is not healing by the normal joining together of skin edges.

Incision: a cut made with a knife.

Infection: morbid state caused by multiplication of pathogenic microorganisms within the body.

Inflammatory process: localized response when injury or destruction of tissue has occurred; destroys, wards off, or dilutes the causative agent or the injured tissue.

Irrigate: to rinse or wash out with a fluid.

Isolation: limitation of movement and social contacts of a client; especially those having communicable diseases.

Keloid: scarlike growth of collagen that results in a rounded, hard, shiny, white benign tumor.

Macrophage: a large monocyte that has left the circulation and settled and matured in tissue and serves as scavenger of the blood, cleaning it of old cells and cellular debris.

Microorganism: minute living body not perceptible to the naked eye.

Monocyte: phagocytic white blood cell that matures into a macrophage.

Monokine: chemical mediator released by monocytes and macrophages during the immune response. They affect growth and activity of other white blood cells.

Myofibroblast: an atypical fibroblast with features of a fibroblast and a smooth muscle cell.

Necrotic: death of a portion of tissue.

Neutrophil: white blood cells responsible for body's protection against infection. Plays a large role in the inflammatory process.

Occlusion: the closure or state of being closed, of a passage.

Organism: a living thing, either plant or animal.

Pathogen: disease-producing organism.

Periwound: area surrounding wound; healthy tissue around wound.

Phagocytosis: ingestion and digestion of bacteria by phagocytes.

Pressure ulcer: a break in the skin caused by pressure and restricted blood flow to the area. The ulcer generally occurs over bony prominences of the heels, sacrum, hip, and shoulder.

Primary healing: minimal tissue loss and edges are closely approximated. Wound heals with minimal granulation tissue and scarring.

Purulent: containing pus, or caused by pus.

Pus: an inflammation containing leukocytes and exudate.

Second intention healing: second stage in wound healing in which granulation occurs.

Semiocclusive dressing: create and maintain a moist environment by holding liquid drainage from wound and moisture vapor at the wound surface.

Tertiary healing: using open method of wound healing; allow granulation to occur.

Vacuum-assisted wound closure: negative pressure applied to wound to promote healing.

Warm-Up® therapy: heat therapy used to stimulate healing process.

Wound dehiscence: the separation of layers of a surgical wound.

Wound evisceration: protrusion of the internal viscera or organs through an opened incisional site.

WOUND HEALING

The three major phases of wound healing are inflammation, proliferation (or granulation), and maturation (or wound remodeling).

Inflammatory Phase

The onset of the first phase of wound healing occurs immediately after an injury and lasts 4–6 days. After the injury, small blood vessels dilate and become more permeable and serous fluid leaks into the traumatized tissue as a result of histamine and prostaglandin release. Plasma and electrolytes leak into the interstitial spaces causing edema. The edema leads to a reddened, swollen, and tender wound. Neutrophils reach the site in about 6 hours. Through the process of phagocytosis, they assist in preventing infection by ingesting and digesting bacteria. Oxygen is necessary for the neutrophils to destroy the bacteria. They survive only several hours after ingesting bacteria and necrotic tissue before releasing their intracellular contents, which forms part of the wound exudate. By the fourth day, monocytes enter the wound and differentiate into macrophages, which digest necrotic tissue, remove debris, and inhibit microbial growth. They also play a role in creating collagen synthesis. If macrophages are depleted, deposition of wound collagen decreases significantly. Macrophages direct healing through the release of monokines.

Proliferative, or Granulation, Phase

This phase begins between 1 and 4 days after the injury and ends 14–21 days later. During granulation there is rapid growth of epithelial cells to produce a protective covering for the wound. The granulation tissue is formed from a rebuilding of the vascular capillary network and collagen tissue. The collagen fibers increase the tensile strength of the wound and provide wound integrity. Collagen fibers fill in the gaps and form the scar. Wound scar tissue is very fragile and susceptible to reinjury. In 6 weeks, the scar is only 10% of the tensile strength of normal skin. Large wounds may take months to build enough granulation tissue to close the wound. Healthy granulation tissue has a healthy reddish-pink color. The color results from increased blood flow that delivers oxygen and nutrients to the newly formed tissue.

Maturation, or Wound-Remodeling, Phase

Wound contraction begins between 14 and 21 days after the injury and can last up to 2 years. During this phase, the scar shrinks and thins. It becomes less red as the capillaries regress. Contraction of the wound occurs as a result of myofibroblasts, which assist in moving the wound edges toward the center of the wound. The skin and fascia of the healed wound achieve only about 70–80% of the tensile strength of normal skin.

WOUND CLASSIFICATION

There are different wound classification systems used to describe wounds. These are useful when the nurse is planning for wound care management. The classification systems include categorizing the wound by cause: intentional or unintentional; cleanliness: clean, contaminated, or infected; depth: superficial, partial-thickness, or full-thickness; and by color. The RYB classification system has been used in wound care classification since the late 1980s. This system classifies open wounds that are healing by secondary or delayed primary intention in both acute and chronic wounds. It is used as an adjunct to other classification systems. It does not lend itself to an in-depth, comprehensive evaluation. It can be used to determine the state of healing. This system identifies what phase a wound is in on the continuum of the wound healing process. Red wounds (R) can be in the inflammatory, proliferative, or maturation phase of wound healing. Yellow wounds (Y) are infected or contain fibrinous slough and aren't ready to heal. Black wounds (B) contain necrotic tissue and aren't ready to heal. Treatment options are based on the color of the wound. Red wounds need to be kept clean and moist. Yellow wounds require the removal of slough or fibrinous tissue. Black wounds must have the eschar removed for healing to take place. If the wound has a combination of colors, the rule is that the most severe color treatment is completed.

TYPES OF WOUND HEALING

Primary Intention

This is the simplest form of healing. The skin is cleanly incised through a surgical incision or a traumatic laceration. The wound can be closed with sutures or staples, which approximates, or pulls together, the wound edges. These wounds close rapidly because there are no gaps in the tissue. The top layer of cells migrate, or epithelize, within 72 hours. The wound surface is "sealed," thus preventing bacteria from entering and fluid from escaping. The tensile strength of the wound is very weak at this stage of healing.

Secondary Intention

These wounds heal by granulation. As granulation tissue builds, it fills the gap under the skin and cells epithelize from the edge of the wound to create the closure. Burns, pressure ulcers, and wounds with large pieces of skin missing heal by this method. In these types of wounds no edges are available to be approximated and sutured. These wounds are at risk for local and systemic infection due to the destruction of the dermis and the increased time necessary for healing to occur.

Tertiary Intention

Healing by tertiary intention is a method that leaves the wound open to heal. These wounds are infected and need frequent irrigations and dressing changes to facilitate healing. Clients with peritonitis, a ruptured appendix, or diverticula frequently require this type of wound healing. After irrigations and dressing changes for approximately 10 days, the wound is sutured and allowed to heal by primary and secondary intention.

MAJOR FACTORS AFFECTING WOUND HEALING

In addition to proper wound care and generally good physical health, nutrition plays a major role in wound healing. Medication use may interfere with wound healing.

Nutrition

Low serum albumin levels slow the diffusion of oxygen and diminish the ability of neutrophils to kill bacteria. Low oxygen at the capillary level diminishes the proliferation of healthy granulation tissue. Zinc deficiency can slow the rate of epithelialization and decrease wound and collagen strength. Adequate amounts of vitamins A and C and of iron and copper are necessary for effective collagen formation. Collagen synthesis also depends on appropriate intake of protein, carbohydrates, and fats. Wound healing requires almost double the usual protein and carbohydrate requirements for age. For the scar to develop adequate tensile strength, the client's intake of vitamin C, iron, and zinc must be increased.

General Physical Health

The major obstacle to wound healing is infection. Infected wounds have friable tissue, bleed easily, and have delayed healing. Immunosuppressed clients have more difficulty healing wounds because the inflammatory phase is impaired. When the blood glucose level is consistently over 200 mg/dL or the hemoglobin is below 10 g/dL, wounds do not follow the usual phases of healing. Any condition that reduces the formation of adequate white blood cells, especially macrophages, adversely affects healing. Such conditions include diabetes mellitus, anemia, uremia, cancer, atherosclerosis, infection, and malnutrition. Older clients, clients who smoke or are obese, and those undergoing radiation or steroid therapy are also prone to delayed wound healing.

Medications

Any medication that reduces the inflammatory response, such as steroids and nonsteroidal medications used to

Nutritional Support for Wound Healing

Nutrient	Food Sources
Protein	Meat, fish, poultry, milk, cheese, eggs, dried beans, peas, peanut butter
Carbohydrates	Legumes, fruits, vegetables, whole-grain cereal, bread, pasta
Vitamins	
Vitamin A	Dark green leafy vegetables, milk, eggs, carrots, liver
Vitamin C	Citrus fruits, vegetables, potatoes
Minerals	
Iron	Meat, eggs, cereal, vegetables
Copper	Seafood, nuts, seeds, organ meats
Zinc	Meat, liver, seafood, eggs

TABLE 25–1 RYB Wound Dressing Guidelines*

Dressings Most Commonly Used to Treat RYB Wounds	
Red Wounds Biologicals Foams Gauze Hydrocolloids Hydrogels Moist gauze Nonadherent gauze Transparent film	Yellow Wounds (fibrinous slough) Alginate Exudate absorbers Foams Hypertonic gauze Hydrocolloid Hydrogel Transparent film
Yellow Wounds (infected) Alginates Impregnated dressings Exudate absorbers Foams Hypertonic gauze Wound pouches	Black Wounds Alginate Hydrocolloid Hydrogel Gauze Transparent film

See: Assessing a wound, p.832.

treat arthritis or respiratory conditions, also impairs wound healing. Anti-inflammatories decrease epithelialization and wound contraction and may also affect fibroblast proliferation and collagen synthesis. Steroids decrease the tensile strength of a closed wound and cause inadequate deposits of collagen. Administration of vitamin A can reverse the processes associated with steroid use.

GOALS OF WOUND CARE

Wound assessment and measures to treat wounds have changed dramatically over the last 10 years. The major trend is to treat wounds using moisture-retentive dressing rather than drying the wound. Wound care specialists also diverge on the use of sterile versus clean technique during dressing changes.

Whatever plan is used in treating a wound, the goals remain the same.

- Remove necrotic tissue to promote wound healing.
- Prevent, eliminate, or control infection.
- Absorb drainage (exudate).
- Maintain a moist wound environment.
- Protect the wound from further injury.
- Protect the surrounding skin from infection and trauma.

To accomplish these goals, a moist wound environment must be maintained to allow tissue to granulate. A wound bed that is too moist or too dry kills healthy tissue and impairs healing. Drainage from the wound site needs to be contained to protect adjacent healthy skin from maceration. All wounds require a dressing that is dry on the air-exposed side to prevent bacterial invasion by downward capillary mobility of contaminants. The dressing should be secured over the wound and taped in place using the "window paning" method of taping if there is not an adhesive backing on the dressing. Using this method, the edges remain taped down and the dressing stays intact.

There are many types of wound care products available, including skin cleansers, skin barriers, irrigants, various types of dressings, gauze dressings, and enzymes. Physician and wound care specialist preferences, as well as type and extent of wound, determine wound care.

Complications Associated with Wound Healing

One complication that may occur after wound healing has seemed to progress satisfactorily is adhesions. Adhesions frequently form in the peritoneal cavity after abdominal surgery and can either constrict or fold around the intestines.

Frequently clients are admitted to the hospital with incisional strangulated internal hernias that may even be gangrenous. Other complications are surgical or incisional hernias that may occur when the intraperitoneal pressure is such that it pushes against the scar tissue and causes a hernia (or outpouching) through the incision.

Contractures, formed as a result of a shortening of scar tissue, can decrease mobility and joint movement. Contractures caused by incisional scars are far less common than those caused by scar tissue from burns.

Excessive collagen formation results in the formation of a keloid, a complication that does not present a serious problem with body function; however, it generally causes an altered self-image if the keloid is large or in a prominent place on the body.

WOUND INFECTIONS

Open wounds of any type provide an environment for bacterial invasion. All wounds may be considered contaminated but not necessarily infected. Wound care must include regular wound cleansing, the use of semiocclusive dressings, using Standard Precautions when providing care to the client, maintaining proper handwashing technique, and following dressing change protocols. Semiocclusive dressings in wound care have reduced the incidence of wound infections by more than 50% compared to gauze dressings. These dressings promote a moist environment, provide a mechanical barrier for bacterial invasion, and reduce airborne dispersal of bacteria during dressing changes.

The clinical symptoms of wound infection generally begin in 3–5 days postoperatively or following injury. When the client's temperature and pulse rate increase, an associated tachypnea occurs. As the inflammatory process proceeds, the wound becomes progressively more tender, painful, and edematous. Erythema surrounds the edges of the wound unless the infection is in the deeper tissues. Abnormal firmness of the wound edge may be present. Usually, a persistent WBC count of 12,000/mm^3 or greater, lasting longer than 72 hours, accompanies the infection. Foul-smelling, purulent drainage may occur. An absence of local signs of infection does not necessarily mean that deep wound infections are absent.

Several microorganisms are responsible for the majority of wound infections. *Staphylococcus aureus* is still a major cause of postoperative infection. *Escherichia coli, Streptococcus faecalis, Proteus vulgaris, Klebsiella, Enterobacter*, and *Pseudomonas aeruginosa* are also closely associated with wound infection. Antimicrobial agents themselves can promote infection by increasing the susceptibility of clients to colonization with nosocomial microflora; these agents also select and concentrate antibiotic-resistant organisms on or in the host.

Maintaining asepsis during dressing changes assists in preventing wound infections. Using sterile equipment, including gloves, is the first barrier against infection. A mask and gown should be worn during dressing changes to prevent the spread of microorganisms to other clients and to the health care worker.

When wounds become grossly infected or are extensive in nature, the physician may order wound irrigations. Normal saline or Ringer's solution are the usual irrigating solutions used for wounds. Most of the agents used in the past have been identified as toxic to the cells generated in the inflammatory phase of healing.

Each hospital has its own protocol for wound irrigation and you should become familiar with the institution's procedure. This chapter presents one method of wound irrigation that is helpful in most clinical situations.

Wound Specimens for Culture

Exudate, or purulent drainage, from infected wounds can contain a variety of aerobic and anaerobic microorganisms. In the majority of wound infections, the causative agent is usually found in the upper respiratory tract, gastrointestinal tract, and genitourinary tract. When these organisms invade other body parts, they can cause severe infections and sometimes death.

Before a wound can be cultured, it should be irrigated with normal saline to remove the surface bacteria. The best method of obtaining a culture specimen is to rotate a swab along the granulation tissue. Refer to Chapter 20, Specimen Collection, for skill. For the most accurate results, the physician should take a biopsy of the tissue.

Wounds Caused by Vascular Insufficiency

There are three types of wounds caused by vascular insufficiency. These include venous insufficiency ulcers, arterial insufficiency ulcers, and pressure ulcers (capillary insufficiency ulcers). There are five major factors that contribute to ulcer formation in vascular insufficiency: poor nutrition and a lack of blood flow causing inability of nutrients to diffuse through the interstitial spaces; continuous pressure on certain areas of the body, such as bony prominences; mechanical, thermal, or chemical insults to limbs, resulting in lack of nutrients reaching the lower limbs; decreased sensation in the lower extremities; and excess moisture from incontinence.

Venous Ulcers

These are mistakenly termed venous stasis ulcers; however, they are not due to a lack of venous blood flow, but rather a diminished ability of nutrients to diffuse through the interstitial space from the capillaries. The usual etiology of this condition includes calf pump failure as a result of outflow tract obstruction, associated with pregnancy, obesity, tumor, or deep vein thrombosis. Insufficient valves, either deep venous valve incompetence or superficial vein incompetence (varicose veins), are causes as well. Peripheral neuropathy and musculoskeletal disorders may lead to venous ulcers as a result of calf muscle disuse.

Compression therapy is used to treat venous ulcers. This therapy includes the use of compression stockings, Unna's boot, or a compression dressing when wound care is included in the treatment. Compression therapy is contraindicated in clients with phlebitis, diminished sensation, and arterial insufficiency, as it will exacerbate the insufficiency.

Arterial Ulcers

Arterial ulcers are often seen in clients with diabetes mellitus and atherosclerosis. Clients with a history of smoking and who sustain mechanical trauma to the extremity are prone to arterial ulcers. In these situations, there is diminished oxygenation and thus, nutrients, to the periphery. Drug therapy with vasodilators, anticoagulants, or thrombolytic agents are part of the treatment plan for these clients. Surgical treatment may be necessary if drug therapy is insufficient to treat the ulcer. Sympathectomy, endarterectomy, or bypass surgery may be necessary treatment modalities.

Pressure Ulcers

Pressure ulcers are defined by the National Pressure Ulcer Advisory Panel as any lesion caused by unrelieved pressure resulting in damage to underlying tissue. Four mechanical factors contribute to the development of pressure ulcers: pressure, friction, shearing, and moisture. Pressure ulcers are usually located over a bony prominence, where normal tissue is squeezed between the bone and pressure or friction caused by the bed or chair. External pressure that lasts long enough to result in decreased blood flow causes altered oxygenation and nutrition to the tissue, resulting in a pressure ulcer. Immobility, especially associated with the elderly, is the primary cause of pressure ulcer formation. In addition to mechanical factors and immobility, aging skin and malnutrition increase the risk of skin breakdown.

Each year 1.5 million hospitalized clients develop pressure ulcers, resulting in 60,000 deaths. Data suggests 25% of these clients develop the pressure ulcer in the operating room, especially when the surgery is prolonged beyond 3 hours. Surgical clients experience periods of prolonged immobility, resulting in unrelieved pressure and decreased blood flow to the skin. In addition to the 9% of hospitalized clients, 23% of all nursing home clients develop pressure ulcers. Elderly clients are affected most often and account for the highest number of cases. A large percentage of the clients who develop pressure ulcers in a nursing home die as a result. These statistics are appalling when one considers that ulcers are preventable and treatable.

Pressure ulcers are classified in stages by the degree of tissue damage observed. See Unit 5 for illustration and description.

Management of pressure ulcers is best accomplished using a team of health care providers, including physicians, nurses, an enterostomal therapist, dietitian, physical therapist, family members, and the client.

Client education should include:

- Discussion of pressure ulcer treatment options.
- Discussion of client's active participation in his or her own care.
- Developing a plan of care that is consistent with the client's goals and desires.

Client treatment plan should include:

- Assessment of the pressure ulcer.
- Managing tissue loads.
- Ulcer care.
- Managing bacterial colonization and infection.
- Operative repair of the pressure ulcer.

Management and prevention of pressure ulcers should begin on hospital admission with a thorough assessment of the client's skin, especially over bony prominences. Preventive steps for high-risk clients include the following:

- Ensure that skin is kept clean, and prevent it from getting too dry by using moisturizing lotions.
- Provide a balanced diet high in protein, vitamins, and minerals for tissue repair.
- Ensure a fluid intake of 2,000 mL/day for adequate hydration.
- Place clients on a pressure-reducing mattress or chair cushion.
- Do not elevate head of the bed more than 30°.
- Reposition a bedridden client at least every 2 hours and a chair-bound client every hour—positioning remains the basic standard of ulcer prevention.
- Complete a risk assessment for the client, evaluating factors for developing pressure ulcers.

ADJUNCTIVE WOUND CARE THERAPY

Three of the more common types of adjunctive wound therapy include electrical stimulation, noncontact normothermic wound therapy, and the vacuum assisted closure system.

Electrical stimulation uses transfer of an electric current through a surface electrode pad that is in contact with external skin surface or the wound bed itself. It influences wound healing by attracting cells of repair, changing cell membrane permeability, enhancing cellular secretion through cell membranes, and orienting cell structure. A moist wound environment must be maintained for this therapy to be successful in healing. Electrical stimulation increases blood flow, oxygen uptake, and DNA and protein synthesis. It can be used in a variety of wound problems including burns, pressure ulcers, vascular ulcers, and surgical wounds.

Warm-up therapy stimulates the healing process through application of infrared heat to the wound. This system uses warmth to help the body heal itself. It also maintains humidity and absorbs exudates, and its transparent window allows the nurse to assess the wound without disrupting wound tissue. Wound cover allows clients more freedom in their movements, as well as an increased comfort level. The heat increases blood flow and oxygen to the wound. It is commonly used for clients with venous ulcers and pressure ulcers. It can also be used for clients with surgical or traumatic wounds and diabetic ulcers.

Vacuum-assisted closure uses a foam dressing applied directly to the wound. This system stimulates growth of granulation tissue while promoting a moist environment. A negative pressure is applied to foam through use of tubing connected to a canister where exudate and wound fluids are collected. This system is used with infected wounds, as well as chronic wounds, acute and traumatic wounds, and dehiscence.

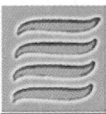

NURSING DIAGNOSES

The following nursing diagnoses may be appropriate to use on client care plans when the components are related to the client requiring wound care.

NURSING DIAGNOSIS	RELATED FACTORS
Risk for Infection	Altered circulation, invasive procedures, trauma Exposure to nosocomial agents, surgical incision, open wound
Chronic Pain	Tissue injury, extensive dressing changes, recent surgery, vascular ulcers
Impaired Physical Mobility	Bed rest, wounds, or pressure ulcers
Impaired Skin Integrity	Mechanical factors (shearing force, pressure), altered circulation due to pressure on a bony prominence, immobility, poor nutritional intake
Ineffective Tissue Perfusion	Interrupted blood supply to site depleting oxygen and nutrients

- The single most important nursing action to decrease the incidence of hospital-based infections is handwashing. **Remember to wash your hands or use antibacterial gel before and after each and every client contact.**

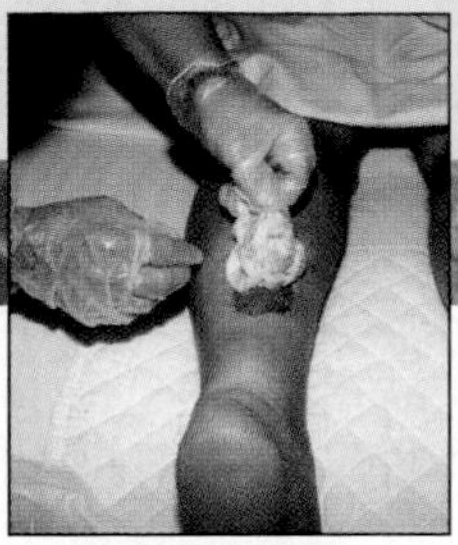

UNIT 1

Measures to Prevent Infection

Nursing Process Data

ASSESSMENT *Data Base*

Identify clients at risk for infection (i.e., diabetics, elderly, malnourished, obese, smokers, immunosuppressed).

Identify length of time client remained in surgery (the more hours in surgery the greater the risk for infection).

Assess incision three times a day.

Identify the components necessary to prevent infection for individual clients.

Assess need for sterile technique compliance in client care.

Assess lab results for abnormal values (i.e., WBC, Hgb, Hct).

PLANNING *Objectives*

To prevent clients with impaired resistance from becoming infected

To prevent microorganisms from entering the wound

To provide a sterile working field for dressing changes

IMPLEMENTATION *Procedures*

Completing a Surgical Hand Scrub

Donning Sterile Gloves

Pouring from a Sterile Container

Preparing a Sterile Field

Preparing a Sterile Field Using Prepackaged Supplies

Preparing for Dressing Change with Individual Supplies

EVALUATION *Expected Outcomes*

Infection is prevented in clients with impaired resistance.

Sterile technique is maintained throughout wound care.

Sterile field is set up appropriately.

COMPLETING A SURGICAL HAND SCRUB

Equipment

Plastic or orangewood stick
Antimicrobial solution
Sterile towel

Procedure

1. Remove all jewelry; rings, watch, bracelets.
2. Turn on water using foot or knee pedal or hand lever. Water should be tepid. **Rationale**: Hot water dries skin and is uncomfortable. Cold water prevents soap from lathering and bacteria is not rinsed away.
3. Wet your hands thoroughly.
4. With your arms held up in front of you, begin to scrub by cleaning your fingernails with a plastic or orangewood stick.
5. Scrub your hands for 10 strokes with an antimicrobial solution (time based on facility policy).
   a. Scrub may be done using brush or friction of hands.
   b. Start at fingertips and with circular motion work around each finger and between each finger.
   c. Scrub back and front of hands using circular motion with scrub.
   d. For 10 more strokes, move to 3 inches above wrist, and then up arm to elbow continuing with circular scrubbing motion. Keep hand higher than arm at all times.
   e. Repeat procedure for second hand and arm.
   f. Placing arms under water faucet, keep fingertips pointed upward and rinse thoroughly with water flowing down toward elbows. **Rationale:** This method keeps fingers and hands free of contamination.

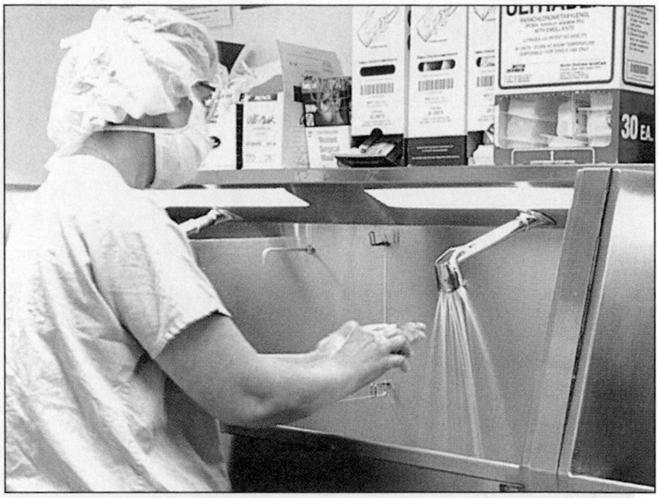
Scrub hands with an antimicrobial solution.

6. Dry your hands with a sterile towel starting at the fingertips and moving toward the elbows.
7. If hand levers are used to control water flow, turn faucets off with sterile towel used for drying hands. Do not touch faucet or sink with hands. **Rationale:** Contamination of hands occurs if objects are touched after handwashing.

CLINICAL ALERT

If hand or arm is contaminated during washing, repeat wash of specific area for 10 strokes.

DONNING STERILE GLOVES

Equipment

Packaged sterile gloves

Procedure

1. Wash and dry your hands.
2. Place glove package on a clean, dry, firm surface which is at waist height (usually an over-bed table). **Rationale:** Objects below waist level are considered to be out of the sterile field.
3. Remove outside wrapper of glove package by peeling the tabs apart where indicated on the wrapper. Pull edges laterally to expose glove package. Ensure that this step is accomplished over the firm surface. **Rationale:** This prevents the glove package from accidentally falling on a contaminated surface.
4. Place the glove package on the firm surface maintaining sterility of gloves by touching only outside of wrapper.
5. Grasp two edges of wrapper and lift wrapper edges up and away from gloves, being careful to not touch gloves as you open the package. **Rationale:** Lifting the edges up and away as you open the package will prevent touching the gloves accidentally and causing contamination.
6. With your nondominant hand, pick up the opposite glove by grasping the section that has a folded edge (inside edge of the cuff). Lift the glove up and away from the wrapper. **Rationale:** This prevents accidental contamination of the glove or inside of glove package.
7. Holding your hands above waist level, insert your dominant hand into the glove opening. Gently pull the glove into place with your nondominant hand touching only the inside of the cuff. Do not attempt to straighten out gloved fingers until both gloves have been put on. **Rationale:** It is easy to contaminate the glove when attempting to adjust the fingers in the glove.

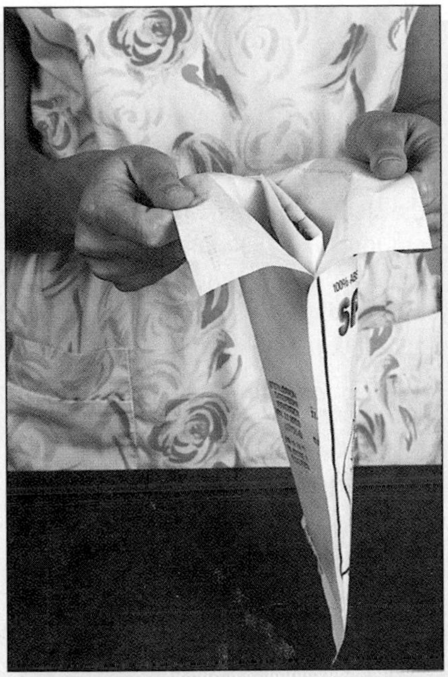

Grasp two upper edges of the glove package and pull laterally to open package.

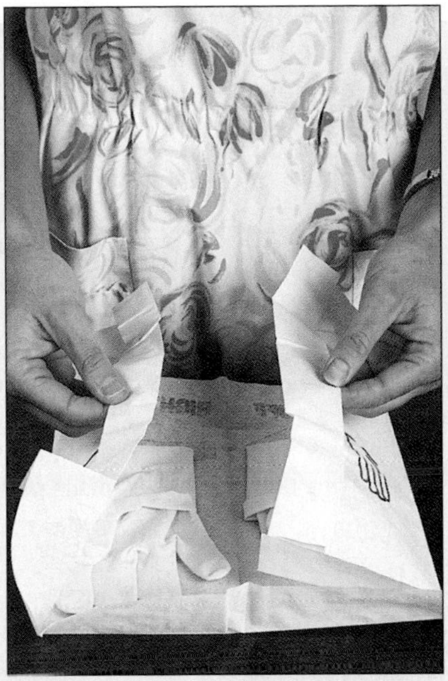

Place sterile glove wrapper on clean, flat surface and lift wrapper edges away from gloves.

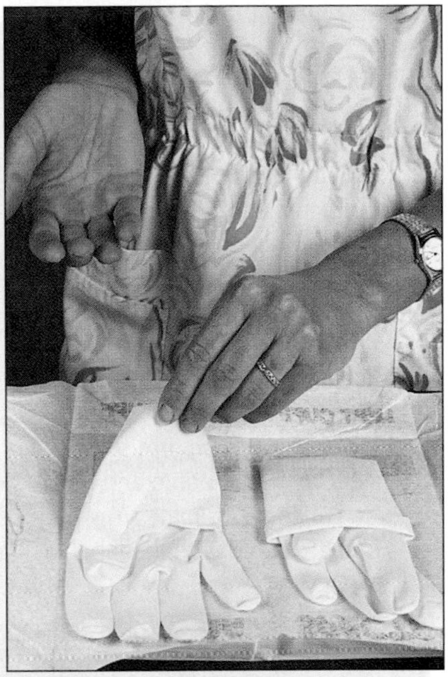

Grasp folded edge of glove with nondominant hand and lift glove away from wrapper.

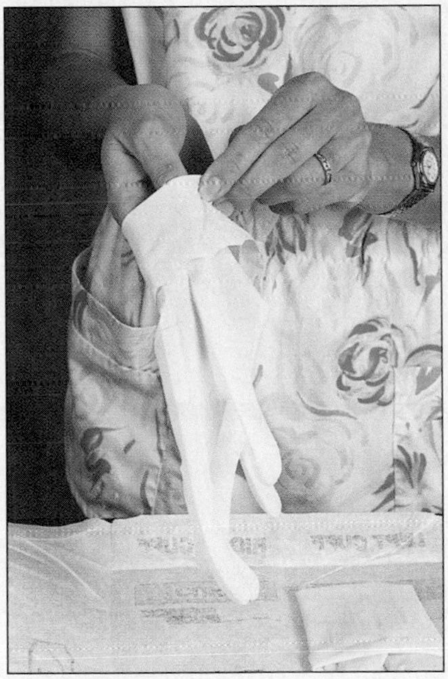

Slip dominant hand into glove opening without contaminating glove.

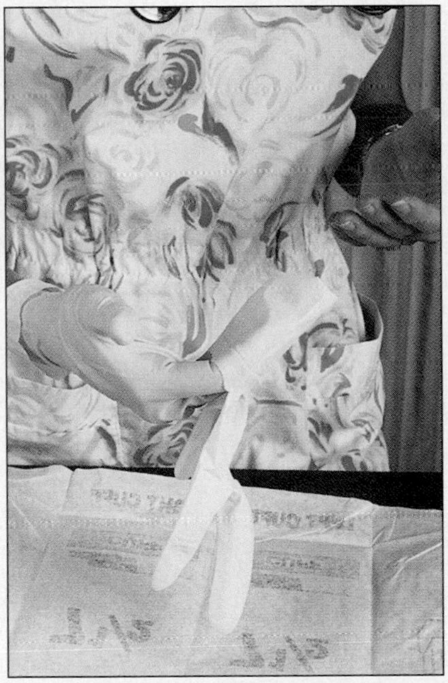

Remove second glove from wrapper by placing gloved fingers under cuff.

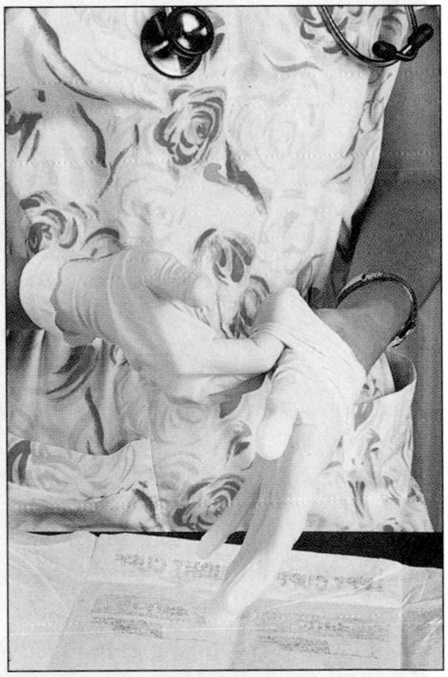

Continue to keep fingers under cuff of glove as the glove is pulled on.

8. With your dominant, gloved hand, remove the other glove from the package, making sure you touch only the inside of the folded cuff. Lift this glove up and away from the wrapper. **Rationale:** This prevents gloves from inadvertently touching wrapper and contaminating gloves.
9. Hold your gloved thumb away from your body to prevent touching your skin.
10. Place your ungloved fingers into the new glove opening. Gently pull the glove over your hand as before.
11. Keeping your hands above waist level, adjust both gloves by touching only your fingers, remembering to touch sterile surfaces with sterile surfaces. **Rationale:** Fingers of gloves are considered sterile; cuff area is considered contaminated.
12. Keep both sterile gloves in front of you above your waist level. **Rationale:** Being able to see gloves at all times helps prevent potential contamination.

POURING FROM A STERILE CONTAINER

Equipment

Sterile container
Nonsterile container
Sterile solution

Procedure

1. Wash your hands.
2. Gather equipment.
3. Open sterile container according to procedure.
4. Place container on firm surface.
5. Take cap off the bottle and invert the cap before laying on firm surface. **Rationale:** This keeps the cap sterile.
6. Hold the bottle with the label facing up.
7. Pour a small amount of liquid into a nonsterile container. **Rationale:** This action cleans the lip of the bottle.
8. Pour the liquid into the sterile container while keeping the label facing up and not touching the container with the bottle. Do not reach over a sterile field if the container has been placed on one. **Rationale:** Crossing over a sterile field can lead to contamination of the field.
9. Replace the cap if liquid remains in the bottle. If total contents have been used, dispose of bottle in trash.
10. Date and initial bottle if reusing.
11. Replace partially filled bottle to storage area if it is to be reused.

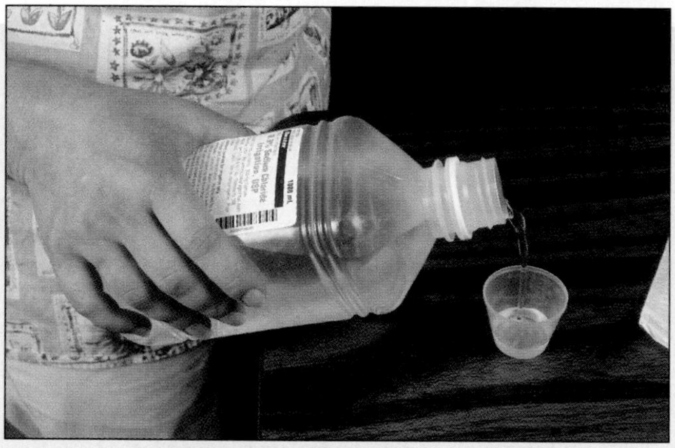

First pour a small amount of liquid into nonsterile container.

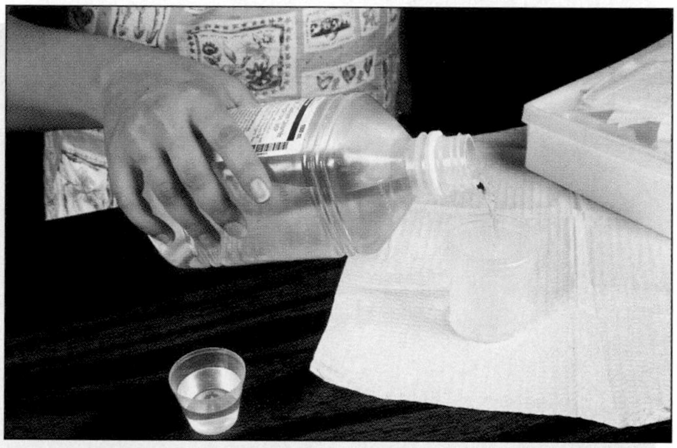

Pour liquid by placing container close to edge of sterile area.

PREPARING A STERILE FIELD

Equipment

Antiseptic cleansing solution, as ordered
Two packages of sterile towels
Number and type of dressings required for dressing change
Tape
Container for antiseptic solution
Paper bag for disposal of soiled dressings
Mask
Sterile gloves

> **CLINICAL ALERT**
>
> Preparing a sterile field is commonly used for burn dressings or large wound dressings. It is not used routinely for other dressings.

Preparation

1. Check physician's orders and client care plan.
2. Gather equipment from supply area.
3. Clean off over-bed table.

Procedure

1. Wash your hands, using aseptic technique.
2. Place sterile towel packages on over-bed table or on another surface close to the table. Place packages so that first wrapper edge can be opened away from the sterile area. **Rationale:** This prevents contamination when crossing over a sterile field.
3. Grasp far edge of the wrapper and open away from you. **Rationale:** This exposes the sterile part of package.
4. Don sterile gloves and mask according to hospital policy.

Gloves and mask are usually used when preparing burn sterile field. This procedure may be performed without gloves, maintaining sterility.

5. Using both hands, pick up the two side edges of the first wrapper and open them away from the middle of the sterile field. Unfold the last edge toward you, without touching the wrapper.
6. Pick up one edge of the sterile towel, and move away from the table. Gently shake the towel open, keeping it away from the sterile area.
7. When the towel is open, use your other hand to pick up the two edges that are away from you. Be careful to not touch towel with clothing.
8. Lower the towel onto the tray or bedside stand so the towel is furthest away from you. Then lay the towel down on the tray by bringing it toward you, covering the entire tray. **Rationale:** This prevents crossing over the sterile field.
9. Repeat the same steps with a second sterile towel.
10. If solutions for cleansing the skin are required, place sterile medicine cups near one side of the sterile towel.
11. Take the cap off the antiseptic bottle.
12. Pour a small amount of solution into a container, not on the sterile field, keeping the label in uppermost position. **Rationale:** This action rinses contaminated particles from the lip of the bottle.
13. Pour the antiseptic solution, from the side of the sterile field, directly into the medicine cup. **Rationale:** Pouring solution from the side prevents crossing over the sterile field.
14. Open sterile packages of dressings, and place on sterile surface.

for Commercially Prepared Packages

a. Open package at designated end by pulling edges apart and downward to expose contents.
b. Grasp the edges of the two sides of the package and invert the package over the edge of the sterile field. Allow the contents to drop onto the sterile field.
c. Repeat procedure for each item to be placed on the sterile field.

for Hospital-Wrapped Packages

a. Hold package in your hand, and securely grasp one edge.
b. Open package wrapper by allowing edges to drop down, away from package.
c. Grasp the edges of the wrapper with your free hand and pull them toward your wrist, thus exposing the sterile contents.
d. Gently drop the contents on the sterile field. **Rationale:** Touching the sterile field with the wrapper contaminates it.
e. Repeat procedure for each item to be placed on the sterile field.

15. If sterile supplies are not to be used immediately, cover with sterile towels.
    a. Open sterile towel package by opening wrapper away from you so that you do not cross over a sterile field.
    b. Pick up one towel at the edge and open towel by moving yourself away from the sterile field and allowing towel to fall open.
    c. Grasp corner of towel opposite one you are holding. Keep towel from touching contaminated areas.
    d. Place towel over sterile field starting at edge nearest you. Lay the towel down without touching the tray with your hand. Move the towel across the tray toward the opposite edge.
    e. Repeat procedure with second sterile towel.

Guidelines for Sterile Field

- Never turn your back on a sterile field.
- Avoid talking, coughing, sneezing, or reaching across a sterile field.
- Keep sterile objects above waist level.
- Do not spill solutions on the sterile field.
- Open all sterile packages away from the sterile field to prevent crossover and contamination.

PREPARING A STERILE FIELD USING PREPACKAGED SUPPLIES

Equipment

Packaged supplies

Procedure

1. Wash your hands.
2. Ensure working surface is clean and dry. Client's over-bed table is frequently used as preparation area. **Rationale:** This prevents contamination of sterile package.
3. Remove outer plastic wrap.
4. Place package in center of work area and position so that you first open package flap away from you. **Rationale:** This prevents reaching across the sterile field as you continue to open package.
5. Grasp edge of the first flap of the wrapper, move it away from you, and place it on the working surface.
6. Grasp the first side flap, lift it up; grasp the second side flap and together move both hands out toward the sides. Place the flaps down on the working surface.
7. Grasp the last flap of the wrapper and open it toward you, taking care not to touch the inside of the flap or any of the contents of the package. **Rationale:** This prevents contamination of the supplies.

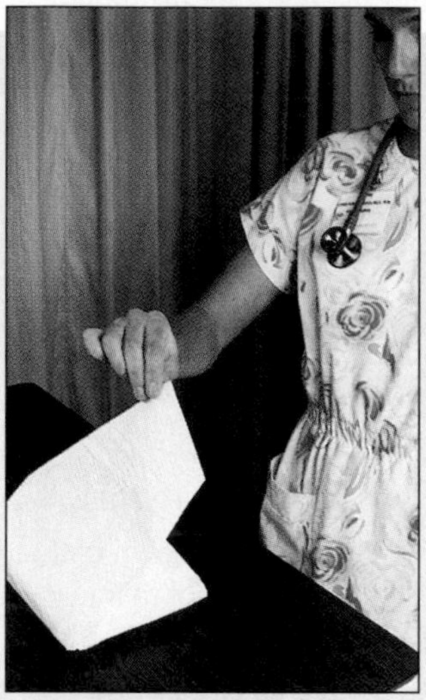

Grasp edge of top flap of wrapper and lift it away from you.

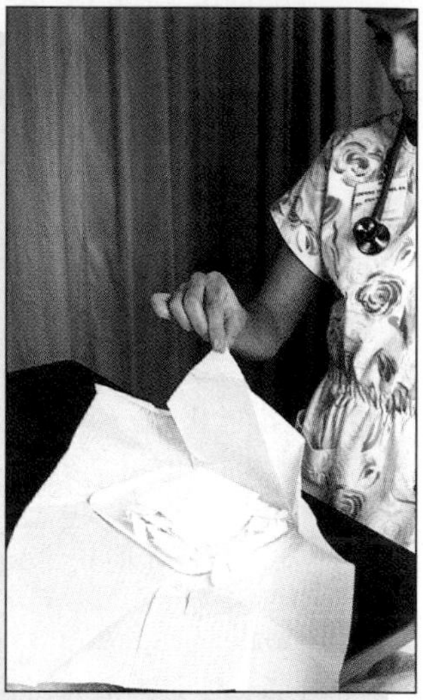

Open last flap toward you—do not cross over sterile field.

PREPARING FOR DRESSING CHANGE WITH INDIVIDUAL SUPPLIES

Equipment

Antiseptic cleaner or cleaning solution
Number and type of dressings needed (i.e., 4 × 4 gauze pads, ABD pads, application sticks, transparent dressings)
Tape
Clean gloves
Sterile gloves
Disposal bag
Mask, if needed

Procedure

1. Wash your hands.
2. Clean off bedside stand and wash thoroughly with antiseptic solution. Dry thoroughly.
3. Place supply packages on table in configuration that allows you to open packages without reaching over sterile field.

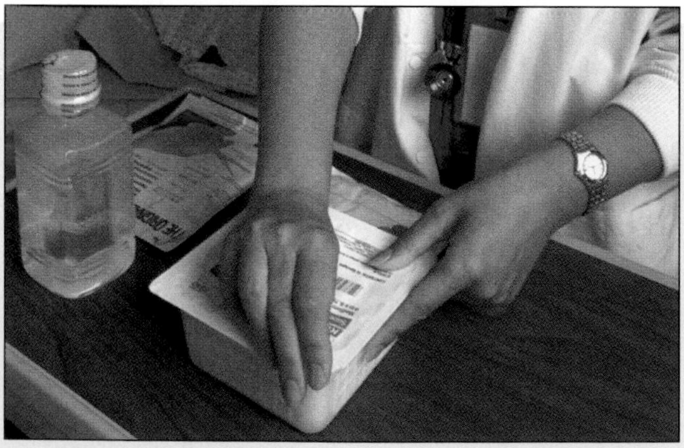

Open sterile 4 × 4 pads container by pulling back on flap.

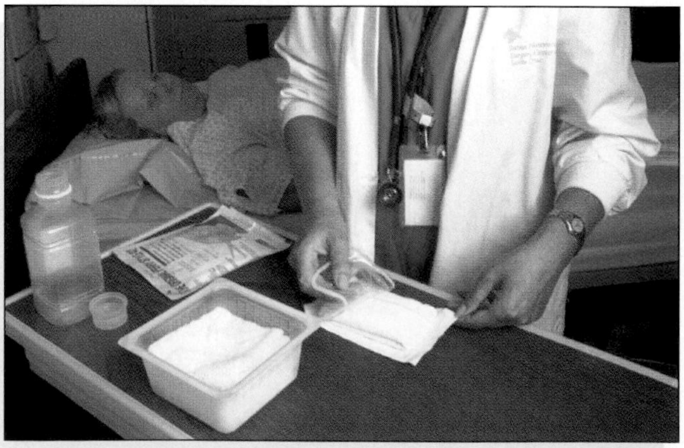

Open transparent dressing packet.

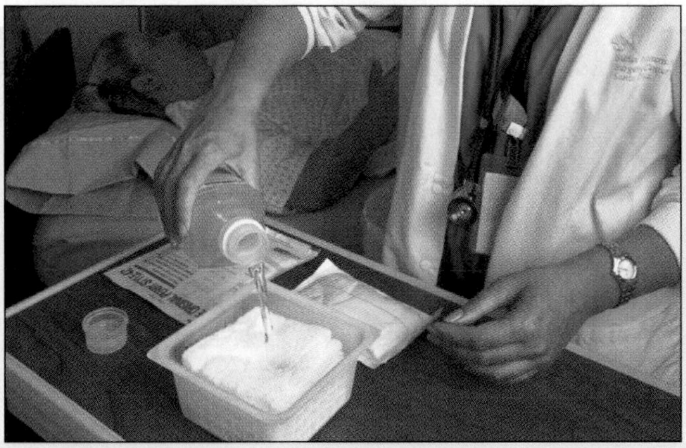

Pour cleaning solution over 4 × 4 pads.

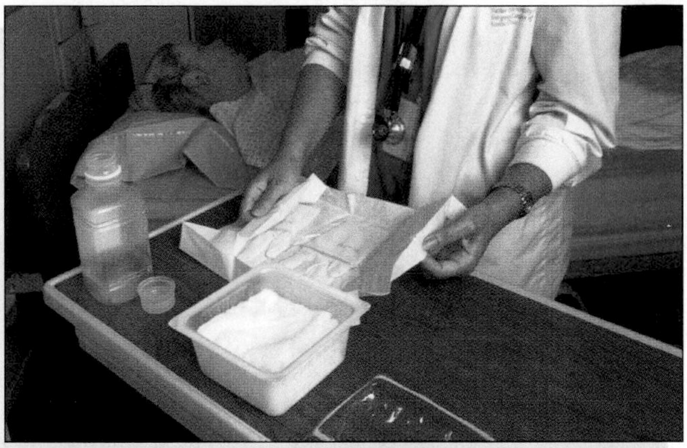

Open sterile glove packet on over-bed table.

Rationale: Reaching over sterile field will contaminate supplies.

4. Grasp cover of 4 × 4 pad plastic container and pull flap back and away from sterile area. Place cover in disposal bag.
5. Grasp edge of transparent dressings package, peel back top covering. Place open package on work surface. Do not cross over any open supply packages.
6. Continue to open all supplies using above steps.
7. Pour solution over pads in plastic container, if ordered.
8. Open sterile gloves. Place in position on table where you do not pass over a sterile field.
9. Tear tape and place on side of over-bed table.

Documentation for Measures to Prevent Infection

- Type and number of sterile dressings used
- Antiseptic solution used

Critical Thinking Application

UNEXPECTED OUTCOMES	CRITICAL THINKING OPTIONS
Hole develops in glove while performing sterile technique.	• Discard gloves and replace with sterile gloves. • Examine hands for cuts if hole caused by sharp object. • If hands are cut, scrub hands and replace sterile gloves.
Sterile field becomes wet or damp.	• Discard supplies on sterile field. • Set up new sterile field.

UNIT 2

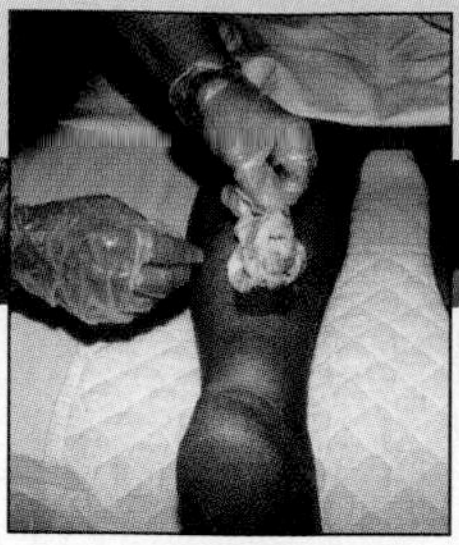

Dressing Change

Nursing Process Data

ASSESSMENT Data Base

Identify type of dressing required.

Determine if sutures or staples need to be removed.

Assess incision for infection.

Assess extent of healing.

Assess nutritional status.

PLANNING Objectives

To promote incision healing

To prevent wound infection

To maintain sterility during dressing change

To remove sutures or staples using appropriate technique

IMPLEMENTATION Procedures

Changing a Dry Sterile Dressing

Removing Sutures

Removing Staples

EVALUATION Expected Outcomes

Incision is healing without infection.

Sterility is maintained throughout dressing change.

Sutures and staples are removed using proper technique.

CHANGING A DRY STERILE DRESSING

Equipment

Sterile gloves
Clean gloves
Mask
Gown
Disposal bag for used dressings
Dressing supplies, as needed
Micropore tape
Sterile normal saline, optional
Package sterile cotton swabs, or 4 × 4 pads
Bath blanket

Preparation

1. Check physician's orders and client care plan.
2. Wash your hands.
3. Gather equipment.
4. Identify the client, and explain procedure.
5. Provide privacy.
6. Clean off over-bed table.
7. Place sterile supplies on over-bed table.
8. Raise bed to HIGH position, and lower side rails, if appropriate.
9. Place bag for soiled dressings near incision site.
10. Fanfold linen to expose incision area.
11. Cover client with bath blanket, leaving incision area exposed.
12. Open sterile packages, and place on over-bed table. Arrange packages to ensure you don't cross over the sterile field when reaching for dressings. **Rationale:** Commercially prepared sterile packages can be opened and used for the sterile field because the inside of the package is sterile.
13. Cut tape into appropriate length strips and place on edge of over-bed table.

Procedure

1. Remove tape slowly by pulling tape toward the wound. **Rationale:** Pulling toward the wound decreases the pain of tape removal by not putting pressure on the incision line.

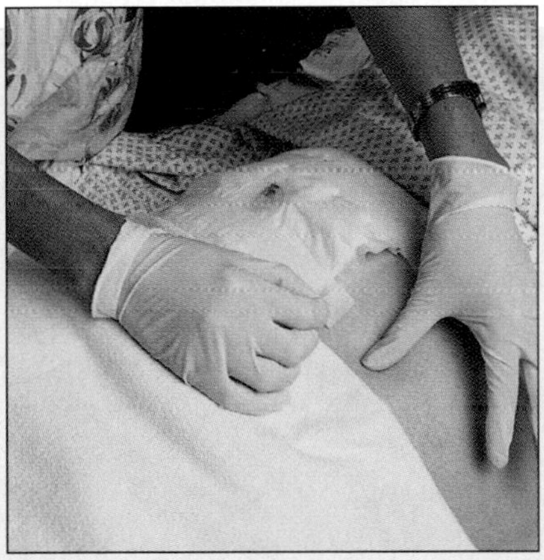
Remove tape by gently lifting toward wound.

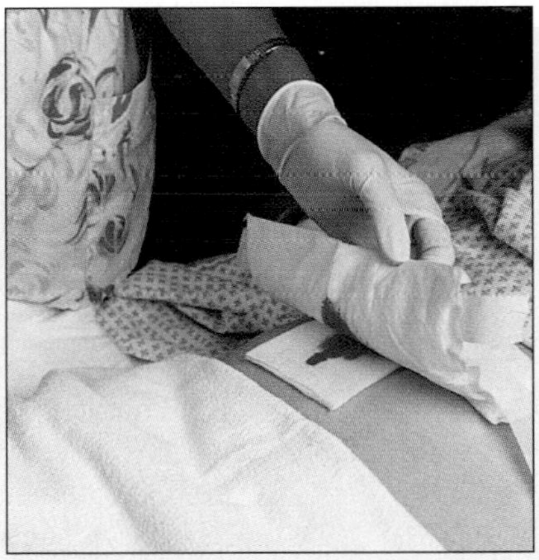
Remove soiled dressing carefully.

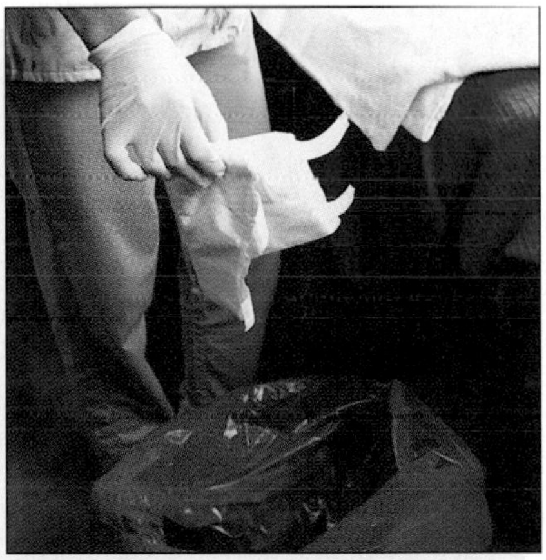
Dispose of dressing in appropriate container.

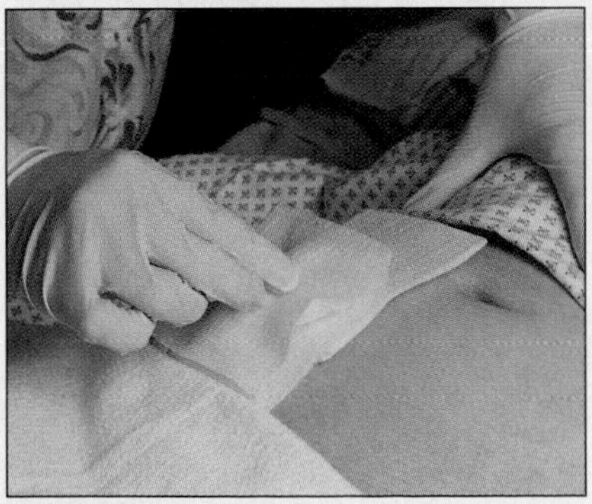
Do not touch incision when applying dressing.

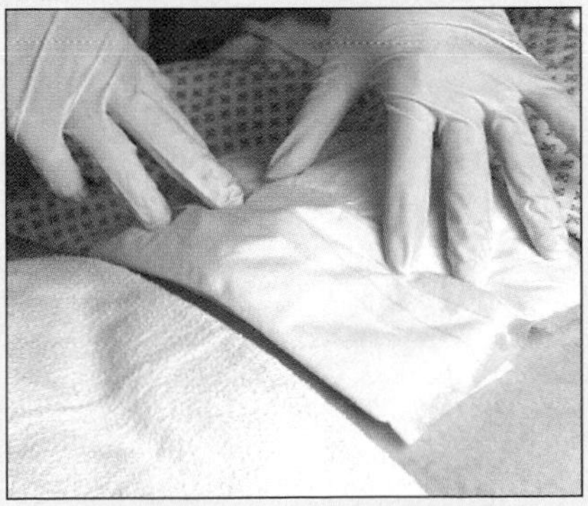
Place abdominal pad over center of incision.

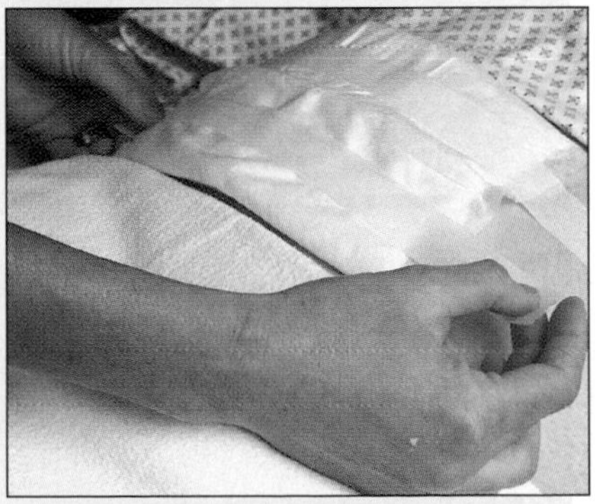
Tape dressing securely to prevent slipping.

2. Don clean gloves.
3. Remove soiled dressings, and dispose of in the proper bag. Wet dressing with sterile normal saline if it adheres to the suture line.
4. Assess incision area for erythema, edema, or drainage. **Rationale:** Persistent drainage, edema, or temperature above 100.4° F 2 days postop indicates a complication is occurring.
5. Assess color of incision. (A healing incision looks pink or red.) **Rationale:** Redness that does not fade 48 hours after surgery may indicate impaired healing.
6. Remove clean gloves, and discard.
7. Move over-bed table next to working area.
8. Don sterile gloves.
9. Cleanse incision area with swabs or 4 × 4 pads soaked in normal saline, according to hospital policy. Cleanse from incision line outward, cleaning from top to bottom, using the swab only once. Discard swabs or 4 × 4 pads in disposal bag. **Rationale:** Cleaning outward from incision cleans from least to most contaminated area. Cleaning from top to bottom prevents contamination from secretions that accumulate at the bottom of the wound.
10. Place 4 × 4 gauze pads over incision area, being careful not to touch incision or client with your gloves. **Rationale:** Touching the incision or client contaminates the gloves. You need to reglove if this occurs.
11. Place abdominal pad over incision, being careful not to contaminate the gloves.
12. Remove gloves and discard.
13. Tape dressing securely.
14. Discard trash in appropriate receptacle.
15. Lower bed and raise side rails. Position client for comfort.
16. Wash your hands.

REMOVING SUTURES

Equipment

Sterile suture removal set
Antiseptic solution
Tape
Butterfly tape
Paper bag for disposal of dressings
Two pair clean gloves (1 pair optional)

Procedure

1. Gather equipment.
2. Wash hands, and don clean gloves.
3. Remove dressing and discard in disposal bag. (Discard gloves only if soiled.)
4. Open suture removal set, and don gloves if second pair needed.
5. Pick up forceps with nondominant hand.
6. Grasp suture at the knot with forceps and lift away from skin.
7. Pick up suture scissors with dominant hand.
8. Place curved tip of suture scissors under suture, next to knot.
9. Cut suture, and with forceps, pull suture through skin with one movement.
10. Discard suture into disposal bag.
11. Check that entire suture is removed.
12. Continue to remove remaining sutures according to hospital policy. Some policies state that every other suture is

Topical Glue for Wound Closure

A new product to replace sutures and staples (estimated at 80–90 million procedures annually) was approved by the FDA after proving itself in clinical trials. This superglue is called *Dermabond.* It is a synthetic, noninvasive glue that mitigates trauma and post-procedure inflammation while providing a waterproof seal and protecting underlying tissue without the need for bandages. *Dermabond* is also painless, fast and simple to apply, and naturally sloughs off in 7–10 days.

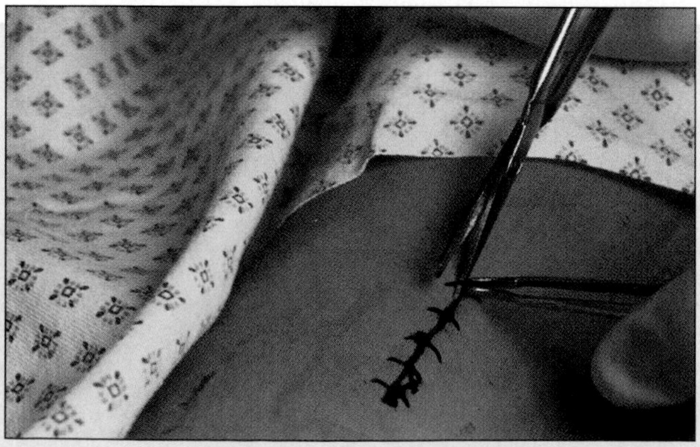
Grasp suture at the knot with forceps and lift away from skin.

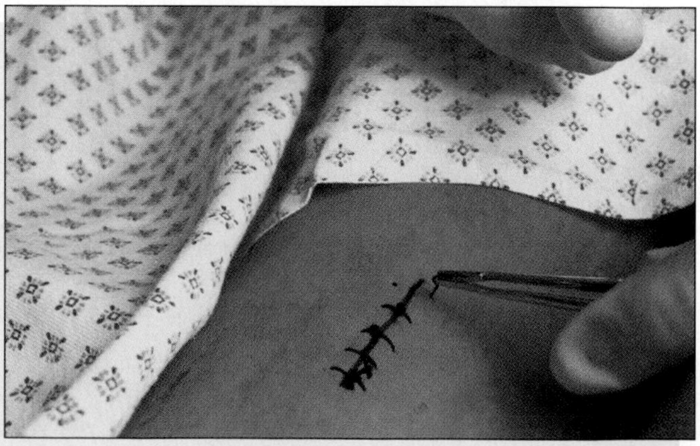
After cutting suture, grasp suture at knot and pull through skin.

removed and then remaining sutures are removed at a later time. **Rationale:** This prevents wound dehiscence.
13. Cleanse suture site with antiseptic solution.
14. Remove gloves, and place in disposal bag.
15. Place dressing or butterfly tape over incision area, if ordered.
16. Discard disposal bag into contaminated waste container.
17. Wash hands.

REMOVING STAPLES

Equipment

Sterile staple remover
Disposal bag
Two pair clean gloves (1 pair optional)
Dressings
Tape or butterfly tape
Antiseptic solution

Procedure

1. Gather equipment, and open sterile staple remover.
2. Wash hands and don clean gloves.
3. Remove dressing, and discard in disposal bag. (Discard gloves only if soiled.)
4. Don gloves if necessary.
5. Place lower tip of staple remover under staple.
6. Press handles together to depress center of staple.
7. Lift staple remover upward, away from incision site when both ends of staple are visible.
8. Place staple removal device over disposal bag and release handles to release staple.
9. Remove all staples or as directed by hospital policy. Some policies indicate every other staple is removed with remaining staples done at a later time. **Rationale:** To prevent wound dehiscence.

CLINICAL ALERT

Steri-strips may be applied over incision to protect incision after staples are removed.

10. Cleanse incision area with antiseptic solution if ordered.
11. Remove gloves, and place in disposal bag.
12. Place dressing over incision and secure with tape, or place butterfly tape over incision.
13. Discard disposal bag in contaminated waste container.
14. Wash hands.

Discharge Client Teaching

- Instruct client to eat foods high in protein, carbohydrates, vitamins, and minerals to promote wound healing.
- Splint wound when coughing or moving from chair or bed to prevent separation of wound edges.
- Provide list of signs and symptoms of wound infection or delayed healing. Include when to notify physician.
- Encourage use of daily showers; water may run over wound.
- Instruct not to use soap, lotions, or vitamin creams on incision.
- Instruct in dressing change procedure.
- Instruct to not lift heavy objects (anything over 10 pounds).
- Instruct in measures to promote elimination.

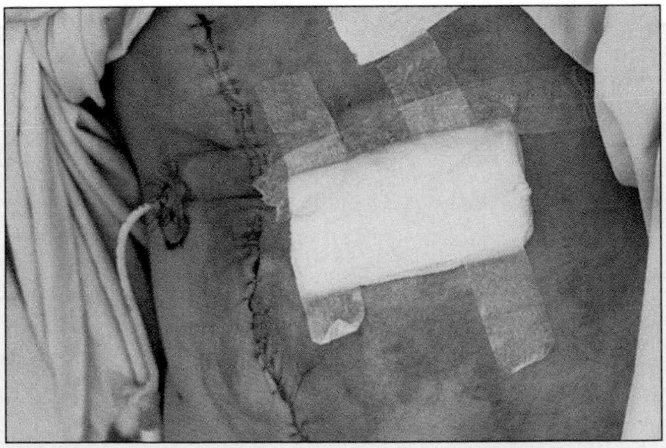
Large abdominal wound with staples closing incision.

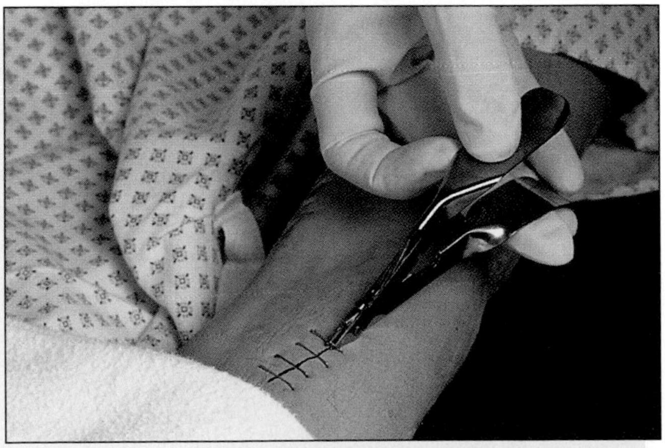
Place lower tip of staple removal device under staple.

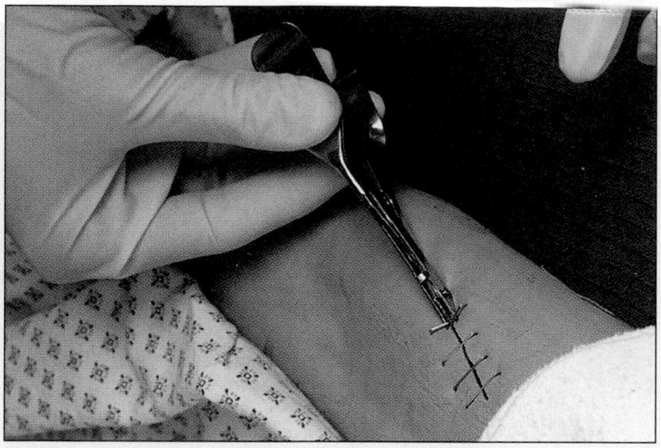

Press handle together to depress center of staple.

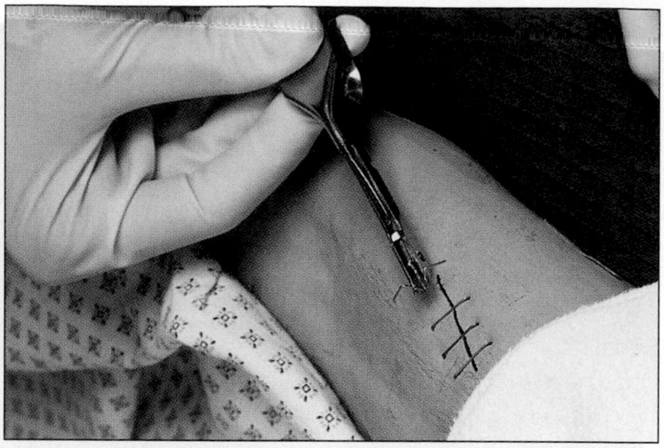

Lift staple remover device upward and away from incision.

Documentation for Dressing Change, Removal of Sutures and Staples

- Conditions of suture line
- Presence of exudate or erythema
- Sutures removed
- Staples removed
- Dressing applied, if appropriate

Critical Thinking Application

UNEXPECTED OUTCOMES	CRITICAL THINKING OPTIONS
Wound appears to be infected.	• Obtain order for wound culture. • Obtain order for different type of dressing. • Document observations.
Client complains of fever, pain in incisional area.	• Check incision for edema, erythema, or drainage; wound could be infected.
Wound edges separate when suture or staple is removed.	• Do not continue to remove sutures or staples. • Place steri-strip over edges. • Notify physician.
Client complains of pain with dressing change.	• Lift small edge of tape or dressing. • Use alcohol pad, wipe area next to dressing with pad. • Remove dressing by wiping, with pad, each time the dressing is lifted up until entire dressing is removed.

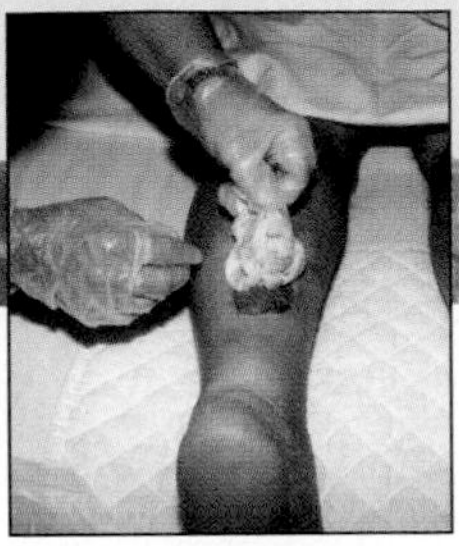

UNIT 3

Wound Care

Nursing Process Data

ASSESSMENT Data Base

Identify type of dressing needed (Table 25–2).
Assess level of pain associated with wound care and dressing change.
Assess wound for color, odor, drainage.
Assess extent of wound.
Assess type of wound.
Assess for function of Hemovac or Jackson–Pratt suction.
Assess for extent of wound healing.
Assess wound.
Assess for arterial insufficiency, claudication, pain, ischemic tissue loss, and functional limitations.

PLANNING Objectives

To assess wound appropriately
To assess for arterial sufficiency
To promote wound healing by first or second intention
To prevent microorganisms from entering the wound
To decrease the presence of purulent wound drainage
To maintain sterility during a dressing change
To maintain patency of Hemovac or Jackson–Pratt suction
To immobilize and support a wound
To assist in removal of necrotic tissue
To apply medication to wound
To pack a wound to promote granulation of tissue

IMPLEMENTATION Procedures

Assessing a Wound
Changing a Wound Dressing
Packing a Wound
Changing a Dressing for a Venous Ulcer
Assessing Ankle–Brachial Index (ABI)
Caring for a Wound with a Drain
Applying an Abdominal Binder
Maintaining Wound Drainage System
Irrigating Wounds

EVALUATION Expected Outcomes

Granulation takes place, and healing occurs.

Sterility is maintained during dressing change.

Drain is advanced appropriately.

Hemovac suction remains patent.

Abdominal binder keeps dressing in place and supports abdomen.

Compression dressing applied to appropriate vascular ulcer.

TABLE 25–2 Moisture-Retentive Dressings

	Advantages	Disadvantages	Clinical Use
Transparent Adhesive Film	• Transparency allows wound visualization • Conforms to area of application • Can reduce friction of area • Promotes autolysis of dry eschar • Semipermeable vapor can escape and environmental oxygen can enter to reduce chance of anaerobic bacterial growth • Barrier to bacterial invasion; can aspirate fluid and patch • Does not require secondary dressing	• Does *not* absorb exudate • Exudate may macerate skin around wound • Edges will roll in friction area • May be difficult to apply • May be too tightly applied • Removal may tear under-lying skin • May increase bacterial growth in infected wounds	• Pressure ulcers, stage I and II • Donor sites • Abrasions • Extend edge to minimum 1¼ inch beyond wound; skin around wound must be dry for adhesion; apply without tension • Change when fluid build-up and leaking occurs and when edges are loosening to potentially expose wound
Hydrogel	• Comes in sheets or gel to conform to the wound • May be soothing • Absorbs some exudate • Provides moist wound healing • Rehydrates dry wound beds	• Expensive • Held in place with gauze dressing or transparent film • May have transparent film on both sides (film next to wound must be removed)	• Wounds with necrosis and slough • Partial thickness (use sheets) • Gel can be used to fill wound cavity • Change every day or twice a day—based on wound exudate
Hydrocolloids	• Use on acute and chronic wounds • Absorbs exudate • Conforms to area • Prevents bacterial invasion	• Not transparent • Melts down with exudate • Characteristic drainage and odor • Edges may need to be taped to prevent rolling • Most do *not* allow environmental oxygen, so growth of anaerobic bacteria may be a problem	• Noninfected dermal ulcers • May leave in place up to 7 days • Change if leaking • Change in clinical signs of infection • Cleanse wound before application • Roll dressing over wound • Do *not* stretch; press securely

ASSESSING A WOUND

Equipment

Pliable disposable measuring device/grid
Cotton-tipped applicator sticks
Saline-filled syringe
Plastic disposal bag
Clean gloves
Sterile gloves if necessary

Preparation

1. Obtain health history, medical diagnosis, and physical examination data from chart or obtain missing information. The health history must include information on the following:
   a. Current medical diagnosis including all disease processes. **Rationale:** Diseases that affect circulation and perfusion of blood can interfere with nutrition and oxygenation of cells. Infection and wounds can result from this pathology.
   b. Medications, both past and current: include anticoagulants, corticosteroids, immunosuppressives, and antineoplastics. **Rationale:** These drugs may adversely affect wound healing.
   c. Nutrition and hydration status: check for signs of malnutrition and assess hydration status of client. **Rationale:** Malnutrition leads to poor cell growth and repair. Both

dehydration and overhydration lead to impaired oxygen and nutrient transportation.
   d. Laboratory data evaluation: albumin, serum total protein, serum transferrin, and total lymphocyte count. **Rationale:** These lab values are used to determine nutritional status and potential for wound healing.
2. Determine type of wound: acute or chronic, and cause of wound. **Rationale:** This information is used to evaluate healing process.

Note: Acute wounds progress through normal process of wound healing in about 1 month. Chronic wounds do not go through normal wound healing phases. Wounds that do not heal within 1 month should be considered chronic.

3. Wash your hands and don gloves.

Procedure

1. Assess location of wound. **Rationale:** Location influences rate of healing. Lower body heals more slowly.
2. Observe color of wound if using this classification.
   a. Black: necrotic tissue/black eschar (inhibits formation of granulation tissue).
   b. Yellow: pus, fibrin, debris (will advance to eschar).
   c. Red: indicates wound ready to heal (granulation tissue present).
3. Assess odor of wound.
   a. Foul: infected (necrotic tissue has an odor even if not infected).
   b. Sweet: Pseudomonas infection.
4. Assess level of moisture in wound. (A moist environment allows wound to heal without forming a scab.)

> **CLINICAL ALERT**
>
> Moist wound environment is essential. Epithelial tissue will not migrate into wounds with necrotic tissue or if deprived of oxygen.

5. Assess wound exudate.
   a. Type: dry or moist.
   b. Amount: minimum, moderate, maximum (copious).
   c. Color of drainage: clear (serous), brown-brown/yellow (slough), yellow-yellow/green (pus from strep, staph), blue-green (Pseudomonas).
6. Assess tissue viability.
   a. Presence of granulation tissue; red, moist, beefy appearance.
   b. Presence of epithelialized tissue; new pink, shiny epidermis.
   c. Absence of necrotic tissue; slough of yellow, gray. Green and brown color or eschar of hard, black, leathery tissue.
7. Assess periwound condition.
   a. Skin nutrition: loss of hair, thickening of nails, atrophy.
   b. Edema of skin or scaly skin.
   c. Skin hydration: skin turgor indicates hydration or dehydration.
   d. Areas of inflammation surrounding wound.
   e. Skin integrity: maceration, induration, crepitus, hematoma, blisters.
   f. Color: red (inflammation), white (arterial insufficiency), blue (cyanosis, severe arterial insufficiency), black (necrosis), brown (venous insufficiency).
   g. Skin temperature: cool, cold, warm, normal temperature.
8. Assess extent of pain, if present.
   a. Determine if pain present during dressing change only or constant.
   b. Use pain scale to determine severity of pain.
   c. Observe for signs of infection.
   d. Arterial insufficiency wounds are very painful.
   e. Venous insufficiency wounds are relatively pain free.
9. Measure the length and width of wound using a disposable measuring device/grid. Measure in cm.
10. Measure depth of wound by placing a sterile cotton-tipped applicator stick into wound in several areas. Measure depth of each area using measuring device/grid. Measure in cm.
11. Check for undermining and/or tunneling or sinus tracts by placing a sterile cotton-tipped applicator stick into suspected areas. Gently probe margins of lesion for extensions into surrounding tissue (undermining) and beyond wound base (sinus tract).
12. Evaluate laboratory values.
    a. Increased white blood cell count indicates infection, usually before other signs and symptoms are evident.
    b. Low hemoglobin and hematocrit indicates anemia which can decrease oxygen transport to the wound.
    c. Altered serum glucose levels may indicate presence of diabetes mellitus which interferes with normal wound healing.
13. Evaluate client's stress level. Increased stress leads to hypermetabolic states, which uses up oxygen and nutrients and affects wound healing.
14. Complete skill by following appropriate steps described in skill *Changing a Wound Dressing.*
15. Document findings and notify physician of any changes or unusual findings in the assessment.

CHANGING A WOUND DRESSING

Equipment

Sterile, prepackaged dressing(s) as needed
Tape; micropore, paper, or Montgomery tie tapes
Clean gloves
Sterile gloves
Sterile normal saline irrigation solution
Wound culture media, as needed
Plastic bag
Bath blanket
Emesis basin

Preparation

1. Complete steps in *Assessing a Wound*
2. Check physician's orders and client care plan.
3. Wash your hands.
4. Gather equipment.
5. Identify the client, and explain procedure.

CLINICAL ALERT

Gauze dressings do not support healing or prevent entry of exogenous bacteria.

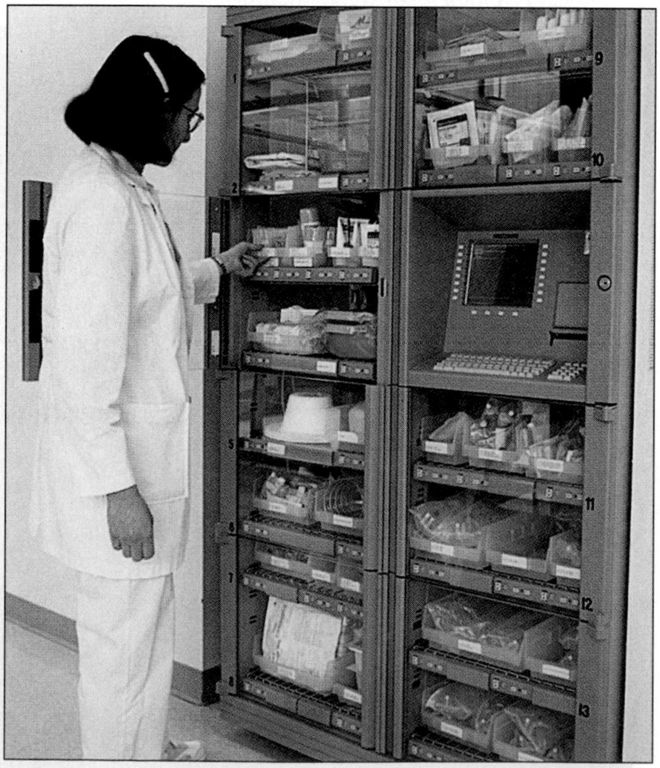

PYXIS supply station provides easy access for dressing supplies.

6. Provide privacy.
7. Clean off over-bed table.
8. Place sterile supplies on the over-bed table.
9. Raise bed to HIGH position, and lower side rails on working side of bed, if necessary.
10. Place bag for soiled dressings near wound site.
11. Open sterile packages and place on over-bed table. Arrange packages to ensure that you don't cross over the sterile field when using dressings. **Rationale:** Commercially prepared sterile packages can be opened and used for the sterile field; the inside of the package is sterile.
12. Fanfold linens to expose wound site.
13. Cover client with bath blanket, leaving wound area exposed.
14. Cut tape into appropriate strips, and place on over-bed table.

Procedure

1. Remove tape slowly by pulling tape toward the wound. **Rationale:** Pulling toward the wound decreases the pain of tape removal by not putting pressure on the incision line.
2. Don clean gloves.
3. Remove soiled dressings, and dispose of in bag. Soaking dressings that are dried to skin or incision with sterile normal saline prevents tissue damage and pain when dressings are removed.

CLINICAL ALERT

Normal saline or Ringer's solution are widely advocated as fluids of choice for cleansing and irrigating wounds. Iodine and chlorhexidine are cytotoxic, particularly to fibroblasts. In severely infected wounds, antimicrobial irrigations may be used.

4. Obtain wound specimen for culture if ordered.
5. Remove clean gloves, and discard into plastic bag.
6. Bring over-bed table close to working area.
7. Open sterile saline solution, and pour over wound. Place emesis basin next to skin surface to catch overflow.

How to Obtain a Wound Culture

- Rinse wound thoroughly with sterile saline.
- Use non-cotton-tipped swab.
- Rotate swab while obtaining specimen.
- Swab edges starting at top, crisscross wound to bottom.
- Do *not* take specimen from exudate or eschar.

Use of Antimicrobial Agents in Wound Care

Antiseptics and antibiotics are two types of antimicrobial agents used in wound care management. Antiseptics, unlike antibiotics, cannot be used exclusively to kill bacteria. Systemic antibiotics should be used only to treat wound infections; however, wounds that have impaired blood flow will not receive the systemic antibiotics. Topical antibiotics are used only for a limited time with infected wounds. These agents are not used as preventative measures; they are used when infection is present.

Antiseptics return the wound back to bacterial balance, promoting wound healing. Cadexomer iodine gel is used to absorb wound exudates and assists in autolytic debridement. Silver nitrate and sulfadiazine are used against many antibiotic-resistant strains of bacteria, as they reduce the number of viable bacteria.

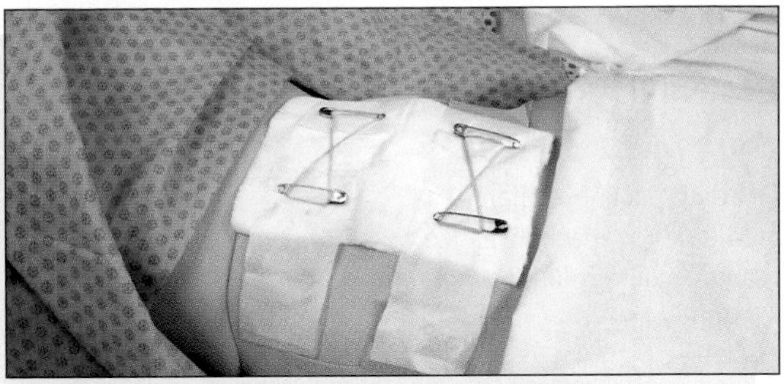

Montgomery straps are used to prevent skin irritation when frequent dressing changes are required.

8. Don sterile gloves.
9. Form a ball with gauze pads by tucking all four corners together. Use the center of gauze pads to cleanse the wound. **Rationale:** This action prevents contamination of your hands during cleansing.
10. Cleanse wound. When cleansing an area, always start at the cleanest area and work away from that area. Never return to an area you have previously cleaned. Usually start at top of wound and work toward bottom. **Rationale:** Prevents contamination of area.
11. Assess the wound, measure, identify type and determine if signs of infection are present. **Rationale:** This allows nurse to determine most effective treatment and type of dressing to be used.
12. Cleanse under the drain and around the site with a 4 × 4 gauze pad and cleansing solution if a drain is present. Do not use a cytotoxic or dangerous chemical. **Rationale:** These agents may harm granulating tissue.
13. Place several gauze pads under the drain.
14. Place several 4 × 4 gauze pads over the wound. Cover with an ABD pad if necessary; remove gloves, and tape securely. Montgomery straps (tie tapes) may be used if frequent dressing changes are required or the client has sensitive skin. **Rationale:** Once a dressing has been placed over the wound it is not to be moved and readjusted, as microorganisms from the skin could be introduced into the wound.
15. Use skin sealants or moisture barrier ointments on intact skin and moisture-retentive dressing over 4 × 4 gauze pad and even over ABD, if used. **Rationale:** Moisture-retentive dressings are flexible and water resistant, which allows clients to move freely and take showers without disturbing the dressing.
16. Cover client.
17. Close the plastic bag, and dispose of bag as isolation material.
18. Remove gloves, and wash your hands thoroughly.
19. Check with client to see that he or she is comfortable before leaving room.
20. Lower the bed and raise the side rail.

EVIDENCE BASED NURSING PRACTICE

Maintaining a Moist Environment

Dressings that promote a moist wound environment stimulate rapid wound healing. Saline soaks are not as effective as moisture-retentive dressings. The type of dressing used is dependent on the type of wound, whether infected or if debris is present, amount of exudates, cost, and client comfort.

Source: Joanna Briggs Institute for Evidence Based Nursing & Midwifery. www.joannabriggs.edu.au/procmana.html.

PACKING A WOUND

Equipment

Dressing pack, optional
Sterile narrow packing gauze or 4 × 4 gauze pads
Normal saline solution
Alcohol wipe
Dressings
Forceps, optional
Sterile scissors
Paper tape
Montgomery tapes
Plastic bag
Clean gloves
Sterile gloves

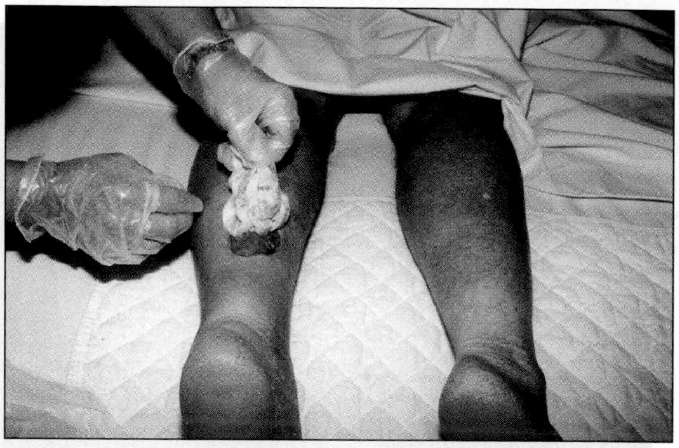

Pack wound dressing in all tunneling and undermined areas.

Procedure

1. Follow steps in *Preparation for Changing a Wound Dressing.*
2. Determine client's need for pain medication before beginning procedure. **Rationale:** Pain can be present particularly when removing old packing that may have become attached to the tissue.
3. Don clean gloves and place plastic bag near wound site
4. Remove tape slowly by pulling tape toward wound.
5. Remove soiled dressings and dispose of dressings and packing into plastic bag. Moisten packing with sterile saline solution if dry.
6. Assess wound site.
   a. Identify location of ulcer: usually medial lower leg superior to medial malleolus.
   b. Observe wound bed and appearance: beefy red, granular appearance.
   c. Check wound size, shape, and margins: usually large with irregular margins.
   d. Observe exudates: usually moderate to heavy.
   e. Assess surrounding skin: brownish discoloration, edematous, macerated.
   f. Evaluate presence of pain: deep ulcers are painful.
7. Remove clean gloves and discard.
8. Don sterile gloves.
9. Clean wound with saline solution and pat wound dry with 4 × 4 gauze pads.
10. Place packing material in wound; pack lightly, filling tunneling or undermined areas. Forceps can be used to place packing material into corners and wound areas hard to reach. **Rationale:** Wound packing is used to facilitate healing by secondary intention. Type of packing material is dependent on type of wound and material available. Gauze pads should be moistened before packing.
11. Cut ribbon gauze with sterile scissors and leave small wick exposed, if used for packing.
12. Cover packing with dressing and tape securely.
13. Dispose of used packing and gloves.
14. Wash your hands.
15. Position client for comfort.

EVIDENCE BASED NURSING RESEARCH

Medieval Remedies

Medieval remedies, like maggots for bedsores, bee stings for MS, and leeches to improve blood flow after surgery, are enjoying a renaissance.

Leeches reemerged a while ago and now have a well-established role in plastic and reconstructive surgery. Maggots are being considered more often for treatment of chronic wounds that do not heal. And bee venom is considered alternative medicine.

Maggots do a better job than more conservative therapy for pressure ulcer treatment. Physicians who use maggots in their practice say they like them because they work.

Source: Wound repair and regeneration. (2002, September) *Archives of Internal Medicine.*

CHANGING A DRESSING FOR A VENOUS ULCER

Equipment

Cleansing solution
Normal saline solution
Sterile 4 × 4 dressings
Moisture-retentive dressings (hydrocolloid, transparent film)
Gel
Compression dressing
Clean gloves
Sterile gloves
Biohazard bag
Scissors
Absorbent pad

Preparation

1. Wash hands.
2. Gather equipment.
3. Explain procedure to client.
4. Provide privacy for client.
5. Raise bed to HIGH position and lower side rails.
6. Open sterile packages, and arrange on over-bed table.
7. Place absorbent pad under wound.

> **CLINICAL ALERT**
>
> The wound bed should be kept moist to promote granulation and reepithelialization and to reduce pain. Ointments provide the most occlusive moisturizer because they contain oil and water.

Procedure

1. Don clean gloves.
2. Remove compression bandage and old dressing, and place in biohazard bag. Compression dressings may be left in place for 3–7 days depending on amount of drainage and type of dressing.

> **CLINICAL ALERT**
>
> Use of semiocclusive dressings reduces incidence of wound infections by more than 50%. They maintain a moist environment, reduce airborne bacteria, and provide a mechanical barrier for bacterial entry.

3. Assess and measure wound. **Rationale:** This determines effectiveness of treatment.
4. Cleanse off debris by pouring cleansing solution over wound.
5. Rinse wound with sterile normal saline.
6. Dry wound using sterile 4 × 4 dressings. Place in biohazard bag.
7. Remove gloves, and don sterile gloves.
8. Apply medicated moisturizer over wound, if ordered. **Rationale:** This keeps wound area moist.

> **CLINICAL ALERT**
>
> **Compression Therapy**
>
> **Inelastic System**
>
> An Unna boot is frequently used to control edema in lower extremities. A zinc oxide–impregnated inelastic bandaging system is applied to the lower extremity. As it dries it becomes rigid and when calf muscles press against the rigid bandage it pumps blood more effectively. This system can be used for both mobile and immobile clients. As edema subsides the boot becomes less effective.
>
> **Elastic Therapy**
>
> Compression stockings and compression pumps are more effective in increasing venous return. Both mobile and immobile clients can use these stockings, although it is more difficult for the client who is mobile. The stockings are available in different pressures.

EVIDENCE BASED CLINICAL PRACTICE

Treatment of Ambulatory Venous Ulcer Patients and Warming Therapy

This was a limited study but other studies indicate the same type of findings. Five clients with a mean age of 65 and pressure ulcers for more than 8 months were treated with Warm-up therapy along with zippered compression stockings for 2 weeks. These clients were monitored for 12 weeks. The therapy consisted of warm therapy three times a day for 1 hour each at a temperature of 38°C. The results indicated that four of five clients increased granulation tissue and decreased pain. Four of five clients were completely healed during the 12-week follow-up.

Source: Cherry, G. C., & Wilson, Dphil J. (1999, September). The treatment of ambulatory venous ulcer patients and warming therapy. *Ostomy/Wound Management 45*(9), 65–70.

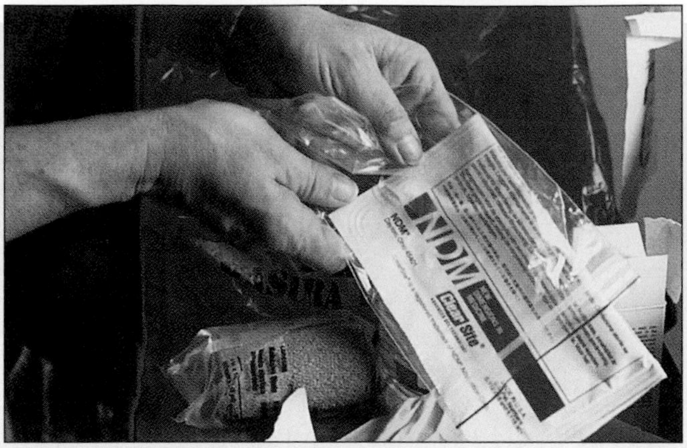

Obtain appropriate wound dressing kit, if available.

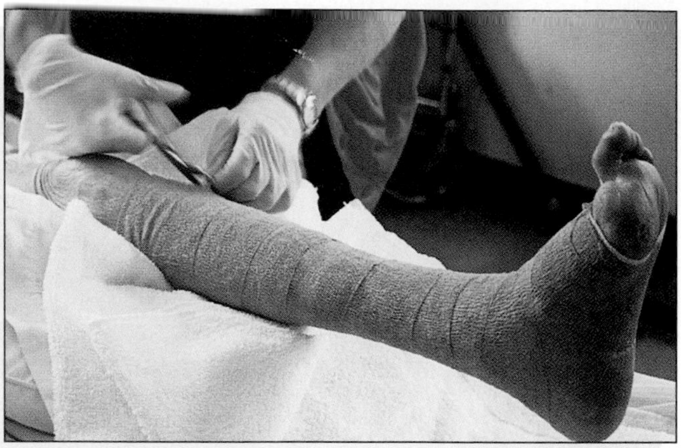
Remove compression dressing being careful not to cut skin.

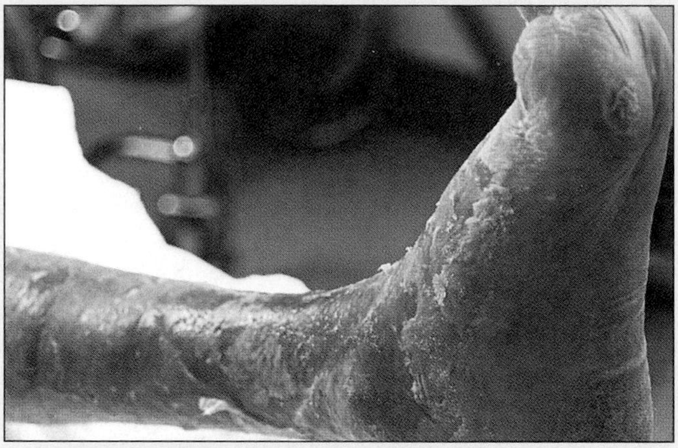
Assess wound healing and evaluate progress (Stage II).

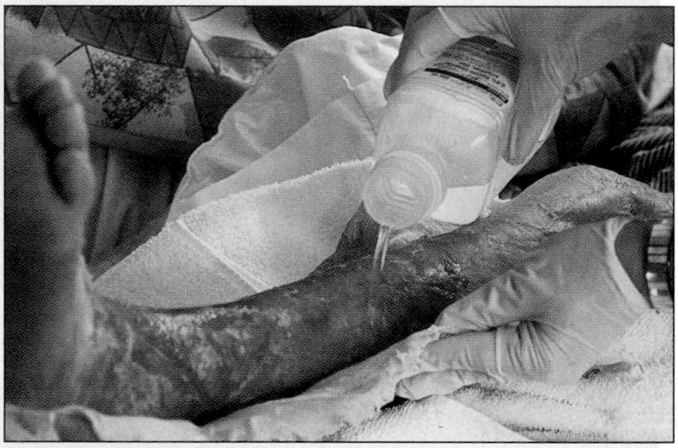
Pour normal saline solution over wound to clean off debris.

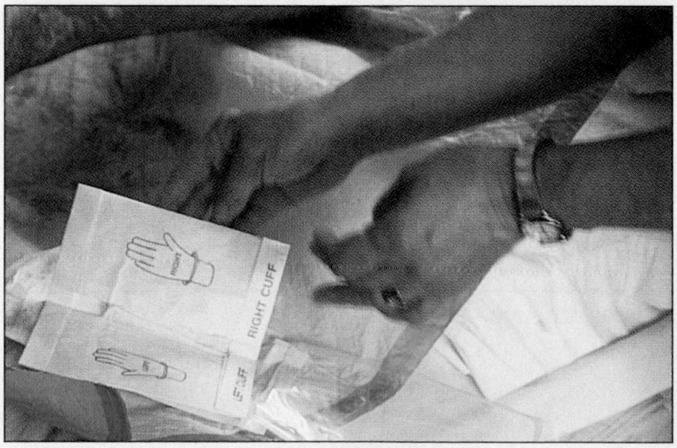

Don sterile gloves before cleaning wound with 4 × 4 gauze pads.

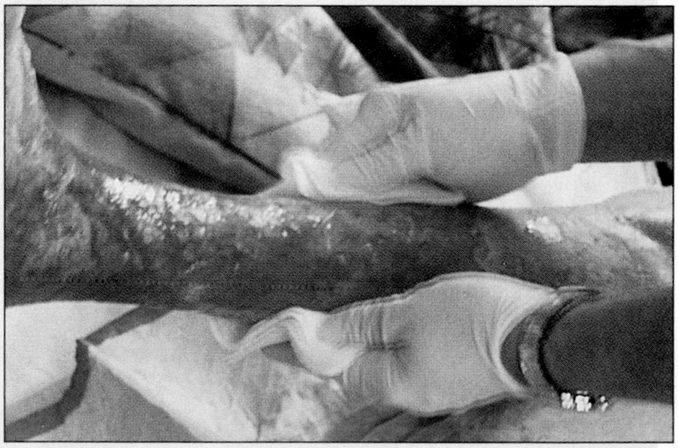
Dry with 4 × 4 gauze pad after cleansing.

9. Remove backing on moisture-retentive dressing, and place over open wound site. These dressings prevent entry of bacteria from surface of dressing.
10. Palpate arterial system; dorsalis pedis, posterior, or tibial pulse. If pulses are nonpalpable obtain an Ankle-Brachial Index (ABI).
11. Apply compression dressing if ABI is greater than 0.6.

    Rationale: Effective compression bandages generate 40–70 mm Hg pressure. If arterial insufficiency is present another ulcer can occur.
12. Reposition leg in elevated position. Leg should be elevated 18 cm above heart for 2 to 4 hours during the day and night. **Rationale:** This prevents edema, venous stasis, and promotes healing.

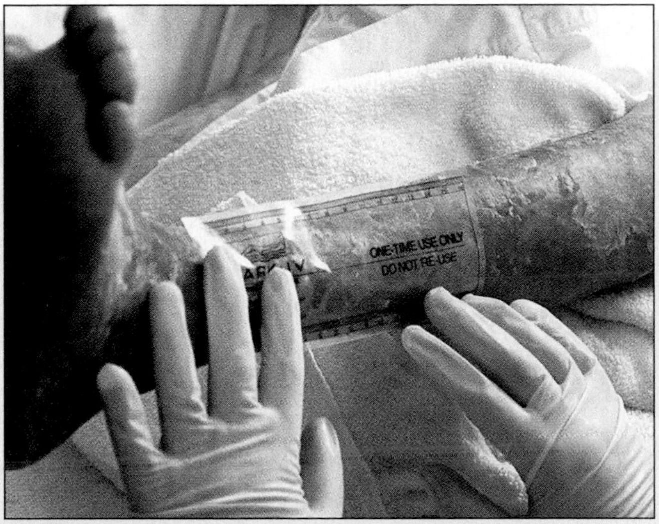

Measure wound to evaluate effectiveness of treatment.

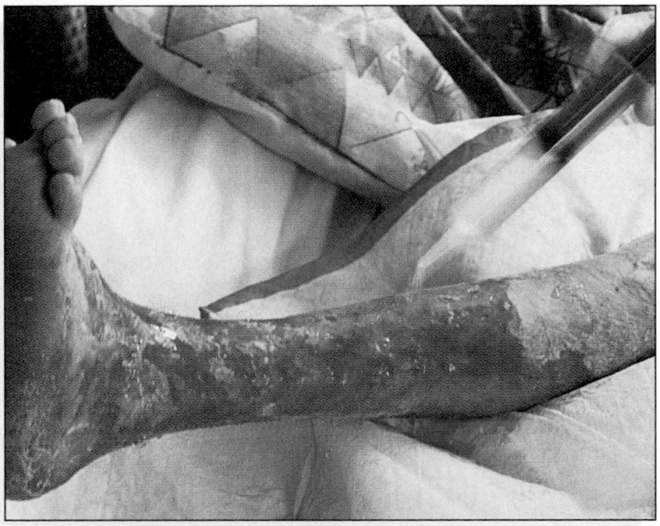
Apply medicated moisturizer on wound, if ordered

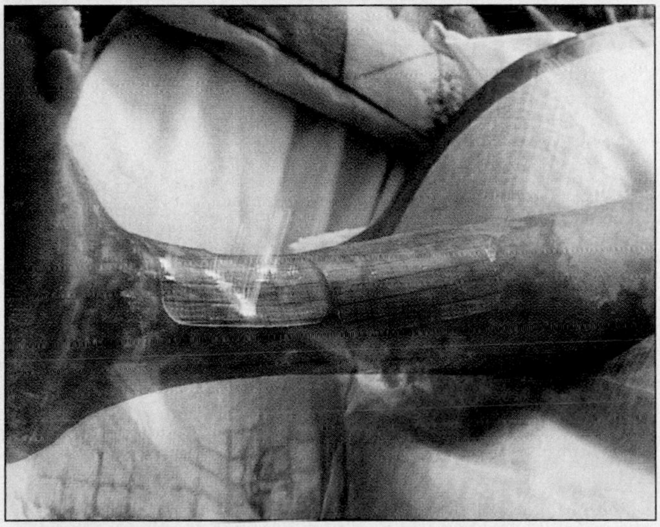
Apply moisture-retentive dressing over wound site.

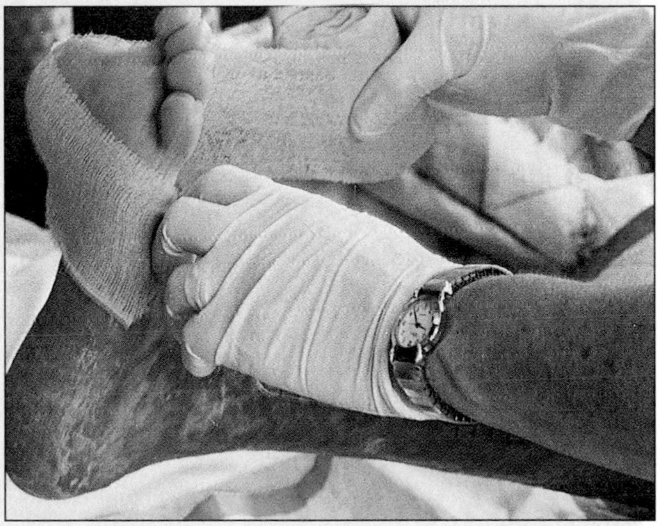
Apply compression dressing for venous or lymphatic conditions.

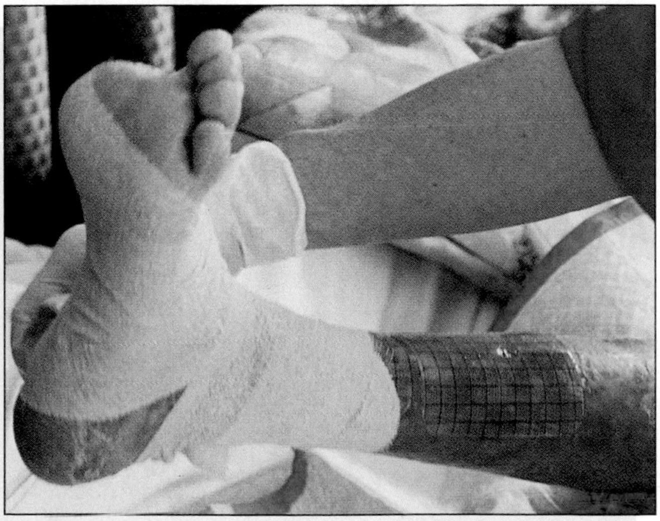
Cover entire area with compression dressing.

13. Remove gloves, and place in biohazard bag. Place all used supplies in bag.
14. Place biohazard bag in appropriate receptacle.
15. Wash your hands.
16. Lower bed and raise side rails.
17. Assess peripheral circulation every 4 hours. **Rationale:** This ensures compression dressing is not too tight.

Arterial Ulcers

Assessment

- Assess arterial flow; dorsalis pedis, femerol, popliteal, or posterior tibial.
- Use Doppler to assess pulses if necessary.
- Assess Ankle–Brachial Index; below 0.5 indicates severe arterial insufficiency.
- Assess temperature of skin.
- Observe color of extremities.
- Assess for presence of pain when client resting.

Treatment

- Keep ulcer moist.
- Use saline-moistened gauze and hydrocolloid dressings.
- Use petroleum jelly on skin surrounding wound to prevent skin maceration.
- Secure dressing with gauze; do not use tape as skin is fragile and tears easily.

ASSESSING ANKLE–BRACHIAL INDEX (ABI)

Equipment

Sphygmomanometer (2 cuffs, one arm and one leg)
Stethoscope
Doppler, handheld

Procedure

1. Review chart to determine if client has diabetes. **Rationale:** The ABI may not be reliable in these clients because arterial calcification causes false readings (high). The ABI is used to indirectly assess lower extremity peripheral blood flow.
2. Explain procedure to client.
3. Place client in supine position. Instruct to lie quietly for 5 minutes.
4. Place cuff above elbow, apply ultrasound gel to brachial pulse area.
5. Hold ultrasound probe at 45° angle. **Rationale:** This position opposes direction of brachial artery blood flow.
6. Inflate cuff pressure and slowly deflate pressure until systolic pulse sound is heard.
7. Obtain blood pressure readings in both arms. Use the higher systolic pressure as the brachial pressure in the ratio.
8. Wrap leg cuff around leg 5 cm above ankle's medial malleolus.
9. Place Doppler probe at a 45° angle to dorsalis pedis or posterior tibial artery.
10. Inflate cuff until Doppler sound stops.
11. Deflate cuff slowly while maintaining Doppler probe in place over artery.
12. Obtain two readings of posterior tibial or dorsalis pedis measurements and select highest value to be used in ABI calculation.
13. Divide ankle systolic pressure by brachial systolic pressure to obtain Ankle–Brachial Index (ABI). Normally, ankle pressure is equal to or slightly higher then brachial pressure.
14. Review ABI guidelines to determine severity of arterial insufficiency.
15. Document findings in nurses' notes and place note on chart for physician.

ABI Guidelines

1.0–1.2 ABI	Normal—No arterial insufficiency
0.8–1.0 ABI	Mild insufficiency
0.5–0.8 ABI	Moderate insufficiency
<0.5 ABI	Severe insufficiency
<0.3 ABI	Limb threatening

CARING FOR A WOUND WITH A DRAIN

Equipment

Same items as for *Changing a Wound Dressing*
Sterile cotton applicators
Sterile safety pin
ABD dressings
Sterile scissors
Sterile gloves
Clean gloves

Preparation

1. Check physician's orders and client care plan.
2. Wash your hands.
3. Gather equipment.
4. Provide privacy.
5. Identify client, and explain procedure.
6. Clean off over-bed table.
7. Raise bed to HIGH position, and lower side rails on working side of bed.
8. Place plastic bag for soiled dressings on bed near wound site.
9. Open sterile packages, and place on over-bed table.

Procedure

1. Remove tape from client's skin by pulling *toward* the incision. **Rationale:** This decreases pain and prevents damage to wound site by preventing a "pull" on the incision.
2. Don clean gloves.
3. Remove soiled dressing.
4. Discard gloves and dressings into plastic bag.
5. Observe wound closely for signs of infection or healing. Don sterile gloves.
6. If pin on the Penrose drain is crusted, replace it with a sterile pin. Be careful not to dislodge drain or suction tubing.
7. Using cotton applicators or gauze pads, cleanse drain site with cleansing solution and then saline.
8. Start cleansing at drain site, moving in a circular motion toward the periphery. **Rationale:** This prevents contamination of the drain site area.
9. Discard applicators in plastic bag.
10. Advance drain if ordered:
    a. Using sterile forceps, pull drain out of wound the ordered number of centimeters.
    b. Reposition the safety pin so it is at the level of the skin. **Rationale:** The pin prevents the drain from slipping back into the wound.
    c. Cut off the excess tubing with sterile scissors. Leave at least 2 inches of tubing on the outside. **Rationale:** This prevents drain from being drawn up into the wound opening.
11. Place several 4 × 4 dressings around the drain.
12. Apply gauze pad with a precut slit under the drain site.
13. Apply dry, sterile gauze pads over drain.
14. Apply ABD pads over sterile gauze.
15. Remove gloves, and dispose of them in refuse bag.
16. Tape dressing or retie Montgomery straps (tie tapes).
17. Remove bag with soiled dressing from room.
18. Wash your hands thoroughly.
19. Position client for comfort.
20. Lower bed and raise side rail.

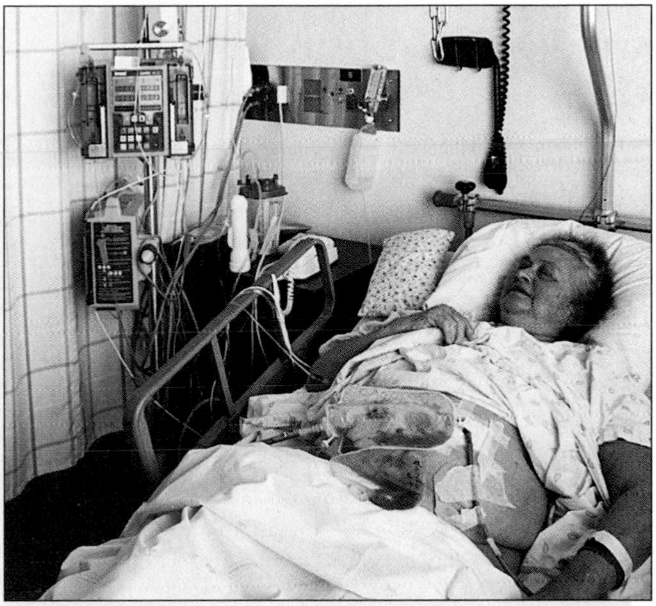

Use drainage pouches for wounds with drains.

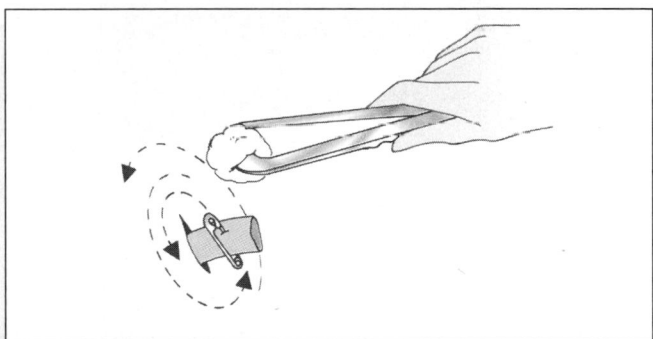

Cleanse the drain site, using a circular motion from the inside to the periphery of the wound.

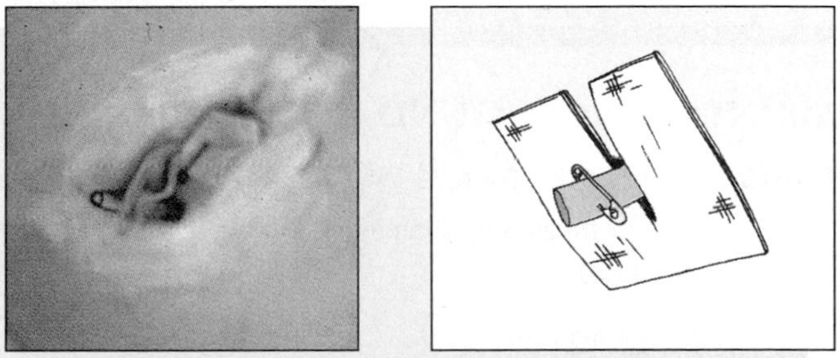

Place a precut sterile 4 × 4 gauze dressing around the drain site to prevent skin excoriation.

Drainage Pouches for Wounds

Apply a pouch to

- Collect drainage
- Measure drainage
- Protect skin from drainage
- Contain drainage
- Contain microorganisms so spread is decreased
- Lessen frequency of care; dressing change is every 24–48 hours

Drainage Systems for Wounds

Open Drains: Discharge flows freely into an absorbent dressing or a drainage bag.

Closed Systems: Remove fluid and debris into a closed container (i.e., Hemovac or Jackson–Pratt). Fewer wound infections occur with this drainage system.

APPLYING AN ABDOMINAL BINDER

Equipment

Abdominal binder: woven-cotton, synthetic, or elasticized material. Most facilities use commercial Velcro binders.

Safety pins for binders without Velcro closure

Procedure

1. Wash hands.
2. Explain use of binder to client.
3. Place client in supine position.
4. Ask client to raise hips, and then slide the binder under client's hips at level of gluteal fold. Place top of binder at client's waist.
5. Bring ends of binder around client, and secure by pressing Velcro surfaces together. If using non-Velcro binder, secure binder with safety pins placed vertically along edges. Start pinning at bottom of binder and pin toward waist. **Rationale:** Pinning binder from bottom to waist provides uplifting support for abdominal muscles.

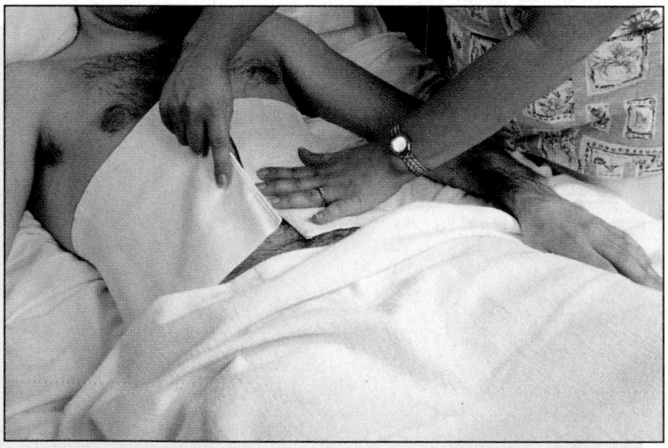

Bring ends of binder around client and secure Velcro surfaces.

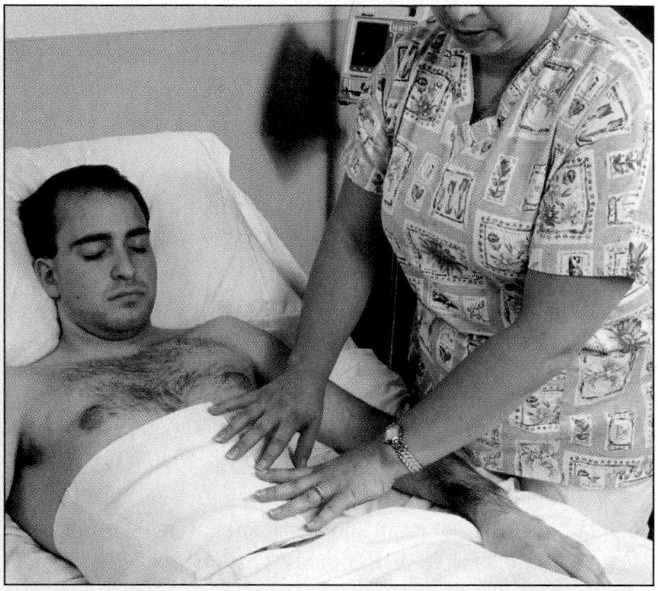

Assess effectiveness of binder every 4 hours.

6. Observe for wrinkles in binder. **Rationale:** Wrinkles can cause pressure areas especially over iliac crest.
7. Assess client's ability to move freely, breathe deeply, and feel secure pressure over abdominal incision. **Rationale:** A binder that is too tight may compromise breathing or place pressure on incisional area.
8. Assess effectiveness of binder every 4 hours, and rewrap every 8 hours if non-Velcro binder is used. Many clients use this binder only when ambulating.

MAINTAINING WOUND DRAINAGE SYSTEM

Equipment

Specimen cup for measuring drainage
I&O bedside record
Absorbent pad
Clean gloves
Hemovac suction or Jackson–Pratt suction drainage system

Preparation

1. Check physician's order and client care plan.
2. Bring specimen cup to bedside.
3. Identify client, and explain procedure, giving client time to ask questions.
4. Provide for comfort and privacy.

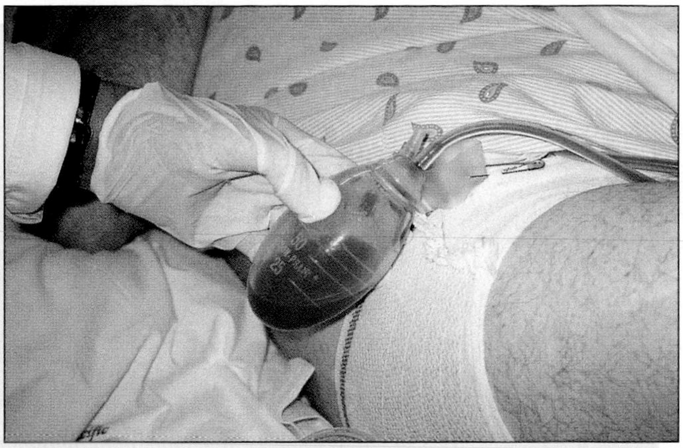

Jackson–Pratt drainage system in place.

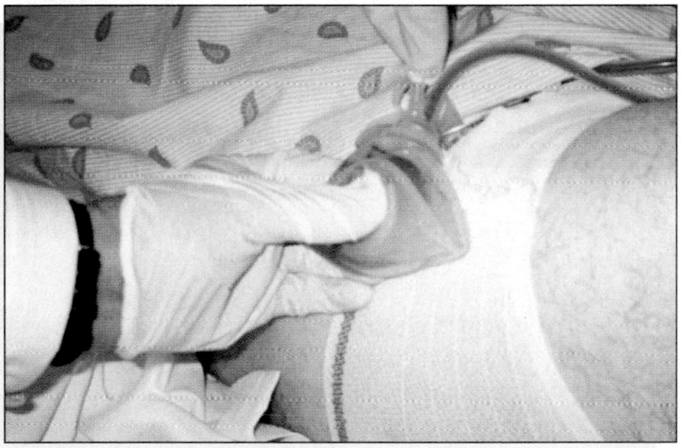

Squeeze bulb and reconnect to drainage tubing after emptying.

5. Wash your hands and don gloves.
6. Elevate bed to workable height.

Procedure

1. Expose catheter insertion site while keeping client draped. Place drainage system on absorbent pad.

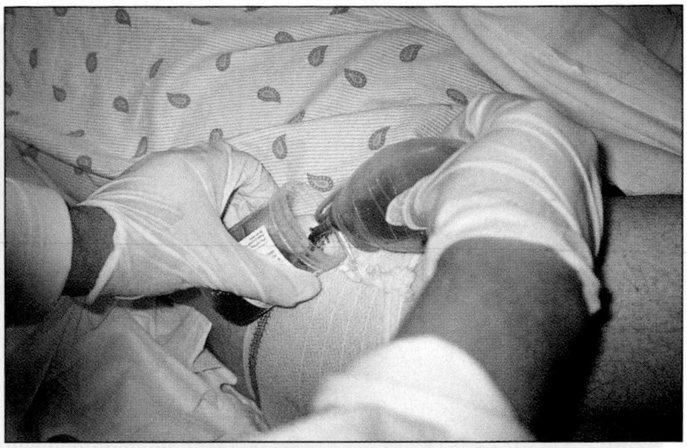

Empty, measure, and record drainage every shift.

2. Examine pump and catheter for patency, seal, and stability. If catheter is occluded, notify physician.
3. Remove Hemovac plug, which is labeled "Pouring Spout," or disconnect tubing from Jackson–Pratt system.
4. Pour drainage into specimen cup.
5. Compress the Hemovac by pushing the top and bottom together with your hands, or compress bulb on Jackson–Pratt.
6. Hold pump or bulb tightly compressed, and reinsert plug or connect tubing to Jackson–Pratt system. **Rationale:** This will reestablish closed drainage system.
7. Position suction devices on bed.
8. Measure and record amount of drainage.
9. Examine drainage for color, consistency, and odor.
10. Discard drainage and container; remove gloves, and wash hands.
11. Send culture specimen to laboratory if ordered.
12. Make client comfortable, and lower bed.
13. Compress evacuator at least every 4 hours to provide suction. Measure drainage at least every 8 hours.

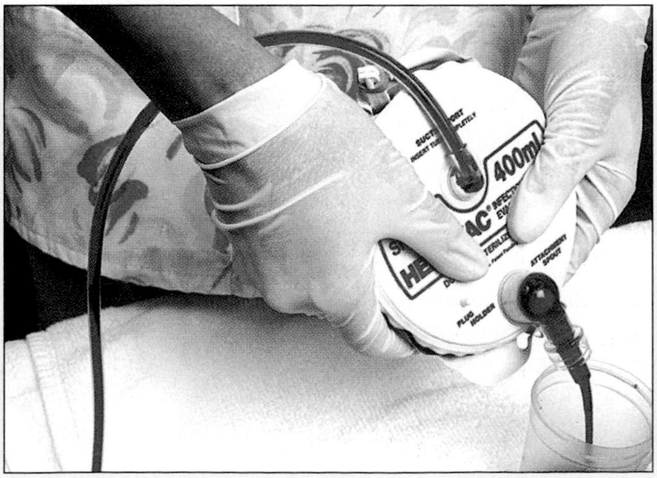

Remove Hemovac plug from "Pouring Spout" for emptying.

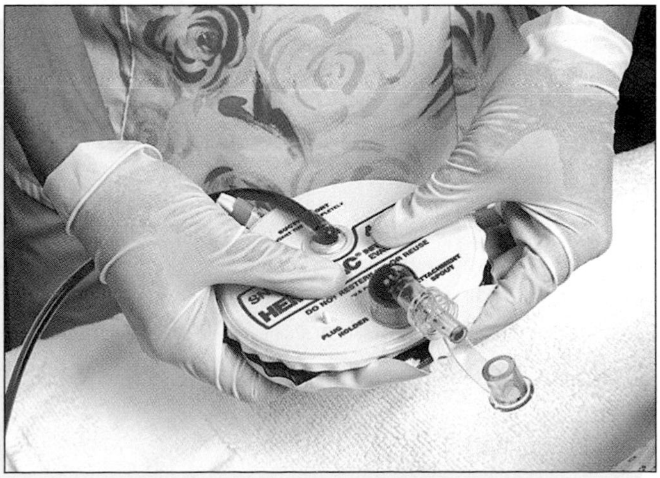

Compress Hemovac by pushing top and bottom together.

IRRIGATING WOUNDS

Equipment

Sterile irrigation solution, preferrably saline or Ringer's solution
Commercial wound cleaner container with nozzle
or
Sterile irrigating set with 35-mL syringe and 19-gauge angiocath tip
Absorbent pad
Sterile gloves
Equipment for dressing change

CLINICAL ALERT

If wound has moderate to heavy drainage, alginate dressings should be used. Alginate forms a gel when it comes in contact with wound fluid. It absorbs up to 20 times its weight in fluid. It can be used in infected and noninfected wounds. It is not to be used in dry wounds, as it can dehydrate the wound.

Preparation

1. Check physician's orders and client care plan.
2. Gather irrigation equipment and dressing material.
3. Check client's identaband.
4. Assemble equipment.
5. Explain procedure to client, and answer any questions.
6. Raise bed and lower side rails.
7. Wash your hands.
8. Open sterile packages on the over-bed table as with dressing change.
9. Pour sterile irrigating solution into container.

Procedure

1. Place absorbent pads under the client. Place a bath blanket under absorbent pads when irrigating a large wound. **Rationale:** This will absorb any spilled irrigation solution.
2. Position client so that solution flows from wound to basin.
3. Don clean gloves.
4. Remove and discard used dressing.
5. Remove gloves, and discard into plastic bag.
6. Place over-bed table near working area with all packages open.
7. Don sterile gloves.
8. Inspect area surrounding wound for redness, tissue integrity, and signs of granulating tissue.
9. Place sterile basin under wound area.
10. Draw solution from sterile container into 35-mL syringe with angiocath tip. Increasing syringe size decreases pressure of stream or increasing bore of catheter tip increases pressure. Open commercial cleaning solution package if using for irrigation.
11. Read directions on commercial wound cleaner container to determine appropriate distance nozzle is positioned from wound during irrigation. If nozzle is too close to the wound, force may be higher than expected If nozzle is too far from the wound, force may be lower than needed. If saline solution is used, deliver irrigant with 8 psi (pounds per square inch) pressure. The 35-mL syringe and 19-gauge angiocath tip delivers this pressure. **Rationale:** Pressures effective in wound cleansing should be between 4 psi and 15 psi in order to effectively clean the wound surface by forcefully loosening foreign materials and nonattached bacteria.
12. Repeat until all irrigation solution has been used.
13. After the irrigation, cleanse client's skin around wound and dry.
14. Apply sterile dressing.
15. Dispose of equipment properly.
16. Remove gloves. Check to see that client is comfortable before leaving the room.
17. Lower bed and raise side rails.
18. Wash your hands.

Debridement

Physical removal of affected tissue by debridement is the most effective method of cleaning the wound. Infected tissue is best removed by surgical debridement. Other methods of debridement include chemical or enzymatic, mechanical, or autolytic. Stage II ulcers can be debrided by gentle mechanical debridement using mesh gauze moistened with saline, hydrocolloid dressings, or enzymatic debriding. Stage IV and large stage III ulcers require surgical debridement. Surgical debridement uses sterile instruments and requires local anesthesia. Only a qualified clinician can use this technique.

Chemical debridement is slower than surgical debridement but is able to be used in home care and long-term care settings. Proteolytic enzymes such as collagenase or papain-urea are commonly used chemical agents. Mechanical debridement is accomplished through whirlpool treatments. Autolytic debridement uses moisture-retentive or moisture-donating dressings to facilitate digestion of tissue by the client's own enzymes and phagocytes.

DOCUMENTATION FOR WOUND CARE

- Observation of wound site, including amount, color, and odor of drainage, as well as appearance of suture site
- Observation of granulating tissue and redness
- Pertinent observations concerning client's tolerance of procedure
- Observation of skin condition around incision site
- Changes in vital signs that indicate possible infection
- Results of Ankle–Brachial Index measurement
- Type of dressing applied
- Material used in wound packing
- Observations on wound irrigation
- Type and amount of irrigation solutions used
- Unusual tension on sutures if present
- Amount and color of Hemovac or Jackson–Pratt drainage
- Document undermining using clock orientation; measure in cm. (i.e., 2 to 5 o'clock)
- Tissue viability; percent healthy and necrotic tissue relative to entire wound.

Critical Thinking Application

UNEXPECTED OUTCOMES	CRITICAL THINKING OPTIONS
Wound becomes infected with multiple microorganisms.	• Notify physician about changes in color or odor of drainage. • Obtain culture and sensitivity if physician orders one. • Wash your hands thoroughly after caring for client to prevent the spread of infection. • Pay strict attention to changing dressings.
Wound does not heal.	• Evaluate use of dressing and perhaps choose a different type of dressing. • Assess nutritional status. Increase protein and carbohydrates if not contraindicated. • Determine availability of a vacuum-assisted closure machine.
Edges of wound split open (wound dehiscence).	• Place client in supine position. Apply butterfly tape to wound edges. Cover opening with sterile dressings. • Apply binder for abdominal incisions after obtaining order. • Notify physician if signs of infection are present. • Obtain culture of drainage if physician orders one. • Observe client for signs of shock. If client in shock, notify physician immediately. • Encourage high-protein diet.
Evisceration occurs (protrusion of bowel contents).	• Institute emergency measures. Place the client in supine position. Cover bowel with sterile gauze moistened with sterile saline. Have IV certified nurse insert IV catheter and infuse normal saline. Reassure client. Obtain vital signs, and treat for shock if present. • After above measures are completed, notify physician, and prepare client for return to surgery. • After surgical repair, notify dietician for diet change to increase protein and vitamin C in diet. • Apply abdominal binder if ordered.

UNEXPECTED OUTCOMES	CRITICAL THINKING OPTIONS
Wound hemorrhages.	• Outline area of blood on dressing with a pen and observe outline to see how quickly the bleeding spreads. • If bleeding is excessive, notify the physician immediately. • Apply pressure dressing to site if there is excessive bleeding.
Skin appears red and broken.	• Clean area with sterile saline and dry thoroughly with sterile 4×4 pads. • Apply moisture-retentive dressing.
Wound is too extensive for application of drainage bag or ABD pads cannot contain drainage.	• Obtain Stomahesive or Hollihesive 8×8 sheets and cut on diagonal $\frac{1}{8}$–$\frac{1}{4}$ inch larger than wound. • If larger barrier needed, Stomahesive may be pieced together to form larger barrier reinforcing juncture points with Karaya paste. • A superadhesive pouch may then be applied. • If dressings are used, they may be secured with Montgomery straps (tie tapes).
Abdominal binder is not effective in supporting incisional area.	• Evaluate the effectiveness of the abdominal binder. • Assess if the binder is properly positioned at the hip level and waist level to provide support. • Assess if the binder is too loose.
Client is too large for the abdominal binder.	• Fold a drawsheet in half lengthwise and place under client. Position the edges at the waist and pubic area. • Pull tightly on the drawsheet, and secure the edges with safety pins.
Drainage system expands quickly after being reconnected.	• Check all connections for an air leak because properly functioning reservoirs expand slowly.
Client is too large for bed.	• Request use of BariAir bed.

UNIT 4

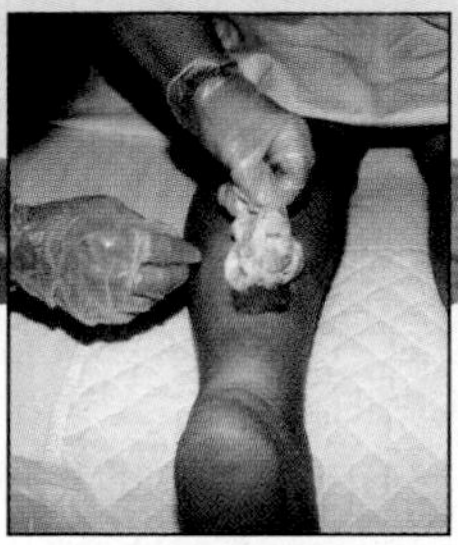

Wet-to-Moist Dressings

Nursing Process Data

ASSESSMENT Data Base

Assess wound edges for presence of granulation tissue.

Assess for changes in amount of drainage.

Assess if necrotic tissue is decreasing in amount.

Identify if appropriate dressing is used for wound care.

PLANNING Objectives

To promote wound healing by secondary intention

To maintain a moist environment conducive to wound healing

To provide the most appropriate treatment for wound care

To enhance local healing

To maintain sterile technique throughout procedure

To remove trapped exudate from wounds

IMPLEMENTATION Procedures

Applying Wet-to-Moist Dressings

EVALUATION Expected Outcomes

Wound heals without complications.

Sterile technique is maintained throughout procedure.

APPLYING WET-TO-MOIST DRESSINGS

Equipment

Sterile 4 × 8 noncotton gauze dressings
Semi-occlusive dressing, optional
Sterile gloves
Clean gloves
Tape
Plastic bag for contaminated dressings
Sterile normal saline solution
Sterile receptacle (round basin or emesis basin)
Montgomery straps, if desired

> **CLINICAL ALERT**
> Wet-to-wet and wet-to-dry dressings are not used today, as they cause tissue damage. Maceration of healthy tissue can occur with dressings that are always wet. Dry dressings cause damage to granulating tissue if removed without first soaking the gauze.

Preparation

1. Check physician's orders and client care plan.
2. Wash hands.
3. Gather equipment.
4. Explain procedure to client.
5. Provide privacy.
6. Raise bed to HIGH position, and lower side rail nearest you.
7. Remove tape by pulling it toward the wound. **Rationale:** This action prevents injury to newly formed tissue.
8. Don clean gloves.
9. Moisten dressing with normal saline before removing if dressing is dry. **Rationale:** Removal of a dry dressing traumatizes granulating tissue and delays wound healing.
10. Remove wound packing by gently grasping the gauze without touching the wound. **Rationale:** Touching only the gauze prevents contamination of the wound.
11. Place soiled dressings in disposable bag.
12. Remove gloves, and dispose of them in bag.
13. Wash your hands.

> **CLINICAL ALERT**
> Heat lamps should not be used to treat pressure ulcers. Preferred wound care is to promote a clean, moist environment.

Procedure

1. Open packages of dressings making sure sterility is maintained.
2. Pour normal saline solution over dressings.
3. Don sterile gloves.
4. Pick up sterile gauze dressings one at a time.
5. Fluff each dressing, and place over wound.
6. Place gauze in the wound, covering all exposed surfaces. Press gauze lightly into depressions or cracks. **Rationale:** Necrotic tissue is more prevalent in these areas.
7. Unfold a moist, sterile, 4 × 8 (ABD pad) dressing into a single layer and place it on top of wet dressings covering the wound area (not on skin).
8. Place a dry 4 × 8 pad over the dressing to hold it in place. Some protocols call for semi-occlusive dressing in place of pad.
9. Remove gloves, and place in plastic bag.
10. Tape only the edges of the dressing. Montgomery tapes may be used to prevent excessive skin irritation and damage due to frequent dressing changes.
11. Position client for comfort. Lower bed, and raise side rail to UP position, if appropriate.
12. Discard soiled material in appropriate container.
13. Wash your hands thoroughly.
14. Observe wound for excessive drainage or drying out of

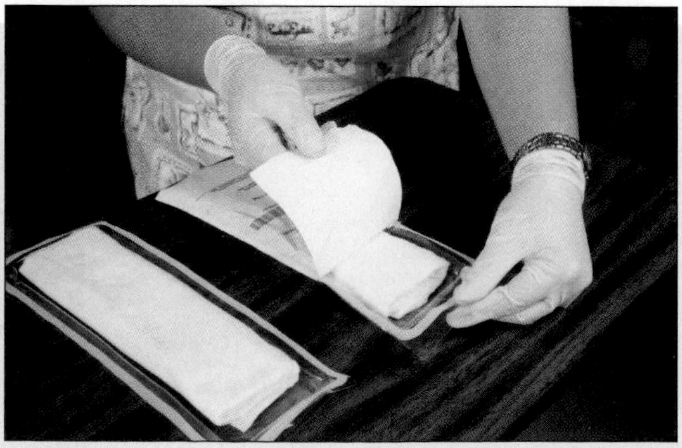

Open sterile packages before beginning dressing change.

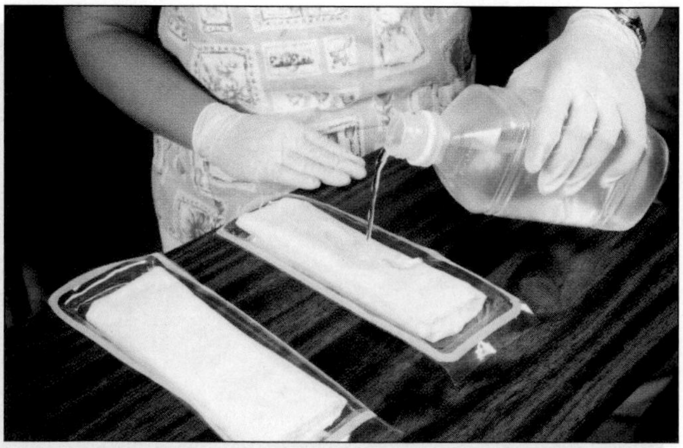

Pour sterile saline solution over dressings to moisten.

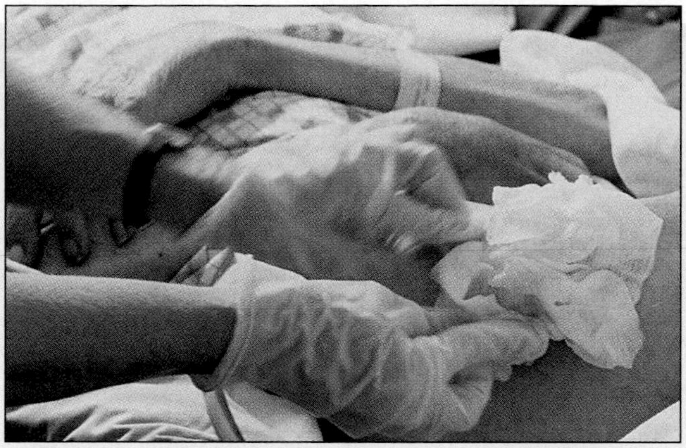

Fluff dressings and apply over wound, covering all exposed surfaces.

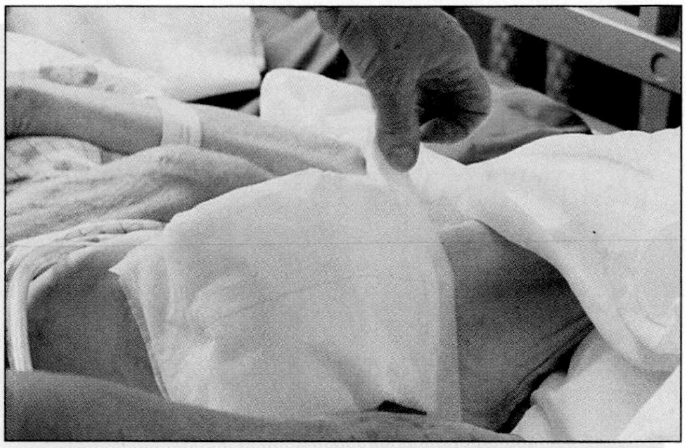

Place moist ABD pad over dressings, then cover with dry pad.

dressing between dressing changes. Remoisten dressing if dry. **Rationale:** Unless excessive drainage occurs, or dressing dries out, dressings are usually changed every 8 hours.

15. Provide client or family teaching regarding wound care, if appropriate.

Note: These dressings function as an osmotic dressing. Normal saline is isotonic. As water evaporates from saline dressing it becomes hypertonic and fluid from wound tissue is drained into dressing.

Documentation for Wet-to-Moist Dressings

- Condition of wound
- Solution used
- Number and type of dressings used
- Signs and symptoms indicative of wound infection
- Color, consistency, presence of odor, amount of drainage on soiled dressings
- Condition of skin surrounding wound
- Client's reaction to procedure

Critical Thinking Application

UNEXPECTED OUTCOMES	CRITICAL THINKING OPTIONS
Wound drainage increases.	• Decrease time between dressing changes. Change every 4 hours. • Obtain order for culture and sensitivity to determine if different microorganisms are present or antibiotic medication is not sensitive to microorganism.
Dressings dry between dressing changes.	• Moisten dressing with sterile normal saline before removing to prevent debridement of granulation tissue. • Ensure that dressing is moist when applied to wound and cover with moist dressing. • Moisten and change dressing more frequently. • Semiocclusive dressing should be considered.

UNIT 5

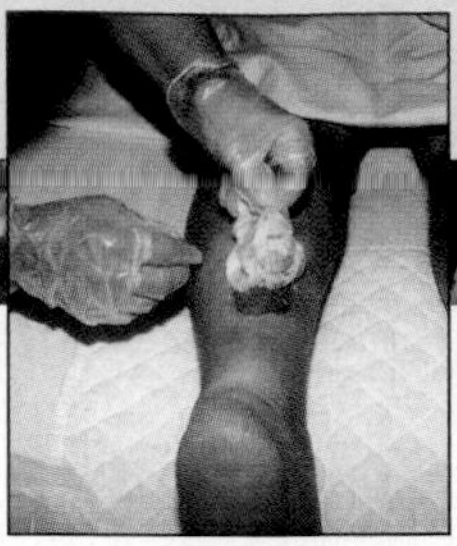

Pressure Ulcers

Nursing Process Data

ASSESSMENT ***Data Base***

Assess stage of ulcer.

Assess size and depth of pressure ulcer.

Assess presence and location of undermining, tunneling, and sinus tracts.

Identify if infection is associated with pressure ulcer.

Assess wound exudate

Evaluate effectiveness of ulcer treatment.

Assess healing process of the ulcer.

Assess other bony prominences for potential formation of pressure ulcers.

Assess for presence of conditions that inhibit wound healing.

Assess wound size for changes.

PLANNING ***Objectives***

To identify the stage of the ulcer

To provide appropriate treatment for specific ulcer stage

To promote healing of established ulcer

To prevent new ulcer formation

To prevent spread of pathogens from ulcerated area

IMPLEMENTATION ***Procedures***

Preventing Pressure Ulcers

Applying Transparent Adhesive Film Dressing

Using Hydrocolloid Dressing

EVALUATION ***Expected Outcomes***

Stage of pressure ulcer is accurately assessed.

Pressure ulcer is treated effectively according to stage of ulcer formation.

Nursing Guide for Assessment of Clients at Risk for Pressure Ulcers

Factors that contribute to development of pressure ulcers:

- Pressure
- Friction
- Shearing
- Moisture

Identify at-risk individuals needing preventative measures:

- Bed- and chairbound individuals
- Clients with impaired ability to reposition themselves
- Clients who are immobilized
- Clients who are incontinent
- Clients with nutritional deficits, such as inadequate dietary intake, malnutrition
- Clients with altered level of consciousness
- Identification of stage I pressure ulcer may be difficult in a dark-skinned client.

A risk assessment tool should be used for all clients admitted to long-term care facilities, an acute care setting, or receiving home care (Braden scale or Norton scale). Systematic reassessments should be done at designated intervals.

- Nursing Homes: Assess on admission and every week for 1 month, then every 3 months. Clients develop pressure ulcers within first month in nursing home.
- Home: Assess on admission and every visit. Instruct family to notify nurse if skin condition changes.
- Acute Care: Assess on admission and every shift for at-risk clients in critical care units or daily to every other day for stable clients.

TABLE 25–3 Pressure Ulcer Staging and Treatment

Stage[a]	Treatment Protocol for Pressure Ulcer Stages
Stage I: Nonblanchable erythema of intact skin, the heralding lesion of skin ulceration.	*Stage I:* Apply an adhesive film dressing over the red area. These dressings are semipermeable to oxygen and prevent bacterial invasion. Healing can occur in 24 hours.
Stage II: Partial-thickness skin loss involving epidermis or dermis. The ulcer is superficial and presents clinically as an abrasion, blister, or shallow crater. Usually caused by friction or moisture plus pressure. Painful and may have minimal drainage.	*Stage II:* Apply a transparent adhesive film dressing if ulcer is not draining. If wound is draining, irrigate with normal saline and apply a hydrocolloid dressing. These occlusive dressings remain in place for 5–7 days, creating a moist environment that promotes epithelialization and restoration of the epidermis.
Stage III: Full-thickness skin loss involving damage or necrosis of subcutaneous tissue that may extend down to, but not through, underlying fascia. The ulcer presents clinically as a deep crater with or without the undermining of adjacent tissue. Usually caused by pressure plus shearing forces.	*Stage III:* Irrigate with normal saline, cover with a hydrocolloid dressing. With excessively draining wounds, absorptive products are placed in the wound for absorption, and then the dressing is applied.
Stage IV: Full-thickness skin loss with extensive destruction, tissue necrosis, or damage to muscle, bone, or supporting structures (tendon or joint capsule are examples). Undermining and sinus tracts may be associated with this stage ulcer.	*Stage IV:* Chemical debridement, autolysis, or surgery are required for treatment of this stage. Wet-to-damp dressing changes are used for small wounds; surgical interventions are used for larger wounds. Negative pressure therapy may be required.

[a] Pressure ulcers are classified in stages by the degree of tissue damage observed. Accurate staging of pressure ulcers is not possible until eschar has sloughed or wound is debrided.

Source: Pressure Ulcers in Adults: Prediction and Prevention, Rockville, MD: U.S. Department of Health and Human Services, Public Health Service, Agency for Health Care Policy and Research.

Assessment for Dark-Skin-Tone Clients

Stage I. Ulcers appear with persistent red, blue, or purple hues. To assess darker skin tones that do not show erythema, shine a light at skin level to check for color change. Palpate area for induration or edema.

Stage II. Solid, smooth, dark pink tissue exposing basal membrane; exposed dermis epithelization.

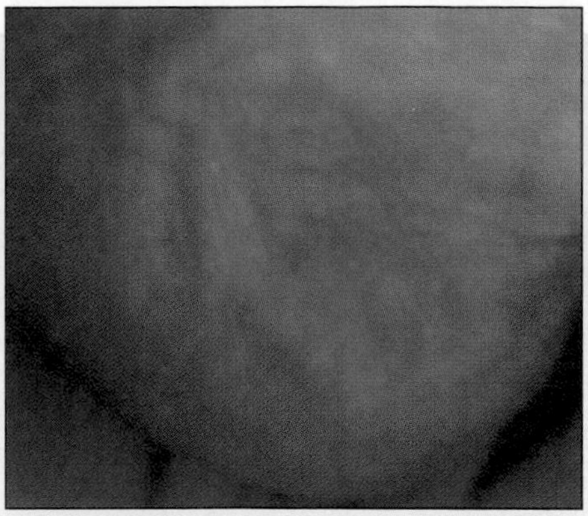

Stage I pressure ulcer.

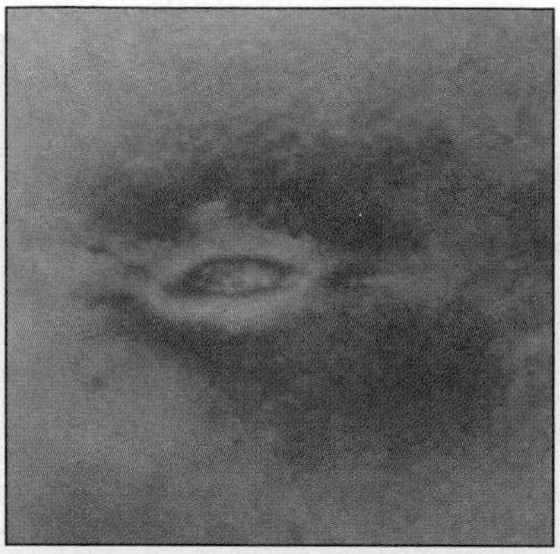

Stage II pressure ulcer.

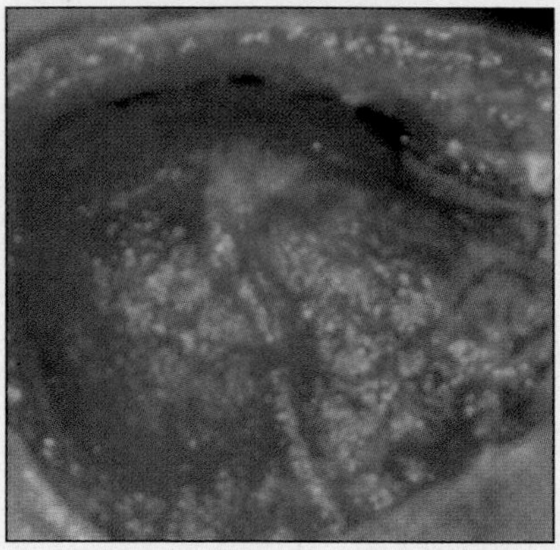

Stage III pressure ulcer.

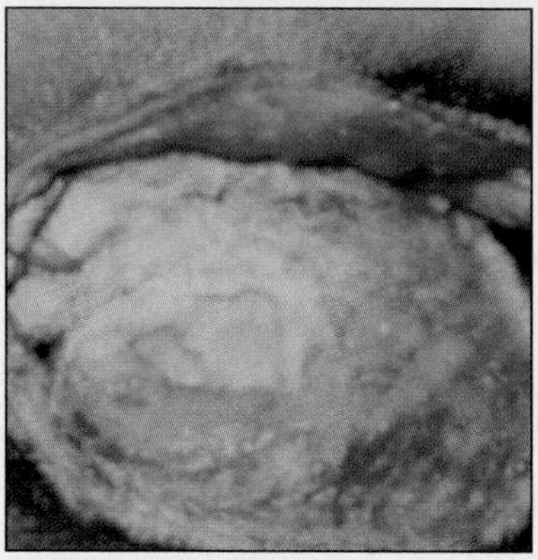

Stage IV pressure ulcer.

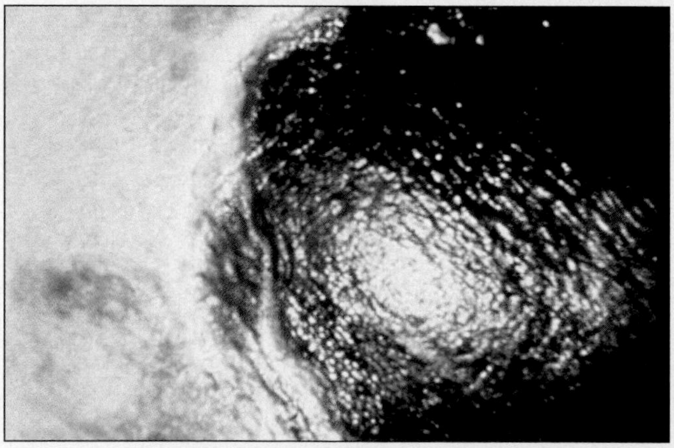

Eschar must be removed by debridement before staging is done.

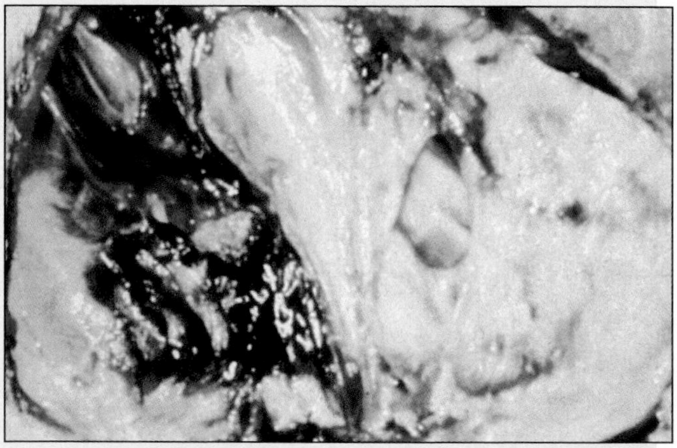

Clinical signs of infection.

TABLE 25–4 Pressure Ulcer Risk Assessment Scales

Norton Scale

Physical Condition		Mental Condition		Activity		Mobility		Continence	
Good	−4	Alert	−4	Walks	−4	Full	−4	Good	−4
Fair	−3	Apathetic	−3	Walks with help	−3	Slightly limited	−3	Occasional incontinence	−3
Poor	−2	Confused	−2	Sits in chair	−2	Very limited	−2	Frequent incontinence	−2
Very poor	−1	Stuporous	−1	Remains in bed	−1	Immobile	−1	Urine and fecal incontinence	−1
Total ____		Total ____		Total ____		Total ____		Total ____	
Grand total = ________									
A score of 14 or less indicates risk of pressure ulcer; a score under 12 indicates high risk.									

Braden Scale

Sensory Perception		Moisture		Activity		Mobility		Nutrition		Friction and Shear	
No impairment	−4	Rarely moist	−4	Walks frequently	−4	No limitations	−4	Excellent	−4		
Slightly limited	−3	Occasionally moist	−3	Walks occasionally	−3	Slightly limited	−3	Adequate	−3	No apparent problems	−3
Very limited	−2	Very Moist	−2	Chairfast	−2	Very limited	−2	Probably inadequate	−2	Potential problem	−2
Completely limited	−1	Constantly moist	−1	Bedfast	−1	Completely Immobile	−1	Very poor	−1	Problem	−1
Total ____		Total ____		Total ____		Total ____		Total ____		Total ____	
Grand total = ____											
Assign a score of 1 to 4 in each category. Total the score; no risk: 19–23; at risk: 15–18; moderate risk: 13–14; high risk: 10–12; very high risk: 9 or below.											

Norton Scale: Adapted from *Pressure Ulcers in Adults: Prediction and Prevention.* AHCRP Publication No. 92-0047 (May 1992), p. 15.
Braden Scale: Adapted from *Pressure Ulcers in Adults: Predictions and Prevention.* AHCRP Publication No. 92-0047 (May 1992), pp. 16–17.
Note: Refer to actual scales for detailed information about both scales.

PREVENTING PRESSURE ULCERS

Procedure

1. Inspect skin at least daily, particularly over bony prominences. Use Braden scale for assessment. Document assessment findings.
2. Individualize client's bathing schedule. Daily baths are not essential. **Rationale:** Daily cleansing can destroy the skin's natural barrier, making it more susceptible to external irritants.
   a. Avoid hot bath water. **Rationale:** Tepid water prevents injury to skin.
   b. Use mild cleansing agents to minimize dryness.
   c. Cleanse skin immediately if urine, fecal incontinence, or wound drainage seeps onto skin.
   d. Provide humidity to prevent drying of skin.
   e. Use cream or thin layer of corn starch to protect skin.
3. Avoid massaging bony prominences. **Rationale:** Massaging can lead to deep tissue trauma.
   a. Keep bony prominences from direct contact with one another.
   b. Use pillow, foam wedges, or other positioning devices.
   c. Use elbow pads and heel elevators
4. Promote adequate dietary intake of protein, calories, and nutrients. **Rationale:** Adequate protein intake in addition to vitamins and minerals help prevent pressure ulcer formation.

CLINICAL ALERT

Air-fluidized beds and low-air-loss beds are recommended to manage pressure ulcers, especially in clients with large or multiple ulcers.

Air-Fluidized

Warm, pressurized air circulates through beads in the bed and creates support surface. Polyester sheet allows for moisture and air to pass through, keeping skin dry. Treatment can take several months. Use of this bed is very expensive.

Low-Air-Loss

Head and foot of bed can be elevated. Bed is a modified standard bed frame, lighter and more portable than air-fluidized bed. Bed circulates cool air.
Urine and feces do not pass through fabric on the bed.
Bed is portable and lighter.
See also section on Special Beds in Chapter 8.

EVIDENCE BASED NURSING PRACTICE

Pressure Relief in Surgical Clients

Pressure ulcers can begin in the operating room. The occurrence of ulcers can be as high as 45% of surgical clients. There are many risk factors leading to ulcer development in as few as 2 ½ hours. Risk factors include position client is placed in during procedure, necessity of positioning devices placing pressure on bony prominences. Medications that constrict blood vessels or lower blood pressure can also lead to pressure ulcers.

Source: Armstrong, D., Bortz, P. An integrative review of pressure relief in surgical patients. *American Organization of Operating Room Nurses Journal, 74*(3), 645.

5. Ensure adequate fluid intake. **Rationale:** Prevent dehydration which is a risk factor for pressure ulcer formation.
6. Reposition bedridden client every 2 hours.
   a. Do not position directly on trochanter.
   b. Do not turn more than 30° angle.
   c. Raise heels off bed by placing pillows under legs; allow heels to hang over edges.
   d. Use trapeze or turning sheet to reposition client.
7. Encourage mobility or range-of-motion exercises. **Rationale:** Range-of-motion exercises promote activity and reduce effects of pressure on tissue.
8. Minimize force and friction on skin when turning or moving client. Use turning sheets or Hoyer lift.
9. Maintain head of bed at lowest degree of elevation consistent with medical problem. Below 30° if possible.
10. Place at-risk clients on pressure-reducing devices, in both bed and chair, such as foam, static-air, alternating gel, water mattress, or air fluidized mattress.
11. Encourage chair-fast clients to shift position every 15 minutes.

APPLYING TRANSPARENT ADHESIVE FILM DRESSING

Equipment

Sterile normal saline
Transparent dressing (e.g., Op-Site, Tegaderm, Bio-occlusive)
Sterile 4 × 4 gauze pads
Scissors
Hypoallergenic tape
Clean gloves
Plasticizing agent (e.g., skin prep [optional])

Preparation

1. Check physician's orders and client care plan.
2. Check type of dressing ordered. **Rationale:** These dressings are very important in preventing pressure ulcers; they prevent friction and shear over bony prominences when moving clients.
3. Gather supplies.
4. Obtain appropriately sized transparent dressing. Dressing can be applied to flat surface. (Coccyx area cannot be treated with this type of dressing.)

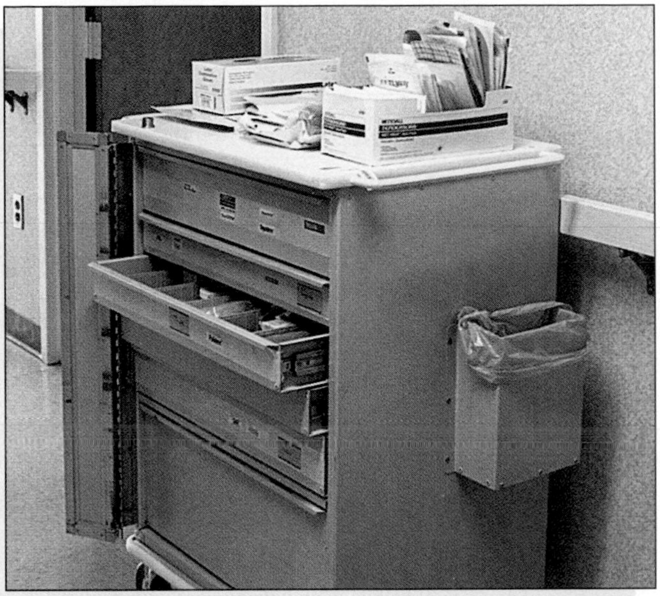

Dressing carts may be used to keep supplies closer to client area.

5. Wash your hands.
6. Explain procedure to client.
7. Provide privacy.

CLINICAL ALERT

Adhesive transparent film dressings remain in place for 5–7 days. These dressings are permeable to moisture, vapor, and atmospheric gases. They are bacteria proof and waterproof. It is imperative to observe the ulcer area daily to determine if a large amount of secretions or serous fluid has accumulated under dressing. If fluid has increased, aspirate with a 26-gauge needle. These dressings are not used for infected areas.

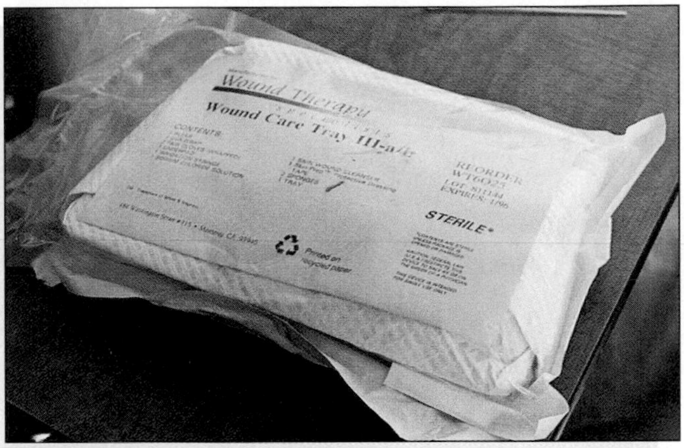

Obtain specific dressing tray for ordered treatment.

Procedure

1. Raise bed to HIGH position, and lower side rail on working side of bed.
2. Don clean gloves.
3. Remove old dressing, "walk off" dressing from one edge to the other, and discard in appropriate receptacle.
4. Wash pressure ulcer with sterile gauze pads moistened with sterile normal saline.
5. Dry thoroughly with sterile gauze pad.
6. Measure wound using pliable device. **Rationale:** Comparison of measurement assists in determining effectiveness of treatment.
7. Apply plasticizing agent (skin prep, skin gel) over surrounding tissue if ordered. **Rationale:** Do not apply directly on ulcer area because the agent contains alcohol, which burns the ulcer area.
8. Loosen transparent dressing from one side of backing paper.
9. "Walk on" dressing: Start at one edge of site and gently lay the dressing down, keeping it free of wrinkles. Allow at least a 1½-inch margin of dressing beyond ulcer margin. **Rationale:** This ensures coverage of entire wound area.

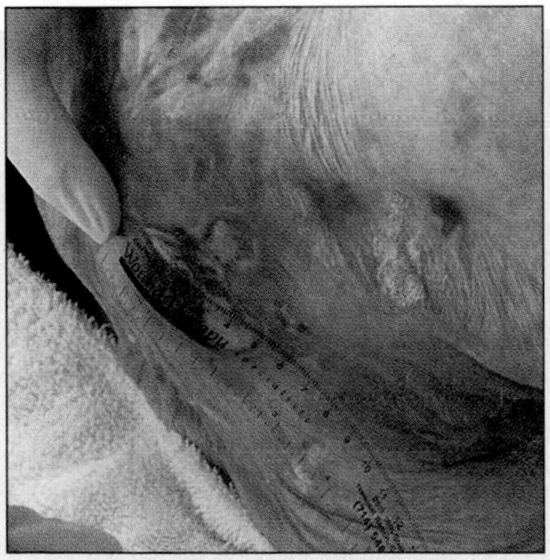

Assess size of wound to determine appropriate size of transparent dressing.

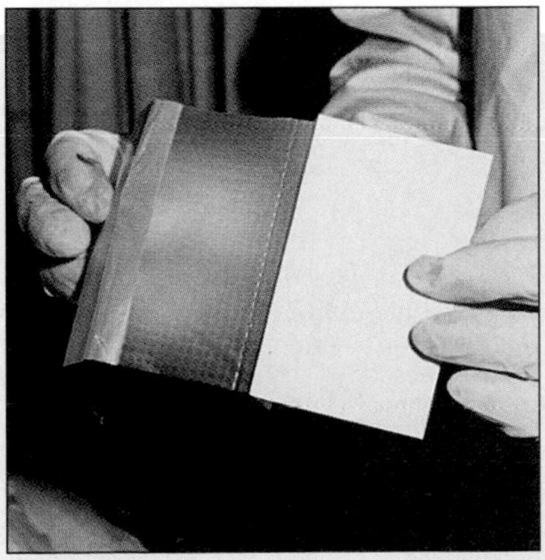

Remove backing from Op-Site dressing before applying.

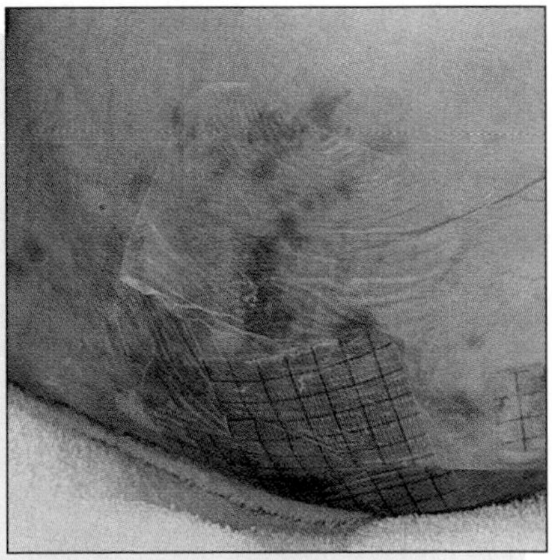

Apply transparent adhesive dressing over wound.

SAMPLE PRESSURE ULCER ASSESSMENT GUIDE

Patient Name: ______________________ Date: __________ Time: __________

Ulcer 1:			Ulcer 2:		
Site ________			Site________		
Stage[a] ______			Stage[a] ______		
Size (cm)			Size (cm)		
Length ______			Length ______		
Width ______			Width ______		
Depth ______			Depth ______		
Sinus Tract	☐	☐	Sinus Tract	☐	☐
Tunneling	☐	☐	Tunneling	☐	☐
Undermining	☐	☐	Undermining	☐	☐
Necrotic Tissue	☐	☐	Necrotic Tissue	☐	☐
Slough	☐	☐	Slough	☐	☐
Eschar	☐	☐	Eschar	☐	☐
Exudate	☐	☐	Exudate	☐	☐
Serous	☐	☐	Serous	☐	☐
Serosanguineous	☐	☐	Serosanguineous	☐	☐
Purulent	☐	☐	Purulent	☐	☐
Granulation	☐	☐	Granulation	☐	☐
Epithelialization	☐	☐	Epithelialization	☐	☐
Pain	☐	☐	Pain	☐	☐
Surrounding Skin:					
Erythema	☐	☐	Erythema	☐	☐
Maceration	☐	☐	Maceration	☐	☐
Induration	☐	☐	Induration	☐	☐

Description of Ulcer(s):

____

____

Indicate Ulcer Sites:

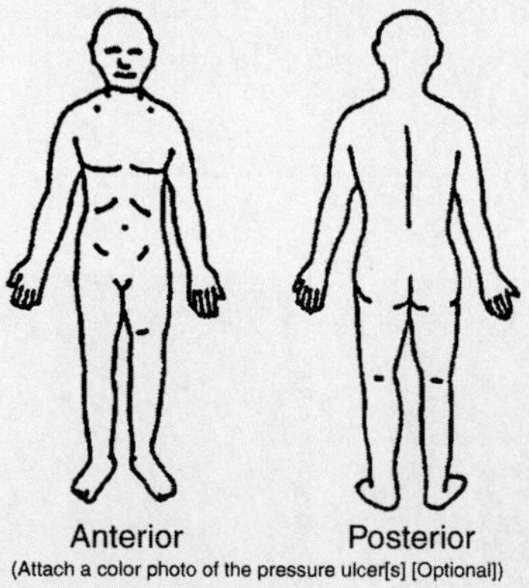

(Attach a color photo of the pressure ulcer[s] [Optional])

[a]Classification of pressure ulcers:

Stage I: Nonblanchable erythema of intact skin, the heralding lesion of skin ulceration. In individuals with darker skin, discoloration of the skin, warmth, edema, induration, or hardness may also be indicators.

Stage II: Partial thickness skin loss involving epidermis, dermis, or both.

Stage III: Full thickness skin loss involving damage to or necrosis of subcutaneous tissue that may extend down to, but not through, underlying fascia. The ulcer presents clinically as a deep crater with or without undermining adjacent tissue.

Stage IV: Full thickness skin loss with extensive destruction, tissue necrosis, or damage to muscle, bone, or supporting structures (e.g., tendon or joint capsule).

Source: Pressure Ulcer Treatment: Quick Reference Guide for Clinicians, No. 15. U.S. Department of Health and Human Services, AHCPR.

CLINICAL ALERT

Film dressings are very useful as a secondary or primary dressing. Examples are alginates, hydrogels, and foams. They hold dressing in place and make it waterproof.

10. Cut off tabs if using Op-Site after wound is completely covered.
11. Tape edges with hypoallergenic tape. **Rationale:** This assists in preventing frequent dressing changes due to loose dressings. These dressings can remain in place for 1 week.
12. Remove gloves, and discard in appropriate receptacle.
13. Position client for comfort.
14. Lower bed, and raise side rails.
15. Remove and discard equipment.
16. Wash your hands.

Using Hydrogel Dressings

- Hydrogel dressings contain 95% water; they are very absorbent and dehydrate easily when not covered with dressing.
- Dressings cannot absorb much exudate; they should be used for dry wounds such as skin tears, surgical wounds, and radiation therapy burns.
- Dressings are nonadhesive, can be transparent and conform to wound surfaces.
- Sterile aqueous hydrogen fiber is used to fill cavity with gel; also used to fill dead space in large wounds.
- Hydrogel sheets are placed in direct contact with wound bed and margins; air bubbles and plastic covering on sheet must be removed.

USING HYDROCOLLOID DRESSING

Equipment

Sterile normal saline
Hydrocolloid dressing (e.g., DuoDERM, Restore, Ultec, Comfeel Plus)
Hydrogel if needed (ClearSite, Aquasorb)
Sterile 4 × 4 gauze pads
Hypoallergenic tape
Clean gloves
Skin prep, optional

Note: These dressings promote a moist wound environment, aid in autolytic debridement, and have no toxic components. They are waterproof and bacteria proof.

Procedure

1. Select dressing size to ensure coverage 1¼ inch beyond ulcer margin. (Dressing available in 4 × 4 to 8 × 8 sizes.) **Rationale:** This ensures complete covering of wound. Use for small ulcers and in Stage II and III.

Note: These dressings can be used for nondressing wounds (i.e., postsurgical incisions, abrasions, blisters, and early stage pressure ulcers).

2. Wash hands and don clean gloves.
3. Cleanse skin with gauze pad moistened with sterile normal saline and pat dry with gauze pad.
4. Measure wound using pliable device.
5. Apply skin prep to surrounding skin to protect, if ordered.
6. Fill ulcer area with Hydrogel if ordered—usually used with Stage III or IV pressure ulcer of the hip when exudate is present. Do not overfill with gel. **Rationale:** Facilitates autolytic debridement of devitalized tissue.
7. Warm dressing by holding in hands. **Rationale:** To increase activity of adhesive.
8. Remove silicone release paper backing from dressing. Minimize finger contact with adhesive surface. **Rationale:** Dressing is sterile and contamination should be avoided.
9. Center dressing over affected area. Gently roll dressing over pressure ulcer—do not stretch dressing. **Rationale:** Stretching the dressing may cause wrinkling of dressing which allows air to enter wound.
10. Placing dressing 1/3 above wound and 2/3 below wound maximizes time between dressing changes. **Rationale:** Increases absorption capacity of dressing.
11. Mold the dressing gently to skin, and hold down with hand for approximately 1 minute.
12. Apply skin prep to area that is to be covered by tape if ordered. Allow to dry. *Do not apply* skin prep under hydrocolloid dressing. **Rationale:** Hydrocolloid dressings are placed over broken skin; skin prep may cause damage to skin.
13. Picture-frame sides of hydrocolloid dressing with silk or hypoallergenic tape.
14. Check dressing each shift for leakage.
15. Change dressing at first sign of leakage. Dressings should not be left on longer than 7 days. Usually left in place for 3–4 days.

Note: Duoderm is removed when exudate seeps from edges of dressing or white blister appears under dressing. Comfeel Plus is changed when dressing becomes transparent or there is leakage.

NUTRITIONAL ASSESSMENT OF CLIENT WITH PRESSURE ULCER(S)

Client Name: ______________________ **Date:** __________ **Time** ________

To be filled out for all clients at risk on initial evaluation and every 12 weeks thereafter, as indicated. Trends will document the efficacy of nutritional support therapy.

Protein Compartments

Somatic:

Current Weight (kg) ______
Previous Weight (kg) ______ (______date)
Percent Change in Weight ______

Height (cm) ______
Height/Weight ______
Current Body Mass Index (BM) ______ [wt/(ht)^2]
Previous BMI ______ (______date)
Percent Change in BMI ______

Visceral:

Serum Albumin ______
(Normal ≥ 3.5 mg/dL)
Total Lymphocyte Count (TLC) ______ (optional)
(White Blood Cell count x percent Lymphocytes/100)

Guide to TLC:

- Immune competence ≥ 1,800 mm^3
- Immunity partly impaired < 1,800 but ≥ 900 mm^3
- Anergy < 900 mm^3

State of Hydration

24-Hour Intake ______ mL 24-Hour Output ______ mL

Note: Thirst, tongue dryness in non-mouth-breathers, and tenting of cervical skin may indicate dehydration. Jugular vein distention may indicate overhydration.

Estimated Nutritional Requirement

Estimated Nonprotein Calories (NPC) ______ /kg Estimated Protein ______ (g/kg)
Actual NPC ______ /kg Actual Protein ______ (g/kg)

Recommendations/Plan

1.

2.

3.

4.

Source: Pressure Ulcer Treatment: Quick Reference Guide for Clinicians, No. 15. U.S. Department of Health and Human Services, AHCPR.

TABLE 25–5 Comparisons of Moisture-Retentive Dressings

	Transparent	Hydrocolloid
Common Brands	Tegaderm Op-Site Bioclusive	Tegasorb DuoDERM Comfeel Restore
Characteristics	Sterile Semipermeable membranes with hypoallergenic adhesive Permeable to oxygen and moisture vapor Allows oxygen exchange Impermeable to bacteria, prevents contamination	Impermeable to oxygen Dressing gel maintains moist environment that promotes autolysis Impermeable to external bacteria and contamination Minimally to moderately absorptive
Function	Provides moist environment Promotes autolysis and protects newly formed tissue Assists with debridement	Dressing contains hydroactive particles that absorb exudate to form a hydrated gel over wound When dressing removed, gel separates from dressing, which protects newly formed tissue
Use	Easy assessment of wound; dressing is transparent Nondraining or minimally draining wounds only, nonabsorbable Pressure ulcers, stage I and some stage II Minor burns, lacerations	Absorbs exudate while preserving moist environment needed for autolysis of slough Irrigate gel with saline to allow for assessing wound Pressure ulcers, some stage III and some clean stage IV Wounds with mild or moderate exudate Wounds with necrosis or slough
Contraindications	Infected wounds Wounds with fragile surrounding skin	Wounds that need frequent assessment, not transparent Wounds with heavy exudate

TABLE 25–6 Additional Moist Wound Dressings

Type of Alternative	Use	Outcome of Treatment	Considerations
Hydrogel Sheet	• Interacts with aqueous solutions • Used with minor wounds with light to moderate drainage • Absorbs minimal to heavy exudates • Nonadherent	Softens necrotic tissue Creates moist environment	Use outer dressing to prevent wound from drying out. Change dressing every 1–2 days.
Impregnated Loose Forms	• Absorbs minimal to heavy exudates • Nonadherent	Conforms to irregular surfaces Eliminates dead space Creates moist environment	Requires outer dressing
Alginate	• Absorbs heavy exudates • Converts to gel when comes in contact with wound drainage • Easily removed from wound • Nonadherent	Maintains moist environment Promotes fast healing of wound	Not to be used on dry wounds
Foams Hydrophilic	• Absorbs minimal to heavy exudates • Nonadherent	Maintains moist environment Decreases tissue trauma when removed. Increases time between dressing changes.	Requires external dressing
Hydrophobic	• Softens necrotic tissue.		
Medical Hydrolysate of Collagen	• Soluble and degrades in wound site • Absorbs wound exudates • Is interactive with wound site to provide mechanical protection against physical and bacterial insult	Absorbs up to 30 times own weight Used in stage I–IV pressure ulcers Accelerates tissue remodeling and reduces scarring	Cover with nonstick dressing Soak dressing in warm water before removing

16. Remove dressing by pressing hand down on adjacent skin surface while carefully lifting edge of dressing from skin. Continue lifting dressing around periphery until all edges are released, then lift dressing carefully away from wound.
17. Remove gloves and wash hands.
18. Record stage, size, and appearance of ulcer; date; and reason for removal of hydrocolloid dressing.

CLINICAL ALERT

Hydrocolloid dressings are occlusive, thus, do not allow water, bacteria, or oxygen into the wound. They are not used if the wound or surrounding skin is infected. They have limited use with heavy exudates wounds.

Note: Although frequently listed as wound care alternatives, topical disinfectant agents such as iodine and silver sulfadiazine are very controversial in wound care. Iodine is cytotoxic to fibroblasts and can impair wound healing. Silver solutions are sometimes used to prevent bacterial colonization in infection prone areas. They do not eliminate existing infections.

DOCUMENTATION FOR PRESSURE ULCERS

- Client's general skin condition
- Periwound assessment
- Assessment of wound (i.e., drainage, evidence of tissue granulation)
- Color, volume, type of exudate
- Type of ulcer care given
- Use of support surface
- Pressure ulcer record completed
- State the exact location of pressure ulcer; if bony prominence involved, use an anatomic name. *Turning* surface involved. (RI, LI, post., ant., medial, lateral)
- *Size:* Indicate size in centimeters
- Identify ulcers by number. Use chart
- Measure depth of ulcer
- Identify undermining and tunneling location
- *Stage:* Write the number of the stage that corresponds to the description of the pressure ulcer (stage I–IV)
- *Treatment:* Chart treatment used (e.g., hydrocolloid dressing applied, transparent adhesive film applied, etc.)
- *Position:* Indicate time client's position was changed

Critical Thinking Application

UNEXPECTED OUTCOMES	CRITICAL THINKING OPTIONS
Client does not have sufficient exercise; appetite decreased.	• Encourage small, frequent feedings • Offer high-calorie drinks like eggnog or Isocal.
Client's wound does not heal with traditional types of treatments.	• In client care conference discuss the following: Is everyone following same treatment? Are causative agents preventing healing? Should treatment be adjusted or changed? Would use of a support surface be effective? Is surgical debridement and grafting necessary for healing?

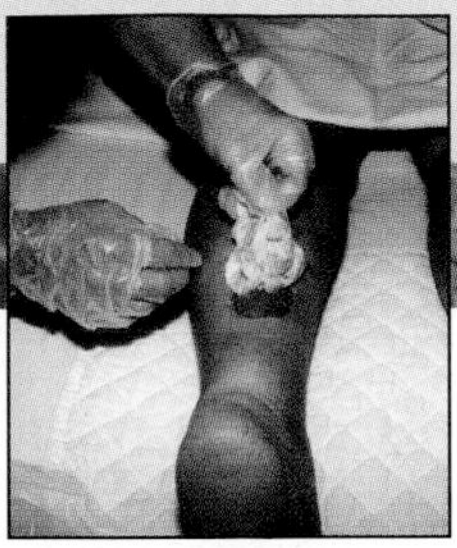

Adjunctive Wound Care Therapy

Nursing Process Data

ASSESSMENT *Data Base*

Identify why usual wound therapy treatments are ineffective.
Identify most effective adjunctive treatment for client.
Assess wound for baseline data before initiating treatment.
Determine if wound is healing using adjunctive therapy.
Assess if client is good candidate for adjunctive therapy.
Assess client's nutritional status to ensure best results from V.A.C.® therapy.
Determine if wound is maintaining a moist environment with adjunctive therapy.
Assess periwound area for signs of maceration.

PLANNING *Objectives*

To assess if adjunctive therapy is providing adequate wound healing
To place client on pressure relief surface if wound is over bony prominence
To determine if client is able to participate in specific therapy
To select appropriate type of dressing for adjunctive therapy

IMPLEMENTATION *Procedures*

Using Electrical Stimulation
Using Noncontact Normothermic Wound Therapy
- *for Using Warm-Up® Therapy System*
- *for Changing Wound Cover*
- *for Charging Batteries*

Using Vacuum Assisted Closure V.A.C.®
- *for Removing Dressing*
- *for Disconnecting V.A.C.® Unit*
- *for Reconnecting V.A.C.® Unit*
- *for Changing Canister*

EVALUATION *Expected Outcomes*

Granulation tissue is evident using adjunctive therapy.
Periwound area remains healthy without evidence of maceration.
Moist wound environment is maintained.
Pain is reduced with adjunctive therapy.
Wound progresses through usual phases with electrical stimulation.
Wound healing occurs faster with radiant heat dressing.
Exudate is removed and wound healing occurs with V.A.C.® therapy.

USING ELECTRICAL STIMULATION

Equipment

Normal saline solution
Bag for soiled dressings
Gauze pads
2 Sterile basins
Hydrogel sheets
Electrode
Bandage tape
Alligator clip
Stimulator
2 Pair clean gloves
Sterile gloves

Preparation

1. Determine if client is candidate for electrical stimulation.
2. Determine phase of wound healing. **Rationale:** This determines the correct treatment protocol.
3. Set the stimulator settings according to manufacturer's directions, based on client's phase in wound healing. The settings include: polarity, pulse rate, intensity, duration, and frequency.
4. Explain procedure to client.
5. Gather equipment.
6. Wash your hands.
7. Provide privacy.

Procedure

1. Raise bed to high position, lower side rails as needed.
2. Place client in position to enable staff to work with wound area and equipment. (Placement depends on wound site.)
3. Place supplies on over-bed table, near working area.
4. Open all supply packages, maintaining sterility.
5. Pour sterile normal saline into one basin.
6. Don clean gloves.
7. Place disposal bag near wound. **Rationale:** For ease in disposing of soiled dressings.
8. Remove dressing carefully to avoid interfering with granulation tissue.
9. Remove clean gloves; place in disposal bag. Don sterile gloves.
10. Place sterile basin next to wound to catch irrigation solution as wound is cleansed.
11. Pour sterile normal saline into wound to cleanse wound. **Rationale:** To remove exudates, slough, and petrolatum products. Current will not be conducted into wound tissue if petrolatum products remain in the wound.
12. Remove excess irrigation solution using sterile gauze pads.
13. Place fluffed gauze pads into normal saline solution, squeeze out excess liquid.
14. Fill wound cavity with gauze including any undermined/tunneled spaces. Pack gently.
15. Place surface (active) electrode in wound bed, over gauze packing. **Rationale:** This transfers electrical energy into wound bed, producing positive effects on necessary components for wound healing (i.e., blood flow, oxygen uptake, DNA, and protein synthesis).
16. Cover with dry gauze pad.
17. Tape dry pad securely.
18. Connect alligator clip to foil.
19. Connect to stimulator lead.
20. Place a wet washcloth over area where dispersive electrode will be placed.
21. Select a dispersive pad that is larger than the sum of areas of active electrodes and wound packing.
22. Place dispersive electrode proximal to wound, over soft tissue, avoiding bony prominences. *Note:* The greater the separation between two electrodes, the deeper the current path. Larger separation space is used to treat deep and undermined wounds. Closer separation space is used for shallow or partial thickness wounds. Ensure electrodes do not touch.
23. Ensure all edges of electrode are in good contact with skin. Hold electrode in place with nylon elasticized strap.
24. Place client in position of comfort. Electrical stimulation treatments usually last 60 minutes.
25. Remove gloves and discard.
26. Wash your hands.
27. Don clean gloves.
28. Remove electrode from wound following treatment.
29. Remove saline soaked gauze and cover wound with occlusive dressing.

Note: Hydrogel sheets or amorphous hydrogel impregnated gauze can be used to conduct current. If hydrogel gauze is the conductor, it is changed BID.

Candidates for Electrical Stimulation

- Pressure ulcers, stage I–IV.
- Diabetic ulcers
- Venous ulcers, ischemic ulcer
- Traumatic wounds
- Surgical wounds
- Wound flap
- Donor site, burn wound

USING NONCONTACT NORMOTHERMIC WOUND THERAPY

Equipment

Warming cover (latex free)
Warming card
Temperature control unit (TCU)
AC adapter
Wound measuring guide
Sterile normal saline solution
Skin scalant
Carrying pouch
Sterile normal saline
Skin sealant
Gauze pads
Moisture proof pad
Sterile basin and irrigating syringe
Sterile gloves
Clean gloves
Disposable bag

Preparation

1. Check physician's orders and client care plan.
2. Gather equipment. Select appropriate sized wound cover and warming card after measuring wound.
3. Check that temperature control unit's battery is charged; if not, recharge with battery pack or wall outlet power source.
4. Explain procedure to client.
5. Provide privacy for client.
6. Wash your hands.

Procedure

1. Place equipment on over-bed table.
2. Open sterile normal saline bottle, gauze pads, and basin with irrigating syringe.
3. Place disposable bag near wound site.
4. Position client for easy access to wound.
5. Remove compression stockings, if used.
6. Don clean gloves.
7. Remove old dressing and place in disposal bag.
8. Remove clean gloves and discard into disposal bag. Don sterile gloves.
9. Fill irrigating syringe with normal saline. **Rationale:** Using the syringe will increase pressure in wound to assist with removing debris and slough.
10. Place moisture-proof pad or sterile basin under wound site.
11. Irrigate wound using the prescribed amount of irrigating solution.
12. Cleanse the surrounding skin with normal saline.
13. Dry periwound skin area.
14. Apply scalant to periwound area. **Rationale:** This protects periwound area from exudates.

The wound cover is sterile and protects wound from contamination and trauma. The cover maintains a moist and warm wound, which creates a healing environment. The cover is a thin shell with a window and a foam frame. The shell has an adhesive border, is water resistant and can be cleaned. It is flexible and moves with the client. The foam cover absorbs excess exudates to protect periwound area from maceration. The foam frame keeps the pocket above the wound surface, so warming card is not in contact with the wound. The window is in the center of the cover and contains a pocket for the warming card.

15. Select wound cover size that is appropriate size for wound. **Rationale:** To ensure that there is adequate healthy periwound skin between edge of foam and wound.
16. Hold wound cover near edges only. Pull away ½ of wound cover liner.
17. Place wound cover over wound, so wound can be seen through window. Do not stretch wound cover over skin while applying. **Rationale:** Damage can occur to skin.
18. Check for holes in wound cover, wrinkling, and folding of its edges. **Rationale:** Wound cover will not be a barrier if this occurs.
19. Press adhesive portion of cover to skin.
20. Pull away other half of wound cover liner and press adhesive portion to skin.
21. Gently smooth adhesive portion of wound cover with your finger tips to ensure adhesive sticks to skin.
22. Instruct the client that wound cover is worn 24 hours per day and requires no additional dressing.
23. Attach wound cover to Warm-Up® therapy system.
24. Remove gloves and discard into disposal bag.
25. Wash your hands.

for Using Warm-Up® Therapy System

1. Select appropriate size warming card based on size of wound cover.
2. Plug warming card into gray socket on temperature control unit (TCU).
3. Insert warming card into wound cover pocket. (Warming card is used throughout warming therapy and is only for one client; it can be cleaned with damp cloth and clean water, if needed. Do not apply the warming card directly to

CLINICAL ALERT

This warming treatment is done three times a day for 1 hour each treatment. Ensure that there is at least 1 hour between treatments. You can expect a significant increase in exudate for at least 7–10 days. This is considered a normal consequence of wound healing process.

EVIDENCE BASED NURSING PRACTICE

Effects of a Normothermic Dressing on Pressure Ulcer Healing

Twenty clients with Stage II and IV ulcers were studied to determine the effects of wound healing when heat was applied. Three groups were treated using three different methods; one group used heating therapy for 4.5 hours each day Monday–Friday for 4 weeks. One group had wounds warmed for two 60-minute periods daily. One group received no heat therapy. Results of the study indicated that the clients who received the most heat therapy healed significantly faster than the others. There were no adverse affects from the heat therapy.

Source: Kloth, Luther, C., et al. (2000, March/April). Effects of a normothermic dressing on pressure ulcer healing. *Advances in Skin & Wound Care, 13*(2).

the periwound area. Always cover the card with the wound cover. **Rationale:** Thermal injury can occur.

4. Turn off TCU.
5. Select mode of power (can use battery or AC adapter wall outlet).
6. Check that battery has sufficient charge for therapy session, usually one hour.
   a. If battery needs charging; plug AC adapter into TCU, then plug the AC adapter into wall outlet.
   b. Charge TCU until amber light on AC adapter flashes rapidly. It takes up to two hours to fully charge battery.
7. Plug AC adapter into black socket on the TCU, if using the TUC with the AC adapter. Plug AC adapter into wall outlet.
8. Position TCU and warming card cable to allow client some movement. Instruct client not to lie on any electronic component, cable, cord, or wound cover.
9. Press the ON button to begin therapy. Follow physician orders for length of time for therapy. The unit will automatically turn off after two hours of continuous use.
10. Shut off TCU and remove warming card by grasping edge of card and sliding it out of wound cover pocket. Place card in plastic pouch for storage between treatments. DO NOT REMOVE WOUND COVER. **Rationale:** Wound cover is replaced if drainage occurs, the cover comes loose, the periwound area becomes macerated, or it has been in place 72 hours.
11. Replace compression therapy if ordered.

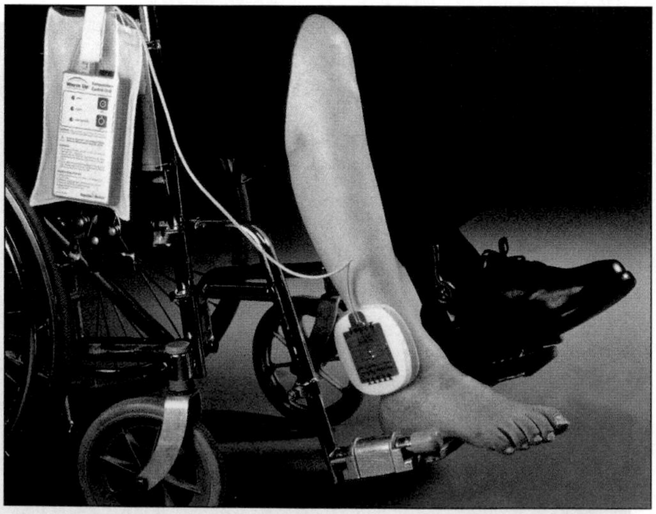

Warm-Up® Therapy unit. (Courtesy of Augustine Medical, Inc., Eden Prairie, MN.)

CLINICAL ALERT

Do not use compression therapy while warming card and TCU are in place. Client injury could occur.

for Changing Wound Cover

1. Check wound cover to ensure it needs to be changed.
2. Gather equipment for new wound cover.
3. Explain procedure to client.
4. Wash your hands.
5. Follow steps in skill *Using Noncontact Normothermic Wound Therapy*, Preparation.
6. Don clean gloves.
7. Place disposal bag near wound.
8. Gently press down on skin along one edge of wound cover.
9. Carefully lift edge of wound cover.
10. Slowly peel away wound cover until all edges are loose.
11. Discard wound cover in disposal bag.
12. Remove gloves, discard, and wash hands.
13. Reapply new wound cover following steps in skill *Using Noncontact Normothermic Wound Therapy*.

for Charging Batteries

1. Plug AC adapter connector into black socket on temperature control unit.
2. Plug AC adapter power cord into AC adapter inlet.
3. Plug AC adapter power cord into properly grounded wall outlet.
4. Observe that green light and a steady amber light on AC adapter panel are on.
5. Charge until amber light is flashing rapidly on AC adapter. Full charge takes 2 hours.

USING VACUUM ASSISTED CLOSURE

Equipment

Foam, Black or White V.A.C.® kit
Gauze pads
Sterile normal saline
Irrigating syringe
Moisture proof pad or sterile basin
Skin prep agent, optional
Razor, optional
Clean gloves
Sterile gloves
V.A.C.® device
Disposal bag
Sterile scissor

Preparation

1. Evaluate if client is candidate for V.A.C.® therapy: nutritionally stable, able to use device 22 hours each day, uses a pressure support surface if wound is over bony prominence.
2. Assess wound to determine if therapy can be implemented.
   a. Wound surrounded by at least 2 cm of intact periwound tissue to maintain air tight seal.
   b. Wound open enough to insert foam dressing that touches all edges.
   c. Wound debrided.
   d. Sufficient circulation to assist in healing process.
3. Select correct foam dressing according to size and type of wound. Black foam has larger pores and is used to stimulate granulation tissue and wound contraction. White (soft) foam is used when granulation tissue needs to be restricted or client cannot tolerate pain associated with Black foam. White foam is used with superficial wounds, shallow chronic ulcers, and tunneling or undermining wounds.
4. Gather equipment and supplies.
5. Provide privacy.
6. Explain procedure to client and determine his willingness to use this therapy.
7. Wash your hands.

Procedure

1. Place disposal bag near wound.
2. Open supplies and place on overbed table. Open kit maintaining sterility.
3. Draw up irrigating solution in syringe.
4. Don clean gloves.
5. Remove old V.A.C.® dressing and place in disposal bag.
6. Place moisture proof pad or sterile basin under wound. **Rationale:** Protects skin and bed during irrigation.
7. Clean wound using aggressive irrigation. If debridement is to be done, only a trained professional can perform the skill. Notify the appropriate person.
8. Remove gloves and place in disposal bag.

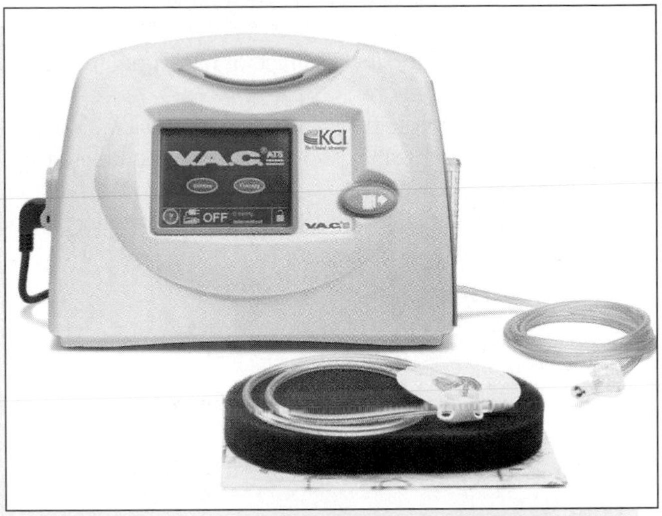

V.A.C.®-ATS machine is placed on level surface or hangs on foot of bed. (Courtesy of Kinetic Concepts, Inc. San Antonio, TX.)

9. Don sterile gloves.
10. Dry wound and prepare periwound tissue with skin preparation agent if necessary. **Rationale:** To promote an airtight seal.
11. Cut the V.A.C.® foam to fit the shape and entire wound cavity, including tunneling or undermined areas.
12. Size and trim drape to cover foam dressing, leaving a 3.5 cm border per wound skin.
13. Gently place the foam into wound ensuring entire wound is covered.
14. Apply tubing to foam. Tubing can be laid on top of foam or placed inside foam dressing. Keep tubing away from bony prominences.

> **CLINICAL ALERT**
>
> For deep wound, reposition tubing to minimize pressure on wound edges every 2 hours. Excess foam can be used to cushion skin under tubing.

15. Cover foam and 3.5 cm per wound area with drape. Do not stretch drape or compress foam with drape. **Rationale:** This ensures a tight seal without causing tension or a shearing force on periwound tissue.
16. Lift tubing and place on drape that has been bunched up to protect skin from pressure of tube.
17. Secure tubing with additional piece of drape or tape several centimeters away from dressing. **Rationale:** This prevents pulling on the dressing, leading to a leak.
18. Remove gloves and discard.
19. Remove canister from sterile package and push it into the V.A.C.® unit until you hear it click in place. Alarm will sound if canister is not properly inserted into unit.

20. Connect dressing tubing to canister tubing.
21. Open both clamps, one on dressing tubing and one on canister tubing.
22. Place V.A.C.® unit on level surface or hang from footboard.
23. Press power button ON.
24. Adjust V.A.C.® unit settings according to physician's orders or Guidelines for Treating Wound Types in the Reference Manual.
25. Assess dressing in 1 minute. **Rationale:** The dressing should collapse unless air leak is present.

for Removing Dressing

1. Wash hands.
2. Don clean gloves.
3. Raise tube connector above level of pump unit.
4. Tighten clamp on dressing tube.
5. Separate canister tube and dressing tubes by disconnecting the connector.
6. Allow pump unit to pull exudates in canister tube into canister; then tighten clamps on canister tube.
7. Press Therapy ON/OFF to deactivate pump
8. Stretch drape horizontally and slowly pull up from skin. Gently remove it from skin. Do not peel if off skin.
9. Discard disposable equipment including gloves in appropriate bag or container.
10. Wash your hands.

for Disconnecting V.A.C.® Unit

1. Turn the unit to OFF.
2. Clamp both clamps on tubing.
3. Press quick release connector to separate dressing tubing from canister tubing
4. Cover ends of tubing with gauze and secure.

for Reconnecting V.A.C.® Unit

1. Remove gauze from ends of tubing.
2. Connect tubing.
3. Unclamp clamps
4. Press V.A.C.® green power button to ON.
5. Select NO at new client prompt. Unit will resume previous settings.
6. Press therapy to ON.

CLINICAL ALERT

Clients should be disconnected from unit for very short periods of time—no more than a total of 2 hours per day.

for Changing Canister

1. Don clean gloves.
2. Assess that canister unit is full. Unit will alarm when full.
3. Tighten clamps on canister tubing from dressing tubing.
4. Pull back on release knob on V.A.C.® unit at same time as you pull canister from slot.
5. Put canister in biohazard disposable bag and place in designated area for disposal.
6. Dispose of gloves.
7. Wash your hands.

CHARTING FOR ADJUNCTIVE WOUND CARE THERAPY

- Wound assessment including location, measurement of wound, presence of tunneling or undermining.
- Color of wound, presence of exudates, color, and odor.
- Wound stage, if appropriate.
- Eschar description if present.
- Presence of pain in periwound area.
- Type, frequency, and duration of adjunctive therapy.
- Date and time of wound cover change in Warm-Up® therapy.
- Clients response to therapy.
- Length of time V.A.C.® treatment is off.

Critical Thinking Application

UNEXPECTED OUTCOMES	CRITICAL THINKING OPTIONS
Warm-Up® Therapy system shows heat light is on and low battery light is flashing.	• Charge battery. • Use TCU and AC adapter together.
Fault light is flashing and an alarm is sounding on TCU.	• Reconnect warming card, it may be disconnected. • Warming card or cable could be bent or damaged. Replace warming card. • TCU is broken. Turn TCU on and off. If light continues and alarm continues, turn off TCU and obtain new unit.
Nothing lights up on TCU panel.	• TCU is not on or battery is low. Turn unit ON or charge battery.
Wound is too large for V.A.C.® kit.	• Use more than 1 foam piece. • Place pieces so they touch each other. • Use only one tubing to one of the pieces.
Periwound skin is fragile.	• Use skin prep prior to applying drape. • Frame wound with skin barrier or Duoderm. • Cut drape large enough to enclose foam dressing and skin barrier layer.
Dressing does not collapse following V.A.C.® application.	• Listen for whistling sound indicating a leak in the system. • Gently press around tubing, check for wrinkles or drape not covering correctly. • Most leaks occur around tubing. • Use excess drape to patch over leak.
Foam is not collapsed in wound bed.	• Ensure therapy is ON. Ensure clamps are open and tubing is not kinked. • Check for leaks and patch.

Gerontologic Considerations

As clients grow older, the usual function of the skin declines leading to major complications. Nearly 40% of clients aged 65–75 have at least one significant problem related to the skin.

- Dry skin is present in 77% of clients over 64.
- Vitamin D deficiency.
- Decrease in sebum production.
- Decrease in sweat production.
- Decrease in thermoregulation.
- Basal cell carcinoma is most common skin malignancy.
- Decrease in sensory perception.

The inflammatory and proliferation phases of wound healing are often defective with elderly clients who have chronic diseases.

- A hemoglobin below 10 g/dL increases susceptibility.
- Uncontrolled diabetes mellitus or a blood glucose level that exceeds 200 mg/dL presents a risk.
- Hyperglycemia retards neutrophil production.
- T and B cells diminish in function and number, indicating a reduced inflammatory response. Elderly clients are at risk for cutaneous viral and fungal infections.

- Clients with rheumatoid arthritis who take steroids or nonsteroidal anti-inflammatory medications are at risk for decreased wound healing. There is a slower rate of epithelialization and severely inhibited contraction.
- Ischemia, anemia, and edema from vascular insufficiency or pressure leads to lack of blood flow to a wound area. Lower oxygen-carrying capacity results from anemia. Edema makes it difficult to transport oxygen and cellular wastes to and from cells. Ischemia leads to diminished oxygen necessary for wound healing.

Nursing actions to counteract risks against wound healing

- All at-risk elderly clients should have a pressure ulcer risk assessment completed at the time of admission and at regular intervals thereafter.
- Use of compression stockings assists in treating both the edema and ultimately the ischemia, therefore increasing blood flow to wound area.
- Turning frequently, at least every 2 hours, for clients free of pressure ulcers and every 1 hour for those at high risk, should be a priority.
- Use of pressure-relieving mattresses decreases risk potential.
- Wound care, including irrigation, use of appropriate dressings, and maintaining aseptic technique with dressing changes, should be priority care for clients with any type of wound.

MANAGEMENT GUIDELINES

Each state legislates a Nurse Practice Act for RNs and LVN/LPNs. Health care facilities are responsible for establishing and implementing policies and procedures that conform to their state's regulations. Verify the regulations and role parameters for each health care worker in your facility.

Delegation of Responsibilities

- Assessment and evaluation of wounds and their management modalities are only RN functions and may not be delegated to other health care workers. The RN in collaboration with the physician develops a plan of care for clients requiring wound management.
- An LVN/LPN may be assigned to complete a sterile dressing change following instructions from the RN and in accordance with the wound care protocol established for the individual client.
- An LVN/LPN may remove staples and sutures after instruction and return demonstrations have been documented. (Most nursing programs include this information in the curriculum.)
- A CNA may apply a dry dressing, but may not perform a sterile procedure.

Information Flow

- Information regarding assessment of the wound should be reported to all staff caring for the client. This can be accomplished during report, documented on the nurses' notes and on client care plans or clinical (critical) pathway documents.
- Wound care procedures (i.e., dressing changes), should be outlined or special wound care steps inserted into computer record. Specific instructions as to type and amount of dressing material needed and specific directions in the application of the dressings must be written clearly so all nurses may follow appropriate directions.
- Specific directions for wound management and use of specialized equipment must be given to the nurse during report from the RN team leader or manager.
- Reports outlining specifics of the wound, such as color, odor, and amount of drainage, must be provided to the RN manager after the dressing change has been completed.
- Any change in wound appearance must be immediately reported to the RN team leader or manager before the dressing change has been completed.

CRITICAL THINKING STRATEGIES

SCENARIO 1

Mrs. Johnson is an 84-year-old retired school teacher who was widowed 10 years ago and now lives alone. She developed diabetes mellitus at the age of 58. She has been in failing health for the last 3 years and has been at home with the assistance of home health aides and weekly visits by the RN. Her coccyx area has had frequent skin breakdown. The Homecare RN determined she now has a stage III pressure ulcer as a result of her being on bed rest the past week. She is being admitted to the hospital for treatment of the ulcer.

1. Identify risk factors for Mrs. Johnson developing pressure ulcers.
2. Describe the stage III pressure ulcer.
3. Identify the most effective treatment for the stage III pressure ulcer.
4. Compare and contrast the two Pressure Ulcer Assessment Scales and identify the score indicating that Mrs. Johnson is a high risk for pressure ulcer formation on one of the scales.
5. In addition to dressing changes, identify a preventative therapy that should be used for clients at high risk for pressure ulcers.
6. Explain why massaging bony prominences should be avoided for clients at risk for pressure ulcer formation.
7. Briefly describe the application of a hydrocolloid dressing.
8. Identify and briefly explain the use of one new advance in the treatment of pressure ulcers.

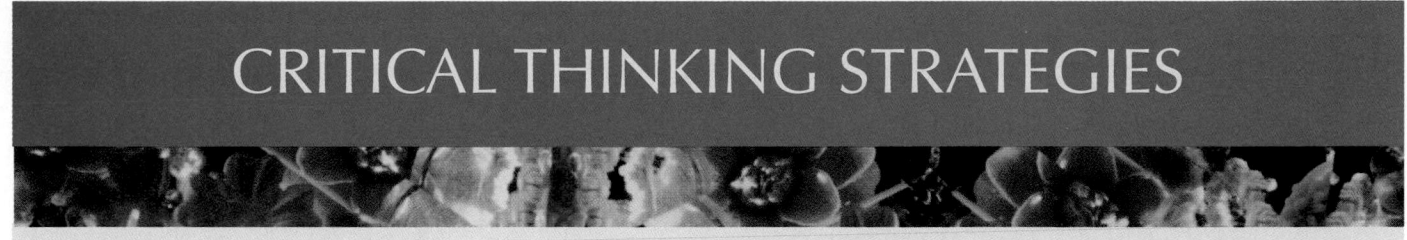

CHAPTER 26

Respiratory Care

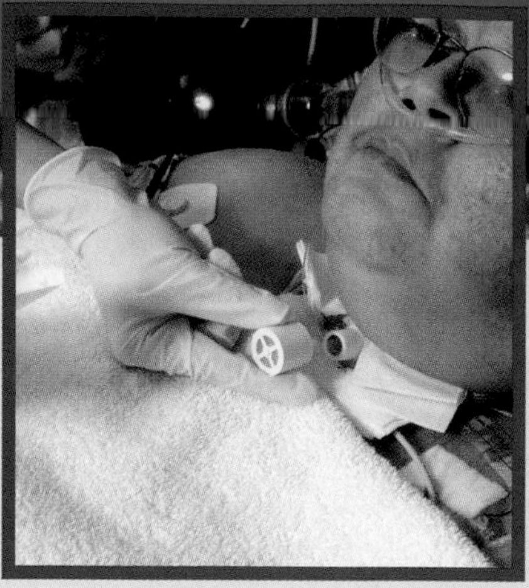

THEORETICAL CONCEPTS

UNIT ONE: Respiratory Preventive and Maintenance Measures 876

Instructing Client to Deep Breathe 877
Instructing Client to Cough 877
Teaching Diaphragmatic Breathing 878
Teaching Use of an Incentive Spirometer (IS) 878
Teaching Peak Flow Measurement 879
Providing CPAP/BIPAP 880
Providing Bag–Valve–Mask Ventilation 881

UNIT TWO: Chest Physiotherapy (CPT) 883

Preparing Client for CPT 884
Performing Postural Drainage 884
Performing Chest Percussion 885
Performing Chest Vibration 885

UNIT THREE: Oxygen Administration 887

Monitoring Clients Receiving Oxygen 888
Using Pulse Oximetry 888
Using an Oxygen Analyzer 890
Using an Oxygen Cylinder 890
Using Nasal Cannula 891
Using an Oxygen Face Mask 892
Providing Oxygen via a Pediatric Tent 894
for Setting Up Pediatric Tent 894
for Monitoring Child in Tent 894
Using an Oxygen Hood 895

UNIT FOUR: Artificial Intubated Airways 897

Inserting an Oropharyngeal Airway 898
Inserting a Nasopharyngeal Airway (Nasal Trumpet) 898
Assisting with Endotracheal Intubation 899
Providing Care for Client with Endotracheal Tube 900
Extubating an Endotracheal Tube 901

UNIT FIVE: Suctioning 903

Suctioning Using Catheter and Gloves 904
Suctioning Using Catheter in Sleeve 906
Suctioning with In-Line Closed Suction System 907

UNIT SIX: Tracheostomy Care 910

Assisting with Tracheostomy Intubation 911
Performing Tracheostomy Suctioning 912
Inflating a Tracheal Tube Cuff 914
Cleaning the Inner Cannula and Ostomy 914
Changing Tracheostomy Tube Ties 916
for Twill Tape Ties 916
Capping with a Passey–Muir Valve 917

UNIT SEVEN: Chest Drainage Systems 921

Maintaining a Two-Bottle Drainage/Suction System 922
for Gravity Drainage 922
for Suction 922
Setting Up and Maintaining a Disposable Water-Seal Chest Drainage System 923
Administering Autotransfusion Using Pleur-Evac ATS 925
Assisting with Removal of Chest Tube 926

GERONTOLOGIC CONSIDERATIONS 929

MANAGEMENT GUIDELINES 929

CRITICAL THINKING STRATEGIES 931

Learning Objectives

- Outline the three processes of respiration.
- Identify three nursing diagnoses for clients with ventilatory dysfunction.
- Describe the steps for teaching a client deep breathing and coughing exercises.
- Discuss the purpose of using an incentive spirometer.
- Describe the steps for peak flow measurement.
- Describe positions for postural drainage and chest percussion and vibration.
- Differentiate modes of oxygen delivery and describe nursing care relevant to each mode.
- Differentiate various modes of airway maintenance.
- Outline the care needs of the intubated client.
- Describe the nursing actions included in tracheostomy care.
- Explain the procedure for inflating a tracheal tube cuff.
- Describe safety measures used when suctioning clients.
- List measures to promote safe, effective care for clients with chest tubes.

Terminology

Acidosis: accumulation of acids (metabolic or respiratory), potentially disturbing acid–base balance and causing acidemia (low pH).

Adventitious: abnormal extra sounds (crackles, wheezes) superimposed on breath sounds.

Alkalosis: condition in which the alkalinity of the body tends to increase beyond normal, potentially resulting in alkalemia (high pH).

Apnea: cessation of breathing, usually of a temporary nature.

Atelectasis: collapse of alveoli, which may lead to hypoxemia, increased PCO_2 and pneumonia.

Auscultation: process of listening for sounds produced by body organs.

Bradycardia: slow heart rate (below 60 beats/min).

Bronchiectasis: dilation of a bronchus or bronchi with production of large amounts of malodorous secretions.

Crackles: discontinuous popping (opening) sounds indicative of hypoventilation of alveoli, usually auscultated at end of inspiration in dependent lung areas.

Cyanosis: bluish or grayish discoloration of the skin resulting from significant reduction of oxygen saturation of hemoglobin (< 85% saturation).

Diaphoresis: profuse sweating.

Dyspnea: a subjective feeling of having difficulty breathing.

Expectorant: an agent that facilitates the removal of airway secretions.

Hemothorax: blood in the pleural space resulting in compression of normal lung tissue.

Hyperventilation: abnormally deep breathing that results in a decrease in PCO_2 (respiratory alkalosis).

Hypoventilation: reduced rate and depth of breathing resulting in retention of carbon dioxide (respiratory acidosis).

Hypoxemia: insufficient oxygenation of the blood (decreased PO_2).

Hypoxia: lack of adequate amount of oxygen transported to the tissues.

Intubation: to insert a tube into a body opening as into the trachea.

Narcosis: unconscious state due to narcotics or other depressing agent (e.g., elevated PCO_2).

Nares: the nostrils.

Percussion: rhythmic striking of the thorax to loosen pulmonary secretions.

Pneumothorax: presence of air in the intrapleural space resulting in lung collapse.

Polycythemia: excess number of red blood cells.

Postural drainage: the use of gravity to drain secretions from the airways.

Spirometer: device used for measuring inhalation and exhalation volumes.

Sputum: substance expelled by coughing.

Tachypnea: increased rate of breathing (over 24 breaths/min).

Tension pneumothorax: lung collapse with potential contralateral shift of mediastinal structures resulting from accumulation of air or fluid in the intrapleural space.

Tracheostomy: surgical opening into the trachea usually for insertion of a tube to provide airway patency.

Ventilation: the acts of inspiration and exhalation for the exchange of oxygen and carbon dioxide between the lungs and the atmosphere.

Vibration: therapeutic high-frequency shaking of a body part.

Wheezes: musical adventitious sounds heard on inspiration and/or expiration due to airway spasm, retained secretions, or other obstruction.

THE RESPIRATORY SYSTEM

The respiratory system provides for the exchange of gases between the blood and the external environment so that cellular respiration can occur. The respiratory structures involved include the nose, pharynx, larynx, trachea, bronchi, lungs, diaphragm, intercostal muscles, and ribs.

The upper respiratory tract includes the nose, pharynx, and larynx. These structures filter, warm, and humidify the air before it passes into the lower airways. When the upper respiratory tract is bypassed by intubation or tracheostomy these protective processes are lost.

The lower respiratory tract is considered a sterile environment. It begins below the larynx. The trachea is composed of smooth muscle reinforced by C-shaped rings of cartilage lined with a membranous sheath. It branches into the right and left mainstream bronchi. The right bronchus extends vertically from the trachea, whereas the left bronchus branches from the trachea at an angle. The right and left bronchi divide further and further into terminal bronchioles and finally into respiratory bronchioles, alveolar ducts, and alveoli.

Because of the anatomical difference of the bronchi, migration of an endotracheal tube (ET) into the right bronchus occurs more frequently. Such a migration would result in ventilation of only the right lung. Chest x-rays are taken to ensure proper placement of ET tubes in the trachea. Auscultation of *bilateral* breath sounds also helps to verify optimal ventilation of intubated clients.

Protective processes of the lower airway include mucus secretion and the presence of special hairlike cells (cilia). This "mucociliary escalator" continuously traps and moves inhaled irritants up toward the pharynx to be removed by swallowing or coughing. Drying pharmacologic agents and pathophysiologic states (e.g., immobility) interfere with these protective processes and place the client at risk for pulmonary complications.

PROCESSES OF RESPIRATION

Cellular respiration occurs when oxygen is transported from the atmosphere to tissue cells, and carbon dioxide is removed and carried from the cells to the atmosphere. RBC hemoglobin is the carrier for these gases. Three processes—ventilation, diffusion, and perfusion—are essential for this to occur.

Ventilation is the mechanical exchange of air between the lungs and the atmosphere. *Inspiration* is the *active* phase of ventilation. It requires contraction of the diaphragm and external intercostal muscles to expand the thorax. When thoracic expansion occurs, intrapulmonic pressure becomes lower than atmospheric pressure, and air flows into the lungs. *Exhalation* is the *passive* phase of

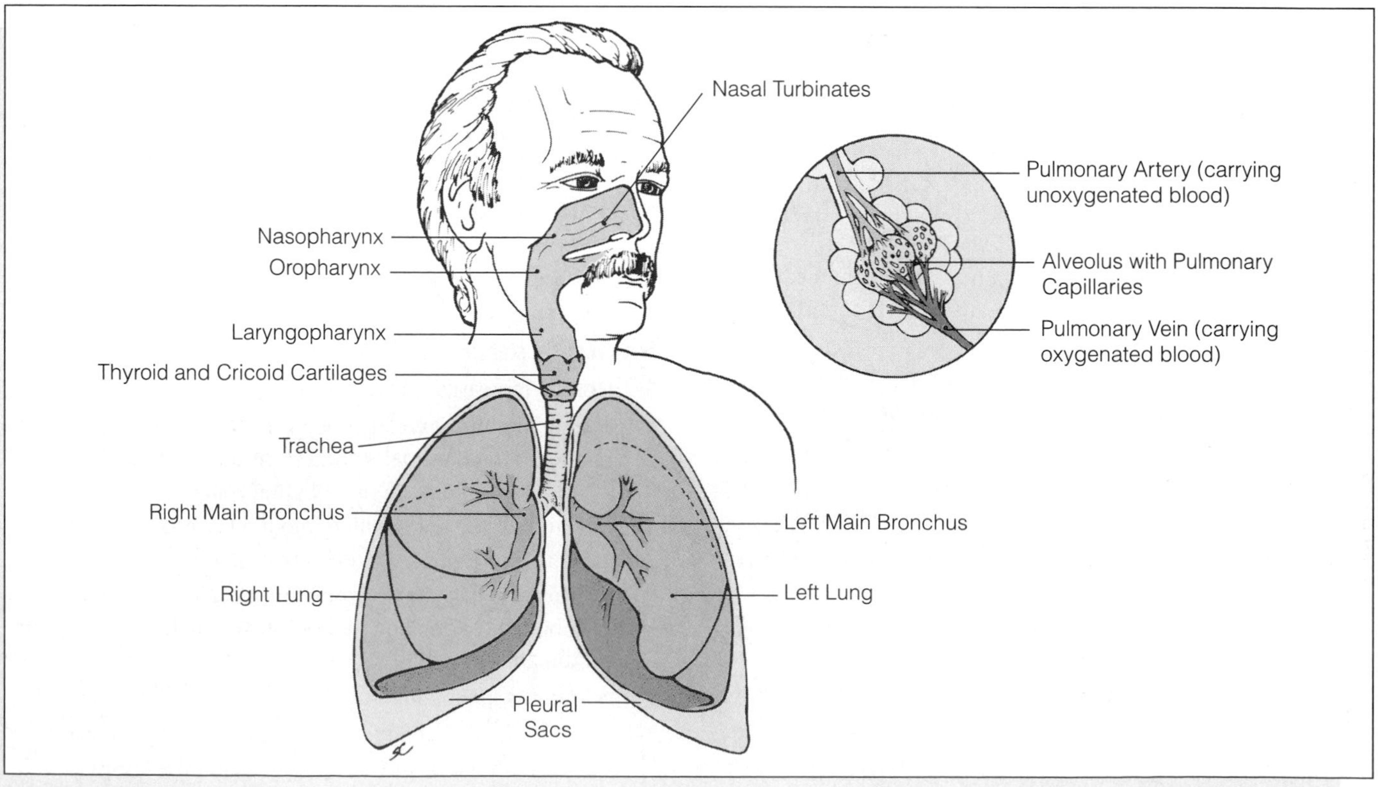

Anatomy of the respiratory system.

ventilation. It occurs when alveolar pressure increases due to elastic recoil of lung tissue and relaxation of the respiratory muscles, and air flows out of the lungs back into the atmosphere.

Ventilation is controlled by the brain stem, which responds to a rise in blood carbon dioxide level (P_{CO_2}). As breathing eliminates CO_2, there is a negative feedback to the brain. Through exhalation of carbon dioxide (which with water forms the volatile acid carbonic acid in the bloodstream) the lungs play a vital role in maintaining the normal alkaline pH of the blood (7.35–7.45). Conditions that result in metabolic acidosis (e.g., diabetic ketoacidosis) make the blood more acidic, also stimulating the brain stem to increase the rate and depth of breathing. The resultant lowering of P_{CO_2} (exhalation of volatile acid or respiratory alkalosis) helps return the blood pH to an alkaline state. This process is called respiratory compensation for metabolic acidosis.

Although CO_2 is the major stimulus for breathing, high sustained levels of carbonic acid depress the respiratory center, and respiratory arrest can occur. Individuals who have chronically elevated P_{CO_2} levels due to chronic obstructive pulmonary disease (COPD) may become insensitive to P_{CO_2} as a stimulus for breathing. Instead, their brain responds to a lower than normal P_{O_2} (less than 60 mm Hg) to stimulate breathing. The administration of high flows of oxygen to such "hypoxic-dependent breathers" can eliminate their stimulus to breathe. Such individuals are at high risk for CO_2 narcosis.

Diffusion is the process of gas exchange between the alveolar air and the blood. The respiratory unit (respiratory bronchiole, alveolar ducts, and alveoli) is surrounded by capillaries, which allow for this exchange of oxygen and carbon dioxide. Alveoli must be ventilated and must remain diffusable for gas exchange to prevent respiratory failure. Oxygen tension in blood flowing through alveolar capillaries is *lower* than the oxygen tension in the alveoli. This pressure gradient causes oxygen to pass from the alveoli to the blood, thus increasing the P_{O_2} and "arterializing" the blood. Conversely, carbon dioxide tension is *higher* in the capillary blood than it is in the alveoli, thus promoting its diffusion into alveoli and the elimination of carbon dioxide on exhalation.

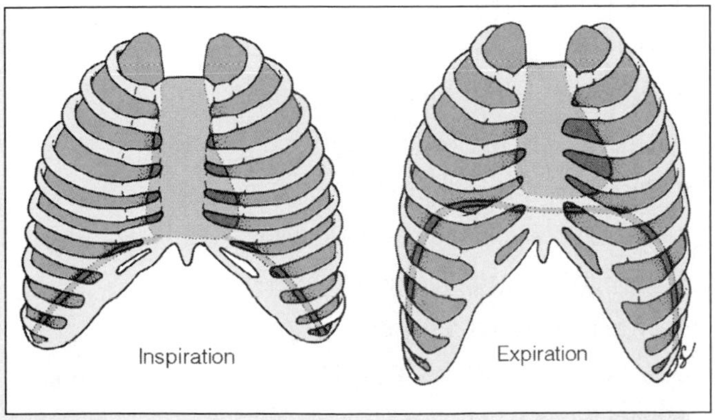

Position of diaphragm at full-end inspiration and full-end expiration.

Perfusion is the process of circulating oxygen and carbon dioxide between the lungs and tissue cells. Without this blood transport and exchange of gases at both the pulmonary and tissue capillary levels, survival is impossible.

Alterations in Respiration

Alterations in tissue respiration can result from dysfunction of any of the three essential processes previously outlined.

Alterations in Ventilation

Ventilation depends on patent airways, the ability to clear airways, chest expansion, and compliant alveoli. Many factors and disease processes can interfere with adequate ventilation, including (a) any limitation in ability to clear airways (ineffective cough, intubation, decreased level of consciousness); (b) any limitation on alveolar expansion (pneumonia, congestive heart failure, fractured ribs, pain, thoracic deformity, neurologic disease, respiratory depressants, immobility); and (c) factors that interfere with surfactant activity, which is essential for alveolar inflation (narcotics, anesthetics, hypoventilation, high oxygen flow rates). Inadequate ventilation results in abnormal arterial blood gases (low P_{O_2} and low Sa_{O_2}, and eventually, an increase in P_{CO_2}).

Pathologic processes that cause ineffective exhalation due to loss of alveolar elastic recoil or decreased airway resistance to increased intrathoracic pressure (as with exhalation or coughing) also result in an increased P_{CO_2} (respiratory acidosis). Chronic obstructive pulmonary disease is an example.

Alterations in Diffusion

Diffusion is dependent on a partial pressure difference in gases and an adequate amount of permeable alveolar surface area. Any disease that thickens the alveolar membrane (fibrosis, congestive heart failure) reduces alveolar permeability and leads to a reduced P_{O_2} (hypoxemia). Alveolar surface area can be reduced by lobectomy or pneumonectomy.

Alterations in Perfusion

For cells to receive oxygen and give off their wastes, blood must flow at both the pulmonary and tissue capillary levels. Adequate perfusion depends on a normal blood volume, an adequate amount of hemoglobin capable of combining with oxygen and carbon dioxide, effective cardiac function, and competent vasculature. Any pathology that interferes with blood cell production, maintenance of blood volume, cardiac function, or vascular patency can result in inadequate tissue perfusion. Likewise, any factor that prevents blood from flowing through pulmonary capillaries (pulmonary embolism) disrupts the process of gas exchange for replenishment of oxygen and the elimination of carbon dioxide.

ASSESSMENT OF RESPIRATORY FUNCTION

Arterial blood gases and pulmonary function tests reflect pulmonary capacity. The pH of the blood is affected by pulmonary function. If carbon dioxide is not eliminated by the lungs due to hypoventilation for any reason, the Pco_2 rises. Since CO_2 creates an acid in the bloodstream, its accumulation (respiration acidosis) causes the blood pH to decrease (acidemia). *Hypoventilation* is the only mechanism for Pco_2 accumulation and is encountered when factors depress the respiratory center, inhibit breathing, or a client has a disease, such as COPD, that prevents efficient exhalation. The peak flow meter measures maximum expiratory flow rates. These units are used by asthma clients to regularly self-assess. A declining flow rate (by 20%) may indicate a worsening condition. Serial measurements help the physician to adjust the client's medical regimen. *Hyperventilation* (due to anxiety, neurologic dysfunction, or iatrogenic overventilation) causes the Pco_2 to fall below normal (respiratory alkalosis) and the blood pH to rise above normal (alkalemia).

Arterial blood gas (ABG) studies also evaluate diffusion and perfusion as reflected by the Po_2 and Sao_2. Pulse oximetry is often preferred over ABGs as a cost-effective laboratory test of Sao_2.

It is essential that ventilation of alveoli is matched with blood flowing through alveolar capillaries. If alveolar ventilation occurs without matched perfusion (e.g., pulmonary embolism), the Po_2 falls, but the Pco_2 remains normal because of the great solubility of CO_2; the Pco_2 may even decrease due to hyperventilation (respiratory alkalosis). Conversely, if the alveoli are perfused but not ventilated (as in atelectasis), the blood is not adequately oxygenated. This condition results in a low Po_2 and a normal Pco_2, because carbon dioxide is highly diffusible. Continued hypoventilation, however, eventually results in an increased Pco_2 (respiratory acidosis).

Normal pulmonary ventilation and perfusion are reflected by *normal blood gas values*: *Note*: Pulse oximetry (Spo_2) allows noninvasive estimation of Sao_2.

pH	7.35–7.45
Pco_2	35–45 mm Hg
HCO_3	22–26 mEq/L
Po_2	80–100 mm Hg (breathing room air)
Sao_2	90–100%

Pulmonary function (spirometry) tests measure lung volume and capacity, and help differentiate restrictive and obstructive defects of ventilation.

VC (vital capacity)	75–80% of that predicted by age, sex, and height (decreased in restrictive disease)
FEV (forced expiratory volume)	65–85% of VC in 1 second and 95% in 3 seconds (decreased in obstructive disease)
FEV_1 (forced expiratory volume in 1 sec)	Normal = 75% VC (decreased in obstructive disease)
FEV 25–75	Measures expiratory flow capacity of small airways; most sensitive measure of small airway disease

Nursing Interventions

The goal of respiratory nursing interventions is to maintain, restore, or to artificially provide the vital functions of the respiratory system.

Nursing interventions are used routinely to help prevent pulmonary complications for clients with known pulmonary problems, for clients who are at risk for pulmonary complications (e.g., immobility), or for surgical clients who have undergone general anesthesia and who experience pain.

These interventions include pain management; maintaining adequate hydration (2–3 L of water/day unless contraindicated); turning to help ventilate dependent lung areas; deep breathing to stimulate surfactant and inflate hypoventilated alveoli; coughing to remove

The most common clinical manifestations indicative of inadequate ventilation are:

- Tachycardia (heart rate over 100/min)
- Tachypnea (breathing rate over 24/min)
- Anxiety reflected in facial expression
- Restlessness or confusion
- Use of accessory muscles for breathing
- Change in cognition or level of response
- Increased blood pressure

Early recognition of these indicators of possible hypoxemia should prompt further investigation and appropriate intervention

retained secretions; and airway suctioning to assist ineffective airway clearance and early ambulation. Protective splinting of operative sites promotes client comfort, adherence, and prevents wound strain.

CPAP/BIPAP is the noninvasive application of positive pressure to upper airways to prevent their obstruction by the soft tissues that surround them. Clients with obstructive sleep apnea, central sleep apnea, or respiratory insufficiency may benefit from this therapy.

Techniques such as postural drainage, chest percussion and vibration (CPT) utilize gravity and mechanical energy to help mobilize secretions. These measures are reserved for the client who produces excessive amounts (> 25 mL/day) of thick secretions that are difficult to mobilize.

A variety of devices are used to deliver supplemental oxygen to the hypoxic client (Sao_2 under 90%). These devices differ in the degree that they control the client's inspired air.

Artificial means to establish and maintain patent airways include oral/pharyngeal and endotracheal devices. Bypassing the body's natural protective airway and communication processes, these devices render the client dependent and at risk for serious respiratory complications. Clients with artificial airways require additional nursing measures to assure ventilation and to protect the respiratory system. Such skills includes suctioning, tracheostomy care, and providing a means for communication.

If air or fluid accumulates in the intrapleural or mediastinal space due to trauma, disease, or surgery, the lung cannot expand. Cardiac tamponade can occur due to decreased venous return secondary to compression of mediastinal structures may compromise cardiac output. Chest tubes are placed to evacuate air and fluid from the pleural or mediastinal space to facilitate lung re-expansion and prevent increased mediastinal pressure. In certain post-operative settings, chest drainage may be reinfused to replace blood lost.

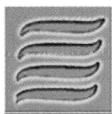

NURSING DIAGNOSES

The following nursing diagnoses may be appropriate to use on client care plans when the components are related to respiratory conditions.

NURSING DIAGNOSIS	RELATED FACTORS
Activity Intolerance	Imbalance between oxygen supply and demand
Ineffective Airway Clearance	Fatigue; excessive secretions; pain
Ineffective Breathing Pattern	Immobility; fatigue, pain; neuromuscular impairment; chronic respiratory disease; pharmacologic agents
Potential for Aspiration	Absence of airway protective mechanisms; presence of artificial airway; enteral feeding
Impaired Gas Exchange	Ventilation/perfusion imbalance; changes in ABGs; hypoventilation
Imbalanced Nutrition: less than body requirements	Fatigue; aerophagia; increased work of breathing
Deficient knowledge	Lack of understanding that chronic condition requires self-monitoring

- The single most important nursing action to decrease the incidence of hospital-based infection is handwashing. **Remember to wash your hands or use antibacterial gel before and after each client contact.**

UNIT 1

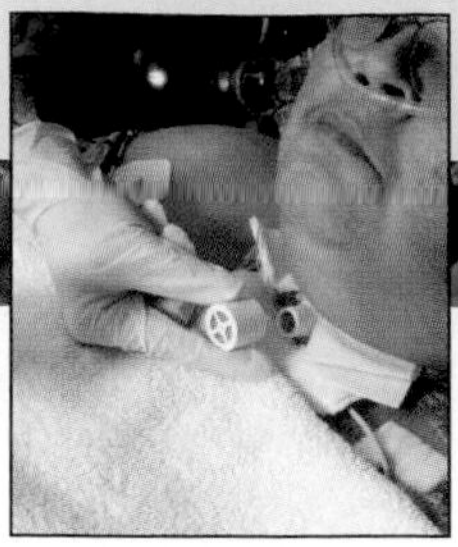

Respiratory Preventive and Maintenance Measures

Nursing Process Data

ASSESSMENT *Data Base*

Observe client's physical ability to perform exercise (e.g., to assume Fowler's position, energy level, degree of pain experienced and need for pain medication).

Observe rhythm, rate, and depth of breathing.

Auscultate breath sounds.

Note client's report of dyspnea or signs of stertorous breathing.

Note presence of adventitious sounds.

Note proximity of incision to muscles necessary for breathing and coughing.

Assess need for supported ventilation/resuscitation.

PLANNING *Objectives*

To improve vital capacity and pulmonary ventilation.

To conserve energy and decrease the work of breathing.

To loosen secretions and promote clear airways.

To prevent hypoventilation and hypoxemia.

IMPLEMENTATION *Procedures*

Instructing Client to Deep Breathe

Instructing Client to Cough

Teaching Diaphragmatic Breathing

Teaching Use of an Incentive Spirometer (IS)

Teaching Peak Flow Measurement

Providing CPAP/BIPAP

Providing Bag–Valve–Mask Ventilation

EVALUATION *Expected Outcomes*

Breath sounds are normal; adventitious sounds are cleared.

Vital capacity, pulmonary ventilation, and gas exchange are improved/supported.

Client reaches predetermined tidal volume level when using incentive spirometer.

Client's energy is conserved and work of breathing is eased.

Secretions are loosened and airways are clear.

Client monitors peak-flow appropriately.

Client experiences an improved sleep pattern.

INSTRUCTING CLIENT TO DEEP BREATHE

Equipment

Straight chair or hospital bed at 90° elevation

Preparation

1. Wash your hands.
2. Provide privacy.
3. Explain the rationale for the procedure.
4. Help client to sit straight up in bed or on side of bed with knees slightly flexed. **Rationale:** This position promotes maximum lung expansion.

Procedure

1. Demonstrate the deep breathing steps, allowing time for client to practice each step.

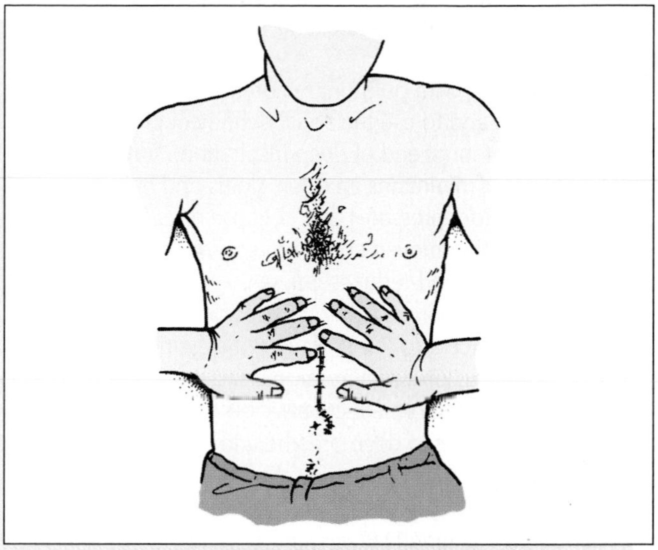

Instruct client in deep breathing exercises to enhance lung expansion.

2. Place your hand or have client place hands palm down around the sides of client's lower ribs. **Rationale:** This action supports deep breathing and assists you to evaluate depth of inspiration.
3. Tell client to breathe in slowly through nose until chest expands and abdomen rises visibly.
4. Have client hold a sustained maximal inspiration 3–5 seconds, then exhale slowly through the mouth.
5. Evaluate client's response to determine how often exercise should be performed—diminished breath sounds or presence of crackles indicates need for frequent deep breathing, turning, and early ambulation.

EVIDENCE BASED NURSING PRACTICE

Improving Oxygenation

Studies show that the Po_2 is lower when the client with unilateral lung disease is positioned on the diseased side. Since the dependent lung has greater blood flow, placing the healthy lung down improves oxygenation.

Source: Bridges, E. (2001). Ask the experts. *Critical Care Nurse, 21*(6), 66.

INSTRUCTING CLIENT TO COUGH

Equipment

Straight chair or hospital bed at 90° elevation
Pillows for positioning and incisional support
Tissues for secretions
Protective gear (gloves, gown, goggles, mask) as indicated

Preparation

1. Premedicate client if indicated for pain-relief.
2. Wash your hands.
3. Provide privacy.
4. Explain procedure to client.
5. Don protective gear if indicated.
6. Provide client with tissues.

Procedure

1. Place client in upright position, upper body positioned slightly forward. **Rationale:** This position assists client to cough more effectively.
2. Ask client to slowly take two or three deep breaths through the nose and exhale through the mouth.

CLINICAL ALERT

Deep breathing is indicated, but coughing is *contra*indicated for the client post-eye, -ear, -brain or -neck surgery, or if efforts are nonproductive.

3. Instruct client to inhale deeply, hold breath for several seconds, lean forward and cough, using abdominal, thigh, and buttock muscles. **Rationale:** This promotes a more effective cough.
4. Instruct client with pulmonary condition to exhale through pursed lips and to use the "huff" while coughing in mid exhalation (not at end of deep inspiration). **Rationale:** The "huff cough" maintains an open glottis and helps prevent high expiratory pressures that collapse diseased airways, thus facilitating movement of secretions along the tracheobronchial tree and reduces fatigue.
5. Support any incision with the palms of your or client's hands, or place a rolled pillow firmly against the incision. **Rationale:** This prevents incisional strain and encourages client to cough more effectively.
6. Encourage client to deep breathe and cough more frequently *if* cough is productive. Explain why coughing is beneficial and keep tissues and disposal receptacle handy. **Rationale:** Accumulated secretions in airways promote bacterial growth and interfere with ventilation.

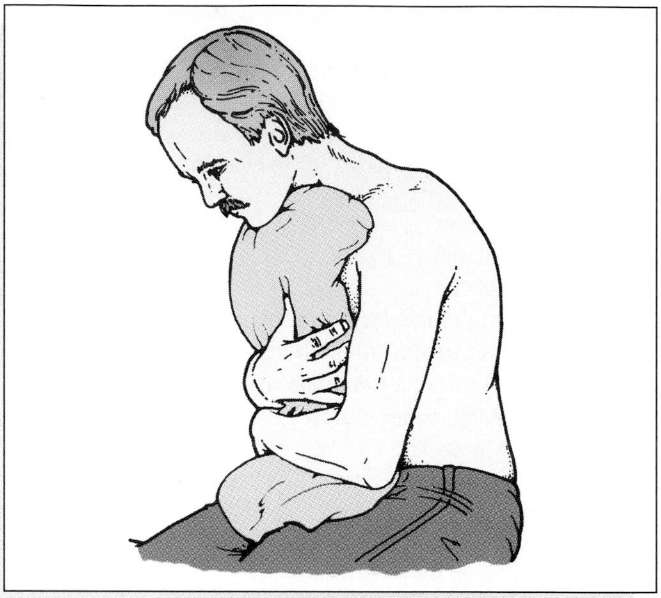

Holding pillow against incision when coughing prevents incisional strain.

TEACHING DIAPHRAGMATIC BREATHING

Equipment

Hospital bed in flat position

Preparation

1. Check physician's orders and client care plan.
2. Wash your hands.
3. Provide privacy.
4. Inform client that the purpose of this exercise is to learn how to breathe by using abdominal muscles.

Note: Clients with COPD tend to overwork the upper chest muscles and suck in the abdomen on inspiration, making it difficult for the diaphragm to descend. This exercise improves breathing efficiency.

Procedure

1. Place your hands on client's abdomen, below ribs.
2. Have client breathe in through the nose and try to push stomach outward against your hands.
3. Instruct client to hold breath for 3–5 seconds to keep alveoli open.
4. Have client breathe out slowly through the mouth as you apply slight pressure at the base of the ribs.
5. Encourage client to practice diaphragmatic breathing frequently, using own hands to feel the abdomen rise.
6. Progressive increments of weight placed on the abdomen (recumbent position) strengthen the diaphragm, while practice improves neuromuscular coordination of diaphragmatic breathing.

TEACHING USE OF AN INCENTIVE SPIROMETER (IS)

Equipment

Hospital bed or straight chair

Incentive spirometer with flow rate indicator; (save bag for storage of device)

Tissues for secretions

Preparation

1. Check physician's orders and client care plan.
2. Gather equipment.
3. Wash your hands.
4. Explain purpose and procedure to client.
5. If preoperative measurement was not done, use guide in spirometer package to determine client's volume goal, and set market at this goal.
6. Attach open end of tubing to stem on front of exerciser.
7. Auscultate lungs before and after using IS. **Rationale:** This evaluates effectiveness of spirometry.

Procedure

1. Instruct client to hold exerciser, place mouth tightly around mouthpiece, and breathe in a trial breath through the mouth. **Rationale:** Client can see the flow rate indicator on side of unit to visualize appropriate rate for inhalation.
2. Explain that a slow deep breath is better than a fast breath.
3. Instruct client to exhale completely, then place mouth tightly around mouthpiece.
4. Instruct client to inhale slowly to raise and maintain flow rate indicator at the "best" flow rate range, and continue inhaling to try to raise piston to prescribed (or preoperative measured) volume level.
5. Instruct client to remove mouthpiece but hold breath at maximum inspiration 3–5 seconds, then exhale through pursed lips. Repeat a few times, then cough.
6. Encourage client to use spirometer hourly, coordinating use with TV program breaks, for instance, as a reminder.
7. Provide positive feedback as client uses IS to reattain predetermined inspiratory capacity using marked goal as an incentive.
8. Replace unit in bag when not in use, and keep in accessible place for client.

Note: Recent studies show that sustained inspiration (breathing in deeply through the nose, holding for 3 seconds, and exhaling) is just as effective as using a commercial incentive spirometer (and more cost-effective) in preventing pulmonary complications.

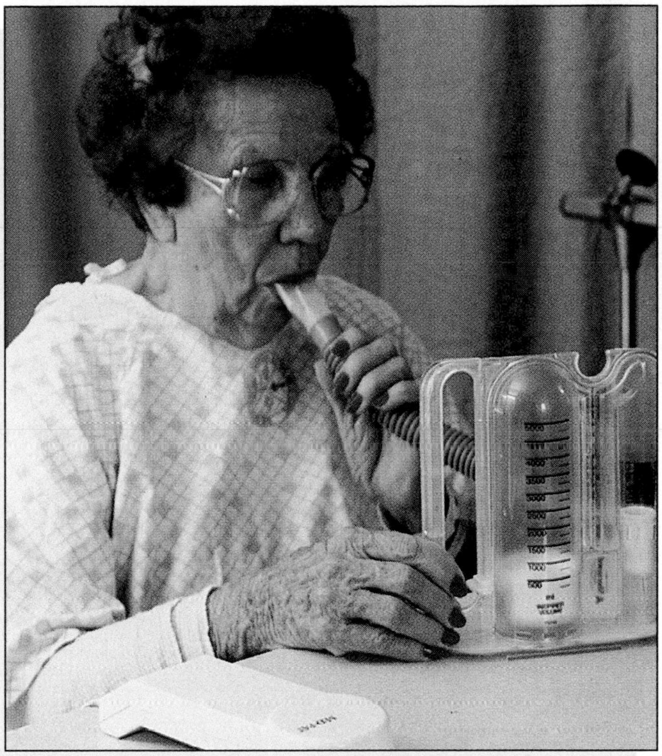

Client places mouth tightly around mouthpiece and inhales slowly, while watching flow rate indicator, to promote lung expansion.

TEACHING PEAK FLOW MEASUREMENT

Equipment

Peak flow meter with instructions for client

Preparation

1. Check physician's orders or client care plan.
2. Gather equipment.

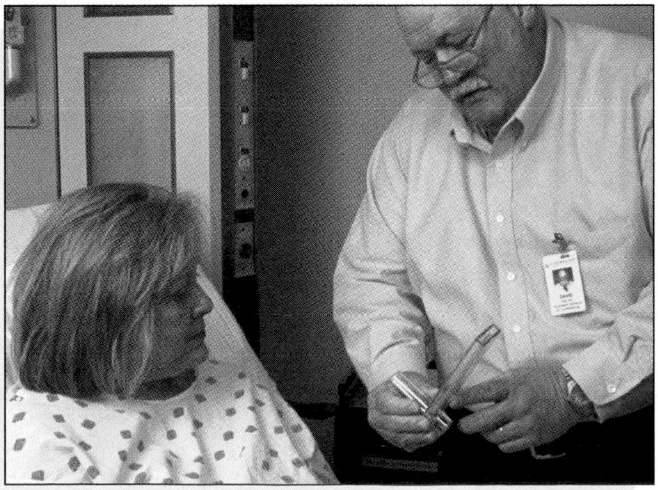

Slide indicator to bottom of meter scale to bring indicator to zero point.

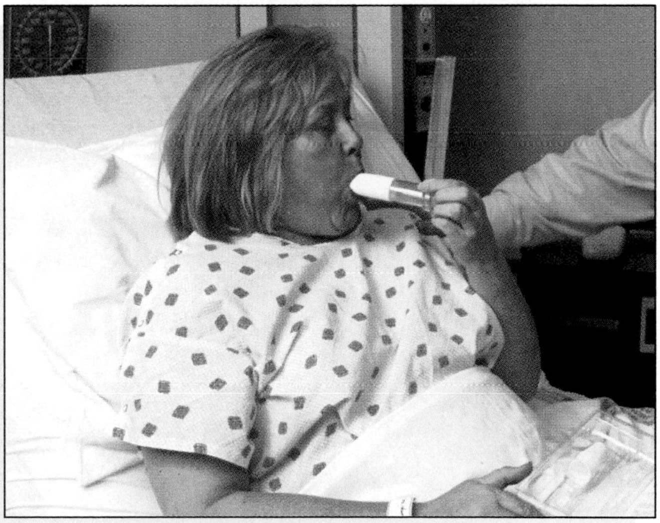

Have client blow out through mouth as hard and fast as possible—indicator moves up scale to record peak expiratory flow (L/min).

3. Wash hands.
4. Explain purpose of procedure and provide instruction sheet to client.

Procedure

1. Assist client to follow product instructions to assemble meter.
2. Instruct client to attach mouthpiece to peak flow meter, if desired. **Rationale:** Most meters can be used with or without mouthpiece.
3. Slide indicator to bottom of meter scale to zero position.
4. Instruct client to inhale as deeply as possible, then place mouth around mouthpiece, forming a tight seal. If possible, client should be standing.
5. Have client blow out through mouth as hard and fast as possible. **Rationale:** As client forcefully exhales, indicator moves up scale to record client's peak expiratory flow (liters per minute).
6. Repeat peak flow measurement three times and record highest value. **Rationale:** Client may keep daily record of peak flow values and report significant changes.
7. Instruct client to clean unit weekly, following manufacturer's instructions.

PROVIDING CPAP/BIPAP

Equipment

Nasal mask, full face mask, or nasal pillows of proper size (S, M, L)
Indelible marker
Airflow generator
Delivery tubing
If ordered:
Oxygen source
Oxygen tubing
Pulse oximetry

Preparation

1. Check physician's orders or client's care plan.
2. Gather equipment.
3. Wash hands.
4. Explain purpose of procedure to client and provide written instructions for home use.
5. Have client wash face.

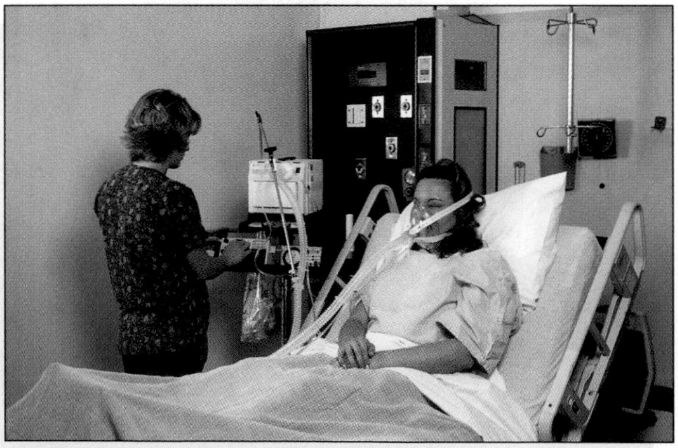

Client receiving CPAP via mask. Machine is capable of CPAP and BIPAP.

Procedure

1. Connect CPAP/BIPAP device delivery tubing to pressure generator.
2. Plug pressure generator into grounded outlet.
3. Connect oxygen delivery tubing into device tubing adapter port (if ordered).
4. Turn on pressure generator.

CLINICAL ALERT

Respiratory therapy and biomedical engineering departments must check to ensure proper functioning and electrical safety of outside equipment (e.g., CPAP) brought from home to be used in an agency.

5. Establish CPAP/BIPAP parameters:
   a. RAMP: time frame for pressure achievement, usually 5–15 minutes.
   b. CPAP or BIPAP setting.
   c. Respiratory rate if applicable.
   d. FIO_2 if applicable.
6. Apply device over client's nose and/or mouth, avoiding tight fit, and mark straps for future proper fit. **Rationale:** Tight fit is uncomfortable for the client and unnecessary for device functioning.
7. Establish continuous pulse oximetry if ordered.
8. Tell client to detach tubing from face device if getting up during the night.
9. Monitor client periodically.
10. Teach client to clean device according to manufacturer's instructions.

- **CPAP** provides single positive pressure to establish minimal airway value (e.g., 5 mm Hg) at end of exhalation.
- **BIPAP** provides two positive airway pressures, one to assist peak pressure on inhalation (e.g., 10 cm H_2O), and a lower one (e.g., 5 cm H_2O) to establish minimal airway value at end of exhalation.
- **BIPAP with Rate Set** provides two positive airway pressures and a set respiratory rate to augment breathing for the client with respiratory insufficiency. This capability qualifies this unit as a "noninvasive mechanical ventilator." The client is spared intubation.

PROVIDING BAG–VALVE–MASK VENTILATION

Equipment

Manual resuscitator bag with nonrebreathing valve.
Oxygen source and tubing
Airway adapter or face mask

Preparation

1. Determine that client's breathing is absent or inadequate.
2. Summon an assistant if client is not intubated. **Rationale:** If no artificial airway present, two responders are essential. Assistant holds masks while nurse compresses resuscitator bag.
3. Gather equipment.
4. Place client in supine position.
5. Connect mask or airway adapter to bag.
6. Connect oxygen tubing and oxygen flow meter to bag inlet.

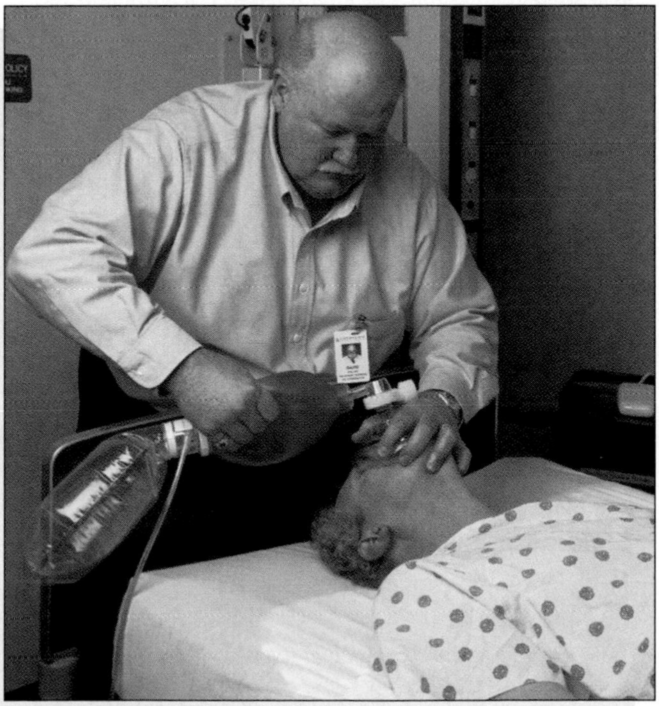
Compress central portion of resuscitator bag until client's chest rises, then allow exhalation.

Procedure

1. Turn oxygen flow meter wide open to 15 L/min ("flush").
2. Stand at client's head and hyperextend client's neck.
3. Place apex of mask over client's nose and place base of mask between client's lower lip and chin. **Rationale:** This ensures a tight seal.
4. Use dominant hand to compress central portion of resuscitator bag until client's chest rises (1–2 seconds), then allow exhalation. **Rationale:** Overinflation may result in gastric distention.
5. Provide ventilations every 5 seconds for an apneic adult, noting that client's chest rises and falls with each compression.

CLINICAL ALERT

If client's chest does not rise with ventilations, suspect foreign body airway obstruction. See Chapter 27 for Heimlich maneuver.

6. Check to see if client breathes spontaneously, then give compressions in synchrony to support ventilation.
7. Observe for possible gastric distention. **Rationale:** Gastric insufflation may result in regurgitation and aspiration.
8. Check if gastric distention is present in the unresponsive client; if so, have assistant provide cricoid pressure to client's airway.

CLINICAL ALERT

Cricoid pressure may be used only if the client
- Is nonresponsive
- Not vomiting
- Does not have a cuffed tracheal tube

9. Notify physician or respiratory care practitioner for further client evaluation.

Documentation for Respiratory Preventive and Maintenance Measures

- Pre- and Post-intervention breath sounds and adventitious sounds
- Frequency of deep breathing exercises or use of IS
- Whether cough is productive or not
- Amount and character of secretions expectorated
- Changes in vital signs, SpO_2, or other client responses
- Inspiratory capacity attained with IS
- Circumstances necessitating use of mask and bag resuscitator
- Client outcome following manual breathing
- Peak flow measurement: highest of three therapy sequential measures

for CPAP/BIPAP

- Type of CPAP/BIPAP device used
- Established parameters
- Respiratory rate if programmed
- FiO_2 if ordered
- SpO_2 findings pre and post therapy
- Client's tolerance of therapy
- Client teaching and return demonstration

Critical Thinking Application

UNEXPECTED OUTCOMES	CRITICAL THINKING OPTIONS
Client is unwilling to complete exercise because of misunderstanding or fear of pain or wound dehiscence.	• Inform client that fresh incision is secure • Instruct again on rationale and necessity for procedure. • Support incision area more fully, using the palms of your hands or a firmly rolled pillow to allay fears of dehiscence. • Medicate 30–60 minutes before using spirometer or participating in breathing exercises.
Nasal congestion inhibits client's breathing capability.	• Ask client to blow nose prior to the breathing exercise. • Check with physician to prescribe medications, such as saline spray to open nasal passages.
Client is unable to master use of incentive spirometer device.	• Instruct client to start slowly and increase volume over several exercise sessions. • Supervise practice with encouragement. • Provide positive reinforcement with increments in volume. • Assure that client does regular deep breathing if device interferes with client adherence. • Turn client q2h and encourage ROM and early ambulation to help stimulate deep breathing and secretion mobilization.
Client doesn't tolerate CPAP therapy.	• Loosen the appliance since some leakage is acceptable and does not compromise function of the device. • Increase RAMP time to improve tolerance/increase comfort. • Use nasal spray (saline solution) to reduce nasal congestion.

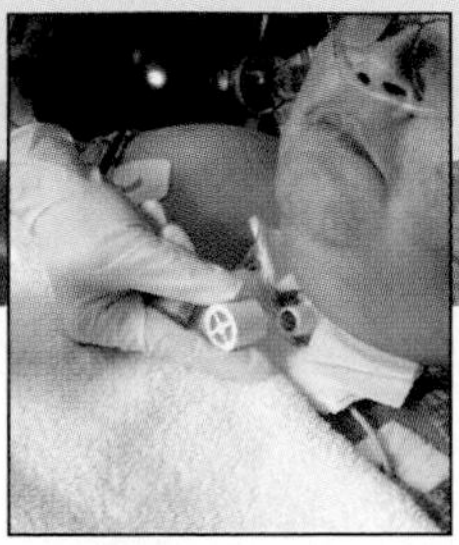

Chest Physiotherapy (CPT)

Nursing Process Data

ASSESSMENT *Data Base*

Note any contraindicating conditions for CPT: acute exacerbation of COPD, pneumonia *without* evidence of significant sputum production, osteoporosis, lung cancer, cerebral edema.

Determine rate and depth of breathing and heart rate/rhythm.

Auscultate breath sounds and check for adventitious sounds or excessive sputum production (over 25 mL/day).

Note time elapsed since eating (perform CPT between meals to prevent regurgitation)

Observe quality of secretions. Thick, tenacious secretions may require aerosol therapy prior to treatment.

Note client's ABGs/SpO_2 and changes on chest x-ray report.

PLANNING *Objectives*

To decrease respiratory rate and improve ventilation and gas exchange

To reduce client's feeling of shortness of breath

To facilitate clearance of retained secretions

To assist client to cough more productively and effectively

To decrease adventitious lung sounds

To decrease risk of infection due to stasis of secretions

IMPLEMENTATION *Procedures*

Preparing Client for CPT

Performing Postural Drainage

Performing Chest Percussion

Performing Chest Vibration

EVALUATION *Expected Outcomes*

Chest x-ray shows improvement.

Breath sounds and adventitious sounds improve on auscultation.

Shortness of breath is reduced.

Sputum production is over 25 mL/day (to justify continuation of therapy).

ABGs/SpO_2 values are improved.

PREPARING CLIENT FOR CPT

Equipment

Hospital bed or other surface to place client in head-down position
Gown or towel (optional)
Tissues
Container for sputum
Gloves
Stethoscope
Pulse oximeter (if indicated)
Mouthwash/oral hygiene product

Procedure

1. Validate physician's order for CPT. **Rationale:** These procedures are tiring to clients, time consuming and contraindicated in cases of osteoporosis, pulmonary embolism, cardiac conditions, lung cancer or other conditions not associated with excessive sputum production.
2. Wash hands.
3. Administer CPT before, or at least 2 hours after meals to prevent vomiting.
4. Establish the location of lung segments if the entire lung field is to undergo CPT, the affected segment should be drained first. **Rationale:** Usually, the lower areas are the most affected.
5. Provide privacy.
6. Prepare client by explaining CPT and purpose.
7. Auscultate chest for breath sounds and adventitious sounds prior to therapy.
8. Obtain pulse oximetry if indicated before therapy.
9. Place towel over skin when performing CPT (optional).

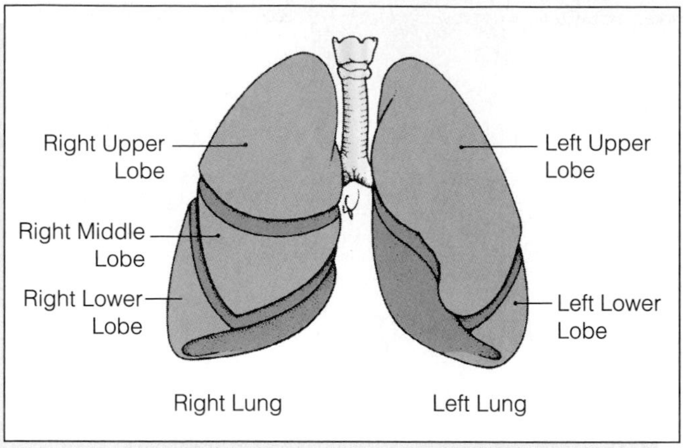

Lobes of the lungs.

PERFORMING POSTURAL DRAINAGE

Equipment

See Preparing Client for CPT.

Preparation

1. See Preparing Client for CPT.
2. Wash hands.

Procedure

1. Loosen any tight clothing.
2. Lower head of bed slowly so that client's head is positioned in no greater than a 25° downward angle. **Rationale:** Gravity helps mobilize secretions.
3. Place sputum container and tissues in client's reach.
4. Tell client to remain in position for 3–15 minutes. **Rationale:** Percussion and vibration may be added to help mobilize secretions *(skills to follow).*
5. Instruct client to expectorate secretions.
6. Instruct client to turn to other side, then to supine position, then repeat procedure.

Note: Clients should deep breathe between position changes.

7. Assist client to slowly return to normal sitting position after coughing in dependent positions.
8. Determine pulse oximetry if ordered.
9. Auscultate chest areas for improved breath sounds
10. Don gloves.
11. Note character and measure sputum, then discard.
12. Remove gloves and wash hands.
13. Offer oral hygiene following secretion expectation.

EVIDENCE BASED NURSING PRACTICE

Bronchial Hygiene Therapy

There is no firm scientific evidence that CPT measures are effective in preventing pulmonary complications. In order to justify continuation of postural drainage the client must demonstrate one or more of the expected outcomes-listed on unit opening page.

Source: Goodfellow, L., & Jones, M. (2002). Bronchial hygiene therapy. *American Journal of Nursing 102*(1), 38.

PERFORMING CHEST PERCUSSION

Equipment

See Preparing Client for CPT.

Preparation

1. See Preparing Client for CPT.
2. Wash hands.

Procedure

1. Cover area to be percussed with gown or cloth towel (optional).
2. Holding arms with elbows slightly flexed, cup your hands with thumbs and fingers closed. Keeping wrists loose and relaxed, rhythmically flex and extend wrists to clap over area to be drained. **Rationale:** This motion produces vibrations that loosen secretions for easier removal with coughing or suctioning.
3. Percuss by alternating hands and listen for hollow sound with strikes.
4. Slowly and rhythmically percuss each area for 3–5 minutes.
5. Do not percuss over bony prominences, breasts, or tender areas. **Rationale:** Vibrations are not transmitted to the chest wall through bone or breast tissue and percussion in these areas can cause discomfort.
6. Encourage client to "huff" cough after percussion of lung areas.
7. Auscultate all lung areas for changes in breath sounds.
8. Don gloves, note character and measure quantity of sputum and discard.

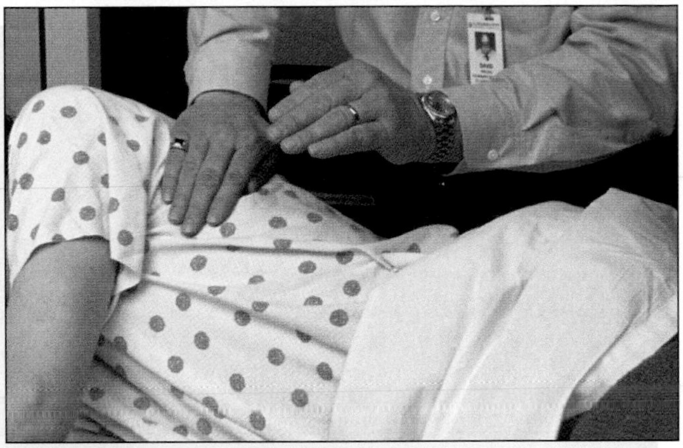

Perform percussion and vibration with each position change.

9. Remove gloves and wash hands.
10. Offer oral hygiene.
11. Document procedure and client's response.

> **CLINICAL ALERT**
>
> Since chest percussion is taxing and time consuming for both client and nurse, it is indicated only in clients with serious secretion retention (e.g., client with cystic fibrosis).

PERFORMING CHEST VIBRATION

Equipment

See Preparing Client for CPT.

Preparation

1. See Preparing Client for CPT.
2. Wash hands.

Procedure

1. Perform vibration following postural drainage and percussion in each position.
2. Cover area to be vibrated with gown or towel (optional).
3. Instruct client to breathe in through nose and exhale slowly through pursed lips.
4. Place your hands flat over area to be vibrated or place one hand on top of the other. Keep your arms and shoulders straight and wrists stiff.
5. Have client inhale deeply.
6. As client exhales through pursed lips, use moderate pressure to vibrate chest by quickly contracting and relaxing your arms and shoulders. **Rationale:** This increases the turbulence and velocity of exhaled air, loosens and mobilizes secretions from peripheral airways.

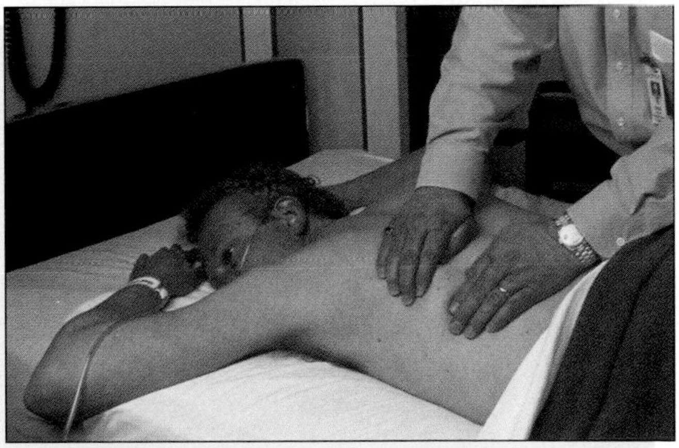

Place hands flat over area to be vibrated, keeping wrists stiff.

7. Vibrate for 3 or 4 exhalations over the area.

8. Encourage clients to "huff" cough before changing positions.
9. Assess vital signs, pulse oximetry and auscultate breath sounds.
10. Don gloves.
11. Measure and note character of expectorated secretions, then discard.
12. Remove gloves and wash hands.
13. Provide oral hygiene.
14. Document procedure and client's response.

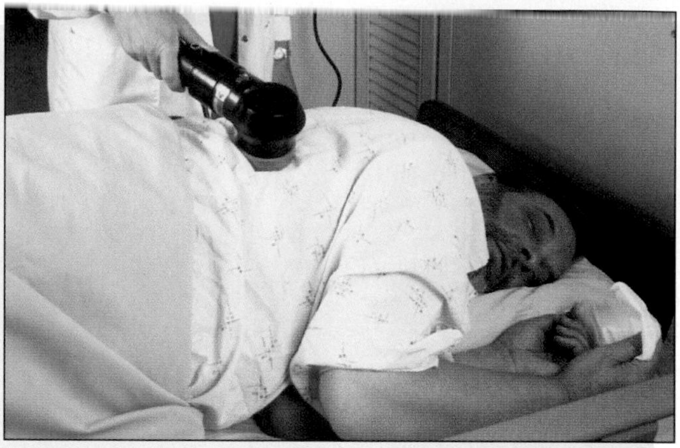
Mechanical device is alternative to manual vibration

CLINICAL ALERT

Strenuous coughing should be avoided with head-down position since it raises intracranial pressure.

DOCUMENTATION FOR CPT

- Time, specific treatment, and duration of therapy
- Pre- and post-therapy vital signs, breath sounds, and pulse oximetry
- Quantity and character of sputum produced
- Client's physical tolerance of procedures

Critical Thinking Application

UNEXPECTED OUTCOMES	CRITICAL THINKING OPTIONS
Client experiences dyspnea during postural drainage.	• Change client's position so head is no lower than 25° below horizontal.
Client is unable to assume position for postural drainage.	• Turn client on side with pillow support to facilitate bronchial drainage.
Client vomits with CPT treatment and coughing.	• Perform treatments between or before meals.
Client tires with manual chest vibration.	• Notify physician to alter therapy with a mechanical device for chest vibration. • Limit total CPT time to less than 40 minutes.
Slapping sounds produced with percussion.	• Cup hands more and assure that clapping is with wrist flexion and extension only.

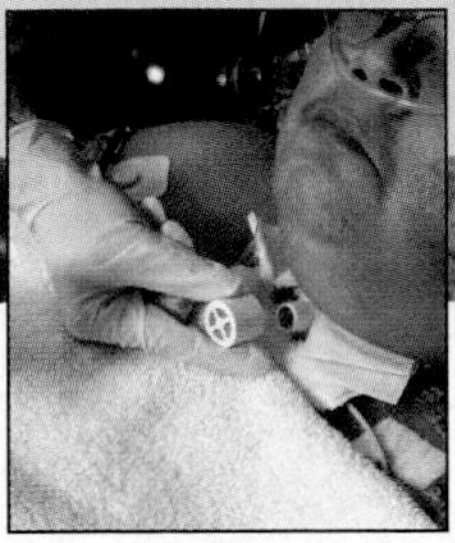

Oxygen Administration

Nursing Process Data

ASSESSMENT Data Base

Review client's ABG results or pulse oximetry for SpO_2.
Assess client's vital signs.
Observe client for signs of increased work of breathing.
Assess skin under oxygen mask for irritation.
Assess for signs of carbon dioxide narcosis.

PLANNING Objectives

To return arterial PO_2 or SpO_2 to normal or acceptable range
To correct hypoxic condition
To assist breathing to return to normal rate and effort
To increase client's comfort, breathing efficiency, and activity tolerance

IMPLEMENTATION Procedures

Monitoring Clients Receiving Oxygen
Using Pulse Oximetry
Using an Oxygen Analyzer
Using an Oxygen Cylinder
Using Nasal Cannula
Using an Oxygen Face Mask
Providing Oxygen via a Pediatric Tent
for Setting Up Pediatric Tent
for Monitoring Child in Tent
Using an Oxygen Hood

EVALUATION Expected Outcomes

Arterial PO_2 and SpO_2 return to normal or acceptable range.
Signs and symptoms of hypoxia are relieved.
Comfort, breathing efficiency, and activity tolerance increased.
Complications of oxygen use do not occur.

MONITORING CLIENTS RECEIVING OXYGEN

Equipment

Oxygen supply source
Oxygen delivery device

Procedure

1. Check physician's orders for mode of oxygen delivery and prescribed oxygen liter flow.
2. Wash hands.
3. Employ safety precautions for oxygen administration.
4. Place client in semi- or high-Fowler's position to facilitate lung expansion.

> **CLINICAL ALERT**
>
> Oxygen is indicated for client's with COPD, but is used conservatively. High levels of oxygen can cause hypoventilation, CO_2 retention, may suppress breathing stimulus and lead to respiratory arrest due to CO_2 narcosis.

5. Turn and reposition client frequently to promote ventilation.
6. Encourage deep breathing and coughing exercises unless directed otherwise.
7. Ensure adequate fluid intake, especially if secretions are thick.
8. If ordered, humidify oxygen when flow rate is greater than 4 L/min.
9. Assess client's progress by frequently checking vital signs, color, level of consciousness, and presence of hypoxia—the best indicator of oxygen delivery problems.

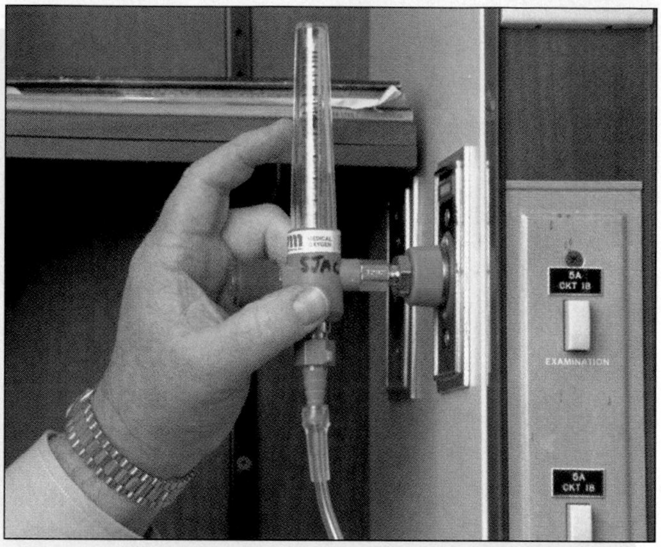

Oxygen flow meter indicates liters per minute delivered to administration setup.

10. Assess clients with COPD frequently for signs of carbon dioxide narcosis:
    a. Bounding peripheral pulses
    b. High blood pressure
    c. Altered sensorium
    d. Increased pulse pressure
    e. Warm, clammy skin
11. Evaluate SpO_2 30 minutes after any change in oxygen flow rate.

USING PULSE OXIMETRY

Equipment

Oximeter (battery or line power operated)
Sensor (clip-on or disposable adhesive sensor)

Preparation

1. Evaluate client's health status before using oximetry. **Rationale:** Inaccurate oximetry readings can be found in clients with
    a. Alkalosis, acidosis
    b. Fever, hypothermia
    c. Poor peripheral blood flow.
    d. Carbon monoxide poisoning
    e. Recent dye injection studies
2. Remove nail polish or artificial nails, if using finger for sensor placement. **Rationale:** These substances can distort readings.
3. Obtain appropriate sensor. **Rationale:** Sensor probes are designated for specific sites, e.g., fingers, toes, earlobes.
4. Wash hands.

> **CLINICAL ALERT**
>
> - Avoid placing SpO_2 sensor on the thumb or edematous site.
> - Avoid extremity with an intra-arterial catheter or non-invasive automatic BP cuff.

Procedure

1. Identify client and explain purpose and procedure for pulse oximetry.
2. Plug unit into electric outlet.
3. Turn on power.
4. Apply sensor probe flush with skin and secure. Make sure both sensor probes are aligned directly opposite each other. **Rationale:** Oximeter sensors contain both red and infrared light-emitting diodes (LEDs) and a photodetector. The photodetector registers light passing through vascular bed, the basis for microprocessor determination of oxygen-saturation.

Safety Precautions for Oxygen Administration

- Set up "No Smoking" and "Oxygen in Use" signs at the site of administration and at the door, according to agency policy.
- Provide cotton gown—synthetics and wool may generate, sparks of static electricity.
- Remove matches, lighters, and ashtrays from bedside (these items should only be present with physician's orders, as hospitals are smoke-free facilities.)
- Remove any friction-type or battery-operated toys devices.
- Disconnect ungrounded electric equipment.
- Remove all volatile or flammable materials (alcohol, oils, petroleum products).
- Make sure that all electrical monitoring equipment is *properly* grounded.
- Locate fire extinguishers and oxygen meter turn-off lever.

5. Set alarms to predetermined saturation levels or pulse rate.
6. Read oxygen saturation level on digital readout monitor.
7. Evaluate findings with previous saturation levels and changes in oxygen therapy.
8. Rotate site of clip-on probes every 4 hours. Replace disposable probes every 24 hours. **Rationale:** Skin irritation can occur with continuous usage.
9. Validate oximeter pulse rate is consistent with manually assessed pulse rate.
10. Document findings on appropriate hospital record.

CLINICAL ALERT

The anemic client may have a normal SpO_2 in spite of inadequate tissue oxygenation because available hemoglobin is maximally saturated with oxygen.

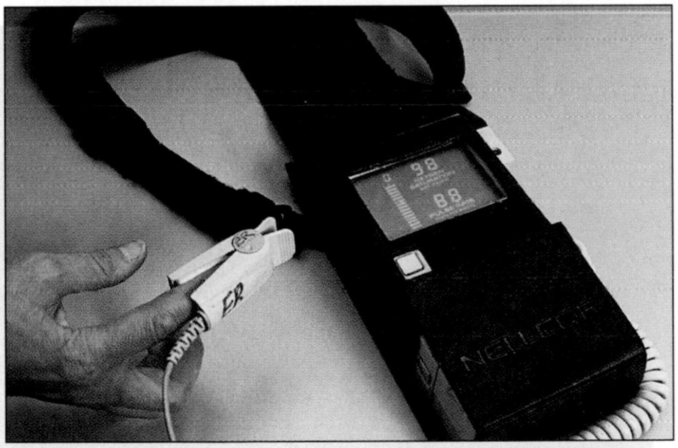

Sensor probe placed on finger for hemoglobin oxygen saturation (SpO_2) analysis and microprocessing unit with digital display.

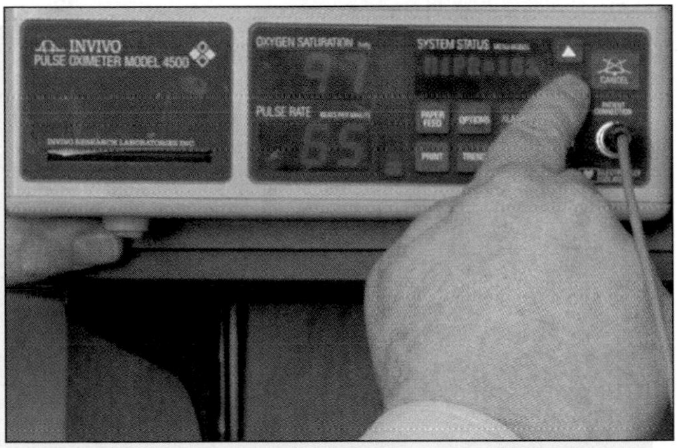

Continuous oximeter unit displays percent of hemoglobin oxygen saturation (SpO_2) and pulse rate. Alarms are set at predetermined limits.

Pulse Oximetry

Arterial blood gas (ABG) analysis has been used for decades to determine a client's gas exchange and oxygenation transport ability. Today, pulse oximetry technology allows for more cost- and time-efficient PRN or continuous monitoring of arterial oxygen saturation (SaO_2). The primary advantages of this method are:

- It is cost-effective.
- It is a noninvasive evaluation tool.
- Minute-to-minute changes in saturation can be assessed and timely intervention made to meet client needs.
- The client's response to treatment can be evaluated immediately and ongoing.

USING AN OXYGEN ANALYZER

Equipment

Analyzer

Procedure

1. Calibrate analyzer with room atmosphere and 100% oxygen.
2. Place sensor in the atmosphere to be monitored.
3. Read and record FIO_2

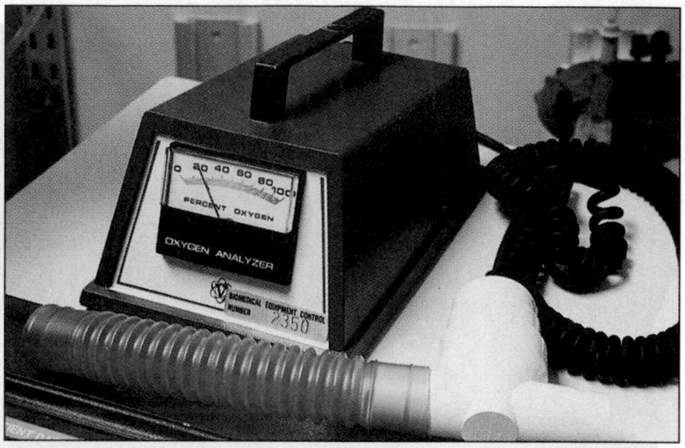

Oxygen analyzer, most often used in pediatrics

USING AN OXYGEN CYLINDER

Equipment

Steel cylinder portable oxygen tank
Regulator/flow meter
Oxygen delivery tubing

Procedure

1. Place oxygen cylinder in carrier in secure upright position. **Rationale:** If cylinder of compressed air falls accidentally, unit becomes a missile with uncontrollable force and direction.
2. Using hexagon key, slowly turn cylinder release valve clockwise (left is loose) to crack tank open for a brief period, then close (right to tighten). **Rationale:** This action removes lint from system.
3. Check pressure gauge on front of tank to determine amount of oxygen pressure in tank. **Rationale:** Full status is 2,200 PSI.
4. Attach flow meter regulator unit over neck of cylinder, aligning pins with green "O" ring openings.
5. Use turn key to tighten regulator to cylinder neck.
6. Connect delivery tubing to "Christmas tree" adapter on regulator unit.
7. Open cylinder release valve using hexagon key on top of cylinder. **Rationale:** This allows oxygen flow.
8. Slowly open regulator/flow meter and adjust to prescribed rate of oxygen delivery in liters per minute.

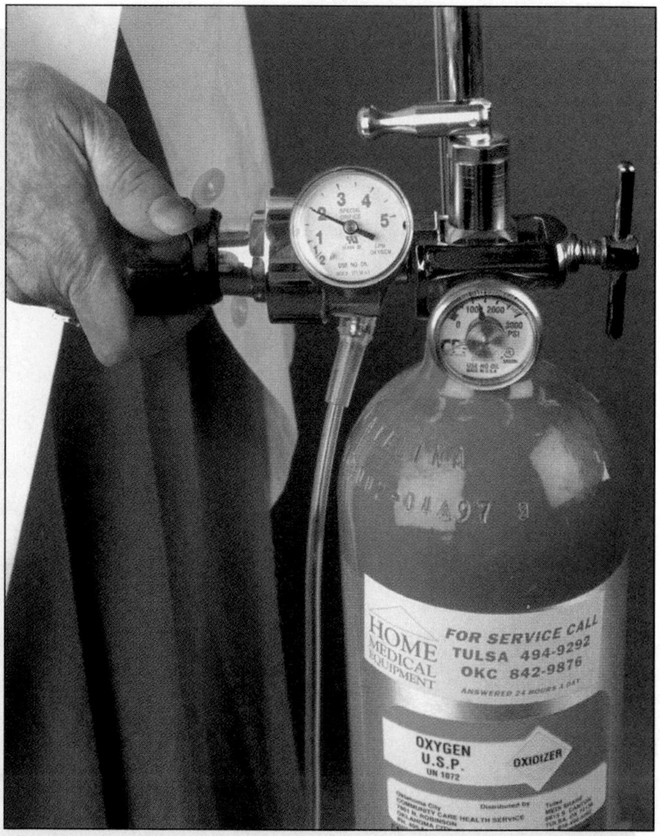

Attach regulator to cylinder neck, attach tubing, open cylinder release valve and adjust oxygen flow rate (L/min) as prescribed.

Signs and Symptoms of Hypoxia

Early Symptoms

- Restlessness
- Headache
- Visual disturbances
- Confusion or change in behavior
- Tachypnea
- Tachycardia
- Hypertension
- Dyspnea
- Anxious face

Advanced Symptoms

- Hypotension
- Bradycardia
- Metabolic acidosis (production of lactic acid)
- Cyanosis

Chronic Hypoxia

- Polycythemia
- Clubbing of fingers and toes
- Peripheral edema
- Right-sided heart failure
- Chronic Po_2 less than 55 mm Hg; O_2 saturation less than 87%
- Elevated Pco_2 (respiratory acidosis)

USING NASAL CANNULA

Equipment

Oxygen source
Oxygen flow meter
Disposable humidifier if ordered (flow rate over 4L/min or per agency policy)
Nasal cannula and tubing

Preparation

1. Check physician's order for oxygen prescription (flow rate).
2. Gather equipment
3. Insert oxygen flow meter into wall outlet.
4. Connect cannula tubing to flow meter.
5. Place disposable humidifier unit between flow meter and cannula tubing if humidification is ordered.
6. Wash hands.

Procedure

1. Explain purpose and procedure of oxygen use to client.
2. Place nasal prongs of cannula into client's nares.
3. Fit cannula tubing around client's ears and adjust tubing slide under client's chin.

CLINICAL ALERT

Humidification of low-flow oxygen through nasal cannulae is not considered essential and is contraindicated because it supports bacterial growth.

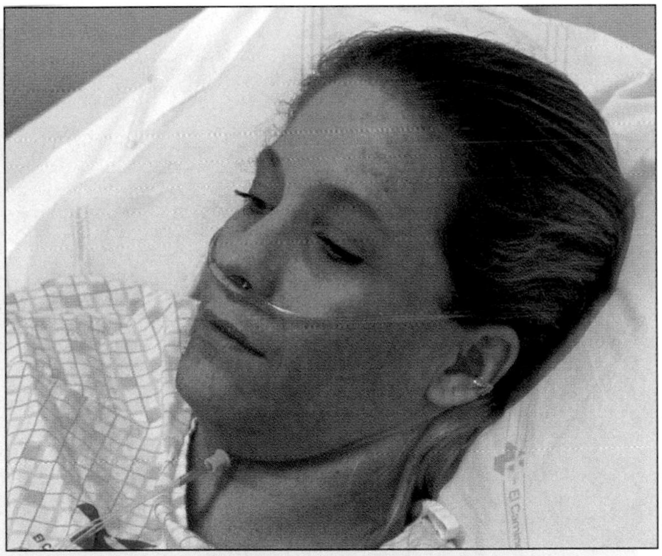

Oxygen administration by nasal cannula.

4. Adjust flow of oxygen. Should be limited to 6 L/min or less, **Rationale:** Since atmospheric air mixes with prescribed oxygen concentration as client inhales, the FiO_2 varies depending on the flow and nature of client's breathing. Deep breathing dilutes rather than enhances the FiO_2 because more room air is inhaled. *Note: Oxygen therapy is not corrective for hypoxia caused by anemia, abnormal hemoglobin, or vascular insufficiency.*

FiO_2: 24–44% Flow: 1–6 L

5. Monitor vital signs and check client's condition regularly.
6. Provide nares care every 4 hours—use ONLY water-soluble products, avoid petroleum products. **Rationale:** Petroleum products are combustible, not absorbed by the body, and difficult to clear from the mucosa.
7. Monitor for pressure around ears and pad cannula tubing for comfort if indicated.

USING AN OXYGEN FACE MASK

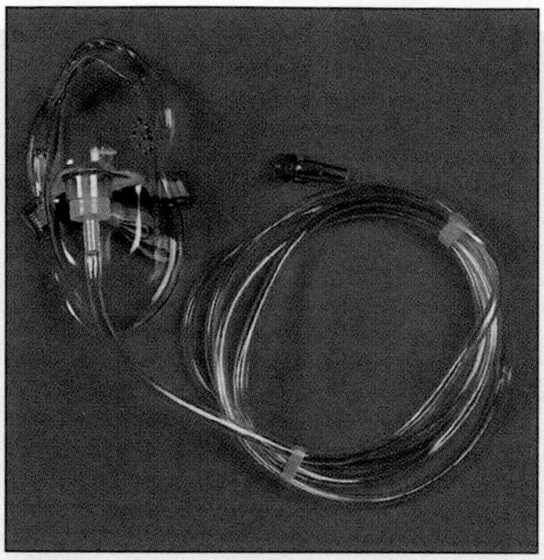

Simple face mask delivers moderately high flow of oxygen

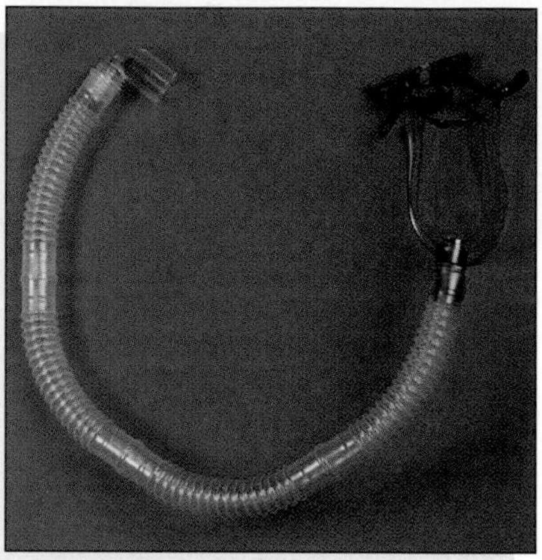

Oxygen face tent delivers unpredictable oxygen flow with high humidity.

Equipment

Oxygen mask
Four types of masks:
- Simple face mask
- Partial rebreather mask with reservoir bag
- Nonrebreather mask with reservoir bag
- Venturi mask used to specifically control oxygen concentration

Oxygen source
Oxygen flowmeter
Disposable humidifier (if indicated)

Preparation

1. Check physician's orders for oxygen.
2. Gather equipment.
3. Wash your hands.

Procedure

1. Explain procedure and rationale for administration of oxygen to client.
2. Check size of face mask to make sure it fits client.
3. Turn on oxygen flow to liters prescribed. If reservoir bag is attached, partially inflate it with oxygen.
4. Place client in semi- or high-Fowler's position.
5. Fit mask to client's face from nose downward during expiration. If reservoir bag is attached, oxygen flow must be at a level to prevent bag from collapsing. **Rationale:** A tight fit prevents oxygen from escaping around eyes or nose.
6. Place elastic band around client's head.
7. Stay with client until client feels at ease with mask. **Rationale:** Clients may be afraid of suffocating.
8. Assess client's condition by checking vital signs and oxygenation status.
9. Change mask and tubing according to agency policy, and provide skin care to face.
10. Check equipment frequently. If humidifier is attached, check water level, dispose and change PRN.

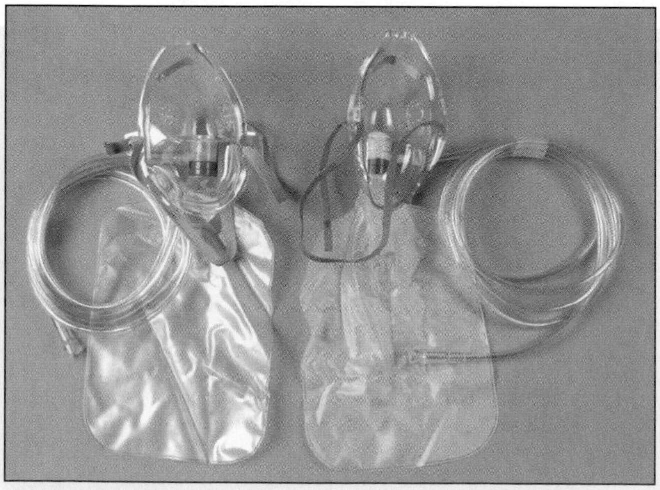

Left: Rebreather mask provides higher FIO_2 than a simple mask.
Right: Nonrebreather mask provides high FIO_2.

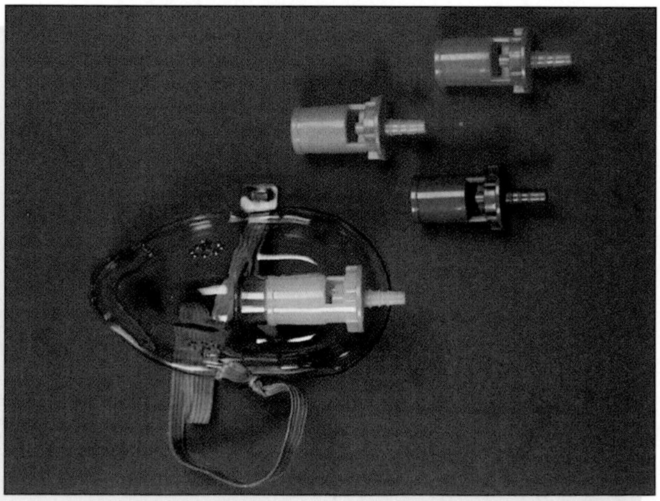

Face mask with oxygen percent control pieces.

TABLE 26–1 Oxygen Delivery Devices

Nasal Cannula

This equipment is easily tolerated by most clients. It is also simpler than a mask. The fraction of inspired oxygen (FIO_2) varies depending on the oxygen liter flow and the rate and depth of client breathing.

FIO_2:	24–38%	Flow:	1–2 L
FIO_2:	30–35%	Flow:	3–4 L
FIO_2:	38–44%	Flow:	5–6 L

Simple Face Mask

This equipment requires fairly high oxygen flow to prevent rebreathing of carbon dioxide. About 75% of the inspired volume is room air drawn in through side holes in the mask. Accurate FIO_2 is difficult to estimate

FIO_2	35–65%	Flow:	8–12 L

Mask with Reservoir Bag

The reservoir allows higher FIO_2 to be delivered. At flows of less than 6 L/min the risk of rebreathing carbon dioxide increases. Two types are available:

Partial rebreathing mask: No inspiratory valve so that the beginning portion of exhaled air returns to the bag and mixes with the inspired air. Ports are present so that most expired air escapes. The reservoir bag remains partially inflated.

FIO_2	40–60%	Flow:	6–10 L

Nonrebreather: Valve closes during expiration so that exhaled air does not enter reservoir and is not rebreathed. Valves on mask side ports allow exhalation but close on inspiration to prevent inhalation of room air.

FIO_2	60–100%	Flow:	6–15 L

Venturi Mask

This system utilizes different sized adapters to deliver a fixed or predicted FIO_2. The FIO_2 is dependent upon liter flow and/or entrainment port size. It is used effectively on clients with COPD when accurate FIO_2 is necessary. Carbon dioxide buildup is kept at a minimum. Humidifiers usually are not used. FIO_2 is dependent upon liter flow and/or entrainment port size.

FIO_2	24–50%

Face Tent

This soft aerosol mask fits loosely around the face and neck. It is an alternative to an aerosol mask for clients who feel claustrophobic, but it is sometimes difficult to keep in place. It is convenient for providing humidification and oxygenation, however oxygen concentration cannot be controlled.

FIO_2:	28–100%	Flow:	8–12 L

Oxygen Hood

This disposable vinyl box fits over a child's head to provide warm humidified oxygen at a controlled temperature.

FIO_2:	28–40%	Flow:	5–8 L
FIO_2:	40–85%	Flow:	8–12 L

Less than 5 L flow may lead to carbon dioxide narcosis.

Oxygen Tent

This canopy encloses the child and is used to provide oxygen, humidification, and/or a cool environment to control temperature.

FIO_2:	Up to 50%	Flow:	10–15 L

PROVIDING OXYGEN VIA A PEDIATRIC TENT

Equipment

Oxygen source
Delivery tubing
Disposable oxygen tent/canopy
Oxygen blender
Oxygen analyzer
Sterile water for nebulizer
Two bath blankets
Ambient thermometer
Pulse oximeter

> **CLINICAL ALERT**
> Avoid use of friction-type toys or battery-operated devices when oxygen is in use.

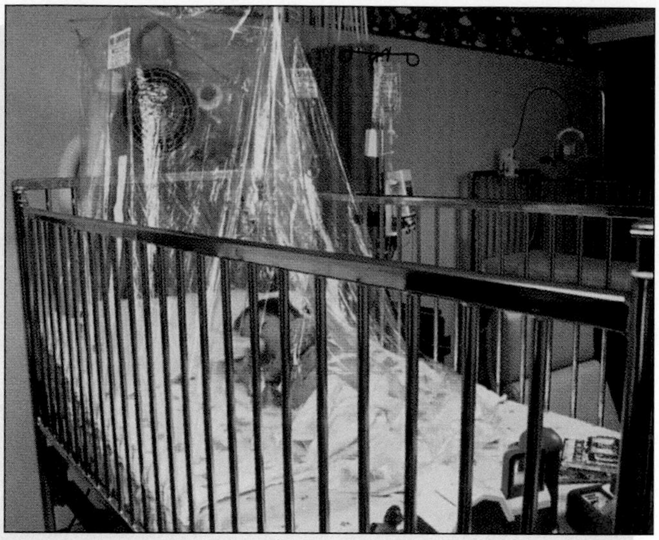

The pediatric tent can be used for oxygen delivery, humidification, temperature control, or a combination of these.

Preparation

1. Check physician's orders.
2. Gather equipment.
3. Explain purpose of tent to child and parents.
4. Provide favorite toy or blanket.
5. Wash hands.

Procedure

for Setting Up Pediatric Tent

1. Secure tent/canopy and place machine at head of empty bed/crib with control knobs on opposite side of working area.
2. Place thermometer in tent.
3. Connect oxygen regulator into oxygen source and select concentration.
4. Connect delivery tubing to canopy.
5. Plug in machine.
6. Set up humidifier/nebulizer and fill tray (at back of machine) with sterile water.
7. Pad crib frame that supports canopy with bath blankets. **Rationale:** Padding protects client from injury and absorbs excess moisture.

for Monitoring Child in Tent

8. Turn on oxygen to prescribed concentration (21–50%) and maintain temperature at 17.8°–21.2° C (64°–70° F).
9. Secure canopy by tucking in all sides under mattress. **Rationale:** To prevent oxygen leak at bottom of tent since oxygen is heavier than air.
10. Monitor temperature regularly. **Rationale:** To determine if temperature goal is achieved.
11. Analyze and record tent oxygen concentration, and check child's vital signs/oximetry as ordered.
12. Keep crib sides up for safety.
13. Select toys that are washable, do not produce static electricity, and are appropriate to the child's age.
14. Check dampness of clothes and change PRN to prevent chilling.
15. Minimize number of times tent is opened to maintain desired (FIO_2).

Note: Frequent linen changes may be necessary to prevent heat loss due to evaporation of moisture.

USING AN OXYGEN HOOD

Equipment

Disposable Oxygen hood
Oxygen source
Oxygen analyzer
Flexible oxygen tubing

Procedure

1. Check physician orders for oxygen level and client care plan.
2. Wash hands.
3. Place hood around child's head and/or upper body and attach tubing to oxygen supply.
4. Close ports and lid, but do not obstruct neck opening. **Rationale:** Obstructing neck opening can lead to carbon dioxide accumulation.
5. Infants are cared for through portholes or lid. **Rationale:** This prevents excessive oxygen leakage.
6. Maintain oxygen levels at 40–50%, and check for moisture that accumulates inside hood.
7. Observe usual oxygen administration precautions.

DOCUMENTATION FOR OXYGEN ADMINISTRATION

- Type of equipment used for oxygen administration, liter flow, FIO_2
- Data from oxygen analyzer
- Arterial PO_2 and SaO_2 or pulse oximetry results
- Vital signs
- Client's tolerance of device
- Client and family teaching and indication of understanding

Critical Thinking Application

UNEXPECTED OUTCOMES	CRITICAL THINKING OPTIONS
Client has difficulty breathing (dyspnea).	• Check ABGs and SpO_2 and compare with previous findings. • Encourage client to describe what he or she is experiencing. • Place client in Fowler's position. • Assist with all ADLs to conserve client's energy. • Employ measures to alleviate pain or anxiety.
Client shows these abnormal signs and symptoms: changes in blood pressure, tachycardia, tachypnea, abnormal color, restlessness, or altered sensorium.	• Check ABGs for drop in blood pH (acidemia) or rise in PCO_2 (respiratory acidosis), and report if found. These conditions can occur if hypoxic drive is blunted by the administration of high oxygen concentration. a. Check oxygen equipment, and use oxygen analyzer to measure oxygen concentration. b. Reduce oxygen concentration as ordered. • Clients who chronically retain carbon dioxide may require controlled oxygen concentration delivery devices (e.g., Venturi mask).
Client develops atelectasis.	• Encourage deep breathing, range of motion, frequent position changes, and early ambulation if possible. • Use sedatives or other respiratory depressants carefully.

UNEXPECTED OUTCOMES	CRITICAL THINKING OPTIONS
	• CPT may be ordered.
	• Check breath sounds. (They are usually decreased with this condition and crackles are frequently heard at the end of inspiration in dependent lung areas.)
Client develops tachypnea.	• Report change and check SpO_2 immediately, since inadequate flow rates may be causing the problem.
	• Increase flow rate as ordered, and monitor.
	• Monitor vital signs and correlate with client findings as pulmonary embolus may be the cause.
	• Check client's breathing pattern and breath sounds and report significant change.
Oxygen toxicity occurs.	• Toxicity occurs soon after initiation of oxygen use and is directly related to the FiO_2.
	• Monitor closely for signs of nausea, restlessness, pallor, lethargy, weakness and dyspnea.
	• Validate that sensor and oximeter are from the same manufacturer.
	• Do not exceed 40% oxygen concentration unless frequent monitoring occurs with pulse oximetry to monitor SpO_2.
Oxygen saturation (SpO_2) findings are erratic.	• Check that sensor probes are aligned to prevent photodetector picking up light from sources other than sensor.
	• Check that appropriate sensor site was selected for specific probes, e.g., finger site for finger sensor.
Pulse oximeter alarm sounds.	• Encourage client to immobilize sensor site. Movement scrambles signals from photodetector, interfering with readings.
	• Place sensor on different site.
	• Avoid placing sensor on hand of arm used for continuous blood pressure monitoring.
Client experiences discomfort with nasal prongs.	• Obtain smaller-gauge pediatric cannula.

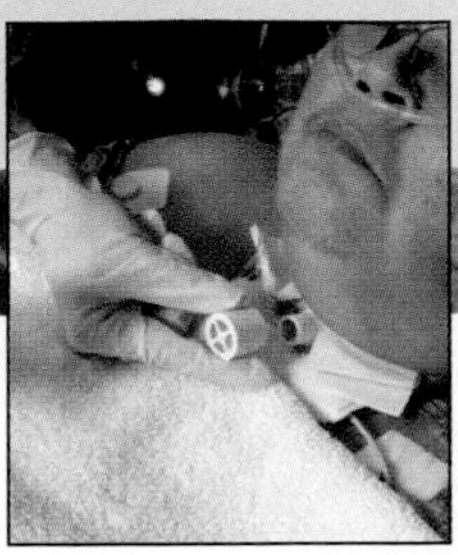

Artificial Intubated Airways

Nursing Process Data

ASSESSMENT ***Data Base***

Assess client's level of consciousness.

Determine if gag/swallow reflex is present.

Assess breath sounds in all lung fields, SpO_2, ABGs

Observe for shortness of breath, labored breathing, tachypnea, or tachycardia.

Note presence of adventitious sounds.

Note character of secretions.

PLANNING ***Objectives***

Oropharyngeal or Nasopharyngeal Intubation

- To provide patent airway

Endotracheal Intubation

- To provide patent airway
- To provide route for mechanical ventilation
- To facilitate removal of airway secretions
- To improve gas exchange

IMPLEMENTATION ***Procedures***

Inserting an Oropharyngeal Airway

Inserting a Nasopharyngeal Airway (Nasal Trumpet)

Assisting with Endotracheal Intubation

Providing Care for Client with Endotracheal Tube

Extubating an Endotracheal Tube

EVALUATION ***Expected Outcomes***

Patent airway maintained

Route established for mechanical ventilation.

Secretions easily suctioned so that pulmonary complications can be treated or prevented.

Breath sounds are present bilaterally.

Removal of artificial airway is tolerated.

INSERTING AN OROPHARYNGEAL AIRWAY

Equipment

Oropharyngeal tube
Tongue depressor
Clean gloves
Suction catheter
Suction source

Procedure

1. Assure that client is *unresponsive* and has NO gag reflex. **Rationale:** Conscious client may vomit and aspirate or develop laryngospasm during tube insertion.
2. Select appropriate size airway—length should be from corner of mouth to corner of ear tragus
3. Wash your hands; don gloves.
4. Gently open client's mouth with crossed finger technique. You may need to use modified jaw thrust to insert tube.
5. Perform oral suctioning.
6. Hold tongue down with tongue depressor and advance airway to back of tongue OR advance airway upside down (curved upward) and, as airway passes uvula, rotate the airway 180°.
7. Check that concave curve fits over tongue. It should extend from the lips to the pharynx, displacing the tongue anteriorly. **Rationale:** Proper positioning helps prevent injury to lips, teeth, tongue, and posterior pharynx.

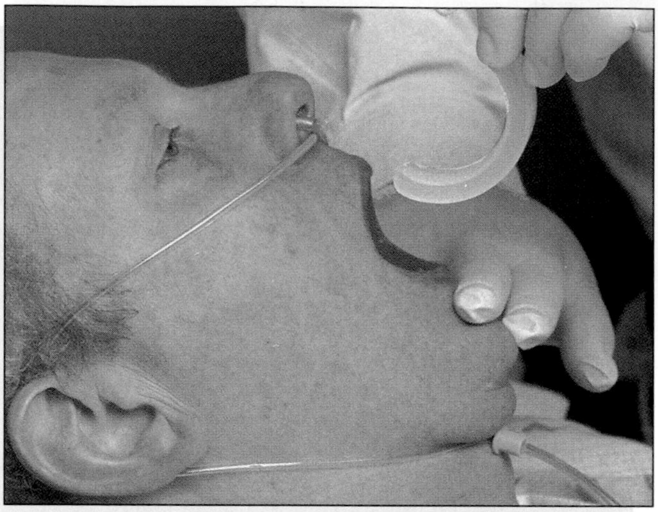

Oral airway is initially inserted upside down (curved upward).

8. Tape top and bottom of airway in position. **Rationale:** Stabilization of the tube prevents injuries.
9. Position client on side to facilitate drainage.
10. Remove gloves and discard.
11. Observe position of airway and evaluate quality of client's spontaneous breathing.
12. Continue to monitor.

INSERTING A NASOPHARYNGEAL AIRWAY (NASAL TRUMPET)

Equipment

Flexible nasopharyngeal airway
Water-soluble lubricant
Clean gloves

Procedure

1. Select appropriate size tube (length from tip of nose to earlobe and lumen slightly narrower than client's naris).
2. Wash your hands; don gloves.
3. Lubricate entire length of tube.
4. Explain procedure to client.
5. Insert entire tube gently through naris, following anatomic line of nasal passage. If obstructed, try other naris.
6. Validate position by
   a. feeling exhaled air through tube opening
   b. Inspecting for tube tip behind uvula.
7. Tape top and bottom of tube in position if necessary to prevent injury to lips, teeth, tongue, and posterior pharynx.
8. Position client on side to facilitate drainage of secretions.

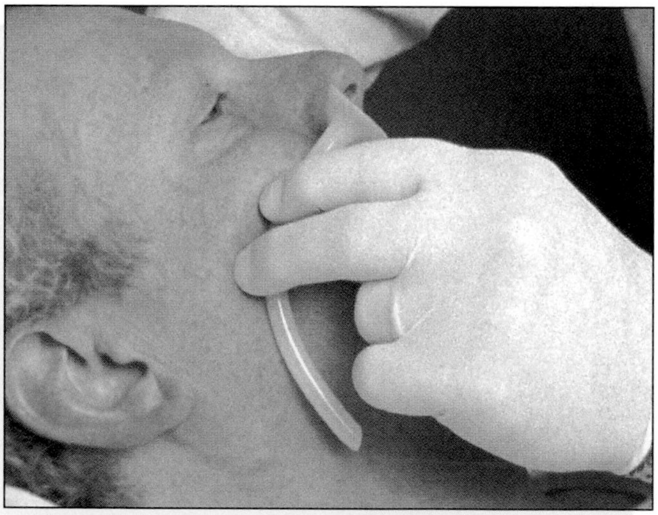

Nasal trumpet protects airway from repeated trauma with upper airway (oropharyngeal) suctioning.

9. Remove gloves and discard.
10. Continue to monitor position of airway and client's response.
11. Suction upper airway PRN using clean technique.

ASSISTING WITH ENDOTRACHEAL INTUBATION

Equipment

"Crash cart" (contains most needed supplies)
Laryngoscope with several blade sizes
Stylet to guide endotracheal tube *(ONLY for oral intubation)*
Endotracheal tubes
Water soluble lubricant
McGill Forceps
Suction Source
Oxygen source
Bag–valve–mask
Twill, adhesive tape, or Velcro holder
Syringe for cuff inflation
Stethoscope
CO_2 detector (for airway placement validation)
Oral airway or bite block
Clean gloves, personal protective equipment
Established pulse oximetry
Wrist restraints (if ordered by physician)
Prepared sedative/neuromuscular blocking agent as ordered

Note: New noninvasive positive pressure ventilation methods using nasal pillows, nasal mask, oral mask or mouthpiece with special head gear provide an appropriate alternative to intubation for many clients with ventilatory insufficiency.

Preparation

1. Determine that client has *no protective airway reflexes.*
2. Bring crash cart to client's doorway.
3. Check that all necessary equipment is functioning: (oxygen/suction source, and delivery systems).
4. Inflate and deflate airway cuff to determine if it is intact. See skill for Inflating a Tracheal Tube Cuff, Unit 6, page 914.
5. Wash hands and don gloves. Don personal protective equipment.
6. Insert stylet into tube (only for oral intubation).
7. Lubricate tube.
8. Administer medication as ordered.
9. Remove client's dentures/bridgework and place in labeled denture cup.
10. Review Procedure for Bag–Valve–Mask Ventilation.

Procedure

1. Place client in flat supine position with pillow under shoulders to hyperextend neck and help open airway. Position so that mouth, pharynx and trachea are aligned. **Rationale:** Proper positioning facilitates intubation.
2. Restrain client's hands only if necessary.
3. Premedicate client as ordered.
4. Preoxygenate client for several minutes, using bag–valve–mask. **Rationale:** To create an "oxygen reserve."

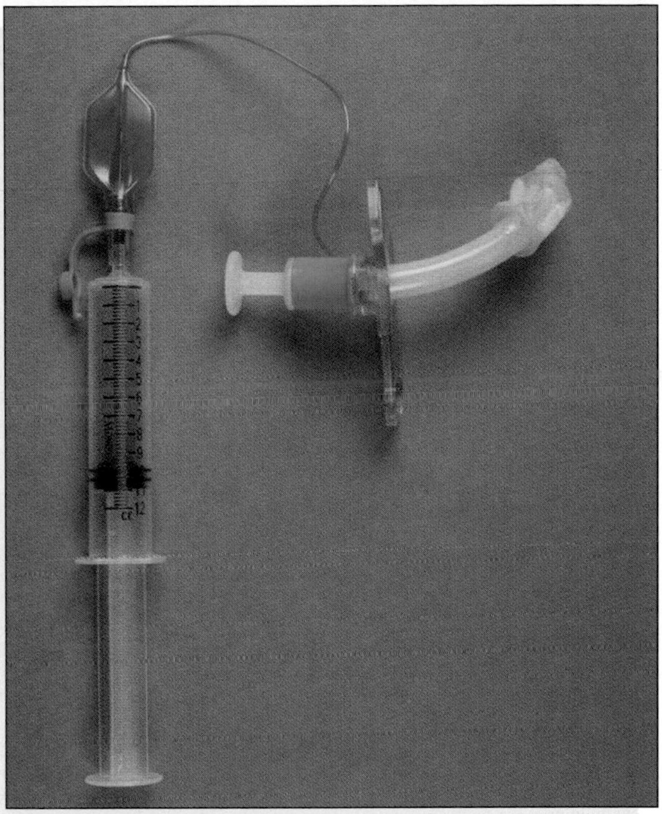

Attach 10-mL syringe to distal end of inflatable cuff. (Tracheostomy tube shown.)

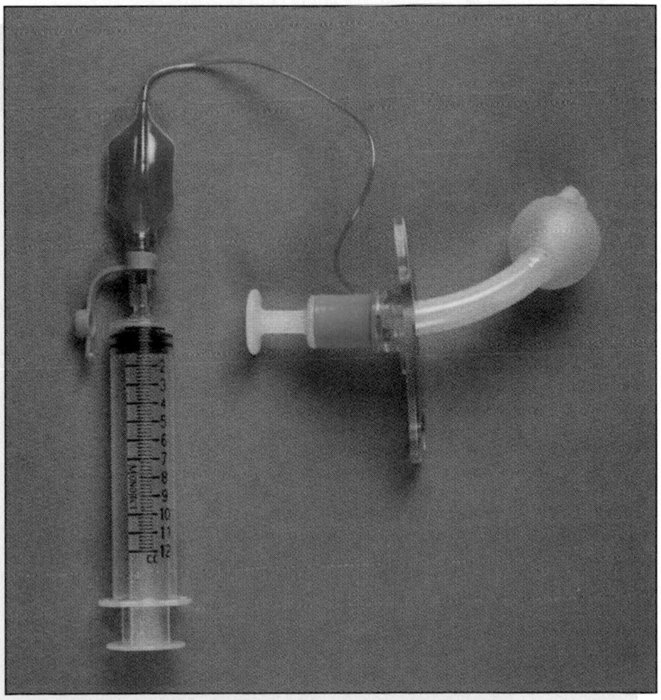

Inflate cuff for minimal leak using minimal occlusive pressure. (Tracheostomy tube shown.)

> **CLINICAL ALERT**
>
> Even if spontaneously breathing, the client should be pre-oxygenated with 100% O_2 for endotracheal tube placement. Ventilation must not be interrupted for over 30 seconds.

5. Using thumb and index finger, apply cricoid pressure during tube insertion. **Rationale:** This facilitates tracheal placement and protects against aspiration of gastric contents.
6. Maintain cricoid pressure while inflating cuff to "minimal leak" inflation by placing stethoscope at client's suprasternal notch and noting a slight hissing sound at peak of inspiration.

Note: For skill "Inflating a Tracheal Tube Cuff, see Unit 6, pg. 914. Tracheal tube cuff inflation is essential for mechanically ventilated clients.

7. Attach bag–valve–mask, provide ventilation and look for chest to rise. **Rationale:** If chest does not rise, esophageal intubation is likely.
8. Check tube placement using CO_2 detector. **Rationale:** Presence of CO_2 indicates tracheal intubation.
9. Place stethoscope over epigastrium. **Rationale:** If gurgling is heard, and abdominal distention noted, esophageal placement is likely.
10. Auscultate lung fields for bilateral breath sounds. **Rationale:** This ensures that accidental right main stem intubation has not occurred.
11. Mark tube at level of client's front teeth and tape securely with twill or adhesive tape or velcro holder. **Rationale:** Secure taping prevents tube displacement.
12. Recheck tube placement with the previous measures (steps 8–10).
13. Place bite block or oral airway if ET tube has been positioned orally.
14. Discard disposable equipment, remove gloves and wash hands.
15. Position client in position as ordered.
16. Obtain chest x-ray to confirm tracheal placement of ET tube.
17. Place call bell and writing material within client's reach (as indicated).
18. Reposition and retape ET tube daily and PRN.

> **CLINICAL ALERT**
>
> Cricoid pressure may be used only if the client:
> - Is nonresponsive
> - Is not vomiting
> - Does not have a cuffed tracheal tube in place

EVIDENCE BASED NURSING PRACTICE

Client's Response to Intubation

Studies show that clients experience anger, worry and fear at being unable to speak, especially in the first few days of intubation.

Source: Menzel, L. (1998). Factors related to the emotional responses of intubated patients to being unable to speak. *Heart & Lung, 27*(4), 245–251.

PROVIDING CARE FOR CLIENT WITH ENDOTRACHEAL TUBE

Procedure

1. Monitor breath sounds every 4 hours. Breath sounds should be heard equally throughout lung fields *bilaterally*.
2. Check marked points on tube at insertion level. **Rationale:** This determines if tube has moved.
3. Inspect positioning and stabilization of tube. **Rationale:** A change of position can obstruct airway or cause erosion and necrosis of tissues.
4. Inspect and clean mouth and nose. Observe for pressure areas or ulceration.
5. Reposition and tape oral ETT to opposite side daily, noting tube depth each time.
6. Provide mouth care every 2 hours. **Rationale:** If client breathes through mouth, mucous membranes become dry.

Note: Providing mouth care reduces pharyngeal bacteria and helps prevent pulmonary infection.

7. Support client's head and tube when turning. **Rationale:** This prevents tube from becoming dislodged or airway from becoming obstructed.
8. Place call bell within reach and provide alternative means of communication when cuffed tube is in place. **Rationale:** No air passes over larynx, so client is not able to summon help or communicate.
9. Support client by spending extra time, using touch, and anticipating client's needs.
10. Ensure adequate hydration. **Rationale:** Artificial airways bypass the humidifying process of normal breathing.

> **CLINICAL ALERT**
>
> Even with appropriate cuff inflation, intubated clients receiving gastric/enteral tube feedings are at high risk for aspiration.

EXTUBATING AN ENDOTRACHEAL TUBE

Equipment

Suction source
Oral suction catheter (or Yankauer)
Sterile suction catheter set
Clean gloves
Sterile gloves
Oxygen source
Postextubation oxygen delivery device
Scissors or syringe for cuff deflation

Preparation

1. Assess client's readiness for extubation.
2. Obtain vital signs.
3. Explain procedure to client.
4. Prepare postextubation oxygen administration device.
5. Place client in Fowler's position.

Procedure

1. Wash hands and don clean gloves.
2. Perform oral or nasopharyngeal suctioning.
3. Have client take several slow deep breaths. **Rationale:** This hyperoxygenates client in preparation for extubation.
4. *Deflate* tube cuff using syringe or cut pilot tubing.
5. *Untie* the tracheal tube.
6. Remove gloves and don sterile gloves.
7. Connect sterile catheter to suction source.
8. Insert sterile suction catheter into airway until resistance is met.
9. Leave suction catheter in place.
10. Have client take a deep breath. **Rationale:** This dilates the vocal cords and makes removal easier and less traumatic.
11. Apply suction while removing catheter and airway at the same time.
12. Immediately apply supplementary oxygen device.
13. Monitor client frequently at first, then regularly.
14. Dispose of equipment and remove gloves.

CLINICAL ALERT

Do not feed client orally immediately post-extubation. Seek consult for a feeding trial for clients at risk for aspiration.

DOCUMENTATION FOR INTUBATION

- Clinical manifestations indicating need for intubation.
- Specific reason for intubation
- Premedication administered
- Size and type of inserted endotracheal, nasopharyngeal, or oropharyngeal tube.
- Minimal occlusive pressure for cuff inflation
- Preoxygenation and postoxygenation when suctioning
- Quantity and character of secretions
- Pre- and post-procedure vital signs
- Client's tolerance of procedure
- Settings of ventilator or other oxygen mode.

Critical Thinking Application

UNEXPECTED OUTCOMES	CRITICAL THINKING OPTIONS
Naso-pharyngeal airway cannot be inserted.	• Change size of tube, change naris. • Relubricate nasopharyngeal airway and attempt to reinsert. • Hyperextend client's neck. • Insert tube at different angle. • Insert oropharyngeal rather than nasopharyngeal airway.
Laryngospasm occurs when endotracheal tube is inserted.	• If not severe, remove tube and wait a few minutes. • If severe, administer muscle relaxant. Physician's orders are required for this action. • If causing respiratory distress, you may need to prepare for immediate cricothyrotomy or tracheostomy.
Prolonged tracheal intubation may cause laryngeal damage.	• A cool aerosol mist is helpful in reducing swelling after intubation. • Prepare for assisting with tracheostomy. • Immediately seek assistance to provide mask and bag resuscitation.
Accidental extubation occurs.	• Call physician immediately. Obtain laryngoscope, blades, and extra endotracheal tubes. • Observe the marking on the tube every 2–4 hours to ensure tube placement and to prevent accidental extubation.
Client is unable to eat when intubated.	• Reduce tube cuff inflation pressure. • Weigh client daily. • Request dietary consult for assessment of nutritional status. • Reassess dietary options for meeting caloric need. • Consider enteral nutrition.
Placement of tube is incorrect.	• Observe for signs of subcutaneous emphysema. • Obtain physician's order for x-ray to verify tube placement in trachea; readjust tube as indicated and tape securely. • Auscultate all lung fields at least every 4 hours to ensure bilateral ventilation.

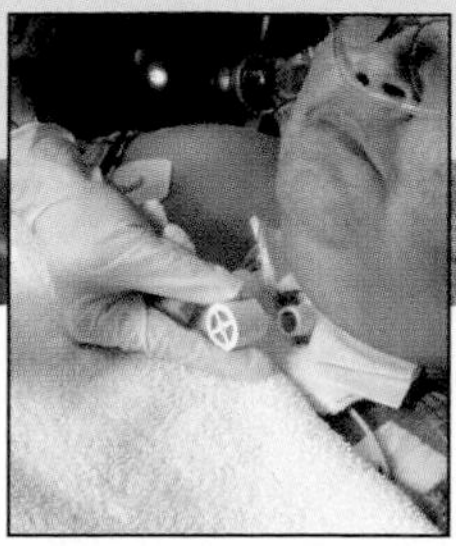

Suctioning

Nursing Process Data

ASSESSMENT Data Base

Assess client's need for suctioning.

Observe vital signs for increases in pulse and respiration.

Auscultate breath sounds for presence of adventitious sounds.

Observe respiratory status for tachypnea, shortness of breath, and restlessness.

Observe for signs of hypoxia.

PLANNING Objectives

To provide patent airway

To remove secretions

To improve ventilation

To decrease breathing rate

To increase tissue oxygenation

IMPLEMENTATION Procedures

Suctioning Using Catheter and Gloves

Suctioning Using Catheter in Sleeve

Suctioning with In-Line Closed Suction System

EVALUATION Expected Outcomes

Secretions removed without complications.

Improved ventilation with increased tissue oxygenation.

Breath sounds clear; no adventitious sounds auscultated.

SUCTIONING USING CATHETER AND GLOVES

Equipment

Portable suction machine or wall suction unit with receptacle and tubing

Oral suction catheter (e.g., Yankauer)

Suction catheter set with: suction catheter, sterile gloves, container for sterile saline

Note: Suction catheter diameter should be no larger than one-half the inner diameter of the client's airway. To determine suction catheter size, multiply the artificial airway's diameter times 2 (e.g., for 8 mm tube, use a 16 French suction catheter).

Sterile saline (mark time and date bottle is opened and discard in 24 hours)

Receptacle

Oxygen source and administration device (e.g., bag–valve device with tracheal tube adapter)

Personal protective equipment—gown, goggles, mask if splash anticipated

Stethoscope

Preparation

1. Check physician's orders and client care plan.
2. Gather equipment.
3. Recruit an assistant for manual ventilation if indicated.
4. Attach resuscitator bag to oxygen tubing, if indicated.
5. Wash your hands.
6. Assess lung sounds, heart rate and rhythm.
7. Open suction catheter package and open saline flush solution container.
8. Set suction control regulator at 80–120 mm Hg.
9. Don protective gown, mask, and goggles. **Rationale:** For self-protection if splash anticipated.

Note: This skill is more safely performed with an assistant who manages the resuscitator bag for hyperoxygenation while the nurse performs suctioning.

Indications for Suctioning

- Ineffective cough
- Client with depressed level of consciousness
- Thick, tenacious mucus
- Impaired pulmonary function

Note: Suction catheter is likely to advance into right bronchus due to greater anatomic angulation of left bronchus. Turning and deep breathing help mobilize secretions from left airways to facilitate their removal.

Procedure

1. Explain procedure and rationale to client regardless of client's level of consciousness.
2. Place client in semi-Fowler's or Fowler's position.
3. Turn on suction.
4. Remove cap from saline bottle.
5. Administer 100% oxygen (oxygen flowmeter to maximum "flush") for 1–2 minutes, or have assistant use resuscitator bag with adapter to hyperoxygenate client. **Rationale:** Suction removes oxygen resulting in hypoxemia and potential cardiac arrest. Hyperoxygenation prevents these complications.

CLINICAL ALERT

Hyperoxygenate the client before and after each time the airway is entered for suctioning, and wait 2 to 3 minutes before suctioning again to prevent severe hypoxemia.

6. Don sterile gloves. *Dominant* hand will remain sterile, *nondominant* hand becomes "clean."

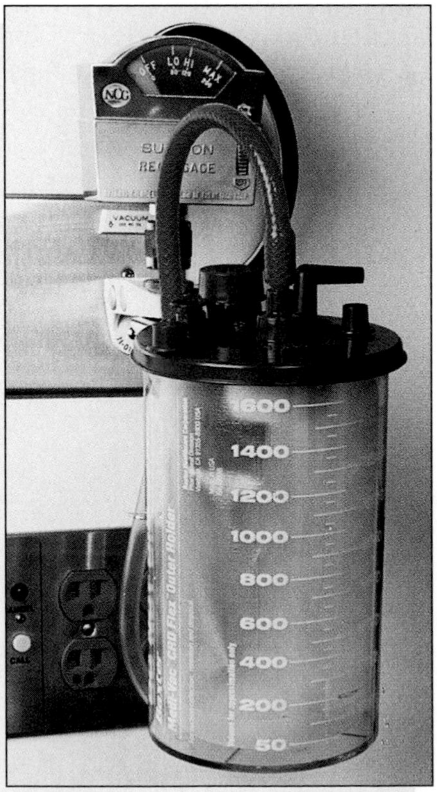

Turn suction source to 80–120 mm pressure.

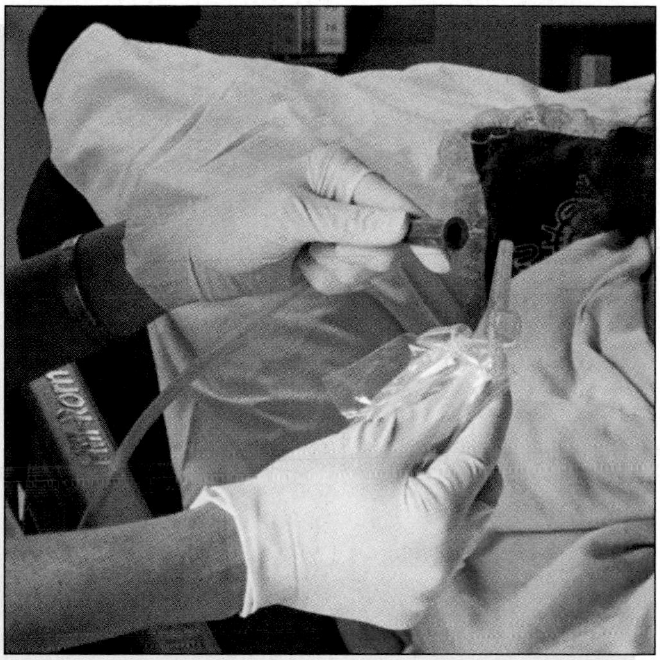

Attach suction catheter to suction tubing, maintaining sterility.

7. Using *nondominant* hand, pour sterile saline into flush solution container (*nondominant* hand is no longer sterile at this point).
8. Holding catheter in protective covering with *dominant* (sterile) hand, attach to suction tubing (held with *nondominant* hand).
9. Hold catheter covering with *nondominant* hand and slip catheter out with dominant (sterile) hand.
10. Lubricate sterile catheter by dipping it into cup with sterile normal saline.
11. Using *dominant* (sterile gloved) hand, insert catheter into client's airway without applying suction. **Rationale:** Suctioning during insertion deprives client of oxygen and inhibits catheter advancement.
12. Continue to advance catheter quickly until resistance is felt, even if client coughs. **Rationale:** Cough is stimulated at the carina (where bronchi divide).

Note: Current studies indicate that instructing the client to turn his or her head left or right to enter opposite bronchus is not effective. It is simply a matter of chance which bronchus is entered.

13. Withdraw catheter slightly, then begin suctioning using a rotating motion as the catheter is withdrawn
14. Suction intermittently by placing and releasing *nondominant* thumb over catheter suction port. **Rationale:** Intermittent vs continuous application of suction may help to reduce airway injury.
15. Limit suction to no more than 5–10 seconds. **Rationale:** This prevents hypoxemic complications induced by suctioning.
16. Reattach oxygen delivery device and have client take several deep breaths, or hyperoxygenate client's lungs with resuscitator bag.
17. Flush suction catheter and tubing with sterile saline.
18. Use same catheter (according to agency policy) and repeat suctioning procedure one time, if necessary. Allow 3 minutes between suctioning attempts for hyperoxygenation.
19. Coil suction catheter around hand and deglove over it to discard.
20. Discard gloves and catheter.
21. Turn off suction source.
22. Cover end of suction tubing connector with sterile gauze. **Rationale:** This prevents contaminating end that connects to suction catheter.
23. Assess lung sounds and heart rate and rhythm for changes. **Rationale:** Suctioning usually causes tachycardia but hypoxemia and vagal response may cause serious bradycardia/cardiac arrest.
24. Wash your hands.
25. Empty suction receptacle PRN or at end of every shift, noting character of secretions.
26. Ensure call bell is within client's reach.

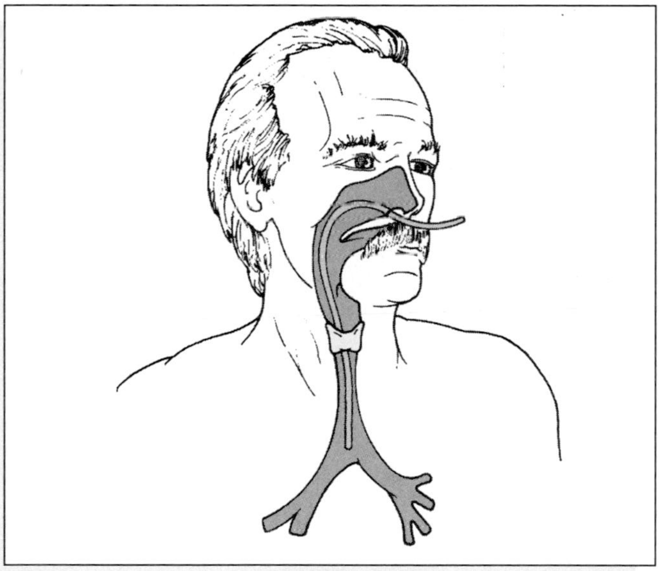

Insert catheter into naris and continue to advance.

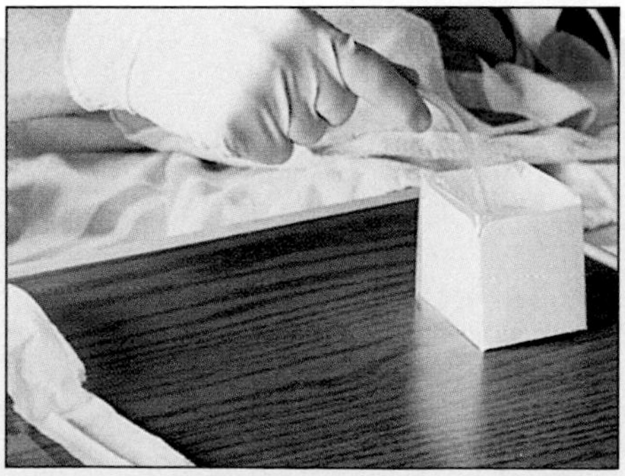

Rinse catheter and connecting tubing with NS to clear tubing.

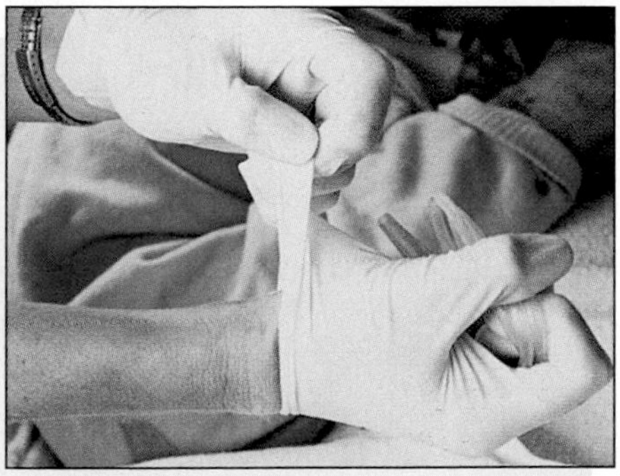

Coil catheter around fingers and pull glove over it to discard.

SUCTIONING USING CATHETER IN SLEEVE

Equipment

Portable suction machine or wall suction unit with receptacle and tubing
Oral suction catheter (e.g., Yankauer)
Suction catheter in protective sleeve
Clean gloves
Sterile saline
Container for sterile saline
Receptacle for used equipment
Oxygen source and administration device (e.g., bag–valve device with tracheal tube adapter)
Personal protective equipment—gown, goggles, mask if splash anticipated.
Stethoscope

Preparation

1. Check physician's orders and client care plan.
2. Gather equipment.
3. Recruit an assistant for manual ventilation, if indicated.
4. Attach resuscitator bag to oxygen tubing, if indicated.
5. Wash your hands.
6. Assess lung sounds, heart rate and rhythm.
7. Open suction catheter package and open saline flush solution container.
8. Set suction control regulator at 80–120 mm Hg.
9. Don protective gown, mask and goggles. **Rationale:** For self-protection if splash anticipated.

Procedure

1. Explain procedure and rationale to client regardless of client's level of consciousness.
2. Place client in semi-Fowler's or Fowler's position.
3. Turn on suction.
4. Remove cap from saline bottle.
5. Administer 100% oxygen (oxygen flowmeter to maximum "flush") for 1–2 minutes. Use resuscitator bag with tracheal tube adapter to hyperoxygenate client. **Rationale:** Suction removes residual lung volume resulting in hypoxemia and potential cardiac arrest. Hyperoxygenation prevents these complications.
6. Don gloves.
7. Use *nondominant* hand and pour sterile saline into flush solution container.
8. Hold catheter in protective covering with *dominant* hand and attach to suction tubing.
9. Hold catheter covering with *nondominant* hand and slip catheter out.
10. Lubricate sterile catheter by dipping it into cup with sterile normal saline.
11. Advance catheter into client's airway while retracting protective sleeve without (or before) applying suction. **Rationale:** Suctioning during insertion deprives client of oxygen and inhibits catheter advancement.
12. Continue to advance catheter quickly until resistance is felt, even if client coughs. **Rationale:** Cough is stimulated at the carina (where bronchi divide).
13. Withdraw catheter slightly, then begin suctioning using a rotating motion as the catheter is retracted back into protective sleeve.
14. Suction intermittently by placing and releasing *nondominant* thumb over catheter suction port. **Rationale:** Intermittent vs continuous application of suction may help to reduce airway injury.
15. Limit suction to no more than 5–10 seconds. **Rationale:** This prevents hypoxemic complications induced by suctioning.
16. Reattach oxygen delivery device to artificial airway and have client take several deep breaths, or hyperoxygenate client's lungs with resuscitator bag.
17. Flush suction catheter and tubing with sterile saline.
18. Reuse same catheter (according to agency policy) and repeat suctioning procedure one time, if necessary. Allow 3 minutes between suctioning attempts for hyperoxygenation.
19. Replace catheter in sleeve at time interval according to agency policy (e.g., 24 hours).
20. Discard gloves.
21. Turn off suction source.

Note: Studies show that instillation of saline into airways has no effect on "thinning" mucus, and leads to greater hypoxemia than suctioning without saline instillation. In addition, bacteria are dispersed through airways with saline instillation.

22. Catheter in sleeve remains attached to suction tubing. **Rationale:** This prevents contaminating end that connects to suction catheter.

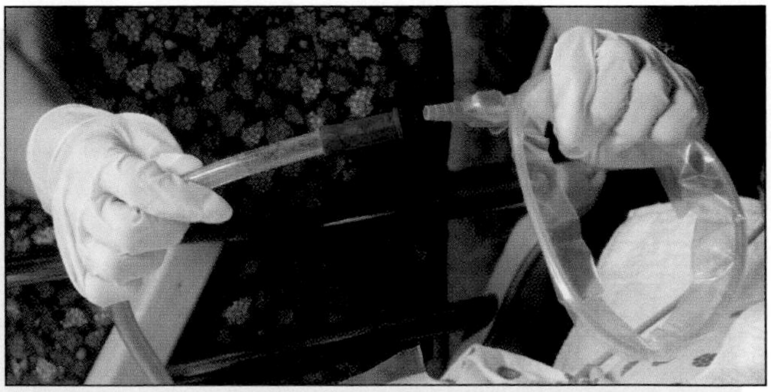

Hold catheter in protective covering with dominant hand and attach to suction tubing.

23. Assess lung sounds and heart rate and rhythm for changes. **Rationale:** Suctioning usually causes tachycardia but hypoxemia and vagal response may cause serious bradycardia/cardiac arrest.
24. Wash your hands.
25. Empty suction receptacle PRN or at end of every shift, noting character of secretions.
26. Ensure call bell is within client's reach.

SUCTIONING WITH IN-LINE CLOSED SUCTION SYSTEM

Equipment

In-line closed system (ET or tracheostomy connected) suction unit with catheter enclosed by plastic sleeve
10 mL normal saline in syringe or unit-dose vial
Suction source
Connecting tubing
Oxygen source and side-arm connector (e.g., bag–valve device or ventilator)
Clean gloves

Note: In-line closed system suctioning allows rapid suctioning for intubated clients and does not interrupt ventilator/client interface.

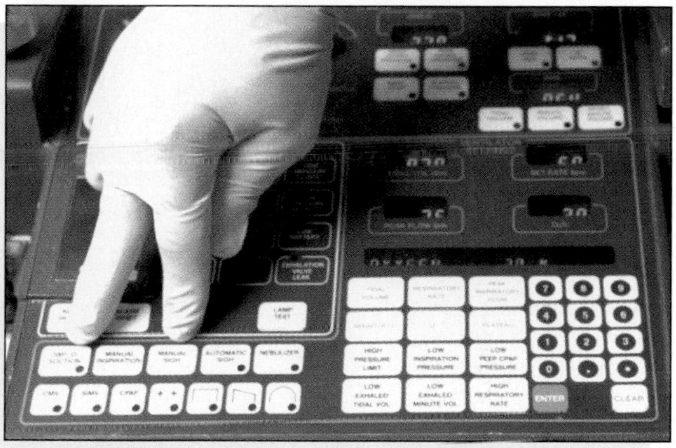

Mechanical ventilator provides 100% oxygen and manual breath.

Procedure

1. Explain procedure and rationale to client regardless of client's level of consciousness.
2. Wash hands and don gloves.
3. Place client in semi-Fowler's or Fowler's position.
4. Turn on suction source

CLINICAL ALERT

Monitor client closely and suction PRN, as coughed secretions may accumulate at the suction catheter/client's airway interface and obstruct airflow to client's lungs.

5. Connect oxygen source to side arm of trach tube connector.
6. Hyperoxygenate client with 100% oxygen, using manual bag or mechanical ventilator (100% oxygen source with several manual sighs, if indicated.)
7. Open access valve and advance catheter within plastic sleeve into client's artificial airway using your dominant hand. **Rationale:** Sterility is maintained because catheter is enclosed by plastic cover and slides within it.
8. With nondominant hand, activate suction valve. Intermittently apply suction (for no more than 5 to 10 seconds) while rotating and withdrawing catheter *completely* back into plastic sheath. **Rationale:** If not totally out of the airway, the catheter impairs client ventilation.
9. Repeat steps 4–6 as necessary to clear secretions; allow time between suctioning for hyperoxygenation. **Rationale:** Repeated suctioning without hyperoxygenation causes complications such as hypoxemia and cardiac dysrhythmias.
10. Attach saline syringe or vial (5–10 mL) to catheter irrigation port; inject saline onto catheter tip while applying suction to rinse catheter and tubing, then close irrigation port and suction valve. **Rationale:** Rinsing prevents catheter occlusion by dried secretions.
11. Remove syringe and turn off suction. Lock mechanism, if appropriate. **Rationale:** Locking catheter prevents inadvertent advancement and occlusion of client's airway.
12. Remove gloves and wash hands.
13. Ensure that call bell is within client's reach.

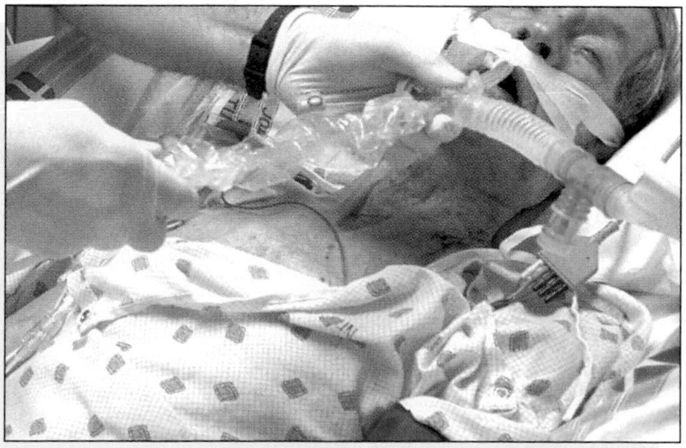

Intubated client with closed system suction catheter being advanced.

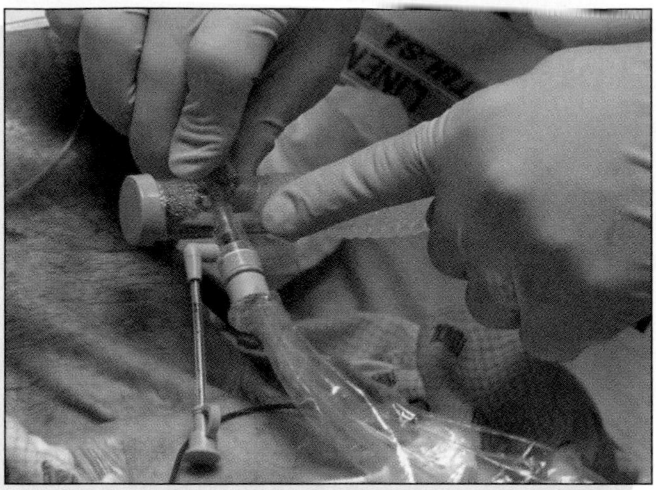

Note black indicator to ensure that catheter is completely withdrawn.

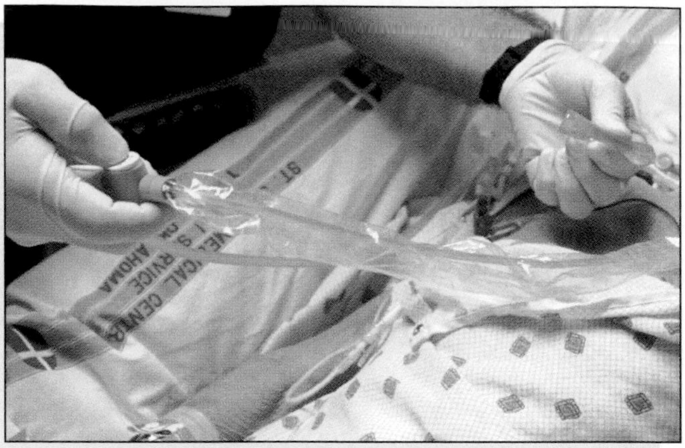

Flush catheter and tubing with saline after suctioning.

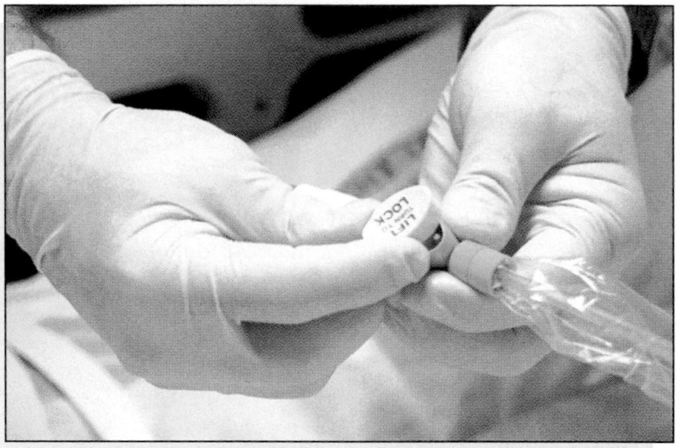

Lock access valve when suctioning is completed.

Documentation for Suctioning

- Frequency of suctioning
- Amount and character of secretions
- Pre- and post-suctioning hyperoxygenation
- Breath sounds, respiratory rate, heart rate and rhythm, and SpO_2
- Client's tolerance of procedure
- Reestablishment of oxygen therapy (e.g., trach mask) and L/minute

Critical Thinking Application

UNEXPECTED OUTCOMES	CRITICAL THINKING OPTIONS
Hypoxemia and bradycardia occur with suctioning	• Preoxygenate before and postoxygenate after suctioning. • Observe for signs of restlessness while suctioning. • Limit suctioning time to no more than 5–10 seconds. • Ensure that catheter is no larger than half the inner diameter of the airway it enters.
Excessive secretions necessitate frequent suctioning.	• Suction more frequently but administer 100% oxygen before and after suctioning. • Establish in-line catheter in sleeve, but check frequently and suction secretions PRN. • Allow rest period before suctioning again (3 minutes). • Turn client regularly to mobilize secretions. • Notify physician for CPT or other therapy. • Maintain adequate hydration.
Aspiration is suspected in enterally tube-fed intubated client.	• Check suctioned secretions for presence of glucose. (Secretions should not contain blood for accurate determination.) • Use only a minimal amount of unit-dose sterile blue dye (as ordered) to tint formula and use with discretion in clients at very high risk for aspiration. • Maintain elevation of HOB. • Monitor gastric residuals regularly. • Advocate small-bore enteral vs NG tube feeding.
ET tube is accidentally extubated.	• Notify physician or call a "code" immediately. • Place client in supine position with head tilt to establish airway. • Provide bag–mask ventilation. • Obtain crash cart for emergency supplies for reintubation.

UNIT 6

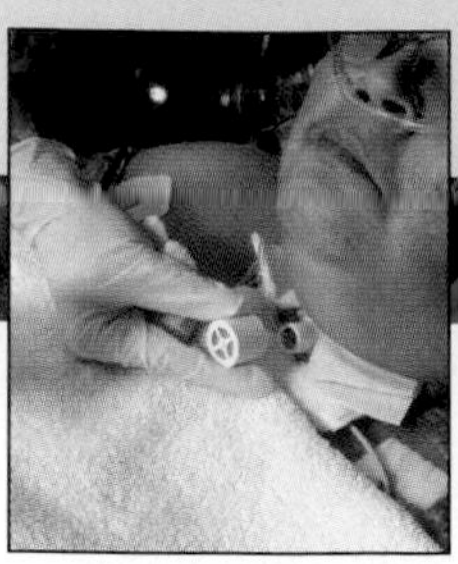

Tracheostomy Care

Nursing Process Data

ASSESSMENT Data Base

Note presence of dried or moist secretions surrounding cannula or on tracheal dressing.

Note excessive coughing or expectoration of secretions.

Assess if routine tracheal care is adequate for this client.

Assess respiratory status: breath sounds, respiratory rate, use of accessory muscles for breathing.

Observe for signs of respiratory distress while tracheal tube is capped: labored breathing, anxious face, flaring of nares, supraclavicular, suprasternal and intercostal retraction while tracheal tube is capped, tachypnea, tachycardia.

Observe vital signs for increased heart rate.

Monitor pulse oximetry (SpO_2).

Auscultate for minimal occlusive cuff inflation pressure.

PLANNING Objectives

To ensure a patent airway

To suction secretions more easily

To improve ventilation

To prevent infection

To prevent tracheal injury

To prevent aspiration while feeding

IMPLEMENTATION Procedures

Assisting with Tracheostomy intubation

Performing Tracheostomy Suctioning

Inflating a Tracheal Tube Cuff

Cleaning the Inner Cannula and Ostomy

Changing Tracheostomy Tube Ties

Capping with a Passey–Muir Valve

EVALUATION Expected Outcomes

Client adequately ventilated and free of respiratory distress.

Secretions easily suctioned.

Tracheostomy site remains free of infection.

Client able to eat without aspirating food.

Client tolerates capped tracheostomy tube.

ASSISTING WITH TRACHEOSTOMY INTUBATION

Equipment

Sterile tracheostomy tray
Antimicrobial solution
Lidocaine for local anesthesia
Sterile tracheal tube with obturator
Sterile gloves
Clean gloves
Suction equipment
Oxygen source
Manual resuscitator bag with adapter
Mechanical ventilator if indicated
Sterile normal saline
Sterile preslit 4 × 4 dressing
Twill (or commercial ties)
Prescribed premedication (e.g., muscle relaxant)
Stethoscope
Soft wrist restraints (if indicated)

Preparation

1. Explain procedure and rationale to client or relatives (or both).
2. If not an emergency situation, obtain permission from client or other legally responsible individual prior to tracheostomy.
3. Wash your hands.
4. Assemble all necessary equipment.
5. Set up tracheostomy tray where sterile field can be maintained; open tray when physician is ready.

Procedure

1. Explain procedure as it is being done.
2. Restrain client, if necessary, with soft wrist restraints. **Rationale:** Interference during insertion can result in injury to client.
3. Open sterile gloves for physician. Don clean gloves.
4. Assist physician by pouring antimicrobial solution into sterile containers on tray. To maintain sterile technique,

Preventing Infection

- Maintain sterile techniques during intubation and suctioning.
- Maintain good handwashing.
- Administer good oral care every 4 hours.
- Avoid instillations of saline into airways.
- Change ventilatory equipment per agency policy.

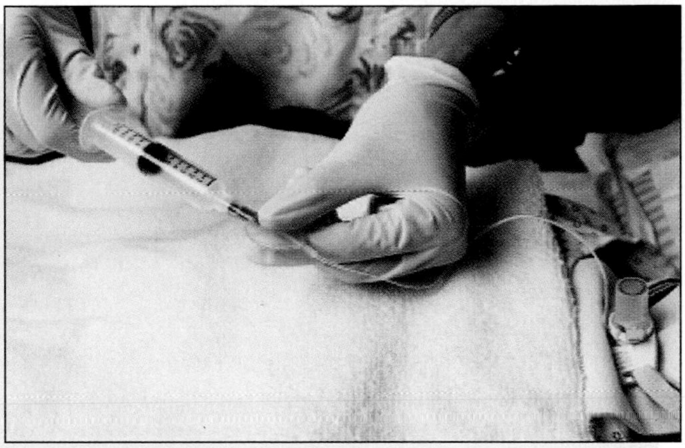

Attach 10-mL syringe to inflate tube cuff.

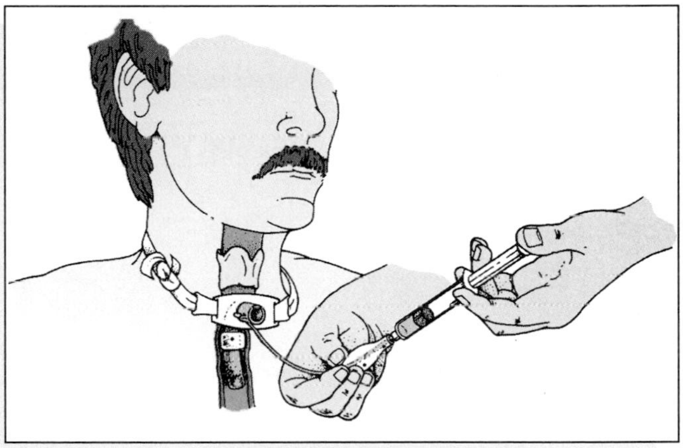

Inflate tube cuff to minimal occlusive volume.

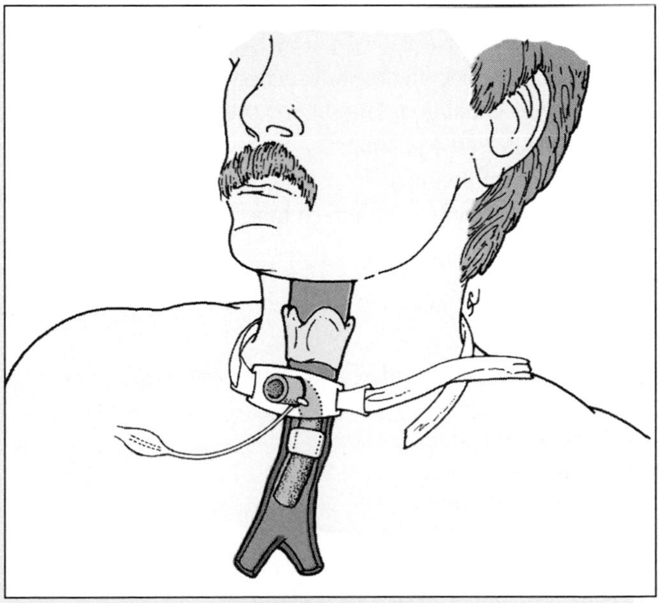

Anatomic placement of a tracheostomy tube.

lidocaine is usually held by the nurse while the physician draws it out of vial.

5. Have suction and oxygen administration equipment ready when trach tube is inserted. (Use suction catheter with diameter half the inner diameter of the tracheostomy tube.) **Rationale:** Introduction of a foreign body increases secretion production. In addition, tube presence hinders effective coughing.
6. Inflate tube cuff. See Inflating a Tracheal Cuff on page 914.
7. Hyperoxygenate client, then, don sterile gloves and, *using sterile technique*, suction when tube is in place. Hyperoxygenate after suctioning.
8. Attach tracheostomy tube with adapter to mechanical ventilator if indicated.
9. Cleanse tracheostomy site with sterile normal saline, secure tube with twill (or commercial holder) and dress site with presplit 4 × 4.
10. Position client for comfort. Semi-Fowler's position makes breathing easier.
11. Tape tube obturator to head of bed. **Rationale:** If tube is inadvertently dislodged, it can be immediately reinserted using obturator.
12. Discard used disposable equipment and remove gloves. Wash hands.
13. Place *call bell* where client can reach it and provide a means of *communication* (e.g., paper and pencil). **Rationale:** Intubation bypasses the upper airway and prevents ability to vocalize.
14. Perform tracheostomy care q4h and PRN.
15. Provide oral hygiene regularly.

> **CLINICAL ALERT**
>
> Suction client's airway PRN. Secretions are usually more copious following the irritation of intubation.

PERFORMING TRACHEOSTOMY SUCTIONING

Equipment

Trach suctioning kit
Bottle of sterile normal saline
2 suction catheters
Suction Catheter Sizes
  Adults: 12–18 French
  Children: 14 French
  Infants: 6–10 French
Sterile gloves, clean gloves
Personal protective equipment—goggles, gown, mask as needed if splash anticipated
Portable suction machine or wall suction with Y-connector or release valve—*maximum* safe suction pressure is −120 mm Hg.
Receptacle for used equipment
Container for sterile saline
Manual resuscitator bag with trach tube adapter
Oxygen source, tubing, and administration device
Stethoscope

Preparation

1. Check physician's orders and client care plan.
2. Gather equipment.
3. Explain procedure to client.
4. Wash your hands.
5. Assess lung sounds.
6. Turn suction on to between −80 and −120 mm Hg pressure. **Rationale:** Higher suction pressure increases risk of mucosal damage.
7. Attach resuscitator bag to oxygen tubing.
8. Turn oxygen flowmeter to maximum (flush).
9. Don clean gloves.
10. Don goggles, mask, and gown as needed.

Procedure

1. Disconnect oxygen source from the tracheostomy tube.
2. Connect oxygen tubing to manual resuscitator bag, then connect to tracheostomy tube.
3. Hyperoxygenate lungs with five breaths using 100% oxygen, or have client take several deep breaths before disconnecting O_2 source from tracheostomy tube. **Rationale:** Suctioning depletes oxygen and causes hypoxia.
4. Disconnect resuscitator bag and place nearby for use after suctioning procedure.
5. Open new suction catheter package. Ensure that catheter size is not greater than half the inner diameter of the tracheostomy tube. **Rationale:** This prevents hypoxia and atelectasis by allowing atmospheric air to be drawn in around catheter.
6. Remove cap from sterile normal saline bottle.
7. Remove clean gloves.
8. Don sterile gloves. Keep dominant hand *sterile* and other hand *clean.*
9. Open sterile container for flushing catheter.
10. Using nondominant (clean) hand, pour saline into container.
11. Holding suction catheter with *sterile* hand, connect it to suction tubing (held in *clean* hand).
12. Grasp vent end of suction catheter with clean hand and guide catheter into tracheostomy tube using sterile hand.
13. Insert catheter, *without* applying suction, quickly and gently into tracheostomy until you feel resistance. **Rationale:** Suction application during insertion may damage tissue.

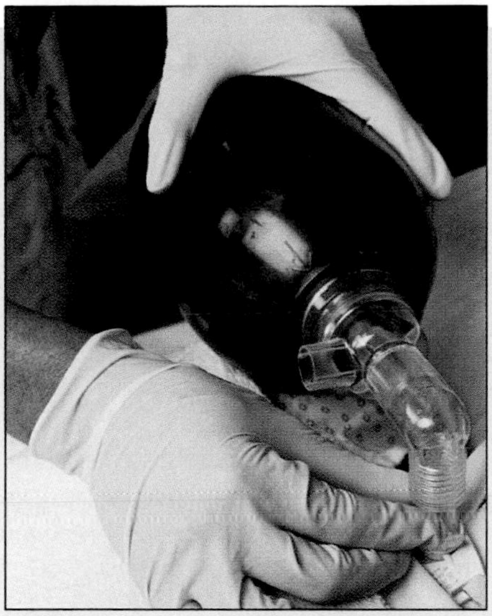

Connect resuscitator bag to hyperoxygenate before and after suctioning.

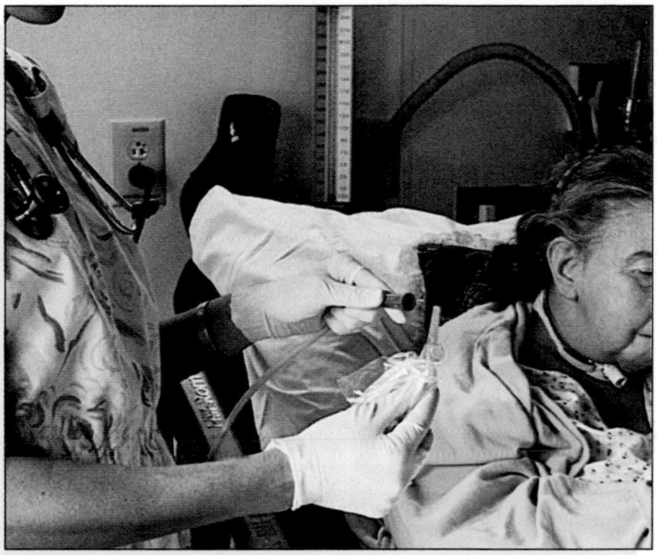

Hold sterile catheter with dominant (sterile) hand and connect suction tubing to catheter.

14. Using *clean* thumb over control opening, apply intermittent suction as you rotate and withdraw catheter from tracheostomy. **Rationale:** Intermittent suction and catheter rotation prevents damage to mucosal lining during suctioning.
15. Suction for no more than 10 seconds. **Rationale:** This minimizes hypoxia and dysrhythmias due to oxygen loss through suctioning.
16. Rinse catheter and connecting tubing with normal saline until clear.
17. Hyperoxygenate lungs with manual resuscitator bag using 100% oxygen, or have client take several deep breaths.
18. Reattach oxygen source to tracheostomy tube.
19. Dispose of catheter by disconnecting it from suction tubing, coiling around fingers, and removing glove back over catheter. Discard the catheter and gloves into appropriate receptacle.
20. Turn off suction.
21. Position client for comfort.
22. Auscultate lungs and check heart rate. Compare to presuctioning data. **Rationale:** Suctioning causes tachycardia but hypoxemia and vagal responses may cause serious bradycardia/cardiac arrest.
23. Wash your hands.
24. Ensure call bell is in client's reach.
25. Empty suction bottle PRN or at end of each shift.

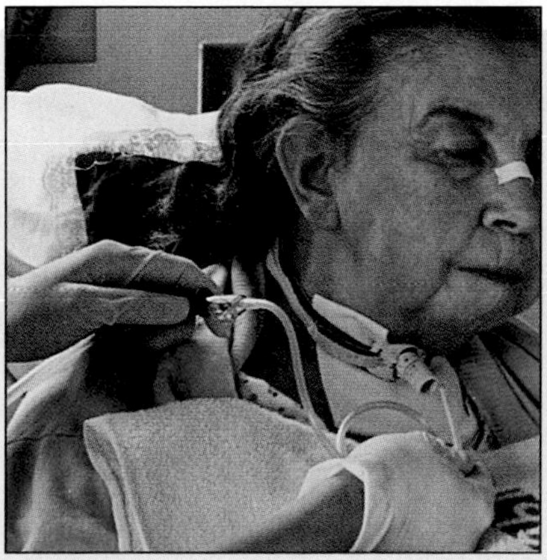

Guide catheter into tracheostomy tube using sterile hand.

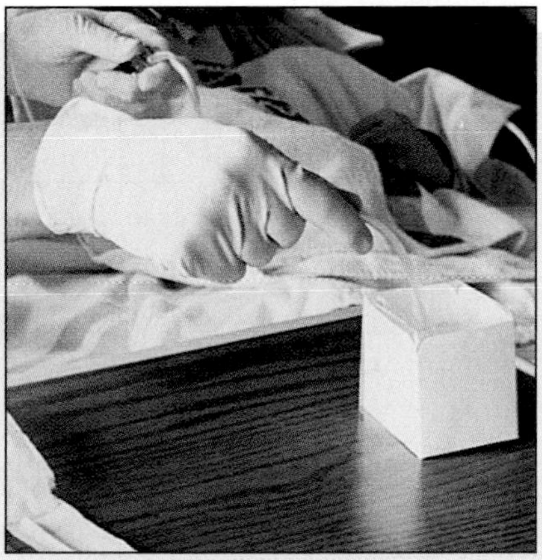

Rinse catheter and connecting tubing with saline to clear.

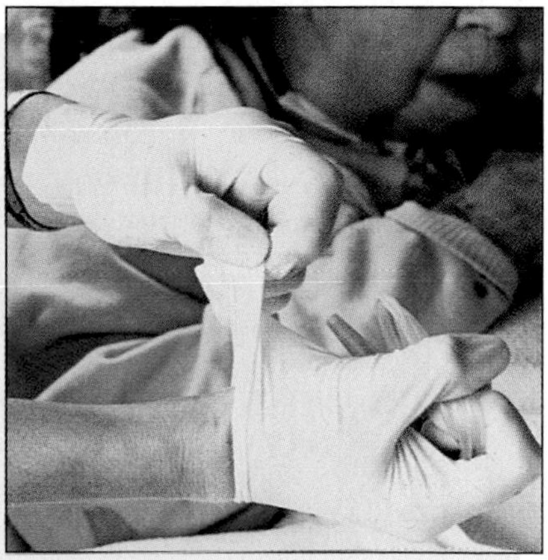

Coil catheter around fingers and pull glove over it for disposal.

INFLATING A TRACHEAL TUBE CUFF

Equipment

10-mL syringe
Suction equipment
Stethoscope
Clean gloves

Note: The foam cuff, a newer type of cuff, does not require injected air. Air enters the balloon when port is open.

CLINICAL ALERT

Low pressure tracheostomy cuffs provide adequate blood flow to trachea, thus decreasing potential of tracheal tissue necrosis. These cuffs do not need periodic deflation.

Procedure

1. Don clean gloves.
2. Attach 10-mL syringe to distal end of inflatable cuff port, making sure seal is tight.
3. Inflate cuff for a minimal leak or minimal occlusive volume. **Rationale:** This provides an adequate seal without risking tracheal pressure necrosis.
4. Ask client to speak—if voice is heard, inflation is inadequate for mechanical ventilation.
5. Connect ventilator or T-piece to tracheal tube opening if indicated.
6. Assess breath sounds every 2 hours. **Rationale:** Presence of bilateral breath sounds indicates proper tube position in trachea.
7. Monitor cuff pressure regularly. **Rationale:** This detects inadvertent cuff overinflation and prevents potential necrosis of tracheal tissue. Pressure is usually maintained at 18–20 mm Hg to prevent tracheal necrosis.

CLINICAL ALERT

Tracheal tube cuff inflation is essential for mechanically ventilated clients. Without cuff inflation, delivered air diverts out through the nose and mouth, and lungs are not ventilated.

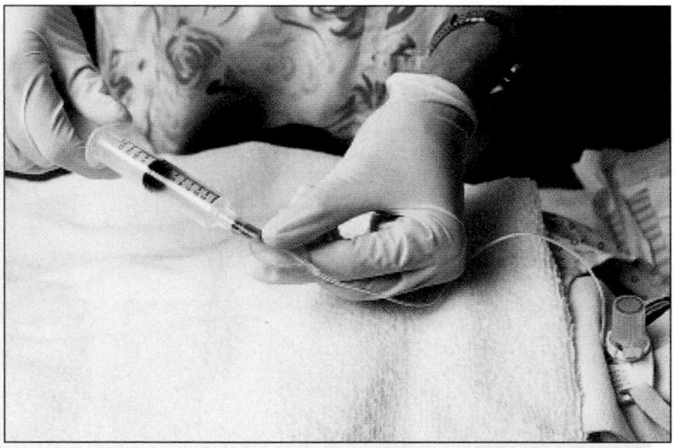

Attach 10-mL syringe to inflate tube cuff.

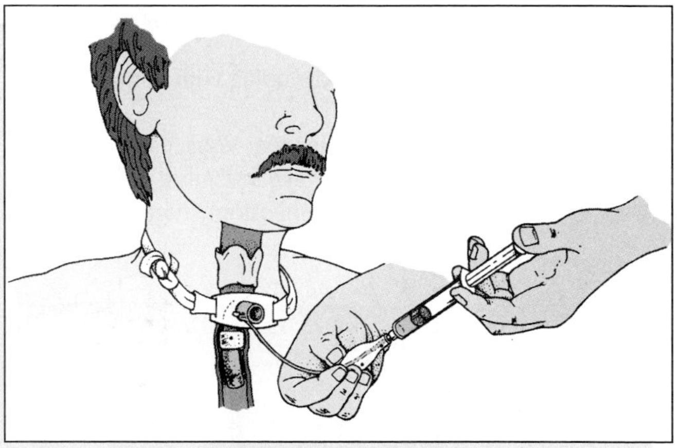

Inflate tube cuff to minimal occlusive volume.

CLEANING THE INNER CANNULA AND OSTOMY

Equipment

Note: Many agencies use disposable inner cannulas that eliminate the need for cleaning.

Tracheal cleaning tray (includes two sterile basins, pipe cleaners, brush, 4 × 4 gauze pad)
Sterile gloves
Suction equipment
Complete tracheal tube set for emergency use
Interchangeable inner cannula of same size
Sterile normal saline
Sterile nonraveling presplit dressings
Clean tracheal ties or commercial tube holder.

Preparation

1. Check physician's orders and client care plan.
2. Assemble equipment.
3. Make sure suction equipment and additional tracheal tubes are available. Suction trach tube before cleaning if indicated.
4. Wash your hands.

Procedure

1. Explain procedure and rationale to client.
2. Open trach tray, and put on one sterile glove.
3. With gloved hand, separate basins; with ungloved hand, pour saline into basin.
4. Don second sterile glove. Secure outer cannula neck plate with index finger and thumb. Unlock inner cannula by turning left about 90°.
5. Gently pull the inner cannula slightly upward and out toward you.
6. Soak nondisposable cannula in sterile basin with saline to remove dried secretions.

> **CLINICAL ALERT**
>
> An obturator is kept at the bedside for emergency use. If the tracheostomy tube is inadvertently dislodged, it can be reinserted immediately using the obturator.

7. Cleanse the lumen and outer surface of the cannula with pipe cleaners or brush moistened with saline. **Rationale:** To remove dried secretions.
8. Rinse cannula thoroughly with saline.
9. Place clean tube on sterile 4 × 4 gauze pad and dry tube thoroughly.
10. Replace inner cannula carefully, stabilizing outer flange of the cannula, with your other hand.
11. Lock the inner cannula by turning the lock to the right so that it is in an upright position.

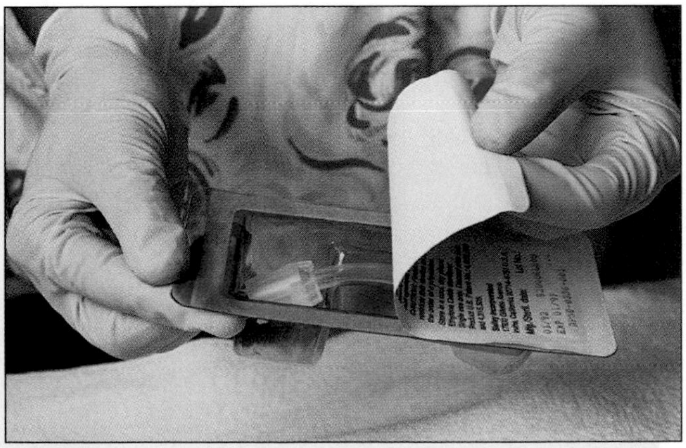

Disposable inner cannula eliminates need for cannula cleaning.

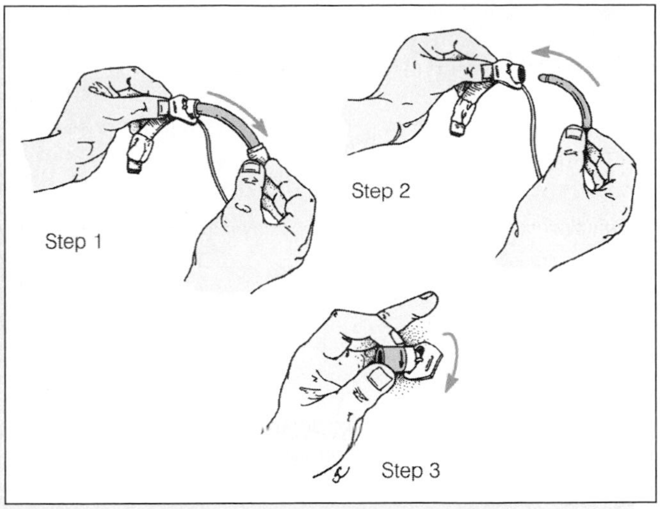

Inner cannula is removed for cleaning. Outer cannula is not.

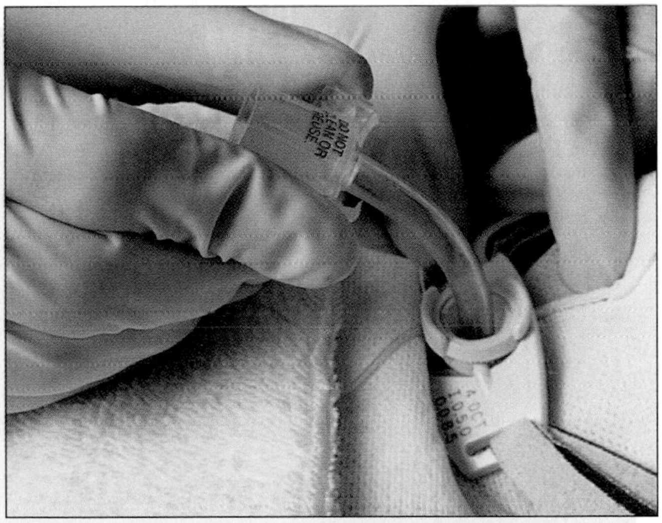

Gently pull inner cannula upward and outward to remove.

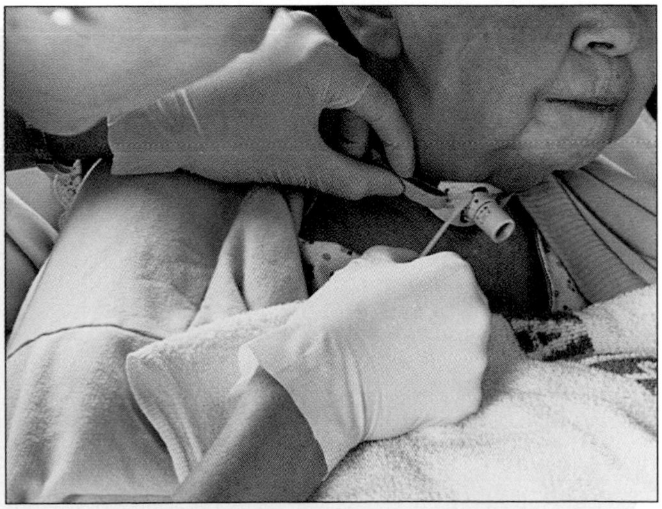

Clean around tracheostomy site and outer cannula.

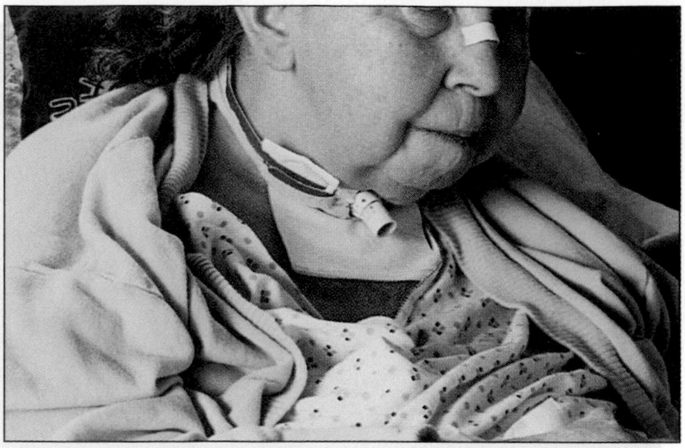

Apply precut nonraveling dressing around tracheostomy.

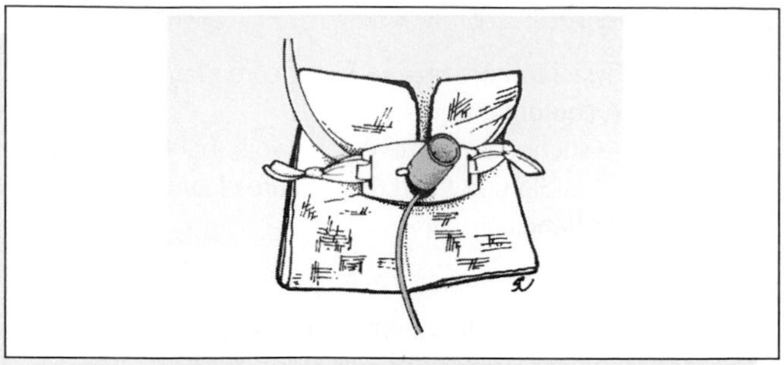

A precut nonraveling sponge is used for the trach dressing to prevent fibers from entering trach site.

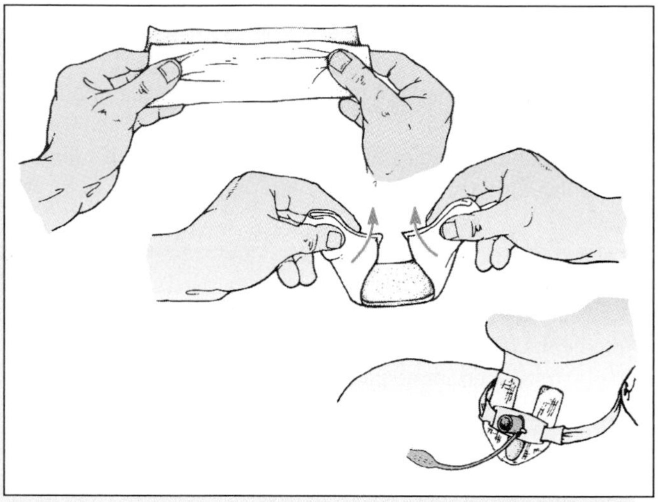

Folded 4 × 4 trach dressing for use if presplit dressing is not available.

12. Cleanse around tracheostomy site with applicator soaked in normal saline.
13. Cleanse outer cannula with separate applicator.
14. Apply precut, nonraveling trach dressing around insertion site (flaps pointing up), and change tracheal ties if needed. **Rationale:** Nonraveling dressing prevents fibers from entering trach tube.
15. Discard soiled dressings, tapes, cleaning equipment, and gloves.
16. Wash your hands.
17. Ensure call bell is within client's reach.

CHANGING TRACHEOSTOMY TUBE TIES

Equipment

Scissors
Forceps
Twill tape or commercial tracheostomy tube holder.

Preparation

1. Seek assistance from another person. **Rationale:** It is safer to have someone hold the trach tube in place when changing ties.
2. Explain procedure to client.
3. Wash your hands.
4. Gather equipment.
5. Place client in semi- to high-Fowler's position.

Procedure

for Twill Tape Ties

1. Cut trach ties length you desire, if not precut.
2. Fold ends of the trach ties over 1½ inches, and cut a slit in the piece starting at the folded edge.
3. If available, have assistant hold the trach tube in place. Cut the old trach ties, remove and discard. **Rationale:** Securing tube helps prevent accidental extubation if client coughs.
4. Pass the slit end of the ties through the flange loop of the trach tube about 2–3 inches (you may use Kelly forceps to grab tie). **Rationale:** Leave the old trach tie in place if you are changing the ties without assistance. This prevents accidental dislodging of the trach tube.
5. Thread the other end of the tie all the way through the slit. Pull it firmly in place. **Rationale:** This action anchors the tie around the flange loop.
6. Repeat steps 4 and 5 on other flange loop.
7. Bring ties around client's neck and tie in a square knot to one side of neck, leaving one finger-breadth slack under tie. **Rationale:** Slack prevents pressure on the neck and jugular vein.
8. Cut off soiled trach ties if not already done, and discard.

9. Position client for comfort.
10. Wash your hands.

Alternate Method

1. Using a long piece of twill, pull end of tape through flange slit.
2. Double tape around back of neck.
3. Thread one end through other flange slit and tie to other end.
4. Apply new tape before old one is cut off and removed (doesn't require an assistant).

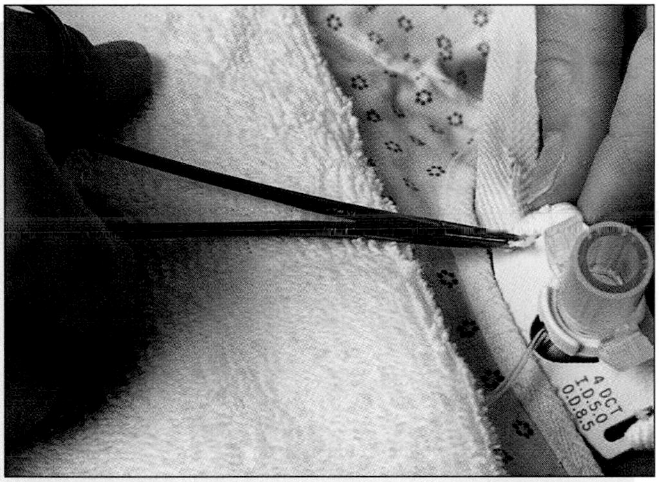

Use forceps to thread tape through tracheostomy neck plate flanges.

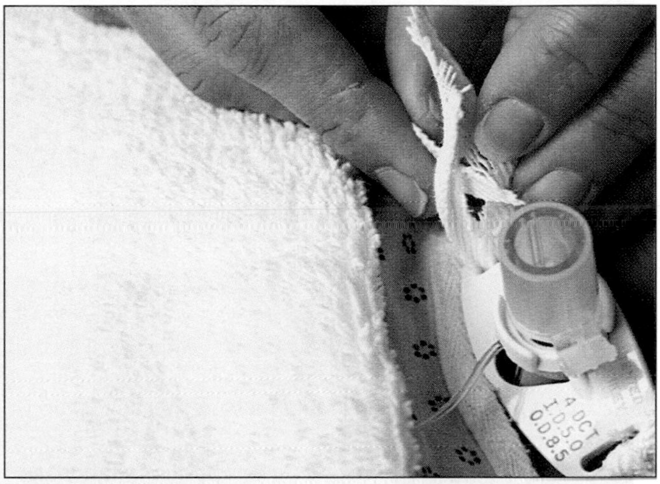

Thread end of tie through slit and pull in place.

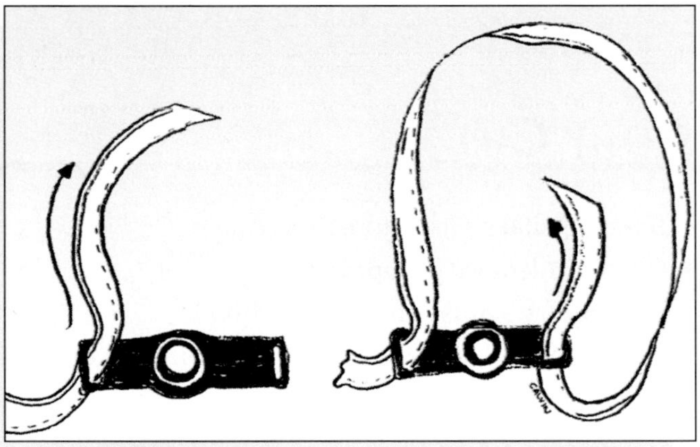

(a) Use a long piece of twill. Pull end through flange slit and double tape around back of neck. (b) Thread one end through other flange slit and tie to other end of twill in square knot.

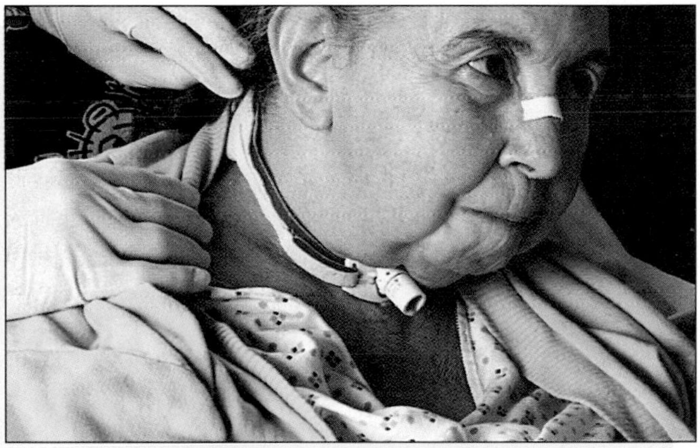

Allow one fingerbreadth slack under trach ties to prevent pressure on neck and jugular vein.

CAPPING WITH A PASSEY–MUIR VALVE

Equipment

Passey-Muir speaking valve or cap
Fenestrated uncuffed tracheostomy tube
Suction source
2 suction catheters
Clean gloves
Sterile gloves
10-mL syringe

Preparation

1. Check physician's orders and client care plan.
2. If client considered to be ready for weaning from airway, obtain order to change to fenestrated uncuffed tube.

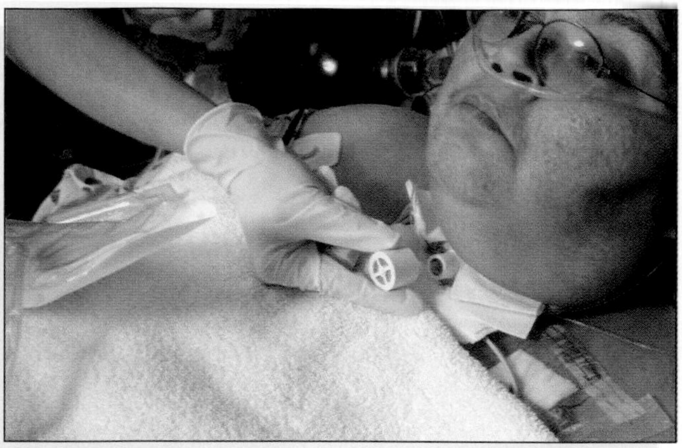

Tracheostomy tube is capped with a one-way valve to allow client to speak.

3. Wash hands.
4. Gather equipment.
5. Explain procedure to client and reassure that suffocation won't occur.
6. Place client in semi- to high-Fowler's position. **Rationale:** This assists with lung expansion and decreases fear of suffocation.
7. Don clean gloves.

Procedure

1. Using clean technique, suction nasopharynx *if cuffed tube in place.* **Rationale:** This removes secretions that have pooled above cuff, preventing their mobilization into lower airways after cuff deflation.
2. Attach syringe and **DEFLATE TRACHEAL CUFF** if present. **Rationale:** If tracheostomy tube is capped and cuff is not deflated, client has no airway. Place speaking valve or cap over opening of tracheostomy tube.
3. Observe client for respiratory distress. **Rationale:** The tube's presence increases resistance to airflow dramatically, thus increasing the work of breathing.
4. Stay at bedside until client is comfortable and exhibits no difficulty breathing.
5. Place notice: "Do not inflate cuff with cap in place" on pilot balloon, over bed, and on client's chart.
6. Discard gloves and wash hands.

CLINICAL ALERT

If tracheostomy tube is capped and cuff is not deflated, client has no airway. Place notice: "*Do not inflate cuff with cap in place*" on pilot balloon, over bed, and on client's chart.

DOCUMENTATION FOR TRACHEOSTOMY CARE

Tracheostomy Intubation

- Clinical manifestations and need for intubation
- Size and type of tube inserted
- Name of physician performing procedure
- Client's tolerance of procedure
- Amount and character of secretions
- Respiratory status before and after procedure
- Any equipment attached to tracheal tube (ventilator or other oxygen delivery device and percent oxygen delivered)
- Provision of means to communicate and summon help.

Cleaning the Inner Cannula and Ostomy

- Time and date of care
- Ostomy site status
- Cannula cleaning or disposable cannula replacement
- Tie or holder replacement

Capping Tracheostomy Tube

- Type of cap utilized
- Tracheal tube DEFLATION status
- Baseline vital signs before procedure
- Client's tolerance of capping
- Respiratory status during procedure
- Vital signs and any indications of respiratory distress postprocedure

Tracheostomy Care

- Trach care completed
- Appearance of site
- Characteristics of secretions
- Trach ties changed
- Client's tolerance of procedure

Tracheostomy Tube Suctioning

- Amount, color, and consistency of secretions
- Changes in breath sounds
- Respiratory and heart rate changes
- Client's tolerance to procedure
- Unanticipated problems and client's response

- Frequency of client suctioning
- Before and after suctioning hyperoxygenation

Tracheal Tube Cuff Inflation

- Cuff inflation auscultated for minimal occlusive pressure.
- Changes in respiratory status after inflation
- Mechanical ventilator settings

Critical Thinking Application

UNEXPECTED OUTCOMES	CRITICAL THINKING OPTIONS
Tracheostomy tube becomes dislodged.	• Notify physician or call a "code" immediately. • Keep second tracheal set available. • Ensure patent airway by one of the following methods: *Note*: It is critical that nurses know what to do if dislodgement occurs, because major complications could occur. a. Immediately insert obturator or sterile forceps into stoma to preserve airway. b. Reinsert old tube using obturator if new one not available. c. Suction stoma, if there is time. Then reinsert new tracheal tube, secure with tapes, and establish ventilation. Oxygenate with manual resuscitation bag if signs of respiratory distress are present. • Establish ventilation by pinching stoma closed and have assistant provide/administer bag-mask ventilation.
Client experiences distress—tracheostomy tube is obstructed; breath sounds not detected.	• Notify physician or call "code" immediately. If no physician available, follow these procedures: Deflate cuff. Cut tracheostomy ties. Remove tube. Insert tracheal dilator (if at bedside) or obturator. Establish airway. Insert new tube, and reestablish ventilation.
Secretions and coughing are excessive while inner cannula is cleansed.	• Perform oral suctioning before removing inner cannula. • Suction lumen, if necessary, while soaking inner cannula. • Place another inner cannula in trach tube, and continue to soak cannula (If not using disposable inner cannula).
Inner cannula is dislodged.	• Insert extra cannula from emergency set if cannulas are interchangeable. If not, insert new tracheal set.
Client unable to be off ventilator long enough for cleansing of inner cannula.	• Insert new inner cannula, and place client back on ventilator • Proceed to clean inner cannula and keep it clean for next change.
for Tracheostomy Tube Suctioning	
Dysrhythmias occur with suctioning.	• Observe for signs of increased restlessness, tachycardia, bradycardia, or other dysrhythmia. • Limit suctioning time to no more than 10 seconds. • Ensure that suction catheter is no larger than half the inner diameter of the artificial airway. • Hyperinflate lungs with 100% oxygen before and after suctioning.

UNEXPECTED OUTCOMES	CRITICAL THINKING OPTIONS
Excessive secretions require frequent suctioning.	• Use catheter in sleeve for convenience and economy.
After suctioning, intubated client still sounds congested.	• Allow rest period before suctioning again (3 minutes). • Hyperoxygenate lungs with 100% oxygen before and after suctioning. • Turn client regularly to mobilize secretions. • Notify physician for CPT or other therapy. • Maintain adequate hydration.
for Tracheostomy Tube Cuff Care	
Balloon ruptures or herniates over the end of the tube. Breath sounds not detected.	• Deflate balloon, remove and replace with new tube immediately and report to physician. • Assess client for respiratory distress. A portion of the cuff may have been aspirated.

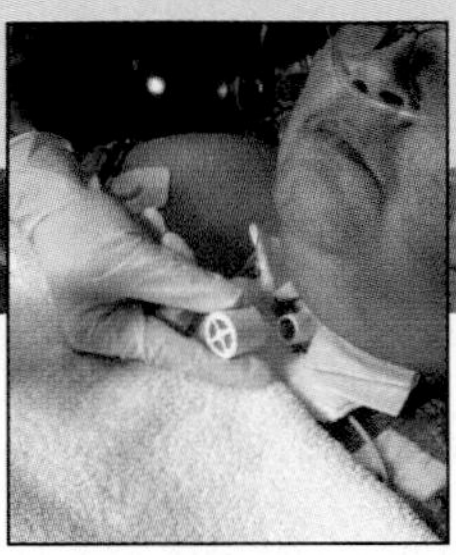

UNIT 7

Chest Drainage Systems

Nursing Process Data

ASSESSMENT *Data Base*
Assess client's respiratory status, vital signs.
Note placement site of chest tube (intrapleural or mediastinal).
Assess that all drainage system connections are securely taped.
Note prescribed amount of negative pressure to be established.
Check patency of chest drainage system.
Assess for signs of mediastinal shift.
Note character and amount of chest drainage.

PLANNING *Objectives*
To evacuate air and/or fluid from intrapleural space to promote lung reexpansion
To reestablish negative intrapleural pressure
To facilitate drainage of fluid from the mediastinum following cardiac surgery
To administer autotransfusion following cardiac surgery

IMPLEMENTATION *Procedures*
Maintaining a Two-Bottle Drainage/Suction System
Setting Up and Maintaining a Disposable Water Seal Chest Drainage System
Administering Autotransfusion Using Pleur-Evac ATS
Assisting with Removal of Chest Tube

EVALUATION *Expected Outcomes*
Water seal drainage or suction is maintained until air/fluid removed from pleural space and client's lung is reexpanded.
Prescribed amount of suction is maintained in system.
Normal respiratory function is restored (breath sounds normal, x-ray shows lung reexpansion).
Mediastinal drainage promotes venous return and cardiac output post cardiac surgery.
Client's blood count improves with postoperative autotransfusion.

MAINTAINING A TWO-BOTTLE DRAINAGE/SUCTION SYSTEM

Equipment

Two-bottle chest drainage system with manufacturer's instructions for use
Tape
Suction source, if indicated (e.g., wall suction or Emerson pump)

Preparation

1. Fill water seal/collection bottle (#1) with 300 mL water to submerge water seal tube.
2. Attach client's chest catheter tubing to water seal tube to establish a seal preventing atmospheric air from entering client's pleural space and to reestablish intrapleural negative pressure.
3. Observe client's chest catheter tubing to check if air/fluid is escaping from client's intrapleural space.
4. Connect water seal bottle to suction regulator (#2).
5. Make sure all tubing and bottle connections are sealed to ensure system is airtight. **Rationale:** System will not function properly if there are air leaks.

Procedure

for Gravity Drainage

1. Check that water seal/collection bottle tube (attached to client's chest catheter tubing) is submerged in 300 mL water. **Rationale:** This prevents air from entering tubing and client's pleural space.
2. Check that air vent tube of second bottle is open to atmosphere and unobstructed.
3. Ensure patency of system by noting tidaling in water seal tube (fluid rises in tube with client's inhalation and descends on exhalation). *Note: Tidaling does not occur with mediastinal tubes.*
4. Note occasional bubbling of air from the water seal tube. **Rationale:** This is a sign that air is being evacuated from client's chest.
5. Report event of continuous bubbling in the water seal bottle. **Rationale:** This is indicative of an air leak. Physician should be notified. See *Steps for Locating Air Leak, p. 925.*
6. Check tubing for obstruction. **Rationale:** Tidaling ceases when lung has reexpanded or intrapleural tube system is obstructed.
7. Assess for return of breath sounds or obtain chest x-ray to determine reexpansion.

CLINICAL ALERT

Chest tubes should not be clamped except briefly while checking for an air leak, or for changing a disposable collection system.

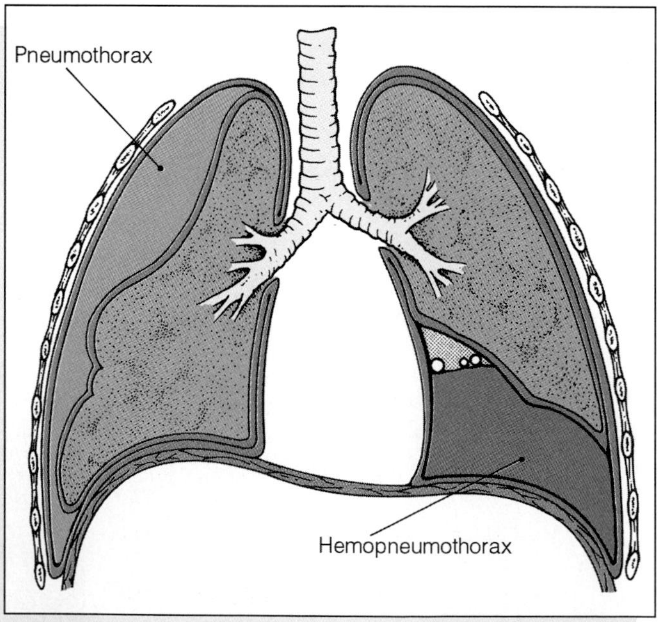

Pneumothorax refers to air in the pleural space and hemothorax to blood in the pleural space around the lung; both conditions lead to build-up of positive pressure and compression of lung tissue and possible compression of medastinal structures with decreased venous return and decreased cardiac output.

for Suction

1. Submerge lower end of suction control tube in prescribed amount of water. **Rationale:** Depth of immersion controls amount of suction applied (20 cm water produces 20 cm suction).
2. Leave suction control tube open at the top. **Rationale:** This provides an outlet of air from client's chest to the atmosphere.
3. Connect air vent tubing to Emerson pump or wall suction.
4. Regulate suction source to point where water in second bottle just bubbles. **Rationale:** This indicates that desired suction has been reached.
5. Note *occasional* bubbling of air in the water seal tube of first bottle. **Rationale:** This indicates that air is being evacuated from client's pleural space. *Continuous bubbling in water seal bottle should not occur.*
6. Note *continual* bubbling of air through open end of control tube in the second bottle (suction source).
7. Note and record fluid level in water seal/collection bottle. **Rationale:** A rise in level represents drainage form client's chest. Notify physician if there is over 100 mL drainage per hour. This amount represents excessive bleeding requiring medical management.

Using a Two-Bottle Chest Drainage/ Suction System

First Bottle

- Functions as a water seal and drainage collection bottle.
- Used mainly to reestablish negative intrapleural pressure to reinflate lung in client with pneumothorax.

Second Bottle

- May serve as an air vent for gravity drainage system, or
- Be connected to suction source (e.g., wall suction or Emerson pump) to establish prescribed amount of negative pressure in system.

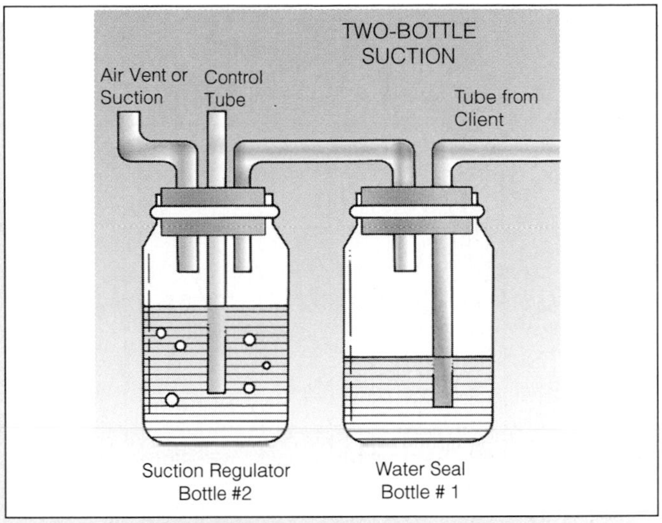

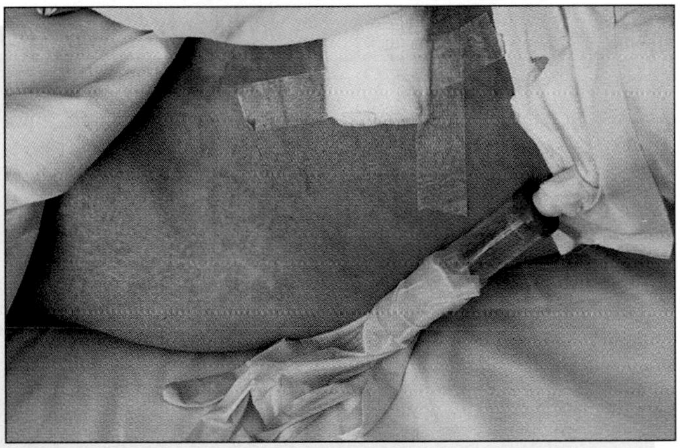

Heimlich valve functions similar to one-bottle suction.

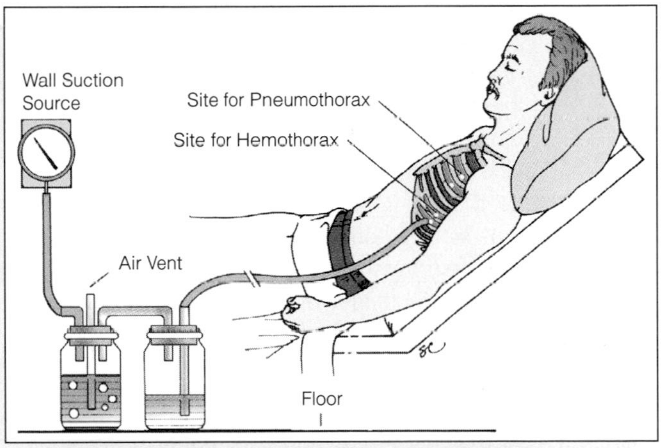

Keep collection system below client's chest.

SETTING UP AND MAINTAINING A DISPOSABLE WATER SEAL CHEST DRAINAGE SYSTEM

Equipment

Disposable water seal chest drainage system and stand
Tubing adapter
60-mL sterile syringe with catheter tip or sterile funnel
Sterile water in pouring bottle
Tape
Suction source

Note: Placement of chest tubes in the mediastinum for drainage following cardiac surgery is common. Intrapleural pressure is not affected.

Procedure

1. Gather equipment.
2. Wash hands.
3. Unwrap water seal chest drainage system.
4. Place unit in stand on floor at bedside.
5. Remove plastic connector on short tube attached to water-seal chamber.
6. Remove plunger from 60-mL syringe and attach barrel of syringe (or funnel) to a short rubber tube.
7. Pour specified amount of sterile water into barrel of syringe, filling water seal chamber to 2-cm level (according to package directions). **Rationale:** This level provides sufficient fluid to create a one-way valve to prevent room air from entering client's intrapleural space.

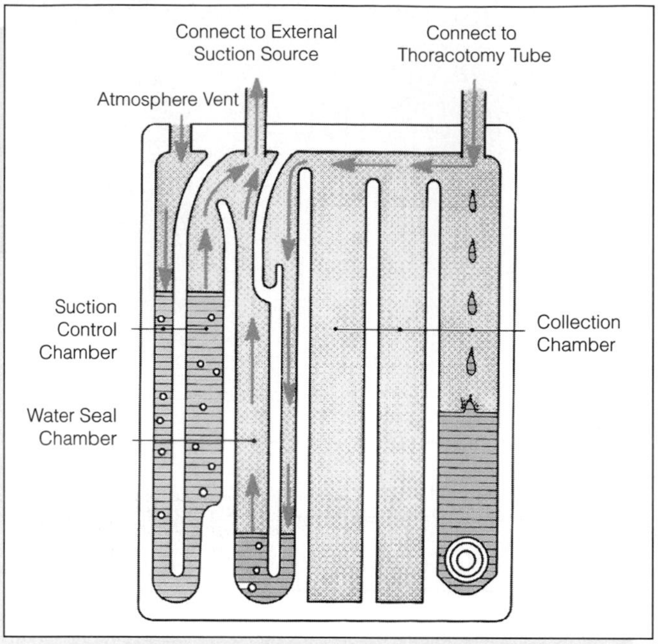

Disposable water-seal chest drainage system.

8. Remove plastic plug from atmosphere vent to suction control chamber.
9. Attach 60mL syringe barrel to atmosphere vent and pour sterile water into chamber.
10. Fill suction control chamber to 20-cm level. **Rationale:** Fluid level controls amount of negative pressure created throughout system.
11. Insert plastic plug to close vent of suction control chamber.

Note: Some chest drainage systems do not require water in either chamber, or only the suction control chamber. See manufacturer's instruction for waterless system use. *Dry suction is quieter and capable of achieving greater degrees of negative pressure (up to -40 cm H_2O). These units may have a "dry suction control" dial usually set at -10 to -20 cm H_2O. Turn on suction source until orange float appears in indicator window to establish suction.*

CLINICAL ALERT

Subcutaneous emphysema (air in tissue) may be felt around the chest tube insertion site, but should be reported if it extends beyond this.

12. Remove long tube adapter from collection chamber and connect it to chest tubes.
13. Tape connection.
14. Coil tubing loosely on the bed, but provide a straight line of tubing from bed to collection system. **Rationale:** Straight-line tubing prevents pooling of fluid.
15. Make sure tubing is free and not kinked. Do not use pins or restrain tubing. **Rationale:** Pins could puncture tubing, causing an air leak.
16. Attach short rubber tube on water-seal chamber to suction source using an adapter connection piece.
17. Turn suction device on slowly until bubbling occurs in suction control chamber.
18. Monitor water levels daily in both water seal chamber and suction control chamber.
19. Maintain pressure.
    a. Keep drainage system below level of bed.
    b. Maintain suction control negative pressure to create gentle bubbling.
    c. Maintain water seal level (2 cm). **Rationale:** Water seal prevents room air from entering pleural space.
    d. Maintain suction control chamber water level at 20 cm or as ordered.

CLINICAL ALERT

Strip and milk chest tubes *only* with physician's orders. Excessive negative pressure created by stripping and milking leads to increased negative pressure in intrapleural space.

20. Maintain chest tube patency. Only if physician orders, milk chest tubes to maintain drainage and tube patency.
    a. Milk tube away from client toward the drainage receptacle (disposable system or bottles).
    b. If ordered, milk tube by alternately folding or squeezing and then releasing drainage tubing. **Rationale:** This provides intermittent suction to the chest tube but generates extreme negative pressure in intrapleural space.
21. Strip chest tubes *only* if physician orders.
    a. To strip chest tube, pinch tubing close to chest with one hand and, using a lubricated thumb and forefinger, compress and slide fingers down tube toward receptacle. (Lubricant material is usually petrolatum or alcohol swab.)
    b. Release pressure on tube and repeat stripping action until reaching receptacle. Increased negative pressure can occur.
22. Keep rubber-tipped hemostat at the client's bedside. **Rationale:** In emergency, tube can be clamped off nearest to chest insertion site.
23. Keep collection system below client's chest level. **Rationale:** This enables fluid to flow by gravity.
24. Mark drainage on disposable system collection chamber every shift. Drainage should be measured at eye level. Report drainage exceeding 100 mL/hr.
25. Assess client's status.
    a. Instruct client to deep breathe and cough at frequent intervals. **Rationale:** Frequent deep breathing helps to expand the lungs.
    b. Encourage client to change positions frequently. Chest tube drainage does not limit client activity.
    c. Observe and report any unusual respiratory signs or symptoms.

Check Points for Chest Tube Air Leaks

Check Insertion Site

- Pinch or briefly clamp with padded hemostat tube at chest insertion site. Bubbling stops in the water seal chamber if there is an air leak at insertion site.

Check Tubing

- Pinch rubber connecting tubing. Bubbling stops if there is a leak at chest tube connector site.

Check Water Seal Drainage System

- Pinch rubber connecting tubing. Bubbling continues if there is a leak in water seal connection.

Observe water seal chamber. There should not be excessive continuous bubbling. A small amount of bubbling is seen in the water seal:

- When suction is first initiated.
- As air is displaced by drainage in the collection chambers.
- As client exhales and coughs and air is forced cut of pleural space.

When lung has reexpanded, the bubbles cease.

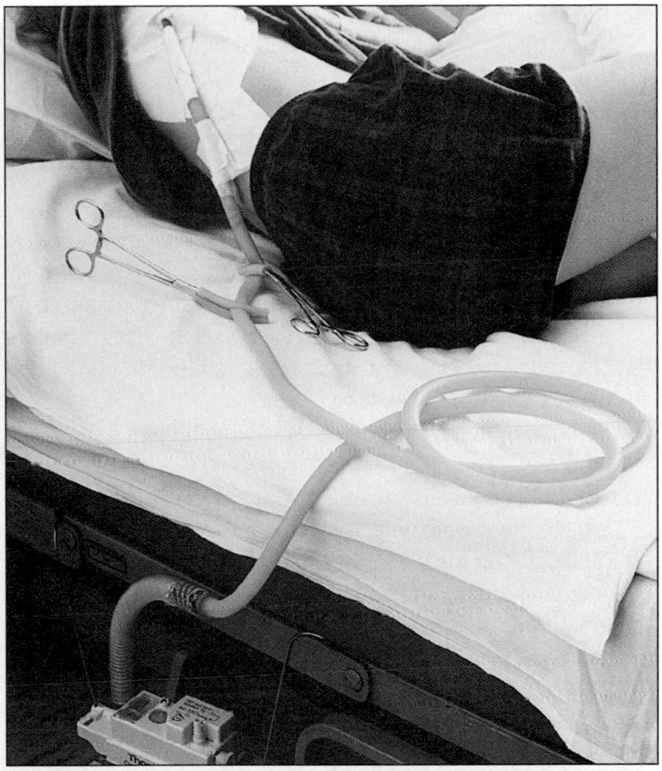

Padded hemostat or plastic tube clamp is used for clamping chest tube. Tube clamped only if ordered.

ADMINISTERING AUTOTRANSFUSION USING PLEUR-EVAC ATS

Equipment

Sterile disposable Pleur-evac ATS including blood collection bag
Replacement bag
Microaggregate filter
Clean gloves
Sterile saline or water in parking bottle

Note: A variety of sterile chest drainage systems provide evacuation of air and/or fluid from the chest or mediastinum. Evacuated blood may be simultaneously reinfused or collected and reinfused in postoperative or trauma cases.

Procedure

1. Wash hands and don gloves.
2. Connect client's pleural or mediastinal chest tube by following steps 1 through 3 printed on Pleur-evac unit. **Rationale:** Tight connection establishes water-seal drainage system.
3. Check that ALL clamps are open on blood collection bag and drainage tubing and that connections are airtight.
4. Check that blood begins collecting in bag.
5. Mark time and amount of drainage on bag.

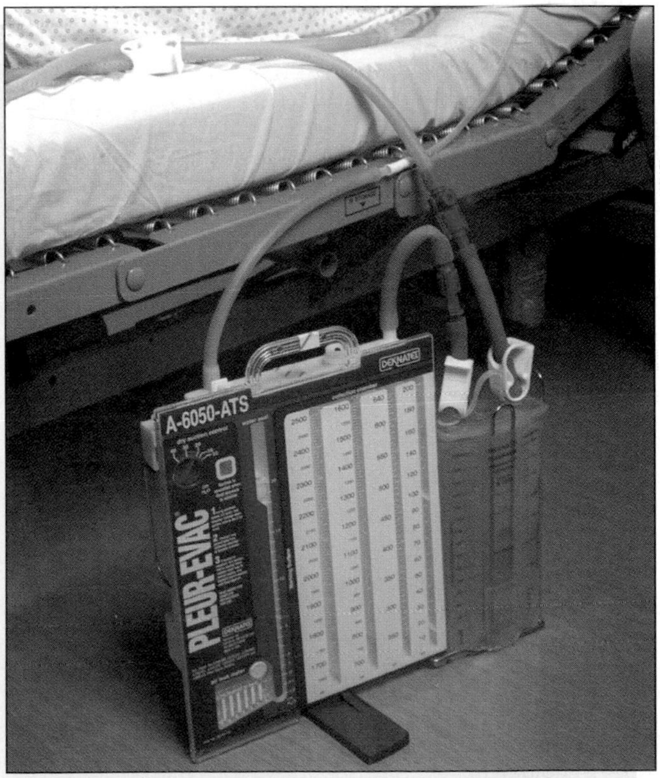

Pleur-evac autotransfusion system (ATS) frequently placed in cardiac surgery.

6. Close clamp on chest drainage tubing and collection bag and connect new bag to drainage system. Make sure all connections are tight.
7. Depress button on high-negativity relief valve, and release it when negativity drops to desired level. **Rationale:** This reduces excess negativity before removing first collection bag.
8. Close white clamp on client tubing, then close two white clamps on top of collection bag, and disconnect all connectors on first bag.
9. Remove protective cap from collection tubing on replacement bag. Maintain aseptic technique when changing tubing.
10. Use red connectors to connect unit's collection tubing to client's chest drainage tube.
11. Remove protective cap from replacement bag's suction tube.
12. Use blue connectors to attach replacement bag's suction tube to Pleur-evac unit.
13. Open all clamps, and check that system is airtight.
14. Attach red (female) and blue (male) connector sections on top of autotransfusion bag.
15. Move out and disconnect metal support arms, and disconnect foot hook. **Rationale:** Releasing these connections allows you to remove bag from drainage unit.
16. Attach replacement bag by using foot hook and support arm.
17. Slide bag off support frame and invert bag with spike port pointing up. **Rationale:** This position allows blood to be reinfused from original collection bag.
18. Remove protective cap from spike port, and insert a microaggregate filter. Twist filter into position. **Rationale:** Filter is essential for reinfusion.
19. Prime filter by gently squeezing inverted bag until drip chamber is half full.
20. Close clamp on reinfusion line, and remove residual air from bag.
21. Invert bag on IV pole.
22. Flush IV tubing to remove air, then reinfuse blood by gravity or pump according to hospital policy. Blood should be totally reinfused within 6 hours from *start of collection.*
23. Remove gloves and wash hands.
24. Assess neurologic signs and pulmonary status every 4 hours. **Rationale:** Microemboli can occur with autotransfusion.

CLINICAL ALERT

Reinfusion is not indicated unless system is primed with drainage, and an additional 50 mL of drainage has been collected for reinfusion.

No more than 6 hours should elapse from time of *beginning* collection to *completion* of reinfusion.

Refer to evacuation/reinfusion system manufacturer's package insert for indications, contraindications, and instructions for use.

ASSISTING WITH REMOVAL OF CHEST TUBE

Equipment

Suture removal set
Rubber-tipped or plastic clamp
Sterile 4 × 4 or petrolatum gauze dressings
Elasticized foam tape
Sterile gloves

Procedure

1. Gather equipment and inform client of the steps of the procedure.
2. Assist client to edge of bed.
3. Don sterile gloves.
4. Assist physician to
   a. Remove dressing.
   b. Clip suture of chest tube.
   c. Place clamp on chest tube.
   d. Instruct client to take a deep breath and hold it or to *hum* during tube removal.
   e. Hold sterile dressing in place while chest tube is being removed. (Petrolatum dressings form airtight seal.)
   f. Apply dressing over wound and tape securely. Remove equipment.
5. Remove gloves and discard. Wash hands.
6. Reevaluate client's status regularly. **Rationale:** Client should be assessed for unstable vital signs, diminished or absent breath sounds, or respiratory distress (pneumothorax, mediastinal shift) following removal of chest tubes.

Note: Chest tubes are usually removed when drainage has been less than 50 mL for 8 hours

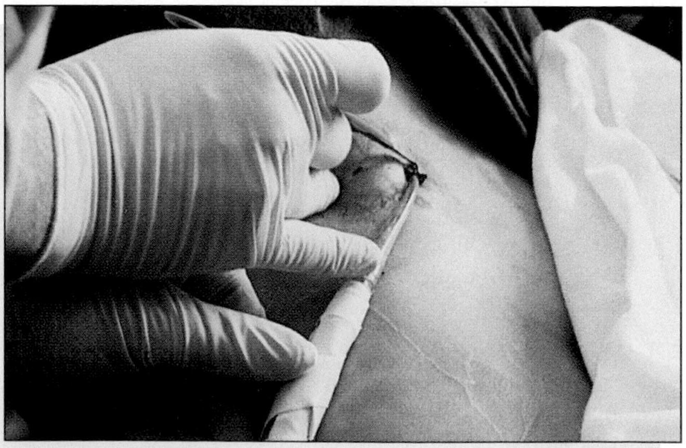

Sutures anchoring chest tube are cut.

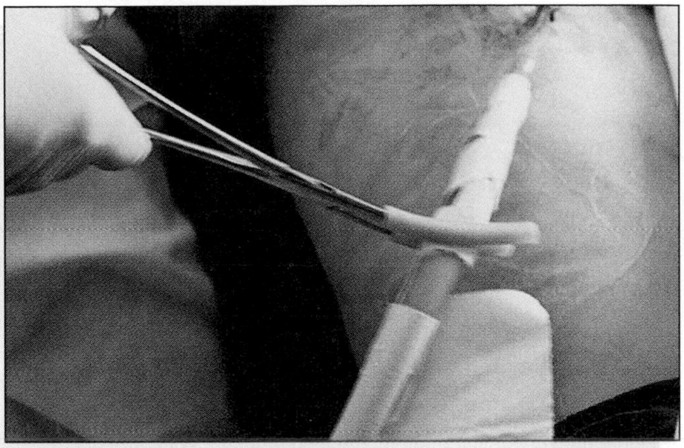

Chest tube is clamped in preparation.

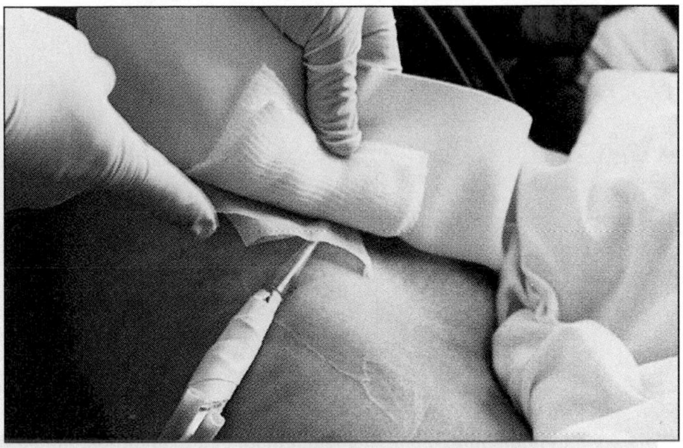

Dressing is applied immediately upon tube removal.

DOCUMENTATION FOR CHEST DRAINAGE SYSTEMS

Chest Drainage System

- Site and size of chest tubes inserted and suction pressure established
- Client's tolerance of procedure
- Vital signs
- Breath sounds
- Drainage—amount, color
- Any problem with the system, and its management
- Client activity (turning, ambulation)
- Respiratory status, including rate, and breath sounds
- Chest-tube milking/stripping if performed

Autotransfusion

- Amount of blood reinfused
- Time collection started to completion of reinfusion
- Signs and symptoms of any complications encountered
- Changes in coagulation times or hemoglobin, hematocrit
- Client's response to treatment

Chest Tube Removal

- Breath sounds
- Premedication administered
- Name of physician removing tube
- Status of insertion site and dressing applied
- Client's tolerance of procedure

Critical Thinking Application

UNEXPECTED OUTCOMES	CRITICAL THINKING OPTIONS
Air leak is present, indicated by continual bubbling in water-seal bottle.	• Check for specific leak area by clamping chest tube (if physician's orders allow) between water-seal bottle or disposable system and client. a. If water-seal bottle continues to bubble, the leak is in the tubing. b. If water-seal bottle stops bubbling, the leak is in the client's chest tube at the site of the insertion. • Secure all connections with tape or wire. • Change tubing if necessary (after obtaining physician's order). • Apply sterile petrolatum gauze or split 4 × 4 and occlusive dressing around chest-tube insertion site if air leak is at insertion site.
Suction control bottle is not bubbling.	• Suction pressure is too low. Increase suction until bubbling occurs.
Chest tube becomes dislodged.	• Instruct the client to exhale. Then compress insertion site and provide tight seal with hand and apply occlusive dressing. • Notify physician.
Client develops signs of mediastinal shift—trachea shifts to unaffected side, paradoxial pulse develops, jugular veins distend, cardiac output decreases.	• Observe for signs of respiratory distress. • Notify physician *immediately*. • Check drainage tube for patency. • Prepare for assisting with possible pericardotomy.
Chest tube becomes disconnected from water-seal drainage system.	• Clamp chest tube near chest insertion site. • Replace the extension tubing leading from the chest tube and insert into open bottle sterile normal saline to create "underwater" seal. • Unclamp chest tube as soon as extension tubing is replaced and placed under temporary water seal or new collection system. • Tape or wire new extension connection sites to prevent disconnection. • Observe for signs of respiratory distress due to pneumothorax and report.
Chest drainage tube becomes obstructed by a clot or obstruction.	• Observe tubing for kinks. Loop tubing on bed and allow straight drainage down to collection system. • Assess tubing for signs of clot, sluggish drainage through tube, visualization of clotted material in tube. • Obtain physician's order to milk or strip chest tubes. • Lift tubing to drain pooled drainage into collection tubing.

GERONTOLOGIC CONSIDERATIONS

The physiologic age changes that occur in the elderly affect the respiratory system.

- The respiratory muscles lose their strength and the rib cage becomes more rigid.
- Lungs lose their elasticity, breathing capacity decreases, and depth of respirations decrease.
- The alveoli increase in size and decrease in number as well as become less elastic and more dilated.
- Gas exchange is reduced; the $Pa{O_2}$ decreases 1 mm/year after age 60, so a reading of 77 mm Hg is not unusual in an elderly client.
- Skeletal alterations affect posture and restrict lung expansion.

Pulmonary disorders occur more frequently in the elderly and are the fourth leading cause of death.

- Functional respiratory reserve is reduced with aging; the elderly are at greater risk for respiratory failure.
- Pneumonia may occur spontaneously or as a complication of other conditions. Because it is frequently a cause of death in the elderly, this condition should be assessed for and monitored aggressively.
- COPD, a broad classification of pulmonary disorders, is a major cause of death and disability, especially among the elderly.
- Asthma may occur as a problem in the elderly who have never had the disease.
- Cancer of the lung is not uncommon in the elderly and is the leading cause of cancer death.

It is important to implement nursing actions that support the respiratory system in the elderly.

- Respiratory activity and exercises are necessary to promote gas exchange; deep breathing, coughing, and moderate exercise.
- Monitor hydration status to liquefy secretions and prevent dehydration.
- Monitor oxygen therapy closely with the elderly—low levels of oxygen with COPD; check for carbon dioxide narcosis.
- The elderly are at especially high risk for hypoxemia with bedrest ($P{O_2}$ may drop to 40 mm Hg even with a night's sleep). Position change (supine to sitting), regular turning, range of motion, and early mobilization all stimulate ventilation and must be encouraged in the bedfast client.

MANAGEMENT GUIDELINES

Each state legislates a Nurse Practice Act for RNs and LVN/LPNs. Health care facilities are responsible for establishing and implementing policies and procedures that conform to their state's regulations. Verify the regulations and role parameters for each health care worker in your facility.

Delegation of Responsibilities

- Each state identifies the scope of practice for RNs, LVN/LPNs, and Respiratory Care Practitioners. States may differ in defining responsibilities of respiratory care by these practitioners. Usually, the respiratory care practitioner is licensed to perform invasive procedures such as suctioning, changing tracheostomy inner cannulas, and administering medication by aerosol. The initiation of oxygen administration by various modes and utilization of biophysical parameters (ABGs, etc.) and standard protocols in decision making and management of the mechanically ventilated client are also within the scope of respiratory care practice.
- All professionals collaborate in the care planning and evaluation of client responses to respiratory care interventions. The nurse must be aware of the unique role competencies, responsibilities, and accountabilities of specialty personnel when a variety of care providers are involved.
- The nurse should ensure that regular turning and deep breathing are encouraged by the CNA/UAP to promote ventilation and prevent complications of immobility in bedfast clients.

- The CNA/UAP should be familiar with appropriate client positioning to promote airway patency and reduce risk for aspiration of oral intake.
- Even though hospitals are "smoke free" today, all personnel must take precautions when oxygen is in use: No petrolatum products around nose or mouth; no battery-operated equipment or friction type toys to be used. The area surrounding the client is oxygen rich and can support combustion.
- All personnel should be able to locate the main oxygen supply valve to the area for discontinuation of oxygen flow in case of fire.
- The nurse must verify that the CNA/UAP understands the importance of oxygen administration so that it is appropriately maintained. The nurse ensures that the CNA/UAP seeks assistance so portable oxygen can be provided if it is required during client ambulation.
- Unlicensed personnel should be informed that aspiration is an ever-present danger for the client with a tracheostomy tube.
- Clients who require oxygen administration may be unable to perform activities of daily living independently. The CNA/UAP providing basic care should be *instructed to assist* the client with these activities (e.g., set up food tray, provide bed or partial bath).
- All care providers must be familiar with the location of emergency supplies and should be prepared to retrieve equipment and assist with manual respiratory resuscitation if necessary.

Information Flow

- The CNA/UAP usually performs routine vital signs assessment and documentation (including respiratory rate). The nurse should request that respiratory rates less than 12 or greater than 20 be reported immediately as more specific assessment may be indicated.
- The CNA/UAP should know to *report* any change in the client's breathing status or tolerance of activity. The character and amount of sputum production should also be reported and saved for the nurse's inspection and documentation.
- While the nurse or respiratory care practitioner is responsible for suctioning clients, the CNA/UAP must recognize the client's need for such and *report* it immediately.
- The PO status of intubated clients must be clearly communicated to all personnel. NPO status should be clearly posted at the bedside.
- All care providers must assure that the intubated client has nonvocal means for summoning help (call bell) and communicating (paper and pencil).
- There should be clear postings at the bedside of the client for: swallowing precautions, oxygen precautions, communication through nonvocal means, intubation precautions.

CRITICAL THINKING STRATEGIES

SCENARIO 1

Mrs. Harvey, age 72, has a history of chronic obstructive pulmonary disease (COPD) with components of emphysema and chronic bronchitis. She has frequent recurrence of respiratory infection requiring hospitalization. With her most recent hospitalization, she has developed pulmonary hypertension and right-sided heart failure with weight gain and systemic edema. After treatment with IV antibiotics, she is ready for discharge, but will be sent home with continuous low-flow (1.5 L) oxygen therapy. Her ABGs at the time of discharge shows elevated Pco_2 (respiratory acidosis), elevated bicarbonate level (metabolic alkalosis), Po_2 of 60 mm Hg, and O_2 saturation of 90% on oxygen. Her blood pH is low normal due to the *compensated* respiratory acidosis.

1. What is the rationale for home oxygen therapy for Mrs. Harvey?
2. What are the hazards that accompany home oxygen therapy?
3. What should the client know about home oxygen therapy?
4. What are the expected outcomes of home oxygen therapy (ABGs)?

CHAPTER 27

Circulatory Maintenance

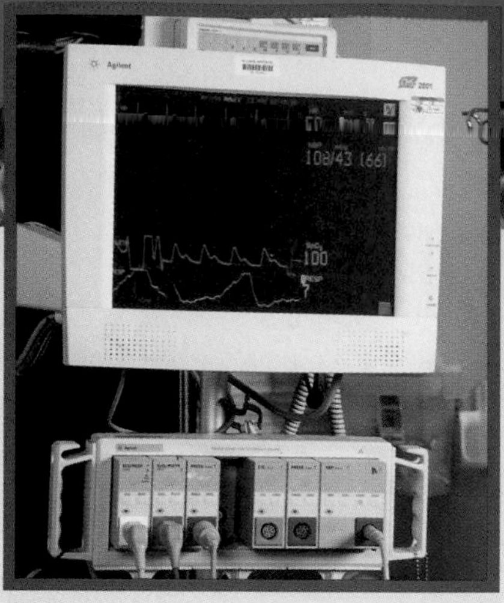

THEORETICAL CONCEPTS

UNIT ONE: **Control of Bleeding 942**

Using Digital Pressure 943

Using Pressure Dressing 943

UNIT TWO: **Circulatory Maintenance 945**

Applying Graduated Compression Stockings 946

Applying Pneumatic Compression Devices 947

UNIT THREE: **Electrocardiogram (ECG) Monitoring 952**

Monitoring the ECG 953

Interpreting an ECG Strip 955

Recording a 12-Lead ECG 956

Monitoring Clients on Telemetry 959

UNIT FOUR: **Emergency Life-Support Measures 963**

Administering Basic Life Support to an Adult 964

Placing Victim in Recovery Position 968

Administering CPR to a Child 968

Providing Bag–Valve–Mask Ventilation 969

Using an Automated External Defibrillator (AED) 970

Administering the Heimlich Maneuver for Conscious Client 971

Administering the Heimlich Maneuver for Unresponsive Client 972

Calling a Code 973

Maintaining the Emergency "Crash" Cart 975

Performing Defibrillation 975

Providing Care Following Code 975

UNIT FIVE: **Pacemaker Management 977**

Assisting with Pacemaker Insertion 978

Maintaining Pacemaker Function 979

Providing Client Teaching 980

UNIT SIX: **Fetal Monitoring 983**

Auscultating Fetal Heart Tones 984

Applying External Electronic Fetal Monitoring 984

Interpreting Electronic Fetal Monitoring Tracings 985

Assessing Periodic Fetal Heart Changes 986

GERONTOLOGIC CONSIDERATIONS 990

MANAGEMENT GUIDELINES 991

CRITICAL THINKING STRATEGIES 992

Cross reference: Chapter 33, Advanced Nursing Skills

Learning Objectives

- Identify three properties of the cardiac muscle and define cardiac output.
- Define the words *inotropic* and *chronotropic.*
- State the reason it is important to minimize the client's stress when hemorrhage occurs.
- Outline the assessment actions for a client who is hemorrhaging.
- Identify two interventions for treating pump failure.
- Define the term *ischemia.*
- List the nine pressure points in the body that can be used to control bleeding if hemorrhage occurs.
- Identify two potential problems that could occur in clients who are bleeding, and state one suggested solution for each problem.
- Describe how to measure appropriately for graduated compression stockings.
- List at least four potential problems for clients requiring CPR and two suggested solutions for each problem.
- Outline the steps in administering CPR with one rescuer and with two rescuers.
- Compare and contrast the differences in administering CPR to an infant or small child.
- Demonstrate the steps in performing the Heimlich maneuver.
- Describe four steps in using the AED.
- State two nursing diagnoses relevant to clients with circulatory dysfunction.
- Differentiate between a normal and abnormal ECG pattern.
- Describe lead placement for a 12-lead ECG.
- Compare and contrast ECG findings for clients with a temporary pacemaker and clients without a pacemaker.
- Evaluate a fetal monitoring tracing.
- Compare and contrast variance decelerations in fetal monitoring strips.

Terminology

Antiembolic: a preventive measure used to help prevent the formation of an embolism, such as elastic hosiery.

Atherosclerosis: a form of arteriosclerosis in which accumulations of lipid-containing material are localized within the surfaces of the blood vessels.

Cardiovascular: pertaining to the heart and blood vessels.

Chronotropic: modification of a repetitive event such as the heartbeat through external causes.

Conductivity: the specific electric conducting capability of a substance.

Congestion: the presence of an excessive amount of blood or fluid in an organ or tissue.

Contractility: having the ability to contract or shorten.

Cyanosis: slightly bluish, grayish, slatelike, or dark purple discoloration of the skin resulting from reduced hemoglobin or oxygen in the blood.

Dilatation: expansion of an organ or vessel.

Dorsiflexion: movement of a part at a joint so as to bend the part toward the dorsum, or posterior, aspect of the body.

Dysrhythmia: an abnormality in cardiac rhythm.

Ecchymosis: a form of macula appearing in large, irregularly formed hemorrhagic areas of the skin; color is blue-black, changing to greenish brown or yellow.

Edema: a condition in which the body tissues contain an excessive amount of fluid.

Embolism: obstruction of a blood vessel by foreign substances or a blood clot.

Endocardial: within the heart or arising from the endocardium.

Endocardium: serous lining membrane of the inner surface and cavities of the heart.

Endotracheal: within the trachea.

Epistaxis: hemorrhage from the nose.

Heart failure: exists when the heart is unable to pump sufficient blood to meet the metabolic needs of the body, provided venous return to the heart is normal.

Hematemesis: vomiting of blood.

Hematoma: a swelling or mass of blood, usually clotted, confined to a specific space and caused by a break in a blood vessel.

Hemodynamic: pertaining to the study of the circulation of the blood.

Hemoptysis: expectoration of blood arising from hemorrhage of the larynx, trachea, bronchi, or lungs.

Hemorrhage: abnormal internal or external discharge of blood.

Homan's sign: pain in the calf when the toe is dorsiflexed. An early sign of deep vein thrombosis in the calf.

Hydrostatic: pertaining to the pressure of liquids in equilibrium and that exerted on liquids.

Hypotension: low blood pressure; due to deficiency of vascular tone.

Immobilize: the making of a part or limb immovable.

Inotropic: influencing the contractibility of muscle tissue.

Ischemia: local and temporary anemia due to the obstruction of the circulation to a part.

Manubrium: the sternum articulating with the clavicle and first pair of costal cartilages.

Pacemaker: a device that provides electrical stimulation to the heart muscle to maintain effective cardiac output.

Perfusion: passing of fluid through spaces.

Petechiae: small, purplish, hemorrhagic spots on the skin, which appear in certain severe fevers.

Phlebitis: inflammation of a vein.

Precordial: pertaining to the precordium or epigastrium.

Purpura: hemorrhage into the skin, mucuous membranes, internal organs, and other tissues.

Resuscitation: act of bringing one back to full consciousness.

Sclerosis: hardening or induration of an organ or tissue due to excessive growth of fibrous tissue.

Shock: term used to designate a clinical syndrome with varying degrees of disturbances of blood flow and oxygen supply to the tissues.

Stasis: standing still; stagnation of normal flow of fluids.

Syncope: fainting, transient loss of consciousness due to inadequate blood flow to the brain.

Thrombosis: formation of a blood clot.

Vertigo: sensation of moving or having objects around you move when they are actually still, due to a disturbance of balance.

Fetal monitoring terminology

Accelerations: abrupt increase in FHR lasting at least 30 seconds and at least 15 BPM greater than the baseline FHR.

Acme: highest point or peak (i.e., uterine contraction).

Amnioinfusion: intrauterine instillation of warm normal saline to reduce risk of cord compression.

Baseline FHR: mean FHR rounded to increments of 5 BPM during a 10-minute segment for a duration of at least 2 minutes; usually 110–160; shown on top portion of EFM graph.

BPM: beats per minute.

Early deceleration: gradual decrease of FHR (onset to nadir at least 30 seconds) in which nadir of decelerations coincides with peak of contractions; often thought to be result of head compression.

Bradycardia: FHR less than 110 BPM.

EFM: electronic fetal monitor that utilizes microprocessors to interpret input from toco and ultrasound transducer; EFM produces a tracing that includes a record of uterine contraction and fetal heart rate.

External monitoring: utilizes an ultrasound transducer to detect sound waves (fetal heart rate) off the valves of the fetal heart and a tocodynamometer to detect pressure changes in the abdomen (uterine contractions).

FHR: fetal heart rate; number of beats per minute of the fetal heart.

Internal monitoring: utilizes a spiral fetal scalp electrode (FSE) attached to the fetal scalp (connected to the FHR monitor) to record FHR and a pressure sensitive tube or intrauterine pressure catheter (IUPC) that senses and records pressure changes inside uterus.

Late deceleration: gradual decrease of FHR (onset to nadir at least 30 seconds) in which the nadir of deceleration occurs after peak of contraction; caused by insufficient oxygenation of uterus and placenta.

Nadir: lowest point; lowest portion of a deceleration.

Tachycardia: FHR greater than 160 BPM.

Tocodynamometer: device for estimating force of uterine contraction.

Tocolytic: drug to inhibit uterine contractions such as adrenergic agonists, magnesium sulfate, and ethanol.

Variability: the irregular fluctuation in the baseline FHR (between uterine contractions); usually at least 2 cycles per minute and between 6 and 25 BPM (jagged line).

Variable deceleration: abrupt decrease (onset to nadir less than 30 seconds) at least 15 BPM, last longer than 15 seconds, and less than 2 minutes. Shape and onset will vary, but decrease from baseline lasts at least 15 seconds and less than 2 minutes.

Periodic or episodic decelerations: decrease in FHR of at least 30 seconds, usually associated with uterine contractions. Three types of decelerations are late, early, and variable.

THE CIRCULATORY SYSTEM

The heart is a three-layered, four-chambered organ, approximately the size of an adult fist. It weighs close to 600 grams in the normal adult. A thick, fibrous sheath, called the pericardium, surrounds about two-thirds of the heart's surface. Most of the mass lies in the heart's middle layer—the myocardium, or cardiac muscle. The endocardium, a thin, inner layer, lines the four chambers.

In considering the heart's chambers, imagine two major pump systems. The right and left atria contract in one phase, and the right and left ventricles contract in the successive phase. The tricuspid, pulmonary, mitral, and aortic valves are the four flow regulators for the chambers.

Three properties of cardiac muscle best illustrate the heart's specialization. Automaticity physiologically differentiates heart muscle from all other muscle tissue. The other two properties—conductivity and contractility—characterize all muscle; however, a cardiac contraction is normally all or none, as opposed to partial contractions in other muscles.

The heart serves as a pump to maintain blood flow and blood pressure. Adequate blood flow perfuses the lungs for oxygenation. Blood pressure is a driving force for that flow and is normally highest during ventricular contractions. The heart pumps 4–7 L of blood per minute. This constitutes a normal cardiac output, formulated by multiplying contraction volume times ventricular rate.

When the heart maintains a safe blood pressure and blood flow, it is in a state of compensation, regardless of cardiac output. If the heart cannot maintain a safe blood pressure and blood flow, it is in a state of decompensation. Three cardiac reserves allow for compensation: inotropic reserve, increased venous filling pressure, and chronotropic reserve.

Inotropic reserve is under the control of sympathetic nerve stimulation. Adrenergic drugs, as well as some others, exert an inotropic effect by increasing the force of the cardiac contraction and therefore stroke volume. Cardiac output also increases with additional filling pressure in the atria. Starling's law of the heart summarizes the relationship by stating that an increased filling pressure causes an increased force of contraction within the elastic limits of the heart. Finally, chronotropic reserve refers to increased heart rate. Atropine-like drugs exert a chronotropic effect by increasing the heart rate.

Blood vessels, together with the heart, form a closed circulatory system unless damage or abnormalities result in leakage. When the ventricles contract, blood leaves the right ventricle through the pulmonic valve into the pulmonary artery. Blood is now in the pulmonary circulation for oxygenation of the red blood cells, or erythrocytes. After gas exchange occurs at the cellular level, the blood is returned to the left atrium through four pulmonary veins. This is normally the most oxygenated blood in the human body.

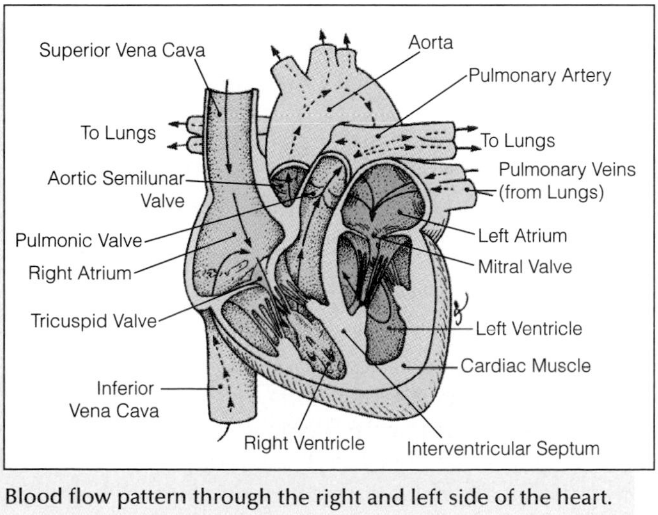

Blood flow pattern through the right and left side of the heart.

On the left side of the heart during a ventricular contraction, blood travels through the aortic valve out of the left ventricle into the ascending aorta. Five percent, or 200–350 mL, of this blood enters coronary circulation for oxygenation and waste removal from the cardiac tissue. Fifteen percent, or 600–1,050 mL, travels to the brain and 25%, or 1,000–1,750 mL, goes to the kidneys, and the same amount to other viscera. The extremities and skin normally receive 30% of the circulating volume.

Arteries carry blood from the heart throughout the body unless obstructed or severed. The largest vessel is the aorta, and the smallest is the arteriole. Similar to the heart, arteries have three layers: endothelium, involuntary muscle, and connective tissue. Capillaries join the arterial system to the venous system and are a single cell layer in thickness. The single layer allows gas, nutrients, and waste exchanges to occur throughout the body. Blood enters the venous system from the capillary beds for eventual return to the right side of the heart via the superior and inferior vena cava.

ELECTRICAL CONDUCTION

Cardiac muscle cells have an inherent rhythm that allows for their spontaneous, repetitive self-stimulation. The rate and rhythm of cardiac contractions are primarily determined by this self-generated impulse. The autonomic nervous system affects the heart rate. Sympathetic stimulation increases heart rate and conduction rate through the atrioventricular (AV) node. Parasympathetic stimulation slows the heart rate by decreasing the firing rate of the sinoatrial (SA) node and the speed of conduction through the AV node.

The electrical impulse starts at the SA node located at the junction of the superior vena cava and the right atrium. It functions as the pacemaker for the heart. The SA node initiates approximately 60–100 impulses each minute. The impulse travels to the AV node, located in the right atrial wall near the tricuspid valve. If there is a problem with the impulse being generated in the SA node, the AV node can actually take over as the pacemaker. Over the long term, this may present a problem because the intrinsic rate of the AV node is only 40–60 impulses per minute. The AV node coordinates the incoming electrical impulse from the atria and relays an impulse to the ventricles. The impulse travels in the septum through the bundle of His specialized muscle fibers, which divide into the right and left bundle branches. The impulse continues to the Purkinje fibers, where it terminates. The right bundle reaches out into the right ventricular muscle. The left bundle divides into the left anterior and left posterior bundle branches. These branches reach out into the left ventricular muscle. Further depolarization of the myocardium takes place by conduction through the muscle fibers themselves. If both the SA and AV node are dysfunctional, the myocardium continues to beat, but at a rate of less than 40 BPM. This rate is the intrinsic pacemaker rate of ventricular myocardial cells.

Pacemakers

When the heart is unable to maintain effective cardiac output, the use of a temporary or permanent pacemaker may be necessary. The main purpose of the pacemaker is to regulate the heartbeat. It paces the heart when inherent electrical system of the heart fails or is inadequate.

Permanent pacemakers are implanted for clients with heart block, sick sinus syndrome, or valvular stenosis. The pacemaker relieves symptoms associated with these conditions and restores normal heart rate. The temporary pacemaker is inserted for temporary conditions, such as severe bradycardia, drug toxicity, myocardial infarction, and in cardiac surgery. The temporary pacemaker is a device that provides a low-voltage electrical stimulus to the endocardial surface of the right atrium or ventricle (transvenous method) or to the epicardium (transthoracic, or epicardial, method). Either chamber can be paced alone, or both chambers paced sequentially. When the pacing lead is attached to the atrium, the pacemaker stimulates it to pump adequate blood into the ventricle. When the lead is attached to the ventricle, it stimulates it to pump an adequate blood supply to the lungs and body. In addition, the pacemaker can be used to suppress or overdrive tachyarrhythmias.

All methods of temporary pacing use a pulse generator with rechargeable or replaceable batteries and some type of electrode or impulse conductor. These electrodes may be either unipolar or bipolar and differ in sensitivity. Unipolar (single-pole) catheter electrodes have a single cathode tip and are more sensitive to the client's generated impulses. The catheter electrode wire fits into the negative output terminal on the generator. Bipolar (double-pole) catheter electrodes have both an anode and cathode at the tip and fit into both positive and negative output terminals on the generator. The pace rate determines the number of beats per minute (BPM) provided by the generator.

Demand (synchronous) pacing is the most frequently used. The electrode is triggered to stimulate the heart only when the heart's intrinsic or natural atrial or ventricular stimulation fails to occur by a predetermined time. The atrial synchronous electrode's discharge is inhibited if natural atrial depolarization occurs, or is triggered to stimulate atrial depolarization if this does not occur naturally within a specified period. The ventricular inhibited pacemaker senses when the ventricle naturally depolarizes, and is inhibited or is triggered to discharge to activate the ventricle if the client's ventricular rate falls below the preset rate.

Pacemaker wires are threaded percutaneously through the subclavian or femoral vein or through a cutdown in the brachial or external jugular vein. The electrode is advanced through the vena cava, to the right atrium, or advanced through the tricuspid valve and positioned at the apex of the right ventricle on the endocardial surface. The electrode is then attached to the generator.

Pacemakers have changed significantly since the early 1950s, when the pacemaker was not fully implanted in the body and the battery-powered pacemaker needed frequent battery replacements. The introduction of lithium iodine batteries and then the titanium battery increased the length of time between battery changes for up to 10 years. Pacemakers went from being "fixed pacemakers," pacing continuously regardless of the client's own pulse rate, to pacemakers with very sophisticated functions. Pacemakers of today adjust to the client's activity by mimicking the natural heart rhythm and adjusting the rhythm according to activity level. Pacemakers can now collect information and store it until the next clinic visit.

ECG

The electrocardiogram (ECG) is used to detect abnormalities associated with the conduction system. The waveforms, which indicate the electrical activity of the myocardium, are analyzed using the ECG printout. The P wave represents atrial muscle depolarization. The QRS complex represents ventricular muscle depolarization. The T wave represents ventricular muscle repolarization. Each segment of the waveform is analyzed for time and configuration of the waveform. Abnormalities in time or configuration indicate a problem is occurring in that specific area of the heart.

Each segment of the heart depicts a different type of waveform termed a dysrhythmia, when abnormalities occur with the myocardial activity in that segment. An atrial dysrhythmia results from a problem with the SA node or atria indicated by an abnormality in the P wave configuration. A ventricular dysrhythmia results from a problem with the ventricle and is indicated by an abnormality in the configuration of the QRS complex. A junctional dysrhythmia occurs when there is a problem associated with the AV node as indicated by a change in the PR interval. A ventricular dysrhythmia is the most life-threatening because it compromises cardiac output.

ALTERATIONS IN CIRCULATION

There are many ways to categorize disorders of the heart, arteries, and veins. Endocarditis, myocarditis, and pericarditis classify cardiac problems according to inflammation of a particular heart layer. Another classification is congenital heart disease, such as tetralogy of Fallot and transposition of the great vessels. For the purpose of this chapter alterations of circulation are divided into hemorrhage, shock, pump failure, ischemia, thrombosis, and embolism.

Hemorrhage

Hemorrhage results when trauma or disease causes leakage in the closed circulatory system. Damage to the heart or arteries usually constitutes the greatest danger because of the high pressure and large volumes. Normally, when a blood vessel ruptures or is severed, compensatory mechanisms protect the body from significant blood loss. The wall of the injured vessel contracts immediately. A platelet plug forms at the site, and blood clotting occurs. New connective tissue penetrates the clot for permanent closure. Interventions for clients who are hemorrhaging are based on one of these compensatory mechanisms.

To prevent, correct, or compensate for hemorrhage, the nurse must assess the client. She identifies the nature of the bleeding as external or internal (or both) and establishes baseline data, which includes blood pressure and vital signs. An assessment is made of the body's response, adaptive, excessive, or deficient, and the nurse assists in formulating and planning appropriate interventions. The first concern is to minimize the client's stress, since sympathetic stimulation of the heart increases heart rate (chronotropic effect) and force of contraction (inotropic effect). Interventions for hemorrhage involve restricting activity, elevating involved body areas above the heart if possible, applying direct pressure, and replacing lost fluid volume. A tourniquet is generally used as a last resort. It is placed proximal to the site of the hemorrhage with the knowledge that the extremity may be sacrificed.

Shock

Unchecked hemorrhage eventually leads to hypovolemic or hemorrhagic shock, a serious state with a poor prognosis. Peripheral resistance is of great significance. In hemorrhagic shock, high peripheral resistance is secondary to pronounced peripheral vasoconstriction in the initial stage. Due to the loss of blood volume it becomes very difficult to start an intravenous line in a superficial vein. Vasoconstrictors, such as Levophed, are undesirable since they cause a further decline in tissue perfusion. Successful recognition and early treatment of hemorrhagic shock depends heavily on sophisticated monitoring devices, the nature of the fluid used for volume replacement, and the use of blood components instead of whole blood. Intervention centers on establishing one or more IV lines for fluid replacement, drug administration, and blood component therapy. Careful monitoring of peripheral pulses, blood pressure, central venous pressure, and even more sophisticated hemodynamic parameters, such as pulmonary arterial wedge pressures, is desirable.

Heart Failure

Heart failure results from any condition that reduces the ability of the heart to pump blood, resulting in inadequate blood flow to tissues. The heart is no longer in a state of compensation, and cardiac output falls. Cardiac arrhythmias and congestion are the most common types of pump failure.

There are many causes of heart failure. Coronary artery disease is the cause of heart failure in about two-thirds of clients with left ventricular systolic dysfunction. Heart valve disease causing heart muscle weakness, hypertension, and primary heart muscle weakness from viral infections or toxins also play a major role in heart failure.

When certain dysrhythmias occur, particularly ventricular tachycardia and ventricular fibrillation, pump failure results due to the inability of ventricles to fill with adequate amounts of blood, leading to insufficient blood supply being pumped to the tissues for oxygenation.

Heart failure may be due to failure of the right or left ventricle or both ventricles, although most heart failure begins on the left side. The cardinal manifestations of heart failure are dyspnea and fatigue, which may limit exercise tolerance and increase fluid retention. This leads to pulmonary congestion and peripheral edema. The buildup of fluid in pulmonary capillaries is termed *pulmonary edema*. Left-sided failure occurs when the left ventricle is unable to pump efficiently. Right-sided heart failure results in diminished circulation into the pulmonary artery, causing a backup of fluid in the systemic circulation. Clinical manifestations associated with left-sided failure include symptoms related to pulmonary congestion: dyspnea; moist, hacking cough; bibasilar crackles; cyanosis; and orthopnea. Clinical manifestations associated with right-sided failure are related to systemic findings: weight gain, oliguria, hepatomegaly, peripheral edema, ascites, and fatigue.

Pulmonary edema, the most common result of pump failure, is a life-threatening condition. Pulmonary edema is a disorder in which alveoli fill with fluid. It produces severe abnormalities in gas exchange and can lead to death if not treated immediately. Several disorders can cause pulmonary edema, all of which produce a high hydrostatic pressure in the pulmonary capillaries. Right ventricular output into the pulmonary capillaries depends in part on the volume of venous return to the heart.

Heart failure should not be confused with circulatory overload, a condition in which cardiac output is adequate but blood volume and/or venous return is excessive. Excessive infusion of IV fluids in too short a period of time results in circulatory overload.

The goal of treatment for heart failure is to reduce workload on the heart, increase efficiency of contractions, and reduce fluid. Both pharmacological and physiological interventions are used to meet the goal. Bed rest during the most critical time may be ordered to promote rest for the heart. Oxygen therapy may be used to promote oxygenation of the tissues; a diet low in sodium and restricted fluids are appropriate. Pharmacological interventions include the use of diuretics, angiotensin-converting enzyme (ACE) inhibitors, beta blockers, digitalis, KCl, and nitrates.

Ischemia

Ischemia is a circulatory condition in which blood supply to a body part or region is reduced to a critical level. Relative ischemia occurs with hypotension or the inability to meet increased metabolic demands. Absolute ischemia is usually a sudden, complete occlusion of a blood vessel, resulting in tissue necrosis. Leaving a tourniquet on an extremity for more than 15 minutes may cause tissue necrosis. Other causes of ischemia include Raynaud's disease, Buerger's disease, thromboembolism, mechanical obstruction, arteriosclerosis, and atherosclerosis. Atherosclerosis is always being studied in relation to hypertension, cigarette smoking, genetic factors, obesity, physical activity, hypercholesterolemia, and emotional stress. The actual cause of coronary atherosclerotic disease (CAD) remains a mystery, and incidence in the United States continues to increase.

Thrombosis and Embolism

Phlebitis is an inflammation of the lining of a vein from an unknown cause. There is pain and tenderness along the vein, edema below the obstruction, mild elevation of the temperature, increased pulse rate, pain in the joint, and discoloration of the skin.

The goal of treatment is toward reducing inflammation and preventing emboli by placing the client on bed rest, elevating the affected limb, and using graduated compression stockings (elastic hosiery) in addition to anticoagulants and analgesics.

There is a risk of thrombus (blood clot) formation along the wall of the vein causing thrombophlebitis. Alterations in venous return; venous stasis, particularly in the lower extremities; and changes in blood viscosity can contribute to the thrombosis. If a thrombus dislodges from the vessel wall and travels in the bloodstream, it is termed an *embolus*. An embolism may be solid, liquid, or air. Liquid emboli are usually injected intravenously by accident, such as during a hyperalimentation procedure (TPN). Similarly, air emboli occur when air is not removed from intravenous or arterial lines before infusion of solutions.

Graduated compression stockings (elastic hosiery TED, Jobst, and others) and sequential stockings are used to prevent venous stasis and avoid thrombus formation and subsequent emboli. They produce compression of peripheral leg veins. This pressure forces the venous blood into deeper, larger leg veins for a more rapid return to the heart. This will decrease venous stasis and reduce the risk of thrombus formation.

ALTERED CIRCULATION

Assessment

Alterations in circulation are indicated by a variety of signs and symptoms. The nurse should not overlook the behavioral manifestations or the more physical signs and symptoms. Systematic client evaluation considers whether or not there is a significant blood loss. If bleeding exists, external and/or internal sites must be identified. Attention is given to the family history for disease conditions of the major organs, and coagulation mechanisms. Baseline data is gathered for vital signs and arterial blood pressures. The color, temperature, and condition of the skin are closely noted. Cyanosis is differentiated as peripheral versus central. Weakness and fatigue is significant, as well as physical discomforts, such as pain, pressure, or numbness. Abnormalities of superficial veins often indicate obstruction or pooling. Impaired renal function, especially related to output, is closely considered. Edema is differentiated as dependent versus generalized. Special observations include such findings as clubbing of the fingers, petechiae, and calf tenderness with dorsiflexion of the foot (positive Homan's sign). Information obtained from the client's drug history and present medications may affect the diagnosis and therefore the nursing intervention. Trauma victims require especially close inspection since more overt signs and symptoms may not appear until days later. Table 27–1 illustrates an assessment of a hemorrhaging client.

Emergency Life Support Measures

Before initiating cardiopulmonary resuscitation (CPR), the emergency medical service (EMS), outside the hospital, or the code team inside the hospital, should be called if you encounter an unresponsive person. In situations such as near drowning or submersion; cardiac arrest associated with trauma; and drug overdoses, CPR is provided for 1 minute before calling for emergency help. Every minute is crucial if the person who is unresponsive is in ventricular fibrillation. This is the most common cause of a sudden, nontraumatic cardiac arrest in adults. Survival decreases 7–10% for each minute that defibrillation is not completed.

Use of the automated external defibrillator (AED) is taught in the Basic Life Support (BLS) class for both laypeople and health care providers. All individuals trained in CPR should be trained, equipped, and authorized to perform defibrillation. New guidelines by the

TABLE 27–1 Assessment Guide for Hemorrhaging

1. Observable bleeding from skin, mucous membranes. Check under the person, clothing, dressing, casts.
2. Observable bleeding into the skin, mucous membranes. Check for petechiae, ecchymosis, hematomas, purpura.
3. Observable bleeding from body orifice. Check for epistaxis, hematemesis, hemoptysis.
4. Observable bleeding from tubes. Check T-tubes, endotracheal tubes, suction drainage, urinary catheters.
5. Generalized signs and symptoms of bleeding.
   a. Low blood pressure (systolic below 90 mm Hg and diastolic below 50 mm Hg).
   b. Progressive drop in blood pressure.
   c. Rapid, weak pulses or absence of pulses.
   d. Clammy skin and central cyanosis.
   e. Deep, rapid respirations (above 24/min).
   f. Low body temperature (one or more degrees below 98.6°F, or 37°C, oral temperature).
   g. Reduced urine output (less than 30 mL/hr).
   h. Behavioral changes.
   i. Syncope and visual disturbance.
   j. Loss of consciousness.
6. Localized signs and symptoms of bleeding.
   a. Painful, swollen, tender, or hot joints.
   b. Soft, spongy uterus high in abdominal cavity during postpartum period.
   c. Pupillary and visual changes, behavioral shifts, tinnitus, vertigo, breathing pattern shifts, loss of consciousness following head injury.

American Heart Association (AHA) indicate that early defibrillation, defined as collapse-to-shock of less than 3 minutes, should be expected for best client outcomes in the hospital or outpatient setting.

Outside the hospital facility, AEDs should be accessible in areas where there is a high probability of cardiac arrest situations and when EMS is at least 5 minutes or more away from the location. Laypersons, properly trained, can recognize signs of cardiac arrest and apply and operate the AED.

The AHA is recommending that even though crash carts are used most commonly in hospitals, if the cart is more than 3 minutes away, AEDs should be available on the nursing units. It is estimated that, in hospitals, time from collapse to first defibrillation shock can be 5 to 10 minutes.

The empirical data regarding use of AEDs in children is still not complete. It is recommended that the AED should be used only in children over the age of 8 years and over 55 pounds (25 kg).

Another change in the AHA guidelines emphasizes the need to use bag–mask ventilations or other airway devices such as laryngeal mask airways or the Combitube, if the BLS rescuer is trained in the use of these devices. Use of these airway devices will deliver air to the lungs rather than the stomach, greatly reducing complications such as aspiration and pneumonia.

The new guidelines have placed a priority on caring for victims of stroke as well as those with an acute myocardial infarction (MI). As with early fibrinolytic treatment for the MI client, those clients with a stroke require treatment within 3 hours of symptoms for quality outcomes. EMS personnel are now trained to provide stroke screening tools and then rapidly transport stroke clients to the nearest hospital where fibrinolytic treatment can be administered within 1 hour of arrival at the facility.

Early Defibrilation Programs in Hospitals

With the new American Heart Association standard-of-care recommendation that the collapse-to-shock interval be less than 3 minutes in all areas of the hospital and ambulatory care facilities, hospitals will need to decide how they will implement this standard of care. Should they still require only physicians and nurses to perform defibrillation in the usual method, or should they implement an early defibrillation program that allows all health care providers to use the AED to deliver defibrillation? Another dilemma is to determine if the usual defibrillation procedures be maintained in critical care situations and use of AEDs in other facility areas. The AEDs are not appropriate for some abnormal rhythm strips that may need defibrillation and they use low current that may not be enough to deliver a functional shock to prevent myocardial damage.

The American Heart Association has now included testing on the use of AEDs as part of the Advance Life Support Course (ACLS) for all health care professionals. In-hospital defibrillation can take as long as 5–10 minutes to be initiated, as it takes the code team that long to reach the client. The availability of the AED in each nursing unit should reduce the time to under 3 minutes.

The AED is a computerized defibrillator that is safe for anyone to use. It analyzes the heart rhythm, recognizes a shockable rhythm, and advises the operator when the victim should be shocked. It is used on unresponsive adults without a detectable pulse.

The AEDs used outside the hospital were designed specifically for that use. They are portable, easy to use, and do not require much maintenance. These same devices may be useful in free-standing clinics. AEDs designed for hospital use have several different features. They have an "override" feature that permits the machine to operate as a manual defibrillator and they provide a comprehensive record of the entire event.

A major benefit for AED usage throughout non-critical care units within the hospital is that other health care providers, and non-critical care nurses can easily provide defibrillation within the new AHA Standard of 3 minutes, without extensive training in defibrillation.

Planning and Intervention

Once an initial assessment of a client for alterations in circulation has been made, the nurse develops a prioritized problem list for planning and intervention. Nurses monitor circulatory status with a variety of sophisticated tools. Again, however, the most valuable approach is direct observation of the client. Blood pressure measurements are usually noninvasive, taken with a blood pressure cuff, stethoscope, and sphygmomanometer. The central venous line and the Swan–Ganz catheter for pulmonary arterial pressures (PAP and PAWP) are invasive methods used under certain conditions and by specially trained personnel.

Interventions for circulatory problems cover numerous therapeutic modalities but usually fall into three broad categories: inputs, outputs, and pressure supports. Inputs include arterial lines, venous lines, drug regimens, transfusions, and blood component therapies. Outputs include suctioning with specialized equipment like hemovacs and procedures like thoracentesis. Pressure supports include dressings, bandages, digital compression, tourniquets, and cardiopulmonary resuscitation.

In coping with alterations in circulation, care should be directed toward promoting, maintaining, or regaining the best possible cardiopulmonary function. The design for nursing action is to assess the situation and client for stressors. The client should be interviewed if possible, observed, and examined to identify actual and/or potential circulatory problems. The client's responses are appropriate, deficient, or excessive, and interventions should be planned accordingly. The nurse attempts to reduce client stress, supports adaptive behaviors, replaces deficiencies, modifies or removes excessive responses, and prevents injury and complications. The nurse should always assist in the evaluation of planned actions, report client responses, and assist in modifying the interventions as indicated.

Fetal Monitoring

Although controversial, the use of continuous electronic fetal heart monitoring (EFM) is very common during antepartum and intrapartum (labor and delivery) periods of pregnancy. Estimates are that about 75% of women in labor utilize EFM, even though there is insufficient evidence to recommend for or against continuous EFM during the intrapartum. The National Institutes of Health (1996) recommendation is to not use routine continuous EFM for low-risk women in labor when adequate clinical management, including intermittent auscultation, is available.

It is important that nurses understand the meaning of fetal heart rate patterns/monitoring and are able to assess the fetal heart rate by auscultation (Doppler or fetoscope) and electronic monitor. The basic reason for EFM is to collect data about oxygenation status of the fetus. The fetus is dependent on oxygenated blood that arrives from maternal circulation, placental perfusion, and the umbilical cord. Any event that decreases the perfusion of the mother's circulatory system, placental circulation, transfer via the umbilical cord, or the fetal circulatory system will affect the oxygenation of the fetus, fetal organs, and fetal brain. The FHR is controlled by the fetus's autonomic nervous system (ANS), comprised of the sympathetic and parasympathetic nervous system. Thus, the increase or decrease in FHR is a reflection of oxygenation in the fetal sympathetic and parasympathetic nervous system. This is depicted as a jagged, oscillating line on the portion of EFM graph that records the FHR.

During a uterine contraction, very little blood passes between uterus and placenta. If the fetus has reserve oxygen to oxygenate the brain, very little change occurs in the function of the ANS, and the FHR remains jagged (variability) and roughly at the same baseline FHR. If there is barely enough oxygen for the fetus without a contraction, then with added stress of a contraction, the fetus becomes deoxygenated, which results in a late deceleration. Late decelerations are often accompanied by a decrease in baseline variability.

A variable deceleration is a periodic change that often is associated with uterine contractions, but may also occur randomly. Because of the sharp drop in baseline (as compared with the gradual declines of early and late decelerations), it is theorized that the cord is compressed, leading to a sudden increase in vascular pressure, which stimulates the baroreceptors. The baroreceptors then initiate the vagal response, resulting in a sharp drop in FHR. Though using similar root words, baseline variability and variable decelerations are very different (refer to Terminology), and the nurse needs to be careful in the use of the proper terminology.

NURSING DIAGNOSES

The following nursing diagnoses may be appropriate to use on a client care plan when the components are related to circulation.

NURSING DIAGNOSIS	RELATED FACTORS
Decreased Cardiac Output	Cardiac disease states, altered electrical conduction, drug side effects, hypovolemia
Deficient Fluid Volume	Blood loss from lacerations, dehydration
Ineffective Tissue Perfusion: Cardiopulmonary	Altered blood supply, arterial or venous, hypovolemia, shock

- The single most important nursing action to decrease the incidence of hospital-based infections is handwashing. **Remember to wash your hands or use antibacterial gel before and after each and every client contact.**

UNIT 1

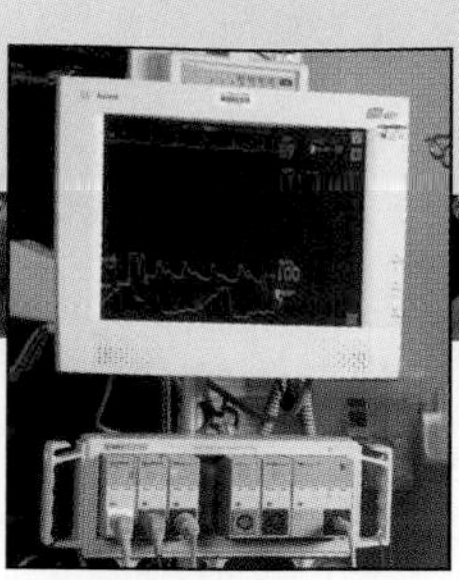

Control of Bleeding

Nursing Process Data

ASSESSMENT Data Base

Observe the amount of bleeding.
Check for the source of bleeding.
Observe the extent of the wound.
Identify familial history of bleeding disorders.
Assess baseline vital signs and arterial blood pressure readings.
Observe color, temperature, and condition of the skin.
Ask about medications taken routinely by client.

PLANNING Objectives

To detect source of bleeding
To stop or control bleeding or hemorrhage before large blood loss occurs
To provide pressure as an assist (adjunct) to stop bleeding
To minimize capillary seepage, hematoma, and serum accumulation

IMPLEMENTATION Procedures

Using Digital Pressure
Using Pressure Dressing

EVALUATION Expected Outcomes

Early detection of bleeding occurs, and loss of blood is minimized.
Pressure dressing is applied, and bleeding is controlled.
Collateral circulation is minimally inhibited.

USING DIGITAL PRESSURE

Equipment

Towels or gauze dressing if available
Gloves

Procedure

1. Wash hands and don gloves, sterile preferred.
2. Identify the closest artery proximal to the bleeding site. **Rationale:** The rapid loss of more than 25%–30% of the total blood volume leads to death.
3. Apply direct pressure to artery, using your gloved finger.
4. If towels or 4 × 4 gauze pads are available, apply direct pressure to site if wound does not contain glass particles. **Rationale:** If pressure is placed on wound when glass is present, additional tissue damage can occur.
5. Raise the affected limb above the level of the heart about 30°. **Rationale:** This decreases arterial blood flow to area and promotes venous return.
6. Maintain direct pressure on site.
7. Do not remove pressure before 5 minutes. **Rationale:** Clot formation has not had an opportunity to stabilize.
8. When bleeding has subsided, proceed to clean and dress the wound.
9. To control nose bleeds (epistaxis), place client in sitting position, with head tilted forward. Pinch nose for 5 minutes. If ordered, apply ice pack to assist in vasoconstriction.
10. Remove gloves when bleeding subsides.
11. Wash hands immediately. **Rationale:** To protect yourself from possible contamination should any leakage have occurred through the gloves.

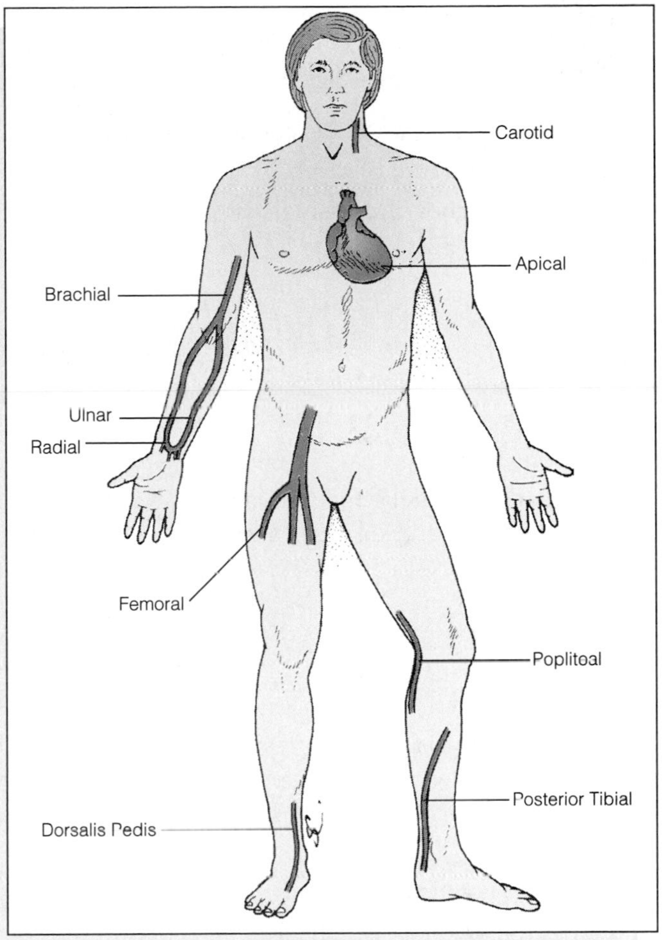

Pulse sites that may be used to control bleeding.

USING PRESSURE DRESSING

Equipment

4 × 4 gauze pad
Sterile dressings—number and size depends on wound
Sterile gloves
Cleansing solution
Tape

Preparation

1. Check physician's orders.
2. Assemble necessary supplies according to extent of wound.
3. If time permits, explain procedure to client and provide light and privacy.
4. Wash your hands thoroughly if time permits.
5. Set up sterile field and prepare cleansing solution if time permits.

Procedure

1. Put on sterile gloves.
2. Cleanse wound and apply dressing. Use several layers of 4 × 4 gauze pads.
3. To provide an occlusive dressing, place tape tightly over entire dressing. Do not completely circle an extremity or the body. **Rationale:** To ensure that collateral blood flow is maintained.
4. Place all soiled materials in biohazard bag.
5. Remove gloves and wash your hands thoroughly.
6. Monitor vital signs, and observe for signs of shock.
7. Position client for comfort.
8. Elevate extremity to prevent bleeding.
9. Monitor frequently for signs of bleeding and hematoma. Hematomas feel spongy even under bandages.

Documentation for Control of Bleeding

- Size, location, condition of wound
- Color, odor, amount of drainage
- Type and number of dressings used
- Approximate amount of blood loss
- Condition of dressing when changed (e.g., soaked with drainage)

Critical Thinking Application

UNEXPECTED OUTCOMES	CRITICAL THINKING OPTIONS
Even with direct pressure and application of pressure dressing, bleeding continues.	• Reinforce pressure dressing. • Monitor IV flow closely. • Notify physician, and be prepared to send client to surgery for wound closure. • Monitor closely for signs of shock. • Aid with placing tourniquets proximal to the site of the hemorrhage to control bleeding if all other actions are unsuccessful.
Wound edges do not approximate.	• Notify physician. • Be prepared to assist with wound closure or to send client to surgery.
Glass particles are evident in wound.	• Irrigate wound profusely with sterile saline solution as ordered. • If large amount of glass or if glass is difficult to extract, notify physician, and be prepared to send client to surgery for wound cleansing and debridement. • Do not apply direct pressure or pressure dressing to wound containing glass. • Apply pressure to vessel above wound or, as a last resort, apply a tourniquet.

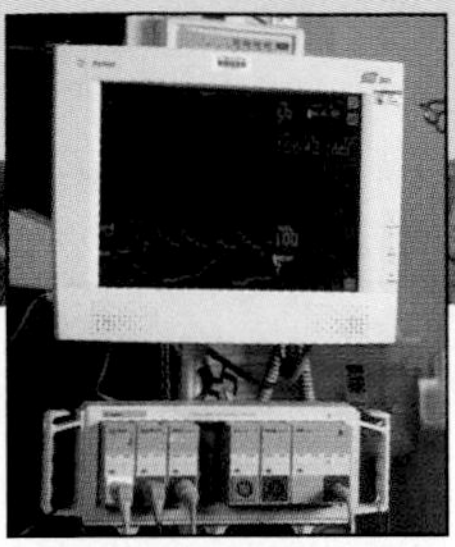

UNIT 2

Circulatory Maintenance

Nursing Process Data

ASSESSMENT ***Data Base***

Evaluate client's overall physical condition, particularly client's cardiovascular status to determine if candidate for compression stockings or devices.

Observe baseline vital signs before procedures are initiated.

Determine if client is at risk for pooling of blood in extremities. Conditions that require use of elastic stockings are leg varicosities, thrombophlebitis, lymphedema, orthostatic hypotension, immediate postcast removal, postoperative venous ligation or stripping, and venous insufficiencies due to muscular inactivity.

Assess for peripheral edema by palpating pulses and observing color and temperature as well as fluid accumulation.

PLANNING ***Objectives***

To prevent venous stasis

To prevent thrombus formation and subsequent emboli

To use elastic hose or sequential stockings to prevent venous stasis

IMPLEMENTATION ***Procedures***

Applying Graduated Compression Stockings (elastic hosiery)

Applying Pneumatic Compression Devices

EVALUATION ***Expected Outcomes***

Elastic stockings remain wrinkle-free, and pressure is evenly distributed.

Peripheral pulses are present throughout use of sequential stockings and elastic hosiery.

APPLYING GRADUATED COMPRESSION STOCKINGS (ELASTIC HOSIERY)

Equipment

Tape measure
Specific type of hosiery (e.g., below-the-knee or above-the-knee)

Preparation

1. Check orders for specific reason client needs elastic stockings.
2. Check physician's orders for type and specifications.
3. Gather supplies, identify client, and explain procedure.
4. Wash your hands, and provide for client's privacy and comfort.
5. Apply drape as top linens are removed. Bathe, dry, and powder client's legs. Ensure legs are dry before applying stockings.
6. Assess lower extremities for edema, dry skin, and palpable pulses.
7. Position client in dorsal recumbent position, and elevate bed to working height.
8. Measure client for hosiery size (Table 27–2).
   a. For below-the-knee stockings, measure from the Achilles tendon to the popliteal fold, and measure the midcalf circumference.
   b. For thigh-high stockings, measure midcalf and midthigh circumference to determine size.
   c. Length is determined by measuring distance from gluteal fold to bottom of the heel.

Note: Review leg measurements regularly to prevent potential complications resulting from edema.

9. Compare your measurements to manufacturer's chart to obtain correct hose size.

Procedure

1. Invert foot of stocking back to heel area.
2. Holding both sides of hose at inverted foot area, pull hose over toes and ease gently toward top of foot.
3. Gather top of hose down to heel area, and with curving motion, cover heel. Pull hose up leg, positioning support section on inner thigh.
4. Reposition client, lower bed, and wash your hands.
5. Observe extremities for edema above level of hose.
6. Observe that stockings are wrinkle free and correctly placed on extremity.
7. Check client in 30 minutes for adequate circulation, assessing for warmth and color of feet.

Effectiveness of Graduated Compression Stockings

Effectiveness of the stockings vary greatly. Data is lacking to support the use of these stockings for clients at high risk for venous thromboembolism, including use alone or in combination with anticoagulant prophylaxis. In moderate-risk clients there is evidence that stockings are effective and should be used. Stockings reduce stasis, and they are inexpensive and free of side effects.

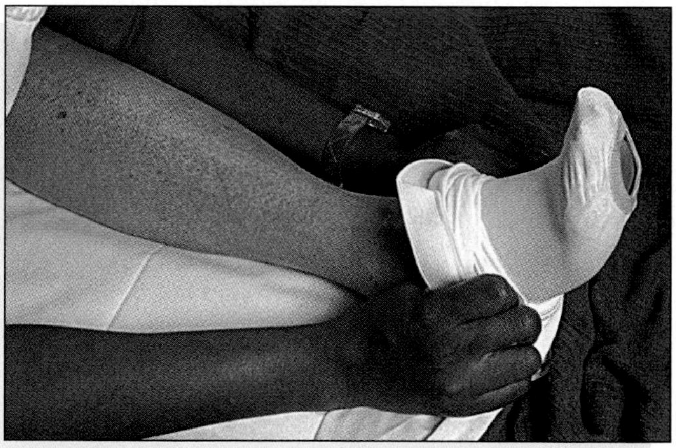

Gather elastic hose and pull over toes and then to top of foot.

TABLE 27–2 Measuring for Graduated Compression Stockings (elastic hosiery)

Thigh-Hi Measuring		Knee-Hi Measuring	
Circumference	**Length**	**Circumference**	**Length**
Measure mid-thigh circumference	Measure leg from bottom of heel to fold of buttocks	Measure calf at largest circumference	Measure leg form Achilles tendon to popliteal fold
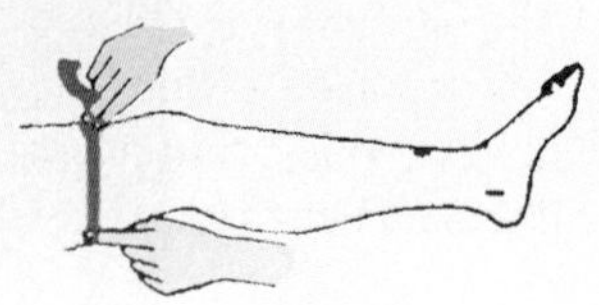	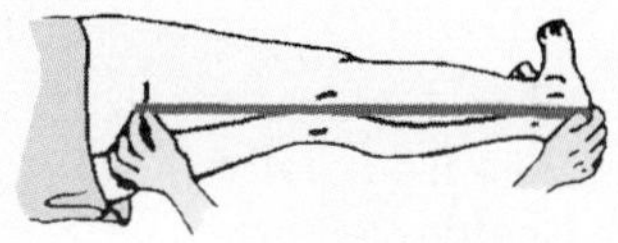	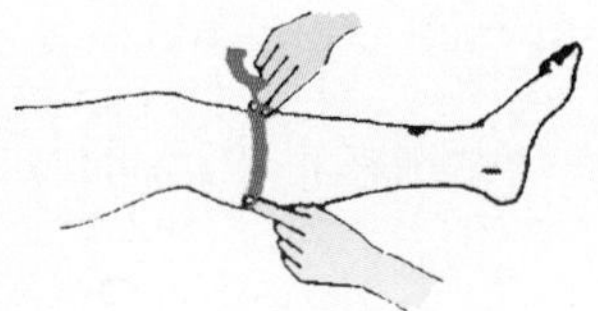	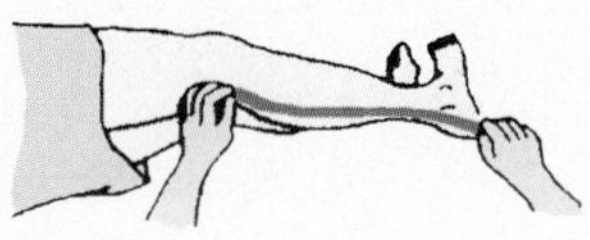

8. Remove hose two to three times daily for 30 minutes. Assess skin integrity and perform neurovascular checks.
9. Wash hose in mild detergent and warm water as needed.

Note: A second pair of hose should be available to use when washing hose.

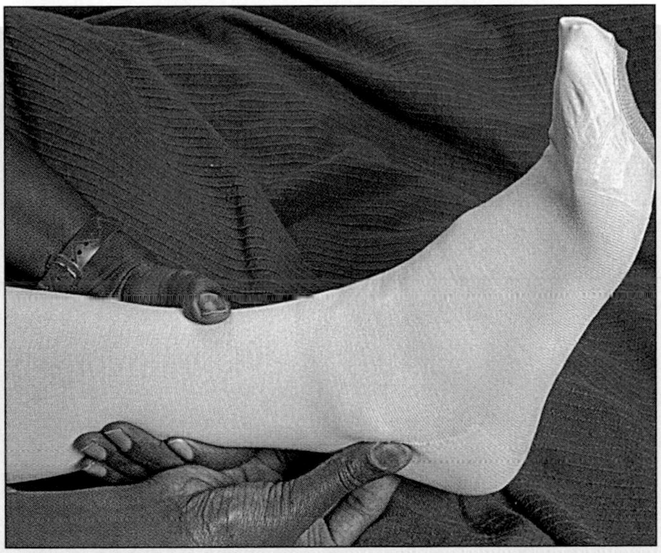

Ensure hose fits properly without wrinkles over toe or heel.

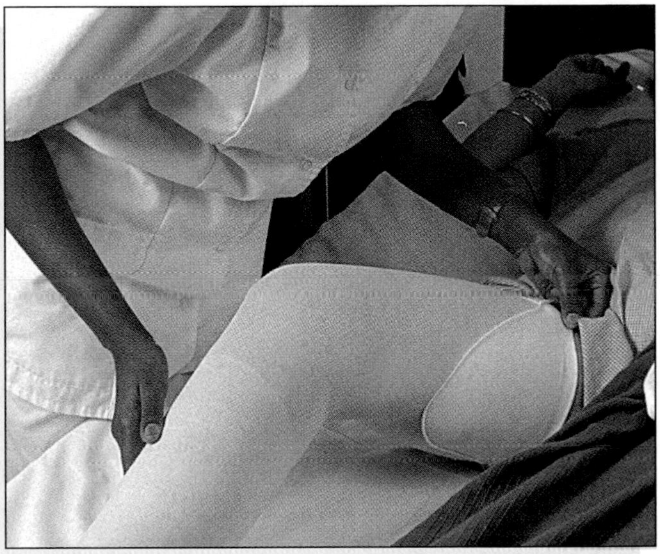

Position support section on inner thigh.

APPLYING PNEUMATIC COMPRESSION DEVICES

Equipment

Disposable leg sleeve(s)
  Knee length or thigh length
Tubing assembly
Compression controller (motor)
Measuring tape

Preparation

1. Review physician's orders for type of disposable leg sleeve needed. **Rationale:** Both knee- and thigh-length sleeves are available.
2. Identify client and explain that this device decreases the risk of developing deep-vein thrombosis (DVT) for clients following surgery or those on long-term bed rest. **Rationale:** This device counteracts blood stasis by increasing peak blood flow velocity. It helps to carry pooled blood from veins and also exerts an anticlotting effect by increasing fibrinolytic activity, while stimulating release of plasminogen activator.
3. Assess client for potential problems, contraindications for use of these devices. **Rationale:** Clients with severe atheroclerosis or other ischemic conditions, massive edema of the leg from pulmonary edema or heart failure, or preexisting DVT within last 6 months are not candidates for these devices, because they could exacerbate the condition. Also, clients with pronounced leg deformities, dermatitis, or gangrene are not candidates. Clients who have been on long-term bed rest prior to need for devices are also not candidates.
4. Measure circumference of upper thigh by placing measuring tape under the thigh and gluteal fold. Hold tape snug, but not tight, when measuring.
5. Note exact measurement and refer to manufacturer's sizing chart to determine exact fit of sleeve.
6. Complete a neurovascular assessment. Include an evaluation of skin color, temperature, sensation, capillary refill, and presence and quality of pedal pulses. Document findings. **Rationale:** This assessment provides baseline data for evaluating neurovascular changes while devices are used.
7. Assemble equipment. Read manufacturer's directions for connecting and operating compression controller and sleeve.
8. Read directions for setting sleeve pressure (between 35 and 45 mm Hg). Maximum pressure should not exceed client's diastolic pressure.
9. Locate and identify the indicator lights on the controller for the ankle, calf, and thigh pressure in addition to the cooling light. **Rationale:** Light is on when the pressure is applied to the three leg sleeves and during the cooling time. Pressure is exerted for a total of 11 seconds. The cooling period lasts 60 seconds, during which time there is no compression by the sleeve.

> **CLINICAL ALERT**
> These devices are used especially if client is not a candidate for heparin infusion.

Procedure

1. Remove sleeve from plastic bag.
2. Unfold sleeve and follow directions to fit sleeve to client's leg. Leg is placed on white side (lining) of sleeve. Markings on the lining indicate the ankle and popliteal area.
3. Place client's leg on sleeve lining. Position back of knee over popliteal opening.
4. Check that back of ankle is over ankle marking.
5. Starting at the side opposite the clear plastic tubing, wrap sleeve securely around client's leg.
6. Attach hook edge securely to the sleeve.
7. Check the fit by placing two fingers between client's leg and sleeve to determine if sleeve fits properly. Readjust Velcro as needed. **Rationale:** To ensure sleeve does not constrict circulation.
8. Remove tubing assembly from package and connect to plugs on leg sleeve by pushing ends firmly together. Arrows on both plug and connector must line up to ensure a proper fit.
9. Connect tubing assembly plug to controller at the tubing assembly connector site.
10. Ensure tubing is free of kinks or twists. **Rationale:** Kinks and twists can restrict air flow through system.
11. Plug controller power cable into grounded electric outlet and attach unit to bedframe.
12. Turn controller power switch to ON. Monitor that alarms are audible.
13. Check that pressure indicator lights and cooling light are functioning properly. When pressure is applied to each segment of leg, specific light is on. When cooling light is on, the compression lights should be OFF, as this is when no compression is applied to leg. Check actual pressure.
14. Monitor that compression and cooling cycles are correct. Ankle pressure is applied first, followed by calf pressure and then thigh pressure.
15. Monitor neurovascular checks every 2–4 hours. Turn machine off immediately if the client complains of numbness other signs of DVT.

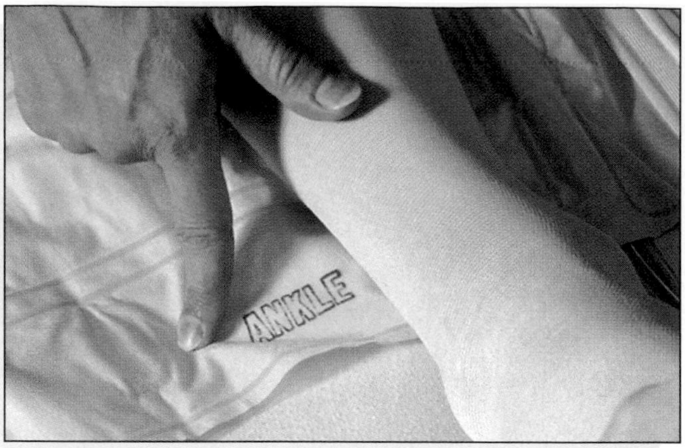

Leg position is indicated on lining of sleeve.

Compression Pattern

Each sleeve in the sequential devices is inflated in sequence. The inflation begins at the ankle and progresses to the knee or mid-thigh. Pressures range from a maximum pressure in the ankle of 45–50 mm Hg, 35 mm Hg at the calf, and 30 mm Hg at the thigh. Compression duration is 11 seconds, with a 60-second relaxation time between compressions.

For intermittent devices, sleeve inflates, then deflates, alternating from one leg to the other.

EVIDENCE BASED NURSING PRACTICE

Preventing Thromboembolic Disease

There is evidence that pneumatic compression devices are significantly more effective than graduated stockings alone at preventing venous thromboembolic disease. Graduated elastic stockings have proven to be effective as an adjuvant to anticoagulant therapy when anticoagulation itself is contraindicated

The American College of Chest Physicians have included a recommendation that prophylactic compression devices with or without the use of compression stockings be ordered for multiple-trauma-injury clients who are at risk for bleeding. This recommendation was based on several clinical trials using clients with hip arthroplasty and neurosurgical clients at risk for thromboembolism. In the neurosurgical trial, the use of compression devices decreased the risk by 60%. Clients with hip arthroplasty had a risk reduction of 63% for deep-vein thrombosis and 48% for proximal-vein throbosis. These devices are used most effectively with preventative drug therapy such as low-molecular-weight heparin or other heparin-type medications.

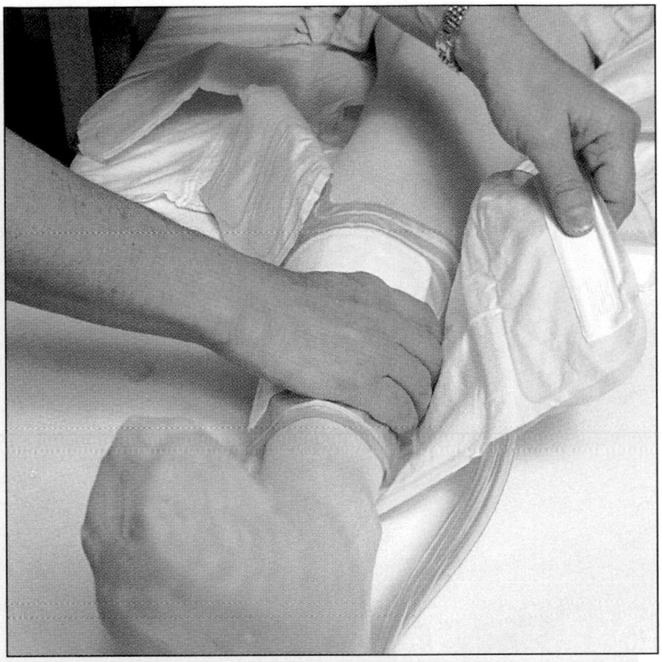
Wrap sleeve securely around client's leg.

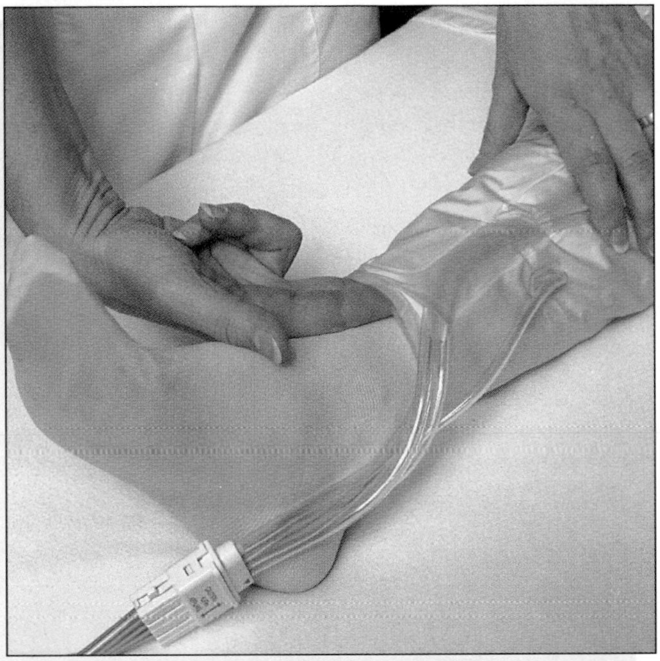
Check for proper fit before inflating compression device.

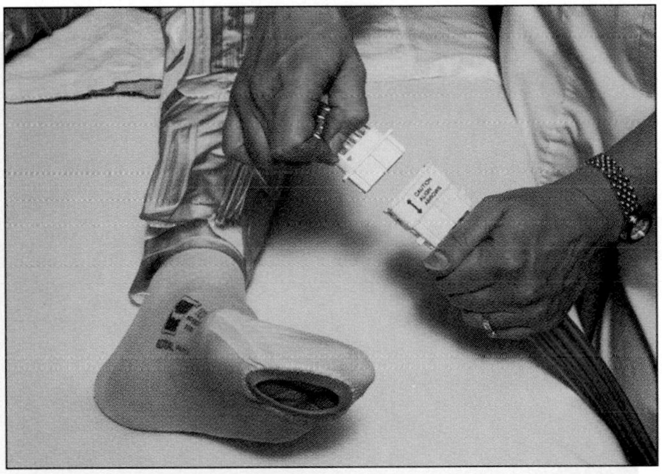
Connect tubing assembly plug to controller.

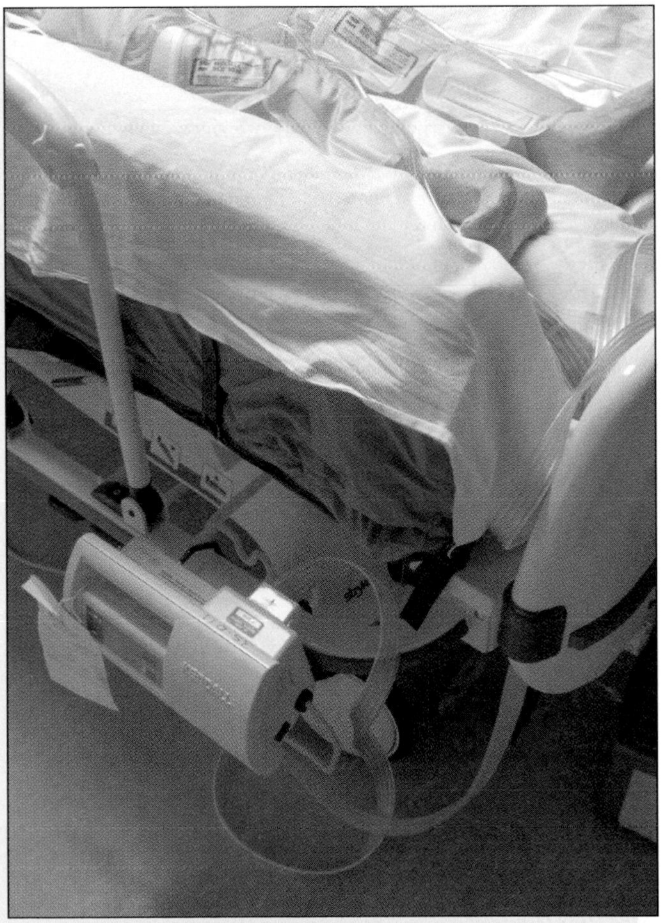
After controller power cable is placed in grounded electrical outlet, place unit on bedframe.

16. Monitor client's tolerance of device.
17. Turn off machine at prescribed time intervals to assess skin and to provide skin care.
18. To remove sleeve, turn power switch OFF, disconnect tubing assembly from sleeve at connection site. Unwrap sleeve from leg.

CLINICAL ALERT

Follow hospital policy for amount of time alternating pneumatic compression stockings are removed during the day. It is important to keep stockings on most of the day to prevent clot formation.

Foot Pumps

Foot pumps gently squeeze the sole of the foot to mimic circulatory effects of walking. The plexus of veins in the foot act as a powerful venous pump in the weight-bearing phase of ambulation. The foot pump is designed to mimic natural effects of walking on blood circulation in feet and legs. These pumps increase circulation and decrease edema and pain to the lower extremities in clients who are not ambulatory.

Example shown is the Kindall Sequential Compression Device (SCD) Foot Pump.

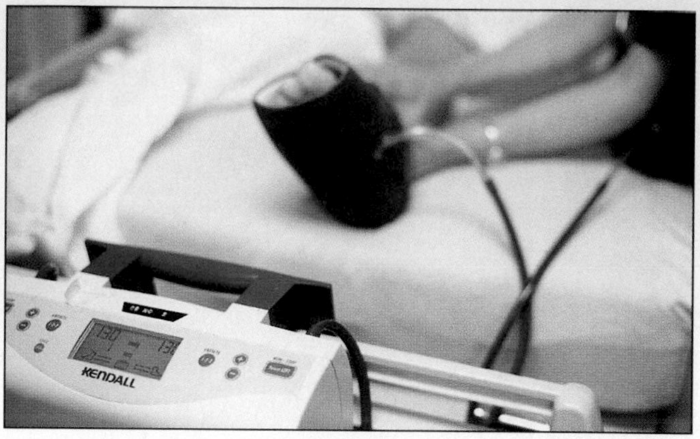

Documentation for Circulatory Maintenance

Elastic Hosiery

- Size and type of elastic hose applied
- Condition of skin
- Presence of pulses
- Edema formation below or above hose
- Time and length of time hose removed

Compression Devices

- Neurovascular assessment baseline data
- Neurovascular assessment during application
- Condition of skin
- Sleeve pressure
- Time compression devices applied and removed
- Type of sleeve used; thigh high, knee high

Critical Thinking Application

UNEXPECTED OUTCOMES	CRITICAL THINKING OPTIONS
for Graduated Compression Stockings	
Graduated Compression Stockings are not available.	• If ordered, use elastic (Ace) bandages. Anchor bandages on top of the foot and and proceed up leg. Bandage should overlap one-third of bandage width; for a 4-inch width each turn overlaps by 1½ inches. Ensure pressure is evenly distributed throughout bandage application.
	• Assess that elastic bandages are tight enough for support but do not obstruct arterial flow. Assess neurovascular status 20 minutes after bandages applied and every 2–4 hours thereafter.
	• While making each turn, place a finger between the bandage and skin to prevent bandage from becoming too tight.
Graduated Compression Stockings are loose and don't provide support.	• Remeasure legs and compare to chart to determine correct size.
	• Hosiery may be old with no elasticity and should be discarded.
Graduated Compression Stockings do not provide support.	• Need to order different knit design and elastomeric yarn denier that will increase pressure. Pressure ranges from less than 15 mm Hg to 30–40 mm Hg at the ankle.
for Pneumatic Compression Devices	
Client complains of numbness or tingling in leg.	• Remove devices immediately.
	• Complete neurovascular assessment.
	• Notify physician of assessment findings.
Buildup of excess sleeve pressure (above 80 mm Hg).	• Check tubing for kinks or twists.
	• Turn power switch to OFF position and then ON to restart system.

UNIT 3

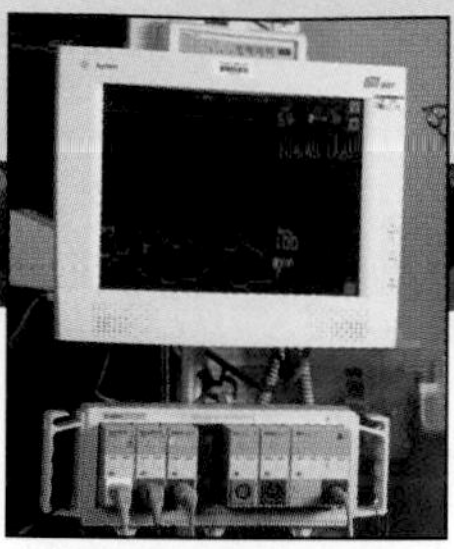

Electrocardiogram (ECG) Monitoring

Nursing Process Data

ASSESSMENT Data Base

Determine if there is preexisting cardiac disease or chest pain.

Assess client's level of understanding and cooperation with procedure.

Determine client's level of fear or anxiety regarding diagnosis, procedure, or outcome.

Identify pharmacologic agents currently prescribed.

Determine other pathologic conditions that may precipitate conditions, such as fever, anxiety, alcohol, tobacco, or caffeine ingestion.

Determine subjective complaints of diaphoresis, palpitations, dizziness, or fainting.

Identify electrolyte abnormalities affecting the electrocardiogram, particularly potassium and calcium deficiencies or excesses.

PLANNING Objectives

To obtain an accurate 12-lead ECG

To clearly display ECG on oscilloscope

To determine ECG changes

To identify ECG abnormalities reflecting electrolyte abnormalities

To determine cardiac irregularities

To identify and treat potentially dangerous rhythms accordingly

To determine if a relationship exists between chest pain and ECG changes

To continuously monitor a client on telemetry

IMPLEMENTATION Procedures

Monitoring the ECG

Interpreting an ECG Strip

Recording a 12-Lead ECG

Monitoring Clients on Telemetry

EVALUATION Expected Outcomes

ECG leads applied appropriately and without difficulty.

Abnormal ECG findings interpreted accurately.

Heart rate calculated correctly.

MONITORING THE ECG

Equipment

Electrode discs
Lead wires
Cardiac monitor and cable
Cassette
Soap and water
Wash cloth or 4 × 4s, soap, and towel

Preparation

1. Gather equipment.
2. Wash your hands.
3. Explain procedure to client.
4. Wipe skin areas on client with soap and water where electrodes are to be attached. Allow to dry. **Rationale:** This removes oily substances and dead skin for better adherence of electrodes. Rub skin until slightly red.
5. Insert ECG cassette into monitor.
6. Check that ECG monitor is plugged in and turned ON.
7. Attach cable to monitor.

Procedure

1. Obtain electrodes (most facilities use disposable electrodes).
2. Check electrode expiration date. **Rationale:** This ensures electrode gel is moist.
3. Select and prepare site for electrode placement.
   a. Select 3 or 5 lead setup: 3 leads provide for a choice of views (but no anterior view); 5 leads allow for 7 views, including anterior view.
   b. Select new site for each electrode application.
4. Apply electrodes.
   a. Peel off paper backing on electrode disc. Check that sponge pad in center of electrode is moist with conductive jelly. Place electrode on skin with adhesive side down. Press edges down to secure.
   b. Apply electrodes in areas where there will not be excessive movement. Do not place over muscular areas or inner arms.
   c. Place near but not directly on bone surfaces, joints, breasts or skin creases. **Rationale:** Placing electrodes on

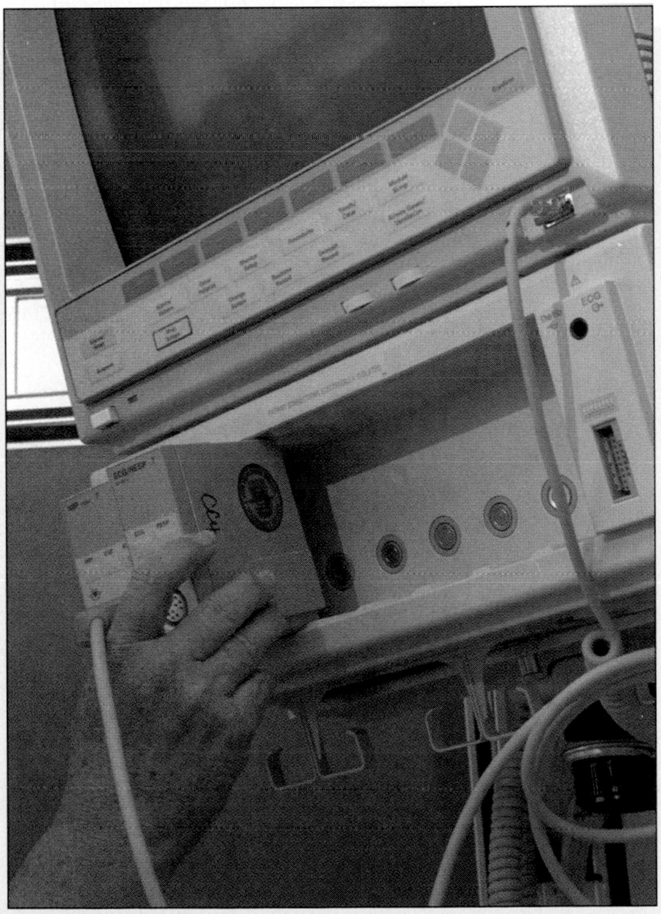

Cassettes are inserted for each function to be monitored.

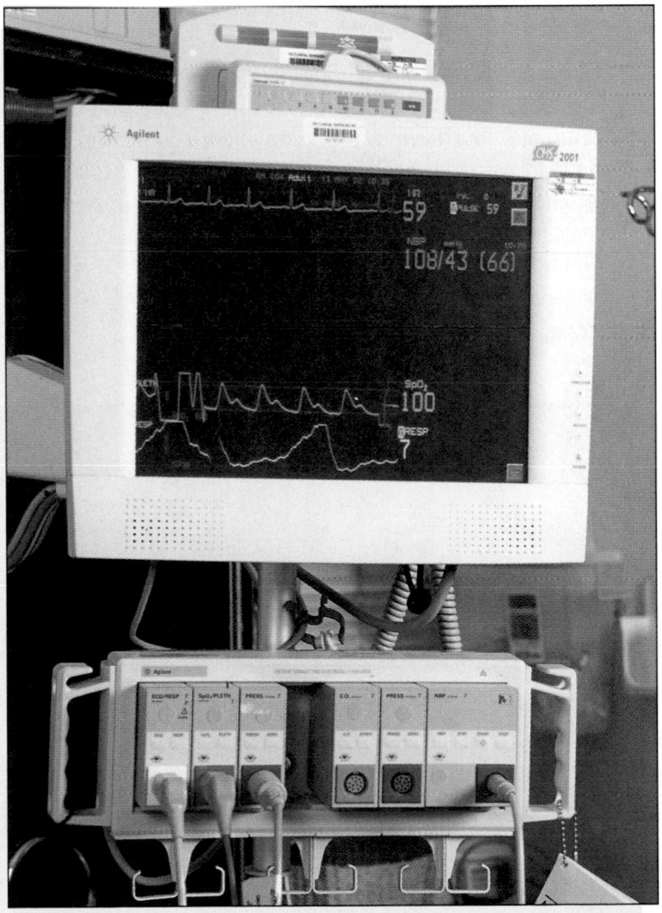

Monitors can record several different sets of data including art line, CVP, O_2 sat, ECG, and respirations.

these areas can lead to artifact on the monitor screen. If client is overly obese, electrodes may have to be placed on the bones, since a large amount of adipose tissue results in a poor image on the oscilloscope.

   d. Avoid placing electrodes over scar tissue, burns, rashes, or other lesions. **Rationale:** These conditions weaken signals or cause wide base-lines on the monitor.

5. Attach the chest electrodes to the lead wires by placing wire level on disc using the appropriate colored lead wires. **Rationale:** The client end of the cable is coded to facilitate connection with the electrodes.
6. Apply five clamp- (or snap)-type electrodes to client's chest:
   a. **White** to right shoulder (negative electrode)
   b. **Black** to left shoulder (lead I positive electrode or MCL_1 negative electrode)
   c. **Red** to left midclavicular upper abdominal area (lead II positive electrode)
   d. **Brown** to fourth intercostal space, right sternal border (MCL_1 positive chest electrode), or left sternal border, or alternatively at 5th intercostal space, midaxillary line (V_6 position)
   e. **Green** to right abdomen or other convenient area (ground electrode)

Note: Limb leads and any one chest lead can be monitored using these electrode positions.

7. If lead wires are snapped onto electrodes, you may want to attach lead wires to electrodes before placing disc on client. **Rationale:** To prevent pushing on client's chest when attaching lead wire to disc. This can cause discomfort to client.
8. Set HIGH and LOW alarm limits on the monitor. Set at 20 beats higher and lower than normal for that client.
9. Turn alarm buttons to ON.
10. Observe pattern to determine clarity of image on oscilloscope.

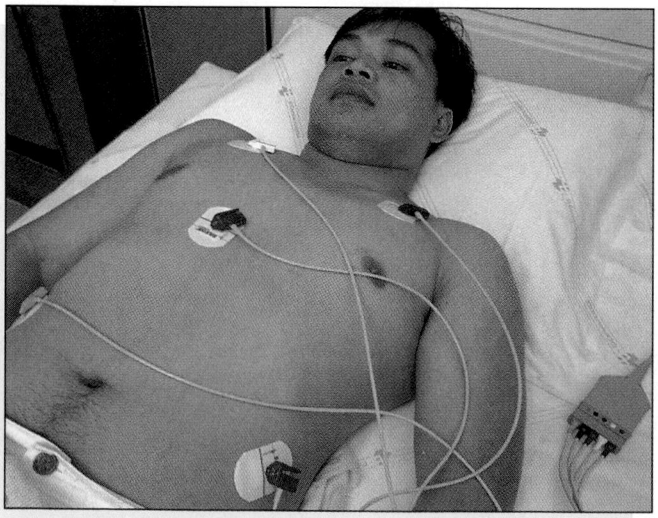

Color-coded lead wires and placement of electrodes for ECG monitoring.

11. Determine best lead image by turning switch on the monitor to appropriate lead.
12. Run ECG strip, and place in nurses' notes. **Rationale:** This provides a baseline record of the ECG pattern at the beginning of monitoring. To run the strip, turn the switch on the monitor to RUN. A strip of ECG paper appears with the wave form printed out.
13. Assess skin surrounding electrode disc for signs of irritation every 4 hours.

Electrode Systems for Cardiac Monitoring

Three-, four-, or five-electrode systems are used in cardiac monitoring. The most popular method is the five-electrode system. This system allows the nurse to monitor any one of the six modified chest leads as well as the other leads without changing electrode placement.

The three-electrode system has one positive electrode, one negative electrode, and a ground.

The four-electrode system has a right leg electrode that becomes a permanent ground for all leads in addition to the three-electrode system.

The five-electrode system has a right leg lead placed on lower chest, just above and to the right of the umbilicus.

In three- and four-electrode systems, lead wires are placed according to the type of monitoring required. Electrical current flows from negative to positive; therefore, each lead has a different configuration for the electrode placement.

- **Lead I:** Used to monitor for atrial rhythms and hemiblocks. Depicts current moving from right to left in the heart. Positive electrode placed on left arm or left side of chest, negative electrode placed on right arm or below right clavicle.
- **Lead II:** Used for routine monitoring and for detection of sinus node and atrial arrhythmias. The positive electrode is placed on the lowest palpable rib at the left midclavicular line and the negative electrode is placed below the right clavicle or on right arm.
- **Lead III:** Used to detect changes associated with an inferior wall myocardial infarction. The positive electrode is placed on the left leg or lowest palpable rib on left midclavicular line. The negative electrode is placed on the left arm or below left clavicle.
- **MCL_1:** Used to assess QRS-complex arrhythmias. This lead is equivalent to the V_1 chest lead on the 12-lead ECG. The positive electrode is placed on the right of the heart at the fourth intercostal space (right of sternum). The negative electrode is placed on the left upper chest below the left clavicle, and the ground electrode is placed on the right upper chest.

INTERPRETING AN ECG STRIP

Equipment

Calipers
ECG rhythm strip

Procedure

1. Assess ECG grid.
   a. Each small block represents 0.04 seconds and 0.1 mV (1 mm).
   b. Each large block represents 0.20 seconds and 0.5 mV (5 mm).
   c. 15 large blocks represent 3 seconds.
2. Determine heart rate by calculating atrial rate (PP interval) and ventrical rate (RR interval). Normal pulse is 60–100.
   Heart rate is calculated by:
   a. Counting the number of cardiac cycles (QRS complexes) in a 6-second strip (30 large blocks) and multiplying that number by 10 to obtain the pulse.
   b. Counting the number of small boxes between R waves, and dividing that number into 1,500. The quotient is the ventricular rate.
   c. Counting the number of small boxes between P waves and dividing that number into 1,500. The quotient is the atrial rate.

NOTE: For accuracy, check the apical pulse and correlate it with the ECG findings.

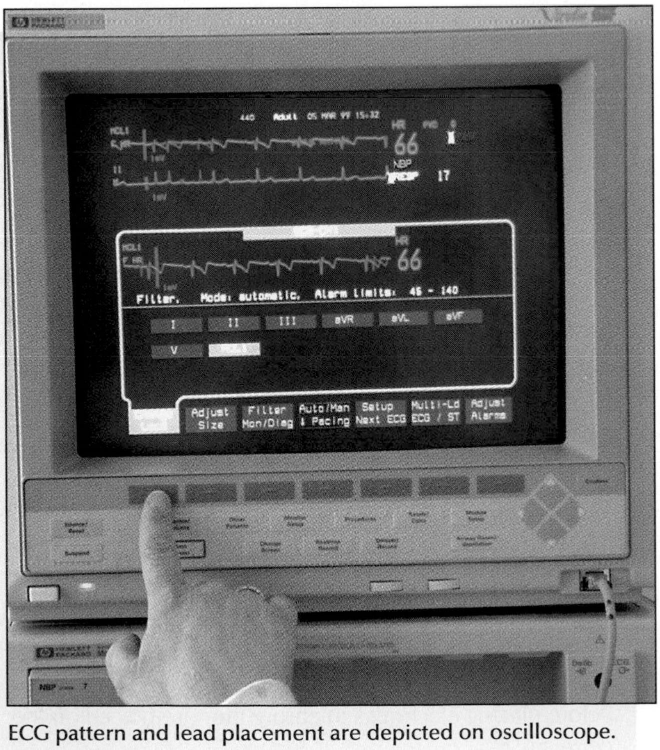

ECG pattern and lead placement are depicted on oscilloscope.

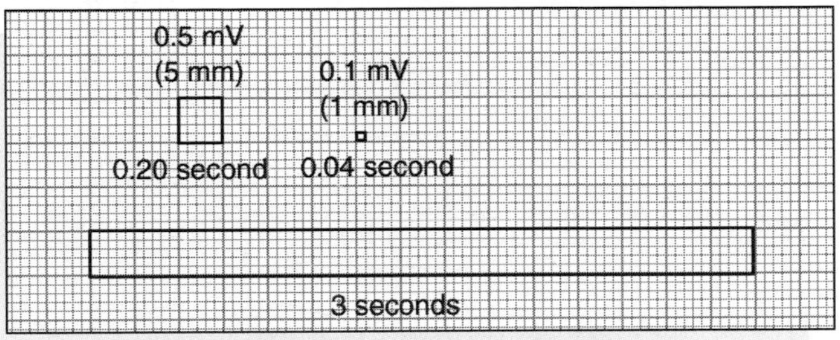

ECG grid.

3. Determine regularity of rhythm (atrial and ventricular). Check if complexes look alike and are equally spaced. Use calipers to check this.
4. Measure PR interval to determine conduction time in atria and AV junction (0.12–0.20 seconds) from beginning of P to beginning of QRS.
5. Measure QRS duration to determine ventricular conduction (QRS = <0.12 seconds duration). There are six complexes.

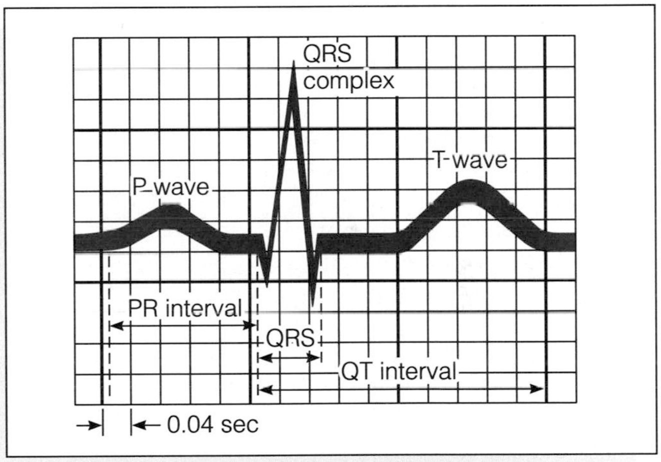

It is important to determine configuration and location of wave pattern to interpret an ECG accurately.

TABLE 27–3 Normal Sinus Rhythm

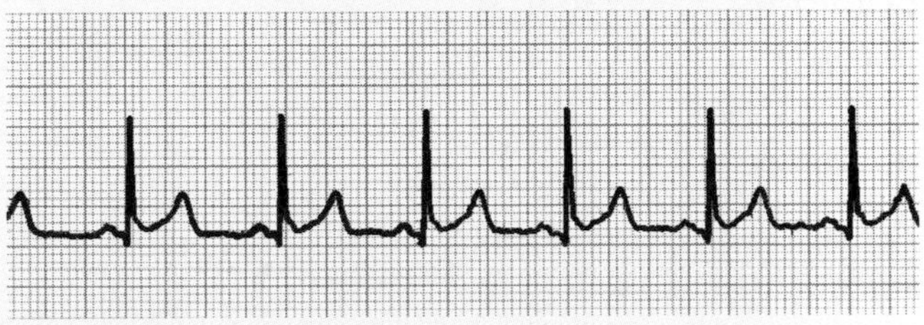

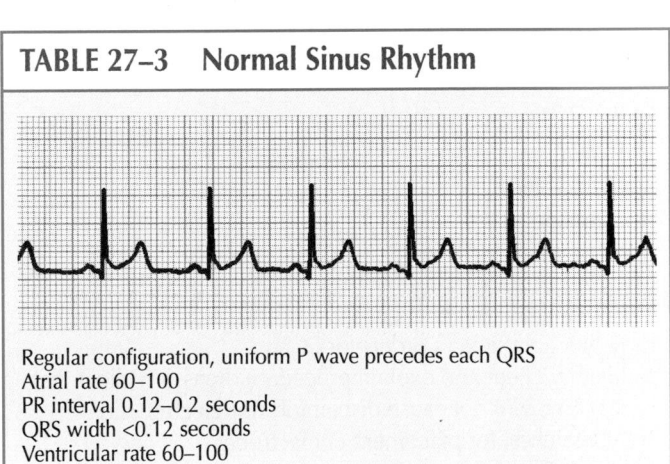

Regular configuration, uniform P wave precedes each QRS
Atrial rate 60–100
PR interval 0.12–0.2 seconds
QRS width <0.12 seconds
Ventricular rate 60–100

TABLE 27–4 Potentially Life-Threatening Arrhythmias

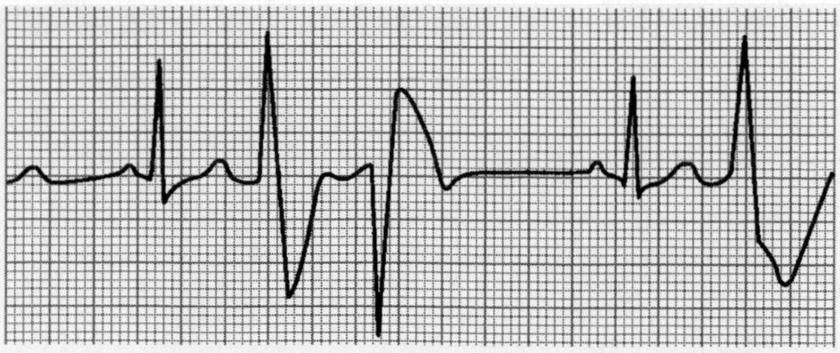

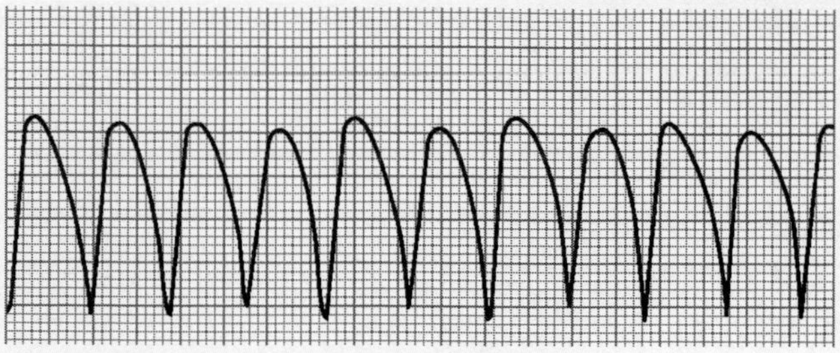

Multifocal Premature Ventricular Contraction (PVCs)	Ventricular Tachycardia
Irregular rhythm P waves—none with premature beat, impulse originates in ventricle Atrial rate—undetermined PR interval—none with premature beat QRS width—greater than 0.12 seconds for premature beat Ventricular rate—varies *Note: Each PVC has different configuration as foci are from different areas of heart.* PVCs are result of increased automaticity of ventricular muscle cells. **Etiology** • Heart disease, MI • Hypoxia • Acidosis • Electrolyte imbalances • Myocardial ischemia • Drug toxicity (especially digitalis) **Initial treatment** • Oxygen • Potassium or magnesium if electrolytes dictate • Lidocaine bolus—1–1.5 mg/kg; may repeat doses of 0.5–0.75 mg/kg every 5–10 minutes up to 3 mg/kg • Continuous IV drip may be started • Correct underlying cause	Regular rhythm Atrial rate—cannot differentiate PR interval—none QRS width—greater than 0.12 seconds Ventricular rate—100–300 *Note: Ventricular tachycardia is a result of myocardial irritability and is life threatening.* **Etiology** • Acute MI • Coronary artery disease, cardiomyopathy • Electrolyte imbalance • Drug intoxication (digitalis) **Initial treatment** • Lidocaine 1.5 mg/kg bolus; may repeat in 3–5 minutes to maximum dose of 3 mg/kg • Cardioversion if cardiac output is compromised • Pulseless ventricular tachycardia—follow treatment for ventricular fibrillation • Insertion of implanted defibrillator • Antiarrhythmic drug regimen, including Amiodarme 150 mg bolus over 10 minutes

6. Measure QT interval (rate of 70 in 1 minute occurring 0.33–0.44 seconds apart).
7. Check configuration and placement of P wave, QRS complex, ST segment, and T wave.
8. Summarize findings to obtain interpretation.
9. Determine if arrhythmias are potentially life threatening. Immediate intervention must be provided to prevent complications.
10. Document interpretation of findings, and place ECG strip in client's chart.

RECORDING A 12-LEAD ECG

Equipment

Electrodes
Soap and water
ECG machine
Cable

Preparation

1. Review physician's orders for ECG.
2. Identify client and explain procedure. Reassure client that machine will not cause discomfort nor electrocution.
3. Assess chest for placement of electrodes.
4. Determine if skin site care is necessary. If so, cleanse areas with soap and water. Allow area to dry thoroughly before placing electrodes. **Rationale:** This will ensure a more secure fit for the electrodes and provide a better ECG tracing.
5. Attach electrodes to wires before pressing onto client's chest. **Rationale:** This prevents pressure being applied to chest area. This is particularly necessary following open heart surgery or chest trauma.
6. Check the color coding on the manufacturer's directions before placing electrodes to ensure they are placed on the correct wires.

TABLE 27–4 continued

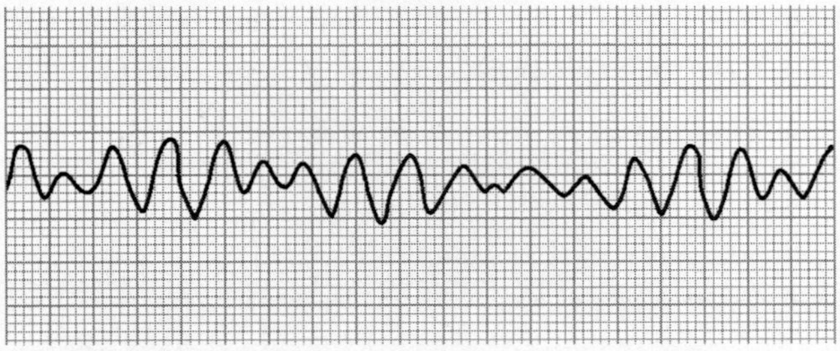

Ventricular Fibrillation

Irregular rhythm
Atrial rate—cannot differentiate
PR interval—none
QRS width—fibrillating waves only
Ventricular rate—cannot differentiate

Note: Ineffective quivering of ventricles with no audible heartbeat, pulse, or respirations.

Etiology
- Myocardial ischemia, Acute MI
- Coronary artery disease
- Cardiomyopathy
- Acid-base imbalance
- Severe hypothemia
- Electrolyte imbalance

Initial treatment
- CPR
- Defibrillate; starting at 200 J, defibrillate up to three times, 200–300 J, 360 J
- Ventricular fibrillation continues—epinephrine 1 mg IV push, repeat 3–5 minutes
- Defibrillate—360 J within 30–60 seconds of drug
- Second-line drugs may be used, such as bretylium and procainamide

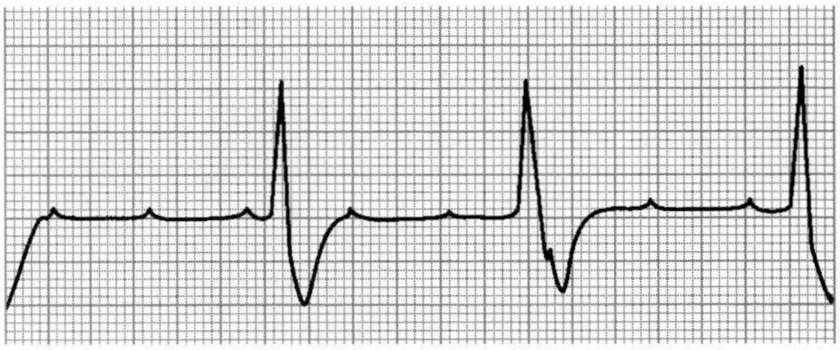

Third-Degree Heart Block

Regular atrial and ventricular rhythm
Atrial rate—greater than ventricular rate
PR interval—varies
QRS width—less than 0.12 second if pacemaker cell in junction; greater than 0.12 seconds if cell in ventricle
Ventricular rate—40–60 if escape pacemaker is from junction; 20–40 if escape is from ventricle

Note: Electrical impulse originates in SA node but is blocked to the Purkinje fibers leading to decreased perfusion of vital organs.

Etiology
- Digitalis toxicity
- Myocardial infarction, anterior
- Organic heart disease

Initial treatment
- Atropine
- Transcutaneous pacing
- Dopamine or epinephrine
- Prepare for pacemaker insertion

TABLE 27–5 Lead Placements

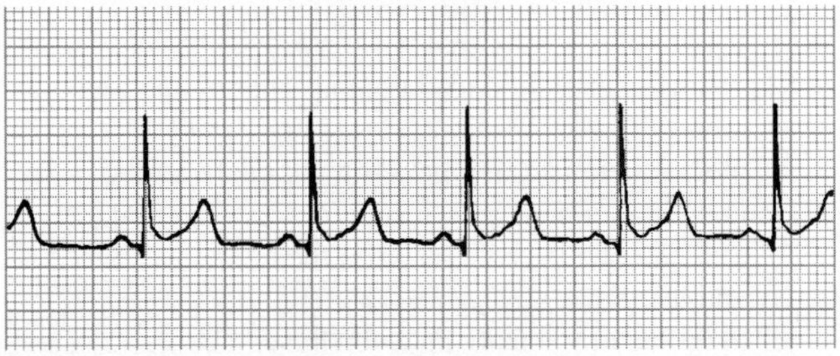

ECG pattern from Lead II placement

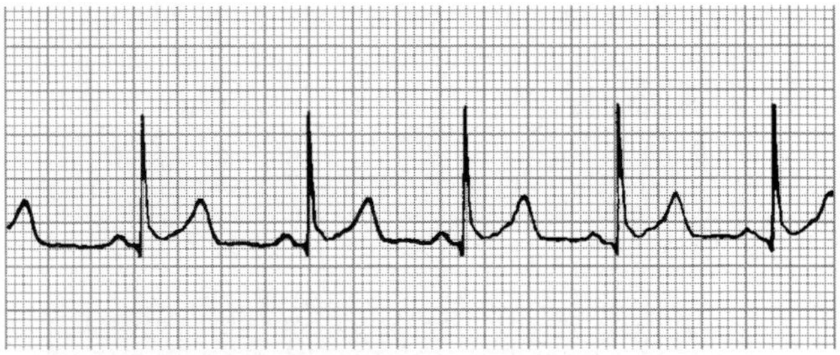

ECG pattern from Lead I placement

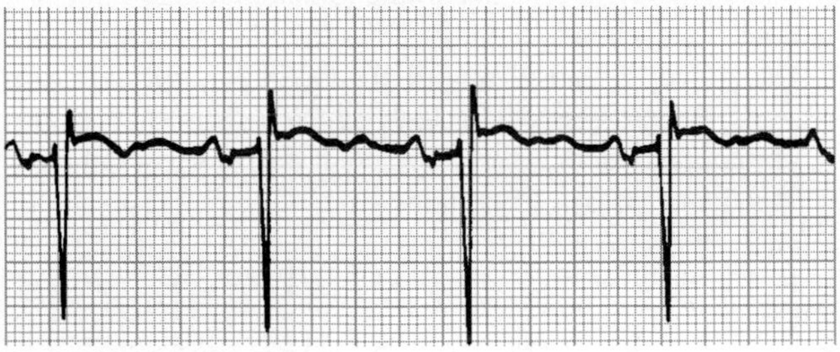

ECG pattern from MCL_1 placement

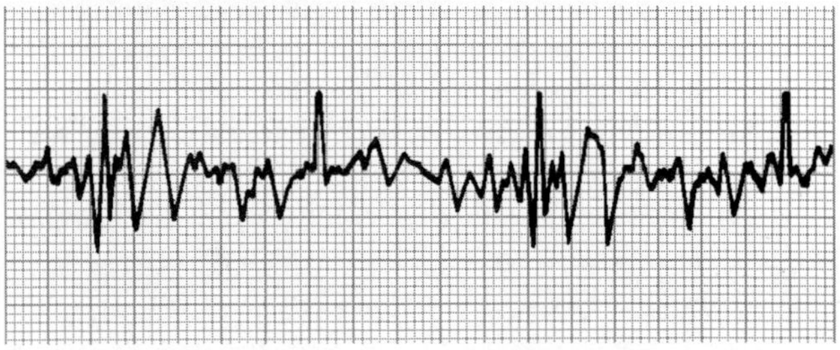

ECG pattern showing artifact

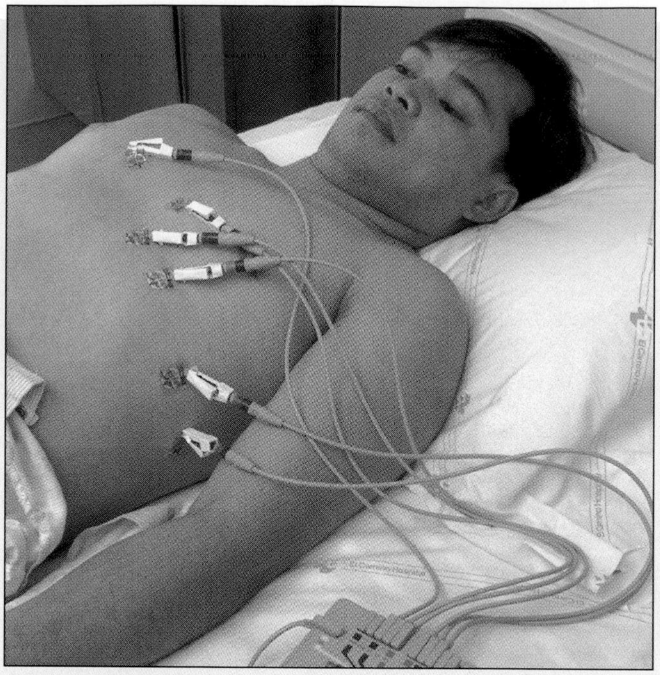

Electrode placement for chest leads V_1–V_6.

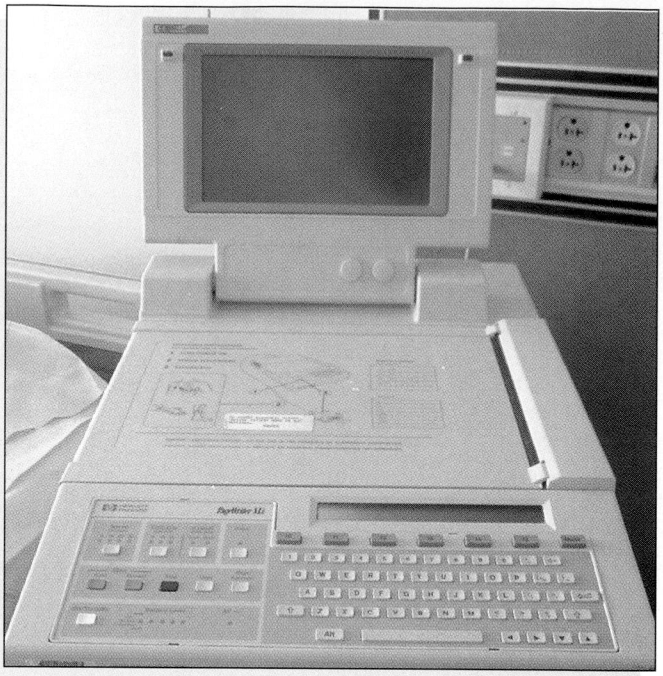

Portable ECG machine for taking 12-lead ECG tracing.

Procedure

1. When placing electrodes, ensure they are all going in the same direction so that lead wires hang at the same angle.
2. Place electrodes on fleshy areas, avoiding bone and muscle. **Rationale:** To ensure good electrical conduction and clear ECG tracings.
3. Place the four limb leads, one on each limb, according to the color coding. Three standard limb leads will be recorded on the 12-lead ECG.
   a. **Lead I:** Right arm (negative electrode) and left arm (positive electrode). Records activity between the two arms.
   b. **Lead II:** Right arm (negative electrode) and left leg (positive electrode). Records activity between arm and leg.
   c. **Lead III:** Left arm (negative electrode) and left leg (positive electrode). Records activity between arm and leg.
4. Place the chest leads as follows. (*See* photo above.)
   a. **V_1:** Fourth intercostal space, right sternal border. Records activity between the center of the heart and the fourth intercostal space; P wave is shown best here.
      (1) Palpare the jugular notch (feels like a depression).
      (2) Move finger down and palpate the manubrium of sternum (feels solid).
      (3) Continue to move finger down to the angle of Louis, which is at the top of the sternal body.
      (4) Move finger to the right of the angle of Louis to the second right rib.
      (5) Below the rib is the second intercostal space.
      (6) Move fingers down, palpating the next two ribs. Below the fourth rib and to the right of the sternal body is the fourth intercostal space. Place electrode in this area.
   b. **V_2:** Fourth intercostal space, left sternal border.
   c. **V_3:** Midway between V_2 and V_4, between 4th and 5th ICS.
   d. **V_4:** Fifth intercostal space, left midclavicular line.
   e. **V_5:** Fifth intercostal space, anterior axillary line, and midclavicular area.
   f. **V_6:** Fifth intercostal space, left midaxillary line.
5. Three augmented limb lead tracings are obtained on the ECG as follows.
   a. **aVR:** Records activity between the center of the heart and right arm.
   b. **aVL:** Records activity between the center of the heart and left arm.
   c. **aVF:** Records activity between the center of the heart and the left leg or foot.
6. Begin taking the ECG according to manufacturer's directions on machine.
7. The above 12 leads (lead I, II, III, aVR, aVL, aVF, and leads V_1–V_6) record electrical activity of the heart and assist the physician to identify the myocardial changes that define specific pathologic conditions.

MONITORING CLIENTS ON TELEMETRY

Equipment

Telemetry transmitter box with 9-volt battery
Electrode pouch
Lead wires
Electrodes
Soap and water
Gauze pad

Preparation

1. Gather equipment.
2. Determine lead placement (Lead II or MCL_1).
3. Explain procedure to client. Radio waves transmit the heart's electrical activity to a central monitoring station. This system allows the client to move around while his/her heart is constantly being monitored.
4. Allay client's fears—the ECG is being monitored at a base station.
5. Explain to client that the telemetry range is limited; therefore, they cannot wander out of the range, which is usually the nursing unit. If they need to go off the unit, they must notify the base station.
6. Instruct the client to notify the nurse if the electrode falls off. Do not attempt to reattach the electrode.

Procedure

1. Check the expiration date on the electrode packet. **Rationale:** The electrode jelly can dry out if old. This can lead to a fuzzy ECG tracing.
2. Select electrode site that is not over bony prominence or over muscular area.
3. Assess skin site before placing electrode. Cleanse area using soap and water if lubricant jelly or topical medicine residue is left on site. Allow site to dry thoroughly before affixing the electrode. **Rationale:** This promotes a secure fit of the electrode.
4. Insert lead wires securely into the transmitter box.
5. Attach wires to electrodes before putting them on the client.

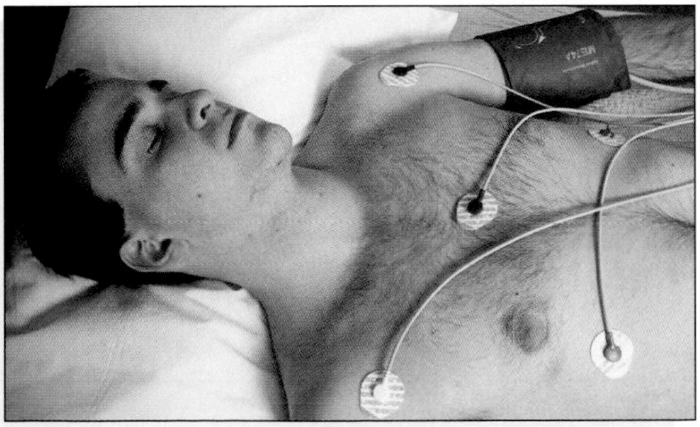

Five-lead placements for telementry monitoring.

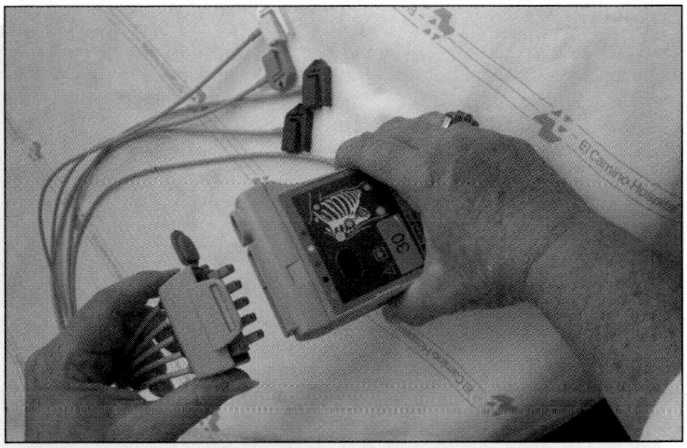

Attach wires into transmitter box.

Rationale: This prevents having to press down on the chest to attach them after the electrodes have been applied.

6. Use the color-coded diagram from the manufacturer to accurately place electrodes on the chest.
7. Have base station run an ECG strip to check clarity of the strip and accurate placement of leads.
8. Place transmitter in the pouch.
9. Check monitor strip at least once a shift or if client condition changes.
10. Switch lead selector on the monitor to obtain a different lead reading if necessary.
11. Check lead placement at least once a shift unless notified by client or base station that electrodes are not functioning properly.
12. Change electrodes at least every 3 days or if ECG strip indicates poor conduction of wave form.
13. Check client at least every four hours or more often if condition warrants.

Note: Review ECG Interpretation and Critical Thinking Application before caring for a client on telemetry.

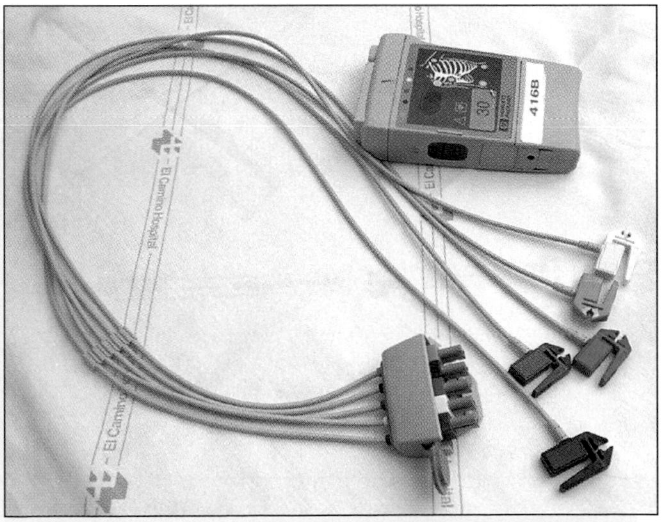

Transmitter box and lead wires for telemetry.

TABLE 27–6 Telemetry Electrode Placement

- **Lead I:** Records activity between a negative electrode (below right clavicle) and a positive electrode (below left clavicle). This lead looks at the heart's left lateral wall. Atrial arrhythmic activity is poorly identified.

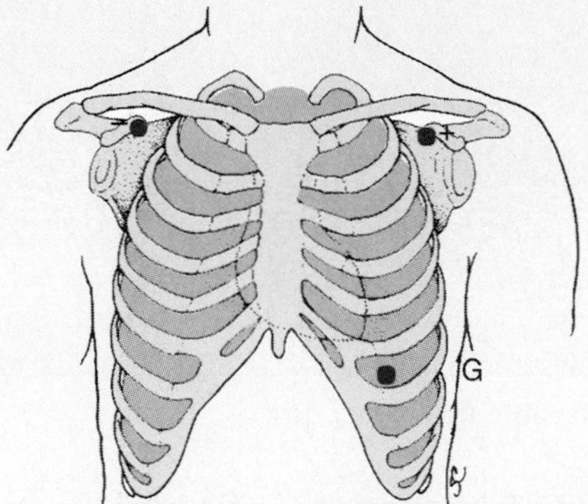

- **Lead II:*** Records activity between a negative electrode (below right clavicle) and a positive electrode (midclavicular line on left flank). This lead looks at left inferior wall. It is used to diagnose supraventricular rhythms which arise from the atrial and junctional nodes. It best detects atrial activity.

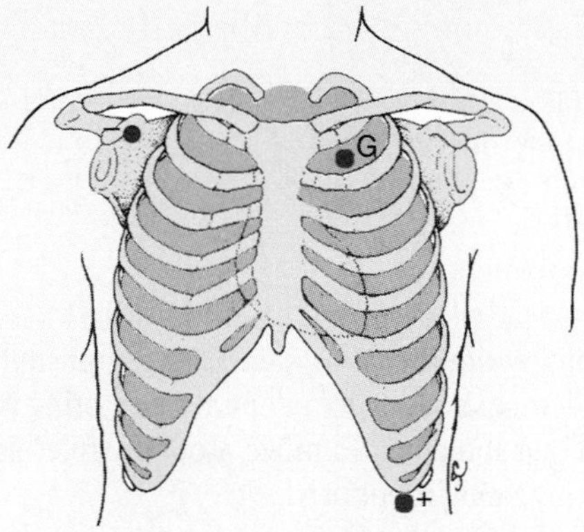

- **Lead III:** Records activity between a negative electrode (below left clavicle) and a positive electrode (lowest rib, left midclavicular line). It looks at left inferior wall.

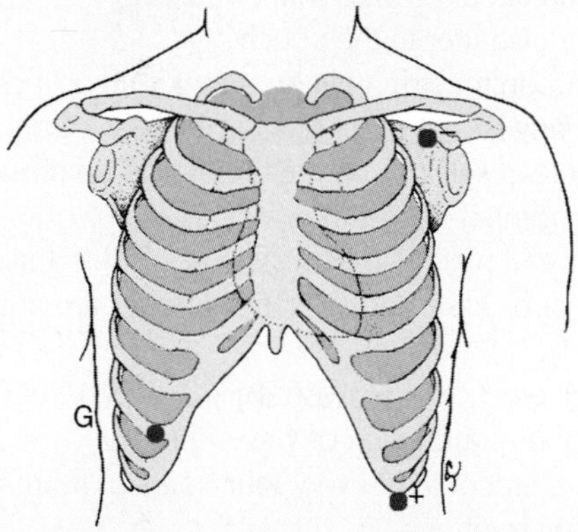

- **Lead MCL$_1$:*** Records activity between a negative electrode (below left clavicle) and a positive electrode (fourth intercostal space, right of sternum). It is used to analyze ventricular activity so it is beneficial for clients at risk for developing ventricular tachycardia or those with bundle branch block.

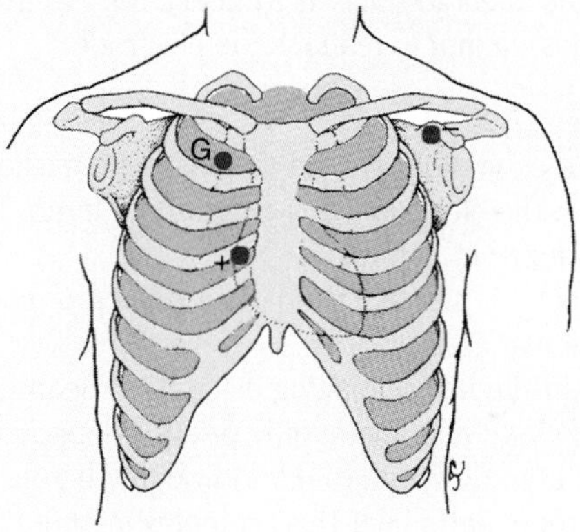

- **Lead MCL$_6$:** Records activity between a negative electrode (below left clavicle) and a positive electrode (fifth intercostal space, left midaxillary line). It monitors ventricular conduction changes much like MCL$_1$.

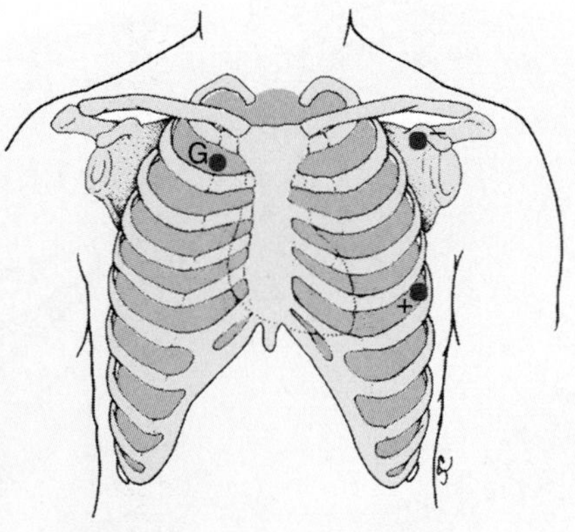

*Most popular leads for telemetry.

DOCUMENTATION FOR ECG MONITORING

- 12-lead ECG taken
- Telemetry initiated
- Findings based on the interpretation of the ECG strip
- Nursing interventions carried out, based on the ECG findings
- Lead placement used in ECG monitoring or telemetry monitoring
- Rhythm strips attached to nurses' notes at least once each shift
- When electrodes were replaced
- Client attitude toward procedure
- Health teaching completed
- When physician was notified of abnormal findings

Critical Thinking Application

UNEXPECTED OUTCOMES	CRITICAL THINKING OPTIONS
for ECG Interpretation	
ECG is not clearly displayed on the oscilloscope.	• Ensure that electrodes are applied in correct position and are securely attached. • Observe for electrical interference resulting in a 60-cycle interference on oscilloscope. • Observe for excessive client activity resulting in artifact display on oscilloscope.
Electrodes do not adhere to skin, and interference appears on oscilloscope.	• Change placement of electrodes to another area. • Put tincture of benzoin on the skin before placing electrodes. • Recleanse skin thoroughly with soap and water.
Alarms ring without change in pattern.	• Check HIGH and LOW parameters. They may need to be changed. • Check GAIN. It may be too low to sense pattern.
ECG pattern is abnormal.	• Recheck each configuration. • Check if pattern is a life-threatening arrhythmia (PVCs, ventricular tachycardia, ventricular fibrillation); if so, notify physician immediately.
Electrical interference continues after lead wires and cable connections are secured.	• Check all other electric equipment in the immediate environment. • Check for proper grounding of monitor. • Change electrodes and cable; sometimes poor conduction results in 60-cycle interference. • Check that monitor is calibrated.
Skin irritation occurs with use of electrodes.	• Remove electrodes, cleanse site, and reapply electrodes on new site.
Chaotic rhythm appears on oscilloscope.	• Check client's other assessment parameters to determine if clinical changes have occurred. • Check electrode contact on skin, and ensure that wires are in contact with cable. • Determine activity level of client.

UNEXPECTED OUTCOMES	CRITICAL THINKING OPTIONS
High or low alarms on monitor continue to sound.	• Check for loose electrodes or try a different lead. • Observe activity level of client. • Check that alarm parameters on monitor are not set too close to client's pulse. • Check client's position. • Reposition electrodes, avoiding large muscle masses or bone.
Electrodes conduct poorly on diaphoretic client.	• Clean skin sites as usual; apply benzoin to the skin and let dry and apply electrodes. • Clean skin sites as usual; apply spray deodorant to the skin, allow skin to dry, and apply electrodes.
Asystole occurs.	• Before beginning CPR, check client's LOC and electrodes, wires, and cables. • If the client has an arterial line, check for an arterial waveform in the absence of an ECG waveform. • Make a note on the rhythm strip if the electrode placement has been altered. The appearance of the waveform may be affected.
ECG tracing is fuzzy.	• Feel that the sponge on the electrode is moist. If not, replace electrode. A dry electrode does not conduct the electrical activity. • Ensure that the electrode placement is on a proper area of the chest, not on a bony prominence or on muscle.
for Telemetry	
ECG only provides partial information on heart activity.	• Obtain 12-lead ECG. It portrays activity in all areas of heart except posterior aspect.
Client experiences life-threatening arrhythmia.	• Begin treatment for arrhythmia. Obtain 12-lead ECG when client is stable.
Telemetry signal not picked up at base station.	• Check that client hasn't wandered to an area where transmission is not available. • Check that transmitter battery is functioning. • Check that transmitter is ON.
ECG tracing is fuzzy.	• Usual cause is a dry electrode. Touch sponge of electrode to determine if it is moist.
ECG tracing is unusual.	• Check color coding to determine if electrodes are placed on correct wires.
for 12-Lead ECG	
Interference apparent on ECG tracing.	• Ensure that lead wires are hanging in same direction on corresponding extremities. • Assess chest to determine if chest dressing is interfering with ECG electrode placement or signal. • Breast tissue may be interfering with ECG signal. Reapply electrodes under the breast as close to the heart as possible.

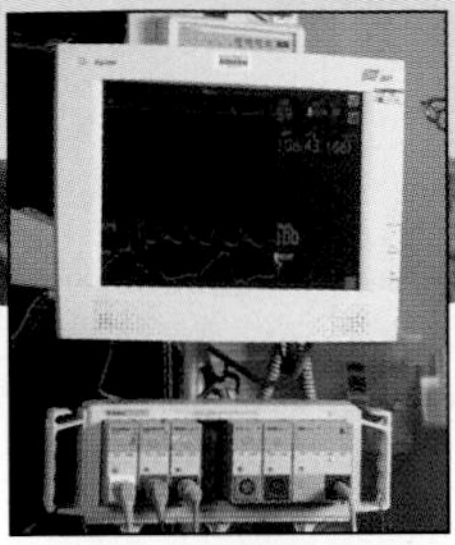

Emergency Life Support Measures

Nursing Process Data

ASSESSMENT *Data Base*

Assess client for signs of cardiac or respiratory arrest.
Know your own responsibilities for an arrest situation.
Identify location of resuscitation equipment.
Identify location of emergency cart, nearest defibrillator, and 12-lead ECG machine.
Identify procedure for activation of cardiac arrest team.

PLANNING *Objectives*

To provide adequate oxygenation of lungs through mechanical support
To provide oxygenated blood to vital organs
To support the client via mechanical intervention or mouth-to-mask ventilation

IMPLEMENTATION *Procedures*

Administering Basic Life Support to an Adult
Placing Victim in Recovery Position
Administering CPR to a Child
Providing Bag–Valve–Mask Ventilation
Using an Automated External Defibrillator (AED)
Administering the Heimlich Maneuver for Conscious Client
Administering the Heimlich Maneuver for Unresponsive Client
Calling a Code
Using an Emergency "Crash" Cart
Performing Emergency Defibrillation
Providing Care Following Code

EVALUATION *Expected Outcomes*

Basic life-support measures established within 3 minutes after arrest.
Emergency measures performed according to established protocol.
Client is adequately oxygenated by use of mechanical adjuncts.
No permanent neurologic damage is sustained.
Foreign body is dislodged.

ADMINISTERING BASIC LIFE SUPPORT TO AN ADULT

Equipment

Cardiac board

Procedure

for Unresponsiveness

1. Assess client as the first step in CPR phase. **Rationale:** Assessment ensures expedient rescue.

> **CLINICAL ALERT**
>
> Institute CPR within 3 minutes. Cardiopulmonary resuscitation is usually not effective in preventing brain damage unless initiated within 4 minutes of an arrest.

2. Quickly approach client.
3. Check responsiveness. Shake shoulders. Shout, "Are you OK?" **Rationale:** To ensure that client has not fainted.

> **CLINICAL ALERT**
>
> **CPR Protocol**
>
> 1. Shake and shout.
> 2. Call for help.
> 3. Open airway.
> 4. Check for breathing.
> 5. Ventilate client with 2 effective breaths.
> 6. Clear foreign body, if necessary.
> 7. Check carotid pulse for 5–10 seconds.
> 8. Initiate CPR at 15 cardiac compressions to 2 ventilations at rate of 100 compressions/minute.
> 9. Check for carotid pulse after 1 minute. If absent, continue CPR.

4. Call out or phone for help. Get AED (should be stored by telephone).
5. Move victim into proper position. Place flat on firm surface and position yourself next to victim, left side near head of victim. **Rationale:** Left side is preferred when using AED.

for Airway

1. Take the following measures if you suspect airway obstruction from food or other foreign body.
2. Press backward on forehead. **Rationale:** This causes head to tilt back and open airway.
3. Lift chin by placing 2 fingers on chin. Lift chin up and forward until teeth are nearly closed.
4. Assess breathing:
   a. Lean over victim's head, and look at chest to determine if chest rises and falls.

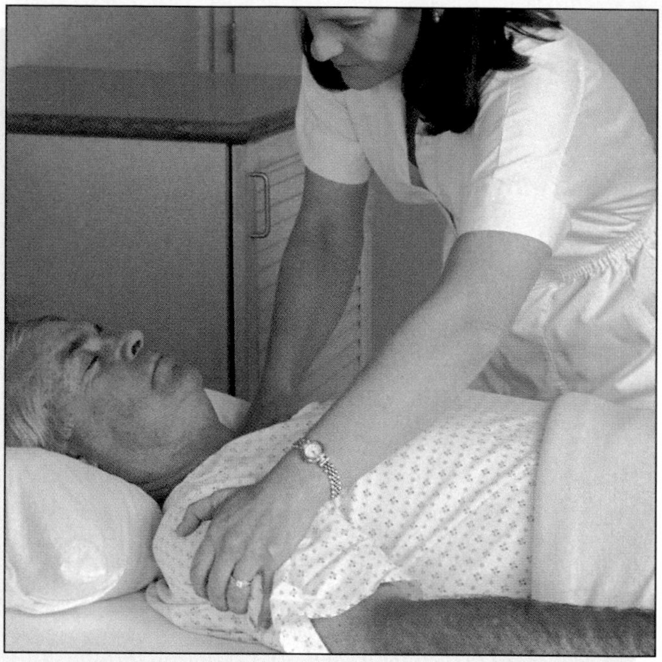

Shake and shout.

   b. Place ear near victim's mouth and nose to listen and feel for air movement. **Rationale:** Reliable indicator of adequate patent airway is feeling and hearing air movement. Chest may actually move but breathing could be obstructed.

> **CLINICAL ALERT**
>
> There have been no documented cases of transmission of HIV, hepatitis, or tuberculosis during mouth-to-mouth or mouth-to-mask ventilation.
>
> *Source:* American Heart Association, *ACLS Provider Manual,* 2001/2002, p. 208.

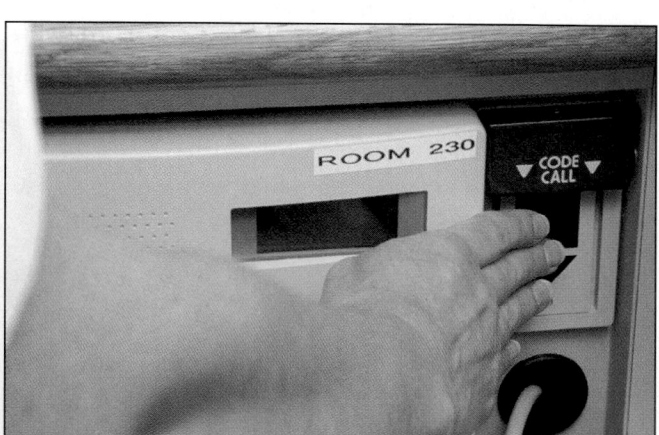

Call for help.

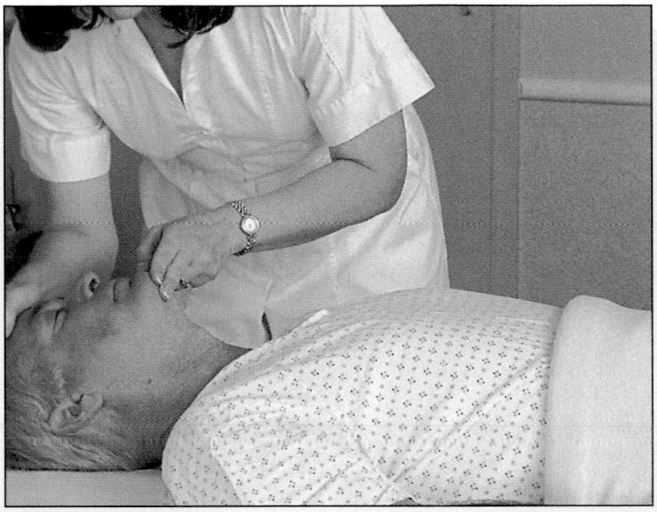

Open airway by tilting client's head back and lifting chin.

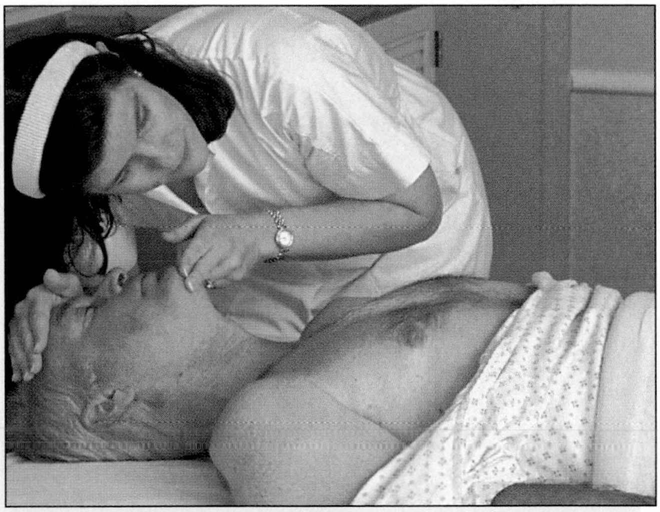

Look, listen, and feel for breathing.

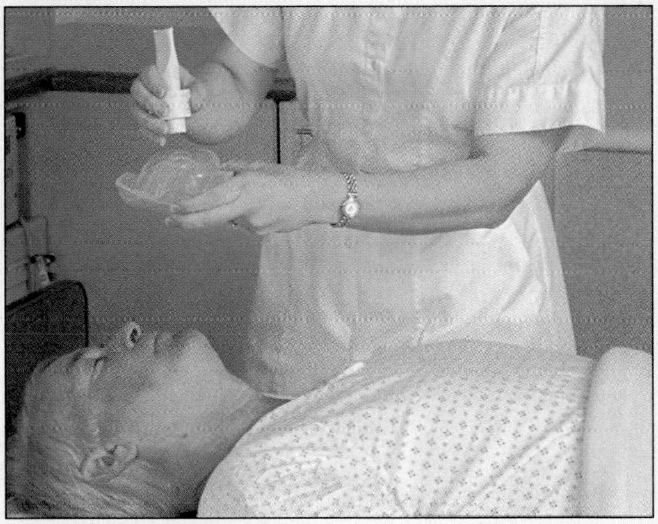

Ventilate with barrier device.

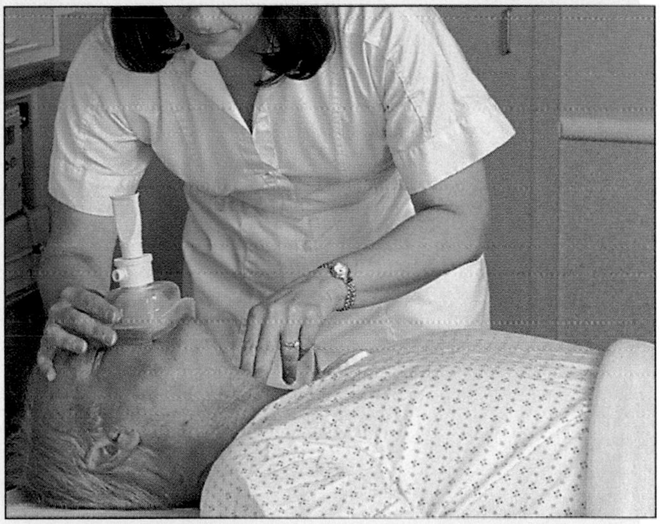

Check for carotid pulse.

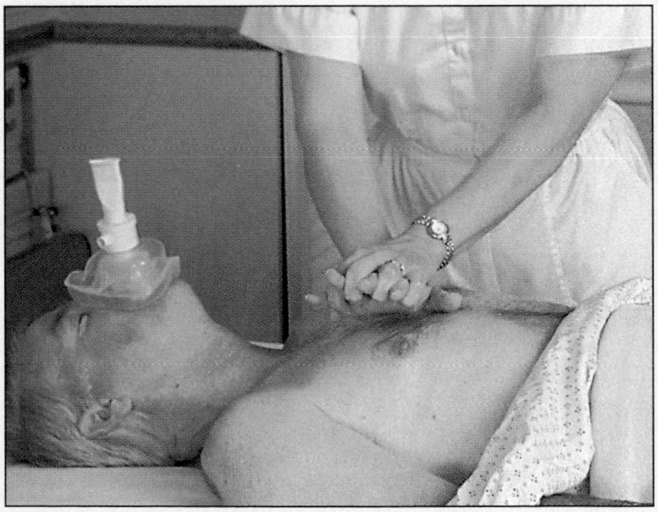

Initiate CPR with cardiac compressions.

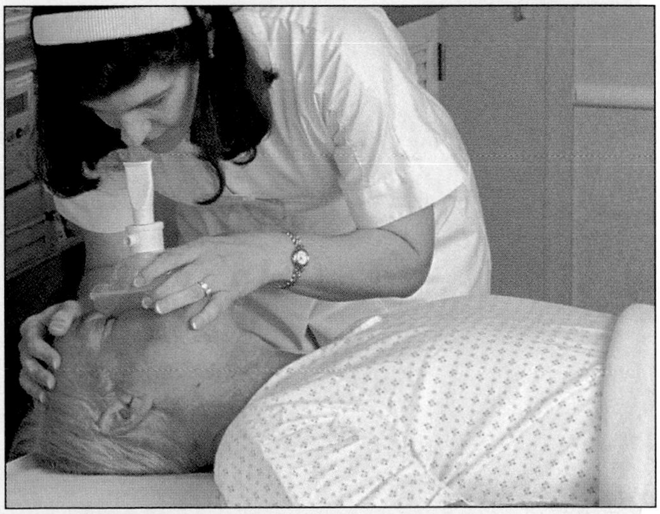

Give 2 ventilations and 15 chest compressions.

for Rescue Breathing

1. Evaluate respiratory function:
   a. Put your ear down near client's mouth and nose.
   b. Look for chest movement. **Rationale:** If chest movement occurs but you cannot feel or hear air, the airway is obstructed.
   c. Feel for air flow against your cheek.
   d. Listen for exhalation of breath.
2. Prepare to ventilate if no respirations are present.
   a. Leave dentures in place. **Rationale:** Facilitates airtight seal.
   b. Pinch off nostrils.
   c. Fully cover victim's mouth to form mouth-to-mouth seal, or place barrier device on victims face and place your mouth on breathing piece or opening.

Note: It is recommended that a barrier device be used when performing rescue breathing.

   d. Continue to tilt head and lift chin before each ventilation.
3. Administer rescue breathing.
   a. Give slow rescue breath, 2 seconds each breath. **Rationale:** Slow ventilation allows time for chest to expand.
   b. Release seal and turn your head.
   c. Take fresh deep breath. **Rationale:** Deep breath is taken before each ventilation to ensure exhaled breath provides more oxygen to victim.
   d. Watch for rise of chest with each breath. If chest does not rise, reopen airway and give another breath.

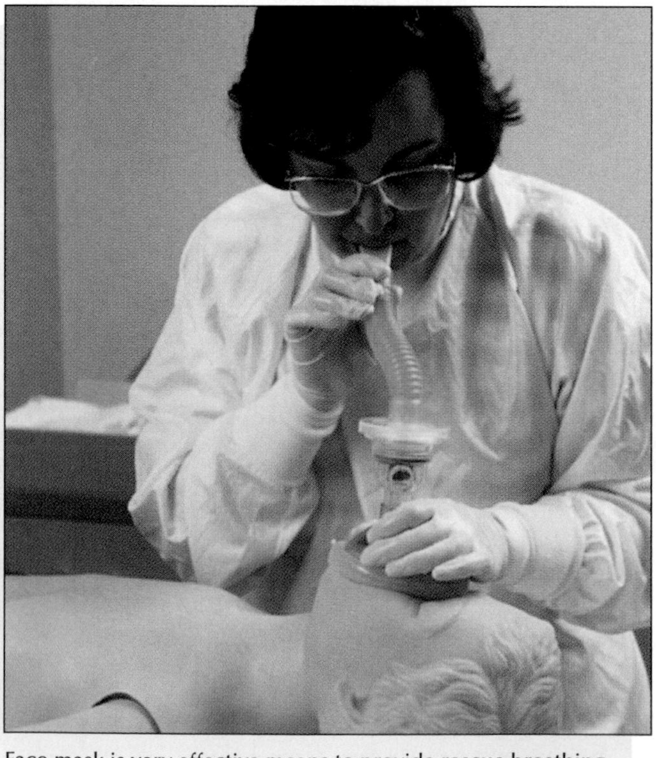

Face mask is very effective means to provide rescue breathing.

   e. Use the least tidal volume necessary to make chest rise.
   f. Check carotid pulse for 5 to 10 seconds.
   g. Continue rescue breaths if pulse is present. Give breath every 5 seconds (12 breaths/min).
   h. If victim has pulse and is breathing, place in recovery position.
   i. If no signs of circulation, no pulse, begin CRP.
4. Alternate method: Perform rescue breathing using barrier device or face mask (in AED box). **Rationale:** This provides infection control barrier.
   a. Assemble equipment.
   b. Place mask over mouth and nose to create a tight seal.
   c. Maintain head tilt and lift chin.
   d. Rescuer blows 2 deep breaths into barrier device.
   e. Take 2 seconds to deliver each breath.
   f. Check for rise of chest.
   g. Reposition device as needed.

for Circulation

Single Rescuer

1. Feel for carotid pulse, and palpate one side with two fingers for 5–10 seconds.
2. Check for other signs of circulation, i.e., normal breathing, coughing, or movement in response to the 2 rescue breaths.
3. If pulse or other signs of circulation are not present, begin CPR.
   a. Position hands lower half of sternum right between nipples. **Rationale:** This location prevents damage to liver.
   b. Place heel of one hand on sternum and other hand superimposed on top of first hand.
   c. Interlace fingers and extend fingers off rib cage.
   d. Position your body directly over your hands. Your shoulders should be above your hands.
   e. Administer 15 compressions at a rate of 100/minute. Compress chest 1½–2 inches. **Rationale:** The rate of 100 is used because studies show that higher compression rates increase coronary blood flow.
   f. Count compressions: Use first 15 letters of alphabet; a, b, c, d, etc., through or "off."
   g. Release pressure between compressions for cardiac refilling but do not take heel of hand off chest. **Rationale:** Leaving the hand on the chest prevents malposition of hands between compressions which could result in injury to the client.

Barrier Devices

Face Shield: Clear plastic or silicon sheet placed over victim's face to prevent direct contact with victim during rescue breathing. Face shields are small, flexible, and portable.

Face Mask: Hard plastic device that fits over mouth and nose. They cost more than face shields and are bulkier, preventing people from carrying them on their person.

4. Continue CPR at the rate of 15 compressions and 2 rescue breaths for a single rescuer.
5. Pause 2 seconds for each ventilation.
6. Check carotid pulse for 5 seconds after 4 cycles of compression and ventilation.

Note: When airway is protected and there is a 2 person rescue, may change to 5:1 ratio.

Two professionals arrive together to do CPR.

1. Rescuer "A" assumes position at head of victim to perform ventilation.
   a. Perform head-tilt/chin-lift maneuver for airway opening.
   b. Assess breathing
   c. Ventilate with two slow breaths of 2 seconds.
   d. Observe for chest rise and fall. **Rationale:** Longer ventilations allow time for chest to expand and reduce potential for abdominal distention.
   e. Rescuer "A" checks for carotid pulse for 5–10 seconds.
   f. Rescuer "B" assumes position of compressor at level of chest and locates site for compression.
   g. If no pulse, Rescuer "A" states "no pulse" and "B" begins compressions.
   h. Rescuer "B" completes 15 compressions (1½–2 inches) at a rate of 100/minute and then pauses after 15 compressions.
   i. Rescuer "A" gives 2 slow breaths.
   j. Rescuer "B" maintains rhythm using alphabet, "a," "b," "c," etc. **Rationale:** Using the alphabet is a faster rate of compressions (100/minute), the currently recommended procedure.
   k. Rescuer "B" begins compressions again at ratio of 15 compressions to 2 ventilations.
   l. Rescuer "A" checks carotid pulse after 1 minute and then after every few minutes.

If AED is used:

- Rescuer who handles AED takes charge of the situation.
- Rescuer B retrieves AED box and summons help.
- Performs defibrillation after assessment.
- Places pocket face mask on client in preparation for ventilations.
- Begins chest compressions.
- Maintains CPR protocol with Rescuer A.

2. When Rescuer "B" becomes tired, a signal to switch is made. (Complete at least 10 cycles before switching.)
   a. Rescuer "B" (compressor) says "switch" and completes the 15th compression. Each rescuer simultaneously switches.
   b. New Rescuer "A," at head, checks carotid pulse for 5–10 seconds. If no pulse, states "no pulse" and gives two slow ventilations.
   c. New Rescuer "B" begins cycle of compressions.

Note: Protocol is based on new American Heart Association Guidelines for Healthcare Providers, 2001/2002.

for Continuing CPR

1. Check carotid pulse and signs of circulation every few minutes of CPR.
2. Check pupils every 4–5 minutes (optional if a third trained person is present)—not always a conclusive indicator.
3. Observe for abdominal distention (all age groups). **Rationale:** Longer ventilations reduce chance of abdominal distention.
   a. If evident, reposition airway, and reduce force of ventilation.
   b. Maintain a volume sufficient to elevate ribs.
4. Ventilator: check carotid pulse frequently between breaths to evaluate perfusion.
5. Ventilator: observe each breath for effectiveness.
6. If respiratory arrest only, check major pulse after each minute (12 breaths) to ensure continuation of cardiac function.
7. If client is breathing, place in recovery (side-lying) position unless you suspect cervical injury.
8. Terminate CPR under the following conditions:
   a. The resuscitation is successful.

CLINICAL ALERT

Studies indicate that chest compressions without ventilations provide significantly better outcomes than no CPR; therefore, if rescuer does not or cannot perform rescue breathing, he or she should be instructed to do chest compressions.

   b. Spontaneous return of vital functions.
   c. Assisted life support measures are initiated.
   d. Client is transferred to emergency vehicle or code team arrives.
   e. Client is pronounced dead by physician.
   f. Rescuer is exhausted and cannot continue.

PLACING VICTIM IN RECOVERY POSITION

Procedure

1. Assess for potential head or neck trauma; if you suspect injury, do not tilt or turn client's head. If no trauma, and client has a pulse and is breathing adequately, place in recovery position.
2. Straighten victim's legs.
3. Place victim's arm nearest to you, at right angles to his/her body with elbow bent and palm upward.
4. Place other arm across chest, and place hand near his/her cheek.
5. Grasp victim's far-side thigh above knee; pull thigh up toward his/her body.
6. Roll victim toward you onto his/her side.
7. Ensure upper leg (including knee and hip) are bent at right angles over the lower leg.
8. Tilt head back to maintain open airway, place hand under cheek to maintain head tilt, if necessary. (This is hand that was placed near cheek.)
9. Monitor victim closely until transported to facility.

ADMINISTERING CPR TO A CHILD

Procedure

1. If you suspect cardiac or respiratory arrest, follow these steps:
   a. Perform CPR for 1 minute unless child is high risk for cardiac arrhythmias or cardiac arrest.
   b. Call for help and get pediatric defibrillator.
   c. Check responsiveness by shaking child, slapping bottom of feet, or gently stimulating to elicit a cry.
   d. Place child on your lap, over your arm, or on a firm surface.
2. If foreign body or aspiration is suspected, follow steps for obstructed airway.
3. For infant: clear airway by administering back and chest thrusts.
   a. Position infant over your forearm, head lower than trunk. Support the head by holding it firmly while resting your arm on your thigh.
   b. With free hand, deliver five sharp blows to infant's back, over spine and between shoulder blades.
   c. Turn infant as a unit to supine position, maintaining head support. Deliver five chest thrusts by placing two fingers over sternum and providing thrusts.
4. Evaluate respiratory function by following these steps:
   a. Place cheek next to child's or infant's mouth and nose.
   b. Observe for chest movement.
   c. Feel for air flow against cheek.
   d. Listen for exhalation.
5. For absent respirations, begin rescue breathing.
   a. Maintain open airway. Tip head back. Lift chin.
   Rationale: Trachea can collapse if neck is hyperextended.
   b. Form tight seal by encircling mouth of child and mouth and nose of infant.
   c. Maintain tight seal.
6. Administer two breaths.
   a. Give breaths slowly.
   b. Fill cheeks with air and use short puffing breaths for infants. Do not use full breaths for children or infants.
   Rationale: Small breaths prevent overinflation of the lungs and abdominal distention.
7. Between breaths, release seal for exhalation, and turn your head to side.
8. Take fresh breath; do not allow complete deflation of lungs (stairstep volume).
9. Do not release the child or infant when giving ventilations; just turn your head to side.
10. Administer ventilations at 20/min (1 to 1½ second per breath for children under 1 year of age, and the same for children over 1 year of age. Neonates are 1 second/breath, then 30–60 breaths min.).
11. Continue ventilations until child or infant is intubated or ambu bag is available.
12. For cardiopulmonary arrest, follow these steps:
   a. Follow procedure for initiating rescue breathing.
   b. After administering two slow breaths, check carotid for presence of pulse. Palpate for 5–10 seconds. (Infant—check brachial pulse, neonate—umbilical).
   c. Begin cardiac compression. Maintain patent airway with your hand on infant's forehead.
13. For infants to 1 year of age:
   a. Grasp both hands behind the infant's back for support and overlap your thumbs at midsternum if two rescuers available.
   b. For one rescuer, place tip of index and middle finger at lower sternum, one fingerbreadth below nipple line.
14. For children 1–8 years of age, use heel of one hand at lower half of sternum.
15. For children over 8 years of age, use two hands over lower half of sternum.
16. Remember that compression depth for children is 1–1½ inches, for infants ½–1 inch, neonates 1/3–1/2 depth of chest.
17. Do not take fingers off infant or heel of hand off child between compressions.

18. Perform cardiac compression and ventilate at the rate of 1 breath to 5 compressions.
    a. For infants under 12 months, administer compression 100 times per minute to depth of $\frac{1}{2}$–1 inch.
    b. For infants over 12 months and up to 8 years, administer compression 100 times per minute to depth of 1–1$\frac{1}{2}$ inches.
    c. For neonates, 120/min (90 compressions to 30 breaths at 1/3–1/2 depth of chest).
19. Compression/ventilation ratio:
    a. Neonate—3:1
    b. Infant under 1 year—5:1
    c. Children 1–8 years—5:1
20. Follow usual steps in CPR for single rescuer until help arrives.
21. Recheck carotid or brachial pulse every 10 cycles.
22. Continue CPR until code team arrives or you are instructed to stop by a physician.

PROVIDING BAG–VALVE–MASK VENTILATION

Equipment

Manual resuscitator bag with non-rebreathing valve
Oxygen source and tubing
Airway adapter or face mask

Preparation

1. Determine that client's breathing is absent or inadequate.
2. Summon an assistant if client is not intubated. **Rationale:** If no artificial airway present, two responders are essential. Assistant holds mask while nurse compresses resuscitator bag.
3. Gather equipment.
4. Place client in supine position.
5. Connect mask or airway adapter to bag.
6. Connect oxygen tubing and oxygen flowmeter to bag inlet.

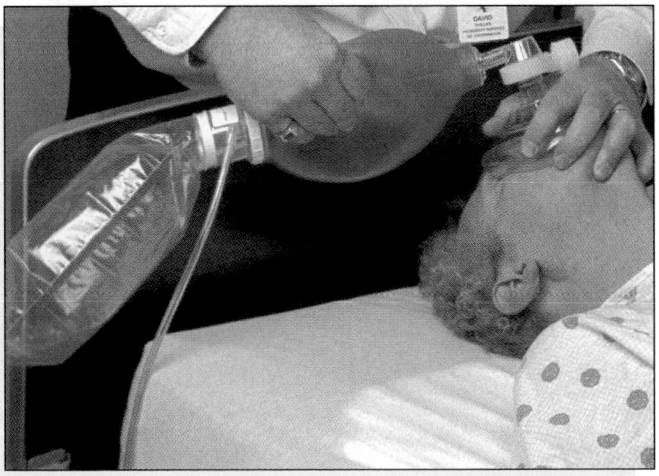

CLINICAL ALERT

If client's chest does not rise with ventilations, suspect foreign body airway obstruction.

Procedure

1. Turn oxygen flowmeter wide open to 15 L/minute ("flush").
2. Standing at client's head, hyperextend client's neck.
3. Place apex of mask over client's nose and place base of mask between client's lower lip and chin. **Rationale:** This ensures a tight seal.
4. Using dominant hand, compress central portion of resuscitator bag just until client's chest rises (1–2 sec), then allow exhalation. **Rationale:** Overinflation may result in gastric distention.
5. Provide ventilations every 5 seconds for an apneic adult, noting that client's chest rises and falls with each compression.
6. If client breathes spontaneously, give compressions in synchrony to support ventilation.
7. Observe for possible gastric distention. **Rationale:** Gastric insufflation may result in regurgitation and aspiration.
8. If gastric distention occurs in the unresponsive client, have assistant provide cricoid pressure to client's airway.
9. Notify physician or respiratory care practitioner for further client evaluation.

CLINICAL ALERT

Cricoid pressure may be used only if the client

- Is nonresponsive
- Is not vomiting
- Does not have a cuffed tracheal tube

USING THE AUTOMATED EXTERNAL DEFIBRILLATOR (AED)

Equipment

AED unit
Face mask

Procedure

1. Open AED. This automatically turns on power in some devices.
2. Press power button on, if not automatically part of opening AED. Sound alerts, lights, and voice prompts will tell you that power is on and will direct you in use of the AED.
3. Place AED near head on left side of victim. **Rationale:** This placement facilitates easy use of machine by rescuer.
4. Remove victim's clothing on torso.
5. Ensure chest is dry. **Rationale:** To ensure electrode pads will stick to chest.
6. Open package of adhesive electrode pads. Some defibrillation electrode pads are preconnected to cables; if not, attach one end of cables to AED and other end to electrode pads. Snap connecting cables to pads.
7. Peel off protective plastic backing from pads to expose adhesive surface.
8. Place 2 adhesive electrode pads directly on skin of chest, following pictures on pads.
   a. First pad goes on upper right side of victim's chest, to right of sternum, with top edge touching bottom of clavicle.
   b. Second pad (marked with a ♥) goes to outside of left nipple, with top margin of pad at anterior axillary line.
   c. Do not place pads directly over nitroglycerin patches or within 5 inches of implanted devices such as pacemakers.

You may receive a voice prompt or alarm if electrode pads are not securely attached to chest or if cables are not fastened properly.

9. Stop CPR if CPR is being performed. Instruct everyone helping to not touch the victim, in order for AED to analyze rhythm. You may need to push ANALYZE button to start the analysis. Some machines begin analyzing rhythm as soon as pads are applied.
10. If analysis indicates need for a shock, push SHOCK on AED. (It may automatically charge when the rhythm indicates the need to shock. A voice message will inform everyone to "*stay clear.*")
11. Press ANALYZE button if necessary or prompted by AED following each shock for follow-up rhythm report.
12. If victim is not in need of shock, rescuer immediately checks for pulse and begins CPR.

CLINICAL ALERT

The number of shocks an AED delivers and the energy level for each shock are preset by the manufacturer. Follow the AED voice and visual prompts. The shock sequence is usually completed three times if the client remains in fibrillation.

13. After three shocks or "no shock indicated" message on machine, check for signs of circulation; if absent, begin CPR for one minute. After 1 minute, press ANALYZE button on AED. Repeat this procedure up to three times.

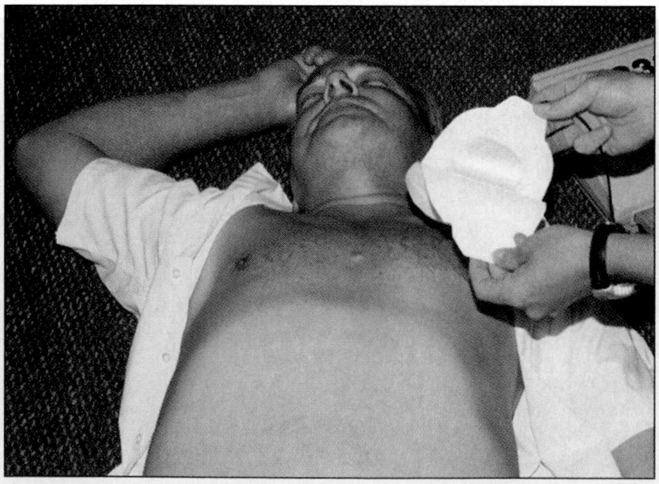
After connecting defibrillator pad to AED unit, remove pad from package.

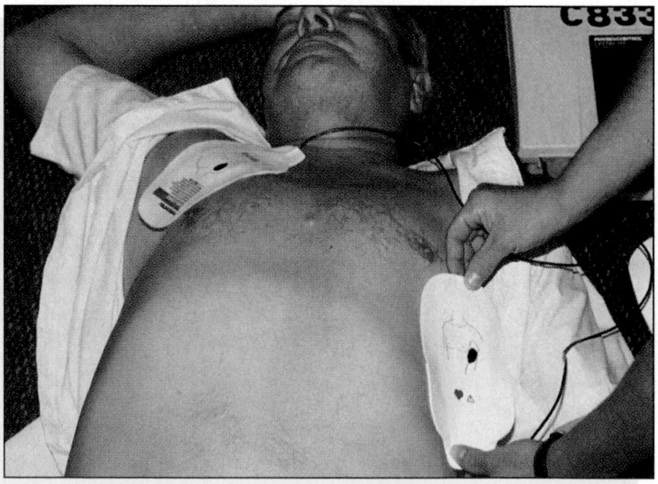
Apply pads to chest according to directions.

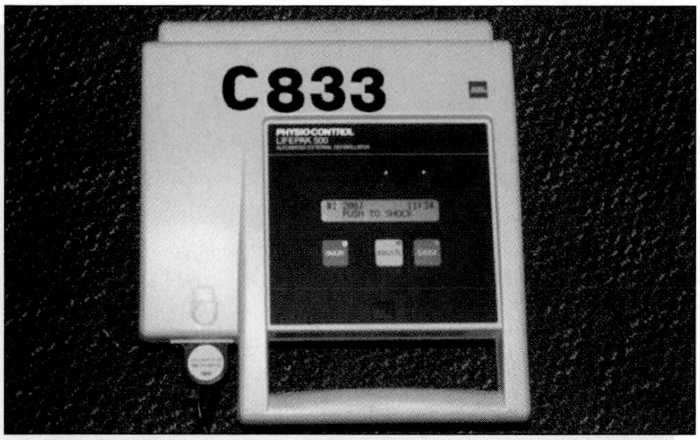

If analysis indicates need for shock, push SHOCK on AED.

14. When victim is no longer in ventricular fibrillation or tachycardia, AED will signal *"no shock indicated"* or *"no shock advised,"* or *"check breathing and pulse."*

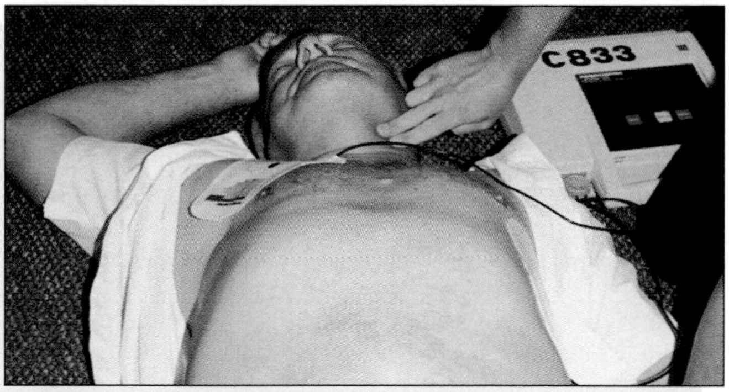

Check pulse when indicated by monitor.

15. Leave AED electrodes attached to victim's chest and leave AED in ON position.
16. Follow protocol for rescue breathing or CPR as victim's condition warrants.

ADMINISTERING THE HEIMLICH MANEUVER FOR CONSCIOUS CLIENT

Procedure

1. Assess choking client for pale color progressing to cyanosis.
2. Be familiar with choking signs.
   a. Ask client if he or she can speak.
   b. Ask client to hold hand on neck if choking. **Rationale:** This is the universal sign for choking.
3. If unable to talk or coughing becomes ineffective, begin abdominal thrusts.

CLINICAL ALERT

Foreign bodies may partially block airway but still allow good air movement. When victim remains conscious and can forcefully cough and speak—do nothing!

4. Stand behind client. Place your arms around the client's waist.
5. Position hands halfway between xiphoid process and umbilicus. (Identify area by placing thumb near xiphoid and index finger on umbilicus.)

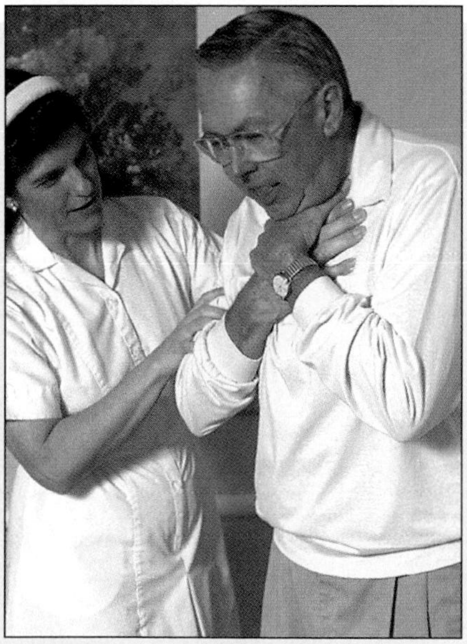

Determine if client is choking.

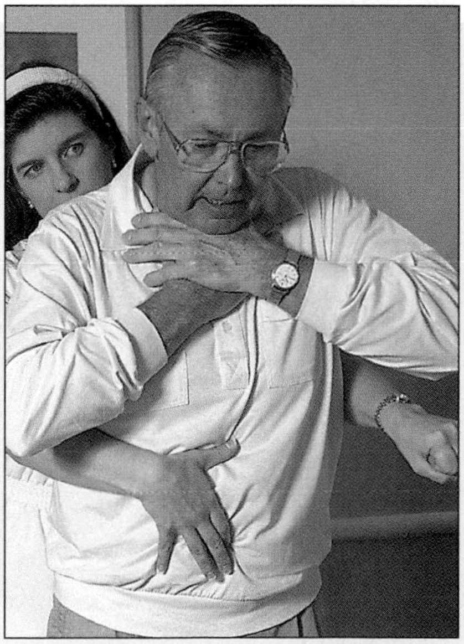

Position hands to perform Heimlich.

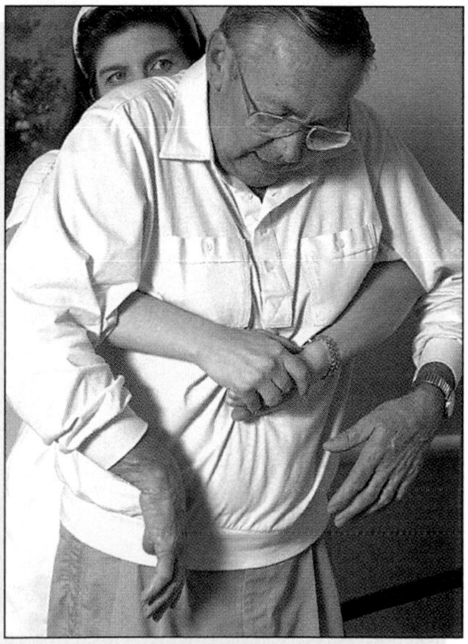

Make fist, and place other hand on top.

6. Make a fist with one hand and press thumb side of fist into victim's abdomen above umbilicus. Place other hand over the fist.
7. Press your fist into client's abdomen.
8. Using a rotating motion of the hands, forcefully thrust your hands in an upward direction to assist in expelling the foreign body. (Client will probably fall over your arms.)
9. Repeat measures until foreign body is expelled.

Airway Obstruction Signs

- Poor air exchange
- Weak, ineffective cough
- High-pitched noise with inhalation
- Cyanosis
- Inability to speak

ADMINISTERING THE HEIMLICH MANEUVER FOR UNRESPONSIVE CLIENT

Procedure

1. Place victim on back.
2. Establish unresponsiveness, shake and shout.
3. Grasp jaw and lift jaw and tongue with one hand.
4. Perform finger sweep with index finger of free hand.
5. Assess breathing.
   a. Lean over client and look at chest to determine if chest rises and falls.
   b. Place ear and cheek near client's mouth and nose to listen and feel for air movement.
6. Pinch nose and attempt to ventilate. Give two long ventilations of 2 seconds duration. **Rationale:** The longer ventilations allow time for chest to rise.
7. Reposition head and attempt to ventilate a second time if chest does not rise and fall.
8. Kneel and straddle client's thighs to prepare for Heimlich maneuver.
9. Place hand just above the umbilicus. Place second hand directly over first hand.
10. Press heel of hand toward head with 5 quick subdiaphragmatic abdominal thrusts.
11. Repeat finger sweep.
12. Repeat abdominal thrusts until foreign object is cleared.
13. Place client in recovery position following removal of foreign body.
14. If pulse is absent but airway is patent, begin CPR.

CLINICAL ALERT

Laypersons performing Heimlich maneuver do not perform finger sweep or abdominal thrusts.

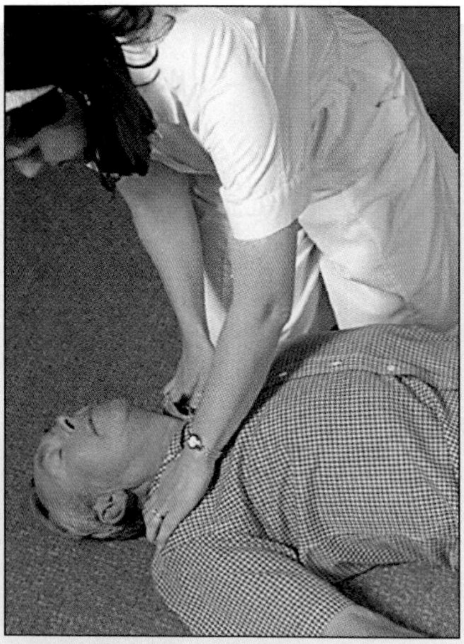

Place victim on back and establish nonresponsiveness.

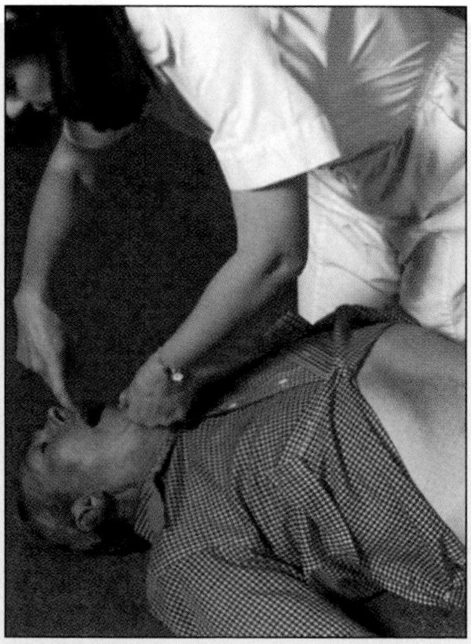

Perform finger sweep to check for a foreign object.

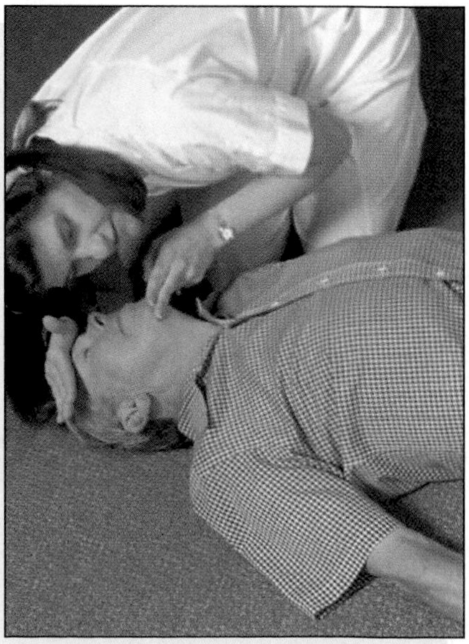

Assess for breathing.

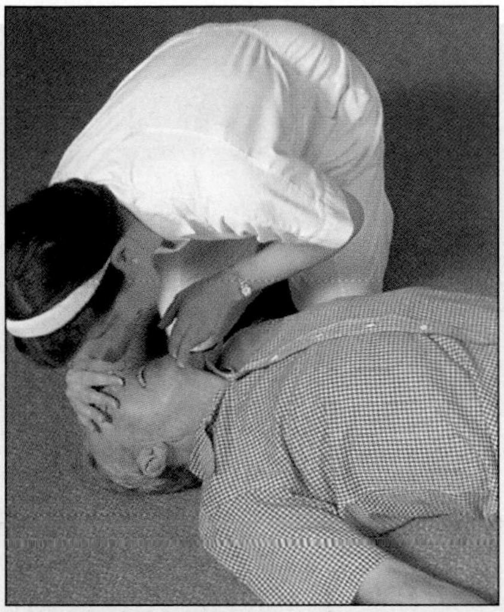

Attempt to ventilate.

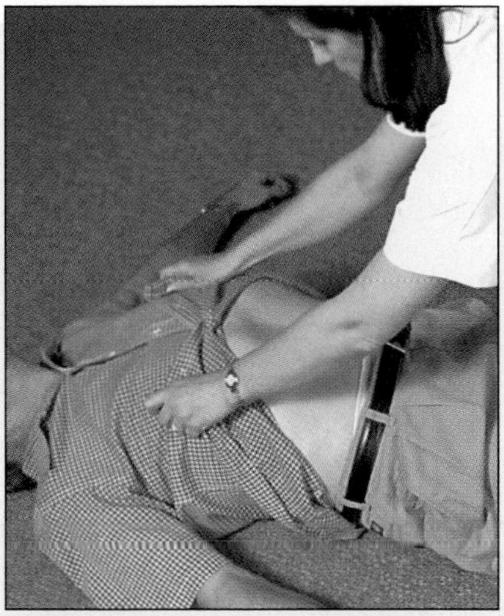

Prepare to administer Heimlich maneuver.

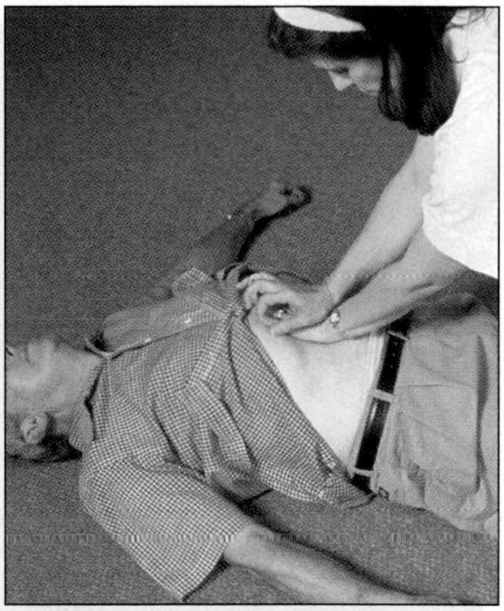

Deliver subdiaphragmatic abdominal thrusts.

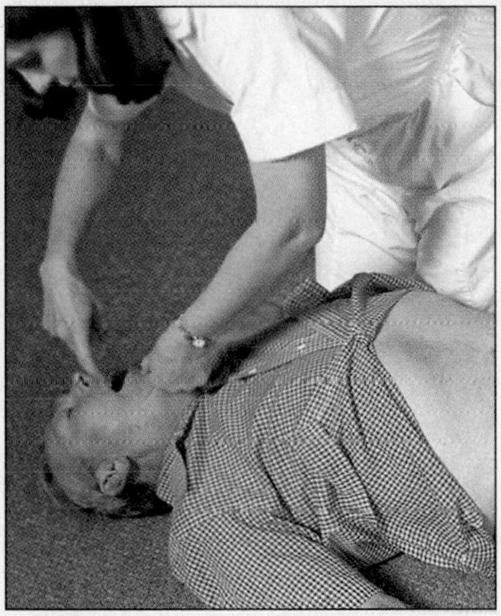

Open mouth and repeat finger sweep.

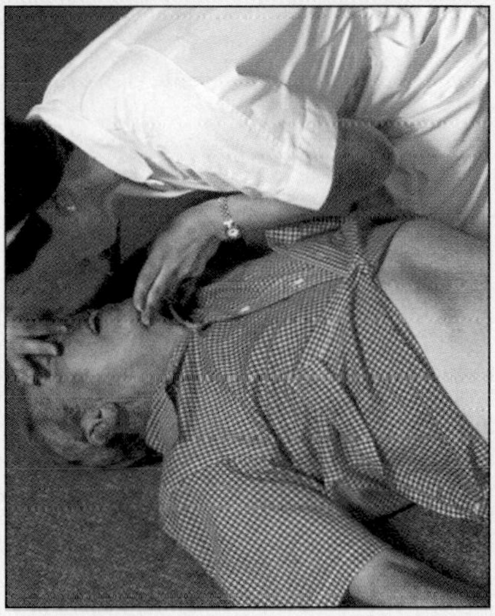

Attempt to ventilate again.

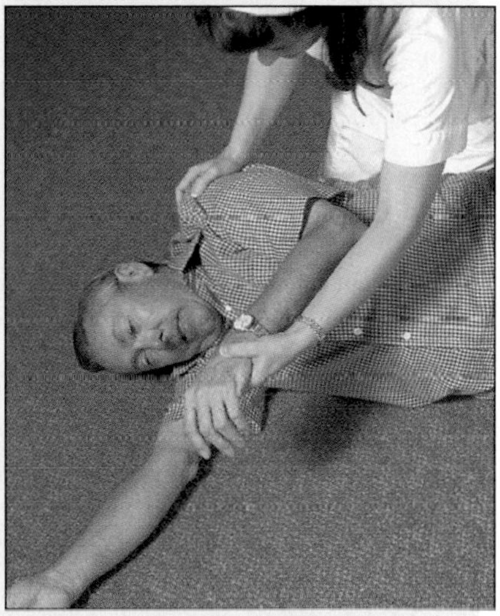

Place on side to assume recovery position.

CALLING A CODE

Equipment

Crash cart
Stethoscope

Preparation

1. Identify clients at risk for coding at the beginning of the shift.
2. Assess breathing for rate, quality, and presence of adventitious breath sounds. **Rationale:** Narrowing of the airways leads to presence of stridor.
3. Evaluate overall color and assess need for oxygen.
4. Assess vital signs and oxygen saturation levels.
5. Palpate for peripheral pulses.
6. Assess extremities for edema and mottled skin.
7. Complete a neurological assessment for baseline data.
8. Check that client has a patent IV. **Rationale:** A venous access is essential for medication administration in the event of a code.
9. Check the code status of the client. Is he or she a full-code, partial code, or do-not attempt-to-resuscitate (DNAR or no CPR) status.
10. Check facility policy for calling a code.
11. Identify location of crash cart.
12. Monitor client for change in status frequently throughout the shift.

Code Team Member Roles

Documentation Nurse

- Communicate findings with code team; last dose of medication, number of doses of each medication, ABCs, ECG findings, length of time since code began.
- Maintain accurate records including code flow sheet.
- Maintain timing of events; time code called, time code terminated and disposition of client.

Crash Cart Nurse

- Set up equipment for code team.
- Set up medications and/or hand to code team member.
- Replace used equipment and medications following code.

Code Team RN or Physician

- Administer medications.
- Defibrillate client.
- Prepare for external pacing as needed.
- Assist with intubation as needed.

Staff Nurse from Unit

- Maintain crowd control. Control number of individuals entering the room.
- Communicate with family members as time allows.
- Make phone calls for additional assistance (lab, ECG, physician) or client arrangements.

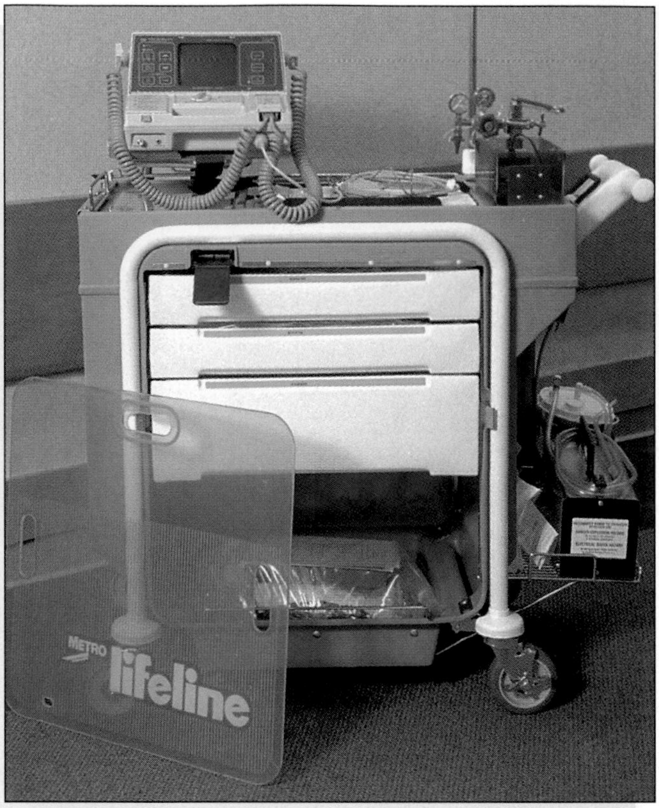

Crash cart with removeable cardiac board.

Note: See Procedure: Maintaining the Emergency "Crash" Cart, Chapter 33, p. 1226.

Procedure

1. Assess if client is nonresponsive.
2. Check for breathing and presence of pulse.
3. Call a code and ask that crash cart be brought into room.
4. Position client in supine position, open airway and initiate breathing. Use barrier device or shield if available. **Rationale:** To maintain standard precautions.
5. Initiate chest compressions if client does not have a pulse.
6. Maintain CPR until code team arrives.
7. Ask unit personnel to clear room of unnecessary equipment to make room for code cart and team.
8. Move other client from the room if possible or close curtain. **Rationale:** To prevent anxiety for other client. Moving the other client also affords more room for code activity.
9. Ask all unnecessary personnel to leave to make room for code equipment and decrease the activity in the room.
10. A team member knowledgeable in CPR should take over for client's nurse to allow her or him to assist code team and provide communication regarding client's condition.
11. When code team arrives, institute bag–valve–mask device immediately. **Rationale:** The mask provides better oxygenation than a barrier mask because the seal is better.
12. Set up flowmeter and oxygen equipment if not already in place. Ventilate client with 100% oxygen.
13. Place client on cardiac board or headboard if not already in place and continue chest compressions.
14. Place client on cardiac monitor.
15. Establish IV of 0.9% sodium chloride or lactated Ringer's solution.
16. Set up suction and intubation equipment.
17. Set up defibrillation and pacing equipment as needed.
18. Assist code team with medication preparation.
19. Act as communicator between physician, lab, family members, and other staff.
20. Prepare to move client to critical care unit or other department as needed.
21. Document the code findings.

Note: See Procedure in Chapter 33: Performing Defibrillation, p. 1228.

MAINTAINING THE EMERGENCY "CRASH" CART

Note: See Procedure in Chapter 33: Advanced Skills, p. 1226.

PERFORMING DEFIBRILLATION

Note: See Procedure in Chapter 33: Advanced Skills, p. 1228.

PROVIDING CARE FOLLOWING CODE

Procedure

1. Remind physician he or she needs to talk with family.
2. Wash client's face and hands, and provide clean top sheet.
3. Escort family in to see client.
4. Assist in transferring client to ICU (or morgue, if necessary).
5. Provide one-to-one nursing care for client until ICU transfer is accomplished.
6. Update charting.
7. If assigned, restock emergency cart or obtain replacement cart.
8. Return all equipment to original location. Remember to recharge defibrillator.
9. Clean room.
10. Allow other clients to return to room.
11. Participate in staff critique of resuscitation management.

DOCUMENTATION FOR CPR

- Time of arrest
- Type of arrest
- Initial resuscitation efforts before arrival of team
- Resuscitation efforts after arrival of team
- Medications administered: name, dose, route, response
- Cardiac rhythm, if on oscilloscope
- Defibrillation: time and number
- Time of cessation of resuscitation efforts
- Outcome of resuscitation efforts
- Outcome of Heimlich maneuver

Critical Thinking Application

UNEXPECTED OUTCOMES	CRITICAL THINKING OPTIONS
Choking client is found on floor, Heimlich maneuver cannot be performed in usual manner.	• Perform procedure for administering the Heimlich maneuver for unconscious client.
Team demonstrates poor coordination efforts.	• Attend practice CPR drills. • Evaluate own performance after every drill.
Client is revived but maintained on life support system.	• Continually reassess CPR protocol. • Assist in preparing client for serial ECGs if brain hypoxia is suspected. • Reassess for developmental level. • Give custodial care if required.
Attempts at ventilation for rescue breathing are ineffective, chest does not rise, no air is felt.	• Perform Heimlich maneuver several times, open victim's mouth, perform finger sweep of mouth (if unconscious), attempt to ventilate; if unsuccessful, try abdominal thrusts.
Rescuer cannot continue efforts at what appears to be unsuccessful CPR.	• Stop CPR if exhaustion or endangerment to you.
AED fails to analyze rhythm after 15 seconds.	• Check that CPR has ceased and no one is touching victim as soon as you activate the ANALYZE function.
Pulse does not return after three AED shocks.	• Resume CPR for 1 minute, reanalyze rhythm, check for pulse, and deliver three more shocks if ventricular fibrillation continues.

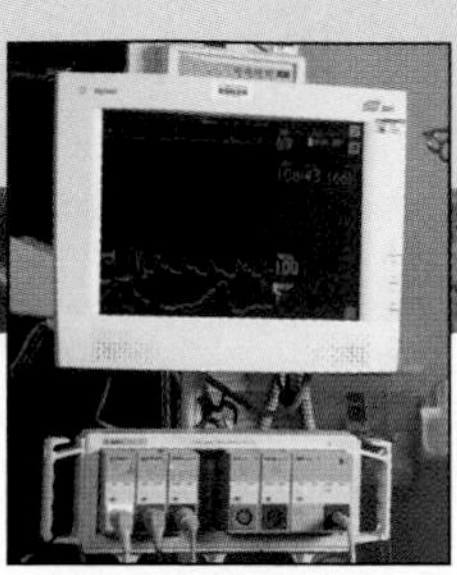

UNIT 5

Pacemaker Management

Nursing Process Data

ASSESSMENT Data Base

Assess preexisting cardiovascular status.

Identify client's or family's knowledge of and cooperation with procedure.

Assess cardiac monitor rhythm and rate.

Assess heart sounds.

Observe client's general appearance for pallor, dyspnea, or edema.

Assess for hemodynamic abnormalities related to low cardiac output, including dizziness, weakness, altered level of consciousness, low blood pressure, and decreased urinary output.

Ensure placement of intravenous route for administration of fluids and drugs during an emergency.

PLANNING Objectives

To provide temporary cardiac electrical stimulation for conditions resulting in alterations of heart rate

To prevent bradycardia

To improve cardiac function, thereby improving cardiac output

To provide a treatment modality for those cardiac dysfunctions impervious to drug therapy

IMPLEMENTATION Procedures

Assisting with Pacemaker Insertion

Maintaining Pacemaker Function

Providing Client Teaching

EVALUATION Expected Outcomes

Client's cardiac rate is maintained through use of a pacemaker.

Client is prepared psychologically and physically for insertion of the pacemaker.

Pacemaker is inserted without complications.

Heart rate and cardiac output improve.

ASSISTING WITH PACEMAKER INSERTION

Equipment

Emergency cart with defibrillator
External pacemaker pulse generator
Pacing catheter electrodes
ECG monitor
Client cable
Rubber glove
Sterile antiseptic solution
Sterile gloves, gown, and mask
Sterile towels
Lidocaine, 1%–2%
Alcohol wipes
Syringe
Needles
Suture with attached needle
Sterile 4 × 4 gauze pads
Tape
Cutdown tray
Gloves

Preparation

1. Wash hands.
2. Provide sedation as necessary. Diazepam (Valium) or Versed is frequently used. Conscious sedation may be used.
3. Connect client to a continuous ECG monitor.
4. Place the client in a supine position with head flat or slightly lower than body.
5. If either the subclavian or external jugular vein is to be used, place a towel roll under the client's shoulders to provide better exposure of the insertion site.

ICHD Pacemaker Coding

A universal code has been developed to communicate the function of pacemakers. The complete code is five letters, but only the first three are used routinely. The 4th and 5th letters are used with permanent pacemakers.

- First letter identifies the chamber(s) being paced (chamber containing the pacing electrode).
  - A = atrium
  - V = ventricle
  - D = dual or both A and V
- Second letter describes chamber being sensed by pacemaker generator. The letters A, V, and D signify the same chambers as in the first letter. An O indicates that sensing function has been turned off.
- Third letter describes type of response by pacemaker to sensing by generator.
  - I = inhibited
  - T = triggered
  - D = inhibited and triggered
  - O = none

Note: Inhibitory-response pacemaker will not function when heart beats. Triggered-response pacemaker will trigger response based on intrinsic heart activity.

Procedure

1. Assist physician as needed.
   a. Physician dons mask, sterile gown, and gloves.
   b. Insertion site is cleansed with sterile antiseptic solution.

Electrical Safety Alert

- Use only grounded equipment; use common ground.
- Remove and tag any defective equipment.
- Maintain environmental humidity at 50%–60%.
- Ground all metal beds.
- Validate electrical safety of beds.
- Avoid placing wet articles on electrical equipment.
- Insulate exposed pacing electrodes at all times.
- Wear rubber gloves when handling pacing electrodes or terminals.
- Do not touch any electric equipment while handling wire or terminals.

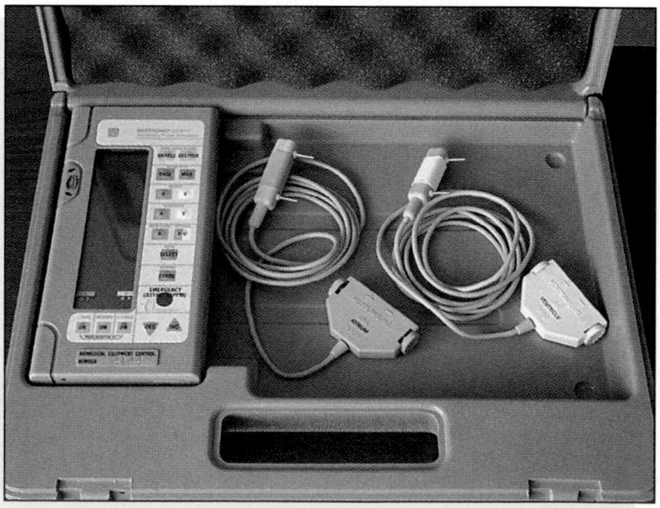

Type of external pacemaker in case.

c. Area is draped with sterile towels.
d. Top of lidocaine is cleansed with alcohol wipe.
e. Physician withdraws lidocaine, and skin is injected with 25-gauge needle.
f. Insertion is accomplished (transvenous method via cutdown or percutaneously). Catheter electrode wires are positioned, and skin sutures are applied.

2. Continuously monitor the ECG and client status during the insertion.
3. Don gloves to prevent microshock to client.
4. Connect the pacing electrode to the appropriate outlet terminal (unipolar to negative and bipolar to both the positive and negative terminals).
5. Turn on power switch on external pacemaker.
6. Set rate according to physician's orders.
7. Set milliamperes (mA) by determining threshold. To do this, observe the ECG while slowly increasing the number of milliamperes from its lowest setting to a point where a QRS complex is detected following each stimulus.
8. Multiply the threshold level according to hospital policy (usually two to four times) to adjust the milliampere setting.
9. Set sensitivity mode according to physician's order (usually 1.5 mV).
10. Secure all connections. Put plastic cover back over pacemaker controls if required.
11. Place external pacemaker and exposed wires in a rubber glove to ensure insulation against electric shock to client.
12. Apply sterile dressings to insertion site, and tape securely.
13. Obtain chest x-ray following insertion to validate lead placement if pacemaker not inserted using fluoroscopy.
14. Obtain 12-lead ECG.

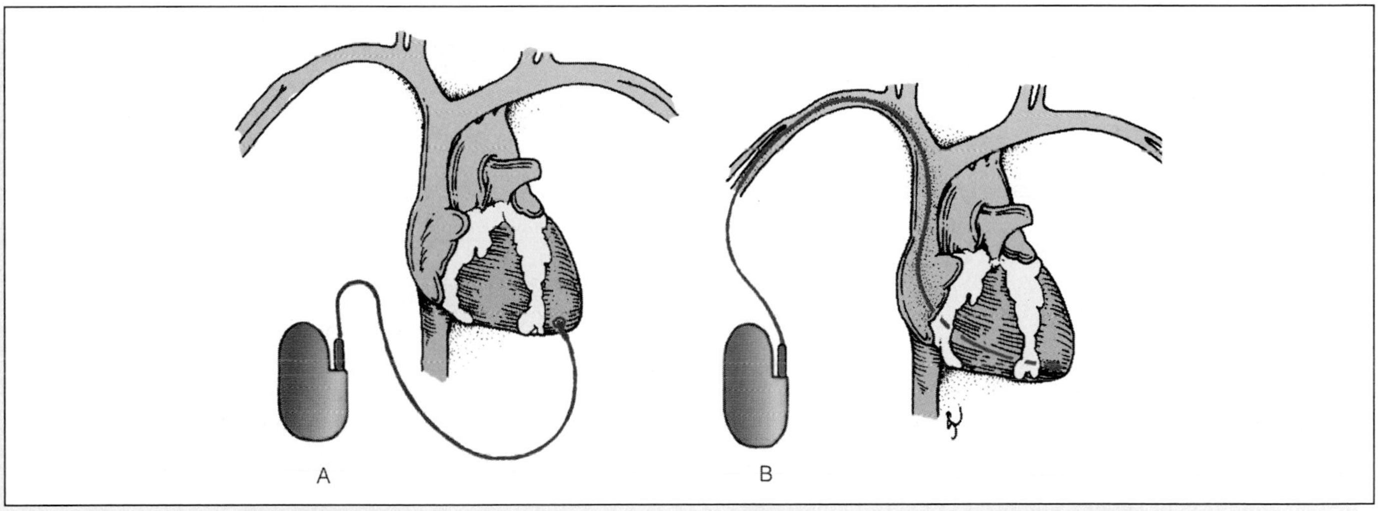

Temporary pacemakers have two parts, the pulse generator and the electrode. The pulse generator is external to the body. (A) Transthoracic pericardial pacemaker. (B) Transvenous pacemaker.

MAINTAINING PACEMAKER FUNCTION

Equipment

Battery
Oscilloscope

Procedure

1. Observe for failure to sense.
   a. Observe the oscilloscope for presence of pacemaker artifact (spikes). Artifact before QRS complex in ventricular paced or preceding the P waves and QRS waves in AV sequential pacing.
   b. Check connections for secure, tight fit.
   c. Observe that pace–sense needle deflects to right, indicating pacing is occurring.
   d. Check sensitivity dial to determine if sensitivity threshold is set correctly.
2. Observe for failure to pace.
   a. Check that external generator is ON.
   b. Check battery to ensure it is functioning.
   c. Check lead connector sites.
   d. Check pace–sense indicator. (Absence of or slight deflection of the pace–sense indicator reveals battery failure.)
3. Observe for failure to capture.
   a. Observe for pacing artifact not followed by QRS complex. **Rationale:** This indicates a failure of the stimulus to trigger a ventricular response.
   b. Check the setting of the mA, or output dial, to determine if setting should be increased. **Rationale:** The myocardial threshold may be altered as a result of disease or drugs.
   c. Check all connector sites for secure, tight fit.

> **CLINICAL ALERT**
> Observe for pacemaker failure:
>
> Decreased urine output
> ECG pattern change
> Decreased blood pressure
> Bradycardia
> Shortness of breath

4. Observe that sutures are intact.
5. Assess insertion site for bleeding, hematoma formation, or infection.
6. Obtain chest x-ray at every observation stage.
7. Monitor client's response to therapy.
   a. Assess urine output. **Rationale:** Decreased urine output indicates poor cardiac output.
   b. Observe for dyspnea, crackles, bradycardia, hypotension.
   c. Monitor temperature.
   d. Observe client for signs of anxiety or fear. Complete pacemaker teaching as necessary.
8. Observe for battery failure.
9. Observe for electrical interference and development of microshocks.
   a. Ground all electrical equipment in close proximity to client.
   b. Cover exposed enclosed wires with nonconductive material.
10. Complete pacemaker teaching as necessary.

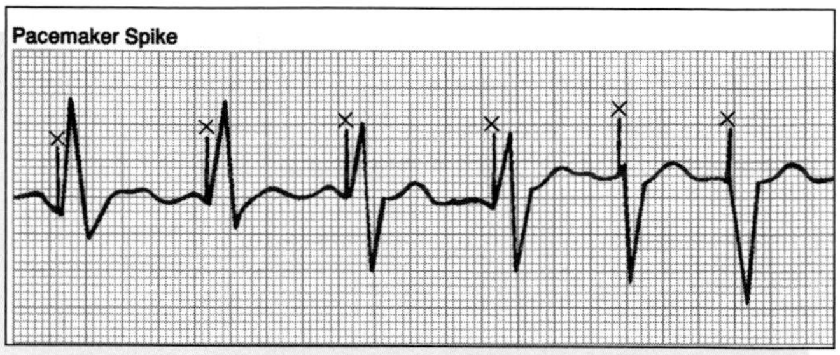

ECG tracing showing pacemaker spike triggering ventricular depolarization (QRS).

PROVIDING CLIENT TEACHING

Equipment

Audiovisual aids
Written material

Procedure

1. Ascertain what client already knows and understands.
2. Determine client's ability and level of interest in learning about pacemaker.
3. Recognize client's fears, and provide opportunity to talk about them. Explain that procedure is temporary.
4. Review facts: heart anatomy and physiology and pacemaker information. Use illustrations and audiovisual aids.
5. Clarify misconceptions and allay fears.
6. Describe insertion procedure.
7. Provide rationale for any mobility restrictions.
8. Answer questions, and provide additional opportunities to discuss impending procedure.
9. Instruct client in clinical manifestations related to pacemaker failure and when to contact physician or pacemaker clinic.

Pacemaker Clinics

Many clients use telephone transmission of the generator's pulse rate to determine status of pacemaker function. Special equipment is used to transmit information concerning function of the pacemaker over the telephone to a receiving system in a pacemaker clinic. The equipment converts information to electronic signals that are permanently recorded on ECG strip. Physicians monitor client's records and can intervene quickly when abnormalities appear on ECG strip. This type of clinic is very common in outlying areas where clients are unable to go to a clinic easily.

Note: Complications related to external pacemaker include: asystole with abrupt cessation of pacing; change in pacemaker function related to electromagnetic changes; high-rate pacing which results in increased tachycardia in a preexisting tachycardia or fibrillation; disconnection or displacement of leads.

Documentation for Pacemaker Management

- Date and time of insertion
- Model and type of pacemaker and generator used
- Type of catheter electrode wires
- Method of insertion
- Mode of pacing
- Location of pulse generator
- Pacemaker settings (rate, outputs, sensitivity, AV interval)
- Client's response to treatment
- Vital signs
- Rhythm strips of pacing obtained during insertion

Critical Thinking Application

UNEXPECTED OUTCOME	CRITICAL THINKING OPTIONS
Client's cardiac rate is not stabilized.	• Check sensitivity setting. (If too high, P or T wave may be sensed; if too low, fixed-rate pacing occurs.) • Check mA setting (may be too high). • Check pace indicator for movement. • Check rate setting. • Check all connections. • Check catheter insertion site. • Check for battery depletion and change if necessary (9-V batteries). • Check for electromagnetic interference. • Insulate generator in rubber glove. • Obtain 12-lead ECG and chest x-ray. • Anticipate repositioning of pacing lead.
Client is unprepared for pacemaker insertion.	• If client is frightened, reassure him or her that a pacemaker is not dangerous. • If client does not understand explanation of how the pacemaker or the heart functions, reexplain the procedure, using illustrated learning aids. • Demonstrate the pacemaker and electrode, and allow time for questions and further explanations. • Describe insertion procedure, allowing time for questions. • Orient your teaching to the client's intellectual and interest level.
Electromagnetic interference occurs.	• Check all electric equipment for proper grounding. Use common ground. • Remove unnecessary electric equipment from vicinity of client. • Insulate generator terminals, and exposed electrodes in a rubber glove.

UNEXPECTED OUTCOME	CRITICAL THINKING OPTIONS
Inflammation occurs at insertion site.	• Provide daily site care using strict aseptic technique. • Keep dressings dry at all times. • Monitor vital signs. • Instruct client to limit extremity movement.
Diaphragmatic pacing occurs.	• Observe for hiccoughs or muscle twitching. • Change client's position. • Decrease the amperage (mA). • Notify physician that endocardial perforation may have occurred.
Failure to capture is suspected.	• Check client's heart rate. If heart rate less than the rate set on generator, and if pace indicator shows firing, suspect failure to capture. • Check all connections. • Anticipate that pacer wires are dislodged. • Check battery. • Change position of extremity. • Turn client on left side; catheter may float back to epicardial wall. • Increase amperage (mA) after checking threshold. • Obtain chest x-ray and 12-lead ECG. • Anticipate change of batteries, electrode terminals, or generator.
Battery depletion occurs.	• Have atropine and isoproterenol on standby. • Anticipate possible CPR. • Turn on power switch, and observe pace indicator. If there is little or no movement, replace battery immediately. • Record clock hours of battery usage. (Record should be taped to back of generator.) • Determine rate fluctuations. • Label each pacemaker with the date battery is inserted. • Store extra batteries in refrigerator, and put new battery in pacemaker before use. • Disconnect catheter from pacemaker before replacing battery. Contact with battery terminal may be dangerous to the client.

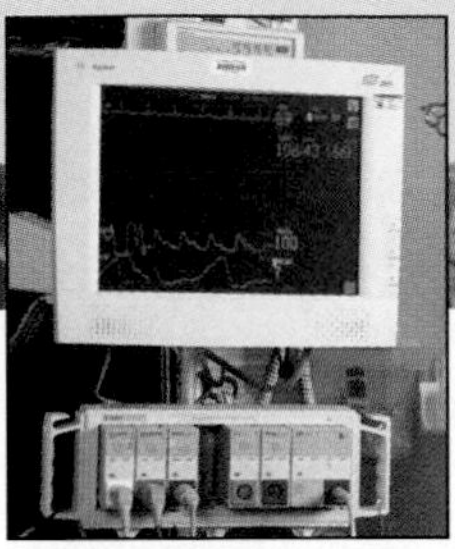

Fetal Monitoring

Nursing Process Data

ASSESSMENT Data Base

Assess client's and family's knowledge or rationale for fetal monitoring.

Evaluate position of fetus using Leopold's maneuver.

Assess characteristics of uterine contractions, fetal heart rate, and relationship to each other and other intrapartal events.

Assess FHR and determine if variability occurs.

Identify changes in the FHR recording over time.

Identify patterns of contractions and determine if complications are occurring.

PLANNING Objectives

To assess well-being of fetus during labor

To monitor fetal heart rate during labor

To provide a measurement of uterine activity during labor

To detect early signs of potential complications related to labor

To ensure fetal heart rate and uterine activity are clearly displayed on monitor

IMPLEMENTATION Procedures

Auscultating Fetal Heart Tones

Applying External Electronic Fetal Monitoring

Interpreting Electronic Fetal Monitoring Tracings

Assessing Periodic Fetal Heart Changes

EVALUATION Expected Outcomes

Fetal oxygenation is improved and adequate

Changes correlate with overall condition of mother and fetus

Monitoring of FHR and uterine contractions is done throughout labor

There is early detection if further intervention(s) (i.e., operative) is necessary; identification of urgency of interventions is recognized

AUSCULTATING FETAL HEART SOUNDS

Equipment

Fetoscope or Doppler
Ultrasound gel if using Doppler

Procedure

1. Wash hands between clients.
2. Introduce self to client and family; check identaband.
3. Explain procedure to client and family.
4. Locate back of fetus, using Leopold's maneuvers and/or ask client which side she usually feels the baby kick.
5. Place bell or diaphragm in quadrant over back of fetus.
6. Evaluate fetal heart rate: is it rapid and does it sound like a horse running? **Rationale:** If you hear a swishing sound along with each beat, it may be the cord (funic soufflé) and the bell or diaphragm should be relocated.
7. Compare mother's pulse with beats you are hearing. **Rationale:** They should not be simultaneous or the same rate. If they are, you should reposition bell to another location.
8. Count fetal heart rate. To obtain rate, count for 30 seconds and multiply by two. Another method is to count for two 15-second periods and multiply by 4. Both numbers should be within 4–8 beats of each other.
9. Auscultate FHR between, during, and for 30 seconds following a uterine contraction.
10. Monitor FHR according to AWHONN* (1998) recommendations.

The Fetoscope

- Place earpiece in ears and curved metal portion over head (if utilizing fetoscope that also has bone conduction).
- Place bell of fetoscope on quadrant of abdomen where back of fetus is located. (Press down sufficiently or tilt direction of bell to hear.)

The Doppler

- Place ultrasonic gel on diaphragm of Doppler. **Rationale:** Gel maintains contact with maternal abdomen and enhances conduction of sound waves
- Place diaphragm on woman's abdomen closest to back of fetus and press down. **Rationale:** Doppler should be tilted to point at which sound waves are most direct.

a. Take 20-minute EFM strip on all clients admitted to labor unit.
b. Low-risk clients: auscultate or assess tracing q 1 hr in latent phase, q 30 min in active phase, and q 15 min in second stage.
c. High-risk clients: auscultate or assess tracing q 30 min in latent phase, q 15 min in active phase, and q 5 min in second stage.

**AWHONN is the Association of Women's Health, Obstetric and Neonatal Nurses.*

EVIDENCE BASED NURSING PRACTICE

Continuous Electronic Heart Rate Monitoring for Fetal Assessment During Labor

In a systematic review of 9 studies (n = 18,561 pregnant women and 18,695 infants) in 7 clinical centers throughout the world, authors concluded that the only clinically significant benefit of routine continuous electronic fetal monitoring was decreased incidence of neonatal seizures. They recommend that because of the increase in cesarean and operative vaginal deliveries, the pregnant woman and her clinician must jointly decide between continuous EFM or intermittent EFM.

Source: Cochrane Library, I, 2002. Thacker, Stroup, and Chang. Oxford Update Software.

APPLYING EXTERNAL ELECTRONIC FETAL MONITORING

Equipment

Two elastic belts
Tocodynamometer
Ultrasound transducer
Ultrasonic gel
Fetal monitor and tracing paper

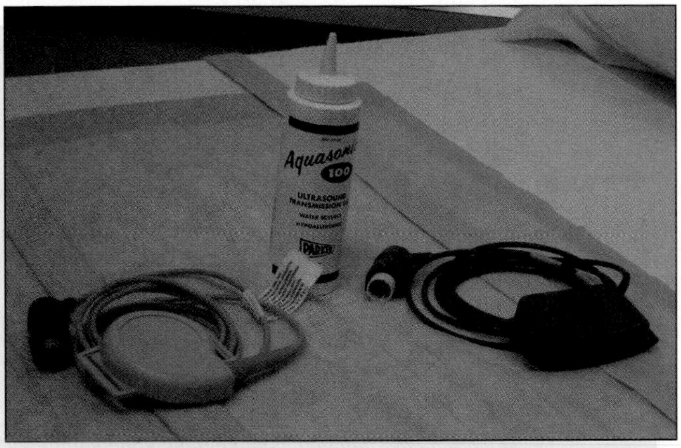

Equipment for external monitoring including belts, gel, and transducers.

Procedure

1. Wash hands and prepare client for monitoring.
2. Explain procedure to client and family.
3. Turn on monitor, calibrate, label (client name, medical record number), and check that monitoring is recording property (e.g., date and time, paper speed).
4. Place two elastic belts around the client's abdomen.
5. Place "toco" over a firm part of uterine fundus, off center. Attach elastic belts snugly. **Rationale:** Uterine contractions start and are strongest in the fundal portion, allowing pressure-sensitive button to better record data.
6. Check and readjust belt periodically. **Rationale:** Elastic belt can cause skin pressure and irritation.
7. Note the uterine contraction (UC) tracing; adjust line to reflect reading. Should be between 10 and 20 mm Hg on the pressure line. The UC tracing reflects onset and duration of contraction, but not intensity. The nurse should assess this with fingers on fundus. **Rationale:** Toco button senses pressure changes, but not actual pressure, which can only be determined by intrauterine pressure catheter (IUPC).
8. Apply ultrasonic gel to diaphragm of ultrasonic transducer. **Rationale:** Gel maintains contact to abdomen.
9. Place transducer on mother's abdomen, usually in the quadrant that the fetus's back is located.
10. When FHR is located and is clear, attach elastic belt snugly to maintain contact.
11. Position mother in side-lying position or posterior position of the fetus. **Rationale:** Placing Doppler toward side of mother's abdomen, directed toward fetus's heart, produces a clearer FHR recording.

Components of FHR Patterns

- Baseline rate
- Baseline FHR variability
- Presence of accelerations
- Periodic or episodic decelerations
- Changes or trends of FHR patterns over time

CLINICAL ALERT

Internal monitor intrauterine pressure catheter (IUPC) and fetal scalp electrode (FSE) are placed by nurses who have clinically precepted according to the individual hospital's policy and procedures.

Usually, information from an external monitor is sufficient. If the tracing is not clear or the information is not consistent, then an internal FSE and/or IUPC should be applied as indicated.

INTERPRETING ELECTRONIC FETAL MONITORING TRACINGS

Equipment

EFH tracing

Procedure

1. Assess if quality and length of recording is adequate to interpret.
2. Determine type of monitor used, external or internal, and paper speed.
3. Evaluate if baseline FHR between 110 and 160.
4. Determine if there is an absent, minimal, moderate, or marked baseline FHR variability.
5. Evaluate if there are accelerations or decelerations from baseline.
6. Determine frequency, duration, and intensity of uterine contractions.

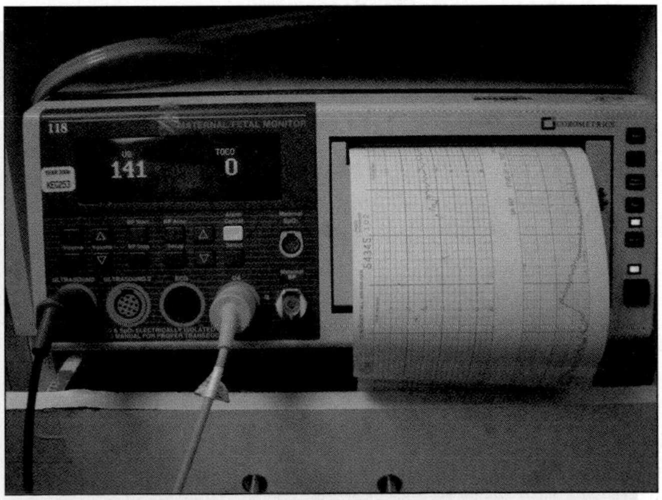

Connect transducers to monitor.

7. Assess if contractions are regular and if there is acceptable relationship to uterine contractions?
8. Evaluate changes occurring over time, which last more than 10 minutes (i.e., baseline changes, uterine contractions, variability).
9. Compare and contrast FHR recording and relate to what is happening clinically (mother and fetus) and to client's history.
10. Determine if FHR is reassuring, nonreassuring, or ominous.
11. Notify clinician with clear description of FHR including: baseline rate, baseline FHR variability, presence of accelerations, periodic changes (decelerations), and change or trends in FHR over time.
12. Document description, interpretation, interventions, and results.

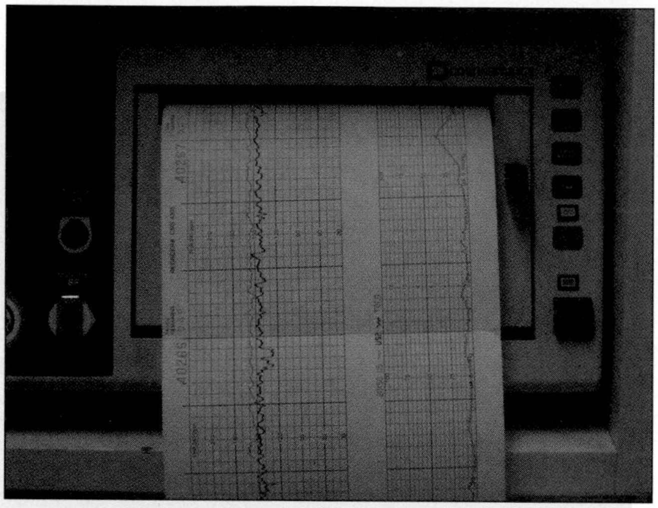

Fetal heart tones and uterine contractions depicted on monitor.

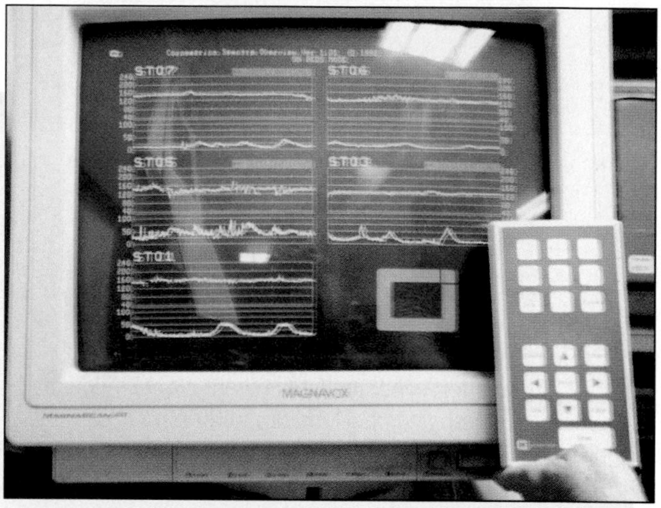

Multiple client monitoring can be accomplished at nurses' station using specific monitor.

ASSESSING PERIODIC FETAL HEART CHANGES

Equipment

Fetal monitoring tracing

Procedure

1. Assess that fetal heart rate and uterine contractions are within normal limits. **Rationale:** This indicates that fetal brain is well oxygenated at this time.
2. Check baseline FHR variability. Normal is between 120 and 160 BPM.
   Rationale:
   a. Bradycardia: FHR between 100 and 120 BPM indicates fetal acidosis. FHR below 100 indicates congenital heart abnormalities. Less than 80 BPM for three minutes, indicates severe hypoxia.
   b. Tachycardia: Mild tachycardia, FHR between 160 and 180. Severe tachycardia is greater than 180 bpm and greater than 200 BPM, usually fatal due to tachyarrhythmias or congenital anomalies.
3. Identify accelerations or decelerations.
   Rationale:
   a. Accelerations: Sign of fetal well-being. Transient increases in FHR are associated with fetal movement, vaginal examinations, uterine contractions, umbilical vein compression, fetal scalp stimulation, or external acoustic stimulation.
   b. Early decelerations: Caused by fetal head compression during contraction that causes vagal stimulation and slows the heart rate. Its image on the tracing is exactly like a contraction.
   c. Late decelerations: Caused by uteroplacental insufficiency resulting from uterine contractions. A decrease in uterine blood flow or placental dysfunction can cause these. Postdate gestation, preeclampsia, chronic hypertension, and diabetes can cause decreased uterine blood flow.
   d. Variable deceleration: Usually a result of premature ruptured membranes and decreased amniotic fluid volume. Caused by compression of umbilical cord. Initial acceleration caused by compression of umbilical vein, followed by occlusion of umbilical artery resulting in sharp downslope. Recovery phase shows sharp return to baseline, followed by brief acceleration.
4. Identify changes in FHR recording over time. **Rationale:** An accurate reading cannot be interpreted on one short review.

TABLE 27–7 Fetal Heart Rate Patterns and Rhythm Strips

Normal Fetal Heart Pattern
Obtained by internal monitoring

Uterine Contractions:
- Frequency: every 2.5–3 minutes
- Duration: 50–60 seconds
- Intensity: mild (25–40 mm Hg) to moderate (50–70 mm Hg)

FHR:
- Baseline: 148 BPM, average
- Variability: moderate
- Periodic changes: none noted
- (Need to note in 10-minute window and over time)

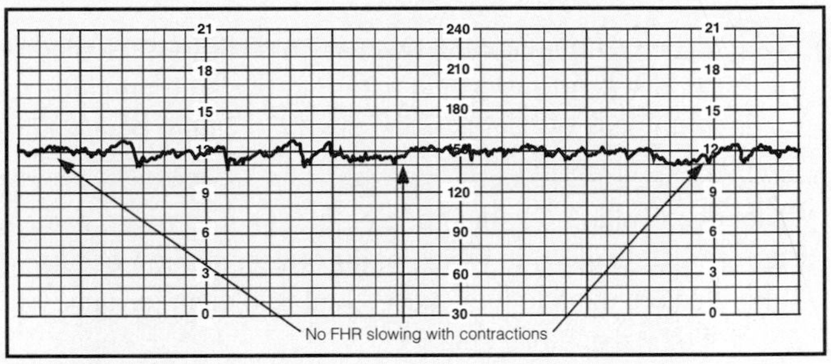

Normal fetal heart rate pattern obtained during internal monitoring.

Early Decelerations
Uterine Contractions:
- Frequency: Every 1.5–2 minutes
- Duration: 40–60 seconds
- Intensity: Mild (30 mm Hg) to moderate (60 mm Hg)

FHR:
- Baseline: 152
- Variability: Moderate
- Periodic Changes: Early Deceleration (nadir 130–145 with peak of uterine contraction)

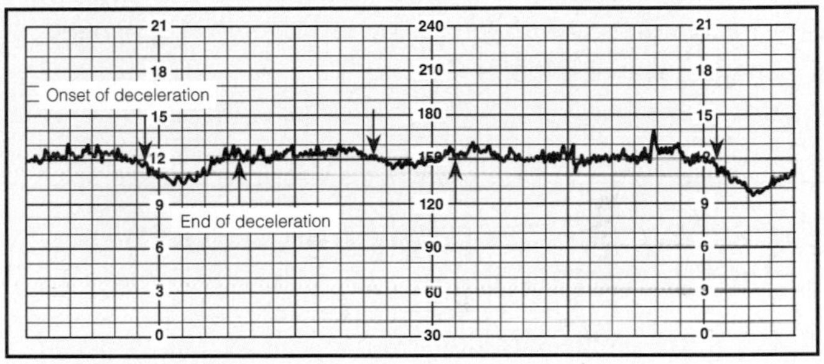

Early deceleration.

Late Decelerations
Uterine Contractions:
- Frequency: Every 40–90 seconds
- Duration: 30–50 seconds
- Intensity: Mild (40 mm Hg) to moderate (60 mm Hg)

FHR:
- Baseline: 132 BPM
- Variability: Absent
- Periodic Changes: Late Decelerations (nadir 110 BPM after peak of uterine contractions)

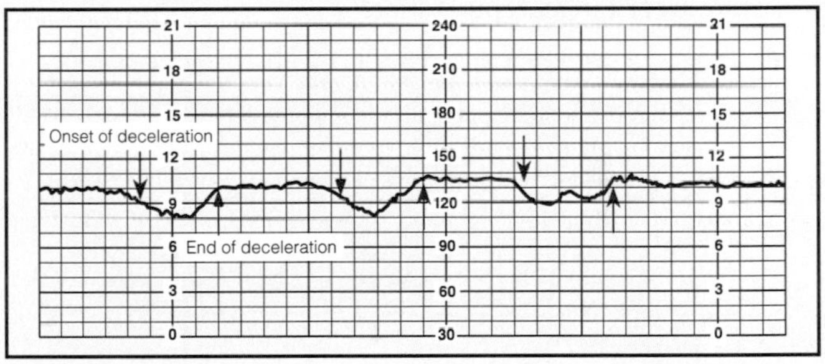

Late deceleration.

Variable Decelerations
Uterine Contractions:
- Frequency: Every 2 minutes
- Duration: 50–60 seconds
- Intensity: Moderate

FHR:
- Baseline: 120 BPM
- Variability: Moderate
- Periodic Changes: Variable Decelerations (nadir 55–80 BPM occurring with uterine contractions)

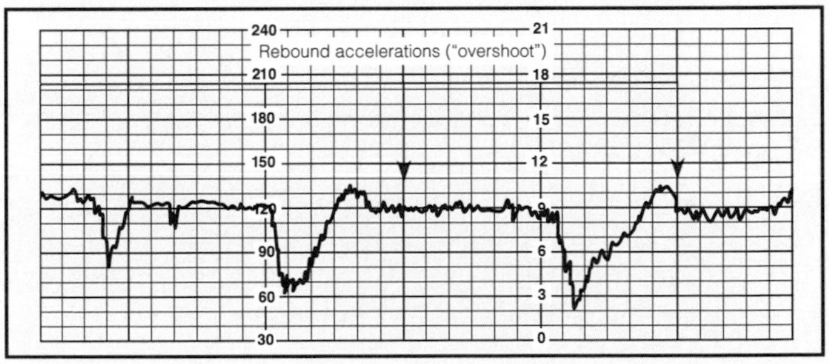

Variable deceleration.

Source: Laedwig, London, Moberly, and Olds. (2002). *Contemporary maternal–newborn nursing care* (5th ed.), (pp. 398, 400). Upper Saddle River, NJ: Prentice Hall.

Types of decelerations: Decreased FHR at least 30 seconds in length, associated with uterine contractions.

- Early deceleration: Gradual decrease of FHR (onset to nadir at least 30 seconds) in which nadir of decelerations coincides with peak of contractions; often thought to be a result of head compression.
- Late deceleration: Gradual decrease of FHR (onset to nadir at least 30 seconds) in which nadir of deceleration occurs after peak of contraction; caused by insufficient oxygenation of uterus and placenta.
- Variable deceleration: Abrupt decrease (onset to nadir less than 30 seconds) of at least 15 BPM, lasts longer than 15 seconds, and less than 2 minutes. The shape and onset will vary, but decrease from baseline lasts at least 15 seconds and less than 2 minutes.

Presumed Fetal Jeopardy (Intrapartum in Full-Term Infants)

- Recurrent late decelerations with absent variability, accompanied by baseline rate outside norm
- Recurrent variable decelerations with absent variability and nadir below 60 beats per minute
- Prolonged severe bradycardia ≤ 60 with absent variability

Nursing Actions for Decelerations

- Treat cause of underlying changes in circulatory or placental changes.
- Early: No changes needed.
- Variable: Relieve pressure on umbilical cord.

  Change position until corrected
  Increase IV fluids
  Administer oxygen (mask at 3–10 L/min) if severe or affecting variability
  Perform vaginal exam to assess for cause of pressure
  Prepare for possible amnioinfusion
- Late: Increase uterine and placental blood flow.

  Increase IV fluids
  Administer oxygen by mask at 8–10 L/min
  Maintain adequate maternal blood pressure
  Increase uterine blood flow
  Decrease frequency of contractions
  Turn to left side
  Discontinue oxytocin if used
  Notify the health care provider immediately
- Document in detail interpretation of FHR, interventions, and effect on maternal and fetal status.

DOCUMENTATION FOR FETAL MONITORING

- Uterine contractions: frequency, duration, and intensity
- Baseline rate
- Baseline FHR variability
- Presence of accelerations
- Periodic or episodic decelerations
- Changes or trends of FHR patterns over time
- Interventions completed and outcomes resulting from changes in monitor or fetal heart rate

Critical Thinking Application

UNEXPECTED OUTCOMES	CRITICAL THINKING OPTIONS
Fetal heart rate baseline is 164 with minimal variability.	• Determine presence of other causes for decreased variability (i.e., fetal sleep cycle, maternal medications, etc.) or if minimal variability is due to fetal hypoxia. • Compare baseline rate with previous rate to determine if there is an increase in baseline lasting more than 10 minutes. If there is an increase, consider possible causes of increased heart rate (maternal medications, maternal fever, maternal blood pressure, fetal anemia, prematurity, fetal hypoxia, etc.). A rise in baseline along with minimal variability can be an ominous sign. • Assess for periodic FHR changes. If associated with late decelerations and caused by fetal hypoxia, prepare for immediate delivery vaginally or surgically (caesarean section birth). • Notify physician and/or nurse-midwife.
Fetal heart rate baseline is 120 with moderate variability. Uterine contractions occur every 2–3 minutes, lasting 60 seconds, moderate intensity. Variable decelerations occur with every contraction, nadir of 70, with a quick return to baseline.	• Determine cause, frequency, and length of time variable decelerations have been present. • Assess for nonreassuring changes (increased severity of decelerations, late onset, and gradual return, etc.). • Perform a vaginal examination to determine if there is a prolapsed cord and progress of labor. • Correlate changes of labor progress. If ready to deliver baby, this may not be a problem, but if mother is in early labor, this could develop into a nonreassuring pattern. • Administer intravenous fluid bolus to increase vascular volume and oxygen carrying capacity. • Change maternal position; may relieve pressure off of cord. • Administer oxygen to mother if variability decreases or variable decelerations change. • Consider amnioinfusion according to physician's orders.
Uterine contractions occur every 1½–2 minutes, duration 60 seconds, strong intensity.	• Reassess uterine contractions, including palpation, rather than electronic monitor.

UNEXPECTED OUTCOMES	CRITICAL THINKING OPTIONS
	• Determine cause of frequent uterine contractions. If client is receiving labor stimulation (prostin or pitocin), discontinue therapy or administer tocolytic after notifying physician and/or nurse-midwife. • Assess fetal status and administer oxygen if nonreassuring patterns. • Increase fluids (intravenous). • Notify physician and/or nurse-midwife.
Fetal heart rate is 100.	• Calibrate and test electronic monitor. • Auscultate fetal heart rate. • Check maternal pulse simultaneously to assure that rate is not maternal heart rate. • Compare with fetal gestation, any anomalies detected by ultrasound. • Determine if any maternal conditions or medications may be influencing fetal heart rate. • Complete a vaginal exam to determine if there is a cord prolapse. • Compare with other information—variability, periodic changes, uterine contractions, maternal status, previous baseline/patterns (i.e., prolonged cord compression).

Gerontologic Considerations

Stressful physical and emotional conditions may have an especially adverse effect on the elderly client.

- The heart may be unable to respond to these changes with an adequate increase in rate, which could precipitate heart failure.
- Changes in the heart lead to decreased myocardial contractility, increased left ventricular ejection time, and delayed conduction, which plays a role in this phenomenon.

Cardiac output is decreased as a result of tachycardia or atrial fibrillation, which is evidenced on the ECG.

- Tachycardia causes a shortened ventricular filling time.
- Atrial fibrillation causes the loss of the atrial kick (blood volume delivered to the ventricle as a result of a coordinated atrial contraction).

ECG may be abnormal due to a chronic disease such as congestive heart failure.

- Assess client for behavioral changes, changes in level of consciousness, palpitations, dyspnea, fatigue, and falls. These are indicators of a dysrhythmic heart.
- Dysrhythmias, such as PVCs and premature atrial contractions (PACs), may be very common and not cause for alarm unless they change in number or configuration.
- Pacemaker spikes are evident on ECGs for clients with pacemakers.

Client requiring CPR has dentures in place.

- Keep dentures in place to provide for good seal around mouth.
- Rescue breathing is more effective when tight seal around mouth is maintained.

Peripheral vascular assessment is essential when an elderly client is using elastic hosiery or sequential stockings.

- Elderly clients may very well have altered peripheral circulation before this treatment is started.
- Stockings that are too tight can interfere with the already compromised vascular blood flow, leading to ulceration of the lower extremity.
- Check color, warmth, capillary refill, and presence of pedal pulses every 4 hours when client using these devices.

MANAGEMENT GUIDELINES

Each state legislates a Nurse Practice Act for RNs and LVN/LPNs. Health care facilities are responsible for establishing and implementing policies and procedures that conform to their state's regulations. Verify the regulations and role parameters for each health care worker in your facility.

Delegation of Responsibilities

- All health care workers are trained in Basic Cardiac Life Support or CPR and Heimlich maneuver; therefore, anyone can initiate CPR or perform the Heimlich maneuver.
- CPR recertification is provided frequently in the health care facility to ensure all employees stay current in the skill.
- RN staff assigned to the critical care units, emergency department, and operating room must also be certified in Advanced Cardiac Life Support (ACLS). These staff members can be delegated as members of the Code Team in the facility. The operating room staff does not respond to codes outside the operating room.
- It is not the usual protocol that LVN/LPNs are assigned to the critical care unit. If they do have responsibility for client care in these settings, additional education regarding ECG monitoring must be provided.
- All health care workers assigned to the team can measure and apply elastic hosiery.
- Ancillary staff members may have additional training in monitoring ECGs (monitoring technicians) and in taking a 12-lead ECG (ECG technician). These individuals can be delegated to perform these tasks.

Information Flow

- If the RN is not directly involved in monitoring the ECG, it is imperative that the technician have specific parameters for reporting the findings. These parameters must be defined during the staff report at the beginning of each shift.
- For clients on telemetry, it is critical that the staff nurse assigned to care for the client on the nursing unit be apprised of any unusual ECG findings. The telemetry nurse must place an ECG tracing on the client's chart according to hospital policy.
- During a code, the nurse caring for the client should be relieved from performing CPR duties to answer questions, obtain information, and assist others in the code team to perform the necessary skills to promote a positive outcome of the event.
- During shift report, ensure that the on-coming shift is apprised of any client who is at risk for developing cardiac complications or is considered a potential "code."
- Orders for a code or no-code status should be addressed so that all staff are aware of the client's status. The code cart should be placed near the client's room if the code is imminent.

CRITICAL THINKING STRATEGIES

SCENARIO 1

You work day shift in the transitional care unit (TCU), and have been assigned two clients who require total care. Each client is on a cardiac monitor.

Client 1: A 65-year-old male in congestive heart failure, responding well to drug therapy of Lasix and digoxin. His lungs are clear, and he has lost 5 pounds since yesterday.

Client 2: A 70-year-female with a myocardial infarction 3 days ago. She is considered unstable and has been place on the TCU for close monitoring.

1. What is your first nursing action of the morning?
2. What alterations will you expect in the assessment of client 2? Provide rationale for your answer.
3. Which client will you attend to first? Provide rationale.
4. Complete the interpretation of the ECG for Client 1.

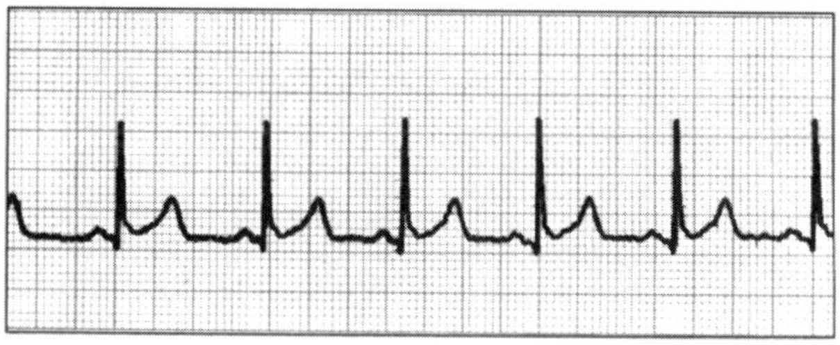

Client 1: ECG Strip

5. Determine the following:
   a. Heart rate
   b. Regularity of rhythm
   c. PR interval
   d. QRS duration
6. Identify the rhythm based on the information in question 5.
7. Is this a life-threatening arrhythmia?
8. What is your priority intervention?

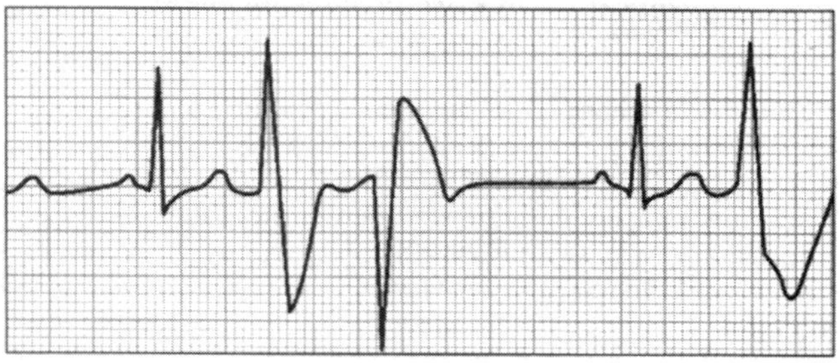

Client 2: ECG Strip

9. Identify the rhythm strip for client 2.
10. What are implications for the condition of this client?
11. Identify why this client may have this type of ECG reading.
12. Identify the most effective drug treatment for this arrhythmia and provide the pharmacologic action to support your answer.
13. Identify the possible side effects of the drug and the clinical manifestations you will be monitoring in your assessment.
14. As you are preparing to provide hygienic care to Client 2, you look at the monitor and see the following ECG findings.

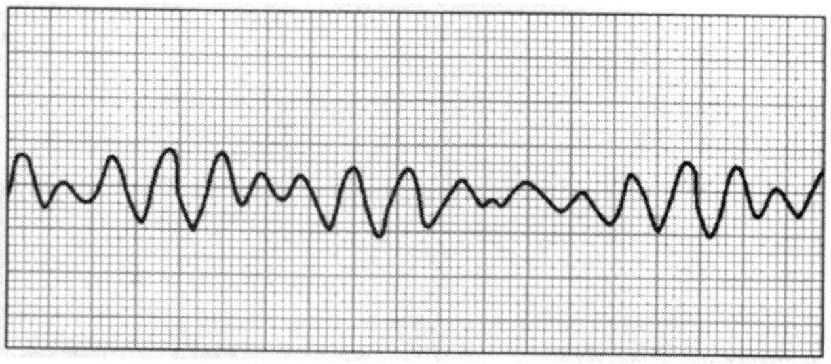

   a. What rhythm is depicted on the above strip?
   b. Describe what is happening to the client in this rhythm?
   c. What priority intervention should be done?
   d. What is the second intervention if the priority intervention is not effective?

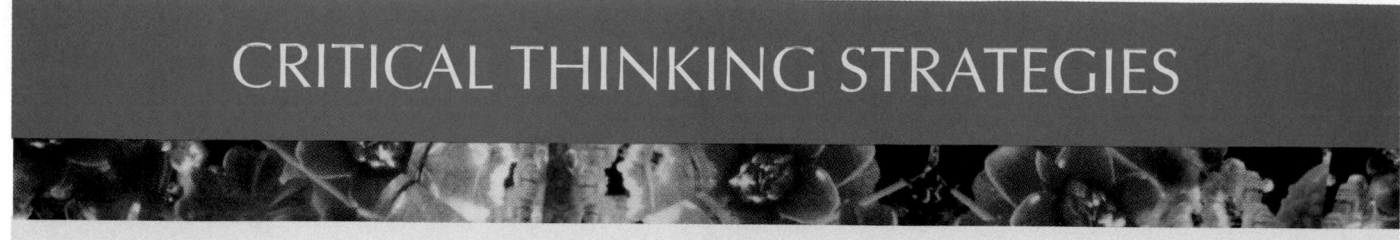

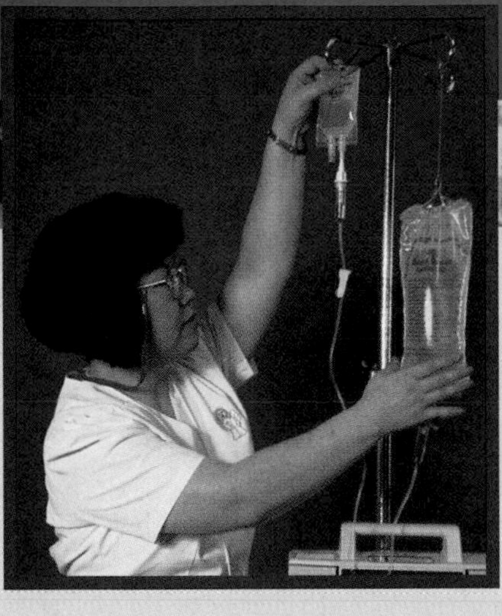

CHAPTER 28

Intravenous Therapy

THEORETICAL CONCEPTS

UNIT ONE: **Initiating Intravenous Therapy 998**

Preparing the Infusion System 999
Adding Extension Tubing 1001
Preparing the Venipuncture Site 1002
Inserting a Winged Needle 1003
Inserting an Over-the-Needle Catheter 1006

UNIT TWO: **Intravenous Management 1010**

Regulating Infusion Flow Rate 1011
Using an Electronic Flow-Control Device 1012
Using a Syringe Pump 1013
Managing the IV Site 1014
Converting IV to Saline Lock 1016
Changing Gown for Client with IV 1017
Discontinuing an IV 1018

UNIT THREE: **Intake and Output 1021**

Monitoring Intake and Output 1022
Monitoring IV Intake 1024

UNIT FOUR: **IV Medication Administration 1026**

Adding Medication to IV Solution 1027
Using a Secondary ("Piggyback") Bag 1027
Using a Volume Control Set 1029
Using a Peripheral Saline Lock 1030
Administering Medications by Peripheral IV Line Injection "Push" 1031

UNIT FIVE: **Blood Transfusions 1033**

Administering Blood through a Y-Set 1034
Administering Blood through a Straight Line 1036
Administering Blood Components 1037
Monitoring for Potential Complications 1037

GERONTOLOGIC CONSIDERATIONS 1041

MANAGEMENT GUIDELINES 1041

CRITICAL THINKING STRATEGIES 1043

LEARNING OBJECTIVES

- Describe the role the kidneys play in maintaining fluid and electrolyte balance.
- Discuss the two hormonal regulatory systems that influence urinary excretion by the kidneys.
- State the major cations and anions in the body.
- Identify the assessment data to determine a client's fluid balance.
- Compare and contrast the client data associated with fluid volume excess or deficit.
- Describe the steps for performing venipuncture using a wing-tipped needle.
- State at least two potential problems that can occur with venipuncture and one suggested solution for each problem.
- Describe the steps for performing vein cannulation.
- Outline the steps in preparing the IV bag for administration.
- Describe the steps for hanging a secondary IV bag.
- Calculate an IV flow rate using a standard formula.
- Describe safety checks utilized to ensure proper blood is administered to the client.
- Differentiate signs and symptoms of hemolytic and allergic blood transfusion reactions.

TERMINOLOGY

Anaphylaxis: a hypersensitive state of the body to a foreign protein or drug.

Antiarrhythmic: an agent used to regulate heart rhythm.

Antidiuretic: hormone that decreases urine production.

Antimicrobic: preventing the development or pathogenic action of microbes.

Ascites: the excessive accumulation of serous fluid in the peritoneal cavity.

Aspirate: to remove material by suction.

Autologous blood transfusion: client's own blood is collected prior to a surgical procedure or future need for transfusion.

Bolus: direct injection of a medication intravenously in order to achieve rapid serum concentrations.

BSI: bloodstream infection.

Cardio: pertaining to the heart.

Cardiovascular: pertaining to the heart and blood vessels.

Catheter-related bloodstream infection: the same organism is found in the blood and catheter segment with clinical symptoms of BSI and no other sources of infection present.

Colonization: growth of an organism from the proximal or distal catheter segment or catheter lumen in conjunction with signs of infection at catheter site.

Cyanosis: slightly bluish, grayish, slatelike, or dark purple discoloration of the skin/mucous membranes.

Diarrhea: frequent passage of watery stool.

Diffusion: passive movement of molecules from an area of high concentration to one of lower concentration.

Directed donation of blood: friends or relatives donate blood for a specific client.

Diuretic: a chemical agent that increases the production of urine.

Dyspnea: a subjective feeling of difficulty breathing.

Edema: an excessive amount of extracellular fluid.

Electrolyte: substance that develops an electrical charge when dissolved in water.

Evaporation: change from liquid to vapor.

Extracellular: outside the cell.

Girth: the distance around something; circumference, as in measuring abdominal circumference.

Granulocytes: a granular leukocyte (e.g., neutrophil).

Hematoma: a collection of blood confined in a space.

Hematuria: blood in the urine.

Hemo-: prefix meaning blood.

Hemolytic: pertinent to the breaking down of red blood cells.

Homeostatis: state of equilibrium of the internal environment.

Homologous blood transfusion: blood from another individual is used for transfusion.

Hydration: the chemical combination of a substance with water.

Hydrostatic pressure: the pressure of liquids during equilibrium.

Hypersecretion: abnormally large amount of secretion.

Hypertonic: solution having greater than 340 mOsm, increased amount of solutes in relationship to plasma.

Hypotonic: solution having less than 240 mOsm, decreased amount of solutes in relationship to plasma.

Hypovolemia: diminished circulating blood volume.

Infusion-related bloodstream infection: the same organism found in the infusion and separate percutaneous blood cultures without an identified source of infection.

Infusion: introduction of a liquid into a vein or other body part.

Interstitial: extracellular fluid found between the cells.

Intracellular: inside the cell.

Intravascular: within blood vessels.

Isotonic: having the same tonicity as plasma, 240–340 mOsm.

Local-catheter-related infection: growth of an organism from the proximal or distal catheter or lumen with accompanying signs of inflammation at the catheter site.

Metabolism: the sum of all physical and chemical changes that take place within an organism.

Nephro: prefix meaning kidney.

Nephrotoxic: damaging to renal cells.

Osmolality: concentration of osmotically active particles per Kg of body water (tonicity).

Osmosis: transmission of water across a semipermeable membrane from an area of low solute concentration to one of higher solute concentration.

Osmotic pressure: pressure exerted on a semipermeable membrane separating a solution from a solvent, the membrane being impermeable to solutes in solution and permeable only to solvent.

Palpate: to examine by touch; to feel.

Pruritis: severe itching.

Purulent: containing pus.

Skin turgor: elastic property of the skin reflecting body fluid status.

Specific gravity: weight of a substance compared with an equal volume of water.

Transfusion: injection of blood or a blood component of one person into the blood vessels of another.

Urticaria: a vascular reaction of the skin characterized by the eruption of pale raised wheals, which are associated with severe itching.

Valsalva's maneuver: attempt to forcibly exhale against a closed glottis.

Venipuncture: puncture of a vein with a needle.

Vesicant: blistering; causing or forming blisters, irritant to blood vessels.

Viscosity: resistance offered by a fluid; property of a substance that is dependent on the friction of its component molecules as they slide by each other.

FLUID AND ELECTROLYTE BALANCE

The body's internal environment is made up of fluids and dissolved substances including electrolytes. Fluids and electrolytes are in a constant state of dynamic equilibrium in order to maintain the delicate balance essential for all the physiologic processes that support life.

Fluids

Body fluid is primarily water. Depending on the amount of body fat, a person's total body weight is usually 50–70% water. Since fat is essentially water-free, an obese adult's body weight is 50% water. In a leaner individual, the percentage of body weight due to body water is closer to 70%. With aging, there is a decrease in lean body mass; therefore, the elderly may have only a 46–52% of body weight as water.

Body water is divided into two main compartments: intracellular and extracellular. The majority of body water (64%) is located inside the cells. The remaining 36% of body fluid is extracellular. Three-fourths of this extracellular fluid is interstitial (surrounding cells), and the remaining one-fourth is intravascular plasma.

Communication between these fluid compartments varies. Intracellular water does not move readily out of the cell. In contrast, in the capillary beds there is constant movement of fluids between the extracellular fluid (interstitial and intravascular) compartments. The movement of body fluid between the intravascular and interstitial space is controlled by two opposing forces: *osmotic pressure* (holding fluid in the vessels) and *hydrostatic pressure* (forcing fluid into tissue spaces). Interstitial and intravascular fluid are similar in composition except for the presence of plasma proteins (which provide osmotic pressure) in the intravascular space.

Body water balance is the result of physiologic homeostatic responses to the fluid gains (intake) and losses (output) that occur on a daily basis. The major sources of intake and output are shown in Table 28–1.

The primary organ of fluid balance is the kidney. The kidneys excrete the end products of cellular metabolism, as well as eliminate excess fluids. In order to clear the blood of wastes, they must produce a minimum of 500–600 mL of urine every 24 hours. To balance a typical amount of fluid intake, however, the usual amount of urine produced on a daily basis varies from 1 to 2 liters.

TABLE 28–1 Average Daily Fluid Gain and Loss

Intake (mL)		Output (mL)	
Oral intake (liquid and food)	2300	Urine	1500
Cellular catabolism		Skin	600 (insensible loss by evaporation)
of proteins, carbohydrates, and fats	300	Lung	300 (insensible loss by vapor)
		Feces	200
	2600		2600

Regulation of the volume, composition, and osmolality of body fluid is controlled by homeostatic mechanisms. A major regulator of intake is thirst. Thirst is stimulated by receptors in the central nervous system. Under normal circumstances, an individual ingests fluids when these receptors are activated. During illness or an altered level of consciousness, and in the aged, the thirst response may be depressed, resulting in hypovolemia and increased tonicity or concentration of the extracellular fluids (Deficient Fluid Volume).

Urine production by the kidneys is influenced by two hormonal regulatory systems, one of which is the antidiuretic hormone (ADH). When extracellular body fluids become concentrated, osmoreceptors located in the hypothalamus stimulate the release of ADH, which stimulates the kidneys to retain more water. As this retained water circulates through the extracellular fluid compartment, the concentration of body fluid is reduced. The osmoreceptors sense this change, slow the secretion of ADH, and the kidneys stop retaining water (negative feedback).

Other conditions that can stimulate the secretion of ADH and lead to increased water retention by the kidneys include hemorrhage, decreased cardiac output, trauma, pain, fear, surgery, and dehydration. Drugs such as morphine, barbiturates, nicotine, and some anesthetics and tranquilizers also increase the secretion of ADH. The secretion of ADH can be inhibited by alcohol, decreased concentration of body fluids and hypervolemic states.

Another major regulatory hormone is aldosterone, which is secreted by the adrenal cortex. Aldosterone regulates fluid volume by stimulating the kidneys to reabsorb sodium and water (an isotonic gain). During this process, sodium is exchanged for potassium or hydrogen; therefore, aldosterone also affects levels of these electrolytes. Secretion of aldosterone is increased in response to several stimuli, which include decreased sodium and increased extracellular potassium, hypovolemia, and stress states.

When blood flow to the kidneys is decreased, a receptorlike area in the glomerulus of the nephron releases an enzyme called renin. As renin circulates in the body, it converts a plasma protein in the liver into a vasoconstrictor substance called angiotensin I. When this substance enters the lungs, it is converted into angiotensin II. Angiotensin II acts directly on the adrenal cortex to increase aldosterone secretion. This then leads to extracellular volume expansion, and even possible fluid volume excess if the cause of decreased renal blood flow was due to heart or liver failure.

Electrolytes

In partnership with body fluids are substances called electrolytes. These substances, mostly minerals, contribute to body function in many ways and are essential to life (Table 28–2). Electrolytes are important components of intracellular and extracellular fluids. The major intracellular electrolytes are potassium, magnesium, phosphate, and sulfate. Major extracellular electrolytes are sodium, chloride and bicarbonate.

TABLE 28–2 Major Electrolytes

Cations		Anions	
Na^+	Sodium	Cl^-	Chloride
K^+	Potassium	HCO_3^-	Bicarbonate
Ca^{2+}	Calcium	HPO_4^{2-}	Phosphate
Mg^{2+}	Magnesium		

Electrolytes are distributed throughout the body, both intracellularly and extracellularly. In the extracellular compartment, the main electrolytes are sodium, chloride, and bicarbonate. Intracellular electrolytes are potassium, magnesium, phosphate, and sulfate.

Electrolytes develop an electric charge when dissolved in water. Electrolytes with a positive charge are called cations. Negatively charged electrolytes are called anions. Positive cations and negative anions are attracted to each other because of their opposite electric charges. When they combine with each other, they form neutral compounds that either remain in body fluids or dissociate and regain their electric charges. When they dissociate, or ionize, they are referred to as ions.

FLUID AND ELECTROLYTE IMBALANCE

Alterations in fluid and electrolytes may occur as a primary event or as a secondary response to a preexisting disease state or to a sudden, unexpected traumatic event. When alterations of fluid and electrolytes exceed the narrow limits consistent with health, the body needs to adjust quickly.

Changes in the composition of body fluid and electrolytes may be relative or absolute. Relative losses or gains can occur when fluids or electrolytes shift from one body space to another. Absolute losses or gains occur when fluids and electrolytes are lost outside the body or added to the overall body stores by IV fluid.

The kidney has an obligatory urine output, and the body has an insensible water loss. A minimum fluid intake of 1500 mL is essential to balance these losses. If the loss of body water is greater than fluid intake (fluid volume deficit), weight loss results. If the gain of body water is greater than output, weight gain results. One kilogram of body weight gain or loss is equal to 1000 mL (1 L) of fluid.

In addition to methods of assessing fluid balance, this chapter discusses interventions for providing fluid and electrolytes to clients who have experienced alterations in their homeostasis. The rationale for interventions associated with alterations in either fluids or electrolytes is to maintain homeostasis.

Clients undergoing major surgery or trauma may be subjected to blood loss necessitating fluid replacement therapy. Clients requiring prolonged intravenous therapy may have associated nutritional losses. Support for these clients must be considered.

IV ADMINISTRATION

Initiating, monitoring, and providing care for clients with IV therapy consumes a large portion of the nurses' time each shift, and requires safe nursing practice to protect the client from complications. Up to 90% of hospitalized clients require some form of IV therapy.

Administering IV drugs can lead to medication errors, even if the nurse does not mix the medication, but hangs and monitors the IV. Whenever the nurse administers an IV both the hospital and federal guidelines must be followed. Guidelines include being properly educated in the use of IV equipment, understanding venous anatomy to ensure proper IV selection sites, and knowing the appropriate catheter gauge and length for the vein selected. In addition, it is imperative that the nurse is knowledgeable about drugs and solutions being administered, the side effects, and treatment if a side effect occurs.

Frequent monitoring of IV infusions is a requisite for safe nursing practice. Knowing the solution infusing, medications added to the solution and rate of infusion, promotes safe care. Monitoring the IV site, proper dressing changes, including tubing changes, within specific time frames helps prevent complications associated with the IV site and cannula.

Intravenous devices are an important part of hospital practice for the administration of fluid, nutrients, medications, blood products, and to hemodynamically monitor unstable clients. These devices are not without problems. Catheter related bloodstream infections can be associated with increased hospital stays, even life-threatening events or death. Peripheral venous catheters are usually not associated with these infections, whereas central vascular devices are the most problematic devices. Phlebitis and infiltration are the most common complications associated with peripheral vein catheters. The risk of phlebitis differs between sites. It is much higher if the lower limb is used as the IV site. Catheters inserted in the hand carry a lower risk of phlebitis than those inserted higher up on the wrist and arm. Providing intravenous therapy for clients is one of the main skills provided by nurses.

This chapter presents skills for providing fluids and electrolytes, blood and blood components, as well as pharmacologic therapy through the intravenous route. Methods for assessing baseline data and evaluating fluid and electrolyte gains or losses are included in this chapter.

NURSING DIAGNOSES

The following nursing diagnoses are appropriate to include in a client care plan when the components are related to intravenous therapy.

NURSING DIAGNOSIS	RELATED FACTORS
Deficient Fluid Volume	Excess fluid loss secondary to vomiting, increased temperature, blood loss, drainage sites or tubes, diarrhea, and diuretics
Excess Fluid Volume	Excessive fluid accumulation secondary to excess sodium intake, medications, renal or cardiac failure; inaccurate IV infusion rate
Risk for Infection	Chronic diseases, invasive procedures, immunodeficiency, tissue destruction and increased environmental exposure
Noncompliance	Inaccurate I&O records, denial, lack of instruction regarding I&O, fluid restriction, care of IV site
Impaired Skin Integrity	Alterations in skin turgor, edema, tissue damage, IV infiltration, infection, immobilization

- The single most important nursing action to decrease the incidence of hospital-based infections is handwashing. **Remember to wash your hands or use antibacterial gel before and after each and every client contact.**

UNIT 1

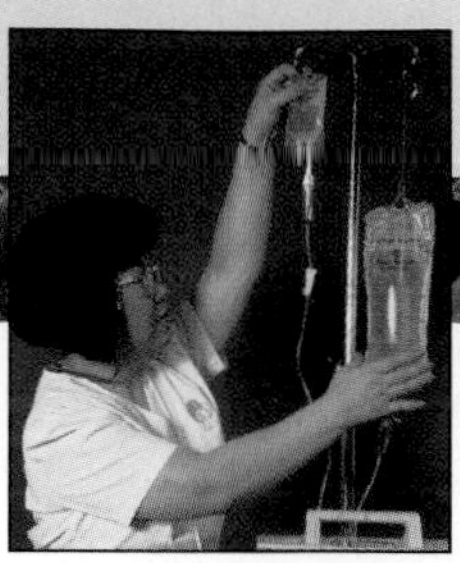

Initiating Intravenous Therapy

Nursing Process Data

ASSESSMENT ***Data Base***

Validate physician's order for IV therapy.

Assess need for client teaching about IV therapy.

Evaluate client for IV site selection.

Select appropriate vessel for venipuncture.

Determine appropriate type and size of cannulation device for client.

Determine IV equipment needed.

PLANNING ***Objectives***

To maintain fluid and electrolyte balance

To aseptically prepare infusion system

To identify and prepare the appropriate site for venipuncture

To perform successful venipuncture using appropriate equipment

IMPLEMENTATION ***Procedures***

Preparing the Infusion System

Adding Extension Tubing

Preparing the Venipuncture Site

Inserting a Winged Needle

Inserting an Over-the-Needle Catheter

EVALUATION ***Expected Outcomes***

Fluid and electrolyte needs are met.

IV fluids infuse without complications.

Vein is cannulated successfully.

Appropriate IV equipment used.

IV site is maintained.

PREPARING THE INFUSION SYSTEM

Equipment

IV solution in bag

Note: The only glass bottles used today are for infusions of certain medications, (e.g., nitroglycerin and amiodarone). Check facility procedures for correct infusion of these medications using the glass bottle.

Primary administration tubing set (compatible with infusion pump)
Add-on particulate filter (according to agency policy) compatible with infusion pump psi
Electronic infusion device or free pole for bag suspension and gravity infusion
Needleless Luer-Lok cannula

CLINICAL ALERT

Take IV solutions out of refrigerator (if stored in refrigerator) and allow to warm to room temperature. This will reduce the number of air bubbles in the IV solution.

It is difficult to detect air bubbles because gas is well assimilated into liquid at low temperatures; thus, air bubbles are fully assimilated into the IV solution when kept in refrigerator. Once solution warms to room temperature, air bubbles appear.

Preparation

1. Wash your hands.
2. Compare the type and amount of solution with physician's order.

Except when infusing TPN or TPN with lipids, PCAs, continuous epidurals, and blood products, in-line filters are not recommended. There is no evidence to suggest that in-line filters prevent infections associated with intravascular devices and infusion systems. Some studies do suggest that they may reduce the incidence of infusion-related phlebitis; however, it has not been proved. Because studies do not justify the cost of the in-line filters, the CDC does not recommend them for infection control purposes.

3. Check pharmacy label for client's identification, solution type, additives, and expiration date.
4. Select IV tubing appropriate for infusion device or rate-controlling tubing (e.g., Dial-a-Flow).
5. Select add-on filter if indicated.
6. Obtain needleless cannula or adapter for established infusion site.

Procedure

1. Remove outer wrap around IV bag if necessary. (It may be wet due to condensation.)
2. Inspect bag carefully for tears or leaks by applying gentle pressure to bag.
3. Hold bag up against both a dark and light background to examine for discoloration, cloudiness, or particulate matter. **Rationale:** Any evidence of change may indicate contamination, and bag should be discarded.
4. Hang the IV bag on the IV pole.
5. Close tubing roller clamp. Affix time strip on bag.
6. Remove plastic protector from tubing spike (end of tubing with drip chamber).

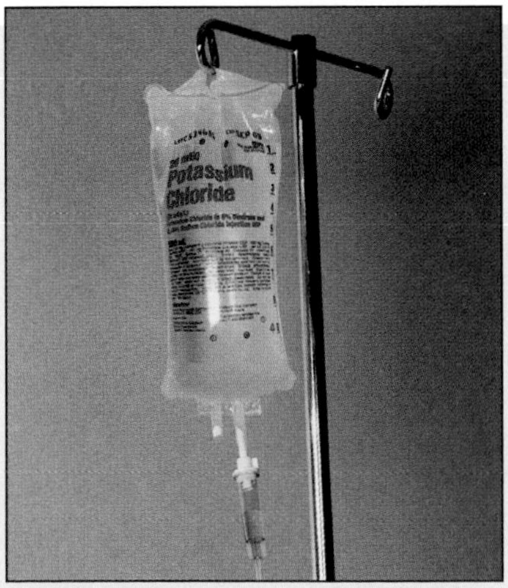

Most hospitals require a "Red Label" if potassium or other drugs are pre-added to the solution.

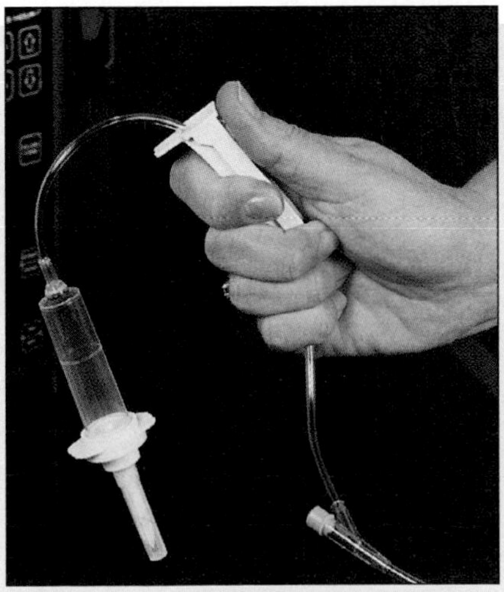
Clamp tubing before spiking IV fluid bag.

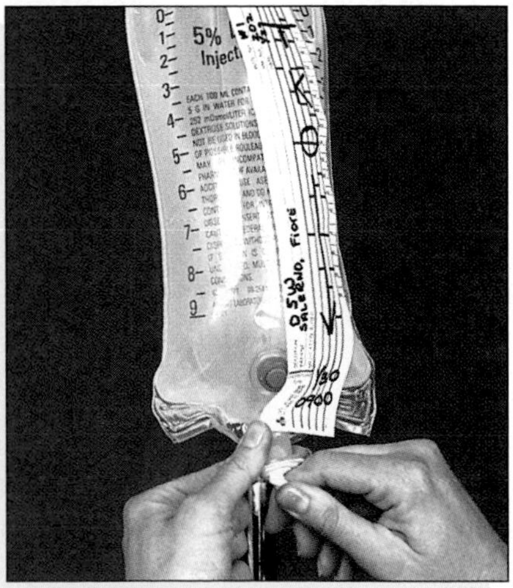
Pull to remove port cap on IV bag.

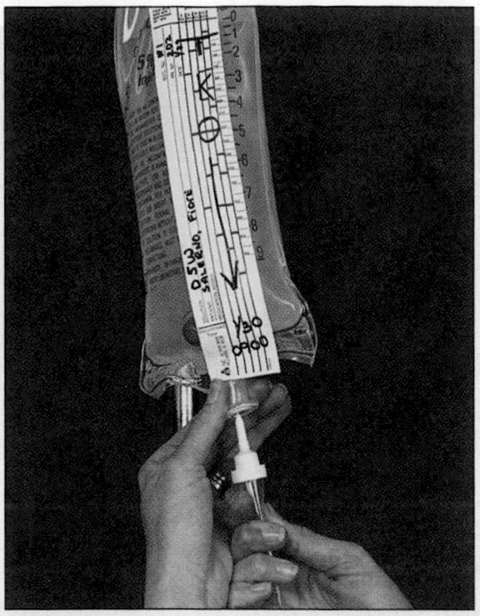

Spike bag port maintaining sterility.

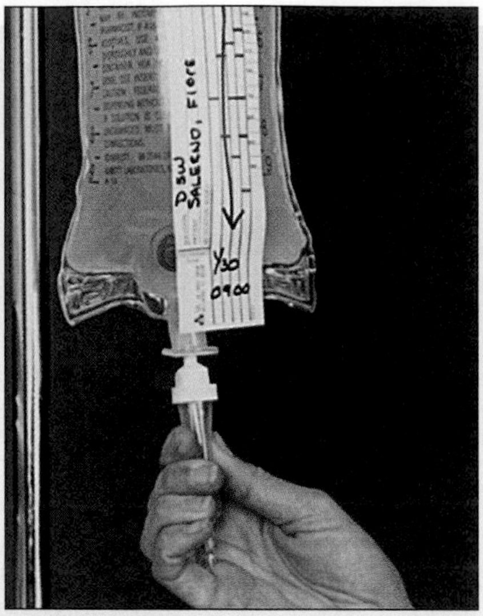

Squeeze and release drip chamber to fill.

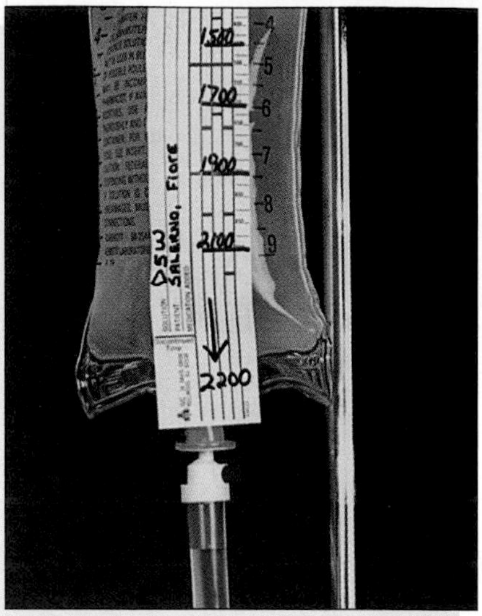

Fill drip chamber one-half full of fluid.

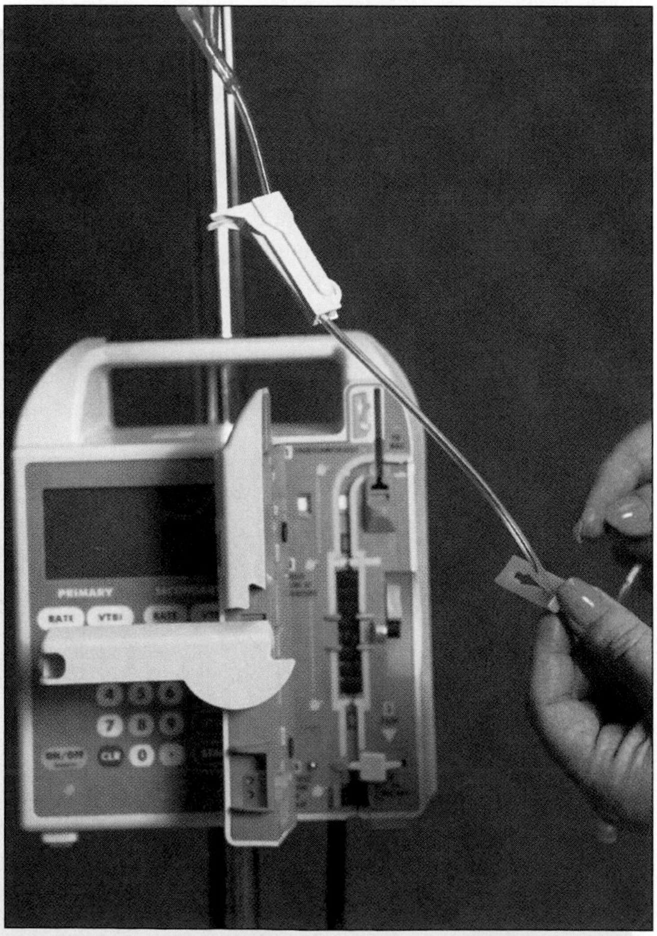

Close tubing clamp when priming is complete.

7. Squeeze drip chamber while inserting tubing spike into bag port, holding port securely to prevent contamination. **Rationale:** Squeezing chamber during insertion prevents air entry into bag.
8. Release pressure on the drip chamber until chamber is partially full.
9. Attach add-on terminal filter (if indicated).
10. Remove protective cap at end of tubing.
11. Open clamp on line to prime tubing and filter.
12. Hold tubing tip higher than tubing-dependent loop while priming. **Rationale:** Air rises and passes out as fluid primes tubing.
13. Invert and tap Y injection sites to remove air as tubing primes.
14. Hold filter (if attached) pointing downward so proximal (closest to client) half of filter fills with fluid first, then invert to complete filter priming, tapping air out as filter primes.
15. Close tubing clamp when primed.
16. Place needleless cannula on end of tubing. **Rationale:** This maintains sterility before infusion is established.
17. Load administration set into electronic pump according to manufacturer's instructions. Most pumps require dedicated tubing and specific loading format.

CLINICAL ALERT

Do not use felt-tip pens to mark IV plastic bag. The ink may leach through the plastic and contaminate the solution.

ADDING EXTENSION TUBING

Equipment

Extension tubing
Antimicrobial swab
Needleless cannula
Injection cap with Luer-Lok adapter, if necessary
Syringe cannula
2 syringes with 1 mL normal saline solution

Procedure

1. Gather equipment and determine type of cap, if needed. Extension tubing may be attached directly to IV catheter.
2. Swab tubing's terminal injection cap and insert syringe cannula.
3. Remove protector at opposite end and prime extension tubing with 1 mL normal saline solution.

> **CLINICAL ALERT**
>
> Peripheral IVs should be started using aseptic technique. IVs started without proper asepsis, for example, in an emergency or outside the hospital, should be replaced at the earliest opportunity, and within 24 hours.

4. Add needleless cannula to tubing if attaching to capped catheter.
5. Swab client's established IV cannula resealable cap and connect extension tubing or insert primed extension tubing directly into client's IV catheter.
6. Flush with 1 mL normal saline solution (optional).

Note: A short extension tubing provides easy access for intermittent infusions and protects IV site from manipulation trauma.

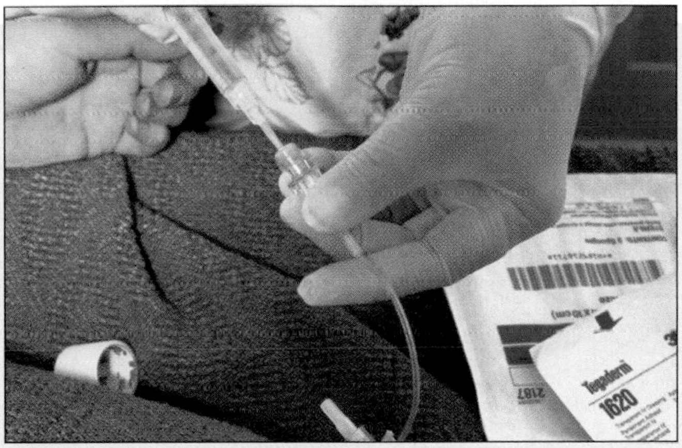

Swab injection cap and insert syringe cannula.

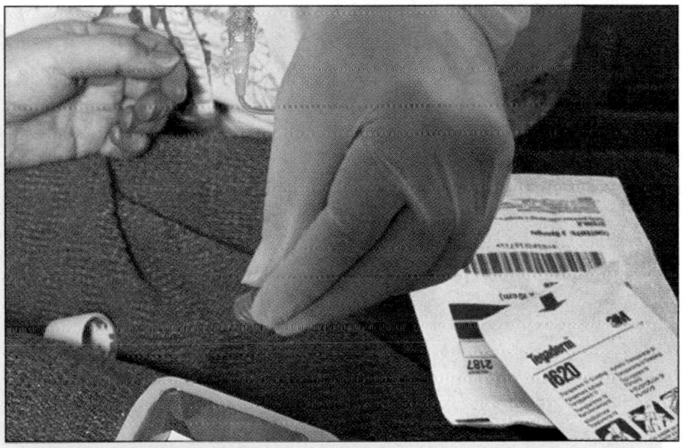

Remove protector at opposite end and prime tubing.

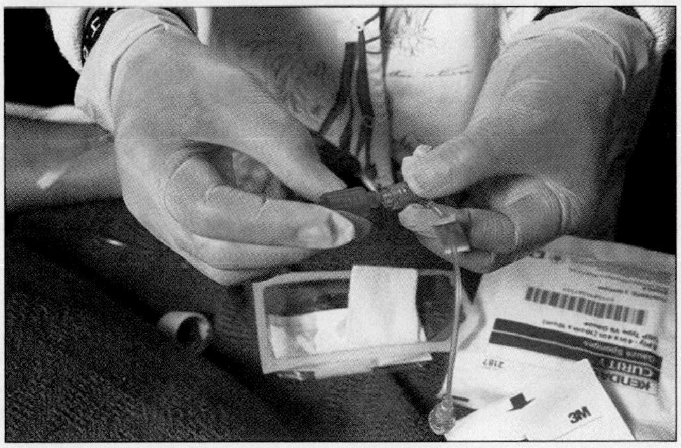

Add needleless cannula to tubing if attaching to capped catheter.

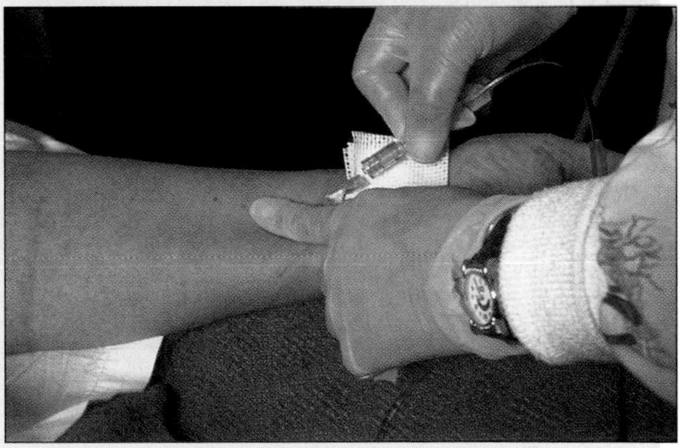
Primed tubing can also be inserted directly into IV catheter.

PREPARING THE VENIPUNCTURE SITE

Equipment

Prepared IV administration setup or sterile needleless access cap
Single use, latex free tourniquet or blood pressure cuff
Antimicrobial wipe: chlorhexadine, 70% isopropyl alcohol, 10% providone iodine, or tincture of iodine—each of these can be used alone
Sterile needle or catheter for venipuncture
½'' wide tape
Transparent semipermeable dressing
Armboard if indicated
Clean gloves
Electronic infusion pump

Preparation

1. Check physician's orders and MAR.
2. Check room number, client's identaband including hospital number, and have client state name.
3. Assemble equipment.

Procedure

1. Explain procedure.
2. Provide privacy.
3. Hang solution bag and primed administration set within easy reach.
4. Position client, and adjust lighting as necessary.
5. Cut pieces of tape and place on edge of clean over-bed table.
6. Wash your hands and don gloves.
7. Select catheter or needle. Catheter gauge should be smallest size that allows greatest flow, without occluding vessel lumen.

Note: Over-the-needle catheters are used most commonly for IV fluid/blood administration. A smaller catheter (22 gauge) may be used for routine antibiotics or maintenance fluids, but a larger catheter (20 gauge) is needed for blood products. For irritating medications, a small-bore catheter is preferable.

CLINICAL ALERT

Do not shave the venipuncture site. Shaving can facilitate the development of infection through the multiplication of organisms in resulting microabrasions. Hairy sites can be clipped with scissors.

8. If possible, select a vein on client's nondominant arm. Also consider client's activity level and expected duration of IV therapy.
   a. Inspect both of client's arms, palpating and visualizing the course of the veins.

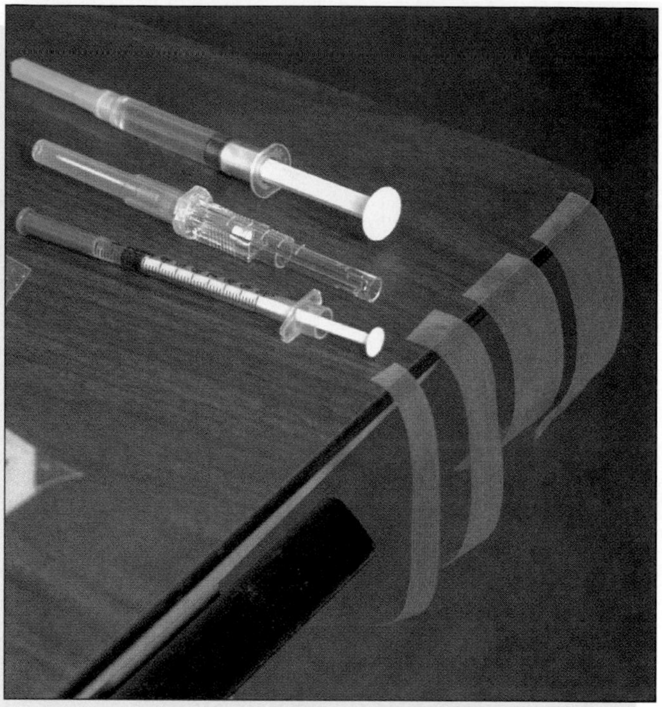

Cut pieces of tape and hang on edge of clean over-bed table.

   b. Vein should be superficial, easily palpated, and large enough for needle insertion and advancement.
   c. Area should be free of lesions or scars and away from joints and areas of frequent motion. **Rationale:** Motion frequency increases the risk of mechanical phlebitis.
   d. Do not use the antecubital fossa except in atypical circumstances.
   e. Do not use the same vein below an infiltrated or phlebitic site.
   f. Select shortest and smallest cannula that will be sufficient to deliver fluids/medications. **Rationale:** The longer the catheter, the greater the risk of infiltration, infection, and thrombus formation. A catheter that is too large does not allow for adequate blood flow around catheter and this can lead to phlebitis.
   g. Distal end of vein should be selected first, reserving more proximal sites for future IV therapy.
   h. Select larger veins for hypertonic solutions, blood, and viscous fluids.
   i. Avoid using veins in affected arm following mastectomy.
   j. Lower extremity sites are associated with complications (e.g., thrombosis) and should be used ONLY if necessary.

CLINICAL ALERT

Some agencies allow only certified professionals to perform venipuncture.

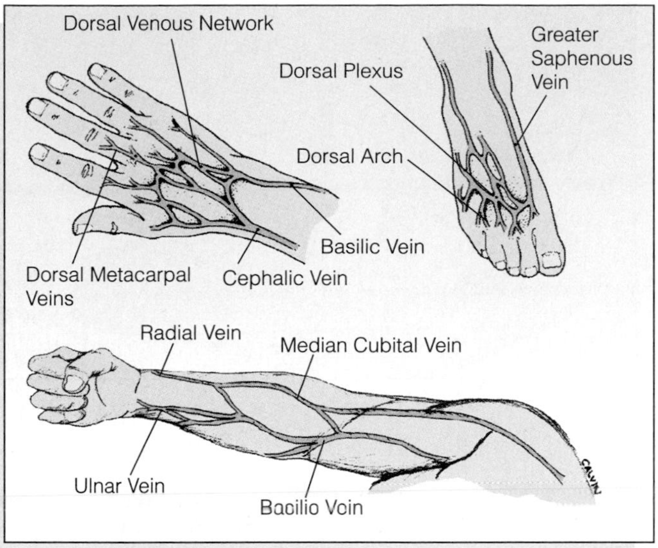

Anatomical sites used for venipuncture.

9. Apply tourniquet 6 inches above the selected site to distend vein. Overlap ends of tourniquet, lift and stretch, then tuck top end under bottom; keep ends pointing away from puncture site. **Rationale:** Tourniquet traps blood and engorges vein for better visibility.
10. If using blood pressure cuff, inflate to pressure just below diastolic reading.
    a. Lightly tap vein. **Rationale:** To distend vein in preparation for venipuncture.

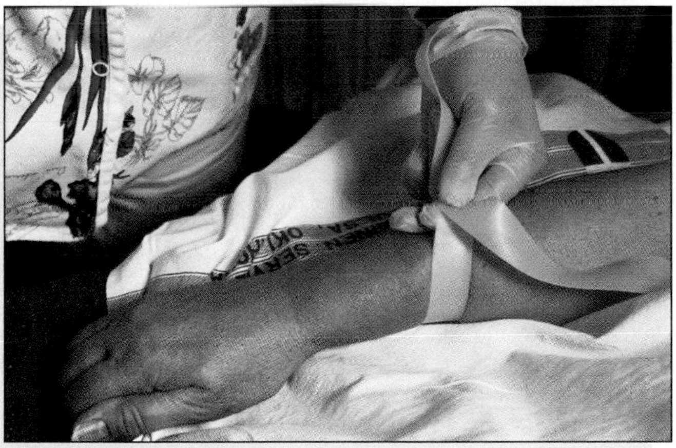

Apply tourniquet 6 inches above selected site.

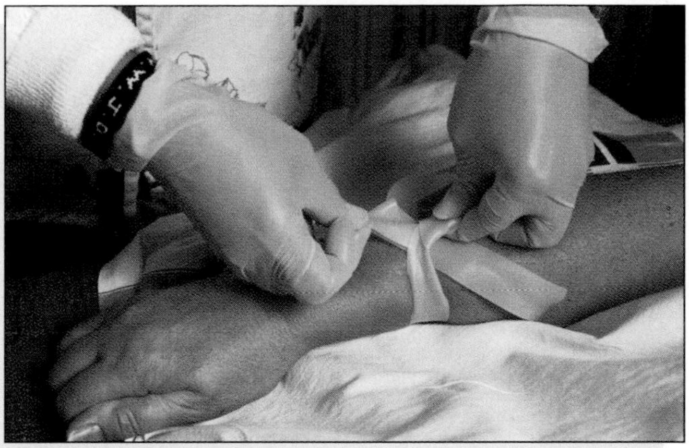

Overlap ends of tourniquet, lift, stretch, and tuck top end under bottom.

> **CLINICAL ALERT**
>
> Latex tourniquets should be used and disposed of after each use.

    b. Ask client to open and close fist several times to help distend selected vein.
    c. If vein is difficult to palpate, release tourniquet and apply warm, moist compresses to arm for 10–20 minutes before reapplying tourniquet.
    d. Position client's arm dependently for a few minutes to promote venous distention before reapplying tourniquet.
11. Prep site with an antimicrobial swab. Cleanse area 2–4 inches in diameter. **Rationale:** Vigorous skin preparation decreases organisms at the venipuncture site.
12. Let prep solution air dry for 30 seconds naturally before continuing with venipuncture. Do not fan to dry skin. **Rationale:** This provides the necessary time for bacteriocidal activity.
13. Do not touch selected insertion site after prepping.
14. Proceed to appropriate procedure for inserting the needle.

> **CLINICAL ALERT**
>
> For antiseptic effectiveness, allow antimicrobial to air dry for at least 30 seconds to provide the minimum time necessary for bacteriocidal activity.

INSERTING A WINGED NEEDLE

Equipment

Prescribed solution, infusion administration set, and electronic infusion pump
Protective resealable injection cap (if indicated)
Syringe with 1 mL NS for locking resealable injection cap
Tourniquet or blood pressure cuff
Sterile winged (small vein) needle (typical hub replaced by two flexible wings) with attached tubing and resealable injection cap or short tubing to affix to infusion administration tubing

Note: Winged needles are available as steel needles or flexible over-the-needle catheter types. The hub is replaced by flexible wings for easier insertion and taping.

Adults use size 16–29 gauge for viscous solutions and 20–25 gauge for less viscous solutions
Neonates use size 25–27 gauge
Older child uses size 21–25 gauge

Antimicrobial wipe
Transparent dressing
Clean gloves
Armboard (if indicated)

Procedure

1. Follow steps in *Preparing the Venipuncture Site* and don gloves.
2. Select a winged needle for adults and for children, infants, and elderly clients who have small or fragile veins.
3. Carefully affix end of IV infusion tubing to end of winged needle tubing. Remove sterile cover from needle and run fluid through needle to prime tubing, then clamp it, and replace needle cover.
4. Apply tourniquet or blood pressure cuff to distend selected vein.
5. Prep the selected site with an antimicrobial wipe. If alcohol is used, it should be applied with friction for a minimum of 30 seconds. Allow to air dry.
6. Remove protective cap from winged needle and hold needle by its wings, anchor vein by placing thumb below client's vein.
7. Place thumb of nondominant hand below selected site and pull skin taut. With needle bevel up, enter client's skin at a 30° angle. You may use either of these methods:
   a. Enter skin next to or along side vein. Flatten angle to 15° once needle is under skin and then enter vein from side.
   b. Insert needle through skin below intended puncture site, then enter vein. **Rationale:** Inserting needle through skin and into small vein with one thrust will result in hematoma formation.

General Time Frame for Tubing Changes

- Primary and secondary tubing—72–96 hours
- Primary intermittent tubing—24 hours
- Extension tubing—replace when vascular device is replaced (it is considered part of the IV system)
- TPN and lipids—every 24 hours
- Blood or blood products tubing—every 4 hours after initiating infusion (new protocol according to American Association of Blood Banks)
- Hemodynamic and arterial pressure monitoring tubing—96 hours

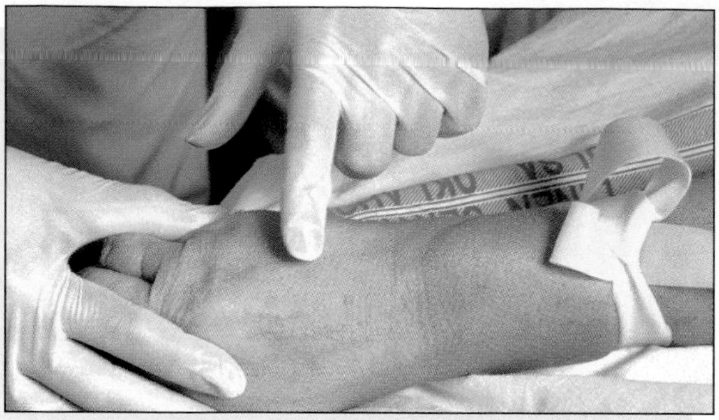

Select site at distal end of vein to preserve future proximal IV sites.

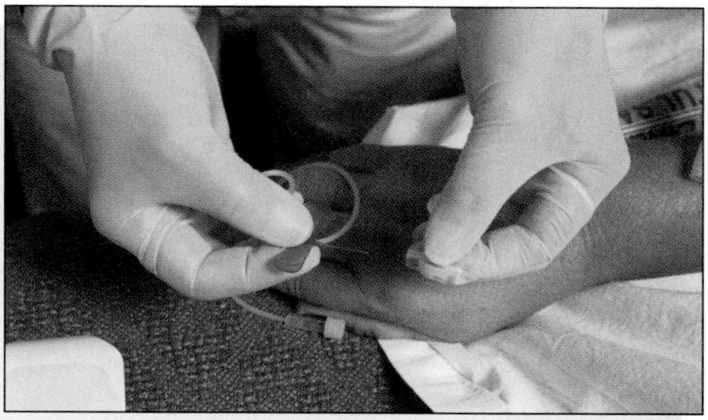

Remove protective cap from winged needle.

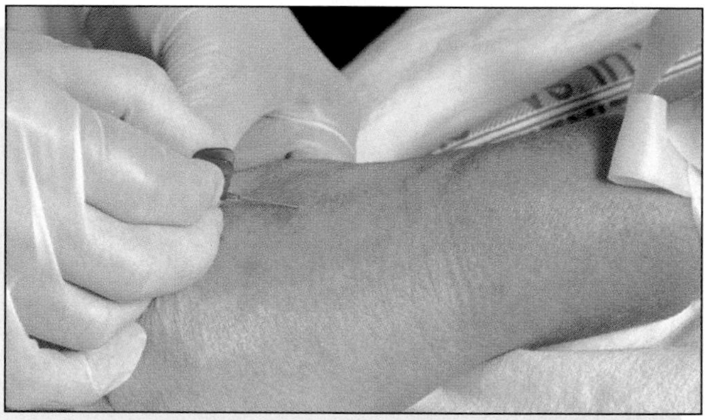

Insert needle at 30° angle through skin below selected vein.

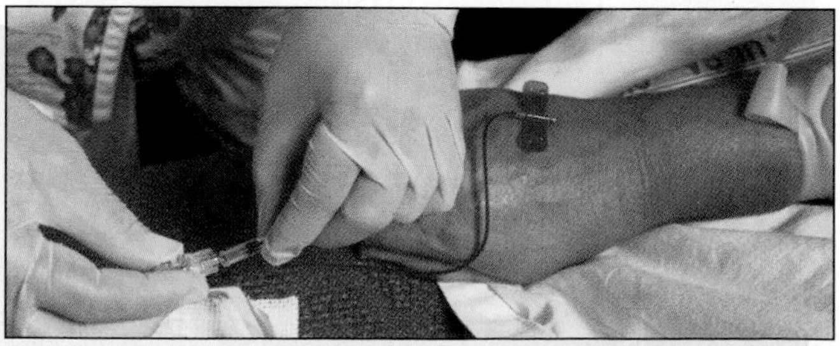

Attach sterile resealable injection cap to end of winged needle tubing.

8. Follow course of vein. Sudden "pop" and lack of resistance is felt when vein is entered.
9. Observe for flashback of blood in needle tubing.
10. Carefully advance needle up course of the vein until it reaches hub.
11. Release tourniquet.
12. Inject normal saline for lock, or affix IV tubing, open clamp and observe drip chamber. **Rationale:** Fluid should flow easily, and there should be no sudden swelling at the IV site.
13. Reduce flow rate to keep open until you have taped needle and tubing in place.
14. Remove gloves (optional, or following dressing, 17) and wash hands.
15. Secure needle with ½″ wide tape (adhesive side up) crossed to chevron over wings. Avoid taping directly on insertion site.
16. Loop and tape IV tubing a short distance from needle.
17. Apply occlusive transparent dressing over infusion site.
18. Label dressing with date, time, and initials, and size of catheter inserted.
19. Establish prescribed infusion rate by pump or calculated gravity flow drips per minute.
20. Immobilize hand in functional position to armboard.
21. Change site every 48–72 hours. **Rationale:** According to studies, an increased risk of thrombophlebitis and bacterial colonization of catheters occurs after 72 hours.

CLINICAL ALERT

Meticulous care must be used to insert the winged-tipped needle because these needles lead to the majority of reported needle stick injuries.

CLINICAL ALERT

The CDC has not established a recommendation for hang time of IV fluids. Follow hospital policy and change fluids accordingly.

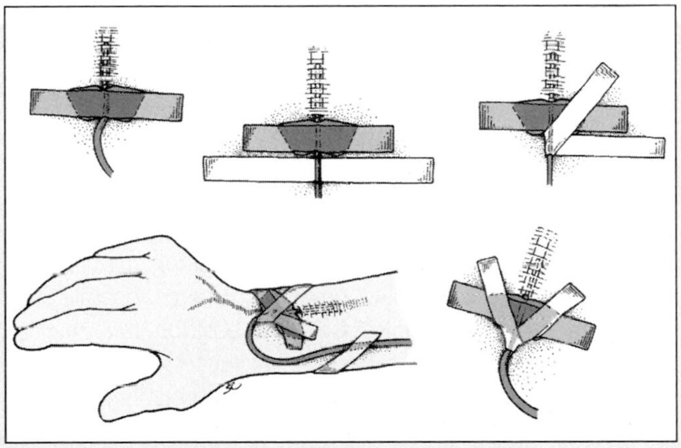

Use chevron method to secure winged small vein needle, then apply occlusive transparent dressing over infusion site.

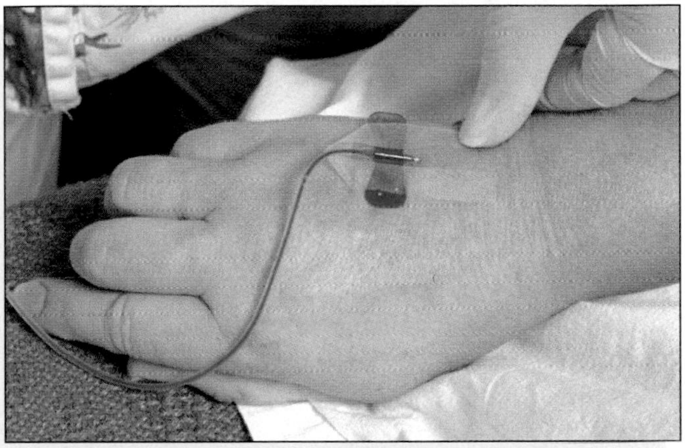

Bring tape over needle and secure needle and wings with chevron method.

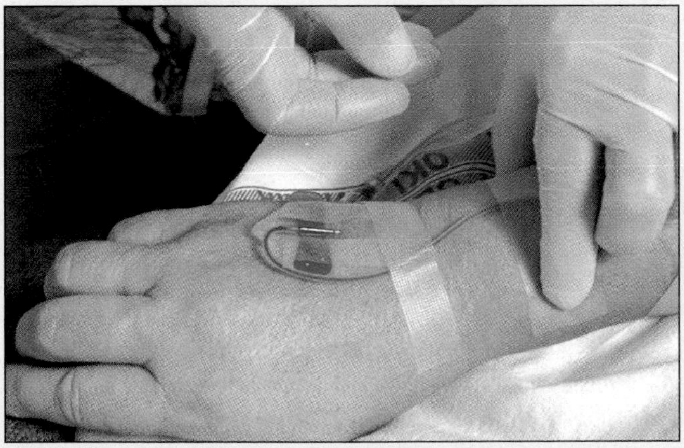

After chevron method secures needle, loop and tape tubing to arm.

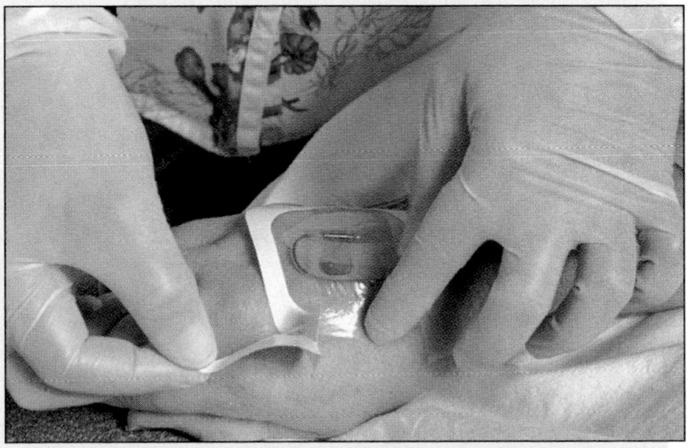

Cover site with transparent dressing; date, time, initials, and size of catheter.

EVIDENCE BASED NURSING PRACTICE

Risks Associated with Peripheral Intravenous Catheter Dwell Times

Even though many studies have been done indicating IV peripheral catheters need to be changed before 72 hours, a retrospective study, using a chart review of 722 clients in a community hospital with peripheral IV catheters for IV fluids or saline locks, indicated that restarting catheters at 72 hours does not reduce risk of complications in the next 24 hours when compared with simply continuing therapy with the original catheter. Additional studies need to be undertaken to justify the policy of automatically restarting the IV after 72 hours.

Source: Homer, L. D., Holmes, K. R. (1998, September–October). Risks associated with 72 and 96 hour peripheral intravenous catheter dwell times. *Intravenous Nursing, 21*(5), 301–305.

INSERTING AN OVER-THE-NEEDLE CATHETER

Equipment

Tourniquet or blood pressure cuff
Antimicrobial wipe
Sterile over-the-needle catheter sizes 14–22 gauge, 1¼–5½ inch long

Note: Some winged devices are over-the-needle catheters.

Syringe with local anesthetic (Lidocaine) and 25–26-gauge needle (check agency policy and client sensitivity before using)
Prepared administration set and infusion solution if ordered
Electronic infusion device
Protective needleless cap
Syringe with 1 mL normal saline for lock (if indicated) ½ inch tape
Clean gloves

Procedure

1. Prepare IV system and follow steps in *Preparing the Venipuncture Site.*
2. Select appropriate size over-the-needle catheter.
3. Don gloves.
4. Position extremity for venipuncture.
5. Inject site intradermally with small wheal of local anesthetic according to agency policy. (Allow 90 seconds for anesthetic to take effect.)
6. Place extremity flat on bed or place in a dependent position. **Rationale:** Gravity will slow venous return and thus dilate the vein. If vein is not distended sufficiently for easy venipuncture, ask client to make a fist or lightly tap on the vein with your fingertips.
7. Hold catheter with bevel up and examine the integrity of end of catheter.
8. Apply traction to stabilize vein.
9. With bevel of needle up, insert needle/catheter unit at a 45° angle into client's skin either:
   a. Along side of vein, or
   b. About ½″ distal to selected puncture site.
10. Revisualize vein; reduce angle of cannula to 30°, pierce vein, a "pop" will frequently be felt. Observe for backflow of blood in plastic hub. Continue to apply traction. **Rationale:** This indicates you are in the vein.
11. Hold needle and gently advance plastic catheter hub over needle and up vein no more than halfway.

CLINICAL ALERT

If no blood is observed and you did not feel the catheter enter the vein, pull back on entire catheter apparatus without exiting skin. Reassess vein position, then reattempt venipuncture. If you are not successful, remove catheter and look for a different site. Remember the catheter is now contaminated and cannot be used again. Most facilitites allow the nurse to attempt two venipunctures; if unsuccessful, they must notify another professional to attempt venipuncture.

Note: Maintain aseptic technique throughout procedure and prevent trauma to site and vein. These catheters are associated with a very high rate of phlebitis—80% in one study.

12. Stop and separate, but do not completely remove, the stylet from catheter.
13. Advance only the catheter until catheter hub meets the skin. The catheter moves over the stylet. If the hub is against the vein valve, you will need to initiate the infusion of IV fluids in order to float catheter to the middle of the vein.
14. Release tourniquet. Leave stylet in catheter while you tape catheter to the skin. **Rationale:** Stylet acts like a plug and by leaving it partially in place you don't have to hurry to tape catheter to the skin.

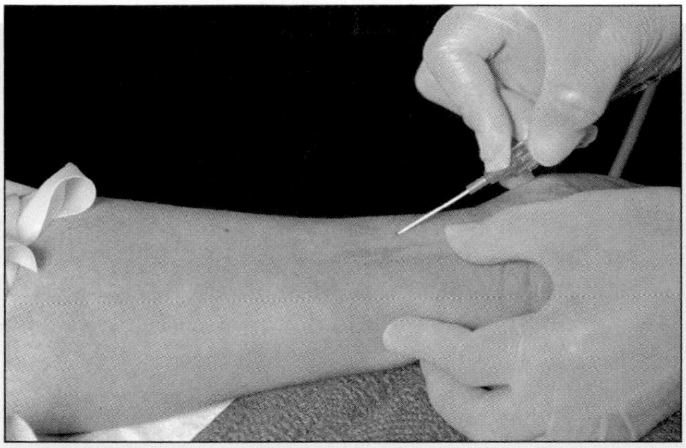

Insert needle with bevel up at a 45° angle along side of vein.

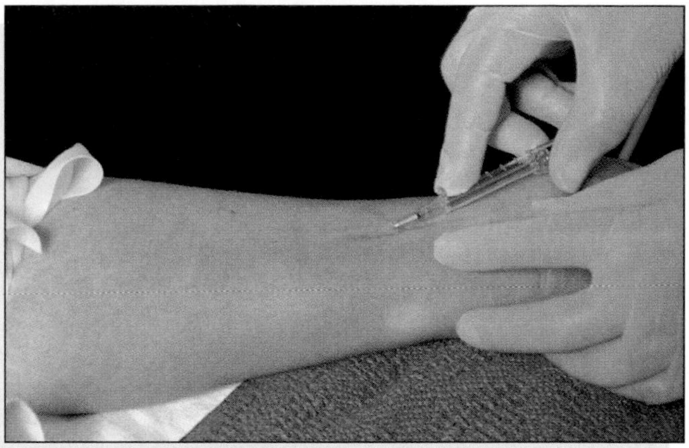

After skin insertion, reduce angle of cannula and advance into vein.

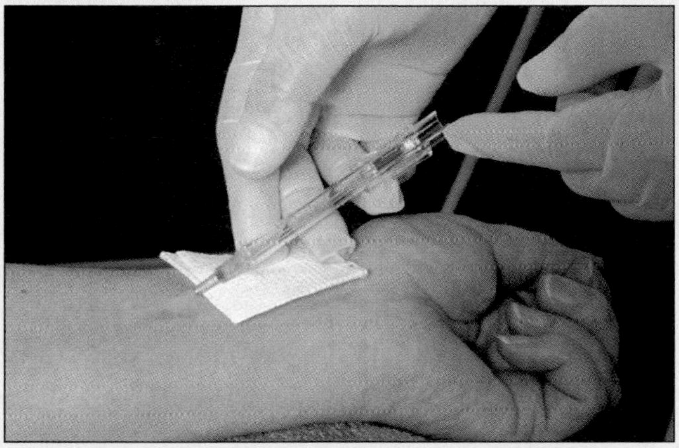

Withdraw needle slightly and observe for blood in the needle hub.

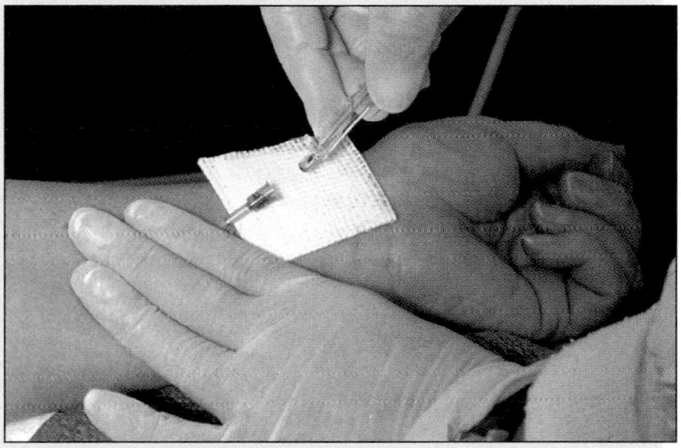

Hold pressure on the vein proximal to catheter to prevent blood loss.

Evaluation Criteria

Catheter sites are evaluated at least each shift for both phlebitis and infiltration using evaluation criteria established by the Intravenous Nurses' Society. The Intravenous Nursing Standards of Practice were revised in 2000.

Phlebitis

0 = no clinical symptoms

1+ = erythema at access site with or without pain

2+ = pain at access site with erythema and/or edema

3+ = pain at access site with erythema and/or edema, streak formation

4+ = pain at access site with erythema and/or edema, streak formation, palpable venous cord > 1 inch in length, purulent discharge

Note: No catheter should remain in place with signs of phlebitis, even with good blood flow and IV infusion rate.

Infiltrations

0 = no symptoms

1 = skin blanched, edema < 1″ in any direction, cool to touch, with or without pain

2 = skin blanched, edema 1–6″ in any direction, cool to touch, with or without pain

3 = skin blanched, translucent, gross edema > 6 inches in any direction, cool to touch, mild-moderate pain, possible numbness

4 = skin blanched, translucent, skin tight, leading, gross edema > 6 inches in any direction, deep pitting tissue edema, skin discolored, bruised, swollen, circulatory impairment moderate-severe pain, *infiltration of any amount of blood product, irritant, or vesicant.*

Note: Infiltrations should be diagnosed well before obvious swelling occurs. Most infiltrations should be warm packed to promote reabsorption of fluid into vascular bed and out of tissues, except in case of infiltration by a vesicant drug, then follow facility policy or drug manufacturer's directions.

EVIDENCE BASED NURSING PRACTICE

Flushing with Low-Dose Heparin

There are many conflicting studies indicating outcomes that are both pro and con for using low-dose heparin with peripheral venous catheters. In one study, low-dose heparin infused continuously through peripheral venous catheters required further study to determine effectiveness in prolonging catheter life. Studies have proven that using heparin in arterial catheters is of benefit. Using intermittent heparin flushes for peripheral IV catheters also requires further validation, as it seems to be no more effective than using NS flushes.

Source: Randolph, A., et al. (1998, May 28) Benefit of heparin in peripheral venous and arterial catheters: Systematic review and meta-analysis of randomized controlled trials. *British Medical Journal, 316*:969–975.

15. Tape catheter wings across body of hub without touching puncture site, and without touching hub/catheter juncture.
16. Place digital pressure over distal end of catheter and carefully remove stylet. Maintaining aseptic technique, connect catheter to IV tubing or place a saline lock on catheter.
17. Connect catheter to needleless cap or insert IV tubing into catheter.
18. Open clamp and observe drip chamber for fluid flow (or preserve patency of system by injecting 1 mL saline through cap). There should not be any sudden swelling at IV site.
19. Observe for signs of infiltration.
20. Reduce flow, and proceed with taping cannula using chevron method.
21. Cover insertion site with sterile transparent dressing.

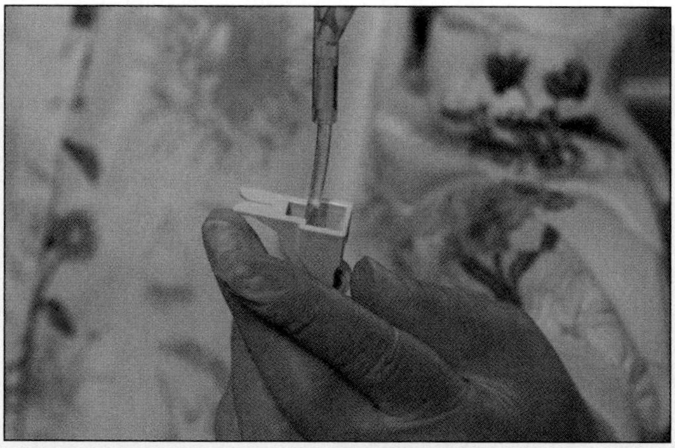
Open clamp and observe drip chamber.

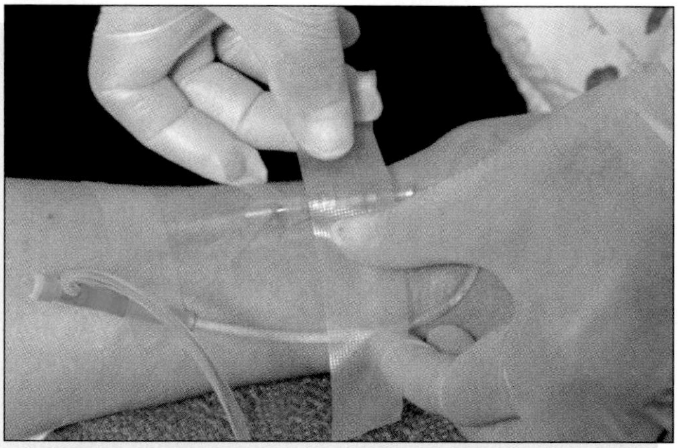
Reduce flow and proceed with taping cannula.

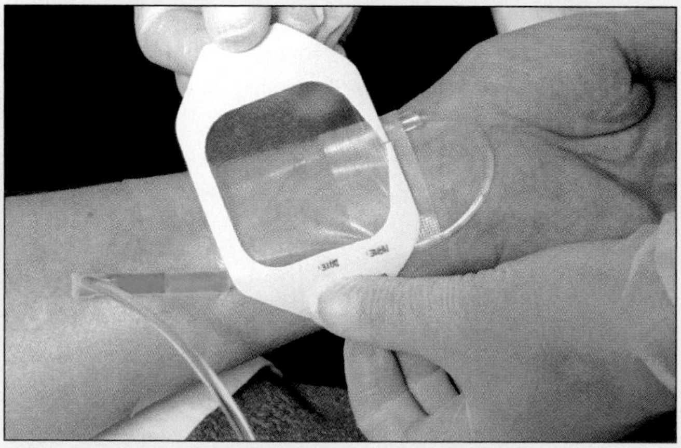
Cover insertion site with transparent dressing.

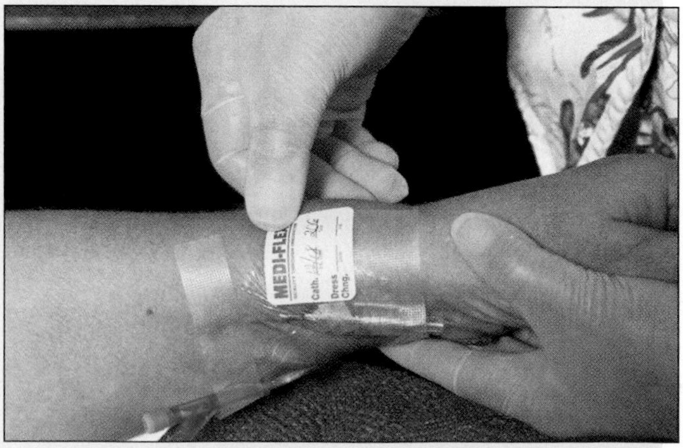
Label IV site with date time, initials, and size catheter.

22. Loop and tape tubing to client's arm a short distance from site.
23. Set drip rate according to physician's order.
24. Label IV site with date, time, initials, and size of catheter.
25. Remove gloves and wash hands.
26. Change cannula and infusion site every 72–96 hours.

CLINICAL ALERT

If using needleless angiocath system, once the "flash" is noted and catheter is advanced, the retract button is pushed and the needle automatically shielded.

DOCUMENTATION FOR IV THERAPY

- Time and date of insertion
- Location of insertion site
- Gauge and type of needle/catheter inserted
- Number of attempts (if more than one)
- Flush administered for cannula patency
- Type, amount, and rate of solution infused
- Status of IV site
- Client response to procedure

Critical Thinking Application

UNEXPECTED OUTCOMES	CRITICAL THINKING OPTIONS
Venipuncture is unsuccessful for needle insertion.	• Remove needle, apply pressure at insertion site until bleeding stops. (This prevents ecchymosis at site.) Apply Band-Aid. • Select another site more proximal in vein, or use another extremity. • Avoid the one-step entry method since this frequently results in a through-and-through vein puncture. • After two failed attempts, seek a more experienced person to perform venipuncture.
Vein rolls and is difficult to enter.	• Apply traction with thumb and index finger to stabilize skin and vein; maintain traction until venipuncture complete. • Select a smaller gauge catheter. • Advance catheter slowly.
Vein is fragile and "balloons" around needle on vein entry.	• Release tourniquet as soon as vein entry is evident. • Avoid use of tourniquet if veins are very fragile or client is taking an anticoagulant. • Enter vein with needle bevel down.
Infiltration occurs.	• Place warm moist pack, using warm towel, enclose area from fingertips to elbow. Place extremity in plastic bag with open end at elbow. Leave in place no more than 10 minutes.
Vesicant drug infuses into tissue.	• Clamp IV tubing. • Infuse antidote for specific medication, according to physician orders.

UNIT 2

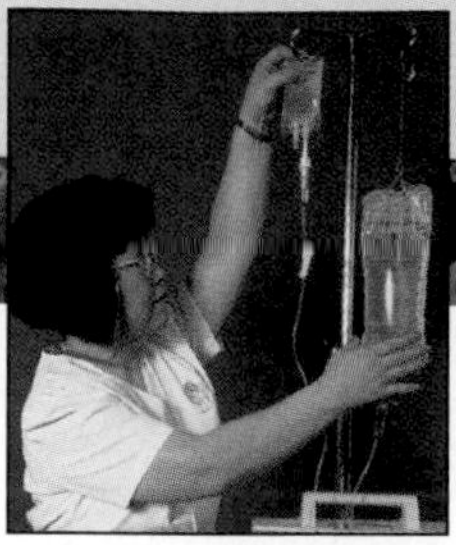

Intravenous Management

Nursing Process Data

ASSESSMENT *Data Base*

Assess site for erythema, swelling, or pain.

Assess infusion for correct solution, amount, and flow rate.

Assess need to change IV to saline lock.

Assess need to change client's gown while IV is infusing.

Assess need to change IV solution/administration set and infusion site.

PLANNING *Objectives*

To maintain the IV site free from erythema, swelling, or pain

To monitor the IV infusion rate accurately

To change a gown while maintaining the IV site

To discontinue IV therapy without complication

To connect IV to saline lock

IMPLEMENTATION *Procedures*

Regulating Infusion Flow Rate

Using an Electronic Flow-Control Device

Using a Syringe Pump

Managing the IV Site

Connecting IV to Saline Lock

Changing Gown for Client with IV

Discontinuing an IV

EVALUATION *Expected Outcomes*

Fluids are administered without adverse effects.

IV site remains free from erythema, swelling, or pain.

IV is infused accurately.

Saline lock is functioning properly.

Client's gown is changed while maintaining IV placement.

IV therapy is discontinued without complications.

REGULATING INFUSION FLOW RATE

Procedure

1. Check manufacturer's drip rate calibration on administration set package. Macrodrip sets vary from 10–15 gtts per 1 mL. Microdrip factor is 60 drops/mL.
2. Check physician's order for amount of fluid to be delivered per unit of time (e.g., 1 liter q8h, or hourly flow rate such as 100 mL/hr).
3. Calculate flow rate.
   a. To find the number of milliliters to be given per hour:

$$\frac{\text{Total solution}}{\text{No. of hours to run}} = \text{mL hour}$$

   b. To find drops per minute:

$$\frac{\text{mL/hr} \times \text{drop factor}}{60 \text{ minutes}} = \text{gtts/minute}$$

IV Calorie Calculation

- 1000 mL D_5W provides 50 g of dextrose.
- 50 g of dextrose provides 4 Cal/g (actually 3.4 Cal); therefore, multiply 50 g × 4 Cal.
- 1000 mL D_5W provides 200 Cal.
- Usual IV fluid maintenance is 2000–3000 mL/day (400–600 Cal/day).

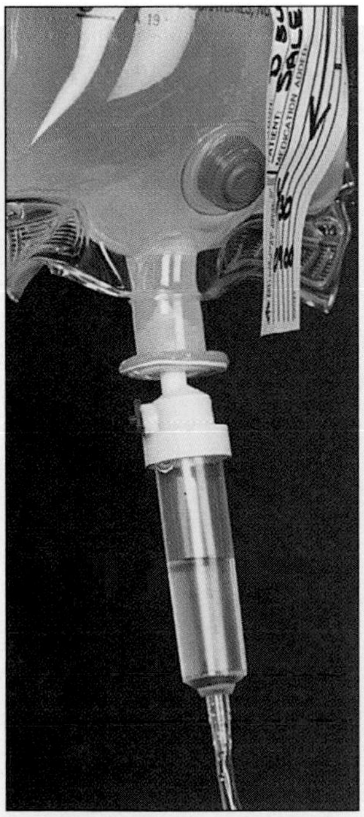

Count drops per minute to check accuracy of drip rate.

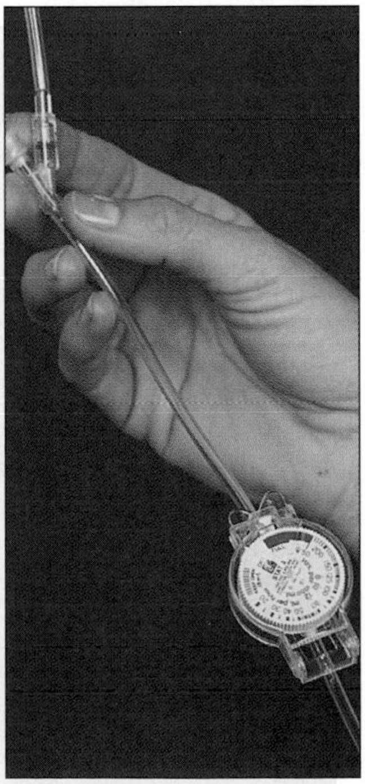

Set dial-a-flow to prescribed mL drip rate per hour.

Electronic Delivery Systems

- IV pump infusions are not absolutely accurate.
- A stable, uniform, IV infusion is more important than accuracy of total amount of fluid infused.
- Place surgical tape on syringe and IV solution bags and mark a scale of every 1–2 hours to confirm accurate infusion volume.
- Warning signs are the biggest problem with IV pumps; it takes only small deviations from normal to sound the warning signal.

Factors That Influence IV Flow Rates When Using Gravity for Infusion

- Warm fluids drip faster than cold fluids.
- The higher the bag is above insertion site, the faster the infusion.
- The more IV administration is tilted, the larger each drop from drip chamber.
- The larger the catheter diameter, the faster the flow rate.
- The longer the catheter, the slower the flow rate because of resistance.
- Increased blood pressure or coughing will slow the flow rate (this is a temporary situation usually).

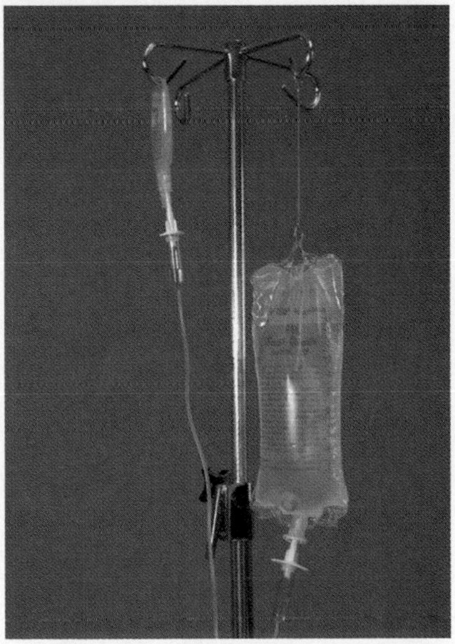

Note: Because of these variables, manual control of IVs is not recommended. IV pumps are the most predictable method of infusing fluids.

4. Note drip chamber; count the drops in one minute (or in 15 seconds and multiply by 4).
5. Adjust tubing clamp until the chamber drips the desired number of drops per minute (or 15 second increment).
6. Monitor flow rate frequently—adjustments to maintain desired delivery are often necessary.

USING AN ELECTRONIC FLOW-CONTROL DEVICE

Equipment

Electronic infusion device (pump)
Device-compatible IV administration set
Needleless cannula
Gloves

Procedure

1. Spike IV solution bag.
2. Close regulating clamp on the set tubing before hanging bag.
3. Fill drip chamber to minimum ⅓ full. **Rationale:** This amount allows sufficient air space in drip chamber.
4. Prime tubing by opening regulating clamp slowly and allowing tubing to fill with IV solution. If using a cassette-type tubing, follow package instructions to correctly prime the cassette portion of the tubing that engages into the control device.

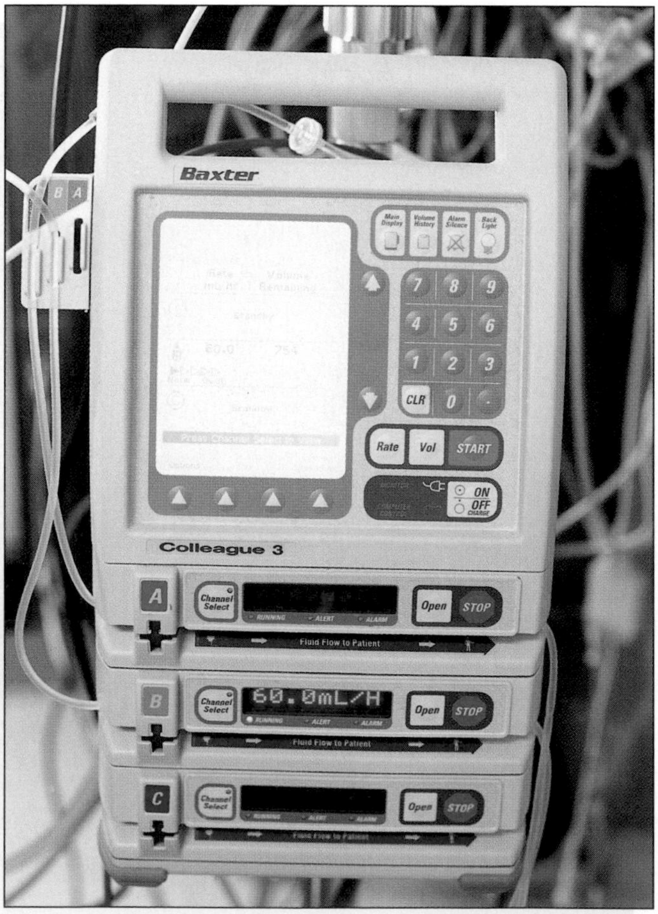

Baxter: Multiple Channel Pump.

If Alarm Sounds, Check the Following

Most devices have a message system that specifies the exact problem. You should be prepared to troubleshoot various components of the system.

- *Infusion Complete:* When the exact volume to be delivered is set and the volume limit has been reached, an alarm sounds and the machine goes to a KVO "keep-open" mode. Establish if the total volume of the container has been delivered; change the solution container if needed, and reset the volume to be infused.
- *Occlusion:* All devices sound an alarm when they cannot maintain delivery in the face of increasing resistance. In this instance, check the insertion site for infiltration, and look for position problems, pinched tubing, closed clamp, turned stopcock, or clogged filter.
- *Other Problems:* Other messages may indicate "air in the line," "low battery," "cassette" (improperly loaded), or "free flow."
- *Nursing Action:* Check trouble spot carefully, readjust, and restart the infusion.

5. Follow manufacturer's instructions to load administration set into device, taking care to fit tubing and cassette into appropriate receptor sites. (The multiple channel pump can infuse 3 different IV solutions at one time.)
6. Close device door and latch.
7. Don gloves.
8. Check that client's venipuncture site is free from signs of vein irritation or infiltration.
9. Connect administration set tubing to established infusion site protective cap using a needleless cannula.
10. Open regulating clamp on administration set.
11. Turn device ON.
12. Set device parameters for operation, again following manufacturer's instructions or machine's setup prompts. Parameters may include:
    a. Infusion (e.g., primary).
    b. Volume to be infused.
    c. Rate (mL/hr).
    d. Pressure (measure can vary; e.g., mm Hg, cm H_2O, or psi).
13. START device when parameters are set.
14. Observe that infusion is running properly.
15. Remove gloves and wash hands.
16. Check client's infusion site frequently.

In contrast to gravity flow devices, positive-pressure infusion pumps are more accurate in the preselected volume delivery by adding pressure to overcome resistance to fluid flow produced by tubing diameter, filter, viscosity of infusing fluid, cannula, etc. Pumps usually require use of specially designed administration sets. When the system is working with normal resistance, delivery pressure is minimal. When resistance (5 psi over baseline) develops in the catheter or tubing, the pump adds pressure (within limits) to maintain infusion. Changes in resistance at an insertion site due to infiltration or thrombosis may not set off the system's alarm, and site problems could become serious. When the pump's maximum pressure limit is reached, an occlusion pressure alarm sounds. The nurse must become familiar with infusion devices by reading the manufacturer's literature and adhering to all instructions to ensure safe, efficient operation.

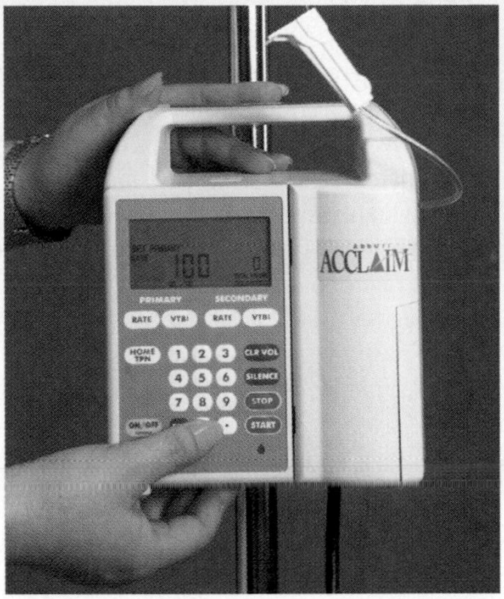

USING A SYRINGE PUMP

Equipment

Battery or electronic operated syringe infusion pump
Pharmacy-prepared and labeled syringe with prescribed medication
Microbore tubing with needleless cannula
Antimicrobial wipe

Procedure

1. Check syringe label with physician's order for drug, dosage, and amount of drug to be delivered over specified time.
2. Assure that medication is compatible with primary infusing solution.
3. Calculate amount of medication to be delivered per minute.

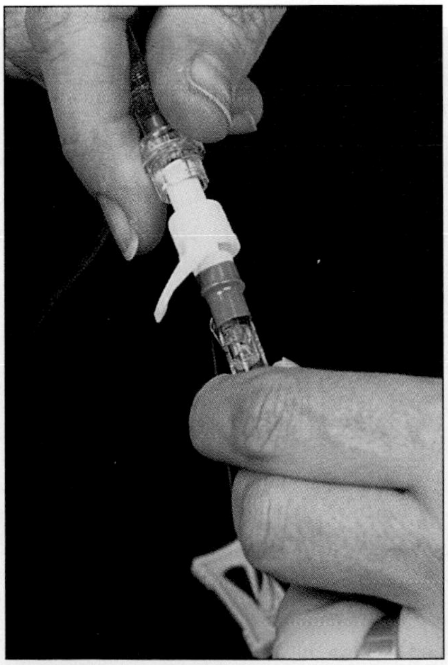
Attach luer access pin to microbore tubing.

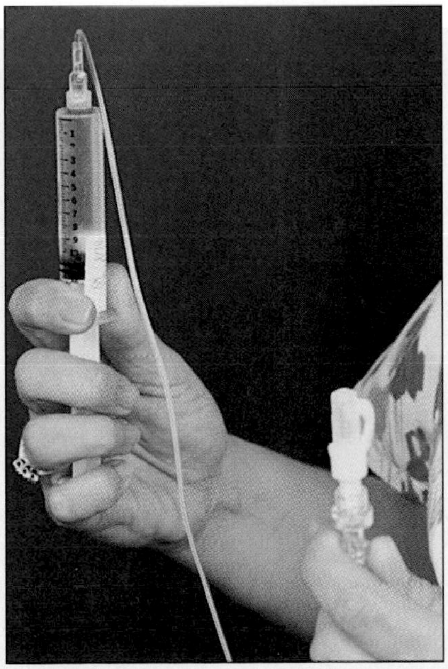
Expel air from syringe before priming tubing.

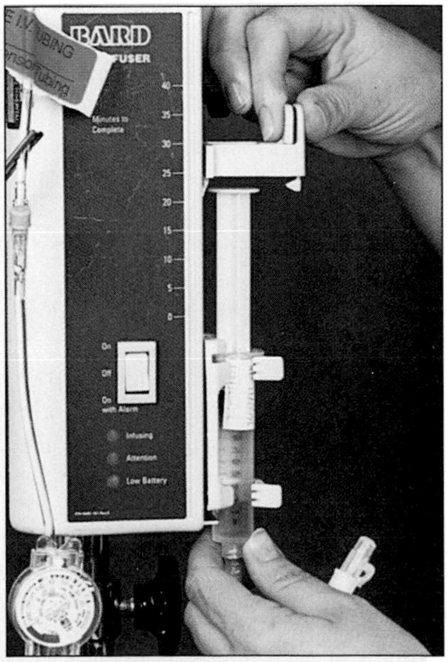

Insert syringe into cradle of pump.

4. Attach microbore tubing to syringe and holding syringe upright, expel air from medication syringe before priming tubing.
5. Holding syringe downward, carefully prime microbore tubing with medication (about 0.5 mL).
6. Insert syringe into cradle of pump, squeezing clamp around designated parts of syringe; attach pusher to plunger.
7. Verify that IV site is free from infiltration or vein irrigation.
8. Swab primary IV tubing port closest to client.
9. Insert microbore cannula into port.
10. Set rate for drug delivery according to pharmacy specifications on syringe label, or as prescribed. Drug will be infused *independent* of the primary infusion rate.
11. Start syringe pump.
12. Check infusion indicator to verify pump is infusing.
13. Monitor site and pump function frequently.
14. For subsequent doses, pharmacy dispenses a new syringe but microbore tubing may be reused for 48–72 hours (according to agency policy). A sterile cap is used each time client's primary tubing is accessed.

Note: For other brands of syringe pumps, follow directions for setup and delivery of meds with their product.

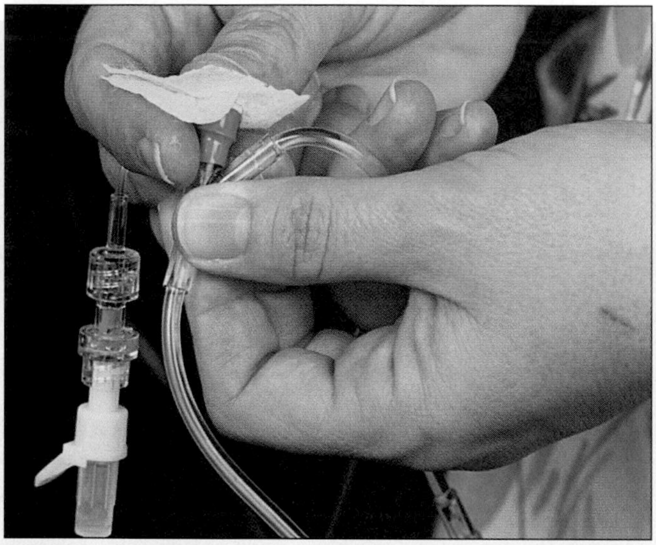

Prep port closest to client before "piggybacking" syringe pump.

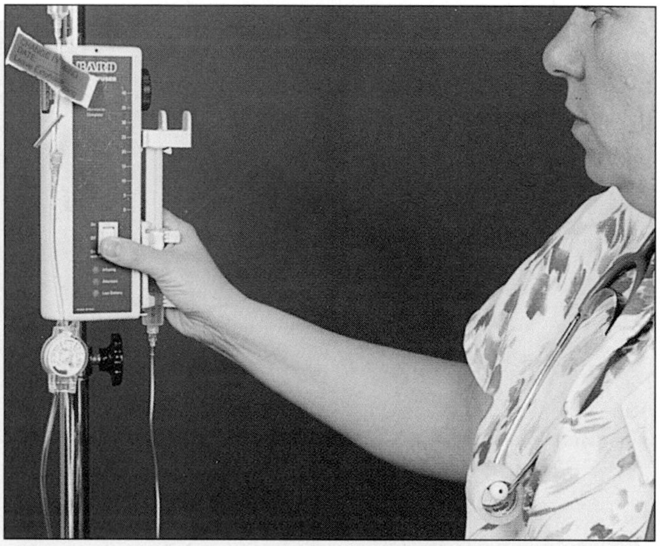

Set infusion rate for drug delivery as prescribed. (Dial-a-flow).

MANAGING THE IV SITE

Procedure

1. Evaluate every 8 hours for site-related complications (Table 28-3).
2. Include gentle palpation through an intact transparent dressing.
3. Remove IV cannula in the periphery, and change to a new more proximal site every 72–96 hours.
4. Assess IV site carefully and frequently if client's status prohibits this change.

CLINICAL ALERT

Clients receiving hypertonic, acidic, or irritating agents, geriatric clients with fragile veins, or pediatric clients who are active are at particular risk for IV site problems.

for IV Administration Sets

1. Change administration sets, including all stopcocks and extension tubings, every 72–96 hours (according to agency policy). This can be done routinely at the same time a new container of IV solution is started.
2. Change IV tubing according to use.
    a. Primary intermittent tubing every 24 hours.
    b. Hyperalimentation every 24 hours.
    c. Secondary infusion tubing every 72–96 hours.
    d. Blood and blood component tubing every 4 hours.
    e. Hemodynamic and arterial pressure monitoring tubing every 96 hours.

CLINICAL ALERT

To check for extravasation, place tourniquet proximal to infusion site tight enough to restrict blood flow through the vein. Set tubing roller clamp to a "keep open" (or slow) rate, and remove tubing from infusion pump. If the infusion continues to drip, fluid is extravasating into the surrounding tissue.

TABLE 28–3 Complications of IV Therapy

Assessment: Signs and Symptoms	Implementation: Nursing Action
Phlebitis	
Pain along the vein, tenderness	Discontinue infusion, and remove needle
Erythema—red streak at vein site	Apply warm compresses
Edema at insertion site	Start IV at another site
	Select a large vein when administering irritating agents
	Anchor cannula to prevent motion in vein
Sluggish flow rate	Do not use positive irrigation with sluggish flow rate—there may be a clot at the end of the needle and it could be flushed into bloodstream
Area is warm to touch	Document description and location of site
Infiltration of fluid	
Edema around insertion site—swelling of cannulated extremity	Discontinue infusion and remove needle
Blanching of infusion site	Apply warm compresses to encourage absorption
Coolness of skin around site	Notify physician if solution contains potassium or other irritating component (e.g., 10% dextrose)
	Do not rely on backflash of blood to determine location of catheter/needle in vein
No backflow of blood when tubing is pinched or fluid container lowered below IV site (tubing must be removed from infusion device)	Lower container below IV site—if blood returns, needle is in vein, *but* fluid may be leaking into tissue if bevel has pierced posterior wall of vein
	Restart IV at another site
Extravasation of medication	
Pain, stinging, or burning at site	Discontinue infusion; attempt to aspirate the drug
Redness and swelling	Apply ice compress to area
	Research the medication—some agents have specific antidotes for extravasation injury
	Notify physician
	Administer irritating or vesicant medications through a central venous device

3. Use separate secondary tubing for each "piggy-backed" agent (do not run an agent through tubing that has been used for a different agent).

for Converting from Continuous IV to a "Lock"

1. Ensure site is patent and functional.
2. Don clean gloves.
3. Clamp infusion tubing.
4. Disconnect IV tubing from catheter.
5. Attach needleless injection cap or primed T connector extension tubing with needleless injection cap to catheter hub.
6. Prep, then inject port with 1 mL sterile normal saline to maintain patency.

for Applying a Transparent Dressing

1. Cover IV insertion site with transparent dressing.
   a. Line up slit in the frame with the catheter hub.
   b. Apply the dressing over insertion site just to top edge of the hub.
   c. Do not stretch the dressing during application.
   d. Firmly smooth down the dressing edges as the frame is slowly removed.

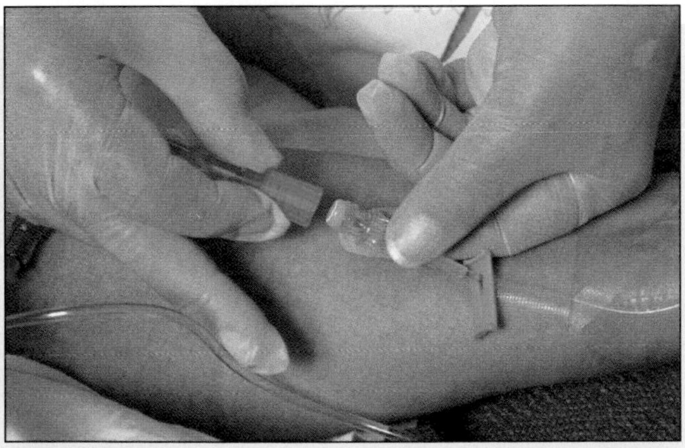

Flush site, then attach needleless cannula into needleless cap.

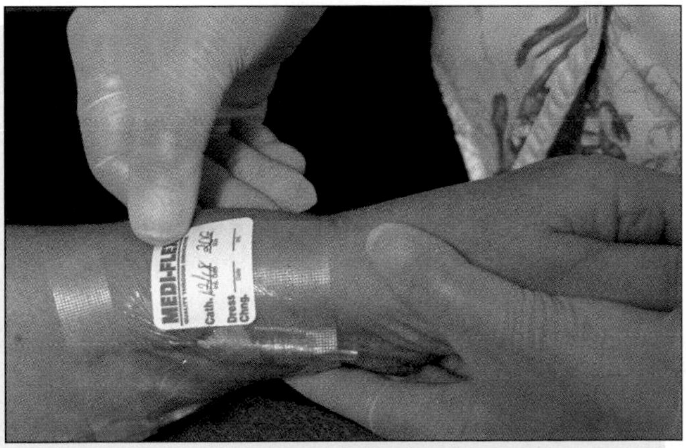

Cover IV site with transparent dressing.

e. Gently pinch and seal the dressing around the catheter hub.
f. Smooth down the entire dressing from the center out to the edges, using firm pressure to enhance adhesion.
2. Document catheter insertion and dressing information.

CLINICAL ALERT

Regard IV systems as closed sterile systems and maintain as such. All entries into the tubing should be made through injection ports that are disinfected just before entry.

Needle-free Devices

Needleless cannula systems are now very available and important for nurses to use because they reduce the risk associated with accidental needle sticks during IV procedures. There are 3 primary types of devices.

1. Blunt Cannula Systems: a rubber injection cap with a slit to accommodate a blunt cannula that attaches to a standard syringe. Accessory products connect the IV set-up to the injection cap. It is used like a heparin lock.
2. One-piece Swabable Adapter: a capless device that opens for fluid flow when a standard syringe or IV set-up is connected. It reseals when the syringe or tubing is removed.
3. Nonswabable Valve System: a special adapter with a reflux valve that opens when the blunt end of a syringe or IV tubing is introduced. When removed, the valve closes and a sterile cap is placed over the end of the adapter.

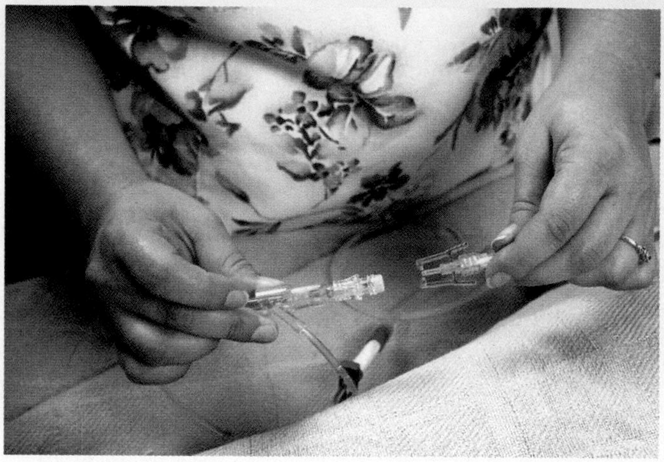

CONVERTING IV TO SALINE LOCK

Equipment

Extension tubing
Lock cannula
Needleless syringe
Clean gloves
Vial of normal saline solution
2 × 2 sterile gauze

Procedure

1. Gather equipment and wash your hands.
2. Assess that IV is infusing and there are no signs of phlebitis or infiltration.
3. Don gloves.
4. Prime extension tubing with normal saline.
5. Turn off IV and disconnect from pump if necessary.
6. Disconnect IV tubing and attach extension tubing to the lock cannula. A 2 × 2 gauze can be placed under IV site to catch drops from IV tubing disconnect.
7. Attach threaded lock cannula to extension tubing.
8. Insert lock cannula into port.
9. Turn threaded cannula until firmly locked in place.
10. Restart IV flow rate. Replace tubing into pump as needed.
11. Redress IV site.
12. Discard equipment.
13. Remove gloves and wash your hands.

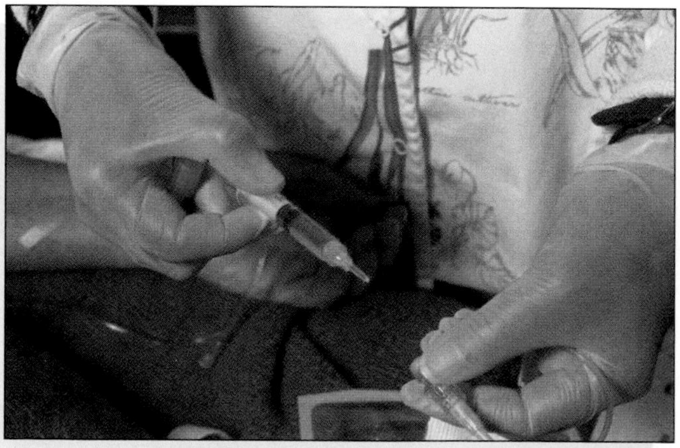

1. Prime extension tubing.

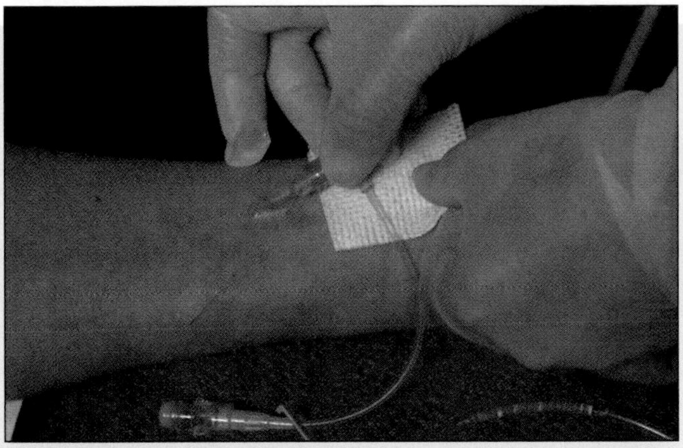

2. Attach extension tubing to IV catheter.

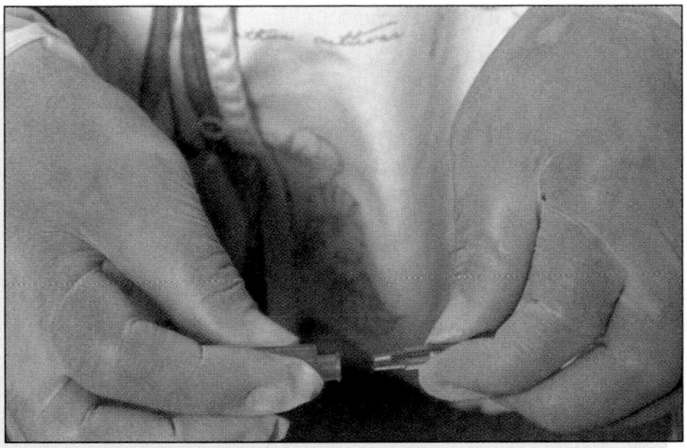

3. Attach IV tubing to threaded lock cannula.

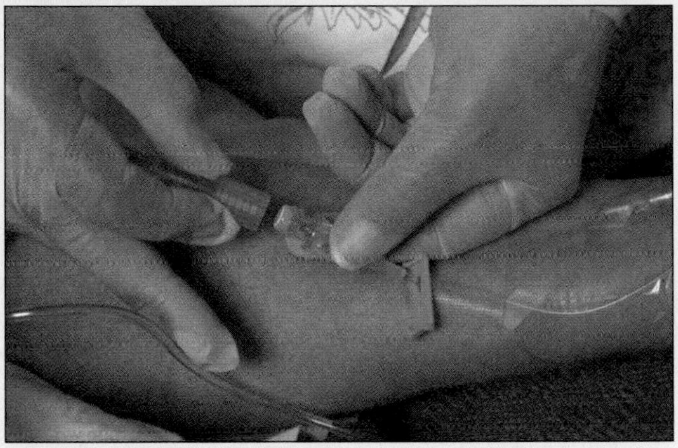

4. Insert threaded lock cannula into port.

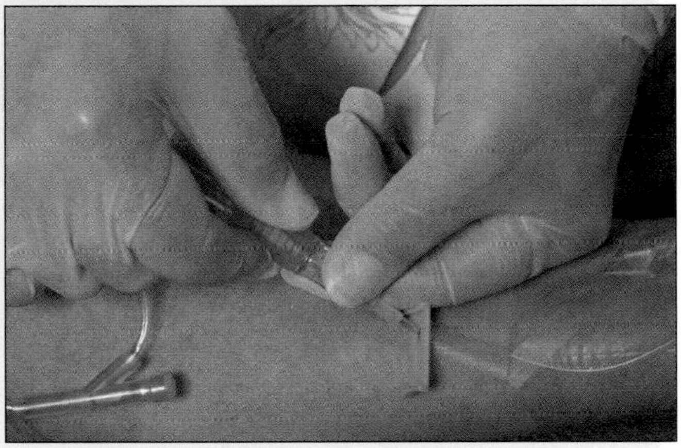

5. Turn threaded cannula firmly.

CHANGING GOWN FOR CLIENT WITH IV

Equipment

Clean gown
Bath blanket
Bathing supplies, if needed

Procedure

1. Check client care plan for infusion drip rate, type of solution, and any special considerations.
2. Wash your hands.
3. Take equipment to client's room.
4. Explain procedure to client.
5. Untie back of gown, and remove gown from unaffected arm. If available, select gown with snap sleeve closure.
6. Support arm with IV and slip gown down arm to IV tubing.
7. Place clean gown over client's chest and abdomen.
8. Use tubing clamp to slow infusion to "keep open" rate and remove tubing from infusion pump if in use.
9. Remove IV bag from hook and slip sleeve over bag, keeping bag above client's arm. **Rationale:** This prevents backflow of blood into tubing. Do not jar or pull tubing. **Rationale:** IV tubing may become dislodged and infiltrate into surrounding tissue.
10. Place your hand up through distal end of clean gown sleeve and grasp IV bag. Pull bag and tubing out through clean gown sleeve.
11. Rehang bag on hook, and check to see that infusion is running according to ordered drip rate.
12. Replace tubing into infusion pump, unclamp and reestablish prescribed infusion flow rate.
13. Guide sleeve of gown up client's arm to shoulder.
14. Assist client to put other arm through remaining sleeve.
15. Tie gown at the back.
16. Check IV infusion rate and IV tubing to determine that solution is flowing unimpeded into client's vein. **Rationale:** Kinks in tubing impede solution flow.
17. Return bed to comfortable position for client, and replace side rails.

18. Remove dirty linen from room.
19. Wash your hands.

Note: Many facilities provide "IV gowns" that snap from the shoulder down the sleeve of the gown for ease in removal without disturbing the IV.

DISCONTINUING AN IV

Equipment

Sterile 2 × 2 gauze pads
Tape
Clean gloves

Procedure

1. Gather equipment.
2. Wash your hands and don gloves.

> **CLINICAL ALERT**
>
> Assess whether client has been receiving antithrombotic (aspirin) or anticoagulant (coumadin, heparin) therapy. Hold pressure for several minutes if client has prolonged bleeding caused by drug therapy.

3. Explain procedure to client.
4. Turn off infusion.
5. Loosen dressing and tape, peeling dressing edges back toward puncture site. **Rationale:** Minimizes trauma to puncture site.
6. Stabilize needle or catheter while removing dressing and tape. **Rationale:** Stabilizing site prevents unnecessary movement that could injure the vein.
7. Hold sterile gauze over site and remove needle/catheter carefully and smoothly, keeping it almost flush with skin. Do not press down on top of needle point while it is in the vein.
8. Quickly press sterile pad over venipuncture site, and hold firmly until bleeding stops.
9. Hold pressure for several minutes if client's drug therapy prolongs bleeding.

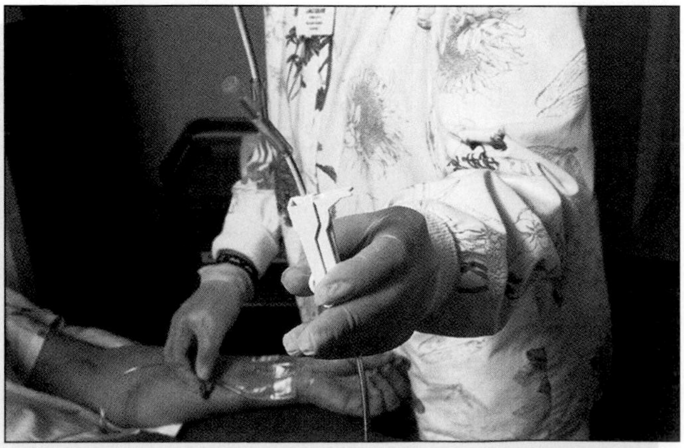

Turn off IV infusion while stabilizing IV site.

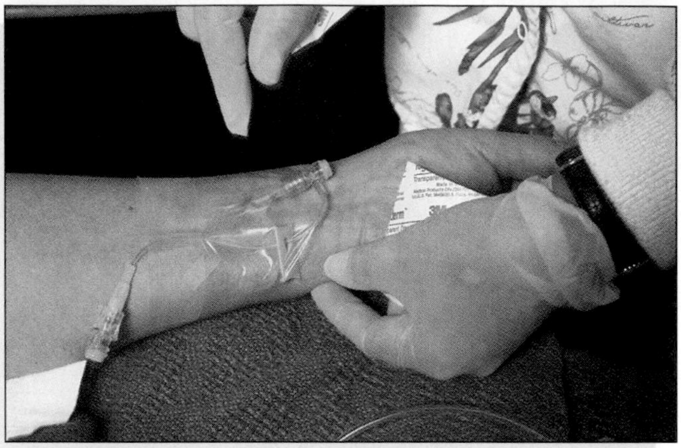

Loosen dressing and tape by peeling dressing edges back toward puncture site.

10. Apply clean pad and tape in place.
11. Elevate arm to reduce venous pressure and help collapse vein to facilitate clot formation. Do not bend arm at elbow. **Rationale:** Bending elbow causes hematoma formation.
12. Observe venipuncture site for redness, swelling, or hematoma.
13. Dispose of equipment and gloves.
14. Wash your hands.
15. Check site again in 15 minutes.
16. Record volume infused on I&O sheet.

Note: If there are signs of infection or inflammation at catheter site or client complains of symptoms related to infection, cut tip of catheter with sterile scissors, place in sterile container, and send to lab for culture.

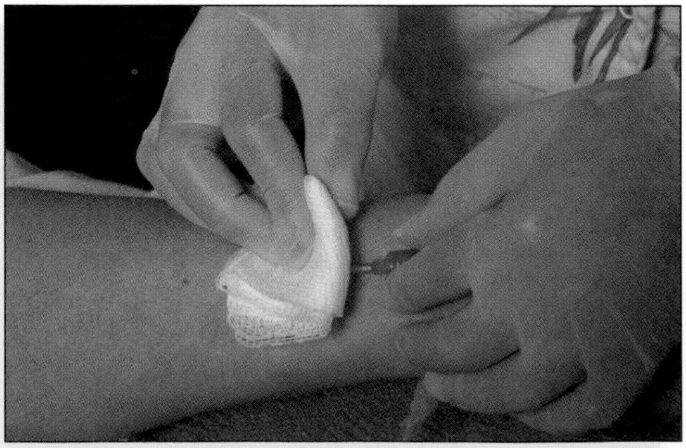

Remove needle/catheter carefully and smoothly, keeping it almost flush with the skin.

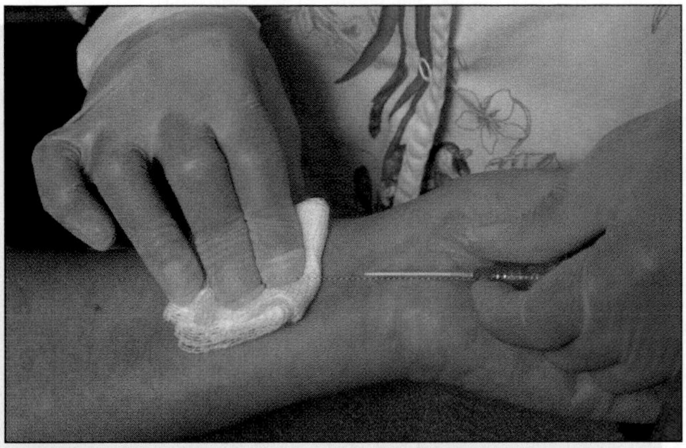

After removing catheter, quickly press sterile pad over insertion site and maintain firm pressure.

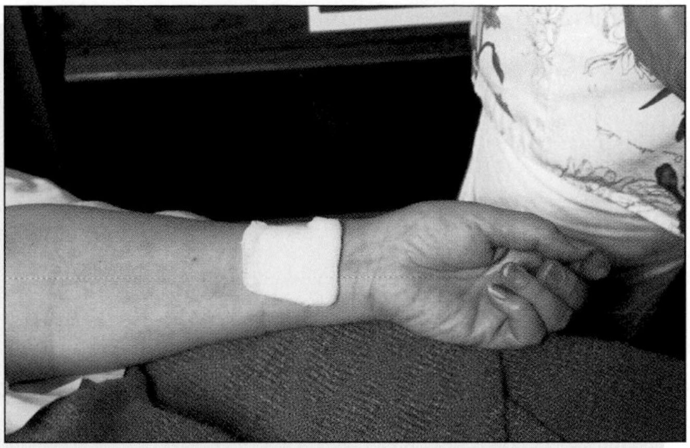

When bleeding ceases, tape sterile pad over insertion site and monitor carefully for oozing or bleeding.

Documentation for Intravenous Management

IV Insertion

- Date and time
- Location of insertion site
- Gauge of needle inserted
- IV solution and flow rate
- Site care given
- Condition of site
- Client response to procedure

IV Discontinued

- Date and time
- Note condition of the catheter—"intact"
- Condition of site
- Client response to procedure
- Catheter tip to lab if appropriate

Critical Thinking Application

UNEXPECTED OUTCOMES	CRITICAL THINKING OPTIONS
Client develops unexplained fever with chills and rising pulse rate.	• Unexplained fever may be associated with catheter-related sepsis. Report to physician. • Ensure that IV solutions hang for no more than 24 hours. • Check client's vital signs: temperature usually above 100°F when caused by IV-related sepsis. • Check for other symptoms of pyrogenic reactions (e.g., backache, headache, malaise, nausea, and vomiting). • Stop the infusion. • Obtain blood specimens, if ordered.
IV solution does not flow properly.	• Ensure that the control clamp is open. • Check that blood pressure readings are not taken on arm in which IV is running, as flow is impeded and a clot can form on the end of the needle. • Ensure that IV administration set is properly loaded. Check pump for flow problem indicator (e.g., cassette seating, air in line). • Check IV tubing from insertion site to IV solution for kinks/obstructions. • Check for extremity causing positional obstruction to flow (e.g., elbow bent, arm rotated).
IV solution appears to be infiltrating resulting in tissue swelling.	• Decrease the flow rate. (Remove from pump for "keep open" rate.) • Lower bag of IV solution; if blood returns, cannula may be in the vein but fluid may be leaking into surrounding tissue via existing puncture in vein wall. • Discontinue infusion and establish a new site.
Phlebitis is suspected at infusion site (tenderness, warmth, erythema, and pain).	• Check infusion solution and medications being administered. (Potassium chloride and hypertonic solutions are particularly irritating to veins.) • Discontinue IV. • Apply warm compress per hospital policy.
Postinfusion phlebitis may also occur after the IV has been discontinued in response to either chemical or mechanical factors of the preexisting IV.	• Check IV solution; hypertonic solution causes irritation necessitating use of large veins and changing IV sites more frequently. • Follow hospital policy for treatment. Warm compresses to the site are generally recommended. • Elevate extremity.

UNIT 3

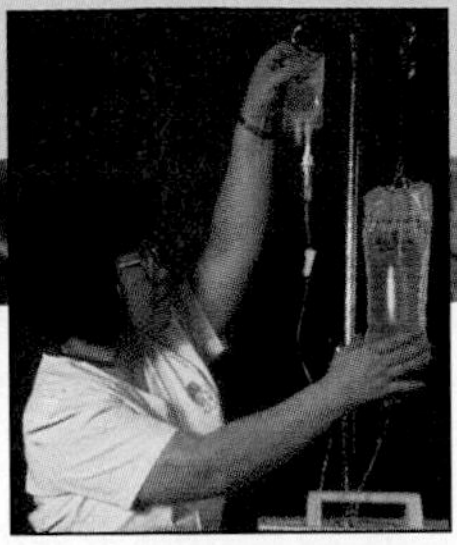

Intake and Output

Nursing Process Data

ASSESSMENT Data Base

Assess client's need for intake and output recording.

Assess client's ability to keep intake and output fluid records.

Evaluate client for any factors that might affect his or her intake and output (e.g., preexisting disease states, concurrent disease, drug therapies, and current physical status).

Determine all measurable sources of fluid intake: fluids with and between meals, tube feeding, liquid medications, IV fluids, and IV medications.

Determine all measurable sources of fluid output: urine, emesis, diarrhea, and drainage sites.

Determine alterations in nonmeasurable sources of fluid intake and loss: food, increased metabolism (e.g., fever), rapid respirations, and perspiration.

Determine balance of daily intake and output.

PLANNING Objectives

To establish a written record of the client's total fluid intake (oral, parenteral, and feeding tubes) and fluid output (urine, wound/tube drainage, diarrhea, and vomiting)

To plan fluid replacement or appropriate therapy by assessing deficits or excesses of fluid and electrolytes

To ensure a fluid intake of at least 1,500–2,000 mL unless contraindicated by diagnosis

To monitor the client's fluid status, vital signs, and mental state to determine homeostasis

IMPLEMENTATION Procedures

Monitoring Intake and Output

Monitoring IV Intake

EVALUATION Expected Outcomes

Intake and output, though not exactly equal, are within 200–300 mL of each other.

Fluid intake is at least 2,000 mL unless contraindicated by diagnosis.

Client's fluid status, vital signs, and mental status are within normal range.

MONITORING INTAKE AND OUTPUT

Equipment

Graduated container in client's bathroom
I&O bedside record sheet (Table 28–6)
Urinal or bedpan; bedside commode or underseat basin for toilet
Hourly in-line urine measurement device for clients requiring frequent monitoring
Posted measurement standards for commonly used drinking and eating utensils (e.g., glasses, mugs, bowls)
Posted signs, dietary slips, and other communication devices to notify hospital personnel about how client's I&O is to be measured

> **CLINICAL ALERT**
>
> Measurement of all fluids is done in milliliters (mLs).

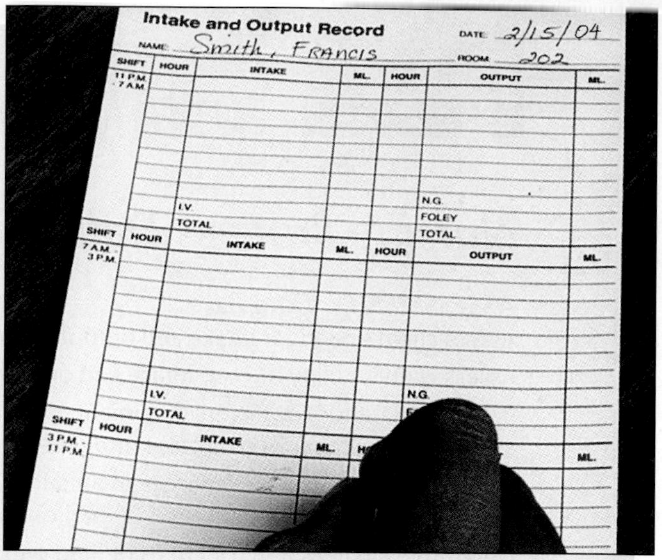

Example of Intake and Output Record.

Procedure

1. Determine if client needs I&O measurements by checking client's chart or care plan. All clients with an IV need I&O measurement.
2. Instruct client and/or family in the need to measure all intake and output.
3. Measure intake from all sources.
   a. Oral fluids.
   b. IV fluids.
   c. Fluid medications (oral or IV).
   d. Tube feedings and water used to clear tubing.
4. Measure output from all sources to establish a record and plan fluid therapy.
   a. Urinary catheters.
   b. Bedpans and urinals.
   c. Nasogastric drainage.
   d. Drainage tubing (e.g., T-tubes, wound, or chest tube).
   e. Diarrheal stools.
   f. Draining wounds.
   g. Emesis.
5. Record I&O on bedside record each time you take a measurement.

TABLE 28–4 Body Sites for Assessment of Fluid Status

Site	Fluid Excess	Fluid Deficit
Head and Neck		
Face	Eyeballs firm or protruding Edema, especially around eyes	Eyeballs soft or sunken Decreased skin turgor over forehead
Mucous Membranes	Excessive salivation Swollen tongue	Dry or sticky mucosa with thick mucous secretions Shrunken tongue with multiple longitudinal furrows Crusted lips
Neck	Jugular vein distention	
Trunk		
Chest	Crackles in lung bases	Decreased skin turgor over sternum Dry, flaking skin
Abdomen	Ascites (measure girth at umbilicus)	
Sacrum	Edema	
Extremities		
Arms	Distended veins Edema, particularly of the hands Delayed capillary refill Pulse bounding	Flattened veins Delayed capillary refill Dry, flaking skin Pulse weak and thready
Legs	Edema Taut shiny skin Peripheral cyanosis	Poor skin turgor, especially across shins Dry, flaky skin, especially on feet Weak pedal pulse or decreased capillary refill

TABLE 28–5 Objective Data Associated with Fluid Status

Data	Fluid Excess	Fluid Deficit
Vital Signs		
Blood Pressure	Increased*	Decreased (especially on standing)
Pulse	Increased rate	Increased rate
Temperature	Unchanged	Elevated
Respirations	Increased rate	Unchanged or increased
Laboratory Findings		
Urine Specific Gravity	Decreased, approaching 1.003	Increased, approaching 1.025 or greater
Blood Hematocrit	Less than three times the hemoglobin	Greater than three times the hemoglobin
Serum Sodium (Na)	Less than 135 mEq/L or normal	Greater than 145 mEq/L or normal
Blood Urea Nitrogen (BUN)	Decreased (except in heart or renal failure)	Proportionately greater than the serum creatinine
Hourly Urine Output	More than 60 mL/hour	Less than 30–60 mL/hour
Weight	A 5% or greater gain	Mild: 2% loss Moderate: 3%–5% loss Severe: 6% or greater loss

*If the heart is unable to pump the increased blood volume, the blood pressure (reflecting cardiac output) may decrease.

Polyuria can also be seen with fluid volume deficit (FVD) as in diabetic states.

6. Correlate intake and output with daily weight. Weight is measured in kilograms (1 pound = 2.2 kg).
7. Record 24-hour totals of I&O on bedside record and place in client's chart.
8. Notify physician of any significant imbalance; more intensive monitoring may be indicated. **Rationale:** Hourly urine output less than 25–30 mL/hour for two consecutive hours or 24-hour urine output less than 500 mL can indicate dehydration or internal bleeding and can result in acute renal failure.

CLINICAL ALERT

Check all drainage receptacles such as Foley bag and NG cannister at the beginning of each shift to ensure they were emptied from the previous shift and that there has not been excessive drainage.

Fluid Replacement Solutions

Hypertonic Solutions—a solution with higher osmolality than blood serum

- Solution causes cells to shrink
- Used in severe salt depletion (very rare)
- Used as nutrient source (10% dextrose)
- Examples of solutions: saline solutions greater than 0.9% (e.g., 3% saline), which can be very dangerous; 10% dextrose in normal saline, D 10% water, D 5% ½NS

Hypotonic Solutions—a solution with lower osmolality than blood serum

- Hydrates cells, causes them to expand
- Used to correct dehydration
- Examples of solutions: hypotonic saline solutions (e.g., 0.45% NaCl, 0.02% NaCl, or 5% dextrose combined with hypotonic saline)

Isotonic Solutions—a solution with the same osmolality as blood serum

- Cells remain unchanged
- Used for replacement or maintenance (expands extracellular volume). Especially used to expand circulating (intravascular) volume.
- Examples of solutions: Lactated Ringer's, 5% dextrose in normal saline (0.9%); 0.9% saline, Ringer's, D .5% water, D .5% ¼NS

Note: One liter of normal saline (0.9% NaCl) meets the usual daily requirement of these electrolytes in an adult.

TABLE 28–6 Intake and Output Flow Sheet

Date	Time	IV No.	IV Started	Description	IV Intake	Oral Intake	Urine Output	Other	N/G
1/9/04	9 A			Full liquid breakfast		620			
	9:45 A			Vomitus				400	
	10:30 A	#1	1000						
	12 N						450		
	2:30 P						400		
				7–3 Total	500	620	850	400	100
	6:30 P	#2	1000						
	9 P						500		
				3–11 Total	1000	NPO	500		350
1/10/04	2:30 A	#3	1000		450				
	5 A						350		
				11–7 Total	1000	NPO	350		375
				24-hour Total	2500	620	1700	400	825

MONITORING IV INTAKE

Equipment

Electronic infusion device
I&O record
Graphic sheet
IV container marked with timed intervals

Procedure

1. Place I&O record at bedside.
2. Determine time interval required for monitoring IV intake.
3. Mark time intervals on IV container according to facility policy (use tape to mark, or use preprinted time strips).
4. Set IV drip rate according to physician's orders.
5. Observe IV container and read IV solution level.
6. Record amount of IV solution infused at prescribed time (e.g., every hour, every shift).
7. If using electronic infusion device, push "total volume infused" for shift amount, then "clear."
8. Record total IV intake on I&O record at end of each shift.
9. Record 24-hour IV total at midnight. Take into account all sources of IV fluid (all IV sites, IV medications).

(For complete I&O Procedure, see Chapter 21.)

DOCUMENTATION FOR INTAKE AND OUTPUT

- Time, amount, and description of all measurable I&O
- Approximate volume of loss when unable to measure contents (e.g., incontinent of urine in bed)
- Dietary intake (food that liquefies at room temperature, as well as liquids)
- 8-hour and 24-hour totals
- Signs and symptoms of client's fluid status, including vital signs, mucous membranes, daily weight, etc.

Note: I&O records are frequently inaccurate due to numerous possibilities for error, estimation being a common source of inaccuracy. It is important to maintain these records accurately.

Critical Thinking Application

UNEXPECTED OUTCOMES	CRITICAL THINKING OPTIONS
Recorded I&O do not balance.	• Emphasize importance of accurate measures to client and family. • Identify possible nonmeasurable sources of I or O. • Report to charge nurse so she can assure that all nurses are keeping accurate records. • Check if client or family can help with keeping the I&O record. • Check the addition on the I&O record to see if an error was made. • Correlate I&O imbalance with weight changes.
Client unable to maintain an intake of at least 1500 mL/day.	• Ensure that fluid restriction is not ordered. • Offer fluids in small amounts more frequently. • Determine client's fluid preferences. • Assess client's ability to use a straw (hemiplegic client is often unable to suck through a straw). • Check if client is able to drink fluids independently or if assistance is needed. • Ensure that adequate fluids are accessible at the bedside for the client. • Do not administer fluids with a bulb syringe. • Address client's toileting needs q 2 hours—some clients restrict their fluid intake for fear of incontinence. • Use a thickening additive to liquids to facilitate swallowing for the client with aspiration precautions.
IV fluids not maintained at appropriate rate to provide adequate intake.	• Monitor IV fluid intake hourly. • Observe IV site for complications. • Restart IV immediately when infiltrated to ensure continuous IV fluid intake. • Document IV fluid intake every shift. • Account for interruption of primary infusion and the delivery of intermittent infusions of medications. • Check accuracy of IV administration equipment: electronic device, dial-a-flow, etc.

UNIT 4

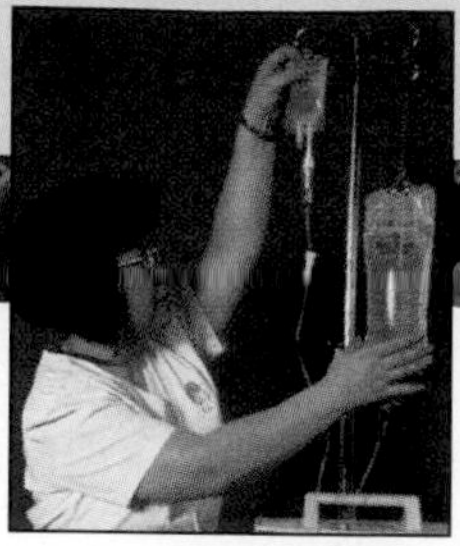

IV Medication Administration

Nursing Process Data

ASSESSMENT *Data Base*

Note client's allergies.

Note any drug or solution incompatibilities.

Assess amount and type of diluent needed to prepare medications.

Assess client's general status to establish a baseline for administering medications.

Assess patency of infusion set and condition of IV insertion site.

PLANNING *Objectives*

To maintain a therapeutic level of medication in the client's bloodstream

To administer medication safely over a specific period of time

To prevent complications associated with medication administration

IMPLEMENTATION *Procedures*

Adding Medication to IV Solution

Using a Secondary ("Piggyback") Bag

Using a Volume Control Set

Using a Peripheral Saline Lock

Administering Medications by Peripheral IV Line Injection "Push"

EVALUATION *Expected Outcomes*

Solutions from additive bottles or bags infuse without difficulty.

Therapeutic blood level of medication is maintained.

Complications of medication administration are prevented.

Medication is infused over appropriate time span.

ADDING MEDICATION TO IV SOLUTION

Equipment

IV solution bag
Syringe with medication
Antimicrobial swab
Label with medication dosage, date, time, and initials

> **CLINICAL ALERT**
>
> Only under unusual circumstances will the nurse be asked to compound a medication with parenteral solution. Refer to the policy and procedure manual to determine which medications can be added by the nurse.

Procedure

1. Check physician's orders, MAR, and agency policy.

Note: The addition (admixture) of medication to an IV solution for continuous administration is usually performed by the pharmacist, according to standards established by the American Society of Health System Pharmacists (ASHP) and Occupational Safety and Health Administration (OSHA). Special precautions for this procedure include preparation in a laminar airflow environment, strict adherence to requirements of asepsis, safety regarding components' stability and compatibility, proper dilution of agents, and control of extraneous particle addition to the admixture.

2. Wash hands.
3. Gather equipment.
4. Draw up medication into syringe according to directions on medication insert (or PDR).
5. Check to ensure that prescribed drug is compatible with IV solution.
6. Wipe injection port on IV bag with antimicrobial swab.
7. Inject medication into bag while maintaining aseptic technique.
8. Squeeze injection port.
9. Mix IV solution and medication by gently agitating bag to mix thoroughly.

> **CLINICAL ALERT**
>
> Some drugs that are incompatible with saline solution include diazepam (Valium), chlordiazepoxide hydrochloride (Librium), and amphotericin B.

10. Affix medication label to IV bag.
11. Hold bag against both dark and light backgrounds to inspect for any precipitate.
12. Insert IV tubing into bag, and proceed with appropriate method or administration as ordered.

USING A SECONDARY ("PIGGYBACK") BAG

Equipment

Primary IV set, consisting of compatible IV solution bag and IV administration set with injection port
Short secondary administration set with needleless cannula and extension hook or lowering hanger for primary bottle (if indicated)
Pharmacy-prepared medication bag with label, including name of medication, date, time, rate for infusion, and client's name
Antimicrobial swab

Preparation

1. Check medication with physician's orders and MAR.
2. Wash hands.
3. Gather equipment.
4. Check client's room number and clients identaband.

Procedure

1. Ensure medication compatibility with primary infusing solution.

Note: If medication is incompatible with primary IV solution, temporarily discontinue primary infusion. Flush client's injection port, initiate a normal saline (or other compatible) solution as the primary, then proceed with "piggyback" into the "new" compatible primary. When complete, restart original primary solution (use new needleless cannula to access client's injection site).

2. Spike bag with secondary administration set. Affix needleless cannula to end of secondary tubing.
3. Cleanse injection port of primary tubing with antimicrobial swab.
4. Insert needleless cannula of secondary "piggyback" tubing into primary tubing port (port above pump).

Note: If using the same tubing from a previous administration, change needleless cannula prior to inserting into primary tubing.

5. Hang the secondary bag on the IV pole.
6. Use extension hook to lower primary bag below secondary

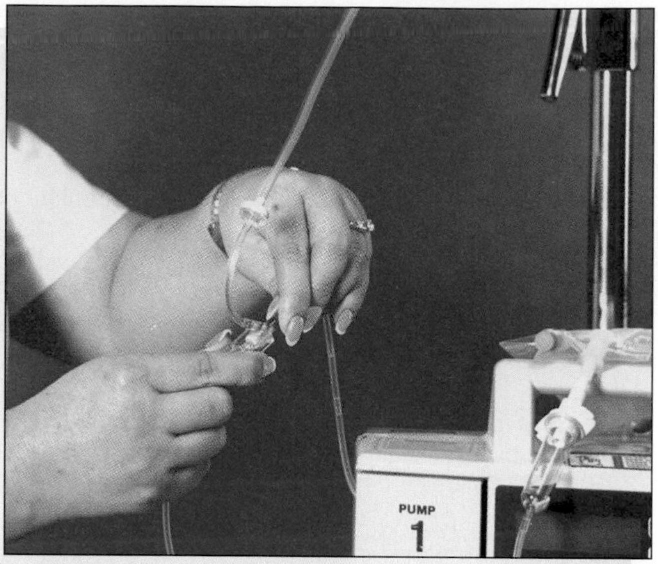

Insert needleless cannula of secondary tubing into distal primary tubing port.

bag if indicated (some infusion devices do not require this). **Rationale:** Primary solution ceases flow because of increased hydrostatic pressure in higher secondary bag.

7. Clear tubing of medication bag by opening clamp, temporarily placing secondary bag lower than the primary solution bag, and allowing primary solution to flow retrograde into secondary bag tubing (back-priming).

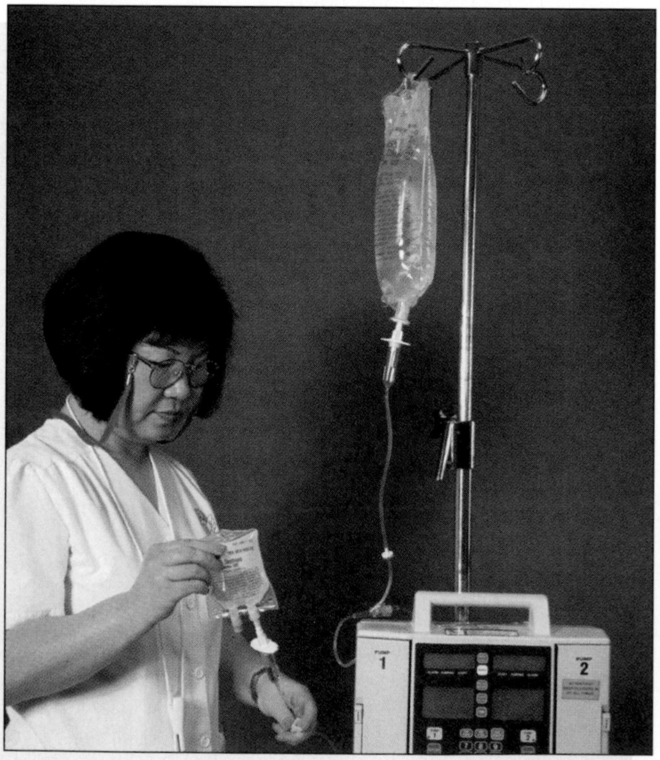

Lower medication bag to clear tubing and back-prime tubing.

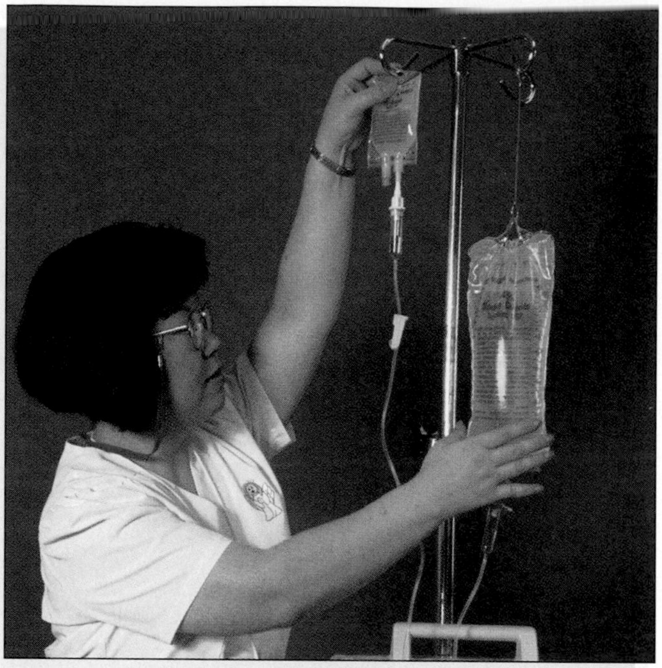

Hang secondary bag on IV pole; lower primary bag.

8. Backfill until secondary tubing chamber is ⅓ full. Clamp secondary tubing. **Rationale:** This ensures that no medication is lost during priming.
9. Program secondary settings into infusion device if used.

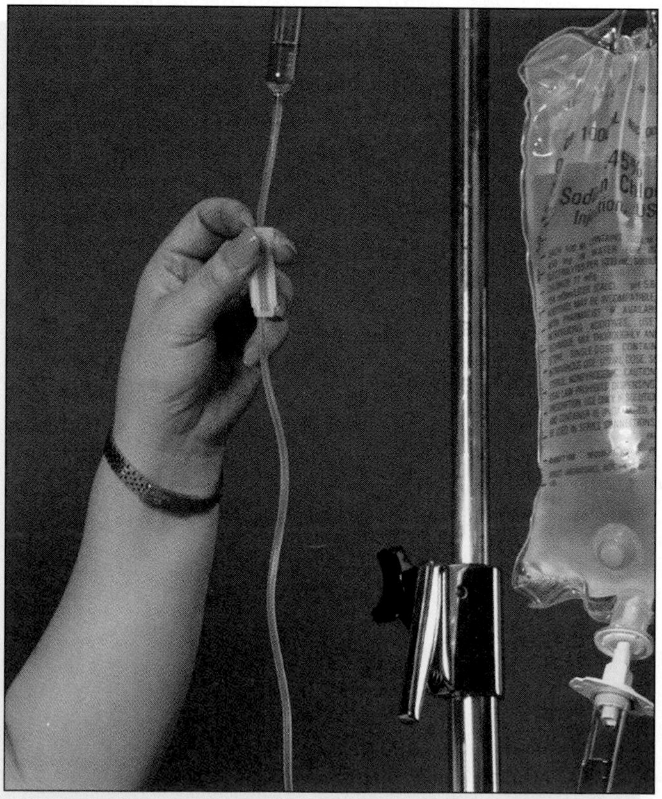

Unclamp secondary tubing.

10. Open clamp on secondary bag tubing. The secondary solution should begin to flow.
11. Check that primary infusion resumes at its "set" rate when secondary volume has been infused.

Note: Some infusion devices control secondary infusions without necessitating bag height differentials.

12. When secondary bag is empty, readjust rate of administration in primary solution to desired flow (unless infusion device controls this).
13. To add a new secondary bag, assure that medication is the same as previously administered since some drug remains in the secondary tubing. A *different* medication requires its own secondary tubing. **Rationale:** This prevents admixture of potentially incompatible drugs.
14. Remove old secondary bag, and spike new "piggyback" medication bag.
15. Lower partial-fill bag below injection port of primary IV.
16. Open clamp on secondary tubing, and allow solution from primary IV set to enter tubing, backfilling the tubing to drip chamber. **Rationale:** This procedure displaces air in the secondary tubing.
17. Replace new secondary bag on IV pole, and proceed with administration.
18. Change secondary tubing every 48 hours.

Using a Mini-Infuser Pump

A mini-infuser pump is a tandem device that allows a small amount of medication to be given (5–60 mL) as a controlled infusion.

- The prefilled syringe is added to the battery-operated mini-infuser and connected to the main IV line.
- A needleless system is the recommended connection to the primary IV line, although a stopcock or port may be used.
- The infusion pump is hung with the primary IV bag and activated by an ON button.
- Following infusion of medication, the primary infusion automatically begins to flow as the pump stops.
- The primary infusion should be checked and the flow regulated when the mini-infusion pump stops.

USING A VOLUME CONTROL SET

Equipment

Primary IV set (IV solution bag and IV administration set)
Calibrated volume control set
Medication prepared in syringe
Antimicrobial swab
Label with medication, date, time, and nurse's initials

Preparation

1. Check physician's orders and MAR.
2. Check client's room number and client's identaband.
3. Determine compatibility of medication with primary infusion.
4. Wash hands.

Procedure

1. Add extension tubing to volume control set if needed and close clamps on volume control set, both above and below volume chamber.
2. Open air vent by turning clamp located on top of volume chamber.
3. Spike IV bag with volume control set, and then hang bag. Attach IV tubing to volume control set.
4. Open upper clamp (between the bag and volume chamber), and fill chamber with IV solution so that chamber is one-third full.
5. Close upper clamp.
6. Open lower clamp, and squeeze drip chamber (located underneath the volume chamber) until it is one-half full.

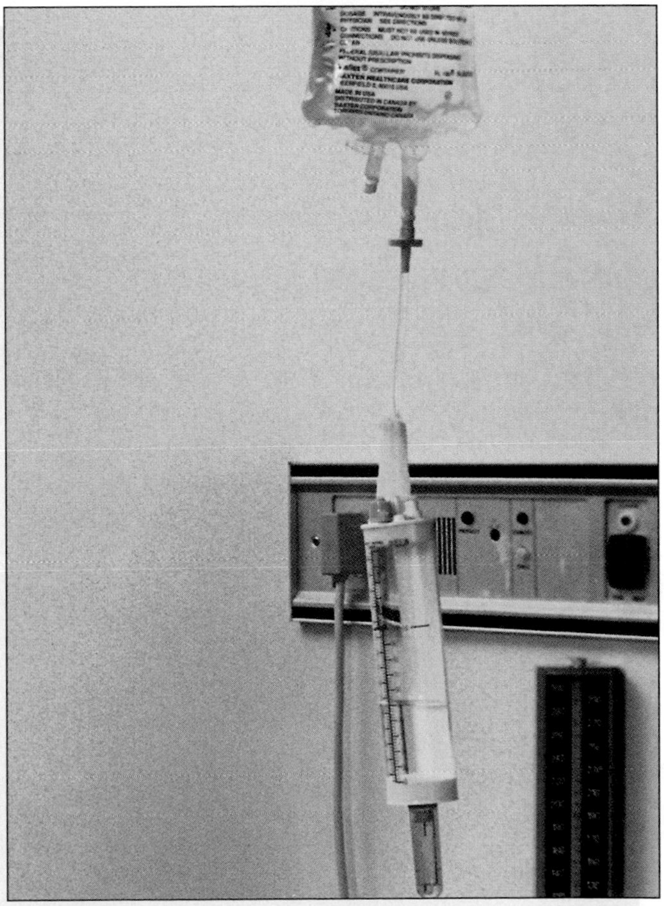

Add extension tubing, if necessary.

7. Allow solution to flow down tubing.
8. Prime tubing and cannula affixed to end of tubing. If volume control set has membrane filter instead of floating valve filter, follow manufacturer's instructions for priming so that you do not damage the filter.
9. Close clamp.

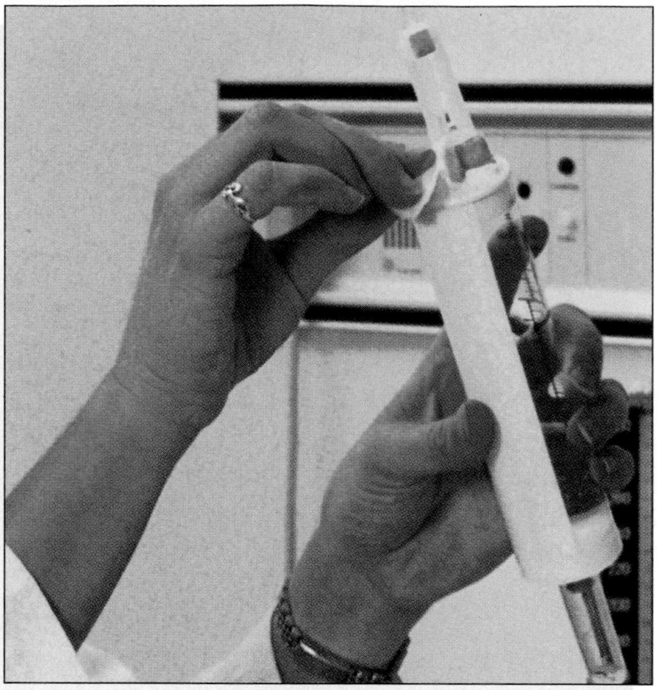

Swab injection port before infusing medication.

10. Swab off injection port (located on top of the volume chamber) with antimicrobial swab.
11. Inject prepared medication into chamber, and agitate gently to mix medication with solution in chamber.
12. Dilute medication, if necessary, by opening upper clamp and adding additional fluid from the IV bag.
13. Open clamp on volume control set and adjust drip rate to desired rate of administration.
14. Place medication label on volume control set. Include client's name, medication, dose, and time medication infusion began.

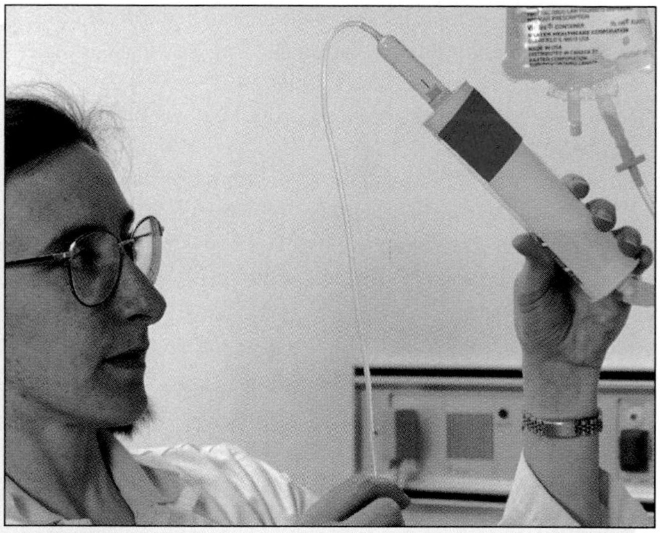

After instilling medication, gently mix with solution in volume control chamber.

USING A PERIPHERAL SALINE LOCK

Equipment

Needleless injection cap with primed extension tubing and port (if one is not in place)
Needleless cannula
Syringe for medication and diluent (if indicated)
2 normal saline prefilled syringes (1 mL each)
Antimicrobial swab
Clean gloves
Stethoscope and sphygmomanometer (if indicated)

Preparation

1. Check physician's orders and MAR.
2. Gather equipment.
3. Wash your hands and don gloves.
4. Check client identaband and ask client to state name.
5. If client does not have peripheral lock in place, proceed with venipuncture, selecting veins that are both large enough to receive the medication and away from areas of movement (e.g., the elbows and wrists).

Procedure

1. Prepare medication with appropriate diluent according to manufacturer's instruction for IV injection and draw it up into syringe. (See drug insert or PDR.)
2. Fill two syringes, each with 1 mL of normal saline.
3. Explain procedure to client.

CLINICAL ALERT

There is no significant difference in using NS or heparin for patency with phlebitis, or to maintain dwell time. Some hospitals however, still use a small amount of dilute heparin for flushing peripheral locks; it is usually prepared with 1 mL heparin (1000 U/mL) added to 9 mL normal saline to produce 100 U/mL solution. Caution should be exercised because heparin-induced thrombocytopenia can occur with as little as 500 U of heparin/day.

4. Check client's vital signs if agent to be given has hemodynamic effects.
5. Prep needleless injection port with antimicrobial swab.
6. Insert first saline syringe into port, briefly aspirate to check patency, then flush system and note for site swelling. **Rationale:** Presence of blood and absence of swelling at site indicate that needle is probably in vein, not in surrounding tissue.
7. Insert medication syringe into port, and inject medication into vein, timing injection administration rate according to drug manufacturer's instruction (see insert or PDR).
8. Observe client for any adverse reactions.
9. Remove medication syringe.
10. Flush with second saline syringe to clear line and maintain patency of lock.
11. Dispose of equipment and gloves and wash hands.
12. Recheck client's vital signs if indicated.

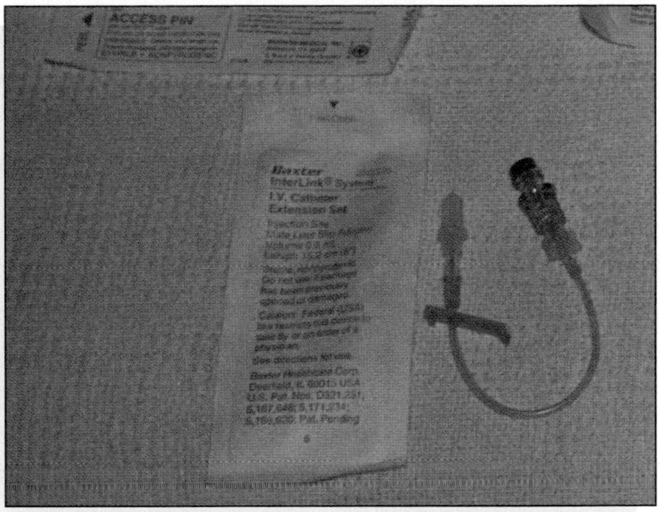
IV extension tubing with saline lock.

ADMINISTERING MEDICATIONS BY PERIPHERAL IV LINE INJECTION "PUSH"

Equipment

Medication prepared in syringe with needleless cannula, according to pharmaceutical instruction for IV *injection*
Antimicrobial swab
Clean gloves
Stethoscope and sphygmomanometer (if indicated by drug action)

> **CLINICAL ALERT**
>
> If drug is irritating, validate intravenous line placement. Place a tourniquet proximal to primary infusion; slow drip rate and remove tubing from pump. Assure that infusion SLOWS or STOPS before injecting the IV medication. This action validates intravenous status of infusion. Blood flashback is not a reliable indicator of such.

Preparation

1. Check physician's orders and MAR.
2. Gather equipment.
3. Wash your hands.
4. Prepare medication according to pharmaceutical company's instructions for IV *injection* in drug insert or PDR.
5. Check insert for drug's compatibility with primary infusing solution. **Rationale:** Flushing the primary infusion tubing will be necessary both before and after administering the drug if incompatibility exists. Alternatively, a secondary "piggyback" bag of normal saline can be hung and used for flushing the primary line during the drug injection.
6. Check medication according to the *Six Rights.*
7. Take medication to client's bedside.
8. Check that client is not allergic to the drug.
9. Don clean gloves.

Procedure

1. Check client's identaband and ask him or her to state name.
2. Obtain vital signs if agent to be given has hemodynamic effects.
3. Prep primary tubing injection port closest to client.

> **CLINICAL ALERT**
>
> In contrast to IV "push," an IV bolus of a drug is rapidly injected in order to achieve an immediate desired drug level—usually for emergency situations. Always refer to pharmaceutical company's instructions for *IV drug injection* before administering.

4. Insert medication syringe cannula into line port.
5. Pinch primary tubing between port and infusion bag while injecting medication slowly in calculated increments (e.g., inject ¼ of medication over a 20-second period).
6. After injecting small increments, unpinch primary tubing to allow flushing of medication.
7. Observe client for any adverse effects.
8. Deliver next increment, using your watch and timing drug injection according to the drug insert instructions.
9. Withdraw cannula when medication injection is complete.
10. Discard equipment.
11. Remove gloves and wash hands.
12. Recheck client's vital signs if indicated.

DOCUMENTATION FOR IV MEDICATIONS

- Amount of medication administered
- Method of drug administration
- Flush (e.g., NS) if indicated for compatibility
- IV site status
- Client's response to medication

Critical Thinking Application

UNEXPECTED OUTCOMES	CRITICAL THINKING OPTIONS
Secondary bag solution does not infuse adequately.	• Check that primary IV bag is lower than secondary bag (if infusion device requires). • Ensure that cannula is positioned properly in the primary injection port and secondary bag is sufficiently spiked. • Check that the roller clamp of the secondary tubing is open fully.
Solution in primary IV tubing is incompatible with medication to be administered via secondary "piggyback."	• Prior to administering medication, flush primary tubing with solution compatible with medication (e.g., normal saline, 5% D/W). • Hang a separate solution compatible with medication and run through line to flush during drug administration.
Solution does not infuse through peripheral lock.	• Gently turn lock to establish flow. • Reposition client's extremity. • Initiate a new IV site.

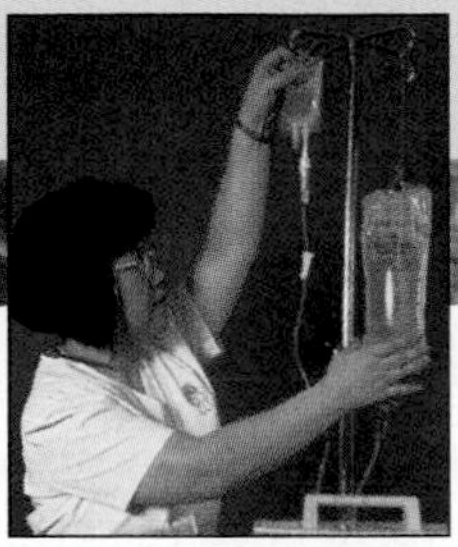

Blood Transfusions

Nursing Process Data

ASSESSMENT Data Base

Assess that client has signed informed consent for transfusion.

Assess if client has an established IV site.

Assess client's vital signs, especially temperature, for baseline data.

Assure that client's number and blood type on unit match client's blood ID bracelet name and number before administration to ensure compatibility. (Validate consistency with another nurse.)

PLANNING Objectives

To provide blood or blood components (e.g., platelets, fresh frozen plasma) for clients with a demonstrated deficiency

To ensure compatibility between client's blood and the blood or blood component to be transfused

To prevent the infusion of microaggregates or leukocytes

To prevent febrile reaction to the transfusion

To monitor and ensure a timely transfusion

To monitor for potential complications during and following the blood transfusion

IMPLEMENTATION Procedures

Administering Blood through a Y-Set

Administering Blood through a Straight Line

Administering Blood Components

Monitoring for Potential Complications

EVALUATION Expected Outcomes

Transfusion of blood is performed in a timely manner.

Client's blood deficiency is corrected.

Transfusion reaction does not occur.

ADMINISTERING BLOOD THROUGH A Y-SET

Equipment

Blood unit (packed RBCs)

Note: Few conditions require the transfusion of whole blood. Most whole blood is used to prepare separate components to meet specific client needs (e.g., RBCs, plasma, platelets).

250 mL bag of normal saline
Y-set blood tubing with filter
Venipuncture supplies if client does not have established site
Needleless injection cap (if not in place)
Needleless cannula
Antimicrobial swabs
Tape
Infusion pump (optional)
Clean gloves

Preparation

1. Check physician's order for number and type of transfusion units (order must dictate "transfusion").

> **CLINICAL ALERT**
>
> In emergency situations, when time does not allow ABO determination, group O red blood cells may be given. *Whole blood*, however, **must** be administered ABO identical. Few conditions require transfusion of whole blood.

2. Check client's room number, identaband, and have client state name.
3. Explain procedure to client and check that client has signed consent form for transfusion.
4. Check that type and crossmatch has been completed and that blood is ready in blood bank.
5. Determine patency of client's IV. Begin infusion of NS with appropriate blood tubing.
6. Obtain client's pretransfusion vital signs. **Rationale:** If client has temperature above 100°F (37.8°C), physician must be notified before proceeding.
7. Obtain ordered typed and matched blood component bag from blood bank, or notify blood bank to deliver unit (according to agency policy). Both nurse and lab tech check transfusion number and sign transfusion form.

> **CLINICAL ALERT**
>
> ALWAYS determine patency of the IV line prior to obtaining blood from the blood bank.

> **Warming Blood for Transfusion**
>
> Routine transfusions are not usually warmed. Warming is required in massive transfusions, or more commonly, may be ordered in maternity or the postanesthesia care unit. A blood-warming device is used. Never warm blood bag in hot water or microwave. Once blood is warmed, it must be used or disposed of, as it cannot be returned to the blood bank. Hemolysis of the blood occurs at temperatures above 104°F.

8. With another nurse, validate that client's blood ID bracelet number matches blood bank number on unit of blood to be transfused. Client MUST have a blood ID bracelet. **Rationale:** If client does not have a blood ID bracelet, return blood product to the blood bank.
9. Validate that client's name, ID number, and blood group/Rh match the blood unit data, and note expiration date.
10. Record client's vital signs on transfusion tag 5 minutes prior to starting, 15 minutes after starting, every 30 minutes until transfusion is completed (1 – 1½ hours), and immediately following the transfusion.

Note: Check hospital policy and procedure for Blood Administration to determine frequency of vital signs as facility may require more frequent monitoring.

Determine hospital policy and obtain informed consent for transfusion.

11. Remember that blood cannot be returned to the blood bank after it has been checked out for 20 minutes.
12. Check blood bag for bubbles, cloudiness, dark color, or sediment. **Rationale:** These signs indicate bacterial contamination.
13. Wash your hands and don clean gloves.

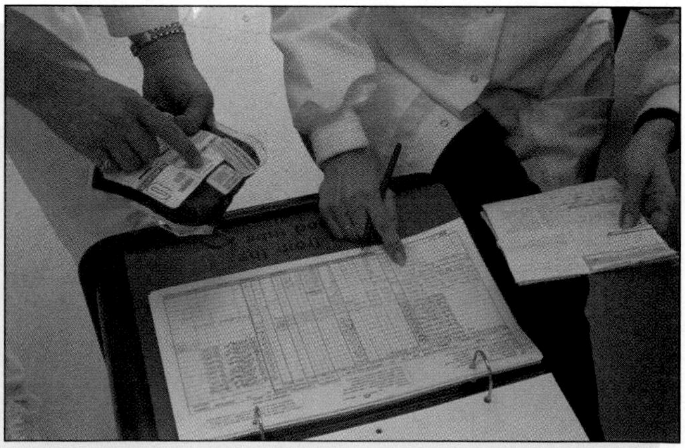

Obtain ordered typed and matched blood/component bag from blood bank.

Procedure

1. Close all clamps on the Y-set tubing.
2. Spike bag of normal saline with one arm of the Y-tubing.
3. Open clamps on both arms of the Y-tubing to flush.
4. Close clamp on free arm of Y-set (blood side) and open clamp below tubing filter to prime main tubing.
5. Close main clamp when tubing is primed and attach needleless cannula.
6. Close clamps.
7. Gently agitate blood unit bag. **Rationale:** Agitation suspends the red cells in the anticoagulant.
8. Pull back tabs on blood unit bag, and expose port.
9. Spike blood bag port with free arm of Y-tubing, then hang unit.
10. Prep client's injection port.
11. Insert cannula into injection port.
12. Load tubing into infusion pump.
13. Open clamp to blood bag.
14. Start blood infusion, administering slowly (25–50 mL of blood) for first 5–15 minutes (rate 100 mL/hr). **Rationale:** Slow administration allows time to observe for adverse reactions. Most reactions occur in the first 15 minutes.

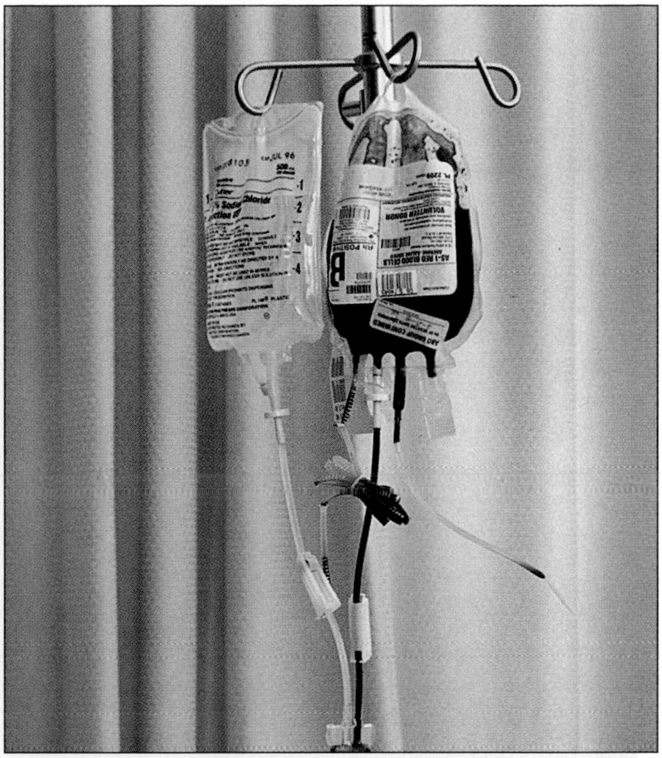

Prime blood administration Y-set tubing with sterile normal saline before starting infusion.

CLINICAL ALERT

Most clients can tolerate a flow rate of one unit of packed cells in 1½–2 hours.

CLINICAL ALERT

Blood must be hung within 20–30 minutes after taking it from blood bank. Usually only 1 unit of blood is dispensed at a time.

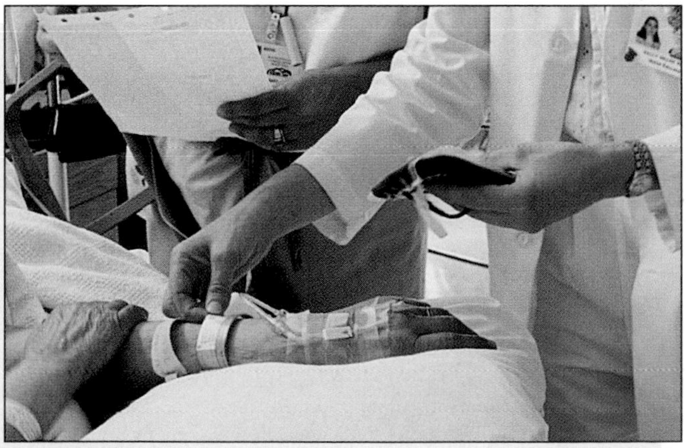

Ascertain that client's name, ID number, and hospital number match number on tag on the blood bag.

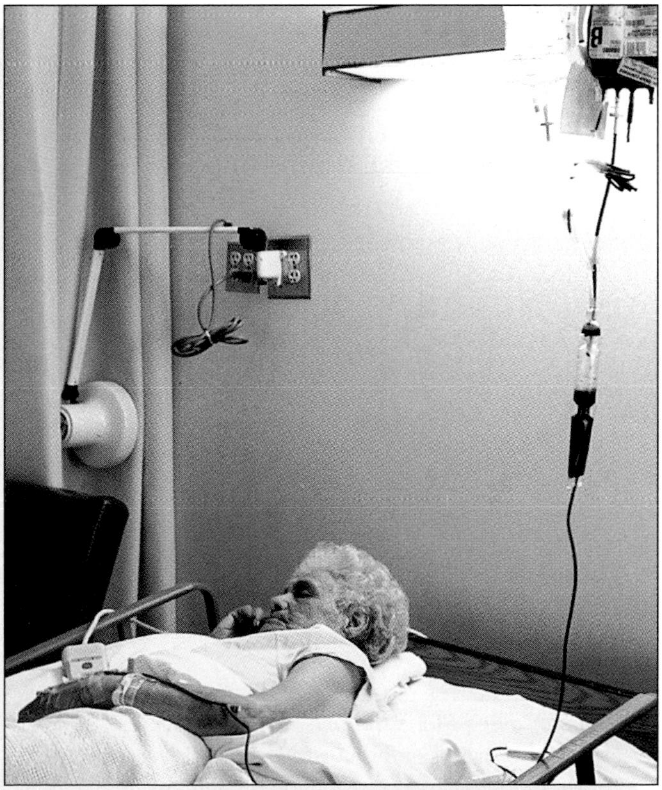

Observe client carefully for first 15 minutes and frequently throughout the blood transfusion.

15. Take vital signs 5 minutes, 15 minutes, and every 30 minutes after starting transfusion and record on Transfusion Log record.
16. Observe client closely for adverse signs: chilling, backache, headache, nausea or vomiting, tachycardia, tachypnea, respiratory distress, skin rash, itching, or hypotension.
17. Agitate blood bag each time the client is checked.
18. If venous spasm occurs with cold blood infusion, apply warm pack to site to improve flow rate.
19. Complete the blood transfusion in less than 4 hours. **Rationale:** Blood deteriorates rapidly after a 2-hour exposure to room temperature and increases risk of bacterial infection.
20. Check that transfusion is completed, then flush line with normal saline.
21. Obtain posttransfusion vital signs.
22. Report a 1°C (2°F) rise in temperature to the physician. **Rationale:** This could be indicative of a transfusion reaction.
23. Complete documentation on the Transfusion Tag: place one copy on client's chart and send remaining copy of the Transfusion Tag to the Blood Bank as soon as transfusion is completed.

Note: Administration set should be changed after each unit, or at the end of four hours to reduce risk of bacterial contamination. Most standard filters are designed to filter 2–4 units of blood.

24. Discard administration set within 4 hours of use.
25. Place all transfusion-related equipment in a biohazard waste receptacle.
26. Remove gloves and wash hands.
27. Continue to observe client for 1 hour.

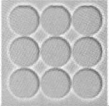

CULTURAL COMPETENCE

Religion and Use of Blood and Blood Products

It is important to know client's religious beliefs about the use of blood and blood products in order to understand their preferences in choosing to allow or not allow transfusions.

- Clients who practice as Christian Science (Church of Christ, Scientist) usually do not accept use of blood or blood products in their medical care.
- Clients who are Jehovah's Witnesses believe blood in any form and agents in which blood is an ingredient is not acceptable. Blood volume expanders are acceptable if they are not derived from blood. Mechanical devices for circulating blood are acceptable as long as they are not primed with blood initially. Their religious belief is based on scripture references and precedents in the history of Christianity. There are times when court orders are obtained for children in life-threatening situations so they may receive blood or blood products.

ADMINISTERING BLOOD THROUGH A STRAIGHT LINE

Equipment

Blood unit

Blood administration straight-line set with 170-μ filter microaggregate or leukocyte-depleting filter

Needleless cannula

Electronic infusion device (optional)

Clean gloves

Procedure

1. Obtain and check blood as stated in *Preparation for Administering Blood through a Y-Set.*
2. Wash your hands and don gloves.
3. Spike blood bag port carefully and hang unit.
4. Gently agitate unit, and suspend.
5. Open clamp and fill drip chamber, making sure filter is totally submerged in the blood.
6. Open clamp on tubing and run blood through tubing, then clamp.
7. Place needleless cannula on end of tubing.
8. Load tubing into infusion pump if used.
9. Carefully connect blood tubing to client's IV site catheter or lock.
10. Begin blood transfusion.
11. Observe client closely for first 5–15, and every 30 minutes.
12. Obtain pre-, intra-, and post-transfusion vital signs.
13. When blood bag is empty, close all clamps and remove blood tubing cannula from IV site.
14. Dispose of equipment in biohazard waste receptacle.
15. Remove gloves and wash your hands.
16. Continue to observe client for one hour.

Blood Transfusion Protocol

The nurse is responsible for early assessment of possible transfusion reactions by completing the following interventions.

- Identify client and blood bag.
  Identaband number matches transfusion record number.
  Name spelled correctly on transfusion record.
  Blood bag number and pilot tube number are the same.
  Blood type matches on transfusion record and blood bag.
- Check blood with an RN before infusing.
- Ask client about allergy history, and report any previous blood reactions.
- Establish baseline vital sign data.
- Start transfusion slowly to observe for severe reactions.
- Maintain aseptic technique during procedure.
- Observe time rules for administering blood. (Hang no longer than 4 hours.)
- Observe blood bag for bubbles, cloudiness, dark color, or black sediment, which is indicative of bacterial invasion.

ADMINISTERING BLOOD COMPONENTS

Equipment

Blood component
Appropriate IV administration set
Clean gloves

Procedure

1. Check physician's orders and client's signed consent for transfusion.
2. Obtain blood component from blood bank.
3. Obtain appropriate administration set.
4. Wash hands and don gloves.
5. Read directions for proper administration of the solution.
6. Identify rate at which blood component should infuse.
7. Check Table 28–8 for appropriate rate, risk factors, and possible complications.

Modified Blood Products

In addition to the usual blood components such as platelets and cryoprecipitate, modified blood products are becoming more popular. Washed, irradiated, or leukocyte-removed blood is being used for clients at risk because of multiple transfusions or a weakened immune system. Testing for cytomegalovirus and matching RBC or human leukocyte antigens is also done to ensure safe transfusions.

CLINICAL ALERT

When infusing a blood product that has undergone leukocyte reduction it still must be filtered again through a standard blood administration set in order to trap cellular debris that may have accumulated since the original filtration.

MONITORING FOR POTENTIAL COMPLICATIONS

Equipment

Sphygmomanometer
Stethoscope
Thermometer

Procedure

1. Check temperature, blood pressure, pulse, and respiration before transfusion is started.
2. Check vital signs every 5–15, and every 30 minutes for the first 100 mL after transfusion has started. **Rationale:** Most blood transfusion reactions occur during this time.
3. Maintain vital sign assessment throughout blood infusion according to hospital policy.
4. Monitor client for possible transfusion reactions.
   a. Hemolytic or incompatibility reaction—most severe reaction
   b. Bacterial contamination
   c. Allergic reaction
5. If any severe untoward sign occurs (increase in temperature, pain in kidney region), STOP transfusion immediately.
6. Remove blood and any blood-filled tubing, and replace with saline bag and new tubing to keep line open. Return blood bag and administration set to blood bank or laboratory.
7. Notify physician immediately after stopping IV for signs of transfusion reaction. Also notify physician if any unusual sign (itching or hives) occurs.

TABLE 28–7 Transfusion Reactions

Type	Clinical Manifestations	Nursing Interventions
Bacterial	Sudden increase in temperature Hypotension Dry, flushed skin Abdominal pain Headache Lumbar pain Sudden chill	Stop transfusion immediately and remove blood tubing. Maintain IV site; change tubing and start infusion of normal saline. Observe for shock. Monitor vital signs every 15 minutes. Insert Foley catheter and monitor urine output hourly. Notify physician and obtain order for antibiotic and steroids/shock management. Draw blood cultures before antibiotic administration. Send remaining blood and tubing to laboratory for culture and sensitivity.
Allergic	Mild: urticaria and hives, pruritus Severe: respiratory distress, wheezing Anaphylactic reaction: shock, loss of consciousness	Stop transfusion immediately if symptoms are severe—immediate resuscitation may be necessary. Monitor vital signs for possible anaphylactic shock. If symptoms are mild, stop transfusion or follow hospital policy and obtain physician's orders. Monitor for signs of progressive allergic reaction as transfusion continues.
Hemolytic	Severe pain in kidney region and chest Pain at needle insertion site Fever (may reach 105°F), chills, flushing Dyspnea and cyanosis Oozing of blood at IV site Headache Hypotension Hematuria Nausea	Stop transfusion immediately and remove blood tubing. Start normal saline infusion at "keep open" rate with a new IV tubing. Obtain vital signs. Notify blood bank STAT. Administer oxygen. Notify physician. Obtain orders for IV volume expansion and diuretic or vasopressor to dilate renal blood vessels to prevent acute renal tubular necrosis. Complete transfusion reaction form. Send two blood samples (from different sites), urine specimen, remaining blood and tubing, and transfusion record to laboratory. Monitor vital signs every 15 minutes for shock. Monitor urine output hourly for possible acute renal failure.

TABLE 28–8 Blood Component Therapy

Type	Use	Alerts	Administration Equipment
Fresh plasma	To replace deficient coagulation factors To increase intravascular compartment	Hepatitis is a risk Administer as rapidly as possible Use within 6 hours	Any straight-line administration set
Platelets	To prevent or treat bleeding problems, especially in surgical clients To replace platelets in clients with acquired or inherited deficiencies (thrombocytopenia, aplastic anemia) To replace when platelets drop below 20,000 mL/mm (normal 150,000–350,000 mL/mm)	Administer at rate of 10 minutes a unit (usually comes in multiple platelet packs)	Platelet transfusion set with special filter to allow platelets to infuse through filter
Granulocytes	To treat oncology clients with severe bone marrow depression and progressive infections To treat granulocytopenic clients with infections that are unresponsive to antibiotics To treat clients with gram-negative bacteremia or infections where marrow recovery does not develop	Administer slowly, over 2–4 hours Give one transfusion daily until granulocytes increase or infection clears Use within 48 hours after drawn Observe for shaking, fever, chills Observe for hives and laryngeal edema (treat with antihistamines)	Use Y-type blood filters and prime with physiologic saline. A microaggregate filter is not used as it filters out platelets
Serum albumin	To treat shock To treat hypoproteinemia	Available as 5% or 25% solution Infuse 25% solution slowly 1 mL/minute to prevent circulatory overload Administer 100–200 mL (25% solution) for shock clients and 200–300 mL for hypoproteinemia	Special tubing accompanies albumin solution in individual boxes
Gamma globulin	To treat agammaglobulinemia To act as a prophylaxis for hepatitis exposure	Pooled plasma contains antibodies to infectious agents Administer 0.25–0.50 mL of immune serum globulin/kg of body weight every 2–4 weeks	Given IM
Coagulation factors	To treat clients with von Willebrand's disease	Made from fresh-frozen plasma	Standard syringe or component drip set only
Factor VIII (cryoprecipitate)	To treat clients with factor VIII, hemophilia A	Administer one unit cryoprecipitate for each 6 kg of body weight initially, followed by 1 U/3 kg of body weight at 6–12-hour intervals until treatment discontinued Administer 1 unit/5 minutes Observe for febrile reactions	
Factor IX	To treat clients with factor IX, hemophilia B	Administer in 12–24-hour cycle Preparation for administration is 400–500 U/vial. Must reconstitute in 10–20 mL diluent One unit/pound of body weight increases the circulating factor activity by 5% Serum hepatitis can be transmitted	Any straight-line set—drip or by IV push—not to exceed 10 mL/min

DOCUMENTATION FOR BLOOD TRANSFUSIONS

- Type, unit number, and amount of blood administered
- Amount of normal saline used
- Time transfusion began and ended
- Vital signs before transfusion begins; 5, 15, 30, and 60 minutes after infusion begins; and then hourly until infusion completed (check hospital blood administration policy and procedure for vital sign frequency)
- Transfusion tag may have space for vital sign information as well
- Client's response to procedure
- Any unusual clinical manifestations; any nursing interventions

Critical Thinking Application

UNEXPECTED OUTCOMES	CRITICAL THINKING OPTIONS
Transfusion reaction or nursing alert conditions occur.	• Stop blood administration. • Check transfusion reaction form for appropriate nursing intervention. • Complete all relevant nursing actions.
Blood does not flow through tubing.	• Check client's IV site. • Gently agitate blood bag to mix blood cells with the anticoagulant. • Raise blood bag higher on IV pole. Squeeze flexible tubing to promote blood flow. • Adjust clamp on tubing. As the blood passes over the filter, more blood microaggregates clog the filter and slow drip rate. • Replace tubing. • Utilize an infusion pump, especially if administering blood through a small catheter or lock.
Blood has been hanging for more than 4 hours.	• Take down blood bag, and send to laboratory. • Maintain IV with normal saline or ordered IV solution. • Monitor vital signs for complications.
Potential circulatory overload occurs.	• Monitor symptoms: sudden dyspnea, tachypnea, tachycardia, chest discomfort, distended neck veins, moist crackles and rales, restlessness, sudden increase in blood pressure. • Stop transfusion and place client in Fowler's position. • Start oxygen at 2 L/min per nasal cannula. • Be prepared for ECG and chest x-ray. • Be prepared to administer Lasix and MS.

GERONTOLOGIC CONSIDERATIONS

Elderly clients' veins are fragile and roll easily, and frequently the needle punctures the wall of the vessel.

- Insert small-gauge winged catheter in distal vein first to preserve proximal vessel.
- Tourniquet may not be necessary for venipuncture. If used, it should be applied loosely.
- If used, release tourniquet as soon as venipuncture yields blood return to prevent excessive pressure in vein.
- Maintain close assessment of IV sites to promote long-term use of vessel.

Elderly clients are prone to fluid and electrolyte disorders as a result of the normal aging process.

- Thirst mechanism is decreased.
- Renal threshold is altered.
- Total body fluid is less due to decreased lean muscle mass.
- Fluid replacement therapy requires close monitoring to prevent fluid overload, leading to pulmonary edema and electrolyte imbalance.
- Dehydration is a common reason for IV therapy.
- When infusing IV fluids, monitor closely for signs of fluid volume overload.
- Monitor BUN and electrolytes regularly for signs of overload.
- Use IV pump whenever infusing fluids into elderly clients. If dextrose solution is being infused, IV pumps *must* be used. Dextrose overload can lead to cerebral edema if infused too rapidly.

Stabilizing IV catheter and dressing is problematic due to client's fragile skin.

- Avoid excessive use of tape.
- Apply skin protector solution before dressing site.
- Use stretch mesh gauze to cover site and tubing to prevent catching on bed (avoid roll-type gauze).

Protect fragile skin that is more susceptible to injury, infiltration, and discomfort from irritating drugs.

- Observe IV site carefully for signs of infiltration. Because of skin's loose folds and decreased tactile sensation, a large amount of fluid can sequester in subcutaneous tissue and go unnoticed before client complains of pain.
- Check IV site frequently when client is receiving drugs that can cause irritation and even necrosis if they infiltrate.
- At first sign of phlebitis or infiltration, remove IV and restart in a new site.
- If client complains of discomfort during IV therapy, apply a moist and warm pack to site, decrease rate of fluid infusion.

MANAGEMENT GUIDELINES

Each state legislates a Nurse Practice Act for RNs and LVN/LPNs. Health care facilities are responsible for establishing and implementing policies and procedures that conform to their state's regulations. Verify the regulations and role parameters for each health care worker in your facility.

Delegation of Responsibilities

- Each state identifies the scope of practice for RNs and LPN/LVNs. Several states have identified that the LPN/LVN has a specific role in IV therapy, but the scope of practice is always dictated by each agency (e.g., initiating, regulating, discontinuing IVs).
- Daily weighing of clients is usually assigned to the CNA or UAP. The RN should verify that weights are taken in the morning before breakfast, using the same scale each time. The client should urinate before weighing for accuracy. Since a client's weight changes are frequently taken into consideration for prescribing fluid allowances or medication adjustments, accuracy in measurement and documentation is imperative.
- All care providers must be aware of clients whose intake and output is monitored and must conscientiously participate in accurate measurement.
- All care providers must be aware of clients for whom fluid restriction is ordered, and carefully adhere to designated allowances.

- CNAs and UAPs report vital data to the professional nurse by monitoring vital signs. This skill can be delegated for the pre-, intra-, and post-blood transfusion, and results should be given immediately to the nurse. The professional nurse then validates and acts upon any abnormal findings accordingly.
- The CNA/UAP providing personal hygiene must understand that the IV system is a closed one and must be able to give care without disrupting this system. The components of the system must never be disconnected for the convenience of care (e.g., changing gown). The CNA/UAP should receive training in changing the client's gown without disrupting the IV system.
- It is the nurse's responsibility to monitor and document intravenous fluid volume administered.
- It is the nurse's responsibility to evaluate the client's total balance of intake and output and to investigate significant imbalances for further decision making.
- While the professional nurse monitors the IV infusion site regularly, the CNA must communicate observations of swelling, client reports of concern (e.g., pain), and infusion device signals that prompt the professional to further assess the client.

Information Flow

- All care providers participate in accurate recording of the client's intake and output. Records are usually kept at the bedside. All must be familiar with the standard capacities for frequently used vessels (bowls, cups) to facilitate accurate recording of intake.
- Likewise, careful recording of measurable output and best estimation of unmeasurable losses (e.g., incontinence) will facilitate care decisions.
- The nurse must ensure that CNA/UAPs know to *report* any unusual fluid loss the client is experiencing (e.g., vomiting). It is the nurse's responsibility to *evaluate* alterations in fluid loss (e.g., vomiting, scant urine output) and act upon these findings accordingly. Knowledge and judgment cannot be delegated.
- It is the nurse's responsibility to document vital client information on the Transfusion Tag record, which is placed into the client's hospital chart.

CRITICAL THINKING STRATEGIES

SCENARIO 1

Mrs. Beatty is a 40-year-old client, 5′1″ tall and weighing 300 lbs. She had emergency abdominal surgery for lysis of adhesions. You are assigned to care for her on her first postoperative day. As you begin your assessment, you note she has an NG tube that is draining bile-colored returns. Her IV is D5% in .45NS infusing at 125 mL/hr. The IV is on a pump. As you observe the IV site, you find it difficult to determine if the site is edematous or it is just her normal appearance. It seems like the area surrounding the site is cooler to the touch than the remaining part of the arm. Mrs. Beatty states the IV area is sore. A gauze dressing is placed directly over the IV site, making it difficult to visualize it. The IV fluid seems to be infusing at the prescribed amount and the IV pump alarm is not ringing.

1. What is your priority action in this situation?
2. After completing the first priority, what is your second priority?
3. While assessing the IV site, what would you look for if you suspect phlebitis or infiltration? With the initial information provided in the scenario, which of these potential complications do you suspect? Provide rationale for your answer.
4. How will you check the IV to determine if the client does have an infiltration?
5. Indicate your priority intervention if you determine the client has an IV that has infiltrated.
6. Indicate your priority intervention if you determine the client has beginning signs of phlebitis.

CHAPTER 29

Central Vascular Access Devices

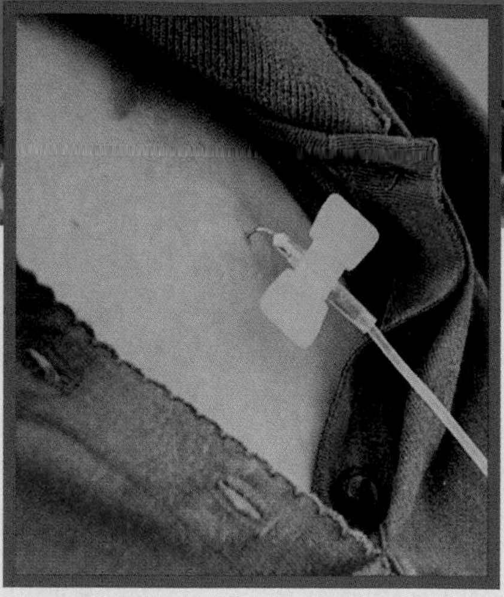

THEORETICAL CONCEPTS

UNIT ONE: Percutaneous Central Vascular Catheters 1049

- Assisting with Percutaneous Central Vascular Catheterization 1050
- Changing a Central Line Catheter Dressing 1051
- Infusing IV Fluids Through a Central Line 1053
- Drawing Blood from Central Line Catheter 1055
- Applying a BIOPATCH 1057
- Changing an Access Cap 1058
- Measuring and Monitoring Central Venous Pressure (CVP) 1059

UNIT TWO: Total Parenteral Nutrition/Total Nutrient Admixture 1063

- Assisting with Catheter Insertion 1064
- Maintaining Hyperalimentation Infusions (TPN) 1066
- Changing Hyperalimentation (TPN) Dressing and Tubing 1067
- Maintaining Hyperalimentation for Children 1068

UNIT THREE: Lipid Emulsion Therapy 1070

- Infusing IV Lipids 1071

UNIT FOUR: Tunneled Central Vascular Access Devices (CVADs) 1074

- Maintaining the Hickman or Broviac CV Catheter 1075
- Changing the Hickman or Broviac CV Catheter Dressing 1076
- Maintaining the CV Catheter with Groshong Valve 1076
- Drawing Blood from the CV Catheter with Groshong Valve 1078

UNIT FIVE: Implanted Subcutaneous Port 1080

- Accessing and Flushing an Implanted Port Using a Huber Needle 1081
- Administering Drugs via a Subcutaneous Implanted Port 1082
- Administering Infusions via a Subcutaneous Port 1083
- Drawing Blood from an Implanted Subcutaneous Port 1084

UNIT SIX: Peripherally Inserted Central Catheter (PICC) 1086

- Maintaining the PICC 1087
- Changing the PICC Dressing 1088
- Drawing Blood from the PICC 1090
- Removing the PICC 1090

GERONTOLOGIC CONSIDERATIONS 1092

MANAGEMENT GUIDELINES 1092

CRITICAL THINKING STRATEGIES 1094

LEARNING OBJECTIVES

- Identify the common types of central vascular access devices (CVADs).
- Discuss the rationale for using central vascular catheters for long-term IV therapy.
- Discuss the special needs of clients with central vascular catheters (prevention of infection, air embolism).
- Explain the nurse's responsibility for assisting the physician with a percutaneous central vascular catheter insertion.
- Compare and contrast features of various central vascular access devices.
- Describe initiation and discontinuation of infusions via CVADs.
- Differentiate protocols for maintaining patency of intermittently used CVADs.
- Outline steps for dressing and protecting the CVAD insertion site.
- Discuss the advantage of using a BIOPATCH at the catheter insertion site.
- Outline the steps in changing an access cap.

TERMINOLOGY

Antimicrobic: preventing the development of pathogenic action of microbes.

Aspirate: application of negative pressure to check for blood return.

Calorie: the amount of heat necessary to raise the temperature of 1 kilogram of water 1° C. One thousand (1 kcal) of these calories equals 1 dietary calorie (or calorie).

Carbohydrates: a group of chemical substances, including sugars, glycogen, starches, dextrins, and celluloses, that contain only carbon, oxygen and hydrogen.

Cardio: word part that pertains to the heart.

Cardiovascular: term that pertains to the heart and blood vessels, as cardiovascular system.

Central vascular access device (CVAD): catheter, centrally placed in the superior vena cava, to provide medication, fluid, and nutrition.

Central venous pressure (CVP) measurement: monitors central venous return (volume) and right ventricular function.

Cyanosis: slightly bluish, grayish, slatelike, or dark purple discoloration due to desaturation of hemoglobin.

Digestion: the process by which food is broken down mechanically and chemically in the gastrointestinal tract.

Dyspnea: a subjective feeling of difficulty breathing.

Electrolyte: substance that develops an electrical charge when dissolved in water.

Erythema: redness of the skin produced by capillary congestion as in a sunburn.

Extracellular: fluid outside the cell (interstitial and intravascular fluid).

Fat: substance made up of carbon, hydrogen, and oxygen, occurring naturally in most foods but especially in meats and dairy products.

Gastrointestinal: term that pertains to the stomach and intestines.

Hemo: prefix meaning blood.

Hemodynamic: study of circulation of blood.

Hemolytic: pertinent to the breaking down of red blood cells.

Huber needle: a right-angled (90°) or straight, noncoring needle.

Hydrostatic: the pressure exerted on liquids.

Hyperalimentation: the process of nourishing the body through parenteral means.

Hyperglycemia: condition characterized by an increase in blood glucose levels.

Hypertonic: solution having a higher osmotic pressure or tonicity than a solution to which it is compared.

Hypovolemia: diminished circulating fluid volume.

Implanted: inserted under the skin.

Implanted infusion port: device placed in subcutaneous tissue with a tunneled catheter that goes into the central venous system.

Infusion: a liquid substance introduced into the body via a vein for therapeutic purposes.

Intracellular: fluid inside the cell.

Intravascular: within blood vessels.

Irrigate: to rinse or wash out with a fluid.

Isotonic: a solution that has the same concentration of salts, or tonicity, as another solution to which it is compared.

Lipids: emulsion containing fats used to correct fatty acid deficiencies via parenteral nutrition.

Lumen: the inner open space of a tube or blood vessel.

Malnutrition: a condition characterized by a lack of essential food substances or improper absorption and distribution of food substances in the body.

Minerals: inorganic elements or compounds.

Nutrient: nourishing food item that supplies the body with necessary elements.

Obstruction: blocking of a structure that prevents it from functioning normally; obstacle.

Osmosis: transmission of water across a semipermeable membrane from an area of low solute concentration to one of higher solute concentration.

Palpate: to examine by touch; to feel.

Peripherally inserted central catheter (PICC): long, soft, flexible catheter placed through an arm vein to the superior vena cava.

Phlebitis: inflammation of a vein.

Polyunsaturate: a long chain of carbon compounds with more than one double bond between the carbons; especially refers to fats.

Port: subcutaneously implanted plastic or metal case that provides access to the venous system.

Protein: substance that contains amino acids essential for growth and repair of tissues.

Sepsis: pathologic state usually febrile, resulting from the presence of microorganisms or their poisonous products in the bloodstream.

Thrombo: a clot of blood; a thrombus.

Thrombophlebitis: an inflammation of a vein due to the presence of a thrombus.

Transfusion: injection of blood or blood component of one person into the blood vessels of another.

Tunneled catheter: a long single or multi-lumen catheter inserted into a central vein, the remainder tunneled subcutaneously to a distant exit site on the chest or abdomen.

Valsalva's maneuver: attempt to forcibly exhale with the glottis closed.

Venipuncture: puncture of a vein with a needle.

Viscosity: resistance offered by a fluid; property of a substance that is dependent on the friction of its component molecules as they slide by each other.

Vitamins: a group of organic substances essential for life.

CENTRAL VASCULAR ACCESS DEVICES

Peripheral Catheters

Intravascular therapy is administered through a variety of catheters and devices. The most common type of intravascular device is the peripheral catheter, inserted into veins of the hands, arms, and antecubital area. These are short catheters, one inch (2.5 cm), intended for short-term IV therapy, usually no more than 5 days. The insertion site needs to be changed frequently, usually every 48–72 hours, according to facility policy. See Chapter 28 for more details on these IV devices.

Midline Catheters

Midline catheters are 3 to 8 inches in length (7.5–20 cm) and are inserted 1 ½ inches (2.5–3.8 cm) above or below the antecubital fossa and terminate in one of the client's arms in a proximal vein. They are similar to the peripherally inserted central catheter (PICC) but shorter in length. Both catheters are used for long-term IV therapy. Midline catheters are used only for administering nonirritating, normal pH solutions or medications, whereas the PICC can be used to infuse vesicants, hyperosmolar solutions and TPN. Clients with midline catheters should not receive any medications or IV fluids where the pH is below 5 or above 10, and osmolarity greater than 600 mOsm/L. Damage to the vessel walls can lead to phlebitis or thrombosis.

Midline catheters, due to their being placed in larger veins, can be left in place for up to 2–4 weeks. Because of the longer dwell time, compared to the peripheral catheter, complications such as thrombosis at the catheter site can occur. Phlebitis, infection, occlusion, clotting, breakage and leakage at the insertion site of the catheter are also associated with use of the midline catheter. Unfortunately, complications are not as easy to assess in clients with midline catheters, as opposed to clients with peripheral lines. For example, it takes longer for symptoms of phlebitis to occur in the client with a midline catheter. The short peripheral or midline catheters are not checked by x-ray for placement because as they do not enter the superior vena cava as do the central vascular catheters.

Central Vascular Access Devices

Long-term intravascular therapy is best accomplished through use of medically placed central vascular access devises (CVADs), which includes subcutaneous ports and catheters, as well as central vascular catheters. The specific type of device used depends on the type and duration of treatment, as well as client variables. CVADs are placed in clients who are actively involved and at home, as well as critically ill hospitalized clients. Clients requiring chemotherapy, nutritional supplements, blood products, and fluids can benefit from CVADs. These devices allow repeated access to the vascular system without venipuncture. CVADs protect clients from vein sclerosis, infection, venipuncture pain, inconvenience, and dependence.

Central vascular catheters are categorized into three types: central catheters, PICC lines, and subcutaneously implanted ports. Central catheters are further classified as tunneled or nontunneled catheters. Nontunneled catheters are large-bore catheters that vary in length from 6–8 inches (15–20 cm) and have one to four lumens. The catheters are made of soft silicone or a polyurethane material. Some of the newer catheters are impregnated with heparin, chlorhexidine, or an antibiotic. In most cases, physicians insert these catheters. Inaccurate placement of any central vascular catheter that is threaded to the superior vena cava can present a potential life-threatening arrhythmia if the catheter lodges against the myocardium.

Central Catheters Central catheters are medically placed percutaneously through the chest wall into the jugular or subclavian vein and are used for fluid or blood administration, obtaining blood specimens, and administering medications. Catheter extension into the superior vena cava minimizes vessel irritation and sclerosis of the vessel due to infusion. Due to the high volume of blood that normally flows through this portion of the superior vena cava (2000 mL/min) the risk of complications is lessened. Central catheters can be single or multilumen catheters.

Tunneled Catheters Hickman, Broviac, and Groshong catheters are tunneled catheters. The closed-ended or Groshong type catheter is designed to prevent backflow into the catheter when it is not in use. In the Groshong, fluids infuse through a slit valve on the side of the tip; when there is not an infusion of fluids into the catheter, the slit valve remains in a closed position. These catheters are never clamped due to this design factor. Pressure related to clamping the catheter or extension tubing can force the slit valve to open, allowing a blood leak back into the lumen. Heparin flushing is not routinely done because of the design of the catheter tip.

Tunneled catheters are used for long-term replacement therapy, medication administration, nutritional supplementation, and blood specimen withdrawal. These catheters can remain in place from months to years. The catheter's tip is inserted into a central vein (e.g., subclavian) and advanced to the distal area of the superior vena cava. The remaining portion of the catheter is threaded subcutaneously to exit at a convenient distal site (chest, abdomen). A dacron cuff on the catheter promotes scar formation to seal the tract to prevent ascending tract infection.

Client Selection for CVADs

- Long-term intravenous therapy
- Need for frequent venous access
- CVP monitoring
- Administration of total parenteral nutrition (TPN)
- Self-administration of intravenous therapies
- Sclerosed peripheral veins
- Limited peripheral venous access

Subcutaneously Implanted Ports

These implanted ports are surgically placed under the skin in a subcutaneous pocket in the chest, arm, abdomen, and occasionally, the back. The attached catheter enters the superior vena cava. Single and dual septal ports are available with open end or closed catheter endings.

Access to the port is by placement of a noncoring needle through the skin, into the self-sealing injection port housed in a plastic or metal case. This needle can remain in place for 7 days, then be replaced. Since the entire unit is implanted subcutaneously, risk for infection and maintenance requirements are greatly reduced.

Peripheral Insertion of a Central Catheter (PICC)

Peripheral (antecubital) insertion of a central vascular catheter (PICC) to the superior vena cava is easier and less risky than entering the central vein through the chest wall or neck. The use of PICC lines presents fewer problems with infection and serious complications; however, they do have infrequent problems associated with bleeding, tenderness, nerve damage, cardiac arrhythmias, chest pain, catheter malposition and catheter emboli. One common problem is that they tend to occlude frequently due to their small diameter. They need to be assessed thoroughly for breakage and phlebitis. Using a PICC line is the most appropriate method for infusing vesicants such as dopamine HCL, hyperosmolar solutions such as TPN or blood products, and antibiotics that are potentially irritating drugs. These drugs and solutions can be infused through the PICC line because the superior vena cava is large and has a large volume of blood by which these medications are diluted before they enter the systemic circulation. Studies have indicated that PICC lines have been in place for up to one year. Current research is looking at the exact time frame for PICC line placement, so this time frame may change. These access devices may be inserted by specially trained nurses who complete a certification process. As with all centrally placed catheters, a chest x-ray is taken to verify placement of the radiopaque catheter to validate that the tip is in the superior vena cava. The catheter must not be used until IV placement is verified.

Sterile technique must be maintained throughout all procedures associated with CVADs and PICC lines. Infection may occur if contamination results from poor technique in maintaining insertion sites, flushing catheters, or inserting the noncoring needle. Transparent dressings are placed over the insertion site for better stabilization and easy assessment and monitoring.

Total Parenteral Nutrition

The gastrointestinal tract is the preferred route for nutrition since it is more physiologic, less expensive, and safe. Parenteral nutrition is a method whereby nutrients are introduced intravenously. Bypassing the normal gastrointestinal system, this route provides a nitrogen source for those with a nonfunctional gastrointestinal tract (enteral starvation), or those with high caloric requirements (burn client), or acute hypoalbuminemia.

Balanced blends of nutrients, including vitamins and minerals, can be administered both by central line and peripherally using isotonic concentrations of glucose (no greater than 10% dextrose). In contrast, hypertonic solutions which are irritating to veins are administered through a central, high-flow vein. Rapid dilution of the solution decreases risk of phlebitis, clot formation, and hemolysis. This technique requires special handling and management, presents greater risk for complications, and is the most expensive method of feeding.

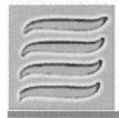

NURSING DIAGNOSES

The following nursing diagnoses may be appropriate to include in a client care plan when the components are related to intravascular therapy.

NURSING DIAGNOSIS	RELATED FACTORS
Activity Intolerance	Change in setting—intensive care, catabolic state Compromised cardiac reserve
Imbalanced Nutrition: Less Than Body Requirements	Chronic fatigue states, fatigue, nausea and vomiting, inadequate absorption, faulty metabolism, eating disorders, side effects of chemotherapy
Anxiety	Lifestyle modification, pain, chronic condition Uncertainty related to illness and diagnosis
Excess Fluid Volume	Excess fluid replacement, medications, renal and cardiac dysfunction
Decreased Cardiac Output	Impaired myocardial function, hypovolemia
Risk for Infection	Invasive procedures, inadequate site care, use of hypertonic glucose solutions, bacterial translocation from the bowel
Ineffective Tissue Perfusion, Cardiopulmonary	Altered blood supply, arterial or venous, impaired myocardial contractility, hypovolemia

- The single most important nursing action to decrease the incidence of hospital-based infections is handwashing. **Remember to wash your hands or use antibacterial gel before and after each and every client contact.**

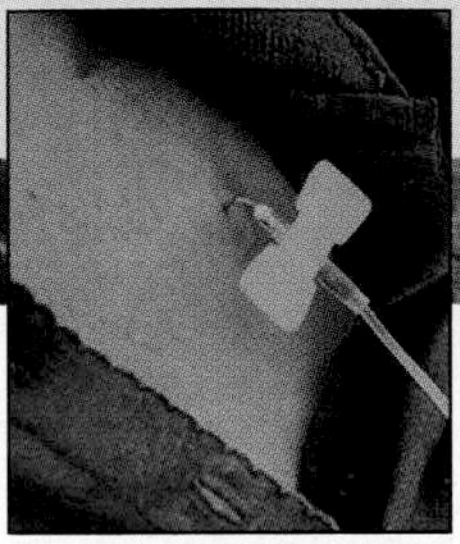

UNIT 1

Percutaneous Central Vascular Catheters

Nursing Process Data

ASSESSMENT Data Base

Determine client's level of consciousness so explanation of procedure can be done to allay anxiety.

Assess level of anxiety to determine need for possible premedication.

Assess skin and surrounding tissue for erythema, edema, and warmth.

Assess circulating volume status and right heart function.

PLANNING Objectives

To assist the physician with percutaneous central vascular catheter insertion

To maintain patency of central vascular catheter

To change central venous catheter dressing without complications

To maintain the insertion site free of infection

To prevent air embolism

To monitor central venous pressure

IMPLEMENTATION Procedures

Assisting with Percutaneous Central Vascular Catheterization

Changing a Central Line Catheter Dressing

Infusing IV Fluids Through a Central Line

Drawing Blood from a Central Line Catheter

Applying a BIOPATCH

Changing an Access Cap

Measuring and Monitoring Central Venous Pressure (CVP)

EVALUATION Expected Outcomes

Central vascular line is properly placed without complication.

Central vascular line remains patent.

Central vascular catheter dressing is changed without complications.

CVP monitoring guides fluid management.

BIOPATCH is applied and potential infection prevented.

Access cap replaced maintaining sterile technique.

ASSISTING WITH PERCUTANEOUS CENTRAL VASCULAR CATHETERIZATION

Equipment

Specific nontunneled catheter
Routine IV setup (tubing and solution)
Through-the-needle radiopaque central catheter
Local anesthetic, syringes, and needles
Sterile gloves, sterile gown, masks, drapes, and sutures
Antimicrobial swabs (prep solution physician prefers)
Intermittent infusion caps
Flush solution and syringes
Transparent semipermeable dressing

Procedure

1. Validate signed consent for catheter insertion.
2. Explain procedure to client, including rationale for mask, positioning and Valsalva's maneuver.
3. Place client in Trendelenburg's position. **Rationale:** This position prevents air embolism and helps distend subclavian and jugular veins.
4. According to physician's preference, extend client's neck and upper chest by placing a rolled pillow or blanket between shoulder blades. **Rationale:** Usual insertion sites are either subclavian or right jugular vein.
5. Place mask on client, and turn client's head away from side of venipuncture. **Rationale:** This facilitates filling the vessel with blood and prevents contamination.
6. Maintain sterility while opening glove packet and sterile drape pack. (Physician must wear sterile gloves, gown, and mask for this procedure.)
7. Open antimicrobial prep pads.
8. Don gloves and assist with central catheter insertion.
   a. Physician dons mask, gown, and sterile gloves for this procedure.

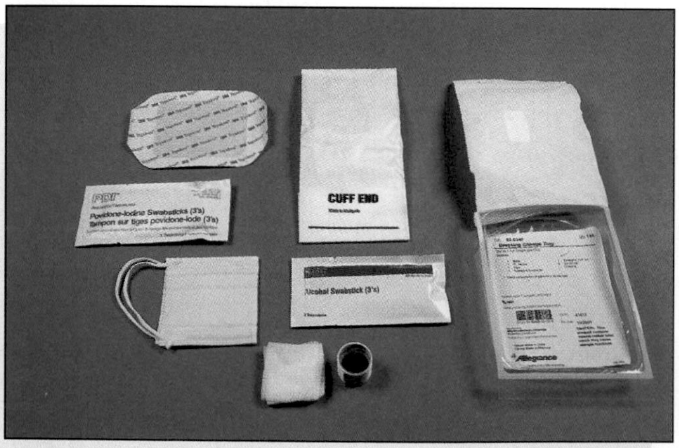

Equipment for changing a central line dressing: gauze and paper tape are used 24 hours and then removed.

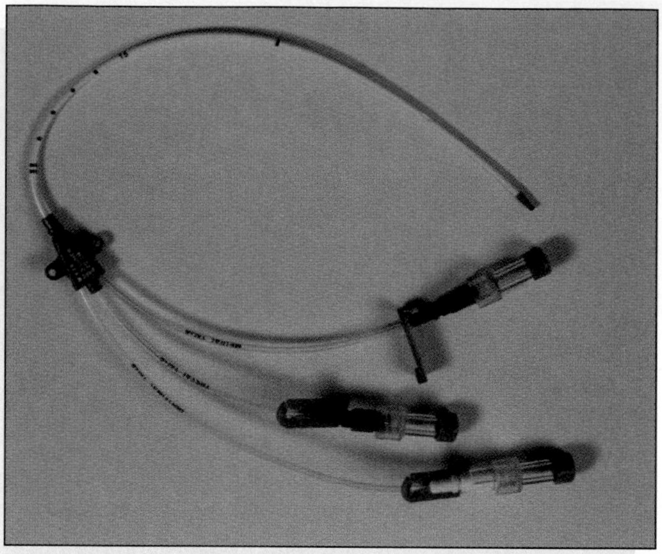
Triple-lumen central venous catheter.

   b. Physician prepares the client's skin, drapes area, and, using a sterile syringe and needle, draws up anesthetic to infiltrate the site.
   c. As physician inserts catheter, have client perform Valsalva's maneuver to prevent air embolism.

Central Catheter Site Preparation

Any one of the following protocols can be used to prepare the site for Central Catheters, PICC lines, and Midline catheters. Based on studies, the most effective site preparation is listed in priority order. Facilities have written policies and should be followed even if they conflict with this priority list.

The priority site preparation is use of a 2% chlorhexidine skin prep applicator. Clean insertion area, starting at the intended insertion site and moving outward in concentric circles for 4–6 inches. Let dry for 30 seconds. For sites that are considered moist, such as the groin, scrub for 2 minutes and let dry for 1 minute.

The second effective method is to clean area with 70% isopropyl alcohol, beginning at intended insertion site and moving outward in concentric circles at least 4–6 inches. Change swabs frequently, using at least 3 swabs. Clean same area with 2% tincture of iodine solution. Follow same steps as cleaning with alcohol. Allow area to dry for 30 seconds. The solution does not need to be removed before completing venipuncture unless the client's skin is irritated from use.

A third method is to clean area with 10% povidone–iodine, beginning at intended insertion site and moving outward in concentric circles at least 4–6 inches. Allow solution to dry for 2 minutes.

(1) Instruct client to exhale against a closed glottis or to hum.
(2) If client is unable to do this, compress client's abdomen. **Rationale:** Both these procedures help to decrease chances of air embolism.

Note: A 14 gauge needle is inserted into the subclavian vein, using the clavicle as a guide. When blood returns in syringe, the syringe is removed from the needle and a wire is threaded through the needle into the subclavian vein. The needle is removed and the catheter is fed over the wire into the subclavian and brachiocephalic vein. The wire is removed when the tip of the catheter rests in superior vena cava.

9. When physician has completed catheterization, insert injection cap, flush with 5 mL NS, then heparinize with 3 mL dilute heparin (according to agency policy). Use 10-mL syringe. **Rationale:** To decrease pressure in catheter.
10. Physician sutures catheter into place.
11. Cover insertion site and sutures with sterile transparent dressing (according to hospital policy).
12. Label insertion site dressing with date, nurse's initials, and time of insertion.
13. Obtain x-ray for validation of placement into superior vena cava before initiating infusion (unless emergency placement performed).
14. Monitor client's vital signs. **Rationale:** Bleeding or pneumothorax may occur.

CLINICAL ALERT

All continuous IV infusions administered via a central line must have an electric infusion controller device in place.

EVIDENCE BASED NURSING PRACTICE

Preventing Intravascular Catheter-Related Bloodstream Infections

Catheter-related bloodstream infection is 2 to 855 times higher with central vascular catheters than peripheral vascular catheters. Approximately 80,000 catheter-related infections occur in the United States each year. These infections are associated with 2,400–20,000 deaths each year. These infections can be dramatically reduced with new products that have been introduced for CVD therapy: The FDA has recently approved the use of catheters impregnated with chlorhexidine. There is still testing being done on the combination of chlorhexidine and silver sulfadiazine because of some anaphylactoid reactions in Japan. Use of minocycline–Rifampin impregnated catheters show promise of even lower infection rates.

- Catheters impregnated with chlorhexidine–silver sulfadiazine or catheters impregnated with minocycline—rifampin
- Catheter hubs containing Iodinated Alcohol
- Chlorhexidine-impregnated sponge dressings placed at the catheter insertion site infection rate decreased from 5.2% to 3% for catheters in place less than 10 days.

Source: Mermel, L. A. (2001, March–April) "New Technologies to Prevent Intravascular Catheter-Related Bloodstream Infections. *Emerging Infectious Diseases*, CDC, *7*(2).

CHANGING A CENTRAL LINE CATHETER DRESSING

Equipment

2% Chlorhexidine, alcohol and 2% tincture of iodine or 10% povidone–iodine
Antimicrobial handsoap
Tape or transparent dressing
Needleless access caps, if also performing IV tubing change
Receptacle for soiled dressing
Clean gloves
Sterile gloves
Mask (according to agency policy)
Sterile long-sleeved gown (according to hospital policy)

Preparation

1. Check physicians orders, MAR, and client care plan for last dressing change (usually changed q 48–72 hrs).
2. Gather equipment.
3. Check client's identaband, ask client to state name and explain procedure to client.

4. Wash your hands for 15–20 seconds with antimicrobial soap.
5. Position client flat on back. **Rationale:** Reduces risk of air embolism.
6. Turn client's head away from the insertion site, and mask the client's nose and mouth if necessary. **Rationale:** Decreases exposure to microorganisms at site.
7. Make sure that all personnel don masks and and/or gloves if client is neutropenic and according to hospital policy.

Procedure

1. Don clean gloves.
2. Carefully remove old dressing or tape without pulling on catheter. Remove edges toward insertion site. **Rationale:** This prevents stress on insertion site.
3. Discard old dressing and gloves in proper receptacle.
4. Remove clean gloves and don sterile gloves.
5. Inspect site for loose sutures, signs of infection, inflammation, or infiltration, and check length of exposed catheter.
6. Cleanse insertion site, sutures, and catheter with chlorhexidine, alcohol or iodine swabs, working from insertion site outward about 4 to 6 inches in a circular motion. **Rationale:** Working from cleanest area outward prevents contamination.

> **CLINICAL ALERT**
>
> Put on mask for dressing change if client is neutropenic or according to facility policy. To determine absolute neutrophil count: Multiply the client's total WBC count (e.g., 0.4) by the percentages of bands plus neutrophils (polys) (e.g., 5%) = 20. If this absolute count is less than 1,000 the client is considered neutropenic and requires special precautions in care.

7. Cleanse site with circular motion three times with three different swabs—allow the agent to dry.
8. Cover site with a sterile transparent dressing.

Gauze dressings are used only if the catheter insertion site is oozing. The dressing should be changed every 48 hours or if soiled.

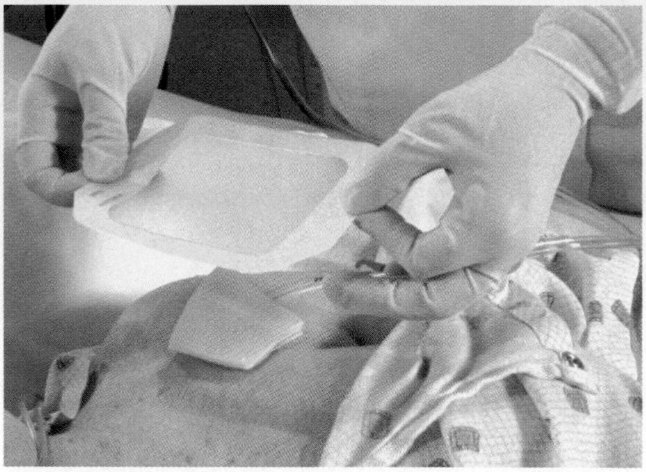

> **CLINICAL ALERT**
>
> Using a transparent dressing alone provides better catheter stabilization; dressing changes are required every 72–96 hours.

9. Change IV tubing according to hospital policy.
   a. Clamp central catheter using on-line slide or squeeze clamp.
   b. Using aseptic technique, change needleless access cap.
   c. Prepare cap with antimicrobial swab.
   d. Insert new tubing with needleless connector.
10. Label dressing and tubing with date and your initials.
11. Change dressing if it becomes loose, wet, or soiled or according to facility policy. **Rationale:** If it is wet, soiled, or loose, it is considered contaminated.
12. Discard equipment and gloves, and wash hands.

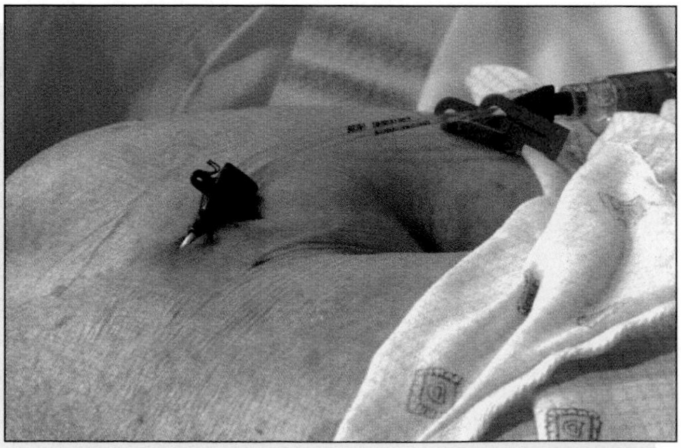

Assess catheter exit site for signs of inflammation/infection (which may be present in this client).

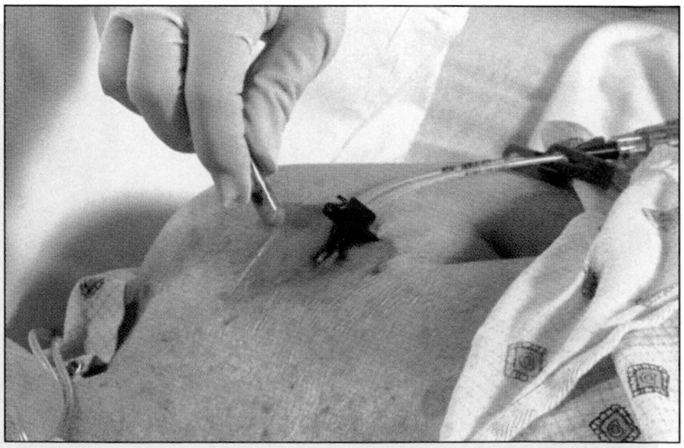

Prep site, starting at catheter exit and cleanse outward in a circular motion.

Infusion Site Complications

Signs & Symptoms	Possible Indications
Redness, swelling at CVAD infusion site	Infiltration, hematoma or sepsis
Crepitus on chest	Subcutaneous emphysema that can lead to respiratory distress
Respiratory distress with recent placement of a central line	Pneumothorax
Arm, shoulder, or neck pain	Infiltration or thrombosis
Temperature elevation	Catheter-related infection

IV Tubing Replacement

Tubing	Replacement Time
Primary and secondary, continuous	72–96 hours
Primary, intermittent	24 hours
TPN and Lipids	24 hours

Prevention of Air Embolism in Clients with Central Lines

1. Clear central line of air prior to insertion.
2. Use IV pumps with in-line air detectors.
3. Use the head-down position and Valsalva maneuver during both insertion and removal.
4. Use screw-on connections and secure with tape. **Rationale:** Hemostats or other clamps can crack hub and open system.
5. Use air-occlusive dressing during use of and after removal of a central catheter. Leave in place for at least 24 hours.

INFUSING IV FLUIDS THROUGH A CENTRAL LINE

Equipment

Primed IV fluid administration set with needleless Luer-Lok connector
Infusion delivery pump
Antimicrobial swabs
10-mL needleless syringe with 5 mL normal saline solution
Clean gloves

CLINICAL ALERT

To minimize pressure on the catheter during injection NEVER use less than a 10-mL syringe for central lines. Smaller syringes increase pressure within the catheter.

Preparation

1. Check physician's order sheet and client's Medication Record for IV order.
2. Check IV order with IV solution bag.
3. Take equipment to client's room.
4. Check room number and client's identaband. Ask client to state name.
5. Explain procedure to client and provide privacy.

Procedure

1. Wash your hands and don gloves.
2. Hang IV solution on IV stand.
3. Wipe access port with antimicrobial swab and allow to dry.
4. Insert needleless cannula from saline flush syringe and unclamp lumen. (Clamp is not found on PICC lines or Groshong valve catheter).
5. Aspirate for blood return, using very little force, to check for lumen patency.
6. Instill saline solution slowly. The CVD and tubing has a volume of 1–3 mL; therefore, about 5 mL should be used to thoroughly flush the catheter. **Rationale:** To clear lumen of inline dilute heparin.
7. Maintain positive pressure when withdrawing syringe by clamping catheter before removing syringe or by maintaining pressure on syringe plunger before you clamp. **Rationale:** This prevents aspiration of blood into lumen and decreases risk of catheter occlusion.
8. Swab access port again with antimicrobial swabs.
9. Insert IV tubing with Luer-Lok connector into access port. Unclamp lumen.
10. Set electronic device to prescribed rate and begin infusing IV fluids.
11. Ensure central line dressing is clean and intact.
12. Remove gloves and wash your hands.

CLINICAL ALERT

Nontunneled central vascular access devices have the highest infection rate of all types of CVADs; therefore, it is crucial that aseptic techniques be used in all aspects of catheter care.

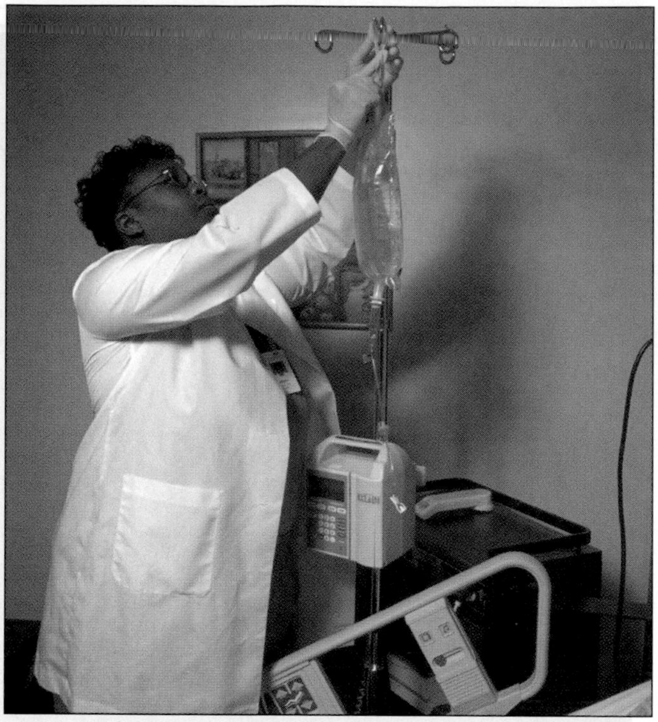

Hang IV solution on IV stand.

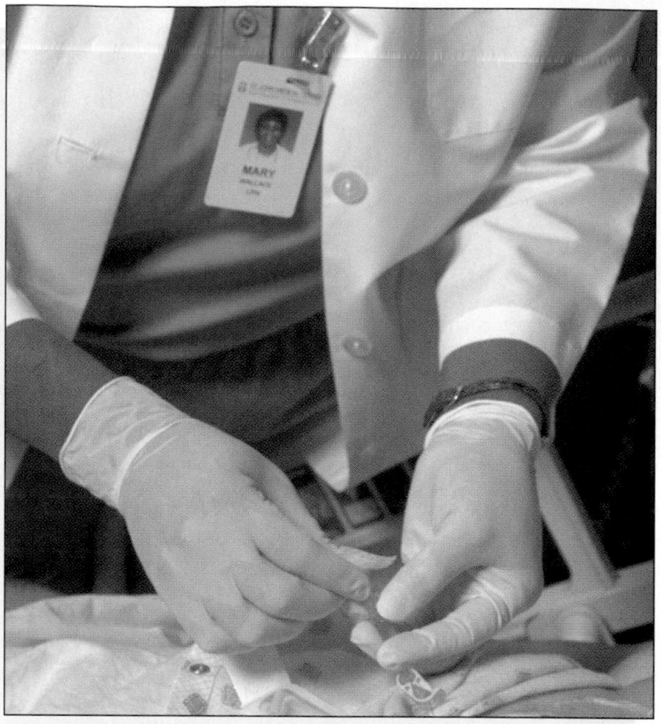

Wipe access cap with antimicrobial swab.

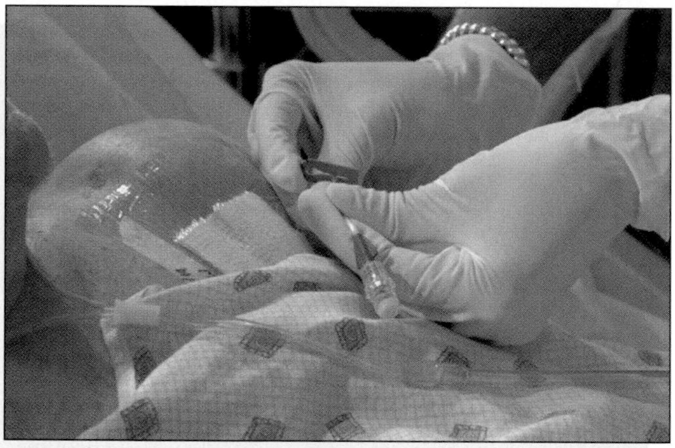

Unclamp lumen to open access to catheter.

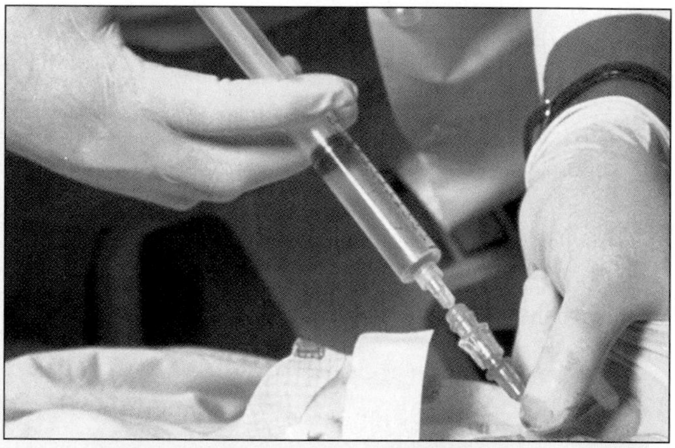

Instant needleless syringe filled with saline solution.

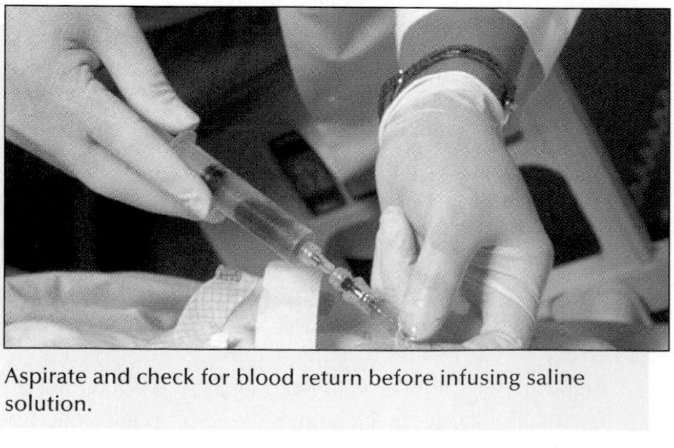

Aspirate and check for blood return before infusing saline solution.

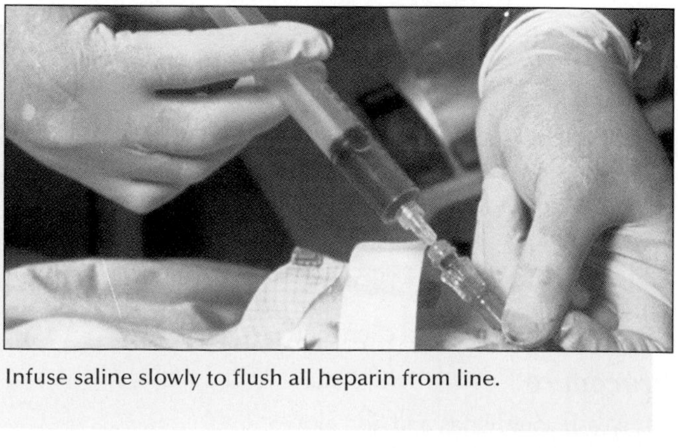

Infuse saline slowly to flush all heparin from line.

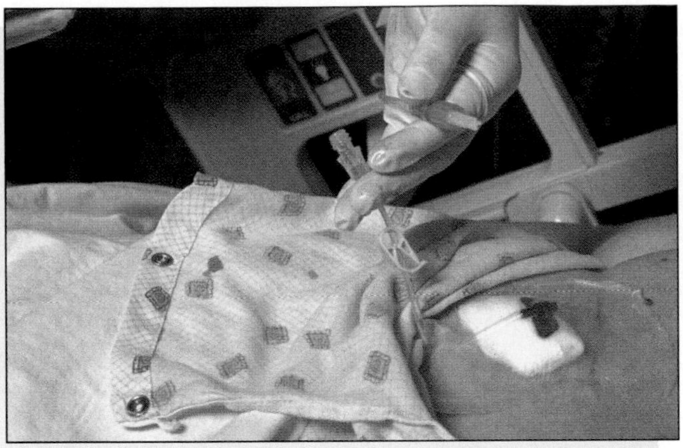

Insert IV tubing into access port.

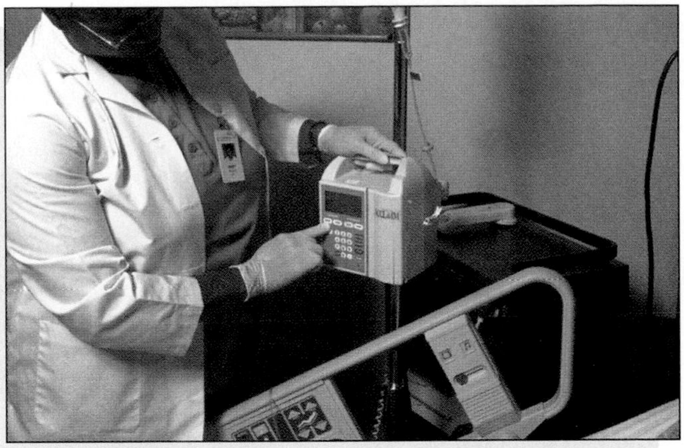

Set electronic device to prescribed IV rate.

DRAWING BLOOD FROM CENTRAL LINE CATHETER

Equipment

2 × 10-mL Luer-Lok syringes filled with sterile normal saline
3-mL Luer-Lok syringe with 3 mL heparinized saline (100 U/mL heparin)
Two 10-mL syringes (or larger if needed) with needleless cannula
Antimicrobial swabs
Blood tubes appropriate for tests ordered
Sterile injection cap
Clean gloves
Mask

CLINICAL ALERT

Some facilities do not allow vacutainers to be used for blood draws from central lines due to increased pressure build up in catheter.

Preparation

1. Check physician's orders and MAR.
2. Check client's room number and identaband.
3. Ask client to state name.

Procedure

1. Explain procedure to client.
2. Wash hands, don gloves and mask.
3. If fluids are infusing through catheter, turn off infusion for at least 1 minute prior to drawing blood specimen.
4. Swab cap and hub with antimicrobial swabs for 30 seconds and allow to dry. Use most proximal lumen of catheter for blood draw. **Rationale:** Proximal port specimen will not be contaminated if fluids are infusing distally.
5. Remove cap from syringe and insert 10 mL saline filled syringe, unclamp catheter.
6. Flush catheter with 5–10 mL normal saline. **Rationale:** To determine patency of catheter.
7. Clamp catheter, remove syringe and attach new 10-mL empty syringe. Unclamp catheter.
8. Withdraw 5 mL of blood from catheter slowly and then clamp catheter. **Rationale:** To clear the catheter of fluids or medications, particularly heparin, before blood samples are obtained.

Note: Withdraw 8–10 mL of blood if coagulation studies have been ordered.

Rationale: To ensure all heparin has been expelled from hub and catheter.

9. Discard syringe in biohazard box.

CLINICAL ALERT

Do not discard any blood if drawing blood for cultures. Blood from the first draw is always used for blood cultures.

10. Again, clean injection cap with antimicrobial swabs and then insert a 10-mL syringe into cap and withdraw required amount of blood. Check lab manual for appropriate blood tube for each test. **Rationale:** Laboratories vary in the amount of blood they require.
11. Clamp catheter, and withdraw syringe. Inject blood into laboratory blood tubes which have a vacuum that draws in blood. Tubes should be secured upright in a wire basket. **Rationale:** Blood cells are easily damaged if put

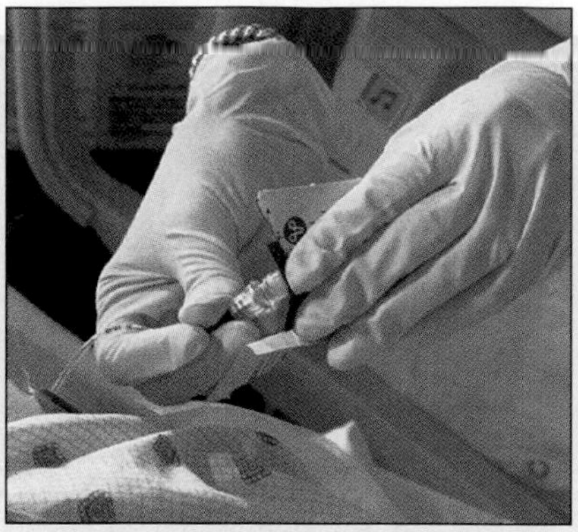

Unclamp catheter; clean cap and hub with antimicrobial swab.

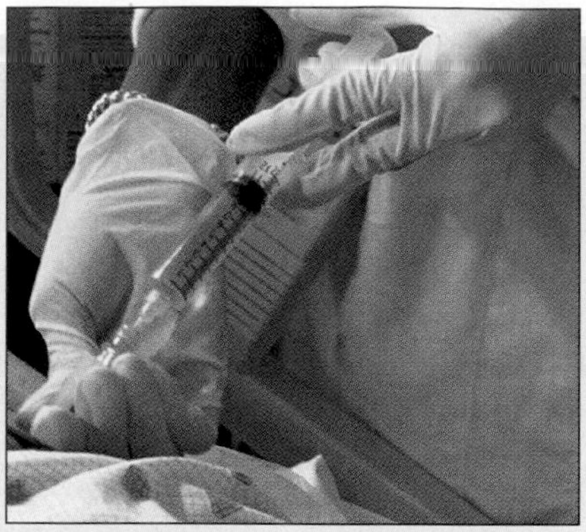

Insert 10-mL syringe into cap and unclamp catheter.

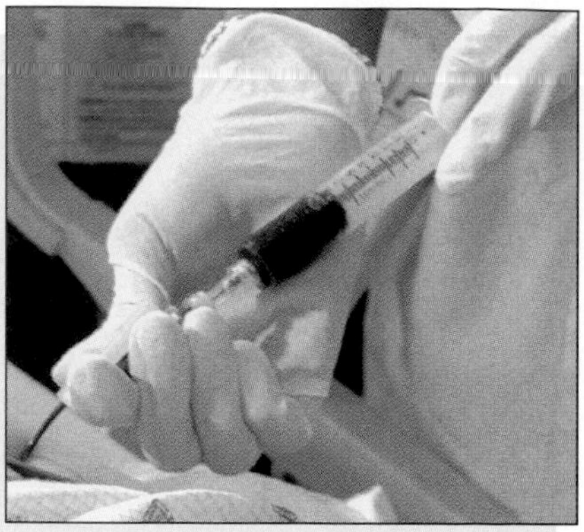

Withdraw 5 ml of blood for discard before drawing blood sample unless specimen is for culture.

through needles smaller than 22 gauge, which causes hemolysis and abnormal laboratory results.

12. Dispose of syringe in biohazard container.
13. Swab cap and insert saline flush syringe, unclamp catheter.
14. Flush catheter slowly with 10-mL saline, clamp catheter and remove syringe or maintain positive pressure on syringe plunger with your thumb while withdrawing syringe from injection cap. **Rationale:** This prevents blood backflow and lowers risk of catheter occlusion.
15. Again, swab cap and insert 3-mL syringe filled with 3 mL dilute heparin solution according to facility policy.
16. Unclamp catheter, gently infuse heparin solution.
17. Clamp catheter and withdraw syringe.
18. Change cap. Cap must be changed every 72–96 hours for continuous infusion, and every 7 days for intermittent infusion. It must also be changed after each blood draw or blood administration or any time the cap is removed for a procedure.
19. Remove gloves and dispose in appropriate container and wash hands.

Note: Newer catheter caps accept a syringe hub for administration of fluids or withdrawal of blood specimens, eliminating need for either uncapping catheter or using a needleless cannula.

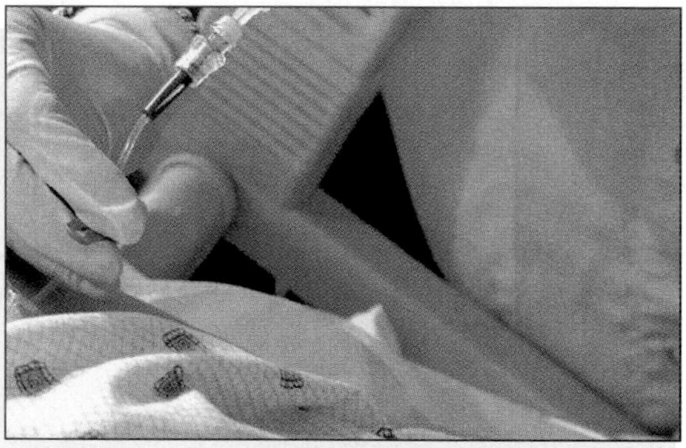

Flush catheter using 10 mL syringe, clamp line and remove syringe.

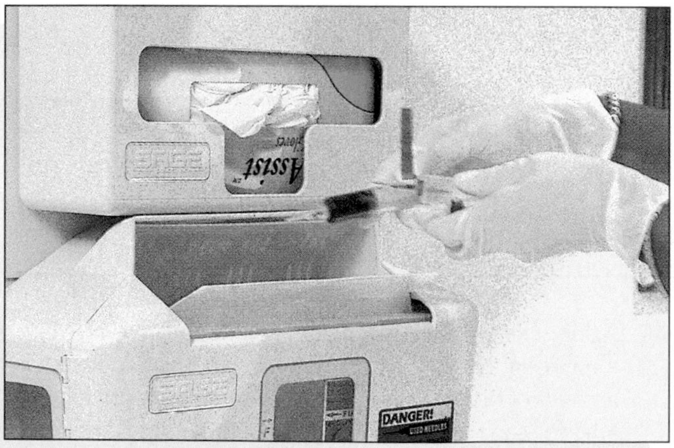

Dispose of blood waste in biohazard container.

CLINICAL ALERT

Specimens obtained from central catheter lines have been reported as inaccurate in some studies. If lab values are significantly different from earlier values or from the normal range, assess client to determine if additional lab tests need to be drawn. In this case, draw specimens from a direct vein, if possible.

APPLYING A BIOPATCH

Equipment

BIOPATCH Antimicrobial Dressing with Chlorhexidine Gluconate
BIOCLUSIVE Transparent Dressing or other similar dressings
Sterile gloves
Clean gloves

Procedure

1. Check the client chart and care plan to determine last dressing change.
2. Gather equipment.
3. Identify correct client (check identaband and ask client to state name) and explain procedure to client.
4. Wash hands and don sterile gloves.
5. Prepare skin surrounding percutaneous device according to hospital protocol. Ensure sufficient space is left between hub of catheter and insertion site for placement of dressing.
6. Remove dressing from sterile package using aseptic technique.
7. Place the BIOPATCH dressing around catheter so catheter rests on slit portion of patch. Ensure GRID side of patch is facing upward. The smooth foam side of patch is next to the skin.

CLINICAL ALERT

The patch is made of a hydrophilic polyurethane absorptive foam with chlorhexidine gluconate (CHG). The patch absorbs up to 8 times its own weight in fluid and the CHG inhibits bacterial growth under dressing.

8. Ensure edges of silt approximate each other to assure efficacy of patch.

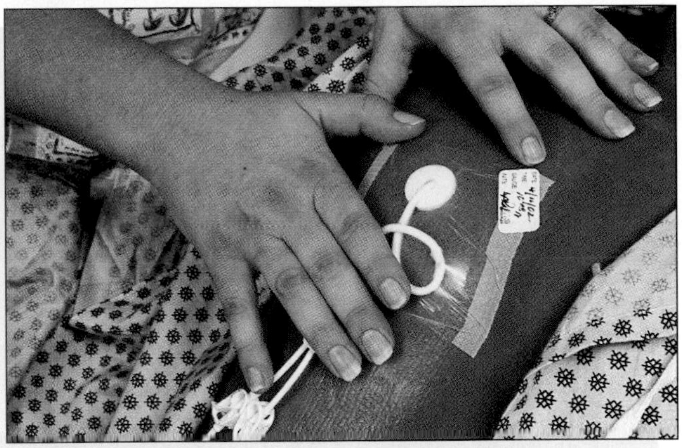

BIOPATCH with transparent dressing over insertion site.

9. Apply transparent dressing over patch and catheter insertion site. Ensure complete contact between skin and transparent dressing.
10. Discard equipment packages.
11. Remove gloves and place in receptacle.
12. Wash hands.
13. Change patch as necessary. Follow facility policy; however dressing change should be at a minimum of every 7 days.
    a. Don clean gloves.
    b. Remove patch by picking up corner of dressing and stretching dressing away from catheter while holding catheter in place. Dressing should partially lift off skin.
    c. Peel back dressing until resistance is felt.
    d. Repeat stretch and peel action until dressing is removed. Both the dressing and the patch will be removed together with this action.
    e. Discard old dressing in biohazard container.
    f. Discard gloves in appropriate receptacle, and wash hands.

EVIDENCE BASED NUSING PRACTICE

Evaluation of BIOPATCH Antimicrobial Dressing

A controlled, randomized study of 687 clients with 1699 central venous or arterial catheter insertion sites was conducted in two centers. Results indicated a 44% reduction in local infections and a 60% reduction in catheter-related bloodstream infections. There were no serious device-related adverse events during the study. Data regarding use of patch on children under 16 is limited. Patch should not be used on premature infants as hypersensitivity reactions and necrosis of the skin has occurred.

Source: Maki, D. G., et al. (2000). An Evaluation of Biopatch Antimicrobial Dressing Compared to Routine Standard of Care in the Prevention of Catheter-Related Bloodstream Infection. Johnson & Johnson Medical Division of ETHICON, Inc.

CHANGING AN ACCESS CAP

Equipment

Antimicrobial swabs
Sterile resealable injection cap
10-mL syringe with 5–10 mL saline for flush
10-mL syringe with 2–3 mL heparin solution for maintenance
Clean gloves

Procedure

1. Check client's chart and care plan to determine time of last access cap change. (Cap is replaced when removed for IV fluid administration.)
2. Check client's room number, identaband, and ask client to state name.

> **CLINICAL ALERT**
>
> The exact time interval is not scientifically known at this time, but it is suggested that the access cap be changed at least every 7 days, when the cap has been accessed more than the manufacturer's recommendations, if the integrity of the port is compromised, or if residual blood remains within the port.

3. Explain procedure to client, and provide privacy.
4. Gather equipment.
5. Wash your hands and don gloves.
6. Open access cap package maintaining sterility and place near working area.
7. Assess access cap to determine if cap should be changed even if time frame is not met.

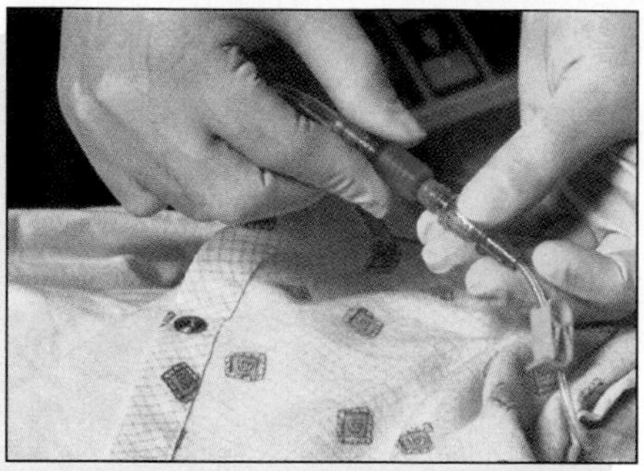

Stop IV infusion and disconnect tubing from access cap.

8. Place client in supine position. Clamp catheter using online slide or squeeze clamp. **Rationale:** To prevent air embolism during cap change. Client can be instructed to perform a Valsalva maneuver during cap change as an alternative to lying supine.
9. Stop any IV infusion and disconnect IV tubing from access cap.
10. Remove existing cap using aseptic technique.
11. Take new access cap out of package, maintaining sterility and place on catheter hub.
12. Cleanse injection cap with antimicrobial swab.
13. Flush catheter using 10-mL syringe with normal saline or insert new IV fluid tubing and begin infusion at prescribed rate.
14. Infuse heparin solution if central line is used for intermittent infusions. Follow directions for infusing heparin solution in Skill: Drawing Blood from Central Line.
15. Remove gloves and wash hands.

TABLE 29–1 Maintaining CVADs

CVAD	Frequency	Flush Solution
Single or multi-lumen Percutaneous Catheter short-term long-term	 q12 h to daily, and after each use daily to weekly and after each use	2–5 mL dilute heparin (250–500 units) per lumen
Implanted Port	monthly and after each use	5 mL dilute heparin
Groshong Valve Device	weekly and after each use	5–10 mL normal saline ONLY in 10-mL syringe
PICC	daily if idle and after each use	5 mL dilute heparin

MEASURING AND MONITORING CENTRAL VENOUS PRESSURE (CVP)

Equipment

Disposable CVP manometer with stopcock
IV solution (5% dextrose in water)
Extension tubing with needleless cannula
IV pole
Carpenter's level
Antimicrobial swabs
10-mL syringe with 5 mL saline solution
Marker

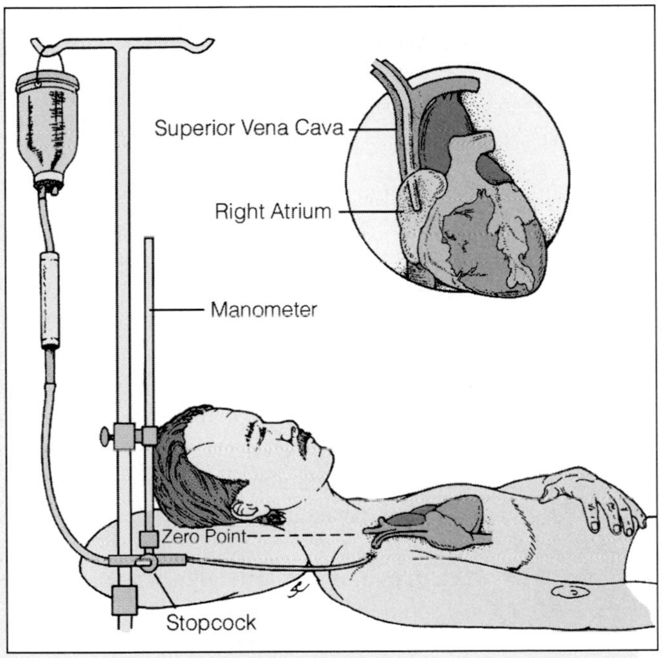

When a CVP reading is taken, the zero of the manometer must be level with client's right atrium, regardless of his position.

Preparation

1. Check client care plan and physician's order.
2. Identify client's room, identaband, and ask client to state name.
3. Explain procedure to client.
4. Provide privacy.
5. Determine client's previous CVP parameters. **Rationale:** Trends are more relevant than isolated pressure readings.

Procedure

1. Wash hands.
2. Spike IV solution bag with IV administration set using sterile technique.
3. Prime tubing with solution.
4. Close clamp on tubing.
5. If you are using a one-piece disposable manometer and stopcock, affix unit to IV pole.
6. Push male end of IV administration set into female end of stopcock, connecting the IV set to stopcock.
7. Turning stopcock so that manometer and IV solution are open to each other, open clamp on IV tubing and fill manometer with IV solution to between 18 and 20 cm. **Rationale:** Overfilling the manometer may expose the client to contamination resulting from overflow.
8. Close clamp, and rotate stopcock so that IV solution is open to client.

CLINICAL ALERT

Central venous pressure (CVP) is a measure of venous return or the pressure of blood in the right atrium. Used to guide fluid administration, it is measured in centimeters of water pressure (normal is 5–10 cm H_2O).

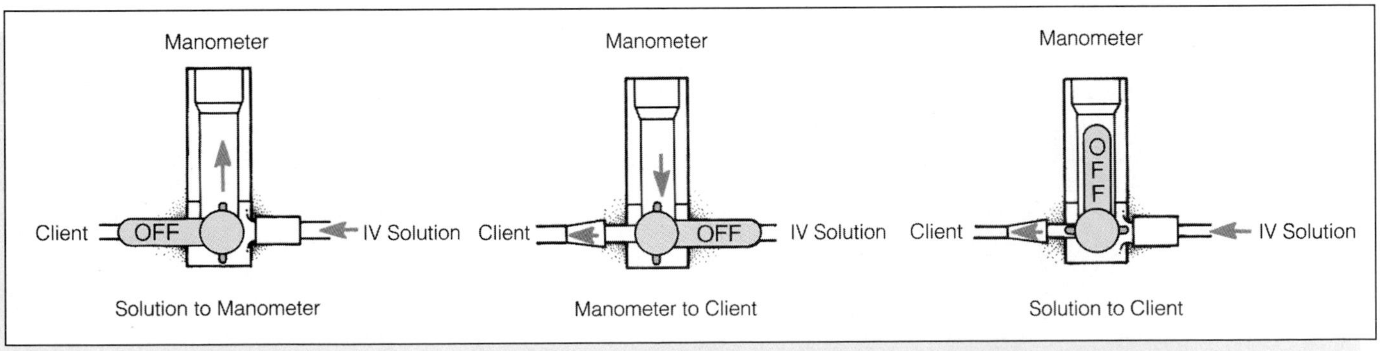

Left stopcock: Fill the manometer by turning stopcock: OFF to the client. This allows solution to flow from the bottle to the manometer. Middle stopcock: Measure CVP by turning stopcock OFF to IV solution allowing fluid to flow from manometer to client. Right stopcock: Reinstitute flow from IV bottle to client by turning stopcock OFF to the manometer.

9. Prime the rest of IV tubing that extends from stopcock to client's central line.
10. Place client flat in bed, without a pillow, if client can tolerate this position. If not, place client in position of comfort (e.g., head of bed at 15°–30°).
11. Record position so that same position can be used each time a CVP reading is made. **Rationale:** This allows accurate CVP trending.
12. Locate client's right atrium (midaxillary at fourth intercostal space). Mark this location on client's skin using marking pen.
13. Adjust level of CVP manometer (using carpenter's level) so that zero on manometer is at the same level as client's right atrium, 5 cm on manometer level to sternal notch. **Rationale:** Using level at right atrium reflects blood volume and cardiac function of client.
14. Turn stopcock to open position for manometer, filling manometer with additional solution if needed.
15. Turn stopcock to the manometer→client position, and watch level of the solution in the manometer fall to the pressure level existing in the right atrium. **Rationale:** Normally this pressure should be between 4 and 11 cm. Remember, however, there are no absolute values and trends—the rise and fall of CVP readings are more important than one isolated pressure reading.
16. Observe meniscus at eye level, and watch rise (with exhalation) and fall (with inhalation) of fluid column in response to client's breathing. **Rationale:** Fluctuations reflect changes in intrathoracic pressures during respiratory cycle and indicate that manometer is functioning properly.
17. Take reading at end of exhalation (rise of fluid in manometer).
18. Turn off stopcock to manometer, and adjust rate of infusion to reestablish IV solution flow to client.
19. Return client to desired position, and record CVP reading.

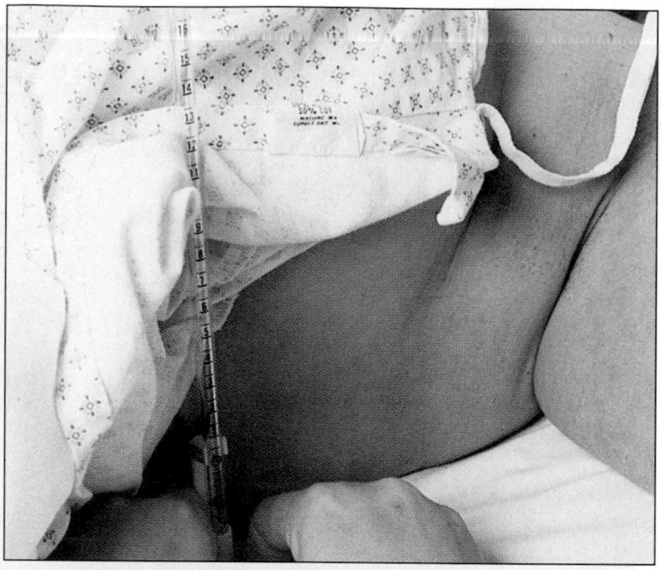

CVP reading is taken with manometer zeroed at client's midaxillary fourth intercostal space.

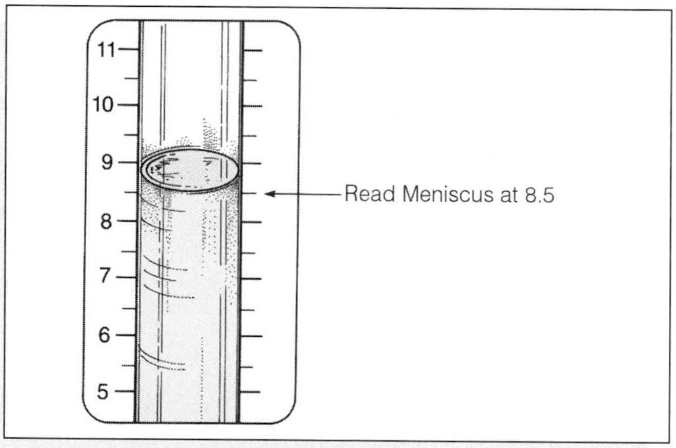

Take CVP reading at base of meniscus and at end of expiration (on higher fluctuation).

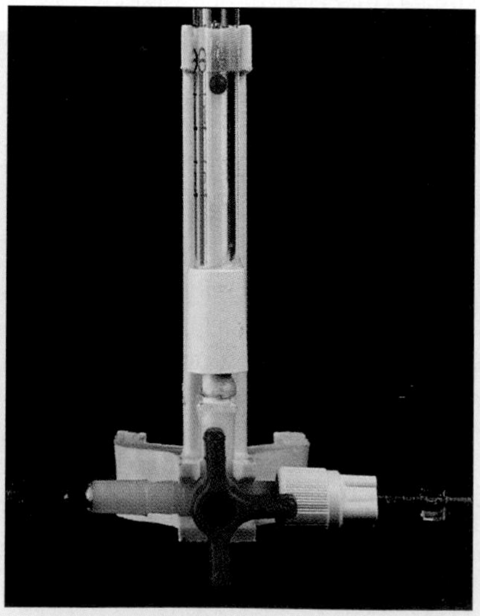

Solution to manometer.

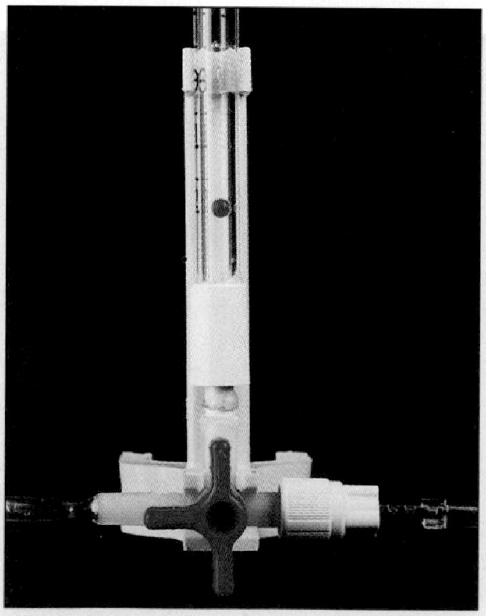

Manometer to client.

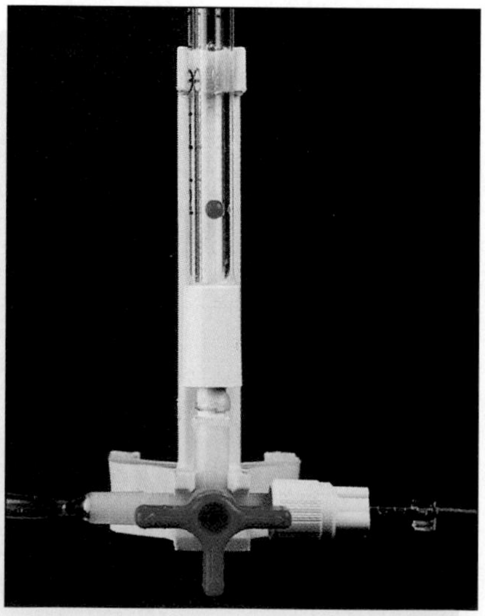

Solution to client.

DOCUMENTATION FOR CENTRAL VASCULAR CATHETERIZATION

- Location of insertion site
- Type and size of cannula used for insertion
- Time of insertion
- Assessment of site and dressing every 8 hrs
- Name of physician performing catheterization
- Types of solutions infused
- Amount of solution infused
- Time x-ray was performed to check position of catheter
- Time, initials, date dressing and tubing changed
- Date and time of CVP reading (record subsequent CVP readings on appropriate flow sheets)
- Client's response to treatment
- Any unusual conditions or reactions

Critical Thinking Application

UNEXPECTED OUTCOMES	CRITICAL THINKING OPTIONS
Air enters central vein, producing air embolism from system being open to atmosphere.	• Immediately clamp catheter and place client in Trendelenburg position (turned to the left so right ventricle is uppermost). • Immediately inform physician and monitor until physician arrives. Assess vital signs and breath sounds. • Administer high-flow O_2 as necessary. • Prevent air embolism by having client perform Valsalva's maneuver any time catheter is open to air, or use in-line catheter clamp. • Ensure client has a patent peripheral IV line.
Infection at insertion site.	• Prepare for catheter removal and possible reinsertion at another site. • If catheter is removed, cut off catheter tip with sterile scissors and place in sterile container, send tip to laboratory for culture. • Administer antibiotics as ordered. • Observe client carefully for signs of systemic infection.
Dysrhythmia detected.	• Change client's position. • Notify physician. • Verify catheter position on chest x-ray (right atrium placement causes dysrhythmias). • Prepare for catheter repositioning or removal of catheter by physician.
Catheter becomes dislodged.	• Check the exact length of catheter to determine extent of problem. • Secure catheter and extension tubing with tape to prevent further migration of tube. • Notify physician immediately.
Catheter appears to be or becomes occluded.	• Reposition client. • Ask client to raise arms overhead.

UNEXPECTED OUTCOMES	CRITICAL THINKING OPTIONS
	• Perform Valsalva maneuver. Turn head to one side. • Attempt to flush catheter with normal saline, using gentle pressure. • Notify physician for order to administer fibrinolytic agent or other agents.
CVP system does not infuse.	• Check line for kinks. Change client's position. Check to make sure the manometer stopcock is in the IV→client position. • Obtain order for placing heparin in IV bottle to maintain patency. • Notify physician and prepare for possible reinsertion.
CVP readings vary greatly.	• Assess patency of setup. • Assess client's level of pain; pain increases the CVP reading. • Assess if position of client has been changed; raising the head of the bed alters the reading unless setup is adjusted. • Check that the marked area at midaxillary level is at the level of the client's right atrium (4th ICS). • If client has COPD, heart failure, or hypovolemia, expect readings to differ from normal range. However, once baseline is established for individual client, trends should be watched and evaluated against goals of therapy.

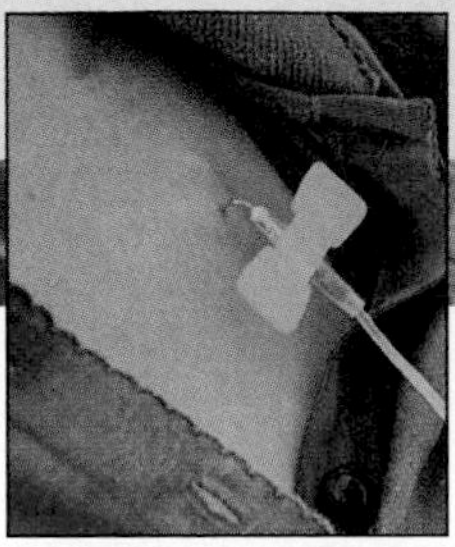

UNIT 2

Total Parenteral Nutrition/ Total Nutrient Admixture

Nursing Process Data

ASSESSMENT ***Data Base***

Complete a physical assessment and client history.

Assess client's nutrition status.

Identify any condition that would affect TPN (renal or cardiac disease).

Assess nutritional needs of clients who are unable to process nutrients normally (gastrointestinally).

Observe for correct additives in each hyperalimentation bag, or container.

Check rate of infusion on physician's orders.

Monitor catheter insertion site for signs of infection or possible infiltration.

Monitor regularly client's blood sugar response to hyperalimentation.

PLANNING ***Objectives***

To provide a nutrition source for clients unable to process nutrients normally

To provide nutrients for clients requiring bypass of the gastrointestinal tract (bowel rest)

To provide increased calories for clients in a catabolic state

To prevent or correct a deficiency of essential fatty acids

To provide a contamination-free mode of delivering parenteral nutrition

To regularly administer sliding scale insulin according to client's glucose level

IMPLEMENTATION ***Procedures***

Assisting with Catheter Insertion

Maintaining Hyperalimentation infusions (TPN)

Changing Hyperalimentation (TPN) Dressing and Tubing

Maintaining Hyperalimentation for Children

EVALUATION ***Expected Outcomes***

Catheter is placed correctly.

Solution is infused at prescribed flow rate and tolerated by client.

Dressing remains dry and intact.

Insertion site remains free of infection and inflammation; sepsis does not occur.

Client receives nutrients necessary for tissue repair.

Client's blood sugar is maintained within normal parameters.

Note: Total Nutrient Admixture (TNA) is being used more frequently in healthcare facilities. Skills are the same as for TPN, only the solution composition is different.

ASSISTING WITH CATHETER INSERTION

Equipment

Multilumen catheter
Antimicrobial swabs
Transparent dressing
Sterile 4 × 4 gauze pads
Sterile gloves
Sterile drapes
Sterile gown
Two masks
3-mL syringe with 25-gauge needle
Lidocaine (Xylocaine—local anesthetic agent)
Suture material
Syringe with 5 mL NS
Syringe with 2 mL dilute heparin
IV administration set with appropriate filter
Hyperalimentation solution
Bath blanket to provide roll under shoulders

Preparation

1. Validate signed consent for catheter insertion.
2. Explain procedure to client to allay anxiety.
3. Teach Valsalva's maneuver for use during catheter insertion procedure. **Rationale:** This maneuver prevents air from entering the catheter during catheter insertion or tubing changes.
   a. Ask client to take a deep breath and bear down without exhaling.
   b. This action produces increased intrathoracic pressure.
4. Review physician's orders for correct hyperalimentation solution.
5. Inspect TPN container for layering, turbidity, or precipitates. If there are layers, return to pharmacy.
6. Assemble IV system with in-line filter. Tubing with a 1.2 micron filter is used for TPN with lipids; a 0.2 micron filter is used for TPN without lipids.

Composition of TPN Solutions

- Amino acid
- Carbohydrates—10%–35% glucose
- Vitamins (become inactive when exposed to light)
- Minerals and trace elements
- Electrolytes (individualized)
- Water
- Hyperalimentation solution is prepared aseptically in the pharmacy under a laminar flow hood

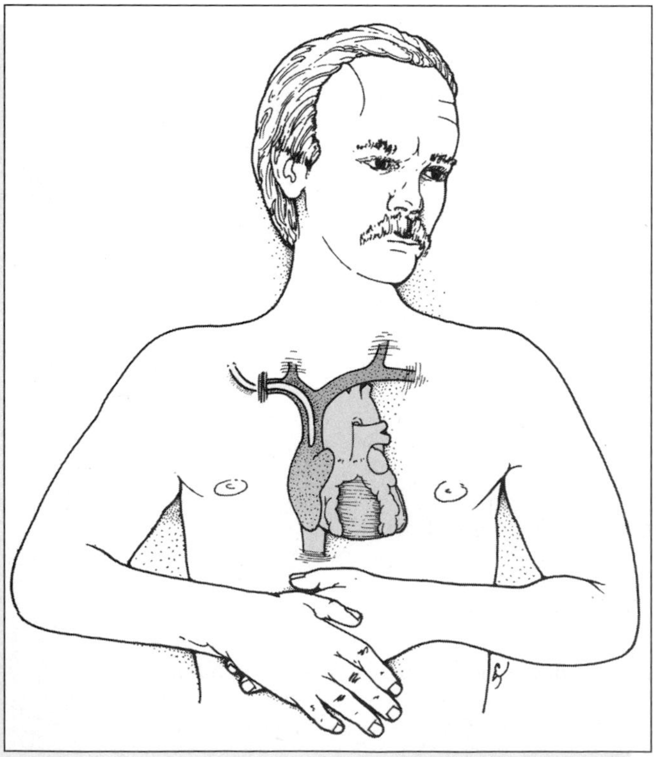
Right subclavian vein is preferred access to right atrium.

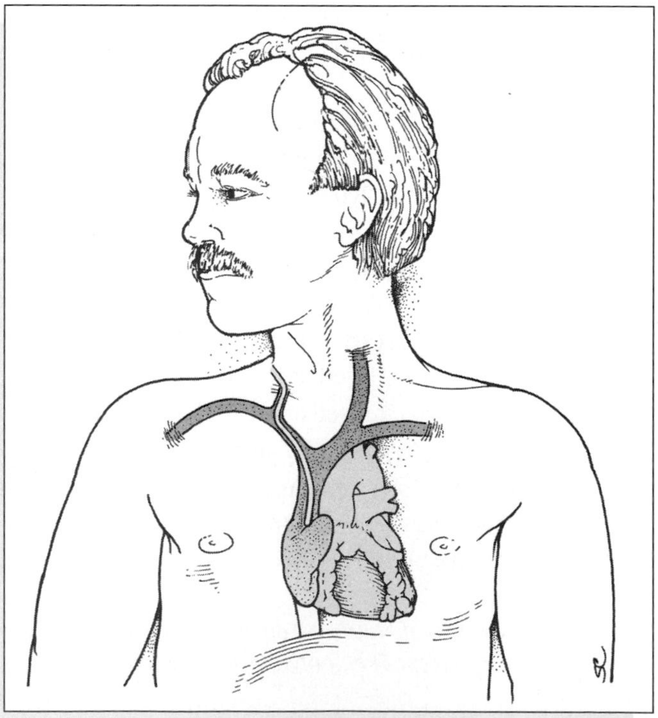
Central venous catheter inserted via right jugular vein.

7. Wash hands.
8. Prime IV tubing and filter with solution.
9. Insert IV tubing into infusion pump.

CLINICAL ALERT

TPN and lipids are frequently infused together in the same bag to prevent microorganism growth from lipid emulsion.

Procedure

1. Position client in head-down position with head turned to opposite direction of catheter insertion site. Place a small roll between client's shoulders to expose insertion site. **Rationale:** This position increases intrathoracic venous pressure and reduces risk of air embolism.
2. Cleanse insertion area with antimicrobial swab.
   a. Cleanse a large area around insertion site.
   b. Use a circular motion to cleanse from insertion site to periphery.
3. Assist physician to put on gown, mask, and gloves prior to beginning procedure.
4. Don mask and sterile gloves.
5. Assist physician as needed during catheter insertion.
6. Instruct client in Valsalva's maneuver when stylet is removed from catheter and injection cap is connected to catheter.
   a. Instruct client to exhale against a closed glottis.

Monitoring Guidelines for TPN

- Monitor for signs of infection or sepsis at the insertion site—the most common complication of TPN.
- Weigh client daily—observe for fluid gain or loss (.5–1.5 kilograms or 1–3 pounds per week). Weight gain may indicate fluid overload rather than nutritional gain.
- Monitor electrolyte and protein levels. Electrolyte imbalances may occur.
- Regularly monitor blood glucose levels observing for hyperglycemia (thirst, polyuria).
- Assess blood urea nitrogen and creatinine levels—increases may indicate excess amino acid intake.
- Check liver function test results—abnormal values may indicate an excess of lipids or problems in protein or glucose metabolism.

TABLE 29–2 Complications with Total Parenteral Nutrition

Complication	Symptoms	Implementation: Prevention	Implementation: Nursing Action
Air embolism Air enters catheter during catheter insertion or tubing changes	Potentially fatal Respiratory distress, apprehension Chest pain, dyspnea Hypotension Pulse weak and rapid Churning heart murmur (classic sign)	Instruct client in Valsalva's maneuver for tubing cap changes Check all catheter connections Place client in head-down position with head turned opposite direction of insertion site (increases intrathoracic venous pressure)	Clamp catheter Place client in left Trendelenburg's position (to trap air in right side of heart) Notify physician Administer oxygen as ordered
Catheter-related infection (sepsis) Because the TPN solution is high-concentrate glucose, it is a medium for bacterial growth	Fever (early sign), chills Insertion site—erythema or drainage Elevated white blood cell count Septic shock	Use strict aseptic technique Change solution every 12 hours Change tubing as ordered (every 24 hours using aseptic technique) Change dressing every 48 hours	Remove tip of catheter, and send to laboratory for culture Administer antibiotics as ordered
Hyperglycemia Increased blood sugar level due to infusion, stress, medications, diabetes	Elevated glucose levels (more than 200 mg/dL) Excessive thirst, fatigue, restlessness, confusion, weakness, diuresis When severe—coma	Check history for glucose intolerance; frequent glucose monitoring—check medications (e.g., steroids) Begin infusion at slow rate (usually 40 mL/hour) Increase proportion of calories as lipids Do not "catch-up" if infusion rate falls behind	Start sliding scale insulin therapy as ordered Monitor blood glucose levels every 4–6 hours Maintain blood glucose <200 mg/dL
Hypoglycemia TPN is discontinued abruptly or client is receiving too much insulin	Client is shaky, weak, anxious, diaphoretic May be hungry Decreased blood glucose (less than 70 mg/dL)	Continue blood glucose monitoring Gradually decrease infusion when discontinuing TPN Use infusion pump	Infuse 10% dextrose in water (50% may be needed) (Restart IV if necessary) Assess blood glucose 1 hour after discontinuing TPN

b. If client is unable to do this, compress client's abdomen. **Rationale:** Both these procedures help decrease possibility of air embolism.

7. After cap is connected, instruct client to breathe normally.
8. Flush catheter with saline, then heparinize with dilute heparin according to agency policy.
9. Apply transparent dressing over insertion site.
10. Obtain portable chest x-ray to verify correct catheter placement.
11. Following confirmation of catheter placement, initiate hyperalimentation solution and adjust flow rate as ordered.
12. Observe for signs of complications.
13. Take vital signs every 4 hours. **Rationale:** If signs change or temperature rises significantly, the client may be developing complications.

MAINTAINING HYPERALIMENTATION INFUSIONS (TPN)

Equipment

Hyperalimentation solution (TPN) (refrigerated)
IV tubing, filter, and infusion pump
Extension tubing
Glucometer
I&O record
Infusion pump

Procedure

1. Store hyperalimentation (TPN) solution in refrigerator until 30 minutes before use. (Some pharmacies deliver the solution before each infusion.) **Rationale:** Solution is refrigerated to prevent growth of organisms, but should be left at room temperature one hour prior to use.
2. Ensure central line is patent when infusing TPN. Check for patency every hour.

CLINICAL ALERT

Do not "catch up" a deficit in infused volume, as doing so could result in complications for the client. To assure constant flow rate, check rate every two hours.

3. Change IV tubing and filter every 24 hours. **Rationale:** This is recommended for TPN infusions to prevent infection.

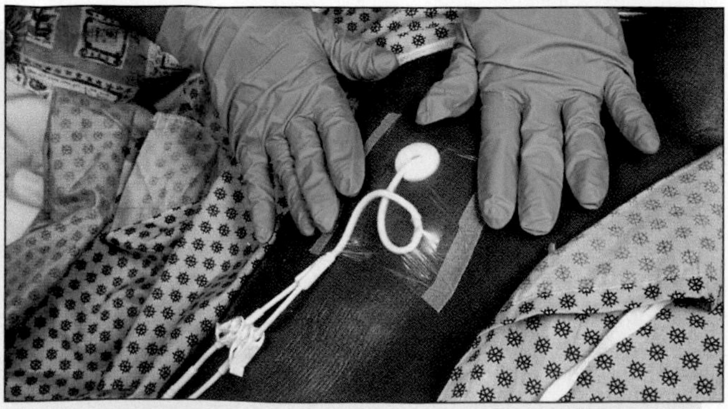

Nontunneled catheter used to deliver parenteral nutrition.

4. Maintain IV flow rate as prescribed. Use infusion pump for infusion.
   a. If rate is too rapid, hyperosmolar diuresis occurs (excess glucose and water is excreted); if severe enough, intractable seizures, coma, and death can occur.
   b. If rate is too slow, little benefit is derived from the calories and nitrogen.
5. Change solution every 12–24 hours. **Rationale:** Changing the solution prevents growth of bacterial organisms that proliferate in sugar solution.

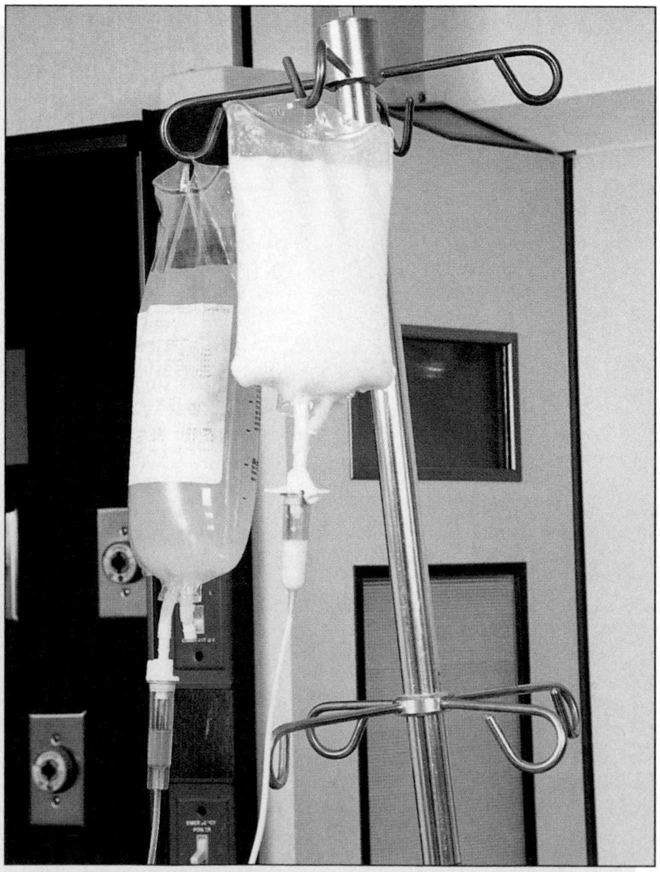

Total parenteral nutrition and lipid solutions infusing separately.

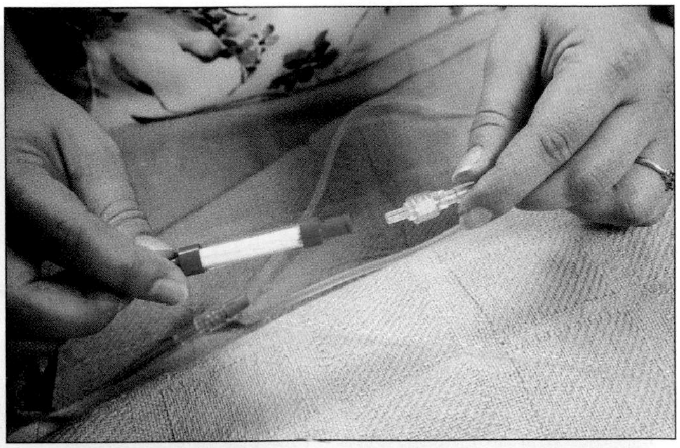

In-line filter used when administering TPN solution.

6. Monitor client's finger-stick blood sugar regularly (e.g., q 6 hrs).
7. If necessary, administer Regular insulin according to prescribed "sliding scale."
8. Maintain accurate I&Q.
9. Observe for complications, such as air embolus, hyperglycemia, osmotic diuresis, infiltration, or sepsis.

CLINICAL ALERT

No medication or blood products are to be added or piggybacked into TPN line.
No blood specimen should be withdrawn from an IV line infusing TPN.
TPN is never stopped abruptly. It should be tapered off.

CHANGING HYPERALIMENTATION (TPN) DRESSING AND TUBING

Equipment

Clean and sterile gloves
Mask
IV tubing and filter (0.22 micron)
TPN solution
2 × 2 sterile gauze pads and tape
Antimicrobial swabs
Transparent semipermeable dressing

Preparation

1. Check when tubing last changed.
2. Gather equipment, and wash hands.
3. Explain procedure to client.
4. Connect IV tubing and filter to parenteral hyperalimentation (TPN) solution container.
5. Flush tubing to clear air.
6. Place IV tubing through infusion pump.
7. Prepare dressing: antimicrobial swabs, sterile 2 × 2 gauze pads and tape, or sterile transparent dressing.
8. Place client supine with head turned in opposite direction of insertion site. Instruct client not to talk or cough. (Place mask on client if client cannot cooperate.) **Rationale:** These instructions reduce risk of contamination.

Procedure

1. Don mask (according to institutional policy), and clean gloves.
2. Remove old dressing and gloves.
3. Put on sterile gloves.
4. Observe insertion site for signs of erythema, drainage, or swelling.
5. Cleanse insertion site with antimicrobial swabs, using a circular movement from inside outward.

CLINICAL ALERT

When central-line dressings are loose, wet, or soiled, they are considered contaminated and must be changed. Dressings are routinely changed 3 times per week.

6. Allow 1 minute for drying.
7. Place sterile transparent dressing over insertion site. Secure dressing.
8. Change IV tubing.
   a. Clamp catheter using slide clamp.
   b. Loosen tubing in catheter hub.
   c. Insert new primed tubing *or*
   d. Cap catheter and insert new IV tubing using needleless connector.
9. Remove gloves and wash hands.
10. Label dressing with date and your initials.

CLINICAL ALERT

If gauze dressings are used, change every 48–72 hrs. Transparent dressing alone can be changed every 72–96 hrs. Transparent dressings are preferred unless site is draining.

MAINTAINING HYPERALIMENTATION FOR CHILDREN

Equipment

Same as for adult hyperalimentation with these additions:

Intracath, 22-gauge needle
Microdrip IV tubing administration set
0.22 micron in-line filter
Restraints, only if necessary and ordered

Procedure

1. Verify solution with physician's orders.
2. Examine solution. Generally, there is a higher concentration of calcium, phosphorus, magnesium, and vitamins. Either a 10% dextrose/2% amino acids or 5% dextrose/4% amino acids solution can be infused peripherally. Higher concentrations are infused centrally, as is long-term therapy.
3. Monitor patency of catheter. Stopcocks are never used. Monitor infusion pump and filter.
4. Obtain finger stick or urine sugar samples every 8 hours. Sugar level rises, but usually exogenous insulin is not required as the pancreas adapts to high glucose loads.
5. Monitor intake and output and daily weight.
6. Change the dressing every 48 hours and the tubing every 24 hours using aseptic technique. Stockinette can be used to keep scalp dressing secure. Tight-fitting T-shirt can keep chest site secure.
7. Monitor for accurate rate of infusion. Do not "catch up" if infusion is behind. Pumps can be used to maintain infusion rates, particularly when small amounts of solution are being infused.
8. If discontinuing, taper infusion for one hour (decrease rate q 30 min). **Rationale:** Abrupt discontinuation may cause a hypoglycemic reaction since insulin production is increased.
9. Observe the child when ambulating for twisting or kinking of tubing, getting the tubing caught in the crib, or stepping on it.
10. Instruct parents on rationale for treatment and methods to prevent accidental dislodging of the tubing.
11. Provide play therapy and sources of stimulation to distract the child from the catheter.

DOCUMENTATION FOR TOTAL PARENTERAL NUTRITION

- Special TPN sheet may be used; if so, charting is done directly on the sheet
- Catheter type, insertion site, physician's name
- X-ray, following insertion
- Type of hyperalimentation solution and flow rate
- Results of blood glucose monitoring
- If insulin administered, type, amount, and site
- Date and time of dressing of tubing change with name or initials of person who did the change
- Condition of insertion site
- Client's tolerance of procedure
- Daily weights
- Intake and output

Critical Thinking Application

UNEXPECTED OUTCOMES	CRITICAL THINKING OPTIONS
Hyperalimentation solution is not infused at the prescribed rate.	• Observe filter to ensure patency. A plugged filter is the most common cause of infusion failure. Change the filter and tubing. • Ensure that the next hyperalimentation bottle is ready to be superimposed. • Observe for signs of hypoglycemia caused by sudden change in dextrose concentration—weakness, trembling, sweating, hunger. Check finger-stick blood sugar. • Adjust flow rate to that which was ordered. Do not attempt to "catch up" the amount not infused as this action could lead to osmotic diuresis from hyperglycemia.
Catheter insertion site becomes inflamed.	• Notify physician immediately so catheter can be discontinued if catheter-related sepsis is suspected. • Cut tip of catheter off with sterile scissors and place in sterile container. Send to laboratory for culture and sensitivity for specific causative organism. • Cleanse site of catheter insertion with antimicrobial swab, and place sterile dressing over site. • Obtain order for and administer antibiotics as needed.
The dressing becomes wet or loose.	• Change the dressing as soon as moisture is observed, using aseptic technique. • If the dressing is exposed to moisture or secretions, cover with transparent dressing (e.g., showering).
TPN solution temporarily unavailable.	• Infuse D10W IV solution at prescribed rate until TPN solution available.

UNIT 3

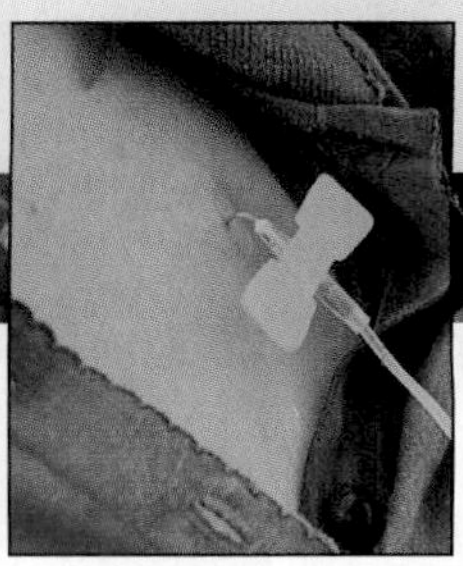

Lipid Emulsion Therapy

Nursing Process Data

ASSESSMENT Data Base

Observe for signs of essential fatty acid deficits; rash; eczema; dry, scaly skin; poor wound healing sparse hair.

Assess pancreatic function.

Assess client for predisposing factors that could promote fat emboli, such as anemia, coagulation disorders, abnormal liver or pulmonary function.

Check IV site for patency, erythema and edema before infusing solution.

Assess vital signs to establish baseline.

PLANNING Objectives

To spare protein in critically ill client

To provide a source of energy for clients with deficient protein intake

To provide essential fatty acids

IMPLEMENTATION Procedures

Infusing IV Lipids

EVALUATION Expected Outcomes

Adequate calories and essential fatty acids are provided to clients unable to ingest them.

Parenteral nutrients are provided without complications.

INFUSING IV LIPIDS

Equipment

IV lipid solution
Nonphthalate IV tubing infusion set (to prevent pooling of fat in IV tubing)
Needleless cannula
Antimicrobial swabs
Volume control device

Preparation

1. Review physician's orders and MAR.
2. Obtain lipid emulsion (refrigerated) from the pharmacy and warm the solution to room temperature.
3. Examine bottle for separation of emulsion into layers or fat globules or for accumulation of froth. Do not use if any of these appear.
4. Label bottle with client name, room number, date, time, flow rate, bottle number, and start and stop times.
5. Identify client and check client's identaband.
6. Explain procedure to client.

Procedure

1. Take vital signs for baseline assessment. **Rationale:** Baseline information is needed because an immediate reaction can occur.
2. Wash hands, and then swab stopper on IV bottle with antimicrobial swab and allow to dry.
3. Attach special IV tubing to bottle, twisting the spike to prevent particles from stopper falling into the emulsion, or spike bag with regular IV tubing.
4. Hang IV bottle at least 30 inches above IV site. **Rationale:** Due to solution viscosity, lipid emulsion needs to be at this height to prevent backing up into infusion tubing.
5. Fill drip chamber two-thirds full, slightly open clamp on the tubing, and prime the tubing slowly. **Rationale:** Priming more slowly reduces chance of air bubbles with this solution.
6. Attach the tubing to the IV site.
7. If piggybacking lipids into hyperalimentation, use port closest to client, below tubing filter.
8. Infuse lipid solutions initially at 1.0 mL/min for adults and 0.1 mL/min for children.

CLINICAL ALERT

Lipid emulsions alone promote growth of specific bacteria and yeasts as soon as 6 hours after the infusion. When lipids are combined with TPN (solution of amino acids, lipid emulsion and glucose) in the same bag, it doesn't appear to support any greater microbial growth than non–lipid-containing TPN fluids. This TPN solution can hang safely for 24 hours.

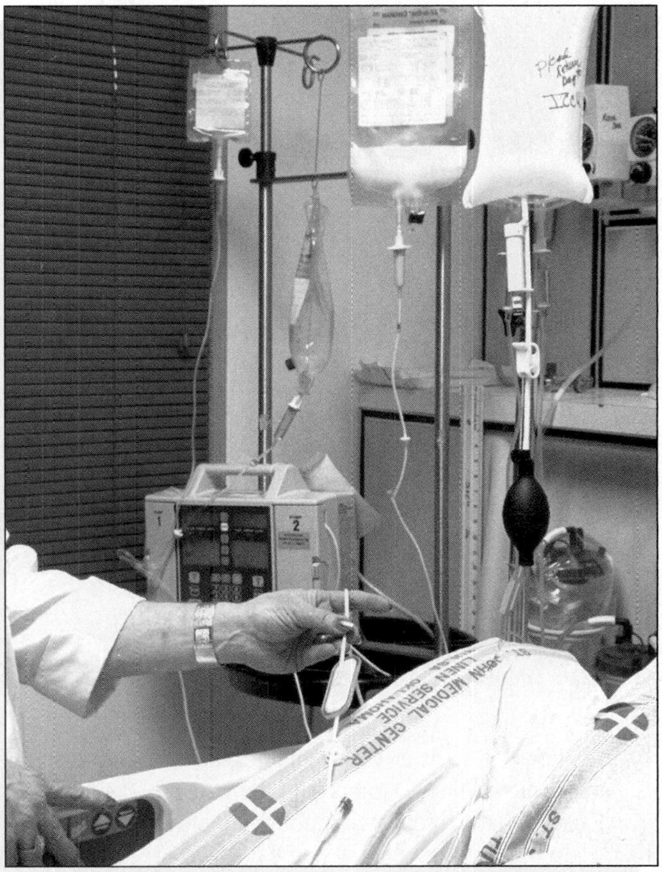

Hyperalimentation solution must be filtered while lipids are not—piggyback lipid solution below filter or use separate line.

Guidelines for IV Lipid Infusion

- IV lipid solutions are isotonic and provide 1.1 Cal/mL of solution.
- Do not put additives into IV bottle.
- Do not use an IV filter because the particles are large and cannot pass through.

for Adults

- Lipid 10%: Up to 500 mL 4–6 hours on first day to maximum of 2.5 g/kg body weight per day. Do not exceed 60% of client's total caloric intake per day.
- Liposyn 10%: No more than 500 mL/day in 4–6 hours.

for Children

- Lipid 10%: Up to 1 g/kg in 4 hours. Do not exceed 60% of total caloric intake.

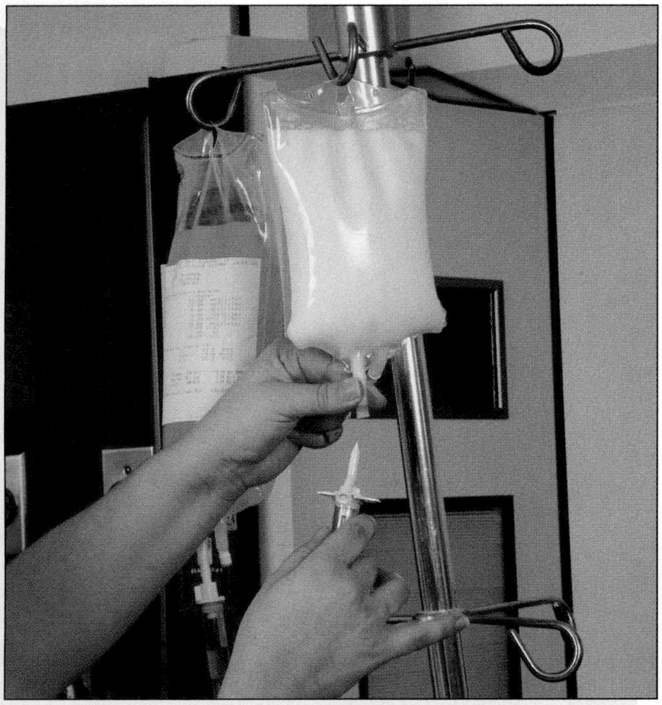

Alternate method to spike lipid solution bag to IV tubing.

9. Monitor vital signs every 10 minutes, and observe for side effects during first 30 minutes of the infusion. If side effects occur, stop the infusion and notify the physician.
10. Adjust flow to prescribed IV rate if no adverse reactions occur.
11. Monitor and maintain the infusion at the ordered rate.
12. Monitor serum lipids 4 hours after discontinuing infusion. **Rationale:** If you draw blood too soon after infusion is completed, incorrect blood values result.
13. Monitor liver function tests for evidence of impaired liver function. **Rationale:** These tests indicate the liver's ability to metabolize the lipids.
14. Discard partially used bottles. **Rationale:** This action prevents contamination.
15. Discard administration set after each unit unless additional units are administered consecutively.
16. Continue to monitor vital signs, and observe client for adverse reactions during the entire process of infusion.
17. Answer any questions the client may have about the procedure, and make client comfortable before leaving room.

CLINICAL ALERT

Observe for IV lipid side effects after starting lipid infusion:

chills	chest and back pain
fever	nausea and vomiting
flushing	headache
diaphoresis	pressure over the eyes
dyspnea	vertigo
cyanosis	sleepiness
allergic reactions	thrombophlebitis

DOCUMENTATION FOR LIPID EMULSION THERAPY

- Type of solution infused
- Rate of infusion
- Site of infusion
- Vital signs monitored
- Adverse clinical manifestations and appropriate nursing intervention

Critical Thinking Application

UNEXPECTED OUTCOMES	CRITICAL THINKING OPTIONS
Client experiences difficulty and cannot continue with lipid infusion.	• Reassess client's ability to tolerate fat solution. • Notify physician for order to discontinue fat solution, and administer hyperalimentation solution. • Monitor liver function test results.
Client develops dyspnea, cyanosis, or allergic reaction, such as nausea, vomiting, increased temperature, or headache.	• Stop infusion immediately, and notify physician.
Client's serum triglyceride and liver function test results remain elevated.	• Hang the solution bottle on an IV stand as you would an IV bottle • Begin the feeding with a weaker concentration of formula, and increase the concentration slowly as ordered.
Client develops hyperlipemia or hypercoagulability.	• Monitor laboratory results, particularly liver function tests, and notify physician when any abnormality occurs.

UNIT 4

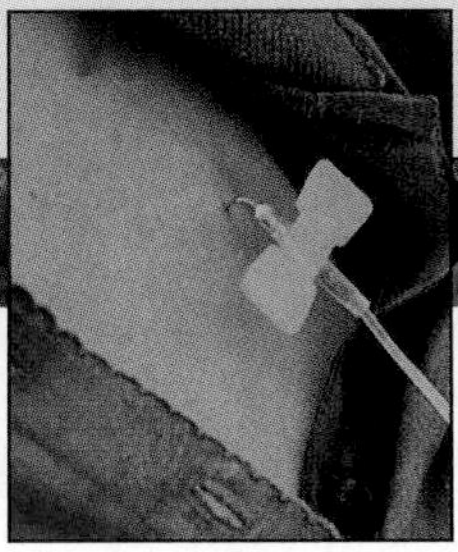

Tunneled Central Vascular Access Devices (CVADs)

Nursing Process Data

ASSESSMENT *Data Base*

Assess patency of catheter.

Assess insertion site for signs of infection.

Assess the tubing for accidental breaks.

Assess injection cap at the end of catheter to ensure tightness.

PLANNING *Objectives*

To provide a patent catheter

To clear a nonpatent catheter

To provide an access for blood drawing

To provide an access for infusions

IMPLEMENTATION *Procedures*

Maintaining the Hickman or Broviac CV Catheter

Changing the Hickman or Broviac CV Catheter Dressing

Maintaining the CV Catheter with Groshong Valve

Drawing Blood from the CV Catheter with Groshong Valve

EVALUATION *Expected Outcomes*

The catheter remains patent.

The catheter site is infection free.

Blood samples are obtained without difficulty.

Infusions of medications or fluids are accomplished without difficulty.

MAINTAINING THE HICKMAN OR BROVIAC CV CATHETER

Equipment

10-mL syringe with needleless cannula with 3 mL dilute heparin (100 U/mL solution)
Antimicrobial swab
Clean gloves
Three tuberculin syringes
10-mL syringe

Preparation

1. Check client care plan, physician's orders and MAR.
2. Prepare syringe with dilute heparin.
3. Explain procedure to client.
4. Provide privacy for client.
5. Wash hands and don gloves.

Procedure

for Flushing Intermittently Used Line

1. Wipe catheter cap with antimicrobial swab.
2. Insert syringe cannula into needleless access cap and unsnap catheter squeeze clamp.
3. Inject heparin solution slowly through catheter until almost empty.
4. Remove syringe while still moving plunger forward or clamp catheter before removing syringe. **Rationale:** This maintains positive pressure in the catheter and prevents clotting by preventing back-flow of blood into catheter.
5. Withdraw syringe.
6. Flush nonused capped lines daily.

for Irrigating a Nonpatent Catheter

1. Prepare three tuberculin syringes with dilute heparin. **Rationale:** The size of this syringe increases pressure exerted in the system.
2. Swab catheter cap with antimicrobial swab.
3. Insert syringe with needleless cannula, and unclamp catheter.
4. Inject heparin from syringes, to a total of 3 mL.
5. Leave heparin in catheter tubing for 1 hour.
6. Check that hour is completed, then use a 10-mL syringe to aspirate solution from catheter by gently pulling back on plunger.
7. Follow with an irrigation of 5–10 mL of heparinized solution if aspiration is successful. Use same dilution factor (100 U/mL) for irrigation solution as with maintenance solution.
8. Repeat procedure once. If unsuccessful, notify physician.
9. Discard equipment, gloves and wash hands.

Tunneled Central Vascular Access Devices (CVADs)

- Tunneled central vascular access devices (CVADs) provide long-term access to a central vein for the purpose of drawing blood, administering drugs (chemotherapy, antibiotics), administering total parenteral nutrition (TPN), or administering blood and blood products.
- Long-term catheters have one, two, or three lumens.
- The tip is inserted into a central vein and advanced to the superior vena cava. The remainder of the catheter passes through a subcutaneous track and exits on the chest wall or abdomen for easy access. A dacron cuff on the catheter elicits scar formation that prevents ascending tract infection.
- Two common tunneled CVADs are the Hickman and Broviac.
- Clients with tunneled CVADs are advised to display medical-alert information.

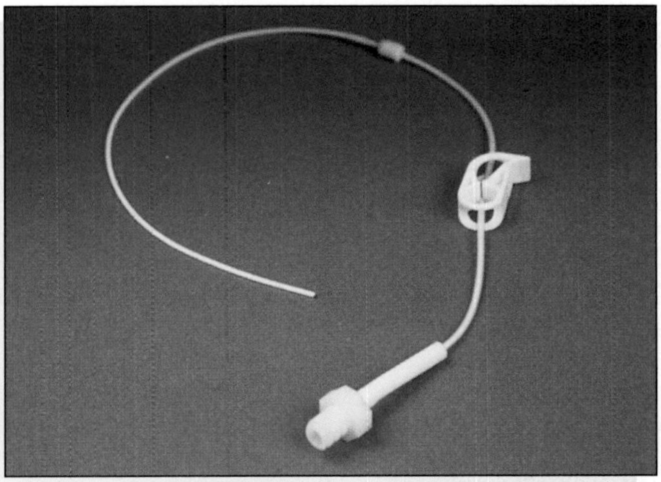

The tunneled Broviac catheter (single, double, or triple lumen) is commonly used for children.

CHANGING THE HICKMAN OR BROVIAC CV CATHETER DRESSING

Equipment

Antimicrobial swabs
Transparent, semipermeable dressing
Tape
Clean gloves
Sterile gloves
Mask (if client is neutropenic and per agency policy)

> **CLINICAL ALERT**
> To prevent a potentially life-threatening mistake, never use scissors near central venous catheters.

Procedure

1. Wash hands and don gloves.
2. Remove old dressing.
3. Observe for signs and symptoms of infection and crepitus at insertion site. **Rationale:** Signs most frequently observed are erythema, edema, and drainage for infection; crackling under the skin denotes crepitus due to air in the subcutaneous tissue—this finding should be reported.
4. Discard dressing and gloves.
5. Set up supplies on a sterile field.
6. Don sterile gloves.
7. Clean exit site using 3 antimicrobial swabs. Start from inner aspect, move out toward periphery approximately 1-2 inches from exit site. Do not go over same area twice with same swab. **Rationale**: This prevents contamination at the insertion site.
8. Clean catheter tubing at exit site. Allow to dry.
9. Apply sterile transparent dressing; change weekly or if soiled. When cuff heals into place, dressings are not necessary.
10. Remove gloves and discard.
11. Sign and date dressing.
12. Secure catheter to prevent dislodging; tape to chest.
13. Wash your hands.

Note: Nonhospitalized clients who are not immunosuppressed may protect exit site with a Band-Aid or leave the site undressed. They should cleanse daily with antibacterial soap and water, palpate site daily to check for signs of infection, and tape catheter to chest to prevent accidental dislodgement.

MAINTAINING THE CV CATHETER WITH GROSHONG VALVE

Note: The Groshong valve is available in a variety of CVADs, including ports and PICCs. The Groshong allows infusion, but prevents backflow of blood unless negative pressure is applied. There is no need for heparin flush, and external clamps are not used. Clamping could force the slit valve open, allowing blood to leak into the lumen.

Equipment

Normal saline
Antimicrobial swab
Chlorhexidine wipe
Sterile injection cap
Appropriate syringe: 10 mL or 20 mL
Clean gloves
Sterile gloves

Preparation

1. Check physician's orders, client care plan, and MAR.
2. Gather equipment.
3. Identify client's room, identaband and ask client to state name.
4. Wash hands, and don gloves.

> **The Groshong Catheter**
>
> The Groshong catheter offers an alternative to the Hickman and Broviac catheters. It is distinguished by a rounded, blunt catheter tip with a three-way pressure-sensitive valve that remains closed at normal vena caval pressure. When closed, it restricts air from entering the venous system or a backflow of blood from the catheter. When a syringe is inserted to create a vacuum, it allows the valve to open inward for blood aspiration. Positive pressure into the catheter by infusion forces the valve to open outward. The primary advantages of this type of catheter are:
>
> - Decreased risk of air emboli or bleeding
> - Elimination of heparin to flush the catheter
> - Elimination of catheter clamping
> - Reduced flushing protocols between use

Procedure

1. Wipe injection cap and catheter connection with antimicrobial swab.
2. While holding catheter, insert flush syringe needleless can-

nula *or* remove catheter cap and attach hub of syringe directly to catheter hub.
3. Inject normal saline rapidly into lumen.
4. Maintain positive pressure on syringe plunger as last 0.5 mL is injected and syringe is withdrawn. **Rationale:** Keeping pressure on the plunger prevents backup of blood into catheter.
5. Attach new, sterile, injection cap.
6. Remove cap by holding catheter connector between thumb and forefinger of one hand and grasping barrel of cap with other hand.
7. Twist and pull counterclockwise to separate cap from connector.

> **CLINICAL ALERT**
>
> Nursing attention to the catheter during dressing change is important to ensure catheter is not pinched, kinked, occluded, cut, or dislodged. It is recommended that the external portion of catheter be coiled and taped to avoid a straight pull on catheter insertion site.

8. Continue to hold connector with one hand. **Rationale:** Holding connector prevents inadvertent contamination by placing connector on dirty surface.
9. Discard old cap.
10. Clean liberally around connector using antimicrobial swab.
11. Holding new injection cap, twist clockwise and insert into connector.

for 10- or 20-mL Irrigation

1. Remove needle from syringe.
2. Remove injection cap carefully from connector and discard.
3. Clean connector with chlorhexidine wipe. DO NOT let go of connector. **Rationale:** Holding connector prevents inadvertent contamination.
4. Insert syringe barrel directly into catheter connector, twisting slightly to ensure good connection.
5. Irrigate lumen with normal saline using stop–start action. **Rationale:** Heparin is not used because clotting is not a factor with catheter tip design of the Groshong.
6. Maintain positive pressure on syringe barrel as syringe is removed from connector. DO NOT clamp the catheter following irrigation. **Rationale:** The Groshong CV catheter does not require clamping to keep blood from entering the lumen. Clamping the catheter damages it.
7. Change injection cap.
8. Remove gloves and wash hands.

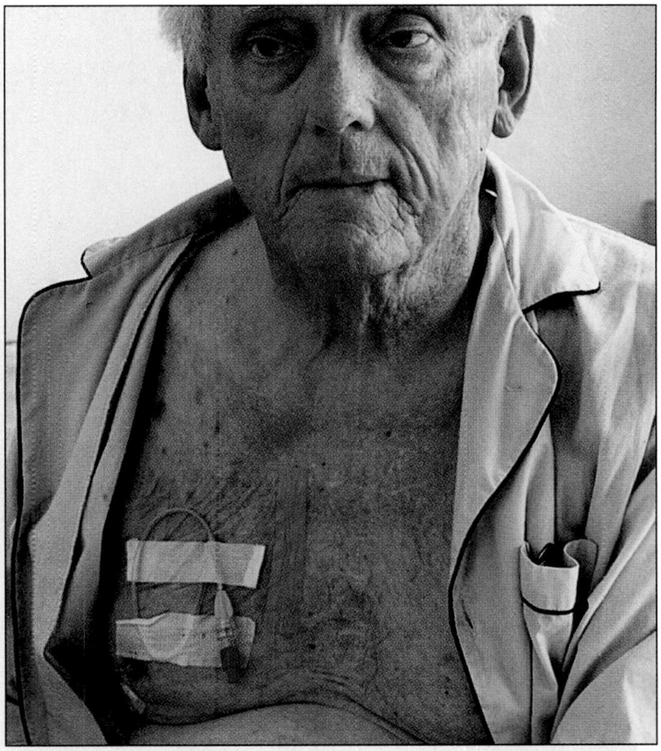

The tunneled CV catheter with Groshong valve is ideal for long-term therapy.

Flushing Tunneled Catheters

Flush catheter with 3–5 mL of heparin (10 units/mL) daily when catheter is not used and before and after each use. The SASH protocol is used (saline, administer drug or withdraw blood, saline, and heparin). This type of flushing is not done with a closed-ended (Groshong) catheter, as its internal valve is designed to prevent blood reflux into the catheter.

Irrigation Protocols

Using 5 mL of Saline

- Irrigate catheter weekly when not in use.
- Irrigate catheter after every use.

Using 20 mL of Saline

- Irrigate catheter before and after any aspiration of blood, after transfusion of blood, or when blood is seen in the catheter (client straining or lifting may cause blood to back up into catheter).
- Irrigate catheter after infusion of lipids or hyperalimentation solutions.

Note: Regardless of the volume of saline used, ALWAYS irrigate in a stop–start action. ***Rationale:*** *This creates a swirling effect at the distal end of the catheter.*

DRAWING BLOOD FROM THE CV CATHETER WITH GROSHONG VALVE

Equipment

Sterile injection cap.
Two 10-mL Luer-Lok syringes for drawing blood
One 20-mL Luer-Lok syringe, filled with normal saline
Blood tubes appropriate for tests ordered
Antimicrobial swabs
Clean gloves

Note: Vacuum tubes should not be used with the Groshong valve.

Procedure

1. Wash hands and don gloves.
2. Clean cap and outside of connector with swabs and allow to dry.
3. Remove and discard injection cap while holding connector so that it does not make contact with any surface.
4. Insert first 10-mL syringe directly into catheter, twisting slightly to ensure connection.
5. Pull back plunger 0.5 mL, pause 2 seconds, and then continue aspirating until 5 mL of blood is in syringe.

CLINICAL ALERT

Groshong catheter MUST BE irrigated with stop–start action with at least 10 mL of NS prior to blood sample removal.

6. Remove syringe, set aside; continue to hold connector.
7. Connect second 10-mL syringe directly to catheter connector, twisting slightly to ensure connection.
8. Proceed to aspirate blood volume needed for sample following same aspiration procedure of pulling 0.5 mL and waiting for 2 seconds.
9. Remove syringe, and continue to hold connector.
10. Flush catheter briskly with 20 mL normal saline and attach new sterile injection cap.
11. Transfer blood sample from second syringe into appropriate tube(s), and label. Do not hold receiving tube during transfer.
12. Discard syringe containing first aspirated blood into biohazard container.
13. Remove gloves and wash hands.

DOCUMENTATION FOR CVADs

- Flush frequency and solution used
- Dressing changes and type applied
- Exit site condition
- Condition and patency of catheter
- Medications or solutions administered through catheter
- Amount of blood withdrawn for testing
- Infusion cap change

Critical Thinking Application

UNEXPECTED OUTCOMES	CRITICAL THINKING OPTIONS
CV Catheter:	
Unable to aspirate blood even though solution flows through the catheter.	• Use less negative pressure on syringe when aspirating blood. Tip of catheter may be sucking against wall of vessel. • Have client raise arms above head. This can alter position of catheter. • Have client perform Valsalva's maneuver. • Change client's position.
Clotting of catheter occurs (client develops arm or neck swelling on catheter side of body).	• Do not force plunger with Groshong, this may rupture catheter. • Make sure clamps are open and tubing is not kinked. • Use irrigating procedure for catheter with a recently developed clot. Instill 1 mL dilute heparin solution followed by 1 mL normal saline. • Allow 15 minutes before aspirating to see if declotting occurs. Repeat if necessary. • Prevent occlusion due to drug sludge by flushing carefully after administration. • Thrombolytic agent is required for fibrinous clot. • FDA approved use of t-PA (tissue plasminogen activator) for thrombolytic protocol. Follow facility policy regarding instillation of drug. • Instill 2 mg of t-PA in a 10-mL syringe. Wait 60 minutes. Aspirate; if unable to obtain blood flow, instill a second dose of t-PA. If this does not produce blood flow, notify physician.
Catheter breaks or is pierced by clamp.	• Immediately clamp catheter proximal to break site, if necessary (Groshong may be clamped using rubber band). • Obtain repair kit for catheter.
Air enters catheter when open to atmosphere; client experiences chest pain, shortness of breath or coughing.	• Clamp catheter (use rubber band if Groshong device). • Turn client on left side with head lower than rest of body to trap air in right heart. • Notify physician immediately. • Administer oxygen.
Signs of infection develop at exit site (redness, pain, fever, chills).	• Catheter will have to be removed and cultures taken.

UNIT 5

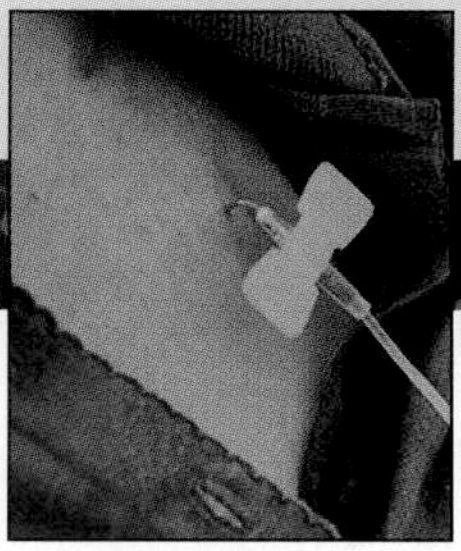

Implanted Subcutaneous Port

Nursing Process Data

***ASSESSMENT* Data Base**

Assess site.

Assess patency of port.

***PLANNING* Objectives**

To provide an access for blood withdrawal

To provide an access for drug or blood/fluid administration

***IMPLEMENTATION* Procedures**

Accessing and Flushing an Implanted Port Using a Huber Needle

Administering Drugs via a Subcutaneous Implanted Port

Administering Infusions via a Subcutaneous Port

Drawing Blood from an Implanted Subcutaneous Port

***EVALUATION* Expected Outcomes**

Implantation site remains free from bruising, swelling, redness, or tenderness.

Port is easily accessed.

Infusions of drugs and fluids are accomplished without difficulty.

Blood samples are obtained without difficulty.

ACCESSING AND FLUSHING AN IMPLANTED PORT USING A HUBER NEEDLE

Note: Implanted venous access ports, such as Port-a-Cath, are usually placed in a subcutaneous pocket on the chest wall, require minimal maintenance, and may be used for months to years before the maximum 2,000 punctures are achieved. Ports are best utilized for cyclic therapies like chemotherapy or antibiotic therapy. They are well suited for care of cancer clients or others with long-term illnesses requiring IV medications. Ports can be used for either bolus or continuous infusions.

Equipment

Noncoring needle (Huber) with attached extension tubing and clamp
Intermittent infusion cap
Two 10-mL syringes with needleless cannula
Normal saline
Heparin (100 U/mL)
Antimicrobial swabs
Sterile gloves
Clean gloves
Mask

Preparation

1. Check physician's orders and client care plan. Review specific hospital policy and procedure for care of implanted port.
2. Gather equipment.
3. Wash hands, using germicide solution.
4. Draw up 10 mL normal saline into 10-mL syringe.
5. Draw up 5 mL dilute heparin (100 U/mL) into 10-mL syringe.
6. Identify client's identaband.
7. Explain procedure to client.
8. Don clean gloves.

Procedure

1. Palpate skin over subcutaneous infusion port. **Rationale:** This identifies location and contours of the device.

- Noncoring needles, such as the Huber needle, are the only ones used to access the port.
- This specially designed needle (bent at 90° angle to its hub or wings) has a sharp-angled bevel and attached extension tubing with clamp and needleless cap.
- Inserted through skin and into rubber septum for central venous access.
- Prevents coring of the port.
- Produces insertion tract that seals itself when it is removed.

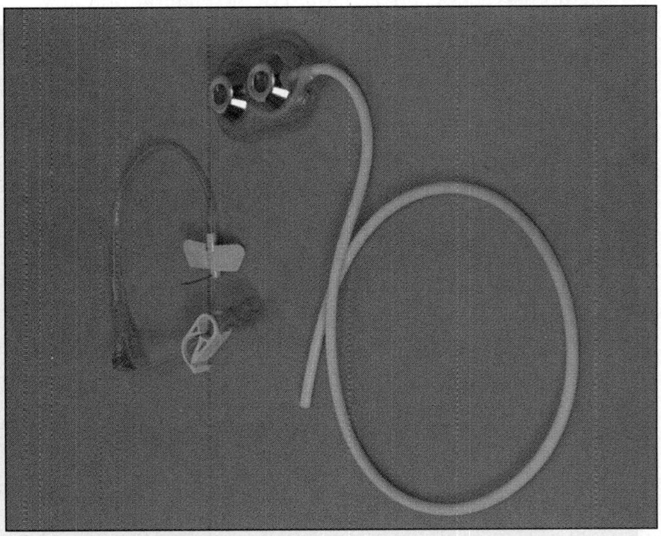

Example of Huber needle and stainless steel housed ports with extension tubing. Ports are surgically implanted under the skin.

2. Place thumb and forefinger of left hand on port (right hand if left-handed) and feel for septum with right hand. **Rationale:** This position stabilizes the port.
3. Numb the area with a topical anesthetic cream or ice, according to facility policy.
4. Clean skin with antimicrobial swab starting from center of septum, working outwards to a diameter of 3 inches. Use circular movement. Scrub for 30 seconds.
5. Allow site to air dry for 30 seconds. **Rationale:** Drying permits solution to work best against bacteria, fungi, and spores.
6. Affix syringe with 10 mL normal saline into Huber needle extension tubing cap and prime tubing; leave syringe attached.
7. Remove clean gloves and dispose in appropriate container.
8. Apply mask according to facility policy and don sterile gloves.
9. Stabilize port using thumb and index finger or index finger and middle finger.
10. Insert needle into port at a 90° angle until it meets resistance from the stainless steel back of the port.
11. Check for correct placement by aspirating for blood return.
    a. Withdraw flash of blood to check needle position. If no blood is obtained, try repositioning client (sit up, raise arms, cough).
    b. If still unable to obtain blood, try flushing port with small amount (2–3 mL) normal saline.
    c. If no blood return, remove noncoring needle and reaccess port.
    d. If still unable to obtain blood, call the physician (x-ray for placement may be required.)

12. If placement is correct, stabilize needle and inject remaining normal saline. There should be no sign of infiltration into surrounding tissue.
13. Close clamp of needle extension tubing.
14. Exchange syringe of normal saline for syringe filled with dilute heparin flush, then open clamp.
15. Instill 5 mL of heparin flush (100 U/mL).
16. Clamp extension tubing before removing needle.
17. Remove needle by pulling straight out from port while stabilizing port with free hand.
18. If needle is to be left in place for intermittent use, place sterile 2 × 2 gauze to fill gap between needle and skin; secure wings with tape for hub, chevron style) and apply sterile transparent dressing over all.
19. Dispose of equipment.
20. Remove gloves and wash hands.

CLINICAL ALERT

Implanted ports have the lowest risk of infection of all chest accessed central lines.

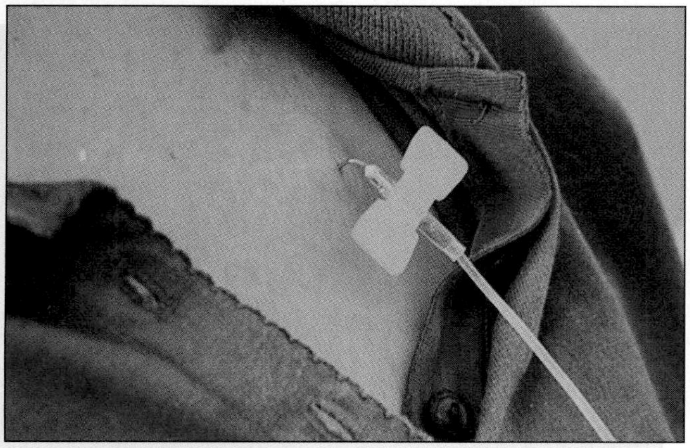

A noncoring 90° angle Huber needle is used to access the port.

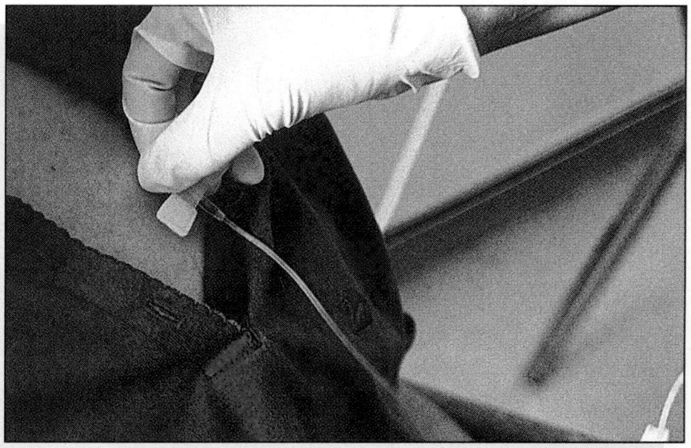

Secure needle in port while flushing. Unused port is flushed monthly.

ADMINISTERING DRUGS VIA A SUBCUTANEOUS IMPLANTED PORT

Equipment

Syringe filled with medication
Equipment as listed in previous skill
Syringe filled with 10 mL saline
Syringe with 10 mL dilute heparin solution

Procedure

1. Follow procedure listed in previous skill. (Using sterile gloves, access port verifying correct placement, i.e., blood return on aspiration, ability to infuse normal saline flush, and no infiltration.)

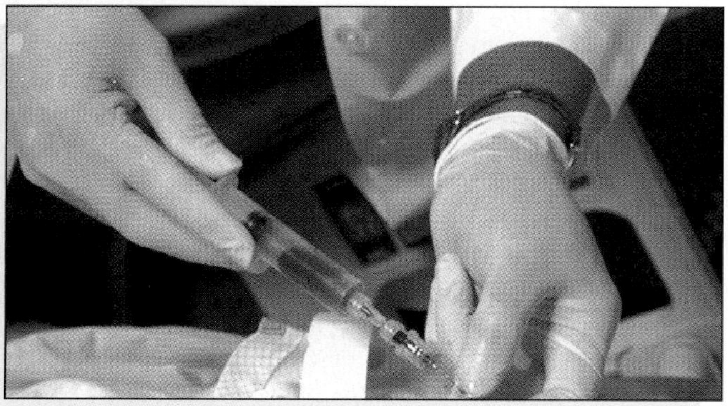

Check for blood flashback when flushing CVAD (unless Groshong valve present).

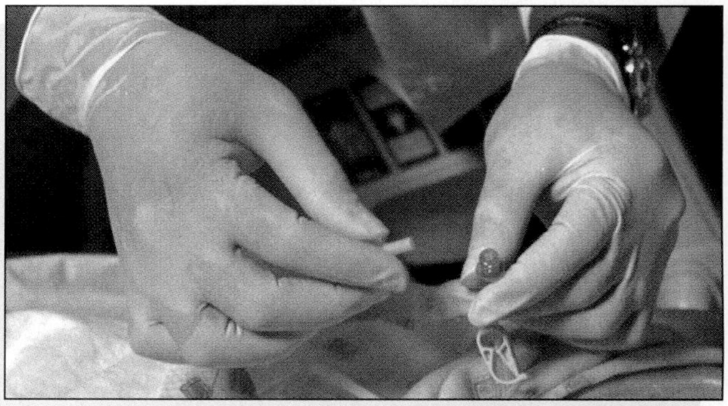

Always have CVAD clamped when changing infusion cap (Groshong valve does not require).

2. Clamp short needle extension tubing.
3. Exchange saline syringe for syringe filled with ordered medication.
4. Unclamp tubing.
5. Administer medication at prescribed rate.
6. Flush port between drugs with 5 mL of saline if giving more than one drug. **Rationale:** This prevents the possibility of drug–drug interactions.
7. Flush system with saline, then with dilute heparin.
8. Inject last 0.5 mL of heparin flush while simultaneously withdrawing needle and stabilizing port.
9. Wipe skin gently with dry swab to remove any solution.
10. If client is to receive intermittent IV drugs or solution, the Huber needle may remain in place for one week. After intermittent administration, clamp tubing, insert new sterile protective cap into extension tubing, open clamp to flush and heparinize, then reclamp tubing.
11. Flush unused port with 5 mL heparin (100 U/mL) daily.
12. Dispose of equipment (including gloves) and wash hands.

Note: Change port dressing weekly or when wet or soiled.

ADMINISTERING INFUSIONS VIA A SUBCUTANEOUS PORT

Equipment

Huber needle with attached extension tubing and in-line clamp
Intermittent infusion cap
5-mL syringe with needleless cannula
Two 10-mL syringes with needleless cannula
Normal saline
Heparin (100 U/mL)
Antimicrobial swabs
Sterile gloves
Mask
Sterile gauze square
Transparent dressing
Tape
Ordered IV solutions, drugs, or blood products

Preparation

1. Check physician's orders, client care plan, and MAR.
2. Gather equipment.
3. Check client's identaband
4. Explain procedure to client.
5. Provide privacy.
6. Raise bed to comfortable working position.
7. Wash hands.

Procedure

1. Remove dressing, prepare site and access port using sterile technique (sterile gloves and mask) as previously described.
2. Secure needle hub with tape, chevron style, or wings with tape or steri-strips—(place folded sterile 2 × 2 gauze to fill gap between needle and skin if necessary).
3. Place transparent dressing over insertion site, needle, and proximal IV tubing; date and initial.
4. Flush port with 10 mL saline solution.
5. Proceed with administration of ordered solution, drug, or blood.
6. Upon completion, flush with 10 mL normal saline, followed by 5 mL dilute heparin flush.

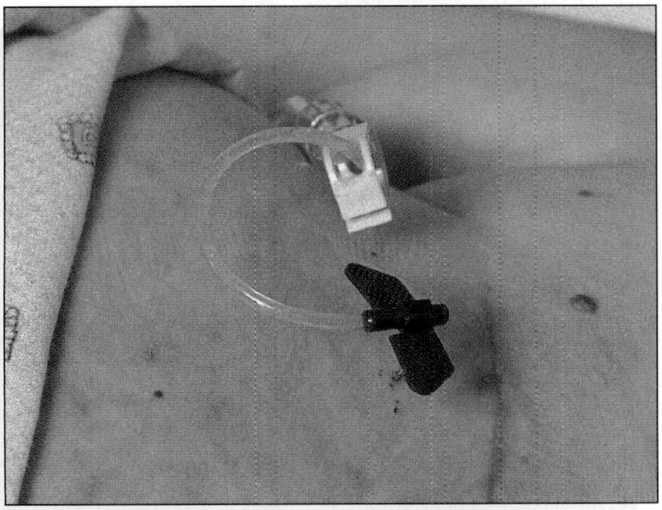

Remove dressing; inspect site for signs of inflammation.

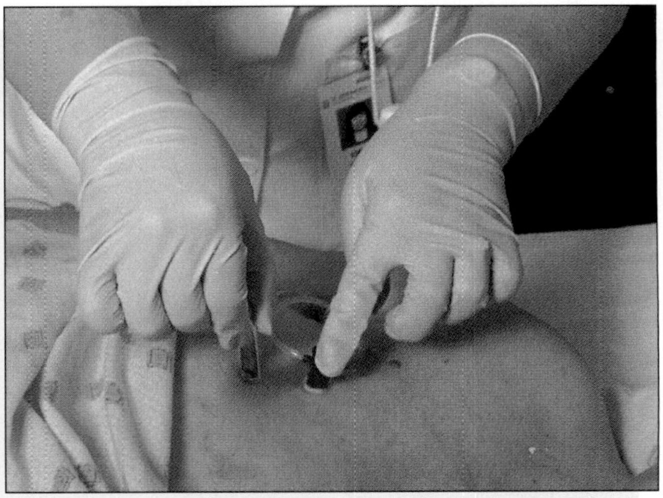

Stabilize Huber needle while prepping outward from insertion site.

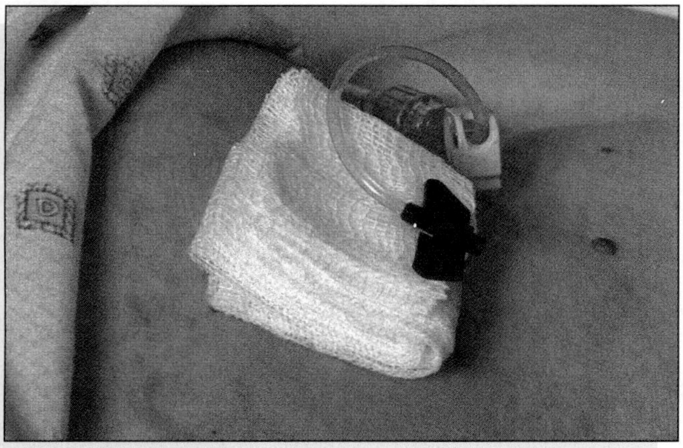

Place sterile gauze under Huber needle and wings for support.

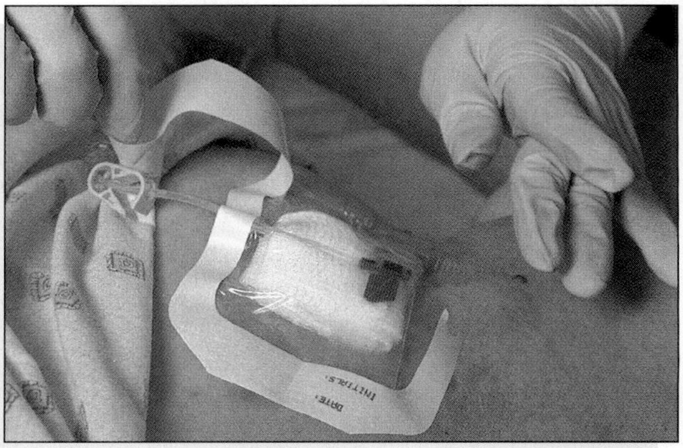

Tape wings and cover all with transparent dressing; tape and initial.

7. Clamp tubing before removing syringe to maintain positive pressure; cap tubing.
8. For continuous infusion, change tubing daily and dressing every 72 hours.
9. Dispose of equipment (including gloves) and wash hands.

CLINICAL ALERT

Electrical controller device (pump) should be used for continuous IV infusion via CVAD.

DRAWING BLOOD FROM AN IMPLANTED SUBCUTANEOUS PORT

Equipment

Huber 19-gauge needle with short extension tubing
Needleless injection cap
Two-10 mL syringes
Blood collection tubes
Heparin 3 mL and normal saline 10 mL flush solutions
Antimicrobial swabs
Tape
Sterile gloves

Procedure

1. Gather equipment.
2. Check physician's orders for type of blood test.
3. Explain procedure to client.
4. Wash hands, and don sterile gloves.
5. Access implanted port using Huber needle with capped extension tubing as discussed previously.
   a. Prep tubing cap with antimicrobial swab.
   b. Clean around junction of cap and hub with antimicrobial swab prior to removing cap.
6. Insert syringe into hub of extension tubing.
7. Unclamp tubing
8. Withdraw 5–10 mL blood, remove syringe and discard.
   Rationale: This discards the filling volume of the catheter.

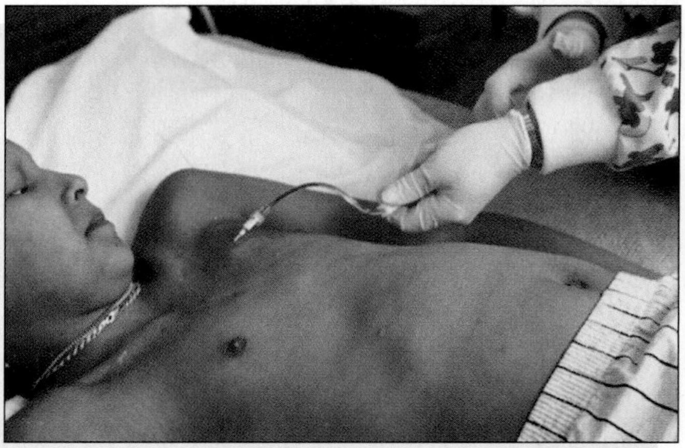

Blood is drawn from an implanted port by piercing the skin directly over the port.

9. Maintain aseptic technique—attach new syringe to hub of extension tubing. Withdraw appropriate amount of blood for tests and remove syringe.

CLINICAL ALERT

When drawing blood, attach syringe directly to hub of extension tubing. Never draw through cap as hemolysis can occur. Always place a new cap on extension tubing after withdrawing blood samples.

10. Fill appropriate type of blood tubing with specified amount of blood according to tests ordered.
11. Flush catheter with 10 mL saline solution after obtaining blood specimens.
12. Place new cap on extension tubing.
13. Discard equipment.
14. Remove gloves and wash hands.

Documentation for Implanted Subcutaneous Port

- Condition of port implantation site
- Frequency and type of flushes
- Name and dosage of drugs or solutions administered
- Presence of Huber needle, if left in place
- Dressing type
- Amount of blood withdrawn

Critical Thinking Application

UNEXPECTED OUTCOMES	CRITICAL THINKING OPTIONS
Needle entry is painful.	• Use topical anesthetic or apply ice before accessing. • Use local anesthetic injected intradermally before inserting needle (check client sensitivity and agency policy).
Occluded catheter.	• Transfuse packed red blood cells along with continuous infusion of normal saline; use an infusion pump; flush catheter well with 20 mL NS following infusion. • Change needle. If no improvement, suspect occluded catheter. • Try gentle aspiration to dislodge clot. • Never try to forcefully flush system—clot may mobilize; catheter may rupture. • Thrombolytic agent may be required to lyse fibrin clot (specialty nurse skill).
Inability to aspirate blood when checking placement.	• Needle may not be in port reservoir. • Tip of catheter may be against vessel wall. Try changing client's position from sitting up to lying or ask client to raise one or both arms. If appropriate, have client bear down or cough using Valsalva's maneuver while irrigating with normal saline. • Heparinize catheter, and return in 40 minutes to aspirate. • Formation of a fibrin clot requires thrombolysis by a certified IV nurse (according to agency policy).
Pain, swelling at site.	• Suspect catheter rupture. Report to physician. • Suspect port migration and infusion infiltrating subcutaneously.
Port becomes movable.	• Port may not be anchored securely. Port could be flipped under skin. • Silicone tubing has separated from port. • Always check for blood return to to ensure accurate needle placement, before injecting medications. • Notify physician and prepare for removing port.

UNIT 6

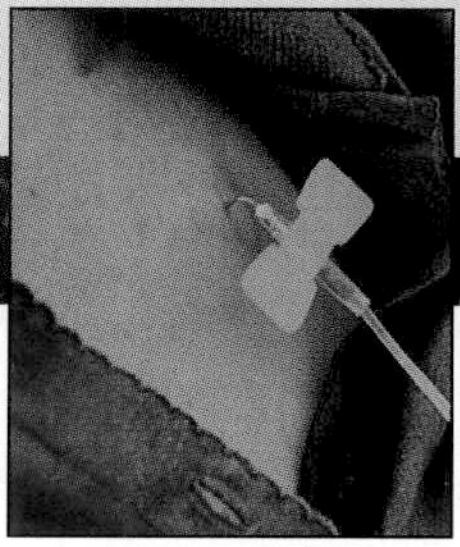

Peripherally Inserted Central Catheter (PICC)

Nursing Process Data

***ASSESSMENT* Data Base**

Assess length of exposed catheter.

Assess that catheter is secure.

Assess insertion site.

Assess catheter patency.

***PLANNING* Objectives**

To provide access for infusion, hyperalimentation, or drugs

To provide access for blood sampling

To provide catheter patency

***IMPLEMENTATION* Procedures**

Maintaining the PICC

Changing the PICC Dressing

Drawing Blood from the PICC

Removing the PICC

***EVALUATION* Expected Outcomes**

PICC remains patent.

Arm vein site remains free of infection.

Dressing secures catheter.

MAINTAINING THE PICC

Equipment

Syringe with 10 mL NS
Syringe with 20 mL NS
Syringe with 3–5 mL dilute heparin (100 U/mL) solution (per hospital policy)
Clean gloves
Antimicrobial swabs

Preparation

1. Check client care plan and MAR.
2. Check client's identaband.
3. Explain procedure to client.
4. Provide privacy for client.

> **CLINICAL ALERT**
>
> If catheter tip is resting in the right atrium or pericardium instead of the superior vena cava, the tip can move across the muscle to the sinoatrial node (SA node) and can cause cardiac arrhythmias, cardiac rupture, or other associated conditions. The PICC catheter must be withdrawn 1 inch (2.5 cm) and a repeat x-ray taken to check for catheter placement.

Procedure

1. Measure external catheter length daily and compare with previous measurements. If it has changed, notify individual who inserted the line. The PICC line is 20–25 inches (50–62.5 cm) long. **Rationale:** The PICC line is inserted into the SVC. If the catheter migrates, it can lead to major cardiac complications.
2. Don gloves.
3. Swab catheter port with antimicrobial swab. Allow to dry.
4. Inject solution (5 mL heparin or 20 mL saline) slowly; flush with minimal force using a *pulsating* motion until syringe is almost empty. **Rationale:** This action creates turbulence for catheter cleansing.
5. Continue to inject flush while removing syringe from catheter port.
6. For intermittent use (e.g., drug therapy).

> **CLINICAL ALERT**
>
> All continuous infusions using a PICC should be connected to an electric infusion device.

   a. Flush catheter with 10 mL normal saline.
   b. Administer infusion or medication.
   c. Flush catheter with 20 mL normal saline.
   d. Flush with 3–5 mL dilute heparin (per hospital policy).
7. Flush nonused catheter daily.
8. Place discarded equipment in appropriate receptacle. Place needle and syringe in sharps container.
9. Remove gloves and wash hands.

Peripherally Inserted Central Catheter

PICCs are long, soft, flexible single or multi-lumen catheters placed in an arm vein and advanced to the middle of the superior vena cava for central venous access. The length of catheter is documented. Placement is less invasive and less expensive than other CVADs since they can be inserted by specially educated certified IV nurses. As with tunneled catheters, exit site below heart level decreases risk of air embolism when system is open to the atmosphere. PICC lines do not need to be checked by x-ray to verify tip placement if inserted into a proximal arm. Clients receiving TPN or vesicants should have tip inserted into SVC, and x-ray should be done to confirm position. Research has shown that PICC lines inserted into SVC have fewer complications such as inflammation or thrombosis.

Some are sutured, but most are secured only with steri-strips to prevent catheter migration. These catheters may be used for long-term therapy if changed every 6 weeks. Dilute heparin is used for maintenance (or saline for the PICC with Groshong valve).

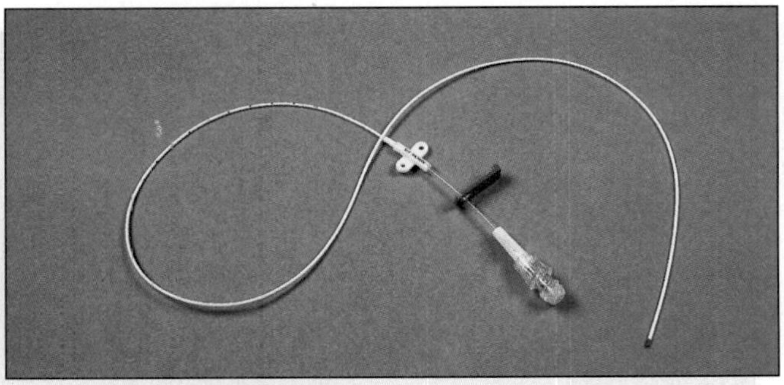

PICC line.

EVIDENCE BASED NURSING PRACTICE

Complication Rates for Valved Versus Nonvalved PICCs

In a randomized study 362 clients (233 men, 129 women; mean age, 44) were given PICC catheters, half of the clients received clamped catheters and half valved catheters. The complication rate for the clamped PICC clients was double for occlusions or infections. (26 for clamped and 12 for valved catheters).

Source: Hoffer, E. K., et al., Comparisons of Valved Versus Nonvalved PICC Catheters. http://www.mcgawexport.com

CHANGING THE PICC DRESSING

Equipment

Antimicrobial swabs
Steri-strip skin closure tape
Transparent semipermeable dressing
Clean gloves
Sterile gloves

Procedure

1. Check MAR and client's identaband.
2. Explain procedure to client.
3. Wash hands, and don clean gloves.
4. Very carefully remove old transparent dressing.
5. Check site for bleeding or signs of phlebitis. **Rationale:** Bleeding may occur with arm use. Phlebitis is the most common complication.
6. Discard old dressing and gloves.
7. Prepare sterile supplies.
8. Don sterile gloves.
9. Clean exit site and catheter with antimicrobial swabs using circular movement from inner to outer edge three times with three swabs. Carefully stabilize catheter with nondominant gloved hand, if necessary.

Note: The catheter is secured by tape only and usually not sutured in place. Approximately 1 inch of catheter extends from the insertion site.

CLINICAL ALERT

Unless absolutely necessary, avoid blood pressure measurement in the arm with a PICC and avoid venipunctures on the extremity with a PICC line.

10. Allow time for antimicrobial solution to dry. Do not blow on arm or wave hand to hasten drying. **Rationale:** Waving hand or blowing may contaminate site—antibacterial action does not take effect until solution is dry.
11. Position external catheter into an "S" shape or loop with steri-strips, if possible. **Rationale:** Catheter is not usually sutured in place, so steri-strips can be used to prevent catheter migration.

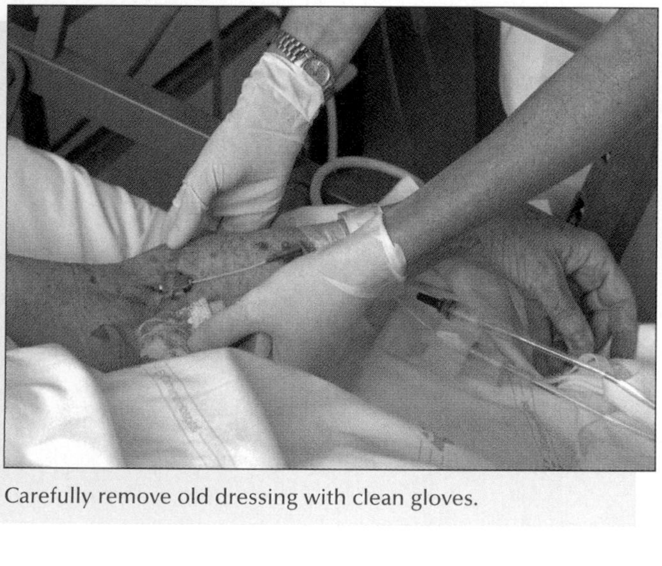

Carefully remove old dressing with clean gloves.

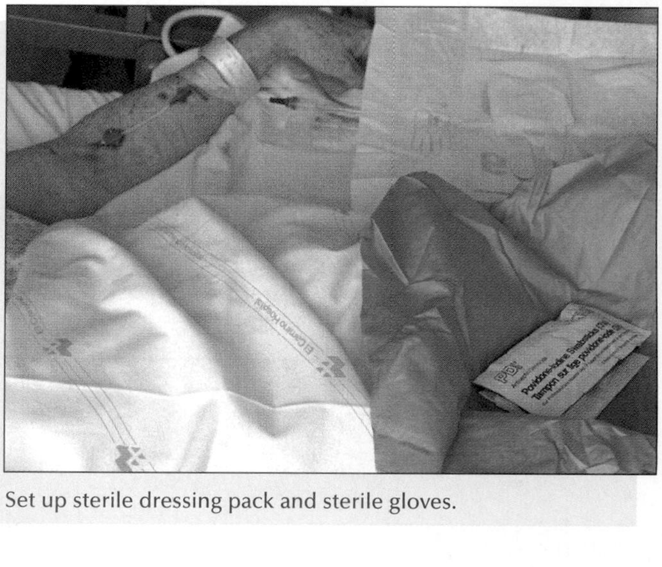

Set up sterile dressing pack and sterile gloves.

Secure PICC Line Using StatLock Securement Device

- Place StatLock pad on client's arm under catheter wings and slide holes of catheter wings into the posts. Close hinged clamps over posts to secure PICC.
- Peel paper liner from device and press StatLock pad onto skin, one side at a time.
- Apply transparent dressing over catheter insertion site.

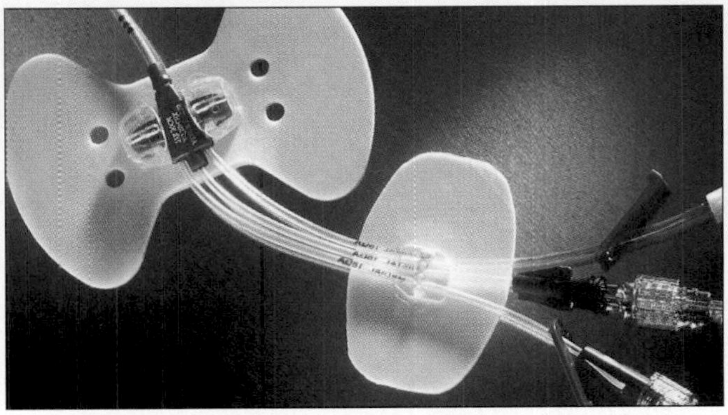

StatLock device. (Courtesy of Venetec, Intl.)

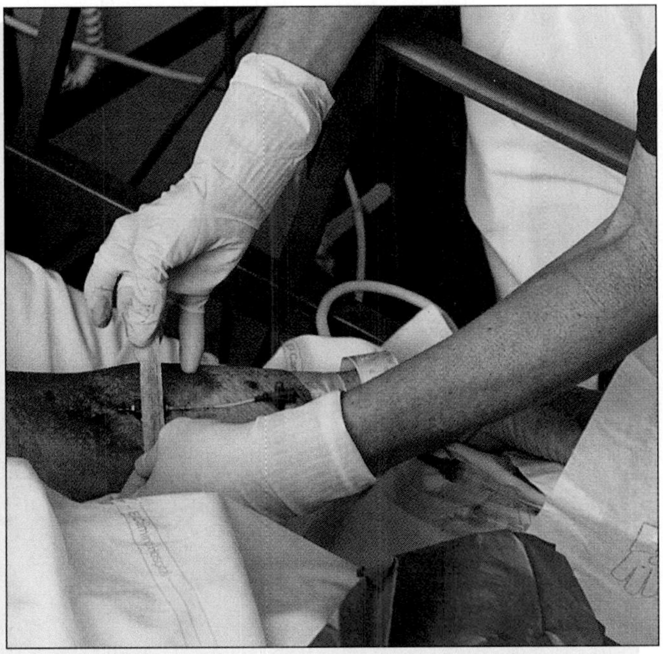

Apply steri-strips to catheter insertion site to prevent migration.

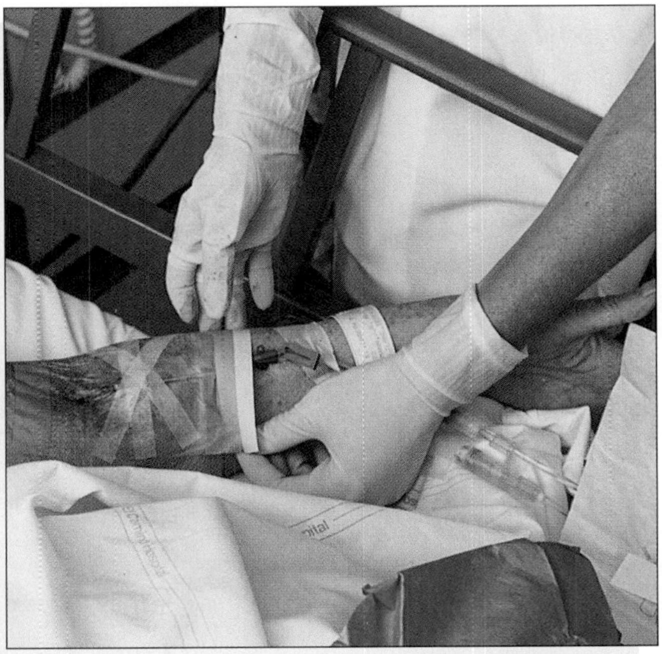

Cover exit site with transparent semipermeable dressing.

12. Cover exit site with transparent semipermeable dressing. No part of actual catheter should be outside transparent dressing.

Note: Transparent dressings are not occlusive, they allow air to circulate through the semipermeable dressing and thus prevent perspiration from collecting under the dressing. To make the dressing occlusive, an antibacterial ointment is applied to the exit site.

13. Remove gloves and wash hands.
14. Initial and date dressing.
15. Change initial transparent dressing in 24 hours and then every 7 days or whenever it is soiled or loose. **Rationale:** First dressing change is done to check insertion site.

DRAWING BLOOD FROM THE PICC

Equipment

Antimicrobial swabs
Two 10-mL syringes with needleless cannula for specimen
20-mL syringe with needleless cannula filled with saline
Syringe with 3–5 mL dilute heparin (per hospital policy) and needleless cannula
Clean gloves

Preparation

1. Check orders and MAR.
2. Check client's identaband.
3. Wash hands and don gloves.
4. Explain procedure to client.

Procedure

1. Stop all infusing fluids for at least 1 minute before drawing a specimen.
2. Swab catheter cap with antimicrobial swab, and allow to dry.
3. Use 10-mL syringe and withdraw 5 mL of blood and discard appropriately in biohazard container. Check facility policy and procedure for amount to discard.
4. Use 10-mL syringe with needleless cannula and withdraw required amount of blood for laboratory tests. Do not use Vacutainer (catheter will collapse with intense vacuum).
5. Change cap after all blood draws and transfusions. Flush with 20 mL saline solution to clear catheter.
6. Complete procedure with dilute heparin flush (unless Groshong valve present).
7. Discard equipment and gloves; wash hands.
8. Handle blood sample appropriately. Transfer to collection tube.

REMOVING THE PICC

Equipment

Suture removal kit if catheter sutured
Clean gloves
Sterile 2 × 2 gauze
Tape

Procedure

1. Check physicians order and MAR.
2. Check client's identaband.
3. Explain the procedure to the client. Client may be in bed or sitting in a chair.
4. Wash hands and don gloves.
5. Carefully remove dressing, loosening edges toward insertion site.
6. Grasp catheter at insertion site.
7. Gradually pull catheter parallel to skin one inch at a time.
8. Continue inching catheter out—if resistance is felt, stop and reposition arm, wait 15 seconds.
9. NEVER FORCE catheter removal (apply warm moist pack to upper arm to relax vein for approximately 15 minutes).
10. After removal, measure length of catheter and compare to documented length on chart.
11. Culture tip according to facility policy. Cut tip with sterile scissor and place in sterile container.
12. Hold gauze at exit site for hemostasis.
13. Apply tape to gauze securely.
14. Dispose of catheter in biohazard container.
15. Document length of catheter removed.

Note: Certified infusion nurses should remove the PICC.

Notify physician or IV therapist if:

- Infusion is leaking from insertion site
- Inconsistent flow rates
- Unable to infuse fluids
- Excessive bleeding or drainage at insertion site
- Chest, neck, ear pain, numbness, tingling of affected arm
- Swelling, pain, redness, palpable cord at or above insertion site

DOCUMENTATION FOR THE PERIPHERALLY INSERTED CENTRAL CATHETER

- Label site "PICC" to ensure proper use of line
- Frequency of flush and type of solution
- Dressing applied. Label date, time, initials, and "PICC"
- Site assessment
- Length of exposed catheter
- Amount of blood withdrawn
- Solutions or drugs administered

for Discontinuing PICC

- Note condition and length of catheter
- Document site assessment
- Client's response to treatment and procedure
- Catheter tip sent to lab for culture, if appropriate

Critical Thinking Application

UNEXPECTED OUTCOMES	CRITICAL THINKING OPTIONS
Mechanical phlebitis (pain, redness spreading to surrounding tissue).	• Apply warm moist compresses for 20 minutes 4 times a day. • Elevate the arm and encourage mild exercise. • Report problem—antibiotics may correct problem and prevent PICC removal.
Bleeding occurs at insertion site.	• Apply direct pressure on insertion site. • Check client's coagulation profile (bleeding time, platelet count, PT, PTT) for coagulation problem.
Exudate occurs at insertion site.	• Notify physician or IV therapist. • Send specimen to lab for culture. • Maintain aseptic technique during site care.
Solution does not infuse.	• Increase volume of flush solution. • Utilize infusion pump or elevate infusion bag for gravity pressure. • Flush with a pulsating motion and clamp catheter before removing syringe. • Report problem—thrombolytic declotting may be necessary.
Pain in shoulder or neck occurs during infusion—or client hears gurgling sound with flush.	• Report so x-ray can validate catheter placement (catheter may have migrated with client maneuvers).
Sepsis occurs (rare).	• Monitor client for fever and assess insertion site for drainage, tenderness, redness. • PICC may be removed—send tip to lab for culture.

Gerontologic Considerations

Elderly clients requiring chemotherapy or parenteral nutrition are good candidates for implanted vascular access devices.

- Decreased amounts of fluids can be administered to prevent fluid overload.
- Risk of infection is decreased, and in the elderly infection is a concern. Frequency and severity of infection tend to increase with age due to a decline in the immune response.
- Repeated IV punctures are not necessary so veins are preserved and discomfort minimized.
- Greater client mobility is achieved.

With aging, epidermal turnover decreases and skin fragility increases. Even minimal trauma may result in serious erosion.

Health care providers or family members can be instructed to provide medication administration, fluid therapy, or parenteral nutrition at home.

Management Guidelines

Each state legislates a Nurse Practice Act for RNs and LVN/LPNs. Health care facilities are responsible for establishing and implementing policies and procedures that conform to their state's regulations. Verify the regulations and role parameters for each health care worker in your facility.

Delegation of Responsibilities

- Each state identifies the scope of practice for RNs and LVN/LPNs. Several states have identified that the LVN/LPN has a specific role in IV therapy, but the scope of practice is always dictated by each agency (e.g., initiating, regulating, discontinuing IVs). The LPN/LVN educated in IV therapy is the minimum level practitioner to assist in tasks delegated by the RN for the delivery of IV therapy. The RN may be assisted by an LPN educated in IV therapy, but the RN remains responsible for the care given.
- Policies outlining the responsibility of the IV nurse vary significantly among agencies. A written policy should clearly outline all aspects of this role, and all staff should be familiar with its scope. Policies and procedures should follow national guidelines and standards of practice established by the Centers for Disease Control and Prevention, the American Association of Blood Banks, and the IV Nurses Society. All nurses must be aware of the many physical hazards associated with IV therapy and related OSHA rules to be observed.
- Central line catheter management must be done by an RN.
- The nurse who delivers IV therapy must be qualified by specific knowledge and experience to perform such highly specialized skills. Many agencies utilize a team of specialty educated and experienced certified IV nurses who focus their attention solely on aspects of IV therapy (initiation, drug preparation, fluid/blood/drug administration, regular client assessment and site care, as well as monitoring product integrity). While these nurses are freed from other care responsibilities, the professional nurse must provide for ongoing client care and ensure client safety.
- TPN and lipids may be administered only by an RN according to specific physician orders.
- The CNA/UAP providing personal hygiene must understand that the IV system is a closed one and must be able to give care without disrupting the system. The components of the CVAD system must never be disconnected. Doing so places the client at risk for infection and air embolism. The CNA/UAP should receive training in changing the client's gown without disrupting the CVAD system.
- For the client with a CVAD allowed to shower, the RN should disconnect infusion lines, place a dry sterile gauze (4×4) over the dressed site and exposed tubing(s), then cover all with a large transparent dressing for waterproofing. Post-shower removal of the covering and inspection of the dressing should also be performed by the RN.

Information Flow

While the professional monitors the IV infusion site regularly, the CNA/UAP provides vital data to the professional nurse by immediately *reporting:*

- Observations of redness or swelling around the CVAD insertion site (signs of possible infiltration, hematoma, sepsis).
- Presence of crepitus (bubble-wrap feeling) on the client's chest (sign of possible subcutaneous emphysema that can lead to respiratory distress).
- Observations of respiratory distress in any client with recent (24 hours) placement of a central line (symptoms of possible pneumothorax).
- Any client complaint of arm, shoulder, or neck pain (symptom of possible thrombosis or infiltration).
- Temperature elevation (fever—sign of possible catheter-related infection if otherwise unexplainable).
- Infusion device alarms to prompt the professional to further assess the client.
- Presence of blood backup in the catheter.
- A loose or soiled/wet dressing.

CRITICAL THINKING STRATEGIES

SCENARIO 1

Mr. John Baker is a 68-year-old retired pharmacist who has just returned from surgery following placement of a tunneled CVAD with a Groshong valve. He will be started on a long-term intermittent chemotherapy regimen for acute lymphocytic leukemia. His wife is a retired RN who worked in the operating room for many years.

1. Identify at least three advantages for inserting the tunneled catheter for his treatment.
2. His wife is very concerned about the initial care of the catheter. What explanation will you give her?
3. After the explanation regarding the care of the catheter, Mrs. Baker asks you how they can prevent an infection of the catheter.
4. The client needs to be instructed on how to flush the catheter. What are the most important directions you should provide to him?
5. Mrs. Baker asks you to describe what symptoms require reporting to the physician. What is your best response to this question?

SCENARIO 2

Seth Eley, age 24, has been admitted to your unit with the diagnosis of inflammatory bowel disease (Crohn's disease) with exacerbation of fever, severe diarrhea, right lower quadrant pain, weight loss, and anemia. Short-term total parenteral nutrition and bowel rest are planned. A triple-lumen central venous catheter has been placed for these purposes.

1. Based on this data, what generalizations can you make about the purpose of hyperalimentation for this client?
2. Why is central venous access necessary?
3. Develop several scenarios about the most common complications of central catheter placement.
4. How does TPN affect fluid and electrolyte balance?

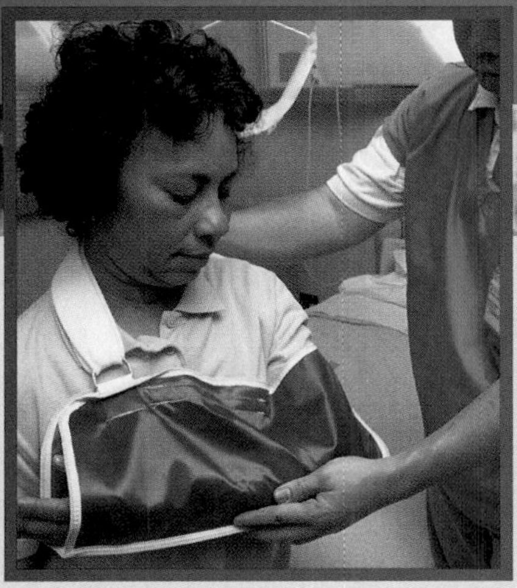

CHAPTER 30

Orthopedic Interventions

THEORETICAL CONCEPTS

UNIT ONE: **Application of Immobilizing Devices 1102**
- Applying a Sling 1103
- Applying a Spiral Bandage 1104
- Applying a Figure-Eight Bandage 1104
- Applying a Splint 1105
- Applying a Cervical Collar 1106
- Applying a Jewett–Taylor Back Brace 1106

UNIT TWO: **Cast Care 1109**
- Caring for a Wet Cast 1110
- Assessing a Casted Extremity 1111
- Instructing Client in Self Care 1112

UNIT THREE: **Traction 1114**
- Maintaining Skin Traction 1115
- Maintaining Skeletal Traction 1117
- Maintaining an External Fixator Device 1119
- Maintaining Halo Traction 1120

UNIT FOUR: **Client with an Amputation 1123**
- Positioning and Exercising the Stump 1124
- Shrinking/Molding the Stump 1125

UNIT FIVE: **Client with Joint Replacement 1127**
- Caring for a Client with Hip Arthroplasty 1128
  - *for Bed Positioning 1128*
  - *for Strengthening Exercises 1128*
  - *for Mobility and Dislocation Prevention 1129*
  - *for Assistive Devices and Adaptive Aids 1129*
- Caring for a Client with Knee Arthroplasty 1130
  - *for Bed Positioning 1130*
  - *for Strengthening Exercises 1130*
  - *for Getting Out of Bed 1131*

UNIT SIX: **Stryker Frame 1132**
- Using a Stryker Wedge Turning Frame 1133
- Turning from Supine to Prone 1133
- Using a Stryker Parallel Frame 1133
- Assisting Client with Bedpan 1134

GERONTOLOGIC CONSIDERATIONS 1135

MANAGEMENT GUIDELINES 1135

CRITICAL THINKING STRATEGIES 1137

LEARNING OBJECTIVES

- Identify nursing diagnoses that apply to care of clients with orthopedic conditions.
- Outline emergency measures for an injured extremity.
- Describe different ways to classify fractures.
- Assess circulation, motion, and sensation in an injured limb.
- Recognize indicators of circulatory compromise in an injured or immobilized extremity.
- Apply a variety of immobilizing modalities (sling, bandage, brace).
- Describe differences between plaster of Paris and synthetic casts.
- Explain the purpose for skin versus skeletal traction.
- Identify types of skin and skeletal traction.
- Develop a teaching plan for the client with a cast.
- Outline the nursing care needs of the client in traction.
- Outline the teaching needs of a client with an amputation.
- Develop a teaching plan for a client undergoing joint replacement (arthroplasty).
- Describe the special needs of the client immobilized on a turning frame.

TERMINOLOGY

Abduction: movement away from the midline of the body or body part, as in raising the arm or spreading the fingers.

Adduction: movement toward the midline of the body.

AKA: above-the-knee amputation.

Alignment: arranged in a straight line.

Amputation: traumatic or surgical removal of a diseased limb or part.

Arthroplasty: repair/replacement of a joint.

Balanced suspension: use of a sling or splint to elevate and support an extremity that is in traction.

BKA: below-the-knee amputation.

Bryant's traction: a type of skin traction used to treat small children with fractures of the femur.

Buck's traction: a type of skin traction used with a hip fracture prior to surgery.

Circulation: movement in a circular course, as the movement of blood.

Comminuted: broken in pieces.

Contusion: soft tissue injury.

Diaphysis: the part of the long bone between the ends, also known as the shaft.

Edema: a condition in which body tissues contain an excessive amount of fluid.

Epiphysis: the end of a long bone.

Extension: a movement that increases the angle between two bones, straightening a joint.

External fixation device: a metal frame with attached metal percutaneous pins that are held in place by the frame. The pins are inserted into or through a bone to maintain alignment.

Exudate: inflammatory response: migration of plasma fluid and circulating components to an injury site.

Flexion: a movement that decreases a joint angle.

Hyperextension: continuation of extension beyond the anatomic position, as in bending the head backward.

Intracapsular: within the joint capsule (e.g., head and neck of the femur).

Metaphysis: wide part of bone at end of shaft adjacent to the epiphyseal disk.

Mobility: state or quality of being mobile; facility of movement.

Musculoskeletal: pertaining to the muscles and bones.

Osteoblasts: immature cell, which on maturation plays a role in bone production.

Orthostatic: concerning an erect or standing position.

Orthostatic hypotension: low blood pressure in a standing or upright position.

Osteoclast: cell that resorbs bone

Paralysis: temporary or permanent loss of voluntary motion.

Paresthesis: pertains to an abnormal sensation.

Pearson attachment: an attachment to Thomas splint that supports lower leg. Used in balanced traction. Allows continuous traction in line of the femur by the use of cords and weights.

Periosteum: connective tissue that covers the bone; contains proliferating cells.

Prosthesis: replacement of a missing part by an artificial substitute.

Restorative: promoting a return to health.

Russell's traction: type of skin traction to treat fractures of the shaft of the femur.

Spica: figure-eight bandage with one of the two loops larger than the other (used for ankle or stump).

Spiral bandage: used to cover a cylindrical part.

Sprain: injury caused by wrenching or twisting of a joint that results in tearing or stretching of the associated ligaments.

Strain: injury caused by excessive force or stretching of muscles or tendons around the joint.

Stryker frame: a special bed used to treat clients with spinal cord injuries.

Syncope: a transient loss of consciousness due to inadequate blood flow to the brain.

Thomas splint: used for balanced suspension along with fracture of the femur.

Torque: a rotary force.

Traction: application of a mechanical pulling force applied to soft tissue.

RESTORING FUNCTION

Orthopedic nursing involves the prevention and correction of alterations in the musculoskeletal system. To help clients achieve and maintain optimal mobility, nurses use preventative, restorative, and rehabilitative methods. Preventative and restorative measures include the use of bandages, positioning, splints, traction, and casts.

The most common cause of injury to the musculoskeletal system is trauma from accidents. These accidents result in soft tissue injuries, fractures, and dislocations. Injuries occurring from falls in the home account for many admissions to health care facilities.

Sprains and strains are the two most common musculoskeletal injuries. The usual treatment is application of a pressure bandage, elevation, and ice.

When sprains, strains, contusions, or dislocations occur, remember the mnemonic RICE. "R" stands for rest the injured part. "I" refers to immobilization, usually with a bandage or by splinting. "C" stands for application of cold treatments, such as ice packs. Cold is applied intermittently. "E" refers to elevation of the affected extremity. These initial interventions prevent edema formation and other complications. Avoid heat for at least 24 hours to prevent edema and pain.

Bandages are used for applying pressure over an area; immobilizing a body part; preventing or reducing edema; correcting a deformity; and securing splints in place. Several types of material are used as bandages. Woven cotton, elastic webbing, and gauze are the most common materials.

Fractures

A fracture is a break in the continuity of a bone that occurs when the bone is subjected to stress forces greater than ordinary. No two fractures are alike since forces occur from different directions and in different amounts and muscle pulls differ in response to injury.

The long bone, the most common type involved in fractures, is composed of the shaft, or diaphysis, and the flared end of the bone, termed the metaphysis. In children the metaphysis is in two important segments: the physis, which is the growth region, and the epiphysis, which is directly adjacent to joints. The epiphysis fuses to the metaphysis at the end of the growth period. Injuries to long bones in childhood can result in growth retardation or arrest in the longitudinal growth of the limb.

When a bone is fractured, a specific repair process takes place, beginning with the formation of a blood clot at the site of the fracture. Once this clot is formed, osteoblasts and fibroblasts converge on the site and start laying down the organic matrix. Together, the fibrin net, the osteoblasts, and the organic matrix form a callus into which calcium salts are deposited. This phase takes 3–6 weeks. This callus evolves into regular bone tissue, which connects the pieces of original bone. In the final stage of the repair process, osteoblasts and osteoclasts remodel the callus area into a permanent and strong bone.

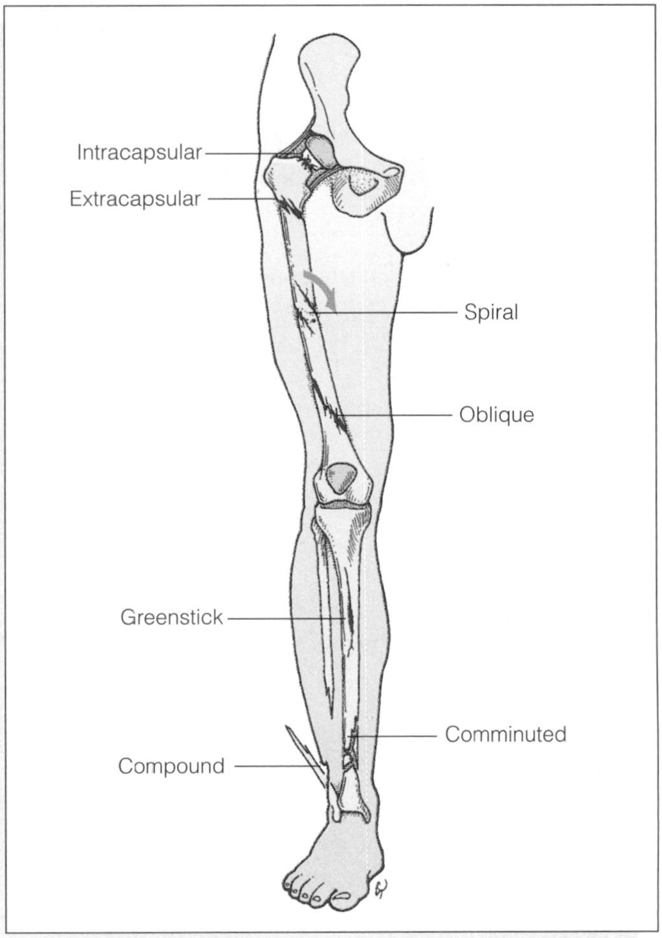

Types of fractures.

Types of Fractures

Greenstick

- A crack; the bending of a bone with incomplete fracture. Only affects one side of the periosteum.
- Common in skull fractures or in young children when bones are pliable.

Comminuted

- Bone completely broken in a transverse, spiral, or oblique direction (indicates the direction of the fracture in relation to the long axis of the fracture bone).
- Bone broken into several fragments.

Open or Compound

- Bone is exposed to the air through a break in the skin.
- Can be associated with soft tissue injury as well.
- Infection is common complication due to exposure to bacterial invasion.

Closed or Simple

- Skin remains intact.
- Chances are greatly decreased for infection.

Compression

- Frequently seen with vertebral fractures.
- Fractured bone has been compressed by other bones.

Complete

- Bone is broken with a disruption of both sides of the periosteum.

Impacted

- One part of fractured bone is driven into another.

Depressed Fracture

- Usually seen in skull or facial fractures.
- Bone or fragments of bone are driven inward.

Pathologic

- Break caused by disease process.

Fractures are classified in a variety of ways. One classification is by the type of injury to the bone or surrounding tissue. Examples of these fractures include a transverse fracture, which proceeds directly across the bone; an oblique fracture, which proceeds at an angle across the bone; and, a comminuted fracture, which results in more than two fragments of bone being displaced.

Fractures can also be classified as open or closed. An open fracture is one in which the skin has been broken due to penetration of a bone fragment or external trauma. An open fracture requires additional treatment to prevent infection as a result of the skin puncture. Surgical debridement and irrigation must be completed within hours of the fracture. A closed fracture indicates that the fracture is contained under the skin surface.

Fractures can be treated by manipulation or closed reduction. This results in manipulating broken bones to return to their normal anatomic position. Closed fractures are treated in this manner.

Open reductions, the correction of bone alignment through a surgical incision, includes internal fixation of the fracture with rods, wires, screws, pins, or nails. An external fixator apparatus is used to compress fracture fragments and immobilize reduced fractures. These are usually used when casts or traction are not appropriate. The fixator is attached to the bone by the use of percutaneous pins. Soft tissue injury is also a probability with fractures. Immediate splinting and elevation of the extremity can prevent complications.

Casts

Casts are generally applied to maintain the reduced fracture in proper alignment. Casts are made from plaster of Paris or synthetic materials, such as polyester, polyurethane, fiberglass, or plastic. The synthetic casts dry faster, weigh less, and can get wet without fear of cracking or disintegration. One major disadvantage of synthetic casts is their cost. Another disadvantage is their inability to mold easily, which prevents their use for immobilizing severely displaced bones or unstable fractures. Casted extremities need to be observed frequently during the drying process. When assessing the client in a cast, remember to check for pulse distal to the cast, pain, pallor, and paresthesia (the four Ps). Casts provide more effective immobilization but are unyielding and can cause injury to underlying skin and tissue. Splitting or windowing may be necessary to release pressure over a specific area, particularly a bony prominence.

Traction

Traction, the application of a mechanical pulling force, can be applied to soft tissue (skin traction) to overcome muscle spasm, to immobilize an injured site, and to relieve pain. It is also another method of treating fractures. It is most effective and useful when reduction of the bone fracture is required. Two types of traction are used: skin traction and skeletal traction.

Skeletal traction is applied directly to bone to reduce a fracture or to maintain a surgically manipulated bone alignment. Significantly greater weight is used with this mode of traction. Pins or wires are inserted through the skin and soft tissue and into bone, then the desired weight is applied to maintain bone alignment. This type of traction is *continuous;* removing or lifting weights displaces fragments and can cause neurovascular damage. Balanced suspension uses splints and slings to support the extremity and weights applied for countertraction (e.g., Thomas splint with Pearson attachment). Suspended support allows greater mobility for the client with skeletal traction.

Tongs are used for fractures or dislocation of the cervical or high thoracic vertebrae. A turning frame or special bed may be used for positioning these clients.

External fixation devices are commonly used for stabilizing a bone or joint. An external fixation device has a metal frame with attached percutaneous pins that are held rigidly in place on the frame. These self-contained devices provide traction without the use of ropes and weights, and therefore, allow client mobility. Similarly, a client with fracture or dislocation of cervical or high thoracic vertebrae can mobilize with a halo ring and vest. Complications of skeletal traction include neurovascular compromise, inadequate bone alignment, skin or soft tissue injury, pin tract infection, and osteomyelitis. Neurovascular function must be assessed every four hours because clients requiring these devices usually have extensive soft tissue, nerve, and vessel damage. Extensive client teaching needs to be accomplished because these clients go home with the devices in place.

Many types of skin traction are used in hospital settings. The oldest and simplest type is Buck's traction. This type of traction is usually applied for short periods, 48–72 hours. Elderly clients may require Buck's traction prior to surgical repair of a fractured hip. Buck's traction is a boot with Velcro straps. Superficial peroneal nerve compression can result if the straps are too tight. Frequent release of the straps prevents this complication.

Bryant's traction, another type of skin traction, is used primarily for children under 3 years of age who have sustained a fractured femur. The foam boot, cervical halter, and pelvic girdle devices are used in skin traction. A rope, pulley, and weight system (5–10 pounds) is attached to the device to provide pulling force to skin and soft tissues. Skin traction for acute muscle spasm (fracture of the femur) should be continuous, but skin traction for chronic problems such as muscle strain is *intermittent*, removed and reapplied as specified by the physician. Complications of skin traction relate to skin integrity and neurovascular impairment.

To be effective, any mode of traction must include *counter*traction. This might be provided by the client's body weight, the pull of weights in the opposite direction, or by elevating the bed under the part in traction. The line of pull must be maintained, weights must hang freely, ropes must be intact and glide freely in the pulley and knots must be secure. Weights and knots should hang far from the pulleys. The system should be free of any impingement such as linens. It is essential that the nurse has a clear understanding of the traction type and purpose, prescribed amount of weight, and client positioning.

Acute Compartment Syndrome

Since muscle groups are bound in a nonyielding fascia and injury causes swelling due to bleeding, edema, and the like, increased pressure within the "compartment" compromises circulation to involved tissues. Similarly, external pressure (e.g., a cast) can cause muscle ischemia and necrosis. As pressure increases within the site, venous return is compressed, leading to increased interstitial fluid (edema), then compression of arterioles and eventual ischemic myositis (necrosis) and contracture formation. The client can nevertheless have intact distal pulses.

To prevent this complication and ultimate loss of limb, immediate fasciotomy is necessary to release the unyielding fascial boundaries. The nurse must be vigilant to early signs and symptoms of acute compartment syndrome:

- Pain on *passive* stretching of the muscle (or distal digits)
- Pain out of proportion to the injury
- Pain that is unrelieved by pain medication
- Pain that increases with *elevation* of the part
- Pain when pressure is applied over the compartment
- Weak active movement of distal digits

Diminished or absent pulses, coolness, and pallor are late signs and unreliable indicators of acute compartment syndrome.

Joint Replacement (Arthroplasty)

Degenerative joint disease of the hip and knee is the number one cause of disability among the elderly. This chronic disease, sometimes called osteoarthritis, has an insidious onset that may progress to pain and stiffness, which impact the client's activities of daily living and role functioning. Elective total joint replacement (arthroplasty) has become increasingly popular because it restores mobility and relieves pain for clients who cannot be managed by medication or physical therapy. Total hip arthroplasty includes replacement of both the femoral and acetabular components of the hip joint. The older procedure for implanting the prosthesis uses polymethyl-methacrylate to "cement" the implant in place which, in turn, bonds to the bone. The newer procedure provides for stability of the prosthesis through a process that facilitates biologic ingrowth of new bone tissue into the porous surface coating the prosthesis. Younger clients with a more active life are candidates for the newer procedure. Following either procedure for replacing a joint, the client's joint alignment must be maintained postoperatively and the client must participate in physical therapy activities to improve function and range of motion of the new joint. Clients may be on long-term anticoagulant therapy and must understand the need for follow-up laboratory appointments. Infections that could affect the prosthesis could lead to the removal of the joint until the infection is dissipated.

Discharge planning begins before admission for elective joint arthroplasty. The client receives education about the perioperative process and "clinical path" expectations, including essentials of self-care rehabilitation. The home is typically equipped with adaptive and safety features before the planned surgery. Prepared clients experience less anxiety, fewer postoperative complications, shorter length of hospital stay, and reduced incidence of hospital readmissions.

Hip Fracture

Hip surgery for the fracture client presents a different challenge. The fracture client is not undergoing *elective* surgery, has had no preoperative preparation and is frequently ill prepared for hospitalization. The emergent hip fracture client may not have the physical health enjoyed by the elective client. The trauma client is more apt to experience serious adverse consequences of emergent hospitalization and surgery, including delirium, and requires vigilant monitoring. Care and teaching for the client with prosthetic replacement for intracapsular hip fracture is identical to care and teaching for the client with total hip replacement.

Hip fracture involving the head or neck of the femur is classified as "intracapsular" (within the joint capsule). Since intracapsular bone lacks periosteum, fracture healing is limited. A hemiarthroplasty is performed whereby the head and neck of the femur are surgically removed and replaced with a *prosthesis*. The client is weight bearing with an assistive device soon after surgery. Because the joint capsule has been surgically disrupted, the hip prosthesis is at risk for dislocation until healing is complete. Specific rehabilitative adherence promotes healing and prevents dislocation of the prosthesis. If the fracture is *extracapsular* (involving the intertrochanteric region) internal fixation with nail, plate, and screws is performed. There is no disruption of the joint capsule, no prosthetic implant, and therefore, no risk of femoral head dislocation, and dislocation precautions are not necessary. On the other hand, a repaired fracture site must heal, so total weight bearing is usually delayed.

Amputation

Amputation of a limb may be due to trauma, in which case the psychological ramifications can be very complex, or it can be a planned reconstructive procedure and a welcome source of relief for the client who has suffered painful vascular insufficiency and tissue necrosis. Regardless, the client who has lost a limb must regain psychological equilibrium and learn new skills. A supportive nurse–client relationship can assist the client to cope with grieving and body image reintegration.

It is normal for amputees to experience phantom sensation, a feeling that the amputated part is still there. Clients should be informed of this before amputation, if possible. Phantom *pain*, however, is a complication thought to be due to referred pain mechanisms that arise from the spinal cord. Signals are generated by intact nerves previously associated with the amputated part and relayed to the cerebral cortex as originating in the phantom limb. Analgesics are effective in managing postoperative stump pain, but have no effect on *phantom* pain. Unfortunately, there is no treatment that is consistently effective. Stress management skills and early ambulation are recommended, and beta blockers, anticonvulsants,

TABLE 30–1 Neurologic Assessment

	Motion	Sensation
Upper Extremity		
Radial nerve	Hyperextends wrist Hyperextends thumb and four fingers	Web space between thumb and index finger
Ulnar nerve	Abducts (spreads) fingers	Lateral aspect of hand and distal end of little finger
Median nerve	Flexes wrist Opposes thumb and little finger	Distal end of index finger
Lower Extremity		
Peroneal nerve	Dorsiflexes ankle Flexes toes	Web space between great and second toe
Tibial nerve	Plantar flexes ankle and toes	Medial and lateral surfaces on sole of foot

neuroleptics, and antidepressants may be helpful, depending on the quality of the pain.

Orthopedic Assessment

All orthopedic clients must be vigilantly monitored for skin and neurovascular status (circulation, motion, and sensation) of the affected part. Assessments should be conducted before, during, and frequently following application of any immobilizing modality. The contralateral extremity and documented baseline findings should be used for comparison.

For circulatory assessment note distal digits or restricted parts for color, temperature, capillary refill, and presence of edema. Inadequate arterial blood flow is characterized by pallor, slow capillary filling (>2 seconds), and coolness to touch. Inadequate venous return causes cyanosis or mottling, increased temperature, and edema with normal capillary filling.

Neurologic function assessment includes motion and sensation.

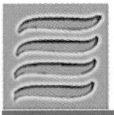

Nursing Diagnoses

The following nursing diagnoses may be appropriate to include in a client care plan when the components related to a client who requires special orthopedic procedures.

NURSING DIAGNOSIS	RELATED FACTORS
Disturbed Body Image	Surgery (loss of limb), chronic illness, chronic pain
Ineffective Coping	Restriction in activity, ability to perform ADLs independently
Pain	Improper position or application of equipment (cast, sling, Stryker frame), surgical procedure, improper alignment, neurologic injury
Impaired Physical Mobility	Decreased motor function or interruption of central nervous system, physical injury, disease process (spinal cord injury or surgical intervention), pain, stiffness, and surgical intervention (joint replacements), joint contractures, inappropriate or inadequately performed range-of-motion exercises
Bathing/Hygiene Self-Care Deficit	Physical limitations, immobilized body or limb, pain, decreased strength and endurance
Impaired Skin Integrity	Pressure points, improper application of cast, sling, or traction, immobility, altered circulation
Social Isolation	Decreased opportunity for communication or interaction with peers, long-term confinement, limited physical ability, lifestyle changes
Risk for Infection	Extended exposure of joint during surgical procedure, presence of environmental pathogens at incisional site, internal fixation device
Risk for Injury	Falls related to weakness, fatigue, pain, ineffective teaching or noncompliance in use of assistive devices
	Malposition of joint following surgery
Ineffective Therapeutic Regimen Management	Lack of knowledge regarding home management or follow-up care
Risk for Peripheral Neurovascular Dysfunction	Surgery, immobility, positioning, inflammatory process

- The single most important nursing action to decrease the incidence of hospital-based infections is handwashing. **Remember to wash your hands or use antibacterial gel before and after each and every client contact.**

UNIT 1

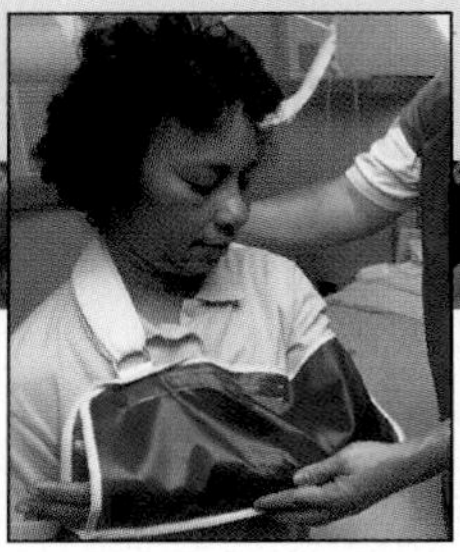

Application of Immobilizing Devices

Nursing Process Data

ASSESSMENT ***Data Base***

Recognize need for site immobilization.

Assess status of surrounding tissues.

Determine type of immobilization required.

Select appropriate immobilizing equipment.

Assess status of surrounding tissue.

Assess affected extremity for circulation, motion, and sensation (CMS) before and after applying modality.

PLANNING ***Objectives***

To immobilize an extremity or body part

To maintain functional alignment

To limit harmful movement

To reduce or prevent pain

To prevent further soft tissue injury and complications

To preserve neurovascular function

To promote healing

IMPLEMENTATION ***Procedures***

Applying a Sling

Applying a Spiral Bandage

Applying a Figure-Eight Bandage

Applying a Splint

Applying a Cervical Collar

Applying a Jewett–Taylor Back Brace

EVALUATION ***Expected Outcomes***

Treated part is effectively immobilized.

Pain is reduced or prevented.

Further injury is prevented.

Edema and bleeding are controlled.

Neurovascular and skin complications do not occur.

Healing occurs without complications.

APPLYING A SLING

Equipment

Commercial sling or
Triangular cloth or bandage
Safety pins

> **CLINICAL ALERT**
>
> Never move an extremity yourself to see if it is fractured. Ask if the client is able to move the limb instead. Always splint the extremity as found.

Preparation

1. Check physician's orders for a sling.
2. Do not remove clothing.
3. Assess injured extremity CMS before sling application.
4. Explain procedure and purpose of immobilization.
5. Remove any circumferential jewelry (ring, bracelet).
6. Have client sit or stand with forearm across chest.

Procedure

1. Place one end of triangular cloth over the shoulder on the unaffected arm.
2. Place cloth against the body and under the affected arm.
3. Place the apex (point) of the triangle toward the elbow.
4. Bring the opposite end of the triangle around the affected arm and over the affected shoulder.
5. Tie the sling at the side of the neck.
6. Fold the apex of the triangle over the elbow in the front, and secure with a safety pin or twist end and tie a square knot.
7. Assess client for comfort and for support of the affected arm.
8. Assess for neck pressure and circulation, motion, and sensation after 20 minutes and then every 2 to 4 hours.

Note: If using commercial sling, check directions on package for proper application.

> **CLINICAL ALERT**
>
> If greater immobilization is indicated (e.g., for shoulder dislocation or fracture), a swathe can be applied over the sling, circling and securing the upper arm to the thorax.

9. Check that hand is supported at a level higher than elbow to prevent dependent edema.
10. Teach client to support the arm higher than heart level and to perform external rotation shoulder exercises to prevent shoulder joint stiffness.

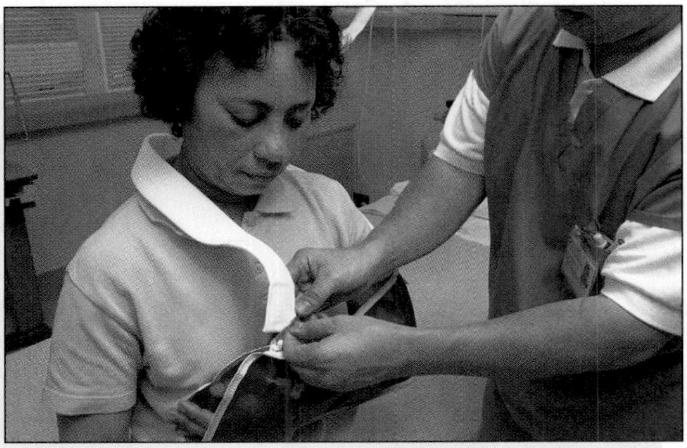

Bring strap over opposite shoulder and pull strap through metal hoops on sling.

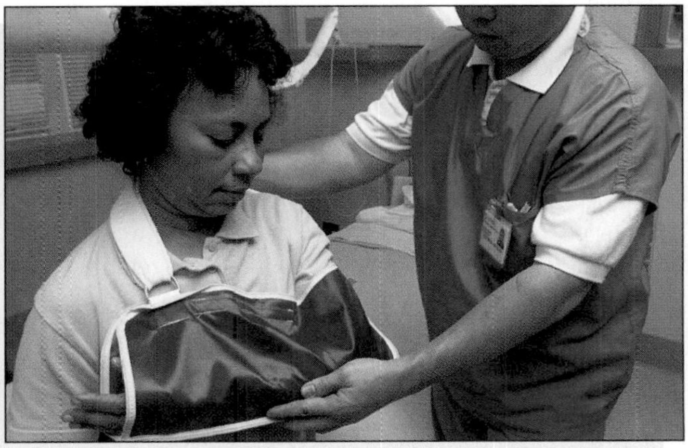

Hand should be supported at a level slightly higher than the elbow to prevent edema.

APPLYING SPIRAL BANDAGE

Equipment

Elastic or gauze roller bandages (width and number required to treat site)
Safety pins or tape
Supplies for wound care if indicated

Preparation

1. Check physician's orders, identify client, and explain procedure and purpose of immobilization.
2. Assess CMS of extremity before bandage application.
3. Remove any circumferential jewelry (ring, bracelet).
4. Have client sit or lie with part elevated.

Procedure

1. Remove existing elastic bandage or use bandage scissors to remove previously applied gauze bandage. **Rationale:** To prevent further injury and allow direct observation of site and wound care if indicated.
2. Remove dressing and redress wound if indicated (See Chapter 25).
3. Place part to be bandaged in an elevated position. **Rationale:** This promotes venous return and facilitates bandage compression to control edema and bleeding.
4. If area is functional or to be exercised, apply bandage with muscle in full contraction. **Rationale:** This prevents bandage constriction with future muscle activity.
5. Hold gauze or elastic roll with loose end outer part of bandage facing client's skin several inches below the site of injury.
6. Unroll bandage twice around extremity to anchor bandage.
7. Continue wrapping extremity upward, using a moderate amount of tension to stretch and apply bandage uniformly. **Rationale:** Unequal pressure can adversely affect circulation.
8. Progress wrapping the extremity *proximally* with spiral or angled turns. **Rationale:** Circular turns create a tourniquet effect. Proximal wrapping promotes venous return.
9. Make bandage turns that overlap by at least one half the previous wrap to prevent bandage separation. **Rationale:** Wrapping distally to proximally promotes venous return. Bandage turn separation tends to pinch the skin.
10. Finish wrap with a couple of wraps directly overlying each other.
11. Secure the bandage by tying or using tape or safety pin.
12. Observe that bandage is snug but not tight, is free of wrinkles, and is not occluding distal circulation.
13. Assess distal digits for CMS in 30 minutes and every 2–4 hours initially.
14. Maintain elevation of involved extremity and encourage active motion of digits. **Rationale:** This helps reduce edema and maintain function.
15. Rewrap bandage at least every 8 hours.

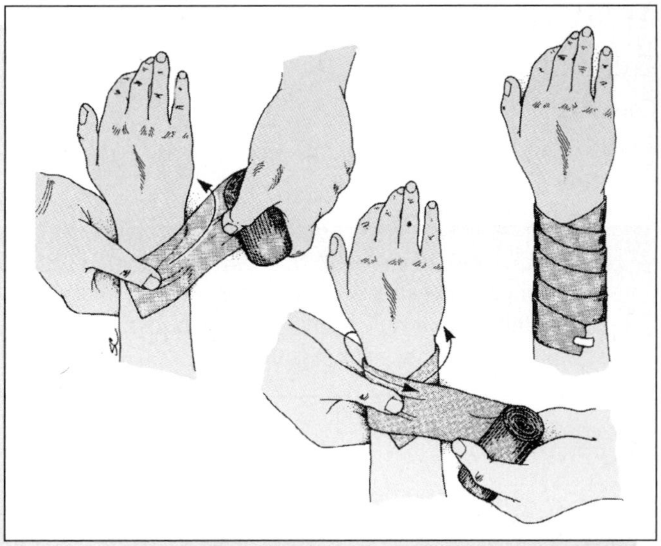
Spiral bandage may be used to secure a wound dressing.

CLINICAL ALERT

Injured tissues swell, but encircling therapies do not expand. For any encircling modality, assess distal digits for circulation, motion, and sensation after the first 30 minutes, and every 2–4 hours thereafter.

APPLYING A FIGURE-EIGHT BANDAGE

Equipment

Roller bandage
Safety pin or tape

Preparation

1. Identify client and explain procedure and rationale.
2. Provide privacy.
3. Position ankle in neutral alignment, neither overflexed nor overextended.

Procedure

1. Gather necessary bandages. The number and width of the bandage depends on the extent and area of the extremity to be bandaged.

2. Hold roll with outer part next to client's skin.
3. Anchor bandage by making a circular turn around instep.
4. Make a circular turn around ankle (heel) and return to starting point.
5. Make a spiral turn down over the ankle and around the foot.
6. Continue to make alternate turns around the ankle and foot. Overlap the preceding turn by at least two-thirds over the preceding layer.
7. Wrap the entire area below and above the involved joint. **Rationale:** This immobilizes the affected area.
8. Assess extremity (exposed digits) for circulation, motion, sensation, and evenness of pressure as well as comfort of client.
9. Assess extremity after 20 minutes and then every 2 to 4 hours, and rewrap every 8 hours.
10. Maintain elevation of extremity.

Note: Edema can result if the heel is not enclosed within bandage. An alternative wrap is to enclose the heel as the bandage is being applied.

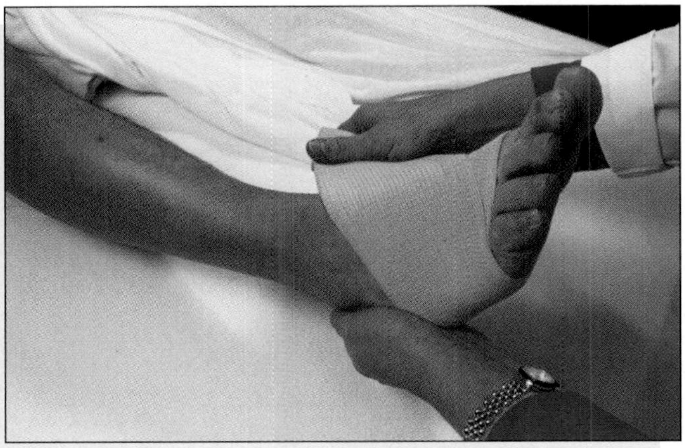

Make a circular turn around instep.

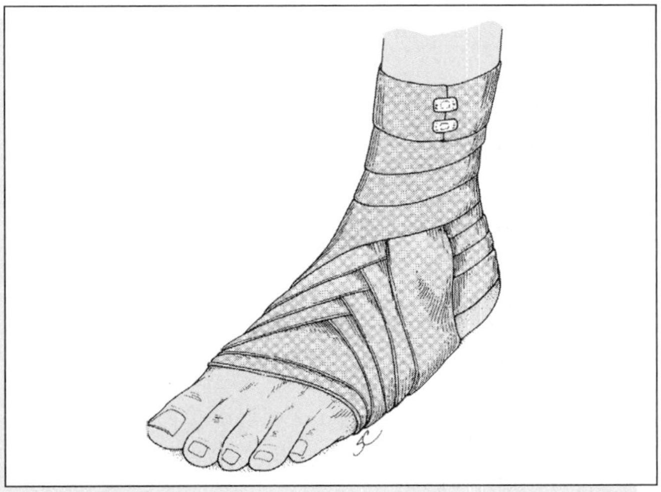

A figure-eight turn is used to support and limit joint movement.

APPLYING A SPLINT

Equipment

Splint materials: pieces of wood or pillows, magazines, blankets
Padding materials: pieces of cloth or towel
Wrapping materials: strips of cloth, rope, tape, elastic bandage

Preparation

1. Assess involved extremity for deformity or soft tissue injury.
2. Do not remove clothing or shoes (except with scissors). **Rationale:** To prevent excessive manipulation of the injured part.
3. Remove any jewelry from extremity to prevent circulatory compromise with swelling.
4. Assess neurovascular status of distal digits.
5. Explain need for and purpose of splint to client.

Procedure

1. Gather needed supplies.
2. Control bleeding by applying direct pressure and by using pressure dressings; apply clean covering to any wound.
3. Explain the rationale for the intervention to client.
4. Move injured extremity as little as possible and splint as it lies.
5. Pad joints, bony prominences, and between digits. **Rationale:** This prevents skin damage. Also make sure that the padding does not affect the client's circulation (e.g., don't put padding in axilla).
6. If splint material is not available, use the client's body for support.
   a. Splint the legs together.
   b. Splint an arm to the torso.
   c. Splint toes or fingers together.
7. Use a spiral (not circular) technique to wrap splint.
8. Strap the splint and extremity together securely so that the extremity is immobile. Try to include the proximal and distal points in the splint.
9. Check the client's distal circulation by assessing pulse, capillary refill, color, and temperature.
10. Elevate part to prevent edema.
11. Arrange to transport client to medical facility as soon as possible.
12. Report specifics to transport personnel.

CLINICAL ALERT

Never straighten an injured extremity or push bone or tissue back into place. Splint a deformed extremity in its deformed shape using a soft support such as a pillow.

APPLYING A CERVICAL COLLAR

Equipment

Measuring tape

Two semi-rigid collars of appropriate size (a spare for alternate use)

Preparation

1. Explain procedure to the client.
2. Ask the client to sit upright and face directly forward.
3. Measure client's neck from bottom of chin to top of sternum.
4. Measure circumference of client's neck.
5. Use client's measurements to select appropriate size collar.

Procedure

1. Follow manufacturer's instructions to apply collar.
2. Place back half of collar on client's neck, centering with the spine, arrow pointing up.
3. Center front half of collar on front of neck so that chin fits into the indentation. **Rationale:** This assures neutral alignment.
4. Lap front half over back half of collar.
5. Adjust side fasteners, if necessary, to assure a secure fit.
6. Inspect skin under collar regularly.
7. Assess neurovascular status of upper and lower extremities every 4–8 hours.

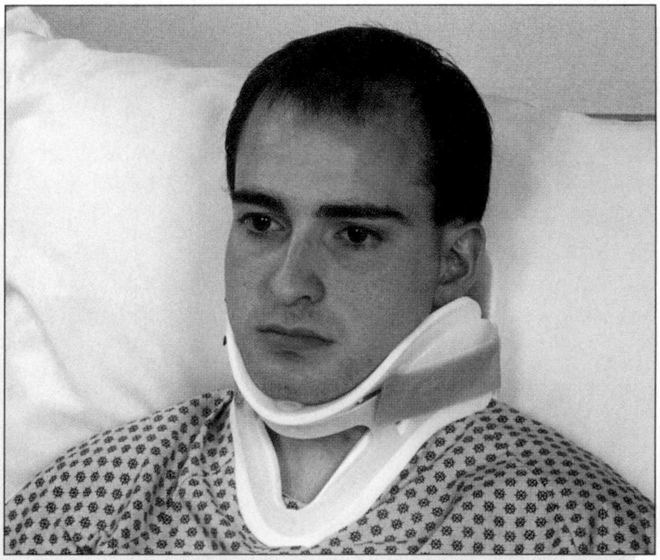

Ensure side fasteners of collar are properly adjusted for a secure fit.

8. Clean collar as needed with soap and water and allow to dry naturally; do not use a hair dryer.
9. Maintain collar use 24 hours/day or as ordered, using alternate collar when necessary.
10. Caution client that without neck flexion, visibility of stairs or objects on the floor is limited.

APPLYING A JEWETT–TAYLOR BACK BRACE

Equipment

Front and back brace with Velcro straps

T-shirt

Preparation

1. Check physician's order and determine rationale for brace application.
2. Determine that client's brace has been fitted by an orthotist (brace fitter).
3. Identify client, explain procedure, or supervise client's application and reinforce previous teaching.
4. Provide privacy.
5. Change wound dressing, if indicated, before applying brace.

Procedure

1. Wash your hands.
2. Put T-shirt on client. **Rationale:** This protects the skin from the brace rubbing on bare skin.
3. Place bed in a flat position. Keep side rail in UP position on side of bed opposite from you.

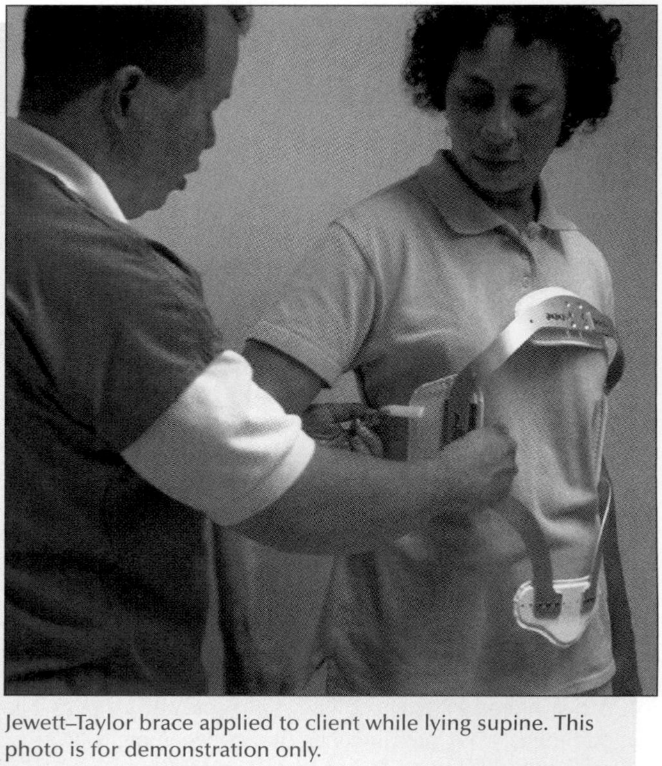

Jewett–Taylor brace applied to client while lying supine. This photo is for demonstration only.

4. Log-roll or ask client to roll to side away from you. **Rationale:** This position prevents torque on the spine.
5. Position brace on back so that struts fit on either side of spine and it fits the natural contour of the back. **Rationale:** Struts provide an open space along the spine so pressure is not exerted on a surgical site or on vertebrae.
6. Log-roll the client back onto brace to a supine position.
7. Place front section of brace over the iliac crest and position iliac wings (made of plastic material). Adjust triangular sternum piece; metal struts will fall into place.
8. Secure brace with Velcro straps.
9. Check under brace for pressure areas. If pressure areas are present, report to orthotist.
10. Provide client with adaptive aids (i.e., reacher). **Rationale:** Client cannot bend forward while wearing brace.

DOCUMENTATION FOR APPLYING IMMOBILIZING MODALITIES

- Time of application
- Site involved
- Skin integrity or wound status
- Type of immobilizing modality applied
- Circulatory and neurologic status of distal parts before and after modality application
- Site positioning or alignment
- Subjective statements of client

Critical Thinking Application

UNEXPECTED OUTCOMES	CRITICAL THINKING APPLICATIONS
Distal edema is noted in bandaged extremity and client is unable to move digits and states sensation is altered.	• Remove bandage and check distal circulation, motion, and sensation. • Keep extremity elevated. • Rewrap bandage with extremity in elevated position. • If edema persists, notify physician for possible addition of cold therapy, anti-inflammatory medication, or further evaluation.
Elevation of extremity increases pain, pain medications are ineffective, and pressure applied to injured site produces severe pain.	• Suspect acute compartment syndrome and notify physician immediately. Fasciotomy may be indicated if tissue swelling compromises circulation within a muscle compartment. • Window or bivalve cast if present. • Loosen external immobilizing device. • Maintain extremity in *dependent* position. • Do *not* apply ice to extremity since this reduces blood flow to area.
Toes become edematous following ankle bandaging.	• Elevate extremity and encourage active exercise of toes to promote venous return. • If area feels warm to touch, consider application of ice to help reduce inflammation. • Loosen bandage.
Bandage securing wound dressing continues to fall off.	• Avoid tape if skin is fragile or area has impaired circulation. • Use expanding "turkey skin" wrap to secure dressing. • Consult wound care specialist for alternative suggestions.

UNEXPECTED OUTCOMES	CRITICAL THINKING APPLICATIONS
Client with neck brace expresses fear of falling.	• Suggest removal of scatter rugs, other obstacles that might cause tripping. • Have client view environment from a distance before advancing into it. • Suggest use of a "blind" cane to scan or tap the area in front of client to warn of potential obstacles or steps.
Client with back brace refuses to eat.	• Loosen brace before and for a while after meals. • Encourage small, frequent meals. • Reduce intake of gas forming foods (cabbage, beans, corn). • Suggest intake of liquid nutritional supplement.

UNIT 2

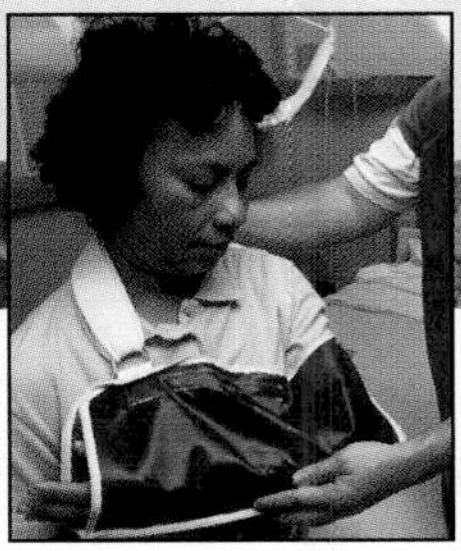

Cast Care

Nursing Process Data

ASSESSMENT ***Data Base***

Identify type of cast applied and rationale for application.

Note condition for which the cast was applied.

Observe condition of the cast.

Assess neurovascular status of involved extremity.

Assess client's understanding of and adherence to care instructions.

PLANNING ***Objectives***

To immobilize a fracture site

To maintain normal sensation, movement, and circulation in a casted extremity

To improve muscle tone and joint flexibility

To promote bone healing

To facilitate self-care following cast application and removal

IMPLEMENTATION ***Procedures***

Caring for a Wet Cast

Assessing a Casted Extremity

Instructing Client in Self Care

EVALUATION ***Expected Outcomes***

Site is adequately immobilized.

Neurovascular complications do not occur.

Cast dries without cracking or indentation areas on the cast.

The client experiences minimal discomfort from pain or swelling.

TABLE 30–2 Comparison of Cast Types

	Plaster	Synthetic
Material	Plaster of paris, comprised of powdered calcium sulfate crystals impregnated into the bandages	Polyester and cotton, fiberglass or plastic. Polyester and cotton is impregnated with water-activated polyurethane resin
Drying time	24–48 hours No weight bearing until dry, 48–72 hours	7–15 minutes for setting 60 minutes for weight bearing
Advantages	Less costly More effective for immobilizing fracture site Smooth surface Doesn't require expensive equipment for application	Less likely to indent into skin Lighter in weight Less restrictive Doesn't crumble Nonabsorbent

CARING FOR A WET CAST

Equipment

Pillows for support
Pen to mark drainage

Preparation

1. Note physician's orders for any client-specific instructions about positioning or cast handling.
2. Identify client and explain all procedures.
3. Recruit assistant(s) to help turn client.

Procedure

1. Explain that the cast feels warm as plaster dries, but urge client to report undue warmth or a burning sensation. **Rationale:** Cast burns can cause serious tissue injury.
2. Until the cast is dry, use *only* the palms of your hands to handle cast when turning and positioning. **Rationale:** Fingers can indent cast and create pressure areas on underlying tissue.
3. Avoid handling over joints where nerves and blood vessels are superficial.
4. Support cast with pillows, with extremity elevated above heart level. **Rationale:** This promotes venous return and reduces edema.
5. Maintain contours built into the cast; support leg so that heel is free of pressure. **Rationale:** To prevent flattening.
6. Keep wet cast uncovered, and turn client to both sides, prone and supine to expose all surfaces, allowing cast to dry by natural evaporation from the inside out.

Note: The wet plaster of paris cast is dry when musty odor is gone, the cast is white and shiny, and it sounds resonant when tapped.

7. Do not try to hasten drying by using artificial measures such as a hair dryer. **Rationale:** Outer layer may dry before inner aspect, resulting in cast weakening.

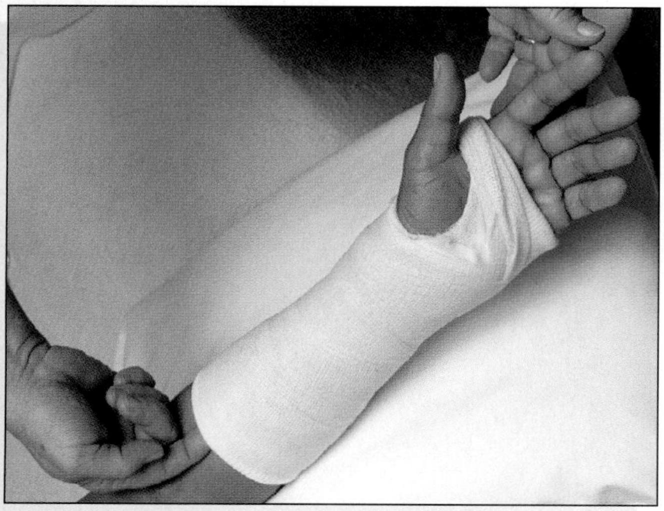

Check cast for tightness. You should be able to insert one or two fingers between cast and skin.

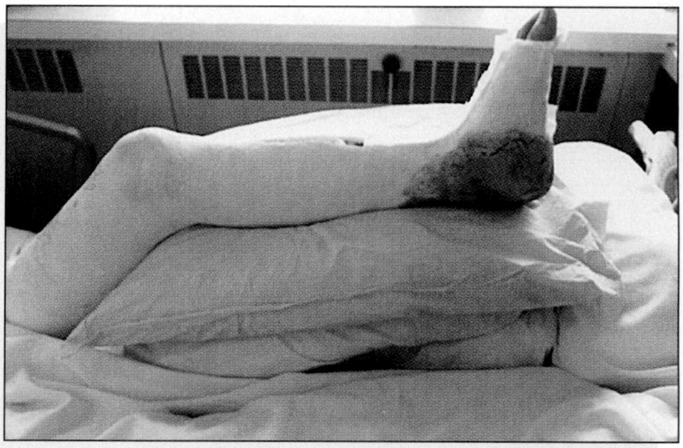

Position casted extremity above level of heart to prevent edema.

8. If ice pack is ordered to reduce edema, place it alongside of cast, not on cast. **Rationale:** Placing ice pack on the cast can cause flattening.
9. If cast edges are rough or crumbly, pull inner stockinette out and over the edge and secure with tape.

CLINICAL ALERT

Injured tissues swell, but encircling therapies do not expand. For any encircling modality, assess distal digits for circulation, motion, and sensation after the first 30 minutes, and every 2–4 hours thereafter. Assessment is ongoing, and continues following discharge.

ASSESSING A CASTED EXTREMITY

Equipment

Pen to mark drainage on cast

Procedure

1. Explain rationale for the procedure to client.
2. Encourage client to notify you of any change in sensation, mobility, or color/temperature in the casted extremity.
   a. Circulation
      - Report if digits are swollen despite elevation and active exercise.
      - Report if digits are pale, blue, or cold to touch.
      - Report delayed (>2 seconds) capillary refill (pinch finger to blanch and determine length of time required for color to return)
   b. Motion
      - *Immediately* report pain on passive movement of digits
      - Report inability to perform range of motion of involved digits (see Table 30–1).
      - Compare strength of action with uninvolved extremity.
   c. Sensation
      - *Immediately* report increasing pain, pain with passive motion of digits, or pain that increases when the extremity is elevated.
      - Report numbness or paresthesia (pins-and-needles feeling).
      - Assess involved nerve sites for sensation (see Table 30–1).
3. Emphasize that a fine margin exists between reversible and irreversible damage to neurovascular structures.

CLINICAL ALERT

When casting material inhibits palpation of peripheral pulses, assess for edema, comfort level, and other parameters of "CMS" as an indication of neurovascular status.

4. Assess for capillary refill by applying pressure to one of the client's digits. After you stop the pressure, observe the area to see how rapidly the color returns. **Rationale:** Comparing your nails to the client's nail is one check on how quickly color should return; it should return in 2 seconds.

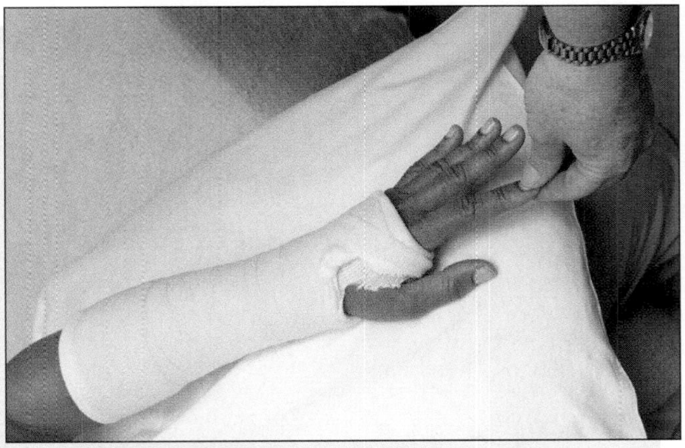

Check fingers or toes for color, temperature, capillary refill, sensation, and motion.

CLINICAL ALERT

Casted extremity should be assessed every ½ hour for 2 hours, then every hour for 24 hours, then every 4 hours for 48 hours.

5. Ask the client to move the fingers or toes that are affected by the cast. The client should be able to move them without difficulty.

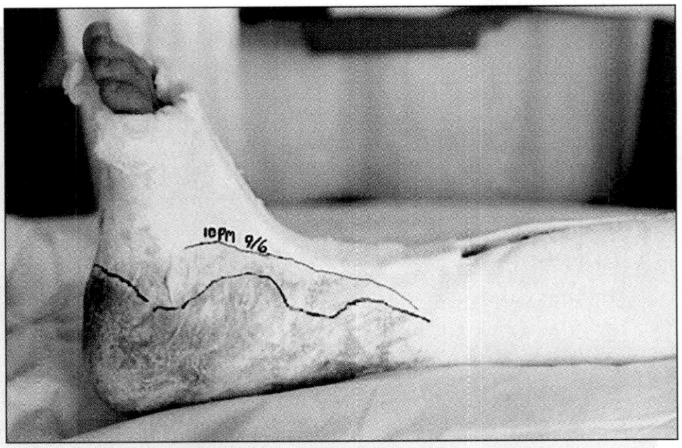

Observe casted extremity frequently to monitor drainage.

6. Check for any wound drainage. Note color and amount of drainage and mark cast.
7. Report any unusual odor or increase in drainage.
8. Check for redness or skin breakdown around casted area.
9. Keep dirt and powder away from cast.
10. Remind client to not stick objects down the cast to scratch skin. **Rationale**: Skin breakdown can occur leading to infection.

> **CLINICAL ALERT**
>
> If the client has had open reduction, wound drainage will be absorbed and spread rapidly, or seep down to back of cast. The visible drainage does not necessarily indicate the amount of actual drainage.
>
> Inspect all cast surfaces and mark drainage regularly if it is increasing. Bleeding should not persist after 24 hours.

> **CLINICAL ALERT**
>
> Diminished or absent pulses, coolness, and pallor are late signs and unreliable indicators of acute compartment syndrome. Always assess active extension, flexion, adduction, and abduction of the fingers, flexion and extension of the toes, and inversion and dorsiflexion of the foot. Pain on passive stretching of the muscle or distal digits is an *early* indicator of circulatory compromise.

INSTRUCTING CLIENT IN SELF CARE

Equipment

Instructions pamphlet
Relevant telephone numbers

Preparation

1. Review client's chart for type of reduction performed (open or closed).
2. Identify client and explain importance of self care to prevent complications.
3. Provide written instructions that reinforce teaching.
4. Provide telephone number of patient care coordinator if relevant for followup concerns.

Procedure

1. Demonstrate and teach importance of regular neurovascular checks, comparing with contralateral extremity. (*See* Assessing a Casted Extremity).
2. Teach client to keep casted extremity elevated and to actively exercise digits. **Rationale:** This reduces stiffness, promotes venous return, reduces edema, and risk of thrombus formation.
3. Report any unusual odor, new drainage, or elevated body temperature. **Rationale:** These are signs of possible infection, especially if client has had open reduction or an object has been placed or fallen into the cast.
4. Remind client to not stick objects into the cast to scratch the skin. Encourage client to blow cool air (hair dryer on "cool" or asepto bulb syringe), or to apply pressure over the area to relieve itching. **Rationale:** Scratching the area abrades the skin and can cause infection.
5. Teach cast protection.
   a. Remove stains with nonabrasive powder cleanser and damp cloth.
   b. Do not shellac or varnish to waterproof the cast. It must "breathe."
   c. Use plastic covering (garbage bag) for showering. Do not cover for prolonged periods as this will cause condensation and weaken the cast.
   d. Report any cracking or softening of cast and redness of skin at cast edges.
   e. Protect cast from urine or stool as odor can't be removed.
   f. Sleep with casted lower extremity next to wall, if possible. **Rationale:** If the casted extremity falls off the bed, the client will go with it.
6. Cast removal.
   a. Inform client that cast saw blade is safe. It does not cut through material, but vibrates.
   b. Prepare client that muscle will have atrophied with disuse, joints will be stiff, and bone is vulnerable to refracture.
   c. Teach client to continue to protect, support, and elevate the extremity following cast removal.

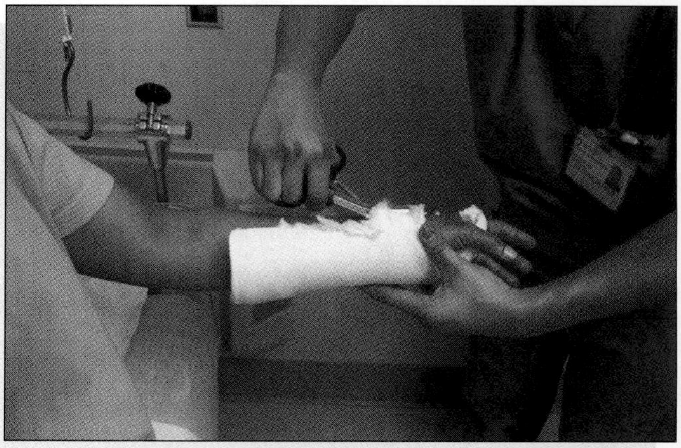

Cast is split with a vibrating blade. Underlying padding is cut with bandage scissors.

d. Teach client that skin will be caked with adherent exudate and not to forcibly remove this. Soften exudate with olive oil, or use full strength cold water wash (e.g., Woolite, Delicare), leave on 20 minutes, then rinse in warm water. **Rationale:** Aggressive removal of exudate can cause bleeding. Enzymes in special cleansers will loosen dead cells and fatty or crusty lesions without injuring underlying cells.

DOCUMENTATION FOR CAST CARE

- Type of cast applied
- Positioning of cast
- Client's complaints and nursing responses
- Color, warmth, movement, and sensation in casted extremity
- Presence, location, and amount of drainage from wound
- Client's acceptance of the cast

Critical Thinking Application

UNEXPECTED OUTCOMES	CRITICAL THINKING OPTIONS
Client complains of numbness, discomfort, or pain.	• Determine when cast was applied. Function should improve over time. • Notify physician immediately. • Reevaluate condition of casted extremity every 15 minutes. • Reassess circulation, motion, and sensation (CMS).
Cast cracks from improper drying or stress.	• Notify physician immediately. • Reassure client. • Do not reposition client until physician assesses.
Synthetic cast has rough edges.	• Smooth edges by filing with nail file if necessary. • Make sure furniture and clothing are protected from scratches and snags by covering cast with stockinette.
Cast edges begin to crumble.	• "Petal" edges of cast with 1- to 2-inch strips of adhesive tape. Place half of tape inside cast, pull tape over cast, and anchor on outside of cast. Continue to petal cast until all edges are covered.
Client immersed synthetic cast in water.	• Immersion should be done *only* with physician's permission. • Flush skin under cast with plain water if it has been exposed to chlorine. • Dry skin under cast thoroughly with hair dryer on LOW. This may require several hours!

UNIT 3

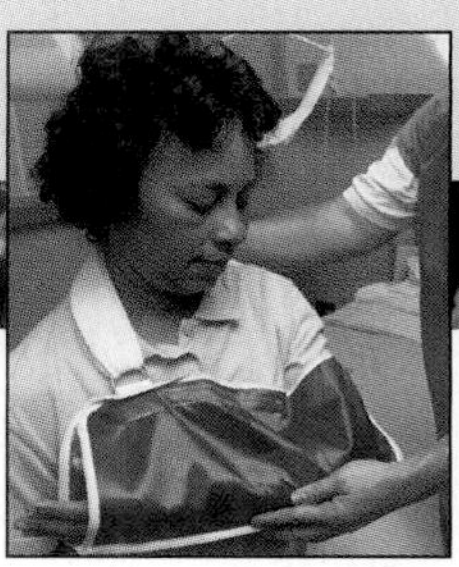

Traction

Nursing Process Data

ASSESSMENT ***Data Base***

Determine type and purpose of traction used.
Note the amount of weight ordered.
Note any conditions requiring special treatment (i.e., continuous or intermittent traction).
Assess circulation, motion, and sensation of affected extremity.
Assess pin site for drainage and signs of infection.
Assess neurovascular status of clients with external fixation devices.

PLANNING ***Objectives***

To relieve muscle spasm
To maintain alignment of fracture site
To prevent unnecessary injury to soft tissue
To prevent neurovascular complications
To use for temporary management of fractures in adults
To maintain pin site free of infection

IMPLEMENTATION ***Procedures***

Maintaining Skin Traction
Maintaining Skeletal Traction
Monitoring External Fixator Devices
Maintaining Halo Traction

EVALUATION ***Expected Outcomes***

Muscle spasm and pain are reduced.
Extremity is maintained in correct alignment.
Neurovascular status is within normal limits.
Skin of affected extremity remains intact.
Pin site remains free of infection.
Fracture healing is facilitated.

MAINTAINING SKIN TRACTION

Preparation

1. Determine if client is preoperative. If so, do not manipulate the extremity.
2. Determine if client has condition (diabetes, peripheral vascular disease) that predisposes to skin damage with traction.
3. Determine if traction is continuous or intermittent.
4. Recruit an assistant to apply manual traction when removing and replacing traction.
5. Explain purpose of traction to client and family.

Procedure

1. Examine type of traction used that attaches weights to the extremity.
   a. Material should be held firmly in place.
   b. Material should fit comfortably, neither too loose nor too tight.
   c. Client should be in functional alignment.
2. Examine all bony prominences of the involved extremity for abrasions or pressure areas.
   a. Traction should be removed at least every 8 hours for skin inspection.
   b. Have an assistant apply manual traction when discontinuing for assessment.
   c. Check for redness, which, if present, indicates excessive pressure on site.

> **CLINICAL ALERT**
> Unless ordered otherwise, the client with Buck's extension should have the knee gatch of the bed elevated 20°–30° to flex the hip in a neutral position.

3. Examine extremity distal to the traction.
   a. Note any presence of edema.
   b. Palpate peripheral pulses.

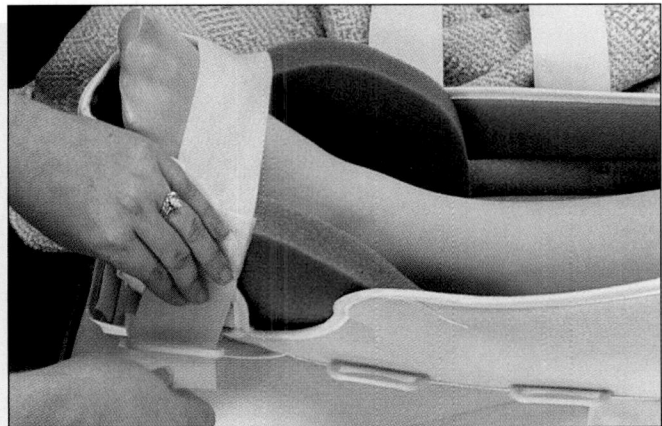

Remove straps on Buck's traction every 8 hours to maintain function and allow inspection.

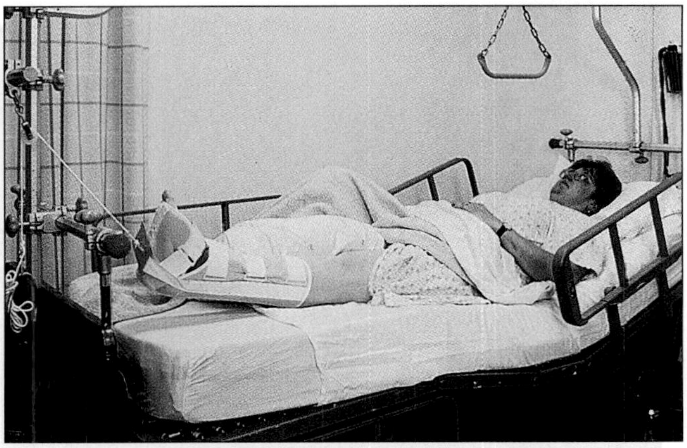

Ensure client is positioned correctly in bed.

   c. Check temperature and color to see if both extremities are normal.
   d. Check time of capillary refill.
4. Assess for possible neurologic impediment from traction slings encroaching on popliteal space or axilla. **Rationale:** Numbness or tingling, if present, indicates neurologic problems have occurred.
5. Examine the rope and weights to see that they hang freely and the pull goes directly through the long axis of the fractured bone.

> **CLINICAL ALERT**
> Do not apply Buck's traction over or under a calf compression device. Foot pumps (only around the foot) are acceptable for deep-vein thrombosis prophylaxis.

6. Check the traction mechanism.
   a. Weights should hang freely, off the floor and bed.
   b. Weights are 5–10 pounds for adult clients.
   c. Knots should be secure in all ropes.
   d. Ropes should move freely through pulleys.
   e. Pulleys should not be constrained by knots.

Principles of Traction Maintenance

- Maintain traction pull by ensuring weights are hanging freely.
- Maintain ropes in pulley system and ensure rope moves freely through system and knots do not interfere with movement.
- Maintain countertraction, client aligned in center of bed.
- Maintain traction either continuous or intermittent, according to physician's orders.

7. Position correctly in bed: the client should be positioned in the center of the bed. Affected leg or arm should be aligned with trunk of body. **Rationale:** Misalignment is the leading cause of pain for traction clients. The client should not be pulled down to the end of the bed because this negates the traction.
8. Place sheepskin or an alternative material under the affected extremity if appropriate. **Rationale:** This helps prevent pressure areas.
9. Provide ordered type of boot to prevent footdrop.

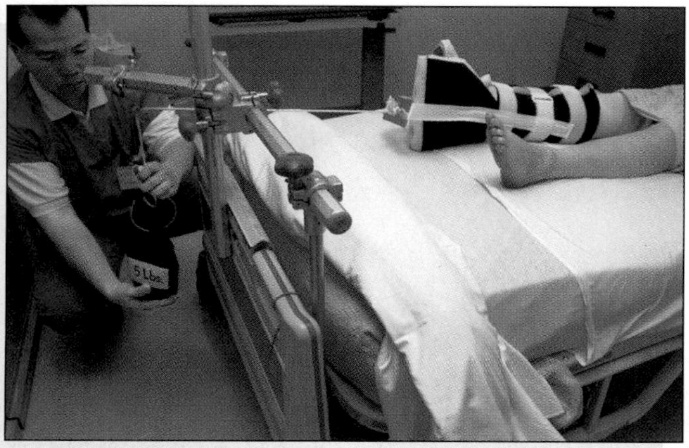
Maintain traction by ensuring that weights hang freely.

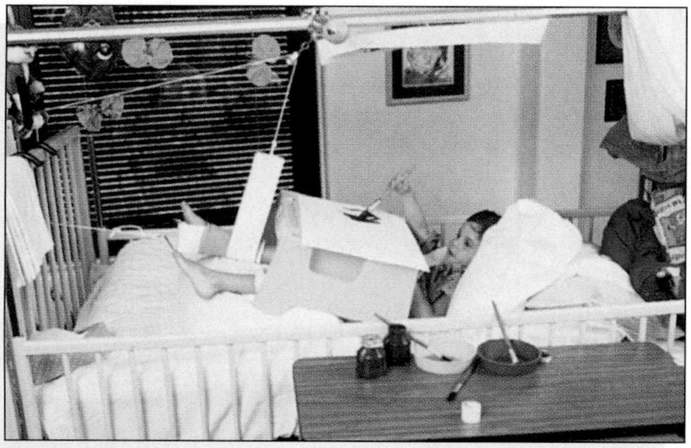
Russell's traction is used for fractures of the femur and lower leg before surgery.

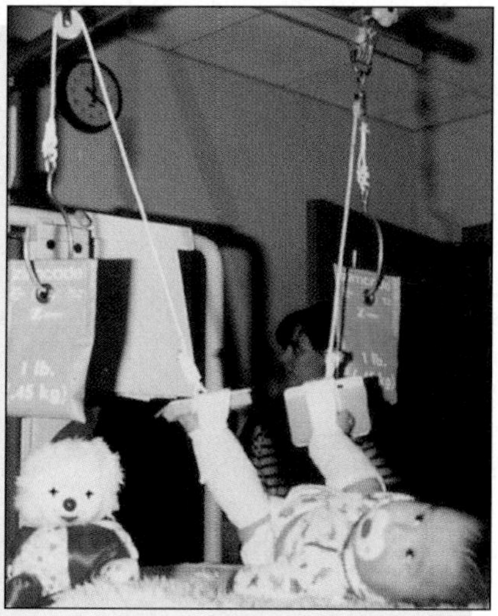
Bryant's traction is used to reduce fractured femur or treat hip dislocation.

TABLE 30–3 Skin Traction

Type	Purpose	Bed Position
Buck's extension	Short-term immobilization of a hip fracture before surgical intervention	Head elevated 10°–20° for ADLs, knee flexed 20°–30°
Cervical	Degenerative or arthritic conditions of cervical vertebrae, neck strain	Flat in bed or head can be elevated 15°–20°
Dunlop	Either skin or skeletal, used for fractured humerus	Flat in bed; arm suspended and flexed
Pelvic girdle	Low back pain, muscle spasm, or herniated disc	Head of bed and knee gatch raised so hips flexed 45° angle (William's position)
Russell's	Used for fractured shaft of femur or lower leg, and some knee injuries	Head of bed elevated 30°–45°
Bryant's	Used specifically for child weighing less than 30 lbs, for fractured femur or hip dysplasia	Flat in bed with both hips flexed at 45°–90°, legs extended and buttocks raised 1 inch from mattress

MAINTAINING SKELETAL TRACTION

Equipment

Sterile cotton-tipped applicators
Prescribed cleansing agent
Sterile cup for solution
Sterile gloves
Sterile 4 × 4 gauze sponges

Preparation

1. Check physician's orders regarding pin site care and client positioning.
2. Check client's identaband.
3. Gather necessary equipment.
4. Wash hands.
5. Provide privacy and explain procedure to client.

Procedure

1. Check pin and site surrounding the pin.
   a. Pin should be immobile.
   b. Pin site should be clean and dry.
2. Assess for infection at the pin site. Note any local pain, redness, heat, or drainage.
3. Provide pin site care if ordered.
   a. Open applicator sticks and gauze package.
   b. Open prescribed cleansing agent and pour into cup.
   c. Don sterile gloves.
   d. Clean area with prescribed cleansing agent. Soak cotton-tipped applicators. Dip stick into solution bottle, or pour solution over sticks.
   e. Clean pin site starting at insertion area and working outward (away from pin site). **Rationale:** To cleanse site from cleanest to dirtiest area.
   f. Use new applicator stick for cleaning each pin site. **Rationale:** This prevents cross contamination of sites.
   g. Loosely dress site with separate gauze sponge.
   h. Remove gloves and discard sticks.
   i. Wash hands.
4. Examine all bony prominences for signs of pressure areas or abrasions.

TABLE 30–4 Skeletal Traction

Type	Purpose	Bed Position
External fixation devices Hoffman Synthes	Manage complex fractures with soft tissue damage; provide stability for severe comminuted fractures	Allows client mobility and active exercise of uninvolved joints
Cervical tongs Crutchfield Gardner–Wells Vinke	Used to immobilize and reduce cervical fractures Tongs maintain alignment of cervical spine	Bedrest, supine position; may turn on special frames or log-rolled
Balanced suspension with Thomas splint and Pearson attachment	Align bone and promote effective line of pull	Bedrest in supine position; may turn side to side for care; knee is flexed

EVIDENCE BASED NURSING PRACTICE

Pin Site Care for Traction

There is no existing standard for traction pin care. Recommended treatments include the use of dressings, cleansing with hydrogen peroxide, alcohol, povidone iodine, normal saline, soap and water or sterile water and chlorhexidine gluconate. Almost all of these preparations are associated with pin corrosion, increased infection rates and delayed healing. Ointments should not be used because they prevent pin site drainage.

Soap and water, sterile water, and normal saline *are useful* because they soften and allow removal of crusts to promote normal pin site drainage (thereby reducing risk of infection), and are not associated with adverse reactions.

Use of sterile technique and loose application of gauze to the site are advocated by the author. Frequency of pin site care should be based on assessment of crusting and need to promote drainage.

Source: McKenzie, L. (1999). In search of a standard for pin site care. *Orthopaedic Nursing, 18*(2), 73–78.

5. Check for circulation, motion, and sensation in the affected extremity.
6. Assess distal extremity for color and edema.
7. Check ropes and weights to make sure pull goes directly through long axis of the fractured bone. **Rationale:** This pull maintains fracture in alignment.
8. Check traction mechanism.
   a. Weights should hang freely, off the floor and bed.
   b. Knots should be secure in all ropes.
   c. Rope should move freely through pulleys.
   d. Pulleys should not be constrained by knots.
9. Instruct client to use trapeze to assist in moving in bed, during linen change and back care.
10. Make sure client is positioned correctly in bed. **Rationale:** If the client is pulled down to the foot of bed, the traction is negated.
11. Check placement of the foot rest. The client's foot should be correctly positioned to prevent footdrop.
12. Check if client has migrated to foot of bed—pull client up using turn sheet. Do *not* release traction during repositioning.
13. Change bed linen in a top to bottom manner while client uses trapeze to lift buttocks.

CLINICAL ALERT

Skeletal traction is never removed without a physician's order.

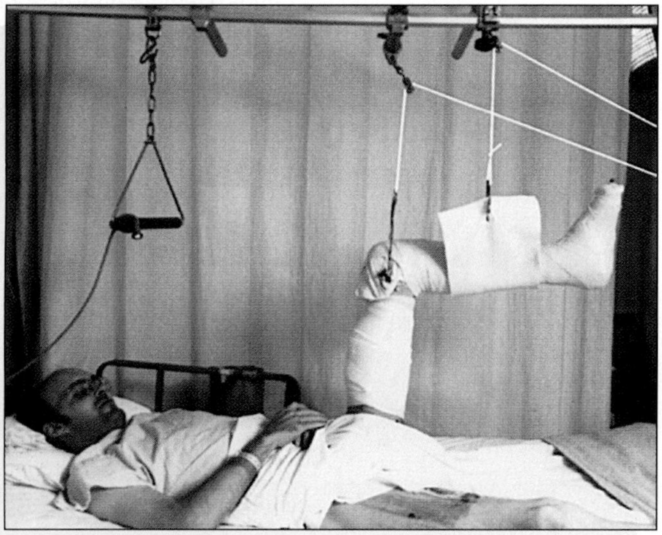

Russell's traction incorporates a sling with ropes and pulleys (this type of *skin* traction may be incorporated with skeletal traction as above).

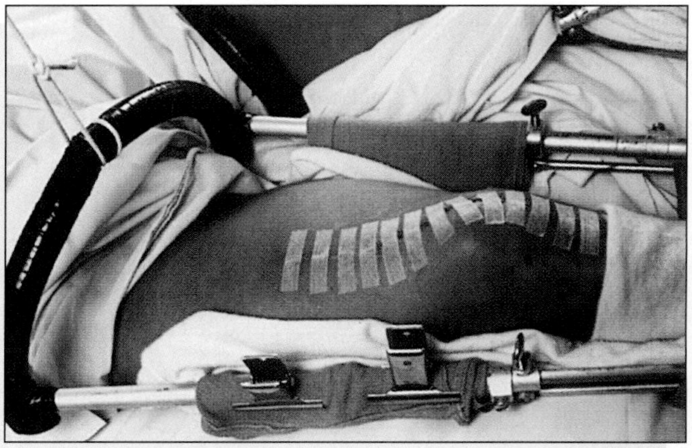

A Thomas *splint* supports the thigh. It is used for balanced suspension along with skeletal traction for fracture of the femur. A Pearson attachment supports the lower leg.

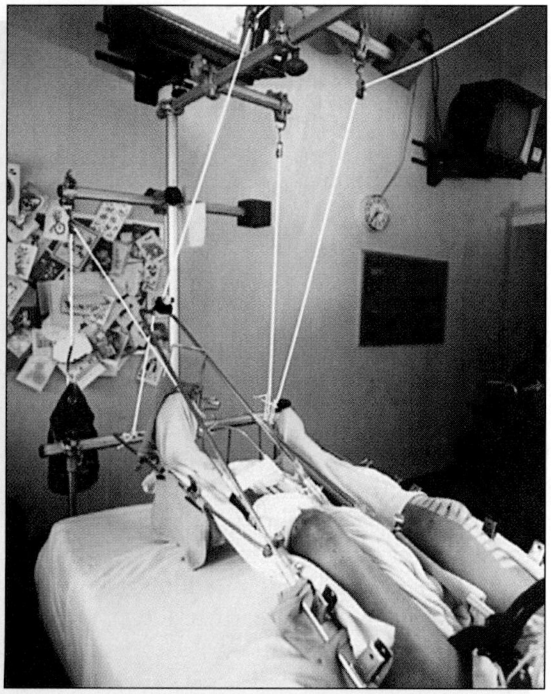

Bilateral Thomas splints with Pearson attachments used for fractured femurs.

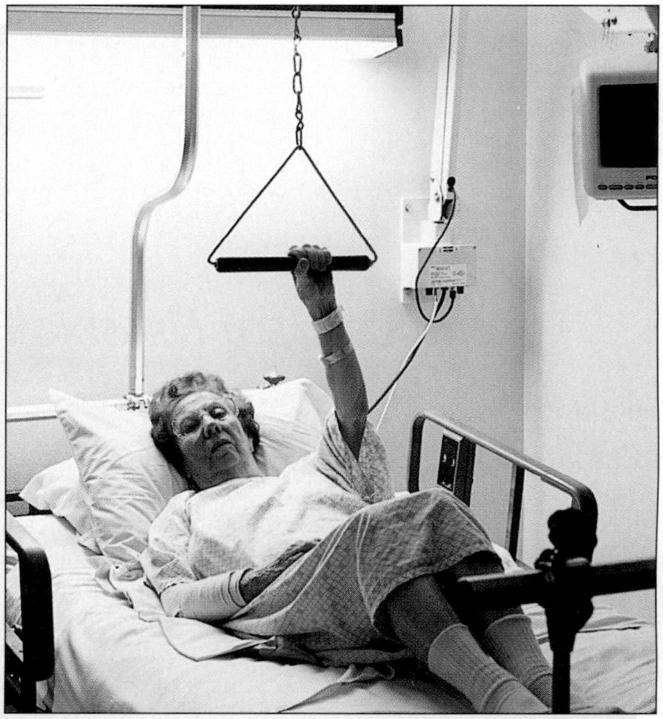

Trapeze is used to assist client to move in bed.

MAINTAINING AN EXTERNAL FIXATOR DEVICE

Equipment

Sterile cotton-tipped applicators
Prescribed cleansing solution
Sterile gloves
Sterile gauze sponges (as ordered)

Procedure

1. Follow steps 1–5 of previous skill.

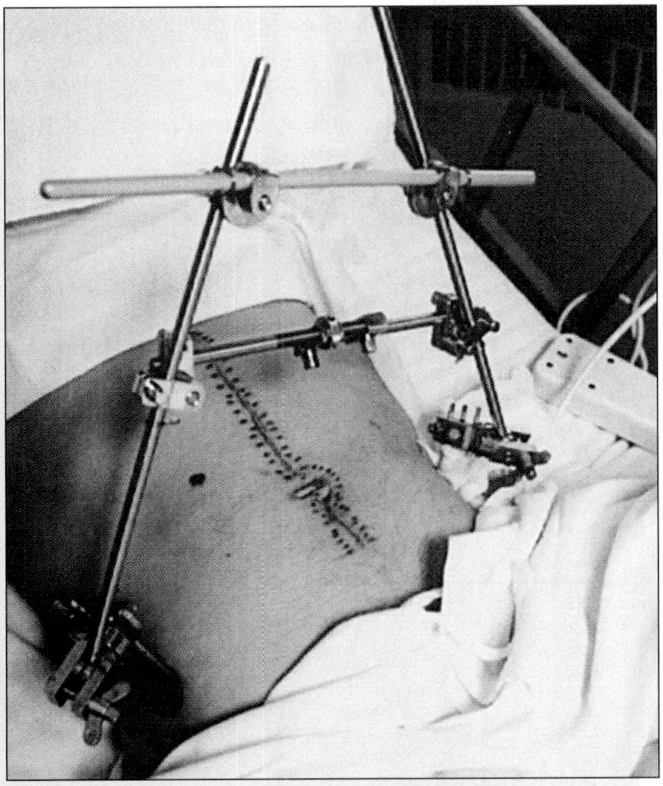

Hoffman frame, external fixator is used for complex fractures, and to allow early mobility.

2. Assess neurovascular status of affected part every four hours. **Rationale:** Clients with external fixation devices usually have extensive soft tissue, nerve, and vessel damage.
3. Provide client teaching before discharge.
   a. Instruct client on the importance of, and how to perform, neurovascular checks and when to call the physician.
   b. Demonstrate pin site care. Have client return the demonstration. **Rationale:** To ensure he or she is using appropriate technique.

Note: Clean technique is used following discharge.

   c. Reinforce physician's instructions regarding activity level. Discuss weight-bearing on affected limb, if appropriate.
   d. Explain that fixator device is not to be used as a handle.
4. Demonstrate range-of-motion exercises, if appropriate, and have client perform return demonstration. **Rationale:** To ensure appropriate exercises are being performed correctly.
5. Instruct client to continue to elevate extremity if edema occurs in affected limb.
6. Teach appropriate use of assistive devices as necessary. **Rationale:** To prevent falls or inappropriate use of the device which could cause accidents.

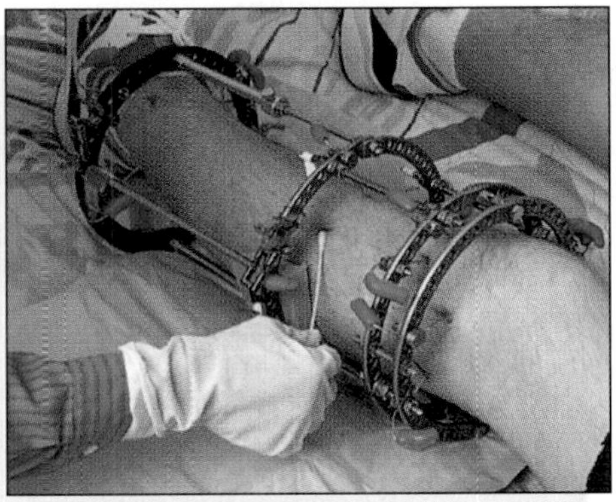

Pin site care for external fixator.

EVIDENCE BASED NURSING PRACTICES

Lifting an Extremity with an External Fixator

A survey of orthopedic surgeons concludes that the best way to lift an extremity with an external fixator is to support the extremity itself, supporting the joint above and below the frame. Repeat lifting and manipulation of the frame itself can lead to pin loosening and fracture malalignment.

Source: DeGeorge, P., & Dunwoody, C. (1995). Transfer techniques of the lower extremity with an external fixator. *Orthopaedic Nursing, 14*(6), 17–21.

MAINTAINING HALO TRACTION

Equipment

Allen wrench
Emergency tracheostomy set (available)
Bag–valve–mask (available)
Bright nail polish
Equipment for pin site care
Prescribed cleansing solution
Sterile cup for solution
Sterile cotton-tipped applicators
Clean gloves

Preparation

1. Review client's history to determine level and type of spinal injury and purpose of halo brace immobilization.
2. Determine specific assessment required for your particular client (depends upon the level of client's spinal injury). **Rationale:** The client with cervical spine injury is at risk for impaired ventilation.
3. Gather necessary equipment.
4. Wash your hands.

Procedure

1. Evaluate client's understanding of halo traction and its purpose.
2. Assess client's respiratory status regularly.
3. Perform complete neurologic assessment (cranial nerves, peripheral nerves, motion and sensation). **Rationale:** Because of their location at the base of the skull, these nerves are prone to injury or excessive stretching with halo traction.
4. Check alignment of traction-brace system. Client's neck should not be flexed or extended.
5. Discuss safety issues.
   a. Client is top heavy and has a limited view of the surrounding environment. Pathways for walking must be clear of obstacles.
   b. Consult PT and OT for adaptive aids and tips for ADLs. **Rationale:** Client should anticipate situations and problems that may occur at home such as sleeping position, bathing, getting in and out of a car.
   c. Keep Allen wrench taped to front of vest. Mark anterior screws that attach vertical bars to brace with bright nail polish. **Rationale:** When marked they are easy to locate. The anterior vest is removed for emergency measures such as CPR.
6. Have emergency tracheostomy tray and bag–valve–mask available on unit. **Rationale:** Endotracheal intubation is contraindicated. A tracheotomy may be necessary for emergency ventilation.
7. Suggest that client cover bolts/screws with moleskin or tape to protect clothing.
8. Inspect anterior (above eyebrows) and posterior (above and behind ears) pin sites for signs of drainage, crusting, or inflammation.
9. Provide skin care under vest:
   a. Open vest at both sides during bath.
   b. Check skin at vest edges and where vest overlaps.

CLINICAL ALERT

Never use the bars of a Halo brace to move the client.

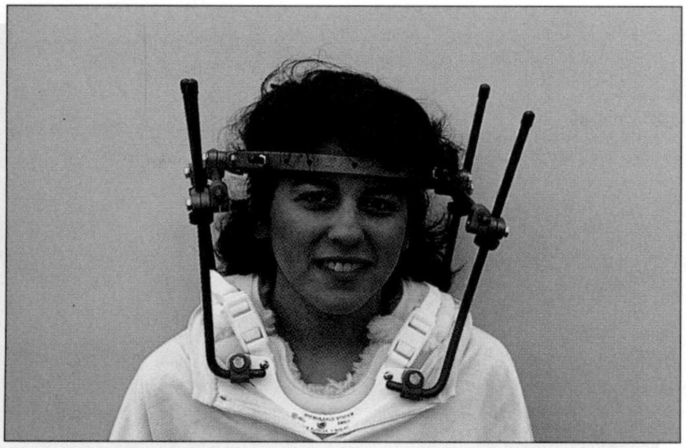

Halo brace traction provides immobilization following cervical or upper thoracic vertebral injury.

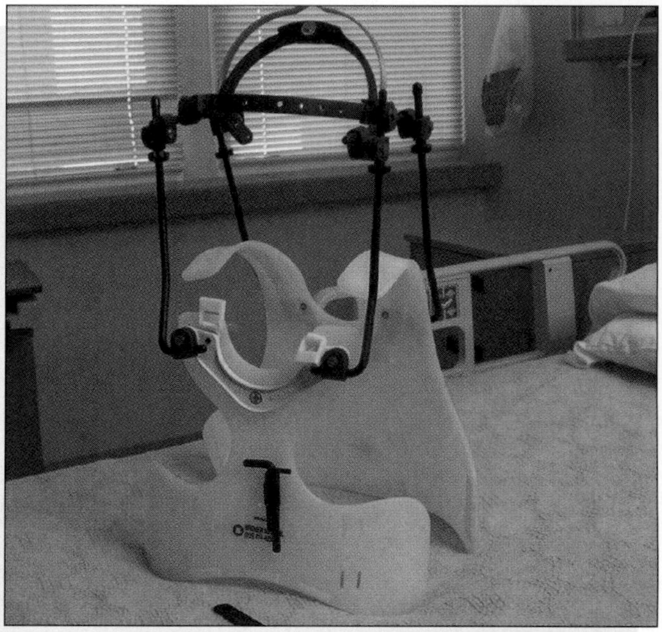

The halo ring is attached to the vest by vertical bars (2 in front and 2 in back). The ring is attached to the skull by 2 anterior and 2 posterior pins. Wrench on vest is for emergency release.

c. Wash and dry skin thoroughly.
d. Do not use lotion or powder under brace. **Rationale:** They combine with perspiration and irritate the skin.
e. Replace vest liner if it becomes wet or dirty.

10. Provide pin site care as prescribed. See steps in previous skill for skeletal traction.

CLINICAL ALERT

If skull pins are loose, keep client immobilized and notify physician immediately.

DOCUMENTATION FOR TRACTION

- Type and location of traction, intermittent, or continuous
- Alignment of traction, client's positioning
- Integrity of the skin
- Circulation, motion, and sensation in extremity
- Specific complaints by client and nursing actions taken to solve problems
- Client's comfort and overall feelings
- Pin site, assessment, and care
- Neurovascular check on clients with external fixator devices
- Client and family teaching
- Client's progress in self-care

Critical Thinking Application

UNEXPECTED OUTCOMES	CRITICAL THINKING OPTIONS
There is a change in the temperature, color, or pulses of the extremity.	• Notify physician at once. • If the client has a fractured femur, measure the circumference of the thigh with a tape measure every 15–30 minutes. Look for areas of ecchymosis; it is possible for several units of blood to be sequestered in the thigh if a major vessel has been involved. • Assess for circulatory shock.
Client requiring Buck's traction has history of venous thrombosis.	• Obtain order for thromboembolic deterrent hosiery or foot compression device. • Do not apply calf compression device under boot. • Encourage client to dorsiflex and plantarflex foot and to do ankle turns.
Client in Buck's traction is unable to dorsiflex the foot.	• Release proximal strap as it may be compressing peroneal nerve over head of fibula. • Assess sensation over dorsum of foot and between big and second toes. • Notify physician.
Client in skeletal traction keeps migrating to foot of bed.	• Without releasing traction, use pull sheet and an assistant to reposition client up in bed. • Elevate lower part of bed with blocks to provide countertraction. • Increase weight of countertraction at head of bed.

UNEXPECTED OUTCOMES	CRITICAL THINKING OPTIONS
Bone in skeletal traction has migrated to end of Kirschner wire.	• Notify orthopedic surgeon. • Pin will be sterilized and moved so that bone centers on wire. • Review ordered mobility restrictions with client.
Halo pin site appears to be infected.	• Notify physician. • Obtain culture of drainage for antibiotic sensitivity studies. • Cleanse pin site as prescribed, using aseptic technique. • Remove crusts to allow drainage. • Monitor systemic signs and neurologic status for possible brain abscess.

UNIT 4

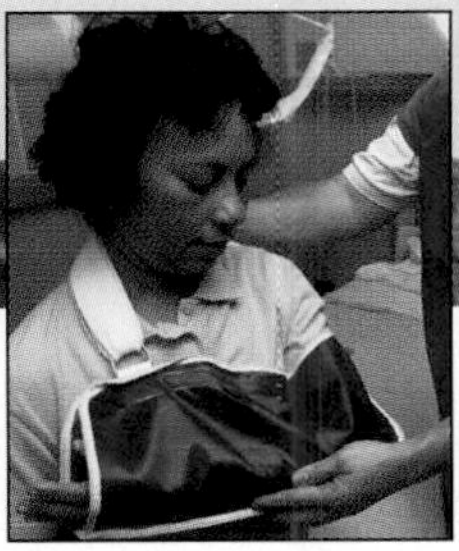

Clients with an Amputation

Nursing Process Data

***ASSESSMENT* Data Base**

Determine whether amputation was therapeutic or traumatic.

Determine rationale for therapeutic amputation (tumor, peripheral vascular disease, diabetes).

Assess status of stump wound.

Assess stump positioning.

Inspect stump for presence of edema.

Assess for phantom sensation or phantom pain.

Assess client's acceptance of amputation.

***PLANNING* Objectives**

To promote wound healing

To reduce edema and discomfort

To prevent contracture development

To mold and prepare stump for prosthesis use

To assist the client in acceptance and self care

***IMPLEMENTATION* Procedures**

Positioning and Exercising the Stump

Shrinking/Molding the Stump

***EVALUATION* Expected Outcomes**

Stump wound heals without complication.

Stump maintains functional alignment.

Stump is prepared for prosthesis use.

Client demonstrates appropriate stump care.

POSITIONING AND EXERCISING THE STUMP

Equipment

Pillows

Preparation

1. Check chart for physician's orders.
2. Identify client and explain purpose of positioning and exercising.
3. Provide privacy.
4. Wash your hands.

Procedure

for Preoperative Care

1. Evaluate nutritional status and request nutritional consult if indicated. **Rationale:** Adequate protein is necessary to promote wound healing.
2. Recruit assistance of OT, PT, physiatrist, psychiatrist (many clients are depressed or in denial about the amputation) and social worker for early multidisciplinary care planning.
3. Explain importance of exercises to client. Tell client that because flexor muscles are stronger than extensors, stump will be permanently flexed and abducted unless the client practices range-of-motion exercises. **Rationale:** Range-of-motion exercises increase muscle strength and improve mobility of amputated extremity.
4. If ordered, teach client quadriceps-setting exercises with a below-the-knee amputation.
   a. Extend leg and try to push back of knee into bed; try to move patella proximally.
   b. Contract quadriceps and hold contraction for 10 seconds.

> **CLINICAL ALERT**
>
> Adequate pain management in the preoperative period can reduce the occurrence of phantom limb pain postoperatively.

   c. Repeat this procedure four or five times.
   d. Repeat the exercise at least four times a day.
5. Teach use of ambulatory aids. **Rationale:** Prepares client for post-surgery mobility.
6. Explain phantom limb sensation; the client may continue to "feel" the lost limb post surgery.
7. Counsel families for they also mourn the loss of a visible body part. **Rationale:** They too need psychological support and education about rehabilitation and necessary skills for self care.

for Postoperative Care

1. Monitor for complications: hemorrhage, infection, unrelieved pain, wound that will not heal.
2. Assess for excessive wound drainage. Keep tourniquet at bedside. **Rationale:** If excessive bleeding occurs, tourniquet must be applied, as hemorrhage is a potentially life-threatening complication.
3. Administer ordered pain medication and continually assess to determine if pain is controlled.
4. Do not place stump on pillow, but elevate foot of bed for first 24 hours ONLY to reduce stump edema and pain. **Rationale:** Elevation on a pillow can promote flexion contracture of stump.
5. Turn client to prone or supine position for at least 1 hour every 4 hours. **Rationale:** This promotes stump extension and helps counteract possible flexion contracture formation.
6. Avoid dependent positioning of stump. **Rationale:** To prevent edema and discomfort. Edema may be present for up to four months after amputation.
7. While washing the stump, tap and massage the stump skin toward the incision line. **Rationale:** To prevent development of painful adhesions.
8. Teach stump extension exercises.
   a. Lie in a prone position with foot hanging over the end of the bed.
   b. Keep stump next to intact leg to extend stump and to contract gluteal muscles.
   c. Hold the contraction for 10 seconds.
   d. Repeat this exercise at least four times a day.
9. Teach adduction exercise.
   a. Place a pillow between the client's thighs.
   b. Squeeze the pillow for 10 seconds and then relax for 10 seconds.
   c. Repeat this exercise at least four times a day.

> **CLINICAL ALERT**
>
> Keep a tourniquet nearby in the event of excessive stump incision bleeding.

10. Have the client keep track of time spent with the stump flexed and then spend an equal amount of time with the stump extended.
11. Encourage appropriate use of trapeze: Use both hands to pull up with trapeze; place foot flat on mattress to lift body. Do not use heel to push in the mattress. **Rationale:** Pushing with the heel can lead to pressure ulcers.
12. After stump incision heals, have client begin to bear weight on stump, initially pressing into padded surface (pillow on chair seat). **Rationale:** To reduce pain and help prepare the stump for prosthesis.

SHRINKING/MOLDING THE STUMP

Equipment

Two elastic bandages: 4 inches for BKA, 6 inches for AKA (if soft dressings are used)
Tape or safety pins
Commercial stump shrinker (sheath)

Preparation

1. Review client's chart to determine date and type of amputation.
2. Gather equipment.
3. Identify client and explain rationale for procedure.
4. Wash hands.
5. Provide privacy.

Procedure

1. Wash stump with soap and water and allow to dry for at least 10 minutes before bandaging. Do not use lotions, powders, or alcohol.
2. Inspect and encourage client to assess stump for circulatory status, pressure areas, wound healing, and edema.

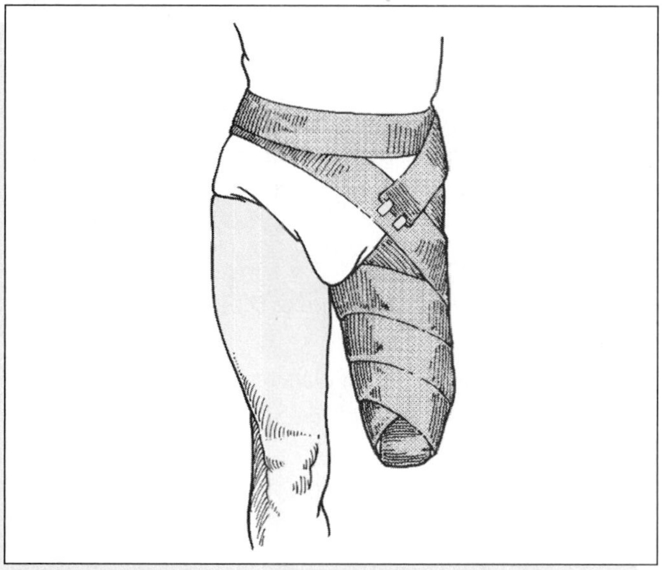

Compression bandage is used following amputation to mold stump in preparation for prosthesis.

3. Explain that purpose of wrap is to form a conical AKA stump to prepare for prosthesis use.
4. Explain that wrap is to be worn at all times except during bathing or when wearing a prosthesis.
5. Start by placing bandage end outer surface on distal stump. **Rationale:** The pressure gradient of the bandage should be greatest at the distal stump.
6. Wrap bandage medially and diagonally around stump. Have client assist by holding turns. Stretch bandages to two-thirds of the limit of the elastic.
7. Continue to wrap smoothly up the stump with medially directed spirals or figure eight turns (not circular). Progress up the stump and well into groin area. **Rationale:** Circular turns constrict circulation. Medial turns help correct stump tendency towards abduction.
8. Finish bandaging with a "spica" turn over and around the client's pelvis, then back down to stump. **Rationale:** Large "spica" turn prevents bandage slipping.
9. Secure the bandage with tape or (*cautiously*) with safety pins. Do not use bandage clips. **Rationale:** Clips can pierce the skin, or easily come loose.
10. Reapply elastic bandage every 4–6 hours, or when loose. **Rationale:** It must never be in place for more than 12 hours without being rewrapped.
11. If client has a stump "shrinker sheath," roll down and stretch the sheath using plastic ring. Fit onto stump end and apply, making sure there are no wrinkles.

CLINICAL ALERT

Amputees use more energy in ambulation than nonamputees. The elderly with an AKA must put forth an effort 100% above normal to walk at a slow rate. The longer the residual limb, the less energy the client must expend for ambulation.

12. Teach client home care of residual limb and prosthesis (washing; assessing for redness, pressure points, irritation, swelling, skin breakdown; socket, stump, socks, liners, mechanical parts, etc.).

DOCUMENTATION FOR CLIENTS WITH AN AMPUTATION

- Time, type, and site of bandage application
- Stump positioning
- Stump and wound assessment
- Exercises performed
- Client teaching
- Client's response to stump and participation in self-care

Critical Thinking Application

UNEXPECTED PROBLEMS	CRITICAL THINKING OPTIONS
Stump edema continues in spite of compression bandage application.	• Intermittently elevate foot of bed to promote venous return and decrease edema. • Assess for possible complication (venous thrombosis). • Evaluate wrapping procedure. Ensure bandages are properly applied with pressure greater at distal stump. • Instruct client to avoid prolonged dependent positioning of stump. • Investigate application of a compression sheath.
Client expresses fear of losing other leg.	• Teach client to care for the remaining extremity. • Inspect for lesions, wash and dry daily, use lotion for dry skin (not between toes), keep nails trimmed straight across, avoid mechanical, chemical, or thermal injury, wear shoes that are wide and deep enough for toes. • Avoid smoking and exercise daily. • Consult podiatrist for individual foot care or shoe orthotic adaptations, especially if diabetic. • Consult physician for management of diabetes or atherosclerosis.

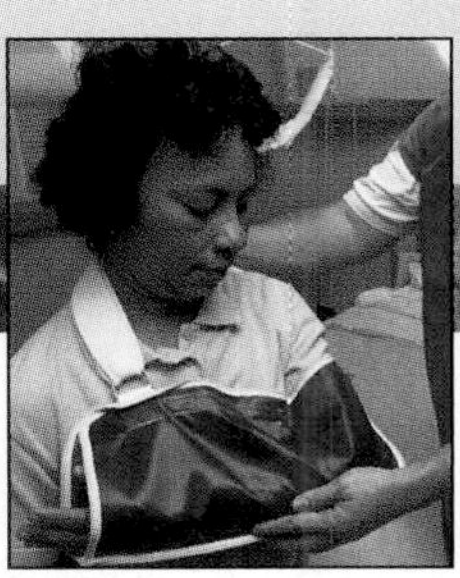

Client with Joint Replacement

Nursing Process Data

ASSESSMENT Data Base

Determine type of joint replacement performed.

Determine if client has had elective surgery with preoperative preparation.

Review client's understanding of protective and preventive self-care measures.

Assess client's progress with clinical path (pain management, activity, client's understanding of expected progress toward discharge).

Assess that leg position is abducted with pillows or splint.

Determine if client uses assistive devices appropriately.

PLANNING Objectives

To assist the client to progress with self-care following elective joint replacement surgery

To promote activities that prevent hip dislocation

To determine that client understands joint motions that could cause joint dislocation

To encourage use of safety and assistive devices in performing activities of daily living

IMPLEMENTATION Procedures

Caring for a Client with Hip Arthroplasty
- *for Bed Positioning*
- *for Strengthening Exercises*
- *for Mobility and Dislocation Prevention*
- *for Assistive Devices and Adaptive Aids*

Caring for a Client with Knee Arthroplasty
- *for Bed Positioning*
- *for Strengthening Exercises*
- *for Getting Out of Bed*

EVALUATION Expected Outcomes

Client actively participates in elective arthroplasty experience.

Client describes positions and activities to avoid in order to prevent hip dislocation.

Client demonstrates safe positioning.

Client performs activities of daily living using adaptive aids.

Complications (infection, dislocation) do not occur.

Client reports pain relief and enhanced joint mobility following joint replacement.

CARING FOR A CLIENT WITH HIP ARTHROPLASTY

Equipment

Abductor pillow ("wedge") or pillows
Non-rotation boot (if ordered)
Bath blanket
Poster reminder for exercises
Walker
Toilet seat extender
Adaptive aids

Preparation

1. Identify client and assess client's understanding of postoperative expectations.
2. Review "clinical path" with client each day.
3. Determine what instructions client has received. **Rationale:** To reinforce and not contradict previous teaching. The client may be included in an acute care group exercise program.

Procedure

for Bed Positioning

1. Maintain body in alignment using abductor pillow or wedge. **Rationale:** The abductor keeps legs in abduction and external rotation to prevent dislocation of the prosthesis.
   a. Place narrow end of wedge between the thighs, above the knees, as high as possible.
   b. Place legs flush with sides of wedge and strap into place above the knee, and above the ankle. **Rationale:** Avoid pressure over joints where nerves and vessels are superficial.
   c. If abductor has separate leg straps, the *unoperated* side may be loosened for comfort and to allow range of motion while client is supine.
2. Place rolled soft blanket or towel under ankles to free heels from the mattress. **Rationale:** To prevent skin breakdown.
3. Turn client every two hours, keeping legs abducted with both legs strapped. *While not generally contraindicated, review surgeon's orders before turning client to operated side.*

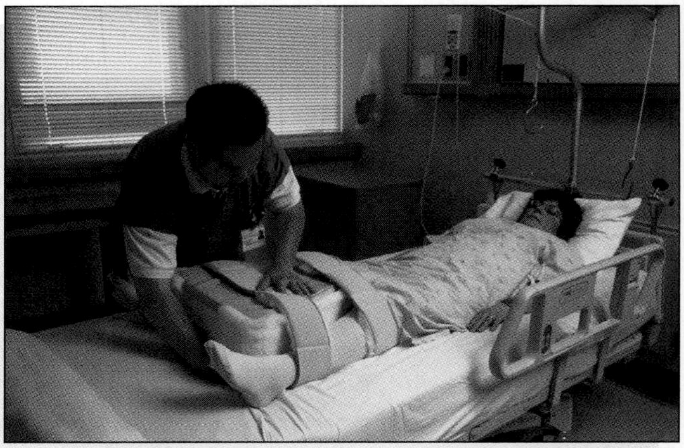
The abductor wedge, or pillows, prevent adduction and internal rotation of the hip.

4. Maintain anti-rotation boot (if indicated) while client is supine, but remove when client is turned. **Rationale:** This boot with bar prevents hip rotation.
5. Encourage standard postoperative preventive measures such as deep breathing, foot pumps, and ankle rotations.
6. Assess CMS and skin integrity at least q4h.

for Strengthening Exercises

1. Place an exercise reminder sign at foot of bed. Have client hold muscle contraction for a count of 5 and repeat 10 times, then increase hold and number of repetitions each day (may do during commercials if watching TV).
2. Quadricep strengthening:
   Have client push back of the knee into bed. **Rationale:** This contracts muscle on top of the thigh. The quadriceps muscle is used to rise to a standing position, to climb stairs, and to walk.
3. Gluteal strengthening:
   a. Have client squeeze buttocks together tightly and hold for a count of 5 and repeat 10 times. **Rationale:** These exercises help strengthen muscles surrounding the hip.

EVIDENCE BASED NURSING PRACTICE

Education for Joint Replacement Patients

This study found that solely providing a preoperative education program is insufficient to ensure performance of postoperative behaviors in total joint replacement patients. Patients with low levels of self-efficacy belief are less likely to perform preventive postoperative behaviors.

Source: Moon, L., & Backer, J. (2000). Relationships among self-efficacy, outcome expectancy, and postoperative behaviors in total joint replacement patients. *Orthopaedic Nursing, 19*(2), 77–85.

b. While standing, move operated leg backward, placing one hand on lower back to prevent arching, then return leg to starting position.
c. While standing, move operated leg laterally (out to the side), keeping foot and knee pointing straight forward, then return to starting position.

CLINICAL ALERT

Hip prosthesis dislocation usually requires a simultaneous combination of contraindicated hip positions, such as crossing the legs and acutely flexing at the same time. Dislocation precautions are continued until the joint capsule has healed. Only the orthopedic surgeon should advise clients when and if precautions are no longer necessary.

for Mobility and Dislocation Prevention

1. Assist client to get out of bed. *Note: A physical therapist usually supervises and assists with the first time out of bed.*
   a. Raise bed to high position. **Rationale:** This allows client to exit bed without acute hip flexion.
   b. Elevate head of bed and instruct client to exit bed from unoperated side. **Rationale:** The stronger side should lead a transfer.
   c. Have client pivot on hips, while keeping legs abducted, and sit on edge of bed with operated leg out in front. Do not allow client to bend forward and push down to stand. **Rationale:** Bending forward may cause prosthesis dislocation.
   d. Assist client by supporting operative leg.
   e. Have client push down with hands on mattress to rise to a standing position. Walker should not be used for support when rising to a standing position.
   f. Walk client first postoperative day (as ordered) with an assistant and a walker with weight bearing as tolerated.
2. Instruct client about positions to avoid.
   a. Do not cross the legs at ankle or knee. Keep knees apart at all times. **Rationale:** Adduction can cause prosthesis dislocation.
   b. Do not stand with toes turned in. **Rationale:** Internal rotation can cause prosthesis dislocation.
   c. Do not flex hips greater than 90°. Always sit with knees lower than hips. Avoid low chairs and do not bend over. Use toilet seat extender (elevator). **Rationale:** Flexion beyond 90° can cause prosthesis dislocation.
   d. Do not sit in bathtub. Use a standing shower or shower/tub chair.
   e. When standing and turning is necessary, turn toward unoperated side. **Rationale:** Turning toward operated hip can cause hip dislocation due to internal rotation.

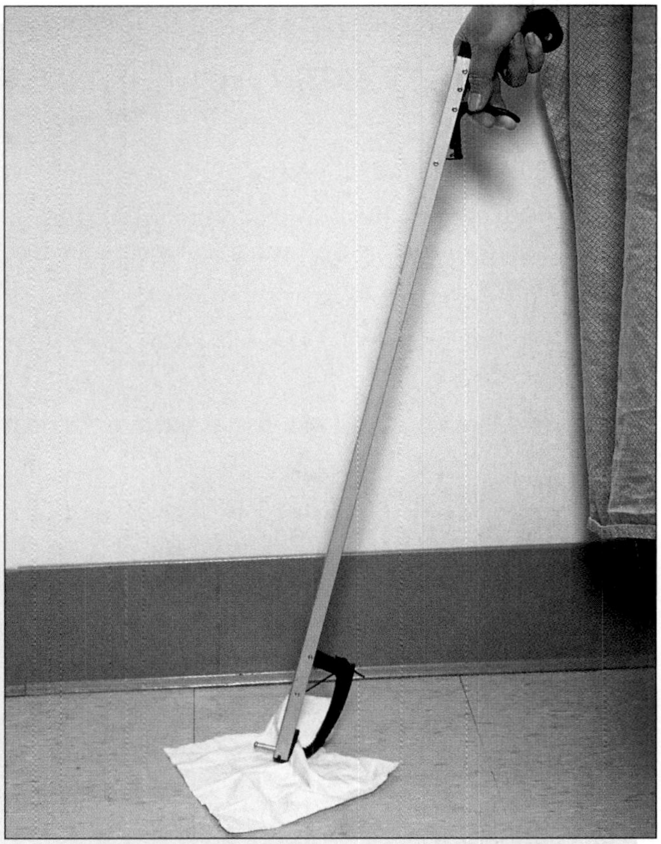

Adaptive aids, such as a reacher, facilitate independence in ADLs.

CLINICAL ALERT

The client undergoing hemiarthroplasty (replacement of the femoral head and neck) for fracture of the femur must adhere to the same precautions as the elective client to prevent prosthesis dislocation. The fracture client has not had the advantage of preoperative preparation and may not enjoy the physical health that is more typical of the elective arthroplasty client.

for Assistive Devices and Adaptive Aids

1. Consult physical therapy to obtain a walker, client instruction, and supervised ambulation.
2. Consult occupational therapy for provision and instruction in use of adaptive aids such as toilet seat extender, reachers, sock aid, long handled sponge, and shoehorn.
3. Discuss home safety adaptations which client may have already installed in preparation for *elective* surgery (pillows to elevate chair seats, shower or tub chair, safety rails, removal of loose rugs and electrical cords, placement of frequently used items within easy reach).

EVIDENCE BASED NURSING PRACTICE

Older Clients at Increased Risk

Because of changes in the skin that occur with aging, older clients are at increased risk for blistering and accidental removal of the epidermis by mechanical means such as tape removal. Tape should be applied vertically only, and without tension.

Source: Blaylock, B., et al., (1995). Tape injury in the patient with total hip replacement. *Orthopaedic Nursing, 14*(3), 25–27.

CARING FOR A CLIENT WITH KNEE ARTHROPLASTY

Equipment

Knee splint immobilizer
CPM device or rocking glider chair

Preparation

See previous skill.

Procedure

for Bed Positioning

1. Assist client to comfortable position. Client may turn from side to side and may have head of bed up or down. There is little risk of dislocation of knee prosthesis.
2. Place pillows lengthwise under lower leg, but not under knee.
3. Apply soft foam knee immobilizer or brace (if ordered).
   a. Place wide strap over knee.
   b. Allow client to direct tightness of fit. If soiling occurs, replace splint with a new one (client will take splint home).
   c. If a hinged splint (Bledsoe) is ordered, do not open, adjust, or remove without a physician's order.
   d. Assess CMS and skin integrity at least q4h.

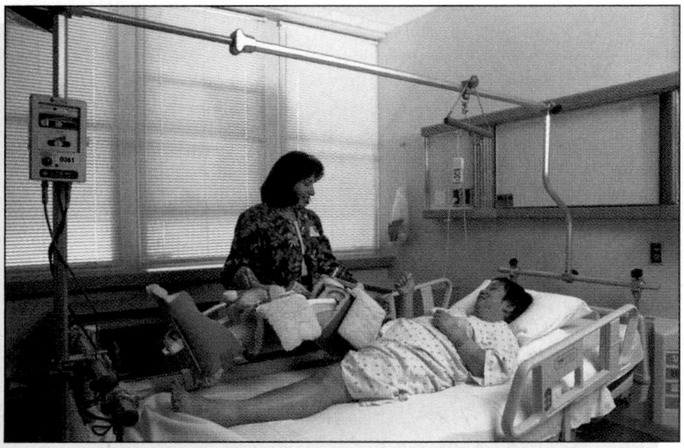

CPM (continuous passive motion) device increases joint mobility following knee surgery.

for Strengthening Exercises

1. Maintain accurate positioning of continuous *passive* motion device, if ordered, to gently flex knee by adjusted increments. Settings start at 10°–30°, and are gradually increased until 90° of flexion is achieved. **Rationale:** CPM prevents adhesion formation and improves range of joint motion during healing.
2. Alternate: Client may use a rocking glider chair. **Rationale:** This encourages independent *active knee flexion and extension,* which has added benefit of improving venous return, reducing edema, and preventing clot formation.
3. Encourage foot pumps, straight leg raising, ankle rotations, quadriceps, and gluteal sets as for client with a total hip replacement.

CLINICAL ALERT

There may be an increase in wound bleeding when initiating knee flexion exercises.

CLINICAL ALERT

Infection is a grave complication with joint replacement surgery. It may occur during the first three months postoperatively, or even after a year. Late infection is usually due to hematogenous spread from a distant site (teeth, GI, or urinary tract).

Clients should remind their physicians and dentists about their prosthesis; antibiotics are usually prescribed before any dental work or other invasive procedure to prevent infection.

for Getting Out of Bed

1. Assist client to pivot and sit on side of the bed, supporting the leg.
2. Unless brace is worn, encourage client to alternate bending and straightening the knee.
3. Weight bearing as tolerated with an assistant and use of a walker is usually allowed first postoperative day.
4. A raised seat will assist client to get in and out of a chair.

DOCUMENTATION FOR CLIENT WITH JOINT REPLACEMENT

- Wound assessment findings
- Character and amount of wound drainage
- Client positioning and frequency of turning
- Neurovascular and skin status of involved extremity
- Placement of abductor splint or brace
- Use of continuous passive motion or rocking glider chair
- Exercises performed: type, duration, and client's tolerance
- Client and family teaching and teaching aids provided
- Client's reflection of understanding of teaching (return demonstration of preventive measures)
- Transfer and ambulation skill
- Use of assistive devices
- Use of adaptive aids

Critical Thinking Application

UNEXPECTED OUTCOMES	CRITICAL THINKING OPTIONS
Client with knee arthroplasty is fearful of dislocation.	• Assure client that, in contrast to hip arthroplasty, knee dislocation rarely occurs. • Encourage client to continue quadriceps setting exercises. • Suggest that client discontinue use of brace as confidence builds. • Suggest use of a cane to relieve weight on knee.
Client with hip arthroplasty asks about adapting ADLs to accommodate hip precautions.	• Suggest purchasing a raised toilet seat before leaving hospital (many places sell these). • Use a standing shower or tub or shower chair for bathing. • Wear lace-up shoes with elastic laces so tying is not required and the foot can be slipped in with a long-handled shoe horn. • Purchase reachers or long barbecue tongs to retrieve things from the floor. • Place frequently used items at arm level so bending down is not required. • Remove scatter rugs, electric cords, and small objects from the floor. • Move car seat back as far as possible, keep operated leg out in front, back into seat, then semi-recline and pivot to face front of car.

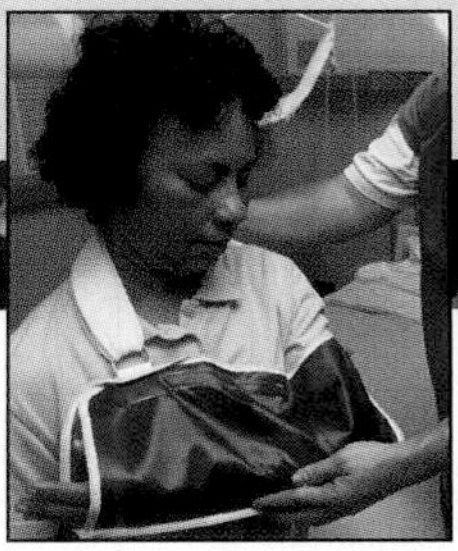

Stryker Frame

Nursing Process Data

ASSESSMENT **Data Base**
Determine client's musculoskeletal and neurologic status.
Evaluate client's understanding of turning procedure.
Assess client alignment and security of device.
Evaluate client's ability to assist with turning.

PLANNING **Objectives**
To turn client horizontally from supine to prone to supine positions
To provide optimal skin care for immobilized clients
To prevent pressure areas and pressure ulcers
To provide optimal nursing care to clients with skin grafts or other conditions that require minimum client movement

IMPLEMENTATION **Procedures**
Using a Stryker Wedge Turning Frame
Turning from Supine to Prone
Using a Stryker Parallel Frame
Assisting Client with Bedpan

EVALUATION **Expected Outcomes**
Client turns horizontally without torsion or abnormal flexion/extension of the spine.
Client receives optimal skin care without developing pressure ulcers.
Client receives optimal nursing care for skin grafts or neurologic condition.

USING A STRYKER WEDGE TURNING FRAME

Equipment

Stryker wedge turning frame
Armrests and footboard
Software: mattress, canvases, linen, straps
Safety straps
Pillows and sheepskin (if used)

Procedure

1. Explain procedure to client.
2. Show client the Stryker frame before placing on the frame.
3. Position the posterior frame at the bottom of the turning circle.
4. Place client supine on the posterior frame (using the three-man carry transfer method, if necessary).
5. If client is on a backboard, place client and board on the posterior frame.
6. Attach the anterior frame.
7. Turn client and remove the backboard.
8. Reverse the procedure, and turn client to his or her back.

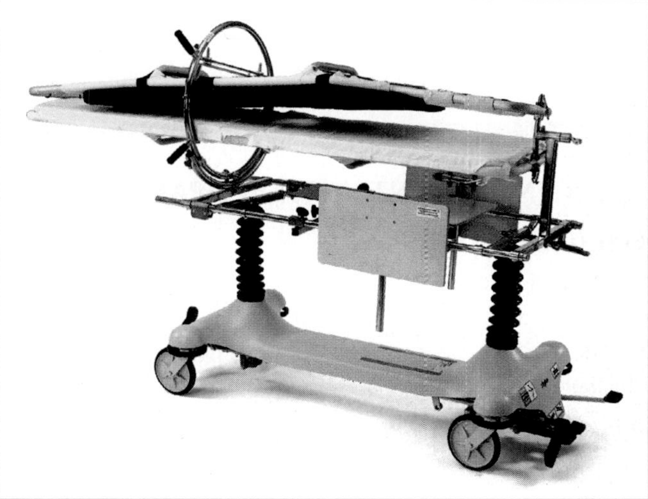

Stryker wedge turning frame.

Note: The Stryker frame has been infrequently used for the past 10 years. However, due to increased numbers of spinal instrumentation procedures, the new Stryker wedge turning frame is again being used following surgery.

TURNING FROM SUPINE TO PRONE

Procedure

1. Explain procedure to client. This procedure requires only one person; however, it is advisable to have two people when possible.
2. Position sheepskin, pillows, or comfort aids on top of client.
3. With client on posterior frame, open the turning circle and put head end of anterior frame on the securing bolt and fasten it with the nut.
4. Fasten the foot end of the anterior frame with the nut, making sure that client's legs and feet are correctly positioned.
5. Have client clasp hands around anterior frame. If client is unable to do this, put a safety strap around the whole frame at elbow level to keep arms contained.
6. Close the turning circle until it locks.
7. Move the armrests down out of the way of the turn.
8. Pull out the bed-turning lock.
9. Turn the frame toward the client's right until it locks automatically. The narrow side of the wedge (at the client's right) always turns down. The frame automatically locks when the bottom frame is horizontal.
10. Open the turning circle, unscrew the nuts, and remove the upper posterior frame. Relock the turning circle for safety.
11. To turn the client on the Stryker wedge from prone to supine, reverse procedure for turning from supine to prone. Remember that the narrow side of the wedge (on client's right) always turns down so client cannot slip out.

USING A STRYKER PARALLEL FRAME

Equipment

Stryker parallel frame
Armrests and footboard
Software: mattress, canvases, linen, straps
Safety straps
Pillows and sheepskins

Procedure

1. Place a pillow lengthwise over the client's legs to prevent moving during turning.
2. Attach the anterior frame to the main frame using the two nuts on the turning circle. Make sure the client is held firmly between the frames.

3. Put three safety straps around the frame at level of knees, waist, and elbows. Tighten securely.
4. With a person at each end of the frame, pull out the locking pins at the center of each end, turn the frame slightly to hold the lock open, and then quickly finish turning the client. The bed automatically locks when the bottom frame is horizontal.
5. Remove the top frame, and reposition the client for comfort.

ASSISTING CLIENT WITH BEDPAN

Equipment

Special bedpan
Plastic drape
Towels
Clean gloves

Procedure

1. Explain procedure to client.
2. Place client in a supine position.
3. Don clean gloves.
4. Drop the center section of the posterior frame by releasing the hooks or rubber bands from the sides of the frame.
5. Protect the linen by putting plastic or towels around the edges.
6. Insert the bedpan into the opening and hold securely with hands or with the arm supports.
7. Remove the bedpan, clean the client, and reattach the center section of the frame.
8. Clean bedpan, and replace in storage area.
9. Remove gloves and discard.
10. Wash your hands.

DOCUMENTATION FOR STRYKER FRAME

- Time and frequency of turning
- How client tolerates turning procedure
- Neuro assessment findings
- Neurovascular status
- Status of the traction apparatus, if indicated
- Vital signs
- Skin assessment

Critical Thinking Application

UNEXPECTED OUTCOMES	CRITICAL THINKING OPTIONS
The client expresses fear of being turned.	• Encourage client to be on frame and be turned before surgery. • Explain each step of the turning process and the use of each piece of equipment. • Allow client to express fears and concerns. • Carefully answer all questions in a way that the client can understand.
The client experiences unusual pain or discomfort when turned.	• Have the client describe details of pain. • Assess the client's neurologic status, and compare it with the client's status before turning. • Ensure that the traction apparatus is intact. • Notify physician if pain persists or if there is a change in neurologic status.

GERONTOLOGIC CONSIDERATIONS

Musculoskeletal integrity can be enhanced and therapeutic goals reached if the aging effect on the musculoskeletal system is appreciated and incorporated into individualized care planning.

Elderly clients generally experience:

- Decreased height
- More brittle bones, decreased density
- Reduced muscle mass
- Diminished strength
- Joint stiffening
- Weakness and slowed movement
- Thinning of the dermis and structures supporting the junction of the epidermis and dermis weaken. Older clients are at increased risk for blistering and epidermal stripping.
- Slower and less effective healing which may result in greater incidence of malunion and nonunion after fracture.

Elderly clients are at high risk for falls and musculoskeletal injury as a result of:

- Weakness and being easily fatigued
- Unsteady balance, gait, and alterations in posture
- Poor eyesight
- Altered mobility resulting from medications or use of assistive device
- Increased time on bed rest, leading to muscle weakness
- Presence of chronic disease

Active elderly clients may seek joint replacement surgery to:

- Decrease pain
- Increase mobility
- Continue an active life

MANAGEMENT GUIDELINES

Each state legislates a Nurse Practice Act for RNs and LVN/LPNs. Health care facilities are responsible for establishing and implementing policies and procedures that conform to their state's regulations. Verify the regulations and role parameters for each health care worker in your facility.

Delegation of Responsibilities

- All health care workers can be assigned to clients with orthopedic conditions for nursing tasks associated with activities of daily living. Occupational and Physical Therapists are assigned to the more complex tasks of ambulating and teaching clients with hip replacements, clients requiring assistive devices to ambulate, etc.
- Some facilities employ orthopedic technicians who set up and monitor traction, assist with cast application, bivalve or removal and help with transfer.

Information Flow

- The RN needs to assess the skill level of all staff assigned to clients requiring assistive devices or special equipment. Documentation of the skill level for the staff should be available on the unit. This is a major safety factor for all staff assigned to orthopedic clients.
- When new equipment is purchased, and before it is put into service, the manufacturer should provide inservice education to all staff to prevent damage to the equipment and promote safety in client care.
- Most orthopedic clients are followed by a multidisciplinary care team, which includes physicians, nurses, physical and occupational therapists, and social workers. The team use the client's DRG related "clinical path" as an action plan for coordinating hospital, discharge, and subacute setting or home care services. Variances can be identified as the client moves through the sequences of specific interventions that promote timely discharge. Such collaboration requires open and ongoing communication among all members of the team. Special documentation forms may be used to facilitate this process.
- The nurse "Patient Care Coordinator" oversees the client's progress and brings multidisciplinary issues

to the physician's attention so that the "path" can be individualized to reflect the client's unique needs.

- Assistive personnel (aides, orthopedic technicians) must be informed of any restriction in client positioning or mobility. They should report any noted changes in the client's condition or problem with any immobilizing device or equipment to the RN so that further assessment and problem solving can be conducted.
- On-coming staff should receive information about the client's progress toward satisfaction of expected outcomes, any unexpected variance that impedes the client's progress toward discharge, and any change in the medical plan of care.

CRITICAL THINKING STRATEGIES

SCENARIO 1

Your orthopedic unit has just admitted an 84-year-old female, Nora James. She was brought to the ED following a fall in the grocery store. Her admitting diagnosis is "intertrochanteric fracture of the left hip." She is scheduled for hip "nailing" surgery as soon as she is cleared by her primary physician, cardiologist, and anesthesiologist.

1. What behaviors would you expect to see upon initial assessment of Miss James?
2. What are the priorities of care in the preoperative period?
3. How will this client's care plan differ from that of the client with hemiarthroplasty replacement of the femoral head and neck?

SCENARIO 2

Mrs. Jacobson, a 73-year-old retired school teacher has been admitted to the hospital for a right total hip replacement as a result of osteoarthritis. She has been very active her entire life, playing golf three times a week, bowling on a team, hiking, and gardening. She is very concerned that she will be unable to continue with these activities if she doesn't have surgery. Her lab work was completed before her admission. She did give 2 units of autologous blood in case she needs it for surgery. Her vital signs are: BP 148/80, P 88, R 26. She uses a cane, which she says is "for balance."

1. Identify the priority preoperative intervention for Mrs. Jacobson. Provide a rationale for your choice.
2. Develop a client care plan: identify short- and long-term goals, state three nursing diagnoses in priority order and provide the rationale for your choices. Describe at least two priority nursing interventions for each nursing diagnosis.
3. Identify two safety issues related to Mrs. Jacobson's care.
4. Describe at least three procedures that need to be discussed prior to her discharge.

CHAPTER 31

Perioperative Care

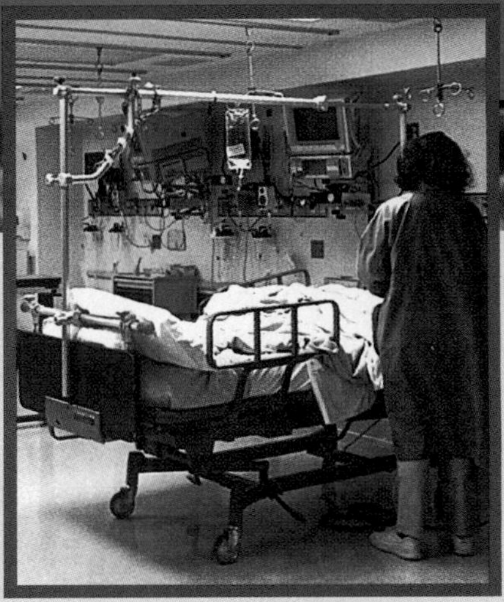

THEORETICAL CONCEPTS

UNIT ONE: Stress in Preoperative Clients 1145
- Preventing Anxiety and Stress 1146
- Reducing Anxiety and Stress 1146
- Assisting the Client Who Uses Denial 1147

UNIT TWO: Preoperative Teaching 1148
- Providing Surgical Information 1149
  - *for the Preoperative Client in the Hospital 1149*
  - *for the Preoperative Client in an Outpatient Setting 1149*
  - *for the Intraoperative Client 1149*
  - *for the Postoperative Client 1150*
- Providing Client Teaching 1150
- Providing Family Teaching 1150
- Teaching for Laser Therapy 1151
- Teaching for Lithotripsy 1152
- Teaching for Diagnostic Laparoscopy 1153
- Teaching for Arthroscopy 1154
- Instructing in Deep Breathing Exercises 1155
- Instructing in Coughing Exercises 1155
- Providing Instruction to Turn in Bed 1156
- Instructing in Leg Exercises 1156

UNIT THREE: Preoperative Care 1158
- Obtaining Baseline Data 1159
- Preparing the Surgical Site 1159
- Preparing the Client for Surgery 1161
- Administering Preoperative Medications 1164

UNIT FOUR: Conscious Sedation 1166
- Preparing Client for Conscious Sedation 1167
- Monitoring Client During Procedure 1168
- Caring for Client Following Conscious Sedation 1169

UNIT FIVE: Postanesthesia Unit Care (PACU) and Discharge 1171
- Providing Postanesthesia Care 1172
- Discharging Client from Postanesthesia Unit to Nursing Unit 1173
- Discharging Client from Phase II Unit to Home 1174

UNIT SIX: Postoperative Care 1176
- Providing Postoperative Care 1177
- Administering Postoperative Medications 1177

GERONTOLOGIC CONSIDERATIONS 1179

MANAGEMENT GUIDELINES 1180

CRITICAL THINKING STRATEGIES 1182

Cross Reference: Chapter 16, Pain Management

LEARNING OBJECTIVES

- Define the word *perioperative.*
- Discuss the nursing care focus in each of the three stages of the perioperative period.
- Identify at least three factors that influence the surgical client's degree of stress.
- Explain why postoperative complications are reduced by decreasing the stress level.
- Describe at least one potential problem and the suggested solution for clients demonstrating high stress levels in the preoperative period.
- State the primary purpose of providing preoperative care for clients.
- Discuss how preoperative teaching can reduce the surgical client's stress.
- Describe the information contained in the surgical permit.
- Outline the essential steps in physically preparing a client for surgery.
- Explain the purpose for administering the three classifications of drugs used for preoperative medications.
- Outline the essential postoperative nursing interventions completed in the surgical unit.
- Summarize the major categories of postoperative pain medications, and describe the general side effects of each category.
- Discuss at least three major postoperative complications and the nursing interventions to prevent and treat the complications.
- Discuss the differences in procedure when a client is discharged to home following outpatient surgery.

TERMINOLOGY

Adaptation: ability of an organism to adjust to a change in environment.

Analgesia: absence of the sense of pain.

Analgesic: a drug that relieves pain without altering the conscious state.

Anesthesia: partial or complete loss of sensation by administration of a drug or gas.

Anxiety: experiencing a sense of dread or fear without a known stimulus. A condition associated with physiologic changes.

Arthrogram: a diagnostic test involving use of dye, which is injected into a joint to visualize tears in ligaments and surrounding tissue.

Arthroscopy: surgical procedure used to visualize, diagnose, and treat problems inside a joint.

Asepsis: sterile; a condition free from germs.

Atelectasis: a collapsed or airless section of the lungs.

Bronchitis: inflammation of the bronchial mucous membrane.

Bronchoscopy: examination of the bronchi with a scope.

Contamination: the introduction of disease, germs, or infectious materials into or on normally sterile objects.

Dehydration: to deprive the body or tissues of water.

Diplopia: double vision.

Egophony: a nasal sound heard while auscultating the lungs of a person as he speaks; a sound heard in pleural effusion.

Emesis: vomiting.

Emphysema: a condition in which the alveoli of the lungs become distended or ruptured.

Enema: injection of water or fluid into rectum and colon to empty the lower intestine or to introduce medicine or food for therapeutic purposes.

Euphoria: an exaggerated feeling of well-being.

Exudate: accumulation of fluid in a cavity.

Hernia: the protrusion or projection of an organ or part of an organ through the wall of the cavity that normally contains it.

Hypertension: higher blood pressure than normal; usually above 140 mm Hg/90 mm Hg.

Hypnotic: drugs that cause insensibility to pain or partial to complete unconsciousness; includes sedatives, analgesics, anesthetics, and intoxicants.

Hypothermia: the state of low body temperature.

Hypovolemia: diminished intravascular volume.

Immunosuppressive: acting to suppress the body's natural immune response to an antigen.

Induction: the process of causing or producing; in anesthesia, the period from the initial inhalation or injection until optimum level of anesthesia is reached.

Intervention: the act of coming in or between so as to modify.

Laparoscopy: a procedure in which a scope is inserted through the umbilicus to detect problems inside the abdominal cavity.

Lethargy: a condition of sluggishness; stupor.

Magnetic resonance imaging (MRI): use of electromagnetic energy in radiography to provide soft tissue images, especially of the musculoskeletal and central nervous system.

Maladaptive: poorly adjusted; inability to adapt.

Mesentery: a peritoneal fold connecting the intestine with the postabdominal wall.

Narcotic: producing stupor or sleep; a drug that depresses the central nervous system.

Neurohormonal: concerning the interaction between nerves and hormones.

Orthopedic: concerning the prevention or correction of deformities of the musculoskeletal system.

Palpitation: rapid, violent, or throbbing pulsation, as an abnormally rapid, throbbing, or fluttering heart.

Perioperative: refers to the three phases of the surgical experience: preoperative, intraoperative, and postoperative.

Peritonitis: inflammation of the peritoneum.

Pneumonia: inflammation of the lungs caused primarily by bacteria, viruses, and chemical agents; can be characterized by chills, high fever, pain in the chest, cough, and purulent and often bloody sputum.

Stress: a mentally or emotionally disruptive or disquieting influence; distress.

Therapeutic: having medicinal or healing properties.

Thrombophlebitis: inflammation of a vein associated with thrombus.

Topical: pertinent to a particular area; local.

Trauma: a physical injury or wound caused by external force or violence; an emotional or psychologic shock that may produce disordered feelings or behavior.

Vasoconstriction: constriction of a blood vessel.

THE SURGICAL EXPERIENCE

Just a few years ago, the surgical experience involved three to ten days in a hospital setting. Now it is often a short hospital stay or an outpatient experience. Many procedures are now performed safely in an outpatient setting and may consist of a same day surgical procedure lasting a few hours. The short stay procedure involves an observation period during an overnight stay in the facility, usually less than 24 hours. In these situations, much of the postoperative period is managed at home. Depending on the protocol, if necessary a home health nurse may visit, or some outpatient facilities provide a postoperative follow-up visit by the nursing staff. In all cases where outpatient procedures are performed, the nurse does phone follow-up within the first one to three postoperative days.

Surgical procedures are classified as either emergency or elective procedures. Elective procedures can be scheduled in advance. This allows the client time to plan for child care arrangements, employment responsibilities, as well as preparing psychologically for the experience. Emergency procedures usually are a result of a life-threatening situation such as hemorrhage, obstruction, malignancy, or body system disruption. Procedures are also termed major or minor according to the degree of risk to the client. Major surgical procedures involve a risk of bleeding and loss of organs or bodily parts. Minor surgical procedures usually involve less risk of bleeding and fewer complications. Examples of these procedures include arthroscopic procedures of the knee, rhinoplasty, and eye surgeries.

Nurse's Role Nurses take an active role in the psychologic and physiologic preparation of the surgical client. Nurses instruct the preoperative client in stress-reduction techniques, explanations of the operating room experience, expectations for the postoperative period, and use of special postoperative equipment. In fact, many hospitals provide time for the operating room nurse to make postoperative visits to clients to assess the client's evaluation of the surgical intervention.

PERIOPERATIVE CARE

Perioperative Areas There are specific physical areas of the hospital where client care takes place during the operative experience.

Preoperative Area Preoperative care can take place in a holding area for invasive procedures and/or the preoperative area of the operating room. Care can also take place in a central testing area, an inpatient room, or clinic examination or treatment room.

Intraoperative Area This includes the operating room suite or a procedure room where invasive surgical procedures occur. The intraoperative area of the operating room suite includes the area surrounding the operating room and the actual operating room suite. Intraoperative care begins when the client enters the invasive procedure area or the operating room suite.

Postoperative area Care can commence in the operating room suite, the procedure room, a recovery room/postoperative area, a client room (ICU), or a treatment room. The postoperative care begins immediately after the completion of the surgical procedure.

Personnel working in these areas must adhere to regulations regarding appropriate attire with personal protective equipment identified for each specific area. Personnel must also follow standard precautions and are not permitted to work if they have open lesions on the hands or arms, eye infections, diarrhea, or respiratory infections.

Preoperative Stage The first stage of the perioperative period is the *preoperative stage*. During this stage, a health history, including identification of all allergies (including latex allergies), medical concerns in other systems, identification of side and site of procedure, a thorough physical assessment, and review of all laboratory tests ordered is completed. Some clients will require an ECG and/or chest x-ray as well. The registered nurse completes the operative check list and notifies the surgeon and anesthesiologist of any abnormal findings according to facility policy and procedures. Infections such as urinary tract infections must be treated before any surgical procedure is done. Some clients receive preoperative IV antibiotic therapy prior to surgery. The nurse must ensure that these orders have been completed before surgery.

Admission to the hospital or outpatient surgery facility and anticipation of surgery result in some degree of anxiety and stress. Stress is a physiologic and psychologic response to a stressor. Anxiety is one of the manifestations of stress. The degree of anxiety and stress depends on many factors:

- The client's likelihood of reacting to anticipated stressors with high anxiety.
- The number of stress-producing events that have occurred recently in the client's life or within the client's family.
- The client's perceptions of the hospitalization and surgical experience.
- The significance of the surgery to the client.
- The number of unknowns that confront the client on admission.
- The client's degree of self-esteem and self-image and perception of how surgery will impact body image.
- The client's belief system and religious conviction.

The body responds physiologically to an actual or perceived threat. The hypothalamus controls a neurohormonal response. The heart rate is increased, and the heart contracts more forcefully. Blood volume is redistributed by vasoconstriction of the vessels in the skin, stomach, mesentery, and kidneys. Increased blood volume increases cardiac output. Increased blood flow to the skeletal muscles results in the muscles becoming tensed for action. The bronchi dilate, and the increased respiratory rate increases oxygenation. Mechanisms that provide energy include increased glucose release and decreased insulin production.

Behavioral responses to stress or anxiety can be adaptive or maladaptive (Table 31–1). Adaptive behaviors are purposeful. The client adapts to a stressful situation by preparing to face it or by removing the threat. Maladaptive behaviors result from the inability to adapt to a stressful situation.

One of the objectives of providing preoperative care is to identify the level of stress present in the client. If nursing interventions can be planned that reduce high anxiety levels, the result is a safer intraoperative period. High levels of anxiety can prevent successful preoperative adaptation and can negatively influence postoperative recovery. Mild anxiety, on the other hand, increases alertness increases the ability to learn, and increases the ability to assess and to adjust to one's environment. Mild anxiety also increases the ability to adjust to several simultaneous stressors. In the preoperative client this level of anxiety is adaptive in nature, while a high level is maladaptive. When levels of anxiety or stress become intolerably high, defense mechanisms are unconsciously implemented to reduce the distress by concealing, falsifying, or distorting reality.

Preoperative anxiety is increased by ambiguity, conflicting perceptions, misconceptions, fears of the unknown, and bombardment by many simultaneous stressors. Ambiguity occurs from uncertainty or vagueness concerning the hospital environment, preoperative procedures, intraoperative procedures, or postoperative events.

Conflicting perceptions occur when preconceived notions about the operative experience are different from those actually encountered. The client who thought that a herniorrhaphy would be a quick, safe cure can become quite anxious after the anesthesiologist informs him or her of potential complications.

Misconceptions arise when inaccurate information is given, or accurate information is misinterpreted, when terminology is not understood, and when events are not explained clearly. A client who is scheduled for a bronchoscopy in the morning, and whose nurse silently places an N.P.O. sign over the bed, may believe that he is destined for the same hospital regimen as his roommate, who had a gastrectomy.

TABLE 31–1 Responses to Anxiety States

Low Anxiety	High Anxiety
Less likely to react with high anxiety to stressors	Likely to react with high anxiety to stressors
Few changes in personal situation in recent past	Many changes in personal situation in recent past
Perceives hospital and surgical experience as beneficial	Perceives hospital and surgical experience as threatening
Believes surgery will end chronic problem	Fears that surgery may lead to pain, disability, and possibly death
Regards admission procedures as friendly and supportive	Regards admission procedures as strange and frightening
Finds hospital conditions comfortable and the nursing staff supportive and informative	Finds hospital conditions unbearable and the nursing staff nonsupportive

TABLE 31–2 Managing Surgical Clients

Conscientious Preoperative Care of Clients Prevents Postoperative Complications	
• Preparing the client psychologically reduces the client's stress level and helps to prevent postoperative complications	• Completing the surgical scrub reduces microorganisms on the body surface and the possibility of wound infections postoperatively
• Teaching coughing and deep breathing exercises, procedures for getting out of bed, and uses of specialized equipment enhance the client's cooperation and prevents postoperative complications	
Scrupulous Asepsis Throughout the Perioperative Period Reduces Complications	
• Maintaining strict asepsis reduces cross-contamination	• Identifying breaks in sterile technique and taking appropriate action decrease the risk of postoperative complications

Stress responses are cumulative. An increasing number of stressors can eventually drain adaptive energy. The newly admitted surgical client who has been confronted with many stressors before admission is more likely to respond with a higher level of stress as each new stressor is encountered.

Preoperative teaching is essential for clients undergoing any surgical procedure. Research studies have repeatedly identified the positive outcomes of client teaching as decreased perception of pain, increased compliance with treatments, decreased postoperative complications, and decreased duration of hospitalization. Of course, fear and anxiety are greatly reduced when explanations are complete and time is allowed during the teaching session to answer questions by both the client and family. The client has the right to know what to expect during the surgical procedure and the postoperative period as set forth in The Client's Bill of Rights.

The teaching plan needs to include the preoperative preparation, time of surgery, and postoperative activities. A tour of the postoperative unit is also an important aspect of the teaching, particularly if they will be going to a critical care or special care unit. A demonstration of specific equipment such as incentive spirometery, PCA pumps, cardiac monitors, and immobilizers should be presented to increase compliance with the equipment postoperatively. Information regarding time of arrival to the hospital and fluid and food restrictions should be provided prior to the hospitalization, whether it be for outpatient or inpatient surgery.

Other areas covered in the preoperative stage are the type of anesthesia (usually described by the anesthesiologist), and the physical preparation of the client, which includes preoperative skin preparation, identifying the correct client in the operating room, and in some cases, the preoperative scrub. This may include the surgical cleansing prep and hair removal. If it must be completed in the intraoperative area, a method that controls aerosolization of hair and epithelium is utilized.

Intraoperative Stage

This stage includes the time the client arrives in the preinduction or holding room until he or she arrives in the recovery room. The client may well complain of being cold. The operating room is kept cool, so offering a warm blanket will make the client more comfortable. During the time the client is in the holding room, the nurse will identify the client, ask the client what procedure is going to be done, determine the side and site of the surgery, and complete an assessment. IVs and Foley catheters may be inserted in the holding room.

Once the client is moved to the operating room itself, the anesthesiologist prepares the client for and administers the anesthesia, while monitoring the client throughout the procedure. The operating room nurses, circulating and scrub, prepare the operating room and provide for client safety. Operating room technicians are used in many facilities in place of scrub nurses. An RN must be assigned to the operating room when an OR Technician is used as a member of the team. In this case, the OR nurse functions as the circulating nurse. The nurse assists in the preparation of the client, positions the client on the operating room table, and ensures that a grounding pad (if electrocautery is used) is securely attached to the client. The circulating nurse also assists the team in gowning for the procedure.

Conscious Sedation Conscious sedation is used for some surgical procedures and for invasive procedures or tests. Procedures once performed only in an operating room can now be safely done in outpatient settings and special procedures rooms. Conscious sedation is the administration of an IV sedative, opioid, or hypnotic drug that produces sedation, analgesia, and amnesia. Clients receiving conscious sedation can respond to commands and maintain their own airway. Clients under light sedation are able to maintain normal respiration, eye movements, and protective reflexes. They usually do not remember the procedure or even the environment. Following the use of conscious sedation, the client may

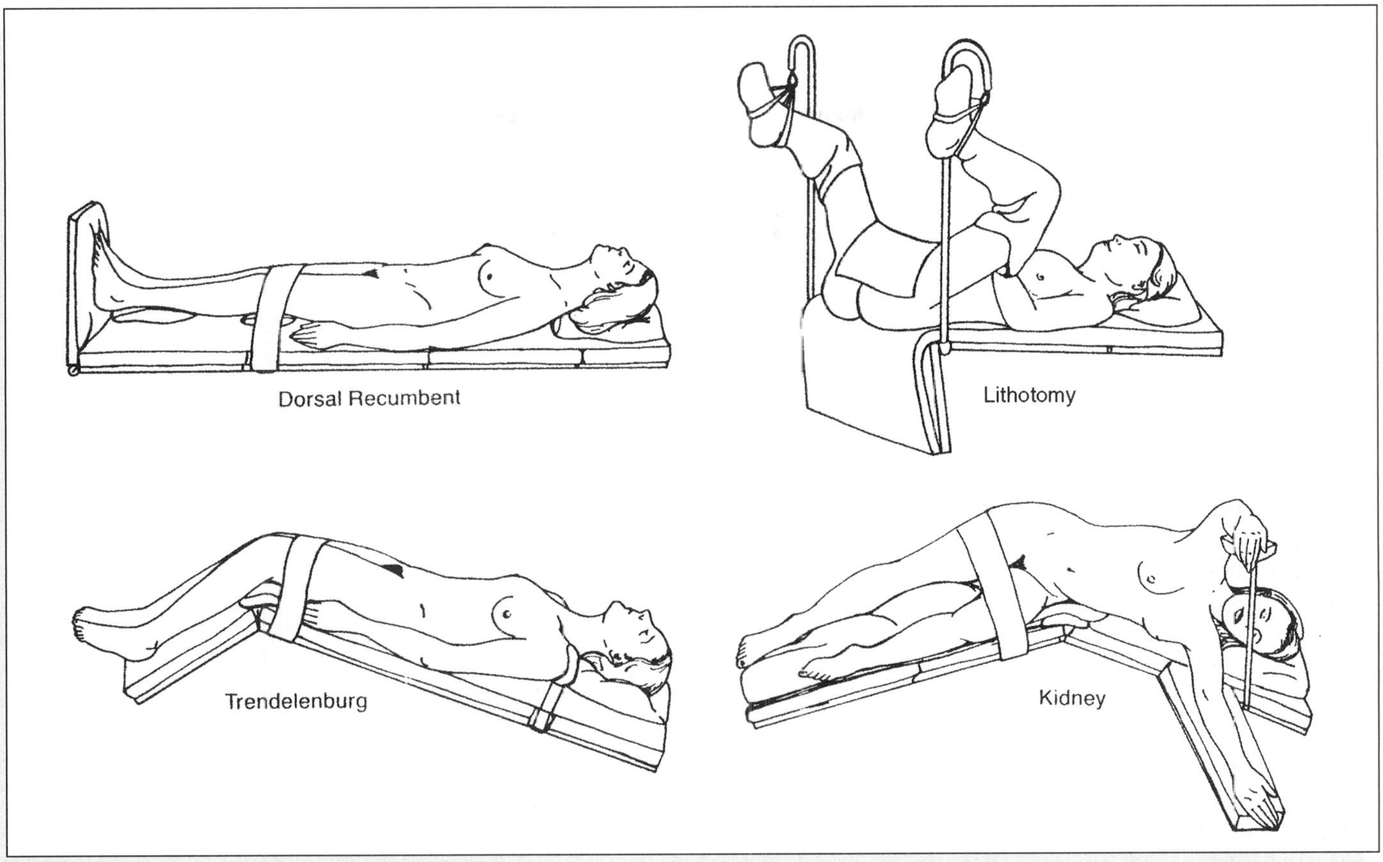

Positions commonly used for surgical procedures.

have slurred speech and nystagmus at the end point of the sedation.

Conscious sedation occurs on a continuum from the state of being alert to being in deep sedation. When the client is in a minimum sedation state, he or she can still be anxious. In deep sedation, the client is in a controlled state of depressed consciousness or unconsciousness and is not easily aroused and does not respond to command. Conscious sedation is considered to be safer than general anesthesia; however, there are risks involved with the use of conscious sedation. As the level of sedation increases, the risk of complications increases as well. Clients can become too deeply sedated and require intervention to maintain a patent airway and breathing. Unlike general anesthesia, conscious sedation allows clients to maintain a patent airway and respond appropriately to physical stimulation and verbal commands. Another benefit of conscious sedation includes a quicker return to baseline neurologic status.

A qualified anesthesia provider must give orders for administration of conscious sedation. Some states and institutional guidelines allow qualified registered nurses to administer sedating drugs. The American Nurses Association and other nursing organizations have written position papers relative to the practice of administering and monitoring clients undergoing conscious sedation. Nurses must be familiar with the state nurse practice act as well as the institutional policies regarding their role in this procedure. Nurses allowed to administer conscious sedation must meet additional criteria and demonstrate proficiency in the skill. The nurses are working under standard procedures in this situation. Nursing students are not allowed to administer conscious sedation or monitor clients while they are receiving conscious sedation.

During the entire procedure the safety of the client is the priority goal for the entire staff assigned to the procedure. All staff assist in monitoring the client, ensure that sterile technique is maintained throughout the procedure, and maintain accurate and complete documentation, including sponge and instrument counts. OSHA guidelines are followed by the staff to protect both the client and the staff from exposure to bloodborne pathogens.

Following the procedure the client is transferred to the postanesthesia room by the anesthesiologist and/or surgeon, and in some facilities the circulating nurse. A complete report of the client's status is provided to the postanesthesia staff.

Postoperative Stage The *postoperative stage* can be divided into three segments. The immediate postoperative period includes the care given to the client in the postanesthesia room and in the first few hours on the surgical floor. The intermediate period usually involves the care given during the course of surgical convalescence to the time of discharge. The third segment in the postoperative stage is discharge planning, teaching, and referral.

Besides nursing care, nursing management during the postoperative period centers on assessing the client's postoperative condition and monitoring for complications. It also includes client teaching, pain control, and psychologic support of both the client and family.

When the client is deemed stable, he or she is transferred to the nursing unit, critical care unit, and in the case of an outpatient client, to home. The nursing care provided in the postoperative period is well described in the chapter.

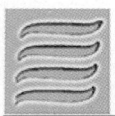

NURSING DIAGNOSES

The following nursing diagnoses are appropriate to include in a client care plan when the components are related to a surgical experience.

NURSING DIAGNOSIS	RELATED FACTORS
Anxiety	Actual or perceived threat to body image, ability to maintain independence, long-term effects of surgical procedure
Impaired Verbal Communication	Inability to speak or understand language, which may result in ineffective client education regarding surgical procedure
Delayed Surgical Recovery	Evidence of interrupted healing of surgical area; difficulty in ambulation, pain, fatigue
Fear	Unknown outcome of surgical procedure, pain, and discomfort from procedure
Ineffective Airway Clearance	Pulmonary secretions, allergic response, medications, suppressed cough reflex, decreased oxygen intake, pain, mechanical obstruction
Ineffective Denial	Impending surgery, diagnosis, and expected outcome
Ineffective Coping	Inadequate support system, change in body integrity, unrealistic expectations regarding surgical outcome, stress from surgery
Deficient Knowledge	Inadequate understanding of surgical procedure, language barrier, incomplete client teaching, lack of motivation, cognitive limitation
Acute Pain	Tissue damage resulting from surgical intervention, ineffective pain relief, psychological factors
Powerlessness	General anesthesia and pain medication leading to temporary or permanent loss of control over self-care, lack of knowledge of surgical intervention

- The single most important nursing action to decrease the incidence of hospital-based infections is handwashing. **Remember to wash your hands or use antibacterial gel before and after each and every client contact.**

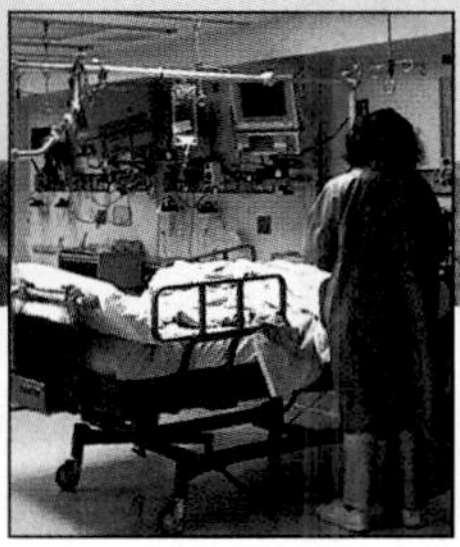

UNIT 1

Stress in Preoperative Clients

Nursing Process Data

ASSESSMENT Data Base

Identify if high level of stress exists.

Assess exaggerated anxiety or stress behaviors.

Evaluate defensive behaviors.

Assess client's vulnerability to number and significance of changes in life before admission.

Evaluate client's level of knowledge and perceptions of the impending surgery and perioperative period.

PLANNING Objectives

To identify the level of stress and anxiety present in preoperative clients

To provide interventions that decrease stress levels and promote optimal preoperative behavioral and physiologic responses

To observe for use of defensive behaviors that mask a failure to adapt appropriately in stressful situations

To prepare the client for a smooth preoperative and postoperative period

To prevent postoperative complications

IMPLEMENTATION Procedures

Preventing Anxiety and Stress

Reducing Anxiety and Stress

Assisting the Client Who Uses Denial

EVALUATION Expected Outcomes

Client's level of stress and anxiety is identified.

Nursing interventions are provided that decrease stress levels and promote optimal preoperative responses.

Denial, as a defense mechanism, is identified in the client and therapeutic interventions are made.

PREVENTING ANXIETY AND STRESS

Procedure

1. Establish a trusting relationship.
2. Encourage verbalization of feelings.
3. Listen attentively.
4. Communicate acceptance of the client as an individual.
5. Identify the client's needs (Table 31–3) and keep the charge nurse informed of them.
6. Give adequate information regarding hospital procedures.
   a. Hospital environment, including sights, sounds, and equipment.
   b. Hospital personnel and routine procedures: mealtimes, telephone usage, call light.
   c. Ordered preoperative procedures: lab tests, diagnostic procedures (explain the sensory experiences that will be encountered).
   d. Scheduled time of surgery.
   e. Hospital regulations: visiting hours, children's age for visiting.
   f. Preoperative procedures: skin preparation, NPO, medications, side rails, dentures, nail polish.
   g. Anticipated intraoperative events: monitors, oxygen mask, intravenous line, etc.
   h. Anticipated postoperative events: recovery room, pain and pain medications, coughing and deep breathing exercises, dressings, IVs, Foley catheter.

TABLE 31–3 Preoperative Stress Assessment

Physiologic Responses	Emotional and Defensive Responses	Anxiety and Activity Responses
Heart rate: rate increases 10 BPM over baseline during these observations Presence of palpitations Blood pressure: increases more than 10 mm Hg over baseline during three observations Respiratory rate: increases more than five per minute over baseline during three observations Vasoconstriction of blood vessels near the skin: cool, pale fingers and toes; increased capillary filling time of more than 3 seconds Vasoconstriction of renal vessels: decreased urine output compared with baseline and fluid intake Vasoconstriction of gastric and mesenteric vessels: anorexia, nausea, vomiting, abdominal distention with flatus, decreased bowel sounds, hyperactivity, diarrhea	Withdrawal: daydreaming, increased time in sleep, unwillingness to talk, disinterest Anger: resentment, aggressiveness, noncompliance, swearing, boasting, attempts to gain control, and independence Denial: joking, carefree attitude, inappropriate laughter, refusal to discuss impending surgery	Hyperactivity: pacing, hand-wringing, lip or nail biting, finger-tapping, impatience, irritability, insomnia Disorganization of thought: repetitive speech, constant conversation, difficulty concentrating Increased sensitivity to environmental noise, light, temperature, activity Increased muscle tensing: furrowed eyebrows, facial tics, clenched jaws, loud or high-pitched voice, stammering, rapid speech, elevated shoulders, clenched fists, urinary frequency, tension, or inability to relax Increased energy and preparedness: restlessness, easily startled, increased activity level

REDUCING ANXIETY AND STRESS

Equipment

Cassette tape player

Appropriate relaxation tape

Procedure

1. Establish a trusting relationship.
2. Encourage verbalization of feelings.
3. Use touch to communicate caring and genuine interest.
4. Avoid false reassurance.
5. Use realistic outcomes.
6. Assist client in exploring effective coping methods to reduce anxiety and/or stress.
   a. Ask the client or the family what method the client normally uses to successfully reduce stress.
   b. Provide activity: walking, range of motion.
   c. Provide a back rub to loosen tense muscles. **Rationale:** Physical relaxation will often lead to mental relaxation.
   d. Teach client relaxation techniques. One technique is to ask the client to picture a blue sky that is clear except for one white, fluffy cloud. Tell client to concentrate on this scene for 10 minutes. This often relaxes the mind and body.
   e. An alternative is to ask the client to picture a favorite place (e.g., a warm, sunny beach with sand and gentle surf).
7. As the client begins to relax, reinforce success. Assist client in recognizing his or her strengths.
8. Encourage self-awareness of increasing tension and immediate reversal of escalation.

ASSISTING THE CLIENT WHO USES DENIAL

Procedure

1. Establish a trusting relationship.
2. Encourage verbalization of feelings and use an interpreter if necessary.
3. Use touch to communicate caring and genuine interest if acceptable to client (i.e., some cultures prefer not to be touched).
4. Do not attempt to enforce reality. The client is denying reality to prevent outright panic. Allow use of this defense.
5. Use techniques to reduce anxiety and stress to manageable proportions.
6. Attempt to determine the cause of the need for denial.
7. Listen for cues that indicate readiness to discuss the stressors causing the need for denial.
8. Notify physician of your findings.

Documentation for Preoperative Stress

- Observed and subjective indications of anxiety or stress levels
- Nursing interventions used to decrease stress and the results of the intervention
- Changes that occurred as a result of the nursing interventions
- Specific fears verbalized by the client
- Nonverbal indications of stress or anxiety

Critical Thinking Application

UNEXPECTED OUTCOMES	CRITICAL THINKING OPTIONS
Anxiety level increases rapidly.	• Maintain calm composure, and speak in a soft caring manner. • Use touch to communicate caring and peacefulness. • Reinforce client self-acceptance as an individual. • If unable to achieve success with stress-reducing techniques, notify physician.
Client becomes angry or hostile.	• Maintain calm composure. • Accept anger, but place limits on how it may be expressed (e.g., no destructive behavior). Understand that anger is usually the result of feeling helpless and powerless to change an intolerable situation. • Do not reward this behavior, but explore other means of meeting client's needs. • Do not isolate client, but continue to respond to needs. • Notify physician of client's behaviors and the actions you used to decrease anger or hostility.
Client becomes depressed because of overwhelming anxiety and feelings of helplessness or hopelessness.	• Convey respect and belief that the client is worthwhile. Question the client's appraisal of reality, and provide support while the client works through his or her feelings. • Provide positive feedback and recognition of strengths, progress, and improved self-esteem. • Spend additional time with the client to allow time to verbalize fears.

UNIT 2

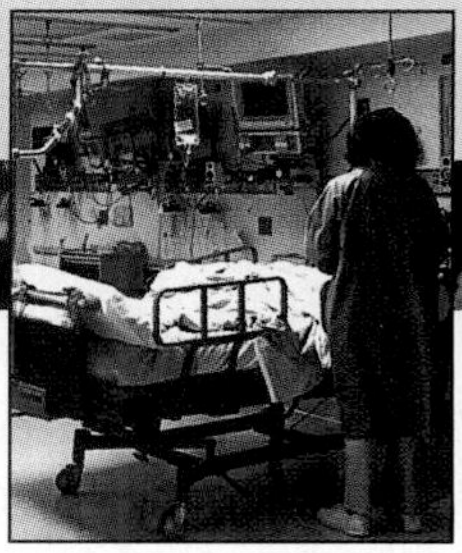

Preoperative Teaching

Nursing Process Data

ASSESSMENT Data Base

Identify type of surgical procedure planned.

Determine if client understands type of anesthesia planned.

Assess client's sociocultural needs.

Assess client's learning needs.

Determine most appropriate method of client teaching.

Assess client's willingness and ability to learn.

Determine availability of prepared audiovisual material or printed information regarding surgical procedure.

PLANNING Objectives

To reinforce physician's explanation of surgical procedure and answer questions regarding treatment

To identify client's readiness to learn about surgical treatment

To select appropriate time and place for client instruction regarding surgery

To provide instruction in measures to prevent postoperative complications

To provide a time for client to ask questions regarding surgical procedure

To instruct client in use of special equipment required during the postoperative period

To provide tour of specialty units, such as critical care unit, lithotripsy, or laser rooms

IMPLEMENTATION Procedures

Providing Surgical Information

- *for the Preoperative Client in the Hospital*
- *for the Preoperative Client in an Outpatient Setting*
- *for the Intraoperative Client*
- *for the Postoperative Client*

Providing Client Teaching

Providing Family Teaching

Teaching for Laser Therapy

Teaching for Lithotripsy

Teaching for Diagnostic Laparoscopy

Teaching for Arthroscopy

Instructing in Deep Breathing Exercises

Instructing in Coughing Exercises

Providing Instruction to Turn in Bed

Instructing in Leg Exercises

EVALUATION Expected Outcomes

Client is psychologically and physically prepared for surgery.

Client is able to demonstrate deep breathing, coughing, turning, and leg exercises accurately.

Client is able to verbalize knowledge of operative procedure, potential problems, and expected nursing actions postoperatively.

Client's family is informed about what to expect during perioperative period.

Appropriate audiovisual and written materials are used for client understanding of perioperative experience.

Client's fears are allayed regarding special equipment used during perioperative experience.

Client is aware of safety precautions used with laser and lithotripsy surgery.

PROVIDING SURGICAL INFORMATION

Equipment

Quiet room for client and family where there will be no interruptions during the teaching program

Equipment that may be used postoperatively by the client (e.g., IV solution, drainage tubes, nasogastric tube, cardiac monitor, and electrodes)

Procedure

for the Preoperative Client in the Hospital

1. Explain necessity for blood work, ECG, urinalysis, chest x-ray.
2. Describe preoperative skin preparation.
3. Discuss placement of nasogastric tube, Foley catheter, as indicated.
4. Describe enema or special bowel preparation as ordered.
5. Explain use of ongoing medications preoperatively and postoperatively.
6. Demonstrate deep breathing and coughing exercises (use of spirometer if indicated).
7. Assess alcohol use and smoking habits. Emphasize smoking cessation techniques.
8. Demonstrate leg exercises, antiembolic stockings, and sequential stockings.
9. Demonstrate turning and moving in bed.
10. Explain use of postoperative medications for pain control; PCA.
11. Discuss reason for NPO, when it begins, and medication schedule.
12. Explain alterations in diet preoperatively or postoperatively.
13. Describe activities and preparation the morning of surgery.
14. State need for quiet environment after medications have been given.
15. State time of surgery to client and family.
16. Describe information usually provided by anesthesiologist and surgeon.
17. Offer tour and explanation of monitoring devices and special equipment in ICU if client is to be transferred there postoperatively.

for the Preoperative Client in an Outpatient Setting

1. Call the client several days in advance if long duration surgical preparations need to be completed before the procedure. If short duration preparations are required, call the client in the afternoon before the procedure. It is best if the nurse who will care for the client during the surgery calls the client. **Rationale:** The call begins the nurse-client relationship and helps decrease anxiety.
2. Assess client's ability to understand instructions. If necessary, ask to speak to someone else in the home. **Rationale:** If instructions are not followed, it could result in unsafe canceled surgery.
3. Review any lab work that needs to be completed before the scheduled surgery. Explain where the lab work is to be done.
4. Answer the client's questions regarding the surgery and the procedures carried out by the staff during the surgery.
5. Arrange for preadmission as needed.
6. Discuss the procedure for admission to the facility; when to check in at the facility (usually 1½–2 hours before the scheduled surgery), and what documents need to be available at the time of registration (e.g., insurance card, and possibly deductible payment).
7. Discuss procedure-appropriate clothing to be worn to the setting. For example, clients having knee surgery should wear loose fitting sweat pants.
8. Explain that all jewelry and valuables should be left at home for safekeeping.
9. Explain that someone needs to be with the client to take them home.

for the Intraoperative Client

1. Describe mode of transportation to operating room.
2. Discuss procedure in preinduction room or operating room suite in relationship to anesthesia.
3. Reinforce physician's explanation of surgery.
4. Describe dressings, tubes, or equipment that will be used postoperatively.

5. Describe postanesthesia room physical environment and procedures.
6. Explain administration of oxygen.
7. Explain administration of medications.

for the Postoperative Client

1. Describe assessment procedures.
2. Provide overview of routine procedures of vital signs.
3. Demonstrate deep breathing, turning, and coughing exercises.
4. Describe IV therapy if indicated.
5. Explain irrigation of tubes when indicated.
6. Discuss catheter care.
7. Review dietary alterations.
8. Describe observation and changes of dressing.
9. State ambulation or restrictions in ambulation.
10. Define type of medications used postoperatively.
11. Provide anticipated discharge and plans for assisted care if needed.

PROVIDING CLIENT TEACHING

Equipment

Prepare teaching aids when available: audiovisual, videos, interactive computer programs, pamphlets, pictures, posters, programmed learning modules, cassette tapes, overhead transparencies

Procedure

1. Assess client's knowledge base and readiness to learn. **Rationale:** This provides framework for client education at the level client can understand.
   a. Determine the information provided to client by physician by reading physician's progress notes and asking client specific questions.
   b. Identify client's psychosocial and cultural status and ability to listen to teaching by communicating with client and asking direct questions.
   c. Be alert for cultural or religious beliefs that may influence client's surgical experience.
   d. Identify client's perceptions of expected surgical experience and preferences for learning.
2. Develop individualized teaching plan based on client's needs.
   a. Choose appropriate equipment for teaching, based on client's level of understanding, knowledge base, and language of preference.
   b. Review information previously provided. **Rationale:** To determine retention of information and needless repetition of information already mastered.
   c. Choose a quiet environment, and provide for sufficient time to allow client to ask questions. **Rationale:** To ensure client understands planned surgical experience.
   d. Be alert for clues indicating client confusion or misunderstanding of information or clients may be nodding "yes," even though they do not understand, especially non–English-speaking clients. **Rationale:** Misunderstanding information can be detrimental to the client's sense of well-being.

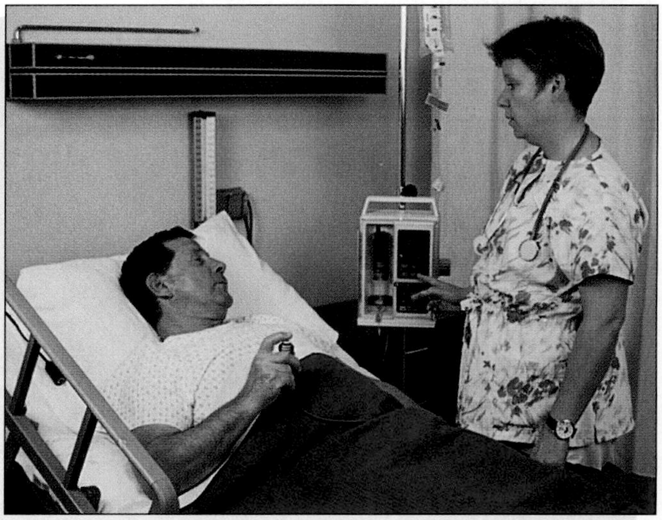

Demonstrate use of special equipment in prospective teaching plan.

3. Select appropriate audiovisual materials to assist with teaching.
4. Demonstrate use of special equipment or devices (e.g., incentive spirometer, chest tubes, suction equipment).
5. Evaluate client teaching by assessing client's ability to return demonstration of exercises and verbally answer specific questions. Reinforce information or provide additional data as needed.

PROVIDING FAMILY TEACHING

Procedure

1. Include family in teaching provided to client.
2. Instructions to family members should include:
   a. Visiting hours.
   b. Where to wait during surgery.
   c. Where the surgeon will meet with them, and when.

d. Where they can find bathrooms, telephones, and food and beverage service.
e. When they can see the client after surgery.
f. How to contact a spiritual or religious resource person.
g. How they can best get information regarding the client's condition while they are at home or in the hospital.
h. Whether they will be called if there is a change in the client's condition.
i. What to expect: client's behavior, which may be regressive; attitude which may be depressed or angry; physical condition, which may appear worse than it is, and postrecovery period. **Rationale:** Some medications may impair client's memory of events.

TEACHING FOR LASER THERAPY

Procedure

1. Determine type of laser (Table 31–4) to be used for surgery.
2. Identify client and introduce yourself.
3. Determine client's willingness to accept instruction.
4. Determine most appropriate time and place for instruction.
5. Identify client's level of understanding of surgical procedure and what information physician has provided (Table 31–5).
6. Reinforce explanation of surgical procedure by physician as needed.
7. Describe operating room setting or outpatient setting, including the environment.
8. Explain that client and operating room staff will wear goggles. **Rationale:** Goggles protect eyes from the laser beam.
9. Explain the use of wet drapes placed over client's skin if required. **Rationale:** Wet drapes prevent skin from burns when some types of laser therapy are used.
10. Describe that laser machine may be very noisy.
11. Describe physician's actions during laser therapy. Physician will discharge laser by using a foot pedal while at the same time issuing instructions to nurses using terms such as *fire, watt seconds,* and *standby.* **Rationale:** Describing these words to client allays fear of unfamiliar terms or actual fire. It also describes nurses' role of regulating power and duration of laser beam use.
12. Caution client, if under local anesthesia, he or she may feel heat and smell smoke and a burning odor from tissue being lased.
13. Instruct client to tell physician if pain occurs. **Rationale:** Additional anesthetic may need to be administered as client should not feel pain.
14. Instruct client to maintain NPO status 6–8 hours before surgery.
15. Instruct client in postoperative care specific to procedure performed.

TABLE 31–4 Types of Laser*

Types	Uses
Carbon dioxide	High-precision cutting instrument used in areas where function must be preserved (e.g., vocal cords, brain, GYN procedures). Also used to treat snoring and for dermatology procedures (e.g., removal of scars and skin cancers)
Holmium	Combines the cutting properties of the CO_2 laser with the coagulation properties of the YAG laser. It is used in targeted tissue affecting adjacent, healthy tissue. Can be used with dense or hard tissue. Used in urology procedures (e.g., laser ablation of the prostate [TLAP], stone fragmentation [lithotripsy], strictures, obstructions, condylomata, bladder and ureteral tumors and contractures)
Nd:YAG	Laser made of a neodymium alloy, vittrium, aluminum, and garnet crystals. Beam penetrates deeply; can be passed through flexible fibers for cardiovascular laser therapy and scopes (e.g., cystoscope, bronchoscope, and endoscope to treat bladder, prostate, and lung tumors and coagulate esophageal varices; also used for eye surgery)
Argon	Used for ophthalmic and dermatologic procedures (e.g., treating glaucoma, cataract, retinal detachment, and removing birthmarks, hemangiomas)
Liquid dye	Used for diagnostic procedures and in conjunction with drugs for photodynamic treatment (e.g., lithotripsy)

*Light amplification by the stimulated emission of radiation. Choice of laser type is determined by procedure required for treatment.

16. Instruct client to notify physician if temperature is above 100°F for more than 24 hours following laser therapy. **Rationale:** Infections are unlikely but can occur; therefore, client needs to monitor for presence of symptoms.

TABLE 31–5 Common Types of Laser Surgical Procedures and Complications

Procedure	Client Teaching	Assessment Findings for Potential Complications
Pulmonary	Gag reflex returns in 2–4 hours Begin taking fluids when gag reflex returns Expect hoarseness, dyspnea, sore throat, difficulty swallowing for 48–72 hours	Bright red blood expectorated related to hemorrhage Fever, shortness of breath Use of accessory muscles for breathing related to tracheal edema Wheezing related to airway obstruction Pneumonia and respiratory insufficiency related to aspiration of secretions Altered arterial blood gases and sudden pain causing altered vital signs related to pneumothorax
Upper GI	May experience burning sensation in esophagus May experience difficulty swallowing Heartburn present for 3 days	Poor skin turgor and decreased urine output related to dehydration that may be caused by dysphagia Vomiting bright red blood related to perforation Abdominal pain related to perforated bowel Vomiting and abdominal distention related to obstruction of GI tract due to edema
Urology	May experience traces of blood, small blood clots, or traces of tissue in urine for 24 hours Catheter may be left in place temporarily for up to 1 week Urinary frequency and urgency may occur for 1 week	Bright red urine related to hemorrhage Abdominal pain related to perforated bladder Fever, increased pulse, malaise related to infection Inability to void related to blood clots
Cardiovascular	May experience slight burning or chest pain over coronary vessels	Arrhythmias related to hypoxia or laser treatment Bleeding at site of percutaneous laser angioplasty; related to catheter insertion Intake and output values altered related to osmotic contrast media used for laser treatment Changes in vital signs (i.e., may become hypotensive with cardiac tamponade)
Eye	Most clients feel no pain because local or topical anesthesia is used Need to remain quiet during procedure	Corneal injury can occur if eye is rubbed or bumped Increased intraocular pressure is unusual but can occur

TEACHING FOR LITHOTRIPSY

Preparation

1. Identify type of extracorporeal shock wave lithotripsy (ESWL) used for kidney stones and occasionally for gallstones.
2. Identify type of anesthesia that will be used: local, epidural, spinal, or general. General anesthesia is usually used to prevent pain as stones are fragmented.
3. Identify if client will have a ureteral stint or Foley catheter inserted after the procedure.

Procedure

1. Identify client and introduce yourself.
2. Determine client's knowledge base and information provided by physician.
3. Reinforce physician's description of procedure, as needed.
4. Answer client's questions regarding procedure.
5. Explain that lithotriptor discharges a series of shock waves through water or water-filled cushion.
6. Describe to client that he or she may feel fluttering or mild blows where shock waves are beamed. From 500 to 2400 shocks are required to disintegrate stones.
7. Discuss use of specialized equipment that will be used. Client may sit in tank of water or lie with water-filled cushion pressed against area of back or abdomen where stones are present.
8. Describe use of monitoring equipment throughout procedure. **Rationale:** The heart rate and rhythm is monitored throughout procedure and shocks may be synchronized with the rhythm to prevent arrhythmias.
9. Explain that the procedure takes 45 minutes to 2 hours, depending on type of procedure.
10. Describe postlithotripsy care.
    a. Following procedure, client is removed from tub, covered with warm blanket, and taken to recovery room.
    b. Vital signs are monitored as with any surgical client.
    c. Urine output is monitored for hematuria. **Rationale:** To determine kidney damage from procedure.
    d. Strain all urine at the facility and at home. **Rationale:** To obtain fragments of the stones in order to send them for analysis. Knowing composition of the stone is essential for altering dietary habits in some cases.

e. Liver function studies are performed following lithotripsy for gallstones. **Rationale:** To assess if shock waves have damaged liver.
f. Pain management is monitored and maintained as gravel is passed following disintegration of stones.
g. Medication is provided for nausea and vomiting. **Rationale:** Nausea and vomiting often accompany pain and postanesthesia.
h. Intake and output measurements are taken. **Rationale:** Fluids are encouraged to hydrate clients with kidney stones to assist in the excretion of gravel.
i. Catheter care is provided for kidney clients requiring indwelling catheters. **Rationale:** Indwelling catheters and ureteral stents, if used, are left in place for 24 hours to assist with passage of gravel or if second ESWL treatment is required.
j. Exercise is encouraged to assist with passing of gravel.
k. Ecchymoses and discomfort may be felt over area of the body that experienced shock waves.

11. Provide tour of lithotriptor room, if possible.

TEACHING FOR DIAGNOSTIC LAPAROSCOPY

Preparation

1. Identify purpose of diagnostic laparoscopy.
2. Identify type of anesthesia that will be used. Usually, it is done under general anesthesia, but can be done under local anesthesia with sedation.
3. Determine if ultrasound, CT scan, and/or MRI was done; if so, have results available for physician.
4. Obtain results of standard blood tests and urine tests if done.

Procedure

1. Identify client and introduce yourself.
2. Determine client's knowledge base and information provided by physician.
3. Reinforce physician's description of procedure as needed.
4. Describe equipment used for procedure: instrument used in procedure is a medical telescope with a light and high resolution television camera so physician can see what is in the abdomen.
5. Describe procedure to client: incision is made into umbilicus; CO_2 gas is infused into abdomen to insert a small air pocket; a small camera and instruments are inserted through incision.
6. Instruct client that procedure is done in a same day surgery setting. Client will go home the same day.
7. Instruct client to not eat or drink for 6–8 hours before procedure.

> A diagnostic laparoscopy is used for the following purposes:
>
> - Diagnose causes of abdominal pain
> - Obtain tissue from an abdominal mass to determine diagnosis
> - Determine cause of ascites
> - Obtain liver tissue for diagnosis
> - Assist in cancer staging or for a "second look" procedure

8. Explain that client should shower evening before or day of surgery with chlorhexidine or agent prescribed by physician. The umbilicus is cleaned with soap, water, and a Q-tip. **Rationale:** Chlorhexidine is well tolerated and does not leave discoloration on skin as a povidone–iodine preparation does.
9. Instruct client to be at the hospital 1–2 hours before the scheduled surgery, according to hospital policy. Tell client to bring someone to drive home.
10. Have client discuss with the surgeon whether to take routine medications the morning of surgery. If medications are taken, only a sip of water is used to swallow pills. Medications used for arthritis, anticoagulants, or aspirin must be stopped before surgery according to physician's orders.
11. Instruct client to follow specific orders from physician's office regarding other preoperative directions.
12. Explain setting where surgery will be performed. If possible, allow client to visit the area if he or she is anxious.
13. Describe post laparoscopy care to client:
    a. Following surgery, client will go to the recovery room.
    b. Vital signs are monitored, dressing will be observed for signs of bleeding, medication for pain may be administered. IV fluids will be infused and monitored until effects of anesthesia have dissipated.
    c. Client is discharged home as soon as he or she is fully awake and able to get out of bed unassisted. Client must be accompanied by someone who can drive him or her home. **Rationale:** The effects of anesthesia may persist for several hours or as long as a day, even if the client feels fully awake.
    d. Instruct client that some soreness around incision is normal. Take pain medications as prescribed by physician.
    e. Notify physician if chills, vomiting, redness at incision site, or worsening pain is not controlled by medication, or if unable to urinate. **Rationale:** These are signs of infection.
    f. Instruct client to schedule a follow-up appointment with physician within 2 weeks.

TEACHING FOR ARTHROSCOPY

Preparation

1. Determine joint on which arthroscopy will be performed. Most common joints: knee, shoulder, elbow, ankle, hip, and wrist.
2. Identify type of anesthesia that will be used. General, spinal, or local anesthetic is used, depending on specific joint involved and suspected problem.
3. Determine if diagnostic tests were done, i.e., MRI, x-rays, or arthrogram. Obtain results for physician.

Procedure

1. Identify client and introduce yourself.
2. Determine client's knowledge base and information provided by physician.
3. Reinforce physician's description of procedure, as needed.
4. Describe equipment used for the procedure: pencil-sized instruments (arthroscope) that contain small lens and lighting system to magnify and illuminate structures inside the joint are inserted through incision.
5. Describe procedure to client: a small incision is made in client's skin to allow instruments to be inserted into the joint so that physician can see the interior of the joint. Several small incisions may be made to see other parts of the joint if needed. The image is projected on a television screen. The surgeon can then determine the amount or type of injury, and repair or correct the problem.
6. Instruct client that procedure is done in an outpatient setting and he or she will go home the same day.
7. Explain preoperative preparation that is completed before the day of surgery:
   a. Diagnostic tests completed.
   b. Operative permit signed.
   c. Physical examination and health history completed.
   d. Physician informed of routine medications and any allergies.
   e. Procedure discussed with physician and anesthesiologist.
   f. Client meets with physical therapist to be fitted with crutches and/or knee brace.
8. Instruct client to not eat or drink anything after midnight unless otherwise instructed by physician.
9. Explain skin prep that is to be completed the night before surgery. A 5-minute scrub with an antiseptic is usually ordered. Follow facility policy for specifics—some physicians order a full shower and some concentrate on the surgical site.
10. Instruct client to follow surgeon or anesthesiologist instructions regarding taking routine medications.
11. Instructions to client before admission:
    a. Remove all nail polish and make-up. **Rationale:** Capillary refill and skin coloration is assessed on all clients receiving anesthesia.
    b. Do not bring jewelry, money, or other valuables to facility. **Rationale:** Facility is not responsible for client's valuables.
    c. Wear comfortable, loose fitting clothes such as loose-fitting shirts or blouses, drawstring shorts, sweat pants, and boxer-style shorts. **Rationale:** This is to make it easier to dress after surgery, especially if a brace or sling has been applied.
    d. Bring crutches, brace, sling, or immobilizer to facility.
    e. An adult must accompany client to facility to provide transportation home. **Rationale:** Even if client feels alert and awake, effects of anesthesia can last up to a day or two.
    f. Arrive at the facility 1½ to 2 hours before scheduled surgery, according to facility policy.
12. Describe post-arthroscopy care to client:
    a. Following surgery he/she will go to recovery room.
    b. Vital signs, circulatory assessments, pain management, IV fluid infusion will continue until client is fully awake and ready for discharge.
    c. A pressure dressing, brace, or ice may be applied to joint.
    d. Discharge instructions are based on joint involved with arthroscopy. Most common joint is knee. Client is to use crutches for short time. Weight bearing is allowed according to physician orders. Brace is worn when walking. Physical therapy will begin within a day or two of surgery.
13. Repeat instructions for home care.
    a. Explain to client that wound and dressing is to be kept clean and dry and changed if it becomes soiled.
    b. Instruct client to place a plastic bag over brace and tape it securely when showering.
    c. Instruct client to apply ice to joint for 24–48 hours after surgery. **Rationale:** To reduce pain and edema.
    d. Demonstrate how to elevate joint (leg, ankle, wrist) to reduce pain and edema.

Conditions usually found and corrected by arthroscopy include:

- **Inflammation:** Synovitis
- **Injury:** acute and chronic:
  Shoulder—rotator cuff tendon tears, dislocation, and impingement syndrome
  Knee—meniscal tears, chondromalacia, and anterior cruciate ligament (ACL) tears and instability
  Wrist—carpal tunnel syndrome
- **Loose bodies of bone and/or cartilage:** knee, shoulder, elbow, ankle, or wrist

e. Explain how pain medication is to be taken: 30 minutes before exercises; tell client to not drink alcohol when on medications.
f. Discuss symptoms that indicate complications and should be reported immediately to physician: swelling; tingling; pain or numbness in extremities; drainage that is yellow, green, or foul smelling; chills or temperature above 38.5°C (101.3°F).

INSTRUCTING IN DEEP BREATHING EXERCISES

Procedure

1. Identify client and introduce yourself.
2. Explain procedure and purpose of exercises. **Rationale:** Deep breathing and coughing exercises promote lung expansion; lower the risk of pneumonia, atelectasis, and pulmonary emboli.
3. Instruct and have client demonstrate deep breathing exercises. **Rationale:** Encouraging the client to practice and return the demonstration before surgery assists him or her to deep breathe more effectively after surgery.
4. Have client sit in upright position.
5. Place client's hands along lower borders of rib cage. Client should feel rib cage expand when breathing in. **Rationale:** This assists client to feel adequate chest movement.
6. Instruct client to breathe through nose slowly, take a deep breath, hold 1–2 seconds, then exhale through mouth. **Rationale:** This expands alveoli and prevents hyperventilation if client is breathing too quickly.
7. Repeat exercise sequence 3–4 times, at least every 2 hours when awake.

INSTRUCTING IN COUGHING EXERCISES

Procedure

1. Identify client and introduce yourself.
2. Explain procedure and purpose of exercises.
3. Instruct and have client demonstrate coughing exercises.
4. Have client sit in upright position.
5. Instruct client to splint incision when deep breathing and coughing.
6. Demonstrate placement of hands on either side of incision. Instruct client to press hands firmly toward incision during exercises. **Rationale:** This prevents tension on the suture line and diminishes pain.
7. Instruct in use of cough pillow. Place folded bath towel in pillowcase. Hold pillow directly over incision and press on pillow when performing exercises. **Rationale:** This prevents pain and discomfort by splinting the incision and reducing stress on suture line.
8. Demonstrate technique for inhaling deeply and holding breath for 1–2 seconds.
9. Instruct client to take 2–3 breaths slowly and exhale passively; on third breath, hold for 2–3 seconds.
10. Encourage client to cough forcefully 2–3 times by using abdominal and other respiratory muscles to assist with coughing. **Rationale:** This extra force provides a more effective cough.
11. Have client cough a second time.
12. Instruct client to do coughing exercises following deep breathing exercises at least every 2 hours when awake.
13. Have tissue available for secretions if client has a productive cough.

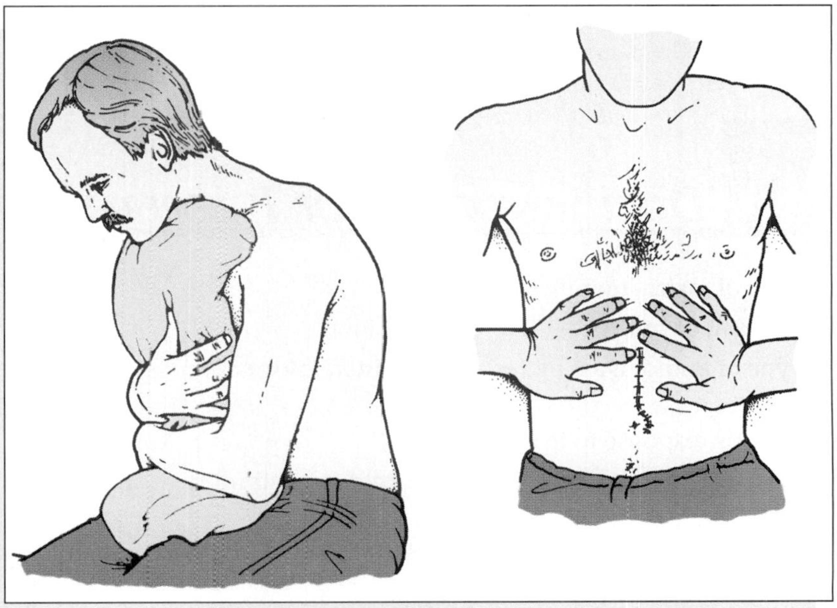

Instruct client in coughing exercises using cough pillow or demonstrate placement of hands on either side of incision for support during coughing.

PROVIDING INSTRUCTION TO TURN IN BED

Procedure

1. Identify client and introduce yourself.
2. Explain turning procedure and purpose. **Rationale:** Turning assists in the prevention of thrombophlebitis, pressure ulcer formation, and respiratory complications.
3. Instruct and demonstrate turning procedure.
4. Instruct client to splint incision whenever turning.
5. Have client move to far side of bed with side rails up. **Rationale:** This position allows client to turn without rolling to edge of bed.
6. Instruct client to splint incision with hand on side toward which he or she will be turning. **Rationale:** This leaves the uppermost hand available to grasp side rail or trapeze to assist with turning.
7. Instruct client to keep leg straight on side to which he or she will turn.
8. Flex other leg over straight lower leg. **Rationale:** Flexing the leg assists in shifting the weight when turning to opposite side.
9. Instruct client to turn on side and grasp side rail.
10. Instruct client to move pillow into comfortable position under head, place arm into comfortable position, or place pillow between legs and behind back (if side-lying position).

INSTRUCTING IN LEG EXERCISES

Procedure

1. Identify client and introduce yourself.
2. Explain exercise and purpose. **Rationale:** These exercises assist in preventing stasis of blood in lower extremities and thus thrombophlebitis.
3. Place client in supine or semi-Fowler's position.
4. Instruct client to bend knee, raise foot in air, and hold this position for 2–3 seconds.
5. Have client extend the leg and lower it to bed.
6. Repeat procedure with other leg.
7. Complete sequence 5–10 times each hour while awake.
8. Have client extend toes (plantar flexion) toward bottom of bed, then flex (dorsiflexion) toward head of bed.
9. Repeat foot extension and flexion with other side.
10. Repeat sequence 5 times each hour while awake.
11. Instruct client to make circles with the ankle moving first to the left and then to the right.
12. Repeat sequence 5 times each hour while awake.

Note: Inhale when extending leg and exhale slowly when lowering leg. This prevents back strain and strengthens abdominal muscles.

DOCUMENTATION FOR PREOPERATIVE TEACHING

- Type of instruction provided
- Amount of time provided for instruction
- Type of audiovisual materials or written information used
- Client's response to teaching
- Accuracy and participation in return demonstration exercises
- Areas of instruction that need to be reinforced
- Psychological response to preoperative teaching and impending surgery
- Preop teaching form if available

Critical Thinking Application

UNEXPECTED OUTCOMES	CRITICAL THINKING OPTIONS
Client refuses to participate in preoperative teaching.	• Encourage client to state reasons for refusal. • Encourage client to discuss knowledge of surgery. • Assess if client is experiencing fear or denial regarding impending surgery. • Ask client to provide a time frame more acceptable for teaching. • Notify physician of client's refusal if facility policy.
Client unable to understand directions.	• Identify client's learning capabilities. • Determine if a language barrier exists. If so, find person who speaks client's primary language and ask for assistance with teaching. • Use different words to explain information. • Determine a different teaching strategy that the client can understand. • Evaluate client's stress level to determine if it is interfering with learning. • Establish a new time for teaching when client may be able to concentrate on teaching. • Develop a slower pace for instruction and present less information at one time.
Client not adequately prepared for surgery.	• Ascertain where data are insufficient or unclear and provide additional instruction in that area. • Use a different approach or teaching style to provide information. • Select different teaching materials that may explain information in a more useful way.
Client becomes angry or hostile.	• Maintain calm composure. • Acknowledge anger, but place limits on how it may be expressed (e.g., destructive behavior). Understand that anger is usually the result of feeling helpless and powerless to change an intolerable situation. • Do not reward this behavior but explore other means of meeting client's needs. • Do not isolate client; continue to respond to needs. • Try to defuse anger, but if safety is threatened, call for assistance.
Client becomes depressed because of overwhelming anxiety and feelings of helplessness or hopelessness.	• Convey respect and belief that client is worthwhile. Question client's appraisal of reality; provide support while client works through feelings. • Provide positive feedback and recognition of strengths, progress, and improved self-esteem. • Spend additional time with the client to allow time to verbalize fears.

UNIT 3

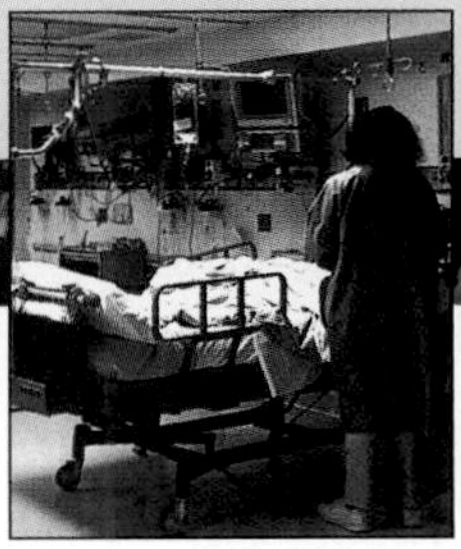

Preoperative Care

Nursing Process Data

ASSESSMENT *Data Base*

Assess type of surgical procedure to be carried out and extent of data base needed.

Evaluate the client's ability to provide accurate information.

Assess level of anxiety present that may interfere in the transmission of information at that moment.

Identify the appropriate physical care needed for the specific surgical intervention.

Assess special needs for the surgical shave.

Check hospital protocol for shaving surgical site or if a special permit is needed for shaving, such as the head for neurosurgical clients, extremities for orthopedic clients, or children.

Check for need for special soap or antiseptic scrub prior to shave.

Check if a policy exists in the hospital for disposing or handling of scalp hair.

Assess surgical site before preparing; observe for unusual cuts, abrasions, or markings, and report findings to charge nurse.

Assess client's knowledge of side and site of surgical procedure.

PLANNING *Objectives*

To assist with monitoring the client's progress through the operative experience

To assist in identifying deviations from the client's baseline data that may occur as a result of anxiety or stress of admission, preoperative events, diagnostic procedures, the surgical trauma, postoperative complications, responses to and side effects of drugs

To provide appropriate preoperative physical care to enable the client to have a safe intraoperative and postoperative period

To report client's statements about allergies or chronic problems that could affect postoperative nursing care

To complete a surgical prep correctly

IMPLEMENTATION *Procedures*

Obtaining Baseline Data

Preparing the Surgical Site

Preparing the Client for Surgery

Administering Preoperative Medications

EVALUATION *Expected Outcomes*

The client's physical or emotional deviations from normal are identified preoperatively.

Preoperative baseline data is obtained.

Explicit preoperative care is provided to ensure a safe intraoperative and postoperative course.

Surgical site is prepared correctly.

OBTAINING BASELINE DATA

Equipment

Thermometer
Sphygmomanometer and stethoscope
Chart for documenting findings

Procedure

1. Establish rapport with the client.
2. Ask about allergies to drugs, food, or latex.
3. Assess for surgical risk: nutritional status, fluid and electrolyte balance, use of prescribed medications, over the counter complementary medications (i.e., herbs), and illicit drugs. **Rationale:** Medications such as anticoagulants, tranquilizers, or CNS depressants can adversely affect surgical experience.
4. Assess for alcohol use and smoking habits. **Rationale:** Complications can arise in clients using these substances particularly with anesthesia.
5. Take and record vital signs and weight of client.
6. Check if client wears dentures, hearing aid, or glasses, or has an artificial eye.
7. Assess mental attitude; record any unusual stress or anxiety exhibited by the client.
8. Complete a physical assessment and health history. Report unusual findings to physician.
9. Evaluate lab values for abnormalities (ECG, x-rays, blood work, and urinalysis). **Rationale:** To detect potential sources for complications, e.g., low Hct, Hgb, urine glucose, lung or cardiac abnormalities.
10. Determine if skin preparation was completed either evening before or morning of surgery. Check if shower or bath with designated antiseptic was completed.
11. Identify topics requiring client teaching.
12. Identify discharge plans.
13. Determine religious or cultural beliefs that may impact surgical experience.

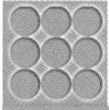

CULTURAL COMPETENCE

Most religions and cultures allow the administration of blood and blood products. The exception is Jehovah's Witnesses who forbid the use of blood and blood products. Christian Science followers ordinarily do not allow blood and blood products either. Surgical procedures are accepted by all religions and cultures with some modification. Buddhists permit surgery, but will avoid extremes in surgical procedures. Roman Catholics do not allow abortion or sterilization procedures.

PREPARING THE SURGICAL SITE

Equipment

Washcloth and towels
Absorbent pad
Bath blanket or drape
Scissors or electric clippers
Disposable prep kit (for shaving)
If kit not available:
- Disposable razor (number according to area to be shaved)
- 2 sterile bowls
- 4 × 4 gauze pads
- Emesis basin
- Applicator sticks
- Cleansing solution
- Sterile water

Clean gloves
Depilatory
Antiseptic solution
Tongue blade
4 × 4 gauze pad

Procedure

1. Refer to physician's orders for specific operative site or area to be prepared. If orders do not state preference for site, refer to procedure manual for appropriate area to be prepared, based on surgical procedure.

Note: Many surgeons do not require hair to be shaved for a surgical site unless it interferes with the surgical procedure or wound closure. Based on clinical research, it has been found that shaving the hair does not prevent surgical site infections, but it does interfere with the client's psychological status. Client's body image can be impaired and he or she senses a loss of control with shaving of the hair, particularly of the head or pubic area.

EVIDENCE BASED NURSING PRACTICE

Surgical Site Infection (SSI)

A preoperative antiseptic shower or bath decreases skin microbial colony count. In a study of over 700 clients who received two preoperative antiseptic showers, chlorhexidine reduced bacterial colony counts nine-fold. Iodine or triclocarban-medicated soap reduced colony counts 1.3– to 1.9–fold, respectively.

Chlorhexidine gluconate–containing products require several applications to obtain maximum antimicrobial benefit, so repeated antiseptic showers are indicated. Even though these showers reduce the colony count, they have not definitively shown a reduction in SSI rate.

Source: Mangram, A. J., et al. (1999). The Hospital Infection Control Practices Advisory Committee. *Infection Control and Hospital Epidemiology, 20*(4), 247–280.

2. Determine type of preparation to be done: clipping of hair, shaving site, or hair removal using depilatory. Gather equipment.
3. Explain procedure to client, and provide privacy.
4. Adjust light to ensure good visualization.
5. Wash your hands.
6. Position client for maximum comfort and site exposure.
7. Drape client for comfort and to prevent undue exposure.
8. Protect bed with absorbent pad.
9. Arrange equipment for your convenience.
10. Put on clean gloves.
11. Assess surgical site before skin preparation for moles, warts, rash, and other skin conditions. **Rationale:** Inadvertent removal of lesions traumatizes skin and may contribute to infection.

Note: CDC standards indicate that clients are to shower or bathe with an antiseptic agent at least the night before surgery. The FDA has also shown that antimicrobial activity of the antiseptic agent prevents skin infections.

12. Prepare site using scissors or clippers.
    a. Use scissors or electric clippers and cut hair 1 cm above surgical site or according to facility policies.

CLINICAL ALERT

If hair must be removed, scissors or clippers should be used and procedure completed before the client reaches the operating room suite. Many hospitals use the minimal shave and scrub preparation approach. The shaved area may be as small as 2 cm surrounding the surgical incision site. Refer to the policy and procedure manual and physician's orders before beginning the surgical prep.

    b. Clip small amount of hair each time.
    c. Cut in direction hair grows.
    d. Remove all hair from site, and discard.
13. Prepare site using depilatory.
    a. Clip hair before applying cream.
    b. Apply cream to designated area using tongue blade or gloved hand.
    c. Leave on skin for designated time, according to directions on package, usually 10 minutes.
    d. Remove cream by rubbing off with tongue blade or moistened 4 × 4 gauze pads.
    e. Wash skin with antiseptic soap; dry area thoroughly.

EVIDENCE BASED NURSING PRACTICE

Use of Hibiclens Preoperatively

In a study conducted in 1988, chlorhexidine gluconate (Hibiclens) was found to be more effective in reducing organisms than povidone–iodine (Betadine). Other studies have also shown Hibiclens to be the preferred agent of choice for preoperative showers. One study compared the results of preoperative baths and showers. Showers were found to reduce more skin bacteria than baths. Two showers were most frequently advised—one the night before surgery and one the morning of the procedure.

Sources: Kaiser, A. B., et al. (1988). Influence of preoperative showers on staphylococcal skin colonization: A comparative trial of antiseptic skin cleansers. *Annals of Thoracic Surgery, 45*(1), 35–38; and Byrne, D. J., et al. (1990). Rationalizing whole body disinfection. *Journal of Hospital Infection, 15*(2), 183–187.

CLINICAL ALERT

Electric or battery powered clippers are preferred to razors to prevent skin irritation and microscopic cuts to the skin. Clippers must have a disposable head that is changed between clients.

f. Remove all hair with washing. **Rationale:** This provides clean, smooth skin, free of abrasions and cuts.

14. Prepare site using razor.
    a. Lather skin with antiseptic soap and 4 × 4 gauze pads. **Rationale:** Wet shave results in fewer microabrasions to the skin. Shaving should be done in direction of hair growth.
    b. Discard soiled sponges frequently.
    c. Using sharp razor, shave hair moving away from incision site. With free hand, stretch skin taut and shave, following the hair growth pattern and using firm, steady strokes. Shave small area at one time. **Rationale:** Shave is closer and nicks are prevented.
    d. Change razor as often as necessary. Avoid nicking the skin. Report if skin is nicked. **Rationale:** Nicks, if severe, can cause infection by bacteria normally found on the skin.
    e. Wash all hair off site with 4 × 4 gauze pads or use sticky mitt or tape to remove hair.
    f. The shave should be completed close to the time of surgery. The shave prep is completed before the client enters the operating room. **Rationale:** Shaving and clipping hair immediately before surgery is associated with a lower risk of infection than if done the night before.
15. After removing hair, apply antiseptic solution with 4 × 4 pads or use disposable prep kit.
16. Begin at incision site and, with light friction, make ever-widening circles, moving outward from the center to the most distant line of area. **Rationale:** Working from most clean to least clean area prevents contamination. Scrub area for 2–3 minutes.
17. Rinse area with warm water and blot dry with 4 × 4 gauze pads.
18. Remove and dispose of equipment; scissors and razors are disposed of in sharps container.
19. Remove gloves, and discard.
20. Wash hands.
21. Assist client to put on clean gown.
22. Position the client for comfort.

EVIDENCE BASED NURSING PRACTICE

Skin Preparation and Surgical Site Infections

Many studies show that hair removal with a razor or clippers can cause skin abrasion, or even nicks in the skin. This can lead to subsequent surgical site infections (SSIs). In a study discussed in the *CDC Guideline for Prevention of Surgical Site Infection*, it was identified that SSIs occurred in 5.6% of clients who had their hair removed by razor shave, compared to an 0.6% rate among those who had hair removed by depilatory, or had no hair removed at all. The CDC advises that if hair is to be removed, it should be done so immediately before surgery, and preferably with electric hair clippers.

Source: Mangram, A. J. (1999). Hospital Infection Control Practices Advisory Committee. *Infection Control and Hospital Epidemiology, 29*(4), 247–280.

PREPARING THE CLIENT FOR SURGERY

Equipment

Preoperative checklist
Operative permit
Specific equipment needed to provide physical care as ordered, such as enema equipment, nasogastric tube, Foley catheter
Antiseptic agent for shower

Procedure

1. Obtain client's signature on surgical consent form and check agency policy.
2. Assist client to complete anesthesia questionnaire if required.
3. Assess if bowel prep was completed at home. **Rationale:** Most clients complete bowel prep before admission to facility. Administer an enema if ordered.
4. Assist client to shower if not completed at home. Instruct on how to shower and specific time guidelines according to facility guidelines.
5. Complete skin prep, if ordered. Follow facility guidelines for skin prep.

CLINICAL ALERT

The Association of PeriOperative Registered Nurses (AORN) recommends preop skin prep should be an antimicrobial agent that has a broad range germicidal action and is non-toxic.

The most common antiseptic agents used for preoperative skin preparation and surgical scrubs include alcohol, chlorhexidine, iodine/iodophors, and Triclosan. Alcohol has the most rapid microbial action, which denatures proteins and is effective against both gram-positive and gram-negative bacteria, viruses, and fungi. Chlorhexidine has an intermediate rapidity of action, disrupting the cell membrane; it works well against gram-positive bacteria, and less well against gram-negative bacteria. Iodine/iodophors has an intermediate action and is acceptable for use against a wide range of bacteria, fungi, and viruses. Triclosan disrupts the cell wall and has an acceptable kill rate against bacteria. Even though alcohol has microbial action, it is not often used as a surgical skin prep because it does not stay on the skin.

Conditions that Place Clients at Risk for Postoperative Infection

- Uncontrolled diabetes
- Renal failure
- Obesity; advanced age
- Receiving corticosteroids
- Receiving immunosuppressive agents
- Prolonged antibiotic therapy
- Protein or ascorbic acid deficiencies
- Marked dehydration and hypovolemia
- Decreased cardiac output
- Edema and fluid and electrolyte imbalances
- Anemia
- Preoperative infection

6. Assess for latex allergy. If present, ensure allergy band is applied, physician is notified, and OR staff are notified. **Rationale:** All latex products must be removed from OR and client must be scheduled for first case in morning.
7. Enquire for symptoms and observe for signs of cold or upper respiratory infection.
8. Explain need for client to be NPO for 8–10 hours preoperatively.
9. Remove lipstick and nail polish.
10. Insert Foley catheter if ordered.
11. Take and record vital signs.
12. Remove earrings, necklaces, medals, watch, rings (ring may be taped to finger in some facilities).
13. Remove contact lenses, glasses, hairpieces, and dentures.
14. Assist client to void if catheter not inserted, and record time and amount.
15. Check identaband, blood band, and allergy bracelet.
16. Put antiembolic stockings on client as ordered.
17. Administer preoperative medications.
18. Place side rails in UP position and bed in low position following administration of medications.
19. Darken room, and provide quiet environment following administration of medications.
20. Check client 15 minutes after medication administered to observe for possible side effects.

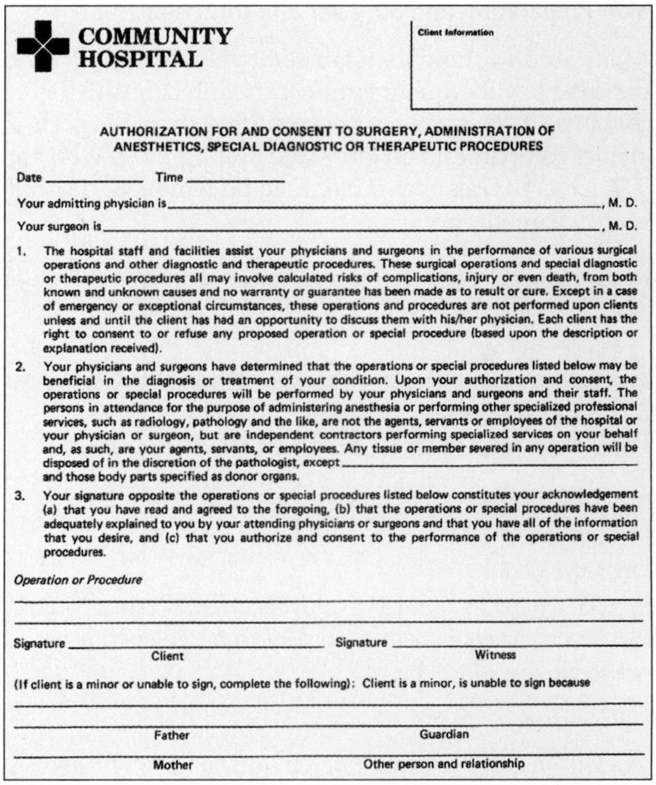

COMMUNITY HOSPITAL

Client Information

AUTHORIZATION FOR AND CONSENT TO SURGERY, ADMINISTRATION OF ANESTHETICS, SPECIAL DIAGNOSTIC OR THERAPEUTIC PROCEDURES

Date ____________ Time ____________

Your admitting physician is ______________________________, M. D.

Your surgeon is ______________________________, M. D.

1. The hospital staff and facilities assist your physicians and surgeons in the performance of various surgical operations and other diagnostic and therapeutic procedures. These surgical operations and special diagnostic or therapeutic procedures all may involve calculated risks of complications, injury or even death, from both known and unknown causes and no warranty or guarantee has been made as to result or cure. Except in a case of emergency or exceptional circumstances, these operations and procedures are not performed upon clients unless and until the client has had an opportunity to discuss them with his/her physician. Each client has the right to consent to or refuse any proposed operation or special procedure (based upon the description or explanation received).
2. Your physicians and surgeons have determined that the operations or special procedures listed below may be beneficial in the diagnosis or treatment of your condition. Upon your authorization and consent, the operations or special procedures will be performed by your physicians and surgeons and their staff. The persons in attendance for the purpose of administering anesthesia or performing other specialized professional services, such as radiology, pathology and the like, are not the agents, servants or employees of the hospital or your physician or surgeon, but are independent contractors performing specialized services on your behalf and, as such, are your agents, servants, or employees. Any tissue or member severed in any operation will be disposed of in the discretion of the pathologist, except ______________________ and those body parts specified as donor organs.
3. Your signature opposite the operations or special procedures listed below constitutes your acknowledgement (a) that you have read and agreed to the foregoing, (b) that the operations or special procedures have been adequately explained to you by your attending physicians or surgeons and that you have all of the information that you desire, and (c) that you authorize and consent to the performance of the operations or special procedures.

Operation or Procedure

____

____

Signature ____________________ (Client)   Signature ____________________ (Witness)

(If client is a minor or unable to sign, complete the following): Client is a minor, is unable to sign because

____

____
Father   Guardian

____
Mother   Other person and relationship

Surgical Consent form.

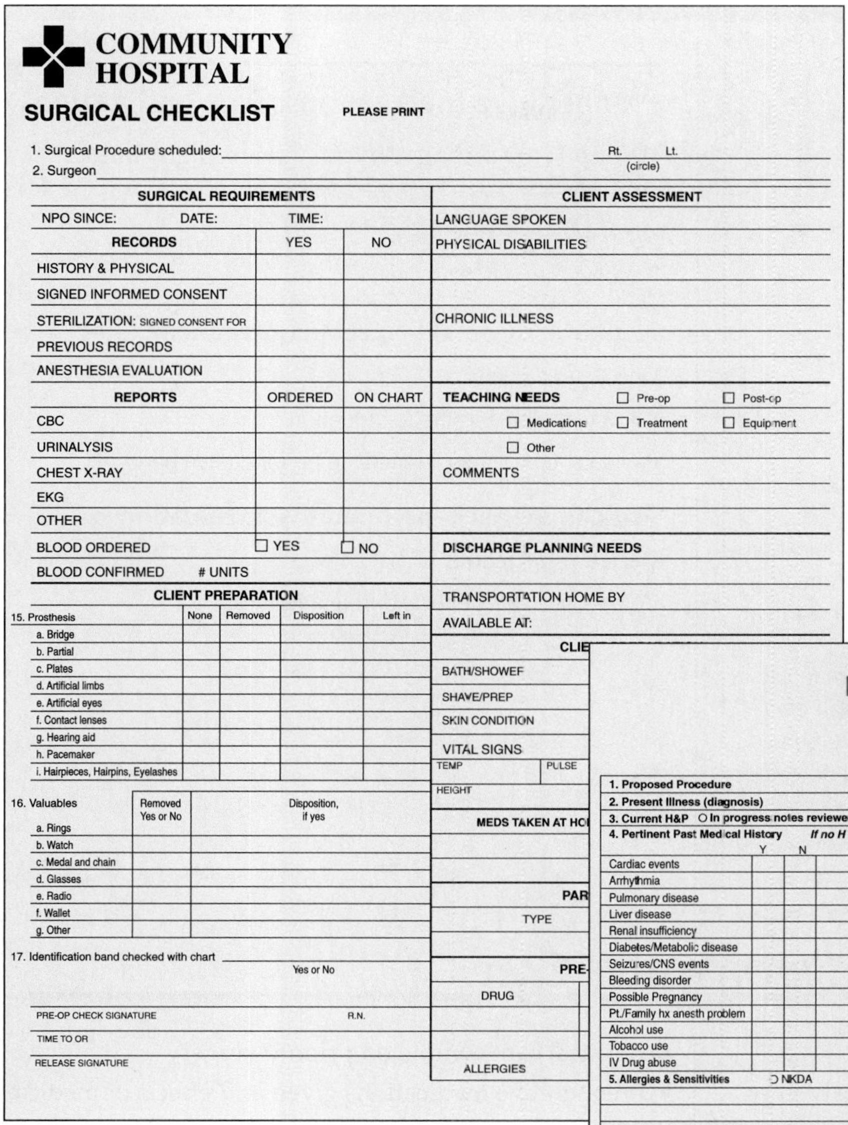

COMMUNITY HOSPITAL

SURGICAL CHECKLIST PLEASE PRINT

1. Surgical Procedure scheduled: ________ Rt. Lt. (circle)
2. Surgeon ________

SURGICAL REQUIREMENTS		
NPO SINCE: DATE: TIME:		
RECORDS	YES	NO
HISTORY & PHYSICAL		
SIGNED INFORMED CONSENT		
STERILIZATION: SIGNED CONSENT FOR		
PREVIOUS RECORDS		
ANESTHESIA EVALUATION		
REPORTS	ORDERED	ON CHART
CBC		
URINALYSIS		
CHEST X-RAY		
EKG		
OTHER		
BLOOD ORDERED	☐ YES	☐ NO
BLOOD CONFIRMED # UNITS		

CLIENT ASSESSMENT

LANGUAGE SPOKEN

PHYSICAL DISABILITIES

CHRONIC ILLNESS

TEACHING NEEDS ☐ Pre-op ☐ Post-op ☐ Medications ☐ Treatment ☐ Equipment ☐ Other

COMMENTS

DISCHARGE PLANNING NEEDS

TRANSPORTATION HOME BY

AVAILABLE AT:

CLIENT PREPARATION

15. Prosthesis	None	Removed	Disposition	Left in
a. Bridge				
b. Partial				
c. Plates				
d. Artificial limbs				
e. Artificial eyes				
f. Contact lenses				
g. Hearing aid				
h. Pacemaker				
i. Hairpieces, Hairpins, Eyelashes				

16. Valuables	Removed Yes or No	Disposition, if yes
a. Rings		
b. Watch		
c. Medal and chain		
d. Glasses		
e. Radio		
f. Wallet		
g. Other		

17. Identification band checked with chart ________ Yes or No

PRE-OP CHECK SIGNATURE R.N.

TIME TO OR

RELEASE SIGNATURE

CLIE…

BATH/SHOWER

SHAVE/PREP

SKIN CONDITION

VITAL SIGNS

TEMP PULSE

HEIGHT

MEDS TAKEN AT HO…

PAR…

TYPE

PRE-…

DRUG

ALLERGIES

Surgical Preoperative Checklist.

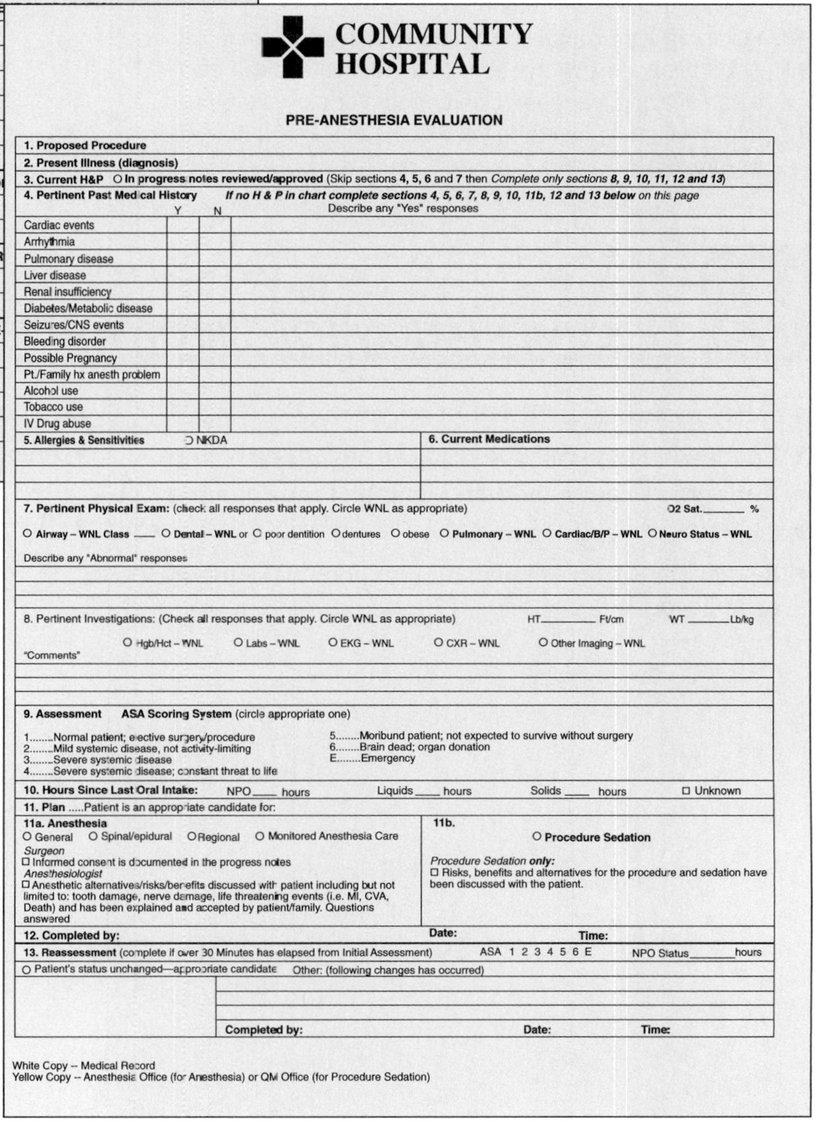

COMMUNITY HOSPITAL

PRE-ANESTHESIA EVALUATION

1. Proposed Procedure
2. Present Illness (diagnosis)
3. Current H&P ○ In progress notes reviewed/approved (Skip sections 4, 5, 6 and 7 then *Complete only sections 8, 9, 10, 11, 12 and 13*)
4. Pertinent Past Medical History *If no H & P in chart complete sections 4, 5, 6, 7, 8, 9, 10, 11b, 12 and 13 below on this page*

	Y	N	Describe any "Yes" responses
Cardiac events			
Arrhythmia			
Pulmonary disease			
Liver disease			
Renal insufficiency			
Diabetes/Metabolic disease			
Seizures/CNS events			
Bleeding disorder			
Possible Pregnancy			
Pt./Family hx anesth problem			
Alcohol use			
Tobacco use			
IV Drug abuse			

5. Allergies & Sensitivities ○ NKDA
6. Current Medications

7. Pertinent Physical Exam: (check all responses that apply. Circle WNL as appropriate) O2 Sat.______ %

○ Airway – WNL Class ___ ○ Dental – WNL or ○ poor dentition ○ dentures ○ obese ○ Pulmonary – WNL ○ Cardiac/B/P – WNL ○ Neuro Status – WNL

Describe any "Abnormal" responses

8. Pertinent Investigations: (Check all responses that apply. Circle WNL as appropriate) HT______ Ft/cm WT______ Lb/kg

○ Hgb/Hct – WNL ○ Labs – WNL ○ EKG – WNL ○ CXR – WNL ○ Other Imaging – WNL

"Comments"

9. Assessment ASA Scoring System (circle appropriate one)

1........Normal patient; elective surgery/procedure
2........Mild systemic disease, not activity-limiting
3........Severe systemic disease
4........Severe systemic disease; constant threat to life
5........Moribund patient; not expected to survive without surgery
6........Brain dead; organ donation
E........Emergency

10. Hours Since Last Oral Intake: NPO____ hours Liquids____ hours Solids____ hours ☐ Unknown

11. Plan .....Patient is an appropriate candidate for:

11a. Anesthesia
○ General ○ Spinal/epidural ○ Regional ○ Monitored Anesthesia Care
Surgeon
☐ Informed consent is documented in the progress notes
Anesthesiologist
☐ Anesthetic alternatives/risks/benefits discussed with patient including but not limited to: tooth damage, nerve damage, life threatening events (i.e. MI, CVA, Death) and has been explained and accepted by patient/family. Questions answered

11b. ○ Procedure Sedation
*Procedure Sedation **only:***
☐ Risks, benefits and alternatives for the procedure and sedation have been discussed with the patient.

12. Completed by: Date: Time:

13. Reassessment (complete if over 30 Minutes has elapsed from Initial Assessment) ASA 1 2 3 4 5 6 E NPO Status______ hours

○ Patient's status unchanged—appropriate candidate Other: (following changes has occurred)

Completed by: Date: Time:

White Copy -- Medical Record
Yellow Copy -- Anesthesia Office (for Anesthesia) or QM Office (for Procedure Sedation)

Preanesthesia evaluation form.

ADMINISTERING PREOPERATIVE MEDICATIONS

Equipment

Preoperative checklist
Preoperative medications

Procedure

1. Complete preoperative checklist.
2. Check orders for medication, dosage, route, and time.
3. Check history for allergy to ordered medication.
4. Explain purpose of medication to client.
5. Warn client that injection may sting or burn.
6. Follow procedure for administration of injections.
7. Administer medication.
8. Raise side rails to UP position and put bed in low position.
9. Explain why client should not get out of bed after medications have been given. **Rationale:** Medication makes client drowsy and affects equilibrium.
10. Place call light within reach, and encourage client to use it.
11. Ask if there are any questions or assistance you can offer before leaving the room. Darken room or close curtains.
12. Inform client of the estimated time he or she will be going to surgery.

Preoperative Medications: Type and Action

Hypnotic or antianxiolytic—given night before surgery

Decreases anxiety

Promotes good night's sleep

Hypnotic or opiate—preoperative medication

Decreases anxiety

Allows smooth anesthetic induction

Provides amnesia for immediate perioperative period

Anticholinergic—preoperative medication

Decreases secretions

Counteracts vagal effects during anesthesia

DOCUMENTATION FOR PREOPERATIVE CARE

- Safety measures carried out preoperatively
- Completion of preoperative shave and area involved
- Antiseptic solution used and length of time of scrub
- Operative checklist completed
- Review physician's explanation of potential surgical complications
- Physical care completed prior to surgery
- Preoperative medications given and effects of medications
- Time and method of transportation to operating room
- Preoperative teaching completed

Critical Thinking Application

UNEXPECTED OUTCOMES	CRITICAL THINKING OPTIONS
Factors that can affect the postoperative course are identified during the preoperative care (e.g., arthritic changes in client's back, history of thrombophlebitis).	• Place information on client's care plan, and inform charge nurse about findings. • Write a note on client's chart, and alert the operating room and recovery room staff of the findings so that they can assess for the problems.
Client refuses to go to operating room without dentures.	• Explain to client that dentures are likely to be lost, broken, or inadvertently pushed to back of mouth if not removed. • If client refuses to remove dentures, alert anesthesiologist that dentures are in place.
Client's skin is cut during shave.	• Notify MD and OR staff of client's condition. • Follow specific directions; surgery may be cancelled as infection could occur as result of break in skin integrity.
Client unable to void before surgery.	• Run water so client can hear trickling sound to stimulate voiding. • Run warm water over perineum. • Place ammonia or oil of wintergreen on a cotton ball in urinal or bedpan.
Client appears to be abnormally stressed.	• Explore feelings and reasons for client's or family's stressed behaviors. • Explore more effective methods to reduce stress for client and family. • Provide additional stress reduction exercises. • Clarify misconceptions and inappropriate perceptions. • Introduce client to another client who has had similar surgery. • Have physician speak to client and answer questions.
Client's preoperative laboratory findings are abnormal.	• Check with laboratory to have them reevaluate if lab results are accurate. • Have laboratory return tests if extremely abnormal. • Notify physician of abnormal findings.
Client states he or she is to have a different surgery or a different surgical side/site.	• Verify with chart and surgeon. • Make sure x-rays are available to verify correct side/site; and mark correct side/site before client leaves preop area.

UNIT 4

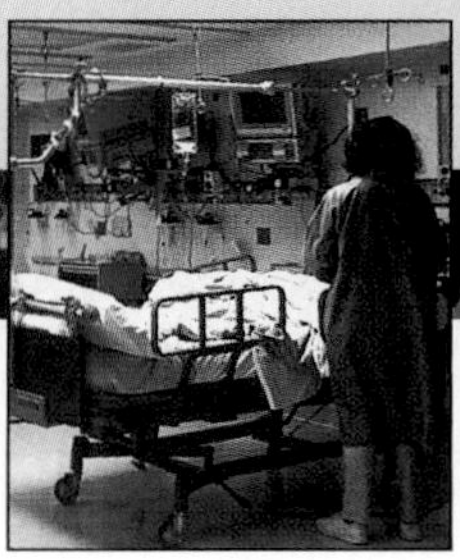

Conscious Sedation

Nursing Process Data

ASSESSMENT Data Base

Assess type of procedure to be done and determine if conscious sedation is appropriate.

Assess type of sedation to be used for procedure.

Determine if medication can be administered by nurse or only by physician.

Check if physician has ordered medication for conscious sedation and if nurse is approved to administer medication.

Determine if history and physical is in client's chart.

Check that signed consent form is in chart.

Assess client's American Society of Anesthesiologists (ASA) Classification of Physical Status

PLANNING Objectives

To determine if client is to receive conscious sedation from nurse or physician

To establish venous access prior to sedation administration

To monitor vital signs throughout procedure

To continuously assess for changes in client's condition and/or untoward responses or effects of medication

To immediately notify physician of changes in client's condition

IMPLEMENTATION Procedures

Preparing Client for Conscious Sedation

Monitoring Client During Procedure

Caring for Client Following Conscious Sedation

EVALUATION Expected Outcomes

Client maintains airway and respiratory status throughout procedure.

Client does not experience anxiety or pain during procedure.

PREPARING CLIENT FOR CONSCIOUS SEDATION

Equipment

Consent form
History and physical
Lab test results, if necessary
Scale

Procedure

1. Ensure that client is candidate for conscious sedation. Use ASA Classification of Physical Status. **Rationale:** Clients in ASA categories 1 and 2 may receive conscious sedation by qualified physicians and nurses. Clients in category 3 or 4 are referred to anesthesia for further evaluation because their condition puts them at risk for complications. Further evaluation of elderly, pregnant or obese clients, and those with a history of substance abuse, sleep apnea, or severe cardiac, respiratory, hepatic, renal or central nervous system diseases are placed at higher risk during the use of conscious sedation.
2. Determine if nurse or physician will administer medication.
3. Check that qualified anesthesia provider has written order for conscious sedation.
4. Check that client has been informed about procedure and use of conscious sedation.
5. Ensure that history and physical has been completed and on client's chart.
6. Obtain height and weight. **Rationale:** To use for drug calculation when administering conscious sedation.
7. Ask about allergies, particularly sedatives.
8. Explain that the medication will relax him or her during procedure, client will feel sleepy but will not be asleep, and will be able to communicate during procedure. **Rationale:** This is necessary to determine comfort and level of sedation during procedure
9. Determine gestures that will be used during procedure to indicate if client is having pain.
10. Ensure that someone is with the client to take him or her home if discharge is anticipated following the procedure. **Rationale:** Residual effects of sedation can last for several hours. Driving can be impaired and thus it is unsafe for the client to drive home.

NOTE: The American Nurses Association and other nursing organizations allow nurses to administer sedating drugs, assess client responses, and monitor vital signs during the use of conscious sedation. Nurses who administer conscious sedation must function within the standard of practice and be allowed to administer conscious sedation according to the nurse practice act in the state in which they are practicing. They must also administer conscious sedation according to policies and procedures of facility in which they are working. At no time will student nurses be allowed to administer conscious sedation.

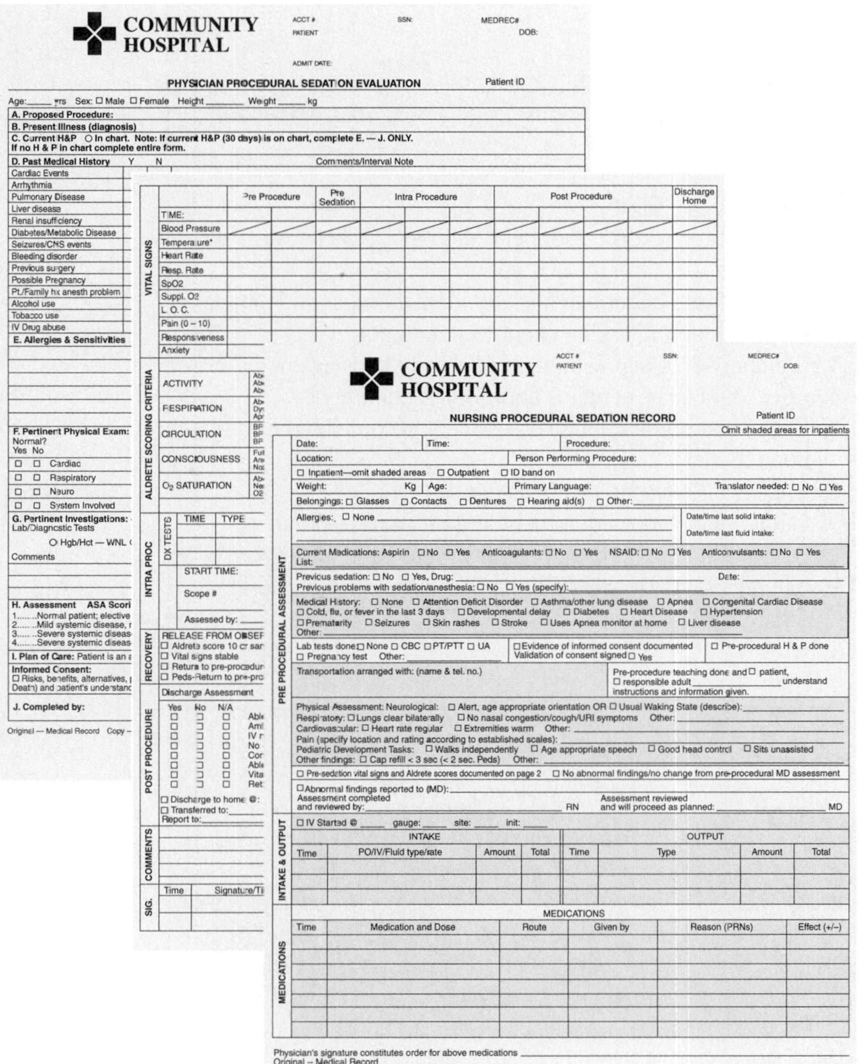

Conscious Sedation Record Samples.

MONITORING CLIENT DURING PROCEDURE

Equipment

Crash cart or following list of equipment:

- Suction equipment; machine, tubing, and suction catheter (tonsil tip)
- Oxygen supply and appropriate delivery system
- Laryngoscope handle and blades of appropriate size
- Endotracheal tubes and stylets in various sizes
- Oral and nasal cannulas
- 3 mL and 10 mL syringes
- Needles, if not using needless system
- IV solution bags
- Reversal drug agents (i.e., Narcan, Romazicon)

Pulse oximeter
ECG machine and defibrillator
Intubation tray and bag–valve–mask device
Vital sign portable machine
Client's chart
Procedural sedation record
Conscious sedation medications; usually benzodiazepines and opioids

Procedure

1. Ensure that backup personnel skilled in ACLS are available if needed.
2. Verify correct client by checking identaband and identification number and asking client to state name.
3. Evaluate ASA Classification of Physical Status again.
4. Check that chart contains appropriate documents.
5. Check that preprocedural assessment is completed on sedation record.
6. Check that consent form was signed.
7. Gather emergency equipment and place near client.
8. Determine if premedication was ordered and given.
9. Obtain vital signs and document findings on procedural sedation record.

Levels of Sedation

Minimal	Client is relaxed and may be awake. Understands direction and can answer questions.
Moderate	Client is drowsy and may sleep through procedure. Easily awakened by touch or voice.
Deep	Client will sleep through procedure. Little or no memory of procedure. Supplemental oxygen is given because breathing slows down.

Conscious Sedation Medications

The most common drugs used for conscious sedation are the benzodiazepines and opioids.

Benzodiazepines	**Opioids**
DRUGS:	
Midazolam, versad, diazepam, lorazepam*	Fentanyl, morphine, meperidine
ACTION:	
Produce anxiolysis and amnesia	Produce sedation, euphoria, pain relief
DISADVANTAGES:	
Lack of analgesic properties	Can cause respiratory depression and decreased level of consciousness
SIDE EFFECTS:	
Decreased blood pressure Increased heart rate	Apnea, hypotension, vertigo, nausea
REVERSAL AGENT:	
Flumazenil	Naloxone

**Frequently administered with narcotics.*

10. Start peripheral IV with ordered solution.
11. Determine gesture to be used for communication regarding pain and sedation.
12. Place ECG leads on, if appropriate.
13. Administer oxygen via nasal cannula at 2 L/min.
14. Begin administration of medication as ordered.
15. Monitor vital signs, oxygen saturation, sedation level, pain level, ECG rate and rhythm every one to five minutes according to facility policy and client condition.

EVIDENCE BASED NURSING PRACTICE

Over- and Undersedation

A survey of critical care nurses and physicians revealed they felt that their critically ill clients were receiving adequate sedation only 50% of the time. Interestingly enough, physicians felt their clients were oversedated and nurses felt clients were undersedated.

Source: McGaffigan. (2000, February), Advancing sedation assessment to promote patient comfort, *Critical Care Nurse* Supplement, 29–36.

Rationale: Close monitoring of these values identifies potential complication such as respiratory depression, oversedation, hypoxia, and hypotension.

16. Continue to monitor client every 15 minutes until stable following completion of procedure using conscious sedation.

CLINICAL ALERT

The sedation assessment parameters that need to be observed during the procedure include: responsiveness, speech, facial expressions, and eyes. Scales available that provide a scoring system are the Ramsay Sedation Scale and the Riker Sedation–Agitation Scale.

CARING FOR CLIENT FOLLOWING CONSCIOUS SEDATION

Equipment

Electronic vital sign machine
Oxygen supply
Oxygen nasal cannula
Procedural sedation record
Aldrete scale
Pulse oximeter
ECG monitor and leads
Emergency equipment

Procedure

1. Observe vital signs, oxygen saturation, respiratory rate and rhythm, and ECG rate and rhythm every 15 minutes unless more frequent monitoring is required according to client condition. **Rationale:** Major complications during the use of conscious sedation and immediately following include respiratory depression, oversedation, hypoxia, and hypotension.
2. Observe client for patent airway if he or she was intubated during procedure and ensure oxygen cannula is in place immediately following extubation.
3. Assess client for pain and medicate accordingly.
4. Monitor client and provide Aldrete Score in preparation for discharge. Client must attain specified score within one hour of completion of procedure. **Rationale:** Client must attain Aldrete score of ±1 point of preprocedure score before discharge. This score should be achieved within one hour of the procedure. A potential complication is occurring if this score is not attained within the specified time.
5. Provide instructions as needed before client is discharged.
6. Ensure client has someone with him or her if discharged to home.
7. Complete documentation on Procedural Sedation Record.

ASA Classification of Physical Status

Class	Definition
P1	A normal healthy client
P2	A client with mild systemic disease
P3	A client with severe systemic disease
P4	A client with severe systemic disease that is a constant threat to life
P5	A moribund client who is not expected to survive without surgery
P6	A declared brain-dead client whose organs are being removed for donor

Source: Adapted from the American Society of Anesthesiologists. ASA Physical Classification System, 1999.

DOCUMENTATION FOR CONSCIOUS SEDATION

- Preprocedural assessment: past medical history, drug allergies, anesthetic history
- Baseline vital signs, particularly respiratory and cardiac findings, ECG findings
- Height and weight
- Teaching provided regarding medication and procedure
- ASA rating
- Continuous documentation of level of consciousness, speech, facial expression, agitation level, pupils, respiratory rate and rhythm, ECG findings if appropriate during procedure
- Score on a sedation scale (Ramsay or Riker)
- Oxygen saturation levels during and following procedure
- Amount and type of medication administered

- Supplemental oxygen, liter flow, and system used
- Aldrete score prior to discharge
- Complications that occurred during the procedure and actions taken
- Complete Procedural Sedation Record

Critical Thinking Application

UNEXPECTED OUTCOMES	CRITICAL THINKING OPTIONS
Client is scheduled to have conscious sedation for procedure but scores above P2 on ASA scale.	• Notify anesthesiologist and physician; nurses may not administer conscious sedation if the client scores above P2 on the scale. • Client is physically compromised and could be unstable during use of conscious sedation medications.
Client does not respond to verbal commands during procedure when using minimal or moderate sedation.	• Notify physician of change in client's status. • Notify anesthesiologist immediately and prepare for intubation. • Have reversal drug available to administer if directed by physician. • Continue to monitor client every one minute for changes in status. • Administer oxygen via nasal cannula if not already in place.
Client experiences airway obstruction or respiratory depression.	• Reposition client's head, lifting jaw and tipping back the head. • Suction client or insert oral airway. • Be prepared to bag client, with bag–valve–mask device.
Client experiences hypoxemia.	• Ensure pulse oximeter is on client. • Check respiratory rate, pattern, and effort. • Increase amount of oxygen delivered. May need to change delivery system to oxygen mask.
Client experiences a 20% drop in blood pressure during procedure.	• Inform physician. • Assess client for potential complications leading to decrease in blood pressure. • Check for presence of hypovolemia. Administer 200 mL bolus of fluid and monitor for response.

UNIT 5

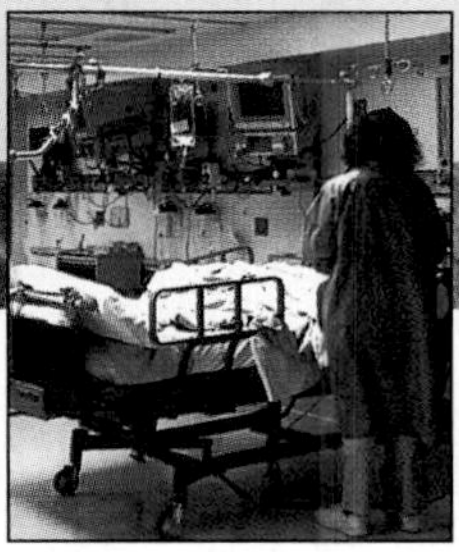

Postanesthesia Care Unit (PACU) and Discharge

Nursing Process Data

ASSESSMENT *Data Base*

Assess for patent airway.

Assess for order and type of oxygen administration set.

Check gag reflex, and remove endotracheal tube as ordered.

Assess vital signs and appropriate pulses.

Assess body temperature.

Check all IVs for type, amount of fluid, and infusion rate.

Observe all dressings, tubes, and drains.

Monitor urine output, color, and consistency.

Assess color, skin temperature, and condition.

Assess monitor findings if ordered.

Assess neurologic status if necessary.

Assess heart and lung sounds.

Assess bowel sounds.

Assess residual anesthetic effect.

Assess for postoperative bleeding.

PLANNING *Objectives*

To provide safe effective nursing care during the immediate postoperative period for clients in the recovery room

To promote and maintain adequate airway function

To monitor and maintain adequate circulatory status

To identify potential postanesthesia complications and initiate nursing interventions to prevent complications

To identify client's readiness to return to nursing unit or to be discharged if an outpatient

IMPLEMENTATION *Procedures*

Providing Postanesthesia Care

Discharging Client from Postanesthesia Unit to Nursing Unit

Discharging Client from Phase II Unit to Home

EVALUATION *Expected Outcomes*

Client experiences no untoward effects during recovery period.

Potential postanesthesia complications are identified early, and appropriate nursing actions are taken to prevent occurrence of complications.

Client is discharged from postanesthesia unit at appropriate time.

PROVIDING POSTANESTHESIA CARE

Equipment

Blood pressure cuff and stethoscope
Pulse oximeter
Oxygen administration device: nasal cannula or mask
Cardiac monitor and leads
IV pole
Suction catheters
Gloves
Special equipment needed—based on surgical procedure

Procedure

1. Identify client and determine surgical procedure performed.
2. Obtain report, and review chart with anesthesiologist and operating room nurse.
3. Connect client to monitoring systems.
4. Assess for patent airway. Leave airway in place until gag reflex returns and client attempts to remove it. **Rationale:** This promotes adequate airway exchange and prevents tongue from falling back and occluding airway.
5. Administer humidified SpO_2 by mask or nasal cannula at 6 L/min or as ordered. **Rationale:** Humidified oxygen prevents drying of the tracheobronchial tree and liquifies secretions to facilitate expectoration.
6. Monitor oxygen saturation using finger probe monitor.
7. Encourage client to cough and deep breathe when awake.
8. Suction client as needed.
9. Position client to ensure adequate ventilation. Side-lying position is best if not contraindicated. Turn every hour if not contraindicated. **Rationale:** This prevents pooling of secretions in lungs and assists with ventilation.
10. Monitor vital signs every 5–15 minutes as condition warrants. Vital signs are sometimes difficult to obtain due to hypothermia and movement from operating room to postanesthesia care unit.
    a. Check pulse rate, quality, and rhythm; include pulse distal to surgical site.
    b. Check blood pressure, pulse pressure, and quality.
    c. Check respiratory rate, rhythm, depth, and pattern.
    d. Assess pain level, determine cause, and medicate as needed.
11. Maintain body temperature by applying warm blankets. **Rationale:** Operating rooms are cold, which promotes vasoconstriction.
12. Observe for adverse signs of general or spinal anesthesia:
    a. Level of consciousness.
    b. Movement of extremities.
13. Monitor IV fluids.
    a. Verify correct type and amount of solution being administered.
    b. Set appropriate flow rate using IV pump or controller if needed.
    c. Observe IV site for signs of infiltration.
    d. Maintain accurate IV intake record.
14. Monitor blood or blood component infusions.
    a. Identify appropriate replacement fluid.
    b. Check client's name and identification number with fluid.
    c. Check blood type, blood bank number, and expiration date.
    d. Check time infusion initiated.
    e. Observe and record amount of fluid remaining in bag when admitted to recovery room.
    f. Determine time frame for completion of fluid.
15. Monitor and measure urine output hourly if indwelling catheter is in place or before client leaves recovery room.

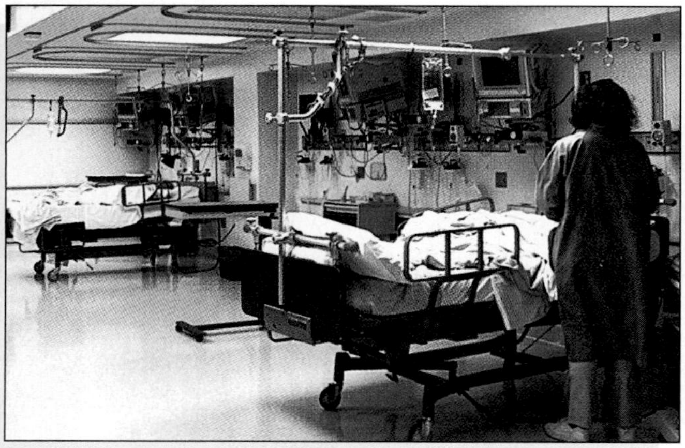

Recovery room is usually an open space for easy observation of all clients.

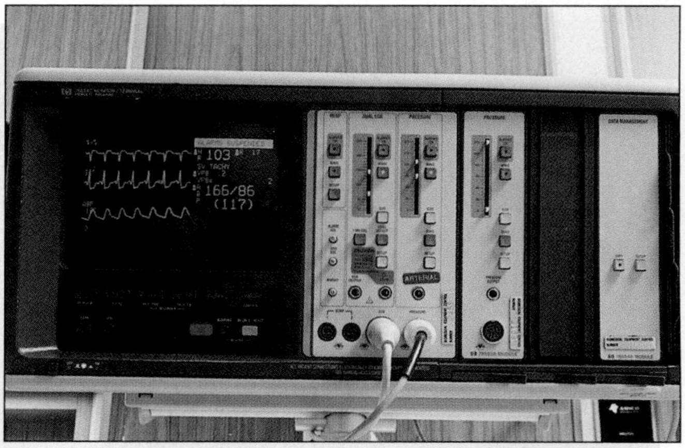

Clients are connected to monitoring system for cardiac surveillance.

16. Observe surgical dressings and drains hourly.
    a. Follow hospital policy for marking drainage on dressings.
    b. Note color and amount of drainage on dressings and from drains or tubes.
    c. Check that dressings are secure.
    d. Reinforce dressings as needed.
    e. Empty drainage collection device as needed.
    f. Report unusual amount or type of drainage to physician before client leaves recovery room.
17. Monitor skin for warmth, color, and moisture.
18. Check nail beds and mucous membranes for color and blanching. Report unusual findings or signs of cyanosis to physician immediately.
19. Orient client to surroundings and relieve anxiety and fear.
20. Observe for return of movement, especially if client received spinal or epidural anesthesia.
21. Monitor for muscle strength/movement.
22. Administer all STAT drugs.
23. Complete PAR record.
24. Assess parameters for discharge from postanesthesia room.

COMMUNITY HOSPITAL

PAR Record

ADMITTED TO PAR AM PM	AWAKE ON ARRIVAL ☐	TIME AWAKE AM PM	RELEASED AM PM	OPERATION
APPARENT CONDITION ON ARRIVAL GOOD FAIR POOR		APPARENT CONDITION ON RELEASE GOOD FAIR POOR		SURGEON
ALLERGIES:				ANESTHEOLOGIST
INTAKE	ADMITTED TO PAR WITH:	RELEASED FROM PAR WITH:		ANESTHESIA GENERAL REGIONAL SPINAL CAUDAL
	IV	IV		OXYGEN NASAL MASK TRACHAEL TENT
				AIRWAY ORAL NASAL TRACHEAL
	BLOOD	BLOOD		MONITORING:
	TOTAL IV FLUIDS OR	TOTAL BLOOD OR		TIME: ON OFF
	TOTAL IV FLUIDS PAR	TOTAL BLOOD PAR		EKG
OUTPUT	TOTAL FLUID LOSS OR	PAR:		CVP
	EBL:			ART
	URINE:			VENTILATOR
	DRAINAGE:			
	NG:			OTHER:
	HEMOVAC:			
	CHEST			

ALDRETE SCORING CRITERIA	Post Anesthetic Recovery Score		TIME	ADM	15'	30'	45'	1'	15'	30'	45'	2'	15'	30'
	ACTIVITY	Able to move 4 extremities voluntarily or on command	2											
		Able to move 2 extremities voluntarily or on command	1											
		Able to move 0 extremities voluntarily or on command	0											
	RESPIRATION	Able to breathe deeply and cough freely	2											
		Dyspnea or limited breathing	1											
		Apneic (needs ventilator or assistance)	0											
	CIRCULATION	BP ± 20% of pre-anesthetic level	2											
		BP ± 20–49% of pre-anesthetic level	1											
		BP ± 50% of pre-anesthetic level	0											
	CONSCIOUSNESS	Fully awake	2											
		Arousable on calling	1											
		Not responding	0											
	O2 SATURATION	Able to maintain O_2 saturation > 92% on room air	2											
		Needs O_2 inhalation to maintain O_2 saturation > 90%	1											
		O_2 saturation < 90% even with O_2 supplement	0											
		TOTAL SCORE												

PAR record.

DISCHARGING CLIENT FROM POSTANESTHESIA UNIT TO NURSING UNIT

Procedure

1. Assess that lung sounds are clear to auscultation and airway is maintained without artificial measures (unless client is to remain on mechanical assistance).
2. Assess that vital signs are within normal range for at least 1 hour and appropriate for client's condition.
3. Observe that client is awake, alert, and responds to commands.
4. Assess that reflexes are present (including gag, swallowing) and that client can move all extremities.
5. Assess skin color and nail beds for signs of cyanosis.
6. Ensure IVs are patent, infusing with correct solution and at prescribed rate. Record total amount of IV fluid infused and amount remaining in bags. Ensure all IVs and irrigating solutions are in sufficient quantity for transfer and immediate continuity of care.
7. Check that all dressings are intact, and there is no excessive drainage from drains or tubes. Reinforce dressings if needed and empty all drainage collection receptables before returning to nursing unit.

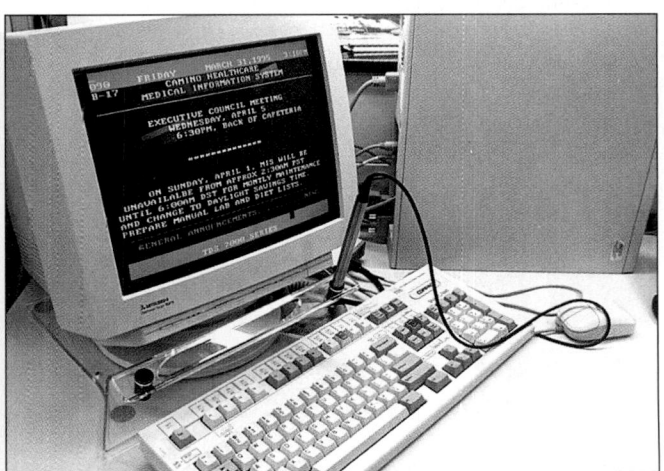

Recovery room documentation is accomplished using computerized system.

8. Ensure urinary output is adequate. Record all urine output and empty drainage bag before transporting to nursing unit.
9. Record all medications administered in recovery room.
10. Medicate client ½ hour before transport if vital signs are stable and client requires pain medication. **Rationale:**

Transporting clients from postanesthesia room can increase pain due to moving and transfer from gurney to bed.

11. Call anesthesiologist for discharge orders or use Aldrete Postanesthesia Recovery Scoring System if used by facility.
12. Call for transport assistance if available. Postanesthesia room nurse accompanies client to nursing unit.
13. Call nursing unit, and provide information on equipment needs for client (e.g., oxygen, IVs).
14. Document all findings in computer or in chart before discharge.
15. Provide report to unit nurse.
    a. Type of surgical procedure performed.
    b. Type of anesthesia and length of procedure.
    c. Length of time in postanesthesia room.
    d. Condition of client at time of discharge from postanesthesia room.
    e. Report on vital signs, IVs, dressings, drains, tubes, need for special equipment, medications received, and time given.

Aldrete Postanesthesia Recovery Scoring System

This is one method for determining if postanesthesia room discharge criteria have been met. In addition to stable vital signs, a total score of 10 for the 5 assessed areas must be achieved for nurses to discharge clients without a physician's order. The areas assessed include:

- Ability to move extremities voluntarily or on command
- Ability to cough and deep breathe freely
- Blood pressure maintained within 20 mm Hg of preanesthesia values
- Fully awake
- Normal skin color

DISCHARGING CLIENT FROM PHASE II UNIT TO HOME

Procedure

1. Follow all actions for Discharging a Client from Postanesthesia Unit to Nursing Unit.
2. Assess for nausea or light-headedness. **Rationale:** These symptoms may be a result of anesthesia or hypovolemia. The client is not discharged until these symptoms have abated or are medically treated.
3. Provide discharge teaching regarding medications, activity, dressing changes, physician office visit, etc. If client is unable to understand instructions, provide information to person taking client home. Send written instructions home with client as well.
4. Assist client to side of bed, feet on floor, and allow to sit for a few minutes. **Rationale:** To prevent a fall when standing as a result of postural hypotension.
5. Assess client's ability to dress self or identify what assistance is needed.
6. Obtain prescriptions from pharmacy if needed.
7. Place client's equipment, supplies, and medications in a plastic bag and hand to person taking client home.
8. Transfer client to wheelchair.
9. Take client to car and assist with transfer.
10. Document all activity related to discharge including person taking client home and method of transport.

DOCUMENTATION FOR POSTANESTHESIA ROOM CARE

for Nursing Unit

- Assessment findings
- Effects of anesthesia
- Status of airway management
- Need for oxygen administration
- Status of neurologic signs and reflexes
- Fluid replacement—type and amount
- Blood and blood product replacement
- Medications administered
- Condition of dressings, drains, and tubes
- Intake and output from all sources: urine, drains, tubes, IVs
- Vital signs: T, P, R, BP, and pain
- Description of pain and interventions for relief of pain
- Response to postanesthesia room activities
- Discharged to room (number) and transporter

for Discharge Home

- Additional charting includes: ability to stand or transfer to wheelchair
- Discharge teaching completed

- Signs or symptoms of nausea, light-headedness
- Discharged to care at home
- Discharged via automobile or other means of transportation.

Critical Thinking Application

UNEXPECTED OUTCOMES	CRITICAL THINKING OPTIONS
Client experiences untoward effects in postanesthesia room	• Contact physician for additional orders. • Complete physical assessment. • Identify and initiate appropriate nursing interventions within allowed guidelines and parameters of the facility.
Client does not awaken easily.	• Retain client in postanesthesia room; check Glasgow scale. • Continue to provide oxygen. • Arouse every 15 minutes. • Check pain medication (may need Narcan).
Client has postoperative hemorrhage.	• Apply direct pressure. • Notify physician immediately. • Assess for signs of hypovolemia. • Assess for signs of overt bleeding, i.e., saturated dressings, large amount of drainage in drainage collection devices, increase in girth of affected surgical area. • Check lab values for hematocrit, hemoglobin and coagulation levels. • Check records for estimated blood loss during surgery.

UNIT 6

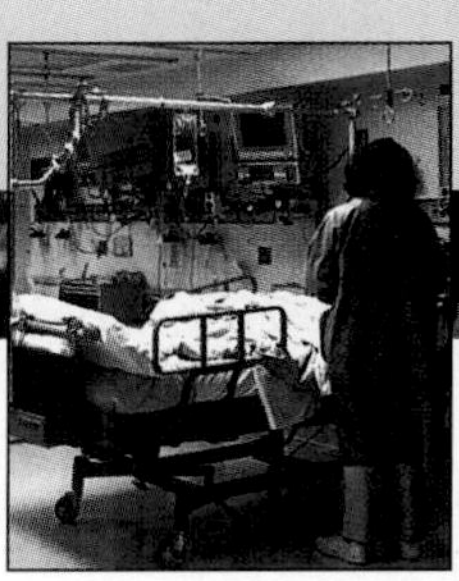

Postoperative Care

Nursing Process Data

ASSESSMENT *Data Base*

Assess for patent airway.

Check if oxygen is ordered.

Auscultate lungs.

Observe for adverse signs of general anesthesia or spinal anesthesia.

Take vital signs (T, P, R, BP, and pain).

Check client's temperature for heat control.

Observe dressings and surgical drains.

Check IVs for type and amount of fluid to be infused.

Observe color and amount of urine.

Auscultate bowel sounds and verify bowel movement and flatus.

Observe client's overall condition.

PLANNING *Objectives*

To ensure that the client experiences an uneventful postoperative course

To provide safe, effective nursing care in the immediate postoperative period

To ensure that postoperative pain is relieved promptly

To be aware of the common postoperative drugs for pain control

IMPLEMENTATION *Procedures*

Providing Postoperative Care

Administering Postoperative Medications

EVALUATION *Expected Outcomes*

Client experiences an uneventful postoperative course.

Postoperative pain is relieved promptly.

Postoperative nursing interventions are carried out effectively and in a timely manner.

Medications control postoperative pain.

PROVIDING POSTOPERATIVE CARE

Equipment

Surgical bed
Absorbent pads
Warm blankets
IV pole
Oxygen source, tubing, and equipment
Emesis basin and tissues
Sphygmomanometer and stethoscope
Thermometer (tympanic, oral, or rectal)
Nurses' notes
Intake and output record
Special equipment depending on type of surgery
Pulse oximeter
Sterile dressings

Procedure

1. Wash hands prior to each client contact.
2. Introduce self to client.
3. Orient client to time, person, and place. Reorient as needed.
4. Assess for patent airway and level of consciousness; administer oxygen if ordered. Attach pulse oximeter if ordered.
5. Assess for effects of anesthesia including general, regional, or local.
6. Take vital signs, including pain assessment: usual orders are every 15 minutes until stable; then every half hour for 2 hours; every hour for 4 hours; then every 4 hours for 24–48 hours.
7. Check pulse oximetry every hour for 4 hours, then every 4 hours. **Rationale:** To detect early signs of hypoxemia.
8. Check for nausea and vomiting.
9. Check IV site and patency frequently.
10. Observe, and record urine output, amount, and color.
11. Measure intake and output.
12. Observe skin color and moisture and nail beds. **Rationale:** To determine adequacy of tissue perfusion.
13. Position client for comfort and maximum airway ventilation according to orders.
14. Turn every 2 hours and PRN.
15. Give back care at least every 4 hours.
16. Encourage coughing and deep breathing every 2 hours (may use spirometer or Triflow if ordered).
17. Keep client comfortable with medications.
18. Monitor for side effects of medications.
19. Check dressings and drainage tubes every 2–4 hours; if abnormal amount of drainage, check more frequently. Empty drainage system when needed.
20. Give oral hygiene at least every 4 hours; if nasogastric tube or nasal oxygen is inserted, give oral hygiene every 2 hours.
21. Bathe client when temperature can be maintained. **Rationale:** Bathing removes the antiseptic solution and stimulates circulation.
22. Keep client warm and avoid chilling, but do not increase temperature above normal. **Rationale:** Increased temperature increases metabolic rate and need for oxygen. Excessive perspiration causes fluid and electrolyte loss.
23. Irrigate nasogastric tube every 4 hours and PRN, as ordered, with normal saline to keep patent and to prevent electrolyte imbalance.
24. Maintain dietary intake: type of diet depends on type and extent of surgical procedure.
    a. Minor surgical conditions: client may drink or eat as soon as he or she is awake, desires food or drink, and has gag reflex present.
    b. Major surgical conditions: NPO until bowel sounds return. Clear liquid advanced to full diet as tolerated.
25. Place client on bedpan 2–4 hours postoperatively if catheter not inserted.
26. Check physician's orders when to begin the client's postoperative activity. Most clients are ambulated within first 24 hours.
27. Observe for signs and symptoms of possible postoperative complications, particularly postoperative bleeding and infection.
28. Dangle or get client up in chair as ordered.

ADMINISTERING POSTOPERATIVE MEDICATIONS*

Equipment

Medication as ordered
Appropriate syringe and needle for parenteral medications

Procedure

1. Evaluate client's need for pain relief.
2. Provide nonmedication measures for relief of pain, such as relaxation techniques, back care, positioning.
3. Identify the pharmacologic action of the ordered medication.
4. Review the general side effects of the medication.

*See Chapter 16, Pain Management, for PCA and epidural.

a. Drowsiness
b. Euphoria
c. Sleep
d. Respiratory depression
e. Nausea and vomiting
5. Administer medications as ordered, usually at 3- to 4-hour intervals for first 24–48 hours for better action and pain relief. Assess for pain relief.
6. Instruct in use of PCA pump, if ordered.
7. Know the action of the following drugs:
   a. Opiates
   b. Synthetic opiate-like drugs
   c. Nonnarcotic pain relievers
   d. Narcotic antagonists
   e. Antiemetics

DOCUMENTATION FOR POSTOPERATIVE CARE

- Postoperative nursing interventions
- Fluid replacement—type and amount of solution
- Condition of dressings and drains
- Urine output, intake, and output
- Orientation to place, person, time
- Vital signs
- Signs and symptoms of potential complications
- Preventive nursing measures
- Client's activity level
- Clinical manifestations indicating pain
- Type, time, and amount of pain medication administered
- Site of injection
- Any side effects of medications observed
- Effectiveness of pain medication

Critical Thinking Application

UNEXPECTED OUTCOMES	CRITICAL THINKING OPTIONS
Client develops abnormal breath sounds.	• Increase deep breathing and coughing exercises to every 2 hours. • Medicate for pain before coughing or ambulating to prevent splinting. • Encourage use of incentive spirometer. • Turn every 1–2 hours, and ambulate if allowed. • Place client in Fowler's position to expand lungs. • Increase fluid intake to liquify secretions, if not contraindicated. • Obtain physician's order for nebulizer treatments if indicated.
Bowel sounds are absent.	• Do not give ice chips or fluids, keep on NPO status until discussed with physician. • Notify physician if client is experiencing nausea and vomiting, or if abdomen is distended and bowel sounds remain absent. It may be necessary to insert an NG tube. • Auscultate bowel sounds q4 hrs. • Encourage frequent turning and ambulation, if allowed.
Deep vein thrombosis (DVT) occurs.	• Place on bedrest. • Remove antiembolic stockings on affected leg.

UNEXPECTED OUTCOMES	CRITICAL THINKING OPTIONS
	• Check for calf pain, discoloration or Homan's sign. • Do not massage legs. • Monitor clotting times and titrate anticoagulants if using Heparin, according to physician's orders. • Measure circumference of both legs each shift to determine effectiveness of treatment. • Encourage leg exercises on unaffected leg.
Temperature increases.	• Day of surgery—check for dehydration. • Day 1 and 2—check breath sounds for potential atelectasis. • Day 2—check for urinary tract infection. • Days 3–10—check for possible wound infection or pneumonia. • Check breath sounds for adventitious sounds or diminished breath sounds. • Fever in first 24 hours is most commonly from atelectasis. • Increase fluids, if not contraindicated. • Monitor temperature frequently, until it returns to normal.
Blood pressure decreases; pulse and respirations increase.	• Check for IV access. • Check skin turgor and urine output and hypovolemia. • Observe dressings and drains for signs of bleeding. • Check intake and output values to determine hydration status.

GERONTOLOGIC CONSIDERATIONS

Statistics for elderly clients requiring surgery are important to consider when providing care.

- Fifty percent of clients over 60 years of age require surgery before they die.
- Forty percent of elderly clients admitted to hospitals undergo a surgical procedure before discharge.
- The most common surgical procedures for elderly clients involve tissue biopsy and pacemaker insertion. Fractures comprise a large percentage of surgical interventions, particularly hip fractures.

Elderly clients are more prone to fluid and electrolyte imbalance.

- Dehydration is the most common cause of fluid and electrolyte imbalance.
- Check IV fluid type and amount to ensure adequate hydration.
- Elderly clients require 1.5–2.5 L of fluid every 24 hours.
- Monitor intake and output carefully to ensure adequate hydration.
- Monitor neurologic status for possible electrolyte imbalance.
- Fluid loss occurs with nasogastric tube placement and preop bowel preparation; clients requiring either of these interventions should be observed for dehydration.
- Evaluate electrolyte lab values for abnormal levels. (Hyperkalemia is common as a response to age-related alterations in the renin–aldosterone system.)

Elderly clients are at risk for complications associated with immobility following surgical interventions.

- Turn client frequently, at least every 2 hours.
- Ambulate as soon as possible postoperatively.

- Encourage deep breathing and coughing exercises every 1–2 hours. Instruct in use of incentive spirometer if ordered.
- Encourage leg exercises every hour when awake.

Preoperative teaching should be individualized keeping in mind the following:

- Elderly clients may have chronic conditions that make movement difficult, altering preventative measures such as turning.
- Clients may have visual or auditory alterations requiring a quiet environment for teaching.
- Larger print or brochures with photos and large print should be used when teaching elderly clients.

Chronic conditions may alter normal vital signs, which may be misinterpreted during the perioperative phases.

- Document abnormalities in vital signs on client care plan so that all health care workers are alerted to client's usual values. Blood pressure and pulse alterations can be different for this age group.
- Monitor peripheral pulses to ensure adequate circulation.

Altered physiologic states need to be communicated to all health care workers.

- Document if client has an artificial eye or other prosthesis.
- Document client's visual or auditory alterations. If hearing aide is necessary for client to hear, indicate clearly on care plan.
- Identify if client has any condition that can interfere with postoperative care.

Elderly clients may not be candidates for conscious sedation.

- Many elderly clients have an ASA reading above 3. This would be considered a contraindication for this sedation.
- Anesthesiologists would most likely have to administer the medication.

Consent forms must be signed by legally competent client.

- Signing of consent form can only be done if client is considered competent to understand directions given and explanation of procedure.
- Signing of consent form must be voluntary.
- Client must be informed about procedure and must understand what he or she is signing.
- A court-appointed conservator may need to be obtained for clients not considered mentally competent to sign for themselves.
- Family members may not sign for client unless they are legally considered the client's guardian or advance directive provides instructions.
- In emergency situations permission may be obtained from family members, but not for routine procedures.
- Two physicians can sign for emergency surgery; however, the surgeon performing the surgery should not sign the permit.

MANAGEMENT GUIDELINES

Each state legislates a Nurse Practice Act for RNs and LVN/LPNs. Health care facilities are responsible for establishing and implementing policies and procedures that conform to their state's regulations. Verify the regulations and role parameters for each health care worker in your facility.

Delegation of Responsibilities

- RNs and LVN/LPNs can complete routine preoperative teaching and care. Anything out of the ordinary would be the responsibility of the RN.
- Postanesthesia Room staff are usually RNs because they need to make quick decisions and use nursing judgment in times of crisis.
- Postoperative care of clients may be provided by both RNs and LVN/LPNs.
- Clients undergoing conscious sedation may be more monitored by RNs if their State Nurse Practice Act and hospital policy allows it, and the clients are in ASA categories 1 and 2 (See section on conscious sedation).
- CNAs can be delegated to take vital signs and do routine hygienic care for clients once they are stable.
- Many facilities use "scrub techs" or OR Techs to perform routine duties such as the preoperative scrub. OR Techs are also assigned to assist the physician during surgery.

Information Flow

- It is very important that all preoperative forms are completed in a timely manner. If data is missing, the client's surgery may be delayed while laboratory tests are taken, history and physical examination reports are found and placed in the chart, or chest x-ray results are placed in the chart.
- Notify OR staff and physician if client indicates he or she has a known latex allergy or does not know of a latex allergy. All latex supplies and equipment must be removed from the OR suite before surgery can commence.
- When the phone call is received from the operating room indicating the nurse should give the preoperative medications or that the OR is ready for the client, ensure the message is relayed immediately to the staff caring for the client. This will allow the nurse to give the medication or complete any last-minute charting and have the client ready for the transporter.
- If there are any client issues or problems that directly affect the surgical procedure, contact the operating room or physician immediately. Surgery may need to be delayed or canceled. Examples of issues that could impact the surgery include an overly anxious client, if the client has a temperature or symptoms indicating an upper respiratory or urinary tract infection.
- Specific report regarding the client's condition will be completed upon admission to the postanesthesia room and again when the client is returned to the nursing unit. The report is given by the RN in the operating room to the RN in the postanesthesia room. The postanesthesia room nurse accompanies the client to the nursing unit and gives report to the RN. The report is outlined as step 15 of the skill *Discharging Client from Postanesthesia Room to Nursing Unit*.

CRITICAL THINKING STRATEGIES

SCENARIO 1

You are assigned to the postanesthesia room on the day shift. You have just arrived on the unit to begin the shift. There are two clients assigned to your care:

- Mrs. Cohen, a 54-year-old client, had an exploratory laparoscopy with general anesthesia and is just arriving in the recovery room.
- Mr. Brewer is a 24-year-old client who had local anesthesia for an arthroscopy of the right knee. He has been in the recovery room for 1 hour.

1. Which client will you see first? Provide rationale for your response.
2. Identify the first action you will take when first seeing each of the two clients. Provide rationale for your response.
3. Identify the priority assessment for Mrs. Cohen and state your rationale.
4. Identify the priority assessment for Mr. Brewer and state your rationale.
5. State nursing interventions that will be provided for all clients in the postanesthesia room.
6. Before discharge from the recovery room, you assess Mr. Brewer on the Aldrete Recovery Scoring System and his score is 7. What is your next action?
7. Mr. Brewer is being discharged home. He tells you he is concerned about going home because he has a dry mouth and is thirsty. What would be an appropriate response to him?

SCENARIO 2

You assess that Mr. Marconi is very anxious while you are admitting him for a surgical procedure.

1. List four priority components of baseline data you need to obtain prior to surgery. Provide a rationale to support this data.
2. What factors might contribute to preoperative stress?
3. Identify a priority intervention to use after assessing that Mr. Marconi is in high-level stress.
4. Mr. Marconi becomes angry and hostile when you attempt to provide preoperative teaching. Describe three possible actions you could take, and state the priority intervention and the rationale for selecting this intervention.

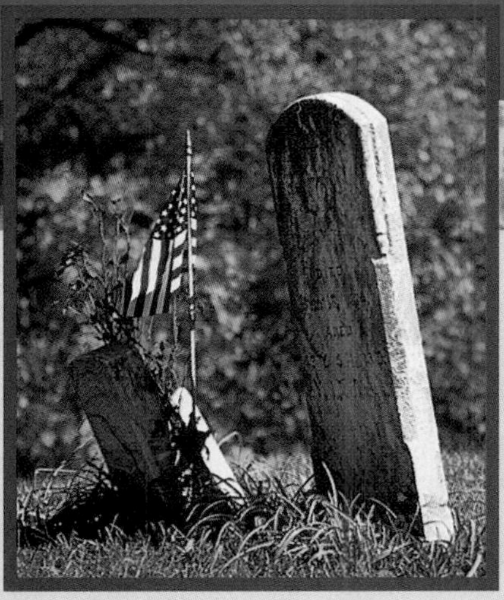

CHAPTER 32

End-of-Life Care

THEORETICAL CONCEPTS

UNIT ONE: **The Grief Process** **1189**
- Understanding Grief 1190
- Assisting with Grief 1190

UNIT TWO: **The Dying Client** **1192**
- Supporting the Client Near the End of Life 1193
- Providing Pain Management at the End of Life 1195
- Assisting the Dying Client 1196
- Supporting the Family or Caregiver 1198

UNIT THREE: **Postmortem Care** **1200**
- Providing Postmortem Care 1201

GERONTOLOGIC CONSIDERATIONS 1203

MANAGEMENT GUIDELINES 1203

CRITICAL THINKING STRATEGIES 1204

Learning Objectives

- Discuss the stages of the grief process.
- State the main characteristics observed in a person experiencing grief.
- Identify the factors that influence the outcome of the grieving process.
- Explain three assessment parameters for observing psychologic and somatic symptoms that accompany the grief process.
- Discuss at least two nursing interventions for each stage of grief.
- Describe the stages of dying outlined by Elisabeth Kübler-Ross.
- Explain what is meant by providing emotional care for the dying client.
- Discuss at least four nursing interventions that assist the client during the end-of-life process.
- Describe the three-step Analgesic Ladder for Pain Control for the Dying Client.
- Describe the steps of providing postmortem care.

Terminology

Adjuvant analgesic drugs: enhance the analgesic efficacy of opioids; treat recurrent symptoms that exacerbate pain and provide independent analgesic effects.

Agitation: excessive restlessness; increased mental and physical activity.

Anger: a feeling of extreme displeasure, hostility, indignation, or exasperation toward someone or something.

Anorexia: loss of appetite occurring from a variety of possible reasons.

Anxiety: a troubled or apprehensive feeling; experiencing a sense of dread or fear.

Cope: to contend with, strive, or handle.

Corneal reflex: closure of eyelids resulting from direct corneal irritation or touch.

Counseling: giving assistance to or guidance.

Crisis: a crucial point or situation in the course of life; turning point.

Denial: refusal to grant the truth of a statement or allegation.

Depression: being dispirited, saddened; low in mood.

Empathy: objective awareness of an insight into the feelings, emotions, and behavior of another person.

Esteem: regard, respect.

Fear: feeling of fright or dread related to a specific source (e.g., fear of pain or dying).

Grief: intense mental anguish, deep remorse, sorrow.

Homeostasis: an internal state of equilibrium or balance.

Hospice: originally a place of shelter for a troubled individual. Now, the term has come to mean more of a concept of care where a dying person can receive care, compassion, support, and treatment.

Idealization: to regard as ideal; to make or regard someone or something as perfect.

Insomnia: inability to sleep; difficulty with sleeping.

Opioids: drugs such as morphine, methadone, and numorphan, used to treat severe pain.

Pain: an unpleasant sensory and emotional experience arising from actual or potential tissue damage or described in terms of such damage; whatever the experiencing person says it is, existing whenever he or she says it does.

Psychosomatic: pertaining to phenomena that are both physiologic and psychologic in origin.

Resolution: the state of having made a firm determination; a course decided on.

Restitution: a return to a former status.

Somatic: referring to the body.

Stress: a mentally or emotionally disruptive or disquieting influence; distress.

Suffering: includes fear of or actual physical distress, fear of dying, changing self perceptions, relationship concerns, the need to find meaning in any given life experience, and past experiences of witnessing another person's distress.

Therapeutic: having medicinal or healing properties.

Withdrawal: to pull back or away.

LOSS AND GRIEVING

Grief is an emotion experienced in relation to loss; it can also be viewed as a behavioral response to death and dying. Human beings experience loss as the emotion of grief and must withdraw from the painful stimulus to recuperate. Emotions allow us to experience our environment—they are the means of cognition. When we are grieving, we experience the emotion of grief; this experience is accompanied by a definite syndrome with somatic and psychologic symptoms.

Stages of Grief

George Engle, in a classic article in the American Journal of Nursing, 1964, describes progression of the grief process in stages. These stages may occur in order, or an individual may skip a stage, become locked in a particular stage, or even return to an earlier stage already worked through.

The first stage is *shock and disbelief*, denial and numbness. The first response on learning of a death is shock and a refusal to accept or comprehend the fact. This reaction is followed by a stunned, numb feeling and does not allow the person to acknowledge the reality of death. This initial phase is characterized by attempts to protect oneself against severe stress by blocking recognition of the death.

Developing awareness is the second stage. Within minutes or hours the individual becomes acutely and increasingly aware of the anguish of loss. Anger may be present during this time and may be directed toward persons or circumstances held to be responsible for the death. Behavior that frequently accompanies this stage is crying and a regression to a more helpless and child-like state. The crying and regression appear to acknowledge the loss, indicating that conscious awareness is now present.

The third stage is *restitution*, in which the various rituals of the culture, such as the funeral, attire, wake, particular folkways, and mores, help to initiate the recovery process. These rituals serve the function of emphasizing the reality of death and the very act of experiencing them assists the mourner to face the loss.

As the reality of death becomes accepted, the *resolution* of the loss begins. This stage involves a number of steps. First, the mourner attempts to deal with the painful void created by the loss of a loved one. At this time the thoughts of the mourner are occupied almost exclusively with the deceased. Then the mourner becomes more aware of his or her own body and bodily sensations. Finally, the mourner begins to talk about the dead person, recalling the dead person's attributes and personality and reminiscing about the memories they shared. Resolving the loss is a long and painful phase that continues until the mourner remembers the positive aspects of the dead person.

The next stage that is frequently experienced is that of *idealization*. All hostile and negative feelings toward the dead person are repressed. As the process proceeds, two important changes are taking place: the recurring thoughts about the dead person bring a distinct image of the loss to mind and these memories serve to bring out the more positive aspects of the lost relationship. At the same time the grieving individual begins to assume certain admired qualities of the dead person through the mechanisms of identification or incorporation. The mourner may begin to dress, speak, or develop mannerisms or beliefs similar to the person who was lost. Often, many months are required for this process to be experienced, and as it dissipates, the mourner's preoccupation with the dead person lessens. It may be at this point that the person begins to reinvest intimate feelings toward other relationships.

Stages of Grief	**Stages of Dying**
• Shock and disbelief	• Denial
• Developing awareness	• Anger
• Restitution	• Bargaining
• Resolution	• Depression
• Idealization	• Acceptance
according to George Engle	*according to Elisabeth Kübler-Ross*

The mourning process usually takes a year or more. The clearest evidence of healing is the ability to remember the deceased comfortably and realistically, with both the pleasures and disappointments of the relationship. At this stage the obsession with the loss is ended and the person accepts the responsibility of living his or her own life.

Each individual who experiences loss moves through at least some of these stages as he or she attempts to cope with loss. The stages of grief are the means human beings have of moving through the loss to resolution.

STAGES OF DYING

Elisabeth Kübler-Ross has described the phases of dying, which mirror those of the grieving process. As a person learns of his or her own impending death, he or she experiences grief in relation to his or her own loss.

The first stage, as Kübler-Ross views this process, is that of *denial*. The denial may be partial or complete and may occur not only during the first stages of illness or confrontation but later on from time to time. This initial denial is usually a temporary defense and is used as a buffer until such time as the person is able to collect him or herself, mobilize defenses, and face the inevitability of death.

The second stage is often *anger*. The person feels violent anger at having to give up life. This emotion may be directed toward persons in the environment or even projected into the environment at random. Kübler-Ross discusses this reaction and the difficulty in handling it for those close to the person by explaining that we should put ourselves in the client's position and consider how we might feel intense anger at having our life interrupted abruptly.

The third stage is *bargaining*. The person attempts to strike a bargain for more time to live or more time to be without pain in return for doing something for God. Often during this stage the person turns or returns to religion.

Depression is the fourth stage. Usually, when people have completed the stages of denial, anger, and bargaining, they move into depression. Kubler-Ross writes about two kinds of depression. One is preparatory depression: this is a tool for dealing with the impending loss. The second type is reactive depression. In this form of depression, the person is reacting against the impending loss of life and grieves for him or herself.

The final stage of dying is that of *acceptance*. This occurs when the person has worked through the previous stages and accepts his or her own inevitable death. With full acceptance of impending death comes the preparation for it; however, even with acceptance, hope is still present and needs to be supported realistically.

Many factors influence how individuals accept death. Personal values and beliefs about life; views of personal successes, both financial and emotional; the way they look physically when experiencing the dying process; their family and friends and their families' attitudes and reactions; their past experiences in coping with difficult or traumatic situations; and, finally, the health care staff who are caring for them during this process—all affect an individual's attitude toward dying.

CORE PRINCIPLES FOR END OF LIFE CARE

The Joint Commission on Accreditation of Healthcare Organizations and a significant number of specialty medical societies have endorsed, modified, or adopted a consistent set of Core Principles for End of Life Care. The overall philosophy was accepted by most societies, but each one amended or expanded certain issues that directly affect their practice.

The Core Principles for End of Life Care—clinical policies and professional practice guidelines for end-of-life care should:

1. Respect the dignity of both patient and caregivers.
2. Be sensitive to and respectful of the patient's and family's wishes.
3. Use the most appropriate measures that are consistent with patient choices.
4. Encompass alleviation of pain and other physical symptoms.
5. Assess and manage psychological, social, and spiritual/religious problems.
6. Offer continuity, the patient should be cared for, if so desired, by his/her primary care and specialist providers.
7. Provide access to any therapy which may realistically be expected to improve the patient's quality of life, including alternative or nontraditional treatments.
8. Provide access to palliative care and hospice care.
9. Respect the right to refuse treatment.
10. Respect the physician's professional responsibility to discontinue some treatments when appropriate, with consideration for both patient and family preferences.
11. Promote clinical and evidence based research on providing care at the end of life.

Source: Principles for Care of Patients at the End of Life: An Emerging Consensus among the Specialties of Medicine, Castle and Foley, December 1999. Milbank Memorial Fund.

Even though many practitioners believe they have explained end of life care options to clients and families, a study of 728 participants in an Oregon study conducted by Silveria, et. al., indicated that there is still a misunderstanding about options for end of life care. This is particularly true with discussion about active euthanasia and assisted suicide. A large percentage of the participants, 69%, did not know about the right to refuse treatment.

MANAGING PAIN

Pain and pain control has been identified as the primary concern of clients as they approach the end of life. Several research studies have identified this aspect of dying as the major concern. Research studies have also indicated that inadequate assessments of pain and poor pain control continue to be an issue even though much research on the topic has been published.

Nurses play a critical role in the management of pain for clients at the end of life. Through adequate assessment on a regular basis, developing a pain control plan, and administering the pharmacologic treatments necessary to provide pain relief, clients can be made more comfortable.

The World Health Organization (WHO) developed a three-step "ladder" that outlines principles of analgesic selection and titration as well as adjuvant drugs that support the effect of the analgesics or counteract adverse side effects. Each step in the ladder defines the type of pain and analgesic most effective for that level of pain.

The foundation for pain management is the use of opioids. In addition to pain medications, assessment and monitoring the client for additional appropriate interventions to relieve pain must also be part of the treatment plan.

In some clients, the pain becomes so severe that even aggressive titration of standard drugs is not sufficient to control the pain. In these cases, sedation should be considered. Sedation for end of life clients is considered a comfort measure when there is intractable pain and other symptoms indicate death is near. When sedation is used in this manner, the client usually loses consciousness. Family members, as well as the client, must be informed of this change in client status before sedation is started.

When sedation is used for end of life clients, the facility must have guidelines in place with parameters for drug selection, dose, and titration. These guidelines are individualized for each client's symptoms.

THE HOSPICE OPTION

Hospice care provides treatment, comfort, and support for the terminally ill client, as well as relief and solace for the family. Hospice care is not only for elderly clients, but for any age client with a life expectancy of less than 6 months. This includes clients with AIDS and ALS, and children with cardiac anomalies or other congenital conditions with limited life expectancy. Hospice can offer any treatment necessary to relieve suffering and allow a client to die peacefully and comfortably. Hospice neither speeds up nor slows down the dying process. It only provides a specialized environment where a dying client may receive medical care in addition to emotional and spiritual support during the dying process.

Facts About Hospice

- Hospice celebrated 20 years of service in 2002.
- There are over 3,100 hospices in the U.S.
- The average daily hospice census is 25 clients.
- Hospice care is a covered benefit under Medicare (and over two-thirds are Medicare certified).
- Many private health insurance policies cover hospice and more and more HMOs offer it as a benefit.
- In 2000, hospices served over 700,000 clients.
- Approximately two-thirds of hospice clients are over age 65.
- U.S. hospices employ over 40,000 professional staff.
- Over 70,000 volunteers (four-fifths of people involved in care) serve in hospice programs, contributing over 5 million hours of service annually.

Hospice Information

For more information, the nurse should contact one of the following organizations:

The National Hospice Organization
1901 N. Moore St., Suite 901
Arlington, VA 22209 Tel: (703) 516-4928

Hospice Foundation of America
777 17 St. #401
Miami Beach, FL 33139 Tel: (800) 854-3402

Choice in Dying
200 Varick St.
New York, NY 10014 Tel: (212) 366-5540

Hospice Hands
Web Address: http://www.hospice-cares.com (Includes a complete index of hospice resources available on the Internet.)

Hospice care can alleviate a great deal of stress on the family when the client is terminally ill and the cold, dispassionate ambiance of a hospital may not be supportive. One of the real advantages of hospice is that the personnel are trained to treat pain aggressively. The underlying philosophy is that the client should be as pain free as possible, while at the same time remaining as alert as possible.

Hospice care includes an interdisciplinary team that includes a Registered Nurse trained in symptom management and pain control, a social worker, a home health aide, a chaplain, and trained volunteers. Hospice care is reimbursed by Medicare in all states and by Medicaid in 42 states. It is less expensive than acute care and it does not require justification of certain treatments (for example, administration of oxygen) that would be necessary in an acute care setting.

If hospice care seems so excellent, why do not more clients and their families elect to use it? Because there are several barriers to hospice care. One barrier is that the client's physician must certify that the life expectancy of the client is six months or less. Often, physicians are reluctant to do this and may not feel comfortable in discussing the fact of dying with the client. Another problem is that some insurance carriers require clients to waive their rights to medical benefits if they are receiving hospice care. Finally, and perhaps the largest obstacle, is that there is a problem with communication—between physician and client, client and family, and family and client. When the finality of dying cannot be discussed, hospice care may not present itself as an option.

NURSING DIAGNOSES

The following nursing diagnoses are appropriate to include in a client care plan when a client is in the process of grieving or dying.

NURSING DIAGNOSIS	RELATED FACTORS
Decisional Conflict	Surgery, diagnostic tests, treatments, perceived threat to value system, lack of experience in making critical decisions
Anticipatory Grieving	Loss of significant other, chronic illness, threat of death, perceived loss of biologic integrity
Health Maintenance, Ineffective	Lack of motivation, lack of education, religious and cultural beliefs, cognitive impairment
Compromised Family Coping	Little support by family, alteration in family role
Spiritual Distress	Hospital barriers to practicing spiritual rituals, loss of body part or function, terminal illness, debilitating disease, death or illness of significant other, challenge to belief or value systems
Death Anxiety	Worry about death's impact on significant others, feeling powerless over issues related to dying, anticipating pain related to death
Chronic Pain	Tissue, organ, or skeletal muscle damage as a result of cancer, severe pain at end of life
Fear	Unknown experience related to death; unfamiliarity with environment

- The single most important nursing action to decrease the incidence of hospital-based infections is handwashing. **Remember to wash your hands or use antibacterial gel before and after each and every client contact.**

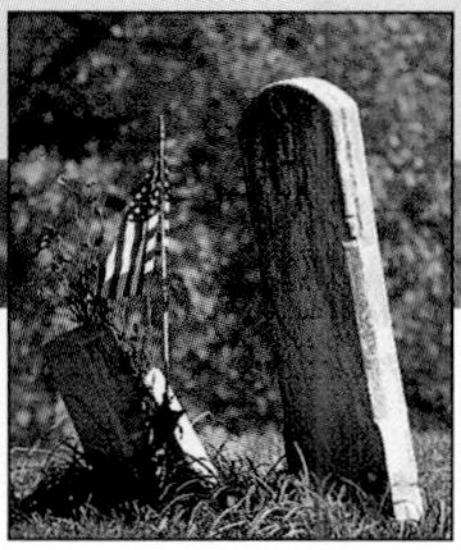

UNIT 1

The Grief Process

Nursing Process Data

ASSESSMENT Data Base

Observe for presence of psychologic symptoms:
- Weeping
- Guilt
- Anger and irritability toward others and the deceased
- Depression
- Inability to initiate meaningful activity

Observe for somatic symptoms:
- Physical exhaustion
- Insomnia
- Restlessness and agitation
- Digestive disturbance
- Anorexia or over eating

Determine client's complaints:
- Sense of unreality
- Sense of detachment
- Lack of strength

Observe stage of grief response client is experiencing:
- Shock and disbelief
- Developing awareness
- Restitution
- Resolution
- Idealization
- Outcome of grieving process—positive or negative

Observe for morbid reaction to grief:
- Delay of reaction
- Distorted reaction—acquisition of symptoms of the deceased (e.g., psychosomatic illness, or disease)
- Atypical grief syndrome manifested by distorted pictures of grief

PLANNING Objectives

To assist the client who is experiencing the grief process

To intervene therapeutically and provide support

To allow the client to express feelings of loss openly

To understand and tolerate client's behavior that is related to loss

To assist the client to move successfully through stages of the grief process

IMPLEMENTATION ***Procedures***

Understanding Grief

Assisting with Grief

EVALUATION ***Expected Outcomes***

Client moves through grieving process.

Client accepts loss, and outcome of grieving process is positive.

UNDERSTANDING GRIEF

Procedure

1. Understand the importance of the deceased person as a source of support.
2. Observe the degree of dependency of the relationship between deceased and others. **Rationale:** The more dependent the more difficult is the task of resolution.
3. Identify the degree of ambivalence felt toward the deceased. **Rationale:** When there are persistent hostile feelings, guilt may interfere with the work of mourning.
4. Check on the number and nature of other relationships the grieving individual has to depend on. **Rationale:** A client with few other meaningful relationships has a more difficult time and is less willing to give up the attachment to the deceased.
5. Check on the number and nature of previous grief experiences. **Rationale:** Losses tend to be cumulative in their effects, and unsuccessfully resolved previous losses only aggravate the current loss.
6. Determine the degree of preparation for the loss. **Rationale:** In terminal illness, grief work may have begun long before the actual death of the person.
7. Determine the capacity to cope with loss. The more inner resources the client has available, the better his or her coping ability. **Rationale:** The physical and psychologic health of the mourner at the time of the loss determines capacity.

ASSISTING WITH GRIEF

Procedure

1. Become familiar with the grief process, stages of grief, and natural responses to grief so you can provide the client with optimal support.
2. Denial stage.
   a. Allow client denial of grief to give him or her time to move through shock and to mobilize defenses.
   b. Encourage client to talk when he or she is ready to do so.
   c. Understand that shock and disbelief may be first response, and anticipate that behavior may be inappropriate or disturbed.
   d. Accept client's inability to face reality, and allow mood swings and expressions of happier times (which may seem inappropriate at this time).
3. Anger stage.
   a. Allow "acting-out" of feelings and verbalization of anger.
   b. Anticipate expression of anger toward others, loved ones, and the environment.
   c. Understand that unreasonable, insatiable demands are an expression of this stage of grief, and attempt to meet the demands. Anticipate client's needs before demanded.
   d. Encourage client to take as much control as possible over care and environment. Avoid criticism and negative feedback at this time.
   e. Avoid false reassurance and false cheerfulness, which lead to distrust. Also, avoid diversion by introducing cheerful activities or stories. These actions lead client to believe you do not care about his or her feelings.
   f. Explain and clarify all procedures and treatments to decrease misinterpretation and expansion of fears.
4. Bargaining stage.
   a. Allow client to move through bargaining stage; listen to verbal expressions without judgment or pointing out reality.
   b. Encourage client to talk about bargaining with God. This may assist client to cope with guilt and not lose faith.
5. Reactive depression stage.
   a. Encourage verbalizations about loss, its meaning in client's life, and feelings about the loss.
   b. Support client's self-esteem and understand that it is affected with awareness of the loss.
   c. Encourage and reassure as appropriate; do not give false reassurance at this stage but assist client to be realistic.

d. Be aware of your own feelings of sadness and loss so that they do not interfere with therapy.
6. Preparatory depression.
   a. Allow client to be quiet and silent in order to internalize feelings.
   b. Remain with client and share on a nonverbal level.
   c. Verbalize feelings to client when they are appropriate; do not deny yourself expressions of sadness or empathy (crying) when appropriate.
   d. Limit association with cheerful, insincere staff, friends, or family.
7. Resolution–acceptance stage.
   a. Allow client to express whatever feelings are present, knowing that he or she has moved through the above stages and may now be feeling totally empty of emotion.
   b. Spend quiet time with client, interacting on a nonverbal, nondemanding level.
   c. Encourage client to make preparations for impending death by supporting requests to finish tasks and discussing options for plans to complete areas in his or her life.
   d. Honor client's requests to be alone, and do not overload client with external information. Client may need a lot of quiet contemplation to prepare for death.
8. Show respect for cultural, religious, and social customs throughout stages of mourning.
9. Offer support and reassurance to family.

Documentation for the Grief Process

- Stage of grief the client is experiencing and client's ability to cope.
- Behavioral manifestations of grief
- Support systems available to client
- Measures nurse has taken to assist client to cope with grief
- Client's response to psychosocial interventions

Critical Thinking Application

UNEXPECTED OUTCOMES	CRITICAL THINKING OPTIONS
The client experiences a morbid reaction to grief.	• Recognize distorted symptoms and be accepting but firm with client. • Request further assistance from the staff.
Family cannot support grief of client or handle their own grief.	• Know the general response to death by recognizing the stages of the grief process. • Understand that the behavior of the mourner may be unstable and disturbed. • Request assistance from nursing staff to cope with the family.

UNIT 2

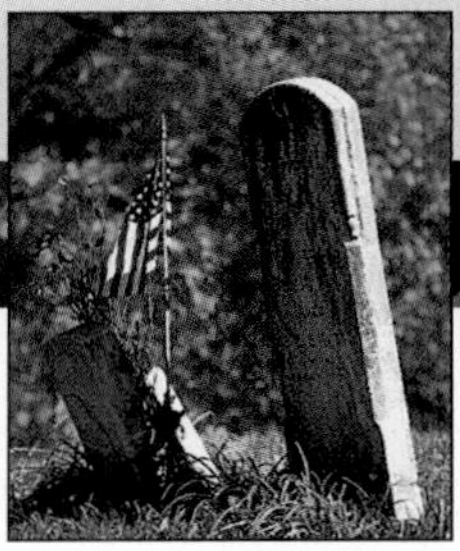

The Dying Client

Nursing Process Data

ASSESSMENT *Data Base*

Observe the physical symptoms.
- Evidence of circulatory collapse
- Variations in blood pressure and pulse
- Disequilibrium of body mechanisms
- Deterioration of physical and mental capabilities
- Absence of corneal reflex

Observe the client's ability to fulfill basic needs without complete assistance.

Assess the nature and degree of pain the client is experiencing.

Observe for impending crisis or emergency situation.

Observe for psychosocial condition.
- Need to establish a relationship for support
- Grief pattern and stage of grief the client is experiencing
- Need to express feelings and verbalize fears and concerns

Determine anxiety level, which may be expressed in physical or emotional behavior.
- Sleep disturbance
- Palpitations
- Digestive complaints
- Anger or hostility
- Withdrawal

Determine depression level that client may be experiencing.
- High fatigue level or lethargy
- Poor appetite, nausea, or vomiting
- Inability to concentrate
- Expressions of sadness, hopelessness, or uselessness
- Assess family members' needs during the loss

PLANNING *Objectives*

To assist client near the end of life to maintain comfort, if possible

To assist the dying client to cope with end of life experiences

To handle own feelings of loss and sadness that arise when caring for a client at the end of life

To provide support for the client and the client's family during the end-of-life process

To complete the actions necessary to care for the client who has died

IMPLEMENTATION *Procedures*

Supporting the Client Near the End of Life

Providing Pain Management at the End of Life

Assisting the Dying Client

Supporting the Family or Caregiver

EVALUATION Expected Outcomes

Client is as comfortable as possible during end of life.

Client finds internal resources to accept death.

Client is able to verbalize feelings and needs.

Family members are supported during end-of-life process.

SUPPORTING THE CLIENT NEAR THE END OF LIFE

Preparation

1. Determine if client has a Do Not Resuscitate (DNR) signed form in chart or as part of informed consent.
2. Determine if client has requested limited support or comfort support rather than CPR. This includes medication administration, airway management, chest compressions or defibrillation, pain control, but not CPR. Ensure physician has documented in client's chart.
3. If client is unable to sign form, ensure that legally recognized surrogate health care decision maker has signed the request. **Rationale:** Without signed DNR orders, staff must perform CPR and begin all lifesaving measures.

Procedure

1. Introduce yourself to client and family members.
2. Determine if client has specific needs for comfort. **Rationale:** Comfort is the primary goal of therapy for dying clients. Provide daily grooming, skin and mouth care, and exercise as client can tolerate.
3. Determine if and how family members may assist client during this stage and assist family members to provide care as requested.
4. Move client's bed near window so he or she can see outside vegetation, flowers, sky, etc.
5. Reduce extraneous noise and odors (perfume, cigarette smoke). Client's room may need to be moved to accomplish this. Do not place bed near nurses' station. **Rationale:** Even if client is not responding they can still hear voices and noises.
6. Display cards, photos, "art work" from children, favorite objects that have special meaning for client in an area where client can see them.
7. Provide room lighting that is muted and soft, not overhead lighting.
8. Encourage client to maintain independence by providing remote controls for TV, radio, lights, and fans. Keep ice and water at the bedside within easy reach by client.
9. Eliminate odors:
   a. Open windows when possible.
   b. Turn on fans.

CARDIOPULMONARY RESUSCITATION

☐ **"FULL SUPPORT"**

☐ **"LIMITED SUPPORT"**

All indicated medical care is provided except that in the event of a cardiac or pulmonary arrest, limitations of therapeutic interventions are indicated:

1. Medications	Routine	☐ yes	☐ no
	Vasopressors	☐ yes	☐ no
	Antiarrhythmics	☐ yes	☐ no
	ACLS drugs	☐ yes	☐ no
2. Airway Management	Intubation	☐ yes	☐ no
	Extubation if patient on ventilator	☐ yes	☐ no
	Reintubate after patient is weaned off ventilator or self extubation	☐ yes	☐ no
3. Chest Compressions		☐ yes	☐ no
4. Defibrillation		☐ yes	☐ no
5. Other		☐ yes	☐ no

☐ **"COMFORT SUPPORT"** *

1. New therapeutic measures contraindicated. Possible reasons may include one or more of the following:
   1.1 Irreversible terminal disease/coma; death is imminent.
   1.2 Brain death (defined by statute).
   1.3 Competent patient or incompetent patient with family or surrogate decision-maker expresses desire that no CPR procedures be instituted.
   1.4 Proposed treatment is disproportionate in terms of benefits to be gained versus burdens caused.
   1.5 Congenital anomalies incompatible with life.
   1.6 Care which is necessary to alleviate pain and suffering shall be provided.

***NOTE:** PHYSICIAN MUST ENTER INTO THE PROGRESS NOTES FOR "LIMITED SUPPORT" AND "COMFORT SUPPORT" ORDERS:

1. Diagnosis / prognosis / code status.
2. Mandatory neurological consultation for diagnosis of brain death.
3. Patient / family / surrogate decision-maker involvement in the decision.
4. Clear documentation of patient or family or surrogate decision-maker approval or support of decision to withhold future CPR procedures.

REASSESSMENT OF CPR STATUS WILL BE DONE WHEN A PATIENT'S CONDITION OR WISHES CHANGE AND/OR A REQUEST IS MADE TO RESCIND THE ORDERS.

PHYSICIAN'S SIGNATURE: ____________ DATE: ________ TIME: ________

NOTED BY: ____________ DATE: ________ TIME: ________

COMMUNITY HOSPITAL

PATIENT I.D. #
NAME
SEX AGE SS#
BIRTH DATE MED REC. #

CPR form.

   c. Use air fresheners.
   d. Use aromatherapy (oils or lotion) for massage.
10. Provide soft music according to client's preference for music.
11. Limit visitors to no more than two at a time, or according to client's wishes. Assess if client needs rest by observing for signs of anxiety, restlessness, and voice trembling. When this occurs, ask the visitors to please leave.
12. Provide touch like Reiki or other therapeutic touch techniques, especially over the area of pain. **Rationale:** This is soothing and relaxing for client.
13. Incorporate the use of relaxation techniques in your daily nursing care of the client.
14. Provide massage with aromatherapy products if client agrees. **Rationale:** Massage reduces stress, decreases pain and discomfort, and stimulates blood circulation.
15. Serve only small portions of food that client requests. **Rationale:** Serving large portions only overwhelms client and he or she will not want to attempt to eat. Encourage clients to take in as much fluid as they are able.
16. Keep lemon drops or mint fresheners at bedside and within easy reach for client. **Rationale:** Breath fresheners make the client feel better especially if they are not eating.
17. Use visualization and guided imagery through audiotapes if client desires.
18. Ensure client has current Advance Directive on file in both the health care facility and physician's office. **Rationale:** Even though Patient Self-Determination Act of 1991 requires health care facilities to inform clients of their right to accept or refuse health care and complete an advance directive, this is not always done.
19. Assist with open communication with clients, family, and health care providers, regarding any cultural, spiritual, or religious issues they wish to discuss relative to end of life. **Rationale:** Understanding the client's religious or spiritual concerns will help support client and family during these times.

The goal of care for the dying client changes from curative to palliative care. Helping the client achieve a measure of comfort and knowing that family members and significant others are being supported during this process is a comfort for the client.

REQUEST TO FOREGO RESUSCITATIVE MEASURES
(Request Made by Patient)

I, ______________________ (name of patient) hereby request to forego resuscitative measures. My physician, ______________________, has explained to me the nature of resuscitative measures, their risks and benefits, the risks and benefits of refusing such resuscitative measures, and the alternatives to such resuscitative measures. I have had all of my questions answered by my physician.

After carefully considering all of the information my physician discussed with me, I request to forego resuscitative measures.

Signature: ______________________

Date: ______________ Time: ________ A.M. / P.M.

Witness: ______________________

REQUEST TO FOREGO RESUSCITATIVE MEASURES
(Request Made by Legally Recognized Surrogate Decision-maker)

NOTE: *If the patient is determined by his or her physician to be incompetent (that is, unable to understand or appreciate the nature and consequences of the medical decision at issue), a legally recognized surrogate health care decision-maker may sign a request to forego resuscitative measures on behalf of the patient.*

I, ______________________ (name of legally recognized surrogate health care decision-maker) hereby request to forego resuscitative measures on behalf of ______________________ (name of patient). The patient's physician, ______________________, has explained to me the nature of resuscitative measures, their risks and benefits, the risks and benefits of refusing such resuscitative measures, and the alternatives to such resuscitative measures. I have had all of my questions answered by the physician.

After carefully considering all of the information the physician discussed with me, I request to forego resuscitative measures on behalf of the patient named above.

Signature: ______________________

Relationship to Patient: ______________________

Date: ______________ Time: ________ A.M. / P.M.

Witness: ______________________

COMMUNITY HOSPITAL

PATIENT I.D. #
NAME
SEX AGE SS#
BIRTH DATE MED REC. # FIN. CLASS

DNR form.

PROVIDING PAIN MANAGEMENT AT THE END OF LIFE

Procedure

1. Assess client for factors that influence management of pain.
   a. Complete detailed history of the client's condition.
   b. Determine effects of pain relief measures and medications client is currently taking.
   c. Have client explain characteristics of pain and have him or her use pain scale to determine severity of pain.
   d. Ask client if there are any cultural issues related to pain that should be known by health care providers.
   e. Assess client's psychosocial needs.
2. Complete physical assessment of client.

> **CLINICAL ALERT**
>
> Most medications for pain are administered via oral or parenteral routes. The use of continuous subcutaneous opioid infusions in clients with chronic cancer pain is becoming more popular. High-concentration opioid medications are used with this method because the amount of drug administered must be limited to prevent tissue trauma.

3. Assess client for nonverbal clues indicating pain: restlessness, grimacing, moaning, irritability, furrowed brow, or crying, particularly if the client is sedated.

WHO-Three-Step Analgesic Ladder for Pain Control

Step 1: Nonopioid with or without adjuvant drugs.

Acetaminophen, aspirin, or another NSAID for mild to moderate pain.

Adjuvant drugs to enhance analgesic efficacy, treat concurrent symptoms that exacerbate pain, and provide independent analgesic activity for specific types of pain that may be used in this step as well as in the other steps.

Step 2: Opioid for mild-to-moderate pain and nonopioid drugs, may or may not use adjuvant drugs.

Add codeine or hydrocodone to the NSAID (do not substitute drugs).

Drugs are administered in fixed-dose combinations with acetaminophen or aspirin. This provides additive analgesia.

Dose-related toxicity might occur with the use of acetaminophen or NSAID.

This may limit the drug combination's efficacy.

Step 3: Opioid for moderate-to-severe pain with or without nonopioid or adjuvant drugs.

This step is used when higher doses of opioids are necessary.

Separate dosage forms of the opioid and nonopioid analgesic are used to avoid exceeding the maximum recommended doses of acetaminophen or NSAID.

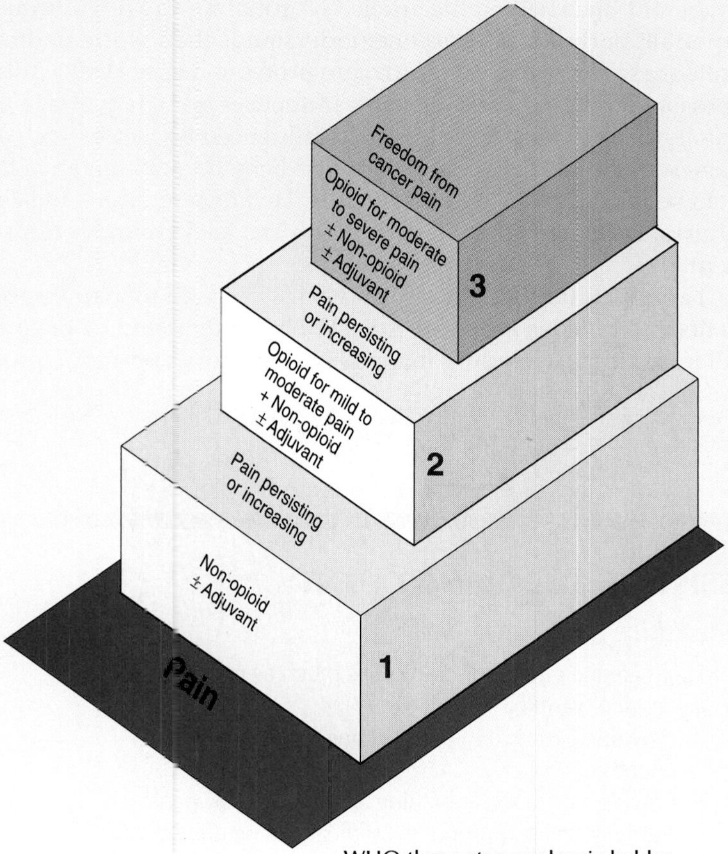

WHO three-step analgesic ladder.

Note: Pain that is persistent, or moderate to severe at the outset, should be treated by increasing the opioid dosage or using a higher potency. Morphine, hydromorphone, methadone, fentanyl, or levorphanol can replace the codeine or hydrocodone when severe pain exists.

Source: Adapted from The World Health Organization, *Cancer pain relief and palliative care*. Geneva, 1996, with permission.

4. Assess client for physiological signs of pain: elevated blood pressure and pulse.
5. After determining appropriate drug, dose, and route, administer drug and observe for effects of medication on pain relief and for potential side effects.
6. Assess client frequently for effects of pain management.
7. Maintain around-the-clock sustained-release medications for continuous pain.
8. Treat break through pain with immediate-release medications.

CLINICAL ALERT

The client's verbal account of his or her pain is accepted for pain measurement. Therefore, it is important to explain the use of the pain scale so the client accurately describes his or her pain as drug therapy is based on the measurement.

CLINICAL ALERT

Medications for persistent cancer-related pain are administered around the clock for best efficacy, not on a PRN basis. Additional PRN medications may be administered as needed.

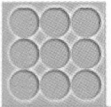

CULTURAL COMPETENCE

Singer and Blackhall, in the article "Negotiating Cross-Cultural Issues at the End of Life," state that culture is an important part of how everyone understands their world and how this impacts their decisions, especially on health care issues. This includes health care professionals as well. Culture influences the way people make meaning out of illness and dying; therefore, it also influences how they utilize the medical community at the end of life. Each individual has a perspective that is also influenced by factors such as personal psychology, gender, and life experiences. There is a wide variation of beliefs and behaviors within any ethnic population. This leads us to realize that each client needs to be treated individually. Health care professionals must not influence clients with their own beliefs or cultures. Failure to take the client's cultural background seriously means we fail to understand the values held by the client.

Lack of cultural sensitivity and skills can lead to inappropriate clinical outcomes and poor interaction with clients and families at a very crucial point in their end-of-life process. Addressing and respecting cultural differences will increase trust, leading to a more satisfactory end-of-life process for both the client and the family.

Source: Kagawa-Singer, M., & Blackhall, L.J. (2001, December 19). Negotiating cross-cultural issues at the end of life. *Journal of the American Medical Association, 286*(23), 2993–3001.

ASSISTING THE DYING CLIENT

Procedure

1. Minimize the client's discomfort as much as possible.
   a. Provide warmth.
   b. Provide assistance in moving, and position client frequently.
   c. Provide assistance in bathing and personal hygiene.
   d. Administer the appropriate medications before the pain becomes severe.
2. Recognize the symptoms of urgency or emergency conditions and seek immediate assistance.
3. Notify the charge nurse or team leader if there is an impending crisis and perform emergency actions until help arrives.
4. Encourage dying clients to do as much as they can for themselves so that they do not just give up—a state that only reinforces low self-esteem.
5. Provide emotional nursing care for the client.
   a. Form a relationship with the dying client. Be willing to be involved, to care, and to be committed to caring for a dying client.
   b. Allocate time to spend with the client so that not only physical care is administered.
   c. Recognize the grief pattern and support the client as he or she moves through it.
   d. Recognize that your physical presence is comforting by staying physically close to the client if he or she is frightened. Use touch if appropriate and nonverbal communication.
   e. Respect the client's need for privacy, and withdraw if the client has a need to be alone or to disengage from personal relationships.

TO MY FAMILY, MY PHYSICIAN, MY LAWYER, MY CLERGYMAN
TO ANY MEDICAL FACILITY IN WHOSE CARE I HAPPEN TO BE
TO ANY INDIVIDUAL WHO MAY BECOME RESPONSIBLE FOR MY HEALTH, WELFARE OR AFFAIRS

Death is as much a reality as birth, growth, maturity and old age—it is the one certainty of life. If the time comes when I, ______________________________ can no longer take part in decisions for my own future, let this statement stand as an expression of my wishes, while I am still of sound mind.

If the situation should arise in which there is no reasonable expectation of my recovery from physical or mental disability, I request that I be allowed to die and not be kept alive by artificial means or "heroic measures". I do not fear death itself as much as the indignities of deterioration, dependence and hopeless pain. I, therefore, ask that medication be mercifully administered to me to alleviate suffering even though this may hasten the moment of death.

This request is made after careful consideration. I hope you who care for me will feel morally bound to follow its mandate. I recognize that this appears to place a heavy responsibility upon you, but it is with the intention of relieving you of such responsibility and of placing it upon myself in accordance with my strong convictions, that this statement is made.

Signed ______________________________

Date ______________________________

Witness ______________________________

Witness ______________________________

Copies of this request have been given to ______________________________

____

____

____

In case of terminal illness, Euthanasia Council's "Living Will" can clarify client's wishes.

f. Be tuned in to client's cues that he or she wants to talk and express feelings, cry, or even intellectually discuss the dying process.
g. Accept the client at the level on which he or she is functioning without making judgments.

6. Provide the level of care that encourages the client to retain confidence in the health care team.
7. Assist the client through the experience of dying in whatever way you are able to do so.
8. Support the family of the dying client.
   a. Understand that the family may be going through anticipatory grief before the actual event of dying.
   b. Understand that different family members react differently to the impending death and support the different reactions.
   c. Be aware that demonstrating your concern and caring assists the family to cope with the grief process.
9. Be aware of your own personal orientation toward the dying process.
   a. Explore your own feelings about death and dying with the understanding that until you have faced the subject of death you will be inadequate to support the client or the family as they experience the dying process.
   b. Share your feelings about dying with the staff and others; actively work through them so that negativity does not get transferred to the client.

SUPPORTING THE FAMILY OR CAREGIVER

Procedure

1. Introduce yourself to the family or caregiver and explain your role in caring for client.
2. Provide honest answers to questions.
3. Reinforce client's wishes for end-of-life care related to DNR orders, living wills, and advance directive.
4. Explain each procedure/intervention you are providing for client.
5. Ask family members or caregiver how he or she wants to participate in client care.
6. Encourage family or caregiver to take time alone to regroup.
7. Provide or obtain psychosocial support and bereavement counseling for family. **Rationale:** Family members may exhaust much of their energy, develop sleep deprivation, and exhibit signs of depression, anxiety, and even chronic health problems during this stressful time.
8. Encourage family members to build a support group of friends or other family members. **Rationale:** No one should be alone during this time.
9. Remind family or caregiver to eat properly and maintain an exercise schedule.
10. Refer family members to support groups as needed.
11. Refer family members to social services for help with issues such as insurance, living wills, funeral arrangement, and other financial constraints.
12. Prepare family for client's death.

EVIDENCE BASED NURSING PRACTICE

Factors Considered Important at End of Life

A cross-sectional, stratified random national survey conducted in March–August 1999 of 340 seriously ill patients, 332 bereaved family, 361 physicians, and 429 nurses and other health care providers studied the importance of 44 attributes of quality at the end of life. Consistently, across all four groups of participants, pain and symptom management, preparation for death, achieving a sense of completion, decisions about treatment preferences, and being treated as a "whole person" were identified as important issues. Pain control was ranked highest among the variables (attributes) and dying at home the least important.

Source: Steinhauser, K.E., et al. (2000, November 15). Factors Considered Important at the End of Life by Patients, Family, Physicians, and Other Care Providers. *Journal of the American Medical Association, 284*(19).

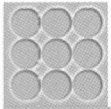

CULTURAL COMPETENCE

Death Rituals Vary from One Culture to Another.

Arab-Americans do not openly anticipate or grieve for a dying person Most of the Arab-American clients prefer to die in the hospital. There are special rituals after the death, such as washing the body and all orifices. The designated head of the family determines how family members will be notified of the death. Organ donation is usually not allowed out of respect for burying the body whole. They will probably not choose a DNR order; in fact, the family may lose trust in the health care system if this option is offered them.

Black Americans vary with respect to dying at home or in the hospital. Many families care for the clients at home until death is imminent, then bring them to the hospital. Some believe it is bad luck to die at home. There are no rituals associated with care of the body. Cremation is usually not done. Organ donation is usually not done except for an immediate family need.

Chinese-Americans may be fatalistic when faced with a terminal illness and death. They usually do not talk about it. Chinese believe that dying at home brings bad luck, but others believe the spirit will get lost if death occurs in the hospital. Each client and family should be supported in their belief. Organ donation and autopsy are generally not accepted, as they believe the body should be kept intact.

Native Americans embrace the present. Some tribes avoid contact with the dying, while others will want to be present 24 hours a day. Eating, playing games, and making jokes in the hospital are seen as appropriate for some tribes. Many of the tribes will bring healers to attend to the spiritual health of the dying client. Some family members will wrap the body for burial and not allow a mortuary to prepare the body, while others may avoid all contact with the body. Organ donation is generally not accepted.

Documentation for the Dying Client

- Client's physical symptoms
- Stage of dying and acceptance of client
- Support systems available to client
- Nursing care measures that make the client the most comfortable
- Family acceptance and interaction with client
- Comfort or limited support measure provided
- DNR orders in place.

Critical Thinking Application

UNEXPECTED OUTCOMES	CRITICAL THINKING OPTIONS
Nurse is unable to care for the dying client due to her or his own emotional reaction.	• Request that other staff members take over, as the objective is to be able to give good nursing care. • Request assistance from skilled professional so you can work through your own feelings about death in order to be able to cope with the next death experience.
Client loses confidence in the health care team.	• Attempt to ascertain exactly what occurred to cause client to lose confidence in the team. • Report to charge nurse so that staff caring for client may be changed. Be sure to choose experienced personnel who are equipped to cope with a dying client.
Client lingers on and does not fulfill expectation that death would occur in the near future.	• Report status to staff so arrangements may be made for respite–supportive care for family who is having a difficult time coping. • Discuss hospice care with the client's family.
Pain cannot be controlled adequately with ordered medication.	• Report to physician so alternative pain relief methods may be used. • Ensure that WHO three-step analysis ladder protocols are being followed. • Ensure that around-the-clock medication administration is occurring. • Assist the client to cope by spending additional time and meeting physical needs.

UNIT 3

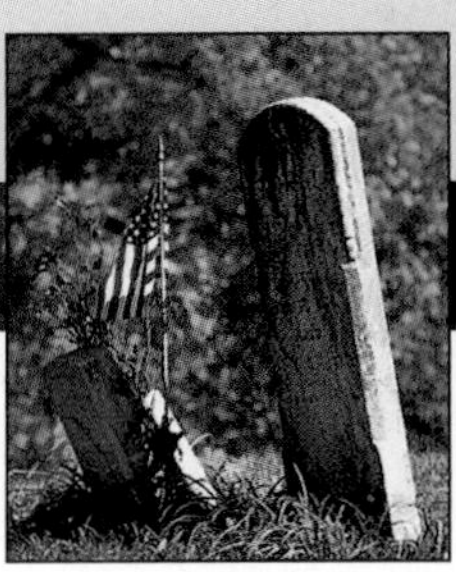

Postmortem Care

Nursing Process Data

ASSESSMENT *Data Base*

Verify that client has been pronounced dead by the physician or other health care provider, as determined by state regulations.

Complete your own observations that client has no observable responses to stimuli.

Identify client by name and client's belongings for labeling.

PLANNING *Objectives*

To prepare body for removal from clinical unit

To protect the condition of the body for the purpose of respect for the deceased and his or her family during final viewing

To document facts and time relating to death

To identify and label client and client's belongings

IMPLEMENTATION *Procedures*

Providing Postmortem Care

EVALUATION *Expected Outcomes*

Postmortem care is completed by assigned staff member.

Client's personal items have been identified and labeled properly.

Family is supported through grief process by staff.

PROVIDING POSTMORTEM CARE

Equipment

Bathing supplies
Shroud or morgue bag
Identification tags
Protective pads, if necessary
Rolls of gauze and abdominal pads, if necessary
Paper bags or plastic bags for personal belongings
Gurney or specialized morgue cart
Clean gloves

Procedure

1. If there are other clients or visitors in the room, carefully explain the situation and ask them to temporarily leave the room if possible. Provide privacy.
2. Collect necessary equipment.
3. Follow hospital procedure regarding notification of various departments and personnel.
   a. Determine if client has signed a donor card and/or has made a decision to donate any organs.
   b. Follow client's advance directive on file at the hospital for donor instructions.
   c. Notify appropriate hospital personnel or local procurement organization (OPO) for assistance with organ donation.
   d. Follow specific procedures for organ transplant according to hospital policy.
4. Maintain proper alignment of the body. Raise the head of the bed 30°. Maintain head elevation throughout care and to morgue. **Rationale:** To prevent pooling of fluids in the head or face.
5. Don gloves.
6. Do not replace dentures. **Rationale:** As facial muscles relax, dentures can fall out and be lost. Leave dentures in a denture cup and send with client to the morgue.
7. Remove any external objects causing pressure or injury to the skin (e.g., oxygen mask).
8. Convert all IV lines to hep loks or intermittent infusion devices. **Rationale:** Removing catheters and IV lines cause fluid to leak into tissues and cause edema and discoloration. Hospital policy may supersede this action; if so, follow hospital policy.
9. Cleanse the body as needed. A partial bath may be required to remove secretions, wound drainage, stains.
10. Close the eyes. If necessary, use paper tape or gauze pads. You may do this after the family has visited the deceased.
11. Place protective incontinent pad under buttocks and between legs diaper fashion.
12. If family is to visit the deceased, provide clean linen and gown for client.
13. Remove equipment used for cleansing client.
14. If previously determined or requested by client or family, notify the appropriate clergy or religious support person.
15. After family and clergy have visited, label the body, attaching ID tags to the big toe, wrist, and morgue bag or as determined by standard procedure.

Signed by the donor and the following two witnesses in the presence of each other:

Signature of Donor | Date of Birth of Donor

Date Signed | City & State

Witness | Witness

This is a legal document under the Uniform Anatomical Gift Act or similar laws.

For further information consult your physician or

National Kidney Foundation
116 East 27th Street, New York, N.Y. 10016

To ensure that organs are donated appropriately, instruct client to fill out and keep donor card available at all times.

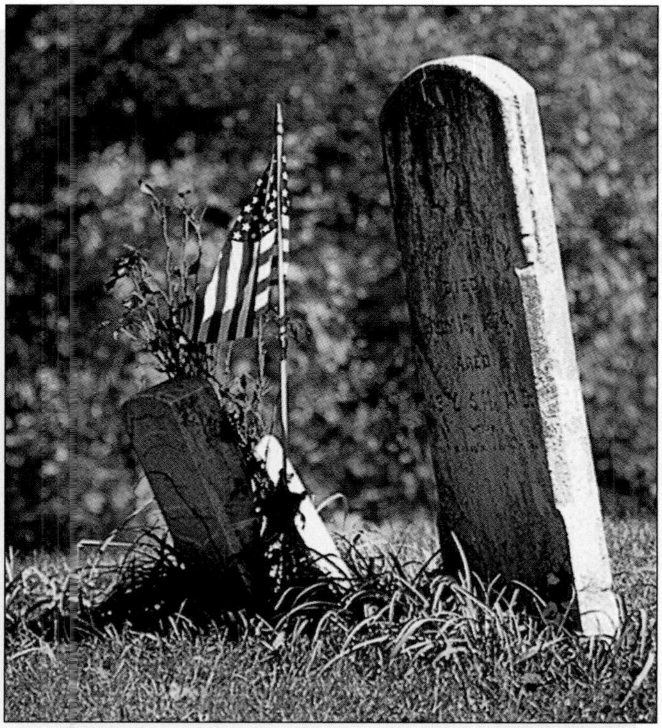

16. Place arms and hands loosely at side or on abdomen. **Rationale:** This prevents discoloration of hands.
17. Place the body in the shroud or in morgue bag.
18. Label all personal belongings, and place them in a bag.
19. Remove gloves and wash hands.
20. Close doors to client's room, and clear hallways in preparation to transfer the body to the morgue.
21. Transfer the body to the morgue on a gurney or a special morgue cart. Keep client's head elevated.
22. Place client's personal belongings in the appropriate place determined by hospital policy.
23. Support family members as needed.

Note: Rigor mortis begins about 4 hours after death and reaches its peak about 10 hours later. It passes from the body after 36 hours. It is best to wait until the body passes through this process before embalming. Therefore, it is not a problem to wait for relatives to view the body within a specified time frame.

CLINICAL ALERT

Inform the funeral home if the client has tuberculosis or any other infectious disease so appropriate care can be taken to prevent contamination of the environment.

CHARTING FOR POSTMORTEM CARE

- The events leading to the actual death (i.e., termination of vital signs)
- The exact time the physician or health care professional was informed and death was pronounced
- When family members or significant others were notified
- Time organ procurement team informed, if appropriate
- Consent forms signed
- Condition of the body and postmortem care delivered
- Time the body and belongings were sent to the morgue

Critical Thinking Application

UNEXPECTED OUTCOMES	CRITICAL THINKING OPTIONS
Client is not identified properly when sent to the morgue.	• Check identaband and shroud label before releasing client to mortician. • Request another nurse to check labels.
Donated organs are needed.	• Provide support to family and give an opportunity for questions. • Obtain signatures for consent form. (Kidneys should be removed within 1 hour after death. Eyes should be removed within 6–24 hours after death.) • Examine reverse side of driver's license, or remind the charge nurse to call mortician if burial plans have been made previously, to check on permission for organ donation through a living will.

Gerontologic Considerations

Three out of four elderly people die of heart disease, cancer, or stroke.

- Heart disease is leading cause of death, although it has declined since 1968.
- Death rates from cancer continue to rise, especially lung cancer.
- Death statistics for people in the 65–74 age group: heart disease accounted for 38%; cancer, 30% of deaths.
- Two thirds of hospice clients are over 65 years of age.

Death in the life cycle.

- In American culture, the obsession with youth often results in denial of death as a natural phase of the life cycle, and death is not considered a positive process.
- Elderly may see death as an end to suffering and loneliness.
- Death is usually not feared if the person has lived a long and fulfilled life, having completed all developmental tasks.
- Spiritual beliefs or philosophy of life are important.

Management Guidelines

Each state legislates a Nurse Practice Act for RNs and LVN/LPNs. Health care facilities are responsible for establishing and implementing policies and procedures that conform to their state's regulations. Verify the regulations and role parameters for each health care worker in your facility.

Delegation of Responsibilities

- Assisting the client to deal with grief may be delegated to any member of the staff who has had experience in working with grief and who has a working relationship with the client. For example, a CNA on the staff may have been a hospice or church worker who has had experience dealing with the grieving process. Assigning staff to work with a dying client will involve similar parameters, with the additional criteria that the nurse or nonprofessional assistant has worked through their own feelings about dying and can deal directly with the subject of death. If a client wishes to discuss dying or fears related to dying, the nurse must be able to listen and appropriately interact with the client. The nurse or CNA/UAP assigned to care for the dying client should be aware of the importance of the family in terms of support and communication.
- The nurse is responsible for checking the advance directives in the client's chart for organ donation or the living will before assigning a nonprofessional member of the team to care for the client.
- Postmortem care may be completed by any of the staff. However, if there are organs to be donated, the professional nurse is responsible for carrying out the hospital policies and/or orders necessary to preserve the organs for organ transplant.

Information Flow

- Because nonprofessional staff are often assigned to care for the basic needs of a dying client, the RN/LVN must set up a channel of communication (both written and verbal) so the nurse is constantly aware of what is happening with the client, and the family is informed of the client's status. The professional nurse should also provide the family with opportunities to discuss the condition of the client and plans (for organ donation), and for the future care of the client (perhaps hospice care). It would be inappropriate for nonprofessional staff to be assigned these activities.

CRITICAL THINKING STRATEGIES

SCENARIO 1

You are assigned to care for Mrs. Garcia, an 85-year-old Hispanic client who speaks limited English. Her caregiver at home has been her daughter, who speaks somewhat more English than her mother. A son and grandson visit her often and both of them speak fluent English. Mrs. Garcia has been brought to the hospital in end-stage renal failure. Her BUN and creatinine are both very high. Her blood pressure is 210/110, pulse 110, and respirations 30 and labored. Her skin has a jaundiced appearance and she has many ecchymotic areas throughout her body. She states she "doesn't want to live like this." She is debating asking to be taken off dialysis, but that decision has not yet been made.

1. Considering her condition, what priority interventions should you consider? What is the rationale for your answer?
2. Considering her limited English skills, how will you carry out your priority interventions?
3. Her daughter asks you how long she will live without dialysis. What is your best response? Provide rationale for your response.
4. In the evening after the son has been to visit his mother in the hospital, the family discussed her wishes. It was decided that they would stop dialysis. What steps will you take to provide end of life care to Mrs. Garcia?
5. Identify at least four interventions you will use to assist the family in coping with the impending death of their mother and grandmother.
6. During the last day, Mrs. Garcia is complaining about mild to moderate pain. What interventions will you use to make her comfortable?

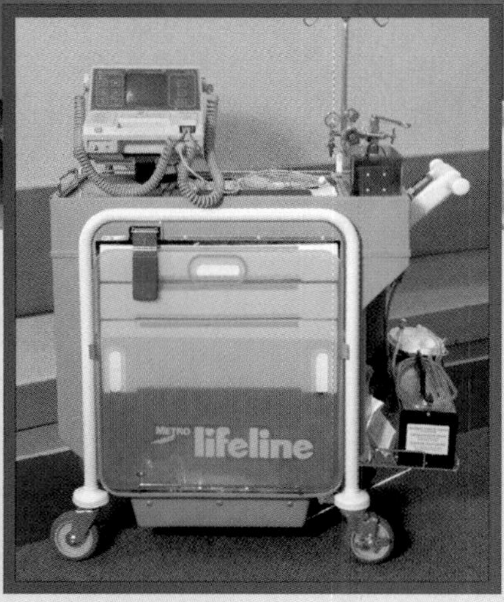

CHAPTER 33

Advanced Nursing Skills

THEORETICAL CONCEPTS

UNIT ONE: **Pulmonary Artery Pressure (Hemodynamic) Monitoring 1209**
- Leveling and Zeroing the Monitor System 1211
- Assisting Physician with Catheter Insertion 1212
- Obtaining Pressure Readings 1214
- Measuring Cardiac Output 1215

UNIT TWO: **Arterial Blood Pressure Monitoring 1217**
- Performing the Allen's Test 1218
- Assisting with Arterial Line Insertion 1219
- Monitoring Arterial Blood Pressure 1219
- Withdrawing Arterial Blood Samples 1221
- Removing Arterial Catheter 1222

UNIT THREE: **Cardiac Emergencies 1225**
- Maintaining the Emergency Cart 1226
- Checking Contents of the Emergency Cart 1227
- Calling a Code 1228
- Performing Defibrillation 1228
- Administering Advanced Life-Support Medications 1230
- Assisting with Elective Synchronized Cardioversion 1231

UNIT FOUR: **Mechanical Ventilation 1235**
- Caring for Clients on Ventilators 1236
- Weaning the Mechanically Ventilated Client 1239

GERONTOLOGIC CONSIDERATIONS 1242

MANAGEMENT GUIDELINES 1242

CRITICAL THINKING STRATEGIES 1244

Cross reference: Chapter 26, Respiratory Care, Chapter 27, Circulatory Maintenance, Chapter 28, Intravenous Therapy

LEARNING OBJECTIVES

- Outline nursing responsibilities in anticipating and responding to cardiac emergencies.
- Ensure client and staff safety during electrical counter-shock procedures.
- Describe the rationale for arterial blood pressure monitoring.
- Outline the steps in performing the Allen test.
- Identify a normal arterial blood pressure waveform.
- Explain the procedure for obtaining a blood sample from an arterial line.
- Outline safety precautions for the client with an arterial line.
- List hemodynamic information obtained by means of a pulmonary artery (balloon-tipped flow-directed) catheter.
- Differentiate waveforms for pulmonary artery and pulmonary capillary wedge pressures.
- Discuss the purpose and method for leveling and zeroing the monitor.
- State three ways to troubleshoot pulmonary artery catheter problems.
- Discuss nursing care needs of the mechanically ventilated client.
- Describe the process of weaning a client from mechanical ventilation.

TERMINOLOGY

Adjunctive: accessory to or assisting with.

Afterload: resistance against which the heart must pump to eject blood during systole. Pulmonary vascular resistance (PVR) presents afterload to the right heart, systemic vascular resistance (SVR) presents afterload to the left heart.

Allen's test: manual test to determine patency of the ulnar or radial artery. Digital pressure is applied directly over the radial and ulnar arteries. When pressure on one vessel is released, blood flow to palm and fingers indicates obstruction is not present in that vessel.

Barotrauma: alveolar injury due to overdistention by mechanical ventilation.

Bipolar leads: electrocardiographic recording in which two poles are used: one positive, one negative. Leads I, II, and III of the 12-lead ECG are bipolar.

Bolus: rapid administration of a volume of fluid or a drug intravenously.

Calibrate: to check or adjust a transducer to a standard measurement.

Cannulation: insertion of a tube into a blood vessel for purposes of invasive pressure monitoring. The cannula is attached to a transducer which in turn converts the pressure to a monitored waveform display.

Cardiac index (CI): the cardiac output in relation to client's body surface area.

Cardiac output (CO): amount of blood ejected by the heart per minute. Determined by multiplying heart rate by stroke volume (HR × SV = CO).

Central venous pressure (CVP): reflects filling pressure of the right heart. Measures central preload.

Diastole: period when ventricles are relaxed; a period of ventricular filling and coronary artery perfusion.

Dicrotic notch: component of the arterial waveform that represents closure of aortic valve at the end of ventricular contraction.

Diffusion: movement of a gas from an area of high pressure to an area of lower pressure.

Distal: area farthest away from point of reference (fingers are most distal part of upper extremity).

Dysrhythmia: abnormality of heart rate or rhythm.

Electrical potential: charges on cell membrane are separated into negative and positive charged particles.

Electrocardiogram (ECG): graphic representation of the variations in electrical potential caused by depolarization of the heart muscles.

Electrode: an adhesive patch applied to the skin to transmit cardiac electrical activity to a machine for display.

Hemodynamic: movement of blood.

Invasive: involves puncturing or incising the skin for insertion of a tube or instrument into the body.

Left ventricular end-diastolic pressure (LVEDP): pressure of blood in the left ventricle at the end of diastole; a measure of left ventricular preload.

Low cardiac output: decreased amount of blood ejected into the systemic circulation due to decreased stroke volume or slow heart rate.

Lumen: the inside, channel, or opening of a blood vessel or tube.

Mean arterial (blood) pressure (MAP): average pressure within the cardiovascular system throughout one cardiac cycle. Determined by adding systolic pressure to two times the diastolic pressure and dividing the sum by three.

Oscilloscope: instrument that displays a visual representation of electrical activity on a monitor screen.

Perfusion: blood flow to tissues.

Phlebostatic axis: the crossing of two reference lines to determine the point at which the zero mark on manometer is level with this axis.

Preload: end diastolic filling pressure (stretch) in the ventricles.

Proximal: refers to an area closest to the point of reference; humerus of upper extremity is more proximal to the body than the fingers.

Pulmonary artery pressure (PAP): waveform representing systolic and diastolic pressures in the pulmonary artery, usually displayed by hemodynamic monitoring. Pulmonary artery diastolic pressure is often used as equivalent to pulmonary artery wedge pressure.

Pulmonary artery wedge pressure: an indirect indicator of left ventricular pressure—normal PAWP is 8 to 13 mm Hg. Elevations are seen in left ventricular failure.

Refractory period: period during which cardiac cells are not responsive to electrical stimulation (QRS and ST segment of the ECG is the refractory period for the ventricles).

Repolarization: restoration of the heart cells to their original resting potential.

Surfactant: a phospholipid synthesized by the lungs; acts to lower alveolar tension and increase lung compliance.

Thermodilution: method of calculating cardiac output by injection of solution into the proximal lumen of a pulmonary artery catheter and determining the solution's temperature change at the thermistor (distal) lumen of the catheter.

Transducer: device that converts one form of energy into another (e.g., biophysical event is converted into electrical waveform, which is displayed on the oscilloscope).

Vasculature: vascular system of the body.

Vasodilator: causes dilation of the blood vessels. A venodilator reduces preload; an arterial vasodilator reduces afterload.

Vasopressor: causes contraction of the muscular tissue of the arteries and veins.

Vasospasm: constriction of a vessel due to spasm.

Ventricular systole: contraction phase of the cardiac cycle during which the ventricles eject blood into receiving arteries.

Voltage: electromagnetic force measured in volts.

Waveform: pictorial representation of a pressure or electrical activity of the heart, depicted on an oscilloscope.

Weaning: gradual withdrawal of mechanical ventilation and the reestablishment of spontaneous breathing.

ADVANCED SKILLS IN NURSING PRACTICE

This chapter presents a nursing process framework for nursing actions used in the maintenance of homeostasis during life-threatening conditions. Provision of competent care during critical periods requires a knowledge of monitoring techniques, skill in the analysis of data, diagnostic reasoning, and decision-making. Working with monitors and providing client care at the same time can be a challenging experience for the nurse.

Monitoring techniques are useful adjunctive tools that provide the practitioner with critical ongoing client information. Interpretation of this information assists in the assessment of the major body systems and recognition of altered hemodynamic states (e.g., fluid deficit or overload). Continuous monitoring of cardiovascular pressure readings serves as a guide for identifying appropriate nursing diagnoses, developing a plan of care, and evaluating the client's response to therapy.

In the clinical setting, nurses are constantly faced with new equipment, new techniques, and better and more sophisticated evaluative methods. To keep pace in the area of technologic advancement can be a monumental task, one that challenges the nurse's energy, patience, and abilities. The nurse's role in assessment, planning, intervention, and evaluation is based in part on the nurse's familiarity with monitoring data.

Hemodynamic monitoring has evolved over the years from continuous ECG monitoring, to measuring CVP (right heart pressure), to direct determination of cardiac output, and indirect measurements of left heart filling pressures. Hemodynamic monitoring techniques require that equipment is properly positioned and functions correctly, that the monitor waveforms are representative of the client's physiologic variables and are interpreted correctly.

A multi-lumen, balloon-tipped, flow-directed catheter (e.g., Swan-Ganz) is used to measure intracardiac pressures. It is inserted into the right side of the heart via a central vein. The catheter is advanced into the pulmonary artery so that individual catheter lumens reflect measures of right atrial pressure (RAP or CVP), pulmonary artery pressure (PAP), and, when advanced briefly to an occlusive position, pulmonary artery wedge pressure (PAWP). Cardiac output (CO) and systemic and pulmonary vascular resistance (SVR, PVR) are other valuable client measures obtained with this catheter. It is simultaneously used for the infusion of fluids and medications.

Waveforms (pressure signals) are transmitted from the catheter to a transducer by means of fluid-filled tub-

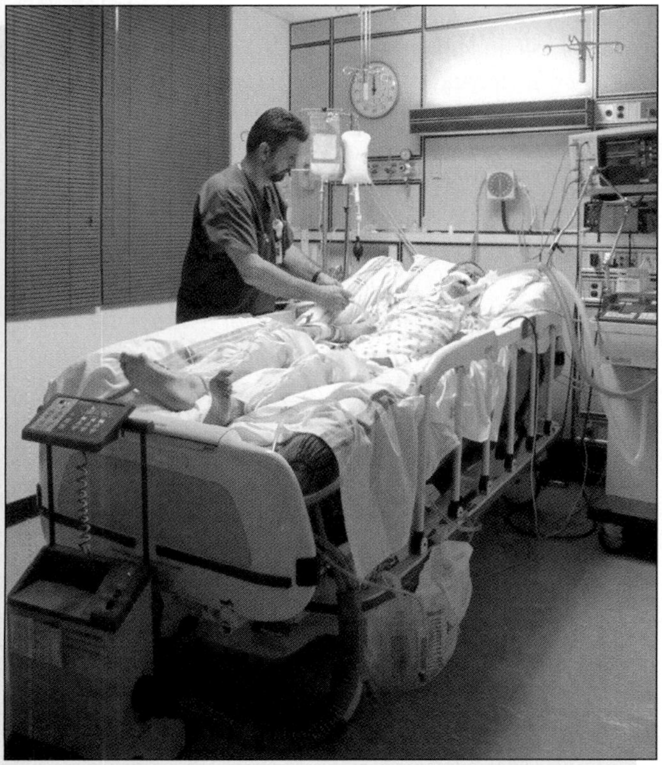

Sophisticated technology facilitates the intensive care of clients.

ing. The signal is then amplified and displayed on an oscilloscope both as a visual (analog) waveform and a digital display. Similarly, a catheter can be placed in a peripheral artery and direct blood pressure can be monitored using these same principles. The client's physiologic pressure signals provide continuous data to help specialized nurses make critical assessments necessary for safe and effective care decisions, such as the titration of drugs and IV fluids.

Ability to integrate all available data is essential to provide excellent nursing care. Advanced technology provides essential measures that augment more overt client data, but it is important that this technology not become more important than the client himself. The first goal is to care for the client, not tend the equipment. One way to achieve a balance of mastery over complex skills and the attainment of high-quality client care is to become familiar with technical equipment so that it no longer causes anxiety and uncertainty. Once this level of confidence is realized, the focus is on the client, rather than the monitoring equipment.

- The single most important nursing action to decrease the incidence of hospital-based infections is handwashing. **Remember to wash your hands or use antibacterial gel before and after each and every client contact.**

Cultural Competence

Some cultures view critical illness as a curse, an imbalance of heat and cold, or disharmony with the universe rather than pathology or injury to an organ system. Western medicine's health care system utilizes much technology and sophisticated equipment. This approach may clash with another culture's beliefs in folk medicine, rituals, and religious healing.

Individuals of the same culture will vary in response to critical illness; therefore, the nurse must explore the meaning of the experience with each individual client in order to provide sensitive care.

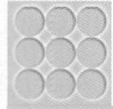

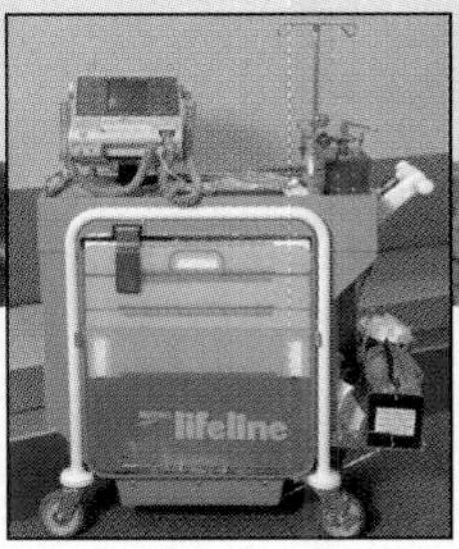

UNIT 1

Pulmonary Artery Pressure (Hemodynamic) Monitoring

Nursing Process Data

ASSESSMENT *Data Base*

Evaluate client's understanding of the procedure.

Assess for preexisting cardiovascular disease.

Determine client's level of anxiety regarding the procedure.

Obtain baseline vital signs and ECG.

Assess insertion site for inflammation or infection.

Assess patency of all lines.

Determine pressure on flush bag.

Level and zero the monitoring system.

Monitor PA systolic, PA diastolic, PA mean, PAWP.

Assess cardiac output using thermodilution technique.

PLANNING *Objectives*

To maintain a patent pulmonary artery monitoring system

To administer intravenous solutions and determine response to fluid therapy

To obtain specific hemodynamic measurements for decision making

To measure cardiac output

To obtain samples of mixed venous blood (mixed due to blood from systemic and coronary veins)

To determine need for drug therapy

IMPLEMENTATION *Procedures*

Leveling and Zeroing the Monitor System

Assisting Physician with Catheter Insertion

Obtaining Pressure Readings

Measuring Cardiac Output

EVALUATION *Expected Outcomes*

Pulmonary artery catheter remains patent.

Pressure on flush bag remains at 300 mm Hg.

Distinct pulmonary artery waveforms depicted on oscilloscope.

Pulmonary artery, systolic, diastolic, and pulmonary artery wedge pressure measurements are measured accurately.

Cardiac output measurements are obtained.

Altered cardiovascular status is detected early.

Hemodynamic information contributes to effective management of the critically ill client.

Tissue perfusion depends on cardiac pump performance, an adequate blood volume and vascular distribution (perfusion). Hypovolemia, cardiac failure, or other conditions (e.g., sepsis) alter intracardiac pressures. Since direct measurement of left atrial or ventricular pressure is not done in the clinical setting, an indication of these measures is obtained by *indirect* means via the right side of the heart.

A balloon-tipped, flow-directed catheter inserted transvenously and advanced into the pulmonary artery permits continuous, *indirect* measurement of left ventricular function for monitoring and assisting care of hemodynamically unstable clients.

Reduced cardiac function is manifested primarily by two hemodynamic abnormalities: decreased cardiac output (or cardiac index) and increased left ventricular end-diastolic pressure (LVEDP). The pulmonary artery catheter indirectly measures the LVEDP by directly measuring pulmonary artery and pulmonary artery wedge pressures. Mixed venous blood monitoring using a fiber optic pulmonary artery catheter provides information about the balance between tissue oxygen delivery and tissue oxygen consumption (SVO_2).

At the end of diastole (ventricular filling), the mitral valve is open, and the left ventricle, left atrium, and pulmonary vasculature momentarily act as a single chamber in which the pressure is equal throughout. Since the normal pressures of these chambers and vessels are known, pressure changes in the pulmonary artery can be used to reflect changes in the LVEDP. The pulmonary artery catheter measures central venous pressure (CVP) or right atrial pressure (RAP), pulmonary artery pressure (PAP), and pulmonary artery wedge pressure (PAWP). Abnormal pressures can indicate changes in a client's fluid balance, vascular tone, or heart pumping action. Cardiac output and other hemodynamic parameters are also calculated using this catheter (Table 33–1). To determine cardiac output, a bolus of cold or room temperature fluid is injected into the right atrial lumen. The fluid's temperature change is then detected in the pulmonary artery by the catheter-tip thermistor. The temperature change over time is computed and represents the cardiac output.

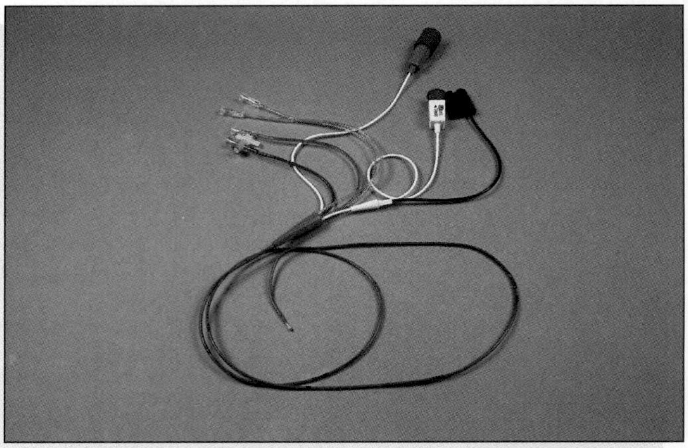
Balloon-tipped catheter has multiple lumens (internal tubes) with openings used to measure intracardiac pressures.

The balloon catheter is inserted into the subclavian vein percutaneously or through a cutdown and threaded *transvenously* to the right atrium. Partial inflation of the balloon at the tip of the catheter allows it to float through the tricuspid valve, the right ventricle, and the pulmonary valve into the pulmonary artery. Here the balloon is *deflated* and pulmonary artery pressure is monitored. If pulmonary artery wedge pressure measurement is required, the balloon is *briefly* inflated and the catheter is

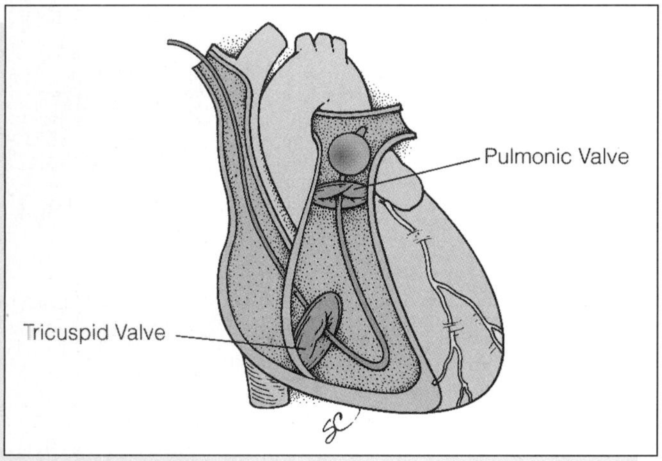

Balloon-tipped, flow-directed catheter with balloon inflated briefly for pulmonary artery wedge pressure determination.

TABLE 33–1 Normal Pressures

Right atrial (RAP): 2–8 mm Hg

Right ventricle (RV): $\frac{25}{5}$ mm Hg

Pulmonary artery pressure (PAP): $\frac{25}{10}$ mm Hg

PA mean $(\overline{PA})$: <15 mm Hg
PAWP: 10
Left atrial (LA): 5–10 mm Hg

Left ventricle (LV): $\frac{130}{5\text{–}10}$ mm Hg

Aorta: $\frac{130}{80}$

Mean arterial pressure (MAP):
70–90 (Diastolic × 2) + (Systolic × 1) ÷ 3 or

$\frac{(SBP) + 2\,(DBP)}{3}$

carried by blood flow through the pulmonary circulation until it wedges. During this brief occlusion (wedge) time, pressure reflected back on the tip of the catheter allows indirect measurement of LVEDP. The balloon is then deflated passively, and floats back to the pulmonary artery.

The pulmonary artery catheter typically has four or five lumens. Two lumens are used for pressure measurements. A proximal lumen is available to measure central venous pressure (right atrial pressure), assist in measuring cardiac output, and to inject selected solutions. The distal lumen is used to measure pulmonary artery pressure and pulmonary artery wedge pressure. A third lumen is used for balloon inflation. A fourth lumen is attached to a thermistor tip that assists in the measurement of cardiac output and blood temperature.

The advantage of pulmonary artery catheter measurements over the CVP reading is that the CVP does not provide information about left ventricular function or pulmonary vascular pressure changes until they are significant enough to be reflected back to the right atrium (CVP).

LEVELING AND ZEROING THE MONITOR SYSTEM

Procedure

1. Wash hands.
2. Reassure client and explain what you are doing.
3. Calibrate system.
   a. Using carpenter's level, adjust height of transducer to level of client's atrium or phlebostatic axis. **Rationale:** Transducer must remain level with client's right atrium for accurate monitoring. Higher transducer position yields low readings and vice versa.
   b. To zero monitor remove port cap (maintain sterility), open stopcock above transducer to air, closing it to the client and the flush system. **Rationale:** This action opens transducer to atmospheric pressure.

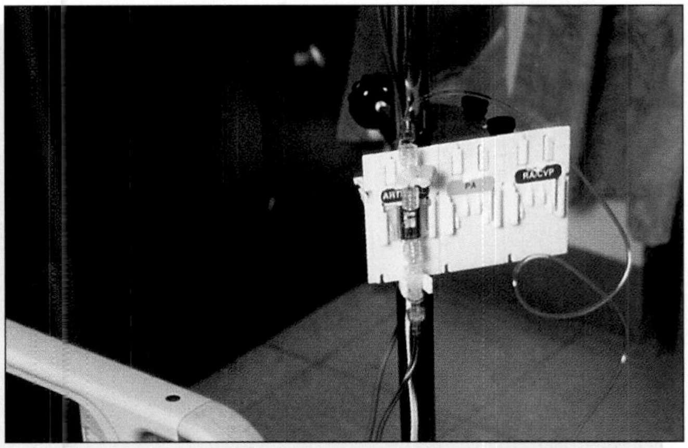

Adjust height of transducer to level of client's phlebostatic axis.

CLINICAL ALERT

Zero the air/fluid interface stopcock (on top of the transducer) to client's phlebostatic axis (intersection of lines at mid anterior–posterior chest and fourth ICS) every 8 hours and any time the bed or client's position is changed.

   c. Push the "zero" monitor button, and check if monitor reading is zero. **Rationale:** When reading is zero, transducer is balanced to atmospheric pressure (actually 760 millibars mm Hg).
4. Check that oscilloscope shows a flat wave at zero line. **Rationale:** This ensures accurate reading as it changes from zero point.
5. Recap port and close stopcock to reestablish flush system.

EVIDENCE BASED NURSING PRACTICE

Determining the Phlebostatic Axis

Since all clients' chests are not equal, the midaxillary line is not an accurate external reference point for the phlebostatic axis. Reference the junction of two lines: one drawn laterally from the fourth intercostal space transecting and one drawn midpoint between the anterior and posterior chest.

Source: McGhee, B., & Bridges, E. (2002). Monitoring arterial blood pressure: What you may not know. *Critical Care Nurse, 22*(2), 60–79.

ASSISTING PHYSICIAN WITH CATHETER INSERTION

Equipment

Sterile gloves
Percutaneous introducer kit
IV pole
Premix flush solution (usually 500 mL D_5W or NS with 1000 U Heparin 2 U/mL)
IV tubing
Pressure transducer system with pressure bag, tubing, flush device, and transducer
Pressure monitor
Clean gloves
Sterile towels
Skin antiseptic solution (povidone–iodine)
Razor
Sterile 4 × 4 sponges
Stethoscope
Lidocaine 1–2%
3 mL syringe with 18- and 25-gauge needle for topical anesthetic
Antimicrobial wipes
Occlusive dressing or tape
Suture with attached needle
Sterile needle holder or clamp
Cutdown tray, sterile gown, mask, and cap
Emergency cart
Sterile syringes filled with 5 mL or 10 mL D_5W (cardiac output)

Preparation

1. Identify client's room, client's identaband, and have client state name.
2. Explain rationale for procedure to client.
3. Verbally reassure client.
4. Wash hands.
5. Connect IV tubing to flush fluid bag.
6. Place prepared flush solution bag in pressure bag, and inflate to 300 mm Hg pressure. **Rationale:** This maintains a rate of flow through the flush device (3 mL/hr).
7. Prepare and assemble pressurized monitoring system (transducer, system flush device, and stopcocks) following manufacturer's instructions. Attach stopcocks to proximal and distal ports. Flush all lumens with flush solution.
8. Attach distal port stopcock to connecting tubing and heparinized flush solution, then attach to pressure monitoring unit, making sure all connections are tight.
9. Place client in Trendelenburg's position and turn client's head to opposite side. **Rationale:** This position distends central veins and prevents air embolism during the procedure.
10. Level and zero system according to manufacturer's instructions. The stopcock on top of the transducer must be at the level of client's atrium or phlebostatic axis (fourth intercostal space at the midchest line).
11. Shave and scrub skin with antiseptic solution.
12. Open sterile gloves for physician.
13. Open drape for physician.
14. Cleanse lidocaine vial with antimicrobial wipe.
15. Continuously monitor client's ECG throughout insertion of catheter. **Rationale:** Dysrhythmias may occur.

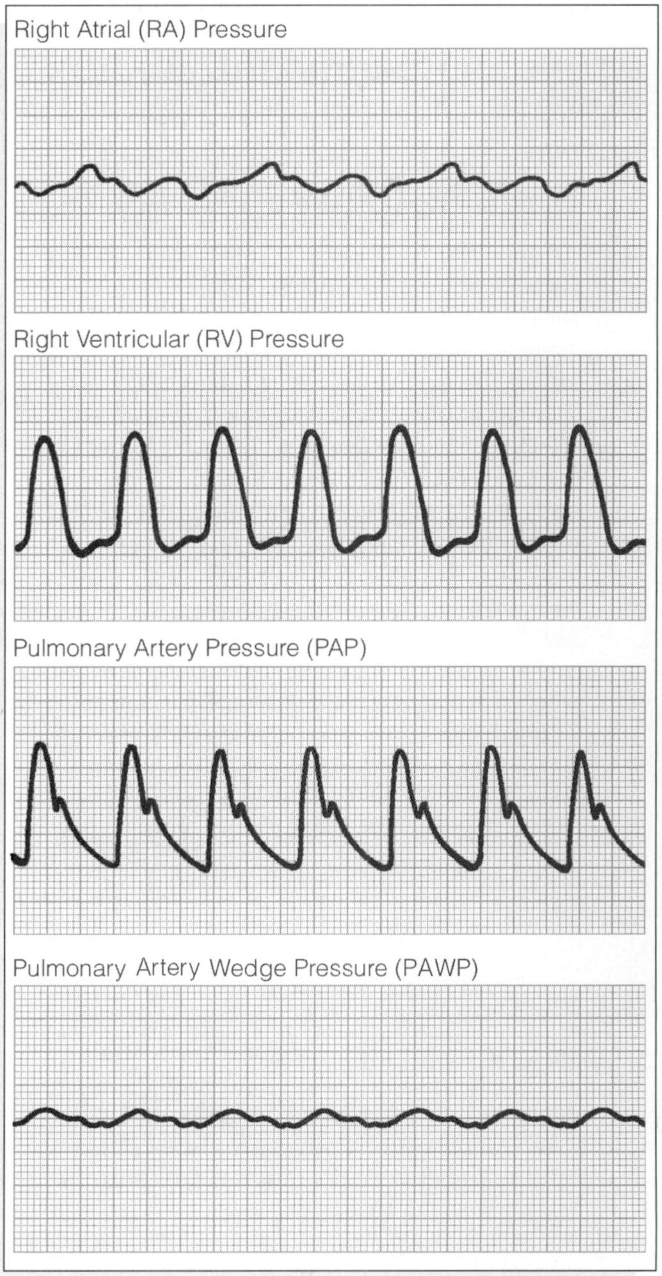

Waveforms depicted on monitor correspond with right heart chambers and pulmonary artery pressures.

Procedure

1. Don sterile gloves to assist physician as necessary.
   a. Physician dons sterile mask, cap, gown, and gloves. Catheter is tested for leaks by inflating balloon with 0.5–1.5 mL (amount determined by catheter size) of *air* while balloon is submerged in sterile basin filled with sterile irrigating solution.
   b. Physician aspirates lidocaine with 18-gauge needle, changes to 25-gauge needle, and injects lidocaine under skin.
   c. Physician performs cutdown or percutaneous insertion. Subclavian vein usually used; however, the jugular or a peripheral vein may be selected.
   d. Physician aspirates and flushes sheath with sterile D_5W or normal saline before inserting catheter. **Rationale:** This clears air and prevents air embolism. The use of D_5W rather than normal saline reduces risk of microshock to the client.
   e. While client performs Valsalva maneuver or hums, catheter is attached to fluid-filled transducer system. **Rationale:** This prevents inhalation and possible air embolism. Continuous pressure monitoring is observed during advancement of catheter.
   f. Catheter is advanced with a balloon partially inflated until correct right axial waveform appears on monitor.
   g. Physician inflates balloon (1–1.5 mL air) to assist in catheter's flow through tricuspid valve into right ventricle.
2. Observe for higher and more pronounced pressure waveform, indicating catheter's presence in right ventricle.
3. Record right ventricular pressure (systolic and diastolic reading), and observe for dysrhythmias: premature ventricular contractions (PVCs) or ventricular tachycardia.
4. Observe monitor for *higher* diastolic pressure and pulmonary arterial waveform. **Rationale:** Right ventricular and pulmonary artery pressures are similar, but pulmonary artery *diastolic* measure "steps up."
5. Remove syringe to allow balloon to deflate passively. (A special syringe is used that prevents overinflation of the balloon.)
6. Record pulmonary artery systolic (PAS), diastolic (PAD), and mean pressures.

Note: Measure all pulmonary artery pressures at end of expiration.

7. Inflate balloon fully (1.5 mL maximum) or until a change is seen in waveform (pulmonary artery to artery wedge pressure). **Rationale:** Inflated balloon assists passage of catheter into distal pulmonary artery.
8. Record PAWP (pulmonary artery wedge pressure).

> **CLINICAL ALERT**
>
> For PAWP (pulmonary artery wedge pressure), inflate balloon *briefly* (8 to 15 seconds), just until PAP changes to PAWP, then allow balloon to deflate by releasing pressure on syringe plunger or removing syringe.

9. Deflate balloon by releasing pressure on syringe plunger or remove syringe to allow passive deflation. **Rationale:** Active aspiration of air from balloon with a syringe plunger can cause balloon damage.
10. Determine balloon deflation by observing return of pulmonary artery waveform. **Rationale:** This assures balloon deflation. Continued occlusion of vessel can cause pulmonary infarction.
11. Repeat steps and measurements to verify function.
12. Leave balloon lumen port open at all times except during wedge placement.
13. Clear catheter using fast flush device.
14. Apply occlusive dressing to site after physician secures catheter with sutures.
15. Reassure client, and position for comfort.
16. Auscultate chest for presence of breath sounds.
17. Validate catheter placement by chest x-ray. **Rationale:** Pneumothorax can occur with jugular or subclavian vein cannulation.
18. Dispose of equipment, remove gloves, and wash hands.

Evidence Based Nursing Practice

Confirming Digital Measurements

This study showed lack of agreement between digital and graphic measurements of CVP and PAD, which ranged from as small as 1 mm Hg to as great as 40 mm Hg, especially in patients with respiratory rate >20. Digital measurements should be confirmed by waveform analysis of a graphic measurement before assuming that the value is accurate.

Source: Ahrens, T., & Schallom, L. (2001). Comparison of pulmonary artery and central venous pressure waveform measurements via digital and graphic measurement methods. *Heart & Lung, 30*(1), 26–38.

OBTAINING PRESSURE READINGS

Preparation

1. Level transducer, and zero (calibrate) monitor at the beginning of every shift. **Rationale:** This ensures accurate and consistent readings.
2. Check catheter, tubing, and connection points to ensure patency and security.
3. Mark client's midchest level at fourth ICS for consistent readings.
4. Place client flat supine or up to 45° elevation.
5. Reassure client.
6. Wash hands.

Procedure

1. Check that air reference port (stopcock) of pressure transducer is at level of client's atrium (phlebostatic axis). **Rationale:** This ensures accurate pressure reading. Level must be adjusted if client's position is changed.

> **CLINICAL ALERT**
> Pulmonary artery diastolic pressure is an acceptable equivalent of PAWP (if correlation determined) and eliminates need for occlusion (wedge) readings.

2. Expose distal port to the transducer. **Rationale:** All pulmonary artery pressure readings are taken from distal lumen of catheter, and right atrial pressures are taken from RA or proximal lumen.
3. Open balloon inflation port-locking device.
4. Attach syringe filled with proper amount of air, and align stopcock to open position.
5. Slowly inject 0.8 or 1.5 mL air into balloon. Inflate sufficient volume only to support float and change in waveform.
6. Observe waveform change from pulmonary artery to pulmonary artery wedge pressure on the monitor.

> **CLINICAL ALERT**
> Suspect balloon rupture if no resistance is encountered on inflation, syringe plunger fails to retract spontaneously, or if blood returns from balloon lumen. Mark stopcock: "DO NOT INFLATE."

7. Balloon should be inflated only long enough to observe PAWP waveform. **Rationale:** Longer inflation can cause overwedging (falsely high pressure readings) and damage to pulmonary tissue.
8. Allow balloon to deflate passively. **Rationale:** Aspirating air with syringe damages balloon.

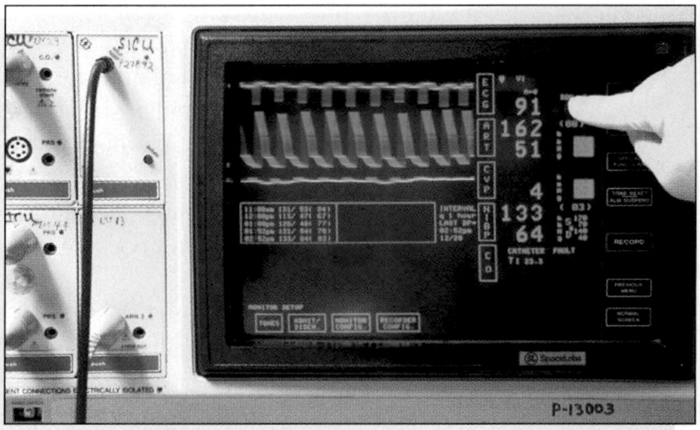

Monitor display of ECG, pressure waveforms, and digital readouts for continuous client assessment.

9. Ensure readings are always taken at end of expiration whether or not client is on ventilator (document if client is on ventilator). **Rationale:** Slightly higher readings are obtained if client is on a ventilator.
10. Use analog strip chart recording to obtain the most valid pressure measurements.
11. Maintain empty syringe on balloon port.
12. Flush line with fast flush device system.
13. Record readings; verify and report unusual findings to physician if they persist.
14. Place client in comfortable position.
15. Change dressings per agency policy, and observe for complications at site of catheter insertion.

> **CLINICAL ALERT**
> Changes in intracardiac pressures and volumes may be altered by changes in myocardial compliance. Any pressure should be interpreted in relation to the client's clinical assessment.

EVIDENCE BASED NURSING PRACTICE

Measuring Hemodynamic Pressures

Analog data (printed strip) rather than digital data or "stop-cursor" freezing the monitor screen remains the recommended method for measuring hemodynamic pressures. Mean pressures are determined by bisecting the waveform (area above and below bisecting line are equal).

Source: Bridges, E. (2000). Monitoring pulmonary artery pressures: Just the facts. *Critical Care Nurse, 20*(6), 59–75.

MEASURING CARDIAC OUTPUT

Equipment

Established pressure monitoring system

Closed system cardiac output set (COSET)

Includes: 500-mL bag of D_5W or NS (injectate), tubing with 3-way stopcock, syringe

Cardiac output cable

Preparation

1. Check physician's orders.
2. Identify client's room, check identaband, and ask client to state name.
3. Wash hands.
4. Spike injectate solution bag with tubing/stopcock.
5. Unclamp injectate tubing, prime tubing and stopcock, then reclamp tubing.
6. Connect primed system to client's PA catheter proximal port.
7. Stop any medication being infused through proximal port. **Rationale:** To prevent medication bolus during cardiac output measurement.
8. Note pulmonary artery waveform on monitor. **Rationale:** To verify catheter position.
9. Connect computer cable to thermistor port of pulmonary artery catheter (according to manufacturer's instructions). **Rationale:** Change in injectate temperature from proximal injectate port to thermistor port at distal lumen is computer calculated and displayed as the cardiac output in L/min.
10. Obtain client's height and weight measures.

Procedure

1. Place client in position used with previous hemodynamic readings; client should be supine, but may be elevated up to 45°.
2. Slowly flush proximal injectate lumen if any medications were being infused. **Rationale:** To prevent bolus medication delivery during cardiac output measurement.
3. Select *cardiac output* on bedside monitor menu.
4. Check and set computation constant to reflect size of catheter, volume (5 or 10 mL) of injectate, client's height and weight (*see PA catheter manufacturer's instructions*). **Rationale:** These are factored into computer derived hemodynamic measures (cardiac index).
5. Unclamp injectate solution tubing.
6. Attach syringe to stopcock and open stopcock to withdraw 5 or 10 mL of injectate into syringe.
7. Ensure that client is quiet. **Rationale:** Movement may cause inaccurate readings.
8. Open stopcock to client and inject rapidly (2–4 seconds). **Rationale:** Slower injectate results in inaccurate readings.
9. Note and record monitor display of client's cardiac output measure.
10. Repeat procedure two more times. **Rationale:** Two most similar readings are averaged to obtain accurate cardiac output measure.
11. Record averaged measure to obtain cardiac output.
12. Clamp injectate tubing.
13. Open stopcock to continue previous infusion to client.
14. Preserve closed cardiac output system by leaving tubing, stopcock, and syringe connections intact. **Rationale:** This eliminates need to open system each time measurements are made.
15. Determine derived values using client's cardiac output measure (stroke volume, systemic vascular resistance, pulmonary vascular resistance).

DOCUMENTATION FOR PULMONARY ARTERY PRESSURE MONITORING

- Physician who placed catheter
- Size of pulmonary artery catheter inserted
- Vessel placement and technique used to insert catheter (cutdown or percutaneous)
- Site care and dressing applied
- Client position during measurements
- Pressure readings obtained (specify digital or analog measures)
- Strip recordings attached
- Client's response to procedure
- Cardiac output results
- Problems arising and interventions performed

Critical Thinking Application

UNEXPECTED OUTCOMES	CRITICAL THINKING OPTIONS
Pulmonary artery catheter not patent.	• Check that tubing is not kinked. • Ensure continuous heparinized flush or normal saline infusion. (Check hospital policy.) Check stopcock connections. • Attempt to aspirate clotted blood through line by pulling back on plunger of a small syringe placed at proximal port. Remove clot, then flush line. • Notify physician if unable to clear line. • Fast flush system and flick tubing to eliminate tiny bubbles.
Pressure waveforms significantly abnormal.	• Check that tubing is not kinked. • Check stopcock level. • Correlate with client for possible change in clinical condition. • Tighten all connections. • Eliminate added stopcocks and tubing extensions. • Ask client to cough or change position to help free catheter. • If condition persists, notify physician to reposition line, and assess client.
Analog waveform inconsistent with digital display.	• Validate leveling at client's phlebostatic axis. • Validate zeroing of system to atmospheric pressure ("0" baseline). • Record analog strips and median measured values on chart—do not rely on digital measures.
No pressure tracing.	• Determine that power is ON. • Check for loose connections. • Check for clotted blood in line (damping is an early sign). Try to aspirate; never flush. • Check stopcocks to make sure they are turned appropriately.
No pulmonary wedge pressure tracing.	• Check and deflate balloon. • Suspect that catheter is not adequately advanced. Chest x-ray may be ordered to check placement of pulmonary artery catheter. • Reposition client. • Suspect possible balloon rupture if no resistance is felt on inflation.

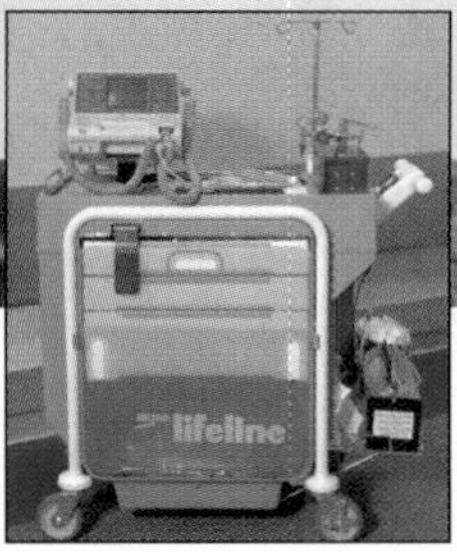

Arterial Blood Pressure Monitoring

Nursing Process Data

ASSESSMENT Data Base

Determine need for intra-arterial blood pressure monitoring.

Determine client's level of anxiety about the procedure.

Assess collateral perfusion of the hand using the Allen's test.

Measure intra-arterial (direct) systolic and diastolic blood pressure readings on the monitor.

Observe the mean arterial pressure on the monitor and validate using analog strip measurement.

Observe for trends in arterial pressure readings.

Evaluate the patency of the arterial catheter.

Validate pressure on infusion system. (Pressure should be 300 mm Hg.)

Assess catheter insertion site for signs of infection or bleeding.

Assess circulation, motion, and sensation of extremity distal to catheter insertion site.

PLANNING Objectives

To maintain a patent arterial catheter

To directly measure systolic, diastolic, and mean arterial blood pressures

To provide essential information regarding fluid volume, cardiac status, and perfusion pressure to vital organs

To assess adequacy of oxygenation

To assess adequacy of alveolar ventilation

To evaluate acid–base balance

To evaluate effectiveness of ventilatory treatment modalities

To provide immediate access for arterial blood gas samples

To allay the client's anxiety, and provide comfort measures

IMPLEMENTATION Procedures

Performing the Allen's Test

Assisting with Arterial Line Insertion

Monitoring Arterial Blood Pressure

Withdrawing Arterial Blood Samples

Removing Arterial Catheter

EVALUATION Expected Outcomes

Blood supply to hand is assessed to be adequate before arterial catheter insertion.

Distinct arterial pressure waveforms are observable on monitor.

Arterial catheter remains patent.

Puncture site remains free of complications (significant bleeding or signs of site infection).

Distal perfusion of extremity remains intact.

Arterial blood samples are obtained.

Blood pressure readings are valid and reliable.

Direct blood pressure monitoring allows continuous measurement of the client's systolic, diastolic, and mean arterial pressures (MAP) to facilitate evaluation of perfusion to vital organs. A short single lumen catheter is placed in the client's radial artery (femoral or brachial artery may be used), then attached to a pressure transducer and high-pressure infusion system and a display monitor.

To preserve the patency of the intraarterial catheter and to prevent thrombosis, a continuous flush of 3 to 10 mL/hr heparinized dextrose or normal saline solution is administered under 300 mm Hg pressure.

Invasive monitoring is appropriate for surgical clients, clients on mechanical ventilators, or those requiring vasodilator or vasopressor drugs, or frequent arterial blood gas studies.

Continuous arterial waveforms are observed on the oscilloscope, and numerical pressures are displayed. Blood pressure deviations can immediately be detected and appropriate therapy instituted without delay. The arterial line also provides easy access to blood sampling for ABGs and other lab values. Arterial blood gas values assist in determining respiratory and metabolic acid–base status (Tables 33-2 and 33-3) as well as lung capacity to provide oxygen. The measurements serve as a guide for implementing and evaluating treatment.

Hemodynamic Monitoring System Components

- Invasive **catheter** with high-pressure tubing connected to transducer
- **Flush/infusion system** with pressure bag at 300 mm Hg maintains patency of system
- **Transducer**—converts physiologic wave to electrical energy
- **Monitor**—converts electrical energy, displays pressure waveform and digital reading in mm Hg

Direct blood pressure waveform correlation to the cardiac cycle is represented by the symbols shown in the figure.

- *a* represents a sharp upstroke correlating with ventricular systole and the QRS complex of the electrocardiogram.
- *b* represents peak systole; its numerical value is the systolic pressure recorded.
- *c* represents the notch on the downstroke of the waveform. This notch is called the *dicrotic notch* and represents closure of the aortic valve.
- *d* represents diastole and is represented by a continuous decline in pressure. The numerical value at the lowest point is the diastolic pressure.

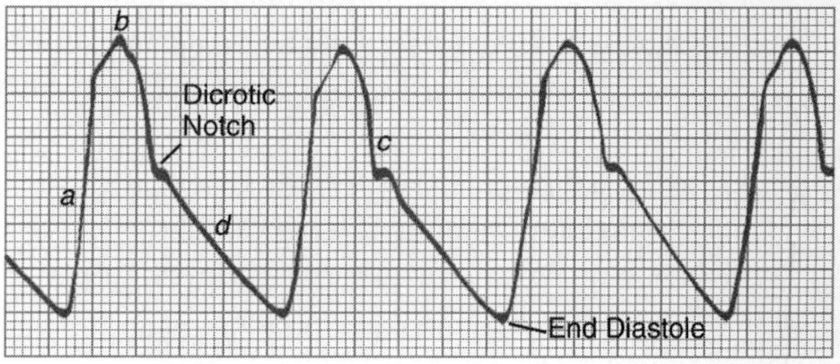

Arterial pressure waveform. The dicrotic notch indicates aortic valve closure.

PERFORMING THE ALLEN'S TEST

Procedure

1. Perform the Allen's test to determine distal peripheral perfusion. **Rationale:** This procedure assesses blood supply to client's hand to determine that radial and ulnar artery status are functioning before an arterial line is inserted.
2. Compress both arteries at client's wrist for about 1 minute.
3. Instruct client to clench and unclench fist several times. **Rationale:** This causes blanching in the hand and palm.
4. With client's hand in open, relaxed position, release pressure on ulnar artery.
5. Observe how quickly the palm color flushes. **Rationale:** If color returns quickly, good collateral blood supply to the hand exists. If normal color does not return, there is insufficient collateral circulation to the hand should radial artery occlusion occur.
6. Repeat procedure with release of the radial artery.
7. Report to physician if collateral blood flow is insufficient.

ASSISTING WITH ARTERIAL LINE INSERTION

Equipment

20-gauge arterial catheter with introducer and flexible guidewire
500 mL D_5W or normal saline for flush
Heparin 1,000 U/mL
One mL unit dose syringe
Pressure bag for flush infusion
IV tubing
Short wide bore, high pressure tubing
Three-way stopcocks
Established pressure monitor system
Clean gloves
Razor
Sterile gloves
Sterile towels and drape
Skin prep solution
Sterile 4 × 4 gauze sponges
Sterile 2 × 2 gauze sponges
Lidocaine 1–2%
3-mL syringe with 18- and 25-gauge needles for *topical* anesthetic
Alcohol wipes
000 silk suture (if used)
Tape or Tegaderm
Atropine for reversal of bradycardia

Preparation

1. Identify client, check identaband and ask client to state name.
2. Explain rationale for procedure and verbally reassure client.
3. Gather equipment.
4. Wash your hands.
5. Add heparin to D_5W or NS solution, and label bag with additive and date (commonly 2 U heparin/mL fluid). Follow hospital protocols.
6. Connect IV tubing to solution bag.
7. Remove *all air* from flush solution bag.
8. Insert flush infusion bag into pressure bag, and hang bag on IV pole.
9. Prepare and assemble pressurized monitoring system (transducer, continuous flush device, and stopcocks) following manufacturer's instructions.
10. Level stopcock above transducer to client's phlebostatic axis (see previous skill).
11. Shave or prepare site as needed.
12. Inflate pressure bag to 300 mm Hg, using hand pump on bag.

Procedure

1. Don gloves, and prepare to assist the physician as needed.
   a. Skin is prepped with skin prep solution.
   b. Lidocaine vial is cleansed with alcohol wipe.
   c. Physician dons sterile gloves.
   d. Sterile drape is placed over arterial insertion site.
   e. Physician aspirates lidocaine with 18-gauge needle, changes needle, and injects client's skin with 25-gauge needle.
   f. Percutaneous insertion is made at arterial insertion site, and arterial catheter is inserted.
   g. Physician advances catheter in artery.
   h. Arterial catheter is sutured in place with 000 silk suture or taped with tape or transparent membrane dressing (Tegaderm).
2. Observe for pulsating bright-red blood spurting retrograde into catheter. **Rationale:** This evidence ensures accurate catheter position.
3. Attach catheter to pressure-monitoring system tubing—make certain all connections are secure.
4. Press fast flush valve to clear system.
5. Observe oscilloscope for arterial waveform.
6. Apply sterile dressing to site.
7. Set monitor alarms for both HIGH and LOW parameters.

MONITORING ARTERIAL BLOOD PRESSURE

Equipment

Disposable pressure transducer, dome, and amplifier
Flush valve with flush system
Display monitor (oscilloscope)
Sterile stopcock cap
2 × 2 gauze sponges
Tape
Gloves
Carpenter's level
Marker

Procedure

1. Leveling and zeroing (calibrating) the system.
   a. Calibrate system at beginning of each shift. **Rationale:** Monitor readings are altered by changes in atmospheric pressure.
   b. Position client with HOB flat or up to 45° elevation.
   c. Using carpenter's level, align stopcock above transducer level with client's left atrium (phlebostatic axis) and mark client's chest for future readings. **Rationale:** Readings will

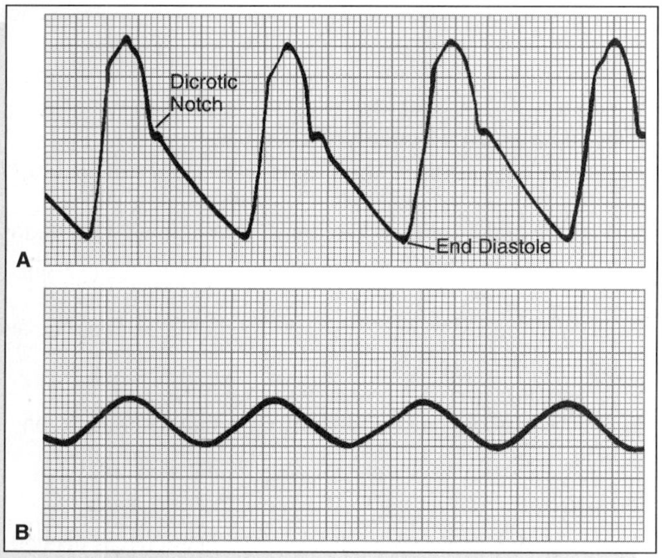

(**A**) Arterial line—normal waveform. (**B**) Arterial line—flattened waveform. Flattened arterial waveform indicates damping. Damping results from obstruction in arterial line or imbalance of transducer.

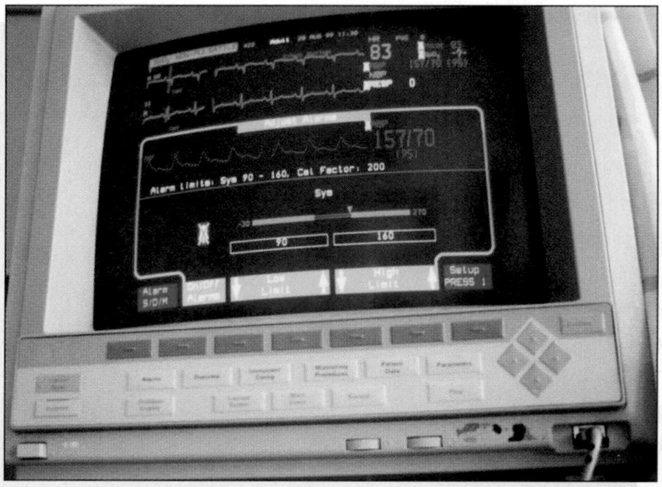

Arterial line allows direct measurement of blood pressure—monitor displays digital and wave form.

be inaccurately high or low if stopcock above transducer is not level with client's phlebostatic axis.

d. To zero ("calibrate") the system, turn stopcock near transducer off to client. Remove cap from stopcock, opening it to air.
e. Depress "zero" button on monitor, release button, and note monitor reading is zero. **Rationale:** Zero reading indicates monitor is calibrated to atmospheric pressure.
f. Replace cap or place new sterile cap on stopcock.
g. Turn stopcock so transducer is open to client.

2. Observe waveform at eye level for the sharp systolic upstroke, peak, dicrotic notch, and end diastole.
3. Compare direct and indirect blood pressure measurements at least every 4 hours. **Rationale:** In normovolemic clients, the direct blood pressure measure is typically 5–10 mm Hg higher than indirect readings. If there is greater disparity, equipment malfunction or errors in leveling and zeroing are likely. Cuff (indirect) measure of blood pressure in the hypovolemic client is unreliable.
4. Fast flush line with valve device. **Rationale:** To keep system airfree.
5. Ensure pressure bag is maintained at 300 mm Hg.
6. Leave cannulated extremity uncovered for easy observation. Assess site for signs of infection every shift.
7. Assess circulation, motion, and sensation of extremity distal to cannulation site every 2 hours initially, then every 8 hours.
8. Immobilize extremity if necessary.
9. Change flush solution and tubing every 24–72 hours.
10. Change dressing every 24–48 hours or if it becomes wet. **Rationale:** Wet dressings increase risk of infection at site.
    a. Put on gloves.
    b. Remove dressing, and discard in biohazard container.
    c. Cover with 2 × 2 sterile gauze sponges.
    d. Tape securely.
11. Remove gloves and wash hands.

Evidence Based Nursing Practice

Monitoring Arterial Blood Pressure

There is no absolute correlation between direct arterial blood pressure monitoring and indirect blood pressure measurement methods. Good correlation between the two methods does not mean the arterial pressure monitoring system is functioning properly.

Source: McGhee, B., & Bridges, E. (2002). Monitoring Arterial Blood Pressure: What you may not know. *Critical Care Nurse, 22* (2), 60–79.

TABLE 33–2 Causes of Acid–Base Imbalance

Acidosis	Alkalosis
Hypoventilation	Hyperventilation
COPD	Hypokalemia
Cardiac arrest	Pulmonary embolus
Diabetic ketoacidosis	Diuretics/steroids
Severe diarrhea	Prolonged vomiting
Renal failure	NG suction
Drug overdose	Dehydration

WITHDRAWING ARTERIAL BLOOD SAMPLES

Equipment

One 5-mL sterile syringe
ABG kit with one 3-mL syringe with dry lithium heparin and 22-gauge needle attached
Air filter device
Gloves
Container with ice (paper cup, emesis basin)
Two specimen labels
Biohazard specimen bag
Gauze sponges/pads

Preparation

1. Identify client, check identaband, and ask client to state name.
2. Gather equipment and explain procedure to client.
3. Attach label to specimen syringe with client's name, hospital number, room number, time, and date. Also add client's current temperature and FIO_2.
4. Fill paper cup or emesis basin with ice.
5. Wash hands and don gloves.

CLINICAL ALERT

"In-line" blood sampling systems eliminate the need for discarding blood, thus reducing blood loss.

Procedure

1. Remove protective cap from open port on three-way stopcock closest to arterial line insertion site.
2. Attach nonheparinized 5-mL sterile syringe without needle to open port of three-way stopcock.

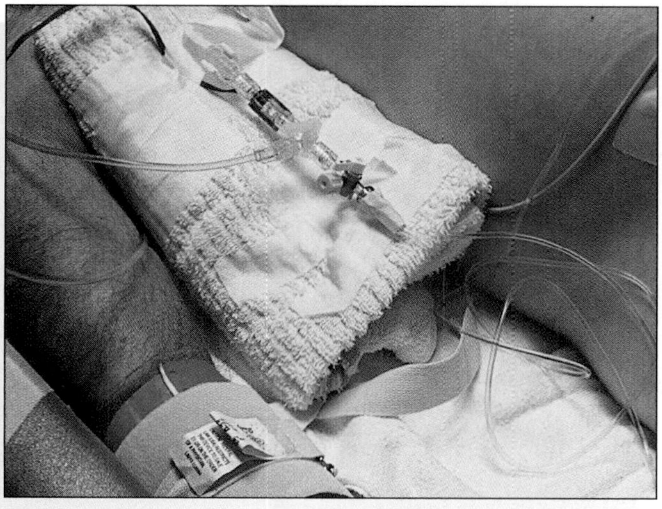

Femoral artery catheter and in-line transducer for monitoring.

EVIDENCE BASED NURSING PRACTICE

Mean Arterial Blood Pressure

In general, the MAP (mean arterial pressure) provides a more accurate interpretation of a patient's hemodynamic status. It provides the best estimate of central aortic pressure and is less sensitive to over- and underdamping distortions.

Source: McGhee, B., & Bridges, E. (2002). Monitoring Arterial Blood Pressure: What you may not know. *Critical Care Nurse, 22*(2), 60–79.

3. Turn stopcock off to transducer.
4. Aspirate 4 mL blood for waste.
5. Turn stopcock midway between open port and tubing. **Rationale:** This prevents escape of blood or introduction of flush solution into line.
6. Discard blood-filled syringe.

TABLE 33–3 Arterial Blood Gas Values in Acid–Base Imbalances

Respiratory Acidosis		Compensation
pH: decreased	<7.35	7.35
Pco_2: increased	>45 mm Hg	
HCO_3^- normal	24	>26 mEq
Respiratory Alkalosis		**Compensation**
pH: increased	>7.45	7.45
Pco_2: decreased	<35 mm Hg	
HCO_3^-: normal	24	<22 mEq
Metabolic Acidosis		**Compensation**
pH: decreased	<7.35	7.35
HCO_3^-: decreased	<22 mEq	
Pco_2: normal	40	<35 mm Hg
Metabolic Alkalosis		**Compensation**
pH: increased	>7.45	7.45
HCO_3^-: increased	>26 mEq	
Pco_2: normal	40	>45 mm Hg
Normal ABG Values		
pH	7.35–7.45	
Pco_2	35–45 mm Hg	
HCO_3	22–26 mEq	

7. Remove needle from ABG specimen syringe.
8. Attach ABG specimen syringe to stopcock.
9. Turn stopcock to open port to syringe.
10. Withdraw 3 mL for arterial blood gas specimen.
11. Turn stopcock off to open port. **Rationale:** This reestablishes flow between flush solution and client.
12. Remove syringe and, holding syringe upright, attach air filter device and activate to expel all air. **Rationale:** Air bubbles interfere with accuracy of specimen analysis.
13. Place arterial blood gas specimen syringe in container filled with ice.
14. Fast flush remaining blood onto gauze pad.
15. Reattach protective cap on open port.
16. Validate good arterial waveform on monitor.

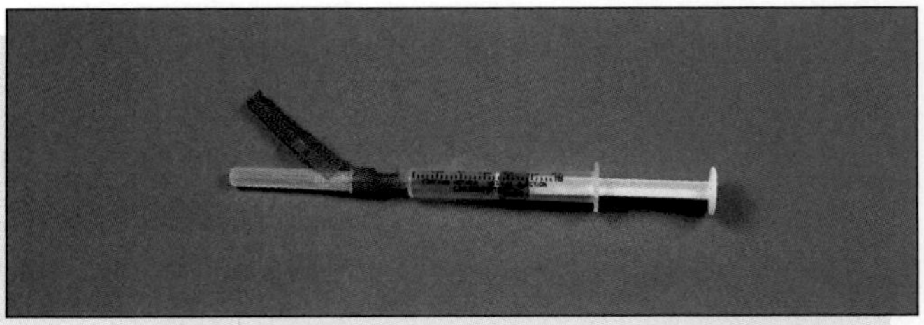

Blood gas sampling syringe containing dry lithium heparin is used for ABGs and electrolyte specimens.

17. Place syringe/specimen into biohazard bag with ice.
18. Remove gloves and wash hands.
19. Send to laboratory immediately.

REMOVING ARTERIAL CATHETER

Equipment

Gloves
Two 4 × 4 gauze pads
Tape
Container for dressing
Laboratory slip

CLINICAL ALERT

Apply pressure to puncture site for at least 10 minutes if client is on anticoagulation or antithrombotic therapy.

Preparation

1. Check physician's orders.
2. Gather equipment.
3. Wash hands.
4. Identify client; check identaband, and explain procedure to client.

Procedure

1. Remove tape from site.

Note: Tape is difficult to remove with gloves on; however, if dressing is soiled, don gloves before removing tape to protect from accidental blood exposure.

2. Don gloves.
3. Remove dressing, and place in appropriate container.
4. Place folded 4 × 4 gauze pad over cannula site with nondominant hand, and apply gentle pressure.
5. Pull arterial cannula straight out of artery with quick, even pressure.
6. Apply firm pressure over or just above cannula site for *at least* 5–10 minutes. **Rationale:** This action achieves hemostasis and prevents formation of a hematoma.
7. Place folded 4 × 4 gauze pad over puncture site, and tape tightly. **Rationale:** This provides additional pressure to site to prevent bleeding.
8. Complete laboratory slip, and send cannula to laboratory for culture and sensitivity if ordered.
9. Check cannulation site frequently. **Rationale:** To observe for bleeding or thrombosis.
10. Check distal extremity for circulation, motion, and sensation intermittently for several hours, then routinely after catheter removal. **Rationale:** Delayed complications (thrombosis) may occur.

Documentation for Arterial Blood Pressure Monitoring

- Size of arterial catheter inserted
- Name of physician inserting catheter
- Pressure readings (systolic, diastolic, and MAP)
- Direct and indirect pressure measurements
- Condition of cannulated extremity: distal circulation, motion, sensation
- Position of client during readings
- Unexpected outcomes and appropriate interventions
- Client response and tolerance of procedure
- Appearance of catheter insertion site

Arterial Blood Sampling
- Time specimen obtained
- Client's temperature and FiO_2 at the time blood was drawn

Dressing Change
- Condition of insertion site
- Dressing applied

Removing Arterial Catheter
- Time of removal
- Condition of insertion site
- Cannula disposal (i.e., to laboratory)
- Presence and quality of distal pulses
- Motion and sensation of involved extremity
- Manual pressure and dressing applied
- Strip recordings

Critical Thinking Application

UNEXPECTED OUTCOMES	CRITICAL THINKING OPTIONS
Absence of collateral circulation noted when performing the Allen's test (negative Allen's test).	• Assess contralateral extremity. • Avoid radial artery. • Notify physician. (An alternate artery may be selected—femoral.)
Hypotension and bradycardia occur during arterial puncture or catheter removal.	• Reverse response with atropine administration.
Arterial waveform loses definition and digital pressures drop.	• Use low compliance (rigid) short (<3–4 ft) monitor tubing. • Check for thrombus formation by aspirating blood through stopcock and then flushing system. • Be sure to fast-flush arterial line thoroughly after arterial blood samples are obtained or system is zeroed. • Make sure all stopcocks are closed to air. • Keep 300 mm Hg pressure in pressure bag. • Ensure secure fit of all stopcocks and connections. Avoid adding stopcocks and line extensions. • Change position of extremity in which catheter is placed.
Hematoma or hemorrhage at arterial insertion site.	• Apply direct pressure over artery while you check for leaks in the system. Check all stopcocks, and see if catheter is inserted in artery as far as it should be. • Remove catheter if oozing or hemorrhage continues.

UNEXPECTED OUTCOMES	CRITICAL THINKING OPTIONS
Infection or inflammation at insertion site.	• Cleanse site, and change dressing every 24–48 hours using strict aseptic technique to prevent infection. • Change tubing every 24–48 hours using sterile technique. • Flush open port after aspirating blood to clear catheter. • Cap open port on stopcock to maintain asepsis. • Prepare for catheter removal if infection occurs. • Notify physician.
Diminished distal perfusion of cannulated extremity.	• Check periphery for changes in color, temperature, movement, and pain resulting from possible thrombus occlusion. • Notify physician immediately. • Prepare for removal of catheter.
Arterial catheter not patent.	• Change position of extremity. • Attempt to aspirate blood from the arterial line. • Check under dressing for kinking in catheter. • Apply gentle traction to catheter at insertion site. • If unable to flush arterial catheter, remove catheter and apply direct pressure over artery for 5–10 minutes. Apply pressure dressing over artery.
Arterial blood sample is unobtainable.	• Release pressure on syringe, allow spasm of artery to stop, and then attempt to aspirate blood with gentle pressure. • Check that catheter is in artery (observe waveform on oscilloscope). If catheter is malfunctioning, attempt to aspirate blood from the catheter. If blood is aspirated, flush the catheter, using valve flush device, then try to obtain the sample again. • Reposition catheter and arm, gently pulling back on plunger. • If necessary, remove dressing, and check if any pressure was applied at the site. • Notify physician, who may need to remove sutures and reposition catheter.
Direct blood pressure readings vary significantly.	• Flick tubing system to remove tiny air bubbles escaping the flush solution. • Recheck transducer and client position to ensure accurate data. • Recalibrate transducer. • Flush system after sampling and zeroing. • Keep flush bag adequately filled and cleared of air. • Maintain bag external pressure at 300 mmHg. • Check that connections are tightly secured.

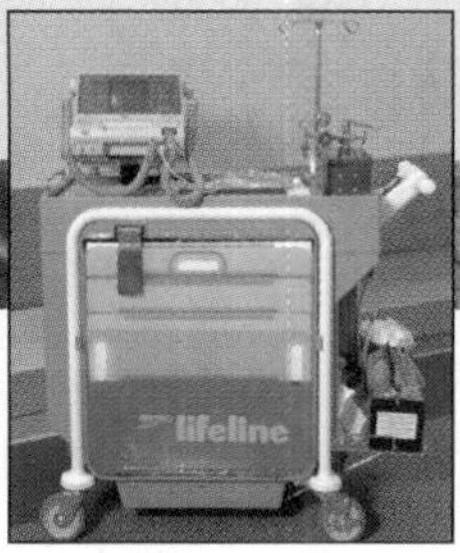

UNIT 3

Cardiac Emergencies

Nursing Process Data

ASSESSMENT Data Base

Assess client's responsiveness and heart rate and rhythm.

Identify lethal dysrhythmias on the ECG recording.

Assess availability of emergency supportive measures and emergency equipment.

Identify appropriate drugs needed for an emergency situation.

PLANNING Objectives

To be prepared to respond to cardiac emergencies

To provide a systematic method of organizing emergency equipment and medications for easy access and use

To identify appropriate drugs used in emergency situations

To provide emergency defibrillation to convert lethal ventricular dysrhythmias to normal sinus rhythm

To assist with elective cardioversion to convert atrial dysrhythmias or unstable ventricular tachycardia to normal sinus rhythm

IMPLEMENTATION Procedures

Maintaining the Emergency Cart

Checking Contents of the Emergency Cart

Calling a Code

Performing Defibrillation

Administering Advanced Cardiac Life-Support Medications

Assisting with Elective Synchronized Cardioversion

EVALUATION Expected Outcomes

Emergency care is provided.

All necessary equipment and medications are easily accessible in an emergency situation.

Client is resuscitated.

Heart rate and rhythm are restored to normal following emergency defibrillation or elective cardioversion.

Early recognition is essential for prompt and effective treatment of cardiac emergencies. Interventions for treating emergencies such as acute pulmonary edema and cardiac arrest include measures to decrease heart work, correct lethal dysrhythmias, and remove excess body fluid.

If left untreated, ventricular dysrhythmias and some atrial arrhythmias can cause reduced cardiac output and inadequate tissue perfusion. One way to restore a normal heart rhythm is to terminate dysrhythmias by delivering an externally applied electrical countershock. This countershock causes simultaneous depolarization of the myocardium, interrupts the dysrhythmia and allows the normal pacemaker (sinoatrial node) of the heart to resume control of the heart rhythm. Two types of electrical countershock applications are used: defibrillation and cardioversion.

Defibrillation is an emergency procedure in which large amounts of electric current are delivered without concern for synchronization with ventricular depolarization (QRS wave) on the ECG. Defibrillation is used to terminate ventricular fibrillation or *pulseless* ventricular tachycardia.

Cardioversion is usually an elective procedure in which an electrical countershock is synchronized with ventricular depolarization (QRS wave on ECG) for the purpose of converting a number of cardiac dysrhythmias, usually atrial in origin, to normal sinus rhythm. Emergency cardioversion is also used to convert "unstable ventricular tachycardia" (severely symptomatic client).

The "crash cart" contains essential life support medications and equipment used in emergency situations in the hospital setting. Familiarity with its location and contents, including typical emergency drugs, will assist the hospital staff to provide quick, competent care to clients during cardiac emergencies. The crash cart should be kept fully stocked, and located in an area that is accessible and obvious to all of the staff. Nurses must have a working knowledge of the contents of each drawer of the cart to quickly find the equipment.

MAINTAINING THE EMERGENCY CART

Equipment

Emergency cart with locking drawers
Emergency cart checklist
Airway equipment
Oxygen equipment
Suction equipment
Monitor leads and electrodes
Defibrillator
Oscilloscope
IV equipment
Emergency drugs

Procedure

1. Identify equipment and medications commonly used in emergency situations.
2. Gather equipment.
3. Maintain equipment in drawers according to priority use in the most commonly occurring emergency situations. Leave defibrillator plugged into electrical outlet at all times or check batteries every shift.
4. Lock drawers when cart is not in use. **Rationale:** This prevents personnel from using equipment for situations other than emergencies and not replacing it.
5. Place emergency cart checklist on outside of cart in visible area. **Rationale:** Cart contents are checked on a daily basis (and every 8 hours in critical care units) to ensure medications are not outdated, equipment is in working condition, and cart is locked.

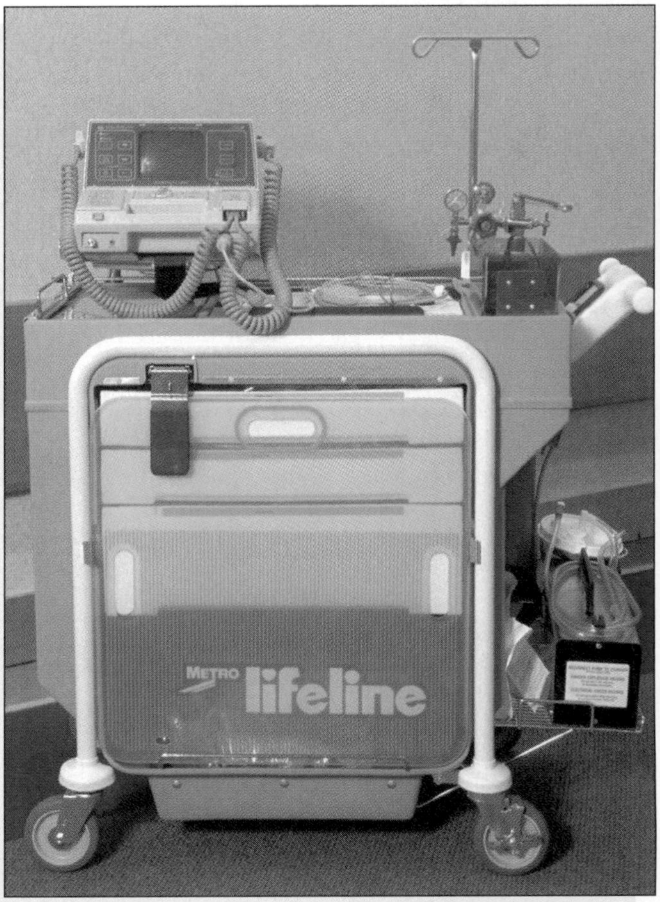

Fully equipped emergency cart is placed in an easily accessible area, visible to staff.

6. Place cart in designated, easily accessible, and visible area of the nursing unit. **Rationale:** Provides for less confusion if the cart is needed.
7. Familiarize all personnel with location and contents of cart, function of equipment, and emergency procedures.
8. Practice retrieving and setting up equipment through mock situations. **Rationale:** This ensures that all personnel are able to use cart during an emergency situation.
9. Check cart daily and document; restock immediately after use. **Rationale:** If cart is not restocked, delays can occur during an emergency situation jeopardizing client care.

CHECKING CONTENTS OF THE EMERGENCY CART

Equipment

Note: Emergency cart contents vary among agencies and among units within agencies.

Top of Cart

Personal protective equipment
Defibrillator/monitor
ECG electrodes, lead wires, and extra roll of recording paper, code record
Defibrillator paddles and conductive pads or "hands-free" pacing/defibrillator electrodes

Front of Cart

Cardiac arrest board

First Drawer

Respiratory supplies

Second Drawer

Emergency medications

Third Drawer

IV supplies: Steel needles, over-the-needle catheters, inside-the-needle catheters, short intracatheters, macrodrop and microdrop IV administration sets, extension tubing, stopcocks, syringes, tape, antimicrobial swabs, tourniquets, tincture of benzoin, gauze pads
Blood sampling supplies: Venous blood tubes, arterial blood gas kits or glass syringes
Spinal needles for intracardiac injections
Scalpels with blades attached
Alligator clips

Bottom Shelf

Tonsil suction
Surgical lubricant
Handheld self-inflating resuscitation bag
Oxygen masks, connecting tubing, flowmeter
Ambu bag
Nasogastric tubes
Tracheostomy tray
Cutdown tray and sutures
IV solutions, armboards
Portable suction device
Pacemaker and electrodes
Small sharps container

Side of Cart

Central venous catheters or long intracatheters
Emergency cart checklist
Cardiac resuscitation recording sheet and clipboard
Suction unit

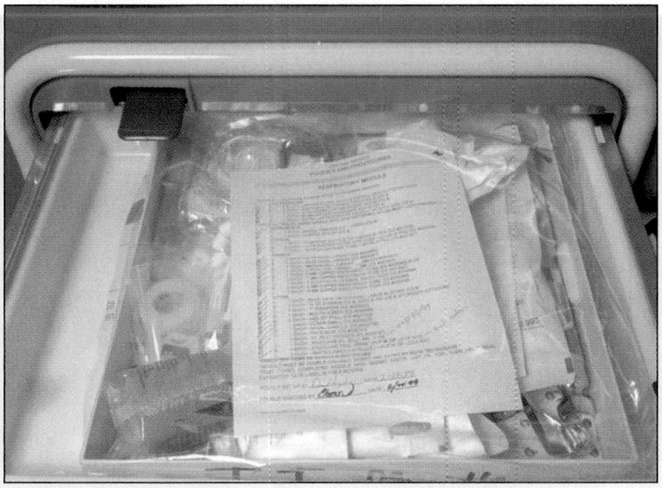

The cart contains equipment for intubating airway.

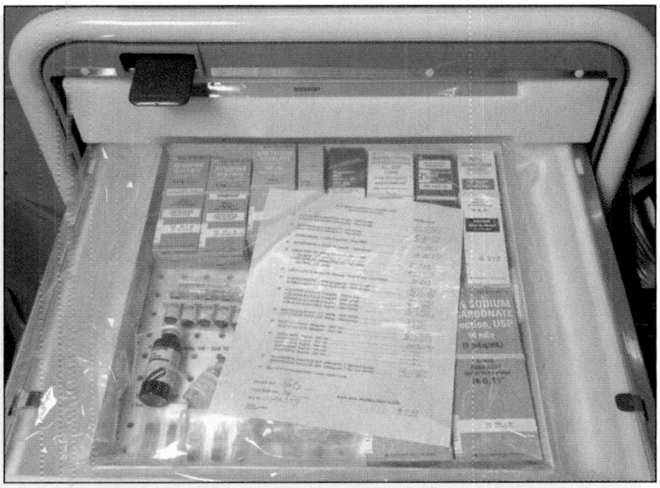

Emergency drugs are checked daily and restocked after use.

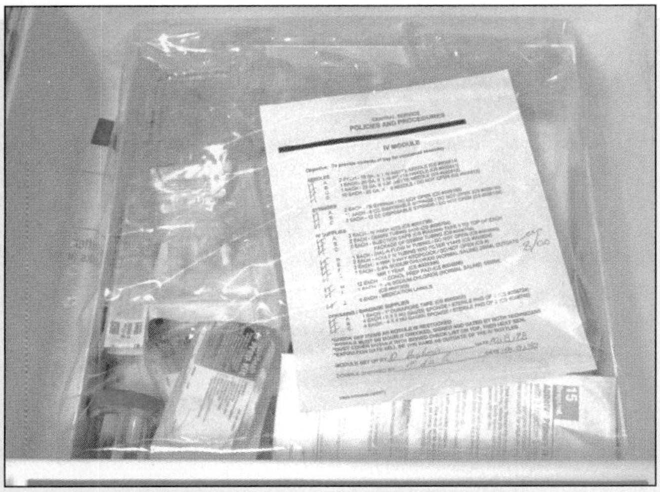

Supplies for initiating IV access are included.

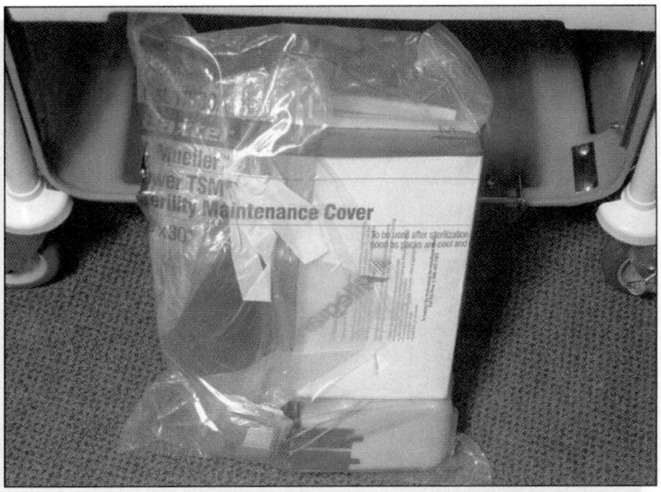

The bottom shelf contains supplies for maintaining client's airway.

CALLING A CODE

See Procedure in Chapter 27: *Circulatory Maintenance*, for CPR/AED skill.

CLINICAL ALERT

Clinically dead clients may be able to hear and remember events occurring throughout resuscitation procedures.

PERFORMING DEFIBRILLATION*

Equipment

Defibrillator monitor
Conducting pads with conducting gel
(or)
"Hands-free" defibrillation electrodes (refer to package for product-specific instructions)
Emergency cart with:
- Airway
- Cardiac board
- Resuscitator bag

Preparation

1. Validate client nonresponsiveness and pulselessness.
2. Call a "code."
3. Verify ECG reading of ventricular fibrillation (or ventricular tachycardia), if client on monitor.
4. Check that crash cart has arrived or begin CPR.

Procedure

1. Plug defibrillator into electric outlet.
2. Turn defibrillator power ON, and allow to warm up.

*Skill only performed by ACLS certified staff.

CLINICAL ALERT

Early defibrillation (within 3 minutes) is the key to successful resuscitation.

3. Place cardiac board under client's back, or convert bed to "cardiac position," if not already present for CPR.
4. Dry client's chest if necessary (do not use alcohol).
5. Place conducting pads on client's chest, or spread thin coat of defibrillation electrode gel to surface of paddles. One pad is placed below right clavicle near sternum and second pad is placed to left of cardiac apex (below and to the left of left nipple) in anterior axillary line. Do not place over broken skin. Press electrode center and edges firmly for complete adhesion. **Rationale:** Conductive medium decreases skin resistance and reduces degree of burns.

CLINICAL ALERT

Before beginning defibrillation or cardioversion procedure, remove any transdermal medication patch on chest. Avoid placing paddles over electrodes/leads; avoid pacemaker by one inch.

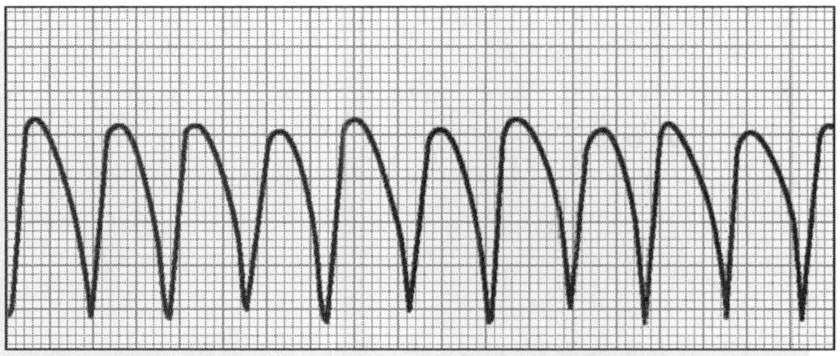

Ventricular Tachycardia

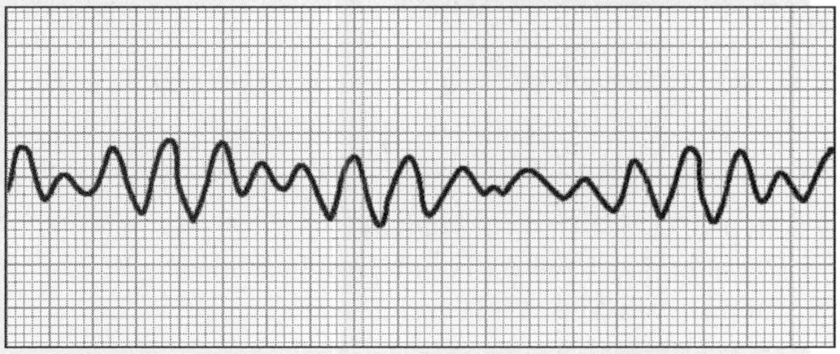

Ventricular Fibrillation

6. *Alternatively*, apply "hands-free" defibrillation pads.
7. Insert electrodes connector into cable. Push firmly for proper connection.
8. Be certain defibrillator is NOT in synchronized mode. **Rationale:** The machine will not respond to ventricular fibrillation if set to synchronized mode.
9. Set defibrillator to charge at 200 watt seconds. **Rationale:** Electric shock is damaging to myocardium. Start with 200 J, then proceed if necessary to 300 J, then 360 J (Table 33–4). *Note:* After identifying urgent situation:
   a. If alone, retrieve AED or defibrillator. **Rationale:** *First responder* defibrillation now has priority over CPR.
   b. If assistance available, call for defibrillation and begin CPR.
10. Command all persons to move away from bed area and any equipment connected to client.
11. Stand away from bed area yourself.
12. Apply paddles with firm pressure (25 lbs).
13. Depress discharge buttons on defibrillator simultaneously to ensure appropriate discharge.

TABLE 33–4 Energy Levels for Defibrillation	
Condition requiring Defibrillation	**Energy Level (J)***
Pulseless ventricular tachycardia, ventricular fibrillation	Stacked shocks of 200 to 200–300J to 360J Alternate with emergency cardiac life support (ACLS) drugs

*1 joule = 1 watt second

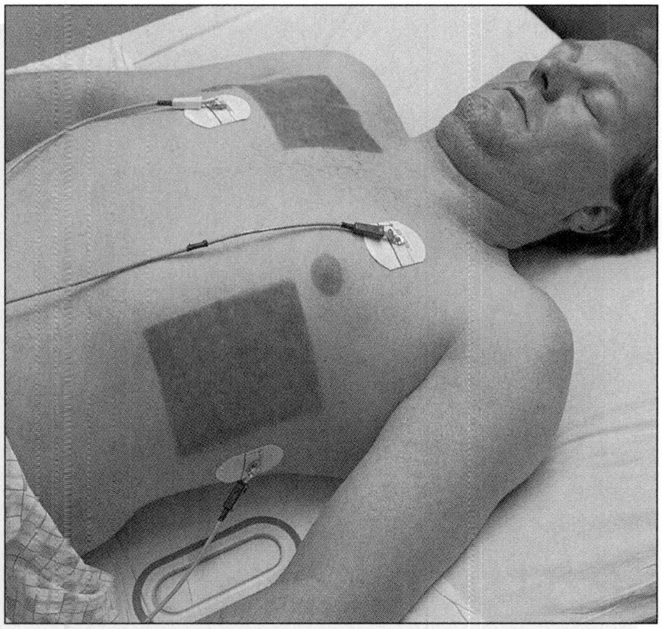

Pads are placed below right clavicle and left of cardiac apex.

14. Deliver 3 stacked shocks (if necessary) in close sequence (200 J, 200–300 J, 360 J). **Rationale:** Escalating current is used with monophasic defibrillators.
15. When using "hands-free" electrodes, activate system by three-step process:
   a. Turn on machine.
   b. Charge.
   c. Push to defibrillate.
   d. Electrodes may also be used for external pacing.
16. Analyze ECG pattern to determine effects of defibrillation. Check for pulse and reinstitute CPR for one minute and administer appropriate medications if indicated.
17. Prepare defibrillator equipment for second attempt at increased shock energy if lethal arrhythmia continues.

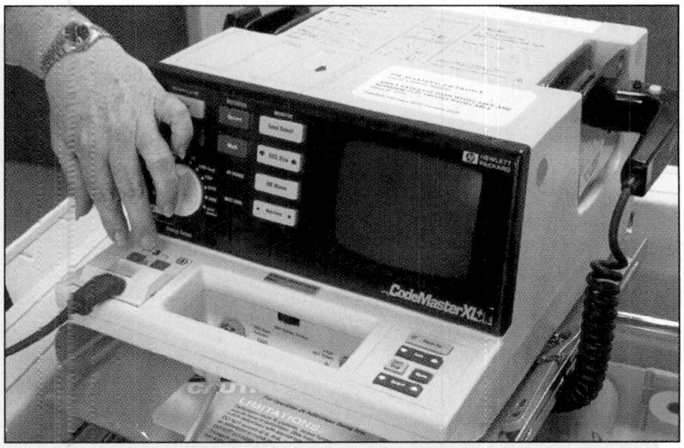

CodeMaster XL^+ Defibrillator can be used as a "hands-free" unit.

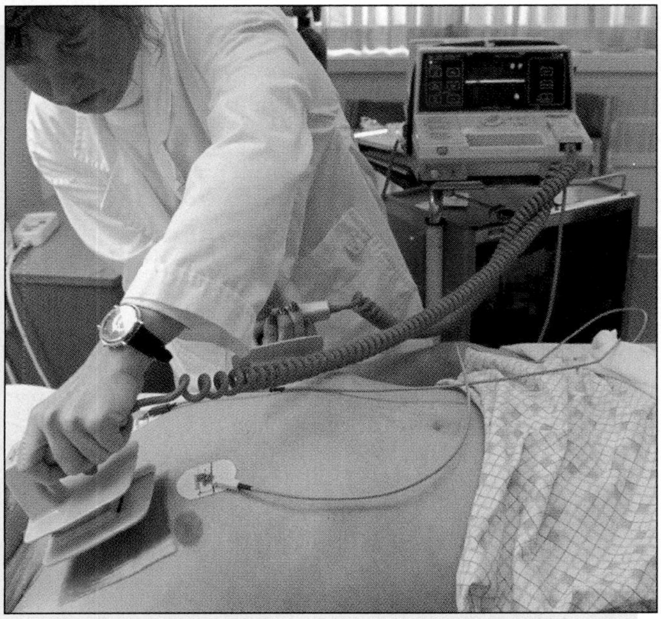

Apply paddles with firm pressure over conducting pads.

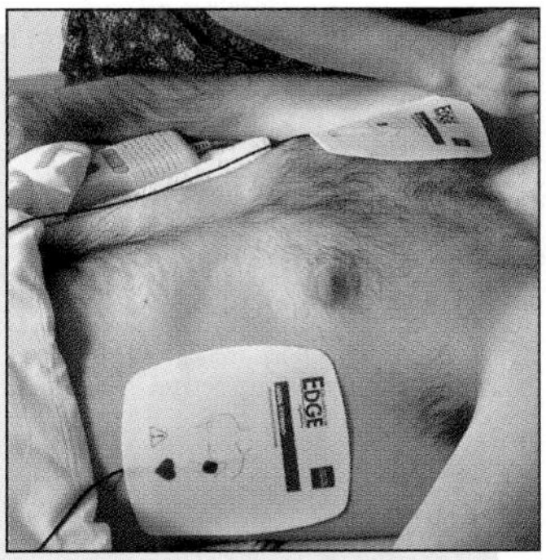

Hands-free pads provide defibrillation and protect provider.

18. Repeat defibrillation procedure.
19. Monitor client every 15 minutes until stable:
    a. Monitored heart rhythm.
    b. Vital signs.
    c. Level of consciousness and neurologic signs.
20. Continue oxygen administration.
21. Continue IV medication administration per ACLS protocol.

ADMINISTERING ADVANCED CARDAIC LIFE-SUPPORT MEDICATIONS

Equipment

Client's medical record (note client's weight for drug dosage determination)

Emergency "crash" cart with medications (may be supplied in ampules, multiple dose vials, or "unit-of-use" containers (cartridge/needle units or cartridge/syringe units)

Preparation

1. Familiarize self with most commonly used medications, their action, usual dose, route and rate of administration, and side effects
2. Review skill for *Administration of Intravenous Medications* (Chapter 28).
3. Client should be intubated and airway placement confirmed (See *Respiratory Care*, Chapter 26).
4. Establish IV access if not already present (intraosseous [IO] or bone access may be necessary in emergency situations).
5. Continue client cardiac monitoring.

Procedure

1. Prepare cartridge/syringe unit by removing caps from cartridge vial and injector.
2. Insert vial into injector, rotating clockwise until medication enters injector needle.
3. Remove protected needle or male Luer-Lok cover and gently press vial to initiate medication flow.
4. Swab needleless IV port with antimicrobial swab and insert system for medication injection.
5. Administer emergency response algorithm as ordered.
    a. If ventricular fibrillation or pulseless ventricular tachycardia persists following the first three shocks, administer

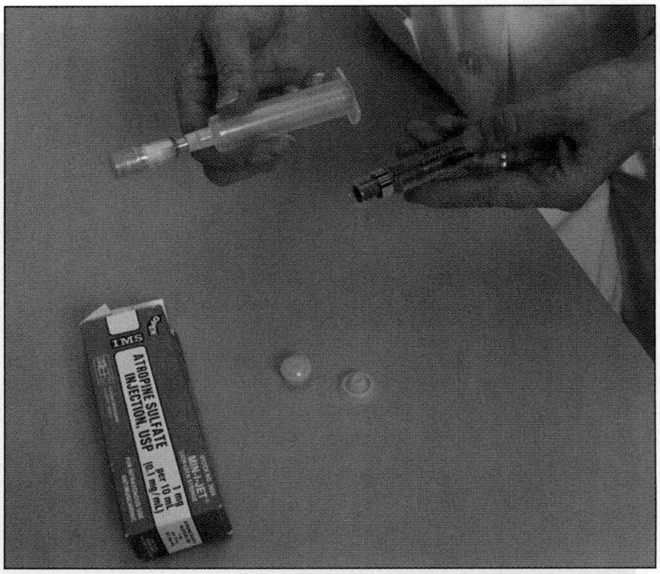

Remove caps from cartridge and injector.

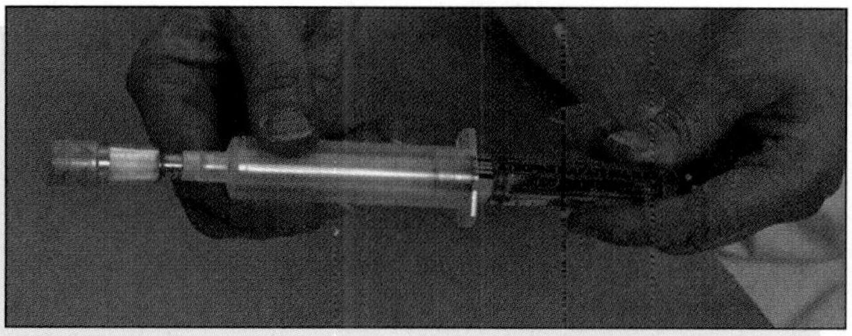

Insert cartridge/vial into injector and rotate clockwise until medication enters needle.

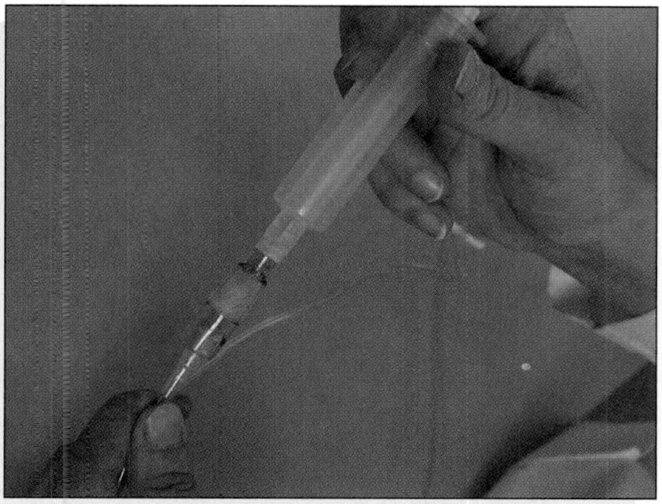

Protected needle or Luer-Lok system may be used for drug administration per IV tubing port.

adrenergic agents as ordered: **vasopressin** (one time only due to longer half-life), or **epinephrine** (repeat every 3–5 minutes between continued shock attempts).

b. Within 30–60 seconds of *first dose* of the medication, three stacked defibrillation shocks of 360 J (or equivalent biphasic) should be delivered, each three shocks followed by 1 mg **epinephrine.**

c. If defibrillation is ineffective, rhythm-appropriate *anti-arrhythmic* agents may be attempted. See Table 33–5.

TABLE 33–5 Advanced Cardiac Life Support Medications

Medication[a]	Dose	Indication
Vasopressin	40 U IV, one time only	For persistent or recurrent VF/VT
Epinephrine	1 mg IV push, or ET*; repeat q 3–5 min during cardiac arrest	Same as above
Amiodarone (a)	300 mg IV push, then 150 mg, max 2.2 g over 24 hrs	Same as above
Lidocaine (indeterminate, b)	1–1.5 mg/kg IV push or ET*, then 0.5–0.75mg/kg q 5–10 min	Same as above
Procainamide (a and indeterminate, b)	30 mg/min to 17 mg/kg max	Recurrent VF/VT
Magnesium sulfate (a)	1–2 g IV push	Known or suspected hypomagnesemia
Atropine	1 mg IV or ET*; repeat every 3–5 min up to 0.04 mg/kg	*Slow* rate pulseless electrical activity (PEA)

* Follow each drug administered with 20 mL NS bolus flush. Shocks and CPR are continued after each drug is administered. Endotracheal doses are 2–4 times the IV dose.
a = acceptable; (*indeterminate,* b) only fair evidence supports possible benefit.

ASSISTING WITH ELECTIVE SYNCHRONIZED CARDIOVERSION

Equipment

Defibrillator set to SYNCHRONIZATION mode
Paddles—anteroposterior or anterolateral or hands-free pads
ECG monitor
Conductive paste or conductive pads
Emergency cart with drugs and equipment

Note: Synchronized cardioversion is used for elective conversion of chronic atrial arrhythmias as well as emergency management of supraventricular and unstable ventricular tachycardia.

Preparation

1. Review cardioversion orders and make sure consent form is signed. Check that equipment is functioning properly.
2. Review precardioversion laboratory values or drug levels, particularly potassium level. **Rationale:** Hypokalemia or drug toxicity may increase risk of dysrhythmias after cardioversion.
3. Bring equipment to client's room.
4. Check that digitalis was discontinued 24 hours or more before cardioversion, or as ordered by physician.

5. Check that client has been receiving anticoagulation therapy for atrial fibrillation.
6. Withhold food and fluids for 6–12 hours before elective cardioversion.
7. Obtain baseline 12-lead ECG, and label it "precardioversion."
8. Obtain baseline vital signs and ECG rhythms.
9. Notify anesthesiologist and physician of readiness.
10. Place emergency cart in room.

Procedure

1. Establish IV line, and administer fluids at "keep open" rate.
2. Administer oxygen as ordered before cardioversion.
3. Plug in defibrillator and turn power switch ON.
4. Turn **synchronizer** switch ON. **Rationale:** Shock delivery synchronized with QRS of ECG reduces possibility of inducing ventricular arrhythmias by the electrical shock being delivered on the "T" wave.
5. Test synchronization by pushing manual synchronization button.
6. Disconnect all electric equipment from client except ECG monitor and cardioverter.
7. Administer sedative as ordered by physician (anesthesiologist may do this).
8. Charge machine to level specified by physician, usually 25–50 J to start (1 joule = 1 watt second). Note that designated charge is reached.
9. Place client in supine position.
10. Make sure client's chest is dry and any transdermal patch removed.
11. Apply conductive gel to surface of paddles, or use "hands-free" defibrillator pads and place on client's chest.
    a. Anterolateral paddles are placed as in defibrillation, one over second intercostal space to right of sternum and other over fifth intercostal space in left midclavicular line.
    b. Anteroposterior paddles are placed with flat paddle posteriorly between scapulae and anterior, handheld paddle over fifth intercostal space in left midclavicular line.
12. Observe ECG rhythm on monitor and start recording.
13. Discontinue oxygen.
14. Ensure that synchronization indicator is superimposed on R wave of ECG.
15. Give command to "stand clear," and stand clear yourself.
16. The **physician** depresses discharge buttons on paddles and keeps them depressed until cardioversion countershock is delivered. The shock may not occur instantly, since machine waits until the next R wave in the ECG to discharge.
17. Observe postcardioversion rhythm.
18. Provide postcardioversion care.
    a. Support airway and ventilation, and oxygenate as needed.
    b. Obtain 12-lead ECG, and label it "postcardioversion."
    c. Monitor heart rhythm continuously.
    d. Evaluate vital signs, ECG, level of consciousness, peripheral pulses, and neurologic status every 15 minutes until stable, then routinely. **Rationale:** Thromboemboli to the lungs or systemic circulation may occur following cardioversion for atrial fibrillation. Coumadin therapy is continued postcardioversion.
    e. Keep client under observation for 12 to 24 hours. **Rationale:** Transient hypotension and minor dysrhythmias may occur.

This skill is usually not done in an acute care setting because of staff time constraints. Client is sent to cath lab where expert personnel use "conscious sedation" for procedure.

TABLE 33–6 Energy Levels for Cardioversion

Cardioversion	Energy Level (J)*
Paroxysmal supraventricular tachycardia	75–100
Atrial flutter	25–50
Atrial fibrillation	100 to 200 to 360J
Unstable ventricular tachycardia	50 to 100 to 200 to 360J

*1 joule = 1 watt second

CLINICAL ALERT

If repeat cardioversion is necessary, reset defibrillator to *synchronize* mode. Most defibrillators default back to unsynchronized mode (immediate shock).

Documentation for Cardiac Emergencies

Defibrillation

- Time of event and call for code
- Client signs (nonresponsiveness)
- Predefibrillation ECG rhythm and vital signs
- Number of defibrillation attempts and watt seconds (Joules) used
- Postdefibrillation rhythm and vital signs
- Other resuscitative measures
- Time resuscitation discontinued
- Outcome of resuscitation
- Drugs administered
- Record responses and interventions (time and personnel) on Code Record

Cardioversion

- Precardioversion client preparation completed
- Precardioversion rhythm and vital signs
- Name of anesthesiologist and physician performing cardioversion
- Number of cardioversion attempts
- Watt seconds for each attempt
- Postcardioversion rhythm with each attempt
- Postcardioversion problems, if any
- Drugs administered
- Postcardioversion monitoring

Critical Thinking Application

UNEXPECTED OUTCOMES	CRITICAL THINKING OPTIONS
for Emergency Cart	
Equipment is missing from cart.	• Immediately notify charge nurse or pharmacist, and obtain replacement from pharmacy, floor stock, or nearby unit. • If any delay in obtaining item, tape warning notice to chart that item is missing.
Equipment cannot be located promptly on cart.	• After resuscitation, suggest more logical placement of item (e.g., alphabetize or place with similar equipment). • After resuscitation, practice mock codes to retrieve items and become more familiar with cart.
Equipment malfunctions.	• Replace malfunctioning equipment immediately. • Obtain cart from the nearest unit.
for Defibrillation	
Carotid pulse is present and client is responsive, although monitor shows pattern of ventricular fibrillation.	• Check monitor electrodes and wires for contact with client, cable, or telemetry connections and adjust or replace as needed.
Electric arc crosses client's chest upon shock discharge.	• Avoid excessive gel on paddles. • Wipe off any conductive gel or perspiration between the paddle sites, and defibrillate again. • Remove transdermal medication patches.

UNEXPECTED OUTCOMES	CRITICAL THINKING OPTIONS
After defibrillation, rhythm changes to standstill or rhythm appears on monitor, but carotid pulse is absent (pulseless electrical activity).	• Call a code and institute CPR. • Intubate client. • Administer IV fluids and oxygen. • Administer emergency medications as ordered by physician.
for Cardioversion	
On precardioversion laboratory assessment there is elevation of serum digitalis level.	• Notify physician of findings. • Reassure client that there is not a life-threatening problem. Procedure may be delayed or postponed.
Asystole appears on ECG.	• Assess client for breathing and pulse. • View a different ECG lead; increase amplitude of lead. • Immediately institute CPR if indicated. • Assist physician in advanced cardiac life-support measures.

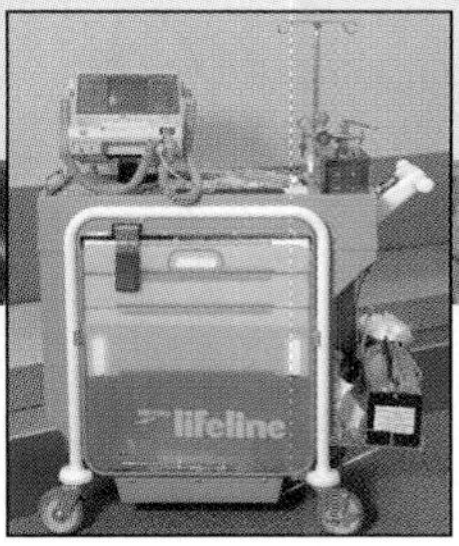

Mechanical Ventilation

Nursing Process Data

ASSESSMENT *Data Base*

Assess client for presence of risk factors for acute respiratory distress syndrome: sepsis, massive trauma, massive fat embolism, aspiration pneumonia, and other disorders characterized by abnormal ventilation and interstitial pulmonary edema.

Auscultate heart and lung sounds for baseline data.

Assess vital signs and measure arterial blood gases and hemodynamic pressures if Swan–Ganz catheter is in place.

Identify if need for mechanical ventilation is present. Criteria for non-COPD clients:

- Vital capacity is less than 15 mL/kg of body weight.
- Negative inspiratory pressure is less than −25 cm H_2O
- P_{CO_2} is below 30 mm Hg or above 50 mm Hg.
- Alveolar–arterial oxygen difference (A–a Δ P_{O_2}) is greater than 350 mm Hg on 100% oxygen.
- Pulmonary shunt is greater than 30%.
- Deadspace-tidal volume (V_D–V_T) ratio is greater than 60%
- P_{O_2} is less than 60 mm Hg on an F_{IO_2} of 1.0 (100%).

Observe for trend of respiratory values (trend is more important than isolated measurements).

Assess client for indications for PEEP:

- Inability to maintain arterial P_{O_2} of at least 70 mm Hg on 50% oxygen during continuous mechanical ventilation.
- Failure of other methods to reduce pulmonary shunt (e.g., treatment of cardiac failure or pneumonia).
- Normovolemia (normal blood volume).

Check physician's orders for ventilator mode and other specified settings.

Assess client's readiness for ventilator weaning.

Assess client's response to ventilator weaning.

PLANNING *Objectives*

To provide or augment pulmonary function

To decrease the work of breathing

To promote gas exchange

To maintain acid–base balance of the body

To assist in keeping alveoli open on expiration, thereby reducing shunt and increasing functional residual capacity (FRC)

To reduce anxiety and resulting physiologic responses to critical illness

To remove the client from mechanical ventilation as safely and quickly as possible

To collaborate with a skilled multidisciplinary team in planning and providing care

To titrate levels of mechanical support to facilitate client's independent breathing

IMPLEMENTATION ***Procedures***

Caring for Clients on Ventilators

Weaning the Mechanically Ventilated Client

EVALUATION ***Expected Outcomes***

Adequate respiratory function is maintained.

ABGs and acid–base balance are improved.

Oxygenation of tissue is improved.

Functional residual capacity and compliance are improved.

Ventilator weaning is assisted by titrating modes facilitating client's independent breathing.

ALTERATIONS OF VENTILATION AND GAS EXCHANGE

Adequate gas exchange in the lungs depends on the effective ventilation of air matched with the perfusion of blood to ventilated alveoli. The thickness and permeability of the alveolar membrane, the amount of surface area available for diffusion, and the pressure gradients are also factors that affect gas exchange. The pressure gradient is the difference between the partial pressures of PO_2 and PCO_2 in the alveolar air and the pulmonary capillary blood. The pressure gradiants drive the inward diffusion of oxygen from alveolar air to the blood and the outward diffusion of carbon dioxide from the blood to the alveolar air for exhalation. These pressures are obtained by arterial blood gas testing.

Ventilation replenishes the supply of oxygen in the alveoli and removes the carbon dioxide released by the capillaries. If ventilation and perfusion are not matched, blood oxygenation is reduced, resulting in a right (heart) to left (heart) "shunt." Right to left shunting is characterized by a low PO_2 (hypoxemia).

Ventilation-perfusion mismatch problems are usually the result of chronic conditions such as chronic obstructive pulmonary disease (COPD). They may also occur acutely due to perfusion failure (e.g., pulmonary embolism), ventilatory failure (e.g., drug overdose, pulmonary disease, sepsis), or pulmonary edema affecting diffusion.

Mechanical ventilation provides support for the work of breathing and assures alveolar ventilation. This intervention, however, may require intubation of the client, interferes with normal airway defenses, and increases the risk of pulmonary injury and nosocomial infection. It is desirable to decrease the level of controlled ventilatory support as soon as possible to assist the client to extubation and the return to independent breathing. Newer techniques of ventilation allow weaning by titrating from high support to minimal support modes to facilitate the transition.

Clients (especially those with underlying disease) who require mechanical ventilation for even a day, may develop ventilator dependence. All efforts focus on identifying and addressing the physiologic and psychological factors that delay successful weaning. This complex process requires the collaborative efforts of a skilled multidisciplinary team including physician, nurse, respiratory therapist, dietitian, and physical therapist. Final clinical outcomes range from successful weaning to incomplete weaning (client remains on ventilatory support at home or in a subacute setting) or terminal weaning at the client's or family's request. Terminal weaning may be facilitated with a continuous infusion of morphine or a sedative to ease the client's death.

CARING FOR CLIENTS ON VENTILATORS

Equipment

Specific ventilator ordered (i.e., Puritan-Bennett 840, Servo 900C, Servo 300/300A, Siemens I, Dräger Evita)

Handheld resuscitator bag connected to oxygen flowmeter

Airway connector

Sterile suction supplies

Ventilator flow sheet

Means for client communication

Preparation

1. Double-check the ventilator settings against those ordered by the physician.
2. Plug the machine in, and turn it ON.
3. Familiarize yourself with location of alarm systems on the ventilator, and turn on all alarm systems.
4. Validate that tube cuff inflation is appropriate with minimal occlusive volume or minimal leak (squeak heard at

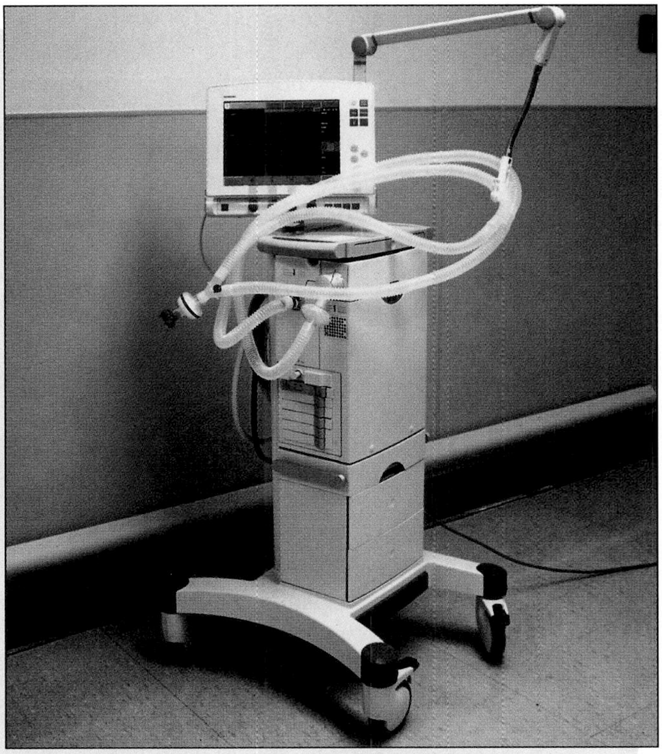

Siemens 300I computerized mechanical ventilator.

end inspiration) while auscultating over suprasternal notch.

5. Connect the ventilator tubing to client's endotracheal tube or tracheostomy tube.

Procedure

1. Monitor client's heart rate and blood pressure until stable.
2. Obtain arterial blood gases 15 minutes after ventilation is established.
3. Monitor ventilator settings and delivered values: tidal volume, inspiratory pressure, peak pressure, rate, FIO_2, inspiratory–expiratory (I:E) ratio, ventilatory modes. Modern ventilators monitor these parameters continuously.
4. Ensure adequate heat and humidification of inspired gases.

CLINICAL ALERT

Many client/ventilator systems include heat moisture filters which replace the need for external humidification of inspired gases. The use of these filters is only safe if pressure monitors are set properly so the machine can warn of impending heat moisture exchange filter occlusion.

5. Check humidifier fluid level every 8 hours, and refill as necessary, if applicable.
6. Record intake, output, and daily weights.
7. Suspend ventilator tubing from an IV hook or support it on a pillow. **Rationale:** This reduces traction on the endotracheal or tracheostomy tube.

Airway Pressure Modes

IPPB—Intermittent positive pressure breathing—inspiration by positive airway pressure; expiration is passive.

CVM/AVC—Invasive or noninvasive continuous mandatory ventilation—total support ventilation with set ventilation rate (e.g., 12) and set tidal volume (e.g., 750 mL). Client-initiated breaths receive set volume and if client does not initiate breath, set rate and volume are guaranteed (sometimes referred to as assist control ventilation).

SIMV—Synchronous intermittent mandatory ventilation—spontaneous ventilation intermittently augmented by positive pressure ventilation.

PEEP—Positive end-expiratory pressure—an expiratory airway pressure modality in which the airway pressure is maintained above atmospheric at the end of expiration. Stimulates surfactant production, increases FRC, functional residual capacity.

CPAP—Invasive or noninvasive continuous positive airway pressure—spontaneous ventilation with maintenance of airway pressures above atmospheric throughout the respiratory cycle.

BIPAP—Spontaneous breathing with maintenance of a bi-positive airway pressure: one set for positive inspiratory pressure and a lesser one set for positive expiratory pressure.

APRV (airway pressure release ventilation)—The ventilator maintains an inspiratory pressure throughout the inspiration time. A short pressure release at the end of the respiratory cycle allows airway pressure to return to zero for a short time.

PSV—Pressure support ventilation—in addition to other ventilator settings, 6–10 cm H_2O pressure support is provided to compensate for the added resistance imposed by artificial airways, making breathing easier. Supports a larger tidal volume with less work of breathing.

PCV (pressure control ventilation)—The ventilator minimizes the pressure used to deliver an acceptable tidal volume. Some machines measure the compliance of the client/ventilator interface and calculate the ideal acceptable minimum tidal volume using the least pressure necessary. The pressure control level is adjusted to some maximum number, then the machine electronically selects the appropriate tidal volume based on PCV value set and previously calculated compliance.

8. Change ventilator tubing if necessary, minimizing frequency of circuit opening. **Rationale:** Epidemiologic studies indicate that maintenance of a closed ventilatory/client interface is desirable.
9. Check vital signs every hour, and auscultate lungs. **Rationale:** Positive pressure ventilation may decrease venous return and cardiac output.

Note: Continuous pulse oximetry facilitates constant assessment of clients receiving ventilatory assistance.

Initial Ventilator Settings

- Tidal volume of 8–12 mL/kg (based on ideal body weight)
- Respiratory rate of 10–15 per minute
- Inspiratory–expiratory (I:E) ratio 1:2. (I:E ratio should be less than 1:1 to prevent air trapping in the lungs.)
- Pressure limit 20% above peak airway pressures delivered.
- FIO_2 of 40%–100%.

10. Observe and listen for possible cuff leaks around tracheostomy or endotracheal tubes.
11. If necessary, discard accumulated water in the ventilator tubing via inline closed circuit drain. **Rationale:** Opening circuit exposes client to environmental pathogens. Frequency of circuit opening should be minimized.
12. Provide client with call bell and method of communication, such as a "magic slate."
13. If ordered, test the gastric fluid pH, and administer medication (antacids) or H_2 antagonists as ordered. **Rationale:** Stress ulcers are frequently associated with mechanical ventilation, so pH should be maintained above 5.
14. Test the nasogastric fluid and stool for occult blood if ordered.
15. Assess lung compliance frequently. **Rationale:** Lung compliance falls before changes are evident in blood gas analysis or clinical manifestations. Compliance is determined by

$$\frac{Vt}{PIP-PEEP}$$

where Vt = tidal volume; PIP = peek inspiratory pressure; and PEEP = positive end-expiratory pressure.

16. Implement methods for stress reduction, such as careful explanation of procedures, pain management, administra-

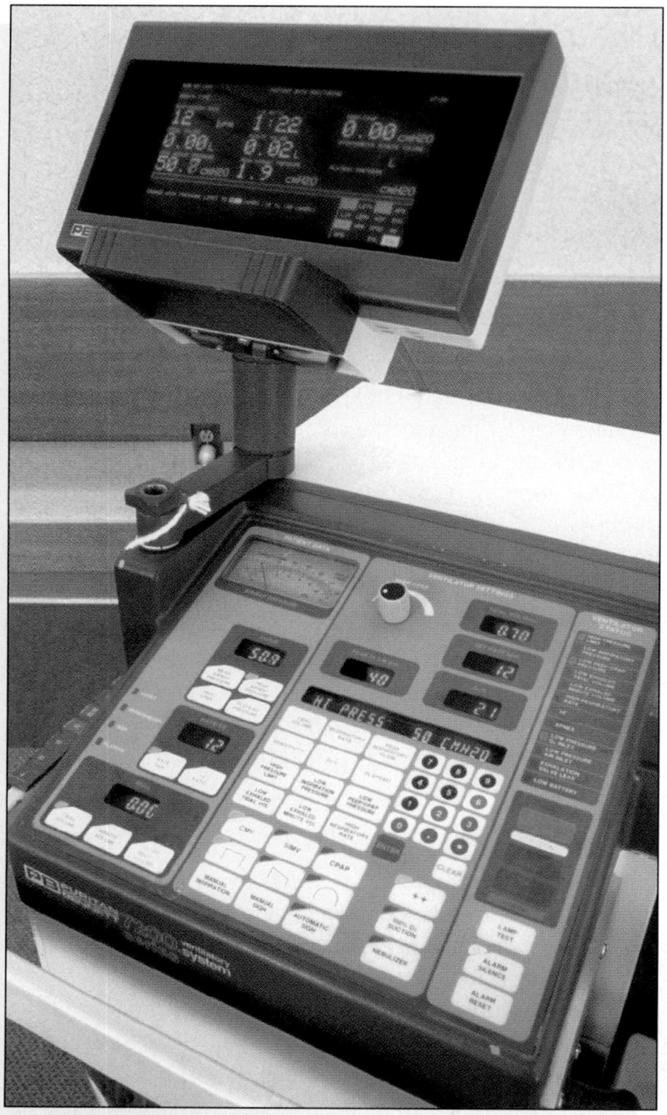

Double-check all ventilator settings with physician's orders.

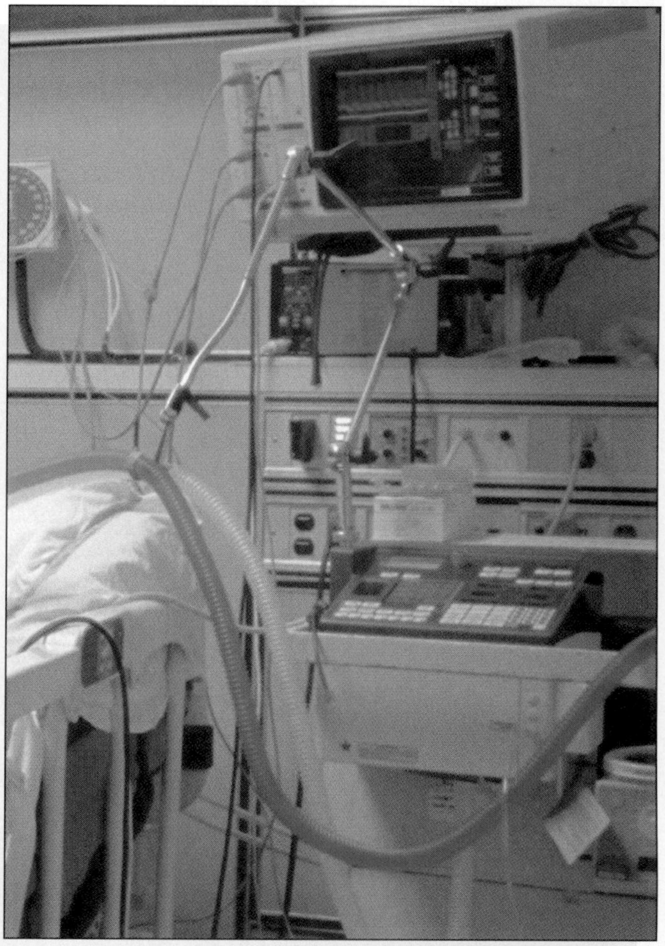

Various machines monitor multiple physiological parameters.

tion of sedatives, or neuromuscular blocking agents, as indicated.

17. Check that ventilator alarm parameters are set.
18. Maintain appropriate "sigh" delivery. **Rationale:** This extra volume breath assists in preventing atelectasis and stimulates surfactant production.

Note: Some newer ventilators do not have "sighs"—they periodically deliver a low-level "PEEP" period to achieve the same result.

19. Monitor client frequently to detect changes in status.

EVIDENCE BASED NURSING PRACTICE

Delirium in Mechanically Ventilated Patients

This study validated sensitivity, specificity, and interrater reliability of an instrument (CAM-ICU) for detection of delirium in mechanically ventilated patients. Delirium occurred in 83.3% of mechanically ventilated patients, 40% of whom were in a neutral level of sedation (neither agitated nor overly sedated), while they were in the ICU.

Source: Ely, E.W. et al. (2001 December). Delirium in mechanically ventilated patients. *Journal of the American Medical Association, 286*(21), 2703–2709.

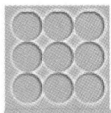

CULTURAL COMPETENCE

Touch button voice systems are available that allow ventilated English- or non–English-speaking clients to tap a touch screen that delivers preprogrammed audible words, phrases or symbols to hold two-way communication with staff.

WEANING THE MECHANICALLY VENTILATED CLIENT

Equipment

Oxygen source
T-piece adaptor or tracheostomy mask if ordered
Suctioning equipment
Arterial blood gas-sampling supplies
Continuous pulse oximetry unit
Stethoscope

Preparation

1. Validate order for weaning trial and assess client's readiness.
   Spontaneous tidal volume ≥ 7 mL/kg/ideal body weight (IBW)
   Respiratory rate between 12 and 20 breaths/min
   Minute ventilation (respiratory rate × TV) ≤ 10L/min
   Vital signs stable (SBP > 90 and < 180, HR > 50 and < 120)
   Vital capacity ≥ 10mL/kg IBW
   Negative inspiratory force is −20cm H_2O or higher
   ABGs: pH 7.35–7.5, PO_2 ≥ 60 mm Hg or FIO_2 ≤ 40%
   Able to protect airway and responsive on minimal sedation
   PEEP < 5 cm H_2O
2. Note client's work of breathing and use of accessory muscles.
3. Note current ECG pattern for baseline.
4. Explain weaning process to client. Reassure client that transition will be based on client's responses. **Rationale:** When client is included in weaning process and rationale for change, anxiety is lessened.
5. Suction client. Hyperinflate client's lungs with 100% oxygen before and after suctioning.
6. Maintain endotracheal or tracheostomy cuff at minimal occlusive pressure (minimal leak) while mechanically ventilated.
7. Establish continuous oximetry. **Rationale:** Client's oxygen status should be continually assessed.

Procedure

1. Elevate head of the bed to facilitate client's diaphragmatic excursion.

2. If physician orders endotracheal tube cuff deflated during weaning, suction secretions that have accumulated above the cuff as follows:
   a. Provide positive pressure to end of tube with a hand-held-resuscitation bag and 100% oxygen.
   b. Place tip of suction catheter in the posterior pharynx.
   c. Deflate cuff, and apply suction to catheter. **Rationale:** Positive pressure blows the secretions into the pharynx, where they can be suctioned out.
   d. Hyperinflate lungs with 100% oxygen for three to five breaths.
3. If ordered, connect T-piece to wide-bore oxygen tubing leading to the gas source.
4. Set oxygen concentration as ordered by physician, usually 10% *higher* than the ventilator FIO_2 the client has been receiving.
5. If appropriate remove ventilator tubing from airway, and connect T-piece to client's airway.
6. Cover end of ventilator tubing with sterile gauze.
7. Observe for vital sign changes, apprehension, diaphoresis, and dysrhythmias. **Rationale:** A mild increase in blood pressure, pulse, and respiratory rate is normal. Mild-to-moderate anxiety is also normal.
8. Measure arterial blood gases 1 hour after initiating weaning if client tolerates.
9. Proceed with weaning procedure as ordered. **Rationale:** Gradual weaning may be necessary.
10. If client tolerates no ventilator support (other than PSV), extubate client. (*See* Chapter 26.)
11. Following weaning, measure vital signs, vital capacity, SpO_2, inspiratory pressure, blood gases, and subjective response.

DOCUMENTATION FOR MECHANICAL VENTILATION

- Type of ventilator or other device used
- Ventilator or device settings; modes used in weaning process
- Time initiated
- Any problems and actions taken
- Suctioning (i.e., frequency, amount, and character of secretions)
- Indicate if client is making spontaneous breathing efforts or is not triggering the machine
- Endotracheal tube location and minimal leak established
- Arterial blood gas and other lab values
- Vital signs and hemodynamic values
- Findings on pulmonary and cardiac assessment
- Ventilator modes utilized in weaning transition process

Critical Thinking Application

UNEXPECTED OUTCOMES	CRITICAL THINKING OPTIONS
Adequate pulmonary function is not maintained.	• Evaluate ventilator settings to see if appropriate. • Check for leaks in system. • Auscultate lungs to determine if air flow is adequate. • Auscultate lungs to determine bilateral ventilation. • Suction airway frequently to improve ventilation. • Validate ET tube placement by x-ray.
Sudden respiratory distress, distended neck veins, and tracheal shift occurs.	• Immediately remove client from ventilator and hand ventilate. • Immediately notify physician as these are signs of a tension pneumothorax. • Prepare equipment and client for emergency chest decompression. • Assist physician with chest tube insertion, if required.

UNEXPECTED OUTCOMES	CRITICAL THINKING OPTIONS
Client experiences signs of decreased pulmonary compliance.	• Check for signs of fluid in lungs (x-ray, increase in PAWP, crackles on auscultation, hypoxemia). • Suction client to maintain a patent airway. • Implement program of chest physical therapy. Provide postural drainage, percussion, and vibration, as ordered. • Turn client frequently. • Turn and deep breathe or sigh client several times an hour to reopen atelectatic alveoli.
Pressure alarm is activated.	• Check for obstructions in tubing and take corrective measures. • Suction client for possible mucous obstruction.
Volume alarm is activated.	• Check for disconnected tubing. • Check for loose connections, and tighten them if present. • Check client for airway displacement and provide emergency measures if indicated. • Deflate and reinflate the airway cuff to minimal occlusive pressure to adjust a possible cuff leak. • If unable to identify and relieve cause immediately, disconnect ventilator tubing, hand ventilate client, and summon help.
Arterial blood gases (ABGs) are not maintained within normal range.	• Notify physician of abnormal ABGs, and obtain order for alteration in ventilator settings, i.e., increased percentage of oxygen. • Maintain mechanical ventilation. Do not attempt to wean or extubate client. • Suction client if secretions are thick or copious.
Client has fever, elevated white blood cell count, or changed odor or color of respiratory secretions.	• Send sputum specimen for culture and sensitivity. • Administer antibiotics as ordered.
Client needs to be transported for diagnostic testing.	• Start oxygen flow through handheld ventilating device. • Attach expiratory resistance, for example PEEP. • Disconnect ventilator tubing from airway at end of inspiration. • Attach handheld ventilator to airway during expiration. • Watch chest, and provide breaths with client's inspirations or at rate of 10–12/min.
Po_2 is not maintained at 80–100 mm Hg.	• Continue delivery of PEEP as ordered. If not effective, notify MD. • Do not attempt to wean client off PEEP until desired parameters are obtained.
Cardiac output decreases significantly.	• Anticipate that client may have difficulty adjusting to increased intrathoracic pressure during weaning process. • Decrease PEEP and notify physician for weaning adjustment.
Weaning attempt is unsuccessful.	• Continue use of ventilator. • If client is extubated, consider noninvasive ventilation (CPAP). • Recruit skilled multidisciplinary team to identify and address physiologic and psychological factors that interfere with weaning success.

UNEXPECTED OUTCOMES	CRITICAL THINKING OPTIONS
Decreased level of consciousness, dyspnea, severe anxiety, or fatigue occurs during weaning process.	• Note client's SpO_2 (anxiety may be due to hypoxemia). • Place client on supportive ventilation. • Provide thorough explanation, and increase reassurance. • Evaluate present use of sedatives or narcotic agents administered.
Client develops unstable vital signs.	• Place client back on more supportive ventilator mode. • Monitor vital signs more frequently, and obtain blood gases to determine oxygen concentration. • Increase FiO_2.

GERONTOLOGIC CONSIDERATIONS

Elderly clients in the critical care unit require more intensive observation and consideration.

- Aging is normally accompanied by a silent physiologic decline and diminished reserve in all body systems. These changes are not pathologic, but do make the elderly less adaptable to stress and illness. The elderly have a greater prevalence of chronic conditions that make them vulnerable to acute exacerbations. Over half of critical care clients are over age 65. Hospitalization is almost twice as long as that for clients under age 65 and survival is 81% compared to 98% in younger clients. However, quality of life post discharge from a critical care unit is not age related.
- Refer to previous chapters for organ systems changes and other functional alterations as well as socioeconomic and lifestyle changes that impact care of the elderly client.

MANAGEMENT GUIDELINES

Each state legislates a Nurse Practice Act for RNs and LVN/LPNs. Health care facilities are responsible for establishing and implementing policies and procedures that conform to their state's regulations. Verify the regulations and role parameters for each health care worker in your facility.

Delegation of Responsibilities

- All personnel in the critical care setting must know how to quickly summon assistance and locate and use emergency/resuscitation equipment.
- In advanced care settings, the RN simultaneously assesses, analyzes, makes decisions, intervenes, and evaluates clients on a continual basis. Complexities of care and unpredictability of outcomes necessitate *intense* ongoing client monitoring and evaluation and personal continuing education. Detection and interpretation of subtle areas of change in the client's status require the knowledge and skill of the professional nurse.
- The RN collaborates with the physician and respiratory therapist for ventilator settings.
- It is the responsibility of nursing faculty to assure that students participating in client care (in any setting) are prepared to do so. Likewise, it is the duty of the student to refuse to perform a function he or she is not qualified or competent to perform.
- The nurse should not assume care for any client who requires care beyond the caregiver's expertise.
- Many agencies provide emergency care protocols or standing orders of action responses to specified changes in client status. The professional nurse must be familiar with conditions for which the nurse is del-

egated medical care decisions guided by such protocols.

- The CNA/UAP must know to leave arterial catheter site uncovered for easy observation.
- The CNA/UAP must not move tubing drainage receptacles (e.g., pleurevac) without supervision.
- The CNA/UAP must understand that IVs, drainage systems, ventilator circuits and systems are closed and must be able to give care without disrupting system integrity or disconnecting components for the convenience of care (e.g., as in changing the client's gown or position).
- The UAP has a limited role in the care of clients who require invasive monitoring. They can offer valued assistance in moving/positioning clients and providing personal hygiene and comfort measures under the direction of the professional nurse.
- The UAP assists the client, preserving an interface between technology and reality, by providing a human dimension of tactile presence while providing basic physical care for clients requiring sophisticated technological monitoring. UAP links to the client assist all caregivers in their attempts to minimize client's feelings of alienation.

Information Flow

While certain tasks may be delegated, the CNA/UAP also can provide vital data to the professional nurse by immediately *reporting*:

- Disconnected systems, loose electrodes, tubing leaks, wet/soiled dressings.
- Subjective or objective change in the client's status (e.g., pain, respiratory distress, acute change in cognition).
- Equipment alarms (e.g., ventilator alarms).
- Near-empty infusion bags.
- Near-full collection devices.
- Collaboration with an interdisciplinary team helps to support clients weaning from mechanical ventilation.

CRITICAL THINKING STRATEGIES

SCENARIO 1

Mr. Jones has a history of COPD and heart failure and has been admitted to your unit with a diagnosis of acute respiratory failure. He has the following arterial blood gas values: pH 7.2, Pco_2 66 mm Hg, HCO_3 25 mEq, and Po_2 49 mm Hg. He is intubated and receiving mechanical ventilation to support his breathing and improve gas exchange, and is being sedated with Versed.

On the third day of hospitalization, he is being weaned from mechanical ventilation, but attempts are unsuccessful due to difficulty breathing and development of pulmonary edema.

1. How does mechanical ventilation differ from the normal physiologic process of breathing?
2. How will resultant changes in intrathoracic pressure affect venous return and cardiac work?
3. What measures should be employed to help achieve successful weaning and extubation in this client?

SCENARIO 2

Mr. Hooper has been admitted to the coronary care unit with the diagnosis of anterior septal myocardial infarction with lateral ischemia and potential for infarct extension. He is being monitored by a balloon-tipped, flow-directed catheter for hemodynamic response to therapy. Myocardial infarction (tissue necrosis) results from an imbalance between heart work (demand for oxygen) and coronary supply of oxygen.

Mr. Hooper's hemodynamic measures include: cardiac index 1.8 (low), blood pressure 94/74, mean arterial pressure (MAP) 80 (normal), stroke volume 21 mL (low), pulmonary artery wedge pressure (PAWP) 24 (elevated), heart rate 110 systemic vascular resistance increased.

1. Explain the relationship between "heart work" and need for oxygen.
2. Discuss the parameters that can be monitored with the balloon-tipped catheter.
3. Identify two drugs that could be used to decrease "heart work" and nursing measures that would enhance their effectiveness.

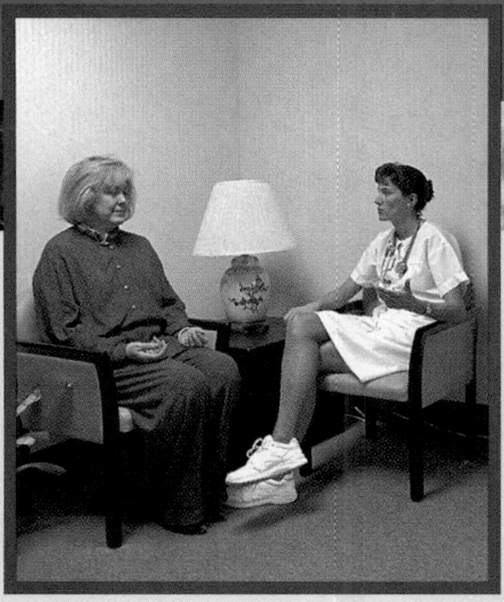

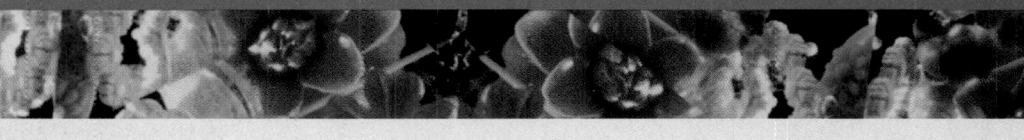

Community-Based Nursing

THEORETICAL CONCEPTS

UNIT ONE: **Admission to Home Care** **1252**

Identifying Eligibility for Medicare Reimbursement 1254
Completing Admission Documentation 1255
Maintaining Nurse's Safety 1255
Assessing Home for Safe Environment 1256
Evaluating Client's Safety 1257
Assessing Caregiver's Safety 1257
Assessing for Elder Abuse 1258

UNIT TWO: **Infection Control** **1259**

Preparing for Client Care 1261
Disposing of Waste Material in the Home Setting 1261
Cleansing Thermometers 1262
Caring for an AIDS or HIV Client in the Home 1262
Cleansing Equipment in the Home Setting 1263
Teaching Preventive Measures in the Home 1263
Teaching Safer Practices to IV Drug Users 1264

UNIT THREE: **Body Mechanics** **1265**

Positioning Nonhospital Bed for Client Care 1267
Moving a Helpless Client Up in Bed Without Assistance 1267

UNIT FOUR: **Hygienic Care** **1268**

Bathing Client in the Home 1270
Transferring Client to Tub or Shower 1270
Adapting Bedmaking to the Home 1271
Providing Pressure Ulcer Care 1271
Preparing Normal Saline 1271
Removing Lice 1272

UNIT FIVE: **Medications** **1273**

Administering Medications 1274
Sterilizing Nondisposable Medication Equipment 1275

UNIT SIX: **Total Nutrient Admixture*** **1276**

Administering Total Nutritional Admixture (TNA) in the Home 1278
Monitoring Client on TNA 1279
Discontinuing TNA Infusion 1279

UNIT SEVEN: **Elimination** **1281**

Using Clean Technique for Intermittent Self-Catheterization 1283
for Female Client 1283
for Male Client 1284
Providing Suprapubic Catheter Care 1284
Administering Continuous Ambulatory Peritoneal Dialysis (CAPD) 1285
Changing Dressing for CAPD Client 1286
Instructing Client in Colostomy Irrigation 1286

UNIT EIGHT: **Respiratory Care** **1288**

Caring for Oxygen Equipment 1290
Teaching Safety Measures for Oxygen Use 1290

Managing Ventilator Equipment 1290
Providing Catheter Care for Transtracheal Catheter 1291
for Heimlich Micro-Trach 1291
for SCOOP Catheter Cleaning in Place 1291
for SCOOP Catheter Cleaning After Removal 1292
Teaching the Client Catheter Care 1293
Teaching Tracheostomy Suction 1293
Cleaning Suction Equipment 1293
Teaching Tracheostomy Care 1294

UNIT NINE: **Circulatory Care 1295**
Monitoring Pacemaker at Home 1297
Checking with Pacemaker Clinic via Telephone 1297
Instructing in Use of Holter Monitor 1298
Teaching Care of Implantable Cardioverter-Defibrillator 1298

LEARNING OBJECTIVES

- Define the criteria for Medicare eligibility.
- Compare and contrast infection control practices in the home and hospital.
- Describe an alternative procedure for handwashing when soap and running water are not available.
- List the contents of the nursing bag carried by home care nurses.
- State at least three safety measures that should be carried out when placing a client into a tub or shower.
- List three areas in the home that should be evaluated for safety.
- Demonstrate at least three improvised nursing actions that promote good body mechanics when providing care in the home.
- Devise a method for assisting the client to remember to take medications.
- Compare and contrast the differences in administering parenteral nutrition in the home and hospital.
- Outline the steps in inserting a straight catheter for a home care client.
- Describe at least six safety measures for home care clients requiring oxygen therapy.
- List the steps for assessing pacemaker function using a pacemaker clinic.
- List two contraindications for using transtracheal oxygen.

INTRODUCTION

Home health care, a rapidly growing field of health care, has developed in response to recent changes in political and social forces in the United States. These changes have demanded that nurses expand their knowledge about home care and acquire skills needed to provide safe, competent care to clients in the home setting.

Several factors have contributed to the emergence of home health care as a primary delivery system. The fastest growing segment of the American population is 85 years of age or older. The elderly constitute the largest proportion of population currently using home health care services. Nine percent of those 65–74 years of age and 25% of those 75 years and older require some type of home care service. Many younger clients are receiving home care visits as a direct result of early discharge from hospitals. Home care visits are funded by private insurance companies and are a cost-effective measure for providing nursing care.

Another factor is the changing structure and role of the American family. Traditionally, women have provided healthcare for the family members at home. With more women working outside the home, the demand for home health services has increased.

Political factors have had an effect on healthcare delivery patterns. A cost-containment measure initiated by the federal government in 1983 to curb rising costs of hospitalized Medicare clients drastically altered the extent of care administered in the hospital setting. A prospective payment system (DRGs), rather than a retrospective payment system, was implemented. This resulted in shorter hospital stays for

Medicare clients. With the shorter stays came a dramatic increase in the need for professional services to care for high acuity clients in the home. Additional types of services have also had to be added to the home care system to meet the needs of these clients. Even more changes occurred with health care reform in the 1990s. Health maintenance organizations (HMOs) and reimbursement policies directly affected the home health care agencies.

The home health care industry has been hit with drastically reduced payments and fewer reimbursable visits as a result of the Balanced Budget Act of 1997. Now home healthcare agencies are required to complete new data collection information forms. The Outcome and Assessment Information Set (OASIS) was instituted in February 1999. The information collected using this tool is in more depth than what was previously being gathered by the agencies. For example, information included regarding the client's health history is far more inclusive when the new forms are utilized. This new system has been developed to measure client outcomes and promote higher quality care. Documentation using OASIS is regulated by HCFA (Health Care Financing Administration). The OASIS system was developed by The Center for Health Policy Research in Denver, Colorado. The new client assessment information was also used to develop a prospective payment system for home health agencies, which went into effect October 2000. Home visits for maternity clients and children under 18 do not require completion of these forms.

Legal Issues in Home Care

Home health nurses are at risk for potential legal liability. Nurses work alone in the home care setting and do not have the advantage of immediately calling on a colleague to collaborate on a client situation. This situation leaves the nurse vulnerable to legal risks. Home health nurses must be extremely skilled in handling equipment of all types, as well as performing specialized procedures without the assistance of another nurse. It is critical that these nurses attend workshops, keep abreast of new equipment and procedures, and continue to read nursing journals on a regular basis. Nurses should know that if equipment is not functioning properly in the home, they should call the agency and report it, fill out an incident report, and not allow the client or themselves to use the equipment.

Home health nurses are also responsible for care provided by unlicensed personnel and LVN/LPNs. It is the responsibility of the nurse to know the competence level of the staff, evaluate their skill level, provide in-service instruction on new equipment or skills, and instruct them to only practice within their specific scope of practice.

Maintaining open communication with other providers is often difficult with the workload of the nurse; however, it is extremely important to keep in contact with physicians and professionals in other disciplines providing care to clients in the caseload. Cell phones and e-mail have improved this aspect of the home health nurse's role. It allows for quick response time and ensures that communication has been maintained.

Another legal issue in home care is appropriate client documentation that supports the need for home care services. If documentation is not accurate, timely, and complete, the client's reimbursement may be denied. This can lead to many hours of valuable time attempting to recover the costs of service or it could lead to legal repercussions. Maintaining appropriate client records is essential to protect the nurse, client, and agency in cases in which there is an investigation of a situation. Writing legibly and neatly, using correct grammar and English, and being succinct and descriptive provides a good legal stance if necessary. Writing notes as close to the time care is delivered is essential so that information is not forgotten. Many agencies now have documentation forms on computer and the nurse enters data as he or she provides care.

The purpose of this chapter is to present clinical skills appropriate for the home setting. Many of the skills used

EVIDENCE BASED NURSING PRACTICE

Percutaneous Injuries in Home Health Care Settings

There is a fast-growing problem with needlesticks in the home setting. There is currently little scientific data to support the extent of the problem. In a study of 290 injuries reported in home care settings, nurses sustained 87% of them. 40% of the injuries are considered "high risk" because they are associated with blood drawing and intravenous access. Most of the injuries occurred from winged steel needles, phlebotomy needles, and lancets. Almost half of the injuries occurred while disposing of equipment.

OSHA does not regulate private homes, therefore the agencies are not held responsible for violations of the Bloodborne Pathogen Standards.

Source: Perry, J., et al. (2001, June). Percutaneous injuries in home healthcare settings. *Home Healthcare Nurse, 19* (6), 342.

in the home are exactly the same as those presented in other sections of this book; therefore, they are not repeated in this chapter. When a specific skill is not included in this unit, refer to a previous unit for that skill. Other skills require minor change for adaptation to the home environment, but, essentially, they are similar. Finally, a few skills are altered for the home setting.

The use of the nursing process is just as important in the home care setting as in the hospital setting. Actually, nursing care plans are required by Medicare regulations and are also used as a justification for skilled nursing services by private insurers. This chapter is presented in the nursing process format to assist in organizing nursing actions and evaluating health care.

Home Care Definition

The term *home health care* refers to all services that promote, maintain, or restore physical, social, or emotional health to clients in the home setting. Home care is provided in the individual's residence. For a smooth transition from hospital to home, the home care coordinator communicates with the family members and the home health nurse.

Home Health Team

A variety of health workers are needed to provide comprehensive home care services to clients and families. The chart below presents an overview of health care providers and their major responsibilities. The list and responsibilities are not inclusive; consult an additional home care reference for more detailed information.

Referral to Home Care

It is necessary for nurses in all settings to be aware of the referral process and the type of client who should be referred for home care services. Although most home care clients have been hospitalized, it is not a prerequisite for service. Physicians, individual clients, families, and friends may refer a client by calling a home health agency and requesting service. A physician's approval is needed for reimbursement. An evaluation visit is made by the RN, PT, or ST to determine if service is needed, and if so, an appropriate plan of care is established.

Most hospitals have a designated protocol for making referrals, which is described in the hospital policy manual. In most hospitals it is the discharge planner or social worker who makes the referral. The nurse may alert the appropriate person to the client's need for home care. It is essential that the nurse provide complete and thorough information about the client's condition, including physical and psychosocial needs. This information is documented on a standard referral form or on an official form from the Department of Health and Human Services and sent to the home health agency. Accurate information and orders are needed to facilitate a smooth transition from

TABLE 34–1 Home Health Team

Health Care Provider	Major Responsibilities
Registered Nurse	Performs as a case manager. Initiates physician ordered plan of care, performs assessment, planning, and interventions for needed home care skills and teaching. Assists in evaluating treatment regimens for all services.
Home Care Aide	Performs hygienic care, skin care, exercise, ambulation, dressing, and elimination skills. Some may prepare and serve meals. They assist in maintaining a clean, safe, client environment (e.g., client's bedroom).
Homemaker	Maintains the home environment, shops for and prepares meals, transports client, and runs errands.
Social Worker	Assists in planning for home care needs, instructs in use of social and community services and resources. Provides information relative to long-term planning and respite care in the home.
Physical Therapist	Evaluates environment in preparation for client's return home. Assists with safety adaptations for the home, instructs in exercise program, gait training, and use of special adaptive equipment.
Occupational Therapist	Instructs in activities of daily living, grooming, upper extremity strengthening, and function activities.
Speech Therapist	Evaluates swallowing and chewing ability; assists with increasing communication techniques for client, family, and health-care provider; and provides speech reeducation program.
Nutritionist	Evaluates and provides for nutritional needs of client. Plans and instructs in appropriate diet.
Physician	Prescribes medical plan of treatment. Writes specific prescriptions for medications, diet, supplies, nursing interventions, and therapist parameters.
Licensed Vocational Nurse	Provides skilled nursing care similar to a Home Care Aide under RN supervision. They are not used by all agencies because of limited independent activities allowed.

hospital to home. Incomplete or inadequate communication could mean a lapse in service and inadequate care for the client.

All age groups use home health services. The criteria for referral depends on various factors, such as client need, agency protocol, and insurance criteria. Since the elderly on Medicare represent the largest segment of the population using home care services, it is important that all nurses know Medicare eligibility criteria for home visits. This ensures that accurate information is given to the client and family. In addition to eligibility criteria, many regulations govern the type and frequency of care. Since these regulations are subject to change and interpretation by the fiscal intermediaries who administer Medicare insurance, frequent review of Medicare regulations should be done. Eligibility for another funding agency, Medicaid, differs from state to state. It is the nurse's responsibility to be familiar with these policies. Each individual insurance company reimburses for services at different rates and for different levels of service. Each insurance plan needs to be reviewed to determine reimbursement.

Transition from Hospital to Home

A smooth transition from hospital to home depends on an appropriate discharge plan. The shorter duration in hospital stay requires a thorough, efficient discharge plan that must be initiated at the time of hospital admission. Identifying the client's needs and resources before planning for discharge results in a realistic plan. Since any illness causes additional stress in the family and necessitates an adaptive coping response, the needs of the family or significant other must be included in the teaching and discharge plan. In addition, accurate and comprehensive documentation must accompany the physician's plan of treatment to ensure a smooth transition. A description of the client at discharge should be provided; include physical assessment findings, ability to assist in ADLs, adaptive devices needed for care, and a brief summary of hospitalization. These data greatly assist in the transition from hospital to home.

Client Teaching

Client teaching is an essential component of both hospital and home care. Since clients are discharged earlier and with a higher acuity level, the client and his or her family are expected to accept more responsibility for follow-up care. It is essential that client teaching begin in the hospital and provide a description of the disease or condition and the treatment regimen. The client and family should be instructed in skills and treatments necessary to restore health and prevent other illness or complications. The home health nurse builds on the teaching plan with the main emphasis on adapting care in the home environment. Continuity of care depends on comprehensive communication between the discharging and home care agencies.

Adapting Care to the Home Setting

The client is often a passive recipient of care in the hospital. In the home setting, on the other hand, the client is in control—it is his or her environment. That is, the environment is determined by the client and family according to their needs, desires, values, and resources. The nurse is a guest in this environment, which requires flexibility in adapting to a variety of situations.

In the hospital, equipment is readily available. Nurses perform procedures or treatments and provide 24-hour-a-day coverage of nursing care. In the home, equipment must be ordered or improvised and the emphasis is on teaching the client or caregiver self-care activities. The home care nurse must become very creative in adapting and improvising equipment and techniques.

When a client referral is received by a home health agency, a nurse, physical therapist, or speech therapist makes an initial admission visit. This visit includes a thorough assessment of the client, family, and home environment. The home environment is evaluated for safety, and the client and family are assessed for knowledge of safety and emergency procedures. Assessment of the client includes physical, emotional, psychologic, and economic status. The home is assessed for any adaptations that must be made to enable the client to function optimally in his or her environment. Family members are assessed for understanding of the client's illness or needs; cultural, ethnic, and health beliefs and values; ability to cope with the current situation; the physical, emotional, and spiritual needs of family members; financial resources; and knowledge of how to use community resources. A complete list of assessment parameters for each of these areas is included on the initial assessment form.

Plan of Treatment

Based on admission findings, a plan of care is established. The Health Care Financing Administration (the federal office that administers the Medicare program) requires that all agencies certified to provide home health care to Medicare clients complete the OASIS forms and the home health certification and plan of treatment form (form H485) within 7 days. These forms must be completed on admission and signed by a physician. The plan of treatment is effective for 60 days, unless the client's condition changes. An updated plan must be signed and submitted to the Medicare office every 60 days.

In addition to form H485 and the OASIS forms, the health care documentation includes admission worksheet, nursing care plan, medication profile, plan of treatment, and consent for admission and service.

Documentation

Accurate documentation of each visit is essential for both legal and fiscal purposes. The same legal considerations for charting apply to home care and the hospital. Legally, the documentation provides proof that care was given. Reimbursement of services is based on documentation. Documentation of visits can be done in a problem-oriented or narrative format, depending on agency policy. Charting must follow the nursing care plan and cover the areas listed in the OASIS documentation system. OASIS is an assessment instrument used to collect specific information when a person is on Medicaid or Medicare and requires the services of a home health agency. OASIS is a key component of Medicare's partnership with the home care industry to foster and monitor improved home health care outcomes. The information is collected in order to improve client outcomes and assist with quality improvement. OASIS data items include sociodemographic, environmental, support system, health status, and functional status attributes of adult clients. Information gathered on the OASIS form is forwarded to the state where it goes to the Health Care Financing Administration (HCFA). There, the information is used for reimbursement purposes for the specific home health agency. This prospective payment system went into effect in October 2000. There are several forms that are required to be completed for each client.

The in-depth assessment is useful in identifying areas in which client status differs from optimal health or functional status. This information leads to improved client care planning.

Documentation takes a great deal of the nurse's time. Because of this, many agencies use standardized care plans and individualize them for each client. Flow sheets are used to expedite charting as much as possible. Use of laptop computers has increased efficiency of documentation.

The independent nature of home health nursing creates potential legal concerns for the nurse. Home care nurses must be adequately prepared and knowledgeable in current treatment procedures, protocols, and teaching modalities and be able to function independently.

Interventions are implemented by the client, family, and part-time caregivers; therefore, all are involved in the treatment plan. The nurse or the case manager is responsible to coordinate and evaluate the care. The speech therapist or physical therapist can also assume the role of case manager. This usually occurs when the client is receiving rehabilitation services only.

Currently, Medicare requires the nurse to make a home visit for the purpose of supervision at least every 14 days to reassess client and family needs and to revise the care plan. One visit each month is to discuss the treatment plan with the family. The nurse also accompanies the home health aide once a month for a supervised visit.

Since home health aides provide care without direct daily supervision of a nurse, it is important that they have thorough training when they begin working for a home health agency and at periodic intervals receive continuing education. If a required course is not needed for employment, on-the-job training will be done. Agencies hire only experienced nursing assistants (in most states, those who have worked in a hospital or nursing home). Home health aide certification is voluntary in some states, and required for others. It is important to check state regulations. The training is completed after they have obtained a CNA certificate in many states.

Currently, home health nurses must meet a national standard of care; no longer does the legal standard of care for nursing practice vary according to locale. Each practicing home health nurse must be aware of the national standards as published by the American Nurses Association. The best preparation for home health nursing continues to be a sound base of nursing skills coupled with a broad knowledge of agency procedures and protocols.

NURSING DIAGNOSES

The following nursing diagnoses may be appropriate to include in a client care plan when the components are related to admitting to the home care setting.

NURSING DIAGNOSIS	RELATED FACTORS
Anxiety	Fear of unknown outcome, actual or perceived threat to self-concept, threat to biologic integrity, change in socioeconomic status
Anticipatory Grieving	Loss of function, change in lifestyle, lack of social support system, change in social role
Impaired Home Maintenance	Unavailable or inadequate support systems (spouse or children not available to provide care), insufficient finances, environmental barriers or physical facilities (lighting, condition of flooring, steps)
Risk for Injury	Impaired judgment, muscle weakness, disease process, safety factors in the home

- The single most important nursing action to decrease the incidence of infection is handwashing. **Remember to wash your hands or use antibacterial gel before and after each and every client contact.**

UNIT 1

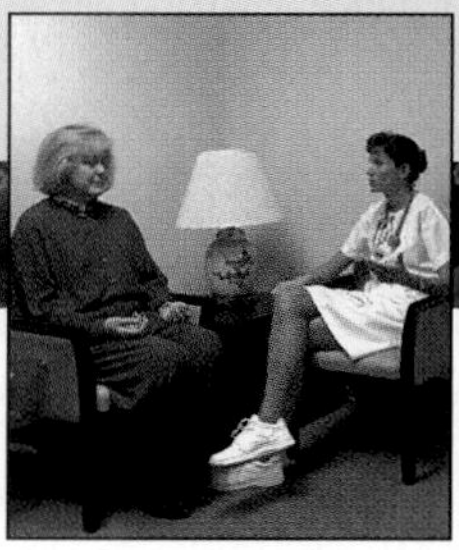

Admission to Home Care

Nursing Process Data

ASSESSMENT ***Data Base***

Assess client's financial eligibility for home care service.
Assess client's care requirements.
Observe client's physical, emotional, and intellectual status.
Observe client's ability to adapt to the home setting.
Assess the client's level of comfort or discomfort.
Determine client's understanding of the disease and its limitations.
Assess home condition prior to client returning home.
Assess safety factors in the home.
Observe equipment for safety features.
Assess nurse's safety for making home visit.
Determine client's safety in home.
Determine caretaker's ability to provide client care and safety.

PLANNING ***Objectives***

To assist client to adapt to home care with minimal distress
To encourage client and family to participate in the plan of care
To provide a comfortable and safe environment for the client
To provide the necessary and appropriate home care treatment modalities
To provide a safe environment for the nurse

IMPLEMENTATION ***Procedures***

Identifying Eligibility for Medicare Reimbursement
Completing Admission Documentation
Maintaining Nurse's Safety
Assessing Home for Safe Environment
Evaluating Client's Safety
Assessing Caregiver's Safety
Assessing for Elder Abuse

EVALUATION ***Expected Outcomes***

Client adapts to home setting with minimal difficulties.
Safe environment is provided for client.
Client obtains necessary home care nursing modalities.
Nurse's safety is maintained during home visit.

DRAFT

Outcome and Assessment Information Set (OASIS-B1)

START OF CARE VERSION
(also used for Resumption of Care Following Inpatient Stay)

Items to be Used at this Time Point-- **M0080-M0325**

CLINICAL RECORD ITEMS

(M0080) Discipline of Person Completing Assessment:

☐ 1-RN ☐ 2-PT ☐ 3-SLP/ST ☐ 4-OT

(M0090) Date Assessment Completed: __ __/__ __/__ __ __ __
month day year

(M0100) This Assessment is Currently Being Completed for the Following Reason:

Start/Resumption of Care
☐ 1 – Start of care—further visits planned
☐ 3 – Resumption of care (after inpatient stay)

DEMOGRAPHICS AND PATIENT HISTORY

(M0175) From which of the following **Inpatient Facilities** was the patient discharged during the past 14 days? **(Mark all that apply.)**

☐ 1 - Hospital
☐ 2 - Rehabilitation facility
☐ 3 - Skilled nursing facility
☐ 4 - Other nursing home
☐ 5 - Other (specify) ________________
☐ NA - Patient was not discharged from an inpatient facility **[If NA, go to *M0200*]**

(M0180) Inpatient Discharge Date (most recent):

__ __/__ __/__ __ __ __
month day year

☐ UK - Unknown

(M0190) Inpatient Diagnoses and ICD code categories (three digits required; five digits optional) for only those conditions treated during an inpatient stay within the last 14 days (no surgical or V-codes):

Inpatient Facility Diagnosis	ICD
a. ____________	(__ __ __ • __ __)
b. ____________	(__ __ __ • __ __)

Effective 10/1/2003

List each Inpatient Diagnosis and ICD-9-CM code at the level of highest specificity for only those conditions treated during an inpatient stay within the last 14 days (no surgical, E-codes, or V-codes):

Inpatient Facility Diagnosis	ICD-9-CM
a. ____________	(__ __ __ • __ __)
b. ____________	(__ __ __ • __ __)

OASIS-B1 SOC (12/2002)

This is the first page (of 9) of the Discharge Documentation Form (OASIS—required by HCFA).

(M0200) Medical or Treatment Regimen Change Within Past 14 Days: Has this patient experienced a change in medical or treatment regimen (e.g., medication, treatment, or service change due to new or additional diagnosis, etc.) within the last 14 days?

☐ 0 - No **[If No, go to *M0220*]**
☐ 1 - Yes

(M0210) List the patient's **Medical Diagnoses** and ICD code categories (three digits required; five digits optional) for those conditions requiring changed medical or treatment regimen (no surgical or V-codes):

Changed Medical Regimen Diagnosis	ICD
a. ____________	(__ __ __ • __ __)
b. ____________	(__ __ __ • __ __)
c. ____________	(__ __ __ • __ __)
d. ____________	(__ __ __ • __ __)

Effective 10/1/2003

List the patient's Medical Diagnosis and ICD-9-CM codes at the level of highest specificity for those conditions requiring changed medical or treatment regimen (no surgical, E-codes, or V-codes):

Changed Medical Regimen Diagnosis	ICD-9-CM
a. ____________	(__ __ __ • __ __)
b. ____________	(__ __ __ • __ __)
c. ____________	(__ __ __ • __ __)
d. ____________	(__ __ __ • __ __)

(M0220) Conditions Prior to Medical or Treatment Regimen Change or Inpatient Stay Within Past 14 Days: If this patient experienced an inpatient facility discharge or change in medical or treatment regimen within the past 14 days, indicate any conditions which existed prior to the inpatient stay or change in medical or treatment regimen. **(Mark all that apply.)**

☐ 1 - Urinary incontinence
☐ 2 - Indwelling/suprapubic catheter
☐ 3 - Intractable pain
☐ 4 - Impaired decision-making
☐ 5 - Disruptive or socially inappropriate behavior
☐ 6 - Memory loss to the extent that supervision required
☐ 7 - None of the above
☐ NA - No inpatient facility discharge and no change in medical or treatment regimen in past 14 days
☐ UK - Unknown

(M0230/M0240) Diagnoses and Severity Index: List each medical diagnosis or problem for which the patient is receiving home care and ICD-9-CM code category (three digits required; five digits optional – no surgical or V-codes) and rate them using the following severity index. (Choose one value that represents the most severe rating appropriate for each diagnosis.) ICD-9-CM sequencing requirements must be followed if multiple coding is indicated for any diagnoses.

Effective 10/1/2003

List each diagnosis and ICD-9-CM code at the level of highest specificity (no surgical codes) for which the patient is receiving home care. Rate each condition using the following severity index. (Choose one value that represents the most severe rating appropriate for each diagnosis.) E-codes (for M0240 only) or V-codes (for M0230 or M0240) may be used. ICD-9-CM sequencing requirements must be followed if multiple coding is indicated for any diagnoses. If a V-code is reported in place of a case mix diagnosis, then M0245 Payment Diagnosis should be completed. Case mix diagnosis is a primary or first secondary diagnosis that determines the Medicare PPS case mix group.

OASIS-B1 SOC (12/2002)

DRAFT

Outcome and Assessment Information Set (OASIS-B1)

DISCHARGE VERSION
(also used for Transfer to an Inpatient Facility or Patient Death at Home)

Items to be Used at Specific Time Points

Transfer to an Inpatient Facility------------------------- **M0080-M0100, M0830-M0855, M0890-M0906**
Transferred to an inpatient facility—patient not discharged from an agency
Transferred to an inpatient facility—patient discharged from agency

Discharge from Agency — Not to an Inpatient Facility
Death at home------------------------- **M0080-M0100, M0906**
Discharge from agency------------------------- **M0080-M0100, M0200-M0220, M0250, M0280-M0380, M0410-M0820, M0830-M0880, M0903-M0906**

CLINICAL RECORD ITEMS

(M0080) Discipline of Person Completing Assessment:

☐ 1-RN ☐ 2-PT ☐ 3-SLP/ST ☐ 4-OT

(M0090) Date Assessment Completed: __ __/__ __/__ __ __ __
month day year

(M0100) This Assessment is Currently Being Completed for the Following Reason:

Transfer to an Inpatient Facility
☐ 6 – Transferred to an inpatient facility—patient not discharged from agency **[Go to *M0830*]**
☐ 7 – Transferred to an inpatient facility—patient discharged from agency **[Go to *M0830*]**
Discharge from Agency — Not to an Inpatient Facility
☐ 8 – Death at home **[Go to *M0906*]**
☐ 9 – Discharge from agency **[Go to *M0200*]**

DEMOGRAPHICS AND PATIENT HISTORY

(M0200) Medical or Treatment Regimen Change Within Past 14 Days: Has this patient experienced a change in medical or treatment regimen (e.g., medication, treatment, or service change due to new or additional diagnosis, etc.) within the last 14 days?

☐ 0 - No **[If No, go to *M0220*]**
☐ 1 - Yes

(M0210) List the patient's **Medical Diagnoses** and ICD code categories (three digits required; five digits optional) for those conditions requiring changed medical or treatment regimen (no surgical or V-codes):

Changed Medical Regimen Diagnosis	ICD
a. ____________	(__ __ __ • __ __)
b. ____________	(__ __ __ • __ __)
c. ____________	(__ __ __ • __ __)
d. ____________	(__ __ __ • __ __)

OASIS-B1 DC (12/2002)

This is the sample first page (of 16) of the Comprehensive Assessment/Evaluation Form (OASIS—required by HCFA).

DEPARTMENT OF HEALTH AND HUMAN SERVICES
HEALTH CARE FINANCING ADMINISTRATION

FORM APPROVED
OMB No. 0938-0357

HOME HEALTH CERTIFICATION AND PLAN OF TREATMENT

1. Patient's HI Claim No.	2. SOC Date	3. Certification Period From: To:	4. Medical Record No.	5. Provider No.

6. Patient's Name and Address

7. Provider's Name and Address.

8. Date of Birth — 9. Sex ☐ M ☐ F

10. Medications: Dose/Frequency/Route (N)ew (C)hanged

11. ICD-9-CM	Principal Diagnosis	Date
12. ICD-9-CM	Surgical Procedure	Date
13. ICD-9-CM	Other Pertinent Diagnosis	Date

14. DME and Supplies

15. Safety Measures:

16. Nutritional Req.

17. Allergies:

18.A. Functional Limitations

1 ☐ Amputation 2 ☐ Bowel/Bladder (Incontinence) 3 ☐ Contracture 4 ☐ Hearing 5 ☐ Paralysis 6 ☐ Endurance 7 ☐ Ambulation 8 ☐ Speech 9 ☐ Legally Blind A ☐ Dyspnea With Minimal Exertion B ☐ Other (Specify)

18.B. Activities Permitted

1 ☐ Complete Bedrest 2 ☐ Bedrest BRP 3 ☐ Up As Tolerated 4 ☐ Transfer Bed/Chair 5 ☐ Exercises Prescribed 6 ☐ Partial Weight Bearing 7 ☐ Independent At Home 8 ☐ Crutches 9 ☐ Cane A ☐ Wheelchair B ☐ Walker C ☐ No Restrictions D ☐ Other (Specify)

19. Mental Status: 1 ☐ Oriented 2 ☐ Comatose 3 ☐ Forgetful 4 ☐ Depressed 5 ☐ Disoriented 6 ☐ Lethargic 7 ☐ Agitated 8 ☐ Other

20. Prognosis: 1 ☐ Poor 2 ☐ Guarded 3 ☐ Fair 4 ☐ Good 5 ☐ Excellent

21. Orders for Discipline and Treatments (Specify Amount/Frequency/Duration)

22. Goals/Rehabilitation Potential/Discharge Plans

23. Nurse's Signature and Date of Verbal SOC Where Applicable:

25. Date HHA Received Signed POT

24. Physician's Name and Address

26. I certify/recertify that this patient is confined to his/her home and needs intermittent skilled nursing care, physical therapy and/or speech therapy or continues to need occupational therapy. The patient is under my care, and I have authorized the services on this plan of care and will periodically renew the plan.

27. Attending Physician's Signature and Date Signed

28. Anyone who misrepresents, falsifies, or conceals essential information required for payment of Federal funds may be subject to fine, imprisonment, or civil penalty under applicable Federal laws.

FORM HCFA-485 (C4) (4-87)

Plan of Treatment—HCFA.

IDENTIFYING ELIGIBILITY FOR MEDICARE REIMBURSEMENT

Procedure

1. Complete OASIS forms.
   a. Integrate information with H485 data.
   b. Complete all sections of document. **Rationale:** Denial of service can result if documentation incomplete.
   c. Complete forms within 7 days.
   d. Ensure information from forms is transcribed accurately onto H485 forms. **Rationale:** To prevent denial of service.
2. Check required criteria for Medicare coverage eligibility. **Rationale:** This prevents administering care for which reimbursement will not be received.
3. Identify client as homebound.
   a. Client's condition severely restricts leaving the home.
   b. Leaving the home requires considerable effort and assistance of another person.
   c. Special transportation is necessary.
   d. Absences from the home are infrequent and short.
4. Check that home service is considered skilled. To be skilled, service must be under the supervision of a registered nurse, a physical therapist, or a speech therapist.
   a. Registered nurse performs specific functions:
      Client teaching.
      Dressings or irrigations.
      Catheterization.
      Parenteral therapies.
      Medication administration and teaching.
   b. Physical therapist performs certain functions:
      Gait training.
      Therapeutic exercises.
      Ultrasound, diathermy, TENS.
      Restorative therapy.
   c. Speech therapist performs certain functions:
      Therapy for clients with certain diagnoses (e.g., CVA, laryngectomies).
      Selected diagnostic and evaluative services.
5. Provide supplemental services from home health aide, social worker, or occupational therapist; care is reimbursed by Medicare only when one of the three skilled services is required.
   a. Supplemental services may be obtained even if one of the skilled services is not needed; however, Medicare does not reimburse, and client is responsible for payment.
   b. Home health aide services are reimbursable only if plan of care is established and supervised by registered nurse.
      Personal care (ADL).
      Light housekeeping (e.g., food preparation, client's laundry).
      Selected semiskilled care (e.g., PROM exercises).
   c. Social worker.
      Interventions must contribute significantly to the improvement of the client's medical condition.
      Indication that social, environmental, or family conditions inhibit progress of recovery from medical condition.
   d. Occupational therapy.
      Design maintenance program.
      Design self-help devices to assist ADL.
      Teach compensatory techniques.
      Provide restorative therapy.
6. Provide care that is part-time and intermittent.
   a. Care must be episodic or acute and not chronic.
   b. Medically predictable recurring need for care must be present.
   c. Knowledge that condition will improve in a limited time frame.
   d. Frequency of service ranges from daily to every 90 days, depending on individual client's need.
7. Check that plan of treatment is authorized by physician and recertified every 60 days.
   a. Health Care Financing Administration form (H485) is standardized for plan of treatment. This form is used by all home health agencies for Medicare clients.
   b. Form must include:
      Identifying data
      Diagnosis (ICD-9CM)
      Start of care
      Types of services required and frequency

CLINICAL ALERT

The Outcome and Assessment Information Set (OASIS-B1) and the Discharge Form in the OASIS paperwork is more extensive than previously gathered information on documentation forms. Be careful to complete all sections of the form.

Guidelines for Home Care

- Take as little with you into the home as possible.
- Use appropriate nursing protocol in home setting.
- Wash your hands on entering and leaving home.
- Maintain clean technique in the home.
- Know the infection control guidelines (CDC).
- Review state and federal guidelines and protocol for reimbursement.

Functional limitations
Activities permitted
Safety measures
Treatments
Medications
Mental status
Nutritional status and diet orders
Medical supplies and DME
Goals and discharge plans
Significant clinical findings
Prognosis
Physician's name, address, signature
Certification of homebound status

8. Assess that care is medically reasonable and necessary.
   a. Entire plan of care must correlate with client's medical problems and client's clinical status.
   b. Each service's goals (client outcomes) must be clearly stated and realistic for the client.

COMPLETING ADMISSION DOCUMENTATION

Procedure

1. Complete all sections of the OASIS document.
   a. Demographic data: address, referring physician, payment source, etc.
   b. Present history.
   c. Present illness.
   d. Living arrangements.
   e. Supportive assistance.
   f. Physical assessment/Review of systems
   g. ADLs
   h. Medications
   i. Equipment management
   j. Homebound status.
   k. Therapy modalities required.
   l. Unmet needs.
   m. Lack of Knowledge section.
   n. Treatment/Procedures Performed.
   o. Response to Teaching/Training Performed.
   p. Patient Rights and Responsibilities.
   q. Coordination of Patient Services.
   r. Discharge Planning.
2. Signed consent forms.
   a. IV therapy.
   b. Consent for treatment.
   c. Consent for service.
3. Signed Advanced Directive document.
4. Signed Patient's Bill of Rights document.
5. Billing Data Base.
6. Discipline Specific Evaluation, if therapy was instituted.
7. Plan of Care.
8. H485 Worksheet.
9. Aide Assignment and Duties, if appropriate.
10. Physician Plan of Care.
11. Home Health Plan of Care.
12. Nurses' Notes as necessary.
13. Identify if prehospital "Do Not Resuscitate" form has been signed.

MAINTAINING NURSE'S SAFETY

Procedure

1. Evaluate safety of nurse prior to the visit.
   a. Call the client before the visit to determine convenient time.
   b. Confirm directions to home.
   c. Determine if household pets are present, if so, ask that they be secured during visit.
   d. Check neighborhood to determine need for assistance from police to make home visit.
2. Wear identifying name badge. Most agencies request that the nurse wear a lab coat.
3. Wear flat shoes to allow you to walk quickly or to run if necessary.
4. Maintain personal safety while traveling in the car.
   a. Keep car in good working order and stocked with necessary equipment.
   b. Keep gas tank at least half full at all times.
   c. Obtain automobile club membership for emergency use. **Rationale:** To call for assistance with car problems.
   d. Keep a windshield cover with CALL POLICE sign available. **Rationale:** To alert neighbors you need immediate assistance.
   e. Have car phone available and charged at all times.
   f. Keep blanket in car. **Rationale:** To keep warm in the winter if you need to wait for assistance.
   g. Keep thermos of water in car at all times. **Rationale:** In case you need to wait for assistance in hot weather.
   h. Keep doors locked and windows up at all times.
   i. Park in full view of neighbors, preferably directly in front of home.
   j. Lock all personal items in trunk of the car before leaving home or office.

k. Keep all equipment in the trunk of the car. Restock the nurses' bag before the visits for the day.
l. Keep nurses' bag on front seat.
m. Keep change in car for phone calls if necessary.
n. Place all valuable objects out of direct sight in car, i.e., laptop computers, phone. Place these under the seat if possible. **Rationale:** To prevent car break-in and theft.

5. Maintain personal safety while walking on the street.
   a. Keep one arm and hand free when walking from car to house.
   b. Walk directly to client's residence.
   c. When approaching a group of strangers, cross the street or walkway, if appropriate.
   d. When leaving a residence, keep keys in your hand with the pointed end of the key facing outward. **Rationale:** The keys can act as a weapon if necessary.
   e. Carry a chemical spray and whistle within easy reach.

CLINICAL ALERT

If your safety is in jeopardy, use one of the following defensive strategies: Scream or yell *FIRE* or *STRANGER.* Kick the person in the shin or groin. Bite or scratch the person. Use chemical spray or blow a whistle. If you feel your personal safety is in question, do not make a visit or stay in the residence.

Note: Attendance at a class is necessary before it is legal to carry a chemical spray such as mace.

6. Maintain personal safety when making home visit.
   a. Use common walkways or hallways. Do not park behind a building or in a dark area.
   b. Knock on the door and wait for permission to enter.
   c. Keep a clear pathway to the door if the situation is potentially unsafe.
   d. Observe home environment for safety hazards, i.e., weapons.
   e. Make a joint visit with another agency staff member or ask for an escort if there is a potentially unsafe situation.
   f. Call for police support if the visit is essential and the situation is unsafe. **Rationale:** There may be times when a visit is essential, but it is unsafe for one individual to make a visit.
   g. Make visit in the morning when good visual support exists if neighborhood is unsafe.
   h. Close the case if the nurse feels the situation is unsafe and there are no alternative actions that can guarantee the nurses' safety.

ASSESSING HOME FOR SAFE ENVIRONMENT

Equipment

Home Assessment Checklist
Outcome and Assessment Information Act (OASIS-B1)

Procedure

1. Identify type of dwelling, i.e., client-owned, boarding home, rental, mobile home.
2. Identify water source.
3. Identify sewer source.
4. Identify type of plumbing available.
5. Determine if any pollutants are present in the environment.
6. Assess exterior of the home for
   a. Condition of sidewalks and steps.
   b. Presence of railings on steps.
   c. Barriers that prevent easy access to the home.
   d. Adequacy of lighting.
   e. Adequacy of roof and windows.
7. Assess interior of the home for
   a. Presence of scatter rugs or worn carpeting.
   b. Uncluttered pathways throughout the house.
   c. Adequacy of lighting.
   d. Doorways wide enough to permit assistive devices.
   e. Cleanliness of house.
   f. Presence of insects, rodents, or infective agents.
   g. Presence of functioning smoke detectors.
   h. Adequate heating and cooling systems.
   i. Presence of running water.
8. Determine if hazardous materials are safely stored.
9. Assess for presence of lead-based paint.
10. Determine if medications can be adequately stored out of reach of children and impaired individuals.
11. Assess stairway and halls for
    a. Adequacy of light.
    b. Handrails that are securely fastened to wall.
    c. Flooring in good repair.
    d. Rugs or carpeting in good repair.
    e. Light switches in easy reach and accessible at both ends of stairs or hallway.
12. Assess kitchen for
    a. Properly functioning stove.
    b. Adequacy of light surrounding stove and sink.
    c. Condition of small appliances.
    d. Accessibility of appliances to clients in wheelchairs.
    e. Adequacy of sewage disposal.
13. Assess bathroom for
    a. Skidproof strips or mat in tub or shower.

b. Handrails around toilet and tub or shower.
c. Accessibility of medicine cabinet.
d. Adequate space if wheelchairs or walkers are used.
e. Temperature of hot water from faucets in sink, tub, or shower.

14. Assess bedroom for
a. Accessibility of closets and cabinets.
b. Ease in getting into and out of bed.
c. Adequate space, if commode or wheelchair is required.
d. Night light availability.
e. Accessibility of medications, water on a night stand.
f. Calling system to alert healthcare provider.
g. Flooring in good repair and nonslippery surface.

EVALUATING CLIENT'S SAFETY

Procedure

1. Evaluate client's cognitive abilities: level of consciousness, orientation, ability to make appropriate judgments, ability to follow commands and directions.
   a. Knowledge of how to operate appliances, e.g., stoves and heaters.
   b. History of alcohol or drug abuse.
   c. Knowledge of medication times and doses to be taken.
   d. Knowledge of how to call for help: physician, nurse, fire, police.
2. Evaluate client's sensory and motor function.
   a. Hearing and vision acuity.
   b. Ability to ambulate with assistance.
   c. Need for assistive devices or support in ambulation.
3. Assess if client needs alternatives to physical restraints.
   a. Determine if environment needs to be modified by removing unsafe objects or barriers.
   b. Remove wheels from chairs or bed.
   c. Install bed check system or alarm device.
   d. Decrease auditory and visual stimuli.
   e. Place supplies close to bed or chair (e.g., tissues, water).
   f. Develop routine for client.
4. Evaluate most effective type of restraint, if absolutely necessary.
   a. Determine that less restrictive methods have been attempted.
   b. Assess purpose of restraint to determine most appropriate type.
   c. Obtain physician's order for restraint. Order must include reason, type, and time of restraints.
   d. Obtain informed consent from client or guardian before applying.
   e. Explain purpose of restraints to client and family members.
   f. Ensure caregiver is instructed on use of restraints.
   g. Evaluate effectiveness and continued need for restraints.

Refer to Chapter 7 for guidelines on use and application of restraints. The safety issues are the same as for clients in the hospital.

5. Determine client's ability to manage self-care.
   a. Bathing, grooming, and dressing.
   b. Preparing food and feeding.
   c. Toileting.
   d. Housekeeping, shopping, transportation to physician and pharmacy.
6. Determine client's financial support.
   a. Determine health care insurance plan, workers' compensation, Medicare, Medicaid.
   b. Determine need for social service intervention.

ASSESSING CAREGIVER'S SAFETY

Procedure

1. Determine caregiver's cognitive function.
   a. Ability to understand and carry out interventions.
   b. Ability to make safe decisions and judgments.
   c. Willingness to care for client.
2. Determine caregiver's sensory and motor function.
   a. Ability to hear client's needs.
   b. Visual acuity to read directions, medication labels.
   c. Ability to feel temperature changes, e.g., water for bathing.
3. Determine caregiver's motor function and strength.
   a. Ability to assist client in transfer, moving, turning, and ADLs.
   b. Ability to provide treatments and care for client.
   c. Ability to prepare food and do housekeeping chores.
   d. Ability to do shopping and provide transportation for physician visits.

ASSESSING FOR ELDER ABUSE

Procedure

1. Assess client for indications of neglect: failure to provide adequate food, clothing, medical assistance, or assistance with ADLs. Check body for signs of cleanliness. Determine if emotional abuse is present. Ask about threats, intimidation, or isolation.
2. Identify if financial abuse has occurred, such as misuse of finances or property.
3. Assess for signs of physical abuse: signs of restraining; hitting, biting, burning; black and blue marks on trunk, abdomen, buttocks, upper thighs; scars, and abrasions. Bilateral bruises or parallel injuries may indicate forceful restraining; shaking may cause parallel injuries of upper arms. Accidental injuries affect knees, back of hands, forehead, and elbows.
4. Assess for signs of malnourishment or dehydration.
5. Check skin for pressure ulcers.
6. Assess for signs of sprains or dislocations from pulling or pushing the client.
7. Ask about visits to the hospital ER. Ask why client sought medical care, how much time elapsed between injury and visit to ER.

Questions to Ask if Suspicion of Abuse

- Who cares for you at home?
- Did someone hurt you?
- Are you happy with where you live?
- Tell me about your daily routine.
- Who assists you with ADLs?
- Do you feel safe living here?
- Who manages your money?
- How did the injury (or bruises) occur?
- Did you receive medical attention?
- Has this type of injury happened before?

8. Assess for signs of emotional abuse. Observe if client is fearful of strangers, becomes quiet when caregiver enters room, craves attention and socialization.

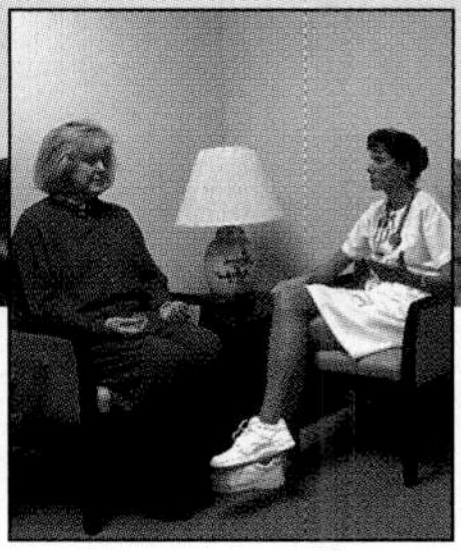

UNIT 2

Infection Control

Nursing Process Data

ASSESSMENT Data Base
Assess need for handwashing.
Identify clients at risk for infection.
Assess need for cleaning equipment and decontaminating equipment.
Identify type of waste material requiring special disposal.
Assess equipment needed to deliver care in the home.
Assess need for teaching preventive measures in the home of HIV or AIDS clients.

PLANNING Objectives
To deliver client care with pathogen-free hands
To clean equipment properly to prevent cross-contamination
To protect client from cross-contamination
To protect the nurse
To properly dispose of contaminated waste material
To protect client's significant others from contamination of infected material

IMPLEMENTATION Procedures
Preparing for Client Care
Disposing of Waste Material in the Home Setting
Cleansing Thermometer
Caring for an AIDS or HIV Client in the Home
Cleansing Equipment in the Home Setting
Teaching Preventive Measures in the Home
Teaching Safer Practices to IV Drug Users
(For additional skills refer to Chapter 15)

EVALUATION Expected Outcomes
Cross-contamination is prevented.
Nurse is protected from infection.
Equipment is cleaned appropriately.
Waste is disposed of in proper manner.
Thermometer is cleaned.

In the home setting, medical asepsis, or clean technique, is often used instead of sterile technique. The major reasons for this protocol change are the nature of the setting and the personnel providing care. The greatest infection control problem in hospitals is nosocomial infections due to the large numbers of antibiotic-resistant organisms present in a hospital setting. Although people are able to survive in what may be considered a less-than-desirable environment without acquiring infections, they would not be protected or possess the acquired immunity to the bacteria in a hospital setting. When clients are in their own environment, however, they tend to develop fewer infections because they are subjected to fewer organisms. In the home setting, focus is on protecting home care staff and family, not other clients. There is minimal data on the incidence of home care acquired infections. Infection preventing strategies in the home should focus on IV therapy, urinary tract care, respiratory and wound care.

Nevertheless, sterile technique and equipment, such as prepackaged catheter and irrigation kits, parenteral fluid equipment, and dressings, are often purchased for home care. When sterile technique is required, it is the responsibility of the nurse to provide the instruction and evaluate the family's ability to perform the skill accurately. Hospital techniques may need to be modified for the home setting, and ideal environmental working conditions may not be present. Therefore, adaptations must be made, but the essential infection control measures must be maintained.

Just as in the hospital, effective handwashing is the *most* effective means of infection control in the home setting. There is one major difference between hospital and home. Equipment (soap, running water, and paper towels) that is readily available to the nurse in the hospital may not be available in the home. Even if running water is available, there may not be soap or clean towels. The nurse must carry handwashing supplies with her or him.

According to the *Home Healthcare Nurse Journal*, (Feb. 2000. "Improving Infection Control in Home Care: From Ritual to Science-Based Practice"), many of the home care infection control practices have been based on ritual, rather than scientific principles. Many changes in infection control procedures in the home are occurring based on a scientific approach. If the home care client is suspected of or diagnosed as having an infectious disease or the client is infected or colonized with VRE or MSRA, the nurse should use the same protective equipment and protocol used in the hospital setting. The equipment includes gloves, disposable gown or apron, mask, cap, and goggles.

Reusable equipment, such as stethoscopes and blood pressure cuffs, should stay in the home and not be used on other home care clients. If possible, these clients should be seen at the end of the day.

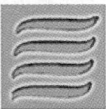

Nursing Diagnoses

The following nursing diagnoses may be appropriate to include in a client care plan when the components are related to clients requiring isolation protocol or sterile procedures.

NURSING DIAGNOSIS	RELATED FACTORS
Ineffective Health Maintenance	Diminished immune system function, steroid and antineoplastic drug therapy, substance abuse
Deficient Knowledge	Lack of access to healthcare facilities, lack of education, cognitive limitation, inadequate explanation or instruction
Noncompliance	Lack of understanding, lack of motivation, education or readiness, information misinterpretation, cultural or religious beliefs

PREPARING FOR CLIENT CARE

Equipment

Community health nursing bag
Liquid soap
Antibacterial gel for handwashing
Disposable gloves
Disposable apron or gown
Goggles
Masks, air-purifying mask
Thermometers (oral and rectal)
Thermometer sheaths
Nex Temp (disposable thermometer)
Vaseline or lubricant
Cotton balls
Alcohol, one small bottle
Antimicrobial wipes
Cotton-tipped applicators
Tongue depressors
Sterile 4 × 4s
Band-Aids
Bandage scissors
Nonallergic tape
Plastic bags with ties
Ketodiastix and chemstrips
Sphygmomanometer
Stethoscope
Paper cups
Bleach, one small bottle

Procedure

1. Arrange equipment in bag prior to making home visit so that handwashing equipment is accessible. Bring only the supplies needed. **Rationale:** This procedure decreases the possibility of cross-contamination.
2. Place bag on flat, dry surface to establish a clean work area during visit.
3. Wash hands.
   a. Use liquid soap and paper towels from bag and client's water supply; or
   b. Use client's soap and towels if you feel comfortable with this and client approves; *or*
   c. Use antimicrobial gel as alternative for handwashing when soap and water are not available. Squeeze small amount of germicide onto palm of hand and rub for 30 seconds along all surfaces of hands, fingers, and nails. Germicide evaporates into air, making towels unnecessary.

> **CLINICAL ALERT**
> If item is soiled and cannot be returned to the bag, place in separate container for transport to agency. Clean item when it is returned to agency.

4. Don disposable gloves when appropriate for infection control, especially when handling blood and body fluids.
5. Take other equipment that will be needed during the visit out of the bag and place on clean work surface.
6. Keep bag closed when not in use to promote cleanliness, safety, and security. Care should be taken not to reenter bag wearing soiled gloves. Washing hands between reentering bag is not necessary unless soiled.
7. Wear disposable apron or gown, goggles, or masks if necessary. **Rationale:** This protects the caregiver from blood or body fluid exposure.
8. Cleanse thoroughly any equipment that left clean area and is to be returned to the bag on completing care.
   a. Rinse equipment (such as bandage scissors, forceps) under *cold* water, wash with soap and water, place in plastic bag, and take back to agency to sterilize.
   b. Return stethoscope and blood pressure cuff to nursing bag. **Rationale:** Clean items can be returned to nursing bag if no visible soiling.
9. Ensure nursing bag is monitored regularly for safety.
   a. Keep bag out of reach of children.
   b. Keep bag in trunk of car or keep in your home overnight. **Rationale:** Unattended bags in cars are more often stolen.
   c. Clean bag monthly and PRN.

DISPOSING OF WASTE MATERIAL IN THE HOME SETTING

Equipment

Plastic bags, heavy duty
Disposable gloves
Receptacle, rigid and puncture-proof
Bleach
Germicide

Procedure

1. Dispose of wastes contaminated with blood or body fluids.
   a. Place waste products in impenetrable, heavy-duty plastic bag.
   b. Remove plastic gloves by rolling inside out (so contaminated side is on inside) and drop into plastic bag.

> **CLINICAL ALERT**
>
> All items contaminated with blood, exudates, or other body fluids should be considered to present a risk of transmission of HIV or hepatitis B. These items should be disposed of by incineration if possible. Use mechanisms for disposal of waste into normal trash only when incineration is not available.

   c. Seal plastic bag with tie.
   d. Discard in client's trash.
   e. Wash hands with soap and water or germicide.
2. Dispose of body wastes, such as urine, feces, respiratory secretions, vomitus, and blood, by flushing them down the toilet. (This is true whether the toilet empties into a septic tank or a sewage system.)
3. Dispose of needles and sharp objects.
   a. Do *not* remove needle from syringe or bend, break, clip, or recap after use.
   b. Drop entire disposable safety syringe intact into rigid, puncture-proof receptacle provided by agency.
   c. Wash hands.
4. Discard other trash.
   a. Place in plastic bag.
   b. Discard in client's trash.

> **CLINICAL ALERT**
>
> Do not use glass bottles or plastic bottles that can be returned to store.
>
> Bleach bottle with screw lid can be left in home for use as a sharp container. Tape closed before disposing of bottle. Small biohazard containers can be obtained from drug stores.

CLEANSING THERMOMETER

Equipment

Two 70% isopropyl alcohol wipes
Green soap or bar soap
Thermometer, preferrably disposable or client owned

Procedure

1. Prepare clean work area.
2. Tear one alcohol wipe in half, and apply soap to each half.
3. Cleanse thermometer with alcohol swab from distal end toward mercury tip using circular movements.
4. Repeat above using second swab.
5. Open remaining alcohol wipe, and wrap it around thermometer, letting it "soak" at least 10 minutes.
6. Discard swabs, and replace thermometer in case.
7. Wipe case with alcohol before replacing.

Note: Using disposable thermometers is preferred. They are one-time use and disposable in the trash. Mercury thermometers may be dangerous if broken.

CARING FOR AN AIDS OR HIV CLIENT IN THE HOME

Equipment

Gloves
Disposable mask, gown, or apron
Protective eyewear
Specimen container if needed
Plastic bag for transport of specimen
Chlorine bleach solution (Clorox)

Procedure

1. Wash hands before and after client care and after disposing of soiled materials.
2. Don disposable gloves for any procedure.
   a. Don double gloves if tearing is likely during the procedure.
   b. If staff member has any type of open wounds or weeping dermatitis, she or he should not administer care (even with gloves) until condition is resolved.
3. Don disposable gown or apron to protect clothing from soilage.
4. Put on mask and protective eyewear if splattering is anticipated during the procedure (e.g., suctioning, wound irrigations).

5. Collect specimens in appropriate containers labeled "Blood and Body Fluid Precautions."
6. Use extraordinary care to avoid puncture wounds with needles and other sharp objects.
   a. If puncture occurs, bleed wound and wash with soap and water.
   b. Notify supervisor immediately, and fill out unusual occurrence report.
7. Clean spills of blood and body fluids with 10% bleach solution (one part liquid chlorine bleach to nine parts water). Make solution fresh each time.
8. Wash eating utensils (dishes and silverware) in hot soapy water. Water should be hot enough to need gloves to tolerate the temperature. No other special precautions are required. It is best to use a dishwasher, if available. It is not necessary to wash client's dishes separately.
9. Store linens and laundry soiled with body fluids in a plastic bag and then wash separately with very hot water. Use a detergent and a 10% bleach solution. (Nonchlorine bleaches such as Clorox II are acceptable for colored clothing.)
10. Dispose of gown or apron in plastic bag after completing care.
11. Take off gloves by peeling them down and turning them inside out so that contaminated side is on the inside. Place in plastic bag.
12. Wash hands.
13. Take off mask and goggles.
14. Wash hands.

CLEANSING EQUIPMENT IN THE HOME SETTING

Equipment

Article to be cleansed	Paper towels
Soap	Plastic bags
Running water	Disposable gloves

Procedure

1. Don gloves when working with equipment contaminated with any body fluid or blood.
2. Rinse article with cold running water. **Rationale:** Cold water releases organic material from the equipment and warm water may make it adhere to the surface.
3. Wash with hot, soapy water using friction.
4. Rinse well with clear water.
5. Dry thoroughly.
6. Disinfect equipment or article as indicated: one part chlorine bleach (Clorox) to nine parts water.
7. Dry thoroughly.
8. Remove disposable gloves.
9. Dispose of gloves (inside out) into plastic bag.
10. Wash hands.

CLINICAL ALERT

If durable medical equipment cannot be sterilized by ethyl oxide or autoclaved, it should be cleaned with 10% chlorine bleach solution after washing with hot soapy water.

Urinary drainage bags can be disinfected in the home. Use soap and water and clean and dry well. Antiseptic solution can be placed in the bag for a few minutes, then rinsed well and dried before attaching to urinary catheter.

TEACHING PREVENTIVE MEASURES IN THE HOME

Procedure

1. Discuss the inadvisability of allowing any person who is ill or who has depressed immune function to come in contact with the client.
2. Teach the client these appropriate hygiene principles:
   a. Wash hands after use of toilet or contact with any body fluids.
   b. Do not share thermometers, razors, razor blades, toothbrushes, douche, or enema equipment.
   c. Do not cough without covering mouth.
   d. Be careful to dispose of nasal secretions in tissue, then in plastic bags.
3. Teach these guidelines for sharing kitchens and bathrooms:
   a. Good household cleaning practices prevent spread of infection.
   b. Don't share eating and drinking utensils. After use, they must be cleaned with hot water (hot enough to necessitate use of gloves) and soap. Use of a dishwasher and soap is appropriate.

c. Kitchen and bathroom surfaces should be cleaned every day with scouring powder or with chlorine bleach solution (10%, one part bleach to nine parts water). Use disposable bathroom cups. Use covered individual toothbrush holders.
d. Clean refrigerators regularly with soap and water; remove old food to prevent mold.
e. Mop floors in bathroom and kitchen weekly. Pour dirty water down the toilet and disinfect with bleach solution.
f. Clean toilet, tub and shower weekly or as often as necessary with 10% bleach solution. If urine or diarrhea spills on toilet or floor, wipe immediately with the 10% bleach solution.
g. Sponges used to clean floors or body fluid spills should be soaked for 5 minutes in a 10% bleach solution.

4. Teach the following principles of food preparation:
   a. Discuss the fact that people infected with HIV may prepare food for others. They should follow usual practices for safe food preparation and be especially diligent about handwashing.
   b. Wash hands thoroughly before any food preparation.
   c. Do not lick fingers or taste from the mixing spoon while cooking.
   d. Avoid unpasteurized milk (danger of contact with *Salmonella*); do not eat old or moldy food (danger of food poisoning); and carefully wash and thoroughly cook chicken.
5. Teach how to care for linens and laundry.
   a. When clothing or linen is soiled with blood or body fluids, it should be stored separately in a plastic bag. Wash separately with very hot water, detergent, and bleach. Use Clorox II for colored clothing.
   b. Wear disposable gloves when touching soiled clothes or linen.
   c. Do not share used towels or washcloths, and wash separately. (Towels and washcloths are, however, safe to use after washing.)
   d. Change towels and washcloths daily.
6. Inform client and family of measures for disposing of trash.
   a. Flush body wastes down the toilet.
   b. Discard dressings, diapers, Chux, or any materials soiled with secretions in a plastic bag. Discard into the regular trash.
   c. Sharp items (e.g., razors, needles) should be placed in a rigid, puncture-proof container with a solution of 10% bleach. Incinerate when container is full. Pharmacy's collect the used containers in some areas.
7. Discuss procedures for caring for pets.
   a. Clean bird cages wearing gloves. Birds can spread psittacosis *(Chlamydia psittaci)* or *Cryptococcus.*
   b. Clean cat litter boxes wearing gloves to prevent spread of toxoplasmosis.
   c. Tropical fish tanks should not be cleaned by the person with AIDS to prevent spread of *Mycobacterium.*
8. Teach general principles of preventing cross-infection.
   a. Wear gloves when handling body fluids, linens, or other objects contaminated with body fluids.
   b. Disposable gowns or aprons protect clothing from becoming soiled.
   c. Caregivers should not provide care when ill themselves. If this is not possible they should wear a mask when in close contact with the person with AIDS. AIDS clients are very susceptible to infections.
   d. Maintain adequate ventilation in the living quarters.
9. Medical supplies should be kept in a clean, dry location. If refrigeration is required, place medications in sealed plastic storage bag.

TEACHING SAFER PRACTICES TO IV DRUG USERS

Procedure

1. Inform persons of risk behaviors and factors associated with IV drug use.
   a. Direct transmission occurs with shared needles and syringes; permits blood-to-blood contact, the most direct method of transmitting the AIDS virus.
   b. Transmission to sexual partners; permits contact of body fluids.
   c. Transmission to fetus during pregnancy.
   d. Suppression of the immune system caused by alcohol or drug use.
   e. Impaired judgment while under the influence of drugs.
2. Teach IV drug users how to reduce the risk.
   a. Do not share needles or syringes with others.
   b. Clean needles and other equipment vigorously. Wash twice with full-strength bleach or alcohol; rinse twice with water.
   c. Boil needles and other equipment for 15 minutes.
   d. Do not borrow or use needles or equipment from others, even if they appear healthy or say that they do not have AIDS.
3. Teach basic health maintenance measures.
   a. Decrease use of all immunosuppressive drugs (marijuana, speed, cocaine, alcohol).
   b. Maintain an adequate, nutritionally sound diet.
   c. Reduce stress on self through stress-reduction practices, or removing self from a stressful situation (living with others who routinely use drugs).
   d. Obtain regular medical and dental care.
   e. Follow lifestyle that provides adequate rest and exercise.
   f. Obtain counseling to assist in living life without dependence on drugs.

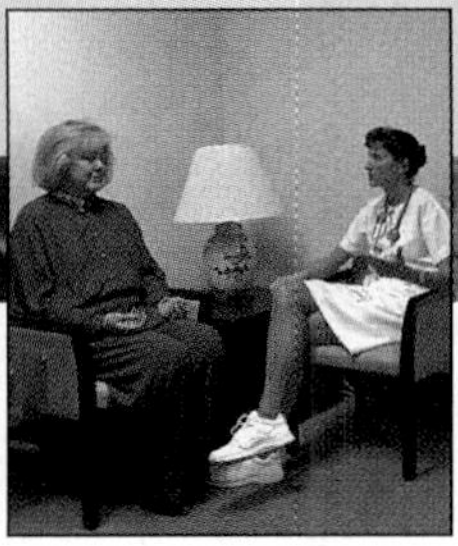

Body Mechanics

Nursing Process Data

ASSESSMENT Data Base

Assess family's knowledge of the principles of body mechanics.

Assess home care provider's knowledge of how to use correct muscle groups for specific activities.

Assess knowledge of how to improvise for a nonhospital bed.

Assess knowledge and correct any misinformation about body alignment and ability to move client up in bed without assistance.

PLANNING Objectives

To promote proper body mechanics while caring for clients

To move clients without assistance, preventing back injury

To provide knowledge of the musculoskeletal system, body alignment, and balance in order to prevent back injury when providing care for a client in the home

To provide methods of improvising for nonhospital bed

IMPLEMENTATION Procedures

Positioning Nonhospital Bed for Client Care

Moving a Helpless Client Up in Bed without Assistance

EVALUATION Expected Outcomes

Correct body mechanics are used in caring for clients.

Injuries are prevented to both nurse and client.

Client care is facilitated by proper body mechanics.

Client is able to move without assistance.

Center of gravity is maintained when lifting objects.

Nonhospital bed is easily adapted for home care.

Knowledge of body mechanics and how to use these principles when giving care is important to both the healthcare provider and the client. Correct use of body mechanics decreases the caregiver's potential for injury and provides safety for the client. Recently, there has been an increase in the number of back injury accident claims among home healthcare providers. One reason for the increase is the improper use of body mechanics while performing skills in the home setting. Also, there may be no one to assist the care provider when lifting and turning clients in the home. The nurse may need to improvise, as the equipment may not be adequate or adjustable. The purpose of this unit is to consider adaptations necessary for providing safe care to the client while using proper body mechanics. In the home setting, much of the care is given by the family; therefore, it is essential that they are also taught good body mechanics.

NURSING DIAGNOSES

The following nursing diagnoses may be appropriate to include on client care plans when the components are related to body mechanics.

NURSING DIAGNOSIS	RELATED FACTORS
Activity Intolerance	Impaired motor function, pain
Risk for Disuse Syndrome	Debilitated state, immobility, muscle weakness, decreased motor agility, joint contractures
Risk for Injury	Altered mobility, impaired sensory function, prolonged bed rest
Impaired Physical Mobility	Trauma or musculoskeletal impairment, surgical procedure, muscle weakness, pain, decreased strength
Caregiver Role Strain	Insufficient resources, time, money, energy; family conflict regarding caregiver issue

POSITIONING NONHOSPITAL BED FOR CLIENT CARE

Procedure

1. Position foam wedges to simulate change in position when head of bed does not move. (High-Fowler's/90°; Fowler's/60°; semi-Fowler's/30°.)
2. Use correct body mechanics to adjust height.
   a. Flex body at knees and keep back straight if bed is only slightly low.
   b. Kneel on pillow by bed or sit in chair alongside bed if bed is extremely low.
3. Lock each wheel or leg of bed in position by securing with bricks or blocks of wood.
4. Make footboard of lumber or item such as a TV tray; position legs of tray under mattress so that tray becomes footboard.

Correct Body Mechanics

- Place both feet flat on the floor, and keep your back straight to prevent back injury.
- Hold objects close to the body to prevent muscle strain and possible back injury.
- Keep body in proper alignment by bending your knees and keeping back straight when lifting objects to prevent injury to back muscles.

MOVING A HELPLESS CLIENT UP IN BED WITHOUT ASSISTANCE

Procedure

1. Lower head of bed, and place pillow at head of bed.
2. Stand at side of client's bed.
   a. Face far corner at foot of bed.
   b. Place one foot behind the other, assume a broad stance, and flex knees.
3. Flex arms so forearms are level with bed. Place one arm under client's head and one under small of back.
4. Rock and shift weight from forward to rear foot; hips will move downward.
5. Guide the client as he or she slides diagonally across bed toward head.
6. Repeat for trunk and leg sections.
7. Move to other side of bed and repeat steps 2 through 5.
8. Repeat until client is satisfactorily positioned in bed.

UNIT 4

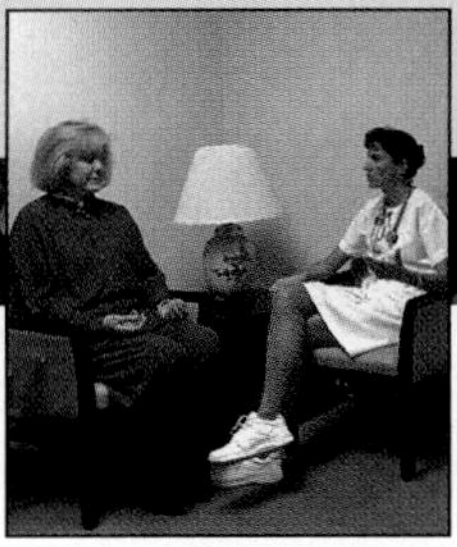

Hygienic Care

Nursing Process Data

ASSESSMENT Data Base

Assess for signs of skin breakdown or stage of pressure ulcer.

Assess color of skin.

Check for alterations in skin turgor.

Assess ability to assist with transfer to tub or shower.

Check general hygienic state.

Assess for presence of lice.

PLANNING Objectives

To maintain intact skin without signs of ischemia, hyperemia, or necrosis

To recognize a break in skin integrity and implement a plan of action

To avoid introduction of pathogens through a break in skin integrity

To prepare sterilized normal saline solution for home care

To promote wound closure for pressure ulcer

To shampoo hair for client on bed rest

To transfer client safely to tub or shower

To eradicate lice from client and belongings

IMPLEMENTATION Procedures

Bathing Client in the Home

Transferring Client to Tub or Shower

Adapting Bedmaking to the Home

Providing Pressure Ulcer Care

Preparing Normal Saline

Removing Lice

(For additional skills see Chapters 8 and 9)

EVALUATION Expected Outcomes

Client's skin remains intact without signs of ischemia, hyperemia, or necrosis.

Client is free of lice infestation.

Pressure ulcer heals.

Bathing and bedmaking are accomplished for client on bedrest.

Client is transferred safely to tub or shower.

In the home care setting most hygienic care is provided by the home health aide (HHA) or the client and family members. The role of the nurse is to (1) assess the personal care needs of an individual client, (2) develop the care plan that is to be implemented by the home health aide, (3) supervise the home health aide, and (4) instruct the family members in how to provide safe, thorough, hygienic care when health care providers are not in the home.

The client care plan is developed by the nurse and implemented by the home health aide or caregiver. Skills include bathing, hair care, oral hygiene, shaving, TPR, toileting, dressing, ambulation, transfers, exercise, range of motion, assistance with assistive devices, feeding, and instructions for any specific observations to be made. The home health aide's responsibilities may include homemaking and supportive assistance activities, such as meal planning, marketing, linen change, light laundry, and light housekeeping. It is important to instruct the client and family that these activities are to be directed toward the client and not the entire household. A copy of the care plan is kept in the client's home for use by the home health aide. A second copy is placed in the permanent client record. The home health aide is responsible for documenting the care provided on each visit to the home. A sample is included in this unit. It is the nurse's responsibility to make sure the documentation is complete and accurate for legal and reimbursement purposes.

BATHING

The type and frequency of bathing depends on the client's condition, personal desires, and family and environmental situation. The client may be bathed in the bed, tub, or shower. The bathing may be done on a daily basis or once, twice, or three times a week. The home health aide may visit two to three times per week for personal care, and the family may perform the care between visits. The nurse's role is to instruct all persons involved in the client's care to perform procedures correctly and safely.

SKIN CARE

Just as in the hospital, skin care is an important component of personal care. The home health nurse must assess the condition of the client's skin and teach skin care techniques to all caregivers. The instructions should include keeping the skin clean and dry, providing special care to buttocks and perineal area, and obtaining available products, such as Chux for incontinent clients, to protect the skin. A skin care program should be initiated by the nurse. All caregivers should follow the plan of action. The program addresses ways to prevent friction, shearing, and pressure.

PRESSURE ULCER CARE

If skin breakdown is present, special treatment is necessary. The stage of pressure ulcer dictates the specific protocol needed. Pressure ulcer treatments for the homebound client are the same as for the hospitalized client. Refer to Chapter 25 for specific protocols.

HAIR CARE

Shampooing the hair of a client on bed rest is similar to the skill in a hospital setting. Rather than using a basin to catch the water, a bucket or pail may be substituted. For long-term bedridden clients, commercial shampoo boards are available.

"Dry shampoo" is available at local pharmacies. This is often used for a client on bedrest for a short time or between regular shampoos. Regular shampooing is necessary to maintain scalp integrity.

Pediculosis is an infestation of lice on the body. It is very contagious by either direct contact with the infected person or by indirect contact with contaminated articles, such as combs, clothing, and bed linen. Although lice can infest the head, body, or pubic area, the head is the most common area of infestation.

NURSING DIAGNOSES

The following nursing diagnoses may be appropriate to include in a client care plan when the components are related to hygienic care.

NURSING DIAGNOSIS	RELATED FACTORS
Activity Intolerance	Prolonged bed rest, surgery, pain, treatment schedule, weakness, fatigue
Ineffective Health Maintenance	Ineffective coping, lack of motivation, motor impairment, lack of financial resources
Self-Care Deficit: Bathing/Hygiene	Dependence on others for assistance, motor impairment, visual disorders, surgery, muscle weakness, pain
Impaired Skin Integrity	Surgery, immobility, prolonged bed rest, mechanical factors (shearing force, pressure), lack of adherence to diet, inadequately prepared caregiver

BATHING CLIENT IN THE HOME

Equipment

Personal care items (i.e., soap, deodorant, toothbrush)
Tray for personal items
Beach towel
Large piece of plastic
Call bell, dinner bell, or smoke alarm
Nonskid strips for tub
Shower chair or suction tips for chair legs

Procedure

1. Keep all personal care items (soap, deodorant, lotion, powder, cosmetics, cologne, hair products, oral hygiene supplies, and other personal items) on a tray or in a handy carry tote (e.g., the type of rubber or plastic tote that can be purchased to carry household cleaning supplies).
2. Use beach towel for bath blanket.
3. Place plastic under towel to protect mattress prior to beginning the bath.
4. Ensure that nonskid strips or mats are on the floor of tub or shower.
   a. Ask family to purchase strips.
   b. Place wet terrycloth towel on floor of tub or shower if strips or mat not available. **Rationale:** A wet towel provides a temporary nonskid surface during bath or shower.
5. Provide tub or shower stool or chair.
   a. Order from supply company, if family desires and can afford.
   b. Improvise shower chair by using straight-backed chair and attaching suction cups to legs to prevent sliding. (Suction cups are available at hardware stores.)
6. Simulate a client call bell by placing dinner bell or battery-powered smoke detector that emits a loud alarm within easy reach of client.

TRANSFERRING CLIENT TO TUB OR SHOWER

Equipment

Towels
Shower or tub chair
Grips in bathtub or bath mat
Safety bars on tub or wall
Assistive devices (e.g., walker, wheelchair, cane) to assist to shower or tub if needed

Procedure

1. Gather equipment.
2. Place wet bath towel on the floor of tub or shower if safety grips or mats are not available.

3. Position chair or shower stool securely in the tub or shower. Place second chair or wheelchair outside tub.
4. Assist client to bathroom.
5. Transfer client to tub or shower chair before putting water in tub.
   a. Stand in front of client.
   b. Lower client into chair, bending your knees and keeping your back straight. **Rationale:** This provides most secure balance and aids in preventing back injuries.
   c. Flex your knees, move to kneeling position, and keep your back straight while assisting client to swing legs over side of tub.

ADAPTING BEDMAKING TO THE HOME

Equipment

Sheets
Pillowcases
Plastic trash bag
Cotton flannel
Plastic shower curtain

Procedure

1. Follow directions for making an occupied or unoccupied bed outlined in Chapter 8.
2. Turn pillowcase inside out and use as laundry bag, or use plastic trash bag.
3. Place one knee on bed if bed cannot be moved away from wall. This is especially useful when making water beds.
4. Make incontinent pads with cotton flannel if commercial pads are not available. **Rationale:** This material is soft and easily laundered.
5. Make bed protectors by cutting a piece of plastic shower curtain or heavy trash bag. Cover with draw sheet or cotton flannel. **Rationale:** This protects skin from direct contact with plastic.

PROVIDING PRESSURE ULCER CARE

Equipment

Normal saline solution
Medicated ointment (if prescribed)
Irrigation set (if needed)
Asepto syringe
Dressings—hydrocolloid or transparent adhesive film
Nonallergic tape
Clean gloves
Plastic bags

Procedure

1. Wash hands.
2. Don clean gloves.
3. Remove dressings. Discard in plastic bag.
4. Cleanse with normal saline solution. Irrigate the wound if excessive drainage is present.
5. Allow to dry or apply medicated ointment, as ordered.
6. Apply dressing as ordered.
7. Dispose of waste according to protocol.
8. Remove gloves and wash hands.

Note: Follow specific directions for pressure ulcer care in Chapter 25.

PREPARING NORMAL SALINE

Equipment

Large pan
Jar with lid
Cold water to cover jar and lid
1 teaspoon salt
500 mL (1 pint) water

Procedure

1. Sterilize jar for storage.
   a. Place cover and jar in large pan of cold water, completely immersing jar and lid in water.
   b. Bring to a boil.
   c. Boil 20 minutes.
   d. Pour off water.
   e. Handle only outside of jar and lid.
2. Add 1 teaspoon salt to 500 mL (1 pint) water.
3. Boil salted water for 20 minutes in covered pan to sterilize.
4. Allow solution to cool in covered pan.
5. Pour water into sterilized jar for storage.

REMOVING LICE

Equipment

Isolation bag or plastic bag
Treatment solution as ordered (i.e., gamma benzene hexachloride [Kwell or Scabene])
Clean linen
Fine-tooth comb
Disinfectant for comb
Clean towel
Spray for fomites

Procedure

1. Obtain order for treatment and notify family members and health care givers. **Rationale:** All household members and caregivers must be treated to prevent the spread of lice to others.
2. Remove and bag client's clothing and linens, and place in plastic bag. Launder these articles separately. Use hot water at 125°F and detergent. **Rationale:** This prevents cross-contamination of lice to other family members.
3. Items that cannot be washed should be dry cleaned. Place in plastic bag, seal, and take to dry cleaner.
4. Begin treatment as ordered by physician. Common treatment is gamma benzene hexachloride applied as a cream, lotion, or shampoo. **Rationale:** Head lice infestation requires shampoo. Body and pubic lice require shower with soap followed by lotion application.
5. Shake lotion well, apply thin film of lotion over entire body, excluding face and urethral meatus. Rub in, allow skin to dry and cool. Leave in place 8–12 hours.
6. Apply shampoo, and leave in place four minutes. **Rationale:** Prolonged use of shampoo can burn scalp.
7. Rinse thoroughly.
8. Comb through hair with fine-tooth comb.
9. Disinfect comb and brushes with Kwell shampoo.
10. Wash your hands.
11. Instruct client to vacuum rugs, upholstery, and furniture. Then, spray with a commercial spray. Empty vacuum cleaner bag into trash bag, and seal.
12. Discuss with client and family the cause, treatment, and preventive measures regarding lice infestation.
13. Instruct client or family to repeat treatment only if living lice are present.

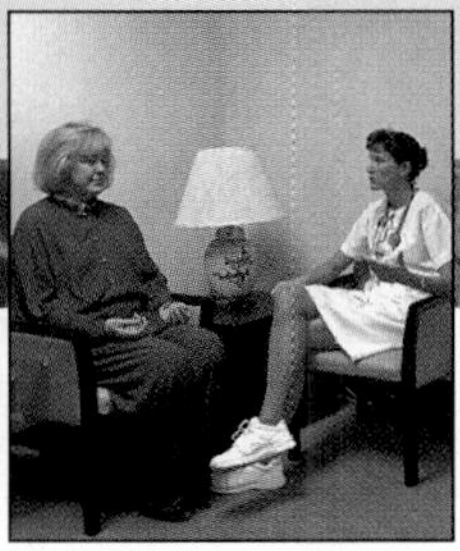

Medications

Nursing Process Data

ASSESSMENT Data Base

Assess that client and family understand time and dosage for medication administration.

Assess most appropriate methods for aiding a client to remember to take medications.

Assess client and family's knowledge and skill in sterilizing medication equipment.

Determine client's physical ability to take medication as ordered.

- Swallow reflex present
- Mental alertness
- Signs of nausea and vomiting
- Uncooperative behavior

PLANNING Objectives

To ensure that medications are taken according to physician's orders

To provide an easy method to sterilize nondisposable medication equipment

To provide client and family education about medications

To determine appropriate aids to assist the client to take medications as ordered

IMPLEMENTATION Procedures

Administering Medications

Sterilizing Nondisposable Medication Equipment

(For additional skills refer to Chapter 18)

EVALUATION Expected Outcomes

Equipment is sterilized and infection prevented.

Medications are taken at appropriate times.

Creative device for remembering to take medications is identified.

In the hospital, medications are given at designated times. The time that the client takes the medication is determined by physician's orders and the hospital, not the client. In the home setting, however, the nurse works with the client and family to establish a medication schedule. This regimen fits their lifestyle, yet comes within the prescribed medication parameters (e.g., number of dosages, blood levels). Since the nurse is not present in the home at all times, the client and family must take responsibility for the routine administration of medications.

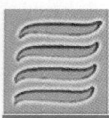

NURSING DIAGNOSES

The following nursing diagnoses may be appropriate to include in a client care plan when the components are related to a client who requires medication.

NURSING DIAGNOSIS	RELATED FACTORS
Ineffective Health Maintenance	Lack of education or readiness to learn, cognitive impairment, lack of equipment, inadequate support systems, inadequate financial resources, religious beliefs, cultural beliefs
Risk for Infection	Contamination of equipment, improper storage, improper technique, traumatized tissue, malnutrition
Deficient Knowledge	Inadequate understanding of condition, misinformation, cognitive impairment
Noncompliance	Impaired ability to perform tasks, side effects of therapy, nontherapeutic environment, denial of condition, lack of information, poor self-esteem, nonsupportive family

ADMINISTERING MEDICATIONS

Procedure

1. Examine all medications taken by the client during your admission visit and subsequent visits. Include all over-the-counter (OTC) as well as prescription drugs. Document on assessment sheet.
2. Discuss lifestyle with client and family as it relates to medication schedule and their beliefs about medications.
3. Establish the medication regimen based on physician's orders or prescribed drugs and client's schedule.
4. Teach client and family the medication regimen.
5. Teach client and family how to monitor for effects and side effects of drugs.
6. Design medication aids, such as a calendar of drugs or daily/weekly pill reminder boxes, to help client and family remember to take medications.
   a. Investigate and share with the client and family those aids that are commercially available.
   b. Improvise using household items, such as egg cartons, tiny paper cups attached together or stacked, or empty match boxes glued together to make a row of pill containers that can be labeled with time and day.

CLINICAL ALERT

Home health aides and homemakers are not allowed to administer medications to clients in the home setting. Families should be instructed not to ask home health aides or homemakers to give medication.

7. Design creative methods to assist client and family to administer medication.
   a. If client has trouble seeing the markings on a syringe or on medication bottles, the nurse may recommend a magnifying glass, magnifying syringe, or marking the bottles or syringes with tape at the appropriate dosage.
   b. If a client lives alone, needs daily insulin, and knows the procedures but cannot see well enough to fill the syringes accurately, the nurse may prefill the syringes and leave them in the refrigerator for use between visits. Check if mixed insulin can be prefilled and is allowed to be refrigerated before using. **Rationale:** NPH or lente insulin mixed with Regular must be administered immediately, otherwise it loses its potency.
   c. Take syringe out of refrigerator 1 hour before administration.

d. If other medications are prefilled in a syringe, determine if any qualifiers exist, such as how long before medication must be administered.

8. Discard uncapped needles and syringes in sharps container.
9. Document all teaching and learning outcomes, administration of medication, and client response to medications.

CLINICAL ALERT

New insulin pens have a magnified dose window for easier viewing of dosage. These dose pens are safer to use for clients with impaired vision.

STERILIZING NONDISPOSABLE MEDICATION EQUIPMENT

Equipment

Large pan or kettle
Jar or container with lid for storage
Equipment to be sterilized
Tongs or forceps for handling sterile equipment

Procedure

1. Place jar, lid, tongs, and equipment in large clean pan.
2. Fill pan with cold water until all equipment is covered.
3. Place pan on stove.
4. Boil water for 20 minutes.
5. Pour off water.
6. Lift equipment out of pan, using tongs. Remove jar from pan by touching only the outside.
7. Position jar so sterile equipment can easily be inserted without touching edges of the jar.
8. Place lid on jar by grasping outside edge and twisting tightly.

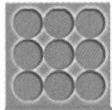

CULTURAL COMPETENCE

Home health care nurses are being asked to decrease the amount of time spent with home care clients. They are also being asked to provide high-quality and culturally competent care and be cost effective. In some areas of the United States, folk remedies are common to the clients but unknown to the nurses. Some clients do not trust nurses who are not of their culture and who do not seem to understand their need for folk remedies. To provide the necessary care and be cost effective, it is imperative that the nurse assess each client's cultural norms and mores, determine their experience with Western medicine and ask about the folk remedies they are currently using. It is very important to identify any herbs or other remedies the client is taking, as it could affect medications being prescribed by the physician. Completing a cultural assessment will provide necessary information for the nurse to develop an effective treatment plan for the client to follow.

UNIT 6

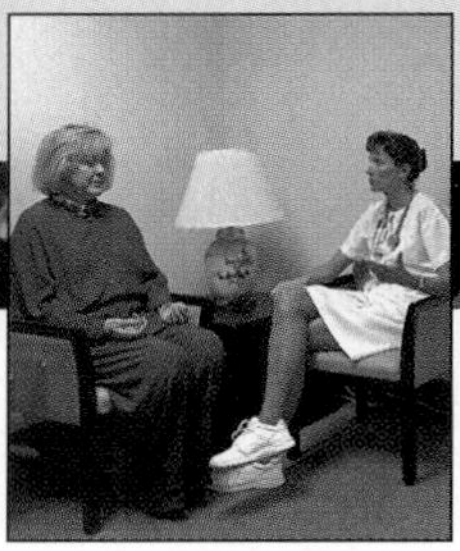

Total Nutrient Admixture

Nursing Process Data

ASSESSMENT ***Data Base***

Observe for correct additives in each hyperalimentation bag.

Check label on solution bag.

Check rate of infusion on volumetric pump.

Assess ability of client to understand instructions during procedure.

Ensure patency of central venous line.

Observe catheter insertion site for signs of infection, thrombophlebitis, or possible infiltration.

Inspect dressing over central line to ensure a dry, noncontaminated dressing.

Identify client and family's ability to provide TNA in the home.

PLANNING ***Objectives***

To provide adequate calories and nutrition for clients unable to tolerate oral feedings

To provide increased calories when oral route is not accessible

To provide a contamination-free mode of delivering the hyperalimentation solution

To heparinize TNA catheter between infusions

To discontinue TNA infusions maintaining sterile technique

IMPLEMENTATION ***Procedures***

Administering Total Nutritional Admixture (TNA) in the Home

Monitoring Client on TNA

Discontinuing TNA Infusion

(For additional skills refer to Chapter 29)

EVALUATION ***Expected Outcomes***

Solution is infused at prescribed flow rate and tolerated by client.

Dressing remains dry and intact during interval between changes.

Insertion site remains free of infection and inflammation.

Client receives nutrients necessary for tissue repair and sustenance.

Client and family understand procedure and infuse TNA correctly.

Heparinization of TNA catheter accomplished.

Nutritional support in the home is not significantly different from that in a hospital setting. Gastrostomy and nasogastric tube feedings are frequently performed in the home setting using small feeding tubes and maintained via continuous feeding pumps. The only difference in the procedure at home is that the family is taught how to provide the feeding. The nurse's role is to change the nasogastric tube and to teach and monitor the family's ability to administer the feeding. Intake and output records are maintained by the family and monitored by the nurse when the client's condition warrants it.

Nutritional teaching principles and information that should be provided to client and family include

- Instruction in positioning client and providing assistance for eating
- Special eating utensils that can be purchased or made for self-feeding
- Instruction in Heimlich maneuver in case of choking
- Method of gently stroking throat if client doesn't remember to swallow
- Resources available in the community to assist with nutritional support:
  Meals on wheels: Meals can be ordered for cardiac and diabetic clients as well
  Food stamps
  Senior nutrition sites that usually serve a hot meal at noon
- Dietary supplements readily available
  Instant breakfast (*not* the diet type) when added to milk provides a less expensive nutritional supplement than some commercially canned ones
  Nutritional supplements frozen into cubes for clients to suck on if they don't like to drink
- Gatorade, a 5% glucose solution, may be used as a supplement if body fluids need replacing

TOTAL NUTRIENT ADMIXTURE (TNA)

Total parenteral nutrition is now being used in the home. The procedure and equipment are similar to that used in the hospital, including the use of sterile technique when preparing and discontinuing the infusion.

Home health agencies have specified policies and procedures for TNA that the nurse must follow to practice within legal parameters. The first infusion of any TNA solution or any IV medication must be given in the hospital or emergency room (where emergency intervention is available if an adverse reaction occurs).

In the home care setting, the client or family is taught how to administer TNA after the first infusion. TNA is also termed 3-in-1 mixture. It is a combination of amino acids, dextrose, and lipids in one container. Many clients prefer to infuse TNA at night while they sleep, since the procedure takes about 12 hours. The client or family must be taught proper storage, fluid administration, electronic ambulatory infusion pump use, and site care. Most people use pre-prepared TNA solutions that are available at the hospital pharmacy. Clients and families must be given careful instruction on sterile technique used in preparing TNA solutions. Catheter site care is performed the same as in the hospital.

Effective management of clients requiring TNA at home includes:

- A nurse who is an expert in all aspects of TNA administration.
- Knowledge of client monitoring, both fluid infusion and potential complications associated with TNA administration.
- Teaching skills are a must as this procedure is very complicated; family and client (or caregiver) must be versed in all aspects of TNA care to prevent complications and infuse TNA appropriately.

Monitoring for complications includes assessment of clinical and therapeutic response to TNA regimen. Assessment involves monitoring nutritional status and monitoring for potential complications. Weight gain or maintenance, increased strength and the absence of complications indicate that TNA has a positive effect on client's condition.

NURSING DIAGNOSES

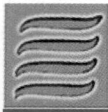

The following nursing diagnoses may be appropriate to include in a client care plan when the components of the plan are related to nutritional problems or nutritional health maintenance.

NURSING DIAGNOSIS	RELATED FACTORS
Impaired Home Maintenance Management	Chronic debilitating disease (cancer, neuromuscular diseases), surgery, injury
Deficient Knowledge	Lack of client and family education, poor understanding of equipment or procedure
Noncompliance	Improper nutritional intake or balance of nutrients, inadequate knowledge base, denial of disease process, chronic illness
Altered Nutrition: Less than Body Requirements	Impaired swallowing, faulty metabolism, dysphagia, altered level of consciousness, inadequate absorption

ADMINISTERING TOTAL NUTRIENT ADMIXTURE (TNA) IN THE HOME

Equipment

TNA solution bag
IV tubing with in-line filter
Volutrol
Controller or pump
Povidone–iodine or antimicrobial swab
Padded Kelly forceps, tape
Sugar and acetone test equipment
Intake and output and TNA record
Clean gloves

> **CLINICAL ALERT**
>
> A 0.2- or 1.2-micron filter is used for PN solutions with amino acids and dextrose. For TNA, a 1.2- or 5-micron filter is used. Filters are changed every 24 hours. If filter becomes occluded, check for precipitation or incompatibility of solutions.

Procedure

1. Remove TNA solution from refrigerator at least 1 hour before using. Parenteral nutrition solutions are stable for 7 days when refrigerated. Without lipids in solution, it is stable for 30–45 days when refrigerated. **Rationale:** Warming the solution prevents venospasm and hypothermia.
2. Gather equipment.
3. Wash hands and don gloves.
4. Inspect TNA solution for cloudiness, clarity, and intact bag. **Rationale:** Contamination of the solution causes a cloudy or milky precipitate.
5. Prepare to administer TNA solution by spiking bag with tubing, adding filter and then flushing tubing of all air.
6. Prepare catheter when solution is ready for infusion by clamping catheter with a padded Kelly forceps and removing injection cap.
7. Cleanse end of catheter with povidone–iodine swab or other antimicrobial swab.

Nutritional Assessment

- Height and weight
- Skin integrity
- Elimination
- Behavioral changes
- Mucous membranes
- Nailbeds
- Oral cavity
- State of edema
- Cardiovascular assessment

8. Remove protective cap from IV tubing and insert tubing into catheter.
9. Tape connection site. **Rationale:** Taping prevents accidental dislodging of the tubing from catheter and lessens chance of contamination.
10. Remove gloves.
11. Thread IV tubing through electronic ambulatory infusion machine according to manufacturer's directions and set machine to deliver appropriate rate.
12. Monitor infusion rate, and assess IV site throughout procedure. Procedure takes about 12 hours; therefore, many clients prefer to infuse the solution during their sleeping hours. **Rationale:** If flow rate is too rapid, excess sugar may cause seizures.
13. Monitor blood glucose daily using Accu-chek or autolet and chemstrips. Report 3+ or 4+ or positive urine acetone findings to physician. **Rationale:** Insulin may need to be ordered.
14. Instruct client to follow physician's directions for lab work. Blood chemistry profiles and liver function tests are done frequently in the beginning of therapy and progress to every 2–4 weeks.
15. Maintain accurate intake and output and TNA sheet.
16. Instruct client to monitor weight and temperature frequently throughout therapy.

NOTE: Pumps can deliver single medication as a continuous infusion or as a dual-therapy pump that delivers single medication as a continuous or intermittent infusion.

MONITORING CLIENT ON TNA

Equipment

Log book
Scale
Blood glucose monitoring equipment
Thermometer

Procedure

1. Instruct client or care giver to document assessment data in log book. Bring book to physician during office visit and share with home health nurse during visits.
2. Instruct client to weigh daily at same time and with same clothing, shoes off.
3. Check glucose when first initiating TNA according to the following guidelines:
   a. Before starting TNA. **Rationale:** To obtain baseline data.
   b. Several hours after starting cyclic TNA. **Rationale:** To assess peak blood glucose.
   c. One hour after discontinuing TNA. **Rationale:** To observe for rebound hypoglycemia.
4. Check glucose every 8–12 hours with continuous TNA.
5. Maintain serum glucose under 200 mg/dL for continuous TNA clients and 240 mg/dL for cyclic TNA clients. Regular insulin on a sliding scale is prescribed for clients on TNA.

> **CLINICAL ALERT**
>
> A sudden increase in blood glucose in a stable client is an indication of impending sepsis.

6. Measure intake and output daily and record in log book.
7. Instruct client or caregiver on signs of fluid volume deficit (poor skin turgor, dry mucous membranes, etc.).
8. Explain signs and symptoms associated with electrolyte imbalance (increased fatigue and muscle weakness).
9. Take temperature daily at same time and record in log book.
10. Monitor any drainage for amount, color, consistency, or any changes from usual.
11. Ensure client has routine blood drawn as scheduled.
12. Instruct client to observe for signs of edema and to report these immediately.
13. Instruct client or caregiver to monitor central venous catheter site for signs of infection. Immediately report to home health nurse and do not infuse TNA until nurse observes site. **Rationale:** Septicemia is a major cause of morbidity in clients on TNA and accounts for 70% of hospital readmissions.

Note: Developing a worksheet and teaching focus sheet will assist client and caregiver in following client education information and documenting pertinent data. A form will also allow the nurse to quickly assess changes in the client between visits.

DISCONTINUING TNA INFUSION

Equipment

Tape
Sterile injection cap
4 × 4 gauze pad
2 mL normal saline
20-gauge needle
25-gauge needle
2-mL syringe

Alcohol swab
Povidone–iodine swab or antimicrobial swab
Padded Kelly clamp
Clean gloves

Procedure

1. Gather equipment.
2. Wash hands, and don clean gloves.
3. Withdraw 2 mL normal saline into syringe.
4. Turn IV solution off by closing roller clamp and turning off controller or pump.
5. Clamp catheter with padded Kelly forceps.
6. Disconnect IV tubing from catheter.
7. Cleanse catheter site with a povidone–iodine swab or antimicrobial swab.
8. Place sterile injection cap on catheter.
9. Wipe injection cap with alcohol swab.
10. Inject 2 mL of normal saline solution through cap.
11. Withdraw needle.
12. Coil catheter and place 4 × 4 gauze pad over catheter and tape catheter to chest or abdomen. Site care is performed every 48 hours using same sterile technique as in hospital. See Chapter 29.
13. Discard used equipment.
14. Remove gloves and wash your hands.

Complications associated with TNA

Nutritional Variations

- Fatty acid deficiency if not receiving lipid emulsions.
- Vitamin deficiency

Metabolic Complications

- Fluid and electrolyte imbalances
- Glucose intolerance, hypo- and hyperglycemia
- Liver complications

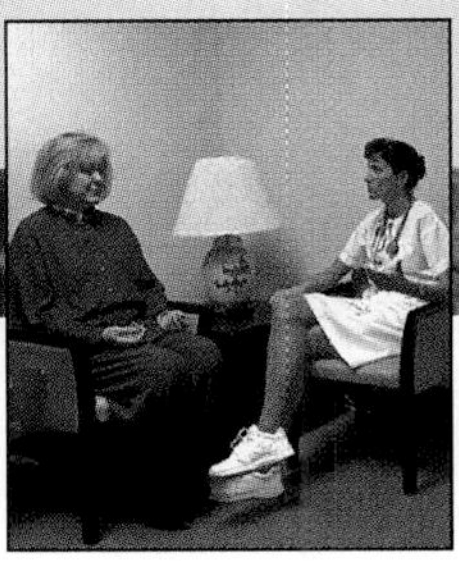

UNIT 7

Elimination

Nursing Process Data

ASSESSMENT *Data Base*

Assess the client's bladder for distention.
Assess the client's physical ability to cooperate with positioning.
Assess urinary meatus and catheter for exudate, edema, inflammation, and general cleanliness.
Assess need for perineal care before catheterization procedure.
Assess condition of skin surrounding catheter or ostomy opening.
Assess dialysate solution for clarity.
Assess dialysis returns for cloudiness.
Assess family's ability to use gloving technique and maintain asepsis.
Assess need for suprapubic catheter care.
Assess need for catheterization procedure.
Assess for proper function of dialysis machine.
Assess client's ability to perform colostomy irrigation.

PLANNING *Objectives*

To prevent or relieve discomfort due to bladder distention
To promote urinary elimination
To identify family's knowledge related to signs and symptoms of dialysis-related infections.
To prevent urinary tract infections through aseptic catheter care
To prevent infection at peritoneal catheter site
To use aseptic technique when instituting CAPD
To identify client's and family's knowledge base regarding CAPD or CCPD
To assist client to feel more confident that bowel will not evacuate at times other than during irrigation.

IMPLEMENTATION *Procedures*

Using Clean Technique for Intermittent Self-Catheterization
- *for Female Client*
- *for Male Client*

Providing Suprapubic Catheter Care
Administering Continuous Ambulatory Peritoneal Dialysis (CAPD)
- *for Draining Fluid*
- *for Infusing Dialysate*

Changing Dressing for CAPD Client
Instructing Client in Colostomy Irrigation
(For additional skills refer to Chapters 22 and 23)

EVALUATION *Expected Outcomes*

Catheterization performed using aseptic technique.

Bladder emptied when client is unable to void.

Urinary tract infection prevented through aseptic catheter care.

Aseptic peritoneal dialysis procedure used.

Catheter site remains free of infection.

Colostomy irrigation will be effective.

Suprapubic catheter care is completed and client is free of urinary tract infections.

URINARY ELIMINATION

Home care clients who require assistance with emptying their bladders are usually placed on intermittent clean catheterization protocols rather than having an indwelling catheter. This procedure assists in preventing penoscrotal abscess formation, overwhelming infection, and altered body image. Fluid intake needs to be monitored and restricted to 1,500 mL per day to avoid bladder distention. If spontaneous voiding returns, frequency of catheterizations can be extended to every 12 hours and discontinued when the residual urine is consistently less than 100 mL in 24 hours.

When an indwelling catheter is used, it is important to be aware that it may lead to urinary tract infection. The nurse must teach the client and family to observe for signs and symptoms of urinary tract infections and sepsis. They should note odor, color, and consistency of the urine. Catheter changes are the responsibility of the nurse and are usually performed once a month. Encouraging fluids becomes a major role assumed by family members and monitored by the nurse. Urinary antiseptics are adjunctive measures when catheterizations are required.

Home care dialysis is common in many areas of the country. The principles and procedures are similar to those in a hospital or free-standing dialysis unit. The major change is the advent of portable dialysis methods such as continuous ambulatory peritoneal dialysis (CAPD) and continuous cycling peritoneal dialysis (CCPD). These procedures allow individuals to participate in a normal lifestyle. However, use of these methods requires monitoring by the nurse and specific teaching of the essential components to prevent complications and promote health. Peritoneal dialysis (PD) reflects more normal kidney function than hemodialysis. Fluid and electrolytes are removed gradually and, therefore, clients have fewer complications with blood pressure alterations and disequilibrium syndrome. There are fewer dietary and fluid restrictions allowing clients to lead a more normal life. PD provides the client with a more flexible schedule allowing him or her to work, travel, and participate in activities. One major restriction, besides ensuring the ordered number of exchanges each day, is the monthly appointment at the dialysis center for lab work and consultation with the physician or nurse.

The catheter is placed in a dependent position in the perineal cavity to minimize the chance of catheter obstruction or erosion into other abdominal organs. The catheter is placed outside of the abdomen to decrease infections. There are several devices that are placed around the catheter that prevent fluid leak from the peritoneal cavity. These devices impede the migration of bacteria.

There are three types of PD; continuous ambulatory peritoneal dialysis (CAPD), continuous cycling peritoneal dialysis (CCPD), and intermittent peritoneal dialysis (IPD). The two most common types for home care clients are CAPD and CCPD.

CAPD does not require a machine and can be done almost anywhere that is clean and well lighted. The client performs 4–5 exchanges daily that take approximately 30–45 minutes for each exchange. Each exchange allows a prescribed amount of a dextrose solution termed *dialysate*, 1500–2000 mL for adults, to flow into the abdomen. The dialysate remains in the abdomen, called dwell time, for approximately 4 hours and then it is drained out of the abdomen for about 10 minutes. The last exchange of the day is before bedtime. The dialysate remains in the abdomen overnight.

CCPD requires a portable machine that connects to the catheter and automatically fills and drains the dialysate from the abdomen at night while the client sleeps. This procedure usually takes 10–12 hours every night.

IPD is similar to CAPD except that is done for about 10 hours each day for 3–4 days each week. The exchanges take place hourly with approximately 2 liters of fluid each exchange. This type of dialysis is usually done in an outpatient setting.

BOWEL ELIMINATION

Most skills involving care of the bowel are the same as those performed in the hospital setting. Please refer to Chapter 23 for information. Colostomy irrigations are usually not taught or initiated in the hospital, as there is little supporting evidence for the need to irrigate a colostomy. It was thought that by irrigating the colostomy it would help regulate the bowel and there would not be bowel eruptions at various times of the day. It has been found that the bowel will return to presurgical habits of elimination. If bowel movements occurred erratically before surgery, this pattern will continue after surgery. To irrigate or not to irrigate is basically a preference by the client.

NURSING DIAGNOSES

The following nursing diagnoses may be appropriate to include in a client care plan when the components are related to promoting elimination.

NURSING DIAGNOSIS	RELATED FACTORS
Disturbed Body Image	Alteration in body appearance, urinary or bowel stoma, presence of stoma, fear of rejection, psychosocial factors
Excess Fluid Volume	Decreased urine output, renal system dysfunction, decreased cardiac output
Ineffective Coping	Poor adjustment to illness or treatment, chronic disease state
Noncompliance	Inadequate knowledge base, inability to manage equipment for irrigation, denial of health status, cultural or spiritual beliefs
Impaired Urinary Elimination	Incontinence, lack of muscle tone, urinary tract infection, motor or sensory impairment, abdominal surgery
Urinary Retention	Inability to void, bladder distention or atony, surgical repair
Anticipatory Grieving	Loss of body contiguity, operative procedure, decreased social interaction as a result of colostomy
Impaired Skin Integrity	Skin irritation or breakdown, poor pouching techniques, incontinence or diarrhea, poor-fitting equipment
Deficient Knowledge	Inability to manage ostomy and unable to understand why and how to irrigate colostomy

USING CLEAN TECHNIQUE FOR INTERMITTENT SELF-CATHETERIZATION

Equipment

Straight catheters in clean container, plastic bag, or wrapped in aluminum foil
Washcloth, soap, water
Water-soluble lubricant (K-Y; Surgilube)
Plastic bags
Basin or container
Mirror

Procedure

for Female Client

1. Attempt to urinate. If unable to do so, continue to follow these steps.
2. Wash hands, and gather equipment. (Keep equipment in one large container.)
3. Assume sitting position on the bed or commode. (Place plastic under towel if bed is used.)
4. Separate labia with one hand while cleaning with soap and water front to back with other hand.
5. Position mirror to visualize urinary meatus.
6. Remove catheter from container (plastic bag or aluminum foil).
7. Lubricate end of catheter with water-soluble lubricant and place other end in container to catch urine.
8. While holding labia apart with one hand, insert catheter about 3 inches or until urine flows.
9. Press down with abdominal muscles to promote bladder's emptying.

10. Pinch off catheter after all urine has drained and withdraw gently, holding tip of catheter upright.
11. Wash and dry perineal area.
12. Wash catheter in warm, soapy water.
13. Rinse with clear water and dry outside with paper towel.
14. Place in plastic bag for storage.
15. Use catheters for 2–4 weeks and then discard.
16. Wash hands.

for Male Client

1. Attempt to urinate. If unable to do so, continue to follow these steps.
2. Wash hands, and gather equipment. (Keep equipment in one large container.)
3. Assume sitting position on the bed or commode. (Place plastic under towel if bed is used.)
4. Retract the foreskin, if present, and wash tip of penis with soap and water.
5. Remove catheter from container (plastic bag or aluminum foil).
6. Lubricate the first 7–10 inches of catheter with water-soluble lubricant. Place other end in container to catch urine.
7. Hold penis at right angle to body, keeping foreskin retracted. Insert catheter 7–10 inches into penis or until urine begins to flow. Then insert catheter 1 inch further.
8. Press down with abdominal muscles to promote bladder's emptying.
9. Pinch off catheter after all urine has drained and gently withdraw, holding tip of catheter upright.
10. Wash and dry area.
11. Wash catheter in warm, soapy water.
12. Rinse with clear water and dry outside with paper towel.
13. Place in plastic bag for storage.
14. Use catheters for 2–4 weeks and then discard.
15. Wash hands.

PROVIDING SUPRAPUBIC CATHETER CARE

Equipment

Catheter plug and clamp
Closed drainage system
Sterile dressings if necessary
Clean gloves
Receptacle to drain urine from drainage bag
Normal saline solution or mild soap and water
White vinegar
Applicator sticks
4 × 4 gauze pads
Paper tape

Procedure

1. Instruct client to gather equipment for specific skill to be done.
2. Wash hands and don gloves.
3. Clean around catheter site with normal saline solution or mild soap and water. Use applicator sticks to remove material from around catheter opening.
4. Ensure catheter is not pulling on exit site. Tape catheter to skin so a gentle curve is present to prevent tugging on catheter.
5. Empty catheter bag. Some clients use regular catheter drainage bags, or leg bags. Empty into container and then dispose of contents in toilet or, if removing bag, empty directly into toilet.
6. Clean drainage bags with warm water and soap every day or two. Place one teaspoon of vinegar in rinse water to reduce odor.
7. Instruct client in bladder testing:
   a. Wash hands and catheter connections with soap and water.
   b. Clamp the SP tube so it does not drain. Use catheter plug or clamp.
   c. Have client attempt to void when client feels urge to urinate. Measure amount of urinate.
   d. Unclamp SP immediately after voiding; empty urine into container and measure residual urine amount.
   e. Instruct client to keep a log of each voiding and residual amount.
   f. Call physician with findings when residual amount is less than 20% voided amount. Usually, this amount is about 60 mL. Usually, SP tube is removed when client is able to urinate without complications.
8. Instruct client to monitor carefully for signs of urinary tract infection and notify physician immediately. Check for bladder pain, bleeding, temperature over 100°F, chills, cloudy urine, drainage or edema around SP tube.

ADMINISTERING CONTINUOUS AMBULATORY PERITONEAL DIALYSIS (CAPD)

Equipment

Sterile dialysate solution, warmed
Transfer set, either Y tubing or straight, and cap
Hook on wall of room used for dialysis
Clamp
Paper towels
Low stool or table
Intake and output record
Clean gloves
Mask
Antibacterial soap

Preparation

1. Wash hands thoroughly, dry using paper towel.
2. Obtain container of sterile dialysate.
3. Check that strength and amount of solution are accurate as ordered.
4. Take equipment to clean area for assembly.

Procedure

for Draining Fluid

1. Don clean gloves. **Rationale:** Infection control precaution for caregiver when there is potential contact with blood or body fluids.
2. Don mask.
3. Uncap catheter maintaining aseptic technique.
4. Attach sterile bag and transfer set to catheter for draining dialysate.
5. Place bag on low stool or table below level of client's abdomen. **Rationale:** This position allows fluid to drain by gravity from client's peritoneal cavity.
6. Unclamp tubing.
7. Allow fluid to drain into bag from abdomen until flow ceases, approximately, 10–20 minutes.
8. Reclamp tubing.
9. Examine drainage for discoloration or cloudiness. **Rationale:** Change in color may indicate presence of infection.
10. Disconnect tubing from drainage bag while maintaining aseptic technique. Unscrew catheter from tubing and attach Mini Cap, according to clinic's instruction. **Rationale:** The glucose in the dialysate solution predisposes the client to infections.
11. Weigh drainage bag on scale. Effluent should weigh at least 4½ pounds. This is equal to 2 liters of fluid. **Rationale:** To ensure all fluid is drained from abdomen.
12. Dispose of effluent into toilet.
13. Double bag tubing and drainage bag. Place biohazardous label on bag. Discard by placing in biohazardous container. Tubing is usually disposed of following each exchange.
14. Remove and discard gloves and mask.
15. Wash hands.
16. Check blood pressure and pulse. **Rationale:** Rapid fluid shift may cause hypotension.

Note: Mini Cap disinfects dialysis tubing between exchanges.

Transfer Sets

Transfer sets are tubing that connect bag of dialysate solution to catheter. There are two types being used for CAPD.

Straight Tubing

Straight tubing stays connected to the catheter. For each exchange, the "free" end is connected to the solution. With this type of transfer set, the empty bag from solution is rolled up and worn under clothing. That bag is then unrolled, placed on the floor, and used to drain dialysate from the abdomen. After draining is completed, tubing is disconnected from the straight transfer set and a new solution bag and tubing are connected to the catheter.

Y-Set Tubing

This type of tubing is disconnected between exchanges. The base of the Y is connected to the catheter. One branch of the Y is connected to a new bag of solution and the other to an empty bag. The base of the Y is closed and a small amount of solution is drained from the full bag into the empty bag. This is done to rid the transfer set of any bacteria that might be in the tubing. The branch that leads to the empty bag is then closed and the solution flows into the abdomen. Once the solution bag is empty, the Y-set is disconnected from the catheter. This deletes the need to wear the bag round the waist while solution is in abdomen. The catheter is then reconnected to the Y-set and solution is drained into an empty bag to discard. A new bag of solution is hung and the process continues. The Y-set is filled with disinfectant when not in use. The disinfectant is flushed out with the used dialysate. The Y-set can be reused for several months.

> **CLINICAL ALERT**
>
> Observe draining dialysate for indications of fibrin, a white gelatin-like material. This indicates a shedding of the peritoneal lining's old skin; an increase in this fibrin indicates potential peritonitis.

for Infusing Dialysate

1. Warm dialysate. The bag can be encased in a heating pad for 1 hour. DO NOT PLACE IN MICROWAVE. **Rationale:** Microwave heating will produce uneven heating and can cause burning in the client.
2. Wash hands for 3 minutes with antibacterial soap. **Rationale:** To prevent contamination.
3. Gather equipment, don gloves and mask.
4. Open plastic wrap on dialysate solution and inspect solution bag for expiration date and color and consistency of dialysate, and assess bag for possible leaks.
5. Add medications as ordered. Maintain sterile technique in this step. **Rationale:** Some clients add routine drugs to dialysate, such as insulin.
6. Connect tubing to dialysate bag by removing protective cover from port and spiking into dialysate bag. Maintain sterility throughout this step. Each manufacturer has a slightly different mechanism for connecting the tubing and bag. Follow manufacturer's directions. *See* box: Transfer Sets.
7. Hang new dialysate bag on hook, which is positioned above client at shoulder height.
8. Open clamp and adjust height to ensure inflow of solution by gravity over a 10- to 20-minute period.
9. Clamp tubing.
10. Discard empty dialysate bag or place in a holding pouch at client's waist, according to type of transfer set being used.
11. Allow fluid to remain in peritoneal cavity approximately 4 hours.
12. Remove mask and gloves.
13. Wash hands.
14. Repeat procedure four times daily, the last time at bedtime, allowing fluid to remain in peritoneal cavity overnight.
15. Ensure that client and caregiver are knowledgeable in strict aseptic technique.
16. Instruct client to notify physician if there is evidence of infection.
17. Document findings and bring to physician at each visit.

CHANGING DRESSING FOR CAPD CLIENT

Equipment

Dressing according to facility policy
Antimicrobial swabs
Sterile saline
Sterile gloves (two pair)
Forceps (optional)

Procedure

1. Wash hands.
2. Don gloves.
3. Remove old dressing with sterile gloves.
4. Inspect site for infection (erythema, edema, warmth, exudate).
5. Remove any dried blood or drainage with normal saline solution.
6. Rinse area with normal saline.
7. Dry area thoroughly.
8. Change gloves.
9. Cleanse area surrounding catheter with antimicrobial swab.
10. Apply dressing according to facility policy.
11. Remove gloves and wash hands.

INSTRUCTING CLIENT IN COLOSTOMY IRRIGATION

Equipment

Solution container with 1,000 mL warm water
Irrigating tubing with cone
Three pair of clean gloves
Irrigating sleeve cut long enough to reach water level in toilet
Items to clean skin and stoma (e.g., washcloths or gauze sponges)
Plastic bag for disposal of used pouch
Clean pouch and closure device
Skin barriers
Water-soluble lubricant
Hook near toilet

Procedure

1. Instruct client in benefits of relaxing and taking periodic deep breaths.
2. Wash hands and don clean gloves.
3. Remove and dispose of used pouch in plastic bag.

4. Clean stoma and skin with warm water and soft cloth. Assess skin for signs of irrigation or breakdown.
5. Apply irrigation sleeve to peristomal skin, and place belt around waist.
6. Fill container with 1,000 mL lukewarm water (500 mL for first irrigation). **Rationale:** Lukewarm water temperature is 105°–110°F. This temperature prevents injury from hot solutions and cramping from cold solutions.
7. Suspend container on bathroom hook at level of client's shoulders (no higher than 18 inches above stoma).
8. Open roller clamp and allow solution to run through tubing; close clamp. **Rationale:** This removes air from tubing and prevents discomfort for client.

CLINICAL ALERT

A distended colon can cause a vagal response resulting in hypotension, bradycardia, and even loss of consciousness.

9. Assist client to sit on toilet or on chair in front of toilet.
10. Place sleeve between client's thighs and direct end into toilet.
11. Lubricate cone tip with water-soluble lubricant.
12. Position cone in sleeve by placing through top opening. If cone cannot be inserted easily do not force it.
13. Hold cone snugly against stoma. **Rationale:** This prevents back flow of solution.
14. Open roller clamp on tubing and allow water to run through cone while inserting cone into stoma.
15. Instill solution (750–1,000 mL) over 5–10 minutes. **Rationale:** The container height and rate of water flow affects results obtained. If client complains of feeling lightheaded or has vertigo, take pulse and stop instillation. **Rationale:** These are symptoms of a vagal response.
16. Clamp tubing for a few minutes if cramping occurs. Instruct client to take a deep breath when solution is instilled. **Rationale:** Deep breathing relaxes abdominal muscles.
17. Remove cone, and close off or fold over top of sleeve after solution is instilled.

CLINICAL ALERT

The danger of perforation of the colon is much greater when irrigating a colostomy with a catheter. The use of an irrigation cone results in safer administration and better water flow.

18. Allow client to remain seated while the majority of stool and solution return, usually 10–15 minutes.
19. Remove gloves and discard.
20. Instruct client to rinse sleeve with water. Dry bottom of sleeve and close end of sleeve.
21. Ask client to wear sleeve in this manner for 30–60 minutes. Client may sit in chair, walk around, or proceed with other activities during this time. **Rationale:** This provides additional time for expelling solution or feces and thus prevents accidental evacuation.
22. Instruct client to remove sleeve, clean, and store in designated area of bathroom.
23. Instruct client to cleanse skin and stoma with warm water and dry thoroughly.
24. Instruct client on how to apply skin barriers and clean pouch.
25. Instruct client to reorder supplies as needed.
26. Place discarded supplies in client's trash.
27. Remove gloves and wash hands.

UNIT 8

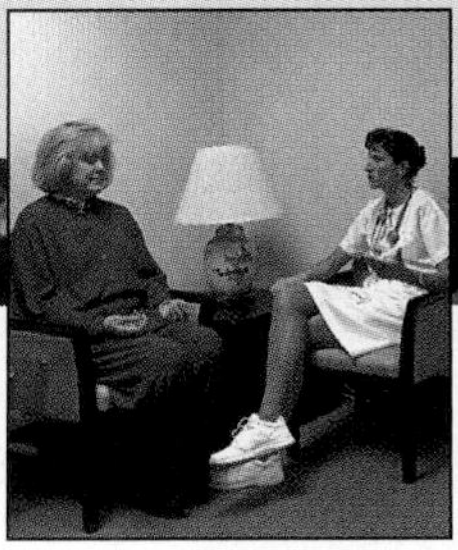

Respiratory Care

Nursing Process Data

ASSESSMENT *Data Base*

Check if client has patent airway.
Assess need for oxygen therapy.
Assess family's ability to suction using aseptic technique.
Observe for cleanliness of equipment (tubing or reservoir).
Assess family's knowledge about safety factors when oxygen is in use.
Assess family's knowledge base related to setup and monitoring of ventilator.
Determine if client has contraindications to using transtracheal oxygenation.
Determine client's willingness to comply with daily routine.

PLANNING *Objectives*

To return or maintain client's arterial Po_2 to normal range
To provide ventilatory assistance for clients with COPD or neuromuscular disorders
To teach safety measures when oxygen is used in the home setting
To promote accurate management of ventilator equipment
To increase client's comfort level when continuous oxygen is required
To prevent nasal irritation or facial skin pressure from continuous nasal cannula use
To promote independence and increase self-esteem in clients requiring continuous oxygenation

IMPLEMENTATION *Procedures*

Caring for Oxygen Equipment
Teaching Safety Measures for Oxygen Use
Managing Ventilator Equipment
(For additional skills refer to Chapter 26)
Providing Catheter Care for Transtracheal Catheter
for Heimlich Micro-Trach
for SCOOP Catheter Cleaning in Place
for SCOOP Catheter Cleaning After Removal
Teaching the Client Catheter Care
Teaching Tracheostomy Suction
Cleaning Suction Equipment
Teaching Tracheostomy Care

EVALUATION *Expected Outcomes*

Safety measures are instituted when oxygen is in use.
Clients are safely maintained on ventilator.
Ventilators are cleaned appropriately.
Arterial PAO_2 is maintained at specified level (usually 65–80 mm Hg).
Client comfort is attained.
Catheter remains patent.
Client is able to provide self-care.

Oxygen therapy is most commonly used in the home situation for clients who have chronic obstructive pulmonary disease (COPD). The type of oxygen equipment used is different from that used in the hospital because there is no "wall oxygen." The systems most frequently used include cylinder tanks, portable walking cylinders, or oxygen concentrators or compressors. If the compressor or concentrator is used, it is plugged into the electrical system. However, it is necessary to have a portable tank or cylinder available in case of power failure. Most people use a portable tank when going outside the home.

Low-flow (2 L) oxygen is usually administered by nasal cannula or Venturi mask. Short and long oxygen tubing is needed to connect the oxygen source to the client. Long tubing is used during the day to allow more flexibility for moving about the house. COPD clients and their families need to be alerted to the signs and symptoms of carbon dioxide narcosis to prevent respiratory distress.

Transtracheal oxygen therapy is provided by the SCOOP system. This method of oxygen delivery is an excellent way to deliver oxygen directly into the lungs and promotes greater oxygenation into blood than oxygen delivery via nasal prongs. Clients report they are much more comfortable and it is more convenient using the SCOOP catheter. This method of oxygen delivery provides required oxygenation throughout 24 hours regardless of the client's other activities. Increased mobility allows them more freedom and the ability to be away from home for longer periods of time. This system uses a lighter and more compact oxygen source than nasal oxygen.

Clients on respirators are now cared for in the home. Since the hospital-type positive pressure machines are too complicated for home use, a more simplified respirator is selected. Positive pressure home respirators have alarms that signal power loss or indicate when pressures are too high or too low. Most respirators function with either electricity or battery power. Each machine has specific operating procedures that must be followed. Before caring for a home care client on a respirator, the nurse must be familiar with the specific equipment.

Clients with neuromuscular diseases can use an external negative pressure ventilator when they do not have an artificial airway and there is no problem with decreased lung compliance. In addition, clients must be able to handle their own secretions to be able to use this type of ventilator. These machines cause the intra-airway pressure to become negative as a result of the pressure surrounding the chest wall. The negative pressure ventilators (Poncho or Pulmo-wrap) are designed to model the old iron lung.

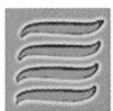

NURSING DIAGNOSES

The following nursing diagnoses may be appropriate to include in a client care plan when the components are related to respiratory conditions.

NURSING DIAGNOSIS	RELATED FACTORS
Activity Intolerance	Fatigue, pain, inadequate oxygenation
Anxiety	Pulmonary congestion, chronic respiratory disorders (COPD), pain
Impaired Gas Exchange	Ventilation–perfusion imbalance, diminished functional lung tissue, changes in arterial blood gases
Ineffective Airway Clearance	Inability to clear secretions, excessive secretions, obstructed respiratory tract, chest trauma, surgical interventions, pain, edema
Ineffective Breathing Pattern	Inability to maintain sufficient oxygen supply to cells, neuromuscular impairment, chronic respiratory disease states
Impaired Oral Mucous Membrane	Prolonged mouth breathing, bypassed airway, disease state, intubation, comatose state
Bathing/Hygiene Self-Care Deficit	Fatigue, hypoxic states (confusion), chronic respiratory disorders, impaired gas exchange

CARING FOR OXYGEN EQUIPMENT

Equipment

Soap
Water
Paper towel
Plastic bag
Distilled water for humidifier

Procedure

1. Obtain order for oxygen therapy.
2. Determine type of oxygen system to be used.
3. Contact inhalation therapy company and ensure company offers 24-hour emergency service. (Usually the company sends a representative to set up the equipment and instruct the client or family on its use and care.)
4. Rinse cannula or mask clean with water and dry with paper towel daily.
5. Wash tubing daily. Hang in bathroom to dry. Store in clean plastic bag when not in use.
6. Wash long tubing weekly. Replace monthly.
7. Clean compressor filter daily with water or according to company instructions.
8. Use distilled water in humidifier. (Store distilled water in refrigerator.) Wash humidifier with soap and water every few days.

Safety Precautions

- Set up "No Smoking" and "Oxygen in use" signs at the site of administration and at the door.
- Remove matches and lighters from bedside.
- Disconnect grounded electric equipment.
- Remove all volatile materials except solutions and equipment to be used during intervention.
- Place fire extinguishers near room where oxygen is in use.

TEACHING SAFETY MEASURES FOR OXYGEN USE

Equipment

"No Smoking" sign
Emergency number of oxygen company
Alternate oxygen supply
Cotton dust cloth

Procedure

1. Post "No Smoking" signs.
2. Keep room temperature at 65°–70°F.
3. Keep an alternative supply of oxygen (e.g., tank) that is not dependent on electrical system.
4. Post emergency number of oxygen company by the phone.
5. Avoid clothing with nylon or wool, which produces static electricity and sparks.
6. Store oxygen away from heat, open flames, or flammable materials.
7. Do not use electric equipment, such as hair dryers and shavers, when oxygen is in use.
8. Keep environment dust free. Damp dust three or four times per week with cotton cloth. Use oxygen equipment in non-carpeted room if possible.

MANAGING VENTILATOR EQUIPMENT

Equipment

Ventilator and accessory equipment (positive or negative pressure ventilator)
Two humidifiers
Distilled water
Sterile tracheostomy tube replacement set as needed
Suctioning equipment
Oxygen or compressed air administration equipment
Tubing
Compressor filter
Bucket or bowl
Weak bleach solution
Plastic bag

Preparation

1. Evaluate home for best room in which to place client and equipment.
2. Order necessary equipment from vendor, based on type of

ventilator being used (positive pressure or negative pressure ventilator).

3. Evaluate client's and family's understanding of principles of ventilator care before client begins treatment.
4. Ensure that fire department, electric company, and telephone company are aware that ventilator-dependent client is in the home. Have electric company place home on high-risk list.
5. Check home environment for cleanliness and safety prevention, such as condition of floors.

Procedure

1. Read manufacturer's directions for setting up ventilator.
2. Attach ventilator to oxygen or compressed air source.
3. Fill humidifier with distilled water.
4. Set ventilator parameters for tidal volume and rate.
5. Set alarm parameters.
6. Analyze oxygen concentration at least every 8 hours or as ordered.
7. Measure tidal volume at least every 8 hours or as ordered.
8. Suction airway as needed.
9. Provide a communication method with the client if tracheostomy tube is in place.
10. Provide oral hygiene for clients with tracheostomy tubes.
11. Force fluids if tolerated. **Rationale:** Fluids aid in liquifying secretions for easy removal.
12. Observe for signs and symptoms of respiratory infection.
13. Drain condensation from tubing by draining fluid into bucket or large bowl. **Rationale:** Draining fluid back into humidifier can lead to bacterial contamination.
14. Change ventilator tubing, compressor filter, and humidifier every 24 hours. **Rationale:** This prevents contamination.
15. Clean tubing and humidifier reservoir using a weak bleach solution (nine parts water to one part bleach).
16. Rinse thoroughly and allow tubing to hang dry.
17. Store clean equipment in plastic bag.

PROVIDING CATHETER CARE FOR TRANSTRACHEAL CATHETER

Equipment

Nasal cannula
Cotton-tipped applicators
Mild bar soap
Antimicrobial soap
Sterile normal saline
Clean gloves
Cleaning rod
Second SCOOP catheter
Sterile water-soluble lubricant

Preparation

1. Cleanse catheter site with cotton swab and tap water twice a day. Use mild bar soap if secretions are thick.
2. Rinse well following use of soap.

Procedure

for Helmlich Micro-Trach

1. Apply nasal cannula oxygen during cleaning procedure.
2. Disconnect oxygen tubing from catheter and connect to nasal catheter.
3. Observe for edema, erythema, or excess drainage around catheter site.
4. Instill 0.5–1.0 mL sterile normal saline into catheter. **Rationale:** Saline stimulates coughing and clearing of accumulated secretions in the lungs. Repeat instillation two to three times each day.
5. Reconnect oxygen tubing to catheter.
6. Reestablish oxygen flow at ordered amount, usually 1–2 L/minute.
7. Replace catheter if dislodged during coughing. Swab catheter with alcohol, and reinsert.

> **CLINICAL ALERT**
>
> Suctioning cannot be done through the SCOOP catheter. The catheter cannot be advanced further toward the lungs.

for SCOOP Catheter Cleaning in Place

1. Gather equipment.
2. Wash your hands.

> **Contraindications for Use of Transtracheal Oxygen**
>
> - Tracheal deformities
> - Disabling anxiety
> - Acute respiratory failure
> - Pleural herniation
> - Arrhythmias
> - Bleeding disorders
> - Severe bronchospasm
> - High steroid dosage

3. Apply nasal cannula oxygen during cleaning procedure.
4. Disconnect SCOOP oxygen tubing from catheter, and connect to nasal catheter. Adjust flow rate to prescribed nasal cannula rate.
5. Observe for edema, erythema, or excess drainage.
6. Don clean gloves.
7. Clean around tract opening using cotton-tipped applicator and mild soap. **Rationale:** Cleans mucous crust from tract opening.
8. Dry area.
9. Wash cleaning rod with antibacterial soap. Rinse under running water.
10. Instill 1.5 mL sterile saline into catheter.
11. Insert cleaning rod into catheter. Pull back and forth three times. **Rationale:** This action removes mucus attached to the catheter.
12. Instill additional 1.5 mL normal saline into catheter.
13. Reconnect SCOOP oxygen tubing to both catheter and oxygen tubing.
14. Return oxygen flow rate to SCOOP resting flow rate.
15. Allow catheter to remain in place for 6–8 weeks. Do not remove or insert catheter until matured. **Rationale:** This allows time for the tract to mature.
16. Replace SCOOP catheter every 90 days. **Rationale:** Catheters are made of plastic so can become brittle, causing tracheal irritation.
17. Clean SCOOP rod with antibacterial soap and store in clean, dry place.

for SCOOP Catheter Cleaning After Removal

1. Gather equipment.
2. Wash hands.

Note: If instructing client in self-care, instruct client to sit in front of mirror near a sink.

3. Apply nasal cannula oxygen during cleaning procedure.
4. Disconnect SCOOP oxygen tubing from catheter and connect nasal cannula to oxygen supply. Adjust oxygen flow rate to prescribed nasal cannula rate.

CLINICAL ALERT

Do not remove or insert catheter while oxygen is flowing through it.

5. Clean mucous crusts from around tract opening using cotton tipped applicator and mild soap. Blot area dry. Do not use ointments or creams around tract opening.
6. Don clean gloves.
7. Apply small amount of water soluble lubricant to tip of clean second SCOOP catheter.

CLINICAL ALERT

If you cannot insert catheter within 5 minutes, replace nasal cannula and call physician. The tract may begin to close within minutes.

8. Disconnect bead chain necklace and remove catheter.
9. Insert second clean catheter. Place tip into tract opening and gently push catheter straight back. Catheter will direct itself into tract. If resistance is felt, twist catheter as it is inserted. (When properly inserted, the SCOOP label will be visible in the upright position.)
10. Reconnect bead chain necklace.
11. Reconnect SCOOP oxygen tubing to oxygen source and catheter. Adjust flow rate to SCOOP resting flow rate.
12. Remove nasal cannula.
13. Rinse mucus off soiled catheter under running water. Clean entire length of catheter, especially tip. Do not soak catheter in disinfectant solutions. **Rationale:** It could damage the plastic catheter.
14. Run cleaning rod through inside of catheter until clean.
15. Wash catheter with antibacterial soap and running water. Rinse thoroughly.
16. Wipe dry and store in clean, dry place.
17. Instruct client to keep oxygen tubing under clothes.

CLINICAL ALERT

Instruct client to call physician immediately if any of the following problems occur:

- Catheter comes out before tract is mature
- Cannot replace catheter within 5 minutes
- Increased coughing or sputum
- Increased shortness of breath
- Cyanosis of lips or nail beds
- Anxiety or severe nervousness
- Edema or erythema around tract opening
- Temperature above 99.5°F

TEACHING THE CLIENT CATHETER CARE

Equipment

Catheter kit
Pulse oximeter
Written information for catheter care

Preparation

1. Ensure client's readiness to learn catheter care.
2. Evaluate client's level of understanding.
3. Determine appropriate time and place for teaching.
4. Arrange for family members to attend teaching session.

Procedure

1. Review verbally and in writing signs and symptoms of infection, bronchospasm, bleeding, respiratory failure, subcutaneous emphysema, and pneumothorax with client and family prior to discharge from hospital. **Rationale:** Understanding catheter insertion complications alert client to notify physician before complications become critical.
2. Instruct client to take oral temperature twice a day for 1 week and to report fever greater than 99.5°F. **Rationale:** Increased temperature indicates possible infection.
3. Review instructions for ordered medications. **Rationale:** Antibiotics are usually prescribed for 1 week to prevent infection. These drugs need to be taken on schedule and for length of time ordered.
4. Instruct client about follow-up hospital and physician visits. Clients with SCOOP catheters have at least two physician visits for catheter change.
5. Instruct in use of pulse oximeter as needed. **Rationale:** Transtracheal oxygen flow rates are adjusted according to these readings.
6. Instruct to return to physician for catheter change every 6 months for Micro-Trach or every 3 months for SCOOP catheter.

TEACHING TRACHEOSTOMY SUCTION

Equipment

Suction machine
Suction catheters
Normal saline
Basin
Water
Second clean tracheostomy tube
Clean gloves
Antimicrobial soap (option)

Procedure

1. Gather equipment.
2. Fill basin with ½ cup water or normal saline.
3. Instruct client to wash hands thoroughly using soap and water. If high risk for infection, use antimicrobial soap. Don gloves.
4. Connect suction catheter to suction machine, turn on, and check that it is functioning properly.
5. Instruct client to take several deep breaths and remove oxygen, if using.
6. Insert catheter 6–8 inches without applying suction.
7. Place thumb over catheter vent and apply intermittent suction, for no more than 10 seconds, as catheter is withdrawn. Rotate catheter as it is being withdrawn.
8. Have client take a deep breath and reapply oxygen source.
9. Repeat procedure if necessary. Clean catheter with normal saline before reinserting into tracheostomy.
10. Suction nasal or oral pharynx, if needed.
11. Rinse catheter with water in basin until clean.
12. Disconnect suction catheter and coil around gloved hand. Catheter is either cleaned and disinfected or discarded. If discarded, when removing glove, enclose catheter in glove.

CLEANING SUCTION EQUIPMENT

Equipment

Clean glass bowl
Distilled white vinegar
Water
Paper towel
Mild detergent soap
Clean gloves

Procedure

1. Gather equipment.
2. Wash hands and don gloves when cleaning equipment.
3. Place suction catheter in bowl with mild soap. Allow to soak in soapy water for 5 minutes. Use bulb syringe to force soapy water through catheter.
4. Rinse catheter with sterile water.

Note: It is best to not reuse suction catheters if possible.

5. Soak catheter for 30 minutes in solution of ½ cup white vinegar and 1 quart water.
6. Rinse thoroughly with water.
7. Dry outside with paper towel, lay catheter down on towel to thoroughly dry inside.
8. Store in clean towel until ready to use.
9. Empty suction bottle, wash with soap and water, and rinse at least once a day. Replace disposable bottles once a week or sterilize nondisposable bottles weekly.
10. Wash connecting tubing daily with soapy water. Discard and replace tubing weekly.
11. Replace solution containers daily.
12. Clean bulb syringe with soapy water and rinse after each use.
13. Discard secretions from suction bottle down toilet every day.

TEACHING TRACHEOSTOMY CARE

Equipment

Clean gloves, 2 pairs
Sterile forceps
Two basins
Twill tape trach tie
Sterile cotton-tipped applicators
4 × 4 gauze sponges
Normal saline or bottled water
Trach brush or pipe cleaners
Warm, soapy water or hydrogen peroxide
Clean trach dressing, optional
Trash bag

Procedure

1. Gather equipment.
2. Wash hands.
3. Pour hydrogen peroxide or warm, soapy water in one container and water or normal saline in second container.
4. Don clean gloves.
5. Remove soiled dressing and place in trash bag.
6. Remove soiled gloves and replace with new gloves.
7. Wash skin around stoma and under trach ties and flanges with presoaked gauze sponges and damp applicators.
8. Dry area thoroughly.
9. Remove inner cannula and place in hydrogen or soapy water basin.
10. Clean inner cannula using brush or pipe cleaners.
11. Rinse cannula with water or normal saline for at least 15 seconds.
12. Replace inner cannula.
13. Change trach ties. Instruct family member to hold face plate of trach tube when removing old ties and applying new ones. Thread ties through opening in trach flange. Tie knot along side of client's neck, leaving one fingerbreadth under tie.
14. Place clean gauze with slit under tracheostomy tube and slip up under tube.
15. Discard disposable items and clean and soak basins and brush in warm, soapy water followed by 30-minute soak in equal parts of vinegar and water. Equipment can be boiled for 15 minutes, air dried, and placed in baggie.
16. Remove gloves and discard in trash.
17. Wash hands.
18. Store reusable equipment in baggie.

UNIT 9

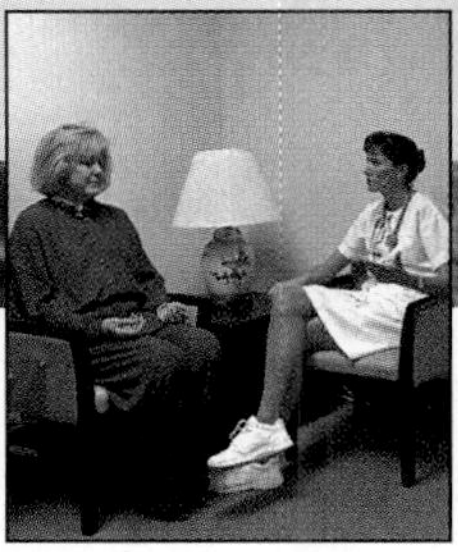

Circulatory Care

Nursing Process Data

ASSESSMENT Data Base

Assess client's ability to monitor pulse accurately.

Identify client's and/or family's knowledge of pacemaker function and safety measures.

Assess pacemaker site for signs and symptoms of infection.

Assess for signs and symptoms related to pacemaker dysfunction, including dizziness, weakness, altered level of consciousness, irregular pulse, low blood pressure, decreased urine output, fatigue.

Assess client's ability and knowledge related to contacting the pacemaker clinic.

PLANNING Objectives

To provide client teaching related to monitoring pulse and use of magnet

To evaluate client's knowledge base about pacemaker clinic

To increase client's knowledge base about pacemaker function

IMPLEMENTATION Procedures

Monitoring Pacemaker at Home

Checking with Pacemaker Clinic via Telephone

Instructing in Use of Holter Monitor

Teaching Care of Implantable Cardioverter-Defibrillator

(For additional skills refer to Chapter 27)

EVALUATION Expected Outcomes

Client is able to accurately monitor pulse.

Client's cardiac rate and rhythm are maintained through use of a pacemaker.

Battery failure is identified early and major complications prevented.

Client is knowledgeable about pacemaker function.

Client is able to contact pacemaker clinic easily and comply with directions for pacemaker check.

Circulatory skills performed in the home setting are similar to those in the hospital. Vital signs are taken using the same equipment and procedures. CPR and the Heimlich maneuver are performed exactly the same way. Care of the pacemaker client, however, is somewhat different.

Clients with permanent pacemakers are expected to monitor pacemaker function on a daily basis. While in the hospital, the client is taught how to monitor pulse, vital signs, symptoms of pacemaker failure, and indications of infection at the pacemaker insertion site. When the client returns home, the home health nurse needs to reinforce the teaching that was initiated in the hospital.

The client should be taught to monitor the pulse daily on awakening to identify altered pacemaker function. This may indicate a need for a battery change earlier than scheduled. Normally, lithium batteries last 6 years or more, whereas mercury–zinc batteries last 5 years. Nuclear-powered pacemakers (plutonium-238) can last 20 years or more. Some batteries can be recharged externally.

The generator is usually placed in the abdominal subcutaneous tissue or under the clavicle on the left side where the outline of the generator can be easily observed. The client must be taught to assess the site during the postoperative period for erythema, edema, and warmth, which may indicate the presence of infection.

A periodic telephone pacemaker check can be used for clients living in rural settings or in areas where a cardiologist is not easily available. Heart sounds are transmitted via telephone signals and recorded on an ECG strip. The technician at the clinic compares a base-line ECG strip that is on file to that of the newly recorded ECG. If there are any alterations from normal, the client is asked to call his physician and the technician also notifies the physician. This procedure identifies early pacemaker dysfunction and aids in preventing complications.

For client safety, it is imperative to stress the importance of having someone present while checking for pacemaker malfunction when a magnet is used. The telephone number of the pacemaker clinic should be kept readily accessible in case of an emergency situation, particularly when testing with the magnet.

NURSING DIAGNOSES

The following nursing diagnoses may be appropriate to include in a client care plan when the components are related to pacemaker function.

NURSING DIAGNOSIS	RELATED FACTORS
Decreased Cardiac Output	Cardiac disease states, altered electrical conduction, drug side effects, hypovolemia
Excess Fluid Volume	Decompensated cardiovascular system, disease states, increased fluid intake secondary to excess sodium, drugs
Risk for Infection	Pacemaker implantation site, altered circulation
Deficient Knowledge	Incomplete understanding or instruction regarding pacemaker function or monitor management

MONITORING PACEMAKER AT HOME

Equipment

Clock or watch with second hand
Daily record
Pacemaker magnet

Procedure

1. Instruct client in care immediately following pacemaker insertion.
   a. Keep site clean and dry for at least 2 weeks.
   b. Demonstrate daily dressing change using sterile gauze and paper tape.
   c. Do not use any ointments on incision site unless physician has instructed to do so.
   d. Assess site daily for signs of erythema, edema, or drainage. Call physician if any of these symptoms occur.
   e. Leave steri-strips in place until physician removes them.
   f. Take a bath, but keep dressing dry.
   g. Limit activity for 4 weeks. **Rationale:** To avoid damaging the pacemaker.
   h. Do not lift arm above shoulder level on side of pacemaker for 4 weeks.
   i. Do not hit or rub insertion site or manipulate pacemaker under skin.
   j. Avoid heavy lifting, running, or contact sports for at least 2 weeks.

> **CLINICAL ALERT**
> Instruct client to notify physician if incision site becomes painful, looks infected, or he or she has a fever of 100.4°F or higher.

2. Establish a daily routine check. **Rationale:** Battery failure can be identified in early stages by routine monitoring of pulse.
   a. Sit on side of bed.
   b. Check pulse for 1 full minute before arising.
   c. Record on daily record.

> **CLINICAL ALERT**
> Pacemaker check with magnet should be done only if someone else is present, never if client is alone, because of possible magnet-induced ventricular arrhythmias.

3. Contact physician if any of these symptoms occur:
   a. Sudden slowing or increasing in pulse rate.
   b. Irregular pulse.
   c. Pain or erythema over incision site.
4. Check with pacemaker magnet if ordered by physician.
   a. Sit on side of bed.
   b. Place magnet over pacemaker generator.
   c. Take pulse for 1 full minute.
   d. Record.
5. Teach safety factors to client and family.
   a. Wear Medic-Alert identification band, and carry pacemaker identification card at all times. **Rationale:** This alerts healthcare providers to the fact that pacemaker is in place and identifies manufacturer's name.
   b. Avoid sources of electromagnetic interference (i.e., large engines, strong magnets, airport screening devices, alarm systems, radio transmitting towers, ham radios, and MRI diagnostic testing). **Rationale:** These devices emit intense magnetic fields that cause temporary pacemaker dysfunction.
   c. Avoid leaning over open hood of running automobile because its electrical field can interfere with pacemaker.
   d. Use microwave ovens in good working order.
   e. Use cellular phones on a different side from pacemaker or place in a shirt pocket.
   f. If dizziness occurs, check pulse. Pulse should return to normal within 5 minutes; otherwise, seek medical attention.

CHECKING WITH PACEMAKER CLINIC VIA TELEPHONE

Equipment

Electrodes (e.g., finger, wrist, underarm)
Telephone
Transtelephonic transmitter
Magnet

Procedure

1. Arrange schedule of calls with nurse at pacemaker clinic.
2. Follow directions of monitoring service.
3. Place electrodes on the skin.
4. Turn on ECG transmitter.
5. Transmitter connects pulse and pacemaker data into a signal. This transmits a single-lead ECG pattern to a monitor in the clinic.
6. Instruct client to contact physician if
   a. Pulse is 5 beats or more per minute less than before magnet use.
   b. ECG pattern is altered from baseline ECG on file in clinic.

Note: Many clinics require that you have a touch tone phone to use services.

INSTRUCTING IN USE OF HOLTER MONITOR

Equipment

Adhesive electrodes and lead wires
Magnetic recorder with cassette tape
Shoulder strap or belt clip
Paper and pencil

Procedure

1. Explain that heart rate and rhythm is monitored during entire time monitor is in place. The Holter monitor is used to obtain a continuous graphic tracing of a client's pulse while ADLs are performed.
2. Explain that Holter monitor will be in place 24–48 hours.
3. Place electrodes at both negative and positive poles, as directed by laboratory staff. There are either 5 or 7 leads.
4. Assist client in strapping monitor in place. Monitor is worn on belt device or over the shoulder.
5. Connect electrodes to recorder.
6. Instruct client to record any unusual pain, abnormal sign, symptom, or activity, stating exact time. **Rationale:** Unusual pain, signs or symptoms or activity are evaluated with findings from ECG tape.
7. Explain that while wearing Holter monitor the following directions must be followed.
   a. Sleep on back, not abdomen.
   b. Take sponge bath only, avoid shower.
   c. Call for instructions if an electrode falls off.
   d. Maintain normal activity level.
8. Explain to client that he or she can call the laboratory or clinic any time during the period the Holter monitor is in place if they have questions. Provide client with phone number of appropriate facility.
9. Instruct client to take recorder, strap, and paper documentation to laboratory as directed.

> **CLINICAL ALERT**
>
> Two new cardiac monitors are currently in use, the Marquette and the King of Hearts recorder. These are smaller monitors, lighter in weight, and have only two leads which provide fewer restrictions for clients.

TEACHING CARE OF IMPLANTABLE CARDIOVERTER–DEFIBRILLATOR

Procedure

1. Instruct client in the following:
   a. Call physician immediately if three shocks in a row are felt, dyspnea develops, or feet or ankle edema occurs.
   b. Take a bath whenever, but don't take a shower until incision is dry and completely healed.
   c. Do not change any medications for treating the arrhythmia unless specifically instructed by the physician.
   d. Take all medications prescribed by the physician. Carry information about medications at all times, including name and dose.
   e. Refrain from wearing tight clothing over defibrillator or lead wires if ICD is in abdomen. (Most ICDs are now implanted in the chest, so clothing restriction is not as much of an issue). Women can wear bras.
   f. Do not participate in contact sports or activities that could damage the defibrillator.
   g. Drink caffeinated beverages in moderation. **Rationale:** Caffeine increases heart rate and could disturb heart rhythm.
   h. Carry medical alert band and ICD number at all times. Know settings on ICD (cutoff points in heart rate that triggers pacing and defibrillation).
2. Explain the symptoms associated with infection and instruct client to phone physician if they occur.
   a. Erythema, edema, or tenderness surrounding incision.
   b. Fluid accumulation around surgical site.
   c. Fever of 100°F or higher.
3. Instruct client to not lift anything over 10–15 pounds the first month after surgery. Do not excessively push, pull, or twist during this time.
4. Instruct client to not exercise arms or overuse them for at least 3 months following surgery.
5. Instruct client not to resume the following activities until approved by physician.
   a. Returning to work.
   b. Doing household chores.
   c. Traveling.
   d. Resuming sexual activity.
   e. Walking, swimming, sports.
   f. Using large electrical appliances or electrical motors in the workplace until they have been tested to determine if there is any effect on defibrillator.
6. Remind client that he or she should not undergo an MRI test. **Rationale:** The equipment has a strong magnetic field and is unsafe for the defibrillator.
7. Remind client that wand metal detectors can affect the ICD, and walking through security checkpoint will set off alarms; therefore, they need to be searched by hand and allowed to enter the search area without going through scanner.

8. Explain that the following devices will not interfere with the defibrillator.
   a. Electrical razor.
   b. Small kitchen appliances, including microwave ovens and small power tools.
   c. Analog cellular phones are o.k., but digital phones may be sensed as abnormal and affect ICD.

CLINICAL ALERT

For an interaction between a small electromagnetic device and the defibrillator to occur, they must be within 10 cm of each other. The greater the output power of the device, the greater the possibility of an interaction with the defibrillator.

BIBLIOGRAPHY

Abrams, A. C. (2000). *Clinical drug therapy: Rationales for nursing practice* (6th ed.). Philadelphia: Lippincott.

Abrutyn, E., Goldmann, D. A., Scheckler, W. E., & Biello, L. (2001). *Saunders infection control reference service.* Philadelphia: Saunders.

Ackley, B. J., & Ladwig, G. B. (2002). *Nursing diagnosis handbook: A guide to planning care* (5th ed.). St. Louis: Mosby.

Acute Pain Management. (1999). University of Iowa Gerontological Nursing Interventions Center, April 6, p. 37.

Aguilera, D. (1994). *Crisis intervention: Theory and methodology* (7th ed.). St. Louis: Mosby.

Ahmed, D. (2000). It's not my job. *American Journal of Nursing, 100*(6), 25.

Alfaro-LeFevre, R. (2001). *Applied nursing process* (4th ed.). Philadelphia: Lippincott.

Alfaro-LeFevre, R. (1998). *Critical thinking in nursing: A practical approach* (2nd ed.). Philadelphia: Saunders.

Alspach, J., & Williams, S. (1998). *Core curriculum for critical care nursing* (6th ed.). Philadelphia: Saunders.

American Diabetes Association Clinical Practice Recommendations. (2002). *Journal of Clinical and Applied Research and Education 25* (Suppl. 1).

American Diabetes Association Position Statement. (1998, January). Insulin administration. *Diabetes Care, 21.*

American Heart Association: ACLS for Healthcare Providers. (2001/2002). Chicago: AHA.

American Hospital Association. (2001). *A patient's bill of rights.* Chicago: AHA.

American Nurses' Association. (1986). *Cultural diversity in nursing.* American Nurses' Association, House of Delegates.

American Nurses' Association. (1991). *Position statements: Nursing and the patient self-determination acts.* Washington, DC: ANA.

American Nurses' Association. (1997). *Unlicensed assistive personnel legislation.* Washington, DC: ANA.

American Nurses' Association. (1998). *Standards of clinical nursing practice* (2nd ed.). Washington, DC: ANA.

American Nurses' Association. (2001). *Code of ethics for nurses with interpretive statements.* Washington, DC: ANA.

Anderson, F., & Maloney, J. (1994, November). Taking blood pressure correctly: It's no off-the-cuff matter. *Nursing94, 24*(11), 34–38.

Anderson, K., Anderson, L., & Glanze, W. (2002). *Mosby's medical, nursing, and allied health dictionary* (6th ed.). St. Louis: Mosby.

Andrews, M., & Boyle, S. (1998). *Transcultural concepts in nursing care* (3rd ed.). Philadelphia: Lippincott.

Angeles, T. (1998, March). Removing a nontunneled central catheter. *Nursing98, 28*(3), 52–54.

AORN (Association of Operating Room Nurses). (2001). *Standards, recommended practices, and guidelines.*

Arbour, R. (1993). Weaning a patient from a ventilator. *Nursing93, 23*(2), 52.

Armstrong, J. (2002, April). Chemical warfare. *RN Magazine, 65*(4), 32–39.

Aronoff, D., & Neilson, E. (2001). Antipyretics: Mechanisms of action and clinical use in fever suppression. *American Journal of Medicine, 111*, 304–315.

Aschenbrenner, D. (2000, April). Skin preps and protocols. *American Journal of Nursing, 100*(4), 78.

Ashworth, L. (1990, July/August). Pressure support ventilation. *Critical Care Nursing, 10*(7), 20–25.

Asselin, M., & Cullen, H. (2001, March). New Guidelines for BLS and ACLS. *Nursing 2001, 31*(3) 48–50.

Asselin, M., & Cullen, H. (2002, February). A new beat for BLS and ACLS guidelines. *Nursing Management 33*(2), 33–35.

Axelrod, P. (2000). External cooling in the management of fever. *Clinical Infectious Diseases, 31*(Suppl. 5), S224–S229.

Ayello, E., & Braden, B. (2001, November). Why is pressure ulcer risk assessment so important? *Nursing 2001, 31*(11), 74–79.

Babcock, D., & Miller, M. (1994). *Client Education: Theory & Practice.* St. Louis: Mosby.

Back, J., (1999, January). Clinical practice guidelines for chronic nonmalignant pain syndrome, *Musculoskeletal Rehabilitation, 13*, 47–58.

Ball, J., & Bindler, R. (2003). *Pediatric Nursing, Caring for Children* (3rd ed.). Upper Saddle River, NJ: Prentice Hall.

Bandman, E., & Bandman, B. (1995). *Critical thinking in nursing* (2nd ed.). Upper Saddle River, NJ: Prentice Hall Health.

Baranoski, S. Skin tears: The enemy of frail skin. *Skin & Woundcare* (www.woundcarenet.com/advances).

Barkauskas, V. H., Baumann, L., & Darling-Fisher, C. (2002). *Health and physical assessment* (3rd ed.). St. Louis: Mosby.

Barnason, S., et al. (1999, February). Does it matter if you use twill or adhesive tape? *RN, 62*(2), 20.

Barry, M. (2001, October). Ankle sprains. *American Journal of Nursing, 101*(10). 40–42.

Basmajian, J. V. (Ed.). (1989). *Biofeedback: Principles and practice for clinicians* (3rd ed.). Baltimore: Williams & Wilkins.

Bates, B. (2002). *Guide to physical examination and history taking* (8th ed.). Philadelphia: Lippincott Williams & Wilkins.

Beare, P., & Myers, J. (1998). *Adult health nursing* (3rd ed.). St. Louis: Mosby.

Beck, V. (1998, January). On the lookout for impaired wound healing. *Nursing98, 28*(1) 32H, 1–4.

Beers, M., & Berkow, R. (1999). *The Merck manual of diagnosis and therapy.* Whitehouse Station, NJ: Merck Research Laboratories.

Beezhold, T., et al. (1996). Latex allergy can induce clinical reaction to specific foods. *Clinical and Experimental Allergy, 26*, 416–422.

Benton, L. (2000, Feb.). DVT prevention. *American Journal of Nursing 100*(2), 84.

Bernzweig, E. (1996). *The nurse's liability for malpractice.* (6th ed.). St. Louis: Mosby.

Best Practice. (2001, February). Graduated compression stockings for the prevention of post-operative venous thromboembolism. *Evidence Based Practice Information Sheets for Health Professionals,* 5(2), 1–6.

Beyea, S. (1996). *Critical pathways for collaborative nursing care.* Upper Saddle River, NJ: Prentice Hall.

Black, J., Hawkes, J., & Keene, A. (2001). *Medical–surgical nursing: Clinical management of positive outcomes* (6th ed.). Philadelphia: Saunders.

Blais, K., Hayes, J., Kozier, B., & Erb, G. (2001). *Professional Nursing Practice: Concepts and Perspectives* (4th ed.). Upper Saddle River, NJ: Prentice Hall Health.

Bloom, B. S. (Ed.). (1956). *Taxonomy of educational objectives, handbook I: Cognitive domain.* New York: McKay.

Boon, T. (1998, February). Don't forget the hospice option. *RN, 61*(2), 30–33.

Boucher, M. A. (1998, February). Delegation alert. *American Journal of Nursing, 98*(2), 26–32.

Bowers, S. (2000, December). All about tubes. *Nursing 2000. 30*(12), 41–47.

Boyer, M. J. (2002). *Math for nurses: A pocket guide to dosage calculations and drug preparations* (5th ed.). Philadelphia: Lippincott.

Braden, B., & Ayello, E. (2002, March). How and why to do pressure ulcer risk assessment. *Advances in Skin and Wound Care: The Journal for Prevention and Healing, 15*(3), 125–131.

Brallier, L., (1982). *Successfully managing stress.* Los Altos, CA: National Nursing Review.

Braunwald, E., et al. (2001). *Harrison's principles of internal medicine* (15th ed.). New York: McGraw-Hill.

Brent, N. (2000). *Nurses and the law: A guide to principles and applications* (2nd ed.). Philadelphia: Saunders.

Brett, A. (2002, June). Therapeutic hypothermia for comatose survivors of cardiac arrest. *Journal Watch, 22*(6), 43.

Bridges, E. (2001, June). Ask the experts. *Critical Care Nurse, 21*(6), 66–68.

Briggs, Joanna (2001, January). Graduated compression stockings for the prevention of post-operative venous thromboembolism. *Best Practice, 5*(1), 1–6.

Brooke, U. (1998, May). Legal risks of alternative therapies. *RN, 61*(5), 53–57.

Brown, L. (2002, January). When your patient wants to leave AMA. *RN, 65*(1), 71.

Brown, S. (2000, November). The legal pitfalls of home care. *RN, 63*(11), 75–80.

Bryant, G. (2001, February). Stump care. *American Journal of Nursing* 101 (2), 67–71.

Bryant, R. (2000). *Acute and chronic wounds* (2nd ed.). St. Louis: Mosby.

Byrne, T. (1999, February). The setup and care of a patient in Buck's traction. *Orthopaedic Nursing, 18*(2), 79–83.

Cameron, M. (1999). *Physical agents in rehabilitation.* Philadelphia: Saunders.

Canavan, K. (1997, May). Combating dangerous delegation. *American Journal of Nursing, 97*(5), 57–58.

Carnevali, D., & Patrick, M. (1993). *Nursing management for the elderly* (3rd ed.). Philadelphia: Lippincott.

Carpenito, L. (1999). *Nursing care plans and documentation: Nursing diagnosis and collaborative problems* (3rd ed.). Philadelphia: Lippincott.

Carpenito, L. (2003). *Nursing diagnosis: Application to clinical practice* (9th ed.). Philadelphia: Lippincott.

Carroll, P. (1996, May). Spotting the difference in respiratory care. *RN, 59*(5), 26–29.

Carroll, P. (2000, October). Exploring chest drain options. *RN, 63*(10), 50–54.

Cerrato, P. (2002, February). RN news watch. *RN, 65*(2), pp. 21–22.

Chapman, G. (1999, November). Documenting a pain assessment. *Nursing 99, 29*(11), 25.

Clinical Update. (2002, April). Hypothermia after brain injury. *Emergency Medicine, 34*(4), 25–27.

Cohen, M. (2000, March). Getting a good mix. *Nursing 2000, 30*(3), 18.

Cohen, M. (2001, August). Medication errors. *Nursing 2001, 31*(8), 22.

Cohen, M. (2002, March). Double checking for errors. *Nursing 2002, 32*(3), 18.

Collins, N. (2001, December). What's in that feeding formula anyway? *Nursing 2001, 31*(12), 32hn1–32hn2.

Colonies, P. (2001, December). Implementing an early defibrillation program. *Nursing 2001, 31*(12).

Cooper, C. (2000). Reducing the use of physical restraints in nursing homes. *Postgraduate Medicine,* 107(2).

Corbett, J. (2000). *Laboratory tests and diagnostic procedures with nursing diagnoses* (5th ed.). Upper Saddle River, NJ: Prentice Hall Health.

D'Arcy, Y. (1999, September). Managing postoperative CABG pain. *Nursing 99, 29*(9), 17.

DeBoer, S. (2001, April). Ipecac syrup or activated charcoal? *American Journal of Nursing, 101*(4), 75.

DeLaune, S., & Ladner, P. (2002). *Fundamentals of nursing: Standards and practice* (2nd ed.). Albany: Delmar.

Denke, M. (2002, January). Dietary retinol: A double-edged sword. *Journal of the American Medical Association 287*(1), 102–103.

deWit, S. (1998). *Essentials of medical–surgical nursing* (4th ed.). Philadelphia: Saunders.

Doenges, M., Moorhouse, M., & Geissler-Murr, A. (2002). *Nurse's Pocket Guide: Diagnosis, Interventions, and Rationales* (8th ed.). Philadelphia: Davis.

Doenges, M., et al. (2002). *Nursing care plans: Guidelines for Individualizing Patient Care* (6th ed.). Philadelphia: Davis.

Dudek, S. (2000, April). Who's assessing what patients eat? *American Journal of Nursing 100*(4), 36–42.

Dunkin, M. (2001, June). Your medicine. *Arthritis Today, 6*(6), 34–64.

Dunn, N. (2001, February). Keeping COPD patients out of the ED. *RN, 64*(2), 33–37.

Ebersole, P., & Hess, P. (1998). *Toward healthy aging: Human needs and nursing responses* (5th ed.). St. Louis: Mosby.

Elder, K., et al. (1998, June). Managed care: The value you bring. *American Journal of Nursing, 98*(6), 34–39.

Eliopoulos, C. (2001). *Gerontological nursing* (5th ed.). Philadelphia: Lippincott Williams & Wilkins.

Ellenberger, A. (2002, February). How to change a PICC dressing. *Nursing 2002, 32*(2), 50–52.

Ernst, D. (1995, October). Flawless phlebotomy: Becoming a great collector. *Nursing 95, 25*(10), 54–57.

Evans, T., & Carroll, P. (2001, May). Rapid sequence intubation. *American Journal of Nursing,* 101 (Suppl.), 16–20.

Fabian, B. (2000, April). Intravenous complication: Infiltration. *Journal of Intravenous Nursing, 23*(4) 229–231.

Fell-Carlson, D. (2003, January). Terrorist Danger. *Nurseweek California*, Sunnyvale, CA.

Fell-Carlson, D. (2003, January). The nurse's role in managing threat. *Nurseweek California*, Sunnyvale, CA.

Fellows, L., et al. (2000, January). Evidence-based practice for enteral feedings: Aspiration prevention strategies, bedside detection, and practice change. *MedSurg Nursing, 9*(1) 27–31.

Fenstermacher, K., & Carter, R. (1998). *Dysrhythmia recognition and management* (3rd ed.). Philadelphia: Saunders.

Ferri, R., & Sofer, D. (2002, March). News. *American Journal of Nursing 102*(3).

Finkelman, A. (2001, January). *Managed Care: A nursing perspective.* Upper Saddle River, NJ: Prentice Hall Health.

Fischbach, F. (2001). *Nurses' quick reference to common laboratory and diagnostic tests* (3rd ed.). Philadelphia: Lippincott Williams & Wilkins.

Fisher, M. (2000, December). Do you have delegation savvy? *Nursing 2000, 30*(12), 58–59.

Fitzpatrick, L. (2002, May). When to administer modified blood products. *Nursing 2002, 32*(5), 36–42.

Forloines-Lynn, S. (1996, March). How to smooth the way for cyclic tube feedings. *Nursing 96, 96*(3), 57–60.

Forloines-Lynn, S. (1996, March). Knowing how to manage complications of tube feeding. *Nursing 96, 96*(3), 32m–32p.

Frankel, E., et al. (1998). Methods of restoring patency to occluded feeding tubes. *Nutrition in Clinical Practice, 13*, 120–131.

Fredrickson, L. (1997). *MiniMed certified pump trainer manual.* Sylmar, CA: MiniMed, Inc.

Freeland, B. (1999, December). More on hypoglycemia. *American Journal of Nursing, 99*(12), 18.

Friedman, L. (2001, November). Where's my hospice moment? *American Journal of Nursing, 101*(11), 25.

Friedman, M. (2000, February). Improving infection control in home care: From ritual to science-based practice. *Home Healthcare Nurse, 18*(2), 99.

Friedman, M. (2000, June). The Joint Commission's "Improving Organizational Performance" Standards for Home Infusion Therapy Providers. *Journal of Intravenous Nursing, 23*(6), 352–357.

Frizzell, J. (1998, February). Avoiding lab test pitfalls. *American Journal of Nursing, 98*(2), 34–37.

Furman, J. (2001, April). Living with dying: How to help the family caregiver. *Nursing 2001, 31*(4), p. 36.

Galvan, T. (2001). Dysphagia: Going down and staying down. *American Journal of Nursing, 101*(1), 37–43.

Gazarian, P. (1997, October). Teaching your patient to use a metered-dose inhaler. *Nursing97, 27*(1).

Gebbie, K., & Qureshi, K. (2002, January). Emergency and disaster preparedness. *American Journal of Nursing, 102*(1), 46–50.

Geier, K. (1998). Perioperative blood management. *Orthopaedic Nursing,* (Suppl.).

Gerber, R. (1988). *Vibrational medicine—New choices for healing ourselves.* Claremont, CA: Bear.

Gerber-Zimmermann, L. (1997, May). Delegating to unlicensed assistive personnel. *Nursing97, 27*(5), 71.

Gever, M. P. (1998, May). Transdermal patches. *Nursing98, 28*(5), 58–59.

Goldberg, Burton Group. (2002). *Alternative medicine: The definitive group.* (2nd ed.) Berkeley, CA: Ten Speed Press.

Goleman, D., & Gurin, J. (1993). *Mind–body medicine.* Yonkers, NY: Consumers Union of United States, Inc.

Goodfellow, L., & Jones, M. (2002, January). Bronchial hygiene therapy. *American Journal of Nursing, 102*(1), 37–43.

Gorski, L. (2001, January). TPN Update: Making each visit count. *Home Healthcare Nurse, 19*(1), 15.

Gray-Vickrey, P. (2000, July). Combating abuse, part I: Protecting the older adult. *Nursing 2000, 30*(7), 34.

Gritter, M. (1998, September). The latex threat. *American Journal of Nursing, 98*(9), 26–32.

Guido, G. (2000). *Legal and ethical issues in nursing.* (3rd ed.) Upper Saddle River, NJ: Prentice Hall Health.

Guyton, A. C. (2000). *Textbook of medical physiology* (10th ed.). Philadelphia: Saunders.

Habel, M. (2001, October 22). Advance directives. *NurseWeek.*

Hadaway, L. (1999). I.V. infiltration: Not just a peripheral problem. *Nursing99, 29*(9).

Haddad, A. (2000). Ethics in action. *RN, 63*, 2124.

Hamilton, S. (2001, December). Detecting dehydration and malnutrition in the elderly. *Nursing, 31*(12), 56–57.

Heineken, J. (2000). Establishing a bond with clients of different cultures. *Home Healthcare Nurse, 18*(1), 45.

Held-Warmkessel, J. (2001). How to make a PICC line stick. *Nursing 2001, 31*(5), 42–44.

Hellwig, K. (2000). Alternatives to restraints: What patients and caregivers should use. *Home Healthcare Nurse, 18*(6), 395.

Henderson, D. (1999, February). The looming threat of bioterrorism. *American Association for Advancement of Science, 283* (5406). 1279–1282.

Herkner, T., et al. (2001). Does bed rest after cervical or lumbar puncture prevent headache? *California Medical Association Journal, 165*, 1311–1316.

Hertz, J., Yocum, C., & Gawel, S. (2000). *1999 Practice analysis of newly licensed registered nurses in the U.S.* Chicago, IL: National Council of State Boards of Nursing.

Hess, C. (1999). Assessing an external fistula. *Nursing 99, 29*(1), 14.

Hess, C. (2000). *Clinical guide: Wound care* (3rd ed.). Springhouse, PA: Springhouse Corporation.

Hess, C. (2000). How to use transparent films. *Nursing 2000, 30*(6), 84.

Hess, C. (1999). Managing an external fistula. *Nursing 99, 29*(3), 18.

Hill, A. (ed.). (1978). *A visual encyclopedia of unconventional medicine.* New York: Crown Publishers.

Hill, J., & Newton, J. (1998). Contrast echo: Your role at the bedside. *RN, 61*(10), 32–35.

Hoffman, R., & Norton, J. (2000, December). Lessons learned from a full-scale bioterrorism exercise. *Emerging Infectious Diseases. 6*(6) 652–653.

Holland, T. (2002). Utilizing the ankle–brachial index in clinical practice. *Ostomy/Wound Management, 48*(1), 38–43.

Holmes, T. H., & Rahe, R. H. (1967). Social readjustment rating scale. *Journal of Psychosomatic Research, 11*, 213.

Holzer, M. (2002). Mild therapeutic hypothermia to improve the neurologic outcome after cardiac arrest. *New England Journal of Medicine, 346*(8), 549–556.

Horattas, M., & Chinnock, B. (2001). Venous access port problems. *EAMedicine Consumer Journal, 2*(7).

How to Perform 3- or 5-lead. (2002). *Nursing 2002, 32*(4), 50–51.

Hrouda, B. (2002). Warming up to IV infusion. *Nursing 2002, 32*(3), 54–55.

Hudak, C., Gallo, B., & Morton, P. (2001). *Critical care nursing* (8th ed). Philadelphia: Lippincott Williams & Wilkins.

Hunt, L. W., Boone-Orke, J. L., & Fransway, A. F., et al. (1996, July). A medical center–wide, multidisciplinary approach to the problem of natural latex allergy. *Journal of Occupational Environmental Medicine, 38*(8), 765–770.

Improved satisfaction through better pain control. (1999, March). *RN, 62*(3), 30–0-P.

ISMP Medication Safety Alert. (2001, December). Handling verbal orders safely. *Nursing 2001, 31*(12), 43.

Jacobson, J. (Ed.). (2002, March). The World Trade Center children's mural. *American Journal of Nursing, 102*(3), 29–33.

Jagger, J., & Perry, J., (2002). Realistic expections for safety devices. *Nursing 2002, 32*(3), 72.

Jarvis, C. (1995). *Physical examination and health assessment* (2nd ed.). Philadelphia: Saunders.

Joint Commission for the Accreditation of Hospitals (2002, February). *Comprehensive Accreditation Manual for Hospitals: The Official Handbook.* Sentinel Events. Chicago: JCAHO.

Joint Commission on Accreditation of Healthcare Organization (JCAHO). (2002). *Comprehensive accreditation manual for hospitals.* Oakbrook Terrace, IL: JCAHO.

Kany, K. (1999). Working with UAPs. *American Journal of Nursing, 99*(10), 71.

Karch, A., & Karch, F. (2001). Take part in the solution: How to report medication errors. *American Journal of Nursing, 101*(10), 25.

Katz, J. (1997, May). Back to basics: Providing effective patient teaching. *American Journal of Nursing, 95*(5), 33–36.

Kaufman, J. (1990, June). Assessing the 12 cranial nerves. *Nursing90, 20*(6), 56–58.

Kee, J. (2002). *Laboratory and diagnostic tests with nursing implications* (6th ed.). Upper Saddle River, NJ: Prentice Hall Health.

Kilpatrick, J. (2002, May). Nuclear attacks. *Nurseweek California*, Sunnyvale, CA, 47–51.

Klein, T. (2001). PICCs and midlines—fine-tuning your care. *RN, 64*(8), 27–29.

Kohn-Keeth, C. (2000). How to keep feeding tubes flowing freely. *Nursing 2000, 30*(3), 58–59.

Kohr, J. (1995, April). Measuring your patient's pain. *RN, 58*(4), 39–40.

Koschel, M. (2001). Rewarming a hypothermic patient. *American Journal of Nursing, 101*(5), 85.

Kost, M. (1999, April). Conscious sedation. *Nursing99*, www.springnet.com.

Kozier, B., Erb, G., Berman, A., & Burke, K. (2000). *Fundamentals of nursing: Concepts, process and practice* (6th ed.). Upper Saddle River, NJ: Prentice Hall Health.

Kruse, L., et al. (1998). Keeping pace with implanted defibrillators. *RN*, 61(8), 30–34.

Kübler-Ross, E. (1993). *On death and dying.* New York: Macmillan.

Kudzma, E. (1999). Culturally competent drug administration. *American Journal of Nursing 99*(8), 46–51.

Kuhn, M. (1998). *Pharmacotherapeutics: A nursing process approach.* Philadelphia: Davis.

Kumar, D. (1998). PET scanning. *American Journal of Nursing, 98*(7), 16G–16H.

Larson, E. (1995). APIC guideline for handwashing and hand antisepsis in health care settings. *Americal Journal of Infection Control, 23*, 251–269.

Lattavo, K. (2001). Pinpointing postoperative hypoxemia. *Nursing 2001, 31*(1), 32hn1–3.

Leahy, J., Kizilay, P., & Eoyang, T. (1998). *Foundations of nursing practice: A nursing process approach.* Philadelphia: Saunders.

Lehman, C. (1998, June). Preventing pressure ulcers with something old and SUMPINU. *Nursing98, 28*(6), 32H, 14–16.

Leininger, S. (1998, April). Caring for a patient with a hip replacement. *Nursing98, 28*(4), 32H, 12–14.

LeMone, P., & Burke, K. (2000). *Medical–surgical nursing: Critical thinking in client care* (2nd ed.). Upper Saddle River, NJ: Prentice Hall Health.

Lewis, S. M., Heitkemper, M., & Dirksen, S. (2004). *Medical–surgical nursing: Assessment and management of clinical problems* (6th ed.). St. Louis: Mosby.

Little, C. (2000). Manual ventilation. *Nursing 2000, 30*(3), 50–51.

Loan, T., Magnuson, B., & Williams, S. (1998, August). Debunking six myths about enteral feeding. *Nursing98, 28*(8), 43–48.

Lo, B., et al. (2002). Discussing religious and spiritual issues at the end of life. *Journal of the American Medical Association, 287*, 749–754.

Lowdermilk, D., Perry, S., & Bobak, I. (1997). *Maternity & women's health care* (6th ed.). St. Louis: Mosby-Yearbook.

Lower, J. (2002). Facing neuro assessment fearlessly. *Nursing 2002, 32*(2), 58–64.

Ludwick, R., Dieckman, B., & Snelson, C. (1999). Assessment of the geriatric orthopaedic trauma patients. *Orthopaedic Nursing, 18*(6), 13–19.

Lueckenotte, A. G. (1998). *Pocket guide to gerontologic assessment* (3rd ed.). St. Louis: Mosby.

Maher, A., Salmond, S., & Pellino, T. (1998). *Orthopaedic nursing* (2nd ed.), Philadelphia: Saunders.

Malseed, R., Goldstein, F., & Baldon, N. (1995). *Pharmacology: Drug therapy and nursing considerations* (4th ed.). Philadelphia: Lippincott.

Mancini, M., & Kaye, W. (1999, May). AEDs: Changing the way you respond to cardiac arrest. *American Journal of Nursing, 99*(5), 26–30.

Maniscalco, P., & Christem, H. (2002). *Understanding terrorism and managing the consequences.* Upper Saddle River, NJ: Pearson Education.

Masoorli, S., & Angeles, T. (2002). Getting a line on central vascular access devices. *Nursing 2002, 32*(4), 36–43.

Matteson, M. A., McConnell, E., & Linton, A. (1997). *Gerontological nursing: Concepts and practices* (2nd ed.). Philadelphia: Saunders.

McCaffrey, M. (1999, July). Assessing pain in a confused, nonverbal patient. *Nursing99, 29*(7), 18.

McCaffery, M., & Pasero, C. (2000, September). Pain control. *Nurseweek*, Sunnyvale, CA.

McCance, K., & Huether, S. (2001). *Pathophysiology: The biologic basis for disease in adults and children* (4th ed.). St. Louis: Mosby-Yearbook.

McConnell, E. A. (1996, March). Administering oxygen by nasal cannula. *Nursing96, 26*(3), 14.

McConnell, E. A. (1999, November). Performing pulse oximetry. *Nursing99, 29*(11), 17.

McConnell, E. A. (2000, January). Suctioning a tracheostomy tube. *Nursing 2000, 30*(1), 80.

McConnell, E. A. (2002, January). Providing tracheostomy care. *Nursing 2002, 32*(1), 17.

McConnell, E. (1996, October). Ensuring electrical safety. *Nursing96, 26*(10), 20.

McConnell, E. (1998, June). Clinical do's and don'ts: Applying cold treatment. *Nursing98, 28*(6), 26.

McConnell, E. (2000, March). Administering an intradermal injection. *Nursing 2000, 30*(3), 17.

McConnell, E. (2000, November). Applying a two-piece cervical collar. *Nursing 2000, 31*(11), 24.

McConnell, E. (2001, December). Applying a hip abduction pillow. *Nursing 2001, 31*(12), 14.

McConnell, E. (2002, February). Teaching your patient to use a metered dose inhaler. *Nursing 2002, 32*(2), 73.

McCormack, B., Cameron, M., & Biel, L. (1995, April). Latex sensitivity: An occupational health strategic plan. *Journal of Occupational Health*, N.J. *43*(4), 190–196.

McKenzie, L. (1999, February). In search of a standard for pin site care. *Orthopaedic Nursing, 18*(2), 73–78.

McKenzie, N. (1998, October). Fever: Uping the body's thermostat. *Nursing98, 28*(10), 41–45.

Mendez-Eastman, S. (1998, January). When wounds won't heal. *RN, 61*(1), 20–23.

Mendez-Eastman, S. (2001, June). Guidelines for using negative pressure wound therapy. *Advances in Skin and Wound Care: The Journal for Prevention and Healing, 14*(6).

Menzel, L. (1998, April). Factors related to the emotional responses of intubated patients to being unable to speak. *Heart & Lung, 27*(4), 245–251.

Messinger, J., et al. (1999, December). Getting conscious sedation right. *American Journal of Nursing, 99*(12), 44–49.

Metheny, N. (2000). *Fluid and electrolyte balance: Nursing considerations* (4th ed.). Philadelphia: Lippincott.

Metheny, N., & Titler, M. (2001, May). Assessing placement of feeding tubes. *American Journal of Nursing, 101*(5), 36–46.

Metheny, W., Wiersema, M., & Clark, J. (1998, January). pH, color and feeding tubes. *RN, 61*(1), 25–27.

Miller, C. (1999). *Nursing care of older adults* (3rd ed.). Philadelphia: Lippincott.

MiniMed. (1996). *MiniMed user's guide: 507 insulin pump.* Sylmar, CA.

MiniMed. (1998). *The MiniMed infusion family.* Sylmar, CA.

Miracle, V., Sims, J. (1999, July). Making sense of the 12-lead ECG. *Nursing99, 29*(7), 34–39.

Mokdad, A. H., et al. (2000, September). Diabetes trends in the U.S. 1990–1998. *Diabetes Care, 23*(9), 1278–1283.

Moon, L., & Backer, J. (2000, February). Relationships among self-efficacy, outcome expectancy and postoperative behaviors in total joint replacement patients. *Orthopaedic Nursing, 19*(2), 77–85.

Morris, M. (2002, January). Advice of counsel. *RN, 65*(1), 71.

Morris, R. (1998, August). Elder abuse: What the law requires. *RN, 61*(8), 52–53.

Murphy, L., & Burke, L. J. (1990, May). Charting by exception: A more efficient way to document. *Nursing90, 20*(5), 65–69.

Moureau, N. (2001, July). Preventing complications with vascular access devices. *Nursing 2001, 31*(7), 52–55.

Navarro, T. (1998, November). Chemotherapy extravasation. *American Journal of Nursing, 98*(11), 38.

Nettina, S., et al. (2001). *Lippincott manual of nursing practice* (7th ed.). Philadelphia: Lippincott.

Newberry, L., (Ed.), (1997). *Emergency nurses association. Sheehy's emergency nursing: Principles and practices.* St. Louis: Mosby.

NICHD Research Planning Workshop (1997, June). Electronic fetal heart rate monitoring: Research guidelines for interpretation. *Journal of Obstetrics, Gynecology, and Neonatal Nursing 26*(6), 635–640.

Nicolson, G. (2001, December). Protection from biological warfare agents. *Townsend letter for doctors & patients.* Port Townsend, WA: 62–67.

North American Nursing Diagnosis Association (2002). NANDA Nursing Diagnoses: Definitions and Classification, 2001–2002. Philadelphia: NANDA.

Olds, S., Landon, M., & Ladewig, P. (2000). *Maternal–newborn nursing* (6th ed.). Upper Saddle River, NJ: Prentice Hall Health.

Ovington, L. (2001, May). Wound care products: How to choose. *Advances in Skin and Wound Care: The Journal for Prevention and Healing, 14*(5), 259.

Ovington, L. (2002, February). Hanging wet-to-dry dressings out to dry. *Advances in Skin and Wound Care: The Journal for Prevention and Healing, 15*(2), 79–84.

Pagana, K., Pagana, T. (2002). *Mosby's manual of diagnostic and laboratory tests* (2nd ed.). St. Louis: Mosby.

Pain Assessment: The Fifth Vital Sign. (2003). *Board of Registered Nursing,* State of California.

Palefski, S., & Stoddard, G. (2001, February). The infusion nurse and patient complication rates of peripheral-short catheters. *Journal of Intravenous Nursing, 24*(2), 113–123.

Panke, J. (2002, July). Difficulties in Managing Pain at the End of Life. *American Journal of Nursing, 104*(7), 26–33.

Parkman, C. (1996, September). Delegation: Are you doing it right? *American Journal of Nursing, 96*(9), 43–47.

Parkman, C., & Calfee, B. (1997, April). Advance directives: Honoring your patient's end-of-life wishes. *Nursing97, 98*(4), 48–53.

Pasero, C. (1996, September). Pain control. *American Journal of Nursing, 96*(9), 22.

Perry, J., et al. (2001, June). Percutaneous injuries in home healthcare settings. *Home Healthcare Nurse, 19*(6), 342.

Phillips, L. (1997). *Manual of IV therapeutics* (2nd ed.). Philadelphia: Davis.

Phipps, W., Sands, J., & Marcek, J. (2004). *Medical–surgical nursing: Concepts and clinical practice* (7th ed.). St. Louis: Mosby.

Physicians' Desk Reference to Pharmaceutical Specialties and Biologicals (56th ed.). (2002). Montvale, MD: Medical Economics Co. Inc.

Pinderman, M. (1994, September). Indwelling urinary catheters: Reducing infection risks. *Nursing94, 24*(9), 66–68.

Pittet, D., & Dharan, S., et al. (1999). Bacterial contamination of the hands of hospital staff during routine patient care. *Archives of Internal Medicine, 159,* 821–826.

Porth, C. (2002). *Pathophysiology concepts of altered health states* (6th ed.). Philadelphia: Lippincott.

Possanza, C. (1997, September). Special delivery: Using a syringe pump to administer IV drugs. *Nursing97, 27*(9), 43–45.

Prentice, W. (1999). *Therapeutic modalities in sports medicine* (4th ed.) Boston: McGraw-Hill.

Purnell, L., & Paulanka, B. (1998). *Transcultural health care: A culturally competent approach.* Philadelphia: Davis.

Raimer, F. (1994, June). How to identify electrolyte imbalances on your patient's ECG. *Nursing94, 24*(6), 54–58.

Randolph, G., et al. (1998). Benefit of heparin in peripheral venous and arterial catheters: Systemic review and meta-analysis of randomised controlled trials. *British Medical Journal, 316,* 969–975.

Rankin, S., & Stallings, K. D. (2001). *Patient education: Principles and practices* (4th ed.). Philadelphia: Lippincott.

Reid, D. (1996, June). Coordinating a successful discharge plan. *American Journal of Nursing, 96*(6), p. 35.

Reid, D. (1998, August). What to consider when developing a safe discharge plan. *American Journal of Nursing, 98*(8).

Rice, R. (1999). *Manual of home health nursing procedures* (2nd ed.). St. Louis: Mosby.

Rice, R. (2001). *Home health nursing practice: Concepts and application* (3rd ed.). St. Louis: Mosby.

Riley, M. (1997, May). Elective cardioversion. *RN, 60*(5), 27–29.

Ritchey, H., & Rice, J. (1998, October). *MIS guide.* Mountain View, CA: El Camino Hospital.

Rivera, P., Kreskow, J. (2000, February). A team approach to managing pain. *Nursing 2000, 29*(2), 32–33.

Roberts, S. (1996). *Critical care nursing assessment and intervention.* Stamford, CT: Appleton & Lange.

Robertson, C. (1998, March). When your patient is on an insulin pump. *RN, 61*(3), 30–33.

Rubenfeld, M. G., & Scheffer, B. K. (1999). *Critical thinking in nursing: An interactive approach* (2nd ed.). Philadelphia: Lippincott.

Ruffolo, D. (2002, February). Hypothermia in trauma. *RN, 65*(2), 46–51.

Safeer, R., & Prabha, U. (2002, May). Cholesterol treatment guidelines update. *American Family Physician, 65*(5), 871–879.

St. John, R. (2000, April). Ask the experts. *Critical Care Nurse, 20*(4), 100–101.

Sakla, S. (2001). Malnutrition: A serious problem in elderly patients. *Family Practice Recertification, 23*(13), 29–39.

Salvatore, T. (2000, March). Elder suicide: A gatekeeper strategy for home care. *Home Healthcare Nurse, 18*(3), 180.

Salvucci, A. (2002, October). Bioterrorism safeguards. *Bottom Line*, Stamford, CT: Boardroom, Inc.

Satarawala, R. (2000, August). Confronting the legal perils of I.V. therapy. *Nursing 2000, 30*(8), 44.

Schears, G., et al. Statlock catheter securement device significantly reduces central venous catheter complications: Patient safety initiative 2000. *Joint Commission on Accreditation of Healthcare Organizations*, 28–36.

Schreiber, D. (2001, July). Trach care at home: A how-to-guide. *RN, 64*(7), 43–46.

Scoble, M., & Kinney, S. (2001, March). Effect of reusing suction catheters on the occurrence of pneumonia in children. *Heart & Lung, 30*(3), 225–233.

Scriven, M., & Paul, R. Definition of critical thinking. National Council for Excellence in Critical Thinking, www.criticalthinking.org/k12.

Selye, H. (1965). *The stress of life.* New York: McGraw-Hill.

Selye, H. (1974). *Stress without distress.* New York: Signet.

Sharber, J. (1997, February). The efficacy of tepid sponge bathing to reduce fever in young children. *American Journal of Emergency Medicine, 15*(2), 188–191.

Sheehan, J. (2001, November). Delegating to UAPs. *RN 64*(11), 65–66.

Sherman, F. (2002, January). Bedside test provides food for thought. *Geriatrics, 57*(1), 3–4.

Skokal, W. (1997, October). Infusion pump update. *RN, 60*(10), 35–38.

Skyler, J. S. (1995). *The insulin pump therapy book.* Sylmar, CA: MiniMed, Inc.

Smeltzer, S., & Bare, B. (2000). *Brunner & Suddarth's textbook of medical–surgical nursing* (9th ed.). Philadelphia: Lippincott.

Smith, J., et al. (2002, February). A randomized, controlled trial comparing compression bandaging and cold therapy in postoperative total knee replacement surgery. *Orthopaedic Nursing, 21*(2), 61–66.

Smith, S. (1998, July). RNs and UAPs: Not much difference? *RN, 62*(7), 37–38.

Smith, S. (2001). *Sandra Smith's review for NCLEX-RN* (10th ed.). Upper Saddle River, NJ: Prentice Hall Health.

Smith, S., Duell, D., & Martin, B. (2002). *Photo guide of nursing skills.* Upper Saddle River, NJ: Prentice Hall Health.

Smith, S., & Smith, C. (1990). *Personal health choices.* Boston: Jones and Bartlett.

Smith-Temple, J., & Young, J. (1998). *Nurses' guide to clinical procedures* (3rd ed.). Philadelphia: Lippincott.

Smith-Temple, J., & Johnson, J. (1998, February). Pressure ulcer management. *American Journal of Nursing, 98*(2), 16D.

Snowberger, P. (1994, October). Premature ventricular contractions. *RN, 57*(10), 59–61.

Sparks, S., & Taylor, C. (2001). *Nursing diagnosis reference manual* (5th ed.). Springhouse, PA: Springhouse.

Spector, R. (2000). *Cultural diversity in health and illness* (5th ed). Upper Saddle River, NJ: Prentice Hall Health.

Stahl, L. (1996, August). How to transfer patients to other units. *American Journal of Nursing, 96*(8), 57–58.

Standards Addressing Discharge Planning. (2001). *Comprehensive Accreditation Manual for Hospitals*, www.jcaho.org.

Stanhope M., & Knollmuller, R. (2000). *Handbook of community based and home health nursing* (3rd ed.). St. Louis: Mosby.

Stanly, M., & Beare, P. G. (1999). *Gerontological Nursing* (2nd ed.). Philadelphia: Davis.

Starkey, C. (1993). *Therapeutic modalities* (2nd ed). Philadelphia: Davis.

Steinhauer, R. (2002, May). Bioterrorism, *RN, 65*(3), 48–54.

Steinhauer, R. (2002, June). The emergency management plan. *RN, 65*(6), 40–45.

Stewart, K., & Murray, H. (1997, May). How to use crutches correctly. *Nursing97, 27*(5).

Stitik, R., & Nadler, S. (1999, December). Sports injuries: When and how to use cold most effectively. *Consultant, 38*(12), 2881–2890.

Stitik, R., & Nadler, S. (1999, January). Sports injuries: When and how to apply the heat. *Consultant, 39*(1), 144–157.

Strevy, S. R. (1998, February). Myths and facts about pain. *RN, 61*(2), 42–46.

Strimike, C., Wojcik, J., & Stark, B. A. (1997, July). Incision care that really cuts it. *RN, 60*(7), 22–24.

Strowig, S. (2001, September). Insulin therapy. *RN, 64*(9), 38–44.

Swackhamer, A. (1995, January). Alternatives—complementary therapies. *RN, 58*(1), 49–51.

Sweha, A., & Nuovo, J. (1999, May). Interpretation of the electronic fetal heart rate during labor. *American Family Physician, 5.*

Taber's cyclopedic medical dictionary (9th ed.). Philadelphia: Davis.

Tate, J., & Tasota, F. (2000, September). Using pulse oximetry. *Nursing 2000, 30*(9), 30.

Taylor, C., Lillis, C., & LeMone, P. (2001). *Fundamentals of nursing: The art and science of nursing care* (4th ed.). Philadelphia: Lippincott.

Taylor, E. (2002). *Spiritual care.* Upper Saddle River, NJ: Prentice Hall Health.

Thacker, S. B., Stroup, D., & Chang, M. (2002). Continuous electronic heart rate monitoring for fetal assessment during labor. *The Cochrane Library*, 1.

Thelan, L., Urden, L., Lough, M., & Stacy, K. (1998). *Critical care nursing* (3rd ed.). St. Louis: Mosby.

Thompson, J. (2000, November). A practical ostomy guide. *RN, 63*(1), 61–68.

Thompson, J., et al. (2002). *Mosby's Manual of Clinical Nursing* (5th ed.). St. Louis: Mosby.

Thurlow, Kate. (2001, June). Latex allergies: Management and clinical responsibilities. *Home Healthcare Nurse, 24*(6), p. 369.

Tiernan, P. J. (1994, October). Independent nursing interventions: Relaxation and guided imagery in critical care. *Critical Care Nursing, 14*(5), 47–51.

Tierney, K., Lindell, M., & Perry, R. (2001). *Facing the unexpected: Disaster preparedness and response in the U.S.* Joseph Henry Press.

Tierney, L., et al. (Ed.). (2002). *Current medical diagnosis and treatment* (30th ed.). New York: Lange Medical Books/McGraw-Hill.

Togger, D., & Brenner, P. (2001, October). Metered dose inhalers. *American Journal of Nursing, 101*(10), 26–32.

Trombley, J. (1996, February). Listen up: Don't trust tympanic thermometers. *Nursing96, 26*(2), 58–59.

Trujillo, E., et al. (2001, April). Feeding critically ill patients: Current concepts. *Critical Care Nurse, 21*(4), 60–67.

UPDATE 96 (1996, September). Heading off brain damage. *Nursing96, 26*(9), 54.

U.S. Department of Agriculture and U.S. Department of Health and Human Services. (1992). *Food guide pyramid—A guide to daily food choices.* Washington, DC: USDA/HNIS.

U.S. Department of Health and Human Services, Public Health Service. (1992, February). *Acute pain management: Operative or medical procedures and trauma.* Pub. No. 920032.

Urben, L., Lough, M., & Stacy, K. (1996). *Priorities in critical care nursing* (2nd ed.). St. Louis: Mosby.

Veenstra, D. L., et al. (1999, March). Efficacy of antiseptic impregnated central venous catheters in preventing catheter related bloodstream infection. *Journal of the American Medical Association, 281*(3), 261.

Walker, B. (1998, May). Preventing falls. *RN, 61*(5), 40–42.

Walsh, S. M., & Banks, L. A. (1990, March). How to insert a small-bore feeding tube safely. *Nursing90, 20*(3), 55–59.

Weaver, S., & Marcus, J. (eds.). (2000). *Dietitian's patient education manual, Vol 2.* Gaithersburg, MD: Aspen Publishers.

Weber, J. (1997). *Nurses' handbook of health assessment* (3rd ed.). Philadelphia: Lippincott Williams & Wilkins.

Weinstein, R. (2001, March–April). Controlling antimicrobial resistance in hospitals: Infection control and use of antibiotics. *Emergency Infectious Diseases Journal, 7*(2).

Weinstein, S. (1997). *Plumer's principles and practice of intravenous therapy* (6th ed.). Philadelphia: Lippincott Williams & Wilkins.

Whaley, L., & Wong, D. (2002). *Nursing care of infants and children* (7th ed.). St. Louis: Mosby.

Whitney, E., Cataldo, C., & Rolfes, S. (2002). *Understanding normal and clinical nutrition* (6th ed.). Belmont, CA: Wadsworth Thomson Learning.

Wigginton, M. (2001, January). Expanded ECGs: Easy As V4, V5, V6. *Nursing 2001, 31*(1), 50–52.

Wilburn, S. (2000, February). Preventing needlesticks in your facility. *American Journal of Nursing, 100*(2), 96.

Wilkinson, J. (2001). *Nursing process and critical thinking approach* (3rd ed.). Redwood City, CA: Addison-Wesley.

Williams, M. (2002). *Nutrition for health, fitness, and sport* (6th ed.). Boston, MA: McGraw-Hill.

Williamson, V. (1997, February). Clinical pathways for a patient with a total joint replacement. *Orthopaedic Nursing, 16*(2), 41–50.

Wilmoth, D., et al. (2001, March). Pulmonary care: Caring for adults with cystic fibrosis. *Critical Care Nurse, 21*(3), 34–44.

Wolfe, S. (1998, August). Look for signs of abuse. *RN*, 61(8), 48–51.

Womac, C., & Thomas, J. (1996, October). Easing the way through an MRI. *RN, 59*(10), 34–37.

Wong, D. (2001). *Whaley and Wong's essentials of pediatric nursing* (6th ed.). St. Louis: Mosby.

Ventura, M. (2000, April). Chemical hazards: How to protect yourself. *RN, 63*(4) 77–80.

Yantis, M., & Nieman, W. (2000, April). Resting easy with PAP therapy. *Nursing 2000, 30*(4), 62–64.

Yocum, F. (2002). Documenting for quality patient care. *Nursing 2002, 32*(8), 58–63.

Zborowski, T. (1992). Cultural components in response to pain. *Journal of Social Issues, 8,* 16–30.

REFERENCES FOUND ON THE INTERNET

American College of Emergency Physicians (2002). NBC Task Force; Office of Emergency Preparedness, Final Report: Resources for Dealing with Stress Brought on by Recent Terrorist Attacks. www.acep.org/Government & Advocacy.

American Hospital Association (2002). Chemical & Biological Terrorism Preparedness Checklist; Policy Forum, Hospital Preparedness for Mass Casualities. www.hospitalconnect.com/ahapolicyforum/resources/disaster.

Association for Professionalism Infection Control and Epidemiology, Inc., Mass Casualty Disaster Plan Checklist: A Template for Healthcare Facilities. www.apic.org/bioterror/checklist.doc.

Army Regulation 40-13 Medical Services. (1985). Medical Support—Nuclear, Chemical Accidents & Incidents. www.cdc.gov/nuclear.

Campbell, A. Improving assessment and decision making in predialysis patients. www.multi-med.com/pdtoday/arto698-6.htm.

Centers for Disease Control and Prevention. AIDS Information: Statistics—Cumulative Cases. www.cdc.gov/nchstp/hiv.cumulati.htm.

Centers for Disease Control and Prevention (2000). Biological & Chemical Terrorism: Strategic Plan for Preparedness and Response. www.cdc.gov/mmwr/preview/mmwrht/rr 4901 al.htm.

Centers for Disease Control and Prevention. Division of HIV/AIDS Prevention, Basic Statistics. www.cdc.gov/hiv/stats.htm.

Centers for Disease Control and Prevention. Emerging Infectious Diseases (2002, September). Preparing at the Local Level for Events Involving Weapons of Mass Destruction. www.cdc.gov/nicdod/EID/vol8no9/01-0520.htm.

Centers for Disease Control and Prevention. Interim Recommendations for the Selection & Use of Protective Clothing & Respirators Against Biological Agents. cdc.gov/niosh/unp-intrecppe. html.

Centers for Disease Control and Prevention. Issues in Healthcare Settings, Part II. Recommendations for Isolation Precautions in Hospitals. cdc.gov/nicdod/hip/isolat/isopart2.htm.

Centers for Disease Control and Prevention. National Center for Infectious Diseases. www.cdc.gov/ncidod/publicat.htm.

Centers for Disease Control and Prevention. National Institute for Occupational Safety and Health. Chemical protective clothing. www.cdc.gov/niosh/npptl/chemprcloth.html.

Centers for Disease Control and Prevention. Office of Communication. CDC Radiation Studies, Nuclear Terrorism & Health Effects. www.cdc.gov/od/oc/media/9-11 pk.html.

Centers for Disease Control and Prevention. Public Health Emergency Preparedness & Response FAQS about Anthrax. www.cdc.gov/documentsapp/faqanthrax.asp#Qr001.

Centers for Disease Control and Prevention. Strategic Planning Workgroup. (2002). Biological & Chemical Terrorism: Strategic Plan for Preparedness Response. www.cdc.gov/mmwr/preview/mmwrhtml/rr 4904al.htm.

Centers for Disease Control and Prevention. Trends. www.cdcnac.org/geneva98/trends/trends_6.htm.

Center for Strategic and International Studies. Combating chemical, biological, radiological, and nuclear terrorism. www.cis.org/home/and/reports contactchembiorad.

Cleveland Clinic Health Information. What you need to know about venous leg ulcers. www.ccf.org/ed/pated/database/docs/0300/0314.htm.

Community Emergency Response Team (CERT). Training: Participant handbook. www.cert-la.com/manuals/tc & intrc.pwf.

Documentation of Wounds. www.uca.edu/glenni/Wounds/wndoc.htm.

Electronic Journal of Biotechnology. (1999). Biological Warfare, bioterrorism, biodefence and the biological antitoxin weapons convention. www.ejb.org/content/vol2/issue 3/full//.

Emergency Weapons of Mass Destruction Responses. (2001). Emergency decontamination triage and treatment. www.2.sbccom.army.mil/hid.

Emerging Infectious Diseases. (1998). Using Nurse Hotline Calls for Disease Surveillance. www.cdc.gov/nicdod/eid/vol4no2/rodman.htm.

Federal Emergency Management Agency. (FEMA). 2001. Federal Response Plan-ESF#8. www.fema.gov/rrr/frpesf8.shtm.

Guidance for Radiation Accident Management. (2002). Managing radiation emergencies. www.orau.gove/reacts/dyndrome.htm.

Guidance for Radiation Accident Management. (2002). Oak Ridge Associated Universities Basics of Radiation Safety Around Radiation Sources. www.orau.gov/reacts/guidance.htm.

Hepatitis Foundation International On-Line. Hepatitis statistics. www://hepfi.org/stats.htm.

Hill, G., et al. Peritoneal dialysis. www.Bgsm.edu/nursing/monitor/1996/SEP-OCT/sep-oct2.htm.

Holter Monitor. Austin Heart. www.austinheart.com/tm_hlt.htm.

Hospital Infection Control Practices Advisory Committee, CDC Issues in Healthcare Settings. Evolution of isolation practices. www.cdc.gov/ncidod/hip/isolat/isopart/htm.

IV Nurses' Society Standards. www.ins1.org.

JCAHO Standards, Security Management Plan. Occupational Safety & Health Administration. (1999, April). Technical information—rubber latex gloves & other natural rubber products. www.osha.gov/as/opa/fol9/TIB 19990412-html.

National Center for HIV, STD, and TB Prevention. Division of HIV/AIDS Prevention. www.cdc.gov/hiv/stats.htm.

OSHA. www.osha.gov/.

Principles of peritoneal dialysis. Fresnius Medical Care. www.fmc-ag.com/daily/pdp_over.htm.

Public Health Service Guidelines for the Management of Health-Care Worker Exposures to HIV and Recommendations for Postexposure Prophylaxis. (1998, May). Reprinted from MMWR Recommendations and Reports. *47*(RR-7). Medical UCSF. http://insite.ucsf.edu/medical/tx_guidelines/2098.3bb2.html.

Recommendations for Chemical Protective Clothing Database. www.cdc.gov/niosh/nepc/ncpc2.html.

Smallpox and Smallpox Vaccines: Adverse Reactions—Thinktwice, Smallpox. www.thinktwice.com/smallpox.htm.

Spiritual Assessment Tool. (1998, June). *American Journal of Nursing, 98*(6). www.nursingcenter.com.

University of Iowa Gerontological Nursing Intervention Center. (1999). Acute pain management. www.guideline.gov/VIEWS/summary.

Weapons of Mass Destruction, Information for EMS First Responders, www.oswegocountyems.org/WMD%20sheet%2ohtml.html.

Wong-Baker (2000). Choosing a FACES Pain Scale, Revised. www.painsourcebook.ca/pdfs/pps92.

Wound Care Communication Network at Springhouse Co. First Annual OR–Acquired Pressure Ulcer Symposium: Highlights and Supplement. www.woundcarenet.com/ulcer_symp98/highlights.htm.

www.acestar.uthscsa.edu Evidence-based practice.

www.artificialeye.net/tears. Artificial eye information.

www.asahq.org/NEWSLETTERS. CDC publishes new guidelines for prevention of intravascular device–related infections.

www.cbhd.org/resources. Advance directives and "Do Not Resuscitate" orders.

www.fda.g.v/cdrh. A guide to bed safety, October 11, 2000.

www.hcfa.gov. Patients' rights, physical restraint, guide for monitoring and evaluating patients in restraints.

www.nap.edu/readingroom. Cultural diversity in decision making about care at the end of life.

www.c.nih.gov/nursing. SOP: Management of the patient in restraints.

INDEX

Page numbers followed by f indicate figure; those followed t indicate table.

A

A-V fistula [*See* Arteriovenous (AV) fistula]
Abdomen
  anatomy of, 295f
  assessment, 295–99
    bowel sounds, 296
    general contour, 296
    gerontologic considerations, 319
    newborns, 310
    in obstetrical assessment, 303
    pediatric, 316
    urinary tract, 297–98
Abdominal binder, applying, 842, 842f
Abducens nerve, 283t
Abduction
  defined, 349, 351, 1096
  range of motion exercises for, 355t, 356t
ABG [*See* Arterial blood gases (ABGs)]
Abortion, defined, 308
Above-the-knee amputation (AKA), defined, 1096
Abrasions, 182t, 195
Abscess, defined, 661
Absorption
  defined, 516
  of medications, 517
  in small intestines, 758
  urinary system and, 700, 701t
  of water, 701t
Abuse
  child, 312, 316
  elder, 1258
Accelerations, in fetal monitoring, 934
Acceptance, defined, 66
Accessory nerve, 283t
Acid–base imbalance
  arterial blood gases (ABGs) associated with, 1221t
  etiology, 1220t
Acidosis
  arterial blood gases (ABGs) associated with, 1221t
  defined, 871
  etiology, 1220t
Acknowledgment, in therapeutic communication, 68
ACLS (*See* Advanced Cardiac Life Support)
Acme, in fetal monitoring, 934
Acne, defined, 161
Acoustic nerve, 283t
Acquired immunodeficiency syndrome (AIDS), 385–87 [*See also* Human immunodeficiency virus (HIV)]
  defined, 385
  epidemiology, 385
  home health care, 1262–63
Activated charcoal, 607
Acuity levels, staffing requirements and, 57
Acuity system, defined, 34
Acupressure, 466, 474
Acupuncture, 474, 502
Acute radiation syndromes, 441–42
Adaptation
  age and, 130
  alcohol and, 131
  anxiety and, 131
  characteristics that influence, 130–31
  defined, 85, 129, 130, 195, 1139
  stress adaptation syndrome, 466, 496, 497f
Adaptive reaction, defined, 466, 495
Addictive, defined, 516
Adduction
  defined, 349, 351, 1096
  range of motion exercises for, 355t, 356t
Adhesions, defined, 812
Adjunctive, defined, 1206
Adjuvant analgesic drugs, defined, 1184
Admission, 85–87, 91
  documentation, 94
  elective, 162
  emergency, 86–87
  equipment, 91
  forms for, 88f
  gerontologic considerations, 102
  to hospital, 85–86
  nursing diagnosis, 89
  to nursing unit, 86–87
  protocol, 86, 91
Admission assessment, 86
Admit, defined, 85
Adrenergics, 1231
Advance medical directives, 9–10, 9f
  durable power of attorney for health care, 10
  end-of-life care and, 1194
  living will, 10
Advanced Cardiac Life Support (ACLS), 964–67, 1225
Advanced nursing skills, 1205–44
  arterial blood pressure monitoring, 1217–24
  cardiac emergencies, 1225–34
  cultural considerations, 1208
  documentation, 1215, 1223, 1233, 1240
  gerontologic considerations, 1242
  hemodynamic monitoring, 1207–8, 1218
  mechanical ventilation, 1235–42
  overview, 1207–8
  pulmonary artery pressure monitoring, 1209–16
Adventitious, defined, 871
Advice giving, in communication, 69
Aerobe, defined, 625, 812
Aerobic wound culture, 655–56, 655f
Aerosol, defined, 414
Affect, assessment of, 301
Afterload, defined, 1206
Against medical advice (AMA) discharge, 101
Age (*See also* Children; Gerontologic considerations)
  and adaptation, 130
  influence on vital signs, 236–37
Agitation, defined, 66, 1184
AIDS [*See* Acquired immunodeficiency syndrome (AIDS); Human immunodeficiency virus (HIV)]
Airborne, defined, 414
Airborne precautions, 283, 384t
Airway, artificial (*See* Artificial airways)
Airway obstruction
  cardiopulmonary resuscitation (CPR)
    for adults, 964, 965f, 966
    for children, 968–69
  Heimlich maneuver for, 971–72, 972f, 973f
  signs of, 972
AKA (above-the-knee amputation), defined, 1096
Alarm reaction stage, of stress, 496, 497t
Albuminuria, defined, 625, 699
Alcohol, and adaptation, 131
Aldosterone
  in fluid balance, 996
  in urine output, 702
Alginate, 859t
Alignment
  defined, 323, 349, 1096
  establishing body, 327, 327f
  maintaining body, 328, 328f
Alimentary, defined, 576
Alkalosis
  arterial blood gases (ABGs) associated with, 1221t
  defined, 871
  etiology, 1220t
Allen's test, 643, 1206, 1218
Allergy
  defined, 516, 661
  latex
    food allergies related to, 596
    management, 395–96, 395f
Alleviate, defined, 466, 495
Alternative medicine, 501 [*See also* Complementary/alternative medicine (CAM)]
Ambiance, defined, 129
Ambient temperature, defined, 786
Ambulance, defined, 129
Ambulation, 352, 360–66
  assistive devices for, 352
  with cane, 364–65, 364f–365f
  defined, 323, 349
  documentation, 366
  falls and, 336f, 363

following surgery, 362
gerontologic considerations, 373–74
minimizing orthostatic hypotension, 361
nursing diagnosis, 353
with one assistant, 362–63, 363f
with two assistants, 361, 362f
with walker, 364, 364f
Ambulatory, defined, 85
American Heart Association (AHA) Guidelines for Life Support, 967
American Hospital Association (AHA), Patient's Bill of Rights, 86–87
American Nurses Association (ANA), standards of practice, 5, 5f
Amino acids, 579–80
Amniocentesis
assisting with, 694
defined, 661
purpose of, 689t
Amnioinfusion, in fetal monitoring, 934
Amniotic fluid, assessment of, 305
Ampule
opening, 553, 553f
withdrawing medication from, 553, 553f
Amputation, 1100–1101
defined, 1096
phantom pain in, 1100
postoperative care, 1124
preoperative care, 1124
shrinking and molding stump, 1125, 1125f
Anabolism, defined, 576
Anaerobe, defined, 812
Anaerobic, defined, 625
Anaerobic wound culture, 656
Anal fissure, defined, 756
Analgesia, defined, 1139
Analgesic, defined, 1139
Anaphylaxis, defined, 516, 994
Anemia, defined, 699
Anesthesia
defined, 516, 1139
postanesthesia care unit (PACU), 1171–75
Anesthesia bed, defined, 160
Anger, defined, 1184
Angina, defined, 466
Angioplasty, 670
transluminal coronary, 670
Anions, 996
Anisocoria, 284
Ankle, range of motion for, 356t
Ankle-brachial index (ABI), 838, 840
Anorexia, defined, 576, 1184
Antagonists, defined, 349
Antepartum assessment, 303–4
Anthrax, 424t–425t, 428–28, 448–49
Anthropometric measurements, 582t
Antiarrhythmics
in cardiac emergencies, 1231, 1231t
defined, 994
Antibacterial, defined, 195
Antibacterial immune mechanisms, infection risk with, 380–81
Antibiotics
defined, 699
in wound care, 835
Antibody, defined, 377
Anticoagulant, defined, 195
Antidiuretic hormone (ADH)
in fluid balance, 996
in urine output, 702
Antidiuretics, defined, 699, 994
Antidote, defined, 414
Antiembolic stockings, defined, 933
Antiemetic, defined, 661
Antimicrobials
defined, 377, 414, 625, 812
in wound care, 835
Antimicrobic, defined, 625, 994, 1045
Antipyretics
defined, 234, 786
for fever, 789
Antiseptics
defined, 377
waterless gel, 378, 392f, 393
in wound care, 835
Anuria, defined, 699
Anxiety (*See also* Stress)
adaptation and, 131
assessment, 301
defined, 66, 495, 1139, 1184
preoperative, 1141–42, 1141t
Aortic valve sounds, 294
Apathy, defined, 495
Apex, defined, 234
Apgar scoring system, for newborns, 311, 311t
Apical pulse, 235, 238
assessment of, 252–53, 252f, 253f, 295
defined, 235
irregular, 295
in neurologic assessment, 281, 281f
Apical–radial pulse, 253–54, 254f
Apnea, 235, 259t, 871
Apocrine glands, 286, 286f
Apothecary equivalents, 574t
Appendicular skeleton, defined, 323
Apprehension, defined, 66, 495
Aquathermic pad, applying, 794–95, 794f, 795f
Arcus senilis, 284
Aromatherapy, 503
Arrhythmia (*See also* Dysrhythmia)
defined, 466
Arterectomy, laser, 670
Arterial blood, collection of, 643
Arterial blood gases (ABGs), 874
assessment of, 281
association with acid–base imbalance, 1221t
gerontologic considerations, 318
normal values, 874
pulse oximetry for, 889
Arterial blood pressure monitoring, 1217–24
assisting with insertion, 1219
blood samples, 1221–22, 1221f
catheter removal, 1222
monitoring arterial blood pressure, 1219–20, 1220f
overview, 1218
performing Allen's test, 1218
Arterial pulse rate, 239
Arterial ulcer, 816–17, 840
Arteriography
defined, 661
preparation for, 669
purpose of, 666t
Arteriosclerosis, defined, 234
Arteriovenous, defined, 699
Arteriovenous (AV) fistula, 699
for hemodialysis, 747, 747f
assessment, 748
safety precautions, 747
Arthritis, defined, 466
Arthrogram, defined, 1139
Arthroplasty, 1099–1100, 1127–31
defined, 1096
hip, 1128–29
knee, 1130–31
Arthroscopy
client education for, 1154–55
defined, 1139
preparation for, 683
purposes of, 683t, 1154
Artificial airways, 875, 897–902 (*See also* Intubation)
documentation, 901
endotracheal tube
care for, 900
extubating, 901
intubation, 899–900, 899f
nasopharyngeal airway, 898, 898f
oropharyngeal airway, 898, 898f
Artificial eye, care of, 227–28, 227f
Ascites, defined, 994
Asepsis
defined, 377, 625, 812, 1139
medical (*See* Handwashing; Medical asepsis)
surgical, 14, 378
in wound care, 816
Aseptic, defined, 129, 516
Aseptic technique (*See also* Medical asepsis; Surgical asepsis)
defined, 377
Aspirate, defined, 516, 576, 994, 1045
Aspiration, defined, 195, 576, 625
Aspiration risk, in enteral feeding, 611, 613
Assessment (*See also* Physical assessment)
abdomen, 295–99
admission, 86
basic nursing, 13–14
of blood pressure (*See* Blood pressure)
body temperature (*See* Body temperature)
breast (*See* Breast)
chest, 288–95
circulatory system, 938
in client care plan, 35
critical thinking and, 25–26
defined, 85, 106, 129, 161
eyes (*See* Eyes)
genitourinary system, 297–99
head and neck, 282–86
health history, 273
of heart, 289, 293–95

Assessment *(continued)*
in home health care, 1249
for elder abuse, 1258
of home, 1256–57
nutritional, 1278–79
mental (*See* Mental assessment)
musculoskeletal system, 14, 316–17, 320
neurologic (*See* Neurologic assessment)
of newborn (*See* Newborns)
in nursing process, 22, 23f
obstetrics, 302–8
pain (*See* Pain assessment)
pediatric, 311–17
respiratory system, 14, 874–75
skin, 181–82
spiritual, 299
Assessment-intervention-response (AIR) charting, 45, 45f
Assistance, defined, 66
Assistive devices, for ambulation, 352
cane, 364–65, 364f–365f
crutches, 367–72 (*See also* Crutch walking)
walker, 364, 364f
Assumptions, in communication, 69
Asterixis, 276
Ataraxia, defined, 495
Ataxic breathing, 280
ATC (around the clock), defined, 466
Atelectasis, defined, 871, 1139
Atherosclerosis, defined, 234, 933
Athetoid movements, 276
Athlete's foot, 196
AtLast Blood Glucose System, for blood glucose testing, 645–46, 645f
Atrial, defined, 234
Atrial fibrillation, defined, 235
Atrial gallop, 294
Atrioventricular (AV) node, 935–36
Atrophy, defined, 349
AT&T Language Line Services, 116
Auditory acuity, assessment, 285, 285f
Auscultation
defined, 871
lungs, 289, 292, 292f
in physical assessment, 273–74, 274f
Autistic, 300
Autogenic training, 505
defined, 466
Autoimmunization, defined, 466
Autoinfections, defined, 377
Autolet, defined, 625
Autologous, defined, 994
Automated dispensing system, using, 524–25, 525f
Automated external defibrillator (AED), 938–39
AHA (American Heart Association), guidelines for, 939
in children, 939
with CPR, 967
using, 970–71, 970f–971f
Autonomic nervous system
control of pulse, 238
defined, 466, 495
Autoregulation
defined, 234
of pulse, 238
Autotransfusion, using Pleur-evac ATS, 925–26, 925f
Awareness, assessment, 301
Axial skeleton, defined, 323
Axilla, defined, 234
Axillary temperature, using digital thermometer, 245
Ayurveda, 503
Azotemia, defined, 699
AZT, defined, 377

B

B vitamins, heart disease risk and, 585
Babinski response, 279, 279f
Back care, 161, 189–90, 190f
Bacteria, defined, 625, 756
Bactericidal, defined, 699
Bacteriostatic, defined, 377
Bacteriuria, 381
Bag–valve–mask ventilation, 881, 881f, 969, 969f
Balance, defined, 323, 349
Balanced suspension, defined, 1096
Balkan overbed frame, 160
Bandage
figure-eight, 1104–5, 1105f
spiral, 1104, 1104f
Barium, defined, 661
Barium studies, 663, 679–81
enema, 680, 680t
small bowel follow-through, 681
swallow, 680–81, 680t
Baroreceptors, 238
Barotrauma, defined, 1206
Barrier nursing, defined, 377
Base of support, defined, 323, 349
Basic life support [*See* Cardiopulmonary resuscitation (CPR)]
Basic nursing assessment, 13–14
Bath
sitz, 796, 796f
tepid, 803, 803f
Bath care, 162–63, 172–78
adults, 174, 175f, 176f
body cleansing systems, 162–63, 176–77
cultural considerations, 175
disposable systems, 162–63, 176–77
documentation, 178
gerontologic considerations, 192
in home health, 1269–70
hydraulic bathtub chair, 178
infant, 177
morning care, 173
therapeutic effect of, 163
types of, 161, 163
washcloth mitt, 173, 173f
Bathtub chair, hydraulic, 178
Battery, defined, 54
Battle's sign, 285
Bedmaking, 165–71
documentation, 171
in home health, 1271
mitered corner, 166, 166f
occupied, 169–71, 170f
pillow case, 166, 166f
sheets for, 160
surgical, 169, 169f
unoccupied, 166–68, 167f–168f
Bedpan
assisting with Stryker frame, 1134
using, 217, 217f
Beds, 133
anesthesia, 160
closed, 160
equipment for, 160
occupied, 160
open, 160
positions for client care, 334, 334f
specialty beds, 162, 184f, 185f, 186t
support surfaces, 162, 184f
types of, 162
Bedside computer-assisted charting, 48, 501
Bedside table, 133
Behavior, defined, 66, 85, 129, 466
Behavioral responses, to stress, 497, 498t
Below-the-knee amputation (BKA), defined, 1096
Belt restraint, 148, 148f
Benzodiazepines, 1168
Best practice, *vs.* evidence-based practice, 30
BID, defined, 195
Bigeminal pulse, defined, 235
Bigeminal pulse rate, 235, 251t
Bile, 584, 757
Biofeedback, 466, 474, 503
Biohazards, 134, 386
defined, 377, 386
disposal precautions, 399
double-bagging, 406–7, 407f
soiled linens, 384
storage, 386
transport, 386
Biologic rhythms (*See* Circadian rhythms)
Bio-occlusive dressing, 854
Biopsies, 664
liver
assisting with, 690, 690f
purpose of, 689t
Biorhythms (*See* Circadian rhythms)
Bioterrorism
agents
anthrax, 424t–425t, 428–28
botulism, 424t–425t, 430
identification, 428–33
pneumonic plague, 424t–425t, 429–30
Q fever, 431
ricin toxin, 432
smallpox, 424t–425t, 432–33 (*See also* Smallpox)
types of, 422–24, 424t
typhoid tularemia, 424t–425t, 430–31
viral hemorrhagic fevers (VHF), 424t–425t, 431
Centers for Disease Control and Prevention (CDC) strategic plan for response, 416–18
decontamination, 451
defined, 414
documentation, 442

infection control, 445
personal protective equipment, 448–49
public policy, 416–18
standard precautions, 446
transporting specimens, 438–39, 439f
Bioterrorism Act, 416–17
Biotransformation, defined, 516
Biot's breathing, 235, 259t, 280
BIPAP, 1237 (*See also* CPAP/BIPAP)
Bipolar leads, defined, 1206
BKA (below-the-knee amputation), defined, 1096
Black wounds, 814, 815t
Bladder, 700
age-related changes, 319
distention, 298
estimating fullness of, 714
in newborns, 310
Bladder irrigation, 726–30
in closed system, 728–29, 729f
continuous, 729–30, 729f
documentation, 730
by opening closed system, 727–28, 727f, 728f
Bladder scanner, using, 713–14
Blanching, defined, 161
Bland therapeutic diet, 592
Bleeding (*See also* Hemorrhage)
controlling, 942–44
digital pressure, 943, 943f
pressure dressing, 943
pulse points for, 943f
signs and symptoms of, 939t
triage, 459
Blink reflex, 279
Blood, directed donation of, 994
Blood-borne pathogens, 384
Blood components, 1037, 1039t
Blood glucose testing, 644–49
AtLast Blood Glucose System, 645–46, 645f
capillary puncture, 645, 645f
Chemstrips, 645–46, 645f
Glucometer, 646
Lifescan one-touch II, 647–49, 648f
principles of, 644
Sure Step Flexx, 646–47, 647f
Blood pressure, 236, 240–42, 935
arterial blood pressure monitoring, 1217–24
assessment of
body position for, 264
continuous noninvasive monitoring, 267, 267f
direct measurement, 241
documentation, 267
evaluation frequency, 263
flush method, 266
frequency, 241
indirect measurement, 241
lower-extremity, 265–66, 266f
procedure, 262–64, 265f
systolic arterial, 265, 265f
children, 239t, 243, 312
factors that influence, 240–41
gerontologic considerations, 269, 318
Korotkoff's sounds, 241–42, 262–63
measurement of, 241–42
in neurologic assessment, 281
in newborns, 237
normal, 241
during pregnancy, 303
pulmonary artery pressure monitoring, 1209–16
Blood pressure cuffs, 262, 262f
Blood specimen collection, 627, 640–49
arterial blood, 643
blood glucose, 644–49
AtLast Blood Glucose System, 645–46, 645f
capillary puncture, 645, 645f
Chemstrips, 645–46, 645f
Glucometer, 646
Lifescan one-touch II, 647–49, 648f
principles of, 644
Sure Step Flexx, 646–47, 647f
central vascular access devices (CVAD), 1055–56, 1056f
Groshong catheter, 1078
implanted subcutaneous ports, 1084–85, 1084f
peripherally inserted central catheter (PICC), 1090
tunneled, 1078
color-identified test tubes for, 627
for culture, 644
vacutainer system, 641–42, 642f
venous blood, 641
Blood transfusions, 1033–40
administering components, 1037, 1039t
complications of, 1037, 1038t
cultural considerations, 1036, 1159
protocol, 1037
through a straight line, 1036
through a Y-set, 1034–36, 1034f, 1035f
warming blood for, 1034
Blood type, 1034, 1037
Blood viscosity, in blood pressure, 241
Blood volume
in blood pressure, 241
urine output and, 702
Bloodstream infection
catheter-related, 994, 1051
defined, 994
infusate-related, 994
Bloody show, 305
Board of Registered Nursing (BRN)
functions of, 5
liability and legal issues, 5–6
state, on delegation, 57
Body alignment
establishing, 327, 327f
maintaining, 328, 328f
Body fluid analysis, 664, 688–94
assisting with
amniocentesis, 694
bone marrow aspiration, 693
lumbar puncture, 689–90, 690f
Papanicolaou (PAP) smear, 693
paracentesis, 692, 692f
thoracentesis, 691, 691f
Body language, 66, 68–69
Body mass index
gerontologic considerations, 620–21
recommended range, 578
Body mechanics, 324–31
back injuries of nurses, 325
basic principles, 329, 329f, 330f, 331
body alignment
establishing, 327, 327f
maintaining, 328, 328f
client falls and, 336f, 363
defined, 323
documentation, 331
guidelines for, 325
in home health care, 1265–67
nursing diagnosis, 325
using coordinated movements, 329, 329f
Body substance isolation (BSI), 382 (*See also* Standard precautions)
Body temperature, 243–49
ambient, 786
assessment of, 238
axillary, 245, 247
in children, 246–47
ear canal, 238
in elderly, 236–37
in newborns, 236, 246–47, 247t
oral, 238, 244–24f
rectal, 238, 246–47
tympanic, 247–48, 247f
using digital thermometer, 244–45, 244f
using electronic thermometer, 245–46, 246f
using heat-sensitive tape, 238, 248, 248f
using infrared thermometer, 247–48, 247f
in children, 246–47, 311
control of
adjustment processes, 787–88
heat transfer, 788
core, 234, 237
documentation, 248
gerontologic considerations, 236–37, 269, 808
hyperthermia, 789
hypothermia, 789–90
inflammatory processes and, 788–90
in neurologic assessment, 281
regulatory mechanisms of, 237
in sensory function assessment, 280
variations in, 238
Body water, 995
Bolus, defined, 994, 1206
Bone cells, 324
Bone densitometry
defined, 661
preparation for, 670–71
purpose of, 666t
Bone marrow aspiration
assisting with, 693
purpose of, 689t
Bone scan
preparation for, 675
purpose of, 675t
Bone(s), 324
alterations in, 324
of skull, 282f

Booster dose, defined, 466
Botulism, 424t–425t, 430, 449
Bounding pulse, defined, 235
Bounding pulse rate, 235, 239, 251t
Bowel
  defined, 756
  obstruction of the lumen of, 579–760
Bowel elimination, 755–84
  alterations in, 759–61
    circulatory deficiencies, 760
    motility, 759
    obstruction, 759–60
    surgical alterations, 760–61 (*See also* Stoma)
  bowel evacuation, 763–67
  colostomy care, 1282–83, 1286–87
  cultural considerations, 762
  documentation, 767, 774, 781
  enema administration, 768–74
  gerontologic considerations, 782
  in home health care, 1282–83
  ostomy pouch application, 775–81, 777f–80f
Bowel evacuation, 763–67
  bowel training, 765
  digital stimulation, 764–65
  documentation, 767
  removing fecal impaction, 764
  suppository administration, 766–67, 766f
Bowel obstruction, 759–60
Bowel sounds, assessment, 296
Bowel training, 765
BPM (beats per minute), in fetal monitoring, 934
Brachial plexus, defined, 323
Braden Scale, for pressure ulcers, 853t
Brady, defined, 466
Bradycardia
  causes of, 239
  defined, 235, 259t, 295, 466, 871
  fetal, 306, 934, 986
Bradypnea, defined, 235
Brain
  anatomy of, 787f
  lobes of, 282, 283f
  segments of, 282, 283f
Brain stem, 282
Breast, assessment of, 289, 291–92, 292f
  in obstetrical assessment, 302
  in pediatric assessment, 315
  postpartum, 307
Breath sounds
  assessment of, 292f, 293, 293f
  bronchial, 293
  bronchovesicular, 293
  vesicular, 293
Breathing (*See also* Respirations)
  deep, 474, 504–5
    instruction for, 877, 877f, 1155
    in stress management, 510–11
  depth of, 240
  evaluation of pattern, 240
  normal rates, 240
  phases of, 240
Breathing pattern, evaluation of, 240
Bronchial breath sounds, 293
Bronchiectasis, defined, 871
Bronchitis, defined, 1139
Bronchodilatation, defined, 516
Bronchoscopy
  defined, 661, 1139
  preparation for, 683–84
  purpose of, 683t
Bronchovesicular breath sounds, 293
Broviac catheter
  changing dressing, 1076
  maintaining, 1075, 1075f
Brucellosis, 449
Bryant's traction, 1096, 1099, 1116t
BSI (bloodstream infection)
  catheter-related, 994, 1051
  defined, 994
  infusate-related, 994
Buck's traction, 1096, 1099, 1115f, 1116t

C

Calcium
  increased therapeutic diet, 591
  restricted therapeutic diet, 590
Calibrate, defined, 1206
Calorie(s)
  defined, 576, 1045
  nutritional recommendations, 581
Calyx, defined, 699
Cancer
  colon, 288, 761
  skin, 288
Candidiasis, of the mouth, 286
Cane, ambulation with, 364–65, 364f–365f
Cannula, defined, 625
Cannulation, defined, 1206
Canthus, defined, 195
Capillary, defined, 195
Capillary puncture, for blood glucose testing, 645, 645f
Caput, 306
Carbohydrate(s), 578–79
  defined, 576, 1045
  nutritional recommendations, 579
  therapeutic diet restricting, 589
(carbon dioxide) CO_2, in respiration process, 873
Cardiac catheterization
  preparation for, 670
  procedures done during, 670
  purpose of, 666t
Cardiac compensation, 935
Cardiac emergencies, 1225–34
  cardiopulmonary resuscitation (CPR)
    adults, 964, 964f, 965f, 966–67
    for children, 968–69
  cardioversion, 1226, 1231–32, 1232t
  "crash cart," 1226–27, 1226f, 1227f, 1228f
  defibrillation, 1226, 1228–30, 1229f, 1230f
  documentation, 1233
  medication administration, 1230–31, 1230f, 1231f
Cardiac index (CI), defined, 1206
Cardiac muscle, properties of, 934–35
Cardiac output
  defined, 234, 240, 1206
  gerontologic considerations, 990
  low, 1206
  normal, 239
  pulmonary artery pressure monitoring for, 1215
Cardinal signs (*See* Vital signs)
Cardio, defined, 234, 576, 994, 1045
Cardiogenic, defined, 234
Cardiology scan, nuclear
  common tests in, 676
  preparation for, 676–77
  purpose of, 675t
Cardiopulmonary resuscitation (CPR), 938
  administering, 964, 964f, 965f, 966–67
  airway, 964
  barrier devices, 966
  for children, 968–69
  circulation, 966–67
  Do Not Resuscitate (DNR) order and, 10
  end-of-life care and, 1193
  protocol, 964
  rescue breathing, 966
Cardiovascular, defined, 349, 466, 576, 933, 994, 1045
Cardiovascular system (*See also* Circulatory system)
  assessment of, 14
Cardioversion, synchronized, 1226, 1231–32, 1232t
Cardioverter-defibrillator, implantable, 1298–99
Care conference, 55
Care plan, 11–12, 12f, 13f (*See also* Client care plan)
  defined, 34
Carina, defined, 576
Caring, defined, 85
Carminative, defined, 756
Carrier, defined, 377
Cartilage, defined, 323
Cast care, 1098
  assessing casted extremity, 1111–12, 1111f
  caring for wet cast, 1110–11, 1110f
  client education, 1112
  documentation, 1113
  plaster of Paris, 1098, 1110f
  removal of, 1112–13, 1112f
  synthetic, 1098, 1110f
Catabolism, defined, 576
Cataract, 284
Cathartic, defined, 756
Catheter
  central line [*See* Central vascular access devices (CVAD)]
  dual-lumen dialysis, 749–50, 750f
  Foley, 699
  Groshong, 1047, 1076–78, 1077f
  Hickman, 1075–76
  midline, 1046
  over-the-needle, 1006–9, 1007f, 1008f
  peripheral, 1046
  suctioning, 904–7, 905f, 906f
  urinary (*See* Urinary catheterization)

Catheter-related bloodstream infection, 994, 1051
Catheterization
cardiac, 666t, 670
central line [*See also* Central vascular access devices (CVAD)]
condom catheter, 709, 709f
defined, 661, 699
retention catheter
females, 717, 717f–19f, 720
males, 721–22, 721f
self-catheterization, 1282, 1283–84
straight catheter
for females, 714–15, 715f
for males, 716–17, 716f
suprapubic catheter care, 732–34, 733f, 1284
total parenteral nutrition (TPN), 1064–66, 1064f
urinary (*See* Urinary catheterization)
Cations, 996
Cecostomy, 760
Cell-mediated immunity, defined, 377
Celsius, Fahrenheit *vs.*, 238, 245t
Center of gravity, defined, 323
Centers for Disease Control and Prevention (CDC)
functions of, 414
strategic plan for bioterrorism response, 416–18
Centesis, defined, 661
Centigrade, Fahrenheit *vs.*, 238, 245t
Central vascular access devices (CVAD), 1044–94
applying BIOPATCH, 1057, 1057f
assisting catheterization, 1050–51
changing cap, 1058
changing dressing, 1051–52, 1052f
client selection for, 1047
complications of, 1088
air embolism, 1053
at site, 1053
defined, 1045
documentation, 1068, 1072, 1078, 1091
drawing blood, 1055–56, 1056f
gerontologic considerations, 1092
implanted subcutaneous ports, 1047, 1080–85
accessing and flushing using Huber needle, 1081–82, 1081f, 1082f
drawing blood, 1084–85, 1084f
infusions, 1083–84, 1083f–1084f
medication administration, 1082–83, 1082f
infection from, 1051
infusing fluids, 1053, 1054f–55f
lipid emulsion therapy, 1070–73
maintenance of, 1058t
monitoring central venous pressure, 1059–60, 1059f, 1060f
nursing diagnosis, 1048
overview, 1046–47
percutaneous central vascular catheters, 1049–62
peripherally inserted central catheter (PICC), 1047, 1086–91
changing dressing, 1088–89, 1088f, 1089f
defined, 1046
drawing blood, 1090
maintaining, 1087, 1087f
removing, 1090
site preparation, 1050
total parenteral nutrition (TPN), 1047–48, 1063–69
tubing replacement time, 1053
tunneled, 1047, 1074–79
changing dressing, 1076
drawing blood, 1078
flushing, 1077
irrigation protocols, 1077
maintaining, 1075
using Groshong valve, 1076–77, 1077f
Central venous dual-lumen dialysis catheter (DLC), 749–50, 750f
Central venous pressure (CVP), 1059
defined, 1045, 1206
documentation, 1061
monitoring of, 1059–60, 1059f, 1060f
in pulmonary artery pressure monitoring, 1210–11
Cerebellum, function of, 282
Cerebral cortex, 282, 283f, 466, 495
Cerebrospinal fluid, leak, ear, 285
Cerumen, defined, 516
Cervical collar, applying, 1106, 1106f
Chain of infection, 378–79, 379f
Change
barriers to, 108
resistance to, 108
Changing the subject, in communication, 69
Charcoal, activated, 607
Charting, 40–53 (*See also* Documentation)
components of
graphic records, 12–13, 16f
laboratory forms, 13, 18f
medication records, 12, 16f
nurses' notes, 12, 15f
physician's history and physical, 13
physician's orders, 13, 17f
physician's progress notes, 13, 17f
computer-assisted, 34, 42, 48–53, 52f
advantages of, 50f
bedside, 48, 501
disadvantages of, 50f
legal considerations, 51, 53
Nursing Retrieval Guides, 50
DAR format, 42
defined, 34
focus, 34, 42
forensic, 41–42
format for, 41
importance of, 40
Joint Commission on Accreditation of Healthcare Organizations (JCAHO) requirements, 40–41
legal considerations, 40–41, 51, 53
nursing process and, 42
for PRN medications, 41
problem-oriented medical record (POMR), 34, 42, 45–48
advantages of, 49f
components of, 46–48
disadvantages of, 49f
PIE format, 45–46
SOAP format, 34, 42
SOAPIE format, 34, 42
source-oriented, 34, 42
narrative, 43–45, 45f
systems, 43, 43f
systems for, 42–48
variance, 39, 39f
Charting by exception, 34, 42–43
Chemical agent exposure
cyanide agents
identifying exposure, 440
treatment, 441
triage, 440
decontamination, 451–52
documentation, 442
identifying exposure, 439–40
nerve agents
identifying exposure, 440
treatment, 441
triage, 440
personal protective equipment, 450
pulmonary agents
identifying exposure, 439
treatment, 441
triage, 440
treatment, 441
triage, 440
vesicant agents
identifying exposure, 440
treatment, 441
triage, 440
Chemical hazards, 134 (*See also* Chemical agent exposure)
Chemical restraint, defined, 129
Chemical terrorism, 414, 423 (*See also* Chemical agent exposure)
Chemoreceptors
in blood pressure, 241
defined, 234
Chemotaxis, defined, 377
Chemstrips, for blood glucose testing, 645–46, 645f
Chest
assessment, 288–95
breast, 289, 291–92, 292f
general appearance, 290
gerontologic considerations, 318
heart, 289, 293–95
lungs, 289, 292–93
newborns, 309
pediatric, 315
tactile and vocal fremitus, 291
flail, 290
percussion of, 885, 885f
vibration, 875, 885–86, 885f, 886f
Chest drainage system, 921–28
Chest excursion, 290, 291f

Chest physiotherapy (CPT), 883–86
  chest percussion, 885, 885f
  chest vibration, 885–86, 885f, 886f
  client preparation, 884
  documentation, 886
  postural drainage, 884
Chest tubes, 875, 921–28
  autotransfusion using Pleur-evac ATS, 925–26, 925f
  check points for air leaks, 925
  disposable water seal system, 923–25, 924f, 925f
  documentation, 927
  removal, 926–27, 926f
  two-bottle system, 922, 923f
Cheyne-Stokes respirations, 235, 269t, 280
Children (*See also* Pediatric assessment)
  automated external defibrillator (AED), 939
  blood pressure, 239t, 243, 312
  body temperature, 246–47, 311
  cardiopulmonary resuscitation (CPR) for, 968–69
  medication administration, 532
  normal breathing rates, 240
  normal respirations, 259
  oxygen tent, 893t, 894, 894f
  pulse, 239t, 311
  respirations, 239t, 312
  restraints
    elbow, 151, 151f
    mummy, 154–55, 154f
  safety precautions, 137
  total parenteral nutrition (TPN), 1068
  Wong-Baker FACES Rating Scale for pain assessment, 469–70, 469f, 470f
Chiropractic, 503
Choking (*See* Heimlich maneuver)
Cholangiography, defined, 661
Cholecystography
  defined, 661
  preparation for, 667–68
  purpose of, 666t
Choreiform movements, 276
Chronic illness, in elderly, 373
Chronic obstructive pulmonary disease (COPD), 873
Chronotropic reserve, 933, 935
Chyme, 756, 758
Circadian rhythms, influence on vital signs, 237, 245
Circulation, defined, 516, 1096
Circulatory care, in home health, 1295–99
  Holter monitor, 1298
  implantable cardioverter-defibrillator, 1298–99
  nursing diagnosis, 1296
  pacemakers, 1296–98
Circulatory overload, 937
Circulatory system, 932–92
  alterations in, 936–38
    assessment of, 938
    embolism, 938
    heart failure, 937–38
    hemorrhage, 937
    ischemia, 938
    planning and intervention, 939–40
    shock, 937
    signs and symptoms of, 938
    thrombosis, 938
  control of bleeding, 942–44
  control of pulse, 238
  documentation, 944, 950, 961, 975, 981, 989
  electrical conduction in, 935–36
  electrocardiogram (ECG), 936, 952–62
  emergency life support measures, 938–39, 963–75
  fetal monitoring, 940, 983–90
  gerontologic considerations, 990
  maintenance, 945–51
    graduated compression stockings, 946–47, 946f, 947f
    pneumatic compression devices, 947–50, 948f, 949f
  nursing diagnosis, 941
  overview, 934–35
  pacemakers, 936, 977–82
Circumduction
  defined, 349, 351
  range of motion exercises for, 355t, 356t
Civil law, 7
Clarification, in therapeutic communication, 68–69
Clarify, defined, 66
Clean-catch urine specimen, 627, 630
Clean technique, 14
Cleaning procedures, in hospital environment, 133
Cliché, defined, 66
Client acuity systems, 57
Client care, outline for, 11
Client care conference, 55
Client care plan, 4, 11–12, 12f, 13f, 35–39
  activating, 37
  components of, 35–38
  computerized, 38
  defined, 85
  evaluating, 37
  future considerations, 37
  inactivating, 37
  individualized, 35
  interdisciplinary, 35
  standardized, 35, 36f
  types of, 35
  updating, 37
  vs. clinical pathways, 35
  vs. protocols, 39
Client education, 107–9, 113–21
  about hospital setting, 135–36
  charting for, 41
  cultural considerations, 110, 111t
  defined, 106
  diagnostic procedures, 662–63
  documentation, 121
  eye care, 229
  gerontologic considerations, 125
  home health care, 1249
    infection control, 1263–64
    nutrition, 1277
  for IV drug users, 1264
  JCAHO on, 107, 109f
  nuclear scanning, 677
  nursing diagnosis related to, 112
  oral hygiene, 200
  ostomy pouch, 780
  pacemaker, 980
  preoperative care, 1142, 1148–57
    arthroscopy, 1154–55
    deep breathing, 1155
    for family, 1150–51
    in hospital setting, 1149
    laparoscopy, 1153
    laser therapy, 1151, 1151t, 1152t
    leg exercises, 1156
    lithotripsy, 1152–53
    in outpatient setting, 1149
    productive cough, 1155, 1155f
    providing, 1150
    turning in bed, 1156
  pressure ulcers, 817
  process of, 113–21
    assess learning needs, 115–17
    data collection, 113–14
    determining teaching strategy, 117–18
    educational setting, 118
    evaluation, 120
    family assessment, 116
    forms for, 120f
    implementation, 119
  readiness to learn, 108, 115
  resistance to change, 108
  student nurse's role in, 109
  tips for client-focused, 108
  tracheostomy care, 1293–94
  urinary diversion, 740
Client's Bill of Rights, 7, 8f
Client's chart
  graphic records, 12–13, 16f
  laboratory forms, 13, 18f
  medication records, 12, 16f
  nurses' notes, 12, 15f
  physician's history and physical, 13
  physician's orders, 13, 17f
  physician's progress notes, 13, 17f
Client's records, 11–12
  care plan, 11–12, 12f, 13f
  critical or clinical pathway, 12, 14f
  Kardex, 11
Clients' rights, 7–10, 8f
  advance medical directives, 9–10, 9f
  consent issues, 7–8
  Do Not Resuscitate (DNR) order, 10
  HIPPA, 7
  Patient Self-Determination Act, 9
  privacy and confidentiality, 8–9
Clinical pathways, 12, 14f, 38–39, 38f
  defined, 34
  vs. client care plan, 35
Clinical practice, 10–14
  basic nursing assessment, 13–14
  client care, 11
  client's chart, 12–13
  client's records, 11–12
  guidelines for, 10–11
  military time, 11, 11t
Closed bed, defined, 160

Closed fracture, 1097f
Clubbing of fingers, 316
CO_2, in respiration process, 873
"Code"
calling a, 973–74, 974f
care following, 975
crash cart in, 974, 974f
team members, 974
Code of ethics
nurses, 2
student nurses, 2, 3f
Cofactors, defined, 377
Cognition, defined, 66
Cognitively impaired, pain assessment in, 470–71, 481
Cold pack
applying, 799, 799f
chemical instant, 800, 800f
Cold therapy, 790, 798–801
benefits of, 790
chemical instant cold pack, 800, 800f
documentation, 801, 806
gerontologic considerations, 808
ice pack/cold pack, 799, 799f
indications for, 790t
nursing diagnosis, 791
physiologic effects of, 788t
systemic cooling therapies, 802–8
Colitis, defined, 756
Collagen, medical hydrolysate of, 859t
Collagen formation, defined, 812
Colon, 758
defined, 756
Colon cancer, colostomy for, 761
Colonic conduit, 741
Colonization, defined, 377, 994
Colonoscopy
preparation for, 684
purpose of, 683t
Colostomy, 760
compared to ileostomy, 761t
defined, 756
descending, 761
double-barrel, 761
end, 761
irrigation, 761
loop, 761
transverse, 761
Colostomy care
in home health care, 1282–83, 1286–87
irrigation, 761, 1282–83, 1286–87
Comatose clients
eye care, 226
oral hygiene, 202, 202f
Comfort, 85, 137
Comminuted fracture, defined, 1096
Commode, using, 218, 218f
Communicable disease, defined, 414
Communication, 67–70 (*See also* Therapeutic communication)
blocks to, 69–70
charting and, 40–41
with clients, 68
defined, 66, 85
in disaster management, 418–20, 419f, 457–58
gerontologic considerations, 81–82
guidelines for effective, 67–68
with hearing impaired, 77
importance in nursing, 67
multicultural health care and, 70–71
nonverbal, 66, 68–69
process of, 67
relationship therapy, 71–72
therapeutic, 68–69
verbal, 67
Community-based nursing, 1245–99 (*See also* Home health care)
overview, 1246–47
Community Emergency Response Team (CERT), 417, 417f
Compartment syndrome, 1099
Compatible, defined, 516
Competency, consent forms and, 54
Complementary/alternative medicine (CAM), 501–5
acupuncture, 502
applied kinesiology, 502
aromatherapy, 503
Ayurveda, 503
biofeedback, 503
chiropractic, 503
classification of, 502
defined, 495
energy medicine, 503
herbal medicine, 503–4
homeopathy, 504
legal considerations in, 502
massage, 504
naturopathy, 504
nursing diagnosis, 506
nutrition, 504
reflexology, 504
relaxation techniques, 504–5
in stress management, 510–12
T'ai Chi Ch'uan, 505
yoga, 505
Complete bed bath, 160
Complete fracture, 1096
Compliance, defined, 106
Compound fracture, 1096
Comprehensive Drug Abuse Prevention Act of 1970, 6
Comprehensive health care, defined, 106, 129
Compress, defined, 786
Compression fracture, 1096
Compression devices, pneumatic, 947–50, 948f, 949f
Compression stockings, graduated, 938
applying, 946–47, 946f, 947f
effectiveness of, 946, 948
measuring for, 946t
Compression therapy, for venous ulcers, 816, 837
Computed tomography (CT scan)
defined, 661
preparation for, 669–70
purpose of, 666t
xenon, 669–70
Computer-assisted charting, 34, 42, 48–53, 52f
advantages of, 50f
bedside, 48, 501
defined, 34
disadvantages of, 50f
legal considerations, 51, 53
Nursing Retrieval Guides, 50
Condom catheter, 709, 709f
Conduction, 788
defined, 786
Conductivity, defined, 933
Conference, client care, 55
Confidential information, 9
Confidentiality, right to, 8–9
Confusion, defined, 66
Congenital, defined, 195
Congestion, defined, 516, 933
Congruence
defined, 66
in therapeutic communication, 69
Conscious sedation, 1142–43, 1166–75
ASA classification system for, 1169
client care following, 1169
client monitoring, 1168–69
client preparation, 1167
gerontologic considerations, 1180
levels of, 1168
medications for, 1168
risks of, 1143
Consciousness
assessment of, 276–77, 300
defined, 130
Consent, 7–8
at admission, 8
age of, 54–55
defined, 8, 66
implied, 54
for invasive testing, 8
Consent forms, 54–55
at admission, 54
mental competency and, 54
nurse's role, 54
Consistency diets, 592–93
mechanical soft, 592–93
pureed, 593
Constipation, 758–59
acute, 759
chronic, 759
defined, 756
gerontologic considerations, 766
Contact lenses, removing and cleaning, 228–29
Contact precautions, 283, 384t
Contagious disease, defined, 377
Contaminate, defined, 516
Contaminated equipment, 409
Contaminated waste, defined, 129
Contamination, defined, 377, 414, 1139
Continuous ambulatory peritoneal dialysis (CAPD), 1282
administering, 1285–86
defined, 699
dressing change, 1286
transfer sets for, 1285

Continuous cycling peritoneal dialysis (CCPD), 699, 1282
Continuous electronic fetal heart monitoring (EFM), 940, 984
Continuous positive airway pressure (CPAP) (*See* CPAP/BIPAP)
Continuous venovenous hemofiltration (CVVH), defined, 699
Contractility, defined, 234, 349, 933
Contractures, in elderly, 345
Contraindication, defined, 516
Contrast medium, 661, 663
Controlling pain (*See* Pain management)
Contusion, defined, 661, 1096
Convection, 786, 788
Conversion tables, for medication administration
  calculating dosages, 523
  converting dosages, 523
Convey, defined, 66
Cooling blanket, administering, 804–5, 805f, 806f
Cooling therapies, systemic, 802–8
  cooling blanket, 804–5, 805f, 806f
  tepid bath, 803, 803f
Coordination, assessment of, 279
Cope, defined, 1184
Coping mechanisms, 66, 302, 466, 495
  for stress, 509–10
Core temperature, defined, 234
Cornea, defined, 195
Corneal reflex, defined, 1184
Corns, 196
Cough, instruction for productive, 877–78, 878f, 1155, 1155f
Counseling, defined, 66, 106, 1184
CPAP/BIPAP, 875, 1237
  administering, 880–81, 880f
CPM machine (*See* Pneumatic compression device, 947)
Crackles, 292
  defined, 871
Cranial nerves, 282
  assessment of, 283t
  function of, 283t
Craniotomy, defined, 661
"Crash cart," 974, 974f
  checking contents, 1227, 1227f, 1228f
  maintaining, 1226–27, 1226f
Crepitus, defined, 661
Criminal law, 7
Criminal negligence, 6
Crisis, defined, 1184
Critical or clinical path, 38–39, 38f
  vs. client care plan, 35
Critical or clinical pathway, 12, 14f
Critical thinking
  competencies for, 24–25
  defined, 24
  nursing process and, 24–27
    assessment, 25–26
    evaluation, 27
    implementation, 27
    nursing diagnosis, 26
    outcome identification, 26–27
  skills for, 25
Crutch walking, 367–72
  documentation, 372
  four-point gait, 369, 369f
  measuring for, 368, 368f
  moving in and out of chair, 372
  muscle-strengthening for, 368
  on stairs, 371, 371f
  swing-through gait, 370, 370f
  swing-to gait, 370, 370f
  three-point gait, 369, 369f
  two-point gait, 370, 370f
Crutches, 352–53
  measuring for, 353
  types of, 353
Cryotherapy (*See also* Cold therapy)
  defined, 786
Cultural assessment, 71
Cultural competence
  defined, 106
  overview, 70
Cultural considerations
  admission and discharge, 93
  bath care, 175
  blood transfusions, 1036
  bowel elimination, 762
  client education, 110, 111t, 116
  critical illness, 1208
  diagnostic procedures, 671
  disaster management, 425
  end-of-life care, 1196, 1198
  illness, 4
  medication administration, 527, 531
  nutrition, 264
  pain management, 478
  perineal and genital care, 222
  personal space, 338
  stress, 511
  therapeutic communication, 75–76
  therapeutic diets, 589, 591
Cultural diversity, defined, 66
Cultural sensitivity, 66, 70–71
Culture, 627–28, 654–57
  blood, 644
  defined, 106, 625
  stool, 638
  throat, 655, 655f
  wound, 816, 834
    aerobic, 655–56, 655f
    anaerobic, 656
CVADs (*See* Central vascular access devices)
CVP (*See* Central venous pressure)
Cyanide agents, 423
Cyanosis, 161, 287, 938
  in children, 316
  defined, 161, 786, 871, 933, 994, 1045
Cystoscopy
  preparation for, 684–85
  purpose of, 683t

D

Dangle, defined, 323
Dangling at bedside, 339–40, 339f–340f
DAR charting format, 42
Data collection, in client education, 113–14
Database, in POMR charting, 46
Death (*See also* End-of-life care)
  due to restraints, 149
  due to trauma, 460
  grief and, 1184–85, 1189–91
    assisting with, 1190–91
    defined, 1184
    stages of, 1185
    understanding, 1190
  rate in smallpox, 425t
Debilitated, defined, 195
Debridement, types of, 844
Debris, defined, 812
Decalcification, defined, 195
Deceleration, in fetal monitoring
  early, 934, 986, 987t, 988
  late, 934, 986, 987t, 988
  periodic, 934
  variable, 934, 986, 987t, 988
Decerebrate posturing, 276, 276f
Decibel, 129, 132
Decompression, in intestinal obstruction, 584–85
Decontamination
  bioterrorism, 451
    sites for, 448
    triage, 447–48
  chemical exposure, 451–52
  defined, 414
  documentation, 454
  radiation exposure, 452–53
  triage and, 421–22
Decorticate posturing, 276, 276f
Decubitus, defined, 195
Decubitus ulcer (*See* Pressure ulcers)
Deep breathing, 474, 504–5
  instruction for, 877, 877f, 1155
  in stress management, 510–11
Deep tendon reflex, 280
Defecation, 756, 758–59
Defense-coping mechanisms, 302
Defense mechanisms, defined, 495
Defibrillation, 1226, 1228–30, 1229f, 1230f
  early, 939
  energy levels for, 1229
  "hands-free," 1229, 1230f
  in hospitals, 939
Defining characteristics, in nursing diagnosis, 29
Dehiscence, defined, 812
Dehydration
  defined, 699, 1139
  urine output and, 702
Delayed gastric emptying, 611, 613
Delegation, 55–59
  Board of Registered Nursing (BRN) on, 57
  client acuity systems, 57
  defined, 34, 57
  Nurse Practice Act and, 55
  parameters of, 58–59
  responsibilities that cannot be delegated, 57–58
  "rights of," 58–59
  unlicensed assistive personnel (UAP), 55, 57

Delegation of responsibilities, management guidelines, 19, 31, 62, 82, 103, 126, 157, 192, 231, 270, 320, 346, 374, 411, 463, 492, 513, 571, 658, 696, 752, 782, 809, 868, 929–30, 991, 1041–42, 1092, 1135, 1180, 1203, 1242–43
Delirium, in ventilated clients, 1239
Deltoid injection site, 551, 567f
Delusions of grandeur, 300
Denial, defined, 1184
Dental plaque, defined, 195
Dentures
  care of, 201–2, 201f
  in elderly, 231
Depression
  and adaptation, 131
  assessment for, 301
  defined, 66, 1184
Dereistic, 300
Dermabond, 828
Dermatitis, contact, 182t
Dermis, 161, 286, 286f, 625, 812
Detergent, defined, 377
Developmental level, 302
Diabetes
  insulin injections, 556–60, 558f, 559f
  insulin pen, 558
  insulin pump, 560–62, 561f
  insulin types, 557t
Diabetic, defined, 576
Diagnosis, defined, 661
Diagnosis-related groups (DRGs), defined, 106
Diagnostic label, in nursing diagnosis, 29
Diagnostic procedures, 660–97 (*See also* Laboratory tests)
  barium studies, 679–81
  cultural considerations, 671
  defined, 85
  documentation, 672, 677, 681, 686, 694
  endoscopic studies, 682–86
  fluid analysis studies, 664
  gerontologic considerations, 695
  magnetic resonance imaging (MRI), 664
  microscopic studies, 664
  nuclear scanning, 663–64, 674–81
  nurse's role
    client education, 662–63
    physician assistance, 664–65
  nursing diagnosis, 665
  as outpatient procedure, 662
  overview, 662–63
  standard precautions, 663
  ultrasound, 663
  x-ray studies, 663, 666–73
Dialysis (*See also* Hemodialysis; Peritoneal dialysis)
  types of, 703
Dialyzer, defined, 699
Diaphoresis, defined, 466, 661, 871
Diaphragmatic breathing, instruction for, 878
Diaphysis, defined, 1096
Diarrhea, defined, 756, 994
Diastole, 234, 240, 1206
Diastolic blood pressure, 241–42
Diastolic heart sounds, 294
Dicrotic notch, 1206, 1218
Diencephalon, 282, 283f
Diet (*See also* Therapeutic diets)
  defined, 576
Dietary fiber, 591
Dietary reference intakes (DRIs), 581
Diffusion, 875, 994, 1206
Digestion, 581, 583–84, 757
  defined, 576, 581, 756, 1043
  gallbladder in, 584
  in large intestine, 583
  liver in, 584
  pancreas in, 584
  parasympathetic nervous system in, 757–58
  in small intestines, 757
  in stomach, 583
Digital stimulation (bowel), 764
Dilatation, defined, 933
Diplopia, defined, 1139
Directed donation of blood, defined, 994
Disability, defined, 85
Disaster
  defined, 414, 416
  impact on infrastructure, 417
  mitigation, 417
Disaster management
  communication matrix, 418–20, 419f, 457–58
    external, 418, 419f, 458
    internal, 418–20, 458
  diversity considerations, 425
  ethical considerations, 424–25
  nursing diagnosis, 426
  psychological reactions, 461
  public policy about, 416–18
    Bioterrorism Act, 416–17
    Community Emergency Response Team (CERT), 417, 417f
    Emergency Medical Treatment and Labor Act (EMTALA), 416
  impact on infrastructure, 417
  JCAHO, 418
  triage, 420–22
  weapons of mass destruction, 415, 418, 422–24
Disaster trauma, psychological, 461
Discharge, 87, 89, 99–101
  to another facility, 87, 89
  defined, 85, 106
  documentation, 101
  form for, 100f
  gerontologic considerations, 102
  against medical advice (AMA), 101
  nursing diagnosis, 89
  procedure, 100–101
Discharge planning, 109–10, 122–24
  client preparation, 123
  defined, 106, 109
  discharge summary, 124
  documentation, 124
  federal requirements for, 110
  form for, 123f
  gerontologic considerations, 125–26
  multidisciplinary approach, 109
  nursing diagnosis, 112
  risk factors in, 110
Discharge summary, 124
  in POMR charting, 47–48, 48f
Disease, stress and, 499
Disinfectants, defined, 377
Disinfection, defined, 377
Disposable system
  bath care, 162–63, 176–77
  shampooing, 205–7, 207f
Dissipate, defined, 661
Distal, defined, 1206
Distensibility, of arteries, 240
Distention, defined, 699
Distribution, of medications, 517
Diuresis, defined, 699
Diuretics, defined, 994
Diverticulitis, defined, 756
Diverticulosis, defined, 576
Diverticulum, defined, 756
Do Not Resuscitate (DNR) or Do Not Attempt Resuscitation (DNAR) order, 10
  end-of-life care and, 1193, 1194f
Documentation, at the end of each unit. *See* Table of Contents
Doppler
  defined, 234
  for fetal heart rate, 984
Doppler ultrasound, 663
Dorsal, defined, 699
Dorsiflexion, defined, 323, 349, 933
Dorsogluteal injection site, 551, 565f, 566f
Dosage
  calculating, 523
  converting systems, 523
  defined, 516
Dose, loading, 466
Double-bagging, biohazard waste, 406–7, 407f
Double-barrel colostomy, 761
Drainage system, wound with
  caring for, 840–43, 841f
  closed systems, 842
  maintaining, 842–43, 843f
  open drains, 842
  pouches for, 841
Draping, a female client, 713, 713f
Dressing wounds, 826–30, 834–35
  applying wet-to-moist dressings, 847–49
  changing, 834–35
  dry sterile dressing, 827–28, 827f
  guidelines for, 815t
  preparation, 824–25, 824f–825f
  pressure ulcer (*See* Pressure ulcers)
  venous ulcer, 837–39, 838f, 839f
Dressings
  applying dry sterile, 827–28, 827f
  BIOPATCH, 1057, 1057f
  hydrocolloid, 857
  hydrogel, 857
  moisture-retentive, 832t, 859t
  pressure, 943
  semiocclusive, 837
  wet-to-moist, 847–49
DRIs (dietary reference intakes), 581
Droplet precautions, 283, 384t

Drug, defined, 516 (*See also* Medications)
Drug administration (*See also* Medication administration)
guidelines for, 6f
Dry skin, 182t
Dual-lumen dialysis catheter (DLC), central venous, 749–50, 750f
Dulcolax tablets, 680
DuoDERM dressing, 857
Dumping syndrome, defined, 576
Durable power of attorney for health care, 10
Dying (*See also* End-of-life care)
stages of, 1185–86, 1190–91
Dynorphin, 469
Dysphagia, 584
assisting with eating, 597
defined, 576
Dyspnea, defined, 516, 661, 871, 994, 1045
Dysrhythmia, 936, 1226
atrial, 936
defined, 933, 1206
emergency treatment, 1226
junctional, 936
life-threatening, 956t–957t
multifocal ventricular contraction (PVCs), 956t
third-degree heart block, 957t
ventricular fibrillation, 957t
ventricular tachycardia, 956t
Dysuria, defined, 699

E

Ear
applying medications, 539, 539f
assessment of, 285, 285f, 314
care for, 229–30
Ear canal, irrigation of, 539–40
Ear canal thermometer, 238
Eardrum, anatomy of, 285t
Eating assistance
for dysphagia, 597
for visually impaired, 596–97
Ecchymosis, defined, 161, 516, 933
Eccrine glands, 286, 286f
ECG (*See* Electrocardiogram)
Echocardiography, 663
Echolalia, 300
Ecosystem, defined, 129
Ectopic beats, 257
Edema
assessment for, 181
in children, 316
defined, 195, 699, 933, 994, 1096
pitting, 287
during pregnancy, 304
pulmonary, 937
in skin assessment, 287
Edematous, defined, 812
Effleurage, 161
EGD (gastrointestinal tract endoscopy)
preparation for, 685
purpose of, 683t
Egophony, defined, 1139
Elastic hosiery, 946–47, 946f, 947f
Elasticity
of arteries, 240, 318
defined, 349
Elbow, range of motion for, 355t
Elbow restraints, 151, 151f
Elder abuse, in home health care assessment, 1258
Elderly (*See* Gerontologic considerations)
Electrical conduction, in circulatory system, 935–36
Electrical injuries, 142–43
Electrical potential, defined, 1206
Electrical stimulation, in wound care, 812, 817, 862
candidates for, 862
equipment, 862
preparation, 862
procedure, 862
Electrocardiogram (ECG), 936, 952–62
12-lead, 957–58, 958f
defined, 1206
electrode systems for, 954
gerontologic considerations, 990
lead placements, 936t, 954
monitoring, 953–54, 953f, 954f
reading strip, 955, 955f, 957, 957f
on telemetry, 950f, 959, 959f
Electrode, defined, 1206
Electrode systems, for electrocardiogram (ECG), 954
Electrolytes, 996, 996t
defined, 699, 994, 1045
gerontologic considerations, 1041, 1179
imbalance, 996–97
Electronic flow-control device, intravenous, 1011–13, 1012f
Emaciation, defined, 576
Embolism, 933, 938, 1053
Emergency (*See also* Cardiac emergencies)
defined, 415
Emergency admissions, 86–87
Emergency life support measures, 938–39, 963–75
automated external defibrillator (AED), 970–71, 970f–971f
bag–valve–mask ventilation, 969, 969f
calling a code, 973–74, 974f
cardiopulmonary resuscitation (CPR), 964, 964f, 965f, 966–67
"code"
calling a, 973–74, 974f
care following, 975
crash cart in, 974, 974f
team members, 974
Heimlich maneuver
for conscious client, 971–72, 972f
for unconscious client, 972, 972f–973f
recovery position for victim, 968
Emergency Medical Treatment and Labor Act (EMTALA), 416
Emesis, defined, 195, 576, 1139
Emollient, defined, 161
Emotion
defined, 66
encouraging client to express, 76
Emotional, defined, 466, 495
Emotional involvement, in communication, 68, 71
Emotional responses, assessment of, 13
Empathy, defined, 66, 85, 1184
Emphysema, defined, 1139
Emulsification, defined, 756
End-of-life care, 1183–1204
core principles, 1186
cultural considerations, 1196, 1198
documentation, 1191, 1199
gerontologic considerations, 1203
grief process, 1184–85, 1189–91
hospice, 1187
nursing diagnosis, 1188
pain management, 1186–87, 1195–96
postmortem care, 1200–1202
stages of dying, 1185–86, 1190–91
supporting client, 1193–94, 1196–97
supporting family, 1198
End-stage renal disease
defined, 699
phases of, 703
Endocardial, defined, 933
Endocardium, defined, 933
Endogenous, defined, 377
Endorphins, 369–470
defined, 466
Endoscopic retrograde cholangiopancreatography (ERCP), 685
Endoscopic studies, 682–86
preparation for various, 683–86
purpose of various, 683t
Endoscopy, defined, 661
Endotracheal, defined, 933
Endotracheal tube
care for, 900
extubating, 901
intubation, 899–900, 899f
Enema, defined, 661, 1139
Enema administration, 768–74
barium enema, 680, 680t
for child, 771, 772f
cleansing, 770
distention reduction, 770
documentation, 774
fluid volume for, 771t
large volume, 769, 769f–770f, 771
medicated, 770
retention, 770, 772–73
return flow, 773
small volume, 772
Energy medicine, 503
Enkephalin, 469
Enteral feedings, 585–87, 610–19
adding blue dye to, 612–13
documentation, 618
for extended nutritional support, 586
formulas for, 585
gastrostomy, 612t, 613–14, 613f, 614f
jejunostomy, 612t
nasogastric (NG) tube, 612t
nasointestinal, 612t
percutaneous endoscopic gastrostomy (PEG), 612t

- small-bore feeding tube
  - continuous feeding, 616–18, 617f
  - inserting, 615–16, 615f
  - safety concerns, 616
- tubes for, 586 [*See also* Nasogastric (NG) tube]
- *vs.* parenteral feeding, 585

Enteral nutrition, defined, 576
Enteral tube, medication administration by, 531–32, 531f–532f
Enteric precautions, defined, 377
Enterostomy, defined, 576
Environment
- defined, 130
- hospital, 131–36 (*See also* Safe environment)
  - food and water, 133–34
  - furniture, 133
  - hazardous material and waste management, 134
  - humidity, 131–32
  - lighting, 131
  - physical and biological dimensions, 131–34
  - sociocultural dimensions, 134–36
  - sound levels, 132
  - space requirements, 131
  - temperature, 131–32
  - ventilation, 132

Environmental orientation, in hospital admission, 86–87, 130, 135–36
Enzymes, in blood pressure, 241
Epidemiologist, defined, 129
Epidemiology, defined, 812
Epidermis, 161, 195, 286, 286f
Epidural narcotic analgesia, administering, 481–83, 482f
Epinephrine, in cardiac emergencies, 1231, 1231t
Epiphysis, defined, 1096
Epispadias, 310
Epistaxis, defined, 933
Epithelium, defined, 812
Equivalent dose, defined, 415
Errors in
- clinical charting, 5, 7
- drug orders, 6, 519

Erythema, 161, 287, 786, 812, 1045
Esophagogastroduodenoscopy (EGD), 685
Esteem, defined, 66, 1184
Ethical considerations, disaster management, 424–25
Ethics, codes of, 2, 3f
Ethnocentrism, defined, 66
Etiology, in nursing diagnosis, 29
Euphoria, defined, 1139
Evaluate, defined, 66
Evaluation
- in client care plan, 37
- in client education, 120
- critical thinking and, 27
- in nursing process, 23–24, 24f

Evaluation tool, defined, 106
Evaporation, 786, 788, 994
Evening care, 160, 188–91
- back care, 189–90, 190f
- documentation, 191
- procedure, 189

Eversion, 195, 349, 351
Evidence-based practice, 30–31
- *vs.* best practice, 30

Evidence-based research, 30f
Evisceration, defined, 812
Excitability, defined, 349
Excoriation, defined, 195, 625, 699
Excreta, defined, 161
Excretion, of medications, 517–18
Exercise(s), 351–52
- active, 351–52
- for crutch walking, 368
- leg, 1156
- nursing diagnosis, 353
- passive, 351
- purpose of, 351
- range of motion, 352
  - active, 359
  - lower body, 356t, 358f
  - passive, 355–56, 356f–358f
  - upper body, 355t, 356f–357f
- resistive, 352
- strength training, 352

Exhalation, defined, 872–73
Exhaustion stage, of stress, 497, 497t
Exogenous, defined, 377
Expectorant, defined, 625, 871
Expectoration, defined, 195
Expiration, 240
Exposure, defined, 415
Extensibility, defined, 349
Extension
- defined, 349, 351, 1096
- muscle, 278
- range of motion exercises for, 355t, 356t

External fixation device, 1096, 1098
External fixation traction, 1099, 1117t, 1119, 1119f
External monitoring, fetal, 934 (*See also* Fetal monitoring)
External rotation, range of motion exercises for, 355t, 356t
Extracellular, defined, 994, 1045
Extremities
- assessment of
  - newborns, 310
  - pediatric, 316–17
- range of motion exercises
  - lower, 356t, 358f
  - upper, 355t, 356f–357f

Exudate, defined, 625, 1096, 1139
Eye care, 197, 225–30
- artificial eye, 227–28, 227f
- client education, 229
- contact lenses, 228–29
- documentation, 230
- postoperative socket care, 226–27
- routine, 226
- for unconscious client, 226

Eye medications
- ophthalmic drops, 537, 537f
- ophthalmic ointment, 537–38, 538f

Eye protection, 383–84, 398, 446
Eyes
- anatomy of, 284f
- assessment of, 284
  - accommodation, 277
  - light reaction, 277
  - newborns, 309
  - pediatric, 313–14
  - pupil, 277, 284, 284f
- irrigation of, 538

F

Face mask
- for oxygen administration, 893t
- with reservoir bag, 893t
- venturi, 893t

Face shield, 383–84, 398f
Face tent, 893t
Facial nerve, 283t
Fahrenheit, Celsius *vs.*, 238, 245t
Fall risk assessment, 137
Falls, 137
- bed siderails and, 137
- body mechanics for client, 336f, 363
- gerontologic considerations, 373–74, 1135
- in hospital, 140
- prevention, 140–42
- risk factors for, 137, 142

False negative, defined, 377
False positive, defined, 377
False reassurance, in communication, 69
Family assessment, in client education, 116
Family history, 273
Fat-soluble vitamins, 579, 580
Fat(s)
- defined, 576, 1045
- nutritional recommendations, 579
- therapeutic diet restricting, 589–90

Fatty acid
- saturated, 577, 579
- trans, 577
- unsaturated, 577, 579

Fear, defined, 1184
Febrile, defined, 234
Fecal impaction, removing, 764
Feces
- altered, 758
- defined, 756
- normal, 758

Federal Bureau of Investigation (FBI), functions of, 415
Federal Emergency Management Agency (FEMA), functions of, 415
Feedback
- defined, 66
- in therapeutic communication, 69

Feeding
- assistance for dysphagia, 597
- assistance for visually impaired, 596–97
- enteral (*See* Enteral feedings)
- total nutrient admixture (TNA), 1276–80
- total parenteral nutrition (TPN) [*See* Total parenteral nutrition (TPN)]

Fetal heart rate (FHR), 940
accelerations, 986
assessing changes, 986, 987t
auscultating, 984
baseline, 934
components of patterns, 985
decelerations
early, 934, 986, 987t, 988
late, 934, 986, 987t, 988
nursing actions for, 988
periodic, 934
variable, 934, 986, 987t, 988
defined, 934
during delivery, 306
normal, 986, 987t
during pregnancy, 304
Fetal jeopardy, 988
Fetal monitoring, 940, 983–90
applying external electronic, 984–85, 985f
assessing fetal heart rate changes, 986, 987t
auscultating fetal heart rate, 984
documentation, 989
external, 934
internal, 934
interpreting electronic tracings, 985–86, 985f, 986f
Fetal position, 304, 304f
Fetoscope, 984
FEV, 874
FEV_1, 874
FEV 25–75, 874
Fever, 789
defined, 786
Q fever, 431
signs and symptoms of, 237–38
viral hemorrhagic fevers (VHF), 424t–425t, 431, 449
ways to reduce, 804
Fiber
high diet, 591
low diet, 591
Fiberoptic scope, defined, 661
Fibrillation, defined, 234
Fibrotic, defined, 349
Fight or flight, defined, 466, 495
Figure-eight bandage, applying, 1104–5, 1105f
Filters
HEPA, 452
IV, 1000
Meds, 553
Filtrate, tubular alterations of, 700, 701t
Fingers, range of motion for, 355t
Fire extinguishers, types of, 143, 143f
Fire procedure, 143
First responder, defined, 415
Fissure
defined, 161, 195
between toes, 196
Fistula
A-V [*See* Arteriovenous (AV) fistula]
defined, 756
mucus, 761
Flaccid, defined, 756
Flaccid posturing, 276
Flaccidity, defined, 349
Flail chest, 290
Flatulence, defined, 756
Flexion
defined, 323, 349, 351, 1096
range of motion exercises for, 355t, 356t
Floss, defined, 195
Flossing, 200–201, 201f
Flow sheets, 12, 15f
defined, 34
in systems charting, 43, 43f
Fluid analysis (*See* Body fluid analysis)
Fluid balance, 995–96
average daily gain and loss, 995t
gerontologic considerations, 1041, 1179
imbalance, 996–97
urinary elimination and, 702
Fluid deficit, assessment for, 1022t, 1023t
Fluid excess, assessment for, 1022t, 1023t
Fluid intake and output, 1021–25
assessment of fluid status, 1022t, 1023t
flow sheet for, 1024t
monitoring, 1021–23
monitoring intake, 1024
Fluid replacement, solutions for, 1023
Fluoroscopy, defined, 661
Flush, defined, 161
Flush method, for blood pressure assessment, 266
Foams, in wound care, 859t
Focus, in therapeutic communication, 69
Focus assessment, 275, 275f
Focus charting, defined, 34
Foley catheter, defined, 699
Fontanels, 308
Food, 133–34 (*See also* Nutritional management; Therapeutic diets)
Food Guide Pyramid, 577–78, 578f, 579f
for the elderly, 620f
Food supplement, defined, 576
Food tray, serving, 596
Foot care, 196–97
documentation, 215
procedure, 214
toe nail care, 214–15
Foot coordination, assessment of, 279
Footboard, 160, 344
Footdrop, defined, 323
Forced expiratory volume (FEV), 874
Forensic charting, 41–42
Four (4)-hour limit (mL), defined, 466
Fowler's position, 323, 334f, 334t
Fractures, 1097–99
casts, 1098
compartment syndrome, 1099
defined, 349
external fixator apparatus, 1098
hip, 1100
repair process, 1097
traction, 1098–99
types of, 1097f, 1098
Fry Formula, 117
Fundal height, 303–4
Fundus, 307
Fungal skin infection, 182t
Fungus, defined, 195
Furniture, in hospital environment, 132, 133

G

Gag and swallow reflex, 279
Gait pattern, in elderly, 373 (*See also* Crutch walking)
Gallbladder, in digestion, 584
Gallium, 664, 675
Gamma Fe-Cult Plus, 637–38
Gangrene, defined, 812
Gardner–Wells cervical tongs, 1117
Gastric lavage, with NG tube, 606
Gastrointestinal, defined, 466, 576, 756, 1045
Gastrointestinal dysfunctions, 584–85
Gastrointestinal hemorrhage, 584
Gastrointestinal intubation (*See* Nasogastric (NG) tube)
Gastrointestinal system
anatomy of, 757, 757f
assessment of, 14, 297–98, 310
components of, 295
functions of, 581, 583
gerontologic considerations, 319
Gastrointestinal tract endoscopy (EGD)
preparation for, 685
purpose of, 683t
Gastrostomy tube, enteral feeding through, 612t, 613, 613f
Gate control theory, of pain, 468–69
Gated cardiac blood pool scan, 676
Gavage, defined, 576
Gender, influence on vital signs, 237
General adaptation syndrome, 466, 495–96, 497f
General appearance, in mental assessment, 299–300
Generic, defined, 516
Genitals
care of (*See* Perineal and genital care)
defined, 195
female, 701f, 715f
male, 701f
Genitourinary, defined, 625, 699
Genitourinary system
assessment of, 14, 297–99
female, 298–99
gerontologic considerations, 319
male, 298
newborns, 310
pediatric, 316
components of, 295–96
female
external structures, 715f
internal structures, 701f
male, 701f
Gerontologic considerations
age-related changes, 81
cardiovascular system, 269
gastrointestinal system, 619–20
hair, 231
musculoskeletal system, 345, 1135
nail, 231
psychosocial, 82, 345–46

respiratory system, 269, 929
skin, 163–64, 184, 191, 867
temperature, 236–37
urinary system, 752
bathing, 192
bowel elimination, 782
central vascular access devices (CVAD), 1092
circulatory system, 990
client education, 125
communication, 81–82
constipation, 766
critical illness, 1242
diagnostic procedures, 695
discharge, 102
discharge planning, 125–26
end-of-life care, 1203
falls, 373–74, 1135
hospital admission, 102
intravenous therapy, 1041
medication administration, 570
nurse–client relationship, 81–82
nutritional management, 619–21
nutritional recommendations, 619
orthopedic interventions, 1135
pain management, 489
personal hygiene, 231
positioning elderly clients, 346
pressure ulcers, 817
respiratory care, 929
safe environment, 157
skin integrity, 191–92
specimen collection, 657
stress, 513
thermal injury, 157
thermoregulation, 808
urinary elimination, 752
vital signs, 269
wandering, 157
wound care, 867–68
Girth, defined, 994
Glossopharyngeal nerve, 283t
Glove use, 398
bioterrorism, 446
CDC recommendations, 383, 384t
donning and removing procedure, 393–94, 394f
donning sterile, 820–21, 821f
glove selection, 395
importance of, 394–95
latex allergies and, 395–96, 395f
protection from toxic materials, 447
Glucometer, for blood glucose testing, 646
Glucose, defined, 625
Glue, for wound closure, 828
Glycogenolysis, 584
Glycosuria, defined, 625
Goals (*See also* Outcome identification)
in client care plan, 36–37
long-term, 37
in nursing process, 23
short-term, 37
Gown use, 384, 384t
bioterrorism, 446
change for IV client, 1017–18
in isolation, 403, 404f, 405
Granulation, defined, 378, 812
Granulation phase, of wound healing, 813
Granulocytes, defined, 625, 994
Graphic records, 12–13, 16f
Gravida, defined, 308
Gravity
center of, 323
defined, 323
line of, 323
Greenstick fracture, 1097
Grief, 1184–85, 1189–91
assisting with, 1190–91
defined, 1184
stages of, 1185
understanding, 1190
Grooming, in mental assessment, 299
Groshong catheter, 1047, 1076
drawing blood from, 1078
maintaining, 1076–77, 1077f
Gross negligence, 6
Guaiac, test for, 637–38

H

Hair
age-related changes in, 231
in pediatric assessment, 313
Hair care, 196, 204–8
documentation, 208
in home health, 1269
procedure, 205
shampooing, 205–7
shaving, 207
Hallucination, defined, 495
Halo traction, 1117t, 1120–21, 1120f
Hand coordination, assessment of, 279
Hand scrub, completing, 820, 820f
Handroll, 344, 344f
Handwashing, 17–18
bioterrorism, 446
CDC recommendations, 383
compliance studies about, 391
in home health care, 1260
importance of, 393
nosocomial infection and, 382
principles of, 383
procedure, 391–93, 392f
waterless antiseptics, 392f, 393
Hazardous material, 134, 415 (*See also* Biohazards)
HAZMAT model, defined, 415
Head, circumference of, newborn, 311
Head and neck, assessment, 282–86
ear, 285, 285f
eyes, 284
gerontologic considerations, 317–18
mouth and lip, 286
newborns, 308–9
nose, 286
pediatric, 313–15
Healing, nutritional requirements for, 592f
Health
defined, 466, 495, 501
holistic approach to, 501–2 [*See also* Complementary/alternative medicine (CAM)]
Health Care Worker Protection Act, 385
Health history, 273
Health Insurance Portability and Accountability Act (HIPPA), 7
Hearing aid
cleaning and checking, 229
documentation, 230
Hearing impairment
communication techniques, 77
gerontologic considerations, 81
Heart
anatomy of, 934
assessment, 289, 293–95 (*See also* Heart sounds)
apical pulse, 295
gerontologic considerations, 318–19
heart murmurs, 294
heart sounds, 293–94
newborns, 310
pediatric, 316
peripheral pulse, 295, 295f
blood flow through, 935, 935f
Heart block, third-degree, 957t
Heart disease, therapeutic diets for, 585
Heart failure, 937–38
defined, 933
etiology, 937
left-sided, 937
manifestations of, 937
right-sided, 937
treatment, 937–38
Heart murmur
assessment, 294
in children, 316
Heart rate, 239
calculation from ECG strip, 955
Heart rhythm, 239
Heart sounds
aortic valve sounds, 294
assessment, 289, 293–95
atrioventricular, 293
diastolic, 294
mitral valve sounds, 293
pulmonic valve sounds, 294
S_1, 293, 294f
S_2, 294, 294f
S_4 (atrial gallop), 294
S_3 (ventricular gallop), 294
tricuspid valve sounds, 293
Heat pack, applying, 793
Heat therapy, 790–91, 792–97
applying heat pack, 793
aquathermic pad, 794–95, 794f, 795f
benefits of, 791
documentation, 797
gerontologic considerations, 808
hot moist pack, 795–96
indications for, 791t
nursing diagnosis, 791
physiologic effects of, 788t
radiant warmer for infants, 793–94, 793f, 794f
sitz bath, 796, 796f
Heat transfer, processes of, 788

Height and weight, 95–98
client preparation, 96
documentation, 97
equipment, 96, 98f
procedure, 96–97
Heimlich maneuver
for conscious client, 971–72, 972f
for unconscious client, 972, 972f–973f
Heimlich micro-trach, 1291
Helping relationship, defined, 66, 106
Hematemesis, defined, 576, 933
Hematoma, defined, 933, 994
Hematuria, defined, 625, 994
Hemo, defined, 994, 1045
Hemoccult test, 638
Hemoconcentration, 627
Hemodialysis, 745–51
for AV fistula of graft, 747, 747f
blood flow for, 747
central venous dual-lumen dialysis catheter (DLC), 749–50, 750f
cultural considerations, 748
defined, 699
documentation, 751
equipment for, 746, 746f
ongoing care, 748
preparation, 746
process of, 747
survival rates of clients, 749
termination of, 748–49, 749f
Hemodynamic, defined, 933, 1045, 1206
Hemodynamic monitoring
arterial blood pressure monitoring, 1217–24
overview, 1207–8
pulmonary artery pressure monitoring, 1209–16
Hemolysis, 627
Hemolytic, defined, 994, 1045
Hemopneumothorax, 922f
Hemoptysis, 933
Hemorrhage, 937
assessment guide for, 939t
defined, 195, 933
gastrointestinal, 584
Hemorrhagic shock, 937
Hemorrhoids, defined, 756
Hemothorax, defined, 871
Heparin
low-dose, 1008
subcutaneous (sub Q) injection, 562–63, 562f
Hepatitis, 388
Hepatitis A (HAV), 388
Hepatitis B (HBV), 51, 53, 388
Hepatitis C (HCV), 388
Herbal medicine, 503–4
Heredity, influence on vital signs, 237
Hernia, defined, 1139
Hickman catheter
changing dressing, 1076
maintaining, 1075
High-Fowler's position, 323, 334f, 334t
Hip
fractures, 1100
range of motion for, 356t
Hip arthroplasty, caring for client with, 1128–29
HIPAA, 7
History, nursing, 91, 92f
HIV infection [*See* Acquired immunodeficiency syndrome (AIDS); Human immunodeficiency virus (HIV)]
Hoffman traction, 1117t, 1119f
Holistic, defined, 495
Holistic medicine, 501 [*See also* complementary/alternative medicine (CAM)]
Holmes and Rahe stress scale (*See* Instructor's Guide), 499
Holter monitor, 1298
Homan's sign, 933, 938
Home care assistance (*See also* Home health care)
defined, 85, 106
Home health care
admission, 1252–58
documentation, 1255
Medicare eligibility, 1254–55
assessment, 1249
for elder abuse, 1258
of home, 1256–57
nutritional, 1278–79
body mechanics, 1265–67
bowel elimination, 1282–83
colostomy care, 1282–83, 1286–87
caregiver's safety, 1257
circulatory care, 1295–99
Holter monitor, 1298
implantable cardioverter-defibrillator, 1298–99
nursing diagnosis, 1296
pacemakers, 1296–98
client education, 1249
infection control, 1263–64
nutrition, 1277
client's safety, 1257
cultural considerations, 1275
defined, 1248
guidelines for, 1254
hygienic care, 1268–72
bathing, 1269–70
bedmaking, 1271
hair care, 1269
nursing diagnosis, 1270
overview, 1269
preparing normal saline, 1271
pressure ulcer care, 1269, 1271
skin care, 1269
sterilizing medication equipment, 1271
transferring, 1270–71
increase in, 1246–47
infection control, 1259–64
AIDs client, 1262–63
cleansing equipment at home, 1263
client education, 1263–64
client preparation, 1261
disposal of waste, 1261–62
nursing diagnosis, 1259–64
legal issues in, 1247
medications, 1273–75
nurse supervision, 1250
nurse's safety, 1255–56
nursing diagnosis, 1251
Outcome and Assessment Information Set (OASIS), 1247
documentation, 1250
forms, 1253f
plan of care, 1249–50
overview, 1246–47
plan of care, 1249–50, 1269
referral for, 1248–49
respiratory care, 1288–94
mechanical ventilation, 1289–91
nursing diagnosis, 1289
oxygen therapy, 1289–90
tracheostomy care, 1293–94
transtracheal oxygen therapy, 1291–93
team for, 1248, 1248t
total parenteral nutrition (TPN), 1276–80
administering, 1278–79
complications of, 1280
discontinuing, 1279–80
monitoring, 1279
nursing diagnosis, 1278
overview, 1277
urinary elimination, 1282
catheter care, 1284
clean technique for catheterization, 1282–84
dialysis, 1282, 1285–86
Homebound, defined, 1254
Homeland security, defined, 415
Homeopathy, 504
Homeostasis, defined, 129, 495, 994, 1184
Homocysteine, 585
Homologous, defined, 994
Hormones, in blood pressure, 241
Hospice, defined, 1184
Hospital
admission to, 85–86
client falls in, 140
early defibrillation programs in, 939
medications from home, 85
nutritional management in, 585–87
smoke-free, 137
Hospital bed (*See* Beds)
Hospitalization
client's role, 3–4
nursing role, 2–3
Host, defined, 378
Hot moist pack, applying, 795–96
Household equivalents, 574t
Hoyer lift
defined, 323
moving clients using, 342, 342f
Huber needle
accessing and flushing using, 1081–82, 1081f, 1082f
defined, 1045
Human immunodeficiency virus (HIV) [*See also* Acquired immunodeficiency syndrome (AIDS)]
computer-assisted charting for, 51, 53
defined, 386
health care worker exposure, 387

PEP protocol for exposure, 387
transmission, 386
Humidity, in hospital environment, 131–32
Humoral immunity, defined, 378
Humulin insulin, 557t
Hydration, defined, 994
Hydraulic bathtub chair, 178
Hydrocolloid dressing, 832t, 857, 859t, 860
Hydrogel dressing, 832t, 857, 859t
Hydrogenation, defined, 576
Hydrostatic, defined, 699, 933, 1045
Hydrostatic pressure, 994–95
defined, 994
Hygiene (*See also* Personal hygiene)
defined, 129, 195, 378
Hyperalimentation [*See also* Total parenteral nutrition (TPN)]
defined, 576, 1045
Hyperamnesia, 301
Hyperemia, defined, 161, 786
Hyperextension
defined, 349, 351, 1096
range of motion exercises for, 355t, 356t
Hyperglycemia, defined, 576, 1045
Hypermotility, 759
defined, 756
Hyperopia, 284
Hyperpigmentation, 287
Hyperpnea, 235, 259t
Hyperreflexia, defined, 756
Hypersecretion, defined, 994
Hypertension, 234, 281, 466, 495, 1139
Hyperthermia, 234, 786, 789
Hypertonic, defined, 576, 756, 994, 1045
Hypertonic solutions, for fluid replacement, 1023
Hypertrophy, defined, 349
Hyperventilation, 874
defined, 871
Hypnosis, 474
Hypnotics, 1139, 1164
Hypoallergenic, defined, 161, 195
Hypoglossal nerve, 283t
Hypoglycemia
defined, 576
risk with insulin, 557
Hypomotility, 756, 759
Hypospadias, 310
Hypotension, 241
defined, 234, 281, 933
orthostatic
in elderly, 269, 319
measuring, 361
minimizing, 361
Hypothalamus
in body temperature regulation, 787
defined, 234
Hypothermia, 789–90
classification of, 805
defined, 234, 786, 1139
medically-induced, 237, 790, 804
Hypotonic, defined, 994
Hypotonic solutions, for fluid replacement, 1023
Hypoventilation, 874
defined, 871
Hypovolemia, defined, 234, 625, 994, 1045, 1139
Hypoxemia, defined (*See also* Hypoxia), 871
Hypoxia
chronic, 891
defined, 871
signs and symptoms of, 891

I

Ice pack, applying, 799, 799f
Idealization, defined, 1184
Identaband, defined, 85
Ileal conduit, 702, 741–42
Ileal pouch, 702
Ileal reservoirs, 702
Ileostomy, 760
compared to colostomy, 761t
defined, 756
Ileus, 576, 611
Illness
and adaptation, 131
defined, 466, 495
Imagery, 474
Immobilize, defined, 933
Immune response, primary, 378
Immunity
acquired, 380
as barrier to infection, 380
natural, 380
Immunization, defined, 415
Immunosuppressive, defined, 1139
Impaction (*See also* Fecal impaction)
defined, 756
removing, 764
Impetigo, defined, 195
Implanted, defined, 1045
Implanted infusion port, defined, 1045
Implementation
in client care plan, 37
critical thinking and, 27
in nursing process, 23, 24f
Incentive spirometer (IS), 878–79, 879f
Incident command system (ICS), 415, 418–19
Incident report (*See also* Unusual occurrence), 53–54, 56f
Incision, defined, 812
Incomplete sentences, in therapeutic communication, 69
Incongruence, in communication, 69
Incontinence, defined, 699
Incontinent, defined, 195
Incubation period, defined, 378, 415
Incurvate, defined, 161, 195
Indiana pouch, 741
Individualized care, in hospital setting, 135
Induction, defined, 1139
Indwelling urethral catheter, defined, 699
Infants (*See also* Newborns)
blood pressure assessment, 266
elbow restraints, 151, 151f
mummy restraints, 154–55, 154f
normal respirations in, 259
oxygen tent, 893t, 894, 894f
radiant warmer for, 793–94, 793f, 794f
skin, 163–64
stool specimen collection, 637
urine specimen collection, 634, 634f
Infarction, defined, 234
Infection
barriers to, 379–80
bloodstream, 994
catheter-related, 994, 1051
infusate-related, 994
chain of, 378–79, 379f
conditions predisposing to, 380–81
defined, 378, 415, 699, 812
fungal skin, 182t
local-catheter-related, 994
surgical site, 1160–62
wound (*See* Wound infection)
Infection control, 376–412
bioterrorism, 445
in home health care, 1259–64
AIDs client, 1262–63
cleansing equipment in home, 1263
client education, 1263–64
client preparation, 1261
disposal of waste, 1261–62
isolation, 402–10
for IV drug users, 1264
medical asepsis, 389–96
nursing diagnosis, 389
standard precautions, 397–401
Infectious agent, in chain of infection, 378–79, 379f
Infiltrations, evaluation criteria, 1007
Inflammation
defined, 161
signs and symptoms of, 789
Inflammatory phase, of wound healing, 813
Inflammatory processes, 788–90
as barrier to infection, 380
defined, 625, 812
Information flow, management guidelines, 19, 31, 62, 82, 103, 126, 157, 192, 231, 270, 320, 346, 374, 411, 463, 492, 513, 571, 658, 696, 752–53, 782–83, 809, 868, 930, 991, 1042, 1092, 1135–36, 1181, 1203, 1242–43
Infusate-related bloodstream infection, defined, 994
Infusion, defined, 994, 1045
Infusions, intravenous therapy, 997
Ingest, defined, 576
Inhalation, defined, 415
Inhaled medications, 545
metered-dose inhaled (MDI) medications, 544–45, 544f, 545f
nonpressurized (nebulized) aerosol, 546
Initial interaction with client, 75, 86
Initiation phase, of nurse–client relationship, 72, 80
Injection sites, 564–67
deltoid, 551, 567f
dorsogluteal, 551, 565f, 566f
vastus lateralis, 551, 566f
ventrogluteal, 551, 564f, 565f

Injections (*See also* Parenteral administration)
disposal of syringe, 550, 550f
intradermal, 551
intramuscular (IM), 551
preparing, 550–54
combining medications in syringe, 552–53
prefilled medication cartridge syringe, 554, 554f
reconstituting powdered medications, 552
selecting needle size, 550, 567
withdrawing from vial, 522f, 550, 552
withdrawing medication from ampule, 553, 553f
sciatic nerve injury, 565
subcutaneous (sub Q), 551
types of, 551
Z-track method, 567–68, 568f
Inotropic reserve, 933, 935
Insomnia, defined, 466, 495, 1184
Inspection, in physical assessment, 274, 274f
Inspiration, 240, 872
Instillation, defined, 516
Insulator, defined, 786
Insulin, 556–60
Continuous Subcutaneous Insulin Infusion (CSII), 561
double checking dose, 559–60
hypoglycemia risk with, 557
mixing two solutions, 559, 559f
premixing, 558
sites for injection, 558f
types and therapeutic action, 557t
Insulin pen, 558
Insulin pump, 560–62, 561f
Integrative medicine, 502
Integumentary, defined, 756
Intelligence, assessment of, 302
Intermittent peritoneal dialysis (IPD), 1282
Internal monitoring, fetal, 934
Internal rotation, range of motion exercises for, 355t, 356t
Intershift reporting, 55
Interstitial, defined, 994
Intervention (*See also* Implementation)
defined, 161, 195, 1139
Intestinal obstruction, 584–85
Intracapsular, defined, 1096
Intracellular, defined, 625, 994, 1045
Intradermal, defined, 516
Intradermal injections, administering, 554, 554f, 555f
Intramuscular, defined, 516
Intramuscular (IM) injections, administering, 563f, 564f, 593–94
Intraoperative care, 1140, 1142–42
Intrashift reporting, 55
Intravascular, defined, 994, 1045
Intravenous, defined, 516
Intravenous pyelography (IVP)
preparation for, 668
purpose of, 666t
Intravenous therapy, 993–1043
blood transfusions, 1033–40
administering components, 1037, 1039t
complications of, 1037, 1038t
cultural considerations, 1036
protocol, 1037
through straight line, 1036
through Y-set, 1034–36, 1034f, 1035f
warming blood for, 1034
complications, 997, 1015t
documentation, 1009, 1019, 1024, 1031, 1040
evaluation criteria, 1007
extravasation, 1014–15
flushing with low-dose heparin, 1008
gerontologic considerations, 1041
initiation, 998–1009
adding extension tubing, 1001, 1001f
over-the-needle catheter, 1006–9, 1007f, 1008f
preparation, 999–1000, 999f–1000f
venipuncture site, 1002–3, 1003f
winged needle, 1003–5, 1004f, 1005f
intake and output, 1021–25
assessment of fluid status, 1022t, 1023t
flow sheet for, 1024t
monitoring, 1021–23
monitoring intake, 1024
management, 1010–20
calorie calculation, 1011
changing gown for client, 1017–18
converting to saline lock, 1016, 1016f, 1017f
discontinuing, 1018, 1018f, 1019f
flow rate, factor that influence, 1011
flow rate regulation, 1011–12
IV site, 1014–16
using electronic flow-control device, 1011–13, 1012f
using syringe pump, 1013–14, 1013f, 1014f
medication administration, 997, 1026–32
adding to IV solution, 1027
mini-infuser pump, 1029
peripheral IV line injection "push," 1031
peripheral saline lock, 1030–31, 1031f
secondary (piggyback) bag, 1027–29, 1028t
volume control set, 1029–30, 1029f, 1030f
needle-free devices, 1016, 1016f
nursing diagnosis, 997
overview, 997
tubing changes, 1004, 1006
Introduction to client, 75, 86
Intubation [*See also* Artificial airways; Nasogastric (NG) tube]
defined, 871
endotracheal, 381, 899–900, 899f
nasopharyngeal, 898, 898f
oropharyngeal, 898, 898f
tracheostomy, 911–12, 911f
Invalidation, in communication, 69
Invasive, defined, 1206
Inversion, defined, 349, 351
Iodine, 664, 675
Ionizing radiation, defined, 415
IPPA sequence, for physical assessment, 273
IR (*See* Incident report)
Iron, increased therapeutic diet, 591
Irrigate, defined, 812, 1045
Irrigation
bladder (*See* Bladder irrigation)
colostomy, 761, 1282–83, 1286–87
defined, 699
of ear canal, 539–40
of eye, 538
wound, 816, 834, 844
Irritation, defined, 195
Ischemia, 161, 234, 933, 938
Ischemic, defined, 466
Isolation room, 402–10
defined, 378, 415, 812
documentation, 410
donning attire, 403, 404f, 405
double-bagging, 406–7, 407f
exiting room, 409
mask use, 405–6, 405f
preparation, 403, 403f
protective, 378
removing items from room, 406
soiled equipment, 409
specimen handling, 408
transporting client, 408, 408f
vital signs assessment, 406
Isotonic, defined, 994, 1045
Isotopes, defined, 415
IVP (*See* Intravenous pyelography)

J

Jackson–Pratt wound drainage system, 842–43
Jaundice, 287
defined, 161
Jejunostomy
defined, 576
enteral feeding through, 612t, 616–18, 617f
Jewett–Taylor brace, applying, 1106–7, 1106f
Joint Commission on Accreditation of Healthcare Organizations (JCAHO), 35, 466
admission assessment, 86
client care plans, 35
documentation requirements, 40–41
Patient and Family Education Standards, 107, 109f, 115
principles of end-of-life care, 1186
restraints, 138
on security management, 418
sentinel events, 136, 137t
smoke-free hospitals, 137
standards for pain management, 471
Joint replacement (*See* Arthroplasty)
Joints, 351
alterations in, 324
defined, 323
movements of, 351
range of motion
in elderly, 320, 345
of various, 355t, 356t
types of, 351
Judgment
assessment of, 301
in communication, 69

K

Kaposi's sarcoma, defined, 378
Kardex, 11, 34
Keloid, defined, 812
Keofeed (*See* Small bore feeding tube)
Kidneys
  age-related changes, 319
  in fluid balance, 995
  functions of, 700–701
  in newborns, 310
Kinesiology, applied, 502
Knee, range of motion for, 356t
Knee arthroplasty, caring for client with, 1130–31
Kock Continent Ileostomy, 760
Kock's reservoir, 741, 760
Korotkoff's sounds
  blood pressure assessment, 262–63
  defined, 234
  phases of, 241–42
Kussmaul's respirations, 235, 259t
Kwashiorkor, defined, 577
Kyphosis, 290, 345

L

Labia, defined, 195
Labor and delivery
  assessment during, 305–7
  first stage, 305–6
  fourth stage, 306–7
  second stage, 306
  third stage, 306
Laboratory forms, 13, 18f
Laboratory tests, 626–28 (*See also* Diagnostic procedures; Specimen collection)
  blood tests, 627
  cultures, 627–28
  nurse's role in, 626
  prehospital, 86
  urine tests, 626–27
Laparoscopy
  client education for, 1153
  defined, 1139
  diagnostic purposes of, 1153
  preparation for, 685
  purpose of, 683t
Large intestine, 583, 758
Laser arterectomy, 670
Laser therapy
  client education for, 1151, 1151t, 1152t
  types of lasers, 1151t
  types of surgery, 1152t
Latex, defined, 378
Latex allergies
  food allergies related to, 596
  management, 395–96, 395f
Lavage
  defined, 577
  gastric, 606
Law (*See also* Legal issues)
  civil, 7
  classifications of, 9f
  criminal, 7
Laxative, defined, 756
Learn, readiness to, 108
Learning
  assessment of needs, 115–17
  defined, 106
Left ventricular end-diastolic pressure (LVEDP), 1210
  defined, 1206
Legal forms, 53–55
  consent forms, 54–55, 56f
  unusual occurrence, 53–54, 56f
Legal issues, 5–6
  in charting, 40–41, 51, 53
  in complementary/alternative medicine (CAM), 502
  in home health care, 1247
  law classifications, 9f
  malpractice, 7
  negligence, 6–7
  professional misconduct, 6
Leg bag, attaching catheter to, 709
Legs
  coordination assessment, 279
  exercises for, 1156
  range of motion exercises, 356t, 358f
Leopold's maneuvers, for fetal position, 304, 304f
Lesion, defined, 195
Lethargy, defined, 1139
Leverage, defined, 323
Liability, 5–6
  consent and, 8
  malpractice, 7
  negligence, 6–7
  professional misconduct, 6
Lice, 210–11, 1269, 1272
Licensed independent practitioner (LIP)
  defined, 129
  restraints use and, 138
Licensure, 4–5
Lifescan one-touch II, for blood glucose testing, 647–49, 648f
Lifestyle, defined, 495
Lifestyle patterns, 302
Lifting, back injury and, 325
Ligament, defined, 323, 349
Lighting, in hospital environment, 131
Limitation, defined, 85, 129
Lindane lotion, 210
Lindane shampoo, 210
Line of gravity, defined, 323
Lip, assessment of, 286
Lipid emulsion therapy, 1070–73
  guidelines for, 1071
  infusing, 1071–72, 1071f, 1072f
Lipids, defined, 1045
Liquid dosages
  calculating, 523
  preparing, 529
Listening, in therapeutic communication, 69
Literacy levels, in client education, 116
Lithotomy, defined, 661
Lithotripsy, client education for, 1152–53
Liver
  age-related changes, 319
  in digestion, 584
  physical assessment, 297
Liver biopsy
  assisting with, 690, 690f
  purpose of, 689t
Living will, 10
  end-of-life care and, 1197f
Loading dose, defined, 466
Local adaptation syndrome, 497
Local-catheter-related infection, defined, 994
Local effect, 517
Lochia, 307
Lockout interval, defined, 467
Logrolling clients, 343, 343f
Low-Fowler's position, 334f, 334t
Lower body, range of motion exercises, 356t, 358f
Lower respiratory tract, 872
Lumbar, defined, 661
Lumbar puncture
  assisting with, 689–90, 690f
  purpose of, 689t
Lumen, defined, 577, 1045, 1206
Lung compliance, 1238
Lung scan
  preparation for, 675–76
  purpose of, 675t
Lung sounds, auscultation, 292–93, 293f
Lungs
  assessment, 289, 292–93
    gerontologic considerations, 318
    newborns, 309
    pediatric, 315
  auscultation, 289, 292–93, 292f, 293f
  lobes of, 884f
  pH of blood and, 240
  relation to skeletal structures, 288–89, 288f, 289f
Lymph nodes, in pediatric assessment, 313

M

Macronutrients, 577–80
  carbohydrates, 578–79
  fats, 579
  proteins, 579–80
  water, 580
Macrophage, defined, 812
Macules, 288
Magnetic resonance imaging (MRI), 664
  defined, 661, 1139
  preparation for, 671–72
  purpose of, 666t
Maladaptation, defined, 85, 129
Maladaptive, defined, 66, 106, 1139
Malnutrition
  defined, 577, 1045
  in elderly, 621
Malpighian corpuscle, defined, 699
Malpractice, 6, 7
Mammography
  defined, 661
  preparation for, 672
  purpose of, 666t

Management guidelines
delegation of responsibilities, 19, 31, 62, 82, 103, 126, 157, 192, 231, 270, 320, 346, 374, 411, 463, 492, 513, 571, 658, 696, 752, 782, 809, 868, 929–30, 991, 1041–42, 1092, 1135, 1180, 1203, 1242–43
information flow, 19, 31, 62, 82, 103, 126, 157, 192, 231, 270, 320, 346, 374, 411, 463, 492, 513, 571, 658, 696, 752–53, 782–83, 809, 868, 930, 991, 1042, 1092, 1135–36, 1181, 1203, 1242–43
Manubrium, defined, 934
MAR (medication administration record), 12, 16f
defined, 516
in medication administration, 518, 521–22, 522f
medications from home, 85
Mask, HEPA or N95 particulate filter respiratory, 446, 448
Mask use, 383–84, 384t, 398
bioterrorism, 446
in isolation, 405–6, 405f
Mass casualty incident (MCI), 415, 416
defined, 415
Massage, 504
in back care, 189–90, 190f
in pain management, 474, 478
Material Safety Data Sheets, 134
Maturation phase, of wound healing, 813
McCaffery, Margo, 467
MDI (*See* Metered dose inhaled medications)
MDR-TB, 378, 387
Mean arterial pressure (MAP), 1206, 1210t, 1218, 1221
Mechanical restraint, defined, 129
Mechanical soft diet, 592–93
Mechanical ventilation, 1235–42
Medical advice, discharge against, 101
Medical asepsis, 389–96 (*See also* Handwashing)
cleaning washable articles, 393
defined, 378
documentation, 396
glove use
CDC recommendations, 383, 384t
donning and removing procedure, 393–94, 394f
glove selection, 395
importance of, 394–95
latex allergies and, 395–96, 395f
handwashing, 14, 17–18, 391–93, 392f
in home health care, 1260
principles, 14, 17, 168
vs. surgical, 14
Medical diagnosis, *vs.* nursing diagnosis, 27, 27f
Medical records, privacy and, 9
Medicare eligibility, for home health care, 1254–55
Medication administration, 518–19
abbreviations and symbols in, 573–74
calculations of solutions, 573
in cardiac emergencies, 1230–31, 1230f, 1231f
conversion tables, 574t
calculating dosages, 523
converting dosages, 523
cultural considerations, 527, 531
documentation, 518, 533, 540, 548
five rights of, 518–19, 526
gerontologic considerations, 570
guidelines for, 6f
intravenous, 997, 1026–32
adding to IV solution, 1027
mini-infuser pump, 1029
peripheral IV line injection "push," 1031
peripheral saline lock, 1030–31, 1031f
secondary (piggyback) bag, 1027–29, 1028t
volume control set, 1029–30, 1029f, 1030f
MAR for, 12, 16F, 85, 516, 518, 521–22, 522f
medication protocol, 526, 526f
mucous membranes, 542–48 (*See also* Mucous membrane medications)
nursing diagnosis, 519
oral, 528–33 (*See also* Oral medications)
parenteral administration, 549–70 (*See also* Injections; Parenteral administration)
postoperative, 1177–78
preoperative, 1164
preparation, 520–27, 521–22
routes of, 517
safety precautions, 517–18, 527
topical, 534–41 (*See also* Topical medications)
using automated dispensing system, 524–25, 525f
using narcotic control system, 524, 524f
Medication administration record (MAR), 12, 16f
defined, 516
in medication administration, 518, 521–22, 522f
medications from home, 85
Medication errors, 526
Medication orders
components of, 518
types of, 518
verbal, 518
Medication records, 12, 16f
Medications
absorption of, 517
administration routes, 517
charting for PRN, 41
defined, 517
distribution of, 517
excretion of, 517–18
gerontologic considerations, 373
from home at hospital, 85
influence on vital signs, 237
metabolism of, 517
side affects, 131
that affect wound healing, 814–15
Medicine, defined, 516 (*See also* Medications)
Meditation, 505
defined, 467, 495
in stress management, 512
Medulla, 282, 283f
Melanoma, 288
Memory
assessment, 301
recall, 301
retention, 301
Mental assessment, 299–302
awareness, 301
consciousness, 300
coping mechanisms, 302
developmental level, 302
expressive aspects of behavior, 300
general appearance, 299–300
intelligence, 302
judgment, 301
lifestyle patterns, 302
memory, 301
mood, 301
purpose of, 299
sensory ability, 302
thought content, 301
thought processes, 300
Mental competency, consent forms and, 54
Mental status, and adaptation, 130–31
Mesentery, defined, 1139
Metabolic acidosis
arterial blood gases (ABGs) associated with, 1221t
respiratory compensation for, 873
Metabolic alkalosis, arterial blood gases (ABGs) associated with, 1221t
Metabolism
defined, 195, 516, 995
of medications, 517
Metaphysis, defined, 1096
Metered-dose inhaled (MDI)
medication administration by, 544–45, 544f
with spacer, 545, 545f
Methicillin-resistant *Staphococcus aureus* (MRSA), 382
Micronutrients, 580–81
minerals, 580–81
vitamins, 580
Microorganism
in chain of infection, 378–79, 379f
defined, 195, 378, 415, 812
Microscopic studies, 664, 688–94
assisting with liver biopsy, 690, 690f
Micturition, 625, 699, 701
Midbrain, 282, 283f
Midline catheter, 1046
Military time, 11, 11t
Minerals
defined, 577, 1045
function of, 581
major, 580
nutritional recommendations, 596
trace, 580
Mini-infuser pump, 1029
Mitered corner, 166, 166f
Mitral valve sounds, 293
Mitt restraints, 150–51

Mobility (*See also* Ambulation)
age-related changes, 320
alterations in, 324
defined, 323, 349, 1096
impaired, in elderly, 345, 373
Monocyte, defined, 812
Monokine, defined, 813
Montgomery straps, in wound care, 835
Mood, assessment, 301
Morning care, 160
Mother–infant bonding, 308
Motor function, assessment of, 278
Mottling, defined, 786
Mouth, assessment of, 286, 309, 314–15
Moving clients, 333–45
with assistance, 337, 337f
from bed to chair, 340–41, 340f–341f
from bed to gurney, 337–38, 338f
dangling at bedside, 339–40, 339f–340f
documentation, 345
gerontologic considerations, 345–46
logrolling, 343, 343f
placing handroll, 344, 344f
placing trochanter roll, 344, 344f
turning to lateral position, 335, 335f
turning to prone position, 335–36, 335f–336f
up in bed, 336, 336f
using footboard, 344
using Hoyer lift, 342, 342f
using safety belt, 341, 341f
using transfer board, 338–39, 338f–339f
MRI (*See* Magnetic resonance imaging)
Mucosa, defined, 161, 196, 756
Mucous membrane medications, 542–48
metered-dose inhaled (MDI) medications, 544–45, 544f, 545f
nonpressurized (nebulized) aerosol, 546
nose drops, 543, 544f
rectal suppositories, 546–47, 547f
sublingual, 543, 543f
vaginal suppositories, 547, 547f
Mucous plug, 305
Mucus fistula, 761
Multicultural health care, 70–71 (*See also* Cultural considerations)
barriers in, 70
cultural assessment, 71
cultural competence, 70
cultural sensitivity, 70–71
defined, 66
religious diversity in, 72t
spiritual assessment, 71
Multidisciplinary Problem Record, 39
Multidisciplinary Team Records, 12, 15f
Multigravida, defined, 308
Multipara, defined, 308
Mummy restraints, 154–55, 154f
Muscle fibers, 350
Muscle strength
assessment of, 278
extension, 278
flexion, 278
Muscle-strengthening, for crutch walking, 368
Muscle tone, assessment of, 278
Muscles
cardiac, 934–35
components of, 350
functions of, 350–51
skeletal, 324
Musculoskeletal, defined, 323, 349, 495, 1096
Musculoskeletal system, 350–51 (*See also* Muscles)
assessment of, 14
gerontologic considerations, 320
pediatric, 316–17
bone, 324
components of, 324
defined, 467
joints, 324 (*See also* Joints)
skeletal muscles, 324
Mutual fit, in therapeutic communication, 69
Myelography
defined, 661
preparation for, 668–69
purpose of, 666t
Myocardium, defined, 234
Myofibroblast, defined, 813
Myopia, 284

N

Nadir, in fetal monitoring, 934
Nails
age changes in, 231
in pediatric assessment, 313
Narcosis, defined, 871
Narcotic control system, using, 524, 524f
Narcotics
addiction, defined, 467
administering epidural, 481–83, 482f
bolus injection, 483
continuous infusion, 483
medications used, 482
defined, 516, 1139
patient-controlled analgesia (PCA), 467, 473, 475
Nares, defined, 871
Narrative charting, 43–45, 45f
advantages of, 44f
assessment-response (AIR) in, 45, 45f
disadvantages of, 44f
Nasal cannula, 891–92, 891f, 893t
Nasal trumpet, inserting, 898, 898f
Nasogastric (NG) tube, 586
administering poison control agents, 607
documentation, 608
enteral feedings, 612t
gastric lavage with, 606
intermittent feedings, 611–12, 611f
intubation, 600–604, 601f, 602f
decompressing GI tract, 603–4
testing blood in gastric specimen, 601–2
testing pH in gastric specimen, 604, 604f
irrigating, 605–6, 605f
medication administration by, 531–32, 531f–532f
removing, 607–8, 607f, 608f
Salem sump tube, 600f
Nasointestinal tube, 586
defined, 577
enteral feeding, 612t, 616–18, 617t
removing, 607–8, 607f, 608f
Nasolacrimal, defined, 196
Nasopharyngeal airway, inserting, 898, 898f
National Nurses Response Team (NNRT), 416
Naturopathy, 504
Nausea, defined, 467, 577
Nebulized medications, 546
Nebulizer, defined, 516
Neck, range of motion for, 355t
Necrosis, defined, 161, 756
Necrotic, defined, 813
Neddle-free devices, 1016
Needle-stick injuries, 384, 387, 550, 1247
Negligence, 6–7
criminal, 6
gross, 6
Neo bladder, 703
Neoplasm, defined, 661
Nephrotoxic, defined, 995
Nerve agent, 415, 423
Neurohormonal, defined, 1139
Neurologic assessment, 14, 276–87, 1100t, 1101
consciousness level, 276–77
gerontologic considerations, 317–18
motor function, 278
pupil assessment, 277
Neutrophil, defined, 813
Newborns (*See also* Infants)
Apgar scoring system for, 311, 311t
assessment, 308–11
abdomen, 310
chest, 309
extremities, 310
genitourinary system, 310
head and neck, 308–9
skin, 308
spine, 310
blood pressure, 237
body temperature in, 236, 246–47, 247t
normal breathing rates of, 240
pulse rate, 237, 310
respirations, 237, 309
NG tube (*See* Nasogastric (NG) tube)
Nitroglycerin (*See* Transdermal medications)
Nocturia, defined, 699
Noise, in hospital environment, 132
Noncompliance, defined, 66
Noncontact normothermic wound therapy, 817–18, 863–94, 864f
Noninvasive pain relief, 471, 474t
Nonpressurized (nebulized) aerosol, 546
Nonverbal communication, 66, 68–69
Nonverbal encouragement, in therapeutic communication, 69
North American Nursing Diagnosis Association (NANDA), nursing diagnoses categorization, 26, 29
Norton Scale, for pressure ulcers, 853t
Nose, assessment of, 286, 309, 314
Nose drops, administering, 543, 544f
Nosocomial, defined, 129

Nosocomial infection, 382
body's natural defenses and, 380
defined, 378, 382
pneumonia, 382
urinary tract, 381
NPO, defined, 661
Nuclear cardiology scan
common tests in, 676
preparation for, 676–77
purpose of, 675t
Nuclear scanning, 663–64, 674–77
client education, 677
preparation for various, 675–77
purpose of various, 675t
Nullipara, defined, 308
Nurse–client communication (*See* Communication; Therapeutic communication)
Nurse–client relationship, 79–81
defined, 71
documentation, 81
facilitation of, 80
gerontologic considerations, 81–82
initiation of, 80
multicultural health care and, 70–71
nursing diagnosis for, 73
phases of, 72
principles for, 71
termination of, 80
therapy, 71–72
Nurse manager, reporting to, 55
Nurse Practice Act, 2, 4, 55
Nurses
code of ethics, 2, 3f
drugs and, 6f, 66
professional role of, 2–4
Nurses' notes, 12, 15f
Nursing diagnosis, 27–30 (*See* opening section in each chapter)
Nursing history, obtaining, 91, 92f
Nursing Interventions Classification (NIC), 29
Nursing Outcomes Classification (NOC), 29
Nursing process
assessment phase of, 22, 23f
charting and, 42
critical thinking and, 24–25
defined, 22, 34
evaluation phase of, 23–24, 24f
implementation phase of, 23, 24f
nursing diagnosis phase of, 22, 23f
outcome identification and planning phase of, 23, 23f
Nursing Retrieval Guides, 50
Nursing unit, admission to, 86–87
Nutrients
assimilation of (*See* Digestion)
defined, 577, 1045
essential, 577–78, 578f, 579f
macronutrients, 577–80
micronutrients, 577, 580–81
Nutritional assessment, 581, 582t–583t
Nutritional management, 504, 577–85 (*See also* Therapeutic diets)
assimilation of nutrients (*See* Digestion)
cultural considerations, 264
documentation, 598
DRIs, 581
enteral feeding, 585–87
essential nutrients, 577–78, 578f, 579f
Food Guide Pyramid, 577–78, 578f, 579f
for the elderly, 620f
gerontologic considerations, 619–21
during hospitalization, 585–87, 595–98
macronutrients, 577–80
micronutrients, 580–81
modified therapeutic diets, 588–94 (*See also* Therapeutic diets)
nursing diagnosis, 587
RDAs, 581
total parenteral nutrition (TPN), 1063–69
in wound healing, 814, 815f
Nutritional recommendations
calories, 581
carbohydrates, 579
fats, 579
gerontologic considerations, 619
for healing, 592f
proteins, 580
vitamins and minerals, 596
water, 580

O

OASIS system, for home health care, 1247
documentation, 1250
forms, 1253f
plan of care, 1249–50
Obesity, health and, 578
Obstetrics, assessment, 302–8
antepartum, 303–4
baseline data, 302–3
intrapartum, 304–5
labor and delivery, 305–7
postpartum, 307–8
Obstipation, defined, 756
Obstructed airway
cardiopulmonary resuscitation (CPR)
for adults, 964, 965f, 966
for children, 968–69
Heimlich maneuver for, 971–72, 972f, 973f
signs of, 972
Obstruction
defined, 577, 1045
intestinal, 584–85
of the lumen of the bowel, 579–760
urinary tract, 702
Occlude, defined, 756
Occlusion, defined, 813
Occult blood
defined, 625, 756
stool specimen for, 637–38, 637f
Occupational Health and Safety Administration (OSHA), 134, 415
Occupied bed, defined, 160
Oculomotor nerve, 283t
Olfactory nerve, 283t
Oligohydramnios, 305
Oliguria, defined, 661, 699
Open bed, defined, 160
Open-ended questions, in therapeutic communication, 69
Ophthalmic, defined, 196, 516
Ophthalmic drops, applying, 537, 537f
Ophthalmic ointment, applying, 537–38, 538f
Opiates, 1164, 1168, 1184 (*See also* Narcotics)
Opioid (narcotic) addiction, defined, 467
Opportunistic infection, defined, 378
Op-site dressing, 854
Opsonin, defined, 378
Optic nerve, 283t
OR care, 160 (*See also* Perioperative care)
Oral, defined, 196
Oral hygiene, 196, 198–203
client education, 200
denture care, 201–2, 201f
documentation, 203
equipment, 199
flossing, 200–201, 201f
toothbrushing, 199–200, 199f, 200f
for unconscious clients, 202, 202f
Oral medications, 528–33
administering to adults, 531
administering to children, 532
crushing, 529–30, 530f
by enteral tube, 531–32, 531f–532f
liquid, 529, 529f, 532
preparation, 529–30
Oral temperature
using an electronic thermometer, 245–46
using digital thermometer, 244–45, 244f
Organism, defined, 813
Orientation, environmental, 86–87, 130
Orientation phase, of nurse-client relationship, 72, 80
Oropharyngeal airway, inserting, 898, 898f
Orthopedic, defined, 1140
Orthopedic assessment, 1100t, 1101
Orthopedic interventions, 1095–1137
amputation, 1100–1101, 1123–26
arthroplasty, 1099–110, 1127–31
casts, 1098, 1109–13
documentation, 1107, 1113, 1121, 1126, 1131, 1134
gerontologic considerations, 1135
immobilizing devices, 1102–8
cervical collar, 1106, 1106f
figure-eight bandage, 1104–5, 1105f
Jewett–Taylor brace, 1106–7, 1106f
sling, 1103, 1103f
spiral bandage, 1104, 1104f
splint, 1105
nursing diagnosis, 1101
Stryker frame, 1132–34
traction, 1098–99, 1114–22
Orthostatic, defined, 1096
Orthostatic hypotension
defined, 1096
in elderly, 269, 319
measuring, 361
minimizing, 361
Oscilloscope, defined, 1206
Osmolality, defined, 995
Osmosis, defined, 995, 1046
Osmotic pressure, 995
defined, 995

Osteoblasts, defined, 1096
Osteoclast, defined, 1096
Ostomy, 757, 760–61
Ostomy pouch
  application, 775–81, 777f–780f
    documentation, 781
    equipment, 776, 776f
  client education about, 780
Otic, defined, 516
Otic medications, applying, 539, 539f
Outbreak, defined, 378, 415
Outcome and Assessment Information Set (OASIS), for home health care, 1247
  documentation, 1250
  forms, 1253f
  plan of care, 1249–50
Outcome identification (*See also* Planning)
  in client care plan, 35–37
  critical thinking and, 26–27
  in nursing process, 23, 23f
Overbed table, 133
Overdependence, defined, 66
Overloading, in communication, 69
Over-the-needle catheter, 1006
Oxygen administration, 875, 887–96
  devices for, 893t
  documentation, 895
  in home health care, 1289–90
    equipment, 1290
    safety precautions, 1290
    transtracheal, 1291–93
  monitoring, 888, 888f
  nasal cannula, 891–92, 891f, 893t
  oxygen analyzer, 890, 890f
  oxygen cylinder, 890, 890f
  oxygen face mask, 892, 892f, 893t
  oxygen hood, 893t, 895
  oxygen tent, 893t, 894, 894f
  pulse oximetry, 888
  safety precautions for, 889
  transtracheal, 1289, 1291–92
    client education for care, 1293
    contraindications, 1291
    SCOOP system for, 1291–92
Oxygen analyzer, 890, 890f
Oxygen cylinder, 890, 890f
Oxygen face mask, 892, 892f, 893t
Oxygen hood, 893t, 895
Oxygen tent, 893t, 894, 894f
Oxygen toxicity, 896

P

Pacemaker, 936, 977–82
  assisting with insertion, 978–79
  client education about, 980
  client self-monitoring, 1296–97
  clinics, 980
  defined, 934
  demand (synchronous), 936
  ICHD pacemaker coding, 978
  maintaining function, 979–80
  permanent, 936
  safety precautions, 978
  telephone check, 1296–98
  temporary, 936, 979f
Pain
  in abdominal assessment, 298
  adaptation and, 131
  breakthrough, 475
  characteristics of, 470, 472
  defined, 467, 495, 1184
  endorphins and, 369–470
  experience of, 470
  as fifth vital sign, 235, 242, 467, 473
  influence on vital signs, 237
  physical sensation of, 467–68, 468f
  referred, 467
  in sensory function assessment, 280
  theories of, 468–69
  types of, 467
Pain assessment, 467
  for children, 69–70, 469f, 470f
  in cognitively impaired, 470–71, 481
  form for, 471f
  gerontologic considerations, 489
  measurement of, 470
  tools for, 469f, 471f
    Wong-Baker FACES Rating Scale, 469–70, 469f, 470f
Pain management, 465–92, 471–75
  for breakthrough pain, 475
  cultural considerations, 478
  documentation, 476, 478, 489
  in end-of-life care, 1186–87
  gerontologic considerations, 489
  guidelines for, 472
  JCAHO standards for, 471
  noninvasive, 471–73
  nonpharmacological approach, 472, 474t, 477–79
    massage, 478
    relaxation techniques, 478
  nurse's role in, 472–73, 473t
  patient-controlled analgesia (PCA), 473, 475
  pharmacological approach, 480–91 (*See also* Pain medications)
  TENS for, 467, 474
Pain medications
  administering, 481
  analgesic ladder, 1195
  epidural, 475
  epidural narcotic analgesia, 481–83, 482f
  intravenous, 475
  options, 481
  patient-controlled analgesia (PCA)
    dose calculation, 486
    form for, 488f
    infuser pump, 485
    preparation, 484–85, 485f
    PRN booster dose, 487
    procedure, 485–86, 486f
    qualifying patient, 483–84
    teaching patient about, 487–88
    terminating, 487
Pain pathways, 470
Palate, defined, 196
Palliative care (*See* End-of-life care)
Pallor, defined, 161, 786
Palpate, defined, 995, 1046
Palpation
  of abdomen, 297
  defined, 234
  in physical assessment, 273–74, 274f
Palpitation, defined, 1140
Pancreas, in digestion, 584
Pancreatic amylase, 584
Pancreatic lipase, 584
Pandemic, defined, 415
Papanicolaou (PAP) smear
  assisting with, 693
  purpose of, 689t
Paracentesis
  assisting with, 692, 692f
  defined, 662
  purpose of, 689t
Paralysis, defined, 323, 349, 1096
Paramnesia, 301
Parasites
  defined, 625, 757
  stool specimen for, 636–37, 636f
Parasympathetic nervous system
  in bowel elimination, 759
  defined, 467, 495
  in digestion, 757–58
  in pain sensation, 467–68, 468f
Parenteral, defined, 516
Parenteral administration, 549–70 (*See also* Injections)
  documentation, 569
  heparin
    subcutaneous, 562–64, 562f
  injection sites
    deltoid, 551, 567f
    dorsogluteal, 551, 565f, 566f
    vastus lateralis, 551, 566f
    ventrogluteal, 551, 564f, 565f
  insulin injections, 556–60 (*See also* Insulin)
  intradermal injections, 554, 554f, 555f
  preparing injections, 550–54
  subcutaneous injections, 555, 555f, 556f
  Z-track method, 567–68, 568f
Parenteral nutrition [*See also* Total parenteral nutrition (TPN)]
  defined, 577
  total nutrient admixture (TNA), 1276–80
  vs. enteral feeding, 585
Paresthesis, defined, 1096
Parietal lobe, function of, 282
Parotid gland, defined, 196
Passey–Muir valve, 917
Patency, defined, 625, 699
Pathogen, defined, 378, 415, 625, 813
Patient and Family Education Standards, by JCAHO, 107, 109f, 115
Patient Care Records, 12, 15f
Patient-controlled analgesia (PCA), 467, 473, 475
Patient rights (*See* Clients' rights)
Patient Self-Determination Act, 9, 87
  advance medical directives, 9–10, 9f
Patient's Bill of Rights, 7, 8f
  American Hospital Association (AHA), 86–87

Pattern theory, of pain, 468
Payne–Martin Classification system, for skin tears, 183
PCA (patient-controlled analgesia), 467
PCO_2, in respiration process, 873
Peak flow measurement, instruction for, 879–80, 879f
Pearson attachment, defined, 1096
Pediatric assessment, 311–17 (*See also* Children)
abdomen, 316
appearance, 312
genitourinary system, 316
head and neck, 313–15
heart, 316
height and weight, 311
lungs, 315
musculoskeletal system, 316–17
skin, 312–13
Pediculosis
defined, 161, 196
home health care, 1269, 1272
removing, 209–12
Pediculus capitis, defined, 161
Pediculus corporis, defined, 161
Pediculus pubis, defined, 161
PEG (*See* Percutaneous endoscopic gastrostomy (PEG))
Pelvic traction, 1116t
PEP protocol, for HIV exposure, 378, 387, 401t
Perceptions
assessment of, 300
defined, 66
Percussion
chest, 871, 875, 885, 885f
in physical assessment, 273–74, 274f
Percutaneous agent, defined, 415
Percutaneous central vascular catheters, 1049–62
Percutaneous endoscopic gastrostomy (PEG), 586
defined, 577
enteral feeding through, 612t, 613–14, 613f
Perforation, defined, 757
Perfusion, 875
alterations in, 873–74
defined, 934, 1207
Perineal and genital care, 197, 220–24
cultural considerations, 222
documentation, 224
females
draping, 221, 221f
procedure, 221–22, 221f, 222f
incontinence care, 222–23
males, 223–24, 223f–224f
Perineum, 196, 307
Perioperative, defined, 1140
Perioperative care
client education, 1142, 1148–57
conscious sedation, 1142–43, 1166–75
documentation, 1147, 1156, 1164, 1169, 1174–75, 1178
gerontologic considerations, 1179–80
intraoperative, 1140, 1142–42
nurse's role, 1140
nursing diagnosis, 1144
postanesthesia room (PAR) care, 1171–75
postoperative, 1140, 1143–144, 1176–79
preoperative, 1140–42, 1142t, 1158–65 (*See also* Preoperative care)
stress and, 1141–42, 1141t, 1145–47
Periosteum, defined, 1096
Peripheral, defined, 234, 662
Peripheral catheter, 1046
Peripheral pulse, assessment of, 239, 295, 295f
Doppler ultrasound stethoscope, 255–56, 255f
palpation, 254–55, 254f
Peripheral vascular disease, defined, 234
Peripherally inserted central catheter (PICC), 1047, 1086–91
changing dressing, 1088–89, 1088f, 1089f
defined, 1046
drawing blood, 1090
maintaining, 1087, 1087f
removing, 1090
Peristalsis, defined, 516, 699, 757
Peritoneal dialysis
continuous ambulatory, 1282
administering, 1285–86
dressing change, 1286
transfer sets for, 1285
continuous cycling, 699
intermittent, 1282
types of, 1282
Peritonitis, defined, 1140
Periwound, defined, 813
Permethrin (Nix), 210–11
Personal care, levels of, 160–61 (*See also* Evening care; Morning care)
Personal hygiene, 194–232
bedpan, urinal, commode, 216–19
ear care, 229–30
eye care, 197, 225–30
foot care, 196–97, 213–15
gerontologic considerations, 231
hair care, 196, 204–8
home health care, 1268–72
bathing, 1269–70
bedmaking, 1271
hair care, 1269
nursing diagnosis, 1270
overview, 1269
preparing normal saline, 1271
pressure ulcer care, 1269, 1271
skin care, 1269
in mental assessment, 299
nursing diagnosis, 197
oral hygiene, 196, 198–203
pediculosis, 209–12
perineal and genital care, 197, 220–24
Personal protective equipment (PPE), 444–54 (*See also* specific equipment)
bioterrorism, 448–49
chemical exposure, 450
defined, 415
documentation, 454
radiation exposure, 450–51
Personal space, cultural considerations, 70, 338
Perspective, defined, 495
PES framework, for nursing diagnosis, 29–30
PET scan
defined, 662
preparation for, 676
purpose of, 675t
Petechiae, defined, 161, 934
pH
of arterial blood gases, 281
of blood and respiration, 240, 873–74
gastric, 604, 604f, 618
of urine, 298
Phagocytosis, defined, 813
Phlebitis, 934, 938, 997, 1007, 1015
defined, 1046
evaluation criteria, 1007
Phlebostatic axis, 1207, 1211
defined, 1207
Phlebotomy, 641
Physical appearance, in mental assessment, 299–300
Physical assessment, 272–321
abdomen, 295–99
chest area, 288–95
examination techniques, 274
focus assessment, 275, 275f
gerontologic considerations, 317–20
head and neck, 282–86
health history, 273
IPPA sequence for, 273
mental, 299–302
neurologic, 276–87
newborns, 308–11
nurses' role, 273–74
obstetrical, 302–8 (*See also* Obstetrics, assessment)
overview, 273
pediatric, 311–17
skin, 286–88
Physical restraint, defined, 129
Physician notification, 55
Physician's history and physical, 13
Physician's orders, 13, 17f
Physician's progress notes, 13, 17f
Physiologic, defined, 129, 467
Physiologic responses, to stress, 497, 498t
PIE charting format, 45–46
Piggyback infusion bag, 1027–29, 1028t
Pigment, defined, 161
Pillow case, 166, 166f
Piloerection, defined, 234
Pinworm, defined, 625
Pitting edema, 287
PKU diet, 589
Plague, 424t–425t, 429–30, 449
Planning (*See also* Outcome identification)
critical thinking and, 26–27
in nursing process, 23, 23f
Plantar flexion, defined, 349
Plantar response, 279
Plantar wart, 197
Plaque, defined, 161, 196
Plasma, blood component, 1039t

Plaster cast, 1098, 1110f
Platelets, blood component, 1039t
Pleur-evac ATS, autotransfusion using, 925–26, 925f
Pleural friction rub, 293
PMI (point of maximum impulse), 235, 252
Pneumatic compression devices, 947–50, 948f, 949f
Pneumonia
  defined, 1140
  nosocomial, 382
  Pneumocystis carinii, 378
Pneumonic plague, 424t–425t, 429–30, 449
Pneumothorax, 871, 922f
Point of maximum impulse (PMI), 235, 252
Poison, defined, 415
Poison control agents, administration with NG tube, 607
Polycythemia, defined, 871
Polydactyly, 310
Polyhydramnios, 305
Polyunsaturated, defined, 577, 1046
Polyuria, defined, 625, 699
Pons, 282, 283f
Port, defined, 1046
Portal of entry, in chain of infection, 379, 379f
Portal of exit, in chain of infection, 379, 379f
Post-traumatic stress disorder, in disaster management, 461
Postanesthesia care unit (PACU), 1171–75
  discharging to home, 1174
  discharging to nursing unit, 1173–74
  documentation, 1174–75
  providing, 1172–73, 1172f
Postexposure prophylaxis (PEP), for HIV exposure, 378, 387, 401t
Postmortem care, 460, 1200–1202
Postoperative care, 1140, 1143–144, 1176–79
  documentation, 1178
  medication administration, 1177–78
  providing, 1177
  surgical site infection, 1160–62
Postoperative diet progression, 591–92
Postpartum, assessment, 307–8
Postural drainage, 871, 875, 884
Postural hypotension (*See* Orthostatic hypotension)
Posture
  defined, 323, 349
  in mental assessment, 300
Potassium
  foods high in, 590
  increased therapeutic diet, 590
Potential, defined, 85
Power of attorney, 10
Practice (*See also* Clinical practice)
  best, 30
  evidence-based, 30–31
  standards of, 4–7
Precordial, defined, 934
Prefixes, listing of, 59–61
Pregnancy, blood pressure during, 243, 303
Prehospital laboratory procedures, 86
Preload, defined, 1207
Premature beats, defined, 235
Preoperative care, 1140–42, 1142t, 1158–65
  checklist for, 1163f
  client education, 1142, 1148–57
    arthroscopy, 1154–55
    deep breathing, 1155
    for family, 1150–51
    in hospital setting, 1149
    laparoscopy, 1153
    laser therapy, 1151, 1151t, 1152t
    leg exercises, 1156
    lithotripsy, 1152–53
    in outpatient setting, 1149
    productive cough, 1155, 1155f
    providing, 1150
    turning in bed, 1156
  client preparation, 1161–62
  documentation, 1147, 1156, 1164, 1169
  medication administration, 1164
  obtaining baseline data, 1159
  stress and, 1141–42, 1141t, 1145–47
    denial, 1147
    prevention, 1146
    reducing, 1146
  surgical site preparation, 1159–61
Preparedness Plan, 417
Pressure dressing, 943
Pressure gradient, in ventilation, 1236
Pressure point, defined, 161, 196
Pressure receptors, 238
Pressure ulcers, 817, 850–60, 854
  classification of, 817
  client education, 817
  in dark-skin-tone clients, 851
  defined, 161, 350, 813, 817
  documentation, 860
  gerontologic considerations, 817
  in hospitalized clients, 817, 854
  management, 817, 851t
    applying transparent adhesive film, 854–55, 855f, 857, 859t
    in home health care, 1269, 1271
    hydrogel, 857, 859t
    ongoing assessment form, 856f
    using hydrocolloid dressing, 857, 859t, 860
  prevention, 817, 853–54
  risk assessment, 851, 853t
  specialty beds for, 162, 184f, 185f, 186t, 854
  staging of, 851t, 852f
  support surfaces for, 162
Primary healing, 813–14
Primary immune response, defined, 378
Prime movers, defined, 349
Primigravida, defined, 308
Primipara, defined, 308
Privacy
  in hospital setting, 135
  right to, 8–9
Problem list, in POMR charting, 46, 46f
Problem-oriented medical record (POMR), 34, 42, 45–48
  advantages of, 49f
  components of, 46–48
    database, 46
    discharge summary, 47–48, 48f
    initial plan, 46
    problem list, 46, 46f
    progress notes, 46–47
    SOAP format, 47, 47f
  defined, 34
  disadvantages of, 49f
  PIE format, 45–46
Problem statement, in nursing diagnosis, 29
Procedures
  defined, 85
  protocols for, 18–19
Professional misconduct, 6
Progress notes, in POMR charting, 46–47
Projectile vomiting, defined, 577
Proliferative phase, of wound healing, 813
Pronation
  defined, 349, 351
  range of motion exercises for, 355t, 356t
Prone, defined, 323, 349
Prosthesis, defined, 1096
Prosthetic devices, implanted, infection risk with, 382
Protein(s), 579–80
  deficiency of, 580
  defined, 577, 1046
  nutritional recommendations, 580
  therapeutic diet restricting, 589
Protocols, 39
  basic, 18–19
  defined, 378
Protraction, defined, 349, 351
Proximal, defined, 349, 1207
Pruritus, defined, 995
Psycho, defined, 129
Psychogenic, defined, 467, 495
Psychological responses
  in pain sensation, 468f
  to stress, 497, 498t
Psychosocial, defined, 129
Psychosomatic, defined, 1184
Ptosis, 284
Pulmonary agents, 423
Pulmonary artery pressure (PAP) monitoring
  assisting with catheter insertion, 1212–13
  leveling and zeroing monitoring system, 1211
  measuring cardiac output, 1215
  normal pressures, 1210t
  obtaining pressure readings, 1214, 1214f
  overview, 1210–11
Pulmonary artery wedge pressure (PAWP), 1210
  defined, 1207
Pulmonary edema, 937
Pulmonary function tests, 874
Pulmonic valve sounds, 294
Pulse
  apical
    assessment, 295
    defined, 235
    irregular, 295
  peripheral, assessment, 2
Pulse deficit, 238
  defined, 235

Pulse oximetry, 888
  arterial blood gases (ABGs) values, 874
  using, 888–89
Pulse pressure, 235, 240
Pulse rate, 238–40, 250–57
  apical, 235, 238
  arterial, 239
  assessment of
    apical, 252–53, 252f, 253f
    apical–radial, 253–54, 254f
    frequency, 239–40
    quality, 239–40, 251t
    radial, 251, 251f, 252f
  bigeminal, 235, 251t
  bounding, 235, 239, 251t
  in children, 311
  circulatory system control of, 238
  documentation, 256
  femoral, in children, 316
  gerontologic considerations, 269
  heart rate, 239 (*See also* Heart rate)
  heart rhythm, 239 (*See also* Heart rhythm)
  in neurologic assessment, 281, 281f
  normal, 235
    in children, 239t
    in newborns, 237
  peripheral
    assessment of, 239
    Doppler ultrasound stethoscope for, 255–56, 255f
    palpation of, 254–55, 254f
  radial, 281
  weak or thready, 235, 251t
Pulsus alternans, 235, 251t
Pupil
  assessment, 277, 284, 284f
  in children, 314
Pureed diet, 593
Purpura, defined, 161, 934
Purulent, defined, 625, 813, 995
Pus, defined, 625, 813
PVCs (*See* Premature ventricular contractions)
Pyelography, defined, 662
Pyrogen, defined, 234
Pyuria, defined, 700
PYXIS system, 524, 527, 834

Q

Q fever, 431
Quadriceps-setting exercises, 1124
Quality assurance, unusual occurrence report and, 53–54
Queckenstedt's test, 690
Questions, open-ended, 69

R

Race, influence on vital signs, 237
AD, 415, 423–24
dial pulse
  assessment of, 251, 251f, 252f
  neurologic assessment, 281
ant warmer, for infants, 793–94, 793f, 794f
Radiation
  background, 424
  defined, 415, 786
  dose meter (film badge), 452–54
  in heat transfer, 788
  ionizing, 415
  as weapon of mass destruction, 423–24, 441–42
    acute radiation syndromes, 442
    controlling contamination, 453–54
    decontamination, 452–53
    external, 423
    health effects, 424
    identifying exposure, 441–42
    internal, 423
    measuring, 423–24
    personal protective equipment, 450–51
Radiation absorbed dose (RAD), 415, 423–24
  defined, 415
Radiation dose, defined, 415
Radiation syndromes, acute, 441–42
Radioactive contamination, defined, 415
Radioactive materials, 144
  implant, 144
  safety for clients receiving, 144
  systemic, 144
Rales, 292
Range of motion, 354–59
  defined, 349
  exercises, 352
    active, 359
    documentation, 359
    lower body, 356t, 358f
    passive, 355–56, 356f–358f
    upper body, 355t, 356f–357f
Rapid Estimation of Adult Literacy in Medicine (REALM), 116
Rapport, defined, 66
RDAs, 581
Readiness to learn, 106, 108, 115
Reality orientation, assessment, 300
Recovery room (*See* Postanesthesia care unit)
Rectal suppositories, administering, 546–47, 547f
Rectal temperature, taking using an electronic thermometer, 245–46
Red wounds, 814, 815t
Referred pain, defined, 467
Reflection, in therapeutic communication, 69
Reflexes, assessment of, 279–80
Reflexology, 504
Reflux, defined, 757
Refractory period, defined, 1207
Regression, defined, 467
Rehabilitation, concepts, 350
Relationship, defined, 67, 106
Relationship therapy, 71–72 (*See also* Nurse-client relationship)
Relaxation
  defined, 467, 495
  techniques, 504–5
    in pain management, 478
    in stress management, 474, 511
Religion, importance of, 76
Religious diversity, considerations for client care, 72t
REM, 415, 424
Renal, defined, 577, 700
Renal replacement therapy (*See* Hemodialysis)
Repolarization, defined, 1207
Report, defined, 34
Reporting, 55
  intershift, 55
  intrashift, 55
  to nurse manager, 55
  physician notification, 55
  shift-to-shift, 55
Reproductive system (*See* Genitourinary system)
Reservoirs
  in chain of infection, 379, 379f
  ileal, 702
  Kock's, 741
  urinary continent, 742
Resident (normal) flora, defined, 378
Resistance, defined, 106, 467
Resistance stage, of stress, 496–97, 497t
Resistance to change, 108
Resistive exercise, 352
Resolution, defined, 1184
Respirations, 236, 240, 258–60 (*See also* Breathing)
  alterations in, 873
  in children, 239t, 312
  control of, 240
  defined, 236
  documentation, 259
  evaluation of, 240
  gerontologic considerations, 237, 269
  in neurologic assessment, 280
  in newborns, 237, 309
  normal, 259
  procedure for assessment, 259, 259f
  process of, 872–73
Respirator use, for bioterrorism protection, 448
Respiratory acidosis, arterial blood gases (ABGs) associated with, 1221t
Respiratory alkalosis, arterial blood gases (ABGs) associated with, 1221t
Respiratory care, 870–931
  artificial airways, 897–902
  bag–valve–mask ventilation, 881, 881f
  chest physiotherapy (CPT), 883–86
    chest percussion, 885, 885f
    chest vibration, 885–86, 885f, 886f
    client preparation, 884
    documentation, 886
    postural drainage, 884
  chest tubes, 921–28 (*See also* Chest tubes)
  documentation, 882, 886, 895, 901, 908, 918, 927
  gerontologic considerations, 929
  home health care, 1288–94
    mechanical ventilation, 1289–91
    nursing diagnosis, 1289
    oxygen therapy, 1289–90
    tracheostomy care, 1293–94
    transtracheal oxygen therapy, 1291–93
  nurse's role in, 874–75

nursing diagnosis, 875
oxygen administration, 887–96 (*See also* Oxygen administration)
preventive measures, 876–82
client positioning, 877
CPAP/BIPAP, 880–81, 880f
deep breathing, 877, 877f
diaphragmatic breathing, 878
documentation, 882
incentive spirometer, 878–79, 879f
peak flow measurement, 879–80, 879f
productive cough, 877–78, 878f
suctioning, 903–9
tracheostomy care, 910–20
Respiratory compensation for metabolic acidosis, 873
Respiratory function, assessment of, 874–75
Respiratory system
alterations in, 873–74
anatomy of, 872, 872f
assessment of, 14
infection risk in, 381
lower, 872
upper, 872
Restatement, in therapeutic communication, 69
Restorative, defined, 1096
Restraints, 138–39, 146–55
assessment for, 146
chemical, 129, 146, 148
deaths due to, 149
defined, 129
documentation, 138, 155
elbow, 151, 151f
form for, 155f
guidelines for use, 139
methods to decrease use, 147
mitt, 150–51
mummy, 154–55, 154f
physical, 129, 146, 148
procedure, 147
regulations about, 138
seclusion, 129, 146
torso/belt restraint, 148, 148f
vest, 152–53, 152f, 153f, 154f
wrist, 149–50, 149f, 150f
Resuscitation [*See also* Cardiac emergencies; Cardiopulmonary resuscitation (CPR); Emergency life support measures]
defined, 934
Retention catheter
females, 717, 717f–719f, 720
males, 721–22, 721f
removing, 723, 723f
Retraction, defined, 349
Retrovirus, defined, 378
Reverse Trendelenburg's position, 323, 334f, 334t
defined, 323
Rh-negative status, 308
Rhonchi sounds, 292
Ricin toxin, 432
"Rights of delegation," 58–59
Ringer's solution, in wound irrigation, 816, 834
Roentgen equivalent dose (REM), 415, 424
Rotation
defined, 350–51
range of motion exercises for, 355t, 356t
external, 355t, 356t
internal, 355t, 356t
Routine Assessment and Care Record, 39
Russell's traction, 1116t, 1118f
defined, 1096
RYB classification system, for wound care, 814, 815t

S

Safe environment, 136–39, 140–45
documentation, 145
fall prevention, 137, 140–42 (*See also* Falls)
fire procedure, 143
gerontologic considerations, 157
nursing diagnosis, 139
radioactive materials, 144
safety precautions, 137
thermal /electrical injuries, 142–43
Safety belt, transfer using, 341, 341f
Safety precautions, 137
Salem sump tube, 600f [*See also* Nasogastric (NG) tube]
Saline
preparing in home health care, 1271
in wound irrigation, 816, 834
SARS, 388–89
Saturated fatty acid, 577, 579
Scabies, removing, 210–11
Scintillation, defined, 662
Sclera, defined, 196
Sclerosis, defined, 934
Scoliosis, 290
SCOOP system, for transtracheal oxygen therapy, 1289, 1291–92
Seclusion, defined, 129
Second intention healing, 813–14
Sedation
conscious (*See* Conscious sedation)
in end-of-life care, 1187
Sediment, defined, 700
Seizures, causes of, 276
Self-catheterization, intermittent, clean technique for, 1282, 1283–84
Self-esteem
defined, 67
using communication to increase client's, 77
Selye's general adaptation syndrome, 466, 496, 497f, 508
Semi-Fowler's position, 196, 323, 334f, 334t
Semiocclusive dressing, defined, 813
Sensory deprivation, defined, 161
Sensory function
assessment of, 280, 302
touch, 287
gerontologic considerations, 317
Sensory overload, defined, 161
Sentences, incomplete, 69
Sentinel event, defined, 129
Sentinel events, 136, 137t
Sepsis
defined, 378, 577, 1046
infusion-related, 381
Septic, defined, 625, 700
Septicemia, 381, 625, 662, 700
Set point, 234, 237
Severe acute respiratory syndrome (SARS), 388–89
Sexuality, age-related changes, 319
Shampoo, Lindane, 210
Shampooing hair, 205–7
on bed rest, 206
in chair, 206
disposable system, 205–7, 207f
on gurney, 206
Sharps containers, 398, 550, 550f, 642f
Shaving, 207
Shearing force, defined, 161
Sheets
for bedmaking, 160
draw, 160
full, 160
incontinent pads, 160
pull, 160
Shift-to-shift reporting, 55
Shivering thermogenesis, defined, 786
Shock
defined, 234, 700, 934
hemorrhagic, 937
triage and, 459
Shoulder, range of motion for, 355t
Siderails, bed, 133
falls and, 137
Sigmoidoscopy
preparation for, 685–86
purpose of, 683t
Signaling system, 133
Silence
of client, 118
in communication, 68
Sinoatrial (SV) node, 935–36
Sinus arrhythmia, defined, 235
Sitz bath, assisting with, 796, 796f
Six rights, the, 518–19
Skeletal muscles, 324
extensors, 324
flexors, 324
Skeletal system (*See also* Musculoskeletal system)
defined, 323
Skeletal traction, 1098–99, 1117–18, 1117t, 1118f
Skeleton
appendicular, 323
axial, 323
Skilled care, defined, 1254
Skin
anatomy of, 286, 286f
assessment of, 13–14, 181–8
gerontologic considerati
lesions, 287
newborn, 308
pediatric, 312–13
sensation, 287

Skin *(continued)*
  as barrier to infection, 379–80
  cancer, 288
  rash, 182t
  turgor, 181, 287, 625, 995
Skin care, 163, 180–84
  in home health care, 1269
Skin integrity, 161, 163–64, 180–87
  documentation, 185
  gerontologic considerations, 163–64, 184, 191–92
  monitoring, 181–82
  nursing diagnosis, 163
  preventing skin breakdown, 182–83, 183f
  preventing skin tears, 183–84
Skin problems, 182t
Skin tears
  defined, 161
  in elderly, 164
  management of, 184
  Payne–Martin Classification system, 183
  preventing, 183–84
Skin traction, 1099, 1115–16, 1115f, 1116f
Skull, bones of, 282f
Sling, applying, 1103, 1103f
Sling lift (Hoyer), moving clients using, 342, 342f
Small bore feeding tube
  inserting, 615
  providing continuous feeding via, 616
Small intestine, 583, 757
Smallpox, 424t–425t, 432–33
  death rate, 425t
  incubation period, 424t, 432
  precautions, 425t, 432–33, 449
  prioritization of high-risk groups, 433
  signs and symptoms of, 424t, 432
  transmission, 424t, 432
  treatment, 425t, 433
Smallpox vaccination
  administration of *vaccinia* vaccine, 434–36, 435f
  dangers of, 432
  documentation, 442
  inadvertent inoculation, 438
  post-vaccination reactions, 436–38, 437f
  prioritization of high-risk groups, 433
  reconstituting *vaccinia* vaccine, 434, 434f
  vaccinia immune globulin (VIG), 433, 438
SOAP format, 34, 42
  defined, 34
  in POMR charting, 47, 47f
SOAPIE format, 34, 42
  defined, 34
  in POMR charting, 47, 47f
Social, defined, 67
Sociocultural dimensions, in hospital environment, 134–36
ocket care, postoperative, 226–27
odium
  foods high in, 590
  estriction therapeutic diet, 590
ium hypochlorite, defined, 415
d linens, disposing of, 384
ic, defined, 1184
Sonic toothbrush, 200
Sonorous, defined, 235
Sound levels, in hospital environment, 132
Source-oriented charting, 34, 42
  defined, 34
  narrative, 43–45, 45f
  systems, 43, 43f
Space requirements, in hospital environment, 131
Spasms, 276
Spasticity, defined, 350
Specific gravity, defined, 625, 700, 995
Specificity theory, of pain, 468
Specimen, defined, 625
Specimen collection, 624–59
  blood, 627, 640–49, 641, 1055–56, 1056f, 1078, 1084–85, 1084f, 1090
  cultures, 627–28, 638, 644, 654–57
  documentation, 631, 639, 649, 653, 657
  fluid analysis, 688–94
  gerontologic considerations, 657
  microscopic studies, 688–94
  nurse's role in, 626
  nursing diagnosis, 628
  sputum, 650–53
  stool, 635–39
  throat, 655, 655f
  urine, 626–27, 629–31
  wound, 655–56, 655f, 816, 834
Specimen handling
  biohazardous agents, 438–39, 439f
  isolation, 408, 408f
Sphincter, defined, 757
Sphygmomanometer, 235, 262
Spica, defined, 1096
Spine, assessment of
  newborns, 310
  pediatric, 317
Spiral bandage
  applying, 1104, 1104f
  defined, 1096
Spiritual assessment, 67, 71, 76, 299
Spirometry, 874
  defined, 871
  incentive spirometer (IS), 878–79, 879f
Splint, applying, 1105
Sprain, defined, 323, 350, 1096
Sputum, defined, 626, 871
Sputum specimen collection, 650–53
  procedure, 651, 651f
  suction trap for, 652, 652f
  by tracheal aspiration, 652
Squamous cell cancer, skin, 288
Stable, defined, 323
Staffing requirements, client acuity systems and, 57
Stamina, defined, 467, 495
Standard precautions, 382–85
  accidental contact with blood or body fluids, 399
  biohazard waste, 134, 386
    defined, 377, 386
    disposal precautions, 399
    double-bagging, 406–7, 407f
    soiled linens, 384
    storage, 386
    transport, 386
  in bioterrorism incidents, 446
  blood-borne pathogens, 384
  client placement, 385
  defined, 415
  in diagnostic procedures, 663
  documentation, 400
  donning protective gear, 398
  exiting client's room, 399
  first tier, 382, 397–401
  glove use, 383, 384t, 398
  gown use, 384, 384t
  guidelines for, 398
  handwashing, 383
  Health Care Worker Protection Act, 385
  mask, eye protection, face shield, 383–84, 398
  transmission-based, 382–283, 384t
Standards of care, 5, 5f, 6f
Standards of practice, 4–7
  American Nurses Association (ANA), 5, 5f
  Board of Registered Nursing (BRN), 5
  liability and legal issues, 5–6
  licensure, 4–5
  Nurse Practice Act, 4
  related to drugs, 6, 6f
Standards of professional performance, 5, 5f
Staphococcus aureus
  methicillin-resistant, 382
  in wound infection, 816
Staples, removing, 829, 829f–830f
Starling's law, 935
START triage system, 415, 420, 421f
Stasis, defined, 934
State statutes
  about charting, 40
  about drugs, 6
  Nurse Practice Act, 4
StatLock securement device, 602, 719, 1089, 1089f
Sterile, defined, 378
Sterile container, pouring from, 822, 822f
Sterile field
  commercially prepared packages, 823–24, 824f
  guidelines for, 823
  hospital-wrapped packages, 823
  preparation of, 822–23
Sterile gloves, 820–21, 821f
Sterile technique, 14
  in home health care, 1260
Stertorous, defined, 235
Stethoscope
  for blood pressure assessment, 263
  in physical assessment, 273
Stockings, graduated compression, 938
  applying, 946–47, 946f, 947f
  effectiveness of, 946, 948
  measuring for, 946t
Stoma, defined, 700, 757
Stomach
  age-related changes, 319
  in digestion, 583

Stool
constipation (*See* Bowel evacuation; Constipation)
defined, 626, 757
Stool specimen collection, 635–39
adult, 636
for bacterial culture, 638
infant, 637
for occult blood, 637–38, 637f
gamma Fe-Cult Plus, 637–38
Hemocult, 638
for ova or parasites, 636–37, 636f
for pinworms, 638–39
Straight catheter
for females, 714–15, 715f
for males, 716–17, 716f
Strain, defined, 323, 350, 1096
Stress, 496, 509
and adaptation, 131
assessment, 1146t
behavioral response to, 1141, 1141t, 1146t
body's response to, 1141, 1141t, 1146t
cultural considerations, 511
danger signals of, 499
defined, 85, 129, 467, 495, 496, 508, 1140, 1184
determining response patterns, 508–9
disease and, 499
documentation, 512
effects of, 496–97, 508
gerontologic considerations, 513
individual responses to, 497–99
management of, 509–11
complementary/alternative medicine (CAM), 510–12
coping strategies, 509–10
deep breathing, 510–11
manipulating environment, 509
meditation, 512
relaxation techniques, 511
nurse's role in relieving, 499, 501
preoperative, 1141–42, 1141t, 1145–47
satisfying life and, 500
signals of, 498f
Stress adaptation syndrome, 466, 496, 497f
Stressor, 467, 495, 498
Stridor, 293
Stroke
emergency treatment of, 939
induced hypothermia and, 804
Stryker frame, 1132–34
assisting with bedpan, 1134
defined, 1096
parallel frame, 1133–34
turning from supine to prone, 1133
wedge turning frame, 1133, 1133f
Student nurses
clinical planning, 59
code of ethics for, 2, 3f
role in client education, 109
Student Clinical Prep Form, 58f, 59
time management, 58f, 59
Stump (amputation) (*See* Amputated limbs)
Subcutaneous, defined, 516
Subcutaneous (sub Q) injections
administering, 555, 555f, 556f
heparin, 562–63, 562f
Subcutaneous tissues, 286, 286f
Sublingual, defined, 516
Sublingual medications, administering, 543, 543f
Subungual, defined, 378
Suction trap, for sputum specimen collection, 652, 652f
Suctioning, 903–9
documentation, 908
with in-line closed system, 907, 907f, 908f
indications for, 904
tracheostomy, 912–13, 913f
using catheter and gloves, 904–5, 905f
using catheter in sleeve, 906–7, 906f
Suffering, defined, 1184
Suffixes, listing of, 59–61
Supervise, defined, 85, 129
Supination
defined, 350–51
range of motion exercises for, 355t, 356t
Support, defined, 67, 106
Suppositories
defined, 757
rectal, 546–47, 547f, 766–67, 766f
vaginal, 547, 547f
Suppuration, defined, 786
Sure Step Flexx, for blood glucose testing, 646–47, 647f
Surfactant, defined, 1207
Surgery
ambulation following, 362
elective, 1140
emergency, 1140
nurse's role, 1140
nursing care for (*See* Perioperative care)
positions used for, 1143f
postoperative diet progression, 591–92
Surgical asepsis
defined, 378
vs. medical, 14
Surgical hand scrub, 820, 820f
Surgical site infection, 380, 1160–62
Susceptible host, in chain of infection, 379, 379f
Susceptible sites, defined, 378
Sutures, removing, 828–29, 828f
Swan–Ganz [*See* Pulmonary artery pressure (PAP) monitoring], 1212
Sweat glands, 286, 286f
Swing-through gait, 370
Swing-to gait, 370
Sympathetic nervous system
defined, 467, 495
in pain sensation, 467–68, 468f
Synchronized cardioversion, 1226, 1231–32, 1232t
Syncope, defined, 934, 1097
Syndactyly, 310
Synergists, defined, 350
Synthetic cast, 1098, 1110f
Synthes external fixation device, 1117
Syringe (*See also* Injections)
disposal of, 550, 550f
prefilled medication cartridge, 554, 554f
safety, 551f
types of, 551f
Syringe pump, using, 1013–14, 1013f, 1014f
Systemic, defined, 196, 516
Systemic effect, 517
Systems charting, 34, 43, 43f
Systolic blood pressure, 241, 265, 265f

T

Tachy, defined, 467
Tachycardia, 295
causes of, 239
defined, 235, 259t, 467, 495, 662
fetal, 306, 934, 986
Tachypnea, defined, 235, 871
Tactile fremitus, 291
T'ai Chi Ch'uan, 505
Tapotement, 161
Taste sense, gerontologic considerations, 317
Taxonomy of Nursing Diagnosis, 29
Teaching (*See also* Client education)
determining strategy, 117–18
Technetium-99m, 664, 675
Technetium pyrophosphate scan, 676
Technology, privacy and, 9
TED hose, (*See* Elastic hosiery)
Teeth (*See also* Oral hygiene)
pediatric assessment of, 315
Tegaderm dressing, 854
Telemetry, electrocardiogram (ECG) on, 950f, 959, 959f
Temperature
body (*See* Body temperature)
in hospital environment, 131–32
Temporal lobe, function of, 282
Tendons, defined, 350
TENS (transcutaneous electrical nerve stimulation), 467, 474
Tension pneumothorax, defined, 871
Tepid bath, administering, 803, 803f
Terminal weaning, 1236
Termination, defined, 67, 85, 106
Termination phase, of nurse–client relationship, 72, 80
Tertiary intention healing, 813–14
Thallium, 664, 675
Thallium scan, 676
with exercise, 676
Therapeutic, defined, 67, 85, 106, 129, 516, 1140, 1184
Therapeutic communication, 74–78
assisting client in describing personal experiences, 76
cultural considerations in, 75–76
defined, 68–69
documentation, 77
encouraging client to express needs, feeling and thoughts, 77
initial interaction, 75
introduction to client, 75
spiritual assessment, 76
techniques for, 68–69
using to increase client's self-worth, 77

Therapeutic diets, 588–94
bland food, 592
calcium restriction, 590
carbohydrate restriction, 589
concepts, 585
consistency diets, 592–93
mechanical soft, 592–93
pureed, 593
cultural considerations in, 589, 591
documentation, 593
fat restriction, 589–90
for heart disease, 585
high dietary fiber, 591
increased calcium, 591
increased iron, 591
increased potassium, 590
low dietary fiber, 591
postoperative diet progression, 591–92
protein restriction, 589
sodium restriction, 590
Thermal, defined, 129
Thermal injuries, 142–43
gerontologic considerations, 157
Thermodilution, defined, 1207
Thermogenesis, 787
defined, 786
shivering, 786, 787
Thermometers
axillary, 245, 247
cleansing, 1262
digital, 244–45
ear canal, 238
electronic, 238, 245–46, 246f
Fahrenheit *vs.* Celsius, 238, 245t
heat-sensitive tape, 238, 248, 248f
infrared, 247–48, 247f
mercury, 245
oral, 238, 244–24f
rectal, 238, 246–47
tympanic, 247–48, 247f
Thermoregulation, defined, 235
Thermotherapy (*See also* Heat therapy)
defined, 786
Thirst, 996
Thomas splint, 1118f
defined, 1097
Thoracentesis
assisting with, 691, 691f
defined, 662
purpose of, 689t
Thorax area (*See* Chest)
Thought content, assessment, 301
Thought processes, assessment, 300
Thready pulse, defined, 235
Threat assessment, defined, 415
Three-point gait, 369
Throat culture, 655, 655f
Thrombophlebitis, defined, 1046, 1140
Thrombosis, 938
defined, 934
Thrush, defined, 196
Thyroid scan, purpose of, 675t
Tidal volume, 240
Time
as environmental factor, 135
military, 11, 11t
Time management, 59
Tocodynamometer, in fetal monitoring, 934
Tocolytic, defined, 934
Toe nails
care of, 214–15
ingrown, 196
Toes, range of motion for, 356t
Tolerance, defined, 467
Tonicity, defined, 350, 516
Toothbrush, sonic, 200
Toothbrushing, 199–200, 199f, 200f
Topical, defined, 1140
Topical medications, 534–41
cream, 535
ophthalmic drops, 537, 537f
ophthalmic ointment, 537–38, 538f
otic medications, 539, 539f
procedure, 535
transdermal medications, 536, 536f
Torque, defined, 1097
Torso/belt restraint, 148, 148f
Total nutrient admixture (TNA) [*See* Total parenteral nutrition (TPN)], 1276–80
Total parenteral nutrition (TPN), 1063–69
catheterization, 1064–66, 1064f
changing dressing and tubing, 1067
for children, 1068
complications of, 1065t, 1280
composition of solutions, 1064
home health care, 1276–80
administering, 1278–79
complications of, 1280
discontinuing, 1279–80
monitoring, 1279
nursing diagnosis, 1278
overview, 1277
infection risk with, 381–82
maintaining hyperalimentation, 1066–67, 1066f, 1067f
monitoring guidelines, 1065
Touch (*See also* Massage)
defined, 467
in sensory function assessment, 280
in skin assessment, 287
Toxin, defined, 415
TPN (*See* Total parenteral nutrition)
Tracheal aspiration, sputum specimen collection by, 652
Tracheal tube cuff, 914, 914f
Tracheostomy, defined, 871
Tracheostomy care, 910–20
capping tube, 917–18, 918f
changing tube ties, 916–17, 917f
cleaning, 914–15, 915f, 916f
documentation, 918
in home health care, 1293–94
client education, 1293–94
suctioning, 1293–94
inflating tube cuff, 914, 914f
intubation, 911–12, 911f
suctioning, 912–13, 913f
Traction, 1098–99, 1114–22
Bryant's, 1096, 1099, 1116t
Buck's, 1096, 1099, 1115f, 1116t
defined, 1097
documentation, 1121
external fixation devices, 1099, 1117t, 1119, 1119f
halo, 1117t, 1120–21, 1120f
Hoffman, 1117t, 1119f
pin site care, 1117
principles of maintenance, 1115f
Russell's, 1116t, 1118f
skeletal, 1098–99, 1117–18, 1117t, 1118f
skin, 1099, 1115–16, 1115f, 1116f
Thomas splint, 1118f
types of, 1116t
Tranquilizer, defined, 495
Trans-fatty acid, defined, 577
Transcutaneous electrical nerve stimulation (TENS), 467, 474
Transdermal medications, 536, 536f
Transducer, defined, 1207, 1211
leveling and zeroing, 1059–60
Transfer, client, 87, 93–94
from bed to chair, 340–41, 340f–341f
from bed to gurney, 337–38, 338f
defined, 85, 106
documentation, 94
equipment, 93
in home health care, 1270–71
nursing diagnosis, 89
procedure, 93
types of devices, 341
using Hoyer lift, 342, 342f
using safety belt, 341, 341f
using transfer board, 338–39, 338f–339f
Transfer board, moving clients using, 338–39, 338f–339f
Transfusion
blood (*See* Blood transfusions)
defined, 995, 1046
Transition, defined, 85, 106
Transitional care, 106, 110
Transitional specialists, 110
Transluminal coronary angioplasty, 670
Transmission-based precautions, 382–283, 384t
airborne, 283, 384t
contact, 283, 384t
droplet, 283, 384t
Transmission mode, in chain of infection, 379, 379f
Transparent adhesive film dressing, 832t, 854–55, 855f, 857, 859t
Transtracheal catheter, 1291–93
Transtracheal, defined, 626
collecting specimen, 652
Transverse colostomy, 761
Trauma
death due to, 460
defined, 415, 577, 1140
Trauma assessment, applied to triage, 459
Treatment directives, 9–10, 9f
Tremors, 276
Trendelenburg's position, 323, 334f, 334t
Triage, 420–22
bleeding, 459
caring for dead, 460
catastrophic, 421, 421f

chemical agent exposure, 420
communication matrix for, 418–20, 419f, 457–58
decontamination and, 421–22
bioterrorism, 447–48
documentation, 462
establishing public health parameters, 456–57
establishing treatment areas, 456
field, 420–21, 421f
life-threatening conditions, 458–59
methods of categorizing, 420, 421f
post-triage assessment, 459–60
post-triage organization, 422
shock, 459
START system, 415, 420, 421f
steps of, 457
trauma assessment applied to, 459
victim flow, 420, 420f
Tricuspid valve sounds, 293
Trigeminal nerve, 283t
Trochanter, defined, 323
Trochanter roll, 344, 344f
Trochlear nerve, 283t
Trypsin, 584
Tube feeding (*See* Total parenteral nutrition (TPN))
Tuberculosis, 387–88
multidrug-resistant, 378, 387
Tumor, defined, 662
Tunneled central vascular access devices (CVAD), 1047, 1074–79
changing dressing, 1076
defined, 1046
drawing blood, 1078
flushing, 1077
irrigation protocols, 1077
maintaining, 1075
using Groshong valve, 1076–77, 1077f
Turgor, 181, 287
defined, 161
Turning clients
to lateral position, 335, 335f
to prone position, 335–36, 335f–336f
Tympanic membrane, anatomy of, 285t
Type A personalities, 499
Type B personalities, 499
Typhoid tularemia, 424t–425t, 430–31, 449

U

Ulcer
arterial, 816–17, 840
defined, 161, 196
pressure (*See* Pressure ulcers)
venous, 816
changing dressing for, 837–39, 838f, 839f
Warm-Up® Therapy for, 837
Ultrafiltrate, defined, 700
Ultrasound, 663
Doppler, 663
Unconscious clients
body temperature assessment, 246
eye care, 226
Heimlich maneuver for, 972, 972f–973f
oral hygiene, 202, 202f
Unconsciousness, 130
Underloading, in communication, 69
Understanding, defined, 67, 105
Universal precautions, 382 (*See also* Standard precautions)
defined, 415
Unlicensed assistive personnel (UAP), delegation and, 55, 57
Unsaturated fatty acid, 577, 579
Unusual occurrence report, 34, 53–54, 56f
Upper body, range of motion exercises, 355t, 356f–357f
Upper respiratory tract, 872
Uremia, defined, 577
Ureterostomy, 702
Urethra, defined, 196, 700
Urinal, using, 217, 217f
Urinary catheterization
attaching leg bag, 709–10, 709f, 710f
documentation, 724
external, 708–10
females
providing catheter care, 722
straight catheter, 714–15, 715f
in home health, 1282
catheter care, 1284
clean technique for self-catheterization, 1282, 1283–84
infection risk with, 381
long term complications, 722
males
condom, 709, 709f
providing catheter care, 722–23
straight catheter, 716–17, 716f
providing catheter care, 722–23
retention catheter
females, 717, 717f–719f, 720
males, 721–22, 721f
removing, 723, 723f
specimens from closed systems, 735–36
suprapubic catheter care, 732–34, 733f, 1284
using bladder scanner, 713–14
Urinary diversion, 702–3, 738–43
applying pouch, 739, 739f–740f, 741
catheterizing continent urinary reservoir, 742
client education about, 740
continent, 702–3
defined, 700
documentation, 743
ileal conduit, 702, 741
ileal pouch, 702
incontinent, 702
Indiana pouch, 741
Kock's reservoir, 741
neo bladder, 703, 741
specimen collection from ileal conduit, 742
types of, 741
ureterostomy, 702
Urinary elimination, 698–743
alterations in, 702–3
related to blood volume, 702
related to end-stage renal disease, 703
related to fluid balance, 702
related to hormones, 702
related to obstructions, 702
bladder irrigation, 726–30
catheterization (*See* Urinary catheterization)
diversion (*See* Urinary diversion)
gerontologic considerations, 752
hemodialysis, 745–51 (*See also* Hemodialysis)
home health care, 1282
catheter care, 1284
clean technique for self-catheterization, 1282–84
dialysis, 1282, 1285–86
measuring intake and output, 704–6, 705f
methods to stimulate voiding, 705
nurse's role associated with, 703
nursing diagnosis, 703
peritoneal dialysis (*See* Peritoneal dialysis)
urinary diversion, 738–43
Urinary retention, risks for, 721
Urinary system, 700–701 (*See also* Genitourinary system)
assessment, 297–98
micturition, 701
structures of, 700
urine production, 700, 701t
Urinary tract infection (UTI)
catheterization and, 1282
defined, 626, 700
Urination, 701 (*See also* Micturition)
Urine
blood in, 298
examination of, 702t
pH, 298
specific gravity, 298
Urine output, 700, 701t
assessment, 297–98
in children, 316
in fluid balance, 996, 1023
measuring, 705–6, 705f
Urine specimen collection, 626–27, 629–31
24-hour, 631
from closed systems, 735–36
from ileal conduit, 742
infant, 634, 634f
midstream, 627, 630
timed tests, 627
Urostomy, continent, 741
Urticaria, defined, 662, 995

V

V.A.C.® (*See* vacuum-assisted wound closure)
Vaccine, defined, 415
Vaccinia vaccine, for smallpox, 433–36, 435f, 438
Vacuum-assisted wound closure (V.A.C.®), 813, 818, 865–66, 865f
Vacutainer system
for blood specimen collection, 641–42, 642f
defined, 626

Vagina
administering suppositories, 547, 547f
age-related changes, 319
assisting with examination, 693
Vagus nerve, 283t
Validate, defined, 67, 106
Validation, in therapeutic communication, 69
Valsalva's maneuver, defined, 235, 995, 1046
Value judgments, in communication, 69
Vancomycin-resistant enterococcus (VRE), 382
Variability, in fetal monitoring, 934
Variance report, 39, 39f, 53–54, 56f
Vascular, defined, 196
Vascular insufficiency, wounds caused by, 816–17
arterial ulcers, 816–17
pressure ulcers, 817
venous ulcers, 816
Vasculature, defined, 1207
Vasoconstriction, defined, 235, 786, 1140
Vasoconstrictor mechanism, in body temperature, 237
Vasodilation, defined, 235, 786
Vasodilator, defined, 1207
Vasomotor, defined, 786
Vasopressin, in cardiac emergencies, 1231, 1231t
Vasospasm, defined, 1207
Vastus lateralis injection site, 551, 566f
Venipuncture, 627
defined, 626, 1046
preparation of site, 1002–3, 1003f
Venipuncture site, sites for, 1003f
Venous, defined, 626
Venous access ports (*See* CVADs)
Venous blood, drawing, 641
Venous filling pressure, increased, 935
Venous ulcer, 816
changing dressing for, 837–39, 838f, 839f
Warm-Up® Therapy for, 837
Venovenous, defined, 700
Ventilation
alterations in, 873, 1236
bag–valve–mask, 881, 881f, 969, 969f
defined, 871–72
in hospital environment, 132
manifestations of inadequate, 874
mechanical, 1235–42
airway pressure modes, 1237
caring for client, 1236–1339, 1238f
delirium and, 1239
documentation, 1240
initial settings, 1238
weaning from, 1236, 1239–40
process of, 1236
Ventilation-perfusion mismatch problems, 1236
Ventricular contraction, multifocal, 956t
Ventricular fibrillation, 957t, 1229f
Ventricular gallop, 294
Ventricular systole, defined, 1207
Ventricular tachycardia, 956t, 1229f
Ventro, defined, 662
Ventrogluteal injection site, 551, 564f, 565f
Verbal communication, defined, 67
Verbal medication orders, 518
Verbalize, defined, 85
Vertigo, defined, 662, 934
Vesicant
agents, 423
defined, 995
Vesicles, defined, 415
Vesicular breath sounds, 293
Vest restraints, 152–53, 152f, 153f, 154f
Vibration, defined, 871, 885
Villi, 757, 758
Vinke skeletal tongs, 1117
Viral hemorrhagic fevers (VHF), 424t–425t, 431, 449
Viral hepatitis, 388
Virulence, defined, 378, 415
Virus, defined, 378, 415
Visceral, defined, 467
Viscosity, defined, 626, 995, 1046
Vision impairment, gerontologic considerations, 81, 373
Visual acuity, assessment, 284
Visual impairment, assisting with eating, 596–97
Visualization, 505
Vital capacity (VP), 874
Vital signs
assessment of, 13
blood pressure, 236, 240–42 (*See also* Blood pressure)
fifth (*See* Pain as fifth vital sign)
for children, 239t
factors that influence, 236–37
in fluid balance, 1023
in focus assessment, 275
form for, 236f
gerontologic considerations, 269
isolation and, 406
in neurologic assessment, 280–81
nursing diagnosis related to, 242
overview, 235–37
pain as fifth, 235, 242, 467, 473
in pain assessment, 236
pulse, 236, 238–40 (*See also* Pulse)
respirations, 236, 240 (*See also* Respirations)
routine, 236
temperature, 236–38 (*See also* Body temperature)
Vitamins, 580
defined, 577, 1046
fat-soluble, 579, 580
nutritional recommendations, 596
water-soluble, 580
Vocal fremitus, 291
Voiding, methods to stimulate, 705
Voltage, defined, 1207
Volunteer, defined, 85
Vomiting, projectile, 577

W

Walker, ambulation with, 364, 364f
Walking (*See also* Ambulation)
with cane, 364–65, 364f–365f
with crutches, 367–72 (*See also* Crutch walking)
with one assistant, 362–63, 363f
with two assistants, 361, 362f
with walker, 364, 364f
Wandering, 157
Warm-Up® Therapy
defined, 813
for venous ulcer, 837
in wound care, 817–18, 863–64, 864f
Wart, plantar, 197
Washable articles, cleaning, 393
Washcloth mitt, 173, 173f
Waste management, 134
in home health care, 1261–62
Water, 133–34
body, 995
as macronutrient, 580
nutritional recommendations for, 580
Water-seal chest drainage system, 921–23
two-bottle, 922–24
Water-soluble vitamins, 580
Waterless antiseptics, 392f, 393
Waveform, defined, 1207
Weaning
defined, 1207
from mechanical ventilation, 1236, 1239–40
terminal, 1236
Weapons of mass destruction, 415, 418, 422–24
biological agents, 422–23 (*See also* Bioterrorism)
chemical agents, 423
identifying exposure, 439–40
treatment, 441
triage, 440
radiation, 423–24, 441–42
acute radiation syndromes, 442
controlling contamination, 453–54
decontamination, 452–53
external, 423
health effects, 424
identifying exposure, 441–42
internal, 423
measuring, 423–24
personal protective equipment, 450–51
Weight (*See also* Height and weight)
chart for desirable, 97f
gain during pregnancy, 303
gerontologic considerations, 621
Wellness, defined, 467, 495
Wet-to-moist dressings, 847–49
Wheals, 288
Wheelchair
for hospital discharge, 100, 100f
vest restraint for, 153, 153f, 154f
weighing client in, 96, 98f
Wheezes, 292, 871
Winged needle, inserting, 1003–5, 1004f, 1005f
Withdrawal, defined, 1184
Wong-Baker FACES Rating Scale, for pain assessment, 469–70, 469f, 470f
Word roots, listing of, 59–61
Wound
caused by vascular insufficiency, 816–17
arterial ulcers, 816–17

pressure ulcers, 817
venous ulcers, 816
classification of, 814
culture of, 655–56, 655f, 816, 834
aerobic, 655–56, 655f
anaerobic, 656
Wound care, 831–46
adjunctive therapy, 817–18, 861–67
defined, 812
electrical stimulation, 817, 862
vacuum-assisted closure (V.A.C.®), 818, 865–66, 865f
Warm-Up® Therapy, 817–18, 863–64, 864f
antimicrobials in, 835
applying abdominal binder, 842, 842f
for arterial ulcer, 840
asepsis in, 816
assessment, 832–33
complications of, 815
documentation, 825, 830, 845, 866
dressings for, 834–35 (*See also* Dressing wounds; Dressings)
gerontologic considerations, 867–68
goals of, 815
irrigation, 816, 834, 844
medieval remedies, 836
nursing diagnosis, 818
packing a wound, 836, 836f
pressure ulcers (*See* Pressure ulcers)
removing staples, 829, 829f–830f
removing sutures, 828–29, 828f
for venous ulcer, 837–39, 833f, 839f
for wound with drain, 840–43, 841f, 843f
Wound classification, 814
Wound dehiscence, defined, 813
Wound evisceration, defined, 813
Wound healing
complications of, 815
in elderly, 191
factors affecting, 814–15
medications, 814–15
nutrition, 814, 815f
physical health, 814
gerontologic considerations, 867–68
moist environment for, 835, 837
phases of, 813
types of, 814
Wound infection, 816–17
microorganisms in, 816
prevention, 819–25
hand scrub, 820, 820f
pouring from sterile container, 822, 822f
preparation for dressing change with individual supplies, 824–25, 824f–825f
sterile field, 822–24, 824f
sterile gloves, 820–21, 821f
signs and symptoms of, 816
Wound irrigation, 816, 834, 844
Wound-remodeling phase, of wound healing, 813
Wound specimen collection, for culture, 816, 834
aerobic, 655–56, 655f
anaerobic, 656
Wrist restraints, 149–50, 149f, 150f

X

X-ray studies, 663, 666–73
preparation for various, 667–72
purpose of various, 667t
Xanthelasma, 284
Xenon computed tomography, 669–70
Xeroderma, 182t

Y

Yellow wounds, 814, 815t
Yoga, 505

Z

Z-track method for injections, 567–68, 568f
Zyvox, 382

SINGLE PC LICENSE AGREEMENT AND LIMITED WARRANTY

READ THIS LICENSE CAREFULLY BEFORE OPENING THIS PACKAGE. BY OPENING THIS PACKAGE, YOU ARE AGREEING TO THE TERMS AND CONDITIONS OF THIS LICENSE. IF YOU DO NOT AGREE, DO NOT OPEN THE PACKAGE. PROMPTLY RETURN THE UNOPENED PACKAGE AND ALL ACCOMPANYING ITEMS TO THE PLACE YOU OBTAINED THEM. ***THESE TERMS APPLY TO ALL LICENSED SOFTWARE ON THE DISK EXCEPT THAT THE TERMS FOR USE OF ANY SHAREWARE OR FREEWARE ON THE DISKETTES ARE AS SET FORTH IN THE ELECTRONIC LICENSE LOCATED ON THE DISK:***

1. GRANT OF LICENSE and OWNERSHIP: The enclosed computer programs and data ("Software") are licensed, not sold, to you by Pearson Education, Inc. ("We" or the "Company") and in consideration of your purchase or adoption of the accompanying Company textbooks and/or other materials, and your agreement to these terms. We reserve any rights not granted to you. You own only the disk(s) but we and/or our licensors own the Software itself. This license allows you to use and display your copy of the Software on a single computer (i.e., with a single CPU) at a single location for academic use only, so long as you comply with the terms of this Agreement. You may make one copy for back up, or transfer your copy to another CPU, provided that the Software is usable on only one computer.

2. RESTRICTIONS: You may not transfer or distribute the Software or documentation to anyone else. Except for backup, you may not copy the documentation or the Software. You may not network the Software or otherwise use it on more than one computer or computer terminal at the same time. You may not reverse engineer, disassemble, decompile, modify, adapt, translate, or create derivative works based on the Software or the Documentation. You may be held legally responsible for any copying or copyright infringement which is caused by your failure to abide by the terms of these restrictions.

3. TERMINATION: This license is effective until terminated. This license will terminate automatically without notice from the Company if you fail to comply with any provisions or limitations of this license. Upon termination, you shall destroy the Documentation and all copies of the Software. All provisions of this Agreement as to limitation and disclaimer of warranties, limitation of liability, remedies or damages, and our ownership rights shall survive termination.

4. LIMITED WARRANTY AND DISCLAIMER OF WARRANTY: Company warrants that for a period of 60 days from the date you purchase this SOFTWARE (or purchase or adopt the accompanying textbook), the Software, when properly installed and used in accordance with the Documentation, will operate in substantial conformity with the description of the Software set forth in the Documentation, and that for a period of 30 days the disk(s) on which the Software is delivered shall be free from defects in materials and workmanship under normal use. The Company does not warrant that the Software will meet your requirements or that the operation of the Software will be uninterrupted or error-free. Your only remedy and the Company's only obligation under these limited warranties is, at the Company's option, return of the disk for a refund of any amounts paid for it by you or replacement of the disk. THIS LIMITED WARRANTY IS THE ONLY WARRANTY PROVIDED BY THE COMPANY AND ITS LICENSORS, AND THE COMPANY AND ITS LICENSORS DISCLAIM ALL OTHER WARRANTIES, EXPRESS OR IMPLIED, INCLUDING WITHOUT LIMITATION, THE IMPLIED WARRANTIES OF MERCHANTABILITY AND FITNESS FOR A PARTICULAR PURPOSE. THE COMPANY DOES NOT WARRANT, GUARANTEE OR MAKE ANY REPRESENTATION REGARDING THE ACCURACY, RELIABILITY, CURRENTNESS, USE, OR RESULTS OF USE, OF THE SOFTWARE.

5. LIMITATION OF REMEDIES AND DAMAGES: IN NO EVENT, SHALL THE COMPANY OR ITS EMPLOYEES, AGENTS, LICENSORS, OR CONTRACTORS BE LIABLE FOR ANY INCIDENTAL, INDIRECT, SPECIAL, OR CONSEQUENTIAL DAMAGES ARISING OUT OF OR IN CONNECTION WITH THIS LICENSE OR THE SOFTWARE, INCLUDING FOR LOSS OF USE, LOSS OF DATA, LOSS OF INCOME OR PROFIT, OR OTHER LOSSES, SUSTAINED AS A RESULT OF INJURY TO ANY PERSON, OR LOSS OF OR DAMAGE TO PROPERTY, OR CLAIMS OF THIRD PARTIES, EVEN IF THE COMPANY OR AN AUTHORIZED REPRESENTATIVE OF THE COMPANY HAS BEEN ADVISED OF THE POSSIBILITY OF SUCH DAMAGES. IN NO EVENT SHALL THE LIABILITY OF THE COMPANY FOR DAMAGES WITH RESPECT TO THE SOFTWARE EXCEED THE AMOUNTS ACTUALLY PAID BY YOU, IF ANY, FOR THE SOFTWARE OR THE ACCOMPANYING TEXTBOOK. BECAUSE SOME JURISDICTIONS DO NOT ALLOW THE LIMITATION OF LIABILITY IN CERTAIN CIRCUMSTANCES, THE ABOVE LIMITATIONS MAY NOT ALWAYS APPLY TO YOU.

6. GENERAL: THIS AGREEMENT SHALL BE CONSTRUED IN ACCORDANCE WITH THE LAWS OF THE UNITED STATES OF AMERICA AND THE STATE OF NEW YORK, APPLICABLE TO CONTRACTS MADE IN NEW YORK, AND SHALL BENEFIT THE COMPANY, ITS AFFILIATES AND ASSIGNEES. THIS AGREEMENT IS THE COMPLETE AND EXCLUSIVE STATEMENT OF THE AGREEMENT BETWEEN YOU AND THE COMPANY AND SUPERSEDES ALL PROPOSALS OR PRIOR AGREEMENTS, ORAL, OR WRITTEN, AND ANY OTHER COMMUNICATIONS BETWEEN YOU AND THE COMPANY OR ANY REPRESENTATIVE OF THE COMPANY RELATING TO THE SUBJECT MATTER OF THIS AGREEMENT. If you are a U.S. Government user, this Software is licensed with "restricted rights" as set forth in subparagraphs (a)–(d) of the Commercial Computer-Restricted Rights clause at FAR 52.227-19 or in subparagraphs (c)(1)(ii) of the Rights in Technical Data and Computer Software clause at DFARS 252.227-7013, and similar clauses, as applicable.

Should you have any questions concerning this agreement or if you wish to contact the Company for any reason, please contact in writing: Prentice-Hall, New Media Department, One Lake Street, Upper Saddle River, NJ 07458.

Health Promotion

Throughout the Lifespan

Carole Lium Edelman, APRN, MS, CS, CMC

Director of Outpatient Programs
Waveny Care Center
New Canaan, Connecticut;
Associate Faculty Member
Yale University School of Nursing
New Haven, Connecticut;
Fellow
Brookdale Center on Aging
Hunter College
New York, New York

Carol Lynn Mandle, PhD, RN, CS, FNP

Associate Professor
Boston College School of Nursing
Chestnut Hill, Massachusetts;
Family Nurse Practitioner
Clinical Nurse Specialist and Scientist
Mind-Body Medical Institute
Beth Israel Deaconess Medical Center
Harvard Medical Center
Boston, Massachusetts

Illustrated

Fifth Edition

Mosby

St. Louis London Philadelphia Sydney Toronto

Mosby

Vice-President and Publishing Director, Nursing: Sally Schrefer
Executive Editor: Darlene Como
Managing Editor: Linda Caldwell
Project Manager: Catherine Jackson
Production Editor: Jamie Lyn Thornton
Designer: Amy Buxton
Cover Designer: Studio Montage

FIFTH EDITION

Mosby, Inc.
11830 Westline Industrial Drive
St. Louis, Missouri 63146

Printed in the United States of America

Library of Congress Cataloging-in-Publication Data

Health promotion throughout the lifespan / [edited by] Carole Lium Edelman, Carol Lynn Mandle.—5th ed.
p. ; cm.
Includes bibliographical references and index.
ISBN 0-323-01484-4
1. Health promotion. 2. Nursing. 3. Medicine, preventive. I. Edelman, Carole. II. Mandle, Carol Lynn.
[DNLM: 1. Nursing. 2. Health Promotion. WY 100 H4343 2001]
RT90.3 .H435 2001
613—dc21 2001044399

01 02 03 04 05 9 8 7 6 5 4 3 2 1

Contributors

Marinda Allender, RN, MSN, CPN
Instructor
Harris School of Nursing
Texas Christian University
Fort Worth, Texas
Chapter 15 *Overview of Growth and Development Framework*
Chapter 18 *Toddler*
Chapter 21 *Adolescent*

Carolyn Spence Cagle, PhD, RNC
Associate Professor
Harris College of Nursing
College of Health and Human Services
Texas Christian University
Fort Worth, Texas
Chapter 16 *The Prenatal Period*
Chapter 19 *Preschool Child*
Chapter 20 *School-Age Child*

Carole Lium Edelman, MS, CS, CMC, APRN
Director of Outpatient Programs
Waveny Care Center
New Canaan, Connecticut;
Associate Faculty Member
Yale University School of Nursing
New Haven, Connecticut;
Fellow Brookdale Center on Aging
Hunter College
New York, New York
Chapter 1 *Health Defined: Objectives for Promotion and Prevention*
Chapter 24 *Older Adult*

Fredric Edelman
Freelance Photographer
Westport, Connecticut

James A. Fain, PhD, RN, FAAN
Associate Professor
Graduate School of Nursing
University of Massachusetts Medical Center
Worcester, Massachusetts
Chapter 1 *Health Defined: Objectives for Promotion and Prevention*

Terry Fulmer, PhD, RN, FAAN
Professor
New York University Division of Nursing
School of Education
New York, New York
Chapter 24 *Older Adult*

Carol Scheel Gavan, EdD, RN
Assistant Professor
Graduate Chair
College of Nursing
State University of New York, Upstate Medical University
Syracuse, New York
Chapter 3 *Health Policy and the Delivery System*

Geraldine V. Go, PhD, RN, CS
ANA Certified Clinical Specialist in Gerontological Nursing
Associate Professor of Nursing
School of Nursing
College of New Rochelle
New Rochelle, New York
Chapter 2 *Changing Populations and Health*

Qalvy Grainzvolt, BS
Dietetic Intern
United States Army
Chapter 11 *Nutrition Counseling*

Philip A. Greiner, DNSc, RN
Associate Professor
Director, Health Promotion Center
Fairfield University School of Nursing
Fairfield, Connecticut
Chapter 1 *Health Defined: Objectives for Promotion and Prevention*

Carolyn Hayes, PhD, RN
Nurse Researcher
Brigham and Women's Hospital
Boston, Massachusetts
Chapter 5 *Ethical Issues Relevant to Health Promotion*

Susan A. Heady, RN, PhD
Associate Professor
Nursing Department
Webster University
St. Louis, Missouri
Chapter 10 *Health Education*

Janice I. Hooper, PhD, RN, CS
Professor and Interim Dean
College of Arts and Sciences
Webster University
St. Louis, Missouri
Chapter 10 *Health Education*

June Andrews Horowitz, PhD, RN, CS, FAAN
Associate Professor
School of Nursing
Boston College
Chestnut Hill, Massachusetts
Chapter 4 *The Therapeutic Relationship*

James S. Huddleston, MS, PT
Physical Therapist/Exercise Specialist
Division of Behavioral Medicine
Mind-Body Medical Institute
Beth Israel Deaconess Medical Center
Boston, Massachusetts
Chapter 12 *Exercise*

Kathleen Huttlinger, PhD, RN
Professor and Chair
Department of Nursing
The University of Virginia's College at Wise
Wise, Virginia
Chapter 25 *Health Promotion for the Twenty-First Century: Throughout the Lifespan and Throughout the World*

Elizabeth C. Kudzma, DNSc, MPH, RNC
Professor
Division of Nursing and Health Studies
Curry College
Milton, Massachusetts
Chapter 22 *Young Adult*

Regina Lowry, RN, MSN
Lecturer
University of Kentucky College of Nursing
Lexington, Kentucky
Chapter 14 *Holistic Health Strategies*

Margaret K. Macali, MS, RN, CS
Director
Public Health Nursing Services
Bergen County Department of Health Services
Paramus, New Jersey
Chapter 9 *Screening*

Carol Lynn Mandle, PhD, RN, CS, FNP
Associate Professor
Boston College School of Nursing
Chestnut Hill, Massachusetts;
Family Nurse Practitioner
Clinical Nurse Specialist and Scientist
Mind-Body Medical Institute
Beth Israel Deaconess Medical Center
Harvard Medical School
Boston, Massachusetts
Chapter 5 *Ethical Issues Relevant to Health Promotion*
Chapter 6 *Health Promotion and the Individual*
Chapter 7 *Health Promotion and the Family*
Chapter 8 *Health Promotion and the Community*
Chapter 13 *Stress Management*
Chapter 19 *Preschool Child*
Chapter 23 *Middle-Age Adult*
Chapter 25 *Health Promotion for the Twenty-First Century: Throughout the Lifespan and Throughout the World*

Susan Pennacchia, ARNP, MSN, MEd
Nursing Program Director
Lake Sumter Community College
Leesburg, Florida
Adjunct Instructor
University of Central Florida
Orlando, Florida
Chapter 17 *Infant*

Arlene Spark, EdD, RD
Associate Professor
Coordinator of Nutrition and Food Science and Public Health Nutrition
University of New York
New York, New York
Chapter 11 *Nutrition Counseling*

Marie Truglio-Londrigan, PhD, RN, GNPC
Assistant Professor
Lienhard School of Nursing
Pace University
Pleasantville, New York
Chapter 9 *Screening*

Meredith Wallace, PhDc, RN, CS
Assistant Professor
Department of Nursing
Southern Connecticut State University
New Haven, Connecticut
Chapter 24 *Older Adult*

Carol L. Wells-Federman, MS, MEd, RN, CS
Co-Director
Chronic Pain Management Clinical Program
Adult Nurse Practitioner
Dartmouth-Hitchcock Medical Center
Manchester, New Hampshire
Chapter 13 *Stress Management*

Acknowledgments for Previous Contributions

Mary E. Abrums, RN, MN
Douglas Bloomquist, PhD
Philip Boyle, PhD
Jacqueline Clinton, PhD, RN, FAAN
Joni Cohen, RN, MN
Rebecca Cohen, RN, EdD
Katherine Smith Detherage, PhD, RN, CNAA
Lea Edwards, BSN, MEd
Gail Park Fast, MN
Marilyn Frank-Stromberg, EdD, NP
Krishan Gupta, MD
Lois Hancock, MSN, ARNP
Dennis T. Jaffe, PhD
Sally Stark Johnson, RN, MSN
Jeanette Lancaster, RN, PhD, FAAN
William Martimucci, MD
Ann Marie McCarthy, RN
Nancy Curro McCarthy, RN, EdD
Nancy Milio, PhD, FAAN, FAPHA
Katherine E. Murphy, MN, FNP
Lisa Newton, PhD
Jean M. O'Connor, MS, MPH, RNC, FNP
Reverend James O'Donahue, SJ, PhD
Ellen F. Olshansky, DNSc, RNC
Johanne Quinn, PhD, RN
Gurpal K. Sandhu, PhD
Jan Schurman, MN, FNP

To our wonderful families, friends, students, and colleagues—
that they promote health in themselves and others.

Preface

PURPOSE OF THE BOOK

The case for promoting and protecting health and preventing disease and injury has been established by many accomplishments throughout the twentieth century. Americans are taking better care of themselves as they enter the twenty-first century. Public concern about physical fitness, good nutrition, and avoidance of health hazards such as smoking has gone beyond a fad and has become ingrained in the American lifestyle.

Encouraging positive health changes has been a major effort of individuals, the government, health professionals, and society in general. In the United States, public and private attempts to improve the health status of individuals and groups traditionally have focused on reducing communicable diseases and health hazards. Now growing concerns exist to improve access to and reduce costs of health services and improve the overall quality of life for all people. Americans also recognize that the health of each individual is influenced by health environments of all individuals worldwide.

Personal lifestyles are known to influence health status and nurses and other professionals can use specific strategies to help individuals, families, communities, and groups maintain and adopt positive lifestyle behaviors. Indirect health information and informed decision or direct health education and resulting health-promotion, health-protection, and disease- and injury-prevention practices can all lead to the adoption of healthy lifestyles.

Health-promotion advances require a better understanding of risk and behavior and intervention measures. Ten categories are identified as important determinants of health status:

1. Smoking
2. Nutrition
3. Alcohol use
4. Habituating drug use
5. Driving
6. Exercise
7. Sexuality and contraceptive use
8. Family relationships
9. Risk management
10. Coping and adaptation

Outcome measures designed to assist individual efforts to change and improve behavior in these areas can lead to a decrease in morbidity and mortality.

Nurses and other professionals who undertake health-promotion strategies also need to understand the basics of health protection and disease and injury prevention. Health protection is directed at population groups of all ages and involves adherence to standards, infectious disease control, and governmental regulation and enforcement. The focus of these activities is on reducing exposure to various sources of hazards, including those related to air, water, foods, drugs, motor vehicles, and other physical agents.

Health care providers present the individual with disease- and injury-*prevention* services, which include immunizations, screenings, health education, and counseling. To implement prevention strategies effectively, it is essential to develop cross-cutting activities targeted to and tailored for all age groups in various settings, including schools, industries, the home, the health care delivery system, and the community.

Throughout the history of the United States, the public health community has assessed the health of Americans. In 1789, the Reverend Edward Wigglesworth developed the first American mortality tables through his study in New England. The *Report of a General Plan for the Promotion of Public and Personal Health* was completed by Lemuel Shattuck in 1880. *Healthy People, The Surgeon General's Report on Health Promotion and Disease Prevention* was first published in 1979 and followed by *Healthy People 2000: National Health Promotion and Disease Prevention Objectives*, which listed three goals to be achieved by the year 2000:

1. Increase the span of healthy life for Americans.
2. Reduce health disparities among Americans.
3. Achieve access to preventive services for all Americans.

This report presented many opportunities in the form of measurable targets, or objectives, which were organized into 22 priority areas within four broad categories: (1) health promotion, (2) health protection, (3) preventive services, and (4) surveillance and data systems.

Healthy People 2000 Mid-Course Review and 1995 Revisions and annual updates evaluated progress in selected areas of health promotion, health protection, preventive services, and surveillance data systems.

In this relatively short time, significant improvements have been made in the health behaviors and health of Americans. Examples of these improvements include reductions in infant mortality; teenage pregnancies; injuries; tobacco, alcohol, and illicit drug use; and death rates from coronary heart disease and cerebrovascular accidents. In addition, childhood vaccination rates are at the highest recorded.

Unfortunately, many more improvements are needed in the health of many Americans. Tobacco use by adolescents continues to increase. Nearly 40% of adults do not participate in leisure-time physical activity and 40% of adults are obese. Violence and other abusive behaviors continue to destroy individuals, families, and communities across the United States. Chronic health problems, such as mental disorders and diabetes mellitus, continue to be undiagnosed and undertreated. Another example of this is the occurrence of HIV and AIDS disproportionately in Black and Hispanic communities, especially in women.

Healthy People 2010 addresses these health problems by establishing goals and objectives for the first decade of the new millenium. The vision for *Healthy People 2010* is "Healthy People in Healthy Communities" because as nursing has long recognized, the health of each individual is inseparable from the health of families, communities, the nation, and the universe. Health is significantly affected by the environments in which each individual lives, works, travels, and plays. Dimensions of the environment are not only physical, but psychosocial and spiritual, including the behaviors, attitudes, and beliefs of each individual. Specific objectives in 28 focus areas support two major goals:

1. Increase quality and years of healthy life.
2. Eliminate health disparities.

These databases continue to provide assessments of health status and risk for evaluations and future planning, not only for health policy makers and health care providers, but for individuals, families, and communities (local, regional, national, and global).

The information in this edition of *Health Promotion Throughout the Lifespan* includes these and other data and recommendations for health promotion, health protection, preventive services, and surveillance data systems, including those in the U.S. Preventive Services Task Force.

APPROACH AND ORGANIZATION

This edition presents health data and related theories and skills that are needed to understand and practice when providing care. This book focuses on primary prevention intervention, based on the Leavell and Clark model; its three main components are (1) health promotion, (2) specific health protection, and (3) prevention of specific diseases. Health promotion is the intervention designed to improve health, such as providing adequate nutrition, a healthy environment, and ongoing health education. Specific protection and prevention are the interventions used to protect against illness, such as massive immunizations, periodic examinations, and safety features in the workplace.

In addition to primary prevention, this book discusses secondary prevention intervention, focusing specifically on screening. Such programs include blood pressure, glaucoma, and diabetes screening and referral. (The acute component of secondary prevention is not addressed in this book.)

This text is presented in five parts, each forming the basis for the next.

Unit One, *Foundations for Health Promotion*, describes the foundational concepts of promoting and protecting health and preventing diseases and injuries, including diagnostic, therapeutic, and ethical decision making based on the nursing emphasis of health patterns as described by Margaret Newman.

Unit Two, *Assessment for Health Promotion*, focuses on individuals, families, and communities and the factors affecting their health. The functional health pattern assessments developed by Gordon serve as the organizing framework for assessing the health of individuals, families, and communities.

Unit Three, *Interventions for Health Promotion*, discusses theories, methodologies, and case studies of nursing interventions, including screening, health education counseling, stress management, and crisis intervention.

Unit Four, *Application of Health Promotion*, also uses Gordon's functional health patterns, emphasizing developmental, cultural, ethnic, and environmental variables in assessing the developing person. The intent is to address the health concerns of all Americans regardless of gender, race, age, or sexual orientation. Although the human development theories discussed are primarily based on the research of male subjects, emerging theories based on female subjects have been included. The hope is to describe human development that more accurately reflects the complexity of human experiences throughout the lifespan.

Unit Five, *Challenges As We Enter the New Millenium*, presents a single chapter that discusses changing population groups and their health needs and related implications for research and practice in the next century. Throughout the text, research abstracts have been added to highlight state-of-the-art and the science of nursing practice and to demonstrate to the reader the relationship among research, practice, and outcomes.

Throughout these units, the evolving health care professions and the changing health care systems, including future challenges and initiatives for health promotion, are described. Emphasis is placed on the current concerns of reducing health care costs while increasing life expectancy and improving the quality of life for all Americans. This promotes the reader's immediate interest in and thoughts about the content of the chapters.

KEY FEATURES

Each chapter starts with a list of **objectives** to help focus the reader and emphasize the content the reader should acquire through reading the book. **Key Terms** are listed at the front to acquaint readers with the important terminology of the chapter.

Each chapter's narrative begins with **Think About It,** the presentation of a clinical issue or scenario that relates to the topic of the chapter, followed by critical thinking questions. This promotes the reader's immediate interest in and thought about the chapter.

Research Highlights provide brief synopses on current health promotion research studies that demonstrate the links between research, theory, and practice.

Multicultural Awareness boxes offer cultural perspectives on various aspects of health promotion.

Hot Topics explores current issues, controversies, and ethical dilemmas with respect to health promotion, providing an opportunity for critical analysis of care issues.

Health Teaching boxes present special tips and guidelines to use when educating people about health promotion activities.

NEW! The **Case Study** highlights a real-life clinical situation relevant to the chapter topic.

NEW! The **Care Plan** details nursing diagnoses relevant to health-promotion activities and the related interventions.

NEW! **Innovative Practice** boxes highlight inventive and resourceful projects, programs, and research studies that are new ways of implementing health promotion.

NEW! A **Glossary** in the back of the book contains the Key Terms from each chapter and their definitions.

ONLINE INSTRUCTOR'S SUPPLEMENT

New to this edition is **Course Resources,** an online supplement for instructors. Accessible at http://mosby.com/MERLIN/Edelman/, this ancillary has many resources to help the instructor present the content of this book. They are:

- Chapter outlines
- Teaching strategies
- Discussion of evaluation and critiquing of research studies
- Approximately 70 figures, boxes, and tables from the book reproduced in an **Image Collection**
- **Test Bank** with questions for each chapter
- **Glossary** of Key Terms and their definitions, reproduced from the book

The current trend to emphasize the developing health of people mandates that health care professionals understand the many issues that surround individuals, families, and communities in social, work, and family settings, including the biological, inherited, cognitive, psychological, environmental, and sociocultural factors that can put their health at risk. Most important is that they develop interventions to promote health by understanding the diverse roles these factors play in the person's beliefs and health practices, particularly in the areas of disease and injury prevention, protection, and health promotion. Achieving such effectiveness requires collaboration with other health care providers and the integration of practice and policy while developing interventions and considering the ethical issues within individual, family, and community responsibilities for health.

Carole Lium Edelman
Carol Lynn Mandle

Acknowledgments

We had the good fortune of receiving much assistance and support from many friends, relatives, and associates. Our colleagues read chapters, gave valuable advice and criticism, helped clarify concepts, and provided case examples.

We also acknowledge the contributions of all the authors. In developing this text, they gave the project their total commitment and support. Their professional competence aided greatly in the development of the final draft of the manuscript. Special thanks go to Mary Toss and Christina Kantzas for assistance with typing the manuscript. Special mention must be given to Zannifer John and Patricia Gomez, PhD, for assisting our explanations of research throughout the world wide web.

The editors worked and learned from each other during the planning and development of this book; throughout the entire process, close contact prevailed. They seemed to become the book and, in turn, the book now reflects them.

Both family and friends helped in the work and fulfilled the many responsibilities requested of them.

I am fortunate to have faith in the Lord, who gives courage and strength to face life's difficulties in a positive manner. My children, Megan, Heather, Deirdre, and John, and my grandchildren, Ryan and Caroline, bring joy to me as an author and editor. Their patience and love are truly appreciated. Lenora Pennacchia provides much encouragement and support. Fredric Edelman gives continued joy and happiness in our marriage.

Carole Lium Edelman

In the continued development of health, I acknowledge our faith in God and the strength of my mother, sister, and aunt; the joy of friends; the love of marriage and family with Robert, Jonathan, David, and Elizabeth; the commitments of nurses to social justice in the care of all people; and the knowledge we are just beginning.

Carol Lynn Mandle

Detailed Contents

Unit One

Foundations for Health Promotion

1 Health Defined: Objectives for Promotion and Prevention, 3
PHILIP A. GREINER, JAMES A. FAIN, and CAROLE LIUM EDELMAN
EXPLORING CONCEPTS OF HEALTH, 4
Models of Health, 5
Health-Illness Continuum, 5
High-Level Wellness, 6
Functioning, 6
Health, 6
ILLNESS, DISEASE, AND HEALTH, 6
PLANNING FOR HEALTH, 7
HEALTHY PEOPLE 2010, 8
Key Features of *Healthy People 2010,* 8
Problem Identification, 12
Planning Interventions, 12
What Was the Actual Cause of Frank's Problem?, 14
Evaluation of the Situation, 14
LEVELS OF PREVENTION, 14
Primary Prevention, 16
Secondary Prevention, 20
Tertiary Prevention, 20
THE NURSE'S ROLE, 20
Nursing Roles in Health Promotion and Protection, 20
IMPROVING PROSPECTS FOR HEALTH, 24
Population Effects, 24
SHIFTING PROBLEMS, 25
MOVING TOWARD SOLUTIONS, 25

2 Changing Populations and Health, 29
GERALDINE V. GO
CHANGING POPULATIONS IN THE UNITED STATES, 30
Immigration to the United States, 30
From Immigrants to Ethnics, 31
THE CONCEPT OF ETHNICITY, 31
The Process of Becoming an Ethnic, 31
Racial, Ethnic, and Minority Groups, 32
Culture, Values, and Value Orientations, 33
HEALTH AS A VALUE, 33
FOLK AND WESTERN HEALTH CARE, 35
ASIAN AMERICANS–PACIFIC ISLANDERS, 36
Prevalent Health Problems of Asian Americans–Pacific Islanders, 36
Selected Health-Related Cultural Aspects, 37
HISPANIC AMERICANS, 37
Prevalent Health Problems of Hispanic Americans, 38
Selected Health-Related Cultural Aspects, 38
BLACK AMERICANS, 39
Prevalent Health Problems of Black Americans, 39
Selected Health-Related Cultural Aspects, 40
NATIVE AMERICANS, 41
Prevalent Health Problems of Native Americans, 42
Selected Health-Related Cultural Aspects, 42
AGING MINORITIES, 43
Health Issues of Aging Minorities, 44
Selected Activities to Address the Health Care Needs of Aging Minorities, 44
THE CHANGING RURAL AND URBAN POPULATIONS: HOMELESS PERSONS, 44
Homelessness and Homeless Persons: Getting to Know Them, 44
Estimates of Homeless Persons, 45
Causes of Today's Homelessness, 45
Health Problems of Homeless People, 45
Selected Strategies to Alleviate Homelessness, 46
PEOPLE LIVING WITH HIV OR AIDS, 47
HIV and AIDS in Ethnic and Minority Groups: Issues and Strategies, 48
HIV and AIDS Prevention in Ethnic and Minority Groups, 48
THE NATION'S RESPONSE TO THE HEALTH CHALLENGES, 49
Healthy People 2010, 49
Nursing's Response to Changing Populations and Health, 49

3 Health Policy and the Delivery System, 55
CAROL SCHEEL GAVAN
HISTORY OF HEALTH CARE, 57
Early Influences, 57
Industrial Influences, 57
Socioeconomic Influences, 57
Public Health Influences, 57

Scientific Influences, 57
Special Population Influences, 58
Political and Economic Influences, 58
Split Between Preventive and Curative Measures, 58
ORGANIZATION OF THE DELIVERY SYSTEM, 60
Private Sector, 60
Public Sector, 62
FINANCING HEALTH CARE, 66
Costs, 66
Sources, 66
Mechanisms, 68
Managed Care Issues, 69
Health Insurance, 70
The Uninsured, 76
THE CANADIAN HEALTH CARE SYSTEM, 77
INFLUENCING HEALTH POLICY, 78

4 The Therapeutic Relationship, 83
JUNE ANDREWS HOROWITZ
VALUES CLARIFICATION, 84
Definition, 84
Values and the Therapeutic Use of Self, 85
THE COMMUNICATION PROCESS, 88
Function and Process, 88
Types of Communication, 89
Functionality of Communication, 90
THE HELPING OR THERAPEUTIC RELATIONSHIP, 94
Characteristics, 94
Ethics in Communicating, 95
Therapeutic Techniques, 95
Barriers to Effective Communication, 97
Setting, 100
Stages, 100
Brief Interactions: The 15-Minute Interview, 102

5 Ethical Issues Relevant to Health Promotion, 107
CAROL LYNN MANDLE and CAROLYN HAYES
TOWARD AN UNDERSTANDING OF ETHICS, 108
The Nature of Ethics, 108
Relationship Between the "Is" and the "Ought", 109
Types of Ethics, 109
Elements of Ethics, 109
Ethical Theory, 110
Feminist Ethics, 112
UNDERSTANDING HEALTH CARE ETHICS, 113
Nature of the Discipline, 113
Professional Oaths and Codes of Ethics, 113
Ethical Principles Currently Stressed, 114
Role of Justice and Rights, 117
Relationship to Civil Law, 118
DECISION MAKING: NATURE AND TECHNIQUES, 118
SELECTED ETHICAL ISSUES, 122
Research, 122
Stewardship over Health, 124
Contraception, 124
Surgical Abortion and RU 486, 127
Genetic Therapy, 128
Reproductive Technology, 129
HIV Screening, 131
CASE STUDY: METHOD FOR ETHICAL ANALYSIS, 131
Gather and Assess Facts, 132
Identify and Characterize Values, 132
Name and Evaluate Method, 132
Integrity-Preserving Compromise, 133
ETHICS OF HEALTH PROMOTION: CASES, 133

Unit Two
Assessment for Health Promotion

6 Health Promotion and the Individual, 141
CAROL LYNN MANDLE
FUNCTIONAL HEALTH PATTERNS: ASSESSMENT OF THE INDIVIDUAL, 142
The Functional Health Pattern Framework, 143
The Patterns, 146
ASSESSMENT PROCESS, 160
Skills, 160
Data Collection, 161
Format, 162
Guidelines, 162
INDIVIDUAL HEALTH PROMOTION THROUGH THE NURSING PROCESS, 163
Collection and Analysis of Data, 163
Planning the Care, 164
Implementing the Plan, 165
Evaluating the Plan, 165

7 Health Promotion and the Family, 169
CAROL LYNN MANDLE
THE NURSING PROCESS AND THE FAMILY, 170
The Nurse's Role, 171
The Family from a Systems Perspective, 171
THE FAMILY FROM A DEVELOPMENTAL PERSPECTIVE, 173
THE FAMILY FROM A RISK-FACTOR PERSPECTIVE, 175

FUNCTIONAL HEALTH PATTERN: ASSESSMENT OF THE FAMILY, 176
Health Perception-Health Management Pattern, 177
Nutritional-Metabolic Pattern, 179
Elimination Pattern, 179
Activity-Exercise Pattern, 179
Sleep-Rest Pattern, 179
Cognitive-Perceptual Pattern, 180
Self-Perception–Self-Concept Pattern, 180
Roles-Relationships Pattern, 180
Sexuality-Reproductive Pattern, 182
Coping–Stress-Tolerance Pattern, 184
Values-Beliefs Pattern, 185
ANALYSIS AND NURSING DIAGNOSIS, 185
Analyzing Data, 185
Formulating Family Nursing Diagnoses, 191
PLANNING WITH THE FAMILY, 192
Goals, 194
IMPLEMENTATION WITH THE FAMILY, 195
EVALUATION WITH THE FAMILY, 196

8 Health Promotion and the Community, 199
CAROL LYNN MANDLE
THE NURSING PROCESS AND THE COMMUNITY, 200
THE NURSE'S ROLE, 201
METHODS OF DATA COLLECTION, 201
SOURCES OF COMMUNITY INFORMATION, 202
COMMUNITY FROM A SYSTEMS PERSPECTIVE, 202
Structure, 202
Function, 203
Interaction, 203
DEVELOPMENTAL FRAMEWORK, 203
RISK FACTOR FRAMEWORK, 204
FUNCTIONAL HEALTH PATTERNS: ASSESSMENT OF THE COMMUNITY, 204
Health Perception-Health Management Pattern, 204
Nutritional-Metabolic Pattern, 204
Elimination Pattern, 211
Activity-Exercise Pattern, 211
Sleep-Rest Pattern, 211
Cognitive-Perceptual Pattern, 211
Self-Perception–Self-Concept Pattern, 212
Roles-Relationships Pattern, 212
Sexuality-Reproductive Pattern, 212
Coping–Stress-Tolerance Pattern, 212
Values-Beliefs Pattern, 213
ANALYSIS AND DIAGNOSIS WITH THE COMMUNITY, 213
Organization of Data, 213
Guidelines for Data Analysis, 214
Community Diagnosis, 216
PLANNING WITH THE COMMUNITY, 217
Purposes, 217
Planned Change, 217
IMPLEMENTATION WITH THE COMMUNITY, 220
EVALUATION WITH THE COMMUNITY, 221

Unit Three
Interventions for Health Promotion

9 Screening, 227
MARIE TRUGLIO-LONDRIGAN and MARGARET K. MACALI
ADVANTAGES AND DISADVANTAGES, 228
SELECTION OF A SCREENABLE DISEASE, 229
Significance, 229
Can the Disease Be Screened?, 229
Should the Disease Be Screened?, 231
ETHICAL CONSIDERATIONS, 234
Health Care Ethics, 234
Economic Ethics, 234
SELECTION OF A SCREENABLE POPULATION, 235
Person-Dependent Factors, 235
Environment-Dependent Factors, 239
COMMONLY SCREENED CONDITIONS, 239
Phenylketonuria (PKU), 239
Breast Cancer, 240
Cervical Cancer, 240
Colorectal Cancer, 241
Prostate Cancer, 241
Cholesterol, 242
Hypertension, 242
Glaucoma, 242
Human Immunodeficiency Virus, 243
Lead, 243
Diabetes, 244
THE NURSE'S ROLE, 244

10 Health Education, 247
SUSAN A. HEADY and JANICE I. HOOPER
NURSING AND HEALTH EDUCATION, 249
Definition, 249
Goals, 250
Learning Assumptions, 251

Family Health Teaching, *251*
Health Behavior Change, *253*
Interventions, *255*
Ethics, *256*
Cultural Considerations in Health Teaching, *257*
SOCIAL MARKETING AND HEALTH EDUCATION, *257*
ADMINISTERING HEALTH EDUCATION PROGRAMS, *258*
The Precede-Proceed Model, *258*
THE TEACHING PLAN, *261*
Assessing Learning Needs, *261*
Determining Expected Learning Outcomes, *263*
Selecting Content, *263*
Designing Learning Strategies, *263*
Referring Individuals to Other Resources, *265*
TEACHING AND ORGANIZING SKILLS, *265*

11 Nutrition Counseling, *269*
ARLENE SPARK and QALVY GRAINZVOLT
NUTRITION IN THE UNITED STATES: LOOKING FORWARD FROM THE PAST, *270*
Classic Vitamin-Deficiency Diseases, *270*
Dietary Excess and Imbalance, *270*
HEALTHY PEOPLE 2010: NUTRITION OBJECTIVES, *271*
Nutrition-Related Health Status, *271*
Nutrition Objectives for the United States, *274*
FOOD AND NUTRITION RECOMMENDATIONS, *275*
Dietary Reference Intakes, *275*
Dietary Supplements and Herbal Medicines, *278*
Dietary Guidelines for Americans, *280*
Food Guide Pyramid, *280*
FOOD SAFETY, *283*
Causes of Food-Borne Illness, *284*
Food Safety Practices, *284*
FOOD, NUTRITION, AND POVERTY, *288*
Poverty and Income Distribution, *288*
Food Assistance for the Poor, *289*
Food Stamp Program, *289*
National School Lunch Program, *290*
School Breakfast Program, *290*
Women, Infants, and Children, *290*
Nutrition Program for the Elderly, *291*
NUTRITION SCREENING, *291*
NUTRITION AND DISEASE, *292*
Cardiovascular Diseases, *292*
Cancer, *297*
Osteoporosis, *299*
Obesity, *303*
Diabetes, *308*
Human Immunodeficiency Virus and Acquired Immunodeficiency Syndrome, *313*
SOURCES OF INFORMATION, *313*

12 Exercise, *310*
JAMES S. HUDDLESTON
HEALTHY PEOPLE 2010, 320
Defining Moment in Health, *320*
Original Physical Activity Goals, *321*
Revised Physical Activity Goals: Making Progress, *321*
HYPOKINETIC STATISTIC, *323*
Coronary Heart Disease, *323*
Obesity, *326*
Aging, *327*
Osteoporosis, *328*
Arthritis, *329*
Low Back Pain, *330*
Immune Function, *331*
Mental Health, *332*
HOW MUCH EXERCISE IS ENOUGH?, *332*
Aerobic Exercise, *333*
Warm-Up and Cool-Down Periods, *336*
Flexibility, *336*
Resistance Training, *337*
EXERCISE THE SPIRIT: RELAXATION RESPONSE, *337*
MONITORING THE INNER AND OUTER ENVIRONMENT, *339*
Fluid News, *340*
What to Wear, *340*
SPECIAL CONSIDERATIONS, *341*
Coronary Heart Disease, *341*
Diabetes, *342*
BUILDING A RHYTHM OF PHYSICAL ACTIVITY, *343*
Adherence and Compliance, *343*
Creating a Climate That Supports Exercise, *345*

13 Stress Management, *353*
CAROL L. WELLS-FEDERMAN and CAROL LYNN MANDLE
SOURCES OF STRESS, *354*
PHYSICAL, PSYCHOLOGICAL, SOCIAL-BEHAVIORAL, AND SPIRITUAL CONSEQUENCES OF STRESS, *355*
Physiological Effects of Stress, *355*
Psychological Effects of Stress, *355*
Social-Behavioral Effects of Stress, *356*
Spiritual Effects of Stress, *357*
HEALTH BENEFITS OF MANAGING STRESS, *357*
ASSESSMENT, *358*
STRESS-MANAGEMENT INTERVENTIONS, *359*
Developing Self-Awareness, *359*

Techniques for Developing Self-Awareness, 360
Healthy Diet, 363
Physical Activity, 364
Sleep Hygiene, 364
Cognitive Restructuring, 365
Affirmations, 366
Social Support, 366
Assertive Communication, 367
Empathy, 368
Healthy Pleasures, 369
Spiritual Practice, 369
Clarifying Values and Beliefs, 370
Setting Realistic Goals, 370
Humor, 370
EFFECTIVE COPING, 371

14 Holistic Health Strategies, 375
REGINA LOWRY
HOLISM, 376
HOLISTIC INTERVENTIONS, 376
Energy Work, 376
Movement Arts, 380
Meditation, 382
Prayer and Distant Healing, 383
Guided Imagery, 384
Music Therapy, 385
Bodywork, 385
Aromatherapy, 386
Presence, 387
SELF-KNOWLEDGE, 393

Unit Four
Application of Health Promotion

15 Overview of Growth and Development Framework, 399
MARINDA ALLENDER
DEVELOPMENTAL PERIODS, 400
OVERVIEW OF GROWTH AND DEVELOPMENT, 400
Concept of Growth, 400
Growth Patterns, 400
Concept of Development, 402
Developmental Patterns, 403
THEORIES OF DEVELOPMENT, 411
Psychosocial Development: Erikson's Theory, 411
Cognitive Development: Piaget's Theory, 412
Moral Development: Kohlberg's Theory, 413

16 The Prenatal Period, 417
CAROLYN SPENCE CAGLE
PHYSICAL CHANGES IN MATERNAL AND FETAL SYSTEMS, 418
Duration of Pregnancy, 418
Fertilization, 418
Implantation, 418
Fetal Growth and Development, 419
Placental Development and Function, 419
Maternal Changes, 421
CHANGES IN TRANSITION FROM FETUS TO NEWBORN, 427
Nursing Interventions, 427
Mucus, 427
Apgar Score, 427
Gender, 427
Race, 428
Genetics, 430
GORDON'S FUNCTIONAL HEALTH PATTERNS, 430
Health Perception-Health Management Pattern, 430
Nutritional-Metabolic Pattern, 430
Elimination Pattern, 434
Activity-Exercise Pattern, 434
Sleep-Rest Pattern, 435
Cognitive-Perceptual Pattern, 435
Self-Perception–Self-Concept Pattern, 438
Roles-Relationships Pattern, 439
Sexuality-Reproductive Pattern, 441
Coping–Stress-Tolerance Pattern, 441
Values-Beliefs Pattern, 442
PATHOLOGICAL PROCESSES, 442
Physical Factors and Diagnostic Tools, 443
Biological Agents, 443
Chemical Agents, 447
Mechanical Forces, 449
Radiation, 450
SOCIAL PROCESSES, 450
Community and Work, 450
Culture and Ethnicity, 451
Legislation, 452
Economics, 453
Health Care Delivery System, 453
NURSING INTERVENTIONS, 454

17 Infant, 459
SUSAN PENNACCHIA
AGE AND PHYSICAL CHANGES, 460
Developmental Tasks, 462

Concepts of Infant Development, 463
Denver Developmental Screening Test, 465
Gender, 465
Race, 470
Genetics, 471
GORDON'S FUNCTIONAL HEALTH PATTERNS, 472
Health Perception-Health Management Pattern, 472
Nutritional-Metabolic Pattern, 472
Elimination Pattern, 476
Activity-Exercise Pattern, 477
Sleep-Rest Pattern, 478
Cognitive-Perceptual Pattern, 480
Self-Perception–Self-Concept Pattern, 482
Roles-Relationships Pattern, 482
Sexuality-Reproductive Pattern, 487
Coping–Stress-Tolerance Pattern, 488
Values-Beliefs Pattern, 489
PATHOLOGICAL PROCESSES, 490
Unintentional Injuries, 490
Biological Agents, 491
Chemical Agents, 493
Motor Vehicles, 496
Radiation, 497
Cancer, 497
SOCIAL PROCESSES, 498
Community and Work, 498
Culture and Ethnicity, 499
Legislation, 501
Economics, 502
Health Care Delivery System, 504
NURSING INTERVENTIONS, 504

18 Toddler, 507
MARINDA ALLENDER
AGE AND PHYSICAL CHANGES, 508
Gender, 510
Race, 510
GORDON'S FUNCTIONAL HEALTH PATTERNS, 511
Health Perception-Health Management Pattern, 511
Nutritional-Metabolic Pattern, 511
Elimination Pattern, 512
Activity-Exercise Pattern, 513
Sleep-Rest Pattern, 515
Cognitive-Perceptual Pattern, 516
Self-Perception–Self-Concept Pattern, 518
Roles-Relationships Pattern, 520
Sexuality-Reproductive Pattern, 523
Coping–Stress-Tolerance Pattern, 523
Values-Beliefs Pattern, 524
PATHOLOGICAL PROCESSES, 525
Unintentional Injuries, 525
Motor Vehicles, 526
Biological and Bacterial Agents, 527
Chemical Agents, 527
SOCIAL PROCESSES, 528
Community and Work, 528
Culture and Ethnicity, 529
Legislation, 529
Economics, 529
Health Care Delivery System, 530

19 Preschool Child, 533
CAROLYN SPENCE CAGLE and CAROL LYNN MANDLE
AGE AND PHYSICAL CHANGES, 534
Gender, 535
Race, 537
Genetics, 537
GORDON'S FUNCTIONAL HEALTH PATTERNS, 537
Health Perception-Health Management Pattern, 537
Nutritional-Metabolic Pattern, 537
Elimination Pattern, 539
Activity-Exercise Pattern, 540
Sleep-Rest Pattern, 541
Cognitive-Perceptual Pattern, 542
Self-Perception–Self-Concept Pattern, 548
Roles-Relationships Pattern, 549
Sexuality-Reproductive Pattern, 551
Coping–Stress-Tolerance Pattern, 551
Values-Beliefs Pattern, 553
PATHOLOGICAL PROCESSES, 554
Injuries, 555
Drownings, 556
Mechanical Forces, 557
Biological and Bacterial Agents, 557
Chemical Agents, 559
Cancer, 559
Asthma, 561
SOCIAL PROCESSES, 561
Community and Work, 561
Culture and Ethnicity, 562
Legislation, 562
Economics, 562
Health Care Delivery System, 562
NURSING INTERVENTIONS, 563

20 School-Age Child, 567
CAROLYN SPENCE CAGLE
AGE AND PHYSICAL CHANGES, 568
Gender, 571
Race, 572
Genetics, 572
GORDON'S FUNCTIONAL HEALTH PATTERNS, 572
Health Perception-Health Management Pattern, 572
Nutritional-Metabolic Pattern, 574
Elimination Pattern, 575
Activity-Exercise Pattern, 577
Sleep-Rest Pattern, 578
Cognitive-Perceptual Pattern, 578
Self-Perception–Self-Concept Pattern, 584
Roles-Relationships Pattern, 586
Sexuality-Reproductive Pattern, 588
Coping–Stress-Tolerance Pattern, 589
Values-Beliefs Pattern, 592
PATHOLOGICAL PROCESSES, 593
Accidents, 593
Mechanical Forces, 597
Biological Agents, 599
Chemical Agents, 601
Radiological Agents, 603
SOCIAL PROCESSES, 603
Community and Work, 604
Culture and Ethnicity, 605
Legislation, 607
Economics, 607
Health Care Delivery System, 609
NURSING INTERVENTIONS, 610
School and the Nurse, 611

21 Adolescent, 617
MARINDA ALLENDER
AGE AND PHYSICAL CHANGES, 618
Scoliosis, 620
Acne, 620
Gender, 621
Race, 623
Genetics, 623
GORDON'S FUNCTIONAL HEALTH PATTERNS, 623
Health Perception-Health Management Pattern, 623
Nutritional-Metabolic Pattern, 624
Elimination Pattern, 627
Activity-Exercise Pattern, 627
Sleep-Rest Pattern, 627
Cognitive-Perceptual Pattern, 628
Self-Perception–Self-Concept Pattern, 630
Roles-Relationships Pattern, 631
Sexuality-Reproductive Pattern, 632
Coping–Stress-Tolerance Pattern, 635
Values-Beliefs Pattern, 636
PATHOLOGICAL PROCESSES, 637
Accidents, 637
Sports, 637
Violence, 638
Mechanical Forces, 639
BIOLOGICAL AND BACTERIAL AGENTS, 639
CHEMICAL AGENTS, 639
Drug Use, 639
Tobacco Use, 641
Cancer, 641
SOCIAL PROCESSES, 643
Community and School, 643
Culture and Ethnicity, 643
Legislation, 644
Economics, 644
Health Care Delivery System, 644
NURSING INTERVENTIONS, 646

22 Young Adult, 649
ELIZABETH C. KUDZMA
AGE AND PHYSICAL CHANGES, 650
GORDON'S FUNCTIONAL HEALTH PATTERNS, 651
Health Perception-Health Management Pattern, 651
Nutritional-Metabolic Pattern, 656
Elimination Pattern, 658
Activity-Exercise Pattern, 658
Sleep-Rest Pattern, 659
Cognitive-Perceptual Pattern, 659
Self-Perception–Self-Concept Pattern, 661
Roles-Relationships Pattern, 661
Sexuality-Reproductive Pattern, 664
Coping–Stress-Tolerance Pattern, 669
Values-Beliefs Pattern, 670
PATHOLOGICAL PROCESSES, 672
Accidents, 672
Pollution, 672
Occupational Hazards and Stressors, 672
Chemical Agents, 673
Cancer, 674
SOCIAL PROCESSES, 675
Community and Work, 675
Culture and Ethnicity, 676
Legislation, 676

Demographics, 676
Economics, 677
Dual Careers, 677
Health Care Delivery System, 677

23 Middle-Age Adult, 681
CAROL LYNN MANDLE
AGE AND PHYSICAL CHANGES, 682
Mortality Rates, 683
Gender and Marital Status, 683
Race and Gender, 684
Genetics, 685
GORDON'S FUNCTIONAL HEALTH PATTERNS, 685
Health Perception-Health Management Pattern, 685
Nutritional-Metabolic Pattern, 685
Elimination Pattern, 690
Activity-Exercise Pattern, 690
Sleep-Rest Pattern, 691
Cognitive-Perceptual Pattern, 691
Self-Perception–Self-Concept Pattern, 692
Roles-Relationships Pattern, 693
Sexuality-Reproductive Pattern, 697
Coping–Stress-Tolerance Pattern, 698
Values-Beliefs Pattern, 699
ENVIRONMENTAL FACTORS, 700
Physical Agents, 700
Biological Agents, 700
Chemical Agents, 701
SOCIAL PROCESSES, 702
Culture and Ethnicity, 702
Economics, 702
Health Care Delivery System, 703
NURSING INTERVENTIONS, 704

24 Older Adult, 709
TERRY FULMER, MERIDITH WALLACE, and CAROLE LIUM EDELMAN
AGE AND PHYSICAL CHANGES, 710
Goals of Health Promotion, 711
Theories of Aging, 711
GORDON'S FUNCTIONAL HEALTH PATTERNS, 711
Health Perception-Health Management Pattern, 711
Nutritional-Metabolic Pattern, 714
Elimination Pattern, 716
Activity-Exercise Pattern, 718
Sleep-Rest Pattern, 719
Cognitive-Perceptual Pattern, 721
Self-Perception–Self-Concept Pattern, 725
Roles-Relationships Pattern, 726
Sexuality-Reproductive Pattern, 727
Coping–Stress-Tolerance Pattern, 728
Values-Beliefs Pattern, 729
PATHOLOGICAL PROCESS, 731
Accidents, 731
Biological Agents, 733
SOCIAL PROCESSES, 736
Environments of Care, 736
Health Care Delivery System, 737

Unit Five

Challenges As We Enter the New Millennium

25 Health Promotion in the Twenty-First Century: Throughout the Lifespan and Throughout the World, 747
KATHLEEN HUTTLINGER and CAROL LYNN MANDLE
HEALTH PROMOTION: PAST DEVELOPMENTS AND FUTURE DIRECTIONS, 749
GLOBAL STRATEGY OF HEALTH FOR ALL, 749
Health for All, 749
Health Care Systems, 750
New Public Health Movement, 751
Ecological Foundations of Health Promotion, 751
Goals and Targets for Health Promotion, 751
Health Rather Than Health Care as a Starting Point, 752
REFORM OF HEALTH PROMOTION AND HEALTH CARE, 753
Clinical Effectiveness of Preventive Health Care, 753
Cost-Effectiveness of Preventive Health Care, 754
Health Promotion and Vulnerable Populations, 755
IMPLICATIONS OF NURSING LEADERSHIP IN HEALTH PROMOTION, 756
Implications for Policy Development, 756
Implications for Practice, 756
Implications for Education, 756
Implications for Research, 757

Unit One

Foundations for Health Promotion

1 Health Defined: Objectives for Promotion and Prevention

2 Changing Populations and Health

3 Health Policy and the Delivery System

4 The Therapeutic Relationship

5 Ethical Issues Relevant to Health Promotion

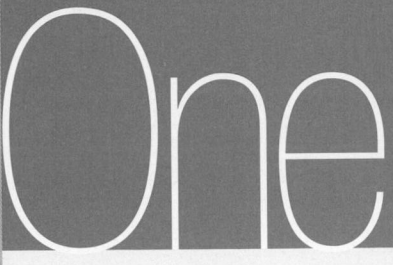

Chapter 1

PHILIP A. GREINER
JAMES A. FAIN
CAROLE LIUM EDELMAN

Health Defined: Objectives for Promotion and Prevention

objectives

After completing this chapter, the nurse will be able to:

- Define the term *health* as it has been used historically and as it is used in this textbook.
- Examine the *Healthy People 2010* commitment to a single, overarching purpose: to promote health and prevent illness, disability, and premature death in the United States.
- Analyze the progress made in this nation from the original *Healthy People* document to the present.
- Explain the differences between health, illness, disease, disability, and premature death.
- Compare the three levels of prevention (primary, secondary, and tertiary) with the levels of service provision available across the lifespan.
- Describe the importance of research and the nurse's role in the research process to the promotion of health for individuals and populations.

key terms

Asset Planning
Case-Controlled Study
Cohort Study
Community-Based Care
Disease
Epidemiology
Evidence-Based Practice
Functioning
Health
Health Promotion
Healthy People 2010
High-Level Wellness
Illness
Levels of Prevention
Randomized Clinical Trials
Research Utilization
Target Population
Wellness
Wellness-Illness Continuum

THINK About It

Use of Nontraditional Therapies

One of the biggest challenges to health care providers is the blending of Western medicine and health practices with the health practices from other cultures and ethnic groups. The federal government recently formed the National Center for Complementary and Alternative Medicine (NCCAM) to conduct and support basic and applied research and training and to disseminate information on complementary and alternative medicine to practitioners and the public. As demographics of the United States shift, more people use a combination of therapies in self-care and for the treatment of specific illnesses.

1. What questions should the student ask to obtain information from people about their use of nontraditional therapies?
2. What are the benefits or drawbacks of using complementary therapists such as acupuncturists, spiritualists, herbalists, chiropractors, among others?
3. What resources should the student trust for informa-

continued

THINK About It

Use of Nontraditional Therapies—cont'd

tion on the efficacy and use of herbal remedies and their relationship to prescription medications?

4 What ideas of health would be most compatible with the use of alternative therapies?

5 How can alternative therapies be integrated into *Healthy People 2010* objectives, given that the emphasis of these objectives is the use of available community resources and the development of partnerships?

A core concept in society is health. This concept is modified with qualifiers such as good, bad, reasonable, or poor, based on a variety of factors. These factors may be age, gender, comparison group, current condition, past conditions, or the demands of various roles in society. This chapter will discuss health as a concept and related concepts such as illness, disease, disability, and functioning. Some motivating factors behind the move to disease prevention and health promotion in society will be examined with an introduction to *Healthy People 2010*. The implementation of these concepts as nursing actions will also be addressed from ideal and pragmatic standpoints. Research supporting these concepts and recommendations for further research will be presented. Nurses need to understand the pivotal role they play in health promotion and disease prevention, the important role of research in the knowledge of what is healthy, and the central role of **epidemiology** (the study of health and disease in society), and public health theory in the everyday practice of nursing.

EXPLORING CONCEPTS OF HEALTH

Newman (1987, 1994, 1995) states that nursing literature can be classified broadly within two major paradigms. The first is the **wellness-illness continuum,** a bipolar interactive portrayal of health and illness in myriad configurations, ranging from high-level wellness to depletion of health (death). **High-level wellness** is further conceptualized as a sense of well being, life satisfaction, and quality of life. Movement toward the negative end of the continuum includes adaptation to disease and disability through various levels of functional ability. The wellness-illness conceptualization is supported by Keller's review of health literature (1981) and is consistent with the categories Smith (1983) identified in her philosophical analysis of health. Research based on the paradigm conforms primarily to scientific methods that seek to control contextual effects, provide the basis for causal explanations, and predict future outcomes (Newman, 1987, 1994, 1995).

The second paradigm characterizes health as a unidirectional development phenomenon of unitary patterning of person-environment. The development perspective of health has been present in the nursing literature since 1970, but it was not identified clearly with health until the late 1970s and early 1980s. It has been conceptualized as expanding consciousness, pattern or meaning recognition, personal transformation, and, tentatively, self-actualization. This shift toward a developmental perspective has had clear implications for the way in which health is conceptualized (Newman, 1987, 1994, 1995). Although not endorsing the development perspective to the extent of Rogers (1970) and Reed (1983), Pender (1987, 1996) has stated that health is an outcome of ongoing patterns of person-environment interaction throughout the lifespan. Research within this paradigm seeks to address the dynamic whole of the health experience; however, the methods by which to accomplish this objective are still in the preliminary states of development.

Health can be better understood if each person is seen as a part of a complex, interconnected, biological and social system. This ecological view is useful to those who promote health.

People involved in health promotion should consider the meaning of health because a focused definition clarifies their work and enhances the quality of the health care system. Health is used to describe a number of entities, such as a philosophy of care (health promotion and health maintenance), a system (health care delivery system), practices (good health practices), behaviors (health behaviors), costs (health care costs), and insurance. The reason that confusion continues regarding the use of the term *health* becomes clear.

Americans born before 1940 have experienced the greatest changes in how health is defined. Infectious diseases claimed the lives of many children and young adults; therefore health was viewed as the absence of disease. The physician was the primary provider of health care services in independent practice, with services provided in the private office. As the national economy expanded during and after World War II in the 1940s and 1950s, the idea of role performance became a focus in industrial research and entered the health care lexicon. Health became linked to a person's ability to fulfill their roles in society. Increasingly, the physician was asked to complete physical examination forms for school, work, military, and insurance purposes as physician practice became linked to hospital-based services more directly. There was the recognition that a person might recover from a disease, yet might not be able to fulfill their family or work roles because residual changes from the illness episode still exist.

From the 1960s to the present, there have been incredible changes in the health care delivery system as federal and state governments have attempted to control spending and health care costs have escalated. The growing number of primary care providers, including nurse practitioners and other advanced practice nurses, now attempt to involve individuals and their families in the delivery of care as individual responsibilities and lifestyle choices have become an important part of care. Health care has become an interdisciplinary endeavor even as managed care companies limit the health promotion options available under insurance plans. During this time, the idea of adaptation has had an important influence on the way Americans view health. Health has become linked to the changing environment to which individuals could react and change rather than becoming a fixed state. Adaptation fit well with the self-help movement during the 1970s and with the progressive growth in knowledge from research about disease prevention and health promotion (Kellogg, 1989).

There has been a more recent emphasis on the quality of a person's life as a component of health. Research on self-rated health (Idler, 1992; Johnson & Wolinsky, 1993) and self-rated function (Greiner, Snowdon, & Greiner, 1996, 1999) indicate that there are multiple factors contributing to a person's perception of his or her health. In addition to the ability to function cognitively and physically, fulfill social roles, and obtain health services, health is related to environment, socioeconomic level, race, and geographic location. Health is directly linked to how providers perceive the recipients of these services and to the options that providers offer.

Throughout history, society has entertained a variety of concepts of health. Smith (1983) describes four distinct models of health.

Models of Health

Clinical Model

The clinical model of health has the absence of signs and symptoms of disease as indicative of health. Illness would be the presence of conspicuous signs and symptoms of disease. People who use this model of health to guide their use of health care services may not seek preventive health services or they may wait until they are very ill to seek care. The clinical model is the conventional model of the discipline of medicine.

Role Performance Model

The role performance model of health has the ability to perform social roles as indicative of health. Role performance includes work, family, and social roles, with performance based on societal expectations. Illness would be the failure to perform a person's roles at the level of others in society. This model is the basis for work and school physical examinations and physician-excused absences. The idea of the sick role, in which people can be excused from performing their social roles while they are ill, is a vital component of the role performance model.

Adaptive Model

The adaptive model is reflective of Rene Dubos' work on adaptation (1980), Hans Selye's research on stress (1950), Jean Piaget's discussion of cognitive development (Piaget & Inhelder, 1975), and Roy's work (1970, 1999). This model of health has the ability to adapt positively to social, mental, and physiological change as indicative of health. Illness occurs when the person fails to adapt or becomes maladaptive to these changes. As the concept of adaptation has entered other aspects of American culture, this model of health has become more accepted.

Eudaimonistic Model

The eudaimonistic model of health has exuberant well being as indicative of health. Derived from Greek terminology, this term indicates a model that embodies the interaction and interrelationships between the physical, social, psychological, and spiritual aspects of life and the environment. Illness is reflected by a denervation or languishing, a wasting away, or lack of involvement with life. Although these ideas may appear to be new when compared with the clinical model of health, there are aspects of the eudaimonistic model that predate the clinical model of health. This model is also more congruent with integrative modes of therapy, which is used increasingly by the majority of people in the United States and the world.

These ideas of health provide a basis for how people view health and disease and how they view the role of nurses, physicians, and other health care providers. For example, in the clinical model of health, a person may expect to see a health care provider only when there are obvious signs of illness. Personal responsibility for health may not be a motivating factor for this individual because the provider is responsible for dealing with the health problem and returning the person to health. Therefore attempts to teach health-promoting activities may not be effective with this person.

Health-Illness Continuum

The health-illness continuum is a traditional depiction of the relationship between the concepts of health and illness. In this paradigm, health is a positive state in which incremental increases in health can be made beyond the midpoint (Fig. 1-1). These increases involve improved physical and mental health states. The opposite end of the continuum is illness, with the possibility of incremental decreases in health beyond the midpoint. This depiction of

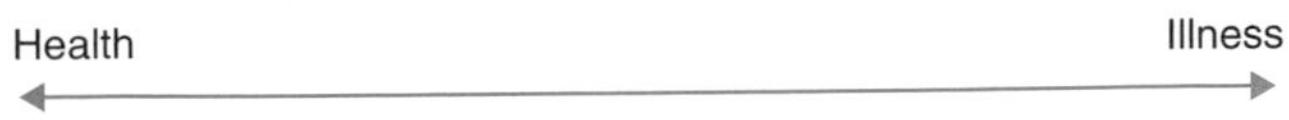

Fig. 1-1 Wellness-illness continuum. Moving from the center to the right shows a progressively worsening state of health. Moving to the left of center indicates increasing levels of health.

the relationship of health and illness fits well with the clinical model of health.

High-Level Wellness

From a dichotomous representation of health and illness as opposites, Dunn (1961) developed a health-illness continuum that would assess a patient based on his or her relative health compared with others and the environment (Fig. 1-2). A second dimension, high-level wellness, was added to the health-illness continuum in which a matrix of a favorable environment allows high-level wellness to occur and an unfavorable environment allows low-level wellness to exist.

With this addition, it became possible to characterize a person based on the clinical model of health and other social and environmental parameters. The concept demonstrates that a person can have a terminal disease and be emotionally prepared for death, while acting as a support for other people and achieving high-level wellness. High-level wellness involves progression toward a higher level of functioning, an open-ended and ever-expanding future with its challenge of fuller potential, and the integration of the whole being (Neilson, 1988). This definition of high-level wellness contains ideas similar to those in the eudaimonistic model of health. Additionally, high-level wellness emphasizes the interrelationship between the environment and the ability of achieving health on both a personal and a societal level.

The second paradigm characterizes health as a unidirectional, developmental phenomenon of unitary patterning of person-environment. The developmental perspective of health has been present in the nursing literature since 1970, but was not identified clearly with health until the late 1970s and early 1980s. This perspective has been conceptualized as expanding consciousness, pattern or meaning recognition, personal transformation, and self-actualization. This shift toward a developmental perspective has had clear implications for the way in which health is conceptualized (Newman, 1987, 1995). Although not endorsing the development perspective to the extent of Rogers (1970) and Reed (1983), Pender (1986, 1987, 1996) has stated that health is a manifestation of evolving patterns of person-environment interaction throughout the lifespan. Research within this paradigm seeks to address the dynamic whole of the health experience; however, the methods by which this objective can be accomplished are still in the preliminary stages of development.

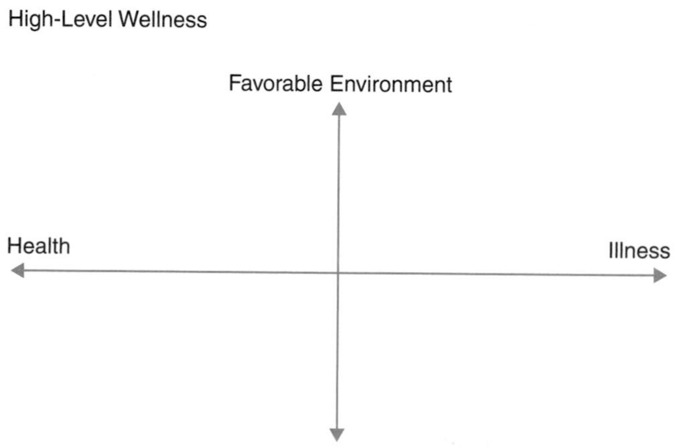

Fig. 1-2 High-level wellness added to the health-illness continuum. (Adapted from U.S. Department of Health and Human Services, Public Health Service, 1982.)

Functioning

One of the defining characteristics of life is the ability to function. Similar to the concept of health, **functioning** can be characterized as being present or absent, high level or low level. Functioning is integral to health. There are physical, mental, and social levels of function reflected in terms of performance and social expectations. Loss of function may be a sign or symptom of a disease. For example, sudden loss of the ability to move an arm or leg may indicate a stroke. The inability to leave the house may indicate overwhelming fear. In both cases, the loss of function is a sign of disease, a state of ill health.

Health

Health, as defined in this text, is a state of physical, mental, and social functioning that realizes a person's potential. Health is an individual's responsibility, but it requires collective action to ensure a society and an environment in which people can act responsibly. The culture and beliefs of the people can also influence health. This definition is consistent with the World Health Organization (WHO) definition of health as the state of complete physical, mental, and social well-being and not merely the absence of disease and infirmity (WHO, 1958) and with Terris' revisions (1975) to that definition. In addition to being measurable in process and outcomes, this definition is applicable across the lifespan, particularly for older adults whose functional abilities may determine needed services.

ILLNESS, DISEASE, AND HEALTH

It is easy to think of health or **wellness** as the lack of disease and to consider illness and disease as interchangeable terms. However, health and disease are not simply antonyms and disease and illness are not synonyms. Disease literally means "without ease." **Disease** may be defined as the failure of a person's adaptive mechanisms to counteract stimuli and stresses adequately, resulting in functional or structural disturbances. This definition is an ecological concept of disease, which uses a multifactorial perspective rather than a search for a single cause. This approach increases the chances of discovering the various factors that may be susceptible to intervention. Health and disease must be inseparable. If disease does not exist, then there is no need to discuss health. **Illness** is a social construct in which people are in an imbalanced, unsustainable relationship with their environment and are failing in their ability to survive and create a higher quality of life. Illness is a response characterized by a mismatch between a person's needs and the resources available to meet those needs. Additionally, illness signals individuals and populations that the present balance is not working. Illness diminishes the ongoing capacity of individuals and the society to respond, limiting an individual's future capabilities. When people can no longer respond and maintain the essential sustaining balance of relationships between their inner and outer worlds, they die (Milio, 1981).

Disease is a biomedical term indicating the presence of a recognizable health deviation, whereas illness is a state of being. Illness has social, psychological, and biomedical components. A person can have a disease without feeling ill (asymptomatic hypertension). The theory that health and illness are dynamic patterns that change with time and social circumstance leads to the conclusion that health assessments must be made frequently during the life cycle. Most health evaluations are relative and based on a series of perceptions and observations rather than a limited standard of measurement. Health arises from a finely graded continuum of functional ability and disability, not from mutually exclusive categories. Health, illness, and disease are neither static nor stationary. Behind every condition is the phenomenon of almost constant alteration. These conditions are continuing processes—a battle by human beings to maintain a positive balance of the biological, physical, mental, and social forces that tend to disturb their health equilibrium (Fig. 1-3).

PLANNING FOR HEALTH

Public health has always had the prevention of disease in society as its focus. However, over the past 30 years, the promotion of health has moved to the forefront within public health and has become a driving force in health care.

A key milestone in promoting health was the advent of *Healthy People* (U.S. Department of Health, Education, and Welfare [USDHEW], Public Health Service, 1979), the first Surgeon General's report on health promotion and disease prevention issued in the waning years of the Carter administration. This document identified five national health goals as:

1. Reducing infant deaths by 35% through preventing low birth weight and birth defects.
2. Reducing deaths in children by 20% through growth and development screening and injury prevention.
3. Reducing deaths in adolescents and young adults by 20% through preventing motor vehicle injuries and decreasing the use of drugs and alcohol.
4. Reducing adult deaths by 25% through screening for and prevention of heart attacks, stroke, and cancer.
5. Reducing sick days in older adults by 20% through maintaining functional independence and preventing influenza and pneumonia.

Further, the document identified three causes of the major health issues in the United States as:

1. Careless habits
2. Pollution of the environment
3. Permitting harmful social conditions to persist (hunger, poverty, and ignorance) that destroy health, especially for infants and children

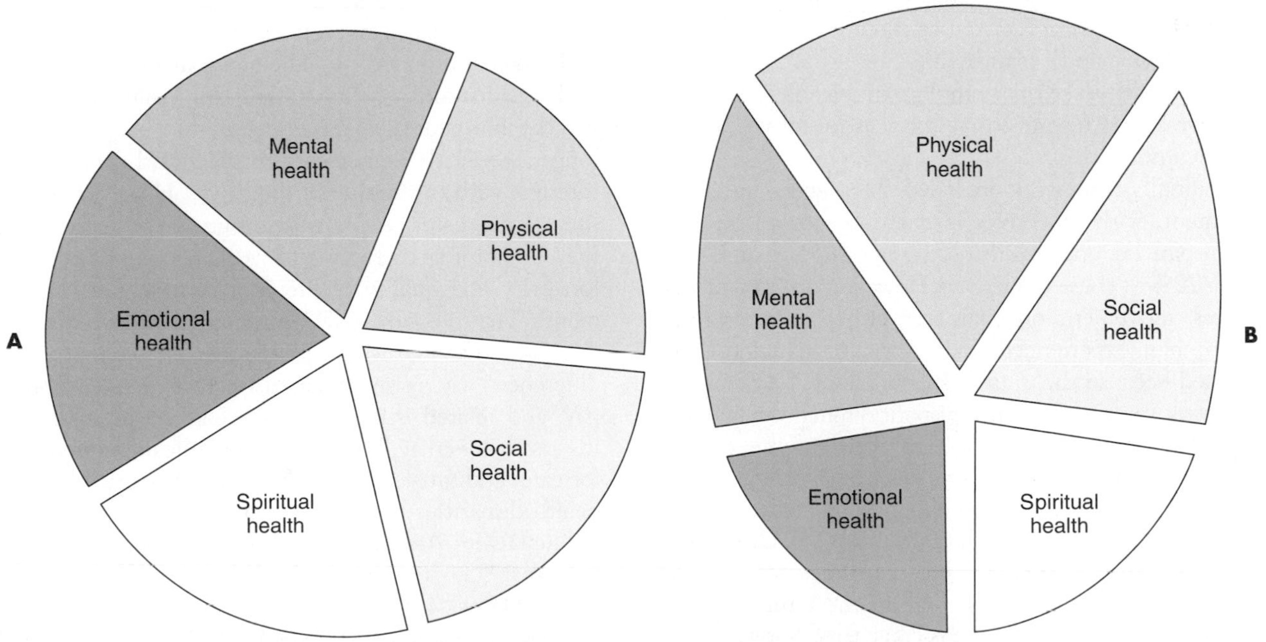

Fig. 1-3 **A,** A single health-illness continuum dot; **B,** The asymmetrical dot on the health-illness continuum. (Modified from Greenberg J., & Dintiman G. [1992]. *Exploring health: Expanding the boundaries of wellness.* Englewood Cliffs, NJ: Prentice Hall.)

Healthy People 2010 was a call to action and an attempt to set health goals for the United States for the next 10 years by issuing 226 health objectives. Unfortunately, a change in political leadership and the spiraling costs of hospital-based health care caused this document to be placed on the back burner for seven years. The need to report on progress toward the national objectives led a larger, renewed effort in the form of *The 1990 Health Objectives for the Nation: A Midcourse Review* (USDHHS, Public Health Service, 1986). This midcourse review noted that, although many goals were achievable, the unachieved goals were hindered by current health status, limited progress on risk reduction, difficulties in data collection, and a lack of public awareness. The work also noted that some of the achievable goals may have been set too low or did not address the complexities of the health problems by addressing only a portion of the problems.

Healthy People 2000 (USDHHS, Public Health Service, 1990) and its *Midcourse Review and 1995 Revisions* (USDHHS, Public Health Service, 1996) were landmark documents in that a consortium of people representing national organizations worked with Public Health Service officials to create a more global view of health. Additionally, a management-by-objectives approach was used to address each problem area. These two documents became the blueprints for each state as funding for federal programs became linked to meeting these national health objectives. As the objectives became more widely implemented, methods for collecting data became formalized and the data flowed back into the system to form the revisions set in 1995. The core of these health objectives remained; that is, prevention of illness and disease was the foundation for health. *Healthy People 2000* set out three broad goals:

1. Increase the span of healthy life.
2. Reduce health disparities among Americans.
3. Achieve access to preventive services for all Americans.

Additionally, the work included 22 specific areas for achievement, with objectives in each area based on age, health disparities, and health needs. By 1995, progress was made on 70% of these objectives. However, on 30% of the objectives, movement on goals was either in the wrong direction, had experienced no change, or could not be determined because the data was insufficient.

Currently, areas of health disparity remain based on race, gender, sexual orientation, disability, income, education, and location (urban versus rural). Access to preventive services remains a challenge as managed care has fought to control health care costs. Additionally, although the span of healthy life continues to increase generally, there are groups of people in the United States for whom the span of health life is considerably lower than the national average and lower than the life expectancy in less affluent countries.

HEALTHY PEOPLE 2010

Healthy People 2010 (USDHHS, Public Health Service, 2000) is the latest of the *Healthy People* documents. This new document sets out 28 specific areas for health improvement in 467 objectives. In her opening remarks, the Secretary of Health and Human Services, Donna Shalala, highlighted some of the key features in this document. She stated:

> Achieving the vision of 'Healthy People in Healthy Communities' represents an opportunity for individuals to make healthy lifestyle choices for themselves and their families. It challenges clinicians to put prevention into their practices. It requires communities and businesses to support health-promoting policies in schools, work sites, and other settings. It calls for scientists to pursue new research. Above all, it demands that all of us work together, using both traditional and innovative approaches, to help the American public achieve the 10-year targets defined by *Healthy People 2010* (USDHHS, Public Health Service, 2000).

Key Features of *Healthy People 2010*

Key features in the development of *Healthy People 2010* include:

- An expanded consortium model involving more than 350 national organizations and 250 state public health, mental health, substance abuse, and environmental agencies.
- National and regional meetings in which the public has an opportunity to ask questions and make further suggestions to consortium members.
- The use of a web site to gather additional information from individuals regarding the objectives.

Healthy People 2010 goals:

1. Increase quality and years of healthy life.
2. Eliminate health disparities.

Each goal is important. The first goal addresses the issues of longevity and quality of life. Increasing the years of healthy life addresses the concern that people are living longer, but with numerous chronic health problems that interfere with the quality of their lives. However, quality of life is an issue for people who are unable to achieve a long life. Combining these two ideas places emphasis on both longevity and quality of life as areas that need improvement. The second goal, eliminating health disparities, addresses the growing problems of access to care; differences in treatment based on race, gender, ability to pay; and related issues such as urban versus rural health, insurance coverage, Medicare and Medicaid reimbursement for care, and satisfaction with service delivery. Eliminating health disparities is one of the key goals of the American Public Health Association (APHA) and is the heart of the Five-Year Plan for the Public Health Nursing Section of the APHA.

Together, these two goals set out the territory in which health promotion and disease prevention efforts take place. Research in a variety of areas has clearly indicated that health disparities are directly and indirectly linked to longevity and quality of life issues. For example, it is known that Black men and women live fewer years than do White men and women, respectively. However, recent research from the Agency for Health Care Research and Quality demonstrates that Black men and women are also provided with less invasive and less expensive interventions for cardiac disease than are White men and women (Canto, Allison, & Kiefe, 2000). By choosing not to offer reperfusion therapy to one racial group when it is warranted and to offer the same therapy to another group contributes to the racial disparity in health care in this country and to the increased mortality of Blacks as compared with Whites (see Multicultural Awareness box).

The *Healthy People 2010* focus areas and objectives become the road map for this territory and a guide for health care research, practice, and communications in a way that should allow the health care community to measure progress on the broader goals.

The detailed objectives can be found on the Internet at www.health.gov/healthypeople. The 28 specific focus areas are listed alphabetically in Box 1-1. A quick look through these focus areas provides an indication of the scope of the *Healthy People 2010* areas compared with earlier versions of *Healthy People*. These focus areas span age categories from conception to death and incorporate prevention, access, treatment, and follow-up at the individual, family, provider, work site, and community levels. As a result, the objectives under each area are more comprehensive and specific than were the *Healthy People 2000* objectives. *Healthy People 2010* is centered on 10 leading health indicators that "reflect the major public health concerns in the United States and were chosen based on their ability to motivate action, the availability of data to measure their progress, and their relevance as broad public health issues" (USDHHS, Public Health Service, 2000, p. 11).

The leading health indicators are listed in Box 1-2. Each indicator was chosen because it is important as a public health concern and because it has the ability to rally support. Each leading health indicator is related to a variety of the health objectives either directly or indirectly. An examination of one objective may help demonstrate this relationship.

Objective 22-2. Increase the proportion of adults who engage regularly, preferably daily, in moderate physical activity for at least 30 minutes per day. This objective directly addresses the first two leading health indicators: physical activity and weight (obesity). Arguably, other indicators such as tobacco and substance abuse and mental health are indirectly related to this objective. If a person smokes or uses drugs regularly, then that person is limited in the ability to meet this objective. Nevertheless, physical activity can contribute to positive mental health through

MULTICULTURAL AWARENESS

Influence of Personal Cultural Values on Health Care Delivery

Culture influences every aspect of human life, including beliefs, values, and customs regarding health care. As health care providers, nurses need to be aware of their beliefs, values, and customs and how these ideas translate into behavior. It is easy to assume that an individual's own perspective is correct and shared by others. This is especially true when working with other health care providers who share the same culture. This concept is referred to as *ethnocentrism* and can lead to a devaluing of the beliefs, values, and customs of others, known as *racism.* Although it is impossible for any person to ignore the cultural influences on their lives, nurses and other health care providers have a special obligation to be aware of their own cultural biases and to focus more on the cultural influences in the lives of their patients. This ability to view another person's situations from their perspective is known as *empathy.* Multicultural health issues will continue to challenge providers to lifelong learning about the persons for whom they provide care.

Box 1-1 The 28 Focus Areas in *Healthy People 2010*

- Access to quality health services
- Arthritis, osteoporosis, and chronic back conditions
- Cancer
- Chronic kidney disease
- Diabetes
- Disability and secondary conditions
- Educational and community-based programs
- Environmental health
- Family planning
- Food safety
- Health communication
- Heart disease and stroke
- Human immunodeficiency virus
- Immunization and infectious diseases
- Injury and violence prevention
- Maternal, infant, and child health
- Medical product safety
- Mental health and mental disorders
- Nutrition and overweight
- Occupational safety and health
- Oral health
- Physical activity and fitness
- Public health infrastructure
- Respiratory diseases
- Sexually transmitted diseases
- Substance abuse
- Tobacco use
- Vision and hearing

From U.S. Department of Health and Human Services, Public Health Service. (1990). *Healthy people 2000: New objectives to promote health, prevent disease.* Washington, DC: Office of Disease Prevention and Health Promotion.

Box 1-2 The 10 Leading Health Indicators in *Healthy People 2010*

- Physical activity
- Overweight and obesity
- Tobacco use
- Substance abuse
- Responsible sexual behavior
- Mental health
- Injury and violence
- Environmental quality
- Immunization
- Access to health care

Data from: U.S. Department of Health and Human Services, Public Health Service. (1990). *Healthy people 2000: New objectives to promote health, prevent disease*. Washington, DC: Office of Disease Prevention and Health Promotion.

stress reduction and physical fitness. Access to health care to obtain a complete physical examination before starting to exercise and the quality of the work or neighborhood environment available for exercise can contribute to success or failure of this objective. This objective is related to other objectives such as nutrition and control of high blood pressure.

Additionally, current knowledge about physical activity and specific populations was considered when creating the *Healthy People 2010* objectives. Women, low-income populations, Black and Hispanic peoples, people with disabilities, and those over the age of 75 exercise less than do White men with moderate-to-high incomes. These health disparities can influence the number of people in these groups who develop high cholesterol or high blood pressure, which further increases their risk of heart disease and stroke. Although this objective addresses adults, other objectives address the need for beginning exercise activities at an early age and encourage young adults to be actively engaged in exercise. How might this objective be adjusted to the needs of an older adult population?

Another important feature of *Healthy People 2010* is its emphasis on responsibility for intervention. Individuals need to accept responsibility for their lifestyle choices and behaviors. Rather than a "repair shop" mentality in which the person waits until something is broken before seeking health care, people need to adopt a "preventive maintenance" approach in which they take responsibility for making good decisions about lifestyle and behaviors that will decrease their need for "repairs." This emphasis on personal responsibility gives each individual a role in the quality of his or her life and the length of healthy life each may have.

Health care providers need to be responsible for offering preventive health services and monitoring behaviors. Unfortunately, many of the incentives for providers are to do tasks and procedures rather than to counsel and help individuals choose between various behaviors. Providers need to take the time to discuss behaviors that may improve the quality of life and extend years of life. For example, the addictive nature of tobacco and its effect on the development and course of a variety of chronic health conditions is now well recognized. Providers should be asking every person if they use tobacco and should be providing them with ways to quit smoking, including economic and social incentives. One individual used the following incentive program to maintain her smoking cessation. Cigarettes cost approximately $4.00 per pack and she smoked one to one-and-a-half packs every day; therefore she allows herself $5.00 per day for each day she is free of tobacco. At the end of each week, she takes one half of the money saved that week ($17.50) and treats herself to dinner at a restaurant. The other half is saved for the year, providing her with over $900 for a vacation. Providers should be using this type of personal incentive to build on successful behavior modification.

Providers also need to look for partnership in the community through which they can better serve the needs of individuals. *Healthy People 2010* emphasizes the efforts of partnerships and partnership building as essential to health promotion. One approach to partnerships is the development and use of community nursing centers. Community nursing centers take two primary forms: primary care programs and health promotion programs. The Health Promotion Center (HPC) operated by Fairfield University School of Nursing in Fairfield, Connecticutis one example of a successful community nursing center. The nurses and student nurses who provide health education and community screening services at the HPC work with existing community organizations to help these organizations better meet the health care needs of underserved people. For example, the HPC works with local Head Start programs to provide education for Head Start staff, parents, and children on a variety of health-related topics. Screening of the children is federally mandated, but not all providers complete the forms or provide a full range of services. The HPC completes the screening activities, referring anyone with positive results back to their primary care provider. Follow-up is provided to ensure that the person receives the needed services or to contact the health care system if services are not obtained. Another approach to partnerships is to have providers serve as active participants on community boards and advisory committees, which enables providers to become more aware of the service needs in the community and the resources available to help meet those needs.

Work sites and communities need to become partners in providing opportunities for people to lead healthy lives through flexible work schedules, work site wellness programs, safe parks, and the availability of exercise facilities. Converting empty lots into community gardens provides beautification of the area, an opportunity for exercise in caring for the garden, and a source of fresh

CASE STUDY

Assessment of Frank Thompson and Family

Frank Thompson's large brick home is located off a sparsely traveled country road. A few yards away stands the uninhabited shack where Frank was born during World War II.

Frank was raised knowing the odds that he faced as a poor tenant farmer. He helped his father Ben with their small tobacco and corn crops. They were unaware that the hazardous chemicals in the pesticides they used would later affect Ben's life. As his father often reminded him, Frank had to do better than others in school so he would not be doomed to the tenant farmer's life. However, Frank's school attendance was erratic because it was interrupted by the frequent demand of tending field crops. Thin and often tired, he had recurrent infections. The school nurse helped the Thompson family obtain the necessary medication for Frank's initial infection, but the family was never able to afford the penicillin that was necessary to prevent recurrent infections.

Inspired by the early work of Martin Luther King, Jr., Frank was intent on helping at home and building something better for his future. Frank managed to more than make up for his lost time at school. He passed his college entrance examinations and was awarded one of the new equal opportunity grants, which offered him a choice of attending any of the Ivy League schools in the Northeast. Instead, he chose the prestigious Southern University and eventually earned a Masters of Business Administration (MBA) degree. He married Sada, his longtime girlfriend, and the two planned their future.

With a good job in a large local sales firm, Frank built his house and started a family. He moved from a salesman to a division head and often traveled to regional meetings, sometimes accompanied by Sada and their three children. Frank's dream of sharing his success with his family included using part of his earnings to help his brothers and sisters with their education.

This new way of life meant little time for relaxation and frequent attendance at business luncheons and career-promoting social occasions. He kept late hours and worked long weekends. Good food, drinks, and cigarettes helped him relax before and after important business and social encounters; these softened the edges of hard bargaining and were status symbols.

Not surprisingly, Frank gained weight. He had a persistent cough, which was probably a result of the smoking habit that developed during the early years of his career. Frank's physician, with whom Frank visited regularly at the corporation's health maintenance organization (HMO), said Frank's blood pressure and serum lipid levels were both higher than normal and that he had chronic bronchitis. The physician urged Frank to do what Frank already knew: cut down on smoking, drinking, saturated fats, and calories; get more exercise; and find ways to relax. However, Frank's life was too busy for exercise. He had to work harder as he moved up in his company, but he also had to appear relaxed, which was an essential characteristic for a prospective vice president. To meet these goals, he tended to drink and smoke more. He also refused to take medication for problems he could not see. Without the outward signs of disease, Frank believed he was out of shape, but generally healthy. Then Sada pointed out that his chance for promotion might actually improve if he lost some weight; therefore he registered for a physical fitness program for executives that he could attend on Sunday mornings and before work during the week. At his first workout, the classic sharp pain gripped his chest and Frank had a massive heart attack.

Weeks later, Frank was convalescing at home after being released from the university's coronary care facility. He was lucky to survive the heart attack, but he was also lucky to have most of the services covered by his medical insurance plan and 80% of his earnings were protected by the company's disability pension. Most people in the United States do not have this protection.

However, Frank's dreams of promotion were shattered. For many months he could go to the office only two or three times a week at most, simply to deal with routine matters. He could not travel, for business or otherwise, for a long time. He was also skeptical about his cardiac rehabilitation program because his heart attack happened during exercise.

vegetables. Providing a work environment that supports positive behaviors benefits everyone. For example, one small insurance company eliminated tobacco use from its building and campus, which was accomplished after months of discussing the idea with employees, limiting smoking to designated areas, eliminating cigarette machines from the building, and offering in-house smoking cessation courses. In addition to favorable comments from employees and individuals after the decision, the company experienced a cost savings in lower premiums for health and fire insurance, less frequent use of the ventilation system, and less smoke and fire damage to furniture and equipment. Additionally, their employees became more receptive to other health messages and generally happier about their jobs than they were in past years.

The health care environment has been slower to adopt healthy employment practices than have other corporations. Imagine a hospital where the staff can set their schedules to accommodate family needs, exercise at an in-hospital exercise facility, eat in an esthetically pleasing environment with relaxing music and healthy food, and participate in other stress-reduction activities and workshops on company time. Hospitals and health care systems have made progress in partnering in their communities, but even in this area, health care providers and their employers should be taking the lead in supporting partnership activities to meet *Healthy People 2010* objectives.

The faith community is a vital partner in meeting *Healthy People 2010* objectives. Faith communities can cut across economic, social, racial, and gender barriers, making them an excellent source for sharing information on health promotion and disease prevention. Parish nurses are becoming increasingly prevalent and they incorporate *Healthy People 2010* objectives into their activities (Berry, 1994).

Public health officials at all levels need to intervene, monitor, and report on each of the objectives and the related focus areas. As part of the core public health functions of assessment, policy development, and assurance, the U.S. Public Health Service and all state, county, and local health departments need to collect data, make information available to the public, create policies that support *Healthy People 2010* objectives, and ensure that needed services are available from a competent workforce. Unfortunately, inadequate funding and lack of focus have left many health departments short of prepared staff and without trained leaders. *Healthy People 2010* provides measurable objectives that can serve as guideposts in reconstructing these health departments.

Healthy People 2010 can form the basis for planning, service delivery, evaluation, and research in every aspect of the health care system. The nurse needs to be familiar with this document and its intent. Nurses should compare their practices with the objective in *Healthy People 2010*. Additionally, the nurse needs to be aware of the research and practice changes that occur as a result of the work toward these objectives.

Problem Identification

How many problems does Frank's situation present? The answer depends on who is asked the question and his or her position in relation to Frank. Each point of view focuses on different aspects of Frank's life. His physician might say that Frank had coronary heart disease with an acute myocardial infarction, hypertension, hyperlipidemia, chronic bronchitis, and obesity. His nurse might add that he paid little attention to his lifestyle, even after being told to make changes. He continued to overeat, drink too much, smoke, not exercise, and live a stressful life. Frank's employer saw a man who had potential, but who was now too disabled to take on new responsibilities and perhaps unable to continue performing his previous duties. Frank's children might feel that he could no longer take them on jaunts or play with them. His wife, Sada, knew that their plans for educating their children and for travel and enjoyment might suffer. The human resource personnel who managed Frank's health insurance and pension programs would say that he had an expensive disease and the state health planner would point out that Frank's problem was only one of a growing number of disabling illnesses that result from preventable causes.

To Frank, the health problems were multidimensional. His initial fear of dying, pain, dependence, and frustration decreased as he began to feel better, but his realization that he might never be able to achieve his dreams for himself and his family haunted him. Although theoretically in his prime, Frank suddenly saw himself as far older than his years, both in body and in social achievement. He believed he had reached his limit and that he would never again have the freedom to choose his future. He and his family needed to evaluate their situation and make alternative plans based on asset planning. A care plan has been developed based on Frank and his family. (See Care Plan box.)

Planning Interventions

Rather than emphasizing the chronic health issues and related problems, the nurse can begin with asset planning within the family. **Asset planning** is a planning approach that, given the realities of the present, helps focus the family and their providers on the building blocks for their future.

Frank's physician and nurse can begin with the fact that Frank survived his first myocardial infarction. The coronary damage resulting from this event becomes the baseline for determining future change in the lives of Frank and his family. Earlier, Frank's physician had taken a broader time perspective when he advised Frank to cut down on smoking, which was contributing to both his bronchitis and his hypertension, and to change his high-fat diet and sedentary habits, which contributed to his weight problem and aggravated his high blood pressure. These lifestyle changes become tools for Frank's recovery and for change within his family. His cardiac event becomes a risk factor for heart disease in the lives of his children.

Looking at the immediate future, Frank's employer saw the effect of the event on Frank's position within the company. Frank would have a long recovery that could be successful if he adhered to his cardiac rehabilitation program. Asset planning at this level meant examining how to move Frank back into his work role without further jeopardizing his health. Frank and Sada also needed to examine if he could continue in this position, given its potential effect on his health.

Frank and his family used a broader perspective than the medical personnel or the corporation. They knew that to achieve the family's economic and educational goals and still spend time together, they made decisions that ultimately affected Frank's health. Similar to many Americans, they had been willing to live with Frank's job pressures and stressful lifestyle. The family members were aware of their impoverished roots and had no wish to go back to them. However, they also recognized that the strength of their family, their ability to work together to achieve goals, and their faith were assets that were missing in other families they knew.

Frank's social network of friends, relatives, and church members became an additional asset. They helped the family through the difficult initial weeks at home by providing meals, taking care of the yard work and laundry, and providing companionship so Sada could shop and have

CARE PLAN

Nursing Diagnosis: Risk for Ineffective Coping Due to Change in Role Performance and Self-Esteem

DEFINING CHARACTERISTICS

- Inability to complete tasks
- Lack of focus on needs
- Feelings of inadequacy
- Inability to make decisions
- Sense of being overwhelmed
- Rest and sleep disturbance
- Frequent stress-related headaches
- Emotional fragility
- Assessment of situations does not match assessments of others

RELATED FACTORS

- Unexpected life changes
- Diagnosis of chronic disease
- Stressful life events
- Unsure of family supports
- Unrealistic expectations of self
- Unpredictable future
- Needs to reassess abilities
- Insecure job status

EXPECTED OUTCOMES

- The person will develop realistic expectations of capabilities based on rehabilitation potential.
- The nurse and person will set mutually agreeable milestones for resuming functions.
- The person will develop a revitalized sense of self.
- The person and family will use available resources to examine social and role shifts that affect the family.
- The person and spouse will express to each other their hopes and fears about the future.

INTERVENTIONS

- Listen to the concerns of the person and spouse regarding job, social, family, and medical concerns.
- Counsel the individual and spouse about realistic goals and expectations of cardiac rehabilitation.
- Assist the individual in setting realistic and reachable short-term goals.
- Assist the individual in developing more effective problem-solving skills.
- Provide support and positive feedback as short-term goals are met.
- Explore available community services that match the goals of the family.
- Facilitate family access to needed services through advocacy and supportive guidance.
- Supervise and teach about the use of prescribed and other medications.
- Coordinate communications between providers, employers, and other organizations to meet coping needs of the individual and his or her family.

time alone. As Frank recovered, they would provide support for the social and lifestyle changes that Frank and his family needed to make.

The visiting nurse played a vital role in Frank's recovery. As the physician continued to monitor Frank's cardiac status, the visiting nurse began the long process of changing Frank's habits. He had stopped smoking while in the hospital, but with more free time than usual, he was craving to smoke again. Using an asset planning approach, the visiting nurse identified the changes that Frank needed to make to decrease the risk of a second heart attack. A plan was developed to help Frank begin to take control of his life through behavior changes. These changes included relaxation techniques, diet modification, smoking cessation, and mild chair exercises. The support of the family was enlisted to reinforce the changes Frank was willing to make. His employer was contacted and agreed to a plan enabling Frank to work from home using a computer as the office became a nonsmoking workplace. Frank became an asset to the workplace, serving as a spokesperson for the benefits of lifestyle change. He was enlisted to talk with other employees about stress management and smoking cessation based on his personal experiences.

Health planners and public health officials used the broadest perspective in asset planning by viewing Frank as an example of a person whose potential shifted as a result of a preventable, disabling illness. The planners looked to public and private community patterns and policies that increase healthful habits and living conditions. These patterns and policies span a wide spectrum. Work schedules and work load; stress and safety in work environments; affirmative action programs for jobs and wages; availability of public transportation systems, recreational facilities, and economically accessible housing; farm price subsidies for food and tobacco crops that affect buying patterns; excise taxes and regulation of health-damaging drugs such as alcohol and nicotine are all taken into consideration (Milio, 1976). The asset planning approach emphasizes the positive actions that can be made to minimize the effects of Frank's illness and related diseases.

What Was the Actual Cause of Frank's Problem?

It is not possible to separate one cause from another because causes are not single factors. In Frank's case, the sources of illness were found in the many interrelationships in his life. Attempting to treat or change each factor as a separate entity can have a limited effect on the improvement of overall health. Frank's health problems were numerous. In addition to a poor diet, weight gain, lack of exercise, and smoking, his hyperlipidemia, an adaptive biological response to the pressures in his life, could not sustain him indefinitely. It eventually clogged his coronary vessels and they became maladaptive. His hypertension, resulting from his diet and time-constrained lifestyle, was also a biological attempt to adjust to a situation that contributed to an imbalance between his personal resources and the demands of his family and the economic world. Frank's smoking was a psychosocial means to help him relieve some of the emotional pressures. It may have served this short-term purpose, but only at a silently rising cost to his health. Cigarette use by persons who have hypertension or high serum cholesterol levels multiplies their risk of coronary heart disease (Logan et al., 1978; Maglacus, 1988; Papenfuss, 1988).

Evaluation of the Situation

The health status of an individual or population depends on a sustainable balance of the complex responses between internal (physiological and psychological) and external (social and environmental) factors. Health was initially conceived as a biological state, with genetic endowment as the starting point. However, health involves psychological and social aspects and is interpreted within the context of the immediate environment.

The interconnections between biophysical, psychological, and environmental causes and consequences did not end with Frank's heart attack. His heart attack was only the most dramatic sign that health-damaging responses outweighed health-promoting ones. The "tip of the iceberg" analogy is frequently used to illustrate the importance of identifying individuals with subclinical symptoms. High blood lipid levels, high blood pressure, obesity, smoking, and persistent worrying were no less important than the infarction in shaping the status of Frank's health. To repair the damage to Frank's heart without changing his lifestyle, habits, and work environment would only buy a brief amount of time before further damage would occur.

The infarction and resulting disability also permanently reshaped Frank's environment. After a few months of working full time, Frank realized that he needed to find a less stressful job. He recognized that his sales administration skills were an asset and began interviewing in the nonprofit sector. Ultimately, he landed a job at half his previous salary, but with excellent benefits and a flexible work environment. His reduced income meant that his children's educational opportunities were more limited than they were before his heart attack, but his family responded by writing for tuition support from community organizations. Frank found that his contacts in both the corporate and the nonprofit sectors increased his value to his new employer. Frank's entire life, internal and external, had changed. He had learned to adapt to his health problems and had developed a more eudaimonistic approach to health and life.

Frank's situation illustrates how causes and effects in life and health tend to merge into constant, inseparable interconnections between individuals and their worlds. A person's health status is a reflection of a web of relationships that characterize that person's life. Health is not an achievement or a prize, but a high-quality interaction between a person's inner and outer worlds that provides the capacity to respond to the demands of the biological, psychological, and environmental systems of these worlds.

After reviewing the list of *Healthy People 2010* Focus Areas listed in Box 1-1, which of the focus areas apply to the promotion of Frank's health? Clearly, the area of heart disease and stroke is most applicable. The *Healthy People 2010* web site has a number of objectives that relate directly to the prevention of heart disease, hypertension, and hyperlipidemia, including objectives that relate to treatment options and training the public to recognize and respond to heart attacks and stroke. Based on the information about Frank and his experience, determine what his children should be taught based on the *Healthy People 2010* objectives in this focus area.

LEVELS OF PREVENTION

Prevention, in a narrow sense, means averting the development of disease in the future. In a broad sense, prevention consists of all measures, including definitive therapy, which limit disease progression. Leavell and Clark (1965) defined three **levels of prevention:** primary, secondary, and tertiary (Fig. 1-4). Each level of prevention occurs at a distinct point in the natural history of a disease and requires specific nursing interventions (Burns, 1976).

Although the levels of prevention are related to the natural history of disease, they can be used to prevent disease and provide nurses with starting points in making effective, positive changes in the health status of their patients. Within the three levels of prevention, there are five steps, as shown in the Leavell and Clark model (1965). These steps include health promotion and specific protection (primary prevention); early diagnosis, prompt treatment, and disability limitation (secondary prevention); and restoration and rehabilitation (tertiary prevention).

Some confusion exists in the interpretation of these concepts; therefore a consistent understanding of primary, secondary, and tertiary prevention is essential. The levels of prevention operate on a continuum, but may overlap in

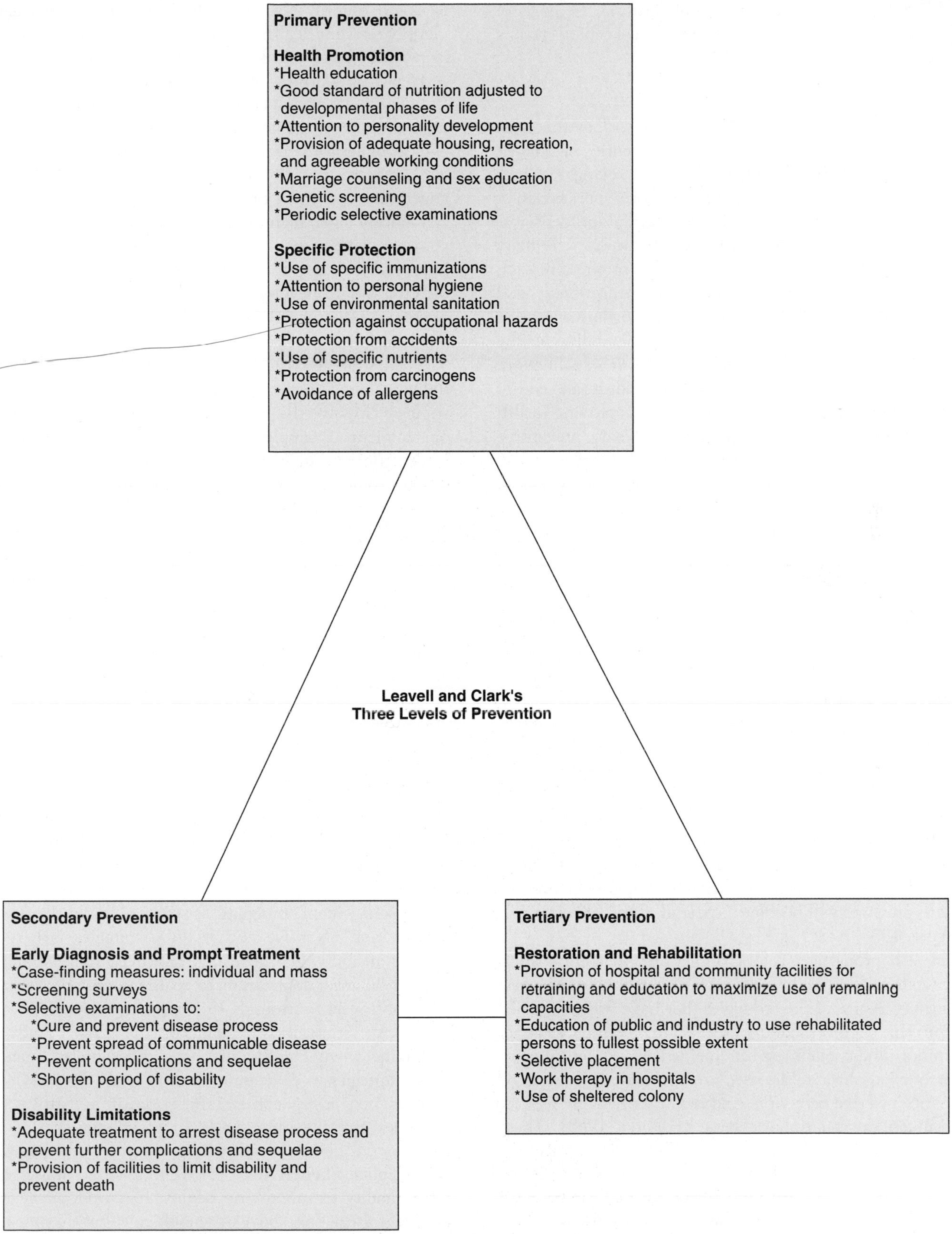

Primary Prevention
Health Promotion
*Health education
*Good standard of nutrition adjusted to developmental phases of life
*Attention to personality development
*Provision of adequate housing, recreation, and agreeable working conditions
*Marriage counseling and sex education
*Genetic screening
*Periodic selective examinations
Specific Protection
*Use of specific immunizations
*Attention to personal hygiene
*Use of environmental sanitation
*Protection against occupational hazards
*Protection from accidents
*Use of specific nutrients
*Protection from carcinogens
*Avoidance of allergens
Leavell and Clark's
Three Levels of Prevention
Secondary Prevention
Early Diagnosis and Prompt Treatment
*Case-finding measures: individual and mass
*Screening surveys
*Selective examinations to:
*Cure and prevent disease process
*Prevent spread of communicable disease
*Prevent complications and sequelae
*Shorten period of disability
Disability Limitations
*Adequate treatment to arrest disease process and prevent further complications and sequelae
*Provision of facilities to limit disability and prevent death
Tertiary Prevention
Restoration and Rehabilitation
*Provision of hospital and community facilities for retraining and education to maximize use of remaining capacities
*Education of public and industry to use rehabilitated persons to fullest possible extent
*Selective placement
*Work therapy in hospitals
*Use of sheltered colony

Fig. 1-4 The three levels of prevention developed by Leavell and Clark. (Data from Leavell H., & Clark A. E. [1965]. *Preventive medicine for doctors in the community.* New York: McGraw-Hill.)

practice. The nurse must clearly understand the goals of each level to intervene effectively in keeping people healthy.

Primary Prevention

Primary prevention precedes disease or dysfunction. However, primary prevention is therapeutic in that it includes health as beneficial to well being, it uses therapeutic treatments, and, as a process or behavior towards enhancing health, it involves symptom identification when teaching stress-reduction techniques. Primary prevention intervention includes health promotion, such as health education about risk factors for heart disease, and specific protection, such as immunization against Hepatitis B. Its purpose is to decrease the vulnerability of the individual or population to disease or dysfunction. Interventions at this level encourage individuals and groups to become more aware of the means of improving health and the things they can do at the primary preventive health level and the optimal health level. People are also taught to use appropriate primary preventive measures. However, primary prevention can also be viewed as advocating for health policies that promote the health of the community and electing public officials who will enact legislation that protects the health of the public.

Health Promotion

Health promotion is a relatively new field; therefore its definitions vary. O'Donnell (1987, p. 4) has defined **health promotion** as "the science and art of helping people change their lifestyle to move toward a state of optimal health." Kreuter and Devore (1980) propose a more complex definition in a paper commissioned by the U.S. Public Health Service. They state that health promotion is "the process of advocating health in order to enhance the probability that personal (individual, family, and community), private (professional and business), and public (federal, state, and local government) support of positive health practices will become a societal norm" (Kreuter and Devore, 1980, p. 26).

Health promotion is not only exercise and nutrition information. It is also proactive decision making at all levels of society. A few of the strategies that have been identified within this decision-making process are screening, self-care of minor illness, readiness for emergencies, successful management of chronic disease, environmental changes to enhance positive behaviors, and health-enhancing policies within an organizational setting (Folding, 1988). These ideals are reflected in the *Healthy People 2010* objectives reviewed earlier in this chapter. Health promotion holds the best promise for low-cost methods of limiting the constant increase in health care costs and for empowering people to be responsible for the aspects of their lives that can enhance well being. Based on the significance of health promotion activities within the health care system, efforts must be made to identify the multiple determinants of health, identify relevant health promotion strategies, and delineate issues relevant to social justice and access to care.

Health promotion efforts, unlike those directed at specific protection from certain diseases, focus on maintaining or improving the general health of individuals, families, and communities (see Health Teaching box). These activities are carried out at the public level, such as government programs promoting adequate housing, at the community level, such as Habitat for Humanity, and at the personal level, such as voting and volunteering for improved low-income housing. Nursing interventions are directed toward developing people's resources to maintain or enhance their well being, which is a form of assets-based planning.

Two strategies of health promotion involve the individual and may be either passive or active. Passive strategies involve the individual as an inactive participant or recipient. Examples of passive strategies are public health efforts to maintain clean water and sanitary sewage systems to decrease infectious diseases and improve health and efforts to introduce vitamin D in all milk to ensure that children will not be at high risk for rickets when there is little sunlight. These passive strategies must be used to promote the health of the public when individual compliance is low. For example, a private well can be an excellent source of water, but the landowner is responsible for monitoring the quality of the water. Contamination of the well by toxins that do not alter the taste or appearance of the water, or by those that do so over time, may go unnoticed and may expose the family to health risks. Municipal water supplies must conform to public health purity requirements and must be monitored routinely for purity.

Active strategies depend on the individual becoming personally involved in adopting a proposed program of health promotion. Two examples of lifestyle change are daily exercise as part of a physical fitness plan and a stress-management program as part of daily living. A combination of active and passive strategies is best for making an individual healthier. However, these strategies depend on mass application to realize economic benefits, and controversy surrounds the optimal balance between these two strategies. Reexamine the Case Study to determine when Frank could have incorporated some of these strategies to decrease his risk of heart disease.

This text is concerned almost entirely with active strategies and the nurse's role in these strategies. Some passive strategies are presented, but they are presented with the implicit belief that each individual must take responsibility for improving health. It is undeniable that passive strategies also have a valuable role, but they must be used within a context of encouraging and teaching individuals to assume more responsibility for their health. For example, the addition of vitamin D to bread should be

HEALTH TEACHING Process for Developing a Workplace Policy on Smoking

I. Planning
   A. Generate support
      1. Top management and administration
         a. Provide rationale for establishing policy
         b. Offer data emphasizing cost effectiveness and benefits
         c. Ask for representatives to serve on advisory committee
      2. Employees
         a. Provide knowledge about health concerns (passive smoking, cardiovascular disease, cancer, and personal hygiene)
         b. Select representatives from nonmanagement to serve on an advisory committee to set policies on smoking
         c. Stress individual, family, and community benefits of a nonsmoking policy
   B. Organize a cooperative process for policy development
      1. Form an advisory committee with one chairperson to develop the policy
      2. Include representatives from all segments of the organization, including smokers and nonsmokers
      3. Review policy options (total ban and designated areas)
   C. Survey management and employees with a questionnaire
      1. Determine prevalence of smoking, introduction to smoking, health risk factors associated with smoking, attitudes about developing and establishing a smoking policy, type of policy, and support services desired
      2. Ascertain the acceptance of and hours for smoking cessation programs
      3. Include demographic information to determine which groups can benefit from health educational programs

II. Policy Content
   A. List level of restriction on smoking
      1. Total ban
      2. Designated smoking areas (specify)
      3. No policy
   B. Address work stations and nonwork areas
      1. Types of walls
      2. Barriers
      3. Ventilation
      4. Air flow
      5. Work patterns
   C. Consider individual wishes of smokers and nonsmokers; when preferences conflict, the nonsmokers prevail
   D. Outline procedures for nonsmokers in facilities that have adopted designated smoking areas in their policies (smoking area with a separate ventilation system, working space located closest to the source of fresh air, and special considerations given to people with a hypersensitivity to tobacco smoke)
   E. Develop simple, written policies
      1. A rationale
      2. A general policy statement
      3. Specific areas affected
      4. A clearly defined complaint-grievance and enforcement procedure

III. Preparation for Implementation
   A. Notify employees individually months in advance of establishment of policy (specify start date)
   B. Offer time for questions, adjustments, and a contingency plan during the transition period

IV. Implementation
   A. Devise a comprehensive plan, including a process for dealing with grievances
   B. Have enforcement policy operational and familiar to the employees when smoking policy is adopted

V. Support for Smokers Trying to Quit
   A. Provide education and behavioral change programs (smoking cessation programs, incentives, supportive pharmaceutical measures, and counseling) to assist employees
   B. Offer education and behavioral change measures before instituting smoking policy and following enactment of policy
   C. Use community resources (speakers or information) to assist in support

VI. Evaluation
   A. Process evaluation questions
      1. How well do the employees feel the smoking policy is working?
      2. Do the employees feel that the smoking policy is easy to understand?
      3. How many of the employees completed the questionnaire?
      4. How many smoking cessation programs were offered?
      5. Were the smoking cessation programs perceived as helpful?
   B. Effect evaluation questions
      1. What percentage of the employees who smoke completed smoking cessation programs?
      2. Contingent on the policy, what percentage of the employees stopped smoking or smoked in designated areas?
      3. How many grievances or complaints were filed?
   C. Outcome evaluation questions
      1. Does a trend toward more smoke-free environments in the workplace emerge as a result?

From Milkanowicz, C. K., & Altman, N. H. (1995). Developing policies on smoking in the workplace, *Journal of Health Education*, 26(3),184.

part of a planned series of activities to teach people to eat foods that are more nutritious and to be more aware of the nutritional value of the foods they eat.

Although health promotion would seem to be a practical and effective mode of health care, the major portion of health care delivery is geared toward responding to acute and chronic disease. Preventing or delaying the onset of chronic disease and adding new dimensions to the quality of life are not as easy to implement because they take time and personal action. These actions are more closely associated with everyday living and the lifestyles adopted by individuals, families, communities, and nations. Habits such as eating, resting, exercising, and handling anxieties appear to be transmitted from parent to child and from social group to social group as part of a cultural, not a genetic, heritage. These activities may be taught in subtle ways, but they influence behavior and have as much of an influence on health as does genetic inheritance. Although the public may not appreciate the causal relationships between behavior and health, it should be apparent to health professionals. Arguably, the concept of risk is the most basic of all health concepts, since health promotion and disease protection are based on this concept.

Health-promotion strategies have the potential of enhancing the quality of life from birth to death. For example, good nutrition, is adjusted to various developmental phases in life, which accounts for rapid growth and development in infancy and early childhood, physiological changes associated with adolescence, extra demands during pregnancy, and the many changes occurring in older adults. Good nutrition is known to enhance the immune system, enabling individuals to fight off infections that could lead to disabling illnesses. Other individual activities are adapted to the person's needs for optimal personality development at all ages. As seen in Unit Four, much can be done on a personal or group basis, through counseling and properly directed parent education, to provide the environmental requirements for the proper personality development of children. Community participation is also an important factor in promoting individual, family, and group health (see Chapters 7 and 8).

Personal health promotion is usually provided through health education (see Chapter 10). As an important function of nurses, physicians, and allied health professionals, health education is principally concerned with eliciting useful changes in human behavior. The goal is the inculcation of a sense of responsibility for an individual's own health and a shared sense of responsibility for avoiding injury to the health of others. This objective implies the encouragement of child-rearing practices that foster normal growth and development (personal, social, and physical). Health education nurtures health-promoting habits, values, and attitudes that must be learned through practice. These must be reinforced through systematic instruction in hygiene, bodily function, physical fitness, and use of leisure time. Another goal is to understand the appropriate use of health services. For example, a semiannual visit to a dentist may teach a child to visit the dentist regularly, although this is not the primary purpose of the visit. Parents, teachers, and caregivers play a vital role in health education. In addition to teaching individuals, nurses need to develop skills in group teaching and in working within community organizations to increase the caregiver's ability to provide health education as part of their services.

Health promotion interventions must continually demonstrate that they are effective and economical to a degree that is rarely or never expected of any acute care intervention (Wamer et al., 1988). Available research clearly shows an increase in longevity, a decrease in mortality and morbidity, and an improvement in the quality of life for individuals who have been involved in health-promotion activities. It must be emphasized that health promotion requires lifestyle change. Once a lifestyle change has been adopted, vigilance is needed to ensure that the lifestyle change is maintained and modified to fit developmental and environmental changes.

Empirical data linking risk factors, health promotion activities, and outcomes are sufficient to drive the development of the *Healthy People 2010* objectives and to be incorporated into quality improvement measures in managed care. Nevertheless, the value of health promotion cannot be based on the idea that these programs save money. In fact, increased health care costs and service use may offset savings realized from health promotion activities. One of the challenges posed in *Healthy People 2010* is the development of measurable outcome objectives that are based on more realistic economic models.

The traditional approach of health promotion is designed to persuade the individual to take responsibility and adopt behaviors that will prevent physical disease; it also generally has an authoritative approach (Beattie, 1991). However, a more recent approach emphasizes positive health; social, spiritual, physical, and mental facets; the acquisition of life skills and self-esteem; and a two-way participatory process (Downie, Fyfe, & Tannahill, 1990). It is also characterized by a negotiated (grassroots and valuing individual autonomy) approach (Beattie, 1991). Both the traditional and the newer approaches are useful. The authoritative approach is useful when local means to promote health are obstructed by powerful gatekeepers such as large corporations or when the mass media is the most effective means of conveying a message. The negotiated approach is useful when individuals are motivated to make positive health changes collectively. For example, a runner may find that he or she is more likely to maintain and improve if running with a group. Motorcyclists may realize that wearing a helmet is more likely to reduce the chances of severe head injury and death, although state law permits them to ride without wearing a helmet.

HOT topics

HEALTH-PROMOTION PROGRAM INCENTIVES

The concept of health-promotion program incentives is multidimensional. Incentives are best defined relative to their purpose, type, and form for either groups or individuals.

An incentive is "an anticipated reward designed to influence the performance of an individual or group," whereas "the perceived positive or negative reward associated with adherence to or avoidance of a specific behavior" is referred to as the "pay value" attached to a particular incentive (Sobel, 1993).

"Incentives can be viewed as formal or informal in nature" (Sobel, 1993). A partial rebate of a program fee for completion of 80% of a smoking-cessation series would be an example of a formal incentive—one that is openly built into the design of a wellness program. An example of an informal incentive would be the chance to spend time with senior management in a company's fitness facility—one that is not openly built into, but is implicit in, the design of the program.

When deciding why incentives should be used in any health-promotion program, the nurse needs to determine the participant's reasons for wanting to adopt any new behavior. For example, the nurse would need to know why the **target population,** a collection of people to which interventions are directed within the broader community population, would want to:

- Wear seat belts.
- Ask their health care providers more questions.
- Get immunized.
- Exercise regularly.
- Stop smoking.
- Have surgery performed in an outpatient setting.
- Use a health care reference book.

Getting answers to these types of questions will help the nurse select the appropriate "pay values" to use in creating an incentive system. It is important to note at this time that incentives are not always advantageous and can therefore have potential disadvantages. However, being cautious and discerning in the design of incentive systems can substantially eliminate the disadvantages.

"Pay values" are the motivators behind the incentive effect. A list of major categories of incentive "pay values" follows:

- Sense of belonging
- Acceptance and approval
- Self-mastery
- Time reward
- Mixing with important people
- Gambling urges
- Fun and lightness
- Financial penalty
- High visibility
- Ease of access
- Good role modeling
- Personal discomfort
- Recognition
- Humor
- Creative outlet
- Material goods
- Financial reward
- Ability to contribute
- Personal challenge
- Group competition

In conclusion, "human behavior is multifactorial in nature, and it is extremely difficult for individuals to change their behavior without clearly perceived reason(s) to change. Incentives help provide those reasons to change" (Sobel, 1993). This statement demonstrates why it is important that nurses supplement wellness program efforts in community and workplace settings by including different types of incentives that will help individuals initiate and maintain specific health behavior changes.

From Connecticut Hospital Association. (1996). *Guidelines for the practice of health promotion*. Wallingford, CT: The Association.

Health promotion is an important concept for nursing because it embodies many other concepts that nursing is concerned with today. As stated, much of the nursing role is involved with health teaching. Nurses take on health-promotion roles and are considered by many to be in an excellent position to do so. Therefore it is vital that nurses consider what health promotion means and what they are being urged to incorporate into their role (see Hot Topics box).

Specific Protection

This aspect of primary prevention focuses on protecting people from disease by providing immunizations and reducing exposure to occupational hazards, carcinogens, and other environmental health risks. Primary prevention intervention is considered health protection because it emphasizes shielding or defending the body from injury. Implementing nursing interventions that prevent a specific health problem may seem easier than promoting well-being among individuals, groups, or communities because the variables are delineated more clearly in prevention than in promotion and the potential influences are less diverse. Two examples may help demonstrate these differences. Immunization for influenza is quite popular and has become a regular activity for older adults each autumn. Nurses participate in this specific protection role by giving the influenza injections in clinics and offices. Creating nut-free schools to protect hypersensitive children from life-threatening allergic reactions to peanut products have largely been the result of grassroots parent organizations working with formal community organizations to adopt policies that protect the health of these children. Nurses may be involved in the parent organizations or the school or public health boards that review the proposed policies. Additionally, nurses must be able to address the need to protect portions of the population at risk.

Secondary Prevention

Although primary prevention measures have decreased the hazards of chronic disease, other conditions that preclude a healthy lifestyle are still prevalent. Secondary prevention ranges from providing screening activities and treating early stages of disease to limiting disability by averting or delaying the consequences of advanced disease.

Screening is secondary prevention because the principle goal is to identify individuals in an early, detectable stage of the disease process. However, screening provides an excellent opportunity to offer health teaching as a primary, preventive measure. Screening activities have become an important aspect in the control of chronic diseases such as heart disease, stroke, and colorectal cancer. Additionally, screening activities provide early diagnosis and treatment of nutritional, behavioral, and other related problems. Nurses play an important role in screening activities because they can provide educationally sound health information during the screening process.

Delayed recognition of disease results in the need to limit future disability in late secondary prevention. Limiting disability is a vital role for nursing. Although certain economic and environmental changes may aid in preventing subsequent problems, preventive measures are primarily therapeutic and are aimed at arresting the disease and preventing further complications. The paradox here is that health education and disease prevention activities are similar to those used in primary prevention. Modifications to the teaching plan must be made based on the individual's current health status and the ability to modify behavior. In the case study, Frank needed secondary prevention after his heart attack. The lifestyle changes needed to prevent a second heart attack were similar to the steps he could have taken to prevent his initial heart attack, but with a recognition that his coronary status was compromised. As a result, exercise had to be increased gradually as part of a cardiac rehabilitation program and diet modifications had to be made with support from a registered dietitian to ensure adequate nutrition and weight loss.

Tertiary Prevention

Tertiary prevention occurs when a defect or disability is permanent and irreversible. The process involves minimizing the effects of disease and disability by surveillance and maintenance activities aimed at preventing complications and deterioration. Tertiary prevention focuses on rehabilitation to help people attain and retain an optimal level of functioning regardless of their disabling condition. The objective is to return the affected individual to a useful place in society, maximize remaining capacities, or both. The responsibility of the nurse is to ensure that persons with disabilities receive services that enable them to live and work according to the resources that are still available to them. When a person has a stroke, rehabilitating this individual to the highest level of functioning and teaching lifestyle change to prevent future strokes are examples of tertiary prevention.

THE NURSE'S ROLE

Evolving demands are placed on the nurse and the nursing profession as a result of changes in society. Emphasis is shifting from acute, hospital-based care to preventive, **community-based care,** which is provided in nontraditional health care settings in the community. This demand for community-based services, with the home as a major community setting for care, is closely related to the changing demographics of America. As the home and community become the existing sites for care, nurses must assume new roles. Nursing role changes must parallel the changes in health care delivery. Nurses are challenged to recognize the distinction between hospital-based and community-based care and they must accommodate this distinction. As the health care delivery system changes, nurses need to be at the forefront. Nurses must assume a variety of roles in health promotion and adopt a view toward future horizons and toward the nurse's roles with the individual and the expanded role in society. A variety of forces have driven the current development of blended roles. Individual needs and the health care system have contributed to the way in which roles have been implemented. Implementation of blended roles provides access to complex care while decreasing costs in a variety of ways. Within these roles, nurses assume a more active involvement in the prevention of disease and the promotion of health. Nurses are more independent in their practice, they place a greater emphasis on promoting and maximizing health, and more than ever, they are accountable morally and legally for their professional behavior.

Nursing Roles in Health Promotion and Protection

Although nurses often work with persons on a one-to-one basis, they seldom work in isolation. Within today's health care system, nurses work with other nurses, physicians, social workers, nutritionists, psychologists, therapists, and individuals. In the role of the caregiver, the nurse is a member of a team and needs to communicate extensively with other team members as a collaborator. As an advocate, the nurse is speaking and acting on behalf of a person or group; the nurse explains and interprets the feelings and positions of the individual or family to others. The nurse may be care managing, facilitating, and coordinating services for the individual to prevent duplication and to ensure that needs are met. Additionally, the nurse may serve as a consultant to other health care providers, persons, or agencies within the community. The nurse may also be a deliverer of services, an educator, and a researcher.

Advocate

The nurse may be an advocate by helping individuals obtain what they are entitled to receive from the system and by trying to make the system more responsive to their needs. One example of individual advocacy involves speaking to a local social service agency before referral to pave the way for family members who need to receive health benefits. In the role of advocate, the nurse strives to ensure that all persons receive quality, appropriate, and cost-effective care. The nurse may spend a great deal of time identifying and coordinating resources for complex cases.

Care Manager

The nurse acts as a care manager to prevent duplication of services and reduce costs. Thorough assessment enables the care manager to help individuals avoid care that is unproven, ineffective, or unsafe. The advent of virtually free Internet access has opened breathtaking vistas of health care information to nurses who are willing to invest a small amount of time and energy learning how to perform searches and organize their findings for future access. The following is a short list of helpful websites that can help the nurse locate health care information, but none of these are specific to care managers:

Medscape, www.medscape.com
Dr. Koop.com, www.drkoop.com
NOAH (New York Online Access to Health), www.noah.cuny.edu (also available in Spanish)
Onhealth.com, www.onhealth.com
Alternative Health News Online, www.altmedicine.com

The first step as an "e-care" manager is to know how to search for and find specific and high-quality information on the Internet. Successful care management depends on a collaborative relationship among the care manager, other nurses and physicians, the individual and his or her family, the payer, and other care providers who work with the person. The wishes of the individual and family need to be clear to the care manager. Facilitating communication among parties is one of the care manager's most important functions.

Consultant

Nurses often mediate the interactions between individuals and others because they are knowledgeable about health promotion and disease prevention. Consultative exchanges can occur with schoolteachers, legislators, or others who maintain a working relationship with the person. Some nurses have specialized areas of expertise, such as gerontology, women's health, or community health, and they are equipped to provide information as consultants in these areas of specialization. For example, a gerontological nurse specialist might be on a community planning board offering advice about what type of health-promotion activities should be considered in planning a new senior citizens' housing development. In contrast to independent consultation, nurses need to develop consultation skills that can be integrated into practice and allow the individual nurse to take advantage of opportunities to provide support on an individual patient level or future development at the organizational level (Berragan, 1998).

Deliverer of Services

The nurse also delivers services such as health education and counseling in health promotion. Visible, direct nursing care is often the foundation of nursing care practice from which the nurse develops clinical skills.

Educator

Health practices in the United States are derived from the theory that health components such as good nutrition, industrial and highway safety, immunization, and specific drug therapy should be within the grasp of the total population. Even with its rich resources, society falls far short of attaining the goal of maximal health for all. The problem is not a lack of knowledge, but rather the lack of application; therefore it is incumbent on nurses to add teaching to their roles. To teach effectively, the nurse knows essential things about the learner and the teaching-learning process (see Chapter 10).

In addition to their storehouse of scientific knowledge, nurses who are committed to their teaching role know that individuals are unique in their response to efforts to change their behavior. To expand the options in teaching methods, nurses explore the literature to find various ways to present health information. Testimonials of personal experiences can also be used for educational purposes. Teaching may range from a chance remark by the nurse, based on a perception of desirable patient behavior, to structurally planned teaching according to patient needs. Selection of the methods most likely to succeed involves the establishment of teacher-learner goals. Health promotion and protection rely heavily on the individual's ability to use appropriate knowledge. Teaching is one of the primary prevention techniques available to avoid the major causes of disability and death today.

Healer

Healing resides in the ability to glimpse or intuit the "interior" of an individual's care, to sense and identify what everyone else has missed or underappreciated, and to incorporate the specific insight into a care plan that speaks therapeutically to the reality of the person's care. Nurses are "artists" who have a special ability to heal. The art of nursing is the extraordinary ability to manage a broad array of clinical, financial, and psychosocial issues—analogous to the way a sculptor might use a wide array of materials—to create something meaningful, sensible, and whole.

Researcher

In today's health care environment, nurses are constantly striving to understand and interpret research findings that will enhance the quality and value of patient care. To provide optimal health care to all people in the United States, nurses need to use research findings as their foundation for clinical decision making. Making care decisions using research findings and clinical expertise enhances the nurse's ability to provide the best practice. When nurses or other clinicians use research findings and the best evidence possible to make decisions, the outcome is termed evidence-based practice. **Evidence-based practice** is defined as the conscientious, explicit, and judicious use of current best evidence in making decisions about the care of individual patients. The practice of evidence-based medicine means integrating individual clinical expertise with the best available external clinical evidence from systematic research (Sackett, Rosenberg, Gray, Haynes, & Richardson, 1996).

Nurses are leaders in providing evidence-based health care. Without a strong commitment to using evidence to guide decisions, nursing would lose credibility as a profession. Nurses need to assess the evidence carefully and focus on answering questions and solving problems about nursing practice. Using clinical expertise and evidence to plan and deliver care for an individual or population leads to evidence-based practice and health care. The notion of evidence-based practice provides a framework for many questions to be asked and answered.

In planning future research for the next five years, goals and strategies were developed by a subcommittee within the National Institute of Nursing Research (NINR). NINR supports clinical research to establish a scientific base for the care of individuals throughout the lifespan, from management of individuals during illness and recovery to the reduction of risks for disease and disability. Additionally, NINR supports research that fosters interdisciplinary collaboration that works toward promoting healthy lifestyles, promoting quality of life for persons with chronic illness, and identifying effective approaches to achieving and sustaining good health. Every 5 years, nurse researchers from around the United States participate in a priority-setting conference during which research priorities are identified and discussed. Specific goals and objectives established for the five-year period from 2000 to 2004 are shown in Box 1-3. Delivery of nursing care and interventions with preventive and health promotion efforts were the focus of these priorities, emphasizing the link between research and practice.

The document *Healthy People 2010,* published by the U.S. Department of Health and Human Services (USDHHS), stresses the national health agenda for the future. This document has formed the basis for the country's health care reform and is a framework for health policy that provides direction for the establishment of programs and services that will meet the health needs of all people in the United States (USDHHS, Public Health Service, 2000). In light of the health promotion and disease-prevention objectives found in *Healthy People 2010,* priority should be given to nursing research that will generate the knowledge to guide the practice. Specifically, health promotion research should focus on health problems and disease-prevention techniques, such as obesity reduction, smoking cessation, and prevention of cancer and heart disease. Traditionally, nurses have provided many health promotion interventions, such as teaching prenatal education classes, stressing prevention of infectious diseases through education and immunizations, teaching hygiene and safety principles in schools and industry, and disseminating information on how to reduce risk factors leading to chronic disease. Research in these areas has fostered a significant improvement in the health status of individuals and families, using aggressive prevention and health-promotion efforts. Two research studies focusing on health-promotion research are displayed in the Research Highlights boxes.

Box 1-3 Research Priorities of the National Institute of Nursing Research (NINR): 2000 to 2004

End of life and palliative care research. NINR is currently the lead institute at the National Institutes of Health (NIH) for this area of research and is focusing on clinical management of physical and psychological symptom management, communication, ethics and clinical decision-making, caregiver support, and care delivery issues.

Chronic illness experiences, such as managing symptoms, avoiding complications of disease and disability, supporting family caregivers, promoting adherence and self-management activities, and promoting healthy behaviors within the context of the chronic condition.

Quality of life and quality of care, to include cost savings for the patient, health care system, and society.

Health promotion and disease prevention research, particularly as it related to lifestyle changes and healthy behavior maintenance across the lifespan.

Symptom management of illness and treatment, such as pain, cognitive impairment, fatigue, nausea and vomiting, and sleep problems.

Telehealth interventions and monitoring or other emerging technologies to promote patient education and treatment.

Implications of genetic advances, including reducing factors that increase risk of disease, issues related to genetic screening, and subsequent gene therapy techniques.

Cultural and ethnic considerations in health and illness, including culturally sensitive interventions to decrease health disparities among groups by focusing on health promotion activities and chronic illness strategies.

Data from National Institute of Nursing Research, National Institutes of Health. (2000-2004). *Research priorities of the National Institute of Nursing Research: 2000 to 2004* [Online]. Available: http://www.nih.gov/ninr.

research highlights

Behavioral Interventions in Health Care

The fields of health education and health promotion and disease prevention have become more widely accepted and the role of the nurse in primary, secondary, and tertiary disease prevention has expanded. Research studies initiated to evaluate the health effects and cost-effectiveness of these programs use both public health and medical models. According to Dr. David Sobel, director of Health Promotion and Patient Education at Kaiser Permanente, Northern California Region, the influence of behavioral interventions in health care may be measured through (1) health improvement, (2) behavioral change, (3) increased satisfaction, and (4) cost savings and cost effectiveness. A review of controlled studies indicates that behavioral and educational interventions significantly decreased the use of more expensive medical treatment, as follows:

- 17% reduction in total ambulatory visits.
- 35% reduction in visits for minor illnesses.
- 25% reduction in pediatric acute illness visits.
- 149% reduction in office visits for acute asthma.
- 140% reduction in office visits for arthritis.
- 156% reduction in cesarean sections.
- 185% reduction in epidural anesthesia in labor and delivery.
- 11.5-day reduction in length of hospital stay for patients requiring surgery.

The literature addressing chronic disease indicates that almost one third of persons visit a physician for bodily symptoms that are a manifestation of psychological distress; another one third have medical conditions resulting from poor lifestyle choices, such as smoking, unhealthy diets, and substance abuse. Therefore the other one third who have disorders such as arthritis, heart disease, diabetes, and asthma should demonstrate significant improvement through educational-behavioral interventions (stress management and relaxation techniques, nutrition education, pain-management strategies).

Data from Connecticut Hospital Association. (1996). *Guidelines for the practice of health promotion*. Wallingford, CT: The Association; Sobel, D. (1993). *Cost effectiveness of health and patient education*. Eighth Annual Interregional Health Education Conference. Berkeley, CA: Kaiser Permanente.

Evidence-based practice involves tracking down the best external evidence with which to answer research questions. Three types of research designs that are considered important when looking at evidence-based practice include randomized clinical trials (RCTs), cohort studies, and case-controlled studies. However, evidence-based practice should not be restricted to using study findings associated exclusively with RCTs. Sackett and colleagues (1996) stressed the use of the best external evidence available to answer clinical questions and explore the next best evidence when appropriate. The next best evidence may include the individual clinical judgment that nurses acquire through clinical experience and clinical practice and other qualitative approaches to research.

Randomized Studies **Randomized clinical trials** (RCTs) are experiments in which individuals are randomly assigned into groups called *study* and *control* groups. The study group receives the intervention and the control group does not receive the intervention. Randomization can be achieved by using computer-generated lists, a table of random numbers, or some other quasi-experimental method. A unique feature of RCTs is the ability to use "blinding." Blinding ensures that subjects in a RCT are unaware of the treatment or intervention to which they are exposed. Double-blinded studies are ones in which neither the researcher nor the subject knows what treatment or intervention they are receiving. This method is often used in many drug studies in which the investigator and subjects are not told what medication, if any, they are receiving so as not to influence the outcome (U.S. Preventive Services Task Force, 1996).

Cohort Studies A **cohort study** differs from a random study in that the investigators do not determine which individuals receive the intervention at the outset. Rather, people who have already been exposed to the risk factor, or intervention, and control subjects who have not been exposed are selected by the investigators to be followed longitudinally over time in an effort to observe differences in outcome. This type of study has the disadvantage of requiring a large sample size, many years of observation to provide adequate statistical power to measure differences in outcome, or both (U.S. Preventive Services Task Force, 1996). Longitudinal studies are typically expensive and time consuming. Additionally, researchers are often faced with subjects who drop out of the study before it is completed. Attrition, or mortality, refers to the loss of subjects from both experimental and control groups for various reasons. Determining whether attrition occurs for random or biased reasons and whether one particular group is affected more than another becomes important (Polit & Hungler, 1999).

Case-Controlled Studies In the **case-controlled study,** both the study group and the control group are selected on the basis of whether they have the disease and not whether they have been exposed to a risk factor or a clinical intervention. Therefore the design is retrospective. The principal disadvantages of this type of study are difficulty identifying important confounding variables and adjusting them for the outcome, difficulty getting the past history of participants, and the improper selection of control groups, which may invalidate conclusions about the presence or absence of statistical associations (U.S. Preventive Services Task Force, 1996).

Although nurses recognize the importance of research as a basis for their practice, they often do not have the time in today's complex health care system to participate in the research process. Several barriers to involvement with research include difficulty reading and understanding research, a lack of relevance of the findings to their practice, resistance to change in many work settings, and increased paperwork responsibilities. Despite these barriers, the role of nursing must include education and research. Nurses must critically read and evaluate research that will contribute to building a sound knowledge base for developing nursing interventions and influencing policy formation. **Research utilization** will provide a firm foundation on which effective health promotion and disease-prevention programs can be instituted.

Reading a variety of research studies on a particular topic helps nurses understand the state of the science within a given area of research and its relevance to their practice. Reading the research also helps nurses identify gaps and controversies and raise new questions for consideration. Chapters 16 to 24 contain specific health promotion research studies. Time should be taken to review these studies and explore the relationship between behavior and disease, to identify which populations groups are at risk, and to discover what types of health-promotion programs work and why they work. Through knowledge of research, nurses can strengthen their confidence in making daily decisions about quality care.

The Pew Health Professions Commission was created in 1989 to focus on the health care workforce. The goal of the Commission was established to help policy makers and educators produce health care professionals who could meet the changing needs of the American health care system. The most significant achievement of the Commission was in raising the awareness of the role of health care professionals in large health care environments. Through the direct involvement of hundreds of individuals playing roles as commissioners, task force members, and staff advanced a comprehensive agenda to understand how the nature of being a health care professional was changing in today's health care environment. In January 1999, the Pew Health Professions Commission closed after 10 years of work and many accomplishments. As the Commission ended its work, it passed many of its initiatives to the Center for the Health Professions at the University of California, San Francisco. The center works today to advance the understanding of issues and develop programs that assist schools and health care professionals in making the necessary accommodation in the changing health care environment. The Commission recommended a list of interdisciplinary competencies for all health care professionals, which is shown in Box 1-4 (Pew Health Professions Commission, 1991, 1998).

IMPROVING PROSPECTS FOR HEALTH

Population Effects

Cultural and socioeconomic changes within the population unequivocally influence lay concepts of health promotion. The myth that all Americans are alike—White and middle class—is no longer the case. By the year 2050, it is predicted that the majority of Americans will not be of White European descent, but rather a mixture of all the people of color in the world. Taken together as a portent for future health promotion strategies, these predictions about the population proclaim that health promotion, as lay people now view it, may not meet the needs of the future American population (see Chapter 2).

Another important factor is the projected age distribution. Considerable growth is expected in the proportion of the population that is 25 years of age and older. For

Box 1-4 Twenty-One Competencies for the Twenty-First Century

1. Embrace a personal ethic of social responsibility and service.
2. Exhibit ethical behavior in all professional activities.
3. Provide evidence-based, clinically competent care.
4. Incorporate the multiple determinants of health in clinical care.
5. Apply knowledge of the new sciences.
6. Demonstrate critical thinking, reflection, and problem-solving skills.
7. Understand the role of primary care.
8. Rigorously practice preventive health care.
9. Integrate population-based care and services into practice.
10. Improve access to health care for persons with unmet health needs.
11. Put relationship-centered care and services into practice.
12. Provide culturally sensitive care to a diverse society.
13. Partner with communities and health care decision makers.
14. Use communication and information technology effectively and appropriately.
15. Work in interdisciplinary teams.
16. Ensure care that balances individual, professional, system, and societal needs.
17. Practice leadership.
18. Take responsibility for quality of care and health outcomes at all levels.
19. Contribute to continuous improvement of the health care system.
20. Advocate for public policy that promotes and protects the health of the public.
21. Continue to learn and help others learn.

Data from Pew Health Professions Commission. (1991). *Healthy America practitioners for 2005: An agenda for action for U.S. health professional schools*. Durham, NC: Duke University Press; Pew Health Professions Commission. (1998). *Critical challenges: Recreating health professional practice for a new century, fourth report*. San Francisco: Center for Health Professions, University of California: San Francisco.

example, the postWorld War II baby boom will increase the number of persons in the 65-and-older age group between the years 2010 and 2030. The drop in births after 1960 will decrease the number of persons entering the 65-and-older age group, resulting in a more stable population pattern by 2050 (Uhlenberg, 1977). Analysis of these population trends and projections helps health professionals determine changing needs. Additionally, analysis of the social environment is necessary for social policy concerning health.

SHIFTING PROBLEMS

The provision of personal health services must be combined with nonpersonal or environmental services. Environmental pollution is a complex and increasingly hazardous problem. Diseases related to industry and technology, including accidents and trauma, have also become important threats to health.

The physical and psychological stresses of a rapidly changing and fast-paced society present daily problems, such as economic pressures and poor health habits. Obesity, especially from the lack of exercise, is at least partly a product of modern technology. The ingestion of potentially toxic, nonnutritious, high-fat foods is another contributing factor to poor health (see Chapter 11). The abuse of tobacco, drugs, and alcohol also negatively affects health.

Environmental conditions produce both physical and socioeconomic limitations. Emphasis on the application of complex technological advancements after the manifestation of disease is not only costly, but it also has minimal effects on improving health. An orientation toward illness clearly focuses on the effects rather than the causes of disease.

A substantial change in wellness patterns has occurred. Infectious and acute diseases were the major causes of death in the early part of the twentieth century, whereas chronic conditions, heart disease, cerebrovascular accident (stroke), and cancer are the major causes today. The diagnosis and treatment of disease, which were highly successful in the past, are not the answer for today's needs, which are closely related to and affected by biochemical make-up, environment, and lifestyle.

In the health belief model, belief in the efficacy of an action implies confidence that it will be beneficial in reducing the perceived health threat. For a health behavior to occur, potential barriers, such as cost and level of complexity of the behavior, must not outweigh the benefits as the individual perceives them. The difference between the individual's perception of the barriers to action and belief in the efficacy of the action influences the state of readiness to take action, thereby influencing the likelihood of action. In addition to perceived susceptibility, severity, efficacy, barriers, and modifying factors, internal (somatic) or external (social or cultural) cues must be present and strong enough to trigger an individual to act (Redeker, 1988).

MOVING TOWARD SOLUTIONS

Solutions are neither simple nor easy, but they can be focused in two major directions: individual involvement and government involvement. The first direction concentrates on actions of the individual, especially actions related to lifestyle beginning early in life with the young child. The learning and the inherent changes that are involved require an attitudinal change, which is perhaps the most difficult requirement. Approximately one fifth of the population is faced with the problem of getting the basic necessities of food and shelter. The other four fifths, whose basic necessities have been met, must overcome problems that result from affluence.

Motivational factors play a large role in influencing attitudinal change. As discussed in Chapter 10, programs for health promotion and health education are only part of the answer. Financial incentives for prevention may be another motivating factor and health advocacy by professionals in the health field is critical. Additionally, private and public action at all levels is needed to reduce possible environmental hazards. toxic agents in the environment can present health hazards that may not be detected for years; therefore it is necessary for individuals to monitor industrial and agricultural production processes to reduce exposure to potentially toxic agents. The government's involvement in health may signal an increasing trend. Health care expenditures have escalated rapidly; illness care is not the answer.

Legislation and financing that relate to primary prevention are discussed in Chapter 3. Government activity, in the form of legislation, is currently increasing in this area. For example, bicycle safety, seat belts, and a graduated tax on cigarettes are specific areas of concern. Health planning presents one of the most important areas of government in the future. The redirection of the existing health care delivery system, putting more emphasis on primary prevention, is probably the most difficult and the most far-reaching goal; however, an emphasis on a wellness system is necessary to improve the health of the U.S. population.

SUMMARY

The way individuals define health and health problems is important because definitions influence attempts to improve health and care delivery. Frank Thompson's health was affected by such obvious, immediate, and personal factors, such as his diet and employment pressures. Nevertheless, his problems had their roots in the social and economic conditions of his parents; in his own early history of illness, education, and work; and in his and his family's hopes and aspirations. His physician, who defined Frank's problem in immediate biomedical terms, used the tools of personal services to help repair the short-term effects of his heart attack. Public health planners, who saw Frank's problem on a longer-term population basis, sought policy solutions to the problem of preventing cardiovascular disease.

The view taken in this text is such that a broad and longer-term perspective of health can guide toward promoting health more effectively, even as nurses deal with individual problems on a day-to-day basis.

Health is a sustainable balance between internal and external forces. Health allows people to move through life free from the constraints of illness, limited only by the winding down of the biological clock's genetically programmed capacity. In this sense, health means keeping in time with the biological clock as individuals and as populations.

Illness is the speeding up of an individual's biological clock as a result of the imbalanced relations that human choices (intertwined social, political, spiritual, professional, and personal choices) create. In the United States, communities may yet have time to slow the onslaught of chronic disability and shift the direction, slow the pace, and humanize the scope of economic and social life.

To shift directions in today's health care, patterns may be possible only when nurses and other health professionals do what is expected of them as leaders in the care of health: to work with others through open processes; to provide leadership in finding the vision and the path; and to inform, educate, and reeducate themselves, their colleagues, the media, and the general public.

The responsibility of nurses as health professionals today calls for seeing the health problem in new ways and helping others to do the same. Responsibility means developing new roles and looking at the problem through others' eyes, including the eyes of individuals, the public, other professionals, and other nations. Responsibility also means evaluating the social and individual consequences, the long-term and short-term effects, and the public and private interests that are involved when deciding on the set of tools to use in the care of health.

REFERENCES

Beattie, A. (1991). Knowledge and control in health promotion: A test for social policy and social theory. In J. Gabe (Ed.), *Sociology of the Health Service*. London: Routledge.

Berragan, L. (1998). Consultancy in nursing: Roles and opportunities, *Journal of Clinical Nursing, 7*(2), 139-143.

Berry, R. (1994). A parish nurse. In Office of Resourcing Committees on Preparation for Ministry, *A day in the life of . . . . A kaleidoscope of specialized ministries*. Louisville: Presbyterian Church Distribution Management Service.

Burns C. R. (1976). The Nonnatural: A paradox in the western concept of health. *Journal of Medical Philosophy, 1*(3), 202.

Canto, J. G., Allison, J. J., & Kiefe, C. I. (2000). Relation of race and sex to the use of reperfusion therapy in Medicare beneficiaries with acute myocardial infarction. *New England Journal of Medicine, 342*(15), 1094-1100.

Connecticut Hospital Association. (1996). *Guidelines for the practice of health promotion*. Wallingford, CT: The Association.

Downie, R. S., Fyfe, C., & Tannahill, A. (1990). *Health promotion models and values*. Oxford, England: Oxford University Press.

Dubos, R. (1980). *Man adapting*. New Haven, CT: Yale University Press.

Dunn, H. (1961). *High-level wellness*. Arlington, VA: R.W. Beatty Co.

Folding, J. (1988). The proof of the health promotion pudding. *Journal of Occupational Medicine: Official Publication of the Industrial Medical Association, 30*(2), 113.

Greiner, P., Snowdon, D., & Greiner, L. (1996). The relationship of self-rated function and self-rated health to concurrent functional ability, functional decline, and mortality: Findings from the Nun Study. *The Journal of Gerontology. Series B, Psychological Sciences and Social Sciences, S 51B*(5), S234-S241.

Greiner, P., Snowdon, D., & Greiner, L. (1999). Self-rated function, self-rated health, and postmortem evidence of brain infarcts: Findings from the Nun Study. *The Journal of Gerontology. Series B, Psychological Sciences and Social Sciences, 54B*(4), S219-S222.

Idler, E. (1992). Self-assessed health and mortality: A review of studies. *International Review of Health Psychology, 1*, 33-54.

Johnson, R., & Wolinsky, F. (1993). The structure of health status among older adults: Disease disability, functional limitation, and perceived health. *Journal of Health and Social Behavior, 34*, 105-121.

Keller, M. J. (1983). Health needs and nursing care of labor force. In M. J. Fromer (Ed.), *Community health care and the nursing process* (2nd ed.). St. Louis: Mosby.

Kellogg. (1989). *Promoting health in America. Breakthroughs and harbingers*. Battle Creek, MI: W.K. Kellogg Foundation.

Kreuter, M., & Devore, R. (1980). Update: Reinforcing the case for health promotion. *Family & Community Health, 10*, 106.

Leavell, H., & Clark, A. E. (1965). *Preventive medicine for doctors in the community*. New York: McGraw-Hill.

Logan, R. et al. (1978). Risk factors of ischemic heart disease in normal men aged 40. *Lancet, 1*(8031), 949.

Maglacas, A. (1988). Health for all: Nursing's role. *Nursing Outlook, 36*(2), 66.

Milio, N. (1976). A framework for prevention: Changing health-damaging to health-generating life patterns. *American Journal of Public Health and the Nation's Health, 66*(5), 435.

Milio, N. (1981). *Promoting health through public policy*. Philadelphia: F.A. Davis.

Milkanowicz, C. K., & Altman, N. H. (1995). Developing policies on smoking in the workplace. *Journal of Health Education, 26*(3), 184.

Neilson, E. (1988). Health values: achieving high level wellness: origin, philosophy, purpose. *Health Values, 12*(3), 5.

O'Donnell, M. (1987). Definition of health promotion. *American Journal of Health Promotion, 1*(1), 4.

Newman, M. (1986). *Health as expanding consciousness*. St. Louis: Mosby.

Newman, M. (1987). Health conceptualizations: Nursing's emerging paradigm—the diagnosis of pattern. In V. A. McLean (Ed.), *Classification of Nursing Diagnosis* (proceedings of the 7th conference). St. Louis: Mosby.

Newman, M. (1994). *Health as expanding consciousness*. New York: National League for Nursing Press.

Newman, M. (1995). *A developing discipline. Selected works of Margaret Newman*. New York: National League for Nursing Press.

Papenfuss, R. I. (1988). Health promotion: Issues for AAHE in the 1980s. *Health Education, 5*, 36.

Pender, N. J. (1987). *Health promotion in nursing practice* (2nd ed.). Norwalk, CT: Appleton & Lange.

Pender, N. J. (1996). *Health promotion in nursing practice* (3rd ed.). Stamford, CT: Appleton & Lange.

Pew Health Professions Commission. (1991). *Healthy America practitioners for 2005: An agenda for action for U.S. health professional schools*. Durham, NC: Duke University Press.

Pew Health Professions Commission. (1998). *Critical Challenges: Recreating health professional practice for a new century, fourth report.* San Francisco Center for Health Professionals: University of California, San Francisco.

Piaget, J., & Inhelder, B. (1975). *The origin of the idea of change in children*. New York: W.W. Norton.

Polit, D. F., & Hungler, B. P. (1999). *Nursing research principles and methods* (6th ed.). Philadelphia: Lippincott, Williams, & Wilkins.

Reed, P. G. (1983). Implications of the lifespan development framework for well-being in adulthood and aging. *Advances in Nursing Science, 1*(18).

Redeker, N. (1988). Health beliefs and adherence in chronic illness. *Image, 20*(1), 18.

Rogers, M. (1970). *An introduction to the theoretical basis of nursing*. Philadelphia: F.A. Davis.

Roy, C. (1970). Adaptation: A basis for nursing practice. *Nursing Outlook, 19*, 254-257.

Roy, C. (1999). *Adaptation model-based research: 25 years of contributions in nursing science*. Indianapolis: Center Nursing Press. Sigma Theta Tau, International.

Sackett, D. L., Rosenberg, W. M. C., Gray, J., Haynes, R. B., & Richardson, W. S. (1996). Evidence of bad medicine: What it is and what it isn't. *British Medical Journal, 312*, 71-72.

Selye, H. (1950). *The stresses of life*. New York: McGraw-Hill.

Smith, J. A. (1983). *The idea of health: Implications for the nursing profession*. New York: Columbia University Teachers College Press.

Sobel, D. (1993). *Cost effectiveness of health and patient education*. Eighth Annual Interregional Health Education Conference. Berkeley, CA: Kaiser Permanente.

Terris, M. (1975). Approaches to an epidemiology of health. *American Journal of Public Health, 65*(10), 1037.

Uhlenberg, P. (1977). Changing structure of the older population of the USA during the twentieth century. *Gerontologist, 17*, 197.

U.S. Department of Health, Education, and Welfare, Public Health Service. (1979). *Healthy people*. U.S. Department of Health and Human Services. Washington, DC: U.S. Government Printing Office.

U.S. Department of Health and Human Services, Public Health Service. (1986). *The 1990 health objectives for the nation: A midcourse review*. U.S. Department of Health and Human Services. Washington, DC: U.S. Government Printing Office.

U.S. Department of Health and Human Services, Public Health Service. (1990). *Healthy people 2000: New objectives to promote health, prevent disease*. Washington, DC: Office of Disease Prevention and Health Promotion.

U.S. Department of Health and Human Services, Public Health Service. (1990). *Healthy people 2000: The Surgeon General's report on health promotion and disease prevention*. U.S. Department of Health and Human Services (Publication No. 7955071). Washington, DC: U.S. Government Printing Office.

U.S. Department of Health and Human Services, Public Health Service. (1996). *Healthy people 2000 mid-course review and 1995 revisions*. Boston: Jones & Bartlett.

U.S. Department of Health and Human Services, Public Health Service. (2000). *Healthy people 2010 (conference edition, in two volumes)*. U.S. Department of Health and Human Services. Washington, DC: U.S. Government Printing Office.

U.S. Preventive Services Task Force. (1996). *Guide to clinical preventive services* (2nd ed.). Baltimore: Williams & Wilkins.

Wamer, K. et al. (1988). Economic implications of workplace health promotion programs: Review of the literature. *Journal of Occupational Medicine, 30*(2), 106.

World Health Organization. (1958). *The first ten years of the World Health Organization*. New York: World Health Organization.

Chapter 2

GERALDINE V. GO

Changing Populations and Health

objectives

After completing this chapter, the nurse will be able to:

- Provide a brief history of immigration patterns to the United States.
- Define the terms *ethnicity, process of ethnicization, ethnic group, minority group, race,* and *culture.*
- Explain the functions of ethnicity, values, and value orientation.
- Contrast the folk health care system from the Western view.
- Identify prevalent health problems of Asian Americans–Pacific Islanders, Blacks, Hispanics, Native Americans, and aging minorities.
- Describe selected health-related aspects of the cultures of Asian Americans–Pacific Islanders, Blacks, Hispanics, and Native Americans.
- Discuss the current status and health problems of homeless persons.
- Explain strategies for alleviating homelessness.
- Describe culturally competent approaches for HIV and AIDS prevention among ethnic minorities.
- Identify global, national, and nurses' work in meeting the challenges of the twenty-first century.

key terms

Acculturation
Acculturation Stress
Antiviral Drug
Assimilation
Assimilation Model
Culture
Ethnic Group
Ethnic Symbols
Ethnicity
Ethnocentric Perspective
Extended Kinship
Folk System
Gene Therapy
Hippocratic Theory
Holistic Approach
Homelessness
Minority Group
Morbidity
Pluralistic
Process of Becoming an Ethnic
Race
Racial Group
Santeria
Shaman
Tao Doctrine
Value Orientations
Western Health Care

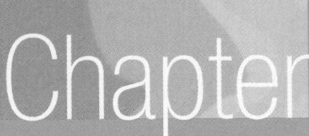

THINK About It

Health Care Practices of Hispanic Americans

In a study of breast self-examination (BSE) practices of Hispanic women, researchers found that only 0.7% of the 1453 Hispanic women who had been taught BSE were actually proficient in the BSE technique. The researchers believed that language and level of acculturation correlated with whether or not a woman performed BSE correctly.

In a study of acculturation and beliefs about AIDS, researchers found that Hispanic parents who were less acculturated had erroneous beliefs about AIDS contagion.

Hispanic Americans' use of health care services is dependent on the level of acculturation, social class, and fluency in the English language.

Language barriers foster powerlessness by limiting the life choices of Hispanic women and their ability to acquire knowledge that will enable them to make decisions to use health care.

1. What thoughts do these cases elicit?
2. Should English be declared the official language in the United States?
3. Is language the strongest factor in acculturation?

In the twenty-first century, the United States continues to experience phenomenal changes including: (1) the downsizing of industries and organizations; (2) advancements in technology, particularly in information processing; (3) exciting developments in research on degenerative and fatal diseases, particularly the Human Genome Project; (4) rapid and continuing growth in ethnic minority populations; (5) an increase in the number of individuals with special needs, such as the elderly, homeless persons, children, and persons afflicted with the human immunodeficiency virus (HIV) and acquired immune deficiency syndrome (AIDS); (6) the emergence of new models of health care delivery; and (7) a wide range of unprecedented changes in the human values that guide everyday life. These changes and situations will be the major challenges of this century.

Good health, well being, and a quality of life in this century will require people to transcend attitudes and behaviors that reflect ignorance, prejudice, and insensitivity to the needs of others. In the United States, a nation of diverse peoples, these attitudes and behaviors can serve as insurmountable barriers in meeting the challenges of the twenty-first century. To meet these challenges, the first and most important step is to overcome ignorance through knowledge that could foster a change in attitudes and behaviors. Appreciation of others' uniqueness will facilitate the collaboration that is necessary to create healthier individuals, families, and communities.

CHANGING POPULATIONS IN THE UNITED STATES

Changes in the size and diversity of the population can be attributed to large-scale immigrations that were mostly voluntary. Voluntary immigrations are generally motivated by the quest of the individual or group for one or more of the following ends:

1. Educational opportunities
2. Economic benefits
3. Social improvements
4. Political and religious freedom (American Immigration, 1999)

A brief look at the patterns of immigration to the United States provides information on the population diversity that has been accomplished over a certain period.

Immigration to the United States

There were two periods of immigration before 1820. The first period, from 1660 to 1775, was called Colonial. The American colonies did not have effective control mechanisms for the immigration of overwhelming numbers of British people, who were mostly Protestant. The second period, from 1775 to 1820, was called the Era of the American Revolution. The first census conducted in 1790 documented 3,929,214 Americans. Approximately 750,000 were Blacks and their descendants. Native Americans were not counted at that time. Approximately 60.9% of the total White population were English. In 1890, New York and Chicago had the largest numbers of foreign-born residents totaling 1.5 and 1.1 million, respectively (American Immigration, 1999). These residents came from Germany, Ireland, Russia, Hungary, and Italy. They assimilated well and reinforced the British Protestant majority, America's predominant population during the Colonial period. One group, the Irish Catholics, came from the southern regions of Ireland and a small number of them were fleeing religious and political persecution under British rule. The great immigration of the Irish occurred when a series of potato crop failures brought famine and other hardships, which forced families to seek economic survival elsewhere (American Immigration, 1999).

The Great Depression and World War II brought drastic reductions in the number of immigrants. At the end of the war, immigration policies were enacted to accommodate refugees, American citizens, and legal aliens who had been separated from their spouses during the war. This period also encompassed the years when the National Origins Quota System (NOQS) reduced the volume of immigration from other countries such as Asia. During this period, most of the immigrants were from the countries of the old immigrants (American Immigration, 1999).

Another type of immigration that changed and increased the population of the United States was the immigration of refugees. From 1951 to 1970, there was an increase in the number of immigrants seeking political asylum. In the 1960s and 1970s, political refugees from

Cuba, Vietnam, and other countries in Southeast Asia were admitted by the thousands. Third World Immigration was facilitated by the abolition of the NOQS. In 1965, President Lyndon Johnson signed the Immigration and Nationality Act. The goals of this Act were to:

1. Provide for the unification of families
2. Increase the pool of skilled and educated aliens
3. Ease population problems caused by environmental and social upheavals
4. Facilitate international exchange programs
5. Prevent entry of poor aliens, persons with health problems, or persons with criminal records (Gonzalez, 1990)

The Immigration and Naturalization Act of 1976 created the Select Commission on Immigration and Refugee Policy. Additionally, the passing of the Refugee Act of 1980 broadened the definition of refugee. This new definition allowed the entry of more Cubans. In 1986, the Immigration Reform and Control Act made an important provision: the legalization of undocumented aliens (Gonzalez, 1990).

The abolition of the NOQS and the series of refugee acts increased the numbers of two groups: Hispanics and Asians. In 1998, there were nine million Asians and 30 million Hispanics (U.S. Census Bureau, 1999).

As immigrants begin to settle in a new land, they are exposed to the host culture. Do they lose their identity? What becomes of their culture, customs, traditions, and values? A look at the processes of **assimilation** (a minority group conforming and modifying its ways of life to conform to the dominant group) and **acculturation** (the process by which a cultural group adapts or learns how to take the behaviors of another group) will provide some answers.

From Immigrants to Ethnics

Two current models of ethnic relations that can be used in understanding how immigrants become ethnic people include the assimilation and the pluralistic models (Queralt, 1996). The **assimilation model** maintains that cultural differences between groups disappear as generations pass. "Persons of diverse backgrounds give up their original cultural identity and language and melt into another group, usually the core group of society" (Queralt, 1996, p. 64). The earliest proponent of this position was Zangwill (1921), who saw all the peoples of Europe coming to the United States, a "melting pot." The melting pot model was the first attempt to analyze what was happening to immigrants in the United States (American Immigration, 1999).

The **pluralistic** view strongly maintains the need for continued persistence of the immigrants' culture. The position of cultural pluralism developed as a response to the question of the relationship between immigrant populations and the host culture (Giddens, 1996; Persell, 1990). This perspective appears to have the stronger support in the literature on immigrant groups. How immigrants maintain their identity can be explained further by an understanding of the concept of ethnicity.

THE CONCEPT OF ETHNICITY

The term ethnicity is derived from the Greek word *ethos*, which originally meant "tribe, race, nation, or people." More recently, ethos has come to be associated with customs, socialization, and cultural patterns rather than biological origins of a given community of people that set them apart from others (Giddens, 1996). Individuals with an awareness of their ethnicity tend to have a sense of belonging or kinship with other members of the same **ethnic group.** This shared sense might be manifested in "kinship patterns, physical contiguity (as in localism or sectionalism), religious affiliation, language or dialect forms, tribal affiliations, nationality, phenotypical features, or a combination of these" (Schermerhorn, 1970, p. 12).

Isajiw (1974, p. 122) suggests that "ethnicity refers to an involuntary group of people who identify themselves and/or are identified by others as belonging to the same involuntary group." Although this definition refers more to an ethnic group than to ethnicity itself, it contains an important element that is also identified in Staiano's definition (1980, p. 29). This author defines **ethnicity** as a process, "an ongoing response, a reaction to the categorical ascription of others, as well as a reaction to the creation and incorporation of symbols into the collective identity." Both definitions incorporate the process of identifying ethnic group members by other individuals. This identification can be clearly understood as the **process of becoming an ethnic**.

The Process of Becoming an Ethnic

DeSantis and Benkin (1980) contended that individuals are perceived as "ethnics" by virtue of their being in a foreign land. Therefore natives are not ethnics in their own countries. The process of becoming an ethnic is initiated by the social results of large-scale emigration—when natives leave their countries with a regional identity rather than a national one (Charsley, 1974). Sarna (1978) proposed a model of ethnicization based on ascription and adversity. He proposed that immigrants, on entry into a new land, are identified by a classification scheme, such as the Immigration Commission's Dictionary of Races. The use of race as a classification criterion is subscribed to and reinforced by the government, schools, churches, the media, and the public at large. As immigrants begin to deemphasize their regional identities and view themselves according to a classification scheme that is intelligible to others, they become ethnics. Through this process of ascription, the immigrants' self-definition and others' definition of them merge into one. This ascribed classification is accepted by the immigrants as "part of defense against prejudice and hostility" (Sarna, 1978, p. 374). Barth proposed that the emergence of a newspaper and of mutual and benevolent societies are two major ethnic symbols, which serve to unite ethnics. **Ethnic symbols** are "routine items internal to the culture and/or race" and are emphasized by ethnics

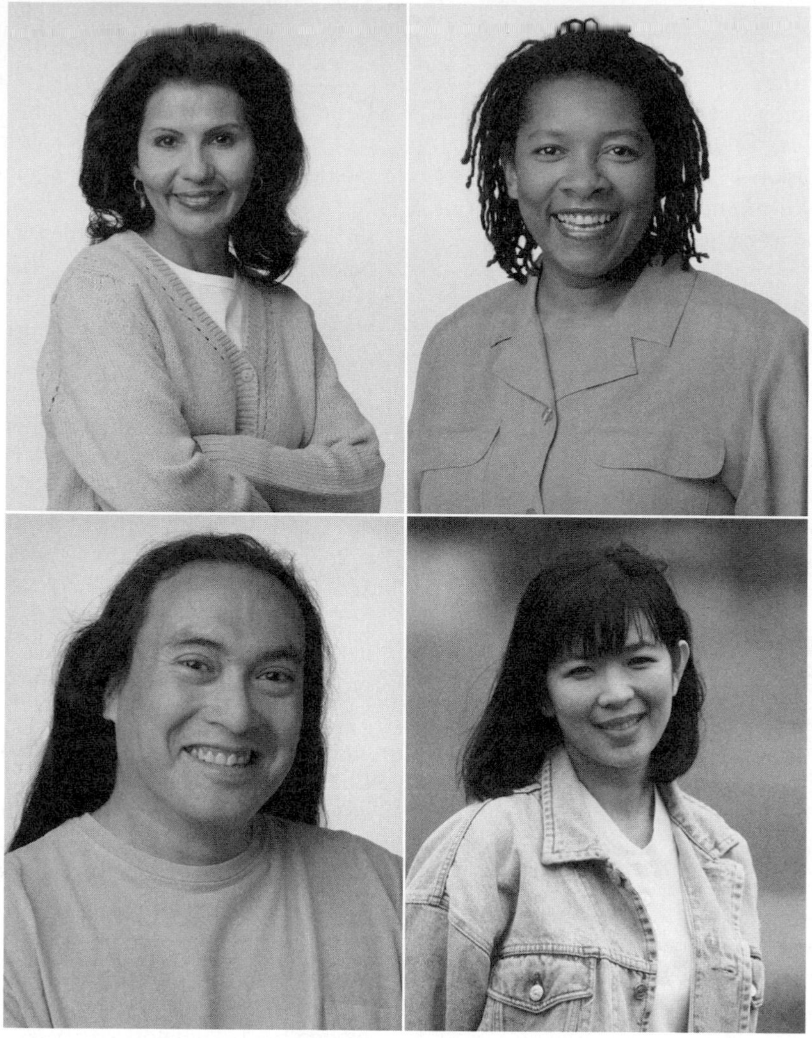

Fig. 2-1 People from different racial origins.

to differentiate themselves (Barth, 1969, p. 54). Furthermore, ethnics create new symbols in an effort to stimulate solidarity and self-consciousness (Sarna, 1978).

Racial, Ethnic, and Minority Groups

Race, a biological term, refers to a grouping of individuals with distinct physical characteristics, such as skin color, hair texture, or facial features (Bauwens & Anderson, 1992; Queralt, 1996) (Fig. 2-1). A **racial group** consists of people of the same race who share some common cultural characteristics (Queralt, 1996). Conversely, an ethnic group is a "collectivity within a larger society" (Feinstein, 1971, p. 4). Its markedly contrasting values, rituals, and maintenance of separate institutions differentiate it from the larger society (Pettigrew, 1971). Both racial and ethnic groups share characteristics that strengthen the individual's sense of identity and belonging.

An ethnic group is often identified as a minority group, but each may be distinct from a sociological perspective. A **minority group** may be perceived as consisting of people who receive less than their share of wealth, power, or social status (Persell, 1990). The identity of the minority group is tied in with the dominant group that is perceived to possess the authority to control the value system and the allocation of resources (Schermerhorn, 1970). Furthermore, a minority may consist of a particular racial, religious, or occupational group (Bauwens & Anderson, 1992). A group may be identified as either a minority group, an ethnic group, or both (see the Health Teaching box).

The process of becoming an ethnic and identifying with an ethnic group serves many functions. Ethnicity plays an important role in the life process of an individual by conveying orientations, values, role expectations, norms, social responsibility, patterns of involvement, commitment, loyalty, and solidarity (Kolm, 1971). Values and perceptions about health and illness evolve from the socialization process within a person's ethnic group. A sense of ethnicity also inspires the person to form a network of individual and

HEALTH TEACHING Working with Diverse Populations

There are many exciting challenges in working with individuals from diverse backgrounds. Communication is critical, even before the interaction. Nurses may have a general knowledge of individuals that should be used in creating positive approaches to care. However, nurses need to be aware that persons are individuals first and avoid categorizing them based solely on their ethnic and cultural backgrounds.

Preinteraction Checklist

What is known about this person?

How can this knowledge facilitate the interaction?

Can anything in the nurse's background influence the impending interaction?

What environmental factors can influence the interaction?

Admission Assessment

How does a person from a different ethnic background perceive health care providers from the mainstream culture?

What strategies can minimize communication barriers?

What techniques can facilitate the individual's acceptance of health care decisions?

What environmental resources can be used?

Working Phase Checklist

What culturally competent nursing care modalities would facilitate goal achievement?

What other resources can be used to augment nursing care approaches?

What are the individual's perceptions regarding illness, the institution, and health care providers?

Discharge Checklist

What resources in the individual's community would facilitate the achievement of the goals of the therapeutic regimen?

What are the individual's plans to maintain health and wellness?

group relationships that are maintained and nurtured by frequent interactions. The importance that individuals place on their families and other relatives as sources of formal and informal support during illness and crisis is a significant aspect of ethnic culture. Ethnicity provides the guidelines for the organization of individual and group life through established and integrated life patterns (Kolm, 1971). Specific roles and expectations regarding different life situations facilitate optimal functioning of individuals. For example, in certain ethnic groups, men and women assume different culturally designated roles to cope with the illness of a parent. Finally, ethnicity provides a basis for assessing the value systems of other groups (Banks & Gay, 1969). This function is operating when ethnics select a health care system that would best serve them; that is, their own **folk system** or the Western system. This concept is discussed more fully in the section entitled, "Health as a Value."

Culture, Values, and Value Orientations

Ethnicity is evidenced in customs that reflect the socialization and cultural patterns of the group. **Culture,** as an element of ethnicity, consists of shared patterns of values and behaviors that characterize a particular group (Marshall, 1990). Culture includes symbols, values, beliefs about the self and others, and perceptions of the external social world and historical and natural events. Values and behaviors that relate to basic areas of life are incorporated into cultural patterns that survive through the teaching-learning process, although innovations may be seen on occasion (Andrews, 1995) (Fig. 2-2). Cultural values determine what behaviors are desirable and how particular behaviors are interpreted and judged. As shared elements of a symbolic system, these values serve as criteria for what is desirable (Kluckhohn, 1953). Additionally, these cultural values determine a person's selection from available modes, means, and ends of action (Persell, 1990).

Value orientations, learned and shared through the socialization process, reflect the personality type of a particular society. The dominant value orientations are shared by the majority of the group. Kluckhohn's model (1953) of value orientations incorporates themes regarding basic human nature, the relationship of human beings to nature, human beings' time orientation, valued personality type, and relationships between human beings. Table 2-1 shows various solutions to the questions proposed by Kluckhohn.

HEALTH AS A VALUE

Leininger (1997) founded transcultural nursing 40 years ago as a "formal area of inquiry and practice to transform nursing and provide culturally congruent and responsible care to people of diverse cultures" (p. 341). Underlying this initiative is the belief that optimal health for all is an essential cultural value. Additionally, society generally believes that all people have a right to health care (Potter, 2001).

However, this value meets complex implementation issues because many barriers exist. For instance, health care for poor Americans and ethnic minorities is less than optimal because they are unable to pay for services (Boyle, 1997). Accessibility therefore has a limited definition for these individuals. Additionally, many barriers exist that hinder people from seeking preventive care. These barriers include difficulties traveling to a facility, long waiting periods in clinics, the unattractive and impersonal surroundings of health care facilities, and lack of understanding of the process of obtaining care by health

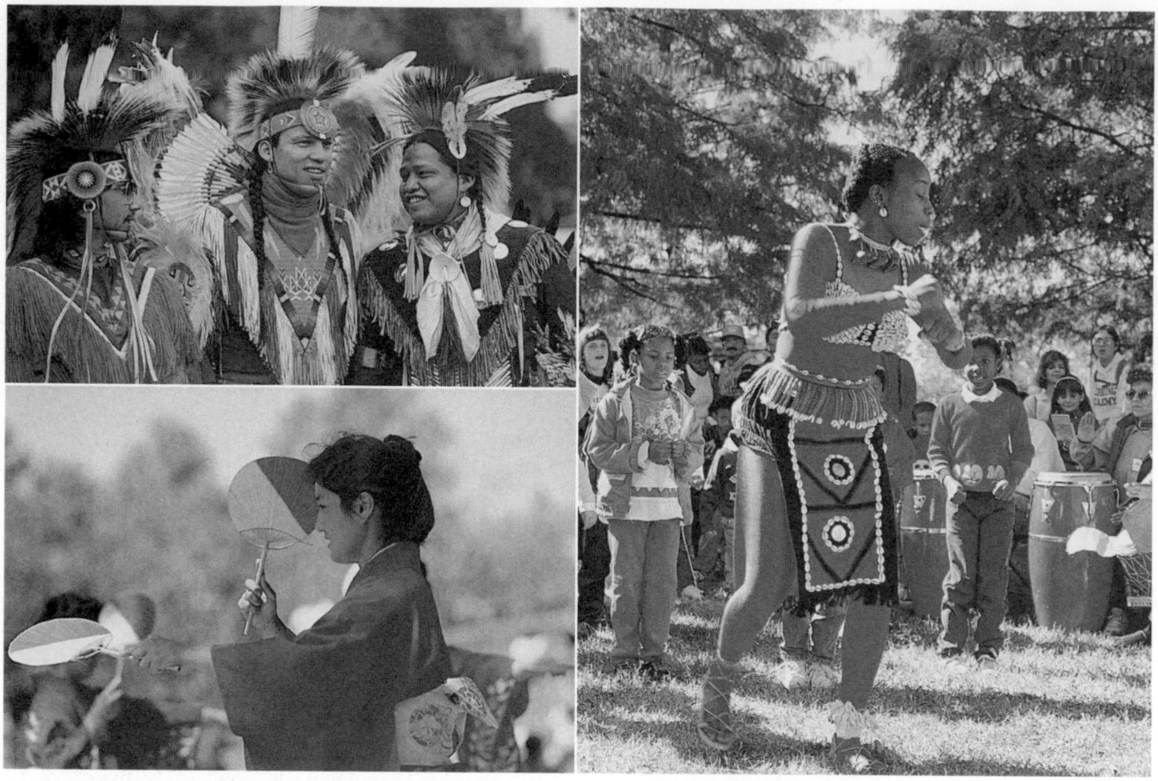

Fig. 2-2 Various cultural groups share and teach their customs.

Table 2-1 **Cultural Value Orientations**

Theme	Solution Types: A	B	C
What is man's innate human nature?	Evil: either unalterable or perfectible only with discipline and effort	Mixed: a combination of good and evil: lapses in behavior are unavoidable, but self-control is possible	Good: unalterable or corruptible
What is man's relationship to nature?	Destiny: man is subjugated to nature: fatalism, inevitability	Harmony: man and nature exist together as a single entity	Mastery: natural forces are to be overcome and put to man's use
What is man's significant time dimension?	Past: focus is on ancestors and traditions	Present: the time is "now"; little attention is paid to the past; future is considered vague or unpredictable	Future: orientation is toward progress and change; not content with present; past considered "old-fashioned"
What is the purpose of man's being?	Being (Dionysian): spontaneous expression of impulses and desires; nondevelopmental in focus	Being-in-becoming (Apollonian): self-contained and inner controlled; detachment that brings enlightenment; development and self-realization paramount	Doing (Promethean): active striving and accomplishment; competition against externally applied standards of achievement
What is man's relationship with his fellow men?	Lineal: continuity through time; heredity and kinship ties; ordered succession	Collateral: group goals primary focus; family orientation	Individual: personal autonomy and independence; authority not absolute; group goals submerged; individual goals dominate

From Kluckhohn, F. R. (1953). Dominant and variant value orientations. In C. Kluckhohn, H. A. Murray, D. A. Schneider (Eds.), *Personality in nature, society, and culture* (2nd ed.). New York: Alfred A. Knopf.

Table 2-2 A Comparison of Folk and Western Health Care Systems

Criteria	Folk	Western
Philosophy of care	"Carative"	Curative
Approach to care	Holistic, personalized	Fragmented specialization
Setting for services	Homes, community, and other social places	Often impersonal institutions
Treatments	Herbs, charms, amulets, massage, meditation	Technology; approved pharmacological agents
Providers of services	Healers, shamans, spiritualists, priests, other lay unlicensed therapists	Licensed professionals
Support for care	Family, relatives, friends	Other ancillary personnel and agencies
Payment for services	Negotiable	Third-party insurers; personal funds
Philosophy of health	Reflected as a quest for harmony with nature	Influenced by the professional's definition; dealt with in terms of illness and treatment
Definition of disease	Illness is an imbalance between the person and the physical, social, and spiritual worlds	The result of cause-effect physical phenomena; the cure is achieved by scientifically proven methods

care consumers (Boyle, 1997; Castillo & Torres, 1995). Fragmentation of care and ethnocentric and impersonal attitudes of some health care providers place individuals in uncomfortable situations when intimate personal information is sought from them. "Cultural diversity raises some very ethnocentric perspectives on people, ideas, action, time, authority, how we think and process information, and more" (Joel, 1998, p. 7). Health care insurance is not affordable for many poor Americans, whose priorities are the basic needs of health: food, clothing, and shelter rather than health care. For ethnic groups, health as a value may have different definitions and their behavior may reflect this. A discussion of the health beliefs and practices of selected ethnic groups later in this text will clarify this statement.

Incongruent beliefs and attitudes about health and health care services among ethnic groups versus the rest of the population, particularly health care providers, are major barriers in improving the health status of ethnic group members. Leininger (1990) believes that although professional nurses and other health care personnel tend to support the cultural value of optimal health, the inconsistency of these values compared with the values of individuals from different cultural groups may serve as a strong barrier. Therefore it is imperative that a closer scrutiny of cultural groups' indigenous health care systems be considered. This closer look may give health care professionals an understanding of the ways in which these health care approaches can coexist with the dominant Western view, providing optimal benefits to individuals.

FOLK AND WESTERN HEALTH CARE

Western scientific principles and values have guided modern health policies and practices in the United States (Adams & Knox, 1988). Therefore differences in the perceptions, orientations, and values of ethnic groups regarding health and illness can create potential difficulties in health care situations.

The practice of **Western health care** is viewed as professional care (Andrews, 1995). Professional care emphasizes approaches that are based on data from the scientifically proven method of research. Methods that do not meet these criteria are negated. Professional care is provided by a group of people who claim to have the authority, knowledge, and skills to determine the experience and needs of others (Starr, 1990). Conversely, a folk system embodies the beliefs, values, and treatment approaches of a particular cultural group that are products of cultural development. Folk health practices are seen in a variety of settings, including community groups, kinship groups, private homes, and healers' shrines. Folk healers range from priests and medicine men and women to fortunetellers, astrologers, and geomancers. Unlicensed practitioners such as lay midwives, bone setters, some dentists, and herbalists are part of the folk sector, as are religious practitioners such as spiritualists, Christian Scientists, and scientologists (Andrews, 1995). Other areas of differences between folk and Western health care systems are summarized in Table 2-2.

The choice of health care system varies among ethnic groups and among individuals within the same group. Lipson, Dibble, and Minarik (1996) provide comprehensive information on the folk healing practices of 24 ethnic groups in the United States. Often, there is a combined use of the services and resources from each system, in different degrees and at different times. One or more situational factors, including access, perceived degree of severity of the illness and its symptoms, previous experiences with each system, and ability to pay for the services and treatments, may influence which system is approached.

Ethnic individuals' preference for their folk healing systems is motivated by their familiarity with the folk healer, who usually speaks the same language and is knowledgeable of the beliefs, customs, and traditions of the ethnic group. Easy access and the individual's ability to pay for the healer's services are real advantages when compared with the difficulty of getting appointments, the long waits, and the unfamiliar institutional settings in the Western system.

When folk healing practices are not effective, the individual may turn to Western health care. Through a culturally sensitive assessment process, nurses can determine what specific folk remedies individuals are using and whether their continued use would interfere with the prescribed medical regimen. Andrews (1995) and Herberg (1995) have developed assessment tools that nurses and other health care providers can use when working with ethnically diverse individuals. Additionally, Geissler (1991) has suggested a taxonomy of nursing diagnoses for culturally diverse persons.

Health care professionals must avoid an ethnocentric perspective when working with ethnic groups. An **ethnocentric perspective,** which views other ways as inferior, unnatural, or even barbaric, can serve as a major obstacle in establishing and maintaining good working relationships with consumers of health care services.

Ethnic groups will continue to use folk remedies and healing. Therefore health care professionals need to take a look at the many positive aspects of folk systems. A **holistic approach**—incorporating family and support systems, consideration of the individual's viewpoint, and caring—is one of the more positive aspects of folk systems that Western health care systems are beginning to recognize. A blend of both systems would optimize health care for ethnic Americans.

Box 2-1 Asian Americans–Pacific Islanders

1998 U.S. population: 10,312,000 (3.3%)
Education (25 years or older):
  High school: 84.9%
  College or higher: 42.1%
Marital status: 81.7% married
Labor force participation (16 years or older): 68.5%
Median household income: $51,850
Poverty level:
  Family: 10.2%
  Individual: 14.0%

From U.S. Census Bureau. (1999). *Statistical abstract of the U.S.* (119th ed.). Washington, DC: Government Printing Office.

ASIAN AMERICANS–PACIFIC ISLANDERS

Asian Americans–Pacific Islanders (AAPIs) comprised 3.3% of the total population of the United States in 1998. In 1996, a total of 128,565 AAPIs entered the United States (U.S. Census Bureau, 1999). It is projected that by 2050, this figure will be 10.1% (Gall & Natividad, 1995). AAPIs include persons from China, Mongolia, Pakistan, Sri Lanka, Maldives, India, Nepal, Bhutan, Bangladesh, Burma, Laos, Thailand, Vietnam, Cambodia, North Korea, South Korea, Japan, Hong Kong, Macao, Taiwan, Philippines, Malaysia, and Polynesia (Kuramoto, 1995). A look at the status of AAPIs reveals that they are doing relatively well in their new home in the United States (Box 2-1).

The importance of education from their perspective is evident in both secondary and higher education. For instance, the 8% dropout rate of AAPIs from 10th grade was the lowest of the ethnic groups (U.S. Department of Education, 1992). A greater percentage earned bachelor's and master's degrees in 1996 compared with Hispanics and Native Americans (Table 2-3). Additionally, AAPIs surpassed all ethnic groups in the number of earned doctoral degrees (U.S. Census Bureau, 1999). Of the ethnic groups discussed in this chapter, AAPIs have the highest percentage of representation in dentistry, medicine, and pharmacology (Prism, 1993).

Prevalent Health Problems of Asian Americans–Pacific Islanders

Variations in the health status of AAPIs are a result primarily of subcultures within the larger group. AAPIs have similar health problems as the White population. Cardiovascular problems are common and they have a high incidence of cerebrovascular accidents. Hypertension is usually the accompanying chronic problem resulting from a high salt intake (Enas, 1996). Cancers are also leading health problems for both women and men. Breast, colorectal, and lung cancers are the leading causes of death (U.S. Department of Health and Human Services, 2000). Liver cancers have a high incidence among foreign-born

Table 2-3 Comparison Among Whites and Ethnic Groups by Higher Education Degrees Conferred

	White	Black	Hispanic	Asian American–Pacific Islander	Native American and Alaskan Native
Total Number in 1998 U.S. Population	270,900,000	34,431,000	29,707,000	10,507,000	2,360,000
Associate's Degree	425,028	51,672	38,163	23,091	5,556
Bachelor's Degree	904,709	91,166	58,288	64,359	6,970
Master's Degree	297,558	25,801	14,412	18,161	6,970
Doctor's Degree	27,756	1,636	999	2,646	158

From: U.S. Census Bureau. (1999). *Statistical abstract of the U.S.* (119th ed.). Washington, DC: Government Printing Office.

Asians with a history of hepatitis B infection. Chinese Americans show a high incidence of nasopharyngeal cancer, whereas Filipino Americans have problems with oral cavity and pharyngeal cancers.

The prevalence of hepatitis B infection among AAPIs ranges from 5% to 15%. Tong (1996) estimates the total number of AAPIs who are infected or who have been exposed among Chinese and Southeast Asians to be approximately 80% and 60% among Koreans. AAPIs have the highest rates of tuberculosis (TB) per 100,000. It is proposed that shame, denial, and anger are barriers to seeking treatment (Choi, 1996). Cultural factors such as language barriers, access, and stigma are major factors that hinder prevention and treatment.

The stress of immigration, acculturation, and adjustment to a new culture may be the predominant factors that affect the mental health and well being of Asians in the United States. Kim (1995) looked at **acculturation stress** (psychological problems experienced by ethnic groups, including language barriers, culture shock, lack of social support, and discrepancies between expectations and achievements following immigration) and cultural influences on depression among Korean Americans. The findings are extremely useful for health care providers.

Selected Health-Related Cultural Aspects

AAPIs share many traditional values. Lipson, Dibble, and Minarik (1996) provide a comprehensive coverage of traditional values in several Asian groups. A list of some of the most important values can be found in Box 2-2.

AAPIs try to inculcate values in their children. Children and their well being are the main concerns of mothers. Children become more cherished when mothers lose their spouses and they look to children as their main resource (Valencia-Go, 1999). However, many people find the task of parenthood in a new country difficult because some of their cultural values conflict with the mainstream cultural values; for example, passivity to avoid conflict versus assertiveness.

Exposure of children to different cultures in schools and in their neighborhood facilitates their adoption of other cultural beliefs and attitudes in their socialization. Additionally, the employment of immigrant women outside the home has exposed their children to other caretakers. The likelihood of the absence of grandparents, who are important transmitters of culture, has contributed to the identification of children with the dominant host culture (Valencia-Go, 1989).

Asian folk medicine and philosophies have a strong Chinese influence as a result of early Chinese migration throughout Asia. Therefore the folk medicines of Filipinos, Japanese, Koreans, and Southeast Asians are all imbued with Chinese principles.

Taoism was the philosophical and theoretical foundation of Chinese medicine. According to **Tao doctrine,** humans are microcosms within the universe. Achieving harmony between the two is essential because the energies of both intertwine. Two forces, Yin and Yang, keep innate energy, called Chi, and sexual energy, called Jing, in balance. Yin is feminine, negative, dark, and cold; Yang is masculine, positive, light, and warm. An imbalance in energy can be caused, for instance, by yielding to strong emotions or eating an improper diet. In their interactions, humans and the universe are both susceptible to the elements of earth, fire, water, metal, and wood (Andrews, 1995).

Asian folk medicine uses a wide variety of herbs for healing purposes: roots, leaves, seeds, tree bark, and parts of flowers. In Chinatown, New York City, there are several drugstores that sell these varieties of folk remedies.

Some aspects of Asian folk medicine have gained popularity within the Western system of health care. Of these, the best known is acupuncture. The acceptance of this treatment, as an adjunct rather than a replacement for Western treatments, may pave the way for the use of other folk remedies. Similar alternative treatment modalities that are slowly gaining wide acceptance are meditation, therapeutic touch, massage, imagery, relaxation, and bipolarity. A recent editorial identified health care consumers' frustrations with conventional medicine as the main reason for the increased popularity of alternative therapies (USA Today, 1996). The College of New Rochelle in New York is the first graduate program that prepares nurses as clinical specialists in holistic nursing. Graduates of this program gain knowledge and skills in a number of alternative, complementary healing modalities (see Chapter 14).

Box 2-2 Selected Cultural Values of Asian Americans–Pacific Islanders

1. The family is extended, with grandparents, uncles, aunts, and cousins as part of the household.
2. Within the family, there is differential treatment based on age and gender. The oldest adult male is usually considered the head of the family.
3. The family's interests and honor supersede those of the individual; therefore every member strives to avoid situations that may bring shame on the family.
4. Older individuals are respected and their authority is unquestioned. Filial piety ensures loyalty and devotion from children.
5. The maintenance of harmony is a priority; therefore there is a strong emphasis on the avoidance of conflict and direct confrontation.
6. Strong values conflict with the mainstream cultural values; for example, passivity to avoid conflict versus assertiveness.
7. Emphasis on respect for authority figures is strong; therefore disagreements are avoided.

HISPANIC AMERICANS

The Hispanic American population in the United States numbered 30,773,000 or 11.1% of the total population of

Box 2-3 Hispanic Americans

1998 U.S. population: 30,773,000 (11.1%)
Education (25 years or older):
- High school: 55.5%
- College or higher: 11.0%

Marital status: 69% married
Labor force participation (16 years or older): 63.1%
Median household income: $28,141
Poverty level:
- Family: 24.7%
- Individual: 27.1%

From U.S. Census Bureau. (1999). *Statistical abstract of the U.S.* (119th ed.). Washington, DC: Government Printing Office.

the United States in 1998 (U.S. Census Bureau, 1999). Hispanic Americans make up the second largest ethnic group in the United States (Box 2-3). The largest Hispanic American subgroups are Cubans, Mexicans, and Puerto Ricans. An estimate of the Hispanic American population in the United States, Alaska, and Hawaii in 1997 was 29.7 million (Hayat, Lucas, & Kington, 2000). Most of the Puerto Ricans (64%) reside in the northeast, most of the Cubans (68%) live in the southern region of the nation, and 57% of the Mexicans live in the west and 35% of the Mexicans live in the south. Overall, Hispanic Americans tend to be urban dwellers.

Hispanic Americans are making educational strides. For example, enrollment rates for children 3 to 4 years of age increased from 47.4% in 1990 to 50.8% in 1997 (U.S. Census Bureau, 1999). They had the same percentage of representation in nursing as Asian Americans. However, in medicine and pharmacology, they were slightly ahead of Native Americans. In dentistry, Hispanic Americans had the second highest percentage representation among the four ethnic groups discussed in this chapter (Prism, 1993). (See Case Study and Care Plan.)

Language often acts as a barrier, as demonstrated by the fact that 50% of dropouts are not fluent in English. This lack of language skill also compromises people's resources, including the ability to find suitable employment (Torres, 1994). The poverty level in 1990 for Hispanic families was 22.3%. This level is not statistically different from the 1980 level (Castillo & Torres, 1995). The most recent poverty levels are 24.7% for the household and 27.1% for the individual (U.S. Census Bureau, 1999).

Prevalent Health Problems of Hispanic Americans

Although cardiovascular disease and cancer are the first and second causes of **morbidity** and mortality among Hispanic Americans, their incidence in the general population is higher. However, they have higher rates of diabetes, alcohol-related problems, and homicide. Among adults 25 to 44 years of age in the Hispanic American population, HIV infection was ranked as the leading cause of death (Suarez & Seifert, 1998; U.S. Department of Health and Human Services, 1996). Among Hispanic American subgroups, socioeconomic status (SES) has been linked to health status. Cubans have a higher percentage (35%) of persons whose families earn $35,000 or more. Additionally, fewer families live below the poverty level. Overall, Puerto Ricans and Mexicans have the lowest incomes and have higher rates of living below the poverty level. Cubans report better health status compared with the other two subgroups. Health care contact and restricted activity days were lowest for Cubans (Hayat, Lucans, & Kington, 2000).

Hispanic Americans receive less preventive health care. This fact can be attributed to employment in occupations that do not provide health insurance (Castillo & Torres, 1995). In 1997, death during the perinatal period for Hispanic infants was 6.5%. Maternal death was 8 per 100,000 (*Healthy People 2010, 2000*). The infant mortality rate is similar to the rate of nonHispanic Whites (Castillo & Torres, 1995). The difficulties experienced by Hispanic Americans in receiving appropriate health care services are identical to those of the poor. Additionally, many Hispanic Americans may not readily seek care because they have continued reliance on their folk system of healing and their difficulties negotiating the health care system because language barriers exist (Cornelius & Altman, 1995; Davis, R. 1996).

Selected Health-Related Cultural Aspects

Each subgroup of the Hispanic American population has distinct cultural beliefs and customs. However, a common heritage determines similar values and beliefs. For instance, the emphasis on family and religion are the two most important aspects of all Hispanic cultures. For older Hispanic Americans, the family is an important component of good health (Ailinger & Causey, 1995). The family is the most important source of support; therefore the needs of the family as a whole supersede the needs of the individual. During times of illness and crisis, the family is there for the individual. Older family members and other relatives are accorded courtesy and respect and are often consulted on important matters (de Paula, Lagana, & Gonzalez-Ramirez, 1996; Juarbe, 1996).

Hispanic Americans' dependence on spiritual strength to aid them in illness and dying is evident in their use of prayer. (See Research Highlights.) They put their trust in God and believe that harmony with God is essential in maintaining health. Furthermore, an offense against God warrants punishment (Queralt, 1996). Hispanic Americans attribute the origins of disease and illness to spiritual or natural punishments, hot and cold imbalances, magic, dislocation of internal organs, natural diseases, and emotional and mental issues (de Paula, Lagana, & Gonzalez-Ramirez, 1996; Juarbe, 1996). The hot and cold concept of disease was derived from the **hippocratic theory**

research highlights

Chronic Illness in Hispanic American Families

The researchers explored Hispanic American family experiences with chronic childhood illness. The purpose of the study was to understand the family's perceptions of the consequences of their faith and its meaning in the face of chronic childhood illness. In this descriptive qualitative study, 25 parents from 19 families provided data about their experience of living with children with a variety of chronic conditions that included genetic syndromes, congenital heart disease, cancer, and sequelae of prematurity.

In their review of the literature, the researchers found that people from Hispanic cultures view and use religion as a source of solace and hope. The researchers cited numerous studies that supported Hispanics' religious beliefs as facilitators, not barriers to seeking health care.

Qualitative data revealed that parents were expressive about their faith and they described how their religion helped them cope with their child's illness. Six dimensions of the experience of chronic childhood illness indicate that faith was considered as a way of life and means to seek beneficial changes for their child's health.

Data from Rehm, R. S. (1999). Religious faith in Mexican-American families dealing with chronic childhood illness. *Image–the Journal of Nursing Scholarship, 31* (1), 33-38.

of pathology. Illness occurs when there is an imbalance. This concept of hot and cold guides Hispanics when they categorize illnesses and select appropriate treatments. For example, rheumatic fever is considered a cold illness. Therefore through the process of neutralization, a hot treatment would correct the imbalance. In this instance, penicillin, considered a hot substance, would be an acceptable treatment (de Paula, Lagana, & Gonzalez-Ramirez, 1996).

Hispanic Americans still resort to many home remedies and consult a folk healer, the curandero. Curanderos use a variety of folk remedies, including prayers, rituals, herbs, and the laying on of hands (Herberg, 1995). Other Hispanic Americans such as Cubans practice Santeria. **Santeria** is viewed as a link to the past and is used to cope with problems. The santero may be consulted or called to assist in balancing or neutralizing various aspects of an illness (Grossman, 1998). Folk remedies are used in combination with Western approaches as long as Western methods do not harm the individual. The individual's belief in the folk remedy can have positive effects on the person's well being. Therefore Western health care professionals need to find ways to blend the two systems to the optimal benefit of Hispanic American individuals and families.

BLACK AMERICANS

In 1998, there were 32,528,000 Black Americans (11.85% of the total population) (U.S. Census Bureau, 1999). The

Box 2-4 Black Americans

1998 U.S. population: 32,528,000 (11.85%)
Education (25 years or older):
High school: 76.0%
College or higher: 14.7%
Marital Status: 47% married couples
Labor force participation (16 years or older): 59.7%
Median household income: $28,602
Poverty level:
Family: 23.6%
Individual: 26.5%

From U.S. Census Bureau. (1999). *Statistical abstract of the U.S.* (119th ed.). Washington, DC: Government Printing Office.

identification of Black Americans as a minority group can be traced to their history of slavery, extreme segregation and exclusion from mainstream society, and discrimination by the majority group.

The immigration history of Blacks to America is significantly different from that of Europeans, Asians, and Hispanics. The beginning of Black America is recorded as the time when Blacks were crew members on a pirate ship that docked in America in 1619 (Bennett, 1992). In their study of Black migration, Johnson and Campbell (1981) noted that although Blacks had participated in many types of migration, the predominant type was forced or impelled, imposed by explorers of the New World from Spain and Portugal. In the New World, many thriving industries had high demands for labor that the Native Americans could not fill; therefore Africans were captured and sold as slaves. In the history of Black slavery, an estimated 6 million Africans were brought to America and enslaved (Bennett, 1992). The saga of centuries of injustice began. This period was only a small part of history, but it was one that had a lasting effect on the current status of Black Americans (Box 2-4).

Educationally, Black Americans have made substantial gains. More Blacks earned high school diplomas compared with Hispanics and Native Americans. Nevertheless, Black Americans still lag behind Whites in all levels of education, as seen earlier in Table 2-3 (U.S. Census Bureau, 1999).

Black American families have a poverty level of 23.6% for the family and 26.5% for the individual, compared with 10% for the family and 11% for the individual in the White population. The median earnings of Black Americans in 1998 was $28,602, compared with $46,754 for Whites (U.S. Census Bureau, 1999). The strong relationship between SES and health points to a bleak profile for Black American health problems.

Prevalent Health Problems of Black Americans

A complex set of social, economic, and environmental factors can be identified as contributors to the current health status of Black Americans. However, poverty may be the most profound and pervasive determinant of health status (Douglas, 1995). In the United States, health care is a commodity that can be purchased according to an individual's ability to pay (Griffin, 1994) and health care is expensive. Individuals and families who are below the poverty level or lack adequate resources are obviously the most affected.

Poor people cannot afford health insurance, which limits their access to health care services such as prenatal and maternal care, childhood immunizations, dental checkups, well-child care, and a wide range of other preventive services. Decreased resources for preventive care may necessitate more expensive services, such as emergency room care and intensive care in times of severe illness.

Two indices of the effects of poverty can be seen in the high rates of infant mortality and maternal mortality. Despite changes in living conditions, advances in infection control, and improved standards in neonatal care, Blacks still experience high infant and maternal mortality rates. In 1997, approximately 12.7% of Black infants died within the first year of life compared with 6.4% for White infants. In 1999, the infant mortality rate for African Americans was 20.3 per 100,000 live births, nearly four times the rate for Whites of 5.1 per 100,000 births (U.S. Department of Health and Human Services, 2000). Life expectancy for Blacks is 70.2 years compared with 76.8 years for Whites (Begun, Klier, & Quiran, 1999).

Black American children living below the poverty level experience numerous health problems, including malnutrition, anemia, and lead poisoning. These problems and the lack of immunizations combine to inhibit normal growth and development and affect school performance.

Poverty-stricken families usually live in depressed socioeconomic areas where housing conditions are unsafe and unhygienic. Unsafe buildings and other environmental structures cause accidents and injuries among young children. Young children have fallen to their deaths from windows that were unprotected by metal railings. Older people have suffered falls and other injuries from poorly lit stairways and hallways. Other hazards include uncollected garbage and abandoned buildings that are used as dumpsites or as meeting places for a variety of illegal activities.

In 1993, the rate of acute conditions per 100 of the population was 23.4% for Blacks and 25.0% for Whites. However, health care dollars spent for Blacks was $894 and $1890 for Whites. Vaccination of children 19 to 35 months of age for Blacks was 48.9% and 62.2% for Whites (Smith & Horton, 1995). High hospital admission rates and stays for all Blacks are attributed largely to adolescent pregnancies and other reproductive conditions. Homicide, motor vehicle accidents, and suicide are also high among adolescent Blacks. The most recent data indicate that HIV infection is the leading cause of death in Black men and women aged 25 to 44 (U.S. Department of Health and Human Services, 1996a).

The Black American population has approximately the same death rates from cardiovascular disease and cancer as the general population (Keller, Fleury, & Bergstrom, 1995). However, Black American men have a 25% higher risk for all cancers and a 45% higher incidence of lung cancer. A higher rate of death for Black Americans occurs after a diagnosis of cancer. Diabetes is 33% more prevalent. Severe high blood pressure is more common for Black Americans in both men and women. In 1997, there were 74 cases of severe high blood pressure per 1000 Black Americans compared with 36 cases among Whites (U.S. Census Bureau, 1999).

It is expected that health issues of Black Americans will receive more attention in the future. Currently, a number of excellent works address health issues and problems. For example, Black American health educators have published a milestone resource, *African-American Voices: African-American Health Educators Speak Out*, which examines major health problems that afflict the Black population (Johnson, R., 1995). The perception and use of health services by Black Americans and their ways of coping with major health problems have been studied by several researchers (Degazon, 1995; Felton & Parsons, 1997). HIV or AIDS experienced by many Black Americans is now slowly being addressed. Researchers such as Jemmott have devoted their professional life to the study of issues in the prevention of AIDS (O'Leary & Jemmott, 1995).

Selected Health-Related Cultural Aspects

Differences in cultural beliefs, attitudes, and practices exist between rural and urban Black Americans; however, they share some basic cultural beliefs. Black American culture is centered on the family and religion. The family, the strongest institution for them, provides strong **extended kinship** bonds with grandparents, aunts, uncles, and cousins. The family is considered the strongest source of support, especially in times of crisis and illness. In a study of elderly Black Americans, the researcher found that the majority discussed their chronic illnesses and problems and managing these with family rather than formal care providers (Jennings, 1999).

Religion and religious behavior are an integral part of the Black American community (Campinha-Bacote, 1998). The church is the second most important institution for Black Americans. Blackwell (1991) identified several important functions of the contemporary Black church, including the following:

1. Provides a cohesive institutional structure within the Black American community
2. Serves as an instrument for the development of leaders
3. Facilitates citizenship training and community social action
4. Performs social and educative roles
5. Acts as a charitable institution

6. Assists in the development of business structures in ventures
7. Serves as an index of social class

Black Americans perceive their church as a place for the inculcation of values and as a refuge from the stresses of daily living (Queralt, 1996). Powell, Gelfand, Parzuchowski, Heilburn, and Franklin (1995) demonstrate that Black American churches are effective avenues for recruiting men into prostate cancer screening. Similarly, a cancer screening program that used church-related resources was well received by a Black American community in South Carolina (Weinrich, S., Holdford, Boyd, Creanga, Cover, Johnson, Frank-Stromberg, & Weinrich, M., 1998).

Black Americans define health as a feeling of well being and the ability to fulfill role expectations. Spiritual balance is a major component. Black Americans continue to use their own traditional health system, especially when they lack access to the Western health care system (Andrews, 1995; Locks & Boateng, 1996). Traditionally, roots, herbs, potions, oils, powders, rituals, and ceremonies are still used in many Southern communities. The use of healers is also common, including the elder, who is knowledgeable about herbs; the spiritualist, who focuses on psychological problems; and the voodoo priest, who is considered to be powerful and can cause desired events (Queralt, 1996).

As noted with the folk health practices of Asian and Hispanic Americans, Black Americans' folk healing beliefs and practices can augment the Western system. Black Americans often find comfort in the support that their religious leader or traditional healer can give them. Health care providers must find an appropriate place for these nontraditional modalities when caring for Black Americans.

NATIVE AMERICANS

Native Americans lived in America for thousands of years before Christopher Columbus arrived (Nabokov, 1991). Nonnative chroniclers of Native-American history believe that these people came to Alaska via land bridges now known as the Bering Strait (Driver, 1964; Embree, 1973; Taylor, 1991), although Native Americans themselves say they have always been here. Native Americans came to be known as Indians, a label given by Columbus when he encountered the native peoples in the West Indies, which he mistook for the East Indies. This label was then extended to all the native peoples of North and South America, from the Arctic to Tierra del Fuego (American Immigration, 1999).

Before 1492 there were an estimated 5 million Native Americans. Columbus' discovery brought colonization and settlement by various European groups, who numbered 75 million by 1890. The ancestral lands of the Native Americans were usurped, and the people were forced to labor on farms and in mines. Thousands died from disease and hard labor or were killed in attempts to escape from slavery (Embree, 1973). Other events, such as the removal of the Southeastern tribes in 1830, the Navajos' Long March to Fort Sumner in 1864, and the massacre at Wounded Knee in 1890 caused the Native American population to dwindle to 250,000 by 1890 (Taylor, 1991). The 1890 census, the first to obtain a complete count of Native Americans, reported an increase from 237,000 in 1900 to 357,000 in 1950. The period from 1950 to 1980 was a time of rapid growth. The Native American population grew to nearly 1.4 million (U.S. Department of Commerce, 1989). Currently, Native Americans are concentrated in Oklahoma, California, Arizona, New Mexico, Alaska, Washington, North Carolina, Texas, New York, and Michigan. Of the total Native American population of almost 2 million, 62.3% live off reservations and 37.7% live on Native American lands. There are 314 reservations and 542 tribes, most of which have fewer than 1000 members. The Cherokees make up the largest tribe (U.S. Census Bureau, 1999) (Box 2-5).

Native Americans, the smallest of the ethnic groups discussed in this chapter, also experience minority group status. In important aspects of life, such as educational attainment and income levels, Native Americans lag behind Whites and major ethnic groups. For example, the percentage of Native Americans in the eighth grade who performed below basic levels of knowledge and skills in mathematics was the highest and the percentage of the same group able to do advanced mathematics was the lowest, compared with Whites, AAPIs, Black Americans, and Hispanic Americans. In 1989, the dropout rate for tenth graders was 36%, which is the highest rate compared with Whites, AAPIs, Black Americans, and Hispanic Americans (U.S. Department of Education, 1991). Native American percentages for higher education degrees are low in proportion to their total number. For example, in 1996 there were only 158 Native Americans who earned doctoral degrees. Native Americans had the lowest percentage representation in nursing, medicine, dentistry, and pharmacology (Prism, 1993). For more information on other higher education degrees, see Table 2-3.

Income levels for Native Americans in 1998 were low, with a median household income of $21,619, the lowest of all ethnic groups discussed. The poverty level for the family

Box 2-5 Native Americans

1998 U.S. population: 2,236,000 (0.7%)
Education (25 years or older):
- High school: 65.6%
- College: 9.4%

Marital status: 65.8% married couples
Labor force participation (16 years or older): 62.1%
Median household income: $21,619
Poverty level:
- Family: 27.2%
- Individual: 31.2%

From U.S. Census Bureau. (1999). *Statistical abstract of the U.S.* (119th ed.). Washington, DC: Government Printing Office.

was 27.2% and 31.2% for the individual (U.S. Census Bureau, 1999). Reported unemployment rates are high and often understated because many Native Americans have given up looking for jobs (Davis, 1996).

Low educational attainment and income levels combined with higher rates of poverty are socioeconomic issues that affect health and the quality of life. Native Americans experience the many negative situations that confront poor people both on the reservations and in the larger society.

Prevalent Health Problems of Native Americans

Many of the health problems of Native Americans can be linked directly to the social and economic conditions described here. These conditions predispose Native Americans to illnesses and health problems that afflict the poor. Some of these problems have been discussed in the section on Black Americans.

Many of the Native American deaths can be attributed to unintentional injuries, cirrhosis, homicide, suicide, pneumonia, and complications of diabetes. Among Native American men under the age of 44, unintentional injuries account for 20% of all deaths each year. Cirrhosis is another chronic problem that afflicts Native Americans more frequently than other groups. Alcohol use affects close to 95% of all Native American families (Davis, M.B., 1996). In 1997, Native Americans had the highest percentage of smoking compared with all groups of people in the United States. There is also a high incidence of noninsulin-dependent diabetes (U.S. Department of Health and Human Services, 2000).

Many mental health problems confront Native Americans. Difficult life situations and stresses of daily life contribute to an array of problems, including feelings of hopelessness, desperation, family dissolution, and substance abuse, specifically alcohol (Davis, M.B., 1996).

The health problems of Native Americans are complicated by difficult access to health care. Persons who live on reservations and are served by the Indian Health Service may find that this federally funded agency does not provide the services they need. Persons who live in rural areas are underserved, with inadequate facilities and a lack of qualified personnel. Among professional-degree graduates in 1989 and 1990, only 52 Native Americans earned the Doctor of Medicine degree compared with 12,127 Whites, 887 Blacks, 554 Hispanics, and 1351 AAPIs (U.S. Department of Education, 1992). Latest data have not specified the type of doctoral degree earned by the 158 graduates in 1998 (U.S. Census Bureau, 1999).

Selected Health-Related Cultural Aspects

Native Americans are generally present-oriented; therefore they emphasize events that are occurring now rather than events that will happen later. They value cooperation rather than competition. Sharing of resources—even among the poor—is an important component of this cultural value (Kramer, 1996). Native Americans place great importance on their families and relatives (Berkram, 1999). Three or more generations form an extended kinship system, which is enlarged by the membership of nonrelatives who are included through various religious ceremonies (Kramer, 1996).

Despite the great diversity among Native American groups in their beliefs and practices concerning health, illness, and healing, they share a common philosophical base. Native Americans believe that a state of health exists when a person lives in total harmony with nature. The earth is seen as a living entity that should be treated with respect; failure to do so harms the body (Blais, 1991). Illness is viewed not as an alteration in a person's physiological state, but rather as an imbalance between the ill person and natural or supernatural forces (Queralt, 1996).

Medicine Grizzlybear Lake (1991), a renowned Native American healer, believes that a person's sickness can be traced directly to having committed a violation against natural and spiritual laws; an individual can also inherit such a violation. The violation causes the person to get out of balance and imbalance causes illness mentally, physically, emotionally, and spiritually. Rituals and healing ceremonies that are believed to restore balance when illness occurs may be carried out by the medicine man or

HOT topics

NEW EYE ON RESEARCH

Undergraduate nursing students in their first research course are often impressed with the initial studies they are taught to critique. When limitations of the study are discussed, students raise the issue of "generalizability."

Recently, the U.S. Census Bureau finally recognized the diversity among people of Hispanic origins. This recognition represents a major breakthrough in survey methodology. Students viewed past U.S. Census Bureau data with a critical eye and questioned the appropriateness of espoused effective nursing interventions with Hispanic individuals. Nurses now have a great deal to consider to revise their perspectives about this ethnic group with its identified subgroups.

Another major breakthrough is the revision of the gender and minority inclusion policy to meet the requirements of the National Institutes of Health (NIH) Revitalization Act of 1993 (public law 103-43). "This law requires recruitment of women and minorities and their subpopulations in all clinical research studies, especially clinical trials" (Harden & McFarland, 2000, p. 83). This revision can only be positive for nursing and health care. Now, practitioners can expect that future research data will have validity for women and minority persons.

woman, who is believed to have hypnotic powers, the gift of mind-reading, and expertise in concocting drugs, medicine, and poisons (Daugherty, 1992). The medicine man or woman, known as the **shaman,** is called to induce a cure. The shaman is usually a powerful individual in the tribe. Although the power and reverence given to shamans may vary among different tribes, they are treated with respect for their role in inculcating religious beliefs and promoting spirituality, good health, and good living for the people (Daugherly, 1992). Acknowledgment of ethnic minorities is slowly increasing, which is evident in research protocols (see Hot Topics box). A more accurate knowledge base about these different groups would only be positive for the nation.

AGING MINORITIES

In 1997, there were 34.1 million people 65 years of age or older, indicating that one in every eight Americans is a senior citizen today, compared with 1 in 25 at the dawn of the twentieth century. The elderly population is expected to double by 2030. In 1997, 15% of the older adults in the United States were minorities; of these, 8% were Black. Projections are that by 2025, elderly minorities will be 24% of the total U.S. elderly population (U.S. Department of Housing and Urban Development, 1999). Elderly minorities are among the poorest persons in the United States. Blacks, Hispanics, and Native Americans have double-digit poverty levels (U.S. Census Bureau, 1999).

CASE STUDY

Mrs. Cruzada

Mrs. Cruzada is a widowed woman from the Philippines. She lost her husband early in their marriage, leaving her with six small children to raise. Her husband served in the U.S. Army in World War II. She was the beneficiary of his pension, paid in U.S. dollars and sent to her in the Philippines. She supplemented this pension with a small business enterprise. She was successful in providing a college education for her children. One of her daughters emigrated to the United States in the 1960s, and when this daughter became a citizen, she petitioned her mother as a resident. This process activated the immigration of all Mrs. Cruzada's children.

Here in the United States, Mrs. Cruzada lives with a married daughter, her husband, and another unmarried son in a house in Queens, New York. Her pension as a widowed soldier's spouse continues and her children provide for some of her financial needs. She is not able to seek employment outside the home because she is unable to speak English. She is visited frequently by her grandchildren, but she feels that they are more American than Filipino in their ways. She still enjoys physical independence and Filipino social activities. As she advances in age, she is concerned about her later years when she can no longer care for herself. She is afraid of living the rest of her life in a nursing home.

- Describe culturally appropriate social activities for her to maintain her ethnic identity.
- Discuss strategies for a healthy lifestyle.
- Explain approaches for close integration with the younger generation.
- Identify community resources that provide support for older members of ethnic groups.

CARE PLAN

Mrs. Cruzada

Mrs. Cruzada is in excellent physical health, but there are potential difficulties in her adjustment to family life here in the United States. Her ability to cope and manage life here could be enhanced by her continued involvement with her family and the community. A few strategies can be implemented to achieve this goal.

- Involve her in a senior citizen center that emphasizes social and health-related activities.
- Engage her as an active member of church groups, such as the Altar Society, or other volunteer groups that work with persons with special needs.
- Secure some part-time employment for her, such as a lunchroom helper at the church school.
- Help create a senior citizen group within the local Filipino association in which she and other older Filipinos could network.
- Provide information on many resources for older people, such as Meals on Wheels, day care, assisted living, and group homes, as alternatives to a nursing home.
- Educate her on the importance of health-promotion activities, such as regular exams, regular exercise, a well-balanced diet, and a positive mental outlook.
- Encourage the Filipino association to conduct activities, such as an annual cultural event, that would bring persons of all ages together.
- Assist her in developing a network of friends who could provide her with socializing when her family is not available.
- Work with her children and grandchildren to help them gain a better understanding of older immigrants such as Mrs. Cruzada.

Health Issues of Aging Minorities

It is difficult to discuss the health issues of aging minorities in depth because there is immense diversity. Not only are these elderly minorities confronting cultural issues relevant to the ethnic group, but they are also facing the issues that are universal to elderly adults. Eliopoulous (1997), a gerontological nursing expert, presents facts that are basic to all older people:

- Growing numbers of Americans are interested in wellness programs that help them stay youthful, active, and healthy.
- More than one third of all surgical patients are over 65 years of age.
- The prevalence of mental health problems increases with age.
- Chronic diseases occur at a rate four times greater in old age than other ages.
- Approximately 40% of all older adults will spend some time in a nursing home during their lives.
- Elderly patients occupy most of the beds in acute medical hospitals.
- Older adults are the most significant users of home health services (pp. 14-15).

Selected Activities to Address the Health Care Needs of Aging Minorities

The health professions have acknowledged the growing numbers of aging minorities in particular. Louie (1999) examined the major health problems of AAPIs and provided information on risk factors and specific culturally sensitive guidelines to assist health care providers in designing health promotion programs. Consistent with the identified growing number of older adults interested in wellness programs, Moneda and Gibson (1999) facilitated the work to establish the Golden Dreamers in the San Francisco Bay area. This successful program addresses "the health maintenance needs of elderly Filipanas and to provide a forum for the expression of Filipino cultural diversity" (p. 17). In its third year of operation, this group has become a strong force for promoting health among the Filipino elderly community.

To address the health care needs of Blacks, nurse researchers and social workers contributed salient works in a wonderful resource described in the section on Black Americans. Health care models and research studies in this resource include cancer, homegrown violence, chronic illness, adolescent pregnancy, stress, care giving, and mental illness.

Access to health care services is an issue with Hispanics. Studies on the use of community-based social and health services (Tran, Dhoopper, & McInnis-Dittrich, 1997) and ethnic and gender differences in perceived needs for social services (Tran & Dhooper, 1996) are useful resources in planning community-based prevention programs.

Research on health outcomes of Native Americans is sparse. Native Americans' health would benefit from nursing research. However, accessing them for research is a major issue. Jacobson, Booton-Hines, Moore, Edwards, Pryor, and Campbell (1998), with support from a grant from the NIH, conducted a study to "implement recommended strategies for successful field research with American Indians" (p. 161). The researchers, from diverse disciplines, focused on Native Americans' beliefs about practices regarding diabetes, a major health problem of this population. Positive outcomes regarding entry into the field, negotiating and maintaining working relationships, and continuing the work, are now solid foundations for future work with Native Americans.

The needs of aging minorities will be addressed increasingly as this population continues to grow. The increase in the numbers of health care professionals, including clinicians, educators, policy-makers, and researchers, would to a great extent, ensure that work will continue toward meeting the health needs of not only aging minorities, but also every older adult.

THE CHANGING RURAL AND URBAN POPULATIONS: HOMELESS PERSONS

Homelessness and Homeless Persons: Getting to Know Them

Homelessness is a complex social and economic problem that affects the individual, family, and society. The Stewart B. McKinney Homeless Assistance Act (public law 100-77) defines homelessness as the lack of a fixed, regular, and adequate nighttime residence. A homeless person's nighttime residence may be a supervised or publicly operated shelter designed as temporary living quarters, an institution serving as a temporary residence for persons who require institutionalization, and any public or private place not intended for regular sleeping accommodations. This definition is extremely limited and presents multiple issues and problems in resolving the homeless situation (Clark, Williams, Percy, & Kim, 1995). The use of this definition would lead to the exclusion of persons in critical need of services. Furthermore, studies on homeless persons have encountered methodological difficulties and therefore accuracy of information is questionable (Reichenbach, McNamee, & Seibel, 1998).

A review of the current literature reveals that there is a nationwide attempt to define homelessness and homeless persons. Marsh (1996) suggested a broader, more comprehensive definition of homelessness and homeless persons, stating "Homelessness is often an on-again, off-again proposition interspersed with periods of low-cost transient living arrangements, institutionalization, or living temporarily with loved ones, friends, and family. Some individuals are the chronic or long-term homeless, while others require shelters only for emergency, temporary, or short-term homelessness" (p. 1). Additionally, women who seek refuge from abusive situations and children who run away from home or from other foster care institutions may also be considered homeless. Vissing (1996) studied the rural homeless and contends that the current definition only has the urban population in mind. This author adds that children living in a marginal existence in housing distress and in poverty and those who have been homeless before and could be easily homeless again must be included. Finally, Walker (1998) offered an important perspective that should be incorporated into the definition, stating "Homeless people are not simply victims of unemployment, recession, racism, or governmental indifference; about 85% are on the streets because they are addicted to alcohol or other drugs, or have some form of mental illness" (p. 26).

Given the multiple dimensions of a comprehensive definition, how many Americans could be considered homeless persons?

Estimates of Homeless Persons

There is no easy answer to the question of how many people are homeless in the United States (O'Toole & Withers, 1998). Although most homeless persons in the 1950s and 1960s were men, the current population consists of men, women, children, couples without children, families with children, and children who are alone or runaways. Estimates of the homeless population range from 250,000 to 4 million persons (Macnee, Hemphill, & Letran, 1996). The subgroup composed of single women with dependent children is the fastest growing subgroup of the homeless population (Gillis & Singer, 1997). Recent estimates put the percentage of homeless women and children fleeing abuse at 25% to 35% of the total homeless population (Vissing, 1996).

The increasing heterogeneity of the homeless population, the difficulty in agreeing on a universal definition, and the methodological process for counting homeless persons are major issues in arriving at a reliable estimate. Most estimates are done by counting persons who use shelters or soup kitchens or those who are found on the streets (Straw, 1995). Persons who are often omitted are the hidden homeless who use their automobiles, abandoned buildings, areas under bridges, and other unaccessible areas (O'Toole & Withers, 1998). Other studies fail to include homeless women with children because these women avoid shelters that do not allow children (Clark, William, Percy, & Kim, 1995). Finally, rural homeless children and families are not counted because many areas do not have shelters or services where homeless persons can be documented (Vissing, 1996).

Causes of Today's Homelessness

In the two previous editions of this book, the author presented brief overviews of the history of homelessness and its causes. In this edition, readers must transcend the past and focus on dealing with the present and changing the future. With *Healthy People 2010* underway, every citizen must have the acuteness of vision and the kindness of heart to help resolve this situation.

Clark, William, Percy, and Kim (1995) explored the health and life problems of 163 homeless men and women in the Southeast. Participants reported more than one reason for being homeless. Family problems and loss of a job were reported by over 40% of the participants. Other problems included alcohol and drug abuse, physical illness, and emotional and mental illness. Marsh's study (1996) found that a majority of the homeless participants in Hartford County, Maryland cited the loss of jobs and the break-up of marriage as the most common causes. Other participants include disability, low income, eviction, alcohol and drugs, jail and prison, and not being able to get along with people in the residence. These causes are consistent with reports by Vissing (1996) in her study of homeless children and families in rural areas. Both Marsh and Vissing (1996) found alcohol abuse to be a major factor in 2% of the study participants. In large areas such as Boston, Chicago, Los Angeles, Minneapolis, New York, Philadelphia, St. Louis, and Washington, DC, there is a relatively high prevalence of mental illness and substance abuse (Kales, J.P., Barone, Bixler, Miljkovic, & Kales, J.D., 1995). A more recent publication by Walker (1998) supports earlier studies that found alcohol and drug abuse and mental illness as predominant causes of homelessness. Similarly, Caton, Shrout, Dominguez, Eagle, Opler, and Cournos (1995) found consistent data among homeless women. Additionally, these researchers found family support to be less adequate, hypothesizing that this aspect would serve as a risk factor for homelessness.

The multiple causes of homelessness that cut across age, gender, and SES make this societal problem a major challenge of this century.

Health Problems of Homeless People

Life as a homeless person generates multiple physical and mental problems because he or she experiences exposure to extremes in temperatures, unsanitary living conditions, crowded shelters, poor nutrition, and unsafe situations, both in the shelters and on the streets. Homeless persons are at greater risk from muggings, beatings, and rape (Gillis & Singer, 1997).

In a clinic for homeless persons, health care providers screened for hypertension, diabetes, anemia, TB, and foot problems. Although the prevalence of diabetes or hypertension is comparable with the general population, the management of these problems is poor because the homeless person is in poverty and experiences a consequent lack of access to a health care provider for monitoring and treatment. Furthermore, homeless persons have no control over their dietary needs including shopping, storage, and the preparation of appropriate foods.

Poor or lack of sanitary facilities predispose homeless persons to a host of infectious diseases such as TB.

Overcrowded living conditions, poor nutrition, and other coexisting problems increase the prevalence of TB. Early diagnosis and prompt treatment are not always possible because the person lives a transient lifestyle and avoids encounters with the health care system. Homeless persons travel almost entirely by foot; therefore they have a high incidence of foot problems, including infections, blisters, ulcers, calluses, and frostbite. Lack of facilities for managing these conditions and worn or ill-fitting shoes exacerbate foot problems (MacNee, Hemphill, & Letran, 1996; O'Toole & Withers, 1998).

Homeless persons who have a drug abuse problem and inject drugs have a high risk for HIV and AIDS (Lebow, O'Connell, Oddleifson, Gallagher, Seage, & Freedberth, 1995). Homeless women often lack prenatal care, which is associated with increased morbidity and mortality rates (Killon, 1995).

Earlier in this chapter, mental or psychiatric problems were cited as causes of homelessness. However, homelessness also creates mental problems. Multiple stresses of living in shelters and on the streets, physical problems, lack of resources, psychosocial issues such as shame and stigma, and feelings of hopelessness and despair often tax the homeless person's ability to cope.

Homeless children suffer from a number of psychological, social, and physical problems. Zima, Wells, and Freeman (1994) identified the problems of children in homeless families who were being served by 22 emergency homeless shelters in Los Angeles County, California. Data from this study were collected from 168 children aged 6 to 12. In this study, 74 children were Black, 59 were Hispanic, 23 were White, and 12 were classified as "other." Approximately 88% of the children were registered in school. However, over a three-month period, about 16% missed more than 3 weeks of school. It is no wonder that 47% scored below the tenth percentile in receptive vocabulary and approximately 40% demonstrated a reading level equivalent to an F grade. Only a small percentage of these children with learning barriers received any help.

Bassuk (1990) documented the effects of homelessness on children in an earlier study. Homeless children showed depression, anxiety, and suicidal tendencies. Sleeping difficulties, shyness, withdrawal, and aggression were common. Wagner, Manke, and Ciccone (1995) assessed 85 rural homeless children and gave them the Denver Developmental Screening Test (DDST). The DDST consists of four categories that must be passed to preclude further evaluation. Data indicated that 41 (48%) of the children passed. The other 44 (52%) children failed at least one of the four tests. The researchers concluded that the children's scores indicated a developmental lag resulting from inadequate environmental stimulation and an identifiable risk for long-term consequences requiring immediate attention.

An important qualitative study by Heusel (1995) on homeless children focused on the experience of being homeless. The multiple losses perceived by these children, including self-respect, security, and the ability to fit in, are valuable perspectives in assisting them to overcome barriers in resolving their homeless situation.

Generally, homeless persons have similar problems compared with the rest of the population. What sets the homeless apart are the many compounding factors and situations that serve as insurmountable obstacles in seeking care. In some states homeless persons do not qualify for Medicaid assistance. Additionally, life as a homeless person limits the support network of family, friends, and neighbors. Furthermore, the emotional stigma and shame place a constraint on the homeless person who is reluctant to seek help or who does not know how to get help (Rosenheck & Lam, 1997).

Selected Strategies to Alleviate Homelessness

Homelessness has long been recognized as a multidimensional problem of modern day society. A review of past strategies would reveal that approaches must go beyond the shelter approach. In addition to shelters, other traditional approaches include (1) community-based residence programs, (2) residential services for the mentally ill, (3) foster family care, (4) halfway houses, (5) community lodges, and (6) satellite housing (Marsh, 1996). Readers are encouraged to seek resources that describe these strategies in depth. Shelters are the predominant temporary residences for homeless persons; therefore a brief discussion is warranted.

Shelters continue to serve homeless persons. Their common purpose is to provide a place to sleep and a refuge from inclement weather and from unsafe streets (Marsh, 1996). Additionally, shelters offer food, showers, laundry facilities, clothing, and television. Some shelter residents are given opportunities for gainful part-time employment by helping in running the day-to-day activities of the shelter. However, some shelters restrict entrance, specializing in certain types of homeless persons because facilities are limited. Some shelters are underused because homeless persons have negative perceptions and are unwilling to abide by the rules of the shelter (Marsh, 1996).

Shelters should be used only as temporary abodes. Strategies must be implemented to prevent the institutionalization of dependency and poverty. Everyone must address this area, especially policy makers and governmental agencies. Work programs, job training, funded education, low-cost housing, and private grants are a few specific initiatives that must be strengthened.

The efforts of nursing and other health care disciplines in addressing the needs of homeless persons are worthy of discussion. A qualitative study by Jezewski (1995) embodies nurses' perspectives about working with homeless persons. This researcher's purpose was to "explain the ways homeless people get health care and to provide insight into the strategies and methods used by nurses and others to facilitate care for homeless people" (p. 203). Using a grounded theory approach, Jezewski identified the core concept of staying connected, which includes "(a) maintaining connectedness to the homeless patient where a trusting relationship is critical, (b) establishing and maintaining a network of providers in the community through active referrals and seeking of available resources, and (c) linking the homeless patient to the health care system in a way that leads to effective treatment and continuity of care" (p. 206).

Recently, more nurses have sustained their involvement in programs for the homeless. Some of these programs include screening clinics established by faculty, students, and their academic institutions. Two nurse practitioners delivering primary care services in two shelters began Health Care for the Homeless (Gillis & Singer, 1997). The Operation Safety Net (OSN) model provides culturally competent care in which homeless people are located and, in the process, avoid frequent trips to the emergency room (O'Toole & Withers, 1998). Additionally, nurse-managed clinics in the community provide entry points into the health care system.

Nurses and other health care professionals have shown active involvement in creating supportive health-related strategies, such as:

- Establishing self-help groups
- Facilitating individual and group therapy
- Providing information for alcohol and drug counseling and job training (Clark, Williams, Percy, & Kim, 1995)

Furthermore, nurses and other professionals have demonstrated their commitment to their excellence in practice by advocating for the training of shelter operators regarding symptoms of mental disorders, referral techniques, and crisis intervention (Kales, J.P., Barone, Bixler, Miljkovic, & Kales, J.D., 1995).

Mentally ill homeless persons have also been the focus. Strategies that are an integral part of their work with these persons include creating a climate of credibility and trust, meeting their basic needs, providing outreach services, and making medication management easier through Depot Dose Pharmacotherapy, which provides long-acting medications given at monthly intervals (Walker, 1998).

Communities also need to continue their in-kind work with homeless persons. Many schools and houses of religious worship have worked with local governments in extending support to the homeless. Food, clothing, night shelter, and short-term socializing have been provided. Parishioners may donate their time preparing meals, preparing the shelter, and serving as chaperones during the night.

Much work is still needed to reduce homelessness. The needs of the recently identified rural homeless must be addressed. Every citizen must be educated so each person can serve as an advocate. Neighborhood coalitions must be established to prevent the increase of homeless persons and to support the return of the homeless person as a dignified, contributing member of society. Health care providers must continue to seek effective ways to coordinate their efforts through the creation of comprehensive resource materials. Technology must be put to its maximal capability to facilitate assessment and monitoring. Preparation for nursing and health care for the homeless in both rural and urban settings should be strengthened as an essential part of the curriculums of the health care disciplines. Finally, more research regarding health care outcomes should be supported and data should be disseminated in a timely manner.

There is a greater degree of optimism today in dealing with the problem of homelessness. Individuals and communities are showing concern through increased involvement. Homelessness is everyone's problem and people can ultimately affect the establishment of priorities to facilitate an improved quality of life. Increasing awareness and knowledge of the current status of homeless people will aid in understanding the problem and its ramifications. This understanding will serve as an excellent guide in providing input, taking necessary action, and making the final decision as to what will make a healthy nation.

PEOPLE LIVING WITH HIV OR AIDS

In an official publication dated June 5, 1981, the Centers for Disease Control and Prevention (CDCP) described the deaths of five individuals who succumbed to severe cases of pneumonia (Grinek, 1990). These five individuals represented the first cases of AIDS. The latest statistics on HIV and AIDS and its continuing devastation of the world's population are frightening (CDCP, 2000). These statistics are presented in Box 2-6.

Some basic facts are extremely important to know when designing appropriate preventive measures. The highest number of AIDS cases can be attributed to a single mode of exposure; that is, men having sex with other men. This activity accounted for 47% of all cases, followed by intravenous drug use at 25%, and heterosexual contact at 10% (CDCP, 2000).

Box 2-6 HIV and AIDS

Estimated deaths of persons, 1993 to 1998: 229,908
Cumulative totals of cases in adults and adolescents through December 1999: 724,656
Pediatric (13 years of age): 8718
HIV infection cases through December 1999:
- Highest: men having sex with men: 39,399
- Heterosexual contact: 19,441
- Injecting drug use: 18,882
- Mothers with or at risk for HIV infection: 1761

Current treatment of AIDS, for the most part, remains ineffective, although there are some encouraging **antiviral drug** combinations (those destructive to viruses) and some progress in **gene therapy** (a procedure that involves the injection of healthy genes into the bloodstream of a person to cure or treat a hereditary disease or similar illness) (Sherman, 1999). Presently, there is no feasible design for an effective vaccine. Even with the discovery of a vaccine, the majority of developing countries, where HIV and AIDS are a raging epidemic, would not have the financial resources for purchase, distribution, and treatment (Schroub, 1999). Furthermore, there is a concern that a single vaccine would not be effective against HIV strains that are resistant (Merson, 1997). The best approach continues to be zealous preventive measures that include serological testing and modification of sexual practices.

To date, education has been the major preventive strategy. High-risk behaviors among sexually active men and women and intravenous drug users have been addressed (Kelly, 1995). However, it is disappointing to know that studies indicate a return to high-risk behaviors "even in groups which had initially responded positively, such as the homosexual and bisexual men of San Francisco" (Schroub, 1999, p. 249).

A statement that could erode all preventive work was made at the recent 13th International AIDS Conference; that is, HIV does not cause AIDS. Poverty was cited as the cause of the deaths of millions and has left nations of orphaned children (Garrett & Sussman, 2000). This position was contradicted by strong leadership and support from many levels of society in attendance at the same conference.

HIV and AIDS in Ethnic and Minority Groups: Issues and Strategies

At the close of 1998 there were an estimated 294,425 persons living with AIDS. In this group, 39% are White, 40% are Black Americans, 19% are Hispanic Americans, 0.78% are AAPIs, and 0.33% are Native Americans (CDCP, 2000). Other important data can be found in Box 2-7. From these data, health care professionals must design and implement aggressive preventive programs to arrest the exposure to and transmission of this disease.

HIV and AIDS Prevention in Ethnic and Minority Groups

Preventive programs for ethnic minorities leave a great deal to be desired. Gutierrez (1997) described his own community in which ethnic minorities made up the majority of HIV-related cases, yet most of the resources went to White Anglo-oriented services staffed by Anglo workers who had little or no training in working with minority groups. Approaches to the research and treatment of HIV is also flawed. For instance, investigators have noted the importance of distinguishing cultural identity or ethnicity from race. "Racial status does not tell us much about the culture from which an individual is derived, yet this consideration is not normally imbedded in research protocols" (O'Connor, 1997, p. xxiv). Furthermore, there is increased distance and potential distrust created when service providers are insensitive to the individual's cultural values.

Box 2-7 Selected HIV and AIDS Data on Ethnic Minorities

PEDIATRIC EXPOSURE (NUMBER OF CASES):
White: 28
Black: 154
Hispanic: 48
AAPI: 0
Native American: 1

MALES AND ADOLESCENTS: MEN HAVING SEX WITH MEN:
White: 8106
Black: 3770
Hispanic: 1899
AAPI: 168
Native American: 63

HETEROSEXUAL CONTACT:
White: 476
Black: 1736
Hispanic: 615
AAPI: 24
Native American: 4

Among Black American men, a complex set of factors interact to complicate the problem of HIV and AIDS. Individual factors include sexual orientation and associated feelings of shame and stigma. Level of education and income are social factors that may interfere with preventive activities and interpersonal factors associated with perceived risks and normative, behavioral, and control beliefs. Finally, sexual venues, social networks and resources for help-seeking and social support are also important considerations (Peterson, 1997). These factors were considered in proposing specific guidelines in designing culturally appropriate approaches (Gutierrez, 1997). Briefly, these guidelines entail (1) reduction of discomfort regarding homosexuality or bisexuality as viewed within the Black American community, (2) increase of racial pride, given that many of these individuals feel ostracized from the Black American community and adopt identities that conform more to the White Anglo gay and lesbian culture to fit into that cultural group, and (3) strengthening of the individual's beliefs that condom use should become normative within the Black American subculture.

Among AAPIs, there was a slow response to the crisis of HIV and AIDS. Yep (1997) maintains that AAPIs have lagged behind other minority groups in terms of education, prevention, service delivery, and advocacy. Incidence for this group is increasing at a higher rate than for Whites. Underreporting may pervade because stigma and the cultural value of preserving family honor exist (Gutierrez, 1997). Prevailing theories now propose that in AAPI communities, the threat of HIV has become a reality. It is suggested that preventive programs consider the diversity of AAPI subgroups, integrate familial values, and avoid direct discussions about sexual practices and homosexuality, topics that are considered taboo. Suggested approaches aimed at prevention should incorporate:

1. Community ownership
2. Increasing knowledge about transmission and perceiving personal risks
3. Changing attitudes toward condoms and other protective devices
4. Disseminating information about resources and support
5. Helping AAPIs learn effective communication techniques to be used in intimate relationships and develop skills in behavioral enactment (Yep, 1997)

HIV and AIDS are affecting Hispanic American men and women at an alarming rate. Heterosexual exposure is a leading cause for Hispanic American womens' dilemma of HIV and AIDS. This trend has enormous implications for persons who are in their childbearing years. A thorough understanding of the cultural issues surrounding HIV and AIDS would facilitate the advocated approaches that need to begin at the individual level. Issues such as masculinity, control of sexuality, and high regard for the family must first be dealt with in an open, nonconfronting manner. Diaz (1997) proposed a strategy of empowerment by which individuals would have the "capacity, ability, and support to formulate and enact their own intentions; empowered people are self-directed" (p. 241). An effective empowerment strategy would consider conversations about sexuality, awareness of cultural values, feeling a sense of community, and acting as change agents.

Black American and Hispanic American women and their high risk for exposure and transmission are paramount in this nondiscriminating disease. The issues related to transmission are major social problems; therefore solutions are difficult.

Poverty and its accompanying evils, such as domestic violence (Goggin & Rabkin, 1997) and coerced sex (O'Leary & Jemmott, 1995), render preventive strategies, such as the use of condoms, useless. Approaches would be beneficial if they concentrated on areas in which an immediate difference can be made (Suarez & Siefert, 1998). Programs for the empowerment of women must include "good negotiation skills and strong confidence or self-efficacy in their ability to persuade partners to use condoms" (O'Leary & Jemmott, 1995, p. 4). More immediate problems besides HIV may confront many women, including drug addiction, poor housing, and the threat of losing custody of their children and welfare benefits. All of these factors must be considered as women's priorities, otherwise HIV prevention may never gain a foothold in their lives.

Although not specific to women from ethnic minority groups, the issue of gender bias must be acknowledged and resolved. Gender bias related to the double standard in sexuality, the victimization of women through prostitution, and the exclusion of women's issues in health care are deterrents to providing effective, humanistic, and quality care.

The HIV and AIDS crisis is beyond ethnic and minority individuals and all people in the United States. It is imperative that everyone treat this crisis as a global problem, where boundaries no longer exist (Mann & Tarantola, 1997; Theodoulou, 1996). The World Health Organization (WHO) has provided the leadership for creating a unique international forum through annual conferences on AIDS, which are cosponsored by WHO and host countries. "It was through these conferences that the dimensions of the pandemic, its commonalities, and diverse features and its scientific, medical, social, economic, and cultural implications emerged" (Sills, 1996, p. 144-145).

Humankind, through the devastation of HIV and AIDS, can hope for salvation only through zealous and continued efforts to protect every human being, regardless of race, color, or creed. Only through this perspective can we be sure of a future for the human species.

THE NATION'S RESPONSE TO THE HEALTH CHALLENGES

Healthy People 2010

Healthy People 2010 outlines a comprehensive, nationwide health promotion and disease-prevention agenda. This initiative is designed to serve as a roadmap for addressing and improving the health of all persons in the United States. *Healthy People 2010* is its foundation. With its 28 identified focus areas, the central goals are to increase quality of life and eliminate health disparities (U.S. Department of Health and Human Services, 2000).

The anticipated success of *Healthy People 2010* would include significant decreases in infant mortality, declines of death rates for coronary heart disease and stroke, advances in the management of cancer. The complex and dynamic interplay of economic, political, social, and technological factors will require active participation in advocating for health, home, community, business, state, and the nation.

Nursing's Response to Changing Populations and Health

Nursing's Code of Ethics explicitly states the profession's commitment to provide service to people regardless of background or situation (American Nurses' Association [ANA], 1985). The ANA's Council on Cultural Diversity supports the work of nurses in their development of culturally competent care. The organization and its leadership, through the Ethnic-Minority Fellowship Program, has had an essential role in supporting the work and efforts of Asian Americans, Black Americans, Hispanic

Americans, and Native Americans with graduate and doctoral work.

Nurses continue to make many positive moves toward understanding culturally diverse populations. One major move has been the formal establishment of the field of transcultural nursing, pioneered by a nurse scholar with a strong interest in anthropology. Leininger's early visions (1990) became reality with the establishment of the Transcultural Nursing Society in 1974. This organization continues to advance the work of transcultural nurses through its sponsorship of conferences that focus on a variety of contemporary issues and practices. The establishment of the *Journal of Transcultural Nursing* in 1989 has facilitated the worldwide sharing of transcultural ideas. More recently, Leininger (1997) provided a historical overview of transcultural nursing over the last 40 years. She reviewed the works of transcultural nurses on health-related issues of minorities. The work of these nurses has advanced the knowledge about nursing care that is culturally congruent and meaningful to the person and his or her family.

There are several other nursing journals that focus on cultural diversity, such as the *Journal of Cultural Diversity* and the *Journal of Multicultural Nursing and Health*. These journals and a variety of other publications are constantly increasing professionals' knowledge of health-related cultural issues. Ethnic nursing organizations are having an effect on greater cultural understanding through their dissemination of important works by clinicians, educators, and researchers.

Major organizations such as the ANA and the National League for Nursing (NLN) publish culturally relevant materials to guide students, clinicians, and educators. Additionally, a cadre of nurses whose research on the cultural practices and beliefs of individuals and families gives professionals a sound base for improving practice and designing cost-effective and humanistic health care strategies.

The quest to deliver culturally competent care has provided the impetus for nursing faculty to require transcultural courses in the nursing curriculum (see the Multicultural Awareness box). Additionally, major textbooks focusing on specific clinical areas of practice devote material on health care issues of ethnic minorities. In the clinical setting, health care workers, through staff development and in-service programs, are provided opportunities to learn and develop culturally sensitive care approaches.

Another undertaking to address the challenge of diversity is the work of nurse researchers in the workforce. Buerhaus and Auerbach (1999) examined minorities in the registered nurse (RN) workforce and found that minorities were underrepresented in all health professions, including nursing. This underrepresentation has long been recognized and governmental response has been positive with the strong lobbying efforts of various nursing organizations and

MULTICULTURAL AWARENESS

Providing a Transcultural Education

Nursing, as a health care discipline, has taken great strides in addressing the issue of multiculturalism. Credit is given to nurse educators who prepare students of nursing to care for persons with diverse backgrounds. There are many excellent resources produced by nurses that address cultural concepts and strategies to facilitate multicultural awareness. Textbooks focusing on clinical areas of practice have integrated cultural diversity in nursing care strategies. However, how can students move above and beyond awareness to provide culturally competent care?

A transcultural course can open a world of knowledge on cultures. Students can get excited knowing about differences and similarities. Students can participate in creative projects such as dress and food presentations. However, do these ensure culturally competent caring?

Clinical courses in nursing must build on the learned transcultural concepts. It is imperative that clinical faculty support students who are caring for persons who are culturally different. The students should implement care modalities that meet the unique needs of the person. For instance, students might want to learn to braid the hair of a Black individual. This aspect of nursing care would also facilitate the establishment of an effective working relationship. Are students able to recognize the hygienic practices of a Filipino person? Faculty should allow students time to think about their care modifications and consider cultural practices and how they fit within standards of care. Faculty should recognize their efforts informally through positive comments and formally through clinical performance evaluations.

As students progress in the curriculum, they will acquire other knowledge and skills essential to the role of a future professional. Courses in research, politics, and leadership may provide other perspectives to advocate for culturally competent care. In each of these courses, faculty can design action projects that will integrate learned transcultural concepts. For instance, students can be directed to assess the health needs of an ethnic community and then design a project with the members of the community to meet a specified need.

Strategies should be selected that involve reviewing the research literature and getting the support of a legislator. Students should be encouraged to build on learned communication skills and to collaborate with a community leader. An example of a community-based project is the transformation of a garbage dump into a small park with benches. People in their neighborhood take care of the annual flowers and plants that local garden shops donate. This park was the collective efforts of students, residents, and legislators.

Students need to see that their efforts to provide culturally competent care is the responsibility of the professional whose mission is to improve health, quality of life, and well being of ethnic minorities in the community.

nurse leaders. For instance, the U.S. Department of Health and Human Services has funded programs for students from ethnic minority backgrounds and who also have economic issues as they pursue their basic nursing curriculums. The author's academic institution was a recipient of a three-year (1997 to 2000) grant for an initiative known as "Growth and Access Increase for Nursing Students" (GAINS). The author served as project director and, with two full-time personnel, college and school administration and faculty, and external consultants, the retention rate of students rose from 50% to 77% (Valencia-Go, 2000). To a certain degree, the success of this grant ensures a return of graduates to their own communities as health care providers.

SUMMARY

Individuals and groups need to collaborate in optimizing the conditions that improve the quality of life. Good health, as a major determinant of the quality of life, should be a right for all, regardless of socioeconomic or cultural background.

The challenge posed by ethnic and minority-group individuals is particularly important as the population of the United States becomes more diverse. The important role of cultural beliefs and practices must be emphasized in health care situations for effective and humanistic care. The United States, and especially the nursing profession, continue to share their vision, creativity, energy, and commitment to ensure health, well being, and quality of life for all in this century and beyond.

REFERENCES

Adams, L. M., & Knox, M. E. (1988). Traditional health practices: Significance for modern health care. In M. Van Horne (Ed.), *Ethnicity and health: Vol. 7. Ethnicity and public policy series*. Milwaukee: The University of Wisconsin System Institute on Race and Ethnicity.

Ailinger, R. L., & Causey, M. E. (1995). Health concepts of older Hispanic immigrants. *Western Journal of Nursing Research, 17* (6), 605-613.

American immigration: Vol. I. (1999). Danbury, CT: Grolier Educational.

American Nurses' Association. (1985). *Code of ethics*. Kansas City, MO: The Association.

Andrews, M. M. (1995). Transcultural nursing care. In M. M. Andrews, & J. S. Boyle (Eds.), *Transcultural concepts in nursing care* (2nd ed.). Philadelphia: J.B. Lippincott.

Banks, J. A., & Gay, G. (1969). Ethnicity in contemporary American society: Toward the development of a typology. *Ethnicity, 5*, 238-251.

Barth, F. (1969). Introduction. In F. Barth (Ed.), *Ethnic groups and boundaries: The social organization of cultural differences*. Boston: Little, Brown.

Bassuk, E. L. (1990). Who are the homeless families? Characteristics of sheltered mothers and children. *Community Mental Health Journal, 26* (5), 425-434.

Bauwens, E., & Anderson, S. (1992). Social and cultural influences on health care. In M. Stanhope & L. Lancaster (Eds.), *Community health nursing* (3rd ed.). St. Louis: Mosby.

Begun, A. M., Klier, B. A., & Quiran, J. F. (1999). *The information series on current topics*. Wylie, TX: Information Plus.

Bennett, L. (1992). *Before the Mayflower: A history of black America* (6th ed.). Chicago: Johnson.

Berkram, P. C. (1999). When God took the reservation by storm. *Journal of Christian Nursing: A Quarterly Publication of Nurses Christian Fellowship, 16* (4), 22-25.

Blackwell, J. E. (1991). *The black community*. New York: Harper Collins.

Blais, K. K. (1991). Ethnic and cultural values. In B. Kozier, G. Erb, & R. Olivieri (Eds.), *Fundamentals of nursing: Concepts, process and practice* (4th ed.). Redwood City, CA: Addison-Wesley.

Boyle, J. S. (1997). Culture and the community. In M. M. Andrews & J. A. Boyle (Eds.), *Transcultural concepts in nursing care* (2nd ed.). Philadephia: J.B. Lippincott.

Buerhaus, P. I., & Auerbach, D. (1999). Slow growth in the United States of the number of minorities in the RN workforce. *Image–the Journal of Nursing Scholarship, 31* (2), 179-183.

Campinha-Bacote, J. (1998). African-Americans. In L. Purnell & B. Paulanha (Eds.), *Transcultural health care: A culturally competent approach*. Philadelphia: F.A. Davis.

Castillo, H., & Torres, S. (1995). Cultural consideration: Providing quality nursing care to Hispanics. *Imprint*, 52-55.

Caton, C. L., Shrout, P. E., Dominguez, B., Eagle, P. F., Opler, L. O., & Cournos, F. (1995). Risk factors for homelessness among women with schizophrenia. *American Journal of Public Health, 85* (8), 1153-1156.

Census figures misleading. (1992). *Lakota Times, 12* (23), A1.

Centers for Disease Control and Prevention, Division of HIV/AIDS Prevention. (2000). *Surveillance report, 11* (2).

Charsley, S. R. (1974). The formation of ethnic groups. In A. Cohen (Ed.), *Urban ethnicity*. London: Tavistock.

Choi, P. (1996). Tuberculosis concerns for Asian Americans and Pacific Islanders. *Asia-Pacific Journal of Public Health/Asia-Pacific Academic Consortium for Public Health, 4* (1,3), 127.

Clark, P. M., Williams, C. A., Percy, M. A., & Kim, Y. S. (1995). Health and life problems of homeless men and women in the Southeast. *Journal of Community Health Nursing, 12* (2), 101-110.

Cornelius, L. J., & Altman, B. M. (1995). Have we succeeded in reducing barriers to medical care for African and Hispanic Americans with disabilities? *Social Work in Health Care, 22* (2), 1.

Daugherty, R. D. (1992). People of the salmon. In M. Josephy (Ed.), *America in 1492: The world of the Indian people before the arrival of Columbus*. New York: Alfred A. Knopf.

Davis, M. B. (1996). *Native America in the Twentieth Century: An encyclopedia*. New York: Garland Publishing, Inc.

Davis, R. (1996). Pearls for practice: The perceptions of Puerto Rican women regarding health care experience. *Journal of the American Academy of Nurse Practitioners, 8* (1), 21-25.

Degazon, C. (1995). Coping, diabetes, and the older African-American. *Nursing Outlook, 43* (6), 254-259.

de Paula, T., Lagana, K., & Gonzalez-Ramirez, L. (1996). Mexican Americans. In J. G. Lipson, S. L. Dibble, & P. A. Minarik (Eds.), *Culture and nursing care: A pocket guide*. San Francisco: University of California, San Francisco, School of Nursing Press.

DeSantis, G., & Benkin, R. (1980). Ethnicity without community. *Ethnicity, 7*, 137-143.

Diaz, R. M. (1997). Latino gay men and psycho cultural barriers to AIDS prevention. In M. P. Levine, P. M. Nardi, & J. N. Gagnon (Eds.), *In changing times*. Chicago: The University of Chicago Press.

Douglas, C. (1995). Cultural considerations for the African American population. *Imprint*, 57-59. Driver, H. I. (1964). *The Americas on the eve of discovery*. Englewood Cliffs, NJ: Prentice Hall.

Eliopoulous, C. (1997). *Gerontological nursing* (4th ed.). Philadelphia: Lippincott.

Embree, E. R. (1973). *Indians of the Americas*. New York: Collier Books.

Enas, E. A. (1996). Cardiovascular diseases in Asian Americans and Pacific Islanders. *Asian American and Pacific Islander Journal of Health, 4* (1,3), 119-120.

Feinstein, O. (1971). *Ethnic groups in the city*. Lexington, MA: Heath Lexington Books.

Felton, G. M., & Parson, M. A. (1997). Health-promoting behaviors of black and white college women. *Western Journal of Nursing Research, 19* (5), 654-664.

Gall, S., & Natividad, I. (1995). *The Asian American almanac*. Detroit: Gale Research, Inc.

Garrett, L., & Susman, T. (2000). Focus on poverty, not on HIV, AIDS. *Newsday*, July 10, pp. A6, A16.

Geissler, E. M. (1991). Nursing diagnosis of culturally diverse patients. *International Nursing Review, 38* (5), 150-163.

Giddens, A. (1996). *Introduction to sociology* (2nd ed.). New York: W.W. Norton.

Gillis, L. M., & Singer, J. (1997). Breaking through the barriers: Healthcare for the homeless. *The Journal of Nursing Administration, 27* (6), 30-34.

Goggin, K. J., & Rabkin, J. G. (1997). Treating HIV-positive women. In T. O'Connor & I. Yalow (Eds.), *Treating the psychological consequences of HIV.* San Francisco: Jossey-Bass Publishers.

Gonzalez, J. L. (1990). *Racial and ethnic groups in America*. Dubuque, IA: Kendall/Hunt.

Griffin, F. N. (1994). Perceptions of African Americans regarding health care. *Journal of Cultural Diversity, 1* (2), 32-34.

Grinek, M. D. (1990). *History of AIDS*, Princeton, NJ: Princeton University Press.

Grossman, D. (1998). Cuban-Americans. In L. D. Purnell & B. J. Paulanha (Eds.), *Transcultural health care: A culturally competent approach*. Philadelphia: F.A. Davis.

Gutierrez, F. J. (1997). Treating ethnic minority individuals. In M. F. O'Connor and I. D. Yalow (Eds.), *Treating the psychological consequences of HIV.* San Francisco: Jossey-Bass Publishers.

Harden, J. T., & McFarland, G. (2000). Avoiding gender and minority barriers to NIH funding. *Journal of Nursing Scholarship, 32* (1), 83-86.

Hayat, A., Lucas, J. B., & Kington, R. (2000). *Health outcomes among Hispanic subgroups: Data from the National Interview Survey, 1992-1995. Advance Data*. Hyattsville, MD: U.S. Department of Health and Human Services.

Herberg, P. (1995). Theoretical foundations of transcultural nursing. In M. M. Andrews & J. S. Boyle (Eds.), *Transcultural concepts in nursing care* (2nd ed.). Philadelphia: J.B. Lippincott.

Heusel, K. J. (1995). *Homeless children: Their perspectives*. New York: Garland Publishing.

Isajiw, W. (1974). Definitions of ethnicity, *Ethnicity, 1*, 111-124.

Jacobson, S. F., Booton-Hiser, D., Moore, J. H., Edwards, K. A., Pryor, S., & Campbell, J. M. (1998). Diabetes research in an American Indian community. *Image–the Journal of Nursing Scholarship, 30* (2), 161-165.

Jennings, A. (1999). Who supports elderly African Americans in adhering to their healthcare regimen? *Home Healthcare Nurse, 17* (8), 519-525.

Jezewski, M. A. (1995). Staying connected: The core of facilitating health care to homeless persons. *Public Health Nursing, 12* (3), 203-210.

Joel, L. A. (1998). Editorial: The upside and downside of cultural diversity. *The American Journal of Nursing, 98* (12), 7.

Johnson, D. M., & Campbell, R. R. (1981). *Black migration in America*. Durham, NC: Duke University Press.

Johnson, R. W. (1995). *African-American voices: African-American health educators speak out.* New York: National League for Nursing Press.

Juarbe, T. (1996). Puerto Ricans. In J. G. Lipson , S. L. Dibble, & P. A. Minari (Eds.), *Culture and nursing care*. San Francisco: University of California, San Francisco, School of Nursing Press.

Kales, J. P., Barone, M. A., Bixler, E. O., Miljkovic, M. M., & Kales, J. D. (1995). Mental illness and substance abuse among sheltered homeless persons in low-density population areas. *Psychiatric Services (Washington, DC), 46* (6), 592-595.

Keller, C., Fleury, J., & Bergstrom, D. L. (1995). Risk factors for coronary heart disease in African-American women. *The Journal of Cardiovascular Nursing, 31* (2), 9-14.

Kelly, J. A. (1995). *Changing HIV risk behavior: Practical strategies*. New York: Guilford Press.

Killon, C. M. (1995). Special health care needs of homeless pregnant women. *Advances in Nursing Science, 18*, 44-65.

Kim, M.T. (1995). Cultural influences on depression in Korean Americans. *Journal of Psychosocial Nursing, 33* (2), 13-18.

Kluckhohn, C. (1953). Dominant and variant value orientations. In C. Kluckhohn, H. A. Murray, & D. A. Schneider (Eds.), *Personality in nature, society, and culture* (2nd ed.). New York: Alfred A. Knopf.

Kolm, R. (1971). Ethnicity in society and community. In O. Feinstein (Ed.), *Ethnic groups in the city*. Lexington, MA: Heath Lexington Books.

Kramer, J. (1996). American Indians. In J. G. Lipson, S. L. Dibble, & P. A. Minarik (Eds.), *Culture and nursing care*. San Francisco: University of California, San Francisco, School of Nursing Press.

Lake, M. G. (1991). *Native healer*. Wheaton, IL: Quest Books.

Kuramoto, F. H. (1995). Who are the Asian Pacific Americans? In S. Gale & I. Natividad (Eds.), *The Asian American almanac*. Detroit: Gale Publishing, Inc.

Lebow, J. M., O'Connell, J., Oddleifson, A., Gallagher, K. M., Seage, G. R., & Freedberth, K. M. (1995). AIDS among homeless of Boston: A cohort study. *Journal of Acquired Immune Deficiency Syndromes and Human Retrovirology: Official Publication of the International Retrovirology Association, 8*, 292-296.

Leininger, M. (1997). Transcultural nursing research to transform nursing education and practice: 40 years. *Image–the Journal of Nursing Scholarship, 29* (4), 341-354.

Leininger, M. (1990). Transcultural nursing: Quo vadis (where goeth the field?). *Journal of Transcultural Nursing: Official Journal of the Transcultural Nursing Society/Transcultural Nursing Society, 1* (2), 33-45.

Lipson, J. G., Dibble, S. L., Minarik, P. A. (1996). *Culture and nursing care*. San Francisco: University of California, San Francisco, School of Nursing Press.

Locks, S., & Boateng, L. A. (1996). Black/African Americans. In J. G. Lipson, S. L. Dibble, & P. A. Minarik (Eds.), *Culture and nursing care*. San Francisco: University of California, San Francisco, School of Nursing Press.

Louie, K. B. (1999). Health promotions interventions for Asian American Pacific Islanders. In L. Zhan (Ed.), *Asian voices: Asian and Asian American health educators speak out*. Boston: Jones and Bartlett Publishers.

Macnee, C. L., Hemphill, J. C., & Letran, J. (1996). Screening clinics for the homeless: Evaluating outcomes. *Journal of Community Health Nursing, 13* (3), 167-177.

Mann, M. M., & Tarantola, J. M. (1997). A global strategy is needed to control the spread of AIDS. In D. A. Leone (Ed.), *The spread of AIDS*. San Diego, CA: Greenhaven Press, Inc.

Marsh, C. E. (1996). *Harford county, Maryland homeless and shelter survey*. Lanham: University Press of America, Inc.

Marshall, P. A. (1990). Cultural influences on perceived quality of life. *Seminars in Oncology Nursing, 6* (4), 278-281.

Merson, M. H. (1997). Society should continue to stress AIDS prevention. In D. A. Leone (Ed.), *The spread of AIDS*. San Diego, CA: Greenhaven Press, Inc.

Moneda, A. G., & Gibson, S. E. (1999). The golden health promotion program for the golden dreamers. In L. Zhan (Ed.), *Asian voices: Asian and Asian American health educators speak out*. Boston: Jones and Bartlett Publishers.

Nabokov, P. (1991). *Native American testimony*. New York: Penguin.

O'Connor, M. F. (1997). Introduction. In M. F. O'Connor & I. D. Yalow (Eds.), *Treating the psychological consequences of HIV*. San Francisco: Jossey-Bass Publishers.

O'Leary, A., & Jemmott, L. S. (1995). *Women at risk: Issues in the primary prevention of AIDS*. New York: Plenum Press.

O'Toole, S. M., & Withers, J. S. (1998). From the streets, to the emergency department, and back: A model of emergency care for the homeless. *Topics in Emergency Medicine, 20* (2), 12-20.

Persell, C. H. (1990). *Understanding society* (3rd ed.). New York: Harper Collins College Publishers.

Peterson, J. L. (1997). AIDS-related risks and same-sex behaviors among African-American men. In M. P. Levine, P. M. Nardi, & J. H. Cagnon (Eds.), *In changing times*. Chicago: The University of Chicago Press.

Pettigrew, T. F. (1971). Ethnicity in American life: A social-psychological perspective. In O. Feinstein (Ed.), *Ethnic groups in the city*. Lexington, MA: Heath Lexington Books.

Potter, P. A. (2001). The health care delivery system. In P. A. Potter & A. G. Griffin (Eds.), *Fundamentals of nursing* (5th ed.). St. Louis: Mosby.

Powell, I. J., Gelfand, D. E., Parzuchowski, J., Heilburn, L., & Franklin, A. (1995). A successful recruitment process of African American men for early detection of prostate cancer. *Cancer, 75* (7), 1880-1884.

Prism. (1993). *The NLN Research and Policy Quarterly* (2), 1.

Queralt, M. (1996). *The social environment and human behavior*. Boston: Allyn and Bacon.

Rehm, R. S. (1999). Religion faith in Mexican-American families dealing with chronic childhood illness. *Image–the Journal of Nursing Scholarship, 31* (1), 33-38.

Reichenbach, E. M., McNamee, M. J., & Seibel, L. V. (1998). The community health nursing implications of the self-reported health status of a local homeless population. *Public Health Nursing, 15* (6), 398-405.

Rosenheck, R., & Lam, J. A. (1997). Client and site characteristics on barriers to service use by homeless persons with serious mental illness. *Psychiatric Services (Washington, DC), 48* (3), 387-390.

Sarna, J. (1978). From immigrants to ethnics: Toward a new theory of ethnicization. *Ethnicity, 5*, 370-378.

Schermerhorn, R. (1970). *Comparative ethnic relations: A framework for theory and research*. Chicago: University of Chicago Press.

Schroub, B. D. (1999). *AIDS and HIV in perspective: A guide to understanding the virus and its consequences* (2nd ed.). Cambridge: Cambridge University Press.

Sherman, D. W. (1999). Essential information for providing care to patients with HIV/AIDS. *The Journal of the New York State Nurses' Association, 30* (2), 8-19.

Sills, Y. G. (1996). The international response. In S. Z. Theodoulou (Ed.), *AIDS: The politics and policy of disease*. Upper Saddle River, NJ: Prentice Hall.

Smith, J. C., & Horton, C. P. (1995). *Statistical record of black America* (4th ed.). New York: Gale.

Staiano, K. (1980). Afro-American identity. *Ethnicity, 7*, 27-33.

Starr, P. (1990). *Social transformation of American medicine*. New York: Basic Books.

Straw, R. B. (1995). Looking behind the numbers in counting the homeless: An invited commentary. *American Journal of Ortho Psychiatry, 65*, 320-329.

Suarez, Z. E., & Siefert, K. (1998). Latinas and sexually transmitted diseases: Implications of recent research for prevention. *Social Work in Health Care, 28*, (1), 1-19.

Taylor, C. F. (1991). *The Native Americans*. New York: Smithmark.

Theodoulou, S. Z. (1996). AIDS equal politics. In S. Z. Theodoulou (Ed.), *AIDS: The politics and policy of disease*. Englewood, NJ: Prentice Hall.

Tong, M. J. (1996). The impact of the hepatitis B infection in Asian Americans. *Asian American and Pacific Islander Journal of Health, 4* (1,3), 125-126.

Torres, S. (1994). A challenge of nursing education: Meeting the needs of the Hispanic community. *Deans Notes, 15* (5), 1-3.

Tran, T. V., & Dhooper, S. S. (1996). Ethnic and gender differences in perceived needs for social services among three elderly Hispanic groups. *Journal of Gerontological Social Work, 25* (3,4), 121-146.

Tran, T. V., Dhooper, S. S., McInnis-Dittrich, K. (1997). Utilization of community-based social and health services among foreign born Hispanic American elderly. *Journal of Gerontological Social Work, 28* (4), 23-42.

USA Today (1996). For frustrated consumers, a welcome trend in medicine. *USA Today*, October 11, 12A.

U.S. Census Bureau. (1999). Statistical Abstract of the U.S. (119th ed.) Washington, DC: Government Printing Office.

U.S. Department of Commerce. (1989). Bureau of the Census. *We, The First Americans*, Washington, DC: Government Printing Office.

U.S. Department of Education. (1991). *Indian nations at risk: An educational strategy for action*. Washington, DC: Indian Nations Risk Task Force.

U.S. Department of Education, National Center for Education Statistics, Office of Educational Research and Improvement. (1992). *Digest of education statistics*. Washington, DC: U.S. Government Printing Office.

U.S. Department of Health and Human Services, Public Health Service, Centers for Disease Control and Prevention, National Center for Health Statistics. (1996). Monthly vital statistics report: Advance report of final mortality statistics, 45 (3), 1.

U.S. Department of Health and Human Services. (2000). *Healthy People 2010. Understanding and Improving Health*. Washington, DC: U.S. Government Printing Office.

U.S. Department of Housing and Urban Development. (1999). *Housing our elders: A report card on the housing conditions and needs of older Americans*. Washington, DC: Office of Policy Development and Research.

Valencia-Go, G. N. (1989). *Integrative aging in widowed immigrant Filipinas: A grounded theory study, order number 8923910*. Ann Arbor, MI: University Microfilms International.

Valencia-Go, G. N. (1999). Elderly Filipino women's adjustment to widowhood: Implications for health and well-being. In L. Zhan (Ed.), *Asian voices: Asian and Asian-American health educators speak out*. Boston: Jones and Bartlett Publishers.

Valencia-Go, G. N. (2000). *Uniform progress report for grants and cooperative agreements for FY 2000*. Arlington, VA: Health Resources and Services Administration Bureau of Health Professions.

Vissing, Y. M. (1996). *Out of sight, out of mind: Homeless children and families in small-town America*. Lexington, KY: The University Press of Kentucky.

Wagner, J. D., Menke, E. M., & Ciccone, J. (1995). What is known about the health of rural homeless families. *Public Health Nursing, 12* (6), 400-408.

Walker, C. (1998). Homeless people and mental health: A nursing concern. *The American Journal of Nursing, 98* (11), 26-32.

Weinrich, S., Holdford, D., Boyd, M., Creanga, D., Cover, K., Johnson, A., Frank-Stomberg, M., & Weinrich, M. (1998). Prostate cancer education in African-American churches. *Public Health Nursing, 15* (3), 188-195.

Yep, G. A. (1997). HIV/AIDS in Asian and Pacific Islander Communities in the U.S.: A review, analysis, and integration. In D. Buchanan & G. Cernada (Eds.), *Progress in preventing AIDS? Dogma, dissent, and innovation*. Amityville, NY: Baywood Publishing Co., Inc.

Zangwill, I. (1921). *The melting pot: Drama in four acts*. New York: Macmillan.

Zima, B. T., Wells, K. B., & Freeman, H. E. (1994). Emotional and behavioral problems and severe academic delay among sheltered homeless children in Los Angeles County. *American Journal of Public Health, 84* (2), 260-268.

Chapter 3

CAROL SCHEEL GAVAN

Health Policy and the Delivery System

objectives

After completing this chapter, the nurse will be able to:

- Discuss key developments in the history of health care that influenced the philosophical basis of American health care and separated preventive from curative measures.
- Differentiate between private and public sector functions and responsibilities in the delivery of health care.
- Describe the mechanisms by which health care in the United States is financed in both private and public sectors.
- Discuss the influence of health legislation on health care delivery.
- Differentiate between the purposes, benefits, and limitations of Medicare and Medicaid programs.
- Discuss the nurse's role in influencing health policy.

key terms

Advocate
Capitation System
Case Management
Fee-for-Service
Health Department
Health Maintenance Organizations
Health Officer
Insurance
Laws
Lobbying
Lobbyist
Managed Care
Nursing Centers
Point-of-Service
Policy Decision Making
Politics
Preferred Provider Organizations
Primary Care
Primary Care Provider
Regulations
Salary System
Sanitarians
Self-Insurance

THINK About It

Making Health Promotion a Reality

The inclusion of health-promotion activities and preventive measures in primary health care is beginning to be realized. Combining clinical preventive services with population-based health-promotion activities, such as group smoking cessation programs, health education programs, and fitness programs in schools and on worksites makes sense. These combined measures are not only cost effective, but they are essential to improve and maintain the health of present and future citizens.

The nurse is a key player in setting up a new health program for her community. She bases her recommendations on a community assessment that shows a need for a worksite fitness program and on research that shows the many benefits for workers in this site. She is a firm believer in the value and ultimate cost-effectiveness of this primary preventive intervention.

1. How can the nurse "sell" the idea of the fitness health-promotion program to her interdisciplinary colleagues?
2. Why is the fitness program cost effective?

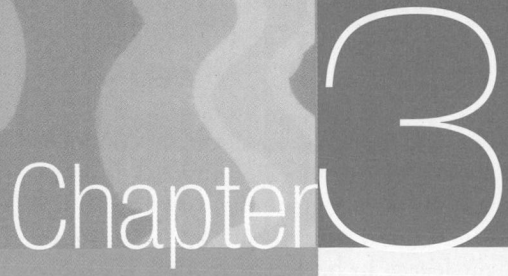

The World Health Organization (WHO) began the "Health for All by the Year 2000" movement in 1977 by setting goals and targets for all member countries to attain a level of health that enables people to live socially and economically productive lives. Internationally, shrinking health care budgets have resulted in a variable level of achievement of these goals.

Over the last 20 years, since the United States began the national health planning process for the *Healthy People* initiative, the nation has made great progress in public health and medicine. *Healthy People 2010* emphasizes the relationship between individual health and community health; that is, the health of the community and the environment in which individuals live, work, and play. Nevertheless, community health is greatly affected by the collective behaviors, attitudes, and beliefs of all individuals who live in a community. The health of individuals is almost inseparable from the health of the larger community and the health of every community in every state determines the health of the nation (USDHHS, 2000c).

The *Healthy People* initiatives are even more important today than they were in the past; the work is not over. Progress toward meeting *Healthy People 2000* objectives indicates that only 15% of the objectives were met, 44% showed movement toward the objectives, and 18% evidenced movement away from the objectives (National Center for Health Statistics, 1999). One of the two overarching goals of *Healthy People 2010* is to eliminate health disparities. There is still racial, ethnic, gender, and socioeconomic inequality; many Americans still do not have sufficient health insurance; people are still homeless; and people are still chronically ill, such as those living with human immunodeficiency virus (HIV) and acquired immune deficiency syndrome (AIDS).

As a nation, the United States has a health care delivery system that boasts some of the best clinicians, hospitals, equipment, and health care facilities in the world (Kovner & Jonas, 1999). For Americans with excellent health insurance or sufficient finances, a wide range of providers and therapies are available to provide comprehensive health care. However, health services are expensive and unequally distributed. America's structural and financing systems for health care are complex and fragmented. The United States spends huge amounts of money on acute care and insufficient amounts on the promotion of health, the prevention of disease, and the provision of chronic care. The other major goal of *Healthy People 2010* is to increase the quality and years of healthy life. This goal can be met only by increased attention to health promotion, disease prevention, and care for people already suffering from chronic illnesses.

Nurses have a long tradition of involvement in health promotion beginning in the time of Florence Nightingale, when activities for health promotion ranged from individuals to communities and from personal care to political activism. Lillian Wald continued to address broad determinants of health to develop community partnerships for influencing health and social policy (Rafael, 1999). Nurses must "reclaim their legacy in health promotion, critically appraise outside influences that threaten to undermine their work, and educate the public and other disciplines about nursing's unique focus on health promotion" (Rafael, 1999, p. 23).

Nurses have a responsibility to understand the system in which they function, not only because of the influence the system has on their professional practice, but also because it has a considerable impact on individuals, the public whom they serve (Maurer, 2000b). Nurses need basic information about the health care system to make informed judgments about the effectiveness of the present system and the effect of suggested reforms (Maurer, 2000).

The health care delivery system in the United States is currently experiencing significant changes. A startling 1998 Institute of Medicine (IOM) study reported that medical errors cause more deaths per year than motor vehicle accidents, breast cancer, or AIDS (44,000 deaths per year) (Kohn, Corrigan, & Donaldson, 1999). The IOM Report concluded that the health care system, not bad practitioners, is the basic cause of this problem. Although health care is often equated with medical care, which focuses on the treatment of illness, this chapter presents the evolution and ongoing development of a broader concept of health based on the definition of health described in Chapter 1.

The complexities of the health care system necessitate an understanding of the system as a whole before focusing on the intermingled causative factors that have created a huge, fragmented enterprise. Many of today's problems have their roots in the decisions and directions of the past. It is not possible to identify and analyze current problems or to devise solutions without first exploring how the system developed to its present state.

The relevance of the split between preventive and curative measures is apparent when the organization and financing of the delivery system is examined. The United States has established a system that uses two basic divisions of society to provide service: the public sector and the private sector. The merger of public health and welfare policies in the public sector is rooted in the Puritan ethic inherent in the historical development of the United States. An understanding of the history and development of the health care delivery system enables the nurse to apply principles to daily care. The focus has shifted to community health care; therefore the nurse must be especially aware of the issues surrounding the developing health care system.

The current focus on managed care as both an organizational strategy and a financing mechanism is highlighted in a discussion of how health care is delivered and financed. This discussion includes the role of the nurse as an advocate in case management and advanced practice and as an influence on health policy development.

HISTORY OF HEALTH CARE

The beginnings of new epochs always go unnoticed. Regardless if the new era is one of light or darkness, it is only after dawn has brightened the sky or deep twilight has fallen that humanity fully comprehends the change that has occurred. Only then can people see in retrospect the point where they turned into a path of no return (Freyman, 1980, p. 381).

Early Influences

Historical records of early civilizations (Egyptian, Indian, Chinese, Aztec, and Greek) show that ancient peoples were concerned with disease and practiced various methods of treatment. The earliest views of health can be viewed as holistic in the sense of having a worldview. Primitive peoples understood illness in mystical terms; sickness and cure theories were tied to the cosmic view of life with natural and supernatural forces often inseparable.

Most of the indigenous peoples of the world practice personal hygiene as part of their religious worldview. For thousands of years, epidemics were viewed as divine judgments on human wickedness with a gradual awareness that pestilence has natural causes such as climate and other aspects of the physical environment.

In the Middle Ages, infectious diseases in epidemic proportions (leprosy, bubonic plague, smallpox, and tuberculosis) were the leading causes of death. A breakthrough in understanding the disease process did not occur until the development of bacteriology in the nineteenth century. In fact, it was not until the twentieth century that infectious diseases were mastered and were no longer the leading causes of death. Details of these influences, including a resurgence of infectious diseases, are presented in the remainder of this section. Clearly, health was viewed in terms of survival and absence of disease until these dreaded infectious diseases were conquered.

Industrial Influences

The population of the Western world began to increase in the 1600s when America was first being explored. The New World had many things to offer explorers. An adequate food supply made it possible for the population to live longer and advances in transportation made distribution of food supplies and other goods and services possible. The influence of manufacturing in the eighteenth century, through the invention of the flush toilet and cast-iron pipe, made sanitary engineering possible, saving many lives by preventing diseases such as typhoid, paratyphoid, and gastroenteritis.

Socioeconomic Influences

Although the Elizabethan Poor Laws (1601) in England provided a system of relief for the poor, which included infants, sick and elderly people, and laborers in the workhouses, a new Poor Law was enacted in 1834 based on the harsher philosophy that regarded pauperism among able-bodied workers as a moral failing. If the worker did not earn a subsistence-level income, then the attitude toward that worker was suspicious and punitive. These Poor Laws are the legal implementation of the Protestant work ethic that the Puritan forebears brought to the United States. People are held directly accountable for their state in life and health maintenance is the responsibility of the individual. The far-reaching implications of this ethic can be seen today in the organization, financing, and delivery of health services.

Public Health Influences

Edwin Chadwick (1800 to 1890) is known as the father of British and American public health. Chadwick established an English Board of Health, which emphasized environmental sanitation, but excluded physicians outside times of crisis. Additionally, he was secretary of the Poor Law Commission, which strove to improve the health of the masses for economic reasons. Chadwick's rationale was that disease among the poor was a major factor in their inability to support themselves. Therefore governmental health and welfare policies have joined in England since the nineteenth century.

In the United States, Lemuel Shattuck began the public health movement. He used the British system as the model, with public health services and welfare combined despite the contradictory emphasis. Public health has focused on improving the health of the poor, whereas welfare has dictated subsistence at the minimal level. The influence of the Puritan ethic on the American health care system is apparent in the emphasis on the value of work and the attitude toward the poor. Today, health and welfare departments continue their contradictory approach to the poor. (See the discussion of Medicaid later in this chapter.)

Scientific Influences

Until the twentieth century, epidemics of infectious disease (plague, cholera, typhoid, smallpox, and influenza) were the most critical health problems and major causes of death and disability for Americans. Scientific advances in the nineteenth century by Louis Pasteur (germ theory), Robert Koch (origin of bacterial infection), Joseph Lister (antisepsis), and Paul Ehrlich (chemotherapy) expanded public health from its earlier concentration on sanitation to control of communicable diseases through a broad biological base. Public health became a major force in decreasing death rates and increasing life expectancy through the application of bacteriology. Environmental conditions were improved by developing systems that safeguard water, milk, and food supplies; promote sanitary sewage disposal; and monitor the quality of urban housing.

The discovery and use of sulfonamides and antibiotics to treat bacterial infections between 1936 and 1954 reduced the death rate to its lowest point in history, with deaths caused by primary infections reduced to 4%, as compared with 33% only 50 years earlier. The death rate did not change significantly between 1954 and the mid1960s. Another decline in the death rate began after the mid1960s. This decline has continued with the exception of a slight increase in 1995. With the control of many infectious diseases and the increasing age of the population, chronic diseases such as heart disease and cancer are now the leading causes of death.

Despite the progress in conquering infectious diseases, for some age groups, infectious diseases are once again among the leading contributors to death in the United States. Diseases that were thought to be under control, such as measles and tuberculosis, are resurfacing and a new group of infectious diseases such as HIV/AIDS and Ebola have emerged. Emerging infectious diseases are those in which the incidence (or number of new cases during a specified time period) has increased significantly in the last two decades or is expected to increase. The incidence of AIDS in the United States rose alarmingly since general reports began in 1984: from an annual incidence of new cases of 1.88 per 100,000 people in 1984 to 40.20 per 100,000 people in 1993. Since that time, the incidence has declined somewhat to 27.20 per 100,000 people in 1995 (Clark, 1999). Combination antiviral therapy and primary prevention of opportunistic infections caused the number of deaths from AIDS to decrease 70% between 1995 and 1998 (CDC, 2000). Incidence rates for tuberculosis increased 20% between 1985 and 1992; in 1999, the incidence rate was more than six times the goal for 2010 (6.4 cases per 100,000 population; the goal is 1 per 100,000) (CDC, 2000).

Drug-resistant strains of organisms (*Staphylococcus aureus*, *Streptococcus pneumoniae*, and *Salmonella typhimurium*) that cause communicable diseases are on the rise. For example, drug-resistant tuberculosis, particularly among high-risk populations, including the homeless, drug abusers, and persons with HIV, has developed to near-epidemic proportions following the elimination of public health appropriations that funded tuberculosis therapy and follow-up for nonadherent populations. This tuberculosis epidemic is a dramatic example of how legislative cuts in funding have cost the nation in both human and financial terms (Mauer, 2000a).

Special Population Influences

The second goal of *Healthy People 2010* is to "eliminate health disparities among different segments of the population" including "gender, race or ethnicity, education or income, disability, living in rural localities, or sexual orientation" (*Healthy People 2010*, p. 17). For many of these disadvantaged people, the issues of preventing disease and promoting good health are often secondary to the problems associated with everyday survival. Additionally, according to the review of *Healthy People 2000*, "Americans who have disabilities, come from low-income families, or are members of minority groups continue to experience disproportionately worse health outcomes than other Americans" (Shalala, 1996). (See Multicultural Awareness box.)

The AIDS epidemic that began in the 1980s will still be a worldwide endemic problem at the end of the twenty-first century, because an effective vaccine has not been developed and successfully implemented worldwide. New, unimagined diseases will arise and, by definition, their effects will be completely unpredictable.

Political and Economic Influences

Political and economic considerations are basic to the health care system. **Politics** determines the decision makers who negotiate a desired outcome. Economics defines what resources are distributed and how they are distributed.

The effect of economics and politics on the delivery of health care is illustrated by the situation in the United States following the Great Depression. The emergence of Roosevelt's New Deal had an effect on health care, specifically in the passage of the Social Security Act in 1935, which authorized grants-in-aid to the individual states to improve state and local public health programs. Funds were available for "categorical assistance" programs, with cash grants first given to needy blind and elderly individuals and later to disabled persons. Medical care was an allowable budget item, but payments often went for food, shelter, or other needs. Additionally, the Social Security Act served as the basis for other assistance programs, such as Medicaid and Medicare, through subsequent amendments.

Split Between Preventive and Curative Measures

An orientation toward prevention has not been a part of the traditional medical education system because physicians were excluded from early public health policies and the nature of medical education. Hospitals have had a monopoly on clinical medical education since the eighteenth century (Freyman, 1980). Hospitals were concerned with the treatment of overt disease, with a focus on activity and observable effects; people attracted to clinical medicine then, as now, were "activists."

The division between clinical medicine and public health is reinforced further by the custom of payment for a measurable act or, in this case, the treatment of visible illness. Monetary value cannot be placed on these "intangibles" as preventive services. Additionally, the

MULTICULTURAL AWARENESS

Transcultural Values and Beliefs About Health Care

WHY DO NURSES NEED TO BE CULTURALLY COMPETENT?

As the demographics of the United States continue to become more diverse, nurses need to be culturally competent or to practice transcultural nursing. The assumption that people are independently oriented and should assume responsibility for caring for themselves is based on Western values of autonomy, self-reliance, individualism, and personal responsibility for health. Some of these Western values are incongruent with nonWestern or minority Western nonAnglo values. For example, cultures that are collectivist rather than individualist in orientation hold what Leininger (1997, p. 342) calls "other-care values" such as interdependence, interconnectedness, and interrelatedness among group members. Other-care values include viewing group needs as more important than those of the individual and promoting group responsibility for others. In some cultures, both group care and the inseparability of the environment and the individual are prominent values. Still other cultures value authoritarianism with specific rules about who has decision-making power or a deterministic view of the cause of illness with reliance on a higher power for matters of health and healing.

THE NURSE'S ROLE

Nurses need to support rather than interfere with family or group roles, challenge religious beliefs, or cause conflict with established lines of authority. For example, in many Middle Eastern countries, family members are expected to care for ill persons and the nurse's role is to educate and support family members. When these people are in the United States alone, they may not be receptive to nurses' attempts to promote their self-care skills (Meleis, 1997).

For nurses to be culturally competent, they must assess cultural values that will enable them to provide culturally congruent nursing care. Unless nurses examine individuals' basic values and beliefs about health and health care, they might assume that all cultures share Western premises and values. Without meaning to impose their values, nurses may unwittingly encourage a behavior that is not culturally congruent for individuals from other-care cultures (see Chapter 2).

Data from Leininger, M. (1997). Transcultural nursing research to transform nursing education and practice. *Image–the Journal of Nursing Scholarship*, 29 (4), 341-347; and Meleis, A. I. (1997). *Theoretical nursing: Development and progress* (3rd ed.). Philadelphia: Lippincott.

Hippocratic oath, the basic philosophy of Western medicine, designates the physician's primary responsibility to the individual. This belief may prevent or prohibit the physician from seeing the broader needs of society, even when these needs coincide with those of the individual.

The advances that conquered infectious disease involved a combination of social, educational, and medical efforts that integrated preventive and curative health care. Nevertheless, the shape of the current health care system stems from the 1850s, when separation of administration and staff for curative services (acute, chronic, and psychiatric illnesses) became the norm (Freyman, 1980).

The link between environmental health and personal medical care developed when **sanitarians** (persons who work to maintain a clean environment) realized that their efforts alone were not sufficient to prevent and cure the diseases of the population as a whole; improvement of personal health was also necessary. Early preventive services directed at individuals originated in medical practice rather than public health, but were limited to welfare medicine (caring for individuals through state programs) or to salaried medical practice in factories. Community health centers that developed in the United States before World War I limited their scope to prevention and health education and, with the exception of some prenatal clinics, were generally located in poor neighborhoods. The delivery of preventive services developed separately from clinical medicine and became associated with public health. The majority of physicians, educated in hospitals, were interested in individuals for whom prevention had failed and whose illnesses brought them to the hospital ward.

Despite the separation of preventive and treatment services, the benefits of prevention were eventually incorporated into clinical medicine for individuals. Preventive and early detection measures became a part of pediatrics and obstetrics in the early part of the twentieth century, when vaccines and vaginal cytology became available and accepted. Later in the twentieth century, internal medicine incorporated early detection of diseases such as diabetes, glaucoma, obesity, and hypertension. A shift to preventive medicine for the individual occurred, but the separate educational programs for public health and medicine still divided these areas. Not until the 1960s did the emphasis begin to turn from individual to societal values (Freyman, 1980). The United States' focus on individual change toward better fitness, stress management, nutrition, and self-administered health care must follow the focus of many other countries' health promotional efforts that call for changing the environment and health behaviors of individuals, families, and communities to promote health.

This new emphasis toward societal values parallels another evolution in the role of health in society. Increasingly, health care is regarded as a right rather than a privilege, with greater governmental involvement in and concern for the protection of that right. The future holds many more changes in the ongoing development of the role of health.

Access to health care is influenced by individual health needs, financial resources, and the health care delivery system. Each of these factors may be affected by the prevailing public policy of federal, state, and local governments. Technological developments, chronic illness,

Table 3-1 Traditional Organization of U.S. Health Care Delivery System

	Private Sector (Independent Practice)	Public Sector (Public Health Agencies)	
	Proprietary	Official	Voluntary
Source of money	Fee-for-service or salary	Taxes	Voluntary contributions or fee-for-service
Accountability	Individual	Citizens	Source of funds
Purpose, duties	Independent contractor operating within professional ethics	Prescribed or mandated by law	Free to experiment and support research

and the aging population each have an independent and interrelated influence on access to health care and the delivery of health services.

ORGANIZATION OF THE DELIVERY SYSTEM

The health care delivery system in the United States has been called a "multiplicity of health care systems (or subsystems)" (Torrens, 1999, p. 21). This complex interrelationship involves providers, consumers, and settings, with both private and public sectors providing services (Table 3-1). The public sector includes voluntary and nonprofit agencies and official or governmental agencies. Delivery of services is organized on three levels in both sectors: local, state, and national. Each of the three levels consists of private providers combined with official or voluntary public agencies. The nurse is often the professional who assists the health consumer through the complex delivery system; therefore a basic understanding of the system's organization is essential.

Private Sector

Independent Practice

Traditionally, a person enters the health care delivery system by contracting directly with a health care provider for individual care based on **fee-for-service.** Free choice of provider has been the hallmark. However, in recent years, more and more physicians are contracting for all or part of their practices with managed health care organizations, particularly independent practice associations (IPAs), **health maintenance organizations** (HMOs), and **preferred provider organizations** (PPOs) (Mezey, 1999).

Although private practice traditionally has been disease oriented, the current emphasis on primary care necessitates a much broader perspective. **Primary care** involves continual and comprehensive care that includes efforts to keep people as healthy as possible and to prevent disease. It is delivered in settings close to where people live and work.

Private care may be delivered in numerous settings, from inpatient (hospital or extended-care facility) to outpatient (ambulatory) settings; the latter is defined as any setting in which the individual is not a bed patient. Ambulatory settings include two major categories: (1) care provided by private physicians (and other providers, such as nurses) in solo, partnership, or private group practice on a fee-for-service basis and (2) organized settings that have an identity separate from the individual providers (Mezey, 1999). These categories overlap because many providers practice in their own offices and contract with one or more managed care organizations (see managed care discussion later in this chapter). Settings in the second category include hospital-based ambulatory services, such as clinics, walk-in and emergency services, hospital-sponsored group practices, and health-promotion centers; freestanding immediate care, same-day surgery, and emergency centers; health department clinics; neighborhood and community health centers; nursing centers; organized home care; community mental health centers; school and workplace health services; and prison health services (Mezey, 1999).

Nursing centers, organizations that give the individual access to professional nursing services, are "strategically positioned to improve the health and well being of vulnerable populations" (Kinsey & Buchanan, 2000, p. 361). Nursing centers trace their origin to the Henry Street Settlement, which was founded by Lillian Wald in 1893 to provide health teaching and nursing care to the sick poor in New York City (Murphy, 1995). The modern movement to establish nursing centers began in 1965 with the establishment of the nurse practitioner role, which allowed nurses to provide primary care to individuals. During the 1970s, university-based centers or academic nursing centers were established to provide nursing services to communities, learning experiences for students, and settings for faculty practice and research. The key components of a community nursing center include: (1) a nurse as chief manager, (2) nursing staff who are accountable and responsible for care and professional practice, and (3) nurses as the primary providers of care. The concept allows for an actual site for care, but may include implementation through nurse-managed services to individuals in their homes, community, hospital, nursing home, or any health care setting (Lockhart, 1995). Using a multidisciplinary collaboration framework, nurses have the opportunity to provide comprehensive primary care services, including a focus on wellness and health promotion; public health programs; and targeted interventions for special needs populations.

CASE STUDY

A Nursing Center

A nursing student is completing her clinical experience in a nursing center. She follows a pregnant diabetic adolescent and her family in the home and for visits with a nurse midwife and dietitian in the center. She has the opportunity to participate in holistic nursing care and observe the delivery of a healthy infant during her clinical stay.

Reflective Questions

1. Compare the philosophy and subsequent care that individuals receive in a nursing center with the illness care they receive in a more traditional outpatient setting.
2. What kind of a role might the nurse pursue within a nursing center after graduation?

The Council for Nursing Centers (CNC), established in 1988 within the National League for Nursing (NLN), promotes the mission and goals of nursing centers through educational programs, publications, research initiatives, and committee work (Murphy, 1995). Members of the CNC also provide mentoring and consultation to support colleagues in developing and advancing nursing centers. Nurses can continue to build community support, trust, and skills needed to make the nursing center model part of mainstream health care delivery in the twenty-first century (Kinsey & Buchanan, 2000).

Managed Health Care Organizations

Managed health care organizations provide for both the delivery and the financing of health care for their members. In fact, "managed health care in its various forms has become the dominant insurance vehicle in the United States" (Thorpe, 1999, p. 452). Overall, 75% of employees were insured through a managed care plan in 1995 (Ballit, 1997). The principal force behind the growth of **managed care** is the belief that health care costs can be controlled by "managing" the way in which health care is delivered.

The foundation of managed care organizations is the **primary care provider** (PCP), who may be a physician, physician's assistant, or nurse. Physician PCPs are usually general or family practitioners, but may also be internists, pediatricians, or obstetrician-gynecologists. Physician's assistants (PAs) are educated and prepared to work under the direct supervision of physicians. Nurses in advanced practice who provide primary care may be nurse practitioners (NPs) or certified nurse midwives (CNMs).

The PCP serves as a "gatekeeper" to coordinate and oversee individual care. The gatekeeper concept is designed to manage the individual's use of resources, to reduce self-referral to specialists, and to ensure coordination, not duplication, of services (Torrens & Williams, 1999). The major areas of cost containment focus on decreasing hospital admissions and costly procedures and limiting referrals to specialists. In fact, PCPs have assumed patient responsibilities previously conferred to specialists, contributing to the oversupply of specialists in some parts of the United States (Mezey, 1999). Box 3-1 provides a glossary of key terms used in managed care.

Box 3-1 A Glossary of Managed Care

Capitation: a preset payment received or paid based on membership rather than services delivered, usually expressed in units of per member per month (PMPM)
Case management: a method of coordinating care to improve continuity and quality of care and lower costs; occurs across a continuum of care
Gatekeeper: a primary care, case management model in which all care, except true emergencies, must be authorized by the primary care provider
HMO: health maintenance organization; the prototypical managed care structure. Encompasses two possibilities: a health plan in which providers assume some of the financial risk and a health plan that uses primary care providers as gatekeepers
IPA: independent practice association; an organization that contracts with a managed care plan to deliver services in return for a single capitation rate
Managed health care: a system that seeks to manage the cost of health care, the quality of that health care, and access to care
Managed competition: a system designed to control costs through competition rather than price controls. Organized groups of providers compete for clients by offering standardized benefit packages
Per diem: reimbursement based on a set rate per day rather than charges
POS: point-of-service; a plan in which members decide how to receive services at the time of service; combines HMO and indemnity features
PPO: preferred provider organization; a plan that contracts with independent providers for services at a discount
Primary care: basic health care that emphasizes general health needs rather than specialized care
PCP: primary care providers; physicians (family practitioners, internists, pediatricians, or obstetrician-gynecologists) or midlevel practitioners (physicians' assistants, nurse practitioners, or nurse midwives) who provide basic health care services
Utilization review: a system used to monitor diagnosis, treatment, and billing practices, the purpose of which is to lower costs by discouraging unnecessary treatment

Adapted from Kongstvedt, P. R. (1996). *The managed health care handbook* (3rd ed.). Gaithersburg, MD: Aspen.

Health Maintenance Organizations

HMOs deliver comprehensive health maintenance and treatment services for a group of enrolled people who pay a prenegotiated, fixed payment. The HMO accepts responsibility for the organization, financing, and delivery of health care services for its members. There are four different HMO models, the major difference being the relationship between the PCP and the fiscal agent (Thorpe & Knickman, 1999). The traditional HMO structure is a *staff model,* in which the fiscal agent employs salaried providers who generally spend all their time providing care to members of the HMO, such as Kaiser Permanente, which also has its own hospital. A *group structure* is a variation of the staff model in which a group of providers contracts with the fiscal agent to provide services. In the *network* and *IPA* models, multiple groups of providers contract with the fiscal agent to provide services to HMO members and to deliver services to nonHMO patients. Network-type HMOs contract with multiple provider groups and IPAs contract with providers in independent or multispecialty group practices to deliver services. Payment arrangements vary from a **capitation system** in which providers are paid a fixed amount per patient to a discounted per diem or per case reimbursement mechanism. Many studies have shown that staff and group models in particular reduce hospital use and total costs (Thorpe & Knickman, 1999).

Preferred Provider Organizations

PPOs, another delivery method in the private sector, are networks of providers who agree to deliver services for a discounted fee. In PPOs, the provider generally incurs no financial risk; the financial burden is on the patient rather than on the provider (Mezey, 1999). Patients may use providers outside the PPO, but must pay extra. The provider must receive prior permission from the PPO, for referral to a specialist and for hospitalization, or the PPO will not pay for the service (Mezey, 1999).

Point-of-Service Plans

Point-of-service (POS) plans combine features of HMOs with some of the individual-choice characteristics of traditional indemnity plans (Thorpe, 1999). As with HMOs, providers are paid through a capitation or risk-based system (see discussion under financing later in this chapter) and, as with PPOs, individuals can choose a nonplan provider by paying extra. For example, the plan may pay only 60% for a nonplan provider. Additionally, as with PPOs, the individual assumes the financial risk (Mezey, 1999).

Public Sector

The public sector contains official and voluntary public health agencies operating at the local, state, federal, and international levels. Health promotion and health protection or disease prevention receive greater emphasis in this sector than in the private sector.

Source of Power

The U.S. Constitution is based on the sharing of sovereign power between federal and state governments. The powers of the federal government in relation to health are not delineated specifically in the Constitution; they are derived from the financial authority to tax and to spend for the general welfare and from powers delegated to the government by the states, which reserve police power. Police power, the basis of the states' role in health, means that the states have the obligation and duty to protect the health, safety, and welfare of their citizens (Bonick, 2000). The state governor or legislature generally delegates police power to a specific health agency, usually the public health department. To protect citizens from the potential risk of contracting a disease, the public health officer can arrest an individual who has a communicable disease, such as tuberculosis, and refuses treatment. Police power also permits states to require the licensing of professionals who deal in the public sector, such as nurses, physicians, and beauticians.

State health authority is based also on the Tenth Amendment, which reserves for the states, or for the people, those powers not delegated to the federal government by the Constitution. The states then use their powers to create local governments and delegate authority to them in health.

Influence of Political Philosophy

The prevailing political philosophy of societal health needs affects the relationship among federal, state, and local governments, such as the 1930 New Deal philosophy. The trend toward increased federal government involvement continued during the Kennedy-Johnson era, when the government focused on societal needs and health care to an unprecedented degree. During the Nixon-Ford era, a New Federalism movement called for less federal encroachment into states' responsibilities and greater state and local responsibility related to the introduction of revenue sharing.

The Reagan-era version of New Federalism included procompetition and deregulation policies as a means of dealing with limited finances (see the financing discussion later in this chapter). Clearly, the federal government's role varies according to political philosophy.

During the 1989 to 1993 Bush administration, little change occurred in moving new legislation toward health care reform. During his 4 years in the Oval Office, President Bush worked toward two principal efforts: the Health Summit convened in 1991 and the report issued by the Social Security Advisory Commission. These efforts provided no concrete solutions for the deep-set problems endemic to the health care system.

In 1993, the Clinton administration proposed a health benefits package for all Americans that included a broad range of preventive services. A health care security card was to guarantee a comprehensive benefits package over the course of an entire lifetime, including coverage when individuals lost their jobs or changed jobs. Congress did not approve the legislation, but the portability of health care coverage bill was passed in 1996 (see discussion later in this chapter). When Clinton was reelected in 1996, the focus shifted to balancing the federal budget by 2002. Legislation included the Balanced Budget Act of 1997, which made significant reforms in Medicare (see discussion about Medicare later in this chapter).

Managed Competition

Although the Clinton health reform plan did not become reality, many changes in the health care marketplace occurred in response to or in preparation for the possible changes. Managed competition, the basis of the Clinton proposal, not only incorporated the coordinated delivery system of managed care, but also encompassed large purchasing groups of businesses, government employees, or individuals. The health care market, not the government, was the driving force behind these networks that were formed in major metropolitan areas. Health care providers and insurers positioned themselves for success under increasing competition and decreasing financial resources in the health care marketplace.

Future Health Policy

Forces that affect future health policy include some that are beyond the control of policy makers, such as the aging of the population, and some that are amenable to direct policy intervention, such as an increase in the supply of physicians and the use of an increasing number of new technologies in health care (Lee & Benjamin, 1999). Agreement on how to contain costs will be needed. Historically, the United States has used both regulation and competition, as discussed in the preceding section. Policy analysts predict that a hybrid of the two approaches to cost containment will continue because there is a "strong role of the private sector, a federalist system of government, the dominance of pluralistic politics" and a preference for gradual rather than drastic reform (Lee & Benjamin, 1999, p. 463).

Nursing's Role in the Search for Health Care Reform

The last decade of the twentieth century was one of great unrest for nurses. Major issues of rising costs, access to care, and accountability for the health care system are addressed in "Nursing's Agenda for Health Care Reform" (ANA, 1991) (Box 3-2). Emphasis on preventive health care rather than high-tech care is featured. Nurses in primary care focus on health promotion and disease prevention; therefore they are in a unique position to open the door to universal, affordable health care. The first major point in nursing's agenda is to provide primary care in convenient, familiar, community settings where individuals live and work, such as schools, work sites, and the home. (See ANA's proposal for universal Medicare later in this chapter.)

Box 3-2 Nursing's National Agenda for Health Care Reform

- Universal access to health care
- Empowerment of consumers
- Wellness and health as priorities
- Integration of public and private resources
- Managed care and primary health care as delivery models of care
- Efficient use of resources
- Direct consumer access to a variety of professional care providers, including nurses
- Mechanisms to protect against catastrophic costs and impoverishment

Reprinted with permission from American Nurses Association. (1993). *The reimbursement manual: How to get paid for your advanced practice nursing services*, Washington, DC, American Nurses Association.

Official Agencies

Official agencies are tax supported and therefore accountable to the citizens through elected or appointed officials or boards. The purpose and duties of official agencies are prescribed or mandated by law. This discussion is from the perspective of the individual gaining knowledge of or access to the health care system.

Local Level The **health department** of a town, city, county, township, or district is the local health unit and is usually the first line of access and health responsibility for the population that it serves. The chief administrator, the **health officer,** is appointed by the mayor, the board of health, or some other executive governing body.

The local health department's role and functions usually center on providing direct services to the public and depend on the state mandate and community resources. The usual range of functions includes basic categories of service that are detailed in Table 3-2.

Local governments, but usually not health departments, have the responsibility to provide general health care services for the poor (see the Medicaid section later in this chapter).

State Level Public health services are organized by each state, with wide variation from one state to another. The chief administrator is usually a state health officer or commissioner appointed by the governor. One agency, typically the state health department, carries out the primary responsibilities in policy, planning, and coordination of programs and services for local units under its jurisdiction.

Federal Level The federal government assumes overall responsibility for the health protection of its citizens. Although all three branches of the government make health-related decisions, the major policy decisions are made by the president and his staff (executive branch) and the congress (legislative branch). These two branches determine health policy. Once policy is determined, other government agencies are responsible for oversight to ensure the implementation of policies.

The U.S. Department of Health and Human Services (USDHHS) is the main federal body concerned with the health of the nation. A 1996 reorganization of USDHHS divided the agencies that were previously under the Public

Table 3-2 Local Health Department: Role and Functions

Category of Service	Basic Functions
1. Vital statistics	Record births, deaths, and reportable communicable diseases
2. Laboratory services	Provide testing: bacteriology, virology, and immunology
3. Communicable disease control	Detect chronic and metabolic disease
4. Environmental health and safety	Investigate outbreaks; maintain free clinics for immunization and early diagnosis and treatment of tuberculosis and venereal disease
5. Personal health services	Supervise food, water, and milk supplies, sanitary conditions in public eating places, and sanitary waste disposal; control water and air pollution; inspect health facilities
	Provide preventive maternal and child health (MCH) services (well-baby clinics, prenatal clinics) and adult health services (health inventories and surveys)
6. Public health education and information	Maintain public health nursing services and health education system, including preventive and rehabilitative services in chronic disease control
7. Research	Engage in research to promote the health of aggregates at risk and the community, such as morbidity, mortality, and program evaluation studies
8. Emergency and special medical services	Provide catastrophic health planning for emergency needs as well as medical care during a natural disaster or an epidemic and care for those involved in serious environmental accidents

Health Service (PHS) into separate individual agencies. The agencies within USDHHS and their major functions are presented in Box 3-3.

USDHHS agencies that relate directly to nursing include the Health Resources and Services Administration (HRSA) and the National Institutes of Health (NIH). The Bureau of Health Professions, within HRSA, contains a division of nursing, which is a source for nursing education and training grants. The National Center for Nursing Research (NCNR), established in 1986, became the National Institute of Nursing Research within the NIH in 1993. "One reason given in Senate testimony favoring the center was the health promotion and illness prevention focus in much of nursing research" (Clark, 1996, p. 41).

Box 3-3 Agencies Within the U.S. Department of Health and Human Services and Their Major Functions

Office of Public Health and Science (OPHS): assumes the prior administrative functions of the Public Health Service and contains the position of Surgeon General of the United States, an appointed position. The office is responsible for formulating and evaluating the *Healthy People* objectives

Health Care Finance Administration (HCFA): oversees the Medicare and Medicaid programs

Food and Drug Administration (FDA): establishes and enforces safe standards for foods, drugs, and cosmetics

Centers for Disease Control and Prevention (CDCP): investigates causes of disease; establishes policies and standards for the prevention, diagnosis, and treatment of health conditions; and provides information on diseases for all health care personnel

Substance Abuse and Mental Health Services Administration (SAMHSA): funds and coordinates programs for each related area, many of which are community based

Agency for Toxic Substances and Disease Registry (ATSDR): works to prevent health-related problems associated with toxic substances

Indian Health Service (IHS): provides health care services to the Native American populations

Agency for Healthcare Policy and Research (AHCPR): conducts research on health care services and delivery; this agency also produces and disseminates information about the quality, cost, and effectiveness of health care

Health Resources and Services Administration (HRSA): conducts health resource planning; funds education of health personnel; and administers the Indian Health Service, the Federal Bureau of Prisons, and the Bureau of Health Professionals

National Institutes of Health (NIH): funds and conducts research, including nursing research

With a budget that has increased from an initial $16 million in 1993 to nearly $90 million in 2000, nurses have increased opportunities to make significant research contributions, particularly related to health promotion (National Institute of Nursing Research [NINR], 2000).

Other departments that are involved in health care at the federal level include: (1) the Veterans Administration (VA), an independent agency directly under the president that provides health care services for four categories of veterans, and (2) the Department of Defense, which sponsors health care for active-duty military personnel. For military dependents and retirees, care is covered through the former Civilian Health and Medical Program for the Uniformed Services (CHAMPUS) insurance program, renamed TRICARE.

Departments engaged in health-related activities include the following:

1. U.S. Department of Agriculture (USDA), which pro-

Table 3-3 Voluntary Agencies, Foundations, and Professional Associations

	Voluntary Agencies	Foundations	Professional Associations
Types/examples	Focus on specific populations (American Red Cross, National Society for Prevention of Blindness, and National Association for Mental Health)	Rockefeller Foundation Ford Foundation	American Nurses Association (ANA), American Medical Association (AMA), American Hospital Association (AHA)
Purpose	Provide public and professional educational programs to improve services and quality of facilities and personnel	Provide support for research	Provide political influence, information, and a forum on current issues; support research and innovation
Financing	Contributions from individual citizens, business, and industry	Private philanthropy	Dues from individual members

vides inspection of and research on crops and animals and also provides food stamps
2. U.S. Department of Housing and Urban Development (HUD), which constructs facilities such as rural hospitals and neighborhood clinics
3. U.S. Department of Labor, which provides preventive services in the workplace through the Occupational Safety and Health Administration (OSHA)

The federal agency that has major accountability for control of the environment is the Environmental Protection Agency (EPA). Established in 1970 as an independent (nondepartmental) government agency, its responsibilities include quality and pollution control of air and water; control of solid waste disposal, radiation hazards, and toxic substances; and pesticide regulation. Functions of the EPA include conducting research on pollution control and the effects of pollution on humans, developing criteria and promulgating national standards for pollutants, and enforcing compliance with these standards.

Despite their need for health promotion and disease prevention, individuals with disabilities face numerous problems gaining access to health-promotion programs and preventive services. The barriers are financial, social, physical, and logistical.

Starting in 1992, health care providers, both as employers and as providers of public services, were required to comply with requirements of the Americans with Disabilities Act (ADA) of 1990. The ADA is considered the most sweeping civil rights legislation since the Civil Rights Act of 1964. The two parts of the ADA that apply most directly to health care providers are the prohibitions of employment discrimination and the requirements for provision of services to persons with disabilities. An example of health care provider accommodation is to install wheelchair lifts in their shuttle bus systems.

In 1990, President Bush signed the Patient Self-Determination Act, which took effect in December 1991. This law was designed to increase individual involvement in decisions about life-sustaining treatment, ensuring that advanced directives for health care are available to physicians at the time that medical decisions are being made and ensuring that individuals who have not prepared such documents are aware of their legal rights. As a condition of Medicare and Medicaid payment, the Patient Self-Determination Act requires health care facilities to have the following: (1) policies and procedures in advanced directives, (2) individual choice in the medical record, (3) individual facility policies and procedures, and (4) facility staff and community education about advanced directives.

International Level The World Health Organization (WHO), which was established as a specialized agency of the United Nations in 1948, directs and coordinates international health. WHO assists governments in strengthening health services, furnishing technical assistance, and encouraging and coordinating international scientific research.

Voluntary Agencies

The voluntary (not-for-profit) health movement, which began in 1882, stems from the goodwill and humanitarian concerns that are part of the nongovernmental, free enterprise heritage of the people of the United States. Powerful forces in the health field, voluntary agencies, foundations, and professional associations are nonprofit entities that maintain a tax-free status (Table 3-3).

Voluntary agencies are influential in promoting health affairs at the national policy level and often have significant influence on health legislation. Their prominent role in public influence was demonstrated by the American Cancer Society's early mass-media announcements about the health hazards of smoking. Additionally, voluntary agencies have stimulated research advances, such as in the development of the polio vaccine by Jonas Salk in 1954 for the prevention of paralytic poliomyelitis.

Philanthropic foundations provide valuable stimulation to the health field and operate under fewer constraints than do other sources in supporting research or training projects. Historically, foundations tend to be less formal in their review and grant procedures and provide support for untried research projects.

Nurses interested in research or advanced clinical study that relates to the special interests of voluntary agencies or foundations may find grant monies available to support their work. Most libraries, available online, contain references detailing specific grant interests and available monies.

Professional associations, organized at the national level with state and local branches, are powerful political forces. For example, the American Medical Association's role in legislation for comprehensive health insurance was in opposition to that endorsed by the American Nurses Association (ANA). Nurses can support their professional organizations (the ANA and the NLN) in influencing the direction of health policy through membership and active participation.

FINANCING HEALTH CARE

Costs

The health care industry is the largest service industry in the United States today (Koch, 1999). In 1997, national health expenditures in the United States totaled $1092 billion, an average of $3912 per person (Levit, Cowan, Lazenby, Sensenig, McDonnell, Stiller, & Martin, 2000). The United States spends far more on health care than any other industrialized country. (See comparison with Canada later in this chapter.)

As a share of the gross domestic product (GDP), national health expenditures rose from 5% in 1960 to 13.7% in 1993 (Levit et al., 2000). Although spending growth has remained relatively stable below 14% of the GDP from 1993 to 1998, projections from 1999 are for a gradual increase to 16.2% of the GDP in 2008 (Smith, Heffler, & Freeland, 1999). Health care analysts credit federal cost-containment measures with this relative "slowing" trend in the rate of increase in health care spending since 1991. (See the discussion of the prospective payment system and the Balanced Budget Act under Medicare later in this chapter.)

The growth in health expenditures, particularly since the onset of Medicare and Medicaid in 1965, is attributed quantitatively to three factors: (1) inflation of the economy in general, (2) medical inflation, and (3) increased "intensity" in health care services provided to patients (Koch, 1999). Some of the qualitative factors that have influenced the increase in health care costs include a growth in the proportion of the elderly, rising expectations about the value of health care services, government financing of health care services, the nature of third-party reimbursement, a lack of competition in the health care system to promote efficiency in the delivery of services, the maldistribution of health care providers, and particularly, the use of medical technology that has expanded the treatment of disease (Koch, 1999). For example, diagnostic and therapeutic techniques, including noninvasive imaging such as magnetic resonance imaging (MRI), cardiac surgery, organ transplantation, and operations on joints (particularly hips and knees) enhance the capabilities of medicine while increasing costs.

Changes in hospital care—more outpatient services, shorter inpatient stays, and more care of chronic illness than acute illness—mean that hospitals have less opportunity to offer prevention or health-promotion education to individuals. Moreover, workforce downsizing, especially in nursing, increased the use of nonprofessional caregivers and inadequate resources or reimbursement and may prevent health care professionals from offering the range of educational efforts called for in the *Year 2010 Objectives*, such as counseling in safety belt use, nutrition education, physical fitness regimens, and stress-coping skills.

Although most industrial countries in the world have adopted some version of a national health care system, the United States has relied on a free-market approach with the private sector, providing insurance coverage and providing for some of those people unable to pay for themselves. Increasingly since the 1980s, with less money available for health care, the nation's employers, who are generally the payers of health care costs, have experimented with different payment mechanisms, such as employee cost sharing, self-insurance, and alternative delivery systems. The effects of this influx of business into health care and the subsequent emphasis on competition to resolve the financial problems are still being realized.

National health expenditures for 1998 are shown in Table 3-4. The largest component is hospital care (33%), although hospital expenditures experienced declining growth between 1990 and 1998. Nearly all hospital care was financed by third parties, with about 6% paid by consumers out of pocket. Spending for professional services totaled 30% of national health expenditures, with physicians accounting for 20%, dental services almost 5%, and other professionals almost 6%. Approximately 16% of physician fees and half of dental fees were paid out of pocket. Another 3% went for home health care and almost 11% went for drugs and durable medical products. Of the nondurable products, two thirds of the expenditures were for drugs and one third for over-the-counter medicines and medical sundries. Durable medical products, such as eyeglasses, wheelchairs, and hearing aids, accounted for about 1% of the total expenditures, with almost 60% paid out of pocket. Spending for nursing home care accounted for nearly 8% of national health expenditures, with Medicaid funding about 46%, Medicare about 12%, and 42% coming from private funding, mostly paid out of pocket by patients or their families (Levit et al., 2000).

Sources

Ultimately, the American people pay for all U.S. health care costs. Money is transferred from consumer to provider by different mechanisms. The major sources are govern-

Table 3-4 National Health Expenditures by Type of Expenditure and Percentage of Total, Billions of Dollars, for Calendar Year 1998

Type of Expenditure	Total	Percentage
National health expenditures	1149.1	100.0
Health services and supplies	1113.7	96.9
Personal health care	1019.3	88.7
Hospital care	382.8	33.3
Physician services	229.5	20.0
Dental services	53.8	4.7
Other professional services	66.6	5.8
Home health care	29.3	2.5
Drugs and other medical nondurables	121.9	10.6
Vision products and other medical durables	15.5	1.3
Nursing home care	87.8	7.6
Other personal health care	32.1	2.8
Program administration and net cost of private health insurance	57.7	5.0
Government public health activities	36.6	3.2
Research and construction	35.3	3.1
Research	19.9	1.7
Construction	15.5	1.3

From Levit et al. (2000). Health spending in 1998: Signals of change. *Health Affairs, 19*(1), 124-132.
NOTE: Numbers are rounded; may not add to totals.

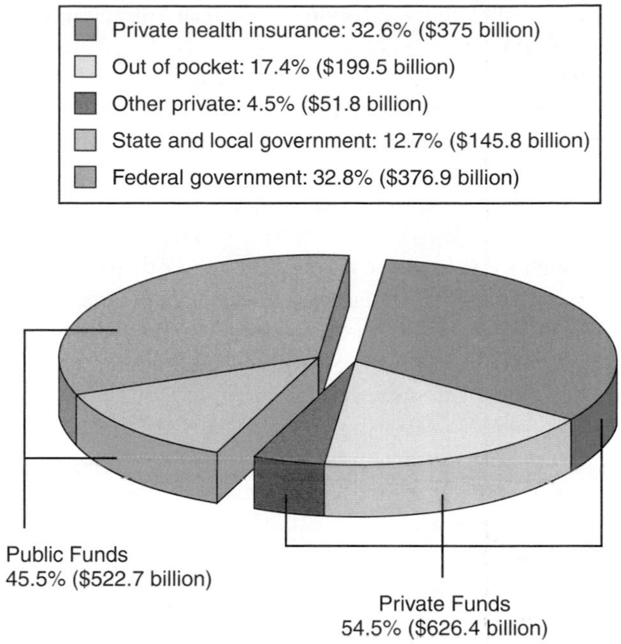

Fig. 3-1 Funding sources for health care in billions of dollars for 1998. (From Health Care Financing Administration, Office of the Actuary, National Health Statistics Group, 2000.)

ment, private insurance, independent plans, and out-of-pocket support (Thorpe & Knickman, 1999).

Figure 3-1 shows funding sources for health care in 1998. Private funding (54.5%) of health care expenditures exceeded that from the public sector (45.5%). Of the private sector's portion, private health insurance accounted for the largest segment, almost one third of all health expenditures. Consumers paid out-of-pocket for 17% and other private sources carried almost 5% of health costs. The federal government paid another one third of health care expenses and state and local governments accounted for almost 13%.

Since 1989, the private share of health care expenditures has increased at a faster pace than the public share. Premiums and benefits paid have increased despite that fact that employees covered by managed care plans accounted for 86% of all insured workers in 1998 (Levit et al., 2000). Enrollees choose from a preapproved list of providers in return for smaller premiums, copayments, and deductibles. The trend is away from HMOs to less restrictive plans, such as POS plans and PPOs (Levit et al., 2000). As the number of consumers enrolled in managed-care plans has grown, the breadth of insurance coverage to more fully cover preventive services has also increased.

Although the public sector's share of health care spending increased from the 1960s through the 1980s, primarily because Medicare and Medicaid costs rose, it has stabilized at approximately 42% of the total costs of health care. Medicare experienced rapid benefit-payment increases (at average annual rates of 13.7%) between 1969 and 1993, with some slowing in growth since that time (down to 2.5% in 1998). Despite the aging of frail older enrollees, Medicare spending in 1998 has experienced "the slowest growth on record" (Levit et al., 2000, p. 130). Medicare costs escalate in the last year of a person's life. This decline between 1994 and 1998 reflects three interacting factors: (1) limits legislated to restrain growth in Medicare payments to providers, including the Balanced Budget Act of 1997 (see further discussion under Medicare later in this chapter); (2) continuing government detection activities for fraud and abuse of Medicare; and (3) a slight slowing of growth in the Medicare population, which is predicted to rise again (Levit et al., 2000). Almost 16% of Medicare recipients were enrolled in managed care plans in 1998 (Levit et al., 2000).

Federal and state Medicaid spending showed an increasing pattern similar to that discussed earlier in this chapter with Medicare until recent years when spending growth rates have become more stable. Welfare-to-work requirements for persons covered under Temporary Assistance for Needy Families (TANF) (1997) was combined with strong job growth to decrease the number of Medicaid recipients (see further discussion of TANF under Medicaid later in this chapter). By 1998, more than half of persons receiving Medicaid, most of whom are poor children and their parents, were in some form of managed care (Levit et al., 2000). The largest share of Medicaid monies goes for institutional services. Namely, two thirds of its benefits go to hospitals and nursing homes. Medicaid is the largest third-party payer of nursing home care, paying about half of the total expenditures for nursing facilities.

Mechanisms

Payment

Although some health care providers and other professionals in the private sector are paid on a fee-for-service basis by individuals or third-party private or public-supported insurance, most health workers, including nurses in institutional or community agencies and in the military, receive salaries. Most nurses are salaried; therefore the separation of nursing costs from all other health-related costs is difficult. Without documentation of specific nursing costs, validating the need for skilled nursing services is also difficult.

In recent years, nurses—especially advanced practice nurses (APNs) nurse practitioners (NPs), clinical nurse specialists (CNSs), certified registered nurse anesthetists (CRNAs), and certified nurse midwives (CNMs)—have entered independent practice to provide direct services. Nurses who are academically prepared for advanced practice represent about 6% of all registered nurses (RNs). In 1998, there were approximately 78,000 NPs, 54,000 CNSs, 34,000 CRNAs, and 8000 CNMs in the United States (Kovner & Salsberg, 1999; Pearson, 2000).

A landmark study in an ambulatory care setting that randomly assigned patients to either NPs (part of Columbia Advanced Practice Nurse Associates, CAPNA) or physicians, confirmed what NPs and their patients have known for a long time: NPs provide effective, quality, primary care. NPs had the same authority, responsibilities, productivity, administrative requirements, and patient populations as physicians and, more importantly, patient outcomes were comparable (Mundinger et al., 2000).

The independent practice of nursing may be viewed as a logical outgrowth of seeking higher levels of professionalism. The Nurse Practice Acts of some states encourage nurses to use their knowledge more comprehensively than many agencies sanction. In independent practice, the nurse is directly accountable to individuals and is paid either directly or by third parties. The philosophical and realistic issues of private nursing practice range from questions about the equity of fee-for-service to the practical problems of setting up this type of practice. Independent practice's ability to become commonplace in nursing's future depends on decisions about reimbursement by third parties in both private and public sectors because reimbursement continues to be a restriction on practice. Although legislation in 1997 included the reimbursement of advanced practice nurses by Medicare, not all plans and provider groups include the use of these nurses as primary care practitioners. Maine passed legislation in 1999 that requires managed care organizations to permit NPs to become credentialed PCPs; other states should follow Maine's lead to give the public a choice of providers (Peters, 1999).

Alternative forms of payment are salary and capitation. The **salary system** involves a set amount for services provided in a specified time frame. This system provides the employer with a fixed nursing income that is protected from changes in supply and demand, includes fringe benefits, and obviates fee-collection problems. The salary system's flexibility makes it easier to fill unpopular jobs or jobs in underserved areas. Disadvantages of this system include a limit on income and constraints on schedules, vacations, and peer review. The nurse may have to meet goals other than personal ones.

In the capitation system, such as in an HMO, each provider receives a flat annual fee for each individual regardless of how often services are used. Individuals who enroll in an HMO pay a fixed amount on a monthly basis whether they use the services or not; prepayment provides an incentive to provide efficient care. The objective is to keep people healthy to prevent costly services. Cost consciousness dictates that illness be treated as early as possible and in the most cost-effective setting. Capitation is simple to administer; no third-party insurance payments are present and the HMO bears the risk of illness. Preventive primary care that deters the need for costly hospitalization keeps costs down and the savings revert to the organization. On the negative side, individuals may make unnecessary visits; the increased number of people necessary to provide more monies may decrease comprehensive care; and there may be limits to quality of care, services, and access to all types of providers.

Cost Containment

The government's interest in hospital treatment cost containment is exemplified by the passage of the Social Security Amendments of 1983 (PL 98-21), which mandate the establishment by the Health Care Financing Administration (HCFA) of a prospective payment system (PPS) for Medicare. This system means that providers are paid at preset rates based on 470 diagnosis-related group (DRG) categories that are used to classify the illness of each Medicare-insured person. Rates for each diagnosis are established according to regional and national amounts based on each hospital's urban and rural cost experience. Average hospital occupancy rates declined by nearly 11% between 1980 and 1990; since the mid-1990s, hospital use has stabilized (Levit et al., 2000).

The revolutionary PPS cost-containment mechanism was the first in a series of changes for the health care industry. The development of managed care plans provided a realignment of the nation's health care system. This variety of forms of prepaid and managed fee-for-service health care is designed to control the use and cost of health care. The intended effects of managed care are more comprehensive care for more people while containing both the use and costs of services. During the 1990s, restrictions on managed care programs have been lifted to allow conversion to for-profit plans. For-profit status allows these plans to contain their costs (Thorpe & Knickman, 1999). The effect on quality and access to care remains to be determined.

Another recent piece of legislation that targets cost containment is the Balanced Budget Act (BBA) of 1997, which also affected Medicare. The 1997 BBA reduced Medicare spending by limiting provider payments, increased options in the choice of managed care plans, and made medical savings accounts an option (Lee & Benjamin, 1999). (See further discussion with Medicare later in this chapter.)

An additional cost-containment method, known as case management, provides a major career opportunity for nurses (May, Schraeder, & Britt, 1996). Essential to the promotion of the health of individuals is an integration of financing, management, and delivery of health care in a continuously changing delivery system (Cary, 2000). Emphasis must be on health management across the continuum of health care delivery. As Medicaid and Medicare managed care systems continue to develop, demand for nurses to fill the case management role will continue.

Case management began through public programs with nurses in public health departments, social workers in public welfare systems, and caseworkers in mental health departments (Evashwick, 1999). Managed-care organizations rely on case management as one method to control costs, reduce inappropriate use of services, and improve quality of care. Case management takes numerous forms, but basic elements involve an individual who coordinates and monitors needed services in a supportive, effective, efficient, and cost-effective way (Cary, 2000). Basic case-management services are described in Box 3-4.

Depending on the case-management model used, services can be implemented in a broad or a narrow manner. For example, assessment broadly defined might include health needs and social and family needs; narrowly defined, assessment might focus solely on individual health concerns. Case managers are particularly important for persons with catastrophic or complex acute or chronic illnesses, disabilities, or injuries, or for members who may experience high risk, volume, cost, or use. The case manager must achieve a balance between cost and quality and must collaborate effectively with all care providers involved, both inside and outside the health plan and with the person's family, to ensure appropriate quality care. Pervasive problems faced by case managers include ethical and liability concerns, such as underservice and barriers to access and practice constraints, emanating from the labor-intensive, time-consuming, and costly nature of case management (Cary, 2000).

An individual with complex chronic health problems requires multiple services from different providers in a variety of settings. For example, under managed care, hospitalizations are reserved for individuals who are acutely ill and require complex technological care. Americans are admitted to hospitals later and sicker, with discharges earlier than ever before. This delayed entry and accelerated community reentry, whether to the home or to a rehabilitative or extended care facility, requires complex coordination of services and providers. The nurse is the key to efficient allocation of resources, coordinated care planning, and documentation of outcomes. To justify the costs associated with quality nursing care, nurses must not only ensure and document positive outcomes of their care, but also show that nursing care is a cost-effective means of achieving desired outcomes (May, Schraeder, & Britt, 1996).

Box 3-4 Case Management Services

1. *Assessment:* evaluating a person's physical, social, functional, psychological, and financial needs, including family situation
2. *Care planning:* setting goals, identifying specific services to meet individual needs, including how to allocate resources
3. *Service coordination and referral:* facilitating and coordinating access to needed providers
4. *Care monitoring and periodic reassessments:* evaluating progress, access to and use of services, and changes in needs

Managed Care Issues

Health care analysts describe several issues for managed care programs and the services they provide to their enrollees. Among these issues are consolidation of health plans, the effect on providers, conflicts of interest, and protection of the public (Torrens & Williams, 1999). As more and more health insurers merge, the tendency is for large organizations to exert more influence in controlling purchasers and payers and providers with subsequent lack of variation and choice in plans in addition to potential monopoly issues. Managed care has created new systems with groups of providers delivering care in more efficient ways. However, with an emphasis on providing fewer services, there may be less humane and compassionate personal care, the opposite of which has been a hallmark of the nation's health care system. Conflicts of interest among and between the many players in a managed care system in reducing the use of various services may affect patients who are unable to get needed services. (See Research Highlights box.)

Protection of the public has reached the legislation stage. Legislation mandating the number of days a woman may stay in a hospital after delivery and prohibiting

research highlights

Perceptions of Nurses, Physicians, and Consumers About Managed Care Experiences

NURSES AND PHYSICIANS

The Kaiser Family Foundation, a nonprofit, independent national health care philanthropy, surveyed nurses and physicians about their perceptions of patients' experiences with managed care plans. The majority of respondents cited one major positive and several negative influences.

The most positive influence of managed care on both nurses and their patients is the emphasis on and access to preventive services, which has always been an important focus for nurses. Nevertheless, the emphasis on short-term cost containment is sometimes at the expense of quality and long-term outcomes. Highlights of the survey's results were:

- Nearly 80% of the registered nurses (RNs) surveyed said that managed care has decreased the quality of care to sick patients
- Almost 50% of the RNs said that specific health plan decisions lead to declining health for patients, and two thirds of these nurses said these adverse decisions occur weekly or monthly
- 69% of RNs saw inadequate staffing as their primary concern
- 58% of physicians were concerned about increased administrative time

CONSUMERS

Consumer Reports surveyed 52,000 of its readers (not a representative sample) about their satisfaction with different types of health care plans comparing experiences of healthy people with those who considered themselves in either fair or poor health. The Kaiser Family Foundation, in conjunction with *Consumer Reports,* surveyed a nationally representative sample of 2500 consumers under the age of 65 in any kind of health plan, focusing on specific ways consumers tried to resolve problems with their health plans.

In both of these consumer surveys, most people rated their health plans highly overall. The results highlighted some important concerns:

- Sick people face obstacles getting appropriate treatment from managed care plans; the more restrictive the plan, the more problems were reported
- Three quarters of the consumers who contacted their plans complained about billing concerns; consumers in health maintenance organizations (HMOs) found lower costs and reported fewer billing concerns than those in preferred provider organizations (PPOs)
- 51% of consumers surveyed by Kaiser reported some problem with their plan during the past year; although most problems were resolved, 40% of consumers with problems said they paid more for treatment or services than expected and 20% said their health declined as a result
- A majority of respondents to the Kaiser survey reported that it would be helpful to be able to appeal health plan decisions to an independent medical expert; although more than 30 states have an appeals process, few consumers were aware of it or had used it (see discussion of Patient's Bill of Rights legislation in this chapter)

Data from Anonymous. (2000). Is an HMO for you? *Consumer Reports, 65* (7), 38-41; Kaiser Family Foundation. (1999). *A view from the bedside: A survey of doctors and nurses on their patients' experiences with health plans.* Menlo Park, CA: The Author; Stewart, M. (1999). Survey highlights nurses' concerns about health care. *The American Nurse, 31* (5), 3.

outpatient mastectomy surgery for breast cancer are two specific examples (Torrens & Williams, 1999). Patient's Bill of Rights proposals have common efforts to restore control over health care decision making to patients and their providers (Angell, 2000). Some versions include language that would allow patients to sue their managed care companies. The argument against this stipulation is that lawsuits would tend to increase costs for the managed care companies, which will be passed along to employers; employers may then decide to reduce or drop health care coverage and indirectly increase the number of uninsured. These bills also provide for appeal mechanisms when services are denied, for treatment in hospital emergency departments when patients believe it is essential, and for referral decisions to be made by providers and patients rather than health plans and employers.

Nurses must be **advocates** to ensure that people receive quality care. The ANA adopted three resolutions related to managed care, namely, to preserve the health care practitioner and therapeutic relationship, to advocate for the rights of individuals enrolled in health plans, and to examine compensation methods that threaten to diminish standards of nursing practice (Canavan, 1996). An information resource for consumers is the National Committee for Quality Assurance's (NCQA) Quality Compass, which is a national database of comparative information about the quality of managed care. Through this database, consumers and employers can compare information such as accreditation status, regional and national averages, and other aspects of various managed care plans' quality measures (Canavan, 1996). (See the Health Teaching box for suggestions for teaching individuals about resources to evaluate managed care plans.)

Health Insurance

Positive elements of the health care system in America were mentioned in the introduction to this chapter—excellent clinicians, health care facilities, and equipment—all of which are available to people with good health insurance or adequate finances (Kovner & Jonas, 1999). The U.S. system exhibits a high degree of technological change and innovation and excellent information, quality, and cost-accounting systems. Financial outlays for education of health care workers; products such as drugs, medical

HEALTH TEACHING Access Health Care Information from the Internet

Mary Jones, age 38, and her family are new in a primary care clinic. Mary asks the nurse for advice in choosing a health plan that will best meet the needs of her growing family. Mary is 4 months pregnant with her third child. She and her husband, Joe, work for a state agency that provides multiple health plan choices. Joe, age 48, has many of the symptoms of coronary artery disease. Their son Billy, age 8, is an asthmatic, and their daughter Laurel, age 4, has Down's syndrome.

The nurse discusses Mary's family's general health promotion and protection needs and the special needs presented by the specific diseases that have been identified. She provides some specific resources for Mary to learn more about the specific plans available in her area. The Jones' have a computer at home and are eager to access the websites you have suggested.

From the Agency for Healthcare Research and Quality (AHRQ), a federal government agency with health information for consumers:

- http://www.ahrq.gov/consumer/hlthpln1.htm: provides guidelines to consumers in choosing and using a health plan
- http://www.ahrq.gov/consumer/qualguid.pdf: "Your Guide to Choosing Quality Health Care" is a comprehensive consumer reference for choosing health plans, physicians, treatments, and hospitals

From the Foundation for Accountability (Facct), a foundation to assist the public in understanding health care quality and making informed choices:

- http://www.facct.org/measures.html: provides quality measures for selected clinical conditions, such as asthma

From the National Committee for Quality Assurance (NCQA), a nonprofit organization that assesses and reports on the quality of managed care plans:

- http://www.ncqa.org/pages/communications/publications/brotext.htm: provides guidelines for consumers in choosing a health plan

From HealthCareReportCards.com:

- http://www./healthcarereportcards.com/index.cfm: provides data on hospital performance, such as rankings for coronary bypass surgery

Data from above websites; Oermann, M., & Huber, D. (1999). Patient outcomes: A measure of nursing's value. *American Journal of Nursing*, 99 (9), 40-48.

equipment, and supplies; and research is second to no other country (Kovner & Jonas, 1999). In 1999, the health care system covered approximately 84% of Americans through health insurance (Thorpe & Knickman, 1999).

This high level of quality does not deny the problems with the system. More than 44.3 million people, or 16.3% of the population, do not have health insurance (O'Grady, 2000). (See the discussion of the uninsured later in this chapter.) These people receive health care, but they do so through the back door of the health care system (the emergency room door), which is the most inefficient and most costly way of providing care.

Health care forecasters and strategists predict that the Internet will change the health system. From its beginnings as an "experimental, Defense Department funded, secure data network," the Internet has become a new "social institution" (Goldsmith, 2000, p. 148). Predictions are that the Internet will accelerate the "virtualization" of health care plans and systems and help with the clerical aspects of caregiving and insurance. Consumer access to information is an ongoing benefit. Privacy concerns and professional resistance are two areas that remain to be solved (Goldsmith, 2000).

Insurance refers to individual payment to a fund to provide protection for each contributor against financial losses resulting from an unlikely but possible occurrence. Medical insurance began in this tradition in 1847, with payments made to offset income lost as a result of an accident. Sickness benefits began as an extra benefit and again emphasized the loss of income. Blue Cross and Blue Shield originated the reimbursement of general health care costs in the 1930s.

The term insurance is really a misnomer because health care is often required and is not a rare occurrence. Assurance is the term used in England to mean coverage for expected happenings (life assurance), whereas insurance covers unexpected happenings, such as fire and theft.

Private Health Insurance

The private health insurance industry in the United States has changed dramatically since the growth of managed care and the consolidation of health plans (Thorpe & Knickman, 1999). Conventional indemnity fee-for-service insurance accounted for less than 15% of employees and 86% of all insured workers were covered by some kind of managed care plan in 1998 (Levit et al., 2000). Managed care approaches to control costs range from measures such as second surgical opinion, preadmission certification review, and length of stay reviews to measures to transfer some of the cost to the enrollee through deductibles and coinsurance costs (Thorpe & Knickman, 1999).

In the private sector, the following five types of organizations provide health care insurance:

1. The traditional insurance companies (including the earliest insurer, Blue Cross and Blue Shield, a nonprofit charitable organization) and for-profit commercial insurance companies
2. PPOs acting as "brokers" between insurers and health care providers
3. HMOs, which are independent prepayment plans

4. POS plans, which combine features of classic HMOs with patient choice characteristics of PPOs
5. Self-insurance and self-funded plans in which either the employer takes on the role of insurer or the enrollee sets up a trust account with tax savings

Traditionally, private insurers charged employers or individuals annual premiums and provided services on a fee-for-service basis. Organized at the state and local level, Blue Cross and Blue Shield generally complement each other, with Blue Cross reimbursing hospitals and Blue Shield covering physicians and other providers. After World War II, insurance companies began to provide health insurance plans in competition with Blue Cross and Blue Shield. Today, more than 800 commercial, profit-making insurance companies, such as Metropolitan Life and Aetna, offer policies that cover hospitalization and in-hospital or office-based physician care, major medical expenses directed primarily at catastrophic illness, or cash payments as a flat sum of money per day of hospitalization. Fewer insurers every year offer insurance coverage for individuals, which is extremely expensive. They contract with employers to offer group plans (Whitted, 1999). Much of the individual insurance sold today is "supplementary," such as that designed to supplement Medicare. Known as *Medigap*, these plans reimburse only deductibles and coinsurance payments associated with Medicare.

The PPO, essentially a fee-for-service arrangement, acts as a "broker" between private insurers and health care providers. Enrollees, who incur either lower premiums or a waiver of cost-sharing requirements, use providers who agree to give price discounts to the insurer (Thorpe & Knickman, 1999).

HMOs attempt to lower health care costs by emphasizing preventive rather than curative care, possibly decreasing the severity of some illnesses. Outpatient care is the focus, with lower hospitalization rates than in the fee-for-service area, almost entirely as a result of lower admission rates. HMOs tend to use fewer services, with emphasis on the least costly means of providing a needed service.

POS plans enable enrollees to choose, at the point of service, whether to use the plan's provider network or seek care from nonnetwork providers. Typically, network providers are paid on a capitated or discounted-fee basis, and nonnetwork providers are paid on a fee-for-service basis. Coinsurance (about 30%) and deductibles (about $300 per year) for nonnetwork providers are high, to dissuade enrollees from choosing this option (Thorpe, 1999).

Another change in the structure of the insurance industry is the growth of self-insured or self-funded plans. **Self-insurance** means that an employer (or union) assumes the claims risk of its insured employees, whereas *self-funding* refers to paying insurance claims from an established fund, such as a bank account or trust fund. Self-insurance gives employers a financial advantage, including an exemption from state taxes on health insurance premiums and interest earnings on reserves before claims payment (Thorpe & Knickman, 1999). Approximately two thirds of firms with 200 or more employees were at least partially self-insured for their employees' health care costs in 1996 (Thorpe & Knickman, 1999).

Public Health Insurance and Assistance

Medicare Medicare is a federal insurance program that provides funds for medical costs to people who are 65 years of age and older and certain people younger than 65 who are disabled. Federal Medicare legislation, Title XVIII of the amendments to the Social Security Act, went into effect in 1966 after decades of debate. The intent was to protect older adults against the catastrophic financial debts often incurred in treating chronic illness. This was the first time that federal legislation was enacted to remove financial barriers to medical care for the elderly. In 1983, Medicare added hospice benefits during the last six months of life to cover services for the terminally ill, of whom nearly 72% are over the age of 65 (Evashwick, 1999). Hospice is based on a philosophy that views death as a normal part of the life cycle and emphasizes living the remainder of life as fully and comfortably as possible. Additionally, Medicare pays about two thirds of hospice care, which is less costly than hospital services (Evashwick, 1999).

Since 1973, two groups of disabled persons under the age of 65 have also been eligible to receive Medicare benefits: persons who are totally and permanently disabled and who qualify for Social Security and those who require hemodialysis or kidney transplantation.

Medicare, Part A, financed by payroll taxes under the Social Security system, covers care rendered in a hospital, an extended-care facility, or a person's home (Table 3-5). Medicare, Part B, is supplementary voluntary medical insurance supported by general tax revenues and by the subscriber or person buying the insurance covers health care provider's services and other medical expenses. Approximately 98% of older adults are enrolled in Part A and 95% of those enrolled in Part A also opt for Part B (Koch, 1999) (see Table 3-5).

Neither Part A nor Part B of Medicare offers comprehensive coverage. Inherent in the program are deductibles, set amounts that the individual must pay for each type of service before Medicare begins to pay, and coinsurance, a percentage of charges paid by the individual. There are also limitations on the amount of coverage. For example, hospital benefits end after 90 days (with a lifetime reserve of an additional 60 days) and extended-care facility benefits last a maximum of 100 days.

Except for end-stage renal disease (ESRD) and some diabetes monitoring (discussed later in this chapter), Medicare does not provide for catastrophic chronic illness. Additionally, continual health needs such as routine physical examinations, vision care (including

Table 3-5 Medicare Insurance-Covered Services for 2000

Services	Benefit	Medicare Pays	You Pay
PART A: HOSPITAL			
Hospitalization			
Semiprivate room and board, general nursing and miscellaneous hospital services and supplies	First 60 days 61 to 90 days 91 to 150 days* Beyond 150 days	All but $776 All but $194 All but $388 a day Nothing	$776 $194 a day $388 a day All costs
Inpatient mental health	190-day lifetime limit		
Skilled Nursing Facility Care			
Semiprivate room and board, skilled nursing and rehabilitative services, and services and supplies (after a 3-day hospital stay and within 30 days after discharge)†	First 20 days Additional 80 days Beyond 100 days	100% of approved amount; All but $97 a day Nothing	Nothing $0.97 a day All costs
Home Health Care			
Medically necessary skilled care	Part-time or intermittent care for as long as Medicare conditions are met	100% of approved amount 80% of approved amount for durable medical equipment	Nothing 20% of approved amount for durable medical equipment
Hospice Care			
Pain relief, symptom management and support services for the terminally ill	If the hospice option is elected and as long as doctor certifies need	All but limited costs for outpatient drugs and inpatient respite care	Limited cost sharing for outpatient respite care
Blood	Unlimited if medically necessary	All but first 3 pints per calendar year	For first 3 pints‡
PART B: HOSPITAL			
Medical Expenses			
Doctors' services, inpatient and outpatient medical and surgical services and supplies, physical and speech therapy, ambulance, diagnostic tests, and more	Medicare pays for medical services in or out of the hospital if medically necessary	80% of approved amount (after $100 deductible)	$100 deductible§ plus 20% of approved amount and limited charges above approved amounts
Outpatient mental health services		50% of approved amount	50% of approved amount‖
Clinical Laboratory Services			
Blood tests, biopsies, urinalyses, and more	Unlimited if medically necessary	100% of approved amount	Nothing for service
Home Health Care			
Medically necessary skilled care	Part-time or intermittent skilled care for as long as conditions for benefits are met	100% of approved amount 80% of approved amount for durable medical equipment	Nothing for services 20% of approved amount for durable medical equipment
Outpatient Hospital Treatment			
Services for the diagnosis or treatment of illness or injury	Unlimited if medically necessary	80% of approved amount (after $100 deductible)	$100 deductible plus 20% of billed charges

From U.S. Department of Health and Human Services, Health Care Financing Administration. (2000b). *Your Medicare handbook*. Washington, DC: U.S. Government Printing Office.

*This 60-reserve-days benefit may be used only once in a lifetime.

†Neither Medicare nor private Medigap insurance will pay for most nursing home care.

‡To the extent that the blood deductible is met under one part of Medicare during the calendar year, it does not have to be met under the other part.

§Once you have had $100 of expenses for covered services in 1996, the Part B deductible does not apply to any further covered services you receive for the rest of the year.

‖If your doctor does not accept assignment.

Continued

Table 3-5 Medicare Insurance-Covered Services for 2000—cont'd

Services	Benefit	Medicare Pays	You Pay
Blood	Unlimited if medically necessary	80% of approved amount (after $100 deductible starting with fourth pint)	First 3 pints plus 20% of approved amount for additional pints (after $100 deductible) 2000 Part B monthly premium: $45.50 (premium may be higher if you enroll late)

From U.S. Department of Health and Human Services, Health Care Financing Administration. (2000b). *Your Medicare handbook*. Washington, DC: U.S. Government Printing Office.

eyeglasses), medication, dental care, and private-duty nursing care are not provided through Medicare. Furthermore, custodial care, whether at home or in a nursing home, is not covered. This is the most costly and financially catastrophic service.

The limits in Medicare coverage mean that older adults pay a substantial portion of their health care costs beyond the expected 20%, especially when they have a chronic illness. Dissimilar to most private insurance, Medicare does not include an annual limit on out-of-pocket spending (Thorpe & Knickman, 1999). The main population at risk, the elderly, may have limited financial access to preventive health services such as periodic examinations or screening for early detection of other diseases such as high blood pressure and glaucoma.

Quality and cost of care have been issues for Medicare for more than 25 years. Numerous pieces of legislation and Medicare amendments have attempted to solve various aspects of the cost and quality concerns.

The Tax Equity and Fiscal Responsibility Act (TEFRA) of 1982 established a case-based reimbursement system, namely DRGs, which was designed to provide cost-containment incentives. Subsequently, in 1983, Title VI of public law 98-21 established a PPS for paying inpatient services for Medicare patients. This legislation also encouraged growth in the number of HMOs and other comprehensive plans enrolling Medicare beneficiaries. Although the PPS system has slowed the growth of inpatient hospital Medicare spending, the growth in outpatient spending continues to rise (Thorpe, 1999).

In 1988, Congress passed the Medicare Catastrophic Act, designed to expand Medicare to shield beneficiaries from catastrophic hospital and physician's costs related to acute illnesses. Although new benefits for long-term care were not provided, the bill included coverage for outpatient prescription drugs. In 1989, before it could be implemented, this bill was repealed as a result of pressure from older adults who objected to the legislation's financial approach. Costs of the program were passed on to the elderly as new premiums and income-related surcharges connected to their federal income tax (Fig. 3-2).

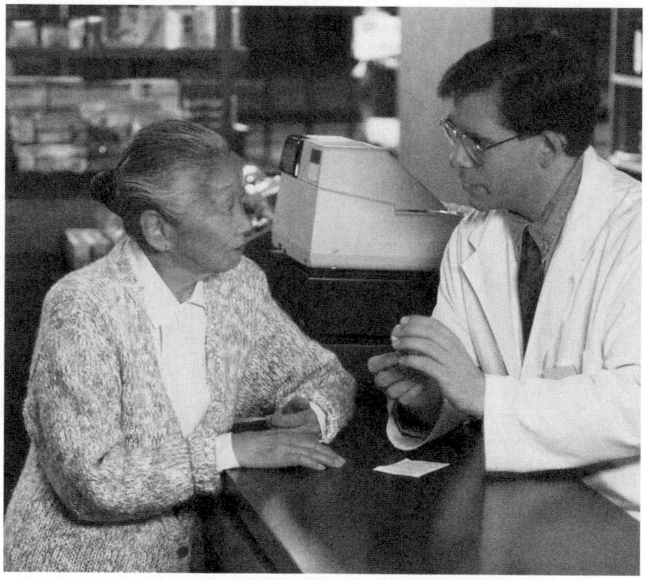

Fig. 3-2 Cost of prescription medication for the elderly can be a substantial portion of their out-of-pocket expense.

In the Omnibus Reconciliation Act (OBRA) of 1989, Medicare revised its payment scheme for physicians. First, a new payment system that went into effect in 1992 assigned relative values to services based on the time, skill, and intensity required to provide them. Second, a limit was set on the amount that physicians could charge individuals above the amount that Medicare pays. This restriction was designed to limit growth of Medicare costs for physician payments.

The BBA of 1997 included *Medicare+Choice*, which offers the option of managed care plans such as HMOs, POS plans, PPOs, or private fee-for-service plans in which the enrollee pays extra when costs for care are higher than Medicare rates. Additionally, medical savings account (MSA) plans are available whereby Medicare pays a health insurance policy putting money into an MSA. Enrollees use

Table 3-6 Comparison of Medicare and Medicaid

Type of Program	Medicare (Title XVIII)	Medicaid (Title XIX)
Source of money	Insurance Part A—Social Security tax Part B—tax revenues and voluntary premiums	Assistance General tax revenues
Level of administration	Federal (same in all states)	Federal and state (varies from state to state)
Eligible people	1. People over age 65 2. Those qualifying for disability under social security 3. People of any age with kidney disease requiring dialysis or transplant	Required: Categorically needy people who receive either of the following (must apply): SSI (Supplemental Security Income) TANF (Temporary Assistance to Needy Families) Optional: Medically indigent person unable to pay for medical care (must apply)
Services	Part A 1. Hospital insurance (compulsory) 2. Posthospital care—ECF (extended care facility) 3. Home health services Part B—voluntary (optional) medical insurance 1. Physicians' services 2. Outpatient hospital services 3. Home health services 4. Other medical services	1. Inpatient and outpatient hospital care 2. Prenatal care 3. Physicians' services 4. Nursing facility services for persons age 21 and older 5. Home health services 6. Family planning services 7. Rural health clinic services 8. Laboratory and radiologic tests 9. Pediatric and family nurse practitioner and nurse midwife services 10. Certain federally qualified ambulatory and health center services 11. EPSDT (early and periodic screening, diagnosis, and treatment) for people under age 21 12. Optional services according to state's choice

the MSA and their own money for care (up to a certain amount per year); when that amount is reached, the insurance covers all Medicare-approved expenses for the rest of the year. If an enrollee has money in the MSA at the end of the year, then the amount is rolled over for the next year (USDHHS, 2000a).

The BBA of 1997 added several new preventive services to the Medicare benefit package. These services included coverage for screening tests for breast, cervical, vaginal, prostate, and colorectal cancer; bone mass measurements; diabetes monitoring and diabetes self-management; and influenza, pneumonia, and hepatitis B vaccinations.

The missing Medicare benefit that is causing great concern currently is outpatient prescription drugs. Americans aged 65 and over account for over one third of all drug spending, but represent only about one eighth of the population (Deets, 2000). Although some HMO plans provide this benefit for seniors, less than 16% of seniors were enrolled in managed care plans in 1998 (Levit et al., 2000). Of the average 19% of older adults' out-of-pocket income ($2430) spent on health care in 1999, 17% of that amount was for prescription drugs (Deets, 2000).

Medicaid Medicaid is an assistance program managed jointly by the federal and state governments to provide partial or full payment of medical costs for categories of individuals and families of any age who are too poor to pay for the care. Medicaid legislation, Title XIX of the amendments to the Social Security Act, went into effect in 1967. The federal government provides funds to states on a cost-sharing basis, with 50% to 83% from the federal government and the remainder from the state, according to the per capita income of each state, to guarantee medical services to eligible Medicaid recipients (Clemen-Stone, McGuire, & Eigsti, 1998). Table 3-6 compares Medicare and Medicaid.

People eligible for Medicaid are those who receive Supplemental Security Income (SSI) and TANF (see discussion of welfare reform). Additionally, Medicaid pays the Medicare premiums, deductibles, and coinsurance for certain low-income Medicare recipients (Koch, 1999). Medicaid is not automatic, as was the case in the past; people must apply for Medicaid.

States administer Medicaid under broad federal requirements and guidelines. Each state establishes its own eligibility standards; determines the scope, type, duration, and amount of services to be provided; sets the rate of payment; and administers its own program. Programs vary widely from state to state in terms of covered services.

For a list of basic health services mandated, see Table 3-6. Included are inpatient and outpatient care; laboratory and radiologic services; prenatal care; family planning services and supplies; rural health clinic services; federally qualified ambulatory and health center services; physician services; nurse-midwife, pediatric and family nurse practitioner services; home health care for persons eligible for skilled nursing services; skilled nursing facility services for people 21 years of age and older; and early and periodic screening, diagnosis, and treatment (EPSDT) of people under 21 years of age. Other services, such as dental care, eyeglasses, or intermediate care facility services, may be added at the state's option.

The EPSDT provision signified the federal government's recognition of the need for primary prevention and health promotion. The emphasis on prevention rather than treatment—the focus of this text—was a positive approach toward health and required the development and implementation of new methods of health care delivery. The EPSDT program has five phases: (1) outreach and case findings, (2) screening, (3) testing, (4) compiling and reporting of results, and (5) follow-up and treatment.

State Medicaid programs must cover all pregnant women and children up to 6 years of age with family incomes less than 133% of the federal poverty level; children below 100% of the poverty level who are age 12 or younger (all poor children under age 19 will be covered by 2002); poor families who lose cash assistance resulting from work earnings (for a transition period); for a 12-month period, two-parent families whose principal wage earner is unemployed; and disabled persons losing eligibility from work earnings (Thorpe & Knickman, 1999).

States have looked to managed care to lower their Medicaid costs. In 1998, more than one half of all Medicaid recipients were in some type of managed care plan, most using the HMO model (Levit et al., 2000). As the number of Medicaid beneficiaries in managed care increases, the effect of these changes must be monitored to determine access to and quality of care for low-income individuals.

Several states are participating in the Robert Wood Johnson model program of purchasing long-term care insurance to protect a specific amount of money. Once the insurance monies are paid out up to that amount, the insured individual qualifies for Medicaid. This program is considered an attempt to cut Medicaid costs for long-term care of individuals over the age of 65.

Traditionally, states determine Medicaid eligibility, covered benefits, and provider-payment mechanisms; therefore Medicaid programs have varied widely from one state to another and may be inadequate to meet the health care needs of covered individuals. The previously discussed legislation that separated Medicaid from the receipt of cash assistance, such as covering low-income pregnant women and children, is meant to produce greater uniformity in Medicaid. However, each state still determines its Medicaid budget and optional services based on its financial status. Despite the program expansions and the fact that Medicaid is the largest program that provides health care services to the poor, it covers only 40% of individuals with income below the poverty level (Thorpe & Knickman, 1999).

Passage of the welfare reform bill in 1996 (Personal Responsibility and Work Opportunity Reconciliation Act of 1996, PL 104-193) reveals a significant philosophical shift in federal thinking about welfare assistance in the United States. For the first time, Medicaid is not linked directly to welfare programs. Ending a 61-year guarantee of federal aid, the TANF program (formerly Aid to Families with Dependent Children [AFDC]), established by this legislation, provides temporary financial aid with a 5-year lifetime limit. Legal immigrants who arrive in the United States after the passage of this bill must wait 5 years to become eligible for programs. The aim is to help parents to become self-sufficient through welfare-to-work programs. Some states have changed the name of their official department of social services (Family Independence Agency) to reflect the change in philosophy from dependency to temporary assistance (Clemen-Stone et al., 1998). As welfare changes dramatically, there is concern about an increase in health disparities among Americans and restriction of resources for children, especially in states with high rates of immigration such as California and Texas. Changes in Medicaid eligibility resulted in an increased number of uninsured (O'Grady, 2000).

The Uninsured

The number of Americans without health insurance of any kind increased 23% between 1979 and 1995; between 1997 and 1998, the number of uninsured Americans increased by one million to a total of 44.3 million people or 16.3% of the population (O'Grady, 2000). The lack of health insurance is greatest for Hispanics and Blacks, younger Americans (18 to 34 years of age), persons with low educational attainment, men more than women, and particularly persons living in the South and the West (Koch, 1999). The majority of the uninsured have at least one family member who is working full time; over one half have family incomes of less than 200% of the federal poverty level (about $33,000 for a family of four) (O'Grady, 2000). Even among the 20% of uninsured who have access to employer-sponsored health insurance, they are unable or unwilling to obtain coverage because the cost of premiums are high (O'Grady, 2000). The highest numbers of the uninsured work in retail, service, construction, and agriculture jobs, with much higher rates among small employers and the self-employed (Billings, 1999). Without solutions, the projection is for the number of uninsured to increase to 55 million by 2010 (O'Grady, 2000).

The uninsured incur increased health risks because they delay care more than three times the rate of people with coverage. They more often need hospital treatment that

HOT topics

MEDICARE FOR ALL AMERICANS?

The American Nurses' Association (ANA) voted at their 1999 House of Delegates meeting to support a single-payer system that would establish health care as a right. The ANA is committed to the idea that all Americans are entitled to accessible and affordable quality health care services. Their 2000 proposal was for a Universal Medicare program, based on the improvement and expansion of Medicare into a universal, seamless program of health coverage for all Americans. The ANA chose to modify the Medicare program because it is "a tested model of social health insurance" that has worked well to ensure coverage for the elderly, permanently disabled, and ESRD patients for more than 30 years (ANA, 2000, p. 5). The proposal *improves* Medicare by providing a shift from illness-focused care to care that addresses the continuum of American health care needs, with an emphasis on prevention and primary care; it *improves* Medicare by including an outpatient prescription benefit, a major economic burden for many Medicare recipients, particularly older adults; and it *expands* the mental health benefits to make them the same as physical health benefits (no lifetime limit, copayments of 20% rather than the current 50%). Additionally, during the phase-in period, children would be the first priority. All children under age 19, regardless of income, would be covered immediately.

Initially, the program would be financed through a payroll tax, general fund revenue, and a trust fund consisting of employer contributions based on existing premium amounts. Then, over a 3-year period, a financing system would be phased in based on payroll taxes and general fund revenues along with limited beneficiary coinsurance requirements. Medicaid would continue, at least initially, to be the primary payer for long-term care.

Questions:

- Is health care a right or a privilege?
- Is the United States ready for universal health care?
- Is a single-payer system, such as Canada's, the best plan?

Data from ANA. (2000). *Achieving access for all Americans: A proposal from the ANA for health coverage 2000* [On-line]. Available: http://www.ana.org/readroom/rwjpaper.htm.

could have been avoided, are more often diagnosed with cancer in a later stage, and more often increase their likelihood of dying in a hospital more than three times the rate of people with health insurance (O'Grady, 2000). Without health insurance, low-income families must rely on a frequently fragmented and difficult-to-use public system of health care. Regular preventive care, including prenatal care, immunization, and well-child care, is sometimes difficult to obtain; and its availability may not be adequately understood. Only when families do not have to make a choice between food on the table and a visit to the doctor or clinic will adequate care for families most at risk be provided.

A plan that targets poor, uninsured, nonMedicaid-eligible children is included as a provision of the BBA of 1997, which established the State Children's Health Insurance Program (CHIP). Implemented at the state level, these programs have experienced problems with lower than expected enrollments, which may be a result of a lack of awareness of the program, eligibility requirements, or other unknown factors (ANA, 2000). (See the Hot Topics box for a discussion of the ANA's plan to expand Medicare coverage to all Americans.)

Another step toward addressing part of the problem for the uninsured and underinsured was the passage of the Health Insurance Portability and Accountability Act (HIPAA) (PL 104-191) in 1996, which took effect in 1997. The portability provision means that individuals with health insurance who lose or leave their jobs can maintain insurance coverage even when they are sick. However, cost may be a prohibitive factor because it does not deal with premium costs. Insurers are also prohibited from refusing coverage based on an individual's health status, although limited waiting periods may apply. Additionally, the bill addresses a project that allows individuals in small firms, uninsured individuals, or self-insured individuals with high-deductible plans to set up a tax-exempt MSA. This MSA allows tax deductions for long-term care insurance premiums and for qualified, nonreimbursed home health and long-term care services; it allows the terminally ill earlier access to earnings built up in life insurance policies without tax penalties; it establishes fraud and abuse guidelines; it provides liability coverage for medical volunteers who provide free medical care to low-income individuals in medically underserved areas; and it mandates that USDHHS develop regulations and standards for the electronic transfer of medical information, confidentiality, and a unique health identifier (Calcagno, 1996; Crowley, 1996). One of the most costly and complicated changes for health care companies to comply with HIPAA is to design interactive data systems that allow the transfer of health data while maintaining patient confidentiality (Goedert, 2000).

THE CANADIAN HEALTH CARE SYSTEM

The Canadian universal coverage and single-payer system has been cited by some health care analysts as a model that the United States should adopt. Contrary to what some in the U.S. health care industry would suggest, Canada does not have "socialized medicine." Medicare, Canada's health care system, is simply a social insurance plan similar to Social Security and Medicare for older people in the

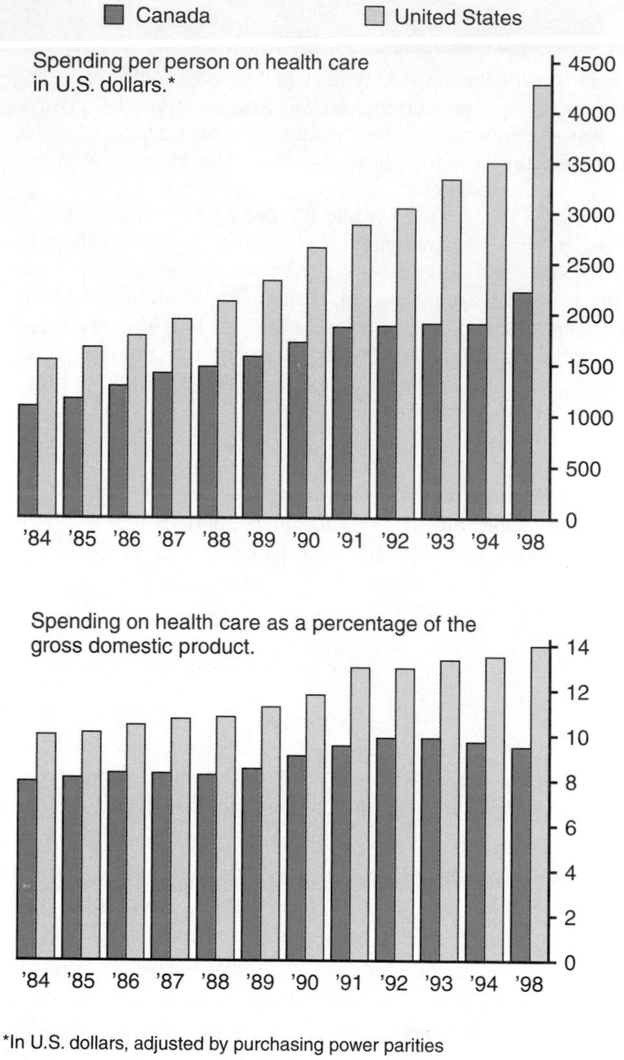

Fig. 3-3 Comparison of the health care spending in Canada and the United States. (From Organization for Economic Cooperation and Development [OECD], Health Data, [1999]. In G. Anderson, J. Hurst, P. Hussey, & M. Hughes (Eds.), [2000]. Health spending and outcomes: Trends in OECD countries, 1960-1998. *Health Affairs, 19* [3], 151.)

United States. Physicians practicing in Canada do not work on salary for the government, but are paid on a fee-for-service basis as in the United States.

Canadians pay for health care through a variety of federal and provincial taxes, just as Americans pay for Social Security and Medicare through payroll taxes (Fig. 3-3). The government of each province pays the medical bills for its citizens with matching federal funds. Because the government is the primary payer of medical bills, Canada's health care system is referred to as a single-payer arrangement. Benefits vary somewhat among the provinces, but most cover—in addition to hospital care, medical care, long-term care, and mental health services—all prescription drugs for people over age 65. Private insurance exists only for services not covered by the provincial plans. Although each province runs its own insurance program as it sees fit, all are guided by the five principles of the Canada Health Act, as shown in Box 3-5. (See the Hot Topics issue about ANA's plan to expand Medicare coverage to all Americans.)

Box 3-5 Five Principles of the Canada Health Act

1. *Universality:* everyone in the nation is covered
2. *Portability:* people can move from province to province and from job to job or onto the unemployment roles and still retain their health coverage
3. *Accessibility:* everyone has access to the system's health care providers
4. *Comprehensiveness:* provincial plans cover all medically necessary treatment
5. *Public administration:* the system is publicly run and publicly accountable

INFLUENCING HEALTH POLICY

The primary responsibility of the nurse is to the individual, family, group, or community served. A major portion of the nurse's role is to advocate not only for the individual, but also for justice in health care delivery. Nurses need to be aware of issues that have an effect on the health of the American people and to know how to work for needed change.

Health cannot be separated from its environment; therefore it is essential that nurses become involved in all aspects of planning for health to maximize the health potential of all Americans. This involvement needs to include attention to policy decisions and political action. Policy affects the broader aspects of environment, the biophysical and socioeconomic conditions of homes, schools, workplaces, communities, and the health care delivery environment. By virtue of their numbers, nurses, who make up the largest group of health care providers in the United States, have tremendous potential to influence decision making.

Participating in **policy decision making** requires the nurse to take a proactive stance to determine needs before a problem arises. Policy development and change take place on many levels from within the nurse's agency or work group to the community, state, and national levels. At the institutional level, clinical decisions influence policy as do management issues. The nurse should examine the rationale behind an existing or planned policy and determine whether or not it is relevant now. Nurses are empowered by their education and experience to use their people skills and to apply change theory to influence policy development and change.

Much health-related decision making is the result of legislation at the local, state, or national level. **Laws,** rules enforced by a ruling authority by which society is governed, and **regulations,** agency or department rules developed for the implementation of laws, define what services are being offered to whom and who will pay how much. Politics, the use of power to promote a needed change, is an arena for nursing's participation that is part of this nation's democratic heritage. The nurse can be politically involved in many ways. Voting, after becoming well informed on current issues and candidates, is a major way for nurses to be actively involved. The nurse should get to know the politically influential people in the community and disseminate information learned from them to others.

The nurse can run for political office (many nurses now represent their local constituencies and they have increasing visibility at the state and national levels) and support colleagues who represent nursing's interests. Financial contributions to Nurses for Political Action Coalition (N-PAC), ANA's political arm, increase the power base of nurses. Membership in professional and community groups provides the nurse with a collective voice to influence legislators. ANA's Nurses Strategic Action Team (N-STAT) network is an organized grassroots effort by nurses to help elect ANA–PAC-endorsed candidates and to inform members of Congress about policy issues of concern to nurses. When nurses join N-STAT, they receive *Action Alert and Legislative Update*, detailing specific legislative issues to enable them to be adequately informed and to respond to legislators in a timely manner.

Legislators are influenced by the information that they receive and the source of that information. Nurses have a wealth of knowledge about health care that legislators need to know. The process of trying to persuade legislators to vote for or against measures important to the interest group represented is called **lobbying.** A **lobbyist** is a registered representative of a special interest group. The ANA, located in Washington, DC, employs nurse lobbyists. The lobbyists need to receive input from nurses individually and as a group. The ANA website contains valuable information about current issues and initiatives important to nurses and links to other websites that contain specific legislative information.

A legislator can be approached personally or via telephone, telegram, electronic mail (e-mail), or regular mail. Legislators have staffs of experts in the applicable areas of their involvement, and each legislator is assigned to certain committees. To understand the legislative process, the nurse needs to follow the progress of a bill. It is essential that nurses become politically aware and active to enable the collective voice of nursing to reach its full potential.

It is the responsibility of nurses to become and remain well informed. As well-informed, empowered professionals, nurses play a significant role in supporting appropriate legislative initiatives that promote and protect the health of the public.

SUMMARY

The health care delivery system in the United States is dynamic, characterized by continuous change and activity. Most of the time it changes slowly, but when significant dissatisfaction with the system occurs, there "exists a window of opportunity for substantive change to occur" (Maurer, 2000, p. 54). Nurses need to be involved in these changes to be proactive; they need to understand the complexity and diversity of the health care system to be able to educate individuals about health care resources and to coordinate services. To accomplish this task, nurses need to become and remain well-informed citizens and health care consumer advocates.

A historical perspective and a description of the present health care delivery system in the United States provide a framework for the analysis of trends, values, and needs related to health. Comprehensive health services exist in the United States, but they are fragmented, unequally distributed, and extremely expensive. Although there is more emphasis on health promotion with health policy attention to its importance in *Healthy People 2010*, the current system continues to concentrate on the delivery and financing of illness care. The real purpose of health care—the promotion of health—needs to be incorporated into the delivery of health care for all Americans. The delivery system needs to move beyond a focus on short-term, episodic disease patterns that were predominant in the first half of the twentieth century and instead to conquer the problems that predominated during the second half of the century and into the twenty-first century. Current and future health problems are chronic in nature, requiring long-term continual delivery and financing mechanisms. A change in emphasis and direction is needed.

The U.S. government provides the legal underpinnings for protecting and controlling the environment for health and delivery of health care services through the enactment of laws and the regulation of financing for the system. Social policy, as a reflection of society's values, has changed from a laissez-faire approach in the 1850s to one in which the central federal government has a prominent role in organizing and financing health care since the 1970s. Health care became a major political issue in 1991 and is likely to remain an issue until the problems of health care cost containment and universal access to health care are solved. Other major industrialized nations have managed to provide universal health care insurance and to control costs. The American public is becoming increasingly dissatisfied with the present system of health care financing and the costs of care. Although cost containment was the primary concern in the 1990s, quality is paramount in this new century. To address both cost and quality is the challenge for the future.

The issue of inequitable access to health care "will not be resolved in the predictable future" (Hofmann, 1999, p. 476). Rationing of health care occurs "silently, insidiously, sporadically, and arbitrarily" (Hofmann, 1999, p. 476). Health care is rationed based on numerous factors: ability to pay; age, in the Medicare program; income, marital status, and having dependent children, in the

Medicaid program; employment; insurance status; type of disease (for example, Medicare covers end-stage renal disease); and geography, for rural and inner-city Americans (Hofmann, 1999). Future decisions will determine how scarce resources are to be distributed.

REFERENCES

American Nurses Association. (1991). *Nursing's agenda for health care reform*. Washington, DC: American Nurses' Association.

American Nurses Association. (2000). *Achieving access for all Americans: A proposal from the ANA for health coverage 2000* [On-line]. Available: http://www.ana.org/readroom/rwjpaper.htm.

Anderson, G., Hurst, J., Hussey, P., & Hughes, M. (2000). Health spending and outcomes: Trends in OECD countries, 1960-1998. *Health Affairs, 19* (3), 150-157.

Angell, M. (2000). Patients' rights bills and other futile gestures. *New England journal of Medicine, 342* (22), 1663-1664.

Anonymous. (2000). Is an HMO for you? *Consumer Reports, 65* (7), 38-41.

Ballit, M. H. (1997). Ominous signs and portents: A purchaser's view of health care market trends. *Health Affairs, 16* (6), 85-88.

Billings, J. (1999). Access to health care services. In A. Kovner, & S. Jonas (Eds.), *Jonas and Kovner's health care delivery in the United States* (6th ed., pp. 401-438). New York: Springer.

Bonick, J. (2000). Policy, politics, and the law. In M. Stanhope, & J. Lancaster (Eds.), *Community and public health nursing* (5th ed., pp. 177-199). St. Louis: Mosby.

Calcagno, A. (1996, Oct.). Kennedy-Kassebaum is signed into law (PL 104-191). *Vital Signs*, p. 5.

Canavan, K. (1996, Oct.). Nursing addresses troubling trends in managed care. *The American Nurse*, p. 1.

Cary, A. H. (2000). Case management. In M. Stanhope, & J. Lancaster (Eds.), *Community and public health nursing* (5th ed., pp. 380-99). St. Louis: Mosby.

Centers for Disease Control and Prevention, National Center for HIV, STD, and TB Elimination, Division of HIV/AIDS Elimination. (2000). *HIV/AIDS surveillance reports* [On-line]. Atlanta: The Author. Available: http://www.cdc.gov/hiv/stats/hasrlink.htm.

Centers for Disease Control and Prevention, National Center for HIV, STD, and TB Elimination, Division of TB Elimination. (2000). *TB surveillance reports* [On-line]. Atlanta: The Author. Available: http://www.cdc.gov/nchstp/tb/surv/surv.htm.

Clark, M. J. (1996). *Nursing in the community* (2nd ed.). Stamford, CT: Appleton & Lange.

Clark, M. J. (1999). *Nursing in the community: Dimensions of community health nursing* (3rd ed.). Stamford, CT: Appleton & Lange.

Clemen-Stone, S., McGuire, S., & Eigsti, D. G. (1998). *Comprehensive community health nursing* (5th ed.). St. Louis: Mosby.

Crowley, S. L. (1996). New law protects workers from losing health coverage, *AARP Bulletin, 37* (8), 6.

Deets, H. (2000, Feb.). Medicare drug coverage: It's smart medicine. *AARP Bulletin*, 28.

Evashwick, C. J. (1999). The continuum of long-term care. In S. J. Williams, & P. R. Torrens (Eds.), *Introduction to health services* (5th ed., pp. 295-348). Albany: Delmar.

Freyman, J. G. (1980). *The American health care system: Its genesis and trajectory*. Huntington, NY: Krieger.

Goedert, J. (2000). The dawn of HIPAA: What the Health Insurance Portability and Accountability Act means to you. *Health Data Management, 8* (4), 84-106.

Goldsmith, J. (2000). How will the Internet change our health system? *Health Affairs, 19* (1), 148-156.

Hofmann, P. B. (1999). Ethics in health care. In A. Kovner, & S. Jonas (Eds.), *Jonas and Kovner's health care delivery in the United States* (6th ed., pp. 474-502). New York: Springer.

Kaiser Family Foundation. (1999). *A view from the bedside: A survey of doctors and nurses on their patients' experiences with health plans*. Menlo Park, CA: The Author.

Kinsey, K., & Buchanan, M. (2000). The nursing center: A model of community health nursing practice. In M. Stanhope, & J. Lancaster (Eds.), *Community and public health nursing* (5th ed., pp. 360-379). St. Louis: Mosby.

Koch, A. L. (1999). Financing health services. In S. J. Williams, & P. R. Torrens (Eds.), *Introduction to health services* (5th ed., pp. 113-150). Albany: Delmar.

Kohn, L., Corrigan, J., & Donaldson, M. (1999). *To err is human: Building a safer health system*. Institute of Medicine. Washington, DC: National Academy Press.

Kongstvedt, P. R. (1996). *The managed health care handbook* (3rd ed.). Gaithersburg, MD: Aspen.

Kovner, A., & Jonas, S. (1999). Introduction: The state of health care delivery in the United States. In A. Kovner, & S. Jonas (Eds.), *Jonas and Kovner's health care delivery in the United States* (6th ed., pp. 3-6). New York: Springer.

Kovner, C., & Salsberg, E. (1999). The health care work force. In A. Kovner, & S. Jonas (Eds.), *Jonas and Kovner's health care delivery in the United States* (6th ed., pp. 64-115). New York: Springer.

Lee, P., & Benjamin, A. E. (1999). Health policy and the politics of health care. In S. J. Williams, & P. R. Torrens (Eds.), *Introduction to health services* (5th ed., pp. 439-65). Albany: Delmar.

Leininger, M. (1997). Transcultural nursing research to transform nursing education and practice. *Image–the Journal of Nursing Scholarship, 29* (4), 341-347.

Levit, K., Cowan, C., Lazenby, H., Sensenig, A., McDonnell, P., Stiller, J., Martin, A., & the Health Accounts Team. (2000). Health spending in 1998: Signals of change. *Health Affairs, 19* (1), 124-132.

Lockhart, C. A. (1995). Community nursing centers: An analysis of status and needs. In B. Murphy (Ed.), *Nursing centers: The time is now*. New York: National League for Nursing Press.

Maurer, F. A. (2000a). Communicable diseases. In C. M. Smith & F. A. Maurer (Eds.), *Community health nursing: Theory and practice* (2nd ed., pp. 523-570). Philadelphia: Saunders.

Maurer, F. A. (2000b). The U.S. health care system. In C. M. Smith, & F. A. Maurer (Eds.), *Community health nursing: Theory and practice* (2nd ed., pp. 53-90). Philadelphia: Saunders.

May, C., Schraeder, C., & Britt, T. (1996). *Managed care and case management: Roles of professional nursing*. Washington, DC: American Nurses Publishing.

Meleis, A. I. (1997). *Theoretical nursing: Development and progress* (3rd ed.). Philadelphia: Lippincott.

Mezey, A. P. (1999). Ambulatory care. In A. Kovner, & S. Jonas (Eds.), *Jonas and Kovner's health care delivery in the United States* (6th ed., pp. 183-205). New York: Springer.

Mundinger, M., Lane, R., Lenz, E., Totten, A., Wei-Yann, T., Cleary, P., Friedewald, W., Siu, A., & Shelanski, M. (2000). Primary care outcomes in patients treated by nurse practitioners or physicians: A randomized trial. *Journal of the American Medical Association, 283* (1), 59-68.

Murphy, B. (1995). *Nursing centers: The time is now*. New York: National League for Nursing Press.

National Center for Health Statistics. (1999). *Healthy people 2000 review, 1998-1999*. Hyattsville, MD: Public Health Service.

National Institutes of Health, National Institute of Nursing Research. (2000). *Strategic planning for the 21st century* [On-line]. Available: http://www.nih,gov/ninr/a-mission.html.

O'Grady, E. (2000). Access to health care: An issue central to nursing. *Nursing Economics, 18* (2), 88-90.

Oermann, M., & Huber, D. (1999). Patient outcomes: A measure of nursing's value. *American Journal of Nursing, 99* (9), 40-48.

Pearson, L. (2000). Annual legislative update: How each state stands on legislative issues affecting advanced practice nurses. *The Nurse Practitioner, 25* (1), 16-28.

Peters, S. (1999, Dec.). Medicare, medicaid, managed care. *Advance for Nurse Practitioners*, 25-28.

Rafael, A. (1999). The politics of health promotion: Influences on public health promoting nursing practice in Ontario, Canada from Nightingale to the nineties. *Advances in Nursing Science, 22* (1), 23-39.

Shalala, D. (1996). *Healthy People 2000: Mid-course review and 1995 revisions*. Washington, DC: U.S. Department of Health and Human Services.

Smith, S., Heffler, S., Freeland, M., & the National Health Expenditures Projection Team. (1999). The next decade of health spending: A new outlook. *Health Affairs, 18* (4), 86-95.

Stewart, M. (1999). Survey highlights nurses' concerns about health care. *The American Nurse, 31* (5), 3.

Thorpe, K. (1999). Health care cost containment: Reflections and future directions. In A. Kovner, & S. Jonas (Eds.), *Jonas and Kovner's health care delivery in the United States* (6th ed., pp. 439-473). New York: Springer.

Thorpe, K., & Knickman, J. (1999). Financing for health care. In A. Kovner, & S. Jonas (Eds.), *Jonas and Kovner's health care delivery in the United States* (6th ed., pp. 32-63). New York: Springer.

Torrens, P. R. (1999). Historical evolution and overview of health services in the United States. In S. J. Williams, & P. R. Torrens (Eds.), *Introduction to health services* (5th ed., pp. 3-35). Albany: Delmar.

Torrens, P. R., & Williams, S. J. (1999). Managed care: Restructuring the system. In S. J. Williams, & P. R. Torrens (Eds.), *Introduction to health services* (5th ed., pp. 151-170). Albany: Delmar.

U.S. Department of Health and Human Services, Health Care Financing Administration. (2000a). *Choices under Medicare, 2000*. Washington, DC: U.S. Government Printing Office.

U.S. Department of Health and Human Services, Health Care Financing Administration. (2000b). *Your Medicare handbook*. Washington DC: U.S. Government Printing Office.

U.S. Department of Health and Human Services. (2000c). *Healthy people 2010: Understanding and improving health*. Washington, DC: U.S. Government Printing Office.

Whitted, G. (1999). Private health insurance and employee benefits. In S. J. Williams, & P. R. Torrens (Eds.), *Introduction to health services* (5th ed., pp. 171-203). Albany: Delmar.

Chapter 4

JUNE ANDREWS HOROWITZ

The Therapeutic Relationship

objectives

After completing this chapter, the nurse will be able to:

- Describe the process of values clarification.
- Examine the elements and process of communication.
- Analyze differences between functional and dysfunctional communication.
- Apply knowledge of values clarification and communication to the development of the helping relationship.
- Develop strategies to promote the therapeutic relationships with a diverse population across clinical settings, contexts, and nursing roles.
- Understand the significance of the therapeutic relationship in all aspects of clinical practice.

key terms

15-Minute Interview
Body Motion or Kinetic Behavior
Communication Process
Countertransference
Empathy
Feedback
Helping or Therapeutic Relationship
Input
Metacommunication
Nonverbal Communication
Output
Paralanguage
Proxemics
Relationship Stages
Self-Disclosure
Therapeutic Use of Self
Transference
Values Clarification

THINK About It

How Does a Nurse Respond When an Individual's Values Conflict with the Nurse's Values of Promoting Healthy Behaviors?

Julie, a 15-year old girl, comes into the health clinic at her school to ask the nurse practitioner to prescribe birth control pills for her and to check her for a vaginal discharge. The nurse begins the appointment by asking Julie about her chief complaint of discharge. Julie answers these questions willingly until the nurse asks about her relationship with her boyfriend. Julie comments, "Don't worry about me. We're in love and I just need birth control pills so I won't get pregnant." When the nurse introduces the topic of health risks associated with unprotected sex, Julie says, "Look, I don't need a lecture. You sound like my mother. I know what I'm doing and I don't need condoms because he's not with anyone else."

1 How can this nurse bridge the apparent gap between the nurse's values and Julie's values?

2 In this brief encounter, how can the nurse begin to establish a therapeutic relationship?

3 What responsibilities does the nurse need to weigh in responding to Julie's request? Might clinic or school policies affect the kind of health services available to a 15-year-old girl? Do laws regarding mature minors apply in this instance so that health services may be provided without parental consent? What health risks exist if the nurse does or does not do what Julie wants at this visit?

4 What strategies could the nurse use to engage Julie in a conversation about her sexual behaviors and related health issues?

The interpersonal context of the therapeutic relationship is the milieu in which nursing care occurs. Practice is shaped by the nurse's one-way interest in the individual, which Peplau (1991) described as the nurse's ability to focus on the interests, concerns, and needs of the individual. The desired outcome is characterized as "knowing the patient": a process of understanding the individual as a unique person (Whittemore, 2000, p. 75).

"Knowing the patient" is embedded in a relational context and provides the foundation for nursing interventions. Even interventions that are characterized as primarily technical in nature are interpersonal events involving the nurse and the individual. When the interactional nature of intervention is recognized, the nurse will not seek to do something to the individual to solve a problem, as defined by the nurse or other health care providers. Rather, the nurse will interact with the individual as a partner. To view nursing as a relational process requires a shift in thinking from the instrumental paradigm that directs the nurse and other providers to define the problem and to intervene to correct it. Liaschenko (1997) has placed knowing the patient at the center of nursing practice.

> The question remains, Why is knowledge of the person important/What is the significance of such knowledge to nursing practice? Nursing is an interventionist discipline; that is, it is aimed at doing something to or for people. Knowing the person becomes critically important when the moral work of nursing practice includes acting for individuals, with the aim of helping them to maintain the integrity of their lives, to take up their lives after disease or injury, and to face progressive deterioration and death (p. 30).

In today's rapidly changing health care environment, relationship-centered care is critical to knowing individuals, families, groups and communities, and colleagues. "A clear goal of relationship-centered care is to promote positive encounters and to diminish negative interactions among health care providers and recipients" (Kowalski, Burton, & Rehwaldt, 1997, p. 220). To achieve this aim, interpersonal skills, personal insight, accountability, mutual respect, and a supportive working milieu are requisite. In addition to developing therapeutic interactions with persons and families, nurses must forge intraprofessional working alliances to provide competent care (DeMarco, Horowitz, & McLoed, 2000).

Clearly, health promotion is essentially an interpersonal endeavor. Essential to this interactional process are values clarification, communication, and the helping relationship.

VALUES CLARIFICATION

Definition

Values are qualities, principles, attitudes, or beliefs about the inherent worth of an object, behavior, or idea. Values guide action by sanctioning certain behaviors and negating others. There are two types of values: cognitive and active. Cognitive values are those that are ascribed to verbally and intellectually. Active values, in contrast, are those that are physically acted out. Judging the power of a given value by its ability to influence action is important. For example, a nurse may claim to value the worth of all people equally, but may treat individuals of various races differently and provide the most time and concern for those who are similar to the nurse. This cognitive value has little power to shape the nurse's behavior. If the nurse treated people of all races with equal respect, then the value would also be active and have great power to motivate behavior.

Many forces shape values. Passed down from one generation to another, values color an individual's identity, goals, and sense of personal meaning. Values are imbedded in the culture and taught within a family and social context, giving meaning to the life events and happenings outside the family's boundaries (Horowitz, 1995; Wright & Leahey, 2000). Values are always linked to culture. Recognition that values are culture bound is a critical step in exploring personal values and appreciating the values held by others. To enter into a partnership with an individual, the nurse must strive to understand how cultural values, traditions, and practices influence caregiving in a multiethnic and multicultural society (Phillips et al., 1996). Without this understanding, the nurse is likely to relate to individuals with a limited awareness of assumptions and inadequate sensitivity to the uniqueness and perspective of the person, family, or community.

A repertoire of conscious and unconscious values evolves over time. However, once established, values are not static. Life events and social processes can spark a reappraisal of personal values. **Values clarification** is a method whereby a person purposely seeks to discover his or her values and the importance of these values (Raths, Harmin, & Simon, 1978). Values clarification does not tell individuals how to act, but assists them in recognizing what values are held to evaluate how they influence action.

The values of the individual and nurse will affect their interaction; for example, how values influence expectations, the norms for interactions, the interpretations of exchanged messages, and established goals all influence their interaction. Sensitivity to possible discrepancies in values and respect for the individual's values are essential if the nurse hopes to engage the person in a therapeutic relationship.

Box 4-1 outlines seven steps in the valuing process. The first three steps of choosing involve a cognitive process, the next two steps involve the affective or emotional domain, and the final steps involve behavior (Raths, Harmin, & Simon, 1978; Stuart & Laraia, 1998).

The nurse uses values clarification to examine personal values and their potential influence on nursing care and to assist people in identifying their values and reflecting on their connection to health-related behaviors. Box 4-2 lists suggestions for putting values clarification into action.

Box 4-1 The Valuing Process

CHOOSING
1. Choosing freely
2. Choosing from possible alternatives
3. Choosing after careful consideration of potential outcomes of each alternative

PRIZING
4. Cherishing and being happy with personal beliefs and actions
5. Affirming the choice in public, when appropriate

ACTING
6. Acting out the choice
7. Repeatedly acting in some type of pattern

Box 4-2 Techniques for Assisting Individuals to Clarify Values

IDENTIFY THE INDIVIDUAL'S VALUES
- "What is important to you?"
- "Which of the following statements sounds most like the way you think?"
- "What do you value most in life?"

USE REFLECTION TO RESTATE THE VALUE AND MAKE IT EXPLICIT
- "In what you've just told me, I hear that it is very important to you that . . . "
- "I understand that you value . . ."

IDENTIFY VALUE CONFLICTS OR CONFLICTS BETWEEN VALUES AND ACTIONS
- "What connection does this value have to your current health or illness and to the healthy behaviors, interventions, or treatments needed to maintain or restore your health?"
- "How does this particular value affect your behavior and health?"
- "What are some ways that you might put your values into action?"
- "Are your actions consistent with your values? If not, then what might you change?"

Values clarification becomes a clinical aim when individuals' values lead to behaviors that conflict with the nurse's value of promoting health. For example, a nurse tells a childbirth education class consisting of pregnant women and their coaches that alcohol use poses serious risks to the fetus. After the class, one woman comments, "Do you really think that having a drink once in a while is bad for the baby? I'm sick of being told that I can't do things because of the baby." In this example, a conflict in values is clear. Intervention would have to be aimed at examining how this woman's wish for freedom from restrictions or for gratification clashes with her desire to have a healthy child. The nurse must also weigh his or her own values related to health promotion for the individual and the fetus against respecting an individual's right to make decisions about his or her own health behaviors. When values conflict, an ethical dilemma results. Resolution of this conflict and success of subsequent interventions rest on the ability of the nurse and individual to examine the conflicting values and their outcomes and to acknowledge responsibility for the decisions.

Values and the Therapeutic Use of Self

The self, the most precious and unique of all human endowments, is a personal concept of individuality as distinct from other people and objects in the world. The **therapeutic use of self** is the application of one's cognitions, perceptions, and behaviors to create interpersonal encounters that promote health in another person, family, group, or community. Without self-awareness and clarification of values, therapeutic use of self is impaired. The terms *self-concept* and *self-esteem* comprise important components of individuals' judgments and attitudes about themselves. Self-concept refers to perceptions of personal characteristics, environment, and goals and comprises a mental picture of the self. Although self-concept is the cognitive self-perception, self-esteem is its affective component. Self-esteem is how an individual feels about the way he or she sees themselves (Seigley, 1999).

Self-concept evolves throughout life. From birth, family experiences and parental identification mold the child's sense of identity. The classic research studies of Coopersmith (1967) and Sears (1970) demonstrate positive relationships between the self-reliance, self-esteem, and self-confidence of parents and children. To cultivate children's self-esteem and enable them to have a realistic perception of their strengths and weaknesses, parents should avoid focusing on negatives, failing to give feedback on abilities and limitations, and leaving the child without a sense of belonging.

Sullivan (1953), founder of the Interpersonal School of Psychiatry, which has influenced the evolution of psychiatric nursing theory and practice, stressed the importance of early parent-child experiences in molding the child's self-concept. Positive, rewarding, anxiety-free interactions contribute to security, esteem, and positive self-view. Negative experiences intensified by a moderate degree of anxiety contribute to the child's sense of "bad me"; that is, a sense of incompetence, insecurity, and negative self-concept. The "bad me" serves a purpose by reflecting a realistic view of particular areas of the self that are not positive. In contrast, the "not me" portion of the self emerges from highly anxiety-laden experiences and represents the dissociation of part of the self. A healthy self-concept would include a large "good me," a small "bad

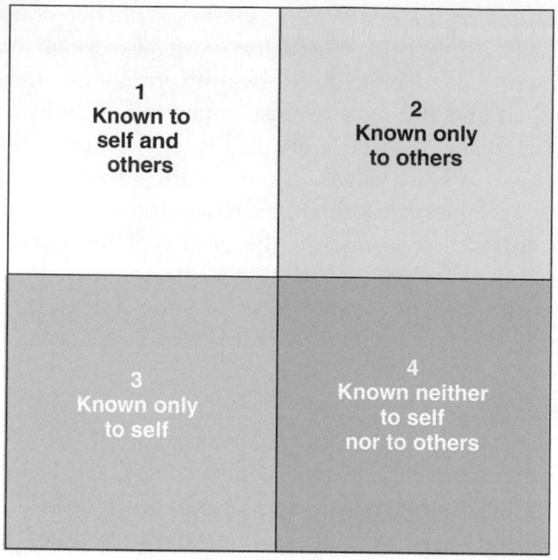

Fig. 4-1 Johari window. (From *Group Processes: An Introduction to Group Dynamics, Third Edition* by Joseph Luft. Copyright © 1984 by Joseph Luft. Reprinted by permission of Mayfield Publishing Company.)

me," and little or no "not me." Multiple positive but realistic appraisals from significant others, especially the parents, help the young child to develop this healthy self-view.

The self does not develop solely in response to the reflected appraisals of others. Genetic endowment, experiential opportunities, and the individual's action shape self-concept. People can accept or reject the appraisals of others and modify their behavior. The ability to control actions and evaluate outcomes of interactions allows individuals to modify and alter their views of self. As such, the self is dynamic, changing through interaction with the outside world and in response to the various maturational and situational crises of life.

The ability to examine, reflect on, and evaluate the self is a uniquely human talent. Self-awareness involves interactions between the self and the external world and the symbolic connections created by the individual. The self includes an unconscious component that is only partially accessible and influences behavior.

Self-awareness is influenced by the degree to which an individual has an accurate concept of all dimensions of the self. The Johari window (Luft, 1984) provides a schema for understanding the various components of the self (Fig. 4-1). Box 4-3 lists these four components of the self.

Together, these windowpanes represent the total self. Three principles guide an understanding of how the self functions in this representation: (1) change in one portion influences all other portions; (2) the smaller the first portion, the poorer communication will be; and (3) interpersonal learning enlarges the first portion and decreases the size of one or more other portions (Luft, 1969). The goal of self-awareness is to increase the size of the first windowpane

BOX 4-3 Components of the Self

1. The public self, which is shown to others
2. The semipublic self, which is seen by others but may be outside the individual's awareness
3. The private self, which is known to the individual, but not revealed to others
4. The inner self, which is the unconscious portion not known even to the individual because it has anxiety-provoking content

while reducing the size of the other three areas (Fig. 4-2) (Sundeen, Stuart, Rankin, & Cohen, 1998).

Consider the differences between windows A and B of Fig. 4-2. Window A represents an individual with little self-awareness. Windowpane number four is large, suggesting that a good deal of the person's experiences, thoughts, and feelings are repressed or suppressed, probably a result of associated anxiety. Additionally, window A suggests a large "not me" portion of the self. In contrast, window B represents a person who is open to the world and is comfortable with his or her self-concept.

The goal of high self-awareness, as illustrated in window B of Fig. 4-2, is reached through three steps (Sundeen, Stuart, Rankin, & Cohen, 1998). The first step is listening to oneself and paying attention to emotions, thoughts, memories, reactions, and impulses. Frequently, people tune out their feelings and thoughts because they are anxious or because they are in a hurry to accomplish some other task. Without self-reflection, people act automatically and lose some of the meaning of living. To improve the ability of self-reflection, ask questions such as the following:

- What am I feeling now?
- What emotions have I experienced today and in the past day or so? What were my thoughts?
- What events led up to these thoughts and feelings?
- What actions did I take? Did my behavior fit with my thoughts and feelings, or was there a lack of harmony?
- Was I aware of my reactions at the time that they took place?
- How have I responded in clinical situations lately? How did I react in response to a particularly happy, sad, or difficult situation? In what way might I alter my actions now? What feelings and reactions did I experience while interacting with this individual?

The second step is listening to and learning from others. Feedback from others can cause anxiety when it conflicts with self-image, even when that image is distorted. In response, the feedback is ignored or translated incorrectly to preserve self-image and reduce anxiety. However, this pattern of responding limits knowledge of the self; it inhibits the ability to examine the appraisals of others and to grow as a result. It is helpful to ask, "What feedback have I received today?" and "What is the other person trying to

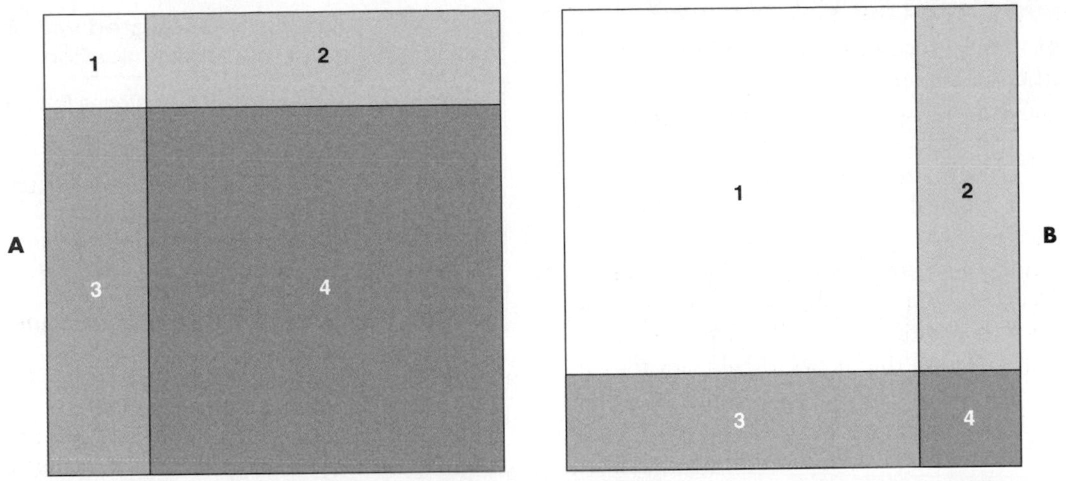

Fig. 4-2 Johari windows illustrate varying degrees of self-awareness. **A,** person has little self-awareness; **B,** person has great amount of self-awareness; *1,* public self; *2,* semipublic self; *3,* private self; *4,* inner self. (From Sundeen S. J., Stuart, G. W., Rankin, E. A. D., & Cohen, S. A. [1998]. *Nurse-client interaction: Implementing the nursing process* [6th ed.]. St Louis: Mosby.)

tell me now?" A person also can ask others directly for feedback. For example, a student nurse might ask another student how he or she comes across. The feedback might be used to alter aspects of behavior that are ineffective or problematic before asking a faculty member for evaluative feedback. Using clinical supervision and consultation with colleagues provides needed opportunity for reflection on practice. "The intensity of interpersonal work necessitates that an arena be provided in which nurses can be helped to reflect on their practice" (DeMarco et al., 2000, p. 172).

The third step is **self-disclosure;** sharing aspects of the self enriches interpersonal life. Through self-disclosure, people come to know themselves better because they have held thoughts, actions, and feelings up to the light for examination with others. Self-disclosure is an indicator of a healthy personality and a strategy for developing one (Jourard, 1971; Stuart & Laraia, 1998). Self-disclosure by one person tends to trigger self-disclosure by another in an interaction; therefore it has been described as a facet of reciprocity, that is, a pattern of interaction in which the two participants perform similar activities within the same or subsequent time intervals (Gilbert, 1993). Therapeutic interactions characterized by reciprocity involve a mutual exchange—a pattern of communication between the nurse and an individual, not a one-way intervention from the nurse to the other person. Traditionally, nurses have been warned to be wary of self-disclosure because it may lead the nurse to cross a boundary from a professional to a personal relationship with individuals. Additionally, the nurse's self-disclosure was thought to burden the individual and shift the focus of attention from the individual to the nurse. Although these guidelines should be kept in mind to prevent excessive or inappropriate self-disclosure, it also is essential for the nurse to appreciate that self-disclosure occurs within human interactions. Nurses are not blank screens, robots, or technicians delivering care; individuals value nurses who engage in interactions as real people and who are willing to share information about themselves.

Why is it important for nurses to clarify personal values and increase self-awareness? The things the nurses value and their ability to understand themselves influence their behavior. The nurse uses behavior in interactions with individuals. The self is the nurse's greatest tool; to use the self effectively, the nurse must be fully aware of how it functions. When unexamined values and aspects of the self, or unconscious material, motivate a great deal of the nurse's behavior, the therapeutic use of self becomes impossible. The nurse's needs must be kept in check so that the other person's needs can be met (Peplau, 1969).

Self-awareness and acceptance of personal beliefs free the nurse to direct energy toward meeting the individual's needs. Openness to the self generates openness to others and acceptance of differences among people. These qualities are essential to the therapeutic use of self. Additionally, the definitions of a situation are derived from active construction and interpretation of experience. These definitions generate actions to follow (Kasch, 1986). The systems of beliefs and values for the nurse and the individual shape their interactions. Moreover, reflection and self-awareness directly influence the nursing framework. Cody (2000) stated, "The selection of a theory base to guide professional practice and research is one of the most profound undertakings of one's life . . . . A central criterion (perhaps *the* central criterion) for selecting a theory base for practice and research is whether or not that theory base offers descriptions and explanations of humans and health in a way that speaks deeply to the nurse and becomes the main lens through which he or she sees himself or herself" (p. 192).

THE COMMUNICATION PROCESS

The **communication process** is far more than simply talking with others or imparting information. Communication is the forum for all thought and relationships shared between people. As such, communication is crucial to human life and growth. In conjunction with the use of scientific and technological advances, communication is an essential tool for the nurse.

Communication is an information exchange between individuals through shared symbols and signs and commonly understood behavior (Ruesch & Bateson, 1987). This exchange involves all the modes of behavior that an individual uses, consciously or unconsciously, to affect another person. Communication includes the spoken and written word and **nonverbal communication** (gestures, facial expressions, movement, body messages or signals, and artistic symbols).

In nursing, communication is essential to the business of treating and caring for individuals. The term "patient-centered communication" refers to a set of communication strategies and actions to enhance reciprocity, mutual understanding, and decision making (Brown, 1999, p. 85-87). Focusing the clinical discussion around the person's story rather than a version reformulated by the provider is essential to patient-centered communication. Box 4-4 highlights strategies associated with patient-centered communication based on Brown's synthesis of the research literature.

Considerable evidence supports the effectiveness of these separate strategies. Investigation of the relationship between comprehensive patient-centered communication and individual outcomes is merited; however, it is likely that accuracy of diagnoses and relevance of treatment plans would be demonstrated. A review of randomized clinical trials of physician-patient communication found that effective communication was associated with improved health outcomes (Stewart, 1995).

Box 4-4 Strategies Associated with Individual-Centered Communication

- Permitting persons to tell their stories in their own words and chronology
- Using a conversational interviewing style
- Eliciting persons' views, perspectives, thoughts, wishes, goals, values, and expectations
- Inquiring about the nature of individuals' lives
- Responding to cues concerning emotional issues and problems
- Giving information about self-care and participation in decision making
- Developing mutual understanding
- Creating collaborative health care plans
- Showing concern for the individual's well being
- Connecting with individuals through humor, touch, and selective disclosure

Adapted from Brown, S. J. (1999). Patient-centered communication. In J. J. Fitzpatrick (Ed.), *Annual review of nursing research: Vol. 17. Focus on complementary health and pain management* (pp. 85-104). New York: Springer Publishing Co.

Function and Process

Ruesch and Bateson (1987) have delineated the following functions of communication:

1. To obtain and send messages and to retain information
2. To use the information to arrive at new conclusions, to reconstruct the past, and to look forward to future events
3. To begin and to modify physiological processes
4. To influence others and outside events

Communication transmits information, both interpersonally and intrapersonally, and it provides the basis for action.

The process of communication consists of four components (Watzlawick, Beavin, & Jackson, 1967). Nurses must be able to diagnose communication difficulties in any of these components. **Input** involves taking in information from outside the individual or group. Once taken in, input must be transformed in some manner to be used. For example, food must be broken down for use as energy and symbols must be translated into ideas. The flow and transformation of processed input refers to the way information is analyzed and stored within the individual or the way it is transmitted from person to person within a human system (group or family) before communication with the external environment occurs. The outcome of information processing, **output,** involves further exchange with the environment or other person. A new information exchange is triggered at this point in the cycle by the response called **feedback,** a monitoring system through which the person or group controls the internal and external responses to behavior (output) and accommodates these responses appropriately. The idea of a feedback loop shows the dynamic nature of communication. Each piece of communication is both a stimulus designed to elicit a response and a response to a different stimulus (Fig. 4-3).

When interpersonal communication is analyzed, two types of feedback can be identified: positive (encouraging change) and negative (encouraging homeostasis or no change). The following parent's commands to a young child illustrate these types of feedback: (1) positive—"Try that again; you almost had it" and (2) negative—"Don't touch that; it's hot." The first statement shows the parent's attempt to encourage the child to continue new behavior; the second illustrates an effort to curtail undesired behavior. Rather than meaning "good" or "bad," positive and negative feedback refer to promotion of system change and stability, which is the process of balancing the direction and magnitude of change. Both types of feedback are needed, depending on the situation.

The notion of the situational context of communication is important. The context of communication is the setting's physical, psychosocial, and cultural dimensions. The

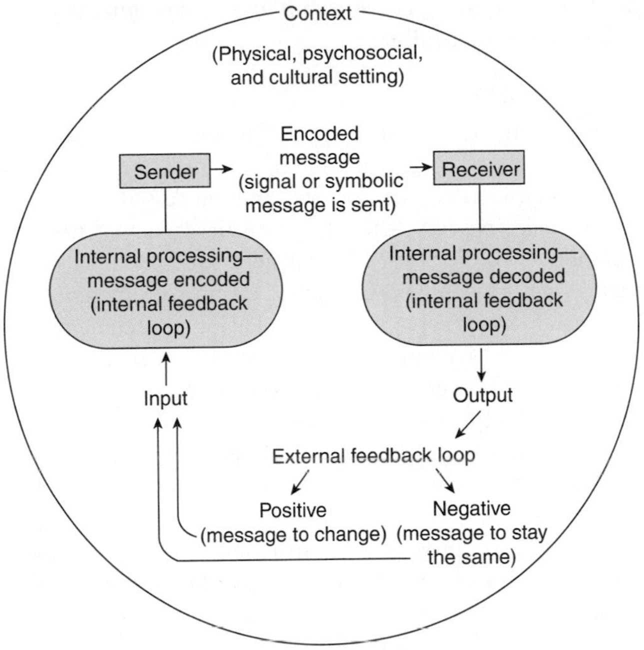

Fig. 4-3 Communication system.

context includes the relationship between sender and receiver; their previous experiences, feelings, values, cultural norms, and age and developmental stage; and the physical location (Kasch, 1986; Stuart & Laraia, 1998).

Types of Communication

All human communication occurs in three forms: (1) verbal, (2) nonverbal, and (3) metacommunication. Each affects the meaning and influences the interpretation of the message.

Verbal Communication

Verbal communication is the transmission of messages using spoken or written words. As symbols for ideas, words impart meaning defined by a specific language. The ability to communicate with language is a uniquely human attribute and a critical ability.

People who are deaf or hard of hearing often use sign language to communicate. Signs, similar to spoken or written words, are used consistently to represent a particular meaning. Words also may be spelled out through finger spelling in a manner parallel to written communication. Braille assists blind and visually challenged people to read. Touch is used to interpret markings that represent letters and words. Sign language and Braille blend aspects of verbal and nonverbal communication.

Verbal communication with people who speak a different language than the nurse does pose a challenge. As societies become increasingly multicultural, assistance from specially trained interpreters is essential to providing culturally competent care (Poss, 1999). Confidentiality issues, the complexity of health information, and the need to validate understandings and reach mutual decisions make it inappropriate to use untrained personnel or relatives to interpret simply because they are available.

The importance of language development is apparent in its three functions: (1) informing the person of others' thoughts and feelings, (2) stimulating the receiver of a message by triggering a response, and (3) serving a descriptive function by imparting information and sharing observations, ideas, inferences, and memories (Watzlawick, Beavin, & Jackson, 1967). The ability of verbal communication to fulfill these functions is influenced by many factors, including the communicator's social class, culture, age, milieu, and ability to receive and interpret messages.

Nonverbal Communication

Nonverbal communication or language encompasses all messages that are not spoken or written. Movement, facial and eye expressions, gestures, appearance, and vocalization or paralanguage all constitute nonverbal modes of communication (Blondis & Jackson, 1982).

Sign language is another form of nonverbal communication because, although it uses symbols communicated through specific signs, these are enhanced by facial expressions and body postures. However, sign language shares many aspects of verbal communication. It has syntax and grammar, words may be spelled out, and a standard meaning is assigned to specific signs to create symbolic language, just as words share common definitions.

Although all communication has the potential of being misunderstood, Blondis and Jackson (1982, p. 96) point out that nonverbal communication is particularly subject to misunderstanding because it does not always reflect the sender's conscious intent. Nonverbal messages also tend to be nebulous, without specific beginnings and endings. Nonverbal communication "is constant, flowing, and dynamic—a two-way mime performed on the stage of the subconscious."

The channels of nonverbal communication are the five senses. The ability to see, hear, smell, touch, and taste assists in the perception of messages. The senses can be tuned to differing aspects of communication; for example, the receiver might hear the sender laugh but see a sad facial expression. Both messages are crucial to interpretation of the communication.

Body Motion or Kinetic Behavior **Body motion** or **kinetic behavior** includes facial expression (or facies), eye movements, body movements, gestures, and posture (Blondis & Jackson, 1982).

When observing facial expression, the nurse notices the affect or emotion that is communicated. Does the person appear happy or sad; alert, distracted, or sleepy; or contented, agitated, or anxious? The degree of emotion expressed should also be noted. Does the person's face express what is generally considered an excessive degree of feeling for the situation, too little, or none at all?

Eye movements are closely related to facial expression. Eyes, in conjunction with the movement of other facial muscles, move in ways that convey effect. Eye contact conveys messages of interest or trust; lack of eye contact can imply lack of interest or anxiety; constant eye contact can send a message of hostility.

It is important to note that all these messages are culturally and situationally bound. Interpretations of nonverbal behavior, particularly facial and eye expressions, are rooted in the context of the communication. For example, avoidance of direct eye contact between some people can be a sign of respect in certain circumstances and cultures.

Appearance Appearance is an overall notion of how people present themselves. The nurse must consider whether the person's appearance seems appropriate to the context.

Paralanguage **Paralanguage** is vocalization other than expression of words and includes many aspects of sound, such as tone, pitch, and tempo of speech. Sounds of crying, groaning, gasping, and grunting are all examples of paralanguage (Blondis & Jackson, 1982). Infants begin their vocal communication with paralanguage. Although paralanguage may be classified as verbal communication (Sullivan, 1953), it seems more appropriate to view paralanguage as nonverbal communication because words, the hallmark of verbal communication, are not used.

Importance Health care providers do not overlook the importance of nonverbal communication. This communication has great power to transmit information about another's thoughts and feelings; therefore the nurse must observe carefully. Even a silent individual can be very revealing. The significance of nonverbal communication is best captured by the axiom, "Actions speak louder than words."

Metacommunication

Besides verbal and nonverbal communication, there is a phenomenon called **metacommunication** that refers to a message about the message. Watzlawick, Beavin, and Jackson (1967, p. 49) describe metacommunication as the impossibility of not communicating; that is, "one cannot not communicate. Persons transmit a message about what is being communicated even when words are not spoken."

Metacommunication is the relationship aspect of communication. In a sense, metacommunication involves reading between the lines or going past the surface content of the message to glean nuances of meaning. When the content and the relationship aspects, or metacommunication aspects, of a message are incongruent, interpreting the communication accurately may be difficult, leaving the receiver uncomfortable and confused.

The importance of metacommunication is particularly clear in relation to communication between adults and children. When nonverbal and verbal messages are conflicting, the young child becomes confused, trust is diminished, and the child's emergent self-concept can be compromised. The child will not learn to trust personal reactions and interpretations and may find communicating to be a risky enterprise.

Group Process

In group settings, a special type of metacommunication is called process. A basic principle of group theory states that all communication has content and process. Content is what is said; process is the relationship aspect of what is communicated. For example, consider two individuals in a therapy group who always support each other by agreeing with each other and offering additional comments or criticism to any group member who disagrees. Although this pairing between the individuals offers them some protection from anxiety that may result from self-examination and feedback, it isolates them and curtails feedback from others. Examination of this group process is an essential task. The nurse leader and participants can transform this problematic situation into a learning opportunity by doing the following: (1) identifying the pattern by pointing out the behavior after it has occurred frequently; (2) helping the pair and other group members consider what needs are being met through this pattern; (3) looking at each person's role in fostering this process (why other group members have failed to confront the pair); and (4) discussing potential outcomes of changing the behavior. The principles embedded in these steps for examining group process can be applied in clinical situations when greater self-understanding is a goal.

Group process occurs during every group encounter. Staff meetings, such as therapy, counseling, and psychoeducational groups, always involve group process. To understand what is being communicated beyond the manifest content or topic of discussion, the nurse must attend to process in every group situation.

Functionality of Communication

Understanding what makes communication functional will improve the nurse's ability to assess needs and to intervene effectively. Steps to functional communication include the following: (1) firmly stating the case, (2) clarifying and qualifying the message, (3) seeking feedback, and (4) being receptive to feedback when it is received.

To state the case firmly, the sender needs to make the content and the metacommunication congruent; when they conflict, the message is confusing. For example, a nurse is angry with a colleague for making statements to an administrator that undermined the nurse's plans for reconfiguring patient discharge planning. When the nurse had a chance to speak with this colleague before a staff meeting, the nurse exchanged pleasantries without mention of what the nurse thought about the colleague's prior statements to the administrator. When the colleague asks whether something is bothering the nurse, the nurse responds that nothing is wrong. The colleague senses that the nurse's verbal and nonverbal communication do not match; in other words, the content of the message and the metacommunication are incongruent. The colleague is left feeling uneasy and the nurse failed to express his or her thoughts or take effective action to rectify what the nurse believed as a problem with the colleague. To make the communication functional, the nurse needs to bring thoughts and feelings into awareness and reflect on the message he or she wants to transmit. Once these steps are accomplished, the message's content and metacommunication can be readily adjusted to match, and the nurse's communication is likely to be effective.

To clarify and qualify the message, the sender must give a complete message. Important features of the message should be emphasized and specifics of any request must be stated, not assumed. The message's importance also must be indicated. To illustrate, a wife mentions to her husband that it is nearly June. The husband responds that he had noticed how warm the weather was becoming. On the surface, this communication may seem functional until the intent of the wife's message is considered. The wife meant to imply that June is the month of their anniversary. She hoped that her husband would somehow know that she wanted him to comment on their anniversary plans. To make this communication functional, she needed to expand the message ("Our anniversary is coming up") and clarify her wish for a response ("What shall we do to celebrate?"). Additionally, she needed to show how important the message was ("I'd really like to do something special this year"). If the husband had been attuned to the metacommunication in this exchange, he could have clarified his wife's intent.

One technique for clarifying and qualifying messages is called the "I" statement in which the sender states what he or she wants, feels, thinks, or plans (including likes and dislikes). For example, "I felt hurt when you forgot our anniversary last year," ("I" statement that the wife could have used).

Questions can clarify and qualify depending on the type of question asked. Open-ended questions tend to elicit descriptive responses rather than one-word answers. For example, "Tell me what you did at school today" is likely to yield a more elaborate description from the child than the question, "Did everything go okay at school today?" However, direct questions that seek a one-word answer are useful when a specific piece of information is sought. "Did you pass your math test today?" may be a better approach than "What was the math test like?" when the issue of passing the test is important to discuss. Also, for individuals having trouble expressing more than the simplest thoughts, asking direct questions that call for brief replies can be helpful, such as, "Did you eat breakfast?" This approach is particularly useful with persons who are depressed, regressed, cognitively impaired, or unable to handle complex information or communication at a particular time.

Seeking feedback is another element of functional communication. Consensual validation, confirming that both sender and receiver understand the same information, calls for the use of the clarification skills just described. In family communication, the parent, as the sender, should model this behavior for children by asking the child, as the receiver, to explain his or her sense of the message and how to ask the sender for further explanation. For example, "I want you to clean your room" (message from parent) can be followed by, "Tell me how you think you will do that" (validating that child and parent agree about what the task entails). This style of seeking validation can be adapted to nurse-nurse/other professional exchanges between colleagues and therapeutic interactions.

It is also crucial for the sender to be open to feedback. A "no questions" attitude blocks functional communication, whether in the home, classroom, or clinical setting. Children, students, individuals, and even other nurses may be afraid to question anyone in authority or may assume that the person should magically know what is intended or expected. For example, one person may avoid confronting a nurse who fails to explain the treatment plan and then communicates that the person should know how to follow through. Statements by the sender such as "Tell me what you think" and "What is your understanding of what I said?" are helpful.

Receiving messages involves many of the same processes as sending. Evaluation of the intent of the message, both the content and the metacommunication, is the first step. Because this task is difficult, particularly when the content and metamessage are not congruent, the receiver frequently must ask for clarification and validate the understanding of the message. The importance of clarifying meaning is underscored by results from a study of health care professionals' experiences of encounters with patients in clinical settings (Takman & Severinsson, 1999). Clinicians' interviews revealed three categories of description: (1) gaining personal knowledge and understanding of patients' different ways of expressing suffering, (2) making patients feel confident, and (3) focusing on medical problems without understanding patients' unique ways of communicating their suffering. Although the first two categories indicated professionals' ability to understand patients' experience of suffering, the third category showed evidence of difficulty reaching such understanding. To increase ability to comprehend patients' expressions of their experience, the researchers recommended that professionals be supported to explore their own feelings and reactions through clinical supervision.

Listening

Effective listening, an important part of communication, is more than passively taking in information; it is actively focusing attention on the message. Asking questions to explore what is meant helps the listener reach an accurate assessment of the message's meaning.

Activities that communicate listening are not universal and are culturally determined; therefore these behaviors are understandable within a context. However, many forms of nonverbal communication have been identified that, from a Western or European perspective, commonly convey that the person is listening. These nonverbal communications include direct gazing and eye contact, head nodding, orienting one's body to maintain interpersonal closeness, leaning forward, facial expressions such as eyebrow animation and smiling, and brief verbal statements that indicate interest, such as "Please go on" or "Tell me more about . . . ." The ability of these behaviors to communicate that the person is listening depends on the context and intensity of the activities. For example, leaning too close to the person might be interpreted as intrusive. Reciprocity, the patterning of similar activities within the same interval by two people, can help the nurse communicate a listening stance in an effective way. When the nurse matches nuances of the individual's type and style of behavior, the chances that the person will interpret the nurse's behavior as an indication of active listening are increased, and the likelihood of misinterpretation is reduced. In an experimental study of nurses' communication, Gilbert (1993) indicated that reciprocity is present even during first encounters. This finding suggests that nurses can enhance the quality of their communication, even when encounters are brief, by attending to reciprocity in their interactions and by validating whether reciprocity is associated with shared interpretations of meaning. Sensitivity to nuances in communication and validation of meaning can be particularly helpful strategies when the nurse and individual come from different cultural backgrounds.

Effective listening is essential if the nurse is to assist the person and to understand him or her as an individual. The nurse's failure to listen may be caused by anxiety; lack of experience, which leads to excessive talking by the nurse; preoccupation with personal thoughts; or lack of practice (Stuart & Laraia, 1998).

Flexibility

In flexibility, a balance exists between control and permissiveness. In overcontrol, every message is monitored. In exaggerated permissiveness, anything can be communicated in any way. For communication to be functional, rules should be laid down as to what is appropriate, without rigid prescriptions that inhibit any meaningful interchange. For example, the rule that nurses will not answer questions concerning intimate details of their lives sets an appropriate limit; however, that does not mean that nurses should refuse to answer any question about themselves.

Silence

Silence between people is often uncomfortable for the nurse who is somewhat insecure about what should occur during a therapeutic encounter. However, silence can be useful when used carefully. When a person is seeking a verbal response, silence can be perceived as a lack of interest. At other times, silence allows individuals to reflect on what is being discussed or experienced, lets them know that the nurse is willing to wait until they are ready to say more, or simply provides them with comfort and support. Each situation needs individual evaluation by the nurse, with sensitivity to the individual's needs. Rather than asking a flurry of questions to break the silence, the nurse should allow the person time to decide when to comment or should make brief comments that do not demand answers, such as "It can be helpful to take time to think about what we've been discussing." Also, comments such as "Try putting your thoughts or feelings into words" can help the person to share these thoughts or feelings when silence is blocking rather than improving the communication.

Humor

Humor is part of being human; it relieves tension, reduces aggression, and creates a climate of sharing (Fig. 4-4). Humor can block communication when it is used to avoid subjects that might be uncomfortable or when it excludes other people. Humor can also inflict emotional pain and communicate negative views or stereotypes about particular individuals or groups through teasing and jokes concerning race, ethnicity, culture, country of origin, occupation, age, gender, sexual activity, or other traits that stand out or are devalued. A direct response to the latent content or message in this type of humor is an effective way to curtail its use and minimize its effect. For example, "That kind of joke makes me very uncomfortable. I don't find it funny to describe [the specific group in question] that way, and I would like you to stop." To be helpful, the meaning of the humor must be understood and its purpose supportive to the individual. Clarification of the meaning should be used when there is doubt or concern.

Touch

Touch is an interesting means of nonverbal communication for nurses, who often touch individuals during administration of care. The nurse's concern can be expressed by a gentle or soothing application of touch. Nevertheless, in

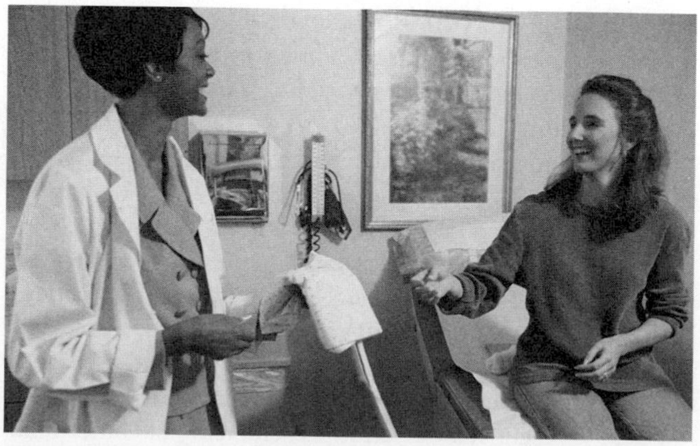

Fig. 4-4 Use of humor helps ease the tension for physical examination.

some instances, touch is inappropriate. For example, in interactions with individuals who have acute psychiatric disturbance, touch might be misinterpreted. A psychotic individual might think that the nurse is attacking him or her; an anxious person might be startled when touched. It is important for the nurse to evaluate the context and meaning of touch to the individual based on knowledge of that person and interpretation of feedback. Appropriate use of touch is illustrated in Fig. 4-5.

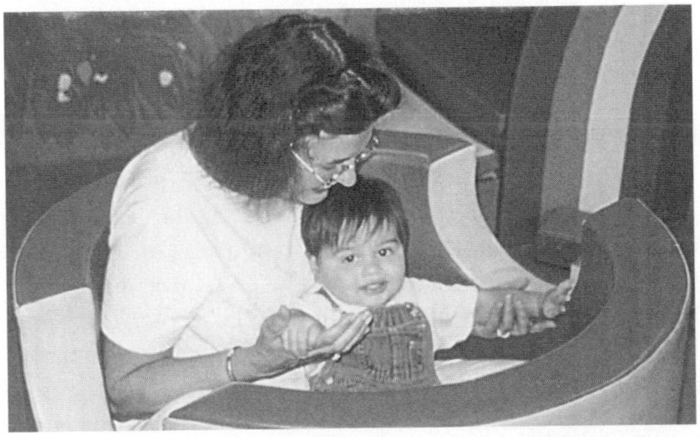

Fig. 4-5 Touch is a powerful form of nonverbal communication.

Space

Space between communicators varies according to the type of communication, the setting, and the culture. Hall (1973) researched **proxemics,** the use of space between communicators, and identified four zones of space commonly used in interaction in North America that are presented in Box 4-5.

Understanding the appropriate distance for a given type of interaction assists the nurse in making nonverbal

Box 4-5 Zones of Space Common to Interaction in North America

1. *Intimate Space:* up to 18 inches (45.5 cm); used for high interpersonal sensory stimulation (Fig. 4-6, *A*)
2. *Personal Space:* 18 inches to 4 feet (45.5 to 120 cm); appropriate for close relationships in which touching may be involved and good visualization is desired (Fig. 4-6, *B*)
3. *Social-consultative Space:* 9 to 12 feet (270 to 360 cm); less intimate and personal, requiring louder verbal communication (Fig. 4-6, *C*)
4. *Public Space:* 12 feet (360 cm) and over; appropriately used for formal gatherings, such as giving speeches (Fig. 4-6, *D*)

Based on data from Hall, E. (1973). *The silent language*. Garden City, NY: Doubleday/Anchor Press.

A B C D

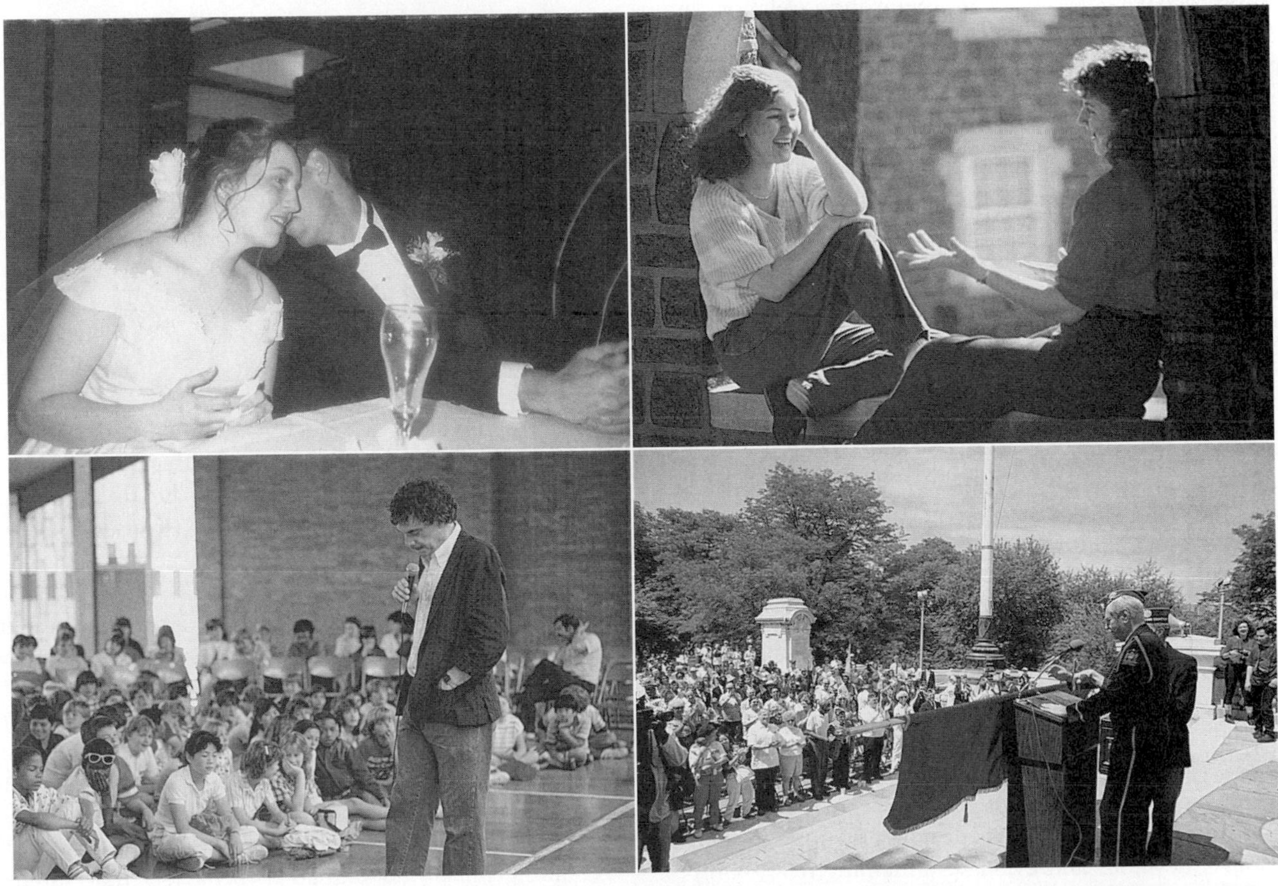

Fig. 4-6 **A,** intimate distance communication; **B,** personal distance communication; **C,** social-consultative distance communication; **D,** public distance communication. (Courtesy Richard B. Levine.)

and verbal communication congruent. Awareness of the cultural norms concerning distance is also important in shaping communication and interpreting the behavior of others. When people from different cultures or groups communicate, there may be a discomfort about the acceptable distance between them when speaking. Recognition of differences helps the nurse adjust the distance and interpret the meaning of this nonverbal communication.

The many traits and components discussed in this chapter characterize functional communication. However, communication is more subtle and intricate. It cannot be reduced to a set of parts and principles; its roles and nuances are far more complex and variable. To communicate by language and symbols is a special human ability. When communication is healthy, it enables people to bridge the gap between themselves, to move from being alone to being together, which is clearly one of the crucial tasks of living. Effective communication is also the foundation for the helping relationship.

THE HELPING OR THERAPEUTIC RELATIONSHIP

A **helping or therapeutic relationship** is a process by which one person promotes the development of another person by fostering the latter's maturation, adaptation, integration, openness, and ability to find meaning in the present situation (Peplau, 1969). The therapeutic relationship emerges from purposeful encounters. This helping relationship is created through the nurse's application of scientific knowledge, his or her understanding of human behavior and communication, and his or her commitment to the individual. The therapeutic relationship is the foundation of clinical nursing practice—the essential element of care with every individual in every situation. Techniques, technology, interventions, and contexts vary, but the relational aspect of nurses' practice produces a cohesive unity, allowing nurses to see individuals holistically and as unique persons.

No perfect profile or personality of a helping person exists. However, certain traits can be nurtured without thwarting the nurse's unique personality. These characteristics enable the nurse to be an agent of therapeutic care (Peplau, 1963; Stuart & Laraia, 1998). Box 4-6 lists characteristics associated with therapeutic effectiveness.

The process of values clarification, as described in this chapter, can assist the nurse to nurture these personal characteristics. Counseling people can serve many purposes and is useful in a variety of settings.

Characteristics

No recipe is available for a successful therapeutic relationship. Techniques and concepts serve only as tools. As a nurse develops and evaluates a helping relationship, the following guidelines may be useful.

Box 4-6 Characteristics Associated with Therapeutic Effectiveness

1. Self-awareness and self-reflection
2. Openness
3. Self-confidence and strength
4. Genuineness
5. Concern for the individual
6. Respect for the individual
7. Knowledge
8. Ability to empathize
9. Sensitivity
10. Acceptance
11. Creativity
12. Ability to focus and confront

Purposeful Communication

Purposeful communication means that the nurse focuses communication for a particular aim. Social chitchat—communication without a goal—should not make up the bulk of therapeutic interaction. This does not mean that the nurse should never discuss a social topic; nonetheless, there should be some purpose. For example, discussing the weather with a somewhat disoriented elderly individual serves the purpose of orienting that person to the environment. Goals guide the nurse in focusing communication.

Rapport

Rapport is a harmony and an affinity between people in a relationship (Rogers, 1965). It is the nurse's responsibility to establish an atmosphere in which rapport can develop, using many of the traits listed for a helping person. To let the person know that his or her concerns interest the nurse and that working together may alleviate some of his or her difficulties and encourage growth, it is important to be genuine, open, and concerned.

Trust

Trust is a necessary component of any helping relationship. Trust involves an affective experience that evolves from rapport and is based on a belief that it is safe to be genuine and honest in a relationship because the other person will respond in a respectful way (Kottler & Brown, 1996; Long, 1996). Trust is the reliance on the ability, character, and behavior of a person; it involves a sense of certainty that the other will carry out responsibilities and promises, and it's an expectation that the outcome of interaction need not be feared (Sundeen et al., 1998). The nurse can promote trust by modeling trust; for example, trusting the individual to do as promised; clearly defining the relationship parameters and expectations, particularly the purpose and specifics of time, place, and anticipated behavior; being consistent; and willingly examining nurse and individual behaviors that interfere with trust.

Empathy

Empathy is feeling with another person and understanding the dynamic meaning of behavior. Empathic nurses experience the individual's feelings by drawing on emotions and experiences that enable them to place themselves in his or her situation. Empathy involves the ability to understand another's feelings without losing personal identity and perspective. It is the critical element in creating a caring atmosphere through therapeutic use of self. The research literature is beginning to build knowledge about the role that empathy plays in outcomes. For example, in a correlational study of relationships among nurse-expressed empathy, patient-perceived empathy, and patient distress, Olson (1995) demonstrates a connection between nurse-expressed empathy and individual outcomes. Empathy has a significant negative effect on patient distress. As the patient's sense that the nurse understands and accepts him or her increases, the patient's feelings of anxiety, depression, and anger decrease. Additionally, two empathy factors that contribute significantly toward patient-perceived empathy are the nurse's acknowledgment of the content of the patient's communication and limited use of "don't feel" statements. Olson's study is one of the first studies to demonstrate a link between behavioral measures of nurse-expressed empathy and individual outcomes.

Nurses can learn behavioral approaches that enhance empathic relations with persons through supervised experiential learning. For example, nurses do not empathize by switching the focus of the interaction to themselves or by sympathizing ("I know exactly how you feel; that happened to me once"); they use personal experience to appreciate the individual's feelings and experiences. Using personal understanding while maintaining boundaries is the essence of empathy in the helping relationship. With empathic understanding, the nurse acknowledges the affective domain of personal experiences and uses this knowledge to appreciate the person's reactions. Empathy enables the listener to share human experiences as the basis for providing care.

Goal Direction

A helping relationship is special in its goal-directed nature. Dissimilar to most human relationships that focus on mutual benefit, a helping relationship exists solely to meet some need or promote the growth of the individual. Although a side benefit is often gratification, learning, or growth for the nurse, the relationship is centered on the individual.

As stated, goals are formulated as desired individual behaviors. Short-term goals are changes likely to be achieved within 10 days to 2 weeks; long-term goals are all others. All goals should be stated in measurable terms and should focus on a positive change or on the decrease of problematic behavior.

Ideally, a person works with the nurse to establish goals. However, some individuals, such as those who are seriously depressed, psychotic, or organically impaired, are unable to establish goals. When an individual is unable to negotiate appropriate goals, the nurse establishes realistic goals and shares them with the person, who is free to participate or to reject efforts to reach these goals.

Ethics in Communicating

Ethical decision making is closely linked with the goal-directed nature of helping relationships. Ethical issues are present in human interactions whenever behavior may affect others, whenever actions involve conscious choices of methods and ends, and whenever actions can be evaluated in reference to standards of right and wrong (Johannesen, 1996). In his examination of various ethical perspectives, Johannesen (1996) discerned guidelines that may be adapted as ethical standards for interpersonal communication. Several guidelines that are most salient to the therapeutic relationship are highlighted in the Hot Topics box.

Frequently, the nurse may wish to set goals that the individual does not want to reach; the nurse must remember that the problem belongs to the other person, as does the choice of care alternatives. The nurse assists the individual in decision making, with the decision based on the individual's value system. However, the nurse should not take a laissez-faire approach and avoid assisting the person. The nurse's responsibility is to help the individual examine values, identify conflicts, and prioritize goals and desired health care outcomes. Action follows from understanding values and the best available information. Both the individual and the nurse must bring interpreted facts and their own clarified values to the interaction to establish goals. Recognizing this interplay, the nurse must clarify personal values, subsequently respect the individual's rights, and act to support and protect the integrity of the person and the family.

Therapeutic Techniques

Occasionally, individuals who are novices in establishing helping relationships assume that they are bound to "say the wrong thing" and cause terrible damage to the person or that they will learn some magical phrases and questions to create instant rapport. No nurse or other professional is so powerful that a "wrong word" will destroy the individual's self-concept or self-esteem. Even persons with physical and emotional problems are resilient and have coped, at least to some degree, with a lifetime of stresses. Alternately, there is no magical saying that the nurse can always plug into an interaction to communicate successfully. Although some techniques are often useful, they must be applied with purpose, skill, and attention to the context and individuality of each person. The following therapeutic techniques therefore should be

HOT topics: GUIDELINES FOR ETHICAL INTERPERSONAL COMMUNICATION

- Share personal views candidly and clearly
- Communicate information accurately with minimal loss or distortion of intended meaning
- Purposeful deception is unethical communication
- Verbal and nonverbal messages should communicate congruent meanings
- Intentional blocking of the communication process is usually unethical; for example, changing subjects when the other person has not finished communicating, cutting a person off, or distracting others from the subject under discussion
- Self-awareness and openness to changing concepts of self and others are needed in conjunction with simultaneous attention to: role responsibilities; individual sacrifice, when it is required to make a "good" decision; and emotions, while guarding against letting them be the sole guide of our behavior
- Avoid scapegoating or unnecessary condemnation of others
- Lying or deceiving can cause intentional or unintentional harm
- Avoid verbally "hitting below the belt" by taking advantage of another's vulnerability
- Communicators share responsibility for the consequences
- Recognize the multicultural context of all communication: express respect for the dignity of every person and excise any elements of your communication that denigrate, stereotype, or devalue others

Modified from Johannesen, R. L. (1996). *Ethics in human communication* (4th ed.). Prospect Heights, IL: Waveland Press.

viewed as guidelines for effectively shaping the therapeutic relationship.

Focus on the Individual

Nurses must first master the ability to focus on the individual's needs by orienting the person toward who she or he is and why the interaction is occurring; nurses should avoid delving into their own personal lives to the extent that it diverts attention from the other person's concern. Avoiding nurse-directed conversation can be difficult; a useful rule of thumb is for nurses to answer or respond to obvious questions and to switch the focus back to clinical concerns when other questions are asked. For example:

Individual (looks at nurse's wedding ring): "Are you married?"

Nurse: "Yes, I am."

Individual: "What does your husband do for a living?"

Nurse: "Rather than get distracted by a discussion about me, let's get back to planning how you will manage at work."

This focus also involves acknowledging the person's intent by stating the portion of the message that is clear, seeking validation, and helping the individual clarify the rest of the message.

Help the Individual Describe and Clarify Content and Meaning

Too often, nurses rush to offer an interpretation of the nature of the problem and quickly follow by offering a solution. Solving problems efficiently makes the nurse feel effective, important, and powerful; however, the person's needs may not be met. A crucial step in using the therapeutic relationship effectively is to assist the individual in describing a particular experience or concern. Description is enhanced when the nurse prompts the person to clarify the description and interpret its meaning.

The use of who, what, and where questions and statements, beginning with phrases such as "tell me," "go on," "describe to me," "explain it to me," and "give me an example," help the person expand and clarify the content and meaning of what is communicated. By seeking feedback, the nurse helps the individual to explain the meaning further.

In clarifying, the nurse should avoid threatening, detectivelike questions. Questions that begin with "why" often increase the person's anxiety because they demand reasons, conclusions, analysis, or causes (Peplau, 1964). Reformulating questions to obtain data first and then helping the individual to analyze links among events, thoughts, feelings, actions, and outcomes is generally more helpful.

Nurses can employ sequential steps for helping the individual to acquire new knowledge and skills, to explain events, to change circumstances and responses that interfere with health, and to solve problems (Peplau, 1963; O'Toole & Welt, 1989). This problem-solving approach can be adapted for use in health promotion to assist the person in problem solving by working through the steps outlined in the Health Teaching box. These steps are a useful guideline for keeping the focus of concern on the individual and his or her definition of the problem. The primary goal is for the nurse to help the person describe the problem and formulate solutions in partnership with the nurse rather than to tell the person what is wrong and how to fix it.

Use Reflection

Reflection is the restatement of what the individual has said in the same or different words. This technique can

HEALTH TEACHING Steps in Promoting Problem Solving

- Describe the experience or event of concern

Helpful Verbal Nursing Strategies:

"Tell me what happened." "Describe the experience to me."

- Analyze the parts of the experience and see relationships to other events

Helpful Verbal Nursing Strategies:

"What meaning does this have for you?" "What pattern is there?"

- Formulate the problem

Helpful Verbal Nursing Strategies:

"In what way is this problematic?" "What do you want to see changed?"

- Validate the formulation

Helpful Verbal Nursing Strategies:

"Do you mean . . . ?" "Let me tell you what I understand you to be saying."

- Use the formulation to identify ways to solve or manage the difficulty

Helpful Verbal Nursing Strategies:

"What would you do the next time?" "In what way has your view changed?" "What actions are needed to solve the problem that you've identified?"

- Try out the solutions, judge the outcomes, and adjust the plan accordingly

Helpful Nursing Strategies:

Encourage application in new situations through role playing or through practice in appropriate settings; assist the individual to cycle through the above sequence as needed to evaluate the outcome and make adjustments to the plan.

Adapted from Peplau, H. E. (1963). Process and concept of learning. In S. Burd, & M. Marshall (Eds., pp. 348-352), *Some clinical approaches to psychiatric nursing*. New York: Macmillan.

involve paraphrasing or summarizing the person's main point to indicate interest and to focus the discussion. Effective use of this approach does not include frequent, parrot-like repetition of the individual's statements. Rather, it is the selective paraphrasing or literal repetition of the person's words to underscore the importance of what has been said or to elicit additional comments.

Use Constructive Confrontation

Confronting an individual means that the nurse points out a specific behavior and then helps that person examine its meaning or consequences. For example:

Nurse: "You missed your appointment for the consultation we had scheduled."

Individual: "Oh, I didn't notice the date."

Nurse: "What do you think was going on with you that you didn't notice the date when you are usually very aware of time and appointments?"

This type of confrontation is not an angry exchange, but a purposeful way of helping the person examine personal actions and their meaning.

Use Nouns and Pronouns Correctly

Some individuals have difficulty separating themselves from others or specifying the object or subject in their language. These individuals misuse pronouns by referring to we, us, they, him, and her, without clearly identifying the referent, making statements such as, "They don't like me. They told me I was useless." Others may use general nouns such as everyone, people, doctors, and nurses, avoiding clear communication about specific persons. The nurse can clarify by asking, "Who are they?" or "To whom are you referring?" Additionally, the nurse must be careful to use separate pronouns when speaking of herself or himself and the individual. For example, when communicating with persons with disordered thinking, the nurse should say you and I rather than us or we to assist these individuals in maintaining personal boundaries (Peplau, 1963).

Use Silence

Allowing a thoughtful silence at intervals helps the individual talk at his or her own pace without pressure to perform for the nurse. Silence also permits time for reflection. Particularly helpful to the depressed or physically ill person, silence can reduce pressure and conserve energy. After several moments, the nurse can help the person by asking him or her to try sharing some thoughts. For example, "Try putting your thoughts into words," "Tell me what are you thinking or feeling now," or "I'll be here when you feel ready to talk."

Accept Communication

Allowing the person to communicate verbally and nonverbally in his or her own fashion makes the person feel safe and respected. This does not mean that the nurse always agrees with the individual or tolerates inappropriate behavior within the established limits of the setting, such as verbal or physical abuse. Acceptance of the person's mode of communication is an important ingredient in a helping relationship.

Barriers to Effective Communication

A number of barriers to effective communication can originate with the nurse, the individual, or both. The most obvious barrier is the nurse's failure to use the types of therapeutic techniques just described. Lack of knowledge or experience can limit the nurse's ability to assess the individual's needs and repertoire of skills. Supervision and study can help the nurse apply the steps of the nursing process by using effective intervention approaches.

Communication is also ineffective when some part of the communication-feedback loop breaks down. Failure to send a clear message, receive and interpret the message correctly, or provide useful feedback can interfere with communication. Diagnosing the source of the communication breakdown, taking steps to correct it, and using knowledge of the communication process and appropriate therapeutic techniques are the nurse's responsibility.

Anxiety

When the nurse or individual is highly anxious during an interaction, perception is altered and the ability to communicate effectively is sharply curtailed. The use of defense mechanisms, such as denial, projection, or displacement, reduces anxiety at the expense of understanding the true meaning of an interaction. Severe anxiety and the use of defenses distort reality and lead to disordered communication. The nurse should identify the feeling of anxiety and its source and use anxiety-reducing interventions to enhance interpersonal communication.

Attitudes

Biases and stereotyped notions can limit the nurse's and individual's ability to relate in both the nurse and the individual. When the problem is the individual's problem, the nurse can assist in examining those views that interfere with the person's relationships. When the problem is the nurse's, openness to examination of personal behavior in the supervisory relationship is crucial. When the nurse fails to examine his or her attitudes toward the person, negativity may be communicated and the interaction may be distorted.

Gaps Between the Nurse and Individual

Related to attitudinal barriers is the idea that gaps in gender, age, socioeconomic background, race, religion, ethnicity, or language can block functional communication between the nurse and individual. These factors can cause differences in perception and block mutual understanding. The nurse can help the person recognize how perceptions may be different and clarify meanings (see Multicultural Awareness box and Chapter 2).

Resistance

Resistance comprises all phenomena that inhibit the flow of thoughts, feelings, and memories in an interpersonal encounter and behaviors that interfere with therapeutic goals. Resistance arises from anxiety when a person feels threatened. To reduce this anxiety, the person implements resistant behavior, most often in the form of avoidance, such as being late, changing the subject, forgetting, blocking, or becoming angry.

Initially, the nurse should first identify the behavior, whether it is the nurse's behavior or the individual's behavior, and then attempt to interpret it in the context of the interaction. Exploration of possible threats in the relationship, goals, or a particular topic can lead to understanding the source of the resistance and finding the ability to handle these difficulties. Anxiety reduction is often a necessary step in dealing with resistant behavior.

Transference and Countertransference

Transference is reacting to another person in an exchange as though that person were someone from the past. Transference may involve a host of feelings that are generally classified as positive (love, affection, or regard) or negative (anger, dislike, or frustration). The usual transference reaction involves an important figure from the past such as a mother or father; however, at times it may be more general and include all authority figures. Something about the other person's characteristics, behavior, or position triggers this response. Persons in a therapeutic relationship often develop strong transference feelings toward the helping professional, arising from the interaction's intensity and the care provider's authoritative or nurturing role.

Countertransference is the same phenomenon, but it is experienced by the health care professional. The nurse experiences many feelings toward the person; these feelings are not problems unless they remain unanalyzed and become potential blocks to the nurse's ability to work effectively with the individual. For example, if a nurse has deep feelings for the person and thinks the person cannot possibly function after discharge without the nurse's aid, then the nurse is likely to distort the individual's abilities, encourage a childlike dependency, and interfere with the person's progress. This nurse needs to examine his or her personal feelings to understand their source. Once understood, countertransference reactions generally cease to interfere with the relationship. Although rooted in psychoanalytic theory, the contemporary meanings of countertransference are germane to today's practice. Ens' cogent analysis (1998) directs nurses to examine their countertransference to know themselves and the individuals they serve. "If nursing is to attain its widely stated and accepted goals of being with the patient, being part of the patient's environment, and providing empathetic caring, it is imperative that nurses examine impediments such as countertransference, which interfere with these stated goals" (p. 280).

In working with an individual's transference reactions, the nurse helps the person examine his or her feelings and thoughts about the nurse. The person can compare and contrast the nurse with persons from his or her past to better comprehend the present reality.

MULTICULTURAL AWARENESS

Multicultural Context of Communication

As health care providers, nurses might believe that they have expert knowledge about health promotion and the treatment of illness that will be beneficial to others. Therefore, it seems logical that nurses would select appropriate information to share with individuals to help them maintain health and manage illness or alterations in health status. However, consider the possible influences of cultural differences between the nurse and individual.

Much of nursing knowledge and knowledge generated from related disciplines and the sciences is rooted in a Western perspective. Particularly in the United States, knowledge is generated and interpreted from the perspective of the dominant cultural group; that is, a White Anglo-Saxon Christian point of view. When this perspective remains unexamined, alternative perspectives are ignored and invisible. Nurses who are members of the dominant cultural group may be well-intentioned, but ineffective when they attempt to engage a person of a different cultural group in a relationship without questioning how culture influences interactions, interpretations of events and information, and beliefs and values concerning health and health care practices. Preconceived ideas about people based on some characteristic or group affiliation, such as racial or ethnic identity, religion, country of origin, gender, or sexual orientation, can interfere with nurses' ability to relate to people as individuals. At the same time, a lack of knowledge of other cultural groups hampers nurses' understanding of the individual's point of view.

Guidelines for recognizing the multicultural context of communication in therapeutic relationships include the following:

- Make ethnocultural assessment a critical component of every clinical evaluation
- Allow other persons to define themselves
- Respect the language of others and do not assume superiority in language
- Collaborate with trained translators and health promoters (persons with the same ethnic or racial background as the individuals)
- Avoid use of racist, sexist, ageist, and other forms of denigrating language
- Do not perpetuate stereotypes in communication
- Adapt communication to the uniqueness of the individual
- Reject humor that degrades members based on gender, race, ethnicity, religion, sexual orientation, country of origin, and so forth
- Respect the rights of others to have different practices and customs
- Do not allow injustice to continue through silence
- Present information clearly to all people to make an informed choice
- Do not judge values, traditions, and practices based on their similarity or difference from personal values, traditions, and practices, but based on whether they facilitate human potential

The following are some issues for the nurse to consider:

- When the nurse works with a person from a different cultural background, what are common barriers to establishing a therapeutic relationship?
- In learning about different cultural groups, is there a risk of creating new stereotypes that interfere with the ability to treat persons as unique individuals?
- If the nurse has little or no knowledge about a person's culture, how can the nurse provide meaningful nursing care?
- Are the two previous questions contradictory? How can the nurse meet the different challenges that they imply?
- Research measurements are typically developed from the perspective of the dominant culture. If the nurse wishes to use a standardized instrument to measure clinical or research variables among members of different cultural groups, then what questions about the instrument should the nurse ask, and what problems might the nurse encounter? What would need to be done to determine whether an instrument truly measures the same phenomenon across different populations?

Consider the possible influences of cultural differences between the nurse and the individual. Think of an example of two people from different cultural groups who developed a relationship. Examine how they got to know each other and what differences and similarities they uncovered. Did barriers to understanding each other exist? If so, then how did they bridge these barriers? What did they learn about themselves? What did they learn about the ways that culture shapes perspective and interactions? Think about how you can apply these insights to your relationships with persons from cultural groups that differ from their own.

- How would a multicultural perspective change the practice?

Guidelines adapted from Byrd, M. L. (1993). *The intracultural communication book*. New York: McGraw-Hill; Johannesen, R. L. (1996). *Ethics in human communication* (4th ed.). Prospect Heights, IL: Waveland Press; Poss, J. E. (1999). Providing culturally competent care: Is there a role for health promoters? *Nursing Outlook*, 47, 30-36.

Sensory Barriers

When the individual has any sensory limitations, the nurse may need to use extra skill in communicating. Use of the other senses to send or receive messages should be attempted. Special help is often available from trained therapists and teachers; for example, many agencies have access to interpreters for deaf persons and visual aides may be useful. Nurses must be as creative as possible, learn from others who are skilled in alternative forms of communication, and make needed referrals.

Failure to Address Concerns or Needs

The failure to meet the individual's needs or to recognize the individual's concerns is the most serious barrier to effective interaction. This failure can arise from (1) inadequate assessment, (2) lack of knowledge, (3) inability to separate the nurse's needs from the individual's needs, and (4) confusion between friendship and a helping relationship, including unrecognized or unresolved sexual issues. To correct this problem, the nurse should recognize that a barrier to relating with the person exists. Using the supervisory process to determine the problem's source, the nurse should then take corrective action, such as obtaining more information or knowledge, performing a self-assessment with values clarification, and examining reactions, biases, and expectations.

Setting

The setting of a therapeutic interaction can affect the goals and the nature of the communication. The most important aspect of any setting is that the nurse and individual are able to attend to each other. The nurse's attention to the person helps create this atmosphere. The nurse should assess the possible influence of factors such as lighting, noise, temperature, comfort, physical distance, and privacy; potentially disturbing factors can be altered or controlled within the limits of the setting. Occasionally, the nurse has only minimal control over the setting, as in a busy clinic, health center, inpatient unit, or the individual's home. Although far from the ideal of a quiet, pleasant, well-lit private office, these typical clinical settings can be used effectively by creating a sense of private space. Curtains can be drawn, doors shut, and two chairs pulled to a corner to shape an environment for interaction. When possible, however, nurses should seek offices or rooms to establish privacy during significant communication or when imparting important or complex health information. The nurse can also acknowledge verbally that some aspect of the environment, such as an interruption or noise, is bothersome. This strategy shows people that the nurse recognizes possible concentration difficulties and is sharing the environment with them.

Stages

Therapeutic relationships follow sequential phases, which may overlap, vary in length, or involve issues that appear over time rather than in a set sequence. Orientation (introductory), working, and termination phases have been identified by researchers and clinicians.

Originally, these stages were identified from therapeutic relationships that developed over time. However, they can be observed in brief encounters that are effective; that is, interactions that meet individuals' needs rather than therapeutic interactions that have been reduced to little more than quick question-and-answer sessions. Whether the nurse is engaged in a long-term or short-term relationship with an individual, attention to the **relationship stages** is important. Brief therapeutic relationships will telescope the stages; therefore it is particularly important that the nurse focus on meeting the key demands of each relationship phase. It is important to note that individuals may move in and out of direct care episodes while a therapeutic relationship is maintained over time. A relationship exists even when the nurse and individual do not see each other for an extended period and each encounter takes place within the trajectory of the relationship stages.

Orientation or Introductory Phase

The orientation or introductory phase begins when the nurse and individual meet. This meeting typically involves some feeling of anxiety; neither party knows what to expect. When the therapeutic relationship is primarily a counseling type of relationship, part of the nurse's role is to help structure the interaction by discussing several topics during the initial and sometimes first few meetings. Box 4-7 lists topics appropriate to this phase of the therapeutic relationship. Discussion of these issues establishes a contract or pact and involves a mutual understanding of the parameters of the relationship and an agreement to work together.

The orientation stage is a critical juncture in any therapeutic relationship. Without successful transition through the orientation phase, no working alliance will exist and treatment goals will remain unmet. In research concerning factors that influenced the progress of the therapeutic relationship during the orientation phase, Forchuk (1995) noted that the duration, but not the frequency, of therapeutic interactions is significantly related to time spent in the orientation phase. This finding has implications for the way that nurses and organizations plan interactions. Frequent, brief encounters may be less effective and more expensive in the long run (by prolonging the orientation process) than fewer sessions scheduled for longer periods. Moreover, assessment of an individual's needs should be the primary guideline for session planning. In a descriptive qualitative study of the nurses' perceptions of their therapeutic relationships, Forchuk and colleagues (2000) identified the following helpful factors during the orientation phase: consistency, pacing, listening, positive initial impressions, and attention to comfort and control. In contrast, factors that hamper relationships include inconsistency, unavailability, individ-

Box 4-7 Key Topics of Discussion During the Orientation or Introductory Phase of the Therapeutic Relationship

1. What to call each other
2. Purpose of meeting
3. Location, time, and length of meetings
4. Termination date or time for review of progress
5. Confidentiality (with whom clinical data will be shared)
6. Any other limits related to the particular setting

ual factors associated with trust, nurses' feelings about the other person, confrontation of delusions, and unrealistic expectations.

When first attempting to establish a relationship with individuals, students and novice nurses may be unsure of what to expect and may feel anxious. To relieve their anxiety, students and nurses may use defense mechanisms such as finding excuses that prevent them from initiating a meeting with the person or becoming angry at the staff, faculty, or individual. When students and nurses are open to examination of their behaviors and feelings in this situation, they are able to manage their anxiety and engage in work with individuals; they are ready to move to the next phase of the therapeutic relationship.

When the therapeutic relationship is not primarily structured as counseling with a specific number of sessions, the orientation phase may appear less distinct and the topics noted may seem irrelevant. In this case, the nurse can adapt the suggested topics to meet the specific situation. However, except in true emergencies, initial encounters should always include introductions by name, discussion of the purpose, and a plan for ongoing care or specific follow-up.

research highlights

Effective Therapeutic Relationships

Using a descriptive qualitative approach, Forchuk and colleagues (2000) examined the evolving therapeutic relationship from the nurses' perspective and compared the patterns described by the nurses with those found in Hildagard Peplau's theory of interpersonal relations in nursing (1969, 1991). In a tertiary care psychiatric hospital in southern Ontario, Canada, 10 nurses participated in audiotaped interviews throughout the orientation phase of their newly formed therapeutic relationships with 10 psychiatric inpatients.

Research questions concerned the nature and progression of the therapeutic relationship and helping and hampering factors. Seven of the nurse-individual dyads established a working relationship during the admission over a period that ranged 2 1/2 weeks and 6 months. Two other dyads failed to develop a working relationship despite efforts over a 6-month timeframe for one dyad and 1 year for the other. The nurses identified consistency, pacing set by the individual, listening, positive initial impression, individual comfort and shared control, and individual factors (active participation, efforts to seek out the nurse, and trust) as helping factors. Hampering factors were composed of inconsistency and unavailability, nurses' feelings and lack of self-awareness, patient factors and trust, confrontation of delusions, and unrealistic expectations. Helping factors that emerged and descriptions of therapeutic relationships are consistent with Peplau's theory. Nevertheless, the dyads who experienced problems during the orientation phase failed to progress to the working phase. Rather, these dyads moved to a "grappling and struggling phase" (p. 9) characterized by mutually frustrating efforts to try out and drop various approaches. Subsequently, these dyads dissolved in the final "mutual withdrawal phase" (p. 9).

This study provides empiric support for Peplau's theory of effective therapeutic relationships. Moreover, the researchers elucidated factors that interfere with establishing therapeutic relationships with selected psychiatric hospitalized individuals. Although additional research is needed that includes greater diversity of settings, individual profiles, and contexts, this study highlights helping and hampering factors that nurses can assess and monitor to promote success when establishing therapeutic relationships.

Data from Forchuck, C., Westwell, J., Martin, M., Bamber-Azzapardi, W., Kosterewa-Tolman, D., & Hux, M. (2000). The developing nurse-client relationship: Nurses' perspectives. *Journal of the American Psychiatric Nurses Association*, 6, 3-10.

Working Phase

The working phase of the therapeutic relationship emerges when the nurse and the individual collaborate as partners in promoting the person's health. The working phase may last for an established number of sessions, as in brief psychotherapy, or it may extend over an extended period if the nurse is the primary care provider for an individual or family.

During this phase, the major tasks of the relationship are met. Goals are set and the nurse and individual work mutually toward their accomplishment. Interventions are tailored to the specific situation and health needs of the person and family. Solving problems, coping with stressors, and gaining insight are all part of the working phase. The nurse and individual recognize each other's uniqueness.

Resistant behaviors may be observed during this phase as the nurse and individual become closer and work on potentially anxiety-producing problems. The person may pull away through the use of defense mechanisms because change can be difficult. Overcoming the resistance becomes an important nursing task.

The working phase is the vehicle for effective nursing intervention. During the working phase, the relationship is the context through which change takes place; it is the context for health promotion.

Termination Phase

Termination marks the end of the relationship established in the therapeutic contract or negotiated in accordance with the limits of the contract. Ending a relationship can cause anxiety for both the individual and the nurse. Termination represents a loss; therefore it can trigger feelings of sadness, frustration, and anger. Termination is the loss of a relationship and the loss of future involvement, with its attendant realistic expectations or fantasies. Termination also reawakens feelings of previously unresolved losses, such as a death or divorce.

It is important that the individual works through any feelings related to the termination. Some individuals require the nurse's assistance to experience the feelings of

Box 4-8 Interventions for Use During the Termination Phase of the Therapeutic Relationship

1. Let the individual know why the relationship is to be terminated
2. Remind the person of the date and how many meetings are left during the latter period of the relationship
3. Collaborate with other staff so they are aware of how the individual is reacting and any special needs the person may have at this time
4. Help the person identify other people with whom it is possible to have a relationship
5. Review the gains and the goals that remain
6. Discuss the pros and cons experienced during the relationship to help the individual develop a realistic appraisal
7. Make any referrals for follow-up care

Box 4-9 Key Ingredients for a 15-Minute Family Interview

1. Use manners to engage or reengage. Make an introduction by offering name and role. Orient family members to the purpose of a brief family interview
2. Assess key areas of internal and external structure and function (obtain genogram information and key external support data)
3. Ask three key questions of family members
4. Commend the family on one or two strengths.
5. Evaluate usefulness and conclude

Adapted from Wright L. M., & Leahey M. (2000). *Nurses and families: A guide to family assessment and intervention* (3rd ed., p. 287). Philadelphia: F.A. Davis.

loss and to connect present reactions to past real or symbolic losses. Box 4-8 lists additional interventions for use during the termination phase.

Both the nurse and the individual can learn much during termination; the process directs both participants to examine problems and progress in the relationship, feelings, and reactions. Termination experience also helps the nurse and individual gain practice in ending relationships and in exploring reactions, which can be most helpful when future losses occur.

Brief Interactions: The 15-Minute Interview

Time constraints in practice are unavoidable. Although challenging, brief therapeutic encounters can be meaningful and useful (Gilbert, 1998). Limited time is not a valid reason to avoid interviewing or interacting with individuals. Rather, nurses can purposefully structure brief interactions to achieve specific clinical outcomes (Wright & Leahey, 2000). Box 4-9 delineates key ingredients for a **15-minute interview** with a family.

These guidelines for brief interactions with families can be adapted for interviews with individuals. An effective 15-minute interview is feasible if nurses plan to introduce themselves, state the purpose of meeting, validate understanding with the person and/or family, clarify parameters such as time, focus and listen, and elicit significant individual and family data. Most importantly, the goal of the interaction must be realistic and clearly defined. For example, the purpose may be to elicit a family's view of the presenting problem or to prioritize problems to be treated.

research highlights

Relational Messages

A relational message framework was used in a study of themes communicated by nurses during brief encounters with patients (Gilbert, 1998). The following research questions were addressed: "(a) What relational message factors, if any, are communicated by nurses' listening behavior during brief patient-nurse interactions? (b) If any are communicated, does their pattern of scores reflect a positive patient-nurse relationship?" (p. 8).

Participants were 173 nonnursing undergraduate students enrolled in an entry-level nursing survey course. Given the possible cultural influences on relational messages, only data from American-born White women were reported. Participants viewed videotaped patient-nurse interactions recorded in a previous study (Gilbert, 1993). The videotapes show White baccalaureate-prepared female nurses dressed in lab coats who were asked to "listen" to the same White actress acting as a patient who described an accident in which her best friend had been killed. After a practice session, participants viewed six segments involving different nurses interacting with the same "patient" describing the same event. Presentation order was varied.

After viewing each videotape segment, participants reported what the nurse's listening behavior communicated on a rating scale of 29 items representative of relational messages. The thirtieth item concerned overall satisfaction with each nurse's communication. Data from each segment were analyzed using principal axis factoring with pair-wise deletion of data and varimax rotation. A seven-factor solution revealed a similar factor structure for each of the six interactions. Explained variance ranged from 57.7% to 65%.

The study's findings revealed the following relational message factors communicated by nurses' listening behavior: "trust/receptivity, depth/similarity/affection, difference, dominance or power, formality, and composure" (p. 18). Gilbert (1998) concluded that the findings supported the relational message framework. The pattern of thematic scores in four interactions suggested communication indicative of a positive nurse-patient relationship. Although implications for practice should be drawn with caution, the findings indicate that communication of positive patient-nurse relationships is not automatically precluded by time constraints common to today's practice arena.

Data from Gilbert, D. A. (1998). Relational message themes in nurses' listening behavior during brief patient-nurse interactions. *Scholarly Inquiry for Nursing Practice: An International Journal, 12*, 5-26.

CASE STUDY

A Home Visit

As part of a clinical nursing experience, Jessica Mills made a home visit to Mrs. Maria Sanchez-Cohen. Ms. Mills had provided nursing care to Mrs. Sanchez-Cohen during her delivery of her first baby 3 weeks earlier. The purpose of the home visit was to conduct an infant assessment, provide breastfeeding support, teach about normal infant development and care activities, and assess Mrs. Sanchez-Cohen's adaptation to motherhood and her postpartum recovery status. Ms. Mills was looking forward to seeing Mrs. Sanchez-Cohen and her baby, Jacob Thomas.

Before making the home visit, Ms. Mills reviewed the clinical information she obtained during Mrs. Sanchez-Cohen's hospitalization. Mrs. Sanchez-Cohen is a 34-year-old Hispanic, primiparous woman who delivered a 7 pound, 10 ounce healthy boy after a 12-hour labor. The labor had progressed well without complication. Mrs. Sanchez-Cohen received epidural anesthesia at 6-centimeter dilation and she delivered vaginally. Her husband, Mark Cohen, provided labor support and was present for the delivery. After a 2-day hospital stay, Mrs. Sanchez-Cohen was discharged breastfeeding. At discharge, the infant had a normal newborn examination and weighed 7 pounds, 5 ounces. Ms. Mills had been impressed by both parents' preparation for the birth; they had attended childbirth classes and read several books about infant development and parenting. Mrs. Sanchez-Cohen planned to take an 8-week maternity leave from her position as a lawyer in a large practice and had arranged for a childcare provider to come to the family's home to take care of the infant beginning 2 weeks before the end of her maternity leave. Mr. Cohen had not planned to take time off from his job because he had recently been promoted to a high-level managerial position in his company that required increased travel and time at work. He was able to postpone a business trip to be present at the delivery and had sent a plane ticket to his mother-in-law so she could come and stay at their home during the first week after Mrs. Sanchez-Cohen and Jacob Thomas came home from the hospital.

During the home visit, Ms. Mills first assessed the infant. She incorporated teaching concerning normal infant development and concluded that Jacob Thomas was a healthy 3-week old infant who was feeding well. Jacob Thomas's circumcision was healing without complication. Mrs. Sanchez-Cohen described the visit to the pediatrician's office the previous week. The pediatrician had said that Jacob Thomas was doing very well and said he was pleased to see that he had regained his birth weight.

When Ms. Mills asked how Mrs. Sanchez-Cohen was doing, Mrs. Sanchez-Cohen hesitated and then responded, "I'm not sure. I'm very glad that Jacob is doing well. I worry sometimes that I'm not going to be able to do everything right for him. It's funny, but I've spent so many years getting an education and establishing my law career. It was hard work, but I managed to do well. Now a little infant overwhelms me. I don't know how I'll manage this." When Ms. Mills asked Mrs. Sanchez-Cohen to talk more about her concerns, Mrs. Sanchez-Cohen described how incompetent she felt while her mother was staying with her. "My mother could do everything so easily. I fumbled with every diaper. It felt like she criticized how I did things. When she told me about postpartum practices she had learned when she had children, I felt pushed to do things 'her way' and not the way that I had planned. She even wanted to give him a bottle when I was trying so hard to get breastfeeding going. At least the doctor said Jacob had gained enough weight. That made me feel like I wasn't a total failure. I couldn't wait for her to go, but I fell apart after she left. I was alone. Mark is out of town until the weekend and I couldn't get Jacob to stop crying yesterday. I thought I would scream so I put him down in his crib and I just sat there crying. What's wrong with me? I've never felt so out of control before. I want to be a good mother, but I feel like I can't give any more right now."

In response to Ms. Mills' follow-up questions about mental status, Mrs. Sanchez-Cohen described the following: frequently feeling irritated and sad, crying a few times over the last several days, difficulty sleeping even when the baby was asleep, feeling fatigue, and being worried about how she would be able to go back to work in only a few weeks. Ms. Mills also inquired about the family's cultural, ethnic, and religious backgrounds. Mrs. Sanchez-Cohen responded, "Interesting that you should ask. That's actually another issue right now. I'm from New Mexico and my family is Hispanic and Catholic. You might guess that I'm Latina from my hyphenated name. I added my maiden name to Cohen when I got married to honor my family. We even put Thomas as a middle name to honor my grandfather. Mark is Jewish and his family comes from New Jersey. They are very nice and were supportive when we got married. We were lucky that our families accepted us together.

I have to admit, though, that we didn't really figure out what we would do about raising the baby. I mean, I told Mark that I thought we could raise the baby Jewish because it's so important to him and we believe some of the same things anyway. I learned a lot of Bible stories growing up and I'm not very religious now. We didn't really take the time to talk it through more than that and didn't talk to our families either. I think I wanted to avoid it. I knew my mother would want to have a Baptism, but I didn't think that would be right. At the same time, I didn't want to disappoint or hurt her. Mark expected that we'd have a bris to circumcise Jacob when he was 8 days old. I didn't realize it was so important to do it then or that it was such an important religious thing for him. My mother was here and got very upset when we told her our plans. I felt like I had betrayed my upbringing and I felt guilty that I hadn't talked it over with her sooner. Mark had wanted to invite his relatives and some friends here to celebrate the bris, but I couldn't handle it. We had a big scene. We still had Jacob circumcised, but we just did it at the obstetrician's office. I felt like I had ruined everything. Mark was so proud to be a father and have our son. He planned this special party and I couldn't do it. My mother was angry with me, too. I think she wanted to plan a Christening party in a few weeks back in New Mexico. She just assumed that we'd have Catholic children. Having different backgrounds has never been a problem for Mark and me. Now everything is a problem. I don't know how to fix things. I've made such a mess. Can you help me? I feel like I'm going out of my mind and I don't know what to do."

This case study raises a variety of clinical concerns. As the

Continued

CASE STUDY cont'd

nurse in this encounter, Ms. Mills might begin by considering the following questions:

- What is the significance of the distress symptoms that Mrs. Sanchez-Cohen reported? Given that the period during which many women experience postpartum blues has passed, what is the most appropriate action to obtain a thorough mental status examination?
- What are my feelings as I listen to her story and her distress? Am I aware of how my values and expectations affect my interaction with this person?
- How can I establish a therapeutic relationship to support Mrs. Sanchez-Cohen during this stressful period? Who is the most appropriate health care provider to evaluate and treat her for the postpartum depression that I suspect she is developing? How can I facilitate getting her the care she needs and can I remain available to her? What risks might exist for the infant and how can these be addressed?
- In what ways do family dynamics, values, and expectations related to differing cultural and religious heritages contribute to the problems described? What can I do to explore these issues further? How can I engage support systems to ameliorate rather than exacerbate the difficulties? What can be done to engage both Mr. Cohen and Mrs. Sanchez-Cohen in a therapeutic relationship to focus on the couple and parenting concerns and to involve both partners in treatment strategies?

HOT topics

THERAPEUTIC RELATIONSHIPS IN THE AGE OF THE INTERNET

Technological advances have produced rapid changes in communication. Automatic teller machines have replaced human tellers at banks for most routine transactions. Libraries have removed card catalogs in favor of online listings of holdings and access to a network of databases and libraries. Voicemail rather than a receptionist is likely to answer calls and messages are electronically recorded. A response may come in the form of another voicemail message. Information in so many areas is now available via access to a computer and an Internet connection. These technologies can speed up work and expand capabilities. Who would prefer to use a traditional typewriter to prepare papers and documents after mastering a word-processing computer program?

Telehealth, the use of "telecommunications equipment and communications networks for transferring health care information between participants at different locations" (Chaffee, 1999, p. 27), is now omnipresent. Telenursing, delivery of nursing care via a telecommunication system (Chaffee, 1999), is a rapidly expanding facet of practice. These technological advances have produced benefits; however, technology can also reduce the need for direct interpersonal contact.

- What effects on the therapeutic relationship results from technological changes?
- Will face-to-face interaction become a rare occurrence? In the future, might therapeutic interactions take place primarily via technology, such as voicemail, the Internet, and video? What advantages and disadvantages will appear in the increasing use of technology in nursing practice?
- What creative approaches may evolve using technology in therapeutic relationships? Consider how to avoid making interactions impersonal when technology is used.

For additional information about telehealth, see: American Nurses Association. (1999). *Core principles on telehealth*. Washington, DC: American Nurses Publishing; Chaffee, M. (1999). A telehealth odyssey. *American Journal of Nursing, 99*, 27-32.

Even when time is limited, the interview is structured to provide opportunity for the person or family to engage in dialogue as an active participant in care and the nurse's attention is completely focused on the individual.

SUMMARY

Relating to individuals offers many challenges and rewards for nurses. Although some aspects of this work are predictable, each person or family is unique and each provides a chance for the nurse to learn, grow, and help in new ways. This chapter provides guidelines for developing therapeutic relationships, but it does not guarantee success or an easy job. The desire and skill of the individual nurse bring this information to life. The blend of the nurse's artistry, humanity, knowledge, skill, and ethics sparks concern and the ability to help another human being communicate effectively.

The therapeutic relationship is the primary arena for health promotion. Values clarification, communication, and the helping relationship are its core components. Knowing how to apply this knowledge to their role beyond the confines of individual therapeutic encounters is useful to nurses.

As technology increases and pressure to provide cost-effective care continues, it is paramount that nurses provide interventions that are embedded in the therapeutic relationship (see Hot Topics box). Without a relational context, the care dimension in health care is lost and health promotion is reduced to standardized recipelike prescriptions. To promote real change in health and health care, nurses can focus on their value of caring, communicate and demonstrate their worth and the importance of their work to others, and nurture their professional nurse-nurse relationships.

REFERENCES

American Nurses Association. (1999). *Core principles on telehealth*. Washington, DC: American Nurses Publishing.

Blondis, M. N., & Jackson, B. E. (1982). *Nonverbal communication with patients: Back to the human touch* (2nd ed.). New York: John Wiley & Sons.

Brown, S. J. (1999). Patient-centered communication. In J. J. Fitzpatrick (Ed.), *Annual review of nursing research: Vol. 17. Focus on complementary health and pain management* (pp. 85-104). New York: Springer Publishing Co.

Byrd, M. L. (1993). *The intracultural communication book*. New York: McGraw-Hill.

Chaffee, M. (1999). A telehealth odyssey. *American Journal of Nursing, 99*, 27-32.

Cody, W. K. (2000). Nursing science frameworks for practice and research as means of knowing self. *Nursing Science Quarterly, 13*, 188-195.

Coopersmith, S. (1967). *The antecedents of self-esteem*. San Francisco: WH Freeman.

DeMarco, R. F., Horowitz, J. A., & McLoed, D. (2000). A call to intraprofessional alliances. *Nursing Outlook, 48*, 172-178.

Ens, I. C. (1998). An analysis of the concept of countertransference. *Archives of Psychiatric Nursing, 12*, 273-281.

Forchuk, C. (1995). Development of nurse-client relationships: what helps? *Journal of the American Psychiatric Nurses Association 1*, 146-153.

Forchuck, C., Westwell, J., Martin, M., Bamber-Azzapardi, W., Kosterewa-Tolman, D., & Hux, M. (2000). The developing nurse-client relationship: Nurses' perspectives. *Journal of the American Psychiatric Nurses Association*, 6, 3-10.

Gilbert, D. A. (1993). Reciprocity of involvement activities in client-nurse interactions. *Western Journal of Nursing Research, 15*, 674-689.

Gilbert, D. A. (1998). Relational message themes in nurses' listening behavior during brief patient-nurse interactions. *Scholarly Inquiry for Nursing Practice: An International Journal, 12*, 5-26.

Hall, E. (1973). *The silent language*. Garden City, NY: Doubleday/ Anchor Press.

Horowitz, J. A. (1995). A conceptualization of parenting: Examining the single-parent family. *Marriage and Family Review, 20*, 43-70.

Johannesen, R. L. (1996). *Ethics in human communication* (4th ed.). Prospect Heights, IL: Waveland Press.

Jourard, S. (1971). *The transparent self* (Rev. ed.). New York: Van Nostrand Reinhold.

Kasch, C. R. (1986). Toward a theory of nursing action: Skills and competency in nurse-patient interactions. *Nursing Research, 35*, 226-230.

Kottler, J. A., & Brown, R. W. (1996). *Introduction to therapeutic counseling* (3rd ed.). Pacific Grove, CA: Brooks/Cole.

Kowalski, K., Burton, L., & Rehwaldt, M. (1997). Revisioning, re-educating, regenerating, and recommitting nursing for the twenty-first century. *Nursing Outlook, 54*, 220-223.

Liaschenko, J. (1997). Knowing the patient? In S. E. Thorne, & V. E. Hayes (Eds.), *Nursing praxis: Knowledge and action* (pp. 23-38). Thousand Oaks, CA: Sage Publications.

Long, V. O. (1996). *Communication skills in helping relationships: A framework for facilitating personal growth*. Pacific Grove, CA: Brooks/Cole.

Luft, J. (1969). *Of human interaction*. Palo Alto, CA: National Press Books.

Luft, J. (1984). *Group processes: an introduction to group dynamics* (3rd ed.). Palo Alto, CA: Mayfield.

Olson, J. K. (1995). Relationships between nurse-expressed empathy, patient-perceived empathy and patient distress. *Image–Journal of Nursing Scholarship, 27*, 317-322.

O'Toole, A., & Welt S. R. (1989). *Interpersonal theory in nursing practice*. New York: Springer.

Peplau, H. E. (1963). Process and concept of learning. In S. Burd, & M. Marshall (Eds., pp. 348-352), *Some clinical approaches to psychiatric nursing*. New York: Macmillan.

Peplau, H. E. (1964). *Basic principles of patient counseling* (2nd ed.). Philadelphia: Smith Kline and French Laboratories.

Peplau, H. E. (1969). Professional closeness: As a special kind of involvement with a patient, client, or family group, *Nursing Forum, 8*, 342-360.

Peplau, H. E. (1991). *Interpersonal relations in nursing*. New York: Springer.

Phillips, L. R., Luna, I., Russell, C. K., Baca, G., Lim, Y. M., Cromwell. S. L., & Torres de Ardon, E. (1996). Toward a cross-cultural perspective of family caregiving. *Western Journal of Nursing Research, 18*, 236-251.

Poss, J. E. (1999). Providing culturally competent care: Is there a role for health promoters? *Nursing Outlook, 47*, 30-36.

Raths, L., Harmin, M., & Simon, S. (1978). *Values and teaching*. Columbus, OH: Charles E Merrill.

Rogers, C. (1965). *Client-centered therapy*. Boston: Houghton Mifflin.

Ruesch, J., & Bateson, G. (1987). *Communication: The social matrix of psychiatry*. New York: W.W. Norton.

Sears, R. R. (1970). Relation of early socialization experience to self-concepts and gender role in middle childhood. *Child Development, 41*, 267-289.

Seigley, L. A. (1999). Self-esteem and health behavior: Theoretic and empiric links. *Nursing Outlook, 47*, 74-77.

Stewart, M. A. (1995). Effective physician-patient communication and health outcomes: A review. *Canadian Medical Association Journal, 152*, 1423-1433.

Stuart, G. W., & Laraia, M. T. (1998). *Stuart & Sundeen's principles and practice of psychiatric nursing* (6th ed.). St Louis: Mosby.

Sullivan, H. S. (1953). *The interpersonal theory of psychiatry*. New York: W.W. Norton.

Sundeen, S. J., Stuart, G. W., Rankin, E. A. D., & Cohen, S. A. (1998). *Nurse-client interaction: Implementing the nursing process* (6th ed.). St. Louis: Mosby.

Takman, C. A. S., & Severinsson, E. I. (1999). A description of health care professionals' experiences of encounters with patients in clinical settings. *Journal of Advanced Nursing, 30*, 1368-1374.

Watzlawick, P., Beavin, J. H., & Jackson, D. D. (1967). *Pragmatics of human communication: A study of interactional patterns, pathologies and paradoxes*. New York: W.W. Norton.

Whittemore, R. (2000). Consequences of not "knowing the patient." *Clinical Specialist, 14*, 75-81.

Wong, D. (2000). *Whaley & Wong's nursing care of infants and children* (6th ed.). St Louis: Mosby.

Wright, L. M., & Leahey, M. (2000). *Nurses and families: A guide to family assessment and intervention* (3rd ed.). Philadelphia: F.A. Davis.

Chapter 5

CAROL LYNN MANDLE
CAROLYN HAYES

Ethical Issues Relevant to Health Promotion

objectives

After completing this chapter, the nurse will be able to:

- Discuss ethics as *humanizing;* that is, pertaining to the development of the whole person.
- Describe the relationship of norm to value.
- Describe three traditional theoretic approaches in philosophical ethics: egoism, Kantianism, and utilitarianism.
- Describe five traditional theoretic approaches in theological ethics: Jewish, Catholic, and Protestant.
- Describe three contemporary theoretic approaches in philosophical ethics: Frankena's theory of obligation, Firth's ideal observer theology, Rawls' justice as fairness, care ethics, and feminist ethics.
- Define the nature of the discipline of health care ethics today.
- Describe the role and limitations of professional codes of ethics in nursing today.
- Identify the principles of ethics stressed in professional codes of ethics for nursing today.
- Contrast the influences of ethics versus laws in the nursing profession and health promotion today.
- Discuss factors to consider in moral decision making.
- Describe the concept of integrity-preserving compromise and its relationship to moral agency of the nurse.
- Delineate a method for analyzing ethical dilemmas in health promotion.
- Discuss paradigmatic cases of ethical dilemmas in health promotion.

key terms

Care-Based Reasoning
Codes
Deontology
Dilemmas
Ethics
Integrity-Preserving Compromise
Morality
Teleology

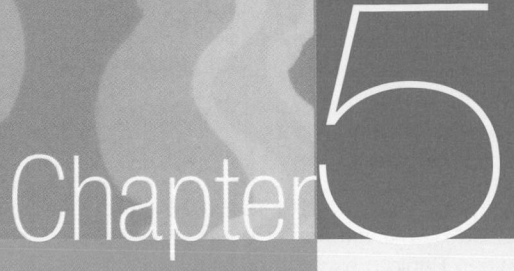

THINK About It: Ethical Issues in *In Vitro* Fertilization

Paula and Greg have been married for over 10 years. They have spent the past 5 years actively trying to have children. They very much want to become parents. Greg's infertility work-up has revealed that he is capable of impregnating a woman. However, Paula's tests have revealed that her best chance at pregnancy is through assisted reproductive technology (ART). In fact, the chances of Paula getting pregnant without ART are considered to be close to zero.

Greg does not believe in "interfering with nature." He considers such extreme measures to be "playing God." However, after 2 years of counseling, he has agreed to donate sperm for fertilization. He agrees because he is committed to Paula and he knows how strongly she feels about birthing her own child. His concession is premised with the condition that Paula will be implanted with all fertilized eggs regardless of how many children that would leave them accountable for raising. He believes the fertilized eggs are the beginning of life. He wants them treated as his children. Greg does not want to create any fertilized eggs that will not be given a chance to be born.

Paula agrees to Greg's condition that every fertilized egg will be implanted. Together they shared this information with the health care team, including the nurse. Paula returned to the clinic alone for a separate appointment to begin hormone injections. During that visit, Paula told the nurse her plan was to be implanted with all the fertilized eggs as she had agreed, but to have a selective reduction procedure should she become pregnant with more fetuses than the physician thought she could carry to term. Additionally, Paula expressed certainty that Greg would change his mind about future pregnancies after one or two children were part of their family. Paula considered this exchange confidential and believes the nurse is not free to discuss her plans with Greg.

1 Who is the patient in this situation? Can there ever be more than one person to whom the health care team must answer equally? Are there legal consequences for any of the possible actions the nurse may take?

2 Does informed consent for Greg's sperm donation include disclosure of the long-term plans should Paula become impregnated with multiple fetuses? Is this matter between the two of them or are the health care team members ethically accountable for actions taken? Could Paula be ethically or legally held to her promise to be impregnated with all the fertilized eggs?

3 Is there an ethical difference between not telling Greg if Paula has a selective reduction in these circumstances versus not telling any father when a mother chooses to have an abortive or selective reduction procedure?

continued

THINK About It: Ethical Issues in *In Vitro* Fertilization—cont'd

4 How can the nurse best anticipate the ethical dilemmas posed by this situation? What should the nurse do when Paula presents her plans? What could the health care team have done when meeting with Greg and Paula together that may have helped avoid the current dilemma?

The previous chapters have examined the biological, psychosocial, economical, philosophical, and theological dimensions of staying healthy. In this chapter, the ethical dimensions of these important issues are discussed. There are many misunderstandings about the discipline of ethics and, before some major ethical issues of interest to healthy people are examined, it is necessary to describe basic ethical notions before presenting a discussion on the specific questions of health care ethics. Additionally, fundamental notions on the nature and techniques of ethical decision making must be set forth. Then specific ethical issues of interest to healthy people can be considered.

TOWARD AN UNDERSTANDING OF ETHICS

The Nature of Ethics

Ethics is concerned with the humanization process. It proclaims its share of "oughts" and "ought nots," enabling men and women to become what they are destined to be: fully developed and mature human beings. Throughout the centuries, many definitions of ethics have been proposed. For some persons ethics is an attempt to discover the behavioral implications of being human. For others it is a study of the origins and nature of "oughts" and "ought nots" that constitute the pursuit of what the classic authors called the *verum humanum*, "that which embodies total humanization." Above all, ethics is a search for what shapes the human being, for what contributes to the growth and development of the person. It is an attempt to discover all those elements that are required to make and keep life human so a person may achieve the goals of the humanization process and live as properly and well as possible (Ladd, 1978; Reich, 1978).

The word *ethics* is derived from the Greek *ethos*, "the customary way of acting," or the manner of action that contributes to the growth of the human person. Often the word *morality* is used as a substitute for ethics. **Morality** is merely a synonym for ethics, derived from the Latin *mosmoris*, which also signifies "the customary way of acting," in the sense of that which "customarily" brings about true humanization. The term *moral ethics* is redundant and should not be used. A person engaged in the study of how human beings should act is involved in the study of "ethics," if one employs the Greek root, or in the study of "morality," if one uses the Latin root.

Relationship Between the "Is" and the "Ought"

The study of ethics is concerned with the discovery of humanizing "oughts" and the discouragement of dehumanizing "ought nots." Where are these found? Most traditional forms of thinking have always located the "ought" in the "is"; what the person ought to do is always rooted in what the person actually is. An automobile ought to be able to transport its owner; a power mower *ought* to be able to cut grass. A car cannot be expected to cut the lawn or a power mower cannot be a means of transportation. What these machines *ought* to do is very much related to what each is.

Ethics is not concerned with any type of ought; rather, it is concerned solely with *humanizing oughts*. Ethics must begin with a consideration of what constitutes the human being, what the individual is. Every system of ethics articulates its "oughts" in the light of and as a consequence of the manner in which it conceives the essence of the human being. Every ethical system proceeds from and is rooted in a basic *anthropology*, an understanding of what constitutes the human being. A system's anthropology constitutes the point of departure for the formulation of its ethics. For example, nursing has a discipline-based conception of the essence of the human person. The American Nurses' Association (ANA) Social Policy Statement articulates this perspective when stating, "Humans manifest as an essential unity of mind/body/spirit" (ANA, 1995, p. 3).

In a pluralist society, a considerable number of ethical systems are met, many of which differ radically from others. As examples, one group favors abortion as a practical and humanizing solution for an unwanted pregnancy and another classifies abortion as the direct taking of an innocent life. One group favors euthanasia for individuals with terminal illnesses; another denounces this action as the unjust taking of human life. One group favors cochlear implants to correct a disability; another views being deaf as a culture, not a handicap (Dolnick, 1993). Differing solutions to human problems are rooted in different understandings of what constitutes the human person. Every ethical system that articulates humanizing "oughts" and dehumanizing "ought nots" finds the source of its teaching in a specific understanding of what shapes that elusive entity known as *human nature*.

Types of Ethics

As stated, all systems of ethics are rooted in a specific anthropology. The "oughts" and "ought nots" that they set forth find their origins in a specific understanding of human nature. The source of such understandings must now be sought by seeking the answer to a specific question: "Where can human beings discover the elements that constitute their nature?" To answer that question, the distinction between philosophical and theological ethics must be made.

Philosophical ethics is grounded in its comprehension of human nature in human reason. Human reason tries to formulate an understanding of human nature by means of a rational and comprehensive examination of the elements that distinguish members of the human race from animals and other forms of subhuman existence. Human reason proceeds from the premise that all things fundamentally reasonable contribute to the humanizing process. Stating that the use of reason distinguishes human beings from all other creatures, this form of ethics teaches that, when properly applied, human reason can determine those elements essential to the growth and development of the person. To accomplish this task in a competent manner, philosophical ethics uses a variety of auxiliary sciences, such as psychology and sociology.

Theological ethics is also based in its comprehension of human nature in the use of reason, but it does so by using human reason enlightened by the means of a religious faith or affirmative acceptance of a divine revelation, which is a sort of divine "breakthrough." By means of this revelation, God communicates some knowledge of the divine nature and that of the human beings whom God has created. For individuals unfamiliar with theology, it is important to point out that the knowledge about God, or God's people with whom God communicates, is in no way contrary to human reason, but it supplements it. Theological ethics therefore attempts to articulate the ethical implications of being a believer: one who accepts and takes to heart the revelatory communications made by a gracious God. These systems include Muslim ethics, Jewish ethics, and Christian ethics, the last of which has been subdivided into Catholic and Reformed (Protestant) ethics, at least since the fifteenth century.

Although the difference between philosophical and theological ethics can be distinguished in theory, it is important to remember that theology cannot be separated from philosophy. Theological ethics is not merely a system of pious platitudes devoid of rational foundation. Rather, it is a science that attempts to articulate accurately a religious faith by using other sciences such as philosophy, psychology, sociology, cultural anthropology, reproductive physiology, and history.

Elements of Ethics

According to Dyck (1977), "Ethics as a discipline . . . is a systematic analysis of what things are right or wrong, good or bad, virtuous or evil (normative ethics); of what is meant or conveyed by these moral terms to see whether or to what extent judgments involving them can or cannot be rationally justified (metaethics); and of specific moral decisions and policies, and what ethics can contribute to such decisions and policies (moral policy)."

Ethics is a normative science. Dissimilar to sociology, ethics is not merely content to observe what human beings are doing; rather, it is especially concerned with what human beings "ought" or "ought not" to be doing. Ethics lays down certain norms that are to be followed if the humanization process is to be accomplished; it is concerned with precepts, rules and regulations, principles, and guidelines. Ethics tries to answer the question: "What should I do and what should I avoid if I am to become a mature human being?" As a normative discipline, ethics tries to point out what human beings should do or refrain from doing if they are to achieve the *verum humanum*.

Ethics is also concerned with *metaethics*. Ethics is not merely content to lay down the "what" concerning human activity; it also attempts to articulate the "why" behind the "what." Ethics tries to show why norms are needed, how they should be formulated, and the type of language that should be used in their formulation. Additionally, ethics endeavors to identify the specific value that underlies the norm. Any humanizing good is called a value; the norm's function is to indicate how to achieve the particular good. Norms are rooted in and dependent upon values. As insights into values change, norms must be modified accordingly. As a metaethical discipline, ethics does not merely articulate norms to achieve humanization, it also explores the "why." As Ladd (1978) writes, "Metaethics encompasses three broad categories of questions. The first . . . concerns the connection between morality and conduct; . . . the second . . . concerns the connection between beliefs about right and wrong and facts about the real world; . . . the third . . . concerns the logical relationship between the ethical propositions of various degrees of generality, for example, all embracing super principles . . . , moral rules and practices, and individual, here-and-now moral decisions."

As a discipline, ethics does not end at setting forth the "whats" and the "whys," it attempts to respond to the "how." How should individuals act if they are to respond to the proposed norms and the justification for them? The function of ethics is to attempt an answer to the following question: "How can I, as the person I am and existing in these specific circumstances, best achieve the purpose for which the norm was set forth?" Besides knowing the norm or appreciating the reasons governing its formulation, the ethical person must also be able to choose the method to use in each existential situation.

In the past, many people believed the work of ethics was completed whenever norms were set forth. Today, people are becoming more aware of the added need to be conscious of values and to be able to formulate an ethical strategy or policy. Just as the metaethical and strategy questions of ethics were neglected in the past, the renewed emphasis on them today may lead to a neglect of the normative question. Keeping these three questions in their proper focus is difficult, but the fact that ethics is not merely about norms, metaethics, and strategy taken singly must never be forgotten. All three elements are correlated and must be seen as essential elements in the study of ethics as a discipline.

Clinical ethics, as defined later in this chapter, examines all three questions. Strategies taken to address an individual case might also be examined in relation to the norms of health care for the situation. These norms should be examined in light of larger metaethical concerns. As a discipline, nursing ascribes to positions on issues such as euthanasia, assisted suicide, cultural diversity, and many more to address the why, what, and how questions in nursing practice (ANA, 1991a, 1991b, 1992a, 1992b, 1994a, 1994b, 1997).

Ethical Theory

Ethical theory refers to a workable system that provides a proper framework within which individuals can determine and distinguish morally appropriate actions. How can individuals discover how to act in the light of the existential situation? Should individuals look merely to the rule, or should they also look to the consequences that can result from keeping or breaking the rule? Should individuals look at the rule or consequences without examining the relationships of the people involved or the context of the situation?

Most ethical textbooks distinguish two types of ethical theory: deontology and teleology. Two aspects should be noted: (1) the deontology-teleology dichotomy was formally introduced into the study of ethics only 50 or 60 years ago and (2) the terms are often used in different senses by different authors. Some ethicists employ them as mutually exclusive, whereas others see them as overlapping, if not at least complementary in most instances. Nursing ethics incorporates ideas from these two theoretical perspectives and ideas from **care-based reasoning.**

Deontology, or formalism, as it is often called, is concerned more with what the act that is to be performed *is* rather than what the act *does*. The basic premise of deontology is that the moral act does not depend entirely on the consequences of the act; there are duties or obligations affecting actions that have ethical validity independent of the consequences. Some deontologists admit that the rightness or wrongness of some actions, under certain conditions, can be determined by some consideration of their consequence. However, they are adamant in maintaining that there are certain actions that are "intrinsically evil"—actions that are always wrong, no matter what the consequences or circumstances (Bai, 1978).

At present, most authors would distinguish four principal paradigms of deontology: (1) Judeo-Christian, (2) Kantian, (3) Oxford Intuitionist, and (4) contemporary version of the contract theory, as formulated by John Rawls.

In the *Judeo-Christian* model the moral life is seen as consisting of the total obedience to the plan of God, as made manifest through revelation or through the positive legislation enacted by the faith community. Consequently, this model holds that certain absolute prohibitions exist that the moral individual will never contravene, no matter what the consequences. This position is evidenced in the writings of the classic Roman Catholic moral theologians, who taught that actions such as direct abortion, direct contraception, direct killing, and active euthanasia can never be permitted, despite the consequences. In the case of actions forbidden but not "intrinsically evil," these same authors teach that some exceptions are permitted through a careful application of the *principle of the double effect*. This principle asserts that individuals may never purposefully do evil, even for a good reason, but they may for a proportionate reason; it permits unintended evil consequences that might flow from a good action. The principle of the double effect is based on many actions having two effects (one good and the other evil) and on a significant difference existing between doing evil and permitting it as a side effect of a good action. Traditionally, the principle is described as follows: it is licit to posit an action that has two foreseen effects (one good and the other bad) if four conditions are verified all at the same time: (1) if the action taken is, in itself, good or at least morally indifferent; (2) if the good effect is not produced by means of the bad effect; (3) if only the good effect is directly intended; and (4) if there is a proportionate reason for placing the action and permitting the bad effect.

One common application of this principle today is the distinction between euthanasia and pain management in a terminally ill person. Aggressive pain management (the good effect) that would have the unintended, albeit foreseeable effect of hastening death (the bad effect), is ethically justifiable if medication is given with the intent and proportion necessary to stop pain. This action would meet all four of the conditions listed. However, injecting the person with an agent, the intent of which is to cause death (the bad effect) as the means to stop pain (the good effect), is not ethically justifiable, because the intent is to stop the life, not ease the pain. The action (injecting a lethal dose of potassium into a vein) is not morally indifferent; the bad effect is the intent and there is no proportionality because the dose is known to be lethal. The ANA position statement on euthanasia supports the principle of double effect (ANA, 1994a).

In the *Kantian* system, the morally upright person is always prepared to do whatever the moral duty requires (Dyck, 1977). This system teaches that all individuals are subject to a "categorical imperative," which is based solely on the formal nature of the law and unconditionally requires every rational being to act only on maxims regarded as universal laws of nature. The Kantian system requires that these maxims be followed, despite the consequences of the act. This system sees all moral imperatives as unconditional and admits to no exceptions.

The *Oxford Institutionists* hold on to the intrinsicalism of the deontologists, but shy away from their absolutism (Dyck, 1977). These theorists hold that the determination of the moral rightness or wrongness of a specific act depends on its intrinsic nature; however, they believe that the consequences of the act are always, but not totally, relevant to its rightness. An act is morally correct when its right-making properties outweigh its wrong-making properties.

Rawls (1977) retains the intrinsicalism common to the Oxford Intuitionists, but he stresses the values that arise from a satisfaction of the proper conditions of human association, such as freedom, autonomy, human rights, dignity, self-respect, and just distribution of jointly produced primary goods.

Before considering teleology, the sizeable group of contemporary Roman Catholic moral theologians who are introducing some modifications of the system proposed by the classic moral theologians is worth noting. The theory that these theologians propose has been given different names by different authors, but it is commonly referred to as "mixed consequentialism," "an ethic of proportionality," or "an ethic of relationality and proportionality." These theories focus on the denial that any action can be intrinsically evil apart from any consideration of consequences and circumstances (Gula, 1982). In determining the morality of any action, consequences must be given due consideration without giving them the entire and sole consideration. These moral theologians evaluate consequences in terms of needs and purposes to be established, not by the subjective preference of the moral agent (subjectivism) or merely abstract laws (legalism), but rather by the nature of the human person considered within the dimensions and implications of individual and communal attributes.

Teleology, or consequentialism as it is sometimes called, is an ethical theory that is more concerned with what the act *does* than with what the act *is*. This theory maintains that no action, as such, can be termed intrinsically evil; the principal determinant of the morality of any act is its *consequences*. The morally good action is one that produces the best consequences, either for the moral agent or for human society.

Teleology manifests itself today in various forms, such as ethical *hedonism* (only the moral agent's good is to be considered), ethical *elitism* (only the good of the people most gifted in society is to be considered), ethical *parochialism* (only the good of the moral agent's appropriate in-group is to be considered), and ethical *universalism* (the good of all humankind is to be considered).

The most common and most widely championed teleological theory is *utilitarianism*, which holds that established rules are "useful rules of thumb," but breakable and with exception prescriptions. The foundation of utilitarianism is the *principle of utility*, which teaches that in all circumstances, the greatest possible balance of value over disvalue for all individuals affected must be sought. This theory is based on an evaluative calculus that would enable an individual to conduct a moral life in a rational manner comparable with that of the efficient businessperson. Just as this person maximizes profits, so the moral person maximizes the net balance of good over bad, pleasure over pain, and happiness over unhappiness. The single, without exception principle for the utilitarian is that the right action is the one that, by means of empirical calculation, produces the greatest amount of good for the greatest number of people.

A perusal of contemporary ethical literature shows that utilitarians make a distinction between *rule* utilitarianism and *act* utilitarianism. In the act form, the rightness of an act is determined by its conformity with all the compulsory social rules that pass the test of utility. In the rule type, the only right-making property is "optimificity": the act has consequences at least as good as those of any other alternate acts open to the agent. Rule utilitarianism is less radical than act utilitarianism and most likely originated to defend utilitarianism against the objection that it pays no attention to moral principles and rules. For this reason, utilitarianism maintains that the correct act is prescribed by a set of rules whose general acceptance in society will produce more utility than the acceptance of any other set of rules.

Closely allied to utilitarianism is *situation ethics*. This system is motivated by concern for human well being, flexible in its decision-making method, and guided in its judgments by the greatest good realized rather than by adherence to prefabricated norms or moral rules. Each case is weighed on its own merits, both clinically and consequentially. For many who profess this method of moral discourse, there is only one serious ethical question: "What is the best thing to do in this case for this particular person and for this particular ethical dilemma?"

Gilligan (1982) first introduced *Care ethics*, or care-based reasoning, in her book, *In a Different Voice: Psychological Theory and Women's Development*. Gilligan's research began the debates that question whether previously established modes of ethical reasoning were gender-specific to men and had excluded examination of relationships and contexts when making ethical decisions. Care ethics includes identifying the moral conflict or problem in context, considering the others who are involved in the conflict and how they are interrelated, and feeling concern for relationships and individuals and identifying oneself in relation to the individuals and problems involved. This theoretical reasoning includes consideration of case-specific relationship factors while allowing for consideration of consequences, duties, and virtues of the moral person making a decision and the others whom the decision would affect. The actions and judgments made using care-based reasoning must be measured against what it means to be "caring" within the context of the responsibilities the moral individual has to others involved in the conflict. Health care professionals in general, and nurses in particular, are attracted to this reasoning because it examines ethical dilemmas and problems in a comprehensive way, accommodating context and relationships (Bishop & Scudder, 2001; Fry & Veatch, 2000).

Care ethics has been criticized for being distracting, counterproductive for professionals, and even antiintellectual, allowing the substitution of feeling for thought (Allmark, 1995; Barker, Reynold & Ward, 1995; Lowey, 1995; Nelson, 1992). Gilligan's movement toward moral reasoning based on caring and context was not intended to exclude justice or any other principle important to patients or providers; rather, this effort merely ascribes value to the context and relationships. Gilligan (1987) wrote, "Justice and care as moral perspectives are not opposites or mirror images of one another . . . these perspectives denote different ways of organizing the basic elements of moral judgment; self, others, and the relationship between them." Fry, Killen, and Robinson (1996) address these cited critics and conclude that care-based reasoning, caring, and the ethic of care provide " . . . contemporary responses to the need for new moral theories adequate for the moral questions we face."

Feminist Ethics

There has been significant illumination of oppressed groups of people in the United States and many other countries during the last 50 years. Oppression has been defined as the interlocking series of restrictions and barriers to reduce the choices of a group of people. These processes are often very insidious and, in fact, become the accepted cultural norms.

"Feminism is the name given to the various theories that help reveal the multiple, gender-specific patterns of harm that constitute women's oppression. It is also the term used to characterize the complex, diverse political movement to eliminate all such forms of oppression" (Sherwin, 1992 p. 13).

The scholarship and application of feminist ethics has been derived from the moral and political perspectives of feminism in which the oppression of women is not acceptable. Feminist ethics are developed from the moral perspective of women that includes the ethics of care, as described in the above discussion. It emphasizes the importance of moral agents' responsibilities to other persons, including themselves, in decision making. The details of experience and context are also evaluated. Therefore traditional ethical theories' commitment to purely abstract reasoning and the paradigm of moral agents being fully developed, autonomous, independent rational beings are rejected in the scholarship and practices of feminist ethics. Most importantly, however, is that feminist ethics is committed to eliminating the subordination of all oppressed persons and the possibilities to be realized when these persons are empowered (Sherwin, 1992, 1998; Tong 1997; Purdy 1996; Chambliss, 1996).

UNDERSTANDING HEALTH CARE ETHICS

Nature of the Discipline

As in other areas of life, the principles and theories of ethics previously mentioned are applied to the human relationships of health care to provide ways by which people can systematically reason through ethical issues and **dilemmas.** Davis, Aroskar, Liaschenko, & Drought (1997) state, "Health care ethics, sometimes also called medical ethics, biomedical ethics, and bioethics, is normative ethics specific to the health *science* in that it raises the questions of what is right or what ought to be done in a health science situation when a moral decision is called for." These authors believe that health care ethics address four interrelated areas: (1) clinical, (2) allocation of scarce resources, (3) human experimentation, and (4) health policy.

The recent expansion in knowledge and its application in technology have increased the complexities of the ethical issues and dilemmas within each of these areas. Consequently, both clinicians and individuals potentially have great power over the quantity and quality of human life. "Health care ethics does not promote a particular moral lifestyle, nor does it campaign for particular life values. Its role has been defined as functioning (1) to sensitize or raise the consciousness of health professionals (and the lay public) concerning ethical issues found in health care settings and policies; and (2) to structure the issues so that ethically relevant trends of complex situations can be drawn out." (Benjamin & Curtis, 1992; Davis, Aroskar, Liaschenko, & Drought, 1997).

Based on the holistic perspective of the person, nursing requires its members to consider the wholeness of each patient and themselves when ascribing to particular theories of ethics. To be a nurse requires the willing assumption of ethical responsibility in every dimension of practice. Nurses cannot act morally unless each has developed a strong moral self and constructed a moral system that supports each act (Fitzpatrick, 1998; Pence & Cantral, 1990; Veatch & Fry, 1987).

In making each decision, a person decides or determines what type of individual he or she is and wants to become. Therefore all nursing judgments are also ethical judgments; no dichotomy exists between nursing or clinical judgments and decisions and ethical decisions. Every nursing decision is either an ethical or an unethical nursing decision. The nurse first needs sensitivity and an ability to recognize the presence of ethical issues (Lauer & Mlecko, 1982).

In addition to personal values and beliefs, the ethics of the profession influences the nurse's development of a moral self. What is a good nurse? How should a good nurse interact? What helps a nurse do what should be done? Perhaps the single greatest cause for confusion, stress, and misunderstanding in nursing today is an inadequate definition of the nursing role, particularly the meaning of professionalism in nursing. What are the roles, rights, and responsibilities of patients? Of nurses? Of other health care providers and agency administrators? The patient, nurse, physician, and administrator are all human beings with relatively unique roles and concurrent, often undefined, but frequently overlapping rights and responsibilities that demand mutual knowledge and respect. Informal and formal professional ethics provide some assistance in addressing these questions (Haering, 1973; Hastings & Hudson Institute of Society, 1948; Leininger, 1990).

Professional Oaths and Codes of Ethics

Informal professional ethics are not readily reduced to writing. The nurse acquires informal ethics through socialization. The content of *ad hoc,* clinical advice from superiors and from peers contains these covert messages of what is right and what is wrong to do in particular situations.

The other classification is *formal* professional ethics, as represented in writings, usually by health care organizations, frequently in the format of codes. The purpose of ethical **codes** is to provide a framework for each nurse to generate personal ethical decisions, but within the guidelines of the profession. Professional codes indicate a profession's acceptance of the responsibility and trust society invests. On entering a profession, each person inherits this responsibility and trust. The ethical codes of a profession provide a primary means for the exercise of self-regulation by the profession and each professional in the profession.

The primary relationship of the nurse is defined to be therapeutic with individuals. Historically, this responsibility has not been clear and frequently, it has been quite different. The nurse has been responsible to the church, to the administration of the health care agency, to other health care providers (especially physicians), and to the socially selected members of the person's family. This multiplication of responsibilities has presented ethical dilemmas to the nurse because there are conflicting demands in deciding who should be the decision makers (Davis & Krueger, 1980; Lanik & Webb, 1989).

These multiple perspectives of responsibilities are particularly evident in the *Florence Nightingale Pledge*. The Farr Training School of Harper Hospital in Detroit, Michigan appointed a committee of people who thereby constructed the oath in 1863 (Box 5-1).

Before the industrialization of the nineteenth century, nursing was practiced primarily within religious communities. In this context, the ethics of the particular denomination guided the ministrations of the nurses. With the social changes of industrialization in England, nurses came from more varied backgrounds and brought with them a wider range of beliefs and abilities; many were even of marginal social development and character. Florence Nightingale organized and developed nurses during the Crimean War. Her ideals are reflected in this pledge, which has been taken by nurses throughout the world.

Box 5-1 Florence Nightingale's Pledge for Nurses

I solemnly pledge myself before God and in the presence of this assembly to pass my life in purity and to practice my profession faithfully.
I will abstain from whatever is deleterious and mischievous and will not take or knowingly administer any harmful drug.
I will do all in my power to elevate the standard of my profession and will hold in confidence all personal matters committed to my keeping and all family affairs coming to my knowledge in the practice of my calling.
With loyalty will I endeavor to aid the physician in his work and devote myself to the welfare of those committed to my care.

Box 5-2 American Nurses' Association Code for Nurses

1. The nurse provides services with respect for human dignity and the uniqueness of the individual unrestricted by considerations of social or economic status, personal attributes, or the nature of health problems.
2. The nurse safeguards the individual's right to privacy by judiciously protecting information of a confidential nature.
3. The nurse acts to safeguard the individual and the public when health care and safety are affected by the incompetent, unethical, or illegal practices of any person.
4. The nurse assumes responsibility and accountability for individual nursing judgments and actions.
5. The nurse maintains competence in nursing.
6. The nurse exercises informed judgment and uses individual competence and qualifications as criteria in seeking consultation, accepting responsibilities, and delegating nursing activities to others.
7. The nurse participates in activities that contribute to the ongoing development of the professional's body of knowledge.
8. The nurse participates in the profession's efforts to implement and improve standards of nursing.
9. The nurse participates in the profession's efforts to establish and maintain conditions of employment conducive to high quality nursing care.
10. The nurse participates in the profession's efforts to protect the public from misinformation and misrepresentation and to maintain the integrity of nursing.
11. The nurse collaborates with members of the health professions and other citizens in promoting community and national efforts to meet the health needs of the public.

From American Nurses Association. (1985). *ANA Publication Code No. G-56 42M11/86R*. Kansas City, MO: ANA.

The *Code for Nurses* (Box 5-2), adopted by the ANA in 1950, has been revised many times, most recently in 1985 and is currently being revised. This revision, less prescriptive than previous revisions, relies more on the individual nurse's accountability to the individual, whose right of self-determination is affirmed (ANA, 1985).

Additionally, in 1953 the International Council of Nurses' (ICN) code (Ethical Concepts Applied to Nursing) was developed and accepted (Box 5-3). This code was revised in 1965 and 1973 and then reaffirmed in 1989 and most recently revised in 2000 (Box 5-3). The extraordinary challenge of the code is to provide guidelines that can be applied to all cultures and to the various developmental stages of nursing in countries throughout the world. The preamble of the ICN Code states, "Nurses have four fundamental responsibilities: to promote health, to prevent illness, to restore health, and to alleviate suffering. The need for nursing is universal. Inherent in nursing is respect for human rights, including the right to die, to have dignity, and to be treated with respect. Nursing care is unrestricted by considerations of age, color, creed, culture, disability, illness, gender, nationality, policies, race, or social status" (ICN Code, p. 2) Fry identifies four ethical concepts described by the international nursing community as essential to nursing practice: (1) advocacy, (2) accountability or responsibility, (3) cooperation, and (4) caring.

Interpretive statements that further explain and illustrate their intent accompany both codes. The welfare of the recipient of nursing care is emphasized in both, demonstrating that they are codes of ethics rather than codes of professional etiquette that exist for some other professions.

Additionally, the ANA has written a position statement and a social policy statement to articulate the framework of responsibilities that nurses have to the recipients of their care (ANA 1991a, 1991b, 1992a, 1992b, 1994a, 1994b, 1995, 1997). For example, to address the need for culturally sensitive nursing practice, the ANA's position statement on cultural diversity in nursing practice was written (ANA, 1997). For another example, the ANA wrote a position statement to address the nurse's responsibilities to the patient in the specific context of the Patient Self-Determination Act (ANA, 1991a).

Ethical Principles Currently Stressed

Beaucamp and Childress (1994) believe that moral principles govern laws of conduct as codes of conduct by which individuals direct their lives or actions, or as generalizations that provide a basis for reasoning. Moral principles are statements that convey a directive or prescriptive force, an internal suggestion that a person can use in guiding behavior.

Rawls (1997) has developed five criteria for moral principles: generality, universality, publicity, imposition of an order, and finality. *General* (versus particular) descriptions of the properties and relations of principles are preferred. *Universality* refers to the application of principles to all people. *Publicity* of principles is needed to ensure public acknowledgment and acceptance by a society. The principle, according to Rawls, also should *impose an order*

Box 5-3 The ICN Code of Ethics for Nurses

PREAMBLE

Nurses have four fundamental responsibilities: (1) to promote health, (2) to prevent illness, (3) to restore health, and (4) to alleviate suffering. The need for nursing is universal.

Inherent in nursing is respect for human rights, including the right to life, to dignity, and to be treated with respect. Nursing care is unrestricted by considerations of age, color, creed, culture, disability or illness, gender, nationality, politics, race, or social status.

Nurses render health services to the individual, the family, and the community, and coordinate their services with those of related groups.

THE CODE

The *ICN Code of Ethics for Nurses* has four principal elements that outline the standards of ethical conduct.

ELEMENTS OF THE CODE

1. Nurses and People

The nurse's primary professional responsibility is to people requiring nursing care.

In providing care, the nurse promotes an environment in which the human rights, values, customs, and spiritual beliefs of the individual, family, and community are respected.

The nurse ensures that the individual receives sufficient information on which to base consent for care and related treatment.

The nurse holds in confidence personal information and uses judgement in sharing this information.

The nurse shares with society the responsibility for initiating and supporting action to meet the health and social needs of the public, in particular those of vulnerable populations.

The nurse also shares responsibility to sustain and protect the natural environment from depletion, pollution, degradation, and destruction.

2. Nurses and Practice

The nurse carries personal responsibility and accountability for nursing practice and for maintaining competence by continual learning.

The nurse maintains a standard of personal health such that the ability to provide care is not compromised.

The nurse uses judgement regarding individual competence when accepting and delegating responsibility.

The nurse at all times maintains standards of personal conduct that reflect well on the profession and enhance public confidence.

The nurse, in providing care, ensures that use of technology and scientific advances are compatible with the safety, dignity, and rights of people.

3. Nurses and Profession

The nurse assumes the major role in determining and implementing acceptable standards of clinical nursing practice, management, research, and education.

The nurse is active in developing a core of research-based professional knowledge.

The nurse, acting through the professional organization, participates in creating and maintaining equitable social and economic working conditions in nursing.

Nurses and Co-Workers

The nurse sustains a cooperative relationship with co-workers in nursing and other fields.

The nurse takes appropriate action to safeguard individuals when their care is endangered by a co-worker or any other person.

ELEMENTS OF THE CODE #1: NURSES AND PEOPLE

Practitioners and Managers

Provide care that respects human rights and is sensitive to the values, customs, and beliefs of people.

Provide continuing education in ethical issues.

Provide sufficient information to permit informed consent and the right to choose or refuse treatment.

Use recording and information management systems that ensure confidentiality.

Develop and monitor environmental safety in the workplace.

Educators and Researchers

Include in the curriculum references to human rights, equity, justice, and solidarity as the basis for access to care.

Provide teaching and learning opportunities for ethical issues and decision making.

Provide teaching and learning opportunities related to informed consent.

Introduce into curriculum concepts of privacy and confidentiality.

Sensitize students to the importance of social action in current concerns.

National Nurses' Associations

Develop position statements and guidelines that support human rights and ethical standards.

Lobby for involvement of nurses in ethics review committees.

Provide guidelines, position statements, and continuing education related to informed consent.

Incorporate issues of confidentiality and privacy into a national code of ethics for nurses.

Advocate for safe and healthy environment.

ELEMENT OF THE CODE #2: NURSES AND PRACTICE

Practitoners and Managers

Establish standards of care and a work setting that promotes quality care.

Establish systems for professional appraisal, continuing education, and systematic renewal of licensure to practice.

Monitor and promote the personal health of nursing staff in relation to their competence for practice.

Educators and Researchers

Provide teaching and learning opportunities that foster lifelong learning and competence for practice.

Conduct and disseminate research that shows links between continual learning and competence to practice.

Promote the importance of personal health and illustrate its relation to other values.

From International Council of Nurses. (2000). *The international code of ethics for nurses*. Geneva, Switzerland: The Author. Reprinted with permission from the International Council of Nurses, revised 2000.

Continued

Box 5-3 The ICN Code of Ethics for Nurses cont'd

National Nurses' Associations

Provide access to continuing education through journals, conferences, distance education, etc.
Lobby to ensure continuing education opportunities and quality care standards.
Promote healthy lifestyles for nursing professional. Lobby for healthy workplaces and services for nurses.

ELEMENT OF THE CODE #3: NURSES AND THE PROFESSION

Practitioners and Managers

Set standards for nursing practice, research, education, and management.
Foster workplace support of the conduct, dissemination, and utilization of research related to nursing and health.
Promote participation in national nurses' associations to create favorable socioeconomic conditions for nurses.

Educators and Researchers

Provide teaching and learning opportunities in setting standards for nursing practice, research, education, and management.
Conduct, disseminate, and utilize research to advance the nursing profession.
Sensitize learners to the importance of professional nursing associations.

National Nurses' Associations

Collaborate with others to set standards for nursing education, practice, research, and management.
Develop position statements, guidelines, and standards related to nursing research.
Lobby for fair social and economic working conditions in nursing. Develop position statements and guidelines in workplace issues.

ELEMENT OF THE CODE #4: NURSES AND CO-WORKERS

Practitioners and Managers

Create awareness of specific and overlapping functions and the potential for interdisciplinary tensions.
Develop workplace systems that support common professional ethical values and behavior.
Develop mechanisms to safeguard the individual, family, or community when their care is endangered by health care personnel.

Educators and Researchers

Develop understanding of the roles of other workers.
Communicate nursing ethics to other professions.
Instill in learners the need to safeguard the individual, family, or community when care is endangered by health care personnel.

National Nurses' Associations

Stimulate cooperation with other related disciplines.
Develop awareness of ethical issues of other professions.
Provide guidelines, position statements, and discussion related to safeguarding people when their care is endangered by health care personnel.

DISSEMINATION OF THE *ICN CODE OF ETHICS FOR NURSES*

To be effective, the *ICN Code of Ethics for Nurses* must be familiar to nurses. We encourage you to help with its dissemination to schools of nursing, practicing nurses, the nursing press, and the other mass media. The *Code* should also be disseminated to other health professions, the general public, consumer and policy making groups, human rights organizations, and employers of nurses.

GLOSSARY OF TERMS USED IN THE *ICN CODE OF ETHICS FOR NURSES*

Cooperative Relationship: A professional relationship based on collegial and reciprocal actions and behaviors that aim to achieve certain goals.
Co-Worker: Other nurses and other health and nonhealth-related workers and professionals.
Nurse Shares with Society: a nurse, as a health professional and a citizen, initiates and supports appropriate action to meet the health and social needs of the public.
Personal Health: Mental, physical, social, and spiritual well-being of the nurse.
Personal Information: Information obtained during professional contact that is private to an individual or family, and that, when disclosed, may violate the right to privacy, cause inconvenience, embarrassment, or harm to the individual or family.
Related Groups: Other nurses, health care workers, or other professionals providing service to an individual, family, or community and working toward desired goals.

From International Council of Nurses. (2000). *The international code of ethics for nurses*. Geneva, Switzerland: The Author. Reprinted with permission from the International Council of Nurses, revised 2000.

on conflicting claims among individuals. *Finality* holds that the reasoning processes from these principles is conclusive in moral decision making.

Meeting these criteria, Davis, Aroskar, Liaschenko, and Drought (1997) suggest principles that nurses can effectively apply to identified ethical issues and dilemmas in direct care and health policy-making levels: principles of respect for individuals, of beneficence, and of justice. The principle of respect for individuals includes not only autonomy and self-determination of the individual, but also recognition of the individual as a member of the human community. This principle adds the dimensions of duties and obligations to others and to the individual in making moral judgments (Ozonoff & Ozonoff, 1977). Dworkin (1977) defines self-determination as an individual's exercise of the capacity to form, revise, and pursue personal plans for life.

Bok (1977) identifies two ways to interfere with legitimate, autonomous choices by patients: (1) overt coercion and (2) deception. Bok defines deception as manipulating the information reaching patients for the purpose of accepting what they would not have chosen had they been correctly informed.

The two principles of doing good and of not doing harm (beneficence and nonmaleficence) are particularly relevant in caring for healthy people. These principles are best developed by Frankena (1973), who has defined four components: (1) one ought not to inflict evil or harm; (2) one ought to prevent evil or harm; (3) one ought to remove evil; and (4) one ought to do or promote good to or for anyone. The duty not to inflict evil or harm takes priority over the other components.

Role of Justice and Rights

Currently, many different perspectives on justice are found in society in general and particularly in nursing care. One particularly strong concern is delivering care in an equitable manner. At present, health care is distributed according to the individual and third-party's abilities to pay. Rawls' principle of justice as fairness (1977) provides assistance in developing a more just allocation of resources. Fairness is based on the perspective of the needs of the least advantaged in society. "Each person participating in a practice, or affected by it, has an equal right to the most extensive liberty compatible with like liberty for all."

The concepts of rights are used in many different ways in society. Currently, the word *rights* is overused to the extent that it is misused. Rights are most effectively understood as rationally demonstrable claims enabling a person to have access to all the things necessary to achieve development as a person. Rights are rooted in needs; specifically, biological (needs for bodily existence and sustenance), psychosocial (needs for love, affection, and respect), ethical (needs for insights into right and wrong), and spiritual (needs flowing from the soul).

The papal encyclical work, *Pacem in tetris*, a document issued by the Roman Catholic Church, describes four kinds of rights: (1) moral (natural), (2) legal (positive), (3) human, and (4) socioeconomic (Gibbons, 1963). *Moral* rights are natural rights that exist before and independent of social conventions or legal rules. A person has a moral right when guided by moral principles or the principles of an enlightened conscience (Frankena, 1973).

All human beings have the right to be shown respect for their persons and for their good reputations. Additionally, everyone has the right to be free in searching for truth, in expressing opinions, and in pursuing art. Moral rights also give the person the right to share in the benefits of culture, including education and truthful information about public events and the right to religious worship both privately and publicly.

In contrast, *legal* or positive rights are recognized, conferred, or protected by law or by some other social or political enactment. For example, the right to private property, even productive goods, is an effective safeguard of the dignity of the individual.

Human rights are moral rights of fundamental importance; for example, the right to food, water, health care, and liberty. These rights are held equally by all human beings and are unconditional and unalterable. *Socioeconomic* rights are claims to have the particular processes that are generally basic to the pursuit of human rights, including the right to free initiative in the economic field, the right to work, and the right to a proper wage.

Moral rights are the source and basis of all rights, including the right to life and to all the means necessary and suitable for its proper development. Some rights are basic because they are necessary for the development of the individual. However, all rights are inseparably connected in the individual who is their subject, with respective duties or responsibilities. For example, the right of every person to life is correlated with the duty to preserve it.

Clearly, a person's right necessitates duties, responsibilities, and obligations of others to acknowledge and respect the right. Societies frequently exercise control over them because rights have social implications. To have a right is one thing; to be able to exercise it is quite another. In certain situations, conflicts in rights can arise (whenever the rights of one individual clash with similar rights of another, especially when both have a legitimate claim on the same object). These conflicts frequently occur in health care decisions. An individual's right to freedom versus society's right to have someone immunized for the safety of others is an example of an ethical dilemma.

However, in society, there is no legally recognized claim or right to health care. An individual may request care, but an individual has no legal right to health care, with the exception that certain states impose legal duties on physicians and hospitals to treat people in life-threatening situations. Affirmations to rights to health care are addressing moral rights and generally have no legal obligations or duties of others.

As managed care becomes increasingly prevalent (versus fee-for-service), this discrepancy between a moral right to health care without a legal right becomes more pressing. Time spent with a health care provider is a resource. In a managed care environment, all resources are to be distributed with consideration of cost for an aggregate population, not necessarily for the individual patient, because in for-profit organizations, there is a conflict in fiduciary responsibilities. On one hand, there is a duty to the patient, and on the other hand, there is a duty to the shareholders. Occasionally, treating the patient comes at the expense of profitability, which means the shareholders lose. Conversely, being profitable may mean not treating patients fully. As a society, the United States is trying to come to terms with priorities in this context. La Puma (1998) argues, "There is hope for justice in managed care if disease prevention, duty to others, and social mission achieve a more prominent place at the managed care planning table." However, La Puma (1998) also states that to promote fairness, physicians in particular must "acknowledge that the conflict between fidelity to an individual patient and the greatest good for the greatest number is part of managed care."

Relationship to Civil Law

Fenner (1980) describes the evolution of contemporary law from two sources: (1) legislation and (2) judicial decision. Law enacted by legislative bodies (federal, state, or local) is termed statutory; law created by judicial decision is termed case law or common law.

The purpose and function of statutory law is to maintain or promote the rights of the state to uphold the social order and to protect the rights of the individual. Law that deals with the protection of the rights of the individual is civil law. Violations of civil law are known as torts and include acts that harm the individual or the individual's property.

As citizens, nurses are subject to the laws of society and laws specific to nurses also govern them. For example, nursing practice acts and the related rules and regulations are the basis for providing nursing care.

Within each state, statutes govern the practice of nursing. These statutes usually delineate minimal educational requirements to apply for registered nurse licensure and the scope and limitations of nursing practice standards and minimal continuing education requirements. Increasingly, the various levels of nursing education and practice are defined.

Other laws also govern the practice of nursing. For example, in 1979, the legislature of the Commonwealth of Massachusetts enacted a patient's bill of rights, Chapter 214, into law. This legislation has since been supplemented into its current provisions. In contrast to other codes of rights, this bill has the power of the law enforcing it.

Fenner (1980) discusses four principles of law that provide the basis on which many of the processes of the legal system function. The fundamental principle on which all law is based is a concern for justice and fairness, the intent of which is to protect the rights of one party from infringement by the actions of another party. The characteristic of change is the second principle of law. As change occurs in society, change in the legal system is also necessary. The recent changes in laws created by the accumulation of health care knowledge and technology are effective examples. The third principle of law holds that an action is judged on the basis of what a similarly trained and experienced, reasonable, and prudent individual would do under similar circumstances. This principle has become increasingly challenging for the nursing profession because it has evolving, multiple levels of nursing education and specialization of practice. The last principle of law holds that each individual has rights and responsibilities. As discussed, the powers or privileges that each person possesses have attendant responsibilities.

Smith and Davis (1980) describe four relationships between ethics and law. An individual's actions can be: (1) ethical and legal, (2) unethical and illegal, (3) ethical and illegal, and (4) unethical and legal. The last two relationships present particularly perplexing situations for nurses.

The requirements of the professional codes of nursing often exceed, but are never in lieu of, the requirements of the law. However, punishments for violations of laws and codes are quite different. Violations of the law can become civil or criminal liabilities and, accordingly, can be punitive. Moreover, professional associations may reprimand, censure, suspend, or expel a professional from membership. For both types of violations, the nurse loses the respect of the community, especially colleagues who share the obligation as peers adhering to legal and professional requirements. Familiarity with appropriate processes to fulfill ethical and legal requirements can enable the nurse to practice more effectively.

Nurses have the ethical and legal right, even in military service, of conscientious objection from participating in any procedure they consider morally objectionable. With this right, as with all rights, there are associated responsibilities. For example, during the hiring process, nurses have the responsibility to inform potential employers of their conscientious moral objections to any moral issues, such as abortion. However, when the nurse is unexpectedly confronted with the moral issue in any emergency, the nurse's responsibility is the patient's safety until the nurse can withdraw from the care when alternate staff becomes available.

DECISION MAKING: NATURE AND TECHNIQUES

Contemporary ethical literature places heavy emphasis on the decision-making process as being vitally important for the moral agent. Primarily, this emphasis is a result of both the present focus on the dignity and freedom of the individual and the personal responsibility demanded by those who possess such dignity and freedom. An individual can speak of morality only when the action under discussion is performed by an individual possessing knowledge and freedom and is capable of using them in a responsible fashion.

As a consequence of this contemporary development, less emphasis appears in ethical writing on the moral *fiat* issued by individuals in authority that they are to be obeyed almost blindly and without questioning by their human subjects. The moral agent has become a decision maker rather than a passive recipient for a neatly packaged moral judgment handed down. This development is as it should be, but it can be counterproductive when decision making is expected of people who were never allowed or taught to make decisions.

Whenever individuals are faced with making a moral decision, they are also faced with making a practical judgment about the rightness or wrongness of a projected action. Considerable effort must be made to decide where the moral obligation is located. Decision making is a process by which individuals, in the throes of a moral dilemma and often in the presence of a series of conflicting opinions about the binding force of a specific ethical rule, attempt to discover where their true obligation resides.

Decision making is a difficult and demanding task. The method by which an individual makes moral decisions will greatly influence the type of person this individual will become (Hauerwas, 1974).

The following guidelines contribute to making a good moral judgment:

- Assemble all the relevant data (facts, norms, principles, rules, and interpretations of the rules)
- Realize that all personal judgments contain subjectivity; on account of personal prejudices and previous history, no one can claim to be totally objective
- Understand that all personal judgments have communal dimensions: human existence is coexistence; consultation of the many voices in the community is essential; and reflection on the possible consequences of a decision on the community is imperative
- Realize that every human judgment is fallible; they are judgments of people who can err and who can both deceive themselves and be deceived in their comprehension of the situation
- Understand that personal judgments do not create the truth in and of themselves, but they are practical judgments of what appears to be the proper procedure in the here and now
- Know the distinction between the superego and the conscience; the superego makes decisions out of a desire to gain approval, whereas the conscience makes decisions out of a desire to do what is just and loving

The last guideline contains an important distinction. Glaser (1971) makes the following observations:

- The basis for action in the superego is the fear of love withdrawal, whereas the basis for conscience is a call to commit oneself in abiding love
- Superego is static (it cannot function creatively in a new situation), whereas conscience is dynamic (it is sensitive to values and grows in each new situation)
- Superego is authority oriented (it responds to command rather than to value), whereas conscience is value oriented (it responds to values as perceived in the here and now)
- Superego is atomized (individual acts are seen in isolation), whereas conscience is global (individual acts are seen as part of a larger pattern)
- Superego guilt depends on the weight of the authority figure rather than on the density of the value in question, whereas conscience guilt depends on the density of the value in question rather than on the weight of the authority figure

Whenever the history of ethical thought is studied, some serious advice on the nature of decision making is usually presented. No advice is more clear and to the point than that offered by Aquinas (1950) in his *Summa Theologiae*. Listed in this work are eight qualities that are essential for what Aquinas calls "the prudent decision":

Memoria: the ability to recall universal principles and commandments and the accumulated wisdom of the past

Intellectus: the ability to penetrate to the central values at stake and the ability to grasp the unique situation in its true meaning

Ratio: the ability to reason from insights and to experience new insights

Docilitas: the ability to be open to new learning and to profit by the experience of others

Solertia: the ability to come to a decision without undo delay

Providentia: the ability to exercise foresight, which gauges the effects or consequences of the decision

Circumspectio: the ability to take into consideration and weigh all possible circumstances

Precautio: the ability to anticipate obstacles and prepare to overcome them

These guidelines provide profound insights into human psychology. Decision making can be greatly enriched if their practical advice is heeded.

From an ethical perspective, addressing the care of self presents many issues. Most prominent is the dilemma of self-determination or autonomy versus the common good. This argument is between the rights and responsibilities of the individual and those of society and is related to discussion of the quality versus the sanctity of life.

A second area of ethical concern is the application of the principles of informed consent, particularly an individual's right to truth. What does an individual need to know to make informed decisions about personal health? A third issue is that of nonmaleficence and beneficence, which is a reminder to prevent harm, remove evil, promote good, and not inflict harm or evil. This principle applies to the care of self and to the care of others. (See Multicultural Awareness box.)

That last area of ethical dilemma for healthy people is the allocation of care resources. Who should receive the money, time, and space allocations for health care in society? Should resources be given to those who are well for increased health when the ill are suffering?

Every individual has the capability of learning about the self. This increased consciousness of self is essential for good stewardship of an individual's life and health. An individual learns self-care through the care received from others. At the beginning stages of life, these significant

MULTICULTURAL AWARENESS

Autonomy and Self-Determination

Respecting autonomy and self-determination is a strong American value. The most common example of this value is in a commitment to the informed consent process. That individuals are given necessary information to make a decision regarding courses of action for their health is part of the moral fiber of the U.S. health care system. However, not every culture places this same priority on autonomy. In fact, for some cultures, this approach to decision making is perceived as harmful.

For example, in some cultures, a belief exists that the family patriarch should make decisions without consulting the recipient of the health care. Other cultures believe it is harmful to use words such as "cancer" or "dying." Subcultures of Americans, the older adults for example, value deference to the physicians' judgments over participation in decision making about their care. In these cases, health care providers who have a modern value for autonomy are confronted with a culture that perceives information as harm. A moral dilemma exists because autonomy and nonmaleficence are in conflict. In these examples, perceptions and realities about legal obligations for informed consent are also in conflict with culturally defined benefits and harms.

As per the 1995 ANA Social Policy Statement, nurses promise to view individuals as culturally and contextually defined (ANA, 1995). A careful assessment of a person's cultural imperatives regarding information and decision making is necessary to proceed with any informed consent processes to avoid harm. For example, care may be compromised if the health care provider is communicating with the "wrong" person, even if this person is the recipient of care. It may be that either the designated family member or community leader is to receive information from the health care provider or it is of no use to the person. It may also be that maintaining family or community order is more valuable to the individual than participation in the decision-making process. In this case, forcing the individuals to participate can be more harmful and disruptive to their life than being excluded from a decision.

Legally and morally, health care providers must provide informed consent. However, because autonomy and informed consent are rooted in the moral obligation to demonstrate respect for the individual, asking individuals how they choose to be respected may be preferable. Is it their self-determination or their autonomous wish that they defer to either the provider or another member of their family or community? Asking these questions enables a nurse to realize that careful cultural assessments and cultural sensitivity are important interventions for preventative ethics.

others are primarily the family. Gradually, they include broader circles of the community, including health care providers. In the context of this organized community, a person grows and develops as an individual. In receiving truthful information from others within this context of a just community, an individual can make well-informed decisions about life. However, there is always an attempt to negotiate the rights and responsibilities of the individual with those of the community by balancing autonomy and self-determination with the common good presented with varying degrees of truthfulness and justice. What then are an individual's rights and responsibilities for health and what are the community's rights and responsibilities for the health of an individual and the health of the community as a whole? Health is of an intimate nature; therefore the primary responsibility for an individual's health rests with that individual, not with the community. It is especially difficult for the nurse or anyone else to acknowledge that an individual's first responsibility is to self; that is, to practice effective health promotion and prevention to avoid illness.

However, this has not been clear in the Western health care system. Health has become so "high tech" that an individual may be more likely to depend on others, such as professional specialists, than the self. Perceiving the body, mind, and spirit is a subjective experience, which is difficult to describe to oneself, let alone to others.

Although difficult, the moral obligation to consider the individual's body, mind, and spirit as a subjective experience is present in nursing practice. The ANA (1995, p. 3) has issued a position statement on the value of respecting cultural diversity and the ANA Social Policy Statement reinforces the position that nurses view human experiences as "contextually and culturally defined." As discussed in Chapter 8, communities, cultures, and religious groups have developed specific guidelines for the promotion of health and prevention of illness. Leininger (1990) and Spector (1991) identify many of these prescribed health practices. Varying cultures and religions emphasize contrasting recommendations for rest, activity, nutritional intake, and so forth.

Some groups prohibit ingesting certain food or drink, such as pork or alcohol. Other groups advise individuals to wear protective metals and jewelry. Although these customs are differences among the health prescriptions of specific cultures and religions, the theme of wholeness is generally included. Clearly, groups throughout the world and history recognize the influence of the body, mind, and spirit on one another and on the promotion of health for the individual.

Nurses can use these culturally and religiously prescribed guidelines for health to anticipate concerns and desired activities of individuals. With the many religious beliefs and practices in society, however, the nurse is advised to explore these issues individually with each person. For example, many religious people believe that disease and trauma are the direct punishments for moral evil and sin rather than the result of physical phenomena.

In making decisions about personal health, an individual is affirming a commitment to health or illness, to life or death. The person who makes a commitment to life strives for wholeness in every dimension of being. Many people decide not to choose, which is a decision for illness and death.

However, the Jewish religion presents strong affirmations. The Old Testament presents the Jewish view as profoundly life affirming. Ashley and O'Rourke (1978) state, "It constantly emphasizes the idea that God gives his friends health, security, children, and long life and God has created men and women for life and wishes to prolong it for them . . . thus disease, aging, and death are not willed by God, but only permitted by Him as . . . the inevitable consequence of human commitments to death rather than to life."

This tradition continues with Christianity. Braaten and Braaten (1976) believe the role of the body is addressed in Christianity. "Energy, courage, zest for life, and willingness to undertake arduous endeavors are all bound up with bodily health. Attempting a harmonious balance of exercise, diet, rest, and positive mental attitude is, therefore, a duty of the human body-person, as it certainly is of the Christian who recognizes the material world and the body as precious gifts from the Creator."

Personal responsibility for health means manifesting a health-affirming lifestyle, which is a rarity today. Stress; insufficient time for rest, exercise, and nutrition; and chemical abuse (cigarettes, alcohol, or drugs) do not provide the individual with the substance for health. Typically, many individuals live without clear commitments or goals, suffering from the emptiness, meaninglessness, and absurdity of life, in a loneliness that never seeks deep level communication with others. To be healthy, other choices need to be made. Unhealthy behaviors have to be rejected for a quality life to be developed.

Stewardship of health involves the mind, body, and spirit and the community and environment. Ashley and O'Rourke (1978) have formulated the following *principles of stewardship and creativity:*

> We are ethically obliged to use our natural environment and our multidimensional human nature as precious gifts, with profound respect for their intrinsic teleology.
>
> We are also obliged to use our creativity as an equally precious gift to improve our environment and our nature, with a caution set by the limits of our actual knowledge and by the risk of destroying that same creativity.

A clear example of the ethical dilemma of self-determination versus the common good can be found in the 1967 federal standard for highway safety, which declared that states require motorcycle riders to wear helmets. A threatened reduction in highway and safety funds encouraged compliance. Although few data were available to document the costs and benefits, preventing injuries and saving lives seemed to be logical. Many individuals believed this legislation was an infringement on their liberties. The ethical controversies are thoroughly discussed by Watson and colleagues (1981). Perkins (1981) attempts to summarize the issues by asking, "What variables are most significant in the cause of motorcycle accidents?" Different answers may be found, such as motorcyclists involved in accidents having inadequate driver training and therefore not able to take appropriate evasive actions.

The quest for greater autonomy in caring for the self is also demonstrated in the currently popular self-help health literature and in the increasing number of people seeking complementary and alternative therapies that promote self-healing. Many of the self-help publications hold the position that the health problems of the individual are interwoven into the health problems of the society. Any interventions that do not consider this relationship are therefore inadequate (McLeroy, Gottlieb, & Burdine, 1987).

Health care providers are concerned that many of these publications do not meet Frankena's (1973) principles of nonmaleficence (not doing harm). For example, several weight-reducing diet manuals have prescribed deficient nutritional patterns. Consumers of these recommended diets have experienced severe complications.

There are many examples of a person's responsibilities for health. A theme throughout these choices is the individual's use of time. Ruthmann (1973) discusses that society's present attitudes toward work and leisure are more utilitarian compared with the Puritan philosophy, which values industry, punctuality, and thrift. As Lauer and Mlecko (1982) state, "Utilitarians live consciously or unconsciously by the principle that only useful activity is valuable, meaningful and moral." In a more psychosocial perspective, Ruthmann (1973) discusses the tendency to assume that the more individuals do, the more they are alive, which is really a subtle way of running away from the self. To develop a more balanced life, Ruthmann believes that individuals must experience acceptance of self as good people, not what they can produce. This concept is similar to Erikson's fifth stage of identity development in adolescence (1997).

Many different criteria are offered to define the quality of life. As discussed, ancient Greek ethical theories proposed two types of standards for evaluating the value of a human life: (1) perfectionist standards and (2) utilitarian standards. The perfectionist standard specifies a given number of qualities, such as the ability to reason, as being necessary for a valuable life. Today's self-actualization theories are derived from this perspective. Utilitarian standards are based on the net utility (utility minus net utility) of a life. Varieties include the consideration of pleasure minus pain and fulfillment of desire minus nonfulfillment of desires.

Another perspective of the quality of life is developed in Judaism and Christianity. The Judeo-Christian, sanctity-of-life ethic appears to be rooted in deontological theory, which gives equal value to each human life on the basis of inherent values, regardless of the condition or abilities of the person. McCormick (1974) describes the Judeo-Christian tradition as being midway between the extremes of medical vitalism, which holds that life is an absolute to be preserved at all costs and medical pessimism, which is based on the premise that only the fittest have a right to life and health care.

However, the danger in current arguments is the polarization of these positions, precluding one from the other. The mixed *consequentialism* approach considers this risk and combines both perspectives for a more balanced approach to the value of a human life.

The Code for Nurses states that nursing encompasses the promotion and restoration of health, prevention of illness, and alleviation of suffering (see Box 5-2). These are partly accomplished by arriving at the best decisions declared by the circumstances, the individual's rights and wishes, and the highest standards of care. The measures used to provide assistance should enable each person to live with as much comfort, dignity, and freedom from anxiety and pain as possible. The varying definitions of quality of life vary with the context and an individual's self-determination to define quality of life to make the corresponding decisions for his or her own life are clearly affirmed (Murphy & Hunter, 1982).

The same answer is given in the study of ethical problems by the President's Commission (1982), which posed the question, "What are the values that ought to guide decision making in the provider-patient relationship or by which the success of a particular interaction can be judged?" The answer was the "promotion of a patient's well being and respect for a patient's self determination." As discussed throughout this text, well being is difficult to define consistently because there is minimal objective criteria and legitimate subjective perspectives of individuals.

In conclusion, optimal health challenges each person to become more fully human, using acceptable means to obtain meaningful ends. Health is a means of living the kind of life and fulfilling the kinds of goals an individual has chosen based on the meaning found in life. The nurse has an opportunity in each phase of the nursing process to help individuals develop meaningful appraisals of their own conditions in life. (Downe, Fyfe, & Tannahill, 1990; Doxiadis, 1985).

SELECTED ETHICAL ISSUES

Research

Confronting the ethical dilemmas of research in health care is not new. What is new is the rapid development of knowledge and technology in society. As discussed, this knowledge gives health care providers great potential for the control over the quantity and quality of human life—areas in which the complexities of ethical issues and dilemmas accelerate. From an ethical perspective, the fundamental dilemma in research with human beings involves individual rights versus societal rights, the right balance between present lives and future lives, individual morality and statistical morality, immediate benefits versus future benefits and science versus therapy.

Experimentation can mean either the use of interventions not adequately accepted or the use of interventions designed to accept or reject a newly posed hypothesis. Generally, the first application allows for greater accuracy in the prediction of the outcomes, including desirable and undesirable effects.

Investigational treatments may also be distinguished according to their therapeutic benefits. In therapeutic research, individuals usually receive direct benefits from a research project, such as increased knowledge about their own health and ways to prevent problems for which they are at risk. Conversely, in nontherapeutic research, the subject generally receives no direct benefits and may actually experience a loss, such as blood for samples, the hope being that the data obtained will benefit people in the future (Jonas, 1977).

A second fundamental ethical issue in human experimentation is the informed consent of the subject. Informed consent is a generally accepted component in health care, especially with procedures that are invasive or are less predictable regarding outcomes. Virtually all codes of ethics affirm the principle of informed consent, which Ramsey (1970) defines as the cardinal canon of loyalty that joins individuals together in health care practice and investigation. However, the problem is actually obtaining informed consent. What does fully informing the subject mean? How can experimenters explain the outcomes when they cannot accurately predict them? Can an individual give truly free and voluntary consent? (ANA, 1975; Fenner, 1980; President's Commission, 1982).

How can a researcher adequately inform an individual about the complexities of current deoxyribonucleic acid (DNA) research, including unknown, irreversible genetic and immunological processes? How does an experimenter describe the potential risks of psychosocial research? Can the benefits and risks to the individual versus society be reasonably predicted? How can altered interventions and experimental interventions be differentiated? Such questions confront today's nurse, whose knowledge base and scope of responsibilities change almost on a daily basis.

Two rights are specified within this document. The first right is the right to freedom from intrinsic risk of injury, which demands that the individual be informed of the extent of potential risks. Occasionally, it is difficult for investigators to explain adequately potential risks because there is inadequate knowledge and anticipated benefits for the individual and humanity.

The second right is the right to privacy and dignity. Estimating a possible invasion of privacy or a threat to the dignity of an individual, especially in today's pluralistic society, is equally difficult for the investigator. Presumptions of an individual's perspectives are inappropriate. All aspects of the investigation (instruments, protocols, and techniques) should be reviewed with the subject. When anonymity or confidentiality may be sacrificed, additional consent must be obtained.

Individuals who are particularly vulnerable to exploitation through research are specifically addressed. The use of captive audiences in research, including prisoners, military personnel, students, children, and fetuses, requires special justification by investigators.

However, the other commitment of the nurse is to society as a whole. Balancing the rights of the individual with the rights and benefits of society has been difficult, especially in preventive interventions such as immunization and fluoridation. For the nurse, these responsibilities most commonly include ensuring that individuals are told that they are taking experimental protocols and that informed consent documents are truly free and informed.

The mechanisms for the protection of rights are identified as being ensured by informed consent, agency review committees, and professional organizations. To fulfill these professional obligations, "each nurse must develop an awareness of the issues and a framework for dealing effectively with emerging human rights problems" (ANA, 1975).

These concerns about individual rights, duty, and autonomy become even more intensified when vulnerable individuals are considered, such as fetuses, children, mentally compromised patients, and prisoners. Some ethicists argue that no experiments should be performed on these groups; it is better to limit health care research than to limit the rights and autonomy of these individuals. However, any new intervention is an investigation in practice, even revised assessment, teaching, or counseling protocols.

Gray (1981) lists five basic principles that are generally accepted in research with human beings:

- A research subject is a person who has volunteered to participate in research on the basis of having all the necessary information so the individual's decision will be a truly informed decision.
- The research subject should be allowed to withdraw from the study at any point if desired.
- All necessary risks should be eliminated in the research design, and, if appropriate, the research design should have been conducted with prior animal studies, which are addressed separately.
- The benefits of the study, either to society or to the individual (preferably both), should outweigh the risks to the subject involved.
- Only qualified individuals should conduct the experimentation.

All professional health care agencies and political codes of ethics generally contain these principles. However, it is worth noting that the protectionist stance (protecting vulnerable people from the exposure to harm in research without offering direct benefit to the individual) has shifted recently to questions of the "right" to be a research participant. For some individuals suffering from a variety of ailments, participating in a clinical trial may be their only access to a hope of cure, either because the drug is not available outside the clinical trial or because the price is prohibitive. The ethical issues here are the questions regarding the coercion of desperation and the possibility of including an individual who does not meet the criteria for the study, which may contaminate the findings. The former issue makes informed consent to participate questionable. The latter issue may indicate that the research offers no benefit to general society and all participants were therefore placed at risk for no benefit.

World War II marked society's formal concern with matters related to human experimentation. The atrocities of the war, particularly those committed by Nazi physicians, necessitated a worldwide response. The results included the Nuremberg and Helsinki declarations, which were landmark documentations in human experimentation that specified the relationship between experimenter and subject. The ethical values of human freedom and the inviolability of the human person are the foundation of these codes (Hastings, 1948).

These efforts were followed by many other codes that were more specific. These codes were also developed from the rapid explosion of knowledge and technology during and after World War II. People needed guidelines to make decisions about the application of massive amounts of data in political, health care, and work environments. Included among these codes are the *Code for Nurses* (ANA, 1950), *The International Code of Ethics for Nurses* (International Council of Nurses, 2000), *Principles of Research and Experimentation* (World Medical Association, 1954), *Principles of Medical Ethics* (American Medical Association, 1971), and *Department of Health, Education, and Welfare Guidelines* (1974), which were revised in the 1981 and titled, *Basic Health and Human Services Policy for Protection of Human Research Subjects*.

The ANA's *Code for Nurses* (1985) also provides contemporary guidelines for nurses participating in research. The value of research and protection of human rights are emphasized. Inherent is "respect for each individual to exercise self-determination, to choose to participate, to have full information, and to terminate participation without penalty" (see Box 5-2).

The ANA's *Code for Nurses* emphasizes the self-determination of individuals:

> Whenever possible, individuals should be fully involved in the planning and implementation of their own health care. Each client has the moral right to determine what will be done with his/her person; to be given information necessary for making informed judgments; to be told the possible effects of care; and to accept, refuse, or terminate care. These same rights apply to minors

and others not legally qualified and must be respected to the fullest degree permissible under the law. The nurse must also recognize those situations in which individual rights to self-determination in health care may temporarily be altered for the common good (1985).

The near impossibility of full and informed consent appears to be reflected in the U.S. Department of Health and Human Services' regulations (1981), which emphasize "reasonably" informed consent in the following guidelines:

- A fair explanation of the procedures to be followed and their purposes, including identification of any procedures that are experimental
- A description of the accompanying discomforts and risks to be expected
- A description of the benefits to be expected
- A disclosure of appropriate alternative procedures that might be advantageous for the subject
- An offer to answer any inquiries concerning the procedures
- An instruction that the person is free to withdraw consent and to discontinue participation in the project or activity at any time without prejudice to the subjects

In 1975, the ANA established the Commission on Nursing Research that developed *Human Rights Guidelines for Nurses in Clinical and Other Research*. This document publicly affirms the nursing profession's obligation to develop scientific knowledge toward improving nursing practice and patient care. Therefore two sets of human rights are addressed with commitments. Supporting qualified nurses to conduct research and to have access to related resources is the first commitment. The second commitment is to the human rights of all people who participate in research, especially subjects who are directly or indirectly involved with nursing care. The right of self-determination of each subject is a critical issue; each nurse has an obligation to support this moral and legal right of the individual (see Research Highlights).

These guidelines emphasize the need for special protection of the human rights of the individual when "the focus of care is not specifically directed toward meeting the needs of the client or subject . . . especially when the probable outcomes are unknown or doubtful" (ANA, 1985). Individual health care agencies are encouraged to develop written statements and guidelines.

The inescapable moral responsibility therefore rests with the nurse who is conducting, participating in, or has knowledge of the clinical investigation. The nurse's level of sensitivity and ability to implement basic ethical principles determine the proper approach to the ethics of the research processes (Fry, 1981; Munhall, 1982).

research highlights

Ethics in Research

Nurses play an active and valuable role in any human subject research with which they or their patients are involved. Nurses are principal investigators, coinvestigators, research assistants, data collectors, and users of and participants in research. Each role has varied responsibilities, but there are common underlying ethical concerns. The following list highlights the most basic concerns for ethical research involving human subjects:

- Research of human subjects should always place the welfare of the individual over the welfare of society and scientific knowledge. Nurses need to ensure that risk will be minimized, consent will be informed, and the knowledge gained will be beneficial. Research is ethical when it is designed; it does not become ethical because it yields valuable results for society.
- Confidentiality is not withdrawn when someone agrees to participate in research; it is still a right and should be protected as such.
- Nurses who participate as data collectors or as an actor in an intervention (draw blood or administer a study drug) are obligated to know the expected consequences of their actions; they must be knowledgeable about the protocol they are implementing. Risks and hazards should be predictable.
- Informed consent means a person understands the risks and benefits of participation. This understanding includes knowledge that the research question is not yet answered and therefore without direct benefit to the research participant. Understanding also includes the concept of being free from coercion. There are legal requirements for age and competency for consent. Literacy levels of consent forms may be problematic, but informed consent always includes a verbal explanation. Participants have an absolute right to have all their questions answered before and during participation in a research study.
- Vulnerable populations (pregnant women, children, prisoners, and minorities) are more likely to have coercion as an impediment to true consent.
- Any suggestion of a breech in protocol or research integrity should be reported to the Institutional Review Board (IRB) that approved the study.
- Nodata can be collected for research before consent.
- Adverse reactions and events experienced by study participants need to be reported to the principal investigator and the IRB. Reactions and events that may be unrelated to the actual study should be included in the report.

Stewardship over Health

The title of a recent movie and play asks the question, "Whose life is it anyway?" This question represents the core issue in approaching the stewardship of an individual's own health. In addition to *who* decides, *what* is health? This question is addressed from multiple perspectives in Chapter 1 (see Research Highlights box).

Contraception

From the beginnings of recorded history, men and women have been interested in the possibility of controlling births while not limiting the pleasure of human coitus. A variety

research highlights

Patient Self-Determination Act

The Patient Self-Determination Act became law in 1990. Since then, the American public and health care providers have had a shared responsibility to review life values and choices as they relate to health care decisions. Although the genesis of this social movement and subsequent legislation were focused on end-of-life scenarios, the onus rests primarily with the health care consumers and providers before these decisions need to be made. The ideal practice for advance directives are discussions with primary care providers during well visits and appointed health care proxies before illness or trauma.

Research has shown that this process is not occurring. Ott (1999) has summarized the body of research concerning advance directives as of 1999. Highlights of that work include the following study findings. Only 2% to 15% of the adults in the United States are believed to have an advance directive document (Emanuel, Barry, Stoeckle, Ettelson, & Emanuel, 1991). In a study of geriatric primary care patients, only 2.3% had named a health care proxy (Meier, Fuss, O'Rourke, Baksin, Lewis, & Morrison, 1996). Even when researching a terminally ill patient population, researchers found only 55.7% of the study population had completed an advance directive (Virmani, Schneiderman, & Kaplan, 1994).

One hypothesis for the reason these numbers are low holds that health care providers are not comfortable having these discussions, in part because they believe the individuals will sense there is something wrong even when there may not be. However, health care providers should be aware that research findings regarding individual perceptions of advance directives are supportive of soliciting this information. In one study population, 88% said they believed being asked about advance directives was evidence of positive concern (Broadwell, Boisaubin, Dunn, & Engelhardt, 1993). In a separate study, 94% of the subjects said they would be comfortable discussing advance directives with their attending physician and 78% reported that they would be comfortable discussing them with a nurse (Elpern, Yellen, & Burton, 1993). Lastly, of the Americans who have completed advance directives, research has shown that they are persons with higher levels of education (Meier, Fuss, O'Rourke, Baksin, Lewis, & Morrison, 1996; Virmani, Schneiderman, & Kaplan, 1994) and higher socioeconomic status (Meier, Fuss, O'Rourke, Baksin, Lewis, & Morrison, 1996; Silverman, Tuma, Schaeffer, & Singh, 1995; Sugarman, Weinberger, & Samsa, 1992). Imbedded in these research findings is a call for nurses working with ill or well populations to engage in advance directive discussions more often and to assess cultural barriers to these discussions.

Data from Broadwell, A. W., Boisaubin, E. V., Dunn, J. K., & Engelhardt, H. T. (1993). Advance directives on hospital admission: A survey of patient attitudes. *Southern Medical Journal, 86* (2), 165-168; Elpern, E. H., Yellen, S. B., & Burton, L. A. (1993). A preliminary investigation of opinions and behaviors regarding advance directives for medical care. *American Journal of Critical Care, 2* (2), 161-167; Emanuel, L. L., Barry, M. J., Stoeckle, J. D., Ettelson, L. M., & Emanuel, E. J. (1991). Advance directives for medical care: A case for greater use. *New England Journal of Medicine, 324*, 889-895; Meier, D. E., Fuss, B. R., O'Rourke, D., Baksin, S. A., Lewis, M., & Morrison, S. (1996). Marked improvement in recognition and completion of health care proxies. A randomized controlled trial of counseling by hospital patient representatives. *Archives of Internal Medicine, 156* (11), 1227-1232; Ott B. B. (1999). Advance directives: The emerging body of research. *American Journal of Critical Care, 8* (1), 514-519; Silverman, H. J., Tuma, P., Schaeffer, M. H., & Singh, B. (1995). Implementation of the Patient Self-Determination Act in a hospital setting: An initial evaluation. *Archives of Internal Medicine, 155* (5), 502-510; Sugarman, J., Weinberger, M., & Samsa, G. (1992). Factors associated with veterans' decisions about living wills. *Archives of Internal Medicine, 152* (2), 343-347; Virmani, J., Schneiderman, L. J., & Kaplan, R. N. (1994). Relationship of advance directives to physician-patient communication. *Archives of Internal Medicine, 154* (8), 909-913.

of methods have been devised, many of which have given rise to some serious ethical problems. As might be assumed, these issues range from the possibility of physical harm to the morality of government intervention in curbing population growth.

In contemporary society, which is marked by a great deal of sexual freedom, contraception has become for many matter-of-fact and devoid of any ethical dimensions. The freedom to procreate is similarly taken for granted in society. Birth limitation is something usually practiced by healthy persons and physically healthy persons are considered free to procreate; therefore both are considered in this text.

Contraception can be defined as the use of any mechanical, chemical, pharmaceutical, or surgical means of preventing sexual intercourse from resulting in the generation of offspring. As such, contraception is distinguished from periodic continence (rhythm) and natural family planning systems, which entail the use of no mechanical, artificial, or unnatural means. Throughout history, discussions about the ethical implications of contraception have been intense, but it is only within the last 100 years with the technological development of more effective and safer methods of contraception and with serious discussions about the problem of world population, has the issue become controversial. The heart of the discussion may be found in the varying understandings of the meaning of human coitus.

The practice of contraception presents a dilemma for many healthy people. A decision to practice contraception is not always taken lightly, because the attitude chosen has a direct relationship with the couple's appreciation of the meaning and purpose of human coitus. For this reason, nurses should assess for the need or desire for a couple practicing contraception to receive competent spiritual counseling and medical advice. Contraception may be particularly important to the patient whenever consideration is being given to the possibility of permanent sterilization (tubal ligation in women and vasectomy in men). Currently, these procedures are practically irreversible and exclude the possibility of future children if there should be a subsequent marriage or if a sudden turn of events, such as the death of an only child, would make a future pregnancy desirable. (See Hot Topics box.)

As stated, the right to procreate is taken for granted in Western culture. Women are free to procreate regardless of marital status, sexual orientation, age, economics, addiction to drugs, and ability to provide for the child. This freedom is based in the values of autonomy and self-determination. Questions of justice and beneficence are asked in many situations. At what point, if any, should society restrict procreation? Should procreation be restricted when it can be reasonably predicted that the mother will harm the child? In the United States, the unborn child has no rights; the mother has many. Whether an individual personally agrees or not, under the constitutional right to privacy and ethical principle of autonomy, the U.S. courts, for the most part, have allowed mothers complete freedom to choose to procreate.

However, there is one circumstance in which health care providers still have questions that explorations of autonomy cannot erase. Sulpizi (1996) explores the issues of sexuality in women with developmental disabilities and concludes, "The reproductive needs of women with developmental disabilities often are overlooked by family, caregivers, institutions, and even health care professionals because these women are regarded as somehow asexual. However, women with developmental disabilities are becoming more active in their communities, leading to greater opportunities for social-sexual interactions and an even greater need for reproductive services." Mentally disabled women are not *necessarily* capable of autonomous decisions about their health care. Is it ethical to use pharmaceutical or surgical contraceptive devices against the will of those unable to make other health care decisions for themselves? If a woman is deemed not capable of refusing other medical treatments, should she be allowed the right to refuse sterilization?

The arguments for "forced" sterilization include the benefits to the woman who may not be capable of understanding changes in her body related to the pregnancy and birthing processes. Additionally, if the woman is incapable of caring for the child once the infant is born, some argue that society has a vested interest in preventing conception since the infant will become a ward of the state. Lastly, it can be argued that noncompliance

HOT topics

GENETIC TESTING

As the culture becomes more and more entrenched in the power and availability of information, individuals wish to have more. Information is perceived by many to be power and control. The advances in genetic testing are a manifestation of these perceptions. In fact, health care providers have gained the ability to reverse, stall, and predict many diseases with this new information. However, these scientific explorations are not pursued without ethical concern.

Genetic testing has forced health care to address new ethical questions. For example, on a personal level, what if individuals could prepare better for their future needs because they know what they are going to face? What if an individual could make a more informed decision about procreation based on the probabilities of having an unhealthy child? What if individuals could alter their future from knowledge about the genes? Ethically, these questions are questions of autonomy, beneficence, stewardship, personal accountability, and respect for persons.

On a societal level, what if individuals could prioritize research based on actual potential effects because researchers know how many individuals are affected by which genetic markers? What if health care costs could be anticipated more accurately? What if resources could be distributed based on these data, saving money because all are better prepared? Ethically, these are questions of social and distributive justice.

Conversely, is it beneficial to know the genetic predisposition of a certain disease, even if the individual cannot alter anything? Would knowledge alter how a sibling is treated versus another if one is a carrier for a deadly disease and one is not? Would individuals forego investing in their future if they thought the future was limited? For example, would an individual go to college, marry, have children, or bother to save for retirement? What if an unforeseen cure is discovered and the individual suddenly has a future? Ethically, these are questions of autonomy, nonmaleficence, stewardship, personal accountability, and respect for persons.

Can insurers have access to the information before accepting a customer? Will there be a time when society decides what treatment options should be taken, based on statistical analyses of genetic make-up and prognoses or costs? Would potential employers gain access to the information? The rationale would be such that employers have a financial interest in the health of their employees. Ethically, these are questions of autonomy, confidentiality, and justice.

If tested, does that not mean that an individual's family gets information concerning themselves that they may or may not wish to have? Does distributing this information violate informed consent? What about information based on race and ethnicity? If statistics are categorized by race or ethnicity, do individuals act differently? Could this genetic information compound already complex social and economic realities around racial and ethnic differences? Ethically, these are questions of autonomy and social justice.

The potential benefits and harms of genetic testing are being debated at the same time the technology is being developed. Individual and collective moral reflection is necessary to avoid as many harms as possible while maximizing the potential goods. Nurses who counsel individuals on genetic testing should reflect on these issues.

with prenatal care may endanger an unborn child, the presumption being that the mentally disabled or mentally ill woman will not comply with recommendations.

The arguments against "forced" sterilization include violating a basic right: the right to procreate. As a society, there has been unwillingness to force drug addicted women or impoverished women to be sterilized against their will. The infants they conceive are as vulnerable to prenatal noncompliance and are likely to become wards of the state. In fact, babies born to drug addicted mothers have many physical complications and are immediately removed from their mothers' care. The issues of autonomy for the mentally disabled are usually dealt with in the same manner as with other incompetent patient issues; that is, the legal guardian is given the power to consent or to refuse treatment. However, it continues to be legally variable state by state and an ethical dilemma for many health care providers who must decide for themselves whether they should participate in a procedure under these circumstances.

Surgical Abortion and RU 486

The Centers for Disease Control and Prevention (CDC) compiled data about legally induced abortions in 1997 from 50 states, New York City, and the District of Columbia. (CDC, 1997). Different states report the data to the CDC in different ways; for example, some states included "early medical abortions" accomplished with methotrexate and misoprostol in their numbers and some did not. Not all states require the reporting of abortions, therefore the reported numbers are considered lower than actual. The number of legally induced abortions reported for 1997 was 1,184,758. The CDC reported that the number of abortions had declined from the previous year and was the lowest on record since 1978.

The basis of the ethical difficulty can be stated as follows: how can the rights of the mother be reconciled, related, and balanced with the rights of nascent life in such a way that this reconciliation can be translated into public policy? Individuals who take a "pro-life" stance on the issue of abortion continue to debate with those who assume the "pro-choice" stance and yet nothing seems to result. No easy solution to this problem exists; it is one of the most complex ethical issues facing contemporary society. The problem was well stated by Glaser (1971), a Roman Catholic moralist in the United States, when he wrote:

> Abortion is a matter that is morally problematic, pastorally delicate, legislatively thorny, constitutionally insecure, ecumenically divisive, medically normless, humanly anguishing, racially provocative, journalistically abused, personally biased, and widely performed. It demands a most extraordinary discipline of moral thought, one that is penetrating without being impenetrable, humanly compassionate without being morally compromising, legally realistic without being legally positivistic, instructed by cognate disciplines without being determined by those informed by tradition without being enslaved by it (p. 30).

In U.S. society, the "abortion debate" occurs within the context of religious and philosophical pluralism; it deeply concerns all people of good will because it goes to the core of the vision of what the human being is and of what constitutes the human being's right to life. A variety of reasons has been proposed to justify abortion: to protect the life of the mother; to safeguard the physical and mental health of the mother; to act as a remedy against injustices caused by rape or incest; to prevent the birth of defective children; to vindicate the right of the woman to determine her own reproductive capacities and have control over her body; to protect the reputation of a violated woman; and to alleviate economical, sociological, or demographical problems.

The ethical issue focuses on the difficult question of the beginning of human life. Many theories discuss the beginnings of human life and each uses differing criteria for arriving at a determination. Generally, these criteria can be reduced to the individual-biological criterion, which places the beginning of human life at conception or at early stages of development, and the relational and conferral-of-rights criterion, which accepts a late point in development for the beginning of a life that can be regarded as truly human.

In contemporary society, four basic stances on the ethics of abortion are offered by people in the tradition of secular humanism and by three major religious groups: (1) Jewish, (2) Protestant, and (3) Roman Catholicism. However, within each of these systems, a number of nuances can be found that give rise to a variety of opinions when it comes to practical cases. This discussion focuses on the principal position of each group.

The U.S. Supreme Court decision handed down in 1973 reflects the basic tenet of the secular humanist group; that is, the individual woman's right to privacy encompasses the decision to terminate a pregnancy and this right to abort is fundamental enough to override any interest the state might have in protecting fetal life. Many of the ethicists who follow utilitarianism or situationism would make this position their own.

Traditional Judaism is cautious about the morality of abortion. Its position can be identified with that of the late Chief Rabbi of Israel, Issar Unterman, who viewed any abortion as "akin to homicide" and therefore allowable only in cases of corresponding gravity, such as saving the life of the mother. Against today's background of more causal abortion, most rabbis adhere to this opinion and allow abortions only for serious reasons (Feldman, 1978).

In American Protestantism, the perspectives on abortion range along a continuum from antiabortion to abortion-on-demand, including perhaps the group affirming the justifiable-but-tragic abortion in certain situations when there is a serious conflict of values. Ramsey (1970), a deontologist, represents the antiabortion position; Gustafson (1978), a mixed consequentialist, holds the justifiable-but-tragic position; Fletcher (1983), taking a utilitarian or situationist approach, favors the abortion-on-demand position.

Among Roman Catholic ethicists, the official opinion on abortion is deontological as stated in the *Declaration on Abortion* issued by the Vatican (Vatican Congregation, 1987):

> The right to life is no less to be respected in the small infant just born than in the mature person. In reality, respect for human life is called for from the time that the process of generation begins. From the time that the ovum is fertilized, a life is begun, which is neither that of the father nor of the mother; it is rather the life of a new human being with his or her own growth. One can never approve of abortion; but it is above all necessary to combat its causes.

This position is totally in conformity with the statement issued in 1965 by the Second Vatican Council: "Life from its conception is to be guarded with the greatest care. Abortion and infanticide are horrible crimes."

However, a growing number of contemporary Roman Catholic theologians are tentatively arguing that there might be some legitimate exceptions to the general rule prohibiting abortions. Arguing from a position of proportionalism or mixed consequentialism, some of these theologians permit what traditional moralists would call "directly forbidden actions" whenever certain disvalues are minimized. Therefore some hold that abortion to save the life of the mother might be permitted, but only in this specific case because no other possible cause could be proportionate to directly taking the life of an unborn child.

For the most part, these debates and positions have focused on surgical abortions because it has been technologically possible. Importantly, with the introduction of "medical" abortions, the major debate is not assuaged, specifically with RU 486, which was recently approved by the U.S. Food and Drug Administration (FDA). The issue is not the method of intervention; rather, the meaning and outcome are the issue. The availability of a different method does not resolve the dilemmas that have been debated for decades.

This section on the question of the morality of abortion is necessarily brief and incomplete. As mentioned, the abortion issue is extremely complex and problematic. However, it must never be forgotten that abortion is a question intimately connected with the meaning and value of human existence. Nurses caring for patients considering abortion need to be sensitive to the many complexities and counsel them accordingly. A nurse who chooses not to participate in abortions is free to choose.

Genetic Therapy

Within the past several decades, advances in molecular biology have enabled scientists to acquire extraordinary insights into genetics and human genetic development. Even at this time, a definite possibility exists that geneticists can eliminate deleterious genes from the human gene pool and add desirable genes that will improve human individuals and the human species. Advances in this area have already begun to affect the manner in which parents, together with their physicians and genetic counselors, make decisions about parenthood and childbearing. These extraordinary developments will have considerable influence on the human race in the future; therefore they are observed with great interest by ethicists who frequently pose the question, "If we can do it, should we?" The possibility of genetic therapy can bring great blessings for the human race, but failing to admit that it can also cause considerable damage would be naive. Consequently, the ethicist must constantly evaluate the advances that genetic therapy can accomplish. In trying to perform this evaluation, the ethicist must ask two questions: (1) To what extent do human beings have the right to interfere in the genetic processes and (2) what effect will this interference have on basic social structures, such as marriage and the family?

Some ideas on the various methods proposed for genetic control should be mentioned. First, there is the phenomenon known as *eugenics*, which can be described as "planned breeding"; it has been used successfully in the development of hybrid breeds of cattle and certain food products. Eugenics involve the selection and recombination of genes already existing in the gene pool. Two types of eugenics are envisioned: (1) positive eugenics, or preferential breeding of superior individuals to improve the genetic stock of the human race and (2) negative eugenics, or discouragement or legal prohibition of reproduction to individuals who carry defective genes. The first type urges the development of sperm banks for the purpose of storing frozen sperm acquired from outstanding people and cloning, the transplantation of nuclei from one cell to another to make an exact copy of a certain perfect specimen of humanity. The second type urges genetic counseling or the provision for abortion or sterilization on either a voluntary or an enforced basis.

A second method proposed for genetic control is *genetic engineering*, or altering the individual's genetic complement. Genetic engineering entails changing a particular molecule in the complex structure of the gene, either to eliminate a certain deleterious trait or to improve the genotype. For example, this process might be used to control genetic diseases such as sickle cell anemia or Tay-Sachs disease.

A final method proposed by geneticists is called *euthenics* or *euphenics*. These terms describe techniques for correcting defects in individuals after they have been born. Consequently, when a person is born with defective liver cells and lacks some needed enzyme, it might be possible to extract one or two liver cells, modify their DNA, and reimplant them (Fletcher, 1983; Shinn, 1978).

Genetic therapy has great possibilities, but it is not without its problems. First, immense disagreement exists on what an ideal genetic inheritance might be. Care must be taken that the concept of genetic illness not be broadened to include genetic liabilities. Second, many modes of genetic therapy involve some of the most radical contemporary scientific experiments and projections and therefore involve serious human risks. Third, by successfully treating some age-old illnesses of genetic origin, modern medicine enables individuals to survive and reproduce in situations in which they could not have done so in the past. Genetic therapy can interfere with the processes of natural selection, which operate in a cruel manner toward many individuals but, at the same time, strengthen the human species. Fourth, genetic therapy can often entail manipulation of individuals. Geneticists need to be careful that they do not attempt to "play God" and they must be careful not to harm the evolutionary process and ecology. Finally, because genetic therapy represents such a major enhancement of human powers, it has the makings of unprecedented totalitarianism within its grasp. Techniques for genetic therapy can become techniques for more ambitious programs of reconstituting the human genetic heritage, producing a super race or even breeding a new race of human chimeras or imaginary monsters who do menial tasks.

Ramsey (1970, 1972), a deontologist, submits that those who would project a program for genetic engineering should seriously consider the implications of two basic ethical principles: (1) the separation of the spheres of procreation and marital love as something forbidden by the nature of human parenthood and (2) the difference between therapy and experimentation and their relationship to informed consent. For these reasons, Ramsey is opposed to techniques that would require artificial insemination from donors and the entire procedure of cloning.

Fletcher (1988), a consequentialist-utilitarian, would permit any form of genetic engineering that could offer an optimal or maximal degree of desirable consequences. For him, to be human is to be a maker, a selector, and a designer; coital reproduction is less human than laboratory reproduction, which is more rationally contrived and hence more human.

Gustafson (1978), a consequentialist-deontologist, believes that societal benefits should count in genetic decisions, but not at all costs, just as individual rights should be respected, but not at all costs. Gustafson thinks that in the processes used by genetic engineering, scientists should try to hold two intransigent elements of moral discourse in balance: (1) the utter complexity of human reality and (2) the abiding need to attempt to bring decisions under objective rational scrutiny to ensure that any resultant moral policies can be kept truly human.

Curran (1970, p. 61), an advocate of an ethics of relationality and proportionality, insists on a proper understanding of "human stewardship"; that is, the ability to control destiny with the context of constitutive principles. Curran disagrees with Ramsey's approach, which the former believes restricts human stewardship unnecessarily; Curran also disagrees with Fletcher, who seems to attribute too much power to human stewardship. Curran suggests that everyone should be highly critical of utopian schemes in the field of genetics because this science will never completely overcome the inherent human limitations. Moreover, Curran warns against any technological practice that ignores the dignity of the human person in the concern for pragmatic adaptability.

Lay people and health care providers question whether knowledge of genetic make-up will unduly influence decisions such as sending a child to college or favoring one sibling over another. Others are concerned that knowledge of genetic test results will constitute a preexisting condition that might cause insurance providers to decline coverage or that might affect the abortion rate. Many ethicists are critical observers of genetic engineering, believing that human persons are witnessing only the beginning of genetic therapy and should be extremely cautious to steer a middle course between enthusiasm and rigid opposition. These ethicists also hold that it is their role to exercise a critical function of the programs suggested by those competent in the field of genetic therapy. The ethicist must be ready to pose hard questions, always keeping in mind not only what the therapy can accomplish, but also what the therapy entails in relationship with the demands of human nature, as properly understood. Ethicists must check on the experimentation that genetic therapy may require. They must demand that any experimentation used respect human dignity, receive informed consent, and not totally subordinate the good of the individual to the goals of scientific advancement.

All individuals involved in the field of genetic therapy should keep two basic ethical principles in mind: (1) the principle of human stewardship over human existence and (2) the principle of nonmaleficence related to testing and results. Genetic therapy has great possibilities for the advancement of the human person, but it also has great potential for harm. Currently, the potential of genetic therapy is largely unknown. It is important to resist the technological enthusiasm that insists everything possible should be tried or is at least desirable.

Reproductive Technology

Many people are plagued with problems of infertility. Individuals are anxious to bear children, but for reasons that include infertility or for those who are partners in a homosexual relationship, conception is physiologically precluded. In the past, little could be done to help these people; today, reproductive technology can come to the rescue by means of artificial insemination and *in vitro* fertilization. Both procedures can help infertile people, but the techniques are not without their difficulties from a moral point of view.

Artificial insemination has two methods: (1) it may be performed by means of sperm taken from a husband, or husband artificial insemination (AIH) or (2) by means of sperm obtained from a donor, or donor artificial insemination, (AID). The discussions about the morality of these procedures focus on the origins of the sperm. Most ethicists would have no difficulty with AIH, but many of them have real difficulty with AID (Robertson, 1978).

With regard to the morality of homologous artificial insemination, all secular humanists, most Protestant and Jewish ethicists, and some contemporary Roman Catholic moralists agree that AIH is a morally legitimate intervention to overcome chronic infertility. The strongest opposition to artificial insemination in the past came from the majority of Roman Catholic moralists who, following the teaching of Pope Pius XII in 1951, held that AIH is immoral because a child born in this manner is the product of a laboratory intervention and not the fruit of an act expressive of the spouses' personal love. This argument is no longer accepted by a number of responsible Roman Catholic theologians who would agree with the majority of their Roman Catholic colleagues that AIH is morally legitimate if procreation occurs in this manner. When artificial insemination is performed by way of exception to help a concerned couple achieve the fruit of their love, it is not contrary to the nature and purpose of the marital act. These theologians base their opinion on the conviction that parenthood is not principally a matter of biologic begetting; rather, it has a broader human function: a man and a wife accepting responsibility to care for and rear a child (Vatican Congregation, 1987).

Ethicists from almost every theological and philosophical persuasion voice strong opposition to AID. With few exceptions, Roman Catholic and Jewish ethicists take exception to this intervention as a legitimate means for overcoming marital infertility. Roman Catholic moralists list the following reasons for their objections: (1) AID violates the marriage contract, in which exclusive, nontransferable, and inalienable rights to each other's bodies for procreative acts are exchanged; (2) it can lead to or at least foster the acceptability of adultery; and (3) it creates a "stud-farm" approach to marriage. Jewish ethicists employ similar arguments: "By reducing human generation to stud-farming methods, AID severs the link between the procreation of children and marriage, indispensable to the maintenance of the family as the most basic and sacred unit of human society. It would enable women to satisfy their craving for children without the necessity to have homes and husbands" (Jakobovitz, 1975).

Protestant ethicists offer more diversified points of view. Fletcher (1983), speaking from the situationist-utilitarian point of view, holds that AID does not violate the marriage bond because the mutual agreement of the spouses to permit the use of sperm taken from a third party in no way constitutes a break in conjugal fidelity. However, Ramsey (1970), writing from a deontologist viewpoint, voices strong opposition to this position. Ramsey believes AID illicitly separates that which God has joined: the spheres of personal love and procreation.

The discussion about the morality of AID and AIH will continue, with the key issue being to what extent such practices can disturb or destroy the connection between the unitive and procreative dimensions of marital sexuality. However, it seems proper to conclude that the pro and con arguments regarding AID have a substantial validity and can be safely followed in practice.

Closely allied to the problem of artificial insemination is the problem of in vitro fertilization. Whereas insemination can be a remedy for male sterility, *in vitro* fertilization can be offered as a remedy for female infertility. Successful attempts at fertilization in this manner have been made, but failures have also occurred. Abundant ethical literature on the subject has been offered. One of these publications is a *Commonwealth* editorial.

The authors of the editorial identify three possible approaches to the problem. First, they cite the "anathema" approach, which evaluates in vitro fertilization as something morally unthinkable, a gross and depersonalizing interference in the natural reproductive process and a procedure that places a severe risk on an unborn individual. It demands a consent that obviously can never be given and inevitably involves the foreseeable rejection of fertilized ova or even the calculated abortion of defective fetuses. Second, the authors cite the "assimilation" approach; neither the ends nor the means involved in this procedure are drastic departures from what people have already been doing. The end and purpose is an ancient one—to help childless couples have offspring—and the means used are merely an extension of the intervention human beings already accept whenever nature proves to be harsh or recalcitrant. Third, they cite the "apprehension" approach; *in vitro* fertilization will loosen human procreation just that much more from the knot of personal determinacy, sexual intimacy, and marital relations. Great possibilities exist for moral and social misuse, and human reproduction is moved one more step toward becoming another form of manufacturing.

Having proposed these three approaches to the issue, the editors of *Commonwealth* offer a critique of each of them. The first approach (anathema) is considered too naïve about "nature" and too negative toward human control. Additionally, the editors believe it was too unrealistic about risks, too certain about possible abortions, and too dogmatic in its tone. The second approach (assimilation) is labeled as "deluding." The authors believe that its attempt to justify today's developments because they are not much different from yesterday's developments is to pile ambiguity on ambiguity and to construct a morality "based on sand." The third approach (apprehension) is the most reasonable and the editors list some of the chief sources of their own concern: (1) the loss of zygotes or miniabortions; (2) the problem of fetal damage and deformity once the transfer has been accomplished, a risk to which the fetus can give no consent; (3) the drift toward donor *in vitro* fertilization and surrogate wombs; (4) the possibility of viewing the zygote as a "product" and the child as a "consumer item"; (5) the restriction of the issue to purely individual benefits—with limited resources we should not be pouring money into life-creating technologies when other more basic health needs are unmet; and (6) the publicity given to these cases can lead people to false hopes, delaying the decision to adopt.

Current ethical questions involving reproductive technology include the rights of individuals with the human immunodeficiency virus (HIV) to have access to fertility treatments. The concerns are threefold: (1) the transfer of the virus to the unborn child; (2) the insurance reimbursement that raises questions of justice; and (3) the creation of a new life that may not have a caregiving parent, considering the health condition of the parent. Advances in medications to reduce transfer to fetuses and to elongate life in a person with acquired immunodeficiency syndrome (AIDS) have diminished some of the moral concern, but not all. In fact, the advancement of medications that significantly decrease transfer of the virus to fetuses has exacerbated the ethical concern of a pregnant woman's right to refuse to be HIV tested.

The morality of reproductive technology is far from totally determined and the weight of contemporary literature on the subject suggests caution. In these matters, as in so many others that influence the pursuit of the *verum humanum*, the role of the ethicist is to keep asking pertinent and substantial questions. If these questions are not asked seriously, publicly, and continually, then there is a real danger that the humanly and morally good will be identified with what is technologically possible.

HIV Screening

The ethical dilemmas between individual liberty and privacy and public health and safety occur in all matters related to HIV infection. For the individual, measures to control the spread of HIV may involve the invasion of privacy in the form of constraints on drug use, sexual conduct, and procreation and limitations on liberty (Bader, 1987). The stigmatization of those at risk for AIDS (homosexuals, bisexuals, drug abusers) has made confidential screening and counseling particular concerns (Durham, 1991). Individual clinicians and staff have a duty to keep all aspects of the screening confidential.

Many organizations such as insurance companies, branches of the military, and prisons have mandatory HIV testing. Some people contend that society has the right to know who is infected and who is at risk; they contend this knowledge would enhance the understanding of the development and spread of HIV and eventually improve the efficacy of prevention strategies.

Others contend that routine testing and screening are not in the interest of the individual or public and the potential consequences (especially discrimination and cost) outweigh the potential benefits from testing asymptomatic persons who lack risk patterns of behavior.

The informed consent process should include pretest and posttest teaching and counseling to ensure that the individual understands the implications and consequences of the testing process. Crisis intervention needs to be provided for individuals who have adverse reactions after being informed of the test results (Silverman & Silverman, 1985; Wold, 1990). Additionally, health care providers are subjected to the specific legal requirements. (See Massachusetts General Law 1 11:70F in this chapter as an example.)

All questions concerning HIV testing revolve around one central moral issue: to what extent should the identification of possible carriers and the undertaking of preventive health measures be a matter of private choice and to what extent a matter of public health responsibility? Ethically, these distinctions should reflect society's concerns for individuals and its concern for the common good (Levine & Bayer, 1985; Shilts, 1987; Wold, 1990).

CASE STUDY: METHOD FOR ETHICAL ANALYSIS

Moral issues, which often seem complex and irresolvable, sometimes leave the nurse overwhelmed, if not paralyzed. Consider, for example, the case of providing adolescents with information about contraception. The issue presents many competing, almost irreconcilable interests to the extent that some nurses might simply avoid addressing this health issue. The nurse is committed to health promotion and has a long-range vision of the health and socioeconomic effects of adolescent pregnancy on both mother and child. Simultaneously, the nurse recognizes that some parents have other interests that resist anyone outside the family from providing information to their children that they find morally objectionable. In these debates, pitting parents, adolescents, and the government against one another, does any means exist for a nurse to sort out the conflict?

Ethical analysis occurs on several levels: levels of facts, values, and reflection on method (Aroskar, 1989) (Box 5-4). To set the stage for analysis of these three levels, a nurse first needs to ask the question, "What issues must be decided?" For example, in the act of providing adolescents with information on contraception, more than one moral issue needs to be decided. Each subissue, alone or together, will help clarify whether a nurse can offer education about

Box 5-4 Ethics Work-Up

GATHER AND ASSESS FACTS

What facts do you see as important?
What facts are needed?

IDENTIFY AND CHARACTERIZE THE VALUES IN CONFLICT

What values are in conflict (autonomy versus beneficence)?
How can each of the values be characterized?
What are the general rules associated with these values (for example, the patient is the primary decider in health care)?
Is there any stronger justification for one or another value?

NAME AND EVALUATE THE METHOD

What method of ethics do you use to resolve your problem (emotivism, divine commands, or legalism)?
Do different theories arrive at similar or dissimilar answers?

contraception. Who should ultimately decide what information an adolescent receives: the parents, the nurse, the government, or the adolescent? What criteria should be used to balance the health prerogative of the adolescent with the interests of the parents to raise a child as they see fit? To what extent, if any, should the common good of society prevail over the rights of the parents?

Gather and Assess Facts

A careful examination of questions at various levels of ethical consideration might resolve any moral conflicts expeditiously. For example, examining whether all facts have been gathered and assessed is important. For example, in initiating an adolescent education program on contraceptives, although the list is not exhaustive, the following questions might be relevant:

Does the nurse positively understand what part of the content is creating the conflict?
Are there any alternatives to providing adolescents with sensitive information?
Are any alternatives free of conflict? If not, then which education options are most effective in reducing teen pregnancy?
What are the risks of not offering the education program?
What programs have other health promoters in similar circumstances elected to use?
What are the views of parents in a given region of the country about providing adolescents with this information?
What are the parents' cultural and religious perspectives?
Other than the parents and the adolescents, who else will be affected by using this health-promotion strategy?

In some cases, facts alone might resolve the conflict. For example, under the assumption that nurses would be required to use their time only on programs proven to show some benefit, nurses should establish which information program is likely to work. If, for example, only one method is proven effective, the moral course of action is certainly indicated. More frequently, the relevant facts, such as the effectiveness of an education program, will be unclear. Nurses may be compelled to act by circumstances beyond their control, but it is preferable that they attempt to identify the facts to the extent possible to claim they have reached a morally adequate analysis.

Identify and Characterize Values

At the values level, a nurse must identify and characterize the ethical values that are in conflict. Occasionally, the conflict may be a communication problem or an administrative or a legal uncertainty rather than a genuine clash of values. In the case of providing contraceptive information to adolescents, values will pull in opposing directions. The value of protecting the health of the adolescent who could become pregnant, the value of "beneficence," pulls in favor of providing education. The value of autonomy or self-determination also has a bearing on this case as an adolescent's ability to consent to a health-promotion strategy is honored. There is also the value society might have in wanting to avoid an unwanted pregnancy that can carry social and economic costs with it. Pulling in the opposite direction is the value of allowing parents to direct and control a child's education and the value of resisting promiscuity. None of these values is likely to be a sufficient justification for a given course of action. Nevertheless, the moral analysis at the values level includes clarifying the meaning of specific value concepts. The term *beneficent,* for example, is ambiguous. There is little shared understanding about whose perspective should be used to judge beneficence; that of the nurse who is committed to avoiding teen pregnancy or that of the parents who want to direct the moral education of their offspring? In addition, beneficence, "doing good for others," can mean, from one perspective, considerate, respectful, and compassionate care. Therefore part of the analysis will entail characterizing a concept and estimating whether there is any consensus in society on the concept.

A good place to start is by looking to national consensus statements on ethics, such as the President's Commission for the Study of Medicine and Biomedical and Behavioral Research (1983) and the ANA codes of ethics or position statements (ANA, 1985, 1991a, 1991b, 1992a, 1992b, 1994a, 1994b, 1997).

Name and Evaluate Method

Once the values in conflict have been identified and characterized, it is sometimes obvious which value or competing interest prevails. For example, ethical and legal consensus, as found in the president's commission, might prefer one value to another, which is a solid indicator that good reasons favor acting in accordance with the regarded value. However, occasionally no clear value preference exists and a nurse must identify alternative courses of action. Each strategy would be evaluated to determine its consistency with moral values. Particularly, strategies must be judged to determine which minimizes damage to cherished values to the greatest extent.

Even when reasonable people reasonably disagree over alternative courses of action, ethical analysis continues. Moving to a final level of ethical analysis (the ethical method level) will provide clarity. This level of analysis focuses on the method nurses use to select the values in conflict. For example, did the nurse use emotions, intuitions, a divine command, prevailing social opinion, a code, or the course of action that produces the greatest good for the greatest number in society? These methods are theories the conscience uses. Although there is no consensus method used by all, some methods are nonetheless more acceptable than others because they are open to rational argumentation.

Integrity-Preserving Compromise

Frequently, there is no single decision that everyone can agree is ethically superior. The concept of dilemma means that at least two ethically justifiable courses of action are inherent. In these situations, integrity-preserving compromise is a useful strategy (Benjamin, 1992). **Integrity-preserving compromise** is the settlement of differences by which each side makes concessions without violating important basic beliefs. This method allows for a distinction between "being compromised" and "compromising," allowing for everyone's sense of moral agency to remain intact. Compromise requires mutual respect among parties involved and thoughtful discussion. It may be the acceptance of a course of action not desirable to one party, but accepted with a time restriction that would facilitate reevaluation. Compromise is driven by situations of factual uncertainty and moral complexity. In this case study, the nurse is uncertain whether the adolescent would refrain from sexual activity regardless of contraception information and the values conflict. The goal of integrity-preserving compromise is a well-grounded, mutually respectful accommodation that preserves the integrity of all parties involved.

ETHICS OF HEALTH PROMOTION: CASES

The following cases are selected from representative situations that provide insight into the common features a health promotion nurse confronts in daily practice and does not attempt to offer an exhaustive set of cases that the nurse will face. Questions are posed at the end of each case to encourage consideration of the essential values, including the responsibilities and relationships involved when making ethical decisions.

CASE 1 Assisted Suicide or Emotional Support?—Ana and Victor

A nurse in a clinic is accountable for ongoing assessments of pain management in a chronic pain population. One of the long-term patients, Ana, has been requiring increasing amounts of narcotics for her pain management over the last year. The nurse has known for over a year that Ana's husband, Victor, has amyotrophic lateral sclerosis (ALS), or Lou Gehrig's disease. Victor's disease adds a great deal of stress to both their lives, which has had a negative effect on Ana's physical health. The nurse assesses the emotional toll of Victor's illness as part of Ana's pain assessment. During one of these discussions, Ana asks the nurse how much of her narcotics would her husband need to take to end his life.

What does it mean to provide someone with the "means" to commit suicide?
What questions would you have for Ana at this point of the conversation?
What would you do with the answers?
Do you have any obligations to Victor?
Do you collaborate with Victor's physician?
What is in Ana's "best interests"?
Who or what are your resources?
What does nursing as a discipline say about assisted suicide?
What is the law in your state?
What should you do?

CASE 2 What Is a Culture?—Mary, John, and Baby Susan

Jane, a nurse practitioner caring for Mary for almost 10 years, is well aware of Mary's feelings about being born completely unable to hear and being raised in a deaf community. Jane knows that Mary has thought long and hard about marrying John because he was not part of that community. His hearing was normal. After they married, Mary and John spent years struggling with infertility. Together they had agreed to adopt a hearing-impaired baby because Mary felt that she could parent the baby better than most adoptive mothers. John agreed, but Baby Susan's postadoption pediatrician told John and Mary that cochlear implants were an option that could restore at least partial hearing to their child. John was all for the procedure. Mary felt it was wrong; she believes deafness is a culture, not a medical condition. John thinks being deaf is a handicap and he owes it to his child to remove the handicap when possible. He wants "to give her every chance at a 'normal' life." Mary asks Jane to "talk John out of this nonsense and make him realize he is violating her culture. Lie to him that the implant is impossible in Susan's case if that is what it takes." John asks Jane to "persuade Mary to give Susan an advantage Mary never had in life."

Who is the patient when discussing cochlear implants? Is it Susan, Mary, or John? Are all three of them your patients? Is being hearing impaired a culture or a medical condition? What resources do you have to decide the issue for yourself? Does the nursing profession take a stand on the issue? Should your matter?

Can you ethically justify misrepresenting information to John?

Would it be culturally insensitive of you to try to persuade Mary?

CASE 3 How Much Money Can One Patient Spend?—Joe Does Not Like Taking Pills

A nurse practitioner is caring for people in an economically poor neighborhood. An older woman, Rose, frequently runs out of inhalers for her asthma. The insurance does not pay enough per month for her to be able to use the inhalers as directed. She struggles along as best she can, but frequently cancels outings with loved ones because she "can't always catch her breath and it scares the little ones." The nurse practitioner has tried to advocate for more medication. Time and time again, the response of the insurance company is, "There is only so much money to spread around."

Across the street is Joe who has been a patient for nearly 3 years. He needs to take his diuretic medications to avoid frequent hospitalizations. He does not like to think of himself as a "man who needs pills." Consequently, he does not take the diuretic medication, resulting in preventable hospitalizations. If he changed his pattern of behavior, then there would be money for Rose to receive more medication.

What are the ethical questions in this scenario?

Ethically, can the nurse practitioner tells Joe about Rose's situation to try to persuade him to take his pills?

Is there anything the nurse practitioner should do individually to resolve this dilemma? Is there anything that nursing as a discipline should do?

What course of action would be in Rose's best interest?

CASE 4 Your Colleague or Someone Else's Nurse?—Jacquie and Beth

You work beside Jacquie every day. You were classmates. Jacquie is a single mother who struggles with sleepless nights and a lack of money. She is a "good nurse" when she is at work. Your supervisor has counseled Jacquie because her sleepless nights have had an effect on her attendance. You are Jacquie's friend and you listen to her with sympathy nearly every day. You know she cannot miss any more work or her life will get worse because she will lose her job.

On Tuesday, you walked into the area where the narcotics are kept under lock and key. Jacquie fumbled a bit when you came in, but you suspect nothing until the next day when the staff was informed that there are drugs missing. Drugs you now suspect Jacquie took to keep her awake while at work. In the staff meeting, the supervisor reminded everyone that substance abuse in colleagues is no less of a problem than it is in patients. In fact, impaired health care professionals are a serious risk not only to themselves, but also to patients. You confront Jacquie, but she emphatically denies your suspicions.

To whom do you have fiduciary relationships?

Which of these relationships pose the highest degree of obligation?

Who or what are your resources?

What should you do?

CASE 5 She's My Patient!—Lilly and "Jake" (a.k.a. Paul)

A nurse practitioner is at a conference when a physician colleague discusses a difficult case. One of his patients, "Jake," is HIV positive, but refuses any treatment. The physician explains that "Jake" fears that his wife will discover and recognize the names of the medications because he knows "these drug names are discussed on television all the time." He has not told, nor does he ever intend to disclose to his wife that he is HIV positive. "Jake" firmly believes his condition is his private information and, for now, the couple uses condoms for birth control anyway. The physician is concerned that "Jake" will not tell his wife. The physician is presenting this case to colleagues to highlight the public awareness campaigns that, to some extent, have affected patient privacy. He argues, "Listen to how they call out your name and the drugs at the pharmacy counter."

The nurse practitioner recognizes bits and pieces of information and come to the painful realization that "Jake" is really Paul, and Paul is the husband of one of her patients, Lilly. Lilly has begun to discuss with you that she wants to get pregnant soon. The town is too small for the nurse practitioner to be mistaken. Or is it?

Is it ethical for the nurse practitioner to ask the physician if Jake is Paul?

Is it ethical for her to tell Lilly you suspect Paul is HIV positive?

Should this information change how she counsels Lilly about a pregnancy?

What is in Lilly's best interests?

What resources are there?

SUMMARY

Perhaps the most crucial theme confronting nurses throughout the ethical issues and decision-making processes is also the single most serious cause of professional burnout: the perception that nurses, although they have tremendous power over the individual, over the most intimate details of an individual's life, and, at times, even over life and death, have little power over the health care system to affect changes in the patient's best interests.

The nurse has the ethical responsibility to *enforce* principles of ethics by addressing and acting against

HEALTH TEACHING Advocacy in Health Care

Nurses have a long-standing tradition of viewing themselves as "advocates" for individuals. Nurses consider sound ethical practice to include acts of advocacy. Nurses also have a long-standing tradition of promoting self-care activities. In today's health care environment, combining the established need for advocacy with self-care activities is an important aspect of nursing practice. Nurses should teach individuals how to be their own advocates or solicit family members. Ethically, this effort promotes autonomy, beneficence, nonmaleficence, and justice.

Nurses should use individual-provider interactions as an opportunity to do the following:

1. Assess the person's comfort level with self-advocacy and the numerous cultural issues. Ask about family members who may advocate for them if and when necessary. If the individual agrees to it, invite an advocate the individual selects to be part of the individual-provider interactions. The friend or family member may be a better resource to recall the conversation after the interaction has ended.
2. Assess for literacy issues or other communication barriers such as language, hearing, and culture that may prevent the individual from understanding information exchanged.
3. Assess for economic limitations that may compromise access to follow-up care or information.
4. Individuals should be encouraged to ask every question they have when interacting with a health care provider. Some people may need to keep notes when the questions come to them because it is stressful during visits and therefore remembering is difficult. Individuals should be encouraged and taught how to request the time they will need to get answers.
5. Individuals should be queried about their values even when they are healthy. Unexpected illnesses and traumas happen. Providing information about their wishes when people have the capacity to do so is important; individuals can never be sure if or when they will lose capacity.
6. Actively listen to the person. Advocacy for individuals must be in pursuit of their goals, not those of the providers. To be a true advocate, the nurse must first hear the individual's wishes. Listening is a strong demonstration of respect for person and autonomy.

injustices in the system and educating peers, individuals, legislators, and society in general about changes needed to improve the quality of health care in a cost-effective manner.

A second theme is the day-to-day value conflicts with physicians and health care administrators. For example, as advocates for individuals, nurses are required to challenge a physician's or administrator's analysis of a situation when, in their professional judgment, the analysis is potentially lethal, dangerous, or counter to the individual's best interest. (See Health Teaching box.) Nurses need to know exactly what to do within and beyond the agency when a conflict with the physician or administrator is irreconcilable. In the end, nurses are ethically and legally responsible for their actions, despite the power of others, including physicians, administrators, and legislators.

Nursing is the study of the whole person and the application of this study as a part of the individual's care. The humanization of the whole person is considered by the discipline of ethics. The nurse's level of sensitivity and ability to implement basic ethical principles through the roles of educator, advocate, and enforcer determine the proper approaches to the study and care of the whole person in developing higher levels of health.

REFERENCES

Allmark, P. (1995). Can there be an ethics of care? *Journal of Medical Ethics, 21*, 19-24.

American Nurses' Association. (1972). *Standards of nursing practice*. Kansas City, MO: The Association.

American Nurses' Association. (1975). *Human rights guidelines for nurses in clinical and other research*. Kansas City, MO: The Association.

American Nurses' Association. (1985). *Code for nurses with interpretive statements*. Kansas City, MO: The Association.

American Nurses' Association. (1991a). *Position statement on nursing and the Patient Self-Determination Act*. Washington, DC: The Association.

American Nurses' Association. (1991b). *Position statement on promotion of comfort and relief of pain in the dying patient*. Washington, DC: The Association.

American Nurses' Association. (1992a). *Position statement on foregoing nutrition and hydration*. Washington, DC: The Association.

American Nurses' Association. (1992b). *Position statement on nursing care and do-not-resuscitate decisions*. Washington, DC: The Association.

American Nurses' Association. (1994a). *Position statement on active euthanasia*. Washington, DC: The Association.

American Nurses' Association. (1994b). *Position statement on assisted suicide*. Washington, DC: The Association.

American Nurses' Association. (1995). *Social Policy Statement*. Washington, DC: The Association.

American Nurses' Association. (1997). *Position statement on cultural diversity in nursing practice*. Washington, DC: The Association.

Aquinas, T. (1950). *Treatise on law* (summa theologica books IA IIAE QQ 90-97). Chicago: Great Books Foundation.

Aroskar, M. A. (1989). Community health nurses: Their most significant ethical decision-making problems. *The Nursing Clinics of North America, 24*, 967-975.

Ashley, B., & O'Rourke, K. (1978). *Health care ethics*. St. Louis: Catholic Hospital Association.

Bader, D., & McMillan, E. (1997). *AIDS-ethical guidelines for healthcare providers*. St. Louis: The Catholic Health Association of the United States.

Bai, K. (1978). Deontological theories. In W. Reich (Ed.), *Encyclopedia of bioethics, Vol 1*. New York: Free Press.

Barker, P. J., Reynolds, W., & Ward, T. (1995). The proper focus of nursing: A critique of the caring ideology. *International Journal of Nursing Studies, 32* (4), 386-397.

Beauchamp, T. L., & Childress, J. F. (1994). *Principles of biomedical ethics* (4th ed.). New York: Oxford University Press.

Benjamin, M., & Curtis, J. (1992). *Ethics in nursing* (3rd ed.). New York: Oxford University Press.

Bishop, A., Scudder, J. (2001). *Nursing ethics-holistic caring practices* (2nd ed.). Boston: Jones & Bartlett.

Bok, S. (1977). The tools of bioethics. In J. R. Stanley (Ed.), *Ethics in medicine: historical perspectives & contemporary concerns*. Cambridge, MA: Massachusetts Institute of Technology.

Boyle, P. J. (1988). AIDS education and parentalrights. *St. Louis University Public Law Review 8*, 45-54.

Braaten, C., & Braaten, L. (1976) *The living temple: A practical theology of the body and the foods of the earth*. New York: Harper & Row.

Catholic Hospital Association. (1975). *Religious aspects of medical care*. St. Louis: The Association.

Centers for Disease Control and Prevention (1997). Report on abortion in U.S. in 1997. Washington, DC: U.S. Government Printing Office.

Chambliss, F. (1996). Beyond caring: hospitals, nurses and the social integration of ethics. Chicago, IL: University of Chicago Press.

Curran, C. (1970). Theology and genetics: A multi-faceted dialogue. *d'Ecumenical Studies, 7*, 61.

Davis, A., Aroskar, M., Liaschenko, J., & Drought, T. (1997). *Ethical dilemmas and nursing practice* (4th ed.). Norwalk, CT: Appleton-Lange.

Davis, A., & Krueger, J. (1980). *Patients, nurses, ethics*. New York: American Journal of Nursing Publications.

Dolnick, E. (1993). Deafness as culture. *Atlantic, 272* (3), 37-53.

Downe, R. S., Fyfe, C., & Tannahill, A. (1990). *Health promotion models and values*. New York: Oxford University Press.

Doxiadis, S. (1985). *Ethical issues in preventive medicine, behavioral and social sciences* (No. 26). Dordrecht, The Netherlands: Martinus Nijhoff.

Durham, J., & Cohen, F. (1991). *The person with AIDS* (2nd ed.). New York: Springer Publishing.

Dworkin, G. (1977). Paternalism. In J. R. Stanley (Ed.), *Ethics in medicine: historical perspectives & contemporary concerns*. Cambridge, MA: Massachusetts Institute of Technology.

Dyck, A. (1977). *On human care: An introduction to ethics*. Nashville, TN: Abington.

Erikson, E. (1997). *The life cycle completed: A review*. New York: W. W. Norton.

Feldman, D. (1978). Abortion: Jewish perspectives. In W. Reich (Ed.), *Encyclopedia of bioethics* (Vol. 1). New York: Free Press, 5-9.

Fenner, K. (1980). *Ethics and law in nursing professional perspectives*. New York: Van Nostrand Reinhold.

Fitzpatrick, F. J. (1988). *Ethics in nursing practice: Basic principles and their application*. London: The Linacre Centre.

Fletcher, J. (1983). Ethical aspects of genetic controls. *New England Journal of Medicine, 285*, 776-783.

Fletcher, J. (1988). *The ethics of genetic control*. Buffalo, NY: Prometheus Books.

Fletcher, J. C. (1997). *Introduction to clinical ethics* (2nd ed.). Frederick, MD: University Publishing Group.

Frankena, W. (1973). *Ethics* (2nd ed.). Englewood Cliffs, NJ: Prentice Hall.

Fry, S. (1981). Accountability in research: The relationship of scientific and humanistic values. *ANS. Advances in nursing science, 4*, 1-13.

Fry, S. (1994). *Ethics in nursing practice*. Geneva, Switzerland: International Council of Nurses.

Fry, S., Killen, A., & Robinson, E. (1996). Care-based reasoning, caring, and the ethic of care: A need for clarity. *The Journal of Clinical Ethics, 7* (1), 41-47.

Fry, S. & Veatch, R. M. (2000). Case studies in nursing ethics (2nd ed.). Boston, MA: Jones & Bartlett.

Gibbons, W. (1963). *Pacem in tetrisencyclical letter of His Holiness Pope John XXIII*. New York: Paulist Press.

Gilligan, C. (1982). *In a different voice: Psychological theory and women's development*. Cambridge, MA: Harvard University Press.

Gilligan, C. (1987). Moral orientation and moral development. In E. F. Kittay, & D. T. Meyers (Eds.), *Women and moral theory* (pp. 19-33). Savage, MD: Rowman and Littlefield.

Glaser, J. (1971). Conscience and the superego. *Theological Studies, 32*, 30-47.

Gray, B. (1981). *Human subjects in medical experimentation: A sociological study of the conduct and regulation of clinical research*. New York: John Wiley & Sons.

Gula, R. (1982). *What are they saying about moral norms?* New York: Paulist Press.

Gustafson, J. (1978). Genetic engineering and the normative view of the human. In P. N. Williams (Ed.), *Ethical issues in biology and medicine*. Cambridge, MA: Schenkman.

Haering, B. (1973). *Medical ethics*. Notre Dame, IN: Fides.

Hauerwas, S. (1974). Toward an ethics of character. *Vision and Virtue*. Notre Dame, IN: Fides.

International Council of Nurses (2000). The international code of ethics for nurses. Geneva Switzerland: ICN.

Jakobovitz, L. (1975). *Jewish medical ethics* (2nd ed.). New York: Bloch.

Jonas, H. (1977). Philosophical reflections on experimenting with human subjects. In J. R. Stanley (Ed.), *Ethics in medicine: historical perspectives & contemporary concerns*. Cambridge, MA: Massachusetts Institute of Technology.

La Puma, J. (1998). *Managed care ethics: Essays on the impact of managed care on traditional medical ethics*. New York: Hatherleigh Press.

Ladd, J. (1978). The task of ethics. In W. Reich (Ed.), *Encyclopedia of bioethics* (Vol. 1). New York: Free Press, 400-407.

Lanik, G., & Webb, A. A. (1989). Ethical decision making for community health nurses. *Journal of Community Health Nursing, 6*, 95-102.

Lauer, E., & Mlecko, J. (1982). *A Christian understanding of the human person*. New York: Paulist Press.

Leininger, M. (1990). *Ethical and moral dimensions of care*. Detroit: Wayne State University Press.

Levine, C., & Bayer, R. (1985). Screening blood: Public health and medical uncertainty. *Hastings Center Report, 15 (4)*, 8-11.

Lowey, E. (1995). Care ethics: A concept in search of a framework. *Cambridge Quarterly of Healthcare Ethics, 4(1)*, 56-63.

McCormick, R. (1974). Notes on moral theology: The abortion dossier. *Theological Studies, 35 (2)*, 312-359.

McLeroy, K. R., Gottlieb, N., & Burdine, J. (1987). The business of health promotion: Ethical issues and professional responsibilities. *Health Education Quarterly, 14*, 91-109.

Munhall, P. (1982). Nursing philosophy and nursing research: an apposition or opposition. *Nursing Research, 31* (3), 176-177.

Murphy, C., & Hunter, H. (1982). *Ethical problems in the nurse-patient relationship*. Boston: Allyn & Bacon.

Nelson, H. L. (1992). Against caring. *The Journal of Clinical Ethics, 3* (1), 8-15.

Hastings & Hudson Institute of Society. (1948). *Nuremberg Code, Readings*. New York: Ethics & Life Sciences.

Ozonoff, V., & Ozonoff, D. (1977). On helping those who help themselves. *Hastings Center Report, 7*, 7-10.

Pence, T., & Cantral, J. (1990). *Ethics in nursing: An anthology*. New York: National League for Nursing.
Perkins, R. J. (1981). Perspective on the public good. *American Journal of Public Health, 71* (3), 294-295.
President's Commission for the Study of Ethical Problems in Medicine and Biomedical and Behavioral Research. (1982). *Report: Making health care decisions: The ethical and legal implications of informed consent in the patient-practitioner relationship (Vol. 1)*. Washington, DC: U.S. Government Printing Office.
President's Commission for the Study of Ethical Problems in Medicine and Biomedical and Behavioral Research. (1983). *Securing access to health care: The ethical implications of differences in the availability of health services (Vol. 1)*. Washington, DC: U.S. Government Printing Office.
Purdy, L. (1996). Reproducing persons: issues in feminist bioethics. Ithica, NY: Cornell University Press.
Ramsey, P. (1972). Genetic therapy: A theologian's response. In M. P. Hamilton (Ed.), *The new genetics and the future of man*. Grand Rapids, MI: Eerdmans.
Ramsey, P. (1970). Parenthood and the future of man. *Fabricated man*. New Haven, CT: Yale University Press.
Rawls, J. (1977). Justice as fairness. In J. R. Stanley (Ed.), *Ethics in medicine: historical perspectives & contemporary concerns*. Cambridge, MA: Massachusetts Institute of Technology.
Reich, W. (1978). *Encyclopedia on bioethics*. New York: Free Press.
Robertson, J. (1978). Reproductive technologies: Legal aspects. In W. Reich (Ed.), *Encyclopedia of bioethics* (Vol. 4). New York: Free Press, 1464-1469.
Ruthmann, M. (1973). Celebrating leisure today. *Review of Religions, 23* (2), 37-41.
Sherwin, S. (1992). *No longer patient: feminist ethics and health care*. Philadelphia: Temple.
Sherwin, S. (1998). *The politics of women's health: exploring agency and autonomy*. Philadelphia: Temple.
Shilts, R. (1987). *And the band played on*. New York: St. Martin's Press.
Shinn, R. (1978). Gene therapy: Ethical issues. In W. Reich (Ed.), *Encyclopedia of bioethics* (Vol. 2). New York: Free Press, 521-527.
Silverman, M., & Silverman, D. (1985). AIDS and the threat to public health. *Hastings Center Report, 15 (4)*, 19-22.
Smith, S. A., & Davis, A. J. (1980). Ethical dilemmas: Conflicts among rights, duties, and obligations. *The American Journal of Nursing, 80*, 1463-1467.
Spector, R. (1991). *Cultural diversity in health and illness* (3rd ed.). New York: Appleton-Century-Crofts.
Sulpizi, L. K. (1996). Issues in sexuality and gynecologic care of women with developmental disabilities. *Journal of Gynecologic and Neonatal Nursing, 25* (7), 609-614.
Tong, R. (1997). *Feminist approaches to bioethics: theoretical reflections and practical applications*. Boulder, CO: Westview Press.
U.S. Department of Health and Human Services. (1981). *Basic HHS policy for protection of human research subjects*. Washington, DC: U.S. Government Printing Office.
Vatican Congregation for the Doctrine of the Faith. (1987, Feb. 22). *Instruction on respect for human life in its origin and the dignity for its procreation*.
Veatch, R. M. & Fry, S. T. (1987). *Case studies in nursing ethics*. Philadelphia: JB Lippincott.
Watson, G. (1981). Helmet use, helmet use laws, and motorcyclist fatalities. *American Journal of Public Health, 71* (3), 297-300.
Wold, J. (1990). AIDS testing, an ethical question. *The Journal of Neuroscience Nursing, 22*, 258-261.

Unit Two
Assessment for Health Promotion

6 Health Promotion and the Individual

7 Health Promotion and the Family

8 Health Promotion and the Community

Chapter 6

CAROL LYNN MANDLE

Health Promotion and the Individual

objectives

After completing this chapter, the nurse will be able to:

- Define the framework of functional health patterns as described by Gordon.
- Describe the use of the functional health pattern framework in assessing the individual throughout the lifespan.
- Give examples of the following categories of behaviors within the health patterns: functional, potentially dysfunctional, and actually dysfunctional.
- Describe aspects to consider while diagnosing the risk factors or the contributing etiological factors of actually or potentially dysfunctional health patterns.
- Discuss planning, implementing, and evaluating nursing interventions in health promotion with the individual.
- Develop a specific health promotion plan based on an assessment of an individual.

key terms

Cultural Competence
Cultural Focus
Expected Outcomes
Functional Focus
Functional Health Patterns
Health Status
Nursing Diagnosis
Nursing Intervention
Pattern Focus
Risk Factors

THINK About It

Assessment of Alcohol Consumption

*When assessing a woman for a problem with alcoholism, it is important to remember that women are more likely to feel guilty about their drinking. This guilt can lead to a false-positive result based on the regular CAGE test (considered **C**utting down on drinking, been **A**nnoyed by criticism of drinking, feeling **G**uilty about drinking, and using alcohol as an **E**ye opener). Instead, women are better assessed according to the T-ACE test:*

- *How many drinks does it **T**ake to make you feel drunk?*
- *Have you ever been **A**nnoyed by people criticizing your drinking?*
- *Have you ever considered **C**utting down your drinking?*
- *Have you ever used alcohol as an **E**ye opener?*

1 Why do nurses tailor their assessments to meet the individual's characteristics?

2 How effectively would this screening tool identify alcohol problems in women within the population?

Sections of this chapter are adapted from the curriculum of the Adult Health Nursing, Master of Science Program, Boston College Graduate School of Nursing, Chestnut Hill, Massachusetts; Gordon M. (1994). *Nursing diagnosis: Process and application* (3rd ed.). St. Louis: Mosby.

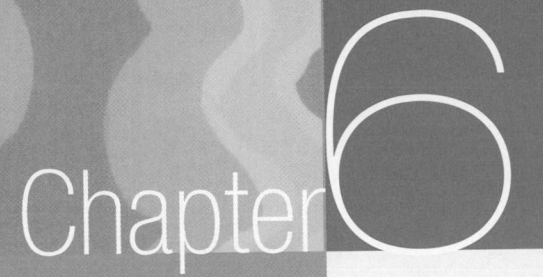

A central unifying theme links all definitions, philosophies, and frameworks of nursing: a holistic examination of person-environment relationships throughout the lifespan, with nursing's purpose being to facilitate these processes.

> Crucial is the idea that health and illness are not separate entities . . . but are reflections of the changing patterns of the life process. The peaks and troughs of this pattern might be considered the times when the pattern and organization of an individual become increasingly inefficient or disorganized, until the situation is regarded as illness . . . [which] can provide the tension or shock, redirecting the energy pattern and thus bringing about a more harmonious, free-flowing pattern . . . better suited to the individual's needs (Newman, 1995; Rogers, 1970).

From Nightingale's belief that the laws of health and nursing are the same and pertinent for both the sick and the well individual (Nightingale, 1861), health promotion continues to be an integral component of nursing practice today.

The American Nurses' Association (ANA) defines the practice of nursing as the performance of services using the nursing process in (1) promoting and maintaining health; (2) case finding and managing illness, injury, or infirmity; (3) restoring optimal functioning; or (4) helping the patient achieve a dignified death (ANA, 1980a, 1980b, 1991). Although this definition was designed to provide a model for state nursing practice acts, the familiar terminology in the ANA social policy statement is more concise: "Nursing is the diagnosis and treatment of human responses to actual or potential health problems" (ANA, 1995, p. 6). This is the definition of nursing used in the majority of nurse practice acts in the United States. These responses are divided into health-restoring responses (reactions to health problems as illness) and health-supporting responses (concerns about potential health problems, such as susceptibility to illness) (ANA, 1995). The nursing process is the organized method of giving individualized nursing care to each individual, family, and community, including assessment, diagnosis, outcome criteria, process criteria (including planned interventions), implementation, and evaluation. These components are explained comprehensively in the ANA Standards of Clinical Nursing Practice (1991).

Based on this definition, primary prevention is a crucial element of nursing and includes generalized health promotion and specific protection from disease. This concept of health promotion connotes an active process involving specific protection (immunizations, occupational safety, and environmental control) along with a lifestyle, value and belief system, and set of behaviors that enhance health. Chapter 1 describes the health of any individual, family, or community as a sustainable balance involving complex responses between internal physiological and psychological systems and the external environment. Many references are available that describe the medical model of assessment of an individual's biophysical states, including the comprehensive review of systems and physical exam conducted by the nurse, physician, or physician's assistant (Bickley, 1999; Jarvis, 2000). Additionally, the nurse needs a framework in which to assess the interactions among a person's biophysical, psychosocial, and spiritual states and the environment because "diagnosis based solely on pathology of systems and parts obscures the total pattern (of the individual). Understanding the total pattern (of the individual) is needed in order to know when and what intervention is indicated" (Newman, 1995).

With health promotion serving as the underlying theme, this chapter focuses on the nursing assessment of the individual. The framework used for assessment is the functional health patterns assessment of the individual described by Gordon. This same framework is used throughout this unit to demonstrate assessment approaches with the family and community (see Chapters 7 and 8). This chapter also discusses components of the nursing process as they relate to health promotion of the individual.

FUNCTIONAL HEALTH PATTERNS: ASSESSMENT OF THE INDIVIDUAL

Nursing assessment's focus is to determine the **health status** of the individual. Table 6-1 demonstrates the aspects common to a complete nursing assessment. Assessment here refers to collection of data only, although an artificial component separation—diagnosis or problem identification—is considered separately for clarity. This process follows guidelines proposed by Bloch (1974) and

Table 6-1 Aspects of a Nursing Assessment

Definition	Deliberate and Systematic Data Collection
Components	Subjective data: health history—subjective reports and individual perceptions Objective data: Observations of nurse Findings of physical examination Information from health record Results of clinical testing
Function	Description of person's health status
Structure	Organization of interdependent parts describing health, function, or patterns of behavior that reflect the "whole" individual and environment
Process	Interview, observation, and examination
Format	Systematic but flexible; individualized to each person, nurse, and situation
Goal	Nursing diagnosis or problem identification Identification of areas of strengths, limitations, alterations, responses to alterations and therapies, and risks

used in the ANA Standards of Care (ANA, 1991). Assessment of health status must consider not only the physiological parameters, but also the entire human being interacting with the environment. Patterns of behaviors, beliefs, perceptions, and values are essential components of a health (nursing) assessment if the maximal health potential of the individual is to be realized. Understanding patterns is basic to understanding the health of an individual (Bramwell, 1984; Newman, 1987, 1994, 1995; Rogers, 1970).

Gordon (1994) has taken a set of health-related behaviors that have been traditional concerns of nursing (Abbey, 1980; Lawton, 1971; McCain, 1965; Mitchell, 1981; Smith, 1968) and developed an assessment framework of 11 **functional health patterns.** Functional patterns interact to make up an individual's lifestyle. Using this framework, the nurse combines assessment skills with subjective and objective data to construct patterns reflective of this lifestyle.

This section expands on functional health pattern assessment as a framework and the assessment process using this framework. Each pattern is presented and includes the following:

1. Definition of the pattern
2. Significance of the pattern to the individual's lifestyle, including developmental focus and environmental influences, when appropriate
3. Assessment objectives
4. Assessment parameters for the health history
5. Pattern indicators within the physical examination
6. Implications for practice, including specific examples for clarification

The Functional Health Pattern Framework

The wholeness of the person and the totality of the person's interactions with the environment are the philosophical foundations of this text. These factors are also the perspective of Gordon's typology of 11 functional health patterns, which provide a mechanism for data collection that encompasses the entire person and all the life processes. By examining the specific functional patterns and the interaction among the patterns, the nurse can accurately determine and diagnose actual or potential problems, intervene more effectively, and achieve outcomes that promote health and well being (Gordon, 1976, 1990, 1994, 1995). In addition to providing a framework for holistically assessing individuals, families, and communities, the functional health patterns provide a strong focus for more effective nursing interventions and outcomes for each individual, family, and community. This focus provides a stronger position from which nurses can make decisions about health care systems at organizational, community, national, and international levels.

Definition

Functional health patterns are an interrelated group of behavioral areas that provide a view of the whole individual. The typology of 11 patterns serves as a useful tool to collect and organize the assessment data and create a mechanism for verifying information with the individual or relaying it to other nurses and members of the health care team.

Each pattern, briefly described in Table 6-2, is a biopsychosocial-spiritual expression of the whole person. Individual reports and nursing observations provide the data for describing the patterns. As a framework for assessment, functional health patterns provide an effective means for the nurse to perceive and record the complex interactions of a person's biophysical state, psychological makeup, and relationship to the environment.

Characteristics

Functional health patterns are characterized by their focus. Gordon (1994) identified five areas: (1) pattern, (2) indi-

Table 6-2 Typology of 11 Functional Health Patterns

Pattern	Description
Health perception-health management pattern	Individual's perceived health and well being and how health is managed
Nutritional-metabolic pattern	Food and fluid consumption relative to metabolic need and indicators of local nutrient supply
Elimination pattern	Excretory function (bowel, bladder, and skin)
Activity-exercise pattern	Exercise, activity, leisure, and recreation
Sleep-rest pattern	Sleep, rest, and relaxation
Cognitive-perceptual pattern	Sensory perceptual and cognitive patterns
Self-perception–self-concept pattern	Self-concept pattern and perceptions of self (body comfort, body image, and feeling state); self-conception and self-esteem
Roles-relationships pattern	Role engagements and relationships
Sexuality-reproductive pattern	Person's satisfaction and dissatisfaction with sexuality and reproduction
Coping–stress tolerance pattern	General coping pattern and effectiveness in stress tolerance
Values-beliefs pattern	Values, beliefs (including spiritual), or goals that guide choices or decisions

Modified from Gordon, M. (1994). *Nursing diagnosis: Process and application* (3rd ed.). St. Louis: Mosby.

vidual-environmental, (3) age-developmental, (4) functional, and (5) cultural.

Pattern focus implies that the nurse explores patterns or sequences of behavior over time. Gordon's (1994) use of the term behavior encompasses biophysical, psychological, sociological, and any other classification of human behavior. The recognition of a pattern by the nurse is a cognitive process that occurs during information collection. As information is collected, a pattern emerges that represents historical and current behavior over time. This pattern is easiest to recognize when behavior or information is quantifiable, as with blood pressure, and is facilitated when baseline data are available for the individual. Patterns within patterns are developed and assessed. Blood pressure, for example, is a pattern within the activity and exercise pattern. The individual baseline and subsequent readings may present a pattern within expected norms. Erratic blood pressure measurements indicate an absence of pattern. This lack of pattern forms a type of pattern in itself. The categories of functional health provide a structure for analyzing a factor within a category (blood pressure: activity pattern) and a structure to focus the search for causal explanations, usually outside the category (excess sodium intake: nutritional pattern) (Gordon, 1994).

The concept of individual-environmental focus can be demonstrated by food intake. Although reference is made within many patterns to environmental influence, it often refers to the physical environments within and external to the individual person. Common to each functional health pattern are environmental influences such as role relationships, family values, and society mores. Personal preference, knowledge of food preparation, and ability to consume and retain food govern the individual's food intake. Cultural and family habits, financial ability to secure the food, and crop availability also influence food intake. Additionally, the person who secures, prepares, and serves the food, such as the mother or father, controls nutritional intake for children.

Human growth and age-developmental focus are reflected in each pattern (Beyed & Matzo, 1989; Burn, 1992; Rengucci, 1992). The previous discussion of health addresses the complex interaction between biopsychosocial-spiritual systems of the individual and the environment. One of the main influences on this dynamic interaction is the development of the person. Fulfillment of developmental tasks increases the complexity of the components and interactions of health. These tasks, however, also provide learning opportunities for the individual to maintain and improve health. Approximately 25 years ago, Bruhn and colleagues (1977) proposed a framework to organize specific health tasks for the individual to accomplish at each developmental phase of the life cycle, as identified by Erikson (1986) and Havighurst (1973) and presented in Table 6-3. Learning these tasks begins at birth and continues to the end of a person's life. By considering current epidemiological data and specifically recommended health behaviors, this framework continues to be useful for health promotion throughout the lifespan. This framework is used throughout Unit 4, which explores each of these developmental tasks and the related learning and practice of these health behaviors that result from appropriate nursing interventions for health promotion.

Functional focus refers to the individual's functional level, a traditional area of concern to nursing. Other disciplines examine functional patterns, but the assessment data vary. Genitourinary functions for medicine refer to frequency or voiding patterns and characteristics of urine, such as color, odor, and laboratory analysis. In addition to these factors, nursing assesses how the particular voiding pattern affects the person's lifestyle, especially the effect of frequency on sleep patterns and the ability to carry out desired activities, such as shopping or socializing. Additional concerns might include whether the individual is able to walk or climb stairs to the bathroom or manage these activities safely at night.

Culturally based age, developmental, and gender norms are important personal and social environmental influences on the development of health patterns. Therefore the **cultural focus** serves as the last area of focus characterizing functional health patterns.

The American Academy of Nursing Expert Panel (1992, p. 227) defines cross-cultural nursing care as "care delivered to individuals, families, or groups that are considered (by self or others) a minority because of race, culture, heritage, or sexual orientation." To possess **cultural competence,** attention to ways of living by a human group that are transmitted to succeeding generations, nurses must be sensitive to the underlying personal and cultural reality of an individual, identifying and using cultural norms, values, and communication and time patterns in collecting and interpreting assessment information (Kelley & Fitzsimmons, 2000).

Rationale for Use

As the discussion of the characteristics illustrates, health is the focus of the functional health pattern framework. The information collected is basic to all nursing assessments of individuals. Although various theoretical and conceptual frameworks of nursing collect holistic data about the person, variations exist in the interpretation of the data and the interventions used to achieve the desired outcomes. The assessment structure of the functional health pattern framework is relevant to all conceptual models.

A distinct advantage in the use of functional health patterns is that they are concise and easily learned. Repeated use facilitates learning; therefore the nurse who is just beginning to use functional health patterns for assessment may find an acronym (SCHREVSNACS) or a

Table **6-3** Relationship Between Selected Developmental Tasks and Wellness Tasks for Each Stage of the Life Cycle

Erikson's Eight Life Stages	Havighurst's Developmental Tasks	Examples of Minimal Wellness Tasks for Each Developmental Stage
1. Infancy (trust vs. basic mistrust)	Learning to walk Learning to take solid foods Learning to talk Learning to control elimination of body waste	Acquiring ability to perform psychomotor skills Learning functional definition of health Learning social and emotional responsiveness to others and to physical environment
2. Early childhood (autonomy vs. shame and doubt)	Learning gender difference and sexual modesty Achieving physiological stability Forming simple concepts of social-physical reality Learning to relate emotionally to parents, siblings, and others Learning to distinguish right from wrong and developing a conscience	Learning about proper foods, exercise, and sleep Learning dental hygiene Learning injury prevention (safety belts and helmets, sunscreen, smoke detectors, poisons, firearms, and swimming)
3. Late childhood (initiative vs. guilt)	Learning physical skills necessary for ordinary games Building wholesome attitudes toward self as a growing organism Learning to get along with peers	Refining psychomotor and cognitive skills Developing self-concept Learning attitudes of competition and cooperation with others Learning social, ethical, and moral differences and responsibilities
4. Early adolescence (industry vs. inferiority)	Learning appropriate gender identity: masculine or feminine role Developing fundamental skills in reading, writing, and calculating Developing concepts necessary for everyday living Developing conscience, morality, and scale of values Achieving personal independence Developing attitudes toward social groups and institutions	Learning that health is an important value Learning self-regulation of physiological needs—sleep, rest, food, drink, and exercise Learning risk taking and its consequences (injury prevention)
5. Adolescence (identity vs. role confusion)	Achieving new and more mature relations with peers and both sexes Achieving gender identity Accepting physique and using body effectively Achieving emotional independence of parents and other adults Achieving assurance of economic independence Selecting and preparing for occupation Preparing for marriage and family life Developing intellectual skills and concepts necessary for civic competence Desiring and achieving socially responsible behavior	Learning economic responsibility Learning social responsibility for self and others (preventing pregnancy and sexually transmitted diseases) Experiencing social, emotional, and ethical commitments to others Accepting self and physical development Reconciling discrepancies between personal health concepts and observed health behaviors of others (use of alcohol, drugs, tobacco, firearms, and violence) Learning to cope with life events and problems (suicide prevention) Considering life goals and career plans and acquiring necessary skills to reach goals
6. Early adulthood (intimacy vs. isolation)	Selecting and learning to live with a mate Starting a family; managing a home Taking on civic responsibility	Learning importance of time to self and world Committing to mate and family responsibilities Selecting a career Incorporating health habits into lifestyle

Modified from Bruhn, J., Cordova, F. D., Williams, J. A., Fuentes, R. G. (1977). The wellness process. *Journal of Community Health, 2*, 209-221; Erikson, E. (1986). *Childhood and society* (35th anniversary ed.). New York: Norton; Havighurst, R. (1973). *Developmental tasks and education* (3rd ed.). New York: David McKay; U.S. Department of Health and Human Services. (2000). *Healthy People 2010. National health promotion and disease prevention objectives* (Conference Edition). Washington, DC: Public Health Service; U.S. Preventive Services Task Force. (1996). *Guide to clinical preventive services: An assessment of the effectiveness of 169 interventions*. Baltimore: Williams & Wilkins.

Continued

Table 6-3 Relationship Between Selected Developmental Tasks and Wellness Tasks for Each Stage of the Life Cycle—cont'd

Erikson's Eight Life Stages	Havighurst's Developmental Tasks	Examples of Minimal Wellness Tasks for Each Developmental Stage
7. Middle adulthood (generativity vs. stagnation)	Accepting and adjusting to physiological changes Achieving adult social responsibility Maintaining economic standard of living Assisting adolescent children	Accepting aging of self and others Coping with societal pressures Recognizing importance of good health habits Reassessing life goals periodically
8. Maturity (ego integrity vs. despair)	Adjusting to decreasing physical strength and health Adjusting to retirement and reduced income Adjusting to death of spouse Establishing an explicit affiliation with own age group Establishing satisfactory physical living arrangements	Becoming aware of tasks to health and adjusting lifestyle and habits to cope with risks Adjusting to loss of job, income, and family and friends through death Redefining self-concept Adjusting to changes in personal time and new physical environment Adjusting previous health habits to current physical and mental capabilities

Modified from Bruhn, J., Cordova, F. D., Williams, J. A., Fuentes, R. G. (1977). The wellness process. *Journal of Community Health, 2,* 209-221; Erikson, E. (1986). *Childhood and society* (35th anniversary ed.). New York: Norton; Havighurst, R. (1973). *Developmental tasks and education* (3rd ed.). New York: David McKay; U.S. Department of Health and Human Services. (2000). *Healthy People 2010. National health promotion and disease prevention objectives* (Conference Edition). Washington, DC: Public Health Service; U.S. Preventive Services Task Force. (1996). *Guide to clinical preventive services: An assessment of the effectiveness of 169 interventions*. Baltimore: Williams & Wilkins.

mnemonic sentence ("However, Never Expect Anticipated Solutions," Cautioned Sister Rose, "Since Cooperation Varies") useful. After the 11 terms are committed to memory, they serve as a guideline for assessment and for retrieving from memory the specific items to be assessed in each area.

Other advantages of a functional health pattern framework specific to the practice of nursing include the following:

- The structure provides a consistent nursing focus through a means of collecting, organizing, presenting, and analyzing data to arrive at a nursing (not a medical) diagnosis
- The format is flexible and can be tailored to the individual, the situation, or the nurse
- The information collected is suitable to any arena of practice, whether in the home, clinic, or institution and whether assessing the individual (adult or child), family, or community

Theoretical components of nursing (education and research) are also facilitated with the use of functional health patterns. The student, educator, or researcher is able to do the following:

- Organize clinical knowledge in a way relevant to the nursing diagnoses, interventions, and outcomes
- Gain advanced knowledge of the individual's problems amenable to nursing care and of diagnosis-specific interventions and outcomes
- Identify areas in which knowledge in nursing requires expansion

Medical science data is incorporated into, but is not the focus for, organizing nursing knowledge.

The Patterns

Each pattern is a biopsychosocial spiritual expression of the individual and reflects lifestyle or life processes from the perspective of both the individual and the nurse. Additionally, this expression reflects (1) a pattern or sequencing of behaviors, (2) the role of the environment (physical environs and family, societal, and cultural influences), and (3) any influences of a developmental nature.

The assessment of each pattern as functional (strengths), dysfunctional (nursing diagnosis), or potentially dysfunctional includes an indication of the individual's level of satisfaction with the pattern. Any problems reported should be further assessed to include the individual's explanation of the problem, remedial actions taken, and the perceived effect of these actions.

A major goal in assessing each pattern is to determine the individual's knowledge of health promotion, the ability to manage health-promoting activities, and the value that the individual ascribes to health promotion.

This section develops each pattern in sufficient detail to allow the nurse to use a functional health pattern framework for assessment and diagnosis in the clinical practice of nursing. Understanding the role that each pattern plays in the individual's life and in the nurse's practice is also helpful; therefore there will be a discussion of individual significance and nursing implications.

Health Perception-Health Management Pattern

This pattern provides an overview of the individual's health status and the health practices that are used to reach the current level of health or wellness. The focus is on the perceived health status and the importance placed on health along with the individual's level of commitment to maintaining health (Gordon, 1994). When eliciting information of this sort, areas will be introduced that will likely need further exploration under another functional health pattern. For example, when an individual says that mowing the lawn in no longer possible without becoming short of breath or suffering severe back pain, this information is stored and retrieved when assessing the activity and exercise pattern or the cognitive-perceptual pattern.

The importance of this pattern area to an individual is apparent. If people do not perceive that health problems are present, if they are unaware of necessary health promotion in the absence of problems, if they do not feel capable of managing their own health, or if they believe that any activity on their part is useless in promoting health, then their lifestyle and ability to function will be affected. Health promoting activities (adequate nutrition, activity and exercise, sleep, and rest), routine professional examinations, self-examinations, immunizations, and safety precautions (auto safety restraints and locked medicine cabinets) have been shown to be instrumental in improving or maintaining an optimal quality of life.

The objective in assessing the health perception–health management pattern is to obtain data about perceptions, management, and preventive health practices (Gordon, 1994). Tentatively, values may lead to identifying potential health hazards such as noncompliance to a prescribed medical or nursing regimen or inability to manage health effectively.* In addition to these clues, the nurse does not overlook unrealistic health and illness perceptions and expectations.

Specific assessment parameters to be explored during the history include the health and safety practices of the individual, previous patterns of adherence or compliance, and use of the health care system—knowledge of the availability of health services, patterns indicating at what point health care is sought, and accessibility to health care through financial resources, health insurance, and transportation.

In addition to methods of health management, the nurse explores health perception as the individual describes current health status, past problems, and anticipation of future problems associated with health or health care. Expectations are indicative of health beliefs, locus of control, and realistic understanding of health state and any health problems (see Multicultural Awareness box).

MULTICULTURAL AWARENESS

Self-Assessed Health Status of Hispanic Americans

	Excellent	Very Good	Good	Fair to Poor
Cuban	38%	22%	26%	14%
Mexican	28%	24%	31%	16%
Puerto Rican	28%	27%	28%	18%
Other (including Central and South American)	33%	28%	28%	12%

Data from National Center for Health Statistics, U.S. Department of Health & Human Services. (2000). *Health outcomes among Hispanic subgroups: Data from the National Health Interview Survey, 1992-1995.* Washington, DC: U.S. Government Printing Office.

Examination of the individual provides limited clues within this pattern because its basis is the individual's perception rather than the actual health status. The general appearance may provide some indication of true health status, but in reality, the entire health assessment, including history and examination, is the best indicator of whether the individual's perception is accurate. General appearance and condition may reveal evidence as to when the individual actually seeks health care or may reveal multiple bruises or cognitive and perceptual disturbances that would be **risk factors** for injury. An inspection of the home environment might uncover additional risk factors.

The significance of this pattern to nursing cannot be overstressed. Health perceptions influence data collection and provide direction for all future planning of care. The individuals' health beliefs, also discussed under the values-beliefs pattern, directly influence their participation in care. Individuals are less apt to engage in self-care or preventive measures when they (1) believe it is the responsibility of health team members to keep them healthy, (2) do not recognize or acknowledge their susceptibility to an impending health problem, or (3) believe that they cannot influence their health status.

Health management in the past serves as a predictor of future health management. If there has been a lack of adherence to a prescribed regimen, a recurrence is likely unless the nurse is able to identify and remedy related causes. An illustration of this situation can be found in an individual with high blood pressure who fails to keep follow-up appointments, often "forgets" to take medication, and eats foods with high sodium content. An assessment must be made to determine whether this evident noncompliance is based on a conflict within the value system of the individual (health beliefs); inaccurate information; misunderstanding; decreased ability to learn, retain, or retrieve information (knowledge deficit); or

*The terms cues or clues to problems mentioned within this section refer to the presence of defining characteristics identified by the North American Nursing Diagnosis Association (NANDA, 2000).

denial of illness (health perception). Variables such as financial resources, transportation difficulties, nutritional preferences, daily activities (individual and family patterns), and ability to read written instructions (literacy or visual acuity), may have affected the individual's behaviors.

The information collected within the health perception–health management pattern depends on the purpose of data collection and the population. Often, problems within this area may not be apparent until other patterns are assessed.

Nutritional-Metabolic Pattern

This pattern describes nutrient intake relative to metabolic need (Gordon, 1994). The focus includes not only the individual's description of food and fluid consumption (history), but also the nurse's observations and perceptions regarding adequate nutrition (physical examination). The nurse should also elicit the individual's satisfaction with current eating and drinking patterns, including restrictions and the individual's perception of problems associated with eating and drinking, growth and development, skin condition, and healing processes.

All bodily functions and the lifestyle of the individual are governed by adequate intake and supply of nutrients to tissues and organs. Sufficient food and fluid intake is necessary to provide the needed energy for performance of all activities, which include both the internal physiological functioning of the body organs and the external gross body movements. Any interruption in the acquisition or retention of food or fluids will offset this balance and significantly alter the person's daily lifestyle. Nutrition and metabolism also govern the rate of an individual's growth and development.

The assessment objective is to collect data about a typical pattern of food and fluid consumption, the adequacy of this pattern of consumption, and as with all patterns, any perceived problems associated with nutritional intake. Specific clues may point to an individual who is overweight, underweight, overly hydrated, dehydrated, or experiencing difficulties in skin integrity, such as breakdown or delayed healing. Individuals may also be at risk for developing these problems.

Parameters for assessment fall into two broad categories: (1) parameters that evaluate nutrient intake and (2) parameters that evaluate metabolic demands. Nutrient intake may be assessed with a 24-hour recall of flood and fluid consumption; a listing of diet restrictions, food allergies, vitamin supplements, caffeine and alcohol ingestion (when not included in the medication history); and a schedule of eating and drinking patterns. Assessment includes screening from problems associated with swallowing or chewing.

When problems seem apparent, the focus assessment might include patterns of food preference, feelings about present weight, and a detail of eating habits. Eating may be affected if the individual eats alone rather than with others. Frequent dining out may be indicative of problems in this or other functional patterns. When the diet consists of fast foods, the consumption pattern may uncover a deficit of essential vitamins or minerals. When appropriate, the nurse assesses areas pertinent to obtaining food. Who purchases it? Is shopping preplanned, as with a grocery list? Are there adequate financial resources and a food budget? Is food stored properly? Who prepares the food? In what manner are most foods prepared (fried, broiled, steamed, boiled, or baked)?

Metabolic demands vary from individual to individual and within the same individual during times of illness, stress, growth, high activity levels, healing, or recovery. Both developmental and environmental conditions may alter the metabolic demands. Appetite and reported changes in weight, skin integrity, and general healing ability are the parameters elicited during the interview or health history. The individual may also note a decreased tolerance for hot and cold weather.

The observations and perceptions of the nurse play vital roles in assessing the nutritional and metabolic pattern. The physical examination allows assessment of both the nutrient supply to the tissue and the metabolic needs of the individual. Objective findings serve as indicators to measure the reliability of the subjective reports concerning nutrient intake.

Gross metabolic indicators include temperature, height, and weight. The physical examination also focuses on the skin, bony prominences, dentition, hair, and mucous membranes. Skin and mucous membranes, in particular, use nutrients rapidly and provide excellent indices for evaluating adequacy of nutrient supply. Assessment of the skin includes color, temperature, turgor, and a description of any skin lesions, areas of dry or scaly skin, rashes, pruritus, or edema. The mucous membranes are also examined for color, integrity, moisture, and lesions. Dentition is evaluated for structure. Are teeth erupted at normal stages of development? Are teeth firmly implanted? Are dentures fitted properly? Additionally, decay and evidence of oral hygiene are evaluated. Healing is assessed when there is evidence of injury.

In assessing the individual, the nutritional-metabolic pattern should naturally follow the health perception–health management pattern. Nutritional intake is often mentioned when describing health practices. By referring again to the individual's initial discussion of "three meals a day," the nurse can direct the interview into more specific details of nutritional intake. Another useful method of leading from one pattern to another without causing disjointedness is to assess drug history at the end of health perception-health management, adding caffeine and alcohol intake, thereby beginning fluid consumption evaluation. If the nurse prefers to begin with food consumption, then a question discussing the use of vitamin supplements bridges the gap between the two patterns. Regardless of the response, the nurse can then ask, "Why do you find that necessary (or unnecessary)?" A description of nutritional intake generally follows with little additional prompting.

Several points need to be emphasized at this time. No matter what the purpose of the particular assessment is—initial screening, follow-up visit, or yearly checkup—the assessment of nutrition versus metabolic need should be a continuing process. Any internally altered chemical state expresses itself outwardly. Pregnancy, for example, may cause increased appetite or weight changes. Appetite and weight changes, along with physical indicators, may also be apparent in a nonpregnant, healthy woman. The nurse notes these changes and checks other patterns that may be the cause, such as decreased activity (activity-exercise pattern) or increased stress (coping-stress-tolerance pattern). Inadequate nutrition (fluid and electrolyte disturbances) may cause decreased mental alertness or increased confusion.

Although problem identification occurs after assessment of all 11 functional health patterns, a problem in any one area serves as a clue to the possibility of other dysfunctional patterns. Assessment of the pattern is facilitated by synthesizing and analyzing data collected in the other 10 functional health patterns. Nutrition and metabolism are especially significant in patterns of health management, elimination, activity, sleep, cognition, roles, and stress tolerance. The values-beliefs pattern may significantly alter all other functional patterns. Sociocultural values and ethnic backgrounds play a major role in determining an individual's pattern of eating.

It is particularly important how patterns of nutrient supply and demand and eating habits and food preferences vary over the lifespan. Raw fruits and vegetables may be fun "finger food" for the toddler, but the older adult, especially one with loose dentures or arthritis of the temporomandibular joint (jaw), may find it impossible to eat these foods.

Implications for practice include a strong focus on educational needs. Assessment aims not only to disclose dysfunctional or potentially dysfunctional patterns, but also to demonstrate functional patterns. When good nutrition is part of the health-promotion activities of the individual, this should be considered a strength. Health promotion in this pattern may provide a stepping stone for similar activities in the other patterns. For example, if a balanced nutritional intake is believed to improve functional level, then that individual may also learn relaxation techniques to decrease the effect of stress. An understanding of the balance of food and fluid intake and body requirements will help the individual adjust caloric intake as growth decreases and prevent overweight problems in the adult years.

Proper education can prevent potential problems. Although an individual may follow a prescribed no-salt diet and demonstrate an understanding of which foods contain significant amounts of sodium, assessing whether the individual also understands why this is important is vital. Potential problems with compliance might be avoided several years later if the nurse includes this education in the plan of care.

Elimination Pattern

This pattern is designed to describe the function of the bowel, bladder, and skin in the excretion of wastes. The nurse measures the regularity, quality, and quantity of stool and urine according to the individual's subjective reporting, assessing any aids that are used to achieve regularity or control, and any pattern changes or perceived problems. Skin is considered during this assessment only in terms of excretory function (the amount of perspiration and associated odor control) (Gordon, 1994).

The significance of the elimination pattern to the whole person may vary on an individual level. Many people view regularity of elimination as a measure of their health and as a sensitive indicator of proper nutrition and stress level. The individual's perceptions are important in determining whether the pattern is problematic and dysfunctional and assessment is based on what is "normal" for each individual. Many misconceptions about regularity exist, especially in the area of bowel function. More than many other areas, bowel function is an area in which individuals often treat themselves when problems are perceived; it is important to collect data about treatment methods used.

Any difficulty in control of excreta has many culturally based implications. When any lack of control exists, body image (self-perception) is frequently altered, and altered modes of elimination may affect feelings of sexuality. Both lack of control and altered modes of elimination impinge on the activity level of the individual, decrease socialization, and even affect sleeping patterns.

Age and developmental levels direct the line of questioning. Assessment of children is geared to toilet-training methods, whereas regularity is more often a concern of adults. In addition to constipation, older adults may begin to develop problems of control. Women past the childbearing age are particularly prone to stress incontinence.

The assessment objective is to collect data about regularity and control of excretory patterns (Gordon, 1994). The nurse investigates clues suggesting constipation patterns, diarrhea, or any form of incontinence through focus assessment. Changes in elimination pattern, pain or discomfort, and any perceived problems are also assessed. Data collection includes an explanation of the problem, methods of self-treatment, and perceived results (Gordon, 1994).

Pattern parameters are data such as quantity, quality (color, odor, and consistency), and frequency or regularity of stool, urine, and perspiration. The nurse assesses excretory mode, time patterns, and control of stool and urine, exploring changes in pattern, perceived problems, and elimination habits with the individual. Examination includes gross screening of specimens, with the nurse noting amount, consistency, color, and odor. Any drainage from wounds or fistulas should be noted when skin is assessed.

The transition from nutrition to the elimination pattern often occurs naturally. Roughage level in the diet affects bowel elimination patterns and urinary elimination problems are frequently linked to fluid intake. Even skin integrity may herald questioning about drainage and lead to discussion of additional elimination patterns.

Many individuals do not consider laxatives as they discuss current medication. The nurse must ask specific questions about any remedial actions taken when constipation is a problem. A perceptive nurse will note discrepancies between dietary intake and reported regularity of bowel movements. Assessment may disclose a dependency on laxatives, suppositories, or enemas and may indicate that the individual has a knowledge deficit regarding bowel elimination. Health education in areas of normal bowel function, nutritional guidelines to assist the individual in elimination, or an exercise program may significantly alter the elimination pattern.

Urinary frequency may also demand further health education. Research indicating that delayed time between urinations is associated with increased incidence of urinary tract infections guides the nurse in helping the individual establish a more suitable elimination routine.

As mentioned, assessment is a cognitive process that collects and organizes data systematically. As the assessment continues, the nurse constructs a pattern from data in all 11 functional health patterns. Detailed exploration of areas is indicated whenever a problem is suspected.

Although the individual claims perspiration is not a problem, further assessment is necessary if the individual obviously exhibits an odor control problem. Activity intolerance may exist that prevents the previously necessary daily shower or toileting facilities may not be readily available. Recent life events may have caused depression and decreased interest in self-care and hygiene. Conversely, if the person claims daily activities include four showers or baths, then the nurse must be alert to the possibility of an elimination problem, even if no problem is evident, or a determination must be made as to whether the pattern merely indicates personal values or frequent vigorous exercising. If excess perspiration and odor control are problems, then a metabolic disturbance needing medical evaluation may exist.

Although any area perceived to be a problem by the individual is a problem, the nursing assessment is also designed to evaluate patterns of dysfunction or potential dysfunction of which the individual is unaware. The nurse then shares the analysis of the data with the individual, basing the care plan on mutually shared goals.

Activity-Exercise Pattern

This pattern describes the individual's activity level, exercise program, and leisure activities. The nurse assesses movement capability, activity tolerance, self-care abilities, the use of assistive devices, changes in pattern, the individual's satisfaction with activity and exercise patterns, and any perceived problems (Gordon, 1994).

Limitations within the individual's movement capabilities or ability to perform activities of daily living significantly alter the individual's lifestyle and may affect every other functional health pattern. The importance of movement and independent functioning in self-care is an almost universally accepted value. Child-rearing practices demonstrate this value; parents boast of their infant who walks early, their toilet-trained toddler, and their preschooler who dresses without assistance. The "devastation of paralysis," even in the older adult, signifies the value society places on independent movement and function.

The activity-exercise pattern provides an effective indicator of the individual's commitment to health promotion and preventive care. The importance of exercise to health status has been thoroughly documented and public awareness has grown tremendously in recent years. The number of people who jog or walk as part of a regular fitness routine has certainly increased, as can be seen at nearly every public park in metropolitan areas (Fig. 6-1).

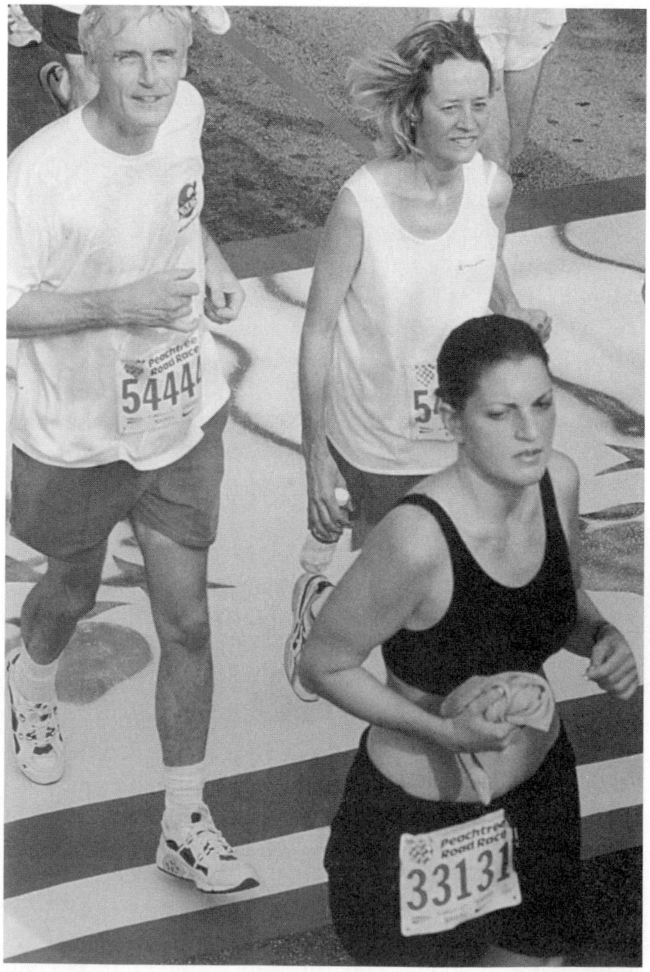

Fig. 6-1 Runners in a road race.

The growing number of health spas demonstrates increased membership and companies involved in selling exercise programming to group consumers (businesses, church and social groups, and housing complexes) claim increasing participation.

In addition to examining exercise and mobility levels, this pattern provides an indication of energy expenditure levels and activity tolerance levels. Leisure activities provide clues to the individual's value system. The American work ethic and competitive nature of many occupations may create a void in leisure or recreational activities. The nurse directs the individual's focus to as many aspects of health promotion as possible. Unless health promotion is brought to people's attention, they may be too busy to realize there is no time for recreation.

The ability to move and perform activities of daily living directly affects the ability to control the immediate environment; therefore an obvious link exists between the activity-exercise pattern and the individual's health. Environment also affects mobility; individuals living alone in high-crime areas may limit activity to the home because they are afraid to leave. The older individual may be too far away from public transportation to shop for groceries; in the past, this walk may have been the major mode of exercise. The number of stairs the individual must negotiate with a cane may restrict activities. Weather may also play a role in altering exercise. For individuals with any neuromuscular or perceptual disturbances, the environmental barriers may be a major handicap. Only recently has legislation faced issues concerning access to public buildings for people in wheelchairs.

The objective of this assessment is to determine the individual's pattern of activities that require energy expenditure. Components reviewed are daily activities, exercise, and leisure activities (Gordon, 1994). The nurse seeks clues to uncover strengths and weaknesses within the pattern. Decreased energy levels, changes within the patterns of activity and exercise, the associated explanation of these changes, perceived problems, and coping strategies to overcome difficulties are all important clues that demand in-depth exploration. Generally, any individual with respiratory or cardiac disease warrants an in-depth assessment and focused assessment is necessary for individuals with neuromuscular, perceptual, or circulatory impairments.

Although many medical conditions may affect the individual's activity-exercise pattern, the nursing goals are designed to help find alternative solutions to limitations, improve activity tolerance levels through planned exercise programs, and prevent further dysfunction by prescribing activities to ensure maximal functioning. Assessment within this area may indicate the need for further medical evaluation to diagnose suggested disease or monitor current disease progression.

Dimensions to be described and assessed include daily activities, leisure activities, and exercise. Daily activities include: (1) occupation (position, hours of work or school, and amount of physical exercise versus cognitive or sedentary activities), (2) self-care abilities (feeding, bathing, grooming, dressing, and toileting), and (3) home-management routines (cooking, cleaning, shopping, laundry, and outdoor activities). Problems within any of these areas require further explanation. Is it a problem of energy expenditure, mobility limitations, or decreased motivation caused by depression, grieving, or incongruent values?

Leisure activities focus on recreational activities, which may be classified according to the degree of energy expenditure and the level of socialization. Breen (1961) describes activities on four levels: (1) active social (organized sports, backyard softball, or golf), (2) active isolate (jogging, walking, or gym workout), (3) sedentary social (bingo, cards, or lecture and discussion groups), and (4) sedentary isolate level (reading, knitting, or coin or stamp collecting). Although not all activities fall into any one category, examining these areas can help the nurse assess recreational activities. Information elicited includes type and frequency of the activity and the value that the individual places on it. The data may prove useful after goals are established and an area of particular interest might be incorporated into the individual's plan of care. For example, a particularly despondent individual who at one time was an avid follower of classical music may be remotivated when this information is properly used. Feelings of heightened self-worth or self-esteem are closely associated with recreational activities, especially in the older individual.

Exercise parameters include type, frequency, duration, and intensity of the individual's regular exercise. The nurse should also assess the importance of exercise to the individual's feelings about exercise.

A 24-hour recall of the previous day's activities provides an initial picture of the pattern; specifics are then addressed as described for each major component. A weekly log is particularly useful for follow-up visits and whenever a problem is suspected. In addition to the weekly log, a focus assessment includes details such as mode of transportation. Does the individual go everywhere in a car? Is public transportation used, and if so, then how far away is the route? Are elevators used rather than climbing a flight of stairs?

Factors interfering with exercise or mobility include dyspnea, fatigue, muscle cramping, neuromuscular or perceptual deficits, chest pain, and angina. As with other patterns, feelings of satisfaction and the individual's perception of problems always provide valuable indications of dysfunctional or potentially dysfunctional patterns.

The nurse carefully evaluates subjective reporting of complaints, such as dyspnea, by noting any difficulty for the individual during the interview and physical examination. Components of the examination assess circulatory, respiratory, and neuromuscular indicators. The nurse measures and records skin color and temperature, heart rate (apical and radial measurement), and blood pressure and notes respiratory rate, rhythmicity, depth of inspiration, and effort involved. Ambulation is observed and a record of gait, posture, and balance is made. Muscle tone, strength, coordination, and range of motion may provide useful clues to validate individuals' reports of activity and exercise. The use of assistive devices or prostheses is evaluated in terms of proper use, proper fit, and degree of assistance or support provided.

The history and the examination are closely linked. Examination alone may not disclose early morning pain and stiffness of the joints and this subjective reporting is invaluable. When appropriate, the nurse may ask the individual to climb stairs or perform self-care activities, which are useful in assessing level of impairment. Various instruments have been designed to quantify level of ability or disability. Gordon (1994) uses an adapted version of work by McCourt (1981) to assess self-care activities and physical mobility. For some individuals, a metabolic activity index, in which each activity is measured according to kilocalories of energy expended per minute, may be a helpful "quantifier" in assessing and planning care.

Developmental norms have been established for the infant and toddler. Childhood development is carefully monitored through milestones such as sitting, crawling, walking, running, and hopping. However, the nurse must remember that some degree of activity is needed regardless of age or health status. Careful assessment of ability, limitations, and interests will guide the nurse in establishing improved patterns of activity and exercise after the whole individual is assessed; the nurse is again cautioned to reserve problem identification until all patterns have been constructed. Useful clues within this pattern may guide the interview in the other pattern areas, but premature closure is dangerous. At this point, only tentative hypotheses are possible and often the explanation of the problem lies in another functional health pattern. For example, when the individual expresses an inability to perform exercise on a routine basis, is it because exercise is associated with knowledge deficit, personal or family value system, overriding priorities, or not valued? Is the inability to perform a result of general fatigue caused by inadequate or decreased sleep time associated with anxiety, nocturia, pain, or an infant waking every three hours for feeding? Are the responsibilities associated with the care of several preschoolers and inadequate financial resources to secure a babysitter the cause? The assessment's purpose is to narrow the scope of possible explanations.

Sleep-Rest Pattern

Perhaps the single most important factor that is assessed in this pattern is the perception of adequacy of sleep and relaxation. Subjective reports of fatigue or energy levels provide some indication of the individual's satisfaction.

Assumed roles that sleep and rest play in preparing the individual for the required or desired daily activities lead this pattern to become extremely important when perceived to be insufficient to promote rest and provide energy. Although the exact function of sleep has not been clearly identified, it seems to serve a restorative function in most individuals. Sleep-deprivation studies provide vivid demonstrations of the need for different types of sleep: light, deep, dream, or rapid eye movement (REM).

Again, problems within this pattern may cause problems in other patterns. A person who has difficulty with sleep may be tense and irritable, unable to tolerate stress, more prone to infectious processes, and incapable of health-promoting relationships. Alterations in appetite, elimination difficulties, and activity intolerance will likely be experienced. Some degree of cognitive dysfunction generally occurs.

Interestingly, sleep researchers note that although people can fool other people and often even themselves, sleep patterns are remarkably accurate indicators of stress tolerance. Sleep is disturbed by strong emotions. Anxiety, for example, frequently makes falling asleep difficult. Depression often causes premature awakening. The inability to initiate or maintain sleep provides clues to other dysfunctional patterns. Sleep problems may be related to physical discomfort, family stress, role or work stress, conflict in the values of the individual or family, nutritional intake (caffeine), activity levels (inactivity or daytime boredom), fears, fluid intake or urinary elimination patterns (nocturia), and schedule of activities associated with role responsibilities (mother and nighttime feedings, 24 hours on call for work, or frequent shift changes). Any change in environment or habit will affect sleep patterns, as does the individual value placed on sleep.

Research studies have linked many variables to sleep disturbances. Age, sex, temperament, individual circadian rhythms, state of mind or emotional state, health status, degree of fatigue, physical condition or comfort, nutritional intake, and many drugs (prescription or over-the-counter drugs, nicotine, caffeine, and alcohol), may cause differences in sleep patterns. The quantity and quality of recent sleep obtained and different forms of exercise govern the amount and type of sleep. However, the single most important determinant of a person's sleep pattern is age. Environment, including noise, lighting, temperature, and barometric pressure, also play a role in the person's ability to sleep.

The objective in assessing a sleep and rest pattern is to describe the effectiveness of the pattern from the individual's perspective. The wide variation in sleep time (from four hours to more than 10 hours) does not necessarily affect functional performance; different individuals require different amounts of sleep. Pertinent information includes data suggestive of difficulties with sleep onset, sleep interruptions, and awakening. The nurse also evaluates disturbances such as dreaming and nightmares, sleepwalking, nocturnal enuresis, and penile tumescence. Counseling, institution of safety measures, or medical referral may be necessary.

In addition to sleep, the nurse assesses rest and relaxation according to the individual's perceptions. Activities of the sedentary isolate type, such as reading or crocheting, may be relaxing for some individuals. Passive involvement, as with television viewing, may provide the only source of relaxation for the individual. Daily naps or various forms of relaxation exercises (meditation, yoga, or breathing exercises) may also be a part of this pattern.

Assessment parameters of the sleep dimension are divided into two parts: (1) sleep quality and (2) sleep quantity. Sleep quality assesses the individual's perception of sleep adequacy, performance level, and physical and psychological state on awakening.

Sleep quantity, in addition to the hours slept each day, is used to disclose a schedule of sleep times. The nurse assesses time of retiring, time of awakening, and additional periods of sleep throughout the day for regularity. Sleep onset and number of and reasons for awakenings provide clues to possible problems. When a problem exists, focusing may evaluate the efficiency of time spent in bed for sleep compared with actual sleeping time.

The dimensions of rest and relaxation include the parameters of type, frequency or regularity, and duration. The perceived effectiveness of methods used to promote rest is also assessed.

The value attributed to sleep by the individual will largely affect both the motivation and the ability to achieve it. Individuals are conditioned to sleep under certain circumstances and maintaining their bedtime rituals is a distinct advantage in sleep promotion. A person who expects to sleep usually will, providing that established patterns are maintained. The nurse should also assess changes in schedule and routines associated with bedtime. When assessing bedtime routines, the nurse includes rituals along with other aids to sleep, such as natural aids (warm milk) or medications (prescription and nonprescription). Physical examination by the nurse includes the individual's general appearance, behavior, and performance changes.

As with pain, sleep is a subjective experience. Comprehensive examination may be performed (for example, with polysomnography), but this is beyond the scope of nursing. Research indicates that subjective reporting of sleep quality and measures of sleep time closely approximate electroencephalographic findings. Most difficulties associated with sleep are amenable to nursing therapies.

Nursing implications focus on the need to be alerted to evidence of sleep disturbances so that proper interventions can be made before sleep deprivation occurs. The nurse concentrates on subjective reports of difficulties or feelings of not being sufficiently rested. Care is taken not to interpret isolated findings; every person has experienced at least one poor night's sleep.

Frequent awakenings do not necessarily imply sleep interruption. Many individuals may awaken numerous times during the night, but return to sleep within seconds. This may be especially true of older adults who generally spend most of the night in stages of light sleep. Their normal developmental pattern does not include deep sleep; therefore awakenings may not affect the sleep cycles and resultant feelings after awakening in the morning. More commonly, however, the older individual experiences difficulty returning to sleep because they experience discomfort, fears, or other variables.

Gaining a sense of the individual's biological rhythm and peak performance time may be helpful to the nurse in planning return visits or providing health education. Individuals commonly refer to themselves as morning people or night owls; the patterns of retiring and arising may provide clues.

Patterns or schedules of sleep and rest in conjunction with subjective reports of physical and mental well being help determine appropriate interventions.

Cognitive-Perceptual Pattern

Cognitive patterns include the ability of the individual to understand and follow directions, retain information, make decisions, solve problems, and use language appropriately. Sensory and perceptual patterns describe auditory, visual, olfactory, gustatory, tactile, and kinesthetic sensations and perceptions. Pain perception and pain tolerance are described within this pattern area (Gordon, 1994).

Thinking and perceiving are major components by which capacity for independent functioning of the individual is measured. Any difficulties in the cognitive-perceptual pattern must somehow be compensated for to ensure the individual's safety. The balance between the individual and the environment that is necessary for health is clearly important; decreasing levels of cognition or perception require increasing levels of environmental control. Sheltered work environments and group living arrangements for the mentally or sensory-impaired individual are examples of this process.

The developmental stage plays a significant role in cognitive and perceptual abilities. Vision and hearing do not reach full potential until school age; 20/30 vision is normal for the preschooler. The ability to problem solve and conceptualize is also marked by developmental stages (Piaget, 1981). As the adult reaches maturity, declines in visual acuity, hearing, touch, and even taste begin and continue through the later years.

The interrelationships among the individual, the developmental stage, and the environment are extremely important. The 20-year-old man who dropped out of high school at age 16 and is now employed in a factory as an assembly line worker and the 20-year-old man who is a second-year premed student at a competitive university will likely exhibit different behavior patterns. The cognitive functioning of the individual must be evaluated within the context of the environment (Gordon, 1994). The complexity of the environment chosen by the individual results in different levels of functioning; the nurse's expectations should reflect this difference.

In addition to the environmental complexity level, the level of sensory input within the environment and the individual's capacity to perceive this input play key roles in determining problem areas. Basic orientation of the individual to the environment is instrumental in determining functional level. Similar to the person on vacation who often cannot remember the date or the day of the week, an individual who recently changed office locations and is now having difficulty concentrating is not unusual. The likelihood of this complaint is at least doubled when the lights flicker or the noise level is significantly different in the office.

The objective in assessing the individual's cognitive-perceptual pattern is to describe the adequacy of language, cognitive skills, and perception relative to desired or required activities (Gordon, 1994). The nurse collects and assesses clues that may indicate potential problems, especially sensory deficits, sensory deprivation or overload, and ineffective pain management. Cognitive dysfunction may cause impaired reasoning, knowledge deficits related to health practices, and memory deficits.

A number of assessment parameters are available. All individuals should be questioned regarding sensory-perceptual problems. Subjective reporting includes whether and when the individual has been routinely tested for hearing and vision. Any changes in the sensation or perception of the individual should be noted. In addition to decreased ability or acuity in hearing, vision, smell, and taste, the nurse evaluates other perceptual disturbances, such as vertigo; increased or decreased sensitivity to heat, cold, or light touch; and visual or auditory hallucinations or illusions. The use and perceived effectiveness of assistive devices, such as hearing aids, glasses, and contact lenses, are noted.

Any discomfort or pain is evaluated further. Useful tools have been designed to record and quantify changes in pain perception (Jones & Lepley, 1992; McCaffery, 1999). Specifically, the location, type, degree, and duration of pain provide indicators of possible causes or sources. Relief measures used to control pain (medication, heat, cold applications, and relaxation) and the effectiveness of each provide additional data and possible areas in which health education may be useful (Caudill, 1995). For all individuals, exploring tolerance to pain is appropriate. "Do you feel you are particularly sensitive to pain?" "What level of pain is associated with your (cut sprain, broken bone, or labor contractions)?"

Areas of cognitive patterning to be explored at this point include educational level, recent memory changes, ease or difficulty in learning, and preferred method of learning. Even when no problems are apparent or suspected, the nurse may assess these areas in more detail if health-teaching plans are to be made.

Objective data are accumulated throughout the entire interviewing or assessment process. This data collection begins with the nurse's perception of the individual's general appearance: hygiene and grooming, proper use of clothing, neatness and appropriateness of dress, and indication that these are appropriate to the individual's developmental stage. Language and vocabulary use, the ability to convey an idea with words or with actions when speech is impaired or not yet developed, and grammatical correctness provide clues to cognitive functioning. Amplitude and quality of speech, affect and mood, and attention and concentration are all indicative of the individual's mental status. For many individuals, this information is sufficient to relay a sense of the level of understanding, memory, and mentation. Problem-solving abilities can usually be determined when the individual is asked to relate any perceived problems, explanation of the problems, actions taken to solve the problems, and results of the actions taken. Because this is a basic assessment in each functional health pattern, the nurse already has an idea of whether thought processes are logical, coherent, and relevant for this individual. The fund of information is generally apparent, at least regarding health promotion, even as the nurse assesses the health perception–management pattern.

When the nurse perceives no apparent problems within the cognitive realm, the information is recorded as part of the objective data or findings of the physical examination. Data to be noted include language; vocabulary; attention span; grasp of ideas; level of consciousness; orientation to person, place, and time; language spoken (whether primary or secondary); and behavior during the interview and examination, including posture, facial expression, and general body movements.

However, when a problem is apparent or even suspected based on age, hereditary factors, or any inconsistencies in the assessment data, a focus assessment is essential. Coma scales or functional dementia scales may be used when appropriate. More commonly, a mental status examination is performed to assess orientation, registration, attention and calculation, language (ability to name objects, repeat abstract ideas, and follow commands), and recall (immediate-term, short-term, and long-term memory). Abilities to read, write, and copy designs can also be assessed.

The examination of a sensory-perceptual pattern evaluates hearing, vision, and areas of pain at a screening level; comprehensive examinations are available and may be indicated. A full neurological assessment is warranted when specific sensory deficits are reported after the examination.

Although these assessment areas may seem overwhelming, the time required is generally less than in most other pattern areas, perhaps because more information relevant to the cognitive-perceptual patterns is available as each pattern is assessed. Transition into the cognitive-perceptual pattern from any other pattern might be facilitated by referring to a problem already described, with the nurse asking, for example, "Do you generally find it easy to solve problems effectively?" The self-perception pattern follows the cognitive pattern particularly well because any measure of mental status includes feelings and perceptions of the individual regarding self. Mood, affect, and responses to the interviewer, such as eye contact, are further indications of the individual's level of esteem. The relationship between cognitive and perceptual ability and the ability to function (self-care) or manipulate within the environment (activity and exercise) is overwhelming.

The placement of each of the patterns in a sequence suitable to each nurse, individual, or situation has been discussed. However, when there is reason to suspect that the individual's cognitive-perceptual pattern may be dysfunctional and that the individual is an unreliable historian, incorporating this pattern into the assessment immediately after the health perception–health management pattern or as soon as reasonable doubt exists as to the individual's ability to describe a pattern would be wise. This course would save valuable time and permit the nurse to identify a more reliable pattern.

The nurse realizes that every person has experienced temporary memory lapses at one time or another. These events alone should not be sufficient to make a judgment. Sequence of behaviors and clustering of appropriate signals (defining characteristics) are necessary to any **nursing diagnosis.** Equally important is the need to assess all pattern areas before data analysis and problem identification.

Cognitive data and sensory abilities guide the nurse in planning care, which is especially apparent in health teaching. The formulation of the health teaching plan should reflect the individual's preferred method of learning, taking into account information storage and retrieval abilities, compensatory mechanisms for sensory deficits, neuromuscular and sensory levels necessary for skills development, and demonstrated developmental level. Goals and short-term objectives are developed in an individually tailored plan. Although self-care might be an outcome for a person newly diagnosed with diabetes mellitus, the plan will reflect different behaviors for the adult than for the child.

Self-Perception–Self-Concept Pattern

This pattern includes the individual's sense of personal identity, goals, emotional patterns, and feelings about the self. Self-image and sense of worth stem from the individual's perception of personal appearance, competencies, and limitations, including the individual's self-perception and others' perceptions. The nurse assesses both verbal and nonverbal cues (Gordon, 1994).

The significance of the sense of self to the whole person is best exemplified by personal experiences. When individuals feels good about themselves, it shows in the way they look and act. Conversely, when individuals feel unable to accomplish anything worthwhile, changes in eating, sleeping, and activity patterns usually follow.

The individual's developmental level affects and is affected by this pattern. Erikson (1986) identifies eight stages of human development, proposing that, with each stage, a central task or crisis must be resolved before healthy growth can continue. According to Erikson, early childhood is the time to develop a sense of autonomy versus shame and doubt. When this development is appropriately achieved or resolved, the child can then develop initiative during the next stage. One of the tasks Havighurst (1973) identifies during this later phase is building wholesome attitudes toward oneself (self-esteem), whereas, Bruhn and colleagues (1977) refer specifically to developing self-concept. Delays in developing or failing to develop a self-concept will affect future development and the ability to accomplish subsequent tasks (see Table 6-3).

Usually, the family climate and relationship pattern influences the environmental effects on the self-concept pattern. Combining the developmental tasks of Erikson and the appropriate stages of the family life cycle (see Chapter 7) clearly demonstrates the family's role in the individual's development (Duvall & Miller, 1985; Newman, 1995).

In addition to the family, all people who are closely associated with the individual affect that person's concept of self-esteem. Most people care what others think of them and the support of significant others affects the self-perception–self-concept pattern (Muhlenkamp & Sayles, 1986).

Achieving a sense of "I" versus "we" is vital for the individual. A sense of "I" as a person, apart from the roles that the person may assume, is important ("me" rather than roles such as mother, father, daughter, son, student, or nurse).

The assessment objective in this pattern area is to describe the individual's patterns and beliefs about general self-worth and feeling states (Gordon, 1994). The nurse looks for clues that indicate identity confusion, altered body image, disturbances in self-esteem, and feelings of powerlessness. Anxiety, fear, and depression are states that can be identified and are responsive to nursing interventions (Calarco & Drone, 1991; Dalton & Busch, 1995).

Erikson's framework is helpful in describing a sequential and healthy developmental pattern as related by the individual. The accomplishment of the wellness tasks may be apparent in other functional health patterns, providing additional indications of developmental level (see Unit 4) (Bruhn, Cordova, Williams, & Fuentes, 1977).

In addition to assessing the individual's developmental level and pattern, feelings about the self are elicited. The nurse must determine what knowledge the person has of individual strengths and limitations along with attitudes toward these strengths and limitations. Questions regarding personal appearance and capabilities in the cognitive, affective, and psychomotor domains are asked. This portrayal provides evidence of a sense of identity and worth, self-image, and body image.

A description of emotional patterns or a general feeling state concludes the history when no problems are indicated. A focused assessment may use specific tools, when necessary, to measure body image (McCloskey, 1976), anxiety (AHCPR, 1993), or depression (Beck, 1972; Zung, 1971, 1973).

The nurse should note general appearance and affect, which may have been assessed as part of a formal mental status examination. A lowered self-esteem may be indicated by head and shoulder flexion, lack of eye contact, and mumbled or slurred speech. Anxiety or nervousness might be revealed through extraneous body movements such as foot shuffling or tapping, facial tension or grimace, rapid speech, voice quivering, twitches or tremors, and general restlessness or shifts in body position. Any of these indicators demand further exploration to determine underlying problems.

Self-concept or lack of it alters the nurse-individual interaction. Assessment within this pattern is particularly difficult because it is of a personal nature. After an individual shares this sort of information with the nurse, which can be facilitated when the nurse possesses strong communication skills and a caring attitude, the individual will be more involved in goal planning and more open to nursing interventions.

Roles-Relationships Pattern

This pattern describes the roles assumed and the relationships engaged in by the individual. As part of the assessment, the individual's perception is the major component and should include the level of satisfaction with roles and relationships.

The need for relationships with other people is universal. Dunn (1972) has identified basic needs for communication, fellowship, and love in high-level wellness. Similarly, Maslow's hierarchy of needs (1983, 1987) includes a sense of love and belonging.

The ability to communicate with other people in a meaningful way greatly affects the whole person. The balance necessary for health between the individual and the environment (anything external to or separate from the individual) is indicative of the major role that relationships with others plays in health status (Bulechek & McCloskey, 1996; Girdano & Eberly, 1986; Newman, 1987, 1994, 1995).

innovative practice

The Humor Potential, Inc.

The Humor Potential, Inc. is a company that provides resources, products, and seminars for stress management with the use of humor. Company president Loretta LaRoche is an internationally recognized expert on stress management, emphasizing the importance of balancing daily living experiences with humor. The Humor Potential, Inc. offers seminars and lectures to health care professionals, schools, corporations, other organizations, and the general public. The corporation also produces television programs that have been shown on PBS, NBC, CNN, and HBO. The first PBS show, "The Joy of Stress," was nominated for a regional Emmy Award.

Ms. LaRoche was chosen by Microsoft as one of America's Most Interesting Women. She is the author of the book *Relax, You May Only Have a Few Minutes Left.* She has contributed to *The Wellness Book,* (Benson & Stuart, 1992) and has published articles in many magazines and newspapers, including *USA Today, The Boston Globe,* and *Atlantic Monthly.* Her company also publishes the *TaDah Gazette,* which includes summaries of research studies on the relationships between stress and health. Loretta also gives her humorous advice at iVillage.com in Channel Highlights.

Recently, the company opened the "Tickle Your Soul Giftshop: A Store for the Mind, Body, and Spirit," located in Plymouth, Massachusetts, which sells books, prints, audiotapes and videotapes, and other products dealing with humor. The Corporation Collection consists of audiotapes and videotapes that have been developed for corporate meetings and training. Examples of these are *Stressbusters!* An audiotape and videotape and action guide that increases productivity by reducing stress. Two other tapes, *Oh No! Not another Meeting,* and *Whoopee! Another Meeting* are meeting openers for staff development programs given to employees to improve communication, productivity, and outcomes within an organization. A catalog is also available for e-mail, fax, phone, and mail orders.

Contact Information:
The Humor Potential, Inc.
URL http://www.lorettalaroche.com
Email: inquires@lorettalaroche.com
Phone: 1-800-99-TADAH (1-800-998-2324)

Courtesy Carol Lynn Mandle.

The role of development is apparent in Erikson's stages of ego development (1986). This series of hypotheses about readiness proposes that attainment of each stage is regarded as necessary for progression toward a later stage. For example, a person can become immersed in a relationship of genuine intimacy only after self-identity has been stabilized.

Certain tasks for family development have been similarly identified by Duvall and Miller (1985) (see Chapter 7). The emphasis here is on the role of the

CASE STUDY

Cindy

Cindy is a single 28-year-old woman. Cindy studies nursing and shares an apartment with two friends. She was having increasing difficulties with her course work and was placed on academic probation. Cindy became concerned about the effect of her stress on her ability to finish her studies and on her future career. She grew increasingly nervous and began to ask, "Will I ever be okay?" and "Will I ever be able to finish school and function as a nurse?" Cindy expressed her fear of weakness and feelings of isolation, loneliness, helplessness, and loss of control. These feelings began to find expression in anger related to this major life disruption. She verbalized her anger at God for allowing this to happen to her. Her incapacity deprived her of her normal outlets for expressing and finding support for such concerns. Cindy was unable to participate in the practices of her faith, where she usually had found strength in facing life's challenges. Her inability to concentrate and her growing feeling of lethargy added to her frustration. Expressing these fears and concerns was difficult for Cindy. The nurse, however, developed a trusting relationship with Cindy, permitting Cindy to express her fears, anxieties, and concerns. Based on the nurse's assessment of Cindy, the nursing diagnosis of "spiritual distress" was formulated and the following plan of care was proposed:

1. What are other differential diagnoses the nurse considers?
2. Describe other individuals you know who have experienced "spiritual distress."

Adapted from McFarland, G. K., & McFarlane, E. A. (1993). *Nursing diagnosis and intervention: Planning for patient care*. St. Louis: Mosby.

individual within the family and within the larger context of society.

The objective of the roles-relationships pattern assessment is to describe an individual's pattern of family and social roles with the associated responsibilities. The individual's perception of satisfaction or dissatisfaction with the established relationship is a component of this area. Loss, change, and threat produce the major problems within this pattern. Clues indicative of impaired verbal communication, social isolation, alterations in parenting, independence-dependence conflicts, dysfunctional grieving, and potential for violence are important.

The assessment focuses on the role and relationships of the individual regarding family, work, and community. Within the family, assessment parameters include the structure, roles, dynamics (decision making, power and authority, division of labor, and communication patterns), and social support systems.

Student and employee roles and relationships assess the specific occupation or position along with work responsibilities and work environment (stress, safety, and health factors) (see the Case Study and Care Plan). Financial concerns, job security, and retirement plans are elicited.

CARE PLAN

Nursing Diagnosis: Spiritual Distress Related to a Threat to Well Being, Loss of Meaningful Role, and Separation from Religious and Family Ties

EXPECTED OUTCOMES

Cindy will have a greater sense of purpose, meaning, and hope in her life and her illness, as evidenced by expressing acceptance of the limitations life has presented to her and by verbalizing that illness is not a punishment.

NURSING INTERVENTIONS

- Take time to be present and available to listen to Cindy's expressions and feelings
- Encourage Cindy to verbalize feelings
- Engage Cindy in value clarification

EXPECTED OUTCOMES

Cindy will express feelings of anger verbally and will discuss anger with another person.

NURSING INTERVENTIONS

- Encourage Cindy to acknowledge feelings of anger and to acknowledge and name any feelings she experiences
- Reassure Cindy that it is okay to feel angry toward God and encourage her to express her feelings directly to God
- Encourage honest dialogue with a peer whom Cindy trusts
- Reinforce that God loves and accepts people as they are

EXPECTED OUTCOMES

Cindy will develop a sense of control despite separation from religious practices as evidenced by her expressing knowledge of available religious resources.

NURSING INTERVENTIONS

- Offer consultation with appropriate spiritual advisor
- Inform Cindy of available religious resources
- Pray with Cindy as indicated

Adapted from McFarland, G. K., & McFarlane, E. A. (1993). *Nursing diagnosis and intervention: Planning for patient care*. St. Louis: Mosby.

Time commitments allowing for leisure and level of physical exercise regarding work were assessed with activity patterns.

Community roles and relationships indicate the individual's involvement within the neighborhood and other social groups. Specifically, the nurse elicits the level of socialization and amount of social support available.

Within all three components (family, work or school, and community) the individual is asked to describe the level of satisfaction with the present roles and relationships. The nurse should explore parenting or marital difficulties and any abuse.

Specific attention is paid to any threat of change, actual change, or loss. Grieving is evaluated as to its appropriateness to health promotion. The nurse also evaluates the relationship among role components. Family or work roles alone may not cause stress, but combining them may cause difficulties, as with the working mother or traveling husband and father.

Unless the nurse sees the individual in the company of significant others, as with a home visit, objective data are not available. When possible, family interaction and communication patterns are noted. Cognizant of the importance of family and meaningful relationships, the nurse will be especially alert to potential problems with the college student away from home, the individual who travels or moves frequently, and sole family survivors (older adults often outlive many of their family members and friends) (Calarco & Drone, 1991; Dalton & Busch, 1995).

The relationship among the different functional health patterns is clearly apparent in the light of developmental stages. When a person has difficulties within the self-concept pattern, difficulties with relationships are a near certainty (Erikson, 1986; Muhlenkamp & Sayles, 1986). Relationships affect the whole person; therefore problems in the roles-relationships pattern may be exhibited in other areas, such as sleep, appetite, and sexuality.

Sexuality-Reproductive Pattern

This pattern describes the individual's sexual self-concept, sexual functioning, methods of intimacy, and reproductive areas. Data collection combines subjective information, nursing observations, and physical examination. Normal development and perceived satisfaction are crucial elements (Gordon, 1994).

Sexuality is the behavioral expression of sexual identity. The importance of this pattern area to the individual's life and health are closely related to the self-perception and the relationship patterns. Body image, self-concept, and role and gender identity are linked to sexual identity. This concept of sexual self and the individual's relationship pattern indicate the level and the perceived satisfaction of sexual functioning achieved. Sexual functioning involves, but is not limited to, sexual relations with a partner. Reproductive patterns are equally significant to this pattern assessment, the whole individual, and the family and community (see Chapters 7 and 8).

As discussed, developmental influence includes the individual's development of reproductive capacities (secondary sex characteristics and genital development), ego integrity (Erikson, 1986), and the family life-cycle stage (Duvall & Miller, 1985).

The role of the environment is instrumental in the expression of a person's sexuality-reproductive pattern. Cultural and family norms may contribute to the expression of sexuality and combine with other factors, such as the family's financial stability, to influence reproductive patterns. The various norms within society may create problems in gender and in expressions of sexuality.

One objective of assessment in this pattern is to describe behavioral problems or difficulties (Gordon, 1994). Equally important is assessing the individual's knowledge of sexual functioning, preventive health practices (breast and testicular self-examinations, Papanicolaou (Pap) smears, and effective contraceptive use), and prevention of infection. Clues are evaluated for any potential or actual sexual dysfunction.

The parameters assessed include: (1) sexual self-concept, which may be derived from information collected in the self-perception–self-concept and the roles-relationships patterns; (2) sexual functioning, with the nurse noting evidence of some form of intimacy, the level of sexual activity or libido, and the effect of health or illness on sexual expression; and (3) reproductive patterns in which the nurse collects data pertinent to menstruation (onset, duration, frequency, last menstrual period, discomfort, and feelings related to aging and menopause), reproductive stage (gravida, para, and use of birth control methods), and health-promotion factors (preventive practices and knowledge of sexual functioning).

The nurse assesses the individual's level of satisfaction with sexual self-concept, sexual functioning, and reproduction. Problems or difficulties (ineffective or inappropriate sexual performance, discharges, infections, venereal disease, discomfort, and history of abuse) are further evaluated. Additional information is collected with sexual dysfunction or trauma.

The physical examination evaluates the development of the genital organs and secondary sex characteristics. The nurse may observe forms of intimacy, such as holding hands and hugging, between partners.

Nursing implications are present for both approach and health teaching as the sexuality-reproductive pattern is assessed. Discussions relating to this pattern area may be threatening; depth of exploration should be governed in part by the individual's wishes, but the nurse encourages discussion, perhaps at a later time, after a firmer and more trusting relationship is established.

A clear picture of the individual's knowledge and practice of preventive practices facilitates health promotion. Although sex education is associated most often with school programs, education on sexual functioning is provided for adults. Sex education is a key element in preparation for parenthood classes. Improved understanding of sexual functioning can only lead to discovering improved methods of sexual performance and a greater satisfaction level (see Health Teaching box).

Coping–Stress-Tolerance Pattern

Gordon (1994) describes this pattern as a description of the individual's general coping pattern and the effectiveness of the pattern in terms of stress management. The pattern

HEALTH TEACHING Sexuality and Aging Women: Common Myths

- Masturbation is an immature activity of youngsters and adolescents, not of older women
- Sexual desire and prowess wane during the climacteric; therefore menopause is the death of a woman's sexuality
- Hysterectomy creates a physical disability that causes the inability to function sexually
- Sex has no role in the lives of older adults except as perversion or remembrance of times past
- Sexual expression in old age is taboo
- Older adults are too old and frail to engage in sex
- The young are considered lusty or virile; elderly adults are considered lecherous
- Sex is unimportant or over
- Older women do not wish to discuss their sexuality with professionals

Modified from Morrison-Beedy, D., & Robbin, L. (1989). Sexual assessment and the aging female. *Nursing Practice, 14,* 35; Ebersole, P., & Hess, P. (1994). *Toward healthy aging: Human needs and nursing response* (4th ed.). St. Louis: Mosby.

includes the individual's ability to handle life crises and to resist factors that disrupt the self-integrity of the ego, mode of conflict resolution and stress management, and accessibility to necessary resources.

The ability to manage stress effectively in life is a learned behavior. Some stress is a necessary part of life; without it, there is no motivation to grow. Stress is a problem only when the ability to tolerate it is too weak, leading to interference with daily activities (Benson & Stuart, 1992; Dixon, Dixon, & Spinner, 1989; Pollock, 1984).

Most stress comes not from great tragedies, but from an accumulation of minor irritations. Stress is not inherent in an event, but in the individual perception of the event. Whereas one individual is "stressed" from missing the bus and can think only of being 10 minutes late, another will consider it an opportunity to spend 10 minutes reading the newspaper. This difference in perception may represent a different set of values used in identifying sources of stress or an effective strategy for dealing with the stress.

For purposes of assessing this pattern, coping (or the individual behavioral response to stress) includes both problem-solving ability and use of defense mechanisms. Coping is viewed not as a single act but as a process incorporating many behaviors. The function of coping is to deal with the threat or emotional distress of an event. The effectiveness of coping is assessed from the individual's perspective and from the nurse's observation of the individual's ability to function in the presence of actual or potential stressors in the environment.

The perception of stress and the ability to manage stress depends on personal development, amount of stress previously experienced, current level of stress within the environment, and available sources of social support. Although an elderly individual may have experienced many stresses during life and managed them effectively, coping may no longer be possible because too many stressors (physical incapacitation, fixed income, fear of illness or injury, and lack of transportation) exist or because a social support system is no longer available (Norbeck, Lindsey, & Carrieri, 1983).

The objective in assessment is to determine the individual's stress tolerance and past coping patterns. The nurse evaluates clues to difficulties in handling past and current stressors and changes in the effectiveness of a coping pattern to determine personal coping capacity.

The assessment parameters include: (1) the coping task, including the physical, psychological, and socioeconomic stimuli with which the individual must cope; (2) coping style, or the tendency to use a specific style, such as approach oriented, avoidance oriented, or nonspecific; (3) coping strategies, including specifics; and (4) coping effectiveness.

Coping strategy or mode of coping may be divided into information seeking, direct action (fight or flight), inhibition of action, or use of social support. Coping effectiveness is best assessed by eliciting the individual resources (variety of coping mechanisms used by the individual, flexibility of these mechanisms, and health promotion value associated with each mechanism) and the individual's functional level (Benson & Stuart, 1992).

Stress tolerance patterns elicit the amount of stress effectively handled in the past. The use of anticipatory coping is assessed along with whether the individual knows how to cope, but does not (production deficit), or simply does not know how to cope (skill deficit).

Other indicators of value within this pattern are discussed under the self-perception–self-concept pattern. The objective data include physical signs of restlessness, irritability, and nervousness (increased heart rate and blood pressure and perspiration).

The nurse is aware that evidence of coping ability and tolerance to stress is found in every other functional health pattern. Evidence of stress also affects the other patterns, thereby resulting in health problems such as insomnia, weight loss, and decreased concentration (Benson & Stuart, 1992; Gordon, 1994).

Health promotion can be greatly assisted through early intervention. Holmes and Rahe (1967) have found a significant relationship between perceived stressful life events and subsequent illness (Holmes & David, 1984, 1989). Coping patterns and stress tolerance in the past may uncover unhealthy behavior, such as smoking and drinking, that needs to be replaced by alternative coping strategies.

Stress-reduction workshops would be helpful for most of the population since it can be predicted with certainty that the future will include stress, some of which may be overwhelming without coping strategies.

Girdano and Eberly (1986) offer specific categories of stress-management strategies: (1) social engineering strategies, such as time management or planned change; (2) personality engineering strategies, such as assertiveness training or cognitive rehearsal; and (3) altered states of consciousness, such as meditation or relaxation. The nurse is alert to the use of any of these strategies while assessing all functional health patterns to help determine a coping pattern. Benson and Stuart (1992) offer specific ways that individuals can develop more effective problem solving and coping strategies when managing stress.

Values-Beliefs Pattern

This pattern describes values (including spiritual values), beliefs, and goals of the individual and includes perceptions of what is right and what is good and any conflicts that beliefs and values may present.

Each pattern has addressed the value system of the individual and society. Life is governed by what the individual believes or values and these values and beliefs are developed over time, reflecting personal experiences and family and societal influences (Brink, 1984; Downing & Kuckelman-Cobb, 1990; Harvey, 1992).

The objective in assessing this pattern is to understand the value and belief basis for the individual's health-related decisions and actions (Gordon, 1994). The individual's health beliefs influence behavior in seeking health care, practicing preventive measures, planning health goals, and undertaking self-care (Harvey, 1992). Rosenstock (1974) suggests that an individual will engage in preventive health behavior according to whether a threat to wellness or health status exists. Several other health belief models expand on this concept by including other motivations, such as personal values and environmental influences. The nurse assesses clues to conflicts within the individual's value system or between the person's value system and that of the family or society.

Dimensions of assessment include the individual's values, beliefs, or goals that guide choice or decisions that are related to health. The nurse collects this information while exploring each pattern and includes it in this pattern to summarize, clarify, or secure any additional information. Specifically, the values and beliefs about self, relationships, and society are assessed. The nurse discusses the individual's beliefs, goals, and purposes of life along with any conflicts the individual perceives as existing between the person's philosophies and those of the family, culture, and society. The individual's source of strength, such as God or significant individual practices, is elicited; religious beliefs and preference are included.

Past goals and expectations are assessed through the individual's satisfaction. The nurse must identify the individual's goals and expectations concerning health; these must be clear to help the individual achieve them. As discussed, health-promotion interventions are based on the individual's value system and health beliefs (Harvey, 1992; Kleinman, 1988; Lau, Hartmen, & Ware, 1986; Pender, 1996; Tompkins, 1992).

The brevity of this discussion is no indication of the importance that the value and belief pattern plays in the assessment of the individual. The development of each pattern indicates the role of individual values.

ASSESSMENT PROCESS

The purpose of this section is to present information about skills needed, types of data collected, and format used as it specifically relates to functional health-pattern assessment of the individual. Additionally, guidelines reviewing crucial issues are presented along with examples of methods available for the assessment of individual's functional health patterns.

Skills

The communication skills outlined in Chapter 4 are all necessary for obtaining a thorough and accurate health assessment. Listening cannot be overemphasized; it is particularly important to avoid missing cues that may indicate a dysfunctional or potentially dysfunctional pattern. Box 6-1 provides an example of basic data to be collected within the functional health patterns.

The use of open-ended questions allows for pattern construction. A nonjudgmental attitude is vital in establishing rapport with the individual and it may directly affect the subsequent amount and type of information the individual is willing to share and data reliability. Many individuals know the "right" answers (types of food to be eaten or recommended amount and frequency of exercise), but knowing does not necessarily imply practicing. A nonjudgmental attitude will allow any answer to be the "right" answer.

Observation and evaluation skills are also essential. The depth of exploration is determined by the situational context and the presence or absence of significant cues. Situational context includes the setting (private office or curtained cubicle), the physiological and psychological comfort of the individual (individual in pain or one concerned that the results of the health assessment may result in loss of job), and the purpose of the assessment (database assessment; problem-focused assessment; emergency assessment; or follow-up, time-lapsed reassessment) (Gordon, 1994).

The clinical expertise of the nurse directs the assessment of each pattern as cues are probed further (branching) and the range of possibilities is narrowed (focus assessment) (Gordon, 1990, 1994; Monninger, Padgett, & Fleeger, 1994; McFadden & Gunnett, 1992). Clinical expertise is

Box 6-1 Functional Health Patterns Assessment (Adult)

HEALTH PERCEPTION-HEALTH MANAGEMENT PATTERN

1. History
   a. How has general health been?
   b. Any colds in past year? When appropriate: absences from work?
   c. Most important things you do to keep healthy? Think these things make a difference to health? (Include family folk remedies when appropriate.) Use of cigarettes, alcohol, drugs? Breast self-examination?
   d. Accidents (home, work, driving)?
   e. In past, been easy to find ways to follow suggestions from physicians or nurses?
   f. When appropriate: what do you think caused this illness? Actions taken when symptoms perceived? Results of action?
   g. When appropriate: things important to you in your health care? How can we be most helpful?
2. Examination—general health appearance

NUTRITIONAL-METABOLIC PATTERN

1. History
   a. Typical daily food intake? (Describe.) Supplements (vitamins, type of snacks)?
   b. Typical daily fluid intake? (Describe.)
   c. Weight loss or gain? (Amount.) Height loss or gain? (Amount.)
   d. Appetite?
   e. Food or eating: Discomfort? Swallowing? Diet restrictions?
   f. Heal well or poorly?
   g. Skin problems: Lesions? Dryness?
   h. Dental problems?
2. Examination
   a. Skin: Bony prominences? Lesions? Color changes? Moistness?
   b. Oral mucous membranes: Color? Moistness? Lesions?
   c. Teeth: General appearance and alignment? Dentures? Cavities? Missing teeth?
   d. Actual weight, height.
   e. Temperature.
   f. Intravenous feeding–parenteral feeding (specify)?

ELIMINATION PATTERN

1. History
   a. Bowel elimination pattern? (Describe.) Frequency? Character? Discomfort? Problem in control? Laxatives?
   b. Urinary elimination pattern? (Describe.) Frequency? Problem in control?
   c. Excessive perspiration? Odor problems?
   d. Body cavity drainage, suction, and so on? (Specify.)
2. Examination—when indicated: examine excreta or drainage color and consistency.

ACTIVITY-EXERCISE PATTERN

1. History
   a. Sufficient energy for desired or required activities?
   b. Exercise pattern? Type? Regularity?
   c. Spare-time (leisure) activities? Child: play activities?
   d. Perceived ability (code for level) for:
      Feeding ______ Dressing ______ Cooking ______
      Bathing ______ Grooming ______ Shopping ______
      Toileting ______ General mobility ______
      Bed mobility ______ Home maintenance ______
      Functional Level Codes:
      Level 0: full self-care
      Level I: requires use of equipment or device
      Level II: requires assistance or supervision from another person
      Level III: requires assistance or supervision from another person and equipment or device
      Level IV: is dependent and does not participate
2. Examination
   a. Demonstrated ability (code listed above) for:
      Feeding ______ Dressing ______ Cooking ______
      Bathing ______ Grooming ______ Shopping ______
      Toileting ______ General mobility ______
   b. Gait ______ Posture ______ Absent body part? (Specify.) ______
   c. Range of motion (joints) ______ Muscle firmness ______
   d. Hand grip ______ Can pick up a pencil? ______
   e. Pulse (rate) ______ (rhythm) ______ Breath sounds ______
   f. Respirations (rate) ______ (rhythm) ______ Breath sounds ______
   g. Blood pressure ______
   h. General appearance (grooming, hygiene, and energy level)

From Gordon, M. (1994). *Nursing diagnosis: Process and application* (3rd ed.). St. Louis: Mosby; Gordon, M. (2000). *Manual of nursing diagnosis: 1995-1996*. St. Louis: Mosby.

discussed later because this sort of diagnostic skill is a major variable in the diagnostic process.

Data Collection

Essential elements of data collection include the method of collection, the nature of the data, and the depth of exploration. Data are collected through subjective reports and objective nursing observations. The subjective data are obtained through reports from the individual (primary source) whenever possible. In assessing the individual, secondary sources (parents or relatives) are used only when necessary, as deemed by age or cognitive functioning ability of the individual, such as a child or a confused individual. This aspect is further discussed as it relates to the type of data being collected (see the section on the cognitive-perceptual pattern earlier in this chapter).

The nature of the data collected may be uncertain in many of the human sciences. The assumption is that the data are reliable, except as previously noted or when the nurse has reason to believe otherwise. Corroborating the subjective reports with objective measures is possible in some instances. For example, when the individual reports a nutritional intake appropriate to metabolic demand and still gains considerable weight in the absence of any medical condition, the nurse is alerted to the possibility of unreliable data.

Using nutritional intake as an example again demonstrates the type of data available. Listing foods prepared for each meal or packed for lunch is not a valid indicator of foods consumed; the school-age child's report of eating all the foods packed may not always be reliable and may require verification by a teacher or classmate. Past and current data are necessary for pattern construction. Foods eaten in the past compared with foods eaten at present provide a more accurate picture of current health status.

Obviously, some patterns are easier to evaluate compared with other patterns. Corroboration of subjective reports in an area such as self-perception is more difficult. Nursing observations should include verbal and nonverbal cues; body language (posture and gestures), eye contact, and displays of emotion (crying or fist slamming) should be noted.

Cues that may indicate the possible presence of problems are significant when they (1) represent an unexpected change in the individual's usual patterns, not a result of developmental norms or previously instituted therapies; (2) deviate from appropriate population norms; or (3) represent a behavior that results in nonproductivity for the individual (Gordon, 1994). Other cues govern the depth of the assessment and represent the characteristics of functional health patterns. Pattern areas are explored at least until a pattern emerges, environmental and developmental influences are apparent, and functional ability is demonstrated. The presence of defining characteristics for a specific diagnosis indicates a need for further assessment. Pattern construction continues until sufficient evidence (cluster of cues) exists to identify a problem (nursing diagnosis) and propose interventions based on contributing etiological factors.

Format

The specific sequencing of patterns in collecting and recording information gathered during a functional health-pattern assessment is flexible. However, the method of recording data should be systematic and consistent. Interviewing the individual first and then performing the physical examination is usually advantageous. That subjective and objective data are separately recorded is vital for clarity. The subjective data are recorded in phrases and each pattern is separately labeled. Information is recorded in concise language and should include at least some direct quotes from the individual. The objective data may follow functional health patterns or a systems ("head-to-toe") approach.

A distinct advantage in the format is the openness of each pattern. In-depth exploration in some areas may be included, whereas screening information may be appropriate in other patterns. The important point is not to collect irrelevant data. The same information is not necessary for all individuals and forms to be filled in for initial databases generally do not include this option. Similarly, checklists and predesigned formats with questions do not provide space for all pertinent data. The functional health-pattern format records all information pertinent to a particular pattern, even when collected after the initial visit. This method prevents important assessment data from being lost among the progress notes.

Guidelines

The development of each pattern in the following section provides dimensions and parameters for assessment. These dimensions and parameters are not inclusive, but provide a base for initial assessment in the absence of problems. Using knowledge of the situation and perception of whether problems exist, the nurse directs the line of questioning to an appropriate depth. Either the physician or the nurse should perform a complete physical examination in the usual manner, as governed by the situation or institutional guidelines.

One method of data collection, the 24-hour recall, is mentioned in several patterns as a way of describing the individual's normal pattern. Obviously, this method is of value regarding aspects such as nutritional intake or daily activities. The nurse may use another version, the weekly log, when problems are apparent or when further description is necessary. A weekly log helps determine patterns such as nutrition, elimination, sleep, and activity and may also be used to discuss self-perception, roles and relationships, and coping with stress. For example, the individual may be asked to record every stressful situation the person encounters. The individual is asked to list thoughts, feelings, and factors preceding and following the stressful event, explain why the event is stressful, list what was done about it, and describe the effects of this action. This type of process helps assess coping-stress tolerance patterns and promotes improved understanding by the individual and the nurse. This understanding is helpful in mutually setting goals and planning appropriate interventions.

Two concepts are crucial elements in discussing the process of assessment. The first concept is that all patterns need to be assessed before forming any diagnosis. Although a tentative diagnosis may occur during the collection of data regarding nutrition, the diagnosis is not definitive until the nurse assesses the other 10 areas. The problem of nutrition alteration, more than body requirements (exogenous obesity), may be related to overindulgence, knowledge deficit regarding proper nutrition in relation to health promotion, inadequate exercising, depression, self-image, family eating habits, or the value placed on eating by the individual or the individual's family, culture, and community. Unless the reason or probable cause is discovered, nursing interventions cannot be focused and evaluation of nursing interventions may demonstrate that none of the outcomes has been achieved.

When potential problems are suspected within any pattern, the nurse may use this suspicion as a guide to direct and complete the assessment. The pattern is then determined to be (1) functional, indicating the individual's strengths and high-level wellness; (2) dysfunctional, indicating the individual's limitations and actual health problems; or (3) potentially dysfunctional, indicating presence of risk factors and potentially problematic areas (Gordon, 1994).

The second concept crucial to assessment is that it be a continual process. Data collection continues during all nurse-individual interactions. The same is true of the overall diagnostic process. The collection of data is only the first step in the process of collecting, interpreting, and clustering information and then naming the cluster through the nursing diagnosis.

INDIVIDUAL HEALTH PROMOTION THROUGH THE NURSING PROCESS

The nursing process—the systematic approach to reduce or eliminate the individual's health problem—is accomplished by first collecting the necessary data. With the individual, the nurse analyzes the data, identifies a nursing diagnosis, projects outcomes, prescribes interventions, and evaluates effectiveness. Reassessment, reordering of priorities, new goal setting, and revising the plan continues as part of the process toward outcome attainment (ANA, 1991; Moritz, 1995).

Collection and Analysis of Data

The assessment is a systematic technique for learning as much as possible about the individual. The main purpose in collecting data from a new individual is to see whether health problems exist and to identify the individual's health goals.

The data collection includes necessary biographical data, such as age, sex, and the purpose of the visit. This process is followed by the assessment of the previously outlined 11 functional health patterns. Subjective reporting, nursing observations and perceptions, and the physical examination are assessed and recorded. The remaining discussion focuses on nursing diagnosis.

Problem Identification

Although the concept of problem identification has been debated in the past, most nurses now have distinguished nursing diagnosis as the problem label. Diagnosis is a careful examination and analysis of the facts in an attempt to explain something. Nursing diagnosis is the naming of an individual's response to actual or potential health problems or life processes (Carpenito, 1999; Gordon, 1994; NANDA, 2000).

Nursing diagnoses provide the basis for selection of nursing interventions to achieve outcomes for which the nurse is accountable (Gordon, 1994, 2000). The North American Nursing Diagnoses Association (NANDA) has provided leadership in developing standardization of the descriptions of human responses that nurses treat. The most recent revision of this taxonomy has been approved for clinical testing and has been endorsed by the ANA (NANDA, 2000).

Gordon (1994) proposed the accepted format of nursing diagnosis, PES, that lists the Problem, Etiology, and Signs and symptoms, or defining characteristics, for each diagnosis accepted for clinical testing.

At the 1998 NANDA conference, a multiaxial framework for nursing diagnoses was proposed, but has yet to be completed and approved by the NANDA Board. This proposed formation for nursing diagnoses is a more detailed clinical language and an improved structure for nursing diagnoses to be included in computerized databases. If approved in the future, then nursing diagnoses will be expressed by six axes: (1) diagnostic concept (parenting); (2) acuity (altered); (3) unit of care (individual); (4) developmental stage (adolescent); (5) potentiality (at risk for); and (6) descriptor, creating the diagnostic statement of risk for altered parenting by an adolescent (NANDA, 2000, pp. 158-159).

In discussions of problems, the meaning of "problem" must be clearly defined and identified. The concept as used in this text refers to Gordon's proposition that a health problem is defined as a dysfunctional pattern and that nursing's major contribution to health care is in preventing and treating these patterns (Gordon, 1994). A pattern is dysfunctional when it represents a deviation from established norms or from the individual's previous condition or goals. (Normative behavior is further discussed in Unit 4.) A dysfunctional pattern is a problem when it generates therapeutic concern on the part of the individual, others, or the nurse and when it is amenable to nursing therapies.

As patterns are assessed, the nurse proposes several hypotheses regarding functional or dysfunctional labeling. At the completion of the assessment, conclusions must be drawn. The possibility exists that all patterns are functional, that some are functional, and that others are dysfunctional or potentially dysfunctional.

Functional refers to wellness and optimal health. Dysfunctional patterns, indicating some health problem, may be present in the absence of disease; that is, nursing care may be needed for health promotion and health maintenance, not health restoration. The case history of Frank Thompson in Chapter 1 effectively illustrates the multiple nursing care needs of an individual who is not ill.

HOT topics

HEART DISEASE IN WOMEN

Contrary to what many people think, heart disease is the leading cause of death in women. Approximately 370,000 American women of all races and ethnic groups die from heart disease each year. Black women have the highest death rate from heart disease (535 deaths per 100,000 population), followed by White women (388 deaths per 100,000 population), Hispanic women (265 deaths per 100,000 population), Native-American women (259 deaths per 100,000 population), and Asian-American and Pacific-Islander women (221 deaths per 100,000 population). Nurses need to assess women for risk factors and symptoms of heart disease.

From U.S. Department of Health and Human Services. (2000). *Women and heart disease: An atlas of racial and ethnic disparities in mortality.* Washington, DC: U.S. Government Printing Office.

In potentially dysfunctional patterns, sufficient evidence exists or enough risk factors are present to indicate that a pattern dysfunction will likely occur if interventions are not made. This early identification of potential problems is possible through systematic data collection and analysis.

Contributing Etiological Factors

To plan care, the nurse must first determine what has caused the actual or potential health problem: its contributing etiological factors. The etiological factors of most dysfunctional patterns lie within another pattern or patterns. Although etiology is never an absolute within human sciences, the projection of outcomes or goals must be based on some probable causes. Interventions then focus on mediating or resolving the probable causes. Most often, multicausal factors are involved and problems are said to "relate to" rather than be a result of these factors.

Potential problems are not actual problems but risk states; therefore they have no specific cause and are identified when risk factors are present. **Nursing intervention** is directed toward risk reduction through education (classes or brochures) to improve nutrition, prevent accidents, and so forth. Risk estimate theory and potential health problems are further developed in Chapters 7 and 8 and Unit 4. (See Hot Topics box.)

Diagnostic Variables

The ability to arrive at an accurate diagnosis, even when all the appropriate information is available, is governed primarily by the nurse's clinical skills. Experience improves the technique when nursing is performed as a scientific process. Nursing requires gathering information, interpreting it based on normative values, organizing and grouping inappropriate findings, identifying the problem, and then planning appropriate goals and interventions.

Difficulties are encountered when there are no available norms, which occur frequently in the psychosocial assessment components. Using the 11 interdependent functional health patterns helps to solve these difficulties. By focusing on each of these areas, recognizing whether a problem does or does not exist is easier. Any change within the pattern may be a sign of dysfunction or an unhealthy but stabilized behavior. This sign might include a two-year-old child who is still not walking; developmental growth is a major factor in activity patterns of infants, toddlers, and children.

The use of physiological parameters clearly demonstrates the idea of a stabilized dysfunctional pattern, but equal care must be given to psychological development. For instance, evidence of a 26-year-old man who lives with his mother and gives no indication of independent decision making should certainly be further explored.

It should be apparent that assessment information primarily comes from the initial contact with the individual and the database, which is generally the case in health-promotion activities. However, in any acute situation or emergency, quick assessment of the major problems is given high priority on a hierarchy-of-needs basis and the full nursing assessment is temporarily postponed.

For further understanding of the nursing diagnosis, the nurse is referred to books discussing the development of diagnoses, the diagnostic process, and specific details of each accepted diagnosis (Gordon, 1994; NANDA, 2000; McFarland & McFarlane, 1993; Sparks & Taylor, 1998).

Planning the Care

Planning, in the nursing process, is the proposal of diagnosis-specific treatment to assist the individual toward the goal, or expected outcome, of optimal health. The individual's goals and the determined nursing diagnosis provide the basis for planning. The clarity of the goals and diagnoses are critical to the development of an effective plan of care.

Yura and Walsh (1988) identify the following purposes of the planning phase: (1) to assign priority to the problems diagnosed; (2) to specify the behavioral outcomes or goals with the individual, including the expected time of achievement; (3) to differentiate individual problems that can be resolved by nursing intervention, those that can be handled by the individual or family member, and those that should be handled with or referred to other members of the health team; (4) to designate specific actions, the frequency of these actions, and the short-term, intermediate-term, and long-term results; and (5) to list the individual's problems (nursing diagnosis) and nursing actions (frequency and **expected outcomes,** or goals) on the nursing care plan or blueprint for action. This plan provides the direction for individual and nursing activities and is the guide for the evaluation. There are many research studies involving outcomes from which nurses can draw to promote the effectiveness of the care they provide.

Implementing the Plan

Implementing is the completion of the actions necessary to fulfill the goals for optimal health; it is the enactment of the nursing care plan toward the behaviors described in the proposed individual outcome.

The selection of a nursing intervention depends on several factors: (1) the desired patient outcome, (2) the characteristics of the nursing diagnosis, (3) the research base associated with the intervention, (4) the feasibility of successfully implementing the intervention, (5) the acceptability of the intervention to the individual, and (6) the capability of the nurse (Bulechek & McCloskey, 1996).

A nursing interventions classification is being developed. As discussed in Unit 1, a critical component of effective communication is the accurate interpretation of the individual's information. This feedback process continues throughout all phases of the nursing process; the nurse continues to collect data to modify the plan as needed and does not blindly implement the care plan. As discussed in Unit 3, the most frequently used nursing interventions in health promotion are screening, education, counseling, and crisis intervention. All of these interventions require strong communication abilities from the nurse.

Evaluating the Plan

The process of analyzing changes experienced by the individual occurs in the evaluation phase of the nursing process, with the nurse examining the relationships between nursing actions and the individual's goal achievement. Yura and Walsh (1988) emphasize that evaluation is always considered in terms of how the individual responds to the planned action. As discussed, the nursing diagnosis, or health problems, and the goal, or expected outcome, guide the evaluation of the nursing care plan.

Many variables influence outcomes: the interventions prescribed by the health care providers, the health care providers themselves, the environment in which the care is received, the individual's motivation and genetic structure, and the individual's significant others. The task for nursing is to define which outcomes are sensitive to nursing care; that is, to identify the expected and attainable results of nursing care for each individual (Bulechek & McCloskey, 1996).

All of these components of the nursing process are correspondingly documented by the nurse on the individual's health care record (DiBlasi & Savage, 1992; Hirshfield-Bartek, Dow, & Creaton, 1990).

SUMMARY

Data relevant to the health promotional activities of the individual focus primarily on the assessment of the current health status so the nurse can identify problem areas, or areas of dysfunction, within the individual's health and lifestyle pattern. This process is a fundamental first step and precedes all other components of the nursing process. Without a clear picture of the problem, nursing activities are fruitless.

Gordon's functional health pattern framework provides the framework for the individual assessment. The focus of each pattern includes the age-developmental influences exerted, cultural and environmental roles played, the functional ability displayed, and the behavioral patterns specific to each individual. The interaction between internal mechanisms and the environment is assessed through these 11 functional health patterns.

When assessing each pattern, the nurse must understand the pattern definition, the significance of the pattern to the whole individual, the developmental influences, the environmental role, the assessment objectives, the assessment parameters and indicators, and the nursing implications. Assessment is essential to all components of the nursing process in health promotion for the individual.

REFERENCES

Abbey, J. (1980). Fancap: What is it? In J. Riehl, & C. Roy (Eds.), *Conceptual models for nursing practice* (2nd ed.). New York: Appleton-Century-Crofts.

Agency for Health Care Policy and Research. (1993). *Depression in primary care: Clinical practice guideline*. Rockville, MD: U.S. Department of Health and Human Services.

American Academy of Nursing Expert Panel. (1992). Culturally competent health care. *Nursing Outlook, 40*, 277-283.

American Nurses' Association. (1980a). *The nursing practice act: Suggested state legislation*. Kansas City, MO: The Association.

American Nurses' Association. (1980b). *Scope of nursing practice: A social policy statement*. Kansas City, MO: The Association.

American Nurses' Association. (1991). *Standards of clinical nursing practice*. Kansas City, MO: The Association.

American Nurses' Association. (1995). *Nursing's social policy statement*. Washington, DC: The Association.

American Nurses' Association. (1996). *Nursing's social policy statement*. Washington, DC: The Association. Beck, A. (1972). Screening depressed patients in family practice. *Postgraduate Medicine, 52*, 81.

Benson, H., & Stuart, E. M. (1992). *The wellness book*. New York: Simon & Schuster.

Beyea, S., & Matzo, M. (1989). Assessing elders using the functional health pattern assessment model. *Nurse Educator, 14*, 32-37.

Bickley, L. S. (1999). *Bates' guide to physical examination and history taking* (7th ed.). Philadelphia: Lippincott.

Bloch, D. (1974). Some crucial terms in nursing: What do they really mean? *Nursing Outlook, 22*, 689.

Bromwell, L. (1984). Use of life history in pattern identification and health promotion. *Advances in Nursing Science, 7* (1), 37-44.

Breen, L. (1961). *The adult years: A report prepared for the Bartholomew Retirement Foundation*. Lafayette, IN: Purdue Sociology Department.

Brink, J. P. (1984). Value orientation as an assessment tool in cultural diversity. *Nursing Research, 33* (4), 198.

Bruhn, J., Cordova, F. D., Williams, J. A., Fuentes, R. G. (1977). The wellness process. *Journal of Community Health, 2*, 209-221.

Bulechek, G., & McCloskey, J. (1996). *Nursing interventions classification: Taxonomy of nursing interventions* (2nd ed.). St. Louis: Mosby.

Burn, C. (1992). A new assessment model and tool for pediatric nurse practitioners. *Journal of Pediatric Health Care: Official publication of National Association of Pediatric Nurse Associates & Practitioners, 6*, 73-81.

Calarco, M. M., & Drone, K. P. (1991). An integrated nursing model of depressive behavior in adults. Theory and implications for practice. *The Nursing Clinics of North America, 26*, 573-584.

Carpenito, L. (1999). *Nursing care plans and documentation: Nursing diagnosis and collaborative problems* (3rd ed.). Philadelphia: Lippincott.

Caudill, M. A. (1995). *Managing pain before it manages you*. New York: Guildford Press.

Dalton, J. R., & Busch, I. D. (1995). Depression: The missing diagnosis in the elderly. *Home Health Nurse, 13*, 31-35.

DiBlasi, M., & Savage, J. (1992). Revitalizing a documentation system. *Rehabilitation Nursing: The Official Journal of the Association of Rehabilitation Nurses, 17*, 27-29.

Dixon, J., Dixon, J., & Spinner, J. (1989). Preceptions of life pattern disintegrity as a link in the relationship between stress and illness. *Advances in Nursing Science, 11* (2), 1-11.

Downing, C. K., & Kuckelman-Cobb, A. (1990). Value orientation of homeless men. *Western Journal of Nursing Research, 12* (5), 619-628.

Dunn, H. (1972). *High-level wellness*. Arlington, VA: Beatty.

Duvall, E., & Miller, B. (1985). *Marriage and family development* (7th ed.). New York: Harper Collins.

Ebersole, P., & Hess, P. (1994). *Toward healthy aging: Human needs and nursing response* (4th ed.). St. Louis: Mosby.

Erikson, E. (1986). *Childhood and society* (35th anniversary ed.). New York: Norton.

Girdano, S., & Eberly, N. (1986). *Controlling stress and tension: A holistic approach* (2nd ed.). Englewood Cliffs, NJ: Prentice Hall.

Gordon, M. (1976). Nursing diagnosis and the diagnostic process. *American Journal of Nursing, 76*, 1232-1234.

Gordon, M. (1990). Toward theory-based diagnostic categories. *Nursing Diagnosis: ND: The Official Journal of the North American Nursing Diagnosis Association, 1*, 5-11.

Gordon, M. (1994). *Nursing diagnosis: Process and application* (3rd ed.). St. Louis: Mosby.

Gordon, M. (1995). *Manual of nursing diagnosis: 1995-1996*. St. Louis: Mosby.

Gordon, M. (2000). *Manual of nursing diagnosis: 1998-2000*. St. Louis: Mosby.

Harvey, R. M. (1992). The relationship of values to adjustment in illness: A model for nursing practice. *Journal of Advanced Nursing, 17*, 467-472.

Havighurst, R. (1973). *Developmental tasks and education* (3rd ed.). New York: David McKay.

Hirshfield-Bartek, J., Dow, K. H., & Creaton, E. (1990). Decreasing documentation time using a patient self-assessment tool. *Oncology Nursing Forum, 17*, 251-255.

Holmes, T., & David, E. (1984). *Life change events research, 1967-1978: An annotated bibliography of the periodical literature*. Westport, CT: Greenwood.

Holmes, T., & David, E. (1989). *Life change, life events and illness: Selected papers*. Westport, CT: Greenwood.

Holmes, T., & Rahe, F. (1967). The social readjustment rating scale. *Journal of Psychosomatic Research, 11*, 213-218.

Jarvis, C. (2000). *Physical examination and health assessment* (3rd ed.). Philadelphia: Saunders.

Jones, D., & Lepley, M. (1992). *Assessment across the lifespan*. New York: McGraw-Hill.

Kelley, M. L., & Fitzsimmons, V. M. (2000). *Understanding cultural diversity: Culture, curriculum and community in nursing*. New York: National League for Nursing.

Kleinman, A. (1988). *The illness narratives*. New York: Basic Books.

Lau, R. R., Hartman, K. A., & Ware, Jr., J. E. (1986). Health as a value: Methodological and theoretical considerations. *Health Psychology: Official Journal of the Division of Health Psychology, American Psychological Association, 5* (1), 25-43.

Lawton, M. (1971). The functional assessment of elderly people. *Journal of the American Geriatrics Society, 19*, 465-481.

Maslow, A. (1983). *The farthest reaches of human nature*. Magnolia, MS: Peter Smith.

Maslow, A. (1987). *Motivation and personality* (3rd ed.). New York: Harper & Row.

McCaffery, M. (1999). *Pain: Clinical manual*. St. Louis: Mosby.

McCain, F. (1965). Nursing by assessment—not intuition. *American Journal of Nursing, 65*, 82.

McCloskey, J. (1976). How to make the most of body image theory in nursing. *Nursing, 6*, 68.

McCourt, A. (1981). *Measurement of functional deficit in quality assurance: Quality assurance update*. Kansas City, MO: The American Nurses' Association.

McFadden, E. A., & Gunnett, A. E. (1992). A study of diagnostic reasoning in pediatric nurses. *Pediatric Nursing, 18*, 517-520, 538.

McFarland, G. K., & McFarlane, E. A. (1993). *Nursing diagnosis and intervention: Planning for patient care*. St. Louis: Mosby.

Mitchell, P. (1981). *Concepts basic to nursing* (3rd ed.). New York: McGraw-Hill.

Monninger, E., Padgett, D., & Fleeger, M. E. (1994). Functional health pattern nursing assessment for BSN students in classification of nursing diagnoses. In R. M. Carroll-Johnson (Ed.), *Proceedings of the 10th conference*. Philadelphia: Lippincott.

Moritz, P. (1995). WSRN state of the science papers. Outcomes research: Examining clinical effectiveness. *Community Nursing Research, 28*, 113-131.

Morrison-Beedy, D., & Robbin, L. (1989). Sexual assessment and the aging female. *Nursing Practice, 14*, 35, 38-39, 42.

Muhlenkamp, A. F., & Sayles, J. A. (1986). Self esteem, social support and positive health practices. *Nursing Research, 35* (6), 334.

NANDA. (2000). *NANDA nursing diagnoses: Definitions and classification, 1999-2000*. Philadelphia: NANDA.

National Center for Health Statistics, U.S. Department of Health & Human Services. (2000). *Health outcomes among Hispanic subgroups: Data from the National Health Interview Survey, 1992-1995*. Washington, DC: U.S. Government Printing Office.

Newman, M. (1987). Nursing's emerging paradigm: The diagnosis of pattern. In A. M. McLane (Ed.), *Classification of nursing diagnosis: Proceedings of the seventh conference*. St. Louis: Mosby.

Newman, M. (1994). *Health as expanding consciousness* (2nd ed.). New York: National League for Nursing.

Newman, M. (1995): *A developing discipline: Selected works of Margaret Newman*. New York: National League for Nursing.

Nightingale, F. (1861). *Notes on nursing*. London: Harrison.

Pender, N. J. (1996). *Health promotion in nursing practice* (3rd ed.). Norwalk, CT: Appleton & Lange.

Piaget, J. (1981). *Intelligence and affectivity: Their relationship during child development*. Palo Alto, CA: Annual Reviews. (Translated by Brown, T., & Kaegi, C.)

Pollock, S. E. (1984). The stress response. *Critical Care Nursing Quarterly, 6* (4), 1-14.

Rengucci, L. M. (1992). Neonatal nursing assessment by functional health patterns critical care. *The Nursing Clinics of North America, 4*, 471-480.

Rogers, M. (1970). *An introduction to the theoretical basis of nursing*. Philadelphia: F. A. Davis.

Rosenstock, I. (1974). The health belief model and preventative health behavior. *Health Education Monographs, 2*, 354.

Smith, D. M. (1968). A clinical nursing tool. *American Journal of Nursing, 68*, 2384-2388.

Sparks, S. M., & Taylor, C. M. (1998). *Nursing diagnosis reference manual* (4th ed.). Springhouse, PA: Springhouse.

Tompkins, E. S. (1992). Nurse/client values congruence. *Western Journal of Nursing Research, 14* (2), 225.

U.S. Department of Health & Human Services. (2000). *Healthy People 2010* (Conference Edition). Washington, DC: U.S. Government Printing Office.

U.S. Department of Health & Human Services. (2000). *Women and heart disease: An atlas of racial and ethnic disparities in mortality*. Washington, DC: U.S. Government Printing Office.

Yura, H., & Walsh, M. (1988). *Human needs and the nursing process* (5th ed.). New York: Appleton-Century-Crofts.

Zung, W. (1971). A rating instrument for anxiety disorders. *Psychosomatics, 12* (6), 371-379.

Zung, W. (1973). From art to science: Diagnoses and treatment of depression. *Archives of General Psychiatry, 29*, 328-337.

Chapter 7

CAROL LYNN MANDLE

Health Promotion and the Family

objectives

After completing this chapter, the nurse will be able to:

- Describe the use of the functional health-pattern framework in assessing families throughout the lifespan.
- Give examples of the clinical data to be collected in each health pattern during the different family developmental phases.
- Give examples of the following behavioral changes within the health patterns of families: functional, potentially dysfunctional, and actually dysfunctional.
- Describe developmental and cultural characteristics of the family to consider while identifying risk factors or etiological factors of potentially or actually dysfunctional health patterns.
- Discuss planning, implementing, and evaluating nursing interventions in health promotion with families.
- Develop a specific health-promotion plan based on a family assessment, nursing diagnosis, and contributing risks or etiological factors.

key terms

Cultural Competence
Developmental Theory
Divergent Family Structures
Ecomap
Family Developmental Tasks
Family Function
Family Health Status
Family Nursing Diagnosis
Family Nursing Interventions
Family Pattern
Family Risk Factors
Family Strengths
Family Structure
Genogram
Risk Factor Theory
Systems Theory

THINK About It

Caring for Older Adults

Today, older family members, who may even have health problems of their own, find themselves caring for their old parents. This type of situation is expected to become more prevalent in the coming years.

1 What are the implications of this growing situation for individuals? Families? Communities? The nation?

2 How will this trend affect life personally and professionally?

How family members behave relative to one another influences the understanding of behavior, which is demonstrated in the family's structural, functional, communicational, and developmental patterns (Dzurec, 1995; Wright & Leahy, 2000). Therefore a primary approach to health promotion and disease prevention is through the family. Within families, children and adults are nurtured, provided for, and taught about health values by word and by example. Also within families, members first learn to make choices that promote their health.

Healthy People 2010 views families as means of providing an important opportunity for health promotion and disease prevention. This report states that beginning a family should be one of the joys of life. Through family planning, parents can ensure that they are ready to assume responsibility to care for and provide for their children. After the choice has been made to begin a new life, the mother has the responsibility to seek prenatal care in the first trimester of pregnancy to ensure a healthy birth. Breast feeding can also help give a child a healthy start. A nutritious diet that supports physical growth and development coupled with physical activity can ensure that a child begins life with healthy habits. Within families, behaviors are first observed and learned. Diet and activity patterns, oral hygiene, and coping skills are established at an early age and are supported by the examples set by family members. Patterns of alcohol consumption and tobacco use are similarly established within families. For adolescents and young adults, learning about physical development can foster positive awareness of their sexuality. Promoting self-esteem and reinforcing positive behaviors also builds the mental health of children. Primary care providers can be supportive by ensuring that family members are provided scientifically sound clinical preventive services, including immunizations, screening to detect asymptomatic disease in its early stages, and appropriate counseling to foster healthy behaviors.

Pender (1996) believes that the family is a logical unit of assessment and intervention for health promotion because it has the primary responsibility for (1) developing self-care and dependent-care competencies of the family, (2) fostering the resilience of family members, (3) providing social and physical resources to the family group, and (4) promoting healthy individuation while maintaining family cohesion. Furthermore, the task of fostering health and healthy behaviors should be an integral part of family functioning.

This chapter uses systems theory, developmental theory, and risk factor theory to guide the nursing process with families. The 11 functional health patterns described in the previous chapter are used for posing questions to obtain assessment data. The analysis phase of the nursing process categorizes these data with stages of family development and, from the analysis, a nursing diagnosis is formulated. **Family health status** is considered functional, potentially dysfunctional (potential problem), or dysfunctional (actual problem) (Gordon, 1994). The planning phase begins with the family when goals and objectives are stated for measuring behavioral change. The nurse, the family, or other health professionals facilitate implementation of the plan. Four types of interventions are discussed for health promotion and disease prevention. Various roles that the nurse may assume through the stages of family development are also listed. Evaluation considers outcomes that are specific, objective, and measurable and that rely on the family's subjective interpretation of concerns and probability of success (McFarland & McFarlane, 1993; NANDA, 2000; Sparks & Taylor, 1998).

THE NURSING PROCESS AND THE FAMILY

The goal of nursing is to facilitate the health of the family (Newman, 1995). The nursing process with the family begins when the nurse and the family meet for the purpose of enhancing wellness or solving a health problem or a potential health problem (Wright & Leahy, 2000). Although this encounter may occur in several settings, the home is a natural environment for families. Members of different age groups (infants, children, and older adults) are apt to be more readily available in the home. The nurse can also observe first hand the physical environment during the home visit (detecting household items that may present a safety hazard). For example, the nurse can see the whole family as a unit and observe mealtime rituals, roles of family members, and interpersonal interactions. Generally, the nurse contacts the family and sets up an appointment for the visit. Including each member of the family in the visit will provide the nurse with a broader perspective than interviewing an isolated member. During the visit, the nursing process is carried out *with* the family and not *for* the family; the family becomes a partner with the nurse in all phases of the process. Guidelines for the home visit are presented in Box 7-1.

A comprehensive family assessment is the foundation of promoting the health of a family (Wright & Leahy, 2000). Several factors influence the assessment of the family: the nurse's perception of what constitutes a family; knowledge of theories, norms, and standards; and an ability to put the family at ease during visits. In addition to factors that pertain to the nurse, familial factors also influence the assessment phase: cooperation from family members, mutual agreement to work toward a desired goal, and the family's ability to see the relevance of nursing actions to their needs and desires. A useful health-promotion (versus illness care) family assessment involves listening to the family, engaging in participatory dialogue, recognizing patterns, and assessing the family's potential for active, positive change (Wright & Leahy, 2000).

The assessment phase of the nursing process seeks and identifies information from the family about its activities in health promotion and disease prevention. To obtain this

Box 7-1 Guidelines for Home Visit to Promote Health and Prevent Disease

PLANNING THE VISIT

- Make arrangements with the family
- Study information regarding the family from agency record, referral forms, and other sources of information
- State the purpose of the visit
- Obtain appropriate supplies and teaching aids for visits

MAKING THE VISIT

- Offer an introduction and explain the purpose of the visit
- Place the nurse's bag in the appropriate location
- Include all family members in the discussion
- Identify the family's request for assistance
- Understand the situation from the family's perspective
- Identify appropriate activities for health promotion and disease prevention
- Identify how the home visit is to be financed
- Make a contract with the family that states specific goals and objectives that the family wants to reach
- Terminate the visit with specific instructions and information on the next visit: when it will occur; what will happen; who will be present; and what the family must accomplish before then

research highlights

Definition of Family Health

An ethnographic study completed in an Appalachian county in southeastern Ohio included eight families and community informants (N = 25). The purpose of the study was to identify ways in which economically disadvantaged families with young children defined family health within household contexts. Families were recipients of public assistance. Home interviews were conducted with multiple family members who had unique perspectives and described family health as a dynamic household construction affected by the community. Subjects described health routines as patterns affected by the household context. Mothers played key roles as health leaders, caregivers, and gatekeepers in family health.

Study implications include: (1) guarding against semantic slippage when using the term "family health"; (2) developing family-focused care models in which mothers are pivotal; (3) identifying the contextual factors most predictive for promoting family health; and (4) including health routines in planning care.

Data from Denham, S. A. (1999b). Family health in an economically disadvantaged population. *Journal of Family Nursing, 5* (2), 184-213.

information, the nurse must know the family's progress through its developmental tasks and its ability to generate low risk-taking behaviors associated with disease prevention. Approaches considered in this chapter are the developmental framework and the risk-factor estimate. Developmental norms as proposed by Duvall (1985) and risk-factor estimates as proposed in *Healthy People 2010* are used to guide the nurse through the steps of the nursing process.

The Nurse's Role

Working with the family from a systems perspective, the nurse understands the ways in which family members interact, what the family norms and expectations are, how effectively members communicate, how the family makes decisions, and how the family deals with needs and expectations. The nurse's role in health promotion and disease prevention includes the following tasks:

1. To become aware of family attitudes and behaviors toward health promotion and disease prevention
2. To serve as role model for the family
3. To collaborate with the family in assessing, improving, enhancing, and evaluating their current health practices
4. To assist the family in growth and development behaviors
5. To assist the family in identifying risk-taking behaviors
6. To assist the family in decision making about lifestyle choices
7. To provide reinforcement for positive health-behavior practices
8. To assist the family in learning behaviors that promote health and prevent disease
9. To serve as a liaison for referral or collaboration between community resources and the family
10. To provide health information to the family
11. To assist the family in problem solving and decision making about health promotion

How the nurse works with families to assist them with health promotion and disease prevention will depend on the framework used to guide, observe, and classify the situation. Table 7-1 presents nursing roles for families in various stages of development.

The Family from a Systems Perspective

The family can be defined as a set of interacting individuals who are related by blood, marriage, cohabitation, or adoption and who are interdependent in carrying out relevant functions through roles. Relevant functions of the family include values and practices placed on health. Health is viewed as any activity undertaken by the family for the purpose of health promotion and disease prevention. The effective execution of health-related functions is based on the way in which the family progresses through its developmental tasks and its ability to generate low risk-producing behaviors associated with disease prevention. Choices regarding health-promotion and disease-prevention behaviors determine the potential for the family to enhance health practices in its members.

Table 7-1 Possible Nurse's Roles in Health Promotion and Disease Prevention Through Stages of Family Development

Stage	Possible Nursing Role
Couple	Counselor on sexual and role adjustment Teacher of and counselor on family planning Teacher of parenting skills Coordinator for genetic counseling Facilitator in interpersonal relationships
Childbearing family	Monitor of prenatal care and referrer for problems of pregnancy Counselor on prenatal nutrition Counselor on prenatal maternal habits Supporter of amniocentesis Counselor on breast feeding Coordinator with pediatric services Supervisor of immunizations Referrer to social services Assistant in adjustment to parental role
Family with preschool or school-aged children	Monitor of early childhood development; referrer when indicated Teacher of first-aid and emergency measures Coordinator with pediatric services Counselor on nutrition and exercise Teacher of problem-solving issues regarding health habits Participant in community organizations for environmental control Teacher of dental hygiene Counselor on environmental safety in home Facilitator in interpersonal relationships
Family with adolescents	Teacher of risk factors to health Teacher of problem-solving issues regarding alcohol, smoking, diet, and exercise Facilitator of interpersonal skills with adolescents and parents Direct supporter of, counselor on, or referrer to mental health resources Counselor on family planning Referrer for sexually transmittable disease
Family with young or middle-aged adults	Participant in community organizations involved in disease control Teacher of problem-solving issues regarding lifestyle and habits Participant in community organizations involved in environmental control Case finder in the home and community Screener for hypertension, Pap smear, breast examination, cancer signs, mental health, and dental care Counselor on menopausal transition
Family with older adults	Facilitator of interpersonal relationships among family members Referrer for work and social activity, nutritional programs, homemakers' services, and nursing home Monitor of exercise, nutrition, preventive services, and medications Supervisor of immunization Counselor on safety in the home Counselor on bereavement

Systems theory perceives patterns of living among the members who make up the family system. Behaviors and responses of family members are seen as influencing the family's pattern and life. Meanings and values are vital components of the family system and provide motivation and energy. Every family has a unique culture, value structure, and history. Values (the means of interpreting events and information) are passed down from generation to generation and are subject to change by continuing interaction with the environment. The family processes information and energy exchange with the environment through values; the values identify the meaning of the information for the family's use.

Systems have boundaries that separate the family system from the rest of the environment and control the flow of information, energy, and matter between the system and the surrounding environment to maintain the system. This characteristic becomes the family's psychic energy and internal manager, made up of interactions and relationships of members with one another and with those outside the family system. The family is considered a unified whole rather than the sum of its parts—an integrated system of interdependent functions, structures, and relationships that reacts as a single whole. Living systems are open systems. As a living system, the family must be open to a constant exchange of energy and information with the environment; the greater the openness of the family is, the greater the possible changes will be. Change in one part or member of the family results in changes in the family as a whole. Change requires the adaptation of every member of the family as roles and functions take on new meanings. After the family has made the change, it does not revert to its former state; the change is incorporated into the system.

Families are composed of both structural and functional components. **Family structure** refers to the family's roles and relationships, whereas **family function** is the process of continual change in the system as information and energy are exchanged between the family and the environment.

THE FAMILY FROM A DEVELOPMENTAL PERSPECTIVE

Building on Erikson's theory of psychosocial development (1986), Duvall and Miller (1985) identify stages of the family life cycle and critical family developmental tasks. Although Duvall's classification has been criticized for its middle-class homogeneity and lack of diversity in family forms, the assessment of families is useful because it provides a way for anticipating what to expect. By knowing the composition of the family, the ways in which the members are related, and the family's particular life cycle, the nurse can predict somewhat reliably what the overall pattern of the family's activities is, what significant elements to seek, and what forces will likely be found. Box 7-2 lists tasks essential to the family's survival and continuity. Duvall maintains that all families in general have these basic family tasks as long as they exist, with each family performing them in its own way. The nurse collects data to ascertain the ways in which the family is meeting each task. In addition to the general tasks of survival and continuity, each family has stages of development and specific tasks related to each stage. A specific task is a growth responsibility that arises at a certain stage in the life of a family. Failure in the tasks may lead to disapproval by society (child abuse or neglect) and possible intervention by police, welfare, health department, or other agencies (see Health Teaching box). Failure early in the life cycle may lead to difficulty with later developmental tasks.

As the family enters each new stage of its development, a critical role transition occurs. Events such as getting married, bearing children, releasing members as adolescents and young adults, and continuing as a couple or single person through the "empty nest" and aging years move the family into and through new stages in its history.

Each new developmental stage requires adaptations and new responsibilities. Concurrently, each developmental stage provides new opportunities for the family to realize its fullest potential. As the family enters each new stage, the nurse is alerted to what may be expected and to an approximate timetable for anticipating change. Each new stage then becomes an opportunity for health promotion and intervention.

Box 7-2 Tasks for Family Survival and Continuity

- Providing shelter, food, clothing, health care, and similar needs for its members
- Meeting family costs and allocating resources, such as time, space, and facilities, according to each member's needs
- Determining who does what in the support, management, and care of the home and its members
- Ensuring each member's socialization through the internalization of increasingly mature roles in the family and in society
- Establishing ways of interacting, communicating, and expressing affections, aggression, sexuality, and similar interactions within limits acceptable to society
- Bearing (or adopting) and rearing children, then incorporating and releasing family members appropriately
- Relating to school, church, work, and community life and establishing policies for including in-laws, relatives, guests, friends, mass media, and others
- Maintaining morale and motivation, rewarding achievement, meeting personal and family crises, setting attainable goals, and developing family loyalties and values

Modified from Duvall, E. M., & Miller, B. (1985). *Marriage and family development* (6th ed.). New York: Harper & Row.

The stages of family development, although reflective of the traditional nuclear family and extended family networks, can be applied to other family configurations. For example, the couple who marries and brings children of various ages from a previous marriage to the union must accomplish the developmental tasks of the couple stage and the specific family stages of the children. The couple and the children bring values and beliefs from past unions that the existing group must integrate and share. In situations in which there are no children, individual development is integrated into the lives of the couple. The childless couple presents a different set of developmental tasks than those proposed for the couple with children.

In assessing a family's developmental stage and its performance of the tasks appropriate to that stage, the nurse uses a guideline for analyzing family growth and health-promotion needs. Table 7-2 summarizes the **family developmental tasks** during critical stages.

Family risk factors can be inferred from (1) lifestyle (habits of overeating, drug dependency, high sugar intake, high-cholesterol diets, or smoking), (2) biological factors (genetic inheritance, congenital malformation, or mental retardation), (3) environmental factors (work pressures leading to stress; anxieties; tensions; or air, noise, and water

HEALTH TEACHING Domestic Violence

- Encourage all women to pursue education, employment, and other means of self-actualization to empower themselves and build self-esteem
- Teach women to control their fertility through available methods of contraception and abortion services; this can have an empowering effect and help them avoid an unwanted pregnancy that might lead to more episodes of abuse
- Inform adolescents and young women that violence and abuse are not a normal part of intimate relationships; help them avoid potential abusers such as men who seem overly jealous, overprotective, or controlling; men who have a history of substance or alcohol abuse; or men who exhibit violent behavior toward animals, objects, or other people
- Let the woman know that she is free to discuss this issue and encourage her to do so
- Assure the woman that she is not alone and that many women share this problem; explore the health consequences of battering for her, her children, and other family-household members
- Educate the woman about the cycle of violence and explain that without intervention, violent episodes will likely increase in both frequency and severity
- Provide the woman with referral information for legal, law enforcement, shelter, financial, and counseling services
  - The Michigan Coalition Against Domestic Violence provides information to health care providers and operates a national hotline: 800-333-SAFE; telecommunications device for the deaf: 800-873-6363
  - The National Coalition Against Domestic Violence provides a network of shelters and counseling programs: P.O. Box 34103, Washington, DC 20043-4103, (202) 638-6388
- Help the woman develop an escape plan

From Star, W. L., Lommel , L. L., & Shannon, M. T. (1995). *Womens' primary health care*. Washington, DC: American Nurses Publishing.

Table 7-2 Selected Developmental Tasks of the Family at Critical Stages

Scope	Position in Family	Developmental Tasks
Couple	Wife Husband	Establishing mutually satisfying marriage Relating to kin network Planning to have or not to have children
Childbearing family	Wife-mother Husband-father Infant daughter or son or both	Having and adjusting to infant and supporting needs of all three family members Renegotiating marital and extended-family relationships
Family with preschoolers	Wife-mother Husband-father Daughter-sister Son-brother	Adjusting to predictable and unexpected costs of family life Adapting to critical needs and interests of preschool children in stimulating, growth-promoting ways Coping with energy depletion and lack of privacy as parents
Family with school-aged children	Wife-mother Husband-father Daughter-sister Son-brother	Adjusting to growing children's activity Promoting joint decision making of children and parents Encouraging and supporting children's educational achievement
Family with adolescents	Wife-mother Husband-father Daughter-sister Son-brother	Maintaining open communication among family members Strengthening marital relationship Supporting ethical and moral values within family Balancing freedom with responsibility with adolescents as they mature and emancipate themselves
Family with young adults	Wife-mother-grandmother Husband-father-grandfather Daughter-sister-aunt Son-brother-uncle	Releasing young adults with appropriate rituals and assistance Reestablishing marital relationship as couple Maintaining supportive home base
Family with middle-age adults	Wife-mother-grandmother Husband-father-grandfather	Preparing for retirement Maintaining kin ties with older and younger generations
Family with older adults	Widow or widower Wife-mother-grandmother Husband-father-grandfather	Adjusting to retirement Adjusting to loss of spouse Closing family home or adapting it for elderly members

Modified from Duvall, E. M., & Miller, B. (1985). *Marriage and family development* (6th ed.). New York: Harper & Row.

pollution), (4) social and psychological dimensions (crowding, isolation, or rapid and accelerated rates of change), and (5) the health care system (overuse, underuse, or inappropriate use of accessibility). (See the Frank Thompson case study in Chapter 1.)

The family's role in reducing risk factors focuses mainly on influencing health behaviors of its members. Individuals are induced to make personal lifestyle choices in a society that glamorizes many hazardous behaviors through advertising and mass media, the health consequences of which may not be immediately visible. Families can be influential in assisting their members to weigh the consequences of risk-taking behavior. Awareness of risk factors may prompt families to make an extra effort to reduce risks more directly under their control and lessen overall risk of disease and injury. Healthy behavior, including judicious use of preventive health care services, is a significant area of family responsibility for the personal health of its members.

THE FAMILY FROM A RISK-FACTOR PERSPECTIVE

Traditionally, epidemiology has used levels and trends of mortality and morbidity rates (death and illness) as indirect evidence of health. Data such as infant mortality rates, stillbirth rates, and leading causes of death have long been used as indicators of the collective health of a community. Healthy family functioning links the stages of the family life cycle and specific risk factors. Epidemiology often describes a disease association in terms of risk. Risks to health can be physiological (genetic in origin) or psychological (low self-image). Risks may arise from the environment, including the physical environment and socioeconomic conditions (U.S. Preventive Services Taskforce, 1996). As a pivotal part of the environment, the **risk factor theory** considers the family to be the most important of the naturally occurring social support systems in lowering risks for its members.

By comparing the frequency of deaths, illnesses, or injuries from a specific cause in a group that has some specific trait or risk factor with the frequency in another group that does not have this trait or in the population as a whole, a risk estimate can be obtained. Some diseases may occur more frequently in certain families, such as sickle cell anemia in Black families and Tay-Sachs disease in Ashkenazi (East European) Jewish families. These high-risk families are not difficult to identify because there is a hereditary association with these diseases.

However, other diseases are not linked so clearly to heredity and are much more difficult to attribute to specific causes. For example, the natural history of chronic disease may predispose individual members to greater risk, but the specific cause may be difficult to identify. Leppink (1982) identifies six progressive stages in the natural history of chronic diseases in Box 7-3.

With lung cancer, for example, the stages of the natural history of chronic disease indicate that individuals may be at no risk until they start to smoke. At some point, the dysplasia of the epithelial cells of the bronchi will indicate that the disease is active. Intervention at stage three will prevent the disease and anatomical changes can be reversed.

Box 7-3 Six Progressive Stages in the Natural History of Chronic Diseases

1. *No-risk stage:* the period in an individual's life when no risk of developing the disease exists, varying from a few to many years
2. *Risk stage:* one or more of the causative agents or factors becomes part of the host's environment
3. *Infiltration stage:* causative agent or agents are active in the individual, although no symptoms or signs of overt disease can be detected by any known diagnostic means
4. *Critical stage:* signs are present. This stage is the transition from wellness to illness. If the risks had been eliminated before this stage, then the disease process might have been reversed or significantly decelerated. The individual is likely unaware that a disease process is underway. Arresting or reducing the seriousness of the disease and enhancing longevity are still possible
5. *Symptom stage:* the individual is now aware of the problem and seeks help from the health care system. Diagnosis may still be elusive. Any behavioral change is likely to have no significant effect on the course of the disease
6. *Overt disease stage:* evidence is seen, and a definitive diagnosis can be established readily

From Leppink, H. (1982). Health risk estimation. In M. M. Faber, & A. M. Reinhardt (Eds.), *Promoting health through risk reduction*. New York: Macmillan.

This model can be used with diseases such as cervical cancer, cerebrovascular accident (stroke), and heart disease. By changing some behavior or activity during the first three stages of the disease, prevention or reduction of morbidity is usually possible.

Throughout the family's life cycle, probabilities of risk change depend on the family's activities in health promotion and disease prevention. The stages of family development are used to classify risk factors. The age-specific developmental stage and the age-specific health problems appear in Table 7-3 and represent periods during which the family may be most vulnerable or sensitive to certain risk factors and the time during which health promotion and disease prevention can be enhanced. Many of the health problems listed are related to excesses, such as smoking, drinking, faulty nutrition, overuse of medications, fast driving, and relentless pressure to achieve. Habits learned in the family setting may cause excesses. At least seven of the 10 leading causes of death listed in the *Healthy People 2010* report might be substantially reduced if the family improves only five habits: (1) poor diet, (2) smoking, (3) lack of exercise, (4) alcohol abuse, and (5) stress.

Table 7-3 Family Stage: Specific Risk Factors and Related Health Problems

Stage	Risk Factors	Health Problems
Beginning childbearing	Lack of knowledge about family planning Adolescent marriage Lack of knowledge concerning sexual and marital roles and adjustments Low–birth-weight infant Underweight or overweight Lack of prenatal care Inadequate nutrition Poor eating habits Smoking, alcohol, and drug abuse Unmarried status First pregnancy before age 16 or after age 35 History of hypertension and infections during pregnancy Rubella, syphilis, gonorrhea, and AIDS Genetic factors present Low socioeconomic and educational levels Lack of safety in the home Home unsafe	Premature baby family Unsuccessful marriage Birth defects Birth injuries Accidents SIDS Respiratory distress syndrome Sterility Pelvic inflammatory disease Fetal alcohol syndrome Mental retardation Child abuse Injuries Birth defects
Family with school-aged children	Home unstimulating Working parents with inappropriate use of resources for child care Poverty environment Abuse or neglect of children Generational pattern of using social agencies as a way of life Multiple, closely spaced children Low family self-esteem Children used as scapegoat for parental frustration Repeated infections, accidents, or hospitalizations Parents immature, dependent, and unable to handle responsibility Unrecognized or unattended health problems Strong beliefs about physical punishment Toxic substances unguarded in the home Poor nutrition (overeating and undereating)	Behavior disturbances Speech and vision problems Communicable diseases Dental caries School problems Learning disabilities Cancer Injuries Chronic diseases Homicide Violence
Family with adolescents	Racial and ethnic family origin Lifestyle and behavior patterns leading to chronic disease Lack of problem-solving skills Family values of aggressiveness and competition Socioeconomic factors contributing to peer relationships Family values rigid and inflexible Daredevil risk-taking attitudes Denial behavior Conflicts between parents and children Pressure to live up to family expectations	Violent deaths and injuries Alcohol and drug abuse Unwanted pregnancies Sexually transmitted diseases Suicide Depression

Modified from U.S. Department of Health and Human Services. (2000). *Healthy People 2010*. Washington, DC: U.S. Government Printing Office.
AIDS, acquired immunodeficiency syndrome; *FAS*, fetal alcohol syndrome; *PID*, pelvic inflammatory disease; *RDS*, respiratory distress syndrome; *SIDS*, sudden infant death syndrome.

Continued

FUNCTIONAL HEALTH PATTERN: ASSESSMENT OF THE FAMILY

The typology of 11 functional health patterns provided by Gordon (1994) helps organize the collection of basic assessment information of the family (Nettle, Pavelich, Jones, Beltz, Laboon, Pifer 1993). The structure of the patterns represents a standardized assessment format that can be integrated into the system's developmental and risk-factor approach to the family (functional health pattern: assessment of the family). Information obtained from the 11 functional patterns is judged against family developmental norms and age-specific risk factors. When a problem in one **family pattern** is diagnosed, the causal factors may be found in that pattern and in one or more of

Table 7-3 Family Stage: Specific Risk Factors and Related Health Problems—cont'd

Stage	Risk Factors	Health Problems
Family with middle-aged adults	Hypertension Smoking High cholesterol level Diabetes Overweight Physical inactivity Personality patterns related to stress Genetic predisposition Use of oral contraceptives Sex, race, and other hereditary factors Geographic area, age, and occupational deficiencies Habits (diet with low fiber, pickling, charcoal use, and broiling) Alcohol abuse Exposure to certain substances (sunlight, radiation, water or air pollution) Social class Residence Depression	Cardiovascular disease, principally coronary artery disease and cerebrovascular accident (stroke) Cancer Accidents Homicide Suicide Abnormal fetus Mental illness
	Gingivitis	Periodontal disease and loss of teeth
Family with older adults	Age Drug interactions Depression Metabolic disorders Pituitary malfunctions Cushing's syndrome Hypercalcemia Chronic illness Retirement Loss of spouse Reduced income Poor nutrition Lack of exercise Past environments and lifestyle Lack of preparation for death	Mental confusion Reduced vision Hearing impairment Hypertension Acute illness Infectious disease Influenza Pneumonia Injuries such as burns and falls Depression Chronic disease Elderly abuse Death without dignity

the other patterns. Problems in one pattern are reflected in other areas because the patterns are interdependent (see Chapter 6).

Problems in functional patterns are identified as a dysfunctional health pattern, not a disease; a potential dysfunction is predicted when risk factors are present. A developmental risk and a risk of change toward a less functional health pattern are types of risk states. If risk factors are present, then a family is said to be susceptible to or at risk for a problem (see Table 7-3).

Gordon (1994) interprets a risk state as a potential problem, which indicates the presence of factors that predispose a family to a dysfunctional health pattern. To formulate a nursing diagnosis, the nurse names the problem and causative factor. Probable causes may be logically related to the problem or may precede or occur with a problem. The nurse identifies causal factors to plan care, then directs intervention toward the causal factors that can be changed and are predicted to have an effect on the problem. Risk factors are the signs indicating a potential problem; in a sense, they are the cause. This potential state is predicted and is not an actual state with an actual cause; therefore the origin may be nonspecific. Intervention in this case is directed toward reducing risk factors.

The sequence of patterns in the history begins with the family's health perception and health management. This pattern gives an overview that can be used to predict where problems may exist in other patterns and it may require in-depth assessment. Additionally, this pattern starts the history taking from the family's perspective and helps the family define the situation. The role-relationships pattern defines the family structure and function. Lifestyle indicators are assessed through the remaining nine patterns.

Health Perception-Health Management Pattern

This pattern identifies characteristics of the family's general health perceptions and management and preventive practices. Pratt (1976) has identified six characteristics of healthy families: (1) members facilitate an interaction process, (2) members enhance individual development, (3) role relationships are structured effectively, (4) members actively attempt to cope with problems, (5) members promote healthy home environments and lifestyles, and (6) members establish regular links with the broader community.

Health practices vary from family to family; each identifies and carries out health-maintenance activities related to what members believe is healthy and what they think is feasible, as demonstrated in their lifestyle practices. In facilitating the health of the family, the nurse helps family members become more conscious of their health beliefs, behaviors, and status. The nurse helps families develop "an increased range of responses of family members to each other and the world outside the family, and in addition, to refine the quality of those responses" (Newman, 1995).

Questions for assessment are as follows:

- What is the family's philosophy of health? Does each family member believe the same? Do family members practice what they believe?
- In what behaviors or lifestyle practices, such as smoking, alcohol, and drug abuse, does the family engage?
- What behaviors are the family exhibiting that point to chronic disease?
- Does the family engage in health-related behaviors, such as eating three meals a day at regular times, eating breakfast every day, exercising a minimum of 2 or 3 days a week, sleeping 7 to 8 hours each night, and abstaining from smoking?
- Are risk factors present for infections, such as lack of immunization, lack of knowledge of transmittable diseases, and lack of personal hygiene?
- Are there risk factors that point to bodily injury, accidents, or drugs? Are chemicals in the home in easy reach of children?
- Do elderly members know what medications they are taking and why?
- Are there medications in the home that are not being used and should be discarded?
- Is nutrition sufficient to maintain adequate energy levels?
- Are any unattended health problems present?
- Is there a history of repeated infections and hospitalization? Is safety lacking in the home?
- Is the home understimulating or overstimulating?
- Where does the family go for health and illness care?
- Is the family engaged in a dental program?
- How does the family describe previous experiences with nurses and other health care professionals?
- Describe the family's previous experience with a nurse and other health professionals.

The environment also influences family health and well being. The home is considered a natural environment of the family; other environmental aspects include the neighborhood and community.

Questions for assessment of the home environment are as follows:

- What type of dwelling is it (condominium, single dwelling, low-income apartment, or temporary shelter)?
- Does the family own or rent?
- Is the interior and exterior in good or poor repair (glass, trash, broken stairs, peeling paint, inadequate insulation, inadequate lighting on stairs, or broken fixtures)?
- Are the number and type of rooms adequate for the size of the family?
- Is there adequate furniture to meet the needs of the family (enough chairs, beds, and a kitchen table)?
- Is the dwelling warm in winter and cool in summer?
- Is the lighting adequate for reading, sewing, and other activities?
- Is there an adequate water supply? Is it fluoridated or polluted?
- Is there a telephone? Are emergency numbers listed?
- Does the kitchen have safe sanitation measures and adequate refrigeration?
- Does the bathroom have adequate sanitation measures, water supply, toilet facilities, and towels and soap?
- Are the sleeping arrangements adequate for family members considering age, gender, relationships, and spatial needs?
- Are there smoke detectors and an escape route and plan inside the home?
- Are first-aid directions posted for poisons, burns, lacerations, and other first-aid needs?
- Are signs of vermin present inside or outside the home?
- What are the family's impressions about their home? Do they consider the living space adequate for privacy, their own interests, and status?

Questions for assessment of the neighborhood are as follows:

- Are the dwellings and streets well kept or deteriorating?
- How and when is the garbage collected?
- What is the incidence of crime (house break-ins or violence) and auto accidents?
- What type of industry is present (does it cause air pollution or toxic waste)?
- What are the social class and ethnic characteristics of the neighborhood?
- What are the occupations and interests of the families in the neighborhood? What is the population density?
- Is public transportation available? Is it used?

Questions for assessment of the community are as follows:

- What resources does the family use (schools, church, transportation, shopping, and recreational)?

- How accessible are the health care facilities used by the family (physician's office, clinic, hospital, gym, swimming pool, natural food store, and weight-reduction clinic)?

By driving or walking around the area, the nurse can obtain the neighborhood and community data. Other sources of information include the family, health professionals, teachers, business people, and others who work in the area. Official resources, such as the U.S. Census Report or statistics from the city or state health departments and libraries, are also helpful in describing a neighborhood and community.

Nutritional-Metabolic Pattern

The nutritional-metabolic pattern describes characteristics of the family's typical food and fluid consumption. Included are child growth and development patterns, pregnancy-related nutritional patterns, and the family's eating patterns. Dietary habits are learned within the context of the family and involve behavioral patterns central to daily life. A useful way to determine a family's pattern of food and fluid intake is to have the family keep a diary of what they eat and drink for a week. Distinctions should be made between family meals and additional consumption by individual members.

Questions for assessment are as follows:
- Does the family eat together?
- Is food used as a reward or punishment?
- Is there adequate storage and refrigeration?

Elimination Pattern

The elimination pattern describes characteristics of regularity and control of the family's excretory functions. This pattern includes human (bowel and bladder) and environmental factors in the home, neighborhood, and community that influence family life. The nurse addresses the habits of bowel regularity in the family members and environmental wastes such as garbage disposal.

Questions are phrased according to the age-specific developmental stage of the family. For example, in determining whether there is a problem in the preschool stage, it would be appropriate to ask whether the child is being toilet trained. In families with adolescents, the nurse may ask how often individuals have bowel movements and whether there have been any changes from usual patterns. The nurse may ask elderly members whether they have any problems with constipation.

Activity-Exercise Pattern

This pattern describes characteristics of the family that require energy expenditure. Components reviewed are daily activities, exercise, and leisure activities. Families set the stage for individual members to be either physically active or sedentary and apathetic toward physical activity.

Questions for assessment are as follows:
- Does the family believe regular exercise and physical fitness are necessary for good health?
- What types of daily activities include physical exercise and who does what with whom?
- What does the family do to have fun (Fig. 7-1)?

Sleep-Rest Pattern

This pattern describes characteristics of rest habits from the family's perspective. Sleep is a restorative function; without it, individuals may exhibit poor performance, bad temper, and overreliance on drugs or alcohol. Regular, sufficient sleep patterns have been linked to improved mental status. Every family has patterns for sleeping, although in some families, these patterns may not be readily apparent. The important point is to elicit the data about sleep and rest from the family's perspective.

Questions for assessment are as follows:
- What are the usual sleeping habits of the family?
- Are they suitable according to age and health status?
- Are regular hours established for sleeping?
- Who decides when children go to sleep?
- Do family members take naps or have other regular means of resting or relaxing?
- Does the family rise early and go to bed early or rise late and go to bed late?

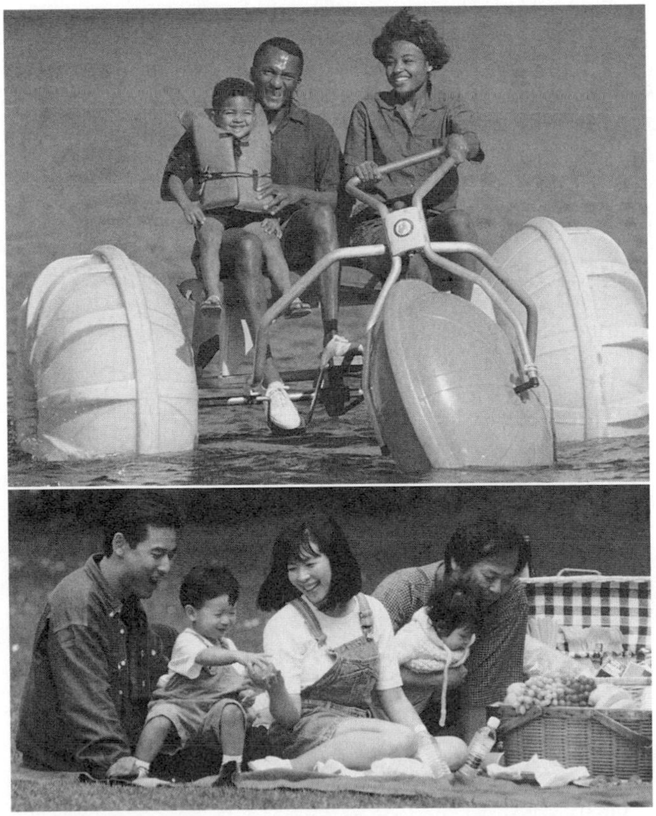
A

B

Fig. 7-1 **A,** Family outings can be adventurous and exciting or **B,** leisurely and restful.

Cognitive-Perceptual Pattern

The cognitive-perceptual pattern identifies characteristics of language, cognitive skills, and perception relative to desired or required family activities: specifically, how family decisions are made, the concreteness or abstractness of thinking, and whether decisions are oriented toward the present or the future. Decision making in the family is associated with power in family functioning. Families that are highly educated have a greater repertoire for problem solving. Power and ability to solve problems are linked to leadership; the family's leader must be acknowledged if nursing interventions are to be implemented.

Questions for assessment are as follows:

- How does the family usually go about making decisions regarding health promotion and disease prevention?
- Do all members contribute to the decision-making process, or is one person responsible for all decisions?
- How knowledgeable is the family in recognizing risk factors and growth and development milestones?
- How and on what information are choices made regarding lifestyle?
- Are family members aware of their health behavior (or destructive behavior)?
- Are signs and symptoms recognized?
- Is medical attention sought immediately when necessary?
- Are over-the-counter medications taken or home remedies prescribed?

Self-Perception–Self-Concept Pattern

The self-perception–self-concept pattern identifies characteristics that describe the family's self-worth and feeling states. A sense of trust between the family and the nurse will assist the family in disclosing this information. Families have perceptions and concepts about their image, their status in the community, and their competency as a unit to deal with life. These perceptions and concepts are often manifested through the family's mutual strivings, values, expectations, fears, successes, and failures, shared in and complemented by the role behavior of the members. The closeness of the relationships in a family promotes the sharing of emotions and experiences. Situations that affect one member have an effect on the entire family group. How each member describes the family often gives clues as to the family's perceptions of itself.

Questions for assessment are as follows:

- What makes this family different from others?
- What special things does each member contribute to the family?
- What would each member like to see changed in the family?
- What kinds of feelings do family members have for each other?
- What is the tone of feelings in the family (indifferent, secretive, angry, or open)?

Table 7-4 Variety of Family Structures

Configuration	Positions in Family
Single parent (separated, divorced, or widowed)	Mother or father Son(s), daughter(s)
Unmarried single parent (never married)	Mother or father Son(s), daughter(s)
Unmarried couple	Two adults
Unmarried parents	Mother and father Son(s), daughter(s)
Commune family	Mothers and fathers Shared son(s), daughter(s)
Stepparents	Mother and father Son(s), daughter(s) from previous marriages
Adoptive parents	Mother and father Adopted son(s), daughter(s)

- How does the family think it fits in with the neighborhood?
- Does the family believe it is operating at its maximal potential?
- How does the family handle crisis situations?
- Has the family experienced changes in the way it feels about itself?
- Can the family relate the events that led to the change?

Roles-Relationships Pattern

This pattern identifies characteristics of family roles and relationships. Structural and functional aspects are assessed.

Structural aspects of the family include each member's name, role (mother, aunt, or sister), age, sex, education, and occupation. The family's origin (ethnic and cultural) and genetic heritage complete the family identification data. Traditionally, families have been described as nuclear (husband, wife, and children) and extended or family of orientation (aunts, uncles, cousins, and grandparents).

The prevalence of the traditional nuclear family has been influenced by societal changes, such as the women's movement, employment of mothers, and divorce and remarriage. This change has resulted in greater recognition of other family structures, such as those listed in Table 7-4. Numerous questions and unresolved issues are related to the specific effects of different family structures on child rearing and individual growth and development and pose a challenge to the nurse in health promotion and disease prevention.

Spradley (1990) has classified **divergent family structures** into three types that are of particular relevance to the nurse. The first type is the growing number of adolescent unwed mothers whose developmental needs and lack of parenting skills pose particular challenges for the nurse (Connelly, 1998). The second type refers to couples who, after widowhood or divorce, have remarried and merged two families. Merged families require considerable adjustment and relearning of roles, tasks, communication patterns, and relationships. The third type is made up of older couples or older individuals (mostly women) living alone. This group of people often needs assistance in understanding the functions and developmental tasks that would help them adjust and experience positive aging (Grabbe, Demi, Camann, & Potter, 1997).

Culin and Thyne (1986), writing about understanding and supporting families in the process of divorce, state that divorce and remarriage as a series of events involving a period of transition is important to appreciate. The process is complex and multifaceted, requiring the disintegration of one family structure and the reorganization of another. The developmental levels of the children, their individual temperaments, and the quality of their environmental support will all play a role in how the children respond. Supporting the children may be difficult for the parents, who are at the same time experiencing an adjustment to each other. How parents handle the situational crisis and accomplish the organization of the family in the post-divorce period is a significant variable in long-term individual and family adjustment.

Dietz-Omar (1991) studied family coping in stepfamilies and traditional nuclear families during pregnancy. In this study, stepfamilies emerge as "evolving" new families; therefore they need more assistance in working out roles, rules, bonding, and boundary issues within their family structures. Traditional nuclear families were experiencing a pregnancy other than a first one with their spouse and may have felt more capable of adding another child. Dietz-Omar (1991) notes that the established families may have acquired satisfactory levels of adaptability and cohesion through negotiation of behavioral and emotional involvement within the family structure.

The way in which the family is organized influences its ability to perform health-promotion and disease-prevention functions. For example, a single parent without an extended family network may be in need of community resources to help raise the children (Butcher & Gaffney, 1995; Ford-Gilboe, 1994) (Fig. 7-2). A two-parent family living near its extended family may have all the support needed to raise children, but may need to become aware of growth and development stages and immunization schedules.

An individual may experience different family forms in one lifetime. A person may be part of a nuclear family as an infant, a single-parent family after the parents are divorced, a stepparent family when the mother or father remarries, and an unmarried-couple family when the person is one of two adults who share a household. The person brings the values and beliefs about disease prevention and health promotion that were practiced in previous unions to each new family configuration. Nonshared values can result in divergent expectations unless they are integrated into a shared set of values and beliefs with the new union.

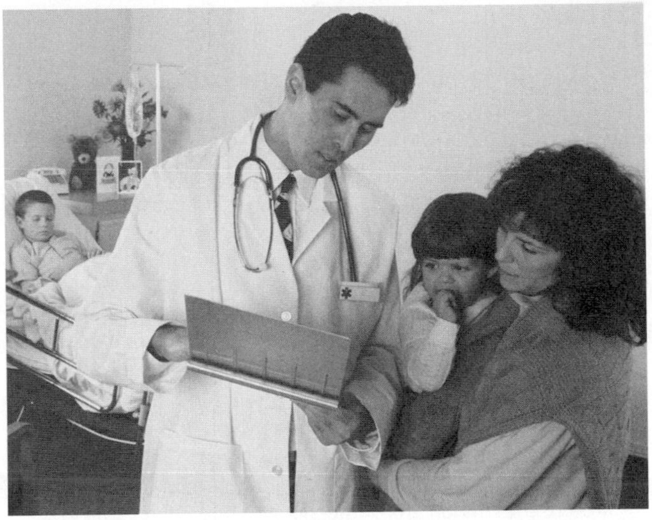

Fig. 7-2 Hospitalization of a child is stressful for any family, but especially in a single-parent household.

Shifting family forms have affected individuals in ways that could well determine the future viability of the family and the direction of the health care system.

Violence is a health problem that specifically threatens the integrity of American families. Family violence includes child abuse, spouse abuse, and elder abuse, with women being victimized especially during pregnancy. Nurses have difficulty assessing this area of family behaviors. By having an "advocacy orientation that avoids victim blaming, nurses can participate in health-promoting disease-prevention approaches to reduce violence-related injuries" (Campbell, Harris, & Lee, 1995) and deaths (Tilden, Schmidt, Limandri, Chiodo, Garland, & Loveless, 1994, p. 126).

Questions for assessment are as follows:

- What formal positions and roles do each of the family members fulfill?
- Are these roles acceptable and consistent with the family's expectations?
- Is there flexibility in roles when needed?
- What informal roles exist? Who plays them and with what consistency? What purpose do the informal roles serve?
- Who were the role models for the couples or single people as parents?
- Who were their role models as marital partners and what were their characteristics?
- How does the family manage daily living? How are the household tasks divided?
- How are problems handled? How are problems with children handled?
- Who is employed outside the home?
- Who takes care of the children when both parents are employed outside the home?
- How does the family care for its ill members? Its elderly members?

research highlights

Domestic Violence

Domestic violence may occur in as many as one of every four families in the United States. Approximately two to four million American women are physically abused each year. In the United States, the assailants of women who are victims of assault, rape, or murder are most often the victim's current or former male partner.

In this study, a cross-sectional, self-administered, anonymous survey was conducted at four community practice settings. Nurses asked 1952 female adult patients of varying ages their marital status, educational status, and economic status to complete the survey's questionnaire.

One of every 20 women in this study had experienced domestic violence within the previous year. One in five had experienced domestic violence during her adult life. One in three had experienced domestic violence either as a child or as an adult.

Women who had been recently abused were more likely to be younger than 35 years of age, single, and separated or divorced. These women were often receiving medical assistance or had no insurance. These women had more symptoms, including higher scores on measurements for depression, anxiety, somatization, and interpersonal sensitivity (low self-esteem). Additionally, these women were more likely to have a partner who was abusing drugs or alcohol and they often exhibited these tendencies also. Although they had made more suicide attempts and more frequent visits to the emergency department, these women had fewer hospitalizations. Using a multiple repression model into which the nine risk factors were entered, the likelihood of current abuse increased with the number of risk factors indicated (70.4% likelihood of current abuse when six to seven risk factors were present). Nurses should ask all female patients about domestic violence, especially when any of these risk factors are present.

Data from McCauley, J. (1995). The "battering syndrome:" Prevalence and clinical characteristics of domestic violence in primary care internal medicine practices. *Annals of Internal Medicine, 123,* 737.

- Are behaviors appropriate for family stages of development?
- Is decision making allocated to the appropriate members?
- Does the family respond appropriately to its members' developmental needs?
- Is there fair distribution of tasks among family members?
- Is the family's emotional climate conducive to growth and development?

Genogram

A useful way of viewing the family from identification data is to draw a **genogram,** or family diagram, that depicts each member of the family and shows connections between the generations. Data are gathered on at least three generations, including the current generation, their parents, and maternal and paternal grandparents, including aunts and uncles and their children. The extent of the family genogram depends on the clues leading to the familial history of health problems. Figure 7-3 depicts the accepted genogram symbols and Fig. 7-4 depicts a sample genogram of the Jeddi family. The genogram shows a variety of family structures, including family changes resulting from marriage, divorce, death, and childbearing. This type of information enables the nurse to highlight a family's health patterns and provide related anticipatory health guidance (strategies to reduce coronary artery disease).

Ecomap

Similar to the genogram, the **ecomap** is an effective form of documentation because it has visual clarity. The family genogram is labeled family or household, preceded by the family name, and placed in a circle in the center of the page. Outside the circle, smaller circles are drawn and labeled with the names of other significant people, agencies, and institutions in the family's social environment. Lines are drawn from the family-household to each circle. Straight lines indicate strong connections; a wider line indicates a strong relationship. Dotted lines reflect fragile or tenuous connections. Slashed lines signify stressful relationships. Arrows can be drawn parallel to the lines to indicate the flow of energy or resources. Figure 7-5 shows an ecomap for the Jeddi family.

Sexuality-Reproductive Pattern

Sexuality is the expression of sexual identity. The sexuality-reproductive pattern describes "patterns of satisfaction or dissatisfaction with sexuality" (Gordon, 1994), including behavioral patterns of reproduction. This pattern also includes perceptions of satisfaction or disturbances in sexuality, sexual relationships, and reproduction, such as developmental changes (menopause) throughout the lifespan (see Hot Topics box). The sexuality-reproductive pattern "includes a couple's level of satisfaction with their sexual relationship, any problems they perceive, how the problems are managed, and the results of actions taken to resolve the problems. When there are children, what information about sexual subjects is taught?" (Gordon, 1994).

Questions for assessment are as follows:

- Is the couple's sexual behavior mutually satisfying?
- Is the couple able to communicate needs to each other?
- Is there a sense of commitment, love, obligation, responsibility, and care for each other?
- Is the couple realistic in their expectations of marriage and parenthood and about their relationship as lovers?
- Are birth control measures used?
- Is the type of contraceptive used satisfactory to both partners?

The nurse takes a complete pregnancy history when indicated, including sexual practices and partners, number and ages of children, number and outcome of pregnancies, and birth control methods in use. The nurse also observes

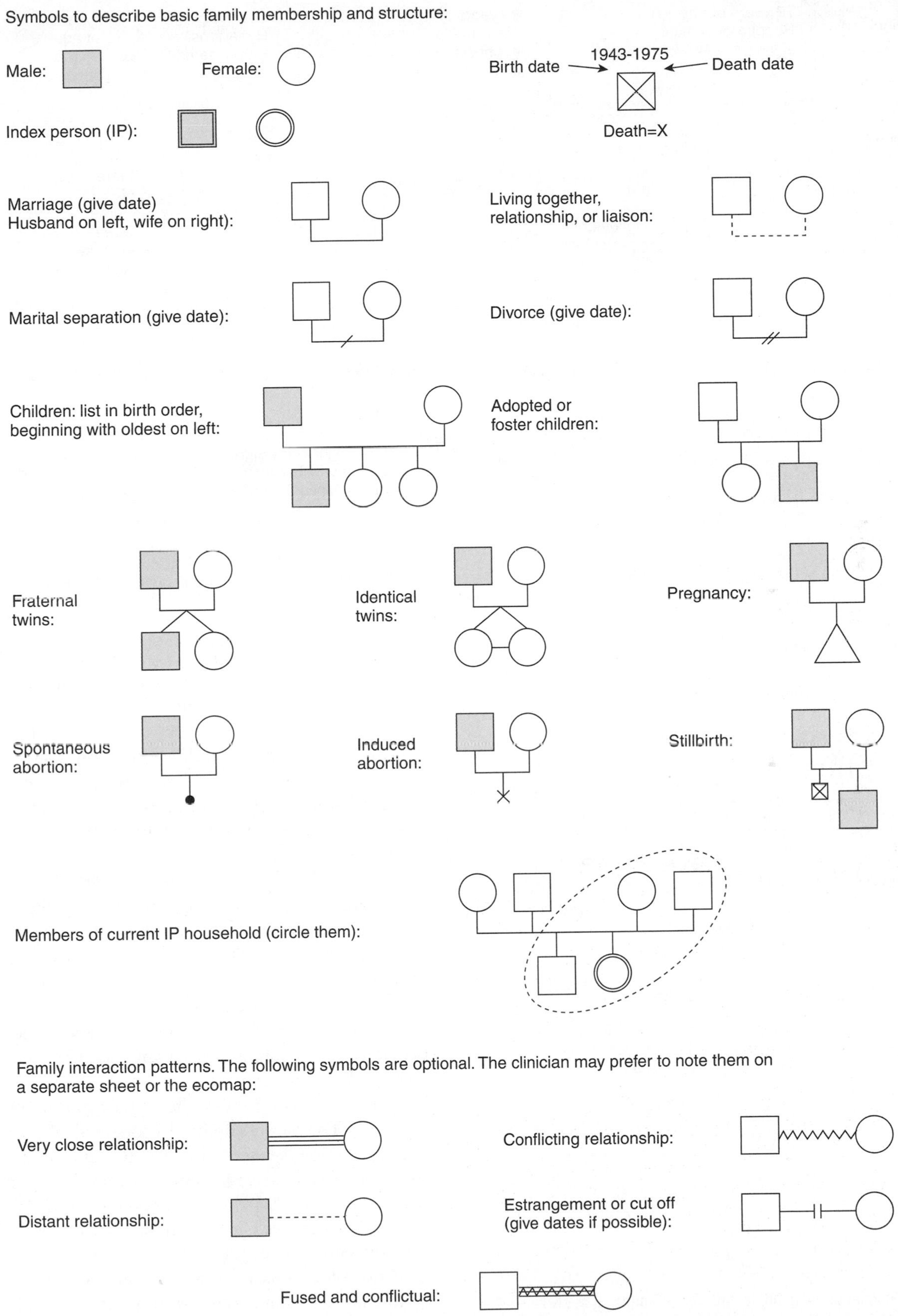

Fig. 7-3 Genogram symbols. (Modified from McGoldrick, M., & Gerson, R. [1985]. *Genograms in family assessment.* New York: Norton.)

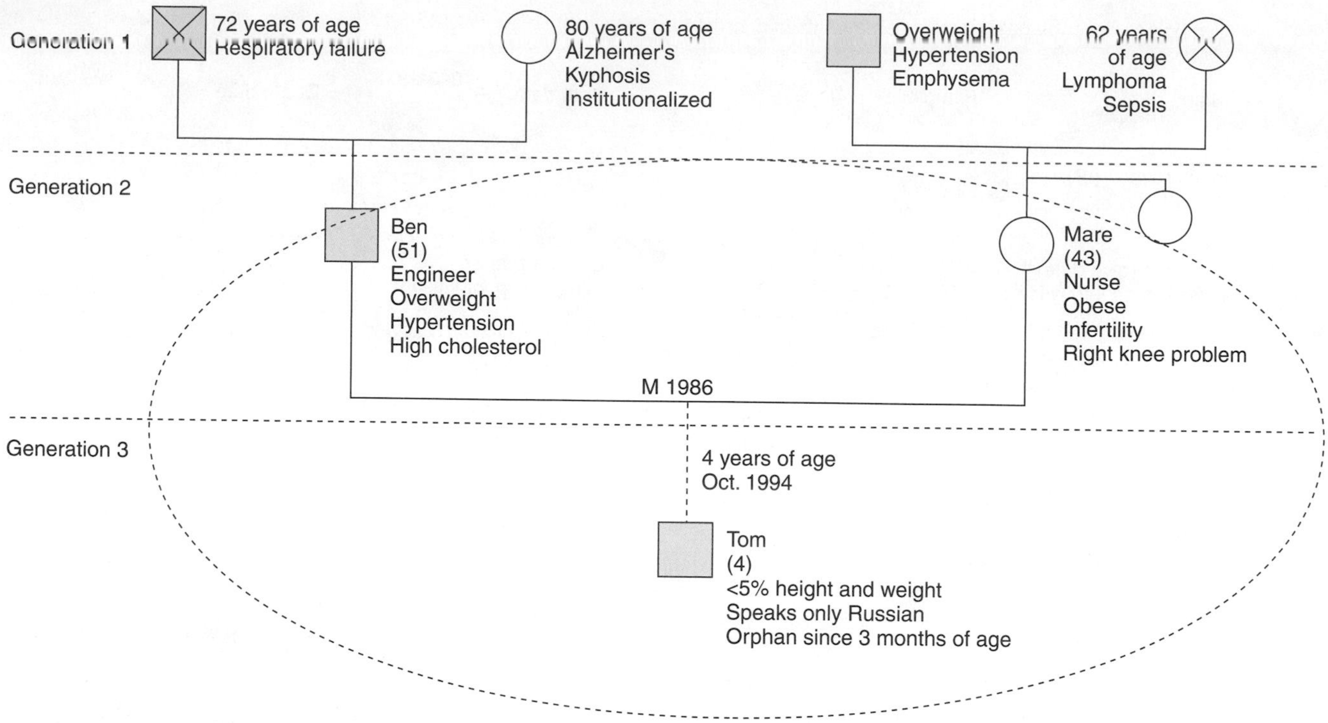

Fig. 7-4 Genogram of the Jeddi family. (From Stanhope, M., & Lancaster, J. [2000]. *Community and public health nursing* [5th ed.]. St. Louis: Mosby.)

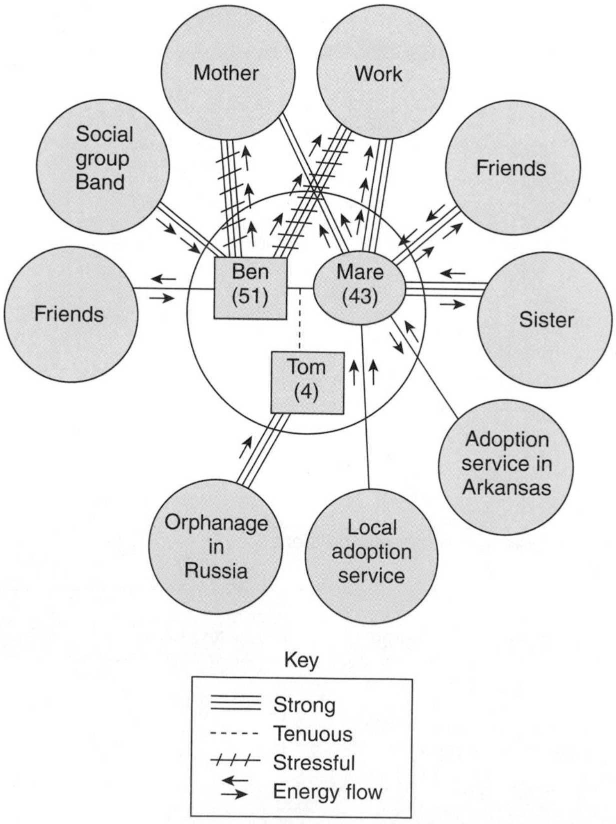

Fig. 7-5 Ecomap of the Jeddi family. (From Stanhope, M., & Lancaster, J. [2000]. *Community and public health nursing* [5th ed.]. St. Louis: Mosby.)

whether the adults seem uncomfortable when discussing sexual subjects about themselves or uninformed when discussing sexual subjects with their children. Particularly important is the nurse's responsibility to provide appropriate health assessment and information considering the variety of sexual practices within heterosexual, homosexual, and bisexual relationships, with one or more partners (Roberts & Sorensen, 1995; Stevens, 1995).

Coping–Stress-Tolerance Pattern

The coping–stress-tolerance pattern describes how the family adapts to the many internal and external changes that impinge on it. The energy for this exchange comes from within family members as they face their normal, continually evolving developmental needs and the unexpected situations that occasionally arise. The external demands on a family for change come from society's interaction with the family during the family's life cycle. The family must cope with these changes if it is to survive and grow. The family's ability to cope with the demands of everyday living is essential to its success. Family relationships can be supportive in coping or they may lead to stress. Life events such as divorce, moving, or developmental stages of the life cycle and economic hardships, such as loss of a job, can be stressful.

Questions for assessment are as follows:

- How does the family cope with stressful life events?
- What strengths does the family have and use to counterbalance the stresses?

HOT topics

TELEVISION AND SEX

Television is one of the most pervasive influences in American society. Sex permeates television programs. During significantly formative stages of sexual development, children and adolescents view thousands of sexual relationships on television that are rapid, casual, frequent, and extramarital. These sexual relationships often convey status, but rarely depict the responsibilities and consequences related to these types of relationships. Although more research is needed, evidence shows that mass media influence beliefs about sex and sexual behavior.

Nurses work with families and educators to (1) inform and provide services to children and adolescents concerning television and sexuality, (2) encourage television producers to develop more health-promoting messages about sexuality and health-related issues, and (3) promote legislation to support more effective resources for health promotion related to sexuality.

- Can the family make a realistic appraisal of the situation?
- Is the family able to make decisions based on an objective appraisal of the situation?
- What are the family's resources (use of knowledge or linkage to family networks or community resources)?
- Is the family using any dysfunctional adaptive strategies (redundant violence)?

Values-Beliefs Pattern

This pattern describes the characteristics of the family's beliefs and values and how these affect the family's behavior. Understanding what is important to a particular family is critical for assessment, diagnosis, and intervention. When values and beliefs are identified, the nurse may better understand the reasons for family dynamics, enhancing the interpretation of family behavior.

Questions for assessment are as follows:

- What are the values and beliefs held by the family? Are they related to aggressive competition and rigid, inflexible rules?
- What is the specific cultural or ethnic group with which the family identifies? Are the family's practices consistent with the norms of the ethnic group?
- What are the family's traditions and practices?
- What cultural beliefs are significant to health and illness?
- Is religion important to the family? Does the family turn to religion when difficulties arise?
- Does the family believe it can handle crisis situations?
- Does the family get what it wants out of life?
- Are there any value conflicts evident within the family?
- How do identified family values affect the health status of the family?

Data collected in the 11 functional patterns give clues to the family's health-promotion and disease-prevention practice. Risks to healthy family functioning may be identified in each pattern and some risk factors may be found in one or more areas. For example, air pollution from cigarette smoking can be easily identified as an environmental factor (home). However, the family's reaction to smoke pollution will determine the extent of the family's susceptibility (genetics). If the family has a high incidence of chronic obstructive lung disease in the nuclear extended family or in past generations and if all adult members of the family smoke (health perception and health management) and ignore the warnings of research (cognitive), then several pattern areas may indicate risk factors. However, the nurse must recognize and identify not only the risk factors, but also the interrelationships of risks and their effects on one another.

ANALYSIS AND NURSING DIAGNOSIS

Analyzing Data

After completing the data collection, the nurse and the family analyze the data. A variety of approaches is used to analyze health data, including systems theory, developmental theory, and risk-estimate theory.

From a systems approach, the family is evaluated as open or closed, with permeable or rigid boundaries in terms of change. The systems approach includes the structural and functional components of the family as a system. The 11 functional patterns are used to obtain baseline data on assessment (Box 7-4).

The **developmental theory** approaches the family from tasks and stages of progression through its life cycle. The nurse analyzes the collected data for cues that identify the stages of the family life cycle and the tasks that need to be accomplished for successful family function. The nurse then notes the family's developmental needs, considering the wide variety of family structures and functions in society. (Although the following section presents a developmental framework based on couples and children, the nurse considers the aforementioned divergent family structures and functions described by Spradley [1990].)

The stages of family development are used as a guide to categorize and analyze the baseline data. If the nurse finds gaps, missing data, or conflicting information, then efforts should be made to obtain the necessary information on the next visit.

Couple Family

The first stage of family development may or may not begin with marriage. In today's society, legal marriage may not be the basis of the relationship; nonetheless, the adults may define themselves as a family unit. Married or not, two individuals move from their family of orientation to an

Box 7-4 Eleven Functional Health Pattern Assessment Guidelines for Families

FAMILY ASSESSMENT

The 11 functional health-pattern areas are applicable to the assessment of families. Families are the focus in community health nursing. In some cases, a family assessment may be indicated (1) in the care of an infant or child whose development is influenced by family health patterns or (2) when an adult has certain health problems that can be influenced by family patterns. The following guidelines provide information on family functioning:

1. Health perception-health management pattern
   History:
   a. How has family's general health been (in last few years)?
   b. Colds in past year? Absence from work or school?
   c. Most important activities to keep healthy? Think these make a difference to health? (Include family folk remedies, when appropriate.)
   d. Members' use of cigarettes, alcohol, or drugs?
   e. Immunizations? Health care provider? Frequency of checkups? Accidents (home, work, school, or driving)? (When appropriate: storage of drugs, cleaning products, or scatter rugs.)
   f. In past, has it been easy to find ways to follow suggestions of physicians, nurses, or social workers (when appropriate)?
   g. Things important in family's health with which I could help?
   Examination:
   a. General appearance of family members and home.
   b. When appropriate: storage of medicines, cribs, playpens, stove, scatter rugs, and hazards.
2. Nutritional-metabolic pattern
   History:
   a. Typical family meal pattern or food intake? (Describe.) Supplements (vitamins, types of snacks)?
   b. Typical family fluid intake? (Describe.) Supplements: type available (fruit juices, soft drinks, or coffee)?
   c. Appetites?
   d. Dental problems? Dental care (frequency)?
   e. Skin problems? Healing problems?
   Examination:
   a. When opportunity available: refrigerator contents, meal preparation, or contents of meal?
3. Elimination pattern
   History:
   a. Family use of laxatives or other aids?
   b. Problems in waste and garbage disposal?
   c. Pet or animals' waste disposal (indoor and outdoor)?
   d. When indicated: problems with flies, roaches, or rodents?
   Examination:
   a. When opportunity available: examine toilet facilities, garbage disposal, and pet waste disposal; indicators of risk for flies, roaches, and rodents.
4. Activity-exercise pattern
   History:
   a. In general, does family get a lot or little exercise? Type? Regularity?
   b. Family leisure activities? Active or passive?
   c. Problems in shopping (transportation), cooking, keeping up the house, budgeting for food, clothes, housekeeping, house costs?
   Examination:
   a. Pattern of general home maintenance and personal maintenance.
5. Sleep-rest pattern
   History:
   a. Generally, family members seem to be well rested and ready for schoolwork?
   b. Sufficient sleeping space and quiet?
   c. Family finds time to relax?
   Examination:
   a. When opportunity available: observe sleeping space and arrangements.
6. Cognitive-perceptual pattern
   History:
   a. Visual or hearing problems? How managed?
   b. Any big decisions family has had to make? How made?
   Examination:
   a. When indicated: language spoken at home.
   b. Grasp of ideas and questions (abstract or concrete).
   c. Vocabulary level.
7. Self-perception–self-concept pattern
   History:
   a. Most of time family feels good (not good) about themselves as a family?
   b. General mood of family? Happy? Anxious? Depressed? What helps family mood?
   Examination:
   a. Mood state generally nervous = 5 or relaxed = 1; rate from 1 to 5.
   b. Members generally assertive = 5 or passive = 1; rate from 1 to 5.
8. Roles-relationship pattern
   History:
   a. Family (or household) members? Member age and family structure (diagram).
   b. Any family problems that are difficult to handle (nuclear or extended)? Child rearing? When appropriate: spouse or parents (should be included if children are interviewed) ever get rough with you? The children?
   Family Assessment:
   c. Relationships good (not good) among family members? Siblings? Support each other?
   d. When appropriate: income sufficient for needs?

From Gordon, M. (2000). *Manual of nursing diagnosis: 1999-2000*. St. Louis: Mosby.

Continued

Box 7-4 Eleven Functional Health-Pattern Assessment Guidelines for Families—cont'd

e. Feel part of (or isolated from) community? Neighbors?

Examination:

a. Interaction among family members (when present).
b. Family leadership roles.

9. Sexuality-reproductive pattern

History:

a. When appropriate (sexual partner within household or situation): sexual relations satisfying? Changes? Problems?
b. Use of family planning? Contraceptives? Problems?
c. When appropriate (to age of children): feel comfortable in explaining or discussing sexual subjects?

Examination: None

10. Coping–stress tolerance pattern

History:

a. Any major changes within family in last few years?
b. Family tense or relaxed most of time? When tense, what helps? Use of medicines, drugs, or alcohol to decrease tension?
c. When (if) family problems, how handled?
d. Most of the time is this way or these ways successful?

Examination: None

11. Values-beliefs pattern

History:

a. Generally, family gets what it wants out of life?
b. Important goals for the future?
c. Any "rules" in the family that everyone believes are important?
d. Religion important in family? Does this help when difficulties arise?

Examination: None

unfamiliar couple relationship. One of the tasks of each individual is to adapt to the role expectations of the other. Analysis of critical family developmental tasks includes establishing a mutually satisfying adult relationship that fits into the kinship network. The major adjustment for the couple is learning how to mesh two personalities, two life histories, and two aspirations of growth. Major decisions in this stage include whether the partners both work, how money (making, spending, and saving) is handled, where they are going to live, how they are going to relate to in-laws and other family members, and if and when to have children. Other decisions, consciously or unconsciously made, are the sharing of the work-load tasks of cooking, washing, cleaning, and shopping.

Integrating health practices and habits into the lifestyle of the couple is a health-related developmental task that requires consideration during analysis. Health behavior constitutes particular actions taken toward promotion of health and prevention of disease; for example, following a hygienic practice; participating in well-balanced programs of rest, exercise, and balanced diet; attending smoking-cessation classes; wearing seat belts; and directing activities toward the attainment of self-actualization. Each individual brings values and beliefs from the family of origin and develops other values and beliefs from personal experiences. Consciously working out health practices that are going to be part of the couple's lifestyle will promote health as a value at the beginning of the family life cycle.

Achieving a mutually satisfying relationship depends on the way the couple is able to handle conflicts and differences. When the method the couple uses to solve problems is congruent with each individual, adjustments can be made that will prove satisfying to both partners. If one individual is in the habit of solving problems by avoiding conflict at any price, then problem solving will tend to be ineffective.

If the decision to adopt or give birth to a child is made, then commitment to long-term responsibilities becomes a focus of family development and a primary health need. The nurse, in analyzing the learning needs of the pregnant couple, considers all aspects of the couple's decision and motivations that may be involved with the pregnancy. With single-parent families becoming increasingly common through divorce, death, adoption, or the choice to have a child out of wedlock, the analysis of data must consider the special needs of these family structures (Rosenwald & Demi, 1993).

The free attitudes and practices in society regarding sexuality have given rise to risks of sexually transmitted diseases such as genital herpes, gonorrhea, and syphilis. Acquired immunodeficiency syndrome (AIDS), the most recent sexually transmitted disease, was first described in 1981. AIDS is a disease with a unique set of problems that poses a threat to the individual and therefore to the family and society. The human immunodeficiency virus (HIV) can be transmitted through heterosexual, homosexual, or oral sexual intercourse and through direct contact with infected blood, shared needles during intravenous drug use, and perinatal transfer from infected mothers to their infants. Prevention of HIV transmission requires either abstinence from or modification of relevant behaviors and adherence to safety precautions for health care workers who handle infectious bodily fluids.

Risk factors associated with sexuality include lack of knowledge about "safer sex," anatomy and physiology of the reproductive system and personal hygiene, lack of prenatal care, pregnancy before age 16 and after age 35, a history of hypertension and infection during pregnancy, and unplanned or unwanted pregnancy.

Risk factors for premature pregnancies and unsatisfying marriage are lack of knowledge about family planning, age (adolescents are more at risk and people in their late 20s are less at risk), and lack of knowledge concerning sexual and role adjustments. In unplanned adolescent pregnancies, the parents place an undue biological risk on their developing child. Lack of knowledge about prenatal care, birthing, and child-rearing practices compounds the risks for both the mother and the child. Parents who are unable to carry out the role functions of parenting are at risk for an unsatisfying relationship and an inappropriate developmental growth at the beginning stage of the family life cycle.

If the couple decides to remain childless, then its learning needs may focus on available methods of contraception.

Childbearing Family

The birth or adoption of a child is the beginning of a new family unit. All members of the family must learn new roles as the unit expands in functions and responsibilities. The parents' history as a dyad and their experiences in other groups, particularly their families of origin, will influence the way the triad develops (see Multicultural Awareness box).

The family may lose equilibrium while the couple is exploring ways to accommodate the new member into the group. As a group, the three explore ways to meet each other's needs, to minimize differences, and to work together. First-time parents often feel a lack of emotional support during the first several months of parenthood. The first days after the birth or adoption can be especially trying when the couple has no network of family or friends on which it can depend for support. Analysis of needs during this critical time can be effective in helping the new parents. Parents may be proficient in caring for the child's needs, but may lack the ability to feel any self-growth in the parenting role. If the mother had been working, then she may find the routines of baby care and being in the house all day boring. The father may be anxious about one income being inadequate to support the family and may increase his workload. Both parents may be exhausted from working full time and providing child care. The demands are even greater for single parents (usually the mother). Neither parent may be able to offer the other emotional support if neither has been able to find satisfaction in parenthood. As the childbearing family struggles to adapt to a new member, the family of origin or other support system (self-help groups, neighbors, or friends) may be called for assistance (Niska, Snyder, & Lia-Hoagberg, 1999; Polomeno, 1998, 1999).

Some parents thrive during the period when an infant needs almost total and constant care and nurturing. These parents are able to find support in each other and in a network of family and friends. The couple who finds satisfaction in parenthood seems to realize that parental influence begins at birth and is the single most important factor in the child's physical, emotional, and cognitive development; they are therefore ready to assume the responsibility. The parents' ability to assume responsibility depends largely on their own maturity; how they were nurtured as children; their conceptions about self, culture, social class, and religion; their relationship with each other; their values and philosophy of life; their perceptions of and experiences with children and other adults; and the life stresses they have experienced. A direct relationship has been found between the degree of emotional health of children and the degree to which the relationship between the parents was positive.

In analyzing child-rearing needs of the family, the nurse considers these factors and the family's developmental task of providing for the physical health, economic support, and nurturing actions vital to the child's learning and social development. In analyzing the couple's needs during this stage, the nurse must be aware of the interactions among the triad. Observing the way decisions are made concerning needs will demonstrate how the family functions, what roles each member has, and how effectively the family meets the needs of all its members.

Risks associated with role relationships include working parents with insufficient resources for child care, abuse or neglect of children, multiple closely spaced children, low family self-esteem, children used as scapegoats for parental frustration, immature parents who are dependent and unable to handle responsibility, and strong beliefs about physical punishment or obedience.

MULTICULTURAL AWARENESS

Preconception Care

Preconception care is a significant health-promotion opportunity for the whole family. The importance of this care has been recognized by *Healthy People 2010,* the Institute of Medicine, and the Public Health Services Expert Panel on the Content of Prenatal Care.

One important area of preconception care is evaluating a couple's genetic history as documented on the standard family genogram. Further evaluation should be considered for couples who are related outside marriage or who have ethnic backgrounds such as Mediterranean, Black, or Ashkenazic Jew and women older than 35 years of age or younger than 16 years of age who have preexisting medical conditions. Couples who have a history of any of the following health problems should be referred for further genetic testing and counseling: cystic fibrosis, hemophilia, phenylketonuria, Tay-Sachs disease, thalassemia, sickle-cell disease or trait, birth defects, or mental retardation.

Family with Preschool Children

This family may have more than one child, each growing and developing at an individual pace. Preschool children place great demands on the family; the family must adjust to each new member who comes into the group and must provide space and equipment for expansion.

The home environment must be adapted to the critical needs and interests of preschool children. In analyzing data about the home, the nurse observes whether the child has stimulation-promoting opportunities to experience and explore. The home should be made safe while allowing for exploration by the child. Rather than keeping children away from the kitchen or garden, ways to include the child into a cooking or planting activity will provide learning experiences for the child. Other environmental influences that will affect the child's rate and style of development include religious practices, ethnic background, education, and disciplinary techniques.

Increasing evidence shows that the onset of ill health is linked strongly to environmental influences. In the home environment, contamination of air, water, and food increases health risks. For example, lead poisoning, a preventable disease that continues to affect thousands of children, can be the result of lead paint and other factors in the home. Although lead-based paint has been restricted to the exterior of homes in the United States, many homes still have it on interior walls. Both the home and the automobile should be considered as possible sources of exposure to the poisonous agent carbon. The nurse also reviews data for safety in the home.

Developmental tasks for the family include adjusting to energy depletion in the couple while they are responding to the demands of parenthood and each other. The nurse may be required to explore alternative means of finding relief from parenting for the couple. Parents need time for themselves and they need to know their children are safe with a responsible person; economic restraints may make this balance difficult.

The family with preschoolers must be aware of the health-promotion habits of proper foods, exercise, sleep, and dental hygiene. Through their example, the routines they provide for the children and their use of positive reinforcement, the parents can do much in teaching the preschooler about health.

Family with School-Aged Children

The family with children in school may have reached its maximal size in numbers and interrelationships. The parents' major problem during this stage is the dichotomy between self-interest and finding fulfillment in rearing the next generation. The family's developmental tasks revolve around the major goals of reorganization to prepare for the expanding world of school-aged children. Promoting school achievement is one of the critical tasks in the socialization of children. Viewing social and educational goals in terms of family culture and the parent's defined goals is particularly important in this stage of development. For example, many opportunities for health education exist in schools for influencing children to develop desirable health habits and to acquire positive health beliefs. However, parental pressure has caused health education in the school to be oriented toward problems such as smoking, drugs, and alcohol abuse. The message given is that health is oriented toward problems and crises when the children should be learning the positive aspects of healthy behaviors. As a result, neither the school nor the home may be providing the school-aged child with skills that involve developing values about health and making decisions about risk-taking behaviors and their consequences. During this period of development, the family can be influential at home and in school in teaching children how to assess risks for engaging in certain behaviors and what benefits to expect when practicing other behaviors.

As activity broadens inside and outside the home, another important developmental task during this stage for both parent and child is letting go. Parents are likely to be involved in community groups such as the parent-teacher association, scout groups, sports teams, and other volunteer organizations. The mother may enter the workforce or renew educational opportunities. Encouraging children to join in the family discussions that establish policies and make decisions fosters a positive self-concept in children. The group's position on health practices is included in family policies and decisions.

During this stage, the family is vulnerable to risk factors such as an unsafe and unstimulating home, repeated infections, abuse and neglect of children, poverty, and low family self-esteem. Children exposed to an unstimulating and unsafe home environment are at risk for behavior disturbances, school problems, and learning disabilities. Parents who cannot manage their children in growth-promoting ways soon experience depletion of energy and may turn to unorthodox ways of finding relief from parenting.

Family with Adolescents

Families with adolescent members may experience a "change-in-life pregnancy," which means the parents are caring for an infant while other children in the family are in school. Having a new member enter the family at this stage may be a source of joy or a source of frustration for the family. The overall goal with adolescent members is loosening family ties to allow greater responsibility and freedom in preparation for releasing young adults. While each member of the family is working through individual developmental tasks in the midst of social pressures, the family as a whole has tasks to accomplish. Strengthening the marital relationship to build a foundation for future family stages is a critical task during this time.

Open communication, a critical developmental task at

this stage, may be difficult between parents and adolescents because there is often mutual rejection by parents and adolescents of one another's values and lifestyles. Family values and standards are questioned and challenged. Although the mother and father clearly hold the balance of power in deciding who will do what (who uses the family car and how the family money is spent), adolescents may want to do what their friends do, have their own car, and make their own money to spend in ways that they see fit. Parents who give adolescent members opportunities to experience social, emotional, and ethical situations with others are providing learning opportunities for enhancing a sense of autonomy and responsibility.

As adolescents mature and emancipate themselves, families must deal with the developmental task of balancing freedom with responsibility. Health problems in this age group include violent deaths, injuries, and alcohol and drug abuse. Contributing risk factors include lack of problem-solving skills, family values of aggressiveness and competition, socioeconomic factors contributing to peer relationships, rigid and inflexible family values, daredevil risk-taking attitudes, and conflicts between parents and children. The family cannot readily decrease many environmental risks to violent deaths and injuries; some responsibility lies with the highway system, automobile manufacturers, and the legislation of standards of safety. The family must rely largely on the efforts of public health officials and others to reduce these environmental risks.

However, the family can be a supportive force for adolescents in this stage of development by including them in the decision-making process and by allowing them to choose alternative behaviors and experience the positive and negative consequences. Having made a choice, a commitment to the chosen behavior will follow. Family values of winning and not losing, aggressiveness, and competition may need to be reexamined during this period; the adolescent may decide that these values are no longer applicable. The change in values in the adolescent may produce conflict and pose a threat to the family, which may respond by placing an undue amount of pressure on the adolescent to conform to family values. In matters of life and death, parents must be firm and take a stand; for example, "No driving when drinking!"

This stage of family development may be viewed as an identity crisis in the adolescent, the adults, and the family as a whole. The adolescent is moving from childhood to adulthood while the adult is passing from parent to nonparent. The adolescent is struggling to find an identity independent of, but connected to, the family. Adults are in midlife and must come to terms with their own adolescent fantasies and decide who they are and who they will be for the rest of their lives.

Family with Young Adults

This family is seen as a launching center because children begin to leave home. In letting their children go, parents are relinquishing many years of the parenting role and returning to their original marital dyad. The couple builds a new life together while maintaining relationships with aging parents, children, grandchildren, and in-laws.

A couple may find it difficult to redefine their relationship. For the woman, her role as mother is changing because the children no longer need her in the same way. If she has devoted the past 20 years to raising children, then she might feel unneeded and lacking in purpose. She may decide to enter the workforce for the first time and might need help in the transition. The man might be at the peak of his career or realize he will not progress further. In addition to individual changes occurring between the couple, the family with young adults can experience other pressures. Aging parents in the extended family might need assistance and children might need financial and emotional support in leaving home for college, marriage, or work. Financial and emotional responsibilities to other members of the family can prevent the couple from focusing on themselves and their marital relationship during this developmental phase.

Health-promoting activities that can be enhanced during this stage include coping with pressures of social and occupational responsibilities and mobility, recognizing the importance of good health habits and practices, accepting aging in oneself and in the marital partner, and reassessing life goals.

Family with Middle-Age Adults

This family may consist of only two members; thinking of oneself and enhancing self-concept and the marital relationship typically occur at this time. Usually the children have all left home and the parents are experiencing a new sense of freedom and well being. Some marriages, having made it to this stage, have a certain amount of security and stability; the couple has reached an understanding about meeting each other's needs. The pressures of parenting have lifted and the couple can enjoy the accomplishments of their children and grandchildren. The couple has probably lived in a neighborhood long enough to have acquired a network of friends. Long-time acquaintances seek their participation in neighborhood rituals and events. Economic security and personal self-esteem may be at a peak for the couple.

By contrast, some marriages that have made it to this stage may be in trouble. The last child departing from home may create the "empty-nest syndrome." If the couple is not prepared for this stage, then the individuals might look elsewhere for opportunities to enhance self-concept. The husband, thinking that his father role is no longer necessary, may look for a younger wife with whom to begin a new family. The wife, no longer feeling needed by her children or husband, may turn to alcohol, drugs, or other self-destructive behaviors. Both husband and wife might be experiencing problems particular to their sex and unable to turn to each other for the necessary support.

Health tasks in this developmental stage require a new awareness from susceptibility or vulnerability to illness and disease in this age group. The couple must become aware of the risks to health and adjust their lifestyle and habits to cope with them. Losses at this stage can also cause health problems; the couple may have to cope with the deaths of family members and friends and a declining income. If the husband or wife has developed a physical or mental illness, then the other may have to adjust to the current physical and mental capabilities. A redefining of self-concept may be necessary.

Middle-age families are susceptible to a host of risk factors leading to the three most prevalent causes of death: (1) heart disease, (2) cancer, and (3) cerebrovascular accident (stroke). The family lifestyle may help to decrease risks by placing a high value on physical activity, not smoking, maintaining adequate and sound nutritional habits, and consuming moderate amounts of alcohol. Lifestyle habits that are transmitted through role modeling have a greater influence on the younger members of the family than any verbal edict. When possible, middle-age members can be instrumental in choosing an environment that is free or low in water pollution and air pollution and free from crippling stress factors such as excessive noise, traffic, and overcrowding. Family members can also apply pressure on key persons in the community to decrease risks in the environment.

Family with Older Adults

Adjustment to retirement is one of the crucial tasks of the family with older adults. Retirement affects many aspects of a person, including relationships with others. Besides a loss of work, retirement also means a sharp reduction in income for most people. Adjusting living standards to retirement income and being able to supplement this income with wage-earning activity is a task of the aging family. Other tasks during this stage include adjusting the home environment to be safe and comfortable and adjusting to the loss of a spouse, which may require the surviving member to look to the family for support and satisfaction (Demi & Miles, 1986, 1987). Illness may create further dependence on family members (Given & Given, 1998).

Health promotion during this stage is directed toward maintaining functional ability, limiting the effects of disabling conditions, and maintaining the quality of life. Older adults may fear being helpless and useless and unable to care for themselves. In analyzing risk factors in the aging family, the nurse looks at the couple's ability to function well enough to carry out normal roles and responsibilities. As with all persons, older adults hope for a state of well being that will allow them to function at their highest capacity physically, psychologically, socially, and spiritually. Many older adults remain in their own homes, and the majority are vigorous and completely independent. Only five percent of older adults reside in institutions and many of these people are temporary residents who are recovering from illness and who expect to return to the community.

Ego integrity (the union of all previous phases of the life cycle) is the challenge in this stage and demands successful aging through continued activity. Having gone through the various stages of family development, the couple accepts what they have done as their own. At this time, they may need family or professional support to pursue other interests or maintain former activities to feel needed and useful.

As another approach to data analysis, the nurse and family compare the information to documented norms of health promotion and disease prevention in older adults. Norms or expected values can be derived from the family's baseline information of 11 functional pattern areas, knowledge of growth and development for all age groups and the family as a whole, risk-factor estimates, and the population norms.

Population norms specify a range of normal limits for these particular groups. For example, age is associated with various risk factors; some disorders are so common that they are called "diseases of the older person." In certain diseases, such as lung cancer, a long period is associated with long-term exposure. When risk increases with cumulative exposure, the frequency of the disease increases with age. Gender is related to various risk factors (breast cancer in women).

Analysis of data on values, beliefs, self-perception, or role relationships with general population norms may not be as easy; the nurse must also consider cultural, ethnic, and religious factors. Analysis may have to be based on whether the family perceives the situation to be a problem or a potential problem. What the nurse identifies as a problem may not be perceived as a problem by the family (Denham, 1999a; Green, 1997; Niska, Snyder, & Lia-Hoagberg, 1999). The family's baseline information is important because it provides comparative criteria in the analysis. Reviewing previous records of the family might also be useful in obtaining this data. When no previous record exists, the information taken on first contact provides criteria for subsequent measurement of progress.

In developing increased awareness or consciousness of a family's health (by the family and the nurse) the nurse may want to reflect on Newman's definitions of family health (1995), which are based on a synthesis of disease and nondisease (Box 7-5).

Formulating Family Nursing Diagnoses

The purpose of writing a **family nursing diagnosis** is to help the family promote health through the life cycle and prevent disease through low risk-taking behaviors. The nurse derives the diagnosis from assessed validated data. As a concise summary statement of a problem or potential problem, the diagnosis provides direction for outcomes and interventions by identifying the negative health state and the factors that must be changed to alleviate or prevent it (see Chapter 6). Table 7-5 provides examples of family nursing diagnoses using developmental and risk factor approaches.

Describing the health of the family and validating the potential or actual health problems with the family are important; cooperation occurs only when the nurse and family agree on the situation. If the family does not agree, then further assessment or negotiation may be needed. The family and the nurse must also agree on the sequence of problem resolution.

The **cultural competence** of the nurse is an essential component of the nursing process. "Within the heterogeneous society our nation has become, a necessary component of cultural competence is an understanding of and respect for the belief and priorities of the families being served" (Yoos, Kitzman, Olds, Overacker 1995, p. 343). This knowledge increases the efficacy of health promotion for all families, especially those from extraordinarily vulnerable populations.*

Box 7-5 Newman's Definitions of Family Health

1. Health encompasses family situations in which one or more family members may be diagnosed as ill
2. The illness of family members can be considered a manifestation of the pattern of the family interaction (the child with anorexia nervosa is often found in a family with an enmeshed pattern of interaction in which the boundaries between family members are unclear) (Minuchin, Rossman, & Baker, 1966)
3. Elimination of the disease condition in the identified ill family members will not change the overall pattern of the family. In some families, when one member changes a behavior, another will assume that role; for example, depression as a result of absorbing conflict by the peacemaker (Swanson, personal communication, to Margaret A. Newman, Sept. 7, 1981)
4. If one person becoming ill is the only way that the family can become more conscious of its pattern, then that is health (in process) for that family (the depression of one family member is not an isolated incident to be viewed as an entity in and of itself, but as a manifestation of the pattern of interaction of the family)
5. Health is the expansion of consciousness (informational capacity) of the family. As the quantity and quality of responses of family members increase, spontaneity within the family increases. Members are no longer locked into limited responses and growth can occur

PLANNING WITH THE FAMILY

A plan of intervention is designed after completion of the assessment, analysis, and nursing diagnosis. The purpose of the plan is to bring about some behavioral change in the family that will promote health or prevent dysfunction. As in the assessment phase, the family is an active participant in the planning process; the degree of responsibility that the family assumes for personal health status is important to the success of behavioral change outcomes. The planning process involves several steps with the nurse and family identifying the following:

1. Order of priority for problems or potential problems
2. Items that can be handled by the nurse and the family and items that must be referred to others
3. Actions and expected outcomes

The planning phase is completed with the nursing plan, which provides direction for implementation of the plan and the framework for evaluation.

*Bailey, 1987; Friedman, 1990; Hill, 1993; Kerr & Ritchey, 1990; McLoyd, 1990; Rorie, Paine, & Barger, 1996; Yoos, H. L., Kitzman, H., Olds, D. L., Overacker, I. 1995.

Table 7-5 Examples of Family Nursing Diagnoses

Theoretical Model	Stage	Health Status	Pattern	Problem
Developmental	Family with preschoolers	Potential for physical injury	Health-perception–health management pattern	Medications and poisonous cleaning substances within reach of children
	Family with adolescents	Potential alteration in parenting	Roles-relationships pattern	Value systems of parents and adolescent members in conflict
	Family with older adults	Grieving	Roles-relationships pattern	Loss of spouse
Risk factors	Young couple	Compromised and ineffective	Coping–stress-tolerance pattern	Teenage marriage Pregnancy before age 16
	Middle-age adults	Reactive and situational depression	Self-perception–self-concept pattern	Feelings of failure Inability to relate to spouse and children Alcohol and drug abuse

As mentioned, a family's health status can be diagnosed as functional, potentially dysfunctional, or dysfunctional. When the family's health status is considered functional, the nurse verifies the situation and a plan for periodic reevaluation of the family's health status is formulated jointly. Plans to continue healthy living behaviors are reinforced and specific information that the family requests or requires is given, such as immunization schedules, growth and development milestones, and recommended dietary allowances. The family is instructed to seek further

CARE PLAN

Nursing Diagnosis: Risk for Caregiver-Role Strain Related to Caring for a Family Member With Alzheimer's Disease

DEFINING CHARACTERISTICS

- Feeling exhausted
- Inability to complete caregiving tasks
- Declining health status
- Feeling depressed
- Feeling loss of usual or expected relationship with care receiver
- Grieving
- Increased stress or nervousness
- Increased emotional liability
- Preoccupation with care routine
- Family conflict
- Withdrawal from social contacts
- Change in leisure activities
- Sleep pattern disturbance
- Low self-esteem

RELATED FACTORS

- Illness severity of care receiver
- Increasing care needs of care receiver
- Addiction or codependency of caregiver or care receiver
- Conflicting role demands
- Caregiver health impairment
- No previous experience in caregiver role
- Discharge of family member with significant home care needs
- Unpredictable illness course or instability in the care receiver's health
- Psychological or cognitive problems in the care receiver
- Caregiver not developmentally ready for caregiving role
- Developmental delay or retardation of the care receiver or caregiver
- Marginal family adaptation or dysfunction before caregiving situation
- Marginal coping patterns of caregiver
- Providing direct, ongoing in-home care
- History of poor relationship between caregiver and care receiver
- Care receiver exhibits deviant, bizarre behavior
- Incontinence in the care receiver

EXPECTED OUTCOMES

- Caregiver describes current obligations and the challenges that lie ahead
- Caregiver distinguishes obligations that must be fulfilled from those that can be controlled or limited
- In conjunction with the nurse, the caregiver develops a plan of care for the patient
- Caregiver demonstrates the ability to follow the plan of care
- Caregiver receives and accepts appropriate levels of support from family members, friends, and others
- Caregiver describes help available from informal and formal support systems in the community and takes steps to obtain help

INTERVENTIONS

- Assess the level of the caregiver's stress. A number of tools are available for this purpose; for example, *Alzheimer's: A Caregiver's Guide and Source Book*, by Howard Gruetzner
- Describe the five stages of Alzheimer's disease (early and late confusional states and early, middle, and late dementia); discuss the characteristics of each stage and ways to respond to the patient's behavioral problems that may occur in each stage
- Assist the caregiver in developing a realistic plan of care, considering the patient's abilities and limitations; the plan will require modification as the patient decompensates
- Instruct the caregiver to encourage the patient to participate, to the greatest extent possible, in social and self-care activities such as bathing, dressing, dining out with friends, and playing cards
- Facilitate a family meeting to help the primary caregiver seek assistance from other family members
- Support the caregiver and family members as they adjust to the degenerative nature of the disease; be aware that over time the stress associated with caring for the patient increases
- Identify community resources that may offer the caregiver relief from constant supervision of the patient (home health aides, respite care, and adult day care)
- Help the caregiver contact informal sources of support, such as church groups, extended family, and community volunteers
- When the patient is taking drugs approved for Alzheimer's disease, ensure that the caregiver understands the dosages, side effects, and signs and symptoms to report to the physician
- Encourage the caregiver to attend an Alzheimer's support group
- Refer the caregiver to The Alzheimer's Association

Adapted from Sparks, S. M., & Taylor, C. M. (1998). *Nursing diagnosis reference manual* (4th ed.). Springhouse, PA: Springhouse.

assistance when necessary. In working with healthy families, the nurse controls the assessment and analysis phases of the nursing process. If the health status is judged functional, then the planning of health education materials, the scheduling of periodic examinations, and the accessibility of the nurse are all professional responsibilities. The implementation and evaluation of the health-promotion activities are the family's responsibilities.

In setting priorities in health promotion and disease prevention, a life-threatening situation is rarely encountered. However, when the family's data reveal this type of situation, the identified problem receives the highest priority of intervention. For other identified potential or actual problems, the nurse relies on the family to decide which problem or potential problem to approach. After the ordering of priorities is established, the family and nurse determine who will work on the problem.

Problems or potential problems that can be resolved by the nurse are identified separately from those that need referral or the family's intervention. Problems that the family can handle or those with which the family is already involved are considered strengths and should be acknowledged and supported by the nurse. For example, when there is consistency among values and actions, physical fitness, weight management, and ability to cope with stress, the family is already taking informed and responsible action in these areas. The extent to which family members can provide their own health promotion and disease prevention will depend on their knowledge, skills, motivation, and orientation toward health.

Problems that need medical, legal, or social attention should be referred to appropriate agencies. The nurse should have a directory of available resources in the community to consult when referrals are needed.

Problems that need nursing interventions must be stated in nursing actions that are clear, purposeful, moral, capable of being accomplished, and adapted to the particular life situation, beliefs, and expectations of the family.

Goals

A goal is a statement describing a desired outcome. Included in the family outcome are expected behaviors of the family, the circumstances under which the behaviors will be demonstrated, and the criteria by which to determine when and how the behaviors will be performed. Health-promotion goals reflect a desire to function at a higher level of health and to grow beyond maintaining health or preventing disease, as illustrated in Box 7-6.

Box 7-6 Nursing Diagnosis Goals and Examples

NURSING DIAGNOSIS	GOAL
Family coping; potential for growth hindered by inadequate understanding of response to stress.	Each family member will observe and record reactions in tense situations for 1 week.
Potential alteration in parents' busy schedules.	All family members will participate in a recreational activity together once a week.

Health-promotion goals reflect a desire to change a health habit that indicates a potential problem before signs and symptoms appear as follows:

NURSING DIAGNOSIS	GOAL
Inadequate coping skills to handle smoking cessation.	Family will support member who enrolls in a smoking-cessation program.
Alteration in nutrition: potential obesity; excessive caloric intake.	Family will reduce caloric intake by 500 calories per day.
Knowledge deficit of relaxation skills.	Family will practice a relaxation response taught by the nurse.

Both the nurse and the individual are partners in goal formation. The nurse contributes knowledge and understanding of the various implications of the nursing diagnosis; the individual brings motivation and the family's unique perspective to the problem. Together their contributions determine the goal outcome and increase the family's level of health.

After goals are established for the appropriate diagnosis, objectives are developed that specify how to reach these goals. Usually a number of objectives are written for each goal because several goals may exist for each nursing diagnosis. For example:

NURSING DIAGNOSIS	GOALS	OBJECTIVES
Potential for health management deficit from sedentary lifestyle.	Decrease risk for hypertension.	Take brisk walk four times a week for 45 minutes each time. Buy blood pressure cuff and learn to take own blood pressure. Have blood pressure checked at clinic every 3 months.
	Maintain desired weight of 190 pounds.	Keep 24-hour record of food intake for 1 week. Cut calories to lose one pound every 2 weeks for 6 months. Plan exercise regimen and caloric intake to maintain weight.

IMPLEMENTATION WITH THE FAMILY

Implementation is putting the nursing plan into action. The implementation phase is not to be considered unchangeable. As the nurse and family work together, new information is used to adapt and change the plan as necessary. **Family nursing interventions** are aimed at assisting the family in carrying out functions that the members cannot perform for themselves. In health promotion and disease prevention, the nurse assists the family in improving their capacity to act on its own behalf (Hatrick, 2000).

Families may know that they are taking risks by smoking, drinking, and engaging in a stressful lifestyle. As the nurse explains the rationale behind the proposed changes, the family may choose to deny that they are jeopardizing their future health and may simply continue with their risk-taking behaviors. This situation tests the nurse's ingenuity; factors that the nurse has not considered may cause the family's resistance. For example, the family may have more pressing basic needs such as food, clothing, and housing. Health promotion and disease prevention may not have been part of the family's life experiences, giving the nurse the educational task of trying to change attitudes and values so that the family will be more open to health needs.

In health promotion and disease prevention, four types of nursing interventions are found: (1) increasing knowledge and skills, (2) increasing strengths, (3) decreasing exposure, and (4) decreasing susceptibility.

Increasing knowledge and skills so that families can improve their capacity to act on health-promotion and disease-prevention behaviors may be the primary strategy. Inherent in this strategy is assisting families to make informed choices about healthful lifestyle behaviors and to eliminate harmful environmental influences that affect their health. The first step is creating awareness, which is accomplished in the first three steps of the nursing process as the nurse and family work together to uncover actual or potential problems. The second step is to recognize particular families at risk. The third step offers families at risk the benefits of nursing knowledge about motivating and supporting behavioral change.

Family strengths, first defined by Otto (1980), are factors or forces that contribute to family unity and solidarity and that foster the development of inherent family potential. These factors include the following:

- Physical, emotional, and spiritual factors
- Healthy child-rearing practices and discipline
- Meaningful and clear communication
- Support, security, and encouragement
- Growth-producing relationships and experiences
- Responsible community relationships
- Growth with and through children
- Self-help and acceptance of help
- Flexibility in family functions and roles
- Mutual respect for individuality
- Crisis as a means for growth
- Family unity and loyalty and intrafamily cooperation
- Adaptability of family strengths

In recent years, a shift of family health care from an illness or problem and deficiency focus to a strength-based focus has occurred. Both the McGill Model of Nursing (Feeley & Gottlieb, 2000) and the Calgary Family Assessment and Intervention Models (Wright & Leahy, 2000) are examples of frameworks used by nurses to assess, develop, and use the strengths and resources of families. For example, Denham (1999a) describes how family members use communication, cooperation, and caregiving to develop and maintain health-promotion behaviors; Niska (1999a, 1999b) and Hatrick (2000) identify corresponding nursing interventions to support and further develop the family dynamics of socialization, support, and nurturance. Additionally, Plager (1999) describes the importance of understanding the significance of family legacy to a family's health and related health practice.

Families with significant strengths may need to learn new, unfamiliar skills for mastering a specific technique, such as meditation, and to apply new tools for decision making. These families rarely require the ongoing supervision or support of sustained interventions aimed at changing their coping patterns, communication, or role behavior. They may be highly capable of seeking and using information.

Assisting functional families may simply involve providing information in terms that can be understood and offering them opportunities to ask questions and clarify information.

Decreasing exposure to risk factors may include making parental behaviors more in tune with the child's behaviors. Less educated parents may respond differently to the child's attempt to communicate and in their behavior toward the child. This tendency may lead to significant differences later in the child's intellectual ability. For example, using adequate restraints in automobiles and protecting the toddler from wandering into dangerous streets or places conducive to falls are means of reducing exposure to fatal accidents.

No substitute can be found for continuous supervision of a child. Homes can be made less hazardous by educated attempts to remove common hazards from children's reach. This effort includes putting all cleaning solutions and medications beyond their reach; erecting barriers in front of exposed heaters, high windows, and stairways; keeping pots and pans turned inward on the stove and out of the child's reach; fencing in a yard or a swimming pool; and teaching children to avoid dangerous areas. Becoming aware of peeling paint and toxic chemicals that parents might carry home from the job on their clothing can also protect the child.

Decreasing susceptibility means educating the family about the principles of prevention. The family must realize how diseases are spread from person to person; through hair, water and food, and by insects and the rodents on which insects live. The role of personal hygiene and cleanliness in avoiding infections must also be recognized. The family should know which signs and symptoms need medical attention and learn how to take care of minor illnesses.

Pender (1996) cites several research studies that support the importance of perceived susceptibility as a predictor of preventive behavior. Perceived susceptibility is the family's estimated subjective probability that a specific health problem will be encountered. Family perceptions of health risks and their susceptibility will determine how they change their behavior. If the overweight family believes obesity to be a threat to their health and if the nurse works with them in changing their eating habits to reduce weight and maintain weight norms, then the family is likely to react positively to the change. Nurses who introduce threat as a motivator to action are morally obligated to reduce the threat by meaningful and purposeful interventions. (See Table 7-1 for various nursing roles used in the implementation stage.)

innovative practice

The Wellness Community

Wellness Communities are located throughout the United States, offering free educational and support programs for people with cancer and their families. Weekly support groups help family members support one another, explore new ways of coping with the stresses of cancer, and learn ways to become the most effective possible partners with their health care team.

Wellness Communities offer a wide variety of workshops and programs (Gentle Strength and Stretch; Meditation and Guided Imagery; Nutrition Matters; Nutrition and the Immune System; Nutrition at Midlife: Preventing Heart Disease and Osteoporosis; Tai Chi; Yoga; Mindfulness and Feng Shui). Social events are organized (Comfort Food Potluck Dinner; Couples Networking Groups; Singles Networking Group; Family and Friends Networking Group).

Although each Wellness Community does not charge for its services, donations are appreciated and necessary to help serve the thousands of people living with cancer and their families. The Wellness Community's mission is to provide hope to these individuals and to help them regain a sense of control over their lives.

Contact Information:
National Headquarters
35 East 7th Street, Suite 412
Cincinnati, OH 45202
toll-free: 1-888-793-WELL
phone: (513) 421-7111
fax: (513) 421-7119
URL: http://www.wellness-community.org

EVALUATION WITH THE FAMILY

The purpose of evaluation is to determine how the family has responded to the planned interventions and whether these interventions were successful. Goals and objectives that are stated in specific behavioral terms will make evaluation much easier than when they are given in general terms. Specific criteria used to evaluate interventions, such as weight changes, increased lung capacity from an exercise program, and lower pulse rate as a result of relaxation exercises, are simple to measure. Other factors of health promotion and disease prevention are not as easy to measure, but must be considered in the evaluation step of the nursing process. As stated, when considering these factors as values, beliefs, self-perceptions, or role relationships, the nurse may base the evaluation on whether the family indicates that the interventions were successful. Additionally, the family's baseline data are used as comparative criteria in evaluation. The nurse reassesses the situation and compares the new information with the information on the original assessment to determine whether change has occurred.

Leavitt (1982) identifies the following five measures of family functioning that can be used to determine the effectiveness of interventions:

1. Changes in interaction patterns
2. Effective communication
3. Ability to express emotions
4. Responsiveness to needs of members as individuals
5. Problem-solving ability

Using these measures, the nurse returns to the original assessment of the family's functioning and compares current observations with previous data in the evaluation.

When the planning phase of the nursing process has identified the criteria (norms and standards) for the desired outcomes, these outcomes are the basis of evaluation. Data from the family that describe their behavior relative to the desired outcomes determine whether the nursing care was successful. With the criteria stated, the goals and objectives outline how the family can demonstrate a successful outcome and the behavior change expected to result from nursing intervention. The more objective and measurable the desired outcome is, the more reliable the results of evaluation will be.

After the goals and objectives are reached, the problem no longer exists. If evaluation shows the nursing actions did not achieve the goals or objectives, then the nurse must review the nursing process to determine whether there were gaps in the assessment data, errors in analysis or nursing diagnosis, or alternative interventions that might have been considered. The nurse also needs to review the process with the family to determine whether they have contributed to outcome failure. Finally, the agency employing the nurse may be another factor; if intervention is costly or a shortage of staff exists, then health promotion and disease prevention may have low priority.

SUMMARY

The family's learning of health promotion and disease prevention begins at birth, with the family providing the stimulus for incorporating health in the value system of its members. From a systems perspective, the family has both structure and function; relevant functions include values and practices placed on health. The effective execution of health-related functions involves the family's progression through its developmental tasks and its ability to generate low risk-producing behaviors associated with disease prevention.

Developmental and risk-estimate theories can be applied effectively to the nursing process with the family. The nurse uses functional patterns (an inherent part of both theories) to collect data for assessment. After organizing information on family life-cycle stages for analysis with the family, the nurse writes the nursing diagnosis and plans, implements, and evaluates the interventions used to promote health and prevent disease in the family.

REFERENCES

Bailey, E. (1987). Sociocultural factors and health care–seeking behavior among Black Americans. *Journal of the National Medical Association, 79*, 389-392.

Butcher, L. A., & Gaffney, M. (1995). Building healthy families: A program for single mothers. *Clinical Nurse Specialist CNS*, 9, 221-225.

Campbell, J. C., Harris, M. J., & Lee, R. K. (1995). Violence research: An overview. *Scholarly Inquiry for Nursing Practice: An International Journal*, 9, 105-126.

Connelly, C. D. (1998). Hopefulness, self-esteem and perceived social support among pregnant and non-pregnant adolescents. *Western Journal of Nursing Research, 20* (2), 195-209.

Culin, R., & Thyne, M. (1986). Understanding and supporting families in the process of divorce. *Nursing Practice*, 37.

Demi, A. S., & Miles, M. S. (1986). Bereavement: Review of nursing research. *Annual Review of Nursing Research, 4*, 105-123.

Demi, A. S., & Miles, M. S. (1987). Parameters of normal grief: A Delphi study. *Death Studies, 11* (6), 387-412.

Denham, S. A. (1999a). The definition and practice of family health. *Journal of Family Nursing, 5* (2), 133-159.

Denham, S. A. (1999b). Family health in an economically disadvantaged population. *Journal of Family Nursing, 5* (2), 184-213.

Dietz-Omar, M. (1991). Couple adaptation in stepfamilies and traditional nuclear families during pregnancy. *Applied Nursing Research: ANR, 4*, 6-10.

Duvall, E. M., & Miller, B. (1985). *Marriage and family development* (6th ed.). New York: Harper & Row.

Dzurec, L. C. (1995). Assessing fit: A key indicator of family health. *Journal of Nurse-Midwifery, 40*, 277-289.

Erikson, E. (1986). *Childhood and society*. New York: Norton.

Feeley, N., & Gottlieb, L. N. (2000). Nursing approaches for working with family strengths and resources. *Journal of Family Nursing*, 6 (1), 9-24.

Ford-Gilboe, M. V. (1994). *Family strengths, motivation and resources as predictors of health promotion behavior in single parent and two parent families*. Unpublished doctoral dissertation, Wayne State University.

Friedman, M. M. (1990). Transcultural family nursing: Application to Latino and black families. *Journal of Pediatric Nursing*, 5, 214-222.

Given, B. A., & Given, C. W. (1998). Health promotion for family caregivers of chronically ill elders. *Annual Review of Nursing Research, 16* (1), 197-217.

Gordon, M. (1994). *Nursing diagnosis: Process and application*. St. Louis: Mosby.

Gordon, M. (2000). *Manual of nursing diagnosis 1999-2000*. St. Louis: Mosby.

Grabbe, L., Demi, A. S., Camann, M. A., & Potter, L. (1997). The health status of elderly persons in the last year of life: A comparison of deaths by suicide, injury and natural causes. *American Journal of Public Health, 87* (3), 434-437.

Green, C. P. (1997). Teaching students how to "think family." *Journal of Family Nursing, 3* (3), 230-246.

Hatrick, G. (2000). Developing health-promoting practices with families. *Journal of Advanced Nursing, 31* (1), 27-34.

Hill, R. B. (1993). Dispelling myths and building strengths and supporting African-American families. *Family Resource Coalition,12*, 2.

Kerr, M., & Ritchey, D. (1990). Health promoting lifestyles of English speaking and Spanish speaking Mexican American migrant farm workers. *Public Health Nursing*, 7(2), 80-87.

Leavitt, M. B. (1982). *Families at risk: Primary prevention in nursing practice*. Boston: Little, Brown.

Leppink, H. (1982). Health risk estimation. In M. M. Faber, & A. M. Reinhardt (Eds.), *Promoting health through risk reduction*. New York: Macmillan.

McCauley, J. (1995). The "battering syndrome": Prevalence and clinical characteristics of domestic violence in primary care internal medicine practices. *Annals of Internal Medicine, 123*, 737.

McFarland, G. K., & McFarlane, E. A. (1993). *Nursing diagnosis & intervention: Planning for patient care*. St. Louis: Mosby.

McGoldrick, M., & Gerson, R. (1985). *Genograms in family assessment*. New York: Norton.

McLoyd, V. C. (1990). The impact of economic hardship on black families: Psychological distress, parenting, and socioeconomic development. *Child Development, 61*, 311-346.

Minuchin, S., Rossman, B., & Baker, L. (1966). *Psychosomatic families: Anorexia nervosa in context*. Cambridge, MA: Harvard University Press.

NANDA. (2000). *NANDA nursing diagnoses: Definitions and classifications, 1999-2000*. Philadelphia: NANDA.

Nettle, C., Pavelich, J., Jones, N., Beltz, C., Laboon, P., Pifer, P. (1993). Family as client: Using Gordon's health pattern typology. *Journal of Community Health Nursing, 10*, 53-57.

Newman, M. (1995). *A developing discipline: Selected works of Margaret Newman*. New York: National League for Nursing.

Niska, K. J. (1999a). Family nursing interventions: Mexican American early family formation. *Nursing Science Quarterly, 12* (4), 335-340.

Niska, K. J. (1999b). Mexican American family processes: Nurturing, support and socialization. *Nursing Science Quarterly, 12* (2), 138-142.

Niska, K. J., Snyder, M., & Lia-Hoagberg, B. (1999). The meaning of family health among Mexican American first-time mothers and fathers. *Journal of Family Nursing, 5* (2), 218-233.

Otto, H. A. (1980). A framework for assessing family strengths. In A. M. Reinhardt, & M. D. Quinn (Eds.), *Family-centered community nursing Vol. 2*. St. Louis: Mosby.

Pender, N. J. (1996). *Health promotion in nursing practice* (3rd ed.). Stanford, CT: Appleton-Lange.

Plager, K. A. (1999). Understanding family legacy in family health concerns. *Journal of Family Nursing, 5* (1), 51-71.

Polomeno, V. (1998). An exemplary service: Health promotion for expectant fathers: Part II. Practical considerations. *Journal of Perinatal Education, 7* (2), 27-39.

Polomeno, V. (1999). Perinatal education and grandparenting: Creating an interdependent family environment. *Journal of Perinatal Education*, 8 (2), 28-38.

Pratt, L. (1976). *Family structure and effective health behavior: The energized family*. Boston: Houghton Mifflin.

Roberts, S. J., & Sorensen, L. (1995). Lesbian health care: A review and recommendations for health promotion in primary care settings. *Nurse Practitioner*, 20(6), 42-47.

Rorie, J. L., Paine, L. L., & Barger, M. K. (1996). Primary care for women: Cultural competence in primary care services. *Journal of Nurse-Midwifery*, *41*, 92-100.

Rosenwald, E., & Demi, A. S. (1993). A primary prevention groups for latency and children with adoption issues. *Journal of Child and Adolescent Psychiatric and Mental Health Nursing*, 6 (1), 15-21.

Sparks, S. M., & Taylor, C. M. (1998). *Nursing diagnosis reference manual*. Springhouse, PA: Springhouse.

Spradley, B. W. (1990). *Community health nursing: Concepts and practice* (3rd ed.). Glenview, IL: Scott, Foresman, Little, Brown Higher Education.

Stanhope, M., & Lancaster, J. (2000). *Community and public health nursing* (5th ed.). St. Louis: Mosby.

Star, W. L., Lommel, L. L., & Shannon, M. T. (1995). *Women's primary health care*. Washington, DC: American Nurses Publishing.

Stevens, P. E. (1995). Structural and interpersonal impact of heterosexual assumptions on lesbian health care clients. *Nursing Research*, *44*, 25-30.

Tilden, V. P., Schmidt, T. A., Limandri, B. J., Chiodo, G. T., Garland, M. J., Loveless, P. A. (1994). Factors that influence clinicians' assessment and management of family violence. *American Journal of Public Health*, *84*, 628-633.

U.S. Department of Health and Human Services. (2000). *Healthy People 2000* (Conference Edition). Washington, DC: U.S. Government Printing Office.

U.S. Preventive Services Taskforce, U.S. Department of Health & Human Services. (1996). *Guide to clinical preventive services*. Washington, DC: U. S. Government Printing Office.

Wright, L. M., & Leahy, M. (2000). *Nurses and families: A guide to family assessment and intervention* (3rd ed.). Philadelphia: F.A. Davis.

Yoos, H. L., Kitzman, H., Olds, D. L., Overacker, I. (1995). Childrearing beliefs in the African-American community: Implications for culturally competent pediatric care. *Journal of Pediatric Nursing*, *10*, 343-353.

Chapter 8

CAROL LYNN MANDLE

Health Promotion and the Community

objectives

After completing this chapter, the nurse will be able to:

- Describe the 11 functional health patterns and explain how they are used as a basis of data collection in assessment of the community.
- Identify characteristics of the community to consider for risk factors and developmental aggregates of potential or actual dysfunctional health patterns.
- Identify methods of community data collection and sources of information.
- Describe a method of planned change for the community.
- Discuss planning, implementing, and evaluating nursing interventions in health promotion with communities.
- Develop a specific health-promotion plan based on community assessment, nursing diagnosis, and contributing factors.

key terms

Community
Community Diagnosis
Community Evaluation
Community Health Promotion
Community Nursing Intervention
Community Outcome
Community Pattern
Community Risk Factors
Demography
Developmental Theory
Function of a Community
Interview
Interview Data
Measurement
Observation Data
Risk Factor Theory
Structure of a Community
Systems Theory
Windshield Survey

THINK About It

Teenagers: Drinking and Driving

In a small rural community, seven teenagers have died in alcohol-related car accidents within the past 3 months. Alcohol and drug education is taught during the first year at the local high school, but driver's education classes are not offered because the school cannot afford the program. Parents within this community are extremely concerned.

1. What other information must be acquired before making a diagnosis?
2. What health-promotion ideas could be recommended, based on the information provided?

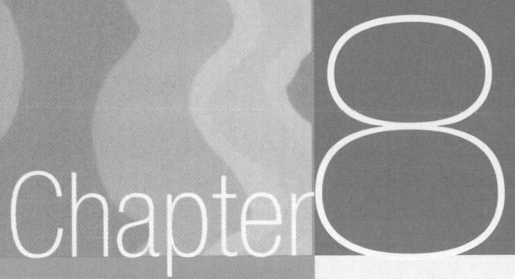

Over the last two decades, several social trends in the United States have increased public interest in health promotion and disease prevention. The landmark documents the U.S. Department of Health and Human Services (USDHHS) published (see Chapter 1) have been helpful in changing the focus of health care from a reactive stance to a proactive stance that emphasizes prevention of disease and promotion of health. By stating national health objectives in relation to age-specific risks to good health, these documents set a course to reduce the percentage of risk factors, thereby reducing the incidence of disease.

Another social trend creating interest in the promotion of health and the prevention of disease is the changing population of the United States. The U.S. Census Bureau estimates that by the year 2025, there will be 60 million people in the United States over the age of 65 (20% of the population) (USDHHS, 2000). Older people tend to have more diseases that are chronic and consume a larger portion of health-care services than do other age groups. It is also anticipated that the aging population will require more home health care and nursing home services than previous generations because they experience increasing longevity and illnesses of a chronic nature. A growing number of articles in the literature propose that the major improvements in the population's health will be derived from self-care and strategies of health promotion and disease prevention, not from medical technology and services.

Understanding the dynamic and complex nature of communities and being able to gather certain facts about them are important prerequisites for effective planning, delivery, and coordination of health-promotion and health-protection activities. Nurses play an important role in collecting information about their communities and they use it to promote and protect community health. Each community's health needs and concerns differ; therefore the type of health-promotion and health-protection activities will vary. As knowledge is gained about the community, the nurse is better able to address a wide range of health-related responses that are observed in the community. These responses can be reactions to actual health-related problems (disease) or to potential health problems. Community responses are frequently multiple, continual, and fluid and they tend to vary. Many potential health concerns are discrete or individually distinct.

The term community is used in various contexts with various meanings, depending on the frame of reference. In this text, the definition of **community** is the same definition used by *Healthy People 2010* and the Health Glossary of the World Health Organization (WHO). "A specific group of people, often living in a defined geographical area, who share a common culture, values, and norms and who are arranged in a social structure according to relationships that community has developed over a period of time" (USDHHS, 2000, p. 7-27; WHO, 1998). The community includes workplaces (Association of Worksite Health Promotion, 1999; Bresler, 1999) and schools (CDC, 1997; Lear, 1996).

For example, school nurses "serve 48 million youth in the nation's schools. School nurses assess student health and development, help families determine when services are needed, and serve as a professional link with . . . community resources" (USDHHS, 2000, p. 7-17). (Bennett, Contessa, & Turner, 1999; Illuzzi & Cinelli, 2000; Opas, 1995; Orpinas, Kelder, Frankowski, Murray, Zhang, & McAlister, 2000). People are assumed to share the need for and use of the resources in their environment that are influenced by the passage of time and the environment in which they are located.

People are important to any concept of community; human beings give it shape, character, and form. An individual's health is reflected in the community through the person's contribution to its statistical rates and cultural and psychological makeup. Conversely, the community is reflected in the individual through similar modes of expression.

This chapter focuses on the application of the nursing process to the community. The nurse's role is inherent in independent, interdependent, and dependent activities. Methods of data collection and sources of information about a community are provided because they may differ from individual sources. Systems theory, **developmental theory,** and **risk factor theory** are used to guide the nursing process. Development theory refers to a variety of explanations of phases of human development—physical, psychosocial, cognitive, and spiritual dimensions—based on descriptive research studies. Similarly, risk factor theory is an identification of human characteristics and behaviors that increase the likelihood of the manifestation of health problems. Gordon's typology (1994) of 11 functional health patterns is used to provide a database for assessment. An example of a data collection guide is presented to facilitate the comprehension, synthesis, and application of observation, interview, and measurement data. A description and examples of data analysis, nursing diagnosis, planning, implementing, and evaluation follow.

THE NURSING PROCESS AND THE COMMUNITY

As stated previously, Gordon's 11 functional health patterns (1994) are used to collect a database for assessment. The health-related patterns can provide a useful framework for collecting observation, interview, and measurement data. The health-related patterns that the nurse chooses for an assessment depend on the community setting, the focus of the assessment, and the nurse's preference. Assessing all pattern areas provides a basic set of data that can be analyzed and used for comparison purposes in evaluation (see Chapter 6).

Risk and developmental age factors also influence health patterns (see Multicultural Awareness box). For example, a health concern might be identified in one pattern area,

MULTICULTURAL AWARENESS

Guidelines for Nursing Interventions for Ethnic Elders

- Respect cultural preferences in food, music, and religion.
- Design teaching to the vocabulary and attitude of the individual.
- Listen attentively to complaints because these may be clues to health problems.
- In Blacks, the signs of some disorders may be masked by color (pallor, cyanosis, and ecchymosis); buccal cavity coloration is significant.
- Base physical assessment on norms for the ethnic group. Adequate light is especially important in skin assessment for turgor, blemishes, and cyanosis; eye lens, nail beds, palms of hands, and soles of feet can be revealing.
- Listen for signs of depression, often in the form of hypochondriasis and apathy.
- Inquire about losses and the individual's adaptation to them.
- Gather information about lifestyle preferences and incorporate into care plans.
- Inquire about health practices that the individual finds effective.
- Identify spiritual resources and incorporate into care plan; contact clergy and church, synagogue, mosque, or friends.

From Ebersole, P., & Hess, P. (1994). *Toward healthy aging: human needs and nursing response* (4th ed.). St. Louis: Mosby.

such as an increase in an age-related factor of teenage pregnancy (sexuality-reproductive pattern). Data from other areas might reveal the containment of sex education in the home (coping–stress-tolerance pattern) and the unacceptability of sex education in the school from parental nonsupport (values-beliefs pattern). Limiting sex education to the home and ignoring it in the school may be factors that young people of childbearing age share in the community, placing them at risk for unwanted pregnancies. Factors from several pattern areas may form a cluster that has the potential for placing certain groups at risk (see Chapter 6).

THE NURSE'S ROLE

Community health nursing is seen as a synthesis of nursing practice and public health concepts applied to promoting the health of populations. It is not limited to any particular individual or group of individuals. The nursing concerns are the community's responses to existing and potential health-related problems, including such health-supporting responses as monitoring and teaching population groups. The nurse may supply a community at risk with the educational information necessary to develop health-oriented skills, attitudes, and related behavioral changes (Sheilds & Lindsey, 1998).

The nurse's role is also concerned with the relationships that are essential to accomplish the community's health-related mission. The complexity and dynamic nature of communities and the increasing public involvement in health and health policy highlight the importance of the human interactions that are inherent in the nurse's responses to potential health problems, needs, and expectations. Therefore nursing practice with communities requires a broad knowledge base derived from the natural, behavioral, and humanistic sciences and the application of intellectual, interpersonal, and technical skills through the nursing process.

The nurse's role can be seen as independent, interdependent, and dependent and these frequently overlap. Independent functions include assessing, analyzing, diagnosing, planning, implementing, and evaluating nursing activities such as health promotion and health education. Interdependent functions include collaboration with community members and interdisciplinary teamwork functions that are crucial to effective community health. Dependent functions include implementing the therapeutic plans of team members.

Community health promotion includes all of the following:

Involved community participation with representatives from at least three of the following community sectors: government, education, business, faith organizations, health care, media, voluntary agencies, and the public.

Community assessment guided by a community assessment and planning model to determine community health problems, resources, perceptions, and priorities for action.

Targeted and measurable objectives to address any of the following: health outcomes, risk factors, public awareness, services, and protection.

Comprehensive, multifaceted, culturally relevant interventions that have multiple targets for change.

Monitoring and evaluation of the processes to determine whether the objectives are reached (USDHHS, 2000, pp. 7, 21-28).

METHODS OF DATA COLLECTION

The nurse obtains community assessment data through observation, interview, and measurement. These three methods are used most frequently in various combinations to ensure the validity of the information.

Obtaining data through observation—often referred to as the **windshield survey** approach to assessment—includes the use of the senses (sight, touch, hearing, smell, and taste) to determine community appearances. These appearances include the type and state of residential dwellings; the people; and the physical and biological characteristics, such as animal and plant life, temperature, transportation, sounds, and odors. Some communities have an observable characteristic "flavor." The community's physical characteristics can influence health. What type of space is available? Children need space in which to run and play; young and middle-age adults require space for recreation and exercise. What spatial barriers exist? The community nurse can obtain a great deal of subjective data just by walking or riding around a community and using the senses. The data obtained by observation can provide important clues about the community, its actual or potential health problems, and its strengths. When **observation data** are analyzed, hypotheses can be generated that are further assessed by using interview and measurement data.

The second method, the **interview,** is probably the most common approach for collecting information from people. **Interview data** include verbal statements from community residents, key community officials, health care personnel, and various community agency staff. This method is a useful way to obtain information about how members perceive their community. Key community leaders can provide important information about community health concerns, necessary health resources, and community strengths. Particular health beliefs and community health goals can also be ascertained.

Community residents can provide useful information about their perceptions of health, health concerns and needs, and the availability, accessibility, and acceptability of health services. Health agency personnel can provide data on available health resources, whom they serve, when they are available, and their perceptions of concerns and needs. Developing a basic set of questions in advance will enhance the relevance of interview data.

Measurement, the third method, uses instruments to quantify data in information collection. Measurement data include population statistics, pollution indices, morbidity and mortality rates, census statistics, and epidemiological data. These data can be found in community libraries; health departments; environmental protection agencies; schools; police and fire departments; local health system agencies; and town, city, or state planning offices. Publicly supported agencies are required by law to share their information with interested people and community nurses should not hesitate to request such data.

SOURCES OF COMMUNITY INFORMATION

Census information found in libraries and public agencies is the most complete source for population information. Because the U.S. Census is completed once every 10 years at the beginning of a decade, the data for most communities become less accurate as the decade progresses. Community agencies, such as the chamber of commerce and local planning commissions, work with census data to develop projection statistics and developmental trends, which the nurse can use to gain an understanding of population patterns and dynamics. Health data are usually available from town, city, or state public health departments and community health-related organizations.

Environmental measurement data can be obtained from the local branch of the U.S. Environmental Protection Agency (EPA). Generally, the sanitation department of the local health department is in charge of monitoring the community's water, food, and sanitation systems. School health information is available from the health department, school nurse, or school administration.

Information on land use, boundaries, housing conditions, utilities, and community services is generally available from the town, city, or county administration. Community newspapers can be an excellent source of information on community dynamics, health-related concerns, cultural activities, and community decision makers. Recording community observation, interview, and measurement data are approached in the same manner as data on an individual or family. A triple-column format that separates the data of each method can facilitate recording.

COMMUNITY FROM A SYSTEMS PERSPECTIVE

Systems theory provides an overall framework in which otherwise unconnected parts can be integrated. A system is an entity composed of interrelated, interacting parts or components within a boundary that filters both the type and the rate of input and output (Von Bertalanffy, 1968). As in family assessment (see Chapter 7), a community that is viewed as a system has both structure and function. These aspects of a population living in a specific geographical area are determined in a community assessment.

Structure

The **structure of a community** system or subsystem can be seen as the formal or informal arrangement of its parts at any given time, including both animate and inanimate properties. The population, schools, fire department, and health resources are examples of structural parts. Nursing, which operates within the context of the health system, can be considered as a component of a community system.

The parts of a community are viewed as subsystems, each of which is in itself a system. The suprasystem, often a county or state, is the larger system of which the community is a part. Figure 8-1 shows a hierarchical arrangement of a community system.

The arrangement and organization of a community system's parts, such as the age distribution of the population and the types of health-promotion and health-protection programs and their availability and accessibility, can change over time. The parts may remain relatively stable for long periods, based on the state of the environment and

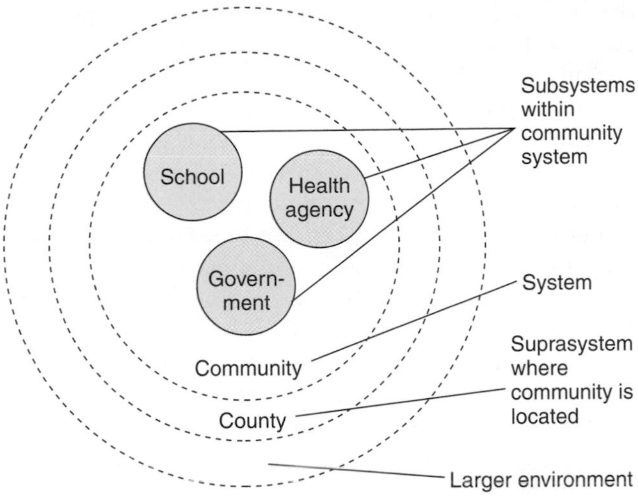

Fig. 8-1 Hierarchical nature of a community system.

the processes that occur within the parts and between the parts and the larger environment.

The existence, arrangement, and assimilation of a community's parts play a major role in providing direction to both health-promotion and health-protection activities. Therefore when conducting an assessment, the nurse must consider the various community parts or systems as they relate to health. Viewing the community structure as a population (collection of people) and considering the arrangement of the community's health care parts (existing health services) are especially important.

The study of a population is referred to as demography. **Demography** provides information on population characteristics (size, age distribution, gender ratio, racial composition, marital status ratio, nationality, language, religious grouping, and educational and occupational distributions).

Obtaining demographic data of a population living in a specific area provides an important basis for analysis and a means for identifying developmental concerns of various population groups who might be at risk. Such information can also provide clues for the direction of health strategies. For example, an examination of age distribution over the past several years reveals important population shifts and a need for additional health-promotion activities; the large increase in the population over age 65 may require changes in community health priorities to reflect this group's needs. Demographic information is so vital that it is generally considered first in any community assessment.

Comparison statistics about population characteristics, which also need to be considered in community structure, enable the nurse to make inferences about the community. Comparisons are made among three systems: (1) the town, which is a part of the county; (2) the county, which is a part of the larger system; and (3) the state. Comparisons are typically made between communities of similar population size.

Function

The **function of a community** refers to the process of dynamic change or adaptation in the system's parts and the way the community system and its subsystems interact. How community members make decisions and allocate health-promotion and health-protection resources are important considerations.

Strategies are processes through which decisions are made to obtain compliance from another system or subsystem. Schaller (1988) has identified the following four general strategies to affect change: (1) coercion, which uses force; (2) co-optation, in which one item is offered for another; (3) conflict, which serves to clarify issues, but may have a negative effect; and (4) cooperation, which obtains compliance with persuasion.

Cooperation requires skill in communication and interpersonal relations; therefore it can be very time consuming, but it can effectively produce change that is readily accepted. With the exception of coercion, the least desirable strategy for change, each of these strategies can be effective. (The four strategies are discussed further in the Community Assessment section of this chapter.)

Interaction

Interaction is an important concept in systems theory. Through dynamic interaction with the environment, a system exchanges matter, energy, and information (in such communication forms as verbal and behavioral) and uses information to make decisions. Interaction is also important if the community system is to survive, protect, and promote the health of its members. Through environmental interactions, a community system uses mechanisms of adaptation. The nurse must determine how the community applies these mechanisms toward health services.

Various health-related patterns also emerge from these interactions. For example, certain human activity patterns can negatively alter the natural environmental patterns, which influence human health patterns. Gordon's assessment framework (1994) focuses on 11 health-related functional patterns; community and environment interaction is assumed in each. The framework used, such as the systems theory described, dictates the approach used in assessing these patterns.

DEVELOPMENTAL FRAMEWORK

A developmental framework can be used to identify existing or potential health problems for a particular age group in a community. A population group is defined as an aggregate of persons who share similar personal or environmental characteristics. Community nurses are interested in the total community population; therefore they use a developmental, age-correlated approach to identify health-promotion and health-protection activities for all age groups.

At each stage of life, age-related risks can be identified and different steps taken to maximize wellness and promote health as a lifelong concern (USDHHS, 2000). For example, adolescent single mothers of infants are at high risk both emotionally and physically and they require help with parenting skills. Accidents are the greatest threat to children's health; therefore accident-prevention activities are a priority for this age group. Many age-related risk factors (see Chapters 6 and 7) associated with individuals and families can be extended to include community groups.

RISK FACTOR FRAMEWORK

Risk factors are associated with a community's disease, illness, and death rates (USDHHS, 2000). A risk factor does not necessarily play a causal role in these rates, but simply helps to predict the likelihood of the development of a particular adverse health condition.

Risk factors may include a combination of demographic, psychological, physiological, or environmental characteristics (or they may include a single characteristic). For example, age, gender, race, geographical location, consumption pattern, or lack of health services may be considered risk factors because one or more may contribute to disease or death and place the population sharing them at risk. (See Research Highlight box.) The degree of influence of various risk factors differs from person to person and group to group from genetic makeup, geographical location, lifestyle patterns, resources, socioeconomic status, level of education, or environmental variation. Some groups may be at high risk from a single risk factor such as insufficient immunizations or exposure to asbestos. However, synergism does operate. A combined potential for adverse health effects exists when many risk factors are present because they interact in different ways and can multiply each other (USDHHS, 2000). As a result, communities can experience substantial variability in both the incidence of and susceptibility to adverse health conditions. The risk factor concept is based on disease and, conversely, health because it is multifactorial in genesis; frequently, the essential cause cannot be attributed to any single risk factor. For example, risk factors such as air pollution, smoking, and forms of radiation in various combinations may be related to high rates of lung cancer, emphysema, and bronchitis in a community. The potential to control many or just a few risk factors and to have relevant health-related resources available is the basis of health-promotion and health-protection activities.

A general description of the 11 functional health patterns and the guidelines for posing questions in observations and interviews are provided in Table 8-1. A variety of functional health-pattern assessments are used with communities. The nurse uses Gordon's functional health reference assessment (1994) as exemplified in this chapter (Decker & Knight, 1990; Kriegler & Harton, 1992) or other assessments in the literature (Clark, 1999; Hitchcock, Schubert, & Thomas, 1999; Reece, 1998; Stanley & Stein, 1998).

research highlights

Preventing Unintentional Childhood Injuries

The purpose of this study was to analyze a "systematic review of the world literature to provide information about the most effective forms of health-promotion interventions to reduce childhood (0 to 14 years) unintentional injuries" (p. 140). Literature was identified through electronic databases, manual researches, and consultations. The interventions described as most effective in the literature are bicycle helmet legislation, area-wide traffic-calming measures, child safety restraint legislation, child-resistant containers to prevent poisoning, window bars to prevent falls . . . provision of home hazard detection, and pedestrian education. For the community-based campaigns, the key to success has been the sustained use of surveillance systems, the commitment of interagency cooperation, and the time needed to develop networks and implement a range of interventions.

The conclusion of the study is, "The design of evaluations in injury prevention needs to be improved so that more reliable evidence can be obtained . . . so that successful strategies can be replicated elsewhere" (p. 149).

Downswell, T., Towner, E. M. L., Simpson, T. G., & Jarvis. S. N. (1996). Preventing childhood unintentional injuries—what works? *Injury Prevention, 2*(2), 140-149.

FUNCTIONAL HEALTH PATTERNS: ASSESSMENT OF THE COMMUNITY

Health Perception-Health Management Pattern

This pattern identifies data about the community's health status, its health-promotion and disease-protection practices, and its members' perceptions of health (Gordon, 1994). Some residents might perceive a substance abuse problem with adolescents or a high rate of unwanted pregnancies, breast cancer, or sexually transmitted disease as a concern. Valuable information can be elicited from interviewing key community persons about their health concerns and issues. Mortality and morbidity statistics and other public health information sources can provide measurement data (see Chapter 2).

Nutritional-Metabolic Pattern

This pattern identifies data relevant to a community's consumption habits as reflected in the accessibility and availability of food stores and subsidized food programs for infants, children, and older adults. Community well being rests on adequate dietary habits, food intake, and supply of nutrients, all of which can be influenced by culture and the presence or absence of kitchen facilities and adequate plumbing.

Obtaining data by a drive or a walk through the community and using the five senses can provide information about grocery stores, fast-food establishments,

Text continued on p. 211

Table 8-1 Functional Health Patterns: Data Collection Guide in Assessing the Community As Client

Pattern	Observation	Interview	Measurement
HEALTH PERCEPTION-HEALTH MANAGEMENT PATTERN	—	How is community health perceived? What are the major health concerns? What health concerns do community residents perceive? What health services do residents believe they need and have? What are the cultural patterns influencing health practices? What languages are spoken? What religious groups are in the community? Do people feel fire, police, and safety programs are sufficient?	What is the population size and age distribution? What is the sex ratio, racial composition, marital status, and nationality composition? What is the education, occupation, and income distribution? What are the statistics regarding mortality, morbidity, and prevalent infectious diseases? What are the motor-vehicle accident statistics? What are the currently operating health facilities (types)? What are the ongoing health-promotion and health-prevention programs and use rates? What is the ratio of health professionals to the population? What are the laws regarding drinking age? What are the statistics for drug use and for drinking and driving, by age group?
NUTRITIONAL-METABOLIC PATTERN	What shopping facilities are visible? Are there grocery stores? Kinds and accessibility? What are the predominant food smells in the area (Asian, Mexican, or other cultures)? Food purchases (observable at food store checkout)? What nutritional services are visible? Are junk food vendors and fast-food establishments near schools and workplaces? What geographical features of community pose a threat to community food and consumption patterns? In general, do most people seem well nourished? Children? The elderly?	What nutritional services are available to community residents? Are there school lunch programs, elderly feeding programs, and special milk programs? Are women, infant, and children feeding programs or summer food service programs available to residents? How are they funded? Is cost of food reasonable in this area relative to income? Does community housing have adequate kitchen and plumbing facilities?	How many food programs are available? How is the water supplied and what is its quality? What are the testing services available (if own wells)? If appropriate: Water usage cost? Any drought restrictions? Any data to indicate community growth will exceed good water supply? Are heating and cooling costs manageable for most programs? What percentage of community housing has no or inadequate kitchen and plumbing facilities?

Continued

Table 8-1 Functional Health Patterns: Data Collection Guide in Assessing the Community As Client—cont'd

Pattern	Observation	Interview	Measurement
ELIMINATION PATTERN	Are chemical dumps or disposal dumps visible? Are they close to waterways or densely populated areas?	How adequate are disposal sites? Are there chemical dumpsites in the community? What efforts are being made to control leached materials?	How many waste-disposal sites are in the community? How many chemical dumps?
Physical Agents	What is visible in the community (waterways, highways, or mountains)? What is the topography? What is the shape of the community? What is the size? What is the location? Near a major harbor or desert? Are major highways evident that allow easy access to community? Are smells present? Are noxious chemicals evident?	Are emission controls enforced?	What is the water quality? What are solium and bacteria levels? Square miles of the community? Population per square mile? Temperature range, humidity range, and altitude of community? Air pollution index?
Biological Agents	What plants are observed? Are they poisonous? Are rats and rodents evident? Are dogs running around unleashed? Is there evidence of defoliation and deforestation?	What chemicals are used to control mosquitoes and other insects? Are food plants contaminated?	—
ACTIVITY-EXERCISE PATTERN	Do children play in streets or vacant lots? What recreational facilities are visible? Are swimming pools, ball fields, and tennis courts evident? Are residents walking, riding bikes, or driving around the community? Are joggers evident? Are there cultural programs? Aids for the disabled? Residential centers or nursing homes? External maintenance of homes, yards, and apartment houses? What is the general activity level (bustling or quiet)?	What diversional activities are available for children, adolescents, middle-aged adults, and older adults? What are the mobility patterns? Are there transient groups? How do people find transportation here? To work? For recreation? To health care facilities?	How many recreational facilities are available and for whom? What are the statistics on repopulation trends? Is the population increasing, decreasing, or stable? Is housing adequate (availability and cost)? Is public housing available? Rehabilitation facilities relative to population needs?

SLEEP-REST PATTERN	What is heard when walking or riding around the community? Is the area quiet? Loud industrial, bus, truck, train, airplane, or construction noises? Is there movement of residents during certain times of day? In what areas of the community is noise loudest? Near an airport?	Are residential areas protected from industrial buildings? Are noise ordinances enforced? What efforts are being made to control noise levels?	How many airports and trucking firms exist in community? What is the noise level in various parts of the community?
COGNITIVE-PERCEPTUAL PATTERN			
Coercion	What are the community's decision-making patterns? Are decisions made by a few people or a group of leaders? Are residents heard regarding health matters or does evidence show that they are forced to comply? Do residents believe they have been deceived about health-related issues?	Do key community leaders and business, religious, and other social groups support health-related activities? Are schools seen as good or needing improvement? Is adult education desired and available?	Education level of population? School facilities? Dropout rates?
Bargaining	Are there negotiations between health-related services to meet community needs and goals? Are there negotiations between health service personnel and community residents to meet community needs and goals?		
Team Cooperation	Do health-related agencies work together or in isolation? Do they think they are working together? Do they have similar services and clientele? Do community residents believe there is a cooperative effort to achieve community health goals?		
Gemeinschaft	Do community residents support health activities for the common good of the community? Do most groups speak English? Bilingual? Community government structure?		

Continued

Table 8-1 Functional Health Patterns: Data Collection Guide in Assessing the Community As Client—cont'd

Pattern	Observation	Interview	Measurement
SELF-PERCEPTION–SELF-CONCEPT PATTERN	What is observed when walking or driving around the community? Are community beautification projects evident? What is the condition of housing and community buildings (in good repair or state of disrepair)? What is the appearance of streets, sidewalks, and yards? Are they clean or littered with rubbish? Is it an old community? Fairly new? Are people's moods, in general, enjoying life, stressed, or feeling down?	Do community residents think it is a good place to live? Do people generally have the kinds of skills needed in this community?	What age group predominates? Any community functions (picnics or parades)? Racial ethnic mix? Socioeconomic level?
ROLES-RELATIONSHIPS PATTERN	Are there newspapers, newsletters, flyers, and bulletins that provide information about community activities and schedules of meetings? What are the meeting places (street corners, bars, laundromats, meeting halls, or parks)? Do residents seem friendly? Do they stop and talk or walk on? Do residents seem to get along well together?	How is health-related information transmitted in the community (newspapers or bulletins)? Do radio or television stations provide public information announcements? Are there public meetings to discuss community concerns? What are the official channels of communication? What is the organizational structure of community? Where is the locus of power? Are key leaders available and easily accessible to residents? What community systems exchange functions, such as the health department, collaborating with schools for screening or immunizations? Do people feel they are heard by the government? Are there enough jobs in the community? Are wages good? Do people seem to like the work they do or is there job stress?	High or low participation at meetings? What is the unemployment rate? Poverty rate? What is the rate of riot, violence, child and elder abuse? What is the divorce rate?

SEXUALITY-REPRODUCTIVE PATTERN	What family planning services are visible? What marital, family, and adolescent counseling services are visible? Are abortion services evident?	Are sex-related crimes a problem? Is spouse or child abuse a problem? What specific family and adolescent services are available? Are they accessible? Are they acceptable to residents? Do people feel there is a problem with pornography or prostitution? Do people support or want sex education in schools and community?	What are the statistics regarding live births by mother's age and marital status? What are the neonatal, infant, and maternal death rates? What are the abortion rates? What are the statistics regarding sex-related crimes and spouse and child abuse? How many family counseling services are available? What is the average family size and type of household? What is the male-female ratio? What is the teen pregnancy rate? Sexual violence statistics? Laws and regulations regarding information on birth control?
COPING–STRESS-TOLERANCE PATTERN			
Obtain	What health-promotion and health-protection services are visible? What educational facilities are visible?	What health-promotion and health-protection services are made available to community? Where are these services located? Are they acceptable to residents? What community residents (groups) have access to these services? What services does the community need to obtain? Are health services public or private? How are they funded or supported? Are they private or public? What health-promotion and health-protection services are available to students? What health knowledge, facilities, or work force is the community trying to obtain? What is the tax structure of the community?	How many health-promotion and health-protection services are available? How many educational facilities are available? How many students attend these facilities? How many elementary school children have their required immunizations? What amount of tax money is allocated for health-promotion and health-protection activities?

Continued

Table 8-1 Functional Health Patterns: Data Collection Guide in Assessing the Community As Client—cont'd

Pattern	Observation	Interview	Measurement
COPING–STRESS-TOLERANCE PATTERN—cont'd			
Contain	—	Is substance abuse a problem? What is being done to contain it? Is crime a problem? What is being done to eliminate it? Is a type of housing, such as low income, being opposed? Is a health facility, clinic, or mental health residence being opposed? Why?	What are the crime statistics?
Retain	—	Does the community strive to maintain specific housing codes, such as type of structure and use of lead-free paint, to maintain a standard of living? Are there specific health problems and services that are valued and maintained? Are specific cultural and ethnic groups valued and maintained? Are health education and family planning supported and maintained in the home? Are specific health-promotion and health-protection services being maintained and supported?	What percentage of housing was built before 1959?
Dispose	—	Is the community trying to get rid of specific health services? Is the community trying to market a specific health service? Is the community trying to market health education programs?	—
VALUES-BELIEFS PATTERN	What have you read about the history of the community? How did it come into being? What are some of its traditions? What changes were made and valued?	What are the community's priorities? Is it receptive to new ideas? What ethnic groups are acceptable? What health services and programs are acceptable? What common values and norms are shared? Are health-promotion and health-protection services available to all groups? What changes has the community supported?	Zoning and conservation laws? Community health committee meeting reports (goals and priorities)? Health budget in relation to total budget?

ethnic shopping facilities, and street corner vendors. Government programs, private soup kitchens, and food donations by houses of worship also provide information about the nutritional pattern of a community.

Elimination Pattern

This pattern identifies data about the environmental factors of a community and includes exposure to pollutants in the community through such media as contaminated soil, water, air, and the food chain. It further classifies two broad areas of environmental factors: (1) physical and (2) biological. Alterations in environmental processes can threaten the health and integrity of a community, necessitating health-promotion and health-protection activities.

Physical agents include geological, geographical, climatic, and meteorological aspects of the community. Certain population groups are particularly susceptible to acute respiratory disease and aggravated asthmatic episodes when the air quality is poor. The geographical location of a community and major waterways, highways, or mountains located within it can act as barriers to health facilities. Inaccessibility of health care services can also be a barrier to groups who are at risk for potential health problems. Knowledge of the community's climatic conditions, though obvious to many, can provide clues to a population's susceptibility to illness resulting from temperature or humidity conditions.

Biological agents include living things, such as plants, animals and their waste products, disease agents, microbial pathogens, and toxic substances that can be potentially hazardous to health. For example, Lyme disease, viral hepatitis, pneumonia, influenza, and the large number of diseases associated with childhood continue to be threats to a community's health.

Information concerning elimination patterns can be elicited through observation and interviews with key community people. The EPA and the Centers for Disease Control and Prevention (CDC) are excellent resources in this area.

Activity-Exercise Pattern

This pattern identifies a community's physical activities and recreational options. In some communities, science and technology have had an increasing influence on productivity while simultaneously reducing and, in some cases, eliminating the amount of physical work required by the labor force. As a result, physical activity can no longer be attained on the job and leisure hours represent the only viable time for its development. During leisure time, choices are available from literally dozens of activities that are sufficiently different from one another so almost anyone can find a physical activity that is enjoyable and challenging. Physical activity reduces the risk of many diseases, including heart disease, hypertension, cancer, osteoporosis, and diabetes mellitus.

Physiological evidence shows that physical activity improves many biological measures associated with health and psychological functioning. Regular physical activity and musculoskeletal fitness are important in the maintenance of healthy independent living as people grow older.

Observation and interviews provide clues to a community's ability to provide cultural and recreational activities.

Sleep-Rest Pattern

This pattern identifies a community's rhythm of sleeping, resting, and relaxing. Some towns never shut down; that is, stores, traffic flow, and recreational facilities are open day and night. These situations can produce disturbances, such as unwanted noise, that are disagreeable or harmful to a community's well being. Excessive noise from highways or airplanes can produce a physiological or psychological problem and can elicit a response ranging from mild irritation to pain or permanent hearing loss. Although noise cannot be eliminated from the community, much can be done to minimize or control it. Observation and interviews will provide clues to this pattern.

Cognitive-Perceptual Pattern

This pattern identifies information about a community's ability to solve problems and make decisions. The process of how a community makes decisions and allocates resources is necessary for a system's survival and relevant to health promotion and protection. Communities must have a functioning decision-making body to ensure that its rules are followed and its goals are achieved. The five transactional strategies—coercion, bargaining, legal bureaucratic, team cooperative, and gemeinschaft—can be assessed to determine how the community interacts with the environment and whether the strategies used are effective in meeting health concerns and needs (Neuman, 1995).

Coercion uses force, fraud, or deception to convince the community to comply. For example, people living in a particular area of a community with high dioxin levels or asbestos may be forced to leave the area to protect their health.

Bargaining obtains compliance by offering the community an exchange. For example, one community may have a radiograph machine for mammography, but no primary care facility; it might negotiate with another community to provide mammographies in return for receiving primary care services.

The legal bureaucratic method ensures compliance by using an outside authority. For example, the state may mandate that the community maintain certain health standards. Therefore all school children must be immunized against specific diseases before entering public school.

The team-cooperative method obtains compliance by persuading members that they share common goals. For example, community residents may oppose a chemical dumpsite within the area because they believe it may be detrimental to their health.

Gemeinschaft plays on community sentiments, convincing people to comply because they hold some loyalty in the situation or relationship. For example, community residents might expend a great deal of effort and money fighting for the retention of a health clinic because they feel loyal to it.

Identifying the various decision-making patterns used by a community can provide clues about its priorities and value system related to health activities, about matches and mismatches between what exists and what are the health goals, and about whether future planning is performed. Data can best be obtained by observation and interviews.

Self-Perception–Self-Concept Pattern

This pattern identifies the self-worth and personal identity of a community. Image, status, and perceived competency to deal with problems are characteristics that can be noted about a community. The image of a community may be reflected in housing conditions, buildings, and cleanliness. What do the images in Fig. 8-2 say about these communities? Community perception of self-worth may relate to school systems, crime rates, accidents, and whether residents and outsiders consider it a good place to live. Competency in dealing with social and political issues and community spirit will create a positive self-evaluation. Knowing the level of community pride may assist in innovative health programs. The emotional tone (fear, depression, or positive emotional outlook) can usually be related to findings in other pattern areas. For example, tensions in the cognitive-perceptual pattern (conflict between groups concerning health issues) may explain a general feeling of fear in the residents. Data are obtained through observation and interviews.

A

B

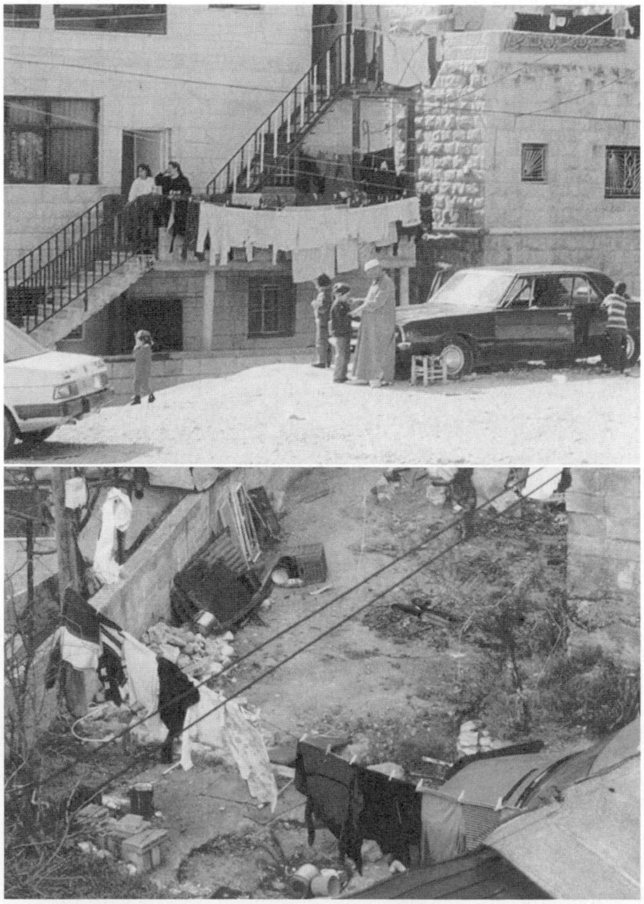

Fig. 8-2 Lack of laundry facilities may require hanging clothes outdoors. **A,** Condition of community street. Note rubbish under car. **B,** Note rubbish adjacent to laundry.

Roles-Relationships Pattern

This pattern identifies communication styles and formal and informal relationships. Of particular concern are roles and relationships that affect the community's ability to realize its health potential. Patterns of crime, racial incidents, and social networks are indices of human relationships in a community. Patterns of official communication are important to know so health-promotion activities can be publicized; major communicators can help make or break a health-related program. Key community leaders may not always be identified easily, but community members can help in this area.

Use of the media and other mass information programs can increase communication, the flow of health information, and the number of community members reached. Interviews, television, and newspapers are examples of ways in which information can be obtained.

Sexuality-Reproductive Pattern

This pattern identifies the reproductive data of a community, as reflected in live birth statistics and the mother's age and marital status. This information provides clues to the health-promotion needs of a particular community group.

The reproductive pattern of a community is also reflected in premature infant rates; abortion rates; and neonatal, infant, and maternal death rates. Such information identifies groups who are potentially at risk based on particular characteristics associated with these rates. Health concerns are also identified when a mismatch is found between existing health services, health education programs, and community health statistics. Other areas to be identified are the availability of sex education in the schools, spouse and child abuse, and sex-related crimes. Minutes of meetings, health records, statistical data, and public documents are examples of where this data can be found.

Coping–Stress-Tolerance Pattern

This pattern identifies the community's ability to cope or adapt. Communities respond in different ways to various events, some of which might threaten its integrity. The way in which a community responds is its coping pattern. The ability of individuals and groups to give and take goods, services, goals, values, and ideals to survive and to promote and protect the community's health is inherent in the community.

Community efforts to obtain goods from the environment, contain goods within the environment, retain goods within the community, and dispose of goods can play a significant role in influencing health. Examples of goods that a community might obtain from the environment to promote health include local, state, or federal funding; health services; a health-related workforce; and new knowledge and technological advances. Some communities have obtained an abundance of health care institutions and services. However, when examined closely, primary services are frequently inadequate or nonexistent. The lack of available health services, or the lack of ability to obtain them, constitutes community health needs.

Examples of goods a community might attempt to contain because a threat to community integrity, values, and health exists include sex-related crimes, various diseases, substance abuse, industry, hazardous wastes in the water supply, and noxious chemicals in the air.

The community's coping efforts might be geared toward retaining within its boundaries certain health-protection services, such as immunization services for children, and adequate health facilities. Coping efforts may also include strict zoning laws and housing codes or certain values such as sex education within the home.

Examples of goods that a community might dispose of into the environment include industrial and human wastes, substance abuse, certain health services or programs, and certain groups. Data can be obtained through minutes of meetings, public documents, health surveys, statistical data, and health records.

Values-Beliefs Pattern

This pattern identifies the values and beliefs of a community. Such information can provide clues to the health-promotion and health-protection efforts that the community values and is willing to support.

Values underlie decisions about whether the community should have health education in the schools, hypertension screening for the general public, prevention programs, or well-child clinics and how much of the community's tax money will be allocated for health-related activities. Traditions, norms, and cultural and ethnic groups all share in identifying the values and beliefs of a community. Data can be obtained through interviews with key community persons and health-related personnel.

ANALYSIS AND DIAGNOSIS WITH THE COMMUNITY

Analysis refers to the categorization of data and the determination of patterns. Once information about a community is obtained, the data must be organized and synthesized in a meaningful way to ascertain patterns of health activities and trends. Decision making and judgment inherent in the nursing process are particularly significant during the analysis and diagnostic phases. Community data can be grouped and organized in several ways (Table 8-2).

Organization of Data

Data can be synthesized through the use of various techniques, such as charts, figures, and tables. Graphic presentations of population distributions, morbidity and mortality data, or vital statistics can be most effective in pinpointing significant community concerns and actual or potential health problems. The data can be compared with the community health-related responses to these concerns.

Mapping is another valuable technique that facilitates data analysis. For example, data that change with time can be followed with a series of maps; several variables that may be spatially identical and contiguous can be analyzed simultaneously, such as the location of environmental hazards, densely populated areas, health-promotion services, and major highways. Poor environmental conditions; the distribution of illness, disease, and death rates; and the accessibility of health-protection and health-promotion activities for the population can be determined at a glance with dotted scatter maps. When maps are used, the population base of the community must be identified. For example, a less populated geographical area might have fewer health facilities for its residents than another area; one community might have fewer neonatal deaths than another because it has fewer women of childbearing age.

The use of theoretical frameworks and the 11 pattern areas will also facilitate the organization and analysis of community data. Several guidelines are presented to help

Table 8-2 Stages of Change

Stages	Interventions
PRECONTEMPLATION	• Provide information (identify risk factors) • Raise doubts about current behaviors and future outcomes
CONTEMPLATION	• Discuss risks of not changing • Discuss benefits of changing
ACTION	• Help plan phases of change • Help implement phases of change
MAINTENANCE	• Help develop strategies to prevent relapse, emphasizing self-efficacy • Offer encouragement
RELAPSE	• Highlight past successes and future benefits

Modified from Prochaska, J. O., Norcross, J. C., & DiClemente, C. C. (1994). *Changing for good.* New York: Avon.

the community nurse analyze community person data. Analysis often supports the need for further data collection.

Guidelines for Data Analysis

Check for Missing Data

The community nurse cannot obtain all the possible facts about the health-related pattern areas because complexity, size, and number of community characteristics must be considered. However, missing or insufficient data that indicate areas in need of further assessment should be identified. Additional assessment may be necessary to determine specific approaches or a particular community diagnosis. Missing data in a community assessment might include pollution indices, links between health resources and population groups, accessibility to resources, and morbidity statistics, all of which may be necessary to determine actual or potential health concerns. Census data may not be current, which should be noted. Missing data are generally indicated in a nursing diagnosis.

The nurse examines community data for incongruities; it is common to obtain conflicting information. For example, a key community official might deny the existence of pollutants in the water supply, whereas newspaper reports of the health department's water analysis findings indicate otherwise. The nurse validates such inconsistencies before identifying existing or potential health concerns.

Identify Patterns

The subjective and objective data of the assessment are examined for clues to determine whether a **community pattern** emerges or a clustering of information occurs. During this stage, the community nurse makes decisions and begins to formulate diagnostic hypotheses (ideas and tentative judgments about possible health concerns), identify possible community groups at risk, and establish probable causes and relationships. This activity further directs the search for additional clues in the data to confirm, reject, or revise the hypotheses generated. Judgments or hypotheses are generated constantly in the selection of clues that could form patterns in the data or relationships. For example, in obtaining interview data, the community nurse may have generated certain hypotheses that directed the search for additional information or may have determined the need for education programs within the community.

Community nurses can become overwhelmed by the data collected. They must narrow the list of the multitude of possible community health-promotion and health-protection concerns. One approach is to formulate broad problem statements based on the health-related pattern areas (Gordon, 1994). For example, does the community have an elimination problem (noxious chemicals), a coping and stress-tolerance problem (inability to obtain a particular health-education program), or a health perception-health management problem (high teenage mortality rate from motor vehicle accidents)? Asking such broad questions will help direct the community nurse to clues in the database.

Apply Theories, Models, Norms, and Standards

Analyzing community data requires a broad knowledge of developmental age-related risks and theories and concepts of nursing, public health, and epidemiology. This base enables the nurse to search for additional clues in the health-related patterns to develop community-nursing diagnoses amenable to nursing interventions.

The developmental approach can be used as a basis for identifying groups with potential health concerns. Different age groups vary in susceptibility; therefore the nurse must examine the community's resources to determine if they are directing services to highly susceptible groups. For example, community data may indicate an increase in live births among older women, which may indicate a need for additional health-promotion services for this group. If community data show an increasing number of aging citizens, the nurse should explore the existing health services that are available and accessible to them.

Data are also analyzed for population groups according to common personal or environmental characteristics. For example, the nurse may identify select groups at risk based on a shared health concern, such as substance abuse, lack of immunizations, unsafe housing conditions, high exposure to asbestos or noxious chemicals, or inadequate health services. A shared characteristic, such as race, may provide clues to susceptible groups in need of particular screening activities; a Black population may need hypertension screening if such services are lacking and children may be susceptible to dental caries and require screening if fluoridated water systems are lacking.

Other groups may have illiteracy in common. The literacy of a community is critical in health-promotion activities because it determines the methods used by nurses in establishing programs for specific health education. "The Internet has increased dramatically access to environmental information. Databases Toxnet, Grateful Med, and the Toxic Release Inventory may provide useful information about environmental hazards or other environmental problems in communities . . . better dissemination of global environmental health information . . . will help develop and achieve effective ways to prevent disease worldwide as well" (Edmondson & Williamson, 1998; USDHHS, 2000, p. 8-11).

Various standards are also used in analyzing data (Association for Worksite Health Promotion, 1999; Preventive Services Task Force, 1996; USDHHS, 2000). For example, community data regarding air can be compared with state or national ambient air quality standards to determine health. The term *ambient* in this context refers to outside air in a town, city, or other defined region. Continual air-monitoring stations are generally located in various urban and rural areas within each state.

The nurse explores the data concerning the health perception-health management pattern and then determines what available community resources are directed toward preventing risk factors and health problems. In this way, gaps in health-promotion and health-protection services can be identified more readily.

Identify Strengths and Health Concerns

Community data are analyzed and interpreted in light of community strengths and concerns and within obtainable limits of certainty. This requires making judgments and inferences about the community's health, responses to health situations and conditions, and population needs. One approach is to assume that health concerns exist unless the assessment data indicate otherwise (Gordon, 1994).

To make a diagnosis, the community nurse first summarizes the data and then makes one or more of the following judgments (Yura & Walsh, 1988):

1. No problem exists, but providing health-promotion or health-protection services may affect a potential health concern. For example, providing health education in the high school could offset *a potential for increased sexually transmitted disease in the high school population.*
2. A problem exists, but is recognized by community members or health-related professionals and is being handled effectively.
3. A problem exists that has been recognized by the community, but resources are inadequate or the community has not responded. Assistance is needed.
4. A problem exists that the community recognizes, but cannot deal with at this time, such as a lack of fluoridated water systems. Dentists, nurses, and nutritionists could be assigned to assist the community in resolving a potential problem of dental caries.
5. A problem or potential health concern exists that needs further study.

A community may have many strengths. Identifying these strengths is important because they can be integrated into plans for health-promotion and health-protection activities. For example, a community may have many nutritional feeding programs for its older adults, women, and children. However, few community members may know about such resources because community communications are lacking. Examples of community strengths and concerns are shown in Box 8-1.

Identify Causes and Risk Factors

In this step, the data are examined for those factors or characteristics that contribute to the list of the identified potential and existing health-related concerns. The nurse makes inferences about various population groups, identifying factors that place them at risk. For example, children entering elementary school may be at risk for rubella and mumps related to inadequate health-protection services in the community (a health-management deficit in the community). The identification of the risk factors gives direction to community nursing actions. Some risk factors may signify an immediate health concern for a population group, such as polluted water supplies; others may indicate a potential health problem if they are not altered, such as a lack of knowledge about childhood disease protection.

In identifying **community risk factors,** the community nurse must consider what risk factors have the potential to be altered, eliminated, or controlled through nursing actions. Some factors, such as the age, race, and gender of a population, cannot be altered; others, such as a lack of health-education programs, can be altered to lower a particular group's risk to potentially harmful health situations or conditions (see Multicultural Awareness box).

Box 8-1 Examples of Community Strengths and Concerns

STRENGTHS	CONCERNS
Well-child clinic available	Unavailable
Elderly feeding program accessible	Inaccessible
Sex education in schools acceptable	Unacceptable
Family planning services accessible	Inaccessible
Fluoridated water system	Nonfluoridated
Open communication	Dysfunctional communication
Interagency cooperation	Dysfunctional transactions
Adequate kitchen and plumbing facilities	Inadequate
High interest of key leaders in health promotion	Lack of interest

MULTICULTURAL AWARENESS

Poverty Among Black Americans

Blacks constitute 12% of the population of the United States. Although Blacks are represented in every socioeconomic group, one third live in poverty. This is a rate three times higher than the White American rate. Although Black Americans live in all areas of the United States, more than half live in urban areas. In these urban settings, they encounter the typical problems of poverty, such as crowded, inadequate housing and schools and high morbidity, crime, and mortality rates.

Community Diagnosis

A community assessment, as previously described, culminates in a nursing diagnosis or diagnoses. The process of determining a **community diagnosis** includes (1) a community situation or state within a population or population group; (2) data collection using some combination of observation, interview, and measurement; (3) a framework; (4) existing or potential health concerns; (5) appropriate risk factors related to the health concerns; and (6) a requirement for nursing actions. A diagnosis becomes the basis for planning and implementing interventions and nursing actions and for making evaluative judgments about health concerns (McFarland & McFarlane, 1993; NANDA, 2000; Sparks & Taylor, 1998). The Hot Topics box and the Health Teaching box discuss a diagnosis of violence and some recommendations to reduce the problem.

A community diagnosis is stated in a clear and concise manner to facilitate communication among community health professionals, team members, and laypersons. Lists of community diagnostic categories specific to certain populations are beginning to be developed (McFarland & McFarlane, 1993; NANDA, 2000; Sparks & Taylor, 1998). Community health nurses need to continue to develop diagnostic statements that are community and population centered, specific, accurate, and amenable to nursing interventions. The diagnosis may be written or stated according to the structural and functional aspects of a community.

Structural aspects include those related to the population, such as the demographic characteristics of groups who have similar characteristics (preschool children, adolescents, or a high school population). The functional aspects include those related to the psychosocial, physiological, or spiritual health patterns, such as decision making (cognitive-perceptual pattern) or communication links among health care resources (roles-relationships pattern). Information about health concerns and risk factors are obtained from the 11 functional health patterns. The structural and functional aspects of the community provide a framework from which diagnostic statements can be made (see Chapter 6).

HOT topics

OCCUPATIONAL SAFETY AND HEALTH ADMINISTRATION TAKES AIM AT WORKPLACE VIOLENCE

The Occupational Safety and Health Administration (OSHA) recently issued the first federal guidelines on preventing workplace violence. A document aimed at health care and social service workers was released in March 1996 and it will be followed by a document specific to retail workers. The new guidelines are not mandatory. They are also not specific because risks vary from site to site. For example, OSHA suggests installing metal detectors and bullet-resistant glass, but acknowledges that these measures are most appropriate for inner-city emergency departments, abortion clinics, and psychiatric facilities. OSHA recommends that every health care setting thoroughly assess security problems and adopt measures based on those findings. Some of the general recommendations are:

To Adopt Policies to

- Thoroughly evaluate risks.
- Train workers in prevention.
- Set up employee buddy systems.
- Encourage workers to report violent episodes.
- Cooperate with authorities.
- Identify visitors who may be prone to violence.

To Install

- Ample lighting
- Barriers that restrict access to work areas
- Deep service counters
- Mirrors at corners and hallway intersections
- Panic buttons to summon help
- Closed-circuit television
- Metal detectors
- Bullet-resistant glass
- Seclusion areas for patients who are violent

From Hinojosa, I. (1996). Taking control of violence in the workplace. *Advance for Nurse Practitioners, 11*, 36.

HEALTH TEACHING Ten Steps to Defuse Potential Violence

1. Make eye contact.
2. Stop what you are doing and give full attention.
3. Create a relaxed environment and speak calmly.
4. Build trust and strengthen the relationship.
5. Be open and honest.
6. Let the person have his or her say.
7. Listen attentively.
8. Ask for specific examples.
9. Carefully define the problem.
10. Explore the issue with open-ended questions.

From Hinojosa, I. (1996). Taking control of violence in the workplace. *Advanced Practice Nurse, 11*, 36.

PLANNING WITH THE COMMUNITY

The community health-planning phase begins with the nursing diagnosis. The desired goals are expected to resolve existing or potential health concerns. For example, if a high rate of childhood diseases in the community is the problem, decreasing the rate is the goal. The identification of the specific or potential health concern and planned actions to achieve the desired **community outcome** become the framework and data for **community evaluation.** Therefore health planning can be viewed as a problem-solving approach that has several purposes.

Purposes

The four major purposes of the planning phase are the following:

1. To prioritize the problems diagnosed from the assessment phase.
2. To differentiate problems that nursing actions can resolve from those that others can handle best.
3. To identify immediate, intermediate, and long-term goals; behavior objectives oriented to community behavior and derived from the goals; and the specific actions to achieve the objectives.
4. To write the problems, actions, and expected behavioral outcomes in a community nursing care plan (see Care Plan).

The planning phase culminates in a nursing plan that provides the framework for evaluation. Once developed, the plan is implemented.

The cost of delivering health services, the kinds of personnel involved, and the financial resources available will influence the priority given to health concerns, as will community values and the nurse's philosophy about people, health, the community, and nursing. Examples of problems to be given high priority in some communities are infectious agents, sexually transmitted disease, alcohol and drug use, smoking, inadequate nutrition, inadequate infant and child care, high death rate from motor vehicle accidents, and unwanted teenage pregnancies.

Community participation in health planning is essential to help assign priorities. As recipients of health-related services, members can also help ensure that the services being planned are of reasonable cost and high quality. Community residents can help ascertain the benefits sought by groups in need and determine whether the planned health services will be responsive to the needs and concerns of the population for whom they are intended. If community members and the nurse differ in setting priorities, mutual communication and a statement of the reasons for designating a particular priority can help resolve the difference.

When planning, the nurse must differentiate those problems that **community nursing intervention,** a behavior implemented by the nurse to fulfill a health goal of the community, can resolve from those health concerns that could best be handled by community members, referred to health-related professionals, or handled with community support. Rodents, poor sanitation conditions, or the absence of community recreational facilities should be referred to appropriate community leaders or agencies.

Developing goals, measurable behavioral outcomes, or objectives and designating those actions that will achieve the expected outcomes are important nursing activities. Outcomes are projected before the actual implementation of planned actions and are stated in terms of the individual behaviors that are expected to result from nursing actions. The effectiveness of nursing actions can be evaluated.

Health planning emphasizes promoting and protecting the health of population groups within the community; therefore problems, solutions, and actions are defined on this level. Community nurses who plan and implement health plans for one community population group, such as school-aged children, help the community begin developing health-promotion services for all residents. Nurses frequently act as agents of change by taking responsibility for influencing and changing existing and potential health patterns and behavior. Decisions and plans for health interventions are based on the community nurse's awareness and understanding of human behavior and principles of planned change.

Planned Change

Planned change is the result of specific efforts by individuals or groups and involves fundamental shifts in their behavior (Prochaska, Norcross, & DiClemente, 1994). Individuals can be the agents of their own health conditions; health is often determined more by what the person does than by what some outside germ or infectious agent can do. Some important community health objectives depend partly on individuals deciding to change their lifestyle (reducing alcohol consumption or giving up smoking).

Efforts to influence and reinforce changes in community health behavior are the central focus if risk reduction programs are to be effective. Any change effort by community nurses and groups can be viewed as a process.

Many studies have tried to explain why some groups of people effectively participate in certain health programs, whereas others do not. The early health belief model proposed by Rosenstock (1974) and more recent models developed by Pender (1996) and Prochaska, Norcross, & DiClemente (1994), among others, identify concepts that are critical to understanding how individuals undergo a change in health behavior. In Rosenstock's model, the following four steps are identified:

1. Perceiving the behavior as a threat to health in terms of susceptibility and seriousness.
2. Believing the behavior is a threat to health.
3. Taking action to adopt preventive health.
4. Reinforcing the new behavior.

CARE PLAN

Nursing Diagnosis: Ineffective Community Coping Related to Increased Levels of Teen Pregnancy

DEFINING CHARACTERISTICS

- Absence of education or support for sexually-active teenagers.
- Absence of programs for pregnancy testing, counseling, or teaching young women to care for infants.
- Absence of sex education in the home, school, and community.
- Community conflicts over what to teach adolescents and preadolescent children about sex.
- Failure of teenagers to perceive long-term effects of having babies.
- High incidence of infants who are born prematurely or with health problems.
- High rate of teen pregnancy.
- Lack of access to birth control pills or devices for teenagers.
- Lack of community support for preventive sex education.

EXPECTED OUTCOMES

- Community members express awareness of the seriousness of the high adolescent pregnancy rate in their community.
- Community members express the need for a plan to reduce the prevalence of teen pregnancies.
- Community members develop and implement plans to reduce teen pregnancy.
- Community members evaluate the success of the plan in meeting goals and objectives.
- Community members continue to revise the plan to prevent teen pregnancy as necessary.

INTERVENTIONS

- Assess teenagers' knowledge about sex and sexuality *to determine their educational needs.*
- Work with schools to develop pregnancy prevention programs *to provide adolescents with information about the risks, problems, and complications of early pregnancy.*
- Work closely with individual adolescents who are pregnant *to assess their needs and provide care.*
- Implement an outreach and health-promotion program to raise community members' awareness of the need *to approach teen pregnancy as a community problem.* Consider taking the following five steps:
    1. Work with teachers, school psychologists, counselors, school nurses, students, and the parent and teacher association *to determine the extent of the teen pregnancy problem.*
    2. Encourage local youth groups, churches, and social service organizations *to feature presentations on pregnancy prevention at their meetings.*
    3. Contact representatives of local corporations *to ask for funding for educational programs.*
    4. Help community members (school nurses, counselors, and teachers) recognize adolescent girls who need counseling regarding such issues as peer pressure to be sexually active and the long-term consequences of pregnancy. Remind community members of the importance of listening attentively and remaining nonjudgmental.
    5. Provide education on preventive birth control measures (including abstinence from sex) and have this information available at school.
- Establish clubs for adolescent girls in the community. *The goal of these clubs is to foster self-esteem.* During club meetings, members should have the opportunity to openly discuss difficult questions, such as why girls consider a baby as a status symbol and how to respond to peer pressure to be sexually active. *Improved self-esteem has been found the most effective way to reduce teen pregnancies.*
- Encourage adolescents to participate in peer support networks where they can openly discuss social and dating pressure and other issues related to teen pregnancy *to allow adolescents an opportunity to openly express their feelings and obtain support from peers.*
- Encourage community members to establish school-based clinics in which teens can have access to reproductive system models, pregnancy tests, and nonprescription birth control measures *to support the teenagers who make the decision to protect themselves from unwanted pregnancies.*
- Develop a list of referrals for teenagers, such as hospitals with human sexuality courses, charities that provide prenatal care and childbirth services, women's clinics, and Planned Parenthood *to compensate for restricted access to information in the adolescent's home or school.*
- Encourage community members to implement an information campaign to educate adolescents, parents, and community members about the problems associated with teen pregnancy.
- Work with community members to evaluate the effectiveness of the teen pregnancy prevention program and assist in modifying the program as needed *to ensure the program's effectiveness and promote use of the program as a model for preventive health.*
- Collect statistical data from the schools to analyze the teen pregnancy rates *to help evaluate the effectiveness of the prevention program.*

Modified from Sparks, S. M., & Taylor, C. M. (1998). *Nursing diagnosis reference manual* (4th ed.). Springhouse, PA: Springhouse.

Table 8-3 Implementation of Community Health Plan with Objectives and Rationale

Nursing Diagnosis: **Potential for increasing the incidence of fatal motor vehicle accidents in high school population related to alcohol use and driving.**
Goal: **North High School population will have reduced incidence (at least 20%) of fatal motor vehicle accidents related to alcohol use and abuse by December.**

Objective	Plans	Rationale
1. Community will have access to information about the incidence of fatal motor vehicle accidents and drunken driving arrests of its high school population for the last five years by March.	Interview local police about the incidence of fatal auto accidents and substance abuse in the community. Interview parents of deceased high school students, students, teachers, physicians, clergy, and emergency-room personnel about the incidence of the problem and suggested measures for decreasing the problem; suggest that interviews be broadcast over the high school radio station. Have several people write to the community newspaper commenting on the broadcast and problem.	*Unfreezing:* For change to occur, the community has to become dissatisfied with status quo and sense a need for change. *Empiric-rational strategy:* People are rational; discussion of facts can bring about support for change. Important elements for preventing the problem include educating the public and having key community leaders discuss their views; concern lends credibility and is necessary for action. People tend to listen to those with informal power. Keeping the issue before the community can raise consciousness.
2. Community will take action to inform the population at risk about responsible drinking and driving by June.	Suggest to school principal and school board the creation of a task force of community residents to plan a health program on individual responsibility and alcohol use in high school. Task force to include teachers, students, parents, clergy, police, nurse, and physician. Task force to: examine ways to determine and teach content, integrate it into the curricula, and recommend that community members, such as a nurse, be involved in teaching content.	*Changing:* Moving to a new level; community involvement will influence acceptability of changes. Community residents like to be involved in decision making. It is important to establish trust and collaboration between community groups; this opens communication channels between adolescents and the health community. Community involvement facilitates acceptance of change.
3. Community will implement an educational program for its high school population related to the use of alcohol and individual responsibility by November.	Implement educational plan.	*Refreezing:* Moving to the level of change brought about by community forces. Educational strategies built around the concept of individual responsibility are essential elements in promoting the health of young adults.

In this model, the consumer at first takes on a passive role; the transition from passive to active occurs between steps two and three (belief to action). If the ultimate goal is to improve the health of a community through risk reduction programs, community members need to be influenced so they will assume more responsibility for their health and become more active in adopting healthy lifestyles and behaviors. In planning health-promotion activities, the nurse must consider effective strategies to motivate and support the community's transition from a passive to an active state.

Once the plan is developed, it becomes a guide to nursing actions. The nurse must make additions and changes based on the community's problems, resources, and resolution of these problems to keep the plan viable. Table 8-3 gives an example of a community-oriented, health-promotion plan based on the goals recommended by the surgeon general's report on health promotion and disease

Box 8-2 Plan Options for Community-Based Action: Alcohol Abuse

COPING–STRESS-TOLERANCE PATTERN

Identify available community alcohol treatment resources.

Regulation and enforcement: Develop local alcohol control laws oriented toward prevention of abuse; develop consistent state regulation and control laws.

ROLES-RELATIONSHIPS PATTERN

Increase communication among community control agencies, the school, residents, and health-related agencies.

Restrict community advertisements for alcohol in community newsletters and newspapers.

prevention. As shown, several specific objectives have been derived from a broad goal. The objectives' direction is based on the nursing diagnosis, which includes risk factors that can be altered.

Examples of various rationales show how the nurse can incorporate major concepts of planned change into a community-based health-promotion plan.

Communicating the plans to other health professionals, community members, and key officials should not be overlooked; this is an essential aspect of planning. An article describing the educational plan can be published in local newspapers and bulletins and school officials can send letters to students' parents.

Other community-based actions in which the nurse may become involved to change alcohol abuse in the community are listed in Box 8-2. The various plans have been categorized according to the health patterns to show that a community problem can be approached from many directions. Plans that are feasible and well formulated help prepare for implementation (CDC, 1995).

IMPLEMENTATION WITH THE COMMUNITY

Once the plan for health-promotion and health-protection activities has been developed, the implementation of the nursing process begins. The plan may be implemented by the community nurse alone or together with team members and community residents and tested for viability. Its success or failure will depend on the nurse's intellectual, interpersonal, and technical skills and the plan's acceptability to community members.

Usually, resistance to change is overcome for the planned intervention to be successful. However, resistance to new health-promotion and health-protection activities is feedback that can be used constructively. In general, people resist change when they are defending something important that appears to be threatened by the change. Table 8-4 lists several factors identified as deterrents to community participation in health programs. An informed nurse takes steps to deal with such factors to ensure the successful implementation of the plan. The nurse recognizes that community members may resist the type of planned activities or the individuals promoting them. Others resist changing their own attitudes or lifestyle behaviors (Fig. 8-3).

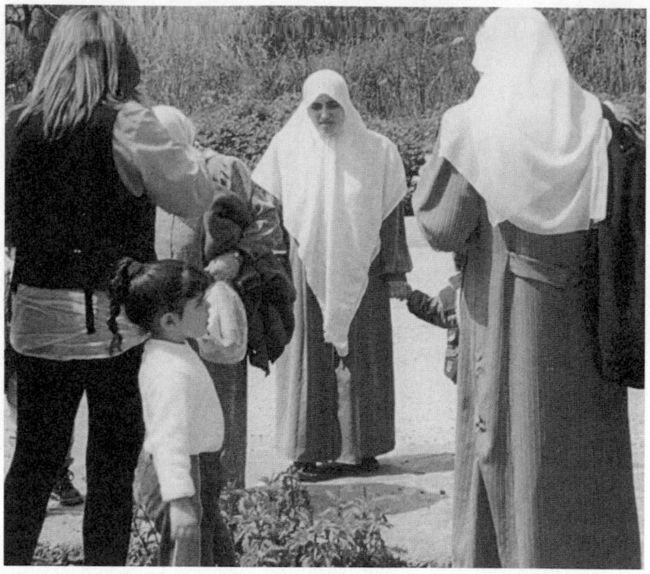

Fig. 8-3 Resistance to change may serve to increase a sense of security.

Table 8-4 Potential Sources of Resistance to Health-Promotion Programs, with Agent Responses

Source of Resistance	Response
Lack of communication about the implementation of the program	Communicate through community newsletter, newspapers, high school radio station, and posters
Misinformation regarding time and place of health activity	Disseminate valid information
Fear of the unknown	Inform and encourage
Need for security	Clarify intentions and methods
No desired need to change behaviors	Demonstrate opportunity for change
Cultural or religious beliefs or vested interests threatened	Enlist key community leaders in planning change
Inaccessibility	Focus activities near the largest potential target population and in an area accessible by public transportation

Community nurses implement health-promotion and health-protection plans in a variety of community settings (including schools, industry, public and private health agencies, and ambulatory care settings) where various population groups are relatively healthy. Nursing centers in communities provide nursing faculty, staff, and students unique opportunities to assess health and plan, implement, and evaluate care (including holistic health promotion and primary health care) to individuals, families, and communities with unmet health care needs (Clear, Starbecker, & Kelly, 1999; Gerrity & Kinsey, 1999; Lundeen, 1999; Taylor, Resnick, D'Antonio, & Carrell, 1997). The simplicity or complexity of implementing health actions will vary from one community or population group to another. However, as the nursing plan is implemented, nurses also learn more about the community and their own responses, strengths, limitations, and abilities to cope and adapt.

Although the implementation phase has an action focus, it also includes assessment, planning, and evaluation activities to monitor the actions taken to resolve, reduce, eliminate, or control the health concern.

EVALUATION WITH THE COMMUNITY

Evaluation is the phase of the nursing process in which the community nurse learns whether the actions designated in the nursing plan actually achieved the desired outcomes. The community and the nurse determine the community's progress or lack of progress toward goal achievement (American Nurses' Association, 1995). The nurse is responsible for the evaluation data, although community members or health-team members may participate in the process. For example, if a reduction in the incidence of fatal motor vehicle accidents is expected to result from nursing actions, the nurse is responsible for obtaining the community's behavioral outcomes, which should show that a reduction has occurred and that nursing actions helped bring about these outcomes.

As previously noted, the nursing plan, which includes the nursing diagnosis, expected outcomes, and interventions, provides the framework for evaluation. The community is the focus; its goals and objectives define what is evaluated and they are considered in terms of how the community responded to the planned actions. For example, if a reduction in childhood disease rates is expected after nursing actions, the nurse compares community responses before and after the actions. This also determines whether nursing actions are completely effective, partly effective, or ineffective in achieving the desired goal.

Evaluation is an ongoing process and is approached in a purposeful, goal-directed manner (Rootman, Goodstadt, & McQueen, 1999; USDHHS, 2000). Determining the effect of nursing actions during and after implementation is an important element in evaluating the degree to which goals are achieved. The frequency of evaluation will depend on the situation, the changes expected, and the objectives. For example, a bleeding individual may need to be evaluated every 15 minutes for signs of change, whereas evaluation of behavioral changes in community groups is not usually so immediate. In any population group, existing or potential health problems will be resolved or controlled within different intervals. Evaluation is determined by immediate, intermediate, and long-range goals; therefore the process is continued until the goals are realized.

The results of evaluating the community-nursing plan are also important because they may indicate the need to reassess, revise, or modify the plan. Community planning and nursing actions are not always effective in achieving the goals related to the health concerns and needs of the community (as noted, resistance to change may play an important role). As a result, the community nurse reassesses the situation and plans a new approach, then implements and evaluates the revised plan. The nursing process is a continual cycle.

Equally important is the community nurse's self-evaluation to determine strengths and weaknesses or how the nursing plan might have been implemented more effectively or efficiently. The quality of health-promotion and health-protection services to a community depends on the professional qualities of those providing the services and their effective use of the nursing process.

Effective programs of community health promotion are needed. However, skyrocketing health care costs limit available community health care resources. During this time of dramatic health care reforms, nurses need to increase the support for community health-promotion programs by demonstrating their effectiveness. Deal (1994) reviews numerous studies of intervention provided by nurses and documents their efficacy as described in a variety of research articles, including descriptive analyses and outcome evaluation studies on home-based and community-centered nursing interventions to meet needs of high-risk families, geographical communities, and vulnerable populations. Recommendations to gain support from legislators for community health-promotion programs are also included. In addition, *Healthy People 2010 Toolkit: A Field Guide to Health Planning* (2000) includes examples of national and state partnerships of setting health objectives and sustaining the initiatives.

SUMMARY

Illness, disability, and disease are not inevitable events that are experienced equally among a community's members. Understanding the dynamic and complex nature of communities is an important function of the community nurse if the planning, delivery, and coordination of health-promotion and health-protection activities for high-risk populations are to be effective.

The nurse uses various theoretical frameworks to assess the community's health-related patterns, health concerns, and health action potential and to implement the nursing process. Community data are collected and analyzed so subpopulations at risk can be identified. The community

innovative practice

The Por Cristo-Boston College School of Nursing Health Project: Collaborative Nursing Education and Practice in Ecuador

Since 1992, Boston College nursing students have participated in a community health clinical experience in Ecuador. This began as a voluntary project between Por Cristo, a medical missionary group, and Boston College School of Nursing (BCSON). It evolved into a credit-granting undergraduate clinical course and provided supervised clinical practice for several family nurse practitioner students. Dr. Ronna Krozy, an Associate Professor of Community Health Nursing at Boston College, developed the project and accompanies each team.

The goals of the Por Cristo-BCSON Health Project are to provide basic health education and service to an underserved population, develop creative teaching approaches, immerse students in a linguistically and culturally diverse community, develop students' sensitivity and awareness of cultural diversity and universality, recognize human dignity without regard to socioeconomic status, empower the community through enhancing their self-help capabilities, directly observe the effects of poverty, and demonstrate the community nurse and family nurse practitioner roles. Student experiences include home visits, family and community assessment, presenting community classes on various health topics, direct care, exchange of classes with Ecuadorian undergraduate and graduate nursing students, and visiting health facilities. Participants are required to have some fluency in Spanish and all materials and presentations are in Spanish.

From the outset, a number of collaborative relationships between faculty, students, and nurses in practice have been associated with the project. Students work with Father Frank Smith, a British missionary priest, who is also a registered nurse. They have assisted Father Frank in training auxiliary health care workers who provide care in their small community clinic and in home visits. The BCSON students present daily health classes to community groups and donate all of their materials for use by the auxiliaries.

Relationships have also been established with two local university schools of nursing: (1) Catholic University (CU) of Guayaquil, which is private, and (2) University of Guayaquil (UG), a public university. Both BCSON and Ecuadorian students present seminars to one another and a small group of Ecuadorian students accompany the BCSON students to work in the assigned community.

In 1996, Dr. Krozy received a Fulbright Scholarship to Ecuador to teach a symposium on AIDS and to assist in curriculum reform at CU. She began working with the nursing programs at both CU and UG to promote the use of Gordon's functional health patterns (FHPs) to assess the individual, family, and community and to expand their understanding and application of nursing diagnosis. She collaborated with faculty in developing workshops for students and nurses in practice, using the bilingual FHPs assessment tools she had developed as a collaborative research project with various Ecuadorian participants (Krozy & McCarthy, 1999). In 1999, Krozy co-facilitated the first Andean conference on nursing diagnosis with the nursing director of UG. Dr. Marjorie Gordon was the featured speaker and over 300 nurses and students attended. A nursing professor from UG was also sponsored as a visiting scholar at BCSON and is furthering the goals of UG to develop both nurse practitioner and doctoral programs in nursing.

Each team of undergraduate students is accompanied by a bilingual nurse practitioner to assist in overseeing students' direct care. For several years, the NP served a dual role in providing approved supervision for FNP students acquiring their clinical expertise. Individuals crossed the entire lifespan and reported conditions ranging from pregnancy to those associated with poverty and unhealthy environments. The experience provided a rich opportunity to address a variety of issues and to demonstrate an ideal advanced practice role for the FNP.

Collaborative international faculty and student experiences allow participants to learn and share with one another; these experiences are a means toward improving nursing as a profession and the care offered to individuals. In addition, collaborative practice promotes global health and international unity in nursing. Ultimately, it broadens the perspective and skills of nurses at all levels of practice.

References: Gordon, M. (2000). *Manual of nursing diagnosis* (9th ed.). St. Louis: Mosby; Krozy, R. E., & McCarthy, N. C. (1999). Developing bilingual tools to assess functional health patterns. *Nursing Diagnosis: The Journal of Nursing Language and Classification, 10* (1), 21-29, 34.

Courtesy Ronna E. Krozy, RN, PhD, Boston College School of Nursing, Boston, Massachusetts.

nurse identifies populations or aggregates at risk so specific health-promotion and health-protection services can be directed most profitably. These activities are be enhanced through the nursing process.

Many communities have obvious deficiencies in health services that warrant health-planning action. Community nurses play a significant role in health planning that is directed toward reducing risks associated with disease, premature death, and injury and promoting the health of community members. Principles of planned change are used to increase the community's awareness of health, healthy behavior, and participation in preventive health services.

The simplicity or complexity of applying the nursing process with a community will vary from one community or geographical area to another. Community nurses must research the relation of particular health-promotion actions to specific community phenomena to provide the necessary scientific evidence to support the benefits of nursing actions.

REFERENCES

American Nurses' Association. (1995). *Nursing a social policy statement*. Kansas City, MO: The Association.

Association for Worksite Health Promotion. (1999). *National worksite health promotion survey*. Northbrook, IL: The Association.

Bennett, J. A., Contessa, S. T., & Turner, L. C. (1999). Parent to parent: Preventing adolescent exposure to HIV. *Holistic Nursing Practice, 14*(1), 59-76.

Brezler, G. D. (1999). Injuries in adolescent workers: Health promotion and primary prevention. *American Association of Occupational Health Nurses, 47*(2), 5764.

Centers for Disease Control and Prevention. (1997). Youth risk behavior surveillance: National college health risk behavior survey/United States. *Morbidity and Mortality Weekly Report, 46*, 55-56.

Centers for Disease Control and Prevention. (1995). *Planned approach to community health: Guide for the local coordinator*. Atlanta, GA: CDC.

Clark, M. J. (1999). *Nursing in the community* (3rd ed.). Stamford, CT: Appleton & Lange.

Clear, J. B., Starbecker, M. M., & Kelly, D. W. (1999). Nursing centers and health promotion: A federal vantage point. *Family and Community Health, 21*(4), 1-14.

Deal, L. W. (1994). The effectiveness of community health nursing interventions: A literature review. *Public Health Nursing, 11*, 315-328.

Decker, S. D., & Knight, L. (1990). Functional health pattern assessment in a seasonal migrant farm worker community. *Journal of Community Health Nursing, 7*, 141-151.

Downswell, T., Towner, E. M. L., Simpson, T. G., & Jarvis, S. N. (1996). Preventing childhood unintentional injuries—what works? *Injury Prevention, 2*(2), 140-149.

Ebersole, P., & Hess, P. (1994). *Toward healthy aging: Human needs and nursing response* (4th ed.). St. Louis: Mosby.

Edmondson, M. E., & Williamson, G. S. (1998). Environmental health education for health professionals and communities: Using a train the trainer approach. *American Association of Occupational Health Nurses, 46*(1), 14-19.

Gerberich, S. S., Sterns, S. J., & Dowd, T. (1995). A critical skill for the future: Community assessment, *Journal of Community Health Nursing, 9*, 239-250.

Gerrity, P., & Kinsey, K. K. (1999). An urban nurse-managed primary health care center: Health promotion in action. *Family and Community Health, 21*(4), 29-40.

Gordon, M. (1994). *Nursing diagnosis: process and application*. St. Louis: Mosby.

Hinojosa, I. (1996). Taking control of violence in the workplace. *Advance for Nurse Practitioners, 11*, 35-38.

Hitchcock, J. E., Schubert, P. E., & Thomas, S. A. (1999). *Community health nursing—caring in action*. Albany, NY: Delmar.

Illuzzi, S., & Cinelli, B. (2000). A coordinated school health program approach to adolescent obesity. *Journal of School Nursing, 16*(1), 12-19.

Kriegler, N. F., & Harton, M. K. (1992). Community health assessment tool: A patterns approach to data collection and diagnosis. *Journal of Community Health Nursing, 9*, 229-234.

Lear, J. G. (1996). School-based services and adolescent health: Past, present and future. *Adolescent Medicine: State of the Art Reviews, 7*(2), 163-180.

Lundeen, S. P. (1999). An alternative paradigm for promoting health in communities: The Lundeen Community Nursing Center Model. *Family and Community Health, 21*(4), 15-28.

McFarland, G. K., & McFarlane, E. A. (1993). *Nursing diagnosis and intervention: Planning for patient care*. St. Louis: Mosby.

North American Nursing Diagnosis Association (NANDA) (2000). *NANDA nursing diagnoses: Definitions and classification, 1999-2000*. Philadelphia, PA: The Association.

Neuman, B. (1995). *The Newman systems model: Application to nursing education and practice*. Norwalk, CT: Appleton-Century-Crofts.

Opas, S. R. (1995). *Exploring the potential for school nurse practice: An ethnographic study of the roles of a school nurse in an elementary school setting*. Unpublished doctoral dissertation, University of California, Santa Barbara, CA.

Orpinas, P., Kelder, S., Frankowski, R. Murray, N., Zhang, Q., & McAlister, A. (2000). Outcome evaluation of a multicomponent violence-prevention program for middle schools: The students for peace project. *Health Education Research, 5*(1), 48-58.

Pender, N. J. (1996). *Health Promotion in Nursing Practice* (2nd ed.). Stamford, CT: Appleton Lange.

Prochaska, J. O., Norcross, J. C., & DiClemente, C. C. (1994). *Changing for good*. New York: Avon.

Reece, S. M. (1998). Community analysis for health planning: Strategies for primary care practitioners: Nurse practitioner. *American Journal of Primary Health Care, 23*(10), 46, 49, 53-54.

Rootman, I., Goodstadt, M., Hyndman, B., & McQueen, D. (1999). *Evaluation in health promotion: Principles and perspectives*. Copenhagen: World Health Organization.

Rosenstock, I. (1974). The health belief model and preventive health behavior. *Health Education Monograph, 2*, 354-361.

Sheilds, L. E., & Lindsey, A. E. (1998). Community health promotion nursing practice. *Advances in Nursing Science, 20*(4), 23-36.

Sparks, S. M., & Taylor, C. M. (1998). *Nursing diagnosis reference manual* (4th ed.). Springhouse, PA: Springhouse.

Stanley, S. A. R., & Stein, D. S. (1998). Health Watch 2000: Community health assessment in South Central Ohio. *Journal of Community Health Nursing, 15*(4), 225-236.

Taylor, C. A., Resnick, L., D'Antonio, J. A., & Carroll, T. L. (1997). The advanced practice nurse role in implementing and evaluating two nurse-managed wellness clinics: Lessons learned about structure process and outcome. *Advanced Practice Nursing Quarterly, 3*(2), 36-45.

U.S. Department of Health and Human Services. (2000, July 25). *Healthy people 2010 toolkit: A field guide to health planning* [On-line]. Available: www.healthgov/healthy people/state/toolkit.

U.S. Department of Health and Human Services. (2000). *Healthy people 2010* (Conference Edition). Washington, DC: The Department.

Von Bertalanffy, L. (1968). *General systems theory*. New York: George Braziller.

World Health Organization, Division of Health Promotion, Education and Communication (1998). *Health promotion glossary*. Geneva: World Health Organization.

Yura, H., & Walsh, M. B. (1988). *The nursing process: assessing, planning, implementing, evaluating* (5th ed.). Norwalk, CT: Appleton & Lange.

Unit Three

Interventions for Health Promotion

9 Screening

10 Health Education

11 Nutrition Counseling

12 Exercise

13 Stress Management and Crisis Intervention

14 Holistic Health Strategies

Chapter 9

MARIE TRUGLIO-LONDRIGAN
MARGARET K. MACALI

Screening

objectives

After completing this chapter, the nurse will be able to:

- Define screening and its relationship to preventive health care intervention.
- Identify the advantages and disadvantages of the screening process.
- Define the specific criteria that determine a screenable disease.
- Discuss the health care and economic issues related to the screening process that result in ethical implications.
- Explain sensitivity and specificity as they relate to the efficacy of screening.
- Identify the broad range of community resources included in and affected by the screening process.
- Describe the nursing role in the screening process.
- Identify critical questions pertaining to culture and ethics within the health care system.
- Discuss how a Collaborative Partnership may assist a community in the attainment of *Healthy People 2010* goals.

key terms

Cost-Benefit Ratio Analysis
Cost-Effectiveness Analysis
Cost-Efficiency Analysis
Ethical Issue
False Negative
False Positive
Group or Mass Screening
Individual Screening
Interobserver Reliability
Intraobserver Reliability
Multiple-Test Screening
Natural History
One-Test Disease Specific Screening
Reliability
Sensitivity
Specificity
Validity

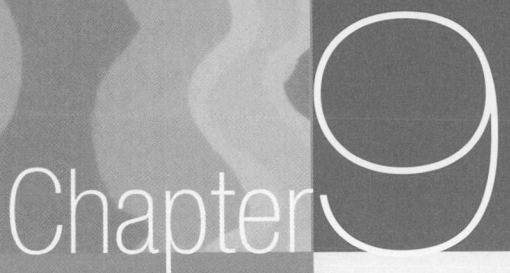

THINK About It

Screening to Identify Risk Factors

Ms. Lukas is a 55-year-old account executive for a leading advertising firm. This is a high-power, high-pressure position that requires her attention from 12 to 14 hours a day. It leaves little time for rest, relaxation, or exercise. She frequents take-out restaurants because she is unable to find time to cook or shop for healthy food. Her job often requires her to take individuals out for dinner and drinks. A recent increase in job pressures has provoked her to resume smoking two to three packs of cigarettes a day.

During a lunch hour, Ms. Lukas and a colleague visited a community health fair and were offered a free health screening. Ms. Lukas' blood pressure was 200/110 mm Hg. Her nonfasting cholesterol measurement revealed a level of 265 mg/dl. Her colleague, who is 20 years younger and leads a similar lifestyle with similar habits, had a blood pressure reading of 130/82 and a cholesterol level of 215 mg/dl. The counselor was very adept at evaluating risk factors for both individuals. This analysis revealed similar risks for each woman.

Although Ms. Lukas did benefit from the early identification of potential hypertension and hypercholesterolemia, she did not reap the benefits of early risk factor analysis like her younger colleague. If counseling and education prove successful, Ms. Lukas' colleague will demonstrate increased wellness through appropriate behavioral changes that could potentially prevent the realization of disease.

1. Recent research has supported the need for screening in an attempt to identify disease at early stages. However, if this were the case, would it not support the notion of screening for the identification of risk factors that have been associated with disease processes?
2. Will this identification of risk factors dramatically affect the onset of disease?
3. How can nurses use their expertise to help individuals achieve the desired behavioral changes necessary for risk factor reduction?

Screening has received growing recognition as a valuable tool for health care professionals, particularly as health care delivery moves toward preventive interventions. Although health education about screening comes under the rubric of primary prevention (see Chapter 1), the actual process of screening is a form of secondary prevention. The primary objective of screening is the detection of a disease in its early stages to treat it and deter its progression. The basic assumption guiding this process is that detection during the early asymptomatic period allows treatment at a time when the course of the disease can be significantly altered. The screening concept is based on the principle that disease is preceded by a period of asymptomatic pathogenesis (disease development) when risk factors predisposing a person to the pathological condition are building momentum toward manifestation of the disease. Screening takes advantage of the early pathogenic state. The administration of tests (often simple in form) during this stage identifies specific variables that distinguish individuals who most likely have the condition from those who do not. Screening is not considered a diagnostic measure; it is seen as a preliminary step to direct a health care provider in assessment of the ostensibly healthy individual's chances of becoming unhealthy. The ultimate goal could be curative, but more often it is to prevent further development of the disease or to ameliorate the possible outcomes. A second, but equally important, objective of screening is to reduce the costs of treating the disease by avoiding the more vigorous interventions required during its later stages. The added attraction of a cost-conscious approach to health care mandates that health care professionals at all levels acquire a basic understanding of the screening process and its application.

This chapter describes the screening process and the strengths and weaknesses of its implementation. The presentation allows the nurse to (1) analyze the screenability of a particular disease and (2) determine the means of implementing a screening program specific to the population, the disease, and the system of health care delivery.

ADVANTAGES AND DISADVANTAGES

Preclinical illness and previously unrecognized disease in individuals may be detected via screening efforts (Anderson & McFarlane, 2000). Screening tests offer several advantages. First, screening tests are often simple and inexpensive and, frequently, a trained technician can administer them. The simplicity of the screening procedure decreases the time and cost of involved health care personnel and enables lesser-skilled technicians to administer the test. This also reduces cost and permits the more appropriate use of highly skilled, costly professionals at the definitive, diagnostic stage. A second advantage is the ability to apply the screening process to both individuals and large groups. In an **individual screening** program, one person is tested by a health professional who has designated the individual as high risk. The practitioner can make this selection independently, the health care agency can define a specific policy, or a legislative body can require the screening by law as in the case of phenylketonuria (PKU) or lead-screening programs. **Group or mass screening** occurs when a target population is selected on the basis of an increased incidence of condition or a recognized element of high risk within the group. An example of this would be lower-income populations or cultural groups that may exhibit a significant prevalence of a particular condition, such as hypertension. The target population may be invited to a central location on a designated day to be tested for the selected disorder. A third advantage is the ability to provide one-test specific screening or multiple-test screenings. A **one-test disease specific screening** is the administration of a single test that searches for a specific characteristic that indicates a high risk of developing a disorder. An example of this would be blood pressure screenings to evaluate the risk of hypertension. **Multiple-test screening** is the administration of two or more tests to detect more than one disease. In some cases, the same sample can be used to evaluate the possibility of several conditions, saving time and money and making the process efficient and economic. For example, a blood sample can be evaluated for both elevated glucose and cholesterol. Ultimately, it is the combination of the relatively low cost of a screening test and flexibility that makes screenings adaptable to all levels of the health care delivery system.

The disadvantages of screening stem largely from the imperfection of modern science, which results in a margin of error for most instruments and tests. In screening, when program effectiveness depends on the test's ability to distinguish those who probably do have the disease from those who do not, the margin of error can precipitate serious consequences. Some individuals who do not have the condition will be referred for further tests and some who do have the disease will not. Those incorrectly referred suffer needless anxiety while awaiting more definitive diagnostic procedures. They must also bear the burden of the cost of follow-up visits, lost time, and inconvenience. The effects on those whose disorders have been missed are even more important. These individuals leave with a false sense of a healthful state that will be shattered eventually. They lose the opportunity to receive early treatment that could prevent irreversible damage. The difficulty of balancing the benefits to some against the losses to others is an **ethical issue** of most screening programs. The significance of this disadvantage can vary; therefore it should be assessed for each project, disease, and population.

SELECTION OF A SCREENABLE DISEASE

The selection of a screenable disease goes beyond examination of the disease alone. The selection process must often encompass less tangible factors, such as the emotional and financial impact of the disease's detection on the screened population. Even after gathering data and reviewing the critical issues, the final decision "to screen or not to screen" must often be reached with incomplete data or with answers that raise highly ethical issues. The potential uncertainties confounding the decision emphasize the need to conduct an exhaustive analysis of available material to obtain a decision that is as objective and scientific as possible. The answers to the following three questions provide a basis for designating a disease as screenable or not screenable:

1. Does the significance of the disorder warrant its consideration as a community problem?
2. Can the disease be screened?
3. Should the disease be screened?

As simplistic as these questions may appear, the answers or lack of answers may expose numerous complex issues that determine whether or not a well-informed decision can be made on screenability.

Significance

The significance of a disease refers to the level of priority assigned to the disease as a public health concern. Although the opinions of political and public interest groups may enter into the evaluation, significance is generally determined by the quantity and quality of life affected by the disorder. The greater the physical and psychological harm experienced by the population, the greater the need to designate the disease as a priority health problem. The first step in assessing screenability is evaluation of this significance to decide if the disorder warrants the time, effort, and funds that must be allocated to a screenable disease.

Estimating the quality of life affected by a disease presents a problem. The perception of quality is subjective and individual evaluations may differ. For example, not all people equally perceive the disability resulting from a disease; some make adjustments and cope, whereas others do not. Those who do not would be more likely to say that the quality of their lives is significantly lower than that of the people around them.

By contrast, measures of the quantity of life affected by the disease are more readily obtainable. Disease-specific mortality rates present one picture of this effect, whereas prevalence and incidence rates provide another. Prevalence defines the number of old and new cases during a specific time; incidence examines only the new cases during a specified period. Usually, chronic conditions are measured by their prevalence, whereas acute conditions are assessed by their incidence.

In this era of cost-conscious health care, a new dimension has been added to the evaluation of significance: the cost required to treat the disease. In some cases, the prevalence of the disorder may not be great, but the problem requires disproportionate amounts spent on maintenance or treatment after the condition is fully expressed. For example, with phenylketonuria (PKU), the incidence is not significant, but the cost of an undetected case at birth is a lifetime of case management across the lifespan. Given the costly outcome if undetected and the reasonable price of the test to detect the disorder, the cost of screening all newborns is nominal.

Can the Disease Be Screened?

With the relative significance of the disease established, the next step is to determine if health professionals can screen for the disease. Do well-documented diagnostic criteria for the disorder exist? Is there a screening instrument? Are sufficient community resources and treatment modalities available to support a screening program?

Diagnostic Criteria

Detection of a disease requires knowledge of characteristics that clearly indicate its presence or, as in screening, its early pathogenic, asymptomatic state. Selected diagnostic criteria should be well documented; it should not be merely accepted or commonly used indicators. The impact of uncertainty in detecting disease is amplified when considering the application of the screening design. Some diseases are defined by the presence or absence of a single, isolated factor, such as sickle cell anemia. Other conditions are indicated by the measurement of statistically derived numerical values for which a normal range has been set, such as hypertension. Disagreement over the parameters of the normal range, combined with contentions that what is abnormal for one individual may not be abnormal for another, makes these conditions more controversial to designate as screenable diseases.

Screening Instruments

The next step is to determine if methods exist to detect the disease during early pathogenesis. If instruments are available, a careful analysis should determine if any of them fulfill the requirements for the screening process: safe, cost-effective, and accurate. Ultimately, the question is how well the instrument can distinguish those individuals who probably do not have and will not develop the condition from those who are likely to develop it. The variables that aid in instrument evaluation include reliability and validity.

Reliability **Reliability** is an assessment of the reproducibility of the test's results when different individuals with the same level of skill perform the test during different periods and under different conditions. If the same result emerges from two individuals performing the test, **interobserver reliability** is shown. If the same individual is able to reproduce the results several times, **intraobserver reliability** is shown. Therefore testing for instrument reliability can yield data on the accuracy of the test (U.S. Preventive Service Task Force, 1996).

From these data, the health professional can determine the amount of training that is required for the health care technicians or personnel who administer the test. For example, if interobserver reliability is low, additional training might be required to work toward a more consistent method of delivering the test. This is frequently necessary in hypertension screening. If intraobserver reliability is low, the health professional might surmise that the instrument, and not the individual, is at fault.

Validity **Validity** measures the test's ability to correctly distinguish between diseased and nondiseased individuals. In a controlled setting, validity is evaluated by testing the instrument on a group of individuals who have positive or negative test reactions. The ideal result is to have the instrument pick out 100% of the diseased people (positive reactions) and 100% of the nondiseased people (negative reactions). Such accuracy rarely occurs in practice; therefore the measure of validity has been divided into two components that quantify the margin of error in the screening instrument. **Sensitivity** measures the first component. This refers to the proportion of persons with a condition who correctly test positive when screened. A test with poor sensitivity will miss individuals with the condition and there will be a large number of **false negative** test results or individuals who actually have the condition, but were told they are disease free. **Specificity** is the second component. Specificity measures the test's ability to recognize negative reactions or nondiseased individuals. A test with poor specificity will result in individuals being told that they have a condition, a **false positive,** when in actuality they do not.

Application of sensitivity and specificity data to the actual outcome of the program raises some interesting points. Consider the issues that a public health nurse must face when given a newly developed screening test with low specificity and moderate sensitivity. Low specificity means few true negative and more false positive test results. The nurse and other health professionals must then consider the cost, inconvenience, and psychological stress experienced by the people with false positive reactions during the period after their incorrect screening test, the unnecessary additional referrals, and the ability of the existing follow-up services to meet these needs.

With only moderate sensitivity, a number of false negatives could occur, which may send away individuals who could benefit from treatment. The issue raised here is ethical; that is, should a screening program be implemented when it is known that individuals who could benefit from treatment will be sent away?

The issues emerging from investigation of the screening instrument demonstrate the significant influence it has on the entire screening process. Data on the reliability and validity of the screening test provide valuable information to evaluate, anticipate, and ideally control these influences, enabling the program to work effectively toward its goal.

Community Resources

Implementing a screening program depends on available appropriate community resources, such as funds, health care workers, follow through, treatment sources, and administrative personnel. The judicious organization of the overall program is key to its success. Knowledge of the disease's characteristics and the screening instrument are useless without financial and organized human support to apply it. The overall approach is complex, requiring intense efforts in the area of partnership development.

A lead agency is identified to oversee the development process of the community health program. Origins of the lead agency vary from a community service organization to the local public health department responding to a mandate from the state. Regardless of its origin, the agency must perform a self-evaluation to compare its level of expertise with that required to oversee the process inclusive of the screening effort. Early identification of the lead agency, with partnership strengths and weakness, allows for the effective use of talents and the division of labor.

For the lead agency to develop and oversee the development process of the community health program and the delivery of a screening program, the development of partnerships is essential. The agency must contract and organize necessary stakeholders, including health and social service agencies, community organizations, and key community individuals. Examples of stakeholders include health and social service agencies, such as a primary health care center, and community organizations, such as houses of worship, community centers, schools, transportation agencies, and volunteer organizations. Key community individuals are those people who are considered leaders within the community. The primary rule is: never assume what is appropriate and effective for one community will be appropriate and effective for another.

Together, the members of the partnership carry out the community assessment. A community assessment is a systematic method of data collection that provides a detailed account regarding the type, quantity, and quality of available resources. This community assessment includes recreation, physical environment, education, safety and transportation, politics, government, health, social services, communications, economics, the core components of demographic, vital statistics, and morbidity and mortality data (Anderson and McFarlane, 2000).

After completing the assessment, the analysis of data will reveal the target community or high-risk population, the available health care resources, and the high-risk population health need. The identified partners collaborate, review, and analyze the data leading to the development of health improvement strategies (in this case, a screening program) with methods of implementation to move the target population smoothly through the screening process. Finally, monitoring and evaluating outcomes is essential to determine the effectiveness of the program and the achievement of stated goals. It is important to note that evaluation is inclusive of monitoring the entire process, including the successful workings of the partnership. Figure 9-1 presents a model of the Collaborative Partnership: Community Health Program Development.

Constraints affecting the operation of a screening program include financial concerns, political issues, cultural constraints, follow-up and referral services, and available treatment facilities. All partners are aware that responses from the target community are affected partly by their experience with other screening programs, such as the means used to inform them, the accessibility of the screening programs location, the availability of transportation, the convenience of the program's hours, and the cultural

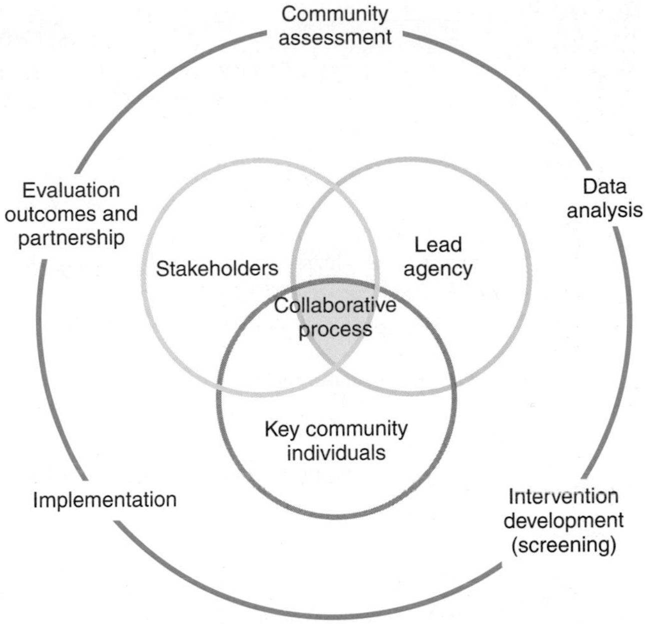

Fig. 9-1 Collaborative partnership: Community Health Program Development.

sensitivity of the delivery and design of the program. A public health nursing approach identifies the necessary community resources and defines how these resources interact and may be mobilized to achieve maximum benefits and positive outcomes. One example of this is presented in the Collaborative Partnership Community Care Plan for a Breast and Cervical Cancer Screening Program.

Financial support of the screening program is a constraint that can influence all points in the system. Although some programs are delivered entirely on a voluntary basis, other program organizers must submit grant proposals to local, state, or federal departments when consideration of medical and economic ethics is involved. Planners must look beyond the screening day and investigate financial resources for follow-up care and treatment.

In addition to financial accessibility, follow-up services should be accessible in terms of convenient locations and open hours. For example, an evening clinic may compensate for those who are reluctant or financially unable to miss work. Development of an efficient referral system links the follow-up resources to the screening program, providing continuity of care. A method must be devised to encourage the participant to take positive action on the referral. Public health nurses will use a variety of communication techniques to facilitate this process, such as telephone or in-person counseling, mailings, and home visits.

Should the Disease Be Screened?

After determining that the disease is significant and can be screened, establishing whether health professionals should screen for the disorder is the final step. Screening for a

CARE PLAN

Collaborative Partnership Community Care Plan: Breast and Cervical Cancer Screening Program

The planning and development of any screening program warrants partners to address and analyze two primary areas of importance:

1. Their working relationship and the problems and potential complications that may have an affect on the successful implementation and outcome of the program.
2. The major health care issues and the special needs of the targeted population.

With this information in hand, partners will know what issues may have to be addressed during the planning process of the screening program so they may assist the individual or individuals using the screening program, enhancing individual health outcomes. (The participant may be an individual, a family, or a targeted group.)

I. DIAGNOSTIC CLUSTERS

A. Collaborative Partnership Problems and Potential Complications
   1. Interagency agreements regarding screening, follow-up, and treatment.
   2. Transportation of individuals as needed.
   3. Movement of individuals through screening process, including follow-up.

B. Participant Problems and Potential Complications
   1. Knowledge deficit.
   2. Language barriers.
   3. Cultural differences.
   4. Anxiety.

II. NURSING DIAGNOSIS

A. Nursing Diagnosis for Collaborative Partnership Problems and Potential Complications
   1. Ineffective management of interagency agreements regarding screening, follow-up, and treatment related to complexity of partnership and communication difficulties.
   2. Lack of transportation services to assist targeted group related to limited resources within targeted community.
   3. Ineffective movement of individuals through the screening process, including follow-up related to complexity of the screening process.

B. Nursing Diagnosis for Participant Problems and Potential Complications
   1. Knowledge deficit and unfamiliarity with breast and cervical cancer screening resources and processes related to unfamiliarity with information.
   2. Impaired communication related to cultural differences (English as a second language or primary communication patterns are in a language other than English).
   3. Anxiety related to unfamiliar routine and environment.

III. GOALS

A. Collaborative Partnership Problems and Potential Complications
   1. Goal #1: Will negotiate the complexity of the partnership.
   2. Goal #2: Will negotiate transportation services with specific collaborative partners.
   3. Goal #3: Will develop policy and procedures that support movement of individuals throughout the screening process seamlessly.

B. Participant Problems and Potential Complications
   1. Goal #1: Will verbalize their understanding of the breast and cervical cancer screening process and the significance of their individual results.
   2. Goal #2: Will verbalize their understanding of the follow-up process and the necessary steps to take to enhance their health.
   3. Goal #3: Will verbalize their comfort with the screening process, environment, and follow-up.

IV. INTERVENTIONS

A. Collaborative Partnership Problems and Potential Complications
   1. Intervention #1
      a. Develop organizational maps outlining lead agency, stakeholders, key community individuals, and documented roles and responsibilities with regard to the collaborative partnership.
      b. Establish clear lines of communication.
      c. Develop technology systems to assist with communication, documentation, and surveillance.
   2. Intervention #2
      a. Develop strategies to enhance and use transportation resources already in place to serve the targeted group.
      b. Develop new transportation systems that will support the targeted group to and from screening sites.
   3. Intervention #3
      a. Develop a program to support availability, accessibility, affordability, appropriateness, adequacy, and acceptability (National Institute of Nursing Research, 1995).
      b. Provide for an environment that supports cultural sensitivity and awareness of culturally specific needs.
      c. Provide for interpreters and materials that are language- and culture-appropriate.
      d. Implement protocols, policy, and procedures related to outreach, advertisement, process of screening, education, documentation (number of screenings, number of positives and negatives, number of borderline cases, number referred,

CARE PLAN

Collaborative Partnership Community Care Plan: Breast and Cervical Cancer Screening Program—cont'd

number who completed follow-up, and number diagnosed), follow-up, referral, and treatment.

B. Participant Problems and Potential Complications
   1. Intervention #1
      a. Provide culturally sensitive, educational material.
      b. Provide educational materials in multiple languages where appropriate.
      c. Provide educational materials that focus on: (1) the disease or specific area on which the screening program is focusing, (2) the steps of the screening process, (3) the results of the test, (4) the meaning of the results, (5) the importance of follow-up, (6) how to access the system for appointments, and (7) how to contact resource persons they may use if unable to follow up and in need of assistance.
   2. Intervention #2 (same as Intervention #1)
   3. Intervention #3
      a. Support individuals in treatment choices and in self-care toward health-promoting behavior.
      b. Create a comforting environment.

V. OUTCOME
A. Collaborative Partnership Problems and Potential Complications
   1. Outcome #1: The collaborative partnership communicates efficiently and effectively and uses resources and information technology.
   2. Outcome #2: Transportation serves the targeted group efficiently and effectively.
   3. Outcome #3: Seamless screening process is in place with individuals moving effortlessly throughout the program.
B. Participant Problems and Potential Complications:
   1. Outcome #1: Describe breast and cervical cancer screening process, the significance of results, and the importance of follow-up.
   2. Outcome #2: Describe health promotion and behavioral change necessary to promote health.
   3. Outcome #3: Describe the screening process.

particular disorder and ultimately treating the individual with the early-identified disorder should improve the chances of a favorable outcome in comparison to those individuals who are not found until actual signs and symptoms become evident. Therefore several questions must be considered. If a test is accurate in the identification of a condition in the early stages, is there any benefit to the individual? Are there effective treatment modalities in place for the identified condition?

Interventions

Screening is based on the disease's asymptomatic period; therefore adequate information must exist concerning: (1) the optimal time for screening, (2) specific intervention during this time, and (3) knowledge as to the effect of early detection and treatment on the prognosis. Without this knowledge, health care professionals are unable to explain how the consequences of the detected disease differ from those of the undetected. They can neither evaluate nor explain the health benefits derived through participation in the screening program.

The absence of any interventions can be almost as detrimental as the presence of adverse effects of a disorder. In this situation, not only has the screening program misled the screened population that a health benefit will result from their efforts, but the development and implementation of the screening program has used both personal and community resources that have no possibility of altering the course of a particular disease.

The first step in a screening program is follow-up with the postscreening referral. The success of this endeavor depends on the accessibility, availability, affordability, appropriateness, adequacy, and acceptability of community health agencies and health care professionals (National Institute of Nursing Research, 1995). Meeting these six challenges is critical for efficient follow-up.

The next step is follow-up with the prescribed regimen, such as diet, exercise, and drug therapy. Evaluation of follow-up may include a review of the literature that discusses former successes or failures in follow-up with a particular drug and the identification of intervention characteristics that impair follow-up, such as cost, inconvenience, or side effects. Consideration must also be given to those factors that enhance follow-up. For example, nurses can provide ongoing counseling and education about a particular drug and assist individuals in a transformation of lifestyle to include health-promoting behaviors.

Safety of the intervention is a particular concern when considering the widespread application of a remedy after a screening program. Risks or harmful side effects can be costly in terms of human health and the increased medical care required to correct the iatrogenic effects resulting from the intervention. Health care professionals must decide if these risks significantly diminish the success of the treatment and outweigh the benefits derived from the treatment.

ETHICAL CONSIDERATIONS

Any step taken toward improving health is usually deemed a just and moral act within the health care system's values. However, when approaching health care practices with a more critical eye and realizing that not all the results of a well-intended practice are beneficial, the need to balance the benefit against the detriment becomes an issue. The resulting decision process becomes a value judgment and an ethical decision.

Health Care Ethics

A screening program is unlike the normal mechanism of the health care system. Rather than receiving those who have performed a self-assessment and elected to enter the system, a screening program invites apparently well individuals to be tested for the determination of disease risk and the need for further follow-up. The request for participation implies that a health benefit will be derived, although at this stage nothing is said about what it will be or what the consumer must do to obtain it. Program planning that attempts to clarify this implication and inform participants of the issues develops the basis for an ethically sound project and enhances the screenability of the disease.

Most screening programs are called *hypertension screening* or *diabetic screening;* therefore it is not surprising that participants enter them assuming the results received are diagnostic and will classify them as disease free or disease laden. This is untrue because the screening goal is only identification and referral of individuals at risk or who may need further follow-up or evaluation. The initial presentation of and contact with the program implies a benefit not being delivered. To alleviate this problem, the planning committee should develop a method of informing participants of the meaning and limitations of the results. Participants need to know whether the ultimate benefit is preventive, ameliorative, or curative and, most importantly, what responsibility they must assume to secure this outcome.

The misinterpretation made by the screening instrument is of even greater ethical concern than human misperception. As the information on sensitivity and specificity indicates, false positives and false negatives occur with any screening instrument. One of the more difficult ethical issues in screening is to evaluate whether the benefits received by those correctly screened are worth the problems experienced by those incorrectly screened. What obligation does the project have to incorrectly screened individuals? What is an acceptable number of people with false negative test results, all of whom will both miss the benefit of early treatment and be misled about the need for tests in the near future? What will be the response of an individual who has a false positive reaction? Answers to these questions are generally value judgments that vary according to the disease.

Additional issues that confound the medical ethics of screening are cutoff points for the screening instrument and borderline cases. How precisely do the instrument's numerical values define the high-risk disease state? The goal of a screening program, identifying an individual as high risk or not, depends on this numerical value. When the parameter for this distinction is not clear, a cutoff point is set. Above this point, the person is considered disease positive; below this point, the individual is disease negative. Consequently, readjusting the cutoff point becomes a highly controversial issue, because it controls the percentage of positive and negative results. If the disease were potentially life threatening, an increase in false positive results (lower cutoff point) would be preferred to missing individuals who may have the disease. In addition, if a disease is relatively benign in terms of potential stigmatization, anxiety, and problems with treatment, lowering the cutoff point could again be safe and ethical. However, if the disease does not satisfy these characteristics, raising the cutoff point would be the answer, referring fewer people, but increasing accuracy and eliminating some of the false positive results.

A problem closely related to the cutoff point is defining a policy for borderline cases. Hypertension is a common disease in which a variance of 5 to 10 mm Hg can make the difference in labeling a person as high risk or not. A more sophisticated approach may be taken to discriminate between a borderline case that should be referred and one that should not. The health professional can specify other risk factors associated with hypertension, such as family history, diet, and smoking, as criteria contributing to the decision to refer an individual. With the increasing interest in and knowledge of risk factors, the effectiveness of this method has improved.

The medical ethics of screening will continue to demand review of the same questions and issues; however, the answers may change as more is discovered about the various conditions and their treatments. An updated literature review is imperative before reviewing these issues in relation to a particular screenable disease.

Economic Ethics

Associating a monetary value with health care outcomes is generally against the nature and ideals of most health care professionals. In the past, the tendency was to place no limits on the cost of promoting a healthy, disease-free or disease-controlled status, resulting in a philosophy that all care should be given to all people at all costs. This philosophy has evolved to one of conscious recognition of the costs pertaining to the implementation of screening programs. Assessing the feasibility of a screening program in which community funds allocated to the program could

HOT topics: ECONOMIC ETHICS OF SCREENING

Economic ethics have been discussed within this text to include the consideration of cost-benefit ratio, cost-effectiveness, and cost-efficiency analyses when developing selective screening programs. Those in the health care system are currently struggling to devise program guidelines that are ethically and economically sound. Questions give way to still more questions as nurses grapple with issues of cost, quality, technological benefits in screening, and service rationing. Managed care models continue to be a key force in major decision making in health care.

- How does this affect a health care provider's decision to deliver care?
- Do health care providers have the autonomy to make decisions that they deem necessary regarding screening and treatment?
- How does this affect screening protocols?
- Will the quality of care deteriorate?

mean a lack of funds for other projects illustrates this point. The persons benefiting from a screening test will be countered by those suffering from a lack of service for other medical or social needs. These trade-offs result in ethical decisions demanding careful analysis by the screening administration (see Hot Topics box).

Screening can be a costly project for both organizers and consumers. Initial operational costs must be considered, including buying or renting the screening instruments, renting floor space, engaging professionals or technicians to administer the tests, and interpreting the results.

These costs are encountered again when people are referred for further evaluation. Consumer costs include follow-up practitioner visits, treatment, time, and income that is lost while complying with each. Given the combined operational and consumer costs, several questions are raised. Do the costs result in the desired health outcome to the individual, group, or community? Are the benefits reaped worth the expenditures required? The answer is determined partly by what values (other than monetary ones) are attributed to the benefit, such as saving a life. However, a strictly economic approach generally eliminates the intangible variables, demanding the use of more objective data for decision making.

When program designs are being considered with screening, three major approaches may be used to direct a thorough evaluation of the economic resources affected: (1) cost-benefit ratio, (2) cost-effectiveness, and (3) cost-efficiency analyses. Once far from the thoughts of health care workers, the current relevance and use of such concepts require a basic understanding of their role in the selection of a screenable condition. Although presented here in successive fashion, they are entirely separate methods and are most frequently used independently of one another.

Cost-Benefit Ratio

Cost-benefit ratio analysis is performed first because it allows the comparison of various outcomes in monetary terms. This comparison is necessary in health planning when the initial consideration is what health outcome, such as reduction of cardiovascular disease, decreased infant mortality, or reduction of a visual problem, will be most beneficial to the community at the most reasonable cost.

Cost-Effectiveness

If the reduction of cardiovascular disease is chosen as the desired outcome, the next step is a **cost-effectiveness analysis**, which determines the optimal use of available resources to reach a predetermined, constant end point (the desired health outcome). The outcome remains the same; the best method of deriving it is the issue. For example, considering the selected health outcome, reduction of cardiovascular disease, the various methods might be screening for hypertension, taking electrocardiograms of all individuals aged 25 or older who are admitted to the hospital, beginning an antismoking campaign, or obtaining nutrition counseling. Implementation of all these options would be ideal, but with limited resources a choice must be made.

Cost-Efficiency

The last approach to help bring the economic resources into perspective is **cost-efficiency analysis.** The purpose is to be efficient and budget a limited amount of money toward achieving as much of the preselected desired outcome as possible. The funds are the central issue, not the health benefit.

SELECTION OF A SCREENABLE POPULATION

The selection of a screenable population is as important as the selection of a screenable disease. The objective is to identify a high-risk group that, when tested, will yield a significant number of diseased individuals. With such results, the efforts and cost of screening the population are minimized and the health benefit received is maximized. The main criterion used to define an appropriate population is the definitive presence of risk factors related to the disorder. To ensure a thorough examination of possible risk factors, both person-dependent and environment-dependent factors should be reviewed.

Person-Dependent Factors

One characteristic related to the person, age, is increasingly important because its distribution changes throughout the population (Tables 9-1 and 9-2). Accepted practice has always placed a high priority on screening the vulnerable, at-risk infant population, partly because health profession-

Table 9-1 **Recommended Guide to Health Tests and Screenings for Females**

Test	Purpose	Age	Frequency
Guthrie	Early detection of PKU	Newborns	Once, unless done before 24 hours of age, when it should be repeated by 2 weeks of age
Blood lead and free erythrocyte (or zinc) protoporphyrin levels	Early detection of lead levels	12 months	At least once for children at risk
Breast examination	Self-breast examination: To detect changes in breast tissue or appearance	18 to menopause	Monthly; 1 week after onset of period
		Postmenopause	Monthly; first day of every month
	Clinical breast examination: To detect changes in the breast that go unnoticed by self-examination	50 to 69	Every 1 to 2 years (recommendations vary depending on professional organizations)
Mammogram	To detect changes in breast tissue that are too small to be felt	50 to 69	Every 1 to 2 years (recommendations vary depending on professional organization)
Pap smear	To detect cervical abnormalities, including cancer	Onset of sexual activity or 18 and over	Every three years; with individual recommendations by primary health care practitioner based on individual risk factors
Digital rectal examination	To detect early signs of colorectal cancer	40 and over	Annually
Colorectal examination (FOBT)	To detect traces of blood in stool, an early sign of colorectal cancer	50 and over	Annually
Sigmoidoscopy	To detect early signs of colorectal cancer	50 and over	Every three to five years
Cholesterol	To determine risk of heart disease	45 to 65	Once every 5 years if levels are within normal range
Blood Pressure	To detect hypertension, a major risk factor for cardiovascular disease	21 and over	Every 1 to 2 years if normal; as directed by health care provider if blood pressure is abnormal
1. Tonometer 2. Ophthalmoscopic evaluation 3. Perimetry	To detect early signs of glaucoma	High-risk individuals	As directed by specialists
Fasting plasma glucose test and oral glucose tolerance test	Early detection of Type 2 Diabetes	Individuals with one or more risk factors	3-year intervals
EIA	Early detection of HIV	Individuals at risk	Individually determined

From American Cancer Society. (2000). *Colorectal cancer: Early detection* [On-line]. Available: www.3cancer.org/cancerinfo/load_cont.asp?ct=28&Language=English; U.S. Preventative Service Task Force. (1996). *Guide to clinical preventive services* (2nd ed.). Baltimore: Williams & Wilkins.

EIA, enzyme immunoassay; *FOBT*, Fecal occult blood test; *PKU*, phenylketonuria.

als are soon faced with the results of negligence, which affects children's growth and development. However, as the average lifespan increases, the effects of longer-range risk factors are becoming apparent, making certain prevalent and costly chronic conditions equally important to control. Therefore ideal populations for screening can be found in senior-citizen housing projects or elderly day-care settings. Middle-age adults are also being recognized as a screenable group for certain conditions; breast cancer, glaucoma, and heart disease commonly appear during this period.

Table 9-2 **Recommended Guide to Health Tests and Screenings for Males**

Test	Purpose	Age	Frequency
Guthrie	Early detection of PKU	Newborns	Once, unless done before 24 hours of age, when it should be repeated by 2 weeks of age
Blood lead and free erythrocyte (or zinc) protoporphyrin levels	Early detection of lead levels	12 months	At least once for children at risk
Prostate digital examination	Early detection of prostate cancer	50 years of age or 40 years of age for those considered at risk	Annually
Prostate-specific antigen (PSA)	Early detection of prostate cancer	50 years of age or 40 years of age for those considered at risk	Annually
Digital rectal examination	To detect early signs of colorectal cancer	40 and over	Annually
Colorectal examination (FOBT)	To detect traces of blood in stool, an early sign of colorectal cancer	50 and over	Annually
Sigmoidoscopy	To detect early signs of colorectal cancer	50 and over	Every 3 to 5 years
Cholesterol	To determine risk of heart disease	45 to 65	Once every 5 years if levels are within normal range
Blood Pressure	To detect hypertension, a major risk factor for cardiovascular disease	21 and over	Every 1 to 2 years if normal; as directed by health care provider if blood pressure is abnormal
1. Tonometer 2. Ophthalmoscopic evaluation 3. Perimetry	To detect early signs of glaucoma	High-risk individuals	As directed by specialists
Fasting plasma glucose test and oral glucose tolerance test	Early detection of Type 2 Diabetes	Individuals with one or more risk factors	3-year intervals
EIA	Early detection of HIV	Individuals at risk	Individually determined

From American Cancer Society. (1997). *American cancer society updates prostate cancer screening guidelines* [On-line]. Available: www.cancer/org/media/story/1jnune12.html; American Cancer Society. (2000). *Colorectal cancer: Early detection* [On-line]. Available: www3.cancer.org/cancerinfo/load_cont.asp?ct=28&Language=English; and U.S. Preventive Services Task Force. (1996). *Guide to clinical preventive services* (2nd ed.). Baltimore: Williams & Wilkins.
FOBT, Fecal occult blood test; *PKU*, phenylketonuria.

Gender has obvious implications for screening programs. For example, women are tested for two commonly screened conditions: (1) breast cancer and (2) cervical cancer. Men are tested for conditions such as prostate and testicular cancer.

A population representing a particular race or ethnic group is also appropriate to consider when planning screening programs (see Multicultural Awareness box). Race is frequently defined as a group that is homogeneous with regard to genetic inheritance (Last, 1997, p. 33). It is known that some disorders do occur more frequently in certain racial or ethnic groups. For example, Blacks have a higher prevalence and mortality rate from hypertension and cancer of the prostate than do certain other cultural groups, whereas Native Americans have higher prevalence rates of diabetes than do other cultural groups (Last, 1997). Although these health disparities are of great concern, their cause is not easy to ascertain. It is believed that these differences are actually the result of complex interactions between genetic variations, environmental factors, and health behaviors (U.S. Department of Human Services, 2000). The need to identify the causes of these health disparities has been of central importance. This is evident by the proliferation of research being conducted to identify and describe the possible reasons for these differences. When health care professionals have a greater understand-

MULTICULTURAL AWARENESS

Eliminating Health Disparities Among Ethnic Groups

Frequently, the United States has been referred to as a melting pot. This diversity has been acknowledged as a strength, but it is apparent that disparities do exist in culture among the various racial and ethnic groups in the attainment and maintenance of health. The minority populations of the United States have been categorized as Blacks, Hispanics, Asian-Pacific Islanders, American Indians, and Alaskan Natives. These categories oversimplify the reality of the multicultural nature in assessing health status, screening, and making plans to improve health. These particular racial groupings are not absolutes because there are subgroups within each (U.S. Department of Health and Human Services, 2000). Over the past decade, it has become increasingly apparent that disparities exist between and among these groups regarding disease and the attainment of health. In fact, the second goal of *Healthy People 2010* is to eliminate health disparities among different segments of the population. Racial and ethnic health disparities need to be taken into consideration when conducting a community health assessment, diagnosis, and intervention plan. To outreach, educate, and screen a target community successfully, the provider must have awareness and respect for differences and incorporate key individuals from the community into the planning and screening process. Throughout the entire process, considerations include, but are not limited to, the following:

- Socioeconomic status
- Environmental factors
- Educational attainment
- Heredity factors
- Values, religious, and cultural beliefs
- Communication styles and language
- Lifestyle choices

The health care provider should realize that these disparities represent a more complex picture than poverty alone. An understanding of this assists the health care provider in identifying those individuals at greatest risk and in developing screening programs for early identification and possible treatment.

From U.S. Department of Health and Human Services. (2000). *Healthy people 2010* (Conference Edition). Washington, DC: The Department.

research highlights

Acculturation and Breast Cancer Screening Among Hispanic Women in New York City

Acculturation has been defined as "the psychosocial adaptation of persons from their culture of origin to a new or host cultural environment" (Burnam, Hough, Karno, Escobar, & Telles, 1987, p. 90).

The authors listed in the following reference investigated whether acculturation was associated with the accepted use of clinical breast examinations and mammograms among Colombian, Ecuadorian, Dominican, and Puerto Rican women aged 18 to 74 in New York City. The authors chose to look at the linguistic aspects of acculturation, such as language and media. This included television, radio, books, magazines, and newspapers that were used in a variety of situations (work, home, neighborhood, and shopping) with different people (spouses, children, parents, and friends). Even after controlling variables such as health status, sociodemographics, source of care, cancer attitudes, and health beliefs, it was found that greater acculturation was significantly associated with higher rates of screening for clinical breast examination and mammogram. In addition, similar to other studies, the authors reported that those with insurance had a greater rate of screening than those without. The findings of this research demonstrated that not only do community-based partnerships need to increase screening among Hispanic women who are less acculturated, but the health care providers who develop, plan, and implement such screening programs must consider the importance of acculturation in the delivery of breast cancer screening.

Data from O'Malley, A., Kerner, J., Johnson, A., & Mandelblatt, J. (1999). Acculturation and breast cancer screening among Hispanic women in New York City. *American Journal of Public Health, 89*(2), 210-227.

ing as to why these disparities exist, it will be possible to develop effective and efficient plans to counteract these problems (see Research Highlights box).

Income level has been associated repeatedly with the presence or absence of a healthy state and it underlies many health disparities. Often lower-income groups have the least education. Such differences in both income and education is associated with disparities in the occurrence of disorders, including heart disease, diabetes, obesity, elevated blood lead levels, and low birth weight (U.S. Department of Human Services, 2000). Poverty accompanies poor environmental conditions, poor nutrition, inadequate housing, poor lifestyle habits, psychological and physical abuse, violence, teenage pregnancy, unemployment, and limited access to health care (Green & Shellenberger, 1991).

Personal behavioral characteristics related to lifestyle may suggest the need to screen an individual or group. When health care practitioners consider lifestyle, they are looking at daily habits that affect health and wellness. Personal behavioral characteristics related to lifestyle include diet, exercise, smoking, alcohol and drug use, stress management, and use of seat belts. Engaging in some of these behaviors while avoiding others is essential for living a healthy life. Therefore screening for those personal behavioral characteristics that are considered risky suggests the likelihood of a longer, disease-free life. Once screening suggests those behaviors that are considered risky, the development of healthy behaviors via programming and a conscious transformation in lifestyle is key.

Once screening is completed, health care providers bear a responsibility to educate individuals about the next step

HEALTH TEACHING Pender's Health Promotion Model

A health care provider's responsibility is not only to assess, develop, plan, implement, and evaluate a screening program, but also to educate individuals, families, and populations about the importance of engaging in such programs and ultimately engaging in behavior that enhances health. The health care provider may find the Health Promotion Model (Pender, 1987) useful to guide his or her practice. The model presents the interrelationship between cognitive and perceptual factors and modifying factors that influence behaviors that promote health. The health care provider may find that the application of this model in practice influences the relationship between the provider and the individual in a positive way. The model provides a framework by which the provider engages in the assessment of factors believed to influence health behavior changes. Once the provider has an accurate assessment, decisions may be made concerning factors that inhibit health-promoting behaviors and, ultimately, potential interventions to assist individuals in achieving positive health outcomes. This information will assist the provider in the development of appropriate teaching methods.

From Tillett, L. A. (1998). The health promotion model. In A. M. Tomey, & M. R. Alligood (Eds.), *Nursing theorists and their work* (4th ed., pp. 529-537). St. Louis: Mosby.

in the evaluation of their potential condition. Those being screened also bear a certain responsibility to seek treatment, follow-up, and ultimately engage in behavioral change toward a healthy lifestyle if the screening is to serve a purpose (see Health Teaching box).

Environment-Dependent Factors

The area of environmental health and protection has expanded over the years and is becoming more complex. Environmental health and protection has been defined as the act of protecting against environmental factors that may have an adverse influence on human health and adversely affect the balance of environmental quality (Gordon, 1997, p. 303). Environmental-related risk factors relevant to screening designs are derived from an individual's physical surroundings. Areas that may be considered include air quality, both indoor and outdoor; water pollution; safe drinking water; noise pollution; hazardous-waste management; vector control; and pesticide control (Gordon, 1997).

In occupational health, a legitimate population for screening is the high-risk work area, where harmful chemicals, airborne particles, or high-decibel machinery put the worker at risk of cancer, respiratory conditions, or auditory problems. At the other extreme is the sedentary executive work life, in which stress and lack of exercise are prevalent. The use of an occupational health nurse to provide individual and mass screening for such problems is recognized as an integral role of both the health professions and the business world.

Environment-dependent factors have long been associated with the presence or absence of certain conditions. Primary prevention would be the preferred mode of protection; however, with the shortsightedness of present society, secondary prevention appears to be the preferred choice. Screening must focus on the short-term results of certain environmental conditions and monitor the development of chronic trends.

COMMONLY SCREENED CONDITIONS

The following section reviews several commonly screened diseases to demonstrate the complexity of issues that may surround the screening process. Ultimately, a systematic approach where decision making is collaborative in nature will move the targeted population toward health improvement and the attainment of the two central goals of *Healthy People 2010* (U.S. Department of Human Services, 2000):

1. Increased quality and years of healthy life
2. Elimination of health disparities

Phenylketonuria (PKU)

PKU is a condition characterized by the genetically determined lack of phenylalanine hydroxylase, an enzyme necessary to metabolize an important amino acid, phenylalanine. In its absence, blood levels of the phenylalanine increase, causing irreversible damage to the brain and central nervous system and resulting in severe mental retardation. The significance of PKU is not so much in the incidence of the condition, which is 1 of every 10,000 births, but in the economic burden associated with lifelong case management and the emotional strain associated with care (Nicholson, 1998).

Knowledge of PKU's **natural history,** or the progression of the specific disease from prepathogenesis to pathogenesis, will define the optimal time to administer the test, which is for all newborns before discharge from the nursery (U.S. Preventive Services Task Force, 1996) (Fig. 9-2). The U.S. Preventive Services Task Force (1996) also recommends a repeat screening test by 2 weeks of age if the infant was tested before 24 hours of age. The effective screening method is an individually administered, disease-specific blood sample test for evaluation of phenylalanine known as the Guthrie test. This sample is often used to test for other conditions, reducing the cost of detecting PKU. Dietary control of phenylalanine intake is a safe, effective treatment for PKU. With this diet, individualized according to the infant's rate and point of growth and

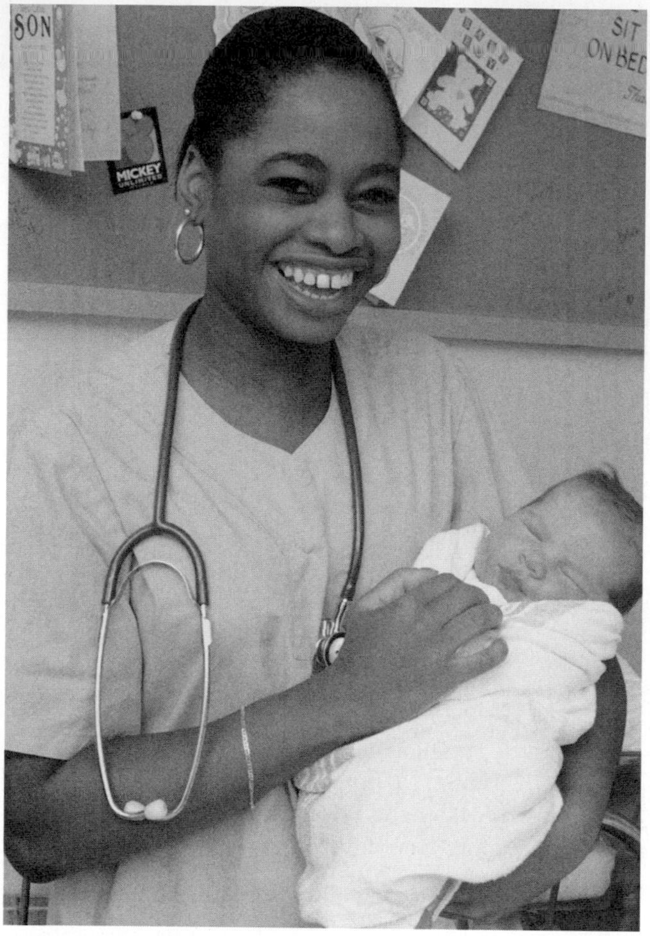

Fig. 9-2 PKU testing is optimally done on all newborns before they are discharged from the nursery.

development, mental retardation can be avoided. PKU therefore fulfills the basic law of screening: Early intervention can affect a disease's progress. Medically and economically, PKU screening is almost a model screenable disease.

Breast Cancer

In the United States, the most common cancer among women is breast cancer (U.S. Department of Human Services, 2000). At present, a lesion in the breast indicates the disease; severity is based on the size of the lesion and the length of time that it has been present. Screening for asymptomatic cases and finding unnoticed and presumably smaller masses permit more successful and conservative treatments because the stage is less severe.

In American women, the incidence of breast cancer increases with age. Nulliparous women, women who have never given birth, run a high risk of breast carcinoma; women who had their first child before the age of 20 constitute the lowest risk group. Women who start menstruating at an earlier age than average and reach menopause at a later age than average are also known to

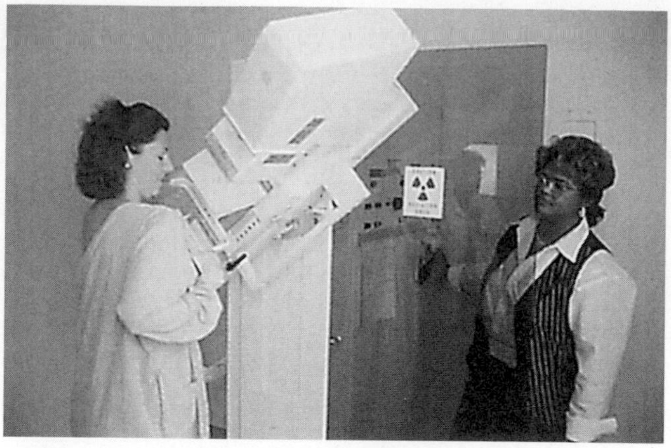

Fig. 9-3 Mammography is used to screen women for breast cancer. (From Edge, V., & Miller, M. (1994). *Women's health care.* St. Louis: Mosby.)

be at a somewhat higher risk, as are those who bore their first child in their late 30s. Additional risks may include women with fibrocystic disease of the breast, family history of breast cancer, extended use of estrogen, obesity, and a diet high in fat.

Three screening tests usually considered appropriate for early detection include: (1) the clinical breast examination, (2) mammography, and (3) self-breast examination (Fig. 9-3). The sensitivity and specificity of these tests depends on multiple factors: the size of the lesion, the characteristic of the breast, the age of the individual being examined, the skill and experience of the examiner, and the quality of the mammography equipment and the skills of the technicians and radiologist (U.S. Preventive Services Task Force, 1996).

The nurse is often the health care provider who teaches a woman how to perform a monthly self-examination of the breasts (Fig. 9-4). Self-examination should be encouraged; in many cases, this practice has proved to be lifesaving. Although breast self-examination is encouraged and considered an important screening test for early detection of breast cancer, data regarding the effectiveness are limited and the accuracy of this self-examination is considered inferior to that of the clinical breast examination and mammography (U.S. Preventive Services Task Force, 1996). Presently, screening for breast cancer every 1 to 2 years, with mammography alone or mammography and annual clinical breast examination, is recommended for women aged 50 to 69 (U.S. Preventive Services Task Force, 1996).

Cervical Cancer

The tenth most common cancer among women in the United States is cervical cancer (U.S. Department of Human Services, 2000). The principal screening test for cervical cancer is the Papanicolaou's (Pap) smear. Although all sexually active women are at risk for cervical

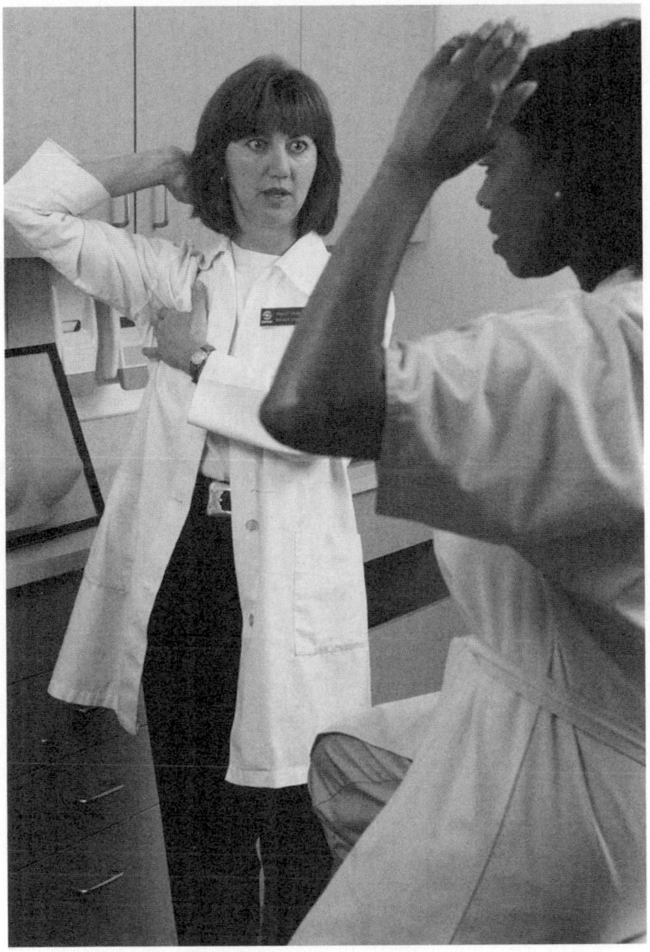

Fig. 9-4 Assisting the individual to demonstrate self-breast examination on herself is an excellent method of teaching self-breast examinations.

cancer, the disease is more common among women of low socioeconomic status, women with a history of multiple sex partners, women with an early first sexual intercourse, smokers, and women with certain types of human papilloma virus and human immunodeficiency virus (HIV).

The incidence of invasive cervical cancer has dramatically decreased since the implementation of early detection programs involving the Pap smear. The official guidelines for Pap smear testing include the following (U.S. Preventive Services Task Force, 1996):

1. Testing should be performed on all women aged 18 years and older, or earlier if sexually active, and those who have a cervix.
2. Pap smear testing should be performed at least every three years. However, the health care provider, based on the risk factors noted earlier, should determine the interval for each person.
3. There is insufficient evidence to recommend for or against an upper age limit for Pap testing, but recommendations can be made on other grounds to discontinue regular testing after age 65 in women who have had regular previous screenings with normal smears.

Colorectal Cancer

Colorectal cancer is the second leading cause of cancer deaths in the United States (U.S. Department of Human Services, 2000). A campaign for early detection of colorectal carcinoma has been widely publicized by the American Cancer Society in recent years. Early detection of colorectal cancer is associated with a better outcome in both morbidity and mortality; the five-year survival rate is over 90% for patients with a localized disease.

The American Cancer Society (2000) developed guidelines for both men and women who, at the age of 50, should follow one of the following procedures: (1) an annual fecal occult blood test (FOBT) plus a flexible sigmoidoscopy every five years; (2) a colonoscopy every 10 years or double contrast barium enema every 5 to 10 years; and (3) a digital rectal examination (DRE) should be performed at the time of each screening. Most organizations recommend the more intensive screening, which includes barium enema and colonoscopy, for those in at-risk groups. Principal risk factors include a history of inflammatory bowel disease; family history of first-degree relative with colorectal cancer; previously diagnosed colorectal cancer; adenomatous polyps; and prior diagnosis of endometrial, ovarian, or breast cancer.

Prostate Cancer

Prostate cancer is the most common diagnosed cancer in males and the second leading cause of death among males in the United States (U.S. Department of Human Services, 2000). Risk increases with age beginning at 50 years and is higher among Black men.

Three principal screening tests are used for prostate cancer. These include DRE, analysis for the serum tumor marker prostate-specific antigen (PSA), and transrectal ultrasound (TRUS) (U.S. Preventive Task Force, 1996). To date, the PSA is controversial. PSA is a protein produced by the prostate. Higher levels in the blood may indicate the presence of prostate cancer, but not always. Sometimes an individual may have a normal PSA level when, in fact, a prostate tumor may be in evidence. Although the PSA test is not 100% reliable, it may be very useful in the early identification of prostate cancer leading to a decrease in mortality rates (Reuters Health, 2000).

The American Cancer Society (1997) recommends an annual digital examination in men 50 years of age and older to screen for prostate cancer along with a PSA. For men at higher risk, such as Black men and those with a family history, screening may be recommended at earlier ages. Ultimately, a TRUS helps determine the mass, size, and consistency of the prostate.

Cholesterol

One of the major modifiable risk factors for coronary heart disease (CHD) is elevated blood cholesterol levels (U.S. Department of Health and Human Services, 2000). Extensive research, educational programs, and media attention have increased the knowledge and understanding of the implications of high-cholesterol levels and of the role of cholesterol in a healthy lifestyle. Cholesterol screening can identify high-risk individuals who are most likely to benefit from individualized risk factor counseling, dietary instruction, and drug therapies. Indeed, the most convincing data that support cholesterol screening is the ability of cholesterol-lowering interventions to reduce the risk of CHD in those with high cholesterol (U.S. Preventive Services Task Force, 1996).

Screening for total cholesterol and high-density lipoprotein cholesterol (HDL-C) can be obtained in fasting or nonfasting individuals from finger stick or venipuncture samples (U.S. Preventive Services Task Force, 1996) (Fig. 9-5). Minor illness, posture, stress, seasonal fluctuation, and technical or laboratory error can all affect the cholesterol values obtained. The U.S. Preventive Services Task Force (1996) advises that because a single cholesterol value does not accurately assess an individuals true cholesterol level, intervention decisions must be based on a minimum of two measurements along with assessment of the individuals cardiovascular risk factors.

Recommendations for cholesterol screening include periodic screening for high blood cholesterol for all men aged 35 to 65 and women aged 45 to 64. Intervals for this periodic screening is not known, but the recommendation remains at every 5 years with longer intervals for those considered at low risk and more frequent for those considered at high risk. Screening of children, adolescents, and young adults is not recommended because there is insufficient evidence as to the effectiveness of such actions; any such considerations must be made on a case-by-case review, depending on presenting risk factors. Screening of persons over age 65 must also be made on a case-by-case review (U.S. Preventive Services Task Force, 1996).

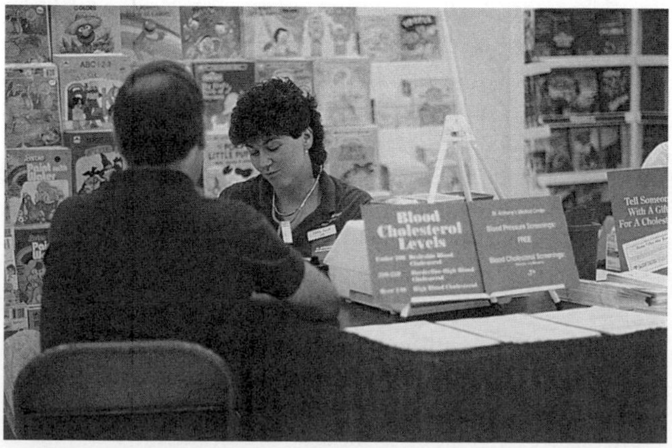

Fig. 9-5 Blood cholesterol screenings are often conducted as mass screenings.

Hypertension

Hypertension is a leading risk factor for CHD, congestive heart failure, stroke, ruptured aortic aneurysm, renal disease, and retinopathy. Heart disease is the leading cause of death in the United States, accounting for nearly 740,000 deaths each year; cerebral vascular disease, the third leading cause of death, accounts for 150,000 deaths each year (U.S. Preventive Services Task Force, 1996). Detecting high blood pressure is a primary prevention strategy for CHD, cerebrovascular disease, and peripheral vascular disease; it is a secondary prevention strategy for hypertension.

Hypertension is currently defined for adults as a diastolic blood pressure reading of 90 mm Hg or a systolic pressure of 140 mm Hg or higher; for children, the criteria for defining hypertension varies with age (U.S. Preventive Services Task Force, 1996). Sphygmomanometry continues to be the most suitable screening instrument, but measuring errors can occur from the instrument, the observer, or the individual so diagnosis must rely on more than one elevated reading (U.S. Preventive Services Task Force, 1996). Criteria for referral may vary according to the screening program and the specific level of elevation. At the very least, the individual will be advised to have a recheck in 2 years; at most they would be referred for follow-up care immediately.

Periodic screening is recommended for everyone 21 years of age and older, but the optimal interval of screening has yet to be determined and is presently left to the clinician's judgment (U.S. Preventive Services Task Force, 1996). Presently, screening recommendations for most adults with a diastolic blood pressure below 85 mm Hg and a systolic pressure below 140 mm Hg is at least biannual.

Recommendations are annual for individuals with a diastolic blood pressure of 85 to 89 mm Hg. Blood pressure screening during office visits is also recommended for children and adolescents (U.S. Preventive Services Task Force, 1996). Assessment of other cardiovascular risk factors may modify these guidelines and clinical discretion is always key.

When hypertension is effectively treated, it has important long-term implications for decreased mortality and morbidity from diminished end organ effects. Therefore it should be a part of any comprehensive screening program.

Glaucoma

Glaucoma is the second leading cause of irreversible blindness and an estimated 2.5 million persons in the United States suffer from this disease (Woolf, 1996). The prevalence of glaucoma is fourfold to sixfold higher in the Black population than the White population and it increases steadily with age. There is an increase in the prevalence of glaucoma in individuals with diabetes mellitus, myopia, and a family history of glaucoma. The natural history of glaucoma is currently explained by the increased intraocular pressure (IOP), which results from an obstruction of the outflow of aqueous humor from the eye's interior and damages the optic nerve, causing loss of vision. Visual deficits that are caused by glaucoma are not generally reversible, but early treatment is widely believed to prevent or delay the progression to more serious problems.

Three diagnostic criteria exist for the screening of glaucoma: (1) an increase in IOP as measured by a tonometer; (2) damage to the optic nerve, which is assessed through ophthalmoscopic evaluation; and (3) visual field loss, as measured by perimetry. Although the presence of all three criteria is indicative of glaucoma, experts disagree whether one variable alone is indicative of the disease. In addition, the accuracy of testing depends of the choice of test, experience of the examiner, and the variables of the individual. Presently, insufficient evidence exists to recommend for or against routine screening. However, recommendations to refer at-risk individuals to specialists for evaluation is noted when the specialist has the experience and the access to the specialized equipment that is necessary to evaluate the optic disc and measure the visual fields.

Human Immunodeficiency Virus

As of November 1999, HIV and acquired immunodeficiency syndrome (AIDS) have been reported in every racial and ethnic population, in every age and socioeconomic group, in every state, and in most large cities throughout the United States (U.S. Department of Health and Human Services, 2000). HIV is now the leading cause of death for those in the Black population, aged 25 to 44, and it dropped to eighth place for all others in this age group by 1997 (U.S. Department of Health and Human Services, 2000). *Healthy People 2010* reports that the infection rates appear to have stabilized to a slower growth rate of approximately 40,000 new infections per year. In addition, recent therapies have reduced illness and improved survival. However, the need for HIV screening to increase the numbers of individuals who know of their HIV status continues to be important. The goal is to detect infection at the earliest possible time and decrease transmission when the potential is greatest and to increase access to early care, prevention, and treatment, including highly active antiretroviral therapy (HAART) (U.S. Department of Health and Human Services, 2000).

Health care providers need to assess the risk factors for HIV infection in all individuals by obtaining a careful sexual history and inquiring about past or present drug use. Periodic screening for HIV should be offered to all individuals who are at increased risk for the infection. Included are those seeking treatment for sexually transmitted diseases, men who have had sex with men, past or present intravenous drug users, individuals with multiple sexual partners, people who engage in sex for money or drugs, persons with a history of transfusion between 1978 and 1985, and men or women whose past or present sex partners were HIV infected (U.S. Preventive Services Task Force, 1996) (Fig. 9-6).

The basic screening test for HIV is the enzyme immunoassay (EIA). Presently, screening for infection with HIV is recommended for all persons at increased risk of infection. There is limited information to recommend for or against routine HIV screening in individuals without risk factors. Screening is also recommended for all pregnant women at risk (U.S. Preventive Services Task Force, 1996).

Lead

During the 1990s, the mean blood lead levels in the United States were reduced to less than 5 ug/dL. Although a known normal blood lead level does not exist, the Centers for Disease Control and Prevention (CDC) has reported that children's blood lead levels less that 10 ug/dL as normal (Durch, Bailey, & Stoto, 1997). Elevated blood lead levels and its threat of lead toxicity continue to be a prevalent, yet preventable, health threat in both children and adults. Childhood lead intoxication can result in serious illness with lifelong consequences, such as developmental delay and reduced intelligence quotient (IQ) scores; it can also lead to anemia, convulsions, and death (Durch, Bailey, & Stoto, 1997). Childhood lead poisoning often

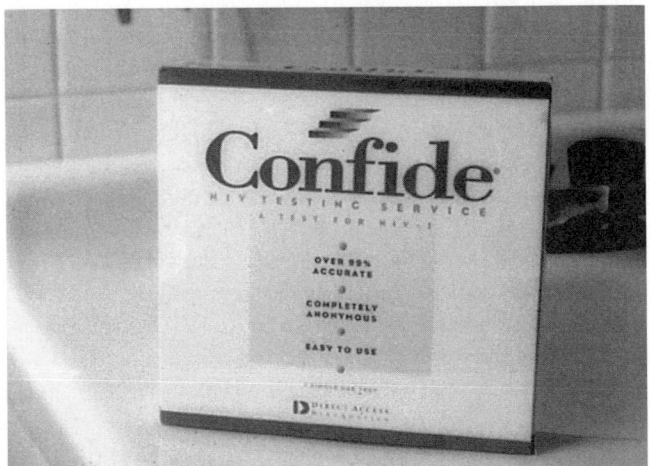

Fig. 9-6 A number of controversial, ethical issues surround the "Confide" HIV test. A person can purchase this test in any pharmacy and then administer the test at home. The sample is sent to the laboratory. After screening is complete, the person calls and receives the results over the phone. Although this manner of screening provides the person with privacy, the person may not receive the counseling and guidance needed, which is provided when a health care provider administers this test.

comes from the home itself, such as lead-based paint and dust, or from items in the home, such as lead-based glass and make-up.

Lead toxicity is not as prevalent in adults and is generally related to occupational risk or a specific hobby. Durch, Bailey, and Stoto (1997) reported on a review of medical literature that suggested adults may also experience serious health consequences from elevated blood lead levels, such as hypertension and adverse neurological reproductive effects.

Two screening tests are used for detecting lead exposure: (1) blood lead and (2) free erythrocyte or zinc protoporphyrin levels. Blood lead is the more sensitive, but can be easily affected by environmental lead contamination during blood collection. Erythrocyte protoporphyrin is an indirect measure of lead exposure and it is not affected by environmental lead contamination. However, it is not as sensitive to modest lead elevations as the blood lead test.

Screening for elevated blood lead is recommended at least once at 12 months for all children at increased risk for lead exposure. In communities where there is a low prevalence of elevated lead levels requiring intervention, a lead risk factor questionnaire would screen out at-risk children for targeted blood testing.

Diabetes

Diabetes mellitus is a group of metabolic diseases characterized by hyperglycemia resulting from defects in insulin secretion, insulin action, or both (American Diabetes Association, 1999). Noninsulin-dependent diabetes mellitus or Type 2 accounts for 90% to 95% of diabetes in the United States, whereas insulin-dependent or Type 1 diabetes accounts for 5% to 10% (Alberti, DeFronzo, & Zimmet, 1995). Type 1 diabetes has an acute onset of symptoms, which are detected soon after the clinical presentations. Screening for asymptomatic individuals for the presence of autoantibodies related to Type 1 diabetes is not recommended presently for many reasons including:

- Cutoff values for some of the immune-marker assays have not been established for the clinical setting.
- There is no agreement as to what actions need to be taken with positive autoantibody test results.
- The low incidence of Type 1 diabetes will ultimately produce a very small number of positively identified individuals at the completion of a screening program (American Diabetes Association, 1999).

Type 2 diabetes is often asymptomatic in its early stages and remains undiagnosed for many years. Undiagnosed Type 2 diabetes is associated with long-term damage to multiple organ systems. Early detection via screening will result in prompt treatment, ultimately reducing the burden of this disease. The risk of developing Type 2 diabetes increases with age, obesity, and lack of exercise. Those individuals with a family history, hypertension dyslipidemia, delivery of babies over nine pounds, or who are members of particular racial or ethnic groups also have increased risk of developing this disease.

Screening for diabetes as part of routine care may be appropriate if the individual has one or more of the above risk factors. However, at this time, mass screening of all individuals (even all individuals considered at high risk) is not recommended. The decision to screen or not to screen should be made based upon expert clinical judgment of the health care practitioner. Screening of high-risk individuals should be considered at 3-year intervals. The fasting plasma glucose test and the oral glucose tolerance test are preferred because it is easy to administer, it is fast, convenient, and relatively inexpensive (American Diabetes Association, 1999).

THE NURSE'S ROLE

The potential and the need for nursing involvement exists at all levels of the collaborative partnership process. Being one of the many important stakeholders, nurses play an important role in every aspect of the program development process, including assessment, analysis of data, planning, implementation, evaluation of the health outcomes, and the evaluation of the process (including the workings of the partnership). One aspect of this health process is the development and implementation of screening programs for targeted groups. As nurses become more involved in decision making they will be faced with the question, "Should this condition be screened or not?" In the role of decision maker and planner, the nurse is responsible for reviewing all the issues concerning a screenable disease, including: (1) the criteria specific to the disease, (2) the medical and economic ethics, and (3) the community resources that are affected. If the choice is to screen, the participation of nurses and other partnering groups is essential in the development of the Partnership Community Care Plan (see the Partnership Community Care Plan). The last step is the planning and development of an efficient referral system to enhance continuity of care and to ensure follow-up with the recommended referral.

Nurses have long been responsible for screening patients, such as giving tuberculin tests and Snellen eye tests or checking blood pressures. As in any nursing intervention, adequate knowledge of the method of administration and the potential side effects is needed. Teaching individuals the meaning and limitation of the test results is an important element of this role, as is informing them of their part in obtaining the implied benefit.

The combined health educator and screener component means that the nurse continues to educate individuals for additional risk factors and teach them ways to alter and reduce risks through lifestyle changes, such as proper diet, exercise, and stress management, and by controlling the use of alcohol, drugs, and tobacco. The role as educator is essential in the screening process because nurses provide individuals with the information necessary for choices that

CASE STUDY

Prostate Screening

A local hospital offered a comprehensive, free prostate screening for men aged 50 and over in a diverse community. The overall goal was to bring in individuals from lower socioeconomic and diverse cultural groups who would not be able to access screening. Publicity, including press releases and screening event advertisements, was run in all the local papers and screenings were conducted at different hours and different days of the week to accommodate the target group. Despite this, the results indicated that the targeted group did not use the service as hoped and the predominant individuals who accessed the service were White, middle class, insured men.

1. What was wrong with the presentation of this screening?
2. What were the possible reasons for this problem?
3. If you are the public health nurse assigned to plan and implement the screening next year, what would you do differently?
4. How would you proceed?
5. What other community organizations and key individuals or groups would you include in the process?

are made regarding healthy behavioral change. The nurse is actually practicing primary prevention interventions, but it is in coordination with a secondary preventive role.

SUMMARY

As a method of preclinical secondary prevention, screening is the rapid administration of a simple test to distinguish individuals who may have a condition from those who probably do not have a condition. It can be an effective, efficient tool in preventive health care if used for conditions applicable to the screening model and directed toward an at-risk population. A unique characteristic and significant advantage of screening is that it can be applied to individuals or groups.

Three questions provide a means of analyzing the screenability of a disease:

1. Is the condition significant?
2. Can the condition be screened?
3. Should the condition be screened?

Screening programs are not appropriate for all conditions or all communities. Alternative methods of reaching the desired health outcome should always be considered. Screening in health care presents numerous roles for nurses and provides them with a valuable preventive tool in the care of healthy individuals.

REFERENCES

Alberti, K. G. M. M., DeFronzo, R. A., & Zimmet, P. (1995). *International textbook of diabetes mellitus*. New York: John Wiley and Sons.

American Cancer Society. (1997). *American Cancer Society updates prostate cancer screening guidelines* [On-line]. Available: www.cancer/org/media/story/1june12.html.

American Cancer Society. (2000). *Colorectal cancer: Early detection* [On-line]. Available: www.3cancer.org/cancerinfo/load_cont.asp?ct=28&Language=English.

American Diabetes Association. (1999). *Clinical practice recommendations: Screening for type 2 diabetes* [On-line]. Available: www.diabetes.org/DiabetesCare/supplemet199/S20.htm.

Anderson, E. T., & McFarlane, J. M. (2000). *Community as partner: Theory and practice in nursing* (3rd ed.). New York: Lippincott, Williams, & Wilkins.

Burnam, M. A., Hough, R. L., Karno, M., Escobar, J., & Telles, C. A. (1987). Acculturation and lifetime prevalence of psychiatric disorders among Mexican Americans in Los Angeles. *Journal Health and Social Behavior, 28*, 89-102.

Durch, J. S., Bailey, L. A., & Stoto, M. A. (1997). Environmental and occupational lead poisoning. In J. S. Durch, L. A. Bailey, & M. A. Stoto (Eds.), *Improving health in the community* (pp. 242-258). Washington, DC: National Academy Press.

Gordon, L. J. (1997). Environmental health and protection. In F. D. Scutchfield, & C. W. Keck (Eds.), *Principles of public health practice* (pp. 300-317). Albany, NY: Delmar Publishers.

Green, J. & Shellenberger, R. (1991). *The dynamics of health & wellness: A biopsychosocial approach*. New York: Harcourt Brace College Publishers.

Last, J. M. (1997). The determinants of health. In F. D. Scutchfield, & C. W. Keck (Eds.), *Principles of public health practice* (pp. 31-41). Albany, NY: Delmar Publishers.

National Institute of Nursing Research. (1995). *Community-based health care: Nursing strategies*. Bethesda, MD: The Institute.

Nicholson, J. F. (1998). Inborn errors of metabolism. In R. E. Behrman, & R. M. Kliegman (Eds.), *Nelson essentials of pediatrics* (3rd ed., pp. 147-166). Philadelphia: W.B. Saunders Company.

O'Malley, A., Kerner, J., Johnson, A., & Mandelblatt, J. (1999). Acculturation and breast cancer screening among Hispanic women in New York City. *American Journal of Public Health, 89* (2), 210-227.

Pender, J. J. (1987). *Health promotion in nursing practice* (2nd ed.). New York: Appleton & Lange.

Reuters Health. (2000). *Studies back use of PSA screening for prostate cancer* [On-line]. Available: www.cancerfacts.com.

Tillett, L. A. (1998). The health promotion model. In A. M. Tomey, & M. R. Alligood (Eds.), *Nursing theorists and their work* (4th ed., pp. 529-537). St. Louis: Mosby.

U.S. Department of Human Services. (2000). *Healthy people 2010* (Conference Edition). Washington, DC: The Department.

U.S. Preventive Services Task Force. (1996). *Guide to clinical preventive services* (2nd ed.). Baltimore: Williams & Wilkins.

Woolf, S. H. (1996). What not to do and why. In S. H. Woolf, S. Jonas, & R. S. Lawrence (Eds.), *Health promotion and disease prevention in clinical practice* (pp. 448-463). Baltimore, MD: Williams & Wilkins.

Chapter 10

SUSAN A. HEADY
JANICE I. HOOPER

Health Education

objectives

After completing this chapter, the nurse will be able to:

- Define health education.
- Describe the aims of health education.
- Discuss learning principles that affect health education.
- Apply teaching and learning concepts to teaching the family.
- Describe the health belief model and behavior-change process.
- Describe the use of social marketing in planning health education programs.
- Describe a system for planning health education programs.
- Identify the steps in administering health education programs.
- Identify the steps in preparing a health-teaching plan.
- Select content and learning strategies appropriate to the health learning needs of a target audience.
- List ways to evaluate a person's progress.
- State personal plans for developing teaching skills.

key terms

Behavior Change
Disease Prevention
Health Behaviors
Health Belief Model
Health Counseling
Health Education
Health Promotion
Precede-Proceed Model
Social Cognitive Theory
Social Learning Theory
Social Marketing

THINK About It

The Challenges of Health

An analysis of a nursing assessment often leads to a nursing diagnosis related to the individual's demonstration of a lack of knowledge in the areas of health promotion or health-promotion strategies. The nurse may recognize certain risk factors in a person, such as a lack of knowledge, possession of incorrect knowledge, misinterpretation of information, or reliance on harmful myths and folk medicine. Additionally, the individual may demonstrate little or no interest in learning, a lack of motivation to learn, or a cognitive or perceptual inability to learn.

The success of any health activity or goal will depend on the individual's perception of the situation and his or her responsiveness to teaching. The success of health teaching depends on a person's ability to learn and process information and the individual's motivation to change behaviors to improve the present condition or move toward better health. The nurse must assist each person in a process of self-understanding and self-direction so the individual will experience the desire and motivation to change. Frequently, the individual must make major life decisions in the process of learning. If the nurse, through education and counseling, can enhance the person in logical and clear thinking, then the individual's decision-making abilities and progress in meeting life's needs will be developed further. To encourage critical thinking by an individual, the nurse may pose some of the following questions:

1. What do you know about the health problem or concern?
2. What were you told?
3. What do you think will help you deal with the problem or concern?
4. How do you explain this problem or concern to yourself?
5. How do you see yourself in six months?
6. What types of efforts have worked for you in the past with this problem or concern?
7. How does the problem or concern affect your daily life?
8. What one aspect would indicate an improvement in your condition?
9. If you could have one question answered about this problem or concern, what would it be?
10. How much control do you think you have over this situation?
11. What is one goal that you would like to set for yourself?
12. Can you see any good coming out of this situation?

Scenario

Ronald is a successful executive in a local business. In his annual physical examination, an irregular heartbeat was noted on the electrocardiogram (ECG). Ronald's father died of a heart attack at age 50; therefore the physician scheduled Ronald for a thallium stress test. The stress test indicated a need for further evaluation through a cardiac catheterization. A 60% blockage in one artery was detected during this process. Ronald's condition will be handled conservatively at this point. He recognizes that some lifestyle behavior changes are necessary. He is overweight and eats in restaurants frequently. He has not been active in regular exercise. He and his wife live in a condominium. They have grown children and grandchildren. They have not seen one of their sons for several years and hear from him rarely because he has a serious drug problem.

1. How might the nurse begin working with Ronald?
2. How likely is he to be motivated to learn and change?
3. What are some barriers to change in his life behaviors?

Healthy People 2010 continues the health initiatives outlined in the previous document, *Healthy People 2000*, to improve the health of all people in the United States in the twenty-first century (U.S. Department of Health and Human Services, 2000). Although it is difficult to separate some health problems from social and environmental influences, many health goals are affected by individual lifestyle changes. Behavioral research indicates that people can make choices that will increase both the quality and the quantity of life. People can be motivated by information, positive influences, assistance in changing health-risking habits or situations, or support to escape victimization and move forward (Sullivan, 1991).

Nursing, with its unique contributions to health care, represents a significant professional resource that can help facilitate these changes through health education strategies. Nurses, in partnership with other health care professionals, can be the link between the philosophy of *Healthy People 2010* and the people who need to hear and act on these messages.

Although the average life expectancy of the American population as a whole has increased, the number of years of healthy living has declined. Morbidity and mortality data point to the continuing need for a better understanding of how to implement health **behavior change** strategies, **disease prevention,** and health-promotion interventions. In the preface to *Healthy People 2010*, Donna E. Shalala, Secretary of Health and Human Services, recognizes the value of the 467 health objectives in guiding efforts to bring better health to all people in this country (U.S. Department of Health and Human Services, 2000). She states that the nation is challenged to continue the commitment to improve the health of the country in the twenty-first century, which involves not only a reduction of premature death, but also promotion of health and prevention of disease and disability (U.S. Department of Health and Human Services, 2000). The nurse, using health education principles, can assist people in achieving these goals in a way that is consistent with their personal lifestyles, values, and beliefs.

NURSING AND HEALTH EDUCATION

Nursing's Agenda for Health Care Reform is a call for consumers to "assume more responsibility for their own care and become better informed about the range of providers and the potential options for services" (American Nurses' Association [ANA], 1991a, p. 4). As a case manager, the nurse can help the individual and family choose wisely as they seek to ensure their health and wellness (National League for Nursing, 1993). The Standards of Clinical Nursing Practice describes nursing responsibilities for all individuals, including educating persons about their illness, treatment, health-promotion or self-care activities, and planning for continuity of care (ANA, 1991b). Health teaching and **health counseling** are also included among the responsibilities of the nurse in the ANA's Nursing's Social Policy Statement, which views the nurse as one who assists people effectively, whether giving physical care, providing emotional support, engaging in health teaching or counseling, or assisting recovery or a peaceful death (ANA, 1995). This responsibility to teach individuals is balanced by their right to know about diagnosis, treatment, and prognosis. Although information about the medical diagnosis is reserved for the physician, the nurse's role is to support the right of individuals to know their medical status and to assess and assist a person's physical, psychosocial, and spiritual response to that knowledge. The nurse also provides appropriate health teaching and health counseling to the individual (Bandman & Bandman, 1995).

Nurses usually function as health care coordinators for individuals in their care. Depending on the interest and needs of a person, nurses establish a partnership to guide the individual in the selection and use of relevant health services. Principles of health education provide the nurse with specific strategies and tools for assessing an individual's readiness for health teaching, with technical information and with help in practicing health care techniques at home. These strategies also help the nurse facilitate behavior change while satisfying the person's right to relevant health information and to the freedom for people to make decisions about their health. Health education encourages self-care, self-empowerment, and, ultimately, less dependence on the health care system.

Nurses have long been involved in public health education, taking on the full-time role of coordinating the educational services provided by a health agency or institution. As a health educator, the nurse may use marketing strategies to enhance the effectiveness of health education programs that are focused on certain target populations. The health education specialist helps other nurses and health professionals improve their skills in developing and delivering teaching plans.

Definition

Health education is "the process of assisting individuals, acting separately or collectively, to make informed decisions on matters affecting individuals, family, and community health" (Aspen Reference Group, 1997, p. 3). This process involves several key components. First, health education involves the use of teaching-learning strategies. Second, learners maintain voluntary control over the decision to make changes in their actions. Third, health education focuses on behavior changes that have been found to improve health status.

Health education facilitates the development of health knowledge, skills, and attitudes through the application of theories or models. Two commonly used theories, behavioral theory and social learning theory, will be discussed later in this chapter. Generally, health education strategies help ensure that individuals, as consumers of health services, are satisfied and have received the health care that is most relevant to their problems. From a public health perspective, health education programs not only attempt to enhance individuals' ability to make positive lifestyle changes, but also to support social and political actions that promote health and quality of life in communities (Green & Kreuter, 1999).

The following scenario is an example of a therapeutic situation in which a health education approach may be used to meet an individual's health needs:

Sada Thompson, a 21-year-old university senior, visits university health services because she wants to change her method of birth control. She has experienced side effects from the birth control pill that she has been taking for the last year and knows little about other options. She has recently started dating John after breaking up with Steven 3 months ago. Having decided to be sexually active with John, Sada is feeling uncertain about what she needs to do to take care of herself and how to discuss this uncertainty with John. She is aware of all the talk about AIDS on campus and she knows that John is popular and has dated several other women in school, which concerns her.

Sada needs to learn new information, she may need to acquire new skills, and she must clarify any feelings or attitudes that affect her decision to use a new birth control method and ensure her continued safety (Fig. 10-1). After recording her health assessment history and arranging for a gynecological examination and laboratory tests, the nurse develops a teaching plan. Selecting one or more strategies for helping Sada review all the birth control options, the nurse establishes an environment in which Sada can voluntarily choose to try a new method or request a change in her prescription for oral contraceptives. Together, they identify actions that Sada can take to use the method properly. They also anticipate and identify ways that Sada can solve problems of adjusting to the new method.

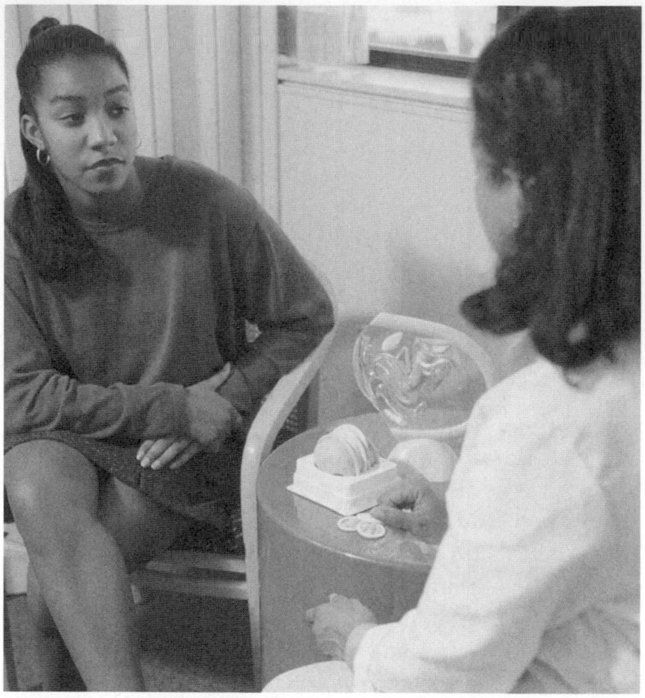

Fig. 10-1 Educating an individual involves not only dissemination of information, but also noting the person's response to that information.

The nurse answers Sada's immediate questions about safe sex, gives her several pamphlets written for college students about this topic, and suggests that she participate in the peer counseling night on sexually transmitted diseases (STDs) that will be held on campus in 2 weeks. The peer counseling hotline number and drop-in hours are given to her and the nurse explains that these students are trained to help other students talk about and deal with this important issue. The nurse invites Sada to call or come back to the office for additional help, information, and problem-solving discussion.

This example illustrates that educational interventions, in addition to direct health services, are necessary to meet the individual's goal. Although health care providers and nurses prefer that people choose to take actions that will promote health and not detract from it, the individual controls the at-home application of health recommendations.

Goals

The goal of health education is to help individuals, families, and communities achieve, through their own actions and initiative, optimal states of health. Health education should facilitate voluntary actions to promote health. **Health promotion** is defined as "the combination of educational and ecological supports for actions and conditions of living conducive to health" (Green & Kreuter, 1999, p. 27).

A broader definition and a goal of health education is the detection of illness, treatment, rehabilitation, and long-term care (Glanz, Lewis, & Rimer, 1997). Health education encourages positive, informed changes in lifestyle behaviors that prevent acute and chronic disease, decrease disability, and enhance wellness. Another goal of health education that may foster successful changes in health behavior is the empowerment of the individual. People who believe that they can make a difference in health are more likely to make changes (Simons-Morton & Crump, 1996). The result of health education should be voluntary behavior changes that are based on the analysis of past and new knowledge, attitudes, personal skills, and environmental conditions. Education enables the individual to lead a normal, healthy life; to rely on self rather than others; to wisely handle daily decisions; and to manage a chronic condition responsibly (DeAlva, 1999).

Box 10-1 Recommendations of U.S. Preventive Services Task Force: Strategies in Health Education and Counseling

1. Frame the teaching to match the patient's perceptions.
2. Fully inform patients of the purposes and expected effects of interventions and when to expect these effects.
3. Suggest small changes rather than large ones.
4. Be specific.
5. Adding new behaviors rather than eliminating established behaviors is sometimes easier.
6. Link new behaviors to old behaviors.
7. Use the power of the profession.
8. Get explicit commitments from the patient.
9. Use a combination of strategies.
10. Involve office staff.
11. Refer.
12. Monitor progress through follow-up contact.

From U.S. Preventive Services Task Force (1996). *Guide to clinical preventive services* (2nd ed.). Baltimore, MD: Williams & Wilkins.

Disease-prevention efforts such as screening tests and immunizations have significantly reduced mortality and morbidity in the United States. However, changes in health behaviors that are related to health education and counseling promise to help prevent disease, illness, and disability on another level. Naturally, this promise is predicated on the motivation and participation of the individual. Two major objectives of health education and counseling, identified by the U.S. Preventive Services Task Force (1996), are to change health behaviors and to improve health status. Information alone does not change behavior (Box 10-1).

Health education and health counseling are mutually supportive activities. Health educators often use one-to-one and group counseling techniques as strategies for active health learning. Counselors may refer people to health education resources or assist them in acquiring health information pertinent to solving a health problem.

The following example helps illustrate the goals of health education:

Kate Hanson, 22 years old, visits the local family health center with the complaint of fatigue and symptoms similar to influenza. During the assessment with the nurse, Kate discloses that she has missed her last two periods.

The physical examination, the laboratory tests, and the health assessment pattern confirm Kate's suspicions of pregnancy. Psychosocial evaluation reveals that Kate works part time as a secretary for a temporary agency and lives in an apartment with her recently unemployed husband, Jim. Further interviewing reveals that Kate has minimal knowledge of prenatal care; she has a diet of take-out food that is high in fat, sodium, and sugar, with infrequent consumption of fresh fruits or vegetables; and she has three or four beers on the weekends. Kate has never taken vitamins, she leads a sedentary lifestyle, and she is obviously overwhelmed by the news that she is pregnant.

The nurse first takes steps to create a safe and trusting atmosphere in which Kate can feel free to share her concerns and apprehensions. Finding that Kate needs counseling for telling her husband about the pregnancy, the nurse discusses this with her. Kate is then taught the importance of taking a multiple vitamin with an iron supplement daily, discontinuing the use of any medications or alcohol, and making time for more rest during the day. Sensing that this is all that can be accomplished at this time, the nurse gives Kate two pamphlets on prenatal care and makes an appointment for her to return in a week with her husband. Kate acknowledges that she understands the instructions and the nurse documents the teaching and recommendations in Kate's chart.

During the next visit, the nurse meets with Kate and Jim, explores the meaning of the pregnancy in their lives, and helps them identify actions they will need to take. The recommendations that were made during Kate's first visit are reviewed and reinforced. The nurse then details specifics of dietary changes and the need for proper rest and exercise and helps them solve problems as they adjust to these new responsibilities. Most importantly, the nurse gives them information on the clinic's weekly prenatal classes and explains that because the classes are partially covered by local community funding, the charge is minimal. The classes include information about physical changes, psychosocial changes, and nutritional needs during the pregnancy, the labor and delivery, and the newborn and postpartum periods. The nurse practitioner conducts the classes at the clinic, which are given in a group format to facilitate social support and problem solving among expectant parents.

The nurse gives them several other pamphlets to read at home, makes an appointment for Kate to see the physician in a couple of weeks, and encourages her to call if she has questions or concerns in the interim. A schedule of the prenatal classes is reviewed and a date for the next session is made. The couple is also encouraged to meet with the social worker to explore their financial needs and options because Jim was recently laid off. Kate and Jim acknowledge that they understand what they need to do and the nurse documents what was taught and discussed in Kate's health care record.

This example illustrates the goal of health education; that is, to help individuals achieve optimal health and well being through their actions and initiative. Through health education, individuals can learn to make informed decisions about personal and family health practices and to use health services in the community. The individual in this example receives educational assistance from the nurse that will promote better health and well being for herself and her baby.

Box 10-2 How to Facilitate Learning

- Use methods that stimulate a variety of senses.
- Actively involve the person in the learning process.
- Establish a comfortable, appropriate learning environment.
- Assess the readiness of the learner, which may be affected by physical and emotional factors.
- Make the information relevant by connecting with the existing needs and interests of the learner.
- Use repetition. Review and reinforce concepts several times in a variety of ways.
- Make the learning encounter positive. Structure it to achieve progress recognizable by the individual and provide frequent, positive feedback.
- Start with what is known and proceed to what is unknown, moving from simple to complex.
- Apply the concepts to several settings to facilitate generalization.
- Pace the learning appropriately for the individual.

Learning Assumptions

Individual chapters in this text address the factors to consider when teaching different age groups and the learners' characteristics to consider when developing a teaching plan. The following general principles of learning are fundamental to the planning of successful health education programs (Aspen Reference Group, 1997) (Box 10-2).

The nurse considers the developmental stage, cognitive level, and interests of the individual. The level of information to be conveyed and the skills and abilities of the individual will guide the methods and resources used. Children deserve special planning for health teaching (see Health Teaching box).

Family Health Teaching

The family is the unit for the caregiving of its members; therefore the family must often learn specific tasks of illness care. The family is also responsible for teaching health

HEALTH TEACHING Teaching Health Promotion to Preschoolers and School-Aged Children

Teaching the principles of health promotion to young children can influence their behaviors now and in the future and may affect family health. Young children are at a receptive age for learning behaviors that will become life habits (Pender, 1996).

Useful Principles for Teaching Children

- Children learn best through all their senses.
- Learning activities should be interesting and meaningful.
- Teachers should show love and respect for all children.
- Good teaching is based on theory, philosophy, goals, and objectives.
- Children's learning is enhanced through the use of concrete materials.
- Teaching should be centered on the child.
- Teaching should move from the concrete to the abstract.
- Teaching should be based on the children's interests (Morrison, 1995).

General Goals for Teaching Health-Related Topics to Children

Social and Interpersonal Goals

- Helping children know how to get along well with others.
- Helping children learn to help others and develop caring attitudes.
- Helping children understand the importance of caring for the environment.
- Helping children value and respect differences among individuals.

Self-Help Skills

- Helping children know appropriate clothing to wear.
- Teaching children hygienic skills (hand washing and oral care).
- Helping children choose positive television programs.
- Teaching children about body parts, functions, and maintaining health.

Self-Esteem Goals

- Promoting skills to help children develop positive self-esteem.
- Teaching children to understand their emotions and other's emotions.

Safety Goals

- Teaching children fire safety.
- Teaching children how to stay safe when outside, when alone, and when approached by strangers.
- Teaching children special safety rules, such as winter safety, Halloween safety, and water safety.

Nutrition, Exercise, and Health Behavior Goals

- Teaching children good nutrition.
- Teaching children the importance of exercise and rest.

Other Factors

In all planning, the children should be considered. When possible, the particular group should be observed and the learning experience should be as individualized as possible. The approach should be planned for the specific group of children with the following factors considered:

- Teaching environment: physical accommodations, equipment, and materials available.
- Readiness of the children: their previous schedule.
- Depth of knowledge of the children on the topic.
- Ability of the teacher to be flexible when plans change.
- Ways to involve as many children as possible.
- Plans to manage discipline.
- Plans to manage children's questions and stories (Seefeldt & Barbour, 1994).

Planning Learning Activities

Considerations in planning the learning activities include the following:

- The children's developmental level
- Any special considerations of the children
- The children's past experiences, interests, and abilities
- Activities that create enthusiasm and interest
- Activities that stimulate many senses
- Activities that leave the child with something to take home (Pender, 1996; Redman, 1997)

Suggested Teaching Activities

- Games
- Dialogue and interaction with children
- Role-playing and dramatic play
- Showing items, objects, and examples
- Puppets, stories, and books
- Artwork or handwork (coloring and drawing)
- Questions

The nurse may wear a costume or a special item of clothing that is related to the topic. The children will enjoy receiving a certificate of completion of a health lesson. Having something to take home to discuss with their parents is also meaningful for the children.

The health teaching should emphasize skills that children can use or develop immediately. Experiences should be selected with children's cognitive abilities in mind. For example, young children cannot understand cause and effect; they cannot anticipate the effects of dangerous situations, poor nutrition, and unsound health practices.

promotion; family members learn healthy behaviors in the home. Skills in family interviewing and family assessment are valuable tools for nurses working with families. Family health assessment and family health teaching are closely related. The family assessment model in the chapter on family health promotion provides a comprehensive approach to identifying family problems, strengths, and health-education needs. The goal of family health education is to help the family achieve optimal states of health while guiding them through problem solving and decision making. This process empowers the family; members believe they can make a difference in their own health.

In clarifying the health teaching needs of a family, the nurse might ask herself, "Who is in this family? What tasks should they be performing? How are they functioning and how are they meeting each others' needs? How well are they communicating? What does this family need to know? What do they need to know *now*? What do they think they need to know? How can they learn what they need to know?"

The nurse sets a broad health-promotion goal for the family, but directs the health teaching toward a more specific area. Most importantly, the family should be in agreement with the goal and teaching needs. As the family participates in the assessment interview, perhaps members can identify their own health teaching needs. Some broad goals for family teaching include:

- Better family functioning
- Achieving developmental tasks
- Better family communication
- Improved self-concept
- Increased self-esteem
- Reduced health risks
- Healthier lifestyle behaviors (improved diet and health habits)
- Improved energy level within the family
- A sense of control
- Adaptation to change in family structure
- Adaptation to change in family situation or life state

Health teaching to a family unit includes all family members, with learning activities appropriate for each individual. The general health-teaching goal will be the same for all family members, but the approaches and specific goals for each member or subsystem will be different. Children, adolescents, and elderly members pose special challenges to the nurse who may be geared toward teaching young or middle-aged adults.

Health Behavior Change

The process of health education directs people toward voluntary changes of their health behaviors. This section examines the use of the health belief model to analyze the probability that a person will make changes for improving health or preventing disease and the application of social learning theory to clarify environmental and social factors that affect the learning of new health behaviors.

Beliefs, attitudes, values, and information contribute to motivation and behavior and are underlying components in making any decision to change behavior (Richards, 1997). **Health behaviors** are any activities that an individual undertakes to enhance health, prevent disease, and detect and control the symptomatic stage of a disease. Identifying and teaching people about lifestyle behaviors that need to be changed is only the first step in the process of assisting individuals in moving from knowledge to action. The nurse uses the health belief model and social learning theory as subsequent steps in formulating an action plan that meets the needs and capabilities of each person in making healthy behavior changes.

Health Belief Model

The **health belief model** is a paradigm used to predict and explain health behavior that is based on value-expectancy theory. The health belief model was developed in the 1950s by social psychologists from the U.S. Public Health Service to describe why people failed to participate in programs to detect or prevent disease. The model has been expanded to explain responses to symptoms, disease, prescribed treatments, and potential health problems (Glanz, Lewis, & Rimer, 1997). The health belief model and social learning theory assist the nurse in formulating an action plan that meets the needs and capabilities of the individual in making health behavior changes.

The following health belief model provides guidelines for nurses to analyze factors that contribute to a person's perceived state of health or risk of disease and to the individual's probability of taking appropriate health plans of action (Becker, 1974; Janz & Becker, 1984; Kolbe, Iverson, Kreuter, Hochbaum, & Christensen, 1981; Rosenstock & Becker, 1988). To assess a person's perceived state of health or threat of disease, the nurse examines the following:

1. Individual perceptions or readiness for change
   a. The value of health to the individual compared with other aspects of living
   b. Perceived susceptibility to a disease and complications
   c. Perceived seriousness of the disease level threatening the achievement of certain goals or aims
   d. Belief in the diagnosis and therapy plan
2. Modifying factors about the person
   a. Demographic variables (age and gender)
   b. Socioeconomic variables (family and peer group characteristics, income, and education)
   c. Previous experience with the disease
   d. Risk factors to a disease attributed to heredity, race or culture, medical history, or other causes
   e. Level of participation in and satisfaction with regular health care
   f. Actual extent of change necessary
   g. Personal aspirations in life and valued social and vocational activities
3. Motivating and environmental factors (cues to action)
   a. Exposure to mass media
   b. Advice from others
   c. Reminders from health professionals
   d. Illness of a family member or friend
   e. Perceived benefits of complying with a treatment plan
   f. Previous success at changing behaviors

To assess a person's likelihood of taking preventive health actions, the nurse compares this picture of perceived threat of disease with the following:

4. Individual-nurse transaction factors
   a. Previous use of health services
   b. Perceived benefits of health action

c. Perceived barriers to promotion action
d. Continued reassessment of the treatment plan by the individual and provider

The health belief model does not specify the interventions that will influence an individual's likelihood of taking action. Rather, the health belief model explains the role of values and beliefs in predicting treatment outcomes and adherence while generating data that guides nurses in choosing effective educational strategies. Developing the most appropriate interventions for a particular person must be negotiated between the individual and the health care professional.

Social Learning Theory

Social learning theory (SLT), recently renamed **social cognitive theory** (SCT), is another model that adds to the understanding of the determinants of health behavior. Bandura (1997) emphasizes the influence of efficacy beliefs and outcome expectations on health behavior.

Efficacy beliefs, or self-efficacy, refer to an individual's perception of self-competence to perform the behavior required to influence outcomes. Efficacy expectation is distinct from outcome expectation (see Case Study). An outcome expectation is the assumed consequences of actions taken. Outcome expectations refer to a person's estimate that a given behavior will lead to a particular outcome.

According to behavioral theory, behavior is regulated by its consequences (reinforcements), but only as these consequences are interpreted and understood by the individual. Incentives are defined as the value of a particular object or outcome. The outcome may be related to health status, physical appearance, approval of others, economic gain, or other consequences. For example, people who value the perceived effects of changed lifestyles (incentives), will attempt to change when they believe: (1) their current lifestyles pose a threat to a personally valued outcome, such as health or appearance (environmental cues); (2) particular behavioral changes will reduce the threat (outcome expectations); and (3) they are personally capable of adopting the new behaviors (efficacy expectations).

Two important contributions have been made by SCT to explain health behavior change (Rosenstock & Becker, 1988). The first contribution is the informational and motivational role of reinforcement and the role of observational learning through modeling (imitating) the behavior of others. Opportunities to observe others performing the behavior in question, such as in a local YMCA risk-factor reduction program in which individuals exercise together and report on health behavior changes of smoking cessation and eating a low-fat diet, can enhance expectations of mastery. For modeling to affect a person's self-efficacy (an individual's perception of confidence in the ability to perform a specific behavior), the model must be similar to the observer in characteristics such as age and gender and must be seen as overcoming difficulties through determined effort rather than ease (Fitzgerald, 1991).

The concept of outcome expectation (a person's estimate that a given behavior will lead to a particular outcome) is similar to the health belief model concept of perceived benefits. Distinguishing between outcome and efficacy expectations is significant because both are required for behavior change. Figure 10-2, Bandura's diagram (1997), shows this relationship. For example, to begin an exercise program (behavior) for health reasons (outcome), a person must believe that exercise will benefit the person's health (outcome expectation) and that the person is capable of exercising (efficacy expectation) (Rosenstock & Becker, 1988).

Regardless of nurses' best assessment methods and educational strategies, research in the area of health education indicates that people do not always make the choices recommended to them by health professionals (Rankin & Stallings, 1996). Nurses often label these people noncompliant, a term that suggests that the individual has not followed their instructions. Naturally, health professionals want people to choose the recommended course of action; however, each individual has the right to choose not to follow advice. Enlisting the individual's partnership or cooperation rather than compliance is important.

CASE STUDY

Alicia

Alicia Gonzalez is a 16-year-old pregnant adolescent who is expecting her first baby in 1 month. She lives in an apartment with her mother, Teresa. Both of them came to the United States from Puerto Rico about 10 years ago. Although their primary language is Spanish, both speak and understand English fairly well. While at the clinic for a prenatal visit, Alicia tells the nurse, "I'm really scared about going into labor. I'm not sure I can handle it." Alicia also expresses concern that her mother doesn't think she will be able to care for the baby properly and that her mother will "take over" the care of the baby.

- How can the prenatal teaching be adapted for her cultural background?
- How can the nurse promote Alicia's self-efficacy in caring for the infant?

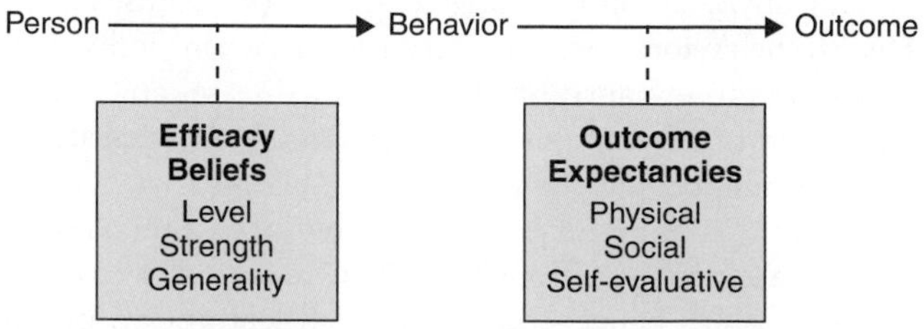

Fig. 10-2 Diagram of self-efficacy concept. (From *Self-Efficacy: The Exercise of Control* by Albert Bandura. © 1997 by W.H. Freeman and Company. Used with the permission of Worth Publishers.)

Attempts to influence a person's behavior through education are not always successful. Attempting to persuade people to change their behavior to something that might make them, their friends, and their family healthier can be discouraging and sometimes futile. An individual's values, beliefs, and life stresses may present obstacles to the adoption of changes in behavior. Effective health education requires an understanding of the influential factors affecting the individual's decision making (values, beliefs, attitudes, current life stresses, religion, previous experiences with the health care system, and life goals).

Many health professionals tend to view a person's cooperation with the medical regimen as a single choice, when in fact, this cooperation often involves many choices every day. For example, following a low-fat, low-cholesterol diet involves constant, and often inconvenient, choices throughout the day. The expectation is that people will do this every day for the rest of their lives, even when the nurse cannot guarantee freedom from angina, myocardial infarctions, or other complications.

Ultimately, the nurse must respect a person's right to choose. However, nurses can increase an individual's motivation and capabilities to change by involving the individual in planning and goal setting, providing information that is understandable and acceptable, and assisting the person in developing new skills for mastery.

After clarifying behaviors that may need to be changed, the nurse can use the following set of questions evolved from SCT to assist in constructing effective educational and motivational interventions for behavior change (Timmreck, Cole, James, & Butterworth, 1987):

- What is the nature of the physical and social environment in which the behavior occurs?
- What are the characteristics of the situation in which the behavior occurs?
- What factors tend to reinforce existing behaviors?
- What rewards or praise would help a person make behavioral changes?
- Do appropriate social models in the environment exist from which the person might learn new behaviors vicariously?
- What opportunities exist for the person to manage personal rewards?
- Does the person have the skills or capabilities needed to make changes?
- What does the person expect to occur as a result of these changes?
- What does the person value as outcomes to practicing new behaviors?
- Will the person be able to monitor the new behaviors and control the reinforcers in the environment?
- Does the person believe in a personal sense of competence to achieve new behaviors?
- In what ways will the environment be influenced by the person's new behaviors?

The information collected by answering the SCT questions forms the basis on which to design educational interventions that are appropriate to the phases of the behavior-change process.

Theories of health behavior change are at the heart of health education. The theories presented in this section help the nurses get started. The goals of teaching plans will differ depending on the individual's stage in the behavior-change process. Ongoing health education courses and programs in the community, school, and worksite will also differ in strategy and style depending on these phases. The next section includes an example of a person working through these phases with educational interventions from a nurse.

Interventions

Interventions are specific techniques used with a person or population to promote healthy changes. In health education, interventions take the form of teaching methods and strategies. The nurse selects a particular teaching method depending on the health behavior involved and the person's (student's) progress through the behavior-change process. Consider the following example:

Mrs. Pat Taylor, recently widowed at age 69, takes several regular medications: a diuretic, potassium tablets, and a high-dose vitamin. She recently had dental work performed and the dentist gave her a prescription for aspirin with codeine phosphate (Empirin with codeine). Mrs. Taylor now has symptoms of a winter cold and is about to decide whether to take a cold capsule, some aspirin, or cough syrup. She has always been somewhat confused as to how to select and schedule regular medications, her diet, and over-the-counter drugs, but she has never had a drug reaction. This time, she decides to call her nurse practitioner for advice.

The nurse, Barbara Crandall, realizes that, gradually, Mrs. Taylor will need various medications; because there is no support person at home, she will need to develop safe habits of taking different medications. This telephone call provides an opportunity for Mrs. Taylor to learn preventive behaviors for both her current symptoms and future conditions. After handling the medical questions according to office protocol and determining that Mrs. Taylor is interested in learning more about the safe use of prescription medications and over-the-counter drugs, Barbara begins the pretraining phase.

During the pretraining phase, the nurse provides information that builds awareness of the health issue and expands his or her options for alternative plans of action. The individual may select interventions such as audiovisual aids, pamphlets, magazine articles, or short presentations (lecturettes). To help analyze options, the health professional may facilitate a question-and-answer discussion or lead value-clarification exercises. The result of the pretraining phase should be a statement of the goals and a list of learning needs developed mutually between the individual and the nurse.

Barbara and the internist with whom she works conduct education programs periodically for many older adults. Barbara invites Mrs. Taylor to participate in a session on medication safety. Using slides and one or two group exercises, the members learn to assess their own level of knowledge on the subject and their behavior patterns. The goals of the session are to improve decision-making habits about medications and to identify changes in the environment and in the activities of daily living that will ensure safety in medication use.

Another useful strategy, health risk appraisal, is both a method and a tool that describes a person's chances of becoming ill or dying from specific diseases (Pender, 1996). The tool used for health risk appraisal should be thoroughly tested so each individual receives an accurate estimate of risk for the current major causes of death and disability. The appraisal tool serves to personalize health risk information in the media and helps individuals list specific behaviors that cause a health risk. As a health education method, health risk appraisal helps participants narrow the focus of their learning needs. Risk factors can be identified in three profile components: (1) behavioral risk, (2) social risk, and (3) environmental (physical, chemical, or biological) risk. Behavioral risk appraisal includes dietary habits, substance use, and physical activity. Social risk appraisal assesses stress associated with work, isolation, education, and social supports and networks. Environmental risk appraisal includes the quality of the environment, such as water, soil, air, climate, and housing (Bracht, 1990).

During the training phase, the decision is made to enter a change program. Programmed learning strategies are appropriate for learning facts and concepts. Skill practice sessions with return demonstration by the participants are effective for developing motor skills. Group discussion and role-playing methods help participants develop problem-solving techniques, a sense of self-confidence, and emotional control skills. During this phase, the nurse also helps people observe their own learning progress and reassess learning needs.

Mrs. Taylor's group decides to meet again to help one another solve the problems that they have identified about taking medications. Barbara is asked to provide information about questionable combinations of medications and a list of books on the subject. After the second session, Barbara stipulates that each group member will have to set personal objectives to practice the new behaviors at home. The group may not plan to meet again, but Barbara will be able to follow up on their new experiences in several ways.

The trial of new skills or behaviors, usually in a setting common to the individual's lifestyle, helps to characterize the initial testing phase. Community weight-control programs, fitness clubs, and self-help groups are examples of programs in which the participant has continued group support while proceeding through the trial period. Educational strategies that facilitate the initial testing phase include guided practice, contracting, self-monitoring, and continued session related to problem solving, values clarification, and role-playing.

Contracting refers to verbal or written agreements to try or practice specific actions within a time frame. The individual and the health professional or other support person negotiates the contract. At the end of the initial testing phase, individuals should be well aware of their records of performance, problems that cause barriers to performance, and aspects of their environments that promote or reinforce the desired behavior, such as rewards and social benefits.

When each group member returns for the next regular visit, Barbara asks what each of them learned during the sessions on medications, what changes each has tried, and the resulting outcomes. She records this information (without names) in a log maintained for evaluating the effectiveness of the group sessions. Depending on the needs of each person, she may suggest different ways to solve problems and monitor medication use.

The end of the behavior-change process occurs when the participant performs the desired behaviors on a regular basis. Intervention strategies during this phase tend to take the form of helpful consultation sessions, periodic progress reports, and the provision of rewards. Some methods used during the pretraining phase might be repeated to demonstrate progress and to assess new learning needs. Tests of the participant's knowledge with verbal or written tests and skill practice and demonstration sessions are not meant to determine whether a person will eventually perform a behavior regularly. However, in individual-oriented health education, these evaluation techniques serve to provide feedback and improve the individual's awareness of progress.

Ethics

The nurse upholds democratic principles such as respect for human dignity and the right to self-determination. However, when selecting health education interventions, nurses experience several ethical dilemmas.

Although the focus of health education may be on the behavior-change process, the nurse must be certain that tactics of coercion, persuasion, and manipulation have not been used to influence the changes (Bandman & Bandman, 1995). The role of the nurse is to facilitate a communicative environment in which people can exercise their right to make informed free choices. Individuals must participate in the decision-making process when their lives may be influenced by a change.

Although each person's state of health affects family members and the community, individuals are responsible for their own health maintenance. Health professionals must accept and welcome individual differences in meeting this responsibility. By selecting interventions that create an environment of open communication and risk taking, individuals can better develop the problem-solving skills to direct their growth and development.

Cultural Considerations in Health Teaching

Another challenge for health professionals is to apply health education strategies with people from various cultural backgrounds, people who do not speak English as their native language, and people who cannot read at elementary levels. The health professional must take the time to assess cultural beliefs that influence social and health practices and must make an effort to analyze educational interventions that are acceptable and satisfying to the individual. Social marketing processes discussed in the next section help identify characteristics, interests, and concerns of target populations.

When teaching persons of different cultural, racial, and ethnic groups, the nurse should endeavor to provide culturally sensitive patient education. The nurse should seek to understand the meanings that different cultural groups attribute to illness. A teaching approach that considers the individual's beliefs about illness will be both acceptable and effective in the areas of compliance and motivation (Rankin & Stallings, 1996). By combining an understanding of the nurse's culture and the culture of the individual, the nurse can adapt and individualize teaching to meet the preferences and needs of the culture (Price & Cordell, 1994) (see Multicultural Awareness box).

MULTICULTURAL AWARENESS

WHEN THERE IS A LANGUAGE BARRIER

- Use courtesy and a formal approach.
- Address the person by his or her last name.
- Introduce yourself, pointing to yourself as you give your name.
- Project a friendly attitude with a smile and a handshake.
- Speak with a moderate tone and volume.
- Attempt to use words in the person's language, which indicates respect for the individual's culture.
- Use simple, everyday words rather than complex words, medical jargon, or colloquialisms.
- Use hand gestures to help the person understand meaning.
- Instruct the person in small increments.
- Have the person demonstrate understanding of the message.
- Write down the instructions for the person to take home.
- Involve others who can serve as interpreters.
- When available, use flash cards and phrase books in other languages (Jarvis, 1996).

AREAS TO CONSIDER IN CULTURAL ASSESSMENT

- Individual's identification with a particular ethnic group
- Racial background
- Place of birth
- Personal history
- Habits, customs, values, and beliefs
- Cultural sanctions and restrictions
- Language and communication patterns
- Healing beliefs and practices
- Cultural health practices
- Nutritional beliefs
- Food preferences and restrictions (Schrefer, 1994)

SOCIAL MARKETING AND HEALTH EDUCATION

When nurses begin to teach groups of people, they automatically enter a program-planning and administrative process. When an organization wants to offer an ongoing health education program for specific target populations, social marketing provides a strategy for reaching members of the group and implementing a service that will satisfy these members as consumers. Principles of social marketing and health education strategies are combined to promote population-based changes in behavior to improve health.

Social marketing is defined as "the application of commercial marketing technologies to the analysis, planning, execution, and evaluation of programs designed to influence the voluntary behavior of target audiences in order to improve their personal welfare and that of their society" (Andreasen, 1995, p. 7). Key aspects of social marketing are: (1) its focus on benefit to individuals and society rather than on profit and organizational benefits as commercial marketing practices, (2) its focus on behavior change rather than awareness or attitude change, and (3) its involvement of the target audience in the process (Lefebvre & Rochlin, 1997).

The practice of social marketing involves developing and implementing integrated elements that have the shared purpose of leading to a specific change in behavior, which is referred to as the program objective. Strategies are then developed to guide program planners in developing specific tactics to meet this objective. A combination of tactics appropriate to the individual and the integration of these tactics constitutes a social marketing program.

Benefits of this consumer-driven approach, as compared with a top-down approach, may include more effective design, delivery, and reception of the message by the public. The effectiveness of social marketing is highly dependent on how well the target audience is understood and addressed, how well barriers and benefits to new behaviors are strategically addressed, and how effectively the program components are integrated and managed. Analysis of the target audience, using a variety of research techniques such as focus groups and pilot testing of strategies, are components of social marketing that enhance the tailoring of the program for specific groups (Lefebvre & Rochlin, 1997).

For example, use of social marketing strategies in designing smoking-cessation programs for ethnic minorities may improve adherence rates (Abrams, Borrelli, Shabel,

King, Bock, & Niaura, 1998). Any information about the target population that is generated by social marketing strategies will improve the nurse's ability to develop effective educational interventions.

ADMINISTERING HEALTH EDUCATION PROGRAMS

A planning model such as the precede-proceed model, which provides a sequence of steps for administering health education programs, can be used to guide program planning. The steps allow for two-way communication between provider and consumer, which is necessary for maintaining consumer satisfaction and for contributing to the reduction of public health problems through health behavior change.

The Precede-Proceed Model

The **precede-proceed model** is a comprehensive planning guide for the administration of health education programs. The first step is to decide whether an educational intervention will contribute to reducing a public health or medical problem. The precede framework, which guides the planner to arrive at a highly focused subset of factors as targets for intervention, examines the multiple factors that shape health status and quality of life. The precede aspect helps generate specific objectives and criteria for evaluation. The proceed framework gives additional steps for developing policy and initiating the processes of implementation and evaluation. These two frameworks work in tandem, providing a continual series of steps or phases in planning, implementation, and evaluation. Precede guides the planner in identifying priorities and setting objectives and further provides the objectives and criteria for policy, implementation, and evaluation in the proceed phases (Green & Kreuter, 1999).

Studying Fig. 10-3, focusing first of the right-hand side, helps develop an overview of the model. Working through the following phases using a familiar community health-promotion project, may help focus the exercise.

Phase 1: Social Assessment

The nurse lists indications of the quality of life from individuals and families in the target population, including social, economic, communication, or spiritual problems. Involving the people in a self-study of their needs and aspirations is the best way to accomplish this task. Situations that involve unemployment, loneliness or isolation, crowded conditions, or crime often have health-related causes; nonetheless, health is often a secondary value to

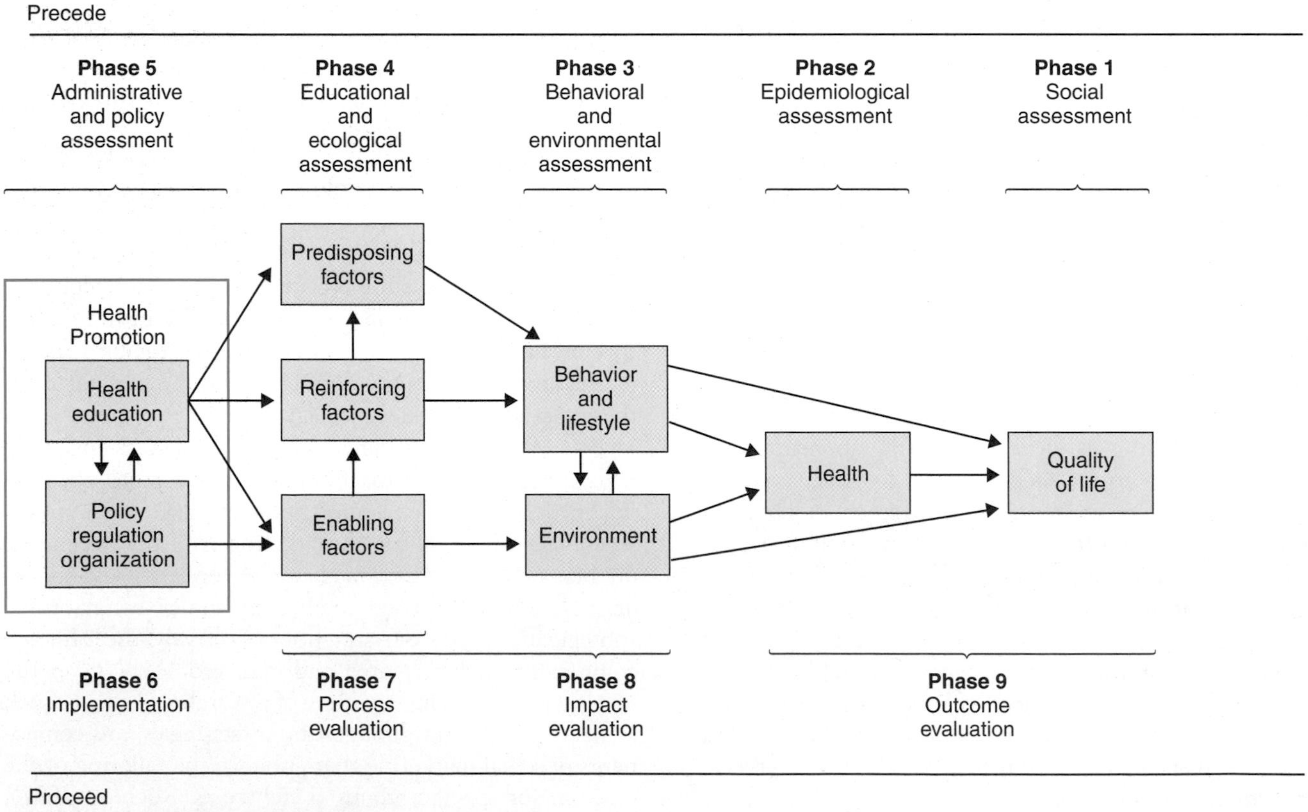

Fig. 10-3 The precede-proceed model of health-promotion planning and evaluation. (Modified from *Health promotion planning: An educational and ecological approach* [3rd ed.]. by Lawrence W. Green and Marshall W. Kreuter. Copyright © 1999 by Mayfield Publishing Company. Reprinted by permission of the publisher.)

social concerns or benefits. Relating health problems to social problems helps the provider and the consumer expand the rationale or justification of a health-education or health-promotion project. Community needs assessment information is especially useful for completing phase 1. Marketing profile information provides subjective indications of the target audience's quality-of-life concerns.

Phase 2: Epidemiological Assessment

The task of phase 2 is to identify specific health concerns that may be contributing to the problems in phase 1. Using data from the needs assessment in phase 1, the planner ranks the health problems and selects the specific health problem that is most deserving of scarce educational and promotional resources. Examples of vital indicators, or physiological measures of health factors on which to measure these, are shown in Fig. 10-4. The nurse differentiates between health problems and nonhealth factors that contribute to the social problems. Epidemiological data, such as morbidity and mortality statistics, suggest health problems of a target population. Data sources may include health insurance and workers' compensation statistics, local and federal public health statistics, and health service plans. These statistics indicate problems such as alcoholism, communicable and chronic diseases, infant mortality, and child abuse. Nonhealth factors include educational or income level, industrial layoffs, and climatic conditions. Analysis of the health problems facilitates the ability to prioritize programs by using rates of prevalence, cost, and so forth. This step also suggests the most appropriate organizations or professional groups for helping resolve the problem. Program goals and objectives indicate the expected influence of a health-education project on the prevalence of a health problem.

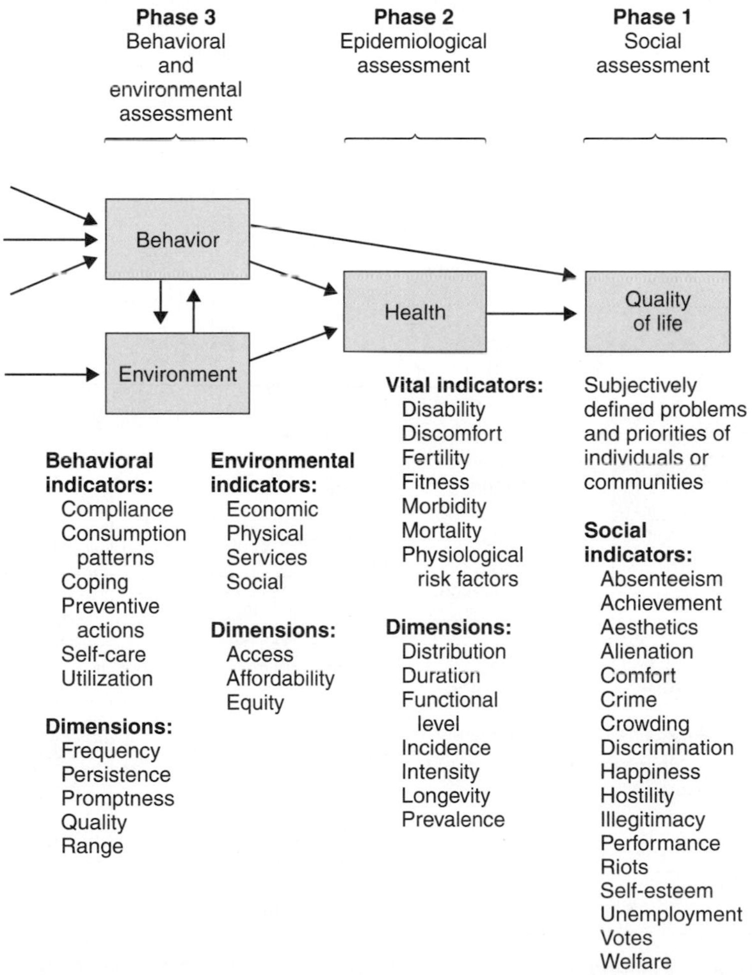

Fig. 10-4 Relationships, indicators, and dimensions of factors that might be identified in phases 1, 2, and 3 of the precede assessment process or evaluated as outcomes in proceed phases 8 and 9. (Modified from *Health promotion planning: An educational and ecological approach* [3rd ed.]. by Lawrence W. Green and Marshall W. Kreuter. Copyright © 1999 by Mayfield Publishing Company. Reprinted by permission of the publisher.)

Phase 3: Behavioral and Environmental Assessment

The nurse determines the behavioral risk factors that contribute to the specific health problems. Some behaviors increase the risk of many diseases. For example, smoking increases the chances of heart disease and cancer. Overeating may contribute to diabetes, high blood pressure, and obesity. The change of an isolated health behavior can help reduce the risk of several diseases.

Nonbehavioral causes of a health problem are not modifiable; they cannot be changed by the individual. A person cannot change age, gender, or ethnic background. Environmental conditions may affect a health problem, but this particular health problem may not be solved by the individual's behavior change. Environmental hazards often need to be managed by community organizations or legislation.

Some categories of changeable behaviors include lifestyle health habits, use of health care facilities, compliance with prescribed treatment plans, accident-prevention behaviors, communication and educational styles between consumers and providers, and personal changes in home, work, and recreational environments. After determining the behavioral causes of a health problem, the nurse then selects several priority behaviors for further analysis with the precede model.

Phase 4: Educational and Ecological Assessment

The nurse lists factors that cause health behaviors in three categories: (1) predisposing, (2) enabling, and (3) reinforcing (Fig. 10-5). Predisposing factors include the characteristics of the person or population (values, beliefs, attitudes, knowledge, age, gender, and family heritage) that influence the tendency to practice a particular behavior. Enabling factors include the resources that are available to an individual to take certain health actions, such as personal problem-solving skills, physical abilities, and community resources. Reinforcing factors are aspects of a person's social environment that support or inhibit behavior change, such as family attitudes and behaviors of health professionals. From the list of factors, the nurse selects those that are most appropriate for a health education program. This constitutes an educational assessment.

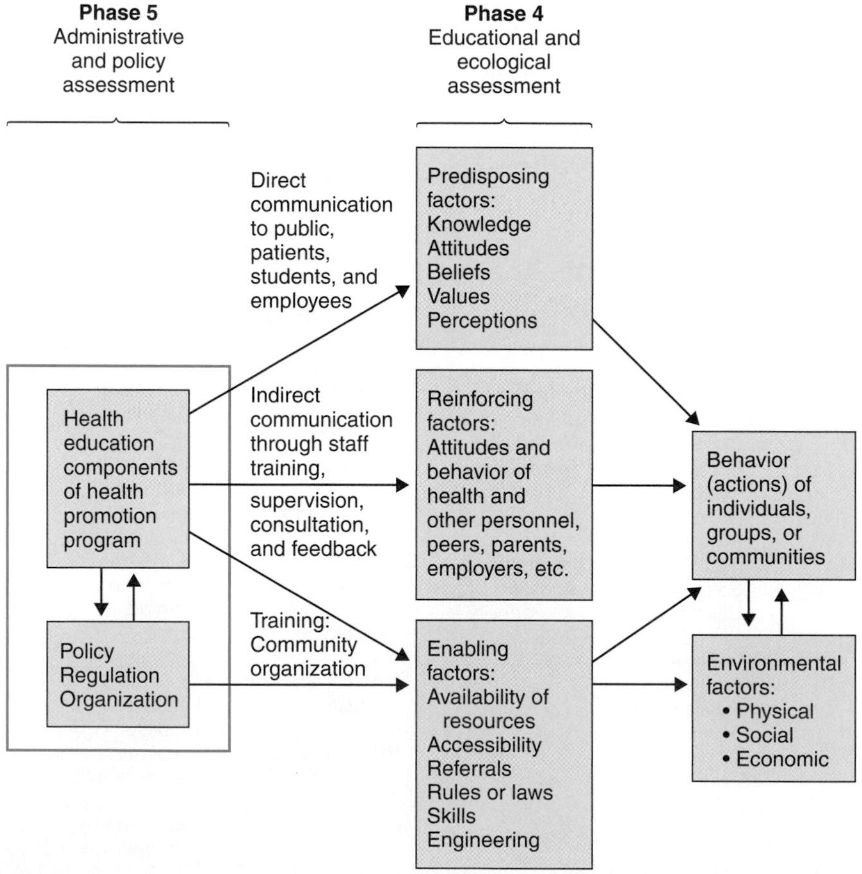

Fig. 10-5 Phases 4 and 5 of the precede process address the strategies and resources required to influence the predisposing, reinforcing, and enabling factors influencing or supporting behavioral and environmental changes. (Modified from *Health promotion planning: An educational and ecological approach* [3rd ed.]. by Lawrence W. Green and Marshall W. Kreuter. Copyright © 1999 by Mayfield Publishing Company. Reprinted by permission of the publisher.)

Phase 5: Administrative and Policy Assessment

Prepared with diagnostic information, the nurse is ready for the assessment of organizational and administrative capabilities and resources for the development and implementation of a program. The nurse selects educational strategies that are suitable for the facilitation of voluntary changes in behavior and, by assessing the organizational problems in implementing the health education program, develops alternatives in evaluation strategies and instruments.

Phases 6 through 9: Proceed

The nurse generates a list of action steps established from the goals and objectives of the program for organizing, promoting, teaching, and evaluating. The implementation of these steps is carried out and followed by an evaluation of the program. Listing evaluation as the last phase is misleading; however, this is the case because evaluation becomes an important and continual part of working with the entire model from the beginning. The criteria for evaluation proceed naturally from the objectives that were defined in the corresponding steps during the diagnostic process.

There are two fundamental propositions emphasized by the precede-proceed model: (1) health and health risks are a result of multiple factors and (2) efforts to effect behavioral, environmental, and social change must be multidimensional or multisectoral (Green & Kreuter, 1999).

Advantages

Advantages of using a planning model such as the precede-proceed model include the ability to connect health and social problems with appropriate and effective educational strategies, to develop a broad perspective about all the factors that influence health behavior and the interaction among the factors, and to select evaluation techniques tailored to assess the achievement of desired objectives. This process improves the chances that an educational intervention will meet the concerns of the target audience; that is, the consumer group.

THE TEACHING PLAN

Preparation for teaching one or more group programs, such as a seminar or course, begins after the marketing and administrative plans are well under way. These activities ensure that there are enough participants for the program, and they provide the structure for developing the teaching plan—the program objectives, available time, human and material resources, and so on. When the marketing and administrative functions have been provided by others and when educational strategies are developed for one person at a time, the nurse can concentrate efforts on developing the teaching plan.

A health-teaching plan may emphasize a phase of the behavior-change process that is related to the individual's medical or health problems. The plan may also follow the sequence of this process from pretraining to the continued performance of a behavior that helps resolve a medical or health problem. The written teaching plan represents a package of educational services provided to a consumer or student. The plan should be written from the student's point of view.

The process of generating a teaching plan helps the nurse recognize and use methods of learning that involve the individual as an active participant. The plan should include a list of specific actions or abilities that the person may perform at intervals during and at the end of the educational intervention. Teaching plans help nurses clarify what individuals as students should be able to do when the educational intervention is completed.

When preparing a teaching plan for one person in a primary care setting, the nurse may learn background information about the individual from that person's record and any agency reports that include descriptions of the person's population group. Often, nurses agree to teach health classes that others have organized. In this case, the nurse should ask for any project reports that provide marketing and needs-assessment information about the students who are expected to attend the classes and that indicate the steps to be taken to administer the entire educational program (see the Care Plan).

Nurses might approach the exercise of preparing a teaching plan in stages. The reader can simulate this by doing the following:

1. Review the chapter subsections that follow and jot down ideas and information about a real or hypothetical teaching project for each subsection.
2. Make a list of the information resources or human resources that are needed to complete the teaching plan.
3. After these resources are collected or consulted, draft a teaching plan. Use any structure for the plan that identifies the educational goal, behavioral objectives, content topics, learning methods, and evaluation strategies.
4. Review the written plan with a focus on whether the plan is an adequate tool to manage the educational intervention.

Assessing Learning Needs

The assessment of learning needs is important in developing health education programs for individuals, families, communities, or organizations. This process involves answering five questions:

1. What are the characteristics and learning capabilities of the individual?
2. What are the learner's needs for health promotion, risk reduction, or health problems?

CARE PLAN

Nursing Diagnosis: Knowledge Deficit (Specify Area)

DEFINING CHARACTERISTICS

- Verbalization of inadequate information or an inadequate recall of information
- Verbalization of misunderstanding or misconception
- Requesting information
- Instructions inaccurately followed
- Inadequate performance on a test
- Inadequate demonstration of a skill

RELATED FACTORS

- Pathophysiological states
- Sensory deficits
- Memory loss
- Intellectual limitations
- Interfering coping strategies (denial or anxiety)
- Lack of exposure to accurate information
- Lack of motivation to learn
- Inattention
- Cultural or language barriers.

EXPECTED OUTCOMES

- The individual will express an interest in learning.
- The individual will correctly state the information on the specific topic.
- The individual will correctly demonstrate skills needed to practice health-related behavior.
- The individual and family will explain how to incorporate new information into their lifestyle.
- The individual will modify health behavior based on the acquisition of new knowledge.
- The individual will list resources for more information or support.

INTERVENTIONS

- Provide accurate and culturally relevant information related to the specific topic.
- Select teaching techniques appropriate to the individual's learning need.
- Explore the individual's interpretation of the information and its meaning to the person in the context of the person's life.
- Demonstrate and have the individual practice new skills.
- Assist the person in identifying and implementing alternative strategies when initial choices are not successful.
- Include the family or significant others as appropriate.
- Provide names and telephone numbers of resource people or organizations.

3. What does the person already know and what skills can the person already perform that are relevant to the health needs?
4. Is the learner motivated to change any unhealthy behaviors?
5. What are the barriers to and facilitators of health behavior change?

Characteristics

Activities to help the nurse identify characteristics of the learner include:

Consideration of the individual's age and developmental stage in the person's life cycle.

Consideration of the individual's level on Maslow's hierarchy of basic human needs (survival, safety, love and belonging, self-esteem, and self-actualization).

Review of marketing profile descriptions of the individual's population segment (demographic, geographical, and psychographic characteristics).

The reader is encouraged to refer to the individual developmental chapters in this text for further information on developmental characteristics.

Health Problems

Information resources on the health problems of a population group include epidemiological reports, community needs assessment reports, insurance statistics, and incident reports. Nursing and medical texts often provide lists of concepts or skills to learn about a health problem and to comply with a treatment plan.

Current Knowledge and Skills

Methods for assessing current knowledge and skills include individual or group interviews, questionnaires or pretests, skill demonstrations, and observations of problem-solving behaviors and competencies. Health-risk appraisals and other tests help the individual become an active participant in assessing learning needs.

Motivation

The health belief model helps assess a person's health problems and the factors that indicate the likelihood of a desire to take preventive actions. When a person appears unmotivated to change, the nurse looks for environmental factors, lack of knowledge or skills, social stimuli, or false incentives that may be inhibiting the person's readiness. One aim of the pretraining phase of the behavior-change process is to create a learning climate that encourages the individual to make decisions for health behavior change.

Barriers and Facilitators

From the precede model, the predisposing, enabling, and reinforcing factors that create health behaviors also provide cues to program promotion and teaching techniques that may inhibit or enhance the learning process (see Fig. 10-5). The teaching plan, to the greatest extent possible, should incorporate activities that facilitate learning for the individual or target population. Readiness to learn new concepts, skills, or attitudes often depends on whether the educational intervention is timed appropriately. People may need time to research information, discuss the topics, or identify the consequences of not changing before they are ready to learn new material. The time of day and sequence of learning activities may also affect readiness.

Determining Expected Learning Outcomes

To determine the expected learning outcomes of a health education intervention, the nurse answers the following questions:

1. What are the broad public health and social goals that guide the proposed educational program?
2. What are the participant's learning goals?
3. What must the learner know, do, and believe to progress through the behavior-change process?

Program Goals

The program goal of a health education project should reflect the desire to facilitate improvement in some health problem or social living condition, as indicated in phases 1 and 2 of the precede model (see Fig. 10-5). Program goals suggest a level of aspiration and are usually qualified; they do not indicate what combination of interventions will solve health and social problems (Williamson, 1980).

Learning Goals

Learning goals are best established through the individual and the nurse working together. These goals reflect the health behavior or health status change that the person will have achieved by the end of an educational intervention. Learning goals should relate to the program goal.

Learning Objectives

Learning objectives indicate the steps to be taken by the individual toward meeting the learning goal and may involve the development of knowledge, skill, or change in attitude. Objectives are most useful when stated in behavioral terms and when they contain the following components: the learner and a precise action verb that indicates what the learner should be able to do, the conditions under which the task is performed, and the specific level of performance expected (Bastable & Sculco, 1997). Learning objectives guide the selection of content and methods and help narrow the focus of a teaching plan to more achievable steps; they also aid in setting standards of performance and suggesting evaluation strategies.

Selecting Content

To select appropriate content for a health education program, the nurse considers what information, skills, and attitudes need to be taught and the level of learning to be achieved (Insel & Roth, 1996).

Three Domains of Learning

Content is commonly divided into three domains: (1) cognitive, (2) psychomotor, and (3) affective. Cognitive learning refers to the development of new facts or concepts, building on or applying knowledge to new situations. Psychomotor learning involves developing physical skills from simple to complex actions. Affective learning alludes to the recognition of values, religious and spiritual beliefs, family interaction patterns and relationships, and personal attitudes that affect decisions and problem-solving progress.

To learn or change a health behavior, a person may need to acquire new information, practice some physical techniques, and clarify the ways in which the new behavior may affect relationships with others. The nurse's role is to select a combination of content from the three domains that is appropriate to meet the behavioral objective. To find samples of content for a teaching plan, the nurse researches resource materials, such as books, teaching guides, journal articles, pamphlets, and flyers printed by nonprofit agencies and professional organizations. The nurse should be careful about using materials with technical vocabulary that is too complex for the person or group.

Level of Learning

The level of learning to be achieved depends on how the nurse anticipates the content will be used. Bloom's taxonomy (1969) is widely accepted as the standard tool for arranging levels of learning objectives according to type and complexity (Bastable & Sculco, 1997). For example, in the cognitive domain, levels of learning include the following:

- Knowledge: person recalls facts and the concept
- Comprehension: person understands the meaning of the concept
- Application: person uses the concept
- Analysis: person can examine or explain the concept
- Synthesis: person integrates the concept with other learning
- Evaluation: person judges or compares the concept

When preparing a teaching plan, the nurse differentiates between information the individual must know and information considered helpful to know to develop appropriate learning objectives. This process provides cues to the nurse for planning effective strategies for the necessary level of learning. As the level of learning to be achieved becomes complex, the educational strategies and methods selected should involve the individuals in more active application and analysis of the content.

Designing Learning Strategies

Designing the learning strategies for an educational intervention means selecting the methods and tools and structuring the sequence of activities. The teaching plan to this point provides the foundation on which to base the activity selection and sequence. The following questions should guide the design of learning strategies:

1. What are some basic considerations for selecting teaching methods for health education programs?
2. How does the nurse, as instructor, establish and maintain a learning climate?
3. What actions can the nurse perform to increase the effectiveness of the learning methods?
4. What are the appropriate methods for each learning domain?
5. What methods tend to promote behavior change?

Considerations for Selecting Methods

First, the nurse considers promoting an environment and using methods that foster self-directed learning, which implies that the individual develops skills in assessing learning needs and deciding how to proceed through the learning process. The self-directed learner can participate in establishing standards of performance and is gradually able to monitor progress. Adult learners must decide whether they want control or whether they prefer to relinquish the right to self-direction (Coates, 1999). Greater learning is usually achieved when the learner is an active participant in the learning process.

There will be many preferred learning styles in a group audience; therefore the nurse varies the teaching methods used in a given session. Taking into consideration the characteristics of the population (developmental stage, age, and knowledge of the topic), the nurse selects teaching methods that best support the goals and theme of the educational program. The flow or order of content should proceed from simple ideas and skills to the more complex concepts, from known material toward the lesser-known data. The nurse must be sensitive to the energy level and anxiety of the audience when presenting content that either requires strong concentration or causes unwanted anxiety.

Learning Climate

For group presentations, the nurse addresses several activities when seeking to establish an environment that is conducive to health behavior change. The first activity is creating a sense of preparedness and organization by providing appropriate physical facilities with adequate furnishings and suitable audiovisual materials and handouts. Even the instructor's appearance will lend credibility or distraction to the presentation.

The second activity involves anticipating the needs of the group and communicating information about the schedule and the facilities. This action alleviates the group's apprehension and makes them more comfortable in the learning situation.

The third activity focuses on the nurse's assessment of the individual and group learning needs, possibly through questions and dialog with the group. Members of the group must believe that the program will be beneficial and relevant to their situations. The instructor should watch for and reinforce signs of motivation to participate in the experience.

Fourth, with a positive learning climate established, the nurse seeks to maintain a high level of motivation, a sense of individualized attention, and ongoing progression. As a reality check, the nurse might ask for periodic feedback from the group about the effectiveness of the program and its relevance to group needs.

Finally, the nurse works with the group to maintain the learning climate. This process involves observing group interactions, helping individuals to participate, intervening to help the group deal with controlling its members, and remaining cognizant of any dynamics in the group process that will facilitate or inhibit learning.

Teaching for Each Learning Domain

As mentioned, teaching is directed toward one or more of three learning domains: (1) cognitive, (2) psychomotor, and (3) affective. Methodologies appropriate for cognitive instruction include lectures, programmed instruction, simulations and games, computer-assisted programs, modules, projects, and role-playing sessions. These methods support teaching that is focused on transmitting information and changing behaviors as a result of greater mental understanding.

Teaching psychomotor skills is directed toward the student gaining physical skills to perform procedures, treatments, or health behaviors independently. Demonstrations, drill and practice times, games, role-playing exercises, and peer teaching represent effective modes for teaching psychomotor skills.

Learning in the affective domain involves a change in attitudes or emotions that will affect behaviors. Suggested teaching methods include discussion, simulations, role-playing, and field experiences (Redman, 1997).

The teacher can evaluate the effectiveness of teaching and learning in all domains through the use of written or oral testing, demonstrations, observation, self-reports, and self-monitoring. Teaching methods for one domain may overlap the teaching methods for another domain.

Instructor Performance Feedback

The nurse can incorporate written, verbal, and nonverbal techniques into the teaching plan for obtaining feedback about teaching performance. Postprogram questionnaires are the usual method for obtaining written feedback. The nurse may ask for verbal feedback at various times from the group, from individual students, and from observers of the class. Nonverbal communication cues from participants may indicate their satisfaction, fatigue, or frustration with the educational intervention.

Implementation Factors

The procedures used to organize and promote an educational program can affect its ultimate success. The nurse (or a program administration committee) records activities such as advertising, registration, fee collection, and availability and repair of equipment and materials. This evaluative information can then be used to improve subsequent programs. Surveys by telephone or by postprogram questionnaires help obtain the consumer's opinion about these implementation procedures (see Research Highlights box). Word-of-mouth referrals to future programs and support from other community agencies and professionals may also indicate approval of the program format.

Program Influence

Occasionally, the nurse is asked to justify a health-education program in terms of its effect on the community's public health goals or social problems. Health promotion involves a combination of health-protection activities, preventive health services, and health-education programs; therefore drawing a direct correlation between an educational intervention and the statistical improvement of the health problem can be difficult.

By working through the precede framework, nurses can often describe the theoretical influence of an educational intervention on health behaviors, health problems, and social problems. Statistics such as the number of people served each year, the percentage of the target population reached, the number of service providers used, and the number and cost of programs are important and must be preserved. As these statistics change over time, the data will provide cues to program successes and problems.

Referring Individuals to Other Resources

The end of a teaching plan should include resources for people to use for continuing education, counseling, peer support, and health services. Nurses should encourage persons to view health education as a lifelong learning process. Each person has different developmental needs and health concerns through the life cycle. Moreover, any one educational intervention may only help a person move from one phase of the behavior-change process to the next. Additionally, many variables aside from learning may exist that influence a person's health practices (see Hot Topics box).

research highlights

Health Promotion via the Telephone

Telephone interventions have been used by nurses, especially ambulatory care nurses, for many years. Current research documents the effective use of telephone nursing interventions in several areas. These interventions include monitoring postoperative cardiac surgery patients after early discharge (Savage & Grap, 1999), providing family grief support following the death of a member (Kaunonen, Aalto, Tarkka, & Paunonen, 2000), enhancing medication compliance in elderly adults (Fulmer, Feldman, Kim, Carty, Beers, Molina, & Putman 1999), and supporting persons with chronic mental illness (Hunter, 2000).

In an experimental study, Thome and Alder (1999) used a brief telephone intervention intended to decrease fatigue and the resulting symptoms of mothers with difficult infants. The intervention was initiated when the infants were between 4 and 6 months of age and was limited to a maximal time frame of 2 months duration and five calls for every mother-infant pair. The intervention was effective in reducing the fatigue and the side effects experienced by mothers caring for difficult infants.

Huber and Blanchfield (1999) conducted an exploratory study to describe telephone nursing practice in ambulatory care. The study compares nursing diagnoses used, nursing interventions performed, and the amount of time spent per call in a pediatric site with the same data in an adult ambulatory care site. The interventions the pediatric site nurses used most frequently were health system guidance and teaching. Interventions the adult site nurses used most frequently were self-care assistance and medication management.

Advantages of telenursing are believed to include decreased cost of therapeutic interaction, increased access to rural and other distant persons (including international), and cost savings resulting from direction of individuals to more appropriate use of health care services such as avoiding unnecessary after-hours visits to the emergency room. With the growth of managed care financing for health care, telephone nursing is expected to increase. Additional well-designed research studies are needed to describe telephone nursing interventions and to evaluate their effectiveness. Standards of telephone nursing practice for telenursing have been developed by the American Academy of Ambulatory Care Nurses (AAACN) (1997). These standards are likely to facilitate studying the outcomes of telephone interventions by nurses.

TEACHING AND ORGANIZING SKILLS

To develop teaching and organizing skills in health education, the nurse must often learn new behaviors. A systematic guide can be used for learning these professional skills. To begin, the nurse seeks self-assessment opportunities. The nurse then identifies, lists, and prioritizes learning needs. Using this list, the nurse begins to identify the resources that are available for reading, instructor training, and practice teaching. Working on steering committees or group projects offers opportunities to develop program-organizing skills. The nurse then drafts an initial set of learning goals.

When starting to teach the first few group programs, the nurse avoids groups that are either too large (more than 20) or too small (fewer than five). These situations cannot provide an optimal learning environment. After selecting the target population and the general topic, the nurse

HOT topics THE INTERNET AS A HEALTH EDUCATION TOOL

The availability of health information on the Internet has far-reaching implications for health education. The Internet provides access to information from numerous sources on a broad range of topics to an increasing number of individuals and families. Examples of these topics include well-child care, women's health, nutrition, and information regarding disease treatment and provision of home care for the terminally ill.

Consumers have access to a wealth of valuable information, but they may be overwhelmed by the amount and types of resources. Some resources may be useful and accurate; others may be biased, inaccurate, misunderstood by individuals, and potentially problematic. Nurses need to develop skill in using the Internet as a patient-education tool and in guiding individuals' selection of health information sources.

The best sources are government and university websites. Websites for individual's and lay organizations may be less objective (London, 1999). Healthfinder (http://www.healthfinder.gov), an online filter created by the U.S. Department of Health and Human Services, provides links to health information from government health agencies, public health and professional groups, universities, support groups, medical journals, and some news sites (Kramer, Bucher, Glassman, & Sui, 1999).

In selecting and evaluating Internet sources, nurses should ask these questions:

- Is the source reputable and reliable?
- Is the information current, accurate, understandable, and appropriate for the target audience?
- Identify sites that may be useful to the target group. Check education sites before recommending them.
- Encourage people to discuss information obtained from Internet resources to establish an opportunity to clarify their understanding and direct them to sources that are more appropriate when necessary.

Two examples of websites containing useful health information are:

- For women's health and other health issues: http://www.mayohealth.org
- For nutrition advice: http://www.navigator.tufts.edu

works through the precede-proceed model as a planning stage and then develops a teaching plan. The nurse identifies other people or an available project team to help.

After implementing the educational intervention, the nurse sets time aside to discuss what took place. Did the program go as planned? What changes were made in the teaching plan? What should be changed for the next program? The nurse reviews the self-developed learning goals and determines new ones.

As additional programs on either an individual or group basis are provided, the nurse will be able to clarify specific instructor teaching and organizing skills that come naturally. These skills tend to improve a program's effectiveness and enable the logistics to run smoothly. The teacher is first a learner; this is true in health education and any other form of education.

SUMMARY

Compared with other health professionals, nurses spend the greatest amount of time in direct contact with individuals; they have many opportunities to recognize a need for knowledge and a readiness to learn new information and behaviors. Nurses often coordinate group programs. The more accurate the analysis of the educational aspects of a health-promotion program and the assessment of characteristics and learning needs of the target audience is, the more effective an educational intervention will be in influencing health behaviors.

The principles of health education form a generic basis for implementing a variety of health topics, such as accident prevention and first aid, expectant parent education, high blood pressure education, nutrition and fitness, stress management, substance abuse, sex education, and patient education in areas including diabetes and arthritis. The three scenarios described in this chapter provide insights into the nurse's role in conducting educational interventions about family planning, high blood pressure, and medication safety.

Differences exist in planning to teach one person and in planning to teach a group. One-to-one interventions tend to follow a counseling or problem-solving approach. Group interventions can range from guided discussions on concerns that evolve from the group to a more structured learning experience involving presentations, skill practice, and attitude-awareness exercises. The range of health education strategies provide nurses and all health care professionals with techniques and methods applicable in health service settings, schools, worksites, and other community facilities.

REFERENCES

Abrams, D. B., Borrelli, B., Shadel, W. G., King, T., Bock, B., & Niaura, R. (1998). Adherence to treatment for nicotine dependence. In S. A. Shumaker, E. B. Schron, J. K. Ockene, & W. L. McBee (Eds.), *The handbook of health behavior change* (2nd ed.). New York: Springer.

American Academy of Ambulatory Care Nurses. (1997). *AAACN telephone nursing practice administration and practice standards*. Pitman, NJ: Anthony J. Janetti.

American Nurses' Association. (1991a). *Nursing's agenda for health care reform*. New York: National League for Nursing.

American Nurses' Association. (1991b). *Standards of clinical nursing practice*. Washington, DC: The Association.

American Nurses' Association. (1995). *Nursing's social policy statement*. Washington, DC: The Association.

Andreasen, A. R. (1995). *Marketing social change: Changing behavior to promote health, social development, and the environment*. San Francisco: Jossey-Bass.

Aspen Reference Group. (1997). *Community health education and promotion: A guide to program design and evaluation*. Gaithersburg, MD: Aspen.

Bandman, E. L., & Bandman, B. (1995). *Nursing ethics through the life span* (3rd ed.). Norwalk, CT: Appleton & Lange.

Bandura, A. (1997). *Self-efficacy: The exercise of control*. New York: W.H. Freeman.

Bastable, S. B., & Sculco, C. (1997). Educational objectives. In S. B. Bastable (Ed.), *Nurse as educator: Principles of teaching and learning*. Sudbury, MS: Jones & Bartlett.

Becker, M. H. (Ed.) (1974). *The health belief model and personal health behavior*. Thorofare, NJ: Charles B. Slack.

Bloom, B. (1969). *Taxonomy of educational objectives*. New York: Longman-Green.

Bracht, N. (1990). *Health promotion at the community level*. Newbury Park, CA: Sage.

Coates, V. E. (1999). *Education for patients and clients*. London: Routledge.

deAlva, M. L. (1999). Editorial: A liberating tool. *Diabetes Forum, 12*(3), 132.

Fitzgerald, S. T. (1991). Self-efficacy theory: Implications for the occupational health nurse. *AAOHN Journal, 39*(12), 552-557.

Friedman, M. M. (1998). *Family nursing: Research, theory, & practice* (4th ed.). Stanford, CT: Appleton & Lange.

Fulmer, T. T., Feldman, P. H., Kim, T. S., Carty, B., Beers, M., Molina, M., & Putman, M. (1999). An intervention study to enhance medication compliance in community-dwelling elderly individuals. *Journal of Gerontological Nursing, 25*(8), 6-14.

Glanz, K., Lewis, F. M., & Rimer, B. K. (1997). *Health behavior and health education: Theory, research, and practice* (2nd ed.). San Francisco: Jossey-Bass.

Green, L., & Kreuter, M. (1999). *Health promotion planning: An educational and ecological approach*. Mountain View, CA: Mayfield.

Huber, D. L., & Blanchfield, K. (1999). Telephone nursing interventions in ambulatory care. *Journal of Nursing Administration, 29*(3), 38-44.

Hunter, E. F. (2000). Telephone support for persons with chronic mental illness. *Home Healthcare Nurse, 18*(3), 172-179.

Insel, P. M., & Roth, W. T. (1996). *Core concepts in health* (7th ed.). Mountain View, CA: Mayfield.

Janz, N. K., & Becker, M. H. (1984). The health belief model: A decade later. *Health Education Quarterly, 11*(1), 1-47.

Jarvis, C. (1996). *Physical examination and health assessment* (2nd ed.). Philadelphia: W.B. Saunders.

Kaunonen, M., Aalto, P., Tarkka, M., & Paunonen, M. (2000). Oncology ward nurses' perspectives of family grief and a supportive telephone call after the death of a significant other. *Cancer Nursing, 23*(4), 314-324.

Kolbe, L. J., Iverson, D. C., Kreuter, M. W., Hochbaum, G., & Christensen, G. (1981). Propositions for an alternate and complementary health education paradigm. *Health Education, 12*(3), 24-30.

Kramer, E. J., Bucher, J. A., Glassman, K. S, & Sui, S. (1999). Strategies for patient teaching: How to seize the teachable moment. In W. B. Bateman, E. J. Kramer, & K. S. Glassman (Eds.), *Patient and family education in managed care and beyond: Seizing the teachable moment*. New York: Springer.

Lefebvre, R. C., & Rochlin, L. (1997). Social marketing. In K. Glanz & F. M. Marcus (Eds.), *Health behavior and health education: Theory, research, and practice*. San Francisco: Jossey-Bass.

London, F. (1999). *No time to teach? A nurse's guide to patient and family education*. Philadelphia: J.B. Lippincott.

Morrison, G. W. (1995). *Early childhood education today* (6th ed.). Englewood Cliffs, NJ: Merrill.

National League for Nursing. (1993). *A vision for nursing education*. New York: The League.

Pender, N. J. (1996). *Health promotion in nursing practice* (3rd ed.). Stamford, CT: Appleton & Lange.

Price, J. L., & Cordell, B. (1994). Cultural diversity and patient teaching. *Journal of Continuing Education in Nursing, 25*(4), 163-166.

Rankin, S. H., & Stallings, K. D. (1996). *Patient education: Issues, principles, policies* (3rd ed.). Philadelphia: J.B. Lippincott.

Redman, B. K. (1997). *The practice of patient education* (7th ed.). St Louis: Mosby.

Richards, E. (1997). Motivation, compliance, and health behaviors of the learner. In S. B. Bastable (Ed.), *Nurse as educator: Principles of teaching and learning*. Sudbury, MS: Jones & Bartlett.

Rosenstock, I. M., Strecher, K. J., & Becker, M. H. (1988). The social learning theory and health belief model. *Health Education Quarterly, 15*, 175-183.

Savage, L. S., & Grap, M. J. (1999). Telephone monitoring after early discharge for cardiac surgery patients. *American Journal of Critical Care, 8*(3), 154-159.

Schrefer, S. (1994). *Quick reference to cultural assessment*. St. Louis: Mosby.

Seefeldt, C., & Barbour, N. (1994). *Early childhood education: An introduction*. New York: Merrill.

Simons-Morton, B. G., & Crump, A. D. (1996). Empowerment: The process and the outcome. *Health Education Quarterly, 23*(3), 290-292.

Sullivan, L. W. (1991). Partners in prevention: A mobilization plan for implementing Healthy People 2000. *American Journal of Health Promotion, 5*(4), 291.

Thome, M., & Alder, B. (1999). A telephone intervention to reduce fatigue and symptom distress in mothers with difficult infants in the community. *Journal of Advanced Nursing, 29*(1), 128-137.

Timmreck, T. C., Cole, G. E., James, G., & Butterworth, D. O. (1987). Health education and health promotion: A look at the jungle of supportive fields, philosophies and theoretical foundations. *Health Education, 18*(6), 23-28.

U.S. Department of Health and Human Services. (2000). *Healthy People 2010: Vols. 1-2* (Conference edition). Washington, DC: U.S. Department of Health and Human Services.

U.S. Preventive Services Task Force. (1996). *Guide to clinical preventive services* (2nd ed.). Baltimore, MD: Williams & Wilkins.

Williamson, F. E. (1980). *Health education and health planning analysis of health systems plans: Focal points*. Washington, DC: U.S. Department of Health and Human Services.

Chapter 11

ARLENE SPARK
QALVY GRAINZVOLT

Nutrition Counseling

objectives

After completing this chapter, the nurse will be able to:

- Recognize *Healthy People 2010* nutrition objectives.
- List the leading nutrition-related causes of death in the United States and identify the dietary factors associated with each cause.
- Summarize the nutrition recommendations contained in the Dietary Guidelines for Americans.
- List the number of servings and serving sizes recommended in The Food Guide Pyramid.
- Discuss U.S. food aid programs for the poor and older adults.
- Plan a 1-day menu that is consistent with recent dietary guidance for a person at any stage of the life cycle.

key terms

Cancer
Cardiovascular Disease
Cholesterol
Coronary Heart Disease
Dietary Guidelines
Fat
Fiber
Food Guide Pyramid
Human Immunodeficiency Virus
Hypertension
Nutrition Screening
Obesity
Osteoporosis
Overweight
Serving Size
Stroke
Sugar
Type 2 Diabetes
Underweight
Vegetarian

THINK About It

Nutritional Self-Assessment

Begin thinking about your food and health and the food and health of people around you. Check the box of each statement that describes the way you usually eat. Add the number of statements that you have checked and compare that number with the scores listed after the questions.

The way I usually eat:

- *I eat whole grain or enriched breads, cereals, rice, or pasta daily.*
- *I eat 2 to 3 pieces or more of fruit daily.*
- *I eat 2 to 3 cups or more of raw or cooked vegetables daily.*
- *I drink skim milk and eat low-fat or fat-free dairy products daily.*
- *I trim fat from meat and take the skin off chicken and turkey or I do not eat meat.*
- *I eat small servings (no larger than the size of a deck of cards) of meat, poultry, and fish or I do not eat meat.*
- *Most food and snacks that I eat are not fried or are made with no added fat.*
- *I add very little fat (butter, margarine, oil, or salad dressing) to my food.*
- *Most desserts and snacks that I eat contain no added sugar.*
- *Most of what I drink is made without sugar or contains no added sugar.*
- *I rarely cook with salt or add salt at the table.*
- *I do not drink alcohol or I drink no more than 1 to 2 beers, 1 to 2 glasses of wine, or 1 to 2 mixed drinks daily.*

continued

Table 11-1 Nutrient-Deficiency Diseases

Key Nutrient Involved	Deficiency Disease	Typical Disease Symptoms	Major Dietary Sources for the Nutrient
Protein	Kwashiorkor, protein-calorie malnutrition (PCM)	Growth failure in children (60% to 80% weight for age), edema, fatty liver, changes in hair texture, apathy, and anorexia	Egg white, beef, fish, poultry, milk, cheese, legumes, and nuts
Thiamin	Beriberi	Nerve degeneration, poor muscle coordination, enlarged heart, and abnormal heart rhythms	Pork, sunflower seeds, dried beans, and wheat germ
Niacin	Pellagra	The 3 Ds (diarrhea, dermatitis, and dementia) and anorexia	Wheat bran, beef, mushrooms, salmon, and tuna
Vitamin C	Scurvy	Impaired wound healing, bleeding gums and skin, and frequent infections	Citrus fruits, broccoli, strawberries, and cabbage
Vitamin A	Xerophthalmia	Blindness, poor growth, increased infections, and cracks in teeth	Liver, fortified milk, sweet potatoes, pumpkin, and mustard greens
Iron	Iron deficiency anemia	Poor growth, reduced resistance to infections, and reduced learning ability in children	Red meats, oysters, clams, tofu (soybean curd), and spinach
Iodine	Goiter and cretinism	Enlarged thyroid gland, weight gain, and mental and physical retardation in infants	Seafood, crops grown in iodine-rich oil (coastal areas), and iodized salt

THINK About It

Nutritional Self-Assessment—cont'd

Number of boxes checked

Score: *9 to 12.* ***Evaluation:*** *Great job!* ***Recommendation:*** *While reading this chapter, you will be reminded of all the things you are doing that contribute to your healthy lifestyle. You are an excellent role model for others. The best nutrition educators practice what they teach.*

Score: *5 to 8.* ***Evaluation:*** *Okay.* ***Recommendation:*** *You do make some good choices, but a number of changes in your food habits would be of great value to you personally and professionally. Hopefully, you will be motivated by some of the ideas presented in this chapter.*

Score: *0 to 4.* ***Evaluation:*** *Improvement needed.* ***Recommendation:*** *The first steps toward good eating are the hardest to take, but making healthy choices is worth the investment. You are investing in your education and planning a career in the health professions. Now, begin investing in your own health also. Improved health is a natural dividend of your training. This chapter will help you focus on improving your own diet and health and the well being of others.*

NUTRITION IN THE UNITED STATES: LOOKING FORWARD FROM THE PAST

Classic Vitamin-Deficiency Diseases

Food and nutrition have always been vitally important to health. Until as recently as the 1940s, many nutrient-deficiency diseases, such as rickets, pellagra, scurvy, beriberi, xerophthalmia, and goiter, were still prevalent in the United States (Carpenter, 2000). Although these conditions still persist in developing countries, they have virtually disappeared from developed areas of the world. *Why?* An abundant food supply, fortification of some foods with critical nutrients, and better methods of determining and improving the nutrient contents of foods have contributed to the decline of the nutrient-deficiency diseases that are summarized in Table 11-1.

The introduction of iodized salt in the 1920s, for example, contributed greatly to eliminating iodine-deficiency goiter as a public health problem. Similarly, pellagra disappeared after the discovery that inadequate niacin levels contribute to the condition. Today, nutrient deficiencies are rarely reported in the United States. The few cases of protein-energy malnutrition that are listed annually as causes of death generally occur as secondary results of severe illness or injury, premature birth, child neglect, problems of the homebound aged, alcoholism, or some combination of these factors. Although undernutrition still occurs in some groups of people in the United States, including isolated or economically deprived people, these once-prevalent diseases of nutritional deficiency have been replaced by diseases of dietary excess and imbalance (Table 11-2).

Dietary Excess and Imbalance

Problems resulting from overconsumption now rank among the leading causes of illness and death in the United States. The four leading causes of death directly associated with diet are **coronary heart disease** (CHD), some types of cancer, **stroke,** and diabetes mellitus. In fact, heart disease, cancers, and stroke account for almost two thirds of all

Table 11-2 Health Problems Related to Poor Nutrition

A number of health problems are caused or exacerbated by poor nutrition. Health care professionals strive to prevent or delay these health problems.

Health Problem	Questionable Practices
Anemia	Inadequate iron and folate intake
Cancer (breast, cervical, and colon)	Excessive fat intake; low fiber intake
Cirrhosis	Excessive alcohol intake
Constipation	Inadequate fiber or fluid intake; high fat intake; sedentary lifestyle
Dental caries	Excessive, frequent consumption of concentrated sweets; lack of fluoride; poor hygiene
Type 2 diabetes	Excessive energy intake
Hypercholesterolemia	Inadequate fiber intake
Hypertension	Obesity; excessive energy intake; excessive sodium intake in sodium-sensitive individuals
Infection	Malnutrition
Obesity	Excessive energy intake; excessive fat intake; sedentary lifestyle
Osteoporosis	Inadequate calcium intake; inadequate vitamin D intake or inadequate exposure to the sun; sedentary lifestyle
Underweight and growth failure	Inadequate energy intake

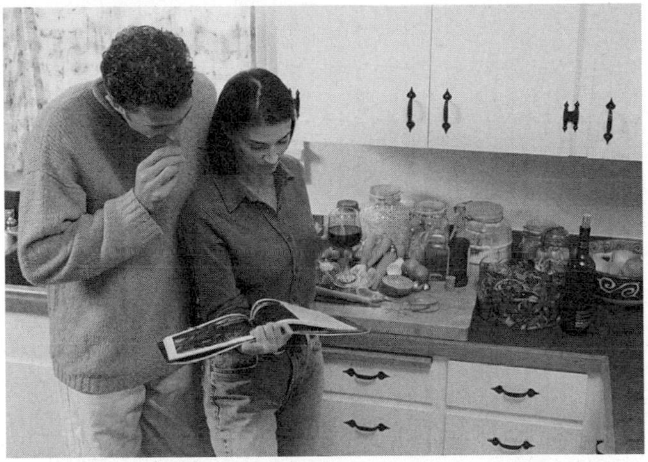

Fig. 11-1 Choosing a healthier diet may mean learning new recipes and new ways of cooking.

deaths every year in America. Four more major causes of death—accidents, cirrhosis of the liver, suicide, and homicide—are associated with excessive alcohol intake.

Encouraging healthy choices in diet, exercise, and weight control is one of the major themes of *Healthy People 2010* (USDHHS, 2000) (Fig. 11-1). As dietary factors contribute substantially to the burden of preventable illness and premature death, *Healthy People 2010* is aimed at bringing American dietary patterns into line with current dietary recommendations, especially the Dietary Guidelines for Americans (USDHHS, 2000).

HEALTHY PEOPLE 2010: NUTRITION OBJECTIVES

As discussed throughout this text, the 28 focus areas in *Healthy People 2010* contain 467 specific national health-promotion and disease-prevention objectives. Many *Healthy People 2010* nutrition-related objectives target interventions designed to reduce or eliminate illness, disability, and premature death among individuals and communities. Each objective has a target for specific improvements to be achieved by 2010. The topics covered by the objectives in *Healthy People 2010* reflect the array of critical influences that determine the health of individuals and communities. For example, individual behaviors and environmental factors are responsible for approximately 70% of all premature deaths in the United States. Understanding these influences and how they relate to one another are crucial for achieving *Healthy People 2010* goals.

The report also contains 10 leading health indicators: (1) physical activity, (2) overweight and obesity, (3) tobacco use, (4) substance abuse, (5) mental health, (6) injury and violence, (7) environmental quality, (8) immunization, (9) responsible sexual behavior, and (10) access to health care. By monitoring these measures, states and communities can assess their current health status and follow it over time. Overweight and obesity is supported by two specific measurable objectives:

- *19-3c.* Reduce the proportion of children and adolescents who are overweight or obese.
- *19-2.* Reduce the proportion of adults who are obese.

These and most of the other *Healthy People 2010* nutrition-related objectives are cited throughout this chapter (Tables 11-3 and 11-4).

Nutrition-Related Health Status

Overweight and high-serum cholesterol levels, hypertension (high blood pressure), and osteoporosis (decreased bone mass) increase the risk of CHD, stroke, and bone

Table 11-3 Nutrition Objectives in *Healthy People 2010*

Objective Number	Objective	Baseline (and Date at Baseline)	Target for 2010
19-1	Increase the proportion of adults who are at a healthy weight.	42% (1988 to 1994)	60%
19-2	Reduce the proportion of adults who are obese.	23% (1988 to 1994)	15%
19-3	Reduce the proportion of children and adolescents who are overweight or obese.		
	3a. 6 to 11 years	11% (1988 to 1994)	5%
	3b. 12 to 19 years	12% (1988 to 1994)	5%
	3c. 6 to 19 years	11% (1988 to 1994)	5%
19-4	Reduce growth retardation among low-income children under age 5 years.	8% (1997)	5%
19-5	Increase the proportion of persons aged 2 years and older who consume at least 2 daily servings of fruit.	28% (1994 to 1996)	75%
19-6	Increase the proportion of persons aged 2 years and older who consume at least 3 daily servings of vegetables, with at least one third being dark green or deep yellow vegetables.	3% (1994 to 1996)	50%
19-7	Increase the proportion of persons aged 2 years and older who consume at least 6 daily servings of grain products, with at least 3 being whole grains.	7% (1994 to 1996)	50%
19-8	Increase the proportion of persons aged 2 years and older who consume less than 10% of calories from saturated fat.	36% (1994 to 1996)	75%
19-9	Increase the proportion of persons aged 2 years and older who consume no more than 30% calories from fat.	33% (1988 to 1994)	75%
19-10	Increase the proportion of persons aged 2 years and older who consume 2400 mg or less of sodium daily.	21% (1988 to 1994)	65%
19-11	Increase the proportion of persons aged 2 years and older who meet dietary recommendations for calcium.	46% (1988 to 1994)	75%
19-12	Reduce iron deficiency among young children and women of childbearing age.		
	12a. Children 1 to 2 years	9% (1988 to 1994)	5%
	12b. Children 3 to 4 years	4% (1988 to 1994)	1%
	12c. Nonpregnant women, 12 to 49 years	11% (1988 to 1994)	7%
19-13	Reduce anemia among low-income pregnant women in their third trimester.	29% (1996)	20%
19-14	Reduce iron deficiency among pregnant women.	NA	NA
19-15	Increase the proportion of children and adolescents age 6 to 19 years whose intake of meals and snacks at school contributes proportionally to good overall dietary quality.	NA	NA
19-16	Increase the proportion of work sites that offer nutrition or weight management classes or counseling.	55% (1998 to 1999)	85%
19-17	Increase the proportion of physician office visits made by patients with a diagnosis of cardiovascular disease, diabetes, or hyperlipidemia, which includes counseling or education related to diet and nutrition.	42% (1997)	75%
19-18	Increase food security among U.S. households and, in so doing, reduce hunger.	88% (1995)	94%

Adapted from U.S. Department of Health and Human Services. (2000). *Healthy people 2010: Volumes I and II* (Conference Edition). Washington, DC: The Department. The entire conference copy of the two-volume report is available on the *Healthy People 2010* web site: http://www.health.gov/healthypeople/default.htm.

fracture, respectively. The following statements describe the health status of Americans:

More Americans are overweight now compared with the late 1970s. Many adults also report sedentary lifestyles. being overweight is associated with many chronic diseases and health outcomes; therefore its increased prevalence is a cause for public health concern.

Although the number of adults with desirable serum total cholesterol levels is increasing steadily, many people still have high levels. A high serum cholesterol is a major risk factor for CHD.

Hypertension remains a major public health problem in middle-aged and older adults. Blacks have a higher age-related prevalence of hypertension than Whites and Hispanic Americans. Hypertension is the most important risk factor for stroke and a major risk factor for CHD.

Femoral osteoporosis in women 50 years of age and older in the United States occurs in 21% of Whites, 10% of

Table 11-4 Nutrition-Related Objectives in *Healthy People 2010*

Chapter Number	Chapter Title	Objective Number and Objective	Baseline (and date at baseline)	Target for 2010
1	Access to quality health services	*1-3.* Increase the number of people appropriately counseled about health behaviors	NA	NA
2	Arthritis, osteoporosis, and chronic back conditions	*2-9.* Reduce the overall number of cases of osteoporosis	10% (1988 to 1994)	8%
3	Cancer	*3-1.* Reduce the overall cancer death rate.	201.4 deaths per 100,000 (1998)	158.7 deaths per 100,000
		3-3. Reduce the breast cancer death rate in women.	27.7 deaths per 100,000 (1998)	22.2 deaths per 100,000
		3-5. Reduce the colorectal cancer death rate.	21.1 deaths per 100,000 (1998)	13.9 deaths per 100,000
4	Chronic kidney disease	*4-3.* Increase the proportion of treated chronic kidney failure patients who have received counseling on nutrition . . . 12 months before the start of renal replacement therapy.	45% (1996)	60%
5	Diabetes	*5-1.* Increase the proportion of people with diabetes who receive formal education.	40% (1998)	60%
		5-2. Prevent diabetes	3.1 new cases per 1000 persons per year (1994 to 1996)	2.5 new cases per 1000 persons per year
10	Food safety	*10-4.* Reduce deaths from anaphylaxis caused by food allergies.	NA	NA
		10-5. Increase the proportion of consumers who follow key food safety practices.	72% (1998)	79%
12	Heart disease and stroke	*12-1.* Reduce coronary heart disease deaths.	208 per 100,000 (1998)	166 per 100,000
		12-7. Reduce stroke deaths.	60 per 100,000 (1998)	48 per 100,000
		12-9. Reduce the proportion of adults with high blood pressure.	28% (1988 to 1994)	16%
		12-11. Increase the proportion of adults with high blood pressure who are taking action (losing weight and reducing sodium intake).	72% (1998)	95%
		12-12. Reduce the mean total blood cholesterol levels among adults.	206 mg/dl (1988 to 1994)	199 mg/dl
		12-13. Reduce the proportion of adults with high total blood cholesterol levels.	21% (1988 to 1994)	17%
16	Maternal, infant, and child health	*16-11.* Reduce all live preterm births.	11.4% (1997)	7.6%
		16-12. Increase the proportion of mothers who achieve a recommended weight gain during pregnancy.	35% (1996)	70%
		16-13. Reduce the occurrence of spina bifida and other neural tube defects.	6 new cases per 10,000 live births	3 new cases per 10,000 live births
		16-16a. Increase the proportion of pregnancies begun with an optimal folic acid level (in the diet).	21% (1991 to 1994)	80%

Adapted from U.S. Department of Health and Human Services. (2000). *Healthy people 2010: Volumes I and II* (Conference Edition). Washington, DC: The Department. The entire conference copy of the two-volume report is available on the *Healthy People 2010* web site: http://www.health.gov/healthypeople/default.htm.

Continued

Table 11-4 Nutrition-Related Objectives in *Healthy People 2010*—cont'd

Chapter		Objective		
Number	Title	Number and Objective	Baseline (and date at baseline)	Target for 2010
		16-17a. (b.) Increase abstinence from alcohol (and binge drinking) among pregnant women.	86% (99%)	94% (100%)
		16-18. Reduce the occurrence of fetal alcohol syndrome.	NA	NA
		16-19. Increase the proportion of mothers who breastfeed their babies:		
		a. In early postpartum period	64%	75%
		b. At 6 months	29%	50%
		c. At 1 year	16%	25%
18	Mental health and mental disorders	*18-5.* Reduce the relapse rates for persons with eating-disorder relapses including anorexia nervosa and bulimia nervosa.	NA	NA
22	Physical activity and fitness	*22-1.* Reduce the proportion of adults who engage in no leisure-time physical activity.	40% (1997)	20%
		22-2. Increase the proportion of adults who engage regularly, preferably daily, in moderate physical activity for at least 30 minutes per day.	15% (1997)	30%
		22-6. Increase the proportion of adolescents who engage in moderate physical activity for at least 30 minutes on 5 or more of the previous 7 days.	20% (1997)	30%
		22-9. Increase the proportion of the nation's public and private schools that require daily physical education for all students.	27% (1997)	50%
		22-13. Increase the proportion of work sites with less than 50 employees (more than 50 employees) offering employer-sponsored physical activity and fitness programs.	NA (NA)	75% (75%)
26	Substance Abuse	*26-12.* Reduce average annual alcohol consumption in people aged 14 years and older.	2.9 (1996) gallons of ethanol per person	Two gallons of ethanol per person

Adapted from U.S. Department of Health and Human Services. (2000). *Healthy people 2010: Volumes I and II* (Conference Edition). Washington, DC: The Department. The entire conference copy of the two-volume report is available on the *Healthy People 2010* web site: http://www.health.gov/healthypeople/default.htm.

Blacks, and 16% of Hispanic Americans. Low calcium intake and lack of weight-bearing exercise, among other factors, contribute to bone loss (FASEB, 1995).

Nutrition Objectives for the United States

Although Americans are slowly changing their eating patterns toward more healthful diets, a considerable gap exists between public health recommendations and consumers' practices. The overarching goal of nutrition in the beginning of the millennium is that food intake change in the direction of the targeted goals recommended in *Healthy People 2010*, the Food Guide Pyramid, and the Dietary Guidelines for Americans. According to a report on nutrition monitoring in the United States, the nutritional quality of the American diet falls short in the following areas (FASEB, 1995):

- Energy balance remains a problem for many Americans, as indicated by an increased prevalence of being overweight in the United States since the 1970s. Approximately one third of adults and one fifth of adolescents in the United States are overweight, suggesting that they have higher energy intakes than expenditures.
- Although intake of total fat, saturated fatty acids, and cholesterol has decreased, it remains above the recommended levels for a large portion of the population.

- Sodium intake from food is higher than is recommended for most Americans over the age of 6 years.
- Calcium intake from food is below the recommended values, particularly for adolescents, women, elderly people, and Black men. Many Americans are not getting the calcium required to maintain optimal bone health and prevent age-related bone loss.
- Iron intake from food is less than is recommended for children 1 to 2 years of age and for women 12 to 59 years of age, among whom the prevalence of anemia is generally higher compared with other groups.
- Less than one third of American adults meet the recommendation to consume 5 or more servings of fruits and vegetables per day. The average intake is approximately 4 servings per day.
- Although the availability of food and nutrients in the U.S. food supply on a per capita basis is generally adequate to prevent undernutrition and deficiency-related diseases, approximately 13% of people living in low-income households or families experience some degree of food insufficiency (not enough to eat because of a lack of money or other resources).

FOOD AND NUTRITION RECOMMENDATIONS

Food and nutrition guidelines are introduced in Chapter 11. A goal of this discussion is to heighten people's interest in the health promotion power of good nutrition to inspire their gradual adoption of the dietary recommendations presented here.

The kinds and amounts of food that are required to obtain the necessary energy and nutrients are defined in these reports:

- Dietary Reference Intakes (NRC, 1997, 2000a, 2000b, 2000c), including the Recommended Dietary Allowances (NRC, 1989)
- *Nutrition and Your Health: Dietary Guidelines for Americans*, fifth edition (USDA, 2000)
- The Food Guide Pyramid (USDA, 1992)

Dietary Reference Intakes

The Dietary Reference Intakes (DRI) is a set of values for the dietary nutrient intakes of healthy people in the United States and Canada. These values are used for planning and assessing diets, including the Recommended Daily Allowance (RDA), Adequate Intake (IA), Estimated Average Requirement (EAR), and Tolerable Upper Intake Level (UL) (Box 11-1).

The DRI recommends intake levels for U.S. and Canadian individuals and population groups and it sets maximal-level guidelines to reduce the risk of adverse health effects from overconsumption of a nutrient. The understanding of the relationship between nutrition and chronic disease has progressed to the extent that intakes can now be recommended that are thought to help people achieve measurable physical indicators of good health. The DRI represents a major leap forward in nutrition science—from a primary concern for the prevention of deficiency to an emphasis on beneficial effects of healthy eating. The new recommendations focus on decreasing the risk of chronic disease through nutrition.

Box 11-1 Dietary Reference Intakes

Recommended Dietary Allowance (RDA). The intake that meets the nutrient needs of nearly all healthy individuals in a specific age and gender group. The RDA should be used to guide individuals in achieving adequate nutrient intake aimed at decreasing the risk of chronic disease. The RDA is based on estimating an average requirement in addition to an increase to account for variations within a particular group.

Adequate Intake (AI). When sufficient scientific evidence is unavailable to estimate an average requirement, AIs are set. Individuals should use AI as a goal for intake when no RDAs exist. AI is derived through experimental or observational data that show a mean intake that appears to sustain a desired level of health, such as calcium retention in bone for most members of a population group. For example, AIs have been set for infants through 1 year of age using the average observed nutrient intake of populations of breast-fed infants as the standard.

Estimated Average Requirement (EAR). The intake that meets the estimated nutrient need of one half of the individuals in a specific group. EAR is used as a basis for developing the RDA and by nutrition policy-makers in evaluating adequacy of nutrient intakes of the group and for planning how much the group should consume.

Tolerable Upper Intake Level (UL). The maximal intake by an individual that is unlikely to pose risks of adverse health effects in almost all healthy individuals in a specified group. UL is not intended to be a recommended level of intake and no established benefit exists for individuals to consume nutrients at levels above the RDA or AI. For most nutrients, this figure refers to total intakes from food, fortified food, and nutrient supplements.

The *old* RDA, which may have been learned before 1997, established the minimal amounts of nutrients needed to protect against possible nutrient deficiency. In contrast, the DRI is designed to reflect the latest understanding about nutrient requirements based on optimizing health in individuals and groups. Collectively called the DRI, the new recommendations include four categories of reference intakes that were established by examining the results of hundreds of nutritional studies on both the beneficial aspects of nutrients and the hazards of consuming too much of a nutrient. Where the scientific evidence allows, recommendations are made to help individuals at different stages of life obtain enough of a nutrient to promote health and to maintain normal nutritional status.

The current DRI and 1989 RDA appear in Table 11-5 and Table 11-6, respectively. The new DRI will be announced soon for the macronutrients (protein, fat, and

Table 11-5 Dietary Reference Intakes (RDAs and AIs): Recommended Intakes for Individuals

Life Stage Group	Calcium	Phosphorous	Magnesium	Vitamin D[a,b]	Fluoride	Thiamin	Riboflavin	Niacin[c]	Vitamin B-6	Folate[d,h,i]	Vitamin B-12[g]	Pantothenic Acid	Biotin	Choline[e]	Vitamin C	Vitamin E[f]	Selenium
	mg	mg	mg	µg	mg	mg	mg	mg	mg	µg	µg	mg	µg	mg	mg	µg	µg
INFANTS																	
0 to 6 months	210*	100*	30*	5*	0.01*	0.2*	0.3*	2*	0.1*	65*	0.4*	1.7*	5*	125*	40*	4*	15*
7 to 12 months	270*	275*	75*	5*	0.5*	0.3*	0.4*	4*	0.3*	80*	0.5*	1.8*	6*	150*	50*	6*	20*
CHILDREN																	
1 to 3 years	500*	460	80	5*	0.7*	0.5	0.5	6	0.5	150	0.9	2*	8*	200*	15	6	20
4 to 8 years	800*	500	130	5*	1*	0.6	0.6	8	0.6	200	1.2	3*	12*	250*	25	7	30
MALES																	
9 to 13 years	1300*	1250	240	5*	2*	0.9	0.9	12	1	300	1.8	4*	20*	375*	45	11	40
14 to 18 years	1300*	1250	410	5*	3*	1.2	1.3	16	1.3	400	2.4	5*	25*	550*	75	15	55
19 to 30 years	1000*	700	400	5*	4*	1.2	1.3	16	1.5	400	2.4	5*	30*	550*	90	15	55
31 to 50 years	1000*	700	420	5*	4*	1.2	1.3	16	1.5	400	2.4	5*	30*	550*	90	15	55
51 to 70 years	1200*	700	420	10*	4*	1.2	1.3	16	1.7	400	2.4g	5*	30*	550*	90	15	55
Over 70 years	1200*	700	420	15*	4*	1.2	1.3	16	1.7	400	2.4g	5*	30*	550*	90	15	55
FEMALES																	
9 to 13 years	1300*	1250	240	5*	2*	0.9	0.9	12	1	300	1.8	4*	20*	375*	45	11	40
14 to 18 years	1500*	1250	360	5*	3*	1	1	14	1.2	400	2.4	5*	25*	400*	65	15	55
19 to 30 years	1000*	700	310	5*	3*	1.1	1.1	14	1.3	400	2.4	5*	30*	425*	75	15	55
31 to 50 years	1000*	700	320	5*	3*	1.1	1.1	14	1.3	400	2.4	5*	30*	425*	75	15	55
51 to 70 years	1200*	700	320	10*	3*	1.1	1.1	14	1.5	400	2.4g	5*	30*	425*	75	15	55
Over 70 years	1200*	700	320	15*	3*	1.1	1.1	14	1.5	400	2.4g	5*	30*	425*	75	15	55

PREGNANCY																	
18 years or less	1500*	**1250**	**400**	5*	3*	**1.4**	**1.4**	**18**	**1.9**	**600**	**2.6**	6*	30*	450*	**80**	**15**	**60**
19 to 30 years	1000*	**700**	**350**	5*	3*	**1.4**	**1.4**	**18**	**1.9**	**600**	**2.6**	6*	30*	450*	**85**	**15**	**60**
31 to 50 years	1000*	**700**	**360**	5*	3*	**1.4**	**1.4**	**18**	**1.9**	**600**	**2.6**	6*	30*	450*	**85**	**15**	**60**
LACTATION																	
18 years or less	1300*	**1250**	**360**	5*	3*	**1.4**	**1.6**	**17**	**2**	**500**	**2.8**	7*	35*	550*	**115**	**19**	**70**
19 to 30 years	1000*	**700**	**310**	5*	3*	**1.4**	**1.6**	**17**	**2**	**500**	**2.8**	7*	35*	550*	**120**	**19**	**70**
31 to 50 years	1000*	**700**	**320**	5*	3*	**1.4**	**1.6**	**17**	**2**	**500**	**2.8**	7*	35*	550*	**120**	**19**	**70**

From Institute of Medicine, Food and Nutrition Board. (1997). *Dietary reference intakes for calcium, phosphorus, magnesium, vitamin D, and fluoride* [Online]. Report of the Subcommittee on Calcium and Related Nutrients. Washington, DC: National Academy Press. Available: http://www.nap.edu/catalog/5776.html; Institute of Medicine, Food and Nutrition Board. (2000a). *Dietary reference intakes for thiamin, riboflavin, niacin, vitamin B6, folate, vitamin B12, pantothenic acid, biotin, and choline* [Online]. Washington, DC: National Academy Press. Available: http://www.nap.edu/catalog/6015.html.

RDAs are presented in bold type and AIs in ordinary type followed by an asterisk (*). RDAs and AIs may both be used as goals for individual intake. RDAs are set to meet the needs of almost all (97 to 98%) of the individuals in a group. For healthy breastfed infants, the AI is the mean intake. The AI for other life-stage and gender groups is believed to cover the needs of all individuals in the group, but lack of data or uncertainty in the data prevent being able to specify with confidence the percentage of individual covered by this intake.

[a]As cholecalciferol. 1 μg cholecalciferol = 40 IU vitamin D.

[b]In the absence of adequate exposure to sunlight.

[c]As niacin equivalents (NE). 1 mg of niacin = 60 mg of the amino acid tryptophan; 0 to 6 months = preformed niacin (not NE).

[d]As dietary folate equivalents (DFE). 1 DFE = 1 μg of food folate = 0.6 μg of folic acid from fortified food or as a supplement consumed with food = 0.5 μg of folate from a supplement consumed on an empty stomach.

[e]Although AIs have been set for choline, there are few data to assess whether a dietary supply of choline is needed at all stages of the lifecycle and it may be that the choline requirement can be met by endogenous synthesis at some of these stages.

[f]As α-tocopherol.

[g]Because 1 to 30% of older people may malabsorb food-bound B_{12}, it is advisable for those over 50 years of age to meet their RDA mainly by consuming foods fortified with B_{12} or a supplement containing B_{12}.

[h]In view of evidence linking inadequate folate intake with neural tube defects in the fetus, it is recommended that all women capable of becoming pregnant consume 400 μg from supplements or fortified foods in addition to intake from food folate from a varied diet.

[i]It is assumed that women will continue consuming 400 μg from supplements or fortified food until their pregnancy is confirmed and they enter prenatal care, which ordinarily occurs after the end of the periconceptual period—the critical time for the formation of the neural tube.

α, alpha; μg, microgram; *AIs*, adequate intakes; *IU*, international unit; *mg*, milligram; *RDAs*, recommended dietary allowances.

Table 11-6 1989 Recommended Dietary Allowances

Age (yr)	Energy (kcal)	Protein (g)	Vitamin A (μg RE)	Vitamin K (μg)	Iron (mg)	Zinc (mg)	Iodine (μg)
INFANTS							
0.0 to 0.5	650	13	375	5	6	5	40
0.5 to 1.0	850	14	375	10	10	5	50
CHILDREN							
1 to 3	1300	16	400	15	10	10	70
4 to 6	1800	24	500	20	10	10	90
7 to 10	2000	28	700	30	10	10	120
MEN							
11 to 14	2500	45	1000	45	12	15	150
15 to 18	3000	59	1000	65	12	15	150
19 to 24	2900	58	1000	70	10	15	150
25 to 50	2900	63	1000	80	10	15	150
51+	2300	63	1000	80	10	15	150
WOMEN							
11 to 14	2200	46	800	45	15	12	150
15 to 18	2200	44	800	55	15	12	150
19 to 24	2200	46	800	60	15	12	150
25 to 50	2200	50	800	65	15	12	150
51+	1900	50	800	65	10	12	150
Pregnancy	+300	60	800	65	30	15	175
LACTATION							
First 6 mo.	+500	65	1300	65	15	19	200
Second 6 mo.	+500	62	1200	65	15	16	200

Adapted from National Research Council, Food and Nutrition Board. (1989). *Recommended dietary allowances* (10th ed.). Washington, DC: National Academy Press.
The values in this table for vitamins A and K and the minerals iodine, iron, and zinc will be replaced by the recommendations that are forthcoming in: National Research Council, Institute of Medicine, Food and Nutrition Board. (2001, in press). *Dietary reference intakes for vitamin A, vitamin K, arsenic, boron, chromium, copper, iodine, iron, manganese, molybdenum, nickel, silicon, vanadium, and zinc*. Washington, DC: National Academy Press.

carbohydrates), trace elements (iron and zinc), electrolytes and water, and other food components (fiber and phytoestrogens). Information will be posted on the Internet by the Food and Nutrition Board as these recommendations are released.

Dietary Supplements and Herbal Medicines

The popularity of supplemental vitamins, minerals, proteins, fiber, and herbs has, in recent decades, earned a high profile in the field of health. A vast array of these products are available without a prescription. All people are entitled to know exactly what they are ingesting, whether it is necessary, and whether it is safe.

Traditionally, dietary supplements were products composed of one or more of the essential nutrients (vitamins, minerals, and proteins) that were ingested to enhance the usual diet. More recently, through the 1994 Dietary Supplement Health and Education Act, the definition of dietary supplement has been expanded to include any product intended for ingestion as a supplement to the diet, including vitamins, minerals, herbs, botanicals and other plant-derived substances, amino acids (individual building blocks of protein) and concentrates, metabolites, constituents, and extracts of these substances (USFDA, 1999).

Similar to supplements, drugs can also be of plant origin. Drugs are used in Western medicine as agents intended to diagnose, cure, mitigate, treat, or prevent diseases. Before marketing, drugs must undergo clinical trials to determine their effectiveness, safety, possible adverse interactions with other substances, and appropriate dosage amounts. The U.S. Food and Drug Administration (FDA) then reviews the data collected on the studied drug and, depending on the outcome of the review, officially authorizes the drug as safe for the general public.

Supplements are sold in the pharmaceutical section of retail stores in a variety of forms (tablets, capsules, powders, soft gels, gel caps, and liquids) that make them resemble drugs. Many people use supplements as drugs because they are marketed in the same manner as over-the-counter medications. Nevertheless, supplements are unregulated by the FDA.

A dietary supplement can be distinguished from an over-the-counter drug by the words *dietary supplement*, which must appear on the product label. A claim that the supplement is formulated to treat or cure a specific disease or condition cannot appear on the label. However, "structure/function claims" about certain common conditions associated with aging, pregnancy, menopause, and adolescence that do not relate to disease are permitted. These include health maintenance claims ("maintains a healthy circulatory system"), other nondisease claims ("for muscle enhancement" or "helps you relax,"), and claims for common, minor symptoms associated with life stages ("for common symptoms of PMS" or "for hot flashes").

Considerable research on the effects of dietary supplements has been conducted in Asia and Europe where these plant products have a long tradition of use. However, the overwhelming majority of supplements have not been studied scientifically. Therefore the National Institutes of Health (NIH) Office of Alternative Medicine and Office of Dietary Supplements are promoting the scientific study of the benefits and risks of dietary supplements (including medicinal herbs) in health maintenance and disease prevention.

Health care professionals are often asked, "Should I take a nutrient supplement?" Many people in the United States take dietary supplements, but not necessarily to meet nutrient requirements. Although the adverse affects of large doses of certain nutrients (such as vitamin A) have been recognized for years, there are no documented reports that daily vitamins and mineral supplements that supply up to the recommended intake for a particular nutrient are either beneficial or harmful for the general population. Low-dose supplements that contain the recommended intakes for micronutrients (vitamins and minerals) appear to be generally safe. Although the desirable way for the general public to obtain recommended levels of nutrients is by eating a variety of foods, when people take dietary supplements, they should avoid taking them in excess of the recommended intake on any given day.

Circumstances When Nutrient Supplementation Is Indicated

Nutrient supplements and/or fortified foods are sometimes necessary for specific populations to obtain desirable amounts of particular nutrients (American Dietetic Association, 2001).

- Folic acid for females who could become pregnant; to help prevent neural tube defects
- Iron during pregnancy
- Calcium for individuals who do not meet the recommended intake of calcium
- Vitamin D for elderly people who do not drink generous quantities of fortified milk or who do not manufacture sufficient vitamin D from sunlight
- Vitamin B-12 for elderly people with atrophic gastritis who do not absorb sufficient vitamin B-12 from the food they eat

Vitamin Toxicity

An important point of concern for many health professionals is the use of vitamin and mineral supplements in excess. Toxic levels of certain micronutrients may result and can cause a host of health problems. For example, it is important to advise patients not to overuse vitamins of the fat-soluble class (vitamins A, D, E, and K). Of particular concern is vitamin A, an excess of which may be teratogenic during pregnancy. On the other hand, water soluble vitamins such as vitamin C and the B-complex vitamins pose less danger because the body is able to excrete them through the urine.

Nutrient imbalances and toxicities are less likely to occur when nutrients are derived from foods. Most nutrient toxicities occur through supplementation. Estimated toxic doses for daily oral consumption of vitamins and minerals by adults are as low as 5 times the recommended intake for selenium, and as high as 25 to 50 times or more the recommended intakes for folic acid and vitamins C and E. The toxicities of high doses of nutrients such as vitamins A, B-6, and D; niacin; iron; and selenium are well established. Iron supplements intended for other household members are the most common cause of pediatric poisoning deaths in the United States (American Dietetic Association, 2001).

Large doses of vitamin A may be teratogenic. Because of this risk, supplementation with preformed vitamin A should be avoided during the first trimester of pregnancy unless there is specific evidence of vitamin A deficiency. Excess preformed vitamin A (more than 10,000 IU) during the first trimester of pregnancy has been linked to the birth of babies with cranial neural crest defects (Rothman et al., 1995). Such a risk in early pregnancy raises a need for caution about general vitamin and mineral supplement use by women of child-bearing age.

Besides problems with direct toxicity of some individual nutrients, nutrient supplementation can cause problems related to nutrient imbalances or adverse interactions with medical care. Many problems associated with high doses of a single nutrient may reflect interactions that result in a relative deficiency for another nutrient. For example, high doses of vitamin E can interfere with vitamin K action and enhance the effect of coumarin anticoagulant drugs. High amounts of calcium inhibit absorption of iron and possibly other trace elements. Folic acid can mask hematological signs of vitamin B-12 deficiency, which, if untreated, can result in irreversible neurological damage. Folic acid can also interact adversely with anticonvulsant medications. Zinc supplementation can reduce copper status, impair immune responses, and decrease high-density lipoprotein cholesterol levels.

Dietary Guidelines for Americans

The influence of the **Dietary Guidelines** for Americans is wide ranging. First issued in 1980 in response to the public's desire for authoritative, consistent guidance on diet and health, the Dietary Guidelines forms the foundation of federal nutrition policy in the United States. Each federally-sponsored nutrition program in the United States uses the Dietary Guidelines as a part of its nutrition standard; therefore every day the guidelines directly influence the lives of millions of Americans in food stamp, school lunch, and school breakfast programs and the women, infants, and children receiving benefits under the Special Supplemental Nutrition Program for Women, Infants, and Children (WIC). These guidelines also form the basis for nutrition education messages for the general public of adults and children beginning at 2 years of age.

The National Nutrition Monitoring and Related Research Act of 1990 mandates that the guidelines be reviewed every 5 years by the U.S. Department of Agriculture (USDA) and the U.S. Department of Health and Human Services (USDHHS). Each edition of the Dietary Guidelines continues to reflect the overwhelming consensus of science to answer the question, "What should Americans eat to stay healthy?" (USDA, 1985, 1990, 1995.)

Consumption patterns based on the Dietary Guidelines for Americans will lead to major improvements in public health and nutrition for the United States (Johnson & Kennedy, 2000). Nursing professionals play a key role in promoting the Dietary Guidelines as one component of healthful lifestyles (see Multicultural Awareness Box). For convenience, the entire Dietary Guidelines report is available on the Internet (http://www.usda.gov/cnpp/DietGd.pdf). Although the document is lengthy (44 pages), the report is an excellent source of background information for health care professionals. Individual sections are available to photocopy for use as education materials.

The most recent edition of the Dietary Guidelines (USDA, 2000) is based on three basic messages: (1) Aim for fitness, (2) Build a healthy base, and (3) Choose sensibly for good health (ABC). The ABCs for good health help organize the guidelines in a memorable, meaningful way.

Aim for Fitness

Aim for a healthy weight.
Be physically active each day.

Build a Healthy Base

Let the Pyramid guide your food choices.
Choose a variety of grains daily, especially whole grains.
Choose a variety of fruits and vegetables daily.
Keep food safe to eat.

Choose Sensibly

Choose a diet that is low in saturated fat and cholesterol and moderate in total fat. Choose beverages and foods to moderate your intake of sugars.
Choose and prepare foods with less salt.
When you drink alcoholic beverages, do so in moderation.

These guidelines for a healthy diet are intended for healthy Americans 2 years of age and older. By following this advice, individuals can benefit from better health and reduce the chance of falling prey to certain diseases such as CHD, high blood pressure, stroke, certain cancers, osteoporosis, and type 2 diabetes. Representing the best and most up-to-date advice from nutrition experts, these guidelines are intended to help people select foods and beverages that will constitute a healthy diet (Box 11-2).

Food Guide Pyramid

The **Food Guide Pyramid** was introduced in 1992 as a means for the USDA and the USDHHS to translate nutrition recommendations into terms that consumers would understand. As the twentieth-century anthropologist Margaret Mead once said, "People eat food, not nutrition." Nutrition recommendations stated in terms of grams of total fat and saturated fat, or milligrams of vitamin C, are useless unless people are advised as to what types and what quantities of foods should be consumed to obtain the recommended nutrients. The Food Guide Pyramid is a graphic representation of dietary balance and variety. Foods are classified into 6 food groups, each of which contains a variety of nutritionally similar foods.

Grains, Fruits, and Vegetables

At the base of the Food Guide Pyramid are breads, cereals, rice, and pasta (foods from grains). According to the pyramid, diets should contain more servings of grain products each day than of any other food group. The level immediately above the grains contains other foods from the plant kingdom, such as fruits and vegetables. Together, the grains, fruits, and vegetables supply fiber, vitamins, and minerals that are almost completely fat free. Potatoes and other starchy vegetables, such as sweet green peas and corn, are classified as vegetables in the Food Guide Pyramid. For weight loss and diabetes meal planning, these starchy foods are counted as servings from the grains group because they are similar to breads and pasta in terms of carbohydrate content.

Overall, Americans eat fewer fruits and vegetables than is recommended. A program called 5 *A Day* is designed to address the goal of making Americans more aware of the way in which fruits and vegetables can improve their health. This program, jointly sponsored by the National Cancer Institute (NCI) and Produce for Better Health Foundation, is the first national effort to focus on the positive role of fruits and vegetables in reducing the risk of cancer and other chronic diseases.

Dairy and Meat

Above fruits and vegetables on the Food Guide Pyramid are two more groups: (1) dairy products (milk, yogurt, and cheese) and (2) protein-rich foods from the animal (meat, fish, poultry, and eggs) and plant (dry beans and nuts) kingdoms.

MULTICULTURAL AWARENESS

Food and Culture

The reasons why people eat the way they do are numerous. Although it is true that without food, people cannot survive, food is much more than a tool of survival. Food is also a source of pleasure ("Let's eat out tonight."), a source of comfort ("Right now, I could use some of my mother's chicken soup."), a symbol of hospitality ("Please come to my house for brunch on Sunday."), and an indicator of social status (consider an expensive T-bone steak versus a hamburger). Food has ritual significance also; for example, drinking champagne to celebrate an important event, the bride and groom saving the top layer of their wedding cake, or people of the Jewish faith sharing *challah* (braided bread) at their Sabbath (Friday evening) meal.

To a large extent, the environment determines what people typically eat. For example, wheat that is plentiful in the heartland of the United States is the principal grain in North America, whereas rice enjoys a similar status in Asian countries. Typical wheat-based staples in the United States and Canada include a slice of wheat bread, a bowl of wheat cereal, wheat crackers, pastries made from wheat flour, and pasta made from wheat. Rice-based foods form the backbone of the Chinese diet.

Every culture has its particular foodways, or activities related to food. Foodways include the activities that surround procuring, distributing, storing, consuming, and disposing of food, all of which define what is fit to eat (what is edible). The factors that affect everyone's food choices and factors that affect food choices of new arrivals to a community should be examined.

Food is often believed to promote health, cure disease, or contain other medicinal qualities. Health beliefs, which can have a great influence on food choices, may be beneficial, neutral, and sometimes dangerous. When actions that are based on these beliefs cause no harm, they should be encouraged. For example, in the United States, Americans consume vitamin C in the belief that it might help prevent or cure the common cold. In fact, although large doses (500 to 1000 mg per day) have no significant effect on incidence of the common cold, vitamin C provides a moderate benefit in terms of the duration and severity of cold symptoms in some groups of people. The often-reported improvement in the severity of colds after ingesting vitamin C may be a result of the antihistaminic action of the vitamin at these large doses (National Research Council, 2000a).

Among traditional Chinese people, health and disease are believed to relate to the balance between the forces of *yin* and *yang* in the body. Diseases that are caused by yang forces may be treated with yin forces to restore balance. Yin foods include low-caloric density, low-protein foods, such as fresh fruits and vegetables. Yang foods are high in calories, cooked in oil, irritating to the mouth, or are red, orange, and yellow in color. Examples include most meats, chili peppers, tomatoes, garlic, ginger, and alcoholic beverages. The hot-cold theory in Puerto Rico follows the same basic principles as do yin and yang, but the food groupings differ somewhat.

Religious beliefs affect the food choices of millions of people worldwide. Many religions, including Buddhism, Hinduism, Islam, Judaism, and Seventh-Day Adventism, specify the foods that may be eaten and how they should be prepared. The following is a summary of the principal dietary practices of these five major world religions (Barer-Stein, 1979; Kittler & Sucher, 2000).

- Many Buddhists practice vegetarianism. Foods of plant origin are viewed as the most appropriate for consumption, except pungent foods (garlic, leeks, scallions, chives, and onions), which are believed to generate lust when eaten cooked and rage when eaten raw. For the majority of Buddhists, however, dietary rules such as these are observed on a voluntary basis. What characterizes *all* Buddhists is the belief that all forms of life share a common link and are thus sacred. Therefore rather than the specific type of food eaten, more important is the attitude of the person receiving the food and the person's sincere gratitude for the lives of the plants and animals contained in the meal that have served to sustain and further enhance the life of the individual.
- Many Hindus are vegetarians, but those who come from the cold northern areas of India eat meat (except for beef, which is prohibited). The expression "holy cow" is derived from the Hindu belief that the cow is sacred.
- Islamic food laws prohibit the consumption of foods believed to be unclean, such as carrion or already-dead animals; swine; animals slaughtered without pronouncing the name of Allah on them; carnivorous animals with fangs (dogs, cats, and lions); birds of prey; and land animals without ears (frogs and snakes). Alcohol is also prohibited.
- Judaism prohibits the consumption of swine, carrion, carrion eaters (scavengers), shellfish, animals without a cloven (split) hoof and those that do not chew their cud (horses), and animals not slaughtered by the appropriate ritual method. According to Jewish dietary laws, meat (beef, lamb, veal, and poultry) and meat products (fish and eggs) cannot be served at the same meal or cooked in the same vessels as dairy products.
- The dietary practices of Seventh-Day Adventists focus on health, with vegetarianism as the foundation of their dietary standard. Seventh-Day Adventists also abstain from alcohol and many do not drink caffeine-containing beverages.

People who are ovovegetarians (eggs are the only animal products eaten) and vegans (pure vegetarians who eat no animal products) will find that the Food Guide Pyramid does not address their special dietary needs. These people will benefit from a **vegetarian** food plan that makes a healthy, balanced diet possible without requiring the intake of animal products. An example of this food plan is the "Traditional Healthy Vegetarian Diet Pyramid," which is available on the Internet (http://www.oldwayspt.org/html/p_veg.htm).

Fats, Oils, and Sweets

The top of the Food Guide Pyramid shows fats, oils, and sweets. A major function of the pyramid is its focus on **fat** because most American diets are high in fat, especially saturated fat. The group containing fats, oils, and

Box 11-2 Rationale for the Dietary Guidelines and Suggestions for Implementing Specific Recommendations

AIM FOR A HEALTHY WEIGHT

The condition of being overweight increases the risk of elevated blood cholesterol, high blood pressure, stroke, heart disease, certain types of cancer, diabetes, arthritis, and breathing problems. Conversely, being too thin is linked with menstrual irregularities and osteoporosis in women and with greater risk of early death in both women and men.

Current research indicates that several factors may work in concert to promote weight gain. These factors range from a genetic inclination toward obesity to an overreliance on time-saving equipment and vehicles that eliminate opportunities for exercise. Weight management is recognized as no easy task, but there are several strategies recommended toward this goal. For example, long-term adjustments in eating behavior and physical activity should be made by choosing sensible foods and gradually building a healthy routine of good nutrition and exercise. A healthful variety of foods should be chosen including vegetables, fruits, grains (especially whole grains), skim milk, fish, lean meat, and poultry or beans. Additionally, foods low in fat and added sugar are recommended because fat and extra sugar contribute calories, which, in excess of metabolic needs, are stored in the body as fat.

Physical activity is another important step toward effective weight management. Adults are encouraged to engage in approximately 30 minutes or more of moderate exercise on most and preferably all days of the week. A healthy weight for adults is a weight that falls within a certain range related to height (see Fig. 11-4). The higher weights in the ranges generally apply to men because men tend to have more muscle and bone compared with women.

BE PHYSICALLY ACTIVE EACH DAY

Compared with being sedentary, being physically active for a minimum of 30 minutes a day produces several health benefits. For children, adolescents, adults, and elderly adults, regular physical activity can improve health and well being in the following ways:

- Increases physical fitness.
- Helps build and maintain healthy bones, muscles, and joints.
- Builds endurance and muscular strength.
- Helps manage weight.
- Lowers risk factors for CVD, colon cancer, and type 2 diabetes.
- Helps control blood pressure.
- Promotes psychological well being and self-esteem.
- Reduces depression and anxiety.

Two types of physical exercise are especially beneficial:

1. *Aerobic activities.* These activities increase heart rate and breathing and they support cardiovascular fitness.
2. *Activities for strength and flexibility.* Cultivating strength can help build and maintain bone density. For example, carrying groceries and lifting weights are 2 strength-building activities. Gentle stretching, dancing, and yoga can increase flexibility.

Physical activity and nutrition work in concert for better health. For example, exercise increases the amount of energy that is needed, which, in turn, balances the amount of energy obtained from food. This balance helps regulate the amount of calories remaining for the body to store as fat. Furthermore, because physical activity burns additional calories, the body can use additional food without gaining weight and can also obtain required nutrients more easily.

CHOOSE A VARIETY OF GRAINS DAILY

Foods made from grains (wheat, rice, and oats), particularly whole grains, help form the pillars of a nutritionally sound diet. Grains provide vitamins, minerals, carbohydrates (starch and dietary fiber), and other protective substances conducive to good health. Grain products are naturally low in fat, unless fat is added at a later stage of production or preparation. Additionally, whole grains, as compared with refined grain products, contain fiber and nutrients, both of which benefit health in several ways. The current recommendation is to eat at least 6 servings of grain or grain products every day. Eating fiber and nutrient-rich foods promotes proper bowel function and imparts a protection against many chronic diseases.

Reading the ingredients label carefully ensures that a whole grain product is indeed what it claims to be. For example, for a whole wheat bread to actually be whole wheat bread, it must list *whole wheat* flour as its first ingredient, which indicates that the ingredient in the highest quantity is indeed whole grain.

In recent years, folic acid (a form of the B-vitamin folate) has been added to all enriched grain products (thiamin, riboflavin, niacin, and iron have been added to enriched grains for many years). Folate has been found to reduce the risk of some serious types of birth defects (namely, neural tube defects) when consumed before and during early pregnancy. Current research is underway to discern whether folate has any protective properties regarding CHD, stroke, and certain types of cancer.

CHOOSE A VARIETY OF FRUITS AND VEGETABLES DAILY

Fruits and vegetables are integral parts of a varied diet contributing an array of vitamins (vitamin C, folate, and the carotenoids, which form vitamin A), minerals (primarily potassium), and fiber. Similar to grains, eating a variety of fruits and vegetables (all fruit and vegetable products are rich in different nutrients) may help protect against certain chronic diseases and will promote healthy bowel function.

Based on data from *Nutrition and your health: Dietary guidelines for Americans* [Online]. Washington, DC: U.S. Department of Agriculture. Available: http://www.usda.gov/cnpp/DietGd.pdf.

sweets makes up the smallest area of the pyramid, indicating that fats and sweets should be eaten in small quantities as compared with the amounts of foods from the other food groups. No specific recommendation is made for the number of servings from the fats and sweets group to be included in the diet daily. This group is included in its conspicuous location at the top of the Pyramid both as a reminder of its importance and to illustrate the concepts of moderation and proportionality.

Box 11-2 Rationale for the Dietary Guidelines and Suggestions for Implementing Specific Recommendations—cont'd

With the exception of avocados and olives, fruits and vegetables are generally low in fat and calories and are filling, which aids people who want to regulate their weight. These foods are also a significant source of folate. Good folate sources include dry beans, lentils, chickpeas, cowpeas, and peanuts; leafy green vegetables (the word folate is derived from *foliage,* which means *leafy*); and fruits, such as oranges, orange juice, strawberries, pineapple juice, and plantains. Consuming a wide variety of produce is important because different fruits and vegetables are rich in different nutrients. As a general rule, juices are not a good substitute for actual produce because juices contain little or no fiber and a high amount of sugar.

KEEP FOODS SAFE TO EAT

For a review of the safety precautions when eating or handling food, see the Food Safety section.

CHOOSE A DIET LOW IN SATURATED FAT AND CHOLESTEROL AND MODERATE IN TOTAL FAT

Fats supply energy and essential fatty acids, which help absorb the fat-soluble vitamins A, D, E, K, and carotenoids. As such, having some dietary fat is necessary. However, certain types of fat, especially saturated fats, increase the risk for CHD by raising the blood cholesterol. Eating a significant amount of fat—any fat—can provide excess calories.

The goals for fat apply to the diet over several days, not to a single meal or food. The total fat goal depends on calorie requirements. An amount that provides 30% or less of calories is highly recommended. Table 11-7 shows the upper limit on the grams of total and saturated fat per day that corresponds to various daily calorie intakes. All fats contain both saturated and unsaturated fats (fatty acids). The fats in animal products are the main sources of saturated fat in most diets, with tropical oils (coconut, palm kernel, and palm oils) and hydrogenated fats providing additional saturated fats.

Trans-fatty *acids* tend to raise blood cholesterol. These foods include sources high in partially hydrogenated vegetable oils, such as many hard margarines and shortenings.

Cholesterol is found exclusively in animal products. Eating less fat from animal sources will help lower the intake of total fat, saturated fat, and cholesterol.

CHOOSE BEVERAGES AND FOODS TO MODERATE SUGAR INTAKE

Sugars and many foods that contain sugars in large amounts supply calories, but are limited in nutrients. Sugar comes in many forms, such as table sugar (sucrose), brown sugar, honey, syrup, corn, sweetener, high-fructose corn sweetener, molasses, glucose (dextrose), fructose, maltose, and lactose. Sugars should be used in moderation or sparingly if calorie needs are low. Diets high in sugars have not been shown to cause diabetes. However, both sugars and starches, which break down into sugars, can contribute to tooth decay (cariogenic sugars). Excessive snacking should be avoided; teeth should be brushed regularly with a fluoride toothpaste and flossed to help prevent tooth decay. A dentist, nurse practitioner, or physician, when needed, can provide advice on supplemental fluoride, especially for children.

CHOOSE AND PREPARE FOODS WITH LESS SALT

Salt contains the mineral *sodium,* which is a substance that affects blood pressure. Most Americans eat more salt and sodium than they need. In populations with diets low in salt, high blood pressure is less common compared with populations with diets high in salt. Eating less salt and sodium will benefit people whose blood pressure increases with salt intake. Some useful food tips to control the use of salt and sodium in the diet are listed on p. 295.

IF DRINKING ALCOHOLIC BEVERAGES, DO SO IN MODERATION

Alcoholic beverages supply calories, but few or no nutrients. Alcoholic beverages are harmful when consumed in excess and some people should not drink alcoholic beverages at all. Although current evidence suggests that moderate drinking is associated with a lower risk of CHD in some individuals, excess alcohol intake alters judgment, can lead to dependency, and raises the risk for high blood pressure, stroke, CHD, certain cancers, accidents, violence, suicide, birth defects, and overall mortality. Excessive alcohol consumption may cause cirrhosis of the liver, inflammation of the pancreas, and damage to the brain and heart. Heavy alcohol drinkers are also at risk for malnutrition because alcohol contains calories that may substitute for those from more nutritious foods. People who drink alcoholic beverages should do so in moderation, with meals, and when consumption does not endanger others.

For women, moderate drinking is no more than 1 drink a day; for men it is no more than 2 drinks a day. A drink may be counted as 12 ounces of regular beer (150 calories), 5 ounces of wine (100 calories), or one and a half ounces of 80-proof distilled spirits (100 calories). Beer labeled *lite* contains fewer calories compared with the same brand of regular beer, but contains an equal amount of alcohol.

Women who are pregnant, who are trying to conceive, or who might conceive because they are sexually active and not using contraceptives should avoid drinking alcoholic beverages. Others who should abstain from drinking alcohol are individuals who use medications (even over-the-counter medications), those who plan to drive or engage in other activities that require skill and attention, and those who are unable to drink moderately. Children and adolescents, obviously, are among this group.

FOOD SAFETY

Food safety is vitally important in promoting health and remains in the limelight as severe food-borne illnesses sweep across the nation. In this section, the importance of safeguarding food, the different types of contamination that endangers the food supply, and steps that can be taken to avoid falling victim to food-borne illness are considered.

Every organization and individual connected to the food chain, from food production to the table, share responsibility for the safety and integrity of the food supply (Institute of Medicine, 1998). This chain includes people who produce or grow, process, ship, sell, and prepare food and the consumer who makes up the final link in the chain. The USDA establishes and monitors guidelines and

Table 11-7 Recommended Total Fat and Saturated Fat Intake for Healthy People

Total Energy (Calories) Per Day	Maximum Total Fat (g)*	Saturated Fat (g) **
1200	40	Less than 13
1500	50	Less than 17
1600	53	Less than 18
2000	66	Less than 20
2200	73	Less than 24
2500	80	Less than 25
2800	93	Less than 31

*Up to 30% of energy
**Less than 10% of energy

standards to be followed by all groups involved. When the safeguards built into this system fail, however, consumers themselves must serve as the final and sometimes most important guardian against unsafe food. Therefore being informed and educated about the potential dangers of food-borne illness and how to avoid these complications to stay healthy is essential.

Causes of Food-Borne Illness

A food-borne illness is classified according to the source of its contamination (the unintended presence of harmful substances or microorganisms). Food contaminants may be categorized as biological, chemical, or physical. *Biological* contaminants include bacteria, viruses, parasites, and fungi (yeasts and mold) unintentionally inhabiting food. *Chemical* contamination refers to the presence of pesticides, kitchen cleaning supplies, and toxic chemicals in food that have been leached out of worn metal cookware and equipment. *Physical* contamination includes dirt, glass chips, crockery, wood, splinters, stones, hair, jewelry, and metal shavings from dull can openers (Table 11-8).

Mad Cow Disease

The highly active surveillance on beef from Europe and specifically the United Kingdom is a prime example of the effect unsafe food can have on entire populations. This particular problem known as *bovine spongiform encephalopathy* (BSE) or more commonly as *mad cow disease* is traced back to unsafe food practices of certain producers in the meat industry. Sheep products and waste meat contaminated with an infectious protein-like particle known as a prion cause a fatal neurological disease in cows. These cows became uncontrollable and wild, much different from their usual docile nature. Humans who eat contaminated beef suffer from a similar fatal neurological degeneration called new variant Creutzfeldt-Jacob disease (nvCJD). This particular contaminant cannot be destroyed by heat, radiation, or disinfectants. Cooperation among the whole food safety network, especially the consumer, is therefore important for special cases like this one to be controlled. To reduce the possible current risk of acquiring nvCJD from food, travelers to Europe should be advised to consider either avoiding beef and beef products altogether, or selecting beef or beef products as solid pieces of muscle meat (versus ground products such as burgers and sausages) that have a reduced opportunity for contamination with tissues that might harbor the BSE agent. Milk and milk products from cows are not believed to pose any risk for transmitting the BSE agent (CDC, 2001).

Food Safety Practices

Hand washing is one of the most important practices in the prevention of food-borne illness. Hands should be washed thoroughly before food preparation and before eating. The accepted method of hand washing entails running warm water over the hands, applying soap, and generating friction and agitation for approximately 20 to 30 seconds. Young children should be taught to wash their hands for as long as it takes them to sing the alphabet song twice. Nearly one half of all cases of food-borne illness might be completely avoided if people were to wash their hands more often when preparing and handling food.

Raw, cooked, and ready-to-eat foods should be separated while shopping, preparing, or storing foods. Separating foods prevents cross-contamination, which is the transfer of harmful substances or microorganisms from one location to another. Cross-contamination can occur when unwashed hands come in contact with food, when a microorganism-carrying food comes in contact with another food, or when a surface comes in contact with a food (Box 11-3 and Fig. 11-2). To prevent cross-contamination, follow these additional safety measures:

- Wash fresh fruits and vegetables thoroughly.
- Drink pasteurized juices.
- Do not consume raw (unpasteurized) milk and or cheeses made with raw milk.
- Eat food that has been chilled and refrigerated properly.
- When eating out, make sure that food requiring refrigeration is served chilled.
- When shopping, buy perishable foods last and take them straight home.
- Follow the label. Always read and follow safety instructions on the package, such as, "Keep Refrigerated" and "Safe handling Instructions."
- Eat food that is served safely. Keep hot foods hot (140° F or above) and cold foods cold (40° F or below). Between these temperatures is the *danger zone* in which harmful bacteria can grow rapidly, even exponentially.
- Whether raw or cooked, never leave meat, poultry, eggs, fish, or shellfish out at room temperature for more than 2 hours (1 hour in hot weather that is 90° F and above). Be sure to chill leftovers as soon as you are finished eating.

These guidelines also apply to carryout meals, restaurant leftovers, and home-packed meals-to-go. If in doubt, throw it out (Box 11-4).

Making a food safe after it has been handled improperly

Table 11-8 Major Biological and Chemical Contaminants Affecting Food Safety in the United States

Contaminant	Mode of Transmission	Symptoms	Typically Affected Foods	Prevention Strategies
Campylobacter jejuni *Bacteria*	The common reservoir for this bacteria is domestic and wild animals.	Although not as deadly as other types of harmful bacteria, it can make humans severely ill with diarrhea, vomiting, abdominal pain, headache, and fever.	Undercooked chicken or foods contaminated by raw chicken is the usual cause of Campylobacteriosis. However, raw vegetables, nonpasteurized milk and dairy products, pork, beef and lamb have also been found to contain this bacteria.	Avoid cross-contamination, cook foods thoroughly, use only pasteurized milk, and wash all produce.
Escherichia coli (*E. coli*) 0157:H7 *Bacteria*	Unwashed hands used to prepare or consume food, animal fecal matter contaminating drinking water or food supplies, *E. coli* 0157:H7-harboring foods contaminating other food.	Most types of *E. coli* bacteria are harmless; however, this is a deadly strain that often causes bloody diarrhea, severe abdominal pain, nausea, vomiting, fever, and sometimes death.	Most often found in undercooked ground beef. However, it is becoming common to find this bacterial strain in vegetables such as lettuce and other produce resulting from breaches of safety protocol from farm to storage to preparation and processing.	Cook beef and red meats thoroughly and adequately, avoid cross-contamination, use safe water and food supplies, avoid possible fecal contamination by food handlers through obtaining food at sanitary and reputable facilities and stores, and cook foods to a high enough temperature to kill bacteria.
Hepatitis A *Virus*	Contaminated water often spreads this virus.	This is a contagious virus that causes inflammation of the liver.	Various types of foods, from produce such as strawberries to animal products, can harbor this particular viral contaminant.	Thoroughly clean and rinse all produce and, when necessary, remove skin or outermost leaves. Cook all foods to a safe temperature. Pay attention to the source of water used to prepare food.
Listeria monocytogenes *Bacteria*	Commonly known as the cold cut or deli meat bacteria, Listeria can survive at refrigerator temperatures and has been found in the feces of humans, sheep, cattle, and poultry. Also detected in cow's milk, unwashed leafy green vegetables, fruit, and soil. Dairy and meat processing factories can also harbor this bacterium.	Listeria can be lethal and is capable of causing miscarriage in pregnant women. It can also cause influenza-like symptoms leading to septicemia, meningitis, and perinatal septicemia.	Cold meats and other cold or refrigerated foods, including unpasteurized milk, soft cheeses, and raw produce.	Use only pasteurized milk and dairy products, cook foods to proper temperatures, reheat foods to at least 165° F, and avoid cross-contamination. Wash all produce well.

Data from Cody, M. M. (1996). *Safe food for you and your family*. Minneapolis: The American Dietetic Association, Chronimed Publishing; Spears, M. C. (2000). *Food service organizations—A managerial and systems approach*. Upper Saddle River, NJ: Prentice Hall.

Continued

Table 11-8 Major Biological and Chemical Contaminants Affecting Food Safety in the United States—cont'd

Contaminant	Mode of Transmission	Symptoms	Typically Affected Foods	Prevention Strategies
Molds *Fungus/spores*	Molds can survive in environments inhabitable to most bacteria.	These organisms can become air borne and be inhaled, thereby causing lung infections and a variety of other complications.	Jams, preserves, jelly, and bread are few of the foods capable of supporting molds.	Follow the proper storage procedures prescribed for the specific type or category of food being handled. For example, foods requiring dry storage should be stored in a cool, dry (low moisture), darkened space.
Norwalk-like *Virus*	As this viral agent is usually found in the human intestinal tract, a route of contamination is human feces from unwashed hands. It is also transmitted by contaminated water.	Symptoms include nausea, vomiting, abdominal pain, headache, and low-grade fever. (Because it is a virus, it can reproduce in food but remains inactive until consumed.)	Commonly affected foods are raw vegetables fertilized with manure, prepared salads, raw shellfish, eggs, icing on baked pastries, manufactured ice cubes, frozen foods and water contaminated with human feces.	Use only water known to be safe or take measures to make water safe (via boiling), be wary of unsafe food handlers that do not practice good hygiene (washing hands), and always cook foods thoroughly.
Salmonella *Bacteria*	Of the 2000 types of Salmonella, only a few strains cause food-borne illness. Tiered chicken cages (stacked one on top of the other).	Abdominal pain, headache, nausea, vomiting, fever, and diarrhea.	Milk, chicken, beef, and eggs are the foods most commonly associated with Salmonellosis.	Avoid cross contamination, refrigerate food, cool cooked meat products properly, combat possible fecal contamination from food handlers by following minimal cooking temperature guidelines and purchasing food from sanitary facilities and stores.
Staphylococcus aureus *Bacteria*	Contaminating food after touching a mucus membrane region of the body, such as nose, scalp, or hair.	One of the main culprits of *nosocomial* infections; often causes nausea, vomiting, abdominal cramps, diarrhea, and dehydration.	All food is at risk of contamination by this bacteria. Most often, however, salad with protein-containing ingredients, meat, poultry, milk, and egg products (including custards).	Avoid contamination from bare hands, exclude sick or unhealthy food handlers from preparation and serving of food, maintain adequate hygiene and sanitary practices, and follow proper heating and refrigeration requirements for various foods.
Trichinella spiralis *Parasite*	This parasite usually gains entrance into the human body when a person consumes the encysted larvae inhabiting poorly cooked pork.	Muscle pain and fever	Raw or undercooked pork or meat of carnivorous animals	Irradiation, freezing pork (5° F for 30 days), and cooking food adequately.
Pesticides *Chemical*	Many ways exist by which chemicals taint food, such as by accidentally spilling kitchen detergents on foods and eating unwashed, pesticide-coated foods.	Depending on the chemical used, any number of side effects can occur, from nausea to cancer.	Mostly produce (fruits and vegetables) that are sprayed with a variety of chemical pesticides.	Wash all fruits and vegetables vigorously under clean running water, peel skins when necessary, and remove outermost leaves when required.

Data from Cody, M. M. (1996). *Safe food for you and your family*. Minneapolis: The American Dietetic Association, Chronimed Publishing; Spears, M. C. (2000). *Food service organizations—A managerial and systems approach*. Upper Saddle River, NJ: Prentice Hall.

Box 11-3 Food Safety Practices

- Keep raw meat, poultry, eggs, fish, and shellfish away from other foods. Also, be sure these foods have separate food preparation surfaces, utensils, and serving plates.
- When buying or storing raw meat, poultry, fish, and shellfish, prevent fluids from passing between foods by using leak-proof bags or containers that keep juices from dripping. Clean food preparation surfaces (such as cutting boards) and utensils (such as knives and food-slicing devices) frequently, especially when preparing animal products.
- Eat food that is cooked to a safe temperature. Uncooked and undercooked animal foods are potentially unsafe; proper cooking makes most raw foods safe to eat. The best way to tell whether meat, poultry, or egg dishes are cooked to a safe temperature is by measuring their temperature with a food thermometer. Inexpensive thermometers are available at many supermarkets and hardware stores. Follow these guidelines:

Reheat sauces, soups, marinades, and gravies, to a boil. Reheat leftovers thoroughly to at least 165° F.

When using a microwave oven, cover the container and turn or stir the food to make sure it is heated evenly.

Cook eggs until whites and yolks are firm. Do not eat raw or partially cooked eggs or foods containing raw eggs.

Do not eat undercooked (rare) hamburger and raw fish (including sushi), clams, and oysters.

Cook fish and shellfish until it is opaque; fish should flake easily with a fork.

Cook Foods to a Safe Temperature

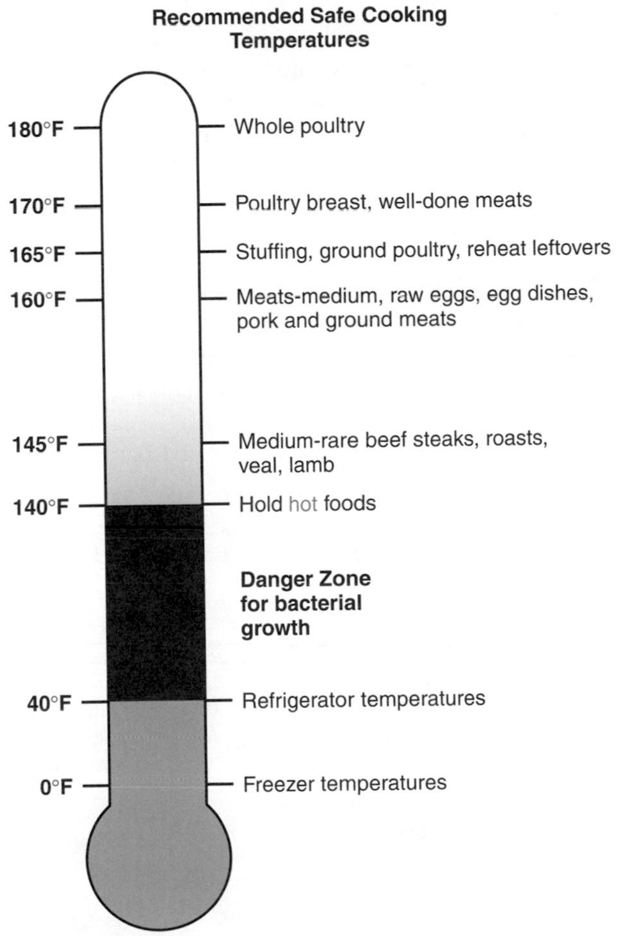

These food temperatures are for home use. They are not intended for processing, institutional, or foodservice preparation.

Fig. 11-2 Temperature range thermometer. (From U.S. Department of Agriculture, U.S. Department of Health and Human Services. [2000]. *Nutrition and your health: Dietary guidelines for Americans* [5th ed.]. Home and Garden Bulletin No. 232. Washington, DC: U.S. Government Printing Office.)

Box 11-4 Food Safety Practices at Home

- Promptly refrigerate or freeze meat, poultry, eggs, fish, shellfish, ready-to-eat foods, and leftovers.
- Refrigerate within 2 hours of purchasing or preparation (within 1 hour when the air temperature is above 90° F).
- Use refrigerated leftovers within 3 to 4 days.
- Always refrigerate at or below 40° F and freeze at or below 0° F.
- Freeze fresh meat, poultry, fish, and shellfish that cannot be eaten in a few days.
- Thaw frozen meat, poultry, fish, and shellfish in the refrigerator, microwave, or cold water changed every 30 minutes. (This process keeps the surface chilled.)
- Never thaw meat, poultry, fish, or shellfish at room temperature.
- Cook foods immediately after thawing.

may not always be possible. Therefore the best practice is to discard food when there is a doubt as to the safety of food preparation, service, or storage. For example, certain bacteria found in food that has been left at room temperature too long may produce a heat-resistant toxin that cannot be destroyed by cooking. Therefore the bottom line is to be careful in preparing food, which includes keeping track of the time the food is exposed to certain temperatures and being vigilant when eating out. If there is any doubt about the safety of the food, then caution is urged; it is better not to eat it.

Without exception, everyone should exercise their best judgment and care when eating out, when handling their own food, or when handling the food of others. Prevention through education is the key to promoting healthy lives that are unscathed by the potentially severe and life-threatening effects of food-borne illness. People who do not have healthy immune systems (individuals with various health problems and many older adults) and people with immune systems that are not fully developed (infants) are at the greatest risk of developing food-borne illnesses.

That food is shipped to the United States from all over the world, coupled with the fact that people do not have effective antibiotics available to meet the challenge of ever-changing and mutating microbial agents, makes it imperative to follow the basic food safety guidelines outlined in this chapter.

On a more positive note, normal healthy adults with a healthy immune system are able to ward off most of the contaminants from the environment and from food without much effort most of the time. Nevertheless, everyone should follow standard safety procedures when eating out and when handling food.

FOOD, NUTRITION, AND POVERTY

Healthy People 2010 Goal: promote health and reduce chronic disease associated with diet.

19-18. Increase food security in U.S. households from 88% in 1995 to 94% by 2010.

Food insecurity and hunger represent extremes of the dichotomy of excess versus deprivation. At a time during which many people are being encouraged to eat moderately, those who do not have enough to eat must also be considered. Concern for the hungry is focused primarily on the quantity of food they eat; sufficient caloric intake to support growth in children and maintain a healthy body weight in adults is the first concern in feeding programs. After caloric sufficiency is achieved, nutritional quality of the diet becomes the primary issue. Nutrient adequacy and caloric sufficiency are equally essential in combating hunger and its long-term effects.

Satisfying hunger is an immediate requirement. Stopgap measures to ease the pain of hunger are justifiable. However, without long-term solutions, hunger will return only to demand another quick fix. The effects of hunger goes far beyond the immediate suffering that it causes. Hunger compromises the ability to learn; therefore hungry children have significantly higher absentee rates and on the days they do spend in school, their powers of concentration are greatly reduced. Even moderate undernutrition can have lasting effects on a child's cognitive development and school performance (CDCP, 1996). Hunger is therefore more than simply an issue of compassion for people who do not have enough to eat; it is an issue of failed beginnings for many children, for the future of the planet.

Additionally, the high prevalence of chronic diseases among the disadvantaged must not be overlooked. Care must be taken to ensure that efforts directed at eliminating hunger do not result in the consumption of foods that exacerbate the incidence of heart disease, stroke, and some types of cancers, which are the leading causes of death in the United States.

Recognizing the need to provide poor people with enough food to eat, the United States allocates billions of dollars for food assistance, 80% of which funds the programs described in this section: the Food Stamp Program, child nutrition programs, WIC, and feeding programs for seniors (which includes congregate meals and home-delivered meals through Meals on Wheels).

Poverty and Income Distribution

For most people in the United States, income has risen over time, providing more options for personal consumption expenditures, including expenditures on food. However, growth in income has not increased for all households equally. Poverty still exists in the United States.

Table 11-9 Federal Income Poverty Guidelines and Income Eligibility Guidelines for Federal Food and Nutrition Programs, 2001 to 2001

Family Size	Poverty Threshold (100%): The 48 Contiguous States and Washington, DC	Hawaii	Alaska	Maximal Income for Residents of the 48 Contiguous States and Washington, DC: 130% of the Poverty Threshold: Eligible for Food Stamps and Free NSLP and SBP	185% of the Poverty Threshold: Eligible for WIC and Reduced-Price NSLP and SBP
1	$ 8590	$ 9890	$10,730	$11,167	$15,892
2	$11,610	$13,360	$14,510	$15,093	$21,479
3	$14,630	$16,830	$18,290	$19,019	$27,066
4	$17,650	$20,300	$22,070	$22,945	$32,653
5	$20,670	$23,770	$25,850	$26,871	$38,240
6	$23,690	$27,240	$29,630	$30,797	$43,827
7	$26,710	$30,710	$33,410	$34,723	$49,414
8	$29,730	$34,180	$37,190	$38,649	$55,001
Add for each additional person	$ 3020	$ 3470	$ 3780	$ 3926	$ 5587

From *Federal Register,* 66(55), 15829.

NSLP, National School Lunch Program; *SBP,* School Breakfast Program; *WIC,* Special Supplemental Nutrition Program for Women, Infants, and Children.

According to official 1998 poverty statistics (Weinberg, 1999), 12.7% or 34.5 million people live below the poverty level—a level of income set annually by the government to determine eligibility for various types of government programs as discussed in this section. As illustrated in Table 11-9, the poverty level in 2000-2001 is indicates an annual income of $17,650 or less for a family of four. Nonmetropolitan populations generally experience a higher poverty rate than metropolitan populations.

Groups with particularly high poverty rates include Hispanics and Blacks, with statistically equivalent poverty rates of 25.6% and 26.1%, respectively (Table 11-10). In contrast, the poverty rate was 8.2% for Whites. Children, who make up 39% of the poor, but only 26% of the total population, have a 18.9% poverty rate, which is higher than the rate of any other age group. In 1998, approximately 13.5 million children were poor. People living in families headed by single women have a poverty rate of over 33%, accounting for one half of all poor children. People living alone or with nonrelatives also have high rates of poverty.

Table 11-10 U.S. Poverty Statistics, 1998

Population	Median Income for Household	Poverty Rate
All	$38,900	About 13%
White	$42,400	8.2%
Black	$25,400	25.6%
Hispanic	$28,300	26.1%
Children (26% of the population)	NA	18.9%
Families headed by single women	NA	33%

From Weinberg, D. H. (1999). *Income and poverty 1998. Press briefing on 1998 income and poverty estimates* [Online]. Housing and Household Economic Statistics Division, U.S. Census Bureau. Available: http://www.census.gov/hhes/income/income98/prs99asc.html.

Food Assistance for the Poor

For people who are poor, obtaining a nutritious diet without assistance can be a challenge. Federal, state, and local governments and private charitable organizations mitigate this problem by providing billions of dollars annually in food assistance. Overall, the bulk of food aid in the United States is financed at the federal level by the USDA. In 1999, federally funded outlays for food assistance programs amounted to almost $33 billion:

- Food Stamps: Almost $19 billion
- Child nutrition (mostly for the School-Based Partnerships [SBP] and the National School Lunch Program [NSLP]): Almost $9.5 billion
- WIC: Over $4 billion
- Food donations (to Native-American communities, the Nutrition Program for the Elderly [NPE], the Emergency Food Distribution Program, etc.): Almost $500 million

One in six people in the United States receives federally funded food assistance at some point every year. The Food Stamp Program, NSLP, SBP, WIC, and NPE are the major programs that provide domestic food and nutrition assistance. Table 11-11 contains information on identifying low-income people who need help getting enough food and referring them to the appropriate program.

Food Stamp Program

Food coupons or food stamps are used to supplement the food-buying power of eligible low-income people. The program provides monthly allotments to low-income families to help purchase nutritionally adequate foods. Although there is no requirement that food stamps be used to purchase food that is healthy, the goal of the food stamp nutrition education program is to increase the likelihood that food stamp recipients will make healthy food choices within their limited food budget. Households can use food stamps to buy any food or food product for human consumption and seeds and plants for use in home gardens. Restaurants can be authorized to accept food stamps from

Table 11-11 Referral Guide for Federal Food Assistance Programs

Program	Target Population	Indicators of Need	Where to Call
School lunch	Children of school age	Poor nutritional status	Local school district
School breakfast	Children unlikely to eat before school	Harried household, low-income, poor nutritional status	Local school district
Summer food program	Children who live in low-income neighborhoods	Economic stress, poor nutritional status	Local social services office
WIC	Low-income pregnant and lactating women; infants and children up to age 5	Risk of existing health or nutritional problem	Local health department or community action agency
Congregate dining	Elderly adults, especially low-income minority and frail	Few social contacts, poor quality or quantity diet	Local office on aging
Home-delivered meals	Frail, homebound, elderly adults	Unable to shop for or prepare food, no available caretaker	Local hospital or office on aging

From Splett, P. L. (1994). Federal food assistance programs: A step to food security for many. *Nutrition Today*, 29 (2): 6-13.

qualified homeless, elderly, or disabled people in exchange for low-cost meals. Among the items that recipients cannot buy with food stamps are alcoholic beverages, tobacco, hot ready-to-eat foods, lunch-counter items, foods to be eaten in the store, vitamins, medicines, and pet foods. Food stamps cannot be exchanged for cash. The program is administered nationally by the Food and Nutrition Service (FNS) and locally by state welfare agencies. To qualify, households must meet eligibility criteria, including a gross income at or below 130% of the poverty guidelines issued by the USDHHS. Most able-bodied adult applicants must also meet certain work requirements. Households may own certain resources. In addition to income, the food stamp allotment is also based on family size. In 1998, the Food Stamp Program provided benefits to 19.8 million people: 58% children, 39% adults, and 8% seniors. In 2000, the average monthly benefit per person was approximately $73 and almost $173 per household (USDA, 2000).

National School Lunch Program

The federally funded NSLP is administered by FNS, an agency within the USDA. On the state level, the NSLP is usually administered by the U.S. Department of Education, which provides school lunches through agreements with local schools to provide balanced, low-cost or free lunches. The NSLP reaches about 24 million children each school day.

- Children from families with incomes at or below 130% of the poverty level are eligible for *free* school meals.
- Children from families at 130% to 185% of the poverty level are eligible for *reduced-price* school meals.
- Children from families at over 185% of the poverty level are eligible for *full-price* school meals.

Schools that choose to take part in the lunch program are provided with cash subsidies and donated commodities from the USDA. Donated foods include meats, canned and frozen fruits and vegetables, fruit juices, vegetable shortening, peanut products, vegetable oil, and flour and other grain products. In return for this financial and food support, the schools serve free or reduced-price lunches to children that meet these federal minimal pattern requirements:

- Must provide one third of the recommend nutrient intake.
- To the extent possible, must be consistent with the Dietary Guidelines for Americans recommendations for reducing sugar, salt, and fat intake.

To help meet the goal of healthier school meals, the USDA launched Team Nutrition, an initiative designed to help make implementation of the new policy in schools easier and more successful.

School Breakfast Program

Skipping breakfast can adversely affect children's performance in problem-solving tasks. A study of low-income elementary school students indicated that children who participated in the school breakfast program (SBP) had greater improvements in standardized test scores and reduced rates of absence and tardiness than did children who qualified for the program, but did not participate (CDCP, 1996). The SBP provides assistance to states to initiate, maintain, or expand nonprofit breakfast programs in eligible schools and residential child-care institutions. The program is administered by the FNS. Any child attending a participating school may receive a free, reduced-price, or full-price breakfast based on the same income criteria used by the NSLP.

Women, Infants, and Children

Food, nutrition counseling, and access to health services are provided to low-income women, infants, and children under the WIC program. This grant program administered by the FNS provides supplemental foods and health care referrals and nutrition education at no cost to the recipient. Low-income pregnant or postpartum women and children younger than 5 years old who are at risk nutritionally are eligible for WIC. The eligibility level is an income less than 185% of the poverty level. Nutritional risk is determined by federal guidelines. Three major types of nutritional risk are recognized: (1) high-priority, medically based risks, such as anemia, being underweight, low maternal age, history of pregnancy complications; (2) diet-based risks, such as inadequate dietary patterns; and (3) conditions such as alcoholism or drug addiction that predispose people to medically based or diet-based risks.

WIC participants receive coupons redeemable for foods that are rich in protein, calcium, iron, vitamin A, and vitamin C. Also included are iron-fortified infant formula and infant cereal, iron-fortified adult cereal, fruit or vegetable juice rich in vitamin C, eggs, milk, cheese, and peanut butter or dried beans. Special therapeutic formulas are provided when prescribed by a physician for a specific medical condition. Each WIC participant is designated to receive 1 of 6 different food packages that is especially designed for: (1) infants from birth through 3 months, (2) infants from 4 months through a year, (3) women and children with special dietary needs, (4) children 1 to 5 years of age, (5) pregnant and breast-feeding women, and (6) nonbreast-feeding postpartum women. More than 1.5 million infants participate in WIC, which is almost one third of the infants born in the United States.

Pregnant or postpartum women, infants, and children up to age 5 are eligible for WIC benefits. Participants must meet income guidelines (applicants before tax income must fall at or below 185% of the U.S. poverty income guidelines). Although most states use the maximal guidelines, states may set lower income limits. A person or certain family members who participate in other benefits programs, such as the Food Stamp Program, Medicaid, or Temporary Assistance for Needy Families, automatically meet the income eligibility requirement. There is also a state residency requirement and the applicant or child must be certified as at nutritional risk. Two major types of nutritional risk are recognized for WIC eligibility:

- Medically based risks, such as anemia, underweight, maternal age, history of pregnancy complications, or poor pregnancy outcomes.
- Diet-based risks, such as inadequate dietary pattern as determined by 24-hour recall, food frequency questionnaire, or diet history.

Children have always been the largest category of WIC participants. An average monthly participation for 1999 was approximately 7.31 million people, approximately half of whom were children, about one quarter were infants, and one quarter were women. WIC serves approximately 45% of all infants born in the United States and is currently estimated to be serving approximately 81% of all eligible women, infants, and children.

All eligible people are unable to be served by WIC; therefore a system of priorities has been established for filling program openings. After a local WIC agency has reached its maximal caseload, vacancies are generally filled in the order of the following priority levels:

- Pregnant women, breast-feeding women, and infants determined to be at nutritional risk from serious medical problems.
- Infants up to 6 months of age whose mothers participate in WIC or are eligible to participate and have serious medical problems.
- Children (up to age 5) at nutritional risk from serious medical problems.
- Pregnant or breast-feeding women and infants who are at nutritional risk from dietary problems.
- Children (up to age 5) at nutritional risk from dietary problems.
- Nonbreast-feeding, postpartum women with any nutritional risk.
- Individuals at nutritional risk only because they are homeless or migrants and current participants who would likely continue to have medical and, or dietary problems without WIC assistance.

In most WIC state agencies, participants receive checks or vouchers monthly to purchase specific foods to supplement their usual diets. Each WIC food is high in one or more of the following nutrients: protein, calcium, iron, and vitamins A and C. These nutrients are frequently missing in the diets of the program's low-income target population. Different food packages are provided for different categories of participants. A few WIC state agencies distribute WIC foods through warehouses; some agencies deliver WIC foods to participants.

WIC foods include iron-fortified infant formula and infant cereal, iron-fortified adult cereal, vitamin C-rich fruit and vegetable juice, eggs, milk, cheese, peanut butter, dried beans or peas, tuna fish, and carrots. Special infant formulas and certain medical foods may be provided when prescribed by a physician or health professional for a specified medical condition. The WIC Farmers' Market Nutrition Program, established in 1992, provides additional coupons to WIC participants to use for purchasing fresh fruits and vegetables at participating farmers' markets. The program has two goals: (1) to provide fresh, nutritious, unprepared, locally grown fruits and vegetables from farmers' markets to WIC participants; and (2) to expand consumers' awareness and use of farmers' markets. In 1998, this program was offered in 32 states, the District of Columbia, and 2 Native-American tribal communities.

The WIC program is effective in improving the health of pregnant women, new mothers, and infants. Women who participate in the program during pregnancy have lower Medicaid costs for themselves and their infants compared with women who do not participate. WIC participation is also linked with longer gestation periods, higher birth weights, and lower infant mortality.

Nutrition Program for the Elderly

NPE helps provide elderly adults with nutritionally sound meals through Meals on Wheels programs, or in senior citizen centers and similar congregate feeding settings in which meals provide the focal points for activities that have the dual objective of promoting better health and reducing the isolation that may occur in old age. Age is the only factor used in determining eligibility. People 60 years of age or older and their spouses regardless of age are eligible for NPE benefits. Native-American tribal organizations may select an age below 60 for defining an *older* person for their tribes. Additionally, disabled people who live in elder-care housing facilities, persons who accompany elderly participants to congregate feeding sites, and volunteers who assist in the meal service may also receive meals through NPE.

There is no income requirement to receive meals in the NPE. Each recipient may contribute as much as desired toward the cost of the meal, but meals are free to people who cannot make any contribution. In 1996, more than three million people participated, about one third of whom received benefits through home delivery. The NPE is administered by the Administration on Aging, a component unit of the USDHHS. However, the NPE receives commodity foods and financial support from the USDA's FNS. This program is administered at the state level; therefore the local state distribution agency should be contacted for information about local programs.

NUTRITION SCREENING

Nutrition screening is the process of discovering characteristics or risk factors that are known to be associated with dietary or nutrition problems. The primary purpose of nutrition screening is to identify individuals (such as older adults and the poor) who are potentially at high risk from complex and involved problems that relate to nutrition. To serve this purpose, screening criteria must be simple, relatively straightforward, and easy to administer. Screening is also helpful in establishing priorities for the most efficient use of available and valuable time and money.

The single largest demographic group at disproportionate risk of malnutrition is composed of elderly Americans. Nutrition screening holds a tremendous preventive health potential for older adults. The nurse should provide nutrition counseling or a referral to a registered dietitian for an older person who has food-related problems. A dietitian or community nutrition program might be appropriate if any of the following are identified in the individual:

- Inappropriate, inadequate, or excessive food intake.
- Problems complying with a specialized diet.
- Need for nutrient-specific counseling or counseling related to a specific disease.
- Weight of more than 20% above what is desirable.
- Serum cholesterol level of more than 240 mg/dl.
- Functionally dependent for eating or for food-related activities of daily living.

The health care professional should refer the individual to a physician when there has been an involuntary decrease in weight of more than 10 pounds in the last 6 months. Additional anthropometric measurements suggesting malnutrition include the following:

- Triceps skinfold thickness less than tenth percentile.
- Midarm muscle circumference less than tenth percentile.
- Serum albumin level less than 3.5 g/dl.
- Evidence of osteoporosis or mineral deficiency (indicated by a history of bone pain or fractures, particularly in housebound older women).
- Evidence of vitamin deficiency (indicated by inadequate fruit and vegetable intake; angular stomatitis, glossitis, or bleeding gums; pressure sores in bedridden individuals).

Otherwise healthy older persons can be provided with the *70+ Pyramid*, which they can use as a quick screening tool to assess their own food intake. The pyramid is available on the Internet (http://commentator.tufts.edu/archive/nutrition/pyramid.html).

NUTRITION AND DISEASE

In any assessment of the role that diet plays in the prevention of heart disease, cancers, stroke, and other diseases, an understanding is required that a combination and interaction of environmental, behavioral, social, and genetic factors cause these conditions. The exact number of factors that can be attributed directly to the diet is unknown. Although suggestions are such that dietary factors overall are responsible for at least one third of all cases of cancer and CHD, these estimates are based on interpretations of research studies that cannot distinguish dietary factors completely from genetic, environmental, and behavioral causes. Many dietary components are involved in the relationship between diet and health. Chief among them is the disproportionate consumption of foods high in fats, often at the expense of foods that are rich in the complex carbohydrates and dietary fibers that may be more conducive to health.

This section examines the role of nutrition in the etiology and prevention of the leading nutrition-related chronic diseases—heart disease, stroke, some forms of cancer, osteoporosis, obesity, and type 2 diabetes, and in the early treatment of people who are recently diagnosed with the human immunodeficiency virus.

Each disease discussed contains references to sites to which patients can be referred if they have access to the Internet, or the information can be downloaded to customize education materials.

Understanding the Hispanic culture is particularly important in any review of nutrition and disease in the United States because Hispanics account for about 13% of the people in the United States (35.3 million from the total population of 281.4 million). Hispanic Americans are the largest minority group, exceeding African Americans who account for about 12.9% of the population (Grieco & Cassidy, 2001). Aside from cultural and language barriers, Hispanic Americans challenge the health care industry because they are twice as likely to have diabetes compared with the White population of similar age. Additionally, since 1989, the rate of acquired immune deficiency syndrome among Hispanic Americans has been higher compared with the White population.

Cardiovascular Diseases

Epidemiology

Cardiovascular disease (CVD), principally CHD and stroke, are among the nation's leading killers of both men and women and among all racial and ethnic groups. Approximately one fourth of the nation's population has some form of CVD, including high blood pressure, CHD, and stroke.

Heart Disease

Healthy People 2010 Objectives

- Reduce CHD deaths.
- *12-12*. Reduce the mean total blood cholesterol levels among adults from 206 mg/dL to 199 mg/dL.
- *12-13*. Reduce the proportion of adults with high total blood cholesterol levels.
- *19-8*. Increase the proportion of persons aged 2 years and older who receive less than 10% of calories from saturated fat.
- *19-9*. Increase the proportion of persons aged 2 years and older who receive no more than 30% calories from fat.

Diet Intervention

In an attempt to reduce CVD, the American Hospital Association (AHA) recommends that people over the age of 2 years adopt an overall healthy diet and achieve and maintain an appropriate body weight, cholesterol level, and blood pressure level (Krauss et al., 2000).

To achieve an overall healthy eating pattern, include a variety of fruits, vegetables, grains, low-fat or nonfat dairy products, fish, legumes, poultry, and lean meats. Specifically:

- Choose an overall balanced diet with foods from all major food groups, emphasizing fruits, vegetables and grains.
- Consume a variety of fruits, vegetables, and grain products.
- Consume at least 5 daily servings of fruits and vegetables.
- Consume at least 6 daily servings of grain products, including whole grains.
- Include fat-free and low-fat dairy products, fish, legumes, poultry, and lean meats.
- Eat at least 2 servings of fish every week.

To achieve and maintain an appropriate body weight, match the energy intake to energy needs, with appropriate changes to achieve weight loss when indicated. Specifically:

- Avoid excess intake of calories.
- Maintain a level of physical activity that achieves fitness and that balances energy expenditure with caloric intake; for weight reduction, expenditure should exceed intake.
- Limit foods that are high in calories and low in nutritional quality, including foods with a high amount of added **sugar**.

To achieve and maintain a desirable cholesterol level, limit foods high in saturated fat and cholesterol and substitute unsaturated fat from vegetables, fish, legumes, nuts. Specifically:

- Limit foods with a high content of saturated fat and cholesterol. Substitute these foods with grains and unsaturated fat from vegetables, fish, legumes and nuts.
- Limit cholesterol to 300 mg a day for the general population and 200 mg a day for people with CVD or its risk factors.
- Limit *trans*-fatty acids. *Trans*-fatty acids are found in foods containing partially hydrogenated vegetable oils, such as packaged cookies, crackers, and other baked goods; commercially prepared fried foods; and some margarines.

To achieve and maintain a desirable blood pressure level, limit salt and alcohol, maintain a healthy body weight, and enjoy a diet with emphasis on vegetables, fruits, and low-fat or nonfat dairy products. Specifically:

- Limit salt intake to less than 6 g (2400 mg sodium) per day, slightly more than 1 teaspoon a day.
- If you drink, limit alcohol consumption to no more than 1 drink per day for women and 2 drinks per day for men. A drink is defined as 12 ounces of beer, 5 ounces of wine, or 1.5 ounces of distilled spirits.

Many children, adolescents, and adults who already have undesirable levels of lipids in their blood should receive nutrition counseling when their total **cholesterol** level is elevated. In children ages 2 to 20, an acceptable level of cholesterol is less than 170 mg/dl.

Individuals with LDL cholesterol levels that are above current (2000) National Cholesterol Education Program (NCEP) targets for primary or secondary prevention should be advised to reduce their intake of dietary saturated fat and cholesterol to levels below the levels recommended for the general population. The upper limit for these individuals is less than 7% of the total energy for saturated fat and less than 200 mg of cholesterol per day. In both cases, however, lower intake levels can be of further benefit in reducing LDL cholesterol levels. After the program is outlined, follow-up sessions are scheduled to monitor lipid levels and dietary compliance. In 3 to 6 months, if acceptable lipid levels have not been achieved, then the individual should be referred to a registered dietitian.

The NCEP develops new guidelines periodically, as warranted by research advances. Their first and second guidelines were issued in 1988 and 1993. The most recent set of guidelines was released in 2001: "Third Report of the NCEP Expert Panel on Detection, Evaluation, and Treatment of High Blood Cholesterol in Adults," also known as Adult Treatment Panel (ATP) III. The report appears online at www.nhlbi.nih.gov. The ATP guidelines are expected to result in about 6.5 million Americans being

Table 11-12 ATP-III Classifications of Serum Lipids* in Adults Age 20 and Above

Classification	LDL-Cholesterol, mg/dL	Total Cholesterol, mg/dL	Triglycerides, mg/dL	HDL-Cholesterol, mg/dL
Optimal/desirable	<100	<200	<150	≥60
Near optimal/above normal	100 to 129			
Borderline high	130 to 159	200 to 239	150 to 199	
High	160 to 189		200 to 499	
Very high	≥190	≥240	≥500	
Low				≤40

From Expert Panel on Detection, Evaluation, and Treatment of High Blood Cholesterol in Adults. (2001). Executive summary of the third report of the National Cholesterol Education Program (NCEP) expert panel on detection, evaluation, and treatment of high blood cholesterol in adults (adult treatment panel III). *Journal of the American Medical Association*, 285, 2486-2497.

*Measured in milligrams (mg) of lipid per deciliter (dL) of blood.

treated for high cholesterol through *Therapeutic Lifestyle Changes (TLC)*.

The ATP recommends that healthy adults have a lipoprotein analysis once every 5 years. A lipoprotein profile measures levels of LDL, total cholesterol, HDL, and triglycerides (another fatty substance in the blood). The level at which low HDL becomes a major *risk factor* for heart disease is <40 mg/dl.

In addition to a low HDL, there are other major *risk factors* for developing CHD:

- Clinical forms of atherosclerotic disease (Peripheral arterial disease, abdominal aortic aneurysm, and symptomatic carotid artery disease)
- Age (≥55 for men and ≥65 for women)
- Cigarette smoking
- Hypertension (BP ≥140/90 mmg Hg, or on antihypertension medication)
- Diabetes (fasting glucose 110 mg/dL)
- Family history of premature heart disease (heart disease in a first-degree relative at age ≤55 for men or at age ≤65 for women)
- (HD+L-cholesterol ≥60 counts as a negative risk factor. Its presence removes one risk factor from the total count.)

The "Therapeutic Lifestyle Changes" Treatment Plan

The *TLC* treatment plan of nutrition, physical activity, and weight control is recommended for treating people who present with type 2 diabetes, elevated LDL, and/or metabolic syndrome.

"Metabolic syndrome" describes the presence of a cluster of risk factors that often occur together, which dramatically increase the risk for coronary events. The syndrome is diagnosed when an individual presents with 3 or more of these factors:

- Excessive abdominal fat, as indicated by too large a waist measurement (>35 inches or 88 centimeters in women and >40 inches or 102 centimeters in men)
- Elevated blood pressure (≥130/≥85 mmHg)
- Elevated triglycerides (≥150 mg/dL)
- Low HDL (<40 mg/dL)
- An elevated triglyceride level, which is significantly linked to the degree of heart disease risk. (The guidelines recommend treating even borderline-high triglyceride levels with therapy that includes weight control and physical activity.)

The dietary component of the TLC includes daily intake of:

- Less than 7% of calories from saturated fat
- Less than 200 mg of dietary cholesterol
- Up to 35 percent of calories from total fat, provided most of the fat is from unsaturated fat, which does not raise cholesterol levels. (A higher fat intake may be needed by some patients with high triglycerides and/or a low HDL to keep their tryglycerides or HDL from worsening.)
- Intake of certain foods to boost the diet's LDL-lowering power: 2 g/day of plant stanols and sterols found in cholesterol-lowering margarines and salad dressings, and 10-25 g/day of foods high in soluble fiber, such as cereal grains, beans, peas, legumes, and many fruits and vegetables

A primary treatment goal of the TLC is reducing elevated LDL to:

- >100 mg/dL in the presence of CHD or other forms of atherosclerotic disease
- >130 mg/dL in the presence of 2 or more risk factors for CHD
- >160 mg/dL in the presence of less than 2 risk factors for CHD

The final goal of the TLC includes weight control (to enhance LDL lowering and raise HDL) and physical activity that lasts at least 30 minutes, expending at least 200 kilocalories per day on most days (to improve HDL and, for some, LDL).

Removing Barriers to Compliance

Compiance with the ATP II guidelines of lipid management in patients with coronary artery disease has not been widespread. Barriers to effective lipid management have been identified at numerous levels of interaction between the patient, provider, and health care organizations (Thomas, 1997). To improve patient adherence to ATP III goals, treatment barriers can be eliminated by developing protocols to encourage long-term patient compliance and follow-up, such as establishing clinic policy and developing computerized patient databases, establishing management algorithms, reinforcing and rewarding adherence, and enhancing third party reimbursement.

Patient Education Materials on the Internet

Patient education materials on CVDs can be found at the following web sites:

- American Heart Association Dietary Guidelines At-A-Glance: http://www.americanheart.org/dietaryguidelines/ataglance.html
- "The Healthy Refrigerator": http://www.healthyfridge.org/mainmenu.html
- National Heart, Lung, and Blood Institute. National Cholesterol Education Program, "Live Healthier—Live Longer.": http://rover.nhlbi.nih.gov/chd/
- National Heart, Lung, and Blood Institute. Latino Cardiovascular Health Resources, Bi-Lingual Booklets on Cardiovascular Risk Factors: http://www.nhlbi.nih.gov/health/prof/heart/latino/lat_8pub.htm
- "Heart Information Network": http://www.heartinfo.org/
- The National Heart, Lungs and Blood Institute: http://www.nhlbi.nih.gov

Hypertension

Blood pressure, the force of blood against the walls of arteries, is recorded as stow numbers—the systolic pressure (as the heart beats) over the diastolic pressure (as the heart relaxes between beats). The measurement is written one above (or before) the other, with the systolic number on top and the diastolic number on the bottom. For example, a blood pressure measurement of 120/80 mm Hg (millimeters of mercury) is expressed verbally as "120 over 80." Normal blood pressure is less than 130 mm Hg systolic and less than 85 mm Hg diastolic. Optimal blood pressure is less than 120 mm Hg systolic and less than 80 mm Hg diastolic.

Epidemiology

Hypertension (high blood pressure) killed 42,565 Americans in 1997 and contributed to the deaths of approximately 210,000 people. As many as 50 million Americans aged 6 and older have high blood pressure, which represents 20% of the total population and 25% of all adults in the United States (based on National Health and Nutrition Examination Survey [NHANES] III data). Of the 50 million people, only two thirds know they have high blood pressure, and of these, only about one fourth receive adequate therapy (diet alone or diet and drugs). Untreated, hypertension can damage arteries and increase a risk for stroke and congestive heart failure. High blood pressure is also responsible for many cases of kidney failure requiring dialysis and increases the risk of kidney failure in diabetics.

Blacks and Hispanic Americans are more likely to suffer from high blood pressure compared with Whites. Additionally, people with lower educational and income levels tend to have higher levels of blood pressure. In 1997, the death rates per 100,000 population from high blood pressure were 14.0 for White men, 50.2 for Black men, 12.8 for White women, and 40.6 for Black women, adjusted to the year 2000 standard (American Heart Association, 2000) (Table 11-13).

Healthy People 2010 Objectives

- *12-7.* Reduce stroke deaths.
- 12-9. Reduce the proportion of adults with high blood pressure.
- *12-11.* Increase the proportion of adults with high blood pressure who are taking action (losing weight and reducing sodium intake).
- *19-10.* Increase the proportion of persons aged 2 years and older who consume 2400 mg or less of sodium daily.

Diet Intervention

The modifiable nutrition-related risk factors for stroke include obesity, habitual high alcohol intake, and high intake of sodium. No certain method exists for identifying susceptible people or ascertaining how many of them become hypertensive as a result of excessive salt intake; therefore the conservative preventive health approach recommends a salt intake limited to 6 g or less per day for adults. Sodium chloride is approximately 40% sodium by weight; therefore a diet with 6 g salt contains about *2.4 g of sodium*. This amount is regarded as *mild sodium restriction*. Table 11-14 lists the approximate sodium content of representative foods.

Table 11-13 Categories for Blood Pressure Levels in Adults Age 18 Years and Older*

Category	Blood Pressure Level (mm Hg)	
Systolic	Diastolic	
Optimal	<120	<80
Normal	<130	<85
High Normal	130 to 139	85 to 89
High Blood Pressure (mm Hg)**		
Stage 1	140 to 159	90 to 99
Stage 2	160 to 179	100 to 109
Stage 3	≥180	≥110

From National Institutes of Health, National Heart, Lung, and Blood Institute, National High Blood Pressure Education Program. (1977, Nov.). *The sixth report of the joint national committee on prevention, detection, evaluation, and treatment of high blood pressure* (p. 11). NIH Publication No. 98-4080. Washington, DC: National Institutes of Health.
*For those not taking medicine for high blood pressure and not having a short-term serious illness. These categories are from the National High Blood Pressure Education Program.
**Based on the average of 2 or more readings taken at each of 2 or more visits after an initial screening.

The three major sources of sodium in the U.S. diet are:

1. Salt added by consumers to food during cooking or at the table.
2. Salt added by food-processing companies as an ingredient in almost all processed foods (including many foods that do not taste salty, such as baked goods). Most processed foods are high in sodium content.
3. Salt from all animal products, which are a natural source of sodium.

The following recommended food tips are designed to reduce salt and sodium intake:

- Sodium occurs naturally in many foods and is also added to most processed foods; therefore salt should be used only sparingly in home cooking and at the table.
- Consume fewer foods that tend to be higher in sodium, such as many cheeses, processed meats, most frozen dinners and entrees, packaged mixes, most canned soups and vegetables, salad dressings, and condiments such as soy sauce, pickles, olives, catsup, and mustard.
- Before warming canned vegetables, rinse them first.
- Salty, highly processed salty, salt-preserved, and salt-pickled foods should be eaten sparingly.
- Check labels for the amount of sodium in foods and choose products lower in sodium when (Fig. 11-3).

According to the study presented in the Research Highlights box, the DASH eating plan makes consuming less salt and sodium easier because the plan includes abundant fruits and vegetables, which are lower in sodium compared with other foods. The DASH clinical study found that elevated blood pressure can be reduced with an eating plan low in saturated fat, total fat, and cholesterol and rich in fruits, vegetables, and low-fat dairy foods. The plan is rich in magnesium, potassium, calcium, and protein and fiber. The amounts of the nutrients vary by caloric intake. At approximately 2000 calories a day, the nutrients include 4700 mg of potassium, 500 mg of magnesium, and 1240 mg of calcium. These totals are approximately 2 to 3 times the amounts most Americans receive.

When blood pressure is normal, the DASH eating plan may help avoid blood pressure problems. If blood pressure is only slightly elevated, then the plan may actually eliminate the need for medication. For more severe high blood pressure, the plan may allow a reduction in medication. Other steps to control or prevent hypertension should continue to be encouraged, including exercising, losing excess weight, not smoking, and limiting alcohol. DASH may improve health in other ways also. Fruits and vegetables may reduce the risk for some cancers; the calcium in dairy products can lower risk for osteoporosis; and a diet low in saturated fat and cholesterol can reduce cardiovascular disease risk.

Patient Education Materials on the Internet

Patient education materials about stroke can be found at the following web sites:

- U.S. Department of Agriculture, "Sodium Content of

Table 11-14 Sodium Content of Food

Food Group	High	MgNa	Low	MgNa
Grain products	English muffin	300	White rice, 1 cup	6
	Waffle, 1 frozen	275	Popcorn, 3 cups	3
	Potato chips, 10	200	Puffed rice, 2 cups	2
	White bread, 1 slice	115	Oatmeal, 3/4 cup	1
	Saltine crackers, 2	70	Wheat germ, toasted, 1/4 cup	1
Meat, poultry, and fish	Herring, 3 oz smoked	5235	Codfish, 3 oz	65
	Frankfurter, 1 oz	310	Chicken, 3 oz	60
	Ham, 3 oz baked	280	Beef, 3 oz	55
	Bacon, 2 strips	275	Turkey, 3 oz	50
	Bologna, 1 slice	220		
	Scallops, 3 oz	215		
	Lobster, 3 oz	180		
	Shrimp, 3 oz	115		
Dairy products	Cottage cheese, 1/2 cup	460	Yogurt, 1/2 cup, frozen	60
	American cheese, 1 slice	405	Ricotta, 1 oz, whole milk	24
	Buttermilk, 1 cup	240	Cottage cheese, 1/2 cup dry curd	10
	Gouda cheese, 1 oz	230		
	Cheddar cheese, 1 oz	175		
	Yogurt, 1 cup lowfat	175		
	Milk, 1 cup	120		
	Butter, 1 tbsp	100		
Fruits and vegetables	Sauerkraut, 1 cup	1555	All fresh fruits	0 to 20
	Mushrooms, 1 cup, canned	800	Brussels sprouts, 1 cup	15
	Spinach, 1 cup canned	780	Mushrooms, 1 cup, fresh	10
	Creamed corn, 1 cup canned	670	Potato, 1 medium	5
	Tomato juice, 1 cup	500	Corn, 1 cup, fresh or frozen	2
	Tomatoes, 1 cup canned	430		
	Peas, 1 cup, canned	490		
	Corn, 1 cup, canned, whole kernel	385		
	Celery, 1 cup, diced	130		
	Orange drink, 1 cup	80		
	Lemonade, 1 cup	60		
Miscellaneous	Garlic salt, 1 tsp	1850	Peanuts, 1 cup unsalted	8
	Dill pickle, 1 large	1430	Jam or jelly, 1 tbsp	2
	Soy sauce, 1 tbsp	1030	Vinegar, 1/2 cup	1
	Baking soda, 1 tsp	1000	Lemon juice, 1 tbsp	1
	Olives, 10 small green	685	Yeast, 1 pkg dry	1
	MSG, 1 tbsp	490	Honey, 1 tbsp	1
	Bouillon, 1 cube	425	Garlic powder, 1 tsp	1
	Baking powder, 1 tsp	370	Vegetable oil, 1 tbsp	0
	Catsup, 2 tbsp	355		
	Margarine, 1 tbsp	135		

Heart Healthy Foods": http://www.nhlbi.nih.gov/health/public/heart/chol/sbs-chol/sodium.htm

- National Heart, Lung, and Blood Institute, "Your Guide to Lowering High Blood Pressure": http://www.nhlbi.nih.gov/hbp/consumer/consumer.html
- "Search in the NHLBI web site." Go to: http://www.nhlbi.nih.gov/search/index.htm and enter the letters DASH.

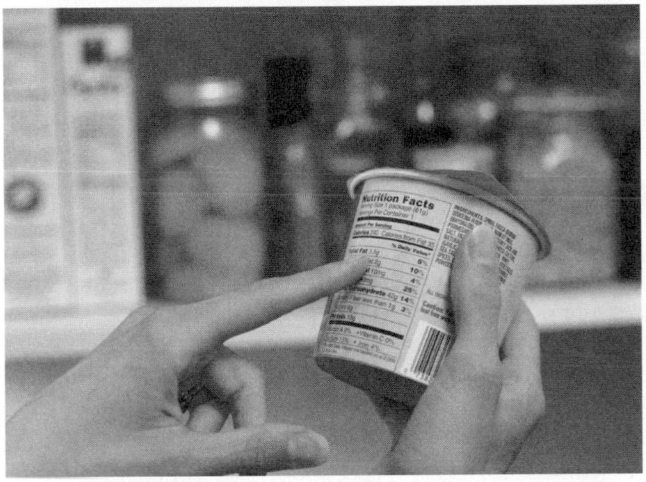

Fig. 11-3 Sodium content is given on the nutrition label. An individual cannot rely on taste to determine the amount of sodium in foods.

Cancer

Epidemiology

In 2000, approximately 1,220,100 cases of **cancer** were diagnosed in the United States and approximately 552,200 Americans died of this disease. Overall, Blacks are more likely to develop cancer compared with persons of any other racial and ethnic group. During the period from 1990 to 1996, incidence rates were 442.9 per 100,000 among Blacks, 402.9 per 100,000 among Whites, 275.4 per 100,000 among Hispanic Americans, 279.1 per 100,000 among Asian Americans, and 153.4 per 100,000 among Native Americans. During these same years, cancer incidence rates decreased among Whites (down 1.2% per year), Hispanic Americans (down 1.7% per year), and Native Americans (down 0.7% per year), and remained relatively stable among Blacks and Asian Americans. The incidence rate of breast cancer in women is highest among White women (113.2 per 100,000) and lowest among Native-American women (33.9 per 100,000). Black women have the highest incidence rates of colon and rectum cancer (44.9 per 100,000) and lung and bronchus cancer (46.2 per 100,000) followed by Whites, Asian Americans, Hispanic Americans, and Native Americans.

Blacks are approximately 33% more likely to die of cancer than Whites and are 2 times more likely to die of cancer than Asian Americans, Native Americans, and

research highlights

Dietary Approaches to Stop Hypertension (DASH)

This research is supported by grants from the NHLBI, the Office of Research on Minority Health, and the National Center for Research Resources of the NIH. From the disproportionate burden of hypertension in minority populations, particularly among Blacks, one of the goals of the trial was to recruit a cohort in which two thirds of the subjects were members of a racial or ethnic minority.

Methodology: This study was a multicenter, randomized controlled, clinical trial of three experimental diets given to 459 adult participants (approximately half of whom were women and 60% were Black). All three diet plans contained about 3000 mg of sodium daily (approximately 20% below the U.S. average for adults). None of the plans was vegetarian or used specialty foods.

For 3 weeks, the subjects consumed a control diet that was low in fruits, vegetables, and dairy products, with a fat content typical of the average diet in the United States. The subjects were then randomly assigned for 8 weeks to receive the control diet; or a diet rich in fruits and vegetables; or the DASH eating plan, rich in fruits, vegetables, and low-fat dairy products with reduced saturated and total fat. All food for the experimental diets was provided to the participants. Body weights of participants were maintained at constant levels.

Results: At baseline, the mean systolic and diastolic (SD) blood pressures were 131.3 ± 10.8 mmHg and 84.7 ± 4.7 mmHg, respectively. DASH reduced SD blood pressure by 5.5 and 3.0 mmHg more, respectively, compared with the control diet; the fruits-and-vegetables diet reduced systolic blood pressure by 2.8 mmHg more and diastolic blood pressure by 1.1 mmHg more than the control diet. Among the 133 subjects with hypertension (systolic pressure greater than or equal to 140 mmHg, diastolic pressure greater than or equal to 90 mmHg, or both), the combination diet reduced SD blood pressure by 11.4 and 5.5 mmHg more, respectively, compared with the control diet; among the 326 subjects without hypertension, the corresponding reductions were 3.5 mmHg (P less than 0.001) and 2.1 mmHg. All results are statistically significant

Clinical application: Both the fruit-and-vegetable and DASH plans reduced blood pressure, but DASH had the greater effect, reducing blood pressure by an average of 6 mmHg for systolic and 3 mmHg for diastolic. The DASH plan worked even better for people with high blood pressure (on average, the systolic dropped 11 mmHg and the diastolic dropped approximately 6 mmHg). Furthermore, the reductions came quickly (within 2 weeks of starting the eating plan). The dietary patterns are constructed with commonly consumed food items; therefore the positive results may be conveniently implemented in dietary recommendations to the general public.

Based on Appel, L. J., et al. (1997). A clinical trial of the effects of dietary patterns on blood pressure. DASH Collaborative Research Group. *New England Journal of Medicine*, 336, 1117-1124.

Hispanic Americans. During the period from 1990 to 1996, cancer mortality rates were 223.4 per 100,000 among Blacks, 167.5 per 100,000 among Whites, 104.9 per 100,000 among Hispanic Americans, 103.4 per 100,000 among Asian Americans, and 104.0 per 100,000 among Native Americans. Cancer mortality rates for many racial and ethnic groups have begun to decline recently. During the period from 1990 to 1996, mortality rates decreased among Whites (down 0.5% per year), Blacks (down 0.9% per year), and Hispanic Americans (down 0.6% per year); remained relatively stable among Asian Americans; and increased slightly among Native Americans (0.9% per year). Black women are more likely to die of breast cancer (31.4 per 100,000) and colon and rectum cancer (20.0 per 100,000) compared with women of any other racial and ethnic group (ACS, 2000b).

Approximately 40% of cancer incidence among men and 60% among women is related to diet. The introduction of a healthy diet and exercise practices at any time from childhood to old age can promote health and likely reduce cancer risk.

Diet Intervention for Risk Reduction

Many dietary factors can affect cancer risk: types of foods, food preparation methods, portion sizes, food variety, and overall caloric balance. An overall dietary pattern that includes a high proportion of plant foods (fruits, vegetables, grains, and beans), limited amounts of meat, dairy, and other high-fat foods, and a balance of caloric intake and physical activity can reduce the risk of cancer. The associations between diet and cancer causation are summarized in Table 11-15.

Based on its review of the scientific evidence, the American Cancer Society (ACS) updated its nutrition guidelines in 1999. The ACS recommendations are consistent in principle with the Food Guide Pyramid, the Dietary Guidelines for Americans, and dietary recommendations of other agencies for general health promotion and for the prevention of coronary heart disease, diabetes, and other diet-related chronic conditions. Although no diet can guarantee full protection against any disease, the ACS believes that the following recommendations offer the best nutrition information currently available to help Americans.

Choose Most of the Foods You Eat from Plant Sources. Eat 5 or more servings of fruits and vegetables every day; eat other foods from plant sources, such as breads, cereals, grain products, rice, pasta, or beans several times every day. Many scientific studies show that eating fruits and vegetables (especially green and dark yellow vegetables, foods in the cabbage family, soy products, and legumes) can protect against cancers at many sites, particularly for cancers of the gastrointestinal and respiratory tracts. Grains are an important source of many vitamins and minerals, such as folate, calcium, and selenium, which have been associated with a lower risk of colon cancer in some studies. Beans (legumes) are especially rich in nutrients that may protect against cancer.

Since 1991, the *5 A Day for Better Health Program* has raised public awareness about the importance of fruits and vegetables in disease prevention. The program is jointly sponsored by the NCI (a division of the USDHHS) and the Produce for Better Health Foundation (a nonprofit consumer education foundation representing the fruit and vegetable industry). Through its unique national public-private partnership, 5 A Day seeks to increase consumption of fruits and vegetables to 5 or more servings each day. The national 5 A Day for Better Health Program gives Americans a simple, positive message: eat 5 or more servings of fruits and vegetables every day for better health.

In *The New American Plate*, the American Institute for Cancer Research (AICR) recommends reducing meat, fish, or chicken to 3 ounces and filling the dinner plate with dishes composed of vegetables, fruits, whole grains, and beans. The program urges people to reverse the traditional American plate and think of meat as a side dish or condiment rather than the primary ingredient. In terms that laypersons can understand, this regimen translates into vegetables, fruits, whole grains, and beans covering two thirds (or more) of the plate, with animal-source foods covering one third (or less) (AICR, 2000).

The NCI recommends that adult diets contain 20 g to 30 g of **fiber** daily (not to exceed 35 g because of possible adverse effects). Typical diets in the United States contain approximately 11 g of fiber. The recommended fiber intake is proportionately lower for children. The recommended fiber intake for children older than 2 years of age can be determined by using the handy formula *age plus 5* (add 5 g of fiber per day to the child's age in years) (Williams, 1995; Williams, Boellella, & Wynder, 1995). Therefore the dietary fiber recommendation for an 8-year-old child is 13 g of fiber per day (8 + 5 = 13). If the child needs more fiber resulting from obesity or hypercholesterolemia, then the

Table 11-15 Associations Between Diet and Cancer

Cancer Site	Dietary Factors
Esophagus	Alcohol (especially with tobacco)
Stomach	Salt-preserved foods; low levels of fruits and vegetables
Colon and rectum	Fat (particularly saturated); low vegetable intake
Liver	Alcohol
Lung	Greens and yellow vegetables believed to be protective
Breast	High-calorie diet (high fat and low fiber suspected)
Endometrium	Diet-related diseases, such as obesity, hypertension, type 2 diabetes
Bladder	Unknown
Prostate	High-fat diets

fiber recommendation may be calculated by adding as much as 10 g to the child's age (age plus 10), which is 18 grams of fiber for an 8-year-old child. By the time a child reaches the age of 18, the fiber recommendation becomes 23 g per day, which is within the range of intake recommended by the NCI. Foods that are high in fiber are usually low in fat; the only source of fiber-containing foods is the plant kingdom. Table 11-16 lists the fiber content of some common foods.

Guidelines for reducing the risk of breast cancer include recommendations for breast self-examination, stress reduction, physical activity, weight control, and diet (Wood & Spark, 1996).

Limit Intake of High-Fat Foods, Particularly from Animal Sources. Choose foods low in fat and limit consumption of meats, especially high-fat meats. High-fat diets have been associated with an increased risk of cancers of the colon and rectum, prostate, and endometrium. The association between high-fat diets and the risk of breast cancer is weaker. Whether these associations are caused by the total amount of fat, the particular type of fat (saturated, monounsaturated, or polyunsaturated), the calories contributed by fat, or by some other factor in food fats has not been determined. Consumption of meat, particularly red meat, has been associated with an increased risk of cancer at several sites, most notably the colon and prostate.

Be Physically Active: Achieve and Maintain a Healthy Weight. Physical activity can help protect against some cancers either by balancing caloric intake with energy expenditure or by other mechanisms. An imbalance of caloric intake and energy output can lead to being overweight or obese and an increased risk for cancers at several sites, such as the colon and rectum, prostate, endometrium, breast (among postmenopausal women), and kidney. Both physical activity and controlled caloric intake are necessary to achieve or maintain a healthy body weight.

Limit Consumption of Alcoholic Beverages. Alcoholic beverages, along with cigarette smoking and the use of snuff and chewing tobacco, cause cancers of the oral cavity, esophagus, and larynx. The combined use of tobacco and alcohol leads to a greatly increased risk of oral and esophageal cancers; the effect of tobacco and alcohol combined is greater than the sum of their individual effects. Studies also have shown an association between alcohol consumption and an increased risk of breast cancer. The mechanism of this effect is not known, but the association may be related to carcinogenic actions of alcohol or its metabolites, to alcohol-induced changes in levels of hormones such as estrogens, or to some other process. Regardless of the mechanism, studies show that the risk of breast cancer increases with an intake beginning at only a few drinks per week. Reducing alcohol consumption is a good way for women who drink regularly to reduce their risk of breast cancer (ACS, 2000a).

Guidelines for reducing the risk of breast cancer include recommendations for breast self-examination, stress reduction, physical activity, weight control, and diet (Wood & Spark, 1996) (Box 11-5).

Table 11-16 Fiber Content of Food

Grams	Food
16 to 20	1 cup baked beans; 1 cup chili with beans
10 to 15	1/3 cup All Bran with extra fiber; 1 cup fresh blackberries
8 to 9	1/3 cup All Bran; 1/2 cup stewed prunes; 1/4 cup dried apricots
5 to 7	1/4 cup shelled almonds; 1 cup lentil soup; 1/2 cup cooked spinach; 1 cup fresh blueberries; 1/2 cup homemade granola
3 to 4	1 small sweet potato or medium baked potato with skin; 1 medium banana, apple, or nectarine; 1 cup fresh raspberries, strawberries, or pineapple chunks; 1/2 cup canned corn or peas; 1/2 cup garbanzo beans (chickpeas) or lima beans; 1/2 cup cooked broccoli or eggplant; 1/4 cup shelled peanuts; 1/2 cup bran cereal; 4 Rye Crisp crackers or 1 oz Kavli, Wasa, Triscuit, or finn crackers; 3 cups popcorn
2 to 3	1 medium tomato or carrot; 1 slice whole wheat bread; 1 small orange or pear; 1/2 cup applesauce or fruit cocktail; 1/4 cup shredded coconut; 1 cup grapefruit sections; 2 tbsp peanut butter; 1/2 cup cabbage; 1/2 cup cooked brown rice; 1/4 cup sunflower seeds; 1tbsp tahini; 1 cup New England clam chowder
1 to 2	1/2 cup cooked white rice; 1/2 cup cooked cauliflower; 2 stalks celery; 1/6 head lettuce; 10 grapes or 1 cup grape juice; 1 plum; 1 cup vegetable juice cocktail; 10 green olives; 1 cup Manhattan clam chowder
>1	1 slice white bread or 1 bagel; 1 cup pineapple juice; dill pickle; 1 cup tomato soup
0	Milk, yogurt, cheese, ice cream, meat, fish, poultry; butter, margarine, mayonnaise, oil

Patient Education Materials on the Internet

Patient education materials about cancer can be found at the following web sites:

- American Institute for Cancer Research, Full-text booklets and brochures: http://www.aicr.org/form1.htm
- National Cancer Institute. National Institutes of Health, Full-text publications: http://www.5aday.gov/5adaymaterials.htm

Osteoporosis

Epidemiology

In the United States, 10 million individuals have osteoporosis and 18 million more people have low bone mineral density (BMD), placing them at increased risk for this disorder. Of the people with hip fractures, 20% die

Box 11-5 Decreasing the Risk for Breast Cancer

PHYSICAL EXAMINATION

- Perform a breast self-examination monthly.
- Obtain a mammogram every 1 to 2 years.

STRESS

- Take at least 15 minutes for yourself each day.
- Learn to say no.
- Get 8 hours of uninterrupted sleep every night.

PHYSICAL ACTIVITY

- Move the body daily while participating in an enjoyable activity.
- Participate in an aerobic activity (take a brisk walk) 3 to 4 times a week.

WEIGHT CONTROL

- Determine your healthy weight.
- When needing to lose weight, decrease daily caloric intake by 250 calories and exercise 25 to 50 minutes each day; ideally, lose one half pound each week.
- When needing to gain weight, increase daily caloric intake by 250 calories (1 serving each of low-fat milk, fruit, and grain) and participate in strength training 3 to 4 times a week to increase muscle mass; ideally, gain one quarter to one half pound each week.

DIET

- Drink at least 8 glasses of water daily.
- Learn to read food labels to make lower fat choices; reduce fat to 20% of daily calories.
- Use olive, canola, or peanut oil rather than corn, sunflower, or safflower oil; choose butter rather than margarine.
- Substitute low-fat dairy, fish, or vegetable dishes for some of the meat meals (spaghetti marinara, bean burritos, vegetable lasagna, or *vegiburgers*).
- Add some soy products to the diet (use soy flour to make muffins); soy products may inhibit tumor growth.
- Eat at least five different types of fruits and vegetables; fruits contain nature's cancer fighters (antioxidants, phytoestrogens and other phytochemicals, and fiber).
- Do not consume excessive amounts of vitamins unless a medical condition requires additional supplements; a low-cost multivitamin and mineral supplement is sufficient. (One tablet is sufficient.)
- Before going to bed each night, take a calcium supplement of at least 500 mg (1000 mg if not consuming dairy products); calcium supplements will aid in more sound sleep.

FRUITS AND VEGETABLES THAT MAY PROVIDE PROTECTION AGAINST CANCER

	CONTAINS FIBER	CONTAINS VITAMIN A OR C	CONTAINS PHYTOCHEMICALS, ANTIOXIDANTS, OR OTHER ANTICANCER AGENTS NATURALLY PRESENT IN FOOD
Fruits			
Avocado	X	X	
Apple	X	X	
Apricot	X	X	
Blueberries			X
Blackberries	X		X
Cantaloupe	X	X	X
Cranberries	X		X
Grapefruit		X	X
Grapes	X		X
Kiwi	X	X	
Oranges		X	
Papaya	X	X	
Prunes	X	X	
Red grapes	X		
Raspberries	X		
Strawberries		X	
Watermelon			X
Vegetables			
Artichoke	X	X	
Bell pepper	X	X	
Beets	X		X
Broccoli	X	X	X
Brussel sprouts	X	X	X
Cabbage	X	X	X
Carrot	X	X	X
Cauliflower	X	X	X
Celery	X	X	
Corn	X		X
Eggplant			X
Kale	X	X	X
Kidney beans	X		
Onions	X	X	X
Potato	X	X	
Iceberg lettuce	X		
Radishes			X
Spinach		X	X
Sweet potato	X	X	
Soybeans	X		X
Tomato	X	X	X
Winter squash	X	X	X
Yellow pepper		X	X

Based on Wood, O., & Spark, A. (1996). Medical nutrition therapy guidelines for treating the breast cancer patient. *Journal of the American Dietetic Association*, 96 (Suppl), A-35.

within a year, and half of the survivors never walk again. Direct financial expenditures for treatment alone of osteoporotic fracture are estimated at $10 billion to $15 billion annually. These figures underestimate significantly the true costs of osteoporosis because they fail to include the costs of treatment for individuals without a history of fractures or the indirect costs of lost wages or productivity of either the individual or the caregiver.

The prevalence of osteoporosis and the incidence of fracture vary by gender and race-ethnicity. The probability that a 50-year-old individual will have a hip fracture during a lifetime is 14% for a White woman and 5% to 6% for a White man. The risk for Blacks is much lower at 6% and 3% for 50-year-old woman and man, respectively.

- White, postmenopausal women comprise almost 75% of all hip fractures and have the highest age-adjusted fracture incidence.
- Black women have higher BMD compared with White women throughout life and they experience lower hip fracture rates.
- Some Japanese women have lower peak BMD compared with White women, but they have a lower hip fracture rate, the reasons for which are not fully understood.
- Hispanic-American women have bone densities intermediate between those of White women and Black women.
- Limited available information on Native-American women suggests they have lower BMD compared with White women.

Healthy People 2010 *Objectives*

Goal: prevent illness and disability related to arthritis and other rheumatic conditions, osteoporosis, and chronic back conditions.

- *2-9*. Reduce the overall number of cases of osteoporosis as measured by low total femur BMD.
- *19-11*. Increase the proportion of individuals aged 2 years and older who meet dietary recommendations for calcium.

Pathophysiology

Osteoporosis is a slowly developing condition that causes loss of bone mass and increased fractures, especially in the wrist, hip, and spinal areas. **Osteoporosis** is defined as a skeletal disorder characterized by *compromised bone strength predisposing to an increased risk of fracture*. Bone strength reflects the integration of two main features: (1) bone density and (2) bone quality. Bone density is expressed as grams of mineral per area or volume and, in any given individual, is determined by peak bone mass and amount of bone loss. Bone quality refers to architecture, turnover, damage accumulation (microfractures), and mineralization. A fracture occurs when a trauma is applied to osteoporotic bone; therefore osteoporosis is a significant risk factor for fracture.

Osteoporosis may be the result of bone loss that commonly occurs as men and women age. However, an individual who does not reach optimal (peak) bone mass during childhood and adolescence may develop osteoporosis without the occurrence of accelerated bone loss. Therefore *suboptimal bone growth in childhood and adolescence is as important as bone loss is to the development of osteoporosis*.

The consequences of osteoporosis include financial, physical, and psychosocial aspects, which significantly affect the individual, the family, and community. An osteoporotic fracture is a tragic outcome of a traumatic event in the presence of compromised bone strength and its incidence is increased by various other risk factors. Traumatic events can range from high-impact falls to normal lifting and bending. The incidence of fracture is high in individuals with osteoporosis and increases with age.

Osteoporotic fractures, particularly vertebral fractures, can be associated with chronic disabling pain. Nearly one third of patients with hip fractures are discharged to nursing homes within the year following a fracture. Notably, 1 in 5 patients is no longer living 12 months after sustaining an osteoporotic hip fracture. Hip and vertebral fractures are a problem for women in their late 70s and 80s, wrist fractures are a problem in the late 50s to early 70s, and all other fractures (including pelvic and rib fractures) are a problem throughout the postmenopausal years.

Hip fracture has a profound effect on quality of life: adverse effects on physical health (effect of skeletal deformity) and on financial resources. An osteoporotic fracture is associated with increased difficulty in activities of daily life because only one third of fracture patients regain prefracture level of function and one third require nursing home placement. Fear, anxiety, and depression are frequently reported in women with established osteoporosis and these consequences are likely underaddressed when considering the overall effect of this condition (Box 11-6).

Men also get osteoporosis and 20% of American men will suffer at least one fracture because their bones have become too thin and weak to withstand the normal stresses of life. One third of the people with hip fractures die within 1 year from complications of the fracture or its treatment. A total of 1.5 million men in the United States already have osteoporosis and 3.5 million more men are at high risk of developing the condition. Men are especially at risk when they have testosterone levels that are low enough to cause impotence and an absence of nocturnal emissions. As with women, lifestyle factors are important contributors; that is, a lifetime of inadequate amounts of calcium and vitamin D.

Factors Involved in Building and Maintaining Skeletal Health Throughout Life. Growth in bone size and strength occurs during childhood, but bone accumulation is not completed until the third decade of life, after the cessation of linear growth. *The bone mass attained early in life is perhaps the most important determinant of lifelong skeletal health*. Individuals with the highest peak bone mass after adolescence have the greatest protective advantage when the inevitable declines in bone density associated with increasing age, illness, and diminished sex-steroid production take their toll.

Genetic factors exert a strong and perhaps predominant influence on peak bone mass, but physiological, environmental, and modifiable lifestyle factors can also play a significant role. Among these factors are adequate nutrition and body weight, exposure to sex hormones at puberty, and physical activity. Therefore maximizing BMD early in life

Box 11-6 Risk Factors for Developing Osteoporosis

PREDICTORS OF LOW BMD

- *Gender.* Women are more at risk than are men. Both men and women experience an age-related decline in BMD starting in midlife, but women experience more rapid bone loss in the early years following menopause, which places them at earlier risk for fractures.
- *Age.* After reaching a peak bone mass in the third or fourth decade of life, all individuals gradually lose bone mass. Decreasing bone mass produces a weaker bone structure that is more susceptible to osteoporotic fractures.
- *Low BMD.* This value is one of the strongest predictors of osteoporosis.
- *Early menopause (before 40 years of age).* The early occurrence of menopause, by natural or surgical means, results in shorter exposure to the protective effect of estrogen.
- *Thin, small-framed body.* A petite, thin person may have a relatively low peak bone mass.
- *Race.* Whites and Asian Americans develop more osteoporosis than do Blacks. Blacks have heavier bone density and Black women have about one half the incidence of hip fractures compared with White women.
- *Lack of physical activity.* Immobilized, bedridden, or extremely inactive individuals may have low muscle and bone mass.
- *Family history of osteoporosis*
- *Cigarette smoking*
- *Dietary excesses of fiber, caffeine, alcohol, and/or protein*
- *Residents of nursing homes and other long-term care facilities.* Most residents have low BMD and a high prevalence of other risk factors for fracture, including advanced age, poor physical function, low muscle strength, and decreased cognition and high rates of dementia, poor nutrition, and often, use of multiple medications.

presents a critical opportunity to reduce the effect of bone loss related to aging. Childhood is also a critical time for the development of lifestyle habits conducive to maintaining good bone health throughout life. Additionally, cigarette smoking, which usually starts in adolescence, may have a deleterious effect on achieving bone mass.

Prevention

Once thought to be a natural part of aging among women, osteoporosis is no longer considered age- or gender-dependent and is largely preventable thanks to the recent progress in the understanding of its causes, diagnosis, and treatment. Optimization of bone health is a process that must occur throughout the lifespan in both men and women. Factors that enhance bone health at all ages are essential to prevent osteoporosis and its devastating consequences. *Calcium is the specific nutrient most important for attaining peak bone mass and for preventing and treating osteoporosis.*

Good nutrition is essential for normal growth. A balanced diet, adequate calories, and appropriate nutrients are the foundation developing all tissues, including bone. Adequate and appropriate nutrition is important for all individuals, but not everyone follows a diet that is optimal for bone health.

Sufficient data that recommend specific dietary calcium intakes at various stages of life include:

- Young children, 3 to 8 years: 800 mg per day.
- Children and adolescents, 9 to 17 years: 1300 mg per day. (Only 25% of boys and 10% of girls meet these recommendations. Supplementation of calcium and vitamin D may be necessary. Excessive pursuit of thinness in particular may affect adequate nutrition and bone health.)
- Adults: 1000 to 1500 mg per day (only 50% to 60% meets this recommendation).

Factors contributing to low calcium intakes are restriction of dairy products, a generally low level of fruit and vegetable consumption, and a high intake of low-calcium beverages, such as soft drinks. Lactose and vitamin D enhance calcium absorption and exercise enhances calcium balance. Calcium is absorbed best from dairy foods, which are the only source of the disaccharide lactose.

Vitamin D is synthesized in the body when the skin is exposed to the ultraviolet rays of the sun. Commonly added to milk, other food sources of vitamin D include fatty fish (salmon and mackerel), margarine, eggs, and some fortified, ready-to-eat cereals. Most infants and young children in the United States have adequate vitamin D intake from the supplementation and fortification of milk. During adolescence, when consumption of dairy products decreases, vitamin D intake is likely to be inadequate, which may affect calcium absorption adversely. Elderly people may be at risk for suboptimal levels of vitamin D when they do not drink milk or when they are housebound or institutionalized and do not get sufficient exposure to the sun (20 minutes a day with hands and face exposed) (Ryan, Eleazer, & Egbert, 1995). A recommended vitamin D intake of 5 to 15 μg per day has been established for adults *who are not exposed to sunlight.*

Other nutrients have been evaluated relative to bone health. High dietary protein, caffeine, phosphorus, and sodium can adversely affect calcium balance; however, their effects appear to be unimportant in individuals with adequate calcium intakes.

Food should be selected to provide adequate calcium, with special attention to adolescents, who normally have high mineral requirements, and women who are susceptible to inadequate dietary calcium because of low caloric intake. Women of all ages should be concerned about adequate calcium intake. A means for increasing individual consumption of calcium includes educating consumers to eat more calcium-rich foods, including calcium-fortified foods such as orange juice, and recommending dietary supplements. Individuals who wish to increase their calcium can consume more low-fat or nonfat dairy products or fortified food products. Taking calcium tablets may be appropriate for people at high risk of health problems from inadequate calcium intake.

Although maintaining a proper daily calcium intake through food is preferable, calcium supplements are available for people who do not get enough of the mineral through their regular diet. Calcium carbonate (40% elemental calcium), calcium citrate (24%), calcium lactate (14%), and calcium gluconate (9%) are preferred. (Dolomite and bone meal are not recommended because they may be contaminated with lead.) Calcium supplement absorption is most efficient at individual doses no greater than 500 mg when taken between meals for individuals with adequate gastric acid production.

The mandate is clear for nursing professionals interested in preventive health: encourage increased consumption of calcium-rich foods. Milk and dairy products deliver the most calcium of any food group, but they are also among the richest sources of fat in the American diet. Low-fat and fat-free milk, yogurt, and low-fat cheeses are the dairy products of choice. Other good sources of calcium include sardines, canned salmon (if the bones are eaten), and some dark green leafy vegetables, especially collard greens. Orange juice and milk fortified with calcium are also good sources. The calcium content of some common foods is summarized in Table 11-17.

Anyone under 25 years of age whose intake is less than the recommended intake of calcium should be urged to develop strategies for increasing calcium. Children, particularly preadolescent girls, should take care to receive the proper amount. By modeling appropriate behaviors, health care professionals can help prevent or delay the onset of osteoporosis in themselves, their families, and the people who are in their care.

Patient Education Materials on the Internet

Patient education materials on osteoporosis can be found at the following web sites:

National Institutes of Health. Osteoporosis and Related Bone Diseases National Resource Center, Fast Facts on Osteoporosis: http://www.osteo.org/osteofast-fact.html

National Institutes of Health. Osteoporosis and Related Bone Diseases. National Resource Center, Alcohol and Bone Health: http://www.osteo.org/newsvol2no2.html

National Osteoporosis Foundation, How Can I Prevent Osteoporosis? http://www.nof.org/prevention/prevention.htm

Table 11-17 Calcium Content of Foods

Calcium Sources	Calcium (Milligrams)
1 cup plain, low-fat yogurt	400
3 oz sardines, with bones	370
1 cup low-fat fruit yogurt	345
1/4 of 14-inch cheese pizza	330
1 cup fluid milk (whole, fat-free skim milk, 1% [low-fat], 2% [reduced-fat], buttermilk)	300
1 cup calcium-fortified soy milk	300
1 cup calcium-fortified orange juice	300
1 oz Swiss cheese	270
1 oz cheddar cheese	200
1/2 cup cooked collard greens	180
1 oz American cheese	170
4 oz tofu (soybean curd)	145
1 tbsp blackstrap molasses	140
1 5-inch stalk broccoli	100
1/2 cup kale, cooked	100
2 oz cornbread, enriched	95

From Pennington, J. A. T. (1997). *Bowes and Church's food values of portions commonly used* (17th ed.). Philadelphia: Lippincott.

Obesity

As almost everyone in health care in the United States knows, a paradox exists in modern America. On the one hand, many people who do not need to lose weight are trying to do so, and on the other hand, many who actually need to lose weight are not trying; those who are trying are unsuccessful in losing the weight and maintaining their weight loss.

Overweight, about 10% to 20% over healthy weight, can seriously affect health and longevity and is associated with the leading nutrition-related causes of death in the United States: type 2 diabetes, CVD, and some cancers. **Obesity,** about 20% or more overweight, is also associated with gout and gallbladder disease and may contribute to the development of osteoarthritis in the weight-bearing joints.

Epidemiology

Overweight and obesity are found worldwide and the prevalence of these conditions in the United States ranks high with other developed nations. Approximately 280,000 adult deaths in the United States each year are attributable to obesity. Almost one quarter of the nation's adults are obese and over one half are overweight (including people who are obese) (Table 11-18).

The prevalence of being overweight has steadily increased over the years among nearly all racial and ethnic groups. From 1960 to 1994, the prevalence of *overweight* increased from 31.6% to 32.6% in adults in the United States. The prevalence of *obesity* during this same period increased from 13.4% to 22.3%—a relative

Table 11-18 Prevalence of Healthy Weight, Overweight, and Obesity in U.S. Adults Age 20 Years and Older

Body Weight Classification	All Adults	Women	Men
Healthy weight (BMI = 19 to 24.9)	41.4%	43.6%	39.0%
Overweight (BMI = 25 to 29.9)	54.9%	50.7%	59.4%
Obese (BMI = >30)	22.3%	25%	19.5%

From U.S. Department of Health and Human Services, National Institutes of Health, National Institute of Diabetes and Digestive and Kidney Diseases, Weight-Control Information Network. (1996). *Statistics related to overweight and obesity* [Online]. NIH Publication No. 96-4158. Available: http://www.niddk.nih.gov/health/nutrit/pubs/statobes.htm.

increase of more than 50%, with most of this increase occurring in the 1990s. The prevalence of overweight and obesity increases with advancing age until people reach their 60s, when it starts to decline. From 1991 to 1998, obesity increased in every state of the United States, in both genders and across all races and ethnicities, age groups, educational levels, and smoking statuses, with the exception of White men in their 20s to 40s, in whom the prevalence of obesity decreased from the early 1970s to late 1970s.

Healthy People 2010 *Objectives*

- Leading health indicators: reduce the proportion of adults who are obese from 23% to 15% and reduce the proportion of children and adolescents who are overweight or obese from 11% and 12% to 5% (objective numbers: *19-2* and *19-3*).
- *19-1*. Increase the proportion of adults who are at a healthy weight from 42% to 60%.

Obesity is more common in women than in men. Among men, there is a modest ethnic variation in the prevalence of being overweight, the greatest difference occurring between White men and Hispanic-American men. Among women, the ethnic variation in being overweight is substantial. Almost 25% of White women are overweight; Hispanic-American and Puerto Rican women have a greater prevalence of being overweight than their White counterparts; and more than 45% of Black women are overweight. Potential contributing factors to the greater propensity for adult Black women to become obese include a more sedentary lifestyle, higher energy intake, earlier menarche, earlier age of first childbirth, and less loss of weight gained during gestation (Burke et al., 1992) (see the Case Study).

Excess body weight is 7 to 12 times more frequent in women from lower social classes compared with women from upper social classes. In men, social class has a significantly less pronounced relationship to being overweight (Bray, 1996).

CASE STUDY

Janie

Janie is a 25-year-old Black woman who works 5 days a week as a kindergarten teacher. She weighs 175 pounds and is 5 feet 4 inches tall. Her father died of a heart attack at 50 years of age. Janie lives with her 55-year-old mother, who is confined to a wheelchair as a result of a massive stroke she suffered 6 months ago. Born and raised in Atlanta, Janie's mother prides herself as an excellent *soul food* cook. In fact, she is still able to prepare most of the family's meals.

Janie recently joined the health maintenance organization (HMO), which covers one complete physical per year. She was referred because she is engaged to be married and wants to lose 25 pounds by her wedding day, which is 2 months from now.

- Can Janie meet her wedding day goal weight? Why or why not?
- If she cannot meet her goal, then what could be recommended instead? Prioritize the recommendations. Set long-term and short-term goals.

Body Mass Index for Adults

Based on an adult's height and weight, body mass index (BMI) (wt/ht^2) is a helpful indicator of obesity and being **underweight** (Garrow & Webster, 1958). A person's BMI can be determined by referring to Fig. 11-4, by using a calculator on the Internet (the CDCP's on-line BMI calculator) (http://www.cdc.gov/nccdphp/dnpa/bmi/calc-bmi.htm), or by using a hand-held calculator and the following formulas:

Body Mass Index Formulas

English Formula

$$\text{BMI} = \text{weight in pounds} \div \text{height in inches} \div \text{height in inches} \times 703.$$

Example: For a 6-foot tall person weighing 210 pounds: BMI = 210 pounds divided by 72 inches divided by 72 inches multiplied by 703 = 28.5.

Metric Formulas

$$\text{BMI} = \text{weight in kilograms} \div (\text{height in meters})^2$$

and

$$\text{BMI} = (\text{weight in kilograms} \div \text{height in cm} \div \text{height in cm}) \times 10{,}000.$$

Example: For a person who is 182.9 centimeters tall and weighs 95.3 kilograms: BMI = 95.3 kg divided by 182.9 cm multiplied by 10,000 = 28.5.

BMI is a good indicator of body fat, but cannot be interpreted as a specific percentage of body fat. Age and gender influence the relationship between fat and BMI. For example, women are more likely to have a higher percentage of body fat than men have for the same BMI. At the same BMI, older people have more body fat than do younger

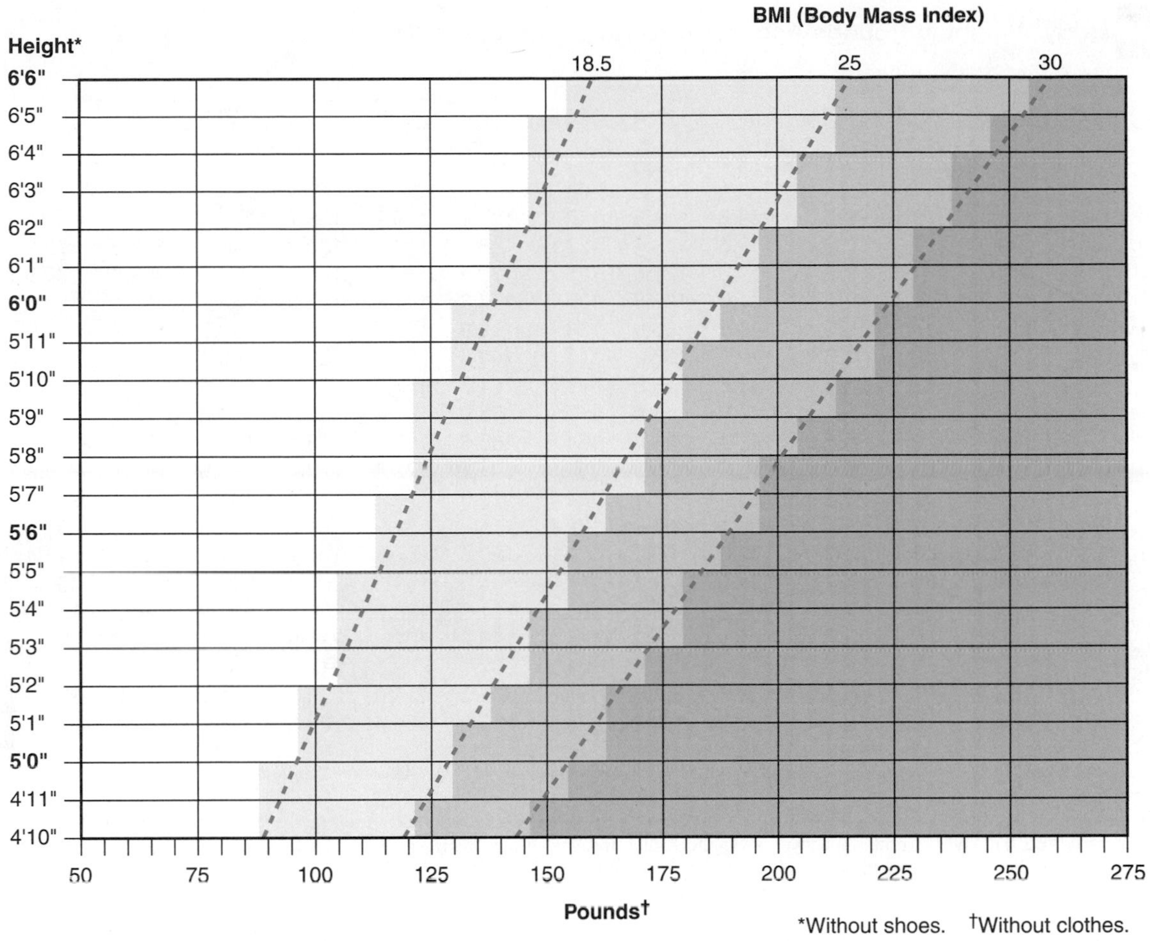

BMI measures weight in relation to height. The BMI ranges shown above are for adults. They are not exact ranges of healthy and unhealthy weights. However, they show that health risk increases at higher levels of overweight and obesity. Even within the healthy BMI range, weight gains can carry health risks for adults.

Directions: Find your weight on the bottom of the graph. Go straight up from that point until you come to the line that matches your height. Then look to find your weight group.

- **Healthy weight:** BMI from 18.5 up to 25 refers to healthy weight.
- **Overweight:** BMI from 25 up to 30 refers to overweight.
- **Obese:** BMI 30 or higher refers to obesity. Obese persons are also overweight.

Fig. 11-4 Body mass index. (From U.S. Department of Agriculture, U.S. Department of Health and Human Services. [2000]. *Nutrition and your health: Dietary guidelines for Americans* [5th ed.]. Home and Garden Bulletin No. 232. Washington, DC: U.S. Government Printing Office.)

adults (Gallagher et al., 1996). BMI is used to screen and monitor a population to detect the risk of health or nutritional disorders. In an individual, other data must be used to determine whether a high BMI is associated with increased risk of disease and death for that person; BMI alone is not diagnostic (Willett, Dietz, & Colditz, 1999).

BMI ranges are based on the effect body weight has on disease and death (WHO, 1995). BMI values of from 19 to 25 is a healthy target range for adults. BMI values greater than 25 are associated with increasing risks for developing cardiovascular disease, gallbladder disease, high blood pressure, and noninsulin-dependent diabetes mellitus. A high BMI value is predictive of death from CVD (Calle, Thun, Petrelli, Rodriguez, & Heath, 1999) (Table 11-19).

BMI values for adults is expressed with one number, regardless of age or sex, using the following guidelines:
Underweight: BMI less than 18.5.
Healthy weight: BMI of 18.5 to 24.9.
Overweight: BMI of 25.0 to 29.9.
Obese: BMI of 30.0 or more.

Researchers suggest that after reaching peak growth at the age of about 21 years, body weight should be stabilized and maintained at a constant, healthy weight (BMI less

Table 11-19 Body Weight in Pounds According to Height and Body Mass Index

	Body Mass Index (kg per m²)													
	119.0	20.0	21.0	22.0	23.0	24.0	25.0	26.0	27.0	28.0	29.0	30.0	35.0	40.0
Height (inches)	Body Weight (pounds)													
58.0	90.7	95.5	100.3	105.0	109.8	114.6	119.4	124.1	128.9	133.7	138.5	143.2	167.1	191.0
59.0	93.9	98.8	103.8	108.7	113.6	118.6	123.5	128.5	133.4	138.3	143.3	148.2	172.9	197.6
60.0	97.1	102.2	107.3	112.4	117.5	122.6	127.7	132.9	138.0	143.1	148.2	153.3	178.8	204.4
61.0	100.3	105.6	110.9	116.2	121.5	126.8	132.0	137.3	142.6	147.9	153.2	158.4	184.8	211.3
62.0	103.7	109.1	114.6	120.0	125.5	130.9	136.4	141.9	147.3	152.8	158.2	163.7	191.0	218.2
63.0	107.0	112.7	118.3	123.9	129.6	135.2	140.8	146.5	152.1	157.7	163.4	169.0	197.2	225.3
64.0	110.5	116.3	122.1	127.9	133.7	139.5	145.3	151.2	157.0	162.8	168.6	174.4	203.5	232.5
65.0	113.9	119.9	125.9	131.9	137.9	143.9	149.9	155.9	161.9	167.9	173.9	179.9	209.9	239.9
66.0	117.5	123.7	129.8	136.0	142.2	148.4	154.6	160.8	166.9	173.1	179.3	185.5	216.4	247.3
67.0	121.1	127.4	133.8	140.2	146.5	152.9	159.3	165.7	172.0	178.4	184.8	191.1	223.0	254.9
68.0	124.7	131.3	137.8	114.4	185.0	157.5	164.1	170.6	177.2	183.8	190.3	196.9	229.7	262.5
69.0	128.4	135.2	141.9	148.7	155.4	162.2	168.9	175.7	182.5	189.2	196.0	202.7	236.5	270.3
70.0	132.1	139.1	146.1	153.0	160.0	166.9	173.9	180.8	187.8	194.7	201.7	208.6	243.4	278.2
71.0	135.9	143.1	150.3	157.4	164.6	171.7	178.9	186.0	193.2	200.3	207.5	214.6	250.4	286.2
72.0	139.8	147.2	154.5	161.9	169.2	176.6	183.9	191.3	198.7	206.0	213.4	220.7	257.5	294.3
73.0	143.7	151.3	158.8	166.4	174.0	181.5	189.1	196.7	204.2	211.8	219.3	226.9	264.7	302.5
74.0	147.7	155.4	163.2	171.0	178.8	186.5	194.3	202.1	209.9	217.6	225.4	233.2	272.0	310.9
75.0	151.7	159.7	167.7	175.6	183.6	191.6	199.6	207.6	215.6	223.5	231.5	239.5	279.4	319.4
76.0	155.8	164.0	172.2	180.4	188.6	196.8	205.0	213.2	221.4	229.5	237.7	245.9	286.9	327.9

From U.S. Department of Health and Human Services, National Institutes of Health. (1992). *Methods for voluntary weight loss and control.* Bethesda, MD: The Institutes.

Note: A body mass index (BMI) of 27.8 for men and 27.3 for women is the cutoff point for obesity used in the National Health and Nutrition Examination Survey (NHANES II). The National Academy of Sciences' diet and health report suggests that a BMI of 22 to 27 is normal for people 45 to 54 years of age, a BMI of 23 to 28 is normal for people 55 to 65 years of age, and a BMI of 24 to 29 is normal for people over 65 years of age.

than 25) throughout life to prevent undesirable weight gain (Meisler & St. Jeor, 1996).

BMI Growth Charts for Children

Many parents are familiar with the original growth charts used by pediatric health care providers since 1977. Those charts were widely used by pediatricians, nurses, and nutritionists to track growth and development in children and assist in signaling potential developmental problems. The charts consist of a series of cures called "percentiles" that illustrate the distribution in growth of children across the United States.

In 2000, the Centers for Disease Control (CDC) released new pediatric growth charts that more accurately reflect he nation's cultural and racial diversity and track children and young people through age 20. The new charts will be used to monitor children's growth and help identify weight problems early during childhood. The charts include an assessment of BMI. The BMI is an early warning signal that is helpful as early as age 2 to help identify children who have the potential to become overweight. Early identification of obesity risk gives parents the opportunity to modify their children's eating habits before a weight problem develops.

The CDC's new charts are based on data gathered through the National Health and Nutrition Examination Survey (NHANES), the only survey that collects data from actual physical examinations on a cross-section of Americans from all over the country. This survey shows that since the 1980s, the number of overweight children and adolescents has doubled. Additionally, it shows that over half of all American adults are overweight and that the number of obese adults has doubled. It is expected that the new BMI charts will help address this nationwide problem. The growth charts indicate that, in general, children are heavier today than in 1977, but height has remained virtually unchanged. The new charts are available on the CDC web site at http://www.cdc.gov/growthcharts.

Diet Intervention

"Please help me lose weight" is one of the most common requests heard in the health field. As discussed, a balanced diet is important and must include the appropriate **serving sizes** for the recommended daily intake of each food group. Additionally, exercise is particularly necessary from the outset because with exercise there is less need to restrict food. Exercise also favors long-term maintenance of body weight (as described in Chapter 12).

Nurses should make referrals to supervised or unsupervised programs as appropriate (see Care Plan). People expect this type of advice on maintaining their health.

CARE PLAN

SOAP Notes

Subjective
Objective
Assessment
Plan

SUBJECTIVE

Person expressed desire to lose 25 pounds in 2 months.

OBJECTIVE

A. Weight: BMI = 30 kg/m^2; healthy body weight = 123 to 127 pounds.
B. Individual presents with multiple risks for
   1. Overweight
   2. Relatives with CVD
   3. High-fat, high-salt diet
   4. Stress

ASSESSMENT

Person should shift focus from unrealistic weight loss expectations to initiating efforts aimed at CVD risk reduction.

PLAN

A. Present weight loss realities.
B. Discuss modifiable CVD risks.
C. Negotiate strategies to decrease individual's CVD risk factors.
   1. Short-term: Establish behavioral objectives that will result in one or more of the following:
      a. Increased physical activity.
      b. Decreased intake of saturated fat.
      c. Decreased intake of salt.
      d. Implementation of DASH plan.
   2. Long-term: Establish evaluation and follow-up activities to evaluate success in achieving objectives *a* through *d* and to reinforce desirable behaviors.
   3. Refer to appropriate health care provider who can support short- and long-term recommendations as outlined.

Therefore nurses can play an important role, although not supervising individuals' weight loss efforts directly. (For more information on obesity among adults, see USDHHS, National Heart, Lung, and Blood Institute, 1998 [http://www.nhlbi.nih.gov/guidelines/obesity/ob_home.htm].)

There are many positive effects of only relatively small amounts of weight loss (5% to 10% of body weight) for people who are obese:

- Decreased blood pressure (decreased risk of a heart attack and stroke).
- Reduced abnormally high levels of blood glucose associated with diabetes.
- Reduced elevated levels of cholesterol and triglycerides associated with CVD.
- Reduced sleep apnea (irregular breathing during sleep).
- Decreased risk of osteoarthritis in the weight-bearing joints.
- Decreased depression.
- Increased self-esteem.

The acronym LEARN has been suggested as a mnemonic device for health professionals. LEARN refers to the steps nurses can take to help the person who needs to improve health-related behavior (Brownell, 2000). LEARN is particularly useful as a guideline for communicating with the clinically obese patient who has indicated dissatisfaction with current weight:

L: Listen with sympathy and understanding to the patient's perception of the problem.
E: Explain personal perceptions of the problem.
A: Acknowledge and discuss differences and similarities.
R: Recommend treatment.
N: Negotiate an agreement.

In 1992, an NIH-sponsored technical support conference identified the following characteristics of voluntary weight loss and weight control in the United States (USDHHS, 1992):

1. Obesity is a chronic disease.
2. Obesity has many causes.
3. Cure is rare; palliation is realistic.
4. Weight loss is slow.
5. Recidivism is common.
6. Weight regain may be slow, but it is often rapid.
7. Treatment is often more frustrating than the underlying disease.

The conference noted significant adverse effects for obese dieters who regain lost weight:

- Repeated weight gain and loss may have adverse psychological and physical effects; for example, evidence suggests that mildly to moderately overweight women who are dieting may be at risk for binge eating without vomiting and purging.
- Although data on the health effects of repeated weight gain and loss (weight cycling) are also inconclusive, weight cycling appears to affect energy metabolism and may cause faster regaining of weight.
- Depression and decreased self-esteem occur.

According to some *radical* nurses, nutritionists, social workers, psychologists, physicians, and lay advocates, a new model for health care is needed for people who *cannot* maintain a BMI under 30. The new paradigm, *health at any size*, is described in the Hot Topics box.

Patient Education Materials on the Internet

Patient education materials about obesity can be found at the following web sites:

- National Institutes of Health. National Institute of Diabetes and Digestive and Kidney Diseases. Weight Control Information Network, On-line publications: http://www.niddk.nih.gov/health/nutrit/nutrit.htm

HOT topics

HEALTH AT ANY SIZE: THE SIZE ACCEPTANCE NONDIET MOVEMENT

Restricting food intake causes many problems. For most people, dieting to reduce weight is ineffective. The majority of obese dieters struggle in vain and blame themselves for relapses. Self-imposed dieting appears to cause eating binges after food becomes available and may cause psychological manifestations, such as preoccupation with food and eating, increased emotional responsiveness, and dysphoria and distractibility (Polivy, 1996). Additional problems associated with dieting include failure of caloric regulation and a heightened response to food palatability and hunger, which are greater under conditions of moderate restriction and unpredictable access to food (Wooley, Wooley, & Dyrenforth, 1979). To add insult to injury, many health care professionals unwittingly contribute both to their obese patients' false hopes for success in losing weight and to the further denigration of their patients' self-esteem (Wooley & Garner, 1991).

The *size acceptance nondiet movement* emerged during the last 2 decades of the twentieth century in response to the ineffective traditional obesity treatment programs. Goals of the movement include improving self-image, normalizing eating behavior resulting in healthful balanced eating *without specific food restrictions,* and increasing physical activity.

The new paradigm has replaced the question, "How can fat people lose weight?" with the question, "How can fat people be healthy?" (Spark, 2001). The following tenets are the foundation of the movement:

- Good health is a state of physical, mental, and social well being. People of all sizes and shapes can reduce their risk of poor health by adopting a healthy lifestyle, which includes (1) eating a variety of healthy foods, (2) being physically active because it is fun and feels good, and (3) appreciating the body as it is now.
- Human beings come in a variety of sizes and shapes; size diversity is a positive characteristic of the human race. Respect the bodies of others, although they might be quite different.
- There is no ideal body size, shape, BMI, or body composition that every individual should strive to achieve.
- Self-esteem and body image are strongly linked. Helping people feel good about their bodies and about who they are can help motivate and maintain healthy behaviors.
- People are responsible for care of their own bodies.
- Appearance stereotyping is wrong. Their weight notwithstanding, all people *deserve* to be treated equally in the job market and on the job, to be treated equally in the media, and to receive competent and respectful treatment by health care professionals.

How to Become a Size-Sensitive Health Professional

- On the intake form, include a question asking whether the person is satisfied with the body size. If the answer is "yes," then try to avoid the issue in the future.
- When the person asks not to be weighed, the request is acknowledged without complaint and automatically taken into account on follow-up office visits. (There are a few cases in which weighing is necessary, such as when administering certain medications, chemotherapy, or anesthesia.)
- A size-sensitive health care professional does not necessarily avoid mentioning weight, but should avoid making an issue of weight, avoid lectures and humiliation, and respect the individual's wishes with regard to weight discussions.
- When weight contributes to a problem, the professional mentions this situation, but also considers other diagnoses and recommends tests to determine the actual diagnosis when appropriate. If weight loss is a recommended treatment for a problem, then the compassionate professional may mention this, but at minimum, and recommend and prescribe other treatments. Accept the individual's wish not to use weight loss as a treatment.
- Some health care professionals believe that overweight and obesity are not necessarily unhealthy. However, other professionals who believe that fat is unhealthy may acknowledge that weight loss is usually ineffective or that the patients have the right to direct their own treatment.
- Ideally, the waiting area, examining suite, and consultation room are equipped with armless chairs, large blood pressure cuffs, large examination gowns, and other equipment suitable for large people. If this is not the case, then the office staff acknowledges the importance of these items when told.

Polivy, J. (1996). Psychological consequences of food restriction. *Journal of the American Dietetic Association, 96,* 589-592; Spark, A. (2001). Health at any size: The size-acceptance nondiet movement. *Journal of the American Medical Women's Association, 56,* 69-71; Wooley, S. C., & Garner, D. M. (1991). Obesity treatment: The high cost of false hope. *Journal of the American Dietetic Association, 91,* 1248-1251; Wooley, S. C., Wooley, O. W., & Dyrenforth, S. R. (1979). Theoretical, practical, and social issues in behavioral treatments of obesity. *Journal of Applied Behavior Analysis, 12* (Spring), 3-25.

- LEARN. The lifestyle company: http://www.learneducation.com/
- Healthy Weight Network, "Shape Up America!": http://www.healthyweight.net/
- American Heart Association, Fad Diets: http://americanheart.org/Heart_and_Stroke_A_Z_Guide/fad.html
- Healthy Weight Network (nondietary approach): http://www.healthyweight.net/

Diabetes

Healthy People 2010 Goal: through prevention programs, reduce the disease and economic burden of diabetes and improve the quality of life for all persons who have or are at risk for diabetes.

- *5-1.* Increase the proportion of persons with diabetes who receive formal diabetes education from 40% in 1998 to 60% in 2010.

HEALTH TEACHING Types of Fad Diets

- *Food-specific diets.* Certain diets focus on one food (such as grapefruit), class of foods (such as fresh fruit), or combination (such as kelp and vinegar) with purported special properties that facilitate weight loss. Following a plan by which only one type of food is eaten while others are excluded results in weight loss, the reason being that eating the same food becomes monotonous and results in reduced eating, causing a loss of weight. These food-specific diets fail to teach healthy eating habits and are usually nutritionally unbalanced.
- *Liquid diets.* Liquid diets include over-the-counter, liquid-meal replacements. Each 8-ounce single serving provides approximately 300 kilocalories and approximately one quarter of the recommended intake for most nutrients. When limited to 4 cans per day, a liquid diet will provide 1200 calories and will therefore result in weight loss. Many people have reported that removing the temptations of usual food and beverages and the social trappings of traditional mealtime makes adhering to a reduced-calorie regimen easier. Liquid diets fail to teach portion control, providing no guidance for healthful eating after the desired amount of weight is lost. Although liquid diets have been used for large weight losses (more than 100 pounds) in clinical settings with medical supervision and psychological support, regaining the lost weight is common.
- *High-fiber diets.* Fiber-rich foods are an essential part of a healthy diet and can be especially beneficial to people trying to lose weight. Fiber-rich foods are filling and because fiber cannot be digested, it contains no calories (which leads to weight gain when eaten in excess). Conversely, eating too much fiber is not necessarily better. Consuming more than 50 or 60 grams of high-fiber foods every day can lead to bloating, cramping, diarrhea, and loss of minerals from the body. However, enjoying 30 to 35 grams per day of fiber-rich foods is likely to result in weight loss because the fiber-containing choices displace other high-calorie foods from the diet.
- *High-protein diets.* High-protein, low-carbohydrate diets lead to weight loss, although the weight loss may be temporary. If an individual needs to lose weight quickly and decides to accomplish this task with a high-protein, low-carbohydrate diet, this is how it will work.
  1. A portion of potential calories from the protein-rich food is absorbed by the process of metabolizing the large amount of nitrogen in the protein; therefore the energy is not available to the body for any other use.
  2. The diet can be monotonous from eating the same high-protein foods over and over again, ultimately leading to a decreased food intake.
  3. High-protein intake causes an increased water loss to carry the nitrogen from the body.
- *Fasting.* Fasting has been recommended for decades to cleanse the body of impurities or to embark on a weight-loss plan. Most people who undergo fasts use their common sense: they drink liquids that can supply some energy and nutrients, set safe time limits as to how long they will abstain from foods, and educate themselves on the basics of safe fasting. However, fasting deprives the body of nutrients. A person undergoing an especially prolonged fast experiences not only weight loss, but also low energy, weakness, poor nutritional status, and lightheadedness. Additionally, when carbohydrates are not available for energy, *ketones* can accumulate (as the body's carbohydrate substitute), causing stress for the kidneys, which can be harmful to overall health.

Adapted from Kirby, R. (1998). *Dieting for dummies*. New York: IDG Publishing.

- *5-2.* Prevent diabetes, from 3.1 new cases per 1000 persons in 1994 to 1996 to 2.5 new cases per 1000 in 2010.

Prevalence and Incidence

Diabetes is becoming more prevalent. The numbers of existing cases (prevalence) and new cases (incidence) of diabetes are increasing and most of this increase is *not* a result of aging of the U.S. population. Trends also show that minority and elderly populations are disproportionately affected by diabetes. In 1996, approximately 3.2% of the population (8.5 million people) in the United States reported that they had diabetes mellitus. Nearly one million new cases of diabetes were reported in 1996. An estimated 16 million Americans have diabetes and approximately one half of them are unaware they have the disease (CDC, 2001).

Previously called noninsulin-dependent diabetes mellitus (NIDDM) or adult-onset diabetes, **type 2 diabetes** accounts for 90% to 95% percent of all diagnosed cases of diabetes. Risk factors include older age, obesity, family history of diabetes, history of gestational diabetes, impaired glucose tolerance, physical inactivity, and race and ethnicity. Blacks, Hispanic and Latino Americans, Native Americans, and some Asian Americans are at particularly high risk for type 2 diabetes.

Type 2 diabetes is one of the leading causes of death among Americans and the leading cause of new cases of blindness, kidney failure, and lower extremity amputations, plus it greatly increases a person's risk for a heart attack or stroke. In 1997, diabetes accounted for more than $98 billion in direct and indirect medical costs and lost productivity. During that same year, the average health care cost for a person with diabetes was $10,071 compared with $2699 for a person without diabetes (CDC, 2001). Much of the burden of diabetes can be prevented with early detection, improved delivery of care, and better education on diabetes self-management.

Type 2 Diabetes in Children

Although diabetes mellitus occurring in children and adolescents was believed to be exclusively type 1 and type 2 diabetes in children and adolescents, it is now considered to be a sizeable and growing problem among Native Americans and an emerging public health problem among other North American ethnic groups. The epidemic of obesity among children and adolescents, the decreasing level of physical activity during adolescence, and the increased exposure to diabetes *in utero* are likely contributors to the increase in type 2 diabetes during childhood and adolescence.

Although some children and adolescents are symptomatic, others are present with severe ketoacidosis and a transient insulin requirement. Diabetic complications (dyslipidemia and hypertension) have been observed among Pima Indians as early as the teenage years. Currently, no evidence-based guidelines for treatment of type 2 diabetes in children and adolescents are available and oral agents have not been specifically tested and approved for this age group. Generally, children and adolescents with type 2 diabetes have poor glycemic control. Population mobility, lack of symptoms and denial, absence of family support, and inadequate health care insurance coverage have all been identified as major barriers to adherence to treatment and follow-up and to successful clinical management. Because of a longer duration of disease (from earlier onset) and because glucose control and compliance are challenging during the teenage years, the lifetime complications (microvascular and macrovascular diseases and decreased quality of life) in this population will probably be very considerable (Fagot-Champagna et al., 2000).

Diet Intervention

MNT is the most critical and pivotal component of diabetes care. At the minimum, MNT involves the team efforts of a physician, a registered nurse or registered dietitian, and in some practice settings, a mental health professional. The purpose of MNT for people with type 2 diabetes is to delay or prevent the development of diabetes complications (blindness, CHD, nephropathy, and neuropathy). No single *diabetic diet* or *American Diabetes Association diet* exists. The recommended diet can only be defined as a nutrition prescription based on assessment and treatment goals and outcomes. Nutrition advice for people with type 2 diabetes is essentially the same as for the general population; they should be following the Dietary Guidelines for Americans. MNT for people with diabetes should be individualized, with consideration given to usual eating habits and other lifestyle factors. Nutrition recommendations are then developed and implemented to meet treatment goals and desired outcomes. Monitoring metabolic parameters, including blood glucose levels, glycated hemoglobin, lipids, blood pressure, body weight, renal function (when appropriate), and quality of life is crucial to ensure successful outcomes. The American Diabetes Association further recommends ongoing nutrition self-management education for individuals with diabetes.

For people with hyperglycemia, hyperlipidemia, obesity, or suboptimal nutrition, start with this nonpharmacological treatment:

1. Recommend an appropriate meal plan: determine daily energy needs based on healthy body weight and then use the patient's daily energy needs to determine the appropriate number of choices from the food groups in the Food Guide Pyramid.
2. Encourage regular aerobic exercise.
3. Evaluate the individual using outcome measures in Table 11-20. People who have been counseled regarding diet and exercise, but who have not responded satisfactorily after 4 to 6 weeks should be referred to a registered dietitian or nurse who is a registered diabetes educator. Refer to a physician a patient with acute complications of diabetes, such as hypoglycemia, exercise-related problems, renal disease, autonomic neuropathy, hypertension, or CVD (Box 11-7).

One step in nutrition therapy that has frustrated many registered dietitians is receiving a nutrition prescription (diet order) based only on a person's height and weight (Powers, 1996). Nurses should know as much as possible about the individual and the condition of the individual before writing a nutrition prescription. (This requirement is

Table 11-20 Desired Outcomes After 4 to 6 Weeks of MNT for Individuals with Type 2 Diabetes

Index	Goal	Desired Outcome After 4 to 6 Weeks of Initial MNT
FBS	80 to 120 mg/dl	Downward trend (down 10%) or at target goal
HbA_{1c}	60% to 75%	Downward trend (down 10%) or at target goal
Weight change	Maintain reasonable weight	Loss of 1.5 to 3 kg (3 to 6 lb)
Food and meal planning	Meals and snacks eaten on a regular basis; appropriate food choices and amounts	Positive changes in food selection and amount, frequency, and timing of meals
Exercise	If no medical limitations, physical activity for at least 10 minutes, 3 times a week	Physical activity level gradually increased or continued at target goal

MNT, Medical Nutrition Therapy.

Box 11-7 Medical Nutrition Therapy for Type 2 Diabetes

The goals are to achieve and maintain glucose, lipid, and blood pressure targets. Although reduced-calorie diets and weight loss usually improve short-term glycemic levels and have the potential to improve long-term metabolic control, traditional dietary strategies (even extremely low-calorie diets) have usually been ineffective in achieving long-term weight loss. Therefore the focus should be shifted to achieving and maintaining near-normal blood glucose levels independent of weight loss. Several additional strategies can be implemented, but no one proved strategy or method can be uniformly recommended.

Recommended are moderate caloric restrictions (250 to 500 calories less than average daily intake, calculated from a food history) and a nutritionally adequate meal plan with a reduction of total fat, specifically saturated fat, accompanied by an increase in physical activity. A reduced-calorie diet (independent of weight loss) is associated with increased sensitivity to insulin and improvement in blood glucose levels. Moderate weight loss (5 to 9kg [10 to 20lb]), regardless of starting weight, has been shown to reduce hyperglycemia, dyslipidemia, and hypertension.

Spacing of meals (spreading nutrient intake, particularly carbohydrate, throughout the day) is another strategy that can be adopted. Regular exercise and learning new behaviors and attitudes can help facilitate long-term lifestyle changes. However, if individuals with diabetes have made all the lifestyle changes they are able to make and metabolic control has not improve, then an oral glucose-lowering agent or insulin may need to be added to MNT.

Many individuals with refractory obesity may have limited success with the these strategies. As new pharmacological agents become available (for people with BMI less than or equal to 27kg/m^2 without other health risks or problems), these strategies may prove to be effective. Gastric reduction surgery is available for people with a BMI greater than 35kg/m^2. Studies on the long-term efficacy and safety of these methods are needed.

PROTEIN

Protein consumption should comprise 10% to 20% of the daily calorie intake derived from plant and animal sources or 25 to 50 g of protein per 1000 calories daily. In the patient with overt nephropathy, a protein intake of approximately the adult RDA of 0.8 g/kg/day (less than 10% of daily calories) is recommended. Further protein-restricted plans should be designed by a registered dietitian who is familiar with all components of MNT for diabetes. For information on nephropathy, see the American Diabetes Association position statement, Diabetic Nephropathy, in *Diabetes Care,* 24(Suppl 1), S69-S72. Also available at: http://www.diabetes.org/linicalrecommendations/Supplement101/S69.htm.

TOTAL FAT, SATURATED FAT, AND CHOLESTEROL

If dietary protein contributes 10% to 20% of the total caloric content of the diet, then 80% to 90% of calories remain to be distributed between dietary fat and carbohydrates. The recommended percentage of calories from fat is dependent on identified lipid problems and treatment goals for glucose, lipids, and weight. People who are at a healthy weight and have normal lipid levels are encouraged to follow the recommendations of the National Cholesterol Education Program (NCEP).

When obesity and weight loss are the primary concerns, a reduction in dietary fat should be considered. When triglycerides and very low-density lipoprotein cholesterol are the primary concerns, a moderate increase in monounsaturated fat intake with less than 10% of the calories from saturated fats and a more moderate carbohydrate intake is one approach that may be tried. However, in obese individuals, care should be taken to ensure that increased fat does not perpetuate or aggravate the obesity. Additionally, individuals with triglyceride levels greater than or equal to 1000 mg/dl (greater than or equal to 11.3 mmol/l) require reduction of all types of dietary fat (less than 10% of calories) in addition to pharmacological treatment to reduce the risk of pancreatitis. Monitoring of glycemic and lipid status and body weight, with any dietary fat modifications, is essential to assess the effectiveness of the nutrition recommendations.

A reduction in saturated fat and cholesterol consumption is an important goal to reduce the risk of CVD. Diabetes is a strong independent risk factor for CVD, over and above the adverse effects of an elevated serum cholesterol. Therefore less than 10% of the daily calories should be from saturated fats and dietary cholesterol should be limited to less than or equal to 1000 mg per 1000 calories daily. However, even these recommendations must be incorporated with consideration of an individual's cultural and ethnic background.

CARBOHYDRATE, SWEETENERS, FIBER, AND MICRONUTRIENTS

The percentage of calories from carbohydrate will also vary and is based on the individual's eating habits and glucose and lipid goals. The use of sucrose as part of the total carbohydrate content of the diet does not impair blood-glucose control in individuals with type 1 or type 2 diabetes. Sucrose and sucrose-containing foods must be substituted for other carbohydrates, gram for gram, and not simply added to the meal plan.

Dietary fructose produces a smaller increase in plasma glucose compared with equivalent amounts of sucrose and most starches. In this regard, fructose may offer an advantage as a sweetening agent in the diabetic diet. However, because there are potential adverse effects of large amounts of fructose on serum cholesterol and LDL cholesterol, fructose may have no overall advantage as a sweetening agent in the diabetic diet. Although people with dyslipidemia should avoid consuming large amounts of fructose, there is no reason to recommend that people with diabetes avoid consumption of fruits and vegetables, in which fructose occurs naturally, or moderate consumption of fructose-sweetened foods.

Nutritive sweeteners other than sucrose and fructose include corn sweeteners, such as corn syrup, fruit juice or fruit juice concentrate, honey, molasses, dextrose, and maltose.

From American Diabetes Association. (2001). Position statement. Nutrition recommendations and principles for people with diabetes mellitus. Clinical practice recommendations 2001. *Diabetes Care*, 24(Suppl 1), S44-S47. Also available at: http://www.diabetes.org/clincialrecommendations/Supplement101/S44.htm.

Continued

Box 11-7 Medical Nutrition Therapy for Type 2 Diabetes—cont'd

Foods sweetened with these sweeteners have no advantage or disadvantage over foods sweetened with sucrose in decreasing total calories or carbohydrate content of the diet or in improving overall diabetes control. The calories and carbohydrate content from all nutritive sweeteners must be accounted for in the meal plan and have the potential to affect blood glucose levels.

Nonnutritive sweeteners approved by the FDA include saccharin, aspartame, and acesulfame K for use in the United States. Fiber recommendations for people with diabetes are the same as those for the general population: 20 to 35 g of dietary fiber daily from both soluble and insoluble fibers from a wide variety of food sources. When dietary intake is adequate, there is generally no need for additional vitamin and mineral supplementation for the majority of people with diabetes.

SODIUM

Sodium recommendations for people with diabetes are the same as those for the general population: 2400 to 3000 mg/day for the general population; less than or equal to 2400 mg/day for people with mild to moderate hypertension; and less than or equal to 2000 mg/day for people with hypertension and nephropathy.

ALCOHOL

The same precautions regarding the use of alcohol that apply to the general public also apply to people with diabetes. The Dietary Guidelines for Americans recommends no more than 2 drinks per day for men and no more than 1 drink per day for women (1 alcoholic beverage is equivalent to 12 ounces of beer, 5 ounces of wine, or one and a half ounces of distilled spirits). Abstaining from alcohol should be advised for people with a history of alcohol abuse or for women during pregnancy.

The effect of alcohol on blood glucose levels is dependent on the amount of alcohol ingested and on the relationship to food intake. Alcohol is not metabolized into glucose and inhibits gluconeogenesis; therefore hypoglycemia can result if alcohol is consumed without food by people treated with insulin or oral glucose-lowering agents. Hypoglycemia can occur at blood alcohol levels that do not exceed mild intoxication. However, when used in moderation and with food, blood glucose levels are unaffected by the ingestion of alcohol when diabetes is well controlled. For individuals using insulin, 1 or 2 alcoholic beverages can be ingested with and in addition to the regular meal plan. No food should be omitted because there is the possibility of alcohol-induced hypoglycemia. When calories from alcohol need to be calculated as part of the total caloric intake, alcohol is best substituted for fat exchanges (1 alcoholic beverage equals 2 fat exchanges) or fat calories. Reduction of or abstention from alcohol intake is advisable for diabetic individuals with medical problems such as pancreatitis, dyslipidemia, and especially elevated triglycerides, or neuropathy.

From American Diabetes Association. (2001). Position statement. Nutrition recommendations and principles for people with diabetes mellitus. Clinical practice recommendations 2001. *Diabetes Care,* 24(Suppl 1), S44-S47. Also available at: http://www.diabetes.org/clincialrecommendations/Supplement101/S44.htm.

Name ________________ DOB________ ☐ male ☐ female
Phone ________________

Referred by ____________ Address ________________
Phone ________________ Date ________________

Diabetes treatment regimen ☐ MNT ☐ MNT + oral hypoglycemic agents
☐ MNT + insulin or combination therapy

Lab Values HbA_{1C} ___ FBS___ BP___ TC___ HDL___ LDL___
Microalbumin___

MD/DO/RN goals for MNT BS___ HbA_{1C} ___
Other ________________________________

Medical Hx ☐ Dyslipidemia or CVD ☐ Hypertension ☐ Renal disease
☐ Autonomic neuropathy, esp. GI
List Meds for Diabetes___ Hypertension___ Lipid-lowering___ GI___
Other ________________________________

Exercise ☐ Medical clearance for exercise ☐ Limitations, if any_____
____

Fig. 11-5 Referring patient with type 2 diabetes to a registered dietitian for medical nutrition therapy (MNT).

comparable with the physician's need to complete a physical and medical assessment before writing a medication prescription.) The nutrition prescription may be general, but it should reflect the person's therapy goals. The following are some sample orders the nurse might write for the dietitian:

- Diabetic meal plan to achieve clinical goals of diabetes MNT.
- MNT to achieve as near-normal blood glucose as possible.
- Meal plan to improve diabetes control and blood lipid levels.
- Diet for improved glycemia.
- Diet for diabetes and hypertension.

The prescription may be further defined by the registered dietitian with a summary of the planned nutrition intervention. For example, the dietitian might write:

- Weight-reduction meal plan based on general eating guidelines, 1200 to 1500 kcals, 3 meals, and 1 snack.
- 2400 mg sodium meal plan with weight maintenance.
- Cholesterol-counting meal plan, adjusting cholesterol and meal-timing to achieve target glucose goals.

When referring people to a registered dietitian, provide the information that is summarized in Fig. 11-5.

Patient Education Materials Online

Patient education materials on diabetes can be found at the following web sites:

- American Diabetes Association, Eating Healthy with the Diabetes Food Pyramid As Your Guide: http://www.diabetes.org/nutrition/article031799.asp
- Diabetes Life Network, Carbohydrate Counting: http://www.diabeteslife.net/living/nutrition/carbo.html
- Joslin Diabetes Center. Carbohydrate Counting: As Easy As 1-2-3: http://www.joslin.harvard.edu/education/library/wcarbsug.html#portion
- U.S. Department of Agriculture, Nutrition and Diabetes Resource List for Consumers: http://www.nal.usda.gov/fnic/pubs/bibs/topics/diabetes/diabetes.html

Human Immunodeficiency Virus and Acquired Immunodeficiency Syndrome

Epidemiology

Since 1981, when it was first identified, almost half a million people have died from the **human immunodeficiency virus** (HIV) or acquired immunodeficiency syndrome (AIDS). Over 13,000 AIDS-related deaths occurred in the United States in 1998, when the prevalence of the disease was estimated at 5 per 100,000 population.

Healthy People 2010 *Objectives*

- *Goal 13:* prevent HIV infection and its related illness and death.
- *13-15.* Expand the interval between an initial diagnosis of HIV infection and AIDS diagnosis to increase years of life of an individual with HIV.
- *13-17.* Reduce new cases of perinatal-acquired HIV infection.

Diet Intervention

Attention to nutrition in early HIV intervention is essential for several reasons. AIDS produces nutritional consequences; therefore good dietary habits early in the disease may have benefits for end-stage developments such as severe weight loss. The person diagnosed as HIV positive usually becomes depressed. Depression leads to loss of appetite; therefore attention to nutrition is critical as soon as a positive diagnosis is made.

An initial nutritional assessment is necessary, suggesting the extent to which nutrition education is needed and providing valuable baseline information for evaluating the disease's progression. Nurses should involve the person's significant others in early discussions of optimal nutrition. A nutrient-dense, protein-rich, well-balanced diet that includes a vitamin and mineral supplement should be stressed. Information on food sanitation should also be provided. Box 11-8 summarizes nutrition intervention for people who are HIV positive.

The aims of nutrition therapy and counseling specifically for HIV and AIDS (Krales, 2000):

- Determine how the person appeared physically before becoming HIV positive. Was the patient obese or heavily muscled? A couch potato or an athlete? On a good diet?
- Help meet or exceed the amount of muscle the person had before becoming HIV positive. Introduce the person to proper eating and exercise.
- Help get the person back to the original weight or maintain the current weight.
- Teach about food and water safety.
- Advise on the ability of food to ease some of the gastrointestinal side effects of medications.
- Teach the importance of maintaining eating and medication schedules to ensure maximal absorption of medications.
- When the individual is diabetic or hyperlipidemic, teach about the dietary management of these conditions. Viewing HIV as a terminal illness is no longer appropriate. HIV is now considered to a chronic disease because people are living many years with the diagnosis.

Breastfeeding should be avoided to prevent vertical transmission of HIV from mother to child. This objective is much easier to implement in the United States, which has had a long history of safe breast milk substitutes in the form of milk-based, soy-based infant formulas. In many developing countries, however, the risks attached to feeding an infant artificially are greater than the 20% risk of vertical transmission of the virus that causes AIDS.

Patient Education Materials on the Internet

Patient education materials on HIV and AIDS can be found at the following web sites:

- Tennessee Department of Health AIDS Program. "Nutrition and HIV: Your Choices Make a Difference": http://www.thebody.com/tdoh/nuthiv/nutix.html
- The Body: An AIDS and HIV Information Resource: http://www.thebody.com/index.shtml
- Nutrition Links and Resources: http://www.hivresources.com/Nutrition.htm

SOURCES OF INFORMATION

Local resources include registered dietitians at local hospitals or in private practice; professors of nutrition, biochemistry, and foods and nutrition at nearby colleges and universities; local newspaper food editors; extension agents; and public health nutritionists who work at departments of health or WIC centers. Excellent sources of nutrition information can be found in print, such as books, journals, and newsletters. Health and fitness magazines for men and women often provide practical applications of current research. However, if a claim promises something that seems too good to be true, then it probably is. Reputable information is available from the following sources:

- Government (tax-supported) agencies, such as the USDA, USDHHS, and the CDCP.

Box 11-8 Nutrition Intervention for People Who Are HIV-Positive

EARLY-STAGE HIV (AT DIAGNOSIS)

- Obtain a nutritional assessment:

Anthropometry: BMI and body composition
Biochemistry: lab values
Clinical: nausea, vomiting, diarrhea, appetite, and oral lesions
Dietary: food frequency or diet history
Economic and educational

- Maximize food intake to grow lean body mass (LBM): 1.5 g protein and 3.5 kcal/kg.
- Encourage exercise.
- Stress food sanitation.
- Introduce the person to a dietitian.

SYMPTOMATIC HIV DISEASE

- Preserve LBM: 2 g protein and 40 kcal/kg.
- Combat anorexia and other symptoms.
- Continue work with registered dietitian.

LATE-STAGE HIV DISEASE: PROVIDE ENERGY AND NUTRIENTS

OVERALL FOOD INTAKE RECOMMENDATIONS

- Recommend a balanced diet.
- Prescribe a daily vitamin and mineral supplement containing 100% to 200% of the RDAs.
- Advise enhancing calories and nutrients by increasing the number and size of meals daily and by substituting nutrient-dense and calorie-rich foods for low-calorie or calorie-free foods and beverages.
- Suggest strategies for fortifying food with protein and calories.
- Advise adding calorie-containing supplements as needed.

EXERCISE RECOMMENDATIONS

- Involve the person in an active resistance exercise program, such as weight lifting, to increase LBM.
- Walking (not running) is recommended as a means of relaxation and to combat depression.

SANITATION RECOMMENDATIONS

- Explain the importance of lowering the risk of exposure to food-borne organisms.
- Provide food safety information.

LEAN BODY MASS CONSIDERATIONS

- Aim for a daily intake of 3000 calories per day.
- 1.5 to 2.0 g protein per kg (for reference, the RDA is 0.8 g protein per kg). In common measures, protein needs are 0.75 to 1.00 g protein per pound of body weight. Useful hint: 1 oz of a protein-rich food such as tuna fish has 7 g of protein (a 6-oz can of tuna delivers 42 g of protein).
- 35 to 40 calories per kg usual body weight or 17 to 19 calories per pound.
- Initiate liquid supplements to provide an additional 360 to 550 calories with an extra 15 to 20 g of protein.
- Appetite stimulant, if necessary, such as megestrol acetate (Megace) or delta 9 THC (Marinol).
- Minimize gastrointestinal symptoms: diarrhea, nausea and vomiting, and oral and esophageal lesions.

INDICATIONS THAT NUTRITIONAL COUNSELING OR THE HELP OF A DIETITIAN IS NEEDED

- A diagnosis (dx) of HIV-seropositivity
- Food intolerances (e.g. lactose intolerance)
- Anorexia
- Nausea and vomiting
- Weight loss (more than 5% premorbid weight)
- Diarrhea (more than 3 stools per day)
- Slow wound healing
- Lab values indicating malnutrition (serum albumin less than 3.5 g/dl; Hgb less than 12 g/dl; Hct less than 40; MCV less than 80 or greater than or equal to 95; serum cholesterol less than 100 mg/dl)
- Dysphagia
- Oral candidiasis
- History (hx) of food faddism
- Dx of type 2 diabetes, hypertension, hepatic or renal insufficiency
- Need of oral nutritional supplements

DIETITIAN SERVICES IN THE MANAGEMENT OF PATIENTS WITH HIV

- Diet history and analysis
- Diet counseling on therapeutic diets
- Counseling on food faddism and *megadosing* of vitamins and minerals
- Individualized instruction on diet supplements
- Information on food and drinking water safety
- Instruction on planning low-cost meals
- Planning of regimens for enteral or parenteral nutrition
- Counseling of family members and other caregivers

Data from Jossey-Bass, R., & Smigleski, C. (1996). *Eat up! Nutrition advice and food ideas for people living with HIV and AIDS*. Boston: Tufts University; McQuiggan, M. M. (1994). Nutritional support of the AIDS patient. *RD, 10* (3), 1; Watson, R.R. (1994). *Nutrition and AIDS*. Boca Raton, FL: CRC Press.

- Professional associations, such as the American Dietetic Association and the American Diabetes Association.
- Voluntary organizations, such as ACS and AHA.

Many of these organizations provide their publication lists on request. All publications can be accessed on the Internet, which has literally thousands of web sites devoted to food, normal and preventive nutrition, and MNT. An efficient way to stay abreast of developments in the field of nutrition is to regularly scan web sites that tackle the particular areas of interest. Generally, web sites that are operated by the U.S. government have the most credibility. Look for addresses (also known as Uniform Resource Locators, or URLs) that end in ".gov." Slightly less credible than tax-supported government sites are those maintained by educational organizations (".edu") and professional organizations (".org"). However, the information they contain is generally good. Sites maintained by the for-profit sector that have addresses ending in ".com" are the least reliable in terms of providing unbiased nutrition information.

The many references from government-sponsored web sites in this chapter are a testament to how useful the Internet can be for accessing timely and reliable information on topics in nutrition. Particularly useful for obtaining nutrition information are:

- U.S. Department of Agriculture: http://www.hhs.gov
- U.S. Department of Health, Education, and Welfare: http://www.usda.gov

Both web sites contain extensive hyperlinks or connections to other related web sites.

SUMMARY

This chapter introduces a wide range of subjects, including the *Healthy People 2010* nutrition objectives, the most current diet recommendations to reduce the risks of developing nutrition-related diseases, FDA regulations for food labeling, government food aid programs for the poor and elderly Americans, and primary and secondary prevention strategies related to the most common nutrition-related chronic diseases. Together, these topics form the basis of what is known as preventive nutrition, a requisite for the promotion of the nation's public health. All of the topics examined in this chapter can be studied further using the Internet. High quality, up-to-date materials, and continuing nutrition education literature for professionals are free and online.

REFERENCES

American Cancer Society. (2000a). *Cancer facts and figures: Nutrition and diet* [Online]. Available: http://www.cancer.org/statistics/cff2000/nutrition.html#choose.

American Cancer Society. (2000b). *Cancer facts and figures: Cancer in minorities* [Online]. Available: http://www.cancer.org/statistics/cff2000/minoritycancer.html.

American Diabetes Association. (2001). Position statement. Nutrition recommendations and principles for people with diabetes mellitus. Clinical practice recommendations 2001. *Diabetes Care*, 24(Suppl 1), S44-S47. Also available at: http://www.diabetes.org/clincialrecommendations/Supplement101/S44.htm.

American Dietetic Association (2001). Position of the American Dietetic Association: Food fortification and dietary supplements. *Journal of the American Dietetic Association*, 101, 115-125.

American Heart Association. (2000). *High blood pressure statistics 2000* [Online]. Available: http://www.americanheart.org/hbp/phys_stats.html.

American Institute for Cancer Research. (2000). *The new American plate, 2000* [Online]. Available: http://www.aicr.org/nap2.htm.

Appel, L. J., Moore, T. J., & Obarzanek, E., Vollmer, W. M., Svetkey, L. P., Sacks, F. M., Bray, G. A., Vogt, T. M., Cutler, J. A., Windhauser, M. M., Lin, P. H., & Karanja, N. (1997). DASH Collaborative Research Group. A clinical trial of the effects of dietary patterns on blood pressure. *New England Journal of Medicine*, 336, 1117-1124.

Barer-Stein, T. (1979). *You eat what you are*. Toronto, Canada: McClelland & Stewart.

Bray, G. A. (1996). Obesity. In E. E. Zeigler, & L. J. Filer, Jr. (Eds.), *Present knowledge in nutrition* (7th ed.). Washington, DC: International Life Sciences Institute Press.

Brownell, K. (2000). *The learn program for weight management 2000*. Dallas: American Health Publishing Co.

Burke, G. L., Savage, P. J., Manolio, T. A., Sprafka, J. M., Wagenknecht, L. E., Sidney, S., Perkins, L. L., Liu, K., & Jacobs, D. R., Jr. (1992). Correlates of obesity in young black and white women: The CARDIA study. *American Journal of Public Health*, 82, 1621-1625.

Calle, E. E., Thun, M. J., Petrelli, J. M., Rodriguez, C., & Heath, C. W., Jr. (1999). BMI and mortality in a prospective cohort of U.S. adults. *New England Journal of Medicine*, 341, 1097-1105.

Carpenter, K. J. (2000). *Berberi, white rice, and vitamin B: A disease, a cause, and a cure*. Berkeley, CA: Berkeley University Press.

Centers for Disease Control and Prevention. (1996, June). Guidelines for school health programs to promote lifelong healthy eating. *Morbidity and Mortality Weekly Report*, 45 (RR-9), 1-33. Available: http://www.cdc.gov/mmwr/preview/mmwrhtml/00042446.htm.

Centers for Disease Control and Prevention, National Center for Infectious Diseases (2001). *Bovine spongiform encephalopathy and new variant Creutzfeldt-Jackob disease*. [Online]. Available: http://www.cdc.gov/ncidod/diseases/cjd/bse_cjd.htm.

Centers for Disease Control and Prevention, National Center for Chronic Disease Prevention and Health Promotion. (2001). *Diabetes: A serious public health problem at a glance, 2001* [Online]. Available: http://www.cdc.gov/diabetes/pubs/glance/htm.

Expert Panel on Detection, Evaluation, and Treatment of High Blood Cholesterol in Adults. (2001). Executive summary of the third report of he national cholesterol education program (NCEP) expert panel on detection, evaluation, and treatment of high blood cholesterol in adults (adult treatment panel III). *Journal of the American Medical Association*, 285: 2486-2497.

Fagot-Champagna, A., Pettitt, D. J., Engelgau, M. M., Burrows, N. R., Geiss, L. S., Valdez, R., Beckles, G. L., Saaddine, J., Gregg, E. W., Williamson, D. F., Narayan, K. M., (2000). Type 2 diabetes among North American children and adolescents: An epidemiologic review and a public health perspective. *Journal of Pediatrics*, 136, 664-672.

Federal Register, 66(55), 15829. *NSLP*, National School Lunch Program; *SBP*, School Breakfast Program, *WIC*, Special Supplemental Nutrition Program for Women, Infants, and Children.

Gallagher, D., Visser, M., Sepulveda, D., Pierson, R. N., Harris, T., & Heymsfield, S. B. (1996). How useful is BMI for comparison of body fatness across age, sex and ethnic groups? *American Journal of Epidemiology*, 143, 228-239.

Garrow, J. S., & Webster, J. (1958). Quetelet's index (W/H^2) as a measure of fatness. *International Journal of Obesity*, 9, 147-153.

Grieco, E. M., & Cassidy, R. C. (2001). *Census 2000 brief: Overview of race and Hispanic origin* (p 11). Washington, DC: U.S. Department of Commerce. Economics and Statistics Administration. U.S. Census Bureau.

Grodner, M., Anderson, S. L., & DeYoung, S. (2000). *Nutrition: A nursing approach* (2nd ed.). St. Louis: Mosby.

Institute of Medicine, National Research Council. (1998). *Ensuring safe food: From production to consumption*. Washington, DC: National Academy Press.

Johnson, R. K., & Kennedy, E. (2000). The 2000 dietary guidelines for Americans: What are the changes and why were they made? *Journal of the American Dietetic Association*, 100, 769-774.

Kirby, R. (1998). *Dieting for dummies*. New York: IDG Publishing.

Kittler, P. G., & Sucher, K. P. (2000). *Cultural foods: Traditions and trends*. Belmont, CA: Wadsworth.

Krales, E. (2000, April 13). Setting standards: The expert panel for developing national HIV/AIDS nutrition guidelines. *Body Positive (13)* [Online]. Available: http://www.thebody.com/bp/apr00/standards.html.

Krauss, R. K., Eckel, R. H., & Howard, B., Appel, L. J., Daniels, S. R., Deckelbaum, R. J., Erdman, J. W., Jr., Kris-Etherton, P., Goldberg, I. J., Kotchen, T. A., Lichtenstein, A. H., Mitch, W. E., Mullis, R., Robinson, K., Wylie-Rosett, J., St. Jeor, S., Suttie, J., Tribble, D. L., & Bazzarre, T. L. (2000). AHA dietary guidelines. Revision 2000: A statement for healthcare professionals from the Nutrition Committee of the American Heart Association. *Circulation, 102*, 2284-2299. Available: http://circ.ahajournals.org/cgi/content/full/4304635102.

Mellin, L., Croughan-Minihane, M., & Dickey, L. (1997). The Solution Method: 2-year trends in weight, blood pressure, exercise, depression, and functioning of adults trained in developmental skills. *Journal of the American Dietetic Association, 97*, 1133-1138.

National Cholesterol Education Program. (1994). Second report of the expert panel on detection, evaluation, and treatment of high blood cholesterol in adults (adult treatment panel II). *Circulation*, 89, 1333-1445.

National Institutes of Health, National Heart, Lung, and Blood Institute, National High Blood Pressure Education Program. (1977, Nov.). *The sixth report of the joint national committee on prevention, detection, evaluation, and treatment of high blood pressure* (p. 11). NIH publication No. 98-4080, Washington, DC: National Institutes of Health.

National Institutes of Health, Office of Dietary Supplements. (2000). *What are dietary supplements?* [Online]. Available: http://odp.od.nih.gov/ods/whatare/whatare.html.

National Institutes of Health. (2000). *The National Institute of Diabetes and Digestive and Kidney Diseases: Statistics related to overweight and obesity* [Online]. Available: http://www.niddk.nih.gov/health/nutrit/pubs/statobes.htm#prev.

National Research Council, Food and Nutrition Board. (1989). *Recommended dietary allowances* (10th ed.). Washington, DC: National Academy Press.

National Research Council, Institute of Medicine, Food and Nutrition Board, Standing Committee on the Scientific Evaluation of Dietary Reference Intakes. (1997). *Dietary reference intakes for calcium, phosphorous, magnesium, vitamin D, and fluoride*. Report of the Subcommitttee on Calcium and Related Nutrients. Washington, DC: National Academy Press. [Online]. Available at: http://www.nap.edu/catalog/5776.html.

National Research Council, Institute of Medicine, Food and Nutrition Board. (2000a). *Dietary reference intakes for thiamin, riboflavin, niacin, vitamin B6, vitamin B12, pantothenic acid, biotin, and choline*. Washington, DC: National Academy Press. [Online]. Available at: http://www.nap.edu/catalog/6015.html.

National Research Council, Institute of Medicine, Food and Nutrition Board. (2000b). *Dietary reference intakes for vitamin C, vitamin E, selenium, and carotenoids*. Washington, DC: National Academy Press.

Powers, M. A. (1996). Medical nutrition therapy for diabetes. In M. A. Powers (Ed.), *Handbook of diabetes medical nutrition therapy*. Gaithersberg, MD: Aspen.

Rothman, K. J., Morre, L. L., Singer, M. R., Nguyen, U. D. T., Mannino, S., & Milunsky, A. (1995). Teratagenicity of high vitamin A intake. *New England Journal of Medicine*, 333, 1369-1373.

Ryan, C., Eleazer, P., & Egbert, J. (1995). Vitamin D in the elderly. *Nutrition Today*, 30, 228.

Spark, A. (2001). Health at any size: The size acceptance nondiet movement. *Journal of the American Medical Women's Association*, 56, 69-71.

Thomas, T. S., (1997). Improving care with nurse case managers: Practical aspects of designing lipid clinics. *American Journal of Cardiology*, 80, 62H-65H.

U.S. Department of Agriculture and U.S. Department of Health and Human Services. (1985). *Nutrition and your health: Dietary guidelines for Americans* (2nd ed.). Home and Garden Bulletin no. 232. Washington, DC: U.S. Government Printing Office.

U.S. Department of Agriculture and U.S. Department of Health and Human Services. (1990). *Nutrition and your health: Dietary guidelines for Americans* (3rd ed.). Home and Garden Bulletin no. 232. Washington, DC: U.S. Government Printing Office.

U.S. Department of Agriculture and U.S. Department of Health and Human Services. (1992). *The food guide pyramid*. Home and Garden Bulletin No. 249. Washington, DC: U.S. Government Printing Office.

U.S. Department of Agriculture and U.S. Department of Health and Human Services. (1995). *Nutrition and your health: Dietary guidelines for Americans* (4th ed.). Home and Garden Bulletin no. 232. Washington, DC: U.S. Government Printing Office.

U.S. Department of Agriculture, Agricultural Research Service, Dietary Guidelines Committee. (1995). *Report of the dietary guidelines advisory committee on the dietary guidelines for Americans, 1995, to the Secretary of Health and Human Services and the Secretary of Agriculture*. Washington, DC: U.S. Government Printing Office.

U.S. Department of Agriculture and U.S. Department of Health and Human Services. (2000). *Nutrition and your health: Dietary guidelines for Americans* (5th ed.). Home and Garden Bulletin no. 232. Washington, DC: U.S. Government Printing Office. Available: http://www.usda.gov/cnpp/DietGd.pdf.

U.S. Department of Agriculture, Food Stamp Program. (2000). *Frequently asked questions* [Online]. Available: http://www.fns.usda.gov/fsp/MENU/faqs/faqs.htm.

U.S. Department of Health and Human Services, National Institutes of Health, Office of Medical Applications of Research. (1992). *Methods for voluntary weight loss and control* [Online]. Bethesda, MD: U.S. Department of Health and Human Services. Available: http://mantis.cit.nih.gov/temp/CDC/consensus/ta/010/010_statement.htm.

U.S. Department of Health and Human Services, National Institutes of Health, National Heart, Lung, and Blood Institute. (1998). *Clinical guidelines on the identification, evaluation, and treatment of overweight and obesity in adults*. Bethesda, MD: U.S. Department of Health and Human Services.

U.S. Food and Drug Administration, Center for Food Safety and Applied Nutrition. (1999). *Dietary Supplement Health and Education Act of 1994* [Online]. Washington, DC: U.S. Food and Drug Administration. Available: http://vm.cfsan.fda.gov/~dms/dietsupp.html.

Weinberg, D. H. (1999). Income and Poverty 1998. *Press briefing on 1998 income and poverty estimates, housing and household economic statistics division, U.S. Census Bureau* [Online]. Available: http://www.census.gov/hhes/income/income98/prs99asc.html.

Willett, W. C., Dietz, W. H., & Colditz, G. A. (1999). Primary care: Guidelines for healthy weight. *New England Journal Medicine, 341*, 427-434.

Williams, C. L. (1995). Importance of dietary fiber in childhood. *Journal of the American Dietetic Association*, 95, 1140.

Williams, C. L., Bollella, M., & Wynder, E. L. (1995). A new recommendation for dietary fiber in childhood. *Pediatrics*, 96, 985-988.

Wood, O., & Spark, A. (1996). Medical nutrition therapy guidelines for treating the breast cancer patient, *Journal of the American Dietetic Association*, 96 (supplement), A-35.

Wooley, S. C., Wooley, O. W., & Dyrenforth, S. R. (1979). Theoretical, practical, and social issues in behavioral treatments of obesity. *Journal of Applied Behavior Analysis*, *12* (Spring), 3-25.

Wooley, S. C., Garner, D.M. (1991). Obesity treatment: The high cost of false hope. *Journal of the American Dietetic Association*, *91*, 1248-1251.

World Health Organization. (1995). *Physical status: The use and interpretation of anthropometry*. Geneva, Switzerland: The Organization.

Chapter 12

JAMES S. HUDDLESTON

Exercise

objectives

After completing this chapter, the nurse will be able to:

- Explain the physical activity and fitness goals of *Healthy People 2000* and the progress made toward these goals.
- Describe how physical activity positively influences physical and psychological health.
- Identify the benefits of physical activity throughout the aging process.
- Describe the prescriptions for and benefits of daily physical activity, aerobic exercise, and resistance training.
- Discuss how exercise can be combined with mindfulness to facilitate body awareness and self-inquiry.
- Explain the interventions to promote exercise adherence and compliance.

key terms

Aerobic Exercise
Anaerobic Exercise
Cardiorespiratory Fitness
Cool-Down Period
Exercise
Flexibility
Muscular Fitness
Physical Activity
Physical Fitness
Relaxation Response
Resistance Training
Warm-Up Period
Yoga

THINK About It

Knowing versus Doing

Having the knowledge about the benefits of exercise does not correlate well with long-term exercise compliance. Confidence in the ability to exercise and a sense of the meaning and purpose (core desire) of exercise in life ensures better success.

1. What motivates putting the effort into developing and maintaining an active lifestyle?
2. Why is being active and physically fit important?

Regular physical activity and exercise enhance both physical and psychological health. Generally speaking, people who exercise regularly, or those who naturally include physical activity in their daily routine, feel better mentally and physically, improve their health profile, and safeguard their functional independence as they go through the aging process. A holistic approach to physical activity involves exercise for cardiorespiratory health (endurance), exercise for musculoskeletal health (strength, flexibility, and bone density), and body awareness. Body awareness and mindfulness during exercise facilitate self-inquiry and self-acceptance, helping to relieve psychological stress and preventing physical injury.

Unfortunately, only 20% to 25% of adult Americans exercise enough to gain significant health benefits. Consequently, approximately 250,000 deaths each year (about 12% of the population) are related to a lack of regular physical activity (Pate et al., 1995). Not only is an active lifestyle an important component of primary prevention, but regular physical activity is also an essential modality in the treatment of chronic disease, which sets up the potential for benefit in all aspects of the biopsychosocial and spiritual model of health (Box 12-1).

Box 12-1 The Gift of Exercise

The other day, I was looking for a gift to give to a friend. This friend is very important to me and I want her to be around for a long time; I want her to live a long and healthy life. I thought how great it would be if I could give her a gift that would improve the quality of her life.

So, I sat down and made a list of what I would look for in this special gift:

- It would help her to be stronger, firmer, leaner, more flexible, and energetic.
- It would help lower her risk of dying from heart disease, lower blood pressure, improve lipid profile, control blood glucose level, fight obesity, and help her to age more gracefully.
- It would help improve immune function, concentration and task performance, and the quality of sleep.
- It would help reduce stress, improve mood, enhance self-esteem, and increase optimism and confidence.
- It would help to increase self-awareness and control over choices in her life.
- It would be fun, but also challenging.
- It would allow for socialization, but also time alone, depending on her needs.
- It would come in all different modes and styles and adapt to various environments and weather conditions.
- Finally, it would have a good *Consumer Reports* rating, supported by scientific data from reputable sources.

After completing my list, I realized that the only gift that meets all these criteria is the gift of exercise. Have a happy and healthy life, my friend.

HEALTHY PEOPLE 2010

Everyone needs physical activity to be healthy. Human physiology has evolved in preparation for physical exertion. Until recently, survival through the vigor of daily living depended on a moderate degree of physical fitness. However, with mechanization and the style of living in today's society, daily life has become too sedentary. The following circumstances have been cited as contributing to a sedentary lifestyle:

- Machines to do the work and provide transportation.
- Increased computer time at work and home.
- Decreased financial resources in schools, colleges, and communities for physical activity instruction, playgrounds, parks and recreation facilities, and after-school sports programs and staff.
- Decreased outdoor activity resulting from fear of crime in neighborhoods.
- Children spending increased time watching television and playing video games (USDHHS, 1995).

A lifestyle of inactivity places the population at risk for disease and the literature supports exercise as an essential protective element in health.

Population studies (Kannel & Sorlie, 1989; Morris, 1973; Morris, Clayton, Everitt, Semmence, & Burgess, 1990; Paffenbarger & Hyde, 1980; Paffenbarger, Wing, & Hyde, 1978; Paffenbarger, Hyde, Wing, & Hsieh, 1986) set the standard for demonstrating a positive correlation between vocational and leisure-time physical activity and decreased rates of morbidity and mortality. Blair et al. (1989) examined the relationship between level of physical fitness (an objective marker for physical activity) and all-cause and cause-specific mortality in both men and women. Higher levels of fitness are associated with a lower mortality rate. Another study by Blair et al. (1995) on men considered solely the relationship between changes in physical fitness over time and the rate of mortality. Men who improved from unfit to fit had a 44% reduction in age-adjusted, all-cause mortality rates and a 52% reduction in age-adjusted cardiovascular disease (CVD) risk compared with their peers who remained unfit. Although the men who demonstrated the greatest increase in fitness had the greatest reduction in all-cause mortality rates, men who initially tested as already fit, but improved their fitness levels over time, lowered their risk of mortality from all causes. Blair et al. (1996) determined that the least fit, 20% of the men and women in this study, had double the risk of death during an 8-year follow-up compared with their fit counterparts. These studies support the philosophy that an active lifestyle improves health and lowers mortality rates for people of all fitness levels.

Defining Moment in Health

To fully understand the *Healthy People 2010* objectives regarding exercise, the following definitions will be used

(American College of Sports Medicine [ACSM], 1998; USDHHS, 2000):

- **Physical activity:** bodily movement that is produced by the contraction of skeletal muscles and that substantially increases energy expenditure; includes transportation and vocational and leisure-time activity. Leisure-time activity can be further categorized into sports, recreational activities, and exercise training.
- **Exercise** (exercise training): planned, structured, and repetitive bodily movement performed to improve or maintain one or more components of physical fitness.
- **Aerobic exercise:** activity that uses large muscle groups in a repetitive, rhythmic fashion over an extended period to improve the efficiency of the oxidative energy-producing system and improve cardiorespiratory endurance; uses stored adipose tissue as major fuel source.
- **Anaerobic exercise:** high-intensity, short-duration activity that improves the efficiency of the phosphocreatine and glycolytic energy-producing systems and increases muscle strength, power, and speed of reactivity; uses phosphagens and glucose-glycogen as major fuel sources.
- **Physical fitness:** a set of attributes (cardiorespiratory fitness, muscular fitness, and flexibility) that people have or achieve that relates to the ability to perform physical activity without undue fatigue or risk of injury.
- **Cardiorespiratory fitness** (aerobic capacity, functional capacity, and oxygen uptake [$\dot{V}O_2$]): the ability to deliver and use oxygen throughout the body to allow physical activity over an extended period without excessive fatigue.
- **Muscular fitness:** the strength and endurance of muscles that allows for participation in daily activities with low risk of musculoskeletal injury.
- **Flexibility:** adequate muscle length and joint mobility to allow free and painless movement through a wide range of motion (ROM).

Original Physical Activity Goals

Unfortunately, only 23% of the adult population perform enough regular, sustained exercise to gain any significant health benefit and slightly over 10% of the population exercises at an intensity necessary to promote cardiorespiratory fitness. A full 70% to 75% of adult Americans are sedentary, reporting no leisure-time activity or are not regularly active (USDHHS, 2000).

Recognizing the importance of physical activity in the nation's health, *Healthy People 2000* (USDHHS, 1990) established physical activity goals. These goals take into account the demonstrated relationship between physical activity and an improvement in the biological markers associated with health and they identify the reasons for the trend toward a more sedentary lifestyle.

Box 12-2 *Healthy People 2000*—Goals for Physical Activity

- Reduce coronary heart disease (CHD) deaths.
- Reduce the prevalence of being overweight.
- Increase the number of people who engage in light to moderate physical activity for at least 30 minutes per day.
- Increase the number of people who engage in vigorous physical activity 3 or more days per week for 20 or more minutes each session.
- Reduce the number of people who engage in no leisure-time physical activity.
- Increase the number of people who regularly perform physical activities that enhance and maintain muscular strength, endurance, and flexibility.
- Increase the number of overweight people who have adopted sound dietary practices combined with regular physical activity to attain an appropriate body weight.
- Increase the number of children and adolescents in first through twelfth grades who participate in daily school physical education.
- Increase the amount of school physical education class time that students spend being physically active.
- Increase the number of work sites that offer employer-sponsored physical activity and fitness programs.
- Increase community availability and accessibility of physical activity and fitness facilities.
- Increase the number of primary care providers who routinely assess and counsel people regarding physical activity practices.
- Increase the proportion of children and adolescents who view television 2 or less hours per day.
- Increase the proportion of trips made by walking and bicycling.

From U.S. Department of Health and Human Services. (1990). *Healthy people 2000: National health promotion and disease prevention objectives* (Pub No 91-50212). Washington, DC: Public Health Service.

Box 12-2 provides a summary of the physical activity goals set for 2000.

Revised Physical Activity Goals: Making Progress

The *Healthy People 2010* objectives (USDHHS, 1995, 1999, 2000) provide evidence of the progress that has been made toward achieving the original objectives. Figure 12-1 shows that progress has been made in decreasing the number of people who die from coronary heart disease (CHD). The number of people who engage in regular moderate and vigorous physical activity and strength training activities has also increased. However, despite the solid gains in these objectives—indicating that the message regarding the benefits of physical activity is reaching some segments of the population—the improvements fall short of the goals set for the year 2000. The new goals set for

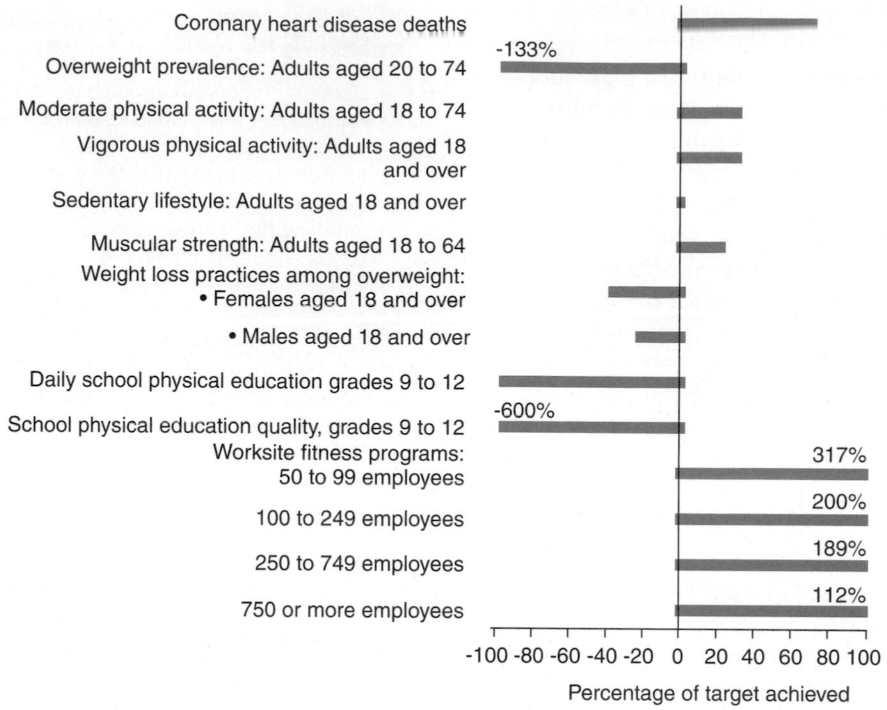

Fig. 12-1 The status of physical activity and fitness objectives. Tracking data for the objective concerning community involvement are unavailable.

Healthy People 2010 reflect the work that remains (USDHHS, 2000).

The one area in which considerable improvement has been demonstrated, and in fact exceeds the goal, is providing work site fitness programs. These programs can increase employee physical activity and fitness and improve employee health (Iverson, Fielding, Crow, & Christensen, 1985). The significant increase in work site programs may be contributing to the increase in the number of people who are performing regular physical activity.

On a less positive note, Fig. 12-1 also indicates that little progress has been made in mobilizing the population out of a sedentary lifestyle. Although only 10.4% of adolescents report no leisure-time physical activity, the percentage increases throughout the lifespan from approximately 31% for men and women 18 to 24 years of age to 65% for individuals 75 years and older (USDHHS, 2000). The tendency to be sedentary continues to increase with age, increasing the risk of premature morbidity, mortality, and disability and limiting functional independence.

The prevalence of obesity has increased in all age groups in the United States. One in five teens and one in three adults are overweight. The number of adults who combine good dietary practice with regular physical activity in an attempt to attain an appropriate body weight has decreased. This decidedly negative trend may be related to the decline in physical activity in the schools. The number of students involved in daily school physical education decreased from 42% in 1991 to 27% in 1997 and only 32% of students are physically active for 20 minutes or more in daily physical education classes (USDHHS, 2000). Physical activity habits tend to track (be consistent) during early childhood and less active children tend to remain less active over time, increasing their risk of becoming sedentary adults (Pate, Baranowski, Dowda, & Trost, 1996). If a standard is to be set for the importance of physical activity throughout the lifespan, then it needs to start with children, who have the potential to develop lifelong healthy habits.

As the health care system moves toward a preventive model, primary care providers must facilitate a wellness attitude in their patients, which involves not only encouraging individuals to be physically active, but also leading by example. Recommending regular exercise and espousing the benefits from personal experience can have a significant influence on individual involvement. Nurses are in a position to inquire about and provide counseling for exercise habits of their patients. Although some progress has been made in providing this service, especially with nurse practitioners, data through 1997 indicate a shortfall in reaching the goal set for 2000 of 50% of patients (USDHHS, 1999). Although there has been some improvement in some areas, overall, the proportion of the population reporting physical activity has remained essentially unchanged and progress is limited. Obviously, the progress that has been made toward physical activity goals for the year 2000 does not reflect a significant shift in the attitude of the general population or the health care profession. This is still a population at risk.

HYPOKINETIC STATISTIC

Although a sedentary lifestyle places the individual at risk for becoming a hypokinetic statistic, regular physical activity is associated with a wide variety of physical and mental health benefits; for example, the prevention and management of CHD, hypertension (HTN), noninsulin-dependent diabetes mellitus (NIDDM), colon cancer, osteoporosis, obesity, and anxiety and depression (NIH, 1996; Pate et al., 1995). Regular physical activity may also be linked to a reduction in back injuries (Cady, Thomas, & Karwasky, 1985). Activity that promotes fitness, builds muscle strength, endurance, and flexibility and expends calories may protect against injury, chronic disease, and disability. Regular physical activity can help maintain functional independence and improve the quality of life throughout the aging process (Astrand, 1992; USDHHS, 2000).

Coronary Heart Disease

Of particular importance is the role of physical activity in preventing CHD, the leading cause of death in the United States. Physical inactivity affects more people in the development of CHD than any other risk factor, making it a significant public health problem. Until recently, physical inactivity was not considered one of the most powerful risk factors; HTN, smoking, obesity, and hyperlipidemia were considered to have greater influence. However, at any level or combination of risk factors, individuals who are sedentary are at an even greater risk (Table 12-1).

Blair et al. (1989) suggests a significant inverse relationship between physical fitness and CHD risk; higher levels of fitness are associated with lower CHD risk. A sedentary lifestyle is now recognized as a major risk factor in the development of CHD (Fletcher et al., 1992). In fact, the relative risk of CHD associated with physical inactivity is comparable to the risk observed for hyperlipidemia, HTN, and cigarette smoking. A study by Paffenbarger et al. (1993) indicates that the reduction in CHD risk associated with increased physical activity is equivalent to the reduction in risk associated with the cessation of smoking. These findings are supported by Blair et al. (1995, 1996), who identify a similar reduction of CHD risk between an increase in physical fitness and the cessation of smoking.

The importance of exercise in the hierarchy of risk factors increases with the knowledge that not only is physical activity identified as a major independent predictor of CHD, but it can also help modify the negative effects of other risk factors in both men and women. Blair et al. (1989, 1996) demonstrate that highly fit men and women with multiple risk factors have lower death rates compared with poorly fit people who have no other risk factors. A large study of over 25,000 men suggests that even in the presence of other CHD risk factors, moderate to high levels of cardiorespiratory fitness provides protection from CHD mortality (Farrell et al., 1998). Data from the Nurses' Health Study indicate that both moderate and vigorous exercise decrease the risk of coronary events in women by 30% to 40% (Manson et al., 1999).

Table 12-1 Major Coronary Risk Factors

Positive Risk Factors	Defining Criteria
Age	Men over age 45; women over age 55 or at early menopause without estrogen replacement therapy
Family history	MI or sudden death under age 55 in father or under age 65 in mother (or other first-degree relative)
Current cigarette smoking	
Hypertension	BP more than 140/90 mmHg (measured on two separate occasions) or on anti-hypertension medications
Hypercholesterolemia	Total serum cholesterol over 200 mg/dl (5.2 mmol/L) (if lipoprotein profile is unavailable) or HDL under 40 mg/dl (0.9 mmol/L)
Diabetes mellitus	People with IDDM 1 to 30 years or who have had it for more than 15 years, and people with NIDDM over the age of 35 years
Sedentary lifestyle	Sedentary job and no regular exercise or leisure-time activity

Modified from American College of Sports Medicine. (1995). *Guidelines for exercise testing and prescription* (5th ed.). Media, PA: Williams & Wilkins.

BP, blood pressure; *HDL*, high-density lipoprotein; *IDDM*, insulin-dependent diabetes mellitus; *MI*, myocardial infarction, *NIDDM*, noninsulin-dependent diabetes mellitus.

All of these studies reveal the value of exercise in the primary prevention of CHD. Exercise also plays a role in secondary prevention (recurrence). Increased physical activity appears to benefit individuals with CVD, including myocardial infarction (MI), angina pectoris, congestive heart failure, their status after coronary artery bypass surgery (CABG), and percutaneous transluminal coronary angioplasty (PTCA) or stent. Benefits include reduction in cardiovascular mortality rates, reduction of symptoms, improvement in exercise tolerance and functional capacity, and improvement in psychological well being and quality of life (NIH, 1996). A review by Thompson (1988) suggests that, by pooling the results of several studies, exercise-treated subjects can experience a reduction in recurrent MI and mortality rates. A review study by Oldridge, Guyatt, Fischer, & Rimno (1988) reports similar findings. In an analysis of 10 major studies involving more than 4000 people who had had an MI, individuals who participated in cardiac rehabilitation exercise programs had 25% fewer deaths from CHD. People who include regular exercise in their lives after an MI have improved rates of survival.

The 1990 statement on exercise by the Committee on Exercise and Cardiac Rehabilitation (McHenry et al., 1990) concurs with these findings. The consensus is that regular dynamic physical activity plays a role in both the primary and secondary prevention of CHD. Evidence suggests that regular moderate or vigorous leisure-time or occupational physical activity may protect against CHD. Additionally, exercise may improve the likelihood of surviving an MI and reduce the chances of recurrence in some individuals. Although heavy physical exertion can trigger an MI, habitual physical activity lowers the relative risk of suffering an MI during heavy physical exertion (Mittleman et al., 1993).

Current literature strongly demonstrates that the risk of CHD decreases as physical activity increases and that a plausible relationship between the decreased risk and a number of potential physiological and metabolic mechanisms exists:

- Increasing high-density lipoprotein (HDL) cholesterol.
- Decreasing serum triglyceride (TRG) levels.
- Decreasing high blood pressure.
- Improving glucose tolerance and insulin sensitivity.
- Decreasing obesity; altering distribution of body fat.
- Reducing the sensitivity of the myocardium to the effects of catecholamines, thereby decreasing the risk of ventricular arrhythmias.
- Enhancing fibrinolysis and altering platelet function (Pate et al., 1995).

High-Density Lipoprotein and Serum Triglyceride Levels

Exercise has a major influence on lipoprotein metabolism, primarily affecting plasma levels of HDL and TRG. There is a powerful negative correlation between CHD and plasma HDL. Increases in HDL lower the total cholesterol-HDL ratio, thereby reducing CHD risk. Exercise also has a potent lowering effect on levels of plasma TRG that is evident within hours after a bout of exercise (Haskell, 1992). Exercise training increases lipoprotein lipase activity, an enzyme that removes cholesterol and fatty acids from the blood (Stefanick & Wood, 1994). TRG levels are lower and HDL levels are higher in physically active people compared with the sedentary population. A dose-response relationship between amounts of physical activity and HDL levels appears to exist, with endurance-trained athletes having 20% to 30% higher HDL levels and lower TRG levels compared with healthy, age-matched, sedentary people (Leon, 1991). In a study of women runners, Williams (1996) identifies a significant incremental dose-response relationship between increased weekly running distance and increased HDL concentrations.

The effect of exercise on lipid metabolism may be related more to the volume (duration and frequency) rather than to the intensity of the exercise. Although single episodes of physical activity result in an improved blood lipid profile that can last for several days (Durstine & Haskell, 1994), regular repeated bouts of activity are needed for long-term benefits. Short periods of exercise training result in modest increases in HDL, but longer periods of training produce larger increases in HDL (Haskell et al., 1992). Exercise's lowering effect on TRG is cumulative; therefore frequent bouts of exercise result in a progressive decrease in TRG. Changes in lipid profiles are most significant with moderate exercise over a prolonged period (1 year). On the average, exercise training has the potential to increase HDL approximately 2 mg/dl. Although this benefit may not appear significant, a 1 mg/dl increase in HDL is associated with a 2% decrease in CHD risk. More exercise may provide even more benefit. In the study by Williams (1996), the 9.6 mg/dl difference in HDL between the groups running the shortest distances and the longest represents a 29% reduction in CHD risk. However, exercise is not a quick fix. At best, exercise appears to involve a commitment to regular, moderately intense physical activity over an extended period—a lifetime commitment to an active lifestyle.

Hypertension

Studies by Paffenbarger, Wing, Hyde, & Jung (1983) and Blair et al. (1989) suggest that habitual activity and physical fitness may reduce the risk of developing HTN. In these studies, people who did not engage in vigorous sports play or who were at low levels of fitness were at 35% to 52% greater risk for developing HTN. Although these studies reflect the chronic effect of exercise on control of HTN, studies by Roman, Camuzzi, Villalon, & Klenner (1981) and Kiyonaga, Arakawa, Tanaka, & Shindo (1985) demonstrate that acute bouts of aerobic exercise (3 times a week for 30 to 60 minutes at a moderate intensity for 3 months) result in a significant reduction of both systolic blood pressure (SBP) and diastolic blood pressure (DBP) at rest. The benefits of aerobic exercise on lowering HTN are supported by two analyses (Arroll & Beaglehole, 1992; Kelly & McClellan, 1994); both SBP and DBP decreased approximately 6 to 7 mmHg with aerobic exercise (of similar parameters as those listed previously). Fagard and Tipton (1994) report that endurance training decreases resting blood pressure (RBP) an average of 7 to 10 mmHg for both SBP and DBP in individuals with HTN. Keleman, Effron, Valenti, & Stewart (1990) suggest that exercise may be as strong a treatment modality for HTN as some medications. The need for making exercise part of a habitual lifestyle change is reflected in the study by Roman et al. (1981); RBP increased again when training was discontinued.

Low- to moderate-intensity endurance exercise appears to be most effective in lowering HTN. Circuit weight training also has a positive effect on HTN, whereas resistance training (designed primarily to increase strength) and high-intensity aerobic training appear to have minimal benefit. Mechanisms underlying the exercise-training effect on lowering blood pressure are not completely clear, but may involve attenuation of sympathetic nervous system (SNS) activity. This attenuation results in the dilation of peripheral blood vessels, which decreases systemic vascular resistance. Decreasing SNS activity may have a beneficial effect on the insulin resistance that is often observed in hypertensive people. Reductions in circulating insulin levels decrease the potential for insulin-mediated sodium reabsorption by the kidneys and increased blood pressure (Tipton, 1984).

Hyperinsulinemia and Glucose Intolerance

Hyperinsulinemia and glucose intolerance account for the following types of diabetes: diabetes mellitus (DM), which encompasses a group of metabolic disorders that have in common an increase in blood glucose levels and associated metabolic dysfunction; insulin-dependent diabetes mellitus (IDDM), which involves elevated blood glucose levels that are a result of a deficiency of circulating insulin caused by destruction of the pancreatic beta cells; and NIDDM, which involves elevated blood glucose levels from insulin resistance (decreased insulin sensitivity)—largely in skeletal muscles—or impaired insulin secretion. Approximately 90% of persons with diabetes have NIDDM.

Exercise training is associated directly with improved insulin sensitivity (Holloszy, 1986). Prospective cohort studies demonstrate that physical activity is related to a reduced incidence of NIDDM (Helmrich, Rogland, Leving, & Paffenbarger, 1991; Manson et al., 1992). These findings are supported by population studies of various ethnic groups (see Multicultural Awareness box). Physical activity is inversely related to the incidence of NIDDM, a relationship that is most evident in men at high risk for developing diabetes (those with a high body mass index (BMI), a history of HTN, or a family history of DM). A dose-response relationship was noted: each 500 kcals of additional leisure-time physical activity per week was associated with a 6% reduction in the risk of developing NIDDM (Helmrich et al., 1991).

During physical activity, contracting skeletal muscles work with insulin to enhance glucose uptake into the cells. Insulin resistance impedes glucose mobilization into cells, increasing plasma glucose levels and setting the potential for developing NIDDM. Although insulin resistance in skeletal muscles may be the primary defect, the development of disease appears to be related to elevated insulin

MULTICULTURAL AWARENESS

Walk Away from Ethnic Glucose Intolerance

The Pima Indians of the Gila River Indian Community in Arizona have the highest documented incidence rates of NIDDM in the world. On the island of Mauritius in the southwest Indian Ocean, all four ethnic groups (Hindu and Muslim-Asian Indians, African Creoles, and Chinese) have been identified with unusually high rates of NIDDM. In the United States, NIDDM is 30% more prevalent in Blacks compared with Whites. The presence of NIDDM in each of these ethnic groups provides strong support for the presence of one or more modifiable risk factors in the cause of the disease.

Excessive weight gain is a strong independent predictor of NIDDM. The development of NIDDM (characterized by insulin resistance, hyperinsulinemia, and glucose intolerance) is related to weight gain in adults, particularly in fat accumulation around the waist, abdomen, and upper body (android or apple shape). This type of fat distribution is also associated with a higher risk of developing CHD. Adipose tissue is a major site for insulin insensitivity and most obese individuals have increased insulin resistance and/or some degree of glucose intolerance.

Physical activity has been identified as having an important role in the prevention and treatment of NIDDM. By helping to maintain a proper lean-to-fat body mass, either by encouraging weight loss or preventing weight gain, physical activity may indirectly protect against the development of NIDDM, and by its modulating effect on fat stores, physical activity helps to improve insulin sensitivity and glucose tolerance. Additionally, physical activity may directly affect glucose metabolism. The acute effect of exercise can lower plasma glucose levels by enhancing the effect of insulin; long-term exercise improves insulin action and glucose tolerance.

Epidemiological studies of ethnic groups indicate that physical inactivity is also a risk factor for NIDDM. In the United States, Blacks and Native Americans have a disproportionate number of poor, unemployed, and disadvantaged individuals who lack access to the health care system. The least active individuals within these populations should be given the most attention because they have the most to gain. The methods and programs that are used to get information on the importance of physical activity out to the public need to be varied, depending on the socioeconomic and cultural factors specific to various ethnic populations. Promotion of physical activity by schools, communities, and government and health agencies, with these factors in mind, will significantly help achieve the goal of improving lifestyles and decreasing the incidence of NIDDM.

Data from Harris, M. I., et al. (1998). Prevalence of diabetes, impaired fasting glucose, and impaired glucose tolerance in US adults. *Diabetes Care, 21*, 518-524; Helmrich, S. P., Ragland, D. R., & Paffenbarger, R. S. (1994). Prevention of non–insulin-dependent diabetes mellitus with physical activity. *Medicine and Science in Sports and Exercise, 26*, 824-830; Kriska, A. M., et al. (1993). The association of physical activity with obesity, fat distribution and glucose intolerance in Pima Indians. *Diabetologia, 36*, 863-869; Pereira, M. A., et al. (1995). Physical inactivity and glucose intolerance in the multi-ethnic island of Mauritius. *Medicine and Science in Sports and Exercise, 27*, 1626-1634.

levels, a result of the body's response to the need to mobilize glucose into the cells. Additionally, this syndrome often also involves elevated TRG and HTN, which contribute to the potential for disease. Exercise increases insulin sensitivity, improves the inherent effect of endogenous insulin, decreases obesity, and plays a role in lowering TRG and HTN; therefore it is recommended in the treatment of NIDDM. With diet, weight control, and exercise, preventing or decreasing the need for oral antiglucolytic agents and insulin is possible while maintaining normal blood glucose levels. Physical activity may be most beneficial in preventing the progression of NIDDM during the earlier stages of the disease process, before insulin therapy is required (Holloszy, 1986). Overall, physical activity has a significant positive effect on a chronic disease that is associated with a high risk of developing CHD. Wei, Gibbons, Kampert, Nichamen, & Blair (2000) reveal that cardiorespiratory fitness and physical activity lower mortality rates in men with NIDDM. Low-fitness men are 7.4 times more likely to die from their diabetes and twice as likely to die from CHD.

Fibrinolysis and Platelet Aggregability

The relationship among physical activity, fibrinolysis, and platelet aggregability suggests that regular physical activity decreases the risk of acute cardiovascular thrombosis (Rauramaa & Salomen, 1994). Regular endurance exercise lowers the risk of CHD through its action on the factors that affect thrombotic function (Morris et al., 1990). However, more research must be carried out for a better understanding of this relationship.

Obesity

Obesity is not often considered as an independent risk factor for CHD because its effects are exerted through other risk factors, such as HTN, hyperlipidemia, and DM. Nevertheless, obesity should be considered an independent target for intervention in health promotion. Being overweight and obese are major contributors to many preventable causes of death. On average, higher body weights are associated with higher death rates (USDHHS, 2000). For men, obesity is closely related to CVD, respiratory disease, NIDDM, musculoskeletal dysfunction, various cancers, emotional stress, and all-cause mortality (Lee, Manson, Hennekens, & Paffenbarger 1993; Manson et al., 1992).

In the United States, the incidence of adult obesity has increased from 25% in the 1970s to 33% in the 1990s (Kuczmarski, Flegol, Campbell, & Johnson, 1994). Obesity is generally defined as an excess of adipose tissue, corresponding to a weight that is equal to or greater than 120% to 125% of the ideal body weight (Kuczmarski, Flegol, Campbell, & Johnson, 1994). Fat mass (body fat percentage) is most important in determining the ideal body weight. The recommended body fat levels for men and women are approximately 15% to 16% for men and 23% to 24% for women (ACSM, 1997). The average American man and woman tend to exceed the recommended body fat level. An increase in fat mass and the development of obesity occur when energy intake exceeds total daily energy expenditure for a prolonged period (Leibel, Rosenbaum, & Hirsch, 1995). Decreased physical activity may be both a cause and a consequence of weight gain over a lifetime.

Maintaining fitness and health is closely related to controlling weight. Literature supports the positive influence that physical activity has on body weight and obesity (USDHHS, 1996). Physical activity does the following:

- Promotes a negative energy balance (burns calories).
- Increases metabolic rate for an extended period after the activity.
- Increases metabolic efficiency for burning calories by increasing lean body mass.
- Helps counteract the decrease in metabolic rate associated with low-calorie diets by preserving lean body mass.
- Is a good alternative to eating when eating is a response to stress rather than to hunger (Williford, Scharff-Olson, & Blessing, 1993).

Unfortunately, most overweight people ignore exercise as a means of weight loss or they exercise at rates below federal health guidelines (CDCP, 2000).

The treatment of obesity involves a comprehensive program of nutrition management, behavior modification, and physical activity or exercise. The key to normalizing body fatness is long-term adherence and permanent lifestyle changes, not from dieting or short-term exercise trials. The combination of increased physical activity and nutrition management appears to be more effective for long-term weight regulation compared with either exercise or dieting alone (Kayman, Bruvold, & Stern 1990; Wallace, 1989). The effectiveness of physical activity is related to the frequency and duration of each activity session and the longevity of the activity program. Recommended thresholds for exercise include:

- A program of low-impact aerobic exercise, increase in daily activities, and resistance training.
- A frequency of 5 to 7 times a week.
- A length of 40 to 60 minutes a day or 20 to 30 minutes twice daily (ACSM, 1997).

As long as calorie expenditure is similar, moderate lifestyle activity may be as effective as structured exercise (Andersen et al., 1999). Moderate intensity appears to be most effective for total and fat calorie consumption during the activity (see Health Teaching box).

Women tend to have a 5% to 10% lower resting metabolic rate compared with men and a higher percentage of body fat compared with men of similar weight. Consequently, women have a lower percentage of lean body mass and may not be as metabolically active as are

HEALTH TEACHING Do Not Myth These Fat-Burning Facts!

Myth: Low-intensity exercise is best for burning fat.

Fact: Low-intensity exercise burns a higher percentage of fat calories than carbohydrate calories. Additionally, as the intensity of exercise increases, a greater percentage of calories burned shifts to carbohydrates from fat. However, although the percentage of fat calories burned during low-intensity exercise is higher than during moderate-intensity exercise, both the absolute number of calories expended and the absolute number of calories derived from fat tend to be higher with moderate exercise. If the ultimate goal is to burn calories to aid weight loss, then low intensity is not the best or the fastest way.

Fact: The bottom line is that people need to start exercising. Some exercise is better than none, especially for people who are uncomfortable with exercising at higher intensities or for those who are at higher risk for injury when doing so. However, the goal of weight loss may be achieved faster by picking up the pace a little. If the pace needs to be slower, then exercise should last longer to achieve comparable energy-expenditure levels. A goal of 30 to 60 minutes, 3 to 5 times a week, creating a 300-calorie expenditure with each session, is recommended to facilitate weight loss. See Fig. 12-3 for suggestions on physical activities to burn calories.

Fact: To further enhance the potential for weight loss, a person should add resistance training to weekly exercise. First, resistance training is a good calorie burner. Second, muscle tissue burns more calories than fat; therefore as muscle mass increases, the resting metabolic rate increases, making the body a more efficient calorie-burning machine. Resistance training 2 or 3 times a week can make a significant difference in long-term weight loss and maintenance.

Fact: Simply being more physically active throughout the day can also help with weight loss. It is easy to find excuses to get up and move around during the day, such as taking the stairs rather than the elevator; parking on the far side of the lot and walking the extra distance; doing house and yard work rather than paying someone else to do it. All of these activities burn calories and, in addition to regular aerobic and resistance exercise, will result in lost pounds of fat.

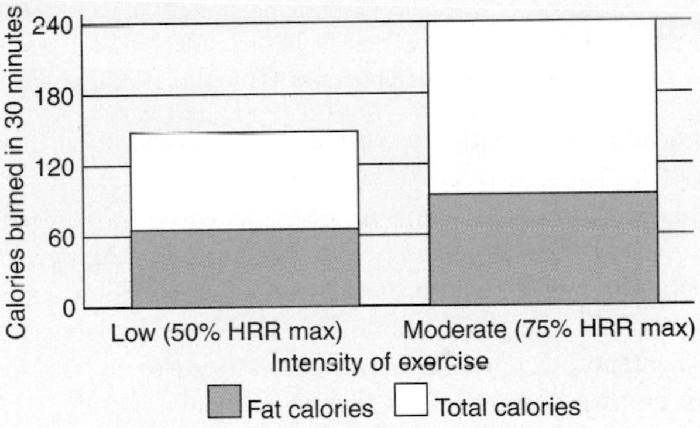

Data from American College of Sports Medicine. (1996). *Guidelines for exercise testing and prescription* (5th ed.). Media, PA: Williams & Wilkins; Bean, A. (1996). The truth about burning fat. *Runner's World, 31,* 47-50; Williford, H. N., Scharff-Olson, M., & Blessings, D. (1993). Exercise prescription for women. *Sports Medicine, 15,* 299-311.

men during exercise. Women may expend up to 40% fewer calories than do men during the same exercise protocol at the same relative intensity (Tremblay, Despres, & Bouchard, 1985).

Fat in men is stored primarily in the upper body or upper abdominal region. Fat in women is primarily stored in the lower half of the abdomen, the hips, and the thighs. Adipose tissue metabolism tends to be different in various regions. The fat-metabolism response to exercise appears to be less in the femoral-gluteal region compared with the upper body-abdominal region. Femoral-gluteal adipose tissue serves as an important source of energy during lactation. Women may not lose fat as easily as do men in response to exercise because genetic differences are related to where and how fat is stored and metabolized (Williford, Scharff-Olson, & Blessing, 1993). Consequently, women who need to lose weight may need to be more diligent about increasing the duration of their exercise training sessions and to make resistance training a priority to facilitate maximal energy expenditure.

Aging

The biological changes attributed to aging closely resemble the effects of physical inactivity. The list for both aging and inactivity includes an increase in body fat and a decrease in aerobic capacity, muscle mass, metabolic rate, strength and flexibility, bone mass, sexual function, mental performance, immune function, and sleep quality.

Although these changes occur with aging, their rate and magnitude are lessened in people who participate in regular exercise (Bortz, 1982). The popular theory that exercise increases the quality of life is based on the rationale that regular exercise maintains function during the aging process. Physical activity has been shown to be associated with reductions in age-related morbidity, improvements in functional capacity, and preservation of independence (Matheson, Macintyre, Taunton, Clement, & Lloyd-Smith, 1989).

A review of the major studies that examine levels of physical activity and life expectancy indicate a 1- to 2-year increased life expectancy for physically active men compared with physically inactive men (Heyden & Fodor, 1988). This fact hardly seems significant considering that life expectancy in the United States has increased from 47 years in 1900 to approximately 75 years in 1988. However, after years of inactivity, a large number of older adults are living at levels of physical ability that are tenuous at best, such that even minor setbacks can force them into a dependent state (Astrand, 1992). Physical training (including aerobics for endurance, resistance training for strength, and Tai Chi and yoga for balance and flexibility) can help maintain and even improve function in older adults, postponing physical deterioration for 10 to 20 years (Astrand, 1992; Fiatarone et al., 1990, 1994; Green & Crouse, 1995; Jackson et al., 1995; Lan, Lai, Chen, & Wong, 1998; Wolf, Barnhart, & Kutner, 1996). Regular physical activity may not necessarily improve the quantity of life, but it can have an enormous effect on the quality of life during the aging process, helping to sustain function and independent living.

All parts of the body that have a function, if used in moderation and exercised in labors in which each is accustomed, become thereby healthy, well-developed, and age more slowly, but if unused and left idle they become liable to disease, defective in growth, and age quickly—Hippocrates (Franklin, 1993, p. 476).

More in keeping with the vernacular of today, "Use it or lose it!"

Making an investment in exercise early in life will produce a better return of health later in life. "Aging is a self-fulfilling prophecy. It is learning how to know what time it is in your life" (Bortz, 1993). Naturally, genetic, environmental, and accidental factors need to be considered, but the bottom line is that people have some choice in how they want to age and exercise can help them age more gracefully.

By maintaining an active lifestyle or by increasing the level of activity in previously sedentary individuals, older people can maintain relatively high levels of cardiovascular and metabolic functions, including skeletal muscle function and aerobic capacity (Kohrt et al., 1991); it is never too late to start. Morganti et al. (1995) demonstrate strength gains in postmenopausal women, with the greatest gains occurring in the first 3 months of training and continuing for at least 12 months. Fiatarone et al. (1990, 1994) indicate that even 80- and 90-year-old seniors have the capacity to increase muscle mass and strength, stair-climbing power, gait velocity, and level of spontaneous activity. Consequently, they can improve functional mobility and the ability to live independently. Elderly people with more muscle mass can eat more calories and take in more nutrients because their metabolic rate is higher. As a result, the potential for malnutrition, a common problem for older adults, is decreased (Fiatarone et al., 1994).

Functional (aerobic) capacity reflects oxygen delivery and use, which normally decreases with age. Aerobic fitness is important for everyone. It helps to lower the risk of CHD and all-cause mortality (Blair, 1989), it enhances the ability to maintain independence in daily activities, and it improves the overall quality of life. Green and Crouse (1995) demonstrate that regular aerobic exercise increases aerobic capacity (fitness) in the older adults. Exercising for approximately 30 minutes, 3 times a week improves aerobic capacity enough potentially to make the difference between independent living and the need for assistance. Cady et al. (1985) found that firefighters who participated in a work-sponsored fitness program over a 10-year period demonstrated a much slower decline in strength and flexibility and a reversal in the decline of exercise capacity that is normally observed with aging. Jackson et al. (1995) shows that change in aerobic capacity in men is related not only to age, but also to level of physical activity and body composition (see Hot Topics box).

Disuse can easily lead to disrepair, which can be seen with the effects of bed rest on aerobic capacity (Saltin, 1968; Shepard, 1994). It can also be seen in the progression of osteoporosis and arthritis, and in the large number of people who suffer from back pain.

The health of the musculoskeletal system depends on movement and activity. Bone is a dynamic tissue, constantly changing and adapting to the stresses to which it is subjected. Bone strength is dependent on stresses applied by muscular and weight-bearing activity (mechanical stress during active movement). Exercise enhances bone mineralization and helps prevent bone loss over time (Aisenbrey, 1987). To stay healthy, joints must do what they are designed to do—move and bear weight. The health of the cartilage covering the joint surfaces is vital for maintaining proper joint function. The only way the cartilage can receive nourishment is through the manufacture and distribution of synovial fluid, which delivers nutrients, removes waste products, and lubricates joint surfaces (Schatz, 1985). Movement is vital for creating this environment of blood and lymph in and out of joint structures and the adjacent soft tissues. Without the stress of weight-bearing activity, normal bone and cartilage metabolism and repair become dysfunctional, resulting in injury and disease.

Osteoporosis

Osteoporosis is the most common bone disease, affecting 25 million Americans, 80% of whom are women. It is characterized by decreased bone mass and structural weakness of bone tissue, leading to bone fragility and increased risk of fractures. Women are more susceptible than men because they tend to have lower peak bone mass, suffer bone mass loss at an accelerated rate as estrogen levels decline, and have a longer lifespan than men (Cummings, 1985). Some loss of bone occurs naturally after age 30, but the severity of this process is increased with reduced levels of calcium, estrogen, and physical activity (Aisenbrey, 1987). In addition to the importance of optimizing physiological intake of calcium, vitamin D therapy, and maintaining normal menstrual cycles for maximizing peak bone mass, physical activity plays a significant role in developing bone mass during childhood and adolescence and in maintaining skeletal mass into adulthood (Lane & Nydick, 1999). In a study of

HOT topics

MESSAGE FROM MISSION CONTROL: BLAST OFF THAT COUCH!

The interrelation of age, body composition, and exercise habits is evident when loss of aerobic capacity is compared in active and sedentary individuals. A study using male employees from NASA suggests that a 30-year-old man who does moderate exercise and has 20% body fat will lose only one half as much of his aerobic capacity by age 70 if he stays moderately active and maintains his percentage of body fat than if he becomes sedentary and increases his body fat to 30%, which is what happens to the typical American man. If he increases his exercise and decreases his body fat to 15%, then he will lose only 7% of his aerobic capacity (Jackson et al., 1995). Age alone need not cause functional disability if adults maintain an active lifestyle and healthy body composition.

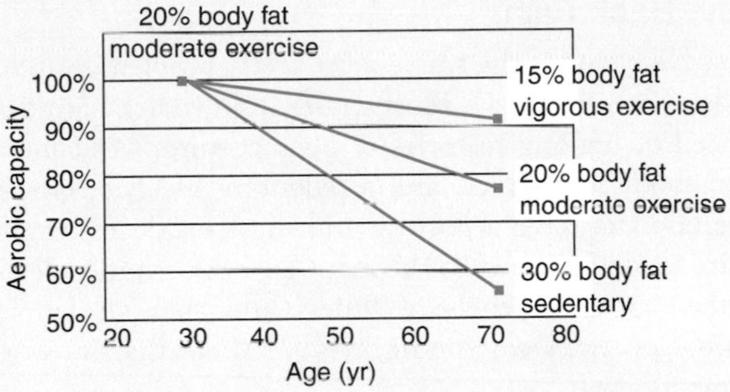

Projected changes in aerobic capacity in men from age 30 to 70 years for different exercise and body composition conditions. (Data from Jackson, A. S., et al. [1995]. Changes in aerobic power of men ages 25-70 yrs. *Medicine and Science in Sports and Exercise, 27,* 113-120.)

Critical Thinking Questions

1. Is it normal for body fat to increase significantly with age?
2. How is body composition related to fitness?
3. What types of exercise are important to help prevent increased body fat and maintain functional independence?
4. Is there a drug that holds as much promise for sustained health as a lifetime program of physical exercise? If not, then why is exercise not prescribed more often?

young women aged 18 to 31, Teegarden et al. (1996) asserts that previous levels of physical activity correlate positively with bone mineral measures. Physical activity increases the potential for increased peak bone mass and provides for a stronger skeletal foundation throughout aging (USDHHS, 1996).

Results from several studies indicate that physical activity can help minimize bone loss and facilitate some gain in bone mineralization (Aloia, 1978; Dalsky et al., 1988; Krolner, Toft, Pors Nielsen, & Tondevold, 1983). Studies with nursing home residents indicate that bone loss in older adults can be reversed with the stress of exercise (Smith, Reddan, & Smith, 1981). Rowe and Kahn (1987) state that the reductions in bone density that are normally seen with aging may be preventable, or at least modifiable, by regular exercise, reduced smoking, and an adequate intake of calcium. Estrogen replacement therapy may also be considered in osteoporosis prevention because the positive effect of physical activity on bone may depend on the presence of estrogen (Kohrt, Sneod, Slatopolsky, & Birge, 1995).

Maintenance of bone mass may be related to the intensity of the physical activity and the degree to which the activity stresses the bone. Although weight-bearing actions that stress the skeleton (walking, stair climbing, and aerobic dance) have a positive effect on bone density, resistance training may be more effective than aerobic exercise in its effects on bone mass. Resistance training also improves muscle mass, strength, and balance, all of which decrease the risk of falls in older adults (Nelson et al., 1994). Nevertheless, even when resistance training cannot increase bone density significantly in osteopenic people, it can help prevent falls and related fractures (Fiatarone, 1994). Whereas in younger women, the goal would be to increase bone density, in elderly women who are already 30 to 40 years past menopause, a more realistic goal would be to decrease the risk of fractures through fall prevention, including exercise (see Research Highlights box).

Arthritis

The process of arthritis upsets the balance of joint health. Although rheumatoid arthritis (RA) and osteoarthritis (OA) have different causes and attack different parts of the joint, impaired joint function is the result. Cartilage is worn away and irregularities occur in the bone ends. As normal movement is altered, proper joint alignment fails, normal ROM is decreased, and, with the imbalance of altered muscle activity, disfigurement and dysfunction occur. Although there is an ongoing progression in arthritis that cannot be healed by exercise, physical activity nevertheless helps to restore health to synovium and cartilage, improve strength and flexibility, decrease joint vulnerability, and delay the onset of dysfunction.

The question is often asked whether exercise causes OA. Cross-sectional and cohort studies suggest that long-term recreational runners have no more risk of developing OA of the hip and knee than do sedentary people. Evidence does not show that recreational walkers with normal joints have an increased risk of OA (Panush & Lane, 1994).

Competitive athletes who participate in activities involving the excessive use of specific joints (a baseball pitcher) have an increased risk of developing OA, especially when the joint has been injured. Joint injury is a

research highlights

Healthy Aging: A Balancing Act

The consequences of frailty are devastating for older persons. Falls and the resulting injuries are among the most serious and common medical problems suffered by older adults, constituting a major barrier to independent living. Deterioration in physical fitness, including the components of strength, endurance, flexibility, and balance, is part of the multifactorial differential that leads to an increased incidence of falling.

Tai Chi, a Chinese traditional conditioning exercise, has been practiced most often in this country by the elderly Asian population to enhance balance and body awareness. Developed more than 700 years ago by Chinese martial artists, Tai Chi combines relaxed, slow movement in choreographed forms, with a calm, alert mental state. The emphasis is on postural alignment; slow, integrated movement; weight shifting (balance); and a focused awareness on breathing.

Recent studies have demonstrated that Tai Chi is effective for improving health fitness in older adults. In a study of 38 men and women aged 58 to 70 years, the Tai Chi group showed significant improvement in aerobic capacity ($p < 0.01$), spinal flexibility ($p < 0.05$), and lower extremity strength (knee flexors and extensors) ($p < 0.05$). The Atlanta study, Frailty and Injuries: Cooperative Studies of Intervention Techniques (FICSIT), evaluated the effects of two exercise modalities on the occurrence of falls. This 15-week study of 200 people aged 70 years and older compared Tai Chi, computerized balance training, and an education group. The Tai Chi intervention reduced the risk of falls by 47.5% ($p = .01$). Additionally, Tai Chi reduced the fear of falling and increase participants' sense of being able to do all that they want to do in their daily lives. This perceived enhancement of mental and physical control and a sense of improvement in overall well being contribute to exercise compliance and motivation.

Although more physically focused methods of exercise (strength training) have been shown to improve strength and balance, Tai Chi affects favorably on both the biomedical and the psychosocial indices of frailty. Its ease of accessibility, low cost, community orientation, and its influence on physical fitness outcomes gives Tai Chi the potential to bring balance to the lives of elderly adults.

Data from Chewning, B., Yu, T., & Johnson, J. (2000, May/June). T'ai Chi: Effects on health. *ACSM's Health and Fitness Journal, 4*, 17-28; Lan, C., et al. (1997). 12-month Tai Chi training in the elderly: Its effect on health fitness. *Medicine and Science in Sports and Exercise, 30*, 345-351; Wolf, S. L. et al. (1996). Reducing frailty and falls in older persons: An investigation of Tai Chi and computerized balance training. *Journal of American Geriatric Society, 44*, 489-497.

strong risk factor for the development of OA; therefore it may not be the physical activity itself, but rather the injury that causes OA (Rangger, Kathrein, Klestil, & Glotzer, 1997). Regular noncompetitive physical activity of the amount and intensity recommended for improving health is not harmful to joints that have no existing injuries (USDHHS, 1996).

One of the chief goals of exercise and physical activity for the individual with arthritis is to counter the effects of inactivity (ACSM, 2000). Although researchers have concluded that regular exercise cannot improve or cure arthritis, exercise has quality-of-life benefits for people with arthritis:

- Improvement in joint function and ROM.
- Increase in muscular strength and aerobic fitness that enhance daily activities of living.
- Improvement in psychological state.
- Decrease in loss of bone mass.
- Decrease in the risk of chronic disease (Nieman, 2000).

Consequently, exercise programs based on individual needs and interests should emphasize exercises to develop joint ROM and flexibility (daily) and should also include muscle strengthening (2 to 3 times per week), aerobic exercise (30 to 45 minutes most days of the week), and recreational activities that are enjoyable (ACSM, 2000).

Low Back Pain

Low back pain is the single most costly problem in industry today (Schatz, 1984). Most causes of low back pain can be traced to lifelong histories of poor posture, weak muscles, poor body mechanics, and a sedentary lifestyle. However, exercise can have a positive influence on decreasing back pain. Cady et al. (1985) report that back injuries decrease with increasing levels of fitness and that an employee fitness program can result in a 25% decline in workers compensation costs.

The spinal column is made up of a series of vertebrae stacked one on another, forming natural curves that allow the bony column to function with the resiliency of a spring. The intervertebral disks help with mobility and shock absorption. The health of the bony vertebrae and the cartilaginous disks depends on movement. The cartilage gets its nutrients from the compression of bearing weight, and this same weight-bearing activity stimulates vertebral bone integrity. Compression fractures of the vertebrae are often the result of osteoporosis. Increases in vertebral bone mass have been noted in women after menopause as the result of an exercise program (Krolner, 1983).

Muscles are intimately involved in the support and function of the spinal column. Maintaining the proper curves (anterior and posterior convexities) of lordosis in the cervical and lumbar vertebrae and kyphosis in the thoracic vertebrae is vital for sustaining the spring and shock-absorption qualities of the spine. The lumbar curve is especially influenced by 3 sets of muscles that are attached to the pelvis and the lumbar vertebrae. By altering the tilt of the pelvis, these muscles can increase (iliopsoas muscle) or decrease (abdominal and hamstring muscles) the lumbar curve (Schatz, 1984). In addition, the deep muscles of the back (paraspinal muscles) work in controlled synergistic and antagonistic fashions to control spinal planes of motion; they are also influential in supporting the spinal curves in posture. Weakness, overstretching, or tightening of any of these muscles can negatively affect posture and increase wear and tear on the back. The result can be back pain from muscle strain, altered joint function (facet joints), and abnormal force on the intervertebral disks.

The goal of exercise programs for individuals with low back pain is to prevent debilitation as a result of inactivity and to improve endurance, strength, and flexibility, allowing for a return to usual functional activities. Exercise recommendations and progression of activity are highly individualized based on origin, duration, and severity of pain. Strengthening exercises for trunk and extremity musculature are useful in persons with chronic—but not acute—low back pain. Aerobic conditioning, such as walking, swimming, and stationary bicycling is recommended to maintain endurance and prevent debilitation from inactivity (ACSM, 1997).

Advanced age, osteoporosis, arthritis, and low back pain are not reasons to exclude exercise from anyone's lifestyle. In fact, the opposite is true. These conditions are reasons to remain as physically active as possible to facilitate the ability to function throughout the aging process.

Immune Function

Establishing the relationship between exercise and immunes function has a fairly long history of study, but renewed interest has grown out of the human immunodeficiency virus (HIV) epidemic. Several studies (LaPierriere, Fletcher, Antoni, Klimes, & Schneiderman, 1991; Rigsby, Dishman, Jackson, MacLean, & Raven, 1992; Spence, Galentino, Mossberg, & Zimmerman, 1990) demonstrate that persons with impaired immune function can exercise safely without risk to their health status and, in fact, can enhance their physiological and psychological well being with regular exercise. Changes in immune markers, such as CD4 and CD8 cell counts and the number and activity of natural killer (NK) cells, indicate that moderate exercise may help bolster an impaired immune system (LaPierriere, 1991).

Evidence also suggests that regular exercisers do not get sick as often as do less active people. Epidemiological studies indicate that a J-curve relationship exists between the intensity of exercise and the risk of upper respiratory tract infection (URTI) (Fig. 12-2).

Moderate exercise may decrease the risk of URTI below that of a sedentary individual, but high-intensity exercise may raise the risk above average. Ultramarathoners and high-intensity marathoners have a significantly higher incidence of URTI symptoms compared with control subjects. Female and elderly subjects who perform moderate exercise have less than half the incidence of URTI compared with sedentary control subjects (Nieman, 1990, 1994).

Immune system changes that are apparently related to the intensity of exercise have been identified. Moderate-endurance exercise stimulates the neuroendocrine system,

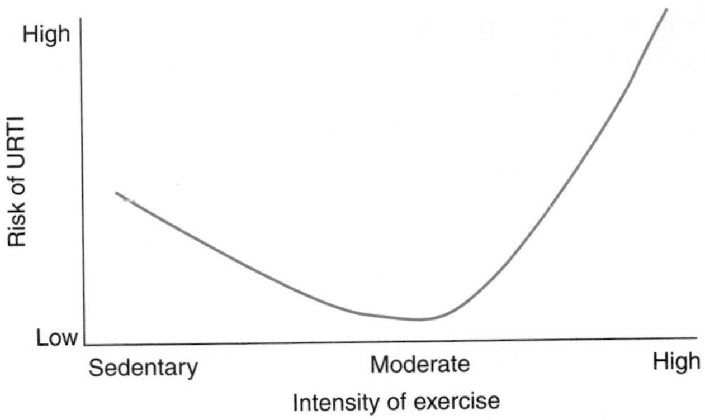

Fig. 12-2 Relationship between exercise and the risk of upper respiratory tract infection (URTI). This relationship is often referred to as a J curve. (Modified from Nieman, D. [1994]. Exercise, upper respiratory tract infection, and the immune system. *Medicine and Science in Sports and Exercise, 26,* 128-139.)

which causes changes in the function and numbers of various immune system cells, such as the NK, CD4, and CD8 cells as mentioned. Evidence also indicates that moderate exercise is associated with a prolonged improvement in the killing capacity of neutrophils (one of the most efficient phagocytes). Several immune marker changes suggest increased risk for high-intensity exercise, including low level of salivary immunoglobulin (antibodies), low serum complement levels, low lymphocyte count, depressed NK cell activity, low helper and suppressor T-cell ratio, and decreased neutrophil phagocytic capacity (Mackinnon, 1992; Nieman, 1994; Pedersen & Ullum, 1994).

Changes in immune cell counts and activity may be related to hormonal immunoregulation. Moderate exercise increases the release of immunostimulatory hormones, such as growth hormone and endogenous opiates (beta-endorphin and methionine-enkephalin). The increase in beta-endorphins with exercise seems to have a positive effect on NK cell activity. Conversely, intense exercise is associated with increases in catecholamine and corticosteroid (cortisol) levels, which have immunosuppressive characteristics (Mackinnon, 1992). High-intensity exercise is also associated with muscle cell damage and inflammation. The immune system is involved in tissue repair. It is theorized that, while immune cells are busy with the repair process, host protection may suffer. A window of opportunity for infection during recovery from high-intensity exercise appears to exist. Accordingly, rest is recommended after vigorous exercise to allow the body to recover, and moderate exercise may be the better choice for enhancing health and well being.

Large-scale epidemiological studies report a reduced incidence of cancer in physically active groups (Albanes, Blair, & Taylor, 1989; Blair, 1989). Research on occupational and leisure-time activity strongly suggests that physical activity has a protective effect against the risk of developing colon cancer (Lee, 1994). Data from the

Nurses' Health Study indicate that women who are more physically active in adulthood have a lower risk of breast cancer compared with those who are less physically active (Rockhill et al., 1999). Possibly, physical activity during adolescence and young adulthood may protect women from the later development of breast cancer (Bernstein, Henderson, Hanisch, Sullivan-Halley, & Ross, 1994). Researchers argue that lifetime physical activity is the critical variable affecting breast cancer risk. A large prospective study of over 12,000 men suggests that cardiorespiratory fitness and higher levels of physical activity may protect against the development of prostate cancer (Oliveria, Kohl, Trichopoulos, & Blair, 1996).

NK cells and microphages are involved in the first-line defense against the development and spread of malignancies. Exercise can help increase NK cell cytotoxicity, change the influx of macrophages into tissue, and promote the release of cytokines with antitumor properties (Woods & Davis, 1994). In helping to prevent colon cancer, exercise increases intestinal motility by altering local prostaglandin synthesis and decreases gastrointestinal transit time, thereby decreasing length of contact between colon mucosa and potential carcinogens (Lee, 1994).

Mental Health

People who exercise regularly generally state that they feel better, have increased self-esteem, and have a more positive outlook on life. Not only do they feel better physically, but they also feel better mentally. Epidemiological research with both men and women suggests that physical activity may be associated with reduced symptoms of depression and anxiety and improvements in positive affect and general sense of well being (Ross & Hayes, 1988; Stephens & Craig, 1990; USDHHS, 2000). A Canadian survey (Stephens & Craig, 1990) suggests that higher levels of daily energy expenditure are associated with a more positive mood compared with lower levels of expenditure and an inverse relationship exists between physical activity and symptoms of depression in people aged 25 years and older. Paffenbarger, Lee, & Leung (1994) revealed the same inverse relationship in a Harvard alumni cohort study.

Intervention studies have supported the positive influence of physical activity on mental health. Folkins (1976) found that after 12 weeks of exercise, the exercise group showed significant improvement in all levels of cardiovascular fitness and decreases in measures of anxiety and depression. In aerobic exercise studies (Berger & Owen, 1988; Blumenthal, Williams, Williams, & Wallace, 1980), the exercise groups experienced reductions in anxiety, tension, depression, and fatigue and an increase in vigor and clear mindedness. A recent study by Blumenthal et al. (1999) demonstrates that exercise is as effective as antidepressant medication in reducing levels of depression in older patients with major depressive disorder. These findings suggest that improvements in physical health are associated with improvements in psychological health.

Jin (1989) found that mood states become more positive during and for a short time after Tai Chi. The psychological changes include a decrease in depression, tension, anger, fatigue, confusion, and anxiety and an increase in vigor. Brown et al. (1995) determined that exercise combined with a cognitive activity (low-intensity walking with the relaxation response, or modified Tai Chi) appears to be more effective in improving mood states compared with exercise alone.

Physical activity helps to improve the mental health of both clinical and nonclinical populations. Although suggestions are that the greatest benefits from conditioning are experienced by the least fit and the most anxious and depressed (Goff & Dimsdale, 1985), Blumenthal et al. (1980) conclude that basically healthy, well-adjusted people who exercise can increase their sense of well being more than healthy people who do not exercise. Even when no change is observed in objective mental health measures with older people in relatively good physical and mental health, they report feelings of improved physical, psychological, and social well being after regular physical activity (Blumenthal et al., 1989).

Kobasa (1985) has performed extensive work on the stress-illness relationship. Exercise is considered one of the moderating variables (resistance resources)—in addition to hardiness and social support—that affects the relationship. Although hardiness (defined in terms of commitment, control, and challenge) is believed to be the most effective buffer against the effects of stress, exercise is associated with lower overall scores in people under stress. Exercise likely protects through decreasing the physical strain of stressful events. In support of these findings, Dyer and Crouch (1988) conclude that exercise not only increases regular participants' feelings about coping with stress, but also enhances their overall feeling of well being. Physical activity and exercise should be encouraged in an attempt to maximize their associated benefits of enhanced sense of personal achievement, self-esteem, and social participation (Goff & Dimsdale, 1985).

HOW MUCH EXERCISE IS ENOUGH?

Literature certainly reflects both the physiological and psychological benefits that can be experienced with commitment to an active lifestyle. In short, regular physical activity or exercise can help people feel better, look better, and perform better. Unfortunately, as discussed, Americans have failed to embrace the concept and health value of an active lifestyle. Many have been overwhelmed by the misperception that to gain health benefits they must perform vigorous, continual exercise. The result has been discouragement in getting started and poor compliance in staying with it. "No pain, no gain" has been an unfortunate, common refrain (see Hot Topics box).

People should be reminded that many of their daily

HOT topics: LESS PAIN, MORE GAIN

In an attempt to encourage increased participation in physical activity, a panel of scientists from the Centers for Disease Control and Prevention and the American College of Sports Medicine came together to review the evidence related to physical activity and to issue a public health message concerning the recommended types and amounts of physical activity (Pate et al., 1995). The evidence clearly indicates that the protective effects of exercise can be achieved at more moderate levels of intensity than had been previously recommended. The health and fitness benefits of exercise appear to be related more to the total amount of exercise accomplished (calories expended) rather than to the specific exercise intensity, frequency, and duration. The recommendations are as follows:

- Adults should accumulate 30 minutes or more of moderate-intensity (brisk) physical activity on most (or all) days of the week, for a weekly total of 3 to 4 hours.
- The activity need not be continuous; benefits can be realized with short bouts of activity (a minimum of 10 minutes) over the course of the day.
- This amount of activity will expend about 150 to 200 calories per day (the equivalent of walking 2 miles briskly) or 1000 to 1400 calories per week.
- All types of activity can be applied to the daily total (raking leaves, dancing, or gardening).
- Lower-intensity activities should be performed more often, or for longer periods, or both. More vigorous activities should be performed for shorter periods or less frequently.

Because most adults do not meet these standards, they have the most to gain by incorporating a few minutes of increased activity into their day, gradually building up to 30 minutes a day. People who are active on an irregular basis should strive to be more consistent. People who prefer more formal exercise can choose to participate in more vigorous, organized exercise regimens, sports, and recreational activities. A dose-response curve best represents the relationship between physical activity (dose) and health benefit (response).

Sedentary individuals gain the most by increasing their activity to the recommended level. However, any person who already meets the standards can derive some additional benefit by becoming more active.

> People who do a little bit of exercise are better off than those . . . who do none. Those who do a little more are better off still (Franklin, 1993, p. 476).

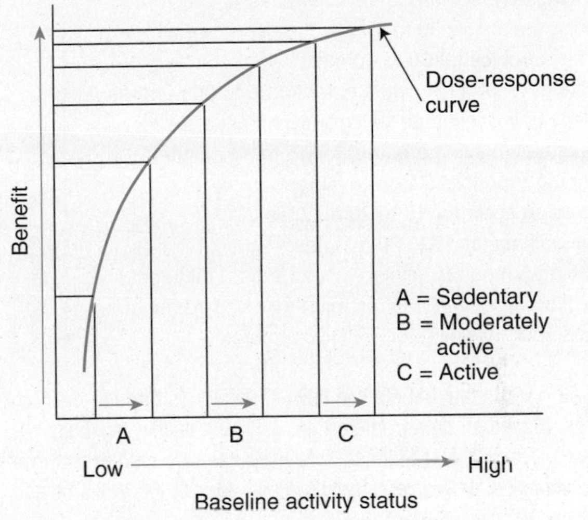

The dose-response curve represents the best estimate of the relationship between physical activity (dose) and health benefit (response). The lower the baseline physical activity status, the greater the health benefit associated with a given increase in physical activity (arrows A, B, and C). (From Pate, R. R., et al. [1995]. Physical activity and public health: A recommendation from the CDC and the ACSM. *Journal of the American Medical Association, 273,* 402-407.)

physical activities are actually forms of exercise (Fig. 12-3). This approach to physical activity serves as a good foundation to a healthy lifestyle. However, when possible, individuals should also be encouraged to include more formal exercise training in their overall activities to promote optimal cardiorespiratory fitness and significantly improve muscle strength and endurance. How much exercise is required to achieve these goals is determined by the parameters of an exercise prescription:

F (Frequency)
3 to 5 times a week of aerobic exercise.
2 to 3 times a week of resistance training.

I (Intensity)
Moderate to vigorous, by heart rate and perceived exertion.
Able to complete each resistance exercise, 8 to 12 repetitions, without strain.

T (Time)
20 to 60 minutes, plus warm-up and cool-down periods.
15 to 30 minutes to complete a series of 8 to 10 resistance exercises.

T (Type)
Aerobic (walking, jogging, biking, swimming, rowing, cross-country skiing, Nordic Track, Stairmaster, aerobics, dancing, skating, or rollerblading).
Resistance training (weight machines, free weights, and calisthenics such as push-ups, sit-ups, or pull-ups) (ACSM, 1998; Westcott, 1993).

Aerobic Exercise

The benefits of aerobic exercise are cumulative; therefore a frequency of 3 to 5 times a week is recommended; every other day is a good frame of reference. The benefits of exercising more than 5 times a week are outweighed by the risk of injury, especially with higher-impact activities. When more frequent exercising is a goal, cross training is recommended. Cross training means performing different types of exercise on different days of the week or performing different types of exercise within one exercise session. The

Ways to burn 150 to 200 calories

Activity	
Walking 2 mph (30 minute mile) for 45 to 60 minutes	↑ Less intense, more time
Washing windows or floors for 45 to 60 minutes	
Domestic housework for 35 to 45 minutes	
Golfing (walk, no cart) for 35 to 45 minutes	
Gardening for 30 to 45 minutes	
Mowing grass (power mower) for 30 to 45 minutes	
Wheeling self in wheelchair for 30 to 45 minutes	
Walking 3 mph (20 minute mile) for 30 to 40 minutes	
Bicycling 10 mph (6 minute mile) for 30 to 40 minutes	
Swimming (moderate crawl) for 30 to 40 minutes	
Dancing fast (social) 30 to 40 minutes	
Raking leaves for 30 to 40 minutes	
Water aerobics for 30 to 40 minutes	
Walking 4 mph (15 minute mile) for 25 to 30 minutes	
Wheelchair basketball for 20 to 25 minutes	
Basketball (playing a game) for 15 to 25 minutes	
Jumping rope for 15 to 20 minutes	
Shoveling snow for 15 to 20 minutes	
Stair walking for 15 to 20 minutes	
Running 6 mph (10 minute mile) 15 to 20 minutes	
Bicycling 12 mph (5 minute mile) for 15 to 20 minutes	
Cross country skiing for 15 to 20 minutes	↓ More intense, less time

Fig. 12-3 Ways that people can burn 150 calories through their daily activities. (Based on data from Lertola, J. [1996, July]. Less pain, more gain. *Time, 7,* 65.; Skinner, J. [1993]. *Exercise testing and exercise prescription for special cases* [2nd ed.]. Media, PA: Williams and Wilkins.)

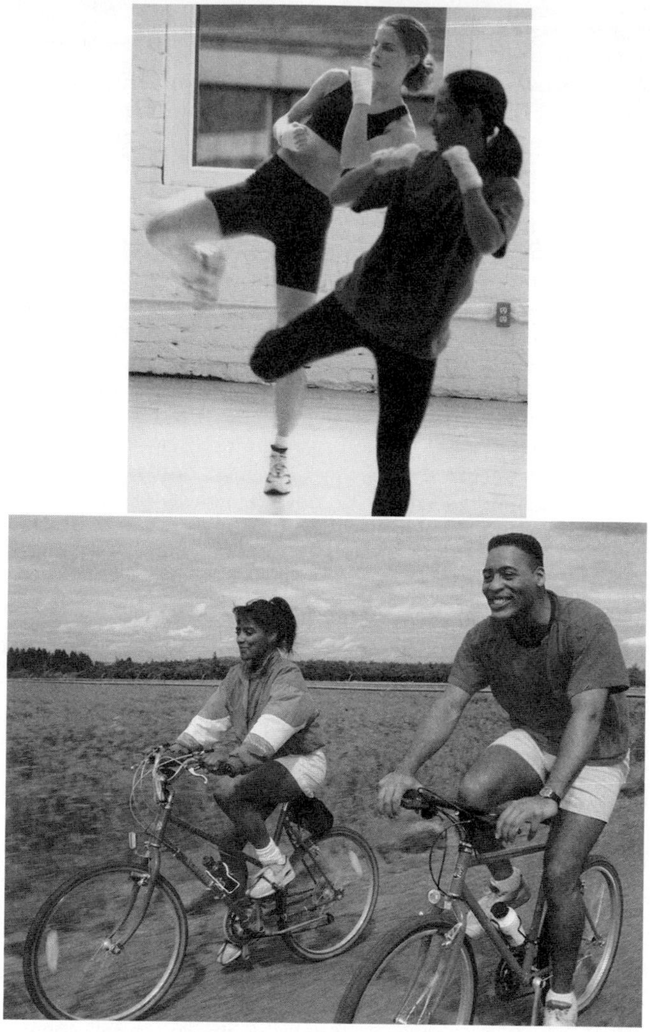

Fig. 12-4 Varying exercise routines from indoors to outdoors can help eliminate boredom.

benefits of cross training include a decreased risk of musculoskeletal injury, an increased potential for total body conditioning, and improved long-term compliance because variety decreases boredom and eliminates the exercise barrier of limited choices (Fig. 12-4).

The intensity of exercise that results in health and fitness benefits ranges from moderate to vigorous and is comfortable, but challenging (brisk). Intensity is defined by the objective measure of heart rate and the subjective measure of perceived exertion.

The increase in heart rate (HR) during exercise has a strong linear relationship with exercise intensity and aerobic capacity. Resting heart rate (RHR) is the HR measured at rest. Maximal heart rate (MHR) is the HR measured at the highest workload tolerated during exercise. MHR also decreases with age; therefore a generic formula for determining MHR is 220 minus age. Formulas for determining appropriate exercise HRs have been developed that take RHR and MHR into consideration.

The difference between MHR and RHR is referred to as the heart rate reserve (HRR). Research indicates that 60% to 80% of the HRR corresponds to approximately 60% to 80% of aerobic capacity (ACSM, 1995, 1998). The recommendation for moderate to vigorous exercise corresponds to 50% to 85% of maximal aerobic capacity (VO_2 max). Therefore the HRR formula for determining exercise heart rate (EHR) is:

$$[(220 - \text{age}) - \text{RHR}] \times \% + \text{RHR} = \text{EHR};\ \% = 50\% \text{ to } 85\%$$

For a 40-year-old person with an RHR of 80 beats per minute (bpm), the EHR would be 130 to 165 bpm.

A more commonly used formula (because less math is involved) takes a fixed percentage of the MHR. This formula is based on the observation that 70% to 85% of the MHR is equal to about 60% to 80% of functional capacity (ACSM, 1995, 1998). Recommended moderate to vigorous exercise corresponds to 60% to 90% of MHR.

$$(220 - \text{age}) \times \% = \text{EHR};\ \% = 60\% \text{ to } 90\%$$

For a 40-year-old person, the EHR would be 108 to 162 bpm.

The HRR method considers RHR; therefore the calculated EHR is more specific to the individual than it is with the MHR method. This factor is especially valuable when setting exercise prescriptions for people with extremely high or extremely low RHRs or for people who are taking cardiac drugs that affect RHR and HR response to exercise (beta blockers).

6	
7	Very, very light
8	
9	Very light
10	
11	Fairly light
12	Somewhat hard
13	
14	Hard
15	
16	Very hard
17	
18	
19	Very, very hard
20	

Fig. 12-5 Borg scale (RPE). (From Borg, G. A. [1982]. Psychophysical basis of perceived exertion. *Medicine and Science in Sports and Exercise, 14,* 377-381.)

Whichever method is used, it is important to remember that the EHR range is only a guideline. The perception of how the exercise feels is as important as the HR response. The goal is to achieve a conditioning effect and to burn a significant number of calories, but the individual must also enjoy the activity enough to be willing to continue exercising on a regular basis. The person should feel challenged by the activity, but also feel comfortable. The Borg Scale for rating perceived exertion (RPE) is a psychophysical category scale for the subjective rating of sensations associated with the intensity of physical work (Borg, 1973, 1982) (Fig. 12-5). The scale uses ratings based on the individual's overall feeling of exertion and physical fatigue. These ratings correspond well with metabolic responses to exercise, such as HR and oxygen consumption. The strong linear relationship between HR and RPE was originally suggested by Borg and has been verified by subsequent studies. Correlation coefficients from 80% to 90% have been consistently reported using a variety of work tasks and exercise conditions (Borg, 1973, 1982; Skinner, Hustler, Bergsteinova, & Buskirk, 1973). However, perceptions of exertion and the relationship to HR are influenced by both physiological and psychological factors (aches, cramps, pain, fatigue, shortness of breath, anxiety, depression, and introversion or extroversion) (Morgan, 1973; O'Sullivan, 1984). Smutok, Skrinar, & Pandolf (1980) note that some subjects are more accurate in regulating exercise intensity by RPE than are others and that this variability may be more the result of psychological rather than physiological factors. Other factors that may alter the strong relationship between HR and RPE are drug-related situations (beta blockers), age, and disease states (O'Sullivan, 1984).

Despite this potential for variability in perception, RPE correlates well with HR clinically, and together, they form a complementary means of helping individuals determine a comfortable, beneficial level of exercise intensity. An RPE of 11 to 14 corresponds well with 50% to 85% HRR. Subjective parameters include being slightly short of breath, but not out of breath; able to talk without difficulty, but unable to sing a song easily; being pleasantly fatigued, but not exhausted; and having mild musculoskeletal discomfort, but no pain.

Attention to RPE helps a person develop a sense of body awareness and an appreciation for the body's response to the stress of activity. Awareness of RPE helps people listen to their bodies and to be aware of how it feels to move, where they carry tension, and where they have discomfort. With this increased awareness, individuals can choose how they want to respond, adjusting their exercise practice on a day-to-day basis, making the activity more enjoyable, decreasing the risk of injury, and improving long-term exercise compliance.

The recommendation for the duration of aerobic conditioning exercise is generally 20 to 60 minutes. Less than 20 minutes usually provides minimal benefit. However, for people who are unaccustomed to exercising or for those who are greatly deconditioned, short durations are permissible, gradually increasing to a beneficial, comfortable level as tolerance and confidence improve. Everyone has to start somewhere and doing a little is much better than doing nothing at all.

The benefit of sessions longer than 45 to 60 minutes is again outweighed by the potential for injury. Exercising more than 60 minutes on occasion (such as an extended bike ride with friends or a leisurely walk on a beautiful day) is certainly not wrong, but a person who increases duration should consider decreasing intensity. Improvements in cardiorespiratory fitness can also be accrued from intermittent bouts of moderate to vigorous exercise (10-minute segments) on a workout day (DeBusk, Stenestrand, Sheehan, & Haskell, 1990; Jakicic, Wing, Butler, & Robertson, 1995). As discussed, longer bouts of exercise are more beneficial for weight loss. The range of acceptable duration allows for greater flexibility, giving reassurance of benefit to the individual who varies exercise choices daily based on capability, interests, and life demands.

As mentioned, many different choices for aerobic exercise are available. The question is often asked, "What is the best aerobic exercise?" The answer is, "The one that the individual is willing to do on a regular basis." Different aerobic exercises have different benefits; they all have their advantages and disadvantages. From a cardiovascular point of view, with relative intensity, frequency, and duration being equal, the benefit is about the same for all modes. Probably the best scenario is cross training, which results in the best all-around benefits. However, the most important recommendation is that people get out and start moving. The type of exercise they prefer and will continue doing is the best one for them to do.

Walking is probably the most accessible and popular form of aerobic exercise. Done briskly, walking provides a good cardiorespiratory challenge in 60% to 80% of the adult population (Blair et al., 1989). Walking is also an activity that nearly everyone can do, requires little equipment or cost, can be done almost anywhere (even on vacation), and can be a social or a solitary activity, depending on individual needs. For people who are unaccustomed to exercising, walking is a great place to start.

Walking is often the recommended exercise of choice for people who are greatly deconditioned or for those who have physical limitations. Considered a low-impact activity, walking can be easily regulated to accommodate a wide range of fitness levels and motor abilities. Cycling, arm ergometry, rowing, and swimming (or water walking or other water aerobics) are also nonweight-bearing activities to low weight-bearing activities that may be good choices for individuals with physical limitations. Water activities are a good exercise alternative for individuals with musculoskeletal limitations who need some weight relief with exercise. Although the buoyancy of the water provides this weight relief, the water also provides resistance to the limbs as they move, encouraging an increase in intensity and conditioning. Individuals should be encouraged to do the types of aerobic exercise that best fit their needs, interests, and lifestyles while providing reasonable benefits.

Warm-Up and Cool-Down Periods

In addition to the endurance phase of exercise, warm-up and cool-down periods should be a regular part of the exercise session. The **warm-up period** usually lasts 5 to 10 minutes and may include light stretching, calisthenics, or performance of the chosen aerobic activity at a low intensity. This approach prepares both the musculoskeletal and cardiorespiratory systems for the transition from rest to exercise by increasing blood flow, respiration, and body temperature and improving muscle flexibility. The warm-up period decreases the risks of injury and potential heart irregularities. Individuals should be encouraged to develop a warm-up practice that involves listening to the body and paying attention to physical and mental cues, which increases awareness of muscle tightness and the general energy level and helps in making exercise goals for that particular session (ACSM, 1995; Huddleston, 1992).

The **cool-down period** follows the endurance phase and usually lasts 5 to 10 minutes. This phase allows the body to readjust gradually from the demands of exercise back to baseline. Stretching and slow, rhythmical movement helps to increase muscle elasticity, prevent blood pooling and potential hypotension, and facilitate dissipation of body heat and removal of lactic acid. The result is the prevention of injury, light-headedness, fatigue, and muscle soreness. Cool-down provides a wonderful opportunity to combine movement with relaxation skills, enhancing mind-body awareness (ACSM, 1995; Huddleston, 1992).

Yoga is an excellent form of exercise to use during warm-up and cool-down periods. The word yoga means *union* or *established in being*, which implies a mind-body connection. Simply defined, **yoga** is *mindful stretching*. The mind is quiet and awareness is focused on feeling the body as it moves. Movement into and out of yoga postures (called *asanas*) provides the necessary stimulation of weight-bearing activity to help keep bones strong, provides the movement to increase joint ROM, and stretches and tones muscles (Fig. 12-6). The Sun Salute (Surya Namaskar), a series of 12 flexion-extension yoga postures linked together as one fluid movement by the breath rhythm, is a wonderful practice to include in the warm-up and cool-down phases of exercise, providing both physiological and mind-body benefits (Douillard, 1995).

Yoga also helps develop an appreciation for the experience of the basic *resting state*—a mindfulness of how it feels to be relaxed physically and mentally during the activity. In this form, exercise becomes an inner experience; that is, quiet and settled on the inside, dynamic and lively on the outside. The yoga philosophy encourages an appreciation of bodily sensations, slow stretching, and maintenance of proper posture, all of which help to prevent injury and promote health. The awareness gained from this slow, controlled form of exercise can help the individual make healthy choices during all types of physical activity (Huddleston, 1992).

Flexibility

Flexibility is a basic component of physical fitness. Warm-up and cool-down periods provide the opportunity to work on stretching muscles and increasing joint ROM.

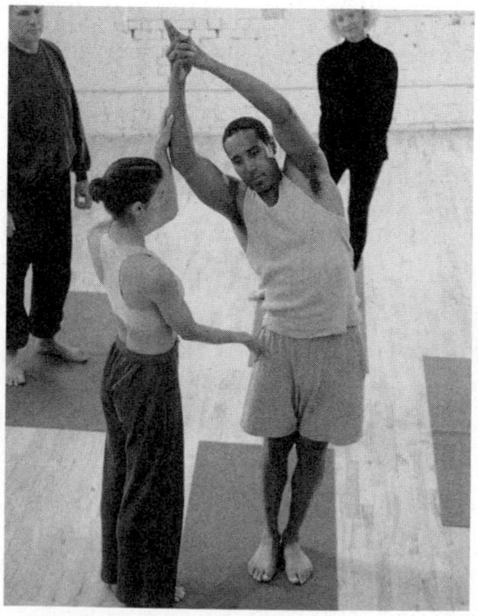

Fig. 12-6 Yoga is an excellent method of stretching and mind relaxation.

A safe stretch is one that is gentle and relaxing; a little discomfort may be felt as the muscle stretches, but the discomfort should never reach the point of pain. Stretching mindfully, as in yoga, will ensure a safe stretch. Holding the position for 10 to 20 seconds and repeating the stretch 3 to 5 times will encourage optimal flexibility (ACSM, 1998).

Resistance Training

Studies suggest that people who maintain or improve their flexibility and strength are better able to perform daily activities and avoid injury and disability (Pate et al., 1995). **Resistance training** increases muscle strength and endurance, increases muscle mass, improves metabolic efficiency, maintains or increases bone density, prevents limitations in performance of everyday tasks, decreases the effort required to perform these tasks, and decreases the potential for injury during physical activity.

On the average, after their early 20s, people lose about half a pound of muscle every year through lack of use. This reduction in muscle mass is largely responsible for a decrease in resting metabolic rate, which may translate into weight gain. Resistance training is recommended for the general population because it has a positive effect on many of the degenerative problems associated with the aging process (Wescott, 1993).

Every individual should try to perform activities throughout the day that stimulate muscle strength and endurance. Activities that involve lifting, carrying, or performing repetitive movement against a resistance (vacuuming, raking, shoveling, or baking bread) help preserve lean body mass. If these types of activities are not performed on a regular basis, then the guidelines for resistance training provided in Box 12-3 are suggested. These guidelines are not meant to represent workouts performed by bodybuilders and competitive weightlifters; they are not meant to result in *bulking up*. The purpose of weight training from a health perspective is (1) to develop toned, healthy muscles that provide the strength to do daily activities without risk of injury and (2) to stimulate healthy bone.

The figures in Box 12-3 demonstrate several suggested resistance exercises for upper-body strengthening. Resistance training for all major muscle groups is appropriate, but individuals often choose to concentrate on the upper body because these muscles tend to be neglected in daily activity and other exercise regimens. Although many people believe that they need to do 3 sets of each exercise, excellent results can be attained by doing one set (Westcott, 1993; Hass, Garzarella, De Hoyos, & Polloch, 2000). The weight that is lifted should result in near muscle fatigue at the end of each set (8 to 12 repetitions) and should be performed without strain and while maintaining proper form. Once 12 repetitions can be completed easily, the resistance can be increased (by 5% or less), or the same weight can be used to do another set of 8 to 12 repetitions (ACSM, 1998). The movements should be made slowly, preferably coordinated with the breath. Slow, controlled movements result in greater benefits, lower risk of injury, and an appreciation of how the body feels as its muscles are challenged.

EXERCISE THE SPIRIT: RELAXATION RESPONSE

Exercise should not be considered merely a physical regimen with objective outcomes (calories burned and repetitions completed). Exercise is also a process of challenging the body and the mind to gain a sense of well being and a feeling of accomplishment, an opportunity to learn about who we really are.

> The body mirrors the mind and soul and is much more accessible than either. If you can become proficient at listening to your body, you will eventually hear from your whole self (Sheehan, 1994).

Most people understand the physical benefits of exercise and some people enjoy the challenge of being physically active, but few realize the learning potential inherent in physical activity. Success in embracing a physically active lifestyle may involve a change in focus from the mechanics of exercise to an appreciation for how it feels and what it means to move. Physical activity can be time spent in meditation that fuels both the body and the spirit.

The **relaxation response** (RR) is an inborn set of physiological changes that offset those of the fight-or-flight (stress) response. When elicited, the RR results in a *letting go* of physical, emotional, and mental tension. The RR is a physiological response inborn in everyone and, although it can sometimes occur without the individual being aware of it, people generally need to develop techniques that help them "let go" on a more regular basis. Some techniques that are commonly used to elicit the RR include diaphragmatic breathing, meditation, imagery, mindfulness, yoga stretching, and repetitive exercise.

The RR can be combined with exercise to facilitate the release of tension and improve self-awareness and the feeling of well being. However, a shift in attitude about exercise is also involved, with the focus becoming the process and awareness of movement. Successful elicitation of the RR involves two basic components: (1) a repetitive focus (the breath, a mantra, and the cadence or rhythm of physical activity) and (2) a nonjudgmental attitude (about everyday thoughts and the quality of performance) (Benson & Stuart, 1992). Berger and Owen (1988) have developed exercise characteristics that facilitate stress reduction and support an exercise environment that allows the successful elicitation of the RR. Activities must:

- Be pleasant and enjoyable.
- Be noncompetitive. Competition implies judgment about the self and others.
- Be predictable. Elicitation of the RR involves a shift in awareness from the external to the internal environment that will take place only with a sense of safety and reliability.

Box 12-3 Resistive Training Exercises

CHEST PRESS (FIGS. 1 AND 2)

a. Lie on bench with feet flat on bench, or lie on the floor with knees bent, feet flat, whichever is more comfortable.
b. Hold weights near shoulders with elbows out and palms facing away from body.
c. Exhale while extending arms straight up, following an "A" pattern with weights touching at peak.
d. Slowly lower weights back down to original position while inhaling.
e. Repeat 8 to 12 times.

1

2
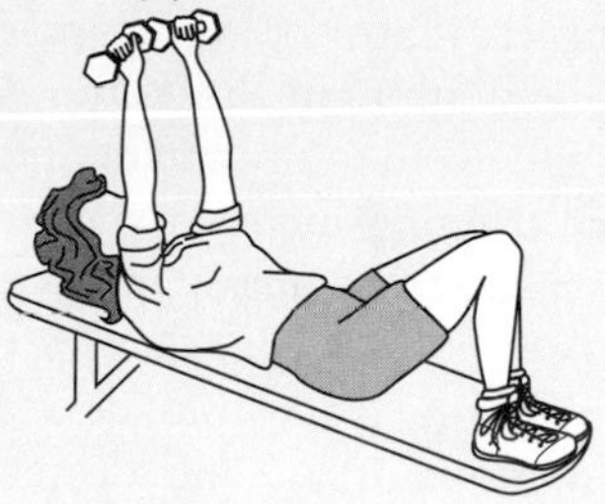

CHEST FLY (FIGS. 3 AND 4)

a. Lie on bench with feet flat on bench, or lie on the floor with knees bent, feet flat, whichever is more comfortable.
b. With palms facing each other, extend arms above chest, keeping elbows slightly bent at all times.
c. Inhale and lower arms perpendicularly away from body until arms are out of peripheral vision.
d. Exhale while returning to starting position by visualizing arms *hugging* a barrel that is lying on the chest.
e. Repeat 8 to 12 times.

3
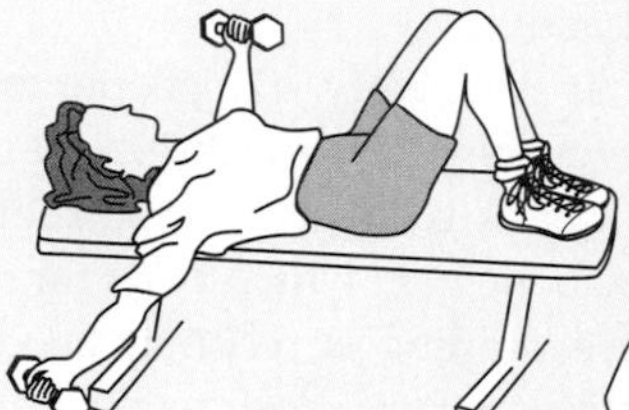
4
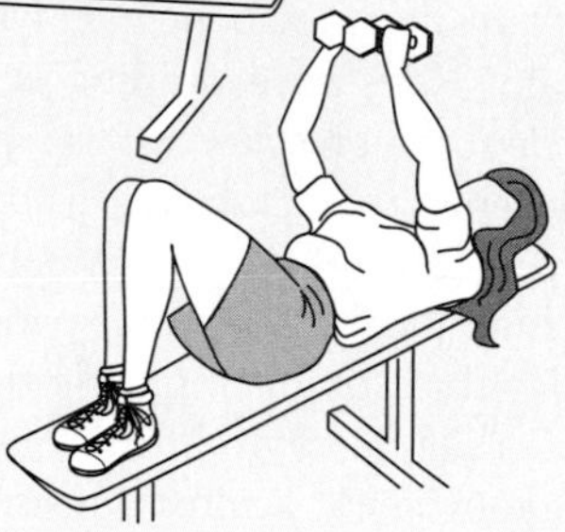

BENT OVER ROW (FIGS. 5 AND 6)

a. Bend at waist while supporting body with one hand (on table, bench, etc.) and holding weight with other hand in an overhand grip.
b. Keep knees bent while weight is hanging perpendicular to torso.
c. Slowly pull weight up to chest as if starting a lawn mower, exhaling and keeping elbow away from body.
d. Slowly lower weight back to starting position while inhaling.
e. Repeat 8 to 12 times on each side.

5
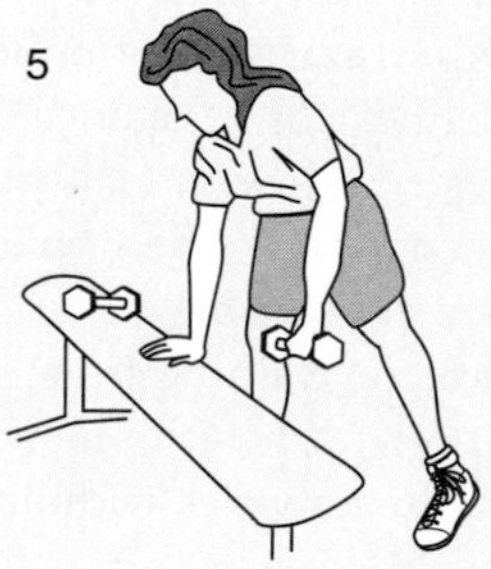
6
 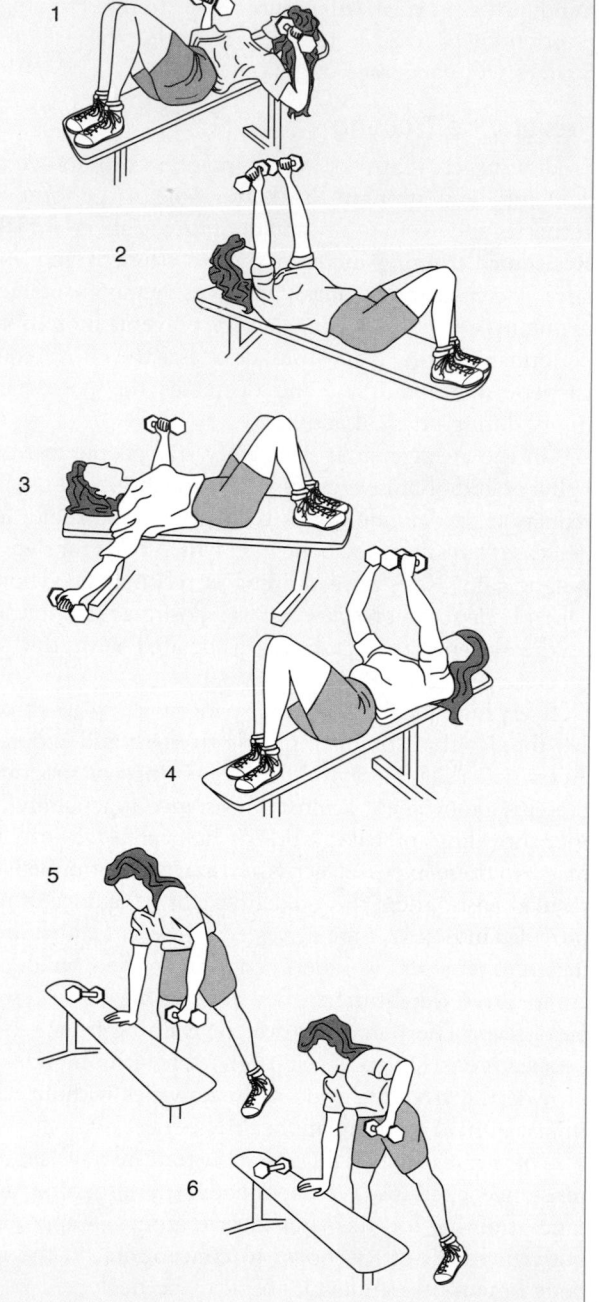

- Be repetitive and rhythmical. The cadence of activity provides a focus for awareness.
- Facilitate abdominal breathing. Watching the breath serves to anchor thoughts in the moment; in combination with cadence, it provides a focused awareness.
- Continue for 20 to 30 minutes at a comfortable intensity on most days of the week. This continuity restores a sense of serenity.

All forms of exercise can be used to gain this experience. As discussed, yoga involves mindful stretching with a breathing focus, providing an environment for successful elicitation of the RR. Tai Chi is another exercise practice with roots in Eastern philosophy. Known as *moving meditation*, Tai Chi combines movement with focused awareness, involving a physical and cognitive focus for moving in choreographed forms that become a meditation.

The quality of body awareness can also be brought into a more traditional exercise practice. Aerobic exercise lends

Box 12-3 **Resistive Training Exercises–cont'd**

DUMBBELL CURL (FIGS. 7 AND 8)

a. Stand or sit with weights held at sides in an underhand grip, keeping elbows close to body and upper arms stationary.
b. Curl weight to chin or upper chest while exhaling.
c. Inhale while slowly lowering weights.
d. Keep back straight through duration of motion.
e. Repeat 8 to 12 times.

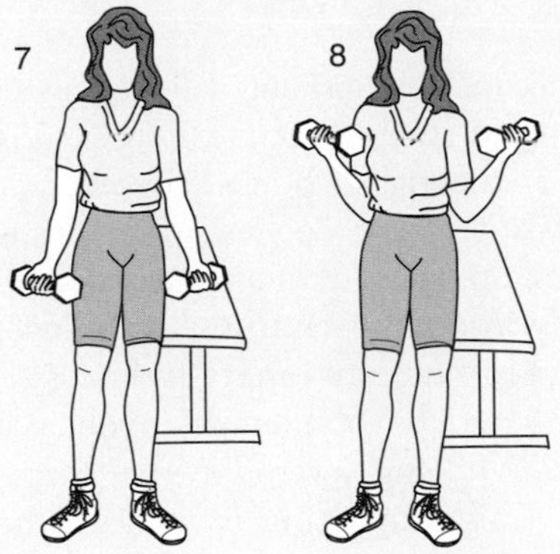

TRICEPS EXTENSION (FIGS. 9 AND 10)

a. While seated or standing in neutral back position, lift hand holding weight straight above head and in alignment with ear.
b. Keeping upper arm tight, slowly bend elbow to lower weight between shoulder blades.
c. Use free hand to support elbow and to prevent movement in upper arm.
d. Raise weight back to its original position by straightening arm and exhaling.
e. Repeat 8 to 12 times on each side.

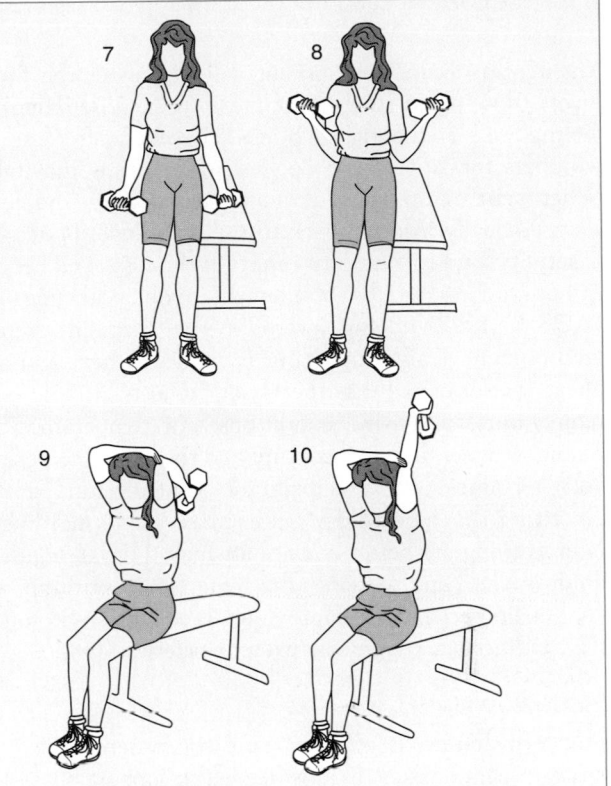

itself well to the elicitation of the RR because it has rhythmical and repetitive form and because it facilitates abdominal breathing. The practitioner can focus on the breath rhythm, the step cadence of walking or jogging, the pedaling cadence of bicycling, or the stroke cadence of swimming. Mantras can be used to create a positive mind-set and to focus the mind in the present moment as the experience unfolds. Resistance training takes on new meaning when coordinated with the breath. Focusing on the muscles and how it feels to move through the ROM enhances the knowledge of what feels good and what does not, providing feedback on accepting physical challenge.

Exercise focus can and should vary on a day-to-day basis depending on need, mood, and intent. Some days it feels right to focus on the more physical aspects of the activity, appreciating the challenge of working harder or longer. Other exercise sessions may be more contemplative, letting creativity run, working through the tension of a lingering stressor, quieting the mind for relaxation, listening to music, or appreciating nature. Focusing on the process rather than the outcomes brings meaning and purpose to the activity and helps achieve something more valuable than mere physical outcomes.

You don't dance to get to the other side of the floor—Watts (Huang & Lynch, 1992, p. 9).

When exercise integrates mind and body, it stops being something that has to be done and instead becomes something desired. Being mindful during physical activity and exercising in the moment increases awareness. With awareness comes choices in the possibilities of self-care. Exercise for fitness of the spirit, walk for the soul, and just let the body do the work.

MONITORING THE INNER AND OUTER ENVIRONMENT

The primary purpose of exercise is to enhance health. However, because exercise involves stress to the body, the potential to cause or exacerbate health problems is inherent. When a person is not feeling well, the exercise effort should be decreased or stopped until the individual is feeling better. With an infection, a cold, or influenza, the body is under stress and overexertion will only increase that stress and possibly lengthen the healing time. The level of activity should be adjusted to accommodate how the individual feels, slowly progressing to normal workout levels until strength and energy return. This philosophy also holds true for chronic diseases such as arthritis and HIV. During an acute exacerbation, activity should be limited to necessary activities of daily living (ADLs); but on a regular basis, staying active is important, adjusting activity levels as tolerated. Exercise can be a useful tool in coping with disease.

The first thing I do when I get up is some stretching, just to get my body moving. It's amazing how much of a difference a tiny amount of exercise makes in how I feel (Roos, 1992, p. 20).

Missing an occasional workout will not affect the fitness level; choosing to stop or cut back on exercise when not feeling well is the right choice. However, after missing workouts for 2 weeks, a decline in fitness is inevitable. When starting up again, resuming the activity should be slow, gradually working back to the usual level of activity. Inactivity for 3 to 5 months results in the loss of all benefits gained and resumption of exercise involves starting over (ACSM, 1998). Being aware of the external exercise environment is also important. Extremes of heat and cold affect performance as the body adjusts to different temperatures and wind conditions. Air temperature and humidity affect muscle flexibility and the ability to perspire and regulate body temperature (Huddleston, 1992). Changing the time of day for exercise (early morning or later evening are better choices for humid days), adjusting fluid intake, and varying the length of warm-up and cool-down periods will improve tolerance for environmental conditions and enhance exercise safety.

Fluid News

Proper hydration is an important component of a good fitness program. Extra fluid is needed to support physiological homeostasis during exercise, especially during hot weather. Drinking a cup of water 15 to 30 minutes before exercise is recommended. If the weather is hot or the indoor exercise area is very warm, then 5 to 12 ounces of fluid should be taken in every 15 or 20 minutes during exercise (Applegate, 1996, 2000). Fitness water is new on the market and is a good fluid replacement during exercise periods lasting less than 1 hour. Propel (Gatorade) and Ultima are low in calories and contain small amounts of electrolytes to help retain fluid, with flavors to encourage drinking more (Applegate, 2000). For exercise routines lasting longer than 1 hour, a sports drink with carbohydrates and electrolytes enhances performance and is recommended. This type of liquid provides muscles with energy and helps delay fatigue while meeting fluid needs. Sports drinks containing a 4% to 6% carbohydrate concentration are designed to replace carbohydrates at the proper rate during exercise. They also contain sodium, which promotes fluid retention, enhances flavor, and protects against hyponatremia, which can occur with lengthy exercise sessions. Most sports drinks provide 14 to 20 grams of carbohydrate per 8-ounce serving. The recommended intake is 5 to 12 ounces every 15 to 20 minutes. Which sports drink is the best? Several brands should be tried to determine personal preference in taste, but one should be chosen that contains approximately 50 to 80 calories per 8-ounce serving; any more and the carbohydrate concentration will inhibit fluid absorption (Applegate, 1996, 2000). Table 12-2 provides choices for sports drinks that both hydrate and energize.

What to Wear

Appropriate foot gear and clothing can enhance comfort and decrease the risk of injury during exercise.

Foot Gear

Although a good all-around shoe with proper support can be adequate for general physical activity, different types of exercise require that the feet be supported in different ways. Whenever possible, jogging shoes should be worn for jogging, walking shoes for walking, and court shoes for tennis and racquetball. For jogging (an activity in which the lower extremities are subjected to high-impact forces with a high risk of injury) having the shoe best suited to accommodate a particular foot structure is important. A normal foot does best in stability shoes with moderate control features. A flat (floppy) foot does best with motion control that reduces pronation. A high-arched (rigid) foot is best supported by cushioned shoes with plenty of flexibility to encourage foot mobility (Wischnia & Brunick, 1996). Any foot or general orthopedic problems that have required medical attention in the past should be discussed with an appropriate health care provider before beginning exercise.

Dress for Success

Cotton T-shirts may be comfortable, but they are not the best choice for exercise. Cotton is great for soaking up sweat, but it also retains the moisture, making the wearer sticky and irritated in hot weather and cold and damp in cooler weather. In warm or hot weather, lightweight, breathable gear made from high-tech fabrics is preferred because it wicks moisture away from the skin to the outer surface of the fabric where it can evaporate quickly, helping the inside surface stay dry. In cold weather, 2 or 3 layers of light clothing that can be removed as the body warms and

Table 12-2 Sports Drinks That Hydrate and Energize

Brand	Calories	Carbohydrates (grams)
All Sport	70	19
Cytomax	80	19
Endura	62	16
Gatorade	50	14
Hydra Fuel	70	17
Isostar	70	16
MetRx ORS	75	19
Perform	60	16
Powerade	70	19
PowerSurge	80	20
Race Day	63	15
XLRB	62	15

From Applegate, L. (2000). Liquid Assets. *Runner's World, 35*, 30-32.

replaced if the body cools off is recommended. The inner layer should be a snug, lightweight, synthetic material that wicks moisture to the outside to prevent chilling. In extremely cold weather, a middle layer is often necessary to provide additional insulation. The outer layer should be a loose-fitting protective shell to shield against cold, wind, rain, or snow while allowing perspiration to evaporate (Portz-Shoulin, 1996).

Wearing a hat helps keep the rest of the body warm, which preserves heat that would be lost through the top of the head and can instead be circulated around the body. For helping to keep the hands and feet warm, wearing a hat is especially beneficial. To further protect the hands, mittens, old socks, or gloves should be worn. Mittens keep the hands warmer than gloves with the shared warmth of the fingers; gloves are good for milder days. Socks that provide warmth, but wick moisture away from the skin, are best for keeping feet comfortable. For hats and hand and footwear, high-tech fabrics that are lightweight and breathable are a better choice than cotton or wool.

SPECIAL CONSIDERATIONS

Most adults do not need to consult a physician before starting a moderate intensity physical activity program. However, men older than 40 years of age and women older than 50 years of age who plan a vigorous program (intensity more than 60% of MHR or V_{O_2} max) or who have either chronic disease or risk factors for chronic disease should consult an appropriate health care provider before starting exercise (Table 12-3 and Box 12-4).

People with CHD and/or diabetes are 2 groups of people with special exercise needs. Earlier in this chapter, the ways in which exercise and physical activity affect positively on primary and secondary prevention in both disease processes were discussed. Limitations in the ability to exercise are related to the severity of the disease and the signs and symptoms of intolerance. For persons with CHD and DM, safety with starting a new exercise program requires supervision and guidance from knowledgeable health care providers. Before starting, these individuals should have a medical evaluation, including an exercise tolerance test (ETT) to determine functional capacity and severity of disease.

Coronary Heart Disease

Exercise plays a strong role in rehabilitation after a cardiac event such as MI, CABG, PTCA and stent, and angina. Increased physical activity appears to benefit individuals from each of these groups. Benefits include the following:

- Reduction in cardiovascular mortality.
- Reduction of symptoms.
- Improvement in exercise tolerance and functional capacity.
- Increase in the confidence and ability to carry out usual ADLs.
- Improvement in psychological well being and quality of life (Friedman, 1973; Oldridge, 1988; Shepard, 1979; USDHHS, 2000; Williams, 1981).

Generally, people with CHD demonstrate a reduction in V_{O_2} max and the ability to do submaximal levels of work. With exercise training, the increase in V_{O_2} max in patients with CHD averages approximately 20% after 3 months. This improvement in conditioning is the result of both central (cardiac) and peripheral (muscular) changes (Thompson, 1988). Some of the most significant improvements in exercise tolerance have been noted in patients with angina. With a decrease in submaximal HR and/or a decrease in SBP resulting from conditioning, myocardial oxygen demand is decreased and patients are able to do a greater amount of work before reaching their anginal threshold. This boost is reflected in an observed increase in rate pressure product (RPP) (HR × SBP) at the anginal threshold (Thompson, 1988). An increase in functional capacity allows for progression of exercise tolerance and progression with daily activities and leisure or vocational activities.

Psychological distress adversely affects the prognosis in patients with CHD (Allison et al., 1995). Episodes of anger

Table 12-3 ACSM Recommendations for Medical Examination and Exercise Testing Before Beginning an Exercise Program

Medical Examination and Clinical Exercise Test Recommended Before:	Apparently Healthy		Increased Risk*		
	Younger‡	Older	No Symptoms	Symptoms	Known Disease†
Moderate exercise§	No	No	No	Yes	Yes
Vigorous exercise¶	No	Yes	Yes	Yes	Yes

From American College of Sports Medicine. (1995). *Guidelines for exercise testing and prescription* (5th ed.). Media, PA: Williams & Wilkins.
*Persons with two or more risk factors or one or more signs or symptoms (see Box 12-4).
†Persons with known cardiac, pulmonary, or metabolic disease.
‡Younger implies ≤40 years of age for men, ≤50 years of age for women.
§Moderate exercise defined by an intensity of 40% to 60% of V_{O_2} max, or if intensity uncertain, an effort well within the individual's current capacity and that can be comfortably sustained for a prolonged period (60 minutes), slow progression, and generally noncompetitive.
¶Vigorous exercise is defined by an intensity >60% of V_{O_2} max, or if intensity is uncertain, exercise intense enough to represent a substantial cardiorespiratory challenge or result in fatigue within 20 minutes.

Box 12-4 Major Symptoms and Signs Suggestive of Cardiopulmonary Disease*

1. Pain, discomfort (or other anginal equivalent) in the chest, neck, jaw, arm, or other areas that may be ischemic in nature
2. Shortness of breath at rest or with mild exertion
3. Dizziness or syncope
4. Orthopnea or paroxysmal nocturnal dyspnea
5. Ankle edema
6. Palpitations or tachycardia
7. Intermittent claudication
8. Known heart murmur
9. Unusual fatigue or shortness of breath with usual activities

From American College of Sports Medicine. (1995). *Guidelines for exercise testing and prescription* (5th ed.). Media, PA: Williams & Wilkins.
*These symptoms must be interpreted in the clinical context in which they appear because they are not all specific for cardiopulmonary or metabolic disease.

are capable of triggering the onset of acute MI (Mittleman et al., 1995) and depression appears to be an important predictor of rehospitalization among persons admitted with CHD (Levine et al., 1996). Exercise plays a significant role in improving negative affective states and may help decrease the onset and recurrence of coronary events and symptoms.

Appropriately prescribed and conducted exercise training programs improve exercise tolerance and physical fitness in patients with CHD. Moderate and vigorous regimens are of value, but care must be taken to determine safe exercise parameters for each individual. The parameters of the exercise prescriptions are the same as those for the general population, including frequency, intensity, duration, and mode of exercise.

Aerobic exercise improves cardiorespiratory fitness and functional capacity. Any of the aforementioned aerobic exercises are acceptable for this population, depending on the level of fitness and musculoskeletal limitations. Traditionally, resistance training has not been commonly recommended for patients with CHD. The belief was that lifting weights resulted in a disproportionate rise in blood pressure, increased the myocardial oxygen demand, and increased risk of angina and MI. However, data from several studies indicate that moderate, supervised weight training is feasible, tolerable, and beneficial for patients with HTN and CHD. Franklin, Bonzheim, Gordon, & Timmis (1991) assert that hemodynamic and electrocardiographic response to mild to moderate weight training is acceptable and similar to traditional forms of aerobic exercise. Stewart et al. (1998) support these findings, suggesting that resistance exercise is safe for patients with an uncomplicated MI. Current belief suggests that strength training can keep the heart healthy by helping to control body weight, reduce cholesterol, and control blood sugar. Guidelines for determination of appropriate individuals include an aerobic capacity of at least 4 to 5 METS, an ejection fraction (EF) of greater than 30%, and no severe, symptomatic aortic stenosis (AS) (Merrill, 1997). However, clinical experience demonstrates that persons with more severe disease can use small hand weights to increase muscle tone without risk of cardiovascular compromise.

The exercise intensity for postevent persons who have not had a symptom-limited ETT should be kept at a low level based on an EHR of 20 to 30 bpm above RHR and an RPE rating of less than 12. After an ETT has been performed, intensity should then be prescribed based on 50% to 85% HRR; an RPE of 11 to 14; and/or below the ischemic, anginal, and/or arrhythmic threshold. Duration and frequency recommendations are similar to those for the general population. People who are the most deconditioned may need to exercise at lower intensities, for short durations, and more frequently throughout the day. Generally, a reasonable goal is 3 to 5 times per week for 20 to 40 minutes, plus 5 to 10 minutes for warm-up and cool-down. Warm-up and cool-down periods are vital components of the exercise session to allow the compromised cardiorespiratory system to adjust hemodynamically and metabolically to the increased and then decreased demands of the conditioning phase of exercise. Emphasis is placed on development of each person's self-monitoring skills for activity tolerance. To continue with safe, progressive exercise on their own, individuals need to develop the ability to monitor pulse rate, RPE, and signs and symptoms of intolerance (Huddleston, 1992).

Diabetes

Exercise has long been regarded as part of the triad in the treatment of diabetes in conjunction with diet and medication (insulin or oral medication). In the early 1900s, it was determined that exercise lowers the blood glucose concentration of people with diabetes. After the introduction of insulin, studies revealed that exercise can potentiate the hypoglycemic effect of injected insulin. More recently, findings suggest that in individuals who are in poor control (excessive blood glucose levels), exercise may induce a further increase in blood glucose levels, resulting in ketoses. On the average, people with diabetes have a lower MHR, achieve a lower cardiac output at maximal exercise, and have a higher blood pressure during exercise, resulting in lower maximal oxygen consumption (McMillan, 1975). However, these individuals can improve their exercise capacity with training and can experience the benefits related to overall fitness and cardiorespiratory training similar to the benefits gained by people without diabetes.

Apparently, both benefits and risks from exercise exist for people with diabetes. The overall goals regarding physical activity should be to teach individuals to incorporate activity into their daily life, pursue an exercise program if they wish, and develop strategies to avoid the complications of exercise (Horton, 1988).

As discussed, in addition to diet and weight loss, regular physical activity is an important modality in the prevention and treatment of NIDDM. People with NIDDM should monitor their blood glucose levels and determine their responses to exercise. However, generally, individuals with NIDDM can follow the same exercise prescription parameters as those of the general population. Although the same exercise benefits can be appreciated by people with IDDM, the inherent behavior and function of endogenous insulin makes exercising a more difficult proposition. The major functions of insulin are to promote glucose uptake into the cells and control metabolic homeostasis during exercise, working in synergy with the counter-regulatory hormones (CRH). With exercise, insulin secretion decreases slightly and the concentration of CRH increases. This increase stimulates hepatic glucose production, which balances the increased use of glucose by the working muscles, maintaining normoglycemia. However, with injected insulin, the plasma insulin concentration does not decrease with exercise, hepatic glucose production does not keep up with glucose use, and a decrease in blood glucose results. In contrast, in poorly controlled diabetes with decreased plasma insulin concentrations, there is already an elevated blood glucose level because there is insufficient insulin to assist glucose transport into cells. During exercise, the liver is stimulated to produce more glucose, which causes a further elevation in blood glucose levels, worsening the hyperglycemic condition. Ketosis may also result from increased mobilization and incomplete combustion of free fatty acids in muscle cells and accelerated ketone body formation in the liver (Franz, 1987; Zinman & Vranic, 1985).

Microvascular changes over time cause people with diabetes to be at risk for developing and should be screened for the presence of retinopathy, nephropathy, cardiovascular disease, and peripheral and autonomic neuropathies (McMillan, 1975), all of which present increased risks with exercise. To prevent rupture of fragile eye vessels in retinopathy, jarring activities and activities that cause a significant rise in blood pressure should be avoided. Initially, vital signs should be monitored and persons watched closely for signs of autonomic neuropathy (hypotension). Individuals with peripheral neuropathy are at risk for decreased sensation and neuropathic joints. Trauma and high-impact activity to the involved extremities should be avoided.

Although each person with diabetes should be evaluated and given individual exercise recommendations, the goals of an exercise program are universal:

1. Maintain or improve cardiovascular fitness to prevent or minimize long-term cardiovascular complications.
2. Improve flexibility that is impaired as muscle collagen becomes glycosylated.
3. Improve muscle strength, which may deteriorate as a result of neuropathy.
4. Allow people with IDDM to safely participate in and enjoy physical activities or sports.
5. Assist with weight control for people with NIDDM.
6. Allow people with diabetes to experience and gain the same benefits and enjoyment from regular exercise as do people without diabetes (Franz, 1989).

Box 12-5 shows a list of recommendations and precautions for people with diabetes who are interested in regular physical activity and exercise.

BUILDING A RHYTHM OF PHYSICAL ACTIVITY

Participation in regular physical activity increased gradually from the 1960s to the 1980s, but seems to have plateaued in recent years. The progress made toward *Healthy People 2000* physical activity goals indicates that the majority of the population has not embraced a physically active lifestyle (USDHHS, 1996, 2000). Although the benefits of physical activity are common to all people, patterns of physical activity vary among population subgroups defined by gender, age, racial background, income, and body fat. The following generalities are true:

- Men are more active than are women.
- Physical activity declines with age.
- Ethnic minorities are less active than are White Americans.
- Higher education and income are associated with more leisure-time activity.
- People who are obese are usually less active compared with their leaner counterparts (Pate et al., 1995).

Adherence and Compliance

Physiological, behavioral, and psychological variables all influence the decision to be physically active. Each person is unique and success with exercise over the long term comes from recognition of personal motivation or *core desire* and support from the social environment. Core desire defines the purpose behind putting the effort into developing and maintaining an active lifestyle; it is what motivates the individual to exercise. People should be encouraged to spend some quiet time meditating on why being physically fit is important to them.

Finding meaning and purpose in an active lifestyle can have a positive influence on enhancing behavior. Biopsychosocial and spiritual variables need to be considered in promoting physical activity. An individual's biopsychosocial factors and spiritual beliefs affect the behavioral and attitudinal factors that influence the motivation and ability to adhere to an active lifestyle. Generally, however, physical activity is more likely to be initiated and maintained if the individual:

- Perceives a net benefit.
- Chooses an enjoyable activity.

Box 12-5 Recommendations and Precautions for People with Diabetes Who Are Interested in Regular Physical Activity and Exercise

1. Notify primary care physician, ophthalmologist, and podiatrist of intent to exercise.
2. Monitor blood glucose level before and 20 to 30 minutes after exercise to determine the response to exercise.
3. Be sure blood glucose level is less than 300 mg/dl IDDM or less than 400 mg/dl NIDDM and urine tests negative for ketones (if blood glucose level is greater than 240 mg/dl). If blood glucose level is consistently equal to or greater than 250 mg/dl, improved control must be established before continuing exercise.
4. If possible, exercise approximately 1 hour after meals when blood glucose level is highest. This plan helps with weight loss because extra food will not have to be eaten to ward off hypoglycemia. When exercising before meals, a snack may be necessary. (See Table 12-4 for suggestions on food adjustments to maintain blood glucose balance with exercise.)
5. Know the action and peak times of insulin dosage and avoid exercising at peak.
6. Consider adjusting oral medication or insulin dosage to prevent low blood glucose level during exercise. Table 12-5 shows several ways to adjust insulin for exercise. The adjustment will depend on the intensity of the exercise, how long the exercise session lasts, and the type of insulin that is acting during exercise.
7. Watch out for the hypoglycemic *lag effect* that may occur 12 to 24 hours after vigorous exercise; an extra snack after exercise will help.
8. Avoid injecting insulin into a muscle area that will be active during exercise; the pumping action of the muscle may speed up absorption of the insulin and cause a rapid decrease of blood glucose.
9. Use proper footwear and make frequent foot inspections.
10. Avoid high-impact activity when prone to neuropathy in the legs or feet or when there is a history of neuropathy.
11. Keep SBP below 180 to 200 mmHg in the presence of eye or kidney disease.
12. Exercising every day is best, but at least 3 to 4 times per week. Start with 10 to 20 minutes and gradually increase to 30 to 40 minutes at 50% to 75% HR. Continuous aerobic activity helps maintain good blood glucose control better than stop-and-go activities. Do not forget the 5- to 10-minute warm-up and cool-down periods.
13. Avoid high-intensity anaerobic exercise, but low- to moderate-intensity resistance training is acceptable.
14. Carry a concentrated form of carbohydrate (sugar packets, glucose tablets, or Life Savers) when exercising.
15. Wear some form of diabetes identification.
16. People with NIDDM need to test blood glucose levels with exercise and potentially adjust oral medications. Consider decreasing medication if blood glucose level is less than 80 mg/dl after exercise. For weight loss, plan the best time to exercise so snacks can be avoided (Beaser & Hill, 1995).

Table 12-4 Food Adjustments

Duration and Intensity	Blood Glucose	Suggested Food Adjustment
< 30 minutes of moderate activity **Examples: Walking a mile or bicycling < 30 minutes**	< 100 100 to 180 > 180	1 fruit + 1 bread +1 meat 1 bread or 1 fruit May not need snack
30 to 60 minutes of moderate activity **Examples: Tennis, swimming, jogging, bicycling, yard work, or housework**	< 100 100 to 180 180 to 240 > 240	1 fruit + 1 bread +1 meat 1 bread or 1 meat 1 bread or 1 fruit May not need snack
60 minutes of moderate to high-intensity activity **Examples: Sports, strenuous bicycling, long-distance running, heavy shoveling**	If doing strenuous activity or playing sports, consult a physician or exercise physiologist for advice on blood glucose management. Insulin adjustment may be required in addition to food adjustments (see Table 12-5). Blood glucose should be tested hourly: 1 bread or 1 fruit per hour unless blood glucose is ≥ 180 (snack may not be needed for that hour).	

Modified from Beaser, R. S., & Hill, J. (1995). *The Joslin guide to diabetes*. New York: Simon and Schuster.

Table 12-5 Insulin Adjustment Guidelines for Exercise

Durations of Exercise	Intensity of Exercise	% to Decrease Peaking Insulin
< 30 minutes	Low, moderate, or high	0%
30 to 60 minutes	Moderate	10%
> 60 minutes	Moderate	20%
	High	30% or more

Modified from Beaser, R. S., & Hill, J. (1995). *The Joslin guide to diabetes*. New York: Simon and Schuster.
Intensity of exercise:
Low = Casual, easy (below exercise heart rate range)
Moderate = Comfortable but challenging, brisk (low end of exercise heart rate range)
High = Challenging, hard (high end of exercise heart rate range)
Regular insulin peak action = 2 to 4 hours
NPH/lente insulin peak action = 6 to 12 hours
Ultralente insulin peak action = 18 to 24 hours (do not adjust Ultralente insulin)

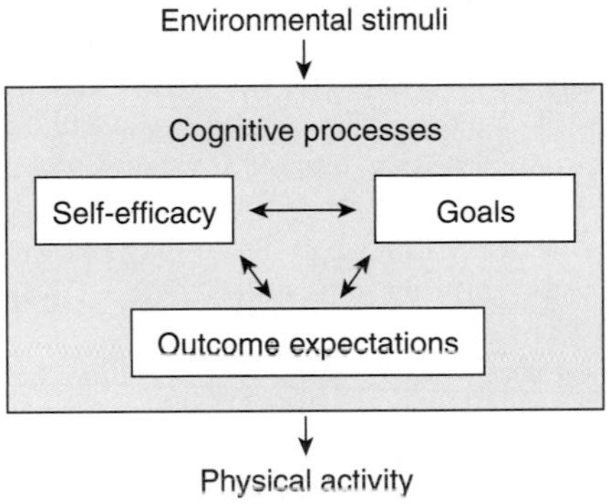

Fig. 12-7 Three interacting cognitive processes of Bandura's social cognitive theory. (Modified from Dzewaltowski, D. A. [1994]. Physical actively determinants: a social-cognitive approach. *Medicine and Science in Sports and Exercise, 26,* 1395-1399.)

- Feels competent doing the activity.
- Feels confident in overcoming barriers that may interfere with the activity.
- Feels safe doing the activity.
- Can easily access the activity on a regular basis.
- Perceives no significant negative financial or social cost.
- Experiences minimal musculoskeletal discomfort.
- Is able to address competing time demands.
- Is readily able to fit the activity into the daily schedule.
- Balances the use of labor-saving devices with activities that involve physical exertion (NIH, 1996).

Educating the public about physical activity helps to provide guidelines for safe and effective exercise, to reinforce potential benefits, and to alleviate misperceptions that may interfere with the decision to change behavior. However, knowledge about exercise and the intent to exercise do not correlate well with long-term compliance. Confidence in the ability to be physically active—and the

CASE STUDY

Ms. G.

Ms. G. is a 53-year-old account executive who is 2 years postmenopausal, complains of insomnia, and has chronic low back pain (LBP) and knee pain.

History: Motor vehicle accident (1970), resulting in bone graft to left leg (her left leg is shorter than her right leg). As part of rehabilitation, Ms. G. started jogging, which was more comfortable than walking with chronic R Sacro-Iliac joint pain. She started running marathons in 1972 and continued until 1988, including a Run Across America *(Guinness Book of Sports Records)*. In 1988, she began to add more variety into exercise and decreased her running, but she still identified herself as being an athlete.

In 1996, she suffered a fall that resulted in chronic LBP and was unable to continue aerobic exercise. She began to experience increased depression and insomnia; exercise had been a significant coping mechanism in the past and now her whole sense of well being is being affected. As Ms. G. attempted to rebuild her exercise practice, she would alternate between doing too much, exacerbating symptoms, and then having to stop and recuperate, reinforcing her negative self-image.

MRI showed mild arthritis in her knees, but not severe.

confidence that overcoming barriers produces positive benefits that are related to personal goals (self-efficacy) (Bandura, 1989)—is strongly related to participation and compliance (Fig. 12-7). Exercise self-efficacy is increased when people perform exercise successfully, receive positive feedback about success, view exercise role models, and learn more about the relationships among exercise, health, and body awareness (Schlicht, Godkin, & Camaione, 1999). (See Case Study and Nursing Care Plan.)

Enjoyment is another strong predictor of compliance and is often associated with low- to moderate-intensity activities versus high-intensity activities; it is also related to increased comfort and decreased incidence of injury (Pate et al., 1995). Additionally, techniques such as goal setting, writing a contract, and self-monitoring progress (keeping an exercise diary) enhance compliance. Conversely, lack of time is the most commonly cited barrier to participation in regular physical activity. However, this obstacle may be a subjective perception that reflects a lack of motivation because population studies indicate that regular exercisers are as likely as sedentary people are to view time as an activity barrier (Dishman, Sallis, & Orenstein, 1985). Embarrassment that is caused by negative self-judgment of ability and appearance often inhibits participation in social physical activities.

Creating a Climate That Supports Exercise

Clearly, exercise and fitness need to be social norms. A climate that supports and encourages physical activity should be fostered. Other people and organizations in the individual's social environment can influence the adoption

CARE PLAN

Ms. G.

MEDICATIONS

Oxazepam 30 mg, 4 to 6 times a week; Gingko Biloba

MAJOR SYMPTOMS

- Insomnia
- Chronic low back and knee pain
- Depression
- Upset about recent weight gain of 10 lbs (61½ inches, 118 lbs); sees ideal body weight as 108 lbs

INITIAL EXERCISE GOALS

- Walking, treadmill (TM), bicycling, and low-impact aerobics (30 minutes, 3 to 4 times per week)
- Weights 3 to 4 times per week
- Stretching 3 to 4 times per week
- Relaxation response (RR) daily
- Build mindfulness into exercise practice

QUESTIONS

- What are some of her barriers to exercise?
- How will a regular practice of mindfulness and the RR benefit her exercise practice?
- How would she benefit from cross training?
- What exercise is she doing that is beneficial for helping to prevent osteoporosis?

ANSWERS TO QUESTIONS

1. Barriers to exercise:
   - Past image of self as high-level exerciser
   - Current negative self-image
   - Musculoskeletal limitations
   - Exacerbation of symptoms with excessive exercise
   - Outcome oriented versus process oriented
2. With practice of RR, mindful stretching (yoga), and being more mindful with regular exercise, Ms. G. is able to gradually accept herself in the present and let go of expectations related to past experiences. She is able to accept decreased level of exercise intensity and to adapt the idea of *less is more*, listening to her body and not to mental messages. She is now enjoying the experience of being physically active rather than focusing on specific accomplishments.
3. Cross training provides overall body conditioning and decreases risk of injury (or exacerbating existing conditions) by decreasing repetitive stress to specific body parts. Cross training also provides a greater variety of choices, eliminating barriers and improving enjoyment and compliance.
4. Weight-bearing activities, such as walking, low-impact aerobics, and weight training, stress the skeleton and help stimulate bone density preservation.

After a 3-month period, she demonstrates the following improvements:

- Decreased frequency of low back and knee pain from constant to 2 to 4 times per week; although she still has some discomfort, the intensity is less and it interferes less with her life.
- Insomnia is decreased from 2 to 3 times per week to once per month; stopped sleep medications.
- Decreased depression and anxiety.
- Less unhappy about weight gain; more accepting of who she is.

EXERCISE PRACTICE

- Treadmill and walking daily for 30 minutes
- Weights: 2 to 3 times per week
- Yoga and stretching daily

and maintenance of physical activity (NIH, 1996; USDHHS, 1996).

Health Care Professionals

People are more likely to increase physical activity if counseled to do so by clinicians. Clinicians should inquire about exercise habits, communicate the benefits of increased activity, assist the person in initiating activity, and provide adequate follow-up. Challenging perceived individual barriers to exercise and offering alternative viewpoints can help create new exercise paradigms. Clinicians should also serve as role models by demonstrating enthusiasm for being physically active.

Recognizing the stages of behavioral change helps in meeting persons at their stage of readiness to change behavior (Prochaska, Norcross, & DiClemente, 1994). Marcus et al. (1992) demonstrate that providing information on physical activity that is designed for specific stages of readiness enables people to move from stages of contemplation and preparation into action. An individual in precontemplation is not ready to actively change behavior. This person may respond better to support and information about the benefits of changing behavior rather than being placed in an action environment. The decision to change may come gradually. After a person has made the commitment to change, the action phase lasts about 6 months. Continued follow-up throughout the action phase into maintenance is valuable in helping the individual stay committed until the termination phase is reached and the behavior is secure.

Family and Friends

Social support can be a valuable resource for behavioral change. Significant others or friends can serve as *buddies*, providing a source of companionship and motivation. These people can offer to share daily responsibilities (household chores) to free up time for exercise. Parents can support their children's activity by having family outings and providing transportation, praise, and encouragement. Joining a fitness club or an exercise group at work provides various forms of stimulation and socialization, which increases the potential for new friendships grounded in an appreciation for the rewards of exercise.

Work Sites

In reviewing progress towards *Healthy People 2000* goals, fitness opportunities at the work site are one of the few bright spots. Employers can provide space for fitness facilities or offer payroll deductions for affiliated health facilities. Companies can make time and programs available to encourage people to be active during work hours. Motivational signs can be placed strategically around the facility that encourage stair climbing and walking or bicycling to work. Secured areas for bikes and shower facilities encourage people to take advantage of building exercise into their work-related schedules.

Schools

Schools are one of the most important resources for increasing physical activity. Strategies must be developed to facilitate increased activity in children because it is clear that children are becoming less active and more obese. Schools are providing less opportunity and poorer quality time for physical activity during school hours. All schools should provide opportunities for physical activity that:

- Are appropriate and enjoyable for children of all skill levels and are not limited to competitive sports or physical education classes.
- Appeal to girls and boys and to children from diverse backgrounds.
- Are offered on a daily basis.
- Can serve as a foundation for activities throughout life (NIH, 1996).

Schools can also serve as a resource for the community. Expanding operating hours at either end of the school day creates a safe, indoor environment for hall walking.

Communities

Participation in regular physical activity at the community level depends in large part on the availability and proximity of facilities and safe environments. Community government agencies, local health agencies, schools, and places of worship have the potential to provide activity resources to the population at large. Churches seem to have been particularly successful in reaching ethnic minorities and elderly adults. Making neighborhoods safe for outdoor activities can have a major effect on improving activity habits, especially among low socioeconomic and disadvantaged populations, who report lower levels of daily physical activity.

Recognizing that many of the previous recommendations require a financial commitment, government agencies must respond to reports by health agencies and establish public policies that support the importance of physical activity for the general population. Individuals should make a personal commitment to be physically active, but that commitment needs to be supported by a social and political environment that values this type of lifestyle choice.

SUMMARY

It is important that people incorporate increased activity into their lifestyles on a long-term basis; exercise in the short term is of little overall benefit. Helping them gain the knowledge (benefits of exercise and recommended parameters for exercise), skills (self-monitoring), and attitude (core desire) improves compliance. People need to be motivated enough to start, enjoy the activity enough to want to continue, and appreciate the value enough to start again if they lapse. Lapses should be anticipated to avoid the unrealistic sense of total success or total failure. Behavioral change is cyclical rather than linear; success often comes with repeated movement through stages of change (Prochaska et al., 1994) and it helps to explore the reasons for the lapse and to view the lapse as a learning experience rather than a failure. The goal is to prevent a relapse that results in a more permanent noncompliance.

The benefits and enjoyment from developing a physically active lifestyle have a significant effect on the quality of life. However, this lifestyle is successful only when it is supported by a degree of self-awareness and self-care. People must realize that they are worth the effort of doing something good for themselves, that they have the perceived right to be happy and healthy, and that exercise can help them achieve that end. By adding a mind-body component to physical activity and not regarding it solely as a physical regime, people can experience *true health* rather than mere *fitness*. A great deal of bodily exercise is not required; 30 minutes a day can make a significant difference. Success comes with building a rhythm of physical activity into everyday life. Suggestions for a lifestyle approach to exercise include:

- Something is better than nothing.
- Attempt small changes over time (gradualism).
- Emphasize moderate intensity.
- Make activity an integral part of life.
- Focus on the process rather than the outcome.

Clinicians can provide a knowledgeable, supportive, and enthusiastic environment to encourage the change to a healthier, more active way of life.

REFERENCES

Aisenbrey, J. (1987). Exercise in the prevention and management of osteoporosis. *Physical Therapy, 67*, 1100-1104.

Albanes, D., Blair, A., & Taylor, P. R. (1989). Physical activity and risk of cancer in the NHANES I population. *American Journal of Public Health, 79*, 744-750.

Allison, T. G., Williams, D. E., Miller, T. D., Patten, C. A., Bailer, K. R., Squires, R. W., & Gau, G. T. (1995). Medical and economic costs of psychologic distress in patients with coronary artery disease. *Mayo Clinic Proceedings, 70*, 734-742.

Aloia, J. F. (1978). Prevention of involutional bone loss by exercise. *Annals of Internal Medicine, 89*, 356-358.

American College of Sports Medicine. (1995). *Guidelines for exercise testing and prescription* (5th ed.). Media, PA: Williams and Wilkins.

American College of Sports Medicine. (1997). *Exercise management for persons with chronic diseases and disabilities*. Champaign, IL: Human Kinetics.

American College of Sports Medicine. (1998). The recommended quantity and quality of exercise for developing and maintaining cardiorespiratory and muscular fitness, and flexibility in healthy adults. *Medicine and Science in Sports and Exercise, 30*, 975-986.

Andersen, R. E., Wadden, T. A., Bartlett, S. J., Zemel, B., Verde, T. J., & Franckowiak, S. C. (1999). Effects of lifestyle activity vs. structured anaerobic exercise in obese women. *Journal of the American Medical Association, 281*, 335-340.

Applegate, L. (1996). Fluid news you can use. *Runner's World, 31*, 26-28.

Applegate, L. (2000). Liquid Assets. *Runner's World, 35*, 30-32.

Arroll, B., & Beaglehole, R. (1992). Does physical activity lower blood pressure? A critical review of the clinical trials. *Journal of Clinical Epidemiology, 45*, 439-447.

Astrand, P. O. (1992). Why exercise? *Medicine and Science in Sports and Exercise, 24*, 153-162.

Bandura, A. (1989). Human agency in social cognitive theory. *The American Psychologist, 9*, 1175-1184.

Bean, A. (1996). The truth about burning fat. *Runner's World, 31*, 47-50.

Beaser, R. S., & Hill, J. (1995). *The Joslin guide to diabetes*. New York: Simon & Schuster.

Benson, H., & Stuart, E. (1992). *The wellness book*. New York: Simon & Schuster.

Berger, B., & Owen, D. (1988). Stress reduction and mood enhancement in four exercise modes: Swimming, body conditioning, hatha yoga and fencing. *Research Quarterly for Exercise and Sport, 59*, 148-159.

Bernstein, L., Henderson, B. E., Hanisch, R., Sullivan-Halley, J., & Ross, R. K. (1994). Physical exercise and reduced risk of breast cancer in young women. *Journal of the National Cancer Institute, 86*, 1403-1408.

Blair, S. N., Kohl, H. W. 3rd, Paffenbarger, R. S., Clark, D. G., Cooper, K. H., & Gibbons, L. W. (1989). Physical fitness and all-cause mortality: A prospective study of healthy men and women. *Journal of the American Medical Association, 262*, 2395-2401.

Blair, S. N., Kohl, H. W., Barlow, C. E., Paffenbarger, R. S., Gibbons, L. W., & Macera, C. A. (1995). Changes in physical fitness and all-cause mortality: A prospective study of healthy and unhealthy men. *Journal of the American Medical Association, 273*, 1093-1098.

Blair, S. N., Kampert, J.B., Kohl, H. W., Barlow, C. E., Macera, C. A., Paffenbarger, R. S., & Gibbons, L. W. (1996). Influences of cardiorespiratory fitness and other precursors on cardiovascular disease and all-cause mortality in men and women. *Journal of the American Medical Association, 276*, 205-210.

Blumenthal, J., Williams, R. S., Williams, R. B., & Wallace, A. G. (1980). Effects of exercise on the type A (coronary prone) behavior pattern. *Psychosomatic Medicine, 42*, 289-296.

Blumenthal, J., Emory, C. F., Madden, D. J., George, L. K., Coleman, R. E., Riddle, M. W., McKee, D. C., Reasoner, J., & William, R. S. (1989). Cardiovascular and behavioral effects of aerobic exercise training in healthy older men and women. *Journal of Gerontology, 44*, 147-157.

Blumenthal, J., Babyak, M. A., Moore, K. A., Craighead, W. E., Herman, S., Khatri, P., Waugh, R., Napolitaine, M. A., Forman, L. M., Appelbaum, M., Doraiswamy, P. M., & Krishnan, K. R. (1999). Effects of exercise training on older patients with major depression. *Archives of Internal Medicine, 159*, 2349-2356.

Borg, G. A. (1973). Perceived exertion: A note on history and methods. *Medicine and Science in Sports and Exercise, 5*, 90-93.

Borg, G. A. (1982). Psychophysical basis of perceived exertion. *Medicine and Science in Sports and Exercise, 14*, 377-381.

Bortz, W. M. (1982). Disuse and aging. *Journal of the American Medical Association, 248*, 1203-1208.

Bortz, W. M. (1993). Dare to be 100. *Cooking Light, 7*, 34-42.

Brown, D. R., Wang, Y., Ward, A. Ebbeling, C. B., Fortlage, L., Puleo, E., Benson, H., & Rippe, J. M. (1995). Chronic psychological effects of exercise and exercise plus cognitive strategies. *Medicine and Science in Sports and Exercise, 27*, 765-775.

Cady, L. D., Thomas, P. C., & Karwasky, R. J. (1985). Program for increasing health and physical fitness of firefighters. *Journal of Occupational Medicine: Official Publication of the Industrial Medical Association, 27*, 110-114.

Centers for Disease Control and Prevention. (2000). Overweight need to step up exercise regimens. *Morbidity and Mortality Weekly Report, 49*, 326-330.

Chewning, B., Yu, T., & Johnson, J. (2000). T'ai Chi: Effects on health. *ACSM's Health and Fitness Journal, 4*, 17-28.

Cummings, S. R. (1985). Epidemiology of osteoporosis and osteoporotic fractures. *Epidemiology Review, 7*, 178-208.

Dalsky, G. P., Stocke, K. S., Ehsani, A. A., Slatoplosky, E., Lee, W. C., & Birge, S. J. (1988). Weight-bearing exercise training and lumbar bone mineral content in postmenopausal women. *Annals of Internal Medicine, 108*, 824-828.

DeBusk, R. F., Stenestrand, V., Sheehan, M., & Haskell, W. L. (1990). Training effects of long versus short bouts of exercise in healthy subjects. *The American Journal of Cardiology, 65*, 1010-1013.

Dishman, R. K., Sallis, J. F., & Orenstein, D. R. (1985). The determinants of physical activity and exercise. *Public Health Reports, 100*, 158-171.

Durstine, J. L., & Haskell, W. L. (1994). Effects of exercise training on plasma lipids and lipoproteins. *Exercise and Sport Sciences Review, 22*, 477-521.

Dyer, J., & Crouch, J. (1988). Effects of running and other activities on moods. *Perceptual and Motor Skills, 67*, 43-50.

Dzewaltowski, D. A. (1994). Physical activity determinants: A social-cognitive approach. *Medicine and Science in Sports and Exercise, 26*, 1395-1399.

Fagard, R. H., & Tipton, C. M. (1994). Physical activity, fitness, and hypertension. In C. Bouchard, R. J. Shephard, & T. Stephens (Eds.), *Physical activity, fitness and health: International proceedings and consensus statement*. Champaign, IL: Human Kinetics.

Farrell, S. W., Kampert, J. B., Kohl, H. W., Barlow, C. E., Macera, C. A., Paffenbarger, R. S., Gibbons, L. B., & Blair, S. N. (1998). Influences of cardiorespiratory fitness levels and other predictors of cardiovascular disease mortality in men. *Medicine and Science in Sports and Exercise, 30*, 899-905.

Fiatarone, M. A., Marks, E. C., Ryan, N. D., Meredith, C. N., Lipsitz, L. A., & Evans, W. J. (1990). High intensity strength training in nonagenarians: Effects on skeletal muscle. *Journal of the American Medical Association, 263*, 3029-3034.

Fiatarone, M. A., O'Neill, E. F., Ryan, N. D., Clements, K. M., Solares, G. R., & Nelson, M. E. (1994). Exercise training and nutritional supplementation for physical frailty in very elderly people. *New England Journal of Medicine, 330*, 1769-1775.

Fletcher, G. F., Blair, S. N., Blumenthal, J., Caspensen, C., Chaitman, B., Epstein, S., Falls, H. Froelicher, E. S., Froelicher, V. F., & Pina, I. L. (1992). Statement on exercise: Benefits and recommendations for physical activity programs for all Americans. *Circulation, 86*, 340-343.

Folkins, C. H. (1976). Effects of physical training on mood. *Journal of Clinical Psychology, 32*, 385-388.

Franklin, B. (1993). How much exercise is enough? *Encyclopedia Britanica*, p. 471-476.

Franklin, B. A., Bonzheim, K., Gorden, S., Timmis, G. (1991). Resistance training in cardiac rehabilitation. *Journal of Cardiopulmonary Rehabilitation, 11*, 99-107.

Franz, M. (1987). Exercise and the management of diabetes mellitus. *Journal of the American Dietetic Association, 87*, 872-880.

Franz, M. (1989). Conclusions. *Diabetes Spectrum, 1*, 247-250.

Friedman, M., Manwaring, J. H., Rosenman, R. H., Donlon, G., Ortega, P., & Grube, S. M. (1973). Instantaneous and sudden deaths: Clinical and pathological differentiation in coronary heart disease. *Journal of the American Medical Association, 224*, 1319-1328.

Goff, D., & Dimsdale, J. (1985). The psychologic effect of exercise. *Journal of Cardiopulmonary Rehabilitation, 5*, 234-240.

Green, J. S., & Crouse, S. T. (1995). The effects of endurance training on functional capacity in the elderly: A meta-analysis. *Medicine and Science in Sports and Exercise, 27*, 920-926.

Harris, M. I., et al. (1988). Prevalence of diabetes, impaired fasting glucose, and impaired glucose tolerance in U.S. adults. *Diabetes Care, 21*, 518-524.

Hass, C. J., Garzarella, L., De Hoyos, D., & Polloch, M. (2000). Single versus multiple sets in long-term recreational weightlifters. *Medicine and Science in Sports and Exercise, 32*, 235-242.

Haskell, W. H., et al. (1992). Cardiovascular benefits and assessment of physical activity and physical fitness in adults. *Medicine and Science in Sports and Exercise, 24* (SVI), S201-S220.

Helmrich, S. P., Ragland, D., Leung, R., Paffenbarger, R. (1991). Physical activity and reduced occurrence of non-insulin dependent diabetes mellitus. *New England Journal of Medicine, 325*, 147-152.

Helmrich, S. P., Ragland, D. R., & Paffenbarger, R. S. (1994). Prevention of non-insulin dependent diabetes mellitus with physical activity. *Medicine and Science in Sports and Exercise, 26*, 824-830.

Heyden, S., & Fodor, F. (1988). Does regular exercise prolong life expectancy? *Sports Medicine, 6*, 63-71.

Holloszy, J. O., Schultz, J., Kusnierkiewicz, J., Hagberg, J. M., & Ehsani, A. A. (1986). Effects of exercise on glucose intolerance and insulin resistance. *Acta Medica Scandinavica Supplementum, 711*, 55.

Horton, E. (1988). Role and management of exercise in diabetes mellitus. *Diabetes Care, 11*, 201-211.

Huang, C. A., & Lynch, J. (1992). *Thinking body, dancing mind.* New York: Bantam Books.

Huddleston, J. S. (1992). Move into health. In H. Benson, & E. Stuart (Eds.), *The wellness book.* New York: Simon & Schuster.

Iverson, D. C., Fielding, J. E., Crow, R. S., Christensen, G. M. (1985). The promotion of physical activity in the U.S. population: The status of programs in medical, worksite, school and community setting. *Public Health Reports, 100*, 212-224.

Jackson, A. S., Beard, E. F., Wier, L. T., Ross, R. M., Stutesville, J. E., & Blair, S. N. (1995). Changes in aerobic power of men ages 25-70 yrs. *Medicine and Science in Sports and Exercise, 27*, 113-120.

Jakicic, J. M., Wing, R. R., Butler, B. A., Robertson, R. J. (1995). Prescribing exercise in multiple short bouts versus one continuous bout: Effect on adherence, cardiorespiratory fitness and weight loss in overweight women. *International Journal of Obesity, 19*, 893-901.

Jin, P. (1989). Changes in heart rate, noradrenaline, cortisol and mood during Tai Chi. *Journal of Psychosomatic Research, 33*, 197-206.

Kannel, W., & Sorlie, P. (1989). Some health benefits of physical activity. *Archives Internal Medicine, 139*, 857-861.

Kayman, S., Bruvold, W., & Stern, J. S. (1990). Maintenance and relapse after weight loss in women. *The American Journal of Clinical Nutrition, 52*, 800-807.

Keleman, M. H., Effron, M., Valente, S., Stewart, K. (1990). Exercise testing combined with anti-hypertensive drug therapy. *Journal of the American Medical Association, 263*, 2766-2771.

Kelly, G., & McClellan, P. (1994). Anti-hypertensive effects of aerobic exercise: A brief meta-analytic review of randomized controlled trials. *American Journal of Hypertension: Journal of the American Society of Hypertension, 7*, 115-119.

Kiyonaga, A., Arakawa, K., Tanaka, H., & Shindo, M. (1985). Blood pressure and hormonal responses to aerobic exercise. *Hypertension, 7*, 125-131.

Kobasa, S. (1985). Effectiveness of hardiness, exercise and social support as resources against illness. *Journal of Psychosomatic Research, 29*, 525-533.

Kohrt, W. M., Malley, M., Coggan, A., Spina, R., Ogawa, T., Ehsani, A., Bourey, R., Martin, W., & Holloszy, J. (1991). Effects of gender, age, and fitness level on response of Vo_2 max to training in 60-71 yr olds. *Journal of Applied Physiology, 71*, 2004-2011.

Kohrt, W. M., Sneod, D. B., Slatoplosky, E., & Birge, S. T. (1995). Additive effects of weight-bearing exercise and estrogen on bone mineral density in older women. *Journal of Bone and Mineral Research: The Official Journal of the American Society for Bone and Mineral Research, 10*, 1303-1311.

Kriska, A. M., LaPorte, R. E., Pettitt, D. J., Charles, M. A., Nelson, R. E., Kuller, L. H., Bennett, P. H., & Knowler, W. C. (1993). The association of physical activity with obesity, fat distribution and glucose intolerance in Pima Indians. *Diabetologia, 36*, 863-6-869.

Krolner, B., Toft, B., Pors Nielsen, S., Tondevold, E. (1983). Physical exercise as a prophylaxis against involuntary bone loss. *Clinical Science, 64*, 541-546.

Kuczmarski, R. J., Flegol, K. M., Campbell, S. M., & Johnson, C. L. (1994). Increasing prevalence of overweight among U.S. adults: The National Health and Nutrition Examination Surveys, 1960 to 1991. *Journal of the American Medical Association, 272*, 205-211.

Lan, C., Lai, J. S., Chen, S. Y., Wong, M. K. (1998). 12-Month Tai Chi training in the elderly: Its effect on health fitness. *Medicine and Science in Sports and Exercise, 30*, 345-351.

Lane, J. M., & Nydick, M. (1999). Osteoporosis: Current modes of prevention and treatment. *The Journal of the American Academy of Orthopedic Surgeons, 7*, 19-31.

LaPierriere, A., Fletcher, M., Antoni, M., Klimas, N., Schneiderman, N. (1991). Aerobic exercise training in an AIDS risk group. *International Journal of Sports Medicine, 12*, 1-5.

Lee, I. M. (1994). Physical activity, fitness, and cancer. In C. Bouchard, R. J. Shephard, & T. Stephens (Eds.), *Physical activity, fitness and health: International proceedings and consensus statement.* Champaign, IL: Human Kinetics.

Lee, I. M., Manson, J. E., Hennekens, C. H., & Paffenbarger, R. S. (1993). Body weight and mortality: A 27 year follow-up of middle-aged men. *Journal of the American Medical Association, 270*, 2823-2828.

Leibel, R. L., Rosenbaum, M., & Hirsch, J. (1995). Changes in energy expenditure resulting from altered body weight. *New England Journal of Medicine, 332*, 621-628.

Leon, A. S. (1991). Effects of exercise conditioning on physiologic precursors of coronary heart disease. *Journal of Cardiopulmonary Rehabilitation, 11*, 46-57.

Levine, J. B., Covinon, A., Slack, W. V., Safran, C., Safran, D. B., Boro, J. E., Davis, R. B., Buchaman, G. M., & Gervino, E. V. (1996). Psychological predictors of subsequent medical care among patients hospitalized with cardiac disease. *Journal of Cardiopulmonary Rehabilitation, 16*, 109-116.

Mackinnon, L. T. (1992). *Exercise and immunology.* Champaign, IL: Human Kinetics.

Manson, J. E., Nathan, K. M., Knolewski, A. S., Stranysfer, M. J., Willett, W. C., & Hennekens, C. H. (1992). A prospective study of exercise and incidence of diabetes among U.S. male physicians. *Journal of the American Medical Association, 268*, 63-67.

Manson, J. E., Hu, F. B., Rich-Edwards, J. W., Colditz, G. A., Stampfer, M. J., Willet, W. C., Speizer, F. E., & Hennekens, C. H. (1999). A prospective study of walking as compared with vigorous exercise in the prevention of coronary disease in women. *New England Journal of Medicine, 341*, 650-658.

Marcus, B. H., Banspach, S. W., Hefebvre, R. C., Rossi, J. S., Carleton, R. A., & Abrams, D. B. (1992). Using the stages of change model to increase the adoption of physical activity among community participants. *American Journal of Health Promotion, 6*, 424-429.

Matheson, G., Macintyre, J. G., Taunton, J. E., Clement, D. B., Lloyd-Smith, R. (1989). Musculoskeletal injuries associated with physical activity in older adults. *Medicine and Science in Sports and Exercise, 21*, 379-385.

McHenry, P. L., McHenry, P. L., Ellestad, M. H., Fletcher, G. F., Froelicher, Hartley, H., Mitchell, J. H., Froelicher, E. S. S. (1990). A special report: Statement on exercise. *Circulation, 81*, 396-398.

McMillan, D. (1975). Deterioration of the microcirculation in diabetes. *Diabetes, 24*, 944-957.

Merrill, J. (1997). Resistance training in cardiac rehabilitation. *Fitness Management Magazine, 13*, 35-37.

Mittleman, M. A., Maclure, M., Tofler, G. H., Sherwood, J. B., Goldberg, R. J., & Miller, J. E. (1993). Triggering of acute MI by heavy physical exertion: Protection against triggering by regular exertion. *New England Journal of Medicine, 329*, 1677-1683.

Mittleman, M. A., Maclure, M., Sherwood, J. B., Mulry, R. P., Tofler, G. H., Jacobs, S. C., Friedman, R., Benson, H., & Muller, J. E. (1995). Triggering of acute myocardial infarction onset by episodes of anger. *Circulation, 92*, 1720-1725.

Morgan, W. (1973). Psychological factors influencing perceived exertion. *Medicine and Science in Sports and Exercise, 5*, 97-103.

Morganti, C. M., et al. (1995). Strength improvements with 1 yr of progressive resistance training in older women. *Medicine and Science in Sports and Exercise, 27*, 906-912.

Morris, J. N., et al. (1973). Vigorous exercise in leisure time and incidence of coronary heart disease. *Lancet, 1*, 333-339.

Morris, J. N., Clayton, D. G., Everitt, M. G., Semmence, A. M., Burgess, E. H. (1990). Exercise in leisure time: Coronary attack and death rates. *British Heart Journal, 63*, 325-334.

National Institute of Health, Consensus Development Panel. (1996). Physical activity and cardiovascular health. *Journal of the American Medical Association, 276*, 241-246.

Nelson, M. F., Fiatarone, M. A., Morganit, C. M., Trice, I., Greenberg, R. A., & Evans, W. J. (1994). Effects of high intensity strength training on multiple risk factors for osteoporotic fractures. *Journal of the American Medical Association, 272*, 1909-1914.

Nieman, D. (1994). Exercise, upper respiratory tract infection, and the immune system. *Medicine and Science in Sports and Exercise, 26*, 128-139.

Nieman, D., Nehlsen-Cannarella, S. L., Markoff, P. A., Balk-Lamberton, A. J., Yang, H., Chritton, D. B., Lee, J. W., & Arabatzis, K. (1990). The effects of moderate exercise training on natural killer cells and acute upper respiratory tract infections. *International Journal of Sports Medicine, 11*, 467-473.

Nieman, D. (2000). Exercise soothes arthritis. *ACSM's Health and Fitness Journal, 4*, 20-27.

Oldridge, N. B., Guyatt, G., Fischer, M., & Rimno, A. (1988). Cardiac rehabilitation after MI. *Journal of the American Medical Association, 260*, 945-950.

Oliveria, S. A., Kohl, H., Trichopoulos, D., & Blair, S. (1996). The association between cardiorespiratory fitness and prostate cancer. *Medicine and Science in Sports and Exercise, 28*, 97-104.

O'Sullivan, S. B. (1984). Perceived exertion: A review. *Physical Therapy, 64*, 343-346.

Paffenbarger, R. S., & Hyde, R. (1980). Exercise as protection against heart attack. *New England Journal of Medicine*, 308, 1026-1027.

Paffenbarger, R. S., Lee, I. M., & Leung, R. (1994). Physical activity and personal characteristics associated with depression and suicide in American college men. *Acta Medica Scandinavica Supplementum, 377*, 16-22.

Paffenbarger, R. S., Wing, A. L., & Hyde, R. T. (1978). Physical activity as an index of heart attack risk in college alumni. *American Journal of Epidemiology, 108*, 161-175.

Paffenbarger, R. S., Wing, A. L., Hyde, R. T., & Jung, D. C. (1983). Physical activity and incidence of hypertension in college alumni. *American Journal of Epidemiology, 117*, 245-257.

Paffenbarger, R. S., Hyde, R. T., Wing, A. L., Hsieh, C. C. (1986). Physical activity, all-cause mortality, and longevity of college alumni. *New England Journal of Medicine, 314*, 605-613.

Paffenbarger, R. S., Hyde, R. T., Wing, A. L., Lee, I-M, Jung, D. L., & Kampert, J. B. (1993). The association of changes in physical activity level and other lifestyle characteristics with mortality among men. *New England Journal of Medicine, 328*, 538-545.

Panush, R. S., & Lane, N. E. (1994). Exercise and the musculoskeletal system. *Bailliere's Clinical Rheumatology, 8*, 79-102.

Pate, R. R., Pratt, M., Blair, S. N., Haskell, W. L., Macera, C. A., Bouchard, C., Buchner, D., Ettinger, W., Heath, G. W., King, A. C. (1995). Physical activity and public health: A recommendation from the Centers for Disease Control and Prevention and the American College of Sports Medicine. *Journal of the American Medical Association, 273*, 402-407.

Pate, R. R., Baranowski, T., Dowda, M., & Trost, S. (1996). Tracking of physical activity in young children. *Medicine and Science in Sports and Exercise, 28*, 92-96.

Pedersen, B., & Ullum, H. (1994). NK cell response to physical activity: Possible mechanisms of action. *Medicine and Science in Sports and Exercise, 26*, 140-146.

Pereira, M. A., Kriska, A. M., Joswiak, M. L., Zimmet, P. Z., Gareeboo, H., Chitson, P., Hemraj, F., Purran, A., & Fareed, D. (1995). Physical inactivity and glucose intolerance in the multi-ethnic island of Mauritius. *Medicine and Science in Sports and Exercise, 27*, 1626-1634.

Portz-Shoulin, E. (1996). Put it to the test. *Runner's World, 31*, 80-87.

Prochaska, J. O., Norcross, J. C., & DiClemente, C. C. (1994). *Changing for good.* New York: William Morrow.

Rangger, C., Kathrein, A., Klestil, T., & Glotzer, W. (1997). Partial meniscectomy and osteoarthritis: Implications for treatment of athletes. *Sports Medicine, 23*, 61-68.

Rauramaa, R., & Salomen, J. T. (1994). Physical activity, fibrinolysis, and platelet aggregability. In C. Bouchard, R. J. Shephard, & T. Stephens (Eds.), *Physical activity, fitness and health.* Champaign, IL: Human Kinetics.

Rigsby, L., Dishman, R., Jackson, A., Maclean, G., Raven, P. (1992). Effects of exercise training on men seropositive for the human immunodeficiency virus. *Medicine and Science in Sports and Exercise, 24*, 6-12.

Rockhill, B., Willett, W. C., Hunter, D. J., Manson, J. E., Hankinson, S. E., & Colditz, G. A. (1999). A prospective study of recreational physical activity and breast cancer risk. *Archives of Internal Medicine, 159*, 2290-2296.

Roman, O., Camuzzi, A., Villalon, E., Klenner, C. (1981). Physical training program in arterial hypertension: A long-term prospective follow-up. *Cardiology, 67*, 230-243.

Roos, R. (1992). Defying the odds with exercise: A physiologist battles AIDS. *Your Patient and Fitness, 6*, 20-23.

Ross, C. E., & Hayes, D. (1988). Exercise and psychologic well-being in the community. *American Journal of Epidemiology, 127*, 762-771.

Rowe, J. W., & Kahn, R. L. (1987). Human aging: Usual and successful. *Science, 237*, 143-149.

Saltin, B. (1968). Response to exercise after bed rest and after training: A longitudinal study of adaptive changes in oxygen transport and body composition. *Circulation, 38* (SVII), 1-78.

Schatz, M. P. (1984). Living with your lower back. *Yoga Journal*, 36-45.

Schatz, M. P. (1985). Yoga relief for arthritis. *Yoga Journal*, 29-34.

Schlicht, J., Godin, J., & Camaione, D. N. (1999). Build self-efficacy to promote exercise adherence. *ACSM's Health & Fitness Journal*, *3(6)*, 27-31.

Sheehan, G. (1994). The best of Sheehan: Changing course. *Runner's World*, *29*, 16.

Shepard, R. J. (1994). *Aerobic fitness and health*. Champaign, IL: Human Kinetics.

Shepard, R. J. (1979). Recurrence of myocardial infarction in an exercising population. *British Heart Journal*, *41*, 133-138.

Skinner, J. S., Hustler, R., Bergsteinova, V., Buskirke, R. (1973). The validity and reliability of a rating scale of perceived exertion. *Medicine and Science in Sports and Exercise*, *5*, 94-96.

Smith, E. C., Reddan, W., & Smith, P. E. (1981). Physical activity and calcium modalities for bone mineral increase in aged women. *Medicine and Science in Sports and Exercise*, *13*, 60-64.

Smutok, M., Skrinar, G., & Pendolf, K. (1980). Exercise intensity: Subjective regulation by perceived exertion. *Archives of Physical Medicine and Rehabilitation*, *61*, 569-574.

Spence, D., Galentino, M. L., Mossberg, K., Zimmerman, S. (1990). Progressive resistance exercise: Effect on muscle function and anthropometry of a select AIDS population. *Archives of Physical Medicine and Rehabilitation*, *71*, 644-648.

Stefanick, M. L., & Wood, P. D. (1994). Physical activity, lipid and lipoprotein metabolism, and lipid transport. In C. Bouchard, R. J. Shephard, & T. Stephens (Eds.), *Physical activity, fitness and health: International proceedings and consensus statement*. Champaign, IL: Human Kinetics.

Stephens, T., & Craig, C. L. (1990). *The well-being of Canadians: Highlights of the 1988 Campbell's survey*. Ottawa: Canadian Fitness and Lifestyle Research Institute.

Stewart, K. (1998). Safety and efficiency of weight training soon after acute myocardial infarction. *Journal of Cardiopulmonary Rehabilitation*, *18*, 37-44.

Teegarden, D., Proulx, W. R., Kern, M., Sedlock, D., Weaven, C. M., Johnston, C. C., & Lyle, R. M. (1996). Previous physical activity relates to bone mineral measures in young women. *Medicine and Science in Sports and Exercise*, *28*, 105-113.

Thompson, P. D. (1988). The benefits and risks of exercise training in patients with chronic coronary artery disease. *Journal of the American Medical Association*, *259*, 1537-1540.

Tipton, C. M. (1984). Exercise and resting blood pressure. In H. M. Eckert, & H. J. Montoye (Eds.), *Exercise and health*. Champaign, IL: Human Kinetics.

Tremblay, A., Despres, J. P., & Bouchard, C. (1985). The effects of exercise training on energy balance and adipose tissue morphology and metabolism. *Sports Medicine*, *2*, 223-233.

U.S. Department of Health and Human Services. (1990). *Healthy people 2000: National health promotion and disease prevention objectives* (Pub No 91-50212). Washington, DC: Public Health Service.

U.S. Department of Health and Human Services. (1995). *Healthy people 2000: Mid-course review and 1995 revisions*. Washington, DC: Public Health Service.

U.S. Department of Health and Human Services. (1996). *Physical activity and health: A report of the surgeon general*. Atlanta: U.S. Department of Health and Human Services, Centers for Disease Control and Prevention, National Center for Chronic Disease Prevention and Health Promotion.

U.S. Department of Health and Human Services. (1999). *Healthy people 2000 review, 1998-1999* (DHHS Pub No 99-1256). Hyattsville, MD: Centers for Disease Control and Prevention, National Center for Health Statistics.

U.S. Department of Health and Human Services. (2000, Jan.). *Healthy people 2010: Vol. 1 and 2* (Conference Edition). Washington, DC: Centers for Disease Control and Prevention, President's Council on Physical Fitness and Sports.

Wallace, J. (1989). Exercise myths. *Diabetes Forecast*, pp. 25-28.

Wei, M., Gibbons, L. W., Kampart, J. B., Nichamen, M. Z., Blair, S. N. (2000). Cow cardioresiratiory fitness and physical activity as predictors of mortality in men with type II diabetes. *Annals of Internal Medicine*, *132*, 605-611.

Westcott, W. L. (1993). Strength for everyone. *Fitness Management*, *32-36*.

Williams, P. T. (1996). High density lipoprotein cholesterol and other risk factors for coronary heart disease in female runners. *New England Journal of Medicine*, *334*, 1298-1303.

Williams, R. S. (1981). Guidelines for unsupervised exercise in patients with ischemic heart disease. *Journal of Cardiopulmonary Rehabilitation*, *1*, 213-219.

Williford, H. N., Scharff-Olson, M., & Blessings, D. (1993). Exercise prescription for women. *Sports Medicine*, *15*, 299-311.

Wischnia, R., & Brunick, T. (1996). Choosing the right shoe. *Runner's World*, 46-47.

Wolf, S. L., Barnhart, H. X., & Kutner, N. G. (1996). Reducing frailty and falls in older persons: An investigation of Tai Chi and computerized balance training. *Journal of the American Geriatric Society*, *44*, 489-497.

Woods, J. A., & Davis, J. M. (1994). Exercise, monocyte/macrophage function, and cancer. *Medicine and Science in Sports and Exercise*, *26*, 147-156.

Zinman, B., & Vranic, M. (1985). Diabetes and exercise. *The Medical Clinics of North America*, *69*, 145-157.

Chapter 13

CAROL L. WELLS-FEDERMAN
CAROL LYNN MANDLE

Stress Management

objectives

After completing this chapter, the nurse will be able to:

- Differentiate stress and stressor.
- Differentiate eustress and distress.
- Evaluate potential physical, psychological, social, and behavioral stressors.
- Identify pathophysiology of the stress response and effects on health and illness.
- Analyze primary and secondary appraisals of stress.
- Discuss the nurse's role in stress management.
- Propose stress-management interventions that can be used in clinical practice.
- Develop a nursing care plan for stress management.

key terms

Affirmation
Assertive Communication
Cognitive Restructuring
Coping
Distress
Empathy
Eustress
Exercise
Goal Setting
Healthy Diet
Healthy Pleasure
Humor
Journal Writing
Mini-relaxation
Primary Appraisal
Relaxation Response
Secondary Appraisal
Sleep Hygiene
Social Support
Spiritual Practice
Stress
Stress Management
Stressor
Stress Warning Signals
Values Clarification

THINK About It

Learning to Swim

Once upon a time, in a land not very far away, there was a community located along the banks of a river. The citizens were distressed because so many people were drowning in the river. So, they developed ambulance speedboats, impressive resuscitation procedures, and intensive care units. Sometimes, the rescues worked, but often, they did not. Either way, their heroic medical efforts fully occupied their time, attention, and resources. Then, one day, someone asked, "Why don't these people learn to swim?"

1. How is this story similar to the way in which people manage stress today?
2. How is this story similar to the way in which the current health care system addresses stress management?

From Sobel D., & Ornstein, R. (1996) *The healthy mind, healthy body handbook.* Los Altos, CA: DRx.

Stress is an excellent paradigm for understanding the relationships among the determinants of health, the leading health indicators, and health outcomes. Stress has been shown to cause or exacerbate many of the leading health problems in the United States today, such as those related to obesity, alcohol and drug abuse, and sexually transmitted diseases (U.S. Department of Health and Human Services [USDHHS], 2000). Consequently, caring for and supporting individuals, families, and communities to help them find more effective ways to respond to stress is important for promoting health.

Stress management has been shown to be an effective intervention for health promotion, disease prevention, and symptom management. Stress-management strategies such as relaxation and imagery, self-monitoring, goal setting, cognitive restructuring, and problem solving have long been the staple of community programs, including Alcoholics Anonymous, Smoke Enders, and Weight Watchers, which help people improve quality of life by modifying health-risking behaviors. However, current data on the health of the nation point to the need for continued and expanded use of these modalities across the lifespan of Americans. Unfortunately, as the previous story points out, although the United States is good at expensive, heroic care, it is poor at low-cost preventive care, particularly stress management (Hoffman et al., 1982). Nursing's unique understanding of the human being as mind, body, and spirit and awareness of looking beyond the symptom to the multiple factors contributing to the development of that symptom, provides a valuable contribution to meeting these health care needs and the goals of *Healthy People 2010*.

Stress-management strategies are beneficial across a broad spectrum of chronological, gender, cultural, and ethnic characteristics. Men and women, young or old, from divergent socioeconomic, cultural, and ethnic backgrounds can benefit from a variety of stress-management interventions. Nurses are sensitive in teaching individuals within high-risk groups, such as immigrants, refugees, and families with few financial resources. Assessment and intervention techniques are modified to meet the special needs and values of each individual. As with all people, nurses use empathic listening, intention, and presence in helping people from diverse populations manage stress.

The goal of **stress management** is to improve quality of life by increasing healthy, effective coping, thereby reducing the unhealthy consequences of distress. This process produces a dynamic interaction of mind, body, and spirit, which affects not only physical health and well being, but also cognitive and emotional states and behavior; therefore it is an essential tool for expert nursing practice. This chapter outlines the psychophysiological aspects of stress, examines strategies shown to mediate the harmful effects, reviews clinical situations in which stress management has been shown to be effective, and explores the unique perspective nurses bring that help patents identify healthy stress-management strategies.

SOURCES OF STRESS

A **stressor** is any experience that disrupts homeostasis (Bartol & Courts, 2000; Chapman & Gavrin, 1999), thereby requiring change or adaptation. Individuals encounter a variety of physical, psychological, social, spiritual, and environmental stressors. Stressors range from physical illness, trauma, or blood loss, to activities of daily living (caring for children, meeting work deadlines, and cleaning or repairing the house), to events such as taking a critical examination, experiencing the death of a relative, losing possessions in a fire, losing a job, getting a divorce, or getting married. Stressors can be categorized as those over which people have no control (extrinsic factors), such as the weather, a traffic jam, or the death of a spouse; stressors that individuals can modify by changing their environment, social interactions, or behaviors; and stressors created or exacerbated (intrinsic factors) by poor time management, procrastination, poor communication, catastrophic negative thinking (expecting the worst), or struggling with self-defeating behaviors. Stress is part of living; it is a complex relationship between a person and the environment in which the person appraises a situation as taxing or exceeding the individual's resources and endangering the individual's well being (Lazarus & Folkman, 1984; Stuart & Wells-Federman, 2000). Appraisal or perception is an important concept because it helps explain why two people react in different ways to the same situation.

The example of Ms. Smith and Ms. Jones represents a case in point. Both individuals are about to become residents of the nursing home in their hometown. Ms. Smith perceives this move as an opportunity to increase the ease of her socializations and activities of daily living and is looking forward to making new friends and participating in new recreational activities. In contrast, Ms. Jones views this move as being abandoned by her family and fears the care will be inadequate. Although the event (moving to a nursing home) is the same for both Ms. Smith and Ms. Jones, the physiological and psychosocial consequences will not be the same because there are differences in the way in which each perceives the situation.

Stress is the negative physical, psychological, social, or spiritual effect of life's pressures and events. More correctly stated, however, the term for the negative effect of stress is ***distress.*** Canadian physiologist Dr. Hans Selye (1982) demonstrates that, to a certain extent, stress can be challenging and useful, which he identifies as ***eustress.*** Selye also observes that when stress becomes chronic or excessive, the body is unable to adapt and maintain homeostasis and thus coined the term *dis*tress. Other researchers have shown that stress is both useful and

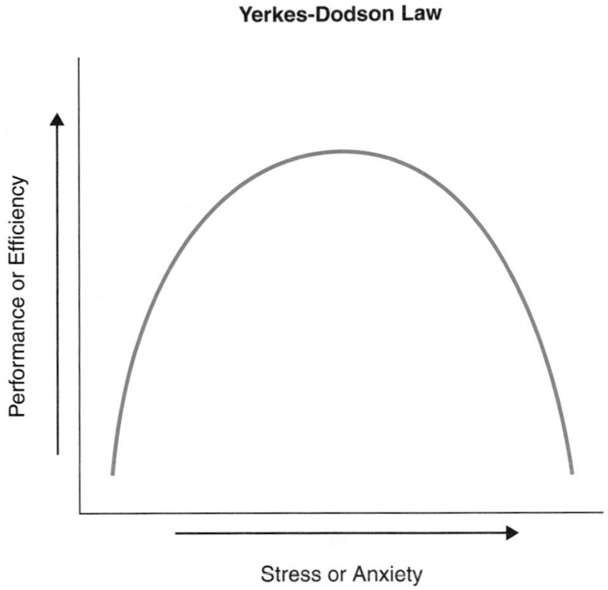

Fig. 13-1 Yerkes-Dodson law. (Adapted from Benson, H. [1987]. *Your maximum mind.* New York: Times Books).

harmful (Yerkes & Dodson, 1908). As stress or challenge increases, efficiency and performance also increase, but not endlessly. As illustrated in Fig. 13-1, at a certain point, performance and efficiency start to decrease significantly if stress continues to build. The multiple causes of stress and the negative physical, psychosocial, and spiritual consequences of distress are important to understand, which, in turn, provides the rationale for a multifaceted approach to management.

PHYSICAL, PSYCHOLOGICAL, SOCIAL-BEHAVIORAL, AND SPIRITUAL CONSEQUENCES OF STRESS

Physiological Effects of Stress

An individual's response to stress provides a model to examine changes across the biopsychosocial-spiritual domains. In response to a perceived threat (stressor), the body prepares to meet the challenge. This perception of threat (stress) stimulates a physiological pattern of neural and endocrine activation and behavioral changes mediated by the central nervous system (Fig. 13-2) (Bartol & Courts, 2000; Chapman & Gavrin, 1999; Wells-Federman et al., 1995). In most cases, this response is an adaptive, short-term, acute response to a stressor. First termed the fight-or-flight response (Cannon, 1914) and later called the stress response (Selye, 1982), the individual's reaction to stress prepares the body for emergency reaction and fosters survival in circumstances of immediate, time-limited threat. This physiological arousal proceeds along three main pathways: (1) the musculoskeletal system (MSS), (2) the autonomic nervous system (ANS), and (3) the psychoneuroendocrine system (PNE).

The MSS responds by increasing tension and tone. At the same time, the ANS, via the sympathetic branch, orchestrates a generalized arousal that includes increases in heart rate, blood pressure, and respiratory rate. Additionally, a heightened awareness of the environment is triggered, blood shifts from the visceral organs to the large muscle groups, lipid metabolism is altered (Grundy & Griffin, 1959), and platelet aggregability is increased (Malkoff, Muldoon, Zeigler, & Manuck, 1993; Shelby & McCance, 1998). Concurrently, the PNE stimulates the hypothalamic-pituitary-adrenal axis and the secretion of glucocorticoids (primarily cortisol) and other neuroendocrine substances into the systemic circulation, increasing glucose levels, influencing sodium retention, and, in the acute phase, increasing the antiinflammatory response. Eventually, however, there is a decrease in immune function (Maier & Watkins, 1998). Additionally, other hormones regulated by the PNE system, such as reproductive and growth hormones, endorphins, and enkephalins, can be affected by chronic stress (Chapman & Gavrin, 1999; Shelby & McCance, 1998).

As mentioned, in most cases, the stress response is a beneficial adaptive pattern, but it can prove maladaptive when a stressor continues indefinitely. Maladaptive stress is an enduring and sometimes self-sustaining cascade of responses that degenerate physical, psychosocial, and spiritual well being. Studies show that maladaptive stress can cause or exacerbate disease or symptoms of diseases, such as angina, cardiac arrhythmias, pain, tension headaches, insomnia, and gastrointestinal complaints. This influence is well documented in comprehensive experimental and clinical literature (Bartol & Courts, 2000; Bryla, 1996; Chapman & Gavrin, 1999; Shelby & McCance, 1998). Not surprisingly, stress has been found to influence the development of coronary heart disease in women (Arnold, 1997), to cause slow wound healing in women caregivers of relatives of dementia (Kiecolt-Glaser, 1995), and to increase the susceptibility of catching the common cold (Cohen, Tyrell, & Smith, 1991) (see Hot Topics box).

Psychological Effects of Stress

The psychological effects of stress are best illustrated by its contributory role in negative mood states, including anxiety, depression, hostility, and anger. For example, approximately 50% of all patients with severe depression show hypersecretion of cortisol (Price & Carpenter, 1997). Cortisol concentration is frequently raised in urine, plasma, and cerebrospinal fluid of patients with depression. Further investigations indicate that when a depressed individual returns to good health, cortisol secretion returns to normal (Chapman & Gavrin, 1999). These observations suggest that continual stress may cause an excessive neuroendocrine response.

At the same time, a growing body of literature documents the relationship between sustained negative mood states and increased morbidity and mortality in certain

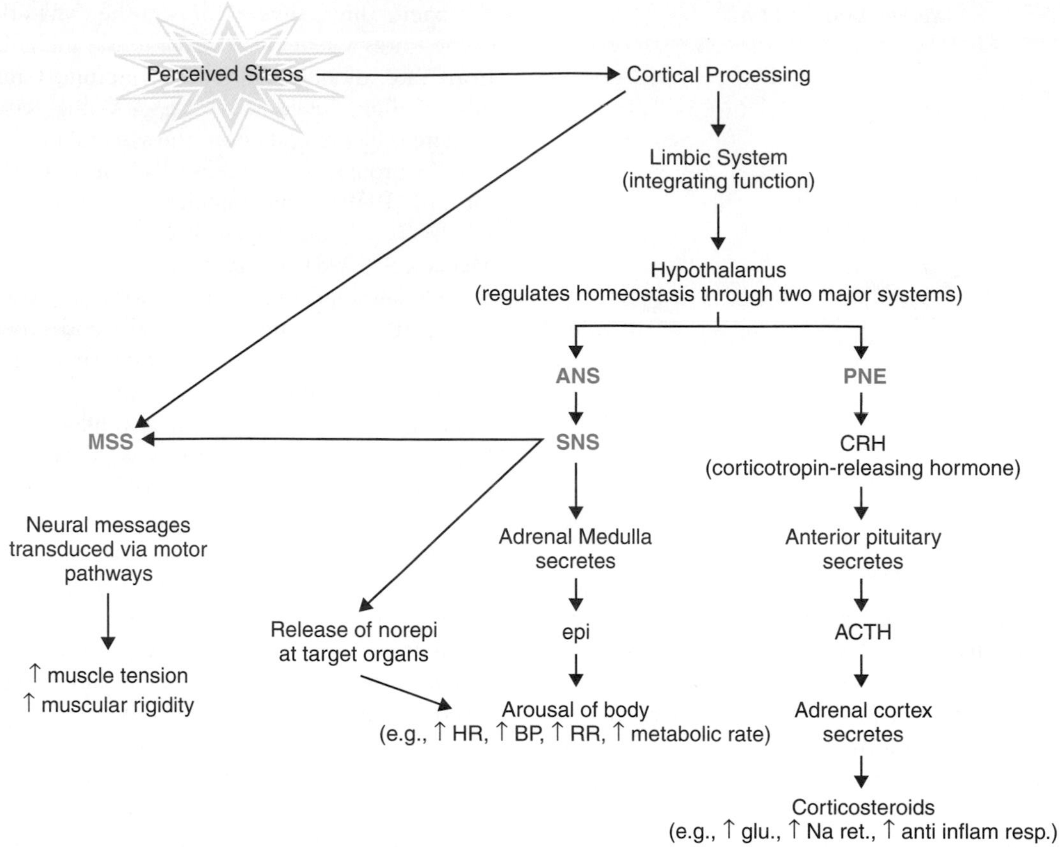

ACTH, adrenocorticotropic hormone; *ANS*, autonomic nervous sytem; *BP*, blood pressure; *epi*, epinephrine; *glu.*, blood glucose level; *HR*, heart rate; *MSS*, musculoskeletal system; *Na ret.*, sodium retention; *norepi*, norepinephrine; *PNE*, pituitary-neuroendocrine system; *RR*, respiratory rate; *SNS*, sympathetic nervous system.

Fig. 13-2 The stress response. (From Wells-Federman, Stuart, Deckro, Mandle, Baim, & Medich. [1995]. The mind/body connection: The psychophysiology of many traditional nursing interventions. *Clinical Nurse Specialist, 9,* 60.)

HOT topics

RELATIONSHIP BETWEEN STRESS AND THE DEVELOPMENT OF BREAST CANCER

Nurses appreciate the multiple factors in the development of breast cancer and other diseases. Studies exploring the relationship between stress and the development of breast cancer demonstrate a relationship among stress (personality traits, the occurrence of stressful life events, and responses to stress), the immune system, genetics, and environmental factors. The physiological influences of stress in breast cancer may be mediated by the immune system.

Although women may be unable to prevent stress in their lives, they can learn stress-management strategies. Dealing positively with stress may improve the quality of life for individuals and their families with or at risk for breast cancer.

From Bryla, C. M. (1996). Relationship between stress and the development of breast cancer: A literature review. *Oncology Nursing Forum, 23* (3), 441-448.

diseases. Frasure-Smith et al. (2000) and Lesperance, Frasure-Smith, & Talajic (1996) report that depression is associated with increased risk for morbidity and mortality from cardiovascular disease. Evidence from the longitudinal Framingham Heart Study, indicating an increased risk for hypertension related to factors such as cigarette smoking, sedentary lifestyle, and family history, also documents a relationship between anxiety and hypertension (Markovitz, Matthews, Kannel, Cobb, & D'Agostino, 1993). Researchers found that among middle aged men, anxiety levels measured 20 years earlier can predict incidence of hypertension. Additionally, Williams et al. (2000) found a relationship between increased anger and increased risk of coronary disease.

Social-Behavioral Effects of Stress

In response to stress, individuals often revert to or increase their reliance on less healthy behaviors, such as overeating, excessive use of alcohol, smoking, sedentary lifestyle (Steptoe, Wardel, Pollard, Canaan, & Davies, 1996), drug use, and an increase in violent behavior. Recognizing that these behaviors are inconsistent with the healthy behaviors needed to cope with stress is easy. This inability to control health-risking behaviors as a result of increased stress is called the *stress-disinhibition effect* (Marlatt, 1985). Health-risking behaviors such as a sedentary lifestyle, obesity, overeating high-fat foods, smoking, drug use, and social isolation have been clearly linked to morbidity and mortality (USDHHS, 2000). Exercise, healthy diet, smoking cessation, healthy weight maintenance, and social interaction have been identified as leading indicators of health in this country (USDHHS, 2000). Stress-management strategies that help break the cycle of stress-disinhibition in response to stress are important to mediate this unhealthy pattern.

Spiritual Effects of Stress

Today, the study of spirituality and health is of significant interest. In response to stress, people often feel disconnected from life's meaning and purpose, which affects spiritual health and well being. A variety of studies have examined the influence of spirituality—defined as connection with life meaning and purpose—on health (Dossey, 1996a; Kass, Friedman, Lesserman, Zuttermeister, & Benson, 1991; Larson & Milano, 1995; Levin, Larson, & Puchalski, 1997; Schlitz, 1996). Additional studies in this area are confirming that prayer can affect healing (Dossey, 1996b). Religious practices are examples of ways in which some people choose to express their spirituality. Koenig et al. (1998) report that Christians who attended religious services at least once per week and those who read the bible or pray regularly have consistently lower diastolic blood pressure readings compared with people who do not engage in spiritual activities. Research now affirms what nurses have known since the writings of Florence Nightingale (1859, 1992) over a century ago; that is, helping people use interventions that influence or restore connection with life meaning and purpose has important health-promoting benefits.

The previous paragraphs have provided information that stress can adversely affect biological activity, cognition, emotions, behavior, and spiritual well being. This understanding of the psychophysiology of the mind-body-spirit connection is fundamental to the application of stress management in nursing and provides an obvious rationale for a multifaceted approach. Further support is provided from research endorsing the health-promoting effects of managing stress.

HEALTH BENEFITS OF MANAGING STRESS

The importance of controlling stress to promote health and quality of life for people with a variety of health problems is highlighted in a continually growing body of evidence. Cancer, human immunodeficiency virus (HIV), and other immune system diseases have been shown to respond to interventions that reduce the stress response (Cruess et al., 2000; Fawzy et al., 1993; Spiegel, Bloom, Kraemer, & Gottheil, 1989). Arthritis (Keefe & Caldwell, 1997; Keefe et al., 1999; Lorig, Mazonson, & Holman, 1993), chronic pain (Caudill, Schnable, Zuttermeister, Benson, & Friedman, 1991; Morley, Eccleston, & Williams, 1999), chronic disease (Lorig et al., 1999), coronary heart disease, (Frasure-Smith & Prince, 1985, 1991; Ornish et al., 1998; Stuart et al., 1997; Toobert, Glasgow, Nettekoven, & Brown, 1998; Ulmer, 1996), and hypertension (Spence, Barnett, Linden, Ramsden, & Taenzer, 1999). Additionally, cardiac arrhythmias, insomnia, premenstrual syndrome, infertility, and the nausea and vomiting associated with chemotherapy (Benson & Stuart, 1993) have also been shown to respond to stress-management interventions.

A recent study by Mendez and Belendez (1997) found that adolescents with diabetes who attended a 12-session intervention program that involved learning a variety of stress-management skills such as relaxation exercises, self-instruction, and problem-solving strategies, showed significant changes in adherence to treatment regimen, daily hassles, skills, and frequency of glycemic analysis. Individuals with osteoarthritis of the knee who participated in a 10-week spouse-assisted coping skills training program were found to have a significantly higher level of self-efficacy for pain and tended to have lower levels of physical disability both at the end of the program and 12-months later as compared with those attending an arthritis education and support group (Keefe et al., 1999). In addition to improving health outcomes, interventions that help counter the negative effects of stress have been shown to be cost-effective (Friedman, Sobel, Myers, Caudill, & Benson, 1995). These studies are only a few of the hundreds of research projects that provide confirmation that helping individuals counter the negative effects of stress improves their health and well being and evidence of the multidirectional relationships among thoughts, feelings, beliefs, behaviors, and physiological activity.

Other research has demonstrated the benefits of developing a positive attitude and approach to coping with stress. Kobasa, Maddi, and Kahn (1982) described individuals with stress-hardy characteristics who, when exercising and accessing social support, were shown to be less vulnerable to stress-related symptoms and diseases. The characteristics of stress-hardiness are control, challenge, and commitment. For stress-hardy individuals, stress is viewed as a challenge rather than a threat; they feel in control of situations in their lives; and they are committed to rather than alienated from work, home, and family.

Recent studies continue to support the role of stress-hardy characteristics in promoting better health. Pengilly and Dowd (2000) found that hardiness moderates the relationship between stress and depression. Conversely, Kenney and Bhattacharjee (2000) found that women with medium or high stressors and low assertiveness, low hardiness, or the inability to express their feelings, are more likely to report physical symptoms compared with women who are stronger in these personality traits. Other research demonstrates the health-promoting effects of a specific clinical nursing intervention (the Wellness Program) in terms of its usefulness in fostering the development of health-related hardiness (Webster & Austin, 1999). Findings demonstrate a significant reduction in symptoms related to obsessive compulsiveness, hostility, psychoticism, and average level of distress after subjects complete this relatively short health-promotion group study.

Investigators have also found a link between better health and an optimistic explanatory style. This link was made by tracking the lives of a group of Harvard graduates from the class of 1945 (Colligan, Offord, Malinchoc, Shulman, & Seligman, 1994). Researchers discovered that by middle age, men who were pessimists in college experienced more health problems. The researchers theorize that a pessimistic explanatory style or attitude weakens the immune system through a sustained increase in sympathetic arousal in addition to negatively affecting behavior. For example, pessimists exhibit more health-risking behaviors, such as smoking, alcohol misuse, and sedentary lifestyles. More recent results (Manuta, Colligan, Malinchoc, & Offord, 2000) indicate that a pessimistic explanatory style is associated with early mortality. Recognizing the influence of explanatory style on health and well being furthers the understanding of how thoughts, feelings, behaviors, and physiological activity interact. Furthermore, nurses can identify people with high stressors and unhealthy personality traits that increase their risk for stress-related illnesses and assist them to modify these factors to enhance their health.

The previous paragraphs describe the bidirectional relationship among thoughts, feelings, behaviors, beliefs, and biological activity and offer a systematic way to understand these interactions. Evidence is presented that perceptions, or the way individuals view situations, can lead to stress and, in turn, adversely affect biological activity, emotions, behavior, and the connection with life meaning and purpose, which, in turn, increases stress and fosters a negative stress cycle. The remainder of this chapter examines the assessment of stress relating to the physical, psychosocial, and spiritual health and well being of individuals and introduces the application of a variety of strategies shown to help break the negative stress cycle and mediate its harmful effects across the biopsychosocial-spiritual domains.

ASSESSMENT

Assessment of the stress-coping abilities of an individual, family, or community is part of the comprehensive health assessment, which includes past and present subjective and objective data. The collection of this data enables the individual and nurse to determine the status of the individual's stress-coping pattern and the actual and potential strengths and weaknesses.

The nurse thoroughly collects data during the history, physical exam, and health patterns assessment (see Chapters 7, 8, and 9). Especially important is identifying the stress-coping pattern. Each individual is the primary data source; no other person can accurately explain the individual's perceptions of the stressors, stress responses, and resources to prevent or alleviate the stress.

Stress is experienced across the biopsychosocial-spiritual domains; therefore all perceptions are important parts in the assessment. Throughout the assessment process, individuals may become aware of information of which they were previously unaware or information that relates to their perceived problems. For example, a man may be aware of the stress of his job, but may be unaware that he now has high blood pressure caused by this stress.

The nurse uses effective interviewing techniques to help individuals describe their evaluations of stressful events, situations, or demands (see Chapter 5). Lazarus and Folkman (1984) have developed a theory that identifies two components of these evaluations: (1) primary and (2) secondary appraisals of the effectiveness of an individual's coping skills.

Primary appraisal of coping includes descriptions of perceived actual and potential positive and negative outcomes. Negative outcomes refer to harm, whereas positive outcomes refer to the challenges that an individual perceives can be achieved as a result of the stressors. Examples of negative outcomes are physical injury, disease, loss of a cherished relationship, position or possession, and death. Positive outcomes include graduation, promotion, and development of important relationships (see Case Study).

Following primary appraisal is **secondary appraisal,** which includes the individual's identification of available choices to cope with the actual or potential harm, threat, or challenge. The choices may be internal or external resources and responses. For example, a social resource in coping with the needs of a toddler might be learning strategies in a parent-effectiveness training course. A coping response to the challenges of parenting a toddler might be restructuring the toddler's and parent's schedules to allow for more frequent cycles of activities and rest.

The individual's primary and secondary appraisals of stress provide opportunities to consider the stress experiences in different ways. Resources may be remembered that had been forgotten or a threat may be newly viewed as a challenge and an opportunity for enhanced development and status.

By using measurement instruments with established validity and reliability, nurses can increase their accuracy of assessing an individual's stress and coping. Using these tools can help nurses distinguish between diagnoses that have many signs and symptoms in common. For example, disturbances in thinking and feeling processes are difficult to distinguish and often confound the presentation of one

CASE STUDY

Mr. John R.

Mr. John R., a 29-year-old separated man, walked into the health maintenance organization (HMO) stating he had a severe sore throat, could not eat, had not worked for a day, and was feeling "awful." He wanted to see the doctor and get a prescription for an antibiotic. The medical record revealed two episodes within the last 9 months of complaints of a sore throat, culture of organism, and antibiotic treatment. The separation from his wife occurred 1 year ago. He had not had a physical in 2 years. During the assessment interview, the nurse gathered the following information: Mr. John R. appeared tired, he presented his problem in short, terse statements, he was irritable about the clinic's slowness, and he expressed a need to get back to work. Within the last 3 weeks, he had been required to work overtime because he faced deadline penalties and his boss said that the patient's promotion, due in 2 months, depended on his performance now. The patient said that, in general, things were fine. His wife was apparently happy without him and he was too busy to care or to think about that relationship now. He made one remark about his boss, "What do you do with a nervous boss?" He described his diet as fast food "taken on the run." He obtains about 6 hours of sleep per night and awakens 1 to 2 times near morning. He has infrequent contact with his family, who lives in the area.

Reflection Exercises

1. Describe how Mr. John R.'s nurse will comprehensively assess his health.
2. Discuss several different diagnoses and possible individual, family, and community causes.

CARE PLAN

Nursing Diagnosis: Ineffective Individual Coping

DEFINING CHARACTERISTICS

The presence of the following defining characteristics indicates that the patient may be experiencing ineffective individual coping:

- Physiological disturbances
- Abuse of alcohol and/or drugs
- Participation in potentially dangerous activities
- Engaging in lifestyle with risk to health
- Impairment of social role functioning:
  - Nonproductive lifestyle
  - Lack of functioning in usual social roles
  - Nonperformance of activities of daily living
  - Inappropriate behaviors in social situations
  - Self-absorption
  - Lack of concern for or detachment from usual social supports
- Poor morale:
  - Unhappiness
  - Lack of future orientation
  - Hopelessness
  - Unacceptable quality of life
  - Pessimism
- Defensive patterns:
  - Inflexibility
  - Hypervigilance
  - Avoidance
  - Inertia
  - Refusal or rejection of help

another. These disturbances can occur separately or simultaneously in the same person. An example of this complexity is the ability to differentiate between depression and dementia. The nurse must determine whether one health problem is actually the cause of the other to develop an effective plan of care (see Care Plan).

A wide variety of tests and questionnaires are available for nurses to assess orientation, attention, cognitive skills and patterns, traits and states of emotions, and overall quality of life. Examples of instruments with widely published validity scores include Folstein's Mini Mental Status Exam, Spielberger's State and Trait Anxiety Inventory, Beck's Depression Inventory, Jalowiec Coping Scale, Pender's Lifestyle Profile, and Padilla's Quality of Life Index.

Not only do instruments promote greater accuracy in developing diagnoses and plans of care, they are also useful in evaluating the effectiveness of care. For example, a nurse may compare an individual's self-evaluation positive scores on a questionnaire before intervention with postintervention scores and revise the plan of care as needed. Additionally, nurses may analyze outcomes of a population and develop programs of research and quality improvements toward generating more effective diagnoses and process and outcome criteria, including standards of practice for stress management.

STRESS-MANAGEMENT INTERVENTIONS

Stress-management interventions are useful across a wide range of chronological, gender, cultural, and ethnic diversities. Assessment and stress-management strategies are modified to meet the needs and values of each individual. When nurses listen carefully to an individual's description of stress in the context of who the person is, with an intention to honor the individual and respect choices or sociocultural differences, the utility of stress-management interventions are less limited. Nurses are sensitive to the needs of individuals in high-risk groups, such as immigrants, refugees, and families with few financial resources. The language, belief system, and cultural distinctions of individuals guide the choice or alteration of stress-management strategies.

Developing Self-Awareness

To help individuals learn to manage stress, one of the most effective and crucial steps is to help them develop self-awareness. Self-awareness helps people learn about the relationship of mind-body-spirit, increase a sense of control, and counter self-defeating perceptions. The purpose of self-awareness interventions is to help people make sense of life events and circumstances that may be bewildering or discomforting. Many experiences in life lead to feelings of emptiness and disharmony because the person is unable to connect the experience with thoughts, feelings, actions, and physiological responses. Self-awareness helps individuals recognize stress that they create through negative, exaggerated, unrealistic thinking. This recognition affords an opportunity to change these negative thought patterns, thereby decreasing stress and increasing control. Using strategies that increase self-awareness can empower individuals to make new connections and to reframe and reinterpret their experiences in light of their own inner strengths and wisdom.

Techniques for Developing Self-Awareness

Monitoring Stress Warning Signs

The negative stress cycle can be difficult to interrupt. Recognizing the warning signs of stress is a necessary first step. Often, individuals have long ignored the **stress warning signs** (physical, emotional, or behavioral cues or reactions to a stressor) that their mind or body gives them. The man suffering from chronic intermittent backaches who ignores the daily muscle tension caused by poor posture, which precedes the backaches, provides an example. If he had attended to his early stress warning signs (poor posture and muscle tension), then he might have avoided the backache that kept him from exercising and socializing. Becoming aware of these stress warning signs is the first step. Attending to these cues is the next step. After this connection is made, developing skills to reduce negative mood states, unhealthy behaviors, and physical symptoms becomes much easier. To continue with the previous example, when the man notices muscle tension and then stops, takes a few deep breaths, corrects his posture, and gently stretches the area rather than waiting for the backache to become incapacitating before acting, it is easier to prevent a backache from becoming disabling.

Nurses teach people to identify their warning signals of stress and to stop, take a few breaths, and break the cycle. Figure 13-3 is a sample form for identifying and recording this information. These signals or cues differ from individual to individual and can be physical, emotional, behavioral, cognitive, relational, or spiritual. When asked to monitor their responses to a particular event, individuals become more consciously aware of these cues. Although this heightened awareness may initially increase an individual's consciousness of physical pain or emotional discomfort, it is a necessary first step in recognizing the negative effects of stress and the relationship of thoughts, feelings, behavior, and biological processes.

Try this: ask an individual to identify a stressful experience and the physical or emotional reaction (stress warning signals) to that particular experience. For example, after being instructed to stop, take a breath and notice the physical and emotional response to a stressful situation, one woman related the following:

> On my way to work yesterday, I sat in a huge traffic jam. I noticed that my heart was racing, my breathing had changed, and my hands were gripping the steering wheel. I felt angry and frustrated because I was going to be late for work.

Although these responses seem quite obvious, most people are unaware of the effects of stress on their mind and body. After individuals become aware of these effects, they may be able to release tension more easily, countering the negative effects of stress and increasing a sense of control.

Learning and Practicing a Relaxation Technique

Another technique to help people develop awareness and counter the negative effects of stress is learning and practicing a technique that elicits the **relaxation response.** Relaxation techniques counter the stress response by reducing sympathetic arousal (Benson, 1975; Wallace, Benson, & Wilson, 1971). The immediate physiological effects of relaxation are decreases in heart rate, blood pressure, respiratory rate, and muscle tension. The long-term physiological effect is a decrease in central nervous system arousal with a concomitant decrease in MSS, ANS, and PNE arousal (Hoffman et al., 1982). To the extent that stress causes or exacerbates a symptom, eliciting the relaxation response can break this stress-symptom cycle. In addition to these physiological changes, psychological changes such as improved mood and behavioral changes, including reduced health-risking behavior, can occur. This relaxed state of mind can also help individuals develop a spiritual perspective that can engender a shift in values and beliefs that are important to personal growth and development. A study conducted by Kass, Friedman, Lesserman, Zuttermeister, & Benson (1991) found that subjects who regularly elicit the relaxation response, regardless of method, report an increase in positive attitudes associated with spirituality. These positive attitudes correlate with an increased incidence of health-promoting behaviors and a decrease in frequency of symptoms.

The relaxation response is an innate physiological response (Benson, 1975); therefore a number of techniques that involve mental focusing can be used (Fig. 13-4). Details on these specific techniques and guidelines for clinical applications can be found in Chapter 14. All of these techniques have two basic components:

1. The repetition of a word, sound, phrase, prayer, image, or physical activity.
2. The passive disregard of everyday thoughts when they occur.

Audiotapes are recommended to help guide this process of focusing, especially in the initial learning phase.

STRESS WARNING SIGNALS

Physical Symptoms

___ Headaches
___ Indigestion
___ Stomachaches
___ Sweaty palms
___ Sleep difficulties
___ Dizziness
___ Back pain
___ Tight neck and shoulders
___ Racing heart
___ Restlessness
___ Tiredness
___ Ringing in ears

Behavioral Symptoms

___ Excess smoking
___ Bossiness
___ Compulsive gum chewing
___ Attitude critical of others
___ Grinding of teeth at night
___ Overuse of alcohol
___ Compulsive eating
___ Inability to get things done

Emotional Symptoms

___ Crying
___ Nervousness and anxiety
___ Boredom (no meaning to things)
___ Edginess (ready to explode)
___ Feeling powerless to change things
___ Overwhelming sense of pressure
___ Anger
___ Loneliness
___ Unhappiness for no reason
___ Easily upset

Cognitive Symptoms

___ Trouble thinking clearly
___ Lack of creativity
___ Memory loss
___ Forgetfulness
___ Inability to make decisions
___ Thoughts of running away
___ Constant worry
___ Loss of sense of humor

Spiritual Symptoms

___ Emptiness
___ Loss of meaning
___ Doubt
___ Unforgiving
___ Martyrdom
___ Looking for magic
___ Loss of direction
___ Cynicism
___ Apathy
___ Needing to "prove" self

Relational Symptoms

___ Isolation
___ Intolerance
___ Resentment
___ Loneliness
___ Lashing out
___ Hiding
___ Clamming up
___ Lowered sex drive
___ Nagging
___ Distrust
___ Lack of intimacy
___ Using people

Fig. 13-3 Stress warning signals. (From *Medical symptom reduction clinic patient notebook.* Division of Behavioral Medicine, Beth Israel-Deaconess Medical Center, The Mind/Body Medical Institute, Harvard Medical School, Boston, MA.)

"What Is Important and Meaningful to You in Life?"

In each of the following areas, what do you want for yourself, today, next week, a year from now?

Under each of the following categories, please ask yourself these important questions.

Professional, educational, and intellectual
Today ______
Next week ______
A year from now ______

Relationships
Today ______
Next week ______
A year from now ______

Creative things
Today ______
Next week ______
A year from now ______

Spiritual
Today ______
Next week ______
A year from now ______

Volunteer and altruistic
Today ______
Next week ______
A year from now ______

Health
Today ______
Next week ______
A year from now ______

Fun and play
Today ______
Next week ______
A year from now ______

Material objects
Today ______
Next week ______
A year from now ______

Fig. 13-4 What is important and meaningful in life? (From *Medical symptom reduction clinic patient notebook.* Division of Behavioral Medicine, Beth Israel-Deaconess Medical Center, The Mind/Body Medical Institute, Harvard Medical School, Boston, MA.)

Nurses can often introduce individuals to the immediate calming effects of the relaxation response in less than 5 minutes. One effective way is to have the person make a fist and notice what happens to the breathing pattern. Most people have a tendency to hold their breath while tensing a body part. Now ask the person to take a few deep diaphragmatic breaths while making a fist. Most people will notice that the tension is much harder to maintain while taking a deep breath. This awareness helps to recognize the relationship between breath and tension. This connection between breathing and relaxation is the principle behind the use of Lamaze techniques for helping mothers control pain during delivery.

Most people hold their breath when they perceive a threat (stress), feel anxious, or become angry. By stopping and taking a few deep breaths when they become aware of

HEALTH TEACHING Mini-Relaxation

Nurses can teach individuals to elicit a mini-relaxation through a variety of suggestions, including:

- Count slowly up to four as you inhale and slowly back down again as you exhale.
- Change your breathing to diaphragmatic breathing. Try inhaling through your nose and exhaling through your mouth. You should feel your stomach rising about 1 inch as you inhale and falling about 1 inch as you exhale.
- Take a few deep diaphragmatic breaths, and as you do so, begin to recall something that would bring a smile to your face, which might be the image of your child's face, your favorite pet, or another loved one; or it could be the memory of a favorite place, food, or event in your life.

Nurses can remind people to notice how quickly *minis* help to relieve tension and worry. People can be asked to practice often throughout the day to counter the harmful effects of arousal from the stress response.

Adapted from Hoblitzelle, O. A., & Benson, H. (1993). Eliciting the relaxation response. In H. Benson, & E. Stuart (Eds.), *The wellness book: The comprehensive guide to maintaining health and treating stress-related illness*. New York: Fireside.

physical changes (holding the breath or clenching the jaw) or emotional changes (feeling anxious or angry), individuals can elicit the relaxation response, reduce sympathetic arousal, calm negative mood states, and increase a sense of control.

Using Mini-Relaxations

Mini-relaxations can also be taught quickly and used throughout the day to help develop awareness and to counter the negative effects of stress on the mind, body, and spirit (Hoblitzelle & Benson, 1993). Individuals can be taught to monitor minor stress warning signs (jaw and shoulder tension) and to use a mini-relaxation to keep these initial symptoms of stress from developing into an incapacitating tension headache. A mini-relaxation response can be anything from a few conscious, deep diaphragmatic breaths to several minutes of sitting quietly (see Health Teaching box).

Journal Writing

Journal writing—more specifically, self-confessional writing—is useful in processing emotions and in measurably improving physical and mental health (Pennebaker, 2000). Pennebaker, Kiecolt-Glaser, & Glaser (1988) report that persons who admit their feelings to themselves and others have healthier psychological profiles and fewer illnesses compared with those who do not admit these feelings. They suggest that when individuals write about personal difficulties, they become their own researchers. Individuals may find resolutions to conflicts in a way that works uniquely for them and not for anyone else, which, in turn, increases a sense of control, mediating the negative consequences of stress.

Nurses can advise people to get a special notebook for a journal and write about a stressful event for 15 minutes a day in a setting in which they will not be interrupted. From a health perspective, people will be more effective when making themselves the only audience. The nurse should warn that the individual may feel sad or depressed immediately after the writing session, but these feelings usually dissipate within an hour. Exploring deep thoughts and feelings on paper is not a panacea. When an individual is coping with death, divorce, or some other major stressor, feeling better instantly after writing cannot be expected. A person can, however, have a clearer understanding of feelings and of the situation through journal writing. In other words, journal writing helps people objectify experiences, identify the influence of stress on symptoms, and develop insights into more effective problem solving. Some individuals may recognize the need for psychotherapeutic support through journal writing and an appropriate referral can then be made.

Healthy Diet

Countering the negative effects of stress requires caring for physical health and well being. The mind and body are connected; therefore people cannot ignore one while paying attention to the other (Wells-Federman, 1996). The body requires rest, a **healthy diet** of balanced food choices from the five food groups, and exercise. Over the last few decades, nutrition has moved to the forefront as a major component of health promotion, disease prevention, and symptom management. Food is now being viewed as having a positive influence on the individual's health, physical performance, and state of mind, not merely as providing substances, the absence of which would produce disease (Luck, 2000). Nutrition is becoming an important component of early intervention strategies to improve physical, cognitive, emotional, and social functioning.

However, the American lifestyle has made practicing healthy eating habits increasingly more difficult. Americans frequently replace nutritionally balanced meals with readily available high-fat, high-calorie foods. Many times, this course of action is an attempt to find immediate gratification to counter feelings of anxiety and depression caused by stress (stress-disinhibition). One of the frustrations that nurses experience is trying to help children and adults develop healthy eating habits. This effort, takes planning and correctly choosing a variety of foods, and choosing a diet low in fat, saturated fat, and cholesterol, with plenty of vegetables, fruits, and grain products. The current U.S. dietary guidelines presented in the Food

Guide Pyramid (U.S. Department of Agriculture [USDA], 1992) emphasize that daily food choices should be made from the five food groups. Research confirms this dietary pattern to be associated with a decreased risk of mortality (Kant, Schatzkin, Graubard, & Schairer, 2000). The pyramid is an outline of what to eat each day, not a rigid prescription, and represents a general guide that lets individuals choose a healthful diet. A detailed discussion of the health benefits of balanced nutrition and guidelines throughout the lifespan can be found in Chapter 11.

Working with individuals to help them make healthier dietary choices provides another opportunity for people to recognize that control over their health and well being is possible. This knowledge, in turn, helps counter the negative effects of stress and lower the stress-disinhibition effect that can influence poor dietary choices.

Physical Activity

Combining a healthy diet with a regular exercise routine has many health benefits and can positively affect quality of life. For example, one of the most effective ways to lose weight and improve self-esteem is to combine exercise with nutritious eating. **Exercise** (physical activity that improves strength, flexibility, and conditioning) and balanced nutrition serve as protective factors against several major chronic diseases. Regular physical activity decreases the risk of death from heart disease, lowers the risk of developing diabetes, and is associated with a decreased risk of colon cancer (Bandura, 1997; USDHHS, 2000). Exercise helps prevent high blood pressure and helps lower blood pressure in persons with elevated levels. Regular physical activity, even at moderate levels, is associated with lower death rates for adults of any age. Psychological well being is enhanced and the risk of developing depression can be reduced; regular physical activity appears to reduce symptoms of depression and anxiety and to improve mood.

Additionally, children and adolescents need weight-bearing exercise for normal skeletal development and young adults need this type of exercise to achieve and maintain peak bone mass (USDHHS, 2000). Older adults can improve and maintain strength and agility with regular physical activity (Fiatarone, 1995), which can reduce the risk of falling, helping older adults maintain an independent living status. Regular physical activity also increases the ability of people with certain chronic, disabling conditions to perform activities of daily living. Chapter 12 provides a comprehensive discussion of the benefits of exercise and clinical application throughout the lifespan.

Regular physical activity helps people adopt a more active lifestyle as they begin to feel better physically and emotionally, helping to break the negative stress cycle. These positive effects can be obtained with exercise of only moderate intensity. For example, a brisk walk of 30 to 60 minutes, 3 to 5 times a week, is sufficient to produce the fitness standard that promotes health and decreases risk of disease. Being physically active on a daily basis is extremely important; therefore nurses can help individuals increase physical activity by suggesting a variety of activities in which they might engage each day (Box 13-1). By simply changing a few daily routines, individuals can gain enormous physical, psychosocial, and spiritual rewards that promote health and break the negative stress cycle.

Box 13-1 Helping Individuals Increase Physical Activity

Nurses can suggest multiple ways individuals can increase physical activity throughout the day, including:
- Have fun and play active games with children.
- Engage in a sport.
- Find a friend with whom to walk or jog.
- Take a class in yoga or Tai Chi.
- Get and walk a dog.
- Garden on the weekends.
- Walk or bicycle to school or work.
- Take the stairs, never the elevator.
- Park the car at the farthest point in the parking lot at work, school, or when shopping.

By simply changing a few daily routines, a person can gain enormous physical, psychosocial, and spiritual rewards that promote health and break the negative stress cycle.

Sleep Hygiene

Good health and the ability to meet life's many demands and manage stress effectively require proper rest. Many people suffer from sleep deprivation that can cause or exacerbate conditions such as depression and fatigue and contribute to poor concentration and ineffective problem solving. Insomnia can be induced by stress or other cognitive-behavioral factors, such as unrealistic expectations, inappropriate scheduling of sleep, trying too hard to sleep, consuming caffeine, maintaining inadequate exercise, and a number of other factors including illness, alcohol use, or drug use. By determining the extent to which sleep disturbance is the result of behavioral or stress-related issues and by counseling people to follow several **sleep hygiene** or behavioral guidelines (keeping a sleep diary, having a regular sleep-wake cycle, and making prudent dietary changes), nurses can help individuals improve their sleep patterns (Jacobs, 1998) (Box 13-2).

Overcoming sleep disturbance cannot be done quickly. Changing these behaviors requires patience and persistence over time. Individuals will often abandon a behavioral technique when it does not produce an immediate improvement in sleep. Nurses can remind individuals that although these changes may be slower than those produced by sleep aides, these techniques are more enduring and effective (Morin, Colecchi, Stone, Sood, & Brink, 1999). Assisting people to make healthy behavior changes in their sleep habits provides another opportunity for them to

Box 13-2 Sleep Hygiene Strategies

Nurses find the following suggestions to be helpful for individuals with sleep disturbance resulting from behavioral or stress-related issues:

- Keep a sleep diary, which helps determine sleep patterns more accurately, assess progress, and reinforce effective behavior change.
- Reduce consumption of alcohol and caffeine. (Chapter 11, *Nutrition Counseling,* gives some tips.)
- Have a regular sleep-wake schedule, even on the weekends.
- If unable to fall asleep within 20 to 30 minutes or if waking up and unable to fall back to sleep within that time, get out of bed and do something until groggy and sleepy again.
- Use a relaxation tape or practice diaphragmatic breathing to help release tension and calm down.
- Limit naps during the day to less than 45 minutes. Longer naps reset the biological clock and disturb nighttime sleep.
- Exercise within 3 to 6 hours of bedtime. Exercise improves sleep by producing a significant rise in body temperature, followed by a compensatory drop a few hours later, making it easier to fall and stay asleep. Furthermore, because exercise is a physical stressor to the body, the brain compensates by increasing deep sleep.
- Take a hot bath 2 hours before bedtime. The temperature drop after the bath helps to induce sleep.
- Sleep in a cool room. Individuals grow sleepier and become less active when body temperature falls.

Adapted from Jacobs, G. D. (1998). *Say goodnight to insomnia*. New York: Henry Holt and Company, Inc.

increase self-regulation, confidence, and control, thereby reducing stress and increasing quality of life.

Cognitive Restructuring

As mentioned, many stressful situations can be created or exacerbated by negative, exaggerated, catastrophic thinking. Cognitive therapy is a conceptual model for a short-term intervention to modify this thinking and reduce stress. In the context of cognitive therapy, **cognitive restructuring** is a technique or series of strategies that help people evaluate their thoughts, challenge them, and replace them with responses that are more rational. Appraisal, or the way in which a situation is viewed, can be a major cause of stress. When situations are viewed in a negative, distorted, or illogical manner, this perception can adversely affect emotions, behaviors, beliefs, and physiological parameters. Cognitive restructuring teaches people to recognize that negative thinking often causes emotional distress. This recognition, in turn, reduces the negative consequences of stress and enhances health (Stuart & Wells-Federman, 2000).

Cognitive restructuring does not gloss over or deny misfortune, suffering, or negative feelings. Many circumstances exist in peoples' lives for which it is appropriate to feel sad, anxious, angry, or depressed. More accurately, cognitive restructuring is a technique that helps people become *unstuck* from these moods so they can experience a broader range of feelings (Wells-Federman, Stuart-Shor, & Webster, 2001).

Box 13-3 The Four-Step Approach to Cognitive Restructuring

To help individuals develop the skill of cognitive restructuring, nurses can teach them to examine a stressful situation using a four-step approach (Stuart & Wells-Federman, 2000).

1. Stop (break the cycle of escalating, negative thoughts).
2. Take a breath (elicit the relaxation response and release tension).
3. Reflect (ask, "What is going on here? What am I thinking? Is the thought true? Is the thought helpful? Am I jumping to conclusions or magnifying the situation?")
4. Choose a more realistic, rational response.

In this structured method, individuals are asked to consider their cognitive appraisal of a situation and how this assessment affects feelings, behaviors, and physiological processes. Reframing, or cognitive reappraisal, educates individuals in monitoring thoughts and replacing those that are negative and irrational with those that are more realistic and helpful.

For example, a woman may have had plans to meet a friend for lunch on a day she woke up with a migraine headache. She might begin to think such thoughts as "This always happens to me when I have plans," "This headache will never go away," "I shouldn't have to deal with this," or "My day is ruined." The result of this negative irrational self-talk is disappointment, frustration, and anger. This emotional arousal will, in turn, increase muscle tension and a variety of other stress-related symptoms, which may exacerbate the headache. To help individuals develop the skill of cognitive restructuring, nurses can teach them to examine a stressful situation using a four-step approach highlighted in Box 13-3 (Stuart & Wells-Federman, 2000).

In the previous example, the woman may reflect that "I am having a migraine headache and I hate that it is on a day that I had made plans, but I will take my medication, listen to my relaxation tapes, and rest. I'll call my friend and see if we can change our plans. Perhaps she can come over to visit me for tea this afternoon if I feel better." Although it is understandable that anyone would be disappointed and upset over this situation, applying the four-step cognitive restructuring technique can help identify healthy choices and gain a sense of control.

For a more comprehensive review of cognitive therapy and its clinical applications, the articles and books of cognitive therapists, such as Aaron Beck (1991, 2000),

David Burns (1993, 1999), Albert Ellis (1997, 1998, 1999, 2000), and Donald Meichenbaum (1993, 1999) are recommended (see Research Highlights box).

Affirmations

Affirmations can be an effective stress-management and cognitive restructuring skill because they are a method of countering self-defeating negative thoughts and attitudes (Stuart & Wells-Federman, 2000) in addition to being helpful in addressing spiritual needs. An **affirmation** is a positive thought, in the form of a short phrase or saying, which has meaning for the individual. By reinforcing new ways of thinking or behaving in the present moment, affirmations are statements that people can use to reaffirm new intentions and to increase clarity of goals.

Nurses can coach individuals to create an affirmation as a way of developing a more helpful, realistic belief system. For example, thoughts such as "I can't handle this" and "My day is ruined" can be countered with "I can handle this" and "I know ways to increase my comfort." Repeating an affirmation often throughout the day, perhaps after eliciting the relaxation response or as part of a breathing exercise, can become second nature and can help to enhance self-esteem and reduce stress.

Social Support

As illustrated by *The Goose Story* presented in Box 13-4, having supportive family, friends, and co-workers for many individuals is important to effective coping and has been shown to contribute to stress hardiness (Kobasa, 1982; Pengilly & Dowd, 2000). Many people believe that confiding in others and *talking out* problems can be a helpful way to get good advice or uncritical support (Pennebaker, 2000). **Social support,** a network of close family, friends, co-workers, and professionals, often protects against the development of dementia (Berkman, 2000; Fratiglioni, Wang, Ericsson, Maytan, & Winblad, 2000) and reduces the incidence of heart disease and other health problems. Social support literature notes that both the numbers of supports and the quality of the relationships are important (Frasure-Smith et al., 2000).

Research confirms the positive effect of social support on health outcome in medical settings. Studies by Frasure-Smith and Prince (1985, 1991) reveal that individuals receiving social support through nurses' visits after discharge following myocardial infarction have a significantly lower risk of a second event relative to persons in a control group. The authors postulate that positive changes in the emotional state of individuals in the experimental group modulate the stress response.

Emotional support during labor and delivery appears to affect positive health outcomes. Delivery by Cesarean (C-section), the most common surgical procedure performed in the United States, increases the risk of complications to mother and child and extends hospital

research highlights

Use of Cognitive-Behavioral Intervention

The purpose of this study is to test the effectiveness of a 6-week cognitive-behavioral group intervention on depressive symptoms, negative thinking, and poor self-esteem in college women at risk for depression. A randomized control trial was conducted with 92 college women (ages 18 to 24) who were randomly assigned to either the control or experimental group. Compared with the women in the control group, the women in the experimental group had a significantly greater decrease in both depressive symptoms and negative thinking and increased self-esteem at both 1 month and 6 months after intervention.

Based on data from Peden, A. R., Hall, L. A., Rayens, M. K., & Beebe, L. L. (2000). Reducing negative thinking and depressive symptoms in college women. *Journal of Nursing Scholarship, 32* (2), 145-151.

Box 13-4 The Goose Story

by Dr. Harry Clarke Hoyes

Next fall, when you see geese heading south for the winter . . . flying along in V formation . . . you might consider what science has discovered as to why they fly that way.

As each bird flaps its wings, it creates an uplift for the bird immediately following.

By flying in V formation, the whole flock adds at least 71% greater flying range than if each bird flew on its own.

People who share a common direction and sense of community can get where they are going more quickly and easily because they are traveling on the thrust of one another.

When a goose falls out of formation, it suddenly feels the drag and resistance of trying to go it alone . . . and quickly gets back into formation to take advantage of the lifting power of the bird in front.

If we have as much sense as a goose, we will stay in formation with those who are headed the same way we are.

When the head goose gets tired, it rotates back in the wing and another goose flies point.

It is sensible to take turns doing demanding jobs with people or with geese flying south.

Geese honk from behind to encourage those up front to keep up their speed.

What do we say when we honk from behind?

Finally . . . and this is important . . . when a goose gets sick or it is wounded by gunshots and falls out of formation, two other geese fall out with the goose and follow it down to lend help and protection. They stay with the fallen goose until it is able to fly or until it dies. Only then do they launch out on their own or with another formation to catch up with their group.

If we have the sense of a goose, we will stand by each other like that.

From Hoyes, H. C. (1992). The goose story. *Beginnings, 12* (7), 3.

stay (USDHHS, 2000). Researchers found that the presence of a supportive woman (Doula) during labor and delivery reduces the need for C-section, shortens labor and delivery, and reduces perinatal problems (Kennell, Klaus, McGrath, Robertson, & Hinkley, 1991; Klaus & Kennell, 1997; Klaus, Kennell, Berkowitz, & Klaus, 1992). The benefits of social support to both an individual's health and health care itself is easily apparent from this evidence.

Social support, provided in a culturally sensitive way, can affect health promotion. Researchers at the University of California School Public Health (Hodge, Fredericks, & Rodriquez, 1996) used a culturally acceptable mode of social support called Talking Circles to promote a cervical cancer screening program for Native-American women. Cervical cancer is important to Native-American women because they have high mortality and low survival rates compared with other ethnic groups (Hodge, Fredericks, & Rodriquez, 1996). This project used the Talking Circle format, coupled with traditional Native-American stories, as a vehicle to provide cancer education and improve adherence to cancer screening. Preliminary results showed that the Native-American women responded favorably to this culturally framed education project by accepting and acting on the information provided. The social support provided within the Hispanic-American culture has been shown to have a positive effect on health (see Multicultural Awareness box).

Nurses can do much to facilitate social support to promote effective coping and reduce stress. Using information available in their local community or through national organizations, nurses can suggest support groups (see Chapter 8), web site chat rooms, educational classes, and exercise facilities, to name a few. Individuals and their families are often referred to organizations such as the American Lung Association, American Heart Association, American Cancer Society, and the Arthritis Foundation for resources related to specific health-promotion needs.

MULTICULTURAL AWARENESS

Hispanic-American Paradox

For nearly 20 years, studies have demonstrated that Mexicans and Mexican Americans typically had lower socioeconomic status (SES), yet their health compared similarly with nonHispanic White individuals with a higher SES—thus the Hispanic-American Paradox.

Experts suggest the most compelling reasons for this paradox might be diet, social support, and location. Hispanic Americans eat more fruits and vegetables than do *typical* Americans. Additionally, strong social supports exist in Hispanic-American families that are more intact and there is a transplanting of the Mexican environment. These factors are easier to maintain when there is a geographical closeness to the country of origin, as there is in Los Angeles County.

As Mexican Americans become more acculturated, rates of smoking, alcohol, and illicit drug consumption tend to increase.

Adapted from Ericksen, A. B. (2000). Separate identities. *Minority Nurse*, 20-23; Hajat, A. (2000). Health outcomes among Hispanic subgroups: Data from the National Health Interview Survey 1992-1995. Vital Health and Statistics of the Centers of Disease Control and Prevention, National Center for Health Statistics.

Assertive Communication

An important stress-management skill is effective communication. Communication is an important coping and problem-solving skill that can be adversely affected by exaggerated negative thoughts and deeply held negative beliefs and assumptions (Stuart & Wells-Federman, 2000).

People who have difficulty with communication usually have one or all of the following problems (Caudill, 1995):

- Disparity between what they say (statement) and what they want (intent).
- Confusion about or resistance to stating clearly how they feel, what they want, or what they need (assertiveness). There is either a tendency to deny their own feelings (passiveness) or indifference toward the feelings of others (aggressiveness).
- Inability to listen.

The importance of matching the statement with intention is illustrated by the following example:

As David is leaving for his basketball game on a Saturday afternoon, his mother tells him, "Remember to be home early tonight." When David arrives home at 9:00 PM, his mother, who is waiting at the front door, yells, "Where were you? Is this your idea of early? You know your father and I had plans tonight. We were counting on you. You only think of yourself. This always happens. You'll never change. You'll always be irresponsible and selfish."

The first principle of effective communication is that people are clear about what they want and what they need (intent) in statements to others. Although it would be wonderful if a son, spouse, friend, or others were great mind readers, assuming that they are does little to help with communication. Nurses can help individuals match statements with intentions. This process requires that individuals recognize distorted, exaggerated thoughts and emotions and take responsibility for their part of the conversation. Communicating effectively is an art and a skill.

Reviewing the previous example, if the mother's *intention* was to have her son home before 8:00 PM, then her *statement* needs to reflect this. She should have said, "I hope you enjoy the game, but remember your father and I are going out tonight. We need to have you home before 8:00 PM to take care of your sister." It is important that the person understand that the other person in the conversation is not obligated to respond as one would wish. However, a request can be much clearer when the statement reflects the intent.

The next principle of effective communication is to be assertive (Caudill, 1995). **Assertive communication,** in most cases, is the most effective way to communicate. An assertive statement is nonjudgmental, expresses feelings and opinions, and reaffirms perceived rights. The general format of an assertive statement is: *I feel* [emotion], *when you* [the behavior] *because* [explanation].

The formula requires that all three elements be included. Cognitive restructuring facilitates assertive communication because it requires individuals to identify their thoughts and feelings. In the previous example, David's mother should:

1. Stop (break the cycle of escalating, negative thoughts).
2. Take a breath (release physical tension; promote relaxation).
3. Reflect:
   How do I feel emotionally? (Frustrated.)
   What are my automatic thoughts? ("If he cared about us, then he would have been home on time. He's always selfish and irresponsible. He's never going to change.")
4. Choose:
   A more realistic, helpful way of thinking. ("He's not always selfish and irresponsible. Even though it feels like he doesn't care about us when he does this, I know he cares.")

Becoming aware of her automatic thoughts and feelings would help David's mother plan an assertive statement when David comes home. She could then say, "I feel *frustrated* [emotion] when you *are late* [behavior] because *I expected you would be home in time to care for your sister while your father and I went out, or that you would have called if you were going to be late* [explanation]." This statement makes both her feelings clear and explains why she feels this way, which, in turn, provides a better opportunity to work on problem solving. When people cannot verbalize both their feelings and their needs, others are forced to figure out what they are. When others fail to do so correctly, individuals may feel victimized and blame the others for not understanding. Nurses help people recognize that they have a right and a responsibility to speak up and to do so in an assertive manner. The nurse can help individuals in matching their emotion with the explanation (frustration equals unmet expectation). It is important to remind them that this way of communicating may feel awkward and uncomfortable at first. Practicing this technique many times may be required before communication improves. Other people need time to become accustomed to the changes. Effective communication takes both practice and patience with everyone involved (Caudill, 1995; Stuart & Wells-Federman, 2000).

Empathy

Empathy is an effective stress-management intervention because it helps communication (Stuart & Wells-Federman, 2000). **Empathy** is the ability to take another person's perspectives into consideration and to communicate this understanding back to that person. Empathy helps individuals become better listeners.

Empathy can be facilitated through the technique of active listening. Active listening requires conscious, empathic, nonjudgmental awareness. Listening also helps clarify the issues involved and can deescalate many emotional exchanges. For example, during a situation in which a spouse announces, "I'm fed up with you always being late," the response may be important to resolving the issues without promoting further miscommunications and increasing problems. Rather than being caught by a defensive emotional reaction, individuals can learn to communicate empathetically using the four-step approach:

1. Stop (break the cycle of escalating, negative thoughts).
2. Take a breath (release physical tension; promote relaxation).
3. Reflect:
   How do I feel emotionally? (Hurt. Angry.)
   What are my automatic thoughts? ("How could [person] say that? It's not my fault. I have things to do. [Person] always accuses me. This is never going to change.")
   What are the thoughts and emotions being expressed by the other person?

The practice of asking this question will provide a different view. The individual can then begin to plan a response:

4. Choose:
   "My feelings are hurt, but I don't have to react defensively."
   "I'm going to try to understand [person's] perspective using this phrase: 'You sound ______ about ______' and listen to [person's] response."

By using this phrase, an individual can gain awareness from another person's perspective (Rogers, 1951). Continuing with the scenario, the response might be, "You sound *upset* about *my being late*." Possible responses to this empathetic statement might include, "It's not just about that. Everything went wrong today and this was just one more thing," or, "You're right. I hate having to wait. It feels like you don't respect or value my time."

By using active listening, the other person often feels *heard*. An opportunity to clarify any misunderstanding becomes available. This exercise may help reduce emotional arousal, defensive behavior, and conflict. Active listening allows the individual to *buy* time and to get a better perspective on what the other person is thinking and feeling. Individuals can then make a choice as to how they want to respond. They may choose to use assertive communication or to step away from the interaction. Active listening promotes empathic, objective, and nonjudgmental communication. Nurses can suggest that individuals use stress-management skills that include active listening techniques to facilitate effective communication, which, in turn, reduces conflict and stress (Stuart & Wells-Federman, 2000).

Healthy Pleasures

Engaging in **healthy pleasures** (activities that bring feelings of peace, joy, and happiness) is, for most individuals, an important part of life and has been known to enhance health (Ornstein & Sobel, 1989; Sobel & Ornstein, 1996). However, for individuals who are feeling overwhelmed with daily hassles, illness, or loss, this practice may have been lost. Individuals may feel that they do not deserve to have pleasure or that they are waiting for happiness until they feel better, until the stressors are resolved, or until they go away. This belief makes breaking the stress cycle even more challenging. By asking people to pursue a healthy and pleasurable activity every week, motivating them to become more involved in their lives and break this cycle is often easier. The activity can be simple and it need not cost money. For example, people often find pleasure in watching a sunset, observing birds at a feeder, calling a friend with whom they have not spoken in years, reading a favorite poem or book, or watching a funny movie (Wells-Federman, 2000). Nurses can suggest that individuals make the activity purposeful and conscious to break the stress cycle.

Spiritual Practice

In response to stress, people can feel disconnected from life's meaning and purpose, which, in turn, affects spiritual health and well being. Meeting spiritual needs may be facilitated by **spiritual practice** or activities that help people find meaning, purpose, and connection. For example, individuals may choose to elicit the relaxation response through prayer. This focused, relaxed state of mind might help individuals develop a spiritual perspective that can engender a shift in values and beliefs to help cope with a stressor they cannot change, such as chronic illness or loss of a loved one. Nurses might suggest a referral to a chaplain or clergy member, provide spiritual music or art work, recommend spiritual reading material, and provide personal presence (Taylor, Jones, & Burns, 1998) (Box 13-5).

Nurses can suggest a variety of activities that provide a sense of meaning and purpose. Keeping a *gratitude* journal can be an important strategy to help individuals focus on aspects of life that are more positive and that become clouded from view when feeling overwhelmed by stress. Finding ways of helping others (tutoring children, reading to the blind, or visiting an elderly adult) can have a positive influence on spiritual health and well being. Altruism, generosity, kindness, and service to others are more than moral virtues. These attributes not only help to make the world a better place, they also help people find meaning and purpose in life (Taylor, Jones, & Burns, 1998).

Box 13-5 A Stress-Management Strategy for Nurses

Develop the skill of personal presence. Presence is a nursing intervention described as a "... physical 'being there' and psychological 'being with' a person for the purpose of meeting the person's health care needs" (Moch & Shaefer, 1998, p.159). Presence is the gift of *self* through availability and attention to needs. To be available to others in this way, first practice the skill of being present with yourself. One effective way of developing this skill is through mindfulness, which is the ability to focus attention on what you are experiencing from moment to moment. Mindfulness encompasses the abilities of slowing down and bringing your full attention (thoughts, feelings, and bodily sensations) to the action in which you are engaged at the moment. The practice can be particularly useful in allowing yourself to extend the benefits of eliciting the relaxation response into more areas of your daily life.

Some ideas for practicing personal presence (mindfulness) are:

- When you awaken each morning, bring your full attention to your breathing. Allow your awareness to gradually expand into the room and then slowly begin to listen to the sounds of the outdoors.
- On your way to work, focus on how you walk, drive, or ride the transit. Take some deep diaphragmatic breaths and relax your body as you travel.
- Take a moment to attend to your breath, relax your body, and focus your mind before entering an individual's room.
- As you eat a meal, carefully examine it through all of your senses, the sight, smell, touch, taste and the sound of each bite. *Mindfully* enjoy this new experience.
- Recurring events of the day can become cues for a *mini-relaxation* (the ringing telephone; auscultating a heart beat; answering a call light; before, during, and after rounds or reports).
- Make the transition home from work *mindful.* Leave thoughts and worries of work at work and be conscious of your home environment each day.
- Once again, focus on your breathing and become completely aware of your surroundings as you go to sleep. Practice *mindfully* letting go of today and tomorrow as you allow your mind and body to get some much needed rest.

Adapted from Hoblitzelle, O. A., & Benson, H. (1993). Eliciting the relaxation response. In H. Benson, & E. Stuart (Eds.), *The wellness book: The comprehensive guide to maintaining health and treating stress-related illness*. New York: Fireside.

When individuals help others, their mood and sense of well being is improved, social isolation is reduced, and coping with anxiety, depression, hostility, and chronic illness becomes a little easier (Sobel & Ornstein, 1996). Elderly or chronically ill people can be encouraged to produce written or oral histories that can be a legacy. Even people who are homebound can write cards to persons needing care or make telephone calls to raise funds for a favorite charity (Taylor, Jones, & Burns, 1998).

Clarifying Values and Beliefs

To manage stress and develop a balanced lifestyle, people must recognize the things that are important to them, reflect on where they are in life, evaluate what needs to be changed, and generate an action plan for that change (Gaydos, 2000). This process is known as **values clarification.** The first step is to identify what is important, meaningful, and valuable so as to assess whether actions are consistent with beliefs. What people believe and value guide their actions by endorsing certain behaviors and changing other behaviors. When people assess their values and beliefs, they employ the ability to make their own choices rather than relying on beliefs and values dictated to them by others.

One method nurses can use to help people identify what they value and, ultimately, to help them clarify the relationship between their beliefs and actions is to ask them to identify what is important or meaningful to them. The form in Fig. 13-4 is an example of questions used in the Medical Symptom Reduction Clinic at the Division of Behavioral Medicine at the Beth-Israel Deaconess Medical Center in Boston. Individuals are asked to identify what is important and meaningful to them in eight different domains. Nurses may change the domains to reflect the values and beliefs of the individuals they are counseling more accurately. After reviewing the results, individuals may find that there are certain things that are important to them (becoming more physically active, eating a healthier diet, volunteering, or spending time with their children) that they have not been doing. When people detect inconsistencies between their values and their actual living habits, they can begin to develop a working plan for correcting these inconsistencies. This process enables individuals to make conscious choices and to have more control.

Setting Realistic Goals

Developing an action plan for change to work toward a more balanced health-promoting lifestyle that is consistent with a person's values and beliefs is an important stress-management strategy. Setting realistic, attainable goals facilitates developing this plan. **Goal setting** is a dynamic process that involves both the individual and the nurse (Stuart & Wells-Federman, 2000). Goals should be specific, concrete, measurable, and achievable. Nurses can facilitate this process by respecting the individual's input, using a values clarification exercise (such as the one mentioned) to facilitate a more complete database to guide individuals to identify and prioritize problems to be addressed, and set mutually agreed upon long- and short-term goals. Nurses should encourage individuals to challenge themselves when their behaviors are not consistent with what they identified as important and meaningful to them. For example, when an overweight man with hypertension and high cholesterol continues to smoke and eat high-fat foods, encourage him to look at these behaviors relative to what is meaningful to him, such as his family. The cost benefit is usually clear and the responsibility for the change is with the individual, not the nurse. Nurses can use the following questions to help individuals clarify long-term goals (Stuart & Wells-Federman, 2000, p. 399):

- What is most important and meaningful in your life?
- What aspects of your life would you like to change most right now?
- How can you begin the first step in that change?
- On what date would you like to achieve that goal?
- How can you reward yourself for success?
- How will your life be different when you succeed?
- How can I help?

When helping people set goals, nurses often advise using the 2 × 50 rule. The individual is asked to state the goal and then multiply the amount of time needed to accomplish the goal by 2, or reduce its difficulty by 50%. For example, losing 10 pounds in the next month is likely an unrealistic goal; losing 10 pounds in 2 months or losing 5 pounds in the next month is a more attainable goal. Setting realistic, attainable goals helps to create a sense of confidence and achievement and to build enthusiasm to set future goals. This, in turn, increases a sense of control and mediates the negative effects of stress (Stuart & Wells-Federman, 2000).

Humor

Humor is not only enjoyable and one of the best antidotes to stress, it has also been found to have significant health-promoting properties (Sobel & Ornstein, 1996; Wooten, 2000). Laughter creates predictable physiological changes in the body. Similar to other forms of exercise, the body responds in two stages: (1) an arousal phase with an increase in physiological parameters and (2) a resolution phase, during which these parameters return to resting values or lower values (Wooten, 2000). Laughter enhances immunity (Berk, 1996; Berk & Tan, 1993), raises pain threshold, improves mood, and reduces stress (Sobel & Ornstein, 1996; Wooten, 2000).

Humor can be empowering; it gives people a different perspective on their problems; and it facilitates objectivity, which increases a sense of self-protection and control in their environment. When individuals can see humor in a stressful situation, the response to the perceived threat can often be changed (Baim & LaRoche, 1993). Today, more and more hospitals are recognizing the value of humor to health promotion. Some hospitals have laughter libraries, humor rooms, comedy carts that can be wheeled into a individual's hospital room, or clowns to bring laughter and joy to the bedside. Humor is a powerful, inexpensive, stress-reduction and health-promotion strategy that can offer a valuable perspective for people on their world and on themselves (Box 13-6).

Box 13-6 Humor Strategies for Stress Reduction

Nurses help individuals use humor for health promotion and stress reduction in a variety of ways, including:

- Keeping a humor journal: look for the unintentional amusing remark, watch for funny things young children say or do, and look in the newspaper for humorous grammatical errors or an inappropriate choice of words and write them down in a journal.
- Looking on the Internet for humorous resources.
- Creating a scrapbook of humorous cartoons, pictures, stickers, poems, and songs.
- Reading a cartoon or joke in the newspaper everyday and sharing it with a friend.
- Watching funny movies or reruns of old television programs.
- Finding and spending time with funny, light-hearted people.

Box 13-7 Individualized Nursing Care Plan for Mr. John R.

Nursing Diagnosis: Ineffective Individual Coping Related to Increased Stress at Work and Limited Coping Strategies

EXPECTED OUTCOMES

Mr. John R. will:

- Report increased information on and consequences to himself of stressors experienced.
- Practice the relaxation response for 20 to 30 minutes every day through prayer and contemplation; use multiple mini-relaxations throughout each day.
- Report increasing weekly exercise or activity and healthy changes in nutrition and sleep or rest patterns.
- Develop effective coping and problem-solving abilities to manage stress beginning with the stress at work.

INTERVENTIONS

- Promote an attitude of openness to new information.
- Enroll in a cognitive behavioral group program to learn stress-management strategies and health promotion.
- Monitor daily practice of relaxation response.
- Monitor changes in exercise or activity, nutrition, and sleep or rest patterns.
- Guide patient to develop two coping strategies through cognitive-behavioral restructuring.

Adapted from McFarland, G. K., & McFarlane, E. A. (1993). *Nursing diagnosis and intervention: Planning for patient care*. St. Louis: Mosby.

EFFECTIVE COPING

When people believe that they can effectively cope, the harmful effects of stress can be minimized. The stressful situation is perceived as a challenge rather than a threat. This often-elusive difference has vital mind, body, and spirit effects. When people believe that their lives are more balanced and under control, they are productive, but not driven; aroused, but not anxious; and may even be physically or mentally tired, but not exhausted.

Effective coping is what helps people face great adversity (such as illness) and recognize the opportunity that the situation often presents (Stuart & Wells-Federman, 2000). Primarily, individuals must recognize that **coping** is the art of finding a balance, the ability to find a balance between acceptance and action, between letting go and taking control. Many stress-management strategies help individuals distinguish these differences by providing a format for observing or objectifying their experiences. Other strategies such as exercise and balanced nutrition help individuals promote physical health and well being to counter the harmful effects of stress.

Nurses can help individuals improve effective coping by guiding them in the art of choosing the right strategy at the right time. In doing so, people gain a sense of control that minimizes or buffers harmful effects of stress.

When individuals cannot control or influence the situation (extrinsic stressors), nurses can advise them to:

- *Take care of physical health and well being:* exercise, eat healthy balanced meals, and practice sleep hygiene.
- *Accept:* learn to accept the fact that some situations or people cannot be changed or avoided. Letting go of resentment and forgiveness are often a part of acceptance.
- *Use distraction:* distraction involves putting a worry aside, when necessary, until the situation can be dealt with directly. This prioritizing is quite different from procrastinating or denial because it is a necessary delay rather than avoidance.
- *Reduce emotional arousal:* practice mini-relaxations, listen to a relaxation tape, use the four-step cognitive restructuring technique, exercise, seek social support, pray, use humor and affirmations, write in a journal, and engage in a healthy pleasure.

When individuals can alter or influence the situation, or when they are contributing to or creating the stress (intrinsic stressors), nurses can advise them to:

- *Take care of physical health and well being:* exercise, eat healthy balanced meals, and practice sleep hygiene.
- *Reduce emotional arousal:* practice mini-relaxations, listen to a relaxation tape, exercise, seek social support, pray, use humor and affirmations, write in a journal, engage in a healthy pleasure, and use the four-step cognitive restructuring strategy:
  1. Stop (break the cycle of escalating, negative thoughts).
  2. Take a breath (elicit the relaxation response and release tension).
  3. Reflect (ask, "What is going on here? What am I thinking? Is the thought true? Is the thought helpful? Am I jumping to conclusions or magnifying the situation?")
  4. Choose a more realistic, rational response.

- Problem solve:
  1. Clarify values and beliefs.
  2. Gather information.
  3. Seek advice, support, assistance, or information.
  4. Use assertive communication and empathy.
  5. Set realistic goals, design action strategies, and determine the best steps to handle the problem.
  6. Take action.

See the Individualized Nursing Care Plan for Mr. John R. in Box 13-7 for an example of a plan for effective coping.

SUMMARY

Good health and the ability to effectively meet the many demands of life require managing stress. Combining careful assessment and choice of strategies, thoughtful and honest feedback, and continued support, nurses can help people cope more effectively with the innumerable stressors they encounter. Stress-management strategies provide an opportunity for individuals to acquire the necessary skills to cope more effectively and become confident in self-managing. From this awareness, the individual is able to challenge and change perception, decrease stress reactivity, increase self-management skills, and minimize the harmful consequences of stress. This process positively influences health promotion, disease prevention, and symptom management.

REFERENCES

Arnold, E. (1997). The stress connection: Women and coronary heart disease. *Critical Care Nursing Clinics of North America, 9*, 565-575.

Baim, M., & LaRoche, L. (1993). Jest 'n' joy. In H. Benson, & E. Stuart (Eds.), *The wellness book: A comprehensive guide to maintaining health and treating stress-related illness*. New York: Fireside, Simon & Schuster.

Bandura, A. (1997). Athletic functioning. *Self-efficacy: The exercise of control*. New York: W.H. Freeman and Company.

Bartol, G. M., & Courts, N. F. (2000). The psychophysiology of bodymind healing. In B. Dossey, C. Guzetta, & L. Keegan (Eds.), *Holistic nursing: A handbook for practice* (3rd ed.). Gaithersburg, MD: Aspen Publishers, Inc.

Beck A. (1991). Cognitive therapy: A 30-year retrospective. *American Psychologist*, 368-375.

Beck, A. (2000). *Prisoners of hate: The cognitive basis of anger, hostility and violence*. New York: Harper Collins Publishers.

Benson, H. (1975). *The relaxation response*. New York: William Morrow & Co.

Benson, H., & Stuart, E. (1993). *The wellness book: A comprehensive guide to maintaining health and treating stress-related illness*. New York: Fireside, Simon & Schuster.

Berk, L. (1996). The laughter-immune connection: New discoveries. *Humor and Health Journal, 5*, 1-7.

Berk, L., & Tan, S. (1993). Eustress of humor associated laughter modulates specific immune system. *Annals of Behavioral Medicine, 15*, S111.

Berkman, L. F. (2000). What influences cognitive function: Living alone or being alone? *Lancet, 355*, 1291-1292.

Bryla, C. (1996). The relationship between stress and the development of breast cancer: A literature review. *Oncology Nursing Forum, 23*, 441-448.

Burns, D. (1993). *Ten days to self-esteem: The leader's manual*. New York: William Morrow and Company, Inc.

Burns, D. (1999). *The new mood therapy: Vol. 1*. New York: William Morrow and Company, Inc.

Cannon, W. (1914). The emergency function of the adrenal medulla in pain and the major emotions. *American Journal of Physiology, 33*, 356-372.

Caudill, M. A. (1995). *Managing pain before it manages you*. New York: Guilford Press.

Caudill, M., Schnable, R., Zuttermeister, P., Benson, H., & Friedman, R. (1991). Decreased clinic use by chronic pain patients: Response to behavioral medicine intervention. *Clinical Journal of Pain, 7*, 305-310.

Chapman, C. R., & Gavrin, J. (1999). Suffering: The contributions of persistent pain. *Lancet, 353*, 2233-2236.

Cohen S., Tyrrell D., & Smith A. (1991). Psychological stress and susceptibility to the common cold. *New England Journal of Medicine, 325*, 606-612.

Colligan, R. C., Offord, K. P., Malinchoc, M., Shulman, P., & Seligman, M. E. (1994). CAVEing the MMPI for an optimism-pessimism scale: Seligman's attributional model and the assessment of explanatory style. *Journal of Clinical Psychology, 50*, 71-95.

Cruess, D., Antoni, M., Schneiderman, N., Ironson, G., McCabe, P., Fernandez, J. B., Cruess, S. E., Klimas, N., & Kumar, M. (2000). Cognitive-behavioral stress management increases free testosterone and decreases psychological distress in HIV-seropositive men. *Health Psychology, 19*, 12-20.

Dossey, L. (1996a). *Prayer is good medicine*. San Francisco: Harper.

Dossey, L. (1996b). What's love got to do with it? *Alternative Therapies in Health and Medicine, 2*, 8-15.

Ellis, A. (1997). Albert Ellis on rational emotive behavior therapy. *American Journal of Psychotherapy, 51*, 309-316.

Ellis, A. (1998). *How to control your anger before it controls you*. New York: Carol Publishing.

Ellis, A. (1999). *How to make yourself happy and remarkably less disturbable*. Lafayette, CO: Impact Publishers.

Ellis, A. (2000). A critique of the theoretical contributions of nondirective therapy. *Journal of Clinical Psychology, 56*, 897-905.

Ericksen, A. B. (2000). Separate identities. *Minority Nurse*, 20-23.

Fawzy F. I., Fawzy N. W., Hyun, C. S., Elashoff, R., Guthrie, D., Fahey, J. L., & Morton, D. L. (1993). Malignant melanoma. Effects of an early structured psychiatric intervention, coping, and affective state on recurrence and survival 6 years later. *Archives of General Psychiatry, 50*, 681-689.

Fiatarone, M. A. (1995). Fitness and function at the end of life. *Journal of the American Geriatric Society, 43*, 1439-1440.

Frasure-Smith, N., Lesperance, F., Gravel, G., Masson, A., Martin, J., Talajic, M., & Bourassa, M. G. (2000). Social support, depression, and mortality during the first year after myocardial infarction. *Circulation, 101*, 1919-1924.

Frasure-Smith, N., & Prince, R. (1985). The ischemic heart disease life stress monitoring program: Impact on mortality. *Psychosomatic Medicine, 47*, 431-445.

Frasure-Smith, N., & Prince, R. (1991). Long-term follow-up of the ischemic heart disease life stress monitoring program. *Psychosomatic Medicine, 51*, 485-512.

Fratiglioni, L., Wang, H. X., Ericsson, K., Maytan, M., & Winblad, B. (2000). Influence of social network on occurrence of dementia: A community-based longitudinal study. *Lancet, 355*, 1315-1319.

Friedman R., Sobel, D., Myers, P., Caudill, M., & Benson, H. (1995). Behavioral medicine, clinical health psychology, and cost offset. *Health Psychology, 14*, 509-518.

Gaydos, H. L. B. (2000). The art of holistic nursing and the human health experience. In B. Dossey, C. Guzetta, & L. Keegan (Eds.), *Holistic nursing: A handbook for practice* (3rd ed.). Gaithersburg, MD: Aspen Publishers, Inc.

Grundy, S., & Griffin, A. (1959). Relationship of periodic mental stress to serum lipoprotein and cholesterol levels. *Journal of the American Medical Association, 171*, 1794-1796.

Hajat, A., Lucas, J. B., Kington, R. (2000). *Advance data from vital and health statistics of the National Center for Health Statistics 310* (pp. 1-14). Washington, DC: U.S. Government Printing Office.

Hoblitzelle, O. A., & Benson, H. (1993). Eliciting the relaxation response. In H. Benson, & E. Stuart (Eds.), *The wellness book: The comprehensive guide to maintaining health and treating stress-related illness*. New York: Fireside.

Hodge, F. S., Fredericks, L., & Rodriquez, B. (1996). American Indian women's talking circle. A cervical cancer screening and prevention project. *Cancer, 78* (Suppl. 7), 1592-1597.

Hoffman J. W., Benson, H., Arns, P. A., Stainbrook, G. L., Landsberg, L., Young, J. B., & Gill, A. (1982). Reduced sympathetic nervous system responsivity associated with the relaxation response. *Science, 215*, 190-192.

Hoyes, H. C. (1992). The goose story. *Beginnings, 12*(7), 3.

Jacobs, G. D. (1998). *Say goodnight to insomnia*. New York: Henry Holt and Company, Inc.

Kant, A. K., Schatzkin, A., Graubard, B. I., & Schairer, C. (2000). A prospective study of diet quality and mortality in women. *Journal of the American Medical Association, 283*, 2109-2115.

Kass, J., Friedman, R., Lesserman, J., Zuttermeister, P. C., & Benson, H. (1991). Health outcomes and a new index of spiritual experience. *Journal for the Scientific Study of Religion, 30*, 203-211.

Keefe, F. & Caldwell, D. (1997). Cognitive behavioral control of arthritis pain. *Medical Clinics of North America, 81*, 277-290.

Keefe, J. F., Caldwell, D. S., Baucom, D., Salley, A., Robinson, E., Timmons, K., Beaupre, P., Weisberg, J., & Helms, M. (1999). Spouse-assisted coping skills training in the management of osteoarthritic pain: Long-term follow results. *Arthritis Care and Research, 12*, 101-111.

Kennell, J., Klaus, M., McGrath, S., Robertson, S., & Hinkley, C. (1991). Continuous emotional support during labor in a U.S. hospital: A randomized controlled trial. *Journal of the American Medical Association, 265*, 2197-2237.

Kenney, J. W. & Bhattacharjee, A. (2000). Interactive model of women's stressors, personality traits and health problems. *Journal of Advanced Nursing, 32*, 249-258.

Kiecolt-Glaser, J. K. (1995). Slowing of wound healing by psychological stress. *Lancet, 346*, 1194-1196.

Klaus, M. K., Kennell, J., Berkowitz, G., & Klaus, P. (1992). Maternal assistance and support in labor: Father, nurse, midwife or doula? *Clinical Consultations in Obstetrics and Gynecology, 4*, 211-217.

Klaus, M. K., & Kennell, J. H. (1997). The doula: An essential ingredient of childbirth rediscovered. *Acta Paedictrica, 10*, 1034-1036.

Kobasa, S. C., Maddi, S. R., & Kahn, S. (1982). Hardiness and health: A prospective study. *Journal of Personality and Social Psychology, 42*, 391-404.

Koenig, H. G., George, L. K., Cohen, H. J., Hays, J. C., Larson, D. B., & Blazer, D. G. (1998). The relationship between religious activity and blood pressure in older adults. *International Journal of Psychiatry in Medicine, 28*, 189-213.

Larson, D., & Milano, M. (1995). Are religion and spirituality clinically relevant in health care? *Mind/Body Medicine, 1*, 147-157.

Lazarus, R., & Folkman, S. (1984). *Stress, appraisal, and coping*. New York: Springer.

Lesperance, F., Frasure-Smith, N., & Talajic, M. (1996). Major depression before and after myocardial infarction: Its nature and consequences. *Psychosomatic Medicine, 2*, 99-110.

Levin, J. S., Larson, D. B., & Puchalski, C. M. (1997). Religion and spirituality in medicine: Research and education. *Journal of the American Medical Association, 278*, 792-793.

Lorig, K., Mazonson, P., & Holman, H. (1993). Evidence suggesting that health education for self-management in patients with chronic arthritis has sustained health benefits while reducing health care costs. *Arthritis and Rheumatism, 36*, 439-446.

Lorig, K., Sobel, D., Stewart, A., Brown, B. W., Bandura, A., Ritter, P., Gonzalez, V. M., Laurent, D. D., & Holman, H. R. (1999). Evidence suggesting that a chronic disease self-management program can improve health status while reducing hospitalization: A randomized trial. *Medical Care, 37*, 5-14.

Luck, S. (2000). Nutrition. In B. Dossey, C. Guzetta, & L. Keegan (Eds.), *Holistic nursing: A handbook for practice* (3rd ed.). Gaithersburg, MD: Aspen Publishers, Inc.

Maier, S. F., & Watkins, L. R. (1998). Cytokines for psychologists: Implications of bidirectional immune-to-brain communication for understanding behavior, mood, and cognition. *Psychological Review, 105*, 83-107.

Malkoff, S., Muldoon, M., Zeigler, Z., & Manuck, S. B. (1993). Blood platelet reactivity to acute mental stress. *Psychosomatic Medicine, 55*, 477-482.

Manuta, T., Colligan, R. C., Malinchoc, M., Offord, K. P. (2000). Optimists vs. pessimists: Survival rate among medical patients over a 30-year period. *Mayo Clinic Proceedings, 75*, 140-143.

Markovitz, J. A., Matthews, K. A., Kannel, W. B., Cobb, J. L., & D'Agostino, R. B. (1993). Psychological predictors of hypertension in the Framingham study. Is there tension in hypertension? *Journal of the American Medical Association, 270*, 2439-2443.

Marlatt, G. (1985). Relapse prevention: Theoretical rationale and overview of the model. In G. Marlatt, & J. Gordon (Eds.), *Relapse prevention*. New York: Guilford.

McFarland, G. K., & McFarlane, E. A. (1993). Planning for patient care. In G. K. McFarland, & E. A. McFarlane (Eds.), *Nursing diagnosis and intervention*. St. Louis: Mosby.

Meichenbaum, D. (1993). Changing conceptions of cognitive behavior modification: Retrospect and prospect. *Journal of Clinical Psychology, 61*, 202-204.

Meichenbaum, D. (1999). *Cognitive behavior modification: An integrative approach*. New York: Perseus Press.

Mendez, F. J., & Belendez, M. (1997). Effects of a behavioral intervention on treatment adherence and stress management in adolescents with IDDM. *Diabetes Care, 20*, 1370-1375.

Moch, S., & Shaefer, C. (1998). Presence. In M. Snyder, & R. Lindquist (Eds.), *Complementary/alternative therapies in nursing* (3rd ed.). New York: Springer.

Morin, C. M., Colecchi, C., Stone, J., Sood, R., & Brink, D. (1999). Behavioral and pharmacological therapies for late-life insomnia: A randomized controlled trial. *Journal of the American Medical Association, 281*, 1991-1999.

Morley, S., Eccleston, C., & Williams, A. (1999). Systematic review and meta-analysis of randomized controlled trials of cognitive behaviour therapy and behaviour therapy for chronic pain in adults, excluding headache. *Pain, 80*, 1-13.

Nightingale, F. (1859, 1992). *Notes on nursing: What it is and what it is not* (Commemorative edition). Philadelphia: J.B. Lippincott Company.

Ornish, D., Scherwitz, L. W., Billings, J. H., Gould, L., Merritt, T., Sparler, S., Armstrong, W. T., Ports, T. A., Kirkeeide, R. L., Hogeboom, C., & Brand, R. J. (1998). Intensive lifestyle changes for reversal of coronary heart disease. *Journal of the American Medical Association, 280*, 2001-2007.

Peden, A. R., Hall, L. A., Rayens, M. K., & Beebe, L. L. (2000). Reducing negative thinking and depressive symptoms in college women. *Journal of Nursing Scholarship, 32*, 145-151.

Pengilly, J. W., & Dowd, E. T. (2000). Hardiness and social support as moderators of stress. *Journal Clinical Psychology, 56*, 813-820.

Pennebaker, J. (2000). Telling stories: The health benefits of narrative. *Literary Medicine, 19*, 3-18.

Pennebaker, J. W., Kiecolt-Glaser, J. K., & Glaser, R. (1988). Disclosure of traumas and immune function: Health implications for psychotherapy. *Journal of Consulting and Clinical Psychology, 56*, 239-245.

Price, L. H., & Carpenter, L. L. (1997). The use of antiglucorticoids for treating depression. *Medscape Mental Health. 2*, 1-23.

Rogers, C. (1951). *Client-centered therapy*. Boston: Houghton Mifflin.

Schlitz, M. (1996). Intentionality and intuition and their clinical implications: A challenge for science and medicine. *Advances. The Journal of Mind-Body Health, 12*, 58-66.

Selye, H. (1982). History and present status of stress concept. In L. Goldberger, & S. Breznitz (Eds.), *Handbook of stress: Theoretical and clinical aspects*. New York: The Free Press.

Shelby, J., & McCance, K. L. (1998). Stress and disease. In K. L. McCance, & S. E. Heuther (Eds.), *Pathophysiology: The biologic basis for disease in adults and children*. St. Louis: Mosby.

Sobel, D., & Ornstein, R. (1996). *The healthy mind, healthy body handbook*. Los Altos, CA: DRx.

Spence, J., Barnett, P., Linden, W., Ramsden, V., & Taenzer, P. (1999). Lifestyle modifications to prevent and control hypertension. Recommendations on stress management. *Canadian Medical Association Journal, 160*, S46-S50.

Spiegel, D., Bloom, J., Kraemer, H., & Gottheil, E. (1989). Effect of psychosocial treatment on survival of patients with metastatic breast cancer. *Lancet, 2*, 888-891.

Steptoe, A., Wardel, J., Pollard. T. M., Canaan, L., & Davies, G. J. (1996). Stress, social support and health-related behavior: A study of smoking, alcohol consumption and physical exercise. *Journal of Psychosomatic Research, 41*(2), 171-180.

Stuart, E., & Wells-Federman, C. L. (2000). Cognitive therapy. In B. Dossey, C. Guzetta, & L. Keegan (Eds.), *Holistic nursing: A handbook for practice* (3rd ed.). Gaithersburg, MD: Aspen Publishers, Inc.

Stuart, E. M., Welty, F. K, Huddleston, J. S., Ennis, M. F., Goyer, L., O'Meara, M. C., Zuttermeister, P. C., Resurrection, L. A., & Friedman, R. (1997). An integrated multiple risk reduction program: Psychosocial and behavioral outcomes. *Circulation 96*, 1-191.

Taylor, E. J., Jones, P., & Burns, M. (1998). Quality of life. In I. M. Lubkin (Ed.), *Chronic illness: Impact and interventions*. Sudbury, MA: Jones and Bartlett Publishers.

Toobert, D. J., Glasgow, R. E., Nettekoven, L. A., & Brown, J. E. (1998). Behavioral and psychosocial effects of intensive lifestyle management for women with coronary heart disease. *Patient Education and Counseling, 35*, 177-188.

Ulmer, D. (1996). Stress management for the cardiovascular patient: A look at current treatment and trends. *Progress in Cardiovascular Nursing, 11*, 21-29.

U.S. Department of Agriculture. (1992). *The food guide pyramid* (Home and garden bulletin, no. 252). Washington, DC: U.S. Government Printing Office.

U.S. Department of Health and Human Services. (2000). *Healthy people 2010* [Online]. Available: health.gov/healthypeople/document/html.

Wallace, R. K., Benson, H., & Wilson, A. F. (1971). A wakeful hypometabolic physiologic state. *American Journal of Physiology, 221*, 795-799.

Webster, C., & Austin, W. (1999). Health-related hardiness and the effect of a psycho-educational group on clients' symptoms. *Journal of Psychiatric and Mental Health Nursing, 6*, 241-247.

Wells-Federman, C. (1996). Awakening the nurse healer within. *Holistic Nursing Practice, 10*, 13-29.

Wells-Federman, C. (2000). Caring for the patient in chronic pain. Part II. *Clinical Excellence for Nurse Practitioners, 4*, 4-12.

Wells-Federman, C., Stuart-Shor, E., Deckro, J., Mandle, C. L., Baim, M., & Medich, C. (1995). The mind/body connection: The psychophysiology of many traditional nursing interventions. *Clinical Nurse Specialist, 9*, 59-66.

Wells-Federman, C., Stuart-Shor, E., & Webster, A. (2001). Cognitive therapy: Applications for health promotion, disease prevention and disease management. *Nursing Clinics of North America, 36*, 93-133.

Williams, J. E., Paton, C., Siegler, I. C., Eigenbrodt, M. L., Nieto, F. J., & Tyrole, H. A. (2000). Anger proneness predicts coronary heart disease risk: Prospective analysis from the Atherosclerosis Risk in Communities (ARIC) study. *Circulation, 101*, 2034-2039.

Wooten, P. (2000). Humor, laughter, and play: Maintaining balance in a serious world. In B. Dossey, Guzetta, C., & L. Keegan (Eds.), *Holistic nursing: A handbook for practice* (3rd ed.). Gaithersburg, MD: Aspen Publishers, Inc.

Yerkes, R. M., & Dodson, J. D. (1908). The relation of strength of stimulus to rapidity of habit-formation. *Journal of Comparative Neurology and Psychology, 18*, 459-482.

Chapter 14

REGINA LOWRY

Holistic Health Strategies

objectives

After completing this chapter, the nurse will be able to:

- Define holistic health.
- Explain how holistic health care differs from conventional health care.
- Describe the philosophical base of energy medicinc.
- Describe the origin and practice of selected holistic health strategies.
- Explain the importance of self-exploration for individuals and health care professionals.

key terms

Acupuncturc
Aromatherapy
Centering
Chi (Qi)
Energy
Holism
Imagery
Meditation
Prana
Prayer
Presence
Qi Gong
Reflexology
Reiki
Subtle Energy
Tai Chi
Therapeutic Touch
Yoga

THINK About It

Can You Answer the Following Questions?

- *What makes my body feel good?*
- *What makes it hurt?*
- *What makes me feel happy, loving, and connected?*
- *What makes me angry, afraid, and sad?*
- *What thoughts make me smile and feel good?*
- *What thoughts make me frown or tense my muscles?*
- *What causes me inner peace or joy?*
- *What makes me feel that all is right with the world?*
- *What is my purpose in life?*
- *Who do I love?*

Adapted from the American Holistic Health Association. (1999). *Wellness from within: The first step* [booklet]. Anaheim, CA: The Author. Available: http://ahha.org/ahhastep.htm.

HOLISM

Too often in recent health care practice, an individual seeking care has been viewed as the sick part (the gallbladder) or the sick function (the insomniac). Consumers are dissatisfied with conventional health care and perceive that, within the conventional model, they are viewed as machines with parts and pieces. Consumers are seeking an alternative style of health care that will focus on wellness and reduce the number of medications taken (Pelletier, Astin, & Haskell, 1999). **Holism** is the theory that people have an existence other than the mere sum of their parts (Dossey, 1997). The holistic movement in the healing arts reflects the theory of holism and recognizes that people are unique, whole beings with biopsychosocial-spiritual dimensions (Dossey, 1997) and that each dimension influences the other dimensions within the human system.

Holistic practitioners believe that health is more than the absence of disease; health is optimal wellness. The individual seeking health defines health. Working toward health and wellness is an ongoing process that includes self-knowledge and self-care. When disease occurs, holistic practitioners seek to support the person's natural healing systems, to consider the whole person, and to consider the environment (both physical and mental) surrounding the person. The holistic practitioner promotes wellness, treats illness, and attempts to look beyond the symptoms to discover the cause of illness (Walter, 2000).

Many of the interventions used in holistic health care practice are backed by centuries of tradition (Thompson, 2000), but are often considered alternative practices; that is, the interventions are not taught in medical schools (Pelletier, Astin, & Haskell, 1999). This view is changing; alternative and complementary practices are moving into the mainstream. Several medical and nursing schools are adding courses on alternative therapies to their curricula. Dr. Dean Ornish's Program for Reversing Heart Disease, which incorporates diet, yoga, and meditation, is now available in eight states, and some people will qualify for Medicare payment for the program (WebMD, 2000). Alternative therapies can be used as an adjunct to conventional medical care. Rapidly increasing numbers of managed care groups, insurers, and hospitals are including holistic health practices because consumers are demanding them (Pelletier, Astin, & Haskell, 1999). Regions Hospital in St. Paul, Minnesota has recently opened a holistic nursing unit. People on the unit can receive massage, aromatherapy, music therapy, meditation, and relaxation therapy as standard nursing care (Horrigan, 2000). Movements are underway to integrate holistic practices with conventional medical practices; this effort may broaden the opportunity for holistic practitioners even further as some people who might not normally visit an alternative practitioner willingly accept a referral within the same group (Thompson, 2000).

Holistic interventions are used to promote wellness and to treat illness. Holistic practices are moving into the mainstream; therefore nurses should understand the interventions that constitute holistic practice. Nurses must be able to discuss these practices with individuals who are using them. Nurses may wish to make referrals to alternative practitioners. Nurses may also find that holistic interventions such as energy work, bodywork, aromatherapy, prayer, meditation, massage, imagery, music therapy, and the movement arts of yoga, Tai Chi, and Qi Gong provide a useful adjunct to current nursing practice.

HOLISTIC INTERVENTIONS

Energy Work

Persons are animate beings with **energy,** a life force present in all living and nonliving elements of the universe. It is the animating force that flows through the body and extends beyond the body to interact with the energy in the environment. The human energy field may be detected, assessed, and manipulated by an energy practitioner. Martha Rogers (1970, p. 92) brought the idea of energy to nursing when she stated, "The fundamental unit of the living system is an energy field." Certain types of body energy are well known. There is an electrical energy in the body as reflected by electrocardiogram (ECG) and electroencephalogram (EEG) tracings. The human energy field extends beyond the body (Krieger, 1998) and interacts with the environment (Rogers, 1970).

People can be affected by the energy of their environments, including the energy of other people. For example, anxiety is contagious and moves readily and quickly from person to person (Stuart, 1998a). There are medical uses for the energy that comes from the environment. The energy of radiation is used to shrink tumors; sound energy is used to break up kidney stones (Bates, 2000). Music, a form of sound energy, can be relaxing or stimulating. Light energy is useful in treating seasonal affective disorder (Stuart, 1998b) and cool lights increase fatigue and irritability (McKahan, 1993). Color, another form of light energy, may have an effect on emotions, behaviors, and metabolism (McKahan, 1993; Valdez & Mehrabian, 1994).

Other energies can affect healing. Many cultures believe that an energy flows through the body; this energy nourishes organs and promotes optimal functioning. The Chinese call this energy **chi** (qi), Japanese call it ki, and Hindus call it **prana.** In the West, this energy is often called **subtle energy,** life energy, or universal energy. Most of the detailed information on this energy system comes from ancient metaphysical texts and from people who have an ability to see the energy as it moves in and surrounds people. Personal experience may reveal the subtle energy in the body, as demonstrated by the exercise in Box 14-1.

Illness, stress, emotional upset, or spiritual distress can affect the flow of life energy; the flow can become blocked,

Box 14-1 Feel Your Own Energy

This exercise will help you feel your own energy, or chi.

- Sit quietly, back straight, feet touching the floor.
- Place your hands in your lap.
- Take a few deep breaths. Become quiet and still.
- Breathe slowly in and out for a few minutes.
- Slowly raise your hands in front of you, palms facing, hands about 15 inches apart. Cup your fingers as though you are holding a basketball between your hands.
- Concentrate on the space between your hands. What is there? Can you feel anything?
- Slowly bring your palms closer together, focusing on the space between your hands.
- Can you feel warmth? Does it feel spongy? Can you move your hands around a shape?
- What you are feeling is the energy coming from the energy centers in your hands. Focus on the energy. Try to increase the sensation of fullness in the space between your hands.
- If you do not feel anything right away, bring your hands back out to 15 inches apart and slowly move your hands together again. Try no more than three times each time you attempt the exercise.

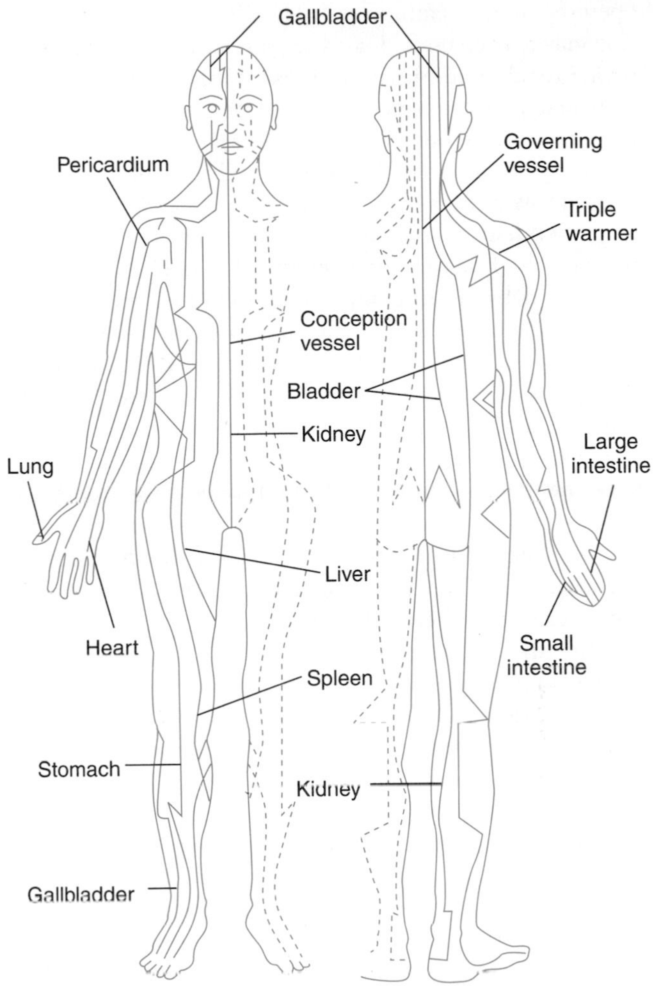

Fig. 14-1 Major body meridians. (Redrawn from Mann, F. [1974]. *The meridians for acupuncture.* London: William Heinemann Medical Books.)

unbalanced, or chaotic. These disruptions in the flow of life energy can cause or exacerbate illness in the physical body and can increase emotional and spiritual distress. The basic premise behind energy work is releasing blockages to energy flow, stimulating deficient life energy, and rebalancing life energy. Various modalities are used to release blockages and rebalance body energies.

Acupuncture, Acupressure, and Reflexology

Acupuncture

Acupuncture manipulates life energy (chi or qi) by stimulating precisely mapped points on the skin surface. The points overlie the channels, called meridians, through which chi travels (Fig. 14-1). The channels are named for the organs they affect, such as the lung meridian, heart meridian, and kidney meridian. Stimulation of the points may be accomplished by inserting fine needles into the points, by electrostimulation, by laser, and by light stimulation. The acupuncture points act as valves in the meridian system. When stimulated, the valve may open to release blocked or excess chi. The valve may close to allow chi to collect if it is deficient. Burning herbs can be used on or over the points to increase point stimulation; this technique is known as moxibustion. Acupuncture is used to diagnose disharmony; the points become tender to palpation in the presence of disturbance. By stimulating points to manipulate chi, acupuncture becomes a treatment modality. Regular acupuncture treatment promotes health by maintaining a balanced flow of chi, helping to keep body, mind, and spirit in harmony (Cohen, 1996).

Acupuncture is a useful treatment for substance abuse; the treatments may be stand alone or combined with other forms of therapy. The National Acupuncture Detoxification Association (NADA) protocol for addiction involves general stimulation of five points in each ear. Treatment goals include symptom palliation during withdrawal and a decreased urge to use the abused substance (Spencer & Jacobs, 1999). Many nurses are trained in the NADA program (Jay Renaud, NADA, personal communication, July 13, 2000). Information on training can be found at the NADA web site (http://www.acudetox.com).

Acupuncture has also been found to be an effective adjunctive treatment for the pain of fibromyalgia (Berman, Ezzo, Hadhazy, & Sawyers, 1999) and other musculoskeletal conditions (Creamer, Singh, Hochberg, & Berman, 1999). Mayer (2000), in a review of the findings of the National Institutes of Health Consensus Development Panel (NIHCDP) on acupuncture, states that the NIHCDP found acupuncture to be effective on postoperative and chemotherapy-induced nausea and vomiting and on postoperative dental pain. The NIHCDP found that acupuncture may also be useful for other pain syndromes, addiction, stroke rehabilitation, and asthma. Acupuncture education is available through many schools of Traditional Chinese Medicine and other sources; a web search of acupuncture schools provides several sources for education.

Acupressure

The meridian points may also be stimulated by hand pressure. Acupressure involves stimulation of the acupuncture points by pressing, knuckling, rubbing, squeezing, and stretching. No oil is used for acupressure and the treatments may be performed with the person fully clothed. Amma therapy and shiatsu are versions of acupressure having Japanese roots (Knaster, 1996). Education in these methods may be acquired through schools of massage. Dibble, Chapman, Mack, and Shih (2000) found that acupressure applied to a point on the inner aspect of the forearm and to a point slightly below the knee decreased the intensity and experience of nausea for the treatment group of patients receiving chemotherapy for breast cancer.

Reflexology

Reflexology is another method of moving energy by using hand pressure. Rather than acupuncture points, the reflexology practitioner applies pressure to mapped points on the feet and/or hands. Pressure is applied with the thumbs, pressing deeply into the point to release tension and stimulate circulation of blood, lymph, and energy. Reflexology is more than massage; practitioners believe that the points correspond to the organs of the body and that stimulating the points will stimulate the organs (Knaster, 1996). There are many web sites related to reflexology. The Association of Reflexologists home page (http://www.aor.org.uk) provides information on the history of reflexology and reflexology training and research.

Touch Therapies

In the touch therapies (Therapeutic Touch, Healing Touch, Reiki, pranic healing, Qi Gong healing, and Polarity Therapy, among others), practitioners use their hands to direct life energies drawn from the environment to the individual in an effort to restore balance and harmony within the human energy system. The mechanism of action for the touch therapies is, at this time, unknown. An actual exchange of physical energy may take place between practitioner and individual (Bruyere, 1994); others believe that the intent and consciousness of the practitioner is the mechanism that causes the effect of the intervention (Quinn, 1996). Still others believe that intention creates an actual exchange of subtle energy (Benor, 1999-2000). During these therapies, the hands can be placed directly on the person's body (contact) or at a distance from the body (noncontact).

Therapeutic Touch

Therapeutic Touch (TT) may be the best known of the touch therapies. TT was developed in the early 1970s by Delores Krieger, a registered nurse and professor of nursing, and her friend Dora Kunz, a lay healer. After observing Kunz and others healing by *laying on of hands* and analyzing their techniques, Krieger trained herself in the technique and began healing patients. Krieger (1979) believes that the ability to transmit universal energy is a natural ability of all humans. She taught a small group of nursing students to perform laying-on-of-hands therapy. This small group became the basis for TT and since these modest beginnings, over 48,000 health care professionals have been trained in the techniques of TT (Krieger, 1998) (see the Hot Topics box).

Three essential elements comprise TT practice. The first element is centering by the practitioner. **Centering** is a process of becoming calm, present in the moment, and connected to the individual being treated. Centering allows the practitioner to connect with the person and give the person undivided attention. The centered practitioner is able to let go of personal feelings and emotions and is more open to inner perceptions (Krieger, 1998). The practitioner remains centered throughout the treatment. During assessment, the second element, the practitioner's hands move over the individual's body at a height of about 3 inches above the skin in an attempt to sense disturbances or imbalances in the person's energy

HOT topics

HOW SHOULD ALTERNATIVE THERAPIES BE EVALUATED?

Those who use Therapeutic Touch (TT) believe strongly that TT is an effective intervention because they have seen it work. Despite an impressive body of research, TT continues to be attacked in the media by people who do not believe that scientific evidence of the effectiveness of the practice exists (Glazer, 2000). Much of the past research on TT has used methods designed to conform to current scientific methods.

Dossey (1995) points out that the double blinded, controlled clinical trial—the current gold standard of clinical research—may not work for many alternative therapies, including TT. Intentionality is involved in TT practice; a TT practitioner cannot be blinded. The standardization of treatment from one study participant to the next may not be possible when studying alternative therapies. A TT treatment is dictated by the needs of the individual and is finished when the practitioner believes that it is finished, not within a rigid time limit imposed by a study protocol. Additionally, healers may be unable to perform identically from day to day and psychological and physical changes within the healer may affect the ability to heal.

1. What standards of proof should the nurse require before adopting a clinical practice?
2. Have all (or even most) of the clinical practices commonly used by nurses today been subjected to these standards?

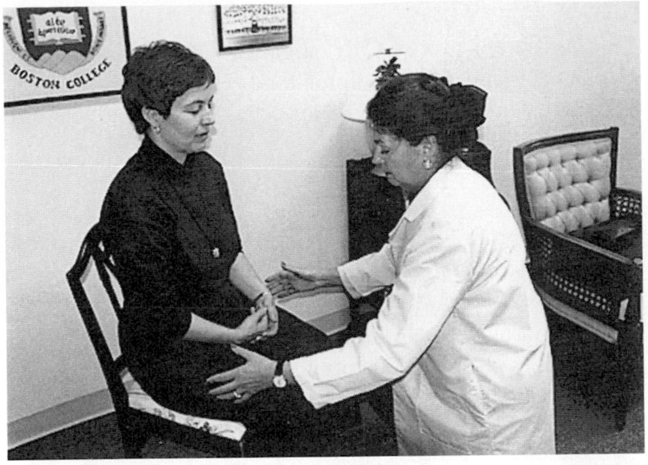

Fig. 14-2 The assessment phase of Therapeutic Touch. The practitioner is attempting to sense disturbances or imbalances in the person's energy field.

field (Fig. 14-2). Assessment is performed before treatment begins and continues throughout treatment. Both Krieger (1993) and Macrae (1999) describe the treatment techniques, the third element of TT practice. These techniques consist of methods to change the patterns in the human energy field (unruffling), to direct energy to the person to replenish depleted energy, and to balance and/or redistribute the individual's energies (modulation). The case study presents the treatment of one person using TT for neck pain.

Healing Touch

A technique known as Healing Touch is a similar modality developed by Janet Mentgen. Healing Touch adds full-body techniques for moving energy and disorder-specific energetic interventions to the modulation phase of TT (Hover-Kramer, 1996). Training in Therapeutic Touch and Healing Touch is readily available. Nurse Healers-Professional Associates (http://www.therapeutic-touch.org) and Healing Touch International (http://www.healingtouch.net) provide information on training programs.

Other Touch Therapies

Qi Gong healing, Pranic healing, and Reiki are similar modalities from the Chinese, Indian, and Japanese traditions, respectively. Yoga practitioners may offer training in Pranic healing during one-day workshops. Qi Gong healing is provided primarily by Qi Gong masters and some Traditional Chinese Medicine doctors (Cohen, 1996), but others who practice Qi Gong regularly may also use the Qi Gong energy to heal (Chuen, 1999).

Reiki healing, from the Japanese tradition, requires training by a Reiki Master. In addition to teaching the hand placements and symbolic gestures used in **Reiki,** the Reiki Master attunes the student. Attunement opens the energy channel, enabling the student to bring universal energy through the body and to the recipient (Knaster, 1996). Further information on Reiki is available at the web site for The International Center for Reiki Training (http://www.reiki.org) and at numerous other web sites.

CASE STUDY

Mr. P.

Mr. P., an 82-year-old White man, came to the clinic reporting neck pain and stiffness of approximately 4 months duration. He was previously treated with Motrin, Percocet, and physical therapy. At the time of the initial clinic visit, Mr. P. was continuing to take Motrin, but had stopped taking Percocet because the pain "isn't bad enough to take drugs [narcotics]." He rated his neck pain as 5 on a scale of 1 to 10. Neck range of motion (ROM) had improved, but still caused Mr. P. problems when driving. Mr. P. lives next to a very busy street and did not feel that he could turn his neck well enough to see the traffic coming. He was afraid to pull out into the street. His daughter drove him to the clinic. She said, "Pop is still in pain. He has little interest in doing anything. He walks like an old man and he can't work in his garden because of the pain." The goal of treatment for Mr. P. is pain relief and increased ROM.

1. What holistic health strategies might be used to relieve Mr. P.'s pain and to help him increase his ROM?
2. After the treatment goals are reached, what holistic health strategies would you recommend to assist Mr. P. in maintaining and improving his health?

Therapeutic Touch (TT) was discussed with Mr. P. Although he was skeptical of the ability of this treatment to be effective, he agreed to treatment to please his daughter. A 30-minute TT treatment was performed with special attention given to the neck and shoulder area. Immediately following the TT treatment, Mr. P. rated his pain as zero on a scale of 1 to 10 and reported that he "couldn't remember when he'd been so relaxed." Mr. P. was also given some simple yoga exercises for the neck and advised to perform the exercises twice a day, five gentle repetitions each time. Mr. P. was seen in the clinic a total of eight times for TT and increasingly more difficult yoga stretches for the neck and shoulders. His pain rating at the end of treatment remained at zero on the scale. He had stopped taking Motrin, saying, "I don't need it anymore." His neck ROM had improved and he was driving and working in his garden again. He continues his yoga stretches and has started performing daily Qi Gong exercises.

Polarity Therapy was created by Randolph Stone, DC, DO. As a combination of energy work, caring intention, movement exercises, and dietary regimens, Polarity Therapy is aimed at cleansing and health building (Burger, 1998). A web search of Polarity Therapy provides many sites for both training and treatment; the American Polarity Therapy Association has a web site (http://www.polaritytherapy.org).

Other people skilled in healing have developed healing schools and training programs. Rosalyn Bruyere and Barbara Brennan are skilled at reading auras (the extension of the energy field beyond the physical body) and the energy flow through the body (Brennan, 1987, Bruyere, 1994). The Brennan school appears to be formally structured; classes, tuition, and other information can be found on the school's web site (http://www.barbarabrennan.com). Rosalyn L. Bruyere, an ordained minister, teaches healing through a series of workshops. Reverend Bruyere also has a web site (www.rosalynlbruyere.org).

Much of the research on touch therapies has examined TT. It has been shown to be effective in treating a wide variety of conditions, including pain (Turner, Clark, Gauthier, & Williams, 1998) (see Research Highlights Box), anxiety (Olson & Sneed, 1995; Peck, 1997), promotion of a sense of well being (Giasson & Bouchard, 1998), and wound healing (Wirth, 1995). Additionally, recipients of therapeutic touch often feel *peaceful* and demonstrate physical signs of relaxation, such as deep sighs, slowed breathing, and drooping shoulders (Heidt, 1990).

Energy healing takes place in many cultures. There are also other types of healing and healers. Shamanism, which arose from the Native-American tradition, is moving into other cultures. As the population of Mexican Americans increases in the United States, the curandero (healer) of Mexico and South-American culture is becoming more familiar. Faith healers are associated with many different religions. The trance surgeons of Brazil are discussed in the Multicultural Awareness Box.

research highlights

Use of Therapeutic Touch for Pain

The pain for patients hospitalized with burns is severe. Burn healing is a slow process that often involves débridement and many painful procedures. Pain and anxiety are frequent companions of the patient hospitalized with burns. Turner, Clark, Gauthier, and Williams (1998) hypothesized that Therapeutic Touch (TT) can help these patients by reducing pain and anxiety.

The study enrolled 99 subjects between 15 and 68 years of age. Subjects were randomly assigned to two groups: (1) one group received five TT treatments from TT practitioners trained in the Krieger-Kunz method; (2) the second group received five sham, or mimic, TT treatments from research assistants (RAs) who were not trained in TT and who did not assess or attempt to manipulate the subject's energy field. Rather than performing TT, the RAs made random, mimic TT movements as they counted backwards from 100.

On day one, baseline data were collected and the first treatment was given. Assessment measures were repeated on day three (pain) and day six (pain and anxiety) following the final treatment. Although no statistically significant difference in the amount of analgesic medication taken per 24 hours between the two groups was demonstrated, the TT group produced a significantly lower pain score compared with the group receiving the sham treatment for three of the indicators on the McGill Pain Questionnaire. The TT group also reported significantly less anxiety after 5 days of therapy.

Data from Turner, J. G., Clark, A. J., Gauthier, D. K., & Williams, M. (1998). The effect of therapeutic touch on pain and anxiety in burn patients. *Journal of Advanced Nursing, 28* (1), 10-20.

Movement Arts

The movement arts of Qi Gong, Tai Chi, and Yoga have also been found to be helpful for body, mind, and spirit. Similar to energy work practices, the movement arts also manipulate life energies.

Qi Gong

Qi Gong (pronounced chee gung), a part of Traditional Chinese Medicine, combines relaxed movements with a meditative aspect and controlled breathing to move Qi energy through the energy channels. The goal of this technique is to balance, smooth, and strengthen the individual's own Qi energy. Many books and videos explain Qi

MULTICULTURAL AWARENESS

Trance Surgery

Two field workers visited Brazil to observe and document the work of healer-mediums who perform surgery while in a state of possession trance (Don & Moura, 2000). The healer-mediums believe that during the surgical procedures, the spirit of an intelligent entity possesses their bodies for its own medical purpose. The first trance surgeon was possessed by Dr. Fritz, a German physician killed during World War I, and began his practice in 1950. He performed surgery and wrote prescriptions under trance until his death in 1971. Since his death, several other mediums have begun to practice trance surgery. Although some mediums are controversial, others have been accepted as being truly possessed by Dr. Fritz, other surgeon spirits, or the spirits of saints.

Don and Moura observed the practice of nine healer-mediums as they treated several thousand patients. Most of the trance surgeons actually cut or pierced the body of the patient and many of the incisions were deep; three incisions entered the peritoneal cavity. Only one of the trance surgeons had formal medical training. Antonio, a former laborer whose education ended after the first grade, practices as Dr. Ricardo. Don and Moura, accompanied by a Brazilian orthopedic surgeon, watched Dr. Ricardo work on 35 patients in a 3-hour period. They report:

> There was no major anesthesia or sterile procedure, and the same tray of instruments was used on all patients. Patients showed no evidence of pain, bleeding was minimal, and no patients went into shock . . . . Major blood vessels were not sutured, although we observed spurting of arterial blood during some procedures . . . . Within 1 hour, all patients were ambulatory; some patients who had been cut deeply were strolling on the town streets . . . . The patients often claim to have been healed (Don & Moura, 2000, pp. 41, 44).

In addition to surgical procedures, Don and Moura report that one healer-medium injected a mixture of alcohol, iodine, and turpentine into both muscles and veins. They witnessed "hundreds of such injections" (p. 41) with no apparent ill effects.

Don and Moura witnessed events that, according to the beliefs of Western medicine, should be impossible. They describe trance surgery as "culturally bounded" (p. 47). Large numbers of Brazilians believe in the reality of spirit possession. It is possible that these witnessed events would not be possible any place other than Brazil.

Gong practice. Qi Gong exercises can be performed by all age groups and all body types, regardless of their state of health (Chuen, 1999). The exercises may be gentle or aerobic (Cohen, 1996). In a randomized, placebo-controlled, clinical trial designed to examine the effect of Qi Gong exercises on pain and anxiety, Wu et al. (1999) found a significant decrease in pain during exercise among participants in the Qi Gong group and a significant decrease in anxiety between sessions.

Tai Chi

Tai Chi (pronounced tie chee) began as a Chinese martial art. Tai Chi combines physical movement, breath control, and meditation in a dancelike sequence of poses based on the movements of animals. One pose flows into the next in a slow, relaxed, gentle, unbroken rhythm. The slowness of movement and focus on breathing brings an awareness of the moment-to-moment state of the body and produces a meditative state. The sequence of poses is called a form; there are both short forms (13 to 18 poses) and long forms. Similar to Qi Gong, the poses and the breathing manipulate and balance chi (Shaller, 1998).

Yoga

Yoga, from the Hindu tradition, originated as a form of spiritual practice. The word yoga means union and the system of **yoga** teaches the methods by which the individual can be joined to the Supreme Being and achieve liberation (Iyengar, 1979). Box 14-2 names and defines these paths to liberation.

The most physical practice, hatha yoga, is most familiar to the Western culture, but ideally, an individual's personal practice of yoga includes all methods. Well-known yoga teacher B. K. S. Iyengar (1979, p. 57) states that without the spiritual aspects of practice, yoga practice of the postures is "mere acrobatics." Iyengar (1979, p. 40-41) defines health as "a state of complete equilibrium of body, mind, and spirit" and states:

> Asanas [the postures or poses of hatha yoga] have been evolved over the centuries so as to exercise every muscle, nerve, and gland in the body. They secure a fine physique, which is strong and elastic without being muscle-bound, and they keep the body free from disease. They reduce fatigue and soothe the nerves. But their real importance lies in the way they train and discipline the mind . . . . The yogi [one who practices yoga] conquers the body by the practice of asanas and makes it a fit vehicle for the spirit.

Box 14-2 The Paths to Union Through Yoga

- Karma yoga: the yoga of right action and good works.
- Bhakti yoga: the yoga of devotional practices.
- Raja yoga: the yoga of meditative practices.
- Jnana yoga: the yoga of the study of spiritual texts.
- Hatha yoga: the yoga of physical practice of various postures called asanas and breath control.
- Mantra yoga: the yoga of repetition of a sacred phrase.
- Laya yoga: the yoga of blending self with the Supreme.

From Sri Swami Sivananda. (1994). Practice of yoga (7th ed.). Himalayas, India: The Divine Life Society.

Yoga asanas often have evocative, descriptive names, such as proud warrior, waterfall, runner's pose, downward-facing dog, mountain pose, and eagle pose. Other asana names are simple descriptions of what the body is doing during the posture, such as standing forward bend and spinal twist. Some of the poses are restful and restorative; some require strength and flexibility, which come with regular practice. Asana practice is a process of effortless effort that often involves a letting go and relaxing into the pose rather than forcing the body into the pose. Asana practice should be noncompetitive. The practice should not be about how the person looks in the pose, but rather, about how the person feels in the pose from the inside out. During asana practice, the breath should flow easily in and out through the nostrils. The body should be active, but the mind should be restful and watching, a witness to your actions. The energies of the body should extend equally through all the limbs and in all directions. Relaxation pose should follow the active asanas to allow incorporation of the work that has been done. (Teri Landers [yoga teacher], personal communication, May 2000).

Hatha yoga also includes breathing exercises known as pranayama. Prana means "breath, respiration, life, vitality, wind, energy, or strength. It also connotes the soul as opposed to the body . . . Ayama means length, expansion, stretching, and restraint" (Iyengar, 1979, p. 43). Control of the breath helps the yogi to control the mind and keep the mind focused on the present moment and/or the Supreme Being. Breathing control also helps move the subtle energy (prana) through channels in the body (nadis) to nourish the body organs and the spirit (Iyengar, 1979). Yoga is an integral part of Dr. Dean Ornish's Program for Reversing Heart Disease (Ornish, 1990). Although there has been little research on yoga in the United States, Ornish states that many well-researched techniques are derived from yoga, including various relaxation techniques, meditation and imagery practice, Lamaze breathing techniques, physical therapy stretches, and athletic stretches (Ornish, 1990). One U.S. study (Garfinkel et al., 1998) found that individuals with carpal tunnel syndrome had significant decreases in pain and increases in grip strength after participating in yoga intervention. The intervention was 11 yoga postures in the Iyengar style designed to strengthen, stretch, and balance the joints in the upper body. Relaxation was included. The intervention was provided 2 times per week for 8 weeks.

Self-instructional videos in the movement arts are available from many sources; however, a well-trained teacher can help refine practice. Qi Gong, Tai Chi, and Yoga classes are available at many fitness centers and community settings. There are different styles of practice within each discipline; therefore experience with different teachers might be necessary to find a teacher whose practice corresponds with the needs of the student.

Meditation

Kreitzer (1998, p. 123) defines **meditation** as a "self-directed practice for relaxing the body and calming the mind." A part of the religious life of many cultures, meditation has become prevalent in the West as a tool to increase physical and mental well being. Sri Swami Sivananda (1994, p. 67) describes the mind as a "mischievous monkey" that jumps from topic to topic causing troubles. He believes that the mind can be controlled through meditation. Generally, meditation involves the focusing of concentration on a single point. When the mind wanders, the individual consciously brings the mind back to the point of concentration. The focus of concentration can be a burning candle, a word, a phrase, the breath, or simply a quiet awareness of what is happening in the present moment. Meditation can be practiced while sitting, walking, or moving.

There are many techniques for meditating. One of the best known is Transcendental Meditation (TM). There are an estimated 2 million TM practitioners in the United States. The Indian spiritual leader Maharishi Mahesh Yogi brought TM to the United States in the 1960s. The TM technique is repetition of a mantra (a word, sound, or phrase). Practitioners repeat the mantra silently over and over again (for 20 minutes, morning and evening). When other thoughts arise during mantra repetition, the practitioner should notice the thought, let the thought go, and return to the mantra. Centering prayer is similar to TM; practitioners are encouraged to focus on a sacred word from the Christian tradition (Kreitzer, 1998).

Mindfulness meditation is a way of paying attention; the point of focus varies. The individual can choose to focus on thoughts, on actions, or on the activity in the environment. Jon Kabat-Zinn (1990, p. 28) believes that "knowing what you are doing while you are doing it is the essence of mindfulness practice." As an introduction of mindfulness meditation in his stress-reduction clinic, Kabat-Zinn asks people to eat three raisins, one at a time. He describes the process of eating a raisin:

> First we bring our attention to seeing the raisin, observing it carefully as if we had never seen one before. We feel its texture between our fingers and notice its colors and surfaces. We are also aware of any thoughts we might be having about raisins or food in general. We note any thoughts and feelings of liking or disliking raisins if they come up while we are looking at it. We then smell it for a while and finally, with awareness, we bring it to our lips, being aware of the arm moving the hand to position it correctly and of salivating as the mind and body anticipate eating. The process continues as we take it into our mouth and chew it slowly, experiencing the actual taste of one raisin. And when we feel ready to swallow, we watch the impulse to swallow as it comes up, so that even that is experienced consciously. We even imagine, or "sense," that now our bodies are one raisin heavier (p. 27-28).

Walking meditation is another form of mindfulness practice; with each step, the person is aware of the movements of the body that make the step possible and of both the external environment and the internal environment. Hanh (as cited in Anselmo & Kolkmeier, 2000, p. 507) believes that the true sense of walking meditation is gained when walking "as if one were planting peace with each step."

One of the simplest methods of meditation is concentration on breathing. With breath meditation, there is no need for a special room, a special mat, or a cushion. The breath is an ever-present tool. Breath meditation can evoke the relaxation response (Anselmo & Kolkmeier, 2000). This technique can be easily taught (see the Health Teaching box) and is useful for anyone who is having a bad day or who wants to be more present with another.

Meditation is an important part of Dr. Dean Ornish's Program for Reversing Heart Disease (Ornish, 1990). The web site for Transcendental Meditation (http://www.tm.org) states that over 500 studies have been completed on TM. Zamarra, Schneider, Besseghini, Robinson, and Salerno (1996) found that TM practice significantly increased exercise tolerance and maximal workload and

HEALTH TEACHING Teaching the Technique of Breath Meditation

- You may stand, sit, or lie quietly as you begin to focus on your breath.
- Inhale and feel the air come into your nostrils, move down your throat, and into your lungs. Do not try to control the breath. Just observe it.

Exhale and feel the air move up from your lungs and into your throat. Feel the warmth of the exhaled air in your nostrils

- Breathe. Feeling the air move in and out. Concentrate on the breath. Do not try to control the breath. Just observe it.
- Continue watching the breath for 5 to 10 minutes. As other thoughts come into focus, notice them and let them go. Focus again on the breath.

As you become comfortable with breath meditation, you may easily add simple imagery to this technique.

- As you inhale, imagine breathing in peace or love or wellness.
- As you exhale, imagine breathing out pain or sorrow or grief.
- As you inhale, breathe in whatever it is that you need.
- As you exhale, breathe out whatever you wish to be free of in your life.

delays the onset of ST-segment depression in people with chronic stable angina using a bicycle ergometer. Wenneberg et al. (1997) found that subjects who practiced TM as recommended show significantly lower ambulatory blood pressures. Smith, Compton, and West (1995) found that a concentration meditation focusing on *peace* increased happiness for people who practiced the meditation more than 3 times a week. Astin (1997) found that an 8-week stress reduction program based on mindfulness meditation produced a significant reduction in psychological symptoms and significant increases in participants' sense of control and spiritual experiences.

Prayer and Distant Healing

Prayer

In the United States, at least 90% of people pray (Walker, Tonigan, Miller, Comer, & Kahlich, 1997). Prayer is one of the oldest forms of therapy (Byrd, 1997; Harris, 1999). People pray for themselves and they pray for others. **Prayer** has different meanings to different people; a prayer may be a request for Divine intervention, a type of meditation (centering prayer), or a form of intentionality that is useful in healing. Prayer is the basis for Christian Science healing practices. Harris (2000) believes prayer facilitates healing by causing changes in consciousness that help individuals recognize their innate wholeness. Recent research on the effect of prayer on health has shown varied outcomes.

Byrd (1997) studied the therapeutic effects of prayer by others (intercessory prayer) on 393 patients in a coronary care unit. The patients were randomly assigned to a prayer group and a control group; patients, staff, and doctors were blinded during the study. People in the prayer group had prayers for rapid recovery and prevention of complications offered on their behalf by 3 to 7 people daily. There was a significant difference between the two groups in several areas. Fewer patients in the prayer group required intubation and/or ventilation, antibiotics, and diuretics. Fewer patients in the prayer group developed congestive heart failure, went into arrest, and developed pneumonia. Severity scores showed that the prayer group had significantly better outcomes. Harris et al. (1999) replicated the Byrd study with 900 patients in a coronary care unit and found similar results.

Walker, Tonigan, Miller, Comer, and Kahlich (1997) examined the effects of intercessory prayer on 40 individuals undergoing treatment for alcohol abuse and found that treatment outcomes were not improved with intercessory prayer. One explanation for this finding is that the subjects may have been less active in their own recovery because they placed their reliance on the efforts of others on their behalf. They found, however, that the subjects who prayed for themselves appeared significantly better early in the study. Meisenhelder and Chandler (2000) examined prayer and health outcomes among 1025 church members. People who prayed most frequently had poorer physical health and were older, yet they experienced better mental health compared with those who prayed less frequently.

innovative practice

The Expanded Care for Healthy Outcomes Model

Since September 1998, the Expanded Care for Healthy Outcomes (ECHO) model project has prepared nurse practitioner students at the Boston College School of Nursing (BCSON) to assess spiritual needs of their patients as part of their overall primary care management. Funded by the Helene Fuld Trust Fund and Teagle Foundation, the ECHO project is a cooperative effort between BCSON and the Pine Street Inn Nurses Clinic, the nation's largest nurse-managed center caring for a homeless population. Four nurse practitioners, one minister, and the nurse practitioner faculty supervise graduate students on site in a transitional shelter clinic for homeless men in recovery from substance addiction.

Before clinical practice, students learn and practice spiritual assessment and receive additional didactic content on spirituality. Students and faculty also participate in monthly seminars to discuss their own spiritual beliefs and values and their clinical experiences with spiritual assessment.

Much of the role of spiritual assessment in primary care is spending the necessary time to develop relationships with patients. The ECHO project emphasizes the holistic dimension of nursing often lost in the push for managed care. Nurse practitioners are particularly vulnerable to the time-management approach of today's primary care marketplace. Helping future nurse practitioner graduates appreciate the role of spirituality in individual's overall health is an important ingredient in understanding the mind, body, and spirit of their patients.

Anecdotally, the ECHO project has been a great success among the 23 students who have been involved with faculty and the hundreds of homeless clinic patients. Nurse practitioners now in clinical practice report that they are transferring the skills learned in the classroom and the supervised clinical placement into other clinical areas. Patients seek out the nurse practitioners and minister regularly and are able to establish more trusting relationships.

As the ECHO project enters its third year of operation, the faculty is beginning to measure the outcomes of spiritual care in the clinic population at Pine Street Inn, specifically, as it relates to rates of relapse and health utilization. Although spiritual care is not limited to homeless populations or individuals in recovery, it has great promise for helping these vulnerable people achieve healthier outcome.

Courtesy Barbara L. Brush, PhD, RN, NP, FAAN, Family Nurse Practitioner Program, Community Health Department, School of Nursing, Boston College, Boston, Massachusetts.

Distant Healing

Praying for others may be a form of distant healing (Targ, 1999); many who practice energy work believe that their efforts are effective over long distances. In two triple-blind studies reported by Targ (1999), people with the human immunodeficiency virus (HIV) were randomly divided into two groups. The exploratory, pilot study contained 20 participants; the second study evaluated 40 participants. Experienced healers were recruited from several traditions and educational backgrounds. The healers included medical doctors, nurses, psychologists, ministers, a Chi-Gong master, a Native-American shaman, and a healer with no formal education who practiced Chinese healing. The healers described their healing practices as energetic (50%), meditative or contemplative (25%), devotional or religious (15%), and shamanic (10%). The healing techniques that were used varied widely.

Each person in the treatment group received healing treatments from one healer at a time, 1 hour per day, 6 days per week, for 10 weeks. A new healer treated the person each week. The participants were followed for 6 months. Although there were no significant differences in the CD4 counts between groups, the treatment group had significantly fewer new diseases, fewer hospitalizations, and lower illness severity scores. This group also demonstrated significant decreases in depression, anxiety, and anger, in addition to significant increases in vigor.

A review of 23 studies involving distant healing and using randomized trials (Astin, Harkness, & Ernst, 2000) concludes that 13 studies (57%) had statistically significant treatment effects, nine studies showed no effect over control interventions, and one study showed a negative effect. Studies involving Therapeutic Touch, prayer, mental healing, and spiritual healing were included.

One method of participating in distance healing is the healing circle (Fig. 14-3). The members of the healing circle join hands. Each member sends healing energy to his or her neighbor on the right until the energy is flowing around the circle. When the energy is flowing readily, each member of the group focuses the energy on one group member who acts to send the energy to someone they know in need of healing. Each member of the circle may, in turn, receive energy from the group and send it to an individual in need of healing.

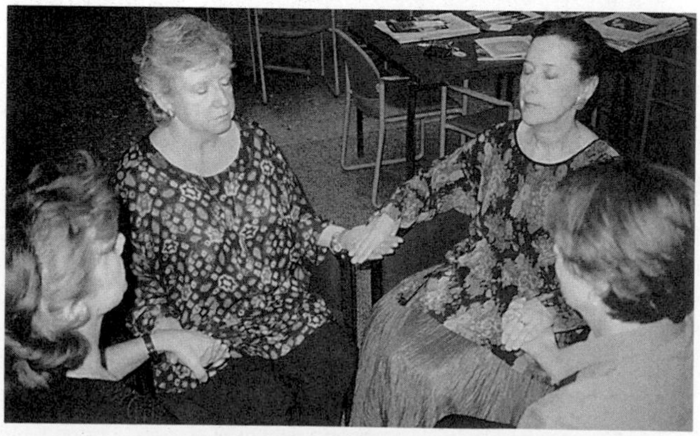

Fig. 14-3 A healing circle.

Guided Imagery

The physical body may react to sensory images in the mind the same way it responds to the real thing (Naparstek, 1994). To illustrate this point, Naparstek uses the example of a woman whose first dose of chemotherapy caused extreme nausea. Traveling to the clinic for the second dose, the individual remembered the experience and formed an image in her mind of the experience. She became nauseated and began to vomit. Serious illness often brings fears of death or disability with it; people imagine the worst and anxiety increases. These examples demonstrate the negative effects of imagination.

Imagination can have a positive influence on health. Imagery can be used to promote a sense of well being and to help cope with stress, diseases, or pain (Schaub & Dossey, 2000). Jeanne Achterberg (1999, p. 77) states, "If the stories in the mind change, thoughts change, emotions change, and the body changes—it's as simple as that."

During **imagery** practice, the person relaxes and focuses attention on the images chosen or presented. Guided imagery scripts are available from several sources; individuals may also work with the practitioners to develop their own script that is specific to their need (Schaub & Dossey, 2000). Generally, the images are presented verbally, but are designed to evoke all the senses. For example, imagery for distraction during a painful procedure might involve asking the individual to identify a special place as a retreat. If the person's special place is a beach, then the practitioner might ask the individual to hear the water softly lapping at the pure, white sand (senses of hearing and sight) and to feel the warm sun falling softly on skin (sense of touch) as the smell of orange blossoms drifts through the air (sense of smell).

When people learn and understand some basic principles of anatomy and physiology, imagery can be used to affect physiological functioning: bone healing, wound healing, and immune system enhancement (Schaub & Dossey, 2000). Tusek, Church, Strong, Grass, and Fazio (1997) examined the use of guided imagery in 130 surgical patients. The patients listened to imagery tapes for 3 days preoperatively, listened to music during the immediate perioperative period, and listened to imagery tapes for 6 days postoperatively. Although there was no difference in overall length of stay or complication rates between the control and treatment groups, the treatment group experienced significant decreases in analgesic use, time to first bowel movement, pain, and anxiety. Kolcaba and Fox (1999) found significant increases in comfort among breast cancer patients receiving guided imagery intervention while undergoing radiation therapy. Decreases in pain, anxiety, insomnia, and fear were especially evident during the first 3 weeks of imagery therapy.

Music Therapy

Music therapy is the use of specific kinds of music (or sounds) to produce desired changes in behaviors, emotions, and physiological processes. Music works as therapy by influencing the area of the brain involved with emotions and feelings, the limbic system (Guzetta, 2000). Music can stimulate the release of endorphins, causing a change in brain receptor sites (McCraty, Barios-Choplin, Atkinson, & Tomasino, 1998), which can change mood. Mental and emotional changes create changes in physiological processes through the autonomic nervous system (McCraty, Barios-Chopin, Atkinson, & Tomasino, 1998).

Different types of music may be used therapeutically. Guzetta (2000) reports that the classical music of Mozart, Haydn, and Bach improves concentration and memory and classical music of the Baroque period (Vivaldi and Handel) gives a sense of safety and stability. Debussy and Ravel, impressionist composers, evoke dreamlike images and open creativity. Gregorian chants ground the individual in the present moment, eliciting feelings of deep peace; they are also useful for releasing pain. Other types of music have different actions. Some music is specifically composed for therapeutic effect; this music is called designer music, which may include sound frequencies that alter brainwave frequencies to achieve a particular brain state or emotion (McCraty, Barios-Chopin, Atkinson, & Tomasino, 1998).

White (1999) examined the effects of investigator-selected classical music on individuals with an acute myocardial infarction. Significant reductions in heart rate, respiratory rate, and oxygen demand were noted immediately after the individuals listened to music for 20 minutes. The reductions continued for 1 hour following the intervention.

Clark, Lipe, and Bilbrey (1998) used the individual's preferred music to affect a significant decrease in aggressive behaviors within the treatment group of persons with dementia when bathing. The caregivers also reported increased cooperation and improved affect during bathing. Ezzone, Baker, Rosselet, and Terepka (1998) found that music therapy produced a significant decrease in nausea and vomiting among persons receiving chemotherapy. The patients listened to self-selected music during peak emetic times during chemotherapy administration. Chlan (1995) examined the effect of music therapy on persons who were mechanically ventilated. Patients listened to classical music of their choice from Chlan's selection of tapes for 30 minutes in the late afternoon or early evening. Significant decreases in heart and respiratory rates and mood scores indicating relaxation and mood improvement occurred during and following the intervention. McCraty and colleagues (1998) found that music can reduce stress, fatigue, and negative affect and can increase emotional well being and mental clarity.

Although music therapy can be used by anyone, the American Music Therapy Association (http://www.musictherapy.org) offers training in music therapy and certifies music therapists who have completed formal education programs.

Bodywork

Massage

Massage is the manipulation of soft tissues of the body. Knaster (1996, p. 143) describes massage as "a primal, instinctive act to make yourself or someone else feel better." Formal massage techniques are variations of rubbing a sore spot after bumping your head or rubbing a friend's back as consolation after a loss. Nurses are advised to give massage (back rubs) to promote sleep and relaxation (Potter & Perry, 1997). Classic Swedish massage contains a variety of hand movements (Table 14-1). During massage, skin lubrication with oil, lotion, or powder reduces friction, pinching, and hair pulling and is generally advised (Knaster, 1996).

The use of massage is supported by research. Among 113 hospitalized patients (Smith, Stallings, Mariner, & Burrall, 1999), massage contributed to increased relaxation, a sense of well being, and positive mood changes in more than 87% of the subjects. More than two thirds of the subjects believed that massage increased their mobility, gave them greater energy, and promoted faster recovery. Richards (1998) found that nurses with no special training in massage could improve the quality and quantity of sleep for critically ill patients by giving a back massage. Corley, Ferriter, Zeh, and Gifford (1995) found that patients receiving back rubs had significant improvement in mood.

A 10-minute foot massage given on 3 consecutive evenings provided significant decreases in pain and nausea and increased feelings of relaxation for patients hospitalized with cancer (Grealish, Lomasney, & Whiteman, 2000). This treatment was not a reflexology treatment. Ironson et al. (1996) found a significant decrease in state anxiety and cortisol levels (a stress hormone) after one massage. Improvement in immune function among immune markers important in HIV disease was evident after 1 month. Ahles et al. (1999) found that 3 weeks of 20-minute daily massage consisting of effleurage, pétrissage, and acupressure to the shoulders, neck, head, and face resulted in a significant reduction in distress, fatigue, nausea, and state anxiety for the treatment group (Fig. 14-4).

In another study (Fields et al., 1998), children with asthma responded to massage with decreased anxiety, decreased cortisol levels, and increased peak airflow. Parents were trained by massage therapists, given written instructions, and given a video. The parents massaged their children for 30 days, 20 minutes each evening.

Knaster (1996) describes several other bodywork

Table 14-1 Techniques of Swedish Massage

Technique	Explanation
Effleurage	Stroking. Use slow, rhythmic, long, flowing strokes. Light or superficial pressure is relaxing. Firm or deep stroking stimulates circulation, moves lymph fluids, and warms the muscle for deeper work.
Pétrissage	Kneading of the muscles. Lift a large skin fold away from the underlying muscle and bone, then squeeze, press, and/or roll the muscles between the hands. Improves circulation, reduces edema, stimulates nerve endings, and cleanses tissues after exercise to present stiffness and soreness. Should be limited to large muscles.
Friction or rubbing	Circular, linear, or transverse strokes that apply constant pressure to one area. May be deep or superficial. May free adhesions and loosen joints and tendons.
Percussion	Series of short, rapid strokes or percussive taps to the fleshy parts of the body. Includes hacking (with the outside edge of the hand), tapping (with the fingertips), plucking (loosely pinching skin between thumb and fingertips and lifting-dropping), and gentle pummeling with the fists.
Vibration	Using the hand or fingertips to create a rapid trembling or shaking sensation in the muscle. Stimulates nerves and releases tight muscles. Mechanical vibrators can be used.
Compression	Rhythmic downward pumping movement on the muscle, which encourages relaxation and increases circulation.
Passive range of motion	Rotation, flexion, and extension of body parts to mobilize joints.

Adapted from Knaster, M. (1996). *Discovering the body's wisdom*. New York: Bantam.

modalities. Two of the most familiar methods are Trager therapy and Craniosacral therapy.

Trager Therapy

Trager Psychophysical Integration involves tissue manipulation, relaxation, and movement reeducation. Practitioners work from a meditative state while they rock, giggle, vibrate, and stretch the body in an effort to set off waves of motion that will lead to deep relaxation and greater mobility. This relaxation and mobility can release long-standing physical and mental patterns. Following treatment, the person is taught a series of exercises and stretches that will reinforce the treatment. Training in Trager therapy is available through schools of massage. A web search for the topic Trager therapy yields a multitude of sites.

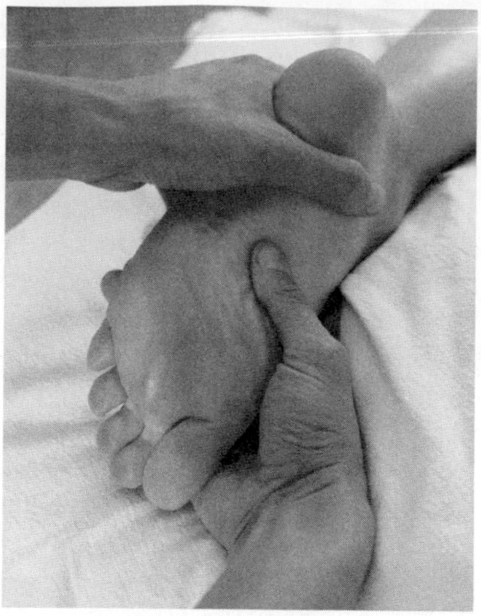

Fig. 14-4 Massage can be effective for many areas of the body.

Craniosacral Therapy

Craniosacral therapy originated in osteopathy, a medical practice that adds manipulation of the bones of the body to conventional medical education. Craniosacral therapists believe that the bones of the cranium, spine, and sacrum are moveable and connected and that the cerebrospinal fluid has a pulse that can be felt. The therapist uses gentle pressure to restore free movement of cerebrospinal fluid, allowing for normal functioning. The therapist also believes that emotions are stored in musculoskeletal system tissue and can be released through manipulation of the craniosacral system. Craniosacral therapy training is provided through the Upledger Institute (http://www.upledger.com).

Many massage therapists, who may be certified by the American Massage Therapy Association after their training, practice a variety of bodywork modalities. Many therapists also include forms of energy work in their massage practices.

Aromatherapy

Aromatherapy uses aromatic plant materials and the essential oils of plants. There is a long history of the use of plant materials in both in Ayurvedic medicine (from the Hindu tradition) and in Traditional Chinese Medicine. The essential oils act on the human body in three different ways:

1. They act pharmacologically when the oils enter the bloodstream either through the lungs or through the skin and act on the body chemistry.
2. They have a physiological effect as they act on body systems to sedate or stimulate.
3. There is a psychological effect when the essence is in-

Box 14-3 Precautions for the Use of Aromatherapy

EXTERNAL USE—INHALATION ONLY

- Generally, essential oils should be restricted to external use and inhalation.

DILUTE OILS

- The oils should be diluted with a carrier oil before direct application to the skin.
- An exception to the dilution rule is oil of lavender. Essential oil of lavender may be applied without dilution to burns, cuts, and insect bites.

AVOID THE EYES AND MUCOUS MEMBRANES

KNOW THE OILS—BE AWARE OF WARNINGS-CONTRAINDICATIONS

- Each essential oil may have specific warnings-contraindications. Have reputable reference material available and refer to it if using essential oils. For example, many of the oils are contraindicated during pregnancy.

WATCH FOR ALLERGIES

- Ask about allergies, preferences, and responses to smells; the sense of smell has a strong association with memory.

Note: Before using aromatherapy in treating patients, professional training is ***strongly*** *recommended.*

Adapted from James, K. (1998). Aromatherapy. In M. Snyder, & R. Lindquist (Eds.), *Complementary/alternative therapies in nursing* (3rd ed., pp. 139-148). New York: Springer; Lawless, J. (1995). *The illustrated encyclopedia of essential oils*. Rockport, MA: Element Books.

haled through the nose and affects the emotions through the limbic system.

Essential oils may used in the following ways:

- They may be added to the bath or used in a douche.
- They may be mixed with carrier oils and used during massage.
- They may be placed on cloth and applied as a compress.
- They may be applied directly to minor injuries to speed healing.
- They may be inhaled after vaporization (Lawless, 1995).

Hay, Jamieson, and Ormerod (1998) studied the effect of a mixture of essential oils on alopecia areata, the sudden, rapid, patchy loss of hair (Seidel, Ball, Dains, & Benedict, 1999), in 86 patients. Oils of thyme, rosemary, lavender, and cedarwood were mixed with carrier oils and massaged into the scalp of the treatment group daily. The control group received massages using only carrier oils. A significant treatment effect was noted for 44% of the treatment group. James (1998) reports that nurses are beginning to use aromatherapy to increase a sense of well being and to promote relaxation and sleep. Oils that are useful for sleep promotion include chamomile, lavender, marjoram, and *ylang ylang*. Oils of bergamot, frankincense, sandalwood, geranium, orange, and patchouli have a sedative effect. Studies have shown that lavender, chamomile, peppermint, and rose in massage oils can be an effective complementary treatment for chronic pain (Buckle, 1999). Box 14-3 lists precautions to keep in mind when using aromatherapy to treat a patient. Alternative use of aromatherapy with individuals is strongly discouraged without professional, clinical training (Buckle, 1999; James, 1998).

Table 14-2 Being There versus Being With

The Nurse Who Is BEING THERE for Patients:	The Nurse Who Is BEING WITH Patients:
Is attentive	Is available with whole self
Is task-oriented	Enters the patient's world
Does the right thing	Becomes vulnerable
Fulfills a role	Is present as a whole person
Assists with coping	Alleviates suffering
Provides security	Enables growth

Adapted from Fredriksson, L. (1999). Modes of relating in a caring conversation: A research synthesis on presence, touch and listening. *Journal of Advanced Nursing, 30* (5), 1167-1176.

Presence

The way people interact with one another can cause pain or promote healing. **Presence** is defined as "being available in a situation with the wholeness of one's individual being . . . of 'being with' rather than 'doing to' " (McKivergin, 2000, p. 208). A study by Halldorsdottir (1991) examined the perceptions of individuals to nurse interactions. Subjects maintained that nurse interactions followed a continuum from *life-destroying* to *life-sustaining* to *life-giving*. Individuals perceived nurses described as *life-giving* as a healing force; they were perceived as being present with—rather than simply being there for—the individuals.

As described by Fredriksson (1999), *being there* would normally be considered acceptable nursing behavior. However, the individuals in the Halldorsdottir (1991) study demonstrate that nurses can be much more than acceptable; the nurse's presence can actually contribute to healing. In examining the differences in *being there* and *being with*, Fredriksson (1999) found that when nurses are *being with* subjects, nurses' attention were focused rather than merely attentive, their touch was caring rather than task oriented, and nurses did not merely hear, they listened. Other differences between *being there* and *being with* are shown in Table 14-2.

When using presence as a holistic intervention and establishing a whole–person-to-whole–person relationship, the nurse becomes vulnerable to the pain of the individual. Nurses may choose to avoid this pain by walking away, maintaining a professional distance, and being too busy with other tasks to be fully present. Nurses may have personal limitations that prevent the use of presence, such

Text continued on p. 393

Section I: Personal Health Habits

What you put into your body—nutrition—how you take care of your body—rest, relaxation, and exercise—and your general level of awareness, love, and acceptance of your body are the major factors important in health. To investigate your health behavior, you might keep weekly diary of food, exercise, sleep, relaxation, and stress. In this way you create an accurate record of your behavior, which is the first step in a program of modification and change. The following pages are *AIDS* for that process and ask important questions about your health behavior.

1. Lester Breslow of UCLA, after observing the health and behavior of thousands of adults, has demonstrated that a person's life expectancy and health are related to the following basic health habits:
   ___Three meals a day at regular times and no snacking
   ___Breakfast every day
   ___Moderate exercise two or three times a week
   ___Adequate sleep (7 to 8 hours, not more or less per night)
   ___No smoking
   ___Moderate weight
   ___No alcohol or only in moderation

Check off how many you observe regularly, giving yourself two checks if you are nearly perfect in that category. Statistically, each habit adds a few years to your life.

Nutrition

2. How much awareness do you have of your particular diet and its effects on your body?
3. In a sentence or two, describe your relationship to food.
4. My favorite foods are:
5. I eat _____ meals a day.
6. My smoking habits are ______________________________
7. My drinking habits are ______________________________
8. Do you see a relationship among stress and tension, emotional upsets, and your diet or eating habits?
   Describe ______________________________

Exercise and relaxation

A person needs to (1) exercise the body regularly to the point of sweating, (2) get adequate rest in the form of sleep, and (3) practice frequently a form of relaxation response, meditation, self-hypnosis, or related technique that elicits deep relaxation. The more stressful and demanding your life, the more you need both relaxation and exercise: the basic pair of methods of keeping the body healthy and in tune.

Exercise

9. I exercise vigorously approximately _____ hours a week.
10. The type of regular exercise in my life are:
    ___active walking
    ___jogging
    ___sport (which) ______________________
    ___heavy labor
    ___other (describe) ______________________
11. Describe your exercise habits and patterns:
12. My attitude toward exercise is:
    ___I love it
    ___I hate it
    ___I'll do it if I have to
    ___other ______________________
13. I would feel better about exercise, or exercise more, if ______________________________
    ____

Sleep

14. I average _____ hours of sleep per night.
15. My sleep is usually
    ___restful and refreshing
    ___fitful
    ___interrupted
    ___other ______________________

Fig. 14-5 An example of a Personal Health Workbook. (Prepared by Dennis T. Jaffe.)

16. I most often awake feeling
 ___refreshed
 ___anxious
 ___exhausted
 ___unfinished
 ___other ______________________
17. I fall asleep
 ___easily
 ___with difficulty
 ___with difficulty when I am under stress
 ___regularly using food _____, drink _____, or medication _____
18. Are there any problems, dissatisfactions, or difficulties connected with your sleep patterns? What aspects would you like to change?

Body awareness

19. I consider my normal energy level to be
 ___high
 ___moderate
 ___adequate for most of what I do
 ___barely adequate
 ___low
 ___other descriptive term that seems appropriate ______________
20. I consider myself to be
 ___tuned into my body's functioning, rhythms, and special needs
 ___unaware of my body's functioning, rhythms, and special needs
 ___other ______________________
21. When I experience my body right now, what does it tell me?
22. How do I feel about my body? (Check all that apply)
 ___I like it
 ___I dislike it
 ___I am proud of it
 ___I am a little ashamed or self-conscious about it
 ___I barely tolerate it
 ___I have no special feelings or awareness
 ___I am not sure I have one
 ___other feelings and attitudes ______________________
23. In a sentence, describe your relationship to your body. ______________
24. The part or parts of my body I like best are ______________
 Why, or what about them? ______________
25. What do you want to change about your body awareness or relationship to your body?
26. Draw a picture of yourself as you see or feel yourself now.

Section II: Health History

How aware are you of your history of illness? How much do you know about what is or was going on physically in your body when you were ill with each of your illnesses? Are you aware of the parts of your body, organs, and organ systems that are weak and tend to be the first to feel the effects of the stress in your life? Each person has one or more target organs, the weak links in his or her physical chain, that are the first to break down.

Knowing your health history, knowing your illnesses and target organs, and looking for patterns can be useful in preparing your own health program. In question 27, fill in as well as you can your personal health history, including dates, severity, organ affected, treatment and also others in your family who may have had that or a similar illness (include the age at which they had it).

27. **Personal Health History** (give most recent first):

Month and year	**Diagnosis**	**Symptoms**	**Severity and duration**	**Organ affected**	**Treatments**	**Other family members with illness and age at onset**

Fig. 14-5, cont'd An example of a Personal Health Workbook. (Prepared by Dennis T. Jaffe.)

Continued

Section III: Family and Life History

28. Please write something about each member of your family of origin, mentioning perhaps such things as how important they were to you, how close or distant you were, where they are now, and the quality of your relationship.
 Father:
 Mother:
 Brothers and sisters:
 Other important family members:
29. Describe the general health or serious illness of each of your parents. If deceased, mention when and the cause of death.
30. Mention something about your childhood home life and family environment, including stressful or traumatic events, family crises, degree of conflict or tension, and any special memories.
31. Do you remember how your family responded to illness? What do you remember about your health or illness as a child and how your family reacted to it?
32. List the most important events, crises, transitions, changes (negative or positive), or developments in your life. Take time to do this, because hopefully it should lead to a period of reflection on your life history and how it created you as you are today. List the events and briefly, in a sentence or two, describe what they were and their effect in you. Place an asterisk or two in front of those events that seem especially central to your life. Some of the important events will be childhood traumas, changes in the family through birth and death, important relationships or emotional changes, and so on.
33. Describe briefly your educational history.
34. Comment on its importance and meaningfulness to your life.
35. Starting with your present work or major life activity (not necessarily for profit), describe the work or jobs you have done.
36. In your life now, what is your most meaningful or central activity?
37. What are the other important jobs or activities that you do?
38. Right now, how do you feel about your work or career? What are your most common feelings about it?
39. How would you like your work or career to change?

Section IV: Leisure and Social Activities

40. Write five things that you do to play.
41. Describe something that you laughed about during the week.
42. What things do you do that make you feel good?
43. How many people, outside your immediate family, do you see in a typical week?
44. What sort of friendships do you have? Are they especially close? Do you have few or many? Are they primarily of the same or opposite sex? Please write about your friendships.
45. Describe your present living conditions—whom you live with, how long you have lived there.
46. Please list some of the main satisfactions and dissatisfactions with your living conditions.
 Satisfactions:
 Dissatisfactions:
47. List the most important people in your life right now and indicate their relationship to you, and in a few words, describe the nature of the relationship or how it feels to you or why it's important in your life.

Person	Relationship

Sex

48. Is sex an important aspect of your life? _____ How important, and what role, would you say sex plays in your current life?
49. Are you currently in a sexual relationship? _____ Please write something about it. How satisfying is it for you?
50. Please write something about your sexual history, attitudes, and feelings about sex in your family, sexual awakening, and previous sexual relationships.
51. Did you feel particularly sexually attractive or unattractive at times in your life? _____ During what periods or times?
52. What would you most want to change about your current sexual relationships?

Fig. 14-5, cont'd An example of a Personal Health Workbook. (Prepared by Dennis T. Jaffe.)

Group or community

53. Every person derives meaning and identity from the human community of which they are a part. A person might identify with many communities—a neighborhood, professional group, friendship network, extended family, religious or ethnic group, political group, and so on. List, in order of their centrality to your life, your communities and affiliations and their importance to you.

Group or community	Importance

54. List some of the ways that you affect your environment or one of your communities. How powerful do you feel in making changes in your world?

Section V: Life Stress and Coping Patterns

Recurrent daily stresses

55. Other specific times, activities, or events are the most regular sources of stress in your life. Think about the past few weeks and which stressful situations occurred regularly, how you usually respond to them (what you did and how you felt), and how you might modify them to make them less stressful or destructive to you.

Description of stressful event	Your response (internal and external)	Potential ways to modify event

56. What seems to be your usual response to stressful situations? For example, do you blow up, withdraw, take it out on others, get sick, get anxious, cry, become afraid, avoid situations, try to forget, or some combination?
57. What situations make you feel calm, relaxed, at peace, or comfortable?
58. What situations make you feel anxious, tense, depressed, fearful, or upset?
59. When you are in such situations, how do you make yourself feel better?
60. Underline any of the following symptoms or difficulties that apply to you:

Headaches	Dizziness	No appetite
Palpitations	Stomach trouble	Insomnia
Bowel disturbances	Fatigue	Alcoholism
Nightmares	Take sedatives	Tremors
Feel tense	Feel panicky	Take drugs
Depressed	Suicidal ideas	Shy with people
Unable to relax	Sexual problems	Can't make decisions
Don't like weekends or vacations	Overambitious	Home conditions bad
Can't make friends	Inferiority feelings	Unable to have a good time
Can't keep a job	Memory problems	Concentration difficulties
Financial problems	Fainting spells	

Others:

61. Which of these symptoms cause you the most concern? Which would you be willing to work on changing?
62. Life change index.

For past and anticipated future life events, add up the mean values assigned to each life event listed in Table 11-1 to get your life change units for both the past year and the coming year. If your total for the past year is over 150, research suggests that you are at risk for a health change or illness, and you need to take steps to counteract the buildup of stress.

Section VI: Personality and Personal Identity

Personality

63. Please write a few words that help to describe you and tell the kind of person you are.
64. What are the most important, or most regular, emotions in your life?
65. What emotions would you say control you?
66. Do you have trouble expressing

___anger	___joy	___happiness
___sadness	___love	___other (specify)
___crying	___sexuality	

Fig. 14-5, cont'd An example of a Personal Health Workbook. (Prepared by Dennis T. Jaffe.)

Continued

67. What do you feel are your major strengths as a person and your most important personal qualities?
68. What are your weaknesses and your negative aspects?

Personal Identity

69. Who am I?

A person has many identities, which embody activities, feelings, and powers within and in the environment and personal relationships. List as many as you can of the ways that you would answer the question, "Who am I?" letting yourself respond freely to any way that you might interpret or experience an answer to that question—in terms of role; in metaphoric or feeling terms; or in terms of job, accomplishment, or the way you think of yourself. Afterwards, go back and rank them, starting with 1, in order of their centrality or importance to you.

Section VII: Values and Inner Life

70. The external events in your life are intimately affected by your inner world, beliefs, and world view. In the first column, write one of the 10 things that you most value in life. Next, describe how you actualize these values or how or why you fail to actualize them. In doing this, you will begin to see how closely you are living your life according to your values.

Value	How actualized	How not actualized

71. In what way would you say you are a religious or spiritual person?
72. What is your religious background?
73. Has your religious or spiritual faith been of help to you during your life? _____ In what ways?
74. Do you meditate, pray, or perform a regular religious ritual? _____ What sort and how frequently?
75. Has your religious or spiritual practice been helpful during times of illness or difficulty? _____ In what ways?

Section VIII: Change Goals and the Future

76. How many more years do you expect to live and how do you expect to die?
77. Please write your own epitaph about how you would like to be remembered.
78. Please write several reasons—things to accomplish, desires, interests, areas of life to explore, realtionships, obligations—that you have to overcome or get relief from your current difficulties. Please do this carefully and be specific.
79. What emotional feeling do you have when you imagine your future?
80. Please write the specific goals and achievements you expect to accomplish in your future.
81. What are some of the specific changes, things you will have to learn or give up, that you will have to make to achieve these goals?
82. How completely do you expect to overcome your current major and minor health, emotional, and life difficulties? (If experiencing any.)
83. How long do you expect this process to take?

Section IX: Inquiry Onto Illness

This section is to be answered if you are currently experiencing an illness or if you want to explore an illness that you had previously.

84. Thinking back to the time of the first onset of the illness or symptoms you wish to explore and your life situation at the time, write down several factors or reasons in your psychological and family life that may have made you susceptible to that illness.
85. Before the initial symptoms or your decision to seek help, did you have any premonitions, dreams, thoughts, expectations, or worries that you might be, or become, ill? _____ Describe them.
86. List a few of the factors in your life today that might tend to maintain you in a state of illness or make it difficult to become well. These may be things that you do, things that you feel, fears of the future, benefits of being ill, feelings about yourself, or things that you can't do. These are the major obstacles to your getting well.
87. Draw a picture that represents to you, either literally or symbolically, and your symptom or illness. Then look at your picture regularly and become familiar with your feelings about it.
88. Draw a representation of the potential healing forces or powers within you that might have an effect on or the power to heal your illness. You might draw the healing forces in action against your illness. Use this image as part of your healing meditation to depict your healing forces in action.

Fig. 14-5, cont'd An example of a Personal Health Workbook. (Prepared by Dennis T. Jaffe.)

as the need to be in control, a lack of patience, a lack of openness, and a lack of desire to be present (McKivergin, 2000). Many of these barriers to the use of presence can be overcome with self-knowledge and self-care.

SELF-KNOWLEDGE

Holistic health involves a personal commitment to wellness and an exploration of what works for the individual and what does not (Walter, 2000). Additionally, holistic health involves:

- Knowing the physical self, the emotional self, the mental self, and the spiritual self.
- Seeking a comfortable balance among these aspects of being.
- Knowing what changes need to be made to achieve this balance (American Holistic Health Association, 1999).

This knowledge is vital to both the nurse attempting holistic practice and the individual interested in pursuing holistic health.

The Think About It questions at the beginning of this chapter can assist both nurse and individual in the exploration of self that begins the process of self-care. Figure 14-5 provides an example of a more detailed assessment instrument. Psychologist and spiritual leader Ram Dass (1976, p. 42) explains the importance of self-knowledge to the nurse when he says, " . . . I could tell you the greatest truths of the world but if I don't understand them inside, forget it, because all I'm doing is taking it from there and giving them to there and I'm not giving you the key that allows you to use it, which is the 'faith' in it, which I can only convey through my own success in whatever I'm doing."

Self-exploration enhances the abilities of the nurse who wants to consider using nursing presence as a holistic healing intervention (McKivergin, 2000). The expanded knowledge of self is valuable because the more that is known about oneself, the more there is of oneself to offer to another, and "the only thing you ever have to offer to another human being, ever, is your own state of being" (Dass, 1976, p. 6).

When self-knowledge is gained, one or more of the holistic health strategies mentioned in this chapter can be useful in helping people achieve optimal wellness. In addition to the strategies mentioned, many other holistic interventions can be helpful. These strategies include homeopathy, flower essences, crystals, and additional forms of bodywork and movement therapies. Every person is a whole, unique being; therefore each person needs to explore the strategies and decide which modalities are the best methods to improve their state of wellness.

People beginning this self-exploration and the practice of holistic health strategies may find that the practice changes their lives. Using presence and giving the gift of self enhance personal growth in the giver (McKivergin, 2000). Nurses who practice TT can experience changes in their perspective on caregiving and increases in inner strength, calmness, self-esteem, self-confidence, spirituality, and sensitivity to others (Cabico, 1992).

SUMMARY

Holistic health strategies are designed to view the individual as a biopsychosocial-spiritual whole being. Many holistic health strategies have been practiced in other cultures for many years; some began as religious practices. As these practices moved to the West, the health-promoting nature of these therapies came to the forefront and the emphasis on religion waned.

A body of research already exists supporting the use of these therapies and more research is being performed. Although the studies that have been made have been unsuccessful in persuading everyone of the utility of the practices, holistic health practitioners are convinced that these practices help promote and maintain health.

Every person is a unique, individual being; therefore some exploration of self, the various strategies, and the practitioner will be necessary before determining which strategy is the *right fit* for the individual. The *right fit* strategy will increase both physical and mental well being. Nurses need to understand holistic health strategies because patients are using these strategies in increasing numbers. Nurses who begin to practice holistic interventions may find these interventions a useful adjunct to their nursing practice. Additionally, nurses may find that beginning to use holistic interventions in their nursing practices changes their practices and their very selves.

REFERENCES

Achterberg, J. (1999). Imagery, ceremony, and healing rituals. *Alternative Therapies in Health and Medicine, 5* (5), 77-83.

Ahles, T. A., Tope, D. M., Pinkson, B., Walch, S., Hann, D., Whedon, M., Dain, B., Weiss, J. E., Mills, L., & Silberfarb, P. M. (1999). Massage therapy for patients undergoing autologous bone marrow transplantation. *Journal of Pain and Symptom Management, 18* (3), 157-163.

American Holistic Health Association. (1999). *Wellness from within: The first step* (booklet). Anaheim, CA: The Author. Available: http://ahha.org/ahhastep.htm.

Anselmo, J., & Kolkmeier, L. G. (2000). Relaxation: The first step to restore, renew, and self-heal. In B. M. Dossey, L. Keegan, & C. E. Guzetta (Eds.), *Holistic nursing: A handbook for practice* (3rd ed., pp. 497-535). Gaithersburg, MD: Aspen Publishers, Inc.

Astin, J. A. (1997). Stress reduction through mindfulness meditation: Effects of psychological symptomatology, sense of control, and spiritual experiences. *Psychotherapy and Psychomatics, 66,* 97-106.

Astin, J. A., Harkness, E., & Ernst, E. (2000). The efficacy of "distant healing": A systematic review of randomized trials. *Annals of Internal Medicine, 132,* 903-910.

Bates, P. (2000). Renal and urologic problems. In S. M. Lewis, M. M. Heitkemper, & S. R. Dirksen (Eds.), *Medical-surgical nursing: Assessment and management of clinical problems* (5th ed., pp. 1261-1298). St. Louis: Mosby.

Benor, D. J. (1999/2000, Winter). Intentionality in wholistic spiritual healing. *Bridges, 10* (4), 15-17.

Berman, B. M., Ezzo, J., Hadhazy, V., & Sawyers, J. P. (1999). Is acupuncture effective in the treatment of fibromyalgia? *The Journal of Family Practice, 48* (3), 213-218.

Brennan, B. A. (1987). *Hands of light: A guide to healing through the human energy field*. New York: Bantam.

Bruyere, R. L. (1994). *Wheels of light: Chakras, auras, and the healing energy of the body*. New York: Simon & Schuster.

Buckle, J. (1999). Use of aromatherapy as a complementary treatment for chronic pain. *Alternative Therapies in Health and Medicine, 5* (5), 42-51.

Burger, B. (1998). *Esoteric anatomy: The body as consciousness*. Berkeley, CA: North Atlantic Books.

Byrd, R. (1997). Positive therapeutic effects of intercessory prayer in a coronary care unit population. *Alternative Therapies in Health and Medicine, 3* (6), 87-90.

Cabico, L. L. (1992). A phenomenological study of the experiences of nurses practicing therapeutic touch [Abstract]. *Masters Abstracts International, 31* (2), 758.

Chlan, L. L. (1995). Psychophysiologic responses of mechanically ventilated patients to music: A pilot study. *American Journal of Critical Care, 4* (3), 233-238.

Chuen, L. K. (1999). *Chi Kung: The way of healing*. New York: Broadway Books.

Clark, M. E., Lipe, A. W., & Bilbrey, M. (1998). Use of music to decrease aggressive behaviors in people with dementia. *Journal of Gerontological Nursing, 24* (7), 10-17.

Cohen, M. R. (1996). *The Chinese way to healing: Many paths to wholeness*. New York: Berkley.

Corley, M. C., Ferriter, J., Zeh, J., & Gifford, C. (1995). Physiological and psychological effects of back rubs. *Applied Nursing Research, 8* (1), 39-42.

Creamer, P., Singh, B. B., Hochberg, M. C., & Berman, B. M. (1999). Are psychosocial factors related to response to acupuncture among patients with knee osteoarthritis? *Alternative Therapies in Health and Medicine, 5* (4), 72-76.

Dass, R. (1976). *The only dance there is*. New York: Jason Aronson, Inc.

Dibble, S. L., Chapman, J., Mack, K. A., & Shih, A. S. (2000). Acupressure for nausea: Results of a pilot study. *Oncology Nursing Forum, 27* (1), 41-47.

Don, N. S., & Moura, G. (2000). Trance surgery in Brazil. *Alternative Therapies in Health and Medicine, 6* (4), 39-48.

Dossey, B. (1997). Holistic nursing practice. In B. Dossey (Ed.), *American Holistic Nurses' Association, core curriculum for holistic nursing* (pp. 4-12). Gaithersburg, MD: Aspen.

Dossey, L. (1995). How should alternative therapies be evaluated? An examination of fundamentals. *Alternative Therapies in Health and Medicine, 1* (2), 6-10, 79-85.

Ezzone, S., Baker, C., Rosselet, R., & Terepka, E. (1998). Music as an adjunct to antiemetic therapy. *Oncology Nursing Forum, 25* (9), 1551-1556.

Fields, T., Henteleff, T., Hernandez-Reif, M., Martinez, E., Mavunda, K., Kuhn, C., & Schanberg, S. (1998). Children with asthma have improved pulmonary functions after massage therapy. *Journal of Pediatrics, 132* (5), 854-858.

Fredriksson, L. (1999). Modes of relating in a caring conversation: A research synthesis on presence, touch and listening. *Journal of Advanced Nursing, 30* (5), 1167-1176.

Garfinkel, M. S., Singhal, A., Katz, W. A., Allan, D. A., Reshetar, R., & Schumacher, H. R. (1998). Yoga-based intervention for carpal tunnel syndrome: A randomized trial. *Journal of the American Medical Association, 280* (18), 1601-1603.

Giasson, M., & Bouchard, L. (1998). Effect of therapeutic touch on the well-being of persons with terminal cancer. *Journal of Holistic Nursing, 16* (3), 383-398.

Glazer, S. (2000, Summer). Postmodern nursing. *The Public Interest, 140*, 3-16.

Grealish, L., Lomasney, A., & Whiteman, B. (2000). Foot massage: A nursing intervention to modify the distressing symptoms of pain and nausea in patients hospitalized with cancer. *Cancer Nursing, 23* (3), 237-243.

Guzetta, C. E. (2000). Music therapy: Hearing the melody of the soul. In B. M. Dossey, L. Keegan, & C. E. Guzetta (Eds.), *Holistic nursing: A handbook for practice* (3rd ed., pp. 585-610). Gaithersburg, MD: Aspen Publishers, Inc.

Halldorsdottir, S. (1991). Five basic modes of being with another. In D. A. Gaut, & M. M. Leininger (Eds.), *Caring: The compassionate healer* (NLN Pub. No. 15-2401, pp. 37-49). New York: National League for Nursing Press.

Harris, V. S. (2000). Christian Science healing practices [Online]. Available: http://www.tfccs.com/GV/harvard/vhtalk.html.

Harris, W. S., Gowda, M., Kolb, J. W., Strychacz, C. P., Vacek, J. L., Jones, P. G., Forker, A., O'Keefe, J. H., & McCallister, B. D. (1999). A randomized, controlled trial of the effects of remote, intercessory prayer on outcomes in patients admitted to the coronary care unit. *Archives of Internal Medicine, 159*, 2273-2278.

Hay, I. D., Jamieson, M., & Ormerod, A. D. (1998). Randomized trial of aromatherapy: Successful treatment for alopecia areata. *Archives of Dermatology, 134* (11), 1349-1352.

Heidt, P. R. (1990). Openness: A qualitative analysis of nurses' and patient's experiences of therapeutic touch. *Image: Journal of Nursing Scholarship, 22* (3), 180-186.

Horrigan, B. J. (2000). Regions Hospital opens holistic nursing unit. *Alternative Therapies in Health and Medicine, 6* (4), 92-93.

Hover-Kramer, D. (1996). *Healing Touch: A resource for health care professionals*. Albany, NY: Delmar.

Ironson, G., Field, T., Scafidi, F., Hashimoto, M., Kumar, M., Kumar, A., Price, A., Goncalves, A., Burman, I., Tetenman, C., Patarca, R., & Fletcher, M. A. (1996). Massage therapy is associated with enhancement of the immune system's cytotoxic capacity. *International Journal of Neuroscience, 84* (1-4), 205-217.

Iyengar, B. K. S. (1979). *Light on yoga: Yoga dipika* (revised edition). New York: Schocken.

James, K. (1998). Aromatherapy. In M. Snyder, & R. Lindquist (Eds.), *Complementary/alternative therapies in nursing* (3rd ed., pp. 139-148). New York: Springer.

Kabat-Zinn, J. (1990). *Full catastrophe living: Using the wisdom of your body and mind to face stress, pain, and illness*. New York: Delta.

Kolcaba, K., & Fox, C. (1999). The effects of guided imagery on comfort of women with early stage breast cancer undergoing radiation therapy. *Oncology Nursing Forum, 26* (1), 67-72.

Knaster, M. (1996). *Discovering the body's wisdom*. New York: Bantam.

Kreitzer, M. J. (1998). Meditation. In M. Snyder, & R. Lindquist (Eds.), *Complementary/alternative therapies in nursing* (3rd ed., pp. 123-137). New York: Springer.

Krieger, D. (1979). *The therapeutic touch: How to use your hands to help or to heal*. New York: Simon & Schuster.

Krieger, D. (1993). *Accepting your power to heal: The personal practice of Therapeutic Touch*. Santa Fe, NM: Bear.

Krieger, D. (1998). Healing with Therapeutic Touch [Interview]. *Alternative Therapies in Health and Medicine, 4* (1), 87-92.

Lawless, J. (1995). *The illustrated encyclopedia of essential oils*. Rockport, MA: Element Books.

Mayer, D. J. (2000). Acupuncture: An evidence-based review of the clinical literature. *Annual Review of Medicine, 51*, 49-63.

Macrae, J. (1999). *Therapeutic touch: A practice guide*. New York: Knopf.

McCraty, R., Barrios-Chopkin, B., Atkinson, M., & Tomasino, D. (1998). The effects of different types of music on mood, tension, and mental clarity. *Alternative Therapies in Health and Medicine, 4* (1), 75-84.

McKahan, D. (1993, Aug.). Healing by design: Therapeutic environments for health care. *Interior Design, 64* (8), 108-109, 118.

McKivergin, M. (2000). The nurse as an instrument of healing. In B. M. Dossey, L. Keegan, & C. E. Guzetta (Eds.), *Holistic nursing: A handbook for practice* (3rd ed., pp. 207-227). Gaithersburg, MD: Aspen Publishers, Inc.

Meisenhelder, J. B., & Chandler, E. N. (2000). Prayer and health outcomes in church members. *Alternative Therapies in Health and Medicine, 6* (4), 56-60.

Naparstek, B. (1994). *Staying well with guided imagery.* New York: Warner.

Olson, M., & Sneed, N. (1995). Anxiety and therapeutic touch. *Issues in Mental Health Nursing, 16* (2), 97-108.

Ornish, D. (1990). *Dr. Dean Ornish's program for reversing heart disease.* New York: Ballantine Books.

Peck, S. D. E. (1997). The effectiveness of therapeutic touch for decreasing pain in elders with degenerative arthritis. *Journal of Holistic Nursing, 15* (2), 176-198.

Pelletier, K. R., Astin, J. A., & Haskell, W. L. (1999). Current trends in the integration and reimbursement of complementary and alternative medicine by managed care organizations (MCOs) and insurance providers: 1998 update and cohort analysis. *American Journal of Health Promotion, 14* (2), 125-133.

Potter, P. A., & Perry, A. G. (1997). *Fundamentals of nursing: Concepts, process, and practice.* St. Louis: Mosby.

Quinn, J. (1996). Therapeutic touch and a healing way. *Alternative Therapies in Health and Medicine, 2* (4), 69-75.

Richards, K. C. (1998). Effect of a back massage and relaxation intervention on sleep in critically ill patients. *American Journal of Critical Care, 7* (4), 288-299.

Rogers, M. E. (1970). *An introduction to the theoretical basis of nursing.* Philadelphia: Davis.

Schaub, B. G., & Dossey, B. M. (2000). Imagery: Awakening the inner healer. In B. M. Dossey, L. Keegan, & C. E. Guzetta (Eds.), *Holistic nursing: A handbook for practice* (3rd ed., pp. 539-581). Gaithersburg, MD: Aspen Publishers, Inc.

Seidel, H. M., Ball, J. W., Dains, J. E., & Benedict, G. W. (1999). *Mosby's guide to physical examination* (4th ed.). St. Louis: Mosby.

Shaller, K. (1998). Tai Chi/movement therapy. In M. Snyder, & R. Lindquist (Eds.), *Complementary/alternative therapies in nursing* (3rd ed., pp. 37-49). New York: Springer.

Sri Swami Sivananda. (1994). *Practice of yoga* (7th ed.). Himalayas, India: The Divine Life Society.

Smith, M. C., Stallings, M. A., Mariner, S., & Burrall, M. (1999). Benefits of massage therapy for hospitalized patients: A descriptive and qualitative evaluation. *Alternative Therapies in Health and Medicine, 5* (4), 64-71.

Smith, W. P., Compton, W. C., & West, W. B. (1995). Meditation as an adjunct to a happiness enhancement program. *Journal of Clinical Psychology, 51* (2), 269-273.

Spencer, J. W., & Jacobs, J. J. (1999). *Complementary/alternative medicine: An evidence-based approach.* St. Louis: Mosby.

Stuart, G. W. (1998a). Anxiety responses and anxiety disorders. In G. W. Stuart, & M. T. Laraia (Eds.), *Principles and practice of psychiatric nursing* (6th ed., pp. 273-298). St. Louis: Mosby.

Stuart, G. W. (1998b). Somatic therapies. In G. W. Stuart, & M. T. Laraia (Eds.), *Principles and practice of psychiatric nursing* (6th ed., pp. 604-617). St. Louis: Mosby.

Targ, E. (1999, Aug. Nov.). Distant healing. *IONS: Noetic Sciences Review, 49,* 24-29.

Thompson, E. (2000, May). The alternative model. *Modern Healthcare, 30* (20), 26-28, 32-34.

Turner, J. G., Clark, A. J., Gauthier, D. K., & Williams, M. (1998). The effect of therapeutic touch on pain and anxiety in burn patients. *Journal of Advanced Nursing, 28* (1), 10-20.

Tusek, D. L., Church, J. M., Strong, S. A., Grass, J. A., & Fazio, V. W. (1997). Guided imagery: A significant advance in the care of patients undergoing elective colorectal surgery. *Diseases of the Colon and Rectum, 40* (2), 172-178.

Valdez, P., & Mehrabian, A. (1994). Effects of color on emotions. *Journal of Experimental Psychology: General, 123* (4), 394-409.

Walker, S. R., Tonigan, J. S., Miller, W. R., Comer, S., & Kahlich, L. (1997). Intercessory prayer in the treatment of alcohol abuse and dependence: A pilot investigation. *Alternative Therapies in Health and Medicine, 3* (6), 79-86.

Walter, S. (2000, July). *Holistic health* [Online]. Available: http://www.healthy.net/pan/chg/AHHA/rosen.htm.

WebMD. (2000, July). *Dean Ornish M.D.'s lifestyle program. Preventive medicine research institute. Dr. Dean Ornish's program for reversing heart disease* [Online]. Available: http://WebMD.lycos.com/content/article/3068.1548.

Wenneberg, S. R., Schneider, R. H., Walton, K. G., MacLean, C. R., Levitsky, D. K., Salerno, J. W., Wallace, R. K., Mandarino, J. V., Rainforth, M. V., & Waziri, R. (1997). A controlled study of the effects of the transcendental meditation program on cardiovascular reactivity and ambulatory blood pressure. *International Journal of Neuroscience, 89* (1-2), 15-28.

White, J. M. (1999). Effects of relaxing music on cardiac autonomic balance and anxiety after acute myocardial infarction. *American Journal of Critical Care, 8* (4), 220-230.

Wirth, D. P. (1995). Complementary healing intervention and dermal wound reepithelization: An overview. *International Journal of Psychosomatics, 42* (1-4), 48-53.

Wu, W., Bandilla, E., Ciccone, D. S., Yang, J., Cheng, S-C. S., Carner, N., Wu, Y., & Shen, R. (1999). Effects of qigong on late-stage complex regional pain syndrome. *Alternative Therapies in Health and Medicine, 5* (1), 45-54.

Zamarra, J. W., Schneider, R. H., Besseghini, I., Robinson, D. K., & Salerno, J. W. (1996). Usefulness of the transcendental meditation program in the treatment of patients with coronary artery disease. *American Journal of Cardiology, 77* (10), 867-870.

Unit Four

Application of Health Promotion

15 Overview of Growth and Development Framework

16 The Prenatal Period

17 Infant

18 Toddler

19 Preschool Child

20 School-Age Child

21 Adolescent

22 Young Adult

23 Middle-Age Adult

24 Older Adult

Chapter 15

MARINDA ALLENDER

Overview of Growth and Development Framework

objectives

After completing this chapter, the nurse will be able to:

- Discuss the importance of development as a framework for assessing and promoting health.
- Contrast the terms *growth* and *development.*
- Discuss factors that can influence the rate and pattern of growth of an individual.
- Describe Erikson's theory of psychosocial development.
- Outline the four stages of Piaget's theory of cognitive development.
- Critique the levels and stages of Gilligan's theory of moral development for women.
- Critique the levels and stages of Kohlberg's theory of moral development.

key terms

Development
Developmental Pattern
Developmental Periods
Erikson's Theory of Psychosocial Development
Gilligan's Theory of Moral Development
Growth
Growth Patterns
Kohlberg's Theory of Moral Development
Piaget's Theory of Cognitive Development

THINK About It

Growth and Development

When Suzi came home from school today, she told her mother all about her exciting day. "Today I got to be Ms. Adams' special helper. Michael was the special helper yesterday, and I don't know who it will be tomorrow. Ms. Adams let me say the Pledge of Allegiance and pass out the cookies, since I was her helper. We had chocolate chip cookies today. At naptime, Lisa forgot her blanket, so I shared mine with her so that she wouldn't be cold. Ms. Adams didn't even have to ask me. At recess, Lisa gave me a flower she found. She is my best friend now. Ms. Adams said I was a great helper today. I wonder who will get to be her helper tomorrow."

1. Which stage seems to describe Suzi's behavior of psychosocial development according to Erikson's theory?
2. According to Piaget's theory, in which stage of cognitive development does Suzi fall?

HEALTH TEACHING Anticipatory Guidance

The nurse is often in a position to provide anticipatory guidance to parents, which involves teaching parents ways to handle a situation *before* it becomes an issue or problem. Knowledge of normal growth and development provides a foundation for this teaching. For example, the toddler period is a period of intense exploration of the environment when locomotion is the major gross motor skill acquired. The nurse provides the following teaching to the parents of a child who is entering the toddler period as a means of injury prevention.

- Always use a federally approved car restraint.
- Supervise closely near any source of water, including the bathtub.
- Turn pot handles toward back of stove.
- Place all toxic substances in a locked cabinet.
- Place gates at the top and bottom of stairs.

Unit 4 focuses on development throughout the lifespan as a framework for health screening, education, and counseling. Assessment strategies may vary, but must be appropriate for individuals at each stage of development. The person may be an individual, such as an independent young adult, or a member of a family, as in the case of an infant with inexperienced or anxious parents.

An understanding of human development can facilitate accurate assessment of health and health practices of people at all ages. Health teaching is more appropriate when the nurse recognizes the individual's developmental level. A mutually acceptable plan for health care and health practices can be determined when the nurse understands the interplay between desire for compliance and the strength of social pressures at each age.

This chapter sets the stage for the study of health promotion at individual developmental levels by exploring basic concepts of growth and development and by presenting an overview of three representative theories of development as applied to specific age groups. Each of the following nine chapters deal with a specific age group. Health assessment and promotion appropriate to each age group are described based on the expected competencies for each group. The developmental periods described are prenatal; infant; toddler; preschool age; school age; adolescent; and young, middle, and older adult.

DEVELOPMENTAL PERIODS

The prenatal period begins at conception and ends with birth and is one of the most important **developmental periods** because development proceeds at an extremely rapid rate. The nurse involved with the care of the expectant parents and fetus will inevitably need to understand the influences of the prenatal period to obtain a meaningful history and to associate relevant factors from the prenatal period with the state of health of the individual and family at any other stage of development. This chapter includes the many changes that the expectant mother and fetus experience and, to some extent, the adjustments of the father and other family members. The health-promotion needs of the expectant mother and the fetus are intimately intertwined to the extent that they must be considered as a unit. Table 15-1 presents each developmental period.

OVERVIEW OF GROWTH AND DEVELOPMENT

In today's world, the concepts of growth and development have expanded in proportion to advances in all fields of science. The increased ability to observe physical and biochemical events scientifically during the intrauterine stage of life has led to increased awareness and knowledge of the effects of fetal events on the individual's later life. The behavioral sciences have contributed to significant changes in the ways in which children of technological societies are reared and taught. Discoveries in the physiological and medical sciences have yielded the ability to alter the course of human life when deformity or debilitating disease occurs.

Research in the area of adult development has revealed that adults experience normative transitions that are as essential to their continuing development as are the developmental landmarks of childhood. Gerontology, the study of the aging process from maturity to old age, has shown that change and development continue through the later years (Erikson, 1986).

Concept of Growth

Growth refers to changes in structure or size. During childhood, the physical changes in weight, height, and body proportion are readily noticeable. During adulthood, continued growth takes place, although more in specific body parts. Metabolic and biochemical processes change as life progresses toward maturity; cells of the central nervous system change as maturity progresses (Guyton, 1996).

Growth Patterns

Expected **growth patterns** exist for all people. Growth is not steady throughout life. The two periods of extremely rapid growth, prenatal through infancy and adolescence, are contrasted with the slower rate of growth during childhood and the almost imperceptible increases after adolescence. These patterns for girls can be seen in the height velocity grid in Fig. 15-1 (see p. 402). The mean increase of 15 cm (6 inches) in height by age 1 and 9.25 cm (3 inches) by age 2 are in marked contrast to the mean of 5.4 or 5.5 cm (2 inches) per year from ages 8 to 10. The adolescent growth spurt, although not of the velocity of infancy, is a dramatic change from the preadolescent pattern.

Table 15-1 **Developmental Periods**

Period	Age	Characteristics
Infancy	0 to 18 months	Infant fully dependent on others for basic needs. Ends when child begins walking alone and possesses the beginning speech sounds of language.
Toddler Period	12 or 18 months to 3 years	Motor development progresses significantly. Child achieves a degree of physical and emotional autonomy while maintaining a close identity with the primary family unit.
Preschool Period	3 to 5 or 6 years	Child has increased interest and involvement with peers and may have social interactions with many people.
School-Age Period	5 or 6 to 10 years	Marked by entrance into elementary school. Interests turn away from family and toward peers.
Adolescence	Onset of puberty; 11 to 14 years	A period of transition, adjustment, and personal exploration. Ends when individual demonstrates readiness to assume full adult responsibilities of financial, emotional, and social independence.
Young Adulthood		Getting started in an occupation or career, finding and learning to live with a partner, and starting and rearing a family.
Middle Adulthood		Being established in a marriage, an occupation or career, and a community. May continue to be a time of transition. Must adjust to physiological changes of middle age.
Older Adulthood		Must adjust to decreased physical strength and health, retirement, reduced income, decreasing independence, and deaths of spouse, friends, and self. May be a time of continued involvement in work and active socializing.

Different parts of the body increase in size at different rates. For example, from conception to birth, the head is the fastest growing section; from age 1 to adolescence, the legs grow the fastest. The changes in proportion of body parts from infancy to adulthood are demonstrated in Fig. 15-2 (see p. 403). Standardized growth grids (see Figs. 17-3 and 17-4) give an indication of the expected flow of height and weight parameters for a given population. Although growth grids often indicate standards to age 18, they are less accurate after the adolescent growth spurt begins. The child's height (or length up to 36 months) and weight are plotted against age and a percentile is obtained. For example, if a 9-year-old girl weighs 30.5 kg (67 lb), she is at the fiftieth percentile for weight. This figure demonstrates that approximately 50% of girls her age will weigh more and 50% will weigh less. Serial measurements plotted on a growth grid indicate a person's pattern of growth and are of greater value than an isolated measurement.

Any dramatic change in percentiles for a child should be investigated. The nurse gathers data on current diet, changes in diet, recent or chronic illnesses, and family stresses to evaluate any significant change in percentile.

Growth refers not only to the obvious changes in height and weight, but also to the increases (and in old age, the decreases) in the size of individual organs and systems. Table 15-2 (see p. 404) outlines the directions of growth changes that take place throughout the lifespan. The growth of some systems, such as the skeletal and muscular, is influenced by the gender of the individual, whereas the growth of other systems, such as the nervous and respiratory, is independent of gender. The changes that take place in middle and old age should particularly be noted. The nurse who has studied growth only from the perspective of children can be missing important differences among adults. The health history and physical assessment of an individual should include all body systems, but should also emphasize systems undergoing the most change.

The rate and pattern of growth can be modified by intrinsic and extrinsic factors, both before and after birth. Genetic endowment, maternal nutrition, disease, birth experience, and emotional factors can all influence an individual's potential for growth from conception through birth.

Some postnatal environmental factors that influence an individual's potential for growth include nutrition, illness, and the opportunity for exercise. Other less obvious influences are climate, air pollution, cultural practices, and child-rearing practices. Although the limits of growth are genetically determined, illness or environmental deficits may hamper a person's growth. A developing individual is most subject to the influence of these factors during periods of rapid growth. The timing of exposure to environmental hazards may determine to a great extent the amount and kind of effect of these influences. For example, if a mother in her first trimester of pregnancy is exposed to the rubella virus, then an abnormality may occur because this period is critical for organ development in the fetus. If, on the other

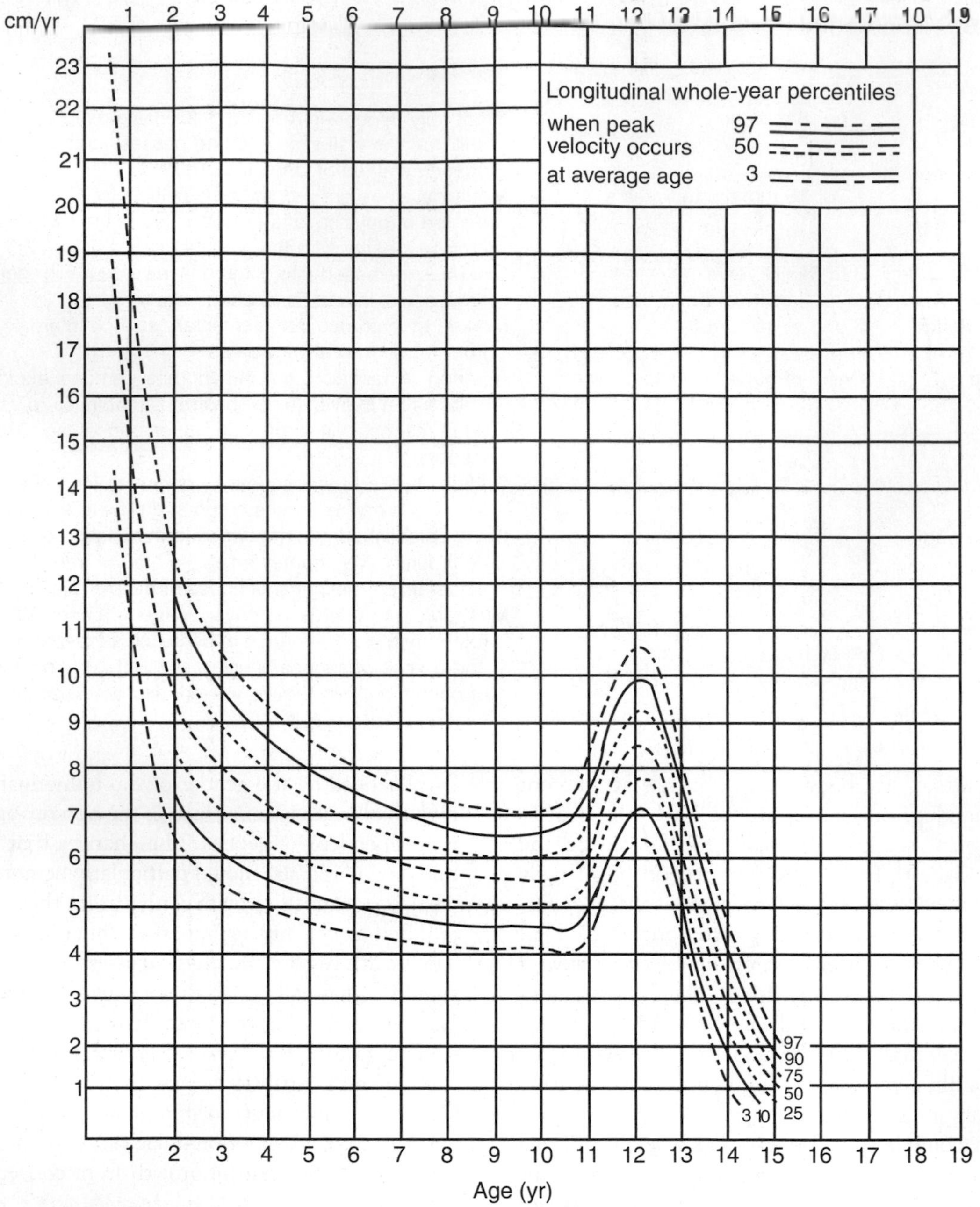

Fig. 15-1 Height velocity grid for girls. (Redrawn from Tanner, J. M., & Whitehouse, R. [1976]. Clinical longitudinal standards for height, weight, height velocity, weight velocity, and stages of puberty. *Archives of Disease and Childhood, 51*[3], 170-179.)

hand, the mother is exposed to the rubella virus during her last trimester of pregnancy, then an abnormality is not likely to occur because this stage is not a time of rapid cell differentiation (see Research Highlights box, p. 411).

Concept of Development

Development refers to changes in skill and capacity to function. In contrast to growth, which is a quantitative or precisely measurable change, development is qualitative. Qualitative changes are more difficult to describe because they cannot be measured in precise units. Development evolves from maturation of physical and mental capacities and learning. The child cannot achieve maturity until physical growth is complete and yet developmental maturity cannot be pinpointed at a particular point in life. Emotional maturity has many interpretations; the close interrelationships of all aspects of life are difficult to describe completely. Physical, emotional, and social factors have made the exact study of human nature elusive and difficult. Philosophy and theology have long

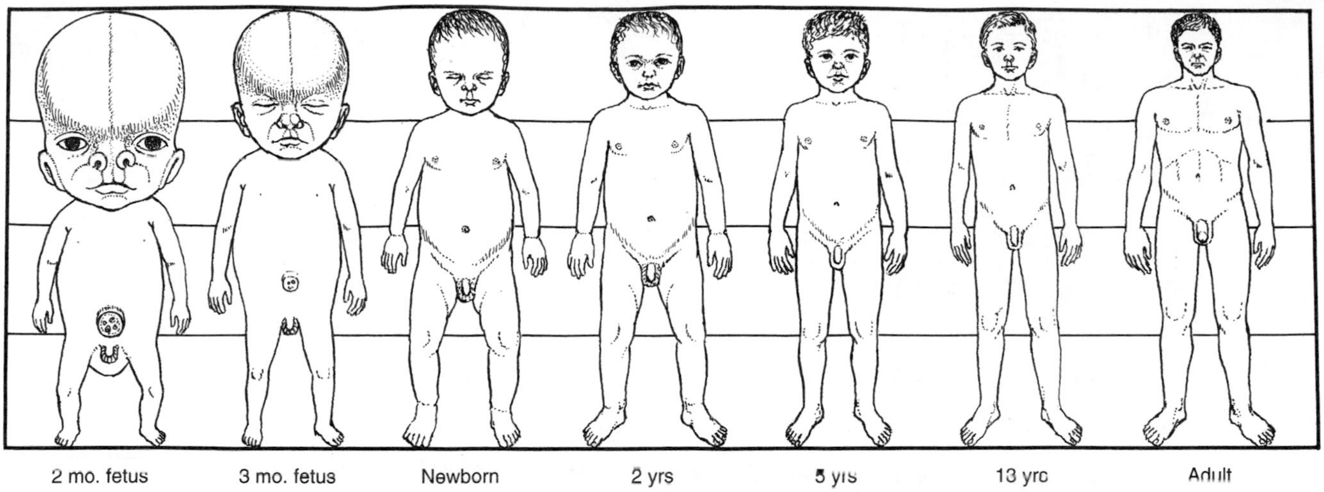

Fig. 15-2 Changes in body proportions from birth to adulthood. (Redrawn from Crouch, J. E., & McClintic, J. R. [1976]. *Human anatomy and physiology* [2nd ed.]. New York: John Wiley & Sons.)

influenced the study of development and the thinking of people most earnestly seeking knowledge of the person. Children and adults are beings with the unique ability to think, feel, ponder, deliberate, and reason; therefore this influence is understandable. The endless quest for understanding of development and life processes is enhanced through the understanding of certain principles and characteristics that can describe, but do not necessarily explain the developmental process.

Developmental Patterns

The pattern of development of physical and mental abilities shows certain common and predictable characteristics. All individuals follow a similar **developmental pattern,** with one stage leading to the next. Early development proceeds as follows:

Pattern of Development
Simple to complex General to specific Cephalocaudal (head to toe) Proximodistal (inner to outer)
Example
An infant makes basic "cooing" sounds before learning to refine those sounds into speech. Infants use the whole hand before learning the finer control of the pincer grasp. Infant gains neck and head control before controlling the movements of the extremities. Infant gains control of structures near the center before those farther away; the infant is able to coordinate the arms to reach for an object before being able to grasp it.

Although developmental sequence is predictable, exact timing of the appearance of skills depends on the individual. Each person follows a predictable pattern in a personal way and at a personal rate. For example, not all infants begin to crawl at the same time, but they do crawl before walking.

Social expectations can influence developmental tasks; society expects an individual to make certain adjustments during each period of development. The ages at which the child is expected to master the developmental tasks are partly determined by the culture. These tasks are similar to lessons that must be learned if the individual is to make a personal and social adjustment to the culture.

Development results from a combination of maturation and learning. Maturation refers to the emergence of the genetic potential that an individual possesses. Learning is the process of gaining specific knowledge or skills resulting from experience, training, and behavioral changes. Maturation and learning are also interrelated; no learning occurs unless the individual is mature enough to be able to understand and change behavior (see Hot Topics box, p. 411).

The foundations laid in the early years often determine the individual's future adjustments to life; therefore early accomplishments in development are crucial to successful later development. Early stages of development set the stage for subsequent steps in the sequence of expected development (Berger, 1998).

Growth and development are complex, interrelated processes that are influenced by and, in turn, can affect the health of an individual. The nurse who understands these relationships is aware of the need for age-specific health screening, nursing history questions, and health teaching.

Text continued on p. 411

Table 15-2 Flowchart Showing Directions of Growth Changes Throughout Life Cycle*

Overview of Developmental Changes	Prenatal→	Infancy→	Childhood→	Puberty and Adolescence→	Adulthood→	Middle Age→	Old Age
HEART AND CIRCULATORY SYSTEM							
Action of heart and circulatory system is under control of autonomic nervous system. Throughout life cardiac rate is responsive to organ needs and emotional states (fear, anxiety, tension, depression).	Heart formed and begins to beat about third week	Heart grows somewhat more slowly than rest of body (weight doubled by 1 yr, body weight tripled) Grows steadily during childhood With birth, considerable change in paths and relative volumes of blood flow, reflected in loss of certain fetal structures and changes in heart and major vessels		At puberty, heart takes part in rapid growth, reaching mature size with rest of body	Heart weight remains relatively constant after age 25 (only organ other than prostate that does not decrease in weight with age) Cardiac output decreases 30% to 40% between age 25 and 65 Cardiac strength lessens with age, whereas expenditure of energy is more than in youth. Capacity to increase rate and strength of beat during physical work is diminished		
	Heart rate high, approx. 150 beats/min	Heart rate falls steadily throughout childhood 130 beats/min Heart rate more variable during childhood—regular	70 to 80 beats/min	60 beats/min in adolescence rate differs with gender	After maturity, women have slightly higher pulse rate than men, 65 beats/min (girls' temperature remains stationary, higher than boys'); men maintain same pulse rate in maturity (slightly lower body temperature than women)		
			Not until midchildhood does peripheral blood picture become same as adult				
URINARY SYSTEM							
Parallels growth of body as a whole. Proportion of bodily water and solids follows pattern related to growth—tendency for human organism to dry out as life progresses. Function of kidneys, with other organ systems, is to help in regulation of internal environment of body	Young fetus is about 90% water Urinary system begins in first month	Newborn is about 70% water Urinary system does not complete full development until end of first year All renal units immature at birth; thus fluid and electrolyte imbalance occurs readily Kidney function adequate at birth if not subjected to undue stress	Composition of urine in healthy child (after age 2) changes very little as child matures; thus renal function and urinalysis can be used as monitor of well-being		Adult is about 58% water Glomerular filtration rate decreases about 47% from age 20 to 90		

DIGESTIVE SYSTEM							
As a whole, grows as total body grows, although evidence suggests that various parts of gastrointestinal system undergo separate periods of growth, maturity, and senescence.	Before birth nutrients are supplied through placental circulation; digestion and absorption do not occur in the gastrointestinal (GI) tract	Stomach size increases rapidly first months, then grows steadily throughout childhood Spurt of growth of puberty Digestive apparatus immature at birth (food passes through rapidly, reverse peristalsis common) Acidity of gastric juices varies over lifespan; low during infancy, rises in childhood, plateau about age 10, rise in puberty Free gastric acid (HCl) more marked in boys			All actions of the GI tract (food intake, digestion, absorption, elimination) not only respond to physiological needs but from birth to old age are sensitive to tensions and anxiety Available data suggest generalized atrophy of entire GI tract with advancing age Nutritional needs vary according to individual variation—decreasing metabolism→ decreasing enzyme production→ HCl→ stomach volume—tone of large intestine may become impaired until decrease with senescence (also diminished taste)		
	Salivary glands small at birth	Increase rapidly during first 3 mo; reach relative adult proportions by age 2					
SPECIAL SENSES							
Most are well developed at birth, although their association with higher centers comes about gradually during early life and diminishes with advancing age.	Begin very early in embryonic development—3 to 6 wk	Sense of touch is developed first, then hearing and vision Vision: infant can perceive simple differences in shape but not complex patterns (greater proportion of total growth before birth); various dimensions of vision develop at various ages, eye muscles function at mature level first year, fusion begins 9 mo until 6 yr; refractive power changes over life cycle—hyperopia increases until eyeball reaches adult size (approx. 8 yr), then reverses trend toward emmetropia—postpubertal years—toward myopia until 30—myopia decreases—hyperopia increases					
ADIPOSE TISSUE							
Although adipose tissue varies greatly from individual to individual, overall lifetime pattern exists. Fat accumulation varies greatly with body build and constitution.	Accumulates rapidly before birth; peak at seventh prenatal month	Increases rapidly during first 6 mo	Decreases from first to seventh year in both genders	Then begins to increase slowly to puberty		Typically both sexes tend to gain weight in 50s and 60s but do not maintain same body contours of earlier years at same at weight (increase deposit on abdomen and hips)	Usually fat stores are lost after seventh decade in both genders Sharpness in contours, increasingly prominent bony landmarks

Adapted from Sutterly, D., & Donneley, G.: Perspectives in human development: Nursing throughout the life cycle, Philadelphia, 1973, JB Lippincott.
*This chart indicates only general trends and directions of growth and development; it is not all inclusive. No distinct ages, absolute values, or ranges of normal variations are intended in this flowchart.

Continued

Table 15-2 Flowchart Showing Directions of Growth Changes Throughout Life Cycle—cont'd

Overview of Developmental Changes	Prenatal→	Infancy→	Childhood→	Puberty and Adolescence→	Adulthood→	Middle Age→	Old Age
ADIPOSE TISSUE—cont'd							
Relationship between caloric intake, amount of exercise, and utilization and/or accumulation of fat is not yet fully understood but is basis of much interrelated research today.	Premature infant may look wrinkled and scrawny because of lack of adipose tissue	(Gender differences are not noted in the body shape of prepubescent children)		Fat begins to accumulate slowly and continues uninterrupted in girls, producing feminine curves, and accounts for much of weight gain	Some girls slim down after full maturation; many maintain about the same amount of adipose as at puberty		
				Deposition of fat differs in body—amount decreases sharply at time of maximum growth spurt (increased weight caused by increase in muscle mass and bones)	After full maturation, fat accumulation begins→	(Continues→)	
LYMPHOID TISSUE							
Lymphoid tissue is scattered widely throughout body and includes lymph nodes, tonsils, adenoids, thymus, spleen, and lymphocytes of the blood; follows unique pattern of growth, rapid in infancy and begins to atrophy at puberty.	Begins in last month of uterine life—immunoglobulins cross placenta at levels equal to mother's and continue for several months after delivery	Grows most rapidly during infancy and childhood, reaching maximum size a few years before puberty; parallels development of immunity Thus increased incidence of disease with increasing age of child		Then atrophies and is smaller in volume at full maturity than during childhood			Thymus so small that it is difficult to locate in older people

RESPIRATORY SYSTEM						
Growth parallels that of total body growth. Respiratory apparatus is a highly organized system of organs under nervous and hormonal regulation, which functions in coordination with rest of body. Gender difference in gaseous exchange becomes apparent during puberty.	Before birth, air sacs do not contain air; oxygen supplied through maternal circulation	When umbilical cord is cut, infant must use own breathing apparatus—breathing irregular at first both in rate and depth—fast in infancy—gradually slowing through childhood until full maturity is reached			No gender difference in respiratory rate at anytime of life	Basal metabolism rate declines (rate higher in men than women)
		Respiratory exchange gradually becomes more efficient as life advances. Actual volume of air inhaled with each breath increases as lung size expands with general body growth. Vital capacity and maximum breathing capacity rise gradual in both genders, increasing more in boys during puberty; adult men have more efficient respiratory exchange, are capable of greater feats of muscular exertion without exhaustion than women.				
SKELETAL SYSTEMS						
Bone growth passes through successive stages of development from connective tissue to cartilage to osseous tissue; completion of calcification indicates end of growing period and is thus a useful measure of growth rate and physiological maturity. Most growth ceases in adolescence.	Follows cephalocaudal law of development		Reserved during growth spurt		Maximum height in early 20s to 30s	Then gradual decline until onset of senescence Thinning of vertebral disk beginning in middle years; most rapid in last decade
		After first year, legs fastest growing, 66% of total increase in height; longer puberty is delayed, greater the leg length				
	70% of head growth before birth; bones of hands and wrist laid down in cartilage	Trunk fastest growing, 60% of total increase		Length of trunk and depth of chest reach peak growth		
		At birth, shafts of metacarpals are ossified (and visible by radiograph); carpal bones begin to ossify	Growth of both genders nearly even until onset of puberty in girls first (approx. 10 yr) Boys begin approx. 2 yr later, but markedly greater Peak in height comes before peak in weight			Spinal column shortens (osteoporosis) with thinning vertebrae—shortening of trunk with long extremities—reversal of growth proportions in infancy

Adapted from Sutterly, D., & Donneley, G.: Perspectives in human development: Nursing throughout the life cycle, Philadelphia, 1973, JB Lippincott.

Continued

Table 15-2 Flowchart Showing Directions of Growth Changes Throughout Life Cycle—cont'd

Overview of Developmental Changes	Prenatal→	Infancy→	Childhood→	Puberty and Adolescence→	Adulthood→	Middle Age→	Old Age
MUSCULAR SYSTEM							
Number of striated muscle fibers is roughly same in all human beings. Tremendous difference in size, not only from fetus to adult, but between adults, is caused by ability of individual muscle fibers to increase in size. Growth potential, however, is influenced by genes, hormones, nutrition, exercise, and possibly other unknown factors as well.	Muscle formation begins early, assuming final shape by end of second month	Increases rapidly during infancy but slowly during childhood	Growth in both genders is same in childhood	With onset of puberty, muscle strength is greater in boys (when muscle growth is stimulated by testosterone)	Muscle mass continues to increase gradually—maximum strength in early adulthood—then declines slightly—according to use and genetic constitution Will increase in bulk and strength as used		
				Greatest increase begins in puberty; muscle size precedes muscle strength in boys			Until onset of senescence—atrophy and loss of muscle tone
			Increase in muscle size means increasing strength in children; increase in skill is more intimately related to maturation of nervous system				
NERVOUS SYSTEM							
Growth and maturation of central and peripheral nervous system (brain, cord, peripheral nerves, many sense organs) reflected by changing size of head.	Growth very rapid during intrauterine development; head increases at greater rate than rest of body	Has all the brain cells of first year, which will continue to increase in size; number and complexity of axons and dendrites will continue to increase			Function continues with use		Possible decrease in size and number of brain cells in senescence (?) (subject of study)
		All neural tissues grow rapidly during infancy and early childhood		(No neural growth spurt at puberty)			Decrease in myelin sheath, impulses decrease; slow down speed of action and reaction
		Brain grows rapidly after birth, reaching 90% of total size by age 2	By midchildhood, almost reaches adult size	Then slow increase to full maturity	Brain weight decreases with age		
	Segmented spinal nerves are mature, fully myelinated, and functioning at term (e.g., knee jerk), but acquisition of myelin in cortex, brainstem, and cord is closely correlated with observed behavior (myelinization of this tract follows cephalocaudal, proximodistal law)					Taste less acute, less discriminatory with advancing age	
		Equipment for sense of taste and smell present at birth and perhaps most acute at that time				Structural changes in CNS result in impaired perception	

REPRODUCTIVE SYSTEM						
Organs of reproductive system show little increase during early life but rapid development just before and coincident with puberty. Maturation and fulfillment of reproductive functions of maturity (in female) are followed by involution in later years.	Genital organs form during uterine life; uterus undergoes growth spurt before birth (hormone stimulation from mother)	Female sex organs well formed but not functioning at birth (but have full quota of sensory nerves)	Quiescent during childhood→	Maturation at puberty (menstruation)→		Involution after menopause
		Uterus undergoes involution to half its birth weight	Regained size by age 10 to 11→	Adult size at puberty→	Maximum increase with pregnancy→	Begin to atrophy with advancing age
		In male—testes, as with ovaries, remain dormant and small, not even growing in proportion to rest of body (with sensory nerves)	Until puberty, interstitial cells of Leydig reappear and secrete testosterone, so testes and penis continue to increase in size (pubic hair appears)			
	Mammary glands develop in both sexes during fetal life	Enlargement of breasts at birth (both sexes)→	Nonsecretory during childhood until puberty→	Development rapid→	Enlarge during pregnancy, developing alveoli→	Atrophy with advanced age
	Sex hormones; until puberty girls and boys produce male hormones (androgens) and female hormones (chiefly estrogens) in small and roughly equal amounts					
INTEGUMENTARY SYSTEM						
Includes skin and its appendages and adnexa (nails, hair, sebaceous glands, eccrine and apocrine sweat glands). Although all skin is similar, this organ shows considerable variability in different parts of body (and from individual to individual) and varies greatly during the lifespan.	Hair, skin, and sebaceous glands fully formed *in utero*	Skin contains all its adult structures at birth but immature in function	Matures slowly until puberty (children prone to rashes)	Rapid spurt in maturation of skin and all its structures		Changes in skin most obvious sign of aging (exposure and environmental conditions)
	Lanugo begins to decrease before birth and continues regression few weeks postnatally→		Replaced by body hair, less extensive distribution; marked difference in type and distribution of hair at puberty→			Regenerative and growth power decreases and skin loses elasticity
	Activity of sebaceous decreases after birth→			Increases rapidly at puberty (more prone to acne)		

Adapted from Sutterly, D., & Donneley, G.: Perspectives in human development: Nursing throughout the life cycle, Philadelphia, 1973, JB Lippincott.

Continued

Table 15-2 Flowchart Showing Directions of Growth Changes Throughout Life Cycle—cont'd

Overview of Developmental Changes	Prenatal→	Infancy→	Childhood→	Puberty and Adolescence→	Adulthood→	Middle Age→	Old Age
ENDOCRINE SYSTEM							
Consists of number of glandular structures scattered throughout the body. Although small in size, their hormones influence all growth and development of whole organism	Immaturity of entire endocrine system puts infant at disadvantage if required to adjust to wide fluctuations in concentration of water, electrolytes, glucose, amino acids. All are interrelated, but each organ develops at own rate; Thyroid—increases from midfetal life to maturity; slightly larger in boys than girls; growth spurt at adolescence Adrenals—after birth decrease in size and continue throughout first year, increase again during childhood (but smaller than birth); spurt at puberty, reaching maturity with rest of body; greater increase in male gonads and testes and female ovaries (endocrine glands as well as reproductive organs), follow genital type of growth pattern Hypophysis, or pituitary gland—produces or stimulates hormones that influence growth Parathyroids—produce hormones that maintain homeostasis of calcium and phosphorus Islets of Langerhans—dispersed through pancreas; produce insulin and glucagon					With age, decline occurs in all endocrine gland functions	

Adapted from Sutterly, D., & Donneley, G.: Perspectives in human development: Nursing throughout the life cycle, Philadelphia, 1973, JB Lippincott.

research highlights

Environmental Risk on Developmental Outcome

For ages, the debate over nature versus nurture has taken place. Is the child born with a *tabula rasa* (blank slate) on which the environment exerts a significant force, or is the child born with all characteristics that determine future development?

There is emerging research that shows that the environment exerts a significant effect on developmental outcome. This effect is often negative when environmental factors such as poverty are considered. Recent studies have shown that biological risks will determine whether a compromised outcome will occur. However, environmental factors will influence the degree of compromise.

Environmental risk factors include quality of the mother-infant interaction and opportunities for age-appropriate stimulation. Biological risk factors include prenatal, perinatal, or postnatal adverse events, such as asphyxia or low birth weight. Frequently, environmental risk factors and biological risk factors occur together. The accumulation of risk factors is the major contributor to developmental morbidity. Environmental risk factors most strongly influence verbal and general cognitive outcome; biological factors are more strongly related to neurological, motor, and perceptual-performance function. Intervention strategies must take in to account the following principles:

- Intervention may not enhance development, but simply prevents a decline.
- Medical-biological risk may produce a *ceiling* that will affect the influence of intervention efforts.
- Individual family participation may be one of the most important factors affecting outcome.
- Intervention foci and techniques must vary, depending on the child's age.

Adapted from Aylward, G. P. (1996). Environmental risk, intervention and developmental outcome. *Ambulatory Child Health, 2,* 161-170.

HOT topics

SELF-ESTEEM IN MALES VERSUS FEMALES

Recent statistics have shown that boys are encountering more difficulties in growing up and succeeding in schools and colleges. Consider the following:

- An increasing number of boys are reared in fatherless homes.
- Boys are less likely to complete high school, attend college, and stay out of jail than are girls.
- Boys commit 75% of suicides in the age group of 10 and 14 years.
- Four times as many boys as girls are prescribed Ritalin for attention deficit disorder.

Years of concern for the self-esteem of girls have paid off. Gender equity programs in school appear to have worked to the benefit of girls. Girls can now be a tomboy or feminine; either role is acceptable. Girls have become empowered to become who they want to be. Should boys be socialized to be more like girls? Is the rowdy, aggressive play of boys normal, or is it something to be reined in with discipline and medication? Some researchers believe that violence is a response to pressure placed on boys to conform to a macho stereotype.

- Should boys be allowed to be boys?
- Should boys be encouraged to express their emotions easily?
- What are the consequences of the current education system that seems suited to girls rather than boys?

Adapted from Leo, J. (2000, July 17). Boys will be boys. *US News and World Report.*

THEORIES OF DEVELOPMENT

Specific aspects of development of the person have been studied for centuries. Many theories of development are used in the study of individuals throughout the lifespan; the nurse may wish to refer to a text on developmental psychology to become familiar with some of these theories. Three widely used theories of psychosocial and cognitive development are employed throughout this unit to gain a holistic view of the progression of individual development throughout the lifespan. These theories were developed by Erikson, Piaget, Gilligan, and Kohlberg.

Psychosocial Development: Erikson's Theory

Erikson (1968, 1993, 1998) described the development of identity of the self and the ego through successive stages that naturally unfold throughout the lifespan. Although he studied with Freud and supported the psychosexual theory of development, **Erikson's theory of psychosocial development** is based on the need of each person to develop a sense of trust in self and others and a sense of personal worth. Erikson described a healthy personality in positive terms, not merely through the absence of disease. Psychosocial adaptation is based on critical steps, each requiring resolution of a conflict between two opposing qualities. The successful outcome of each stage results in specific, lasting outcomes. Accomplishment of each successive task provides the foundation for a healthy self-identity. Each stage depends on the stage before it and must be successfully accomplished for the person to proceed toward successful accomplishment of the next. The influence of other people and the environment is significant, but the motivation to achieve the challenges of identity arises from within.

Although each of the conflicts is predominant at a certain stage in life, recognizing that all the conflicts exist

CASE STUDY

Samantha

Samantha is a 2-month-old infant who is admitted to the children's hospital for meningitis. She must receive 10 days of intravenous antibiotics as the standard treatment. Her mother lives 100 miles away and is a single mother with other children at home. The mother must continue to work to support her family and provide the insurance. Samantha will therefore be alone in the hospital except on the weekend. As a nurse, consider the promotion of normal growth and development as part of your nursing care.

1. What stage of psychosocial development is Samantha experiencing according to Erikson?
2. What are important nursing interventions to facilitate a successful outcome of this stage?
3. What are some developmentally appropriate toys and play that the nurse can provide?

MULTICULTURAL AWARENESS

Cultural Differences in Child-Rearing Practices

Nurses can play a key role in enhancing positive parenting practices that improve the well being of children. Culture plays an important role in the socialization of children. Activities such as feeding, toileting, discipline, and seeking health care are all influenced by culture.

Having an understanding of and respect for the beliefs of others is important in the increasingly multicultural society. Much of the research on which professionals rely on has been carried out by and within the dominant North American, White culture. This research may not represent the actual concerns of people from minority cultures.

The Black population is the largest minority group in the United States. Nurses need to become more familiar with child-rearing beliefs and practices within this community to develop strategies for anticipatory guidance.

In the European-American research, much importance has been placed on the theory of attachment and need for the development of a close relationship with a consistent mother figure. In the Black community, a baby may not have one consistent caregiver. The responsibility for infant care may be dispersed among family members, especially when the mother is an adolescent. The extended family is extremely important because there are a large number of single-parent households. Informal adoption and shared parenting are common.

Black families use a discipline style that places more emphasis on obedience and parent-defined rules than does the mainstream culture, which values the child's autonomy and individuality.

For Black adults, there is greater emphasis on group loyalty, interdependence, and conformity, which is in direct contrast to the North American, White orientation toward competition, autonomy, and self-reliance.

In the North American, Anglo-Saxon parenting style, emphasis is placed on early learning, and parents often begin a programmed learning environment when the child is still a fetus. In the Black culture, less emphasis is placed on the parent as teacher. The child is expected to learn by observation of adults and through participation in daily activities.

Teaching and anticipatory guidance are framed within these expectations. The nurse must be aware of motivators in the culture. The context within which parenting is accomplished must also be considered.

Modified from Yoos, H. L., Kitzman, H., Olds, D. L., & Overacker, I. (1995). Child rearing beliefs in the African-American community: Implications for culturally competent pediatric care. *Journal of Pediatric Nursing, 10*, 343.

in each person, to some extent, at all times and that a conflict, once resolved, may emerge again in appropriate situations is important.

These stages are summarized in Table 15-3. Each of these psychosocial stages is discussed more fully in the specific chapters on each developmental age.

Cognitive Development: Piaget's Theory

Another aspect of development is the progressive acquisition of higher levels of cognitive skills. Jean Piaget, a Swiss psychologist trained in zoology, viewed the child as a biological organism acting on the environment. The child's main goal is to master the environment or, in other words, to establish harmony or equilibrium between the self and the environment.

Piaget's theory of cognitive development is concerned primarily with structure rather than content; that is, with how the mind works rather than with what it does. The concern of this theory is more with understanding than it is with predicting and controlling behavior (Phillips, 1969). Piaget uses the word *scheme* to describe a pattern of action or thought. A scheme is used to take in or assimilate new experiences or may be modified or accommodated by new experiences. Each person is striving to maintain a balance, or equilibrium, between assimilation and accommodation (Phillips, 1969, Piaget, 1950).

Piaget described the stages of cognitive development throughout the developmental years. Through a natural unfolding of ability, the child acquires sequentially predictable cognitive abilities. Given adequate environ-

Table 15-3 Erikson's Eight Stages of Human Development

Stage (approximate)	Psychosocial Stages	Lasting Outcomes
1. Infancy	Basic trust versus basic mistrust	Drive and hope
2. Toddler stage	Autonomy versus shame and doubt	Self-control and willpower
3. Preschool stage	Initiative versus guilt	Direction and purpose
4. Middle childhood stage (school age)	Industry versus inferiority	Method and competence
5. Adolescence	Identity versus role confusion	Devotion and fidelity
6. Young adulthood	Intimacy versus isolation	Affiliation and love
7. Middle adulthood	Generativity versus stagnation	Production and care
8. Older adulthood	Ego integrity versus despair	Renunciation and wisdom

Modified from Erikson, E. H. (1993). *Childhood and society* (35th ed.). New York: W.W. Norton; Erikson, E. H., & Erikson, J. M. (1998). *Life cycle completed*. New York: W.W. Norton.

Table 15-4 Piaget's Stages of Cognitive Development

Stage	Age	Characteristics
Sensorimotor	0 to 2 years	Thought dominated by physical manipulation of objects and events
Substage 1	0 to 1 month	Pure reflex adaptations
Substage 2	1 to 4 months	Primary circular reactions
Substage 3	4 to 8 months	Secondary circular reactions
Substage 4	8 to 12 months	Coordination of secondary schemata
Substage 5	12 to 18 months	Tertiary circular reactions infancy, rise in childhood; plateau about age 10, rise in puberty
Substage 6	18 to 24 months	Invention of new solutions through mental combinations
Preoperational	2 to 7 years	Functions symbolically using language as major tool
Preconceptual	2 to 4 years	Uses representational thought to recall past, represent present, and anticipate future
Intuitive	4 to 7 years	Increased symbolic functioning
Concrete operations	7 to 11 years	Mental reasoning processes assume logical approaches to solving concrete problems
Formal operations	11 to 15 years	True logical thought and manipulation of abstract concepts emerge

Modified from Schuster, C., & Ashburn, S. (1992). *The process of human development: A holistic lifespan approach*. Boston: Lippincott.

mental stimuli and an intact neurological system, the child gradually matures toward full ability to conceptualize. Piaget's theory of cognitive development encompasses the time from birth to approximately 15 years of age. Four distinct stages are divided into a number of substages (Piaget, 1950, 1976). These stages are summarized in Table 15-4 and discussed more fully in the specific chapters on each developmental age.

Piaget suggests that quantitative, but no further qualitative, changes in cognitive function take place after approximately age 15. This cognitive theory of development has far-reaching implications for the nurse in assessing health status and in teaching health promotion. Even the concept of health may not be understood by the child or adult who is unable to grasp abstract ideas.

Moral Development: Kohlberg's Theory

A specific aspect of cognitive development is the development of moral thinking and judgment. **Kohlberg's theory of moral development** is based on interviews with young people from school age through young adulthood. These interviews are focused on hypothetical moral dilemmas; for example, should a man steal an expensive drug that would save his dying wife?

The responses to these moral dilemmas indicate that there are distinct sequential stages of moral thinking. These stages depend greatly on cognitive development and always follow the same sequence. There are three levels of moral judgment and each level consists of two stages. These levels and stages are outlined in Table 15-5 (Kohlberg, 1981; Kohlberg & Kramer, 1969).

In society, progression through the successive stages of moral development generally takes place during the school age, adolescent, and young adult years. Not everyone progresses through all stages. In fact, only a minority of adults operates in stage six or even stage five (Kohlberg, 1981). Beyond the young adult years, a stabilization or increased consistency of thought and perhaps an increased correlation between moral judgment and moral action can occur (Kohlberg, 1981).

CARE PLAN

Nursing Diagnosis:
Altered Family Processes Related to Grandmother Taking Up Residence in the Family Home

DEFINING CHARACTERISTICS

- Expressed concern regarding disruption of family routine
- Expressed differing expectations for behavior of children
- Increased stress or nervousness
- Verbal hostility between husband and wife

RELATED FACTORS

- Change in family roles
- Change in family structure
- Change of environment for maternal grandmother

EXPECTED OUTCOMES

- Family members will acknowledge change in family roles.
- Family members will identify coping patterns.
- Family members will develop plan for communicating expectations to children.

NURSING INTERVENTIONS

- Assess individuals' perceptions of the problem.
- Evaluate strengths, coping skills, and current support systems.
- Encourage family to verbalize feelings.
- Phrase problems as *family* problems as they are owned and dealt with by the family.
- Assist family in breaking down problems into manageable parts.
- Assist with problem-solving process, with delineated responsibilities and follow-through.
- Identify community resources that may be helpful.

Adapted from Gulanick, M. (1998). *Nursing care plans: Nursing diagnosis and interventions*. St. Louis: Mosby.

Table 15-5 Kohlberg's Stages of Moral Development

Level and Stage	What Is Right	Reasons for Doing Right
Level A: Preconventional		
Stage 1: Punishment and obedience	Avoiding breaking rules, obey for obedience's sake, and avoid doing physical damage to people and property	Avoiding punishment and the superior power of authorities
Stage 2: Individual instrumental purpose and exchange	Following rules when it is in someone's immediate interest Using fairness equal exchange, agreement	Serving one's own needs or interests in a world where one must recognize that other people have interests as well
Level B: Conventional		
Stage 3: Mutual interpersonal expectations, relationships, and conformity	Living up to what is expected by relatives and friends or what is generally expected in one's role as son, sister, friend, and so on *Being good* is important	Needing to be good in one's own eyes and those of others Following the *golden rule*
Stage 4: Social system and conscience maintenance	Fulfilling actual duties to which one has agreed Laws are to be upheld except if they conflict with other fixed social duties and rights Contributing to society, the group, or the institution	Keeping institution going as a whole Using self-respect or conscience to meet one's defined obligations
Level B/C: Transition	—	Basing reasons on emotions; conscience is arbitrary and relative
Level C: Postconventional and principled		
Stage 3: Prior rights and social contract or utility	Being aware that persons hold a variety of values and opinions, most of which are relative to one's group Realizing that some nonrelative values and rights, such as life and liberty, must be upheld in any society	Feeling obligated to obey the law because one has made a social contract to make and abide by laws for good of all; the greatest good for the greatest number
Stage 6: Universal ethical principles	Acting in accordance with the principle when laws violate universal ethical principles Understanding the equality of human rights and respecting the dignity of human beings as individuals	As a rational person, seeing validity of principles and becoming committed to them

Compiled from Kohlberg, L. (1981). *The philosophy of moral development, vol. 1*. San Francisco: Harper & Row.

Table 15-6 Gilligan's Model of Moral Development in Women

Level	Characteristics
1. Individual survival	What is practical and best for self, realizing connection to others
2. Goodness as self-sacrifice	Sacrifices wants and needs to fulfill others' wants and needs
3. Nonviolence	Moral equality of self and others

Others studies on moral development in women and men by Gilligan have demonstrated gender differences in describing high morality. Women discussed issues of selfishness versus responsibility, of exercising care, and the avoidance of hurting. Men described terms of justice, fairness, and the rights of individuals. **Gilligan's theory of moral development** suggests that there is a different process of moral development in women in society (1982, 1990). This model is summarized in Table 15-6.

These theories of development provide the nurse with a framework for observations, interactions, and health care planning for individuals and their family members. Each person and family exists in a larger community; this community, whether on a local, state, or national level, can greatly influence the availability of health care and the climate of health promotion versus a disease focus of care.

SUMMARY

Individuals make many choices that affect their health each day and multiple factors may influence how these choices are made. The stage of motor, social, and cognitive development can greatly influence how the person perceives a situation and the choices arising from that situation. The nurse who has studied development has a clearer idea of how a person may respond to a given idea or situation at a specific age or stage of development.

REFERENCES

Berger, K. S. (1998). *The developing person through the life span* (4th ed.). New York: Worth Publishers.

Erikson, E. H. (1986). *Childhood and society* (35th anniversary edition). New York: Norton.

Erikson, E. H. (1968). *Identity, youth and crisis*. New York: Norton.

Erikson, E. H., & Erikson, G. M. (1998). *Lifecycle completed*. New York: Norton.

Gilligan, C. (1982). *In a different voice: Psychological theory and women's development*. Cambridge, MA: Harvard University Press.

Gilligan, C. (1990). *Mapping the moral domain*. Cambridge, MA: Harvard University Press.

Guyton, A. C. (1996). *Textbook of medical physiology* (9th ed.). Philadelphia: WB Saunders.

Kohlberg, L. (1981). *The philosophy of moral development: Vol. 1*. San Francisco: Harper & Row.

Kohlberg, L., & Kramer, R. (1969). Continuities and discontinuities in childhood and adult moral development. *Human Development, 12*, 93.

Phillips, J. R. (1969). *The origins of intellect: Piaget's theory*. San Francisco: W.H. Freeman.

Piaget, J. (1950). *The psychology of intelligence*. London: Routledge and Kegan Paul.

Piaget, J. (1976). *The grasp of consciousness, action and concept in the young child* (translated by S. Wedgwood). Cambridge, MA: Harvard University Press.

Seidel, H. M., Ball, J. W., Dains, J. E., & Benedict, G. W. (1999). *Mosby's physical examination handbook*. St. Louis: Mosby.

Yoos, H. L., Kitzman, H., Olds, D. L., & Overacker, I. (1995). Child rearing beliefs in the African-American community: Implications for culturally competent pediatric care. *Journal of Pediatric Nursing, 10*, 343.

Chapter 16

CAROLYN SPENCE CAGLE

The Prenatal Period

objectives

After completing this chapter, the nurse will be able to:

- Discuss fetal development and the newborn transition to extrauterine life.
- Outline changes in the maternal system during pregnancy and their influence on pregnancy adaptation.
- Discuss the role of the nurse in promoting the physical, mental, and spiritual health of the childbearing family.
- Discuss possible fetal problems caused by maternal drinking, smoking, drug use, and viral exposure of the fetus during pregnancy.
- Discuss the nursing role during labor and delivery with a focus on the physical, emotional, and educational needs of the delivering woman and her family.
- Analyze the influence of factors such as ethnicity, legislative priorities, and practices of the current health care delivery system on childbirth care and the needs of families.

key terms

Acquired Immune Deficiency Syndrome
Amniocentesis
Apgar Scoring System
Bradycardia
Candida Albicans
Cervix
Chlamydia
Chorionic and Amniotic Membranes
Chorionic Villi
Colostrum
Congenital Defect
Cytomegalovirus
Decidua
Down Syndrome
Embryo
Endometrium
Episiotomy
Estrogen
Fertilization
Fetal Heart Monitor
Fetus
First Stage (of Labor)
Fourth Stage (of Labor)
Fundus
Gonococcus
Group Beta Streptococcus
Hepatitis B
Herpes Simplex Virus
Human Chorionic Gonadotrophin
Infant Mortality Rate
Intervillous Spaces
Lamaze
Lecithin-Sphingomyelin Ratio
Meconium
Moro Reflex
Pica
Placenta
Positive Signs of Pregnancy
Probable Signs of Pregnancy
Progesterone
Quickening
Rubella
Second Stage (of Labor)
Sexually Transmitted Disease
Spontaneous Abortion
Syphilis
Tachycardia
Teratogen
Thalidomide
Third Stage (of Labor)
Toxoplasmosis
Trimester
Ultrasound
Zygote

THINK About It

First Pregnancy Labor

Laura, currently at 41 weeks of her first pregnancy, is admitted at 2:00 AM to St. Jude's Medical Center with uterine contractions occurring every 8 minutes since midnight. Her cervix is 2 cm and 80% effaced with a station of -3. Her husband is out of town on a business trip and Laura's neighbor has accompanied her to the hospital. Despite the fact that Laura attended Lamaze classes with her husband, she is anxious about the labor. She says to the nurse, "My back is about to break, I have so much bottom pressure, and I wanted to go natural, without medication and all this high-technology stuff, including the monitor."

1. Based on your knowledge of ethical and legal principles of care, how would you as a caregiver approach Laura to support her needs appropriately with labor and delivery?
2. What factors in your database would support the use of the fetal heart monitor? What factors would not support use of the monitor?
3. What political, legal, ethical, and other factors might be relevant to the wide-range use of monitors in American maternity units today?
4. How does the use of fetal heart rate monitoring involve a health-promotion approach to labor and delivery?

The mystery of life before birth has fascinated scientists, philosophers, and theologians for centuries. With the conception of a child, a miraculous series of events occurs that influence the entire life of the developing individual. Some of these events are presently beyond human control and understanding; others have been discovered and described only recently. This new knowledge has led to speculation about and experimentation with ways to ensure a better life for the child and eventually for all human beings.

The process of conception, pregnancy, and birth involves a complex interaction of many factors, including the physiological and psychological changes in the woman and her family and the development of a fetus into a viable newborn. The focus of this chapter is on the pregnant woman, her family, and the developing fetus; discussing one without the others is impossible. The nurse must consider all three entities when seeking to promote a healthy pregnancy and a healthy family system after birth.

PHYSICAL CHANGES IN MATERNAL AND FETAL SYSTEMS

The physical changes during pregnancy discussed here include natural processes involving fertilization of the egg by the sperm, implantation of the fertilized egg into the uterus, embryonic or fetal growth and development, placental development and function, and maternal changes related to the pregnancy process.

Duration of Pregnancy

Pregnancy begins with the union of a sperm and egg, a process called **fertilization.** Under normal healthy circumstances, a pregnancy lasts approximately 9 (solar) months, or 10 lunar months. The last normal menstrual period (LNMP) is a more certain date than the precise moment of conception; therefore calculation of the estimated date of birth occurs by considering the LNMP as the beginning of the pregnancy. Determining the estimated date of delivery (EDD) involves using Nägele's rule: adding 7 days to the date of the first day of the LNMP and subtracting 3 months. Therefore if a woman's LNMP began on July 13, then the EDD would be determined by adding 7 days to July 13 (July 20) and subtracting 3 months, arriving at the date of April 20. If the LNMP occurred late in a year, the EDD will, of course, fall in the following year. A normal pregnancy consists of 9 months and three equal time periods or **trimesters,** which are used to discuss expected fetal and maternal changes during pregnancy.

Fertilization

The union of sperm and egg requires the existence of several crucial factors, many of which are not fully understood. When a sperm cell successfully penetrates an egg in the fallopian tube, the beginning of a human being called a **zygote** results. Additional division of zygotic cells results in more differentiated structures that eventually produce an embryo and a fetus, which will be discussed later in this chapter.

Various factors must be in place for fertilization to occur and absence of one or more of these factors may cause infertility (the failure of the couple to achieve a pregnancy despite sexual intercourse over time). For example, both a sperm cell and an egg cell must be in a proper state of maturity and in the fallopian tube for approximately 5 hours for union to occur. The sperm must possess high motility and the ability to secrete an enzyme or enzymes that aid in the dissolution of the membrane that surrounds the egg at the point of entry. Although the process of sperm formation (spermatogenesis) requires a low temperature in the man's testes, fertilization requires a certain basal body temperature in the woman. The sperm must be of uniform size and shape and be normally formed. The fallopian tube must be free from adhesions or obstructions to permit transportation of the egg and the zygote. A woman will likely conceive within 24 hours after ovulation. However, because sperm live for up to 72 hours in the female reproductive tract, fertilization may take place if intercourse has occurred up to 3 days before ovulation.

Implantation

Transplantation of the fertilized egg into the uterine cavity through the fallopian tube usually requires approximately 6 days (Georges, 2000). The zygote continues to develop through exposure to secretions from the glands that line the tube. After the zygote reaches the uterus, it remains unattached for an additional 2 to 5 days, but receives nutrition from secretions of the **endometrium,** the inner lining of the uterus (Guyton & Hall, 1997). The cells around the developing zygote secrete enzymes that begin to digest and liquefy the endometrial lining and initiate the conditions required for attaching the zygote to the uterine wall and beginning development of the **placenta.** The placenta provides primary nourishment to the baby and protects the baby throughout the pregnancy process.

Fertilization triggers the production of large amounts of **progesterone** (Georges, 2000; Solomon, 1992). This hormone has already stimulated the formation of endometrial cells rich in glycogen, proteins, lipids, and minerals; the extra supply of progesterone stimulates further development of fetal nourishing cells in the uterus, known as **decidua.** The decidua provides nutrition for the **embryo,** the term defining the growing baby from 2 to 8 gestational weeks. The placenta begins to function within a week after implantation and also helps to nourish the developing organism throughout the pregnancy.

Fetal Growth and Development

The stages of physical development during embryonic life have been defined for each structural system of the body. Metabolic functions, particularly endocrine and neurological, are less well defined. The following description of embryonic development is for normal conditions. Appropriate fetal development depends on these events occurring in a specified period and order during each trimester of pregnancy. When cells do not develop adequately at the necessary point in time and sequence, abnormality in structure or function occurs in the **fetus** and potential newborn. This abnormality has been called a **congenital defect.** This defects may be noted at birth, did not occur at conception (as do genetic defects), but most likely resulted because some disruption occurred during fetal development and after conception. Box 16-1 summarizes growth and development of the fetus during each trimester.

Placental Development and Function

The placenta begins to develop at implantation with integration of the embryonic and decidual cells. The **chorionic and amniotic membranes,** which surround the fetus throughout gestation, also begin to form along with the placenta. Additionally, the manufacture of amniotic fluid by the amniotic membrane occurs to support the developing infant and to protect it from injury.

The basic structure of the placenta (Fig. 16-1) allows interchanges between the mother and the fetus to provide

Box 16-1 Summary of Fetal Growth and Development During Pregnancy

FIRST TRIMESTER

- Very rapid cellular growth occurs.
- Distinct tissue layers for organs needed for extrauterine life develop.
- Rudimentary respiratory, neurological, gastrointestinal, skeletal, muscular, and blood systems exist.
- By sixth week, four-chambered heart and basic circulatory system present.
- Recognizable arms and legs, large head, and protuberant abdomen noted on sonogram.
- By eighth week, embryo becomes fetus and reflects well-formed fingers and toes, a more erect posture, and more humanlike features.
- By tenth to twelfth week, facial structure differentiates, oral palate fuses, and nasal septum forms nasal passages.
- By end of first trimester, able to discern physical differences of male and female fetus.
- At 12 weeks of pregnancy, fetus approximately 10 cm in length.

SECOND TRIMESTER

- At 16 weeks, eyes move closer to nasal bridge, trunk and limbs become more proportional to head, hair growth occurs on head.
- **Meconium** (fecal matter) occurs in fetal intestine.
- Lungs structurally complete, but functionally immature.
- Entire skeletal system exists.
- *Quickening* (intrauterine movements of fetus felt by the mother) occurs approximately 20 weeks.
- Fetus lacks subcutaneous fat and is wrinkled and lean in appearance.
- Myelinization of spinal cord occurs.
- Lanugo (fine distribution of hair to insulate fetus) appears.
- By twentieth week, 25 cm in length and approximately 1 lb in weight.

THIRD TRIMESTER

- Pulmonary function reflects immaturity because of evolving formation of alveoli, pulmonary branching, and low surfactant levels; maturity reached by end of third trimester when these processes are more developed.
- Mature lung status (adequate surfactant development) assessed by measuring **lecithin-sphingomyelin ratio** (L/S) in amniotic fluid of pregnant woman.
- Rapid weight gain and refinement of body systems: fetus weighs 3 lb at 28 weeks and 7 lb at 40 weeks of gestation.
- All sensory organs functional and myelinization of brain begins.
- Reflexes begin to appear (**Moro reflex**, rooting, sucking, and startle) for extrauterine adaptation; reflexes more mature at latter parts of pregnancy.

Adapted from Georges, J. M. (2000). Female genital and reproductive function. In L. C. Copstead, & J. L. Banaski, *Pathophysiology: Biological and behavioral perspectives* (2nd ed., pp. 742-781). Philadelphia: W.B. Saunders; Guyton, A. C., & Hall, J. E. (1997). *Human physiology and mechanisms of disease* (6th ed.). Philadelphia: W.B. Saunders.

nourishment for the fetus and the excretion of fetal waste matter. Throughout most of gestation, increasing complexity of the placenta allows maternal blood to flow through the **intervillous spaces** and for fetal circulation to flow through the **chorionic villi** (Georges, 2000; Guyton & Hall, 1996). The unique structure of the tissues between the maternal and fetal circulatory systems permits the exchange of certain molecules, but prevents the two blood supplies from mixing for most of the pregnancy.

The placenta supplies the fetus with essential nutrients, provides for the excretion of wastes, and protects the fetus from harmful substances. However, additional research continues to predict particular substances that will cross the placenta. Larger and heavier molecules normally do not pass, whereas lighter molecules (such as anesthetic gases, oxygen, carbon dioxide, and electrolytes) cross the placenta readily. Other processes, such as diffusion, pinocytosis, facilitated diffusion, and active transport, have also been implicated as transfer mechanisms (Guyton & Hall, 1997). As there is difficulty predicting exactly which substances cross the placenta, pregnant women need to be informed that they should avoid any agent that might be potentially dangerous to the fetus early in pregnancy and preferably before conception.

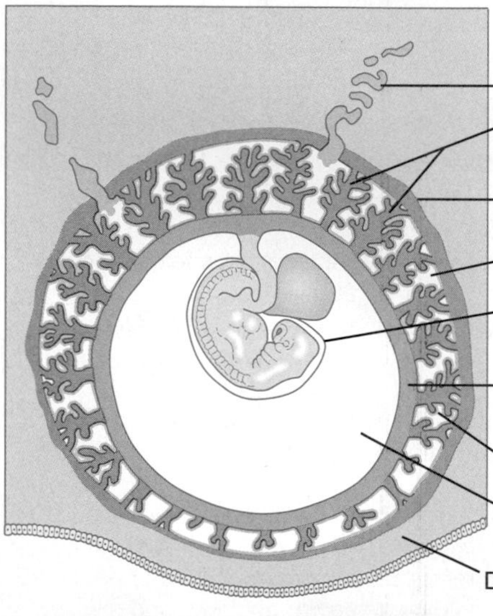

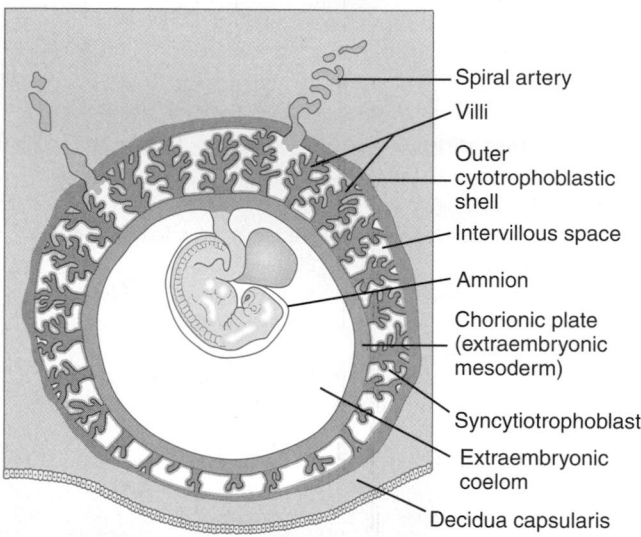

Fig. 16-1 Structure of placenta. (From Carlson, B. M. [1999]. *Human embryology and developmental biology.* St. Louis: Mosby).

Inspection of the placenta after birth reveals important clues that can help interpret the adequacy of gestational life. The placenta contains 14 to 30 distinctive lobules that are separated from one another by thin, septal partitions. The maternal side of the placenta appears dark red and spongy and the fetal side is shiny gray and glassy in consistency. The umbilical cord normally rises from near the center of the placenta and the membranes rise smoothly from the rim. Abnormal insertion of the cord, necrotic areas of the placenta, abnormal insertion of the membranes, or two umbilical vessels rather than three may cause possible problems during gestation, which may not be immediately apparent in the infant at birth.

The fetus, which has continued to gain strength and maturity during the later weeks of gestation, generally assumes a dependent position, with the head resting in the lower maternal pelvis. Figure 16-2 illustrates the relationship of the developing fetus to the placental and membranous structures. The membranes provide fetal protection from infection and act as a container for the amniotic fluid. As birth begins, the membranes may rupture, causing the loss of amniotic fluid and increased uterine contractions or *tightenings* of the uterus, reflective of the labor process. When the rupture of the membranes occurs more than 24 hours before delivery, infection and potential fetal harm are possible. A rupture may cause significant concern in a preterm pregnant woman who may require hospitalization for the remainder of her pregnancy because of concerns about maternal and fetal health.

As gestation nears completion, placental function gradually decreases, which may serve as one possible stimulus for the onset of labor. When pregnancy continues beyond 42 weeks or 2 weeks beyond the calculated due date, placental function decreases even more, posing concerns about the well being of the fetus.

This discussion of fetal development provides only half of the story about the prenatal period. Maternal changes and culmination of the prenatal period, labor, and birth are also important to address.

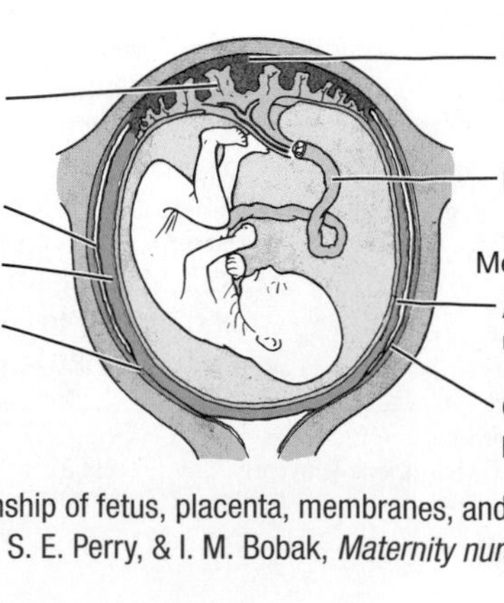

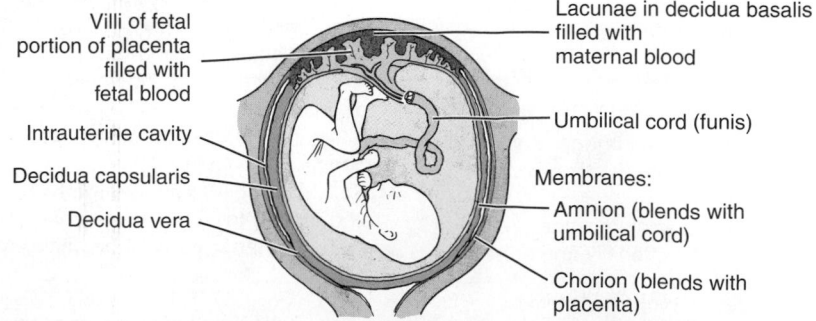

Fig. 16-2 Diagrammatic representation of relationship of fetus, placenta, membranes, and uterus during gestation. (From Perry, S. E. [1999]. Conception and fetal development. In D. L. Lowdermilk, S. E. Perry, & I. M. Bobak, *Maternity nursing* [5th ed., p. 162]. St. Louis: Mosby).

Maternal Changes

A combination of hormonal and mechanical changes creates the physiological effects that a woman experiences during gestation. The hormonal influences tend to increase as the pregnancy progresses. The mechanical (hemodynamic) changes reach a peak in the seventh or eighth month and then gradually decline as the pregnancy nears completion (Guyton & Hall, 1996).

Signs of Pregnancy

The woman may first assume that she is pregnant because she has skipped a menstrual period and may have nausea and vomiting, changes in breast sensations and size, and/or increased urinary frequency (presumptive signs of pregnancy). When these signs are present, the woman should seek a pregnancy test. A number of over-the-counter pregnancy tests are available without prescriptions, but women should be cautioned against relying on these tests because concurrent medication or substance use can cause a false reading. A home pregnancy test that is performed too early may create a false-negative outcome because the woman has not yet produced enough **human chorionic gonadotropin** (HCG), a hormone of pregnancy produced by the placenta, detected in her urine.

Probable signs of pregnancy, objective changes that carry a high degree of probability of pregnancy, may also be observed by the health care provider after a woman seeks care because she suspects pregnancy. These probable signs predict with greater certainty that a pregnancy exists than do the presumptive signs (Box 16-2).

Until recently, the **positive signs of pregnancy,** which diagnose fetal existence, did not usually occur until the second trimester (see Box 16-2). However, with the advent of first-trimester, real-time **ultrasound** (sonogram) testing, health care providers can now often determine fetal and placental adequacy early in pregnancy. This technology, using high frequency sound waves that bounce off the fetus and interpreted by a computer, allows defined visualization of the fetus and gestational structures throughout pregnancy (Fig. 16-3).

Adaptive Changes of Other Systems

In addition to the obvious changes in the reproductive system, adaptive changes in other bodily systems occur during the three trimesters of pregnancy.

The urinary system undergoes dramatic changes during gestation, with a 50% increase in glomerular filtration rate (GFR) (Georges, 2000). Starting in early pregnancy, the renal collecting structures become dilated, creating a physiological hydronephrosis of pregnancy. In all probability, the hormones of estrogen and progesterone create these changes (Guyton & Hall, 1997). The pregnancy hormones influence smooth muscle tone and glandular and mucosal secretions within the gastrointestinal tract; constipation, heartburn, and increased salivation may occur. Although these symptoms do not usually result in serious problems, they can be annoying for the pregnant woman.

Circulatory system changes begin early in pregnancy, as demonstrated by an increase in cardiac output from 30% to 40% by the end of the first trimester. An increase of 30% in total blood volume also takes place during pregnancy (Georges, 2000; Guyton & Hall, 1997). Physiological anemia of pregnancy may result, with a greater proportion of plasma than red blood cells being produced at this time.

Respiratory changes include a considerable increase in the volume of air breathed per minute, which results from the increased tidal volume. Increased alveolar ventilation leads to a more efficient distribution and mixing of gas during late pregnancy (Guyton & Hall, 1996). However,

Box 16-2 Signs of Pregnancy

PROBABLE

- Enlargement of the uterus
- Softening of the uterine isthmus (Hegar's sign)
- Bluish or cyanotic color of cervix and upper vagina (Chadwick's sign)
- Softening of the cervix (Goodell's sign)
- Asymmetrical, softened enlargement of the uterine corner caused by placental development (Piskacek's sign)
- Positive test for HCG in the maternal urine or blood serum
- Changes in skin pigmentation (chloasma and linea nigra)

POSITIVE

- Detection of fetal heart tones by auscultation, sonography, or use of a Doppler instrument
- Palpation of fetal parts through Leopold's maneuvers
- Objective detection of fetal movements
- Radiological or ultrasonic demonstration of fetal parts

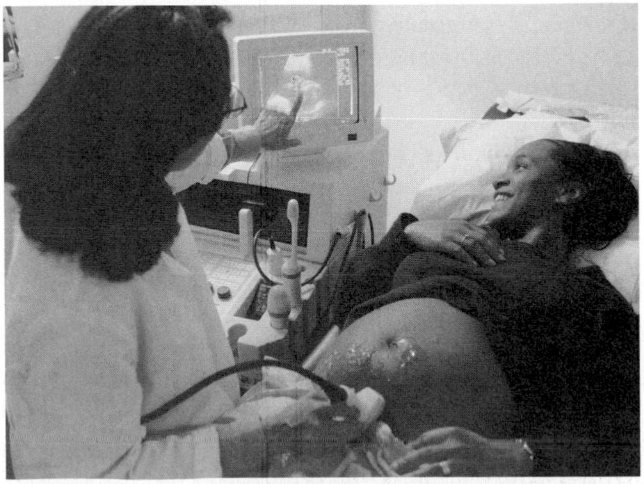

Fig. 16-3 Although an ultrasound examination is not always indicated, seeing normal development of the fetus via ultrasound is reassuring to parents and provides valuable information to health care providers.

enlarging uterine size toward the latter phases of pregnancy causes some shortness of breath (SOB) for many women until the baby descends into the pelvis during the final weeks of pregnancy.

Increased elasticity and softening of connective tissue of the musculoskeletal system results in relaxation of the joints, especially the pelvic joints. This increased flexibility allows the pelvic outlet to stretch for labor and delivery. Lumbar and dorsal curves of the spine increase late in pregnancy and contribute to the *waddle* of pregnancy. This characteristic gait may contribute to the low back pain often expressed by pregnant women.

Dramatic metabolic and endocrine changes occur with pregnancy. Increased basal metabolic rate, radioactive iodine uptake, and thyroid size all reflect increased thyroid gland activity as a response to a hormone called **estrogen.** Similarly, adrenal function increases in pregnancy and parallels fetal adrenal function. Both parathyroid hormone and pituitary production from the anterior lobe increase with pregnancy (Guyton & Hall, 1996).

Reproductive System

Pregnancy changes in the reproductive system include changes in the uterus and in the breasts, vagina, vulva, and ovaries. The prepregnant uterus is approximately the size of a closed fist. The uterus at term has the capacity to contain a 3.2 to 4.5 kg (7 to 10 lb) infant and the placenta. As the uterus enlarges, the **fundus,** the upper uterine segment, moves higher in the abdomen. Figure 16-4 illustrates the placement of the fundus as the pregnancy progresses. The breasts begin enlarging early in the pregnancy and in late pregnancy they may secrete small amounts of **colostrum** (breast milk) that precedes mature breast milk. The vagina and vulva receive a greater blood supply and may appear darker (cyanotic) as a result. Some women will notice an increase in vaginal secretions.

Hormones such as HCG and estrogen, which are secreted by the placenta and the fetus, create an optimal intrauterine environment for the fetus and stimulate many changes in the pregnant woman's body. The developing fetus contributes to the provision of an adequate environment for its own growth and nourishment, despite the possibility of creating discomforts for the pregnant woman.

Normal Discomforts

The many changes in the woman's body can cause the normal discomforts experienced by some women at various times during the pregnancy and support a nursing diagnosis of *alteration in comfort*. Table 16-1 lists these discomforts, the possible causes, and the nursing interventions to facilitate individual coping. Many women feel a sense of relief about the commonality of these complaints and about useful interventions for decreasing these concerns at various points during gestation. Particularly for the woman experiencing her first pregnancy, the nurse serves a valuable educational and support role to help expectant couples adjust to the challenges and discomforts of pregnancy, a goal for the earlier stated diagnosis.

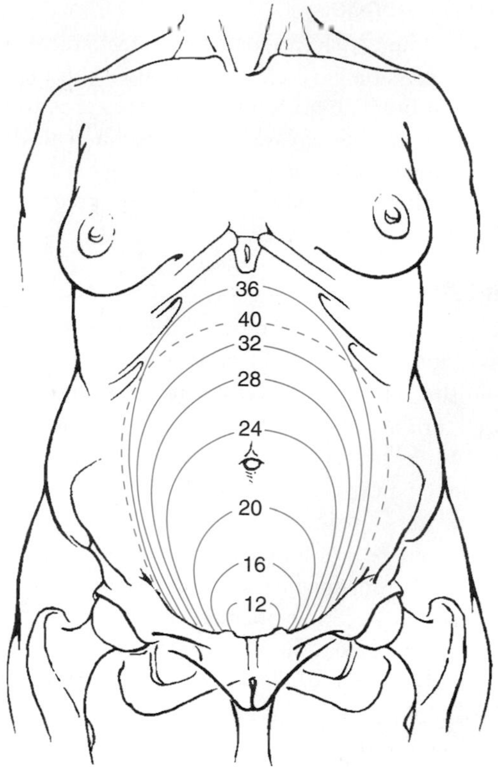

Fig. 16-4 Upper level of enlarging uterus by weeks of normal gestation with a single fetus. (From Barkauskas, V. H., Stoltenberg-Allen, K., Baumann, L. C., & Darling-Fisher, C. [1994]. *Health and physical assessment* [p. 723]. St. Louis: Mosby).

Teaching Throughout Pregnancy

In addition to serving as a caregiver, advocate, and support person, the nurse serves as a teacher throughout pregnancy and during each individual or family interaction. Active teaching that is relevant to individual concerns and gestational issues may occur in the clinic, physician's office, or other care environments. Nursing intervention should address recommended professional practice guidelines for education during the prenatal period to prevent complications during this time for each pregnant family seen by the nurse (see Research Highlights box). For example, the nurse may also offer textbooks, pamphlets, videotapes, and referrals to web sites and other instructional media to increase a couple's knowledge of fetal, maternal, and family changes during gestation and then encourage questions based on these sources. Going beyond one-to-one teaching, the nurse may also refer couples to early pregnancy and **Lamaze** childbirth preparation classes to increase the social support network and to help couples increase their knowledge about labor and delivery. Throughout the

Table 16-1 **Normal Discomforts Experienced During Pregnancy, Probable Cause, and Nursing Suggestions for Relief**

Discomfort	Known or Probable Cause	Nursing Suggestions for Relief
Backache	Changes in posture such as increased lumbar curve Excessive bending or lifting	Practice good posture Perform pelvic rocking Wear comfortable, low-heeled shoes Apply ice or heat to lower back Massage Squat to lift Avoid prolonged sitting Sleep on firm mattress Avoid fatigue Do Kegel exercise during day
Constipation	Pressure of enlarging uterus Slowed peristalsis caused by progesterone Side effect of iron therapy and increased calcium with pregnancy	Increase intake of fruits and vegetables Eat high-fiber foods Exercise Drink warm water first thing in morning Only as last resort, take laxative, stool softener, or suppository with doctor's permission
Fatigue	Decreased metabolic rate with pregnancy Extra weight of pregnancy to carry during day	Get full night's sleep Increase exercise over time Share workload when possible Nap or rest during day Eat healthy diet Usually better after first trimester
Hemorrhoids	Constipation Pressure of enlarged uterus Straining with bowel evacuation	Relieve problem with measures discussed previously Take sitz baths Use ice pack or witch hazel for local relief Do perineal tightening exercises Seek out physician advice for problem
Leg cramps	Pressure of uterus on blood vessels Fatigue or chilling Lack of calcium Sudden stretching or overextension of foot Excessive phosphorus in diet	Take calcium supplement or increase calcium-rich foods Practice steady, gentle stretch to relieve cramp Never massage a cramping muscle Avoid toe-pointing when exercising If negative Homan's sign, dorsiflex ankles throughout day to prevent cramps
Leukorrhea	Increased vascularity of cervix and vagina	Wear cotton-crotch underpants Wash genital area frequently When infection develops (itching and profuse drainage), call physician Do not douche
Nausea and vomiting	Increase in estrogen and progesterone Changes in blood glucose levels	Eat small, frequent meals Eat dry crackers in the morning before arising Snack at bedtime Drink camomile or ginger tea Avoid greasy, fried foods
Varicosities	Increased vascularity of pelvic organs Venous return slowed by pressure of uterus Familial tendency Progesterone effect on smooth muscles	Avoid knee socks and tight elastic on underwear Elevate feet 10 to 15 minutes several times a day Avoid long periods of standing Avoid crossing legs when sitting Wear support stockings Engage in consistent walking during pregnancy
Urinary frequency	Pressure of uterus against bladder in first and third trimesters Nocturia may result from increased extremity venous return when lying down	When interfering with sleep, limit amount of fluids in evening Rest during the day

provision of care, the nurse must be sensitive to the cultural and ethnic beliefs and behaviors of the individual or family in an effort to provide quality care to people with different needs.

Total Weight Gain

Total weight gain during pregnancy reflects not only the growth of the baby and placenta, but also that of the uterus, breasts, maternal fat for storage, and increases in blood and other body fluids. Many practitioners currently recommend for most women a weight gain of 25 to 35 lb for a pregnancy involving one fetus (Institute of Medicine, Subcommittee on Nutritional Status during Pregnancy and Lactation, 1990; U.S. Department of Health and Human Services, 2000; Worthington-Roberts, 1995). Additionally, a consistent pattern of gain with most weight gain in the final two trimesters has also been recommended (Georges, 2000; U.S. Department of Health and Human Services, 2000).

research highlights

Prenatal Care: Successes and Obstacles

The purpose of this study was to educate prenatal and other health care providers on the specific components of the Prenatal Care Initiative, using a comprehensive public health model. Under the Minnesota Prenatal Care Initiative (MPCI), health care providers who offered prenatal care services to Medicaid-enrolled women were asked to complete a prenatal risk assessment provided by the Minnesota Department of Health. A modified version of the Creasy Risk Assessment was selected that included medical, obstetric, and psychosocial factors.

The project spanned 3 years. Phase I (year one) included 12 educational workshops for medical and public health prenatal care providers. The curriculum included information on the coordination of care between medical clinics and community services for hard-to-reach pregnant women. Phase II (years two and three) were designed to follow up and reinforce the initial educational interventions. Additionally, selected sociodemographic variables were examined.

Successes in the first year were a twofold increase in the number of Medicaid-enrolled women who received risk assessment and enhanced services. Similarly, provider participation increased, with greater collaboration among interdisciplinary providers at the community level. Obstacles included provider resistance to changes in practice and dissatisfaction with the enhanced services package and the level of reimbursement. Overall, this study has provided evidence to other states as plans to improve their prenatal services are made. This unique effort provided a model for an effective strategy to promote support and cooperation in the implementation of new health care initiatives.

Data from Skovholt, C., Lia-Hoagberg, B., & Mullett, S. (1994). The Minnesota prenatal care coordination project: Successes and obstacles. *Public Health Reports, 109*, 774-781.

Labor and Delivery

Pregnancy culminates with labor and delivery. The process of giving birth creates a significant emotional response by the delivering family and will be discussed in the next section. However, a description of the events of a normal labor and delivery must occur here to establish a background for considering the physiological changes in the mother and the infant during this time.

The precise cause of the onset of labor remains undefined, although several theories have offered explanations. Several factors likely interact, including distention of the uterus, mechanical irritation, progesterone deprivation, posterior pituitary action, and localized progesterone activity. Labor usually begins around the fortieth gestational age week, or the equivalent of 10 normal menstrual cycles. This factor suggests that some hormonal control, which participates in controlling menstrual cycles, also contributes to the onset of labor (Guyton & Hall, 1997).

The placenta may also play an important role in labor onset. Special hormones may be produced when the placenta has reached term and may be responsible for inducing labor. Placental aging, which results in a decrease in the blood levels of estrogen and progesterone, may also be an influential factor. This process parallels the events of the menstrual cycle, during which deterioration of the corpus luteum and decreased blood levels of estrogen and progesterone initiate menstruation a few days later.

Labor may be conveniently divided into four distinct stages. The **first stage of labor** starts with regularity of uterine contractions and ends with complete dilation and effacement of the cervix. Signs of beginning labor include those listed in Box 16-3. The **cervix,** the lower portion of the uterus, must *open up*, or dilate, from a closed position to one encompassing an opening of about 4 inches (10 cm) in diameter. During the first stage, the cervix must also *thin out*, or completely efface or shorten, from a length of 1 to 2 inches to a barely palpable (*paper thin*) length. Usually, pregnant women will have started the cervical dilation and effacement process because they experience painless Braxton-Hicks contractions during pregnancy and before the active onset of labor. Few women come to the delivery setting without some degree of dilation and effacement.

In the first stage, the presenting part of the fetus begins to press on the cervix and lower uterine segment and on

Box 16-3 Signs of Beginning Labor

- Bloody show or loss of the mucous plug that has sealed the cervical canal during pregnancy.
- Regular uterine contractions.
- Contractions increasing in intensity, duration, and frequency over a specific period.
- Palpable hardening of the uterus during contractions.
- Pain in the lower back and front of abdomen.

the nerve endings around the cervix and vagina. Women vary in their response to the discomfort caused by this process; pain thresholds and cultural perceptions of and responses to pain differ among laboring women. The upper uterine segment (fundus) represents the active contractile portion of the uterus. The fundus becomes thicker as labor progresses and helps to retract the lower uterine segment and cervix, pushing the fetus downward toward the cervix and eventually through the vagina for birth. Stage one of labor lasts an average of 12 hours for women experiencing a first birth and somewhat less for women having a second or additional child. Based on a laboring woman's needs, various medications, Lamaze breathing, and other distractive techniques may be used to alleviate the discomfort associated with first stage of labor.

During the first stage of labor, sterile vaginal examinations by the nurse or other health care provider indicate each laboring woman's progress related to cervical dilatation and effacement and descent of the fetus into the birth canal. In 25% of women, the fetal membranes or amniotic sac ruptures, either spontaneously or artificially, during the first stage of labor (Piotrowski, 1999). Loss of the amniotic membrane normally increases pressure of the fetal head against the cervix. Additionally, loss of the amniotic fluid generally represents the irreversibility of the labor process because labor frequently becomes more intense with a lack of fetal membranes.

During the **second stage of labor,** the baby descends through the birth canal. The upper uterine segment greatly thickens and the abdominal muscles assist in the fetus' descent and expulsion. Women who have attended childbirth classes often actively participate in pushing the baby down toward the perineum and toward birth. For many women, an overwhelming urge to push down during uterine contractions occurs at this time. Pushing occurs at varying intervals and with ever-increasing force and strain. With pressure by the doctor or midwife applied to the fetal head, the fetal spine tends to straighten, adding power to the push of the head downward. With the fetal spine normally parallel to the midline axis of the mother's abdomen or slightly to one side, the fetal head accommodates to the mother's pelvis as it passes through the vaginal

CARE PLAN

Nursing Diagnosis: Ineffective Individual Coping Related to Active Labor Status

DEFINING CHARACTERISTICS

Initiation of labor at 2:00 AM with SROM
First-time childbearing mother without prepared childbirth classes
Supportive spouse
Current gestational age of 36 weeks
Contraction pattern defined as moderate contractions, frequency every 2 minutes, 60 seconds in duration
After 6 hours of labor, 4 cm dilated, 100% effaced, and -2 station
Moaning, moving around in bed, and stating, "I can't take this much longer; it hurts too bad!"

RELATED FACTORS

Prenatal history of URI and UTIs, currently diagnosed with strep throat
Prenatal care since 12 weeks pregnant
History of depression in college
Works as engineer with large manufacturing firm
Gravida 3, para 0 (two losses at 6 to 8 weeks of gestation before current marriage)
Recent resident of city, moved from other part of country approximately 4 months ago
22 years of age, Asian family history, married 1 year

EXPECTED OUTCOMES

Mother will state level of pain to be less than 4 on a scale of 1 to 10 during labor.
Mother will successfully use visual imagery techniques, massage, and slow deep breathing during labor for relaxation during labor.
Mother will state early in labor at least three ways she effectively deals with pain and will be able to implement these strategies in labor as relevant.
Fetus will experience average LTV and no compromise during labor.
Mother and family will verbalize needs during labor and delivery to health care team.

INTERVENTIONS (BY L & D NURSE)

Assess level of labor discomfort every 20 to 30 minutes and PRN according to pain scale rating of 1 to 10.
Implement and document nursing interventions (backrubs, heat and cold, position changes, back pressure and massage, and Jacuzzi therapy, among others) to deal with labor discomforts as needed.
Assess cultural beliefs with labor and delivery management and implement interventions as needed to meet practice standards.
Provide teaching about labor and delivery progress and breathing, visual imagery, and massage techniques that may decrease labor discomfort.
Provide verbal and nonverbal reassurance during labor.
Teach fetal response during labor and rationale for nursing interventions to support fetal health, such as left side position to increase placental blood flow.
Throughout labor, answer any questions from mother and family members about needs and responses to labor process.
Involve family members as much as possible during labor and as requested by mother to increase her coping.

canal by turning first to one side, then to the other. The head becomes flush with the vaginal opening on the woman's perineum and the physician or nurse-midwife may perform an **episiotomy,** a surgical incision into the perineum, to assist the baby's head to deliver.

Finally, the head appears, with the diameter of the occiput visible at the level of the perineum; then the neck straightens, turning the head to one side in alignment with the position of the shoulders. When the shoulders pass through the pelvis and accommodate to the shape of the birth canal, the body continues to rotate. The posterior shoulder normally delivers first over the perineum and the anterior soon follows under the symphysis pubis. The body quickly follows and the infant is born. Women birthing their first baby may push for up to 2 hours; however, women bearing a second or additional baby or those who are more educated about pushing may bear down for significantly less time.

The **third stage of labor** begins after the birth and lasts until placental expulsion. Placental separation usually takes place within 5 to 30 minutes after completion of the second stage. Signs of placental detachment are listed in Box 16-4. After delivery, the placenta must be examined by the doctor or midwife to determine whether all placental tissue has been delivered and to detect any abnormalities that could affect the infant's condition and adaptation to extrauterine life.

The **fourth stage of labor** generally consists of the first 2 hours after delivery, during which the mother faces the greatest danger of postpartum hemorrhage. An expected blood loss varying from 250 to 500 ml may cause the mother to experience a moderate decline in both systolic and diastolic blood pressure. She may also demonstrate tachycardia or increased heart rate as a compensatory mechanism in the early postpartum period based on this blood loss. The Care Plan deals with active labor status.

Overview of Care

Professional members of the health care team play an important role in labor and delivery, but a woman's family or significant others can also be an important part of her care during labor and delivery. Many practitioners suggest that the expectations and beliefs of a couple, particularly those of the delivering woman, have a great effect on how she fulfills the mothering role. Therefore the nurse needs to collaborate with the people who are caring for the pregnant woman to meet that family's needs during pregnancy, labor, and delivery.

The importance of the nurse's caregiving and support cannot be underestimated during the first stage of labor. Independent nursing interventions to increase comfort, such as giving backrubs, massages, offering ice and fluids by mouth, assisting with ambulation and position changes, and providing a clean and dry environment, may allow the woman and her coach to cope with the challenges of labor. Many women will request medication to deal with the pain of delivery, and the nurse may need to review options for medication for each couple. Active emotional and physical support by the nurse may enable a pregnant woman to relax, meet her labor and delivery goals, and support the well being of the fetus. During the first stage, the mother must not *bear down* because this may cause cervical swelling; often, active nursing support and distractive techniques, such as breathing and visual refocus, can prevent pushing before the second stage of labor. A woman may need modeling by the nurse to use the prepared childbirth breathing techniques successfully, which are intended to decrease pain perception during labor. During the first stage of labor, the nurse will need to teach the laboring couple about any interventions used to monitor the progress of labor and the well being of mother and fetus. These interventions may include the use of a **fetal heart monitor** (FHM) (a machine detailing fetal heart rate and activity during labor), intravenous fluids, automatic blood pressure machine, and urinary catheterization. Open and clear communication among health care provider and the laboring woman and her significant others, particularly during frequent and difficult uterine contractions, will increase the coping of the laboring members before the pushing stage begins.

During the second stage of labor, the woman needs to be reassured and supported in the *pushing work*. Constant reinforcement and education by the nurse about labor progress, fetal heart monitor tracings, and other interventions will give the mother and her support system the energy needed to reach the delivery process. Throughout labor, the nurse considers the cultural and ethnic needs of each system to support individualized assessment and a positive perception of labor by the childbearing woman and her family.

Active nursing support during the third and fourth stages of labor includes observing for excessive vaginal bleeding after placental discharge, assisting the woman in breast feeding of her new baby, monitoring vital signs, and implementing uterine massage if the uterus becomes *boggy* or fails to contract over the placental site. Emotional support during assessments and giving information to explain the rationales for assessments are also important roles of the nurse that have been supported by professional standards of practice.

Throughout the entire labor and delivery process, the nurse makes careful observations of the laboring woman to identify unexpected events. These events may signal

Box 16-4 Signs of Placental Detachment

- Rushing of blood from the vagina.
- Lengthening of umbilical cord outside of vulva.
- Rising of uterine fundus and abdomen as placenta passes from uterus into vagina.

difficulties with the progression of labor or with maternal or fetal health during this time. Assessment to identify these possible problems should include the following:

1. Precise description of any unusual fetal or uterine activity.
2. Presence of meconium when the membranes rupture or at any point thereafter.
3. Fetal heart rate decelerations related to uterine activity.
4. Duration of any **tachycardia** (fetal heart rate above 160 beats per minute) or **bradycardia** (fetal heart rate below 120 beats per minute) with labor based on assessment of the gestational age of the fetus (Association of Women's Health, Obstetrical, and Neonatal Nursing [AWHONN], 1998).

When observing an unexpected event, the nurse immediately reports this to the physician, midwife, or appropriate health care provider with a complete oral and written description of the event. The nurse must be aware that abnormal fetal and maternal signs and patterns may be related to the following conditions and therefore should intervene appropriately to support a positive labor and delivery outcome (Piotrowski, 1999):

1. Maternal physical condition such as diabetes or hypertension.
2. Timing and type of medications administered.
3. Frequency, type, and duration of uterine contractions.
4. Intactness of the membranes and the presence or absence of meconium-stained fluid.
5. Bleeding in the pregnant woman or the fetus.
6. Gestational age of infant.

CHANGES IN TRANSITION FROM FETUS TO NEWBORN

A relatively orderly continuum of adaptation occurs from fetal to extrauterine life. The events pass unnoticed and with relative ease in most cases. When difficulty occurs, however, care of the infant depends on understanding the normal events of adaptation occurring in various newborn body systems during this period (Box 16-5). Normal transition depends on a fine balance of chemical, physiological, and anatomical changes; therefore newborn stress is ultimately hazardous (Hammond, 1999). Although newborns have demonstrated a relative resistance to the stress of anoxia, health care providers caring for neonates must have the skills to detect impending dangers to the neonate and to prevent stress that may cause difficulties in newborn adaptation to extrauterine life.

Nursing Interventions

The nursing activities during this adaptation process include assessment and interventions aimed at specific protection of the infant and prevention of complications related to newborn adaptation to extrauterine life. Cold stress should be avoided by keeping the newborn dry, warmly wrapped, and by avoiding environments causing heat loss in the newborn. Overall, the nurse should minimally disturb, but maximally observe, the newborn during reactive periods. Bathing and feeding, for instance, should be delayed until behavior and physiological mechanisms stabilize, usually between 4 and 8 hours of age. The nurse assesses and documents newborn responses to interventions with the realization that newborns of the same age may respond differently to nursing care early in the neonatal period.

Mucus

Newborns tend to regurgitate during this period. Mucus is a normal product of intrauterine life and probably originates in the lung and gastrointestinal tissues. The amount of mucus that is produced varies greatly. Some controversy remains about the efficacy of gastric suctioning to alleviate or prevent mucus regurgitation into the upper esophageal tract, creating a danger for aspiration. When mucus production reaches a level at which aspiration becomes an obvious hazard, suctioning should be employed. When vomiting occurs, suctioning of mucus from the mouth with a simple bulb syringe may help, but the more effective approach is to remove material from the esophagus, then the stomach.

Apgar Score

Assessment of the newborn after the first few hours is essentially the same as assessment of the young infant (see Chapter 17). One technique, specific to timing after birth, is the **Apgar scoring system.** Apgar scoring, used for over 50 years in delivery rooms, provides a simple clinical measure to evaluate an infant's general condition at birth. The scoring, made at 1 minute and 5 minutes of age, may be repeated until the infant's condition has stabilized. Determination of the total score is accomplished by adding the values allotted to observations of heart rate, respiratory effort, muscle tone, reflex irritability, and color, as indicated in Table 16-2. The highest possible score is 10. A score of 8 to 10 indicates that the baby is adapting well. Hammond (1999) notes that the Apgar score does not predict the future neurological development of an individual, important information to convey to parents who may have delivered an infant with a low Apgar value.

Gender

Gender differences also occur in fetal growth. Generally, boys grow faster than girls in the third trimester and after 26 weeks boys are larger. At birth, boys are slightly heavier and longer and have a larger head circumference than do girls (Guyton & Hall, 1997).

Gender differences occur in the number of conceptions and births. Although more boys are conceived, they tend to be spontaneously aborted more often than do girls. The exact cause of this greater loss of male embryos remains

Box 16-5 Systemic Adaptation of Fetus to Extrauterine Life

RESPIRATORY SYSTEM

- Initiation of independent respiration is newborn's greatest challenge soon after birth.
- Pressure changes within newborn's chest; light, sound, and blood gas changes stimulate newborn's initial respiratory activity.
- Lung expansion increases absorptive surface area of alveolar sacs (lung capillaries) to facilitate gas exchange.
- Healthy newborn breathes shallowly and irregularly, approximately 30 to 60 times per minute; may have short apneic spells (less than 15 seconds in duration) early in extrauterine life.
- Newborns are obligatory nose breathers.

CIRCULATORY SYSTEM

- Placental circulation stops with cutting of placental cord.
- Closure of foramen ovale (fetal connection between atria) generally occurs in first 24 hours of life.
- Transient murmurs may be heard because of incomplete or lack of closure of foramen ovale and/or ductus arteriosus (fetal connection between pulmonary artery and aorta).
- Newborn's usual heart rate varies from 120 to 160 beats per minute; blood pressure approximately 78/42 based on newborn activity.
- Increased plasma protein level and hemoglobin concentration occurs because of loss of fluid from RBCs and vascular compartment; may cause common edema found in presenting parts of term newborn.

GASTROINTESTINAL SYSTEM

- Digestive and absorptive mechanisms to handle various types of foods intact at birth.
- Carbohydrates provide newborn's primary source of energy in first few hours of life; fat sources become more important in second day of life; protein metabolism generally occurs on third day of life.
- Brain depends on sufficient carbohydrate to meet energy needs throughout life.
- Live immaturity causes buildup of hemolyzed RBCs, producing jaundice in many term newborns about the third day of life.
- Cold stress may increase expected relative newborn acidosis and contribute to jaundice.
- Active bowel sounds heard by first 24 hours; first bowel movement expected by second day of life.

RENAL SYSTEM

- Immature kidneys in term newborn prevent concentration of urine.
- Rate of fluid intake and excretion many times that of an adult; dehydration and overhydration a concern during newborn period.

NERVOUS SYSTEM

- Although system immature, functions fairly well to meet body requirements.
- Autonomic nervous system most crucial to transition and integrates respiration, acid-base balance, and temperature control of newborn.
- Protective reflexes (Moro, swallow, sucking, Babinski, and rooting) are intact in term infant.
- Sympathetic nervous system functions in infant's ability to increase respiratory rate and to discharge urine, stool, and oral mucus.
- Periods of reactivity occur in the first 24 hours of life to allow infant to breast feed and to experience the extrauterine environment.

Adapted from Guyton, A. C., & Hall, J. E. (1997). *Human physiology and human disease*. Philadelphia: W.B. Saunders; Hammond, B. B. (1999). Immediate care of the newborn. In D. L. Lowdermilk, S. E. Perry, & I. M. Bobak, *Maternity nursing* (5th ed., pp. 489-509). St. Louis: Mosby.

Table 16-2 Apgar Scoring

Sign	Score 0	1	2
Heart Rate	Absent	Slow (under 100)	Over 100
Respiratory effort	Absent	Weak cry, hypoventilation	Good strong cry
Muscle tone	Flaccid, limp	Some flexion of extremities	Active motion, extremities well flexed
Reflex irritability	No response	Grimace	Cry
Color	Blue, pale	Body pink, extremities blue	Completely pink

From Hammond, B. B. (1999). Immediate care of the newborn. In D. L. Lowdermilk, S. E. Perry, & I. M. Bobak, *Maternity nursing* (5th ed., p. 501). Thousand Oaks, CA: Sage.

unclear. Male embryos may succumb to Y-linked recessive conditions during this time, or the female embryo, having two X chromosomes, may have more protection from some of the early hazards of pregnancy. After birth, boys continue to have a lower survival rate than do girls and by middle age, women are more numerous than are men.

Race

Race can affect the fetus' health in several ways. The first is in the rate of twinning. In the United States, nonWhites (mainly Blacks) have more twin pregnancies than Whites (Perry, 1999). Twin fetuses are at increased risk for premature delivery and also place higher nutritional

Box 16-6 Selected National Health-Promotion and Disease-Prevention Objectives for the Prenatal Period

THE PRENATAL PERIOD

- Reduce the infant mortality rate (28 weeks to 7 or more months after birth) to no more than 4.5 per 1000 live births (baseline: 7.2 per 1000 live births in 1998)

Special Population Targets

Infant mortality	1997 baseline	2010 target
Blacks	13.7	4.5
Native Americans-Alaskan Natives	7.9	4.5
Asians	4.6	4.5
Hispanics-Latinas	6.5	4.5

- Reduce the fetal death rate (20 or more weeks of gestation) to no more than 4.1 per 1000 live births plus fetal deaths (baseline: 6.8 per 1000 live births plus fetal deaths in 1997)

Special Population Target

Fetal deaths	1997 baseline	2010 target
Blacks	12.5*	6.8*

- Reduce low birth weight to an incidence of no more than 5% of live births and very low birth weight to no more than 0.9% of live births (baseline: 7.6% and 1.4%, respectively, in 1998)

Special Population Target

	1998 baseline	2010 target
Low birth weight		
Blacks	13.0%	5.0%
Very low birth weight		
Blacks	3.0%	0.9%

- Reduce the number of unintended pregnancies to no more than 30% (baseline: 51% of pregnancies for females 15 to 44 years of age in 1995 were unwanted or earlier than intended)
- Reduce the number of pregnancies occurring in girls ages 15 to 17 to no more than 46 per 1000 (baseline: 72 pregnancies per 1000 girls of this age in 1995)
- Increase the number of women who breast feed in the early postpartum period to at least 75% and increase the proportion who breast feed for 5 to 6 months after birth to at least 50% (baseline: 64% of women chose to breast feed in the early postpartum period in 1998; 29% chose to breast feed for 5 to 6 months in 1998)
- Increase abstinence from tobacco use by pregnant women to at least 98%, increase abstinence from alcohol to 94%, and illicit drugs (cocaine and marijuana) to 100% by pregnant women (baseline: 87% of pregnant women abstained from tobacco use, 86% abstained from alcohol, 98% abstained from cocaine, and 98% abstained from marijuana in 1996 to 1997)
- Increase the number of women who receive prenatal care in the first trimester of pregnancy to at least 90% (baseline: 83% of live births in 1997)

Special Population Targets	1997 baseline	2010 target
Native Americans-Alaskan Natives	68%	90%
Asians	85%	90%
Blacks	72%	90%
Whites	85%	90%

- Increase the proportion of mothers who achieve a recommended weight gain during their pregnancies (baseline: 75% of married women delivering at term gained the recommended weight of 25 to 35 lb with pregnancy in 1988)
- Reduce the cesarean delivery rate to no more than 15 per 100 deliveries (baseline: 17.8 per 100 deliveries in 1997; a rate of 15.5 for primary cesareans and 71 for repeat procedures in 1997)

From U.S. Department of Health and Human Services. (2000). *Healthy People 2010: Vol. 1* (Conference edition). Washington, DC: U.S. Government Printing Office.

demands on the mother. Any premature baby is at higher risk for death or morbidity because of less mature organs. Currently, the United States is twenty-fifth in the world ranking for **infant mortality rate** (IMR) (National Center for Health Statistics, 1999), a statistical reflection of the number of infants dying before their first year of life and the leading indicator of a nation's health. This rate most likely is a result of higher IMRs of Blacks, Hispanics, Native Americans, and Alaskan Natives as compared with Whites in this country. For example, Blacks continue to experience twice the IMR of Whites (Hoyert, 1996; Ventura, Anderson, Martin, & Smith, 1997), a problematic situation that America must confront in the coming years to create a more healthy society (U.S. Department of Health and Human Services, 2000).

Race is also a factor in the frequency of certain genetic and congenital malformations that occur. For example, cleft palates (an opening in the oral palate) are more common among Whites compared with Blacks (Carlson, 1999), whereas sickle cell anemia (abnormally shaped red blood cells) is higher among Blacks. Interestingly, the total number of malformations tends to be about the same in all races that have been studied (Whites, Blacks, Hispanics, and Asians) (Creasy & Resnik, 1999).

An ethnic group may affect fetal outcome from its link to socioeconomic status. For increasing numbers of homeless pregnant women, finances and support services that prioritize prenatal over family survival needs remain limited. Pregnant women of minority groups may have fewer economic resources to obtain a nutritious diet or early and consistent quality prenatal care. These outcomes may be related to access factors or to cultural beliefs that do not support recommended foods or prenatal care in pregnant women. Box 16-6 presents the *Healthy People 2010* objectives.

Genetics

Genetic influences during the prenatal period affect the survival and later well being of the child through several known mechanisms. Abnormal chromosomal number or structure, a mutant (abnormal) gene, and polygenetic inheritance create a significant percentage of congenital malformations or defects. **Down syndrome** (trisomy 21) remains the most recognized and most commonly occurring example of an extra chromosome. Extra chromosomes, deleted chromosomes, or translocations usually result in multiple malformations. Single malformations in an otherwise normal fetus, such as clubfoot, cleft palate, and neural tube defects, probably result from the combined effect of many genes (Askin, 1999).

Many spontaneous abortions have a chromosomal abnormality; natural forces stop the development of many abnormal fetuses. Some genetic problems fail to become apparent until later in life, but the basic defect was present from conception.

Not all malformations and multiple-defect syndromes have a genetic origin. Negative environmental influences can cause fetal abnormalities. These influences, including infectious agents, drugs, radiation, chemicals, alcohol, and nicotine, will be discussed later in this chapter related to environmental processes.

Modern techniques of **amniocentesis,** chorionic villi sampling (CVS), and chromosome analysis have expanded the possibilities for genetic counseling in the prenatal period. The nurse knows where these resources are available in the community and can direct individuals to these resources when family history, previous pregnancy history, race, maternal age, or other factors that a genetic defect or syndrome may be likely for the fetus.

GORDON'S FUNCTIONAL HEALTH PATTERNS

Box 16-7 provides an example of a pregnancy assessment using Gordon's functional health patterns (1995).

Health Perception-Health Management Pattern

A woman may view pregnancy as an illness, as a completely natural and healthy state, or as a combination of the two. This perception will influence her view of her changing body, her attitude toward the usual discomforts of pregnancy such as fatigue or backache, her choice of health- or illness-oriented care, and her decision of whether to seek prenatal care. The woman who sees herself as ill wants a care provider who will accept this view. The woman who sees herself as healthy and as experiencing a normal part of life wants a care provider with a similar outlook. The pregnant woman who sees herself as healthy may have a more positive view of the minor discomforts of pregnancy and may continue active participation in her social circle and her career. The woman who sees her pregnancy as a time of illness may use this as a reason to withdraw from her work and social obligations. Another woman may seek help from a socially approved group, as defined by her culture, and avoid standard Western medicine during pregnancy (Roma Gypsies).

A woman's acceptance of her pregnancy influences her health-management practices. The woman who denies or has strong negative feelings about her pregnancy may fail to eat properly, get enough rest and exercise, breast feed, or seek prenatal care. A woman may deny a pregnancy because she never intended to become pregnant despite having sexual intercourse without birth control. Approximately 50% of American pregnancies are *unintended* and many occur among women 20 years of age and younger; women 40 years of age and older; and among low-income and diverse women who lack access, cultural acceptance, education, and financial resources to purchase or use protection against pregnancy (Brown & Eisenberg, 1995; Kost, Landry, & Darroch, 1998a, 1998b; U.S. Department of Health and Human Services, 2000). This value is 39% in Canada and 6% in the Netherlands (1994 and 1995) (Delbanco, Lundy, Hoff, Parke, & Smith, 1997). American women, faced with an unplanned pregnancy, may expose a fetus to alcohol, tobacco, and sexually transmitted diseases and may later abuse a child who was never wanted (Brown & Eisenberg, 1995; Dye, Wojtowycz, Ambry, Quade, & Kilburn, 1997). A woman who experiences difficulties in accessing contraception and understanding its use may also have closely spaced pregnancies; these repeated pregnancies have been shown to result in more preterm births and low birth weight (LBW) infants needing high risk follow-up after birth (Alan Guttmacher Institute, 1994; U.S. Department of Health and Human Services, 2000; Zhu, Rolfs, Nangle, & Horan, 1999).

To work effectively with each woman seeking pregnancy care, the nurse must assess the meaning of pregnancy for each woman early in the pregnancy process. For example, the woman who views her pregnancy as an illness may demand medication for every discomfort. The nurse should be sensitive to a wide range of views expressed by women who are pregnant and assist each in discussing her thoughts and reaching solutions that will benefit the individual and her family in coping with pregnancy. For example, Hispanic women are less likely to get early prenatal care based on a belief that pregnancy is not an illness. The nurse must target interventions that focus on this group's needs and adherence to professional practice standards.

The dramatic physical and emotional changes that occur in a pregnant woman support the optimal development of the fetus. In addition to considering these changes, the nurse must be aware of the many environmental influences that can affect the mother, the fetus, and the quality of life for both.

Nutritional-Metabolic Pattern

Massive amounts of literature support the importance of optimal nutrition during pregnancy for proper fetal health

Box 16-7 Assessment for Pregnancy According to Gordon's Functional Health Patterns

Health perception-health management pattern: aware of and/or participates in management of pregnancy; expects an uncomplicated pregnancy based on the woman's or significant other's active involvement in her own care; is able to state complications of pregnancy that mandate physician notification; engages in health promotion behaviors specific for pregnancy

Nutritional-metabolic pattern: follows diet changes of pregnancy as recommended by nurse; has appropriate weight for height and has gained adequate weight for gestational age of pregnancy; eats three meals a day and two snacks (afternoon and evening), focusing on increased vegetables, fruits, and *good* fluids involving at least 8 glasses of water per day; has elastic skin turgor

Elimination pattern: experiences occasional constipation from iron therapy of pregnancy—usually corrected by increased fluids, nightly walking, and more diet roughage; voids 7 to 10 times a day, depending on amount of fluids consumed; no known hemorrhoids or difficulty in elimination; voiding without excess frequency, urgency, or burning; understands signs of urinary tract infection (UTI)

Activity-exercise pattern: walks 3 times a week for 20 minutes without complaints of unusual fatigue or soreness; is active at home with housework and at work teaching primary school; swam 2 times a week before pregnancy and move to current residence

Sleep-rest pattern: generally sleeps 7 to 8 hours a night; has increased total daily sleep somewhat with fatigue of pregnancy—naps for 1 hour on weekends and 30 minutes after work; sleeps on side and with two pillows for comfort; uses no sleep aids; is generally able to relax and initiate sleep without difficulty; occasionally has headache at end of workday and takes Tylenol for relief or listens to soft music after work to enhance relaxation

Cognitive-perceptual pattern: realizes the need to decrease work activity and increase rest periods as she nears end of pregnancy; answers questions in appropriate tone and words during pregnancy visits; has intact memory (alert and remote); reads about pregnancy and early parenthood to prepare for the event

Self-perception–self-concept pattern: states she is excited about the pregnancy after a year of trying to conceive; is well-groomed, wears maternity clothes because "I want to"; believes she looks "nice" as a result of pregnancy

Roles-relationships pattern: lives with husband of 3 years; visits extended family, 60 miles away, every month; shares family roles with husband, accepts this balance; has many friends who are supportive of her pregnancy; perceives extensive employee and employer support with pregnancy and time off after delivery

Sexuality-reproductive pattern: states, "I have a satisfying love life and enjoy my husband"; before pregnancy, engaged in sexual intercourse 4 to 5 times a week from desire to become pregnant; with pregnancy and fatigue, has intercourse generally 2 to 3 times a week, with pattern acceptable to both partners; no known sexually transmitted diseases (STDs) in past or present

Coping–stress-tolerance pattern: is concerned about fatigue affecting performance as primary school teacher; walks 3 times a week for 20 minutes to "center myself and feel good"; smiles often, has good sense of humor; has supportive family excited about her pregnancy

Values-beliefs pattern: Protestant religion; prays daily, gains strength from religion

Other Data:

- Medication history:
  Materna, 1 tablet each morning
  Ferrous, SO4 1 tablet each morning
  Tylenol gr. X for occasional headaches
- Physical exam:
  5 feet 4 inches tall
  Weight 140 lb (at 14 weeks pregnancy; weight gain of 5 lb with pregnancy)
  29 years of age
  PERRLA
  TPR 98.2-76-16
  BP 114/78 RA (sitting)
  Peripheral pulses equal, strong bilaterally
  Skin warm, dry, elastic turgor, mucous membranes intact, moist, alert, oriented x 3

Adapted from Gordon, M. (1995). *Nursing diagnosis: 1995-96*. St. Louis: Mosby.

and well being. Maternal malnutrition before and during pregnancy may exert a possible teratogenic effect on the fetus. A **teratogen** is an agent that causes either a functional or structural disability to the organism based on exposure to that agent (Perry, 1999). Teratogens principally affect the central nervous system (CNS) of the fetus, leading to impaired intelligence performance later in life (Worthington-Roberts, 1995) (see Fig. 16-5 later in the chapter).

Fetal development suffers the most in cases in which the mother is an adolescent with poor nutrition or a woman who has had poor nutrition between and during several pregnancies. Nutritional deficiencies of the mother during her own fetal, infant, and childhood periods contribute to the development of structural and physiological disadvantages for supporting a growing fetus. Maternal stature and pelvic development, which evolve from previous nutritional status and genetic endowment, may also influence the difficulty of labor (Worthington-Roberts, 1995).

Studies also suggest that improving the diet of pregnant women who have been poorly nourished throughout their lives does not always appreciably improve their ability to produce healthy offspring. For example, severely underweight women, such as adolescents, before pregnancy may experience higher rates of LBW and preterm labor than do women with appropriate weight before pregnancy

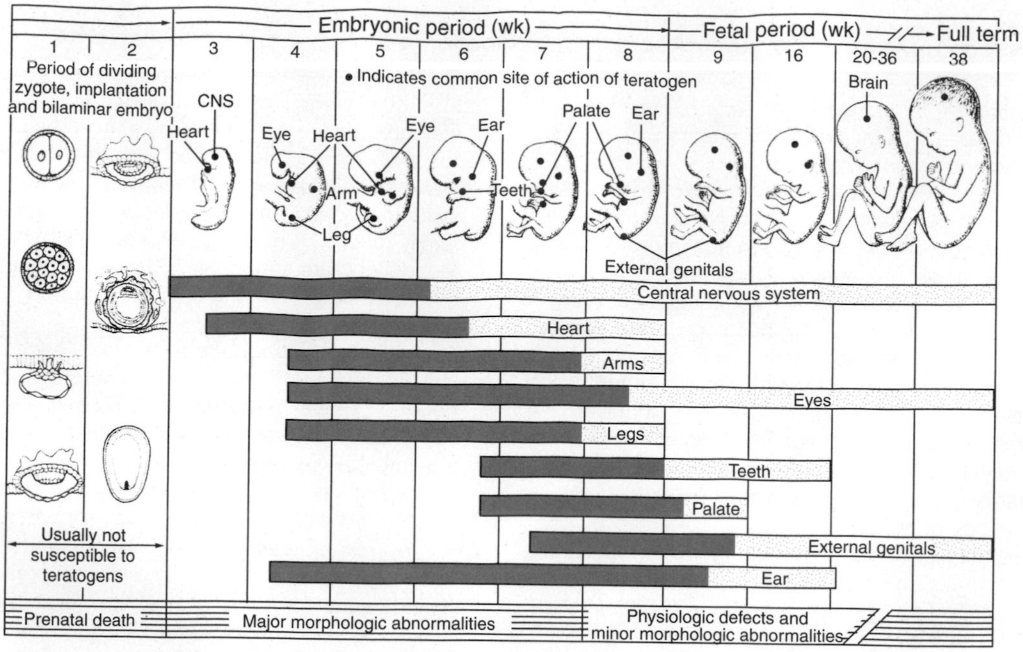

Fig. 16-5 Effects of teratogens on embryo and fetus. Dark color indicates highly sensitive periods; light color indicates less sensitive stages. (From Moore, K. L. [1998]. *Before we are born: Basic embryology and birth defects* [3rd ed.]. Philadelphia: W.B. Saunders).

(Cogswell & Kip, 1997). This statistic appears to conflict with the evidence that supports the proposition that the fetus derives most raw materials for development from the maternal diet and not, as formerly believed, from the mother's body structure and reserves. Maturity and development of all functional systems, such as essential enzyme systems, appear to depend heavily on a lifetime of adequate nurturance. The fetus's ability to use dietary elements effectively may be impaired in a poorly nourished mother. Further study is required to fully understand this aspect of nutrition.

A major proportion of families who eat poorly also suffer from socioeconomic limitations and the dietary practices of a subculture may also strongly influence these families. These factors compound efforts to understand the influence of poor nutrition on fetal well being. Although cultural beliefs may dictate appropriate food habits, poverty can contribute to a diet that is inadequate in basic nutrients in some subcultures. However, in families of cultural groups who are relatively affluent, choosing and eating foods from each of the six basic food groups occurs, although the manner of preparation and seasoning continues to vary according to cultural practices.

The additional dietary demands of the mother, which exceed those of the nonpregnant woman of comparable age, have been estimated based on studies that identify the normal physiological adjustments required during pregnancy. Continuing studies in this area have produced different recommendations for pregnancy nutritional intake based on the recognition that the pregnant woman requires more metabolic energy and structural resources to support pregnancy adequately than does the nonpregnant woman (Institute of Medicine, Subcommittee on Nutritional Status during Pregnancy and Lactation, 1990; Worthington-Roberts, 1995).

Caloric requirements during pregnancy exceed those of the nonpregnant woman by approximately 200 to 300 kcal each day, resulting in a weight gain of about 25 to 35 lb. If, at the end of 20 weeks of gestation, the woman has not gained at least 10 lb, then she should be considered a high-risk mother for delivering an ill infant and an intrauterine growth-restricted (IUGR) infant (Worthington-Roberts, 1995). Although the rate of gain and the total gain during pregnancy varies among women, a correlation exists between an erratic pattern of weight gain and/or too-rapid weight gain and a lack of fetal well being. Low maternal weight gain or being underweight at the onset of pregnancy frequently correlate with newborns who are underweight for their gestational age and who risk the hazards of impaired neonatal adjustment that accompany LBW. The overweight woman at conception also risks endangering the fetus when she attempts to lose weight during pregnancy. The effects of ketoacidosis, which occurs as a result of caloric limitation, have been associated with neuropsychological defects in infants. With the exception of considering specific disease states, the nurse should advise the mother to eat a well-balanced diet from all six food groups and according to her appetite (Worthington-Roberts, 1995).

The well-balanced diet for a pregnant woman parallels the diet that is needed by all human beings, with specific increases of certain components as recommended by the Food and Nutrition Board of the National Academy of Science (Institute of Medicine, Subcommittee on National Status during Pregnancy and Lactation, 1990; U.S. Department of Health and Human Services, 2000). The nurse should approach the diet of a pregnant woman in terms of the food that is offered to the entire family. Additionally, as there are physical demands of pregnancy, the nurse should encourage the pregnant woman to drink at least 8 glasses of water per day and to modify her diet to meet the common complaint of constipation during pregnancy.

Protein requirements during pregnancy increase to about 60 g per day over the amount required during nonpregnancy. Four glasses of milk a day, which have 32 g of protein, can easily meet one half of this increased requirement. Other milk sources, such as cheese, cream soups, puddings, tofu, and yogurt, may be tolerated better and meet the increased requirement. Animal protein and less expensive legume sources provide protein and can be combined to provide easily used protein-source meals, such as tuna and rice, cereal and milk, spaghetti and meat sauce, peanut butter and bread. Protein sources are normally more expensive than other foods; therefore nutritional counseling on how to meet protein needs during pregnancy remains an important teaching role of the nurse in prenatal care.

Mineral intake must also increase during pregnancy. An increase in protein foods usually provides the extra essential minerals that are needed, particularly phosphorus and calcium. Calcium deposit occurs mainly in the fetus during the last month of gestation; therefore calcium stores and intake must be adequate at this time to meet fetal bone needs. The rapid deposit of calcium in fetal bones during the third trimester of pregnancy requires adequate calcium stores from early pregnancy and continued calcium intake by the pregnant woman to prevent maternal bone demineralization. One quart (4 cups) of cow's milk each day supplies adequate calcium during pregnancy; the requirement of the pregnant woman is about 1.2 g daily (Worthington-Roberts, 1995). Other protein foods consumed in adequate amounts supply the extra amount of calcium needed during pregnancy.

Vitamin supplementation, a practice commonly recommended by American physicians, is of unsubstantiated value. With the exception of iron and when the woman's diet is well balanced, the food sources of vitamins and minerals should be adequate to meet the needs of pregnancy. Supplementation with 30 to 60 mg of iron during the last 3 to 4 months of pregnancy can be beneficial in building and protecting maternal iron stores to meet maternal and fetal needs (Worthington-Roberts, 1995). Some evidence points to the desirability of folic acid supplementation, particularly in the case of potential or real anemia or multiple pregnancy. Based on recent research supporting a correlation between low serum folic acid levels and fetal neural-tube defects, many physicians recommend that women who are trying to get pregnant and women in the early stages of pregnancy should take 0.4 mg of folic acid in a daily multivitamin (1 month preconception and 3 months postconception) (Rayburn, Stanley, & Garrett, 1996). However, recent research has shown that only 25% of women of childbearing age consume this amount of folic acid, which is known to be critical for early fetal development (U.S. Department of Health and Human Services, 2000).

Fats and carbohydrates must supply the caloric requirements during pregnancy. Although increased protein provides more calories, the body-building requirements of pregnancy and fetal growth demand most of the added protein. Fats and carbohydrates remain the most important sources of energy and they also supply essential vitamins and minerals. Supplemental vitamins and minerals, though not known to cause harm to the mother or fetus when taken within reasonable limits, cost more to achieve nutritional improvement compared with the cost involved in improving the dietary intake of the mother and her family.

The frequent practice of **pica,** or eating nonfood substances (especially by economically deprived, pregnant Black women) warrants special consideration. This phenomenon also occurs among small children who may have poor nutrition and experience frequent hunger. This situation, combined with normal cravings for food or nonfood substances, can lead to a culturally acceptable practice of eating materials such as starch, mud, clay, soap, or plaster. Although this practice has been known to exist for centuries among many groups of people, the possible harm and the reasons that this practice occurs more commonly during pregnancy remain undefined. The nurse should complete a nutritional assessment on any pregnant woman to identify instances of pica because it contributes to iron deficiency anemia, particularly among women of lower economic status.

The best time to teach a woman about prenatal nutrition is before she discovers that she is pregnant. Most women do not seek prenatal care until they suspect pregnancy; therefore giving information about optimal nutrition generally occurs after critical fetal development has already begun. Although 40% to 50% of primary health care providers supply nutritional counseling (U.S. Department of Health and Human Services, 1995), primary prevention intervention in this situation should begin with high school health classes. Although women may not remember the details of the recommended prenatal diet that are taught to them in high school, they may remember that good nutrition is vitally important at this time and may seek further information when they are planning to become pregnant. Secondary prevention intervention occurs during the pregnancy through laboratory monitoring of iron levels, assessment of the woman's feelings of well being and her actual intake of essential nutrients, and assessment of her pattern and total weight gain during the pregnancy. More pregnant women work outside the home and may reflect the increasing numbers of American families who spend 40% of their food budgets on food eaten away from home (Manning, 1999). With this food containing high amounts of cholesterol, sodium, and fat and little iron and calcium, the nurse should emphasize to the pregnant family the need for an overall plan for healthy food intake during pregnancy.

Elimination Pattern

Fetus

The fetus accomplishes all essential elimination functions through the placenta. Carbon dioxide, water, urea, and other waste products pass through the placenta to be eliminated through the mother's body. By the end of the first trimester, the fetus swallows, makes respiratory movements, and urinates. However, these abilities become truly functional only after birth.

Pregnant Woman

The pregnant woman experiences changes in her elimination pattern because the enlarging uterus causes hormonal influences and mechanical forces. These changes (urinary frequency in the first and third trimesters, constipation, and hemorrhoids) are usually normal, minor discomforts (see Table 16-1). Anticipatory guidance by the nurse assists the pregnant woman in coping with these changes and in preventing complications of pregnancy. For example, teaching the pregnant woman some commonsense measures (see Health Teaching box) may prevent urinary tract infections (UTIs), typically a greater problem with pregnancy. As there is a correlation between UTIs and premature labor, prevention and treatment of these infections must occur during pregnancy.

Activity-Exercise Pattern

Fetus

Early spontaneous movements of the fetus may be reflexive, may be stimulated by passive uterine movement, and may be present as early as 8 gestational age weeks. Ultrasound observation of fetal movement shows that repetitive movements occur by 12 to 16 weeks, *locomotive movements* of arms and legs by approximately 16 weeks, and hand-to-face movements by 24 to 26 weeks (Rubin, 1967; Schuster & Ashburn, 1992). By the end of the second trimester, fetal movement becomes more restricted because of lack of space in the uterus. The pregnant woman feels the fetal movements (**quickening**) that have been shown to be a good indicator of fetal well being. A dramatic decrease in or absence of fetal movements for more than 8 hours may indicate fetal distress. In many instances, the nurse can teach a pregnant woman to count the number of fetal movements occurring each day and to report to the health care provider if these movements decrease or stop entirely.

Pregnant Woman

The physical changes during pregnancy and the rigors of labor and delivery would seem to require that the pregnant woman be in the best physical condition of her life. Fortunately for today's woman, many people view pregnancy as a normal, natural state, and the pregnant woman often actively participates in any physical activity or sport that she enjoyed before pregnancy. Generally, avoidance of high-risk sports, such as sky diving and high-altitude climbing, is recommended during pregnancy because there could be trauma to the fetus from low oxygen availability or a maternal fall. Nurses encourage women to choose activities based on their interests. Comfort and good judgment enable the woman to pursue these activities. When a sport or activity causes undue exhaustion, muscle cramps, or joint pain, it should obviously be modified or discontinued. The pregnant woman may want to choose different sports or exercises or a different level of participation later in the pregnancy because she experiences normal changes in her musculoskeletal system and the shift in her center of gravity as the uterus enlarges.

The woman with a sedentary lifestyle before pregnancy should actually increase her activity level during pregnancy within moderate limits. A 30-minute walk or swim each day is a good introduction to a regular exercise program.

HEALTH TEACHING Suggestions for Preventing Urinary Tract Infections and Promoting Genitourinary Health

- Increase fluid intake to approximately 8 to 10 glasses per day; plain water is best to flush the body's systems of potential toxins; drink a glass of water before sexual intercourse to allow urinary output afterward and to prevent UTIs.
- Avoid bladder irritants such as caffeine products, alcohol, artificial sweeteners, spicy foods, and carbonated beverages.
- Make urination a regular habit; avoid waiting to urinate with a full bladder.
- Urinate before and after sexual intercourse to cleanse the urethra and empty the bladder.
- Be aware that vigorous or frequent intercourse may contribute to increased risk of UTIs.
- Maintain consistently good perineal hygiene, including wiping from front to back after urination and bowel movements.
- Complete all prescriptions given for UTIs, even when the symptoms of the infection have been alleviated.
- Drink cranberry or blueberry juice to acidify the urine or take cranberry pills; these products may relieve some of the symptoms of a UTI.
- Seek health care advice for a vaginal infection, which may contribute to later development of a UTI.
- Assess increased risk for development of a UTI: congenital or structural abnormalities of the genitourinary system, previous surgery to the genitourinary system; pregnancy, previous UTIs, and high fluid intake of carbonated beverages and low fluid intake of water.

Regular exercise contributes to joint flexibility, improved cardiovascular and gastrointestinal fitness, toning of the uterus for eventual labor, and overall feelings of well being in the pregnant woman. Exercises beyond walking can be taught in prenatal classes and many have been illustrated in popular books to educate consumers. For the self-directed woman, a book of exercises can provide enough stimulus to begin and maintain an adequate exercise program. For most women, group exercise can be more helpful because the support of other pregnant women encourage others to exercise. The nurse may want to refer a pregnant woman to a well-managed exercise program for pregnant women. Overall, a consistent exercise program enhances the pregnant woman's ability to cope with the expected discomforts of pregnancy to allow her more control of her body during pregnancy changes.

In a normal pregnancy, sexual activity that is comfortable for the pregnant woman and her partner may occur. Threatened abortion or history of abortion in the first trimester, early rupture of membranes, and some other complications of pregnancy call for restriction of sexual intercourse or orgasm in some pregnant women. In some cases, the enlarging uterus later in gestation will require some modifications in positions for intercourse. The couple's feelings about the woman's changing body can pose a barrier to their sexual relationship (see the section on roles and role changes later in this chapter). The nurse's first step in primary prevention intervention in this area is to support the couple's needs related to sexuality and to relate, in a sensitive fashion, accurate information that facilitates couple intimacy during pregnancy.

Sleep-Rest Pattern

Fetus

Electroencephalogram studies have shown that the fetus has cyclical activity patterns. Four states of activity and alertness have been identified: (1) complete wakefulness, (2) drowsy wakefulness, (3) rapid eye movement (REM) sleep, and (4) quiet sleep. Evidence suggests that during the fetal period, a diurnal (day-night) pattern exists. Generally, fetal activity occurs approximately 3 times per hour during waking periods, activity that reflects a healthy baby.

Pregnant Woman

The exact cause of fatigue during the first trimester remains unknown; therefore no preventive measure for it exists. The nurse can counsel a woman that this fatigue usually subsides by the fourth month. Rest breaks during the day and a full 8 hours of sleep at night can increase comfort during this time. The pregnant woman must be encouraged to rest *when her body says so* because of the rapidly growing fetus and her needs for physical renewal.

Many pregnant women have difficulty getting a full night's sleep because they need to urinate several times throughout the night during the first and third trimesters and some women experience positional discomfort during the third trimester (see Table 16-1). The pregnant woman who experiences fatigue because she is not getting sufficient sleep may find that she has more negative than positive feelings about her pregnancy. The nurse should explore this and help the woman express her thoughts and feelings and find ways to support better sleep and rest patterns. For example, some women may need to take a short nap at work and others may need to sleep in an upright, comfortable chair during the later phases of pregnancy.

Many psychological changes in the way in which the woman thinks about herself, her role, her body, her beliefs, and many other aspects of her life are combined with the dramatic physiological changes during pregnancy. These changes and responses often relate to the culture of the woman and her life experiences that lay the foundation for her childbearing and childrearing behaviors (Lipson, Dibble, & Minarik, 1996). The nurse, in providing prenatal care and assessment, should consider these factors to understand fully and intervene with individual coping during the challenges of pregnancy.

Cognitive-Perceptual Pattern

Fetus

Little information exists about the cognitive and other psychological processes of the fetus. Occasionally, anecdotal reports occur of people *remembering* events that happened or music that was repeatedly played during their gestation, but these instances need further study before they can be accepted as evidence of prenatal learning and memory. During the prenatal period, all sensory systems function or nearly function. These systems include vision, hearing, taste, smell, touch, and the proprioceptive and vestibular senses (Schuster & Ashburn, 1992).

Tactile, proprioceptive, and vestibular responses have been demonstrated in the first trimester. Hearing functions after 20 weeks, as shown by monitoring changes in the fetal heart rate in response to pure tone audiometry. After approximately 25 weeks, the fetus will be startled by a loud, sudden noise; many pregnant women can attest to this. Although capable of seeing by 28 to 32 weeks of age, the fetus has little opportunity to use this ability *in utero* (Guyton & Hall, 1996).

Some pregnant women offer natural sensory stimulation to the fetus by singing or rubbing their abdomen. These actions may indicate a woman's desire to interact with her child; knowledge about her baby's sensory abilities may help her visualize and accept the fetus as a separate person. As a means of assisting in the bonding process of mother and baby, the nurse can include this kind of information in prenatal teaching sessions.

Pregnant Woman

Physical and psychological processes remain closely intertwined as pregnancy progresses. Psychological stresses and problems and normal emotional growth can affect the physical status of the pregnancy, the interactions of the family members, and the eventual relationship between mother and infant. When considering the emotional aspects of pregnancy, the nurse must recognize that the woman's personality, environment, physical state, family, and sociocultural and spiritual background affect the ways in which she handles the psychological changes of pregnancy.

Two major categories of psychological influences are (1) the normal psychological growth that is required of parents to prepare them physically and emotionally for their new child and (2) the major internal or external stressors on the pregnant woman that can detract from her ability to provide the best environment for the developing fetus. The pregnant woman undergoes many cognitive changes that ultimately result in psychological readiness for motherhood.

Emotional Changes

Hormonal and other physical changes assist the woman in the psychological *work* of pregnancy. An increase in progesterone levels affects the woman's general mood, causing her to be more introverted, passive, and somewhat self-absorbed. These mood changes help the woman focus her energy on the growing child and on her own growth and development as a person. In addition to the hormonal changes, the actual presence, growth, and movements of the fetus become more and more a part of the woman's *experiential self*. According to Rubin (1984), the classic researcher on maternal-infant bonding, the pregnant woman receives immediate sensations of touch, motion, and weight that she can only partially share with others, which results in a feeling of separateness and uniqueness. This awareness of the child can cause the woman to turn inward. She frequently worries that the shift in energy away from the world toward herself and the child may cause her to lose contact, drift away from valued relationships, and lose feelings of competence in her areas of achievement.

According to Rubin, as the woman withdraws during pregnancy, she also feels a sense of oneness with all life. Occasionally, the world appears to recede and yet it encompasses the woman in new ways. Her introversion, as disconcerting as it can sometimes be to her, her family, and her friends, allows her to prepare herself for the child. She spends her time analyzing her experiences and their possible influence on her effectiveness as a future parent. She constantly studies the qualities of human relationships and intently learns about the meaning of behavior. This absorption in meaning causes an increase in sensitivity and perceptiveness; to others, she may seem *overly sensitive* and analytical during pregnancy (Rubin, 1967, 1984).

Although the *mood of pregnancy* can vary in women based on a variety of factors and at different times in the pregnancy, many pregnant women experience emotional changes such as wide mood swings, emotional lability, irritability, and changes in sexual desire. These experiences are likely related to endocrine changes. Physical discomforts, feelings about changing body image, cultural considerations, adjustments to work and relationships, and demanding cognitive maturational processes can also illicit these emotional changes.

Factors Influencing Development

By drawing into herself, the woman works through the meanings of actions, studies relationships, experiences mood swings, and fantasizes, accomplishing the developmental tasks of pregnancy. She then experiences a growing sense of adulthood, fulfillment, and integration, developing a new maturity.

Although these tasks may not reach closure during pregnancy, certain elements may need to be completed in the early postpartum period or even in the first few months of the baby's life. Her age, fears about a previous fetal loss (O'Leary & Thorwick, 1997), her general feelings about the pregnancy, her life situation and culture, her degree of stress, the presence of other children, and the influence of her loved ones all strongly influence the ways in which a woman experiences these developmental tasks. A young pregnant woman facing the developmental tasks of adolescence may be searching for her own identity and may have difficulty incorporating the pregnant body or the role of mother into her self-image. Cognitively, she may still be in Piaget's stage of concrete operational thought and unable to think through new problems, such as making plans for the baby or even accepting the pregnancy until she feels the baby move. Nursing teaching interventions are needed when an adolescent faces both age and pregnancy developmental challenges that overlap.

A woman older than age 35 who is experiencing her first pregnancy may feel more isolated by her situation than does the pregnant woman in her 20s. Even the woman who greatly desires a pregnancy may feel ambivalence. Frequently established in career and family, the older pregnant woman should learn how to balance her growth and development in these valued areas with her new sense of changing self. Fears related to being at high risk because of her age may increase her anxiety. She may worry about managing physical demands of labor and delivery, the sleeplessness of motherhood, the possibility of having an abnormal child, and the need to juggle conflicting responsibilities.

A woman with other children moves through the developmental tasks differently than does a woman who is pregnant for the first time. The former may worry about how to incorporate the new infant into all her ongoing relationships and whether she will have time to care for both the new baby and the older children as much as needed. She may have fears and anxieties about labor and delivery because of a previous negative experience. She may be much more aware of the problems involved with caring for a new infant and may not be as excited about a repeated experience of impending motherhood. Developmentally, she may have already worked through some of the tasks with her previous pregnancies, but now she must incorporate new dimensions into her role as mother.

Other factors affect a woman's response to pregnancy. For example, was the pregnancy desired? How supportive or welcoming is the woman's family? What effect will this baby have on her career aspirations? If the woman is under stress from finances, family, work problems, or poor health, then she may be inhibited from doing the work of pregnancy as she copes with day-to-day living and prioritizes basic survival needs above the emotional needs of pregnancy.

Developmental Tasks Rubin (1967, 1977, 1984) describes four major developmental tasks that the woman seeks to accomplish as she learns to become a mother:

1. Ensuring safe passage through pregnancy and childbirth.
2. Ensuring the acceptance of the child by significant people in her family.
3. Binding in to her unknown child.
4. Learning to give of herself.

According to Rubin, all four tasks must be confronted simultaneously, but each task assumes greater priority at certain times than do other tasks. By the end of pregnancy, however, all tasks have become interwoven to create a presentation, similar to a tapestry (Rubin, 1984).

Each woman works through these tasks based on her unique style, cultural values, and life priorities. Many manifestations of the psychological work will be observed in the woman's fantasies and dreams, her interactions with others, her verbal comments, and her behavior (see Research Highlights box).

Ensuring Safe Passage The woman attempts to ensure safe passage for herself and her infant in many ways. Generally, she seeks prenatal care in all forms (from health care professionals, books, videos, television shows, and advice from friends and family) as congruent with her culture and needs. For example, Cambodian women rely on elderly same-cultural women to give prenatal advice, but there is little emphasis on the need for prenatal classes or checkups. Hispanic-American women generally perceive pregnancy to be a healthy, natural experience not mandating prenatal care, but a strong matriarchal support system for a positive outcome of pregnancy.

The folklore of pregnancy becomes extremely important to some women and they attempt to avoid activities that they believe may be detrimental to the baby. Examples of this type of folklore are myths that the cord will strangle the infant if the mother raises her arms above her head or that viewing a disabled person will cause the baby to be abnormal. Chinese-American women may avoid the zoo during pregnancy for fear that the baby will resemble one of the zoo animals.

Activities such as falling, experiencing a blow to the abdomen, or undertaking strenuous exercise involve new risks; normal, everyday events can seem dangerous and threatening. In her growing protectiveness for herself and the fetus, the woman feels more and more vulnerable and may avoid crowds, revolving doors, small spaces, and active children. She often desires peace and serenity and yet hates to be alone.

In her third trimester, the pregnant woman becomes exceedingly anxious about the delivery of her child. She tires of being pregnant, but fears the effect of delivery on her and her child's safety (Rubin, 1972, 1984). Her dreams and fantasies echo her fears and desires, particularly as the pregnancy draws to a close. Frequently, the woman in the later gestation period needs to discuss any negative dreams or thoughts with her health care provider and her family because these may affect the feelings of control that she will need to meet labor and delivery demands (Rubin, 1977).

When able to discuss and work through distressing dreams or thoughts during pregnancy, the woman may gain insight into herself and her ability to succeed in delivery and parenting. She tries to avoid harmful places and behaviors, she attempts to prepare herself for delivery, and she seeks reassurance from friends and health professionals about the probability of having a normal child. However,

research highlights

Guidelines for Prenatal Care

The purpose of this study was to examine the relationship between compliance with the U.S. Public Health Service guidelines for prenatal care and the rate of prenatal hospitalization.

All women admitted to a Boston referral center during January and February 1993 with a pregnancy of at least 18 weeks gestation were included in the study (n = 1453). Of the 1453 eligible women, medical records for 1400 (90%) were located for review and included the prenatal record. The primary outcome variable examined was the rate of prenatal hospitalization. Other variables included age, race, marital status, parity, occupation, current cigarette use, preexisting medical or obstetrical conditions, history of infertility, insurance status, and previous spontaneous abortions or fetal death.

Prenatal hospitalizations occurred during 248 (17.7%) pregnancies. Common causes included preterm labor, pregnancy-induced hypertension, diabetes, vaginal bleeding or placenta previa, premature rupture of membranes, and pyelonephritis. Mean gestational age at the time of prenatal hospitalization was 30.7 weeks (range = 18 to 41 weeks). The median length of stay for all prenatal admissions was 4 days; the median total charge was $5667. Prenatal hospitalization is a significant public health problem and a costly complication of pregnancy. Given the cost and morbidity associated with prenatal hospitalization, interventions should be designed to improve the adequacy of prenatal care.

Data from Haas, J. S., Berman, S., Lee, L. W. K., Goldberg, A. B., & Cook, E. F. (1996). Prenatal hospitalization and compliance with guidelines for prenatal care. *American Journal of Public Health, 86*, 815.

nothing that the woman does during her pregnancy will completely free her from her fears. Only the safe delivery of a normal child can fully accomplish this task (Rubin, 1972).

Ensuring Acceptance of the Child The woman must believe that her child will be accepted into her family based on her definition of family (Zachariah, 1994). According to Rubin (1984), the partner's receptivity to the child is particularly important; the woman may show new concern for the man's acceptance of his role as father and for his dependability in all situations. Many fantasies about the gender of her child revolve around her partner's preference. The woman frequently judges his degree of receptivity to the infant by the amount of love and attention that she herself receives from him during her pregnancy. She accepts these inputs as messages that the child, as part of herself, is welcome. The desirability of one support group, such as other women, may be considered greater than another, such as the father of the baby, based on the individual's background; therefore the nurse must be sensitive to the meaning of support in various cultures.

Binding In to Her Unknown Child This task is the most complex, cognitive process for the pregnant woman (Rubin, 1984). To accomplish this task, she takes two basic steps: (1) incorporating and integrating the fetus as an integral part of herself, then (2) growing in her perception to see the infant as a separate being. This task is not completed until after the birth of the baby. The pregnant woman's fantasies clearly demonstrate her growing awareness of the child as a person. Many early fantasies are fleeting, highly changeable images. The woman may experience associative fantasies: when she eats an egg, for instance, she may think of the baby. Fantasies in the second and third trimesters relate more specifically to what the child will be; the woman may use clothing, imagining placing the baby in little girl or little boy clothes. During the eighth month, she is ready to begin nesting activity. She thinks of the baby as an external reality and starts preparing the environment by readying the crib and the nursery.

Learning to Give of Herself Although the actual mothering activity occurs after the birth, the learning process begins during pregnancy. The woman begins the task by examining what she will gain and lose by becoming a mother. She then explores the meaning of giving by examining how others give to her, how other mothers give to their children, and how she has given to others in the past (Rubin, 1984). If this is her first pregnancy, then she may be concerned about this ability. If she has other children, then she may fear that she will not have enough to give or will give unequally. Outward manifestations of giving are important; the woman values gifts of companionship and concern and needs to have others give gifts to the baby. Gifts for herself and the baby represent meaningful manifestations of her own and others' acceptance and ability to give to the child (Rubin, 1967, 1972).

The woman, according to Rubin (1972), has much ambivalence about the central task of giving birth. She prays for safe delivery and "for the true gifts of living—time, interest, companionship, concern and relief" during a time of anxiety and stress.

Extensive cognitive growth and development occurs in the pregnant woman, which allows her to focus on and accomplish the developmental tasks of pregnancy. The last two tasks (binding in and learning to give of herself) demand that the woman change her self-concept to see herself first as a pregnant woman and then as a mother, making pregnancy a kind of identity reformation.

Self-Perception–Self-Concept Pattern

To develop a maternal identity, the woman must first accept the pregnant body image. Early in the pregnancy, the woman accepts the infant as part of herself; then gradually, she begins to see the baby as a separate individual, simultaneously taking on the new role of mother.

In the developmental task of binding in to the child, the woman first incorporates the infant into her self-image. Ambivalence in the first trimester results partly from the woman's need to make the pregnancy compatible with her perception of herself as a woman. Some women dislike the physical changes of pregnancy, whereas others feel a passive acceptance or love their pregnant bodies and enjoy showing them off.

In the second trimester, the woman frequently begins to feel more positive about her changing womanly image as she feels the baby move; as the increased estrogen and progesterone work to increase her sense of vitality, inner peace, and acceptance; and as her body begins to look pregnant and others respond positively to this change. Some women describe this time of pregnancy as living in anticipation of joy.

During the third trimester, however, the woman frequently tires of the pregnancy. Her sense of awkward moments supersedes feelings of well being; she experiences uncomfortable sleepless nights, the constant need to urinate, Braxton-Hicks contractions, and other discomforts. Some women experience infant movement or mild contractions as pleasurable, sensual sensations, whereas others find them extremely uncomfortable. By pregnancy's end, these women yearn to have their former bodily boundaries back, to hold the baby in their arms, or to have someone else carry the baby.

The nurse realizes that although the woman gradually sees the infant more and more as a separate individual, she continues to perceive the baby as part of her, as can be seen in her bodily sensations postpartum. Some women experience *phantom limb* sensations and continue to feel the baby moving inside; many cannot lie on their stomachs. Another manifestation of this continuing identification can be seen in the way in which the mother treats her baby. When she feels good about herself, she will feel loving toward the infant; when she feels ugly or unlovable, she may make uncomplimentary remarks about the infant's appearance (Rubin, 1984).

Maternal Role

The pregnant woman's personality, level of maturity, and psychological development will influence her readiness to assume the role of mother. The way in which society in general and her culture in particular perceive motherhood and the role of women and the way in which her own views mesh with these perceptions will affect the ease of the transition. The family situation, the availability of peer role models, and her relationship with her mother are also significant. The internalization of the mother role occurs only after the birth, as the woman changes her behavior and interacts with the infant in a reciprocal relationship. The mother claims the infant in a social context rather than as a component of her bodily system (Rubin, 1977).

Nursing Interventions

The woman may feel overwhelmed by her feelings and thoughts during pregnancy. Although the physical changes are visible to and acknowledged by others, the psychological changes are more hidden, especially when the woman feels guilty about her ambivalent or confused feelings. The nurse includes a discussion of cognitive changes and self-image in prenatal teaching. Whether in one-to-one sessions or group prenatal classes, women and their partners should be encouraged to discuss their ideas and feelings relating to the emotional and relationship changes that occur during pregnancy. The woman's self-image and thoughts and feelings about the pregnancy have a strong influence on this intimate relationship; therefore both the pregnant woman and her partner should be involved in any discussion. The nurse is open and nonjudgmental when the pregnant woman reveals ambivalent or negative feelings about her pregnancy and should make referrals to appropriate mental health professionals when a woman demonstrates significant stress.

Roles-Relationships Pattern

The *pregnant family* changes throughout the pregnancy and postpartum period as each family member explores and responds to new roles created by the baby. Role relationships occur as each member explores the interaction of new roles with the changed roles of other family members. A pregnant woman without a partner can feel isolated during her pregnancy. She may look to family members or friends to fill new roles as she adjusts to her situation. Cultural beliefs and traditions can produce stresses during pregnancy and change roles and relationships for the individuals of that cultural group. Conversely, a person's cultural connection can increase available emotional and physical support to the pregnant family as it changes roles to prepare for the new baby.

The partner of the pregnant woman faces many new situations that influence that person's development as a parent. The pregnant woman may appear different to him because of her emotional response to the pregnancy, her introspection, her fantasies, her need for more rest, and her change in sexual drive. He may feel a rivalry with the fetus and later the baby because the woman has a need and desire to divide her time between him and the baby. He may resent the attention that she receives during the pregnancy and the additional demands the she may make on his time. He may experience more financial pressure because there are anticipated needs of the baby and the woman's need to stop working on a short- or long-term basis. These perceptions can lead him to batter or otherwise abuse the woman, which can lead to loss of the fetus, preterm labor, or injury of the fetus. This strong emotional response from the partner must be considered by the nurse to identify priority-nursing interventions for the safety and health of the family during gestation.

The man may be concerned about his ability to fulfill the father role and to be strong and supportive to his wife or significant other. His role models for fathering may be limited because there is a lack of contact with his own father or because he spends his time with men his own age who are not fathers. He may never have even held a baby before and may worry that he might drop or harm his own child. If his wife is ill during the pregnancy or experiencing complications, then he may feel guilty about having caused the pregnancy. Table 16-3 gives a more complete list of both the father's and the mother's emotional responses to a first pregnancy. Adaptation to the first pregnancy and first-time experience as parent affects subsequent coping with future pregnancies and babies; therefore fathers and mothers must be assisted in framing a first pregnancy in a positive manner.

Other children in the family also experience role changes during and after the pregnancy. The very young child, although not having a concept of a *new baby* until the infant arrives, can experience a change in interaction with the pregnant mother, who may have less time for playing or be more irritable from fatigue. Later in the pregnancy, the types of activities that the child and mother enjoy together can change. The mother may limit or stop active play because of her increased awkwardness and concern about her safety. After the baby arrives, this child may be kept away from both baby and mother by well-meaning friends and relatives or may want to breast feed from the mother as the baby does. When permitted to see the newborn, the child may be constantly admonished to "be careful," "don't touch the baby," and "be quiet." The child also quickly comes to realize that the parents must be shared with this new arrival. Understandably, the young child may not accept the baby with open arms.

Table 16-3 Possible Responses to First Pregnancy

Phase of Pregnancy	Father's Response	Mother's Response
First trimester	Fear of losing wife or child Self-doubt as a future father	Loss of interest in coitus Possible less sexual effectiveness Sleepiness and chronic fatigue Nausea Increased dependence
Second trimester	Increased respect Awe as *quickening* comes Names for fetus coined	Solemnity, hilarity, and playfulness about fetal movements Talk about and with fetus Increased eroticism
Third trimester	Fear of coitus hurting fetus Abstinence difficult Envy and/or pride at wife's creativity Worry about birth Keen awareness of male-female differences	Lessened sexual activity Continence (often recommended by physician) Sleepiness Backache Abdominal discomfort Sexual isolation Heightened sense of femininity
Postpartum	Eagerness to resume marital relations Concern over endangering wife's recovery Sense of triumph in becoming a father Tenderness toward wife and baby	Pain and fear of harm from too early coitus Low eroticism Concern about effect on husband of continued abstinence Sense of completion as a mother
Pregnancy as a whole	Increased romanticism Increased nurturance Increased family life participation Anxiety about costs Concern about lack of skills in baby care	Increased romanticism Increased optimism Family roles replacing marital emphases Fear of miscarriage or problems with baby Pride of accomplishment

Adapted from Gorrie, T. M., McKinney, E. S., & Murray, S. S. (1994). Psychosocial adaptations to pregnancy. In T. M. Gorrie, E. S. McKinney, & S. S. Murray, *Foundations of maternal newborn nursing* (pp. 160-167). Philadelphia: W.B. Saunders.

Box 16-8 Nursing Strategies to Help Parents Prepare Siblings for the Neonate

- Explain the pregnancy and birth in a way that is appropriate for the child's age.
- Answer all the child's questions.
- Use relevant literature to educate the child about the coming baby.
- Encourage discussion and questions by talking about the new baby during relaxed family times rather than during busy, rushed times.
- Have the child participate in decisions, such as a name for the baby, clothes, and toys.
- When sibling classes are available as part of the childbirth education process, encourage the parents and the child to attend.
- Suggest that the child go with the mother during clinic or office visits.
- Allow and discuss negative comments about the pregnancy or baby.

The older child understands the newborn's significance more clearly, but still experiences apprehensions about the effects of the baby on the family. The parents must now be shared; therefore the older child may wonder whether they will have time. Older children may have been told that they will now be a big brother or big sister; does this mean giving up toys, their private rooms, and their friends? Older children may also wonder at the changes in the mother, who seems more tired, less available, and perhaps even *sick* at times. Her enlarging abdomen may appear frightening.

The pregnancy can be a difficult time for children in the family, or it can be an exciting time of learning and growing. What happens greatly depends on the parents. The nurse can help the parents make this a positive experience for the newborn's siblings (Box 16-8). Chapter 18 discusses the sibling relationship in greater detail.

Although the extended family does not usually live together in American society, the expectant grandparents also experience changes during the pregnancy of their daughter or daughter-in-law. The maternal grandmother, seeing her daughter assume the mother role, may view her daughter as more of a rival now that they are both mothers. The grandparents may be reminded of their own aging, resenting when their advice about pregnancy and parenting is unheeded. A positive outcome of the pregnancy may be a new closeness between a woman and her mother if the daughter turns to her mother to seek advice and share feelings. The nurse can encourage expectant parents to realize that this time is also one of transition for their own parents, which can enhance extended family cohesion in the future.

Each family member also begins to establish an

emotional attachment to the fetus or the imagined new baby. Maternal attachment to the fetus has been studied more than that of other family members. When the mother has deep feelings of attachment to the fetus and adjusts well to the pregnancy, she will most likely attach to the baby postpartally. Studies suggest that strong social support remains a major factor in the woman's development of a high level of attachment to her fetus. Therefore when working with pregnant families, the nurse should assess the following to help the pregnant couple adapt to pregnancy (Zachariah, 1994):

1. The woman's feelings of support from her family.
2. The effect of the pregnancy on the woman and her family.
3. Conflicts that the woman and her family experience regarding their new roles.
4. Coping strategies of family members.
5. Information that the family requires to facilitate role transition and relationships.

Sexuality-Reproductive Pattern

The pregnant woman's body image and the congruence of this body image with her definition of femininity greatly influence the woman's feelings about her sexuality. For some previously infertile women, achieving pregnancy may be a *blessed* event, despite the need for technology that affects a woman's concept of self and femininity. Many women, despite pregnancy, may still perceive themselves as *infertile* (Schoener & Krysa, 1996). The reflections of others, particularly a pregnant woman's partner, also influence the feelings of pregnant women. However, many women develop a more positive sense of femininity during their pregnancy, which assists them in accepting their bodies. This acceptance can lead to a greater adjustment in their sexual interactions.

Women experience different feelings about their sexuality during pregnancy. Some women experience an increase in desire, whereas others experience a decreased need for sexual activity. Many women worry about the appropriateness of intercourse during pregnancy, fearing that it will cause miscarriage, infection, early delivery, or harm to the baby. Sexual dissatisfaction of the couple may occur from restrictions in sexual positions, pain on penetration, increased vaginal discharge, breast tenderness, or the other physical discomforts of pregnancy, such as fatigue or heartburn. Many women experience a decreased need for sexual intercourse, but an increased desire for holding, touching, and other signs of physical affection.

Coping–Stress-Tolerance Pattern

Physical and psychological adaptations of the woman affect the resulting amount of stress in the pregnant woman's life and her ability to cope. Every pregnant woman experiences certain stresses, as discussed. Many women also have one or more ongoing stresses, such as poverty, marital difficulties, or unsatisfactory living or working conditions. Even the *normal discomforts* of pregnancy, such as fatigue, nausea, or frequent urination, are stresses that call for modifications in the woman's routine and inherently affect her coping ability. Anxiety tends to be high in the first trimester as the woman makes her initial adaptations to her pregnancy and the anticipated life changes. Feelings of anxiety that are related to the pregnancy itself tend to decrease during the second trimester and then increase during the eighth and ninth months as labor and delivery become imminent.

A pregnant woman's anxieties may be represented in her dreams and fantasies. Many pregnant women report having dreams about their baby being deformed or dead, themselves dying, or a family member being injured. Expressing fears about body mutilation with delivery is common for women at the end of pregnancy. Other women may manifest their anxiety by increased reliance on smoking, drinking, or drug use, all of which can harm the fetus. A person who is using illegal drugs, such as cocaine or marijuana, to increase coping during pregnancy must be appropriately advised to protect the growing fetus and the mother's health. The nurse assesses each woman's progress in taking on the mothering role as the pregnancy nears term. This information can be shared with the postpartum nursing staff so they can continue to encourage discussion in this important area. Other women demonstrate their anxieties through psychosomatic complaints and behaviors, such as nausea and vomiting after the first trimester, excessive eating, food cravings, sleeplessness, and fainting.

The pregnant woman's stress and her responses to this stress affect the fetus. Adrenocorticosteroids produced by the mother may cross the placenta to the fetus. Emotional disturbances and severe fatigue of the mother during the third trimester may cause increased motor activity in the fetus and increased irritability and higher heart rate in the fetus. Excessive nausea and vomiting or food cravings for nonnutritious substances can result in insufficient fetal growth. Maternal hypertension associated with stress may also create placental vasoconstriction, which decreases oxygen and food transmission to the fetus (Piotrowski, 1999).

The pregnant woman may perceive a decrease in her ability to cope with not only the stresses specific to pregnancy, but also the everyday crises and stresses that she has managed in the past. She feels more vulnerable to risk and injury, especially in the third trimester. Her new feelings of ambivalence can make it difficult for her to make decisions in her daily life.

To deal with stress, some women use tension-relieving strategies such as listening to soft music, using humor, crying, sleeping, talking to a friend, meditating, exercising, swearing, and fantasizing. These strategies are safe for the fetus and can provide relief for many normal tensions and anxieties during pregnancy and afterward. For women with strong spiritual needs related to their cultural backgrounds, the nurse should consider spiritual interventions in her care. Spiritual interventions allow women to integrate various dimensions of their lives and to find meaning in the changes and goals of pregnancy. The nurse who includes spiritual interventions also respects the need for a holistic approach to health promotion of the expecting family (Lipson, Dibble, & Minarik, 1996).

The nurse plays a key role in health promotion that increases the pregnant woman's coping abilities, whether in the office or clinic setting or during prenatal classes (Box 16-9). Provision of nonjudgmental physical and emotional care during pregnancy will assist the pregnant woman in developing a positive perception of her care and her ability to parent successfully.

Values-Beliefs Pattern

Pregnancy has been described as the fulfillment of the deepest and most powerful wish of a woman, an expression of self-realization. A woman's joy in creating and producing a child is often accompanied by a fear that arises from her feelings of losing part of herself. She gives up some relationships and pleasures to take on other anticipated satisfactions. She may find that she values friendships with other mothers now, whereas in the past, many of her friendships focused on work or school colleagues. She may find, much to her husband's confusion, that she values different qualities in him than she did before anticipating birth. Her husband may also experience a shift in his values.

Pregnant women and their partners may also experience changes in their spiritual values. Seen as a mystical event or miracle, conception may lead to an increased faith in God or a favorite saint. Couples who have not attended a religious service in years may begin attendance after the baby is born because they want religion to be part of their child's life. Religious beliefs can influence a woman's decision to undergo certain tests or procedures, such as amniocentesis or abortion. Some women may feel forced to reproduce because their religion or cultural mores forbids contraception or encourages large families. In these groups, each pregnancy may be seen as another unwanted, but unavoidable, burden or may be valued because more children signify a stronger family.

Box 16-9 Nursing Interventions to Promote Coping During Pregnancy

- Supply accurate information about pregnancy, labor, birth, and parenting. For many women this information will dispel some of their fears that are based on lack of understanding or misinformation. Some women may want to read extensively on these topics and should be given a list of resources. Other women prefer a verbal method of learning and may need more extensive informational sessions with the nurse.
- Discuss the normalcy of anxiety, fear, and tension during pregnancy. Encourage each woman to express some of her own anxieties and discuss these in detail.
- Be nonjudgmental about a woman's negative thoughts and ideas.
- Support each woman in her self-initiated coping strategies unless they are harmful or potentially harmful to herself or the fetus.
- Monitor and document each woman's progress in recognizing and coping with the stress in her life.
- Refer the woman who is not developing adequate coping strategies for more extensive psychological care.

PATHOLOGICAL PROCESSES

A healthy infant is the usual result of most pregnancies. Certain genetic abnormalities and environmental hazards can cause fetal harm, **spontaneous abortion** (natural loss of conceptive products), or minor or serious congenital defects. The availability of current diagnostic methods that allow early identification of a pregnancy or spontaneous abortion, known to affect about 20% of all pregnancies (Woods & Woods, 1997), can assist couples in practicing healthy decisions to prevent early fetal loss or congenital abnormalities. Wardinsky (1994) notes that congenital defects affect 3% to 4% of all live births and these defects contribute to infant mortality rates by causing structural or functional disability incompatible with life. Real-time ultrasonography allows visualization of approximately 85% of fetal anomalies at 36 weeks of gestation (Manning, 1999). This knowledge, gained before delivery, permits expectant couples and the health care delivery team to access resources aimed at improving the life of the affected baby or to start the grieving process for a baby not expected to live. With recent progress made in the Human Genome Project, some couples may be able to prevent fetal defects at conception and during pregnancy and improve the quality of their baby's life after birth (see Hot Topics box). Unfortunately, even when no genetic or congenital defects are apparent, the fetus may still be injured during the process of labor and delivery and face a lesser quality of life because of this injury.

Harmful environmental agents known as teratogens cause spontaneous abortions or congenital defects, either by mutating genes or directly affecting the embryo or fetus. Dissimilar to genetic abnormalities, which occur only at conception, environmental agents can affect the developing infant at any point during gestation, creating a congenital problem at birth. Fetal organs have critical periods of development, and when affected at that time by a teratogen, the infant can then have a defect in that organ system (Fig. 16-5). Teratogenic agents normally do not affect the embryo during the first 14 days after conception to cause a congenital defect; however, in some cases teratogenic agents cause embryonal death early in gestation, resulting in a spontaneous abortion. Therefore anyone contemplating or attempting pregnancy should be counseled to avoid (practice primary prevention) potentially toxic teratogenic agents that might cause fetal loss or damage.

Teratogens have been divided into six groups: (1) infections, (2) maternal diseases or metabolic imbalances, (3) drugs, (4) substance abuse, (5) environmental chemicals, and (6) radiation (Scialli, 1997). Discussion of each of these groups will occur after a review of some common prenatal tools that are used for diagnosing genetic abnormalities or fetal problems.

Physical Factors and Diagnostic Tools

Current diagnostic tools, such as ultrasound (sonography), amniocentesis, CVS, and alpha-fetoprotein (AFP) screening, have been used to identify a number of fetal problems. Box 16-10 presents an explanation of these tools. Certain risk factors, such as family history or maternal age, often indicate the need for the use of these diagnostic tools. These procedures can identify problems that include abnormal size or rate of growth of the fetus; chromosomal abnormalities, such as Down syndrome; sex-linked disorders; inborn errors of metabolism, such as Tay-Sachs disease; and other disorders, such as neural tube defects and the maturity of fetal lungs. The nurse, in consultation with the health care team, must participate in providing informed consent to women who receive high-tech procedures as part of their pregnancies. Collaboration between health care providers and couples will assist both groups in reaching goals for an optimal pregnancy outcome.

> **HOT topics**
>
> **PREDICTION OF HUMAN DISEASE**
>
> Recently, the federal government and a private agency focused on genetic research have released initial information on progress made on the Human Genome Project, a federally-funded, coordinated effort to map the genetic instructions found on human DNA and within the DNA of several model organisms. The hope is that this knowledge will allow prediction of human diseases such as diabetes, hypertension, many types of cancer, and mental illness. Although this knowledge holds much hope for predicting fetal defects and future disease in children, concerns have been voiced by many ethicists about the use of this information. Can this material be used to discriminate against individuals with predisposition to genetically related diseases? Will couples wanting the *perfect baby* seek genome technology to decide whether to maintain a pregnancy or to abort a fetus if a child has a disease perceived as causing a lesser quality of life? Can this information be made available to employers and health care insurers who might then decide to deny insurance to persons with existing or future disease that may increase the health care costs? Although the Human Genome Project will provide information intended to help individuals have a better quality of life, many ethical questions remain for society to address concerning the use of this information.

Biological Agents

Biological processes in the fetal environment, which include infections and other health problems of the mother, can affect fetal growth and development. The mother with a health problem, such as diabetes mellitus, can prevent fetal damage by adhering to a conscientious prenatal plan of care developed by a specialist in the field of diabetes. However, many pregnant women who acquire a viral infection can be asymptomatic or believe their minimal symptoms cannot harm their fetus; therefore they choose not seek health care, particularly in the early portions of pregnancy when fetal damage from viruses occurs most readily.

When discussing the effects of biological processes on the fetus, the nurse must remember to correlate the time of infection or illness with prenatal fetal development to understand the possible congenital defects. Maternal infections that occur during the first trimester of pregnancy often result in severe defects. Infections later in pregnancy can also seriously affect the fetus, but usually occur less frequently. Fetal death and malformations correlate with certain infections, particularly viral illnesses. Pregnancy appears to render many women more susceptible to viral illness. Most viruses travel through the placenta and the embryo (the first 8 weeks of gestation) appears to be more vulnerable to viral attack than the fetus. Only the infections that tend to cause the most serious problems will be discussed.

Toxoplasmosis

Toxoplasmosis, a protozoan, infects people through undercooked meat and handling of cat feces. The infected pregnant woman can have symptoms of toxoplasmosis infection or can have mild to severe upper respiratory symptoms believed to be unrelated to an infection. Most affected fetuses show no signs of the infection at birth. However, about 30% of infants exposed during pregnancy have symptoms ranging from skin rashes, hepatosplenomegaly, lymphadenopathy, myocarditis, pneumonia, jaundice, and severe CNS damage (Remington, McLeod, & Desmontes, 1995). Some infants show clinical symptoms months or years later, whereas others have no clinical symptoms. Although this infection is rare, the results to the infant can be severe. The pregnant women should avoid eating raw meat, handling cats, or cleaning kitty litter boxes to avoid exposure to toxoplasmosis.

Syphilis

Syphilis, a **sexually transmitted disease** (STD) caused by the spirochete *Treponema pallidum*, can be transferred to the fetus from an infected mother. Although preventable and treatable, the number of congenital and neonatal syphilis cases has increased over the last several years, with two to five infants contracting the disease for every 100 women identified as having the disease (Askin, 1999). Approxi-

Box 16-10 Physical and Diagnostic Tools Used with Pregnancy

ULTRASOUND (SONOGRAPHY)

Procedure using high-frequency sound waves that bounce off fetal tissue to produce a fetal image called a sonogram.

- May be used to confirm a pregnancy or to evaluate fetal or placental growth during pregnancy.
- Useful with multifetal pregnancy and complications of pregnancy (such as excess amniotic fluid, fetal anomalies, fetal death, and abnormal fetal position).
- Deemed safe, noninvasive, and lacking risks of radiological examinations.
- May foster maternal-fetal attachment because mother can see infant before birth.

AMNIOCENTESIS

Procedure involving insertion of sterile needle into amniotic sac to withdraw fluid for examination.

- Used to identify abnormal chromosomal number or arrangement indicative of fetal genetic defect, such as Down syndrome or Tay-Sachs' disease, or to identify fetal lung maturity (FLM).
- Usually performed in second trimester when uterus has grown into abdomen and sufficient amniotic fluid exists.
- Performed under ultrasound guidance to prevent potential damage to fetus and/or placenta.
- Involves less than 1% risk, but may cause spontaneous abortion, infection, hemorrhage, premature labor, or maternal-fetal blood mixture.
- Because of potential maternal-fetal blood mixture, Rh-negative woman receives RhoGam (immune globulin) before procedure.
- Because of invasive nature, requires informed consent form to be signed before procedure.

CHORIONIC VILLUS SAMPLING (CVS)

Procedure involving collection of cells from portion of placenta used to identify fetal genetic abnormalities.

- Performed approximately 10 to 12 weeks gestation through abdominal or vaginal collection of placental cells.
- Involves slightly higher risk of bleeding, spontaneous abortion, fetal-maternal mixture of blood, and intrauterine infection than does amniocentesis.
- Because of potential feto-maternal hemorrhage and isoimmunization with pregnancy, Rh-negative women usually take RhoGam before procedure.
- Because of invasive nature, requires signing of informed consent permit before procedure.

MATERNAL SERUM ALPHA-FETOPROTEIN LEVEL (MSAFP)

Procedure involving collection of maternal blood to identify common central nervous system abnormalities.

- Recommended at 16 to 18 weeks of pregnancy to identify common congenital malformations of CNS (anencephaly, spina bifida, and encephalocele) (ACOG, 1996).
- Level may vary with maternal age, gestational age, multiple births, weight, and race of mother (Covington, Gieleghem, Board, Madison, Need, & Miller, 1996).
- Abnormal value in maternal serum normally dictates additional monitoring of potential fetal problems (repeated MSAFP, specialized ultrasonography, and amniocentesis).

CONTRACTION STRESS TEST (CST)

Test evaluating placental functioning and fetal ability to cope with labor and delivery.

- Fetal response to oxytocin (a synthetic hormone used to induce uterine contractions) or breast stimulation occurs in hospital setting.
- External fetal heart monitor used to assess fetal and uterine response to uterine contractions.
- Fetal heart rate decelerations may occur related to poor placental perfusion found in maternal hypertension, diabetes, and other high-risk conditions.
- Usually completed after the thirty-fourth week of pregnancy.
- Expensive and time-consuming test; woman may go into premature labor during test.
- Not commonly performed because of existence of less invasive Biophysical Profile test.

BIOPHYSICAL PROFILE (BPP)

Procedure assessing fetal activity within intrauterine environment.

- Noninvasive test that evaluates fetal breathing movements, fetal tone, amniotic fluid amounts, fetal heart rate, and reactive nonstress test to produce a score indicative of positive fetal outcome.
- Abnormal BPP may dictate need for labor induction to support positive fetal outcome.

NONSTRESS TEST (NST)

Procedure assessing fetal response to fetal movement.

- Commonly used with high-risk pregnancies because of lack of risks, ease of administration.
- Involves external fetal heart rate variability (alternations of fetal heart rate) and uterine contraction activity.
- Desire for a reactive NST: baby accelerates its heart by at least 15 beats per minute, sustains this increase for at least 15 seconds, and shows this pattern at least twice in a 30-minute period.

FETAL HEART RATE MONITORING (FHRM)

Procedure involving belts placed on a pregnant woman's abdomen to identify FHR patterns in response to uterine activity.

- External monitoring accepted standard during labor for many women (Association of Women's Health, Obstetrical and Neonatal Nursing, 1998).
- Internal monitoring through use of scalp electrode to fetal head may be used for high-risk pregnancies (meconium-stained fluid, maternal hypertension, and postmaturity of fetus).
- Need to evaluate necessity for long-term monitoring because may influence ambulatory and coping abilities of laboring women; monitoring should never replace nurse's personal *hands-on* assessment of laboring women's progress physically and emotionally.

Based on data from American College of Obstetricians and Gynecologists. (1996). *Management of isoimmunization in pregnancy* (Educational Bulletin 227). Washington, DC: The Author; Association of Women's Health, Obstetrical, and Neonatal Nursing. (1998). *Standards and guidelines for professional nursing practice in the care of women and newborns* (5th ed.). Washington, DC: The Association; Covington, C., Gieleghem, P., Board, F., Madison, K., Need, D., & Miller, L. (1996). Family care related to alpha-fetoprotein screening. *Journal of Obstetric, Gynecologic, and Neonatal Nursing, 25* (2), 125-130; Garrett, C. (1999). Assessment for risk factors. In D. L. Lowdermilk, S. E. Perry, & I. M. Bobak, *Maternity nursing* (5th ed., pp. 578-600). St. Louis: Mosby.

mately 30% of all affected fetuses die and the symptoms of those who survive vary widely. When the disease is not treated during pregnancy, 40% to 50% of newborns will have active symptoms of the disease (Carlson & Dattel, 2000). The infant can be born with localized mucocutaneous lesions, coryza, anemia, and generalized septicemia. Frequently, however, the infant appears healthy at birth and the symptoms appear during the second to sixth week of life. Occasionally, a child survives without symptoms for 2 or more years. When symptoms start at age 2, relating the illness to prenatal infection can be difficult. Routinely checking for syphilis prenatally and treating mothers with this disease with penicillin or other antibiotics has reduced the number of infants with congenital syphilis. Treating and curing the infected mother usually cures the fetus when intervention occurs in the first 18 weeks of the pregnancy (Askin, 1999).

Rubella

Despite the broad use of the measles, mumps, and **rubella** (MMR) vaccine and the resulting immunity to rubella, approximately 20% of women reach their childbearing period without having had German measles or developing adequate antibodies to the disease (U.S. Department of Health and Human Services, 2000). The symptoms of rubella infection may cause the mother to think she has a minor virus. However, infection in a pregnant mother in the first trimester can be devastating to the developing fetus affected by this known teratogen. The organ systems most often disrupted include the ears, eyes, and heart, with deafness being the most common clinical manifestation in the infant. No treatment exists for an infected fetus; however, rubella can be prevented. Current standards call for children to be immunized against rubella at 12 to 15 months of age and at approximately 12 years of age through the MMR shot. Adult women who are unsure whether they have immunity to rubella should have a rubella titer performed. Women with low titers can then be immunized, but they should also be cautioned to avoid pregnancy for at least 3 months to avoid fetal harm from the vaccine.

Cytomegalovirus

Cytomegalovirus (CMV) represents the most common infection that exerts possible serious complications for the fetus. CMV infects an estimated 1% to 2% of all infants born in the United States. Most mothers infected with CMV have mild, often nonspecific symptoms. The clinical manifestations of CMV appear consistent with those of toxoplasmosis, such as hepatosplenomegaly, cerebral calcifications, mental retardation, chorioretinitis, deafness, and microcephaly. Deafness has been found in many infants with CMV (Fanaroff & Martin, 1997). Unfortunately, at present, no means exist to prevent or treat this viral infection. Perhaps an immunization similar to that for rubella will be developed in the future.

Herpes Simplex Virus

Herpes simplex virus infections remain extremely common today, with many people unaware of having the disease. This infection can be devastating to the newborn. Herpes simplex can produce spontaneous abortion or neurological damage. Infants who are infected at birth can have localized or disseminated disease reflective of clinical manifestations such as vesicular skin lesions, conjunctivitis, seizures, respiratory distress, gastrointestinal bleeding, and a fatal outcome (Fanaroff & Martin, 1997). Most infants who become infected in the newborn period acquire the virus from the mother's infected birth canal. An infant delivered vaginally by a woman with active genital herpes has a 40% to 60% chance of being infected (Fanaroff & Martin, 1997). This problem can be greatly reduced by cesarean delivery. Difficulties occur, however, in identifying women with genital herpes who may benefit from an operative delivery.

Chlamydia, Gonococcus, Group Beta Streptococcus, and Candida Albicans

Chlamydia, gonococcus (GC), **group beta streptococcus** (GRAM B STREP), and **Candida albicans** (yeast) can be present in the woman's vagina or cervix, infecting the infant during a vaginal delivery. Chlamydia, the most common STD, present particularly among poorer women who have little access to care with early or no symptoms, can cause conjunctivitis or pneumonia in the newborn. The newborn's eyes are often treated with erythromycin after birth to destroy any Chlamydia infection. GC can infect the newborn's eyes and has been commonly prevented by treating all newborns with either silver nitrate or erythromycin eye drops at birth. A gram B strep infection can cause preterm rupture of the amniotic membranes, causing preterm labor, respiratory distress syndrome, and fetal septicemia or meningitis. Candida albicans, a common vaginal fungal infection, can cause an oral infection thrush in the newborn. Antibiotic or antifungal treatment must be prescribed during pregnancy to prevent transmission of infection to the fetus or newborn during birth.

Acquired Immunodeficiency Syndrome

Acquired immunodeficiency syndrome (AIDS) has become more common among women; during 1994 and 1995 alone, the rate of American women with this disease increased 63% (Watts, 1997). With more women testing positive for AIDS, the Centers for Disease Control and Prevention (CDCP) has recommended screening and counseling for this disease both before and during pregnancy (CDCP, 1998). Any woman in a high-risk group (an intravenous [IV] drug user, one who has bisexual partners, one who has multiple sexual contacts, or Black or Hispanic women living in poverty) should be tested for antibodies to the human immunodeficiency virus (HIV). For the HIV-positive woman or one who engages in high-risk sexual practices, counseling must occur before conception. Counseling should include both the effect of the virus on pregnancy and the effect of a pregnancy on HIV disease progression. The relationship of HIV and pregnancy remains somewhat unclear, although it appears that HIV disease progresses during pregnancy because of the altered immune status. A number of risks have been documented. Possibly, some of the early pregnancy discomforts, such as fatigue, anorexia, and weight loss, mask the early symptoms of HIV infection and thus postpone a definitive diagnosis. Additionally, the treatment of HIV-precipitated infections can be contraindicated during pregnancy, which forces an ethical choice between treatment and continuation of the pregnancy by the affected woman.

Infants born to HIV-positive women have an infection rate of 20% to 30% (Watts, 1997). Affected infants may not be seropositive for HIV for many months after birth; therefore exposed infants may not be free from developing the disease until later in life. Recent use of zidovudine (AZT) can improve the prognosis of an HIV-positive woman and her fetus, although the drug remains expensive and is sometimes inaccessible to all women who need it for fetal protection from maternal infection with AIDS.

HIV is often sexually transmitted; therefore affected women should be screened for other STDs. Because of the alteration in immune response (the classic sign of AIDS), the pregnant woman who has AIDS or who is HIV positive should be carefully monitored for the opportunistic infections that frequently occur. She should be monitored closely by both an obstetrician and an infectious disease specialist. The nurse is instrumental in helping this woman coordinate her many contacts with care providers, answering her questions, and working as a member of the team to provide optimal care for her and her child. Frequently, the pregnant woman with AIDS does not seek care based on fears of being reported for her disease. However, involving the woman in continuous prenatal care is important to decrease her risk of preterm rupture of membranes, problems with fetal growth, postpartum infection, and continued sociocultural barriers to a better life.

Although important in decreasing the transmission of any disease, especially astute preventive measures must be practiced by the nurse in this case to minimize contact with infected body fluids, such as blood, amniotic fluid, and vaginal secretions (*universal precautions*). Hospitals and birth centers have policies regarding the use of gloves, gowns, and the disposal of needles and other potentially contaminated equipment to prevent the transmission of this disease in particular.

Hepatitis B

Hepatitis B viral (HBV) infection remains a significant concern with pregnancy because it has a major effect on the maternal liver and a high transmission rate (60%) to fetuses from infected women in their third trimester. Various population groups have an increased risk of acquiring Hepatitis B and include women from Asia, Pacific Islands, Subsaharan Africa, health care workers, IV drug users, and women with multiple sex partners (CDCP, 1998). Based on concern about the large number of women exposed to the virus and not showing symptoms until liver damage has occurred, early routine screening of pregnant women and groups perceived as high risk has been recommended. Hepatitis B immunization (three shots over a period of 6 months) can be given before pregnancy or during pregnancy for a mother who is HBV negative (CDCP, 1998). According to Fanaroff and Martin (1997), most women harboring the virus transmit it through the placenta to the fetus, via a vaginal birth, or through contaminated urine, feces, or saliva during birth. Many women carrying the virus deliver prematurely and some infants can have acute hepatitis or later develop liver cancer.

Other Health Concerns

Pregnant women can also have any of the infections of nonpregnant women. Viruses can usually cross the placenta; therefore fetuses can be exposed to many other viruses, with varying results. To date, evidence does not exist that viruses that cause the common cold have a teratogenic effect on the fetus.

A common symptom of many illnesses is fever. A high fever (hyperthermia) over a prolonged period in a pregnant woman can harm the fetus, especially in the first trimester. Whether the high fever or an underlying illness causing the fever has created the problem must be determined. Some reports have found a correlation among prolonged use of a sauna or hot tub, hyperthermia, and resulting birth defects. The defects from hyperthermia, such as microcephaly, anencephaly, and hypotonia, primarily occur in the CNS. Miscarriages, stillbirths, and premature deliveries have also been associated with high fever. Until health care providers understand this issue better, the nurse should advise pregnant women to avoid prolonged sauna or hot tub use. When a pregnant woman develops a high fever, she should be advised to contact her health care provider immediately.

Immunizations of women before pregnancy prevent many infections. Women may ask about immunizations when they are pregnant because they want to protect their unborn child or they may need them for travel. Immunizations such as those for MMR and poliomyelitis, however, are contraindicated because of the potential (although unproven) risk to the fetus. Vaccines from killed bacteria (cholera) or toxoids (tetanus and diphtheria) are likely safe. No conclusive data currently exist; therefore pregnant women should generally not receive these immunizations. Passive immunization with serum or gamma globulin remains safe in situations that mandate individual protection.

Pregnant mothers can have other health problems that can alter their own physiological processes and cause harm to the developing fetus. Black women experience twice the rate of hypertension and diabetes mellitus compared with White women. These higher rates may account for the three to four times higher maternal mortality rate seen among pregnant Black women compared with White women (U.S. Department of Health and Human Services, 2000).

Diabetes

Diabetes can be present before pregnancy or can develop during pregnancy, affecting both mother and fetus. Pregnancy increases the need for insulin. Currently, most women complete a glucose tolerance test (GTT) at 28 weeks of pregnancy based on the recommendation of the American College of Obstetricians and Gynecologists (ACOG, 1996); this blood work identifies abnormal blood glucose utilization and the need for additional monitoring during pregnancy. Complications from diabetes during pregnancy include polyhydramnios, acidosis, increased incidence of infection, vascular complications, and an increased chance of toxemia. Because of an increased incidence of intrauterine death after 36 weeks of gestation, delivery of these infants often occurs before 40 weeks and often by cesarean section. Neonatal complications from diabetes include hypoglycemia, respiratory distress syndrome, hyperbilirubinemia, and hypocalcemia. Infants of mothers with diabetes also have a higher incidence of congenital anomalies, such as a heart lesion or meningocele (Creasy & Resnik, 1999). The pregnant mother with diabetes needs close medical supervision and ongoing health teaching in an effort to control the diabetes as much as possible.

Heart Disease and Hypertension

Heart disease and hypertension are the two major maternal cardiovascular problems during pregnancy. Rheumatic heart disease, a common problem, may contribute to congestive heart failure, threatening the mother's life. The fetus may be premature because of the need for early delivery. Chronic hypertension, seen more frequently in mothers who become pregnant for the first time after age 35, increases the chance of stillbirths, premature delivery, and the development of preeclampsia, which increases the mortality rate for both mother and infant. Mothers with either of these problems must be monitored closely to prevent potential complications (Garrett, 1999).

Rh-Blood-Group Incompatibility

Maternal-fetal disorders sometimes occur and affect fetal development, such as Rh-blood-group incompatibility. The problem usually occurs when the mother has Rh-negative red blood cells and the fetus has Rh-positive blood cells. Maternal antibodies develop and oppose the Rh-positive blood cells. The mother's antibodies to the fetal blood cells cross the placental membranes and destroy the circulating fetal cells, with devastating effects on the fetus. The severity depends on the mother's isoimmunity and complex, inadequately understood factors, which appear to be described best as maternal idiosyncrasies. The results include varying levels of hyperbilirubinemia and erythroblastosis fetalis after the infant has been delivered.

This Rh incompatibility between the mother and the fetus can be prevented by administering Rho (D) immune globulin (RhoGAM) to an Rh-negative mother at 28 weeks of gestation and within 72 hours after birth. The immunization prevents the mother's sensitization to fetal Rh-negative cells by inactivating fetal red blood cells in the mother before the mother can develop an antibody response. The ideal injection time is after the mother's first delivery of an Rh-positive infant or after a miscarriage or a therapeutic abortion. The incompatibility generally does not occur during the first pregnancy, but appears later; RhoGAM prevents this incompatibility from occurring in subsequent pregnancies.

Chemical Agents

Drugs ingested by the mother may contribute chemicals or teratogens to the fetus. The tragic experience with the tranquilizing drug **thalidomide** in the early 1960s has led to a recommendation that medications be avoided almost completely during pregnancy, unless a physician or a midwife approves their use. The fact remains, however, that during the most critical early weeks of fetal development, when drugs can have a serious effect on the fetus, many women are unaware of their pregnancies and thus may not have stopped their drug use.

As illustrated by the thalidomide incident, drugs ingested during the first trimester can seriously interfere with normal fetal growth and development. As the fetus matures during the second half of pregnancy, fetal response to drugs that cross the placental barrier appears to resemble closer the neonate's response. The mechanisms of absorption, distribution, metabolism, and excretion of drug substances occur according to the ability of the fetal organs to perform these functions adequately. Differences in drug action at different fetal stages can depend on the maturity level of interdependent mechanisms that develop at different rates during fetal life. Drugs can also alter the placenta itself, or the placenta can react differently to chemical influences at various stages of pregnancy. The most common drugs that can cause congenital defects are prescription drugs, over-the-counter (OTC) drugs, street drugs, nicotine (cigarettes), caffeine, and alcohol. The U.S. Food and Drug Administration has classified some of these drugs with an "X," an indication of scientific studies showing negative effects of these drugs on fetal development.

Prescription Medications

Women frequently become pregnant while on medications for illnesses diagnosed before pregnancy, such as hypertension, or they may receive medication to treat an illness acquired during pregnancy, such as UTI. Some of the more common drugs that have been studied for fetal effects include antibiotics, anticoagulants, and anticonvulsants.

Most antibiotics have not indicated harm to the fetus. Tetracycline that is given to a pregnant mother between the fourth month of pregnancy and delivery, however, will cause abnormalities in tooth development, including brown spotting and enamel hypoplasia (Gorrie, McKinney, & Murray, 1994). Most teeth affected will be baby teeth, but when the antibiotic is given near the time of delivery, the permanent teeth can be damaged also.

The oral anticoagulant warfarin sodium (Coumadin) has been found to cause defects in the developing fetus, including nasal hypoplasia, small size for gestational age (SGA), skeletal defects, retardation, and blindness (Gorrie, McKinney, & Murray, 1994). Although not normally used in the childbearing years, warfarin sodium can be given to women who have had artificial heart valves or who have thrombophlebitis. A woman who takes this drug during pregnancy or while attempting conception should consult her physician.

The effects of anticonvulsants on the fetus have been thoroughly documented. Women with seizure disorders have conceived and carried infants to term while being treated with hydantoin, barbiturates, and other antiseizure medications. Infants born to mothers taking hydantoin (Dilantin) can have fetal hydantoin syndrome, with symptoms such as microcephaly, retardation, cleft lip and palate, and congenital heart disease. Barbiturates, such as phenobarbital, can cause newborn addiction. Trimethadione (Tridione) causes spontaneous abortions, stillbirths, and fetal malformation syndrome in 80% of the pregnancies during which the drug has been taken. The fetal trimethadione syndrome includes growth deficiency and mental retardation, with possible cleft lip and palate and heart defects. Women with seizure disorders should discuss their medication requirements and other available drugs with their physicians before becoming pregnant and should be closely monitored by both a neurologist and an obstetrician throughout their pregnancies (Gorrie, McKinney, & Murray, 1994).

Over-the-Counter Drugs

Pregnant women, as with virtually all Americans, frequently choose to treat minor illnesses with OTC drugs. Research on acetylsalicylic acid (aspirin) and acetaminophen (Tylenol) indicates that both of these medications are safe, although toxic effects can occur. For example, aspirin alters platelet function and can cause maternal and newborn bleeding when taken close to delivery. Acetaminophen can be toxic to the liver. Certain ingredients in common cold remedies have been associated with some fetal irritability (Gorrie, McKinney, & Murray, 1994). Ibuprofen can prolong labor based on its antiprostaglandin effect. Generally, because any drug has the potential for harming the fetus, all drugs should be avoided during pregnancy.

The nurse includes information on the known and probable effects of medications on the fetus in prenatal teaching. Herbal treatments should also be considered, particularly because little research exists on their effects during pregnancy. The nurse must be sensitive to the use of nontraditional agents that are acceptable to certain cultural groups during pregnancy, but should intervene in a sensitive manner when a woman uses an agent that is known to be harmful to the fetus or pregnant woman. Most pregnant women who are aware of the risks to their baby will avoid medications to promote a good pregnancy outcome. Increasingly, with more herbal therapies for common complaints available to pregnant women, the nurse should address the use of these herbs and possible interaction of prescribed medications and herbs during each prenatal care visit.

Drug Abuse

The use of narcotics, tranquilizers, cocaine, amphetamines, marijuana, and other drugs represent a serious health problem to both the mother and the unborn child. All of these drugs cross the placenta and can harm the fetus. These drugs represent an enormous cost to society also. For example, the cost of alcohol-induced problems for the fetus alone has been estimated to be between $75 million and $9.7 billion annually (Stratton, Howe, & Battaglia, 1996). Much of this cost results from the high rate of LBW, preterm birth, and resulting deficits in child development caused by maternal ingestion of drugs during pregnancy (Sable & Herman, 1997).

Narcotics

The narcotics heroin and methadone cause problems such as prematurity, intrauterine growth restriction (IUGR), respiratory distress at birth, fetal addiction *in utero*, and neonatal withdrawal at birth. Signs of narcotic withdrawal in the newborn include tremors, irritability, hyperactivity, vomiting, diarrhea, sweating, poor feeding, and possibly, convulsions. A neonatal syndrome similar to narcotic withdrawal has been reported in newborns whose mothers have taken tranquilizers, such as diazepam (Valium). No evidence suggests withdrawal in infants whose mothers took cocaine or amphetamines, although some animal experiments indicate that these drugs are teratogenic and cause impaired fetal growth and increased rates of spontaneous abortion (American Academy of Pediatrics, 1995). Frequent marijuana use with pregnancy may cause fetal immunological problems. To avoid these problems, nurses must recognize women who abuse drugs and assist them in seeking appropriate help. This task may be difficult because drug abusers often try to hide their habit, they fear being reported to the police, and they are unable to change their lifestyle without extensive intervention.

Alcohol

Many women in today's society drink alcohol regularly. Alcohol crosses the placenta and reaches the same blood levels in the fetus as in the mother; it has been clearly shown to affect the developing fetus by causing infant death at higher rates than when the fetus was not exposed to the drug (Hoyert, 1996). Studies have shown that no safe level of alcohol use during pregnancy exists; therefore alcohol should be avoided during pregnancy and during the time of attempting conception. Infants who are exposed to alcohol during gestation develop fetal alcohol syndrome and can have IUGR, increased risk of anomalies, structural brain abnormalities, attention deficit hyperactivity disorder (ADHD), retardation, and other characteristic manifestations of the syndrome. Particularly among Blacks, Native Americans, and Alaskan Natives, rates of fetal alcohol syndrome have increased over the last decade (U.S. Department of Health and Human Services, 2000).

Nicotine

Since the 1940s, evidence has existed that cigarette smoking by pregnant mothers causes fetal problems. Today, the effects of maternal smoking include an increase in the rate of spontaneous abortions, LBW for age, preterm delivery, placenta previa, abruptio placentae, vaginal bleeding, congenital anomalies, and premature rupture of the membranes. All of these conditions can place the fetus at risk for illness or death. Long-term effects may include learning difficulties in the school years. The more the woman smokes, the more harm occurs to the infant. Even secondhand smoke, which is gained by exposure to someone else's smoking, may create fetal problems. The best advice for pregnant mothers or women considering pregnancy is not to smoke at all. Responding to this message may be difficult for the woman who has smoked for a long period or who has a partner who smokes.

The nurse plays a major role in preventing potential problems to the fetus by supporting and helping a pregnant woman stop smoking. The nurse may also need to provide referrals to other family members to programs aimed at smoking cessation. Some suggestions of the Florida and American Lung Associations that the nurse can offer to help the woman decrease and ideally stop smoking include the following:

- Extinguishing each cigarette after the first puff.
- Buying only packs and not cartons of cigarettes.
- Changing brands of cigarettes with each pack.
- Putting a cigarette down after each puff.
- Refusing any offered cigarette by saying, "My baby and I don't smoke."

Caffeine

Coffee, cocoa, tea, cola, and chocolate contain caffeine, another addictive drug. Mutations have been found in laboratory animals that were exposed to moderate amounts of caffeine; however, these mutations, congenital defects, or cancers have not been found in human beings. At least one study has implicated excess caffeine intake (more than 300 mg or more than three cups of coffee per day) during pregnancy with problems such as spontaneous abortions, IUGR, and prematurity (Hinds, West, Knight, & Harland, 1996). Until additional research is conducted to uncover the relationship between caffeine intake and fetal effects, prenatal caregivers should teach the avoidance of excess caffeine intake.

Environmental Chemicals

Most environmental chemicals that can pose a threat to the fetus have only been tested in the laboratory on animals, therefore their human teratogen potential remains unclear. Some natural substances found to be teratogenic in animals, but not necessarily in human beings, include insect and bacterial toxins, insecticides, herbicides, and fungicides, including dichlorodiphenyltrichloroethane (DDT). Studies on metals indicate that arsenic, nickel, and cadmium are teratogenic only in animals, but mercury and lead are human teratogens. Some studies have reported stillbirths, abortions, and mental retardation in fetuses exposed to lead. This area needs significantly more study, particularly with more women working in traditional male workplaces involving possible environmental contaminants. Generally, nurses should provide pregnant women with information on potentially damaging environmental agents throughout gestation. This precaution may prevent the situation in which the mother is unaware that she has come in contact with anything unusual.

Medications Given During Delivery

The final time that the fetus can encounter drugs through the mother is during delivery. Increasingly, women desire few drugs with labor and delivery, but many receive medications to help cope with labor discomforts. Understanding of specific drug actions remains limited; therefore practitioners use only a few drugs and with varying degrees of confidence. Drugs administered during labor affect the fetus primarily by exaggerating the degree of fetal asphyxia or by influencing the rate and quality of the infant's recovery, adaptation, and neurological behavior. Studies of visual attentiveness, sucking behavior, and neurological and electroencephalographical features suggest that depressant effects may last as long as days after birth.

One of the nurse's roles during labor and delivery involves monitoring fetal response to medications. The nurse is familiar with the drugs administered to the mother and their effect on the newborn after delivery; any therapeutic agent has a potential for adversely affecting the fetus and the newborn. Additionally, carefully documented observations of infants exposed to maternal drugs during labor contribute significantly to understanding the long-term effects of drugs, which may be observed for several days after birth.

Mechanical Forces

Generally, mild to moderate trauma from minor injuries to the abdomen rarely injures the fetus, who is thoroughly protected by the amniotic fluid. However, major trauma, such as a severe car accident, can cause problems. The nurse should instruct the pregnant woman in the proper way to wear both a lap belt and a shoulder harness to protect her and her fetus when she is in a car.

The uterus is another mechanical force that may affect the fetus. Near the end of pregnancy, the fetus outgrows the uterus and becomes molded by it, which may be more pronounced in a multiple pregnancy. Positional deformities (usually of the head or extremities) may result. Most deformities return to normal either naturally or with some repositioning after birth. Some children have congenitally dislocated hips from this type of positioning. Fetal malpositioning cannot be prevented; therefore assessment of the neonate after birth to identify problems and support of the parents about the newborn's appearance should occur.

The actual labor and delivery process, involving cervical dilation and effacement and pushing of the baby through the vagina toward the mother's perineum, represents the final mechanical force. Few newborns are actually injured in this process and those who are usually recover with no effect. Some of the more common injuries that occur from birth trauma are the following:

1. Molding: changes in the shape of the newborn's head to match the birth canal shape and allow its passage (incompletely fused fetal head sutures allow this to occur).
2. Caput succedaneum: edema of the scalp from the head pushing against and dilating the cervix.
3. Cephalohematoma: blood from ruptured vessels collected under the skull.
4. Forceps marks: abrasions caused by the pressure of forceps used to assist in delivery.
5. Subconjunctival hemorrhages: ruptured scleral capillaries resulting from changes in the neonate's intracranial pressure during delivery.
6. Fractures: broken clavicle, humerus, femur, and skull, most often resulting from the general trauma of birth.
7. Paralysis of areas from nerve damage: weaknesses or lack of function of muscle body resulting from nerve damage from birth (may involve brachial plexus palsy, causing limited use of an arm, and facial paralysis, causing one-sided decreased tone and movement; both conditions are temporary).
8. Other injuries: lack of expected function from trauma from CNS damage, intracranial hemorrhage, and spinal cord injury.

Predicting and preventing traumas during birth is difficult. For example, a large infant or one who requires forceps to be delivered faces the potential for damage. In these cases, based on medical and nursing assessment, cesarean delivery to protect the mother and fetus provides the best option.

Radiation

Scientific evidence indicates that fetuses exposed to x-rays, especially early in pregnancy, can experience chromosomal changes and malignancy leading to fetal loss or alterations in usual cellular structure necessary for life. Studies suggest that the chance of chromosomal changes increases in children of women who have received significant amounts of radiation to the ovaries. Several reports reveal that the fetus absorbs diagnostic radiation during pregnancy and can have an increased chance of developing malignancies later in life. Reports have surfaced in literature about the greater incidence of leukemia in children of women exposed to x-rays during pregnancy compared with children not exposed. Unless the benefits of having x-ray information clearly outweigh the risks of exposing the fetus to x-rays, radiographic examinations should not be performed during gestation unless absolutely necessary. In the latter case, a lead apron, as low a radiation dose as possible, and other recommendations made by the National Council on Radiation Protection and Measurements should be used to protect the developing fetus.

SOCIAL PROCESSES

Community and Work

Many more women are now working outside the home either in careers or in jobs needed for family economic survival. As these women contemplate pregnancy or experience a pregnancy, they may want to ask the following questions to optimize their pregnancy outcome:

1. Is my work strenuous and possibly dangerous to the fetus?
2. Does my job involve exposure to toxic substances that could be teratogenic to the fetus or cause premature fetal loss?
3. Do I work double shifts or unusually long shifts that will interfere with needed rest?
4. Does my job involve exposure to viruses or other organisms that may be harmful to the fetus?
5. Do workplace stresses influence my overall coping with pregnancy and with family needs?

With a safe workplace environment (one that does not involve exposure to hazardous substances or organisms and that provides adequate breaks for rest and body movement), the pregnant woman can continue working until her baby is due, unless her health becomes impaired. Each working woman planning a pregnancy should evaluate her workplace for any possible hazards related to a current or future pregnancy. These hazards may include exposure to viruses, fungi, industrial products (hydrocarbons or pesticides), smoking, medical-diagnostic equipment emitting radiation, air pollutants, asbestos, possibility for workplace violence, mental and physical stress, and even noise pollution. Work ergonomics must also be considered: how will the current work space meet the changing physical needs of pregnancy?

Professional career women, in particular, may choose to continue working throughout most of their pregnancy in *family friendly* work environments. Employers of these women have found that by prioritizing family and pregnant women's needs, health care costs related to pregnancy complications have decreased, and work productivity has increased. These employers might offer health-promotion programs focusing on healthy nutrition, stress management, and exercise topics for salaried employees. However, too few employers support flexible schedules for prenatal care visits, time during the day for rest or physical activity, or removal of vending machines to support more optimal nutrition during pregnancy for working-class women. Some working women, regardless of status, believe that after they announce their pregnancy, they will encounter social pressure at the workplace to stop working or will need to change positions in the company based on their needs during gestation. Based on past experience, perhaps some employers fear that their pregnant employees will overuse sick time or seek a reduced workload. The pregnant woman must deal with these specific situations by being factual and assertive about her ability to continue working. National law dictates that it is illegal to discriminate against a woman because she is pregnant. If a woman believes that she has been unfairly treated because of her pregnancy, then she can legally pursue the issue or become active in local women's rights organizations. When a woman decides to leave a job, this may mean giving up accrued leave time or taking a lower salary. The woman needs to consider the outcomes of this decision and how it will influence her family, career goals, and parenthood goals.

Workplaces vary greatly in allowing leave time during and after pregnancy. Recently, the federal government implemented the Family and Medical Leave Act, which obligates employers of at least 50 people to provide up to 12 weeks paid leave for individuals who have delivered babies or have medical problems. Ideally, a woman who desires children should explore the issue of leave when she interviews for her position, but many women fail to consider this option until they are already pregnant. A woman often requires written verification from her physician that she must have leave time before delivery. Although she may plan to return to work shortly after delivery so as not to lose seniority or for some other reason, the woman should be counseled to allow sufficient time to regain her strength and prepregnant sense of well being. She may be unaware of the demands of infant care or breast feeding, especially the night awakenings. The nurse can help women make reasonable decisions related to working by identifying the potential hazards of the workplace and providing information about the demands of and resources for child care. The National Association for the Education of Young Children and many agencies interested in child care publish pamphlets for parents on choosing quality child care; these publications can be given to working women who are attempting to balance child care with career.

Culture and Ethnicity

Every cultural group has specific ideas and beliefs related to pregnancy, childbirth, and childbearing. The nurse and other health care providers are aware of the beliefs of a particular group to provide appropriate, usable information. Generally, childbearing concepts focus on the following four aspects of a cultural system:

1. *Moral and value system*. What are the duties and obligations of each person involved in the pregnancy, birth, and childbearing? Who monitors this system? What are the repercussions for deviating from expected norms?
2. *Kinship system*. What are each person's rights, duties, and obligations based on their relationships to each other?
3. *Knowledge and belief system*. How does this culture define and understand the processes of conception, labor, and delivery?
4. *Ceremonial and ritual system*. What rituals or ceremonies are viewed as essential to the child's acceptance into the family and community? Who must perform these rituals? Do the requirements of a particular prenatal care setting or hospital interfere with these rituals?

Information and advice given to the expecting couple should be based on their cultural background. The nurse has an obligation to seek out information on the cultures represented in the community through community ethnic organizations, individuals from the community, and culturally focused professional literature. Above all, the nurse must be open to a variety of viewpoints, judging them not against personal beliefs, but rather, in relation to the general concept of health promotion and today's goal to provide culturally competent care (see Multicultural Awareness box).

Before approaching the family, the nurse might consider the following questions to clearly understand culturally determined behaviors specific to the pregnancy and birth and to help intervene more effectively in a particular family's birth experience:

1. Who may have a child? How often?
2. Who may father a child?
3. Is birth control permitted?
4. Is sexual activity limited during pregnancy for a certain period or after delivery?
5. What is acceptable behavior during labor?
6. Who may be present during labor and delivery?
7. Are certain foods restricted during pregnancy?
8. Who cares for the child?
9. What is the value of a child?

The nurse must also determine how engrossed the woman is in her culture. Does she think that some or most of the childbearing ideas of her culture are old fashioned, but does she feel obligated to follow these ideas, at least superficially, because of family pressure? This situation can

MULTICULTURAL AWARENESS

Nursing Roles in Providing Culturally Competent Care

Delivery of culturally competent care implies that a nurse acknowledges and acts on the unique history that a pregnant woman and her family bring to a health care interaction. The nurse supports culturally competent care by:

- Recognizing that cultural diversity exists and the way in which it affects the process and outcome of health care.
- Respecting people as unique individuals who, by their differences from the majority, bring a broadened definition of appropriate health care.
- Using data gained through a cultural assessment for completion of a care plan.
- Encouraging cultural behavior that protects the biopsychosocial, spiritual, and safety needs of the individual.
- Gaining insight into the nurse's own beliefs and values about people who may be different or have different needs than the majority or those within the nurse's own culture; understanding how these beliefs and values influence the outcomes of health care delivery with childbearing families.
- Recognizing the values of the health care system reflected in the current customs and practices of birthing facilities and responding to these facilities based on one's value system.
- Providing interpreters to improve communication between the individual and health care providers.
- Becoming literate in languages, customs, and cultural practices of people commonly seen in the health care environment.

be difficult; therefore the nurse can sometimes be a confidant for the woman who needs to vent her frustrations about cultural restrictions. This release may assist the individual in adjusting her mode of action to meet her needs and the standards of her cultural group.

Legislation

Both legislative actions and social movements influence childbearing. In some countries, such as China, the government decrees how many children a couple can have and imposes economic or social sanctions to enforce these restrictions. Although Americans can have as many children as they desire, the general social trend in this country today is toward smaller families. Various coalitions lobby strongly for restriction of family size and for *desired children* in families. The recent Family and Medical Leave Act validates the federal government's commitment to prioritizing family issues by giving new parents time off from work in the early months of parenthood, while still supporting these individuals' professional goals and needs.

The U.S. government remains concerned about the health of pregnant women and ways to decrease fetal and infant morbidity and mortality. Historically, Medicaid and Title V maternal and child health grant money has been used by states to upgrade services for pregnant women and children relevant to local needs. National governmental decisions determine the amount of money that is sent to states, which can determine how money will be allocated. Current concern focuses on whether this money will be used for women and children's programs when there are so many competing health needs of society. Many community health centers depend totally on this federal money and often must close or drastically reduce services when less money is allocated to states from the federal level. Local health departments usually offer free or low-cost prenatal care for women who are pregnant, but again, the extent of services depends on state government allocation of funds. Despite this free or low-cost care, 20% of the American rural population and 16% of the urban American population have no health insurance to cover significant health care costs (U.S. Department of Health and Human Services, 2000). Ethnically diverse populations and, in particular, Hispanic groups, frequently lack insurance and may also lack a level of education that increases their chance of understanding health-related information for family health promotion. Educating women during the childbearing cycle seems particularly important because greater education of these women increases the chances of their families obtaining and understanding health promotion information for more healthy behaviors (U.S. Department of Health and Human Services, 2000).

The nurse must stay informed to teach pregnant women about pending legislative action on health care issues related to the expecting family. A well-written letter from a nurse to the local representative or a television appearance by a nurse supporting universal prenatal care for every women in the United States can influence decisions on health care issues and change health care policies that focus on pregnancy (Cobb, 1998). Additionally, individuals should be encouraged to express their views and questions to their governmental representatives. This expression indeed works; because there is public sentiment against early hospital discharge of recently delivered mothers (a decision mandated by managed care systems to save money), many states have passed legislation that supports hospital stays of at least 48 hours for women who have vaginal deliveries and even longer stays for women who have cesarean deliveries. Longer stays may allow the identification of potential problems in the mother or the baby before discharge, such as difficulty breast feeding. Legislation in this area may ease concerns about evidence that more mothers and infants experience significant complications at home because of the lack of observation by a health care provider in the delivery agency. Continued legislative work in the areas of insurance reform may support that more health maintenance organizations (HMO) cover family planning services so couples can plan pregnancies to meet their sociocultural and financial goals and needs (U.S. Department of Health and Human Services, 2000). Insurance reform may also improve health care coverage for insured individuals who lack a consistent source of care or report difficulties in receiving care because of communication, structural, or personal barriers within their insurance system (Weinick, Zuvekas, & Drilea, 1997).

Economics

When the pregnant woman begins prenatal care, personal financial resources can influence the kind of care she receives, whether she works during or after a pregnancy, her acceptance of a pregnancy, her nutritional status, and many other aspects. The expenses of the pregnancy itself may be the determining factor in placing the woman or her family in a financial crisis. Couples who have planned a pregnancy have often, but not always, considered the financial implications of the decision. The nurse must understand the financial history and priorities of the couple, because this information will affect prenatal care use.

The nurse inquires about finances to make appropriate suggestions to each family. The Title V maternal-child programs or the local health department may be a resource for families. Until recently, Medicaid provided no family planning services for adolescents, a situation that may have influenced high rates of pregnancy in some sectors of this country (U.S. Department of Health and Human Services, 2000). Many low-income women qualify for the U.S. Department of Agriculture's supplemental feeding program for women, infants, and children (WIC). This program provides essential foods such as milk, cheese, and eggs to the pregnant and lactating woman. The nurse can assist with planning a budget for food and other essential requirements based on what the individual family members need for good health rather than what they are in the habit of eating. Cultural practices must also be considered. Local food banks and secondhand clothing and baby supply stores may provide needed items for these families. Occasionally, free transportation and child care are available to help women get to and from prenatal care and to allow the woman to be focused during her prenatal visits.

Financial need is a sensitive topic for many pregnant women. The nurse must inquire in a caring and sensitive manner, involve relevant family and support people, and offer suggestions similar to other needs of the pregnant woman.

Health Care Delivery System

Options for care during pregnancy range from medical-based care by an obstetrician or general practitioner to more health promotion-focused care by a nurse or lay midwife. A few women will choose to be assisted only by an untrained family member or friend, but this is uncommon. Geographical availability of options, finances, previous experience, partner's preference, cultural or social acceptability of certain options, and preexisting or newly recognized risk factors can influence a woman's choice of care. Progress made in the Human Genome Projects can help identify risk factors more easily and can influence care during and after pregnancy (see the Hot Topics box earlier in the chapter). Based on their culture and the belief that pregnancy is not an illness, some women will not seek Western medical prenatal care, but rather, will rely on individuals within their culture to provide care until the actual labor, for which they will go to a hospital.

A woman can also choose where she will labor and deliver and how much intervention she desires. The movement toward home birth that began in the early 1970s continues to meet many consumer needs for a more family-oriented, natural, health-focused experience. Some couples consider home delivery, but choose a hospital because of available emergency equipment and personnel in case of unexpected complications. Some insurance companies will cover only hospital deliveries. In-hospital delivery can be in the traditional delivery room, a more homelike birthing room, or a birth center attached to the hospital. The woman may also choose to go home within a few hours after the birth or stay for several days. Pros and cons exist for both hospital and home deliveries. The nurse helps expectant couples become aware of the available care and delivery alternatives to make an informed choice and have a positive labor and delivery experience. Women who lack resources to access the health care delivery system and the teaching provided by the nurse during regular prenatal visits have fewer chances to make these informed decisions affecting the perceived quality of their childbearing experience.

Expectant couples also must make an informed choice about the actual process of labor and delivery. A birth plan developed by the couple during pregnancy should identify the components of care and intervention that the couple desires for the birth experience, if no complications arise. A pregnant woman may choose natural childbirth or a method of analgesia or anesthesia related to the methods available in her community. The nurse can help the pregnant woman and her partner choose the most appropriate method by providing information about all the options in the community and encouraging questions about each one. Collaboration between the nurse and the couple in meeting as many birth plan goals as possible is important because research shows that women remember their labor and delivery experiences for a long time (Simkin, 1996).

Prenatal classes that focus on individual behavioral styles in labor and birth provide valuable information for many expecting couples. The International Childbirth Education Association, the American Society for Psychoprophylaxis in Obstetrics (ASPO), and many local groups offer a variety of classes for the expectant couple. These classes may include information on early pregnancy, Lamaze-ASPO or Bradley, cesarean birth, breast feeding, infant cardiopulmonary resuscitation, and parenting. Classes for the siblings of the newborn are also available.

Throughout the prenatal course, the nurse collaborates with the woman and her partner to assess their needs and choose the appropriate care options. For example, literature on breast feeding may be provided that helps a woman decide to use that feeding method. Information through many formats, such as books, videos, and web sites, creates power and direction for individuals. The well-informed woman and her partner can plan a childbearing experience that satisfies their needs and desires and allows for a safe, healthy experience.

NURSING INTERVENTIONS

Teaching the pregnant woman and her partner during the prenatal course is the most important role of the nurse who is providing care during the maternity cycle. Even the woman who has childbearing experience or who has a high degree of education may need or want to learn information from the health care team that will assist her family in effectively adapting to the changes of pregnancy and in supporting a healthy birth outcome (Fig. 16-6).

A

B

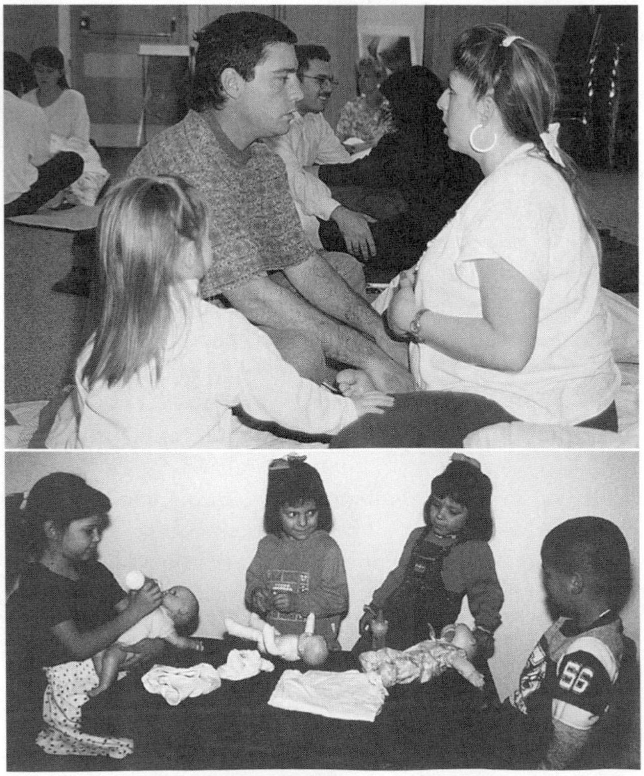

Fig. 16-6 **A,** Expectant parents learning relaxation techniques. (Photo courtesy Marjorie Pyle. In D. L. Lowdermilk, S. E. Perry, & I. M. Bobak. [2000]. *Maternity nursing and women's health care* [7th ed.]. St. Louis: Mosby). **B,** Sibling class of preschoolers learning infant care using dolls. (Photo courtesy of Michael S., Clement, M. D., & Mesa, A. Z. In D. L. Lowdermilk, S. E. Perry, & I. M. Bobak. [2000]. *Maternity and women's health care* [7th ed.]. St. Louis: Mosby).

To provide appropriate teaching, the nurse must perform a comprehensive assessment that involves the entire family (Box 16-11). Assessment, the first step in the nursing process, allows the nurse to determine maternal and fetal physical and psychological risk factors, the woman's informational base for pregnancy and birth, and family needs. Donovan (1996) notes that relating to the pregnant woman and family on their cultural level is important to teach and intervene effectively. Assessment should also include physical, spiritual, emotional, and sociocultural inspection and recognition of abuse. Battering increases during pregnancy and may be detected by physical, emotional, and history assessment of the woman. In cases of suspected abuse, the nurse provides support to allow the woman to make an informed decision about protecting herself and her fetus during pregnancy. The nurse may also want to refer the person to a professional counselor who can help the pregnant woman increase her decision-making abilities and recognition of her power to deal with the situation.

As discussed in this chapter, assessment may also occur by using Gordon's functional health patterns, a common conceptual framework for clinical assessment (see Box 16-7). Data used in the assessment process will likely be collected over the prenatal-visit time and will change based on life occurrences of the pregnant woman. A woman may be defined as high-risk during her pregnancy if she experiences heavy bleeding, premature labor, elevated blood pressure, shows extreme anxiety over the pregnancy, has a fetus that shows signs of distress (lack of growing, fetal tachycardia, or does not respond to a nonstress test), or reflects behavior or symptoms unexpected with pregnancy. After noting these high-risk conditions, the nurse should refer the pregnant woman to an obstetrical specialist or other resources for pregnant women and their families (see the Case Study, p. 457).

After a complete assessment during each prenatal visit, the nurse arranges a teaching plan for the individual. If the woman will be attending group prenatal classes, then the nurse should coordinate her teaching with what is covered in the classes, thereby preventing undue repetition. The nurse who is teaching prenatal classes should provide a list of topics to participants in the class to share these with their own health care providers. A woman may be knowledgeable in some areas, but rather than deciding that a particular woman does not need prenatal teaching, the nurse should develop a more individualized program for her. The following topics may be covered in prenatal teaching sessions:

1. Interpretation of physical findings and laboratory results
2. Value of keeping appointments
3. Danger signs that should be reported
4. Breast care
5. Breast feeding versus bottle feeding

Box 16-11 Prenatal Assessment Guide

ASPECTS OF ADAPTATION

Age
Initial response to pregnancy
Planned or unplanned pregnancy
Feelings about pregnancy and stressors related to pregnancy
Desired family size
Perception of pregnancy affecting present activities and responsibilities
Perception of parenthood affecting future goals
Current developmental task of pregnancy; coping mechanisms, fantasies about pregnancy, and changes in mood and effect on others
Sexual functioning before and during pregnancy; changes, feelings, and problems
History of STDs
Nature of verbal interest expressed about self and fetus
Preparations for prenatal classes (type, when completed), place of delivery, other children in mother's absence, and new sibling
Menstrual history: problems, LNMP, EDD
Height and prepregnancy weight
Obstetric history: dates, course, and outcomes
Present obstetrical status: course, abdominal assessment, quickening fetal heart sound, blood pressure, urinalysis, weight and pattern of gain, and signs of any major complications of pregnancy
Medical history: illness, date, treatment, outcome, surgery, childhood diseases, current immunization status, allergies, venereal disease, and emotional problems
Family medical history: illnesses, emotional problems, and genetic defects (both sides of family)
Loss of significant other in previous year
Food intolerances (lactose, nausea, and vomiting), food cravings, and pica
Vitamin, mineral, and other supplements or medications (OTC) used
Elimination patterns: changes, problems with remedies used
Pattern of rest, sleep: difficulties and remedies used
Exercise patterns before and during pregnancy
Educational background and interests

ASPECTS OF PERSONAL BELIEF SYSTEM AND LIFESTYLE

Date first sought prenatal care for this pregnancy and for previous pregnancies
Reasons for seeking and receiving prenatal care
Beliefs about pregnancy and childbirth; cultural beliefs about childbearing (antepartum, intrapartum, and postpartum)
Racial, ethnic, and religious group beliefs
Beliefs about role of father and family members during pregnancy and labor and in child care
Perception of needs of fetus
Perception of needs of infant and proposed methods to meet these needs
Contraceptive history: methods used, failures or problems, knowledge of alternative methods, and willingness to use
Patterns of use of tobacco, alcohol, prescription and nonprescription drugs, illegal drugs; perception of effects on health of self and fetus
Patterns of nutrient intake: food dislikes and history and method of dieting
Planned method of infant feeding; why chosen
Occupation: present, former, how long, work requirements, hazards, amenities, and work stressors
Recreational activities related to lifestyle
Health-promotion practices (use of seat belt in car, handling of kitty litter in home, and smoke detectors)
Community activities
Perception of and previous experiences with health care personnel and agencies
Date of last physical examination, including breast examination, Pap smear, chest x-ray films, and dental checkup
Breast self-examination practices and needs for education

ASPECTS OF SUPPORT

Address: how long there, housing accommodations, phone, and plans to move (when, where, why?)
Level of education and future plans regarding education
Religion: preference and normal or active involvement
Marital status; years married
Father of baby: age, occupation, educational level, racial and ethnic group, and religious preference
Family composition: household members
Communication patterns with significant others
Communication patterns with health personnel
Perception of emotional and physical support system (mate, family, friends, and community agencies) available and willingness to use
Perception of meaning of this pregnancy to significant other's and mate's response to news of pregnancy and indicators of abuse
Type of prenatal service receiving and perception of its adequacy
Available transportation
Social service and community agencies involved; how long and contact person
Self-concept and perceived ability to cope with life situations
Body-image concept: prepregnant and current and response to physiological changes of pregnancy
Mate's response to body changes in pregnancy
Feelings about parenting the woman received as a child and history of separation from mother
Experience with infants, knowledge of infant care
Feelings about previous pregnancies, labor, puerperium, and mothering skills
Knowledge of reproduction, labor and delivery, and puerperium

Modified from Wheeler, L. (1995). Well women assessment. In C. I. Fogel, & N. F. Woods, *Women's health care* (pp. 144-149). Thousand Oaks, CA: Sage.

innovative practice

Abuse, Women's Self-Care, and Pregnancy Outcomes

The problem of domestic violence is such that reducing physical abuse directed at women by male partners is one of the nation's *Year 2010* health objectives. Problematic pregnancy self-care health behaviors, suboptimal pregnancy outcomes, and psychosocial distress have been linked to pregnancy abuse in some studies.

The nursing faculty from Boston College, the University of Massachusetts, Lowell, and the University of Massachusetts, Boston are conducting a study about this issue. The objectives of this study: (1) determine the prevalence of abuse during pregnancy in selected populations; (2) explore women's appraisal and perceptions of abuse during the perinatal period; and (3) determine whether severity and frequency of abuse affect pregnant women's self-care during pregnancy, perinatal health, and birth outcomes. Self-care behaviors during pregnancy include use of drugs, alcohol, smoking, weight gain, and prenatal care. Perinatal health and birth indicators and outcomes include various deviations from obstetrical norms for maternal blood pressure, weight gain, hematocrit-hemoglobin, neonatal birth weight, and Apgar score at 5 minutes gestational age.

Participants include all women enrolled for care at one of three prenatal health care settings over a specific period. These settings serve women from Hispanic backgrounds and Black, Asian, and White women. The women are recent immigrants and long-time residents of the United States.

Data are being collected in cooperation with participating prenatal nurse providers who have been oriented to the study instruments, the research protocol, informed consent materials, and Safety Protocol by the study team. These nurse providers screen pregnant women between 28 and 40 weeks gestation for emotional and/or physical abuse using the brief five-question Abuse Assessment Screen (McFarlane, Parker, Soeken, & Bullock, 1992). Women who reveal abuse are offered resources and given a brief explanation of the study. The nurse providers inquire as to the women's willingness to participate in Phase 1 of the study. These providers refer interested women to a member of the research team.

A member of the study team interview women who agree to participate. Three instruments are administered in a structured interview format by the team member: (1) the Severity of Violence Against Women Scale (SVAWS) (Marshall, 1992), (2) the Appraisal of Violent Situation (AVS) (Dutton, 1992), and (3) a demographic form. The SVAWS is used to assess symbolic abuse and both physical and sexual abuse. The AVS is a measure of women's appraisal of abuse severity.

Trained research assistants (baccalaureate, master's, and doctoral students from the school of nursing) are reviewing records of all women enrolled for prenatal care at each site for the study period to document the presence or absence of the study's dependent (outcome) variables, which include self-care behaviors, perinatal health, and birth outcomes. Women who do not acknowledge abuse will constitute the control group.

This study is an important example of the cooperation and collaboration of many clinical colleagues and students across all levels of the curriculum in the School of Nursing. Having a research team has been important to the conduct of this research and to the dissemination of findings.

References: Dutton, M. A. (1992). *Empowering and healing the battered woman*. New York: Springer; Marshall, L. L. (1992). Development of the severity of violence against women scales. *Journal of Family Violence, 7*, 103-121; McFarlane, J., Parker, B., Soeken, K., & Bullock, L. (1992). Assessing for abuse during pregnancy: Severity and frequency of injuries and associated entry into prenatal care. *Journal of the American Medical Association, 267*, 3176-3178.

Courtesy Joellen W. Hawkins, RNC, Ph.D., FAAN, School of Nursing, Boston College, Boston, Massachusetts.
Study Team: Joellen W. Hawkins, RNC, Ph.D., FAAN; Joyce Dwyer, RN, MS, MPH, Associate Professor; Lois A. Haggerty, RNC, Ph.D., Associate Professor; Loretta P. Higgins, RN, Ed.D., Associate Professor; Margaret H. Kearney, RNC, Ph.D., Associate Professor; Barbara H. Munro, RN, Ph.D., Dean and Professor; Sharyl Durno, RN, CS-FNP, Ph.D.(c); Ursula Kelly, RN, CS-ANP, doctoral student, Boston College School of Nursing; Carole W. Pearce, RNC, Ph.D., Associate Professor, University of Massachusetts, Lowell; Cynthia S. Aber, RN, Ed.D., Associate Professor; Deborah Mahony, RN, PNP-CS, Dr.PH, Assistant Professor, University of Massachusetts, Boston; Margaret Bell, RN, CS, MS, Project Director, 1996-1999.

6. Exercise and activity
7. Clothing
8. Fetal growth and development
9. Physical and psychological changes during pregnancy
10. Discomforts of pregnancy and relief measures
11. Effects of smoking, drinking, and drugs on the fetus
12. Nutrition
13. Rest
14. Work
15. Body mechanics
16. Personal hygiene
17. Sex during pregnancy
18. Specific preparation for labor and birth
19. Superstitions and *old wives' tales*
20. Signs of impending labor
21. Supplies and preparations for the baby
22. Husband's responses
23. Siblings' responses

Many of these general categories have been examined in the identification of nursing interventions earlier in this chapter. Basic handouts detailing information such as danger signals during pregnancy provide information that the woman can post at home and have accessible should unexpected variations in the pregnancy occur.

SUMMARY

Dramatic changes occur during pregnancy; a new life forms and develops and the expecting family members (mother,

CASE STUDY

Ms. James

Ms. James, a second time 38-year-old Black mother, had elevated blood pressure with her first baby 6 years ago. Because of this problem and the fact that the baby weighed 9 pounds, she delivered by cesarean route that time. She is interested in having a vaginal delivery this time, but recently has had increasing blood pressure values and an abnormal AFP level at 16 weeks of pregnancy. She is currently 18 weeks pregnant and has been scheduled for an ultrasound to visualize the fetus for the possibility of an open spine defect or a Down syndrome baby. Ms. James and her boyfriend disagree about what to do (keep or terminate the pregnancy) if the ultrasound indicates this spinal problem.

1. As the nurse, what priority data would you collect from this couple to help define relevant interventions to meet the needs of this couple?
2. How can you help this couple in deciding about termination or maintenance of the pregnancy? What are your personal views on both options? How does the database influence your views?
3. With the influence of the recent Human Genome Project and the possible ability to predict open spine defects earlier in pregnancy, how will maternity care change in the future?

father, siblings, and other close members) experience major changes in their roles and relationships with each other. Although all fetal-development processes, changes in pregnant women's bodies, and role transitions among family members share common elements, each family experiences pregnancy differently because of experience and culture and therefore has a unique experience. The focus is the entire family, although the nurse most often deals directly with the pregnant woman. The nurse provides valuable resources and information that the family can use to meet its specific needs. The overall nursing goal involves assisting each family in having a healthy pregnancy and childbearing outcome to lay the foundation for effective parenting and family life.

REFERENCES

Alan Guttmacher Institute. (1994). *Sex and America's teenagers*. New York: The Institute.

American College of Obstetricians and Gynecologists (ACOG). (1996). *Management of isoimmunization in pregnancy* (Educational Bulletin 227). Washington DC: The Author.

Askin, D. (1999). The newborn at risk: Acquired and congenital conditions. In D. L. Lowdermilk, S. E. Perry, & I. M. Bobak, *Maternity nursing* (pp. 772-806). St. Louis: Mosby.

American Academy of Pediatrics, Committee on Substance Abuse. (1995). Drug exposed infants. *Pediatrics*, 96 (2), 364-367.

Association of Women's Health, Obstetrical, and Neonatal Nursing. (1998). *Standards and guidelines for professional nursing practice in the care of women and newborns* (5th ed.). Washington, DC: The Association.

Brown, S. S., & Eisenberg, L. (1995). *The best intentions: Unintended pregnancy and the well-being of children and their families*. Washington, DC: National Academy Press.

Carlson, B. M. (1999). Developmental disorders: Causes, mechanisms, and patterns. *Human Embryology and Developmental Biology*. St. Louis: Mosby.

Carlson, E. J., & Dattel, B. J. (2000). Infectious disease complications. In A. T. Evans, & K. R. Niswander, *Manual of obstetrics* (pp. 163-198). Philadelphia: Lippincott-Williams & Wilkins.

Centers for Disease Control and Prevention. (1998). Guidelines for treatment of sexually transmitted diseases. *Morbidity and Mortality Weekly Report*, 47 (R-R 1), 1.

Cogswell, M., & Kip, R. (1997). The influence of fetal and maternal factors on the distribution of birthweight. *Seminars in Perinatology*, 19 (3), 222-225.

Cobb, M. A. (1998). CNS role in women's health promotion and maintenance in a collaborative practice. *Clinical Nurse Specialist*, 12, 112-115.

Creasy, R., & Resnik, J. *Maternal-fetal medicine: Principles and practices* (4th ed.). Philadelphia: W.B. Saunders.

Delbanco, S., Lundy, J., Hoff, T., Parke, M., & Smith, M. D. (1997). Public knowledge and perceptions about unplanned pregnancy and contraception in three countries. *Family Planning Perspectives*, 29 (2), 70-75.

Donovan, P. (1996). Taking family planning services to hard-to-reach populations. *Family Planning Perspectives*, 28 (3), 120-126.

Dye, T. D., Wojtowycz, M. A., Aubry, R. H., Quade, J., & Kilburn, H. (1997). Unintended pregnancy and breastfeeding behavior. *American Journal of Public Health*, 87 (10), 1709-1711.

Fanaroff, A., & Martin, R. (1997). *Neonatal-perinatal medicine: Diseases of the fetus and infant* (6th ed.). St. Louis: Mosby.

Garrett, C. (1999). Assessment for risk factors. In D. L. Lowdermilk, S. E. Perry, & I. M. Bobak, *Maternity nursing* (5th ed., pp. 578-600). St. Louis: Mosby.

Georges, J. M. (2000). Female genital and reproductive function. In L. C. Copstead, & J. L. Banaski, *Pathophysiology: Biological and behavioral perspectives* (2nd ed., pp. 742-781). Philadelphia: W.B. Saunders.

Gordon, M. (1995). *Nursing diagnoses: 1995-96*. St. Louis: Mosby.

Gorrie, T. M., McKinney, E. S., & Murray, S. S. (1994). Effects of drug use during pregnancy and breastfeeding. In T. M. Gorrie, E. S. McKinney, & S. S. Murray, *Foundations of maternal newborn nursing* (pp. 973-977). Philadelphia: W.B. Saunders.

Guyton, A. C., & Hall, J. E. (1996). *Textbook of medical physiology* (9th ed.). Philadelphia: W.B. Saunders.

Guyton, A. C., & Hall, J. E. (1997). *Human physiology and mechanisms of disease* (6th ed., pp. 670-683). Philadelphia: W.B. Saunders.

Hammond, B. B. (1999). Immediate care of the newborn. In D. L. Lowdermilk, S. E. Perry, & I. M. Bobak, *Maternity nursing* (5th ed., pp. 489-509). St. Louis: Mosby.

Hinds, T. S., West, W. L., Knight, E. M., & Harland, B. F. (1996). The effect of caffeine on pregnancy outcome variables. *Nutrition Review*, 54 (7), 203-209.

Hoyert, D. L. (1996). Medical and life-style risk factors affecting fetal mortality, 1989-90. Vital and health statistics. *Data National Vital Statistics System*, 31, 1-32.

Institute of Medicine, Subcommittee on Nutritional Status during Pregnancy and Lactation. (1990). *Nutrition during pregnancy*. Washington, DC: Institute of Medicine, National Academy of Sciences.

Kost, K., Landry, D., & Darroch, J. (1998a). Predicting maternal behaviors during pregnancy: Does intention status matter? *Family Planning Perspectives*, 30 (2), 79-88.

Kost, K., Landry, D., & Darroch, J. (1998b). The effects of pregnancy planning status on birth outcomes and infant care. *Family Planning Perspectives*, 30 (5), 223-230.

Lipson, J. G., Dibble, S. L., & Minarik, P. A. (1996). *Culture & nursing care: A pocket guide*. San Francisco: University of California, San Francisco Press.

Manning, F. (1999). General principles and application of ultrasonography. In R. Creasy, & J. Resnik, *Maternal-fetal medicine: Principles and practice* (4th ed., pp. 169-206). Philadelphia: W.B. Saunders.

National Center for Health Statistics. (1999). *Health, United States, 1999*. Hyattsville, MD: U.S. Department of Health and Human Services.

O'Leary, J. M., & Thorwick, C. (1997). Impact of pregnancy loss on subsequent pregnancy. In J. R. Woods, & J. L. E. Woods, *Loss during pregnancy or the newborn period* (pp. 431-451). Pitman, NJ: Jannett Publications.

Perry, S. E. (1999). Conception and fetal development. In D. L. Lowdermilk, S. E. Perry, & I. M. Bobak, *Maternity nursing* (5th ed., pp. 158-184). St. Louis: Mosby.

Piotrowski, A. (1999). Nursing care during labor and birth. In D. L. Lowdermilk, S. E. Perry, & I. M. Bobak, *Maternity nursing* (5th ed., pp. 348-406). St. Louis: Mosby.

Rayburn, W. F., Stanley, J. R., & Garrett, M. E. (1996). Preconceptional folate intake and neural tube defects. *Journal of the American College of Nutrition, 15* (2), 121-125.

Remington, J., McLeod, R., & Desmontes, G. (1995). Toxoplasmosis. In J. S. Remington, & J. O. Klein, *Infectious diseases of the fetus and newborn infant* (4th ed., pp. 240-267). Philadelphia: W.B. Saunders.

Rubin, R. (1967). Attainment of the maternal role. Part I. Processes. *Nursing Research, 16*, 237-245.

Rubin, R. (1972). Fantasy and object constancy in maternal relationships. *Maternal and Child Nursing Journal, 2*, 101-111.

Rubin, R. (1977). Binding in the postpartum period. *Maternal and Child Nursing Journal, 6*, 67-75.

Rubin, R. (1984). *Maternal identity and the maternal experience*. New York: Springer.

Sable, M. R., & Herman, A. A. (1997). The relationship between prenatal health behavior advice and low birth weight. *Public Health Reports, 112*, 332-339.

Schoener, C. J., & Krysa, L. W. (1996). The comfort and discomfort of infertility. *Journal of Obstetric, Gynecologic, and Neonatal Nursing, 25* (2), 167-172.

Schuster, C. S., & Ashburn, S. S. (1992). *The process of human development: A holistic life span approach* (3rd ed.). New York: J. B. Lippincott.

Scialli, A. (1997). Protocols. High-risk pregnancy. Toxicology. *Contemporary OB GYN 42* (5), 15-16, 19.

Simkin, P. (1996). The experience of maternity in a woman's life. *Journal of Obstetric, Gynecologic, and Neonatal Nursing, 25* (3), 247-252.

Solomon, E. P. (1992). *Introduction to anatomy and physiology*. Philadelphia: W.B. Saunders.

Stratton, K., Howe, C., & Battalgia, F. (1996). *Fetal alcohol syndrome: Diagnosis, epidemiology, prevention, and treatment*. Washington, DC: National Academy Press.

U.S. Department of Health and Human Services (1995). *Healthy people 2000: Mid-course review and 1995 revisions*. Washington, DC: U.S. Government Printing Office.

U.S. Department of Health and Human Services. (2000). *Healthy people 2010: Vol. 1* (Conference ed.). Washington, DC: U.S. Government Printing Office.

Ventura, S. J., Anderson, R. N., Martin, J. A., & Smith, B. L. (1997). Births and deaths: Preliminary data for 1997. *National Vital Statistics Report, 47* (4), 1-42.

Watts, D. H. (1997). Care of the HIV-positive pregnant woman. In D. J. Cotton, & D. H. Watts, *The medical management of AIDS in women* (pp. 193-204). New York: Willey-Liss.

Weinick, R. M., Zuvekas, S. H., & Drilea, S. K. (1997). *Access to health care—sources and barriers, 1996. MEPS research findings No. 3* (AHCPR Pub. No. 98-0001). Rockville, MD: The Agency for Health Care Policy and Research.

Wheeler, L. (1995). Well-woman assessment. In C. I. Fogel, & N. F. Woods, *Women's health care* (pp. 141-187). Thousand Oaks, CA: Sage.

Woods, J. R., & Woods, J. L. E. (1997). *Loss during pregnancy or the newborn period*. Pitman, NJ: Jannett Publishers.

Wardinsky, T. (1994). Visual clues to the diagnosis of birth defects and genetic disease. *Journal of Pediatric Health Care, 8* (2), 63-73.

Worthington-Roberts, B. (1995). Nutrition. In C. I. Fogel, & N. F. Woods, *Women's health care* (pp. 221-260). Thousand Oaks, CA: Sage.

Zachariah, R. (1994). Maternal-fetal attachment: Influence of mother-daughter and husband-wife relationships. *Research in Nursing and Health, 17* (1), 37-44.

Zhu, B., Rolfs, R., Nangle, B., & Horan, J. (1999). Effect of the interval between pregnancies on perinatal outcomes. *New England Journal of Medicine, 340* (8), 589-594.

Chapter 17

SUSAN PENNACCHIA

Infant

objectives

After completing this chapter, the nurse will be able to:

- Define the infant's health status and give examples of basic growth and developmental principles.
- State the developmental tasks for the infant and the behavior indicating that these tasks are being met.
- Explain the immunization schedule and other safety and health-promotion measures to a parent.
- Identify common parental concerns about infants and describe a model for parent education to allay these concerns.
- Describe accidents that occur during infancy and recommend appropriate counseling for accident prevention and safety.
- Specify ways in which nurses can be active in making major policies and influencing legislation concerning health.
- Describe governmental strategies to meet the goals of improving infant health.

key terms

Active Immunization
Birth Defect
Denver Developmental Screening Test
Failure-to-Thrive Syndrome
Growth Index
Passive Immunization
Reflexes
Sensorimotor Period
Sudden Infant Death Syndrome
Weaning

THINK About It

Car-Safety Seats

Infants are at particular risk from automobile accidents. The proper use of occupant protection systems (infant car-safety seats with seat belts) can reduce the risk of death and injury significantly. Although many public service campaigns encourage parents to restrain their infants while riding in automobiles (and all states have laws requiring some type of passenger safety restraint for infants) some parents remain negligent or unaware of the importance of providing safety for their vulnerable infants.

Nurses must remain abreast of car occupant protection systems and the proper use of these protection systems to help parents find new products and obtain the most current information available. Parents often rely on the salesperson of the infant car seat for their information about protection systems and the proper use of car seats. Informational brochures and media campaigns fall short because they usually fail to provide explanations or demonstrations. As a result, parents may misinterpret the information that they receive.

1. What type of program might you develop to reach and inform parents about the importance of car-seat safety?
2. In what settings might such a program be implemented?

continued

THINK About It

Car-Safety Seats—cont'd

3 How would you modify your teaching plan to meet the needs of illiterate parents?
4 How would you modify your program to ensure that parents who come from cultural backgrounds different than your own would respond well to the information?

Providing a safe and sound source of attachment and contact interaction is paramount to the development of a healthy infant. Caregiving and mothering activities are the primary ingredients of an infant's preparation for life and ultimate independence. Nurses play a vital role in influencing this positive interaction through health promotion and education.

This chapter focuses on the infant and family during the infant's developmental period of 1 to 18 months. Because the infant is completely dependent, this chapter addresses the infant's parents and significant others in terms of health-promotion activities. The relationship initiated at birth between parents and infant is the basis for the interdependence that is required for the proper psychological and physical development of the infant. Health care professionals must focus on parent education as a means of fostering healthy, satisfying relationships within the family unit and promoting the development of healthy future generations.

The principles of normal growth and development are used as a structural framework for this chapter. Understanding these principles helps the nurse identify deviations from the norm and institute appropriate preventive measures.

To promote and maintain health during infancy, a balance between the infant's internal and external environmental forces must be established; any disruption places the infant in jeopardy. Several processes that greatly influence this balance are identified and appropriate nursing interventions are outlined to assist the nurse in promoting a healthy infant population (Box 17-1).

AGE AND PHYSICAL CHANGES

Human development begins when a single sperm penetrates a mature ovum. The developmental changes that follow are undeniable and wondrous (Box 17-2).

During this early period of growth and development, the infant depends completely on others to meet all personal needs within the environment. The major resources to

Box 17-1 Selected National Health-Promotion and Disease-Prevention Objectives for Infants

- Reduce iron deficiency to less than 5% among infants age 1 to 2 years. (Baseline is 9% for children age 1 to 2 years. Note: iron deficiency is defined as having abnormal results for two or more of the following tests: serum ferritin concentration, erythrocyte protoporphyrin, or transferrin saturation.)
- Reduce nonfatal poisonings to no more than 292 nonfatal poisonings per 100,000 population. (Baseline is 348.4 nonfatal poisonings per 100,000 population in 1997.)
- Reduce growth retardation among low-income children age 5 and younger to less than 5%. (Baseline is 8% of low-income children under age 5 years were growth retarded in 1997, depending on race and ethnicity. Note: growth retardation is defined as height-for-age below the fifth percentile in the age-gender appropriate population using the NCHS-CDCP growth charts.)
- Reduce infant deaths to no more than 4.5 per 1000 live births by the year 2010. (Baseline is 7.2 per 1000 live births in 1998.)
- Reduce deaths from sudden infant death syndrome (SIDS) to less than 0.30 deaths per 1000 live births by the year 2010. (Baseline is 0.77 deaths per 1000 live births were from SIDS in 1997.)
- Increase the percentage of healthy full-term infants who were put down to sleep on their backs to 70% by the year 2010. (Baseline is 35% of healthy full-term infants were put down to sleep on their back in 1996.)
- Reduce or eliminate indigenous cases of vaccine-preventable disease through universal vaccination by the year 2010. (Target: total elimination for congenital rubella syndrome, diphtheria, *Haemophilus influenzae* type b, measles, mumps, polio, rubella, and tetanus; 41% improvement for pertussis; 99% improvement for hepatitis B; and 99% improvement for varicella.)
- Increase the number of infants age 18 months and younger who have a specific source of ongoing primary care to at least 96%. (Baseline is 93% in 1997.)
- Increase the number of mothers who breast feed their infants in the early postpartum period to at least 75% and the proportion who continue to breast feed until 6 months of age to at least 50%. (Baseline is 64% breast fed in early postpartum period in 1998; 29% breast-fed infant until 6 months of age in 1998.)
- Eliminate elevated blood lead levels in children age 1 to 5 years by the year 2010. (Baseline is 4.4% of children age 1 to 5 years with blood lead levels exceeding 10 μg/dl during 1991 to 1994.)
- Increase the use of occupant child restraints by the year 2010 to 100%. (Baseline is 92% of motor vehicle occupants aged 4 years and under used child restraints in 1998.)

From U.S. Department of Health and Human Services. (2000) Healthy *People 2010: Vol. 1 and 2* (Conference edition). Washington, DC: U.S. Government Printing Office.

Box 17-2 Growth and Development During Infancy

ONE MONTH
Follows and fixes on bright object with eyes when it moves within field of vision
Still has head lag when pulled to sitting position
Displays tonic neck, grasp, and Moro reflexes
Turns head when prone, but unable to support
Displays sucking and rooting reflexes
Holds hands in fists
Make small, throaty sounds
Gains 5 to 7 ounces weekly for 6 months
Grows 1 inch monthly for 6 months
Cries when hungry or uncomfortable
Lifts head momentarily when prone

TWO MONTHS
Has closed posterior fontanel
Listens actively to sounds
Lifts head almost 45 degrees off table when prone
Follows moving object with eyes
Recognizes familiar faces
Pays attention to speaking voice
Assumes less-flexed position when prone
Vocalizes; distinct from crying
Turns from side to back
Begins to have social smile

THREE MONTHS
Visually inspects object and stares at own hand with apparent fascination when either appears in field of vision
Have longer periods of wakefulness without crying
Laughs aloud and shows pleasure in vocalization
Holds head erect and steady; raises chest, usually supported on forearms
Smiles in response to mother's face
Begins prelanguage vocalizations (coos, babbles, and chuckles)
Carries hand or object to mouth at will
Actively holds rattle, but will not reach for it
Turns eyes to object placed in field of vision

FOUR MONTHS
Begins drooling, indicating appearance of saliva; does not know how to swallow it
Holds head steady when in sitting position
Recognizes familiar object
Shows almost no head lag when pulled to sitting position
Rolls from back to side and abdomen to back
Inspects and plays with hands; pulls clothing or blanket over face in play
Begins eye-hand coordination
Chews and bites
Enjoys social interaction
Demands attention by fussing
Reaches out to people
Is aware and interested in new environment
Grasps object with two hands
Squeals

FIVE MONTHS
Reaches persistently; grasps with entire hand
Plays with toes
Smiles at mirror image
Begins to postpone gratification
Shows signs of tooth eruption
Sleeps through night without food
Weighs twice the birth weight
Sits with slight support
Vocalizes displeasure when desired object is taken away
Is able to discriminate strangers from family
Makes cooing noises
Squeals with delight
Looks for object that has fallen
Rolls from back to stomach or vice versa

SIX MONTHS
Gains approximately 3 to 5 ounces weekly during the second 6 months
Grows approximately 1 inch monthly for 6 months
Is able to lift cup by handle
Begins to *hitch* in locomotion
Sits in high chair with straight back
Begins to imitate sounds
Vocalizes to toys and mirror image
Babbles with one-syllable sounds: "ma; ma; da; da"
Has definite likes and dislikes
Likes to be picked up
Plays peek-a-boo
Makes "guh" and "bah" sounds

SEVEN MONTHS
Has eruption of upper central incisors
Bears weight when held in standing position
Sits, leaning forward on both hands
Fixates on one very small object
Produces vowel sounds: "baba" and "dada"
Shows fear of strangers
Displays emotional instability by easy and quick changes from crying to laughing
Repeats activities that are enjoyed
Bangs objects together
Approaches toy and grasps it with one hand
Imitates simple acts

EIGHT MONTHS
Feeds self with finger foods
Sits well alone
Stretches out arms to be picked up
Greets strangers with bashful behavior
Begins to show regular patterns in bladder and bowel elimination
Responds to "no"
Makes consonant sounds: t, d, and w
Dislikes dressing and diaper change
Releases object at will
Shows nervousness with strangers
Pulls toy toward self

Continued

Box 17-2 Growth and Development During Infancy—cont'd

NINE MONTHS
Creeps and crawls (backward at first)
Shows good coordination and sits alone
Responds to adult anger; cries when scolded
Explores object by sucking, chewing, and biting it
Responds to simple verbal requests
Drinks from cup or glass with assistance
Pulls self to standing position
Begins to show fears of going to bed and being left alone
Imitates waving "bye-bye"
Releases object with flexed wrist
Repeats facial expressions of adults
Uses thumb and index finger in pincer grasp

10 MONTHS
Sits by falling down
Says "da-da" and "ma-ma"
Understands "bye-bye"
Looks at and follows pictures in book
Crawls and cruises about well
Pays attention to own name
Picks up object fairly well
Extends toy to another person without releasing
Pulls self to standing position and stands while holding onto solid object

11 MONTHS
Is able to push toys and place several objects in container
Attempts to walk without assistance
Begins to hold spoon
Stands erect with help of person's hand
May have lower lateral incisors erupting
Holds crayon to mark on paper
Imitates definite speech sounds
Reacts to restrictions with frustration

12 MONTHS
Loses Babinski's sign
Develops evident hand dominance
Weighs triple the birth weight
Has equal-circumference head and chest
Walks with help
Knows own name
Has slow vocabulary growth because of increased interest in walking
Develops lumbar curve
Uses spoon in feeding, but often puts it upside down in mouth
Drops object deliberately for it to be picked up
Shakes head for "no"
Plays pat-a-cake
Recovers balance when falling over
Tries to follow when being read to
Does things to attract attention
Imitates vocalization lead

15 MONTHS
Creeps up stairs
Uses "da-da" and "ma-ma" labels for correct parents
Tolerates some separation
Drinks from cup well, but rotates spoon
Asks for object by pointing
Plays interactive games such as peek-a-boo and pat-a-cake
Expresses emotions; has temper tantrums
Walks without help

18 MONTHS
Has closed anterior fontanel
Has long trunk, short and bowed legs, and protruding abdomen
Walks up stairs with help
Turns pages of book
Has short attention span
Begins to test limits
Has bowel movements at appropriate time when placed on potty
Indicates wet pants
Gets into everything
Fills and handles spoon without rotating it, but spills frequently
Runs clumsily and falls often
Is extremely curious
Places object in hole or slot
Becomes communicative, social being
Imitates behavior of parents, such as mimicking household chores

meet these needs are the parents. To assist the parents in their understanding of their infant's progress, the nurse must know what behaviors to expect at certain age levels. These developmental landmarks serve as a basis for giving parents anticipatory guidance regarding their infant (Table 17-1). Parents must be aware of age-appropriate behavior to anticipate and facilitate these developmental landmarks. This knowledge, along with the nurse's anticipatory guidance, can also promote closer family relationships.

In addition to the growth landmarks, the infant must achieve several developmental tasks to facilitate a healthy personality progression.

Developmental Tasks

Everyone faces developmental tasks and must accomplish them individually. Different practices in various societies affect the perception and resolution of the tasks, but all must be faced (Pillitteri, 1999).

The infant's first and most basic task is survival, which includes the physical tasks of breathing, sucking, eating, digesting, eliminating, and sleeping. Because many of these tasks involve the infant's mouth, this stage of life is often referred to as the oral stage of development, reflecting the primary importance of the mouth as the center of pleasure. Duvall and Miller (1984) outline several more develop-

Table 17-1 Parenting Tasks for Developmental Landmarks in Infancy

Age (months)	Landmark	Parenting Task
1	Lifts head when prone	Place infant in prone position and dangle colorful object above head
2	Has social smile	Promote by talking to infant and allowing opportunity to smile
4	Squeals	Encourage and praise for doing
5	Rolls from back to front	Place infant in protected area (crib or playpen) and encourage to move by placing toy out of reach
8 to 9	Uses pincer grasp to feed self	Make finger foods available
10	Pulls self to standing position	Provide safe environment; place chair or object of appropriate height within reach
11 to 12	Initiates vocalization	Talk to infant frequently and include in family gatherings
12 to 15	Walks	Encourage and provide clutter-free, safe walkway; praise for attempts
15	Drinks from cup	Supply cup with appropriate drink; do not scold for clumsiness in handling cup or spills
18	Mimics household chores	Give rags to help with chores, dusting, allow to fold clothes, and so on

mental tasks that must be accomplished during infancy (Box 17-3).

To assist the infant's parents in encouraging achievement of these developmental tasks, the nurse should discuss the importance of stimulation and environmental interactions. Recent information indicates that genetic potential, in terms of the development of the anatomical structures of the brain, is not reached at birth; many of these structures are far from complete (Silberg, 1999). To continue growing, the brain depends not only on internal, embryological, and maturational forces, but also on the interaction of external stimulation with these forces. Stimulation, as provided by the parents, is necessary for a child to develop fully. This external stimulation appears to influence the internal, anatomical, and maturational processes by at least three different mechanisms (Fabes, 1999):

1. Stimulation favors progressive complex arborization of dendrites (the connection between nerve cells).
2. Stimulation increases the degree of vascularization of certain anatomical structures of the brain, such as the centers associated with vision.
3. Stimulation increases the process of myelinization, which is closely related to the rate of development of a variety of functions. Myelin coats the brain and nerve tissue, which then become activated (McKinney et al., 2000).

When counseling parents, the nurse stresses the importance of a variety of stimuli within the infant's environment. Several auditory and visual stimuli should be available, such as colorful mobile, television, radio, spoken voice, and toys, to assist the infant in achieving developmental tasks. The sense of touch is an extremely important stimulus, bringing the infant in tune with the external environment, making it a reality. These parenting tasks are vital to the infant's developmental progression (Pillitteri, 1999).

Box 17-3 Developmental Tasks Accomplished in Infancy

1. Achieves physiological equilibrium after birth.
2. Establishes self as a dependent person, but separate from others.
3. Becomes aware of animate versus inanimate and familiar versus unfamiliar and develops rudimentary social interaction.
4. Develops a feeling of affection for others and the desire for affection from others.
5. Manages the changing body and learns new motor skills, develops equilibrium, begins eye-hand coordination, and establishes rest-activity rhythm.
6. Learns to understand and control the physical world through exploration.
7. Develops a beginning symbol system, conceptual abilities, and preverbal communication.
8. Directs emotional expression to indicate needs and wishes.

Concepts of Infant Development

The study of how a helpless infant grows and develops into a fully functioning, independent adult has fascinated many researchers. Their theories are descriptions of the development of human behavior as overlapping stages that occur in somewhat predictable patterns in an individual's life (U.S. Census Bureau, 2000b). Because these developmental theories are presented in Chapter 15, only their specific application to the infant is discussed here.

Psychosocial Development

Erikson's psychosocial developmental theory is concerned primarily with a series of tasks or crises that each individual must resolve before encountering the next one. The central task during infancy is the development of a sense of trust versus mistrust. Establishing this basic trust or mistrust determines the manner in which the infant approaches all future stages of growth. The infant first develops a sense of trust in the mother (or other caretaker) and then in other significant people in the environment. Trust influences the infant's future relationships, allowing for deeper commitment and intimacy. The infant requires maximal gratification and minimal frustration to provide the balance between inner needs and outer satisfaction, which results in the development of trust.

Prompt, skillful, and consistent response to the infant's needs helps foster security and trust; the mother is essentially relieving the infant's tension. Part of developing trust depends on the infant's ability to predict what will happen within the environment. When no predictability and disorganized routines exist, the infant will develop fear, anger, and insecurity, which eventually lead to mistrust. The infant can demonstrate desire by crying, but depends on the sensitivity and willingness of others to provide relief. If the most important people fail to do this, then the infant has little foundation on which to build faith in others or self when adulthood is attained.

Cognitive Development

Piaget's cognitive developmental theory focuses on intellectual changes that occur in a sequential manner as a result of continual interaction between the infant and the environment (Wong, 1999). Piaget's **sensorimotor period** (up to age 18 months) describes the infant's involvement in mastering simple coordination activities to interact with the environment. The infant solves problems using sensory systems and motor activity rather than symbolic processes that develop later.

Research has shown that fetuses are able to distinguish light from dark and that sight is present at birth. Rod cells in the retina of the eyes, which are responsible for light perception, are functional at birth; the retina (the organ of visual perception) is not fully developed until approximately 4 months of age. However, the infant can perceive color and shape. Because infants are startled by loud noises and are soothed in response to soft voices, their sense of hearing is also functioning, which can be tested with audio equipment at birth. Babies cry when pricked with a diaper pin and fuss when too hot or too cold; therefore the senses of pain and temperature are operative also. Touching, stroking, and rocking typically soothe a fussing infant. Infants will also react to different odors and tastes.

In addition to perceiving stimulation, the newborn is capable of reflexive behavior. **Reflexes** are responses that are normally exhibited after a particular type of stimulation (Pillitteri, 1999). Because the response occurs after the stimulus, reflexes are unlearned. Some infant reflexes have survival value, such as rooting and sucking reflexes. The rooting reflex, activated by lightly stroking the angle of the lips or cheek, helps the infant locate the food source. The infant will turn toward the side that is being stroked and will open the lips to suck. The sucking reflex is initiated when an object is placed in the infant's mouth. Together, these reflexes ensure that the infant can obtain food. Infants also have reflexes for grasping, yawning, hiccoughing, coughing, and sneezing.

Armed with these reflexes and sensory capabilities, the infant is ready to begin interacting with the environment (seeing, hearing, touching, tasting, and smelling) to acquire valuable information.

The infant progresses in various ways between birth and age 18 months, with early capabilities changing and becoming intentional. Piaget outlines five stages within the sensorimotor period that describes the infant's development from the early reflexive behavior to differentiation between self and environment (Table 17-2).

The infant in the sensorimotor period uses behavioral strategies to manipulate objects, to learn some of their properties, and to reach goals by combining several behaviors. The infant's behavior is tied to the concrete and

Table 17-2 Piaget's Five Stages of Infant Development

Stage	Description
Stage 1: birth to 1 month	Modification of reflexes Infant practices and perfects reflexes present at birth. Sucking reflex becomes more refined and voluntary.
Stage 2: 1 to 4 months	Primary circular reactions Infant repeats behavior that previously led to an interesting event. Activities involve only the infant's own body.
Stage 3: 4 to 10 months	Secondary circular reactions Repetitions involve events or objects in the external world. Infant appears to perform actions with a purpose. Hand-eye coordination begins.
Stage 4: 10 to 12 months	Coordination of secondary reactions Infant combines two or more previously acquired strategies to obtain a goal.
Stage 5: 12 to 18 months	Tertiary circular reactions Infant uses active experimentation to achieve previously unattainable goals. Infant purposely varies movements to observe results.

the immediate; schemes can be applied only to objects that can be perceived directly.

Kohlberg, a leading theorist in the area of moral development, states that moral development is prefaced by the child's ability to reason and is part of a sequence that corresponds with the development of intellect. The nurse recognizes the interrelationship between the developmental phases in the different dimensions (physical and psychosocial) of each individual.

Knowledge of the child developmental theories is extremely valuable to the nurse during interactions with infants. Understanding the infant's level of cognitive thought and emotional and social development helps the nurse decipher a child's communications more meaningfully and interpret behaviors and the processes that motivate the child more accurately. This knowledge can be incorporated in the nurse's anticipatory guidance to the parents. The nurse should stress that a variety of sensory and motor stimuli will foster learning within the infant's environment.

Denver Developmental Screening Test

The **Denver Developmental Screening Test** (DDST) is a standardized tool that screens for developmental problems in children from birth to 6 years of age. The original DDST was revised, restandardized, and released in 1990 as the Denver II (Frankenburg & Dodds, 1992). Three purposes have been identified for administering the Denver II: (1) screening apparently healthy infants for developmental problems, (2) validating intuitive concerns about an infant's development with an objective test, and (3) monitoring high-risk children for developmental problems.

Four areas of development are screened: (1) personal-social, (2) fine motor-adaptive, (3) language, and (4) gross motor. Unique features of the Denver II are its recent and sophisticated standardization and its inclusion of norms for various subgroups based on place of residence, ethnicity, and mother's level of education.

The Denver II includes four *test behavior* descriptors to rate the infant's behavior during the test, reflecting the screener's subjective impression of the infant's overall behavior. Behavioral ratings are established for compliance with the examiner's requests for alertness and interest in the surroundings, fearfulness, and attention span.

Although administration of the DDST is not difficult, only nurses or other personnel trained specifically in its procedures and interpretation should make the attempt. This precaution is necessary to ensure the validity of the developmental norms established for the test.

The nurse tells the parents before the test that the DDST is not an intelligence test, but rather, a test of the child's developmental level. By adding the number of accomplished and unaccomplished items on the test form (Fig. 17-1), the screener estimates the child's developmental level. By referring to guidelines on the instruction sheet (Fig. 17-2, p. 467), the child is scored P (passed) or F (failed) on each item. The DDST can be administered with minimal materials and time and, ideally, should be administered to an infant at approximately 3 or 4 months of age, again at 10 months, and again at 3 years (Wong, 1999).

The infant's **growth index,** height and weight measurements plotted on a standard growth chart to assess for normal progression, is also important. Physical growth (height and weight) is a valid health-status indicator that should be measured during each routine office or clinic visit. In the first year of life, growth is rapid. An infant who is growing properly is at low risk for developing a chronic disease (Gullotta, 1999).

The nurse plots the infant's length and weight measurements against exact chronological age on growth grids. In 1986 the National Center for Health Statistics (NCHS) published growth grids that have been standardized to the present growth charts for female and male infants from birth to age 36 months (Figs. 17-3 and 17-4, pp. 468 and 469). Body Mass Index (BMI) is a feature of the new pediatric growth charts recently released by the Centers for Disease Control and Prevention (CDCP). The charts now in use by most pediatricians were developed in 1977 and adapted by the World Health Organization for international use since 1978. With the addition of BMI indices to the charts, the CDCP significantly increased the usefulness of this tool as an early warning signal regarding potential obesity as early as 2 years of age. Parents have an opportunity to change their children's eating habits before a weight problem develops. The revised pediatric growth charts more accurately reflect the United States' cultural and racial diversity and can track children and young people through age 20. Generally, the growth charts indicate that children are heavier today than they were in 1977, but height has remained virtually unchanged.

An infant's growth index, as determined by length and weight, is only one factor in assessing health status. The nurse must have an overall understanding of growth and development principles to counsel parents regarding their infant's progress (Tables 17-3 and 17-4, pp. 470 and 471).

Gender

The infant's gender is determined at the moment of fertilization. Immediately after delivery, the parents usually ask, "Is it a girl or a boy?" The answer has far-reaching implications for many family units. The infant's gender is one of the many important factors that influence the parents' way of relating to the infant to create a healthy environment.

Studies have revealed many biological and behavioral differences between male and female infants. Boys are, on average, larger and have proportionately more muscle mass at birth. Girls are generally smaller, but physiologically more mature at birth and are less vulnerable to stress. Boys show more motor activity, whereas girls display a greater

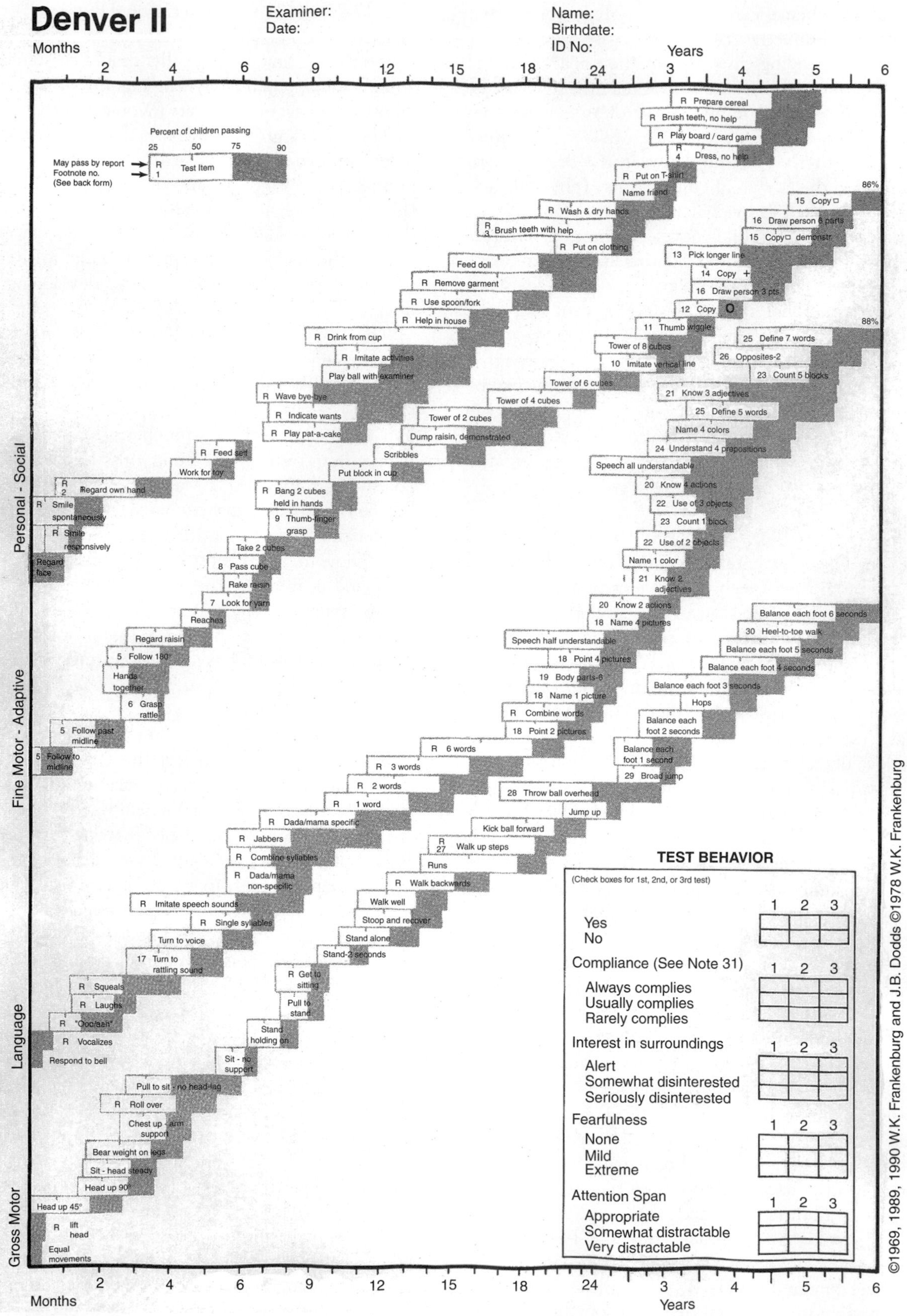

Fig. 17-1 The Denver II. (Courtesy Frankenburg, W. K., & Dodds, J. B. [1990]. University of Colorado Medical Center, Denver.)

Application of Health Promotion

1. Try to get child to smile by smiling, talking or waving to him. Do not touch him.
2. When child is playing with toy, pull it away from him. Pass if he resists.
3. Child does not have to be able to tie shoes or button in the back.
4. Move yarn slowly in an arc from one side to the other, about 6" above child's face. Pass if eyes follow 90° to midline. (Past midline; 180°)
5. Pass if child grasps rattle when it is touched to the backs or tips of fingers.
6. Pass if child continues to look where yarn disappeared or tries to see where it went. Yarn should be dropped quickly from sight from tester's hand without arm movement.
7. Pass if child picks up raisin with any part of thumb and a finger.
8. Pass if child picks up raisin with the ends of thumb and index finger using an over hand approach.

9. Pass any enclosed form. Fail continuous round motions.
10. Which line is longer? (Not bigger.) Turn paper upside down and repeat. (3/3 or 5/6)
11. Pass any crossing lines.
12. Have child copy first. If failed, demonstrate

When giving items 9, 11 and 12, do not name the forms. Do not demonstrate 9 and 11.

13. When scoring, each pair (2 arms, 2 legs, etc.) counts as one part.
14. Point to picture and have child name it. (No credit is given for sounds only.)

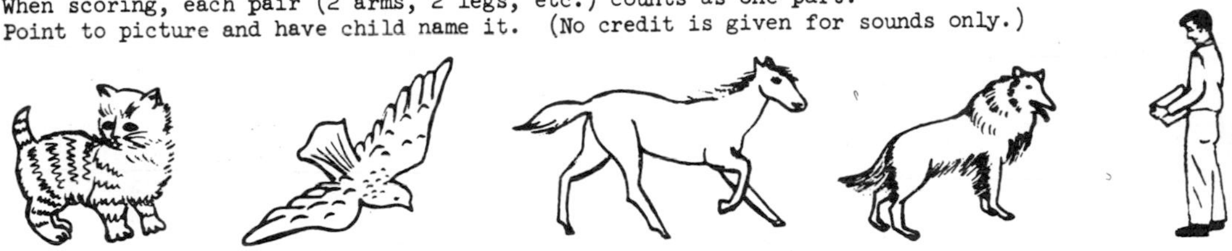

15. Tell child to: Give block to Mommie; put block on table; put block on floor. Pass 2 of 3. (Do not help child by pointing, moving head or eyes.)
16. Ask child: What do you do when you are cold? ..hungry? ..tired? Pass 2 of 3.
17. Tell child to: Put block <u>on</u> table; <u>under</u> table; <u>in front</u> of chair, <u>behind</u> chair. Pass 3 of 4. (Do not help child by pointing, moving head or eyes.)
18. Ask child: If fire is hot, ice is ?; Mother is a woman, Dad is a ?; a horse is big, a mouse is ?. Pass 2 of 3.
19. Ask child: What is a ball? ..lake? ..desk? ..house? ..banana? ..curtain? ..ceiling? ..hedge? ..pavement? Pass if defined in terms of use, shape, what it is made of or general category (such as banana is fruit, not just yellow). Pass 6 of 9.
20. Ask child: What is a spoon made of? ..a shoe made of? ..a door made of? (No other objects may be substituted.) Pass 3 of 3.
21. When placed on stomach, child lifts chest off table with support of forearms and/or hands.
22. When child is on back, grasp his hands and pull him to sitting. Pass if head does not hang back.
23. Child may use wall or rail only, not person. May not crawl.
24. Child must throw ball overhand 3 feet to within arm's reach of tester.
25. Child must perform standing broad jump over width of test sheet. (8-1/2 inches)
26. Tell child to walk forward, ⟶ heel within 1 inch of toe. Tester may demonstrate. Child must walk 4 consecutive steps, 2 out of 3 trials.
27. Bounce ball to child who should stand 3 feet away from tester. Child must catch ball with hands, not arms, 2 out of 3 trials.
28. Tell child to walk backward, ⟵ toe within 1 inch of heel. Tester may demonstrate. Child must walk 4 consecutive steps, 2 out of 3 trials.

<u>DATE AND BEHAVIORAL OBSERVATIONS</u> (how child feels at time of test, relation to tester, attention span, verbal behavior, self-confidence, etc,):

Fig. 17-2 Directions for administration of numbered items on the Denver II. (Courtesy Frankenburg, W. K., & Dodds, J. B. [1990]. University of Colorado Medical Center, Denver.)

response to tactile stimulation and pain (Bee, 2000). As the infant develops, further differences are noted. By 6 months, girls respond to visual stimulation with longer attention spans and are more socially responsive than are boys; girls also tend to sit up, walk, and crawl earlier than do boys. Female infants develop language earlier and respond to speech better than do boys. Therefore from an early age, female infants learn to communicate with language, whereas male infants use their bodies (Pillitteri, 1999).

The gender of the infant, a major concern of many expectant parents, may well influence parental relationships and expectations. The infant's gender can evoke disappointment; in some cases, a woman may feel disappointed in a girl only because she knows that her

Birth to 36 months: Girls
Length-for-age and weight-for-age percentiles

Name ______________________

Record # ______________

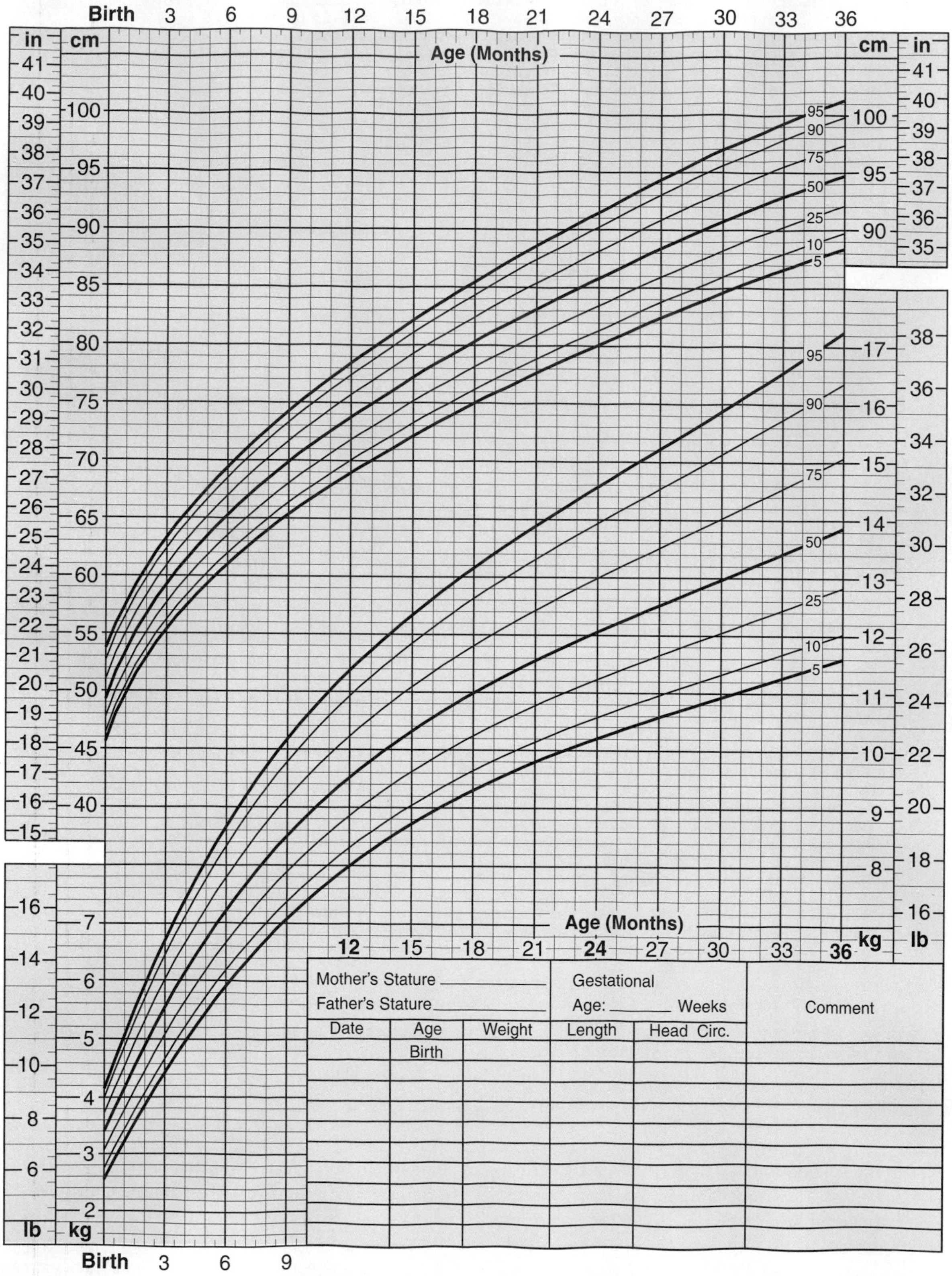

Fig. 17-3 Female infant growth chart. (From National Center for Heath Statistics, Centers for Disease Control and Prevention, 2000.)

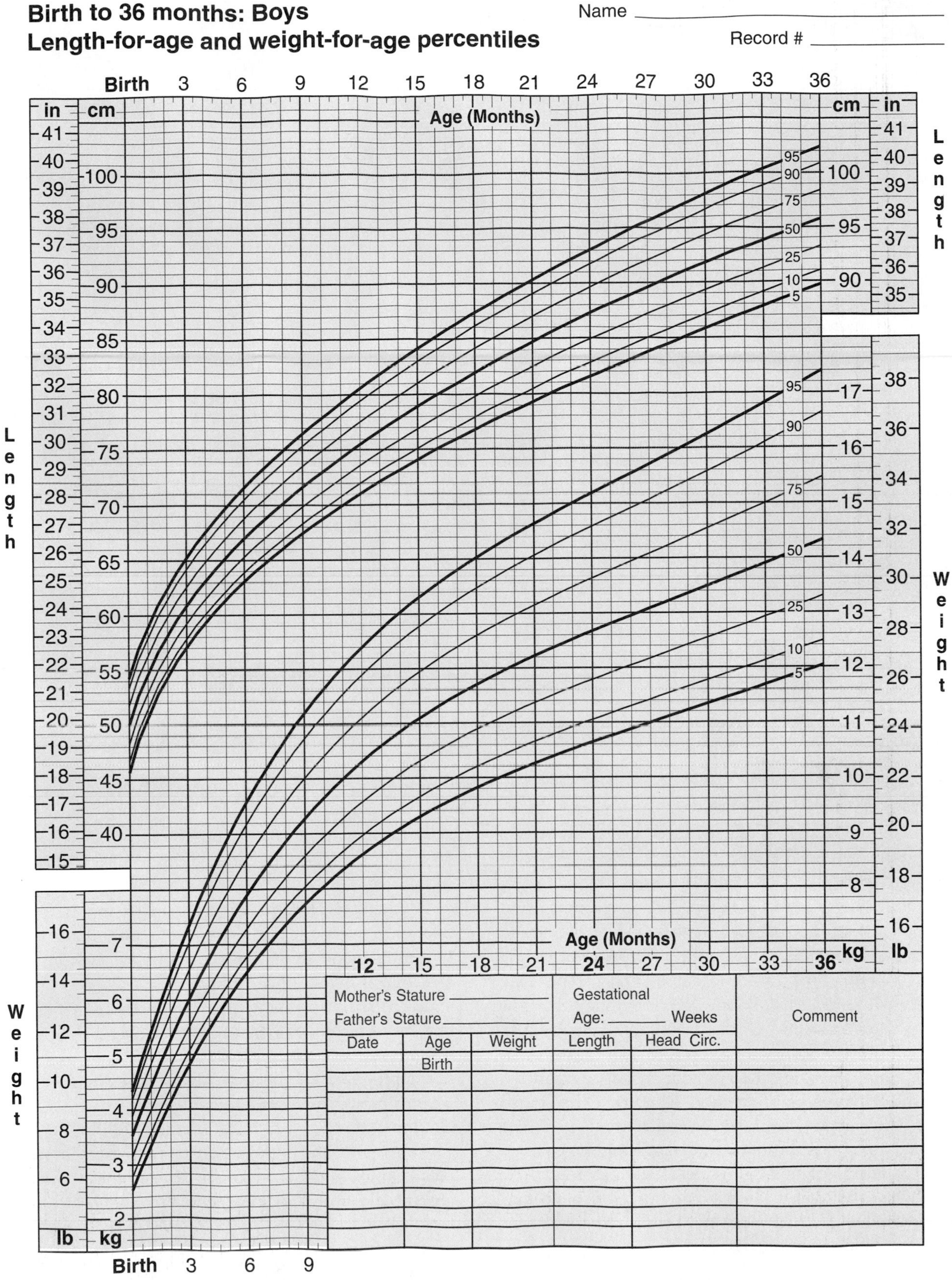

Fig. 17-4 Male infant growth chart. (From National Center for Heath Statistics, Centers for Disease Control and Prevention, 2000.)

Table 17-3 Height and Weight Measurements for Girls

	Height by Percentiles						Weight by Percentiles					
	5		50		95		5		50		95	
age*	cm	inches	cm	inches	cm	inches	kg	lb	kg	lb	kg	lb
Birth	45.4	17¾	49.9	19¾	52.9	20¾	2.36	5¼	3.23	7	3.81	8½
3 months	55.4	21¾	59.5	23½	63.4	25	4.18	9¼	5.4	12	6.74	14¾
6 months	61.8	24¼	65.9	26	70.2	27¾	5.79	12¾	7.21	16	8.73	19¼
9 months	66.1	26	70.4	27¾	75.0	29½	7.0	15½	8.56	18¾	10.17	22½
1	69.8	27½	74.3	29¼	79.1	31¼	7.84	17¼	9.53	21	11.24	24¾
1½	76.0	30	80.9	31¾	86.1	34	8.92	19¾	10.82	23¾	12.76	28¼
2†	81.6	32¼	86.8	34¼	93.6	36¾	9.95	22	11.8	26	14.15	31¼
2½†	84.6	33¼	90.0	35½	96.6	38	10.8	23¾	13.03	28¾	15.76	34¾
3	88.3	34¾	94.1	37	100.6	39½	11.61	25½	14.1	31	17.22	38
3½	91.7	36	97.9	38½	104.5	41¼	12.37	27¼	15.07	33¼	18.59	41
4	95.0	37½	101.6	40	108.3	42¾	13.11	29	15.96	35¼	19.91	44
4½	98.1	38½	105.0	41¼	112.0	44	13.83	30½	16.81	37	21.24	46¾
5	101.1	39¾	108.4	42¾	115.6	45½	14.55	32	17.66	39	22.62	49¾
6	106.6	42	114.6	45	122.7	48¼	16.05	35½	19.52	43	25.75	56¾
7	111.8	44	120.6	47½	129.5	51	17.71	39	21.84	48¼	29.68	65½
8	116.9	46	126.4	49¾	136.2	53½	19.62	43¼	24.84	54¾	34.71	76½
9	122.1	48	132.2	52	142.9	56¼	21.82	48	28.46	62¾	40.64	89½
10	127.5	50¼	138.3	54½	149.5	58¾	24.36	53¾	32.55	71¾	47.17	104
11	133.5	52½	144.8	57	156.2	61½	27.24	60	36.95	81½	54.0	119
12	139.8	55	151.5	59¾	162.7	64	30.52	67¼	41.53	91½	60.81	134
13	145.2	57¼	157.1	61¾	168.1	66¼	34.14	75¼	46.1	101¾	67.3	148¼
14	148.7	58½	160.4	63¾	171.3	67½	37.76	83¼	50.28	110¾	73.08	161
15	150.5	59¼	161.8	63¾	172.8	68	40.99	90¼	53.68	118¼	77.78	171½
16	151.6	59¾	162.4	64	173.3	68¼	43.41	95¾	55.89	123¼	80.99	178½
17	152.7	60	163.1	64¼	173.5	68¼	44.74	98¾	56.69	125	82.46	181¾
18	153.6	60½	163.7	64½	173.6	68¼	45.26	99¾	56.62	124¾	82.47	181¾

Modified from National Center for Health Statistics, Health Resources Administration, U.S. Department of Health, Education, and Welfare. (1982). *Height and weight measurement for girls*. Hyattsville, MD: National Center for Health Statistics. Conversion of metric data to approximate inches and pounds by Ross Laboratories.

*Years unless otherwise indicated.

†Height data include some recumbent length measurements, which make values slightly higher than when all measurements had been of stature (standing height).

husband wanted a boy. Today, the trend is to want one child of each gender. Because the birth rate is down in comparison with the 1950s and inflation rates are up, families are having fewer children. The importance and stress of producing the *right sex* infant is evident. Being the *wrong sex* can be combined with other factors to place the infant at potential risk for child abuse. The parents may find fault with and place blame on the infant for not meeting this expectation (Olson, 1999).

Health intervention focuses on the identification of high-risk families and the promotion of a positive relationship between infant and parents. The nurse promotes the good health, appearance, and potential developmental ability of the infant. Increasing the parents' feelings of adequacy and self-esteem will promote their acceptance of the infant. Most importantly, follow-up care for these families is a high priority to ensure that adequate support and help are available.

Race

Race refers to the classification of human beings into groups based on particular physical characteristics, such as skin pigmentation, head form, and stature. Caucasoid, Mongoloid, and Negroid are the three racial types generally recognized.

A range of physical variation exists among people of different races with regard to growth rate, dentition, body structure, blood group, susceptibility to certain diseases, and a great many other variables.

In assessing an infant, the nurse not only collects data, but also compares the data with established norms, such as a standardized growth chart. When the norms chosen are not appropriate for the individual (for example, an Asian infant's growth is assessed based on norms for Caucasian children) the comparison information will not be accurate.

The nurse who works with families from a variety of racial groups must have an understanding of each background and how it relates to health and health care. To facilitate nursing care for a family from a racial group different from the health care provider's, effective communication must be established. This communication will help foster an understanding of the other's point of view and frame of reference. Each family member should be viewed as an individual and there should be no stereotyping of

Table **17-4** Height and Weight Measurements for Boys

	Height by Percentiles						Weight by Percentiles					
	5		50		95		5		50		95	
age*	cm	inches	cm	inches	cm	inches	kg	lb	kg	lb	kg	lb
Birth	46.4	18¼	50.5	20	54.4	21½	2.54	5½	3.27	7¼	4.15	9¼
3 months	56.7	22¼	61.1	24	65.4	25¾	4.43	9¾	5.98	13¼	7.37	16¼
6 months	63.4	25	67.8	26¾	72.3	28½	6.20	13¾	7.85	17¼	9.46	20¾
9 months	68.0	26¾	72.3	28½	77.1	30¼	7.52	16½	9.18	20¼	10.93	24
1	71.7	28¼	76.1	30	81.2	32	8.43	18½	10.15	22½	11.99	26½
1½	77.5	30½	82.4	32½	88.1	34¾	9.59	21¼	11.47	25¼	13.44	29½
2†	82.5	32½	86.8	34¼	94.4	37¼	10.49	23¼	12.34	27¼	15.50	34¼
2½†	85.4	33½	90.4	35½	97.8	38½	11.27	24¾	13.52	29¾	16.61	36½
3	89.0	35	94.9	37¼	102.0	40¼	12.05	26½	14.62	32¼	17.77	39¼
3½	92.5	36½	99.1	39	106.1	41¾	12.84	28¼	15.68	34½	18.98	41¾
4	95.8	37¾	102.9	40½	109.9	43¼	13.64	30	16.69	36¾	20.27	44¾
4½	98.9	39	106.6	42	113.5	44¾	14.45	30¾	17.69	39	21.63	47¾
5	102.0	40¼	109.9	43¼	117.0	46	15.27	33¾	18.67	41¼	23.09	51
6	107.7	42½	116.1	45¾	123.5	48½	16.93	37¼	20.69	45½	26.34	58
7	113.0	44½	121.7	48	129.7	51	18.64	41	22.85	50¼	30.12	66½
8	118.1	46½	127.0	50	135.7	53½	20.40	45	25.30	55¾	34.51	76
9	122.9	48½	132.2	52	141.8	55¾	22.25	49	28.13	62	39.58	87¼
10	127.7	50¼	137.5	54¼	148.1	58¼	24.33	53¾	31.44	69¼	45.27	99¾
11	132.6	52¼	143.3	56½	154.9	61	26.80	59	35.30	77¾	51.47	113½
12	137.6	54¼	149.7	59	162.3	64	29.85	65¾	39.78	87¾	58.09	128
13	142.9	56¼	156.5	61½	169.8	66¾	33.64	74¼	44.95	99	65.02	143¼
14	148.8	58½	163.1	64¼	176.7	69½	38.22	84¼	50.77	112	72.13	159
15	155.2	61	169.0	66½	181.9	71½	43.11	95	56.71	125	79.12	174½
16	161.1	63½	173.5	68¼	185.4	73	47.74	105¼	62.10	137	85.62	188¾
17	164.9	65	176.2	69¼	187.3	73¾	51.50	113½	66.31	146¼	91.31	201¼
18	165.7	65¼	176.8	69½	187.6	73¾	53.97	119	68.88	151¾	95.76	211

Modified from National Center for Health Statistics, Health Resources Administration, U.S. Department of Health, Education, and Welfare. (1982). *Height and weight measurement for boys*. Hyattsville, MD: National Center for Health Statistics. Conversion of metric data to approximate inches and pounds by Ross Laboratories.

*Years unless otherwise indicated.

†Height data include some recumbent length measurements, which make values slightly higher than when all measurements had been of stature (standing height).

families within a racial group. Despite common language, color, or historical background, not all members of a particular racial group are alike. This diversity presents, without doubt, considerable challenges for nurses who work with families with infants (Schwartz, 1999). Universal norms by which to measure one's growth and skill capacity do not exist. The nurse must recognize the differences and intervene appropriately. The orientation of health maintenance and disease prevention is basic to good health practices, regardless of racial makeup. This concept should be the major focus of all health care.

Genetics

The desired and expected outcome of any pregnancy is the birth of a healthy, *perfect* baby. Unfortunately, a small, but significant, number of parents experience disappointment when they discover that their baby has been born with a defect or genetic disease. A **birth defect** is an abnormality of structure, function, or metabolism as a result of a genetic or environmental influence on the fetus, but often a combination of both. Many couples may refrain from having another child because they have had one with a serious birth defect and do not want to risk another. In these situations, genetic counseling provides information that is needed to understand a hereditary disorder. The major goal of counseling is to explain birth defects to affected families and to allow prospective parents to make informed decisions about childbearing.

Using the basic laws governing heredity and knowing the frequency of specific birth defects in the population, the genetic counselor can often predict the probability of recurrence of a given abnormality in the same family (Jarvis, 1999). An important aspect of primary prevention is identifying families at increased risk and referring them for counseling (Baker, 1998). Aspects to be reviewed in the initial interview are:

1. *Maternal age*. The risk of having a child with Down syndrome increases significantly for the woman over 35 years of age. In this syndrome, three chromosomes appear in the 21 chromosomal group (trisomy 21). Characteristic features include: upwardly slanting eyes; small, malformed ears; large, protruding tongue; broad

hands and feet; and some degree of mental retardation.

2. *Ethnic background*. Several genetic disorders occur with higher frequency in certain groups. Eastern European Jews have a 10 times greater chance of carrying the Tay-Sachs gene compared with the general U.S. population. Abnormal deposits of lipids (fats) in the cells of the cerebral cortex, spleen, liver, and lymph nodes are characterizations of Tay-Sachs disease. An autosomal recessive gene transmits the disease. Blacks have a much greater chance of carrying the sickle cell trait compared with the general population. Sickle cell anemia is an autosomal recessive condition occurring in 1 out of every 400 Black births and causing severe hemolytic anemia crisis episodes.
3. *Family history*. Certain diseases, such as Huntington's chorea, hemophilia, or mental retardation, are often hereditary. Huntington's chorea (an autosomal dominant disease involving the brain) is characterized by deterioration of intellectual functions and involuntary movements of the limbs, face, and trunk. Once manifested, a steady deterioration leads to death after some years. Hemophilia is a sex-linked recessive coagulation disorder caused by a functional deficiency of a certain plasma-clotting factor; bleeding is prolonged. Hemophilia passes from an unaffected carrier mother to her male offspring and occurs in 1 out of every 10,000 births.
4. Reproductive history. Spontaneous abortions, stillbirths, and previous liveborn children with birth defects or slow development may indicate an increased risk.
5. Maternal disease. Several maternal disorders are associated with a higher frequency of birth defects, including diabetes mellitus, seizure disorder, mental retardation, and phenylketonuria.

Prenatal diagnosis offers the couple the option of aborting a fetus that is affected with certain genetic disorders. For many people, this option is unacceptable. Chapter 16 discusses the various tests used for prenatal diagnosis.

The nurse's role throughout the genetic counseling process is to provide the vital link between the counseling team and the high-risk couple. The nurse is involved in case finding, referral, and family education. The nurse has a sound background in the principles of genetics to provide families with appropriate information as part of preventive health care guidance.

GORDON'S FUNCTIONAL HEALTH PATTERNS

Health Perception-Health Management Pattern

Health promotion is aimed at assisting the infant and family in changing behavior to produce greater physical and emotional health in adulthood. To reach this goal, the nurse encourages child-rearing practices that promote normal growth and development, fosters attitudes and values compatible with health, and teaches appropriate use of health services (Chitty, 2001). The nurse promotes the infant's health through the parents, who then determine the care practices for the dependent infant.

Health is largely a subjective judgment; each person's perception of health is related to physical and mental capabilities, self-concept, relationships with others and the environment, and personal goals and values in life (Jarvis, 1999). With this understanding, the nurse uses every opportunity to convey confidence in the parent's health perception-health management pattern and their ability to act to enhance the infant's health. When parents learn and adopt behaviors that improve their own health, they are more likely to ensure that the health needs of their infant are met. Parental modeling increases the chances of good health practices being retained throughout the child's life.

The goals of nursing practice with infants and their families are to promote individual motivation for health, to assist the family to identify health needs, and to develop problem-solving skills using the family's own resources. To meet these goals, the nurse must identify the family's perception of good or bad health practices, which greatly influences participation in health-promoting activities. Age, gender, educational level, cultural orientation, financial status, and occupation combine to influence health perception. When parents believe that the infant is more susceptible to a health problem if promotional behavior is not enacted, they become more motivated to adopt the behavior.

The nurse's task is to help the parents recognize the infant's susceptibility and the potential consequences when healthy practices are not instituted. The nurse works within the family's health-perception framework to become acquainted with the characteristics that strongly influence the infant's health. Unless caregivers meet their own personal needs, they will be unable to meet their infant's developmental needs (Stanhope, 2000).

The nurse supports the parents, strengthening their parental confidence and self-esteem, providing information on meeting their infant's needs and reinforcing their health perception-health management pattern.

Nutritional-Metabolic Pattern

One of the most important aspects of health promotion in the infant is nutritional status. Many opinions have been expressed about the infant's nutritional needs. As research in this area continues, recommendations and opinions will change; however, some basic facts about nutrition remain fairly consistent. Infant nutritional requirements are based on what is considered necessary to (1) support life, (2) provide for growth, and (3) maintain health.

Essential Nutrients

Water, proteins, fats, carbohydrates, vitamins, and minerals are the essential nutrients in any diet. Because the first year of life is a period of rapid growth, nutritional needs during this period are especially important and always changing.

Water is vital to survival. A person can live for several weeks without food, but can survive only a few days without water. Because the infant's body weight is approximately 75% water, the baby must consume large amounts of fluid to maintain water balance. Water requirements average between 125 to 150 ml/kg body weight per day in the first 6 months of life and 120 to 135 ml/kg per day in the second 6 months (Grodner, Anderson, & DeYoung, 2000). The sources of water are fluids (primarily milk) and food; most strained foods are 75% to 85% water. Most infant diets meet the basic water requirement.

The infant must also consume sufficient high-quality protein to facilitate growth and development. Recommended protein requirements are 2.2 g/kg per day during the first 6 months and 2.0 g/kg per day in the second 6 months (Cataldo & Debruyne, 1998).

Carbohydrates should supply 30% to 60% of the energy intake during infancy. Approximately 37% of the calories in human milk and 40% to 50% of the calories in commercial formulas are derived from lactose or other carbohydrates (Dietz & Stern, 1999).

A minimum of 3.8 g/kcal and a maximum of 6.0 g/100 kcal of fat (30% to 54% of calories) are recommended for infants (Dietz & Stern, 1999). This quantity is present in human milk and in all formulas prepared for infants. Significantly lower intakes, such as in skim milk feedings, can result in an inadequate energy intake.

Vitamins are essential nutrients in the infant's diet that regulate metabolism and allow more efficient use of carbohydrates, fats, and proteins within the body. Breast milk, or prepared fortified formula consumed in appropriate amounts, generally meets the infant's needs.

Minerals are found in relatively small amounts in the infant's body, but are vital elements in body structure and control of certain bodily functions. Mineral intake for infants appears to be adequate, except for iron and fluoride.

The full-term infant is born with adequate stores of iron to meet bodily needs for hemoglobin production for up to approximately 4 to 6 months of age. After this time, body stores may need to be replenished to ensure adequate levels. Although iron in human milk is bioavailable, both breast-fed and formula-fed infants should receive an additional source of iron by 6 months of age. Iron-fortified formula and cereals are the most commonly used food sources.

Fluoride, concentrated in the bones and teeth, helps reduce dental caries. The Committee on Nutrition of the Academy of Pediatrics has recommended that optimal fluoride for infants is 0.25 mg per day (Dietz & Stern, 1999). Supplementation is necessary when the diet contains insufficient fluoridated water.

A review of these requirements shows that milk (breast or formula) meets most of the infant's nutritional needs when consumed in adequate amounts. No data support the theory that solid foods are needed to meet these nutritional needs, at least in the first 6 months of life. Despite this fact, many parents introduce semisolid foods to their infants as early as 2 weeks of age.

Breast Feeding

Research throughout the years has demonstrated unequivocally that exclusive breast feeding is the preferred method of infant feeding for the first 4 to 6 months of life. Breast milk is often called the perfect food for the infant and for the mother, because she does not have to buy it, cook it, store it, or clean up after it. Both the American Dietetic Association and the American Academy of Pediatrics have position statements in support of breast feeding. This realization has influenced a number of health-promotion strategies in the United States. The Surgeon General has recommended that by the year 2010, 75% of all women should be breast feeding when they leave the hospital and 50% should still be breast feeding 6 months later (see Research Highlights box). If the nation is to meet the Surgeon General's goal by the year 2010, then efforts to promote breast feeding must be strengthened in hospitals, health maintenance organizations, private health care offices, and public health clinics.

The World Health Organization (WHO) and the United Nations Children's Fund (UNICEF) have jointly adopted the Baby-Friendly Hospital Initiative (BFHI) in attempting to establish a global effort to increase breast

research highlights

Pacifiers and Breast Feeding

In an observational study involving 265 breast-feeding mothers, investigators interviewed the mothers at 2, 6, 12, and 24 weeks postpartum and every 90 days thereafter until breast feeding ended. By the time these infants were 6 months of age, 74% of mothers had begun offering a pacifier. These pacifier users tended to breast feed their infants less often than did mothers who did not introduce a pacifier. At 12 weeks of age, mothers whose infants used pacifiers were more likely to report that breast feeding was inconvenient and that they had trouble producing enough milk (problems consistent with infrequent nursing). These findings suggest that women who introduce pacifiers to their infants at an early age tend to breast feed for fewer months than do women who do not introduce a pacifier at this time, because the early pacifier users breast fed less frequently compared with other breast-feeding mothers. Early pacifier use does not affect whether a mother continues to breast feed during the first 3 months of her infant's life; however, the effect is primarily on long-term breast feeding.

Data from Howard, C. R. (1999). Pacifiers and breastfeeding. *Contemporary Pediatrics, 16* (6), 150.

Box 17-4 Baby-Friendly Hospital Initiative Breast-Feeding Guidelines

1. Have a written breast-feeding policy that is routinely communicated to all health care staff.
2. Train all health care staff in the skills necessary to implement this policy.
3. Inform all pregnant women about the benefits and management of breast feeding.
4. Help the mother initiate breast feeding within 30 minutes after birth.
5. Show mothers how to breast feed and how to maintain lactation even when they are separated from their infants.
6. Give newborn infants no food or drink other than breast milk unless medically indicated.
7. Practice rooming-in; allow mothers and infants to remain together 24 hours a day.
8. Encourage breast feeding on demand.
9. Give no pacifiers to breast-feeding infants.
10. Foster the establishment of breast-feeding support groups and refer mothers to these groups on discharge from the hospital or clinic.

From Pillitteri, A. (1999). *Maternal and child health nursing: Care of the childbearing and childrearing family* (3rd ed.). Philadelphia: Lippincott-Williams & Wilkins.

Box 17-5 Advantages of Breast Feeding

BREAST MILK IS:

- The correct balance of all essential nutrients for infants.
- Full of immunological agents to protect against disease.
- Easier to digest than is formula.
- Contains antiinflammatory properties.
- Promotes growth of *Lactobacillus bifidus.*

BREAST FEEDING:

- Is cheaper and more convenient than formula.
- Provides a unique bonding experience for both infant and mother.
- Assists in process of uterine involution for mother.
- Promotes weight reduction for new mother.

feeding. To become a *baby-friendly* health care facility, the 10 steps to successful breast feeding must be implemented, as shown in Box 17-4.

Nurses can be instrumental in working toward the national goal to increase breast feeding by educating all women about the advantages of the practice (Box 17-5). Nurses in the community who are caring for breast-feeding mothers should stress the following tips to increase the duration of this activity:

- Drink up to eight glasses of fluids daily to produce sufficient quantity of breast milk.
- Consume the proper amount of calories to avoid excessive weight loss.
- Educate nursing mothers about the appropriate interventions for engorged breasts, sore nipples, plugged ducts, infection, and leaking (see Health Teaching box).
- Instruct employed nursing mothers about the use of breast pumps and milk storage.
- Encourage participation in breast-feeding support groups for continued help within the community.
- Advise nursing mothers of the effects of drugs, environmental pollutants, alcohol, and nicotine on breast milk.

Introduction of Solid Foods

No scientific evidence is available on the best time to introduce solid foods during infancy. At approximately 4 to 6 months of age, the infant is usually physiologically and developmentally ready to have solid foods, either commercial or home prepared. Some authorities believe that waiting until the child is 4 to 6 months of age to introduce solid food decreases any tendency toward food allergies. Essentially, the introduction of various foods was recommended to (1) supply a more appealing, diversified diet for the infant; (2) supply energy, iron, and vitamins; and (3) provide needed trace elements (Calamaro, 2000). The decision to start solid foods at 4 to 6 months of age has been found to be based more on neuromuscular and developmental readiness of the infant rather than on any hard scientific data.

All infants develop according to their own schedules and some are ready to start eating solid foods before others are ready. The addition of foods should be governed by an infant's nutritional needs and readiness to handle different forms of foods (Bush, 1999). The order of food introduction and specific amounts to be given are based on tradition rather than on scientific fact. No scientific studies have been performed to determine whether there is a specific order or infant food introduction necessary or amounts needed for optimal development. The sequence of solids typically recommended by the American Academy of Pediatrics is cereal, fruits, vegetables, and meats. Traditionally, the sequence in which specific foods are introduced is shown in Box 17-6, p. 476.

A few tips to assist the parents in making the introduction of solid foods to their infant's diet a smooth process are listed in Box 17-7, p. 477.

A potential list of foods to be introduced is shown in Table 17-5, p. 477.

Weaning

Weaning is a gradual, caring process that introduces the infant to a cup that replaces the bottle or breast. When the infant is ready, weaning should be started. Developmentally, the infant can usually learn to use a cup by age 5 to 6 months; however, many children continue to nurse after they start using a cup. The American Academy of Pediatrics recommends breast feeding for at least the first

HEALTH TEACHING Breast Feeding

How to Hold Your Baby for Feedings

- Sit or lie down comfortably with your back supported.
- Make sure your baby has one arm on either side of your breast as you pull the baby close.
- Use firm pillows or folded blankets under the baby as a means of support during the feeding. As your baby gets older, the extra support will likely be unnecessary.
- Support the baby's back and shoulders firmly. Do not push on the back of the baby's head.
- After the baby's mouth is open wide, pull your baby quickly to your breast.

Four Common Breast-Feeding Positions

Football

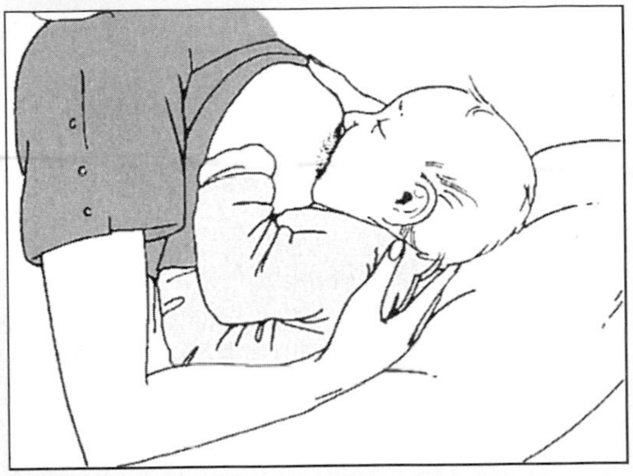

- Hold the baby's back and shoulders in the palm of your hand.
- Tuck the baby up under your arm, keeping the baby's ear, shoulder, and hip in a straight line.
- Support the breast. After the baby's mouth is open wide, pull the baby quickly to you.
- Continue to hold your breast until the baby feeds easily.

Lying Down

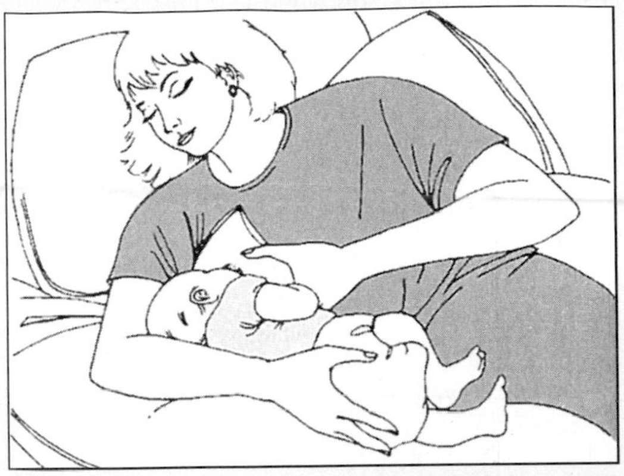

- Lie on your side with a pillow at your back and lay the baby such that you are facing each other.
- To begin, prop yourself up on your elbow and support your breast with that hand.
- Pull the baby close to you, lining up the baby's mouth with your nipple.
- After the baby is feeding well, lie back down. Hold your breast with the opposite hand.

Cradling

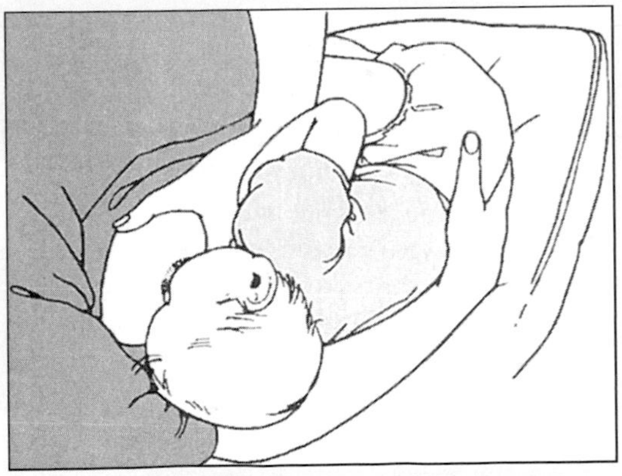

- Cradle the baby in the arm closest to the breast with the baby's head in the crook of your arm.
- Have the baby's body facing you, tummy to tummy.
- Use your opposite hand to support the breast.

Across the Lap

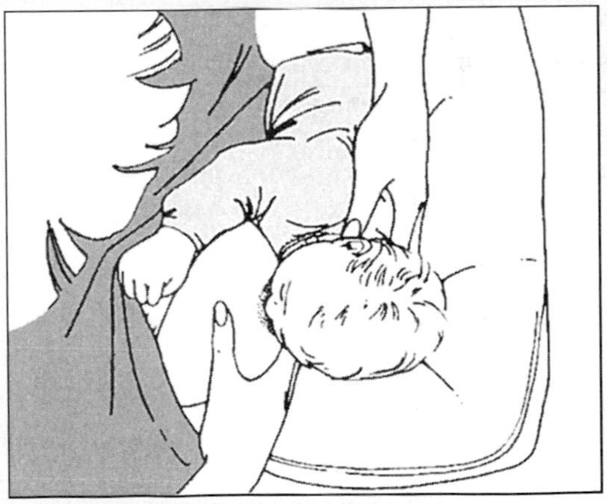

- Lay your baby on firm pillows across your lap.
- Turn the baby, facing you.
- Reach across your lap to support the baby's back and shoulders with the palm of your hand.
- Support your breast from underneath to guide it into the baby's mouth.

Used with permission of Lactation Consultants of North Carolina. Illustrations from a handset accompanying the video, *Breastfeeding: A special relationship*. Courtesy of Eagle Video Productions.

Continued

HEALTH TEACHING Breast Feeding—cont'd

Breast Feeding Is Going Well When . . .

- Your newborn is feeding approximately eight times in 24 hours for 30 to 40 minutes at each feeding. Some newborns need to eat more frequently until they learn to breast feed efficiently. Other babies gain weight while feeding less often.
- At least one breast softens well at each feeding.
- You feel a tug, but not pain, when the baby sucks.
- The baby's arms and shoulders are relaxed during the feeding.
- The baby has bursts of 10 or more sucks and swallows at the beginning of each feeding.
- As your breast softens, the baby slows down to two to three sucks and swallows at a time.
- Your baby is content when you finish breast feeding.
- By the time the baby is 4 days old, you should see at least six wet diapers and two bowel movements every 24 hours.

Box 17-6 Solid Food Introduction Sequence

1. Cereals, particularly rice because of nonallergenic property
2. Fruits such as peaches, pears, and applesauce
3. Vegetables; begin with yellow vegetables (squash and carrots) given before green vegetables (peas or beans)
4. Strained meats, such as nonallergenic lamb or veal

year of life. WHO and UNICEF suggest that the health benefits of breast milk are important throughout the second and third years of life. The infant should be started at this age by periodically taking sips of water or juice. Initially, the infant may not be eager to do so and should become accustomed to this new experience.

Some infants accept the cup readily; other infants are extremely reluctant to give up the bottle, especially the bedtime bottle. Allowing infants to sleep with propped bottles can lead to the need for aspiration if the milk flows too rapidly or the infant becomes too sleepy to coordinate sucking and swallowing. Another potential problem that parents should consider is *baby bottle tooth decay:* decay for all upper teeth and some of the lower posterior teeth from direct contact with sugar, syrup, honey-sweetened water, or fruit juice. Tooth decay occurs when the infant falls asleep and stops sucking on the bottle. The sugary solution pools around the infant's teeth and remains there all night. The carbohydrate of the solution is fermented into organic acids that demineralize the teeth until they decay. By not using the bottle as a pacifier, agents can prevent this condition.

Some additional tips for counseling parents are as follows:

1. Keep a calm, relaxed attitude throughout the weaning process.
2. Do not force an infant to use a cup; it is more detrimental to wean sooner rather than later.
3. Introduce the cup for one feeding per day and progress from there until the breast or bottle is surrendered.
4. Put only purified tap water into the bottle and give the infant juice and milk from a cup.
5. Remember that infants enjoy the accomplishment of using a cup; it is one of their first steps toward independence.

Anticipatory Guidance

The infant progresses from a diet of milk alone to a diet of milk and solid foods within a short period. The nurse, in an attempt to guide the parents in meeting their infant's nutritional needs, understands these needs, developmental capabilities, and helps foster family-infant relationships. The health-promotion activity used in meeting proper infant nutrition focuses on parent education and positive reinforcement of parenting abilities.

Elimination Pattern

The infant develops an elimination pattern by the second week of life, usually associated with the frequency and amount of feedings. Both breast-fed and bottle-fed infants progress to a pattern of fewer stools per day after the first few months of life.

A breast-fed infant's stools have an orange-yellow color and a soft, even consistency, with a *sourish,* but *clean* smell, dissimilar to stools passed later in life. A bottle-fed infant's stools are harder, smellier, and resemble those of an infant eating solid food. The breast-fed infant has many daily stools in the first and second months of life, progressing to one stool per day or even every 4 to 5 days in the later months before solid foods are introduced. The bottle-fed infant has two to four stools per day in the first month, tapering to one a day or even fewer at the end of infancy (Bengson, 1999).

For the first year of life, an infant cannot control the bowels. Bowel evacuation remains under involuntary, reflexive control until myelination of the spinal cord is complete, usually by 14 to 18 months of age (Pillitteri, 1999). Nurses advise overanxious parents to delay toilet training until the infant is developmentally ready.

The stress in American culture on daily bowel movements makes many mothers concerned about their infant's elimination patterns. The breast-fed infant may go for several days without having a bowel movement, which is usually not a problem. When the infant's behavior and feeding and sleeping patterns are normal, no elimination

Box 17-7 Tips for Introducing Solid Foods

1. The infant's first solid foods should be smooth and runny. Gradually, the infant will be ready to accept a slightly rougher texture.
2. Pureed foods are used until the infant has teeth; chopped foods are used when the infant can chew.
3. Introduce only one new food at a time and in small amounts. When the new food is not tolerated or the infant is allergic to it, the new food can be identified quickly and discontinued.
4. The infant must learn how to handle solid foods. Because infants use sucking movements, part of the food is ejected from the mouth. With time and practice, the infant learns how to take solid food from a spoon.
5. Do not mix solid foods together; the infant should learn to appreciate different tastes and textures.
6. Do not add solid foods to the infant's formula bottle; do not make a larger hole to allow *drinking* of foods.
7. Do not start to reduce the milk supply until the infant is taking food successfully from the spoon.
8. Until 1 year of age, feed the baby milk before solid foods.
9. Look at, smile at, and talk to the infant during feeding.
10. Do not give honey to infants less than 12 months of age*

*Honey has been credited throughout the centuries for therapeutic and medicinal uses. However, honey should not be given to infants under 1 year of age. Honey is a known source of bacterial spores that produce a toxin, which can cause infant botulism. This rare, but serious, form of food poisoning affects the nervous system of infants and can result in death. Researchers also suspect a link between infant botulism and some cases of sudden infant death syndrome (SIDS) because breathing is affected in the most severe stages of food poisoning. Botulism spores are quite common, found in dust, soil, and uncooked food. Honey is the only food implicated in infant botulism. Because honey is not essential for the nutrition of infants, parents and caregivers should be reminded not to feed honey to infants younger than 1 year of age. Honey should never be added to baby food or placed on the nipple of a pacifier.

problem exists. A breast-fed infant rarely becomes constipated when consuming adequate amounts of breast milk. Usually, the nurse only has to reassure the parents and discuss normal elimination patterns.

Urination increases as fluid intake increases. An infant who voids 6 to 12 times a day in the first few months of life is usually healthy and well hydrated. Voiding is involuntary until sometime during the second year of life, when bladder sensation develops. Irregular patterns of voiding characterize the remaining period of infancy.

Anticipatory Guidance

Anticipatory guidance and health promotion concerning elimination patterns of the infant should consist of parental teaching and reassurance, with special emphasis on good hygienic practices. Reassuring the parents about the infant's inability to control elimination is important, so their expectations are not unrealistic. Despite what might happen, the infant does not *save it up* until just after a clean diaper was put on the infant.

Table 17-5 First Foods for the Infant

Age (month)	Addition
4 to 6	Iron-fortified rice cereal, followed by other cereals
5 to 7	Strained vegetables and fruits and their juices
6 to 8	Protein foods (cheese, meat, fish, chicken, and yogurt)
9	Finely chopped meat, toast, teething crackers
10 to 12	Whole egg, whole milk, (allergies less likely now)

Activity-Exercise Pattern

Physical activity and exercise contribute to development and coordination throughout the lifespan; infants receive their exercise through play. Initially, infants engage in play with themselves with their hands or feet, with sounds, and by rolling and getting into various positions. By manipulating objects and achieving pleasurable sensations, infants learn about themselves and the objects in the environment.

Activity Through Play

Although the word *play* suggests physical activity, the infant's first play is actually an exercise of the senses. The infant's first toys are visual in nature. Through play, infants learn to hone their senses, to exercise their physical abilities, and to relate to other people. Most of the infant's play is solitary and repetitious. As each discovery is made, self-confidence and pride in the achievement are reinforced (as is the skill) through repetition.

As the infant enters the second half of the first year and becomes mobile, the family should provide the infant with increasing opportunities for spontaneous play and exploration. A planned play period in an environment that is safe for the infant should be established. The infant should have unrestrictive clothing so movement can be free and unhampered. The caregiver should not interfere directly with the play, but be attentive to the infant's needs.

A major nursing role in this area is assisting parents to promote play. The importance of providing opportunities for play that is appropriate for the infant's age should be stressed. Buying expensive toys is unnecessary; common household items, such as pots, pans, lids, and spoons, provide excellent objects for play purposes.

Activity Through Stimulation

Parental stimulation of the infant is an important developmental technique; the infant needs stimulation to learn about the world. This activity does not require expensive objects, but rather, it involves experiences in sight, sound, and touch, which are free and can be provided by any parent (Fig. 17-5). Examples of stimulating experiences for infants include the following:

- Having lullabies sung to them.
- Listening to tape recordings of a heartbeat.
- Seeing colorful mobiles in crib.
- Being rocked in a rocking chair.
- Having a familiar face smiling close by.
- Having space to wander when developmentally ready.
- Looking at themselves in mirrors.
- Listening to music played in the household.

Anticipatory Guidance

Knowledge of developmental landmarks allows the nurse to guide parents in proper play and stimulation for infants. Handing a 15-month-old child a ball and placing the child in a fenced-in back yard to *play* is not enough. These activities must provide interpersonal contact, activity, and exercise. Activity and exercise through stimulation and play are extremely important for adequate and healthy development.

Sleep-Rest Pattern

The amount of sleep that infants need is closely related to their rate of growth. Initially, infants sleep approximately 80% of the time, as demanded by their rapid growth. As growth begins to slow toward the middle of the first year of life, less sleep is needed. The 12-month-old infant sleeps only 12 of 24 hours, a pattern that remains essentially unchanged through the second year (Moore, 1999). To assist parents in understanding normal sleep and rest patterns, the nurse should stress that no set schedule exists (Table 17-6).

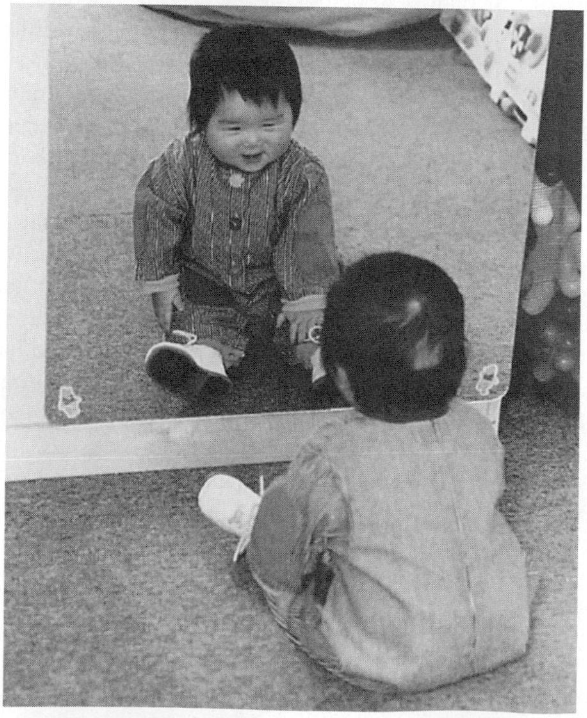

Fig. 17-5 Nine-month-old infant enjoying own image in a mirror. (From Wong, D. L. [1999]. *Whaley & Wong's nursing care of infants and children* [6th ed.]. St. Louis: Mosby.)

Nursing Suggestions

Health-promotion activities can also help the parents determine the individual needs of their infant. The nurse should stress that longer sleep patterns are signs of maturation in the infant and that sleep and rest are recognized as having a significant influence on the infant's growth and development. The nurse may offer the parents helpful comments for promoting infant sleep patterns, such as the following:

1. Provide a quiet room for the infant that is separate from the parents' room.
2. Learn behavioral clues that signal that the infant is going to sleep and is not interacting socially.
3. Learn to become sensitive to sleep cycles and rest periods that the infant is establishing and base care accordingly.
4. Attempt to schedule feeding times during wakeful rather than drowsy periods.
5. Learn that certain cycles are intrinsic to infants and that each infant is unique.
6. Perform rituals for the infant, such as being rocked or reading a bedtime story, to provide comfort and security, and let the infant know the expected behavior.

If parents express a sleep concern, the nurse must assess their reactions to consider their definition of the concern, assess the sleep environment, and observe the infant's own unique sleep patterns. Only then can the nurse's health-promotion approach be individualized to assist the family in caring for the infant.

Sudden Infant Death Syndrome

Recent studies of infant sleep have focused on the abnormal patterns associated with **sudden infant death**

Table 17-6 Normal Sleep Patterns for Infants

Age (month)	Hours in 24-Hour Period
2 to 3	Low: 10 Average: 16½ High: 23 (2 to 4 naps)
3 to 4	Low: 8 to 10 nightly High: 11 to 12 nightly (2 or 3 naps daily)
6 to 12	11 to 12 nightly (2 or 3 naps daily)
12 to 18	8 to 12 nightly (1 or 2 naps daily)

syndrome (SIDS). SIDS is the sudden, unexplained death of an infant younger that 1 year of age. Current research focuses on sleep pathophysiology, particularly in relation to apneic spells that last longer than 10 seconds. The carotid body network and brainstem reflexes normally control physiological variations in heart and respiratory rates during sleep. The mechanism of the relationship between apnea and SIDS is unsubstantiated. Currently thinking is such that a sleeping infant can become hypoxic with positional narrowing of the airway and respiratory inflammation. For unexplained reasons, in SIDS cases, these mechanisms likely fail to work during sleep, and respiration ceases.

SIDS refers to the sudden and unexpected death of an infant who has been previously healthy, with the cause of death unexplained after a thorough postmortem examination (see Hot Topics box). Extensive research, debate, and uncertainty surround this phenomenon; its etiological factors remain a mystery.

The American Academy of Pediatrics Task Force on SIDS recommends the following: (1) healthy infants should be placed to sleep in the supine position in a crib that meets Consumer Product Safety Commission and American Society for Testing and Material standards; (2) avoid placing infants to sleep on soft bedding (including waterbeds, sofas, and soft mattresses) or with pillows, soft comforters and coverings, loose bedding, or stuffed toys; (3) avoid overheating that occurs, for example, by placing excessive clothing or blankets on infants or by keeping the room temperature too high; (4) stop maternal smoking within the infant's environment; and (5) avoid bed sharing (Kennedy, 2000).

Infants who are considered to be at high risk for SIDS include survivors of SIDS, subsequent siblings of SIDS victims, and premature infants with recurrent apneic episodes during sleep. From a preventive perspective, apneic monitors have been used in certain cases. However, controversy remains over this type of respiratory monitoring at home; parents face a heavy psychological responsibility when left in charge of their extraordinarily vulnerable young infant's life and it increases their anxiety and protectiveness of the infant. Nevertheless, as a prevention measure, apneic monitors may save the infant's life (Sears, 1996).

When an infant dies suddenly, unexpectedly, and for no apparent reason, a crisis occurs. The parents are devastated and completely unprepared for the shock, reacting with intense guilt, blaming themselves and each other, and agonizing over the part they may have played in the infant's death. Because many unanswered questions remain, these feelings are universal. Parents think there is something they could have done to prevent the tragedy. In the majority of cases, nothing could have been done. Too frequently, the first sign that something was wrong is death.

The nurse is in an excellent position to help the family through this crisis period. Box 17-8 provides some helpful guidelines.

Dealing with the family's grief is not an easy task. Many families find strength in God to help them through this difficult time. Other family members and close friends can assist the family in their grieving process.

Many receive solace and support from talking to other parents who have lost an infant to SIDS. Several parent

HOT topics

INFANT SLEEP POSITION AND SUDDEN INFANT DEATH SYNDROME

SIDS is the leading cause of infant mortality between 1 month and 1 year of age in the United States, occurring in approximately 4 per 1000 live births. SIDS, defined as the sudden death of an infant under 1 year of age, remains unexplained after a thorough investigation. SIDS tends to occur at a higher-than-usual rate in the infants of adolescent mothers, infants of closely spaced pregnancies, and underweight male infants. However, even these profiles are inconsistent.

A variety of population characteristics have been explored, such as families with smokers, breast-feeding versus bottle-feeding practices, or side or back sleeping positions for the infant. The primary contributor to a 50% decline in SIDS deaths in seven countries, including the United States, over a 12-year period was a decline in the facedown sleeping position of infants. The studies indicate that infants being put down to sleep should be positioned on their sides or backs.

SIDS Facts

1. Incidence is highest between 1 and 8 months of age, with peak incidence at 2 to 3 months.
2. Families of low socioeconomic status with a history of heavy smoking or drug abuse are at greater risk.
3. Infants with low birth weight are at greater risk of dying from SIDS than are term infants.
4. SIDS occurs most often during the infant's sleep cycle.
5. Peak incidence is during the fall and winter seasons.
6. SIDS affects more male infants than it does female infants.
7. SIDS is a specific disease entity.
8. No evidence to date suggests hereditary or contagious causes.
9. SIDS is unexpected and unexplained.
10. No sign of distress, crying, or coughing is apparent at the time of death.
11. A mild upper respiratory infection may be present in some infants, but not all.
12. Autopsy findings are remarkably similar, including pulmonary congestion, intrathoracic petechiae, edema, and inflammatory infiltrates in the upper airway.

Box 17-8 Parental Grieving Guidelines

1. Allow the parents and other family members to mourn in their own way.
2. Let them know that help is available when needed.
3. Present the factual information available about SIDS to help alleviate guilt.
4. Inform the parents that their reactions to the loss are not abnormal and that many other parents have had similar experiences.
5. Review the autopsy findings with them to substantiate the definite cause of death and to reduce guilt.
6. Reassure the parents that accepting the reality of the loss takes time.
7. Stress that communication is important in the adjustment process that follows a crisis.
8. Give the parents and other family members the opportunity to share the experience of losing an infant to SIDS by being a good listener.

groups are available from local chapters of the SIDS Foundation; the nurse can refer them to the foundation in their area.

The nurse's major supportive role with families coping with SIDS is listening and offering compassionate guidance through the weeks and months that follow. The nurse encourages parents to talk about their infant. Too soon, family and friends expect the surviving family to get *over it*. A parent is never *over it;* it is only put in perspective and not so near the surface.

Nursing assessment of the infant at risk for SIDS includes observing the infant for apneic episodes. Usually, however, nursing assessment consists of observing for appropriate grief patterns in the family. Nursing diagnoses for sudden infant death might include the following:

- Spiritual distress related to coping with death.
- Ineffective family coping related to the loss of an infant.
- Dysfunctional grieving related to the parents' inability to cope.

Nurses also discuss feelings about caring for future children with the family. Life can appear out of control and parents may believe that they cannot care for another infant. These feelings must be resolved before another pregnancy is contemplated.

When dealing with the families of SIDS victims, nurses can feel uncomfortable and helpless. As health professionals, they might speak in terms of easing the pain or alleviating the guilt of these families, but many times, simple nonverbal human contact is sufficient to express concern and understanding.

Cognitive-Perceptual Pattern

Cognition is the process by which an individual recognizes, accumulates, and organizes the knowledge of the environment, beginning with the perception or recognition of an event within that environment. Cognitive development is concurrent with biological, adaptive, and psychosocial achievement. The infant's biological and cognitive developmental patterns (Piaget's sensorimotor period) are discussed earlier in this chapter. The focus of this section is on the infant's sensory and language development and the importance of infant stimulation to both developmental areas.

From birth, infants possess sensory capabilities; all sensory organs are well developed and functioning. As the infant is cared for and handled, the special senses become organized neurologically into a pattern of behavior that will greatly influence subsequent development.

Table 17-7 Visual Development During Infancy

Age	Behavior That Indicates Vision
1 to 3 months	Fixes gaze on object 12 to 24 inches away Takes interest in bright colors and faces Follows objects in field of vision
3 to 6 months	Begins to show interest in hands Follows in range of 90 degrees Recognizes familiar objects Able to see full color by now
6 to 9 months	Visual scanning becomes more integrated Capable of organized depth perception Begins to perceive distances accurately Both eyes should focus equally now
9 to 12 months	Able to look for concealed items Converges on objects in close proximity Peripheral vision is well developed Judges distances well
12 to 18 months	Eye-hand coordination develops Depth perception more refined Ability to identify forms and shapes

Vision

The infant's initial visual impressions are unfocused, bizarre, unfamiliar, and without meaning. Because everything is new and only somewhat significant, visual stimuli must be moving, bright, or flashing to capture the infant's attention. The infant's eyes are well developed at birth, but the muscles that attach the eyes to their sockets are weak. This weakness may be stressful to parents because the infant's eyes do not appear to function together. Parents can be assured that most infants coordinate their eye movements by the age of 3 months; by 6 months, this function is mature. Table 17-7 summarizes visual developmental milestones for the infant.

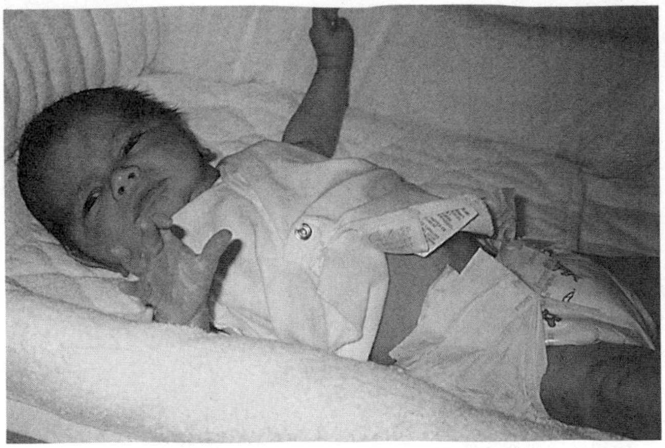

Fig. 17-6 Babies respond to startling loud noises, confirming their sense of hearing.

Table 17-8 Normal Development of Hearing

Age	Behavior That Indicates Hearing
1 to 3 months	Is startled by loud noises Stops activity when spoken to
3 to 6 months	Turns eyes and head toward sound Responds to mother's voice Imitates own noises: oohs and ba-ba's
6 to 9 months	Responds to own name Locates sounds above Recognizes familiar sounds
9 to 12 months	Points to familiar objects or people Imitates simple words and sounds Locates a sound in any direction
12 to 18 months	Follows simple spoken directions Distinguishes between sounds Spoken words are well on their way

Hearing

After the amniotic fluid drains from the middle ear several days after birth, the infant's hearing becomes acute. Hearing is one of the better-developed senses in the infant; the fetus can even hear *in utero* and responds to loud sounds (Fig. 17-6). The newborn can distinguish sound frequencies and turns toward a voice or another sound. The infant may be familiar with the mother's voice early in life. Sounds gradually gain significance and meaning when they are associated with caregivers, food, and pleasure.

The ability to listen and discriminate among sounds is an important task during infancy. The closer the infant is to the sound, the easier the sound can be discriminated.

The groundwork for verbal ability begins to develop long before words appear and many believe that infants whose mothers talk to them tend to speak earlier compared with infants who are not exposed to these sounds (Bee, 2000). Table 17-8 summarizes the infant's auditory development.

Smell

The ability to smell is fully developed at birth. The infant has many receptors in the nose, but lacks the cilia that line the inside of the adult's nose. As a result, the infant has a keen sense of smell, because odors reach the receptor cells easily. Within 2 weeks after birth, an infant can differentiate the odor of the mother's milk from others', an ability developed when the infant is held close (Wong, 1999). At this time, the infant begins associating the parents by detecting their body odors, a perception that is important to infant-parent bonding.

Taste

The sense of taste is present at birth and salivation begins at approximately 3 months of age. The four primary sensations are sour, salty, sweet, and bitter. The taste buds for sweet tastes are more abundant during early life than they are in later life, which may account for the preference for sweets that is characteristic of infants and children.

Touch and Motion

Tactile sensation is well developed at birth, particularly on the lips and tongue. Perceptions of motion and touch are perhaps the most important of all senses. Rocking and other motion are sensations of equilibrium picked up by the middle ear. Skin-to-skin touching should be performed regularly; documented evidence shows that touch helps relieve the unspent tensions that infants develop and accelerates neuromuscular development (Gorrie, 1998). Infants respond with pleasure to rocking and other motion and to tactile sensations of warmth, closeness, and cuddling.

Language Development

Language development, an important aspect of the infant's cognitive and perceptual pattern, is affected by intellectual development, maturation of the central nervous system, development of the organs of speech, and exposure to human verbalization.

Similar to other areas of development, the acquisition of language follows a definite sequence. During the first 2 months, most of the infant's sounds are vowels and are made primarily in the front part of the mouth (Wong, 1999). Crying is the means of communication during this period. Cooing sounds are heard at approximately 2 to 3 months, usually in response to an adult's voice. By 6 months, babbling sounds are heard, and by 9 to 10 months, the infant forms two-syllable sounds. By 12 months, words such as "ma-ma," "bye-bye," and "da-da" are emerging. From 15 to 18 months, an expressive jargon with rhythmic intonations develops, but words are recognized only rarely. The infant uses jargon along with pointing to express wishes.

Nursing Suggestions

The nurse's knowledge and understanding of an infant's cognitive and perceptual behavior facilitates interaction with infants and serves as a guide in parental counseling. The major focus centers on stimulation, because each of the infant's senses is receptive to environmental stimulation. This activity helps the infant learn from the environment. When an infant is exposed to appropriate sensory stimulation, greater curiosity, improved mental capabilities, accelerated neuromuscular growth, enhanced gastrointestinal functioning, quicker weight gain, more rapid language development, and pleasing mother-infant interactions are likely to occur (Erickson, 1999).

Parents are the primary providers of pleasurable and stimulating experiences for the infant. The nurse assists them by offering suggestions about suitable stimuli for each sensory modality.

Self-Perception–Self-Concept Pattern

Self-perception has a pervasive influence on all aspects of life. Self-concept consists of a set of attitudes regarding what each person thinks, believes, and feels about the self. These attitudes form a personal self-belief that is an abstraction referred to as *me*. Many researchers believe that the infant determines self-existence by first noting that actions such as crying or smiling have an effect on others, which depends on receiving feedback (Klaus, Kennell, & Klaus, 2000).

Studies confirm that infants have the ability to identify themselves and therefore form a self-concept. Infants at 4 months of age were found to be particularly fascinated with their images in mirrors and smiled more at themselves than they did at pictures of other infants (Karmiloff & Smith, 2001).

As the infant continues to grow and mature, many circumstances combine to influence self-concept. How others relate to the infant's body and the continuing messages that the infant receives from the body lead to knowledge of a physical self. The ability to use the body to influence others in the environment can lead the psychological self to conclude that someone cares about the infant (Ball & Bindler, 1998).

The infant's development of body image is gradual. At birth, the infant has diffuse feelings of hunger, pain, anger, and comfort, but no body image. Initially, all the infant knows is the self and regards the external world as an extension of the self. Only when infants begin to experience the environment through sensory modalities are they able to distinguish their bodies from animate and inanimate objects.

Nursing Suggestions

The nurse plays a vital role in assisting parents to foster the development of a positive self-concept and a good body image in their infant. The nurse first identifies personal self-concept and how it influences individuals (Fogel, 2000). The nurse stresses that the way in which parents treat the infant influences the infant's self-concept. Basically, infants and young children incorporate their parents' interactions with them (good or bad) into their own view of self. Parents must understand that their infant's self-concept is an important, continuing event. What the infant knows and later believes about the self will affect all interactions with others, and by influencing what the infant will later attempt, the self-concept may have broad effects on the development of new skills (Hoekelman, 1996).

Roles-Relationships Pattern

Literature has extensively explored the effect of early bonding between parents and their infants, emphasizing that this initial attraction sets the stage for the later development of love and affiliation (Staso, 1999). The bonding process has many other implications for the infant's future development as well (Klaus, Kennell, & Klaus, 2000).

Attachment and Bonding

The parent-infant relationship does not begin with the birth of the infant; many aspects have been molded by the life experiences of the parents long before they reach parenthood. The kind of mothering that a woman received as an infant and the concept of *mother* that she developed as she grew represent the early effects that can determine the mother-infant relationship. The mother's overall self-concept as a person will affect her ability to relate to her infant, as will her relationship with the infant's father.

The establishment of this emotional bond between the mother and her infant is known as *attachment*. This emotional bond is considered crucial for the optimal physical and emotional development of the infant. Maternal behaviors such as how the mother holds, feeds, and looks at the infant demonstrate the process of attachment (Brazelton, 1994).

Various theories have attempted to explain the basis for attachment behavior. Freudian psychoanalytical theory emphasizes that the bond between child and mother develops as a result of the mother's satisfying the infant's innate desire to socialize and the physical requirements for survival. Social learning theory contributes the principles of reinforcement to the attachment process; as the mother meets the infant's needs, discomfort is reduced or removed. The infant associates the pleasurable feeling of being satisfied with the mother, who becomes a *significant other* in the infant's life. The bonding process is the basis for the mother-infant relationship, which, in turn, forms the basis for the interdependence that is necessary for the infant's psychological and physical development (Korones, 1998).

In early studies on attachment, Klaus, Kennell, and Klaus (2000) have formulated the following seven crucial principles in the process of attachment:

1. A sensitive period appears to exist in the first minutes

and hours after birth during which it seems necessary for the mother and father to have close contact with their infant for later development to be optimal.

2. Species-specific responses to the infant appear to exist in the human mother and father when the infant is first given to them.
3. The attachment process seems to be structured such that the parents become attached to only one infant at a time.
4. For attachment to occur appropriately, the infant must respond to the mother and father by some signal, such as body or eye movements. This principle has been called the *you can't love a dishrag* phenomenon.
5. Individuals who witness the birth process become strongly attached to the infant.
6. Some adults find it difficult to go through the processes of attachment and detachment simultaneously. Becoming attached to an infant while mourning the loss or threatened loss of another person is difficult for parents.
7. Some early events may have long-lasting effects. For example, anxiety over an infant with a transient disorder in the child's early days may result in long-term concerns or behavior that will have implications for future development.

Just as the infant's behavior influences attachment, it also continues to influence the evolving maternal-paternal-infant relationship as the infant develops. Studies have shown that if the process of attachment is encumbered, later problems are more likely to occur, such as child abuse, failure-to-thrive syndrome, and behavioral problems (Kessler & Dawson, 1999).

Many factors are present when a relationship is being established and maintained. Most people enter a relationship with unrealistic expectations; parents are no exception—they are going to be wise, patient, and devoted, and they will nurture their infant. Because the parents' self-esteem is closely associated with their infant's interactions and accomplishments, when parents' self-esteem is low, disappointment, anger, and a disturbance in their infant's relationship can occur. In some instances, this disturbed parent-infant relationship is short-lived and nothing harmful develops. When a disturbed parent-infant relationship continues, however, the infant is at risk for abuse and other behavioral problems.

The process of bonding is also important for fathers. Recently, a process called *engrossment* has been used to describe the behavior pattern of fathers when they interact with their infants. The major characteristics of engrossment include: (1) visual awareness of the infant; (2) tactile awareness, often expressed in a desire to hold the infant; (3) awareness of distinct characteristics, with emphasis on the features that resemble the father; (4) perception of the infant as *perfect;* (5) development of a strong feeling of attraction to the infant that leads to intense focusing of attention; (6) a feeling of extreme elation; and (7) a sense of deep self-esteem and satisfaction (Brazelton, 1994) (Fig. 17-7).

Child Abuse

Infant and child abuse has always been a part of human history. Acceptable behavior toward infants is largely a learned phenomenon; the art of parenting is not instinctively acquired, as many people believe. Abusing parents are seldom *monsters;* they are merely individuals who are attempting to cope with the demands of parenthood for which there are little or no preparation.

The scope of the problem is extensive: estimates indicate that more than three million infants and children in the United States are victims of abuse (U.S. Census Bureau, 2000b). Children under 3 years of age are the most frequent victims. Women are more frequent abusers than are men because they are the primary caregivers. Men abuse more severely and commit sexual abuse more frequently. Child abuse does not discriminate; it occurs in families of every race, creed, and socioeconomic class.

The child-abuse syndrome is a clinical condition in infants who have suffered serious active or passive abuse at the hands of their parents or other caregivers. Physical trauma is not the only facet, but it is the most overt indicator of a dysfunctional family unit and a disturbed parent-infant relationship (Paulk, 1999).

Active manifestations of abuse include the following:

1. Brain injuries, subdural hematomas, and skull fractures
2. Soft-tissue injuries, such as bruises, lacerations, or burns
3. Fractures of the long bones and ribs; multiple fractures in varying stages of healing

Passive manifestations of abuse include the following:

1. Poor nutrition, failure to thrive, and severe malnutrition
2. Poor physical condition: neglected safeguards against disease, poor skin condition, and lack of medical attention
3. Emotional neglect: rejection, indifference, and deprivation of love
4. Moral neglect: allowing the infant or child to remain in an immoral atmosphere

Abusing parents often have common patterns of behavior. As children, their own parents may have abused them. In this way, child abuse is recycled from generation to generation. The development of the maternal role on which the infant depends for health, progress, and survival begins in the early childhood of the mother. Unless she received love and proper mothering, she will have difficulty with a relationship that entails the complete dependency of another person. She may find the relationship with her own infant to be unrewarding, threatening, and frustrating. Feelings of inadequacy and guilt in the mother and father roles compound the problems.

innovative practice

Promoting Healthy Responsiveness Between Depressed Mothers and Their Infants

Postpartum depression can adversely affect babies and their mothers. In addition to threatening infant health and development, postpartum depression can interfere with the developing mother-infant relationship. Depression compromises mothers' sensitivity to infants' cues. When interacting with their infants, mothers who are depressed tend to withdraw and show little emotion, or they may intrude by poking, handling babies roughly, or speaking in an angry tone. Infants typically respond with distress and protest or withdrawal. These patterns disrupt infants' developing capacity for social interaction and sense of mastery, trust, and control over events. Clearly, research is needed to explore ways to mitigate the consequences of postpartum depression.

A two-phase study on postpartum depression, "Promoting Healthy Responsiveness between Depressed Mothers and their Infants," was recently completed by June Andrews Horowitz, PhD, RN, FAAN, Associate Professor, Boston College School of Nursing. This study involved mothers who delivered at Brigham and Women's Hospital in Boston, Massachusetts and at Brockton Hospital in Brockton, Massachusetts.

The purpose of the study was to test the efficacy of an interactive coaching intervention in promoting maternal-infant responsiveness between mothers with depression symptoms and their infants.

A group of 1215 mothers who consented to be in the study was screened for postpartum depression at 2 to 4 weeks after delivery. From this group, 122 of mothers who showed symptoms of depression agreed to participate in the second phase of the study. These mothers were randomized to either the treatment or the control group. Mothers in both groups received three home visits over a 2-month period from study nurses who videotaped the mothers while they played with their babies. Women in the treatment group were coached to play with their babies using techniques designed to promote increased responsiveness between mother and infant. A team member who did not know which mothers received the intervention later coded the videotaped interactions.

Two important findings with implications for clinical practice resulted from this study. First, 18% of the mothers who participated in the study experienced mild to severe depression symptoms at 2 to 4 weeks after delivery, a finding consistent with other reports in the literature. This number supports the need for routine screening for postpartum depression and for increased parental education about this common problem and what to do when symptoms occur. The second important finding indicated that maternal-infant interaction was significantly higher among mothers in the treatment group. The cost-effective coaching strategy used in this study (teaching mothers how to talk and play with their babies) appeared to have had a positive effect on maternal-infant interaction for vulnerable mothers who experience postpartum depression. This project also represents an example of collaboration among faculty, clinical nursing staff, and students. By participating, nurses were able to identify relevant clinical nursing research in action, and they realized that their effort was critical to the project's success. Students gained first-hand knowledge about research-based practice and developed valuable research skills.

"Promoting Healthy Responsiveness between Depressed Mothers and their Infants," was funded by the March of Dimes Birth Defects Foundation, grant number 12-FY98-0014, and supported by a Boston College Research Incentive Grant. June Andrews Horowitz, Boston College, was the Principal Investigator. Detta Quigley-Lavoie, RN, MA, Nurse Manager, Brigham and Women's Hospital, and staff nurses from both institutions collaborated and provided invaluable assistance in advising patients of the study opportunity. Students from Boston College School of Nursing helped in all phases of the project from recruitment and screening of participants to data analysis.

Courtesy June Andrews Horowitz, PhD, RN, FAAN, Associate Professor, School of Nursing, Boston College, Boston, Massachusetts.

Abusing parents are often socially isolated and have few people to whom they can turn during times of crisis; they also cannot support one another emotionally. These parents may view the infant as the person who can provide the love, support, and nurturing that is lacking in their own lives. When the infant does not fulfill their expectations, the risk of abuse becomes acute (Paulk, 1999).

The abused infant or child is usually singled out as someone who is different. This infant may be chronically ill, may have been premature, may be hyperactive, may have been the product of a difficult and complicated pregnancy, or may have an obvious birth anomaly. Early bonding disturbances (inadequacies in feeding, holding, and caring for the infant) are characteristic signals.

The long-term effects of child abuse are profound. The victims lack basic trust (a major task of infancy) and confidence and self-worth. These deficits follow the victims into adulthood and parenthood and the vicious cycle continues. One of the discouraging findings is that infants and children who were abused frequently grow up to be abusing parents themselves (Murry, Baker, & Levin, 2000).

Across the United States, great interest has been generated in attempts to identify parents in the prenatal and perinatal periods who have significant potential for child abuse. The following measures have been undertaken to help prevent child abuse:

1. Predictive questionnaires to be given to parents on postpartum units.
2. Recognition of parents who have difficulty relating to their infants through body language clues or verbalizations.

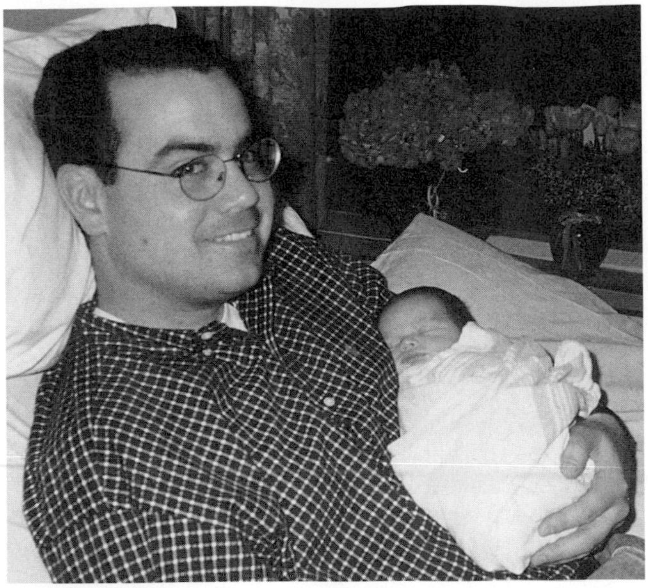

Fig. 17-7 The process of bonding is also important for fathers.

3. Closer follow-up in the postpartum period by the public health nurse.
4. Crisis hot lines made available to parents in distress.

Before focusing on nursing interventions (Box 17-9), the nurse can make several observations by using the following questions to assist in identifying a high-risk infant:

- Does the mother hold the infant close and establish eye contact?
- Does the mother speak negatively about the infant?
- Does the mother intensely dislike the duties of motherhood, such as diapering, feeding, and so on?
- Does the mother expect too much of the infant at a particular stage of development?
- Does the mother focus her attention on the infant rather than on her husband?
- Does the mother have a good support system available?
- Does the mother act overly concerned about the infant's gender?

Most communities are seeking ways in which child abuse can be prevented through educational efforts, improved agency coordination, and development of new collaborative efforts and services for parents and infants. Laws for reporting abuse have been enacted in every state. Reporting all cases of suspected abuse and neglect is mandatory. Everyone must assist in this endeavor to prevent continued abuse.

Failure-to-Thrive Syndrome

Another problem that may stem from a disturbed parent-infant relationship is **failure-to-thrive syndrome** (FTT). There is no consensus definition of FTT. The term is used to describe infants who fail to gain weight resulting from the failure to obtain or use necessary calories. A weight that is persistently below the percentile on a standard growth chart characterizes the FTT infant. Although FTT can result from an organic disease, the most common cause is a disturbance in the relationship between the primary caregiver and the infant.

Five principal factors in the infant's growth and development are adequate nutrition, sleep and rest, activity, adequate secretion of hormones, and a satisfactory relationship with a significant other who provides loving contact and stimulation. When the last of these factor is missing, the infant's growth is disturbed and development is delayed (McKinney et al., 2000).

The nurse realizes that the parent-infant relationship is reciprocal. The mother's failure to provide adequate emotional care and adequate nutrition can result in an infant who fails to gain weight. This failure may be interpreted by the mother as a rejection of her mothering efforts and this interpretation naturally reduces her self-confidence. This lack of self-confidence is, in turn, reflected in her care; therefore a negative pattern of interaction is established between mother and infant (Brazelton, 1994).

The infant who is failing to thrive displays malnourishment and growth failure. The infant may have poor muscle tone, lethargy, an inability to cuddle, and delayed or absent speech patterns (Brazelton, 1994).

The mothers of FTT infants often show many of the characteristics listed in Box 17-10. The first nursing intervention is to assess the family relationships by asking questions and observing interactions (Giddens, 1998). Box 17-11 lists guidelines that can be helpful in the assessment

Box 17-9 Nursing Interventions to Prevent Abuse of Infants

- Promote and facilitate early parent-infant bonding.
- Promote a trusting relationship.
- Provide more frequent office visits and be available by phone.
- Provide infant care instructions to enhance mothering ability.
- Provide for community health person to make home visits.

Box 17-10 Profile of Mother with FTT Infants

1. Disrupted and disorganized home situation.
2. Unable to assess the infant's needs.
3. Unable to think about the future.
4. Lack of proper nurturing as a child.
5. Low self-esteem and feelings of inadequacy.

From Bush, D. (1999). *Growing healthy babies: The growing family's guide to nutrition and wellness*. Humble, TX: Baby Cottage, LLC.

Box 17-11 Family Assessment Process

- Do the parents and infant have eye-to-eye contact frequently?
- How much body contact is present?
- Does vocalizations by the parents evoke a smile from the infant?
- How much does the infant cry? What is the mother's reaction? What is the father's reaction?
- How does the mother describe the infant's feeding and sleeping patterns?
- Does the mother describe her mothering tasks positively or negatively?
- How do the parents perceive this problem? As the infant's fault? As the mother's fault?
- Ask the parents about their own health and its influence on caring for the infant.
- Elicit what family support systems are present. Is the mother isolated?
- Have the mother describe her home life and what changes have taken place within it.

process. The goals of nursing intervention after the assessment of family dynamics are listed in Box 17-12.

Homelessness

Along with food, health, and personal safety, probably no greater basic need for human beings exists than shelter. The loss of shelter is detrimental to the health and well being of all people. Homelessness in the United States is a national disgrace. Most estimates place the number of homeless at three million. One of every four homeless people is a child (Vostanis, 1999).

To say that the well being of the next generation is being jeopardized by homelessness is not an exaggeration. Homelessness devastates every aspect of a child's life, doing damage with long-term implications that remain unknown. Homelessness endangers a child's health throughout childhood. Homeless infants are often exposed to unsafe and unsanitary conditions in shelters in which infectious diseases thrive. These dangers are combined with a lack of access to regular health care; common childhood ailments such as ear infections become extremely serious and sometimes life-threatening illnesses before they are treated.

Ear infections are among the most common health problems encountered in children. Usually, a 10-day course of antibiotics relieves the condition. Rarely are long-term complications encountered. For the homeless infant, however, the story is different. Families are cut off from their regular clinics and providers. The struggle for basic life needs is intense. The poverty, isolation, and disorientation of prolonged homelessness can be complicated by drug or alcohol abuse, provoked, at least in part, by situational despair. The fundamental ability of a family to function is hampered or paralyzed.

Box 17-12 Nursing Interventions to Prevent Failure-to-Thrive Syndrome in Infants

- Improve family interactions and relationships.
- Improve family's ability to cope with stress.
- Increase parental self-esteem.
- Discuss age-appropriate feeding techniques.
- Praise positive parenting behaviors.
- Review growth and developmental behaviors and encourage parents to foster these behaviors.
- Provide adequate nutrition for the malnourished infant.
- Teach parents their infant's nutritional requirements.
- Demonstrate infant feeding positions, formula preparation, and age-appropriate foods.
- Help parents learn and interpret their infant's cues during interaction.
- Promote adequate environmental stimulation.
- Demonstrate techniques of stimulation that will improve growth and development.
- Teach reasons why stimulation is necessary for health promotion.
- Improve family's awareness of and insight into problem areas.
- Allow parents to vent their feelings about the infant.
- Assist in identifying the infant's attributes and unique qualities.
- Discuss stress within the family unit and assist the parents to use support systems within the community: family, friends, clergy, social worker, nurse, and so on.
- Continue counseling efforts at home through a public health agency.
- Refer to appropriate agency for financial, social, or other family needs.

For the homeless family, the fever caused by an infant's acute ear infection may not have the highest priority. Availability, accessibility, and affordability of medical care are serious concerns. As a result, the infection is never treated, and the problem becomes prolonged (the infection evolves to a chronic state). Hearing and language development can be impaired.

Overall, these children simply do not receive routine, reliable health care. They remain at high risk for many health problems. Their health problems remain undiagnosed and undertreated, if they receive health care attention at all. Complications and secondary problems abound. Furthermore, the conditions under which they live (the squalor, the lack of safe food storage and preparation facilities, and the drug-infested and physically dangerous environments) predispose children to a substantially increased rate of disease and injury (Allahyari, 2000).

The pioneering work of Erik Erikson has defined the necessary stages of human development. Each level of maturation must be sequentially mastered; but to do so takes a secure environment, opportunities to succeed, and emotional support. The hidden tragedy for homeless children is the stifling of their personal growth. These losses, dissimilar to the loss of a home, may be irrevocable.

CASE STUDY

Homeless Infants

As a community health nurse in an inner-city health center, you are increasingly aware that the homeless population in your city appears to be the *forgotten aggregate.* Your community health center provides primary care to a culturally diverse and indigent population. As a nurse, you believe that the homeless population within your city has numerous health needs. Beyond the basic requirements, many homeless people have mental and substance abuse problems, lack of life skills, poor family support, and most of all, no child health access.

The homeless population has all of the usual health problems you would expect in the general population in addition to other problems resulting from their homeless lifestyle. Although there are several glaring concerns, you plan to focus your attention first on securing immunizations for the homeless infants and, secondly, to obtain formula for them.

Questions:

1. In planning health services for this special population, what facts do you need to know?
2. What barriers to accessing health care for infants confront the homeless family?
3. How can you overcome some of the barriers in developing your plan for health care?

Discussion:

1. In planning health services for this special population, what facts do you need to know? Some of the first questions that should be asked are:
   - How many homeless infants are in this aggregate?
   - Where are they?
   - How can they access health care in the city?

   To answer these questions, it might be prudent to collaborate and partner with other health and social service agencies, local hospitals, and the state health and human services agency. Collaboration and partnering can bring in additional resources and reduce duplication and gaps in services.
2. What barriers to accessing health care for infants confront the homeless family?
   - Lack of transportation to access health care
   - Lack of trust in the medical establishment
   - Judgmental care on the part of health care providers
   - No health insurance to cover medical visits
   - Preventive care, such as immunizations, is not a priority when you are hungry
   - No money to get prescriptions filled
   - Waiting until condition is serious before seeking treatment
3. How can you overcome some of the barriers in developing your plan for health care?
   - Provide health care in the city shelters for use by homeless families.
   - Set up a mobile health care team and visit the shelters to provide care.
   - Offer free immunizations for all family members.
   - Set up educational sessions within the shelters to provide information.
   - Stress importance of preventive measures to reduce illness in infants.
   - Obtain free formula from company and/or hospitals to give to homeless infants.
   - Work closely with other health care interests within the community.

Theoretically, homelessness can be eliminated. The key factors are increased affordable housing, increased income for low-income families, and strengthened service and support for families at risk of homelessness. Families at risk of homelessness for solely economic reasons can often be helped with short-term loans and grants. Community-based programs can help identify these families before they lose their homes.

Efforts should be made to link the homeless with all available programs and services, such as the Special Supplemental Nutrition Program for Women, Infants, and Children (WIC), food stamps, Head Start, and housing subsidies. These programs should continue to provide assistance after the family is resettled in permanent housing. These families will need more comprehensive services with special problems such as domestic violence, mental illness, or substance abuse.

Because there is a multitude of needs, a partnership that provides a multitude of resources must be developed. Nurses can take a leadership position in helping the homeless achieve a sense of security and adequate health care. Getting involved in community health care for the homeless and providing compassionate care gives the homeless a clear signal of hope and concern about their plight. Bringing attention to this social problem by speaking to various community groups to obtain their support is another way that nurses can help the homeless. Volunteering time in community shelters and organizing health care days through the local health department is another way to address the problem. Nurses can become active in raising the nation's conscience and helping to call attention to this national disgrace. Housing and support services must be provided to assist the homeless in regaining a foothold in society. With the right support services and health care, many homeless people can be stabilized and integrated back into the community. These families with infants are not *throwaways*, but people who have fallen on hard times and need someone to offer a helping hand. Through this help, the nation's health can improve (see Case Study and Care Plan box).

Sexuality-Reproductive Pattern

An infant's identity begins at birth, when the child is named and caretakers act a certain way toward the infant because of its gender. The infant's sexuality gives direction to its physical, emotional, social, and intellectual responses throughout life. Infants have a great oral sensitivity, enjoy skin-to-skin contact, and explore their own bodies for pleasure in the first year of life. A healthy, accepting attitude by caretakers is important in an infant's evolving sexual development.

Coping–Stress-Tolerance Pattern

The term stress implies intense reaction to an experience and changes in usual behavior. Stress is a normal phenomenon that occurs throughout the lifespan when an individual experiences a developmental or situational crisis.

Developmental Crisis

Developmental crises are turning points or periods of great change. Most stressors that the infant experiences are a necessary part of growth and development. For example, learning new skills creates stress. The infant who is unable to move forward while learning to crawl experiences stress. The infant expresses this stress by crying for help. Other

CARE PLAN

Homelessness is a community dilemma and an example of an economic problem that places infants at risk. Families are the fastest growing group of homeless people. Homeless families do not have health insurance; infants within these families are more likely to lack immunizations, proper nutrition, safe environment, and a stable family situation. The community health nurse in this chapter's case study wanted to address two aspects of homeless infants: (1) immunizations and (2) nutrition.

Nursing Diagnosis: Altered health maintenance related to nonadherence to appropriate immunization schedule as manifested by increased incidence of communicable diseases

DEFINING CHARACTERISTICS

History of lack of health-seeking behavior by caregiver, lack of financial, and/or other resources; reported or observed impairment of personal support systems; lack of knowledge regarding health promotion practices; inability to access health care; limited basic personal resources

RELATED FACTORS

Ineffective family coping; perceptual-cognitive impairment; lack of material resources; ineffective individual coping

EXPECTED OUTCOMES

Caretaker of infant will:

- Begin health-seeking behavior on behalf of infant.
- Increase health-promotion and health-maintenance knowledge.
- Gain access to available health care resources.
- Participate in life change to improve health status; meet goals for health care maintenance.

NURSING INTERVENTIONS

- Assess caretaker's feelings, values, and personal situation
- Assess for family patterns, economic issues, and cultural patterns that influence compliance
- Assist caretaker and family to access health care resources available to them
- Refer caretaker and family to community agencies to address social and economic issues
- Educate caretaker and family on the importance of immunizations and disease prevention
- Provide for follow-up to increase chance of health status change taking place

Nursing Diagnosis: High risk for altered nutrition—less than body requirements; related factors and social-economic factors as manifested by low height and weight measurements on growth chart for chronological age

DEFINING CHARACTERISTICS

Pale conjunctival and mucus membranes; poor muscle development; inadequate food intake to maintain body weight; weight loss, fatigue, frequent irritable, fussy, crying behavior; growth and development milestones not met; frequent illnesses suggesting depressed immunity

RELATED FACTORS

Inability to obtain adequate food and/or fluid to nourish body because of social-economic factors

EXPECTED OUTCOMES

Infant will demonstrate the following:

- Progressive weight gains toward desired goal.
- Weight is within normal range for height and weight.
- Infant will consume adequate nourishment.
- Infant will be free of signs of malnutrition.

NURSING INTERVENTIONS

- Assess healthy body weight for age and height
- Observe infant's ability to consume food and fluids
- Monitor food and fluid intake weekly
- Access nutritional resources for the caretaker or family
- Refer to appropriate community agencies to meet needs
- Assist the caretaker or family to identify area needing change, which will make the greatest contribution to improve nutrition
- Implement instructional dialog that is appropriate for their level
- Provide for follow-up care to assist them in changing their health status

stressors are more psychosocial in nature, such as being left with a babysitter or in an unfamiliar place.

Situational Crisis

Situational crises are not anticipated easily and do not occur necessarily as part of the normal growth and development process. One major situational crisis during infancy is separation from the significant other. The following three distinct phases are evident in the reaction to separation (Wong, 1999):

1. Protest. Infant cries loudly, screams for the mother, and refuses attention of the substitute caregiver.
2. Despair. Infant stops crying and becomes less active, withdraws, and becomes apathetic.
3. Withdrawal. Infant takes an interest in surroundings, but tends to ignore or reject the mother when she returns because she failed to meet the infant's needs.

Initially, with no time framework and no understanding of waiting, the infant has little ability to cope with stress. As maturity and a sense of security provided by the caregiver increases, the infant begins to wait a short time to have needs met without protest. An infant who experiences stress reacts by crying, the main tool of communication. The infant gradually learns to tolerate greater stress as time progresses.

Nursing Interventions

Nursing suggestions to assist the infant and family in stressful situations are listed in Box 17-13. By allaying anxiety in the infant's caregiver, the nurse facilitates coping behaviors in the infant. The stressful situation and the problem-solving activities can be turned into growth-producing experiences for the family, with coping capacities strengthened for the future.

Box 17-13 Nursing Interventions to Assist in Stressful Situations During Infancy

- Attempt to meet the infant's needs promptly.
- Allow favorite toy or item of security to be present during stressful experiences.
- Allow familiar caregiver to be present to calm the infant.
- Attempt to keep the number of strangers interacting with the infant to a minimum.
- Attempt to provide a warm and accepting environment for the infant.
- Allow freedom of expression (crying) to reduce tension in the infant.
- Identify the infant's established daily routine and try to follow through with it.
- Reinforce the infant's need for expression.
- Establish a trusting relationship with the infant.
- Provide opportunity for play so the infant can *vent* fears.
- Provide emotional support for the parents so they can, in turn, give support to their infant.

Values-Beliefs Pattern

A value is a standard or principle that is considered to be good or proper. When people communicate, they send both the content message of the spoken words and the unspoken message of who they are and what they believe. Values are pervasive and important and give a focus to people within a particular culture. Because values are attitudes learned from significant others within the environment, the values-beliefs pattern is undeveloped in the infant. The infant has yet to reach the cognitive level of incorporating the parents' values into the behavioral system. The parents, through parenting behaviors, serve as a model as the infant develops into a boy or girl.

Nursing Interventions

By understanding and respecting the parents' value system, the nurse works within their framework of values in the counseling situation. The nurse communicates personal values to the family. To work successfully within a different value system, the nurse should incorporate the following attitudes concerning the values-beliefs pattern into the nursing process (Stanhope, 2000):

1. Believe in the ultimate worth of the infant and the family, regardless of their behavior or situation.
2. Grant families the freedom to make their own informed choices and to experience the responsibilities and consequences of their decisions.
3. Use knowledge of the family's value system in specific ways to reward and reinforce positive health practices.
4. Value the growth potential inherent in developmental and situational crisis situations.
5. Recognize your own value system and its influence on your behavior.
6. Work with families without applying your personal value system in judging their behavior.
7. Broaden your value system by accepting lifestyles different from your own.

The nurse influences the behavior of the parents, who have the greatest influence on developing their infant's values-beliefs pattern. The nurse accomplishes this task by modeling (living congruently with professed values), acting as a consultant by sharing pertinent information with parents, and modifying one's own values (Schlef, 2000).

Modeling can be a potent influence on another individual's behavior. In the counseling situation, the family looks to the nurse for guidance and assistance in promoting healthy child-rearing practices. The methods by which the nurse interacts with the infant, listens to the parents' concerns, and demonstrates respect for the family unit are influencing factors in changing behavior.

Second, the nurse acts as a consultant to influence values. Advice on child-rearing practices is overwhelming to parents; everyone has opinions. The nurse listens before giving advice to determine whether parents will accept the advice and to allow them to decide whether the advice can be useful. Repeated attempts to convert parents to the nurse's value system can make them defensive and resistant to the advice.

Third, by expressing values and attitudes, but remaining open to other approaches, the nurse influences the values-beliefs pattern. Parents should realize that they are free to change and are not bound to traditional values that others outside their value system express (Andrews & Boyle, 1995).

The nurse who uses these communication skills can deal with families more effectively. The nurse's open attitude increases the likelihood that the parents will discuss their concerns and adhere to the health-promotion guidelines that the nurse has offered.

PATHOLOGICAL PROCESSES

This section discusses various factors within the environment that can affect the infant's health status. The entire realm of accident prevention and safety promotion is applicable here.

Accidents are always unexpected and, in retrospect, usually could have been prevented. Adults take for granted that they are living in a world designed by adults for adults. They must remind themselves constantly that infants also live in this complex world and, although they learn at a remarkable rate, infants are unaware of most environmental dangers. This inexperience renders them extremely vulnerable to accidents, a major problem and a challenging field for preventive measures.

Accidents occur in many situations: in the home, in the street, on the playground, and in automobiles. Regulation car seats prevent infant injury in some car accidents (Fig. 17-8). The majority of accidents, however, occur in the home. Their number and seriousness are closely linked to the infant's developmental stage. Accidents tend to increase with the mobility of the infant, but even a 2-month-old can wiggle or fall from a high place.

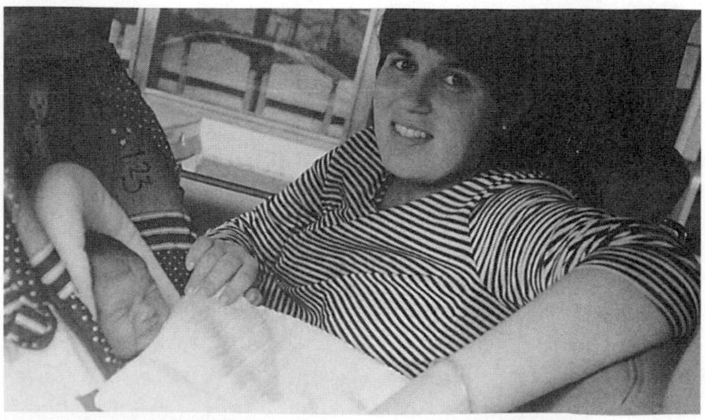

Fig. 17-8 Federally approved infant car restraint. Note the placement of the infant in the middle of the back seat.

Nurses have the opportunity to help parents and caregivers anticipate and understand the common hazards of early life and provide specific guidance for accident prevention.

Unintentional Injuries

Falls

Falls are most common after 4 months of age, when the infant has learned to roll over, but they can occur at any age. The best advice is never to place an infant unattended on a raised surface that has no type of guardrails. When in doubt, the safest place is the floor (Fig. 17-9) (Fogel, 2000). Safety tips to assist parents in preventing falls are listed in Box 17-14.

Burns

Burns are the most frequent and frightening of all accidents during infancy. Because nearly all burns are preventable, the attendant caregiver can experience severe guilt.

Fire from matches or other sources, hot liquids, ultraviolet light from the sun, electricity or electrical outlets, and heating elements such as radiators, registers, and floor heaters can all result in burns. Box 17-15 lists safety tips to assist parents in preventing burns.

Swallowing Foreign Objects

Any small object that an infant puts in the mouth has the potential to be swallowed. Parents should be advised that objects such as safety pins, peanuts, beads, coins, hot dogs, paper clips, nuts, corn, buttons, popcorn, chips, apple with peel, and parts of broken toys are frequently swallowed. Many objects can fit into this category and into the infant's mouth. The carelessness of a caregiver, relative, friend,

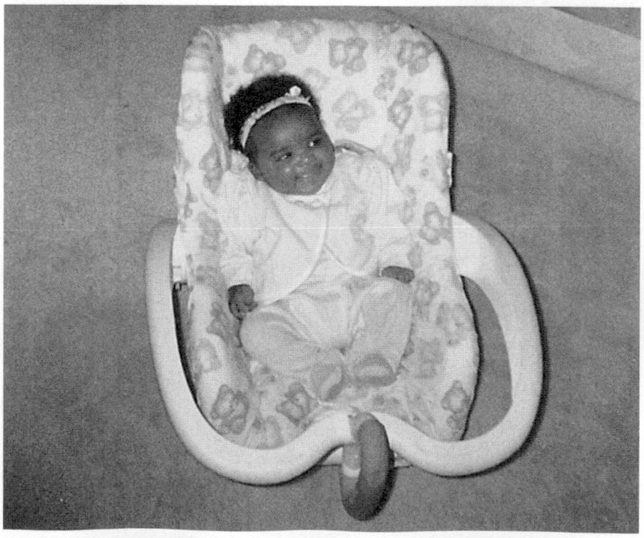

Fig. 17-9 When in doubt, the safest place for an infant is on the floor.

babysitter, or toy manufacturer in leaving small objects available and within reach, or giving toys unsuited to the infant's stage of development, frequently cause these accidents.

When choking occurs, the infant should be placed across the adult's knees (facedown on an incline, with the head at the lower end) and thumped sharply between the shoulder blades (Shelov, 1998).

The nurse gives parents another basic method to prepare them for an incident of choking. The Heimlich maneuver should be learned and used in a life-threatening situation caused by swallowing a foreign body (Fig. 17-10) (Daly, 2000).

Prevention of swallowing foreign objects is the best *treatment*. Some safety measures for parents and caregivers of infants are listed in Box 17-16.

The entire balance of safety for infants rests on allowing them plenty of opportunity to explore and play within the environment while protecting them from harmful physical agents. According to the American Academy of Pediatrics, the greatest threat to the health of infants is not illness, but injuries, many of which can be prevented. The nurse should inform the infant's primary caregivers about ways to childproof their home (Box 17-17).

Biological Agents

The fetus is protected from biological agents in the environment by the placental barrier and the mother's defense system. After birth, however, the infant is thrust into an environment that is filled with infectious, disease-causing agents. These bacterial or viral organisms can be found in food, cribs, the air, pets, the parents, and the sibling—literally everywhere. Even the healthiest environment harbors disease-causing agents. Although the infant cannot escape exposure to these pathogens without being completely isolated, immunizations are given to assist the infant's defense against communicable diseases.

Acquired Immunodeficiency Syndrome

Acquired immunodeficiency syndrome (AIDS) is spread by contact with the human immunodeficiency virus (HIV) through blood and bodily secretions. The virus attacks the T-cell lymphocytes, affecting formation of T4 (T-helper or T-inducer) cells, the cells responsible for directing the immune response. The infant with HIV infection is unable to resist normal infection. Transmission of HIV from mother to infant is the most likely reason for childhood HIV. Transmission of the virus can occur during pregnancy, at delivery, or during breast feeding (Koop, 2000).

Because infants can retain maternal antibodies for HIV infection for as long as 18 months, the diagnosis of HIV infection in an at-risk infant (one whose mother is infected) is extremely difficult. In the last few years,

Box 17-14 Safety Tips to Prevent Falls

1. Whenever the infant is in the crib, keep sides up and securely fastened.
2. Place the infant seat in the playpen or on the floor; always strap the infant in securely.
3. Check high chairs, strollers, and carriages for safety, and restrain the infant who is active.
4. Lock windows if the infant is capable of climbing on the windowsill.
5. Clean up food or liquid spills immediately from the floor.
6. Remember that polished floors are hazardous, especially when throw rugs are present.
7. Close off stairways with doors, gates, or some other safety device as the infant becomes mobile.
8. Do not leave items that the infant might use to climb out of the crib.
9. To prevent falls, set the crib mattress at the lowest adjustment level after the infant can pull up and stand.
10. Strap the infant into a shopping cart to prevent falls.

From Wootan, G. (2000). *Take charge of your child's health: A parent's guide to recognizing symptoms and treating minor illnesses at home* (2nd ed.). New York: Marlowe & Company.

Box 17-15 Burn Prevention Guidelines

1. Keep the infant out of the sun when ultraviolet rays are strongest, generally from 10:00 AM to 3:00 PM.
2. Sunscreen, clothing with long sleeves, pant legs, and a brimmed hat are essential to prevent sun overexposure.
3. Remember that fireplaces can be a serious hazard. Fine-mesh screens attached to a frame are safer compared with freestanding screens. Never leave an infant alone in a room where a fire is burning; make sure the fire is out before going to bed.
4. Avoid bathing the infant in a sink or adult tub near hot water faucets. Test the bath water temperatures before placing the infant in it; keep one hand on the infant at all times during the bath.
5. Be sure that all infant's clothing is made of nonflammable materials.
6. Avoid handling hot liquids near the infant.
7. Turn the handles of cooking utensils toward the back of the stove.
8. Keep all electrical cords taut, especially those for coffee pots; keep cords out of the infant's sight.
9. Cover electrical outlets with protective plastic caps.
10. Place a barrier in front of any heat-producing element, especially floor heaters.
11. Keep all matches and lighters out of the infant's reach.
12. Teach the older infant the meaning of hot.
13. Close oven doors when the oven is in use or when cooling.
14. If you must smoke, keep the heat of cigarettes or cigars away from the infant.

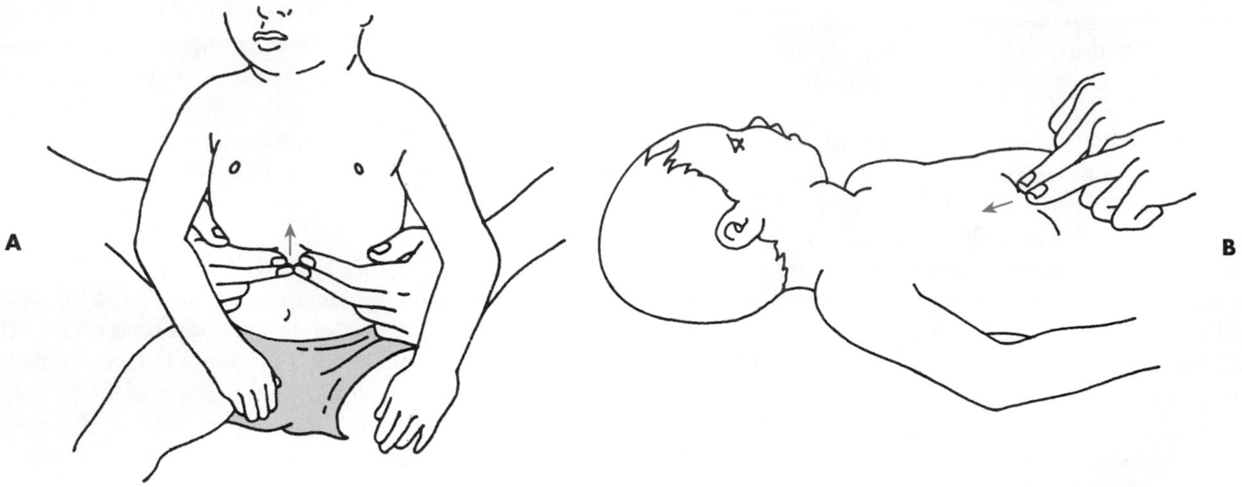

Fig. 17-10 The Heimlich maneuver for infants can be performed two ways. **A,** Place infant in lap, reach around with index and middle fingers of both hands placed against abdomen (above navel and below rib cage), and give quick, upward thrust; **B,** Position infant face upward on firm surface, face infant, and deliver upward thrust with index and middle fingers. Repeat either maneuver if necessary.

Box 17-16 Nursing Interventions to Prevent Swallowing of Foreign Objects by Infants

- Keep small objects out of an infant's reach.
- Avoid propping bottles and making large holes in nipples to prevent aspiration of formulas into the infant's lungs.
- Discourage the use of powder on infants to reduce the risk of pneumonia from inhaling zinc stearate.
- Burp the infant thoroughly before placing in the crib; place on the infant's side.
- Older children should not give food to the infant, who may choke on it. An adult should be near to supervise children around infants.
- Adults should not set a bad example by putting pins or other objects in their mouths; older infants like to mimic adults.
- Inspect toys for loose, removable parts that could potentially reach the infant's mouth.

investigators have demonstrated the utility of highly accurate blood tests in diagnosing HIV infection in infants 6 months of age and younger (Koop, 2000). Although signs and symptoms of illness can occur at any time, they usually begin in the first year of life. In infants, the symptoms of the disease include FTT, oral candidiasis, recurrent bacterial infections, persistent pulmonary infiltrates, delays in reaching important milestones in motor skills and mental development such as crawling, walking and speaking, and chronic diarrhea (Betz & Poster, 1999). Early diagnosis is essential for effective treatment.

Nursing assessment focuses on a careful and complete history of the infant and mother, signs and symptoms of the disease, growth and development history, and psychosocial concerns. Parents must be carefully assessed to determine their level of anxiety; knowledge of the disease process, including prognosis, treatment, and transmission; and awareness of resources, support systems, coping strategies, and perception of the infant's needs.

No other disease causes as much public awareness and panic as does AIDS. Part of this behavior is ignorance. Nurses play a major role in educating the public about the disease process, its mode of transmission, and most of all, preventive measures. Preventive education should begin with young children. Most school health programs include information on AIDS. School nurses can contribute to the success of these programs, as can nurses working in prenatal clinics, to spread the *prevention word.* Nurses in all settings can engage in research related to AIDS to gather further clarification of this fatal disease.

Although the infant is not an active participant in the spread of HIV, parents should understand the mean by which the virus is transmitted and not allow their infant to become a passive participant because of their own high-risk behaviors.

Immunization

The two types of immunization are active and passive. In **active immunization,** a substance is introduced into the body that stimulates the production of antibodies to a specific antigen. This substance is generally a toxin of the disease organism; depending on the virulence and certain other characteristics of the organism, it is used in the vaccine in a live, killed, or attenuated form (D'Lugoff & Schalla, 2000). The attenuated form is alive, but its virulence has been reduced significantly by treatment with laboratory procedures that use, for example, heat or chemicals. Examples of active immunizations include diphtheria, tetanus, and acellular pertussis (DTaP); inactivated polio vaccine (IPV); and measles, mumps, and rubella (MMR). Active immunization affords lifelong immunity.

Box 17-17 Home Childproofing Tips

1. Remove any heavy, sharp, or breakable objects from tables and low shelves.
2. Bolt bookcases to the wall and remove heavy books to prevent falls.
3. Test floor and table lamps to make sure they cannot be pulled over.
4. Disconnect unused appliances and wrap up cords. Secure all other cords to prevent appliances from being pulled down.
5. Close reachable outlets with safety covers.
6. Tie drapery and blind cords out of the infant's reach.
7. Choose stair gates with openings too small for an infant's head and child-resistant fasteners such as pressure bars. Avoid accordion or expandable gates with openings that can trap an infant's head.
8. Install smoke detectors and check the batteries at least once a month.
9. Use sturdy screens in front of fireplaces.
10. Place crib, play yard, and high chair well away from heaters, fans, and electrical outlets to prevent injuries.
11. Install childproof latches on drawers and cupboards. Store all cleaning compounds and detergents in a high, locked cupboard.
12. Buy all medicines in bottles with childproof lids and keep them in their original labeled containers for identification in case of accidental ingestion.
13. Install lids on garbage pails and never leave any harmful materials in them, such as sharp can lids or spoiled food.
14. Check the floor regularly for objects small enough to be swallowed.

Passive immunization consists of the injection of already-formed antibodies. After an individual has been exposed to a disease, a passive immunization is given to prevent contracting the disease. Passive immunizations provide a short immunity, usually 1 to 6 weeks, which will protect the person until the danger of contracting the disease from exposure to it is passed. Passive immunization also helps reduce the severity of the disease when it is contracted. Because of the short duration, active immunization is still needed to remain permanently immune. Passive immunity occurs naturally in newborns by maternal antibodies passed through the placenta or in breast milk.

The Committee on Infectious Diseases of the American Academy of Pediatrics (2000) recommends immunization schedules, which are revised periodically as new information arises. Table 17-9 lists the current recommendations for healthy infants.

Immunization provides one of the most cost-effective means of preventing infection in infants. The importance of immunization is accentuated by the fact that currently available antibiotics cannot destroy viruses; therefore immunization offers the only means of control. Emphasis must be placed on educating parents about the importance of immunization. To motivate them to have their children immunized, the nurse can work toward increasing health education to achieve greater health-maintenance knowledge, providing health services that make immunizations feasible and available, developing a close relationship with the family, and continuing the surveillance of the immunization status of every infant in the health care system.

Table 17-9 Recommended Immunization Schedule for Infants

Age	Immunization
Birth	HBV-1
1 month	HBV-2
2 months	DTaP-1, Hib-1, IPV-1
4 months	DTaP-2, Hib-2, IPV-2
6 months	HBV-3, DtaP-3, Hib-3, IPV-3
12 to 15 months	Hib-4, MMR
15 to 18 months	DTaP-4, Varicella

Modified from the American Academy of Pediatrics. (2000). Recommended childhood immunization schedule: United States. *Pediatrics, 105* (1), 148-151.

DTaP, diphtheria, tetanus, acellular pertussis vaccine; *HBV*, hepatitis B vaccine; *Hib*, Haemophilus influenza type b conjugate vaccine; *IPV*, inactivated polio vaccine; *MMR*, measles, mumps, rubella vaccine.

Nutrition Problems

These problems include undernutrition, in which infants do not receive an adequate supply of an essential nutrient, and overnutrition, in which they receive more of a certain nutrient than is needed for healthy growth and development (Mahan & Escott-Stump, 1999). For infants in the United States, both of these problems are present.

As an alternative to commercial baby food, a parent who wants the infant to have family foods can *blenderize* a small portion of the table food at each meal. This choice necessitates cooking without salt or sugar as is the practice of baby food manufacturers. Making baby food is easy and economical. Several written resources are available for parents who are interested in more details about home-food preparation for infants.

Parents should be encouraged to read baby food labels carefully. Nurses can obtain lists of baby foods and their ingredients from the manufacturers. The best overall recommendation that nurses make to parents is to provide their infants with a well-balanced diet and avoid excesses.

Chemical Agents

Drugs

Aspirin is the medicine most commonly ingested, with acetaminophen and vitamins close behind. Acetaminophen, the active ingredient in Tylenol and other aspirin substitutes, is becoming increasingly popular with parents as an effective antipyretic. Vitamins themselves are usually harmless; however, many vitamins contain iron, making them potentially lethal. Infants are attracted to vitamins because of their appealing colors and flavors.

Recent changes in packaging and limits on the number of tablets contained in each bottle have reduced deaths resulting from overdose. Drug manufacturers are using childproof caps increasingly as a safety measure. Despite a concerted effort by manufacturers, childproof bottle caps vary in their effectiveness (Selxas, 1999). Frequently, the safety caps are *adultproof,* whereas children can readily open them.

This points to the dangers of medications, regardless of the bottle. All medications still must be kept locked away when infants are in the home. Some additional guidelines to help prevent accidents involving drugs include the following:

1. Use a prescription drug only for the purpose for which it is intended. Do not *prescribe* the medication for a similar condition in the infant.
2. Discard unused drugs by flushing them down the toilet; many infants have been poisoned from eating tablets found in the trash.
3. Request safety caps on all prescription drugs.
4. Keep all medicines under lock and key.
5. Have the telephone number of the nearest poison control center readily available.

The major points to be emphasized in giving parents guidance in accident prevention are (1) eliminating specific environmental hazards, such as drugs, from exploring infants and (2) supervising infants while they play, gradually replacing supervision with safety training (Hanley, 1998).

Plants

Houseplants are another source of poison for infants. Most people fail to think of houseplants as potential poisons because people do not consider eating them. However, infants test almost everything by putting it in their mouths and a number of plants can be deadly when eaten. As a result, plants are one of the leading poisons of infants and amateur foragers must learn the hard way that not everything that looks good can be eaten.

Household plants are frequently placed on the floor, where the leaves or flowers are easy to pull off and taste. The best treatment for plant poisoning is prevention, which, in this case, means previous knowledge. Table 17-10 identifies several common household and garden plants that are poisonous. Knowing which plants are harmful when ingested and informing parents of the potential dangers to infants is essential for the nurse.

The National Clearinghouse for Poison Control Centers lists plants as the third most commonly ingested poison after aspirin and household cleaning agents. Safety education should be stressed at all well-baby conferences beginning in the first 6 months of life. Prevention of plant

Table 17-10 Poisonous Parts of Common House and Garden Plants

Plant	Toxic Part	Symptoms
Apple	Seeds	Releases cyanide when ingested in large quantities; can be fatal
Azalea	All parts	Nausea, vomiting, dyspnea, paralysis; can be fatal
Buttercup	All parts	Inflammation around mouth, stomach pains, vomiting, diarrhea, and convulsions
Castor bean	Seeds	Burning of mouth and throat, excessive thirst, and convulsions; one or two seeds are near the lethal dose for adults
Croton species	Plant juice	Gastroenteritis
Daffodil	Bulb	Nausea, vomiting, and diarrhea; can be fatal
Dieffenbachia	All parts	Intensive burning and irritation of the mouth and tongue; death can occur when base of tongue swells enough to occlude air passages
English holly	Berries	Nausea, vomiting, diarrhea, central nervous system depression; can be fatal
English ivy	Leaves and berries	Dyspnea, vomiting, diarrhea, coma, and death
Hyacinth	Bulb	Nausea, vomiting, and diarrhea; can be fatal
Iris	Underground stems	Digestive upset
Jasmine	All parts	Hallucinations, elevated temperature, tachycardia, and paralysis
Lily of the valley	All parts	Arrhythmia, mental confusion, weakness, shock, and death
Mistletoe	Berries	Acute stomach and intestinal irritations with diarrhea; can be fatal
Oak tree	Acorns	Kidney failure, gastritis
Oleander	All parts	Digestive upset, bloody diarrhea, respiratory depression, cardiac arrhythmia, blurred vision, coma, and death
Philodendron	All parts	Burning of lips, mouth, and tongue; swelling of tongue; dyspnea, kidney failure; death
Poinsettia	Leaves	Severe irritation to mouth, throat, and stomach; can be fatal
Potato	All green parts	Cardiac depression; can be fatal
Tomato	Green parts	Cardiac depression; can be fatal
Violet	Seeds	Taken in quantity, cathartic effects can be serious to infant
Yew	Foliage, seeds, bark	Nausea, vomiting, diarrhea, dyspnea, and dilated pupils; death is sudden

poisoning and other accidents depends on a reciprocal relationship between protection and education that must be related to age. Safe behavior is a learned behavior, gradually acquired in a progressive process with increasing age. Box 17-18 lists specific safety measures for parents to prevent plant poisoning for infants (Broome, 1998).

Food Additives

In addition to their questionable nutritional value, additives in commercial baby food can negatively influence an infant's health status. The purposes of food additives vary, including (1) addition of nutritional value, (2) preservation or extension of shelf life, (3) aid in processing preparation, (4) improvement of flavor, color, and texture, and (5) help in keeping flavors and textures consistent (Dietz & Stern, 1999).

Commercially prepared baby foods are generally safe, nutritious, and of high quality. In response to consumer demand, baby food manufacturers have removed much of the added salt and sugar that their products once contained and have eliminated most food additives.

Toxins

Infants are at particular risk from toxic factors in the environment; as dependent, developing organisms, they are inherently vulnerable. Generally, the exposure of infants to potential toxins is quite different from that of adults because of differences in physical environment, activities, and diet. Daily activities of infants such as proximity to the floor or carpet inside the home and the lawn or soil outside, hand-to-mouth behaviors, and smaller body size and composition place them at great risk for environmental toxins. Infants are exposed to a host of environmental pollutants on a regular basis. These exposures occur through all possible environmental media: air, water, soil, and food. Infants have a unique exposure pattern and unique vulnerabilities when exposed to many environmental toxins. For example, the oral habits of infants and their unique diet (ingesting more fruits, vegetables, and water than do adults) magnify their exposure to certain agents. Finally, because infants have a longer lifespan, toxins with effects have a long latency or cumulative toxicity (such as certain carcinogens), which poses a greater risk of harm to the infant (Shannon, 2000).

Certain pesticides that are used to control insects that feed on cereal grains, fruits, and vegetables are notorious for their slow accumulation in human tissue. Over sufficient time, exposure to relatively small amounts of pesticides can result in the buildup of toxic doses and lead to chronic disease in humans.

Lead is another environmental toxin that has no known physiological role in the human body. Although lead is essentially a contaminant, most people absorb a certain amount daily through air, food, and drink. Studies have revealed a high lead content in dust, dirt, and soil. Lead in the air comes primarily from automobile emissions (Huebner & Chilton, 1999). Absorption of lead is closely related to particle size. Airborne lead of small particle size is readily absorbed through the lungs, whereas larger particles fall to the ground. Lead affects practically all systems within the body. At high levels, lead can cause convulsions, coma, and even death. Lower levels of lead can adversely affect the brain, central nervous system, blood cells, and kidneys.

Infants are vulnerable to lead exposure for several reasons. In proportion to their weight, infants breathe in more air and more lead than do adults. Additionally, infants breathe closer to the ground, where a higher concentration of lead is located. Their dust-raising play and habit of putting their hands in their mouths add to an infant's consumption of lead; they also have a greater rate of gastrointestinal absorption of lead and other chemicals. Both exercise and blockage of the nasal passages increase mouth breathing and the mouth is a far less capable filter compared with the nose. Mouth breathing, coupled with their greater frequency of respiratory tract infections, expose infants to a greater amount of environmental toxins. The growing prevalence of asthma is also evidence of environmental exposure to lead and other pollutants. Approximately 5 million children have asthma. Statistics show that asthma rates have doubled in the last decade and death rates have increased in recent years. The reality is that science does not know why asthma is becoming more prevalent, but the link to air pollution is a contributing factor (Huebner & Chilton, 1999).

Human potential and development are clearly important natural resources and a growing body of evidence now links increased exposure to lead in the environment with an impaired intellectual performance and potential. Clinical lead poisoning affects many children, but it is preventable; excess lead in the infant's environment is made by, and should be eliminated by, human beings. Progress has been made in reducing blood lead levels in

Box 17-18 Nursing Interventions to Prevent Plant Poisoning in Infants

- Keep plants out of reach of infants and young children.
- Never eat any part of a plant except the parts that are grown or sold as food.
- Keep jewelry made from unknown seeds or beans away from exploring infants.
- Learn to identify poisonous plants around your house and garden.
- Do not use unknown plants as medicines or teas.
- Pay close attention to infants at play inside and outside.
- Seek help whenever anyone chews or swallows a poisonous plant.
- Be aware that infants are more susceptible than are adults to the effects of poisonous plants.

Table 17-11 Major Pollutants and Their Health Effects

Pollutants	Major Sources	Effects
Carbon monoxide	Vehicle exhaust	Replaces oxygen in red blood cells; causes dizziness, coma, or death
Lead	Antiknock agents in some gasolines, old paint chips, metal pieces, pottery, and soil	Accumulates in the bones and soft tissues; affects blood-forming organs, kidneys, and central nervous system
Nitrogen dioxide	Industrial wastes, vehicle exhaust	Causes structural and chemical changes in lungs; lowers resistance against upper respiratory infection (URI)
Radon	Earth and rock beneath homes, well water, and building materials	Lung cancer
Ozone	Formed when hydrocarbons and nitrogen dioxide react	Produces smog; irritates mucous membranes, causing coughing, choking, and impaired lung function; contributes to asthma and bronchitis
Sulfur dioxide	Burning coal and oil, industrial processes	Increases colds, coughs, and asthma; contributes to acid rain
Passive smoking	Tobacco products	Causes high incidence of URI, pneumonia, bronchitis, and asthma; linked to cancer

From the Environmental Protection Agency. (2000). *Air quality* [Online]. Available: http://www.epa.gov/iaq.

infants and young children. The following factors have contributed to these improvements (U.S. Department of Health and Human Services, 2000):

- Decline in lead used in gasoline.
- Decline in manufactured food and soft-drink cans containing lead solder.
- Ban on leaded paint for residential (indoor) use.
- Established standard for lead exposure in industry.
- Ban on lead-containing solder in household plumbing.
- Implementation of lead poisoning-prevention programs.

Parents need to be educated to take steps to reduce their infant's exposure to lead:

- Keep areas in which infant plays as dust-free and clean as possible.
- Do not remove lead paint yourself.
- Do not bring dust into the home.
- If their work or hobby involves lead, change clothes before entering the home.
- Do not burn painted wood in fireplace.
- Eat a balanced diet, rich in calcium and iron.

Infants do not necessarily escape noxious chemicals when they are indoors. The contaminants that cause air pollution are approximately the same indoors as the are outdoors, with perhaps more carbon monoxide, nitrogen dioxide, and various hydrocarbons from tobacco smoke, poorly ventilated heating and cooking equipment, and aerosol sprays. Many air pollution aftereffects may not be observed during infancy, but can surface in problems that affect both physical and mental well being over a lifetime.

Among the acute illnesses of infancy, respiratory disease is ranked number one, representing between 50% and 75% of all childhood diseases (Wootan, 2000). In addition to the inconvenience and incapacity induced by respiratory diseases, medical costs are high. Dirty air aggravates, and in some cases, causes nearly all respiratory problems. Infants with chronic respiratory disease can become adults with respiratory problems.

Water pollution causes gastrointestinal disturbances in the infant. Parents and health care providers are quick to blame food, teething, or a virus for simple diarrhea, when the underlying cause may come from the kitchen tap. Numerous strong chemicals are used today to help purify drinking water. These chemicals can irritate the delicate lining and cause disturbances in the infant's gastrointestinal tract. Nurses should encourage parents to boil all water before they give it to their infant to help eliminate any potential problem. Table 17-11 lists major pollutants and their health effects.

Motor Vehicles

This section refers to the effects of motion or action of forces on the infant; the focus here is on motor-vehicle accidents.

Automobiles present a danger to people of all ages, but especially to infants. Usually, the problem is improper restraint of the infant inside the automobile. Many parents have been misled by thinking that it is better to be thrown clear of an accident than it is to be restrained. Many also think that is safer to hold an infant on the lap in the front seat rather than to have the infant restrained in the back seat. On the contrary, these practices tempt fate and increase the probability of a fatality. A free-moving child not only distracts the driver, but is also in a more vulnerable position to be thrown.

Adult seat belts are unsuitable for infants or children

Box 17-19 Automobile Safety Precautions

1. Never leave a child unattended in a parked car.
2. Never hold a child in the lap in the front seat.
3. Always use an infant car seat that is properly installed.
4. Keep car doors locked.
5. Use safety restraints for passengers and driver.
6. Continue to use car seats until the child reaches 40 lb and then use adult seat belts.
7. Do not be distracted by an infant while driving.

Pillitteri, A. (1999). *Maternal and child health nursing: Care of the childbearing and childrearing family* (3rd ed.). Philadelphia: Lippincott-Williams & Wilkins.

under 4 years of age because their pelvic structure is small; the American Academy of Pediatrics recommends that safety seats for infants be used (U.S. Department of Health and Human Services, 2000). A variety of car seats is available: for infants up to 20 lb., the recommended type is the rear-facing, molded plastic shell seat, which includes a shoulder restraint and employs the adult seat belt (Wong, 1999). The shield-type car seat, for the child weighing 24 to 48 lb, offers maximal protection for the older infant. All children should be in the back seat because of the potential danger of air bags. Infant safety in motor vehicles depends entirely on the responsible adults.

The nurse can also suggest the automobile safety precautions listed in Box 17-19.

Much of automobile safety is common sense, but the nurse must cover all areas in anticipatory preventive teaching. The importance of automobile safety cannot be overemphasized.

Radiation

Radiation, in its broadest sense, means the transfer of electromagnetic waves through space (Bee, 2000). Radiation of all types presents a potential hazard within the infant's environment. The risk is proportional to the amount of radiation and the length of exposure and to the particular tissues involved. The infant's rapidly growing and immature cells are especially vulnerable.

The infant is exposed to two basic categories of radiation: (1) natural background radiation, which comes from cosmic rays and radioactive material existing naturally in the soil, water, and air, and (2) man-made radiation, which includes x-rays and radiation from nuclear power plants, microwave ovens, and other electronic devices found in the home (U.S. Department of Health and Human Services, 2000).

Cancer

Most people think of cancer as a disease of adults. Cancer, however, is the leading cause of death from disease in children over 1 year of age. The most common cancers found from infancy to age 5 years are Wilms' tumor, retinoblastoma, acute lymphocytic leukemia, neuroblastoma, and rhabdomyosarcoma. Because most childhood cancers' peak incidences occur during other developmental age groups (toddler, preschooler), only retinoblastoma and neuroblastoma are discussed here.

Retinoblastoma

This is a rare malignant tumor involving the retina of the eye, with both genders affected equally in terms of incidences. The majority of these tumors are diagnosed before the child is 2 years of age. The tumor can result from genetic transmission of a defective gene or from spontaneous cell mutation. Autosomal dominance is responsible for the hereditary forms of the disease. Retinoblastoma occurs most often as a spontaneous development rather than as a hereditary incidence. Infants with the inherited type tend to develop a bilateral disease; cases with the spontaneous type may not have the tumor in both eyes.

Perhaps because retinoblastoma is a rare tumor, many health professionals fail to recognize the ominous significance of early clues, usually first noticed by the parents. The result, frequently, is a delay in diagnosis and treatment.

Nursing intervention to identify risk factors includes taking a careful history, which usually reveals a slow progression of symptoms (cat's eye reflex, strabismus, painful red eye, and blindness). The nurse should ask the following questions to identify risk factors:

- Are tumors of the eyes common in your family?
- If so, can you identify which relatives had this and what was done for these tumors?
- Have you noticed your child having any eye problems, such as crossed or lazy eyes, or difficulty seeing?
- Have you noticed any changes in your child's eyes?

Nurses with physical assessment skills can perform screening and ophthalmoscopic examinations on high-risk infants and children. These eye tests include checking for the following:

1. Visual acuity, which can be determined by the fixation test, used to screen vision in infants and children 6 months to 5 years of age.
2. Red reflex, which appears whitish in the infant with retinoblastoma (the cat's eye reflex, the most common presenting sign of this cancer).
3. Lid lag, which is found in exophthalmos.
4. Strabismus, which is determined by giving the cover-uncover test (National Cancer Institute, 2000).

Neuroblastoma

Characterized as a solid cancerous tumor, neuroblastoma begins in nerve tissue in the neck, chest, abdomen, or pelvis, but usually moves into the tissues of the adrenal gland. Neuroblastoma is a disease primarily of infancy and early childhood; approximately one third of all children are under 1 year of age at the time of diagnosis; more than 80% are recognized by 5 years of age. By the time it is diagnosed,

Box 17-20 Nursing Interventions to Prevent Cancer in Infants

- Identify high-risk infants from family history, physical examination, screening programs, and so on.
- Educate parents, caregivers, and day care personnel about the warning signs that may indicate the presence of cancer.
- Refer and provide follow-up care for high-risk infants.
- Update your knowledge concerning cancer and its continuing effect on the environment.
- Be aware of the benefits and risks of x-ray examinations to reduce unnecessary exposure.
- Promote parents' personal habits that are favorable to their own and their infant's health.

the cancer usually has spread most commonly to the lymph nodes, liver, lungs, bones, and bone marrow. Frequently, the symptoms or signs arising from the secondary spread will bring the infant to the attention of health professionals (National Cancer Institute, 2000).

Neuroblastoma is an embryonal childhood cancer that appears to follow both hereditary and nonhereditary patterns. The literature has identified a number of families with more than one affected sibling. Importantly, survivors of neuroblastoma may develop subsequent tumors, necessitating continued medical surveillance. Some experts recommend monitoring the children of individuals with neuroblastoma and examining them carefully for any evidence of reoccurrence. Screening is performed through biochemical tests for metabolites of norepinephrine and dopamine (vanillymandelic acid [VMA] and homovanillic acid [HVA]). Neuroblastomas secrete excessive amounts of these substances into the urine, which can be measured in urine specimens. VMA and HVA in excessive amounts in the urine can indicate a tumor (National Cancer Institute, 2000) (Box 17-20).

SOCIAL PROCESSES

Community and Work

As infants grow and develop, their boundaries may extend beyond the home environment. Many mothers return to the work force while their infants are still young, placing them in community day care centers.

Today, few young families can escape financial burdens. The two-income family is now a way of life and the trend will continue. With more than half of all American mothers working outside the home, the need for a day care service is growing.

This situation is usually an emotional issue for families; the separation process can be traumatic for both infant and parent. The comforting realization in this dilemma is that most studies agree that the quality of time spent with an infant is important, not the quantity (Ball & Bindler, 1998).

The findings from social science research regarding the effects of day care on an infant's development and health can be summarized as follows: (1) little evidence suggests that day care permanently enhances or slows intellectual development; (2) day care can be used, even from earliest infancy, without damaging the mother-infant relationship; and (3) day care can lead to a slight increase in minor illnesses, but excluding ill infants from the center is not an effective means of reducing the spread of illness (Zimiles, 1998).

The question of how old an infant should be before being placed in day care is a frequently asked question of health professionals. Many experts believe that a mother and infant should have 4 to 6 months together before the mother goes to or returns to work. Brazelton (1994) makes a good case for the mother and infant going through four stages of attachment together before the mother goes to work. In the first stage, which takes 10 to 14 days, the infant learns to be attentive to the mother, and the mother learns cues from the infant about being both ready for and tired of attentiveness. The second stage, which lasts 8 weeks, is a stage of playful interaction, when the mother learns how to recognize the infant's nonverbal cues and helps the infant maintain the alert state. The third stage, from the tenth week to the fourth month, is when the mother and infant learn to play games together. In the fourth stage, which occurs in the fourth month, infants rapidly learn about themselves and their world. Brazelton suggests that a mother, when possible, should spend the first 4 months with her new infant; however, every mother must make her own decision.

A nationwide survey of family day care found that nearly 50% of all infants in day care centers in the United States are cared for in one of three types of family arrangements (Broude, 1996):

1. Private homes that provide informal day care to infants of relatives, friends, and neighbors
2. Regulated independent care licensed by state agencies
3. Regulated, sponsored care provided by licensed workers operating as part of home networks under umbrella agencies

The nurse has a vital role in assisting families with infants who need day care. Many factors are reviewed when a family is looking for an appropriate day care program; the nurse can counsel and guide the family in its search. The means by which the nurse counsels and guides the family in selecting a day care center are as follows:

1. Promote awareness of the three types of day care available in their local communities.
2. Counsel parents on what to ask a prospective day care facility (Box 17-21).
3. Help parents to deal with the separation behaviors that are manifested by their infant:
   - Remain calm in the situation.
   - Attempt to reduce number of *strange* adults who interact with the infant and always introduce them.
   - Encourage the parents to bring an infant's special

Box 17-21 Prospective Day Care Facility Questions

- Licensed by the state?
- Open all year?
- Number of children present?
- Age range of children?
- Teacher-to-child ratio? (For infants, 1:3 is recommended.)
- Describe day care program.
- What meals are served?
- What is the cost?
- Are there openings?
- What are the qualifications of caregivers?
- Are the caregivers happy and interacting with the infant?
- Are infants contented?
- Are parents welcome to drop in?

cuddly toy from home to the day care facility to promote security.
- Elicit the parent's understanding of the processes.
- Reassure parents that it takes time for the infant to make the transition from parent to another caregiver and vice versa.
- Emphasize that at certain developmental levels *stranger anxiety* may be heightened (8 months) and separation behaviors of crying and clinging may be repeated.
- Work toward promoting a good relationship among parents, infant, and caregiver by providing opportunities for open discussions of concerns.

Culture and Ethnicity

The developing infant is subject to the influences of culture from the moment of conception. Partly because of the long dependency period, the family environment is the setting within which the infant experiences overall cultural attitudes. The parents' perceptions of illness, wellness, roles, patterns of child-rearing practices, religious values, language, and health practices are all modeled for the infant. In short, culture helps form the infant's view of the world (Schwartz, 1999).

The family's ethnicity includes ideas about health, illness, food preferences, moral codes, and family life that persist across generations and survive even the upheaval of coming to a new country. All cultural groups confront repeated challenges as they transfer their families from familiar to unfamiliar surroundings. Infants are exposed to an appropriate mode of behavior that is in accordance with their family's cultural standards. By observing and imitating family members, infants take cues for behavior. These perceptions are then incorporated into their own self-concepts (Andrews & Boyle, 1995).

To assess and plan appropriate interventions for different ethnic groups, nurses must be aware of their own cultural

Box 17-22 Factors That Facilitate Multicultural Health Care by Nurses

- Knowledge of the historical experience, recent and long-term, of ethnic groups that live in the community.
- Demographic data that include family size, socioeconomic status, and future expectations that are characteristic of diverse ethnic groups.
- Recognition of folk beliefs and cultural attitudes toward health and illness.
- Awareness of the nature of problems encountered by ethnic group members when they enter the health care system, including fear and distrust of health care professionals, language barriers, and discrimination by caregivers.

From Andrews, M. M., & Boyle, J. S.(1995). *Transcultural concepts in nursing care* (2nd ed.). Philadelphia: J.B. Lippincott.

backgrounds. An important consideration is to examine all customs and values in relative terms, seeing none as altogether good or bad. Change is inevitable in family life, whether it is resisted or welcomed. An important function of the nurse is to help families monitor the rate of change that is acceptable to various members and reach a consensus (Box 17-22).

The nurse identifies the power structure within a given cultural group. This knowledge may help dictate which family member to approach with the health teaching. Although the nurse might assume it would be the infant's mother, this may not necessarily be the case. Among some Native-American tribes, the grandmother, not the parents, has the authority over the grandchildren. In many Latin cultural groups, the infant's father, not the mother, makes decisions about the infant's welfare. The nurse assesses the cultural groups' practices and beliefs before planning interventions. Approaches to infant care practices vary among cultural groups (see Multicultural Awareness box).

In American culture, the number of women choosing to breast feed has steadily increased in recent years. Many factors are involved in the decision-making process, such as cultural beliefs and nurses' attitudes while working with the mother and infant. Nurses who deal with mothers must be aware of the multiplicity of factors influencing feeding choice and should encourage and support parents in their decisions.

The family is the primary health care provider for the infant. The family determines when an infant is ill and decides when to seek help in managing an illness. Many cultural groups choose between components of the traditional or folk beliefs that they believe to be appropriate to them and Western medical treatment. The Vietnamese use both. For example, to decrease an infant's fever, a basil leaf is tied to the wrist with a piece of cheesecloth. For colic, a silver coin is dipped in wine and rubbed or scratched on the infant's back. Nurses must be cautious in imposing their own values, beliefs, and attitudes

MULTICULTURAL AWARENESS

Quick Guide for Cross-Cultural Nursing Care

The dominant American attitudes about infants and approaches to infant care have undergone many changes in the last several years. With the increase of women in the work force, fathers are becoming more involved in infant care and day care for infants is increasing. Although children are valued, and raising children within the nuclear family remains a priority, an increasing number of American women are focusing on careers, delaying childbirth, and limiting family size.

Members of some cultures view childbearing and child rearing differently. The birth of a child is crucial for many Hispanic, Navajo, Black, Middle Eastern, and Mormon women, whose social role and status are attained through reproduction within the marital relationship. Preference for a male child exists among families of many cultures, particularly Middle Eastern and Asian (Andrews & Boyle, 1995).

In the dominant American culture, an infant is frequently wrapped warmly in blankets, placed in an infant seat or stroller, and put to sleep in a crib in a separate room from the parents. Mothers of other cultures may choose to carry or wrap their infants differently; women from some cultures carry their infants with them at all times and sleep with them. Southeast-Asian infants may be carried in a hip sling or a blanket carrier; Native-American infants are often carried in cradleboards. A cradleboard is a traditional wooden frame into which an infant is bundled and tied. The cradleboard is properly blessed before it is used and can be carried, attached to the mother's back, hung from a tree, or propped up to keep the infant comfortable, safe, and secure (Andrews & Boyle, 1995).

Different cultural beliefs and practices are continually evolving and changing. Nurses acknowledge and explore their meanings with all the families with which they meet. Nurses work actively to reduce the experience of culture shock for ethnic-minority families, remembering that American medical beliefs and practices may appear strange to others. All behavior must be evaluated from within the context of the family and their cultural background and experience.

Nurses must facilitate health-promoting attitudes and practices and show empathic concern and respect for individuals of all cultural backgrounds. By incorporating the assessment of cultural beliefs and practices into the individual's plan of care, nurses can demonstrate respect and take a step forward in developing culturally appropriate patterns of caring.

on others. Rather than judging people by the nurse's cultural standards, the family should be viewed as a member of a different culture and the nurse should ascertain how this family's culture influences its health practices and outcomes.

Nurses actively work to reduce the experience of culture shock for families raising infants, remembering that American beliefs and behaviors may appear strange to others. The nurse should remember that all behaviors must be evaluated from within the context of the family's cultural background and experiences. Nurses who strive to foster health-promoting attitudes and behaviors must begin at the most basic level: empathic concern and respect for the individual. By incorporating the assessment of cultural beliefs and practices into the infant's plan of care, nurses demonstrate respect, reduce alienation, and take a step toward developing culturally appropriate patterns of health promotion. Respecting another's language and religion is extremely important.

Language

Language is an important medium to understanding and working together. The nurse may avoid or tend to mumble a person's name when it is foreign; people hesitate to express themselves when the material is unfamiliar. The nurse must consider how the individual who speaks a different language feels about being unable to express thoughts and feelings or to understand what is being said. Both parties may play the avoidance game.

The nurse must make provisions to remove communication barriers, including the following:

1. Using a family member as an interpreter to help in the communication process
2. Using pictorial flash cards in the individual's native language to assist in explaining instructions
3. Sending a health care worker to school to learn the basics of the language to help in the interpreting process in the health care facility

Even when a person speaks the nurse's language, understanding and comprehending instructions does not necessarily follow.

Religion

In this pluralistic and democratic society, Americans are confronting the ethical and religious values that impinge on health care services. Interestingly, some health providers believe that religion plays no role with individuals in health care practices; therefore they eschew the persons' religious or ethical concerns and deal mainly with the physical or psychological problems at hand. The individual's religious and ethical concerns are generally the major source for human values when evaluating health care services.

Religious beliefs as risk factors focus primarily on decisions concerning treatment. An example may be the parents who refuse a blood transfusion, surgery, or other medically indicated treatment required to save their infant's life. A court order is needed in many instances to treat these infants. The decision is the parents' responsibility, based on their customs and beliefs, and should be respected. Deciding not to intervene with an opinion may be extremely difficult, but usually, the opinion is unwanted. Religion is often a powerful force, and when the nurse causes conflict and interferes, a gap can be formed. This gap may force the parents to seek nonprofessional health care to help them with their health-related and religious-related ideas about birth, death, stress, birth control, and other matters. To work successfully with an individual, the person's religious background should be investigated and understood thoroughly.

Legislation

Health and well being have become generally accepted rights of everyone, without regard to color, gender, age, economic or social status, or creed. The federal government has pledged to promote the general welfare of the United States in the belief that it belongs to everyone.

To fulfill this pledge, several goals were established to address areas of health concerns. One of these concern is infant health. The goal, as described by the U.S. Department of Health and Human Services is, "To continue to improve infant health, and, by 2010, to reduce infant mortality" (U.S. Department of Health and Human Services, 2000, p. 16-8).

The infant mortality rate has been on a steady decline since the turn of the century, a result of better infant nutrition, improved housing, and improved prenatal, obstetrical, and pediatric care (U.S. Department of Health and Human Services, 2000). To meet the goal of improving infant health, major health problems in this age group must be reduced. A major hazard for infants is low birth weight. To address this problem, associated factors that increase the risk of low birth weight in infants must be identified (Box 17-23).

Many of these factors can be prevented, or risks can be identified early and treated to prevent low birth weight in infants. The major focus for prevention is prenatal care for all women.

Another major threat to infant survival is congenital disorders, such as malformations of the brain and spine (microcephaly and myelomeningocele), congenital heart defects (ventricular septal defects), and combinations of several malformations, such as Down syndrome or Tay-Sachs disease. Some congenital abnormalities cannot be prevented, but many can be through prenatal screening and research to discover the *why* in the development of these birth defects.

Other factors identified by the U.S. Department of Health and Human Services (2000) that contribute to the high infant mortality rate are (1) injuries at birth, (2) SIDS, (3) accidents, (4) respiratory distress syndrome, and (5) inadequate parenting.

Box 17-23 Low Birth Weight Risk Factors

MATERNAL FACTORS:

Low socioeconomic status
No prenatal care
Preeclampsia and eclampsia
Hypertension
Chronic renal disease
Advanced diabetes
Malnutrition
Cigarette smoking (10 per day or more)
Drug addiction
Maternal age (under 15 or over 35)
Alcohol abuse
Marital status

FETAL FACTORS:

Multiple gestation (twins)
Congenital malformation
Chromosomal abnormality
Chronic intrauterine infection
Placental insufficiency

The federal government's plans to attain the goal of healthy infants are the following:

1. Promote family planning services such that all pregnancies are planned and all infants are wanted.
2. Provide pregnancy and infant care services through Maternity and Infant Care (MIC) projects to high-risk populations. The Special Supplemental Nutrition Program for Women, Infants, and Children (WIC) increases the nutritional status of both mother and infant.
3. Encourage educational efforts by schools, health providers, and the media to promote prenatal care.
4. Promote massive immunization efforts such that each infant is protected from communicable disease.

Nursing's Role

The nurse plays a tremendous part in bringing about change in response to a continually expanding knowledge base, consumer health care needs, and governmental legislation. The nurse can play a tremendous part in bringing about change in policies related to health care by actively participating in groups involved with health planning.

The nurse's role in the development of health care policies has three stages: (1) identifying resources for the community to meet its specific need, (2) planning for resources not available to the community, and (3) coordinating the resources available to the community to promote better use of them.

The nurse can become a member of a health planning council, a concerned citizen's group, or an advisory group to

Box 17-24 Nursing Interventions to Help Economically Deprived Families and Infants

- Contact resource agencies (Aid for Families with Dependent Children [AFDC], WIC programs, MIC programs, and Medicaid) to ascertain available services for the family.
- Assume the role of advocate for the deprived family to help members interact with the array of health and social welfare agencies.
- Participate in supporting legislation to reduce the social and economic stresses that affect deprived families.
- Use the knowledge of healthy infant-parent interactions to foster this relationship within the family unit.
- Be aware of a different value system when working with low-income families and do not let this difference interfere with developing a trusting relationship.
- Offer the parents helpful hints as to how they can facilitate their infant's development by using common household items: measuring spoons, plastic cups, and so on.
- Emphasize the need for protecting the infant's health by fostering safety measures within the home environment and receiving immunizations.

a local legislator or to a state health department grant task force. In this capacity, the nurse's responsibility is to inform the other committee members. Because nurses have first-hand experience with many community needs, they are in a good position to speak out and inform others of the issue.

The nurse within the community also has several resources available to assist when a need is identified to promote the infant's health, including resources on the federal level (U.S. Department of Health and Human Services), state level (public health department), local level (MIC clinics and well-baby clinics), and community groups (Parents Anonymous, hot lines, La Leche League, March of Dimes, and SIDS groups).

Coordinating for resources, the nurse actively participates in assessing the availability of services within the community and makes recommendations to consolidate or expand existing services. To make the public aware of community resources, their services, and existing needs is the basis of the nurse's role in developing policy.

Economics

Even in a society of considerable affluence, many people live below the poverty level. These poor families tend to be characterized as having a lack of education, high unemployment rates, large size and female heads, residential crowding, and a lack of adequate bathroom facilities (U.S. Census Bureau, 2000a). Virtually every major health problem is found more frequently in segments of the population with low income compared with high-income groups. The infant mortality rates in low-income families remain significantly higher than do rates in high-income families, despite an overall decrease in infant mortality rate nationally (Gullotta, 1999).

Studies have demonstrated that parents with low incomes are often unaware of their infant's developmental needs; they are frequently faced with many environmental and social stresses that demand their time, energy, and other resources (Harrison, 1999). Many parents have so many unfulfilled needs of their own that they cannot meet their infant's needs.

Box 17-25 Infant Health Care Programs

GOVERNMENT AGENCIES

U.S. Department of Health and Human Services, Office of Child Development (responsible for nationally funded health programs)
U.S. Food and Drug Administration (regulates any ingested substances)
U.S. Public Health Service (responsible for community's health)
State health departments (establish immunization requirements)

VOLUNTARY AGENCIES (NATIONAL FOUNDATIONS)

March of Dimes (goal is to prevent birth defects)
Sudden Infant Death Syndrome Foundation (information, research, and education regarding SIDS)
Child Abuse Prevention Foundation (promote public awareness of the problem)
Childbirth education associations (provide education to expectant parents)

INTERNATIONAL AGENCIES

World Health Organizations
United Nations Children's Fund (goal is to improve children's health worldwide)

LOCAL AGENCIES

Parenting Education:

College or school courses
Hospital and clinic classes
Cooperative extension services
Social health department
Childbirth education classes

Financial Assistance (Reduced-Fee Health Care):

City or county health department
WIC program
Well-baby clinic
Immunization clinic
Prenatal clinic
Family planning clinic

Ambulatory Care:

Pediatrician
Family practice
Pediatric nurse practitioner
Public health nurse

Table 17-12 Suggested Schedule for Health-Promotion Infant Care

Age (Months)	Promotional Activity
1	Complete physical assessment PKU test Immunizations: HBV-2 Parent discussion includes: • Basic infant needs: to be touched, held, fondled, rocked, and talked to • Appropriate toy: colorful mobile • Nutrition: formula or breast milk
2	Complete physical assessment Immunizations: DtaP-1, Hib-1, and IPV-1 Parent discussion includes: • Placing infant in prone position to allow lifting of head • Need of infant to be exposed to variety of stimuli within environment • Need of infant for change of scenery • Colic and other common problems
4	Complete physical assessment Immunizations: DtaP-2, Hib-2, and IPV-2 Parent discussion includes: • Stimulation of infant • Providing a mirror in which the infant can see reflection • Being talked to and played with • Appropriate toy: rattle
6	Complete physical assessment Immunizations: DtaP-3, Hib-3, DTaP-3, HBV-3, and IPV-3 Laboratory work: hematocrit levels Parent discussion includes: • Accident prevention • Teething and use of coal rings • Allowing infant to crawl to explore environment • Stranger anxiety
9	Complete physical assessment Parent discussion includes: • Accident prevention • Dental caries prevention: cleaning teeth with gauze daily • Infant's need for space to crawl about • Use of cup if weaning • Use of finger foods • Paying games with infant: pat-a-cake, peek-a-boo, waving bye-bye, and shaking hands • Appropriate toys: blocks, stack toys, and jack-in-the-box • Fear of strangers
12	Complete physical assessment Immunizations: TB test Laboratory work: CBC Parent discussion includes: • Accident prevention • *Getting into things* • Infant's need to touch and investigate environment, with supervision • Parent's need to read, show pictures, and repeat body parts to infant • Infant's need for limited independence • Sleeping patterns • Appropriate toy: sets of measuring cups, nesting toys, pots and pans, and wooden spoons
15	Complete physical assessment Immunizations: MMR and Hib-4 Parent discussion includes: • Negativism as normal aspect of development • Age of curiosity in infant • Toys appropriate for age: push-pull toys and ball • Accident prevention • Elimination patterns • Discipline: stress positive aspects of behavior, when possible
18	Complete physical assessment Immunizations: DTaP-4 and Varicella Parent discussion includes: • Accident prevention • Begin toilet training, if child is ready • Encourage vocalization • Socialization with other small children • Importance of reading to child • Setting limits on behavior • Coping mechanisms of parents

CBC, complete blood count; *DTaP*, diphtheria, tetanus, acellular pertussis vaccine; *HBV*, hepatitis B vaccine; *Hib*, Haemophilus influenza type b conjugate vaccine; *IPV*, inactivated polio vaccine; *MMR*, measles, mumps, rubella vaccine; *PKU*, phenylketonuria; *TB*, tuberculin.

In many cases, infants from families in poverty have delayed language development. Their parents, with limited educational and life experiences, limit the amount of vocalization that the infant will hear. Infants learn early language sounds from their parents, but their attempts at language must be reinforced.

Armed with the knowledge of how economics can affect the infant's growth, development, and health status, the nurse, before deciding interventions (Box 17-24), must assess the family situation by performing the following tasks:

1. Establish a relationship with the family to obtain pertinent information.
2. Evaluate the home environment in which the infant interacts.
3. Elicit the parents' health perceptions about their own health and that of the infant.

innovative practice

The Touchpoints Model

The birth of a baby is a life-changing event for a couple and family. Although most infants develop through predictable yet individual patterns of development, parents, especially first-time parents, are usually unaware of these patterns and or have difficulty assessing their individual infant's progress and problems. All of these processes can be stressful for the parents, the entire family, and the infant.

The Touchpoints Model Program at Children's Hospital in Boston, Massachusetts delivers a training model for practitioners, emphasizing the building of supportive alliances between parents and professionals around key points in the development of young children. The model is an outgrowth of Dr. T. Berry Brazelton's book, *Touchpoints* (1992), and research at Children's Hospital in Boston. The Touchpoints model provides a form of outreach through which multidisciplinary practitioners can engage parents around important, predictable phases of their baby's development. The Touchpoints model stresses preventive health through development of relationships between parents and providers; acknowledges that developing and maintaining relationships is critical to appreciating cultural, religious, and societal family dynamics; and encourages the practitioner to focus on strengths in individuals and families. Touchpoints is not a stand-alone model; it is intended to be integrated into ongoing pediatric, early childhood, and family intervention programs.

Contact: The Touchpoints Project, Child Development Unit, Children's Hospital, 1295 Boylston Street, Boston, MA 02215. Touchpoints has gone online. Parents and professionals can get advice and information from Dr. Brazelton at: www.Touchpoints.org.

Courtesy Carol Lynn Mandle.

research highlights

Infants at High Risk

The purpose of this study was to evaluate the implementation of a statewide program to meet the needs of infants at risk for developmental delay. Data on infants enrolled in North Carolina's High-Priority Infant Program (HPIP) between July 1983 and June 1988 were examined. Information on the characteristics of the program, types and volume of its services, and follow-up findings at 1 year of age for infants at greatest risk were assessed to indicate whether the program was meeting its objectives. The total number of infants enrolled in the program climbed steadily from 1013 to 4868. Information about the infant's developmental status was collected according to a tracking protocol. The most common health indicators for tracking visits were very low birth weight, gestational age at 34 weeks and below, and respiratory distress syndrome. Evaluation of the program emphasizes health-promotion efforts early in life to maximize the child's emotional and physical growth and functional abilities.

Data from Cilenti, D., & Farel, A. M. (1991). Identifying infants at risk: North Carolina's high-priority infant program. *Public Health Nursing, 8*, 219-222.

4. Complete a thorough physical examination of the infant to identify any problem areas.
5. Identify community resources that are available to the low-income family.

Health Care Delivery System

The U.S. health care delivery system is diverse and large; many different sectors merge to provide infant care. The nurse within this enormous, multidisciplined system is a family advocate to facilitate its passage through the many facets of care. Box 17-25 lists health care programs that have been established for the infant and the family for the purpose of disease prevention and health promotion and maintenance.

The value of preventive health care has been validated; it is cost-effective and is here to stay. As nurses' roles continue to expand within the various parts of the health care system, their duty is to keep pace with the needs, concerns, and available strategies (Hull, 1999). Because many conditions that cause morbidity or mortality in infants are preventable when health-promotion practices are employed, nurses have the mission of working within the health care system to promote healthy infants.

NURSING INTERVENTIONS

Health maintenance, promotion of wellness, and prevention of illness and injury are the goals that have been emphasized throughout this chapter. The federal government has identified areas of concern and made recommendations to promote a healthy infant population. Table 17-12 lists a suggested schedule for health-promotion infant care.

Nurses are the *agents of prevention* within the health care system (McKinney et al., 2000). The increased opportunities for nurses to share in this major health care responsibility are exciting and challenging. If health promotion and disease prevention are to become national realities in the future, then nurses must take the initiative now to preserve the United States' most precious natural resource: its future generations (see Research Highlights box).

SUMMARY

Society is changing, as are people's needs and ideas. Families today want more information and knowledge and they demand that health care professionals be more responsive to their needs. Their demand has been a catalyst for the nurse's expanded health care role and responsibility for health maintenance.

Health-promotion and disease-prevention practices that are applicable during infancy can be used in the nurse's expanded role. A three-pronged approach is stressed:

1. Giving anticipatory guidance to the family unit as the infant grows and develops.
2. Teaching and counseling to ensure the infant's optimal development.
3. Being a family advocate to ensure the safety and future development of the family unit.

Anticipating potential health problems during infancy and effectively intervening to avert these problems are nursing processes that are used to promote health. Early detection and reduction of risk factors avoid many health problems, such as abuse. By anticipating problems and helping families to avoid them, the nurse promotes health maintenance.

Using the infant's normal growth and development, psychosocial tasks, identified common health problems, and health-maintenance strategies, the nurse can make an assessment of the infant, the family, and the infant's developmental status to provide anticipatory guidance.

In teaching, an essential component of the nursing process, the nurse transmits knowledge to families to ensure continuity of care and long-term health maintenance. In counseling, the nurse listens to the identified problem, helps the family to recognize the real issues, and allows the family to make its own decisions regarding health care.

Because the infant is in no position to advocate effectively, the nurse assumes this role to help ensure health maintenance. The ultimate goal of nursing intervention in maintaining the infant's health is future self-care. As the infant grows and matures, well-established family health-maintenance habits can only enhance healthy future generations. The nurse is challenged to join this effort of investment in the future.

REFERENCES

Allahyari, R. A. (2000). *Visions of charity: Morality and the politics of homelessness*. Berkeley: University of California Press.

Andrews, M. M., & Boyle, J. S. (1995). *Transcultural concepts in nursing care* (2nd ed.). Philadelphia: J.B. Lippincott.

Baker, D. L. (1998). *A guide to genetic counseling*. New York: John Wiley & Sons.

Ball, J., & Bindler, R. (1998). *Pediatric nursing: Caring for children*. Norwalk, CT: Appleton & Lange.

Bee, H. (2000). *The developing child* (9th ed.). New York: Allyn & Bacon.

Bengson, D. (1999). *How weaning happens*. Schaumburg, IL: LaLeche League, International.

Betz, C. L., & Poster, E. C. (1999). *Pediatric nursing reference* (3rd ed.). St. Louis: Mosby.

Brazelton, T. B., & Sparrow, J. A. (1994). *Touchpoints: Your child's emotional and behavioral development*. Cambridge, MA: Perseus Publishing.

Broome, M. E., & Rollins, L. A. (1998). *Core curriculum for the nursing care of children and their families*. Pitman, NJ: Jannetti Publications, Inc.

Broude, G. J. (1996). The realities of day care. *Public Interest, 125* (96), 95-105.

Bush, D. (1999). *Growing healthy babies: The growing family's guide to nutrition and wellness*. Humble, TX: Baby Cottage, LLC.

Calamaro, C. J. (2000). Infant nutrition in the first year of life: Tradition or science? *Pediatric Nursing, 26*, 211-215.

Cataldo, C. B., & Debruyne, L. K. (1998). *Nutrition and diet therapy* (5th ed.). Bellmont, CA: Wadsworth Publishing Company.

Chitty, K. K. (2001). *Professional nursing: Concept and challenges* (3rd ed.). Philadelphia: W. B. Saunders.

Cilenti, D., & Farel, A. M. (1991). Identifying infants at risk: North Carolina's high-priority infant program. *Public Health Nursing, 8*, 219-225.

Committee on Infectious Diseases, American Academy of Pediatrics. (2000). Recommended childhood immunization schedule-United States. *Pediatrics, 105* (1), 148-151.

Daly, S. (2000). *Nursing procedures* (3rd ed.). Philadelphia: Springhouse.

Dietz, W. H., & Stern, L. (1999). *American Academy of Pediatrics' guide to your child's nutrition*. New York: Villard Books.

D'Lugoff, M. I., & Schalla, K. M. (2000). Vaccine guide: Demystifying childhood immunizations for nurses. *Pediatric Nursing, 26* (1), 69-75.

Duvall, E., & Miller, B. (1984). *Marriage and family development* (6th ed.). New York: Harper & Row.

Environmental Protection Agency. (2000). *Air quality* [Online]. Available: http://www.epa.gov/iaq.

Erickson, M. F. (1999). *Infants, toddlers and families: A framework for support and intervention*. New York: Guilford Publications.

Fabes, A. (1999). *Exploring child development: Transactions and transformations*. New York: Allyn & Bacon Publishers.

Fogel, A. (2000). *Infancy: Infant, family and society* (4th ed.). Pacific Grove, CA: Brooks/Cole Publishing Company.

Frankenburg, W. K., & Dodds, J. (1994). The Denver II: A major revision and restandardization of the Denver developmental screening test. *Pediatrics*, (1), 89-91.

Giddens, J. (1998). *Health assessment for nursing practice*. St. Louis: Mosby.

Gorrie, T. M. (1998). *Foundations of maternal-newborn nursing* (2nd ed.). Philadelphia: W.B. Saunders.

Grodner, M., Anderson, S. L., & DeYoung, S. (2000). *Foundations and clinical applications of nutrition* (2nd ed.). St. Louis: Mosby.

Gullotta, T., Hampton, R., Adams, G. R., & Ryan, B. A. (1999). *Children's health care: Issues for the year 2000 and beyond*. Thousand Oaks, CA: Sage Publications, Inc.

Hanley, K. (1998). *A-to-Z guide to your new baby*. Chicago: Contemporary Books.

Harrison, V. C. (1999). *Handbook of pediatrics* (5th ed.). New York: Oxford University Press.

Hoekelman, R. A. (1996). *Primary pediatric care* (3rd ed.). St. Louis: Mosby.

Howard, C. R. (1999). Pacifiers and breastfeeding. *Contemporary Pediatrics, 16* (6), 150.

Huebner, S., & Chilton, K. (1999). Environmental alarmism: The children's crusade. *Issues in Science and Technology, 15* (2), 35-38.

Hull, D., & Johnson, D. I. (1999). *Essentials, pediatrics* (4th ed.). London, UK: Churchill Livingstone.

Jarvis, C. (1999). *Physical exam and health assessment* (3rd ed.). St. Louis: W.B. Saunders.

Karmiloff, K., & Smith, A. (2001). *Pathways to language from fetus to adolescent*. Cambridge, MA: Harvard University Press.

Kennedy, M. S. (2000). Changing concepts of sudden infant death syndrome: Implications for infant sleeping environment and sleep position. *Pediatrics, 105* (3) 650-656.

Kessler, D. B., & Dawson, P. (1999). Failure to thrive and pediatric undernutrition: A transdisciplinary approach. *Archives of Pediatrics and Adolescent Medicine, 153* (10), 1109-1114.

Klaus, M. H., Kennell, J. H., & Klaus, P. H. (2000). *Bonding: Building the foundations of secure atttachment and independence*. New York: Perseus Book Group.

Koop, C. E. (2000). *Pediatric AIDS* [Online]. Available: http://www.drkoop.com/conditions/AIDS.

Korones, S. B. (1998). *Neonatal decision making* (2nd ed.). St. Louis: Mosby.

Mahan, L. K., & Escott-Stump, S. (1999). *Krause's food, nutrition and diet therapy* (10th ed.). Philadelphia: W.B. Saunders.

McKinney, E. S., Asheville, J. W., Murray, S. S., James, S. R., Gorrie, T. M., & Droske, S. C. (2000). *Maternal-child nursing*. Philadelphia: W.B. Saunders.

Moore, K. L. (1999). *The developing human* (6th ed.). Philadelphia: W.B. Saunders.

Murry, S. K., Baker, A. W., & Levin, L. (2000). Screening families with young children for child maltreatment potential. *Pediatric Nursing, 26* (1), 47-54.

National Cancer Institute. (2000). *Cancer network* [Online]. Available: http://www.cancernet.nci.nih.gov/cancerlinks.

National Center for Health Statistics, Health Resources Administration, U.S. Department of Health, Education, and Welfare. (1982). *Height and weight measurement for girls*. Hyattsville, MD: National Center for Health Statistics.

Olson, D. H., & DeFrain J. D. (1999). *Marriage and family: Diversity and strength* (3rd ed.). Mountain View, CA: Mayfield Publishing Co.

Paulk, D. (1999). Recognizing child abuse, child abusers, and individuals who are likely to abuse. *Physician's Assistant, 23* (15), 38-42.

Pillitteri, A. (1999). *Maternal and child health nursing: Care of the childbearing and childrearing family* (3rd ed.). Philadelphia: Lippincott-Williams & Wilkins.

Schlef, C. (2000). *Mosby's maternal-newborn patient teaching guide*. St. Louis: Mosby.

Schwartz, M. A. (1999). *Marriage and the family: Diversity and change* (3rd ed.). Paramus, NJ: Prentice Hall.

Sears, W. A. (1996). *SIDS: A parent's guide to understanding and preventing sudden infant death syndrome*. Philadelphia: Lippincott-Williams & Wilkins.

Seixas, J. S., & Youcha, G. (1999). *Drugs, alcohol, and your children: What every parent needs to know*. New York: Viking Penguin.

Shannon, M. W. (2000). Risk assessment of children exposed to environmental pollutants. *Journal of Toxicology: Clinical Toxicology, 38* (12), 201.

Shelov, S. P. (1998). *American academy of pediatrics: Caring for your baby and young child: Birth to age 5* (5th ed.). New York: Bantom Books.

Silberg, J. (1999). *Brain games for babies*. Beltsville, MD: Gryphon House, Inc.

Stanhope, M. (2000). *Community and public health nursing* (5th ed.). St. Louis: Mosby.

Staso, W. H., & Banter, T. (1999). *Neural foundations: What stimulation your baby needs to become smart*. Santa Maria, CA: Great Beginnings Press.

U.S. Census Bureau (2000a). *Characteristics of the population below the poverty level* (pp. 755-757). Washington, DC: U.S. Government Printing Office.

U.S. Census Bureau (2000b). *Statistical abstract of the United States: 2000. Child Abuse*. (120th ed., pp. 365-366). Washington, DC: U.S. Government Printing Office.

U.S. Department of Health and Human Services. (2000). *Healthy People 2010: Vol. 1 and 2*. (Conference edition). Washington, DC: U.S. Government Printing Office.

Vostanis, P. (1999). *Homeless children: Problems and needs*. Philadelphia: Taylor & Francis, Inc.

Wong, D. L. (1999). *Whaley & Wong's nursing care of infants and children* (6th ed.). St. Louis: Mosby.

Wootan, G. (2000). *Take charge of your child's health: A parent's guide to recognizing symptoms and treating minor illnesses at home* (2nd ed.). New York: Marlowe & Company.

Zimiles, H. (1998). Untangling the web of infant care advocacy. *Phi Delta Kappa, 79* (8), 590-591.

Chapter 18

MARINDA ALLENDER

Toddler

objectives

After completing this chapter, the nurse will be able to:

- Discuss the physical changes that occur during the toddler period and relate these changes to health hazards for this age.
- Discuss with a parent the common behavioral problems related to eating during the toddler period.
- Discuss an appropriate plan with a parent for toilet training a 30-month-old toddler.
- Develop a teaching plan for discussion of sleep disturbances during toddlerhood.
- Explain to a parent why temper tantrums are age-appropriate behavior for toddlers.
- Prepare for parents of toddlers a handout on injury prevention in the home.
- Outline the recommended schedule of preventive health visits for the toddler and appropriate subjects for the nurse to discuss with parents during each visit.

key terms

Amblyopia
Child Abuse
Denver Developmental Screening Test II
Egocentric
Night Terrors
Object Permanence
Otitis Media
Preconceptual Phase
Regression
Ritual
Sensorimotor Period
Separation Anxiety
Strabismus
Toddler
Toilet Training

THINK About It

Where Does Limit Setting Begin and End?

Hannah has always been a happy baby. Now that she is entering the toddler stage, she is asserting herself and her will more frequently. Occasionally, she throws temper tantrums in an effort to make her will known and to test the limits that her parents have set. Her parents do not know how to react to these tantrums. They do not want to discourage Hannah from asserting herself, but they want to teach her that tantrums are inappropriate.

1. Why do toddlers throw temper tantrums?
2. What suggestions would you give Hannah's parents as they face this confusing time?

Box 18-1 Selected National Health-Promotion and Disease-Prevention Objectives for Toddlers

- Reduce iron deficiency to less than 5% among children between ages 1 and 2 (baseline is 9% among children between ages 1 and 2 in 1994).
- Reduce drowning deaths among children ages 4 and younger to no more than 0.9 per 100,000 (adjusted baseline is 1.5 per 100,000 in 1997).
- Increase use of child restraints to 100% of children ages 4 and younger (baseline is 92% in 1998).
- Reduce number of courses of antibiotics for ear infections for young children to 88 antibiotic courses per 100 children under age 5 years (baseline is 108 courses of antibiotics per 100 children in 1996 and 1997).
- Reduce nonfatal poisoning among children ages 4 and younger to no more than 292 per 100,000 (baseline is 348.4 per 100,000 in 1997).
- Total elimination of blood lead levels exceeding 10 mg/dl among children ages 1 to 5 years (baseline is 4.4% of children ages 1 to 5 years had blood level exceeding 10 mg/dl in 1994).

From U.S. Department of Health and Human Services. (2000). *Healthy people 2010*. Washington, DC: U.S. Government Printing Office.

The beginning of the **toddler** period is described as the time during which the child is becoming secure in the ability to walk and run and achieving language ability sufficient to express most needs and desires. During this time, the body structure continues to resemble that of an infant more than that of an adult and the child is primarily involved in developing a separate sense of self.

The toddler can be quite isolated from traditional health care supervision because the toddler is past the age of frequent immunizations, but not yet in school, a setting in which periodic screening may be required. Parents may fall into a pattern of illness care rather than periodic preventive visits and health promotion for their toddler. A child from 18 to 36 months of age is not of an age to be an active participant in personal health practices (Box 18-1).

AGE AND PHYSICAL CHANGES

The 24-month-old toddler appears chubby, with relatively short legs and a large head. Over the next 18 months, the growth of subcutaneous adipose tissue decreases and the extremities grow more rapidly compared with the trunk (Seidel, Ball, Dains, & Benedict, 1999).

The toddler has a marked lumbar lordosis and a protuberant abdomen. The 24 month old still has a wide stance and a slight outward rotation of the legs at the hip. By 36 months, the toddler may be *knock kneed* and the fat pad in the instep gives a flat-footed appearance. These conditions are not pathological, but normal characteristics at this age. Intervention is needed only when the child does not progress to a more straight-legged, toes-forward position by school age (Hoekelman, 1997).

The growth rate, which has slowed during late infancy, continues to decelerate until approximately 24 months of age and then remains relatively steady throughout the third year and until school age. Average gains during the second year of life are approximately 2.5 kg (5 lb) in weight, 12 cm (4 inches) in length (height), and less than 2.5 cm (1 inch) in head circumference. The anterior fontanel usually closes by 18 months and the skull becomes thicker. By 24 months, the head is 80% of adult size and height is approximately 50% of final adult height for the individual (Wong, 1999).

The toddler's stature may be measured as length, as is the infant, or as height, as is the older child and adult. The nurse must note which measurement was used in standardizing the growth grid and measure the child in a recumbent position for length or a standing position for height. The difference in measurements is small, but can cause confusion in interpreting the child's pattern of growth.

The kidneys become well differentiated by the toddler years and specific gravity and other urine findings are similar to those of adults (Grodner, Anderson, & DeYoung, 1996). The daily excretion of urine for the 2-year-old child is 500 to 600 ml (15 to 18 oz); for 3-year-old toddlers, the amount is 600 to 750 ml (18 to 22 oz) in 24 hours. The toddler empties the bladder less frequently than does the infant and has more voluntary control of urination because of maturation of the neurological pathways to the bladder and sphincter.

The toddler's gastrointestinal tract reaches functional maturity and can handle most adult foods. The organs of the gastrointestinal tract continue growing to adulthood. The toddler tends to need meals and snacks more frequently than does the older child or adult. Many older toddlers have sufficient voluntary control of rectal sphincters to accomplish successful bowel training.

Basically, no difference exists in lung topography or function after infancy. Lung capacity, however, continues to increase as the toddler grows and the respiratory rate decreases from a mean of 30 breaths per minute at 1 year to 25 breaths per minute at 3 years. The diameter of the toddler's upper respiratory tract is small when compared with an older child or adult. This small diameter, coupled with the toddler's lack of judgment in deciding what to place in the mouth, can result in airway obstruction, which demands emergency action.

The anatomy of the ear and the throat continues to resemble that of the infant more closely than that of the adult, but gradual increases in the size of the structures lessen the probability of spreading infection from one area to another. The tonsils and adenoids remain large during the toddler years (Seidel, Ball, Dains, & Benedict, 1999).

With the exception of reproductive endocrine functions, most endocrine organs become functionally mature during the toddler and preschool years, although function continues at a minimum. The production of glucagon and insulin can be limited or labile, producing variations in blood glucose levels that can be demonstrated throughout early childhood. The production of cortisol, aldosterone, and deoxycorticosterone by the adrenal cortex likely remains somewhat limited, but appears to function more effectively in protecting the young child from the hazards of fluid and electrolyte imbalance than it did during infancy. Secretions of epinephrine and norepinephrine from the adrenal medulla increase sufficiently to perform homeostatic functions of the autonomic nervous system and to mediate certain aspects of increased emotional components of behavior. Regulation of growth during early childhood remains one of the most important functions of the endocrine system. Growth hormone, thyroid hormone, insulin, and corticoids are probably the most vital hormones for normal growth and development during this period (Falkner & Tanner, 1986; Guyton, 1996).

Permanent circulatory pathways are fully established when the child reaches later infancy or toddlerhood. Changes in the system's function, including decreases in heart rate, increases in blood pressure and changes in vascular resistance of various body areas in response to growth in the size of the vessel lumen continue gradually. Heart rate is variable throughout life and the normal range is wide at all ages. The range for toddlers is 110/40 mm Hg (two standard deviations); the mean blood pressure is 99 to 100/60 to 65 (Wong, 1999). Getting the toddler to sit still for a blood pressure reading can be difficult, but worth the effort to obtain several baseline readings for future reference.

The capillary beds gradually increase their capacity to respond to heat and cold in the environment, participating more effectively in thermoregulation. Autonomic control of this function becomes integrated more fully into the total functioning of the central nervous system; the child can now begin to take voluntary measures to relieve the discomfort of heat or cold. For example, the older toddler can put on clothing or move to warmer or cooler areas, assisting physiological efforts in maintaining a constant internal thermal environment.

The immune system of specific antibodies continues to become established. Some common organisms of the environment have been encountered and immune responses have begun to function adequately. When toddlers enter the world of nurseries and day care, exposure to new and different organisms is greatly increased, and they may experience a period during which they appear to succumb to many minor respiratory and gastrointestinal infections. As immunity begins to develop against the organisms of the new environment, their resistance similarly increases. Despite environmental exposure, however, increases in immunoglobulin levels have been demonstrated to follow a well-defined pattern during early childhood. Immunoglobulin G (IgG) continues to rise sharply, immunoglobulin M (IgM) reaches an adult level during later infancy or early childhood, and immunoglobulin A (IgA) demonstrates a gradual increase during these toddler years (Falkner & Tanner, 1986).

Passive immunity to communicable disease acquired through transfer of maternal antibodies during fetal life has disappeared by this time and active immunity to certain communicable diseases through the initial immunization series is usually completed by the age of 18 months. The next scheduled immunizations (booster diphtheria tetanus pertussis [DTP] and oral poliovirus vaccine [OPV]) are during the preschool period (Committee on Infectious Diseases, American Academy of Pediatrics, 1997).

During the second year of life, the last of the 20 primary or deciduous teeth erupt. The sequence is generally as follows: the mandibular cuspids at 16 months, maxillary cuspids at 18 months, mandibular second molars at 20 months, and the maxillary second molars at 24 months. Timing of these eruptions for an individual child can vary widely, but a difference in sequence should alert the nurse to inquire about early trauma to the mouth or familial traits for out-of-sequence tooth eruption.

A mature swallowing pattern (without a forward tongue thrust) and permanent lip and tongue habits, which influence the occlusion and development of arch and jaw relationships, are formed during the second and third year.

Fluoride is an important aspect of preventive dental care and its use should be continued throughout toddlerhood. Families who move to a new community as their child gets older may not know whether the water in that new community is fluoridated, so the nurse makes this information available. Other important aspects of dental care at this age that are included in health teaching are listed in Box 18-2 (Schor, 1995).

Ossification of the skeletal system gradually declines during the toddler years as the process becomes more advanced in many areas of the body, but it continues until full stature is reached.

Increases in the size and strength of muscle fibers also continue. During this period, as during infancy, the use of muscle tissues is the primary stimulus for increased size and strength. Children who tend to develop a significant amount of muscle mass during toddlerhood are responding to a combination of genetic inheritance and stimulation through use. Boys demonstrate this pattern more often than do girls, but this characteristic is not a true gender difference; differential hormonal control of body growth and development is not operative during early childhood (Falkner & Tanner, 1986).

Full development of voluntary motor movement during early childhood is not presently understood. Myelination of the corticospinal tract is functionally advanced sufficient to support most movement, but achievement of full control does not occur until much later in life.

Throughout early childhood, voluntary motor movement is often accompanied by involuntary movements on the other side of the body. This mirroring of action is more pronounced in children who suffer some damage of the central nervous system, but the mechanisms by which this occurs are unknown. The toddler generally does not show

Box 18-2 Nursing Interventions to Promote Dental Health Care for Toddlers

BRUSHING

- Use a soft-bristled brush. The gauze method used during infancy is no longer adequate because the teeth are too close together to allow a finger wrapped in gauze to reach all surfaces.
- Introduce only a moist toothbrush at first. After the toddler has accepted the toothbrush, begin using toothpaste. A pea-size amount is adequate. If the child does not like the taste of the toothpaste, then use plain water.
- Toothpaste should contain fluoride.
- Toddlers do not have the motor coordination to brush their own teeth. They may enjoy *imitating* parents and put the toothbrush in their mouths, but an adult should be responsible for the actual brushing.
- Brush daily; for many toddlers, this practice becomes part of the bedtime routine. When the child appears too tired to cooperate in the evening, the parent should choose some other time of day when this important task will not be ignored.
- Sitting down and placing the toddler on the lap while brushing is likely easiest method for the parent.

FOODS

- Limit high-sugar foods.
- When the young toddler still drinks from a bottle, only plain water should be given; the bottle should be eliminated as soon as possible.

VISITS TO THE DENTIST

- The first visit to the dentist should occur immediately after all 20 primary teeth have erupted and never later than age 3 years.
- Many dentists suggest an inspection-consultation type of visit when the child is approximately 18 months of age. This type of visit provides an early, enjoyable introduction to the dental examination.

complete dominance of one-sided body function. The toddler may still switch hands when eating, throwing a ball, or engaging in other *handed* activities.

Gender

Throughout infancy and childhood, boys are more likely to show atypical development and to be affected by some common childhood illnesses more compared with girls. For example, during the toddler years **otitis media** is a common infection, affecting more than two thirds of children by age 3. Many studies have shown that boys are affected more often than are girls (Guyton, 1996). Boys are also physically handicapped more often than are girls, with a 5:4 ratio for hearing problems and a 3:2 ratio for speech deficits. The reason for this difference is unknown precisely, but one hypothesis suggests that having two X chromosomes protects girls not only from recessively inherited diseases, but also from commonly encountered organisms. Another possibility is that, because of cultural expectations for boys to be *strong, brave*, and so on, even at young ages, boys are exposed to more potential dangers and stresses earlier.

Race

Some differences in the rate of physical growth between races occur during the toddler years, precisely as they do during infancy. During toddlerhood, the most noticeable difference may be the earlier eruption of teeth in Black and Asian children compared with Whites. Blacks continue to be slightly taller and demonstrate some motor tasks somewhat sooner than do White toddlers.

The issue of race's effect on health is complex (see Chapter 15). Is race a major reason for which certain toddlers have more illnesses, or is it a cumulative function of nutrition, living conditions, socioeconomic status, family structure, and availability of health care resources? More study is needed in this area. The nurse should examine socioeconomic factors and race and adapt health teaching to the individual family's situation.

Genetics

Most genetic problems are noted and diagnosed during infancy. These problems can influence the health status of the toddler, but management has been instituted ideally during infancy. Some genetic problems can be detected during the toddler years. The most frequent problem is a mild developmental delay, which is partly or fully genetically determined. Frequently, these delays are not diagnosed in infancy because the subtle language, motor, or cognitive deficiencies do not interfere with expected performance and behavior. If the nurse detects subnormal performance in a standard age-appropriate developmental screening test during the toddler years, then the child should be referred for diagnostic testing.

Other genetic problems that are occasionally recognized during the toddler years include some hematological conditions, such as sickle cell disease resulting from homozygous sickle genes, or spherocytosis, an autosomal dominant trait. These conditions can be detected during routine screening or when the child becomes ill and diagnostic laboratory tests are ordered. The toddler who shows slowed growth or failure to thrive (FTT) may have a growth-hormone deficiency of genetic origin. The nurse recognizes this late onset of FTT during routine screening of growth parameters.

Another genetic problem that is sometimes unidentified until after infancy is cystic fibrosis, an autosomal recessive trait. This condition might appear as a persistent or repeated respiratory infection or gastrointestinal disturbances. The nurse then teaches about or conducts the sweat chloride test, which is diagnostic for cystic fibrosis.

All of these conditions should be referred to a pediatrician or appropriate specialist for definitive diagnosis and medical management. The nurse continues to care for these families by providing health teaching and screening for related problems and complications and the usual childhood guidance.

GORDON'S FUNCTIONAL HEALTH PATTERNS

Health Perception-Health Management Pattern

The toddler develops a sense of body image by seeing its parts, learning how to use them for locomotion, and exploring and observing others.

The toddler is exposed to concepts of health, illness, and related actions by the parents and others, but they may not develop any real understanding of these ideas. The child may come to know that being *sick* means feeling bad or not going to day care, but has little if any understanding of the meaning of health. The toddler may perform or request some health-promotion activities, such as brushing teeth, not because this will prevent caries, but because it is part of the evening **ritual.** Toddlers depend on their parents for health management.

Nutritional-Metabolic Pattern

By the beginning of toddlerhood, weaning from the breast or bottle has usually occurred. Similarly, milk intake has decreased in proportion to solid or table foods.

The primary dietary concern in American society is the prevention of iron-deficiency anemia; adequate iron intake must be ensured, especially as the toddler changes from iron-fortified milk formula to whole milk. Other food sources of iron, such as meat, may be avoided or rejected by the toddler and the family's resources may limit its provision. Eggs, specifically the yolk, offer a valuable source of iron that can be incorporated easily into the toddler's diet, particularly when the family is aware of the child's need for this important nutrient. Iron-enriched cereals are palatable, low-cost sources of iron.

The continued use of a bottle has been associated with iron-deficiency anemia. A toddler who continues to ingest whole milk from a bottle can drink up to 32 oz per day. This practice blunts the child's appetite for other foods that contain iron. Cow's milk is low in iron and may cause microscopic bleeding in the intestines.

From 18 to 24 months of age, the toddler can still be in transition from infant to adult foods. The use of prepared toddler foods during the transition from infancy to early childhood presents a special concern; these products may not provide optimal nutrition or the food range that the child requires. Helping parents understand the information labels on prepared foods is valuable in conveying both the principles of nutrition, sound marketing, and consumer protection. Additionally, parents may not realize the expense of these foods, and when convenience in preparation is not a major consideration, the child can be fed more economically and nutritionally with the regular family diet. Little extra preparation is needed by the time the child's first molar teeth appear.

Similar to other periods of life, the Food Guide Pyramid is used as a source for estimating the adequacy of the toddler's intake of all essential nutrients and the family is counseled accordingly. The decreased rate of growth during later infancy and toddlerhood results in a decrease in necessary calories and therefore a decreased appetite. Toddlers need approximately 102 cal/kg of body weight. Parents who express concern about their toddler's intake should be reminded of this requirement. Table 18-1 lists the recommended food pattern for the toddler.

Table 18-1 Food Pattern for Toddlers, Ages 2 to 4 Years*

Food Group	Examples	Number or Serving Size
Bread	Bread, cereal, rice, spaghetti, noodles, muffin, pancakes	6
Vegetable	Carrots, greens, tomatoes, broccoli	2
Fruit	Orange, strawberries, peach, watermelon	2
Milk	Milk, cheese, yogurt	2 to 3
Meat	Fish, chicken, beef	5 oz
Total fat		53 g
Total sugars		6 tsp

*One tablespoon of solid food per year of age or one fourth to one third of an adult serving of milk is considered one serving.

One difficulty in obtaining an adequate dietary assessment is the difference between what is offered and what is actually consumed. This problem is particularly true for toddlers, who may at times be more interested in playing with a particular food rather than in eating it. A prospective record, such as the one in Fig. 18-1, yields a highly accurate record. A 3-day or 4-day record presents an effective picture of a particular child's intake.

The eating behavior and habits of the young child present one of the major barriers in providing adequate nutrition. The toddler often begins to use mealtime as an occasion to assert individuality, to control the environment, and for simple exploration of food textures and qualities. Definite food preferences and food fads emerge.

The nurse uses the lifestyle of the family as a basis for offering counseling and guidance related to feeding; families vary greatly in their expectations of feeding behavior and mealtime routines. For example, when the adults in the family consistently eat a wide variety of foods and enjoy mealtime together, their expectations of the young child will differ greatly from family members who eat meals individually or have a limited variety of foods.

The parents should explore their fundamental expectations of the toddler's mealtime behavior and determine which expectations are appropriate at different developmental levels. If the parents want the child to learn to eat the foods served at mealtime, then they may need assistance in anticipating the necessary adjustments for the toddler to acquire these feeding behaviors. If the parents find that the toddler is disruptive of family interactions during mealtime, then they may prefer to

Instructions

1. Record all foods and beverages immediately after they are consumed.
2. Measure the amounts of each food carefully with standard measuring cups and spoons. Record meat portions in ounces or as fractions of pounds: 8 ounces of milk, 1 medium egg, ¼ pound of hamburger, 1 slice of white bread, ½ small banana.
3. Indicate method of preparation: medium egg, fried; ½ cup baked beans with 2-inch slice of salt pork; 4 ounces of steak, broiled.
4. Be sure to record any condiments, gravies, salad dressings, butter, margarine, whipped cream, relishes: ¾ cup of mashed potatoes with 3 tbsp of brown gravy, ¼ cup of cottage cheese salad with 2 olives, ½ cup of cornflakes with 1 tsp of sugar and ⅓ cup of 2% milk.
5. Be sure to record all between-meal foods and drinks: coffee with 1 ounce of cream 12 ounces of cola, 4 sugar cookies, 1 candy bar (indicate brand name).
6. If you eat away from home, please put an asterisk (*) in the food column beside the food listing.

Day 1

Date ________ Day of week ________ Weight ________

Time	Food	Amount	How prepared

Fig. 18-1 Food diary for children. (From Trahms, C. M., & Pipes, P. L. [1997]. *Nutrition in infancy and childhood* [6th ed.]. New York: McGraw-Hill.)

continue feeding the toddler separately except for one meal each day.

Within the limits of family resources, the parents understand the need to provide a sufficient variety of foods to ensure adequate nutrition. The family may need specific directions and assistance in selecting this variety and in preparing these foods such that the toddler will accept and be able to chew and swallow them adequately.

Nursing Interventions

1. Offer simple, single foods; toddlers often reject mixtures of foods.
2. Offer a variety of foods, but repeat the same foods to the extent that the toddler recognizes them.
3. Encourage the use of utensils, but accept that toddlers still often need to use their fingers.
4. Do not offer snacks within an hour before a meal.
5. Mealtime should be a pleasant time, free of distractions and discussion of previous *bad* behavior.
6. Do not use food as a reward or punishment for behavior.
7. Schedule meals and sleep periods such that the child is awake and alert during mealtime.
8. Serve small portions and offer seconds after the first portion is consumed.
9. Do not offer raw carrots, celery, or other foods that can easily cause choking. Cut hot dogs lengthwise.

An important point to discuss with parents is that the toddler may at times refuse a meal altogether. The reasons for this refusal range from the assertion of independence to simple fatigue. Parents should not be concerned or punish the child for this behavior. If a major family crisis follows, then the toddler may learn how easily the parents can be controlled by refusing food and may continue this behavior. The nurse helps to avert this situation by explaining that a well-nourished child who skips an occasional meal is not in danger of malnutrition.

The use of a prospective food record for several days can reveal a typical toddler pattern of a hearty breakfast, medium-sized lunch, and a small or no dinner. This routine is common in this age group and is a problem only because it is the opposite pattern for most adults. When the evening meal is considered as *the main meal*, and the toddler does not eat it, parents might think their child will be poorly nourished. The nurse demonstrates the adequacy of the nutrients that the toddler is already receiving during the first two meals of the day and helps the parent work out a plan to offer more of the essential foods during these meals.

The family who has a vegetarian diet may need some assistance in offering a diet adequate in protein for the toddler. Plant proteins must be offered in appropriate combinations and proportions for the amino acids to be complementary. The toddler may not accept sufficient plant foods or the correct proportions to meet protein needs. If the nurse is not sufficiently informed to discuss the details of a vegetarian diet with parents, then the parents should be referred to a nutritionist or written information sources. Vegetarian diets that include prudently chosen plant foods and a reasonable amount of dairy foods are adequate to support normal growth and development (Grodner, Anderson, & DeYoung, 1996).

Elimination Pattern

Toilet training is often a major family concern as the infant grows into toddlerhood. For the family who has never experienced this challenge, toilet training can be a major dilemma, and yet many families are reluctant to seek advice and assistance. The nurse anticipates this developmental task toward the end of infancy and initiates discussion with the parents to determine their understanding of the child's developmental signs of readiness for toilet training and discuss their attitudes and plans well in advance of their early trials.

The child's ability for toilet training depends on

HEALTH TEACHING Initiating a Toileting Program for Toddlers

- When the child shows an awareness of elimination, usually between 12 and 18 months of age, casually and consistently use the words chosen to describe the action. The child therefore begins to associate a word with the appropriate action.
- At approximately 18 to 20 months of age, check for the prerequisite skills for toileting. The toddler should be able to walk well, stay dry for at least 2 hours during the day, and communicate the need for assistance.
- When these prerequisites are present, introduce the child to the potty chair. The potty chair should provide secure seating with the child's feet touching the floor. Initially, the toddler can sit on the potty chair with clothes on.
- A week or so later, remove diapers and have the child sit on the potty chair. Encourage the toddler to stay on the chair for 3 to 5 minutes and always explain what to do ("Go potty") rather than what not to do ("Don't wet your pants").
- Because of the gastrocolic reflex, defecation is more likely after a meal; therefore this is a good time to place the toddler on the potty. When a pattern of defecation or urination is noticed, use this pattern as a guide for placing the child on the potty.
- Praise the child for desired behavior; do not withhold praise until urination or defecation occurs. Although this action is the desired end, positive steps such as sitting on the potty or grunting should also be acknowledged.
- Ignore undesired behavior and never punish the child by scolding, spanking, or other punitive measures.
- As the toddler achieves success, strive for more independence by dressing the child in easy-to-remove pants, keeping the path from usual play areas to the bathroom clear, and providing a secure step-up to hand-washing supplies.

sufficient neurological and psychological maturation, including the following:

1. Local conditioning of reflex sphincter control (approximately 9 months of age).
2. Completion of myelination of pyramidal tracts (12 to 18 months).
3. The ability to cooperate voluntarily (12 to 15 months).

Psychological readiness and desire to control urination and defecation do usually not develop until between 18 and 30 months of age and are significantly affected by parental expectations and attitudes.

Frequently, parents begin toilet training before their child is ready, resulting in months of frustration. The nurse responds to this frustration by discussing the usual periods of readiness and assisting them in planning approaches to use when they are not successful. When the child responds favorably to the toilet-training plan, the parents should be encouraged to continue with the established routine. When the child does not respond as desired, the parents should stop efforts for a few weeks and resume toilet training later.

The following points can reassure parents who are beginning the toilet-training process:

1. The average age for completion of daytime training is 28 months.
2. The majority of children achieve bowel and bladder training simultaneously.
3. The average age for completion of both bowel and bladder training is 33 months, 10 days.
4. Approximately 80% of children are completely trained after 3 years of age.
5. Girls are completely trained an average of 2 months earlier than are boys.

Nursing Interventions

By suggesting the sequence listed in the Health Teaching box, the nurse can help parents with toilet training. The parent who can approach toilet training with a relaxed attitude and accept some delays and frustrations will have a better chance of success and more positive feelings toward the toddler.

Activity-Exercise Pattern

The toddler always seems busy: emptying wastebaskets, rearranging the contents of shelves and drawers, building towers, throwing and running after a ball, or removing and putting on clothes. Many activities are repeated, time and time again, and many provide practice of newly realized motor skills.

The 18-month-old child runs, pulls a toy, climbs, stacks three blocks, walks up steps, and *helps* around the house by running simple errands, dusting, or pushing a broom. This toddler uses a spoon, with moderate to good success, and scribbles, mainly off the paper.

The 24-month-old child kicks a ball, throws a ball overhand, removes and, perhaps, puts on some clothing, and may enjoy some interactive games such as tag (Fig. 18-2, A). This child is skilled in eating with a spoon, turns pages one at a time, and is able to keep the lines on the paper when scribbling (Frankenburg, 1994).

By the end of the toddler period, at 36 months, the child can pedal a tricycle, jump, stand on one foot briefly, wash and dry hands, and put on all clothing. This child can copy a circle, use a fork for some foods, and build a tower of eight blocks (Frankenburg, 1994).

The toddler spends most waking hours playing, which encompasses a variety of activities, from exploring traditional toys and games to imitating *work* and repeating

A

B

C

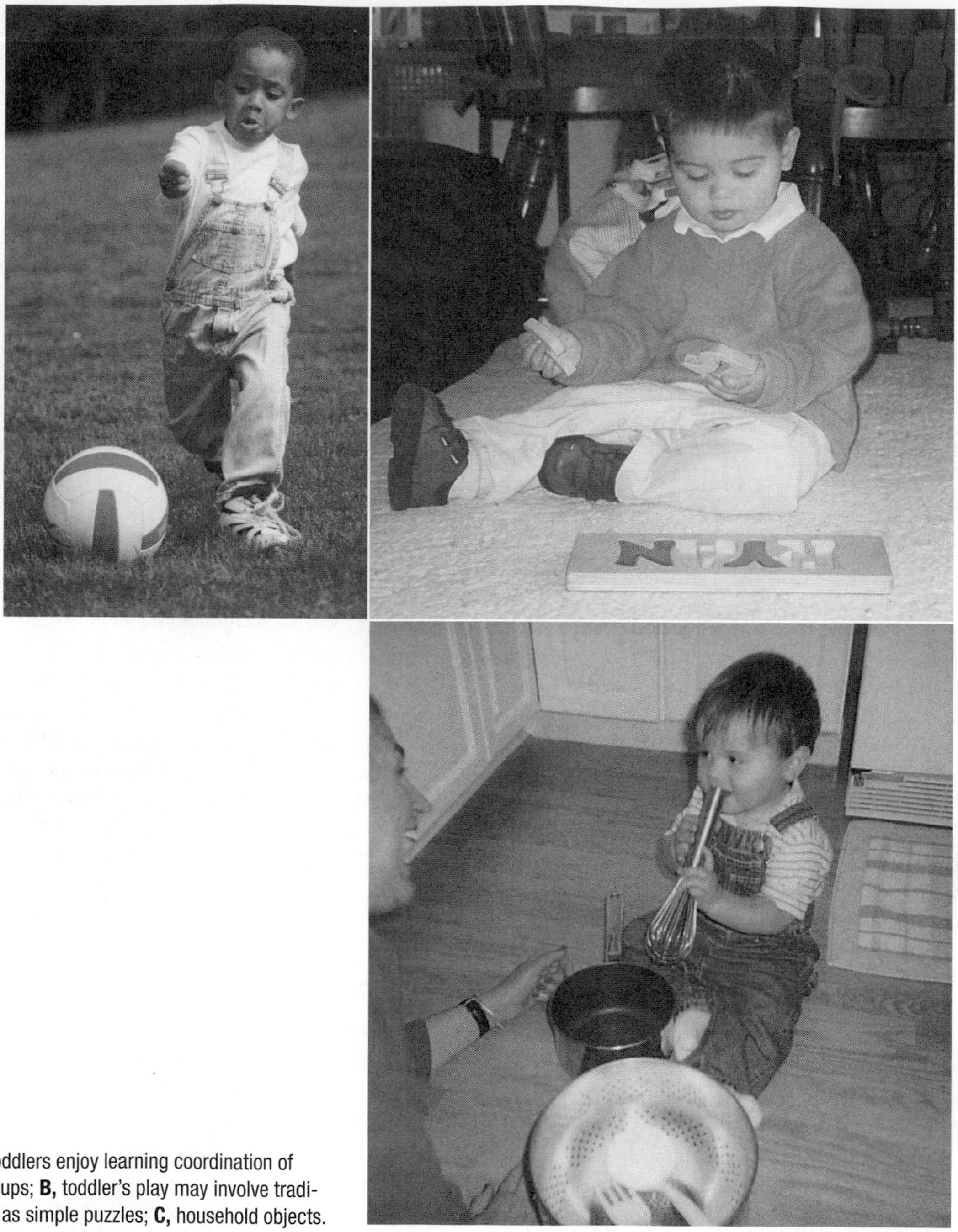

Fig. 18-2 **A,** toddlers enjoy learning coordination of large muscle groups; **B,** toddler's play may involve traditional toys, such as simple puzzles; **C,** household objects.

motor activities (Fig. 18-2, *B*, *C*). Through imitation, the older toddler can *try out* many roles and situations. This imitation, and fantasy play later, becomes prominent during the preschool years (see Chapter 19). Toddlers delight in their own skills and love repeating actions for an appreciative adult. Verbal praise, smiles, or hand clapping are effective reinforcers at this age. In their enthusiasm to try many activities, toddlers invariably take on tasks that are beyond their abilities, which can result in frustration and, occasionally, the well-known temper tantrum.

By 2 years of age, most toddlers are interested in other children, which is manifested by looking at one another, exchanging toys, and saying *hi* or the equivalent. These social overtures are more common in toddlers who spend more time with other children. Despite this interest in each other, play before age 3 is not really shared. Play is described as *parallel play;* that is, toddlers may be doing a similar thing with the same toy, but each is working independently (Berger, 1998).

Nursing Interventions

When parents inquire about what toys and activities to provide their toddler, the following is suggested:

1. Provide toys that challenge the child to develop new skills: toys that require skills slightly above the child's present level, but not advanced such that the child cannot achieve some success. For example, the toddler who has mastered pushing a hobbyhorse is ready for a tricycle.
2. Provide opportunities for new learning, which may be as basic as a book with pictures of new animals or a walk through the produce section of the grocery store to point out several fruits or vegetables.
3. Provide opportunities for social interaction, but do not force *playing together*. An hour in the park close to other toddlers provides the opportunity for looking at other children or offering a toy.
4. Follow the child's lead. Let the toddler choose and explore new toys or objects, within safe limits.

The desire of some parents is to raise the smartest, most coordinated, or most musically talented child. These *super kids* receive intense instructions and practice in a subject or area chosen by their parents. This instruction, occasionally started before age 1, is nearly always underway by the early toddler period. Some of these children have indeed shown the ability to learn at a younger age than was ever considered in the past. The main concern among child development specialists is that the time commitment and intensive drill may interfere with the child's need for self-structured play and exploration. Many unanswered questions remain about the long-term effects on these children (Fraiberg, 1959). The nurse encourages parents who are considering this approach to consult with a child psychologist.

Sleep-Rest Pattern

Sleep Patterns

The toddler requires less sleep time than does the infant. Night sleep averages between 8 and 12 hours at age 2 and naps become less frequent. Total nap time for the 2-year-old child is approximately 30 minutes less than it was for that child at 1 year. Although the need for actual sleep has decreased, the toddler may need *quiet time* (brief periods to unwind from a busy or noisy activity). Occasionally, the mother needs these rest breaks more than the toddler needs them and sitting together in a rocking chair for a soothing song or quiet music can be a calming experience.

The toddler may be highly involved in an activity and not realize that fatigue is present, especially when visitors are in the home or some interesting new toys have been discovered. All parents are familiar with the overtired child who is exhausted, but unable to relax enough to sleep. Parents can avoid this dilemma by scheduling nap and rest breaks even when there are houseguests or holidays that may preempt the toddler's routine.

Rituals are characteristics of this age. Many toddlers have a bedtime ritual. A typical pattern might be a snack, bath, brush teeth, story time, kiss parents, and lights out. Following this ritual is important because the toddler appears to get a sense of security when ending the day. Changing this ritual can be upsetting to the toddler. The nurse should encourage parents to follow the presleep ritual as closely as possible, even when visitors, family illness, or travel makes the routine more difficult.

Many toddlers will try to delay sleep by calling for water, another story, another kiss, or by making other requests. Parents should be certain that the toddler has ample opportunity for interaction with them during the day, follow the usual bedtime ritual, and be firm and consistent in resisting any requests for attention after the final *good nights* have been said.

Sleep Disturbances

Some toddlers, from age 2 on, are fearful of the dark. A night-light or a favorite toy can help to allay this fear.

Night terrors may also occur in the 2- to 4-year-old child. These events are different from nightmares, which generally start at approximately age 3 and result in the child awakening and being able to recall the frightening dream. The child who experiences night terrors does not waken completely, but cries out, looks terrified, and cannot be aroused for several minutes. The child may believe that animals or strange people are in the room or may be disoriented and not recognize the parents. After 5 to 30 minutes, the child falls back into quiet sleep (Hoekelman, 1997).

Night terrors are more rare than nightmares. The parents must be assured that these episodes will stop spontaneously if not too much attention is focused on them. The parents should go to the toddler and talk in a soothing voice, but should not waken the child. If the child does waken, then the parents should provide comfort and tuck the child back in bed.

Repeated requests for attention after bedtime, fear of the dark, and night terrors can precipitate the practice of bringing the child to the parents' bed. The toddler who is allowed to sleep with the parents after a frightening episode comes to expect to stay with them after any frightful incident. This habit can soon result in the youngster spending every night with the parents. Although parents may resent the loss of privacy and restricted sleep space, they can feel trapped in this situation by fear of doing harm resulting from having the child sleep alone.

Nursing Interventions

The nurse helps parents avoid these difficult situations through counseling in late infancy, before these toddler-age problems arise. Important points to discuss with parents are as follows (Fraiberg, 1959):

1. These sleep disturbances result from the developmental level as the child begins to deal with the ideas of separation and aggression.
2. Illness, a new sibling, moving, or a frightening television show or movie can be precipitating factors.
3. The toddler needs sufficient interaction with the parents each day to decrease the likelihood of demanding this attention after bedtime.
4. Parents should be firm, fair, and consistent at bedtime and adhere to the expected ritual.
5. Excessive stimulation in the form of boisterous physical activity, arguments, or frightening stories should be avoided before bedtime.
6. A night-light, favorite toy, or soft music can help the toddler fall asleep.
7. The toddler should not be moved from the bed after night terrors or nightmares, but should be comforted and reassured that the parents are in the house.

Bedtime or nighttime disturbances can be difficult to manage because they occur when the parents are tired and, likely, less patient. Parents may need extensive reassurance that the child will outgrow these problems if they maintain a firm, caring attitude.

Cognitive-Perceptual Pattern

The toddler is intensely active and interested in the environment (poking, prodding, and sampling everything, even other human beings). The child gathers a great deal of data, which form a basis for beginning problem solving and symbolic thinking. Although age ranges are stated, an important aspect to remember is that each toddler is an individual and may not match the description for the age precisely. Additionally, as is true for all ages, the toddler may demonstrate certain cognitive skills in some situations, but not in others. Although not totally understood, this concept may relate to certain circumstances and stresses.

Piaget's Description

The young toddler, from age 18 to 24 months, is in the last substage of the **sensorimotor period** in Jean Piaget's description of cognitive development. The 12- to 18-month-old child in stage 5 solves problems through a process of trial-and-error experimentation (see Chapter 17). The toddler in stage 6 has advanced to solving problems by mental rather than physical experimentation. Faced with a new object, this toddler does not immediately begin a series of physical manipulations to discover the way in which this new thing works. The child may pause, look intently at the object, nearly as though analyzing it, and then proceed to *solve the problem*. Although not always succeeding on the first attempt and doing some analysis by physical manipulation, this child will do more and more problem solving on a mental level, manipulating images rather than real objects.

Object permanence is developed further during early toddlerhood. The older infant who fails to find a hidden object in the original hiding place will abandon the search. The child of 18 to 24 months of age who fails to find the object in the original hiding place will search in several possible hiding places. The toddler remembers that the object exists and that it has permanence and knows that it can be made visible again.

From approximately 24 months of age until the early preschool years, the toddler enters the **preconceptual phase** of Piaget's preoperational period. This phase heralds the beginning of symbolic thinking by which a word, gesture, or image (the *signifier*) stands for an object, person, or event (the *significate*).

The development of language plays a vital role in the cognitive development of symbolic representation. For Piaget, this type of symbolic act greatly enhances the act of internalizing, or mediating, the symbolic functions of the intellect.

Language does not fully represent the thought processes of human beings; it does not fully express the richness or symbolic possibilities in cognitive capacity. The ability to consider the relationships between the signifier and the significate exists before the ability to represent each in the form of language. The signifiers become internalized as images and then a word is found that represents the meaning already acquired.

The toddler's language often reflects acquired meanings. For example, the word *mommy* may be used to represent a wide range of behaviors and actions in addition to its noun sense (the mother). The context and differential vocalization inflection give it the intended meaning; *mommy* may mean *help me* on one occasion and *pick me up* on another. The continuing adaptive functions of assimilation and accommodation provide the child with the means to gradually acquire internalized, differentiated, and precise meanings between signifiers and significates.

Between 18 and 24 months of age, the toddler experiences a major transition in imitation and play. Piaget has labeled this stage *the invention of new means through mental combinations*. The child develops the capacity to imitate models that are not immediately present without using extensive trial and error. Imitation of nonhuman and nonliving objects occurs, which serves the important function of direct experience with object events in the world that are difficult for the toddler to understand. The relative absence of trial and error in imitation is indicative of the child having developed the ability to work out the pattern of experience before engaging in the activity. Play assumes increasingly symbolic functions and meanings. The toddler engages in repeating actions for fun and pleasure as mentioned; but now, there is increasing symbolic meaning in the activity. An object such as a stone or a block of wood can now symbolize, in the child's mind, a person, animal, or any other object.

This make-believe form of play, or *ludic symbolism,* predominates throughout early childhood. Between ages 2 and 4 years, the toddler spends a significant portion of time acting out whole scenes of imagined events. Imaginary companions are frequently present who serve the important function of mirroring the child's self or being a sympathetic audience for the child as the self is allowed full, unrestrained expression and experimentation through play. During this period, the child uses play to act out what is forbidden in reality. This process provides important trial experiences with taboo behaviors and offers an essential means of expressing socially unacceptable parts of the self that require some acceptable outlet. For example, the child may pretend to eat an infant sibling for dinner, expressing a dimension of ambivalent feelings toward the infant in a manner that is not punished and that provides a discharge of hostile or angry feelings (Phillips, 1969).

Toddlers are **egocentric,** seeing everything through their own perspectives, with no realization that other ways of viewing things might exist. This trait is reflected in language and activities.

Although not purposely being selfish, toddlers have no concept that another child or adult may have thoughts or perceptions different from their own. The 2-year-old toddler may come running into a room and ask the parent, "Where is it?" The parent's response, "Where is what?" This response can be confusing to the toddler, who assumes the parent must be having the same thought.

This overview of Piaget's description demonstrates that the toddler is becoming more proficient as a problem solver and is using some symbolic thinking. These skills enable the toddler to mentally manipulate reality and begin to contemplate the future and recall the near past (Berger, 1998).

Vision

The toddler's sensory abilities develop from infantile levels to adultlike ranges. From 18 to 24 months of age, visual acuity is 20/40, and accommodation is well developed. Depth perception is still immature, although better developed when compared with the infant. From 2 to 3 years of age, visual acuity is 20/30, and convergence is smooth. This older toddler is able to recall visual images, which contributes to an increasing skill in describing past events. The child is able to fixate on small objects or pictures for up to 30 seconds.

The possibility of the development of **amblyopia** is greatest from infancy through the fourth year. Amblyopia is loss of vision or diminished vision caused by the disuse of one eye. This disuse usually results from **strabismus,** a deviation of the line of vision from the midline resulting from extraocular muscle weakness or imbalance. Marked and continuous strabismus is usually noticed early by the parents and health care provider and is therefore treated early; the more subtle deviations are often unnoticed until older toddlerhood or the preschool years. Every toddler should be screened for strabismus as part of the routine eye examination that is performed by the physician or nurse practitioner during well-child visits. Strabismus can be treated by patching the unaffected eye or by corrective surgery. Best results are obtained when the condition is diagnosed and treated during the infant or toddler years (Calhoun, 1997).

Other signs of possible visual problems that the nurse observes or parents report in their toddlers include the following *red flags:*

1. Rubs eyes excessively
2. Shuts or covers one eye, tilts head, or thrusts head forward
3. Has difficulty doing work that requires close use of the eyes
4. Blinks more than usual or is irritable when doing close work
5. Holds books close to eyes
6. Is unable to see distant things clearly
7. Squints eyelids together or frowns
8. Has red-rimmed, encrusted, or swollen eyelids
9. Has inflamed or watery eyes
10. Develops recurring styes

Hearing

The development of the hearing capacity, which is critical for the development of speech and language, reaches essential maturity by 3 to 4 years of age. However, during this period, the child begins the lifelong process of learning to listen and comprehend.

Studies estimate that all human beings listen to 50% of what they hear and comprehend only 25%. Parents will express concern that their older toddler or young preschooler must have a hearing problem because the child fails to respond to being called. This concern should be investigated, but the nurse will frequently conclude that this is *selective inattention* to parental requests, which is typical at this age.

Listening ability includes attending to what is heard, discriminating between the various qualities of sound, cognitively associating what is heard with previously learned experiences, and remembering what is heard. The quantity and quality of language that is used in the home is thought to be more important for the development of listening ability and therefore receptive language skills than it is for the development of expressive language skills. Toddlers often seek repetition of auditory input, as observed in their seemingly endless repetition of sounds, words, or combinations of words. This repetition may be their way of organizing and practicing new language.

Taste and Smell

The capacities for taste and smell, which have reached an optimal level of functioning during infancy, are influenced by voluntary control and associated with other sensory and motor areas. Toddlers begin refusing to taste something that looks displeasing to them. These toddlers are able to react accurately to the sensation that a taste or smell arouses them and they begin to learn conditioned associations between certain smells and culturally acceptable values. The foods of the culture become palatable and those that are unacceptable become displeasing. For example, children raised in a family that does not eat a certain meat will learn that this meat tastes bad; they may even be unable to develop a pleasurable association with the taste later in life. Odors of body processes, such as sweating and elimination, become extremely offensive for children in some cultures, whereas these odors are not considered unpleasant in other cultures.

Language and Memory

The toddler's cognitive abilities and increased sensory capabilities are demonstrated in language, memory, and decision-making abilities. Both receptive and expressive language skills are developing rapidly during the toddler period. From 18 to 24 months of age, the transition from single words to short phrases occurs. These 2- and three-word phrases are related most often to present events, describing an action ("daddy go"), a desire ("more cookie"), or possession ("my doggie"). Some landmarks of language for the child from 18 to 36 months of age are listed in Table 18-2. At all ages, the ability to express words and ideas is not as advanced as is the ability to understand language; the 30-month-old child can understand up to 2400 words, but only use approximately 425 in speech.

By age 3, children have mastered the basics of language function, form, and content; these fundamentals will continue to be refined throughout childhood and adolescence. Language development proceeds at an uneven rate; plateaus, spurts, and hesitations occur in the toddler's progress. Parents are generally the most significant people to the toddler and often provide much of the stimulation for language development.

Nursing Interventions

Some suggestions that the nurse can provide to parents to facilitate their toddler's use of language include the following:

1. Allow the child to make decisions about play.
2. Allow the child to initiate verbal interactions.
3. When the toddler says a sentence that is partly unintelligible, the parents can repeat the understood part as a question; this process may help the toddler respond more clearly.
4. If the toddler does not understand a question or direction, rephrase it.
5. Expand on the toddler's phrases: when the child says, "Daddy car," the parents can say, "Daddy gets into the car."
6. Do not criticize or make fun of the toddler's expressions.
7. Do not constantly correct the child's verbalizations; this action may result in decreased verbalizations.

Memory in the toddler is demonstrated by recall of recent events or the need for exact repetition of rituals. Older toddlers can sing a simple song, but, typically, they do this by rote and may be unable to say the words by themselves. Visual and auditory images can be recalled and are important for language development. The toddler is more skilled at recognition memory than recall memory; that is, the child can pick out objects that were seen earlier when they are placed with new objects.

Screening

During the toddler years, routine assessment does not necessarily include testing of intelligence or specific cognitive skills. One of the most frequently used screening tools used during these years to assess overall developmental level is the **Denver Developmental Screening Test II** (DDST II).

The DDST II provides a means of screening for physical developmental problems (Frankenburg, 1994) (see Chapter 17). This tool provides an estimate for the adequacy of motor skills that the child should be able to perform by a given age; however, its usefulness decreases during the fourth and fifth years. Because some items appear biased toward the dominant U.S. culture, difficulties may arise when the tool is used with children who are bilingual or members of a minority subculture. Insightful nursing judgment and further assessment may be needed to determine the accuracy of the test for a given child.

When using any developmental screening tool, the nurse must be fully prepared in the standardized techniques for administration, appropriate approaches to the child, and skill in scoring and interpreting results. The tool loses its effectiveness when inappropriate methods are used in administration, when the child's behavior is adversely affected by the approach of the nurse or when the test is scored incorrectly. Anyone who anticipates using this tool for clinical practice must study the standardized methods, practice with supervision, and have the initial scoring validated by an experienced user (Frankenburg, 1994).

Self-Perception–Self-Concept Pattern

Erikson's Description

According to Erikson (1986, 1997), the developmental task of toddlers is to acquire a sense of autonomy while overcoming a sense of doubt and shame. The toddler's developing cognitive, language, and motor skills provide the means for developing self-concept and self-esteem.

The toddler is discovering that one's behavior is one's

Table 18-2 Landmarks of Speech, Language, and Hearing Ability During the Toddler Period

Age (months)	Receptive Language	Expressive Language	Related Hearing Ability
18	Up to 50 words; recognizes between 6 and 12 objects by name, such as *dog, cat, bottle, ball;* identifies three body parts, such as *eyes, nose, mouth;* understands the concept *now* and simple commands unaccompanied by gesture, such as *give me the doll, open your mouth, stick out your tongue*	Up to 20 words and 21 different phonemes; jargon and echolalia are present; uses names of familiar objects and one-word sentences, such as *go* or *eat;* uses gestures; uses words such as *no, mine, eat, good, bad, hot, cold,* and expressions such as *oh-oh, what's that, all gone;* use of words can be quite inconsistent, 25% of speech intelligible	Has begun to develop gross discrimination by learning to distinguish between highly dissimilar noises, such as doorbell and train, barking dog and auto horn, or mother's and father's voices
24	Up to 1200 words; knows *in, on, under;* identifies *dog, ball, engine, bed, doll, scissors, hair, mouth, feet, nose, cup, spoon, car, key;* distinguishes between one and many and formulates a negative judgment (a knife is not a fork); understands the concept *soon;* understands simple stories; follows simple directions; is beginning to make distinctions between *you* and *me*	Up to 270 words and 25 different phonemes; jargon and echolalia almost gone; averages 75 words per hour during free play; talks in words, phrases, and two- to three-word sentences; averages two words per response; first pronouns appear, such as *I, me, mine, it, who, that;* adjectives and adverbs are only beginning to appear; names objects and common pictures; enjoys Mother Goose; refers to self by name, such as *Bobby go bye-bye;* uses phrases such as *I want, go bye-bye, want cookie, ball all gone;* 60% of speech intelligible	Refinement of gross discriminative skills
30	Up to 2400 words; identifies action in pictures and objects by use; carries out one- and two-part commands, such as *pick up your shoe and give it to mommy;* knows what is used to drink liquids, what goes on the feet, what is used to buy candy; understands plurals, questions, difference between boy and girl, the concepts *one, up, down, run, walk, throw, fast, more, my*	Up to 425 words and 27 phonemes; jargon and echolalia no longer exist; averages 140 words per hour; names words such as *chair, can, box, key, door;* repeats two digits from memory; average sentence length is approximately two and one-half words; uses more adjectives and adverbs; demands repetition from others, such as *do it again;* nearly always announces intentions before action; begins to ask questions of adults; 75% of speech intelligible	—
36	Up to 3600 words; understands *both, two, not today,* what to do when thirsty (hungry, sleepy), why people have stoves, understands *wait, later, big, new, different, strong, today, another,* and taking turns at play; carries out two- and some three-item commands, such as *give me the ball, pick up the doll, and sit down;* identifies several colors; is aware of past and future	Up to 900 words in simple sentences, averaging three to four words per sentence; averages 15,000 words per day and 170 words per hour; uses words such as *when, time, today, not today, new, different, big, strong, surprise, secret;* can repeat three digits, name one color, say name, give simple account of experiences, and tell stories that can be understood; begins to use more pronouns, adjectives, and adverbs; describes at least one element of a picture; is aware of past and future; uses commands such as *you make it* and expressions such as *I can't, I don't want to;* verbalizes toilet needs; expresses desire to take turns; communication includes criticisms, commands, requests, threats, questions, answers; 85% of speech intelligible	Starts to distinguish dissimilar speech sounds, such as the difference between *ee* and *er,* although there may be some difficulty with the concepts of *same* and *different*

Modified from Chinn, P. L. (1976). *Child health maintenance: Concepts in family-centered care* (2nd ed.). St. Louis: Mosby; Weiss, C. E., & White, H. S. (1976). *Communicative disorders.* St. Louis: Mosby.

own and that it has an effect on others. To exert autonomy, the child must relinquish the dependence on others that was enjoyed as an infant. Continued dependency can create a sense of doubt regarding the ability to control one's own actions. Children need appropriate limits on what is acceptable versus unacceptable behavior to establish the boundaries of the ability to control.

The toddler can separate from others by walking away and may no longer quietly cooperate when told to do something. Cognitive and language skills have resulted in the ability to say "no" and to think of things to do independently.

The toddler must explore the world, not only the physical aspects, but also the interpersonal aspects of relationships to develop a true sense of independence. Exploring the physical world involves poking into, climbing onto, crawling under, tasting, smelling, and taking apart the objects encountered. The child explores relationships with others by searching for the limits of the child's power: if a "no" or a temper tantrum means control of another person's behavior, the child learns that one's own *self* is more powerful than the other person's *self*. The toddler continually practices separateness to develop a sense of autonomy.

This process can be trying and confusing for parents. Their baby, who happily followed along at one time, is suddenly saying "no" to requests, even when treats are offered. The toddler may say a vehement "no" when offered a cookie and then scream and cry when the cookie is put away; the parents may wonder if the toddler wants the cookie or not. Likely, the answer is "yes," but the toddler may also need to express autonomy by refusing it. These conflicting desires can be confusing to both the parent and the toddler.

Occasionally, the same toddler who displays this strong need for independence may cuddle and even cling to the parents, realizing that independence can be frightening. The toddler must initiate this closeness; the parents must not force it.

The toddler's need for more autonomy may conflict with parental expectations, safety limits, or the rights of other children or adults. Any of these conflicts results in feelings of frustration. A typical toddler response to frustration is the well-known temper tantrum. Parents can feel unable to cope with these displays of frustration and may give in to the child's desire, even when the desire is potentially unsafe or beyond the family budget. Independence must be practiced, but the toddler must not think that a tantrum behavior can be used to control the environment and other people.

Nursing Interventions

The nurse assesses the toddler-parent relationship to determine the following:

1. How the toddler is expressing the need for independence.
2. How the parents perceive these actions.
3. How the parents respond to the toddler's independence.
4. What the toddler does when frustrated in exploring the environment or controlling personal and other's actions.
5. How the parents respond to the toddler's display of frustration.
6. What provisions the parents are making to allow safe choices for the toddler.

The nurse's teaching focuses on the aspects that are troublesome for an individual toddler-parent pair. Some general concepts to include are:

1. Match the environment to the child's needs and abilities. Childproof the home such that the child can explore safely. Provide toys that the child can master. Give opportunities to play with more challenging toys, but do not make these toys the rule.
2. Give advance notice (approximately 5 minutes) of a change in activity, such as lunchtime, nap time, and so on. Use simple games as a transition.
3. Make positive suggestions rather than giving commands.
4. Give two safe and acceptable choices when possible.
5. Let the toddler be *in charge* during play periods with the parents, choosing the book or game, and deciding when to move on to another activity.
6. Allow the toddler to say "no" in play situations and, when appropriate, in real situations.
7. When a command must be given, state it firmly, and do not give in.
8. Set and enforce consistent limits such that the toddler will come to develop control within these limits.
9. If temper tantrums occur, glance to make sure that the child is safe, then ignore the child until the behavior is acceptable. Give immediate attention when acceptable behavior is shown.
10. Praise the toddler's skills and abilities.

The toddler who is not allowed to develop a sense of autonomy experiences shame and doubt in oneself and one's abilities, missing an important step in the development of a positive self-concept.

Roles-Relationships Pattern

By toddlerhood, the child has learned who the mother, father, and older siblings are and has established some form of reciprocal relationship with each of these people. The toddler may see one family member as the *fixer* of broken toys and bruised knees, another as the troublemaker who always takes away toys, and someone else as the peacemaker who *smoothes things out* after fights. By discovering who can be manipulated and who has the ability to set limits on behavior, the child begins to establish a place in the line of family power. The toddler's

HOT topics

COPING WITH A CHILD'S TEMPERAMENT

Temperament is defined as the style of behaviors that a child habitually uses to cope with the demands and expectations of the environment. Chess and Thomas (1986) have described the three common temperament patterns that they believe are innate: (1) the easy child, (2) the difficult child, and (3) the slow-to-warm-up child.

The easy child is cuddly, affectionate, and easy to manage. The way in which a child with an *easy* temperament elicits positive reactions from adults is obvious.

Children with a *difficult* temperament, however, are less adaptable, are more intense and active, and have more negative moods. These behaviors can be distressing to parents and caregivers and they may cause them to feel ineffective in their role.

Temperament affects development through the lifespan, but is especially significant for toddlers when placed in the context of development. Toddlers are increasingly more mobile and are striving for independence at a time when parents become more demanding. Various approaches to parenting, teaching, and providing health care, including the adults' own temperament styles, culture, and gender-related biases can influence the way in which the child's behavior is viewed.

According to the goodness-of-fit interactive model of temperament, adults can accommodate their demands and expectations in ways that match the child's behaviors, including learning strategies to help toddlers adapt positively to social expectations.

1. What are the consequences of labeling a toddler as a *difficult child*?
2. How would adults react to a 2-year-old girl who was extremely active and highly distractible?
3. What strategies would adults suggest to the parents to manage this behavior?
4. How would adults react to a 3-year-old boy who rarely sleeps, cries whenever he does not get his way, and rarely smiles or laughs?
5. What strategies can be suggested to the parents for managing these behaviors?

Data from Chess, S., & Thomas, A. (1986). *Temperament in clinical practice*. New York: Guildford Press; Gross, D., & Conrad, B. (1995). Temperament in toddlerhood. *Journal of Pediatric Nursing, 10*, 146.

strongest motivator is the love and affection of the parents, which can be difficult for parents to recognize when their toddler is in the midst of asserting independence (see Hot Topics box).

Toddlers are more interested in the parents and siblings than they were as infants; they are curious about what these family members are doing and often imitate their actions (see Research Highlights box). Toddlers are likely to prefer parents' or siblings' possessions to their own. Research demonstrates that young toddlers are most responsive to playful social interaction initiated by the father. At 2 years of age, children are more cooperative, close, involved, excited, and interested in play with their fathers than they are with their mothers or siblings (Berger, 1998).

Sibling Rivalry

Frequently, a toddler must deal with a new member of the family (a tiny, sometimes loud creature who is unable to play, practically untouchable, and demanding of mother's time) (Fig. 18-3). A new baby presents a dilemma for the toddler, who is curious about this *thing*, but is frequently admonished to "don't hit," "don't poke," or "don't be so loud." Is it any wonder that love is not the emotion foremost in the toddler's heart?

Regression may occur in the toddler's skill level in response to a new sibling. **Regression,** or reverting temporarily to an earlier, previously abandoned developmental stage of behavior to retain or regain mastery of a stressful situation, can be beneficial to the toddler and

research highlights

Maternal Employment

Because more than 50% of mothers of toddlers are employed outside the home, questions have been raised about the effects of maternal employment on young children. Some people believe that children of mothers who work will be more insecure and have less maternal attachment. The effect of children and employment on the marital relationship is also debated.

A recent study compared marital quality, psychological well being, and parental sensitivity of single-earner and dual-earner parents when their first-born children were 3 months of age and 2½ years of age. Because marital relations and employment influence parents' psychological well being, the parenting behavior is also influenced.

Results of this study showed that employed mothers were more sensitive to their 3 month olds than were unemployed mothers. When children were age 2½ years, dual-earner parents had lower marital quality than single-earner parents. Marital quality was positively associated with parental sensitivity at both ages. Parents' marital quality declined during the study interval regardless of maternal employment.

This study has implications for anticipatory guidance that the nurse can provide to families who are considering maternal employment or for cases in which the mother must return to work.

Adapted from Broom, B. L. (1998). Parental sensitivity to infants and toddlers in dual-earner and single-earner families. *Nursing Research, 47*, 162-170.

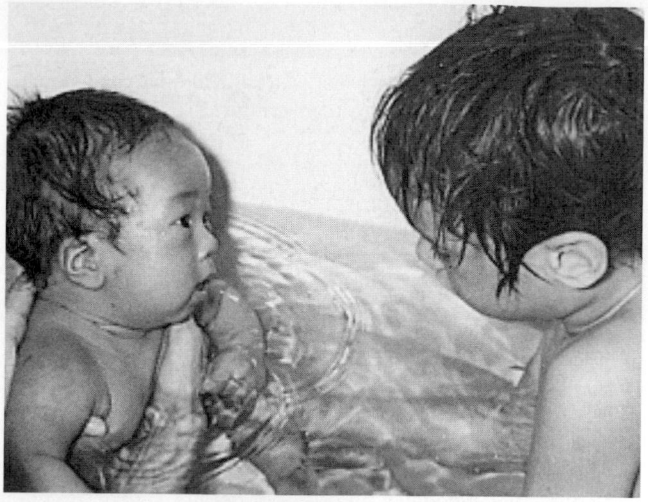

Fig. 18-3 Toddlers might have to learn to deal with a new family member. (From Chinn, P. L. [1979]. *Child health maintenance: Concepts in family-centered care* [2nd ed.]. St. Louis: Mosby.)

distressing to the parents. Toddler regression may take the form of losing toileting skills, crying more, wanting to be fed and dressed after mastering these skills, or reverting to *baby talk*.

When the parents are caring and understanding, the toddler will regain the former skill level within a short time. This process is not the end of sibling rivalry; however, it will continue, but take other forms. All siblings feel competition with each other and all siblings fight. Some competition is subtler than other forms of competition. Parents must recognize that sibling rivalry exists and that it can be most pronounced in the first 4 to 5 years of life. In these early years, siblings need adults to settle conflicts. Later, the adults can step back a little and help the siblings settle their conflicts among themselves.

Occasionally, parents decide to treat siblings the same to avoid any jealousy or rivalry. This tactic does not necessarily solve the problem because the uniqueness of each child is unrecognized. Children, as with adults, have different likes and dislikes. To have particular likes and dislikes recognized and respected is important to a child's self-image; it lets toddlers know that they are regarded as individuals.

Parents cannot stop sibling fighting by forbidding it, but reasonable limits can be established. One way to tone down fighting is to remove the gain. Generally, the desired outcome in the toddler's mind is to see the self rewarded and the sibling punished. When parents do not reward or punish, or when they do not take sides, the gain is missing and fighting becomes less satisfactory. This approach does not mean that all fighting will stop, but the child will look for some other ways of getting approval (Colson & Dworkin, 1997).

Parents and young children must realize that not all family members are equal. Parents, because of their life experiences, should have more authority to make important decisions for the family and individual members. As children get older, they can share in the decision-making process, but expecting or allowing toddlers to make important decisions is ludicrous for parents.

The toddler, dissimilar to the infant, demands some independence; this presents the first conflict in the parent-child relationship. Parents who have had experience with other toddlers or who have read about or discussed their behavior may be better able to deal with this new situation.

Sibling relationships and parent-child relationships can be difficult subjects for parents to discuss. Parents may think that any hint of discord indicates an unhealthy family. The nurse should include discussion of family relationships in the developmental teaching. Sibling rivalry and parent-child conflicts should be anticipated before they become major stresses. For example, sibling rivalry should be discussed before the new baby arrives and the toddler's need for more independence should be discussed in late infancy.

Box 18-3 Warning Signs of Child Abuse

1. Inconsistencies in the history of the injury
2. Child is developmentally incapable of causing injury
3. Multiple healed fractures on x-rays
4. Bruises on face, lips, mouth, buttocks, or genitalia
5. Regular pattern descriptive of object used to inflict injury (belt, shoe, or hand)
6. Burns with sharply demarcated edges, such as a socklike burn from immersion of a foot into hot water

From Cheung, K. K., & Yetman, R. (1999). Practice guidelines: Identifying and documenting findings of physical child abuse and neglect. *Journal of Pediatric Health Care, 13*, 142-143.

Child Abuse

A major disruption in family relationships is **child abuse.** This tragic situation is not limited to a particular age and is more likely to occur with major change or turmoil in the family. The most frequent victims are boys under the age of 3 years. The actual incidence of child abuse is unknown, because many cases are unreported.

Young toddlers are unable to verbalize about abusive situations; therefore health care providers must be alert to signs of abuse. Many of these situations may be difficult to differentiate from accidents (Box 18-3).

The nurse observes the child's attitude and behavior; children who have recently been abused may be hesitant to return home. Some children may withdraw from all adults or be excessively clinging out of fear of complete rejection. Another way to assess potential abusive behavior is to differentiate the behavior of the parents toward children's injuries according to typical reactions and attitudes versus reactions of battering or neglecting parents.

Typically, parental responses to childhood injuries include spontaneous reporting of the details of the illness or injury accompanied by concern, questions about progress and discharge, difficulty in leaving the child, and an attempt to identify with the child's feelings. These parents may also experience guilt for not protecting the child from the accident and may offer gifts to compensate for these feelings of guilt.

In contrast, neglecting or abusing parents are often hesitant to provide information about the illness or injury; they may be evasive or even contradict themselves. Additionally, abusing parents tend to be irritated at the inconvenience of being asked questions, appear angry with the child, or show little or no concern for the injury, prognosis, or discharge plans. Abusing parents tend to visit the child less and may even disappear during the examination. These parents may not exhibit guilt feelings and will generally contend that the child was solely responsible for the injury. Rather than mentioning any good qualities about the child, the abusing parents are highly critical.

Although these signs of potential abuse are certainly not present in all abusive parents and no one exhibits all of these symptoms, their presence should alert the nurse to assess and observe further. The nurse must also remember that some of these signs may be found in nonabusive parents; therefore their presence serves only as a cue for further assessment, not as a conclusive diagnosis (see Multicultural Awareness box). Nurses are required by law to report suspected child abuse to the local Child Protective Services Agency.

Sexuality-Reproductive Pattern

The toileting process, during which attention is focused on the genital area, may precipitate an increased interest in masturbation or curiosity about other's genitals. The nurse should include this aspect in early teaching about toilet training, giving parents time to consider their feelings and decide on the method by which they will deal with these behaviors. Some parents accept the child's curiosity, whereas others may feel obligated to introduce sexual values and taboos.

The nurse helps parents approach the issue reasonably by explaining that nearly all toddlers engage in masturbation occasionally and that it is not harmful. Masturbation provides a means for the toddler to become better acquainted with the body. Parents should not punish their toddler for masturbation, but they can suggest or offer other activities as a distraction. The older toddler can understand the concepts of privacy during elimination and for special body parts.

Many parents are uncertain about the words they should use for the sex organs and elimination; *cute* words that are unrelated to the correct anatomical name or function are sometimes invented to avoid *embarrassing* words. The nurse encourages the parents to teach their toddlers to use correct terminology so toddlers can be understood.

MULTICULTURAL AWARENESS

Evaluating Abuse with Cultural Awareness

Nurses are required by law to report cases of suspected child abuse to the Child Protective Services agency in their state. Although child abuse laws can vary from state to state, generally, abuse is defined as a physical injury that is nonaccidental. Increasingly, nurses are being urged to incorporate culturally based nursing interventions into their care. Occasionally, the nurse may encounter a folk healing practice that produces a nonaccidental physical injury.

The following are two examples found in Southeast-Asian populations:

COINING (CAO GIO)

The edge of a coin is rubbed over the painful or symptomatic area of the body. The appearance of a deep red-purple skin color is confirmation that the person had *bad wind* in the body. The use of the coin produces superficial ecchymotic areas between the rib bones on the front and back of the body. These areas may resemble strap marks.

CUPPING (VENTOUSE)

A vacuum is created inside a special cup by igniting alcohol-soaked cotton inside the cup. When the flame extinguishes, the cup is immediately applied to the skin of the painful site. Suction is created and the skin is pulled up inside the cup. This process creates circular, ecchymotic burn marks approximately 2 inches in diameter.

The nurse who sees this type of injury to the child's skin should discuss the folk healing practices with the parents and encourage them to discontinue their use. If the parents refuse to stop, then the nurse should consult with Child Protective Services. The nurse must always be an advocate for the child.

Coping–Stress-Tolerance Pattern

An infant copes primarily through motor activity; the toddler may continue to use some of these strategies, such as body rocking, change in position, restlessness, and turning away from a stimulus, but is also developing many new ways to respond to stress. The toddler begins to use basic problem-solving strategies as new situations are encountered, many of which result from environmental exploration. Other stresses may include a new sibling, new day care arrangements, increased parental expectations related to toilet training, or changes in parental relationships, such as divorce or separation (see Care Plan box). Although older children and adults can recall past stressful situations and their responses, the toddler cannot draw from this store of memories or think of a wide range of possible responses.

Variables that influence a toddler's response to stress include the child's health status, the nature and timing of

CARE PLAN

Nursing Diagnosis: Altered Parenting Related to Situational Crisis

DEFINING CHARACTERISTICS

- Verbalized concerns about changes in parental role, family function, or family communication
- Inattentiveness to child's needs
- Reluctant or inappropriate caretaking behaviors
- Compulsive seeking of role approval from others
- Disruption in caretaking routines

RELATED FACTORS

- Financial difficulties
- Recent move
- Change in marital status
- Dysfunctional relationship between parents

EXPECTED OUTCOMES

- Parent verbalizes increasing confidence in care of the child
- Parent verbalizes increasing confidence in parenting abilities
- Parent demonstrates nurturing behaviors toward child
- Parent identifies effective ways to express negative emotions
- Parent identifies community resources

INTERVENTIONS

- Help parent identify deficits in parenting skills
- Encourage expression of feelings
- Initiate a plan to assist parent in developing appropriate parenting skills
- Explore available resources with parent

information in preparation for the stressful experience, the observed parental coping patterns, and opportunities for autonomy and freedom of movement that are usually available to the child.

The ill child lacks the same energy to deal with stresses compared with the child in a healthy state. The toddler should be prepared for stressful events shortly before they happen. The parent should not say to a 2-year-old child, "You will get a shot tomorrow"; the toddler's understanding of tomorrow is vague and the imagination has too much time to deal with the host of ramifications of a shot. The parent should tell the toddler directly before this painful event occurs and then help the toddler through the experience by being close and reassuring. Avoiding the term "shot" altogether, because of its association with guns and being injured or killed, is probably best; "injection" can be used with the toddler. The child who is ill and requires a sequence of injections needs more ongoing preparation and opportunity to express fear and other feelings. The child sees the parents' methods of dealing with stress and may adopt or imitate these methods.

CASE STUDY

Grandparents Provide Care

Mary and John are the parents of 18-month-old Jeremy. They plan to take a week-long vacation while leaving Jeremy with his grandparents at their house. Because Jeremy is the first grandchild, the elderly couple is eager to spend time with him, but have expressed concern about caring for a toddler.

1. What should the parents discuss with the grandparents concerning safety issues?
2. What psychosocial issues of a toddler are important to consider for both the parents and the grandparents?
3. Do you think the parents should take this vacation?

Separation anxiety—feelings of anxiety and sadness and not being in control when separated from familiar people, especially the mother and father—and regression are the two most characteristic toddler responses to stress. The child may also use denial, repression, and projection to relieve stress.

Nursing Interventions

Parents may need assistance in understanding and accepting their toddler's coping responses. A typical instance is the regression that is often a response to a new sibling in the family. The nurse helps parents recognize this reaction as a normal response of the toddler who is seeking to reaffirm a place in the family. This toddler needs verbal and physical demonstrations of the parents' love and the opportunity, through verbal play and motor activity, to work through these feelings (Dixon & Stein, 2000).

These early efforts at dealing with stress are essential steps to a more mature coping response as the child grows.

Values-Beliefs Pattern

Conscience

Dissimilar to the infant, whose behavior is largely unrestricted, the toddler is subjected to many limits, which are often stated in the form of a moral dictum from an adult: "Good boy, you ate all your meat," or "No, don't hit your brother; that's bad." Limits are occasionally enforced through punishment, stern reprimands, or ignoring. The toddler is socialized into acting in accordance with adult wishes. The toddler develops some self-control through the efforts of parents and others, but this control continues to depend on their approval or disapproval. This concept does not foster an internally mediated conscience. Conscience (standards and prohibitions that have been adapted by the personality and that govern behavior from within) does not emerge until age 5 or 6 and is rudimentary until age 9 or 10 (Fraiberg, 1959). This theory does not mean that toddlers should not have limits set and enforced, but it does have implications for how limits should be set.

The young toddler may not have a good understanding

of "no." Parents should continue to use the word "no," but it should combine with redirecting the child's attention to another activity that is acceptable. The toddler is helped to channel action and inquisitiveness into more socially acceptable activities. Studies have shown that physical punishment or withdrawal of parental love does not lead to the development of a conscience. The most effective conscience-building technique is an inductive explanation of the consequences of the toddler's action. After the toddler has sufficient receptive language skills, the parent can give a brief, clear description of the outcome: "When you hit me, I hurt." Another effective technique is to explain rules and rights to the toddler: "You can play with the cars and trucks; you mustn't touch the TV." This approach helps the toddler develop acceptable moral feelings (Berger, 1998).

Toddlers' moral behavior also is influenced by what other people do. If toddlers see others (family members, playmates, television characters) doing certain things, they will assume that action is acceptable. A problem is presented when a toddler has been told, for example, "No, don't touch the stove, it will hurt you," but sees the parents and older siblings touching it all the time.

The toddler is more likely to *remember* rules and prohibitions when the parent or another adult is present; left alone, the child is more likely to try the forbidden act. Parents may need assistance in understanding that their toddler is not purposely being *bad,* but rather, moral behavior, because of the child's level of cognitive and emotional development, tends to be influenced by situation, circumstance, and the presence of people. The ability to recite a rule does not mean that the toddler has integrated the rule into a repertoire of actions.

Spiritual Values

Toddlers from families with religious backgrounds are often taught prayers and songs with a spiritual theme, which are sometimes tied into *right* and *wrong* ideas. Toddlers may be able learn the words to these simple prayers and songs, but parents should be cautioned that knowing the words does not mean that toddlers understand the full meaning of what is said. This early introduction into the family's religious beliefs is important as a socialization factor, but should not be assumed to produce a *good* child.

An important aspect of teaching young children what is right and wrong has been mentioned briefly, but should be a major focus for the nurse. This aspect involves is the technique of stating what is acceptable behavior and then reinforcing this behavior. Occasionally, parents find themselves constantly telling children what not to do. Is it possible that children have been given so many prohibitions that they cannot think of other alternatives? Another common mistake of parents is to *not disturb* toddlers when they are being *good*. Therefore they receive no attention for acceptable behavior, but attended to only when they misbehave.

Nursing Interventions

The nurse teaches parents the following points:

1. State briefly and clearly the desired or acceptable action.
2. Praise desired behaviors.
3. Praise attempts at acceptable behavior, even when imperfect.
4. Vary the style of praise, but always be enthusiastic and sincere.
5. Praise the child in front of others.

These techniques must be used repeatedly to produce the desired result: more frequent socially acceptable behavior.

PATHOLOGICAL PROCESSES

Many environmental processes can affect people at every age. Toddlers, because of their lack of judgment related to rudimentary problem-solving skills, level of physical coordination, lack of experience with many types of situations, and high level of curiosity about the environment, are at higher risk than are other age groups.

Unintentional Injuries

Injuries are the most frequent cause of childhood disability and death. In emergency rooms each year, 1 out of every 10 toddlers is treated for trauma or poisoning. The number of unintentional injuries for girls peaks in the toddler years, whereas for boys, two peaks occur (toddlerhood and adolescence). As is true for all ages, boys have more unintentional injuries compared with girls in the toddler period. Motor-vehicle accidents are a major cause of injuries at all ages and are considered in a section that follows. Other agents that are discussed are related to structural elements or materials in buildings, fixtures, and furniture; toys; hazards from sports and recreational equipment or situations; drownings; and burns.

Structural Hazards

Houses and other buildings can be hazardous for toddlers. Their desire to explore places them in locations in which older children or adults would not consider going. The toddler will climb onto furniture or fixtures, out windows, or into small spaces. Falls or injuries that result from these explorations can range from minor scrapes and bruises to fatal head injuries. One study estimates that there are 580 head injuries per 100,000 toddlers from furniture- or fixture-related accidents and 451 head injuries per 100,000 toddlers related to structural hazards. This number is only for head injuries; many more injuries affect other parts of the body from these causes (Hoekelman, 1997).

This discussion is part of the larger concept of *toddler proofing* the home or other settings in which toddlers spend time. Ideally, homes are *baby proofed* before the infant begins scooting and crawling. *Baby proofing* or *toddler proofing* refers to the practice of removing all potential hazards from the child's environment. Hazards are related to motor and cognitive skills, which change as the child matures. Therefore parents should reassess the safety of their home as their child acquires new skills. Child proofing also includes removing or protecting those few irreplaceable or sentimental objects on display in the home. These objects may not be real safety hazards, but they can represent an emotional loss when accidentally destroyed by the exploring child.

When the child or family visits the home of a friend or relative, that dwelling must be inspected for hazards, or the toddler must be confined to one *safe* room. Many injuries occur in unfamiliar environments.

Preventive measures for structural hazards include the following:

1. Have a locking gate or door on all stairs.
2. Carpet stairs to provide some padding in case the child falls.
3. Use furniture with rounded edges.
4. Anchor or temporarily move bookcases, tables, or lamps that can be pulled over.
5. Keep chairs away from counters or tables to prevent providing *steps* for the toddler.
6. Have windows screened and made of safety glass.

Toys

Toys are another source of injury to toddlers. Hazardous elements of these objects include toys or parts of toys that are small enough to be swallowed, flammable toys, toys coated with poisonous paint, stuffed animals with glass or button eyes or toxic stuffing, and toys with sharp edges.

Parents should inspect not only the toys that are in their own homes, but also the toys given to the toddler outside the home by relatives, friends, baby sitters, or day care personnel. Many toys are likely to be safe for the older child in these settings, but extremely hazardous for the toddler. This instance in one in which *sharing* should be discouraged.

Sports

Although sports and recreational equipment are recognized as a major source of accidents during childhood and adolescence, parents and health care personnel occasionally forget that these items can also be hazards to toddlers. A primary danger is the improper storage of sports and recreational equipment. Firearms that are left loaded and not locked away are an obvious hazard. Bodybuilding weights and other heavy equipment look interesting to toddlers, who may pull these objects down on themselves. Unfenced playing fields close to toddlers' play areas present a hazard when the youngsters wander into a soccer or football game. Toddlers should be supervised closely on swings and jungle gyms. When playing alone, toddlers may be safe; but when other youngsters are present, they can be hazardous to one another.

Drownings

Drownings are a major cause of death in toddlers. For the child under 3 years of age, the bathtub is a primary site of drownings. The toddler should never be left alone in the bathtub nor be permitted to lean over the bathtub to play with water toys, the potential is such that the toddler might topple in, hit the head, and be unable to get out. Toilet lids should remain down. Other water risks include swimming pools, natural bodies of water, and boats. All swimming pools should be fenced and have self-closing gates and latches. All children should wear a properly fitting life jacket when in a boat. Toddlers must be supervised constantly and competently whenever they are near any body of water. The American Academy of Pediatrics recommends that a parent accompany children younger than 3 years of age at all times during any swimming lessons. Children should never be forced to put their faces in the water.

Burns

Burns, especially scalds, are another major cause of injury in this age group. A toddler or playmate may turn on a hot water tap and be unable to turn it off. This hazard can be lessened by keeping hot water heater temperatures set below 130° F (54° C). In 1980, Florida was the first state to pass legislation limiting new water heaters to a preset temperature of 125° F (52° C). Other states have passed legislation that specifies a maximum water temperature in all rental units. Additionally, curiosity can cause the toddler to overturn a pot of hot liquid on the stove. This accident can be avoided if family members place panhandles toward the back of the stove and do not leave cords from electric pots hanging within reach of the toddler.

Nursing Interventions

Occasionally, teaching injury prevention is not well-received by parents responding that their child *has to learn sometime* that water is hot and so on, or that a child who has been hurt once *won't do that again*. These statements indicate a lack of understanding of the toddler's cognitive level.

In these cases, the nurse begins accident-prevention teaching with a discussion of the toddler's developmental level. Written handouts can be a helpful way to make this information available to families and people involved in child care.

Motor Vehicles

Motor-vehicle injury is the leading cause of death in children from 1 to 4 years of age. These accidents include passenger and pedestrian injury; for the toddler, passenger injury is more frequent. Many factors affect the risk of passenger injury: speed of the car, highway and road construction, type of vehicle, age of driver, alcohol intoxication of driver, position in the car, and restraint.

Parents can definitely control some of these factors. Speed and alcohol use depend on the good judgment of the driver. Statistics indicate that cars with a wider wheel base provide greater protection for passengers in the event of an accident. Parents should consider this factor when purchasing a new car. Rear-seat position is safer than is front-seat position; therefore children should always be in the back seat.

Recent studies have shown that children under 12 and babies in rear-facing car seats are at risk for injury or death from passenger-side airbags during even low-speed crashes. Therefore children under 12 and all infants should not be allowed to ride in the front seat of a car equipped with a passenger-side airbag.

The most effective preventive measure is the use of a crash-tested and approved toddler car seat. The nurse provides a list of approved car seats and local retail outlets or agencies that lend or rent car seats. Parents must be made aware that some infant seats are not appropriate for toddlers (see Chapter 17). The American Academy of Pediatrics has published a comprehensive pamphlet on choosing a car seat (AAP, 2000).

Unfortunately, not all families who own car seats use them consistently. Primary prevention must include the concept that car seats must be used every time the child is in the car. Most states have passed legislation requiring the use of approved child restraints. The nurse is active in private and community action to get this type of legislation passed and enforced.

Biological and Bacterial Agents

The toddler is susceptible to the same organisms as any other person would be, but may succumb to common illnesses more frequently than would an older child or adult, because the toddler has not built up specific resistance to many common organisms. A classic example of this vulnerability is the annual number of upper respiratory infections (URI), or common colds, in toddlers. Parents often become concerned because their toddler gets more URIs than does anyone else in the family; it is not unusual for the toddler to have 6 to 10 colds every year. This situation can be especially true for the toddler who is exposed to other young children in a group care setting or older siblings.

The URI itself, although troublesome to the child and the caretakers, is not a major concern. However, one of its common results, otitis media, can produce long-term effects. The concern is decreased hearing acuity at a time when the youngster is acquiring many new language skills. Decreased hearing results from a buildup of secretions in the middle ear chamber in which secretions or edema blocks the Eustachian tube. The child with acute otitis media needs appropriate medical management. The child with serious chronic otitis media (fluid in the middle ear) needs careful monitoring of hearing status (Hoekelman, 1997).

This secondary prevention of complications of an existing condition is within the scope of the nurse's role. Hearing can be tested by using pure tone audiometry in the cooperative older toddler. For the younger toddler, more complex methods of conditioned response audiometry or brainstem-evoked response may be required. These children should be referred to an audiologist. Tympanometry is a method of assessing the pressure in the middle ear chamber, which provides valuable information about the progress of serious otitis media. Tympanometry is an easy technique to learn and the equipment is relatively inexpensive and widely available.

Chemical Agents

The toddler is exposed to the same pollutants in the air and water as is any other person; these pollutants are discussed in detail in other chapters of this unit. Chemical agents of particular concern for this age group are ingested poisons, such as household products, lead paint, drugs, cosmetics, pesticides, and plants (Fig. 18-4). The toddler, because of limited experience and cognitive level, is unaware that

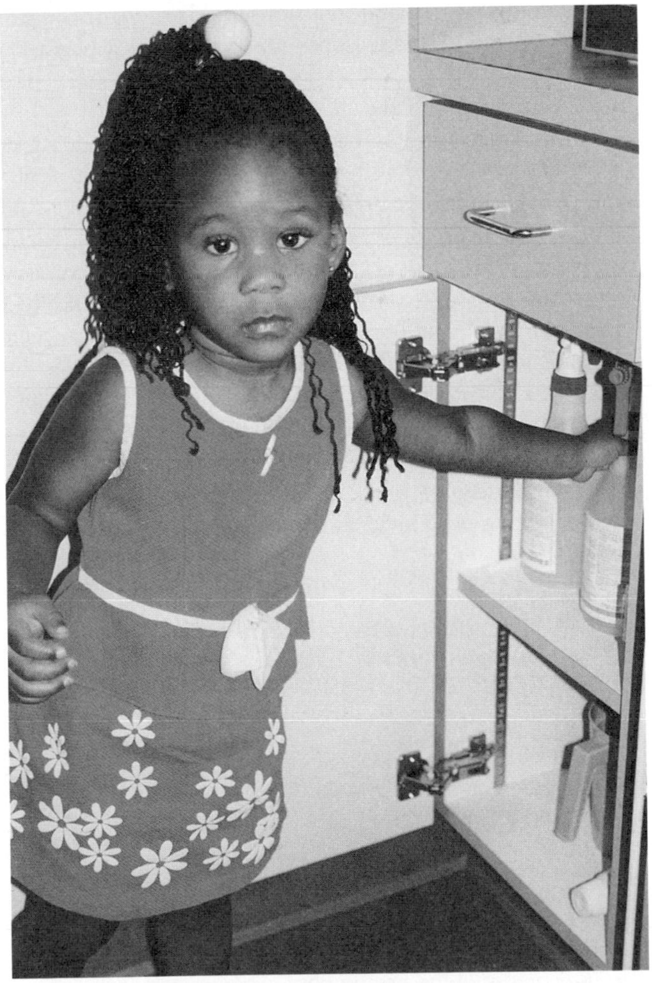

Fig. 18-4 Household cleaning supplies can be extremely dangerous to toddlers and should be out of reach and locked.

these items are harmful. Many emergency room calls and visits are precipitated by a toddler's ingestion of a questionably or actually harmful substance. These acute ingestions are likely to occur in the kitchen, bathroom, bedroom, or work area and are usually discovered by the parent or caretaker because of an open or empty container or a half-eaten leaf or other substance.

When parents or caregivers suspect that a toddler has ingested a poisonous substance, they should call the poison control center, even when the child appears perfectly healthy. Each poison control center is part of a nationwide effort to provide immediate information about poisonings. Parents must not apply any first aid, such as inducing vomiting, without specific instructions. Vomiting can cause further harm if the child is drowsy, unconscious, or convulsing or if the substance ingested is a corrosive, such as lye or a strong acid (Guyton, 1996). When vomiting is recommended by the poison control center, instructions are often given to use ipecac syrup to stimulate the vomiting rapidly. Because ipecac in large doses can be harmful, parents must follow the administration instructions carefully. This medication should be stored as carefully as any other medication or hazardous household product is stored.

The nurse discusses poisoning before the child begins to crawl or walk and then reviews this information when the child begins to ambulate (Box 18-4).

Chronic poisonings (those that occur when a child sucks on an object coated with lead-based paint or eats lead-based paint chips) are often undetected until irreversible damage has occurred. Primary prevention involves teaching parents the dangers of lead-based paint; secondary prevention involves doing periodic screening of blood lead levels on all young children at risk. In certain settings, such as urban areas with older housing, all children should be screened. Consumer protection laws require that all toys and furniture manufactured for small children be free of lead-based paint products. However, many families paint their own furniture and the child's play objects and may be unaware that the paint they have chosen has a lead base.

Box 18-4 Nursing Interventions to Prevent Poisoning in Toddlers

- All household products, such as cleaning products, paints, drugs, cosmetics, and garden products, should be in securely locked locations.
- A child should never be told that medicine is *candy*.
- All products should be kept in their original containers for easy identification.
- No poisonous plants should be kept in the house. (A list is available from local poison control centers.)
- The child should never be left alone in an outdoor setting in which there are potentially poisonous plants.
- The number of the poison control center should be posted next to every telephone.

Carcinogenic agents are essentially the same for toddlers and preschoolers and are discussed in Chapter 19.

SOCIAL PROCESSES

Community and Work

The toddler's world can expand rapidly when entering a day care setting. The toddler years are those during which many parents decide that some experience in a group setting would be beneficial for their child. The nurse can provide counseling about the decision to place a child in day care and the resulting emotions. Topics to consider include the following:

- Feelings of ambivalence or guilt after enrolling a toddler in a day care setting
- Selection of a day care setting
- Ongoing evaluation of the day care setting
- Anticipatory provisions for the toddler's care during episodes of illness
- Planning for the parents' physical and emotional resources
- Anticipation of separation protest

Regardless of the reasons for the parents wanting or needing day care for their child, the traditional expectation of caring for the young child at home continues to influence the parents' concept of what they *should* do for their child. Parents must be reassured that a day care environment congruent with the family environment is not detrimental to the child, that they are not neglecting their parental duty, and that their choice or necessity arises out of achieving goals that will ultimately benefit the child. For example, if the parent must work to earn an income, requires obtain job training or education, or simply needs outside activity and stimulation for self-development, then the child will benefit (Wong, 1999).

Several factors must be considered in selecting the day care center. The economic factor is often the determining variable, but when possible, the family also should include factors such as convenience of location, range and flexibility of hours and services available, quality of the facility, and congruence of the center's philosophy of child care with that of the family. The parent may need assistance in determining the quality of day care and in estimating whether the day-care service follows the parent's philosophy. If a child has been placed in a setting that is detrimental to physical or emotional development, then the parent may need assistance in selecting an alternative setting. Additionally, community action must be taken to intervene at the setting to protect the health of all other children involved (Wong, 1999). Parents can be directed to a local day care referral agency or family day care association for free pamphlets on choosing a child care setting.

Changes in caregivers are difficult for children; therefore parents must make careful selections. However, making the initial choice of care setting is only the first step. Parents should be encouraged to reevaluate the care setting as their child matures. Some settings are wonderful for infants and young toddlers, but cannot offer the range of activities and stimulation needed by the older toddler or preschooler.

Parents must monitor the ongoing safety and quality of their child's care setting. Parents should be concerned about whether they are not welcome to drop in and visit their child at any time, whether the caregiver frequently seems overwhelmed, or whether their child begins to exhibit unusual behaviors (anxious, withdrawn, tearful, or constantly fatigued).

When toddlers first enter a day care setting in which other children are present, the frequency of episode illness usually increases dramatically until the child develops immunological defenses against the infectious organisms that are encountered. The family should anticipate this probability and know what provisions will be made under similar circumstances. Some large cities have one or more day care centers that accept only children with short-term acute illnesses or common infectious diseases, such as chickenpox. Because illness can place an additional financial burden on the family resulting from a of loss of income when the parent remains home from work to care for the child or makes alternative paid arrangements, planning for this added expense can ease the financial burden (Honig, 1995).

Frequently, when parents work and then return home to the demands of caring for an active, dependent young child, their own physical and emotional capacity is rapidly depleted, and their ability to cope with the young child's demands wanes. The nurse guides parents in recognizing their own limits of energy and helps them identify ways in which they can conserve energy, obtain relief during difficult periods, and plan for their own restoration needs.

An initial or transient recurring separation protest can be anticipated in the toddler period. The parents should understand that this is a normal reaction. Armed with firm intentions, the parents should plan to leave the child soon after arriving at the day care setting and clearly inform the child of their intentions, saying that they will return later in the day.

Culture and Ethnicity

The toddler continues to be shaped by the cultural values and beliefs of the parents and begins to be introduced to the more ritualistic family practices. The way in which holidays, holy days, and birthdays are observed is, largely, culturally determined. The toddler is socialized into these rituals and taught to accept them.

Setting limits and establishing discipline are also often culturally determined. Certain cultures expect even extremely young children to show unquestioning respect for adults. In the independent toddler, this expected *respect* for the parents may rarely be seen.

Health care practices are also culturally influenced. When the family views immunizations as dangerous or unnecessary, the child will be unprotected from certain communicable diseases. When medication is unacceptable, the child may be forced to rely on the strength of the immune system for all healing.

Culture also influences people's views of the toddler's curiosity about the body, especially genitals. When this sexual curiosity is considered *bad*, toddlers may be punished for this developmentally normal action.

Dissimilar to the older child, the toddler does not question the cultural practices of the family. The toddler may refuse to do certain expected things, but this is out of a need for independence, not a questioning of beliefs.

Legislation

Local and state legislation specific to the toddler is directed primarily at safety. As mentioned, some states have passed laws on approved car seats and limiting temperature in hot water heaters.

A major legislative issue for this age group is the child abuse and neglect laws in each state. These laws generally state their purpose: to provide protection for a child or developmentally disabled adult, to define *abuse* and *neglect*, to require that a report be made to a designated agency in the case of actual or suspected abuse or neglect, and to define the responsibility of the protecting agency. These laws may also provide for a central registry of reported cases of abuse. Nurses should be aware of the child abuse and neglect laws in their states and make this information available to others involved in child care.

Another key legislative issue for the toddler is the Education of the Handicapped-Act Amendment of 1986 (P.L. 99-457). This law creates programs that assist states in planning, developing, and implementing systems within states for handicapped children from birth to 3 years of age. Nurses who work with young children with disabilities can investigate available programs in their states.

Other legislation pertinent to toddlers involves regulations concerning day care settings. These rules usually pertain to size of facilities and fire prevention and may not deal with the qualifications of persons actually caring for the children. Copies of these regulations can be obtained from the state licensing agency.

Economics

Toddlers from low-income or unemployed families suffer the same effects of poverty that any child would encounter. The toddler is completely incapable of contributing to the economic resources of the family. Economic resources can greatly limit parents' range of child care choices. Some services are available to this age group, such as public assistance, Aid for Families with Dependent Children, and the Special Supplemental Nutrition Program for Women, Infants, and Children (WIC). The nurse helps families obtain these services for their toddler by making resource information available and directing the families to appropriate personnel.

Health Care Delivery System

As mentioned, the nationwide system of poison control centers is a health care resource available to and often used by families with toddlers.

Private physicians or nurse practitioners and public well-child clinics are the most frequently used resources for ongoing health maintenance or illness care for toddlers. Some public clinics sponsor special immunization days for young children who do not receive routine health care.

Another program that serves the older toddler is Early and Periodic Screening Diagnosis and Treatment (EPSDT). Typically, this program focuses on the preschooler (see Chapter 19).

Nursing Interventions

The toddler period presents one of the most interesting challenges in relation to approaching and relating to the child as an individual. Toddlers' reactions to health care workers often become conditioned as feelings of fear and apprehension and their limited experience with people outside the family render them doubtful and uncertain of encounters with strangers. An effective approach to a child of this age requires knowledge of the developmental characteristics of the child and the incorporation of nursing behaviors that are personally comfortable and successful in establishing rapport.

Each of these factors influences the manner and order in which the nurse conducts the health assessment of the toddler. The nurse should not follow a predetermined pattern; rather, each component must be approached according to readiness cues from the young child. Frequently, developmental screening that involves play activities and motor movement is used initially to promote the child's familiarity with the environment and to help establish interaction with the nurse. Assessment procedures that require restraint or discomfort should be integrated into the assessment after the child is at ease and has established a sense of confidence. Activities that restore the child's comfort and sense of security are planned to follow these procedures such that the toddler does not leave the encounter with a negative feeling of being manipulated into a frightening or uncomfortable situation.

The child's imaginative abilities can be used effectively when the nurse approaches the child with an age-appropriate toy, book, or game. Speaking in language that is appropriate, but not demeaning assists in establishing contact. Kneeling and approaching the toddler at eye level can overcome the overwhelming size difference between an adult and a young child. Colors in the nurse's clothing and pictures and toys in the setting all contribute to providing a sense of familiarity that may be missing from the white, polished environment of an office or clinic.

Toddlers need time to explore, to become familiar, and to *settle in* to a new environment; they may need time simply to watch or stare at a new person. Having time to play with toys, listening to the parents interact with people who are unfamiliar, and becoming accustomed to the smells and feels of the environment are important to children. Additionally, toddlers need evidence that they can trust this new environment and the people in it. When painful, discomforting, or threatening procedures must be performed, time must be devoted to establishing a sense of trust and confidence. When children are warned immediately in advance of painful procedures, undue anxiety and fear are produced to the extent that the safe and adequate administration of the procedure is hampered by the child's resistance.

Each protective health visit should include an interval history, measurement of growth parameters, physical assessment, developmental assessment, and discussion of age-appropriate developmental concerns. Immunizations should be given according to the current Recommended Childhood Immunization Schedule: United States, which is published every January and available on the Internet (www.aap.org).

During the 24-month visit, the toddler is screened for anemia and tuberculosis and has a urinalysis performed. The nurse assumes the responsibility for a major portion of each of these visits, the primary objective being health teaching and disease prevention. The health teaching and discussion of toddler development can be on an individual or group basis with parents. An advantage of the group approach is that parents can benefit from one another's experience with similar situations. Specific suggestions and

innovative practice

The Hodman Square Project

The Hodman Square Project is a collaborative community development effort based on the World Health Organization's model for cities. This project is a collaborative effort of Rush University College of Nursing in Chicago, the Rush Primary Care Institute, and the North Lawndale Community Coalition to provide health care programs and services to the residents of the North Lawndale inner-city community on Chicago's West Side. The project's emphasis is on the health promotion of women and children. A primary health care clinic and a wide range of family educational and counseling programs, such as classes on parenting skills and family health screenings, are offered.

Services are provided by a variety of clinicians, including Rush University nurse practitioner faculty, with the common goal of improving the quality of life for this inner-city community.

For more information, contact Rush Primary Care Institute at Kidston Building, 1653 West Congress Parkway, Chicago, IL, 60612 (312) 942-3567. Email rpci@rush.edu or visit online at http://www.rpci.rush.edu/index.html.

Courtesy Carol Lynn Mandle PhD, RN, CS.

information for many concerns of parents of toddlers have typically been discussed.

The nurse contributes to the health of toddlers as a consultant to a day care center, a leader of a toddler-parent discussion or playgroup through a community agency, or a speaker at a parents' organization. As always, the nurse looks beyond the needs of individual families and toddlers and becomes involved with community agencies and local and state legislative bodies that are charged with passing laws related to the health and welfare of these young children. This approach is the only way in which adequate health-promotion opportunities for all children can be ensured.

SUMMARY

The toddler period can be an exciting, challenging time for parents and their child to establish healthy and satisfying interactions and for the toddler to grow and develop into a more independent individual. By screening for developmental delays and signs of disease and by providing ongoing information to parents about their toddler's needs and new skills, the nurse promotes this healthy, satisfying outcome.

REFERENCES

American Academy of Pediatrics. (2000). *2000 family shopping guide to car seats, AAP safe ride program*. Elk Grove, IL: The Academy. Available: AAP, 141 Northwest Point Blvd., P.O. Box 927, Elk Grove, IL 60007-0927, www.aap.org

Berger, K. S. (1998). *The developing person through the life span* (4th ed.). New York: Worth Publishers.

Broom, B. L. (1998). Parental sensitivity to infants and toddlers in dual-earner and single-earner families. *Nursing Research, 47,* 162-170.

Chess, S., & Thomas, A. (1986). *Temperament in clinical practice*. New York: Guildford Press.

Cheung, K. K., & Yetman, R. (1999). Practice guidelines: Identifying and documenting findings of physical child abuse and neglect. *Journal of Pediatric Health Care, 13,* 142-143.

Chinn, P. L. (1976). *Child health maintenance: Concepts in family-centered care* (2nd ed.). St. Louis: Mosby.

Calhoun, J. H. (1997). Eye exams in infants and children. *Pediatrics in Review, 18,* 28-31.

Colson, E. R., & Dworkin, P. H. (1997). Toddler development. *Pediatrics in Review, 18,* 255-259.

Committee on Infectious Diseases, American Academy of Pediatrics. (1997). *Red book: Report of the committee on infectious diseases* (23rd ed.). Elk Grove Village, IL: AAP.

Dixon, S., & Stein, M. (2000). *Encounters with children: Pediatric behavior and development* (3rd ed.). St. Louis: Mosby.

Erikson, E. H. (1986). *The magic years* (35th anniversary edition). New York: Norton.

Erikson E. H. (1997). *The life cycle completed*. New York: Norton.

Falkner, F., & Tanner, J. (1986). *Human growth* (2nd ed.). New York: Plenum.

Fraiberg, S. (1959). *The magic years*. New York: Charles Scribner's Sons.

Frankenburg, W. K. (1994). Preventing developmental delays: Is developmental screening sufficient? *Pediatrics, 93,* 586-589.

Grodner, M., Anderson, S. L., & DeYoung, S. (1996). *Foundations and clinical applications of nutrition: A nursing approach*. St. Louis: Mosby.

Gross, D., & Conrad, B. (1995). Temperament in toddlerhood. *Journal of Pediatric Nursing, 10,* 146.

Guyton, A. C. (1996). *Textbook of medical physiology* (9th ed.). Philadelphia: W.B. Saunders.

Hoekelman, R. A. (1997). *Primary pediatric care* (3rd ed.). St. Louis: Mosby.

Honig, A. S. (1995). Choosing childcare for young children. In M. H. Bornstien, *Handbook of parenting: Vol 4*. Hove, UK: Lawrence Erlbaum.

Phillips, Jr., L. J. (1969). *The origins of intellect: Piaget's theory*. San Francisco: W.H. Freeman.

Schor, E. L. (1995). *Caring for your schoolage child*. New York: Bantam.

Seidel, H. M., Ball, J. W., Dains, J. E., & Benedict, C. W. (1999). *Mosby's guide to physical examination* (4th ed.). St. Louis: Mosby.

Trahms, C. M., & Pipes, P. L. (1997). *Nutrition in infancy and childhood* (6th ed.). New York: McGraw-Hill.

Wong, D. L. (1999). *Whaley and Wong's nursing care of infants and children* (6th ed.). St. Louis: Mosby.

U.S. Department of Health and Human Services. (2000). *Healthy people 2010*. Washington, DC: U.S. Government Printing Office.

Weiss, C. E., & White, H. S. (1976). *Communicative disorders*. St. Louis: Mosby.

Chapter 19

CAROLYN SPENCE CAGLE
CAROL LYNN MANDLE

Preschool Child

objectives

After completing this chapter, the nurse will be able to:

- Describe the physical and psychosocial changes that occur during the preschool years as they relate to child and family health needs.
- Relate the cognitive development of the preschooler to Piaget's theory.
- Describe typical sleep disturbances of the preschooler that are relevant to family teaching and nursing support.
- Discuss appropriate vision and hearing screening tools for the preschooler and the nursing roles regarding their use.
- Compare the coping skills of the preschooler with those of a younger child.
- Outline the immunization requirements of the preschooler that are relevant to primary prevention.
- Identify warning signs of cancer in the preschooler.
- List risk factors of asthma in the preschooler.
- Identify causes of injuries in the preschooler.

key terms

Acquired Lactase Deficiency
Acute Lymphocytic Leukemia
Amblyopia
Asthma
Bender Copy Forms
Centering
Chloroma
Doll or Puppet Play
Draw-a-Person and Draw-a-Family Tests
Early and Periodic Screening, Diagnosis, and Treatment
Egocentrism
Expressive Language
Heterophoria
Heterotropia
Homeostasis
Inductive Explanation
Irreversibility
Ishihara's Test
Lanoue Water Survival Technique
Mnemonic Strategies
Mutual Storytelling
Myopic Vision
Neuroblastoma
Nightmares (Anxiety Dreams)
Night Terrors
Otitis Media
Parental Divorce
Peabody Picture Vocabulary Test
Preoperational Stage
Preschool Readiness Experimental Screening Scale
Receptive Language
Refractive Errors
Retinoblastoma
Snellen E Chart
Strabismus
Transductive Reasoning
Vineland Social Maturity Scale
Wilms' Tumor

THINK About It

Aggressive Behavior

Phillip, age 4, started preschool 2 weeks ago after spending his early years at home with his mother and his 18-month-old sister. His mother recently returned to her job as an accountant, works 9 hours a day, and is fatigued when she picks up Phillip at 5:00 PM. Phillip's father travels for his job, but is home on weekends to spend time with his family. Although Phillip's mother always believed that he was shy because he was quiet, in the last week at child care, he started hitting his peers and becoming vocally loud at story time. His mother, believing that her return to work is related to Phillip's behavior, feels frustrated and embarrassed by his behavior, especially because she enjoys her new job and the extra income.

1 What factors might be contributing to Phillip's changed behavior?
2 How might you define Phillip's temperament? Why?
3 What specific discussions might you have with Phillip's parents to help them understand, respond to, and change their son's behavior for the better?

The preschool child (ages 3 to 6) has a more mature body structure, an ability to control and use the body, and a facility with language that more closely resembles that of the adult when compared with the toddler. The major psychological thrust of this period of development is mastery of the self as an independent human being, with a willingness to extend experiences beyond those of the family. With more families being headed by the mother, more reliance has been placed on child-care settings that expose children to learning opportunities beyond the typical family. Although increasing numbers of children are currently starting formalized schooling in their preschool years, historically, the end of early childhood in the Western world was marked by entrance into the formalized educational system (Box 19-1).

AGE AND PHYSICAL CHANGES

The protuberant abdomen of the toddler disappears in the preschool years as the pelvis begins to straighten and the abdominal muscles become developed. The hips gradually rotate inward, replacing outtoeing with straight or slight intoeing. Mild intoeing (metatarsus adductus) can remain during the preschool years, but anything beyond a mild level should be investigated and treated.

Growth rate remains relatively steady from ages 3 to 6 years. The average preschooler gains approximately 2 kg (4 lb) of body weight and 7 cm (2 inches) of height each year. Head circumference increases less than 2 cm during the entire preschool period.

As early childhood progresses, the skin matures significantly in protecting the child from outer invasion and loss of fluids. The skin's ability to localize infection increases, but remains less than mature. Negligible secretion of sebum makes the skin fairly dry. Changes occur in both color and curliness of the hair, usually becoming darker and straighter than is the hair during infancy. The

Box 19-1 Selected National Health-Promotion and Disease-Prevention Objectives for Preschool Children

- Increase the proportion of persons who have a specific source of ongoing care to 96% (baseline is 93% for children and youth in 1997).
- Reduce the proportion of families that experience difficulties or delays in obtaining care or do not receive needed care to 7% (baseline is 12% in 1997).
- Establish a single toll-free telephone number for access to poison control centers on a 24-hour basis throughout the United States to 100% (baseline is 15% of poison control centers shared a single toll-free number in 1999).
- Increase the number of tribes, states, and the District of Columbia with trauma care systems that maximize the prevention, survival, and functional outcomes of trauma patients to 100% (baseline is five states in 1998).
- Increase the number of states and the District of Columbia that have statewide pediatric protocols for on-line medical direction to 100% (baseline is 17 states in 1997).
- Eliminate elevated blood lead levels in children (baseline is 4.4% of children age 1 to 5 years who had blood lead levels exceeding 10 µg/dl in 1994).
- Reduce indoor allergen levels to 29 million homes with dust mite allergens exceeding 2 µg of dust in the bed (baseline is 36.3 million homes in 1999).
- Increase the proportion of persons visiting primary health care who receive mental health screening and assessment.
- Reduce the proportion of children and adolescents who have dental caries to 11% (baseline is 18% of children age 2 to 4 years in 1988 to 1994).
- Increase the proportion of children and adolescents who view television two or fewer homes per day.
- Increase the proportion of preschool children age 5 years and under who receive vision screening.
- Increase the proportion of persons who have hearing examinations on schedule.
- Reduce otitis media in children and adolescents to 294 per 1000 (baseline is 344.7 per 1000 in 1997).
- Reduce the rate of death for children age 1 to 4 years to 25.0 per 100,000 (baseline is 34.2 per 100,000 in 1998) and for children age 5 to 9 years to 14.3 per 100,000 (baseline is 17.6 per 100,000 in 1998).
- Reduce deaths from asthma to one per million children under age 5 (baseline is 1.7 per million in 1998).
- Reduce hospitalization rates for pediatric asthma to 17.3 per 10,000 (baseline is 23 per 10,000 in 1996).

From U.S. Department of Health and Human Services. (2000). *Healthy people 2010: Mid-course review and 1995 revisions*. Washington, DC: U.S. Government Printing Office.

function of the eccrine sweat glands gradually increases, but the quantity of eccrine sweat produced in response to heat or emotion remains minimal. Apocrine sweat glands remain nonsecretory during this period.

The kidneys have reached full adult maturity by the end of infancy and early toddlerhood. The only change during the preschool years is in size. By the end of this period, daily excretion of urine is 650 to 1000 mL (19 to 30 oz). Under normal homeostatic conditions, the renal system conserves water and concentrates urine on a level that approximates adult abilities. However, under conditions of stress, the preschooler's kidneys lacks the ability to fully respond and maintain **homeostasis** when compared with the more rapid response of the adult system.

Growth of the various gastrointestinal organs continues through the preschool years, but no basic changes in function occur. Children who did not achieve full voluntary control of elimination during the toddler period generally attain this function by the end of the preschool period. **Acquired lactase deficiency,** an intolerance to milk products manifested by diarrhea, can develop during the preschool years. This condition occurs most often in Black, Asian-American, and Native-American children, but can be successfully treated by eliminating lactose from the diet.

Lung capacity continues to increase and the respiratory rate gradually decreases. The preschooler makes better decisions than does the toddler about what things are safe to put in the mouth, thus, generally, fewer instances of choking and obstruction occur. As the ears gradually increase in size, the incidence of **otitis media** decreases slightly. The tonsils and adenoids remain relatively large and can become subject to upper respiratory infections.

The cardiovascular system enlarges in proportion to general body growth. Heart rate for the preschooler is 70 to 40 beats per minute (two standard deviations). The mean blood pressure is 100/60.5 mm Hg. Early hypertension can develop in the preschool years; therefore monitoring blood pressure during this time becomes important, particularly in instances of a strong family history of hypertension (see Chapter 20). The preschool child can maintain adequate levels of hemoglobin when sufficient dietary intake exists. The bone marrow of the ribs, sternum, and vertebrae becomes fully established as the main site of formation of red blood cells, but the liver and spleen maintain the capacity to form erythrocytes and granulocytes during hematopoietic stress.

The immune system gradually continues to develop. The preschooler builds up increased immunity to common pathogens as exposure occurs. Children who join a new preschool or play group can experience an increase in common contagious illnesses for a time. Later, these children may be less prone to disease because of their early exposure to infectious illnesses and their consequent development of immunity.

All the primary teeth have erupted by late toddler or early preschool years. The first permanent tooth can erupt during the end of the preschool period. On average, girls tend to begin permanent tooth eruption approximately 6 months earlier than do boys. Older preschoolers usually take responsibility for dental hygiene, although they may need gentle guidance about proper brushing and appropriate nutritional intake for healthy teeth. Parents should continue to assist with and supervise flossing. Because this is an age of caries formation, regular dental checkups remain essential (Fig. 19-1). If regular dental checkups have not started, then parents should be encouraged to take their preschooler to the dentist for preventive and secondary care. (Suggestions for promoting good oral hygiene as part of general health-promotion teaching can be found in Chapter 20.)

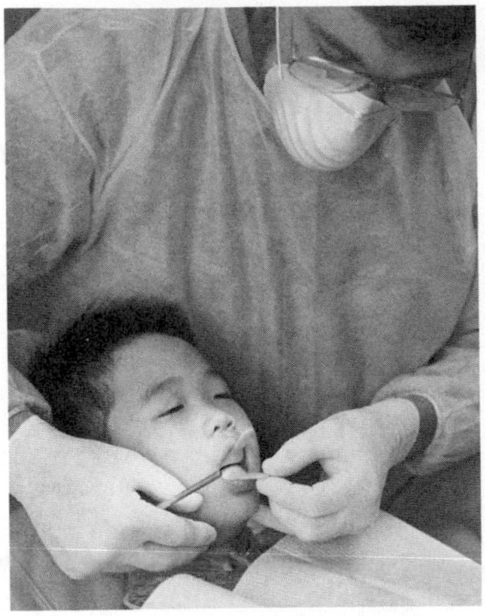

Fig. 19-1 Routine dental checkups should begin during the early preschool period.

Musculoskeletal and neurological system development reaches a level that allows for seemingly effortless walking, running, and climbing. Older preschoolers' ability to copy figures and draw recognizable pictures indicates their advancing fine-motor abilities and their eagerness to demonstrate these skills to others. Practice, increases in muscle size, continuing associations between existing neural pathways, and the establishment of new pathways for already accomplished tasks are a few of the many complex factors that contribute to the advances in functioning observed during early childhood. These advances in fine- and gross-motor development skills are outlined in Table 19-1.

Gender

Boys tend to experience more common childhood illnesses than do girls during ages 3 to 6 (see Chapter 18). Preschoolers are more aware of their sexual identity compared with toddlers and may imitate societal stereotypes more closely than do toddlers. Traditionally, boys have been encouraged to take more risks than girls have been and they have more accidents than do preschool girls,

Table 19-1 Developmental and Behavioral Milestones

Age	Expectations
3 years	At this age, the typical child: Opens doors Builds a tower of nine cubes; imitates bridge made from three cubes Demonstrates speech that is mostly intelligible. (The child who fails to speak in sentences or whose speech is unintelligible to strangers should be referred for speech, language, and hearing evaluation.) Knows own name, age, and gender May comprehend *cold, tired, hungry;* may understand the prepositions *over* and *under;* differentiates *bigger* and *smaller;* can convey the use of scissors, key, and pencil Copies a circle, may imitate a cross, and begins to visually discriminate colors Describes action in picture books Puts on some clothing and shoes Eats without assistance
4 years	At this age, the typical child: Alternates feet when descending stairs; jumps forward; can stand on 1 foot for up to 5 seconds Climbs a ladder Rides a tricycle Can walk on tiptoes Holds and uses a pencil with good control Builds a tower of 10 or more cubes Is able to cut and paste Engages in conversational give-and-take Asks, *why*, *when*, *how*, and inquires about meanings of words Can name three or four primary colors Can count from 1 to 5 and sing a song Enjoys jokes Washes and dries hands and brushes teeth Dresses and undresses with supervision, except for handling laces and buttons, when allowed sufficient time to dress; begins to be selective about clothes Initiates dramatic make-believe and dress-up play during which the child assumes a specific role Is imaginative and intensely curious Has formed gender identification Copies a cross and circle Draws a person with two to three parts Enjoys the companionship of other children, plays cooperatively, and shows interest in other children's bodies Meets the challenges of kindergarten class
5 years	At this age, the typical child: Skips, can walk on tiptoes, and broad jumps Can cut and paste Names four or five colors and can identify coins Tells a simple story and knows several nursery rhymes Defines at least one word (*ball, shoe, chair, table, dog*) Dresses and undresses without supervision Copies a triangle from an illustration Recognizes most letters of the alphabet Draws a person with a head, body, arms, and legs Begins to understand right and wrong, fair and unfair Engages in dramatic make-believe and dress-up play during which the child assumes a specific role; engages in domestic role playing Enjoys the companionship of other children; plays cooperatively Has formed gender identification ("Are you a boy or girl?")
6 years	At this age, the typical child: Bounces a ball 4 to 6 times; throws and catches Skates Rides a bicycle Ties shoelaces Counts up to 10; prints own first name; prints numbers up to 10 Understands right from left Draws a person with six body parts, with the figure depicted wearing clothing

Modified from American Academy of Pediatrics. (1998). *Guidelines for health supervision II*. Chicago: AAP.

who may have been encouraged to choose more sedate activities. In today's society, boys and girls have similar opportunities to choose the same activities. Whether this change will reflect accident statistics in the future will be interesting to observe.

Race

Race, with its related economic and cultural issues, can influence health care practices at this age, as is the case during all ages. Race can also influence dietary choices because of cultural preferences and economics.

Genetics

Signs and symptoms of most genetic problems appear during infancy or the toddler years, whereas other genetic problems will be noted during adolescence. Although genetic conditions diagnosed earlier in life can affect the preschooler's health, the nursing role focuses on continuing parent education, screening for complications of these conditions, and interventions related to improving the family's and child's coping with the genetic condition (Ettner, 1996; Forrest & Starfield, 1998; Gidding, 1999; Guyer, Hughart, Strobino, Jones, & Scharfstein, 2000).

GORDON'S FUNCTIONAL HEALTH PATTERNS

Health Perception-Health Management Pattern

Preschoolers have a fairly accurate perception of the external parts of their own bodies based on what they can see and do; they may be extremely curious about the body of a member of the opposite sex. Their concept of what is inside the body and how the internal functions of the body operate are vague and inaccurate. Preschoolers view the internal part of the body as hollow. Most preschoolers can name one or two items inside the body (blood, bones). Many of their questions about body function involve "having babies."

By age 4 or 5, children have amassed many beliefs about health from the family. An understanding begins that they are partly responsible for their own health. The preschooler often becomes upset over minor injuries. Pain or illness is frequently viewed as a punishment. The preschooler's declaration, "If you don't brush your teeth, your teeth will rot and fall out," is probably a statement of expected immediate and absolute cause and effect. Dental caries in children have declined dramatically in recent years because of preventive measures such as toothbrushing with fluoride toothpaste, community water fluoridation, sound dietary practices, and dental sealants. Approximately 80% of dental caries today is concentrated in 25% of children, especially children in low-income families (Tang et al., 1997; Vargas, Crall, & Schneider, 1998). Oral health promotion involves not only self-care and population-based initiatives, but also professional care. Adequacy of professional dental care varies significantly by age, race, level of education, family income, and dental status (U.S. Department of Health and Human Services, 2000, p. 21-27).

Although preschoolers are not completely responsible for their own health management, they certainly contribute by brushing their teeth, taking medication, wearing appropriate clothing for inclement weather, and performing other actions. Preschoolers' memory for these activities can be sporadic, but they are, at least, beginning to be health care agents for themselves (Mobley & Evashevsk, 2000).

Reinforcement of health-promotion activities can occur in the home and the child care environment, which includes behaviors that affect self-esteem, safety, and an individual's overall balance with life (American College of Preventive Medicine, 1998; Athey & Milner, 2000; Klerman, 1997; Sword, 1997; Cagle & Keen-Payne, 1996; Wood, 1995). Many community bookstores carry health promotion-focused books appropriate to the preschooler population; these references can provide special times and information for interesting discussion among parents, caregivers, and children on the importance of healthy behaviors for success in life (Box 19-2).

Nutritional-Metabolic Pattern

Establishing a balance between healthful nutritional behaviors and physical activity begins in childhood. The Dietary Guidelines for Americans (2000) recommends that children 2 years of age and older should eat a variety of foods plentiful in vegetables, fruits, and grains; moderate in salt and sugar; and low in fat, especially saturated fats (see Table 19-2). The guidelines also advise adequate consumption of calcium-rich and iron-rich foods. The prevalence of iron deficiency anemia continues to be higher in low-income families compared with moderate- or high-income families (McBean & Miller, 1999; Williams, Bollella, & Wynder, 1995).

The average preschooler needs approximately 90 kcal/kg of body weight per day for health maintenance, activity, and growth. Table 19-2 lists a typical daily distribution of foods that provides the essential calories and nutrients for the preschooler. As early childhood progresses, intense expressions of food preferences emerge. This behavior is a natural outgrowth of the increased physical capacity to react to the taste and textures of foods and the realization that expressing an opinion about food is a way in which a person can control the environment. Preschoolers are likely to reject cooked vegetables, mixed dishes, and liver. Older preschoolers are likely to refuse to try new foods. Favorite foods for this age are meat, cereal grains, baked products, fruits, and sweets. Parents should provide nutritious foods, avoid offering salty foods (especially when a family history of hypertension is present), and sweet foods. Parents should encourage good nutritional habits to help establish healthy eating behaviors in preschoolers

Box 19-2 Preschooler Health Promotion: Literature for Children and Parents to Share

SELF-SUFFICIENCY AND INDEPENDENCE

Bingham, M. (1987). *Minou.* Santa Barbara, CA: Advocacy Press.

Dickson, A. H. (1986). *Grover's bad, awful day.* Racine, WI: Western.

Elliott, D. (1982). *Grover goes to school.* New York: Random House, Children's Television Network.

Johnson, C. (1955). *Harold and the purple crayon.* New York: Harper & Row.

Kingsley, E. P. (1980). *I can do it myself.* Racine, WI: Western.

Munsch, R. N. (1980). *The paper bag princess.* Toronto: Annick Press.

Tyrrell, A. (1987). *Elizabeth Jane gets dressed.* New York: Barron's.

BEDTIME

Geisel, T. S. (1962). *Dr. Seuss's sleep book.* New York: Random House.

Mayer, M. (1968). *There's a nightmare in my closet.* New York: Dial.

LOVE, FAMILIES, AND BELONGING

Berenstain, J., & Berenstain, S. (1974). *The Berenstain Bears' new baby.* New York: Random House.

Brown, M. W. (1942). *The runaway bunny.* New York: Harper & Row.

Caines, J. (1982). *Just us women.* New York: Harper & Row.

Munsch, R. (1986). *Love you forever.* Willowdale, Ontario: Firefly Books.

SELF-ESTEEM

Balter, L. (1989). *Linda saves the day.* New York: Barron's.

Brainard, B. (1992). *You can't sell your brother at the garage sale: The kids' book of values.* New York: Dell.

Larche, D. (1985). *Father gander nursery rhymes: The equal rhymes amendment.* Santa Barbara, CA: Advocacy Press.

Lobel, A. (1979). *Days with frog and toad.* New York: Scholastic.

Navarra, T. (1989). *On my own: Helping kids help themselves.* Hauppauge, NY: Barron's.

Sendak, M. (1963). *Where the wild things are.* New York: Harper & Row.

DISCIPLINE

Berenstain, J., & Berenstain, S. (1990). *The Berenstain Bears and the slumber party.* New York: Random House.

Potter, B. (1986). *The tale of Peter Rabbit.* New York: Scholastic.

Scarry, R. (1989). *Richard Scarrey's naughty bunny.* Racine, WI: Western.

Sendak, M. (1961). *What do you do, dear?* New York: Addison-Wesley.

(Variyam, Blaylock, Lin, Ralston, & Smallwood, 1999; Troiano & Flegal, 1998).

Improper nutrition (including increased consumption of fats and processed foods) and diminished physical activity (including increased television watching) contribute to the emergence of obesity and type 2 diabetes in children and adolescents (U.S. Department of Health and Human Services, 2000; Fagot-Campagna, Rios-Burrow, & Williamson, 1999; Rosenbloom, Joe, Young, & Winter, 1999; Cristoffel & Ariza, 1998; Troiano & Flegal, 1998).

Families vary in their tolerance for expressed individual food preferences and children vary in their tendency to develop strong likes and dislikes. When a family and a child reach extreme differences over this matter, major conflicts arise and insightful counseling and support may be needed until some mutually satisfying solution is reached. The nurse provides assessment of the nutritional adequacy of the foods preferred and required by the child, collaborates with the family to discover comfortable approaches to handle the situation, and maintains a flexible approach to the wide range of possibilities that exist for all families of varying cultures in providing the essential nutrients for growth and development (Henchy, 1993).

Many preschoolers eat at least one meal a day at the baby-sitter's house, day care facility, or school. Licensed child care centers and preschools are required to serve approved foods that provide a required percentage of the recommended daily allowances of basic nutrients. Parents should inquire periodically about the foods their child eats while away from home to understand the child's food habits and to provide a varied diet important for growth. Preschoolers in group settings can learn positive or negative eating skills and food preferences from the teacher and other children; communication of these habits from the child's caregiver to the parents allows reinforcement or discouragement of the negative habits at home.

The young preschooler still struggles with the intricacies of using silverware. The older preschooler is skilled with a spoon, demonstrates fair proficiency with a fork, and manages a knife for spreading soft foods on bread or crackers. However, the child may still need help cutting meat and pouring from a large, heavy container.

Preschoolers may enjoy helping to prepare family meals and may be capable of making their own sandwiches. Involvement of young children in meal preparation serves as a valuable parental opportunity to teach children about "good" foods that support health. Working with a family member also nurtures preschoolers' self-esteem and sense of value primarily because they are completing an important duty for their family.

Table 19-2 Food Pattern for Preschool Children, Ages 4 to 6*

Food	Portion Size	Number of Recommended Portions
MILK AND DAIRY PRODUCTS		
Milk†	4 oz	3 to 4
Cheese	1/2 to 3/4 oz	May be substituted for 1 portion of liquid milk
Yogurt	1/4 to 1/2 cup	May be substituted for 1 portion of liquid milk
Powdered skim milk	2 tbsp	May be substituted for 1 portion of liquid milk
MEAT AND MEAT EQUIVALENTS		
Meat,‡ fish,§ poultry	1 to 2 oz	2
Egg	1	1
Peanut butter	1 to 2 tbsp	
Legumes: dried peas and beans	1/4 to 1/3 cup cooked	
VEGETABLES AND FRUITS		
Vegetables‖		4 to 5; includes 1 green leafy or yellow
Cooked	2 to 4 tbsp	
Raw	Few pieces	
Fruit		1 citrus fruit or other food rich in vitamin C
Canned	4 to 8 tbsp	
Raw	1/2 to 1, small	
Fruit juice	3 to 4 oz	
BREAD AND CEREAL GRAINS		
Whole-grain or enriched white bread	1/2 to 1 slice	3
Cooked cereal	1/4 to 1/2 cup	May be substituted for 1 serving of bread
Ready-to-serve dry cereals	1/2 to 1 cup	
Spaghetti, macaroni, noodles, rice	1/4 to 1/2 cup	
Crackers	2 to 3	
FAT		
Bacon	1 slice	
Butter or vitamin A-fortified margarine	1 tsp	3 to 4
DESSERTS	1/4 to 1/2 cup	
SUGARS	1/2 to 1 tsp	2

*Diets should be monitored for adequate intake of iron and vitamin D.
†Approximately 2/3 cup can be incorporated easily in the child's food during cooking.
‡Liver once a week can be prepared as liver sausage or cooked liver.
§Should be served once or twice per week to substitute for meat.
‖When child's preferences are limited, use double portions of preferred vegetables until appetite for other vegetables develops.
From Pipes, P. L. (1993). *Nutrition in infancy and childhood* (4th ed.). St. Louis: Mosby.

"Although most food-borne illness results from a microbial or chemical contaminant in food, a food itself can also cause severe adverse reactions. In the United States, food allergy is an important problem. Two to four percent of children under the age of 6 years . . . are allergic to specific foods. The foods most likely to cause allergic reactions are milk and milk products, eggs and egg products, peanuts and peanut products, tree nuts and tree nut products, soybean and soybean products, fish and fish products, shellfish and shellfish products, cereals containing glutens, and seeds. Allergic reactions to natural rubber latex from food handlers' gloves also occur" (U.S. Department of Health and Human Services, 2000, pp. 10-15). Clear food labeling and education are essential for preventing these allergic reactions. Many preschools have banned foods, such as peanut products, as a precautionary measure.

Elimination Pattern

By the end of the preschool period, most children are capable of and responsible for independent toileting, although they can forget to flush or wash their hands because of being in a hurry rather than lacking the skills. Preschoolers who have occasional "accidents" should not be teased or punished; they should be responsible for changing their clothes and gently reminded that they can do better next time. (Enuresis and encopresis are discussed in Chapter 20.)

Activity-Exercise Pattern

Play continues to be the primary activity of the preschooler and toddler group. The preschooler explores intently and motor activities begin to demonstrate coordination and confidence. The child ventures farther from home than can the toddler. Many play activities involve other children and may involve modeling the behavior of others. Particularly in group care settings, children should be monitored for safe activities that will enhance their gross- and fine-motor skills and create fun in movement.

Most 4-year-old children separate easily from their parents, play simple interactive games, dress themselves, copy a number of basic geometric figures well, and draw recognizable people. Preschoolers enjoy using language skills in telling stories and asking questions and they can balance on one foot, jump, and run well (Frankenburg, Dodds, Archer, Shapiro, & Bresnick, 1990; Health Education Authority, 1997). Generally, these children love an audience and they enjoy practicing new skills and demonstrating mastered skills to others.

Play constitutes an important role in preschoolers' social and inner development. Play serves as a vehicle for exploring and experimenting with the ways of the world, for determining who they are, who they might become, and how they relate to others socially. The drama of play allows them to get outside of themselves and comprehend themselves momentarily from another perspective. Play often reveals the child's inner reality and perception of the world.

Children "act out" the behavior of people familiar to them, rehearsing what has been demonstrated to them as appropriate behavior. Young children seldom assume the role of a younger child or infant in playing "house"; more frequently, they assume mommy or daddy roles and use a doll for the younger child. Through play, preschoolers learn to exert control over their own behavior; in voluntarily assuming an adultlike role, children consciously adopt a more mature form of behavior than is typical for their age. Children can be observed expressing displeasure and anger in a play situation by vocalizing their distress, scolding the offending party, or using withdrawal of attention. When confronted with a similar, but real, anger-provoking situation, these children would more likely respond with aggression, crying, or tantrum behavior. Observation of play reveals children's physical capacities in a natural setting better than that of the examination or testing environment and provides further evidence of their social and inner development.

Social competency can be estimated by observing a child's play in peer groups or through observing imitation play. The new child in a peer group may be expected to stand back and simply observe other children for a time and then approach and begin manipulating a toy object. During the preschool period, the child engages in more interactive play, particularly make-believe play. Two or more children may become involved in a make-believe plot, especially when toys and equipment support a particular plot, such as toy kitchen equipment. Much of the preschooler's play involves fantasy. The 4- to 5-year-old child frequently invents an imaginary companion who plays, eats, and sleeps with the child. (The primary aspects of fantasy and the preschooler are discussed in the section on cognition and perception.)

Most preschoolers spend time in a group setting at least several times a week. Generally, some ground rules at these facilities govern sharing of play materials, quiet times, and group activities. The preschooler appears able to regulate bodily activity better than does the toddler and does not become as frustrated by basic rules compared with the toddler.

Although the concept of time remains incompletely developed in preschoolers, they have an idea of the passage of time and of past and future. Children can enjoy planning activities with their parents for the future. A trip to the zoo may be prefaced by getting library books about wild animals, selecting and helping to pack lunches the night before, and discussing what clothes to wear.

Many preschoolers spend long periods each day watching television. Occasionally, parents who need time to themselves use the television inappropriately as a quasi-babysitter. Although some excellent television shows are available for preschoolers, a significant amount of air time focuses on adult themes and violence. Many experts agree that television watching cannot engage the child's mind in the same way as can participatory involvement with play activities and people. Therefore watching television supports less learning (see Chapter 20). Parents should remember that preschoolers who watch television (1) do not have enough life experiences to interpret many of the issues presented in adult shows (violence, interpersonal relationships, moral decisions), (2) might be missing opportunities for interacting with other children or adults and other opportunities for active learning, and (3) cannot judge which shows are appropriate for them.

Parents should choose which shows are appropriate for their child and, when possible, watch these shows with the child, which provides an opportunity for discussion and for the child to ask questions (American Academy of Pediatrics, 1999a, 1999b; American Academy of Pediatrics, Committee on Public Education, 1999; Strasburger & Donnerstein, 1999). Nurses also explain to parents and preschoolers the relationships between watching television and physical activity leading to health problems such as obesity (Anderson, Crespo, Bartlett, Cheskin, & Pratt, 1998).

Sleep-Rest Pattern

Most preschoolers sleep from 8 to 12 hours during the night, with wide variation from child to child. For many older preschoolers, a nap is not necessary. The preschooler who still naps usually requires only 30 to 60 minutes a day (Berger, 1991). Similar to some toddlers, a "quiet time" in the afternoon can provide a welcome respite for the parent and a change for the active preschooler to relax before afternoon activities. Many child care environments routinely provide these rest periods, enhancing rest and sleep with soft music and a story before sleep. This afternoon rest can also allow the preschooler to work better within the family later in the day, when family members have other duties beyond work and school.

Bedtime Ritual

Many preschoolers require a ritual of activities at bedtime to help them make the transition from playing and being with others to being alone and falling asleep. The 4- and 5-year-old child is more likely than is the toddler to prolong the bedtime routine, insist on sleeping with the light on, take a treasured object to bed, request parental attention after being told good night, and experience delays in falling asleep. The bedtime ritual can take 30 minutes or longer. Rituals that appear reasonable should be honored by the parent; repeated requests for attention after the ritual has been completed should generally be handled firmly and consistently by the parent. Based on the child's temperament, vigorous resistance to bedtime can be more of a problem in the preschool period compared with the toddler period. Preschoolers may learn to act a certain way to meet their needs and control the family by their bedtime behavior, despite the family disruption that this behavior creates.

Nursing Interventions

When bedtime behavior has been a problem for a year or more or lasts longer than 1 hour, the nurse gathers a comprehensive history, which includes the following:

1. Description of early episodes
2. The manner in which these early episodes were managed and the progression of events since the first episodes
3. Current bedtime behaviors of the child and siblings
4. Identification of parental temperament and the resulting responses of parent and family members
5. Feelings of the parents and child about each other and about the bedtime situation
6. Stressful events and changes that have occurred over the last several years
7. Behavior of the child at other times of the day
8. Parents' thoughts on the reasons for which this episode has continued this long
9. Parents' ideas on the ways in which they can deal with the situation now

The nurse then observes interactions between the parents and child; an excellent way to accomplish this task is to go into the home and observe active interaction, such as that during mealtime. In the office or clinic setting, the nurse can ask the parent to teach the child a task or give directions. The nurse is as unobtrusive as possible while observing the interaction. The first-hand observation of parent-child interaction, along with the detailed history, usually provide the nurse with adequate baseline information to decide whether this situation can be managed in a primary care setting or should be referred to a child behavior specialist. Nurses may wish to refer parents to recent literature on management techniques for children with differing temperament characteristics; research has shown that these techniques help parents reach their goals for managing bedtime concerns with preschoolers (Melvin, 1995).

Discipline and management of misbehavior, which includes long-term bedtime resistance, is discussed in the roles and relationships section later in this chapter.

Sleep Disturbances

Nighttime wakening occurs often in the preschool years and are of two types: (1) night terrors and (2) nightmares (anxiety dreams). **Night terrors** appear to be frightening dreams that cause the child to sit up in bed, often scream, stare at an imaginary object, breathe heavily, perspire, and appear in obvious distress (see Chapter 18). The child, who is generally not fully awake and can be inconsolable for 10 minutes or more, then relaxes and returns to a deep sleep. The child, in many cases, does not recall the dream and in the morning does not remember the incident. These night terrors can start at approximately age 2, but are more common during the preschool years. Night terrors rarely occur in older children and adults and only approximately 6% of preschool children have night terrors. When these events occur, they can be extremely upsetting for the parents.

Nightmares (anxiety dreams) represent a much more common cause of night wakening. Although infants and toddlers likely have nightmares, their limited verbal skills make it difficult to document. From age 3 on, children have fairly frequent nightmares. Approximately 20% of the night is spent dreaming; not surprisingly, many dreams are frightening for preschoolers, who have become connected to the larger world and have many fantasy ideas and active imaginations. These children usually fully waken and can feel fearful and helpless; usually, they can vividly describe the dream at the time; and they frequently remember the event in the morning. Parents or baby-sitters should go to the children, listen to their descriptions and fears about the dream, and then reassure them that they were only dreaming and that they need to return to sleep.

Use of the words "pretend" and "real" can be helpful at this age. When the parent reads a story to the child or the child tells a make-believe tale, the parents can specify that these are "pretend" and did not really happen. The parent relating a true event can say, "This is real." As the child differentiates these two concepts, nightmares and fears related to sleep can be defined according to whether they are real or pretend.

Recommendations

Parents of a preschooler can benefit from knowing the following facts:

1. Bedtime rituals of 30 to 45 minutes are common for preschoolers. These rituals, because of their importance to children, should be respected within reasonable limits.
2. Night-wakening events are common in the preschool years. Children who waken at night should be reassured and encouraged to remain in their own beds. Parents should have clear rules about children sleeping with them if the children will not stay in their own beds.
3. Restricting frightening television shows and stories and discussing "real" versus "pretend" ideas and stories can help lessen the incidence of nightmares.

Cognitive-Perceptual Pattern

During the preschool years, the child makes great gains in conceptual and cognitive capacity; this is often enhanced by time spent in a quality child care environment. Concepts of time emerge and the child gradually differentiates today from yesterday and defines tomorrow and the future. The child becomes more oriented in space and develops an awareness of the location of the home within the neighborhood. The child also begins to structure daily activities and to value certain activities, objects, and people above others.

Piaget's Theory

The older toddler enters the first substage of the **preoperational stage** described by Jean Piaget (see Chapter 18). The hallmark of this preconceptual substage includes the ability to function symbolically using language. The preschool child demonstrates increased symbolic functioning during the intuitive substage, from age 4 to 7 years. The predominant feature of this and the following period is the concreteness of the thought processes in comparison with adult thinking. Preschoolers, who begin to experience symbolic mental representations, simply run through all the occurring mental symbols as though they were actually participating in the event. An adult analyzes and synthesizes symbolic information, making the mental connection with the real event unnecessary. At this stage, preschoolers cannot perform mental gymnastics, such as skipping from one part of an operation to another, reversing the operation mentally, or thinking of the whole in relation to the parts.

Preschoolers' concreteness of thinking shows in their limitation of **egocentrism.** At this stage, children cannot conceptualize another person's point of view; they can only consider meanings relative to their own attached meanings and symbols and cannot understand why another person fails to follow these idiosyncratic communications.

Furthermore, the child is unable to shift attention from one part of an object or event to another part when attention is focused on a particular aspect. This behavior, termed **centering** by Piaget, illustrates the child's inability to consider more than one factor in solving a simple problem. For example, a child can be given two identical cups containing equal amounts of water and asked which cup contains the greater amount of water. During the preoperational stage, the child responds that they contain the same amount of water. The child is then asked to pour the water from each cup into two different containers (one flat and wide, the other tall and narrow). When asked which container has more water, the child always identifies one, usually the taller, narrower container in which the water reaches a higher level. When the water is again transferred to the equal cups and the experiment repeated, the child continues to respond precisely as before.

This experiment also illustrates the trait of **irreversibility.** The child is unable to connect the reversible operation, the transfer of the water back into the original cup, and make the logical conclusion that the differently shaped containers hold the same amount of water. The child cannot mentally associate that the transformation from one state to another does not relate to the amount of water, but of the shape of the container.

Finally, Piaget describes the preoperative stage of thinking as using **transductive reasoning.** The child is unable to proceed from general to particular (deduction) or from particular to general (induction); rather, the child moves only from particular to particular in making associations and solving problems. For example, Piaget relates an association made by one of his children between being hunchbacked and being ill. When a hunchbacked neighbor was unable to visit one day because he had a communicable illness, the child understood that the neighbor was ill. However, when the child was told later that the neighbor was better and that she could go see him, her conclusion was that now his hunched back was straight and well. She thought in terms of the man being well or ill, but she placed the man in one or the other category and assumed that he possessed all the attributes and meanings that she linked symbolically with either trait.

The cognitive development of preschoolers is reflected in their play with symbolic games, which becomes significantly more orderly and representative of reality (Box 19-3). Children begin to incorporate the reality of the world as it exists outside the self; they increasingly seek play

Box 19-3 Play As a Method of Learning: Preschool-Age Child

Throughout life, play develops cognitive, affective, and psychomotor skills that are important to the effective performance of life skills. For the preschool-age child, the following play activities provide the foundation for later competency and socialization-skill refinement:

- Arts and crafts (jewelry making, painting, drawing, ceramics, printmaking)
- Group sports (softball, volleyball, soccer, swimming)
- Skating, skateboarding
- Bicycling
- Puzzles
- Gymnastics
- Games (board, card, knock-knock jokes, computer)
- Secret clubs
- Imaginary play (being in playhouse productions)
- Horseback riding

objects that represent models of authentic objects in the environment and increasingly imitate the social rules of society. Social interactive play becomes more predominant as they develop a more secure sense of self.

The preschooler may have one or more imaginary companions who exist for varying periods. These fantasy companions can take the form of another child, an animal, or some other friendly or fearsome creature. The preschooler may save special chairs, insist that an extra place be set at the table, and talk at length to this companion. Imaginary companions serve an important function; they are totally controlled by the child and are not a threat. The preschooler can practice social interactions, control a fearsome beast, or blame someone for naughty behavior without fear of scolding, shame, or attack, primarily because the imaginary companion can do and say only what the child wills. Sensory abilities contribute to the preschooler's skills in perceiving and interacting with the world.

Vision

Vision capabilities, which are well developed by 2 years of age, continue to undergo refinement during the early childhood period; by approximately age 6, the child should approach a 20/20 visual acuity level. The possibility of developing **amblyopia** decreases, which appears most frequently during infancy through approximately the fourth year (see Chapter 18). Depth perception and color vision become fully established; the child recognizes subtle differences in color shading by the sixth year. Maximal visual capability is usually achieved by the end of the preschool years.

Visual capacity throughout the rest of life deteriorates rather than improves. This phenomenon relates partly to changes in the refractive power of the lens and developmental changes that occur in the shape of the eyeball. In the normal sequence of growth, the eyeball becomes increasingly spherical, losing the short shape typical of infancy and progressing to the point at which light converges accurately on the surface of the retina. This change occurs at approximately 6 years of age. When this change occurs before the sixth year, growth continues past the point of ideal light conversion, the eyeball lengthens, and the child may develop early **myopic vision,** which will progress with age. Glasses are always indicated for the child who develops myopia before approximately age 8.

The preschool child's vision must be screened on a regular basis, usually by using the Denver Eye Screening Test or the Snellen Screening Test. The Denver Eye Screening Test was designed particularly for preschool children and includes detection of the commonly occurring visual problems, such as **refractive errors, strabismus** (crossing of the eyes), and amblyopia.

The Snellen screening test, when administered under standardized procedures, has the advantage of rendering a reliable estimate of the actual visual acuity of the child. The child must be able to understand the test requirements of either pointing in the direction of the Es or naming the letters.

The **Snellen E chart** is designed for preschool children; a version for home testing is available from the National Society for Prevention of Blindness. Home testing has been demonstrated to be reliable and offers the advantage of obtaining an estimate for younger children who might not cooperate with this type of testing in a strange environment.

The pupillary light reflex provides a screening approach for **heterotropia,** a condition in which the child's eyes do not focus together to transmit effective, coordinated binocular vision. When the child has developed heterotropia, the light from a penlight held approximately 20 inches from the eyes reflects off the pupil slightly off center. Consistent and observable strabismus may be noted. The cover test provides further evidence of a tendency for the child's eyes to cross, known as **heterophoria.** The child focuses on a spot 14 inches away, then 20 feet away. As the child gazes at the designated spot, one eye is covered completely for several seconds (the eye and eyelashes must not be touched), and then the cover is removed abruptly. If the covered eye moves from the line of vision of the uncovered eye, that eye has a tendency toward muscle imbalance and must be evaluated further (Seidel, Ball, Dains, & Benedict, 1991).

Color blindness presents a particular problem for younger children, particularly in relation to school, because many cues that are encountered in the school setting depend on the ability to distinguish colors. Early detection can result in the child receiving some assistance with learning to interpret visual perceptions; therefore the disadvantage is minimized. The nurse screens for certain types of color discrimination difficulties by asking the child to respond to various colors in the environment; however, adequate testing for all types of color blindness requires the use of a specialized test, such as **Ishihara's test,** which uses a series of cards with color-tinted letters and figures.

The preschooler may be aware of some discomfort or limitations with vision. The nurse gathers history from the parents, including the questions listed in Chapter 18 about signs of eye problems. The preschooler is asked questions to elicit information about the following:

1. Itching, burning, or "scratchy" eyes
2. Poor vision
3. Dizziness, headaches, or nausea after close eye work
4. Blurred or double vision

Hearing

During the preschool period, hearing develops to its optimal level and listening (the ability to attend to and interpret what is heard) becomes more refined compared with the toddler period. The 4-year-old preschooler begins to make fine discriminations among similar speech sounds, such as the difference between sounds made with f and th or f and s. Adequate hearing ability of the preschooler can be hindered by repeated ear infections (otitis media). Parents who notice language delays because of ear infections should be referred to their health care provider for appropriate follow-up (Yoshinaga-Itano, Sedy, Coulter, & Mehl, 1998).

Audiometric methods detect the child's ability to hear most accurately. Without an audiometer, a rough estimate of hearing capacity can be made by whispering instructions when the child's back is turned and observing the ability of the child to hear and respond accurately (Joint Committee on Infant Hearing, 2000).

Most preschoolers enjoy demonstrating their abilities and cooperate easily during vision and hearing screening. The nurse ensures that screening will be a positive experience by following certain points (Box 19-4).

Box 19-4 Nurse's Interventions for Screening the Vision and Hearing of Preschoolers

- Being skilled in the use of the equipment
- Avoiding the term test, because even some preschoolers have come to associate test with anxiety and possibly failure
- Allowing the child to ask questions and examine the equipment
- Performing vision and hearing screening early in the visit before anything intrusive or painful
- Performing screening in a quiet, private area such that the child is not distracted by people or noises
- Praising the child for cooperating
- Taking a brief break when the child becomes distracted or tired
- Discussing the results of the screening with the child using simple, positive terms

Sensory Perception

As vision and hearing acuity reach more mature levels during the preschool years, visual and hearing perception also become more mature. The preschool child may perceive visual stimuli in a diffuse, global manner or in a detail-specific manner. The nature of the stimulus appears to be the primary factor in determining which response will occur. The preschooler is highly susceptible to visual illusions and has difficulty discriminating right and left mirror images, which explains the confusion with letters such as b, d, p, and q.

Auditory perception is at the level of accepting whole words or phrases without analysis or the level of selecting only certain sounds within the whole.

Language

All of these cognitive and sensory abilities contribute to the preschooler's language development. By the time the child reaches the end of the preschool period, **expressive language** may be similar to that of adults except for minor deficiencies in refinement, vocabulary, and structure. The degree to which a child fulfills this ability depends on the aptitude for language, the opportunity for using the language, the quality and quantity of language used at home, and the range of experiences of the child. Regardless of the child's expressive capacity, the development of **receptive language** during the preschool years is believed to be vital, particularly because this ability provides the foundation for later expressive ability. Throughout early childhood, receptive capacity exceeds expressive capacity; children can comprehend the meaning of words and phrases that are not a part of the expressive vocabulary and can make associations between concepts although they are unable to explain these concepts. Table 19-3 outlines the receptive and expressive language skills of the preschooler.

During the early childhood years, the development of rhythm is an important dimension in the development of speech capacity. Between ages 3 and 5, children begins to practice talking as adults; this serves to develop neuromotor capacities for adult language, to stimulate verbal interaction, and to develop vocabulary and a sense of grammatical structure. These attempts are reflected in hesitations, repetitions, and frequent revisions in speech, which may be labeled by adults as stuttering, but actually represent normal speech immaturity. Many authorities believe that stuttering originates during this developmental period, arising not from an inadequacy in the child, but rather, from the response of adults to this normal broken pattern of speech. These reactions can include impatience in waiting to listen to the child's lengthy attempts to express thoughts, which decreases the child's opportunities to use language and the insistence that the child correct this pattern of speech before the capacity for fluent speech is developed. Suggestions for the nurse to give parents to facilitate the preschool child's language development are listed in Box 19-5.

Table 19-3 Landmarks of Speech, Language, and Hearing Ability During the Preschool Period

Age (months)	Receptive Language	Expressive Language	Related Hearing Ability
42	Up to 4200 words; knows words such as *what, where, how, funny, we, surprise, secret;* knows number concepts to 2; knows how to answer questions accurately, such as, *do you have a dog, which is the girl, what toys do you have?*	Up to 1200 words in mostly complete sentences averaging four to five words per sentence; uses all 50 phonemes; 7% of sentences are compound or complex; averages 203 words per hour; rate of speech is accelerating; relates experiences and tells about activities in sequential order; uses words such as *what, where, how, see, little, funny, they, we, he, she, several;* can recite a nursery rhyme; asks permission; 95% of speech is intelligible.	—
48	Up to 5600 words; carries out three-item commands consistently; knows why people have houses, books, umbrella, key; knows nearly all colors; knows words such as *somebody, anybody, even, almost, now, something, like, bigger, too,* full name, one or two songs, number concepts to 4; understands most preschool stories; can complete opposite analogies, such as *brother is a boy, sister is a girl* and *in daytime it is light, at night it is dark.*	Up to 1500 words in sentences averaging five to six words per sentence; averages 400 words per hour; counts up to 3, repeats four digits, names three objects, and repeats nine-word sentences from memory; names the primary colors, some coins; relates fanciful tales; enjoys rhyming nonsense words and using exaggerations; demands reasons why and how; questioning is at a peak, up to 500 a day; passes judgment on own activity; can recite a poem from memory or sing a song; uses words such as *even, almost, something, like, but;* typical expressions might include, *I'm so tired, you almost hit me, now I'll make something else.*	Begins to make the fine discriminations among similar speech sounds, such as the difference between *f* and *th* or *f* and *s.* Child has matured enough to be tested with an audiometer. At this age, formal hearing testing usually can be carried out. Not only has hearing developed to its optimal level, but listening has also become considerably refined.
54	Up to 6500 words; knows of what a house, window, chair, and dress are made and what people do with the eyes and ears; understands differences in texture and composition, such as *hard, soft, rough, smooth;* begins to name or point to penny, nickel, dime; understands *if, because, why, when.*	Up to 1800 words in sentences averaging five to six words; now averages only 230 words per hour—is satisfied with less verbalization; does little commanding or demanding; likes surprises; about 1 in 10 sentences is compound or complex, and only 8% of sentences are incomplete; can define 10 common words and counts up to 20; common expressions are *I don't know, I said, tiny, funny, because;* asks questions for information and learns to manipulate and control people and situations with language.	—
60	Up to 9600 words; knowsnumber concepts to 5; knows and names colors; defines words in terms of use, such as *a horse is to ride;* defines *wind, ball, hat, stove;* understands words such as *if, because, when;* knows for what purpose *horse, fork,* and *legs* are used; begins to understand *right* and *left.*	Up to 2200 words in sentences averaging six words; can define *ball, hat, stove, policeman, wind, horse, fork;* can count five objects and repeat four or five digits; definitions are in terms of use; can single out a word and ask its meaning; makes serious inquiries—*what is this for, how does this work, who made those, what does it mean;* language is now essentially complete in structure and form; uses all types of sentences, clauses, and parts of speech; reads by way of pictures, and prints simple words.	—

Modified from Chinn, P. L. (1979). *Child health maintenance: Concepts in family-centered care* (2nd ed.). St. Louis: Mosby.

Box 19-5 Nursing Suggestions to Encourage Language Development in Preschoolers

- Read to the child. Encourage the child to be an active listener by pausing at times during the story to ask questions, such as, "What do you think will happen next?" and "Why do you think the boy said that?" and "What would you do now?"
- Praise the child's storytelling and creativity with stories.
- Always respond to the child's questions. Occasionally, a response must be delayed; for example, when the parent is driving in heavy traffic and the child asks a question that requires a complex answer, the parent might say, "That's a very good question; let's talk about that as soon as we get home." The parent should remind the child of the question later and respond if the child still expresses interest.
- Never tease or criticize a child about talking style. If the child speaks so fast as to be fumbling over words, then the parent might say, "I can't listen that fast. Slow down a little for me." This is much more encouraging than is the statement, "You talk too fast. No one can understand you."
- Play games that are language-focused, such as naming the colors of houses or kinds of flowers as parent and child walk to the store.

Memory

Memory makes up an important component of language development and of learning in general. At the preschool level, the child can label pictures, group objects, or mimic others as ways to aid memory, although the preschooler does not perform these tasks with the precision of the school-age child. The younger child benefits when an adult suggests the stimuli or the characteristics of an object or action that should be used for grouping. Preschoolers can remember pictures better by saying the name of the picture rather than simply hearing the name when the picture is first shown.

Preschoolers do not use rehearsal or other **mnemonic strategies** (techniques for remembering things) spontaneously, but they use and benefit from rehearsal when suggested (Berger, 1991). The nurse tests memory by asking the child to repeat an arbitrary sequence of numbers. By approximately age 5, children should be able to repeat four consecutively named numbers easily.

Testing of Developmental Level

Parents of preschoolers frequently ask how to determine whether their child is ready for school or for a particular school program. School readiness can be considered as the "fit" among the child's skill level, the child and family's psychosocial status, and the characteristics of the particular school program. Any questions about an individual child's readiness should be answered only after all of these components have been addressed. The developmental testing used during the toddler years appears less accurate as the child approaches school age. Some appropriate tools can help identify the child's skill level.

A widely used tool is the **Preschool Readiness Experimental Screening Scale** (PRESS) (Fig. 19-2). Based on research, the PRESS shows reliability in assessing school readiness. The nurse administers the test easily during a child's health assessment to screen for developmental lags or abnormalities that might interfere with the child's ability to succeed in the academic and social world of school. The tool was constructed for the average capabilities of 5-year-old children, but can be useful in estimating readiness in children slightly older or younger. The test does not measure intellectual level.

When obtaining more specific scores of developmental age becomes necessary, the nurse uses one of the screening tools specific to the preschool child. These screening tools provide only a rough estimate of ability, but can be useful in identifying children who need further extensive evaluation of intellectual capacity.

The **Bender Copy Forms** provide an estimate of the child's visual-motor perception. The child responds to standard figures by reproducing the figures in a timed situation; scoring of the child's responses occurs against normative data supplied with the test. This test does not depend on concepts or language peculiar to any cultural group; it is based on visual and motor perception of figures common to the experience of children in many cultural groups.

The **Peabody Picture Vocabulary Test** examines verbal intelligence, but is useful only with predominantly middle-class children who have acquired standard English-speaking ability. The score, when obtained reliably, estimates verbal intelligence ability when the child fits into this cultural group. For children who have received insufficient language stimulation or for those who come from another cultural group, a false low score can be obtained.

Draw-a-Person and Draw-a-Family tests are used to provide estimates of intelligence and interpretations of a child's emotional development; however, scoring of figure drawings requires administration under standardized conditions and evaluation by a qualified psychometric specialist. The nurse uses these drawings to assess general developmental expectations, fine-motor control, and evidence of concept formation. The child's perceptions of family relationships can also be assessed. The 4-year-old child is able to draw a person with at least six body parts that are placed in proximity to one another and in the appropriate locations. The child is able to name the parts; these need not be accurate representations, but should resemble the actual body parts and be drawn with strong, evenly flowing lines. The family drawing may not include all family members and the drawing of each figure may not be as sophisticated as is the child's actual figure-drawing capacity. The child is able to name the family members shown and describe any of their unique characteristics from the child's

Name ______________________ Birth Date ______________

School ______________________ Date ______________

1. a. What color is grass? ______
   b. What color is the sky if there are no clouds? ______

2. a. Repeat four numbers (one success in two tries): 4-1-7-3 or 3-8-6-4 ______
   b. Recognize four tongue blades. ______

3. a. Does Christmas come in the winter or the summer? ______
   b. Where is your heel? ______

4. Draw a square (best success in two tries). ______

5. a. Comprehension and performance ______
   b. Personal-social maturity ______

Total ______

Comments

PRESS General Outline and Record Form. The children were asked to reproduce a standard 1-inch square.

Introduction

As the child is placed on the examining table and the records and equipment are organized, the nurse says:

1. "Mrs. Smith, as I examine Johnny I will be asking him a few questions, so please don't talk to him for a few minutes." The nurse smiles and asks: "OK?"
2. "Johnny, I hear you're going to start kindergarten soon. Do you think you'll like that?"

Knowledge of colors

These questions are asked during the eye, ear, nose, and throat (EENT) examination:

1. "I hear your teacher will want you to know colors. Do you know any colors yet?"
2. "If she asks you to color a house, what color should you make the grass?"
3. "And what color should you make the sky if there are no clouds?"

Knowledge of numbers

1. "If the teacher tells you some numbers, could you remember them and repeat them back to her?"
2. "I'm going to tell you some numbers. Now you remember them and say the same number right back to me." (4-1-7-3 and 3-8-6-4)
3. "If the teacher asks you to count, could you do that?"
4. "Tell me, how many tongue blades are there?" At this point place four tongue blades on the table beside child.

General knowledge

These are asked as the abdomen, genitalia, and extremities are examined:

1. "I'm going to examine your tummy. You know where your tummy is, don't you?"
2. "Tell me, does Christmas come in the winter or summer?"
3. "Can you show me where your heel is?"

Fig. 19-2 Administration and scoring of the Preschool Readiness Experimental Screening Scale (PRESS). (From Rogers, Jr., W. B., & Rogers, R. A. [1972]. *Clinical Pediatrics, 11,* 10; Rogers, Jr., W. B., & Rogers, R. A. [1975]. *Clinical Pediatrics, 14,* 253.)

Continued

Drawing coordination

This is usually done at the end of the examination:

1. "If the teacher asked you to draw a square like this one (indicate the sample square), let's see you draw one just like it right beside mine. Take your time and make a good one."

General assessment: performance and maturity

These are best evaluated following the hearing and visual acuity tests when everything else is finished.

Scoring

Colors. 1 point for knowing grass is green. 1 point for knowing the sky is blue. Any other answer, such as white, blue and white, or black gets no point.

Numbers. 1 point for repeating the four numbers in the same sequence. If the child misses the first set of numbers, try the second set. Score 1 point for *either* set of numbers repeated back correctly. 1 point for answering the correct number of tongue blades as four. If the child only counts "one, two, three, four," this is not given a point. You may then ask the child *one time only*, "Yes, but how many are there all together?" If the child does not answer four at this time, score 0.

General Knowledge. 1 point for answering *winter*. It is important to suggest winter first. Most children will give the second of two choices if they do not know the correct answer. 1 point for knowing the heel. The child must point to the heel or the Achilles tendon, not to the malleolus.

Drawing Coordination. Allow the child to draw a second square if the first one is poorly done. Encourage the child to make the second more like the sample. Choosing the best square, score in the following manner:
- 2 points for drawing a good, readily recognizable square
- 1 point for drawing a fairly recognizable square
- 0 points for drawing a poor, unrecognizable square

Comprehension and Performance. 1 point for those who reply promptly and follow instructions well (for example, during the hearing and visual acuity tests). 0 points for those who have to be coaxed, need frequent repetition of instructions, or need repeated clarification of what you ask.

Personal-Social Maturity. 1 point if the child seems reasonably mature and self-confident. 0 points for:
- Excessive silliness or playing around
- Overtalkative or hyperactive
- Uncooperative, evasive, no interest
- Unduly attached to mother
- Generally immature compared with most 5-year-olds

It should be evident that the PRESS is not so much a standardized test with strict rules of administration as it is a set of standardized questions that can be blended into a physical examination. The nurse should note that it includes a few questions that are asked but not scored. These questions establish rapport and put the child at ease. They also serve as a lead-in to the test questions and serve indirectly in assessing the child's general maturity. Nurses may intersperse or substitute other lead-in questions if they think these would better express their method of dealing with children. It is important to ask the parent not to speak; an oversolicitious parent may interfere by offering help and encouragement.

Rating system

1. A score of 9 or 10 indicates high average to above average school readiness. A child in this score range should have no difficulty doing average or above average school work.
2. A score of 7 or 8 indicates average school readiness. A child in this score range should have little difficulty doing average school work.
3. A score of 6 indicates borderline school readiness. About half of the males and about a fourth of the females with this score may have difficulty in school. It is recommended that close liaison be maintained with teacher. If any time the child is not functioning at class level, further study should be made at once.
4. A score of 5 or less indicates insufficient school readiness. Such children should be referred to a school psychologist or diagnostic center for further psychological evaluation.

Fig. 19-2, cont'd Administration and scoring of the Preschool Readiness Experimental Screening Scale (PRESS). (From Rogers, Jr., W. B., & Rogers, R. A. [1972]. *Clinical Pediatrics, 11,* 10; Rogers, Jr., W. B., & Rogers, R. A. [1975]. *Clinical Pediatrics, 14,* 253.)

point of view. The child is also able to identify which figures are big or little, as drawn on the sheet of paper.

The nurse provides a pencil and plain sheet of paper and asks the child to draw the best picture possible. The child is informed that the nurse will keep the picture, but that another may be drawn to take home.

Self-Perception–Self-Concept Pattern

The preschooler starts with a basic concept of self that has emerged out of the personal struggle for autonomy as a toddler. The child continues to develop and refine this sense of self through both task-oriented and socially oriented experiences. By reinforcing the preschooler's skills and capabilities and successfully accomplishing tasks, self-esteem is built, enhancing overall health. Social experiences of acceptance help the child feel successful in the role of child, sibling, friend, and so on. The preschooler can try out other roles through a rich imagination. Pretend play of being the parents or baby allows the preschooler to imagine and act out the feelings of others, a safe way to experiment with new ideas (Cole & Cole, 1996; Crain, 2000).

In many child care environments, preschool children learn about their role as manager of the environment and

HEALTH TEACHING Health Promotion with Preschoolers: Environmental Accountability

Rationale in Teaching Preschoolers about the Protection of the Environment

- Environmental education at an early age will produce environmental practitioners of the future.
- Preschoolers can learn basic concepts of environmental accountability and gain a sense of empowerment when they perceive that they make a difference to the future world.
- Health care providers, in consultation with child care settings, can promote environmental education that is based on their knowledge of child growth and development and concerns about overall health.

Basic Ways for Preschoolers to Help the Environment and Promote Overall Societal Health

- Use water wisely.
- Use electricity only when necessary.
- Recycle all acceptable products.
- Avoid using balloons.
- Plant trees, protect plants, and grow a garden.
- Create a compost pile.
- Care for birds.
- Clean up the neighborhood.
- Decrease the amount of trash, say "no" to Styrofoam and plastic garbage bags, and use paper cups and reusable cloth bag for groceries.
- Recycle old toys by giving them to less fortunate people.
- Buy and use only earth-friendly school supplies.
- Walk rather than ride in the car.
- Save Christmas trees and replant.

learn that being accountable for the world is important. When children perceive their value in improving the world in which they live, they experience good feelings about themselves and, ultimately, demonstrate improved mental and physical health. Many simple ways to improve the environment are available and when children learn ways to contribute to environmental health, they often reinforce these behaviors to their parents (see Health Teaching box).

Erikson's Theory

Preschoolers develop a sense of initiative through their vigorous motor activity and active imaginations. Erikson views this development as the central developmental task in the emerging concept of self in the preschool years. By praising the preschooler's efforts to try new actions and ideas and by providing the opportunity for the child to see and try new things, parents can promote the development of initiative. This approach does not mean forcing preschoolers to do something new, but rather, providing options that allow them to choose to experiment. The preschooler must have a feeling of mastery, which implies the need for repetition. When preschoolers achieve mastery over some actions, they become more confident about trying new actions.

Preschoolers remain sensitive to criticism by others. When ridiculed for their ideas or behaviors, preschoolers can develop feelings of guilt and inadequacy. Parents, caregivers, and health care professionals should nurture the ideas of preschoolers and mentor and encourage behaviors that support a positive self-concept in these young children.

Roles-Relationships Pattern

Family members are important to the preschooler, but peers become increasingly important as well. Preschoolers receive ideas and information from their peers that they then introduce into family situations. The preschooler may question why rules or expectations at home are different from those at a particular friend's house. Discussion about different family values and behaviors that are acceptable one place and not another can help the preschooler understand these differences.

Preschoolers understand gender expectations regarding jobs, activities, and competencies of people in their lives. Ideas of what is "girl's work" or "boy's work" are based on models in the home, at child care or preschool centers, and on television. Parents and caregivers should be aware of the powerful influence that these environments have on role perceptions of preschoolers (Box 19-6); when inaccurate portrayals of male and female roles exist, parents and caregivers should discuss more accurate depictions of men and women with their children. The preschooler tries out many roles through play, including family roles. As the mother or father in a play situation, the preschooler can set limits, punish, praise, and make outlandish demands on the "child" of the family. This play represents an important way in which the preschooler can alleviate stress and try out new roles. By playing different roles, preschoolers can safely experience the effect of their role on others' responses to that role and perhaps understand the roles of others more clearly. Parents can also understand the effect of their own behavior on their preschooler more clearly when they see that behavior rehearsed by their child, which can "encourage" parents to positively change their interaction with their child.

Preschoolers now relate to older children in the family on a more equal basis. Although the cognitive, motor, or language skills to keep up with these older siblings and their peers are unrefined, preschoolers are able to participate in some of their activities. These children may admire an older sibling to the point of wanting to do

Box 19-6 Evaluating a Child-Care Setting

Child care that meets the needs and expectations of parents will most likely ensure a happy preschooler as well. Questions that parents should consider in evaluating and choosing the best child care setting for their child include the following:

- Will my needs and those of my child be best met with a caregiver in a family day home, commercial center, or preschool or by having a person come to my home to care for my child?
- What kinds of "backup" plans will I need or will be available if the provider in the setting becomes ill?
- What are my standards for nutrition, safety, sanitation, and health, and can these standards be met at the chosen child care setting?
- How important is it to my child to be with other children? How many children would be ideal for my child's socialization needs?
- What personality and educational preparation attributes do I desire in caregivers of my child? What attributes do I dislike and how will I deal with these attributes to maximize the care given to my child? How important is caregiver stability to me? Can I comfortably communicate with the staff of the setting to collaborate with my child's learning?
- What educational philosophy do I want in the setting to assist my child's learning? What involvement do I wish to have in the educational mission of the setting?
- Do the hours of the setting meet my personal and professional needs? Is close access of the setting to my job or home important to me?
- How are the children grouped and what is the caregiver-child ratio?
- Does the cost of the setting meet my financial needs? Can I pay part-time fees during vacation or when my child is ill for a lengthy period?
- Is accreditation of the setting mandatory for me to use it?
- What is my "internal response" (instinct) to the setting when I visit it before my child's enrollment? Are the caregivers interacting and responsive to the children? Are the children happy and interactive? Are the children's individual needs addressed appropriately? Is the environment supportive of my child's care? Is discipline appropriate for the children?

everything exactly as the sibling does them. This action may be flattering to the older child for a brief period, but generally becomes frustrating to when the activity persists.

The goal of social interaction during this period is to prepare the preschooler for school. Through experience within the family, with peers, and with other adults, the preschooler generally acquires readiness to interact in a group situation, follow directions, take turns, recognize others' rights, channel thoughts and actions to an assigned activity, and demonstrate increasing independence. School readiness can be assessed by using several relevant texts, as discussed in this chapter. The nurse who sees a preschooler over time in an office, clinic, or group care or preschool setting assesses the child's progress in development of social competencies. Comparing the child's current, more mature behavior with previous behavior provides insight into the preschooler's readiness for school. This evaluation outweighs comparison with other children of the same age, particularly because wide variations normally occur among children, but can lead to undue concern for extreme behaviors that may be within normal limits. For example, a child who reflects a quiet temperament and is introverted or subdued can appear more attached to the mother as school approaches in comparison with other children the same age. However, when comparing the child's social behavior with that of earlier years, the nurse may note progress toward independence. When the mother is not available, the child makes sufficient adaptations to remain comfortable and secure.

Evidence of the preschool child's social competency can be obtained by discussion and evaluation of the child's drawing of the family. The nurse observes the drawing and responds to any comments or questions that the child volunteers. When the child asks for advice or assistance, the nurse encourages the child to proceed with the drawing "any way you want to do it." Positive encouragement and praise for the child's efforts can be made, particularly when the child becomes uninterested or reluctant. After the child finishes the drawing, the nurse asks the child to identify the people in the drawing and to describe individual characteristics. The names of each family member appear on the drawing and any specific perceptions of the person that the child relates. Other questions such as, "What do you like best about your brother?" or "When do you get angry with your sister?" can be posed to encourage the child to describe the nature of family interactions. When an adult family member is present, the nurse explains the purposes of the drawing and interview, requesting that the adult not participate until afterward. Any areas of concern or questions should be discussed and the parent should be reassured of confidentiality. The child's perceptions can be verified with the adult at the conclusion of the interview, or further information can be sought to clarify them.

The **Vineland Social Maturity Scale** provides an objective, standardized estimate of social maturity. This tool provides a profile of the child's self-help skills, self-direction, locomotion, communication, and social relations. Designed as a means to measure the child's progression toward independence, the investigator collects data by observing the child's behavior and interviewing the mother or primary caregiver. This tool may employ only interview data when needed, but direct observation of the child's behavior appears to provide a clearer picture of the child (Doll, 1965).

Parental divorce creates a disruption in family relationships for the preschooler. Children's response to this change in family circumstances depends primarily on their developmental stage and on the type of relationship that they had with each family member before the divorce. The nurse realizes that a divorce represents a final decision of the parents, usually culminating from a period of conflict, stress, changing relationships, and "hiding the problem from the kids." Although preschoolers are definitely aware of stress in the home, they cannot name this uncomfortable feeling or find its origin. The children react to the changes in their parents in various ways, including regression, confusion, or irritability. Asking the same questions repeatedly, such as, "Is Daddy coming home for supper tonight?" or "Why doesn't Daddy stay here anymore?" can be a child's way of expressing difficulty in comprehending the situation.

Parents in the midst of marital problems or divorce frequently lack the psychological energy or patience to deal with the preschooler's questions and altered behavior. Nonetheless, children desperately need closeness, patience, and consistent responses from their parents. The nurse serves as an advocate for children by helping parents explore ways to deal with children's regression and irritability, develop skills in explaining the situation to children, and realize that even when the children are not currently manifesting problems in dealing with the family disruption, they are deeply affected (Hetherington & Arastik, 1998). Parents should spend emotionally connected time with their child to show that their love will continue despite the dissolution of the marriage. In many cases, books that are appropriate to the preschooler's cognitive and emotional level can help parents address the feelings and needs of children involved in a divorce.

Child Abuse

Complex social processes within the family and community often create child abuse. Parents and caregivers who experience workplace stressors, financial worries, and other frustrations in their life may project their anger about their life on their children by physically, emotionally, or sexually abusing them. In some communities, hitting children as a form of discipline remains acceptable; however, in instances of apparent child abuse, witnesses must report the abuse to the legal system in the United States. Current research focuses on the complexity of the abuse cycle and the challenges involved in resolving abuse. Possible effective interventions might involve promoting awareness of violence as a social problem, opposing violence to women, and offering community and school programs to teach nonviolent conflict-resolution skills to persons of all ages.

Sexuality-Reproductive Pattern

The role of the preschooler as a girl or boy can also define the self-concept of individuals in this group. The preschooler recognizes that there are two genders and identifies the self with the correct gender. Appropriate and positive representation of both genders on television and in role models, such as working mothers, allows preschoolers to interpret gender roles broadly and define their gender role more realistically.

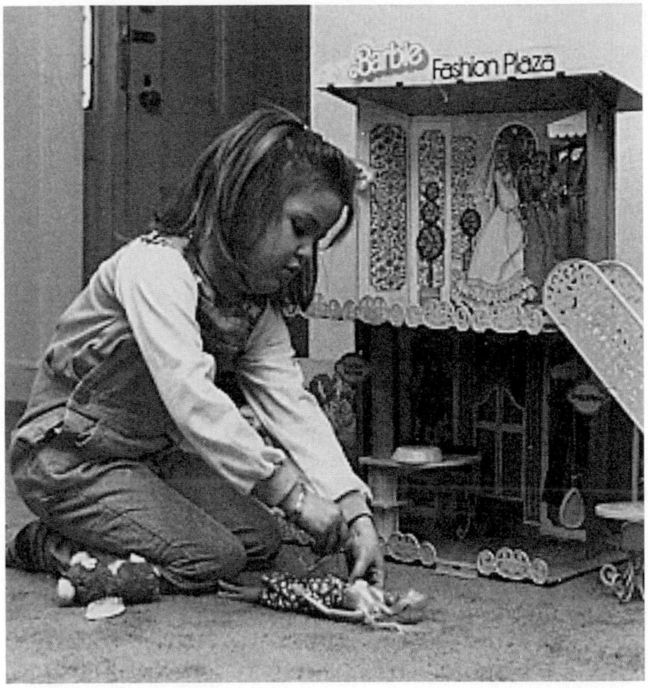

Fig. 19-3 Doll play often reflects child's sense of self. (Photograph by Douglas Bloomquist.)

Body image, a part of gender identity, also includes perception of sex organs. Preschoolers can be curious about other persons' bodies and sexual functions; their questions should be answered simply and factually. Parents and others should avoid teasing the preschooler about this interest or implying that sexual information is "dirty" or "bad." A positive feeling about all aspects of the self (including gender role) creates positive self-esteem. Many recent children's books address the self-esteem of young children and provide interesting and informative approaches to nurturing the overall health promotion of this age group (Downie, 1998) (see Box 19-2).

Coping–Stress-Tolerance Pattern

Play Approaches

Assessing self-concept can be difficult for the nurse dealing with a preschool child who has difficulty defining feelings about the self. Various play approaches may be useful in eliciting behavior that is indicative of the child's sense of self and self-esteem, future success or failure, sense of acceptance, and competence.

Doll or puppet play provides valuable insight into a child's sense of self (Fig. 19-3). Dolls or puppets, including one that represents a young child of the same gender as the preschooler, should be the only toy objects available with this kind of play. If the child spontaneously begins to engage the dolls or puppets in make-believe activity, then no further guidance should be given. If the child-seems reluctant to begin play, then the nurse begins a make-believe situation, such as going to the store, moving the dolls or puppets through the related activities, and then involving the child. Frequently, a preschooler continues the scenario for a time to tell a personal story.

A related technique is **mutual storytelling.** The nurse begins a story and the child finishes it. The nurse might begin with a standard line, such as, "Once upon a time there lived a [girl, boy, cow, monkey, etc.] who . . . " The nurse then pauses to indicate that the child can continue the story. If the child is reluctant to participate, then the nurse might continue the story for another sentence or two or ask the child what the figure in the story is doing. As the child begins to supply details of the story, the nurse asks questions that encourage the child to fill in details or continue with the story, such as, "And then what happened?" or "How did the child feel?"

The child's story then becomes the focus of an evaluative process of several dimensions that may indicate the child's inner nature. First, the emotional theme of the story should be noted and should be congruent with the child's tone and expression. For example, if the child focuses on a theme of aggression and destruction, but describes anger expressed by one of the characters in an emotionless monotone, then the child has shown an incongruence of content and expression. This response may suggest that the child has difficulty in expressing feelings. Second, possible meanings of characters can be revealed by asking children whether they are similar to any of the characters at the conclusion of the story or whether they would like to be any of the characters rather than who they really are.

However, interpretation of a child's behavior and responses in these play situations remains highly speculative and several encounters may be needed to determine possible themes or to estimate the child's self-esteem. Additionally, the nurse's personality and approach to the child have a significant influence on the child's ability to tell a story and on the spontaneity with which the child responds. The actual observed behavior and responses of the child should be recorded for future reference; interpretations are avoided until validated by an experienced specialist.

Coping Mechanisms

The preschooler uses similar types of coping mechanisms as does the toddler (separation anxiety, regression, denial, repression, and projection). Protest behavior in the form of temper tantrums normally disappears as a common stress response in the older preschooler. If temper tantrums persist through the fifth year, then the child may not have developed more mature coping responses because the child has found that tantrums gain the desired result.

In several ways, preschoolers lack the cognitive awareness, social abilities, and motives for communication of adults and older children. Preschoolers may display temperaments and tantrums that appear oppositional to older individuals. Through positive interactions with parents and caregivers, preschoolers frequently learn how to organize their bodies, abilities, and environment to move successfully to the next stage of development (Chess & Thomas, 1986). This "goodness of fit" between the child's temperament and the demands and expectations of the child's environment can be attained by social interaction, which can, in turn, prevent the development of child problem behaviors later (see Hot Topics box).

The preschooler has a larger range of experiences and memories form which to draw and may therefore have more response options than does the toddler when a stressful event occurs. Some variables that determine positive coping resources in children include the following (Berger, 1991):

1. The range of gratification usually available to the child, which helps the child accept substitute gratifications and find alternative solutions
2. The child's positive attitude toward life, including self-pride, resilience, and capacity to mobilize resources
3. The range and flexibility of the child's coping mechanisms and defenses
4. The capacity to regress and retreat to a level of function with fewer demands

Although the types of coping mechanisms appear to be similar for toddlers and preschoolers, the preschooler should show greater ability to verbalize frustration, less temper tantrum behavior, and more patience in trial-and-error experimentation to resolve a situation compared with the toddler. The preschooler's problem-solving skills are more refined than are the toddler's. Through fantasy play, the preschooler may be able to look at and try out solutions or responses to stressful events and find inner control for challenging situations.

Occasionally, projection and fantasy in the preschooler lead parents to think that their child lies. When faced with

> **HOT topics**
>
> **THE CHALLENGE OF TEMPERAMENT AND PRESCHOOLERS**
>
> Temperament describes the way in which an individual behaves or responds to new situations and to overall life occurrences. Some children can be defined as easy, difficult, or hard-to-warm-up-to, based on the way in which they react to their surroundings and to people. For many adults, the challenge in parenting is to learn how to work with a child's temperament, which can vary from the parents' or other children's temperaments, in efforts to attain family happiness.

the question, "Did you break this dish?" the preschooler might respond, "No, Teddy did it." The child might even relate a detailed story of the toy bear's mishap. Preschoolers tend to project the blame away from themselves and active fantasy thoughts help them tell the story. Parents should not accuse preschoolers of lying, but rather, they should help them decide whether the story is "pretend" or "real." These concepts of pretend and real can be helpful in encouraging children to talk about nightmares, television shows, stories, and in dealing with their own active imaginations (Webster-Stratton, 1992).

The preschooler has a greater perceived ability to control and manage situations than does the toddler. Strict adherence to rituals or game rules is one way of controlling situations. As discussed, the preschooler has a longer and more rigid bedtime ritual than does the toddler. The preschooler also dislikes "losing" and may control this situation by structuring the rules to ensure winning. Older children and adults may be able to accept this structuring, but other preschoolers might become upset, particularly because they also need to win. Gentle and consistent direction by parents and caregivers about how to play games "fairly" and to be partially responsible for a positive group outcome assists the preschooler in developing a sense of morality, which is important for later life success and happiness. See the Case Study and Care Plan for a situation of ineffective coping in a preschool child.

Values-Beliefs Pattern

Preschoolers, similar to toddlers, lack a fully developed conscience, but begin to demonstrate some internal controls on their actions. These internal controls may not always be consistent or effective, but they can be strict and the preschool child can feel overwhelming guilt when behavior does not match the internal controls. Fluctuations in behavior and the preschooler's feelings about this behavior depend, largely, on cognitive development, which experiences dramatic growth during ages 3 to 6 years.

Modeling and **inductive explanations** (from specific to general) given by parents and caregivers significantly influence moral behaviors. Modeling can come from many sources, not all of which are positive or which parents desire. Therefore parents should exert some control over what models are available to the child by screening television shows, carefully selecting child-care and baby-sitting situations, and monitoring play sessions. This approach does not mean that the parent constantly plays warden with the child, but rather, that the parent verifies that the models for the child are acceptable. Inductive explanations can be more detailed for the preschooler than they are for the toddler, but should be based on the individual child's cognitive level.

Preschoolers control their behavior because of their supreme desire for parental love and approval. Disapproval from parents does not mean being unloved, but may represent to preschoolers that their parents think less of them. These children therefore suffer a decline in positive self-esteem, which motivates children to change their behavior. The resulting guilt from the perceived reduction of positive self-esteem provides a critical step in the development of a conscience in the preschooler.

Moral actions for the preschooler can be linked to simple activities, such as taking turns and sharing. These actions stem from the assumption that other people have rights and desires that are as important as the rights and desires of the preschooler.

Preschoolers frequently express their values by stating who or what they like or what they want to be when they "grow up." These values can change frequently, even within a few minutes. Preschoolers occasionally use these statements of value as punishment for playmates or family members and display insensitivity to the effect of their remarks on others.

Typically, preschoolers ask endless "why" questions. When they ask these questions about moral actions or feelings, they may simply be asking, "How does this work?" and not questioning the underlying parental value. The same intent exists when the child asks about the spiritual values that the parent may be teaching. Parents may enroll their child in Sunday school or other faith-oriented classes or activities. The preschool child generally enjoys the social aspects of these activities and receives some important modeling of values from the involved adults and from working with peers as they struggle to develop morality.

Preschoolers can also be as fascinated by the end of life as they are with the beginning of life. Because of their lack of emotional connection to the topic, preschoolers ask about dead bugs and the process of death with great interest and, occasionally, with insensitivity. Other preschoolers become upset with the idea of dying,

CASE STUDY

Mark

Mark, age 3, was brought to the clinic by his mother from concerns about his small size, small appetite, and food rituals. Mark lives with his mother, father, and two older sisters. The family moved to the area 6 months ago. Both parents and sisters are of average height and in good health. Mark's mother comments that the girls have always done what the parents requested, but Mark has always had a "strong will." Mealtime is a battle to get Mark to eat, unless his mother feeds him. For a time, the girls could coax him to eat, but that approach no longer works.

Through a comprehensive health assessment, the nurse determines that Mark is at or above average in all areas except social and affective development.

From Mott, S. R., Fazekas, N. F., & James, S. R. (1995). *Nursing care of children and families: A holistic approach*. Menlo Park, CA: Addison-Wesley Publishing.

CARE PLAN

Nursing Diagnosis: Ineffective Coping Related to Positive Feedback for Regressive Behaviors and Lack of Consistent Limits and Fulfillment of Appropriate Responsibilities

EXPECTED OUTCOMES

- Mark will separate from his parents without incident (tantrum, crying).
- Mark will join a community or church peer group activity.
- Mark will perform one household task (picking up his toys) before bedtime every evening.
- Mark will demonstrate independent self-care behaviors (feed himself).
- The parents will have clear, consistent, and age-appropriate expectations for Mark's behavior.
- The parents will explain to Mark the rationale for limiting a socially unacceptable or unsafe behavior as soon as it is displayed.

INTERVENTIONS

- Discuss with the parents the process of growth and development and the child's needs to learn how to compromise, take turns, and channel energy appropriately.
- Use the Prescreening Developmental Questionnaire to validate general assessment data.
- Encourage the parents to leave Mark with his sisters or a baby-sitter to go shopping or to see a movie.
- Encourage the mother to formulate a bedtime ritual with Mark that does not include her sitting in his room until he falls asleep.
- Discuss with the parents and Mark what "jobs" he can do at home and the expectation that they be performed daily.
- Suggest laying out Mark's clothes so that he can dress himself. Set a time to be dressed, such as before or after a certain television program in the morning.
- Explore with the parents the availability of playgroups or community activities for children Mark's age.
- Encourage the parents to take Mark to the neighborhood playground so that he can meet and play with other children.
- Have Mark help around the house alongside his parents. Specify "work" and "play" times.
- Praise Mark for age-appropriate behaviors, being careful not to bribe him to perform.
- Discuss the principles of discipline consistency, immediacy, realistic expectations, and clear explanations.
- Recognize the parent's frustration and encourage them to try different approaches, such as limited choices, diversion, and incentives (when you finish your meat, we'll play a game).
- Suggest that the parents keep a diary of how long an approach was tried and how consistently Mark responded.
- Discuss the decrease in appetite and reliance of food fads that typify Mark's age. Review the principles of nutrition, timing of snacks, and ways of making food attractive to children.
- Refer the parents and Mark to a nutritionist for nutrition counseling.

From Mott, S. R., Fazekas, N. F., & James, S. R. (1995). *Nursing care of children and families: A holistic approach.* Menlo Park, CA: Addison-Wesley Publishing.

assuming that when someone becomes angry and wishes them dead, they will cease to exist. Many children worry about who will care for them if their caregivers die, whether pain comes with death, what causes death, and what happens after someone dies (Neville & Halaby, 1984). Children who actually lose a loved one to death can experience sleep disturbances and other behavioral changes as part of the grieving process. Parents, based on their own religious and cultural values, should respond to children in a supportive and open manner to allow an accurate interpretation of death. In some cases, counseling may be needed if the parents are unable to cope with parenting duties or if the child has significant behavioral problems as a result of the family disruption. Increasingly, books appropriate to the preschooler's level of understanding are available to help deal with this delicate issue within the family (Seibert & Drolet, 1993).

PATHOLOGICAL PROCESSES

For many children, normal development is disrupted by physiologic, psychosocial, and environmental factors that create health problems that interfere with physical, social, and educational activities. Major disruptions can even limit fulfillment of the child's potential in adulthood (Chasan-Taber & Tabachnick, 1999; DiFranza & Lew, 1996; U.S. Department of Health and Human Services, Administration on Children Youth and Families, 1999; Institute of Medicine, Committee on Injury Prevention and Control, 1999; Klassen, MacKay, Moher, Walker, & Jones, 2000).

The environmental processes that affect toddlers also affect preschoolers. Occurrence rates and outcomes of health problems differ in this age group, likely because of developmental differences (U.S. Department of Health and Human Services, Administration on Children Youth and Families, 1999). Preschoolers have more refined problem-solving skills, are more coordinated, and have more experience with a variety of situations compared with toddlers. Although preschoolers can be expected to recognize and avoid some environmental hazards, they are still impulsive and immature in many ways and cannot be expected to recognize or avoid all dangers (Fig. 19-4, Box 19-7, and Research Highlights box.)

As a result of many preschoolers attending child care settings, many young children have been trained to use 911

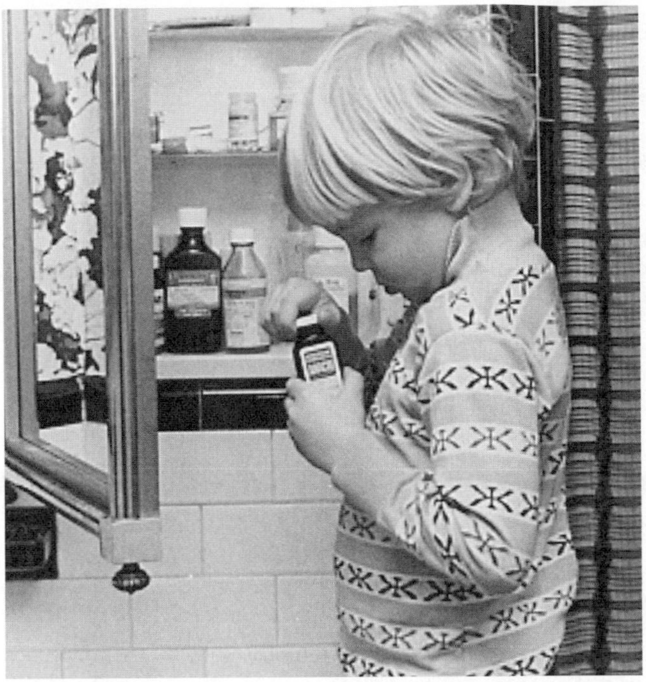

Fig. 19-4 Preschoolers are still impulsive and curious and cannot be expected to avoid all dangers. (Photograph by Douglas Bloomquist.)

and they can access help in emergencies where this phone code exists. At this age, children need to know their name, address, and the way to say "no" to strangers to be safe in their environments.

Injuries

Approximately 55 American children die every day from injuries; 43% of the deaths of children age 1 through 4 years are a result of injuries, "4 times the number of deaths due to birth defects, the second leading cause of death for this age group" (U.S. Department of Health and Human Services, 2000, p. 15-4).

"Many injuries are not accidents" or uncontrollable acts of fate; rather most injuries are predictable and preventable (U.S. Department of Health and Human Services, 2000, p. 15-3). Causes of injuries such as motor vehicle crashes, firearms, falls, abuse, fires, drownings, suffocation, and poisonings are closely associated with violent and abusive behaviors. Youths are both the perpetrators and the victims of violence (National Center for Injury Prevention and Control, 1999). In 1997, nearly 19,000 children aged 19 years and under were victims of injury (33% from violence and 67% from unintentional injury) (U.S. Department of Health and Human Services, 2000, p. 15-7).

Although preschoolers have fewer accidents compared with toddlers, motor vehicle accidents continue to be a major cause of fatalities for this age group. Despite many state laws mandating federally approved car seats for children under 4 feet in height and/or less than 40 lb in weight and booster seats for children up to the age of 6, many parents fail to place their children in appropriate restraint systems. Even children riding in restraint systems in the front seat of a motor vehicle face danger. Recently, federal investigations have concluded that children under age 13 should ride in the back seat of a motor vehicle particularly because of potential child injury or death from a passenger seat air bag that could become activated in a severe car accident (Grossman & Garcia, 1999). Preschoolers can also be injured by running into the street and need to be monitored by an adult when near streets.

Household furniture and fixtures also remain a hazard for preschoolers, as do structural features, such as stairs and windows (Harker & Moore, 1996). The occurrence rates for injuries in these categories remain nearly the same in both age groups. Nursery and toy injuries decrease during the preschool years. Sports and recreational injuries increase markedly, from 8% to 21%, during the preschool years. This increase likely reflects preschoolers' increased involvement in group sports, riding bicycles, and playground equipment. Parents should realize that preschoolers need a broader range of play area and experiences, but providing age-appropriate limits and supervision is essential.

Preschoolers lack the skill or judgment to ride bicycles in the street; at this age, they need to learn about and deal with the hazards of sidewalk cycling and roller-skating. Preschoolers need instruction in the safe use of playground equipment and require adult supervision. Group sports should be under adult supervision as well.

Preschoolers can begin to learn safe ways to handle basic tools, kitchen equipment, and cleaning supplies; they usually take pride in participating in household projects with a supervising parent. "Schools are second only to homes among the primary places that children spend their time and thus are one of the significant places where children may be exposed to potentially harmful environmental conditions" (U.S. Department of Health and Human Services, 2000, p. 75).

Recent concern has focused on firearm safety in homes with small children. Several states have passed legislation allowing handguns for individual protection, but this action has resulted in creating increased numbers of handgun accidents resulting from improper storage and locking of firearms. For example, among 5- to 14-year-old children, firearms remain the fourth leading cause of unintentional injury (U.S. Department of Health and Human Services, 1995, 2000). In response to this societal concern, the Texas Nurses Foundation, in consultation with a broad-based nonpartisan group of organizations, has launched "Gun-Safe" to encourage consumers to secure safer storage and locking of firearms to protect Texas children (American Academy of Pediatrics, 1997; Avens, 1996; Cummings, Grossman, Rivara, & Koepsell, 1997).

Burns

Scalds and direct flame burns are major hazards for the preschooler. "African-American, Hispanic, and Native-

Box 19-7 Environmental Safety with Preschoolers

A safe and developmentally stimulating environment allows children of all ages to explore without negative consequences. When teaching parents how to modify their homes for preschoolers, the following requirements for child safety should be considered:

SAFE SLEEP ENVIRONMENT

Provide beds with guardrails (as needed), soft corners and appropriate bedding to avoid suffocation dangers.

WELL-VENTILATED, BUT OPTIMAL TEMPERATURE ENVIRONMENT FOR PLAY

Provide safe play areas by using electrical outlet covers, stairwells with handrails, toy boxes with lids that securely lock, nonslip floor materials, well-anchored furniture, and appropriate soft ground coverings and padding for outdoor play equipment.

AVOIDANCE OF CHILD BURNS

Use only cool mist humidifier for treatment of upper respiratory infections; dress only in flame-retardant clothing, particularly at bedtime.

APPROPRIATE INSTALLATION AND USE OF EMERGENCY HOME EQUIPMENT

Discuss the importance of properly operating smoke detectors, fire extinguishers in the home, and the practice of an escape plan from the home in case of emergency.

CONNECTION TO EMERGENCY SERVICES

Post 911 on all phones; teach the child how to use 911 and how to report the child's name and address over the phone; parents should be trained in cardio pulmonary resuscitation and the Heimlich maneuver.

PREVENTION OF ASPIRATION

Monitor safe use of balloons and eating habits of the preschooler during meals.

SAFE DAILY HOME ENVIRONMENT

Close doors of dishwasher, oven, washer, and dryer; mark all glass doors with decals to delineate doors; use gates at the top and bottom of stairs for the younger child; set hot water heater temperature at a maximum of 125° F to avoid burns; store all poisonous substances away from the reach of children; discourage running in the house; avoid throw rugs on bare floors.

PREVENTION AND RECOGNITION OF SIGNS OF POISON INGESTION OR EXPOSURE

Know how to use syrup of ipecac and have the nearest poison control center phone number within easy access; learn how to evaluate burns or blisters around the mouth, odor of poisons, empty containers around the child, stomach distress, or changes in normal activity level relevant to poison ingestion.

WATER SAFETY

Monitor bathtub and pool activity; teach preschooler swimming skills (usually by age 4); ensure that all pools are fenced.

BICYCLE SAFETY

Ensure that the child is riding a developmentally appropriate bicycle with a federally approved safety helmet and is schooled in the rules of riding in the street and interacting with strangers.

LEAD CONCERNS

Avoid items with a high poisoning potential in home (paint, wrapping paper, earthenware, colored newspaper); ensure that children are monitored when lead exposure is a concern.

ENVIRONMENTAL CONTAMINANTS HAZARDOUS TO THE CHILD'S HEALTH

Avoid exposure to environmental tobacco smoke, nitrous oxide from wood, burning stoves, asbestos, pesticides, radiation, and factory-produced irritants.

American children are at higher risk for home fire deaths" (U.S. Department of Health and Human Services, 2000, pp. 15-16). The measures discussed in Chapter 18 to reduce scald burns in the home apply to this age group as well. Preschoolers should be taught about the dangers of matches, open flames, and hot objects. Parents and caregivers should also role model (appropriate use of active and potentially dangerous burning devices in the home and child care environments).

Drownings

The child over 3 years of age is at lower risk for drowning in the bathtub, but at greater risk for drowning in swimming pools or natural bodies of water compared with the toddler. In every age group, drowning deaths are significantly greater for boys than they are for girls. In children 1 to 4 years of age, the drowning rates are slightly higher for White children, but twice as high in Black children throughout the rest of childhood. Preschoolers should receive instruction in water safety and swimming and always swim with a trained adult or older person. For children under age 5, drowning represents the major cause of injury death in the United States; fewer children die in motor-vehicle accidents because of greater social awareness of that area (Wintemute, 1992).

A preschooler has the cognitive ability to learn the **Lanoue water survival technique**, a method of floating based on the principle that the body is naturally buoyant when the lungs are filled with air and that the natural floating position is face downward, beneath the surface of the water. Children learn this technique even before learning to swim. Preschoolers should always wear life jackets when they are on boats, even when they know how to swim, and they must be supervised when around water, even in shallow water.

research highlights

Lead Testing and Preschoolers

The purpose of this study was to estimate the percentage of young children in the United States who have been tested for lead and the percentage of dwellings in the United States in which the paint has been tested for lead. A national, random-digit-dial telephone survey was conducted. Of the 22,435 numbers attempted, 12,725 were working, residential numbers. Of these potentially valid numbers, 2182 were called six or more times with no response, 918 did not meet eligibility criteria, and in 283 instances, selected subjects were unable to be reached, leaving 9342 eligible households. The survey resulted in 5238 completed usable interviews, which translates into a response rate of 56.1%.

Of 1626 children 6 years of age and under, 395 were reported to have been tested for lead exposure (U.S. estimate = 23.9%). Higher testing rates were reported for children residing in homes constructed before 1960, those living in rental units, those living in homes with a low household income, and those living in the Northeast.

Of the subjects, 4864 (92.9%) provided information about whether lead testing had been performed on the paint in their homes. Of these subjects, 505 (8.9%) of homes in the United States were reportedly tested for lead.

Despite recommendations for universal screening, this study suggests that only 24% of children age 6 years and under have been screened for lead. Even among children living in the highest risk (pre1960 homes), only an estimated 29% have been screened. The preferred approach to childhood lead poisoning is primary prevention. Screening children for lead poisoning and evaluating homes for the presence of lead paint remain critical efforts.

Data from Binder, S., Matte, T. D., Kresnow, M., Houston, B., Sacks, J. J. (1996). Lead testing of children and homes: Results of a national telephone survey. *Public Health Rep, 111*, 342.

Mechanical Forces

As mentioned, bicycle accidents begin to be a greater source of injury in the preschool years. Many bicycle accidents involve automobiles and most of these result from the child's errors, such as going through a stop or yield sign. Parents should set reasonable and age-appropriate limits about bicycle use. The transition from tricycle to bicycle provides an excellent time to begin the use of a bicycle helmet. Federally approved bicycle helmets are 85% to 88% effective in reducing head trauma, a major cause of death among young children (U.S. Department of Health and Human Services, 1995, 2000). In many communities, bicycle helmets must be worn by all bicyclists and rollerbladers, regardless of age, because of the effectiveness of helmets in reducing head trauma (Wesson, Spence, Hu, & Parkin, 2000).

The preschooler, as a passenger or pedestrian, is at great risk for an auto-related accident. At this age, pedestrian injury is more likely to occur than is passenger injury. Preschoolers should be taught proper street-crossing techniques and, generally, should be supervised when crossing streets. Approved car-seat restraint systems should be used by young children at all times during car travel. Older and heavier preschoolers who have outgrown their booster riding seat by age 6 or 7 years can often sit on a pillow in a car and use both the shoulder and lap restraint systems to ride safely. The back seat is safer than the front seat and all car doors should be locked. If the preschooler refuses to use the seat belt or appropriate restraint, then parents must insist that the outing be postponed. Parents must provide a good example by using their seat belts every time they are in the car. This role modeling directly influences the child's acceptance of "buckling up" as part of riding in the family's car, van, or truck, and it meets the child's desire at this age to imitate the parent. The child who has used a car seat from infancy on will generally accept the seat belt quite well.

Biological and Bacterial Agents

The preschooler may appear healthier to the parents because of fewer respiratory and gastrointestinal illnesses compared with a toddler. The child has built up antibodies to many common organisms through exposure to them during the toddler years or perhaps as a result of attending child care. Children who were not in group settings as toddlers and who begin preschool at age 3 or 4 years usually experience an increase in these common illnesses, particularly because they lack immunity from previous exposure. This factor may be of great concern to parents and should be discussed by the nurse before the child begins attending a group setting. Increasingly, child care settings provide instruction to children about appropriate hand-washing techniques, which may decrease disease transmission, and address relevant health-promotion teaching in that setting (Curry, Andrews, & Daniel, 1997).

Biological agents that are important during this age include the recommended immunizations (CDCP, 1999a, 1999b, 1999c, 1999d; Hoekstra, Le Baron, & Mega-Ioeconomou, 1998; Waterman et al., 1996). For the child who received the full course of immunizations as an infant, a booster dose of the diphtheria, tetanus, and pertussis (DTP) vaccine is given in the fourth year. A second measles, mumps, and rubella (MMR) injection is recommended between ages 4 and 6 years. Many states currently require that all children in a school setting be fully immunized, or parents must present a statement indicating why their children have not been immunized. Parents who have strong religious or other reasons for not accepting immunizations can continue to refuse for their child, but must realize the consequences of the decision. However, many children have been protected only partly from these diseases because of parental forgetfulness or procrastination. Mandatory immunization provides an effective incentive for these parents and may be easier because community drives make immunizations inexpensive and accessible in many communities.

"As of November 1, 1999 all children born in the

United States should be receiving 12-16 doses of vaccine by age 2 years to be protected against 12 vaccine preventable childhood diseases [Table 19-4]. . . . National coverage levels in children are now greater than 90% for each immunization . . . except for Hepatitis B and varicella" (U.S. Department of Health and Human Services, 2000 p. 43). Additional information on infections diseases and immunization can be obtained through www.health.gov/healthypeople/ or 1-800-336-4797 (CDCP, 1999a, 1999b, 1999c).

Financing for childhood vaccinations has improved significantly as a result of two initiatives: (1) Vaccines for Children and (2) the Children's Health Insurance Program and the Public Health Service Act, Section 317. Continued efforts to vaccinate all children are needed, especially children living in poverty, particularly in large cities, with traditionally undervaccinated children (Hoekstra, Le Baron, & Mega-Ioeconomou, 1998). Preschoolers who have received some of their immunizations need not repeat doses that have been received, but must continue immunizations from the time that the vaccinations stopped in infancy. Parents of preschoolers who have failed to receive immunizations should follow the schedule in Table 19-4, as recommended by the American Academy of Pediatrics. The possible side effects of these immunizations are presented in Chapter 18. Parents should be fully informed about the potential side effects. In most office and clinic settings, parents must sign informed-consent documents that address their understanding of side effects.

Preschoolers with disabilities may not attend preschool because the parents wish to protect the child from inadvertent harm or even ridicule from the other children. Financially and socially disadvantaged children are occasionally kept out of preschool because of either lack of money or parents' lack of knowledge about the advantages of preschool to prepare children for school. The nurse helps

Table 19-4 Recommended Immunization Schedules for Children Not Immunized in First Year of Life

Recommended Time/Age	Immunizations*	Comments
	Younger than 7 Years	
First visit	DTP, OPV, MMR	MMR if child ≥ age 15 mo; tuberculin testing may be performed during same visit
	HbCV	For children ages 15 to 59 mo, can be given simultaneously with DTP and other vaccines (at separate sites)
Interval after First Visit		
2 mo	DTP, OPV (HbCV)	Second dose of HbCV is indicated only in children whose first dose was received when younger than 15 mo
4 mo	DTP	Third dose of OPV is not indicated in the United States, but is desirable in other geographic areas where polio is endemic
10 to 16 mo	DTP, OPV	OPV is not given if third dose was given earlier
4 to 6 yr (at or before school entry)	DTP, OPV	DTP is not necessary if the fourth dose was given after the fourth birthday; OPV is not necessary if third dose was given after the fourth birthday
11 to 12 yr	MMR	At entry to middle school or junior high
10 yr later	Td	Repeat every 10 yr throughout life
	7 Years and Older	
First visit	Td, OPV, MMR	
Interval after First Visit		
2 mo	Td, OPV	
8 to 14 mo	Td, OPV	
11 to 12 yr	MMR	At entry to middle school or junior high
10 yr later	Td	Repeat every 10 yr throughout life

DTP, diphtheria, tetanus, pertussis; *OPV*, oral poliovirus vaccine; *MMR*, measles, mumps, rubella; *HbCV*, Haemophilus influenzae b conjugate vaccine; *Td*, tetanus, diphtheria.

*The initial three doses of DTP can be given at 1- to 2-month intervals; for the child in whom immunization is initiated at age 24 months or older, one visit can be eliminated by giving DTP, OPV, and MMR at the first visit; DTP and HbCV at the second visit (1 month later); and DTP and OPV at the third visit (2 months after the first visit). Subsequent DTP and OPV, 10 to 16 months after the first visit, are still indicated. HbCV, MMR, DTP, and OPV can be given simultaneously at separate sites if return of vaccine recipient for future immunizations is doubtful.

From Committee on Infectious Disease, American Academy of Pediatrics. (2000). *Report of the committee (The Red Book)*. Elk Grove Village, IL: AAP; Center for Disease Control and Prevention. (1999c). Recommended childhood immunization schedule-United States. *Morbidity and Mortality Weekly Report, 48*, 12-16; Atkinson, W., Humiston, S. G., & Pollard, B., U.S. Department of Health and Human Services, Centers for Disease Control and Prevention. (1997). *Epidemiology and prevention of vaccine-preventable diseases*. Washington, DC: U.S. Government Printing Office.

these families explore the pros and cons of preschool for their child and ensures that these families obtain information about opportunities in their community and possible assistance with cost.

Chemical Agents

The preschooler faces exposure to the same environmental pollutants as does any child or adult living in the same area. Specific chemical agents of concern during the toddler years continue to merit consideration, although the preschooler can be expected to understand the concept of safe versus poisonous more clearly. "In 1996 more than 1.1 million poisonings among children aged 5 years and under were reported to U.S. poison exposures at a residence" (U.S. Department of Health and Human Services, 2000, pp. 15-20; Litovitz, Smilkstein, & Felberg, 1996). Household products, drugs, pesticides, and poisonous plants should remain in adequately locked places or kept out of the house. Even secondary smoke from parental smoking or lead exposure represents negative chemical influences on the growing child. Preschoolers should receive verbal explanations that something is poisonous or dangerous and why, but parents cannot rely on the preschooler to always remember these precautions. The preschooler can identify certain visual warning symbols, such as "Mr. Yuk" stickers, which can prevent exploration of dangerous substances. Increasingly, preschools and child care settings have incorporated the topic of environmental pollutants and dangerous substances into a health-promotion curriculum to educate preschoolers about this area. Communication with parents about the environmental dangers to their children and the solutions available to create a healthier living environment remains a major role of the child care provider.

Cancer

From infancy to 5 years of age, the most common cancer is **acute lymphocytic leukemia** (ALL), which accounts for over one third of the cases of cancer in this age group. Other cancers commonly seen in this age group affect the eye (retinoblastoma), the kidney (Wilms' tumor), and the sympathetic nervous system (neuroblastoma). Cancer is the leading cause of death from disease among children over 1 year of age. Remarkable progress has been made in treatments that result in long-term survival of children with cancer. Early detection remains the key to successful treatment.

Leukemia

ALL is the most common leukemia of childhood and accounts for about 70% of all cases. The incidence of ALL rises from age 2, peaks at age 5, and diminishes through later childhood and adolescence. The risk factors for ALL are as follows:

- Sibling with leukemia
- Identical twin of a child with leukemia
- Bloom syndrome
- Fanconi syndrome (anemia)
- Immune deficiency disease
- Down syndrome

The dominant signs and symptoms of ALL appear suddenly, but the child may have a prodromal period of weakness, malaise, anorexia, fever, and tachycardia. Bone pain, petechiae, and hemorrhages after minor procedures such as dental extractions are frequently encountered. Another suspicious finding is an unexplained infection that does not respond to treatment. Early detection and treatment of ALL has resulted in a marked increase in 5-year survival rates.

Whenever leukemia is suspected because of the individual's age, symptoms, or known risk factors, the nurse should practice secondary prevention intervention by including the following in the assessment of the child:

1. Examination of the cervical and peripheral lymph nodes.
2. Palpation and percussion of the liver and spleen.
3. Inspection of the skin for systemic signs of leukemia, such as pallor, purpura, petechiae, and **chloroma.** Chloroma is a localized tumor mass that has a greenish appearance and may be found in the skin, orbits, or other tissues in granulocytic forms of leukemia.
4. Inspection of the mouth for enlarged tonsils; hyperplasia of the gums; and red, friable gingivae.
5. Palpation of the sternum, bones, and joints for tenderness and pain.

School nurses and public health nurses working with Down syndrome patients are aware of the relationship between this genetic condition and increased risk for leukemia (approximately 20% higher compared with other population groups). Individuals with Down syndrome should be monitored closely for the early signs and symptoms of leukemia, particularly because they have a twenty-fold increased risk of leukemia.

Wilms' Tumor

The majority of all cases of **Wilms' tumor** (cancer of the kidney) occur in children under 5 years of age. Girls experience the disease approximately twice as often as do boys. A strong correlation exists between Wilms' tumor and several congenital malformations. The strongest association is with sporadic aniridia (congenital absence of the iris). One of every three children with this congenital malformation has developed Wilms' tumor. Other risk factors for Wilms' tumor are as follows:

- Family history of Wilms' tumor (autosomal dominant)
- Previous history of Wilms' tumor
- Trisomy defects (additional chromosome in an otherwise diploid cell)
- Hemihypertrophy (muscular overgrowth of one half of the body or face)
- Genitourinary anomalies

Box 19-8 Warning Signs That May Indicate the Presence of Childhood Cancer

Cancer remains a leading cause of death (one in five) in children under 15 years of age, second only to injuries. In the United States each year, 12.5 of 100,000 children develop cancer.

GENERAL

- Documented weight loss without explanation, failure to thrive
- Persistent poor appetite
- Easy tiring or lack of energy

LEUKEMIA OR LYMPHOMAS: "LIQUID TUMORS," (CANCER OF THE BLOOD, BLOOD-MAKING SYSTEM, LYMPH NODES)

- Persistent fever (more than 2 weeks)
- Bruising without injury and purple or red patches appearing on the skin
- Swollen glands (lymph nodes) unrelated to infection
- Persistent bone pain or limping
- Paleness of the lips, skin, nails, or lining of the eyes

BRAIN TUMOR

- Recurrent headaches, especially accompanied by vomiting, particularly in the morning
- Reflection in the pupil of the eye (eye tumor)
- Unexplained, persistent changes in behavior

KIDNEY TUMORS

- Lump in the abdomen or enlargement of the abdomen
- Blood in the urine
- Bulging of the eyes
- Unexplained, persistent cough or chest pain
- A firm mass in the muscles

MAKE BATH TIME EXAMINATION TIME

- These complaints or physical findings should be interpreted only as warnings of possible serious disease. When these warnings are present, you should consult your physician at once.
- Do not forget that your children must be examined by a physician every year. The earlier that cancer is detected, the better the chances are for a cure. With current treatment methods of surgery, radiation therapy, and chemotherapy (administration of anticancer drugs), the survival rate of children with certain forms of cancer has improved dramatically.

Modified from the Cancer Association of Greater New Orleans, Inc., 211 Camp St., Room 600, New Orleans, LA 70130.

- Hypospadias (urethra on underside of penis)
- Cryptorchism (undescended testes)

A precise history is collected when attempting to identify the high-risk population associated with the development of Wilms' tumor. Children identified as high risk should be referred for continual evaluation and examined closely for any renal masses. Wilms' tumor usually occurs in one of the upper abdominal quadrants. The nurse or trained parent obtains periodic abdominal girth measurements on high-risk children for monitoring early abdominal changes.

An excellent booklet designed to inform parents about the early warning symptoms and signs of childhood cancer is Know the Warning Signs of Cancer in Children, produced by the Cancer Association of Greater New Orleans. This booklet suggests performing routine procedures, such as a bath, as an opportunity for parents to examine the child for physical symptoms of disease and it outlines the issues to discuss with the physician (Box 19-8).

Retinoblastoma

Although **retinoblastoma** (cancer of the eye) is the most common intraocular tumor in younger children, only 1 in every 20,000 to 30,000 live births is affected. This form of cancer can occur spontaneously or can be inherited as a genetic mutation that is transmitted as an autosomal dominant characteristic. Familial retinoblastoma patients are especially at risk for secondary bone and soft tissue sarcomas.

The most important nursing action is to take a careful history, which usually reveals a slow progression of symptoms. Questions that help reveal risk factors are as follows:

- Do tumors of the eyes run in your family?
- If tumors of the eye run in your family, which relatives were affected and how they were treated?
- Have you noticed your child having any eye problems (crossed or lazy eyes or difficulty seeing)?
- Have you noticed any changes in your child's eyes?

Screening eye examinations for high-risk children include:

1. Visual acuity
2. Red reflex; in the child with retinoblastoma, this appears whitish (cat's-eye reflex), the most common sign of this cancer
3. Ophthalmoscopic findings
4. Lid lag, which is found with exophthalmos
5. Strabismus, by doing the cover-uncover test

The cat's-eye reflex and strabismus are the most common signs of retinoblastoma. When the nurse discovers any suspicious findings on the history or screening eye examination, the family is referred for medical evaluation.

Neuroblastoma

Neuroblastoma is cancer of the sympathetic nervous system. Approximately 70% of these tumors begin in the abdomen, primarily in the adrenal gland. The remaining 30% originates in cervical, thoracic, or pelvic areas.

innovative practice

Healthy Start

Risk factors for cardiovascular diseases are prevalent by 3 years of age, the most common of which are hypercholesterolemia and obesity. Healthy Start, a project located in Valhalla, New York, sponsored by the Child Health Foundation and the American Health Foundation, is a 3-year demonstration and research program to evaluate the effectiveness of interventions for reducing cardiovascular risk factors in preschool centers. Two major interventions are recommended. The first major intervention is the preschool food service, which is designed to reduce the total fat in the preschooler's meals and snacks to less than 30% of calories and to reduce saturated fat to less than 10% of calories. The second major intervention is a comprehensive preschool health education curriculum, which focuses on nutrition and exercise.

The effectiveness of this program is evaluated using many components. Changes in the nutritional behaviors (including dietary intake of school snacks and meals of the preschoolers) are being recorded, as are those in snacks and meals consumed at home. Special attention is being given to the intake of total and saturated fat.

Additionally, changes in the health knowledge of preschoolers are being assessed to evaluate the education component. Physical examination data include semiannual assessments of growth and body weight and blood lipid levels.

The specific details of rationale and methods of the randomized control trial studies within the Healthy Start project are described in the following publication: Williams, C. L., Squillace, M. M., Bollella, M. C., Brotanek, J., Campanaro, L., D'Agostino, C., Pfau, J., Sprance, L., Strobino, B. A., Spark, A., & Boccia, L. (1998). Healthy start: A comprehensive health education program for preschool children. *Preventive Medicine, 27* (2), 216-223.

Courtesy Carol Lynn Mandle.

Approximately one half of all individuals are younger than 2 years of age at diagnosis; more than 90% of diagnoses occur by age 5. Unfortunately, two thirds of the children have metastases when this cancer is first observed and frequently, the symptoms of the secondary spread are those that bring the child to the attention of health professionals.

Approximately 22% of all neuroblastomas follow a hereditary pattern. The literature reports that many families with this cancer have more than one child with the disease. Neuroblastoma may be related to some anomalies of neutral crest origin (neurofibromatosis, aganglionosis coli). Despite treatment, survivors of neuroblastoma may develop subsequent tumors necessitating continued medical supervision. Because nearly one fourth of neuroblastomas appear to follow a hereditary pattern, some experts recommend monitoring the offspring of individuals with neuroblastoma and examining them carefully for evidence of neural crest abnormalities. Neuroblastoma produces excessive amounts of neuroactive catecholamines found in the urine of people with this tumor. Therefore vanillylmandelic acid (VMA) in excessive amounts in the urine may indicate neuroblastoma.

Secondary prevention intervention includes the simple procedure of screening children at risk for catecholamines in the urine and for neurofibromatosis.

Asthma

The **asthma** rate is rising more rapidly in preschool-age children compared with any other group (Mannino et al., 1998). Asthma is a chronic inflammatory disorder of the airways. The inflammation contributes to hyperresponsiveness, limited airflow, and respiratory symptoms, including breathlessness, wheezing, cough, and chest tightness. Etiologies include genetic predisposition, specific allergens (animals or dust mites) and nonspecific precipitants (infections, exercise, weather, or stress). The rates are higher in boys compared with girls and in Blacks and Hispanics compared with Whites. Asthma hospitalization rates have increased dramatically for children under age 5 years. Poverty is a significant contributing factor to asthma illness disability and death (Kreiger, Song, Takaro, & Stout, 2000). "Although reasons for these differences are unclear they likely result from multiple factors: high levels of exposure to environmental tobacco smoke, pollutants, and environmental allergens . . . for example, house dust mites, cockroach particles, dog, cat, and rodent dander . . . lack of access to quality medical care; and a lack of financial resources and social support to manage the disease on a long-term basis" (U.S. Department of Health and Human Resources, 2000, pp. 24-26). Two 1996 studies found that secondhand smoke worsens asthma and other respiratory diseases in children (Mannino, Siegel, Husten, Rose, & Etzel, 1996; DiFranza & Lew, 1996).

SOCIAL PROCESSES

Community and Work

Some preschoolers have had a variety of experiences outside their families by age 3. This experience may be in group child care settings, in church play groups, or through family involvement in other activities. Some 3- and 4-year-old children have had limited experience outside the family (Yen & Syme, 1999) and a preschool setting can be their introduction to a wider social arena. This is a time for parents to learn to "let go" in the sense of encouraging more independent activity in a safe, supervised setting. Preschoolers must test their independence, interactive skills, and self-discipline as they learn to function in a group. Preschool provides a transition into kindergarten and first grade in which more group interaction skills are expected. Parents often select a preschool based on geographical closeness to their home or a friend's recommendation. This approach is practical and appropriate for many children. With many child care facilities and options now available, parents frequently need to visit and evaluate the settings to determine which setting will best meet their needs.

Culture and Ethnicity

The cultural heritage of the family continue to shape preschoolers. Dissimilar to the toddler, preschoolers might ask why their family follows certain practices; they also are likely to notice that not all people have the same practices. Their playmates may not celebrate the same holidays or have the same family rituals as does their own family. As preschoolers have more experiences outside their own families, these differences become more obvious. Discussion between the parents or caregivers and the preschoolers about the strength of cultural differences provides an excellent learning opportunity (Carillo, Green, & Bentancourt, 1999; Resnicow, Baranowski, Ahluwalia, & Braithwaite, 1999).

Preschoolers also notice ethnic differences in people's appearance and may decide that certain skin colors, eyes, and hairstyles are "pretty" or "ugly." These children will likely develop prejudices similar to those of their family or playmates because of the socialization process. Parents and caregivers should teach and role model positive behaviors that allow children to see differences in others as being positive rather than negative. This approach includes monitoring mass media influences on physical attractiveness, which will become significant to the child as a teen.

Certain cultures apply more pressure on the child to develop prosocial behaviors or take on more responsibility for younger siblings or household tasks as the school year approaches. The preschooler can become confused if the family's culture varies from that of most playmates. Disciplinary approaches for the same behavior varies from culture to culture. Confusion can also result when the child's parents have integrated their cultural background into the community standards, but the grandparents have maintained strict adherence to traditional cultural practices, rituals, and child-rearing ideas.

Legislation

Many safety-focused legislative bills have affected the preschooler (see Chapter 18). The child also is beginning to be influenced by the school-focused issues discussed in Chapter 20. With current concern about the high cost of health care, the federal government may increase block grants to states, which will need to allocate funding to various competing groups. Concern remains that financial programs that focus on children will lose in the competition. Overall funding for vulnerable populations such as the homeless and the poor will decrease and this reduction will have a negative effect on child health care in general in this country. Because 20% children in the United States live in poverty and more than 50% of all homeless children are under the age of 6, this outcome may become more evident (Bassuk & Rosenberg, 1988; Miller & Lin, 1988; Kemsley & Hunter, 1993).

Economics

Poverty influences the preschooler as it does any child. Dissimilar to the toddler, however, the preschooler is likely more aware of the family's economic status. The preschooler may be aware that the family lacks the money to buy some toy, but does not recognize the more comprehensive idea of the way in which limited economic resources influence the family's basic lifestyle. In some cases, the family's financial history prevents attendance at preschool or child care or influences the ability of the parents to expose their preschooler to extra activities for learning. Preschoolers realize that money or the special plastic card that the parent carries acquires food, toys, and clothes, but they do not yet have a concept of economic values. The preschooler might trade an expensive item for a trinket that happens to look more interesting at the time. By being paid to complete chores around the house, using their earnings to buy a treat for themselves, and then realizing that they must earn more money to buy future treats, preschoolers can be introduced to the concepts of earning money.

Health Care Delivery System

The preschooler has essentially the same resources for health care as has the toddler. As preschoolers enter a school setting, they are likely to be seen by a health care worker for physical and developmental screening as a requirement for admission to the school. For the child from a low-income family, this visit may come under the auspices of **Early and Periodic Screening, Diagnosis and Treatment** (EPSDT), a Medicaid program. This screening is available to any child under age 21 who meets the economic criteria for Medicaid. Private offices, local health departments, and community clinics can provide an EPSDT examination. A preschool child can have one screening per year, which includes the following:

1. Medical history
2. Assessment of physical growth, nutritional status, and mental development
3. Inspection of ears, eyes, nose, mouth, teeth, and throat
4. Vision screening
5. Auditory screening

6. Screening for cardiac abnormalities
7. Screening for anemia
8. Screening for the sickle-cell trait
9. Urine sampling
10. Blood pressure reading
11. Assessment and updating of immunizations
12. Tuberculosis screening, when indicated
13. Referral to a dentist for diagnosis and treatment for children 3 years of age and older

Any health or developmental concerns identified during this screening is further addressed in a complete physical examination. EPSDT is a comprehensive service that is presented as a resource for eligible children.

Box 19-9 Health-Promotion Interventions

SCREENING
- Height and weight
- Blood pressure
- Vision screen (age 3 to 4 years)

COUNSELING
- Child safety car seat (age less than 5 years)
- Lap shoulder belt (age 5 years and older)
- Bicycling: use helmet and avoid traffic
- Smoke detectors, flame retardant sleepwear
- Hot water temperature less than 120° F
- Window stair guards, pool fence
- Safe storage of drugs, toxic substances, firearms, matches
- Close availability: syrup of ipecac, poison control phone number
- Cardio pulmonary resuscitation training of parents and caretakers

NUTRITION AND EXERCISE
- Limit fats, maintain caloric balance, emphasize grains, fruits, vegetables
- Regular physical activity

SUBSTANCE USE
- Effects of passive smoking
- Anti-tobacco messages

DENTAL HEALTH
- Floss; brush with fluoride at least daily
- Regular visits to dentist

IMMUNIZATIONS
- Ensure currency
- Diphtheria, tetanus, pertussis
- Oral poliovirus
- Measles, mumps, rubella
- H influenzae type b
- Hepatitis B
- Varicella

NURSING INTERVENTIONS

Preschoolers show much interest in the tools and procedures of a health screening examination (U.S. Department of Health and Human Services, 1996) (see Box 19-9 and Table 19-5). These inquisitive children may ask to see and try the stethoscope, otoscope, and other diagnostic instruments. The nurse explains the tests in age-appropriate terminology and expects the child to be cooperative for most of the visit. The preschooler may even show self-control during injections, but definitely needs a parent close by to offer support and encouragement. The nurse includes the preschooler in the history by directing questions about dietary-intake and health practices, such as tooth brushing, favorite activities, and friends. This age is optimal for the child to begin taking some interest in health. Developmentally, preschoolers have the cognitive maturity to learn many health-promotion skills that will be important for the rest of their lives.

SUMMARY

The American Academy of Pediatrics' and the United States Task Force suggest schedules for preventive health care during the preschool years that includes visits at 4 and 5 years of age. Each visit includes an ongoing history; growth, physical, and developmental assessment; and discussion of age-appropriate developmental concerns.

In addition to contact with preschoolers in an office or clinic, the nurse can be a consultant to a preschool or a nurse for a primary school and preschool. Early exposure to and reinforcement of health care information to preschool children as part of their education can lay the foundation for later healthy lifestyle habits, which can influence overall societal health. Attention to health as a curricular subject during the school-age years, much as traditional

Table 19-5 Potential Additional Health Promotion Interventions for High-Risk Children and Families

Population	Potential Interventions
Low income, immigrants	Hemoglobin, hematocrit
Native American/Alaska Native	Hemoglobin, hematocrit Hepatitis A vaccine Pneumococcal vaccine
Increased lead exposure	Blood lead level
Inadequate water fluoridation	Daily fluoride supplement
Family history of skin cancer, nevi, fair skin, eyes, hair	Avoid excess and/or midday sun, use protective clothing

From American Academy of Pediatrics. (1998). *National prevention in primary care study*. Washington, DC: AAP; U.S. Preventive Services Task Force, U.S. Department of Health and Human Services. (1996). *Guide to clinical preventive services* (2nd ed.). Washington, DC: U.S. Government Printing Office.

academic subjects, can continue this focus. The school nurse's role in health promotion and prevention of illness is discussed in Chapter 20.

REFERENCES

American Academy of Pediatrics. (1997). *Injury prevention and control for children and youth* (3rd ed.). Elk Grove Village, IL: AAP.

American Academy of Pediatrics. (1999a). *Television and the family*. Elk Grove Village, IL: AAP.

American Academy of Pediatrics. (1999b). *Understanding the impact of media on children and teens*. Elk Grove Village, IL: AAP.

American Academy of Pediatrics, Committee on Public Education. (1999). *Media Education, 104* (2), 341-343.

American College of Preventive Medicine. (1998). *National prevention in primary care study*. Washington, DC: The College.

Anderson, R. E., Crespo, C. J., Bartlett, A. A., Cheskin, B. B., & Pratt, M. (1998). Relationship of physical activity and television watching with body weight and level of fatness among children: Results from the 3rd National Health and Nutrition Survey. *Journal of the American Medical Association, 279*, 938-942.

Athey, K., & Milner, S. (2000). Influencing practices of mothers with pre-school children. *Community Practitioner, 73* (6), 638-640.

Atkinson, W., Humiston, S. G., & Pollard, B., U.S. Department of Health and Human Services, Centers for Disease Control and Prevention. (1997). *Epidemiology and prevention of vaccine-preventable diseases*. Washington, DC: U.S. Government Printing Office.

Avens, S. (1996). Preventing burn injuries among children. *Health Visitor, 69* (3), 105-106.

Barkauskas, V. H., Stoltenberg-Allen, K., Baumann, L. C., & Darling-Fisher, C. (1994). *Health and physical assessment*. St. Louis: Mosby.

Bassuk, E. L., & Rosenberg, L. (1988). Why does family homelessness occur? A case-control study. *American Journal of Public Health, 78*, 783-788.

Berger, K. S. (1991). *The developing person through childhood and adolescence* (3rd ed.). New York: Worth.

Binder, S., Matte, T. D., Kresnow, M., Houston, B., Sacks, J. J. (1996). Lead testing of children and homes. Results of a national telephone survey. *Public Health Report, 11*, 342.

Cagle, C. S., & Keen-Payne, R. (1996). Health promotion teaching in preschools. *MCN. The American Journal of Maternal Child Nursing, 21*, 96-99.

Carillo, J. E., Green, A. R., & Bentancourt, J. R. (1999). Cross-cultural primary care: A patient-based approach. *Annals of Internal Medicine, 130* (1), 829-834.

Centers for Disease Control and Prevention. (1999a). Achievements in public health, 1900-1999. Impact of vaccines universally recommended for children—United States, 1990-1998. *Morbidity and Mortality Weekly Report, 48* (12), 243-248.

Centers for Disease Control and Prevention. (1999b). Notice to readers: Recommended childhood immunization schedule-United States, 1999. *Morbidity and Mortality Weekly Report, 48* (1), 8-16.

Centers for Disease Control and Prevention. (1999c). Recommended childhood immunization schedule-United States. *Morbidity and Mortality Weekly Report, 48*, 12-16.

Centers for Disease Control and Prevention. (1999d). *State immunization requirements*. Washington, DC: U.S. Government Printing Office.

Chasan-Taber, L., & Tabachnick, J. (1999). Evaluation of a child sexual abuse prevention project. *Sex Abuse, 11* (4), 279-292.

Chess, S., & Thomas, A. (1986). *Temperament in clinical practice*. New York: Guilford Press.

Cole, M., & Cole, S. R. (1996). *The development of children*. (3rd ed.). New York: Freeman.

Crain, W. (2000). *Theories of development: Concepts and applications* (4th ed.). Saddle River, NJ: Prentice Hall.

Cristoffel, K., & Ariza, A. (1998). The epidemiology of overweight in children: Relevance for clinical care. *Pediatrics, 101*, 103-105.

Cummings, P., Grossman, D. C., Rivara, I. P., & Koepsell, T. D. (1997). State gun safe storage laws and child mortality due to firearms. *Journal of the American Medical Association, 278* (13). 1084-1086.

Curry, M. D., Andrews, A. W., & Daniel, H. J. (1997). A community-based nursing approach to the prevention of otitis media. *Journal of Community Health Nursing, 14* (2), 81-110.

DiFranza, J. R., & Lew, R. A. (1996). Morbidity and mortality in children associated with the use of tobacco products by other people. *Pediatrics, 97*, 560-568.

Doll, L. A. (1965). *Vineland social maturity scales*. Circle Pines, MN: American Guidance Service.

Downie, J. (1998). Parents as sexuality educators: The challenge for nurses. *Neonatal Pediatric and Child Health Nursing, 1* (1), 12-17.

Ettner, S. L. (1996). The timing of preventive service for women and children: The effect of having a usual source of care. *American Journal of Public Health, 86*, 1748-1754.

Fagot-Campagna, A., Rios-Burrows, N., & Williamson, D. (1999). The public health epidemiology of type 2 diabetes in children and adolescents: A case study of American Indian adolescents in the Southwestern United States. *Clinica Chimica Acta; International Journal of Clinical Chemistry, 286*, 81-95.

Forrest, C. B., & Starfield, B. (1998). Entry into primary care and continuity: The affects of access. *American Journal of Public Health, 88* (9), 1330-1336.

Frankenburg, W. K., Dodds, J., Archer, P., Shapiro, H., Bresnick, B. (1990). *Denver II screening*. Denver: Denver Materials.

Gidding, S. S. (1999). Preventive pediatric cardiology, tobacco, cholesterol, obesity and physical activity. *Pediatric Clinics of North America, 46* (2), 253-262.

Grossman, D. C., & Garcia, C. C. (1999). Effectiveness of health promotion programs to increase motor vehicle occupant restraint use among young children. *American Journal of Preventive Medicine, 16* (Suppl 1), 12-22.

Guyer, B., Hughart, N., Strobino, D., Jones, A., & Scharfstein, D. (2000). Assessing the impact of pediatric-based development services on infants, families and clinicians: Challenges to evaluating the health steps program. *Pediatrics, 105* (3), 1-33.

Harker, P., & Moore, L. (1996). Primary health care action to reduce child home accidents: A review. *Health Education Journal, 55* (3), 322-331.

Health Education Authority. (1997). *Young people and physical activity: A literature review*. London: The Authority.

Henchy, G. (1993). *WIC works: Let's make it work for everyone*. Washington, DC: Food Research and Action Center.

Hetherington, E. M., & Arastik, J. D. (1998). *Impact of divorce, single parenting and step-parenting on children*. Hillsdale, NJ: Laurence Erlbaum.

Hoekstra, E. J., Le Baron, C. W., & Mega-Ioeconomou, Y. (1998). Impact of a large scale immunization initiative in the Special Supplemental Nutrition Program for Women, Infants and Children (WIC). *Journal of the American Medical Association, 280* (3), 1143-1147.

Institute of Medicine, Committee on Injury Prevention and Control, Bonnie, R. J., Fulco, C. E., & Liverman, C. T. (1999). *Reducing the burden of injury: Advancing treatment and prevention*. Washington, DC: National Academy Press.

Joint Committee on Infant Hearing. (2000). Year 2000 position statement: Principles and guidelines for early hearing detection and intervention programs. *American Journal of Audiology, 9* (1), 9-29.

Kemsley, M., & Hunter, J. (1993). Homeless children and families: Clinical and research issues. *Issues in Comprehensive Pediatric Nursing, 16*, 99-108.

Klassen, T. P., MacKay, J. M., Moher, D., Walker, A., & Jones, A. L. (2000). Community-based injury prevention intervention. *Future Child, 10* (1), 83-110.

Klerman, L. V. (1997). Promotion the well-being of children: The need to broaden our vision-the 1996 Martha May Eliot Award Lecture. *Maternal Child Health Journal, 1* (1), 53-59.

Kreiger, J. W., Song, L., Takaro, T. K., & Stout, J. (2000). Asthma and the home environment of low-income urban children: Preliminary findings from the Seattle-King County healthy homes project. *Journal of Urban Health, 77* (1), 50-67.

Litovitz, T. L., Smilkstein, M. S., & Felberg, L. (1996). 1996 annual report of the American Association of Poison Control Centers Toxic Surveillance System. *American Journal of Emergency Medicine, 15* (5), 447-500.

Mannino, D. M., Homa, D. M., Pertowski, C. A., Ashizawa, A., Nixon, L. L., & Johnson, C. A. (1998). Surveillance for asthma-United States 1960-1995. *CDCP. Morbidity and Mortality Weekly Report, Surveillance Summaries, 47*, 1-27.

Mannino, D. M., Siegel, M., Husten, C., Rose, D., & Etzel, R. (1996). Environmental tobacco smoke expose and health effects in children. *Tobacco Control, 5*, 13-18.

McBean, L. D., & Miller, G. D. (1999). Enhancing the nutrition of America's youth. *Journal of the American College of Nutrition, 18* (6), 563-571.

Melvin, N. (1995). Children's temperament: Interventions for parents. *Journal of Pediatric Nursing, 10*, 152-159.

Miller, D. S., & Lin, E. H. (1988). Children in sheltered homeless families: Reported health status and use of health services. *Pediatrics, 81*, 668-673.

Mobley, C. E., & Evashevsk, J. (2000). Evaluating health and safety knowledge of preschoolers: Assessing their early start to be health smart. *Journal of Pediatric Health Care, 14* (4), 160-165.

Mott, S. R., Fazekas, N. F., & James, S. R. (1995). *Nursing care of children and families-a holistic approach*. Menlo Park, CA: Addison-Wesley Publishing Co.

National Center for Injury Prevention and Control. (1999). *Best practices for preventing violence by children and adolescents: A source book*. Atlanta, GA: The Center.

Neville, H., & Halaby, M. (1984). *No-fault parenting*. Tucson, AZ: The Body Press.

Pipes, P. L. (1993). *Nutrition in infancy and childhood* (5th ed.). St. Louis: Mosby.

Resnicow, K., Baranowski, T., Ahluwalia, J., & Braithwaite, R. (1999). Cultural sensitivity in public health defined and demystified. *Ethnicity & Disease, 9* (1), 10-21.

Rosenbloom, A., Joe, J., Young, R., & Winter, W. (1999). Emerging epidemic of type 2 diabetes in youth. *Diabetes Care, 22*, 345-354.

Seibert, D., & Drolet, J. C. (1993). Death themes in literature for children ages 3-8. *Journal of School Health, 63* (2), 86-90.

Seidel, H. M., Ball, J. W., Dains, J. E., & Benedict, G. W. (1991). *Mosby's guide to physical examination* (2nd ed.). St. Louis: Mosby.

Strasburger, V. C., & Donnerstein, E. (1999). Children, adolescents and the media: Issues and solutions. *Pediatrics, 103* (1), 129-139.

Sword, W. A. (1997). Enabling health promotion for low-income single mothers: An integrated perspective. *Clinical Excellence for Nurse Practitioners, 1* (5), 324-332.

Tang, J. M. H., Altman, D. S., Robertson, D. C., O'Sullivan, D. M., Douglas, J. M., & Tinanoff, N. (1997). Dental caries prevalence and treatment levels in Arizona pre school children. *Public Health Reports, 112* (4), 319-331.

Troiano, R. P., & Flegal K. M. (1998). Overweight children and adolescents: Description, epidemiology and demographics. *Pediatrics, 101*, 497-504.

U.S. Department of Agriculture (2000). *Nutrition and your health: Dietary guidelines for Americans* (5th ed.). Home and Garden Bulletin 232. Washington, DC: U.S. Government Printing Office.

U.S. Department of Health and Human Services. (1995). *Healthy people 2000: Mid-course review and 1995 revisions*. Washington, DC: U.S. Government Printing Office.

U.S. Department of Health and Human Services. (1996). *US Preventive Services Task Force guide to clinical preventive services* (2nd ed.). Baltimore: Williams & Wilkins.

U.S. Department of Health and Human Services. (1999). *Vital statistics mortality data, underlying cause of death 1962-1997*. Hyattsville, MD: U.S. Government Printing Office.

U.S. Department of Health and Human Services, Administration on Children, Youth and Families (1999). *Child maltreatment 1997: Reports from the states to the national child abuse and neglect data system*. Washington, DC: U.S. Government Printing Office.

U.S. Department of Health and Human Services. (2000). *Healthy People 2010*. Washington, DC: U.S. Government Printing Office.

U.S. Preventive Services Task Force, U.S. Department of Health and Human Services. (1996). *Guide to clinical preventive services* (2nd ed.). Washington, DC: U.S. Government Printing Office.

Vargas, C. M., Crall, J. J., & Schneider, D. A. (1998). Socio-demographic distribution of pediatric dental caries: NHANES III. *Journal of the American Dental Association, 129*, 1229-1238.

Variyam, J. N., Blaylock, J., Lin, B. H., Ralston, K., & Smallwood, D. (1999). Mother's nutrition knowledge and children's dietary intakes. *American Journal of Agricultural Economics, 81* (2), 373-384.

Waterman, S. H., Hill, L. L., Robyn, B., Yeager, K. K., Maes, E. F., Stevenson, J. M., & Anderson, K. N. (1996). A model immunization demonstration for pre-schoolers in an inner-city barrio, San Diego, California 1992-1994. *American Journal of Preventive Medicine, 12* (4), 8-13.

Webster-Stratton, C. (1992). *The incredible years: A trouble-shooting guide for parents of children aged 3-8*. Toronto: Umbrella Press.

Wesson, D., Spence, L., Hu, X., & Parkin, P. (2000). Trends in bicycling-related head injuries in children after implementation of a community-based bike helmet campaign. *Journal of Pediatric Surgery, 35* (5), 688-689.

Williams, C. L., Bollella, M., & Wynder, E. L. (1995). A new recommendation for dietary fiber in childhood. *Pediatrics*, 96 (5, pt. 2), 985-988.

Williams, C. L., Squillace, M. M., Bollella, M. C., Brotanek, J., Campanaro, L., D'agostino, C., Pfau, J., Sprance, L., Strobino, B. A., Spark, A., Boccia, L. (1998). Healthy start: A comprehensive health education program for preschool children. *Preventive Medicine, 27* (2), 216-223.

Wintemute, G. J. (1992). From research to public policy: The prevention of motor vehicle injuries, childhood drownings, and firearm violence. *American Journal of Health Promotion*, 6 (6), 451-464.

Wood, M. L. (1995). Preschool children's assessment of health values related to selected non-health values. *Health Values*, 6, 11.

Yen, I., & Syme, S. (1999). The social environment and health: A discussion of the epidemiologic literature. *Annual Review of Public Health, 20*, 287-308.

Yoshinaga-Itano, C., Sedy, A., Coulter, D., & Mehl, A. (1998). Language of early and later identified children with hearing loss. *Pediatrics, 102* (5), 1161-1171.

Chapter 20

CAROLYN SPENCE CAGLE

School-Age Child

objectives

After completing this chapter, the nurse will be able to:

- Discuss expected variation in physical changes that occur in the child during the school-age years.
- Screen the school-age child for health risk factors.
- Discuss with families some of the common sleep-related problems that occur in school-age children, including enuresis, sleepwalking, and sleep talking.
- Describe the school-age child's cognitive stage of development relative to academic skills learned in school.
- Discuss with parents ways in which they can enhance their child's self-concept and decrease stress in the school-age child.
- Delineate agents that are responsible for the most common accidents during the school-age years.
- Explain to parents the school-age child's need for social and peer relationships as part of school-age cognitive development.
- Discuss cultural and societal influences, including affluence and poverty, on the school-age child.

key terms

Achievement Tests
Astigmatism
Attention Deficit Hyperactivity Disorder
Braces
Caries
Chronic Serous Otitis Media
Collective Monologs
Concrete Operations
Conservation
Conventional Level
Coping Strategies
Depression
Dyslexia
Encopresis
Enuresis
External Locus of Control
Hyperopic (Farsighted)
Intelligence
Intelligence Quotient
Internal Locus of Control
Learning Disabilities
Limit Setting
Magical Thinking
Menarche
Myelinization
Myopia (Nearsightedness)
Ossification
Peabody Picture Vocabulary Test
Pediculosis
Peers
Phonics
Positive Reinforcement
Preconventional Level
Puberty
Public Law 94-142
Punishment
Rehearsal
Self-Esteem
Semantics
Sexual Abuse
Sleep Talking
Sleepwalking
Socialization
Somatization
Stanford-Binet Test
Syntax
Tympanograms
Wechsler Series

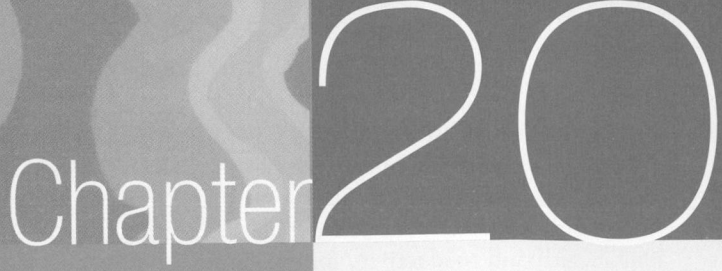

THINK About It

Homework Procrastination

Sally Paul, 9 years of age, has shown a pattern of homework procrastination since the third grade. She has performed reasonably well in school, primarily because of the pressure from her parents to complete her homework and other projects. This pressure has created an intense homework environment that has left Sally and her parents feeling frustrated about Sally's ownership of the problem.

Sally says, on occasion, that she has no homework because she had finished it at school. She is active, wants to go outside to play after school when the weather is good, and therefore must be encouraged to finish her homework completely and neatly after dinner. Her parents, both with full-time jobs, are available to help Sally, often working closely with Sally, to get a project completed because she whines that she "can't do it." This collaboration helps Sally, but leaves her parents wondering who did the work. Additionally, helping Sally decreases the time that her parents have to complete their own work in the evenings.

1. Is Sally's behavior typical for a 9-year-old child?
2. Discuss the values inherent in Sally's and her parents' behavior and how these might be related to the scenario as described.
3. How might you, as the health care professional, guide this family in finding specific ways to increase Sally's ownership of the homework duty and the quality of her work and to decrease family stress related to completion of homework? These ways might include structuring the homework environment, timing the homework, defining the value of homework, and supporting parent and child needs on the matter.
4. How might a behavioral contract be effectively used in improving homework completion?

The school-age years, ages 6 to 12 years, are frequently called the period of calm before the storm of adolescence. Changes do occur in this period, many of which are impressive when the size and skills of a beginning school-age child are compared with a child entering adolescence. Growth in height and weight is slower than it was in infancy and slower than it will be in adolescence, but continues at a steady pace. The child develops new motor skills and perfects them through repeated practice. Mental abilities grow remarkably, with the child able to learn reading, writing, mathematics, and a variety of other subjects. As the child's motor and mental abilities develop, a sense of competence develops. Competency also develops with a child's positive emotional connections to peers and others outside the family.

For most people, the school-age years are the healthiest time of their lives. Their capacity to recover from injury or infection is rapid and relatively complete. Their energy level is high and can appear endless as they engage in socialization and learning activities. However, school age children face challenges in meeting health promotion goals (Box 20-1). Nursing interventions, both in clinic and in school care, can facilitate this population's attainment of adult health and productivity for the future.

AGE AND PHYSICAL CHANGES

Compared with the preschool child's body proportions, the school-age child has an overall slimmer shape, a result of changes in the amount and distribution of fat on the child's body, and longer legs relative to the rest of the body. The gradual decrease in fat stored from ages 1 to 6 years is followed by a reaccumulation and redistribution of fat from age 7 to **puberty,** a time in life during which each gender is capable of sexual reproduction (Wong et al., 1999).

During the school years, growth is relatively steady, with an average weight gain of 3 kg (6 lb) per year and a gain in height of 6 cm (2 inches) per year. However, many children have "spurts" of growth alternating with periods of minimal growth. During these years, girls and boys are similar in size, but Black children tend to be somewhat larger and Asian-American children somewhat smaller than White children (Andrews, 1995; Jarvis, 2000). During puberty, a preadolescent increase in growth tends to occur in girls around age 10 and in boys around age 12 (Wong et al., 1999). Many girls tower over their male classmates during this time. However, many variations still occur, with some late-maturing girls not beginning this growth spurt until ages 12 to 14, whereas early-maturing boys can enter this growth state at age 10. A classroom of 10- to 12-year-old children has a wide range of sizes of both genders.

The child's head continues to grow, but again, at a much slower rate when compared with, for example, the preschooler. After 5 years of age, the head circumference grows only minimally until full adult size has been reached during puberty. This change is usually one of measurement from approximately 51 cm (20 inches) to 53 or 54 cm (21 inches), indicating that the brain has reached its adult size (Wong et al., 1999). The child's hair often darkens, and skin continues to mature and become less sensitive, approaching adult appearance and texture. Sebum and eccrine sweat production is minimal throughout childhood.

Most body systems reach an adult level of functioning during this age if they have not already done so. The gastrointestinal system's maturity is apparent in the child's ability to eat adult foods on a schedule close to that of an adult's, with fewer needs for the frequent snacks of the preschooler. By puberty, all endocrine functions, except those regulating reproduction, approach adult capacity.

Differences in lung capacity occur during this period because of differences in size, but this variation is negligible. Respirations become slower, deeper, and more regular, changing from the 20 to 30 breaths per minute of the preschool child to 17 to 25 per minute for the school-age child. The heart increases in size, and the heart

Box 20-1 Selected National Health-Promotion and Disease-Prevention Objectives for School-Age Children

- Reduce proportion of children and adolescents who experience dental caries in their primary or permanent teeth to 42% for all children in 2010 (baseline is 52% of children ages 6 to 8 in 1988 to 1994).

Special Population Targets

Dental Caries Prevalence	1999 baseline
Native American-Alaska Native	90%
Asian American-Pacific Islander*	90%
Black	50%
White	51%
Mexican American	68%

*1993 to 1994 baseline

- Reduce untreated dental caries such that the proportion of children with untreated caries (in permanent or primary teeth) is no more than 21% among all children ages 6 through 8 and no more than 15% among adolescents age 15 (baseline is 29% of children ages 6 to 8 in 1988 to 1994; 20% of adolescents age 15 in 1988 to 1994).

Special Population Targets

Untreated Dental Caries	1988 to 1994
Children ages 6 to 8 whose parents have less than a high school education	44%
Native American-Alaska Native (ages 6 to 8)	69%
Black (ages 6 to 8)	36%
Mexican American (ages 6 to 8)	43%

- Increase the proportion of children who have received protective sealants on surfaces of molar teeth to at least 50% (baseline is 23% of children age 8 and 15% of adolescents age 14 in 1988 to 1994).
- Reduce physician visits for otitis media among children and adolescents to 294 in 1000 visits (baseline is 344.7 in 1000 visits in 1997).
- Reduce the proportion of children and adolescents regularly exposed to tobacco smoke at home to 10% (baseline is 27% of children 6 years and younger in 1994).
- Increase the proportion for persons age 2 and older who consume less than 10% of their calories from saturated fat to 75% (baseline is 36% of all children in 1994 to 1996).

Special Population Targets

Hispanic-Latino	39%
Mexican American	37%
Black	31%
White	35%

- Reduce the number of asthma deaths among children ages 5 to 14 years to 1% (baseline is 3.2% in 1998).

Special Population Targets

	In 1997
Black	9.7%
White	1.8%

- Increase the proportion of the Nation's public and private schools that require daily physical education for all middle and junior high students to 25% (baseline is 17% in 1994).
- Reduce the proportion of children and adolescents ages 6 to 11 years who are overweight or obese (defined as at or above gender- and age-specific ninety-fifth percentile) to 5% (baseline is 11% in 1988 to 1994).
- Decrease the number of children the incidence of maltreatment of children under age 18 to less than 11.1 per 1000 (baseline is 13.9 per 1000 in 1997).
- Increase the proportion of children and adolescents who view television 2 or fewer hours a day to 75% (baseline is 60% of children ages 8 to 16 years in 1988 to 1994).
- Increase the use of helmets by motorcyclists and passengers to at least 79% (baseline is 67% of motorcyclists and passengers in 1997).
- Reduce deaths caused by motor vehicle crashes to no more than 9 per 100,000 people (baseline is 15 per 100,000 people [age adjusted] in 1998).

Special Population Targets

Children 14 years and younger	4.2

From U.S. Department of Health and Human Services. (2000). *Healthy people 2010: Vol 1 and 2* (Conference ed.). Washington, DC: U.S. Government Printing Office.

rate slows to the average adult heart rate of 70 to 100 beats per minute. Mean blood pressure, however, is not as high in this age group compared with adults (Jarvis, 2000).

The long-term effects of hypertension in adults are well known. The realization that hypertension in adults can begin in childhood, combined with elevated blood pressures (BPs) in children that may potentially indicate other diseases, have encouraged efforts to screen for elevated BP pressure in children early in life. Recent reports from the American Academy of Pediatrics (1995a) and the National High Blood Pressure Education Program (NHBPEP) (1996) define expected BP readings for children and recommendations for checking children's pressures. Both groups support the thesis that children should have their BP measured and plotted yearly, beginning at 3 years of age, and caution that BPs within school-age children can vary greatly. Black children should be screened closely because hypertension occurs earlier with more organ damage compared with White, Hispanic, or Native-American children (American Heart Association, 1996; Saunders, 1995). With a family history of elevated BP, a child should be monitored closely during well-child checkups in the school-age years. If an elevated BP, defined as greater than the ninety-fifth percentile, is obtained in an otherwise normal child, the BP should be repeated (usually twice) over a short time to discern a pattern. The child's height and weight should also be noted. If a child is tall and lean or proportional for one's

Table 20-1 Classification of Hypertension by Age Group

Blood Pressure	Age (yr)	Height Percentile for Boys				Height Percentile for Girls			
		5th	25th	75th	95th	5th	25th	75th	95th
Systolic (mm Hg)	3	104	107	111	113	104	105	108	110
	6	109	112	115	117	108	110	112	114
	10	114	117	121	123	116	117	120	122
	13	121	124	128	130	121	123	126	128
	16	129	132	136	138	125	127	130	132
Diastolic (mm Hg)	3	63	64	66	67	65	65	67	68
	6	72	73	75	76	71	72	73	75
	10	77	79	80	82	77	77	79	80
	13	79	81	83	84	80	81	82	84
	16	83	84	86	87	83	83	85	86

From Sinaiko, A. R. (1996). Henshaw: Hypertension in children. *New England Journal of Medicine, 335* (26), 1968-1973.
Height percentiles were determined with standard growth curves. Data are adapted from those of the Task Force on High Blood Pressure in Children and Adolescents.

height, then an elevated reading can be normal (Sadowski & Faulkner, 1996; Sinaiko, 1996). Table 20-1 illustrates expected BP values for ages within the school-age group.

Although the school-age child experiences many physical changes before adolescence, changes in the three physical areas of oral development, lymphoid tissues, and motor skills are particularly noteworthy.

Throughout childhood, the lymph tissue grows rapidly, reaching its maximal size before puberty, after which it begins to decrease in size, likely because of sex hormones. The lymphoid tissues of a 12-year-old child often exceed those of adult size (Jarvis, 2000). The larger lymphoid tissue in this age group can be apparent in the size of many children's tonsils. What appears pathologically enlarged to a parent can be normal for the child's age. The value of additional lymphoid tissue during the school-age period allows this group to have a greater immunity response than do younger and older children (Wilson, Lewis, & Penix, 1996).

The school child appears to be constantly losing or gaining a tooth. The first permanent teeth to erupt are the 6-year molars, followed by the loss of the deciduous (baby) teeth, usually in the same order in which they erupted, and the appearance of the permanent teeth. Fig. 20-1 shows the 32 adult teeth and their average time of appearance. The child between ages 6 and 13 loses and gains approximately four teeth per year. A 13-year-old child should have 28 teeth to replace the 20 deciduous teeth that are lost (Wong, et al., 1999). When deciduous teeth come out, only the crown is lost; the root has been reabsorbed in the developing permanent tooth. As the child's mouth becomes filled with the larger, permanent teeth, the shape of the jaw and the child's facial appearance normally changes.

Dental problems, primarily **caries** (cavities), periodontal disease, and malocclusion, are among the most common health problems in school-age children today. By the second grade, 50% of school-age children have caries (National Center for Health Statistics). Caries occur more frequently in poor and ethnically diverse children and in those who lack insurance or access to care for preventative dental care (Vargas, Crall, & Schneider, 1998). The nurse can implement an educational program within the school

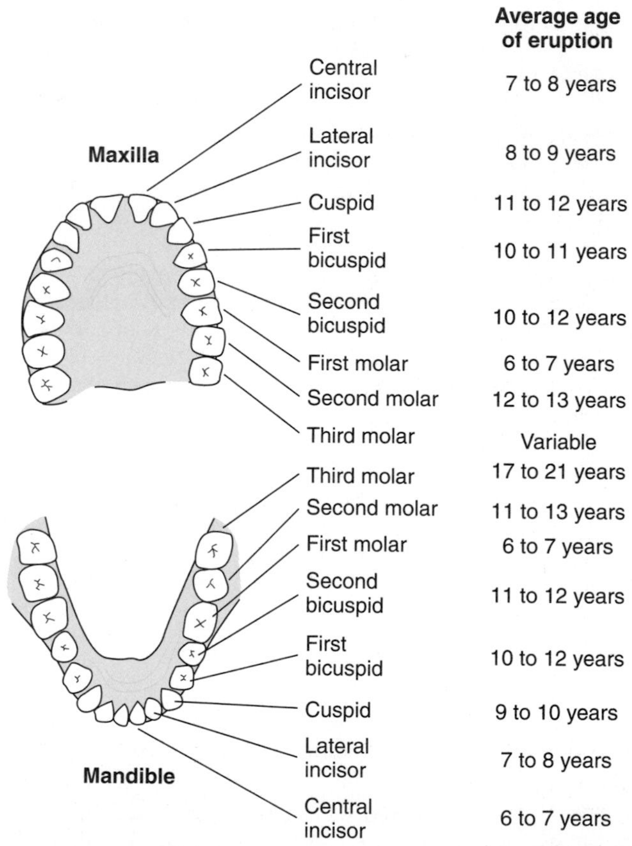

Fig. 20-1 Sequence of eruption of secondary teeth. (From McDonald, R. E., & Avery, D. R. [1994]. *Dentistry for the child and adolescent* [6th ed.]. St. Louis: Mosby.)

and provide the following information to help the child and family improve their dental health:

1. Children in this age group should be responsible for brushing and flossing their own teeth to remove plaque at least twice a day. Although brushing once a day helps remove plaque, brushing after each meal improves plaque removal. The American Dental Association (ADA) has several excellent pamphlets on the appropriate brushing and flossing of teeth, which can be obtained from a local dentist or from a state dental association. Many local dentists are willing speak to children about dental health and often provide free toothbrushes and toothpaste to school-age children.
2. Children must continue daily use of fluoride to protect their teeth; this mineral can be found in fluoridated toothpaste, fluoride rinses, and fluoridated water.
3. Personal toothbrushes should be replaced every 3 months to allow effective brushing.
4. A toothbrush with a straight handle, flat brushing surface, and soft, rounded bristles works best for school-age children; children younger than 8 years frequently need help brushing teeth, and children younger than 10 years may need help reaching back teeth during brushing (Wong et al., 1999).
5. Occasionally, an electric toothbrush makes brushing fun and entices the school-age child into brushing more frequently and more conscientiously.
6. Parents and caregivers should inspect children's teeth frequently to make certain that teeth brushing is being done well; disclosing tablets can allow detection of oral areas not being brushed well.
7. Dental visits every 6 months for preventive care (x-rays, sealants) and treatment should be encouraged.
8. When teeth brushing cannot occur after meals, children should rinse their mouths with water to help clean the teeth.
9. An appropriate diet that is low in sugar and snacks should be encouraged for school-age children's dental health.

With the rapid change in the number and type of teeth and the uneven growth in the child's jaw, malocclusion (an unacceptable relationship of the teeth in one jaw to those in the other) may be noted. A dentist should evaluate children with overbites, gaps in teeth, and other alignment problems. Some children will grow out of their problems, but others may need orthodontic care to correct developing problems, prevent potential problems, or, in some cases, improve appearance. Children frequently have short-term orthodontic appliances (**braces**) during the school-age years and then experience a second phase of appliances after jaw growth has slowed during adolescence. Peer reaction to braces should be addressed as part of the teaching about body changes, which can decrease problems with the affected child's self-concept or body image as a result of looking "different." Conscientious teeth care with braces must be encouraged because the appliances frequently make teeth brushing and flossing more challenging for the school-age child who may lack manual dexterity to complete the task.

Neurological, skeletal, and muscular changes combine to increase the child's overall motor abilities. In the nervous system, **myelinization** (process of acquiring a myelin sheath for nerve fibers) increases, allowing the child more control over and more coordination with motor tasks. The connection between the brain's two hemispheres matures in both structure and function at approximately 7 to 8 years, increasing brain function and integration (Wong et al., 1999). The child grows in height because of increases in the long bones; this growth continues into adolescence. **Ossification,** replacement of cartilage with bone, occurs throughout childhood, but is not complete until adulthood. Therefore special attention must be paid to well-fitting shoes, appropriately sized chairs or desks, and backpack loads to avoid strain on an evolving musculoskeletal system. The child's constant building of new bony tissue during the entire period of childhood generally allows for rapid repair of any fractures.

Muscle mass also increases with muscle strength. During the school-age years, boys are slightly stronger than are girls because of their physical activity, but this difference is not significant until adolescence. With these changes, the child now has the potential to perform more complex fine- and gross-motor functions, but must practice to perfect these skills throughout the school-age period (Table 20-2). Children willingly exercise their newfound skills repeatedly and receive rewards when others see their improved skill level. School-age children enthusiastically ride their bicycles, tie their shoes, throw the ball with their friends, and participate in a number of other activities requiring greater motor skills, such as team sports.

Gender

Girls tend to mature, enter puberty, and stop growing earlier than do boys. Overall, girls' physical growth is more regular, with fewer spurts and plateaus compared with boys. Girls' teeth erupt sooner, and their bones ossify sooner compared with boys. From birth, girls have more fat than boys have, and after puberty, they have a great percentage of body weight devoted to fat. Most physical differences between boys and girls become more pronounced after puberty. This earlier maturing process of girls occurs in many mammals and nearly all primates. Beginning toward the end of the school-age period for most children, this maturation process involves development of sexual characteristics that become more evident during adolescence.

Two other areas of differences in the genders are discussed in detail later in this chapter. First, girls tend to mature faster than do boys in many psychological and physical processes. Many psychological processes, such as cognitive abilities and language skills, depend primarily on

Table 20-2 Motor Development of the School-Age Child

Age (Years)	Gross Motor	Fine Motor
6 to 7	Balances on one foot for 10 seconds Can perform tandem gait Hops 25 times on one foot, 12 times on the other Pedals a bicycle	Spreads with knife Holds pencil with fingertip Draws a person with 3 to 6 parts Cuts with a knife Aligns letters horizontally Ties a bow Draws a triangle Knows right from left
8 to 9	Has good body balance Enjoys vigorous activities Throws objects farther	Spaces words and letters with writing Draws a diamond Draws a 3-dimensional geometric figure Has good eye-hand coordination Bathes self Sews and builds models
10 to 12	Balances on one foot for 15 seconds Catches a fly ball Has some awkwardness because of prepubertal growth spurt Possesses all basic motor skills	Has skills similar to adults

physical maturation of the nervous system. Second, boys tend to have certain problems more frequently than girls have, such as enuresis, encopresis, learning disabilities, and other school difficulties. These concerns are addressed later in this chapter.

Race

Black and Asian-American children mature at a faster rate than do White children, including earlier dental development and **menarche,** the advent of monthly bleeding or menses. Body proportions vary, with Black children being somewhat heavier and taller than are White children during the school-age period. Blacks also have longer and more dense bones than do White and Asian-American children (Garn, 1964; Jarvis, 2000). Blacks tend to have slimmer hips and more muscle and less fat in the limbs compared with more central body fat (Jarvis, 2000).

Determining whether physical differences among White, Black, and Asian-American children relate to racial characteristics or exist as products of the socioeconomic climates in which these diverse groups live is difficult. Most likely, the physical differences reflect the interaction of both factors. However, although differences appear based initially on race, the major issue of poverty among diverse groups influences the physical development of Black children and the growing number of Hispanic children. Certainly not all Blacks are poor, but the number of poor Blacks in proportion to the overall number of Blacks is greater than the same ratio in Whites (U.S. Department of Health and Human Services, 2000).

Limited data exist in this area for Asian-American children. However, one might guess that many new Asian refugee groups in the United States have fewer socioeconomic resources. This economic fact exposes these children to malnutrition, overcrowded housing, school deficits, and health problems based on low access to care, all of which influence the future health and societal productivity of children of diverse groups.

Genetics

School-age children tend to be concerned about their rate of growth, weight, time of menarche, and final height. The nurse is unable to provide exact answers to these questions, but knowledge of genetic influences helps in responding. Both parents contribute an equal number of genes to the final height of their children, but genes for being tall are dominant and genes for being short are recessive. When assessing a child's height, even before referring to standardized growth charts, the nurse should examine the child's family. The child who plots on the third percentile for height compared with all the other children may have parents who are shorter than average; therefore shorter height can be expected because the child represents the genetic lineage of the family.

Rate of growth also appears to be genetically influenced. For example, many girls find their average age of menarche to be 12.8 years, approximately the time when their mothers began their monthly periods. After they have sufficient body fat to stimulate hormones needed for menses, girls can have their first menstrual period anytime between age 11 and 15 and still be "normal." Likely because of better nutrition and differences in lifestyle, girls appear to be experiencing menarche earlier than did girls only 30 years ago.

Generally, most acute, life-threatening diseases of a hereditary nature become evident before the school-age years. Some health problems that occur at this time appear in certain families most likely because of chromosomal contributions at conception of the school-age child. However, environmental influences also contribute to diseases believed to have a genetic component. These conditions include obesity, cardiovascular disease, learning problems, and enuresis (see Research Highlights box).

GORDON'S FUNCTIONAL HEALTH PATTERNS

Health Perception-Health Management Pattern

The school-age child understands what health is and what causes illness, but this understanding is different from that

research highlights

Risk Factors for Cardiovascular Disease in School-Age Children

The purpose of this longitudinal study was to examine the nongenetic (environmental) effects of obesity (defined by body mass index and triceps skinfold thickness) on risk factors for cardiovascular disease (CVD) during the school-age years, adolescence, and the transition between these two developmental phases. A total of 73 pairs of twins were identified as potential subjects in phase 1 (school-age years). The twins were 6- to 11-year-old White children who were free of chronic illness and lived with at least one biological parent. Pairs were evenly distributed by age and predominantly middle-income, two-parent families. In phase 2, 56 twin pairs (77%) of the original phase-1 cohort were retained in the study. In both phases of the study, data were collected by one or two nurse clinicians during one or two home visits. Measures included obesity, lipid profile, and systolic and diastolic blood pressure. Results of the matched-pair T test indicated significant environmental influences on obesity in both phases and during transition. Intraindividual associations of obesity and levels of atherogenic lipids (total and low-density lipoprotein [LDL] cholesterol) emerged during the school-age years. During adolescence, obesity was associated with high-density lipoprotein (HDL) cholesterol and total triglyceride levels. Changes in obesity from the school-age years to adolescence was associated with total triglyceride levels. Results of this study emphasize obesity as part of CVD risk-factor management in children, highlighting the importance of primary prevention.

Data from Hayman, L. L., Meninger, J. C., Coates, P. M., & Gallagher, P. R. (1995). Nongenetic influences of obesity on risk factors for cardiovascular disease during two phases of development. *Nursing Research*, 44, 277-283.

of an adult. Some researchers assert that for younger school-age children the concept of health remains abstract. However, these children perceive symptoms and causes of illness and can participate in health-promoting behaviors early in life to prevent illness. Health teaching is appropriate to the preschooler and school-age child's cognitive level (concrete operations) and moral level (external rules and forces); therefore many educational materials have been developed that focus on cognitive, psychomotor, and affective methods for teaching school-age children about health. Children frequently know more about health than adults have acknowledged and this knowledge serves as a foundation for health-promotion teaching during the child's elementary and middle school years.

School-age children, when asked for their ideas about what causes illness, usually state the *germ theory*, the *punishment theory*, or the *external forces theory*. Many younger school-age children can state that germs play a role in illness, but have limited understanding of germs. Other children believe their behavior causes a resulting punishment (an illness). Closely tied to this concept is the belief that outside elements or people cause illness, such as "the rain gives you a cold." Although these beliefs can make the child feel helpless, they can play a role in teaching these children health-promotion concepts.

Parents teach health-promotion concepts when they spend time monitoring and reinforcing preventive health practices, such as personal hygiene, dental care, and good nutrition. Most children in this age group still need some adult supervision in these areas, and the school environment can also provide this supervision on a daily basis. Some children can become confused about the relationship between these preventive measures and how they work to prevent illness. Therefore role playing, reading in age-appropriate books, and modeling of health-promotion behaviors frequently help children make the link between behavior and improved health. Unfortunately, by modeling some caregivers, children in society can become passive health care consumers, asking few questions and doing as they are told. This unfortunate circumstance is caused partly by their obligation to obey authority figures and partly by the fact that many adults that mentor children are not assertive health care consumers. Generally, parents and teachers must make a commitment to demonstrate and teach healthy behaviors at home and in school; this collaborative effort helps children develop health values as part of their educational process to reach a healthy adulthood (Cagle & Keen-Payne, 1996; Elias & Kress, 1994).

An awareness of the school-age child's normal perceptions of health is important to the nurse in counseling the child and the family on health promotion. *Health* should be broadly defined to include personal and environmental health and safety, all of which allow an individual to optimally contribute to society and to reach human potential. Some suggestions to help the nurse in this area include the following:

1. Assess the child's understanding of the cause or causes of illnesses. Discussion in this area can be part of language arts, social studies, or science discussions and therefore easily integrated into the regular academics of the school program.
2. Before teaching prevention, the nurse must first teach an understanding of the cause of illness.
3. Health-promotion and illness-prevention measures, when properly understood, give the child a heightened sense of control and decreased anxiety over health issues.
4. Parental education on health care issues and health promotion can occur with the support of the school; educational materials can be sent home with children on issues such as immunizations, head lice problems, and other health care issues that may be of concern to parents. This approach helps form a health-focused connection between the school and the parents of the school-age child.

5. Children can be taught during school to be appropriately assertive heath care consumers; they may refuse to buy products that are unsupportive of health, for example.
6. Each interaction of the child with the nurse should be used to teach health-promotion concepts.

Nutritional-Metabolic Pattern

School-age children, similar to all children, need a well-balanced diet. An average of 2400 calories per day meets growth requirements; normally, these calories are provided through three meals and one or two snacks. As the child grows, more food is required and consumed. Extensive recent concern has focused on the nutrition habits of school-age children who appear to have less nutritious food intake patterns, fewer quality snacks, and higher fat intake than their parents had at the same age. These behaviors place children at risk for poor nutritional habits later in life, iron deficiency anemia, and chronic illnesses later in life (U.S. Department of Heath and Human Services, 2000). Apparently, mass media and contemporary busy lifestyles play a role in poor food choices as well. A multitude of television messages pressure children to eat certain foods, many of which contain high amounts of salt, sugar, and calories. Dining outside the home consumes 40% of family budgets (U.S. Department of Heath and Human Services, 2000) resulting in many children frequently eating "fast food" that has poor nutritional quality. Successful interventions that consider these economic, social, and cultural factors must be developed to improve this country's nutrition. These factors must also be considered with increasing concerns about the nutrition of homeless children, children in child care centers, and the high level of obesity found particularly among Hispanic, Black, and Native-American children, all of whom may lack access to safe and nutritious food. This deficit has been related to undernutrition, growth retardation, and iron deficiency anemia among these populations (U.S. Department of Heath and Human Services, 2000).

Although some children in this age group are willing to try new foods, many continue to dislike foods such as vegetables, fruits, casseroles, spicy foods, and iron-rich foods, preferring only a small range of foods. Some children who will not eat cooked fruits or vegetables will eat them raw; they may go through a period of wanting to eat only one food, such as peanut butter sandwiches, every day at lunch. This practice seldom hurts the child nutritionally and usually lasts only a short time. Children frequently make their own after-school snacks and need supervision regarding the content. Foods high in vitamin A and C, fruits, and vegetables should be encouraged. With parental or caregiver help, school-age children can calculate nutritious needs, plan family meals, and eat better because of this involvement. These activities also assist them in fostering wise decision-making practices, math skills, and feelings of empowerment about health. Generally, the responsibility of being involved in meal preparation helps school-age children develop healthy food habits for the rest of their lives. Positive reinforcement by parents, teachers, and caregivers to the school-age child can also increase healthy food choices.

Families generally eat only one meal a day together, most frequently dinner; therefore a positive environment for nutrition and socialization during this shared time is important. Parents and other family members play a role in shaping the child's food preferences and habits. Positive food habits should be encouraged, and pressure to eat certain foods should be avoided to prevent power struggles between caregiver and child. A child's nutritional pattern usually reflects family patterns. For example, parents who skip breakfast tend to have trouble convincing their children to eat breakfast. Educating children as a group to eat healthy foods also seems successful because of the powerful influence of **peers** (people of the same age, experience, and usually gender) during the school-age period. The child whose friend is eating a candy bar usually prefers the same rather than an apple for a snack.

Despite evidence that the school can serve as an environment for nutritional health-promotion education (U.S. Department of Health and Human Services, 1995a), only 69% of states require nutritional education during the kindergarten through twelfth grade (Collins et al., 1995). Nutritional education, as part of the core concepts usually taught in school, teaches students about choices related to weight control and health and help students understand the role of media and culture in nutritional choices (Centers for Disease Control and Prevention, 1996). Schools that offer nutritious foods for lunch and healthy foods that reflect different cultures encourage the use of the Food Guide Pyramid published by the U. S. Department of Agriculture (1992), and discourage the use of vending machines for nonnutritious intake by students help foster appreciation of diverse cultures and healthy food choices for life. Teachers should also serve as role models for optimal eating and exercise habits for the children in their charge. School lunch programs are available in most school systems and range from those that receive federal support for milk alone to programs in which children with financial need receive both breakfast and lunch. These meals must meet the guidelines established by the National School Lunch Program, administered by the U.S. Department of Agriculture in 1992. The guidelines are based on the needs of a 10- to 12-year-old child and include the following requirements:

1. 8 ounces of unflavored, fluid, low-fat milk; skim milk; or buttermilk (whole milk or flavored milk may be offered as a substitute, but low-fat milk must be offered)
2. 2 ounces of protein-rich canned or cooked meat, fish, or poultry; one egg; 1 cup cooked dry peas or beans;

4 tbsp. peanut butter; or equivalent combinations of these foods
3. Two or more portions of vegetables and fruit totaling 1 cup
4. Bread or a bread substitute made with enriched flour

Television, radio, and billboards have a strong influence on children's eating habits. A large percentage of the advertisements that children see and hear are devoted to sugary, nonnutritious "junk" foods. Without parental guidance, school-age children frequently make poor food choices. The nutrients that children tend to consume in amounts less than the recommended amounts are iron and vitamin C. Although this age group is increasingly less willing to be guided by the parents, parents should discuss with their children what they want to eat, need to eat, and will eat to influence the eating habits of school-age children.

Box 20-2 Nursing Interventions to Prevent Obesity During the School-Age Period

- Parents should evaluate their own nutritional values and patterns. Some parents use food as a reward or as an expression of caring and need help to find more appropriate behaviors.
- Meal patterns may need to be assessed and altered. One family may eat only in front of the television, whereas another family may use mealtime as a period of confrontation.
- Family snacking habits can lead to poor snacking habits for the child; therefore the type of food available for snacking may need to be altered.
- The child's snacking habits should be reviewed and changes made as needed.
- Regular exercise is important to everyone and should be encouraged for the child.

Obesity

A major nutrition problem among adults and children in the United States is obesity. Obesity has increased over the last 40 years with 11% of children ages 6 to 19 years now classified as obese (weighing above the ninety-fifth percentile for height) (U.S. Department of Health and Human Services, 2000). Some evidence suggests that obesity in adulthood begins in infancy or childhood. Boys and girls with two slim parents tend to be slim, and boys and girls with two obese parents tend to be obese. This tendency may be the result of a combination of genetic determinants and familial environmental patterns. For example, a child whose overweight parents constantly use food as a reward has a greater tendency for obesity than does a child of thin parents who do not reward with food. The majority of obese children become overweight because of excessive food intake. A lack of physical activity also contributes to a child's being overweight, and obesity tends to reinforce a pattern of decreased activity. The obese child experiences greater risk for a number of physical problems, such as hypertension, diabetes, and coronary heart disease. Obesity tends to occur more with Black children compared with White children, often a reflection of less physical activity because of environmental living conditions and the inability to purchase higher cost healthy food choices (U.S. Department of Health and Human Services, 2000).

The obese child faces ridicule by peers in school and discrimination later in life by others. These responses by the obese individual's peers only reinforce an already low self-esteem and body image. A cycle of personal isolation and poor performance occurs for the obese school-age child that influences that child's future success.

Helping the obese child change lifestyle patterns requires intensive intervention. Treatment of obese children can be discouraging and significant weight loss, especially maintained weight loss, is a rare occurrence because of the complexity of factors (environmental, cultural, economic, and psychological) involved. Programs of treatment have included caloric restriction, anorectic drugs, physical exercise, bypass surgery, and habit pattern changes with varying degrees of success or failure. School-age children are a difficult group with which to work because these children are frequently not ready to be concerned about being overweight.

The age of the child notwithstanding, any program that is instituted must involve the entire family. Family eating patterns or styles frequently must be adjusted, and other family members must be willing to eat many of the same foods that the child must eat. Unfortunately, even the best weight-reduction programs for children demonstrate poor long-term success. Prevention of obesity is significantly more desirable and involves parental teaching early in the child's life and care agencies that reinforce behaviors focused on appropriate weight for height. According to the U.S. Department of Agriculture and the U.S. Department of Health and Human Services (1995), prevention of obesity focuses on the following: eating a variety of foods every day; balancing food intake with physical exercise; and eating a diet focused on fruits, vegetables, high-protein grains, moderate salt and sugar, and low cholesterol and fat for all persons over the age of 2 years. Evidence indicates that children will eat low-fat lunches (Borja, Bordi, & Lambert, 1996), and the influence of peer and teacher encourages reluctant children to eat more healthy foods early in life. Some suggestions that the nurse might give to parents who are interested in preventing obesity in their school-age children are listed in Box 20-2.

Elimination Pattern

Most children have full bowel and bladder control by 5 years of age. Control involves the ability to undress and dress and the wiping, flushing, and cleaning of hands required in toileting. The child's elimination patterns are similar to adult patterns, with urination occurring 6 to 8 times a day and bowel movements averaging 1 or 2 times a day (Wong et al., 1999). For some school-age children, however, elimination continues to be a problem. White children generally assume earlier control of their elimination habits than do Black children, likely based on cultural factors of appropriate timing for this type of control.

Enuresis

The involuntary passing of urine at an age when control should be present is called **enuresis.** *Primary enuretic* children have never achieved bladder control, and *secondary enuretic* children have periods of dryness, usually for several months, and then display enuresis again. Enuresis should not be considered as a disease, but rather, as a variation of normal development.

Urinating at night (bedwetting) is called *nocturnal enuresis*, and wetting during the day is called *diurnal enuresis*. Bedwetting occurs in 7% of boys and 3% of girls at age 5, but only 3% of boys and 2% of girls by age 10 (American Psychiatric Association, 1994). Because both boys and children born prematurely experience higher rates of this problem than do girls, maturational immaturity appears to be related to nocturnal enuresis (Friman, 1995).

Nocturnal enuresis is involuntary wetting during sleep at least once a month. An organic cause is found in few children; the cause, typically, is a urinary tract infection. For the remainder of cases, the origin is likely a combination of factors, including genetic predisposition, neurological developmental delay (including both inhibition of the bladder contraction reflex and the child's slow waking response to a full bladder) reduced bladder capacity, and environmental factors, including family stress.

The school-age child with nocturnal enuresis faces a variety of problems. The child frequently experiences teasing from classmates and siblings. A night away from home appears impossible because of fear of wetting. Parents may be angry at the constant bed changes and washes and may try punishments, thinking that the child should be able to control the problem. Parents and caregivers may become abusive to the child based on their belief that the child should be able to control this behavior (Wong et al., 1999). Parental stress places additional pressure on the child who often has low self-esteem and lacks self-confidence.

Frustrated families frequently seek help with this problem. After a physiological problem, such as urinary tract infection, has been ruled out through a complete evaluation, various treatments can be considered. These treatments include wet alarm systems, retention control, waking schedules, drug therapy (tricyclic antidepressants, antidiuretics, antispasmodics), and hormonal therapy (desmopressin). Friman (1995) notes that imipramine (a tricyclic antidepressant) quickly remedies the problem, but has more side effects than antidiuretic medication. Overall, each method has advantages, disadvantages, and cost considerations, most of which require a commitment of consistency and time from the child and the parents to reach a successful outcome.

With many cases of enuresis spontaneously resolving on their own, explaining the problem to the family and waiting for time to cure it may be the best method of treatment. The treatment regimen notwithstanding, the nurse includes certain information when counseling the parents and child (Box 20-3). By providing information, supporting treatment, and encouraging expression of the child's and the family's feelings, the nurse plays a vital role in helping a family deal with nocturnal enuresis.

Diurnal enuresis is often called *daytime dribbling*. This term accurately describes the pattern of urination for children who have this problem, most of whom are girls. These children demonstrate "holding on" behaviors, such as not voiding first thing in the morning, voiding only 2 to 3 times a day, and voiding exceptionally quickly. The reasons for which these children delay going to the bathroom and only partially empty their bladders, thus precipitating overflow incontinence, remain unclear. Evaluation of these children begins with a urine culture to rule out urinary tract infection. If symptoms persist after an infection is treated or if no infection is found, then the "daytime dribbler" is treated by increasing fluids to prevent "holding" and establishing a voiding routine that includes voiding every 2 hours, with a conscious effort to empty the bladder completely. The nurse remains instrumental in helping the child and parents understand the problem and the treatment.

Box 20-3 Nursing Counseling for Families About Nighttime Enuresis

- Enuresis is a common problem.
- No serious physical problem is present, although the child may have a small or immature bladder.
- Enuresis is often inherited; other family members may have had the same problem. With time, the child will be cured, usually by adolescence.
- The child is not wetting the bed intentionally; it is not a conscious act.
- The parents are not at fault.
- When a treatment is tried, the child should be responsible for dealing with both the problem and the treatment.
- Punishment when the child is wet should be replaced with praise when dry (positive reinforcement).
- Parents might wake the child to urinate before they go to bed.
- A family plan for dealing with the wet bed and child can decrease family arguments. The plan might include deciding who strips the bed and where the sheets go. The child should play a major role in this process to understand the effect of this behavior on the family and to learn responsibility for the act.

Encopresis

Another elimination problem that can occur in children is **encopresis,** defined as the persistent passing of stool into the child's underpants after age 4. A common time for this event to occur is late afternoon. The incidence of encopresis is approximately 1.5% in second-grade children (American Psychiatric Association, 1994). The vast majority of children with encopresis are boys of average or above-average intelligence. These children retain stool at least part of the time, which leads to complaints of recurrent abdominal pain and, for many, a practice of enuresis as well.

These children commonly have emotional difficulties, either before or resulting from the problem of encopresis. Nurses should be aware of this childhood problem to identify the affected child, refer the child for treatment, and support the child and family during treatment. Treatment usually requires a specific bowel program coupled with family and individual counseling.

Activity-Exercise Pattern

Generally, the school-age child is physically active, although one report notes that Hispanic and Black children are less active than are White children (U.S. Department of Health and Human Services, 2000). As discussed, impressive changes in motor skills occur between the ages of 6 and 12 years. The child normally engages in physical exercise or activities to enhance the development of strength, balance, and coordination. Exercise typically occurs through group activities and organized sports, such as Little League baseball and soccer; through activities of individual skill, such as gymnastics and ballet; and through unorganized play, such as bike riding, sledding, rollerblading, and imaginary play. Typically, play provides important learning for the school-age child and, for this reason, should be encouraged as part of the school-age years. For many children, involvement in physical activities is fun and connects them to their peers, important persons in the school-age child's life. As mentioned, daily physical activity helps to prevent health problems later in life.

The play and activities of this age group incorporate other areas of the child's development, including social, personal, and cognitive aspects. The social aspects are of major importance. School-age children frequently prefer interacting with peers rather than with family. This desire is not completely satisfied in the structured time of school and carries over to play and outside activities; many school-age children prefer to be with children of their own gender. Skill in motor tasks can both win the respect of other children and provide a feeling of self-accomplishment. Organized sports such as baseball teach team cooperation, competition, and other social skills. Organized activities such as scouts and 4H clubs teach children about functioning as part of a group, processes in carrying out a task, and the power of social relationships to create change. These lessons can prepare them for the discipline that will be needed for a job later in life.

Children who perform well in these activities, especially when they receive prizes or trophies, feel good about themselves, their competence, and their sense of industry. This feeling of self-accomplishment is also enhanced in simple games played alone or with others, such as hopping or jumping rope. Additional commendation by parents and teachers when children perform well in physical activities facilitates self-esteem as well.

New cognitive skills are incorporated into the child's activities. The abilities to count, sort, and group objects are apparent in the pleasure that children of this age receive from their collections of stamps, rocks, or other objects. Understanding the concepts of fair and consistent rules requires memory, logical reasoning, and the desire to work with others. Many games, such as board games, puzzles, and computer games, integrate several intellectual skills. Daily reading brings enjoyment to the child and provides ideas about life and cultures that are different from those of the child, thereby enhancing the child's acceptance of human diversity.

The nurse helps parents promote healthy activities for children with some of the following suggestions:

1. Encourage reading. Parents can continue to read aloud with children and model reading as a routine leisure activity. Children can obtain library cards, providing both a variety of books and an added responsibility. Children enjoy books that have been written as a series. Receiving their "very own" magazine, such as *Electric Company, Ranger Rick, Highlights for Children*, or *Zillions* can stimulate reading skills on a frequent basis. The magazine *Jack and Jill* has stories with a health-promotion focus; these stories facilitate the school-age child's understanding of health important to the growing years.
2. Monitor television use, particularly because of its passive nature; encourage physical activity as an alternative.
3. Support the child's outside interests. Some children prefer organized group activities, others prefer individual pursuits, and still others prefer a balance of solitary and group activities.
4. Praise the child's success in a variety of activities to encourage further development and a sense of self-worth.
5. Help children recognize both their strengths and their weaknesses so they can learn to deal with both success and failure.
6. Encourage the child to participate in both group and individual activities to perfect a variety of skills.
7. Encourage family activities that focus on physical activity and togetherness.

Sleep-Rest Pattern

Sleep Patterns

The majority of school-age children have no difficulties with sleep; their sleep requirements and patterns are more similar to the adult than those of a younger child. Individual needs vary, but most children sleep between 8 and 12 hours a night without naps during the day. The difficulties frequently encountered in earlier childhood with going to bed occur much less frequently. Most children and parents are able to agree on a bedtime, allow some flexibility on nonschool nights, and keep to that agreement. When problems arise regarding the time set for going to bed, the children may be testing parents who have not been clear and firm about their expectations or who have not been willing to discuss the arrangement with their children.

Children, similar to adults, experience rapid eye movement (REM) sleep alternating with nonREM sleep, with nonREM sleep consisting of four substages.

Sleep Disturbances

The most common sleep problems that occur in the preschool and school-age years are night terrors (see Chapter 19), **sleepwalking, sleep talking,** and enuresis. As a group, these disturbances have been called *disorders of arousal* because they tend to occur between stage 4 and stage 1 of nonREM sleep, as the child is progressing toward waking up (Rosen, Mahowald, & Ferber, 1995). According to these authors, the disorders generally share the following characteristics:

1. They occur immediately before a switch to the REM state.
2. Most occur 1 to 2 hours after going to sleep.
3. The same child may have more than one sleep problem.
4. A positive family history may accompany the problem.
5. Boys have these problems more often than do girls (4:1 ratio).
6. The child does not recall the episodes.

Stages 3 and 4 during nonREM sleep can be affected by fatigue and stress, factors that are common in this age group. Combined with the normal central nervous system (CNS) immaturity and the normal developmental changes in stages 3 and 4 of nonREM sleep, these factors may account for the increased occurrence of sleep problems in children.

Approximately one out of six children between ages 5 and 12 has walked in their sleep at least once, but far fewer children experience persistent sleepwalking (Rosen, Mahowald, & Ferber, 1995). Sleepwalking is occasionally associated with enuresis. Typically, shortly after going to sleep, the child suddenly sits up in bed and moves awkwardly. The type and amount of movement can vary from simply sitting in bed to making repetitive finger and hand movements or getting up and walking. However, the child usually stays in bed. When talking to the child, the child may mumble. In most cases of sleepwalking:

- The episodes last approximately 30 minutes.
- The child avoids being hurt despite the lack of awareness of the situation.
- Onset of the episodes occurs before age 10, but few children still sleepwalk by age 15.

As with sleepwalking, sleep talking is not purposeful. The words tend to be simple, but difficult to understand and the child quickly falls back to sleep. With CNS maturation, both sleepwalking and sleep talking tend to be outgrown.

Parents who are concerned about sleepwalking or sleep talking can be reassured to know that most children outgrow these episodes. However, parents should watch sleepwalking children and protect them from hurting themselves. Gates should be placed at the top of stairs and sharp objects moved from the child's path. Most parents find that the easiest solution is to direct the sleepwalker back to bed, where the child will return to a normal sleep. Trying to wake the child is difficult and can cause more confused behavior or loss of coordination in the child. Occasionally, parents can effectively intervene by implementing relaxation techniques for their child before bedtime, avoiding stressful and fatiguing situations, and providing consistency with sleep preparation patterns (Wong et al., 1999). If a child is having many episodes or if parents are particularly concerned, then the child may need further evaluation and treatment by health care professionals.

Cognitive-Perceptual Pattern

The school-age child spends extensive time in settings that require the mastery of new ideas and concepts. Many elements contribute to the child's ability to learn; only a few are discussed here. The child must continue to develop cognitive skills for success later in life. Basic senses such as vision and hearing must be intact, language skills must expand, and memory capabilities must increase to allow cognitive development. These elements, along with basic intelligence and the child's heredity and environment, encourage or discourage the child's learning. Unfortunately, many children in society have difficulties in these and other areas, which result in learning problems if not identified early through parental awareness, school observations, or routine health care assessments.

Piaget's Theory

Piaget (1969) refers to the span from ages 7 to 11 years as the period of **concrete operations,** a stage when children learn by manipulating concrete objects and lack the ability to perform thinking operations that require abstraction. During this time, the child moves from egocentric interactions to more cooperative interactions, to increased understanding of many concepts associated with objects, such as **conservation** (certain characteristics of objects remain constant, are "conserved"). Children increasingly can change reasoning from intuition to logical or rational operations and engage in serial ordering, addition, subtraction, and other basic mathematical skills. The term *operation* refers to rule-governed actions carried out in the mind, such as ordering and relating. The operations of this period are termed *concrete* because the child's mental operations or actions still depend on the ability to perceive specific examples of what has happened. The ability to perform abstract thinking remains developed. Older children during this period are able to use both types of mental operations, which adds flexibility and control to their thinking and to meet developmental needs of adolescence.

Interestingly, children are not deliberately taught the concepts and operations that are discussed here. These concepts and processes emerge; they are constructed by the environment and by experience, but they are not taught. This is a process, and some aspects of the preoperational preschool child can still occur in the school-age child. For example, some younger school-age children use **magical thinking** (beliefs inconsistent with reality) and are still egocentric in their social behavior.

The preschool child's egocentric thoughts, actions, and understandings in social and perceptual situations change in the school-age child, forming the groundwork for the concepts and operations that develop. For example, the preschool or preoperational child, when talking with another child of similar age, engages in **collective monologs,** a behavior identified when a child pursues a private conversation and talks "at" rather than "with" another person. During the concrete operations period, a school-age child begins to take the other child's point of view into account, incorporating the partner's conversation into the child's own discussion. These traits do not emerge suddenly and completely; they tend to flow into one another, with the new skill being demonstrated initially in behavior only occasionally and then emerging with increasing frequency as the child's mental capacity and experience grow (Piaget, 1969; Wong et al., 1999).

The change away from egocentricity shows in the child's perceptual abilities as well. An experiment in which the child sits at a square table with three molded mountains of varying heights on it illustrates this point. Three empty chairs are placed on three sides of the table. A doll is placed in each of the three chairs sequentially, and each time, the child is asked what the doll sees when looking at the mountains from that side of the table. Before the concrete operations period, the child cannot conceive of what the doll's view might be, and the problem then fails to engage the child's interest. However, after approximately age 7, the child begins to show some interest in the problem and shows the ability to represent the doll's point of view, albeit erratically. Toward the latter part of this period, the child begins to accurately represent the doll's view from all sides of the table (Piaget, 1969; Wong et al., 1999).

During this period, the child understands a number of expanding concepts regarding objects, including the concept of conservation of substance (see Chapter 19). For example, two identical glasses are filled with the same amount of liquid and shown to a child. The liquid from one of the glasses is the poured into a third glass with a different shape. The child is asked whether a difference exists in the amount of liquid between the two glasses. The preschool, preoperational child focuses on the different shapes and says "yes." The concrete operational child realizes that no change has occurred in the substance despite the change in shape. Conservation of numbers, required to understand basic mathematics, emerges at approximately age 7, with some cultural variations from exposure to learning concepts. Conservation of quantity (substance, amount of space occupied by an object) emerges at approximately age 7 or 8. Conservation of weight emerges at approximately age 9, whereas conservation of volume emerges close to the end of the concrete operational period.

The concept of time also develops during this period. Children begin to learn to tell time and to understand the passage of time during the early school years. By age 8, most children understand the difference between past and present; history becomes meaningful. The concept of human aging becomes increasingly understandable, and the child can comprehend the difference between an 18-year-old and an 80-year-old person (Wong et al., 1999).

Two major operations of the period are classifying and ordering. The child now classifies or groups objects by their common element and understands the relationship between groups or classes. For example, when given 12 wooden beads, some brown and some white, this child can understand that the beads can be grouped by their color and by their material. Conversely, the preschool child would be able to focus only on one property of the beads, such as the color. The newfound ability to classify is apparent in the school-age child's interest in collections, such as stamps or coins.

Ordering things requires skill in recognizing the relationships within a group or class. The child with a coin collection first groups all the quarters, nickels, and dimes together and then groups the coins according to another criterion (dates, weight, and so on). Children in school are frequently ordering their world; they line up in school according to height, they repeat numbers and letters in their classic order, and they might be numbered in school to reflect an alphabetized surname. These two operations are important in learning to read, in understanding the concepts of numbers, and in learning subjects based on relations, such as history (the relation of events in time) and geography (the relation of places in space).

During the concrete operations period, the cognitive

abilities required to learn the basic concepts of mathematics, language, science, humanities, and social studies are developed. The child thinks differently now than this same child did as a preschooler. The child considers others' views, can reverse thought processes, recognizes the relationships between objects and within a system, and can classify and order. These same mental abilities can be used to teach health-promotion concepts and content in the school-age years as part of a health-promotion curriculum.

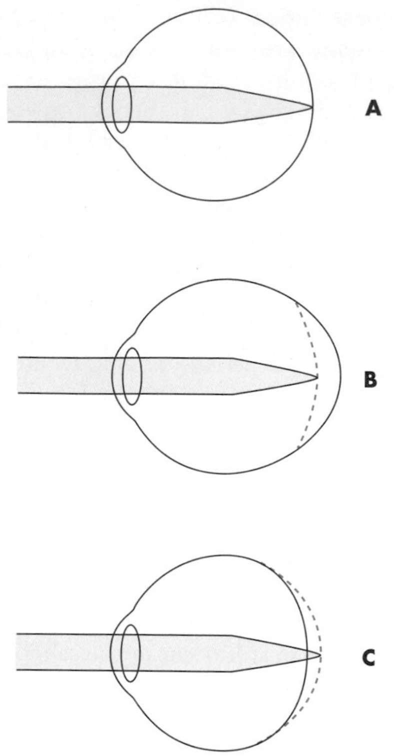

Fig. 20-2 **A,** Normal eye, no accommodation necessary; **B,** Myopia (nearsightedness); eyeball is longer, and distant images fall in front of the retina; many school-age children inherit myopia; **C,** hyperopia (farsightedness); eyeball is shorter, and near images fall behind the retina.

Vision

The child's sensory abilities also continue to develop during the school-age years. Visual capacity should reach optimal function by the sixth or seventh year. The child's peripheral vision should be fully developed, and the ability to discriminate fine differences in shading of colors also develops fully. Acuity should be at maximal development or at least 20/30 in each eye, as measured by the Snellen E Chart, an assessment tool for children who can read some letters (Jarvis, 2000). The child is able to coordinate eye movements, see a single image, and associate incoming visual stimuli with past and present mental images and functions. Throughout childhood, further development of full visual potential occurs through use and practice.

Physiological changes occur in the eye during the school-age years. Eyes in the preschool years are normally **hyperopic (farsighted),** a condition where the visual image of an object falls behind the retina. However, dissimilar to older individuals, preschool children do not need glasses because they normally accommodate their eyes by adjusting their own lenses. For most children, as the shape of the eye changes and grows in length and there is neurological and behavioral maturation, their vision becomes normal (Fig. 20-2, A). However, many school-age children do not have normal vision, and many deficits are not detected in time to prevent academic difficulties. Routine eye screening by a school nurse, as required by many states and as part of a school's approach to health promotion, identifies vision defects early. Parents of children with identified deficits are then encouraged by the nurse to seek further care to correct these defects, allowing these children to learn more effectively.

Although hyperopia is no longer a developmental issue as it was for the preschooler, two other visual problems are common in this age group (Fig. 20-2, C). Many school-age children inherit **myopia (nearsightedness),** a condition where the visual image of an object falls in front of the retina, and have difficulty seeing distant objects (Fig. 20-2, B). The other condition, **astigmatism,** reflects blurred vision caused by a poorly focused image on the retina and changes in the curvature of the cornea and lens of the eye. Glasses identify the defects, but the problem can be in identifying the defects. For example, a child with myopia in the school-age years likely has never experienced maximal visual acuity and does not realize that the visual images are inadequate. Children with corrective lenses often express delight and surprise when they first see the fully focused and rich detail of the world after experiencing less refined visual acuity for some time.

Hearing

The child's hearing ability, or auditory acuity, is nearly complete by 7 years of age, although some maturation continues into adolescence. Hearing deficits are less common than are visual deficits in childhood, but hearing loss affects over 1 million children from birth to age 21 years in the United States (Wong et al., 1999). This hearing deficit can be severe to the extent that it interferes with school. **Chronic serous otitis media,** or long-term fluid in the middle ear, remains a common cause of a hearing deficit in both the preschool and the early school-age years (U.S. Preventive Services Task Force, 1996). All school-age children should have periodic hearing evaluations performed as part of a health-promotion program in school and as required by many states. Periodic evaluations are particularly important to evaluate children who have a history of recurrent ear infections, which can cause persistent fluid in the middle ear that prevents sound waves from traveling for effective hearing. Various treatments exist for treatment of acute otitis media, including antibiotics and the recent discovery that Xylitol gum may be of some benefit (Parker-Pope, 2000). Additionally, work continues on a vaccination for otitis media in the future. **Tympanograms,** used to measure the sensitivity of the tympanic membrane to vibrations induced by pressure and sound waves, are also a valuable tool in detecting and monitoring this problem as part of well-child and ill-child care by the health care team (see Chapter 18).

Sensory Perception

Children learn through many senses simultaneously and teaching approaches use this fact. For example, young school-age children see a letter, hear its sound, and feel the shape of the letter. With this approach, children learn a number of ways to interpret an event and learning generally occurs. For some children, one of the senses becomes more effective than the others for learning, whereas other children learn easier with many senses stimulated. For example, some children learn best by listening, others by doing, and still others by seeing (auditory, psychomotor, and visual learners, respectively). During later childhood, the child begins to use these perceptions to form increasingly complex concepts and understandings of the world. Because no two children have exactly the same sensory acuity, sensitivity, or discrimination, all children build slightly different perceptions and conceptions of the world around them. Therefore teaching approaches must be individualized to meet identified learning needs of most children.

The area of perception that has been studied more than has any other area is visual perception, primarily because of its role in helping children to learn to read. Studies have examined children's abilities to discriminate parts of an entire picture (to see a figure within a picture). Children usually progress from the preschool years, during which they perceive visual stimuli more as a whole, to the school years, during which they perceive more details, and finally to the point at which they perceive and integrate both. The role this process plays in developing children's ability to recognize letters has been hypothesized. Children may first be able to differentiate between obviously different letters, such as *h* and *o*, but may have difficulty with letters similar in appearance, such as *b* and *d*, until they can discriminate details more effectively.

Language

Language develops rapidly during the school years. Most school-age children enter this period with the ability to understand and speak a language, but with only a rudimentary knowledge of reading and writing. By the end of the school-age period, most children have acquired at least a functioning ability in both areas. Many skills are involved in the development of language, including visual perception for reading, auditory acuity and perception for understanding spoken language, and fine-motor skills for both articulation and handwriting.

The full capacity to imitate sounds linguistically develops during the childhood years. Between 6 and 7 years of age, the child shows the ability to produce proper sounds for *v, ch, l, sh, z, s, r,* and *th*. However, children tend to have the most difficulty verbally expressing sounds for *s*, *l*, and *r* (Wong et al., 1999). By 7 years of age, the child should be able to articulate all sounds. The 6-year-old child usually has an expressive vocabulary of at least 2000 words, which then doubles by the sixth grade. The school-age child continues to develop in understanding the **syntax** (grammar) and **semantics** (meaning) of language. Sentences that are more complex are used, and multiple meanings for the same word and the use of metaphors are increasingly understood. The child should be able to recognize and correct spelling and grammatical errors by 8 or 9 years of age. The capacity to learn foreign languages is at an optimal level and provides the rationale for foreign language instruction in the school-age years. Foreign language instruction also provides information about various cultures and an opportunity for school-age children to accept people who are different from themselves.

The ability to read and write fosters the basic academic skills of a literate society. Much of the school-age child's time in school focuses on learning these two skills. Learning to read is a complex process, beginning with recognition of letters and their sounds. Letters are then combined to form words that the child must learn to decode. Words combine to form sentences, and so on. Few children learn to read without assistance. Most children need help from teachers, peers, parents, or older children. The best way for a child to learn to read is controversial. Some researchers believe children learn best by a process involving sounding out the individual letters of a word (**phonics**), whereas others think that learning the word as a whole unit is better. Both processes have value, and likely, a combination of both is most effective. Considering the wide range of processes that are involved in reading (conceptual, perceptual, verbal, and motor), not surprisingly, many children have at least some difficulty in learning to read.

Handwriting requires eye-hand coordination, motor control, and perceptual abilities. Primarily a motor skill, handwriting is not necessarily reflective of mental capacity. Many bright children and adults have poor handwriting, and vice versa. Boys tend to have more problems with legible handwriting than do girls. Writing style does not approach adultlike maturity until the end of late childhood, but the child's handwriting should reflect the child's handedness. No reversal of letter outlines should occur by age 7 or 8, and the relative size of letters should be uniform. By age 8 or 9, letter strokes should be firm, even, and flow with ease. For the individual who has difficulty with handwriting, learning to use a typewriter or computer and graphics can be valuable in producing a satisfactory written product. Tutoring by a specialist in handwriting can help children with **dyslexia,** a term often associated with the tendency to reverse the normal appearance of letters and numbers.

Memory

Memory abilities, both short- and long-term, improve for the school-age child. Strategies used to remember information include organizing, classifying, and labeling information (skills that the child has recently acquired in this stage of concrete operations). **Rehearsal,** repeating an item to be learned, is also a helpful memorization strategy. At age 5, children use rehearsal when it is suggested or modeled; at age 10, they rehearse spontaneously. Memory abilities can be improved through practice and rehearsal and by increasing the child's repertoire of strategies, such a placing the words that need to be remembered in a song or rhyming words.

Intelligence

The concept of intelligence has been used in a variety of ways and is often confusing. People who developed intelligence tests used **intelligence** to indicate the quantity of information that people possessed, their ability to think, and how they compared with others at the same time, chronological age, and experience level.

Scores on an intelligence test should measure the child's basic abilities and, ideally, should predict the child's future performance in school or society. However, this is not always the case. Intelligence test scores tend to differ because each test, or each form of the same test, measures slightly different samples of abilities. Additionally, the type of test tends to reflect the author's philosophy of the nature of intelligence. For example, the **Stanford-Binet Test** places a heavy emphasis on abstract thinking; the **Wechsler Series** emphasizes aggregate, or global, knowledge; and the **Peabody Picture Vocabulary Test** emphasizes verbal skills. The younger the child is, the less developed these skills are and the more difficult they are to measure. As language ability and mental functioning increase during later childhood, the measurement of intellectual capacity is more reliable and valid. It is important to note that many tests used to define intelligence can be culturally insensitive. For example, the protectionism of the Asian culture can cause lower scores on self-help skills and socialization among Asian children who demonstrate that they are good students in other areas of testing.

Children also take **achievement tests** that measure the amount of information learned in a specific area. Although intelligence and achievement tests should measure different issues (basic ability versus learned achievement) their results correlate greatly. Some researchers believe this correlation exists because both tests actually measure the same thing (achievement, not ability).

The results of these tests are reported differently. Intelligence tests usually give an **intelligence quotient** (IQ); that is, the ratio of the child's performance compared with other children's performance, calculated by dividing maturational age (MA) by chronological age (CA) and multiplying by 100 ($MA/CA \times 100 = IQ$). An IQ of 90 to 110 is average. Achievement tests compare the child's performance with other children and report scores as percentiles. A score in the fiftieth percentile means the child is average in that skill, whereas a score in the twentieth percentile means the child is better than only 20% of other children of the same age in that skill, with 80% better than the child. Some of the tests used for this age group to measure intelligence and development are listed in Table 20-3.

A discussion of intelligence must include a discussion of the role played by heredity and environment. Historically, basic intelligence was believed to be inherited and therefore fixed. However, current beliefs accept that some aspect of intelligence is inherited (the extent of which is unclear), but many environmental factors also influence intelligence. Environmental opportunities for learning and the nature of these experiences greatly influence children's learning skills. Most likely, the greatest environmental influence is socioeconomic; children from low-income families tend to score lower on intelligence tests than do children from middle- or high-income families. The reason for this probably relates to many subfactors, such as nutrition, language, parental reinforcement and encouragement, and sociocultural environmental resources. Society has tried to equalize some of these factors through nutrition programs such as the Special Supplemental Nutrition Program for Women, Infants, and Children (WIC) and preschool stimulation programs such as Head Start. Many people have suggested that the use of IQ tests be discontinued, primarily because these tests tend to label children early in life and influence, often negatively, their self-perception and their performance. The controversy of the influence of heredity and environment on overall intelligence will continue for some time.

As outlined, many elements combine to allow a child to learn. Because of the many interactive elements involved, it is not surprising that some children have problems learning. Learning problems may be a result of a health problem, such as poor vision or hearing; an emotional problem, such as anxiety or depression; a cognitive problem, such as retardation or a learning disability; or a complex mixture of many problems. The child who comes into the health care system with a learning problem must have a detailed, extensive evaluation by educational specialists in the field to identify the cause of the problem and strategies to address the child's needs.

Learning Disabilities

Some children with learning problems have **learning disabilities.** One author notes that 20% of America's

Table 20-3 **Common Developmental and Cognitive Tests**

Test	Age (years)	Areas Tested	Methods Used to Test	Comments
Bender-Gestalt (Bender Visual Motor Test)	3 to 4 to adult	Perceptual motor skills	Child copies geometric designs (nine in total), standard criteria for evaluating	
Goodenough-Harris Draw-a-Person Test	3 to 15	Gross mental age	Child asked to draw a person; give points for body parts; evaluate according to criteria	Culture-free test
Peabody Picture Vocabulary Test (PVVT)	2½ to 18	Verbal intellectual capacity	Child told a word, then picks one picture out of four that corresponds	No reading needed
Stanford-Binet Intelligence Scale	2 to adult	Intelligence (global ability, not discrete areas of intellectual ability)	Series of standardized tests	
Wechsler Intelligence Scale for Children (WISC)	5 to 15	Intelligence; two groups of tests (verbal and performance); gives verbal, performance, and full-scale IQ	Standardized tests	Verbally oriented
Vineland Social Maturity Scale	1 to adult	Behavior to meet needs and responsibilities, including self-help in eating and dressing, self-direction, occupation, communication, locomotion, and socialization	Direct observation; directed interview of child or caregiver	Gives social age quotient

children struggle with disabilities, such as learning or behavioral difficulties that inhibit school and life success (Goldstein & Mather, 1998). Many terms and definitions have been used to describe the impairments of these children, who have normal or above normal intelligence and do not have visual, hearing, or motor handicaps or emotional problems.

The American Psychiatric Association classifies many learning disabilities as Specific Developmental Disorders. Examples include developmental arithmetic disorder, developmental expressive writing disorder, developmental reading disorder, and developmental receptive language disorder. All of these specific developmental disorders cause some impairment in academic functioning and are usually diagnosed after the child has experienced difficulty in the school setting. Some children have minor difficulties that are practically unnoticeable, whereas other children are impaired to the extent that they may actually appear to be mentally retarded until appropriately diagnosed. An individual child may have more than one specific developmental disorder. Some of these children will develop behavioral problems as a response to their inability to function satisfactorily (American Psychiatric Association, 1994).

Another condition that causes difficulty in the child's adjustment to the school setting is **attention deficit hyperactivity disorder** (ADHD), a behavior that reflects developmentally inappropriate degrees of inattention, impulsiveness, and hyperactivity (American Psychiatric Association 1994; Hallowell & Ratey, 1994). Frequently, these children have high energy, intuitiveness, and creativity, personal characteristics that help them succeed in some facets of their lives (Hallowell & Ratey, 1994). Historically, ADHD has been given a wide variety of names (minimal brain dysfunction, attention deficit disorder with and without hyperactivity) and has been difficult to assess, primarily because the child can manifest symptoms in varying degrees in different settings and with different people. The American Psychiatric Association has detailed the diagnostic criteria for ADHD (Box 20-4). Treatment of children with ADHD has been controversial and currently includes behavioral management, nutritional therapy, schooling alteration, and medication. These interventions may also be successful in offering behavioral management for ADHD for affected adults.

The nurse's role with the child who has a learning disability is varied. Detection of the problem, consultation during evaluations, and support and counseling for the child and family are all possible nursing contributions. School nurses in particular play a vital role in assessing and

Box 20-4 Diagnostic Criteria for Attention Deficit Hyperactivity Disorder

Note: Consider a criterion met only when the behavior is considerably more frequent than that of most people of the same mental age.

1. A disturbance of at least 6 months is present during which at least six of the criteria for either inattentive behavior or hyperactivity-impulsivity behavior are met.*
2. Some inattentive or hyperactive-impulsive symptoms that caused impairment were present before age 7 years.
3. Some impairment for the symptoms is present in two or more settings (at school or at home).
4. Clear evidence of clinically significant impairment exists in social or academic functioning.
5. The symptoms do not occur only during the course of a pervasive developmental disorder, schizophrenia, or other psychotic disorder and are not more indicative of another mental disorder (mood disorder, anxiety disorder, dissociative disorder, and personality disorder).

*Refer to *Diagnostic and Statistical Manual of Mental Disorders* (4th edition) for the specific criteria.

Modified from American Psychiatric Association. (1994). *Diagnostic and statistical manual of mental disorders* (4th ed.). Washington, DC: The Association.

managing learning disabilities and in serving as a liaison between the school and home environments.

Nurses also play a vital role in promoting a child's overall cognitive and perceptual health, helping to prevent problems in these areas. The following list outlines some general considerations and suggestions for nurses:

- Nurses help parents understand the child's level of cognitive ability to set realistic learning expectations. For example, the child who has a limited understanding of conservation of numbers is not ready for advanced mathematical skills.
- School-age children are in the process of becoming less egocentric, and people working with them must remember that this process remains incomplete; children must understand the consequences of not working well with others and learn from these consequences to improve future interactions with others.
- Vision and hearing are frequently taken for granted. Parents and professionals must remember that during the school years, a child depends on these senses for learning, but that this is also a time when many changes are occurring. School-age children need frequent evaluations of their vision and hearing to allow optimal learning to occur.
- Language development and skills must be monitored. Frequently, parents are conditioned to a child's speech pattern to the extent that they fail to recognize deviations from the norm. The child who has articulation problems beyond approximately age 6 or 7 should be evaluated (Jarvis, 2000).
- Children in school undergo a variety of intelligence, achievement, and aptitude tests. Nurses working with these children must be familiar with the common tests that are used (see Table 20-3) and how to interpret results. This information allows nurses to converse with other professionals about the child and to interpret information for parents and counsel them on meeting their child's needs.
- When assessing a child's cognitive abilities and learning potential, the nurse must perform a thorough assessment of the child's family history and environment. Collaboration with the school learning specialist also helps define an effective learning plan for the child. Many problems associated with learning difficulties tend to recur in families, including myopia, delays in speech, and learning disabilities. Factors in the child's environment, such as divorce or poverty, can interfere with learning and should be considered for any plan dealing with learning difficulties.
- The first person to recognize or assess the child with a learning problem is, in many instances, the nurse. Before jumping to the diagnosis of a learning disability or issues such as a vision or hearing deficit, the nurse and learning specialist team should evaluate any health problem, general immaturity, and environment deficit of the child who is experiencing problems in school.
- The child and family who are dealing with a learning disability need extensive support and counseling. Help may be required in interpreting test results and educational plans, in providing suggestions for dealing with behavioral problems and support in following appropriate medication or diet regimens, and in counseling on how to cope with this typically hidden handicap.

Self-Perception–Self-Concept Pattern

Through each of the developmental processes of physiological growth, cognitive development, learning capacity, and social development, children engage in an important process of self-discovery. Through these processes, children also build and create their own personalities, increase their ability to relate to others, and become exposed to a wide range of possibilities for their own behavior, attitudes, and values (Beck & Myers, 1996). Although a significant foundation for personality develops during infancy and early childhood, late childhood offers a valuable time during which children begin to participate actively in assuming specific traits and choosing values and attitudes.

Erikson's Theory

The stage of personality development described by Erikson for the school-age child is industry versus inferiority. The major task to be accomplished is full mastery of whatever the child is doing (sense of industry). The child's concerns tend to focus on success in personal and social tasks. Erikson calls this desire a sense of industry; the primary

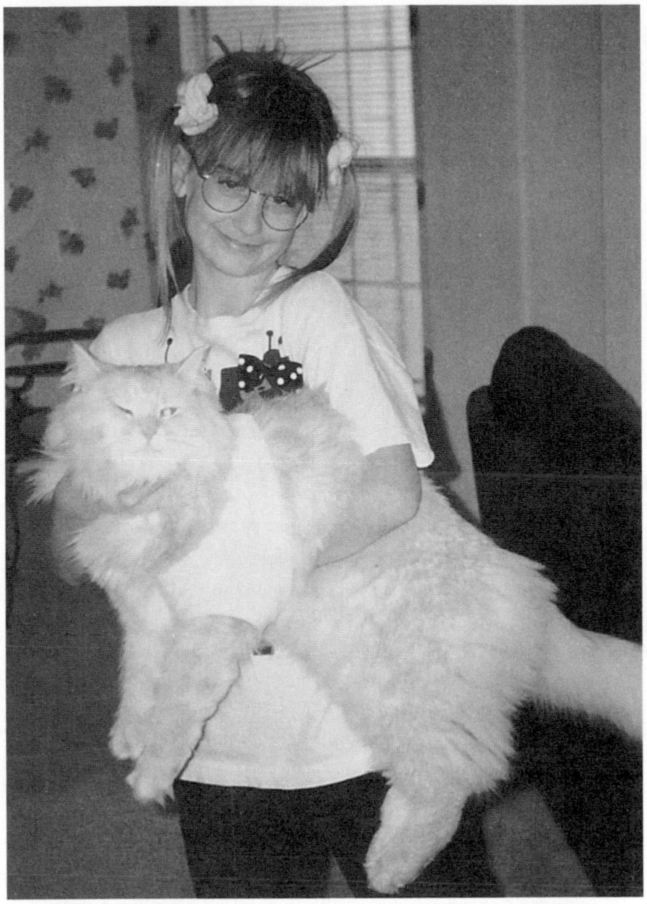

Fig. 20-3 Responsibility for pets during the school-age period nurtures self-esteem of the child.

hazard is the development of a sense of inferiority. Inferiority occurs with repeated failures at attempted tasks and with little encouragement or trust from important people in the child's life. The child can experience mastery through personal accomplishment and interaction with peers. From these dynamics, an intense devotion to and preoccupation with the peer group grows. The child is intense, interested, and involved, concentrating on developing knowledge and skills relevant to the development of peer relationships. As the child gains mastery of the tools of the culture in relationship to those of the peer group, a sense of worth and of understanding of the self develops (Erikson, 1986a, 1986b).

Self-Concept

A child's self-concept develops over time and through a variety of experiences and relationships. For example, by being responsible for a pet's care and by showing love to this animal, the older school-age child nurtures a positive self-concept (Fig. 20-3). The way in which others, especially peers, "see" the child influences the sense of self within the child. With increasing cognitive abilities, the child has a better understanding of the identifying factors of others (race, ethnicity, disability, or gender) and how those others compare to him or her. Self-concept includes self-esteem, sense of control, body concept, and gender role.

Self-Esteem **Self-esteem** has been defined as the extent to which an individual believes oneself to be capable, significant, successful, and worthy. The younger school-age child has a limited self-concept, but this develops as the child successfully completes the tasks of this period (Erikson's sense of industry).

Although the school-age child engages in more activities outside of the home compared with the younger child, the school-age child still depends on the family to foster personal development of high self-esteem. Family involves extended family members (grandparents, aunts, and uncles) and close people in the cultural community. Literature indicates that parents with high self-esteem freely express their affection for each other and their children; they are also supportive and firm in setting behavior guidelines for children (Goldstein & Mather, 1998). For children to appreciate and understand feelings of success fully, there must be approval and reinforcement by others (parents, family, and teachers) and by themselves. Support must also exist for children when they are not successful because of the reality that not all skills can be mastered. Parents must verbalize their pleasure when the child has completed a job well. Other adults should do the same, particularly because the child experiences many learning environments outside the home. Teachers or group leaders frequently reward the child who has succeeded in a task with badges, stars, or privileges (tangible objects that validate success). The idea that "success breeds success" should be implemented by others who deal with school-age children to build their self-esteem early in life.

The peer group's influence on the school-age child's self-esteem is unquestionable. Acceptance by a peer group contributes to the child's feeling of self-worth and sense of belonging to a desired group. Competition with peers also influences the child's feelings of adequacy. For example, the child who faces a bully (a child who lacks social skills to be part of a group) can become frightened when little peer group support for the child's beliefs or behavior exists. Children work and play with their peers through school, organized sports or clubs, and after-school activities. For some children, little time is available for them to focus on their own individual interests. Parents must be encouraged to expose their school-age children to interesting activities of their choice to nurture self-esteem and a sense of uniqueness in the child.

Increasing concern has been voiced recently about school-age girls suffering a decline in self-esteem that affects their achievements. Literature appears to indicate that girls experience greater competition in current environments than they did in the past, and they need strong adult support to realize the importance of their ways of thinking and behaving in a world often built on male values. Elium and Elium (1994) and Bingham and Stryker (1995) note that girls of late school-age need strong role models and harmony between parents to allow perceptions of balance within themselves. Self-esteem appears to be strong in school-age girls with fathers who routinely encourage them to take risks, to question traditional behaviors, and to "listen to their souls" with music and art. Overall, these authors and Rutter (1996) note that girls in the late school-age period must have education that nurtures their independence, assertiveness, analysis, curiosity, and innovation. Teachers who nurture these qualities and serve as role models can increase the chances of female student success. Many proponents of education believe that these qualities can be best met with female-only schools rather than a coeducational approach.

In encouraging the development of self-esteem in all school-age children, the nurse remembers that a child needs to experience success with tasks, and completely structured activities may not provide this opportunity for some children. A child who succeeds in some things and is accepted by peers gains a sense of competence and worth, is self-confident, and has high self-esteem, which are important qualities for life survival (Cagle & Keen-Payne, 1996).

Sense of Control As the school-age child matures, a sense of control is developed over the self and the environment. The child begins to make choices and to feel in charge of the self. *Locus of control* refers to the source of the control, either within the child or outside in the environment. Children with an **internal locus of control** believe they are responsible for their behavior and accomplishments and tend to have higher levels of achievement than do children who believe in an **external locus of control.** These children think that less reason exists for them to try hard at a task because the results are determined not by them, but rather, by others or fate. Older children and girls tend to have a more internalized locus of control than do younger children and boys.

Body Concept The school-age child's concept of the body and its functioning also changes from the preschool period and adds to overall self-concept. By ages 8 to 11, children are aware that the parts of the body are a related whole (Wong et al., 1999). The 11-year-old child can name twice the number of internal bodily structures as can the child who is 6 years of age. The most common structures named are parts of the cardiovascular (heart), musculoskeletal (bones), and nervous (brain) systems. Older children are more accurate in describing the location and function of the structures than are younger children. For example, the child who is age 7 knows that the heart is important and that it beats, whereas the 13-year-old child knows that the heart pumps blood. Changes or differences in the body can be frightening to the school-age child. Loss of baby teeth can be upsetting at first until the child realizes that this is a normal process and that new teeth will grow. Bodily differences, even something as simple as freckles, can provoke ridicule and isolation. Children in this age group frequently feel threatened by others with deformities (Wong et al., 1999). Learning about bodily differences through reading and discussion helps decrease this type of anxiety, increases knowledge of the body and ways to attain and maintain health, and helps the child understand the value of each person, despite any differences that the individual may have from the larger group. Ways in which the nurse can help children develop positive self-concepts are listed in Box 20-5.

Roles-Relationships Pattern

Families provide the child with a sense of security. From this safe setting, the child begins to cope with the external environment. Families encourage children's cognitive growth by exposing them to a variety of experiences and by instilling in them a desire to achieve. By accepting their values that predict behaviors, viewing the world through their glasses, and communicating that acceptance, families also nurture their children's self-esteem (Goldstein & Mather, 1998; Vannoy, 1994).

Parents and children play many roles with each other

Box 20-5 Nursing Interventions to Help Develop a Positive Self-Concept During the School-Age Period

- Remind people working with school-age children that a sense of success is important for a child. All children must believe that they are good at something. Because not all children can succeed at all tasks, a variety of experiences should be provided so they can succeed as much as possible and identify their personal strengths. This approach helps them deal with failure; therefore they will try for more accomplishments and successes.
- Parents should learn the importance of giving positive feedback to their children, of setting realistic goals, of spending quality time with their child, and of helping their child attempt realistic tasks.
- Children should have some control over their lives and environment. School-age children should be encouraged to make choices to develop their sense of control and their decision-making skills and to experience consequences of their choices.
- The many questions that children have about their bodily changes, including sexual changes, should be acknowledged and sensitively discussed at home or at school. Families frequently have strong feelings as to where and when these discussions should occur. Open discussions between parents and educators can determine a solution about the proper timing and place of teaching. Some parents who remain unsure can benefit from the nurse's help to deal with these issues. School nurses should play a vital role in developing, teaching, and evaluating appropriate sex education programs in the school.

and interact in a variety of ways; attachment, love, and companionship usually exist between parents and children. Parents protect the dependent child and teach the learning child. The parent-child relationship is not equal, primarily because parents are usually the authority figures that establish the rules needed for the functioning of the family and the safety and growth of the child. During the school-age years, the child's increasing maturity, independence, and responsibility begins to reduce the amount of parental authority and structure.

School-age children also begin to broaden their interests outside the home, often encouraged by parents. Unfortunately, children can become involved in activities to the extent that it becomes stressful for both them and their parents. The child's changing world frequently alters family schedules and patterns. Studies have found that both mothers and fathers find this period difficult for the family and parents express the least amount of parental satisfaction when their oldest child is between the ages of 6 and 13. The relationships between siblings vary, depending on birth order, gender, and age differences. Sibling interactions have been studied in terms of outcomes such as intelligence and power. Siblings interact with one another in a number of roles, such as playmates, teacher-learner, protector-dependent, and adversaries. The latter role is expected, a result of feelings of jealousy and rivalry that often occur in families (see Chapter 18). School-age children cope with these feelings better than do preschool children because they have outlets outside the family, including school and friends. Parents can minimize these conflicts by recognizing each child's needs and level of maturity.

As children mature, they take on more responsibilities within the family and the community. School-age children can learn responsibility for money, household chores, self-care, or pets, and acquire a sense of empowerment as an integral part of the family; their health may actually improve with responsibilities associated with pet caregiving (Beck & Myers, 1996). This age is the period during which families often give allowances or children earn money through chores or small jobs such as paper routes. School-age children receiving these awards learn valuable lessons later by learning how to spend their allowances efficiently.

The purpose of **limit setting** (defining expected behavior and consequences when limits are not honored) with children is to teach them which behaviors are acceptable in society. Parents can implement many methods based on philosophies of limit setting with varying degrees of effectiveness. However, some generally accepted concepts are applicable to the school-age child. Clear limits and expectations make compliance easier for the child. Violent behavior must be discouraged, and nonviolent methods to reach resolutions for personal problems should be encouraged. Parents who express their feelings, explain why things happen, and listen to their children encourage the development of self-control (see Health Teaching box). Constructive limit setting and parental guidance nurture a child's self-esteem. Behavioral contracts between parent and child provide direction for the child's behavior and encourage improved child behavior by delineating favorable consequences when the child follows the terms of the contract.

Children frequently model their behavior after the behavior of people they love or admire (parents, friends, and other adults). **Positive reinforcement** (rewarding the child for good behavior) is an effective form of limit setting. **Punishment,** a negative reinforcement, can stop an undesired behavior, but, in many instances, only until the child can repeat the action and not be caught. Some families with school-age children find it helpful to have periodic family meetings during which everyone discusses

HEALTH TEACHING The School-Age Child: Points for Effective Discipline

Effective discipline is essential to family harmony and individual child growth. The goal of discipline is to encourage and reinforce positive child behaviors and to eliminate inappropriate behaviors. According to one author (Lighter, 1995), effective discipline involves avoiding conflict with a child, improving communication, optimizing the child care environment, delivering consequences for inappropriate child behavior, and meeting parental needs. The specifics of discipline include:

- Ignoring the misbehavior and acknowledging the appropriate behavior
- Using distraction or substitution to avoid a problem situation
- Offering choices to prevent inappropriate behavior such as whining or an emotional outburst
- Using humor to decrease the intensity of a situation
- Modeling the appropriate behavior
- Setting age-relevant limits
- Giving specific and clear commands for behavior
- Talking calmly, being a good listener, and encouraging negotiation within the family for problem resolution
- Holding family meetings to collaborate on solving a problem
- Limiting a child's environment (distractions such as music and television)
- Setting clear and consistent consequences for misbehavior
- Providing one-to-one time, focusing on positive attention
- Taking time for oneself to replenish one's energies as a parent and as an individual

From Lighter, D. (1995). *Gentle discipline*. New York: Meadowbrook Press.

family issues, rules, and responsibilities. This cooperative effort fosters increased understanding.

Recently, a resurgence of spanking has taken place, and several states, including Oklahoma and Nevada, have passed legislation permitting parents to spank their children. Historically, many cultures have disciplined their children by spanking, but, as recently as 1998, the American Academy of Pediatrics has not supported spanking or any kind of physical punishment directed against children. Despite this stand, many parents say they believe methods such as "time out" and "living with the consequences of poor choices" have been unsuccessful in "out-of-control" children (Costello, 2000). Recent school shootings involving young adolescents have concerned many parents who believe that the return of spanking as a disciplinary method can prevent these occurrences in the future.

Child Abuse

Child abuse and neglect (the physical, sexual, or emotional exploitation of children) continues to be a significant societal problem. Abuse and neglect from primary caregivers directed at children under age 14 is the second leading cause of death among children (Osofsky, Cohen, & Drell, 1995). Abused children sustain fractures, hematomas, skin bruising, and encounter failure to thrive, all indicators of trauma inflicted by a more powerful person. Abused children have an increased likelihood of becoming violent adults and of abusing their own children. The combined factors of family poverty, culture, single-parent status, and teenage parenthood increase the rate of abuse. Cultural factors must also be considered in defining the presence of abuse. For example, coin rubbing of the chest (used in the Asian ethnic group for treatment of respiratory infections) leaves abrasions that can be perceived as abuse by a nurse assessing an ill child. Generally, children who need more attention, resources, or patience also receive more abuse from caregivers. Health care providers must report suspected abuse and participate in preventing, assessing, and treating victims of abuse. In many states, the Nurse Practice Act requires nurses to report suspected cases of abuse. Ultimately, nurses must interrupt the vicious cycle of abuse by becoming involved in community coalitions that support families that face the risk of abuse and by intervening in cases in which abuse has occurred or suspicion of abuse exists.

Unfortunately, relationships between children and adults, even their parents, are not always positive. **Sexual abuse,** use of a child for sexual exploitative purposes, is a serious health problem that has become more prevalent. The problem frequently remains hidden, partly because (1) the child may be too frightened to talk about the situation, (2) families and society are reluctant to admit its existence, and (3) fewer agencies exist to respond to these cases. Statistics on the number of American children who are assaulted are only estimates, but the number of abuse cases appears to be increasing. Only about a third of cases are reported and the victims are more likely to be girls than boys (U.S. Department of Health and Human Services, National Center on Child Abuse and Neglect, 1995b; Wong et al., 1999).

Sexual abuse includes any sexual contact with a child; intercourse per se need not occur. The child is coerced through verbal threats or physical force or seduced by offering treats. Many of the victims know the abuser (the majority of abusers are parents, according to Wong et al., 1999), although persons in positions of authority (doctors, therapists, clergy, and coaches) have also been identified as abusers. The combination of the adult's force and authority makes the child believe that no power or choice is available. The child may comply for a variety of reasons, such as a need to be good, a need for affection, or a need to keep the family together. Emotions are complex and change as the child grows. Fear may give way to embarrassment, shame, and anger. The long-term effects of abuse are usually serious. In adulthood, these children often become chronically ill with anxiety, depression, and multiple physical symptoms and illnesses.

As in any type of suspected abuse, nurses assist these children by recognizing those who are possibly experiencing abuse and helping them to obtain assistance. All persons who work with young children must acknowledge the warning signs of abuse (Box 20-6). When sexual abuse is suspected, an in-depth interview and examination must be conducted by a professional who is sensitive to the needs of the child and understands appropriate ways to examine the child for evidence of abuse. Most authorities believe that children who describe sexual abuse are telling the truth, primarily because the details are usually specific, and the trauma is evident. *Therefore a child's story should be believed unless it is disproved.* This extremely complicated problem is managed most effectively by a multidisciplinary team approach.

Sexuality-Reproductive Pattern

The preschool child learns about gender, its constant nature, and begins to model the general societal behaviors that are expected related to a child's gender. The child enters the school-age years with a strong identification with the parent of the same gender. The child continues to learn the concepts and behavior of the gender role and to incorporate these into the self-concept. This challenge is significant for all children, but more so for homosexual children.

An increasing number of people appear to be aware of societal stereotypes related to gender roles. However, society has begun to narrow the dichotomy between gender roles and no longer encourages vast differences between men and women in occupation, interests, behavior, appearance, or personality traits. Teaching about gender

Box 20-6 Warning Signs of Child Abuse

- Physical evidence of abuse and/or neglect, including previous injuries
- Conflicting stories about the "accident" or injury from the parents or others
- Cause of injury blamed on sibling or other party
- An injury inconsistent with the history, such as a concussion and broken arm from falling off a bed
- History inconsistent with child's developmental level, such as a 6 month old turning on the hot water
- Complaint other than the one associated with signs of abuse, such as a chief complaint of a cold when there is evidence of first- and second-degree burns
- Inappropriate response of caregiver, such as an exaggerated or absent emotional response, refusal to sign for additional tests or to agree to necessary treatment, excessive delay in seeking treatment, or absence of the parents for questioning
- Inappropriate response of child, such as little or no response to pain, fear of being touched, excessive or lack of separation anxiety, or indiscriminate friendliness to strangers
- Child's report of physical or sexual abuse
- Previous reports of abuse in the family
- Repeated visits to emergency facilities with injuries

From Wong, D. L., Hockenberry-Eaton, M., Wilson, D., Winkelstein, M. L., Ahmann, E., DiVito-Thomas, P. A. (1999). *Whaley and Wong's nursing care of infants and children* (6th ed.). St. Louis: Mosby.

roles and emphasizing that gender does not determine one's choices in life starts as early as preschool in many parts of the country. The effects on children with this educational information are interesting to watch. Children are increasingly choosing occupations that are based on their skills and interests rather than on what appears "appropriate" because of their gender.

The school-age child's increasing awareness of the body, its functioning, and a need for sexual identity combine to give the child a desire for knowledge about the biological aspects of sexual function. Late in the school-age period, during which the physical changes of puberty have begun, children frequently become increasingly concerned and curious about sexual issues. Children, especially between ages 9 and 12, are extremely attached to children of the same gender, and for them to explore each other's sexual organs is common. This activity is not true homosexuality, although parents and children may have concerns that it is. The onset of changes varies for each child. Therefore one girl might begin menstruating at 10 years of age and another at 13 years based on genetics, nutrition, and environmental factors.

Children are frequently unsure of whom to question about sexual matters; therefore misinformation is passed throughout the peer group. Parents are frequently uncomfortable or unsure of what information to give to their children and when to give it. Many health care agencies sponsor short programs that focus on bodily changes; these programs can be important for educating parents and later school-age children about bodily and mental changes during preadolescence and puberty in a nonembarrassing environment. An increasing number of age-appropriate books that focus on emotional and body changes can be used at home and in school to increase understanding of children in these areas. Particularly with girls starting their menstrual cycle earlier now than 50 years ago, education of bodily changes and puberty appears appropriate as part of later school-age education.

Nurses play an important role in the area of sex education in health care and education settings. When children are seen for routine health maintenance, the nurse should ask both the child and the parents questions about sexual development and concerns. The school is an ideal setting for group education programs. Children at this age appear to respond favorably with gender segregated classes based on their general discomfort with sexual topics and because they have unique needs and questions that are best addressed in same-gender classes. Some schools have appropriately incorporated these classes into school curricula to reflect the school's acceptance of its role in health teaching; other schools have special programs. Particularly for disabled children, the nurse may need to offer special classes to focus on unique body changes and concerns and ways to express affection, but also to avoid sexual abuse and strategies for gaining independence in personal care despite disability (American Academy of Pediatrics, 1996a).

Perhaps as a result of greater societal acceptance of sexuality teaching to the school-age population, more games, appropriate literature, and creative methods are available to teach children responsibility about sexual health. With parental approval, a sensitive program on responsible sexuality (including abstinence and condom use, pregnancy, sexually transmitted diseases, and the human immunodeficiency virus) can be offered to older school-age children to lay the foundation for later discussions (U.S. Department of Health and Human Services, 2000). In many cases, parents possess special skills to contribute to a linguistically and culturally appropriate sexual education program and to a general health-promotion curriculum throughout the school-age years.

Coping–Stress-Tolerance Pattern

An important aspect of development for the school-age child is that he or she must learn to cope with stress as part of the developmental process. Through a health-promotion program, children learn to identify symptoms of stress (pounding heart, stomach "butterflies," and sweaty hands) and ways to deal with these perceived stresses (deep breathing and walking). Ways to solve complicated problems before they cause physical symptoms of stress can

Table 20-4 The School-Age Child's Coping Strategies and Nursing Interventions to Promote Coping

Coping Strategies	Nursing Interventions
Use of defense mechanisms (regression, denial, repression, projection displacement, sublimation)	Accept child's use of defense mechanisms as temporary, healthy coping responses; provide child options for moving to more age-appropriate ways of responding to stressors
Cognitive mastery (problem solving, communication)	Ask child what they know of situation and how they might handle it; encourage questions; use diagrams and models to help explain; encourage child to verbalize feelings and use past successful strategies that might help deal with present stressors; try personalized approaches, such as books, puppets, manipulation of equipment, to increase feelings of control for child faced with stressful situation; encourage praying and other communications to a chosen deity as appropriate
Controlling, holding behaviors	Encourage child to participate and to make decisions; accept child's need to direct as appropriate; set consistent age-appropriate limits; respond to child signals for help; let child be responsible for self-care
Use of repetition	Use books, games, and other communication media to work through feelings; emphasize "ok" for child to continue to ask questions and to receive answers that assist in coping
Use of humor	Be a good listener and participate in riddles and jokes used by child; be a good sport with school-age children's desire to play jokes on each other; share stories and cartoons with child
Motor activity, aggression, protest behavior	Encourage physical activity to deal with stress; accept appropriate behavior; establish limits on behavior for group safety
Withdrawal (resurgence of separation anxiety)	When child is separated from family, may have separation anxiety; encourage close emotional contacts between child and significant others (friends, family, church); allow favorite objects from home to be brought to hospital or new environment for child

also be part of a health-promotion program taught in the school. Although some adults may believe that this child "has it made" (by being cared for, going to school, and playing), the child actually faces many experiences in life that can be stressful, but must be confronted. These experiences include issues of change, competition, frustration, and failure. Threats to the child's security, or stresses, cause feelings of helplessness and anxiety that can affect the child's ability to function successfully. School-age children may become concerned over pressure to take drugs, cheat, or steal, as noted in at least one study (Neff & Dale, 1996). Grief over the death of a loved one, loss of a favorite activity because of misbehavior, expulsion from a favorite peer group, and a variety of other losses can create negative behavior. Occasionally, this child might "act out" the frustration. Parents can respond to this behavior by disciplining the child, but should also listen and then analyze the factors that might be creating the problem. Constructive parental behaviors serve to increase the child's feelings of control and to decrease the child's stress (see Health Teaching box).

A list of common **coping strategies** (behaviors intended to buffer perceived stressful events) of children are outlined in Table 20-4. These mechanisms are often healthy, adaptive behaviors for the child. However, a child may become overwhelmed by a particularly stressful situation and be unable to move beyond the coping behaviors. Both in the school environment and in conversations with parents, nurses offer a variety of strategies for dealing with a school-age child's problems, enabling the child to learn from others and to move on. Referral to literature on this topic can be helpful in preventing school-age children's misbehavior and in interrupting a negative behavior cycle to allow family health (Box 20-7). Referring these children to their religious and spiritual leaders may also be appropriate; many school-age children believe that prayer to God or their religious deity will help them cope with an otherwise uncontrollable situation (Wong et al., 1999).

Parental Divorce

If current statistics are correct (57% of marriages end in divorce), then many school-age children face the stress of their parents' marital separation. The crisis aspect of divorce is time limited, with much of the disorganization and readjustment occurring in the first 18 months. Children experience a feeling of loss, although they may hope that their parents will reunite at some point. This reaction can delay their acceptance of the situation. Children's responses vary with their level of development. Factors such as economic security, availability of both of their parents, other family, church, and school supports, and quality of interactions with their parents can influence the child's ability to cope with divorce.

Unfortunately, many parents are so involved in their

Box 20-7 Health-Promotion Literature: The School-Age Child

American Girl Library. (1996). *The care and keeping of friends.* Middleton, WI: Pleasant.
Amery, H., & Songi, J. (1994). *The human body.* New York: Western Publishing.
Brainard, B. (1992). *You can't sell your brother at the garage sale.* New York: Dell.
Brown, L. K., & Brown, M. (1990). *Dinosaurs alive and well.* Boston: Little, Brown.
Burnett, F. H. (1962). *The secret garden.* New York: Harper Collins.
Cleary, B. (1979). *Ramona forever.* New York: Yearling Books.
Cohen, B. (1990). *Molly Pilgrim.* New York: Bantam Skylark.
Conford, E. (1991). *Can do, Jenny Archer.* New York: Little, Brown.
Golant, M. (1987). *Sometimes it's ok to be angry!* New York: RGA Publishing Group, Inc.
Holyoke, N. (1995). *Help.* Middleton, WI: Pleasant.
L'Engle, M. (1962). *A wrinkle in time.* New York: Yearling Newberry.
Madaras, L., & Madaras, A. (1993). *My body, my self for girls.* New York: Newmarket Press.
Navarra, T. (1989). *On my own: Helping kids help themselves.* Hauppauge, NY: Barron's.
O'Dell, S. (1960). *The island of the blue dolphins.* New York: Yearling Books.
Schwartz, L. (1990). *Earth book for kids.* Santa Barbara, CA: The Learning Works.
Shannon, J. (1994). *Why it's great to be a girl.* New York: Warner Books.
Stoppard, M. (1997). *Sex ed: Growing up, relationships, and sex.* New York: DK Publishing.
Weston, C. (1998). *For girls only: Wise words, good advice.* New York: Avon Books.

own feelings related to divorce that they are unable to support their children. Conflicts over custody, child support, and visitation rights add to the child's difficulty in coping. Frequently, the school system must become the child's advocate by encouraging the parents to provide a supportive environment for the child's development, despite a concurrent focus on divorce proceedings.

Some children are unable to cope well with their parent's divorce and have emotional after effects that can result in juvenile behavior problems or require long-term counseling. When school system personnel are aware of this history, dealing with these behavioral problems can be less challenging.

Somatization and Depression

Children, similar to adults, use defense mechanisms to cope, with varying degrees of success. What works for some children may not work for others; what is healthy in one situation may not be healthy in another. When a child misbehaves many times and causes harm to self and others, the child may be perceived as mentally ill and in need of therapy. In any given year, 20% of children between ages 9 and 17 receive a diagnosis of mental disorder (Friedman, Katz-Leavy, Manderscheid, & Sondheimer, 1996). Two strategies used by the school-age child to respond to uncontrollable situations are **somatization** and **depression**.

Some children who are unable to cope with a situation and the resulting anxiety will transfer their feelings to a physical problem (somatization). In this phenomenon, school-age children, unable to discuss or even admit their concerns, may complain of stomachaches or headaches, symptoms reflective of functional or psychogenic pain. Children may also develop discrete, repetitive-movement habits, called tics, which are usually a manifestation of anxiety or tension. In many cases, the child with these problems must first be evaluated to determine whether an underlying physiological cause is present. The child and the family will then need assistance in understanding the child's concerns and defining successful ways to deal with the behavior.

Depression also occurs in children, although many people, both professional and laypeople, have found this difficult to accept. Depression reflects a disturbance of mood where a child displays sadness, guilt or worthlessness, and other unusual behaviors that disengage the child from peers and family. The incidence has been difficult to determine, but estimates ranging from 2% to 15% of school-age children have been quoted (American Psychiatric Association, 1994). In trying to define depression in children, most authors point out that they are not referring to the periodic sadness or disappointment that all children experience, but to a more long-term syndrome in which the child's normal development and functioning become impaired. Factors that can place a child at risk for the development of childhood depression include the following (American Psychiatric Association, 1994):

- Death of a parent or significant other
- Divorce
- Long-term hospitalization
- Foster home placement
- Absence or chronic separation of parent and child
- Parents with psychopathology
- Learning problems
- Chronic illness or physical deformity
- Family history of depression
- Rigid parents with uncompromising standards
- Emotional turmoil at home

The manifestations of childhood depression can be difficult to recognize. Behaviors that a depressed child might demonstrate include the following (American Psychiatric Association, 1994; Goldstein & Mather, 1998):

- Anorexia
- Lethargy
- Change in affect (flat to agitated; happy to sad or hopeless)
- Aggression
- Frequent crying

- Propensity of being hurt
- Irritability
- Nonspecific somatic complaints
- Feelings of frustration
- Excessive self-criticism
- Frequent daydreaming
- Low self-esteem
- Antisocial behavior
- School difficulties
- Vacillating hostility toward parents and teachers
- Loss of interest in previously pleasurable activities
- Loss of energy
- Expression of suicidal thoughts

When identifying depression, nurses must recognize that many of these behaviors can be symptoms of other problems or can be normal for the child's level of development. Working within the school and other environments of the school-age child, nurses can be instrumental in observing these behaviors, recognizing that a child may be depressed, gaining parental input, and implementing strategies early in the depressant cycle to help that child and family. Depending on the child and the situation, varying amounts of counseling will be required. Nurses in schools and outpatient settings are often the ideal practitioners, having the skill and time that are necessary to help a child cope with a helpless feeling and its cause. Frequently, this counseling is performed along with other psychologically oriented measures and includes methods of play therapy, family counseling, and individual guidance.

Values-Beliefs Pattern

Children make decisions related to moral and ethical issues every day. Should they tell the teacher which classmate broke the rule? Should they share their candy with a younger sibling? Should they take the small toy that is just sitting on a friend's desk? For all these situations, the child makes a decision based on the level of moral development.

Moral development includes moral behavior, feelings, and judgment. Behavior refers to children's actions; children may know that they should not take a friend's toy, but will they? Feelings refer to how children emotionally respond when they do something that they perceive is wrong. For example, will they feel guilty if they take their friend's toy? The child's behavior and feelings are strongly influenced by environmental processes, the type of discipline used by the family, the role models that the child observes, people with whom the child identifies, and the child's rehearsal and practice of moral behavior. Judgment refers to the child's ability to determine whether something is right or wrong, which is primarily a cognitive, internal process (Wong et al., 1999).

Kohlberg's Theory

The stage of moral judgment in the school-age child is somewhat controversial. Generally, most researchers agree that the younger school-age child is at the **preconventional level,** a stage of moral development characterized by self-interest only. Some children are in stage 1 of this level, punishment and obedience, but many are primarily in stage 2, which consists of individualism, instrumental purpose, and exchange. The child continues to do many things simply to avoid getting in trouble (stage 1), but now also performs actions that will be of benefit (stage 2). During later childhood, most children progress to the **conventional level,** a stage of moral development defined by concern about group interests and values, which includes stage 3, "good child, bad child," and stage 4, "law and order." The age at which the conventional level first occurs varies, but is typically between ages 10 and 13. The conventional level of moral judgment demonstrates a switch in focus, with the child looking to others for approval and to authority in society for a definition of rules. This level coincides with Piaget's cognitive level of concrete operations and with the child's increased social involvement with people outside the home (Kohlberg, 1981; Murray, 2001).

The following six aspects of moral development have been identified by Kohlberg as developing during the school-age years in Western societies:

1. The child enters this period judging behavior relative to real outcome or physical consequences. If children of this age are asked whether it is worse to break five cups while helping mother set the table or to break one cup while stealing a cookie, most children would think that breaking five cups is worse. As the school-age child progresses, the act begins to be judged in terms of the intention of the offender, and the stealing incident is considered the worse of the two acts.
2. Younger children view behavior as completely right or completely wrong. Later they begin to weigh several aspects of the situation and to use judgment with regard to the relative rightness or wrongness of the act.
3. Early in the middle years, children state that an act is wrong because it brings punishment or displeasure from an adult. Later, they develop insight that an act is wrong because it breaks a rule, violates another person's rights, or harms another.
4. Reciprocity is used in defining what will happen when the child offends or is offended. In other words, children are able to calculate that they would hit back when hit and that they would be hit if they were to hit someone else. By age 10 or 11, children can place themselves in another's position and begin to exercise the Golden Rule of "doing unto others as you would have them do unto you." Increasingly, relational ethics (the influence of one's behavior in relationships with others) becomes important, especially with girls, who have been raised to focus on the affective aspect of relationships. This approach con-

trasts with rational ethics, which is concerned with the moral rules of what is right and wrong without consideration of the definition of a caring behavior.

5. Younger children usually recommend severe punishment for the misdeeds of others. Later these same children begin to recommend a milder form of punishment and then an approach that would lead to the reform of the offender.
6. Younger children tend to view accidents or misfortunes as punishment for wrongdoing. Later, this naturally occurring misfortune is not confused with punishment.

Moral Behavioral Problems

Some moral behavioral problems, such as lying, stealing, or cheating, are common during the school-age years. Preschool and younger school-age children who lie frequently do so because of fantasy, exaggerations, or inaccurate understanding. As children grow, they typically use the defense mechanism of denial to block upsetting situations and to maintain self-esteem. The resultant lie then becomes an unconscious act. Older children often lie because they are afraid of being punished or ridiculed. Children may cheat because of a desire to win or to do well in competitive society; peer pressure can be an added stress that causes this tendency. Children usually steal when they think they will not be caught and when they believe that there is no other way to get what they want (Wong et al., 1999). Although these actions can be quite upsetting for the child's parents, they are common developmental behaviors, and parents frequently need reassurance that the child is normal. When confronted with their behavior, children will frequently inflict self-discipline that is tougher than that which the parents might have recommended. Generally, parental support to help the child learn more appropriate ways of dealing with the stressor that is causing the lying or cheating will usually prevent further incidents.

Nurses rarely address the development of morality in children, although it is frequently an area of concern for families. Nurses help families with moral development through the following interventions:

- Help parents and those dealing with school-age children recognize the normal level of moral development in this age group, the importance of being accepted, the ways in which a child's behavior affects others, and the rules of the group or society.
- Support parents in developing fair rules and methods of discipline that are consistent with the child's moral expectations. Family meetings can be effective by the end of the school-age period to allow each family member's input into decision making.
- Counsel parents in ways to deal with the minor behavioral problems of this age and in recognition of the need for more in-depth counseling or treatment. One way to deal with minor problems is to read with children about situations involving moral decisions and to talk with them about preferred choices for behavior.
- Support families in their personal choice of religion and religious education related to the moral teaching of their children.

PATHOLOGICAL PROCESSES

School-age children, similar to all other age groups, are exposed daily to agents and factors in the environment that have the potential of causing injury, illness, or death. Many of these agents and factors are harmless when used appropriately or when exposure is minimal. Examples include physical agents such as fires, mechanical agents such as bicycles and cars, biological agents such as bacteria, chemical agents such as asbestos, and radiological agents such as x-rays. Death rates from these factors vary among ethnic groups because of access to health care and environmental issues. For example, Native Americans and Alaska Natives experience higher death rates than do other groups from motor vehicle accidents, residential fires, and drownings (U.S. Department of Health and Human Services, 2000). Blacks also experience higher death rates than do other ethnic groups for unintentional injury (Centers for Disease Control and Prevention, 1999a).

Accidents

Accidents are the leading cause of death in children over age one in the United States and Great Britain (Cole, Naidoo, & Wills, 1998; U.S. Department of Health and Human Services, 2000). Most accidents do not result in death, but many serious accidents can cause significant morbidity and disability for children involved. Because of the effect of accidents, the nurse has a significant role in educating parents and school system personnel on ways to prevent dangers to school-age children and in becoming involved in public initiatives to create a safer society for children (see Hot Topics box).

The agents, host, and environment are considered in accidents that occur in school-age children. The type of *agents* has been found to vary with the child's age; the most frequent fatal accidents during the school-age period are from motor vehicles accidents, fires and burns, bicycle accidents, pedestrian injuries, falls, drownings, and firearm accidents (Crawley, 1996). The most common nonfatal accidents tend to be caused by simple agents and produce simple injuries. Of the 550,000 emergency room visits made between 1984 and 1988, many involved children and adolescents either become injured or die because of bicycling accidents (Sacks, Holmgreen, Smith, & Sosin, 1991). Despite helmet laws in several states, many children between ages 6 to 11 years continue to experience injuries related to recreational equipment, such as bicycles, swings, and skateboard accidents. Slightly older children have an increased number of accidents from contact sports and cuts, falls, burns, and injuries from firearms.

HOT topics

SAFETY CONCERNS SPECIFIC TO THE SCHOOL-AGE CHILD

Because of increased independence, school-age children face significant exposure to situations that can pose a threat to their health. Consequently, parents of these children must be involved in community and legislative activities that provide safe play environments for their children. Additionally, at appropriate health visits, health care workers should provide anticipatory guidance to parents in the following areas:

- Bicycle safety (have a well-maintained bicycle, ride only in safe areas approved by parents, observe rules for vehicle traffic, ride on side of road with traffic, and "bike defensively") and use of a federally approved helmet while riding
- Street safety (child should look right, left, then right again to check safety of crossing a street; cross only at safe and well-monitored intersections, preferably with an adult present; ensure parental supervision when children are playing close to streets and heavy traffic areas)
- Motor-vehicle safety (child should wear seat belt or be in age-appropriate booster seat as needed; older child should ride in back seat with restraint system until age 12)
- Pool safety (all children should have swimming lessons, swim with a buddy or an adult who can swim well in safe pools with drain covers; child should avoid swim ming after a heavy meal and avoid "roughhousing" behavior around the pool; insure parental supervision with child swimming)
- Firearm safety (adults are responsible for locking away guns, insuring intact gun safety locks, and securing guns in a safe environment; children must be instructed never to touch guns if found in home)
- Playground safety (all playground equipment should meet federally approved standards; children should be trained on how to use equipment safely; equipment should be evaluated for safety and repaired before children's use)
- Fire safety (child has working smoke detector in home and school; family practices fire evacuation plan to prepare for a fire emergency; fire-retardant clothing is worn at night; children do not play with matches, open fires, fireworks, or open wires that can cause injury and fire)
- Toxin safety (child should avoid insecticides, radiation sources, inappropriate use of medications that might cause an overdose, and pollution sources; all known toxins, chemicals, and household cleaning agents should be stored in adequately ventilated location that is inaccessible to children and with childproof lids or tops)
- Stranger safety (child should play with a friend, have a plan for returning home, play in a safe and known area, and report any suspicious activity threatening child safety to an appropriate adult; child should know how to say "no" and how to locate assistance when placed in an unsafe situation)

Specific accident factors relate to the *host,* in this case, the school-age child. Children in this age group tend to become hurt because of their "happy-go-lucky" attitude, curiosity, love of mimicking older persons, and their intense oral tendencies (Hoekelman, Friedman, Nelson, & Siedel, 2001). Typically, accidents occur more frequently in school-age boys than they do in girls. The reason for this tendency is undocumented, although one can hypothesize that it is caused by differences in personalities, societal expectations, child-rearing practices, and the greater risk-taking behaviors of boys compared with girls. The agent varies with the gender of the host. For school-age boys, drowning is the most common fatal accident, and automobile accidents are second; for girls, automobile accidents are the most common, and drowning is the fourth leading cause of death (Centers for Disease Control and Prevention, 1999b).

The physical *environment* of the child dictates the type or frequency of accidents, which occur in settings that include the home, neighborhood, and school. The majority of accidents happen outdoors, which means that school-age children are at greater risk for automobile or bicycle accidents than they are for poisoning or falls that occur predominantly indoors to the younger child.

The incidence of accidents is higher in the summer than it is in the winter, which may be a result of children being outside more, with an increase in accidents such as drowning and pedestrian motor-vehicle accidents. Socioeconomic level affects children's physical environment, making them more likely to suffer from one type of accident more than from another. Space heaters place children in low-income families at risk for burns, whereas a private swimming pool places wealthier children at risk for drowning.

The social environment, which includes the family, school, and playmates, also plays a role in accidents. Although little research has focused on the physical trauma caused by heavy backpacks that many school-age children use, appliances such as these exert significant pressure against muscles of the back and torso that are functionally immature during the school-age period. Muscles that are overused with daily carrying of "bulging" backpacks can cause muscle strain, headaches, improper posture, and other physical problems for children exposed to this trauma on a consistent basis.

As part of the social environment, many studies have shown that stress in the child or the family can increase the likelihood of accidents. Many families have chronic stress (parental unemployment) or a sudden acute stress (parental illness) that results in an increased risk for accidents. This

Box 20-8 Water-Safety Practices

1. School-age and younger children should be taught to swim. Lessons can be incorporated into school gym classes or into outside recreational activities. Continued refinement of swimming skills through repeated swimming lessons can also decrease the chances of a school-age child becoming injured or dying in a swimming accident.
2. Children should not swim alone; preferably, children should swim only in areas in which lifeguards are present.
3. School-age children should be taught basic lifesaving cardiopulmonary resuscitation (CPR) skills through the American Red Cross or other school or community programs.
4. Backyard pools, when unattended, should be protected by high fences and locked gates and be visible to an adult.
5. Handrails and ladders in pools should be in good repair; drains in pools should be covered with appropriate equipment to prevent the overpowering suction that can cause the drowning of a child.
6. Areas around pools and diving boards should be constantly maintained.
7. Children should be cautioned not to run or "fool around" along the edge of pools.
8. Swimming too soon after eating heavy meals should be avoided to decrease the possibility of abdominal cramps.
9. Children should be encouraged to recognize their own swimming abilities and not to be pushed by their peers beyond these abilities.
10. When on boats, children and adults should wear life jackets.

stress has contributed to homicide as the third leading cause of death among children ages 5 to 14 years (Osofsky, Cohen, & Drell, 1995; U.S. Department of Health and Human Services, 2000) and as a greater cause of death among Black and Hispanic children compared with White children (Anderson, Kockanck, & Murphey, 1997). Another vulnerable period for increased accidents is any time that parental supervision is minimal, such as during holidays, a move to a new home, or family crises, during which adults are preoccupied with other matters and fail to monitor their children adequately.

Drownings

Fewer school-age children than infants and adolescents die from drowning. However, for every child who drowns, 14 are taken to the emergency rooms because of near-drowning each year (Wintemute, 1990). Water-safety measures can help reduce this number, along with the many other injuries that occur around water, such as falls in slippery areas (Box 20-8). Environment and safety teaching can also influence the number of school-age children dying as a result of drowning. For example, more Black children of this age die from this cause than do White children (U.S. Department of Health and Human Services, 2000).

Burns

Each year, many Americans become victims of house fires, many of which occur in the winter months from Christmas tree, space heater, and fireplace malfunctions. Many homes lack working smoke detectors because of incorrect installation or inadequate testing. The majority of burned children survive, frequently with physical and psychological scars of varying severity. Children can be accidentally burned through scalds or flame burns. Scalds are more common in the infant, whereas flame burns are more common in the school-age child.

Children in this age group receive their burns by house fires associated with parental smoking. Other potential problem areas involve playing with gasoline, firecrackers, matches, or chemistry sets; space heaters; helping with barbecues or cooking; making candles; or simply watching others involved in these activities. Electrical burns occur in this group when children climb near high-voltage wires and inadvertently grab one. Other burns, such as those from an electrical storm, can be encountered when children fail to take appropriate shelter during bad weather. School-age children generally lack the maturity to handle flammable materials adequately, resulting in many burns and some deaths.

Several measures can be taken to prevent burns in children. One government intervention has been the Flammable Fabrics Act, which requires that fabrics used in children's sleepwear (sizes up to 14) be flame retardant (the material can still burn, but at a slower rate). Children's sleepwear labels should be read to learn the appropriate ways to wash the garment. Through parental written information and seminars, nurses can offer suggestions to decrease the possibility of an accidental burn to the school-age child (Box 20-9).

Firearms

People using firearms frequently cause fatal injury in the United States, including homicide, suicide, and accidents. According to *Healthy People 2000: Mid-Course Review and 1995 Revisions* (U.S. Department of Health and Human Services, 1995a), accidents from the use of firearms remain the fourth cause of unintentional injury among 5- to 14-year-old children. With many U.S. homes containing a handgun, concern about children's safety remains well founded. Possibly the best means of preventing accidents with firearms is to ban them from private ownership (see Chapter 19). For example, the experience of not allowing private handguns in England has led to a decrease in deaths and injuries. However, because handgun ownership is an important individual right in this country, several states have passed legislation that allows handguns for individual protection. With recent school shootings by young adolescents, this discussion has taken on a new fervor for gun activists and those who believe guns should be more highly regulated to protect children of all ages. Much of this discussion has focused on better ways to properly store and lock firearms. Families with firearms in the home should be encouraged to do the following:

1. Store them safely in a locked area
2. Store weapons and ammunition in separate areas
3. Consider using nonlethal (wax) bullets

Sports and Recreation

Accidents from sports and other recreational activities increase during the school-age years. The types of injuries vary and include lacerations, contusions, hematomas, concussions, sprains, and fractures. Children use a variety of equipment, including playground equipment, and are increasingly involved in contact sports, such as football, hockey, soccer, and basketball. Intense social pressure for children to participate in team sports today means that school systems must respond to children's and parents' needs for physical and psychological protection during participation in sports. For example, all schools that engage in team sports must insure that body devices to decrease injuries and appropriate emotional support for winning and losing records exist to foster the developmental needs of children involved in competitive sports.

Injuries that occur in recreation areas can be prevented by several measures. The National Bureau of Standards set guidelines in 1976 for home playground equipment, regulating areas such as sharp edges, moving parts, and equipment design. Nurses can help prevent accidents in this area through school education programs by participating in decisions about school playground equipment and by counseling families on a variety of issues (Box 20-10). Attention to playground safety has become an important issue with 200,000 children injured to the extent that they must go to an emergency room each year (*Healthweek*, 2000). Many of these injuries occur in Hispanic and Pacific Islander students who live in areas where playgrounds fail to meet safety standards (U.S. Department of Health and Human Services, 2000). Counseling by the nurse in clinics and schools should include the need for parents to monitor their children during play, to assess the age-appropriateness of equipment, and to use playground equipment properly.

Nursing Interventions

Nurses offer suggestions to parents to improve children's safety in their play environments and to prevent childhood accidents. Unfortunately, studies in this area of health education have shown varying results (some parents follow the suggestions, but many, although they understand the validity of the suggestions, fail to follow them). Some reasons for which people fail to follow through are difficulty in completing the required frequent assessments, amount of

Box 20-9 Fire-Prevention Practices

1. All homes should have working smoke detectors and fire extinguishers; parents should check the operation of these devices at least twice a year, such as during daylight savings time changes in April and October.
2. All families should have planned escape routes from the home in case of a fire and should practice using these routes frequently.
3. Family members should never smoke while in bed.
4. Appropriate fire escapes and plans should be provided for persons sleeping on upper floors.
5. Children should be taught how to react in case of fire, including how to use the home fire extinguisher, how to call the fire department (911), and how to put out clothing fires.
6. Flame-retardant clothing should be properly used and maintained (read labels).
7. Night clothes that quickly catch fire should be avoided, such as loose, flimsy nightgowns for girls.
8. Children should be cautioned to avoid using matches, cigarette lighters, or flammable liquids and materials. These materials should be stored safely.
9. Open fires, such as fireplaces, should have protective gratings.
10. Children should use stoves and other cooking facilities only with adult supervision.
11. Children should not be allowed to play with fireworks. Although each state regulates the use of fireworks, parents should monitor their children when fireworks are present.
12. Children should be cautioned to avoid touching wires that they encounter on the ground or when climbing.

Box 20-10 Playground-Safety Practices

1. Playground equipment should meet federal and state standards and be age-appropriate. Sharp, protruding, or potentially injurious parts of any equipment should be eliminated.
2. The area surrounding playground equipment should be adequately cushioned for falls.
3. Equipment should be located such that injury to other children can be avoided.
4. Children should be trained to use any new equipment that they obtain safely, such as a skateboard or a fishing pole.
5. Equipment should always be kept in good working order and securely fastened.
6. When children are involved in contact sports, appropriate protective equipment should be worn.
7. During contact sports, rules should be followed and adults should monitor the game for safety violations.

effort involved, high cost, and discomfort in the use of equipment. Most of these factors are perceived differently by different people. This type of education requires increased study to learn the approaches that obtain the best results. Nurses offer general strategies to provide guidance to parents and school personnel on child accident prevention, particularly because individual counseling is an integral part of health promotion and illness prevention. Increasing use of rollerblades means the nurse must address with parents the need for child safety helmets and knee-elbow-wrist guards to prevent muscle sprains and bone fractures. Additional on-site opportunities for teaching children accident prevention are available in the school setting (the proper way to carry a backpack). In addition to providing guidance for accident prevention, nurses can participate in legislative and educational actions to increase community consciousness (Box 20-11). For example, the nurse can become involved in programs aimed at decreasing violence and offering alternative ways to deal with disputes that are more common in low-income neighborhoods, perhaps as a response to perceived discrimination and challenges to survival of these communities.

Box 20-11 Nursing Interventions to Prevent Accidents During the School-Age Period

STRATEGIES FOR COUNSELING

- Discuss accident prevention at optimal times, such as during prenatal visits, well-child visits to the physician, the arrival of a new sibling, or after an accident.
- Rather than discussing all topics at once, pick the major concerns for the development level of the child at each well-child visit. For the school-age child, these topics include motor-vehicle, water, fire, and bicycle safety.
- Repeat information at other visits to emphasize its importance.

COMMUNITY ACTIONS

- Use supplemental materials, such as written pamphlets, to reinforce the verbal information.
- Support local and national legislation that sets standards for potentially harmful agents. Mandating standards has been one of the most successful accident preventives, as seen in the Poison Prevention Packaging Act and the Flammable Fabrics Act.
- Wear a bicycle helmet and other protective gear when appropriate. Many nurses have been active in lobbying for bicycle helmet requirements in their states.
- Consult with manufacturers on safe designs of materials used by children.
- Report any objects that are potentially hazardous.
- Participate in local activities that stress accident prevention, such as local offices of the National Safety Council.
- Educate groups, such as school children and parent organizations.

Mechanical Forces

Motor vehicles and bicycles represent the two most common mechanical agents that cause injury to school-age children.

Motor Vehicles

The leading cause of death in all groups of children from age 1 to adulthood is motor-vehicle accidents (Aetna/U.S. Healthcare, 1998). These groups include children who are passengers in cars, pedestrians, and bicycle riders. Another 145,000 suffer annual injuries in motor vehicles (Hoekelman, Friedman, Nelson, & Siedel, 2001). In the United States, deaths from pedestrian accidents outnumber deaths from passenger accidents among children aged 3 to 12 years. Accidents between automobiles and bicycles account for one sixth of the injuries from motor vehicles in children between ages 5 and 14, but more than 90% of the people killed in bicycle accidents are children (Hoekelman, Friedman, Nelson, & Siedel, 2001). Although not all motor-vehicle accidents result in death, many children are left with long-term disabilities that affect their quality of life.

Injuries to passengers in automobiles can be prevented, or the severity reduced, by altering some aspects of the physical environment. Lower speed limits, not allowing someone to drive after drinking alcohol, better automobile and highway designs, and seat belt requirements in all states have all been shown to reduce the severity and number of accidents and injuries. Increased injuries have been correlated to the higher speed limits instituted in the United States several years ago. Although the American Academy of Pediatrics (1996b) has recommended seat belts for all school buses, many children remain at risk because various school districts and states do not require seat belts for student school and field trip transportation.

Studies have shown that federally approved car seats and belts used consistently and appropriately can decrease the likelihood of a child's death by 70% to 95% and decrease serious injury by 50% to 60% (Hancock, 1987; American Academy of Pediatrics, 1996b). Despite these impressive statistics, a large percentage of school-age children do not appropriately use seat belts and younger, lower weight school-age children do not use booster seats correctly. Educational programs that encourage children to use their seat belts are not always effective. Reasons given by parents and children for not using seat belts include forgetting to replace the seatbelt, difficulty reaching and fastening the belt, discomfort experienced from wearing the belt, and driving short distances. Studies have found a strong correlation between parental and children's use of seat belts; if parents wear their seat belts, children are more likely to use them. Clearly, consistent use of seat belts by children will occur only when these and other safety devices are legally required and parents cooperate and provide role modeling. Recently, the federal government recommended that all children under the age of 12 sit, appropriately restrained, in the back seat of motor vehicles because of the potential of death incurred by activated passenger-seat airbags during a motor vehicle accident (Morbidity and Mortality Weekly Report, 1995) (see Fig. 17-6). Many families will have difficulty meeting this recommendation because of long-term acceptance of older children riding in the front seat after they have outgrown booster seats.

For children under 15 years of age who live in an urban area, more than one half of all the deaths from motor vehicle accidents are caused by pedestrian-automobile accidents. These accidents include those with rollerblades, skate boards, and skate scooters. The injuries from these accidents tend to be more severe than do passenger injuries, with a high percentage of head injuries. Many factors are involved in pedestrian accidents; children often have difficulty interpreting traffic signs, judging how fast cars are going, and forgetting to look "right to left to right" before crossing the street. Other researchers have suggested that overcrowding, poverty, high volume of traffic, stress, and unsafe play areas have an influence. Supervision by adults decreases the likelihood of this type of accident, but effective preventive measures have yet to be clearly documented. Educational safety programs for children have been unsuccessful in changing pedestrian behaviors. Prevention lies in a better understanding of the causes and in an age-appropriate approach to the problem. However, most people agree that parents should teach their children basic street-safety principles, such as how to cross the street and how to obey traffic lights. Box 20-12 lists some preventive measures.

Bicycles

Many accidents occur each year with young children on bicycles and tricycles. According to Tinsworth, Polen, and Cassidy (1994), 71% of bicyclists treated in emergency rooms were under 15 years of age. The majority of accidents are generally not serious, but deaths occur among young children who have suffered head trauma or significant bodily injury. In 1990 approximately 31,000 children under age 15 were killed or injured in bicycle-related accidents, which does not include unreported incidents (California Highway Patrol, 1991). The following list highlights the risk factors associated with bicycle accidents:

1. Reckless riding and lack of control (riding double and trying stunts) are associated with a majority of accidents.
2. Mechanical or structural problems with bicycles (brakes failing and chains slipping) account for approximately 20% of children's accidents (Hancock, 1987).
3. Bicycles that are not the right size for the child, primarily those that are too large, cause added risk.
4. Bicycles with elongated handlebars and low seats add to risk.
5. Hand brakes cause more problems than foot brakes.
6. Typically, boys have more bicycle accidents with cars than do girls.

Bicycle accidents occur most frequently near the child's home and during the day, when the bicycle is being ridden for pleasure. Accidents increase when bicycles are frequently used (during the summer and after Christmas). Children frequently receive injuries from the spokes of their bikes, primarily when they are riding behind the bike seat. These injuries include cuts, bruises, sprains, and fractures.

To prevent bicycle accidents, teaching must encompass safety factors for both the bicycle and the rider. Parents should be cautioned to follow certain guidelines when obtaining a bicycle. The bicycle should be the appropriate size for the child and contain accessories that the child understands (the rider should be able to use the horn properly). When the child sits on the bicycle, the feet should be flat on the ground. When the child is standing, there should be at least an inch between the child and the center bar of a boy's bicycle. There should be easy access to the brakes. Bicycles with sharp, protruding parts or with slippery foot brakes should be avoided. Although only 2% to 5% of children wear helmets during bicycling (Rodgers, 1996), documentation demonstrates that all children should wear helmets approved by the American National Standards Institute (ANSI) to significantly decrease the risk of head trauma with a fall (see Chapter 19). This percentage has increased with many jurisdictions now mandating helmets for both child and adult bicyclists and those using rollerblades. An ANSI-approved helmet has the following features:

- The outer shell is made of hard plastic or fiberglass.
- The helmet liner is made from polystyrene foam and does not feel spongy when pressed.
- The helmet is adjustable to the size and shape of the child's head; as the child gets older, the size can be adjusted by changing to appropriately sized fitting pads.

Box 20-12 Street-Safety Principles

1. Older children and adults can provide supervision as guards to help and educate younger children in crossing streets.
2. Education programs for groups of children should involve parents and consistent adherence to learned behaviors.
3. Streets in communities should be evaluated for areas at high risk for accidents; stop signs, reduced speed signs, speed bumps, or adult supervision may be needed in these areas.
4. Areas of greatest risk are frequently those with a large number of children, such as playgrounds and schools. Children in these areas need adult monitoring and guidance, along with traffic controls, such as reduced speed.

- The helmet does not limit hearing or vision.
- When adjusted properly, the chin strap should hold the helmet securely on the head.

Nurses should encourage parents to teach and reinforce safe bicycling habits to their children throughout their lives. Suggestions for safe bicycling in general and safe bicycling in traffic, based on the American Academy of Pediatrics, Child Safety Suggestions, are listed in Box 20-13.

Biological Agents

School-age children are constantly exposed to bacterial, viral, and other biological agents that are potential threats to health. Compared with the preschool child, the school-age child has fewer illnesses. The most frequent illness continues to be respiratory infections, most commonly upper respiratory infections (URIs). Many of these illnesses cause loss of school days and increased physician visits. Most URIs result from viruses, but bacteria can play either a primary or a secondary role. Two problems associated with URIs are streptococcal infection and otitis media.

Strep throat from group A beta-hemolytic streptococcus is a well-known problem, is diagnosed by a throat culture, and is treated with an antibiotic, most commonly penicillin. Strep throat can occur at any age, but is most common in school-age children. A child with an infection from this strain of streptococcus may have a severe sore throat, fever, and malaise or may have only a minor sore throat.

The concern with group A beta-hemolytic streptococcal infections lies with the risk of secondary complications and potential results. Most serious is the possible development of rheumatic fever or acute glomerulonephritis in a child after streptococcal pharyngitis. Areas in which close person-to-person contact occurs, such as schools, are prone to outbreaks. School nurses should be alert to children with possible streptococcal infections and recommend throat cultures and treatment as needed for children with positive cultures. Children treated for strep throat with an antibiotic are usually noninfectious after 24 hours of treatment and can then return to school (American Academy of Pediatrics, Committee on Infectious Diseases, 1997). Children with throat infections caused by other strains of streptococcus, such as group B, do not usually require treatment, primarily because these infections are not usually associated with the same serious complications.

The frequency of gastrointestinal infection (influenza and gastroenteritis) decreases in the school-age years, although this type of infection is still the second most common acute condition of childhood after URIs. Most

Box 20-13 Bicycle Safety for School-Age Children

SUGGESTIONS FOR SAFE BICYCLING

1. Parents should acquaint the child with a new bicycle, including braking, steering, and balancing, and the appropriate surfaces on which to ride.
2. The child should demonstrate a basic ability in bicycle riding to the parents before being allowed to use it without supervision. This includes the ability to stop the bicycle quickly using the brakes, start riding without wobbling a path 1 yard wide, stop and dismount without falling, and ride in a straight line close to the curb.
3. Parents should discuss locations that the child is permitted to ride. Safe areas for riding can be established and safe routes to and from school, friends' homes, and other locations can be mapped.
4. Families should agree on some general rules for safe riding, such as not riding in the dark, while barefoot, with someone else on the bicycle, in bad weather when brakes might not work, or with loose pants that can get tangled.
5. Bicycles should be inspected regularly to ensure that they are in safe and good working condition, including properly inflated tires.
6. Children should wear ANSI-approved helmets.

SUGGESTIONS FOR SAFE BICYCLING IN TRAFFIC

1. Bicycle riders are subject to the same rules as are automobile operators. *All* traffic signs and signals must be observed.
2. Local and state regulations must be observed, including licensing, registration, and ordinances related to bicycle traffic.
3. When bicycle riding at night, the bicycle should have lights and reflectors, as required by local and state regulations.
4. Both hands should be on the handle bars at all times; sturdy shoes should be worn to secure feet to the bicycle pedals.
5. A basket or backpack should be used if objects must be carried; backpacks and other heavy or bulky materials should be avoided because they can throw off the child's center of balance.
6. Children should ride on the side of the road traveling with traffic, keeping close to the side of the road; they should not ride two abreast, but rather, ride single file.
7. Intersections should be approached with caution and may require walking the bike in the crosswalks.
8. Children should ride bicycles defensively, watching and listening for cars, pedestrians, street dangers, and car doors opening (large hats, earphones with compact disc players, and other items obstructing vision and hearing senses are to be avoided!).

Based on data from Betz, C. L. (1983). Bicycle safety: Opportunities for family education. *Pediatric Nursing*, 9 (2), 109-111; American Academy of Pediatrics. (1978). *Child safety suggestions*. Elk Grove Village, IL: The Academy.

commonly caused by a virus, gastrointestinal infection causes vomiting and diarrhea. Older and larger school-age children are in less danger of rapid dehydration; they basically react to the illness the same as do adults and need to be treated similarly. Gastroenteritis can affect several age groups; therefore children in school should be monitored for outbreaks.

A skin disorder that is commonly found in this age group is infestation with either scabies or lice (**pediculosis**), both of which cause extreme itchiness of either the body (scabies) or the hair (lice) and can spread to other children. School nurses must be aware of these two conditions, primarily because they occur in epidemic proportions in schools. These problems should be identified quickly to allow parental notification. Then, referral to a physician or a nurse practitioner for appropriate treatment can be made, and spread of the infection can be avoided.

A biological agent that many children know about is HIV, the cause of acquired immunodeficiency syndrome (AIDS). Of all age groups, the young school-age child is at the lowest risk for contracting AIDS, because perinatally-acquired AIDS emerges in infancy and toddlerhood, and most young school-age children are not taking intravenous drugs or engaging in high-risk sexual practices. The school-age child may know a person with AIDS and has certainly heard something about AIDS from adults, older children, or the news media. The school-age child should know basic facts about AIDS, its transmission, and, most importantly, the fact that it cannot be transmitted through casual contact, such as being in the same classroom with a child with AIDS. Because of widespread misinformation and fear about AIDS, the United States Surgeon General has called for mandatory, explicit AIDS education beginning with children 8 years of age. Parents remain concerned about the transmission of AIDS to their children primarily because of a lack of knowledge about its route of communication. Involving parents in AIDS-education programs to increase their information base and to assist them in accepting AIDS children frequently helps decrease their initial concern (Lavin et al., 1994; Osborne, Kistner, & Helgemo, 1995). Parents who accept AIDS children also assist their own children in learning to accept children with special needs and to define their own health.

Children with AIDS may attend school as long as it has been determined that they are not in a period of heightened risk for contracting an illness from the other children. With new treatments dramatically improving the lifespan of these children, many will be in school for longer periods and will face exposure to the usual childhood diseases. During outbreaks of chickenpox, measles, or other illnesses, the child with AIDS should have home tutoring to decrease morbidity. The child with AIDS needs continual evaluation of the risks versus benefits of school attendance. Certainly, long periods of isolation from peers will contribute to feelings of loneliness in the child with AIDS and may even appear to be a punishment for being ill. The school nurse will undoubtedly have an important role in facilitating the multidisciplinary care inherent in AIDS care while maximizing the learning environment of affected children.

Box 20-14 Resources for AIDS Educational Materials

American Academy of Pediatrics
Publications Department
P.O. Box 927
Elk Grove Village, IL 60009

American Red Cross
800-342-2437

Kidsrights
3700 Progress Blvd.
P.O. Box 851
Mt. Dora, FL 32757
800-892-5437

Network Publications
P.O. Box 1830
Santa Cruz, CA 95061-1830

San Francisco AIDS Foundation
333 Valencia St.
P.O. Box 6182
San Francisco, CA 94101-6182

AIDS Hotline (U.S. Department of Health and Human Services)
800-342-AIDS

The Multicultural AIDS Coalition
Douglas Park
801-B Tremont St.
Boston, MA 02118
617-442-1622

The school nurse can be instrumental in providing age-appropriate educational materials on AIDS to school-age children, school staff, and parents. Some of this information can be provided in health-promotion classes held throughout the elementary school years or in sex education classes in the later school-age years. Some resources for the nurse on AIDS are listed in Box 20-14.

By school age, most children have received their basic series of immunizations. Most states require that the child's immunizations are current before entering kindergarten or the first grade and additional immunization for tetanus be given every 10 years or with an unclean wound. Although 95% of American children receive immunizations by the time they enter school (U.S. Department of Health and Human Services, 2000), concern remains that an increasing number of immigrants and transient workers in the economy may bring previously conquered diseases and affect overall immunity in this country. Therefore the nurse must inspect immunization records of all students in the school or clinics to ensure that these people are up to date with their "shots" and to inform parents of immunization requirements and resources available in the community.

The child with only a few needed immunizations need not start from the beginning of the immunization schedule, but can pick up where shots were stopped. The child beyond age 6 should be given the adult vaccine tetanus-diphtheria (TD) rather than the diphtheria, tetanus, pertussis vaccine (TDP). Immunization to pertussis (whooping cough) is no longer needed because the risk of the disease decreases with age and the risk of immunization reaction may increase with age (American Academy of Pediatrics, Committee on Infectious Diseases, 1997). The strength of the diphtheria antigen portion (*D* to *d*) decreases, because more reactions to this component of the immunization have been noted with older children. Table 19-4 shows the recommended schedule by the American Academy of Pediatrics for children who were not immunized in early infancy. The Academy recommends a measles, mumps, and rubella booster (MMR) immediately before entry into fifth grade. Research has shown that the immunity that develops after the toddler dose of MMR frequently does not last beyond 10 years. The fifth-grade dose ensures adequate levels of immunity for these youngsters and covers young women as they enter their childbearing years. School-age children who sustain injuries placing them at risk for tetanus should receive prophylaxis according to the guidelines developed by the Academy (American Academy of Pediatrics, Committee on Infectious Diseases, 1997) (Table 20-5).

Table 20-5 Guide to Tetanus Prophylaxis in Wound Management

History of Absorbed Tetanus Toxoid (Doses)	Clean (Minor Wounds)	All Other Wounds#
Unknown or less than 3 doses	Use Td^	Use Td^ and TIG*
Three or more doses##	No need for Td^ or TIG* except for$	No need for Td^ or TIG* except for%

From American Academy of Pediatrics, Committee on Infectious Diseases, Report of the Committee. (1997). *1997 Red Book* (24th ed.). Elk Grove Village, IL: The Academy.

DtaP, diptheria/tetanus/acellular pertussis; *DTP,* diptheria/ tetanus/pertussis; *DT,* diptheria/tetanus; *Td,* tetanus and diptheria toxoid

^For children less than 7 years of age, DTaP (or DTP) recommended; when pertussis is contraindicated, use only DT; for children older than 7 years of age, Td recommended

*For children less than 7 years of age, DTaP (or DTP) recommended; when pertussis contraindicated, DT is given; for children older than 7 years of age, Td is given

$Yes, when more than 10 years since the last dose

%Yes, when more than 5 years since the last dose

#Such as, but not limited to, wounds contaminated with dirt, feces, soil, and saliva; puncture wounds and wounds resulting from missiles, crushing, burns, or frostbite

##Fec soil, saliva; puncture wounds; and wounds resulting from missiles, crushing, burns, and frostbite

Chemical Agents

A number of potentially toxic chemical agents are present in the environment, and the child is exposed to them through inhalation, ingestion, or direct contact. Children are thought to be particularly susceptible to chemical hazards. Two sources of chemicals ingested by children on a regular basis are foods and drugs. Additionally, an increasing number of older school-age children ingest tobacco as a result of cigarette smoking. Although normally safe, some foods and drugs can be harmful when used inappropriately. Other environmental hazards include exposures to pollution, heavy metals (lead and mercury), and pesticides.

The nutritional needs of the school-age child are reviewed earlier in this chapter. As stated, children frequently eat foods with high sugar, salt, and fat quantities and with chemical additives. The effects of some of these additives have been questioned, and recent concern has been expressed about the effect of biochemically altered food on children and future generations. On a short-term basis, some foods are thought to cause allergic reactions; on a long-term basis, some are implicated in the development of coronary disease, hypertension, and cancer. Nurses are aware that the child's diet can be a source of some health problems and should assess the child's intake and counsel the child and parents accordingly.

The incidence of poisoning decreases in the school-age years, primarily because children are more aware of the appropriate uses of drugs and other agents around the home. Childproof containers have helped decrease exposure of children to dangerous poisons and chemicals in the home. However, drug concerns (alcohol and glue inhalants) remain with less parental monitoring because of parental work outside the home. Older school-age children are increasingly exposed to recreational drugs, primarily through their peers and older children (see Chapter 21). In the school environment, wise decision making about using recreational drugs and their effect on the body should be addressed as part of a health-promotion approach specific to the developmental needs of school-age children.

With 25% of 12- to 13-year-old children reporting that they smoke cigarettes and 4% noting they are "regular" smokers (Moss, Allen, Giovino, & Mills, 1992), health-promotion attention must be paid to effective strategies to prevent smoking among children because of health risks identified earlier. This attention appears merited because many authorities on addiction believe that nicotine in cigarettes is highly addictive and leads people to experiment with more risky drugs (cocaine and methamphetamines). Various efforts such as the Tobacco Act of 1991 that focused on this aim by policing businesses selling cigarettes to minors have so far been ineffective because youthful cigarette smoking rates have remained unchanged since 1998 (Recer, 2000). In one study, 75% of children under the age of 16 got weekly cigarettes at stores, and 50% of retailers sold cigarettes to obviously underage children (Stead, Hastings, & Tudor-Smith, 1996). Proponents of antismoking campaigns support higher excise taxes and less media support for smoking behavior. Smoking behavior has been found to be higher in diverse communities in which billboards advertise the attractiveness of smoking, there is greater access to cigarettes, and peer pressure and lowered parental involvement have opposed antismoking efforts by those interested in children's welfare (U.S. Department of Health and Human Services, 2000). The recent Tobacco Settlement Project (1998) forbids tobacco advertisements on television; therefore some progress may occur in decreasing tobacco media messages to children who use television as an information format.

Pollution has become a fact of life for many Americans and, particularly, for the 25% of urban dwelling children who must breathe air that exceeds federal government levels for acceptable ozone (U.S. Department of Health and Human Services, 2000). Air pollution irritates the eyes and the respiratory tract, causing URIs, ear infections, and allergies. Children with allergies, including asthma, can be particularly compromised when exposed to air pollution. More children currently experience asthma that many believe reflects children's exposure to secondary smoke and poor air quality. Death rates from this illness escalated 67% from 1980 to 1993, and 40% of all activity restrictions of children result from asthma (U.S. Department of Health and Human Services, 2000). Knowing the negative effects of air pollution, smoking, and a lack of recycling efforts, school-age children are increasingly participating in school projects that aim at improving society's environmental health.

Metals to which children can be exposed include lead (Fig. 20-4) (see Chapter 17), cadmium, mercury, arsenic, and asbestos. Children exposed to these metals in toxic doses develop a variety of short- and long-term symptoms, with the type and severity varying with the metal. Mercury is particularly toxic to the developing CNS. Asbestos causes lung difficulties, but the response can be delayed for years. Children are exposed to these toxic metals through a variety of sources, including materials carried home from work on parents' clothes, from shoes contacting lead-infused soil, from lead in older residential water pipes, culturally relevant medications, or in school building structures (Wolfe, 2000). The long-term effects of these metals on children are still not completely known, but some evidence indicates children suffer neurotoxic effects from this type of exposure. Moss, Lanphear, and Auinger (1999) also point out that high lead levels in children

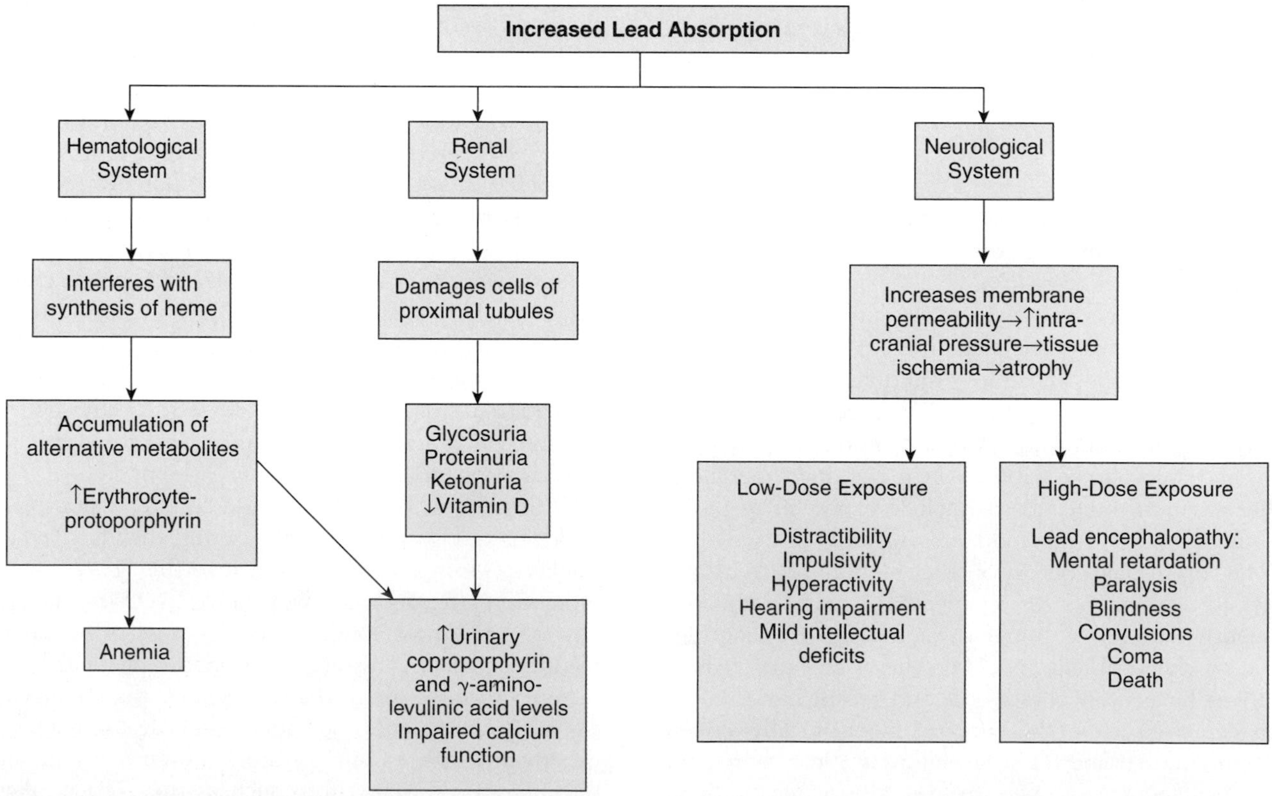

Fig. 20-4 Algorithm showing the main effects of lead on body systems. (Redrawn from Wong, D. L., et al. [1999]. *Whaley & Wong's nursing care of infants and children* [6th ed.]. St. Louis: Mosby.)

contribute to dental caries, and other researchers have supported that hearing loss and even criminal behavior can result from early and consistent child exposure to lead.

The use of pesticides to control insects and undesirable weeds in landscaping has led to increased concerns about exposure to these agents by children. Animal experiments have led to the recent withdrawal of a common pesticide, Dursban, from the marketplace. With increased interest in more natural substances to control insects and gardening problems, perhaps less reliance will be placed on biological chemicals for these problems in the future.

Radiological Agents

The child receives exposure from both naturally occurring radiation and man-made ionizing radiation. Radiation exposure occurs in varying degrees in the x-ray films taken for dental, bone, and other routine examinations; from nuclear power plants and explosions; and in the treatment for many childhood cancers. Children exposed to high levels of radiation have been found to be at risk for developing cancer in the future, with the risk of developing leukemia, thyroid cancer, and breast cancer greater for children compared with adults. Other problems that have been documented after radiation exposure include mental deficiencies and compromised growth.

Nurses and other professionals are active in the prevention of chemical and radiation hazards to children. This is an area in which much work remains to be done. Box 20-15 provides suggestions for ways to begin.

Box 20-15 Nursing Interventions to Prevent Chemical and Radiation Hazards During the School-Age Period

- Become aware of the potential environmental chemical and radiation hazards in general and for a local area in particular. For example, rural areas may have insecticide spraying, factories may emit heavy leads, cities may have serious smog problems, and any area may have chemical waste dumps with potential leaks.
- Know family members' occupations and living situations and their potential hazards. Consider that some previously unexplained illnesses can be caused by these hazards; participate in collecting a complete assessment of an individual's lifestyle to explore reasons for illness.
- Monitor the amount of radiation to which children are exposed through x-ray films and the precautions to be taken, such as covering the genital area to protect future reproductive capability.
- Work with community officials to locate potential hazards.
- Know federal and local regulatory agencies and the roles that they play in monitoring the environment (Environmental Protection Agency [EPA], Department of Labor, Occupational Safety and Health Administration [OSHA], Nuclear Regulatory Commission [NRC]).

Cancer

The cancers most common in this age-group include leukemia (see Chapter 19), brain tumors and lymphomas, and CNS tumors. Primary brain tumors are the most common solid tumors that occur in children, second to the most common childhood cancer, leukemia (Wong et al., 1999). Many brain tumors occur in children less than 15 years of age. The cause of CNS tumors is unknown. In children, dissimilar to adults, most brain tumors are infratentorial in location (brainstem and cerebellum). When the nurse suspects an intracranial lesion, the first step in assessment includes recording detailed history. Increased intracranial pressure is an early symptom in infratentorial tumors. The most common symptoms, however, are vomiting, headache after awakening, and disturbances of gait and balance.

The lymphomas include Hodgkin's disease and non-Hodgkin's lymphoma. The incidence of Hodgkin's disease peaks from age 15 to 24 (see Chapter 21). NonHodgkin's lymphomas have a peak incidence in the school-age years. Boys are affected approximately three times more often than are girls, and mortality rates in the United States tend to be increased in densely populated areas, particularly in higher education and income levels. The most common symptom is abdominal pain caused by intestinal obstruction and symptoms resulting from organ compression. With effective treatment regimens, children with limited disease involvement can be cured; 75% to 80% of children with extensive disease are cured with evolving medications used for nonHodgkin's lymphoma (Reiter et al., 1995; Wong et al., 1999).

Because of the dramatic increase in life expectancy after treatment for some childhood cancers, an increasing number of children return to school after successful treatment. These children present a challenge to the nurse because they are in various stages of recovery or may enjoy full health. However, most children fear some threat of recurrence. Therefore the nurse must provide psychological and emotional support to affected children and help them develop the peer relationships that are important to them at this age.

SOCIAL PROCESSES

The daily life of the school-age child requires frequent interactions with other children and adults. Friends are important, and parents should collaborate with their children to allow them to become independent during the school-age period. Mutual problem solving frequently occurs at this age related to a higher level of maturity in social relationships and concerns. Adequate social functioning with peers, family, and community is vital to the child's well being during these years, specifically because it is often the foundation for future relationships (Vannoy, 1994). The child is exposed to a variety of societal roles and interactions, the process of **socialization.** As socialization occurs, the child develops social competence (the ability and skills to participate effectively in the social interactions of society). Social competence includes both the obvious social behaviors and an inner understanding of the appropriateness of behaviors.

Several elements play a role in the development of the child's social competence. The child's desire for a sense of industry encourages interactions, positive relationships, and accomplishments within society. Cognitive development must exist to understand relationships and to solve problems. Moral judgment helps the child to understand consequences and fairness in relationships. Understanding and obeying authority helps to maintain order in society. Social sensitivity is a result of social interactions and requires the child's ability to perceive the social cues of others, to understand the roles of others, and to communicate verbally with them. Social behaviors are also a part of social competence; these are learned most frequently through the imitation, role modeling, and reinforcement of others' behaviors. The interaction of all these elements produces a level of social competence in the child and simultaneously plays a role in the child's self-perception. Individuals frequently see themselves as others see them. Social competence and self-identify are closely related as discussed in this chapter.

Community and Work

The strongest relationships that school-age children develop outside their families are with their peers (other children who they encounter in their neighborhood and at school). The peer group acts as a new social system, becoming increasingly influential in the child's life. Children learn values, behaviors, and attitudes from their peer group as they did from their families. All children continue to be influenced significantly by the family, the culture of the family, and many other environmental factors, but the peer group now begins to influence lifestyle, habits, and speech patterns and to formulate standards of behavior and performance. The standards of the peer group become vitally important, and all efforts are made to conform. Being accepted by the peer group becomes more important than being accepted by anyone else. Conforming to the pressures of peers becomes an issue, especially when it interferes with the parents' expectations.

Children begin to realize that their own goals, desires, and aspirations might be quite different from those held by the peer group or the school, and they must find some way to cope and to perform according to the new standards if they are to succeed. School-age children's definition of success or failure can be defined more by their peers than by their family. Whereas the devastation of failure with the peer group can be more severe than any experienced before, the sense of success that comes with group approval is powerful and gratifying. The degree to which children are able to fit in socially, make the adjustment, learn to cope, and receive satisfaction from the group is a powerful determinant of healthy socialization.

One type of relationship that develops between children is friendship. Three stages of friendship development have been described and include choosing friends based initially on specific acts that a child believes someone does well. When the child becomes older (9 or 10 years of age), the child has gained trust with friends, which serves as the foundation for friendships. Toward the end of the school-age period, friendships continue because each child in the relationship has a mutual understanding and willingness to help the other as each faces challenges to their lives.

A child may have one best friend or several important friends. Groups that form during this age may change and be goal directed, such as a sports team. These groups frequently have set rules or rituals that connect the members. One notable aspect of the friendships and groups that develop during the school-age years is the tendency toward same-gender relationships. Videos, songs, and books are shared, and media messages become important to define the "best" objects for play. Certainly, children have friends of the opposite gender, but the focus is clearly on friendships of the same gender. Later in the school-age years, the development of sexual relationships changes with the first signs of dating and mixed parties.

School-age children become increasingly involved with adults outside the family, including teachers, coaches, and others who become role models, all of whom influence the child's view of the world and the self. Although this influence may not appear to be as significant as is that of the child's peers, long-term ideas and beliefs frequently develop from these relationships. Children usually perceive some similarity between themselves and their models, those that reflect the same gender with similar physical or behavioral traits. During these years, children may not maintain a strong identification with the parent of the same gender, but they also tend to adopt other adult models with whom they can identify.

Working Parents

Studies have shown that over 50% of mothers with children between ages 6 and 17 work outside the home, the majority of whom work full time. Many of these women work out of economic necessity, but remain concerned about the welfare of their children during work hours. Both dual-career couples and single-mother families influence children's accessibility to parental assistance; it also influences their safety when no adult is present to monitor the environment after school. Many children who are left alone until their parents return from work follow specific directions from their parents. These directions may include beginning dinner in anticipation of their parents' return or completing homework while remaining inside the home with the doors locked.

Parents and school-age children are often in conflict

Box 20-16 After-School Considerations for Latchkey Children

- Each child should be assessed to determine the appropriate after-school supervision. One 10-year-old child might be able to be alone for a short time; another might not be ready for this responsibility. The child should play a role in this discussion, but the parents should make the decision.
- Alternatives should be considered, such as day care, neighbors, other family members, older siblings, or after-school programs. Many public schools are beginning to develop day care programs for older children before and after school.
- When the child is alone, a set schedule should be discussed. This schedule might include the time at which the child should be home and whether a parent should be called.
- Specific guidelines should be discussed, such as after-school activities, use of television, whether playmates can enter the home, and places that the child may go.
- Emergency measures should be planned with the child, such as what to do in the event that the child is sick, loses the key, or has a problem at home. Plans should include how to reach both a parent and another responsible adult in the neighborhood who has agreed to help as needed. The family should discuss situations defining an emergency and the ways in which parents can be most easily notified (cellular phone and pager) when these situations occur.
- The child should be cautioned about strangers, including those encountered while coming home from school, those who knock on the door, or those who call on the telephone.
- Time should be set aside for the parents and child to discuss the arrangements periodically to assess whether they are still appropriate for the child and the family.

about how old is "old enough" to be at home alone or home with an older sibling. Although the school-age child might consider being at home alone to be a real mark of maturity, recent research has raised some issues for consideration. Children who must look after themselves after school can become more isolated, reporting fewer opportunities to play outside or have friends visit until their parents are at home.

Nurses give guidance to families who must deal with the issue of after-school care for school-age children (Box 20-16). If parents believe that their child is too young or too immature to be alone at home, then they should search for a quality after-school program for their child. Nurses assist parents in finding a program that meets their needs and those of their child (see Chapter 19).

Culture and Ethnicity

The school-age child focuses more on the culture in which he or she lives than does the younger child. Aspects of American culture that the child must confront include poverty and affluence of ethnic and racial groups, ethnic and racial differences, acceptance of these differences, and the power of television as a cultural phenomenon in American society.

Ethnic Groups

Whereas preschool children notice racial and ethnic differences, school-age children are increasingly aware of these differences. This is a time during which attitudes toward race develop based on family and community attitudes. Studies of children 5 to 7 years of age show that the majority already identify with and prefer to play with members of their own race. Nurses are aware of this identification and help each child to appreciate other's differences and uniqueness. Nurses must also be culturally sensitive to the various methods of child rearing among ethnic groups that reflect positive parenting by those groups (Yoos, Kitzman, Olds, & Overacker, 1995) (see Multicultural Awareness box). Although prejudice exists, school-age children can be helped with adult guidance to see people of different cultures and values in a favorable perspective. Many schools focus on the uniqueness of other cultures by having multicultural awareness weeks. During these times, children dress, eat, and live as do those of other cultures; this focus allows children to recognize the uniqueness of individual cultures, but also the similar core beliefs and values that all people share. The emphasis on a global economy mandates that schools and adults involved in children's lives must expose children to opportunities that will help children appreciate diversity as part of their lives.

Television

Television is an integral part of and a major influence in the culture. Unfortunately, many television programs and commercials are harmful to children because of the messages and also because television prevents children from being physically active, which is important to their health. In recent years, consumer groups and health professionals have looked critically at television's effect on children through various research studies. Areas of major concern have been the violent themes of television programs, persuasive commercials during children's programming, the unrealistic depiction of the world, and the passivity of television viewing.

Violent acts are certainly a part of society, according to Osofsky, Cohen, and Drell (1995), who note that 90% of American elementary school children have witnessed at least one violent event in their lives. These events include the large numbers of violent acts, including sexually violent acts, projected on the daily television screen. Children see violent acts on computer games, in video arcade games, and on accessible Internet sites. Many times, certain ethnic and racial groups implement the violence in these media sources, leading children to stereotype these groups as the contemplators of violence. By the time the average child is 18 years of age, more time has been spent watching

MULTICULTURAL AWARENESS

Parental Teaching Creating Child Competency: Black Focus

Compared with the majority culture, Black parents may show different parenting beliefs. To reach effective and acceptable child care outcomes, health care providers should consider the following cultural variations generally found among Blacks:

- Children learn best by watching and listening to adults and by playing with and being entertained by children.
- Despite inconsistencies in the role demands of school, home, and community, children must find a balance among these role demands to solve problems in life successfully.
- Early learning as a foundation for later competency may not be considered important.
- Collection of a family's cultural beliefs about their children's cognitive styles and needs forms a foundation for effective teaching by the health care provider.
- Child competence may be defined as the ability to navigate a course of behavior acceptable to school, home, and neighborhood rather than the ability to succeed at various opportunities.
- Black parents may have had negative school experiences as children and may perpetuate this negativity with their children.

To respond to these differences, nurses must provide both formal and informal teaching about the cognitive, physical, and interaction needs of children of Black parents. Additionally, nurses must involve parents in the schools so they can help educate themselves and their children about the positive influence of school achievement on child self-esteem.

From Yoos, H., Kitzman, H., Olds, D., & Overacker, I. (1995). Child-rearing beliefs in the African-American community: Implications for culturally competent pediatric care. *Journal of Pediatric Nursing, 10* (6), 343-353.

television than the time spent sleeping. Derksen and Strasberger (1994) found that television facilitates negative attitudes and values among children, and identification of violent behaviors as appropriate can occur more commonly among young children than it does among adults. Researchers have come to the following conclusions in this area:

1. Watching television violence results in increased aggressive behavior in children. Compared with other age groups, school-age children appear to be more affected by aggressive actions.
2. Children learn new forms of violence from violent programs.
3. As a result of the extensive exposure to television violence, children begin to show less emotional sensitivity when aggressive acts occur in their lives.
4. Children become socialized to expect and accept aggressive behavior.

One positive note is that adults who discuss violence with children, pointing out that these acts goes against their own principles and results in pain, can help inhibit some aggression. Discussion of recent school and church shootings by adolescent boys can help identify the effect of this behavior on individuals, families, and society. Anger control programs, as part of a school health-promotion program, can also help decrease societal violence and produce more collaborative workers for the future (American Academy of Pediatrics, 1995b; Goldstein & Mather, 1998).

The average child in the culture views an overwhelming number of television commercials by age 18, and these commercials influence daily and future choices and behaviors. Leading products that are advertised during children's shows are toys, cereals, candies, and fast-food restaurants. The majority of these commercials are for food, many of which "push" purchase of sugared foods that are potentially harmful to teeth and overall nutrition. Young children cannot always separate the program from the commercials and believe that they must buy what the television people tell them to buy. Many families experience conflict between children who want the things they see on television and parents who do not want to support these advertisements. Authorities question the ethics of exposing children to any type of advertising. Interestingly, many of the earliest children's shows had no advertising, but were instead supported by the stations. Some improvement has been made in decreasing the number of suggestive commercials during Saturday mornings, the time during which many young children are watching television, but more work must be done in this area to send more socially responsible messages to children.

The world as presented on television does not accurately reflect the real world. Despite an increasing diverse and aging population, most actors and actresses are young, White, and depict middle-class values and behaviors. Many others, including women and racial minorities, are stereotyped in their roles; occupations tend to be oriented toward business, health, and law enforcement. Children identify their role models through play and fantasy with adults. Unfortunately, to make money, some television shows present inappropriate role models as a realistic representation of society. Parents and health care providers should monitor television commercials and programs, respond to the television stations about inaccuracies in the content presented, and write letters to their newspaper or the television networks to express concerns about the material that their children watch. Nurses and parents can also become involved in groups that focus on presentation and development of children's television, such Action for Children's Television in Austin, Texas and in groups devoted to monitoring toys, games, and Internet sites for appropriateness to school-age children.

Some positive aspects of television viewing exist. A number of children's programs, such as "Mr. Rogers' Neighborhood" and "Reading Rainbow" for younger children and "Call It Macaroni," "Seventh Heaven," and

"Full House" for older children, have been evaluated as developmentally appropriate for children. Unfortunately, these programs are too few, and many are seen only on public broadcasting stations.

Nurses and other health professionals must consider assessment of television consumption and promotion of good viewing habits as part of health care. The nurse can make the following suggestions to help promote healthy viewing habits and to teach critical viewing:

- Parents should be encouraged to watch television shows with their children and discuss learning and moral points about what was watched. Discussions can focus on nonviolent ways to resolve problems rather than through violent methods.
- Parents should play a guiding role in deciding what programs children can watch.
- Parents should evaluate programs for age appropriateness, positive role models, values, and social issues. Parents and children should discuss television shows and these values regularly.
- The amount of time spent viewing television should be limited, primarily because other activities, including school work, may suffer.

Legislation

Throughout this chapter, laws that are beneficial to the health and well being of the school-age child have been discussed. These laws include guidelines for the safe use of products, flame-retardant clothes, mandates against tobacco advertisements, and the nutritional guidelines for federally supported school lunch programs. Another major law affecting school-age children is mandatory public education for disabled children.

Public Law 94-142, established in 1977, states that all disabled children must receive appropriate public education. Children served range in age from 5 to 21 years, with many states beginning services at 3 years of age. Each child with special needs has the right to have an evaluation by school and/or health professionals, who then develop an individualized educational plan (IEP) for that child. This law has accomplished a great deal in responding to the educational needs of many children who had been lost in the past.

Problems with Public Law 94-142 include the following:

1. The cost of truly meeting all the needs of identified children can be overwhelming.
2. Too much paperwork is frequently involved.
3. School systems may not have the appropriate qualified professionals or the money needed for many of the support services.

Other problems exist in defining "handicap" or "disability" and an "appropriate education." Disability can be defined as a limitation in one or more functional areas (U.S. Department of Health and Human Services, 2000). These limitations affect as many as 10% of all children ages 5 to 17 who have learning disabilities, 6% who have communication limitations, and 1.3% who have mobility limitations in 1994 (Hogan, Msall, Rogers, & Avery, 1997). After an IEP has been developed, some parents become overwhelmed in the process of implementing an IEP for their child. Others worry that the education of their normal or gifted children will suffer because of the time and money committed to new initiatives devoted to the disabled. However, the value of this law has helped people affected by disability believe strongly that the problems can be managed with the educational arena.

Nurses involved with school-age children, especially school nurses, have been active in implementing Public Law 94-142. Some suggestions for nurses specific to Public Law 94-142 are as follows:

- Know the process involved for the individual state.
- As early as possible, help identify children who require special educational services.
- Know the local school personnel who work with special educational placements.
- Become involved in assessing, taking histories, interviewing parents, and observing in the classroom.
- Know the local support services that are available for referral.
- Help parents understand the problems that their child is having and the IEP for their child.
- Become involved in local groups that are associated with children who have disabilities or learning problems.

With the recent emphasis on managed care to decrease health care costs in the larger society, costs of implementing Public Law 94-142 will continue to undergo inspection to meet the educational need of children with disabilities. Support for this type of law exists. As recently as 1996, the Developmental Assistance and Bill of Rights (the Developmental Disabilities Act), as amended by Public Law 104-183, supported and directed assistance be given to states and public and private agencies to insure that all persons with disabilities receive services and opportunities to achieve their maximal potential. The Act partners with various groups to help diverse and minority populations in particular to overcome barriers to health care access related to disability.

Economics

Poverty

In the United States, more than 18% of children under 18 years of age live in families whose incomes are below the poverty level (Recer, 2000). Family conditions that are frequently associated with poverty include unemployment, inadequate housing, poor housing sanitation, poor nutrition, low educational levels, and limited access to health and social services. The numbers of uninsured children continued to be high, particularly among Hispanics (30%), which influences the low number of children and their families receiving primary health care (U.S. Department of Health and Human Services, 2000) (see Box 20-1). Recent concerns about the number of children who are homeless (estimated to be one in five) also relate to family poverty (Kemsley & Hunter, 1993) (see Research Highlights box). The effects of few financial resources on children include higher mortality rates at all ages compared with those who are not poor and more days lost from school for poor children because of illnesses. Because of poverty, these children receive sporadic health care with no consistent coordination. For the school-age child, poverty can influence all aspects of life, including the following:

- Physical processes
  1. Poor nutrition and undernutrition, which can result in iron deficiency anemia, retarded growth, and developmental delay
  2. Poor dental care, which can result in caries and other diseases of the mouth
  3. Limited or no primary or secondary care, which can result in undetected or untreated problems, such as otitis media or strep throat
- Psychological processes
  1. School difficulties resulting from a variety of problems, such as poor health, sensory deficits that are not corrected, turmoil at home, or peer rejection
  2. Poor coping strategies, such as depression or aggression from overwhelming stresses at home (often a single-parent or violent family environment)
  3. Poor self-perception resulting from lack of positive adult reinforcement or positive life experiences
- Environmental processes
  1. Accidents from unsafe home and neighborhood conditions
  2. Other potential health hazards from environmental conditions, such as peeling paint and lead poisoning
  3. Abuse or neglect from parents

Nurses interacting with poor families and their children should be familiar with the many resources that are available to help them, several of which have been discussed in previous chapters. Additionally, the nurse will want to refer parents of uninsured children to the Children's Health Insurance Program (CHIP), a federally supported insurance project implemented at the state level. The intent of the program is to provide care to all uninsured children under the age of 18 years and to deal effectively with problems preventing quality health care (communication and language barriers, confidentiality with those with immigrant alien status, etc.) (U.S. Department of Health and Human Services, 2000).

Other referrals may be needed if the nurse notices signs of abuse, neglect, coping difficulties, and other concerns influencing the health of individual children. The nurse who works with these children intervenes by helping these children succeed in something that will give them a positive feeling about themselves. A relationship with a good adult role model or strong peer interactions can help accomplish this task. Children from poor families who have strong family relationships and committed support systems outside the family that help them develop a positive self-image tend to do better socially over time than do children without such support.

Affluence

The social milieu opposite poverty, affluence, has not been examined or discussed with the same frequency as has poverty. Children of the extremely or moderately rich are also potentially at risk for problems with development or health. Children who stay at home (latchkey children) because both parents work can face increased risk of injury as a result of inadequate parental monitoring. The nurse can offer ideas that will help decrease risk-taking behavior and allow parental-child connection until a parent is in the home. Some aspects of wealth that might have negative effects on the child include the following:

1. Frequent substitute caretakers of varying degrees of quality because of parental absence
2. Extremely high and often unrealistic parental expectations for a child to excel in sports, academics, and social standing
3. Availability of many material possessions with little awareness of responsibilities for these possessions; occasionally, giving material possessions serves as a substitute for emotional giving by the parents

research highlights

Barriers to Well-Child Care among the Homeless in School-Age Children

The purpose of this study was to identify the barriers perceived by families that prevent the homeless child from receiving preventive health care. This study was based on the concept of barriers found in the health belief model. A convenience sample of 53 homeless families with 120 children was drawn from the population of residents at three transitional homeless shelters in two neighboring southern California counties. All shelters were church-affiliated having 35 to 40 beds available. Shelters differed only in ethnicity. A modified version of the Barriers Scale developed by Melnyk was used. Four barriers were cited most frequently by subjects as greatly affecting their children's care: provider-selection difficulties, waiting for well-child appointments, waiting during well-child appointments, and the high cost of transportation and/or parking. Findings confirm the reality of potential barriers to care suggested by earlier studies. Innovative forms of health care delivery, such as shelter-site clinics, mobile units, and the use of a nurse liaison between family shelters and hospital-based clinics, can help reduce or eliminate these barriers.

Data from Riemer, J., Van Cleave, L., & Galbraith, M. (1995). Barriers to well child care for homeless children under age 13. *Public Health Nursing, 12* (1), 61-66.

4. Easy access to cars, drugs, and alcohol, including their potential dangers

Nurses have an opportunity to intervene with these families to promote child and family health. When possible, guidance for these parents should include the following:

1. The importance of the parental role, including demonstration of consistent love, support, and availability to children
2. The need to set realistic limits for appropriate behavior
3. The need to give children clear directions and responsibilities
4. The value of recognizing an individual child's abilities and needs and responding accordingly

When discussing the children raised in poverty or affluence, two points are important to remember. First, many variables are involved for each child; all children are not influenced in the same way by their circumstances. Second, although personality and support networks allow a child in a socially poor environment to excel later in life, overall, most authorities believe that problems of affluence are probably easier to overcome than are the all-pervasive problems of poverty.

Health Care Delivery System

Well-Child Care

The American Academy of Pediatrics recommends that children 6 years and older have a well-child examination at least every two years conducted by either a physician or a nurse practitioner. In the ideal situation, the child has a primary health care provider (one person or practice from which the child receives wellness care and the majority of illness care, coordinated by members of a health care team). Unfortunately, many American children still do not have this quality of care (see the earlier section on economics). With the increasing number of children living in poverty because of family violence, single parenthood, and divorce, accessible health care for physical and dental care is unavailable. Frequently, because of lack of insurance coverage and/or cultural issues, these children do not receive primary preventive care and they receive attention for their health care needs only when they become ill.

Table 20-6 provides an example of a possible health-maintenance protocol for this age group. Certainly, not all areas are covered for each child during every visit. This protocol can be used by providers as a guide to the most important age-related issues. The health history, physical examination, developmental tests, laboratory tests, and other observations can be shared with others (teachers and counselors) to make informed decisions about individual child's care.

The nurse encourages the school-age child to be an active member of any health evaluation along with the parents. Children may give some of their own history, answer questions, and discuss their health concerns. During the history, the child's privacy should be respected. Some children in this age group want a parent present during their examination; others do not. When possible, the nurse should spend at least some time alone with the child to allow discussions that the child may not feel comfortable completing if parents are present. The

Table 20-6 Health Maintenance During the School-Age Period*

Age (years)	Physiological Processes	Psychological Processes	Emotional-Social Processes
6 to 9	Height, weight	School adjustment, level, and progress	Safety: use of seat belts, water safety, bicycles
	Blood pressure	Developmental level, including speech/cognitive level	Immunizations reviewed or updated
	Dental: caries, bites, use of fluoride	Stresses in child's life, coping patterns	Responsibilities for household tasks, money, school work
	Diet: snacks	Self-care, hygiene	Relations with parents, siblings, peers, other adults
	Enuresis	Masturbation, homosexual play	Family activities
	Exercise: motor skills, level of activity, attention		Discipline
	Sleep patterns		After-school work
	Vision and hearing screening		Use of television
			Outside activities
9 to 12	Same as ages 6 to 9 plus:	Same as ages 6 to 9 plus:	Same as ages 6 to 9 plus:
	Posture, scoliosis screening	Habits: drugs, alcohol, smoking and other risky behavior	Time and place for privacy
	Menarche, stage of sexual development	Sexual activity	

*Includes areas for which information should be obtained through history, examination, observation, tests, and so on.

CARE PLAN

Nursing Diagnosis: Isolation Related to Placement in New School and Neighborhood and Single-Parent Family

DEFINING CHARACTERISTICS

- Change in quality of schoolwork; currently, 10-year-old child failing school work with previous history of doing well in school
- Frequent crying at school; visits school nurse to complain of headaches and stomachaches; usually asks to stay at school after dismissal time
- Increased daydreaming behavior, according to most of the teachers
- Aggressive behavior shown at school and on the playground
- Mother unavailable for school meetings to deal with child's behavior at school

RELATED FACTORS

- Child new to area; has attended local school for only 3 months
- Mother works from 8:30 AM to 5:30 PM, 4 days each week; child has to stay at home alone for 2 hours on these days until mother arrives
- Only sibling is 8 years older
- Parents recently divorced

EXPECTED OUTCOMES

- Child will decrease number of visits to school nurse for physical complaints
- Child will display fewer emotional outbursts (crying, aggressive behavior) during school time
- Grades of child will improve for next 9-week period
- Family will become more involved in school setting to allow effective working relationship between family and school to focus on child's needs
- Child will work with student mentor to increase comfort and satisfaction with new school setting

INTERVENTIONS (SCHOOL NURSE)

- Assess level of family problems and concerns with child's visits to nurse
- Over the next 9-week period, document the number of visits the child makes and the physical or other complaints
- Communicate child's concerns to mother and father (if available) enabling strong family-school relationship to be established
- Work with parents to develop a plan for meeting academic and emotional needs of the child
- Offer local resources available for child support, for latchkey children, and, perhaps, for shared, after-school care with another parent of a child in the same grade
- Offer tutoring support after school for child as desired
- Seek out a mentor who is a year older than child to provide friendship and guidance in personal and academic life of child
- Involve child's teachers in identifying ways to increase child's self-esteem and to nurture child's strengths for improved academic performance

examinations can also be a time for education on how the body works and ways to keep it healthy. Preventative information on diet and exercise can be offered relevant to prevention of obesity, cardiovascular disease, and diabetes later in life (Fryer & Igoe, 1995). Information also must be obtained on the child's school adjustment and performance, particularly because this is a major portion of the child's life. School performance can reflect the child's cognitive and general development. If there are any concerns, then the nurse should obtain more information through separate testing or discussion with school officials. Health education should be directed to both the child and the parents for the best results. Activities that the child performs alone and together with the family can give a picture of relationships and adjustments that relate to the child's health (see Care Plan box).

NURSING INTERVENTIONS

The challenge for nurses who work with school-age children is to maintain the children's normally healthy status and prevent the development of illness when possible. This task is accomplished through a variety of health-promotion mechanisms, such as examination, guidance, education, and legislation. The school-age child is capable of playing an active role in personal health care and should be motivated to seek health and use various resources to attain, maintain, or regain optimal health (Cagle & Keen-Payne, 1996). Aspects of the nursing process can be used effectively in various situations to maintain the child's health (assessing immunization status), promote health habits (teaching bicycle safety), and prevent illness (obtaining throat cultures for strep throat).

Nurses have many opportunities and settings to help carry out their interventions. For example, nurses and school-age children interact during well-child evaluations and at school. Nurses in other roles, such as public health nurses and hospital nurses, also play a role in health promotion, although these nurses must often focus more on helping the child and family respond to an illness or a crisis. Local and national groups influence the health of children through their activities and regulations and include organizations such as Boy and Girl Scouts, Big Brothers and Sisters, charities such as the Red Cross, and government agencies such as the Consumer Product Safety Commission. All of these groups have a place for active nursing involvement, as consultants, board members, or as child advocates.

School and the Nurse

As an integral part of the total community, the school system has specific responsibilities in health care and planning to provide a healthy school environment, an adequate school health service, and a comprehensive health education program. School systems vary greatly in the extent to which they fulfill these roles, but agree that these are real functions of the school. Most schools take specific steps to ensure a level of safety and cleanliness in the environment, but an individual school can represent either extreme in providing a healthy physical and emotional environment for children's overall health. School health service in the United States and other countries also varies greatly. In some areas, nurses, physicians, and other health care workers are integrally involved in the school health program, which includes health care and maintenance and education. In other areas, the school health program considers only educational aspects. Programs range from an occasional mention of body care and the changes of puberty to a full program, integrating physical and mental health principles into all aspects of the educational experience as recommended by the Institute of Medicine (1997) (Table 20-7).

Although the ideal role of the school in implementing health care remains a matter of debate, the school, nonetheless, influences and participates in children's health and well being. As children begin to spend an increasingly greater percentage of their waking hours in and around the school, this environment begins to exert an influence on their lives that, at times, outweighs the current influence of the home. The attitudes that the school conveys with regard to health and well being begin to influence children's attitudes, contributing to the shaping and formulation of the concept of health for the rest of their lives (Cagle & Keen-Payne, 1996).

Comprehensive school health services require an interdisciplinary, coordinated effort between health care providers and educators. With many schools forced to share nurses because of cost-cutting measures in education, many current schools simply do not have on-site nurses to conduct and mentor students and faculty in health-promotion areas (U.S. Department of Health and Human Services, 2000) (see Innovative Practice box). However, when available, nurses, by virtue of their training, offer educational and interpersonal skills to initiate health-promotion teaching that can improve the overall health of consumers.

The nurse, either from the community or within the school, is frequently in a position to plan and direct comprehensive health care services for school-age children (Rhodes, 1997). These services should include the following:

1. Planning direct health maintenance
2. Screening and providing health care for problems that interfere with the learning process
3. Providing nursing services for children with health problems
4. Coordinating referral services
5. Planning and implementing actions to ensure a healthy physical and emotional milieu for the school
6. Planning and participating in the health education curriculum that teaches children skills and methods for making wise decisions about their health and about their environment

The role and responsibilities of each nurse depend on many factors in the particular setting, but some or all of these services are included in most roles of school nurses.

Table 20-7 Topics for Health Education During the School-Age Period

Topic	Specific Discussion Areas
Nutrition education	Concept of six basic food groups; foods associated with dental caries; essential nutrients and their function; healthy snack foods
Body hygiene	Value of skin care, bathing, and grooming; care of minor skin injuries; hair care; dental care
Exercise and physical fitness	Physical fitness and sports program; body mechanics and coordination; sleep and rest needs; prevention of injuries
Prevention of illness and accidents	Accident prevention with burns; water safety; lifesaving instruction; bicycle and pedestrian safety; concepts of viral and bacterial diseases; body defenses against disease; protection of vision and eye strain; protection of hearing and screening to assess hearing ability and to monitor exposure to loud noises
Human sexuality	Community and parental awareness; consideration of gender role bias in society; preparation for changes related to puberty; life cycle changes; age-appropriate information on AIDS
Prevention of drug abuse	Information on drugs, specifically tobacco, alcohol, street drugs; reasons people use drugs to feel "grown up"; healthy alternatives to drug use that can be used for coping

innovative practice

Telehealth in a Rural School-Based Health Center

Health centers in schools have been developed specifically to offer a continuum of health care interventions, including health-promotion and disease-prevention strategies, to children. As part of health care delivery in schools, telehealth is a new technology that allows delivery of health care services to school-age children by a nurse who connects through computer and video technology with a physician or other expert in children's health. This expert can, through telehealth methodology, see and talk with the child and school nurse caring for an ill child. The care is often traditional in that a physician and nurse communicate about the child's problems and develop a plan of care based on standards of practice for both the medical and nursing professions.

An example of important nursing involvement in telehealth technology has been found with the collaboration of four clinical and academic institutions (the University of Texas Medical Branch in Galveston School of Nursing, Lamar University Department of Nursing, the University of Texas Medical Branch in Galveston Division of Pediatric Special Services, and the East Texas Area Health Education Center). The collaboration began in the mid 1990s and has expanded to provide telehealth care services to six public schools in Texas. Additionally, the University of Texas Medical Branch provides family nurse practitioner education to Lamar University through this telehealth infrastructure.

Courtesy Carol Lynn Mandle, PhD, RN.

Planning the health maintenance for the children of a school varies, depending on the type of health-maintenance program. In one system, the school nurses may try to ensure that each child has a primary source of health care, whereas in another system, the school's nurse practitioners may be the primary providers. School nurses, for example, have monitored and updated the immunizations of children and identified children with potential health problems, such as scoliosis, strep throat, or child abuse. In either setting, the school nurse must work collaboratively with the school's physician, community physicians, and parents in meeting children's health needs. In most school settings, school nurses can work with community leaders and parents to improve the quality of education, including health education, for all children.

For many years, school nurses have screened children for vision and hearing problems at regular intervals to detect children who were at a disadvantage in the classroom. Many states have laws mandating this type of assessment at intervals during the elementary school years. With the passage of Public Law 94-142, nurses have expanded their role in identifying and caring for children with learning problems. Currently, school nurses frequently work closely with other school professionals in evaluating children whose school performance appears to indicate a problem that is physical in nature. The evaluating team includes teachers, educational specialists, psychologists, physicians, and nurses. The role the nurse plays with the team in developing and implementing the child's IEP varies. Some school nurses have developed assessment tools that provide information to the team on the child's health, family interactions, and the family's perceptions of the problem. Interviews and home visits with the parents and child have been incorporated into these assessments.

Nurses in schools frequently see children with minor illnesses. Policies regarding the management of minor illnesses and accidents at school vary widely from state to state, community to community, and school to school. The nurse should be aware of all state and local laws and policies that affect the scope of nursing activity in the school and consider the legal implications of all nursing activities. Some systems allow only first-aid treatment by the school nurse and then referral to the child's physician. Other schools have developed standard protocols for the management of common problems. These protocols include guidelines on performing an adequate history and physical assessment, developing an acceptable plan of management, and consulting with the school physician. Whatever intervention the nurse takes, collaboration with the child's parents effectively enables the needs of the school and family to be met.

Not all health problems of children in school are minor. With the mainstreaming of children with disabilities, nurses are now involved in administering prescribed medications, watching for side effects, reinforcing diet modifications, monitoring skin care, implementing respiratory treatments for respirator-dependent children, and performing various other nursing care acts with children with special needs.

Children with multiple health problems and other children frequently require the many services they receive to be coordinated. Because children spend extensive time in schools and school professionals and families frequently recognize children's needs, the school nurse is an ideal person to make referrals and follow up on the recommendations. This process is most valuable when the parents are involved, allowing them to take the primary responsibility while the nurse acts as a resource and advocate.

The school nurse can also play a role in developing a healthy environment for children at the school. A specific program aimed at the prevention of accidents in and around the school should be planned by the school health care team. The school environment must be periodically evaluated for sources of health hazards, including pedestrian and automobile traffic patterns, broken playground and classroom equipment, ice and snow, poorly maintained toilet facilities, and inappropriately prepared food. Fire prevention is usually mandatory by law and includes regular fire drills to acquaint teachers and students with the procedures to be used in the event of fire. Chemical hazards should be anticipated as well.

The social environment of the school is also important in providing a healthy environment. The social interactions of the children should be watched and positive social relationships promoted. However, despite all of the efforts to provide for optimal social interactions and reinforcement from the group and assistance with group interactions and coping with group stress, social problems continue to constitute a major concern for many children during this period. Children can experience difficulty in making the initial transition away from the family and in establishing dependency on and satisfaction from the group of peers. Children may make the initial adjustment, but then continue to interact with friends and adults in a relatively immature fashion, failing to form increasing mature social judgments and ways of interacting. When problems such as these arise, an evaluation of the underlying cause is needed. Nurses frequently find that these problems require the evaluation and support of a team of the school's health and educational professionals.

Encouragement of the school-age child's growing ability to serve as the child's own agent in health care provides the major thrust for health education programs in schools. The child requires adequate knowledge of all dimensions of health to make responsible choices to protect it and to seek health care services when needed. Health education programs vary greatly, although all should be comprehensive, interesting, and age appropriate. Whatever program is implemented in a school, the nurse should play an active role in developing, presenting, and evaluating the agenda. Areas frequently covered at the school-age level are presented in Table 20-7.

SUMMARY

Many changes occur in children during the exciting period of the school-age years. The child's overall development progresses from the immaturity of the preschooler to the beginning of adolescence and eventual adulthood. The child's cognitive abilities increase dramatically, adding to the desire to master tasks and the ability to develop moral judgment. The child's world expands beyond the family unit as school and peers begin to exert a major influence. Opportunities for nurses to aid children during this period occur primarily in ambulatory settings, with the school nurse frequently the most effective and influential health care provider for children of this age group and their families (Fig. 20-5).

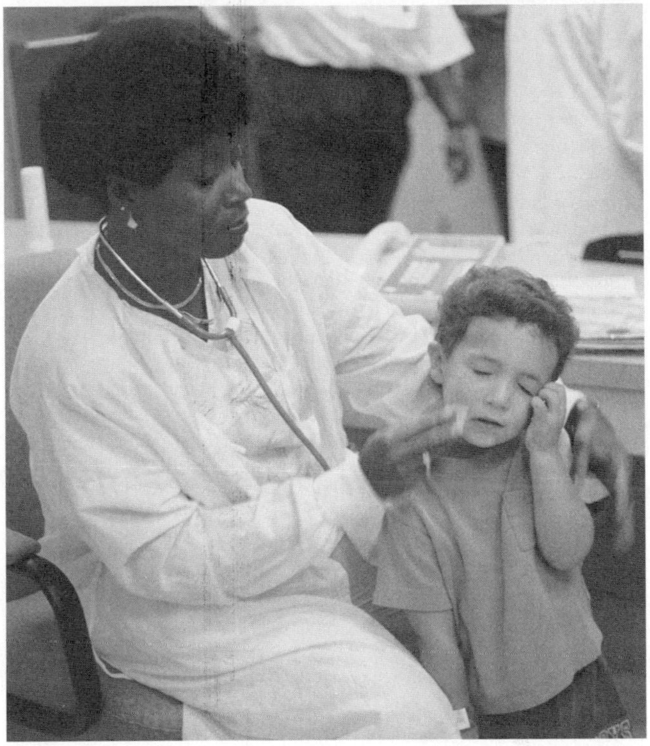

Fig. 20-5 School nurses play a valuable role in forming children's views of health and illness.

CASE STUDY

Jack

Jack, a 10-year-old fifth-grade student, has been caught stealing expensive books from his school library. At first, he denies his involvement in this activity until his best friend Joey tells Jack's teacher that Jack had three of the missing books under his bed. The books cost the library $150.00 when they were purchased 2 years ago for a new curriculum offering in art. To avoid being caught, Jack throws the books into a river near his home. After several days of questioning, Jack admits his guilt to the school principal and to his parents. His parents are angry, and his father does not understand why his son is interested in art, a field of study not meant for boys.

1. If you were the principal and parents, what form of disciplinary approaches would you devise to respond to Jack's behavior?
2. Jack's parents do not understand their son's behavior, and his father is so angry that he says he will spank Jack until "he learns his lesson." As a nurse, how might you respond to this decision made by Jack's father?
3. Is this behavior appropriate for a 10-year-old boy?
4. What interventions might be effective in preventing possible misbehavior by Jack in the future?

REFERENCES

Aetna/U.S. Healthcare. (1998). *Caring for your children's health* (Publication No. 12669-8/98). Hartford, CT: Aetna/U.S. Healthcare.

American Academy of Pediatrics. (1995a). Recommendations for preventive pediatric health care. *Pediatrics*, 96, 373-374.

American Academy of Pediatrics, Committee on Communications. (1995b). Children, adolescents, and television. *Pediatrics*, 96, 786-787.

American Academy of Pediatrics, Committee on Children with Developmental Disabilities. (1996a). Sexuality education of children and adolescents with developmental disabilities. *Pediatrics*, 97, 273-278.

American Academy of Pediatrics, Committee on Poison Injury and Prevention. (1996b). Selecting and using the most appropriate car safety seats for growing children: Guidelines for counseling parents. *Pediatrics*, 97, 761-763.

American Academy of Pediatrics, Committee on Infectious Diseases. (1997). *1997 Red Book*. Elk Grove Village, IL: The Association.

American Heart Association. (1996). *Heart and stroke statistical update*. Dallas: The Association.

American Psychiatric Association. (1994). *Diagnostic and statistical manual of mental disorders. DSM-IV* (4th ed.). Washington, DC: The Association.

Andrews, M. A. (1995). Perspectives in the nursing care of children and adolescents. In M. A. Andrews, & J. S. Boyle, *Transcultural concepts in nursing care* (2nd ed., pp. 128-129). Philadelphia: J.B. Lippincott.

Anderson, R. N., Kockanck, K. D., & Murphey, S. L. (1997). Report of final mortality statistics, 1995. *Monthly Vital Statistics Report, 45* (Suppl 2), 11.

Beck, A. M., & Myers, N. M. (1996). Health enhancement and companion animal ownership. *Annuals of Review of Public Health, 17*, 247-257.

Bingham, M., & Stryker, S. (1995). *Things will be different for my daughter*. New York: Penguin Books.

Borja, M. E., Bordi, P. L., & Lambert, C. U. (1996). New lower-fat dessert recipes for the school lunch program are well-accepted by children. *Journal of American Dietetic Association*, 96 (9), 903-910.

Cagle, C. S., & Keen-Payne, R. (1996). Health promotion teaching in preschoolers. *American Journal of Maternal and Child Nursing, 21*, 96-99.

California Highway Patrol. (1991). *Statewide integrated traffic records system: Annual report of fatal and injury motor vehicle and traffic accidents*. Sacramento, CA: The Patrol.

Centers for Disease Control and Prevention. (1996). Guidelines for school health programs to promote lifelong healthy eating. *Mortality and Morbidity Weekly Report, 45* (RR-9), 1-33.

Centers for Disease Control and Prevention (CDC), National Center for Health Statistics (NCHS) (1999a). Deaths: Final data for 1997. *National Vital Statistics Reports, 47*(19).

Centers for Disease Control and Prevention. (1999b). *Deaths: Final data for 1997. National Vital Statistics Report, 47* (10), 1-104.

Cole, J., Naidoo, J., & Wills, J. (1998). Reducing accidents. In J. Naidoo, & J. Wills, *Practicing health promotion: Dilemmas and challenges* (pp. 187-200). London: Bailliere Tindall.

Collins, J. L., Small, M. L., Kann, L., Pateman, B. C., Gold, R. S., & Kolbe, L. J. (1995). School health education. *Journal of School Health, 65* (8), 302-311.

Costello, D. (2000). Spanking makes a comeback. *Wall Street Journal*. CV (114), W1, W16.

Crawley, T. (1996). Childhood injury: Significance and prevention strategies. *Journal of Pediatric Nursing, 11* (4), 225-232.

Derksen, D. J., & Strasberger, V. C. (1994). Children and the influence of the media. *Primary Care, 21* (4), 747-759.

Elias, M. J., & Kress, H. S. (1994). Social decision-making and life skills development: A critical thinking approach for health promotion in the middle school. *Journal of School Health, 64* (2), 62-66.

Elium, J., & Elium, D. (1994). *Raising a daughter*. Berkeley, CA: Celestial Arts.

Erikson, E. H. (1986a). *Childhood and society* (2nd ed.). New York: W. W. Norton.

Erikson, E. H. (1986b). *Identity, youth and crisis* (35th ed.). New York: W. W. Norton.

Friedman, R. M., Katz-Leavy, J. W., Manderscheid, R. W., & Sondheimer, D. L. (1996). *Prevalence of serious emotional disturbance. An update. Mental health, United States, 1996* (U.S. Department of Health and Human Services Publication [SMA] No. 96-3098). Rockville, MD: U.S. Department of Health and Human Services, Public Health Service, Substance Abuse and Mental Health Administration, Center for Mental Health Services.

Friman, P. C. (1995). Nocturnal enuresis in the child. In R. Ferber, & M. Kryger, *Principles and practices of sleep medicine in the child* (pp. 107-113). Philadelphia: W.B. Saunders.

Fryer, G. E., & Igoe, J. B. (1995). A relationship between availability of school nurses and child well-being. *Journal of School Nursing, 11*, 12-18.

Garn, S. M., Pao, E. M., & Rihl, M. E. (1964). Compact bone in Chinese and Japanese. *Science, 143* (3613), 1439-1440.

Goldstein, S., & Mather, N. (1998). *Overcoming underachieving: An action guide to helping your child succeed in school*. New York: John Wiley & Sons.

Hallowell, E. M., & Ratey, J. J. (1994). *Driven to distraction*. New York: Simon & Schuster.

Hancock, L. (1987). Safe biking: A bike helmet. *Journal of Pediatric Health Care, 1* (6), 344.

Hoekelman, R., Friedman, S. B., Nelson, N. M., & Siedel, H. M. (2001). *Primary pediatric care* (4th ed.). St. Louis: Mosby.

Hogan, D. P., Msall, M. E., Rogers, M. L., & Avery, R. C. (1997). Improved disability population estimates of functional limitations among children 5-17. *Maternal and Child Health Journal, 1* (4), 203-216.

Institute of Medicine. (1997). *Schools and health: Our nation's investment*. Washington, DC: National Academy Press.

Jarvis, C. (2000). *Physical examination and health assessment* (3rd ed.). Philadelphia: W.B. Saunders.

Kemsley, M., & Hunter J. K. (1993). Homeless children and families: Clinical and research issues. *Issues in Comprehensive Pediatric Nursing, 16* (2), 99-108.

Kohlberg, L. (1981). *The philosophy of moral development*. San Francisco: Harper & Row.

Lavin, A. T., Porter, S. M., Shaw, D. M., Weill, K. S., Crocker, A. C., & Palfrey, J. S. (1994). School health services in the age of AIDS. *Journal of School Health, 64* (1), 27-31.

Morbidity and Mortality Weekly Report. (1995). Air bag associated fatal injuries to infants and children riding in front passenger seats-United States. *Morbidity and Mortality Weekly Report, 44* (45), 845-847.

Moss, A. J., Allen, K. F., Giovino, B. A., & Mills, S. L. (1992). *Recent trends in adolescent smoking, smoking update correlates, and expectations about the future. Advance data from vital and health statistics* (No. 221). Hyattsville, MD: National Center for Health Statistics.

Moss, A. J., Lanphear, B. P., & Auinger, P. (1999). Association of dental caries and blood lead levels. *Journal of the American Medical Association, 281* (24), 2294-2298.

Murray, R. B. (2001). Overview: Theories related to human development. In R. B. Murray, & J. P. Zentner, *Health promotion strategies through the life span* (7th ed., pp. 213-277). Upper Saddle River, NJ: Prentice-Hall.

National Center for Health Statistics. *National Health and Nutrition Examination Survey III, 1988-1994*. Hyattville, MD: Centers for Disease Control and Prevention (unpublished data).

National High Blood Pressure Education Program (NHBPEP) (1996). Update on the 1987 task force report on high blood pressure in children and adolescents. *Pediatrics*, 98(4), 649-667.

Neff, E. J., & Dale, J. C. (1996). Worries of school-age children. *Journal of the Society of Pediatric Nurses, 1*, 27-32.

Osborne, M. L., Kistner, J. A., & Helgemo, B. (1995). Parental knowledge and attitudes toward children with AIDS: Influences of educational policies and children's attitudes. *Journal of Pediatric Psychology*, 20 (1), 79-90.

Osofsky, J., Cohen, G., & Drell, M. (1995). The effects of trauma among young children: A case of 2-year-old twins. *International Journal of Psychoanalysis, 76*, 595-607.

Parker-Pope, T. (2000). A sugarless gum may help prevent ear infections in kids. *Wall Street Journal*, CCXXXV (129), B1.

Piaget, J. (1969). *The theory of stages in cognitive development*. New York: McGraw-Hill.

Recer, P. (July 14, 2000). Study finds children's status in the U.S. is improving. *Fort Worth Star Telegram*, 8A.

Reiter, A., Shrappe, M., Parwaresch, R., Henze, G., Muller-Weinrich, S., Sauter, S., Sykora, K. W., Ludwig, W. D., Gadner, H., & Reihm, H. (1995). NonHodgkins lymphomas of childhood and adolescence: Results of a treatment stratified for biologic subtypes and state-A report of the Berlin-Frankfurt-Munster Group. *Journal of Clinical Oncology, 13* (2), 359-372.

Reuters Health. (June 26, 2000). Playground ratings show kids at risk. *Healthweek*, 5 (13), 8.

Rhodes, A. M. (1997). Legal issues: Liability for unlicensed assistive personnel. Part I. *Maternal Child Nursing Journal, 22* (5), 269.

Rodgers, G. B. (1996). Bicycle helmet use patterns among children. *Pediatrics*, 97, 166-173.

Rosen, G., Mahowald, R., & Feber, R. (1995). Sleepwalking, confusional arousals, and sleep terrors in the child. In R. Ferber, & M. Kryger, *Principles and practices of sleep medicine in the child* (pp. 99-106). Philadelphia: W.B. Saunders.

Rutter, V. B. (1996). *Celebrating girls: Nurturing and empowering our daughters*. Berkeley, CA: Conair Press.

Sacks, J. J., Holmgreen, P., Smith, S. M., & Sosin, D. M. (1991). Bicycle-associated head injuries and deaths in the United States from 1984 through 1988. How many are preventable? *Journal of the American Medical Association, 266* (21), 3016-3018.

Sadowski, R. H., & Faulkner, B. (1996). Hypertension in pediatric patients. *American Journal of Kidney Disease, 27*, 305-315.

Saunders, E. (1995). Hypertension in minorities: Blacks. *American Journal of Hypertension*, 8 (Supplement 12), 112S-119S.

Sinaiko, A. R. (1996). Hypertension in children. *New England Journal of Medicine, 335* (26), 1968-1973.

Stead, M., Hastings, G., & Tudor-Smith, C. (1996). Preventing adolescent smoking: A review of options. *Health Education Journal*, 55 (1), 31-54.

Tinsworth, D. K., Polen, C., & Cassidy, S. (1994). Bicycle-related injuries: Injury, hazard, and risk patterns. *International Journal of Consumer Safety, 1*, 207-220.

U.S. Department of Agriculture. (1992). *The food guide pyramid* (USDA Home and Garden Bulletin, No. 252). Washington, DC: USDA.

U.S. Department of Agriculture and U.S. Department of Health and Human Services. (1995). *Dietary guidelines for Americans* (4th ed., USDA Home and Garden Bulletin, No. 232). Washington, DC: USDA.

U.S. Department of Health and Human Services. (1995a). *Healthy people 2000: Mid-course review and 1995 revisions*. Washington, DC: U.S. Government Printing Office.

U.S. Department of Health and Human Services, National Center for Child Abuse and Neglect. (1995b). *Child mistreatment 1993. Reports from the states to the National Center on Child Abuse and Neglect*. Washington, DC: U.S. Government Printing Office.

U.S. Department of Health and Human Services. (2000). *Healthy people 2010: Vol 1 and 2* (Conference ed.). Washington, DC: U.S. Government Printing Office.

U.S. Preventive Services Task Force. (1996). *Guide to clinical preventive services*. Baltimore, MD: Williams & Wilkins.

Vannoy, S. W. (1994). *The 10 greatest gifts I give my children*. New York: Fireside.

Vargas, C. M., Crall, J. J., & Schneider, D. A. (1998). Sociodemographic distribution of pediatric dental caries: NHANES III, 1988-1994. *Journal of American Dental Association, 129*, 1229-1238.

Wilson, C. B., Lewis, D. B., & Penix, L. A. (1996). Immunodeficiency of immaturity. In E. R. Stiehm, *Immunologic disorders in infants and children* (4th ed., pp. 253-295). Philadelphia: W.B. Saunders.

Wintemute, G. J. (1990). Childhood drowning and near-drowning in the United States. *American Journal of Disease of the Child. 144*, 663-669.

Wolfe, C. A. (2000). Pediatric alert: Access to lead. *RN*, 63 (8), 26-30.

Wong, D. L., Hockenberry-Eaton, M., Wilson, D., Winkelstein, M. L., Ahmann, E., & Divito-Thomas, P. A. (1999). *Whaley and Wong's nursing care of infants and children* (6th ed.). St. Louis: Mosby.

Yoos, H. L., Kitzman, H., Olds, D. L., & Overacker, I. (1995). Child-rearing beliefs in the African-American community: Implications for culturally competent pediatric care. *Journal of Pediatric Nursing, 10* (6), 343-353.

Chapter 21

MARINDA ALLENDER

Adolescent

objectives

After completing this chapter, the nurse will be able to:

- Explain to a group of young adolescents the expected body changes of puberty.
- Describe the stages in the development of secondary sexual characteristics of adolescents.
- Discuss the course and treatment of acne with a group of adolescents.
- Contrast the cognitive abilities of the adolescent with those of the school-age child.
- Contrast the adaptive and maladaptive coping mechanisms commonly used by the adolescent.
- Contrast the various stages of moral development that can be represented in a group of adolescents.
- Discuss the pros and cons of sexual activity, pregnancy, and contraception with a group of adolescents.

key terms

Acne
Adolescence
Amenorrhea
Anorexia Nervosa
Argot
Bulimia Nervosa
Contraception
Depression
Dysmenorrhea
Emancipated Minor
Fable of Immunity
Formal Operations
Identity
Menarche
Primary Sex Characteristics
Puberty
Role Confusion
Scoliosis
Secondary Sex Characteristics
Sexually Transmitted Disease

THINK About It

Risk Behaviors in Adolescents

Approximately 33% of adolescents are sexually active by the age of 15 without using any form of contraception.

The mortality rate for teens between 15 and 19 years of age is three times higher than is the rate for children between ages 10 and 14.

Adolescents spend more time watching television than they do in the classroom.

Suicides among teenage boys, both Black and White, are increasing.

1. What growth and developmental factors make adolescents susceptible to these problems?
2. What facts put adolescents at risk for these health problems?
3. What health promotion might be offered to prevent some of these problems?

The period of adolescence, similar to other developmental stages, is impossible to define in exact chronological terms; it is often defined as beginning with the onset of puberty and ending with the achievement of a certain level of independence. These landmarks are difficult to identify, however, and do not adequately describe the many complex factors that make up adolescence in many cultures. Adolescence can be conceptualized most appropriately as the period during which independence from the primary family unit becomes the central task of the individual.

The term **puberty** denotes the period that involves the development and maturation of the reproductive, endocrine, and structural systems. **Adolescence,** conversely, refers to the period characterized by the psychological, emotional, social, and spiritual changes that result in the transition from child to young adult. Adolescence usually begins immediately before puberty and continues until young adult roles and responsibilities are assumed. Cultural and social-class variations become evident at the end of adolescence. The college-bound adolescent typically holds a moratorium on adulthood and has an extended adolescence while in school. The adolescent who is not college bound enters the adult world more quickly than does the college-bound adolescent. The adolescent is in some ways a child and in other ways an adult and can therefore present the greatest challenge to the nurse in providing age-appropriate health care guidance and teaching. (See Box 21-1 for selected national health-promotion and disease-prevention objectives for adolescents).

Box 21-1 Selected National Health-Promotion and Disease-Prevention Objectives for Adolescents

- Reduce the proportion of adolescents with dental decay in their permanent teeth to no more than 15% (baseline is 20% of adolescents in 1988 to 1994).
- Reduce the prevalence of being overweight among adolescents ages 12 through 19 to no more than 5% (baseline is 10% for adolescents age 12 through 19 in 1988 to 1994).
- Reduce suicide among adolescents ages 15 through 19 to no more than 6 per 100,000 (baseline is 10.8 per 100,000 in 1998).
- Reduce the incidence of injurious suicide attempts among adolescents age 14 to 17 to 1.0% (baseline is 2.6% in 1997).
- Reduce deaths among youth ages 15 through 24 caused by motor-vehicle accidents to no more than 9 per 100,000 (baseline is 25.4 per 100,000 in 1998).
- Increase the proportion of high school seniors who associate risk of physical or psychological harm with heavy use of alcohol to 80%, regular use of marijuana to 80%, and experimentation with cocaine to 80% (baseline is 47% for alcohol, 31% for marijuana, and 54% for cocaine in 1997).
- Increase the proportion of adolescents grade 9 through 12 who abstain from intercourse or use condoms if sexually active to at least 95% (baseline for adolescents grades 9 through 12 is 52% who never had intercourse, 13% who had intercourse, but not in the past 3 months, and 20% who currently active and used condoms during last intercourse in 1997).

From U.S. Department of Health and Human Services. (2000). *Healthy people 2010*. Washington, DC: U.S. Government Printing Office.

AGE AND PHYSICAL CHANGES

In contrast to the slow, steady growth of the child, the adolescent experiences markedly accelerated growth. During a 2- to 3-year growth spurt, dramatic alterations in the adolescent's body size and proportions occur. The magnitude of these changes is second only to the growth rate from conception to birth and during infancy.

During this time, sexual characteristics develop, and reproductive maturity is achieved. Physiological functioning of adolescence occurs in a predictable sequence. The age of the onset, magnitude, and duration of growth can vary greatly from individual to individual. Generally, girls enter puberty earlier than do boys (ages 9 to 10 for girls and 10 to 11 for boys). The growth spurt for girls is generally early in puberty, whereas for boys, it is a late pubertal event.

The physical changes experienced during adolescence are regulated by the endocrine system; the hypothalamic-pituitary-gonadal axis is particularly important. This system operates through a negative-feedback mechanism. The hypothalamus responds to drops in circulating sex steroids by secreting gonadotropin-releasing factor (GnRF). This releasing factor stimulates the anterior pituitary gland to release gonadotropins, follicle-stimulating hormone (FSH), and luteinizing hormone (LH). The gonadotropins stimulate the male and female gonads, which, in turn, secrete sex steroids, estrogen, and progesterone from the ovaries and testosterone from the testes. This hormonal interaction is illustrated in Fig. 21-1. During childhood, the hormonal system remains dormant. The immature hypothalamus appears to be extremely sensitive to low levels of circulating sex steroids, which inhibit the release of GnRF. The factors responsible for the changes in this system at puberty are not fully understood; immediately before puberty, the extreme sensitivity of the hypothalamus to sex hormones is believed to diminish. The hypothalamus initiates pituitary secretion of gonadotropins, which then stimulate maturation of the gonads (Hoffman, 1997).

The sex steroids produced by the maturing gonads are primarily responsible for the biological changes of puberty. Sex hormones replace growth hormone as the major regulator of adolescent growth. Recent evidence suggests, however, that growth hormone may play a synergistic role in the growth spurt with the sex steroids (Guyton, 1996).

Acceleration of growth during adolescence is first noted in the musculoskeletal system. During the growth spurt, the average girl gains about 8 cm (3 inches) in height per year. The average boy, in whom the growth spurt is more dramatic and lasts longer than it does in girls, grows at least 10 cm (4 inches) per year during this phase.

Changes in body proportion occur in a predictable pattern. The head, hands, and feet are the first structures to reach adult status. Growth of the extremities precedes growth of the trunk, resulting in the leggy, awkward appearance characteristic of the young adolescent. Increases in shoulder, chest, and hip breadth follow (Guyton, 1996).

Although the size of the brain does not increase significantly during adolescence, the skull and facial bones undergo changes in proportion. Initially, the forehead becomes more prominent. Later, the maxilla and mandible develop, and the jaw assumes its adult character. Dramatic changes in an adolescent's facial appearance within a few months is common.

Ossification of the skeletal system remains incomplete until late adolescence in boys. In girls, ossification is more advanced throughout childhood and is completed at an earlier age compared with boys.

Muscle mass and strength increase during the growth spurt. Muscle development is generally greater in boys than it is in girls at similar stages of development.

Before the growth spurt, many children experience a temporary increase in body fat. During puberty, the proportion of total body weight composed of fat declines, particularly in boys. At the end of the growth spurt, fat again begins to accumulate in both genders. After puberty, girls have proportionately more body fat than do boys. This fat is distributed over the thighs, hips, breasts, and buttocks, contributing to girls' more rounded body contours. Research has shown that 18% to 20% adiposity is required in the adolescent girl for menarche to occur.

Changes in the proportion of body fluids reflect general changes in the proportions of bone, muscle, and adipose tissue. The percentage of total body weight composed of fluid decreases throughout childhood. Boys and girls remain essentially the same in percentages until the changes in body composition occur. Then, boys reach fluid composition of approximately 60% of total body weight, reflecting an increased percentage of muscle tissue, and girls reach an average of about 50% of total body weight in fluid, reflecting an increased percentage of body fat.

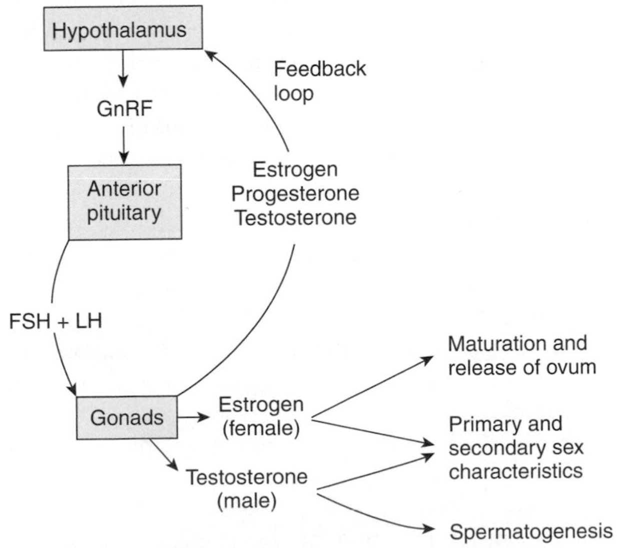

Fig. 21-1 Hormonal interaction between hypothalamus, pituitary, and gonads. (From Wong, D. L., et al. [1999]. *Whaley & Wong's nursing care of infants and children* [6th ed.]. St. Louis: Mosby.)

The basal metabolic rate (BMR) declines over childhood until it reaches an adult level during adolescence. Throughout life, boys have a slightly higher BMR than do girls, which is thought to be a result of the hormone androgen (Guyton, 1996).

During adolescence, the heart grows in size and strength. Blood volume and blood pressure increase, whereas the heart rate declines to adult levels. These cardiovascular changes occur early in girls, consistent with overall growth patterns. Adolescent girls generally have a higher pulse rate and slightly lower systolic blood pressure than do boys.

Blood pressure may fluctuate from time to time in an adolescent, but a systolic or diastolic pressure above the ninety-fifth percentile for age and gender should never be disregarded. Primary hypertension is found more frequently during adolescence than it is during the preschool and school years (Report of the Joint National Committee on the prevention, detection, evaluation, and treatment of high blood pressure, 1997) (see Chapter 20).

Adult levels of all formed elements of the blood are found in adolescents. Hemoglobin levels are higher in postpubertal boys (14 g/dl) than it is in girls (12 g/dl). These are minimal levels for each gender.

Respiratory rate decreases over childhood, reaching an average rate of 15 to 20 breaths per minute during adolescence. Respiratory volume and vital capacity increase, particularly in boys because of their greater shoulder width and chest size. The laryngeal cartilage, larynx, and vocal cords grow, which produces the characteristic voice changes of puberty. Both male and female voices become deeper, with the effect more pronounced in boys than it is in girls (Guyton, 1996).

The liver, kidneys, spleen, and digestive tract enlarge during the growth spurt, but do not change in function; they are already functionally mature by the early school years.

With the exception of the last four molars, which erupt between ages 17 and 21, a full set of permanent teeth is expected by age 12. Dental caries are a significant problem during adolescence, particularly for teens who have not had access to adequate dental care during childhood. Because of the changes in facial structure and proportions during the growth spurt, orthodontic bracing and repair is occasionally started in the adolescent years. As discussed in Chapter 20, good dental hygiene (at least daily brushing and flossing and a visit to the dentist twice a year) continues to be essential for maintaining dental health during the teenage years (Greydanus & Sloane, 1997) (see Box 21-1).

The skin becomes thick and tough during puberty. Under the influence of androgen in both boys and girls, the sebaceous glands become active, particularly on the face, neck, shoulders, upper back, chest, and genitals. These sebaceous glands can become clogged and inflamed, leading to the common teenage condition **acne**.

The exocrine and apocrine sweat glands become fully functional during puberty. The exocrine glands, which are found over most of the body, produce sweat, which helps eliminate body heat through evaporation. The exocrine glands on the palms, soles, and axillae also produce sweat in response to emotional stimuli. The apocrine glands develop in relation to hair follicles and occur in the axillae, genital, and anal areas; in the external auditory canals; around the umbilicus; and around the areolae of the breasts. Apocrine sweat is produced continuously, stored, and released onto the skin in response only to emotional stimuli. The secretion is odorless when it reaches the skin surface, but skin bacteria acts on the fat content, producing characteristic odors.

The noticeable changes in body hair that occur during puberty are discussed in the section on sexual development.

Scoliosis

A common skeletal deformity found in adolescents is **scoliosis,** a lateral S-shaped curvature of the spine. Scoliosis is a progressive disease stimulated by the adolescent growth spurt; the curve is typically convex to the right. Adolescent scoliosis is significantly more prevalent in girls than it is in boys (Friedman, 1998). Some evidence suggests that scoliosis is a genetic disorder. Early intervention is important because untreated scoliosis can result in disfigurement, impaired mobility, and cardiopulmonary complications (Fig. 21-2).

The nurse includes scoliosis screening in the assessment of older school-age children and adolescents. Referral for further orthopedic assessment should be made when any signs of scoliosis are detected.

Acne

Adolescents are typically concerned about their skin changes, which result from the hormonal changes of puberty. The sebaceous glands increase their production of sebum in response to a rise in circulating androgen. This increased sebum is a primary factor in the pathogenesis of acne vulgaris. The sebaceous follicles become clogged with sebum and debris, forming comedones (blackheads or whiteheads). Comedones are a productive environment for propionibacterium acnes, which, when metabolized, release fatty acids that irritate the wall of the sebaceous follicle. Inflammation occurs when closed comedones rupture, spilling their contents into the dermis (Neinstein, 1996).

An estimated 80% of all teens suffer from acne; the degree can range from a few comedones to a severe inflammatory reaction. The incidence of acne within families suggests that hereditary factors are involved.

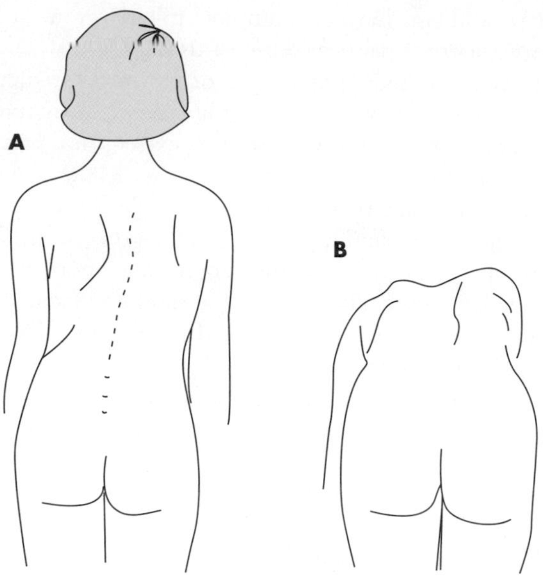

Fig. 21-2 So that the entire back can be seen, the adolescent should remove all clothing from the upper body when being assessed for scoliosis. **A,** While the adolescent stands up straight, check for any asymmetry; palpate for differences in shoulder or scapular height, a prominence of either scapula or hip, waist asymmetry, and misalignment of the spinous processes. Lateral curvature and thoracic convexity of the spine indicate scoliosis. **B,** With feet together, legs straight, and arms hanging freely, the adolescent bends forward until the back is parallel with the floor. Check for prominence of the ribs (rib hump) on one side only and hip and leg asymmetry. With scoliosis, the chest wall on the side of convexity is prominent, and the scapula on the side of convexity is elevated.

Because acne can have severe physical and emotional consequences, aggressive nursing intervention is required. Although the disease is incurable, control is possible. Thorough examination of the adolescent's skin and a discussion of the young person's perceptions of the problem are necessary to determine appropriate management strategies. Intervention should include teaching the individual about the pathophysiological nature of acne. Knowledge allows the adolescent to become instrumental in its management and helps dispel common myths about acne and its care.

The adolescent knows that washing with plain soap and water two or three times a day is the best way to remove dirt and oil. Vigorous scrubbing should be discouraged, because the skin can become irritated, leading to follicular rupture. The adolescent should not attempt to remove the pustules and papules that form. Squeezing the lesion can result in further irritation of the gland and permanent injury to the tissue.

Many nonprescription topical medications are available that contain benzoyl peroxide, such as Oxy-5, Epi-Clear,

Table 21-1 Developmental Stages of Secondary Sex Characteristics*

Stage	Male Genital Development	Pubic Hair Development	Female Breast Development	Other Changes
1	Prepuberty	Hair over pubic area similar to that on abdomen	Increased pigmentation of papillae only	—
2	Initial enlargement of scrotum and testes; reddening and texture changes of scrotum	Sparse growth of long, straight, downy hair at base of penis or along labia	Enlargement of areolar diameter; small area of elevation around papillae	Usual time of peak height velocity for girls
3	Initial enlargement of penis; further growth of testes and scrotum	Hair becomes dark, coarse, and curly; spreads sparsely over entire pubic area	Further elevation and enlargement of breasts and areolae, with no separation or contours	Usual point of onset of menstruation; facial hair begins to grow and voice deepens for boys
4	Further enlargement of penis, testes, and scrotum; growth in breadth and development of glans	Further spread of hair distribution, not extending to thighs	Areolae and papillae project from breast to form secondary mound	Usual time of peak height velocity for boys; axillary hair begins to grow
5	Adult in size and contour	Adult in amount and type	Adult, with projection of papillae only; recession of areolas into general breast contour	—

From Chinn, P. L. (1979). *Child health maintenance: Concepts in family-centered care* (2nd ed.). St. Louis: Mosby.
*As defined by Tanner, J. M. (1990). *Fetus into man: Physical growth from conception to maturity*. Cambridge, MA: Harvard University Press.

and Persadox, which is also bacteriostatic and comedolytic. Unfortunately, these agents cause drying and peeling; therefore therapy is begun with application of 5% strength once a day and after 2 weeks (if tolerated) is increased to twice a day. The nurse refers the adolescent with extensive lesions to a nurse practitioner or physician for prescription medication, which is effective in severe cases.

Adolescent girls should be careful when selecting makeup. Most preparations, when applied extensively over the face, prevent adequate exposure to air and light, causing accumulation of dirt particles on the skin. Any cosmetic that has a grease or fat base should be avoided. Sunlight can have a beneficial effect on acne; however, prolonged sunbathing should be avoided. Stress can also exacerbate acne in some adolescents. In these cases, stress-management techniques should be considered. The effect of diet on acne is a highly controversial issue. Current evidence indicates that dietary restrictions specific to acne are unnecessary, although the adolescent is encouraged to adhere to the age-specific guidelines.

Adolescents with acne need support and understanding. The nurse can help adolescents and their families understand that treatment does not result in immediate improvement. In fact, topical agents may initially make acne appear worse, and improvement occurs slowly over several months.

Clearly, the responsibility for management of the problem should be assigned to the adolescent. The nurse has periodic contact with the adolescent and the family to answer questions, reinforce teaching, and provide positive reinforcement.

Gender

Gender has a profound influence on the physical changes experienced by adolescents. The most obvious differences occur with maturation of the reproductive system. During puberty, both primary and secondary sex characteristics develop. **Primary sex characteristics** involve the organs necessary for reproduction, such as the penis and testes in boys and the vagina and uterus in girls. **Secondary sex characteristics** are external features that differentiate boys from girls, but are unessential for reproduction. Breast development, pubic hair growth, and lowering of the voice are examples of secondary sex characteristics (Table 21-1).

Boys

Sexual development in the male adolescent begins with enlargement of the testes. As the testes grow, the scrotum also enlarges, and the scrotal skin becomes darker. Soon, the penis grows larger and longer, and more hair appears at its base. The development of pubic hair is frequently the first noticeable sign that puberty has begun. During this period, growth in overall body height begins to accelerate.

As maturation proceeds, growth of the penis, testes, and scrotum continues. Pubic hair becomes thick and curly. Adult distribution of pubic hair includes its extension to the inner upper thigh.

Facial hair appears first at the corner of the upper lip. Body proportions change as shoulder breadth increases. The voice begins to deepen. Some degree of bilateral or unilateral breast enlargement, called gynecomastia, may appear and is frequently discovered during peak growth rates. In the United States, this growth is most prevalent at

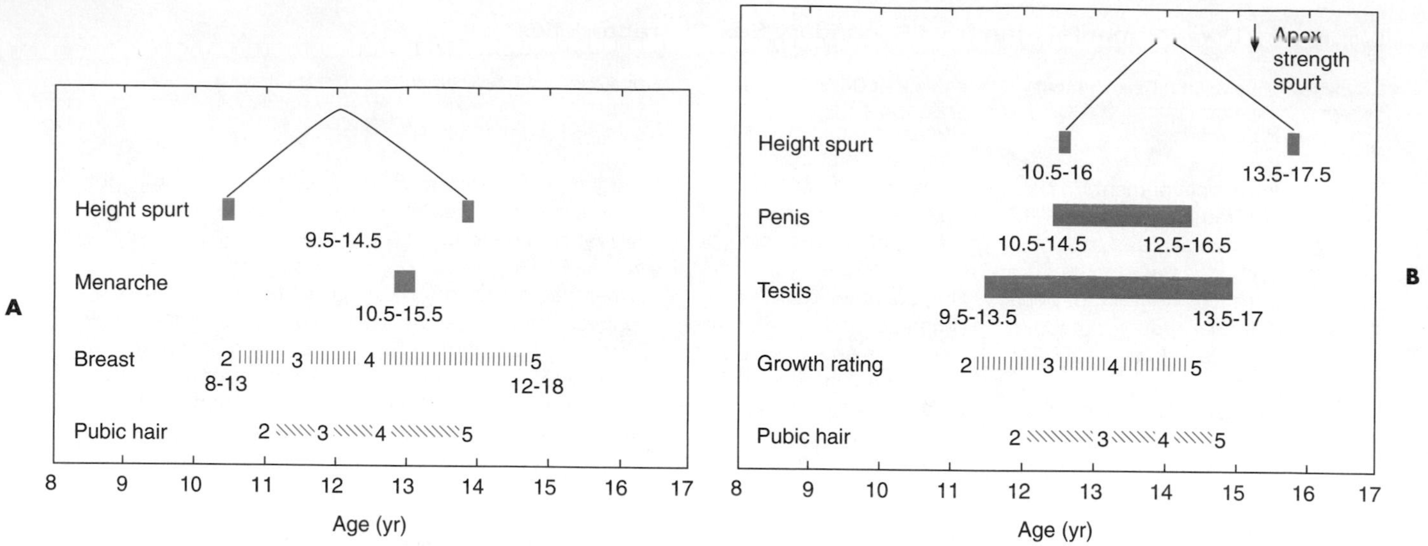

Fig. 21-3 Diagram of sequences of events at adolescence in girls **(A)** and boys **(B)**. Single numbers (2, 3, 4, 5) indicate stages of development. The average is represented. A range of ages when each event may begin and end is indicated by inclusive numbers listed below each event. (Modified from Marshall, W. A., & Tanner, J. M. [1969]. *Archives of Disease in Childhood, 44,* 291; Wong, D. L., et al. [1999]. *Whaley & Wong's nursing care of infants and children* [6th ed.]. St. Louis: Mosby.)

13 years of age. Gynecomastia is temporary and typically disappears by age 17.

In boys, ejaculation is widely considered as the milestone of puberty. In the United States, boys experience their first ejaculation at an average age of 14. Ejaculation precedes fertility by several months (Guyton, 1996).

The primary and secondary sex characteristics continue to develop until late adolescence. In the average boy, the height spurt has decelerated, and sexual maturity has been achieved by age 18.

Girls

In female adolescents, development of the breast bud is usually the first sign that puberty has begun. The appearance of sparse hair along the labia follows, although on some girls it may precede breast bud development. During this stage, the height spurt begins accompanied by the deposition of fat in the characteristic pattern described. Over the next year, pubic hair becomes curly and abundant. Axillary hair appears, and the breasts continue to develop.

The internal reproductive organs grow throughout adolescence, reaching adult size between ages 18 and 20. The onset of menstruation, known as **menarche,** occurs approximately 2 years after the appearance of the breast bud. The average age of menarche in the United States is 12.8 years, with a normal range between ages 10 and 16. Initially, menstrual periods are irregular and scanty and may not be accompanied by ovulation. A consistent pattern of ovulation is generally not established until 1 or 2 years after menarche.

The relationship of the stages of development of the secondary sex characteristics in boys and girls is illustrated in Fig. 21-3. Familiarity with these relationships and stages can help the nurse accurately assess an adolescent's level of development.

Nursing Interventions

The adolescent needs a great deal of support and information during the changes of puberty and the onset of reproductive function. Intellectual knowledge about the events of puberty should be obtained during later childhood. The nurse never assumes, however, that an adolescent has this information. In a tactful and unobtrusive manner, the nurse should assess the teen's knowledge of sexual functioning for both sexes and offer further explanation and clarification as appropriate. Boys particularly should be prepared for erections and nocturnal emissions. Many adolescent boys are concerned about their height and the size of their genitals, linking these physical attributes to their attractiveness and virility. Early adolescence is an excellent time to begin to dispel cultural myths about male sexuality.

As with their male counterparts, adolescent girls have many questions about the physical changes that they experience during puberty. Menarche is perhaps the most significant event of female development; it signals the physical transition from "girl" to "woman." Menarche has not only physiological ramifications, but also psychological and social effects as well.

Preparation for menarche should begin in late childhood. Girls should understand that the timing of menarche varies widely. **Amenorrhea,** the absence of an expected menstrual period, is relatively common in early adolescence. Stress, rigorous athletic training, or a low proportion of body fat can also affect the menstrual cycle, causing missed periods (Reider, 1996). The nurse can encourage a girl to seek health care for these concerns. The sexually active girl can experience a great deal of anxiety when she misses a period. The possibility of pregnancy must be considered along with the other causes of missed periods.

Dysmenorrhea is a common complaint of menstruating women. Characterized by a cramping, lower abdominal pain during menses, and often accompanied by nausea, vomiting, diarrhea, and headaches, dysmenorrhea can last from a few hours up to 3 days. The onset of pain usually precedes or coincides with the onset of bleeding. In primary dysmenorrhea, no evidence of pelvic pathology exists; this disorder does not occur until cyclic ovulation has begun (Emans & Goldsteen, 1998).

Research demonstrates that women who experience discomfort during menstruation have excessive uterine muscle activity. Powerful uterine contractions cause ischemia, which, in turn, causes cramping pain. Evidence suggests that a relationship exists between prostaglandin levels and excessive myometrial activity. This hypothesis has led to the successful use of prostaglandin synthetase inhibitors such as ibuprofen (Motrin) and naproxen (Naprosyn) in the management of this problem (Emans & Goldsteen, 1998; Neinstein, 1996).

Dysmenorrhea is highly prevalent among adolescents and is the leading cause of recurrent short-term school absenteeism. Few adolescents who suffer from dysmenorrhea actually seek help for the problem. Communication with these girls about the causes and options for treatment of dysmenorrhea is important.

Race

Analyzing the relationship between race and the health of adolescents without considering environmental variables is impossible. Proper nutrition, economic stability, and access to health care services are examples of the many environmental resources that are necessary to ensure optimal development and health. Unfortunately, these resources are not equally distributed among the U.S. population. Racial minorities are more likely to grow up in impoverished environments than is the majority population.

Poverty, more than any racial or cultural factor, disturbs family functioning and health. The consequences of poverty among adolescent minorities include increased homicide and other violence, increased incarceration rates, premature pregnancy, substance abuse, and drug trafficking. These psychological and social problems lead to increased morbidity and mortality found in this segment of the population.

A growing number of refugees from Indochina is present in the United States. A recent study of adolescent refugees from Southeast Asia showed that 52% had positive tuberculosis tests, 38% lacked some immunizations, and 10% were anemic. Many other physical and emotional problems were also identified.

Race cannot be isolated as the primary factor responsible for these different risk factors; however, nurses are aware that a relationship between race and certain health problems is likely to exist.

Genetics

Most genetic problems are discovered during infancy and early childhood. Some syndromes, however, may not be diagnosed until adolescence. These genetic disorders are frequently discovered during the assessment of a child with delayed pubertal development.

Turner's syndrome is caused by the absence of one of the X chromosomes in girls, diagnosed most frequently during adolescence because of three outstanding features: (1) short stature, (2) sexual infantilism, and (3) amenorrhea. The incidence is estimated at 1 in 1500 to 1 in 10,000 live female births. Only a few girls with Turner's syndrome manifest all the possible characteristics, which include a webbed neck; low-set ears; a shield-shaped chest with widely spaced, hypoplastic nipples; cardiac anomalies; learning disabilities; and ovarian hypoplasia. Treatment consists primarily of hormonal therapy and ongoing emotional support for the girl and her family (Friedman, 1998).

Klinefelter's syndrome, also seldom diagnosed before puberty, is caused by the presence of one or more additional X chromosomes in boys. This syndrome is the most common of all chromosomal abnormalities; the incidence is estimated to be 1 in 500 live male births. Characteristic features include a tall, eunuchoid figure; sparse facial and pubic hair; gynecomastia; firm, insensitive testes; a small penis; and sterility. Klinefelter's syndrome is associated with learning and/or behavior problems during childhood. As with Turner's syndrome, treatment typically involves hormonal therapy and counseling.

When the nurse recognizes signs of either of these syndromes during routine screening, the child should be referred to specialists who are qualified to diagnose and manage the physical, social, spiritual, and emotional aspects of these problems.

Most adolescents with delayed development do not have a genetic disorder; their pattern of growth merely falls at the far end of the normal curve. Some cases of delayed growth result from inadequate nutrition. Whatever the cause may be, developmental delays can have a tremendous effect on the psychosocial development of the child. This effect is also true of children who mature earlier than do their peers. These adolescents need ongoing assessment and support to promote development of positive self-esteem.

GORDON'S FUNCTIONAL HEALTH PATTERNS

Health Perception-Health Management Pattern

An important task during adolescence is to develop a stable, positive self-image. Young people are concerned about their physical development, appearance, and emotions. Does this egocentrism include an interest in health? If this is the case, then how do adolescents define their unique health care needs?

Box 21-2 Interventions Recommended for the Periodic Health Examination: 11 to 24 Years of Age

SCREENING:

Height and weight
Blood pressure*
Papanicolaou (Pap) test† (girls)
Chlamydia screen‡ (girls under age 20)
Rubella serology or vaccination history§ (girls over age 12)
Assessment for problem drinking

COUNSELING:

Injury Prevention

Lap and shoulder belts
Bicycle, motorcycle, all-terrain vehicle helmets||
Smoke detectors||
Safe storage and removal of firearms||

Substance Use

Avoid tobacco use
Avoid underage drinking and illicit drug use||
Avoid alcohol or drug use while driving, swimming, boating, and so on||

Sexual Behavior

Sexually transmitted disease prevention: abstinence||; avoid high-risk behavior||; condoms; female barrier with spermicide||
Unintended pregnancy; contraception

Diet and Exercise

Limit fat and cholesterol; maintain caloric balance; emphasize grains, fruits, vegetables
Adequate calcium intake (girls)
Regular physical activity||

Dental Health

Regular visits to dental care provider||
Floss and brush with fluoride toothpaste daily||

IMMUNIZATION:

Tetanus-diphtheria (Td) boosters (ages 11 to 16)
Hepatitis B¶
Measles, mumps, and rubella (MMR) (ages 11 to 12)#
Varicella (ages 11 to 12)**
Rubella (girls under age 12r)§
Chemoprophylaxis
Multivitamin with folic acid (girls planning or capable of pregnancy)

*Periodic BP for persons age ≥ age 21.
†If sexually active at present or in the past, q (intercourse, anal or oral sex, or mutual masturbation) ≤ last 3 years. If sexual history is unreliable, begin Pap tests at age 18.
‡If sexually active.
§Serological testing, documented vaccination history, and routine vaccination against rubella (preferably with MMR) are equally acceptable alternatives.
||The ability of clinician counseling to influence this behavior is unsubstantiated.
¶If not previously immunized, current visit, 1 and 6 months later.
#If no previous second dose of MMR.
**If susceptible to chickenpox.

The needs of this age group have been determined largely from an analysis of morbidity and mortality rates. Using these measures, the health of adolescents appears to be good. Teens have fewer acute illnesses than do children and the prevalence of chronic disease among teens is lower than it is among adults. Adolescents are seen in health care facilities less frequently than are children or adults and are rarely hospitalized. Box 21-2 provides a recommended periodic examination schedule for adolescents.

A crucial component of an integrated understanding of adolescent health is consideration of the adolescent's own perceptions of health, illness, and health care services. Classroom discussions about health and health activities and utilization are excellent opportunities for the nurse to address these issues with adolescents.

Although adolescents are able to identify the health problems that concern them most, they are frequently reluctant to seek health care. Some teens deny signs and symptoms of an illness in an effort to maintain their activities of daily living, especially contact with their peers. The following factors influence adolescents' health care service utilization:

1. Severity of the illness
2. Duration of signs and symptoms
3. Restrictions on daily routine
4. Cost of care
5. Availability of a competent, sympathetic provider
6. Awareness of the need for care

Proximity to health care is also an important variable for adolescents. Health clinics located within schools are emerging as a way to reach more teens. Both family and peers can serve as advisors in seeking health care, although peers become more important as the adolescent grows (Neinstein, 1996).

Adolescents are in the process of developing patterns of problem solving and health habits that are likely to last a lifetime. The cognitive and psychological changes that adolescents experience can affect their adherence to preventive health care practices. Teens do not always consider the risks of their behavior and are unlikely to act differently than do their peers. In striving for independence, adolescents will frequently reject adult values and beliefs. An adult who advises an adolescent to seek health or illness care may be met with great resistance. Parents, teachers, and nurses will be more successful in assisting teens to manage health needs wisely if they treat them as partners in planning the care for which the adolescents themselves will assume responsibility (Hoffman, 1997) (see Research Highlight box).

Nutritional-Metabolic Pattern

A balanced diet is essential for optimal growth during adolescence; poor nutrition can retard growth and delay sexual maturation. The Food and Nutrition Board of the National Research Council has recommended dietary

research highlights

Health-Promotion Needs of College Students

The purpose of this study was to investigate the health-promotion needs of students in a college environment. A simple random sampling technique was used to recruit subjects from two college campuses in a metropolitan southern city. Subjects included male and female students, 18 to 21 years of age, enrolled in a full-time program of study. One of the schools was a 2-year state-affiliated community college with a 1992 enrollment of 3492 students. The other institution was a private 4-year coeducation university with a 1992 enrollment of 1928 undergraduate students. Data were collected using a modified version of the Health Promotion Needs Assessment. Data collection was accomplished through a mailed survey; no direct contact was made with subjects.

The greatest number of subjects identified personal health care as the first-priority health-promotion need. Mental health was a first-priority health-promotion need for 20-year-old individuals, Blacks, sophomores, and married participants at the 2-year college, and 19-year-old persons, Asian Americans, and sophomores at the 4-year college. At both colleges, 18-year-old students identified nutrition as their first-priority health-promotion need. Physical fitness was given a first-priority rating by men at the 4-year college. Tobacco, alcohol, and other drugs were consistently given a low ranking by all subjects. An important implication of these results is that the health-promotion needs identified as high priority are not identical to the high-risk behaviors that are cited in the literature for this population. Identification of these needs may contribute to the development and implementation of programs that help students adopt healthy lifestyle behaviors throughout the lifespan. Failure to do so can lead to misdirected priorities in preventive efforts.

Data from Fish, C., & Nies, M. A. (1996). Health promotion needs of students in a college environment. *Public Health Nursing, 13*, 104.

allowances of the nutrients that are necessary to support adolescent growth (Marina & King, 1981). These recommendations are considered as average daily requirements for boys and girls in the given age ranges.

Using age as a basis for determining the nutritional requirements of adolescents has limitations. Because wide variability exists in the timing of pubertal growth, the individual's level of development should be considered when calculating specific nutritional requirements for each adolescent (Spear, 1996).

The highest nutrient and energy demands occur at the peak velocity of growth. For example, a 13-year-old boy in the middle of his growth spurt has different nutritional demands from a 13-year-old boy who has yet to experience pubescent changes. Participation in sports or other forms of intense physical activity also increases nutrient and caloric requirements.

In striving to become interdependent individuals, most adolescents spend increasing amounts of time involved in activities outside the home; their lifestyles often include irregular eating habits, skipping meals, and snacking. Snacking can be a help or a hindrance to good nutrition based on the nutrient content of the snack. The adolescent should be encouraged to select nutritious snacks such as fresh fruit and vegetables, juice, cheese, whole-grain crackers, and nuts. Eating at fast-food restaurants is popular in this age group. Fast foods tend to be high in calories, fat, and sodium and low in iron, calcium, and vitamins A and C (Spear, 1996).

Adolescents are frequently dissatisfied with their appearance. Our predominant cultural ideals, as reflected in mass media, influence this dissatisfaction with body image. Many adolescent girls consider themselves to be too heavy and want to lose weight, although only 15% are actually obese. Many adolescent boys think of themselves as being too thin and want to gain weight, although only 25% are below average in weight.

The desire to be attractive and to "fit in" with peers can lead to unhealthy dietary practices. Fad diets are popular with teens. Rigid diets, however, can result in malnutrition or other serious harm. Typically, adolescent diets are deficient in calcium, iron, zinc, folic acid, and vitamins A and C (Spear, 1996). Adolescent girls, who diet more frequently than do boys, are more likely to ingest insufficient calories and calcium.

Eating Disorders

At one end of the spectrum is **anorexia nervosa,** which affects primarily adolescent girls, although recent studies suggest that the incidence among boys may be higher than was previously suspected (Neinstein, 1996). This complex problem has underlying developmental and psychological disturbances. Symptoms can include self-starving with significant weight loss, amenorrhea, compulsive physical activity, preoccupation with food, and a distorted body image. Typically, the person with anorexia is described as a perfectionist or overachiever who has always performed well academically. This person's family also tends to be achievement oriented, and marital discord is frequently present (Kreipe & Dukarm, 1999).

The onset of the anorexic behavior is typically initiated in response to real or imagined obesity. With dieting, the adolescent begins to lose weight. Personal pride and positive reinforcement from others lead to continued dieting, which becomes the primary focus of the teen's life. Any feelings of hunger are rigidly denied. Eventually, the adolescent becomes dangerously malnourished. Common complications of this type of severely limited intake are fluid and electrolyte imbalances, hypotension, and constipation. Untreated, this disorder can progress to starvation and death. When anorexia is suspected, the nurse refers the individual to a specialist in this complex problem. Recovery is a long process that involves ongoing treatment, including psychotherapy for the entire family. Hospitalization is frequently necessary to prevent physical deterioration.

Another frequently occurring eating disorder is **bulimia nervosa,** a pattern of binge eating followed by forced vomiting and/or laxative use, accompanied by a general sense of a lack of control of eating. This is another complex situation that the nurse refers to a specialist for comprehensive evaluation and management. (See Box 21-3 for the diagnostic criteria for eating disorders.)

Obesity

Obesity is defined as weight that is 20% over the ideal weight for a particular height. Although the etiological factors of this problem are complex, recent evidence suggests that a primary factor is inactivity (Fig. 21-4). Approximately 15% of adolescents are obese. Obesity is more common among girls than it is among boys. The obese adolescent consumes too many calories for the amount of energy expended. Some individuals may not be consuming excessive calories, but skipping breakfast and eating throughout the afternoon and evening is common (Kligh, 1998).

Recent studies have shown a strong correlation between the time viewing television and the tendency to be overweight. The findings indicate that teens who watched more than 5 hours of television each day are 4.6 times more likely to be obese than are those who spend 2 hours or less in front of the television (Gortmaker, et al., 1996).

Obesity can be detrimental to the adolescent's self-esteem and social development. These teens tend to become trapped in a vicious cycle of social rejection, isolation, inactivity, and greater obesity. Unfortunately, obesity during adolescence has a poor prognosis; most obese adolescents become obese adults (Kligh, 1998).

Some methods for treating adolescent obesity are more successful than are others. A holistic approach that addresses environmental, psychosocial, and physiological factors is likely to be most successful. Dietary regimens that include rigid restrictions should be avoided to ensure that

Box 21-3 Diagnostic Criteria for Eating Disorders

ANOREXIA NERVOSA

- Refusal to maintain body weight at or above a minimally normal weight for age and height (weight loss leading to maintenance of body weight less than 85% of that expected or failure to make expected weight gain during period of growth, leading to body weight less than 85% of that expected).
- Intense fear of gaining weight or becoming fat, even when underweight.
- Disturbance in the way in which one's body weight or shape is experienced, undue influence of body weight or shape on self-evaluation, or denial of the seriousness of the current low body weight.
- In postmenarcheal girls, amenorrhea—the absence of at least three consecutive menstrual cycles. (A woman is considered to have amenorrhea when her periods occur only after hormone [estrogen] administration.)

Specify type:

Restricting type: during the current episode of anorexia nervosa, the person has not regularly engaged in binge eating or purging behavior (self-induced vomiting, the misuse of laxatives, diuretics, and enemas).

Binge eating-purging type: during the current episode of anorexia nervosa, the person has regularly engaged in binge eating or purging behavior (self-induced vomiting, the misuse of laxatives, diuretics, and enemas).

BULIMIA NERVOSA

- Recurrent episodes of binge eating. An episode of binge eating is characterized by both of the following:
  1. Eating, in a discrete period of time (within any 2-hour period), an amount of food that is definitely larger than most people would eat during similar period and under similar circumstances.
  2. A sense of lack of control over eating during the episode (a feeling that one cannot stop eating or control what or how much one is eating).
- Recurrent inappropriate compensatory behavior to prevent weight gain, such as self-induced vomiting; misuse of laxatives, diuretics, enemas, or other medications; fasting; or excessive exercise.
- The binge eating and inappropriate compensatory behaviors both occur, on average, at least twice a week for 3 months.
- Self-evaluation is unduly influenced by body shape and weight.
- The disturbance does not occur exclusively during episodes of anorexia nervosa.

Specify type:

Purging type: during the current episode of bulimia nervosa, the person has regularly engaged in self-induced vomiting or the misuse of laxatives, diuretics, or enemas.

Nonpurging type: during the current episode of bulimia nervosa, the person has used other inappropriate compensatory behaviors, such as fasting or excessive exercise, but has not regularly engaged in self-induced vomiting or the misuse of laxatives, diuretics, or enemas.

Modified from American Psychiatric Association. (1994). *Diagnostic and statistical manual of mental disorders* (4th ed.). Washington, DC: The Association.

the nutritional demands of adolescent growth are met (see Case Study).

Nursing Interventions

Through periodic assessment of height and weight, nurses are typically the first to identify obesity; their role in prevention is even more important than that of the family. The suggestions for parents who are interested in preventing obesity in their children that were presented in Chapter 20 are also relevant for parents of adolescents, even though teens assume greater responsibility for their own eating and exercise patterns than do younger children. Limiting television viewing to no more than 2 hours a day and participating in vigorous activities are two suggestions that can be adopted by nearly any family. Health classes in school are appropriate forums for discussion of nutrition and its related problems, such as obesity and anorexia.

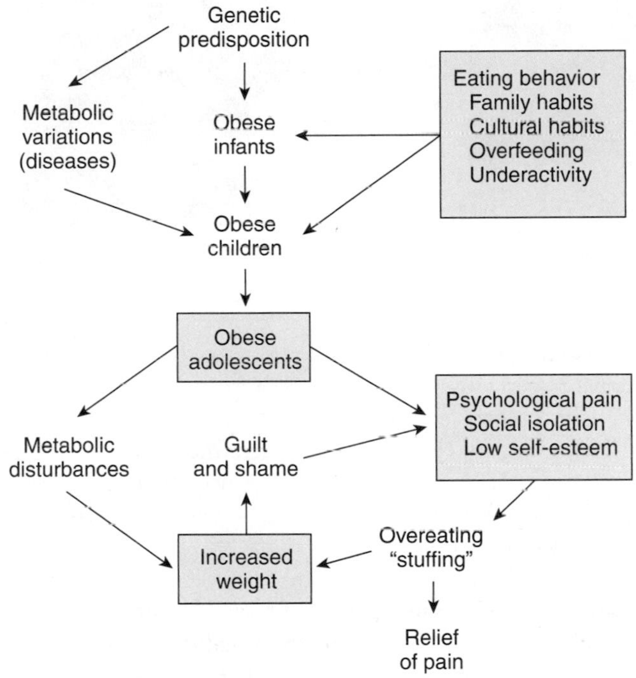

Fig. 21-4 Complex relationships in adolescent obesity. (From Wong, D. L., et al. [1999]. *Whaley & Wong's nursing care of infants and children* [6th ed.]. St. Louis: Mosby.)

> **CASE STUDY**
>
> ***Mary***
>
> Mary, a 16-year-old high school sophomore, expresses concern to the school nurse that she is "too fat." She is trying several fad diets and exercising several hours a day. According to height and weight charts, Mary is in the ninety-fifth percentile for her weight.
>
> What developmental factors are influencing Mary?
>
> What health-promotion strategies might the school nurse use to assist Mary?
>
> At what point should the nurse be concerned about eating disorders?

Elimination Pattern

The renal and gastrointestinal systems are functionally mature by adolescence. Elimination patterns are consistent with those found in adults.

Activity-Exercise Pattern

During adolescence, the alterations in body composition and growth of lean muscle mass allow the teen to experience increased physical strength and endurance. For the first time, the young person has the ability to adapt to strain or stress that is equal to or in excess of that of an adult. This ability results from an increased capacity of the lungs and accompanying structures, which serves to restore oxygen to the tissues after intensive exertion and to facilitate recovery of normal function following the exercise. Heart rate, respiratory rate, reflexive shunting of blood from resting to working muscles, blood pressure, and electrolyte and fluid responses are among the many complex reactions to exercise that reach their full capacity.

Many adolescents enjoy vigorous physical activity; participation in organized, competitive sports is popular. Activity levels vary greatly, however; some adolescents lead active lives and others are sedentary. The nurse who works with this age group should assess the individual's patterns of activity periodically to determine appropriate strategies for health promotion and specific protection.

Adolescents who participate in athletic activities are examined to ensure that they are physically able to cope with the demands of the sport (Reider, 1996). Many schools require a yearly physical examination before participation in athletic programs is allowed. The stage of physical maturity is an important consideration in evaluating teen athletes who will participate in competitive sports, specifically because increased strength accompanies sexual maturity. The Tanner scale, which characterizes sexual maturity into specific stages, is a useful tool for sports-participation physical examinations. Athletes must also be taught ways to strengthen and condition themselves to prevent injuries.

All young people should be taught that good nutrition and regular exercise can improve their endurance, appearance, and general state of health and that these positive effects can extend into adulthood.

Sleep-Rest Pattern

During adolescence, the amount of time spent each night in sleep declines. Although sleep patterns vary greatly among individuals, on average, adolescents sleep 8 hours each night. Working adolescents are most at risk for sleep deprivation and daytime sleepiness. Nurses can help employed adolescents deal with the challenge of balancing

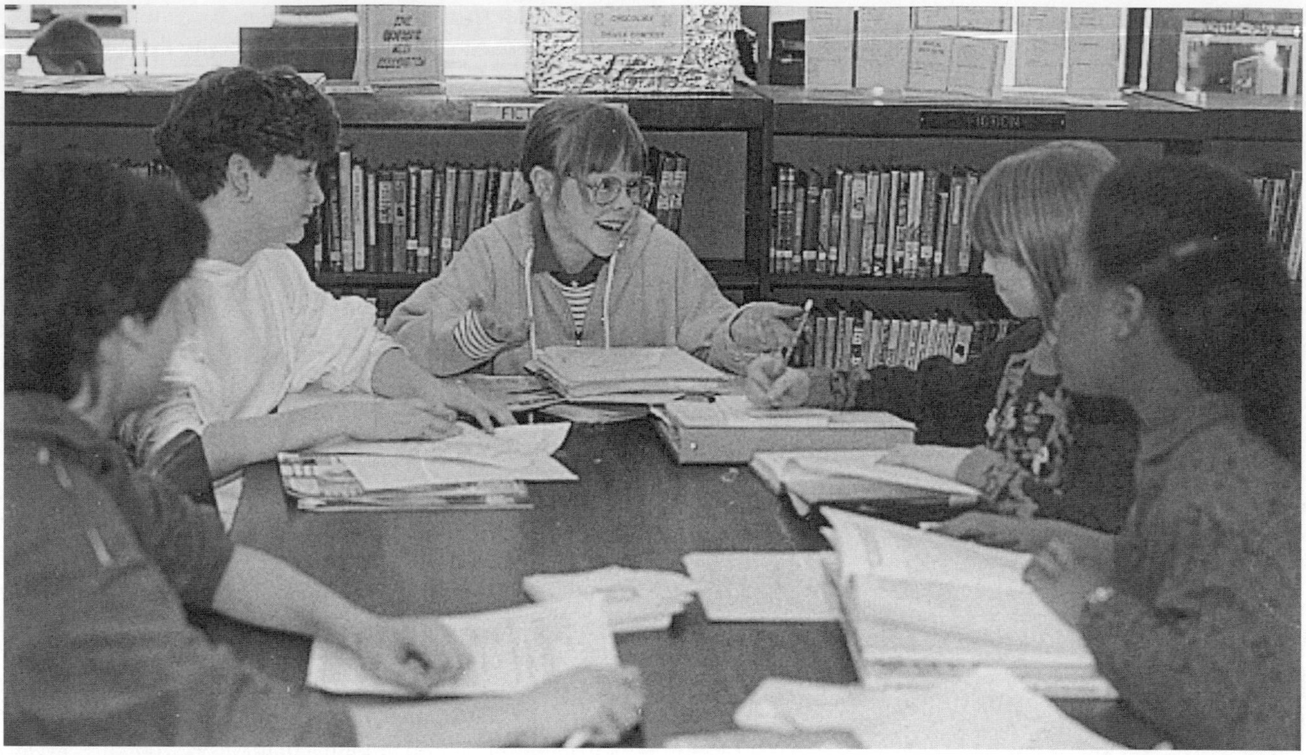

Fig. 21-5 An opportunity to work in a group on a research project encourages adolescents to express their thoughts in more abstract terms and solve problems together.

work, school, leisure time, sleep, and responsibilities to their families.

The physical changes of puberty, as dramatic as they are, appear almost inconsequential when compared with the psychological and social changes that occur during adolescence. The young person moves from being a relatively dependent member of society to taking on full responsibility for oneself, one's actions, and, occasionally, another person, if parenthood should occur. By the end of adolescence, the young person is expected by society to assume a full adult role.

Cognitive-Perceptual Pattern

Piaget's Theory

The early part of adolescence, ages 11 to 15, is the period during which Piaget's stage of **formal operations** begins. Thought processes develop into mature, adultlike patterns, with specific traits that allow for adult accomplishments in thinking. An important point to remember is that not all individuals achieve this advanced thinking capability at the same time. Piaget believes that cognitive development evolves as a result of the maturation of the cerebral structures.

The primary feature of this period of thought is that children can enter into possibilities beyond the world of reality; they are able to think beyond the present and to consider things that do not exist, but that might be. This type of thinking involves real logic and an organized, consistent approach to thinking. Piaget uses the term *formal* to represent the adolescent's focus on the "form" of thought, objects, and experiences rather than on the exact content. When they have attained the level of formal operations, adolescents think in a way that determines possibilities, ranks probabilities, solves problems, and makes decisions (Fig. 21-5).

Nonetheless, adolescents incorporate certain traits of cognition from earlier periods of life. Young people are capable of the fantastic flights from reality that are typical of the preoperational period and yet order their ideational material in a manner that is similar to the organizational patterns used for sensory reality in the operational periods. Reality is recognized, but becomes only a subset of many other possibilities.

As these patterns of thought emerge, adolescents tend to be extremely idealistic, to constantly challenge the way things are, and to consider the way that things can be or should be. What actually is may be completely discarded. During the early part of the formal operations period, young people demonstrate a kind of egocentrism in thinking; their propositions and flights from reality allow them to see themselves as omnipotent and to bring reality in line with their own thinking. Although this trait can be irritating to adults, it is a necessary stage for the completion of the formal operations period. After this characteristic has been mastered, adolescents can move on to thought patterns that are more mature, making use of the propositional, organized approach, but that more fully account for the social and cosmic universe to which they are applied.

In solving a problem, adolescents in the formal operations period can try out a variety of solutions in their minds without having to actually manipulate materials; they can operate solely through symbolism (Pruitt, 1999). Several relevant variables can be held constant while one variable is systematically manipulated, enabling the adolescent to hypothesize about the outcome under each condition. This approach is the classic method of experimental science, but young people rarely realize that they are using this approach with such sophistication.

These new cognitive abilities are reflected in the teen's behavior in several ways. The first change is that because of their new ability to "think about their thinking," adolescents become highly introspective. By middle adolescence, this introspection is quite marked, and the individual may assume that others are equally interested and nearly or actually know what the other is thinking. Elkind (1985) points out that this type of thinking gives rise to the teen's "imaginary audience." The imaginary audience provides the adolescent with a means of evaluating the question, "How do others see me?" and leads to a sense of being the focus—special, unique, and exceptional. Being exceptional to the adolescent means being the exception, and this **fable of immunity** gives rise to the risk-taking behavior for which adolescents are well known:

- "I can get drunk on weekends and not develop a drinking problem."
- "I won't get pregnant; after all I've had sex for 6 months and haven't gotten pregnant."
- "I can take those hairpin turns at 50 miles per hour and not have a wreck."

Another behavioral manifestation of the adolescent's formal operations ability is an intolerance of things as they are. The adolescent can conceptualize things as they might be rather than how they are and they can think of elaborate means for achieving these changes. Teens can be vehement in trying to convince others of their viewpoints and untiring in the support of causes that appear to agree with their ideas. This idealism can also lead to rejection of family beliefs, religion, or social causes, which do not appear to be working fast enough to solve the problems of society. This process can result in major disagreements between parents and adolescents (Pruitt, 1999). Through teaching and counseling, the nurse helps the family develop through this phase.

Erikson's Theory

The central task of adolescence is the establishment of **identity,** with the primary risk being **role confusion,** including identity diffusion and negative identity. Erikson conceptualizes the youth culture that has developed in technological societies as an attempt to establish identity formation. Although it may appear that the young people who create the culture are involved in a final rather than a transient or initial identity formation, dedication to the adolescent culture provides a means of moving into and through the identity crisis of the period. Through the group, individuals find support and help with the many inner problems of developing a new body image, finding sexual identity, establishing intimacy with the opposite sex, and dealing with the many conflicting possibilities and choices of the present and future. Erikson views the adolescent clique as a means of testing the ability to remain constant and loyal in the midst of inevitable conflicts of values (Erikson, 1993, 1997).

The adolescent identity crisis involves a restaging of each of the previous stages of development. The stage of infancy, with the development of trust in self and others, is again encountered as the adolescent searches intently for people and ideals in which to have faith. Adults and peer groups can serve this function.

Although the stage of developing autonomy is reestablished to express individuality, adolescents simultaneously avoid the hazard of behaving in a manner that would expose them to self-doubt or ridicule from others. Young people intensify their search for roles through which they can express themselves in directions that are effective. The accomplishment of this task and the avoidance of shame lead to an interesting paradox: adolescents would rather behave shamelessly in the eyes of their parents than be forced into behavior that would bring ridicule from their peers.

The third stage of life, when a sense of initiative develops, is also reenacted as adolescents seek identity. Their unlimited imagination over what they might become is tempered only by a sense of guilt over the excessiveness of their ambition. Adolescents aspire to great accomplishment at one point, then loudly denounce themselves for exceeding the possible.

The school-age period of developing a sense of industry is carried into the adolescent period as teens make choices in social, recreation, volunteer, academic, familial, and occupational activities. The confusion and hesitation in making these choices arise from fears of participating in activities that will not afford them the opportunity to excel.

The extent to which earlier tasks were successfully completed or resolved influences adolescents' success in finding an identity. Young people who have experienced success tend to be resourceful during adolescence in finding ways of making up any gaps in earlier stages of development. Erikson states that when adolescents believe that society is depriving them of all forms of expression that permit them to integrate the various steps of their previous development, they resist violently and feel forced to defend their development of identity. When the threat of identity confusion is exceedingly great, delinquent behavior and potential alterations in mental health frequently occur. This threat is enhanced by conditions of poverty, racism, sexual orientation, the dysfunctional family, chronic illness, and personal losses and grief. Erikson views society as posing special problems for young people by insisting on self-made identities that are characterized by strength, tolerance, and the readiness to take advantages of opportunity and to adjust to change. Society must present adolescents with ideologies that can be shared by a highly diverse young population while maintaining the ideals of freedom of self-realization and choice (see Hot Topics box).

The pursuit for something to which to be devoted and the search for a meaningful ideology frequently create a puzzling combination of shifting devotion and sudden extremes in action. Erikson views this behavior as an attempt to try various roles and to search for some stable principle that might last through the testing of extremes and into adulthood. Erikson devoted much of his work to finding interpretations of teen behavior that could be related to the entire life history of the individual and to differentiating truly pathological behavior during adolescence from that which is normal and useful in completing life's stages (Erikson, 1993, 1997).

HOT topics

TATTOOING

Adolescence can be a time for experimenting and risk-taking behaviors. Teens may begin cigarette use and alcohol abuse. They are involved in more motor-vehicle accidents than is any other age group. Sexually transmitted disease and pregnancy are also problems associated with adolescence. These behaviors may be explained developmentally as adolescents strive for independence and identity. Today, tattooing is on the rise and has become a popular form of expression for many people.

Tattooing is associated with three areas of risk according to recent research. The risks of purchase and possession include whimsical decision making, the young age of tattooing, the short time frame for decisions, the visual messages in their tattoo designs, the exposed body locations, and the lack of support by parents, siblings, and the public (Armstrong & McConnell, 1994). The third risk involves health concerns, including potential disease, allergies, or infections after tattooing. A second study (Armstrong & Murphy, 1997) found that adolescents who want a tattoo will obtain one, regardless of the costs, regulations, or risks. Tattoos are viewed by adolescents as objects of self-identity and body art. Adults view tattoos as deviant behavior.

Nurses should develop health education programs to allow the adolescents to make informed decisions about tattooing. Information about the transmission of blood-borne disease and the permanency of the markings should be provided.

Adapted from Armstrong, M. L., & McConnell, C. (1994). Tattooing in adolescents, more common than you think: The phenomenon and risks. *Journal of School Nursing, 10*, 22-29; Armstrong, M. L. & Murphy, K. P. (1997). Tattooing: Another adolescent risk behavior warranting health education. *Applied Nursing Research, 10*, 181-189.

Time Orientation Older adolescents look at time differently than they did as children. Young people realize that the response to a problem can and should be delayed to think through the possibilities for approaching the problem. Additionally, teens develop a future orientation and are able to delay immediate gratification to gain more satisfaction in the future.

Sensory Perception The adolescent has a mature sensory repertoire. Touch, taste, smell, vision, hearing, and proprioception have reached full development by this period.

Language Advances in cognitive skills are reflected in an increased understanding of language. Formal operations and more abstract thought processes require expression in different words than did the more concrete thoughts of younger children. Adolescents give complex definitions, frequently including all possible meanings or uses. Interpretations of pictures or stories are complex and abstract. Older teens are capable of using and understanding complex sentence structure, although they, similar to adults, may not use these complex sentences routinely in their speech.

Both receptive and expressive vocabularies increase during adolescence. As with all ages, receptive vocabulary far exceeds expressive vocabulary. Vocabulary tests are used to estimate intelligence quotient (IQ). The adolescent vocabulary frequently includes **argot** (words devised and used by participants in a certain subculture). Adults frequently call this word use slang. Argot may be centered on topics such as drug use, popular dress, music, or certain activities, or it may be more pervasive, in which case adults or "outsiders" may have difficulty following a conversation between two teens.

The level of abstract thinking of the older adolescent is reflected in writing style. The younger adolescent is likely to use a flamboyant, dramatic style, whereas the older adolescent's written expression tends to be objective and controlled.

Intelligence By the end of adolescence, adult IQ tests are used to evaluate level of cognition. IQ tests are based on thought processes and actual experiences in the real world. For adolescents from a limited, restricted background, some of the situations presented or questions asked can be difficult because of their unfamiliarity. Additionally, adolescents of a minority culture may perceive a situation or question from the perspective of their own culture and give an answer that may appear wrong, but is actually correct based on their experiences. The nurse considers differences in the background in evaluating the intellectual capacity of the adolescent.

Self-Perception–Self-Concept Pattern

Body Image

Self-image and self-esteem are tied, to a great extent, to body image, and adolescents who perceive their bodies as being less ideal than those of their peers have less favorable feelings about themselves. As mentioned, adolescent girls frequently view themselves as being overweight, and adolescent boys tend to view themselves as being too thin. These girls want small hips, thighs, or waists; the boys want broader shoulders and more muscular arms (see Care Plan box).

An important aspect of body image during adolescence is sexual characteristics. Boys are concerned with the size of the penis and with body and facial hair. A larger penis and more and early appearance of body and facial hair is viewed as desirable. Girls are concerned with breast size and the onset of menstruation. Larger breasts are viewed as more feminine; the onset of menstruation is one rite of passage into adult femininity. Because many sexual characteristics are primarily genetically determined, adolescents feel as though they are observing their bodies, waiting for the final result.

CARE PLAN

Nursing Diagnosis: Risk for Low Self-Esteem Related to Poor Body Image

DEFINING CHARACTERISTICS
- Verbalizes negative feelings about self
- Expresses inability to deal with events
- Self-destructive behavior (alcohol, drug abuse, promiscuous sexual behavior)
- Lack of eye contact
- Rejection of positive feedback
- Excessive passivity

RELATED FACTORS
- Poor body image
- Poor school performance
- Single-parent family
- Ethnicity
- Recent loss in family

EXPECTED OUTCOMES
- Individual acknowledges personal strengths
- Individual decreases verbalization of negative feelings about self
- Individual develops plan for decreasing self-destructive behavior
- Individual accepts positive feedback

INTERVENTIONS
- Actively involve individual in developing a plan of care
- Assist individual in identifying personal strengths
- Give specific feedback regarding observed positive behaviors
- Set limits about negative verbalization
- Identify positive coping behaviors
- Teach positive behavior skills through role playing, role model, and discussion
- Provide information about available community resources and counseling

Roles-Relationships Pattern

Until adolescence, the child is highly dependent on the parents and other adults. Striving for self-identity and increased independence, an adolescent begins to spend increased time away from the family. Parents sense a narrowing of their influence as their child spends more time with peers and other adults, questions their basic beliefs and values, and becomes more mobile. This is a time of crisis for families, and they may respond by setting unreasonably strict limits or asking intrusive questions about their teen's activities, friends, and ideas. Another typical, but more uncommon, response is for parents to drop all rules and limits and assume that the adolescent can manage alone. Both responses increase tension in the family.

The family with an adolescent also goes through a period of development. The adolescent is striving for a sense of identity and independence within society. The family is learning to let go; parents are focusing on their marital relationship, their aging parents, and their satisfaction with their work and attainment of life goals. The family can be described as being in disequilibrium or in a normative developmental crisis.

Each member is temporarily unsure of the relationship with other family members. The family unit may undergo more stress than at any previous time (Emans & Goldsteen, 1998). Specific issues of conflict may involve the following:

1. The adolescent becomes less psychologically, socially, and physically dependent on the family (while frequently maintaining economic dependence).
2. The adolescent becomes increasingly mobile, spending far longer periods of time away from the family.
3. Power struggles develop over family rules, money, school performance, religion, privacy, or choice of college or career.
4. New roles develop for other family members.

Some families experience better outcomes than do other families. Families in which parents maintain a willingness to listen and demonstrate an ongoing affection for and acceptance of their adolescent have a more constructive, positive outcome during this adjustment period. This situation does not mean that parents necessarily agree with their teens ideas or actions, but rather that they are willing to hear what the adolescent has to say and to negotiate some limits (Pruitt, 1999).

Parents may be worried about substance abuse, early sexual experience, or other actions of their teen, but hesitate to verbalize their concerns. Parents may need assistance in determining negotiable versus nonnegotiable rules and in developing ways to voice their concerns in an honest, open way. Even when teens do not want to discuss these topics, at least they should know the reasons for which their parents are concerned.

Siblings also experience changes in their relationships at this time. Older adolescent siblings withdraw from the child who is just entering adolescence, adult siblings may empathize with the adolescent or assume a "parent" role, and younger siblings may emulate the older adolescent. Conversely, when there is prolonged, heated conflict between the parents and the adolescent, a younger sibling may regress in an attempt to escape the conflict.

Nursing Interventions

The nurse practices primary prevention of undue adolescent-parent and family conflict during this time by encouraging open communication among family members through family meetings during which each member is able to state views without criticism from others. The nurse provides information to both parents and teens about the conflicts that are common at this time and the needs of family members during this transition. Secondary prevention for families that are experiencing unmanageable conflicts includes referral for family or individual counseling through an agency or a practitioner who is experienced in dealing with adolescents and their families.

Peers

Faced with the need to become autonomous, to achieve sexual function and identity, and to become economically self-sufficient and productive, the older adolescent turns from the family to peers and intimate relationships.

Belonging to an informally organized clique, crowd, gang, or specific group is the primary means in Western societies for an adolescent to make the transition from primary allegiance as a child in the family to a colleague in the peer group. A sense of commonality develops within the group and follows no set rules or regulations, but demands loyalty and group solidarity. This type of group membership requires that the individual lay aside personal goals and learn to achieve objectives that are desired for the group as a whole. Identification with the group is proclaimed through conformity to standards of clothing, behavior, language, and values. This feature of the adolescent subculture persists despite the strong inclination in society as a whole toward greater levels of individuality. The adolescent group is a vehicle for movement out of and away from the family unit, and as such, provides a means of achieving the goals of individualization (Pruitt, 1999) (Fig. 21-6).

Adolescents talk a great deal with their peers. Whether on the phone or in person, they can discuss a 10-minute situation for hours on end. This sharing of thoughts and impressions is important for adolescents to orient themselves to the norms of the group. The telephone can provide a "safe" mechanism for the young person to converse with members of the opposite sex.

A same-sex best friend is important, especially in early adolescence. Best friends share their most intimate ideas and concerns and begin to experience closeness and caring that will develop into the capacity to form a future intimate sexual relationship.

Dating is a social custom developed by middle-class youth. *Going with* means an exclusive dating situation.

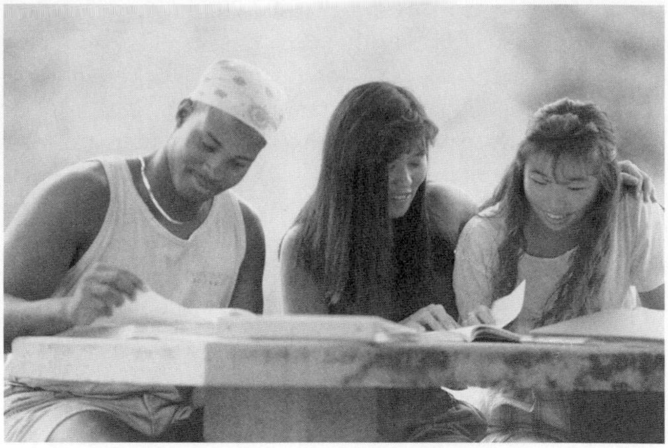

Fig. 21-6 Adolescents commonly trust information from their peers more than that from their parents or health care providers.

Some young teens use the phrase "going with" to indicate their relationship with a member of the opposite sex with whom they have never had a date, but only talked to on the phone on a regular basis. Controversy surrounds young adolescents' dating; certain religious groups disapprove of early dating, whereas some people believe that early dating is a valuable educational experience in social skills and human relationships. Dating clearly improves the adolescents' status among their peers, but parents worry that dating might lead to an early sexual relationship.

Sexuality-Reproductive Pattern

The physical changes of sexual characteristics stimulate a change in the adolescent's concept of sexuality. Young people first fantasize about the pleasures of sex and then gradually experiment with dating, petting, and noncoital and coital contact according their values, beliefs, and customs.

Older adolescents who have had opportunities to work through their sexual roles become comfortable with who they are and what their possible roles may be. Establishing intimacy with a partner or partners begins. This approach forms groundwork for the long-term commitments of young adulthood. Sexual experimentation as a way of being accepted into a specific group or clique does not fall into the concept of true intimacy. As a final step in the acquisition of sexual identity, intimacy frequently includes sexual activity.

Teens become sexually active for a variety of reasons, which vary as the adolescent matures. Adolescents have sex for affection, because of peer pressure, as a symbol of maturity, as spontaneous experimentation, to feel close, and because sex feels good.

Adolescents who are 15 to 18 years of age may take fewer risks and be more thoughtful about the reasons for having sex. Unfortunately, many teens fail to use **contraception** or consider the possible outcomes of sexual activity any more than they did during younger ages. Older adolescents, ages 18 to 20, are more likely to plan for sexual intercourse by obtaining information about and using effective contraception and protection against infection than are younger adolescents.

Sexual activity is no longer the exception for teens; it has become nearly a norm. Although gathering sexual activity data on younger adolescents is difficult because of parental objections to surveys, several studies indicate that this younger group is also sexually active. An indication of this trend is apparent in the number of teen pregnancies: 32.5% of sexually experienced 15- to 19-year-old girls have already had an unmarried pregnancy.

The first step in primary prevention is to involve parents and schools in the provision of accurate information on sexuality, sexual decision making, contraception, and prevention of **sexually transmitted diseases** (STDs).

Sensitivity to sexual preference is an important consideration in working with adolescents. Not all teens are heterosexual, and the nurse has an open, accepting approach to elicit an accurate sexual history and respond to the individual teen's needs (Perrin, 1996).

Because of persistent widespread homophobia, gay, lesbian, and bisexual adolescents tend to be reluctant to discuss their same-sex orientation. Homosexual and bisexual adolescents experience rejection by the people on whom they depend for support: families, siblings, peers, schools, places of worship, and other community organizations, including health care organizations. The nurse helps homosexual and bisexual adolescents achieve a secure, healthy identity to minimize negative health outcomes, including those from victimization.

Contraception

Adolescents should become thoroughly acquainted with the available methods of contraception. Nurses put aside moral judgments in counseling individual teens and in recognizing a health need. Both boys and girls should understand the methods of contraception, and they should know where to obtain help and advice when needed. The community and the family of an individual teen can have reservations or strong objections to the availability of this type of information, and the effect of these preferences must be understood and respected. The individual teen, however, has the right to obtain information and to make a confidential choice that includes the consequences and the inherent responsibilities of the choice. Adolescents can be encouraged to know and understand the teachings of their culture, family, and religion about family planning and to make their own choices based on each aspect of the situation.

The rhythm method of contraception involves determining the time of ovulation during the female cycle and abstaining from coitus during the normal lifespan of sperm before ovulation and for the lifespan of the ovum after ovulation. Ovulation typically occurs 14 days after menstruation begins, but variation in the timing of ovulation from cycle to cycle and from individual to individual makes exact timing of this event difficult to predict. To use the rhythm method, the woman's cycle must be fairly regular from month to month. Because adolescents commonly experience irregular menstrual cycles, this method is not recommended for contraception. However, many teens are unaware of ovulation patterns, fertile periods, and the lifespan of sperm, clear discussion of these issues can increase the teen's reproductive knowledge base.

The diaphragm is small, rubber dome molded onto a circular rim, which is fitted between the posterior fornix and the pubic bone to prevent the entry of sperm into the uterus. Used in combination with a spermicidal cream or jelly, the diaphragm provides both a mechanical and a chemical barrier. The device must be obtained from a health care agency and is not available in drugstores because it must be individually fitted. Use of the diaphragm requires some manipulation, which may be troublesome and inconvenient for the adolescent. The overall failure rate is approximately 12%. The diaphragm has become increasingly popular, however, because of the relative safety of this method over all other forms of contraception for the woman's health.

The U.S. Food and Drug Administration has recently approved a new barrier form of contraception, the cervical cap. This thimble-size device is held in place over the cervix by suction.

The condom is used to provide a mechanical barrier to the entry of sperm into the uterus. Most young adolescent boys likely attempt this method of contraception, and the peer-group sources of sex information usually include some description of the use of condoms. Condoms are recommended as a protection from STDs, but because the sheath covers only a portion of the skin area, protection is limited. The sheaths are made of rubber or plastic and are usually supplied in a rolled form, ready to be unrolled onto the erect penis. A small portion at the end of the sheath acts as a receptacle for the seminal fluid. The actual failure rate is approximately 10%.

Chemical contraceptives are readily available in drugstores without a prescription. In the form of sponges, creams, jellies, and foams, their use is relatively simple and inexpensive. These preparations contain nonoxynol 9, which kills and immobilizes sperm and may provide some protection against STDs. However, these chemical contraceptives must be applied immediately before coitus, may be considered "messy," and involve touching the genital area. The actual effectiveness varies widely depending on use technique. When foam is used with a condom, the effectiveness is nearly 100% and is as effective as oral contraceptives, with the added benefit of reducing transmission of STDs.

The female oral contraceptive pill prevents ovulation by chemically altering the usual endocrine cycle. Most forms contain estrogen, which raises the circulating level of this hormone early in the menstrual cycle. Because high levels of estrogen prevent the release of FSH by the pituitary gland, ovarian follicles are not stimulated to maturity, and ovulation is prevented. When progesterone is added to the estrogen preparation, the endometrium of the uterus is stimulated to develop as during a normal cycle, and cessation of taking the pill causes a menstrual period to occur, which stimulates the normal ovulatory cycle.

The pill has certain bothersome side effects for many women, including weight gain, nausea, breakthrough bleeding, and breast tenderness, all of which simulate a pregnant state. Other side effects include headaches, regression of gum tissue around the teeth, eye complications, and an increase in blood pressure. Serious side effects that have been substantiated are the risks of thromboembolic disease, heart disease, hypertension, and cancer. The pill is never recommended for an adolescent who has had prior blood-clotting problems or who has a family history of these problems. The risk of serious illness or death from the use of the pill is less than that expected from normal pregnancy and childbirth, and the pill is still considered as a safe, convenient, and reliable form of contraception. The adolescent who uses the pill enhances the safety of its use through regular evaluations of her health by her health care professional. This approach frequently involves annual examination before the prescription is refilled. Adolescents who find it difficult or impossible to remember to take the pill daily should use another form of contraception. The failure rate of the pill itself is approximately 0.6%, but most instances of failure result from forgetting to take it regularly.

Progestin-only hormonal injections have been used worldwide for many years as a safe and effective method of contraception. Injections of medroxyprogesterone acetate (Depo-Provera) inhibit ovulations, cause atrophy of the endometrium and thickening of the cervical mucus, and can cause vaginal pain. The effectiveness is similar to that for over-the-counter products and must be given every 90 days. This method provides long-acting contraception, causes amenorrhea or oligomenorrhea, and is an alternative for poor pill takers or to coitus-dependent methods. The use of injections has been associated with a decreased risk of pelvic inflammatory disease, possibly because of the barrier action of the thickened cervical mucus. One of the main disadvantages and most common reason for its discontinuation is menstrual irregularity and spotting (Khoiny, 1995).

Norplant is a Silastic capsule that is placed subdermally in the medial area of the upper arm, slowly releasing levonorgestrel into the bloodstream. This low-dose progestin provides contraception by thickening cervical mucus, reducing peristalsis of the fallopian tube, and causing the endometrium to be inhospitable for implantation. Ovarian follicles develop, and ovulation can occur. The actual failure rate is less than 1%, but of those pregnancies, 25% may be ectopic. Because ovarian estrogen is not suppressed, the endometrium will proliferate and shed unpredictably. Many adolescents find the unpredictable vaginal bleeding unacceptable. The capsules are relatively invisible and easy to place; removal can prove more challenging.

Pregnancy

When contraception fails or is not used and an unwanted pregnancy occurs, the problems for the adolescent become complex. Secondary prevention focuses on providing correct information about the options for continuing or terminating the pregnancy and referral to competent counselors or practitioners. Ideally, the adolescent, her family, and her partner should be involved in the decision of continuing or terminating a pregnancy; frequently, the adolescent makes the decision alone. Her partner may have been a one-time or casual sexual encounter, and she may be afraid to confide in her family because she has never told them that she is sexually active (see Multicultural Awareness box).

The adolescent of any age, but especially the young adolescent, who is pregnant needs skilled counseling and support during this stressful time; she should be strongly encouraged, but not forced to involve her parents. The adolescent who chooses to terminate the pregnancy should be referred to a clinic or a private physician who is experienced with adolescents, and follow-up counseling should be arranged. The adolescent who chooses to continue the pregnancy should be referred to a practitioner who can provide not only the physical monitoring and care during pregnancy, but also the emotional and developmental support that is essential for a positive experience with the pregnancy.

Table 16-3 outlines the developmental tasks of the pregnant adolescent. The nurse should be familiar with these developmental tasks and the possible range of their

MULTICULTURAL AWARENESS

Body Image Perception in Mexican-American Adolescents

Several studies have demonstrated the relationship between body image and self-esteem. A recent study used a self-report survey to obtain data regarding body image, self-esteem, and physical activity involvement of a group of Mexican-American adolescents. The researchers also measured body fat composition. Results demonstrated a positive relationship between body-image perception and self-esteem. Additionally, the study reported that a positive body image increases the likelihood of physical activity. Adolescents with the highest body fat composition had a more negative body image. Self-esteem was the strongest factor in predicting positive body-image scores. Therefore emphasis should be on building esteem and physical activity to promote a healthy body image.

Adapted from Guinn, B., Semper T., Jorgensen, L., & Skaggs, S. (2000). Body image perception in female Mexican-American adolescents. *Journal of School Health, 67,* 112-115.

manifestations to interact with the pregnant adolescent. Many physical risks to the pregnant adolescent and her baby can be reduced or recognized and problems adequately treated through appropriate prenatal care.

Coping–Stress-Tolerance Pattern

Each physical and psychological change of adolescence produces some stress. When all of these changes appear to be happening simultaneously, the stress is compounded. Other stresses include competition, whether in sports, relationships, or school achievement; frustration involved in attempting new activities and new ways of interacting; and the uncertainty of the future combined with the need to make major life decisions about future education and relationships. Although parents are involved in some decisions and changes, the adolescent must become decreasingly dependent on parents, believing that many choices must be made alone. Frequently, the need to separate from the parents and gain a sense of independence is expressed as the time spent away from home, alone in one's bedroom, or absorbed in music.

The adolescent may use egocentric behavior as a way of dealing with the stresses of increasing independence. The older adolescent is capable of using any defense mechanism that adults use. These forms of coping, when not used to excess, can be highly adaptive; they allow the adolescent to move away from the stress briefly to approach the stressor again, with a fresh outlook, possibly turning the stressful situation into a constructive learning experience. Other coping mechanisms of adolescence and ways that the nurse can help the teen use them in adaptive ways are listed in Box 21-4.

Box 21-4 Coping Mechanisms of Adolescents

COGNITIVE MASTERY

The adolescent attempts to learn as much as possible about the situation or stressor. This strategy is common for the adolescent with a chronic illness. The nurse can assist by clarifying any misinformation, sharing findings, and encouraging discussion of feelings, in addition to providing facts.

CONFORMITY

The adolescent attempts to be a mirror image of peers, which includes dress, language, attitudes, and actions. The nurse must respect this need for sameness and can also encourage discussion of feelings about differences between teens.

CONTROLLING BEHAVIOR

The adolescent must be in charge of some aspects of life and can no longer accept family and school rules without question as they did in the past. This need to control extends to health care. The nurse cannot simply give directions or instructions, but rather, present the options and allow the adolescent to state preferences. Together, they can work out an acceptable plan.

FANTASY

The younger adolescent may use this mental exercise more. The nurse can encourage the teen to use fantasy thinking to develop creative plans to deal with the stressful situation.

MOTOR ACTIVITY

Engaging in sports, dancing, running, or other high-energy activity can be an effective tension-releasing strategy. The nurse can encourage safe activities and offer information about community resources for these motor activities.

Depression

All adolescents feel sad at times. **Depression,** however, is an all-pervasive sadness that is present a majority of the time and is more common in adolescents than it is in school-age children. Nurses ask adolescents whether they are depressed as part of a routine history. Teens know what depression means and typically welcome the opportunity to discuss the situation.

Depression is suspected when the adolescent uses words such as *low, blue, hopeless, worried,* or *discouraged* and exhibits several of the following symptoms:

- Change in weight or eating habits (more or less intake)
- Insomnia or hypersomnia
- Loss of energy or fatigue
- Change in motor activity, such as from inactivity to constant motion
- Loss of interest in usual activities
- Out-of-proportion feelings of self-reproach or guilt
- Decline in school performance
- Preoccupation with death

Suicide

A severe maladaptive coping behavior often related to depression is suicide, which is the third leading cause of death in teens ages 15 to 19. However, many adolescents who are suicidal do not have the characteristics that are symptomatic of depression and can easily be overlooked when assessing suicidal risk. Between 1970 and 1980, nearly 50,000 young people between the ages of 15 and 24 committed suicide. The suicide rate among adolescents increased 40% during the last decade, whereas the rates for other age groups remained stable. This dramatic rise was primarily among boys (Friedman, 1998).

These figures may not reflect the full scope of this problem. Many actual suicides are likely classified as accidental deaths. Suicide attempts are not included in these statistics, although estimates show that 50 to 200 attempts occur for every successfully completed suicide. Suicide attempts are three to nine times more common in girls compared with boys, but boys succeed three times as often as do girls because male adolescents use more effective methods (American Academy of Pediatrics, 2000).

No single comprehensive theory adequately explains adolescent suicide. Many researchers believe suicide has developmental dimensions, primarily because it is such a significant problem during middle and late adolescence. Adolescence is certainly a period of considerable stress; when the adolescent's coping mechanisms and social supports are inadequate, suicide may be an outcome. Many researchers who study the problem are convinced that suicide during adolescence is not an impulsive or spontaneous act and is selected only after other problem-solving methods have failed. Problems that lead to suicide attempts begin in early childhood and frequently include one or more of the following:

1. One or both parents absent from the home because of separation, divorce, or death
2. Parent, relative, or close friend who attempted suicide
3. Extreme family conflict, neglect, or abuse
4. Living with a person who is not a biological parent
5. Frequent changes of residence
6. Parental alcoholism

These problems can cause the child great unhappiness and can lead to progressive isolation from satisfying social relationships. During adolescence, the long-standing problems of childhood continue or worsen while the new problems of adolescence are added. Unable to resolve these escalating difficulties, the adolescent develops a sense of helplessness and hopelessness. Before the suicide attempt, the adolescent perceives a rapid dissolution of any meaningful relationships. This circumstance may be precipitated by an event that is often mistaken as the reason for a suicide, such as a pregnancy, school failure, a family fight, or a terminated romance. The adolescent feels completely isolated. Because previous attempts to resolve the problems have failed, suicide is viewed as the only option.

Fortunately, some adolescent suicides can be prevented. Distressed adolescents tend to give clues, both verbally and nonverbally. Any single clue may mean nothing, but when several clues are noted, particularly in an adolescent facing difficult circumstances, they should be recognized as important warning signs. Clues of suicidal risk can be classified into three groups: (1) depressive equivalents, (2) verbal clues, and (3) behavioral clues (Jellinek & Snyder, 1998) (Box 21-5 outlines specific signs and symptoms of suicide).

Identifying and treating these clues as serious forms of communication are essential. The nurse should not be fearful of asking adolescents whether they have been contemplating suicide. If they have, then the teens may be relieved to be able to talk about it; if not, then asking them will not plant the idea. When the nurse suspects that an adolescent is suicidal, immediate referral should be made to a specialist in suicide intervention. A suicide threat should never be ignored. The adolescent who is in immediate danger of committing suicide should not be left alone.

Box 21-5 Clues of Suicidal Risk in Adolescents

Depressive equivalents are symptoms associated with depression: delinquency, aggressiveness, sexual promiscuity, running away, drug or alcohol use, headaches, abdominal pain, accident proneness, fatigue, slow speech, anorexia, sloppiness, and preoccupation with death.

Verbal clues are statements that indicate that the adolescent is thinking of suicide, such as, "This world would be better off without me" or "I won't be around anymore."

Behavioral clues are actions that indicate that the adolescent might be contemplating suicide: resigning from organizations, giving away cherished belongings, writing suicide notes, or exhibiting sudden changes in usual patterns of behavior (the good student who begins to fail or the quiet student who becomes aggressive).

A growing problem in some communities has been the phenomenon of "cluster" suicides (those that occur within a limited period and specific location or suicides in which victims share their thoughts together before the actual suicide). In response to the growing problem of youth suicide and the fear of cluster suicides, some schools have developed suicide-prevention programs. Nurses who work in junior and senior high schools play an important role in development, implementation, and evaluation of suicide-prevention programs. Treatment for the adolescent who attempts suicide involves psychotherapy for both the adolescent and the family.

Drug Use

Other maladaptive coping behaviors are excessive use of drugs of any kind. Teens often see adults using drugs to relieve tension; it is not surprising that they should adapt this socially sanctioned activity. (Drug use and misuse are discussed later in this chapter.)

Exposure to stress and the resulting need to cope is a lifelong process. The adolescent who learns adaptive ways to cope has a strong base on which to build in the adult years.

Values-Beliefs Pattern

During adolescence, young people acquire an intense sense of ideals—a system of values derived from what they believe might be, not necessarily what is. Teens occasionally align their beliefs with a particular religion, philosophical school of thought, social movement, or some other formal system that provides a basis for the formulation of the ideals. The adolescent uses these ideals in weighing decisions of right and wrong, best and worst, important and trivial. The ideal system can change drastically several times during adolescence, and this changing process provides the young person with different ranges of experience on which to base lasting choices in the future. Most adolescents assimilate the values and beliefs of their family systems; occasionally, their values are different from those of the family. When these new values conflict with parental ideas and beliefs about religion, social norms, and proper behavior, parents may demand certain behaviors, such as attending church services, that the teen believes are hypocritical. This conflict creates a great deal of tension between adolescents and parents.

The ability to think abstractly allows adolescents to consider many moral issues that they did not consider or question in the past; it is as though these issues never existed. Young people struggle with issues such as, "Is war justified?" "Is abortion moral?" "Is casual sex wrong?" "Is lying ever justified?" "Are the rich obligated to care for the poor?" Some of these issues form the basis of political and societal standards. When teens question these issues and discover that they cannot justify society's position, they can develop a sense of alienation.

Kohlberg's Theory

Kohlberg's research on the moral development of adolescents closely followed Piaget's work on cognitive development. Older children and young adolescents uphold a morality of law and order to determine right and wrong (Kohlberg, 1981).

As teens move into the transitional level, they begin questioning the status quo. Choice is based on emotions, and morality is situational. At this point, adolescents begin questioning societal standards and standing outside society while deliberating moral dilemmas, with no set principles for their choices and decisions.

Not all adolescents move through the successive stages of moral development, during either the adolescent or the young adult years. Even many adults operate at a conventional (law and order) stage of moral decision making. Adolescents pass through these stages at different rates and frequently discover that they and their friends, who used to think alike about certain moral questions, now differ in their assessment of a situation.

The adolescent who advances to the postconventional and principled level of moral development discovers that moral decisions are based on rights, values, and principles that are theoretically agreeable to a given society. These rights and values, however, can conflict with the stated laws and rules of the society. This person is able to understand and enter into contracts and agreements, recognizing the legal and moral points of view and seeing the conflict between the two. The teen, for example, may engage in peaceful protest demonstrations.

In the final stage of the postconventional and principled level (universal ethical principles) the person bases correct action on the recognition of the validity of the universal principles underlying laws and social agreements. When laws violate these principles, the individual follows the principle, not the law (Kohlberg, 1981).

Adolescents are able to advance through these stages because of their ability to think abstractly about the human effects of certain values and because of their growing experience with different ways of thinking. The school-age child has neither this wealth of experience nor the cognitive skills to view morality in this manner.

Gilligan, Lyons, and Hammer (1990) point out that Kohlberg's theory of moral development is based on research with an all-male population and does not necessarily reflect the development of girls. Girls move from the generic platform of "good is rewarded" to the ability to define "good" as a relational attribute of caring for others. The young female adolescent acquires the ability for self-sacrifice, seeing "good" as caring for the relationships in her life. As her moral reasoning matures, she achieves a balance between what is good for her and what is good for others in her network of relationships. Maturity in moral reasoning is situational and relational. Extensive research is currently being conducted on the topic of gender differences in adolescents' cognitive, emotional, and moral development. Through the process of evaluating this research, the nurse becomes aware of new findings in these areas to work effectively with all teens.

The nurse assists adolescents by being open to their ways of thinking about moral issues and offering opportunities for dialog between teens and adults and between teens and other young people.

Moral thinking is not necessarily reflected in action. An adolescent may think something is wrong and be able to explain this feeling. Under pressure from peers or other stresses, however, the adolescent may act contrary to this expressed belief. This difference between knowledge and action is present throughout life.

PATHOLOGICAL PROCESSES

Accidents

Accidents continue to be the leading cause of death and injury in the adolescent population, as is the case for all children over 1 year of age. The causes of these injuries differ, with nonmotor-vehicle accidents decreasing and motor vehicle-related accidents increasing sharply. The nonmotor-vehicle injuries, such as drowning, burns, and falls, have been discussed in previous chapters.

Sports

Sports activities are extremely important during adolescence; they provide a means for physical, moral, social, and personality development not afforded by any other activity. In addition to valuable exercise, sports activities provide experience in competition and team effort, mature, acceptable conflict resolution, and a way to develop self-esteem.

However, adolescents are particularly prone to sports

injuries because their coordination skills are not fully developed, their judgment is often immature and inadequate, the epiphyses are not yet closed, and the extremities are poorly protected by stabilizing musculature. Additionally, health care workers, who can provide consultation in prevention of sports-related injuries and offer immediate care to injured players, are frequently not a part of school athletic programs.

Sports-related injuries are likely to involve the head, spine, and extremities. Injuries to the head and brain are of special concern because of possible long-term neurological damage or death. Spinal cord injuries can also result in long-term disability or death; cervical spine injuries are the most common and are related to hyperflexion, hyperextension, or flexion compression of the vertebral column. Adolescents are prone to knee injuries because of the lack of strength and flexibility of the musculature and connective tissue surrounding the joint. Injuries tend to occur when the foot is locked to the ground or otherwise immobilized, and a lateral force causes the femur to adduct while the tibia rotates externally, with a medial hinging action between the femur and the tibia. Ankle injuries, particularly sprains, are also common. Foot injuries include puncture wounds, lacerations, and tendinitis.

The nurse practices primary prevention for sports injuries by advocating proper safety equipment and instruction, a sports-focused physical examination for all participants, and strict regulations prohibiting an injured player from further participation until appropriate rehabilitation is complete.

Violence

After teens pass their fifteenth birthday, their risk of dying as a result of violence greatly increases. The mortality rate for people between 15 and 19 years of age is three times higher than the rate is for people between ages 10 and 14 (Fig. 21-7).

Becoming increasingly independent, adolescents test the limits of authority, experiment with a variety of roles, question adult values and authority, and look to peers for affirmation. Teens also have a sense of invulnerability and a limited capacity for abstract thinking. These factors, combined with fluctuating self-esteem, depression, anger, poverty, economic privilege, and the breakdown of social controls, can lead to aggressive behavior and violence.

Many studies suggest that watching violent television programs is associated with a higher incidence of violent behaviors, especially among boys. The graphic violence in music videos and in films may also have an influence.

Nursing Interventions

Nurses challenge adolescents to examine the messages inherent in videos, songs, and television shows with a critical eye. Adolescents are encouraged to limit their

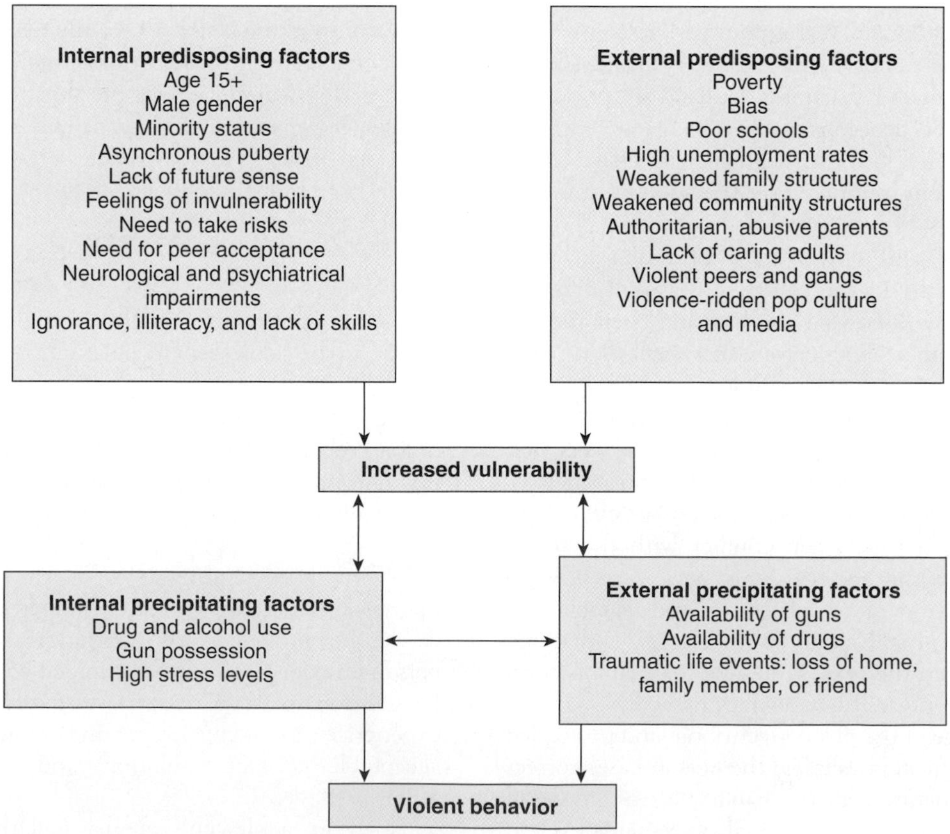

Fig. 21-7 Factors attributing to adolescent violence.

television viewing and maximize the quality of programs and movies that are viewed. Teens who are nurtured by caring adults have the best chance of successfully emerging from adolescence unscathed.

Mechanical Forces

Motor Vehicles

Adolescents become increasingly mobile as they become progressively independent. This increased mobility typically involves the use of motorcycles and other motor vehicles. Teen drivers are overrepresented in fatal crashes, with the death rate for 18-year-old drivers greater than that of any other age group. Beginning at age 13, teen passengers' death rates rise sharply and peak between ages 16 and 19. Nearly two thirds of these deaths occur in cars driven by an adolescent, and 45% to 60% of these accidents are alcohol related. Teens who drive must be aware of traffic regulations and observe the speed limit. Knowledge of limits and regulations, however, does not prevent the young person from surrendering to peer pressure in an attempt to set a record or perform other experimental maneuvers. The teen may use driving as an outlet for stress or as a way to assert increased independence.

Driver-education classes offered through the school can teach adolescents about proper driving techniques and regulations. Unfortunately, the availability of these classes may encourage more adolescents to drive at a younger age compared with those who depend on family members or private driving classes. Communities that have eliminated high school driver-education programs have seen a sharp decline in teen driving accidents. Each young person is evaluated on an individual basis regarding demonstrated level of responsibility, common sense, and ability to resist peer pressure. The teen and the parents should discuss these points and decide whether the adolescent is sufficiently responsible to drive. Age alone does not determine readiness for this significant responsibility.

Adolescents who ride motorcycles are also at risk for injury or death. Because head injury is a frequent outcome of motorcycle crashes, some states have passed strict laws requiring the use of a protective helmet by any motorcycle driver or passenger. These helmets laws have been effective in reducing motorcycle injury and death, but have met much resistance. Unfortunately, because of public pressure, some states have repealed their mandatory helmet laws and have seen a sharp rise in fatalities and injuries among motorcyclists who are not wearing helmets.

Nursing Interventions

Teens who have learned to drive still need some limits on automobile use. Some families have made use of a contract between the parents and the adolescent. This contract includes stipulations concerning safety, such as seat belt use and drinking and driving. The agreement may also include maintenance and upkeep issues as well. Parents and teens should negotiate these limits and periodically review and revise them based on an adolescent's safety record. Adolescents should continually, but gradually assume increasing responsibility for their actions, especially when the consequences can be serious injury or death in an motor-vehicle accident.

BIOLOGICAL AND BACTERIAL AGENTS

By adolescence, a person has built up immunity to many organisms that cause common childhood illnesses. However, the sexually active teen may come in contact with new groups of organisms through STDs, including gonorrhea; syphilis; genital warts (condyloma acuminatum); genital herpes virus type 2; Chlamydia, Trichomonas, and Candida infections; and human immunodeficiency virus (HIV) infection.

Many adolescents over age 15 are at least occasionally sexually active. Young people should be aware of the prevalence of these infections and the means of prevention, detection, diagnosis, and treatment. Prevention is accomplished primarily through avoidance of sexual contact with an infected person; however, a partner's state of infection is not always recognizable. Many teens have heard of the more common STDs, but may not realize that these diseases are practically epidemic in the young population (Holmes, 1999).

Viral STDs, such as venereal warts (human papillomavirus [HPV]) and herpes simplex virus type 2 (HSV-2), have been recognized as serious and, to date, incurable infections that are associated with the occurrence and transmission of HIV (Gortmaker, et al., 1996). HPV is recognized as an oncogenic factor in the evolution of cervical dysplasia (Emans & Goldsteen, 1998; Friedman, 1998).

CHEMICAL AGENTS

Drug Use

Drug abuse (substance abuse) does not start abruptly in adolescence and end before adulthood begins, but it is more widespread during the adolescent years (Box 21-6).

Box 21-6 Signs of Substance Abuse

Appetite loss	Muscle weakness
Blackouts	Nausea
Bleeding gums	Nervousness
Depression	Rash
Diarrhea	Seizures
Dyspnea on exertion	Somnolence
Faintness	Sore tongue
Hangover	Stomach pain
Headache	Taste loss
Indigestion	Tiredness
Insomnia	Vomiting
Memory loss	

From Payne, W. A., & Hahn, D. B. (1995). *Understanding your health* (4th ed.). St. Louis: Mosby.

School-age children may try alcohol or tobacco or other easily available drugs; the use of these substances has been starting at younger ages in recent years. Adults frequently use certain chemical substances to excess, but they are more likely to restrict their use to several agents rather than trying a variety of drugs as adolescents are likely to do. The following four factors should be considered when discussing the causes of substance abuse in teens:

1. Society is oriented to using chemicals such as medications, alcohol, and tobacco to feel better, look better, look and act more social, have more energy, stay awake, go to sleep, be "sexy," and so on. One evening of television viewing illustrates this orientation. Some of the most famous music, theater, and sports stars have openly modeled substance abuse for their fans.
2. Dysfunctional families (characterized by substance abuse, poor communication, rigidity, isolation, divorce, or physical or sexual abuse) produce a higher percentage of teens who are substance abusers (Heischober & Hoffman, 1997).
3. The individual teen may be predisposed to substance abuse because of depression, low self-esteem, pervasive anger, or excessive dependence.
4. The peer group becomes important in the middle teen years and may provide an overwhelming push toward drug use (Fishman, Bruner, & Adger, 1997).

Many adolescents use drugs once or on an infrequent basis; this is called experimental use. Other teens use drugs on a more regular basis, and a small percentage are compulsive users who are drug dependent.

Some of these agents are easy to obtain, whereas other agents require a major risk because of legal ramifications or places where the teen must go to obtain them. Ethnic, geographical, and socioeconomic variables also influence choice of substance among teens. For example, White urban middle-class teens are more likely to choose alcohol and marijuana as "gateway," or initial, substances. Rural and minority teens tend to use inhalants as gateway substances (Heischober & Hoffman, 1997).

Although drugs are usually taken for the pleasurable or positive effects, they can also produce many negative effects (see Research Highlights box).

research highlights

Alcohol and Marijuana Use by Students

A recent research study examined the patterns and predictors of the onset of alcohol and marijuana use. This was a longitudinal study in which 808 students from approximately age 10 until age 18 years were studied. Half of the group received a preventive intervention strategy in the first 2 years of the study. Participants were from relatively low-income and high-crime neighborhoods.

Results showed that at the age of 10.5 years, 25% of the students reported that they had tried alcohol and 3% had tried marijuana. By age 13 years, 64% had used alcohol and by age 18 years, 88% had used marijuana. Marijuana use did not increase as quickly. At age 13 years, only 13% had tried marijuana, with 50% of the students initiating use by age 18 years.

Initiation of alcohol use can be predicted by Asian-American ethnicity, parents' alcohol use norms, and alcohol use by close friends. Beginning the use of marijuana was linked to sex, ethnicity, and marijuana use by friends or siblings. Exposure to other people who use substances was a high risk factor for initiation and has implications for educational programs.

Results of this study underscore the need for early educational programs designed to help delay alcohol and marijuana initiation and help children learn to make healthy choices. Parents and friends must be proactive and make the family standards for use of these substances clear.

From Grunbaum, J. A., Lowry, R., Kann, L., & Pateman, B. (2000). Prevalence of health risk behaviors among Asian American/Pacific Islander high school students. *Journal of Adolescent Health, 27* (5), 322-330.

Nursing Interventions

Nurses must carefully assess their role in teenage drug use. If they believe that their role is to prevent any use of drugs, then the approach will be more rigid than it would be if the goal is to prevent regular drug use and dependence while accepting experimentation.

Primary preventive intervention for chemical use should start in the school-age years. Establishing an open dialogue among school-age children, their teachers, and the health care team is essential in providing openness and trust and these children can seek sound answers to their questions and discuss their concerns; of particular concern is the use that may be modeled in their homes. Nurses should discuss the underlying reasons that people, including their own parents, might use drugs to cope with stress and fear, discuss healthy alternatives that can be used for coping, and experience the use of these alternative methods in the school setting. Young teens must learn self-control skills and effective social skills to deal with peer pressure (Box 21-7). The use of alcohol and tobacco as a way of feeling "grown up" should be discussed, and children should be encouraged to discuss and consider behavior that is more indicative of being "grown up."

During the adolescent years, the health education program continues to inform teens of the hazards of drug misuse and abuse. Special attention is directed at the

Box 21-7 Ways to Cope with Peer Pressure

- Decide what you really think about the situation and stand up for your opinion.
- Say no. Say it over and over again, if necessary.
- Do not make excuses. Simply assert your opinion and repeat it, if necessary.
- Recruit a friend to support your refusal.

misuse of the socially sanctioned alcohol and tobacco products that are available to adolescents. The influence of health education on tobacco and alcohol use has not been confirmed as effective. Teens and children report, however, that drug education has influenced their decisions regarding the use of drugs, alcohol, and tobacco, and the related health hazards are accurately perceived by these groups that have been surveyed. The young person tends to view the adverse health effects as affecting the future, indicating an intention to "worry about that later."

Primary prevention is focused on providing information to help the young person make a responsible decision about drug use before experimentation. Age at first use is a critical risk factor for the development of substance abuse problems. The earlier the experimentation with drugs begins, the more likely it will be that this teen is dealing with a dysfunctional family or social environment (Heischober & Hoffman, 1997). Secondary prevention includes watching for indications that a particular adolescent may be using or abusing a drug (see Box 21-6).

The nurse who suspects that a teen is using or misusing drugs approaches the topic in a nonjudgmental way and attempts to determine the individual's motivation and extent of use. These two factors will help the nurse make the best decision about referral for treatment or more information.

Because drug use is so common in the adolescent population, the nurse routinely asks school-age children and adolescents about drug use. The young person may choose to withhold information, especially when this is the first encounter with the nurse. Conversely, the adolescent may be relieved to know that the topic of drugs is acceptable in the health care setting and may have been wanting to discuss the subject with a knowledgeable adult.

Tobacco Use

The nurse asks adolescents about their tobacco use habits, occupational history, and general respiratory environment at both the workplace and the home. "Smokeless" tobacco, such as snuff and chewing tobacco, is becoming popular among boys. Surveys have shown that from 8% to 30% of high school boys are regular users. Smokeless tobacco has been shown to cause oral-pharyngeal cancer. Although the teen may not have used tobacco for long or worked in an environment in which there is asbestos or other respiratory carcinogens, identifying and informing the adolescent of these risks is important.

Nursing Interventions

The nurse's primary prevention focus is on helping tobacco users stop and keeping nonusers from starting. Adolescents begin using tobacco for a variety of reasons: to appear older, to surrender to peer pressure, or to imitate adult role models. Antismoking discussions should start during the preadolescent years and continue through adolescence. One of the nurse's most important roles in helping young people stop smoking is to serve as a role model. Nurses who smoke contradict all the media coverage and scientific research that point to the physical harm of smoking. Nurses cannot persuade individuals to stop smoking when they have failed to do so themselves. Research indicates that fear tactics, nagging, preaching, and threats are ineffective in convincing people of any age to stop smoking. Basic fear tactics have proved to be ineffective in changing smoking behavior; serious efforts are currently being made to create a social climate in which smoking is an unacceptable behavior.

The nurse helps teens to make rational decisions about tobacco use and occupational exposure to carcinogenic agents in several ways:

1. Conduct educational programs that unemotionally detail the known hazards of tobacco use.
2. Provide adolescents with educational material that further explains the health hazards of tobacco use or high-risk occupations.
3. Provide specific measures for adolescents who desire to stop using tobacco or decrease occupational risk factors.

Many teens who want to stop using tobacco products lack the information to help themselves stop. Nurses must be familiar with the antismoking resources in their communities so appropriate referrals can be made.

Cancer

Radiation and temperature carcinogenic agents have been discussed in previous chapters. Adolescents are affected by many of the same cancers as are younger children, such as leukemia, osteogenic sarcoma, lymphomas, and central nervous system tumors.

Adolescents begin to be at risk for some of the more typical adult-onset cancers because of tobacco use and exposure to carcinogens at a workplace.

Older adolescents are entering the period of their lives during which cancer of the reproductive and related organs is more common. For girls in their teens, the focus is on cervical and breast cancer; for boys, testicular cancer is the area of concern.

Peak incidence of breast and cervical cancer is during middle age and is actually rare in the teenage years. Breast self-examination (BSE), which has been highly recommended for over 30 years, has recently been questioned as a routine practice for most adolescents. The extremely small incidence of breast cancer in teens, weighed against the anxiety that is caused when a girl discovers a "normal" lump in her breast, has caused some health care providers to deemphasize this practice for teens. Because a genetic predisposition exists for breast cancer, the nurse inquires into family history with the adolescent. Certainly, any adolescent with a positive family history should be taught BSE.

HEALTH TEACHING Performing Breast Self-Examination

Breast self-examination (BSE) should be performed once a month, so you become familiar with the usual appearance and feel of your breasts. This regimen makes noticing any changes in the breast from 1 month to another easier. Finding a change from "normal" is the main idea behind a BSE. The best time to perform a BSE is 2 or 3 days after your period ends, when your breasts are least likely to be tender or swollen.

Here is how to do it:

1. Stand in front of a mirror. Inspect both breasts for anything unusual, such as any discharge from the nipples, puckering, dimpling, or scaling of the skin.

The next two steps are designed to emphasize any change in the shape or contour of your breasts. As you perform these actions, you should be able to feel your chest muscles tighten.

2. While watching closely in the mirror, clasp your hands behind your head and press your hands forward.
3. Next, press your hands firmly on your hips and bow slightly toward the mirror as you pull your shoulders and elbows forward.

Some women perform the next part of the examination in the shower. Fingers gliding over soapy skin make concentrating on the texture underneath easier (Fig. 1).

4. Raise your left arm. Use three or four fingers of your right hand to explore your left breast firmly, carefully, and thoroughly. Beginning at the outer edge, press the flat part of your fingers in small circles, moving the circles slowly around the breast. Gradually work toward the nipple. Be sure to cover the entire breast. Pay special attention to the area between the breast and the armpit, including the armpit itself. Feel for any unusual lump or mass under the skin (Fig. 2).
5. Gently squeeze the nipple and look for a discharge. Repeat the exam on your right breast.

Steps 4 and 5 should be repeated lying down (Fig. 3). While lying flat on your back, place your left arm over your head and a pillow or folded towel under your left shoulder. This position flattens the breast and makes examining the breast easier. Use the same circular motion described in step 4. Repeat on your right breast.

1

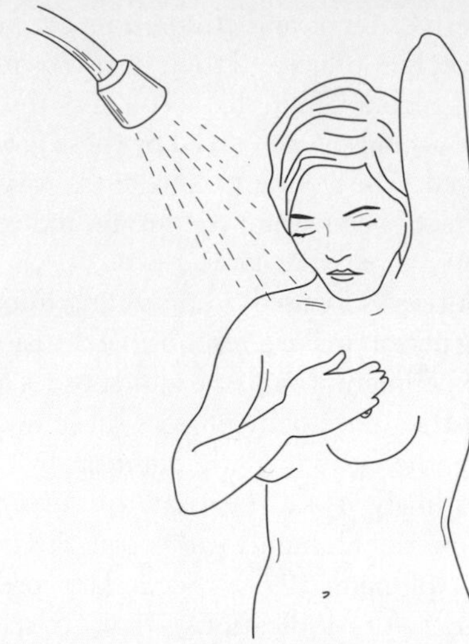

2

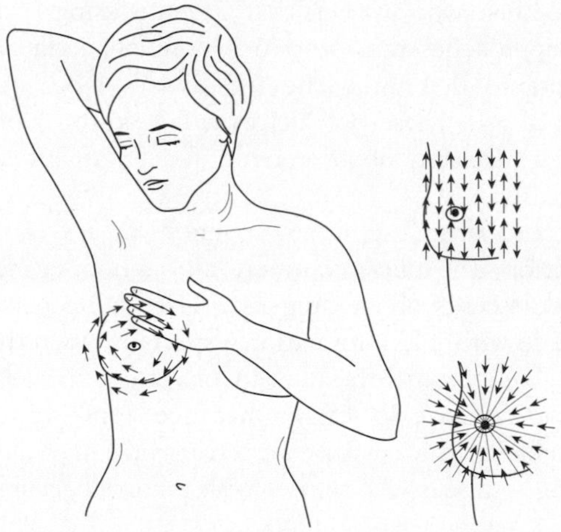

3

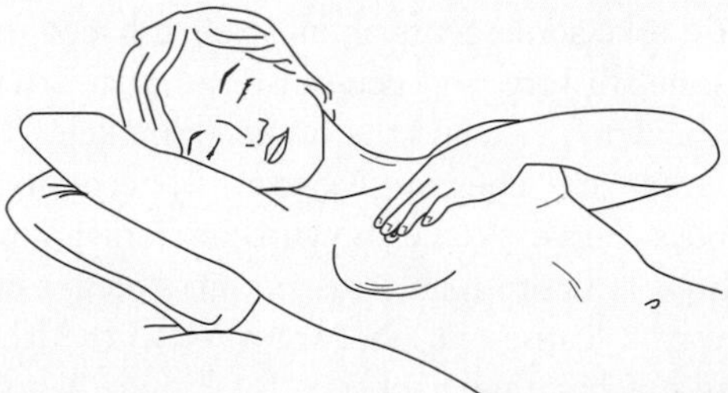

From Lowdermilk, D. L., Perry, S. E., & Bobak, I. M. (1999). *Maternity nursing* (5th ed.). St. Louis: Mosby.

After maturation of the breasts, girls can be taught how to examine themselves for early signs of cancer. Regular examination of the breasts should follow each menstrual period. BSE can be taught during the physical assessment, but films and group discussions are helpful in reinforcing the importance and acceptability of this self-care responsibility (see Health Teaching box). The nurse reminds girls to make an immediate appointment with their health care provider for a breast examination if they feel a breast mass.

Cervical cancer can be detected through a Pap smear; that is, a procedure performed during a pelvic examination to obtain and examine cells from the uterine cervical os. Sexually active girls should have a Pap test performed annually. The American College of Obstetricians and

Box 21-8 Factors That Increase the Risk for Cervical Cancer

- Sexual intercourse before age 20
- Multiple sexual partners
- A sexual partner who has had many partners
- Any history of STDs
- Any exposure to exogenous hormones (DES *in utero* or oral contraceptives)
- History of smoking or current smoker

Adapted from Emans, S. J., & Goldsteen, D. P. (1998). *Pediatric and adolescent gynecology* (4th ed.). Boston: Little, Brown.

Gynecologists recommends annual examinations to begin by age 18, even when the young woman is not sexually active. Adolescent girls are often reluctant to have these checkups because of fear of pain, embarrassment, and the public acknowledgment of being sexually active. By explaining the purpose of the examination, the Pap test, and cultures to teens, and by strongly encouraging them to comply with this preventive measure, the nurse alleviates these concerns. The nurse can reassure the girl that the examination will be performed gently and with sensitivity and that the sensation is one of pressure rather than pain (Box 21-8).

Testicular cancer is one of the most common cancers in men between the ages of 20 and 35. The men themselves first discover most testicular cancers. When treated early, the chances for a total cure are excellent. Adolescent boys should learn to do a testicular self-examination and continue this practice once a month for the rest of their lives.

The best time for self-examination of the testes is immediately after a bath or shower. While each testicle is rolled gently between the thumb and fingers, any abnormal lumps should be noted. The epididymis, located at the back of each testicle, should be identified and not erroneously labeled as an abnormal lump.

Although most adolescents tend to think that they will never have a cancerous lesion, the nurse introduces this concern and teaches the common methods of self-examination and the warning signs of cancer. This is an excellent time to begin a lifelong habit of self-examination.

SOCIAL PROCESSES

Community and School

The school setting provides many important positive experiences for the adolescent: contact with peers, intellectual stimulation, and resources. Schools can also provide negative experiences: overwhelming competition, exposure to drug sellers and users, and peer pressure to rebel against parents, teachers, and other authorities.

Adolescents must experience some degree of success in their academic lives. Young adolescents are particularly vulnerable to slumps in relation to school achievement, primarily because they are dealing with massive changes in their bodies, new social accomplishments, new school situations, and the need to establish new peer relationships. Adolescents' uncertainty about their abilities and their identities is significant, whether it causes poor school performance or correlates with other events with no cause-and-effect relationship. Teens who excel in school can find themselves in a particularly uncomfortable relationship with peers who envy their academic success. Failure to achieve in school may result from the overwhelming need to experience group approval.

Additionally, teens frequently experience conflicting messages about what is considered adequate achievement in school. The teachers in a junior high or middle school may define achievement in ways that are slightly different from those that the child experienced in elementary school. Parents may begin to express increased concern as adolescents approach the stage when grades are important for college entry. Students who are not college bound must develop future life goals in a system that has been ineffective in developing vocational and skill training alternatives.

Teachers and parents can contribute significantly to the nurse's understanding of the total situation of adolescents, and together, they may be able to distinguish a serious problem from one that is within the range of normal adolescent behavior.

Culture and Ethnicity

The family's cultural and ethnic influences that operate throughout childhood continue into adolescence. The adolescent may question or reject these influences more strongly than does a younger counterpart, but the effect, especially when ethnically based, still exists because others can see it. Adolescents with immigrant parents must negotiate two cultures, languages, and sets of expectations. Essentially, these adolescents live a double life, resulting in increased stress that can pervade all aspects of their lives.

The "**emancipated minor**" provision of certain laws recognizes that some adolescents become independent from their families at an early age and assume adult responsibilities. An emancipated minor is an adolescent who has not reached the standard legal age for certain activities, such as consenting to marriage or seeking certain kinds of health or illness care, but who is permitted to accept full responsibility for these decisions because the individual is economically and emotionally separate from the family.

As a separate segment of society, adolescents have a great deal of influence on the rest of society. Advertisers recognize the economic influence of this group and direct much of their strongest propaganda to them. The adolescent is mobile and frequently controls the money for clothing and entertainment needs and desires. This control may result from working or being given an allowance, with few guidelines on ways to allocate it for needs versus desires. Adolescents are particularly vulnerable to advertising that stresses looking or acting similar to other teens or to famous role models. As discussed, adolescents are peer oriented and have an aversion to being different.

Young people from a minority group have a particular problem in relation to the culture of adolescence. These teens may desire strongly to "fit into" the predominant adolescent culture, which in society is often middle class, White, and Protestant, and they may be able to meet one or two of these criteria, but be unable to meet the others because of economics, different appearance, or different education and experiences. Advertising does not emphasize the economically depressed or ethnic-looking model, and the teen's peers are trying every means possible to look and act similar to the majority adolescent. Further pressure comes from their own minority culture when they emulate the majority culture in ways that the family views as offensive to their ideas and beliefs.

The nurse is constantly aware of the current adolescent norms of behavior and accepts the teen's real need to emulate the chosen role models. Some effective health-promotion campaigns, such as cessation of smoking, have used famous role models. The nurse uses a similar strategy in promoting health care ideas to individual adolescents.

Legislation

Many laws and regulations are aimed at the adolescent and deal with the minimal age at which the adolescent may assume adult responsibilities. The traditional rationales for these restrictions are that teens lack the experience, perspective, and judgment to recognize and avoid choices that might be detrimental to them and that teens require protection against exploitation by unscrupulous persons. A question that is frequently raised when considering minimal age and the emancipated or "legally mature" minor is whether strict age criteria are appropriate for any adolescent, particularly because development is variable and experiences are diverse.

Minimal-age requirements for driving a motor vehicle and purchasing firearms, alcohol, and cigarettes affect the health of adolescents, not because these agents cause illness or death to every user, but rather, because of the increased risk of illness or accidents related to the use (and definitely the misuse) of these agents. These restrictions are questioned periodically by groups of adolescents and adults, but have not stirred the same emotional controversy as have the restrictions related to health care and information.

The restrictions that have recently been questioned most strongly deal with issues related to sexual activity. The Supreme Court of the United States has affirmed the right of all individuals to have equal access to contraceptive services, regardless of age or marital status, and the right of a minor to make decisions governing pregnancy termination. Despite these and other court rulings, the federal government, through certain members of Congress, has attempted to deny funding to agencies that provide family planning (contraceptive services and abortion) to any person under age 16 unless the parents are notified in writing by the agency. Advocates of this restrictive approach insist that teens are incapable of making these decisions by themselves. Opponents of this parental notification requirement insist that adolescents are not going to decrease their sexual activity if these resources are withheld, but will instead seek this information and help from unsafe, irresponsible sources. The consequences could be increased unwanted pregnancies, with all the physical, emotional, spiritual and psychological risks, and increased illegal and likely improperly managed abortions. The adolescent is trapped in the midst of these controversies.

The nurse may also feel trapped by the controversy and unsure as to the best way to deal with individual cases. An important point to remember is that the laws related to these sexual issues are in flux. The staff of any health care setting that deals with adolescents must develop policies that are compatible with its knowledge of adolescent development, ideal and actual parental roles, the range of community attitudes toward teens, and the services that are available to them.

Economics

The identification with peers, the essence of self-image during adolescence, includes dressing alike, having similar possessions, doing the same activities, and going to the same places. All of these activities require a fund of economic resources. Parents may give young adolescents and some older adolescents an allowance that covers these desires. Many adolescents work to have money for these expenses, and some, especially older adolescents, support themselves entirely. Money can be a major conflict between parents and teens. Parents may think that they should have the power to decide how their child spends money. Adolescents may believe, just as strongly, that they know the best ways to allocate resources and determine the amount of money they need.

Adolescents vary greatly in the ability to manage money. Ideally, parents and adolescents should negotiate economic questions, with the parents becoming less controlling as the teen gains more experience and expertise in these matters. Unfortunately, the emotional issue of holding on versus letting go frequently interferes with economic discussions.

Some adolescents work not out of need for money, but because they view work as a means of gaining experience and independence. Increased status among peers may also be a reason to work.

Health Care Delivery System

Many health care resources are theoretically available to the adolescent. A basic problem in availability is that young people may be unaware of all of their choices. Teens can continue to see their child health care provider in a pediatric center as they did as children, but this setting is usually rejected because of the young-child atmosphere at most of these centers.

innovative practice

Boston College Health Fair

A health fair is a combination of intertwining relationships among students, faculty, environment, and community. The purpose of a health fair is to enhance lifestyle choices and health promotion in an individual by encompassing aspects of their physical, mental, and spiritual well being. Creating a health fair in a university setting directs health education toward young adult health issues and concerns. In addition to providing university students with information on healthy behaviors and strategies, a health fair also provides information on disease prevention and health promotion. The primary goal is to teach correct and positive health techniques to a younger age population, enhancing healthy lifestyle choices. Because current health behaviors have a direct influence on future diseases, targeting education about health screenings and early detection is invaluable to this population.

The greatest amount of work and planning is directed at establishing the health care needs and issues of the college-age population. At the Boston College's Health Fair, each individual who attends the health fair completes a five-page health questionnaire. This health questionnaire is the fundamental basis for the planning and development of each individual health fair (the answers on the questionnaire are incorporated into the topics at the health fair). The objective data collected from the questionnaire include general health-related questions, the vendors that were visited by the individual and the reasons for which the person visited those particular vendors, which vendors were most or least helpful, and recommendations for the following year. A comment section is also included to encourage individuals to give their opinions on health concerns and identify health-related issues they believe are most prevalent within their population.

The Boston College Graduate Nurses Association (GNA) sponsors an annual health fair with this specific purpose. The Health Fair of the Millennium, held in May of 2000, was designed to include holistic health practices that encompass the full essence of the individual. In addition to traditional philosophies of health-promotion behaviors, new alternative approaches were also included.

One of the most important aspects to consider when developing a health fair is the identification of individuals willing to coordinate the fair and the designation of a Chairperson who acts as a team leader and oversees the group's progress. Each individual focuses on a designated area in which the person has a special interest. This individual will then act as a liaison between the specific volunteer group of interest and the Boston College health fair committee. For example, an individual may choose to coordinate a booth on smoking cessation. This person contacts appropriate company representatives and acquires available printed literature to be accessible at the fair. The Boston College GNA was able to coordinate the *Smokefree Communities Project* with the local Department of Public Health, which provided assistance at the fair. In return, certified smoking cessation counselors volunteered their time and provided printed brochures to those who attended the health fair.

In analyzing the previous years' student health questionnaires, stress and stress-related symptoms were identified as a major concern of the student population. Ideas pertaining to stress reduction and management, it was decided, would be beneficial. A Boston College Graduate School of Nursing professor, who is also codirector of the Medical Symptom Reduction Program at the Mind-Body Medical Institute in Boston, provided information on stress-symptom analysis and biofeedback. The students actively participated in a stress-symptom survey in which they identified stressors directly related to activities of daily living. This activity heightened students' awareness of physical and psychological symptoms associated with stress and common relaxation techniques effective in alleviating various symptoms.

Other booths at Boston College's Health Fair of the Millennium were chosen to represent both female and male members of the student body, community safety and awareness, cultural diversity, and alternative lifestyles. The areas of interest included aromatherapy, domestic violence, testicular and breast cancer screening techniques, skin analysis, blood pressure screening, body fat analysis, anemia and blood glucose testing, eating disorder awareness, yoga and Tai Chi, massage demonstrations, and spinal nerve stress tests. The Boston College community enthusiastically supported the health fair by donating space, food, and beverages, and audio-visual equipment used by various vendors to display their information. Undergraduate nursing students volunteered clinical time to measure blood pressure, faculty members volunteered time to supervise and answer any questions, and members of the Graduate School of Nursing hosted booths and monitored the efficiency of the health fair.

In summary, an efficient and informative health fair benefits the entire school and surrounding community in a holistic manner. Focusing on holistic well being encourages positive health behaviors for all individuals and a healthy environment. The initial process takes a great deal of time and dedication in planning, but with effective communication and available resources, the effort evolves into a productive and valuable learning experience for all who attend and participate.

Courtesy Christine Holborow and Dawnmarie C. Pelrine. Christine Holborow, MS, RN, CS, is a recent graduate of the Boston College Graduate School of Nursing and is currently practicing as a geriatric nurse practitioner for New England Geriatrics in the Boston area. Dawnmarie C. Pelrine, MS, RN, CS, is a recent graduate of Boston College Graduate School of Nursing and is currently practicing as an adult nurse practitioner in an acute care cardiology practice at Massachusetts General Hospital in Boston, Massachusetts.

School health programs are frequently available in junior high, high school, and college. Some of these programs are limited to mass screenings for certain high-risk physical diseases and emergency care. Other settings offer a more comprehensive program of health promotion.

Adolescent-focused clinics are available in many communities through both public and private agencies and, most recently, within schools. These clinics serve only adolescents, and the staff is oriented to the needs of this age group. Adolescents frequently have a higher sense of comfort in these settings compared with those in which young children or adults are also served.

Adolescents can also make use of services such as family planning clinics. These settings may designate certain days and hours for younger individuals, whereas other facilities integrate teens into the adult-oriented protocols. The pregnant adolescent typically finds prenatal care in a basically adult-focused setting, although more adolescent-specific programs are being developed. The basic physical needs of the pregnant adolescent may be the same as those of the pregnant adult, but the psychological needs are different and should be approached by a professional who has a comprehensive knowledge of adolescent development and responses to stress.

NURSING INTERVENTIONS

The adolescent is a rapidly changing individual. The nurse who works in an adolescent-focused practice should be well prepared in both child and adult health-promotion strategies, primarily because these overlap in the adolescent years. The nurse should have a thorough understanding of adolescent development and a recognition of the inherent dignity of each adolescent as a person.

The adolescent tends to be fearful about the procedures or possible diagnosis during a clinic or office visit, but also must be in control of the situation. These conflicting feelings can be difficult to manage simultaneously. By establishing that the adolescent is a partner with the health care providers in promoting good health and screening for health risks, the nurse can facilitate the adolescent's functioning in a health care setting.

The adolescent's questions should be answered thoroughly and honestly. Because in many instances the adolescent is hesitant to voice concerns, information should be offered even when questions are not asked. An effective approach to learning about a particular adolescent's concerns, especially about potentially embarrassing or stressful topics, is to say, "Many teenagers ask me about [a topic]. Have you ever thought about this?" or "A lot of young people want to know about [a topic]."

Asking direct questions is important, even about sensitive topics: "Have you ever thought about suicide?" "Are you depressed?" "Are you sexually active?" "Do you use birth control?" Vague or circuitous questions imply a discomfort or lack of understanding and may cause the adolescent to be equally vague when responding.

Correct anatomical terms and descriptions of laboratory tests, disease processes, and possible outcomes are essential components in treating adolescents as individuals who are capable of being responsible for their own bodies. Nurses should avoid stereotyping adolescents because of their dress or behavior. People are unique individuals, despite striving to be similar to their peers.

Nurses should encourage, but never force, adolescents to share their health care concerns with their parents. Nurses must clearly establish to themselves, the adolescent, and the parents that the adolescent is the client and that family members are viewed as supportive to the client, but not necessarily privy to all the information exchanged between the nurse and the client.

SUMMARY

Adolescence is a period of dramatic change. At times, these teens appear and act as though they are children, and at other times, they act as though they are adults, but usually they are in a category by themselves. This dichotomy can challenge the most experienced nurse. The many theories about adolescent development should form a foundation by which the nurse views each adolescent as a unique, dynamic individual.

REFERENCES

American Academy of Pediatrics, Committee on Adolescence. (2000). Suicide and suicide attempts in adolescence. *Pediatrics, 105*, 871-874.

American Psychiatric Association. (1994). *Diagnostic and statistical manual of mental disorders* (4th ed.). Washington, DC: The Association.

Armstrong, M. L., & McConnell, C. (1994). Tattooing in adolescents, more common than you think: The phenomenon and risks. *Journal of School Nursing, 10*, 22-29.

Armstrong, M. L. & Murphy, K. P. (1997). Tattooing: Another adolescent risk behavior warranting health education. *Applied Nursing Research, 10*, 181-189.

Chinn, P. L. (1979). *Child health maintenance: Concepts in family-centered care* (2nd ed.). St. Louis: Mosby.

Elkind, D. (1985). Egocentrism redux. *Developmental Review, 5*, 218.

Emans, S. J., & Goldsteen, D. P. (1998). *Pediatric and adolescent gynecology* (4th ed.). Boston: Little, Brown.

Erikson, E. H. (1993). *Childhood and society* (35th anniversary ed.). New York: W. W. Norton.

Erikson, E. H. (1997). *The life cycle completed*. New York: W. W. Norton.

Friedman, S. B. (1998). *Comprehensive adolescent health care* (2nd ed.). St. Louis: Quality Medical.

Fish, C., & Nies, M. A. (1996). Health promotion needs of students in a college environment. *Public Health Nursing, 13*, 104.

Fishman, M., Bruner, A., & Adger, H. (1997). Substance abuse among children and adolescents. *Pediatrics in Review, 18*, 394-403.

Gilligan, C., Lyons, N., & Hammer, T. (1990). *Making connections: The relational worlds of adolescent girls at Emma Willard school*. Cambridge, MA: Harvard University Press.

Gortmaker, S. L., Must, A., Sobol, A. M., Peterson, K., Colditz, G. A., & Dietz, W. H. (1996). Television viewing as a cause of increasing obesity among children in the United States, 1986-1990. *Archives of Pediatric and Adolescent Medicine, 150*, 356.

Greydanus, D. E., & Sloane, M. A. (1997). Disorders of the ears, eyes, nose and throat. In A. D. Hoffman, & D. E. Greydanus, *Adolescent medicine*. Stamford, CT: Appleton and Lange.

Grunbaum, J. A., Lowry, R., Kann, L, & Pateman, B. (2000). Prevalence of health risk behaviors among Asian American/Pacific Islanders high school students. *Journal of Adolescent Health, 27*(5), 322-330.

Guinn, B., Semper, T., Jorgensen, L., & Skaggs, S. (2000). Body image perception in female Mexican-American adolescents. *Journal of School Health, 67*, 112-115.

Guyton, A. C. (1996). *Textbook of medical physiology* (8th ed.). Philadelphia: W. B. Saunders.

Heischober, B. S., & Hoffman, A. D. (1997) Substance Abuse. In A. D. Hoffman, & D. E. Greydanus, *Adolescent medicine*. Stamford, CT: Appleton and Lange.

Hoffman, A. D. (1997). Adolescent growth and development. In A. D. Hoffman, & D. E. Greydanus, *Adolescent medicine*. Stamford, CT: Appleton and Lange.

Holmes, K. K. (1999). *Sexually transmitted diseases* (3rd ed.). St. Louis: McGraw-Hill.

Jellinek, M. S., & Snyder, J. B. (1998). Depression and suicide in children and adolescents. *Pediatrics in Review, 19*, 255-264.

Khoiny, F. E. (1995). Use of Depo-Provera in teens. *Journal of Pediatric Health Care, 10* (5), 195-201.

Kligh, W. J. (1998). Childhood obesity. *Pediatrics in Review, 19*, 312-315.

Kohlberg, L. (1981). *The philosophy of moral development*. San Francisco: Harper & Row.

Kreipe, R. E., & Dukarm, C. P. (1999). Eating disorders in adolescents and older children. *Pediatrics in Review, 20*, 410-420.

Lowdermilk, D. L., Perry, S. E., & Bobak, I. M. (1999). *Maternity nursing* (5th ed.). St. Louis: Mosby.

Marina, D. D., & King, J. C. (1981). *Pediatric Clinics of North America, 27*, 125.

Marshall, W. A., & Tanner, J. M. (1969). *Archives of Disease in Childhood, 44*, 291.

Neinstein, S. (1996). *Adolescent health care: A practical guide* (2nd ed.). Baltimore: Urban & Schwarzenberg.

Payne, W. A., & Hahn, D. B. (1995). *Understanding your health* (4th ed.). St. Louis: Mosby.

Perrin, E. C. (1996). Pediatricians and gay and lesbian youth. *Pediatrics in Review, 17*, 311-317.

Pruitt, D. B. (1999). *Your adolescent*. New York: Harper Collins.

Reider, B. (1996). *Sports medicine, the schoolage athlete*. Philadelphia: W. B. Saunders.

Report of the Joint National Committee on the prevention, detection, evaluation and treatment of high blood pressure. (1997). *Archives of Internal Medicine, 157*, 2413-2446.

Spear, B. (1996). Adolescent growth and development. In V. I. Ricker, *Adolescent nutrition assessment and management*. New York: Chapman & Hall.

U.S. Department of Health and Human Services. (2000). *Healthy people 2010*. Washington, DC: U.S. Government Printing Office.

Wong, D. L., Hockenberry-Eaton, M., Wilson, D., Winkelstein, M. L., Ahmann, E., & Divito-Thomas, P. A. (1999). *Whaley and Wong's nursing care of infants and children* (6th ed.). St. Louis: Mosby.

Chapter 22

ELIZABETH C. KUDZMA

Young Adult

objectives

After completing this chapter, the nurse will be able to:

- Identify the attitudes, behaviors, and habits that regulate the lifestyles of young adults.
- Identify tasks that are consistent with the adult maturity achieved during this period.
- Differentiate the disease processes that affect the "younger" young adult and the "older" young adult.
- Describe the specific health requirements of the young adult.
- Analyze the cultural and ethnic risk factors that affect young adults.
- Identify the physiological, psychological, and environmental factors that contribute to health concerns for young adults.
- List the occupational hazards that infringe on the young adult's welfare.
- Describe the nurse's role in reducing the rate of unintentional pregnancies in young adult women.
- State the ways in which the nurse can help reduce the risks that are associated with young adult behaviors of smoking, alcohol consumption, and drug use.
- Differentiate the nursing roles in preventive intervention for healthy young adults in home and community environments.
- Delineate the specific nursing interventions that can help ameliorate the effects of environmental factors that impinge on the health of young adults.

key terms

Achievement-Oriented Stress
Aerobic Exercise
Basal Metabolic Rate
Breast Self-Examination
Coronary Artery Disease
Environmental Tobacco Smoke
Epstein-Barr Virus
Genetic Impairment
Genital Herpes Virus
Hepatitis B
Human Immunodeficiency Virus
Human Papilloma Virus
Hypertension
Infertility
Maternal Mortality
Papanicolaou (Pap) Smear
Postconventional Level of Moral Reasoning
Rubella
Stress
Sun Exposure
Testicular Self-Examination

THINK About It

Assessing College Drinking Behaviors

You are the clinic director and nurse practitioner at a small liberal arts college. In addition to seeing students for various health issues during the academic year, you also run a number of health-promotion and health-prevention programs for the college. Mary, a 19-year-old freshman, has generally been a good student, easily making the adjustment to living away from home during her first 2 months in the dormitory. She comes to you because she had an episode that frightened her last weekend. On Saturday night, she was at a party at a private residence in a rural wooded setting away from the campus. Many people attended the party, most of whom were college students; many were from her dormitory. She remembers consuming five or six alcoholic drinks; however, any memory after midnight is missing. She woke up in a fellow female student's dormitory room without any memory of leaving the party or returning to the dormitory. She was able to piece together information from her friends, who told her that she consumed at least nine alcoholic drinks that night and that she left the party with others who were returning to the dormitory, but were not the friends with whom she had been seen all evening. She is concerned that she may have been drugged or that she may be having memory lapses. Assessment of her use of alcohol in the past reveals that she can recount at least four occasions during which she drank more than seven drinks at a party or family gathering. She describes her family as "social drinkers." After her graduation from high school last June, she reports, she was involved in a minor car accident that might have been related to the fact that she had consumed at least three drinks that afternoon.

1. Do you believe that Mary has a problem with drinking?
2. As what kind of an alcohol user would you classify her?
3. What kind of physical symptoms might assist you in making a determination that Mary has a drinking problem?
4. What kinds of physical examination and observation techniques might be helpful?
5. How do you establish appropriate therapeutic communication that would enable Mary to voice her genuine concerns?
6. Do you know what types of community resources and treatment facilities are located in your area or state that might help Mary?
7. What kinds of monitoring and follow-up mechanisms might be put in place to assist Mary in keeping her behavior consistent with any treatment plan?

The young adult period encompasses the ages between 18 to 35 years, a time that ranges from the end of adolescence to the beginning of middle adulthood. The major task of this period is preparing for the assumption of adult responsibilities, rights, and privileges.

AGE AND PHYSICAL CHANGES

Young adults make up a diverse segment of the population. The young adult period is a time of many physical and emotional changes and is an opportunity for learning by experience and experimentation. All phases of adult development garner considerable interest. Judging by the increase in books about adult self-development, more adults are exploring topics in holistic healing and spiritual health and development. Health behaviors, safety practices, diet, exercise, sexuality, and addictions are widely discussed topics. The preventive health concerns of young adults can be separated into two basic categories: (1) developing behaviors that promote a healthy lifestyle and (2) decreasing the incidence of accidents, injuries, and acts of violence. Death rates related to traffic and motor-vehicle injuries are highest in the age group of 15 to 24 years (U.S. Department of Health and Human Services, 2000).

Approximately 25.6% of the population is composed of adults ages 18 to 35 (U.S. Department of Commerce, 1999). The young adult population is expected to be approximately 23.2% of the general population by the year 2000 and 22.8% or less by the year 2010. Overall, the percentage of individuals who are young adults in the United States has been decreasing. The percentage of young adults ages 20 to 24 years dropped from 9.4% in 1980 to 6.5% in 1998 (U.S. Department of Commerce, 1999). The decline in this age group also affects birth rates. The U.S. Census Bureau reports that the birth rate per 1000 people for women of all ages in 1997 was 14.6; the rate has been dropping slightly since 1988 when it was more than 16 live births per 1000 people. Health-promotion efforts (Box 22-1) are particularly important for young adults because the nurse's health education activities directly influence the next generation (Kulbok & Baldwin, 1992).

Young adulthood is generally the healthiest time of life. Physical growth is complete by the age of 20; most concerns related to physiological development are focused on ensuring the optimal functioning of body systems.

The young adult's physical abilities are in peak condition, and compensatory mechanisms operate optimally during illness to provide minimal disruption in health patterns. Nursing goals for individuals of this age group are oriented toward prolonging this optimal period of physical energy; developing the mental, emotional, and social potential; encouraging proper health habits; anticipating and observing the onset of chronic disease at an early stage; and treating disease when appropriate.

The physical attributes of height, strength, endurance, coordination, and speed of response are at their maximal

Box 22-1 Selected National Health-Promotion and Disease-Prevention Objectives for the Young Adult

Increase the proportion of adults who engage regularly, preferable daily, in moderate physical activity for at least 30 minutes per day. (In 1997 and after, 15% of adults performed the recommended amount of physical activity and 40% of adults engaged in no leisure-time physical activity.)

Reduce the proportion of adults who are obese. (From 1988 through 1994 23% of adults age 20 and older were considered obese.)

Reduce cigarette smoking by adults. (In 1997 24% of adults were current smokers.)

Reduce the proportion of adults using any illicit drug during the preceding 30 days. (Illicit drug use in adults age 18 or older has remained fairly stable at the present rate of 6% since 1980; men continue to have higher rates than do women.)

Reduce the proportion of adults engaging in binge drinking of alcoholic beverages during the preceding month. (Binge drinking remains fairly stable in adults with the highest current rates of 32% among adults ages 18 to 25 years.)

Increase the proportion of sexually active persons who use condoms (In 1997 23% of sexually active adults used condoms.)

Increase the proportion of adults with recognized depression who receive treatment. (In 1997 and after, 23% of adults who were diagnosed with depression received treatment.)

Reduce deaths caused by motor-vehicle crashes. (Death rates associated with motor-vehicle-traffic injuries are highest in the age group 15 to 24 years; the highest intoxication rates in fatal crashes in 1995 were recorded for drivers ages 21 to 24 years.)

Reduce homicides. (In 1997 32,436 individuals died from firearm injuries; 42% of these individuals were homicide victims.)

Reduce the proportion of nonsmokers exposed to environmental tobacco smoke. (Exposure to environmental tobacco smoke among nonsmokers is widespread, with 65% of nonsmokers exposed during the years 1988 through 1994. The overall death rate from asthma increased 52% between 1980 and 1993.)

Increase the proportion of people who have a specific source of ongoing care. (In 1997 86% of all individuals had health insurance and a usual source of health care; individuals ages 18 to 24 years were the most likely to lack a usual source of primary care.)

Increase the proportion of pregnant women who begin prenatal care in the first trimester of pregnancy. (In 1997 83% of pregnant women received prenatal care in the first trimester of pregnancy.)

U.S. Department of Health and Human Services. (2000). *Healthy people 2010* (Conference ed.). Washington, DC: U.S. Government Printing Office.

levels. Physical appearance is determined by genetic endowment; structural differences are evidence of familial genetic contributions. Full adult stature in men is reached at approximately age 21; in women, full growth occurs earlier, typically by age 17.

Optimal muscular strength occurs during ages 25 to 30, then gradually declines by approximately 10% from ages 30 to 60. Most of this decline occurs in the muscles of the back and legs, with less of a decline occurring in the arms. Manual dexterity peaks in young adulthood and declines into the mid30s.

Women have greater longevity than do men. Women are considered biologically stronger than men, outlive men, and naturally outnumber men; however, the woman who neglects her health loses this special edge. On the average, women live 6 years longer than do men in the United States (U.S. Department of Commerce, 1999). This statistic may be a result in part of female genetic composition or men's greater exposure to environmental and occupational hazards. Men also seek health care services less frequently than do women. In 1992 the average use of primary care services by women was 66% higher than for it was by men in similar age groups (U.S. Department of Health and Human Services, 1996). More deaths in men can be attributed to accidents, suicides, and homicides (U.S. Department of Commerce, 1999), and men have higher death rates for each of the 10 leading causes of death (U.S. Department of Health and Human Services, 2000). The maternal mortality rate is a classic public health indicator of a nation's health resources and services. **Maternal mortality,** the number of maternal deaths in a year from causes associated with pregnancy and childbirth within 42 days after delivery, divided by the number of live births in the same year, usually written as deaths per 100,000 live births, includes all deaths related to pregnancy, delivery, and the postpartum period. Since 1980 maternal mortality has been fairly stable in the United States. In 1980 the rate was 9.2 per 100,000 live births; then mortality dropped to 6.6 in 1987, rose to 8.4 in 1988, and decreased slightly to 7.6 in 1996. Although U.S. maternal mortality rates are relatively low (compared with 21.5 in 1970, for example), considerable concern exists about whether it should be lower given the health care resources of this country. By comparison, the Canadian maternal mortality rate in 1991 was 3 per 100,000 (Olds, London, & Ladewig, 1996).

GORDON'S FUNCTIONAL HEALTH PATTERNS

Health Perception-Health Management Pattern

Because possession of excellent physical health is frequently taken for granted, concern about health and well being is relatively low in individuals in their 20s, but begins to increase in individuals in their 30s. However, health monitoring is both necessary and appropriate to determine health needs and incipient problems. After the mid30s, an increased sense of the finiteness of life develops with limitations imposed by work choices, well being, monetary resources, and the deterioration of physical abilities. For health care management, the young adult age span is split into two age groups (18 to 24 and 25 to 35), according to the preventive services that are required.

The assumption that all adults should have an annual physical examination has been supplanted by increased scientifically based information about health screening measures. Services provided in a health monitoring program should meet particular cost and effectiveness criteria. The most important of these criteria are as follows (Frame, 1992):

1. The condition for which screening is offered has a serious effect on the quality or quantity of life.
2. Methods of treatment must be available and effective.
3. The condition must have a latency or asymptomatic period during which the disease can be detected with screening procedures, and recommended treatment, when begun promptly, will reduce morbidity or mortality.
4. Treatment begun during the earlier asymptomatic period is more likely to be effective than is treatment started after symptoms emerge.
5. The cost of screening tests and programs must be acceptable and justifiable in terms of decreasing morbidity and mortality from the disease.
6. The prevalence of the condition must be sufficiently common to warrant the cost of screening procedures and programs.

The inability to satisfy each of these criteria means that the particular screening procedure is likely to be less effective. The next part of this chapter presents health maintenance and screening procedures that many experts agree are effective (Frame, 1992).

Behavioral Health History

A behavioral health history is important for young adults. Particularly, the behavioral history focuses on risk factors for unintentional injuries, such as alcohol consumption and seat belt use, which are major causes of death and disability in this age group (O'Sullivan & Apriceno-Tesoro, 1993). Other health risk factors, such as the consumption of caffeinated beverages, drugs, and tobacco, should be noted. After age 25, concern about emphasizing coronary risk factors increases, which include smoking, obesity, inadequate exercise patterns, and hypertension.

Because many of the health problems that young adults encounter originate from their own actions, a behavioral health history is most useful for examining and exploring the problems of young adults in a systematic manner. Figure 22-1 lists questions and content that might be included in a health history for young adults that focuses on their age-specific behaviors. This list incorporates the Social Readjustment Scale, which rates life changes and occurrences for potential contribution to mental and physical disease.

Preventive Care

Basic goals of preventive care are to maximize the period of optimal health status and detect incipient health problems at an early stage. At age 18 (approximately the time of graduation from high school), a full health appraisal is recommended. This clinic visit should include a family health history, the individual's medical and behavioral health history, and an exploration of the life changes and stress to which the individual has been exposed.

Table 22-1 illustrates preventive care that is important in the young adult period, along with recommended frequency of screening. As a rule, the recommendation for most procedures is a repeat health history and visit at approximately 2-year intervals. Appropriate intervention in the younger age group is directed toward correcting problems through history assessment and counseling about avoidance of adverse health behaviors. Subsequent counseling sessions focus on rechecking and updating earlier meetings.

A physical examination includes a check of height, weight, and blood pressure, with an emphasis on the need to avoid obesity and (for women) education about the importance of **breast self-examination** (BSE), including the importance of repeating the technique monthly. **Testicular self-examination** (TSE) should be taught to men, including what findings to report. Papanicolaou (Pap) smears of sexually active women are generally performed; the incidence of carcinoma in situ, a precursor of invasive cervical and uterine cancer, is high in this group (1 in 1000 women). A rectal examination is not recommended unless symptoms are present. After age 25, the emphasis is on modifying coronary risk factors.

There has been controversy about recommended cholesterol screening intervals for young adults as more physiological information becomes available about the interactive risks of high cholesterol, familial high lipid levels, diabetes mellitus, and smoking. The current recommendation is that total cholesterol should be measured at least once in young adulthood. Individuals with elevated cholesterol levels should be further screened for low-density lipoproteins (LDL), high-density lipoproteins (HDL), and triglycerides (see *Healthy People 2010* target in the following paragraph). Lipid-lowering medications may be considered with diet and lifestyle modifications. Subsequent recommended screening intervals for young adults with normal cholesterol levels is at least every 5 years (Bassetti, 1996).

Cardiac output and efficiency peak during the young adult years. Aging will be responsible for degenerative changes in heart size and cardiac functioning (Schroeder, Tierney, & McPhee, 1992), but during the young adult

Well Young Adult Behavioral Health History Content

Sociodemographic content and questions:

What organizations (community, church, lodge, social, professional, etc.) are you involved in?______________________________

____

How would you describe your community?______________________________

____

Hobbies, skills, interests, and recreational activities?______________________________

Military service? No_____ Yes_____ From ____to_____

Overseas assignment? No_____ Yes_____

Close friends or immediate family members who have died within the past two years? ______________________________

____

Names and addresses of relatives or close friends in the area. ______________________________

____

____

Marital status: S M D W Length of time ___________

Environmental content and questions:

Do you live alone? No_____ Yes_____

When did you last move? ______________________________

Describe your living situation. ______________________________

Number of years of education completed: ______________________________

Elementary?_____ High school?_____ College?_____

Occupation?______________________________ Employer?______________________________

How long have you worked for this employer? ______________________________

Are you satisfied with your work situation? No_____ Yes_____

Do you consider your work risky or dangerous? No_____ Yes_____

Is your work stressful? No_____ Yes_____

Biophysical content questions:

Have you smoked cigarettes? No_____ Yes_____

How much? Less than ½ pack per day? About one pack per day? More than 1½ packs per day?

Are you smoking now? No_____ Yes_____ Length of time smoking?_______________

Have you ever smoked cigars or a pipe? No_____ Yes_____

If yes, how long?_____________ Do you smoke cigars or a pipe now? No_____ Yes_____

Do you drink alcohol (wine, beer, or whiskey)? No_____ Yes_____

If you do, how much each day on the average?___________ Each week?___________

Do you consume large amounts occasionally (binge drinking)? No_____ Yes_____

Have you been drunk on work days? No_____ Yes_____

Have you had alcoholic drinks in the morning sometime in the past year? No_____ Yes_____

How much coffee, tea, or cola do you drink? ______________________________

Do you use seat or lap belts? No_____ Yes_____

What type of exercise do you do each week? Describe type and amount. ______________________________

____

Do you use a bicycle or motorcycle helmet? No_____ Yes_____ Helmet and pads while roller blading? No_____ Yes_____

How much sleep do you usually get each night? ______________________________

Meals: Do you generally eat: three regular meals per day? two meals per day? irregular meals?

Are you sexually active? No_____ Yes_____

If so, are you aware of the risks of sexually transmitted diseases? No_____ Yes_____

For women: Do you perform breast self-examination (BSE) each month? No_____ Yes_____

For men: Do you perform testicular self-examination (TSE) regularly? No_____ Yes_____

Fig. 22-1 Common well young adult behavioral health history content. (Adapted from U.S. Preventive Services Task Force. [1996]. *Guide to clinical preventive services* [2nd ed.]. Baltimore: Williams and Wilkins; Somers, A. R., & Breslow, L. [1979]. Lifetime health monitoring program. *Nurse Practitioner, 4,* 40, 50, 54.)

Table 22-1 **Well Young Adult Health Monitoring**

Health Issue	Ages 18 to 24 Intervention	Ages 18 to 24 Frequency (Years)	Ages 25 to 35 Intervention	Ages 25 to 35 Frequency (Years)
Smoking	History and counseling	Each visit	History and counseling	Each visit
Obesity or poor nutrition	History, weight, and counseling	Each visit	History, weight, and counseling	Each visit
Avoid alcohol, while driving, swimming, etc.	History and counseling	At least once	History and counseling	Every 2
Accidental injury, lap/shoulder belts, bicycle/motorcycle helmets, smoke detectors, safe firearm use	History and counseling	At least once	History and counseling	Every 2
Unintended pregnancy	Counseling	At least once	History and counseling	Every 2
Illegal drug use	History and counseling	At least once	History and counseling	Every 2 to 4
Regular physical activity	History and counseling	At least once	History and counseling	Every 2 to 4
Blood pressure/hypertension	Blood pressure measurement	Every 2	Blood pressure measurement	Every 2
Breast/testicular cancer	BSE or TSE counseling	Every 1 to 2	BSE or TSE counseling	Every 1 to 2
Vision defects	Examination	Once	Examination	Every 4
Tetanus-diphtheria	Booster	Once if 10 yrs since last one	Immunization	Every 10
Hepatitis B	Immunization	If not immunized	Immunization	If not immunized
Cervical dysplasia	Pap smear	Every 2 to 3	Pap smear	Every 2 to 3
Diabetes, proteinuria, bacteriuria	Urinalysis	Once	Urinalysis	Every 4
Coronary artery disease	Serum cholesterol determination, triglyceride level	Once	Serum cholesterol determination	Every 4
Dental care	Dental examination and cleaning	Every 1 to 2	Dental examination and cleaning	Every 1 to 2
Tuberculosis	Skin test/PPD	Once	Skin test/PPD	Every 2 to 3
STD prevention	Counseling determined	Individually	Counseling determined	Individually
Chlamydia	Chlamydia screen	At Gyn exam, if sexually active	Chlamydia screen	At Gyn exam, if sexually active
Contraception	Counseling determined	Individually	Counseling determined	Individually

Modified from U.S. Preventive Services Task Force. (1996). Guide to clinical preventive services (2nd ed.). Baltimore: Williams and Wilkins; Frame, P. S. (1992). Health maintenance in clinical practice: Strategies and barriers. *American Family Physician, 45 (3),* 1192-1200; Bassetti, M. (1996). An ounce of prevention: Updating clinical practice guidelines. *Advanced Practice Nurse, 5,* 37-40: Somers, A. R., & Breslow, L. (1979). Lifetime health monitoring program. *Nurse Practitioner, 4,* 40, 50, 54.

years, this decline amounts to less than 1% per year. Because cardiovascular disease (along with cancer and cerebrovascular disease) is a primary cause of death in American adults (accounting for more than one third of all deaths annually), cardiovascular assessment of the young adult includes determining the presence of hyperlipidemia, hypertension, diabetes, chest pain, or heart disease. A *Healthy People 2010* target is to reduce the mean total blood cholesterol levels among adults to 199 mg/dl; the baseline between 1988 and 1994 for adults 20 and older was 206 mg/dl (U.S. Department of Health and Human Services, 2000).

Parental hypertension is a risk factor for the development of hypertension in young adults; health history questions should elicit pertinent information about hypertension and **coronary artery disease** (CAD) in parents and relatives.

Hypertension, having a systolic blood pressure of 140 mmHg or greater or a diastolic blood pressure of 90 mmHg or above, is a prominent problem for young Black adults, especially men. Hypertension can result from a combination of factors—high-sodium diet, obesity, smoking, or high stress levels, and biological inheritance (salt sensitivity and high renin levels)—but many of the causes for this higher incidence of hypertension are unknown. Hypertension can lead to severe complications; more young Black people than young White people die as a result of chronic heart disease or stroke (cerebrovascular accidents). Although for the entire population, deaths attributable to coronary heart disease and stroke have declined, the mortality rate remains higher for Blacks (U.S. Department of Health and Human Services, 2000). For the overall population, high blood pressure levels and cholesterol levels have been declining because of increased screening and treatment, in combination with changes in lifestyle and nutrition. A target of *Healthy People 2010* is to reduce the proportion of adults with high blood pressure; in 1988 through 1994, 28% of adults age 20 years and above had high blood pressure. Hypertension incidence is highest (40%) in Black or African-American adults. The literature also describes a "stroke belt" in the southeastern states, where the incidence of stroke is reported to be above the national average (60 deaths per 100,000 population) (U.S. Department of Health and Human Services, 2000). A target goal of *Healthy People 2010* is to reduce stroke deaths to 48 deaths per 100,000 population (U.S. Department of Health and Human Services, 2000).

Development of CAD as an older adult is greatly reduced when coronary risk factors are minimized during young adulthood. Known risk factors for cardiac disease are smoking, drug abuse, hyperlipidemia, sedentary lifestyle, poor dietary habits, emotional stress, genetic endowment, and other contributing systemic illnesses, such as diabetes. One study indicates that clues to the later onset of CAD and hypertension can be clearly related to tracking blood pressure levels, obesity, and serum lipid and lipoprotein levels, in addition to understanding the relationship between the development of CAD and gender or race (Nicklas, Webber, Johnson, & Srinivasan, 1995). Young adult women who use oral contraceptives are at risk for cardiovascular disease (specifically blood clots, heart attacks, and strokes) especially when they are smokers (Hatcher et al., 1998). Because young adulthood is a particularly healthy time of life, the difficulty for young adults is to understand that they might develop CAD in the future and that avoidance or modification of coronary risk factors such as obesity, lack of exercise, high blood pressure, and smoking is necessary in the young adult years. Keller (1993) notes that the maintenance of important health behaviors related to the reduction of CAD in young Black women involves developing valued health behaviors, making appropriate decisions, and staying "on track," which means continuing the health-promoting change.

Diabetes is seventh on the list of leading causes of death in the United States. Minority populations (Blacks, Native American-Alaska Natives, and Hispanics) are disproportionately represented in persons afflicted by this disease. The incidence of diabetes, especially type 2 diabetes (adult onset) and related complications (cardiovascular disease, blindness, and end-stage renal disease) are increasing in the United States (U.S. Department of Health and Human Services, 2000). Because improved disease control can delay the beginning and progression of long-term diabetic complications, early detection and monitoring of diabetes is important.

Decision Making and Risk Taking

The decision making of a young adult can directly affect individual health and well being. Peak physical skills stimulate young adults to be venturesome, daring, enterprising, and aggressive. Young adults frequently have less experience with the death of significant others; therefore they tend to take inordinate risks. The young adult is at greater risk for sudden death from accident, suicide, or homicide. Morbidity and mortality statistics for young adults illustrate disturbing trends; youth are increasingly involved in violent acts. If these trends continue, then deaths from firearms will overtake deaths from motor-vehicle crashes. The prevalence of adverse behaviors associated with sudden death illustrates a developmental lack of fear in young adults. Underuse of seat belts and helmets by motorcyclists and bicyclists is a cause of many accidental injuries and deaths.

Sports that involve physical contact are a common source of injury. Popular sports that can cause injury in the young adult include football, soccer, boxing, and bicycling. Some young adults are involved in even more risky activities, such as flying, scuba diving, or hang gliding. Any of the many physical activities in which young adults are involved can expose them to opportunities for injuries and accidental death.

Communicable Disease and Adult Immunization

Communicable (infectious) disease affects young adults with varying degrees of severity. Although the availability of better drug treatments, vaccines, improved hygiene and food handling, and cleaner water supplies have promoted prevention and control of infectious disease, new disease threats are continually emerging. These new threats include Lyme disease, diarrhea borne by *Escherichia coli* 0157:H7, and hantavirus pulmonary disease. In 1997 approximately 39% of tuberculosis cases occurred among foreign-borne persons living in the United States (U.S. Department of Health and Human Services, 2000), even as the incidence of this disease declined for the fifth consecutive year (to 7.4 cases per 100,000 of the population). An increase in tuberculosis rates, particularly in some minority groups (Asian American-Pacific Islanders, Blacks, and Hispanics), illustrates that preventive activities must be reinforced and constant vigilance maintained over monitoring and effectiveness for all communicable diseases.

Approximately 65,000 new cases of **hepatitis B** (HB) were reported in the United States in 1996 (U.S. Department of Health and Human Services, 2000) and many of those affected were young adults. To reduce HB transmission in the United States by 2010, vaccination programs must be targeted to adolescents and adults in high-risk groups. Most of these infections can be traced to blood or sexual contact. High-risk groups include health care workers, others at occupational risk, hemophiliacs, hemodialysis patients, international travelers, and injectable drug users. A primary way of achieving high levels of vaccination coverage is to identify settings in which individuals can be vaccinated, such as correctional facilities, drug treatment centers, and clinics treating sexually transmitted diseases (U.S. Department of Health and Human Services, 2000). HB is a serious infection because of the high incidence of chronic complications, which include chronic carrier state, cirrhosis, and liver failure. Approximately 25% of HB carriers develop chronic active hepatitis.

Hepatitis vaccine is reported to be 95% effective in preventing the disease. Two types of recombinant vaccines are available and licensed for use in the United States; they are given in a three-dose series and recommended for all health care providers and others at occupational risk. Many states are requiring immunization of infants and school-age children. Although antibody titers drop significantly 7 years after the last dose, the belief is that people with normal immune systems continue to be protected from infection. Ultimately, routine infant vaccination will produce a U.S. population with a high immune level sufficient to eliminate HB spread (U.S. Department of Health and Human Services, 2000).

Rubella in young adults is generally a minor disease; however, when the disease is contracted during the first trimester of pregnancy, miscarriage, stillbirth, or congenital rubella syndrome (CRS) can result. Major problems associated with CRS are loss of hearing, ocular defects, developmental delay and growth retardation, and cardiac malformations. The rubella vaccine was first introduced in 1969, and rubella incidence decreased significantly until approximately 1988. After that time, many new cases rubella have developed, which increased the incidence of CRS by 15 times. Most of these new cases occurred in settings in which young adults gathered, including colleges, prisons, and religious communities; large state public health efforts have begun to ensure immunization among these groups, particularly in the college population.

All women of childbearing age should be screened for rubella, and those who are not immune should be immunized. Nurses inform women of childbearing age that antibody testing is recommended before pregnancy and that vaccination is available. A health care provider administers the vaccine as part of a preconception visit or after delivery. Women who are vaccinated should not become pregnant for 3 months after the vaccination; when pregnancy occurs, they may be counseled that termination of the pregnancy is not recommended because studies have indicated few reports of vaccine-related CRS.

Public health authorities have reported rubella among young adults who were immunized only as young children and never contracted the disease. The history of the disease is frequently unreliable because of its minor presentation. Wide-scale immunization without antibody screening might be considered in places in which high-risk individuals congregate, including college and military settings. Nursing activities should be directed toward identification of individuals who have lowered immunity to the disease, such as immunocompromised individuals, excluding persons who test positive for **human immunodeficiency virus** (HIV).

Another target of *Healthy People 2010* is to reduce the incidence of hepatitis C to one case in 100,000 population from the 2.4 new cases per 100,000 population occurring now (U.S. Department of Health and Human Services, 2000). Although new infections with hepatitis C dropped during the previous decade, approximately 4 million Americans remain infected (1.8% of the population), making hepatitis C the most common blood-borne infection in the United States. Individuals most at risk are those who have injected illicit drugs, received clotting factors before 1987, are on hemodialysis, are HIV positive, or have elevated liver function test values (Dieterich, 2000).

Although most outbreaks of meningococcal disease are sporadic, concern is rising among college staff and medical authorities that young adults may be more susceptible. Between 1994 and 1997, 4 of 42 meningococcal outbreaks occurred in colleges. Although meningococci are sensitive to penicillin and many antibiotics, the case fatality rate is 10%, and approximately 15% of survivors will have neurological disabilities or loss of hearing (*Consultant*, 2000). Most at risk are college freshmen living in dormitories who have a higher case ratio (4.6 per 100,000) than that of noncollege students 18 to 23 years of age (1.5 per 100,000) or children 2 to 5 years of age (1.7 per 100,000) (*Consultant*, 2000).

Other viral agents, such as **genital herpes virus, human papilloma virus** (HPV), and **Epstein-Barr virus** (EBV), commonly affect young adults. Genital herpes virus infections occur frequently in young adults because of the escalation of sexual activity during this period. HPV is spread through sexual contact, and some forms of the virus in combination with smoking are strongly related to the later development of cervical dysplasia and cancer. EBV is the cause of mononucleosis, a common infection of young adults.

Nutritional-Metabolic Pattern

Good nutrition is essential for maintaining physical fitness. Young adults tend to devote hours to attaining fitness, requiring discipline and determination. Because young Americans learn to value slimness, defined muscle tone, and athletic ability, healthy eating habits and physical exercise are a necessity.

Box 22-2 Major Principles Regulating Energy and Nutritional Needs of Young Adults

1. Activity level: active individuals need more food energy.
2. Body size: heavier individuals require more nutrient intake.
3. Growth: growing individuals require more food and diversity of nutrients.
4. Temperature: individuals in the tropics require less food than do individuals in colder climates.
5. Pregnancy: pregnant women require more nutrients to meet the needs of the developing fetus.

An optimally functioning **basal metabolic rate** (BMR) in the young adult permits adequate oxygen intake during normal activity and rest periods. Compensation for disturbances requires little disruption of normal functioning. Poor eating practices, however, can place the young adult at risk of being overweight.

Major principles regulating energy and nutritional needs that affect young adults are reviewed in Box 22-2.

A young man requires approximately 1600 to 1800 calories a day to meet his body's basal metabolic needs; a young woman requires only 1200 to 1450 calories a day to meet her needs. In addition to basal metabolic needs, other calories are required for digestion and activity. When a young adult consumes more calories than those that are used, obesity results. When growth stops in the late teens, the BMR declines. When activity slows as well, more weight is gained.

During the young adult years, caloric intake increases substantially, particularly in men. Although White men need a higher caloric intake than do Black men, the caloric intake of all men levels off after age 25. Increased caloric intake without a corresponding energy requirement can lead to obesity, which is a precursor to hypertension, coronary disease, and diabetes.

According to data shown in Fig. 22-2, 11% of children and adolescents ages 6 to 19 years are overweight and 23% of adults age 20 and older are obese (U.S. Department of Health and Human Services, 2000). This information illustrates that the number of overweight individuals continues to rise. Obesity is more frequent in certain ethnic and racial groups; approximately one half of Black women and Mexican-American women are defined as overweight. To stop or decrease the trend of overweight individuals, new behaviors must be learned for nutrition and physical activity. Specifically, decreasing fat intake, increasing fruit and vegetable intake, and increasing physical activity must be emphasized. Food labeling information (particularly for calories, fat, and cholesterol) is now required for many processed and packaged foods.

Proper nutrition is particularly necessary during the childbearing years. Prospective mothers should be con-

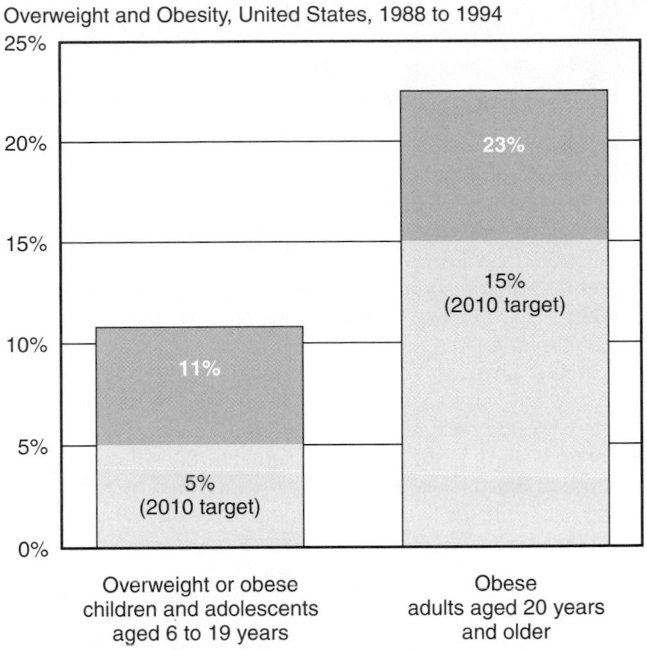

Fig. 22-2 Overweight and obesity, 1988-1994. (From U.S. Department of Health and Human Services. [2000]. *Healthy People 2010* [Conference ed.]. Washington, DC: U.S. Government Printing Office.)

cerned about high-quality nutrition and avoidance of food additives. Iron deficiency anemia is common in young adult women (see Case Study). Contributing factors in this age group are continuous loss of blood (during menses) and pregnancy. A blood loss of 2 to 4 mL per day (1 to 2 mg of iron) can cause iron deficiency anemia. Insufficient iron intake and medications that cause gastrointestinal bleeding can exacerbate the problem. Iron supplementation is recommended during pregnancy for optimal growth of the fetus and supporting structures (Olds, London, & Ladewig, 1996). Folic acid supplementation during the preconception period and early pregnancy reduces the risk of neural tube defects, including spina bifida. The Centers for Disease Control and Prevention recommends that all women of childbearing age consume 0.4 mg of folic acid daily to reduce the possibility of neural tube defect complications during pregnancy; supplementation should include the month before pregnancy and the first trimester during pregnancy.

Osteoporosis is a significant health problem for older women who do not consume adequate amounts of calcium during the young adult years. Osteoporosis is common among older adults and strongly predicts subsequent fractures. The majority of adolescents and adult women fail to meet their calcium requirement, which places them at risk of osteoporosis in later life. This failure is a result of lower food consumption and low consumption of milk relative to soft drink products. Between 1994 and 1996, the amount of soft drinks consumed was twice that used in the 1970s. An increase in calcium-containing foods is therefore

CASE STUDY

Kirsten

Kirsten is healthy, 20-year-old young adult whose favorite sport is running. Since this spring, Kirsten believes that her breathing capacity is diminishing and her levels of energy are decreasing. During her period, these symptoms appear to worsen. Last week, while running up a rather steep course, Kirsten became much more weak, dizzy, and fatigued than usual, and her best friend and running partner recommended that she make a doctor's appointment for a physical. Kirsten's running partner also noted that she appeared pale lately.

In the physician's office, Kirsten is noted to have a normal temperature, an elevated heart and respiratory rate, and a blood pressure of 90/60. Kirsten's description of her period is that it tends to be heavy and has been this way for 5 years. For muscle aches and pains caused by running, she usually takes two aspirin tablets every 3 to 4 hours for as long as 7 days. When her running increases during the summer, she takes aspirin continually for 2 to 3 months. Diagnostic testing indicates that her hemoglobin is 7 g/dl, and her red blood counts are pale and small.

What common health alteration in young adult women is most likely for Kirsten?

What are the contributing factors that place Kirsten particularly at risk?

What lifestyle modifications can Kristen implement to decrease her risk?

recommended, particularly for teens and young women (U.S. Department of Health and Human Services, 2000).

Elimination Pattern

Patterns of elimination are generally well established by young adulthood; however, health problems related to the gastrointestinal tract, including ulcers and colitis, can result from emotional stress. Although eating disorders (anorexia and bulimia) typically begin at an earlier stage of development, they can persist during young adulthood. The fashion industry has been thoroughly criticized for employing underweight waifs as models, thereby emphasizing excessive thinness as the ideal standard for attainment.

In pregnant women, decreased bowel motility is a common disorder of elimination. Constipation (frequently aggravated by iron supplementation) and hemorrhoids are commonly treated conservatively by increasing fluids and roughage in the diet.

Activity-Exercise Pattern

Sufficient physical exercise is required to maintain physical fitness. A physically fit individual has physical adaptability, a greater capacity to respond to increased activity, the additional energy that is needed to perform the skills associated with daily living with sufficient reserve, and the ability to live an active life with minimal risk of injury or disability. Inactivity is a predisposing factor to cardiovascular disease and obesity. A major goal of *Healthy People 2010* is to reduce the proportion of adults who engage in no leisure time activity to 20% from approximately 40% in 1997 and to increase the proportion of adults who engage in moderate physical activity for 30 minutes a day to 30% from 15% in 1997 (U.S. Department of Health and Human Services, 2000).

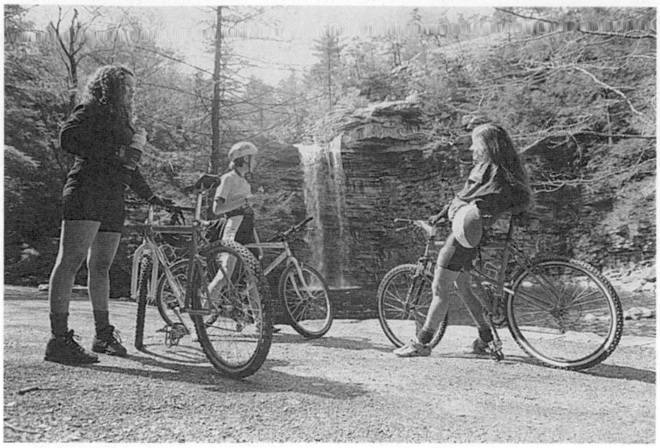

Fig. 22-3 Bicycling and other sports activities provide young adults with needed exercise.

Aerobic exercise, exercise in which oxygen is metabolized to produce energy, develops an optimally functioning cardiovascular-respiratory system. Aerobic conditioning achieves cardiovascular fitness through three periods of intense exercise for 30 minutes or more at a heart rate of approximately 220 minus the age of the person. Depending on inspired air to burn calories and produce energy, aerobic exercise develops muscular fitness, endurance, tone, strength, and flexibility (Cooper, 1992). Young adults are encouraged to engage in fitness activities that increase the heart rate to approximately 150 beats per minute. After 5 minutes of activity at this rate, the body is required to make adjustments in cardiovascular capacity by enlarging the lungs and the capillaries in the muscles and the heart (Cooper, 1992). Repeated aerobic exercise, such as cycling, running, skipping rope, and walking (at least 4 times a week) produces physical fitness and decreases the likelihood of problems caused by inactivity (Fig. 22-3).

Radiation and Excessive Sun Exposure

Involvement in outdoor activities can result in excessive **sun exposure.** Exposure to natural radiation from sunlight is directly linked to skin cancer. Artificial tanning centers are also popular, but these can lead to health problems similar to those encountered from natural radiation.

Nurses teach about the risks of sun exposure and tanning, the preventive use of sun-blocking agents, and the skin symptoms that might indicate cancer. The use of sun-blocking agents, such as paraaminobenzoic acid (PABA), is recommended, particularly because it is rated based on skin type and sensitivity to burning. Choices range from lotions or creams with double protection to those that completely block all burning radiation; choices for children are also available. Many makeup foundations now include sun-blocking agents. Young adults should avoid sunbathing during the 2-hour period around noon, because two thirds of the day's ultraviolet light comes through the earth's atmosphere during this time.

Sports

Bicycling and motorcycling are encouraged by environmentalists to decrease automobile pollution; however, this trend is also promoted as a result of traffic congestion, the high costs of fuel and car maintenance, and an increased interest in healthy exercise. Cyclists are likely to be involved in accidents with automobiles. Older cyclists now represent two thirds of bicycle-related fatalities, when the highest rate of fatalities was, at one time, found in school-age riders. Head injury is responsible for approximately 62% of bicycle-related fatalities. In 1997 only 11 states had mandatory helmet requirements for riders under 15 years of age (U.S. Department of Health and Human Services, 2000). Bicycle helmets are effective in decreasing the incidence of brain and head injury; in fact, helmets are believed to be the single most effective preventive measure available to decrease the incidence of head injury. Bicycle helmets reduce the risk of bicycle-related head injury by 85% (U.S. Department of Health and Human Services, 2000).

Motorcycles are less stable and have less occupant protection than do automobiles, but are appealing to young adults, primarily because they have high performance capabilities. Using a motorcycle helmet reduces the chance of dying in an accident by 29% (U.S. Department of Health and Human Services, 2000). A target of *Healthy People 2010* is to increase the proportion of motorcyclists using helmets from 67% in 1997 to 79% (U.S. Department of Health and Human Services, 2000).

Accidental deaths from drowning are also common in young adults. Swimming, boating, and scuba diving are associated with the high number of water-related fatalities. Hang gliding, parachuting, and flying small aircraft are responsible for a large number of outdoor fatalities. Mountain climbing, hiking in poor weather conditions, downhill ski racing, and bobsledding are other hazardous activities.

Amateur and professional sports activities generally pose few hazards when rules and safety precautions are observed. Relatively few fatalities are associated with the professionally organized contact sports, such as football, hockey, or boxing, but chronic injuries frequently cause discomfort. Foot, ankle, and knee injuries are common in football and hockey; brain damage can result from repeated head injuries in boxing. Some of these injuries can become chronic, or a length of time may be required for symptoms to manifest.

Box 22-3 Nursing Suggestions to Assist the Young Adult in Relaxing

1. Find a quiet environment and assume a comfortable position.
2. Close eyes to block extraneous stimulation.
3. Relax all muscles, starting with toes and feet and progressing toward head. Continue to keep them relaxed.
4. Become aware of breathing pattern. Breathe slowly in and out while counting slowly. Maintain this pattern for 10 to 20 minutes. Sit quietly after this process is finished, first with eyes closed, then with eyes open. Stand only at the conclusion.
5. Do not worry about the success or failure of the relaxation. Maintain an attitude of indifference toward the environment and ignore all distractions.

A comprehensive history of recreational activities will alert the nurse to specific needs about safety education. Young adults are encouraged to learn and abide by the rules of the sport in which they are engaged. Rules in many sports have evolved from health and safety concerns, enabling the individual to learn the sport well under appropriate instruction while promoting patterns of good sportsmanship.

Sleep-Rest Pattern

Young adults are subject to fatigue induced by work, stress, or inactivity. Changes in activity or stressors can help reduce fatigue. Trying out new and challenging tasks can help reduce mental stress. New physical activities, such as learning a new sport or form of exercise, can also provide stimulation.

Relaxation reduces tension, which, in turn, decreases anxiety and fatigue. Relaxation relieves fatigue; assists in coping with anxiety; relieves stress, which contributes to many disorders such as high blood pressure, arteriosclerosis, heart attack, and stroke; aids in sleep; maintains alertness; and reduces the tendency to smoke or use drugs.

Nursing activities to assist young adults in relaxing consist of initial teaching and demonstration of the activity and observing return findings (Box 22-3). Relaxation activities can help individuals with anxiety-provoking situations, hospitalization, and overall lifestyle stress (Box 22-4).

Cognitive-Perceptual Pattern

Physical and Mental Patterns

The physical senses are at their peak during young adulthood. Visual acuity is highest at approximately age 20 and begins to decline at approximately age 40, when farsightedness frequently develops. Hearing is also best at age 20; the ability to distinguish high-pitch tones decreases with age. The other senses (taste, smell, touch, and awareness of temperature and pain) remain stable until age 45 to 50.

Intellectual maturity is necessary for adult decision

Box 22-4 Four Techniques to Induce Relaxation

1. Nonstimulating environment: an ideal environment is free from noise and other distractions. A quiet environment makes repetitive thoughts and actions more effective.
2. Mental stimulus: a word or phrase can be used to shift the activity of the mind away from an organized thought that is directed toward the external environment.
3. Quiescent attitude: adopting an attitude of removal from external sources of stimulation and of passivity toward the environment will induce relaxation
4. Posture: appropriate positioning, with a reduction in muscular tension, will induce relaxation.

making. The maturation process requires young adults to learn skills and behaviors that improve the performance abilities gained as adolescents. Factors that an individual young adult will perceive as essential to learn will depend on specific goals, values, attitudes, and practices as influenced by intrinsic (constitutional) and extrinsic (environmental or community) factors. The development of intellectual maturity influences the selection of behaviors and attitudes that affect health and well-being practices.

Piaget's Theory

Development of adult mental abilities is an important goal for many young adults. Jean Piaget's stage of formal operational thought evolves from concrete operational thought in adolescence and extends through the reasoning process of young adults (Piaget, 1972).

Achievement of formal operational thinking allows a person to analyze all combinations of possibilities and construct hypotheses that are capable of being tested. Young adult thought becomes more perceptive and insightful; issues can therefore be evaluated realistically and objectively. Young adults are energetic and can therefore contribute substantially to social and occupational decision making. Although they tend to take greater risks, young adults typically demonstrate the use of appropriate reasoning and analytical approaches.

Intellectual Growth

Young adults use formal operational reasoning as long as the social environment and acquired experience provide sufficient cognitive and intellectual stimulation (Piaget, 1972). Young adult intelligence is an excellent predictor of older adult performance.

Organization of information influences memory. Evidence shows that recall performance diminishes with age; at its peak in the 20s, memory starts to diminish in the 30s. Improved strategies for organization of information, however, can enhance recall, and limitation of memory with increasing age is likely a result of retrieval rather than storage mechanisms.

Erikson's Theory

A major goal for young adults is the development of an increased sense of competency and self-esteem (Erikson, 1993). Self-esteem appears to develop fairly consistently from adolescence to young adulthood, based on personality traits acquired during early adolescence (Block & Robbins, 1993). In developing self-esteem, the individual learns to be truly open and capable of trust through the formation of intimate relationships, which are characteristic of this period. Erikson has described this stage of psychosocial development as intimacy versus isolation and loneliness (Erikson, 1993).

Passage through the adult years involves dynamic change in which the achievement of intimacy depends on the existence of a strong sense of self-accomplishment in the adolescent years. Erikson's concept of genuine intimacy extends beyond sexual relations to a broader view of mutual psychosocial intimacy with a spouse or lover, parents, children, and friends (Coles, 1978). Characterized by the reciprocal expression of affection, intimacy requires mutual trust. These interchanges are spontaneous for the young adult; relationships should be free and allow for self-disclosure. Young adults who are unsure of their identity may avoid intimate contact or engage in promiscuous behavior lacking in true intimacy, which can result in isolation and consequent self-absorption. Healthy adults search for continuity, regularity, or unity of meaningful relationships, while avoiding situations of little commitment.

Moral Development

Young adults who have successfully mastered the previous cognitive, social, and moral stages are usually able to recognize or use principled reasoning. Lawrence Kohlberg identifies this ability as the **postconventional level of moral reasoning** (Kohlberg & Lickons, 1986). During this phase, the individual is able to differentiate the self from the rules and expectations of others and to define principles regarding rights in terms of self-chosen principles. The individual at the postconventional level understands society's rules, but goes beyond them. When society's rules or practices conflict, the morally developed person judges by principles rather than rules. Therefore the interests of individuals can be weighed against the needs of society and the state, and violations of law can be justified when individual interests are in accord with principles. Gilligan (1982), who studied the development of moral reasoning in women and girls, asserts that their moral judgments reflect less of a "rights" perspective and more of an emphasis on relationships.

Although development of principled moral reasoning is possible in young adulthood, it may never occur if the cognitive and social factors that stimulate increased reasoning are not present. Acts of personal violence representative of lower moral reasoning should not be present; however, such acts do occur during this period, illustrating the need for addressing moral development concerns at earlier stages of education and socialization. One recent study indicates that engaging in wellness behaviors may have moral implications. Data from 54 young adults illustrate that individuals who actively seek wellness identify it as a virtue, with associated "good" and "bad" behaviors. Participation in wellness activities is viewed as intrinsically moral and virtuous (Conrad, 1994).

Self-Perception–Self-Concept Pattern

In nonWestern cultures the entrance to adulthood is generally defined and marked by social events such as marriage. In Western societies, maturation is defined through the individual's achievement of financial and residential independence. In contemporary society, maturation is therefore a more drawn-out, gradual process (Arnett & Taber, 1994). Two emotional themes regarding the value of work become evident in young adulthood. In their 20s, young adults yearn to explore and experiment, keeping structures temporary and reversible. These individuals may move from job to job and relationship to relationship, remaining in a transient state. At the opposite extreme is the urge to prepare for the future by making firm commitments. During this period, both men and women question their value to society, the merit of their accomplishments, their success as sexual beings, and the probability of attaining their unfulfilled goals.

More than 65% of women ages 25 to 35 are employed. As more mothers enter the labor force, the need for adequate child care is increased. The gap in earnings, or pay differential, between men and women continues to grow. Access to insurance and pension benefits is not always available, especially to high-risk groups such as minorities or people receiving the minimum wage. Even when there is sufficient access to health care, some types of employment expose individuals to occupational risks and hazards.

Many young adults are high achievers and seek opportunities to be challenged. Employment problems can be stressful and traumatic to an individual's self-esteem and self-worth. The failure to receive a promotion or a pay raise can accelerate the degree of stress. The loss of their first job, especially when it is an unexpected termination, can shatter the lives of both young and older adults. Employment is more than a source of income; it provides self-esteem and social interaction. Because the adjustment to the job market influences many other aspects of daily living, young adults frequently require assistance in developing coping mechanisms to manage stress. Properly managing the initial stress prevents further complications that can arise if the young adult uses unhealthy stress relievers such as alcohol or drugs.

Young women have many of the same concerns about employment and success as do young men. Many young women postpone childbearing until they have established their careers; many are absent from the job for only a standard maternity leave. Women who return to work when their children are very young frequently risk the emotional strain caused by guilt feelings. In addition to helping parents cope with the stress of being absent from their children, nurses can help them identify ways to provide quality supervision in their absence, either through private baby-sitters, day care programs, or through neighbors, friends, and relatives.

Work dissatisfaction is a potential threat to well being. The U.S. workforce is dramatically changing as companies restructure, downsize, "right size," and shift employees around to meet changing market conditions. White-collar workers are reported to be more satisfied with career choices and work-related environments; they are professionally educated and are usually afforded a high job satisfaction that increases with age until later in life. Lack of work or job satisfaction is a major cause of stress-related illness. Job stress can lead to increased absenteeism, which is more common in young adults. Nursing interventions in industrial settings are directed toward improving both working conditions and employer-employee relationships.

Roles-Relationships Pattern

Young adults interact with people daily in their work, school, or community environments. By establishing relationships, they counteract social isolation. Typically, young adults venture into their relationships with enthusiasm and passion; they are frequently vulnerable to conflict or stress when relationships do not precede in a smooth fashion. Dating, a stressful work environment, or an unfriendly neighbor is a situation capable of creating anxiety and maladaptation.

Young adult friendships are more enduring than are earlier relationships. The focus of the relationship is the sharing of feelings or confidences. True friendship is characteristic of a person who wants to give rather than receive. Friendships are necessary in a constantly changing society; they provide a source of emotional support and a basis of stability for developing the self-concept.

Establishing interpersonal relationships involves agreeable and purposeful interactions with others. Interpersonal relationships can be created with people of the same or the opposite sex; age is typically a less important factor than it was during adolescence. The formation of intimate relationships develops within or outside a family context and occasionally in the work environment.

In addition to achieving intimacy, the young adult must accomplish other developmental tasks to achieve true psychosocial maturation. One of the principal tasks of maturation is the selection of a career. Decision making about life and career directions is the developmental milestone that heralds the transition from adolescence to adulthood. Decisions usually entail establishing independence from the family of origin. This transition may involve an actual physical move from the parent's home (going away to college, joining the military, or getting an apartment) however, movement away is not the sole indicator of independence. Young adults frequently remain in their parent's home for economic reasons, particularly when life choices involve continued schooling or remaining unmarried. In some cultures, unmarried adults live with their parents until they are married, and newly married young adults share the home of their parents until they start their own family.

Exhibiting maturity by taking on adult roles and responsibilities is a developmental process. Most young men and women have the intellectual and emotional solidity to take on new social roles and venture into challenges with eagerness and a desire for mastery. Young adults frequently speak out for causes that affect society; they tend to remain committed to ideas and ideals until resolutions are identified.

Young adults who are striving to accomplish psychosocial maturation are aware that they have many common bonds and goals with their peers. All young adults experience similar conflicts, hopes, desires, disappointments, and urges in the process of change. Dissimilarity exists only in the timing and sequence of age-expected behaviors. Young adulthood is a time of transition and constant psychosocial growth.

Individuals in this age group typically choose life partners and begin families; they make decisions about childbearing and the number and education of children. Additional consideration must be given to decisions related to childbearing, such as finances, safety, family support, housing, the relationship with extended family members, and the roles and responsibilities within the nuclear family unit. Young adults who are establishing a family must have open communication about self-development, which includes issues of dual careers, child-rearing practices, and domestic duties (Fig. 22-4).

Family harmony and development are major goals for many young adults. Although family size and structure have undergone dramatic changes in previous decades, concern about each member's health and safety continues to be a primary focus. Family life is influenced by the qualities of individual family members. Typically, economic security, status, place in the community, and healthy patterns of living, such as good nutrition, personal hygiene, and physical fitness, are associated with healthy family adjustment.

Separation and Divorce

Divorce rates have been rising steadily in the last few decades, but show some indication of leveling off. Rates are high among young adults (Lander, Foster, & Jones, 1992). Many stressors contribute to divorce. Socioeconomic factors often place unreasonable stress on marriages. Age at the time of marriage is correlated with duration of marriage, and young adults whose parents have divorced have an increased frequency of divorce (Lander, Foster, & Jones, 1992). Additionally, the increased employment of women have allowed more women to leave unhappy marriages that they formerly would have been forced to tolerate.

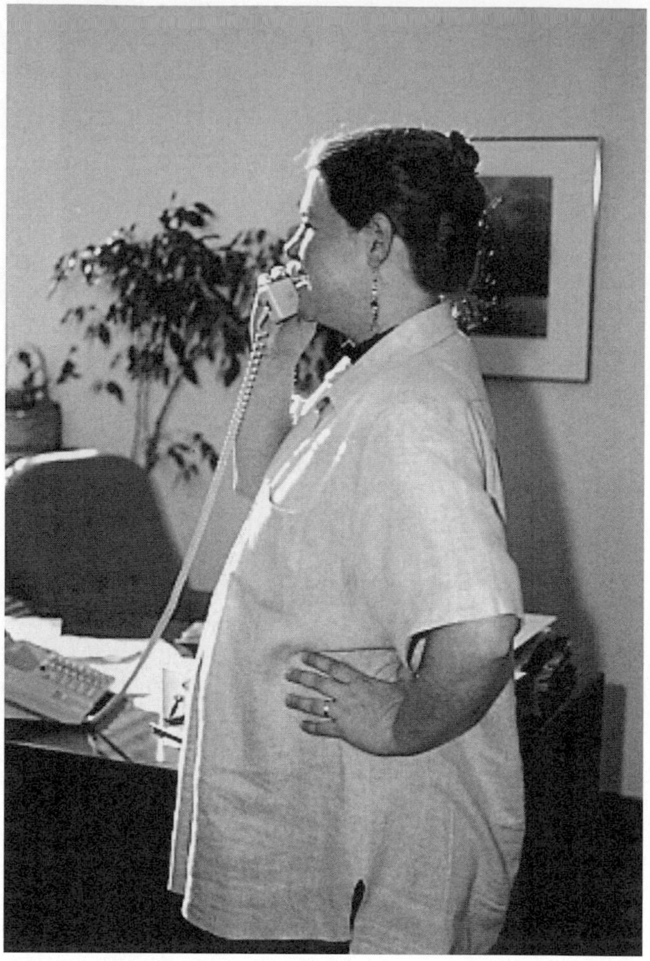

Fig. 22-4 Planning pregnancy and timing this event properly are critical decisions for many young adults.

Although dissatisfaction and unhappiness are frequent precursors to separation and divorce, the decision to dissolve a marriage is not easy either. Considerable emotional strain exists for both partners, their children, their families, and close friends. Divorce requires that young adults reevaluate their basic values, individual personality and ego strength, future job potential, and socioeconomic factors to ensure future security for themselves and their children. Divorced young adults frequently suffer severe emotional strain and depression. Some young adults are unable to adjust to role and status changes and to threats to self-concept. For these reasons, support systems in the form of groups, individual counseling, or special social activities are critical. As a result of divorce, many women and their young children are

HEALTH TEACHING Assessment and Education Regarding Firearm Safety

Nurses are taught to perform community and environmental assessments; however, most fail to incorporate assessment of the presence of firearms in the home.

- Firearm accidents are the fifth leading cause of accidental death for children under the age of 14.
- More than 100 firearm-related deaths occur in the United States each day.
- The risk of suicide is increased nearly 5 times in homes with firearms.
- Approximately 38% of families keep at least one firearm in the home, and approximately 55% of those families report that they normally keep the gun loaded.
- Firearm presence in the home is a risk for violence against women.

Guidelines for Firearm Safety

McClelland, Thompson, Prete, and Hatcher (1996) developed five principles for firearm safety after analyzing current information on the subject, most of which were not developed for use in the home. This model would allow community health nurses to inquire about the personal safety of family members in the home, community, occupational setting, and school. The anagram CARES provides a helpful way of remembering the essential elements of appropriate home firearm assessment.

The CARES of Firearm Safety

1. **C**ommunicate the risks of keeping a firearm in the home for all family members, particularly children and adolescents.
2. **A**dvise that it is safest not to keep a firearm in the home.
3. **R**eview safe methods of storage if a firearm is kept at home (store gun in a locked box; store ammunition separately, preferably locked and in a different room; use trigger locks, childproof safety catches, and loading indicators).
4. **E**ducate parents to teach children about the dangers of firearms, not to touch or handle firearms, and the differences between media violence and real-life violence.
5. **S**hare with the family your state or city laws concerning the presence of a loaded gun in the home that is accessible, particularly to minors.

From McClelland, C., Thompson, P., Prete, S., & Hatcher, P. (1996). Assessing firearm safety. *Nursing & Health Care, 17* (4), 174-178.

forced to seek emergency shelter in publicly operated homes, including welfare hotels and group shelters.

The nurse working with young adults who are considering separation or divorce recognizes the crisis that exists. Many people need support from the nurse to help them work through this difficulty. Nurses help to identify the feelings of guilt, grief, and loss that young adults experience during a separation or divorce. Suggesting that young adults read articles or books on issues related to divorce is helpful, because they provide a reference point for their experiences. The nurse recommends marital counseling by a qualified professional; this may be the most beneficial source of support for guidance of well being.

Male and Female Risk of Violence

Youth are involved as both the perpetrators and the victims of violence. Their targets tend to be elderly, children, and women with whom they are familiar (U.S. Department of Health and Human Services, 2000). Homicide is the second leading cause of death in the 15- to 24-year-old age group and the leading cause of death for Black men in the same age category (U.S. Department of Commerce, 1999). Firearms are involved in approximately two thirds of these deaths, and men have twice the risk of dying than do women. When compared with the general population, mortality statistics are higher for men of poorer populations, in urban areas, and with less formal education. Homicide is closely associated with alcohol and drug abuse and is frequently related to other violent acts, such as robbery. Other risk factors include history of detention or prison experience, access to firearms, abuse in the home, various forms of mental illness, social isolation, and homelessness. The presence of firearms in the home is associated with the increased risk of unintentional and intentional firearm injury to children and increases the risk of suicide in adolescence by nearly five times (McClelland, Thompson, Prete, & Hatcher, 1996) (see Health Teaching box). A target of *Healthy People 2010* is to reduce firearm-related deaths from 11 deaths per 100,000 population in 1998 to 4.9 deaths per 100,000 population and also to reduce the proportion of people living in homes with firearms loaded and unlocked from 19% to 16% (U.S. Department of Health and Human Services, 2000). The firearm-related death rate for young Black men and boys was nearly five times the rate for young White men and boys. although there has been a substantial decline of 10% per year in the death rate between 1993 and 1997 for young Black men and boys 15 to 24 years of age (U.S. Department of Health and Human Services, 2000).

Suicide rates are higher for men than it is for women; approximately four to five times as many men than women take their own lives (Table 22-2). However, more women are known to suffer from depressive disorders and to unsuccessfully attempt suicide than do men. In 1996 approximately 12% of all deaths in the 15- to 24-year-old age group were classified as suicides (U.S. Department of Commerce, 1999). In one study of 694 college freshmen ages 18 to 24, 54% reported that they had considered suicide at least once, 26% had considered suicide during the last 12 months, and 10% reported that they had attempted suicide (Meehan, Lamb, Saltzman, & O'Carroll, 1992). Suicide continues to be a major health problem; annual rates, especially for men, continue to remain high.

Abuse of women is one of the nation's most common health problems; however, because of social and legal factors, it is probably the most underreported (see Hot

Table 22-2 U.S. Suicide Rates for Young Adults by Sex, Race, and Age, 1980 to 1997 (Rates per 100,000 Resident Population)

	Male						Female					
	White		Black		Hispanic		White		Black		Hispanic	
Age	1980	1997	1980	1997	1980	1997	1980	1997	1980	1997	1980	1997
All	19.9	20.2	10.3	10.9	—	9.8	5.9	4.8	2.2	1.9	—	1.6
15-24	21.4	19.5	12.3	16.0	—	14.4	4.6	3.8	2.3	2.4	—	2.4
25-44	24.6	25.3	19.2	17.0	—	13.9	8.1	6.4	4.3	2.7	—	2.2

From U.S. Department of Health and Human Services. (1999). *Health, United States 1999*. Hyattsville, MD: U.S. Government Printing Office.

Topics box). Abuse crosses all socioeconomic, racial, ethnic, religious, and age boundaries. Approximately one half of the women who knew their assailant were murdered by a husband, boyfriend, or former husband (U.S. Department of Health and Human Services, 2000). The rate of violent attacks by individuals known intimately by the victim is highest among women with family incomes of less than $10,000 a year and reported the least in those with family incomes of more than $50,000 a year (U.S. Department of Health and Human Services, 1996). In 1994 approximately one half million women were seen in emergency rooms for violence-related injuries (U.S. Department of Health and Human Services, 2000), and although most women survived, they suffer needless physical and emotional pain. Nurses and other primary health care providers fail to assess, detect, or treat violence or abuse in an optimal manner, and more efforts must be made to recognize the scope of the problem and to provide appropriate counseling.

Sexuality-Reproductive Pattern

By young adulthood, the menstrual cycle is generally well established in the woman. Cyclical hormonal functioning is responsible for regularity in the menstrual cycle and normal functioning of the ovaries and uterus. The normal duration of menses is 5 days, and the usual interval of each menstrual cycle is 25 to 32 days. Menstrual irregularities such as painful menstruation, premenstrual syndrome, intermenstrual bleeding, and prolonged or heavy bleeding can occur. Although the appearance of these problems is not always abnormal, these symptoms and the individual's reaction to them can signal functional disorders and the need for further investigation. Other problems typical of this age group for both genders are infertility, infections of the reproductive tract, and complications associated with contraceptive methods.

Reproductive Problems

Infertility is defined as the lack of conception in the presence of unprotected sexual intercourse for a period of at least 12 months. Approximately 10% to 15% of couples in the United States are believed to be infertile (Olds, London, & Ladewig, 1996). Infertility has become more of a public issue since the advance of assistive reproductive technologies, such as *in vitro* fertilization and gamete intrafallopian transfer, which can enable couples with known reproductive problems to deliver children. These technologies frequently create great stress for the couple and often result in marital conflicts and distress. Generally, infertility is not an issue for the 18- to 25-year-old individual; however, after the age of 25, the diagnosis increasingly occurs. In 1995 approximately 1.8% of the 15- to 24-year-old age group were surgically sterile; by the age of 25 to 35, this number had jumped to 23.6% (U.S. Department of Commerce, 1999). Infertility is an increasingly stressful problem for couples in the middle adult years.

Common reproductive problems in men include external conditions, mumps, orchitis, epididymitis, and the occurrence of varicoceles and hydroceles. External conditions such as fungal infections, contact dermatitis, and eczema; parasites such as scabies and lice; and nonvenereal diseases such as erysipelas, abscesses, and fistulas can occur in the scrotum. Mumps orchitis is a complication of mumps that occurs in 18% of cases in adult men; it can cause sterility and impotence. Epididymitis is a common infection caused by organisms that move from sites or established infections in the urine, urethra, prostate, or seminal vesicles. A hydrocele is swelling in the testicle caused by an abnormality in lymphatic drainage; 90% occur after age 21. A varicocele is an abnormal dilation or twisting of the veins of the testicle that occurs most frequently up to age 25. Varicoceles can cause subfertility by affecting the number and mobility of sperm.

Unintended Pregnancy

Unwanted or unplanned pregnancies can be a considerable source of stress to young adults. Most of these unintended pregnancies are the result of contraceptive method failure or improper use. Unintended pregnancy is an important public health issue related to increased infant mortality and morbidity, and increased risk of parental neglect, child and wife abuse, and emotional deprivation. Despite the advent of modern contraceptives, unintended pregnancy remains a persistent problem. Approximately one half of all pregnancies are unintended (U.S. Department of Health and Human Services, 2000). Although the proportion of unintended pregnancies has declined from 57% to 49%, other industrialized countries report a smaller number, suggesting

HOT topics

VIOLENCE AGAINST WOMEN

Assessing the Problem

Women are victims of domestic violence at a rate of 3.8% to 44%. Quillian (1996) found an 8.4% rate of wife abuse in 2410 women. More than one third of women who are murdered are killed by their male partners, and approximately 6% of emergency room visits are a result of domestic violence. Domestic violence is a problem in all age, ethnic, and religious groups; in some cultures, attitudes toward women can even legitimize the practice.

Are Nurses Willing to Take Action?

Some studies indicate that nurses have been reluctant to take action regarding violence against women. Some of the traditional reasons for not taking action are based on paternalistic attitudes, in which the victim is blamed for her part in the social situation that is the setting for abuse. Yam (1995) found that professionals often failed to recognize abuse and may be unhelpful and untherapeutic. Campbell and associates (1995) noted that nurses should take a stronger role in identifying violence against women; particularly, nursing's strong advocacy stance and emphasis on the communication of nonjudgmental, genuine concern should provide a strong foundation to avoid blaming the victim and to focus on pathological factors that typifies much of the health profession's research in this area.

How Can Nurses Recognize Abuse of Women?

Some research (Ratner, 1995) in this area has demonstrated that nurses are aware of potential indicators of wife abuse. These include the presence, in a health history, of separation or divorce, a visit to the emergency room, hospitalization, or contact with public health nurses and mental health professionals in the preceding year. Abused women had an increased incidence of complaints about headaches, backaches, psychiatric illness, alcoholism, and the acquiring of bruises, sprains, and lacerations. Other indicators demonstrated the probability to have a husband who was unemployed and one who had a higher educational level than that of the wife (Ratner, 1995). Assessment tools are being developed to help nurses detect victimization in diverse settings (Hoff & Rosenbaum, 1994).

What Do You Think?

1. Are nurses less than helpful in their detection and management of violence against women? Why do you think this occurs?
2. Are nurses, because of their education and sensitization to persons with mental problems, more or less likely than others to experience violence in their own domestic settings? Explain.

From Campbell, J. C., Harris, M. J., & Lee, R. K. (1995). Violence research: An overview. *Scholarly Inquiry for Nursing Practice*, 9 (2), 105-126; Hoff, L. A., & Rosenbaum, L. (1994). A victimization assessment tool: Instrument development and clinical implications. *Journal of Advanced Nursing, 20* (4), 627-634; Quillian, J. P. (1996). Screening for spousal or partner abuse in a community health setting. *Journal of the American Academy of Nurse Practitioners*, 8 (4), 155-160; Ratner, P. A. (1995). Indicators of exposure to wife abuse. *Canadian Journal of Nursing Research, 27* (1), 31-46; Yam, M. (1995). Wife abuse: Strategies for a therapeutic response. *Scholarly Inquiry of Nursing Practice*, 9 (2), 147-158.

that more education is needed. Unwanted pregnancies lead to most if not all of the abortions induced each year; in the United States, one abortion occurs for every three live births, a ratio two to four times higher than that of other developed countries (U.S. Department of Health and Human Services, 2000). Although many young adults would consider family planning services as an essential basic health service, health insurance plans have traditionally excluded payment for family planning services (U.S. Department of Health and Human Services, 2000). A target of *Healthy People 2010* is to increase the proportion of pregnancies that are intended from 51% in 1995 to 70% (U.S. Department of Health and Human Services, 2000).

The ability to control the timing of births is an important consideration, particularly for young women. Women frequently have goals for schooling or career that take precedence over family development; interference in these goals can affect a woman's future relationships, including those with her future children. In the traditional order of events, schooling precedes marriage, which precedes the birth of the first child. Premature arrival of the first child forces the parents to alter their activities; for the young man, pregnancy can impose an increased financial burden before schooling is complete or before the first "real" job is secured.

The scenario for an unmarried couple is not different from that of a married couple; however, there may be less stability to the couple relationship, which therefore may not survive the unplanned pregnancy. Difficult decisions about child custody and child support frequently exist.

Eliminating unwanted childbearing is a healthy goal; for many young adults, this entails making active decisions about pregnancy prevention. Both married and unmarried young adults need information about contraceptives to decrease the number of unwanted pregnancies and the need for abortions (Table 22-3). The nurse's role in contraceptive counseling involves helping individuals to choose the method most appropriate to match their needs. Education about the risks, side effects, and complications associated with a specific method and the effective use of the method is vital. Nurses who engage in contraceptive counseling should consider the following: (1) positive decision making and healthy family relationships are vital to emotional security and (2) individual acceptability and skill must be considered when suggesting contraceptives (Hatcher et al., 1998). Laws in some settings restrict nurses and other health providers from engaging in certain types of counseling, including abortion counseling.

Some evidence suggests a decline in unintended pregnancy. Between 1994 and 1997, the birth rate for unmarried

Table 22-3 Summary of Effectiveness, Risks, and Noncontraceptive Benefits of Selected Contraceptive Methods

Contraceptive Method	Risks of Use	Noncontraceptive Health Benefits
Oral contraceptives (OCS) (combined and progestin only)	Thromboembolic disorder, cerebrovascular accident (CVA), coronary artery disease, especially in presence of smoking, hypertension, diabetes	Reduced risk of pelvic inflammatory disease, endometriosis, uterine fibroids, endometrial cancer, ovarian cancer, iron deficiency anemia, ectopic pregnancy
Diaphragm	Toxic shock syndrome, allergy to latex or spermicide, urinary tract infection	Reduced risk of STDs
Condom	Must be used consistently, allergy to rubber or latex or spermicide	Reduced risk of the sexual transmission of HIV and other STDs
Spermicides*	Spermicide sensitivity	Antiviral activity against HIV, decreased activity of other STD organisms, reduced risk of PID
Intrauterine contraceptive device	Bleeding, anemia, difficult removal, pelvic inflammatory disease (PID), ectopic pregnancy, cramping	—
Injectable progestin (Depo-Provera)	Limited data	Limited data indicates reduced risk of anemia, PID, cancer of endometrium and ovary
Implants (rods or capsules) (Norplant)	Data limited, but possibly similar to OCS	Limited data indicates reduced risks of PID and endometrial cancer
Sponge	Toxic shock syndrome	Decreased activity of other STD organisms
Female sterilization (tubal ligation)	Anesthesia, infection, hemorrhage	—
Male sterilization (vasectomy)	Complication rates low, reversal may be difficult	—

Modified from Hatcher, R., Trussell, J., Stewart, F., Cates, W., Stewart, G., Guest, F., & Kowal, D. (1998). *Contraceptive technology* (17th ed.). New York: Ardent Media; Grimes, D., & Wallach, M. (1997). *Modern contraception*. Totowa, NJ: Emron.
*Often used in combination with other methods.

women dropped nearly 11% for Black mothers and nearly 10% for unmarried Hispanic mothers (U.S. Department of Health and Human Services, 1999). Approximately one half of the unintended pregnancies are the result of contraceptive failure. Emergency contraception can reduce the number of unintended pregnancies by a 50% (Morris & Young, 2000) Three hormonal and one nonhormonal methods of emergency contraception are currently available in the United States (Morris & Young, 2000).

Maternal Mortality

Maternal mortality rates have risen slightly and continue to be of concern. The maternal mortality rate has remained between 7 and 8 per 100,000 live births since 1987 when it was 6.6 per 100,000 live births (U.S. Department of Health and Human Services, 2000). A number of factors in the United States influence the provision of sufficient prenatal care that keep maternal mortality rates high compared with those in other developed countries.

Access to prenatal care and financing of sufficient care are critical concerns. High-risk and minority women do not receive sufficient prenatal care. A lack of necessary insurance coverage and less-than-adequate referral mechanisms exist. Between 1990 and 1997 the proportion of mothers receiving care in the first trimester of pregnancy increased from 76% to 83%; the largest changes were seen in mothers of racial and ethnic groups with traditionally low levels of use. However, in 1997 a wide variation in receipt of care remained, ranging from 68% for Native-American mothers to 90% for Cuban-American mothers (U.S. Department of Health and Human Services, 2000).

Measures that are known to contribute to a decline in maternal deaths include the following (Olds, London, & Ladewig, 1996):

1. Compliance with prenatal counseling
2. Better knowledge and management of prenatal complications, labor, and delivery
3. Comprehensive childbirth information
4. Improved monitoring of the postpartum period to prevent complications (hemorrhage or infection)

Sexually Transmitted Disease

Sexually transmitted diseases (STDs) are a leading cause of infection and reproductive dysfunction in adults between ages 15 and 80. Young women ages 15 to 19 report the highest incidence of chlamydia and gonorrhea among women of all ages; men ages 20 to 24 have the highest reported rates of chlamydia and gonorrhea in the male population (U.S. Department of Health and Human Services, 2000). The list of STDs (Table 22-4) now

Table **22-4** **Summary of Sexually Transmitted Diseases**

Disease	Causative Agent	Diagnostic Methods	Treatment	Risks or Complications	Focus of Nursing Teaching
Vulvovaginal candidiasis (VVC)	*Candida albicans*	Wet mount-evidence of hyphae and spores	Antifungal topical medication	Recurrence of disease	Recheck for evidence of disease in 14 days, reduce moisture/heat in genital area
Trichomoniasis	Trichomonas vaginalis	Wet mount-observation of protozoa	Metronidazole (Flagyl)	Recurrence, excoriation of genital area	Understand medication regimen, use condoms to prevent new infection
Bacterial vaginosis (BV)	Gardnerella vaginalis	Wet mount-presence of "clue cells"	Metronidazole (Flagyl)	Asymptomatic infection	—
Chlamydia	Chlamydia trachomatis	Chlamydia monoclonal antibody test	Doxycycline	Infertility, urethral scarring, pelvic inflammatory disease (PID), endocervicitis, neonatal infection	Understand medication regimen, return for test of cure, refer partners for evaluation, use condoms to prevent future infections
Genital herpes	Herpes simplex virus	Herpes culture	Acyclovir at first diagnosis or first episode	Urethral stricture, lymph node enlargement	Examine partners, abstain from sex while symptomatic, annual Pap smears
Genital warts	HPV	Pap smear, observation of warts, colposcopy, biopsy	Podophyllin, trichloroacetic acid (TCA), cryotherapy	Cervical dysplasia	Return for treatment, examine partner
Acquired immunodeficiency syndrome (AIDS)	HIV	ELISA and Western blot	Current recommendations	Opportunistic infections	Monitor lymphocyte count, educate for current treatment recommendations
Gonorrhea	Neisseria gonorrhoeae	Culture	Ceftriaxone, doxycycline	PID, infertility, ectopic pregnancy	Monitor antibiotic treatment, examine partner, reculture
Syphilis	Treponema pallidum	Venereal Disease Research Laboratory (VDRL) test, rapid plasma reagin (RPR) test	Penicillin G benzathine	Secondary or late syphilis	Monitor antibiotic treatment, test and monitor partners

Data from Donovan, P. (1993). *Testing positive: Sexually transmitted disease and the public health response*. New York: Alan Guttmacher Institute; Hatcher, R., Trussell, J., Stewart, F., Cates, W., Stewart, G., Guest, F., & Kowal, D. (1998). *Contraceptive technology* (17th ed.). New York: Ardent Media.

includes HIV, *Chlamydia trachomatis* infections, genital herpes, HPV, chancroid, genital mycoplasmas, cytomegalovirus infections, HB, and vaginitis, in addition to the more widely known diseases of syphilis and gonorrhea. The presence of other STDs increases the risk of HIV transmission (U.S. Department of Health and Human Services, 2000). HPV is the most commonly occurring STD (5.5 million cases per year in 1996) followed by trichomoniasis, Chlamydia, herpes, gonorrhea, HB, syphilis, and HIV. STDs cost millions of dollars in screening, treatment, and reporting. In addition to creating a substantial problem for young adults, STDs impose tremendous demands on health care facilities. Many cases are unreported and untreated for lack of screening or failure to recognize symptoms.

The individual who seeks care frequently has symptoms of vaginal or urethral discharge associated with itching, dysuria, a rash, or the appearance of specific lesions. Many STDs of lesser severity remain unrecognized because of a lack of apparent symptoms. Consequently, STDs are responsible for complications detected later. Women suffer more serious STD complications than do men (U.S. Department of Health and Human Services, 2000). The most serious complications are pelvic inflammatory disease (PID), greater risk of cervical cancer, infertility, ectopic pregnancy, congenital infections, and low birth weight infants. PID is responsible for many cases of infertility, which occurs because pelvic infections tend to be asymptomatic, therefore they remain undiagnosed and untreated and are still able to cause significant scarring in the pelvic organs. PID is responsible for over 50,000 surgical procedures annually. For many women, the outcome of PID is sterility because total removal of the pelvic organs may be necessary. In men, gonorrheal complications can include disseminated gonococcal infection or epididymitis, prostatitis, and urethral stricture.

Condylomata acuminata (genital warts) are caused by HPV and are common in sexually active individuals. Untreated warts can grow into large masses and are a risk factor for cervical cancer. During pregnancy, these warts become especially exuberant and can develop into sites of secondary infection. Infants born to mothers with vaginal warts can develop laryngeal warts. Education about unprotected sexual behavior and the use of condoms is necessary to prevent transmission and to make susceptible individuals aware of health behaviors that decrease exposure (see Research Highlights box).

research highlights

Safer Sexual Behaviors

The purpose of this exploratory study was to examine variables characterized as predisposing to the practice of safer sexual behaviors. A sample of 227 male subjects from a state-supported university in southeastern New England returned questionnaires anonymously containing demographic questions and instruments to measure knowledge of HIV and AIDS, health locus of control, perceived susceptibility to AIDS, attitudes toward condoms, and safer sexual behaviors.

Results indicated that attitudes toward condoms were positively related to safer sexual behaviors. The more positive a subject's attitudes were toward condoms, the higher the score was on safer sex behaviors. As seen in prior research, adolescents and young adults are deficient in knowledge about HIV and AIDS. Although the level of knowledge is increasing, knowledge alone continues to be necessary, but not sufficient, for the practice of safer sexual behaviors. Because knowledge alone is insufficient, programs to prevent HIV transmission through sexual behavior must be specific and relevant to the population that they want to reach. Psychosocial factors that influence the practice of safer sexual behaviors must be targeted.

Data from Cole, F. L., & Slocumb, E. M. (1995). Factors influencing safer sexual behaviors in heterosexual late adolescent and young adult collegiate males. *Image: Journal of Nursing Scholarship*, *27* (3), 217-223.

Human Immunodeficiency Virus

HIV, which was first identified in 1983, causes acquired immunodeficiency syndrome (AIDS). The number of persons estimated to be infected with HIV in the United States ranges from 650,000 to 900,000 (U.S. Department of Health and Human Services, 2000). Although AIDS occurs much later in the infective process, only AIDS cases are formally reported by state health departments. HIV is transmitted by sexual intercourse, shared needles, and infected blood. Another less common source of transmission is from mother to baby across the placental barrier or through breast milk. There are two categories of HIV disease: (1) demonstration of infection with the virus through increased antibody titers (HIV positive) with the individual currently asymptomatic and (2) clinical AIDS, which causes severe immunodeficiency and the inability to combat common environmental and opportunistic infections. Other signs are weight loss, loss of appetite, weakness, lymphadenopathy, and muscle wasting. Definition of the clinical classification of HIV infection is continually undergoing revision as new information and testing become available. Since 1993 the classification has included the CD4 lymphocyte count as an indicator of immunosuppression (Centers for Disease Control and Prevention, 1993). A CD4+ lymphocyte count of under 200 cells per microliter of blood indicates AIDS; this level is one fifth that of a healthy adult. A recent study also indicates that measurement of plasma virus levels, which indicate viral reproduction, is even more accurate than lymphocyte count in predicting the course and progression of the disease (Ferri, 1996). The higher level of worry about contracting an STD in young adults is correlated with the implementation of risk-reduction behavior. Mortality from HIV infection declined 48% in 1997 after a decline of 29% in 1996. This recent decline is in sharp contrast to the period between 1987 and 1994 during which HIV mortality increased at an average rate of 16% per year (U.S. Department of Health and Human Services, 1999).

Nurses are aware that the incidence of STDs is greatly reduced with proper use of condoms. In 1997 only 23% of sexually active adults reported using condoms (U.S. Department of Health and Human Services, 2000). The *Healthy People 2010* target for condom use is 50%. Therefore all sexually active individuals should be counseled on the hazards of unprotected sexual activity and on the effective use and limitations of condoms, stressing that they must be used properly and can fail. Other than abstinence, latex (not natural) condoms provide the best protection from STDs. However, condom failures occur at an estimated rate of 10% to 15%; therefore counseling should stress that condom use is not foolproof.

Another AIDS-prevention success is the 66% decline between 1992 and 1997 in perinatal transmission. Rates of HIV transmission are greatly reduced by zidovudine therapy during pregnancy. Therefore the U.S. Public Health Service recommends voluntary testing for HIV and counseling as a part of basic prenatal care (U.S. Department of Health and Human Services, 2000).

The nurse's role in intervening for STDs includes providing treatment and education. Early diagnosis and treatment are essential for treatment to be the most effective. When an individual is suspected of having an STD, the nurse obtains a complete history, including sexual history, sexual contacts, previous treatment and test results, any signs or symptoms of a present infection, recent use of antibiotics, and allergic reactions to antibiotics. When treatment is required, the nurse ensures that the person understands the goals of treatment in an attempt to gain cooperation and adherence to the plan of care.

The nurse is an educator not only of the individual, but also of the general public. Appropriate health education for the individual with an STD includes modes of transmission, incubation periods, signs and symptoms, methods of treatment, complications derived from lack of treatment, and signs of repeat infections. Assessment of a person's knowledge helps to determine the understanding of all aspects of the health education effort. The hope is that the nurse can promote change in the individual's behavior and improve knowledge about behaviors that prevent STDs.

Coping–Stress-Tolerance Pattern

Assessment of Stress Levels

Stress, the result of forces operating on the individual that disrupt physiological or psychological equilibrium, is an integral part of young adulthood; therefore a comprehensive health assessment should include questions to determine stress levels. Increased anxiety, nervousness, depression, or somatic complaints are indicators of stress-related problems, as are divorce, loss of employment, failure to be promoted, or financial difficulties. The role of the nurse is to listen, offer support, and demonstrate concern. The nurse also suggests referrals to appropriate health providers and support groups.

Achievement Stress

Achievement-oriented stress differs from the stress of situational crises in that the stress of an overachiever is derived from internal pressures to succeed as measured by self-defined goals. Achievement-oriented stress frequently causes workaholic habits, including loss of sleep and omission of meals. When this behavior becomes extreme, serious physical and emotional consequences can occur, such as nutritional problems or burnout, which, in turn, leads to severe emotional and physical exhaustion. Workaholic behaviors may not be perceived by the individual and may not be apparent until changes in bodily functions or behavior occur. Young adults are generally health conscious and willing to alter personal lifestyles and behavior patterns to reduce stress and become healthier. Many people have responded to campaigns for physical fitness, exercise, and nutritional adjustment, which should increase their well being and life expectancy.

Suicide

Suicide is a leading cause of death in the young adult age group. Suicide occurs because many young adults are unable to cope with the pressures of adulthood. For some people, pressure arises when dealing with interpersonal conflicts: marital problems, family discord, or the loss of a close relationship; for others, the precipitating event is a lack of personal resources, unemployment, or dissatisfaction with work or school. Many young adults try to solve their problems before the fatal incident, but see no positive solutions; in many cases, a previous suicide attempt was their signal for help.

Women make suicide attempts more than do men, but men succeed more often. Suicide is more common among single or widowed individuals and divorced people. Young adults are more likely as a group to attempt suicide than are older individuals, and professionals are more likely to attempt suicide than are nonprofessionals. The age-adjusted rate for suicide declined approximately 2% between 1996 and 1997, and it remains the eighth leading cause of death overall. In 1997 the female young adult population exhibited more consistent declines than did the male population, which demonstrates some declines and some increases in suicide rates (see Table 22-2).

Nursing interventions are directed toward identifying behaviors in individuals who may be contemplating suicide. Physical clues to be noted include self-neglect, depression, slowed gait, slumped shoulders, and drooped faces. Presuicidal individuals also tend to exhibit impaired reality testing; feelings of hopelessness, helplessness, and rejection; impaired judgment and decision making; anxiety; weight loss; insomnia; or a radically changed affect.

The nurse working with young adults is aware of suicide as a potential problem. In addition to identifying presuicidal behaviors, the nurse also investigates relationship patterns to determine behaviors that are complicated by feelings of worthlessness and defeat. When the nurse identifies a young adult at risk for a suicide attempt, referrals to other professionals are indicated.

Values-Beliefs Pattern

Developing values and beliefs is part of maturing as an adult. Values, which are lifelong interests expressed in terms such as good or bad, frequently, but not always, predict behavior. Attitudes, frequently described as likes or dislikes, are changed most easily by influence. Beliefs, which are special attitudes based more on faith than on fact, are usually part of the background culture.

Young adults enter their 20s with habits, values, and beliefs acquired during childhood and adolescence. Many acquired habits foster continuance of practices that are hazardous to health and well being in later life. Irregular eating patterns, smoking, excessive use of alcohol, drug abuse, and reckless driving can result directly in obesity, hypertension, cardiovascular disease, cancer, and accidental death. Many adverse health habits and behaviors result from an inability to cope with life stressors.

Whether behavior patterns emanate from earlier periods or emerge during young adulthood, their long-range effects warrant prevention or early intervention in health management. Prevention is directed toward altering value and belief patterns that encourage poor health practices to those that support optimal health behaviors. An understanding of the difference among values, attitudes, and beliefs is important such that the nurse can distinguish one from the other and make a prediction about the relative difficulty of change; for example, attitudes can be revised more easily than values. Nursing interventions are more effective when the nurse can describe, discriminate, identify, and align value and belief patterns consistent with practices known to maximize health.

Values Involved in Parenting

Parenthood is envisioned by a majority of young adults; therefore health-promotion and health-protection activities to ensure healthy offspring are crucial (see Care Plan box). **Genetic impairment,** congenital defect caused by abnormal genes, is responsible for approximately one fourth of serious malformations in newborns (Olds, London, & Ladewig, 1996) and 2% of all newborns are afflicted with congenital malformations. Abnormal genes may result from heredity, environmental exposures, or abnormal cell divisions. Approximately 2000 genetic disorders are known, but only a few are responsible for most genetic diseases. The U.S. Public Health Service recommends that women who are capable of becoming pregnant should supplement their diet with folic acid to reduce the incidence of spina bifida and other neural tube defects.

Better treatment of many genetic diseases means that more individuals will live a normal adult lifespan. Young adults with a genetic disease must make many important decisions; predicting the transmission of the disease to potential offspring is a key factor in childbearing decisions. Diseases with a hereditary or genetic component, such as sickle cell disease and diabetes, frequently pose special problems during childbearing. In sickle cell disease, the carrier state occurs in approximately 1 of 12 Black births; additionally, women diagnosed as having sickle cell disease have decreased fertility and concerns about low oxygen levels, dehydration, and acidosis, all of which can contribute to sickle cell crisis. When pregnancy does occur, spontaneous abortion is common, and the risk of maternal mortality is high (approximately 2%) (Olds, London, & Ladewig, 1996).

Values Regarding Prenatal Diagnosis and Genetic Impairment

Specific prenatal diagnostic procedures have been available since the mid1960s. This capability has enabled the identification of high-risk pregnancies and requires the cooperation and education of childbearing women and their partners, both of whom must provide accurate family health and obstetrical histories and comply with suggested screening and follow-up measures. Decisions about the advisability of reproduction are based on current information on genetics and known deleterious genetic factors.

The finding of a malformed or genetically impaired fetus may result in a parental decision to terminate the pregnancy. The decision of whether to abort becomes a religious, ethical, and legal issue.

Theological and political debates and legislative mandates have greatly influenced family control over many of these decisions. Genetic counseling is an important nursing intervention for young adults. When a nurse suspects based on a health assessment that a family is at risk for producing a child with a genetic impairment, genetic screening should be discussed with the individual. A genetic specialist gives technical explanations of genetic disorders; however, nurses have a supportive role in helping young adults decide whether to have children or to carry through a pregnancy that is at risk.

Ethnicity, Race, and Culture

Ethnicity and culture characterize a person's differences and place within a particular race or subgroup of people. The young adult whose ethnic background is different from the that of the dominant culture is more likely to encounter prejudice and discrimination, which can occur because of specific differences in race, creed, language, attitudes, values, preferences, or behaviors. The young adult is suscepti-

CARE PLAN

Nursing Diagnosis: Health-Seeking Behaviors Related to Preconceptual Assessment and Preparation for Childbearing

DEFINING CHARACTERISTICS

- Expressed desire to improve overall health to prepare for childbearing
- Expressed thoughts about planning for pregnancy in the near future
- Desire to improve nutritional status before childbearing
- Desire to improve nutritional intake of essential vitamins (B_6) and minerals (iron and calcium)
- Plan to take multivitamin each day
- Plan to limit foods high in sodium and fat
- Plan to limit alcohol consumption
- Plan for overall exercise program to increase stamina and flexibility
- Seek physical examination to rule out problems that might negatively affect pregnancy; update immunizations
- Seek laboratory tests to rule out problems that might have negative influence on pregnancy (rubella titer)
- Seek information on possible pregnancy risk factors (biophysical, psychosocial, sociodemographic, and environmental)

RELATED FACTORS

- Expressed desire to improve the quality of relationships with husband or partner
- Desire to attend education classes to improve knowledge of childbearing and good health practices
- Plan for room or housing to accommodate children
- Plan for employment arrangements that accommodate child care

EXPECTED OUTCOMES

- Increase in indices of well being in patient
- Healthy pregnancy and future child
- Increase in self-confidence and awareness preparation for childbearing
- Manage possible pregnancy risk factors before becoming pregnant
- Make the person aware of resources available for pregnancy and child care

INTERVENTIONS

- Assess current level of wellness regarding preparation for childbearing
- Identify community resources that provide information regarding preconceptual planning and preparation
- Identify community sources of education
- Identify primary health provider, midwife or obstetrician, hospitals with delivery services
- Assess for possible biophysical risk factors (genetic disorders, nutritional problems, and current medical problems)
- Assess for history of pregnancy loss
- Test for blood type and Rh
- Screen for sexually transmitted disease, tuberculosis, rubella titer, sickle cell
- Review immunization history, including hepatitis B
- Assess nutrition by using a 3-day review of diet
- Assess need to augment diet, particularly to increase intake of calcium and iron
- Take a multivitamin daily
- Assess for psychosocial risk factors (mental problems, use of drugs, alcohol, caffeine consumption, and smoking)
- Avoid alcohol consumption
- Assess for possible sociodemographic risk factors (poverty, first pregnancy risks of dystocia or PIH, residence [rural or urban], and ethnicity)
- Assess for possible environmental risks (exposures to chemicals, drugs, pesticides, pollution, smoke, stress, and radiation)
- Assess current employment situation
- Identify possible child care arrangements

ble to these prejudices at work, at school, in health care delivery systems, and in the community. Young adults must meet not only personal needs, but also the needs of children or elders; therefore nurses must consider the values that are common to specific cultures and ethnic backgrounds.

Race and ethnicity are important influencers of health for young adults. Longevity for nonWhite men and women has increased recently, the result of a decrease in birth-related fatalities and in deaths caused by specific systemic disabilities. Blacks remain at risk for specific health problems, and the life expectancy of the average Black person is shorter than that of the average White person. Race and ethnicity can also influence the clinical response of an individual to drug therapy; unfortunately, many drug investigations underrepresent minority subjects in their samples, thus drug recommendations may be incompletely studied for some minority groups (Kudzma, 1999).

Race and ethnicity are closely connected to educational and work-related decisions, which subsequently affect choice of residence. Many Blacks must accept substandard housing or crowded living spaces. A lifestyle of this type, when combined with insufficient economic resources, frequently affects health. Couple instability and divorce can be an outgrowth of lifestyle patterns and socioeconomic conditions. Compared with the general population, divorce rates are proportionately higher among younger White women and older Black women; remarriage occurs less frequently for Black women than it does for White women in the same age ranges (U.S. Department of Commerce, 1999). Poverty is more frequent in Black families, which often leads to unmet basic needs of food, clothing, and housing and, in turn, leads to decreased regard for health needs.

Values and Minority Care

Obstacles and perceived barriers hinder entry into the health care system, especially for members of minority groups and recently arrived immigrants. In a study of 75 Vietnamese refugees (the largest group of Southeast Asians in the United States), new arrivals were significantly concerned about having a translator present in the health care facility, being understood by the health care provider, being able to understand oral and written instructions, and comprehending qualities related to the primary provider. Study subjects were also willing to be relocated to another clinic in which a translator was available and to seek more frequent care if a translator could be present (D'Avanzo, 1992).

PATHOLOGICAL PROCESSES

Accidents

Physical injury resulting in the disability or death of young adults can be caused by motor-vehicle accidents, misuse of firearms, falls, drowning, fires, and poisoning. The largest percentage of accidents occurs before age 35; ages 18 to 21 are peak years.

Motor-vehicle accidents are a leading cause of death among young adults; motor vehicles are involved in more fatal accidents that all other causes of death combined. Reducing speed limits contributes to lower fatality rates; however, much of this decrease in deaths is attributed to better use of automobile occupant protection and restraint systems. Approximately 48 states have seat belt laws and all states have seat belt requirements for children. The continued high incidence of vehicle accidents in this age group is related to accessibility of cars to young adults and peer pressure on driving behavior; reckless driving and driving under the influence of alcohol and drugs is now viewed as closely connected to violent and abusive behavior. Death rates for injuries are three times higher in the least educated adults as compared with the more educated adults (U.S. Department of Health and Human Services, 1999).

Accident-prevention education, long considered appropriate for young children, should be an important part of young adult instruction. Most young licensed drivers have participated in driver education courses; current educational programs that encourage the use of seat belts are extremely effective. The young adult must understand the potentially fatal consequences of aggressive tendencies or thoughtless risk-taking. When young adults are encouraged to reflect on the consequences of their actions, they tend to be more willing to control and change unsafe driving behaviors.

Pollution

Noise

Young adults are exposed to high levels of noise in occupational and recreational settings. Exposure to loud noise over time is directly related to impaired hearing and can also increase irritability and stress. Young adults can be exposed to noises in the work setting from industrial machinery and equipment. Noisy conditions are costly to industry in terms of mistakes, absenteeism, decreased efficiency, and lowered employee retention. Although industrial exposure to noise can be difficult to decrease, many young adults worsen the situation through further recreational exposure by listening to music or videos at excessively high-decibel levels.

Moderation in exposure to noise should be encouraged. Ear protection is necessary in some situations to prevent hearing disability. Recognition of noise hazards and corresponding appropriate preventive education are early nursing strategies for decreasing excessive noise exposure.

Air

Young adults are exposed to numerous pollutants in the environment. In industrial societies, pollution can be added to the air faster than natural forces can dilute or remove it. Air is defined as polluted when gases and particulate matter are incorporated to the extent that health, safety, comfort, and outdoor employment are negatively affected.

Motor vehicles are the largest source of air pollution; vehicles release over 90 million tons of particles and noxious gases each year, most of which is either carbon monoxide or hydrocarbons. Carbon monoxide in high concentration is deadly; in lower concentration it causes headaches, dizziness, and heart palpitations. In sunlight and low-lying areas, automobile exhaust becomes photochemical smog that contains ozone, which irritates the eyes and the respiratory tract.

Legislation, including the second Clear Air Act (1970), requires states to submit a plan to the Environmental Protection Agency to achieve air quality standards. Industries have been slow to respond to pollution-removing legislation because the cost of removing pollutants must be passed on to the consumer. Although air pollution is not a problem only for young adults, they frequently work in dirty, entry-level jobs in industrial settings and may be the age group that is most affected.

Occupational Hazards and Stressors

Occupational hazards pose a threat of illness, injury, or death in all age groups, and occupational safety standards have contributed greatly to the reduction of work-related accidents. Legislation, including the Occupational Safety and Health Act (1970), has resulted in the improvement of work conditions, along with the provision of health care facilities, in many companies.

Young adults should not be allowed to work in certain industrial settings without vocational training to reduce hazards. Young adults frequently want a challenge and high wages; therefore they work at hazardous jobs, for example, on offshore drilling rigs, on high bridges, or in nuclear plants. Because of their age, physical stamina, and agility, young adults are suitable candidates to be hired for positions that require physical ability. Occupational training should include education about personal exposure risks, identification of work-related hazards, and identification of situations in which the severity of accidents is connected to personal behaviors or habits. For example, drivers of heavy construction machinery should be particularly observant and avoid reckless behaviors and fast driving.

Routine physical evaluation and surveillance of the work site should be performed by employers. Examination of workers in certain industries is important. Known conditions such as asbestosis, byssinosis, silicosis, and pneumoconiosis (black lung disease) have been greatly reduced because of better knowledge of causative conditions, the process of disease, and protective activities. Working women who are pregnant can also expose their fetuses to industrial substances. Proper evaluation and temporary reassignment may be necessary.

Occupational preventive intervention requires that known work hazards and risks be identified early. Health histories should include questions about the place of work, type of work, and young adults' understanding of the risks associated with their occupations. Occupational risk and health are closely related; stress associated with work, the use of alcohol or drugs, and a negative attitude toward work are predictive of occupational injuries. Job counseling aimed at changing the nature of employment can be an appropriate referral for some health conditions. Employees in industrial settings should visit a health care provider on a periodic basis for health assessment, update of the health history, and counseling.

Chemical Agents

Drug Use

Misuse of drugs, a major risk for young adults, is associated with injury, disability, violence, homicide, and suicide and is related to social problems (various criminal behaviors and maladjustment to accepted norms). Drug abuse may be closely related to an inability to cope appropriately with adult responsibilities. The resulting physical health problems associated with drug misuse account for more than 50% of the major acute and chronic problems of young adults. Heroin users have increased mortality rates because of overdosage or chronic disability associated with hepatitis infections. Drug use is an independent risk factor involved in approximately one quarter of HIV infections.

Use of prescription drugs, such as anabolic steroids, to improve athletic performance is increasing. The risks of using steroids are enormous, and preventive education should focus on more realistic sports and exercise values.

Drug abuse in pregnant women directly affects fetal outcomes. Use of prescription medications during pregnancy requires close professional health care monitoring and strict compliance to the prescribed regimen and dosage. Gestational period is an important consideration when prescribing drugs. Fetal complications can also occur with over-the-counter drug use and drugs taken before the woman is aware that she is pregnant.

Nursing activities include preventive strategies to curb the problem of drug misuse. Distribution of information on drugs, early treatment of complications, and drug treatment centers are only part of the answer. Nursing efforts aimed at increasing individual awareness and altering drug-taking attitudes and behaviors are of critical importance (see Multicultural Awareness box).

Alcohol Use

Alcohol-related accidents among individuals ages 15 to 24 continue to be a leading cause of preventable morbidity, disability, and death. Heavy alcohol use, that is, consuming five or more drinks on at least one occasion within a month, is more common in the 18- to 25-year-old group than it is for younger or older people (U.S. Department of Health and Human Services, 1999). Raising the legal drinking age to 21 reduces not only deaths and injuries connected to motor-vehicle accidents, but also homicides and other violent deaths (Jones, Piper, & Robertson, 1992). Alcohol abuse is directly related to later chronic conditions affecting adults, such as cirrhosis of the liver; alcohol is also a contributing factor in cancer of the esophagus, larynx, and oral cavity. Modifying alcohol consumption in young adults can decrease the frequency of chronic and disabling conditions in later life.

Alcohol consumption is increasing in the young adult population. The best predictor of adult alcohol dependence or abuse is the number of times that an individual was intoxicated before the sixteenth birthday (Clapper , Buka, Goldfield, & Lipsitt, 1995). Although young adults drink less regularly than do older adults, they tend to consume larger amounts of alcohol at one time; the tendency is toward binge drinking, which causes an increased loss of control and is related to an additional risk of accidents.

Women who work outside the home have increased opportunities for social drinking. Pregnant women who drink alcoholic beverages have additional risks for pregnancy complications, including fetal alcohol syndrome, noted by central nervous system manifestations and gastrointestinal alterations in the baby. The number of infants identified as having fetal alcohol syndrome has increased, although the increase may result from more vigilant case finding. Nursing interventions include early

MULTICULTURAL AWARENESS

Racial and Ethnic Variations in Drug Response

Nurses understand that weight, height, age, and gender are important influences of drug response and effectiveness. Various studies, although limited, indicate that race and ethnicity may also be important factors to consider when prescribing certain drugs. Different genetic types tend to metabolize drugs differently, have different binding receptors, or have different environmental influences that change the utilization and uptake of drugs. Several studies indicate that drug effectiveness can vary according to race.

In studies of people with hypertension, Black individuals responded with a greater decrease in systolic pressure to thiazide diuretics (hydrochlorothiazide) and calcium channel blockers. Black patients have a blunted response to beta blockers, which can be improved by adding a diuretic.

The situation in Asian patients appears to be the exact opposite. In a study of the effectiveness of propranolol in Chinese and White men, the Chinese men had at least a twice as much sensitivity as did the White men to propranolol administered at several dosage levels (10, 20, 40, and 80 mg every 8 hours). Compared with the White men, the Chinese men experienced a 20% greater reduction in heart rate and a 10% greater reduction in blood pressure. These findings may explain the low number of prescriptions of propranolol in China.

In another example of a commonly used substance, studies indicate that Asians are more sensitive to alcohol and its drug effects than is the White population. The most outstanding difference was in the amount of facial flushing, which was experienced by 47% to 85% of Asians compared with 3% to 29% of a White sample. The Asians also experienced other undesirable discomforts attributable to alcohol, including palpitations, tachycardia, head pounding, and muscle weakness, to a greater degree than did the White subjects.

These examples suggest that nurses should be aware of racial and ethnic issues in drug metabolism and effectiveness. In individuals who do not respond to certain drugs as expected, the nurse may consider whether this might be related to constitutional factors within the person's genetic makeup. Nurses are aware that height and weight affect drug dosage and utilization, which should indicate that there may be differences in drug effectiveness that are solely attributable to racial and genetic distinctions. This research also has implications for sample selection in clinical drug trials and invites rethinking of managed-care practices that restrict diversity of drug use with prescribed drug formulary listings.

Data from Hall, W. D. (1999). A rational approach to the treatment of hypertension in special populations. *American Family Physician, 60* (1), 156-162; Matthew, H. W. (1995). Racial, ethnic and gender differences in response to medicines. *Drug Metabolism and Drug Interactions, 12* (2), 77-91; Wood, A. J. (1998). Ethnic differences in drug disposition and response. *Therapeutic Drug Monitoring, 20* (5), 525-526; Zhou, H., Kosharji, B., Silverstein, D., Wilkinson, G., & Wood, A. (1989). Racial differences in drug response: Altered sensitivity to and clearance of propranolol in men of Chinese descent as compared with American whites. *New England Journal of Medicine, 320* (9), 565-570.

identification of pregnant women who are heavy alcohol users. Some evidence suggests that a tendency exists for primary care providers to underdiagnose alcohol abuse problems; in some studies, detection rates for alcohol and drug abuse problems appear too low.

Tobacco Use

Smoking is a leading cause of preventable death in the United States; therefore smoking cessation is the single most important counseling topic for all people because of its potential to lower the risk of contracting many preventable diseases. The prevalence of current cigarette smoking in individuals 18 years of age and older is 22% for women and 27% for men (U.S. Department of Health and Human Services, 2000). Evidence suggests that smoking rates in young adults are abating. In 1998 cigarette smoking in high school seniors declined slightly after 5 years of increases (U.S. Department of Health and Human Services, 1999). In later adulthood, the incidence of smoking declines: 28% for persons 18 to 24 years of age, but only 12% for those over age 65 (U.S. Department of Health and Human Services, 2000).

Nurses serve as role models to help people stop smoking. Nurses relate information on the disease consequences of smoking whenever possible. Individuals employed in high-risk occupations should be informed of the synergistic relationship between smoking and occupations involving asbestos and radiation exposure. Fear tactics, nagging, preaching, and threats are generally ineffective in convincing people to stop smoking (see Research Highlights box).

Serious legislative and environmental efforts are currently underway to create a social climate in which smoking is unacceptable; this approach reflects the concept of smoking as a social disease. In one study, the relationship between smoking and the attainment of adolescent and adult roles was investigated. The acquiring of the smoking habit was positively related to pseudomaturity, which was related more to the adolescent social role than it was to the adult role, in which smoking was viewed as an incompatible behavior with adult status (Chassin, Presson, Sherman, & Edwards, 1992) (Box 22-5).

Nurses are familiar with the antismoking resources in their communities, enabling them to make the appropriate referrals. Recommending or prescribing nicotine gum or a patch is particularly useful for highly habituated individuals.

Cancer

Environmental Carcinogens

Exposure to environment carcinogens is a potent stressor. Exposure to carcinogens in young adults is frequently

research highlights

Smoking Cessation in Young Adults

The purpose of this longitudinal epidemiological study was to examine the relationship between age of smoking initiation and age of smoking cessation. A simple random sample of 1200 individuals was selected from 400,000 members of a health maintenance organization in southeastern Michigan. Of those selected, 1007 individuals (84%) were interviewed at their homes by phone. A follow-up phone call was conducted 3½ years after baseline with 979 (97%) of the original individuals. The median age of respondents was 26 years; 61.7% were women, 80.7% were White, and 45% were married. A small percentage (3.7%) had less than a high school education, whereas 46% had some college and 29.3% were college graduates.

With potential confounding variables accounted for, the likelihood of cessation was significantly higher in smokers who initiated smoking after age 13 compared with those who began before this age. Additionally, findings indicated that the potential for quitting was markedly higher in smokers with a college education compared with smokers with no college education. Factors that decreased the likelihood of cessation were nicotine dependence and low education. The generality of the findings is limited to young adults.

Data from Breslau, N., & Peterson, F. L. (1996). Smoking cessation in young adults: Age at initiation of cigarette smoking and other suspected influences. *American Journal of Public Health*, 86 (2), 214-220.

Box 22-5 Three-Pronged Unified Approach Recommended to Decrease the Prevalence of Smoking in the United States

1. Youth antismoking programs to prevent the acquisition of the smoking habit
2. Smoking-cessation programs to help current smokers quit
3. A less harmful cigarette for those who cannot or will not quit smoking

associated with work setting, smoking habit, and alcohol consumption. Although environmental protective controls have limited exposure to some hazardous chemicals, the effects on health of many industrial chemicals remains unknown. For example, latex, long considered inert and safe, has now been shown to cause long-term immune disease in some nurses exposed to the agent (or the chemicals that bind it) in surgical gloves.

Breast cancer, a leading form of malignancy in women, has only recently been surpassed in incidence by lung cancer. Although age-adjusted mortality rates have remained stable, the upswing in the incidence of breast cancer that was detected in the 1980s is the result primarily of an increase in the detection of smaller tumors (Harris, Lippman, Veronesi, & Willett, 1992); this trend is believed to reflect the wider use of screening mammography. Alcohol may act as a carcinogen with regard to breast cancer; an increase in alcohol consumption by younger women may have contributed appreciably to the increased breast-cancer incidence currently observed (Harris, Lippman, Veronesi, & Willett, 1992).

The recent high incidence of lung cancer in women is a consequence of women's delayed, but relatively high smoking rate. **Environmental tobacco smoke** exposes individuals to nicotine and carbon monoxide, which causes endothelial injury, vasospasm, increased platelet aggregation, and atheroslerotic plaques that affect oxygenation of all body cells. It increases the risk of heart disease, asthma, and bronchitis (U.S. Department of Health and Human Services, 2000) and is a potential hazard for infants and young children in the household. Smoking is a potent carcinogen and a smoking history is found in most individuals who develop lung cancer. Cervical cancer has decreased steadily over the years, likely because of the effective use of screening methods, such as **Papanicolaou (Pap) smear** testing. HPV and smoking are known environmental carcinogenic factors that are associated with the development of cervical cancer.

Screening for Malignancies in Women

All adults are likely to contract malignant disease as they age. However, in two prominent ways, earlier detection of malignancies has decreased mortality ratios for women. Two key screening tests are recommended for young adult women: (1) BSEs or mammograms, when necessary and (2) Pap smears. Women in this age group are counseled to perform BSEs and have regular breast examinations by a health care provider. Rates for cervical dysplasia and cancer peak in both White and Black women between ages 20 and 30. The rate for Black women increases faster than it does for White women over the age of 25. Known risk factors for cervical cancer include smoking, early age of first intercourse, increasing number of sexual partners, and infection with HPV.

SOCIAL PROCESSES

Community and Work

Neighborhood Resources

The environment of the community strongly influences the well being of the young adult and sets the standard for the health of people and families living within a neighborhood. Neighbors can be an excellent source of support, which can be especially important to a young mother who does not have immediate family nearby. Nurses working in the community facilitate the contact of individuals with common interests through community and religious activities and support groups.

Community resources for exercise and recreation can make important contributions to the young adult's physical and emotional health (Fig. 22-5). When these resources are

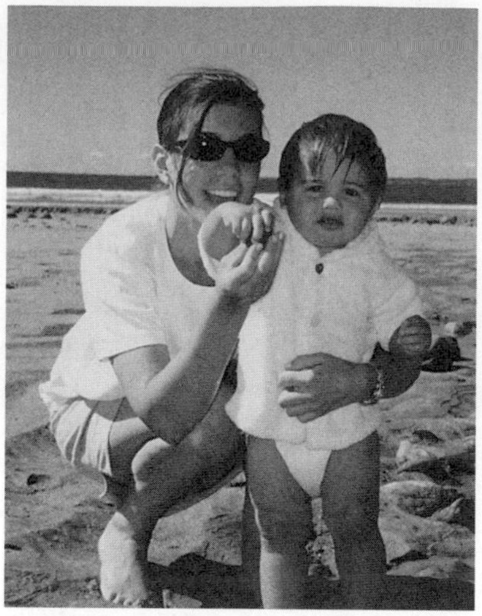

Fig. 22-5 Young adults' need for recreation with their family members can make important contributions to their physical and emotional health.

available, the young adult can have the opportunity to exercise and release stress in a positive fashion. In one study, access to a campus health-promotion program that included aerobic fitness, stress management, interpersonal counseling, and nutrition information had a lasting influence on 90% of 233 young adults who were studied and monitored for at least 2 years (McClary, Pyeritz, Bruce, & Henshaw, 1992).

Schools within the community are a concern for parents; parents who are dissatisfied with the public school system can experience additional stress. When economic resources are available, private schooling becomes an option. This approach can add additional financial burdens to the young family who is already financially troubled. When there are inadequate resources, the family can feel frustration and despair.

Health Service Availability

The availability of health services within a community is important. Economic realities, however, influence the effectiveness of resources, particularly for the young adult who lives in an economically depressed area. In some communities, health services are lacking or, when available, are not culturally sensitive or adapted to the customs and beliefs of the people who are served. In other communities, access to public transportation can be a critical problem affecting the ability of the young adult to make appointments for health care. Young adults ages 18 to 24 years are the least likely of any age group to have a usual source of care, thus a target of *Healthy People 2010* is to increase the proportion of persons with a usual primary care provider (U.S. Department of Health and Human Services, 2000).

Culture and Ethnicity

Cultural beliefs and health practices of young adults, particularly for young women of childbearing age, are a major nursing concern. Young mothers occasionally use inappropriate health practices because of beliefs that are based on historical customs.

Health delivery methods in the United States are based on Western belief systems, which tend to be rigid in their applications for specific individuals. For example, women seeking birth control information and prescriptions are expected to use health clinics and keep to their schedule of return visits. Because health care provider systems have removed many traditional barriers once assumed to be responsible for poor utilization of services by low-income or minority groups (location and scheduling), nonattendance at scheduled clinic visits is frequently interpreted as noncompliance. Among Native Americans, contraceptive education has gained little acceptance, and fertility rates remain high, primarily because conception control is both culturally and religiously objectionable.

Appropriate health strategies and interventions require that nurses identify cultural beliefs and health care practices that are harmful to people. Many cultural practices may be allowed because they do not affect appropriate health care. For example, food cravings are common among many pregnant women. In moderation, following dietary patterns directed by these cravings is not harmful. When the craving leads to an unbalanced diet or to pica (eating nonfood substances), however, the pregnancy can be affected (Olds, London, & Ladewig, 1996).

Legislation

Young adults comprise one of the major political constituencies in the United States; they support many causes and provide the time and energy to publicize issues related to the common good. Some of these issues involve the environment, nuclear energy, war, and pollution. Relative to health, predominant issues have involved housing and health care in neighborhoods and rural areas and health, agricultural, and sanitation concerns in foreign countries. Through these efforts, young adults can influence and improve living conditions for future generations.

Demographics

To ameliorate health problems for an entire population, nurses concentrate on the entire societal environment that influences personal behavior and lifestyle. Thought and planning must be devoted to variables such as world population, food supplies, air, water, energy consumed, technological advances, transportation, schools, housing, and health services. Resources must be protected for future generations such that the land will be kept aesthetically acceptable and family life will continue to nurture the young. The population must simultaneously correct past pollution mistakes and consider the current environment. The future must be prepared by designing ways to preserve energy sources, control the economy, and ensure freedom as a peaceful nation. Many threats to national survival can be protected through the efforts of young adults.

Economics

One of the young adult's age-related tasks is to choose and develop a lifelong career. This choice is directly related to economic factors; young adults want satisfying occupations that also yield adequate economic returns. To manage financially and maintain a lifestyle in which personal needs can be met, young adults may elect to have fewer children. Caring for aging parents can also cause physical, psychosocial, spiritual, and economic stress.

Although goals vary greatly among young adult couples, they are generally concerned with acquiring material comforts; the desire for housing, transportation, clothing, or recreation generally necessitate that both partners work to meet financial obligations. This desire necessitates the changing of roles and the sharing of responsibilities, and open communication becomes a crucial component. For single parents, these challenges can appear insurmountable.

New career opportunities and the more stable economic expansion in the United States during the 1990s have allowed young adults more career choices. During the later part of the 1990s, young adults who are college graduates have had the best choice of employment opportunities in decades. The booming technical industry has provided employment in a wide variety of technical occupations and start-up companies. Work styles within these companies tend to be different from that in the traditional workplace, including an expectation of longer and more fluid workdays. "Dot.com" computer or Internet-based companies provide young adults with jobs that have the potential to give them rapid financial rewards at the cost of long-term job stability. Young adults are becoming accustomed to the idea that long-term employment is less available in the economies of the future.

Homelessness

Homeless people were, at one time, primarily single men; today, entire families account for approximately one third of the estimated homeless population. Five factors are known to contribute to homelessness: (1) the shortage of affordable housing, (2) poverty, (3) mental illness, (4) alcoholism, and (5) family disruption. The process of becoming homeless can be divided into two phases: (1) displacement from current housing and (2) an inability to relocate in substitute housing. In one study, women and their families stayed an average of 2 to 11 months in shelters before locating housing. The study also showed that poverty was a key factor; welfare benefits were generally too low to cover high rents, and long waits for public housing were common. Adequate housing may be located away from transportation and health care facilities, hindering access to health care (Francis, 1992). Men tend to use shelters only for night residence. The proportion of homeless people with high school diplomas has increased over the last few years; many homeless people hold jobs, at least on an intermittent basis, approximately 10% to 20% of the time. Minorities are significantly disproportionately represented among the homeless in larger cities, reflecting the large number of minority people who live below or near the poverty level.

Box 22-6 Important Nursing Activities for Young Adults

1. Publicizing known health risk factors of this age group to young adults at schools, at work sites, and in the community
2. Providing specific techniques and methodologies to alter lifestyles, lowering or decreasing health risks
3. Identifying the signs and symptoms of health problems specific to this age group that merit further medical investigation
4. Finding opportunities for health promotion and protection in the many settings in which young adults are found
5. Broadening the focus of health-promotion efforts to address the role of social inequities on influencing health outcomes

From Minkler, M. (1994). Challenges for health promotion in the 1990s: Social inequities empowerment, negative consequences and the common good. *American Journal of Health Promotion*, 8 (6), 403-413.

Dual Careers

For many young adult couples, different careers, friends, and varying maturity levels place additional strains on their relationship. These circumstances can provide a basis for domestic difficulty. Domestic quarreling tends to precede family disruption, leading to marital separation or divorce. In addition to the emotional strain placed on family members, domestic arguments can result in aggressive acts of abuse and personal injury. Young adults can also be faced with decisions about day care facilities; the couple or mother may need support to resolve guilt feelings related to the separation from her child.

Alternative lifestyles include living arrangements with individuals of the same gender or the opposite gender. Although these lifestyles are becoming more acceptable in today's society, attitudes toward various lifestyles contribute pressures that lead to further stress and uncertainty in the future.

Health Care Delivery System

For the young adult, the principal settings for health care delivery are schools, work sites, and the community. Additionally, many traditional health care settings, such as hospitals and clinics, have programs specifically designed to meet the needs of young adults who frequently perceive themselves as too healthy to use health care services. Between 1990 and 1997 injuries that caused work absenteeism declined 21% to 3.1 per 100 workdays in private sector employment (U.S. Department of Health and Human Services, 1999).

U.S. goals for "younger" young adults focus on improving health and health behaviors that will reduce mortality rates by approximately 20% by the year 2000

(U.S. Department of Health and Human Services, 1996). Specific goals are directed toward promoting healthy lifestyles, reducing fatal motor vehicle and other accidents, reducing alcohol and drug abuse that leads to death, and improving mental health status to reduce suicide and homicide.

SUMMARY

Nurses promote health care measures and behaviors at all places where young adults come into contact with the health care delivery system. In community colleges and university settings, efforts can be directed toward health education curricula with emphasis on positive health behaviors, establishment of peer counseling groups, and better utilization of sports and exercise facilities. Workshops on alcoholism, drugs abuse, sports or exercise, mental health and self-expression, relationships, and various aspects of sexual care have been effective in college populations. At the work site, programs of employee counseling, blood pressure monitoring and treatment, exercise, smoking reduction, cafeteria nutrition management, and stress reduction have also been effective. Employee monitoring and commitment to a safe and healthy work environment should be promoted. Employee insurance programs should undergo continual review to determine an appropriate level of integrated care and

innovative practice

Gay and Lesbian Wellness Series

The Gay and Lesbian Wellness Series is a multidisciplinary educational program offered through the collaborative efforts of the Be Well! programs of the Tanger Center for Health Management and the Lesbian and Gay Advisory Committee at Beth Israel Deaconess Medical Center (BIDMC) in Boston, Massachusetts.

The program was developed to address health and wellness issues of interest to the gay and lesbian communities. The clinician-teachers encourage patients and employees of the hospital and ambulatory care centers and members of the community, whether gay, straight, or bisexual, to come together in these educational, free programs.

"Beth Israel Deaconess Medical Center's mission is to deliver high-quality clinical care, lead research and teaching efforts, and invest in our surrounding communities. The Medical Center is fully committed to meeting the health and wellness needs of the gay and lesbian community. In addition to serving our patients and communities, we also have a strong commitment to celebrating diversity in our workplace. This *new* series represents these strong commitments."

The following examples are indicative of the educational topics that are offered:

SEXUAL ORIENTATION AND THE WORKPLACE: CREATING AN OPEN ENVIRONMENT

Understanding the dynamics of the work environment, whether as a clinician, manager, or support staff, can be challenging when issues of sexual orientation in the workplace are examined. As a gay or lesbian employee, how comfortable do you feel being "out" at work? Alternatively, as a manager of gay and lesbian employees, how successful are you in creating an environment in which staff members feel safe, comfortable, and valued? This class is a discussion of this topic aimed at creating an open environment for all.

A WELCOMING PLACE FOR ALL: IMPROVING ACCESS AND QUALITY FOR GAY AND LESBIAN PATIENTS

Underestimating the power of a simple word or gesture in providing care for individuals is easy. Sensitivity to the wording of materials and forms, and the way in which questions are asked can help gay and lesbian patients feel safe and comfortable. This class offers the opportunity to learn more about steps you can take to make your department, unit, or practice a welcoming place for all. Special emphasis will be placed on standards of practice developed by the Department of Public Health.

SELECTING AND COMMUNICATING WITH YOUR HEALTH CARE PROVIDER

Asking the right questions and developing a comfortable and trusting relationship with a primary care provider are important challenges for everyone. For gay and lesbian patients, the task can be especially difficult. This class is a discussion for patients and providers on the challenges and successes of choosing a health care provider. BIDMC's Gay and Lesbian Provider Network is available for discussion and as a resource. Tips are available for enhancing the lines of communication between the patient and health care providers.

SUPPORTING AND COMMUNICATING WITH YOUR GAY OR LESBIAN CHILD: UNDERSTANDING GAY AND LESBIAN ISSUES IN THE FAMILY

Parents of gay and lesbian children frequently have few places to which to turn for support and information. Struggling with love for one's child and the challenges of accepting the child's sexual orientation can be an overwhelming dilemma. This two-part series offers support and guidance for parents wanting to do their best.

Be Well!
Tanger Center for Health Management
Beth Israel Deaconess Medical Center
Boston, Massachusetts
617-667-4695

Courtesy Carol Lynn Mandle, PhD, RN.

coverage for the insured group. Mental health, dental health, and maternity benefits should be analyzed and increased when necessary.

Nurses must be increasingly active in the development of health policy, which includes identification of resources, planning for resource use, and coordination of services. Because national objectives to promote health affect the lives of all young adults, available resources that provide services to meet these objectives must be identified. Accurate planning of services is essential, primarily because resources for health promotion and disease prevention are limited.

Young adults are generally healthy, which challenges the nurse to be even more sensitive, insightful, and creative in implementing care for individuals within this age group (Box 22-6).

REFERENCES

Arnett, J. J., & Taber,. S. (1994). Adolescence terminable and interminable: When does adolescence end? *Journal of Adolescence, 23* (5), 517-537.

Bassetti, M. (1996). An ounce of prevention: Updating clinical practice guidelines. *Advanced Practice Nurse, 5*, 37-40.

Block, J., & Robbins, R. W. (1993). A longitudinal study of consistency and change in self-esteem from early adolescence to early adulthood. *Child Development, 64*, 909-923.

Breslau, N., & Peterson, F. L. (1996). Smoking cessation in young adults: Age at initiation of cigarette smoking and other suspected influences. *American Journal of Public Health, 86* (2), 214-220.

Campbell, J. C., Harris, M. J., & Lee, R. K. (1995). Violence research: An overview. *Scholarly Inquiry for Nursing Practice, 9* (2), 105-126.

Centers for Disease Control and Prevention. (1993). CDC revises AIDS definition. *American Nurse, 25* (3), 20.

Chassin, L., Presson, C., Sherman, S., & Edwards, D. (1992). The natural history of cigarette smoking and young adult social roles. *Journal of Health and Social Behavior, 33* (4), 328-347.

Clapper, R., Buka, S., Goldfield, E., & Lipsitt, L. (1995). Adolescent problem behaviors as predictors of adult alcohol diagnoses. *International Journal of Addictions, 30* (5), 507-523.

Cole, F. L., & Slocumb, E. M. (1995). Factors influencing safer sexual behaviors in heterosexual late adolescent and young adult collegiate males. *Image: Journal of Nursing Scholarship, 27*, (3), 217-223.

Coles, R. (1978). Work and self-respect. In E. Erikson, *Adulthood*. New York: W. W. Norton.

Conrad, P. (1994). Wellness as virtue: Morality and the pursuit of health. *Culture, Medicine and Psychiatry, 18* (3), 385-401.

Cooper, K. (1992). *Aerobics*. New York: Bantam Books.

D'Avanzo, D. (1992). Barriers to health care for Vietnamese refugees. *Journal of Professional Nursing, 8* (4), 245-253.

Dieterich, D. (2000). Chronic hepatitis C: Update on diagnosis and treatment. *Consultant, 40* (9), 1590-1596.

Donovan, P. (1993). *Testing positive: Sexually transmitted disease and the public health response*. New York: Alan Guttmacher Institute.

Erikson, E. H. (1993). *Childhood and society*. New York: W. W. Norton.

Ferri, R. S. (1996). AIDS update: Viremia—best predictor of AIDS progression. *AIDS Clinical Review, 6* (7), 120-122.

Frame, P. S. (1992). Health maintenance in clinical practice: Strategies and barriers. *American Family Physician, 45* (3), 1192-1200.

Francis, M. B. (1992). Eight homeless mothers' tales. *Image: Journal of Nursing Scholarship, 24* (2), 111-114.

Gilligan, C. (1982). New maps of development: New visions of maturity. *American Journal of Orthopsychiatry, 52* (2), 199-212.

Grimes, D., & Wallach, M. (1997). *Modern contraception*. Totowa, NJ: Emron.

Hall, W. D. (1999). A rational approach to the treatment of hypertension in special populations. *American Family Physician, 60* (1), 156-162.

Harris, J. R., Lippman, M., Veronesi, V., & Willett, W. (1992). Breast cancer. *New England Journal of Medicine, 327* (5), 319-328.

Hatcher, R., Trussell, J., Stewart, F., Cates, W., Stewart, G., Guest, F., & Kowal, D. (1998). *Contraceptive technology* (17th ed.). New York: Ardent Media.

Hoff, L. A., & Rosenbaum, L. (1994). A victimization assessment tool: Instrument development and clinical implications. *Journal of Advanced Nursing, 20* (4), 627-634.

Jones, N. W., Piper, C. F., & Robertson, L. S. (1992). The effect of legal drinking age on fatal injuries of adolescents and young adults. *American Journal of Public Health, 82* (1), 112-115.

Keller, C. (1993). Developing and sustaining valued health behaviors in young African-American women. *Journal of Health Education Promotion, 17* (3), 49-56.

Kohlberg, L., & Lickons, T. (1986). *The stages of ethical development: From childhood through old age*. San Francisco: Harper.

Kudzma, E. C. (1999). Culturally competent drug administration. *American Journal of Nursing, 99* (8), 46-51.

Kulbok, P. A., & Baldwin, J. H. (1992). From preventive health behavior to health promotion: Advancing a positive construct of health. *Advances in Nursing Science, 14* (4), 50-64.

Lander, A., Foster, C., & Jones, H. (1992). *Women's changing roles*. Wylie, TX: Information Plus.

Matthew, H. W. (1995). Racial, ethnic and gender differences in response to medicines. *Drug Metabolism and Drug Interactions, 12* (2), 77-91.

McClary, C., Pyeritz, E., Bruce, W., & Henshaw, E. (1992). A liberal arts health-promotion course. *Journal of American College Health, 41* (2): 71-72.

McClelland, C., Thompson, P., Prete, S., & Hatcher, P. (1996). Assessing firearm safety. *Nursing & Health Care, 17* (4), 174-178.

Meehan, P., Lamb, J., Saltzman, L., & O'Carroll, P. (1992). Attempted suicide among young adults: Progress toward a meaningful estimate of prevalence. *American Journal of Psychology, 149* (1), 41-44.

Minkler, M. (1994). Challenges for health promotion in the 1990s: Social inequities empowerment, negative consequences and the common good. *American Journal of Health Promotion, 8* (6), 403-413.

Morris, B., & Young, C. (2000). Emergency, emergency contraception. *American Journal of Nursing, 100* (9), 46-48.

Nicklas, T., Webber, L., Johnson, C., & Srinivasan, S. (1995). Foundations for health promotion with youth: A review of observations from the Bogalusa Heart Study. *International Journal of Health Education, 26* (2), S18-26.

Olds, S. B., London, M. L., & Ladewig, P. W. (1996). *Maternal-newborn nursing: A family-centered approach*. Menlo Park, CA: Addison-Wesley.

O'Sullivan, A. L., Apriceno-Tesoro, T. (1993). Prevention: Adolescent health. In R. N. Knollmueller, *Prevention across the life span*. Washington, DC: American Nurses Publishing.

Piaget, J. (1972). Intellectual evolution from adolescence to adulthood. *Human Development, 15*, 1-12.

Preventing and controlling meningococcal disease: Latest guidelines. (2000). *Consultant, 40* (9), 1654-1657.

Quillian, J. P. (1996). Screening for spousal or partner abuse in a community health setting. *Journal of the American Academy of Nurse Practitioners, 8* (4), 155-160.

Ratner, P. A. (1995). Indicators of exposure to wife abuse. *Canadian Journal of Nursing Research, 27* (1), 31-46.

Schroeder, S., Tierney, L., & McPhee, S. (1992). *Current medical diagnosis and treatment*. Norwalk, CT: Appleton & Lange.

Somers, A. R., & Breslow, L. (1979). Lifetime health monitoring program. *Nurse Practitioner, 4*, 40, 50, 54.

U.S. Department of Commerce, Bureau of Census. (1999). *Statistical abstracts of the United States: National data book* (119th ed.). Washington, DC: U.S. Government Printing Office.

U.S. Department of Health and Human Services. (1996). *Health, United States, 1995* (PHS Pub. No. 96-1232). Washington, DC: U.S. Government Printing Office.

U.S. Department of Health and Human Services. (1999). *Health-United States, 1999*. Hyattsville: MD: U.S. Government Printing Office.

U.S. Department of Health and Human Services. (2000). *Healthy people 2010: Vol 1 and 2* (Conference ed.). Washington, DC: U.S. Government Printing Office.

U.S. Preventive Services Task Force. (1996). *Guide to clinical preventive services* (2nd ed.). Baltimore: Williams and Wilkins.

Wood, A. J. (1998). Ethnic differences in drug disposition and response. *Therapeutic Drug Monitoring, 20* (5), 525-526.

Yam, M. (1995). Wife abuse: Strategies for a therapeutic response. *Scholarly Inquiry of Nursing Practice*, 9 (2), 147-158.

Zhou, H., Kosharji, B., Silverstein, D., Wilkinson, G., & Wood, A. (1989). Racial differences in drug response: Altered sensitivity to and clearance of propranolol in men of Chinese descent as compared with American whites. *New England Journal of Medicine, 320* (9), 565-570.

Chapter 23

CAROL LYNN MANDLE

Middle-Age Adult

objectives

After completing this chapter, the nurse will be able to:

- Name three psychosocial and spiritual changes that frequently occur during middle age.
- Explain two normal biological changes that occur as a result of the aging process.
- Identify the major causes of mortality in the middle-age adult.
- Describe the health patterns of middle-age adults.
- Discuss the unique health problems related to the occupations of the adult between ages 35 and 65.
- Discuss the influence of psychosocial stressors on the middle-age adult and the ways the individual's culture and occupation can affect these stressors.

key terms

Advance Directive	Functional Aerobic Capacity	Obesity
Calcium	Generativity	Osteoporosis
Cardiac Output	Gingivitis	Periodontitis
Constipation	Kyphosis	Presbycusis
Degenerative Joint Disease	Menopause	Presbyopia
Durable Power of Attorney	Midlife Crisis	Stagnation

THINK About It

Terminal Illness

Charlie Shelton is dying of lung cancer. His wife, Sarah, finds that she must manage a household and provide for their two children (ages 15 and 18) on her own. The elder child plans to enter college next fall, but the Sheltons wonder whether they will be able to afford this. Although Charlie and Sarah worked hard and saved money all their lives, Charlie's long illness continues to deplete their savings. Their parents are helping as best they can, but they live on limited incomes themselves. The hospital bills continue to come, and the Sheltons are overwhelmed.

1. What can health providers do to help the Sheltons during this stressful time?
2. What health-promotion strategies might be suggested and implemented to help them?
3. What community organizations might the health care provider recommend to meet the needs of this family?
4. What responsibilities do health providers and policy makers have to provide health promotion to middle-age adults?

Middle adulthood is defined as the period between 35 and 65 years of age. In this dynamic time, the adult experiences biological, physiological, social, psychological, and spiritual changes (Berger, 1998; Rowe & Kahn, 1998). The middle years represent a stage of development set within major economic productivity and family responsibility. A significant group of society (middle-age adults) makes up nearly one half the population of the United States (U.S. Department of Health and Human Services, Centers for Disease Control and Prevention, & National Center for Health Statistics, 1998).

AGE AND PHYSICAL CHANGES

Although their onset is insidious, biological changes come to the forefront during the middle years, affecting most bodily systems. The hair of the adult begins to thin and turn gray. The skin's moisture and turgor decreases, and with the loss of subcutaneous fat, wrinkling occurs. Excessive sun exposure through the years makes this process more pronounced. The result can be a coarseness of the facial features.

Fat deposition increases during these years with increases in weight gain. The body contour changes as "love handles" and "saddlebags" appear. Sedentary lifestyles and unchanged dietary habits contribute a great deal to these changes. The inactive lifestyle is further compromised by a decrease in energy; "I'm not as young as I used to be" is a common retort. This proclamation is legitimate because the capacity for physical work actually decreases. The **functional aerobic capacity** decreases, with a resulting decrease in **cardiac output.**

In the musculoskeletal system, bone density and mass progressively decrease. When 55-year-old adults say that they were an inch taller when they were 18, the observation is likely to be true. A 1- to 4-inch (2.5- to 10-cm) loss in height occurs as a person ages; thinning of the intervertebral disks accounts for approximately 1 inch. However, dramatic losses in height (as much as 4 inches) can occur with thoracic **kyphosis,** an aggeration or angulation of the posterior spine (commonly know as "hunchback"). The wear and tear on joints predispose the adult to **degenerative joint disease,** deterioration of the joint(s), with more frequent annoying backaches. The general decrease in muscle tone is categorized by many as "flab," which reduces physical agility.

The functional capacity of all organ systems generally decreases. For example, in the gastrointestinal tract, the following chain of events occurs: decreased metabolism leads to less enzyme production, resulting in lower hydrochloric acid levels, decreasing tone in the large intestine. As a result, the middle-age adult may complain of acid indigestion with increased belching.

When the adult leads a sedentary lifestyle as well, the effects of the diminished motility through the gastrointestinal tract can be more pronounced. That Americans eat more refined foods (foods that are low in bulk) compared with third-world nations is well known. A low-bulk diet can contribute to the problem of **constipation,** a change in bowel habits characterized by decreased frequency and/or passage of hard, drier stools and difficult defecation, and is even believed to be a primary contributor of the increased incidence of colon cancer in the United States.

Between ages 25 and 85, a 35% loss of nephron units occurs. The remaining nephrons increase in size and undergo degenerative changes. The entire weight of the kidneys decreases. Because blood supply is also diminished, the glomerular filtration rate is decreased by nearly one half.

Significant changes occur in the cardiovascular system as the blood vessels lose elasticity and become thicker. This process predisposes middle-age adults to coronary artery disease, hypertension, myocardial infarctions, and strokes. Heart disease is the leading cause of death in middle-age adults (U.S. Preventive Task Force, 1996; U.S. Department of Health and Human Services, 2000).

When a previously menstruating woman does not have a period for 1 year, she has reached **menopause.** Menopause usually occurs between ages 45 and 55. A great deal more must be learned about what exactly causes many of the symptoms that women frequently report. During this time, production of ovarian estrogen and progesterone ceases; the remaining estrogen is produced by the adrenal glands. As a result of the diminished estrogen level, a woman's secondary sex characteristics regress, such as loss of pubic hair and decrease in breast size. The female reproductive organs shrink in size, and vaginal secretions decrease. Importantly, however, no decline in libido occurs if a good sexual relationship is maintained.

Box 23-1 Leading Causes of Death in Adults

AGES 25 TO 44 YEARS

Unintentional injuries 27,129
Cancer 21,706
Heart disease 16,513

AGES 45 TO 64 YEARS

Cancer 131,743
Heart disease 101,235
Unintentional injuries 17,521

AGE 65 YEARS AND OLDER

Heart disease 606,913
Cancer 382,913
Stroke 140,366

From Centers for Disease Control and Prevention, National Center for Health Statistics, National Vital Statistics Systems. (1999). Washington, DC: Centers for Disease Control and Prevention/U.S. Government Printing Office.; U.S. Department of Health and Human Services. (2000). *Healthy people 2010* (p. 23). Washington, DC: U.S. Government Printing Office.

Men experience change in their sexual response cycle as testosterone levels plateau, then decrease, as they approach the end of the middle years. The testes undergo degenerative changes, the viable spermatozoa diminish, and the volume and viscosity of semen decrease. In men, sexual energy gradually declines; achieving an erection takes longer, but it is sustained longer. Stress, however, can significantly diminish functioning (Berger, 1998).

Mortality Rates

The leading causes of death in middle adulthood are heart diseases, lung cancer, cerebrovascular disease, breast cancer, and colorectal cancer (Box 23-1). Reducing disabilities and deaths from these chronic conditions are national health-promotion and disease-prevention objectives (U.S. Department of Health & Human Services, 2000) (Box 23-2).

Many of these diseases are preventable, entirely or in part, through behavior changes. Middle adults can influence their own health and their children's health through a healthier lifestyle and primary care (Buttaro, Trybulski, Bailey, & Cook, 1999).

Gender and Marital Status

Male mortality rates have always been higher than female rates for the leading causes of death, with the exception of diabetes. Currently, women live approximately 6 years longer on average than do men. White women have the greatest life expectancy and Black women's life expectancy is now higher than that of White men. Adults in households with annual incomes greater than $25,000 live 3 to 7 years longer on average than do those in households with less than $10,000 income (U.S. Department of Health and Human Services, 2000). The death rates of middle-age men from cardiovascular diseases plays a major part in this disparity. The incidence of lung cancer, however, continues to slowly decrease for men (81.6 per 100,000) and increase for women (41.4 per 100,000), primarily because of the changing smoking and work patterns of women. Mortality rates also vary with gender. Death is lowest among married men and highest in divorced men. Single, widowed, and divorced middle-age men generally demonstrate a higher mortality rate than do those who are married (see Hot Topics box).

Box 23-2 Selected National Health-Promotion and Disease-Prevention Objectives for the Middle-Age Adult*

OVERALL GOALS:

1. Increase quality of life and years of healthy life.
2. Eliminate health disparities.

OBJECTIVES AND GOALS:

1. Improve access to quality health services.
   - Increase the proportion of persons with health insurance to 100% (baseline is 86% of adults).
   - Increase the proportion of adults who have a specific source of ongoing care (baseline is 84% of adults).
2. Reduce the overall cancers death rate to 158.7 per 100,000 population (baseline is 201.4 per 100,000 population).
3. Prevent new cases of diabetes to 2.5 per 1000 persons (baseline is 2.1 new cases per 1000 persons).
4. Increase the proportion of adults with disabilities reporting satisfaction with life to 96% (baseline is 87%).
5. Increase the quality, availability, and effectiveness of educational and community-based programs designed to prevent disease and improve health and quality of life.
6. Promote health for all through a healthy environment.
7. Increase the proportion of pregnancies that are intended to 70% (baseline is 51% of pregnancies were unintended).
8. Reduce increases in food-borne illness.
9. Use communication strategically to improve health.
10. Reduce coronary heart deaths to 166 per 100,000 population (baseline is 208 deaths per 100,000 population).
11. Reduce new cases of AIDS among adolescents and adults to 1 per 100,000 population (baseline is 19.5 new cases per 100,000 population).
12. Reduce indigenous cases of vaccine-preventable diseases.
13. Reduce injuries, disabilities, and deaths from accidents and violence.
14. Improve the health and well being of women, infants, children, and families.
15. Improve mental health and ensure access to appropriate, quality mental health care.
16. Increase the proportion of adults who are at a healthy weight to 60% (baseline is 42% of all adults).
17. Reduce work-related injuries for full-time workers to 4.6 per 100 (baseline is 6.6 injuries per 100 workers) and deaths to 3.2 per 100,000 workers (baseline is 4.5 deaths per 100,000 workers).
18. Increase the proportion of adults who engage regularly, preferably daily, in moderate physical activity for at least 30 minutes per day to 30% (baseline is 15%).
19. Reduce asthma deaths of adults ages 35 to 64 years to 9 per 1 million (baseline is 17 asthma deaths per 1 million).
20. Promote responsible sexual behaviors, including preventing sexually transmitted diseases.
21. Reduce substance abuse to protect the health, safety, and quality of life for all people.
22. Reduce tobacco use by adults to 12% (baseline is 24% of adults).
23. Increase the proportion of persons who have a dilated eye examination at appropriate intervals.

From U.S. Department of Health and Human Services. (2000). *Healthy people 2010*. Washington, DC: U.S. Government Printing Office.
*Target and baseline data identified when available.

HOT topics

HEALTH CARE FOR MIDDLE ADULT WOMEN

Middle-age and older women are the fastest growing segment of American society. At the beginning of the twenty-first century, more than 50 million American women are older than 50 years of age and, when combined with men of the same age group, will represent over 43% of the U.S. population. What are the implications for these women, their families, health care providers, and the health care system as a whole?

research highlights

Health Care of Women in Rural Areas

Over 14,000 Australian women ages 45 to 50 are participating in the Australian Longitudinal Study on Women's Health. The purpose of this study was to track the health of these women for 20 years. Women from rural and remote areas are deliberately overpresented in the sample.

To date, the women living in the rural and remote areas rate their health similarly to that of women in urban areas, but they have (1) significantly fewer visits to general practitioners, (2) significantly more visits to alternative health care providers, (3) lower levels of stress, (4) higher frequencies of being overweight, and (5) fewer gynecological surgeries compared with women from urban areas.

Future follow-up studies will continue to explore the health and health care of these women.

Data from Brown, W. J., Young, A. F., & Byles, J. E., (1999). Journey of distance? The health of mid-age women living in five geographical areas of Australia. *Australian Journal of Rural Health, 7* (3), 148-154.

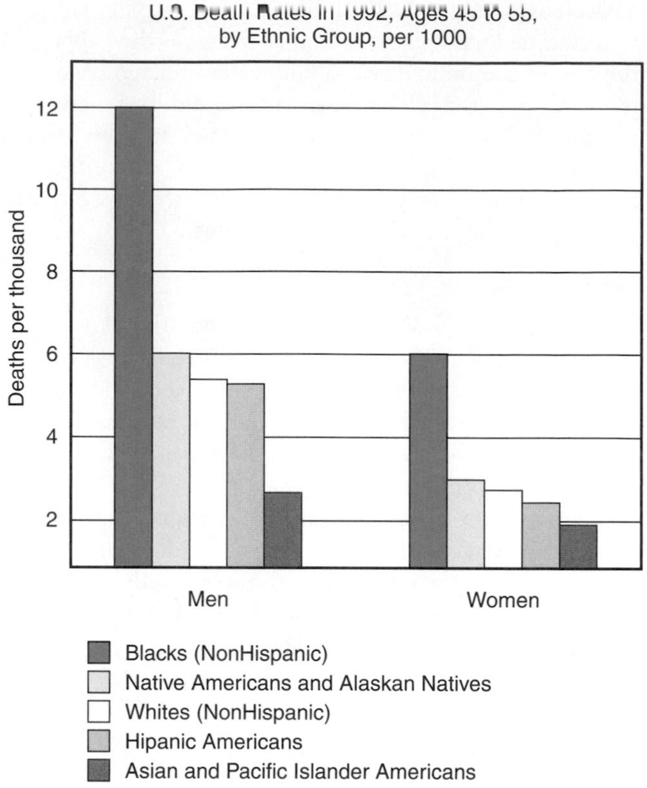

Fig. 23-1 U.S. Death Rates in 1992, ages 45 to 55, by ethnic group, per 1000. (From U.S. Department of Health and Human Services. [2000]. *Healthy people 2010.* Washington, DC: U.S. Government Printing Office.)

Chronic and degenerative diseases are less pronounced in women. The primary cause of death for both genders over age 45 is heart disease. Compared with men, women are more likely to have arthritis, colitis, and gallbladder disease. Men, conversely, have an increased likelihood of developing ulcers, hernias, and emphysema. Injuries are also more common in men (see Research Highlights box).

Race and Gender

Black Americans are the largest minority race (12.8 %) in the nation. Many risk factors are increased in Black adults. Blacks between ages 25 and 64, for instance, have a cerebrovascular accident (CVA) (stroke) rate nearly 2.5 times that of White adults (U.S. Department of Health and Human Services, 2000). Race is also considered to be one of the risk factors in hypertension (U.S. Department of Health and Human Services, 2000; U.S. Preventive Services Task Force, 1996). Black men have an increased incidence and mortality rate in cancers of the lung, colon and rectum, prostate, and esophagus. Black women are more likely to die of breast and colon cancer than is any other group. Hispanics have higher rates of cervical, esophageal, gallbladder, and stomach cancers (U.S. Department of Health and Human Services, 2000). The differences between the cancer rates in Blacks and Whites have been related partly to Blacks residing in lower socioeconomic areas, which tends to increase their exposure to industrial carcinogens. The educational opportunities available to Blacks in urban areas may also be limited, contributing to a lack of knowledge of risk factors, significant signs and symptoms of disease, preventive self-care, and the location of health care resources.

In looking at the major causes of death in middle-age adults, the three leading causes in both White and Black populations are the same: heart disease, cancer, and CVA. Although the primary cause of death for both genders over age 44 continues to be heart disease, the death rate is declining. Women continue to have poorer outcomes than do men. The rate of women who die within a year after a myocardial infarction (heart attack) is 44%, whereas only 27% of men die. The heart disease death rate is higher in Black Americans than it is in White Americans (U.S. Department of Health and Human Services, 2000). Blacks have the highest rate of stroke among all population groups, with a death rate approximately 80% higher than that of White Americans (U.S. Department of Health and Human Services, 2000) (Fig. 23-1).

Genetics

The middle-age adult is at greater risk than is the young adult for diseases known to be associated with genetics (familial characteristics), including diabetes, hypertension, Huntington's chorea, arteriosclerosis, gout, obesity, heart disease, and alcoholism.

Some malignancies tend to be hereditary; for example, women with a personal or family history of breast cancer have a increased risk. Additionally, individuals with a family history of colorectal cancer, rectal or colon polyps, or ulcerative colitis are at high risk for colorectal cancer. The use of diethylstilbestrol (DES) has been linked with the development of cervical cancer and reproductive abnormalities in both sons and daughters of women who took DES while pregnant.

GORDON'S FUNCTIONAL HEALTH PATTERNS

Health Perception-Health Management Pattern

To promote health in the middle-age adult, the nurse performs a health assessment that includes the person's values and beliefs, lifestyle patterns, general perceptions of health, and health practices.

Habits

The self-destructive habits of the middle-age adult that have been practiced for years (cigarette smoking, excessive alcohol use, and overeating) begin to have visible consequences. As pressures increase, adults are tempted to turn to substances such as these as a crutch for coping with multiple stressors. Prevention is extremely important, primarily because withdrawal from any of these substances is a difficult process (Morgan, 1999).

Risk Factors

The major risk factors for adults in the middle years are environmental and behavioral; they can be changed through teaching, counseling, and other nursing interventions (U.S. Department of Health and Human Services, 2000). Helping adults to take care of themselves and to change, when indicated, can be accomplished on an individual or group basis. Whether the nurse interaction is one-to-one or in a group depends largely on the setting and the ways in which the needs are identified (Hartweg & Berbiglia, 1996).

Some of the health-promotion needs of the middle-age adult include acceptance of aging, the need to exercise, and weight control. Decreasing or stopping cigarette smoking and alcohol consumption can also be identified needs. Preventive health screening is vital. The adult needs input into and control of as many of these behaviors as is possible (Browder, 1998).

Total health risks of middle-age adults are composed of group risks (age, gender, race) and personal risks (Flowers & McLean, 1996; Pender, 1996a, 1996b). Precritical secondary prevention includes periodic selective screening for the detection of disease before becoming clinically apparent, such as performing a breast self-examination. A suggested screening examination appears in Box 23-3.

Chronic conditions are defined as those that last for more than 3 months. Approximately 20% of the population ages 45 to 64 reports limitations caused by chronic conditions (Lubkin, 1998). A significant increase is seen between the ages of 45 and 64 (Berger, 1998). Chronic conditions found in the middle-age adult include heart conditions, arthritis, impairments of the back and spine, chronic obstructive lung disease, diabetes, mental and nervous conditions, and dental disease (Philipp, 1999). Diseases and behaviors for which screening is recommended in the middle-age adult are listed in Box 23-4.

Nutritional-Metabolic Pattern

Dietary factors are correlated with 5 of the 10 leading causes of death in the United States: coronary heart disease, some cancers, stroke, noninsulin-dependent diabetes mellitus, and atherosclerosis (U.S. Department of Health and Human Services, 2000).

Physical activities and nutritional patterns are frequently correlated. The middle-age adult typically leads a more sedentary lifestyle than does the young adult, primarily because of increased responsibilities at work and home and the many convenient devices that infiltrate homes and workplaces. This is especially true for middle-age women. Unfortunately, the less active adult usually fails to alter any dietary habits to compensate. Consequently, one of the major health problems of the middle years is obesity (Brown, Young, & Byles, 1999; Willett, Dietz, & Colditz, 1999).

Obesity

Obesity is defined as a body mass index (BMI) of 30 kg/m^2 or more, and being overweight is a BMI over 27.8 kg/m^2 for adult males and 27.3 kg/m^2 for adult females. At least 107 million American adults (23%) are overweight or obese. The proposed target for 2010 is 15% of American adults (U.S. Department of Health & Human Services, 2000).

"Overweight and obesity substantially raise the risk of illness from high blood pressure, high cholesterol, type 2 (noninsulin-dependent) diabetes, heart disease and stroke, gallbladder disease, arthritis, sleep disturbances and problems breathing, and endometrial, breast, prostate and colon cancers. Obese individuals may also suffer from social stigmatization, discrimination, and lowered self-esteem" (U.S. Department of Health and Human Services, 2000, p. 29).

Women with less education and low incomes and Black and Hispanic women are at an increased risk for being overweight. In addition to gender, race, and socioeconomic status, genetics may also be a contributing factor. The most significant variables, however, are health behaviors, particularly food intake and exercise and activity patterns of behavior. Although an abundance of health information is available, these challenges persist.

Box 23-3 Screening Examination: Ages 35 to 65

DATABASE

Health history: initial update with nurse or physician examination (PE)
Health hazard appraisal: initial screening
Psychological inventories as needed

PHYSICAL EXAMINATION (EVERY 3 TO 5 YEARS UNTIL AGE 40, THEN ANNUALLY) EMPHASIZING

Weight and height
Blood pressure, pulse
Breasts
Pelvis
Prostate
Testicles
Eyes
Mouth
Skin

LABORATORY PROCEDURES

Pap smear
Hemoccult: three stools for Hemoccult with PE after age 50
Colonoscopy or sigmoidoscopy every 3 to 5 years after age 50 as indicated
Mammography screening at age 35 every 2 years, then yearly after age 50
Urinalysis: examined at the time of PE
Lipid profile (men ages 35 to 65; women ages 45 to 65)
Chest x-ray film with PE if heavy smoker
Tetanus and diphtheria booster every 10 years
Influenza vaccine: follow current recommendations
Counseling and testing for HIV as indicated
Rubella serology (women of childbearing age)

SELF-CARE EDUCATION AND COUNSELING

With physical examination; individualized according to individual's risk factors
Injury prevention: seatbelts, helmets, firearms, smoke detectors
Stress reduction
Exercise
Diet: cholesterol, fat, sodium, fiber, multivitamins with folic acid (women of childbearing age)
Calcium
Breast self-examination
Testicular self-examination
Dental care
Mouth care
Sexually transmitted diseases
Contraception
Skin protection from ultraviolet light
Alcohol and other substance abuse
Smoking cessation
Discuss hormone prophylaxis (perimenopausal and postmenopausal women)

Based on data from American Cancer Society (Massachusetts Division); U.S. Department of Health and Human Services. (2000). *Healthy people 2010*. Washington, DC: U.S. Government Printing Office; U.S. Preventive Services Task Force. (1996). *Guide to clinical preventive services: An assessment of the effectiveness of 169 interventions* (2nd ed.). Baltimore: Williams and Wilkins.

As much as 40% of a typical American family's food budget is spent on food in restaurants or for "take out" foods, both of which are usually higher in fat than foods prepared at home (U.S. Department of Health and Human Services, 2000). Losing and maintaining weight may require not only an individual to change eating and activity behaviors, but also the social and food preparation and consumption behaviors of the family must change as well.

The prevention of obesity is the goal of weight management in the middle years. When the adult is obese, a clear-cut history of the onset is imperative. A lifelong history of obesity is significantly more arduous to alter than that of adult-onset obesity. A decrease in calories should be accompanied by at least 30 minutes of exercise three to five times a week. When calories are reduced and exercise is increased, weight loss is achieved and maintained (Nelson & Wernick, 1998).

Weight-management resources available to the adult are plentiful. Weight-management programs using behavior modification can be found in varied settings, such as universities and work sites, Weight Watchers, Overeaters Anonymous, and Take Off Pounds Sensibly (TOPS). After the nurse identifies a need for weight management and no program is available, a self-help group can be initiated. Input should be solicited from concerned individuals regarding time and location of meetings. A suggested list of topics generated by the group can be assembled. A discussion of basic nutrition with appropriate handouts is a good place to start. Having adults write down their individual goals and keep a 1-week diet log is nonthreatening and helpful for future planning and also gives them some responsibility in the program.

High-Saturated-Fat Diet

Lipid levels and ratios also have a significant influence on cardiovascular and cerebrovascular morbidity and mortality rates. The National Heart, Lung and Blood Institute regards a blood cholesterol level below 200 mg/dl as desirable. However, the mean cholesterol level for American adults is 206 mg/dl, and approximately 50 million adults in this country are estimated to have blood cholesterol levels that place them at high risk for coronary heart disease and cerebrovascular disease. The Coronary Primary Prevention Trial demonstrates that men at high risk are able to reduce coronary heart disease by approximately 2% for every 1% lower blood cholesterol level. By reducing their intake of saturated fat, total fat, and

Box 23-4 Screening Requirements for Middle-Age Adults

SMOKING HISTORY

Heavy smoking increases the risk of carcinoma, chronic obstructive lung disease, arteriosclerosis, and coronary artery disease. Smoking cessation markedly decreases morbidity and mortality from these diseases.

ALCOHOL SCREENING

Alcoholism is found most frequently in men over age 30. A positive family history is a key risk factor. Approximately 70% of deaths from cirrhosis of the liver are related to heavy alcohol use.

OBESITY

Approximately 23% of Americans are obese. Obesity is especially prevalent among women with lower incomes. Adults who are 20% or more over their ideal weight have a 50% greater mortality rate, primarily from cardiovascular disease, type 2 diabetes, stroke, gallbladder disease, arthritis, sleep disturbances, and various cancers.

HEART DISEASE AND STROKE

Despite dramatic declines in mortality from heart disease and stroke in the last 2 decades, approximately 7 million Americans are affected by coronary artery disease, and cardiovascular diseases still cause more deaths in the United States than do all other diseases combined. Reductions in major risk factors (high blood pressure, high blood cholesterol levels, and smoking) are having a significant effect on cardiovascular mortality.

LIPID PROFILE

A baseline blood test is performed. Studies have shown that a correlation exists between hyperlipidemia and myocardial infarction in men between ages 30 and 59. Approximately 28% of adults in the United States have high blood pressure. People with uncontrolled high blood pressure are at three to four times the risk of developing coronary heart disease and as much as seven times the risk of developing a stroke as are those with normal blood pressures. Overall, Blacks have a higher prevalence of high blood pressure than do Whites (40% versus 27%). Although surveys indicate that most adults with high blood pressure are aware of their condition, only 18% have their blood pressure under control. This negligence remains a problem despite the fact that many can reduce their blood pressure to normal through programs of physical activity and weight loss, reduced sodium and alcohol consumption, and stress management. Medications are available for those who cannot reduce their blood pressure.

BREAST CANCER

Breast cancer is a leading cause of cancer deaths (175,000 newly diagnosed cases and 43,700 deaths in 1999), involving approximately one of every nine women in the United States. Risk factors include female gender, being overweight, reproductive history, previous breast disease, Black and White races, family history of breast cancer, and age over 50 years. In the United States, the incidence of breast cancer rapidly increases from 127 per 100,000 during ages 40 to 44 to 348 per 100,000 during ages 60 to 64. A family history of premenopausal-diagnosed breast cancer in a first-degree relative, such as a mother or sister, is a risk factor of approximately two to three times that of the average women in the general population. Other risk factors include history of benign breast disease nulliparity, first pregnancy after age 30, menarche before age 12, menopause after age 50, obesity, high socioeconomic status, and a history of ovarian or endometrial cancer. Because the 5-year survival rate for localized breast cancer is 90%, early detection is critical. The recommended screening tests for breast cancer are monthly breast self-examination, annual nurse or physician examination, and mammography.

OVARIAN CANCER

Approximately 26,600 new cases and 14,500 deaths from ovarian cancer occurred in 1995. Risk factors include age over 60, nulliparity, late first pregnancy, late menopause, and family history of ovarian cancer. Women who have endometrial or breast cancer have twice the risk of developing ovarian cancer. Jewish women have higher rates than do nonJewish White women. Because symptoms usually do not manifest until the tumor presses on other structures, the overall 5-year

Data from U.S. Department of Health and Human Services. (2000): *Healthy people 2000: National health promotion and disease prevention objectives*. Washington, DC: U.S. Government Printing Office; U.S. Preventive Services Task Force. (1996). *Guide to clinical preventive services: An assessment of the effectiveness of 169 interventions* (2nd ed.). Baltimore: Williams & Wilkins.

Continued

dietary cholesterol and by normalizing their weight and increasing physical activity, most people can lower their high blood cholesterol levels. Medications are available for those whose blood cholesterol levels remain significantly elevated despite diet modification (Benson et al., 1989; U.S. Department of Health and Human Services, 2000; Cleeman & Lenfant, 1998).

Calcium

An adequate **calcium** intake is essential in developing and maintaining bone mass. Additionally, calcium is needed for other physiological processes, including muscle contraction and blood pressure regulation. Men and women need a minimal daily intake of 1000 mg of calcium. Pregnant and nursing women need 1200 mg, and postmenopausal women need either 1000 mg (when taking estrogen) or 1500 mg (when not taking estrogen). Vitamin D enhances the absorption of calcium (Bronfman & Bronfman, 1998). "Taking calcium at bedtime may enhance bone turnover that occurs while the individual is recumbent" (Buttaro, Trybulski, Bailey, & Sandburg-Cook, 1999, p. 776). When the daily intake of calcium is less than 400 mg per day, an adequate serum calcium level will be maintained by leaching calcium from bone, resulting in **osteoporosis.**

Box 23-4 Screening Requirements for Middle Age Adults—cont'd

survival rate is approximately 36% with regional metastases. Women over age 40 with an enlarged abdomen or unexplained digestive symptoms, such as distention, discomfort, or gas, should be examined. No official recommendations have been established to screen for ovarian cancer in asymptomatic women.

UTERINE CANCER

Approximately 46,500 new cases and 10,000 deaths resulting from uterine cancer were reported in 1999. Endometrial cancer affects primarily women between ages 50 and 64. Risk factors include a history of infertility, estrogen therapy, late menopause, and a combination of diabetes, hypertension, and obesity. (The postmenopausal woman should be strongly encouraged to report any vaginal bleeding.)

TESTICULAR CANCER

White men entering their middle years are at lower risk than are young adult men, although a tumor can occur at any age. Early detection and treatment, including testicular self-examination, decrease mortality rates appreciably. The major risk is a history of cryptorchidism.

COLORECTAL CANCER

Colorectal cancer is second only to lung cancer as the leading cause of cancer-related deaths. Approximately 95% of colon cancers are found in adults over age 45. A positive family history is significant as is family or personal history of bowel syndromes. Because some evidence indicates that diets high in fat, alcohol, and/or low in fiber are contributing factors, dietary patterns should be assessed. Fecal occult blood testing every 1 to 2 years and sigmoidoscopy as indicated are important in the early diagnosis of colorectal cancer.

ORAL CANCER

Oral cancer is most common in men over age 40; smoking combined with alcohol account for 90% of all oral cancers. Assess for any mouth pain, sores, or lumps and encourage regular dental care, which includes a comprehensive oral examination twice a year.

TUBERCULOSIS

Tuberculosis (TB) is a highly contagious disease. *Mycobacterium tuberculosis* infects 10 to 15 million Americans. The incident of TB is increasing in the United States. Over 24,000 cases of TB were reported in 1994. Approximately 33% of these cases occurred in Blacks, 20% in Hispanics, and 14% in Asian-Pacific Islander immigrants. TB is 150 to 300 times more common in the homeless than it is in the general population. Compromised immunity resulting from infection with the human immunodeficiency virus (HIV) greatly contributes to the increased incidence of TB. Tuberculin skin testing with the Mantoux test is the primary means of identifying TB in asymptomatic persons. Early detection is important because of the efficacy of isoniazid (INH), although multidrug-resistant TB reports are increasing.

SYPHILIS, GONORRHEA, AND HIV

Rates of sexually transmitted diseases are growing in commercial sex workers and intravenous (IV) illicit drug users. Blacks and Hispanics have up to 60 times the rates of syphilis infections as do Whites. Congenital syphilis causes fetal or perinatal death in 40% of affected pregnancies. Up to 80% of women infected with pharyngeal or anorectal gonorrhea are asymptomatic. The highest rates of infection occur in poor minority communities of large cities and the rural Southeast. As many as 1.2 million Americans are infected with the HIV virus and approximately 80,000 new infections occur each year. IV drug users and men who have sex with men accounted for 80% of reported HIV infections in 1994. Comprehensive sexual histories should be documented and at-risk adults tested.

GLAUCOMA

The American Academy of Ophthalmology recommends a comprehensive eye examination, including examination of the optic disc and tonometry, for all adults beginning at age 40 and periodic reexaminations thereafter. Also recommended is an examination every 3 to 5 years for Black adults between the ages of 20 and 39 because of their greater risk for glaucoma as compared with White adults.

Data from U.S. Department of Health and Human Services. (2000): *Healthy people 2000: National health promotion and disease prevention objectives*. Washington, DC: U.S. Government Printing Office; U.S. Preventive Services Task Force. (1996). *Guide to clinical preventive services: An assessment of the effectiveness of 169 interventions* (2nd ed.). Baltimore: Williams & Wilkins.

Exercise also contributes to bone mass by increasing mechanical stress on the bones.

Food Additives

A great deal of controversy has recently surrounded food additives and their relationship to disease, specifically cancer. Sodium nitrate, for example, is used in the preservation of bacon, ham, and smoked meats; butylated hydroxytoluene (BHT) is found in cereal and potato chips. Saccharin, used in low-calorie foodstuffs, carries a warning label and has been determined to cause cancer in laboratory animals. Studies thus far have been conducted only on laboratory animals and are inconclusive. Importantly, malignancies can take years to develop; many additives have been in use for short periods, so long-term outcomes are unknown (U.S. Department of Health and Human Services, 2000).

Caffeine

Caffeine is a popular stimulant found in coffee, tea, and some soft drinks, such as colas. Caffeine prolongs the amount of time that physical work can be performed and appears to decrease boredom and increase attention span. On the negative side, coffee has come under significant scrutiny from the media recently, with reports of a link between cancer of the pancreas and coffee consumption.

Ray (1982) reports that caffeine increases the blood levels of lipids and glucose. The elevated serum fat levels act on the cardiovascular system to the extent that heavy coffee users may have a higher incidence of angina and myocardial infarction than do moderate users.

Similar to alcohol and nicotine, caffeine is readily available and has become an accepted part of daily living. Because caffeine is a major stimulant with effects that are typically taken for granted, the importance as an addictive substance must be emphasized. Ingestion of 0.5 g of caffeine (3 to 4 cups of coffee) can increase the basal metabolic rate an average of 10% and possibly as much as 25% for some people.

Chronic stimulation of the central nervous system results in restlessness, sleep disturbances, cardiac stimulation, and withdrawal effects. Nurses' assessment should screen for the stimulating and addicting substances that may be producing any of these symptoms.

High-Sodium Diet

High-sodium diets play a significant role in hypertension, especially when consumed over many years. The result may be an increase in total body fluids, which increases peripheral vascular resistance. Salt contains approximately 40% sodium and is a contributing factor in 10% to 20% of Americans who are at risk for hypertension. On average, Americans consume at least 4 to 5 g of sodium per day. The National Research Council of the National Academy of Sciences reports that between 1.1 and 3.3 g are adequate and safe (Joint National Committee, 1997b). A major contributor of dietary sodium is the salt found in processed foods.

Over the last 3 decades, many clinical studies have demonstrated the effectiveness of lowering dietary sodium to lower blood pressure. Other studies have described the relationships between urinary and sodium excretion and the change of blood pressure with age. "However, controlled prospective studies will ultimately be necessary to provide definitive evidence that normotensive persons who practice dietary sodium restriction are at lower risk for developing hypertension over time than are those with more typical sodium consumption" (U.S. Preventive Services Task Force, 1996, p. 629).

Alcohol Abuse

Substance abuse can be a devastating habit. The adult can abuse agents such as prescription and illicit drugs and/or, especially, alcohol. The alcoholic person is at greater risk for cancer of the larynx, oral cavity, and liver.

Initially, alcohol appears to be a stimulant, but actually is a central nervous system depressant and anesthetic. Chronic alcohol use produces tolerance, thereby necessitating gradually increasing doses to achieve the same effect. Alcohol contributes to problems with safety because of the decreased reaction time and depression of the central nervous system.

Alcohol is frequently treated as a nondrug, but alcohol addiction is second only to nicotine. Alcohol is readily available, reasonably inexpensive, and considered as a part of social exchange; its long-range physiological and psychological effects are well documented. In the United States, two thirds of adults consume alcohol, and 18 million are problem drinkers; of this number, an estimated 5% of adults are problem drinkers. Presently, men outnumber women as alcohol abusers by approximately 5:1, but this ratio is decreasing. Alcohol abuse is associated with motor-vehicle accidents, homicides, suicides, drownings, heart disease, cancers, liver disease, pancreatitis, and fetal alcohol syndrome, a major cause of mental retardation in children (U.S. Department of Health and Human Services, 2000). People who abuse alcohol also have higher rates of divorce, depression, domestic violence, risky sexual behaviors, unemployment, and poverty (U.S. Preventive Services Task Force, 1996).

Since World War II, the number of female alcoholics has doubled (Joint National Committee, 1997b). Women drink primarily in relation to life crises to relieve loneliness, feelings of inferiority, and gender role conflicts at home and at work. This situation occurs in all social classes and crosses all lifestyles. Interestingly, 9 of 10 husbands leave alcoholic wives, whereas 9 in 10 wives remain with their alcoholic husbands. The alcoholic woman is likely to abuse other substances as well; her family is also likely to protect her and themselves from public exposure, delaying necessary treatment. "An estimated 27 million American children are at risk for abnormal psychosocial development due to the abuse of alcohol by their parents" (U.S. Preventive Task Force, 1996, p. 568).

The alcoholic may complain of symptoms such as heartburn and gas; stomach distention; poor eating habits; nausea and vomiting; gastric pain; irritation of the mouth, throat, and esophagus; and hepatic pain. Two additional subtle findings are spidery angiomata and palmar erythema.

Primary prevention for substance and alcohol abuse is complex, especially because adults consume these agents for many reasons, including peer pressure, loneliness, alienation, frustration, anxiety, and low self-esteem. Heavy drinkers may also be following the example established by influential people in their lives. Merely telling people about the potential physical, emotional, and legal hazards appears to have little effect as a preventive measure. Natural channels for primary prevention of substance abuse include the media, peers, and family. Promoting more realistic portrayals of substance abuse through the media is difficult to implement. Although techniques such as assertiveness training and teaching adults to resist persuasion are helpful, more useful approaches might include helping them learn to manage anxiety and increase their self-esteem. Less anxious and more confident people have greater skills in resisting peer influences to participate in substance abuse; they also are more likely to have fewer episodes of isolation and loneliness.

Early detection and intervention can decrease ongoing and future physical and psychosocial problems resulting from alcohol abuse. Nurses use a variety of screening strategies to identify individuals' perceptions and consequences of drinking. The CAGE questionnaire is the most popular screening tool used in primary care (U.S. Preventive Services Task Force, 1996). The Michigan alcohol-screening test and alcohol use disorders identification test are examples of other screening instruments. No single tool, however, is sufficiently sensitive to detect levels of drinking that are considered dangerous during pregnancy (U.S. Preventive Service Task Force, 1996).

Laboratory tests, including elevations in aspartate aminotransferase, erythrocyte mean corpuscular volume, and serum γ-glutamyltransferase, are not adequately sensitive and specific and may be a result of other causes including trauma, disease, and medications.

A variety of treatments are known to be effective; but no single "best" intervention has been identified. Effective treatments may include the treatments of other problems, such as stress management, individual and family therapy, and supportive environments.

Although alcohol consumption per person has gradually decreased since 1981, 72% of adult women and 74% of adult men continue to exceed the recommended guidelines for low-risk drinking, with the 2010 target projected at 50% (U.S. Department of Health and Human Services, 2000).

Gingivitis

Gingivitis is common among adults who fail to brush their teeth and use dental floss regularly. Redness and swelling develops around the teeth that becomes more apparent. Bleeding of the gums while brushing the teeth is an early sign of gingivitis. The gums may or may not be tender. When inflammation is not adequately treated and controlled, **periodontitis** involving bone destruction can develop, in addition to tooth loss.

Regular oral hygiene and care are major factors in maintaining oral health. However, less than one half of Americans receive regular oral health care. Middle-age adults have responsibility not only for their own care, but also for the care of their children and elderly parents. Low income is a risk factor (U.S. Department of Health and Human Services, 2000). Untreated dental decay and tooth loss are higher in Blacks, Hispanics, Native American-Alaska natives compared with the total American adult population (U.S. Department of Health and Human Services, 2000; U.S. Preventives services Task Force, 1996). Oral cancer is also a major problem that is not detected in the absence of good dental care, including professional examinations.

Elimination Pattern

Aging brings a gradual decrease of tone in the large intestine. As mentioned, this change, accompanied by a sedentary lifestyle and lack of bulk in the diet, predisposes the adult to constipation. Mass media reports strongly encourage the population to rely on external controls rather than on exercise and dietary means to solve this problem. Consequently, many adults are dependent on laxatives for normal bowel function.

As discussed, degenerative changes in the nephron units occur during the middle-age years. Usually, however, the middle-age adult does not have any appreciable kidney malfunction.

When a woman has had multiple births and little exercise, she may begin experiencing stress incontinence during this time, which can be socially embarrassing (Newman & Dzurinko, 1997).

Activity-Exercise Pattern

Regular physical activity increases life expectancy and quality of life. Regular physical activity can help prevent and manage coronary heart disease, hypertension (National Institutes of Health, 1998), diabetes, osteoporosis, and depression. Physical exercise has been correlated with lower rates of osteoporosis (Bonnick, 1997; National Osteoporosis Foundation, 1998), back injury, stroke, and colon cancer. Effective weight-loss programs that incorporate physical activities also make significant contributions to increased life expectancy and quality of life. (Kriketos, Sharp, Seagle, Peters, & Hill, 2000; U.S. Department of Health and Human Services, 2000).

Despite these benefits, few American adults engage in regular physical activity for 30 minutes, three to five times a week, as recommended. In the United States, 56% of men and 61% of women report they either "never engaged in physical activity or did so on an irregular basis" (U.S. Preventive Services Task force, 1996, p. 611) and only 15% of adults perform the recommended level of physical activity, and 40% of adults report no leisure-time, physical activities. By age 75, one in three men and one in two women engage in no regular physical activity. No regular physical activity and the prevalence of sedentary behavior increases with age (U.S. Department of Health and Human Services, 2000). Continuous, rhythmic exercise maintained for a sufficient period to stress the cardiac system is desirable (Dunn et al., 1999). Some suggested activities include brisk walking, jogging, swimming, bicycling, and skipping rope. Activities that focus on skill and coordination should be attempted by the adult over age 40 rather than activities necessitating speed and strength. Moderation is the key, along with increased caution as the adult approaches age 65. Overexertion, evidenced by symptoms of dizziness, tightness in the chest, and unresolving breathlessness, should be avoided (see Chapter 12).

The nurse initiates an exercise program with the middle-age adult by asking what activities have been enjoyed in the past. When these activities are realistic today, the nurse encourages the individual to rediscover them; when they appear unrealistic, new options should be explored with the individual. Additionally, activities are selected with consideration of the potential for injury. Anyone at risk for heart disease (heavy smoking, high blood pressure, family history, diabetes, or prolonged lack of exercise) should have a complete history and physical examination before developing a rigorous activity program. For some of these individuals, an exercise test is recommended. Proper equipment, including supportive shoes and thermally appropriate clothing, is also important.

To be health promoting, physical exercise involves as many muscles as is possible, performed on a regular basis, preferably three to four times a week, for a minimum of 30 minutes each time. The appropriate level of performance for aerobic exercise is determined by achieving a pulse rate that is established for each individual: taking the number 220, subtracting the person's age, and then computing 75% of that number. A 50-year-old person, for example, should not exceed a pulse rate of 128 ([220 − 50] × .75 = 128).

Despite all these considerations, the choice of activities and style should be an individual choice and approached as something done for oneself and for fun, not as another chore or responsibility of middle age (Brownson et al., 2000).

Sleep-Rest Pattern

Rest is a frequently omitted consideration for middle-age adults, who spend less time in deep sleep and need less sleep overall than do young adults. This change may be interpreted as insomnia; therefore middle-age adults may need reassurance that this is common. Regularly scheduled, quality sleep and occasional napping, when fatigued, are healthful guidelines (Jacobs, 1998; National Sleep Foundation, 1998).

Cognitive-Perceptual Pattern

The notion that at age 21 adults reach their peak and that "it is all downhill after that" is a myth (see Chapter 15). Continued learning is found throughout adulthood in such areas as reasoning, vocabulary, and spatial perception. Decreases can be observed, however, in reaction time and cognitive flexibility.

Intellectual Ability

"Learning" intelligence accumulates through education and life experiences and continues to increase throughout life, as evidenced by the many scholars and artists who are more productive in their middle years than they were as young adults.

The theories of Havighurst, Piaget, and Bloom are relevant to the middle-age adult. The adult in the middle years as the learner-performer is a case in point. These individuals conclude that the prime time to be in the learner role is when the developmental task for that role is to be accomplished. For example, to balance the responsibilities of caring for children and parents and working, the adult may explore new career options or creative endeavors.

Havighurst defines developmental tasks as the basic tasks of living that must be achieved if the adult is to live successfully. These tasks are dictated by the expectations of society, the physiological changes of the body throughout life, and the individual's own value system and goals. Although initially described in the 1950s, Havighurst and Orr's developmental tasks of middle age remain timely (Havighurst & Orr, 1956) (Box 23-5).

If career goals have been previously identified, then reaching them can be highly rewarding, both psychologically and financially. In addition to career activities, the mature adult has an increased social awareness and assumes more civic responsibility.

In Piaget's theory of cognitive development, formal operations is the final period. This stage begins at approximately age 12 and continues throughout life. Piaget describes the thoughts of adults as being both flexible and effective. The adult can deal efficiently with complex problems of reasoning to include hypothesis testing (Piaget, 1970).

Bloom (1984) developed a hierarchy of cognitive levels in the adult learner. Knowledge is the simplest cognitive level; the adult learner understands and can recall specifics. For example, the individual defines high blood pressure in lay terms.

Comprehension is the second level, as indicated by the learner grasping the meaning of the communicated message and relating it to other material. For example, the individual can state one way that obesity influences high blood pressure.

The third level is application. At this level, the learner applies knowledge in the form of abstractions and ideas to concrete situations. For example, the hypertensive person begins a weight-reduction and exercise program.

In analysis, in the fourth level, the adult breaks down material into its constituent parts while noting their relationship. For example, the individual identifies values

Box 23-5 Developmental Tasks of Middle Age

1. Helping children become responsible, happy adults
2. Rediscovering or developing new satisfaction in the relationship with one's spouse (for the single adult, this can occur in a relationship with a sibling or significant other)
3. Developing an affectionate, but independent, relationship with aging parents
4. Reaching the peak in one's career
5. Achieving mature social and civic responsibility
6. Accepting and adapting to biological changes
7. Maintaining or developing friendships
8. Developing leisure-time activities

and life goals in determining actions to be taken for meeting health care needs.

The final levels (synthesis and evaluation) are at times difficult to achieve. The person is able to combine various elements to form a plan and then judge the extent to which the ideas, materials, and so on satisfy the established criteria. For example, people may develop plans to improve their health care and increase their self-care responsibilities. In turn, they may validate their ongoing health care programs in relation to the expected outcomes that they formulated. Genetic, environmental, and personality factors in early and middle adulthood account for the large difference in the ways in which individuals maintain mental abilities. Schaie (1994) has identified seven of these factors that maintain cognitive function in later life:

1. Absence of chronic diseases
2. Living with favorable socioeconomic factors, including maximal occupational complexity, a low degree of routine, and an intact family
3. Involvement in complex social activities
4. Flexible personality style
5. Marriage to a spouse with high cognitive function
6. Maintaining high levels of performance speed
7. Personal satisfaction with accomplishments in midlife and early old age

Perceptual Changes

Presbyopia (farsightedness) is common in middle-age adults, even in individuals who have had no previous vision problems. This condition is easily corrected with corrective lenses, which may only be needed for reading or close work. Other visual conditions that may not allow for ready correction include decreased peripheral vision and decreased visual sensitivity in the dark. Both conditions are a result of the cornea becoming less transparent, and both are slow and subtle in development. Because all of these conditions are not readily detected by the individual, middle-age adults should establish a routine professional eye examination every year.

Another common perceptual change in middle age is **presbycusis** (impaired auditory acuity). The first sounds to be lost are higher sound frequencies, such as a woman's voice. Because this process is also subtle, but important, to the work environment and social interaction, middle age is also a time for auditory evaluations as a part of routine examinations.

Beginning in the middle years, the sense of taste also diminishes. A progressive loss of taste buds occurs, first affecting those located more anteriorly, which detect sweet and salt, and then the posterior taste buds, which detect bitter and sour. Consequently, this change can alter a person's food preferences and present problems for people who insist on adding salt to make up for the deficit. Nurses can suggest using various herbs and spices to enhance flavor.

Self-Perception–Self-Concept Pattern

Levinson's Theory

In Levinson's research on men (1986a, 1986b) and women (1996), a theory on "individual life structures" is posed. Levinson describes age-associated "seasons" or "eras." The midlife transition, beginning at ages 38 to 40 years appears to include reappraising one's life, integrating the polarities, and modifying one's life structure toward being who one wants to be. Middle-age adults struggle with meaning, value, and direction of their lives (Roundtree, 1993).

Erikson's Theory

In Erikson's eight stages of the life cycle (1986), the last three stages are related to adulthood. Stage 7 (generativity versus stagnation or self-absorption) is most frequently associated with the middle-age years.

Erikson identifies generativity as the primary task during this stage. **Generativity** includes a sense of productivity and creativity, as evidenced by reaching previously established goals (Thomas, 1995; Hornstein, 1986; Reifman, Biernat, & Lang, 1991). Generativity also encompasses a desire to care for others and is the opposite of **stagnation,** which is the result of a lack of accomplishment during middle-age's developmental tasks, and self-absorption, the tendency to direct most of one's interest and attention to oneself, thereby excluding others.

Middle age is a time of critical self-review, and some people are sad and disappointed in themselves and their accomplishments. Both women and men question their value to society, the merit of their accomplishments, their success as sexual beings, and the probability of attaining unfilled life goals. Women generally make this life assessment between ages 35 and 50, whereas men do not usually begin until approximately age 40. Because the male life assessment tends to come late, there is a potential problem for couples of approximately the same age. Women begin looking at changes they may want to make in their lives, whereas men remain content with the status quo. This type of self-evaluation and lack of effective communication of personal needs to the spouse is a primary irritant to marriage stability (Burgel, 1993; Erikson, 1986; Valliant & Valliant, 1990).

Physiological Changes

The effect of physiological changes on mental health is nearly as critical during middle age as it is during adolescence. Some of the most obvious changes that influence self-esteem are graying hair, wrinkles, decreased visual and auditory acuity, and changes in body shape. The extent to which these changes are tolerated depends largely on the person's level of self-satisfaction and acceptance. Some people try to "hold on" to youth by dressing as more youthful counterparts dress, whereas others adapt their attire to their age and position in life (Erikson, 1986; Schiff & Parson, 1996; Lancaster & King, 1985).

Although controversial, some researchers believe that hormonal changes during middle age lead to behaviors in men that represent what menopause does to women. In women, decreased supplies of estrogen begin to occur; the loss of estrogen is thought to be responsible for the "hot flashes" and the mood changes that often occur (Futterman & Jones, 1997). The concomitant emotional aspect of menopause appears to be related to the personality of the individual. Women who have a positive self-concept and have coped effectively in the past are less prone to experience the full range of psychological symptoms that are often associated with menopause (The Boston Women's Health Book Collective, 1999; Ben-Kiki & Herman, 1998). The most common changes include emotional lability (excessive or frequently changing emotions), nervousness and anxiety, insomnia, fatigue, and depression. Women need information in making decisions about estrogen supplements, including research on cardiac health, osteoporosis, and breast cancer (Shandler, 1997; North American Menopause Society, 1998; Landau, Cyr, & Moulton, 1995).

Similarly, men frequently experience physical and psychological reactions to middle age. The hormonal changes in men are gradual, typically beginning between ages 40 and 55. The symptoms are similar to those experienced by women, with the emotional effects related to other life events, past coping patterns, and general feelings of self-esteem.

Roles-Relationships Pattern

Craig (1989) notes that middle age is frequently a time of reassessment, turmoil, and change. This time has been called **midlife crisis.** The turning point occurs for several reasons. Middle-age adults recognize that their physical agility is decreasing; the inevitability of one's own death is recognized, perhaps for the first time. Lifestyle choices have been made and are less flexible than are those made at age 25. The adult identifies mistakes made in the past.

Family

Duvall and Miller (1984) delineate eight stages of the family life cycle, with stages 5, 6, and 7 in the middle years (see Chapter 7):

Stage 5: families with children, with the oldest child age 13 to 20; lasts approximately 7 years

Stage 6: families launching young adults, from the first leaving until the last; lasts approximately 8 years

Stage 7: families from empty nest to retirement; lasts approximately 15 years

The developmental tasks identified for the families in stages 6 and 7 are similar to those of Havighurst; they focus on changes from a nuclear family to a marital couple. For example, in stage 6, the parents who are helping their children become independent may also be caring for their aging parents (Friedman, 1986). Additionally, middle-age adults fulfill multiple complex responsibilities within a variety of career, social, and civic positions.

These transitions can be even more challenging for the family headed by a single parent (most typically the mother), which exists in over 10 million American households (out of a total of 35 million). The single most significant health risk in families headed by a single mother is poverty. Nearly one half of all of these families live in poverty, and the median family income for families with two parents is three times that of a family headed by a single mother. These inadequate resources make it extremely difficult for middle-age mothers, who are frequently raising grandchildren as well, to fulfill their responsibilities.

Families with young adolescent or young adult children have been described in research studies as both "postparental" and "launching" families. In contrast, increasing criticism exists of this emphasis on the separation of children (regardless of age) from their families. Gilligan (1982) criticizes the work of many human-development theorists who identify human development in terms of separation from the family. Apter (1991) also challenges the conventional view that adolescent girls must reject their mothers as part of a healthy development. Middle-age parents are encouraged to continue to care for and nurture their adolescent and adult children while recognizing the increasing interdependence of their relationship.

Although many adolescent and young adult children move out of their homes of origin to complete educational or career training, create their own living arrangement, or pursue a career, 54% of 18- to 24-year-old young adults were living in the home of their parents in 1992. Many children of families in these age groups remain dependent on parental help for many more years.

By supporting their children's efforts, parents can increase the self-esteem of their children while being effective role models. The parent assumes less of a parent-child relationship, interacting more on an adult-adult level. As the children are "launched," the parents may have uninterrupted time alone and time to share activities. Parents who remove too much care too quickly place their children at risk for depression, substance abuse, violence, and suicide (Silverstein & Rashbaum, 1995).

Family life may also be threatened by older children living at home, opposition to a child's partner, or the inability to establish satisfactory relationships with potential or actual partners or sons- and daughters-in-law (Bischof, 1989). For many parents, the idea of their children leaving home is anticipated with relief that the heavy care responsibilities of parenting are over or with dread over having to fill the void of time and inactivity. The empty nest syndrome may be exacerbated if the husband and wife have never learned to communicate effectively and to enjoy each other's company without the children.

At the other end of the family spectrum, aging parents can place demands on the adult child, primarily because elderly adults are frequently beset with health problems. A caring relationship is needed in which the need of the aging parent for independence is recognized (Burgel, 1993).

Because of the society's emphasis on youth, the adult must associate feelings of self-worth with personal integrity rather than with bodily appearance or physical prowess. Friends of both genders can be invaluable support systems. With the newly found free time after children have left home, the middle-age adult can share favorite activities and learn new ones. Middle-age adults should remind themselves how much and how well they are doing, especially considering the complexity of the demands placed on them. Never before in history have families pursued such varied and individual-oriented goals as they do today.

Although for many Americans the concept of family remains of major importance, the perceptions are different from those held by previous generations. Parents and children in most families are involved in numerous activities, as evidenced by a "let's-hurry-or-we'll-be-late" orientation. Even younger children frequently have schedules that must be met if they are to get to their dance, drama, play, or enrichment classes. None of these activities necessarily has a negative effect, but the cumulative influence places heavy demands on all family members. Additionally, many activities in which both children and adults are involved have a certain degree of competitiveness. For example, parents frequently get emotionally involved in the athletic activities of their children to the extent that the failure of a 6-year-old to play a winning softball game causes a great deal of parental anguish. One only has to listen to the cheering of parents at a little league baseball game to note whose self-esteem is at stake. Shouts of "Kill her," "Grab the third baseman," and so on do not tend to engender feelings of team spirit or a notion of playing for the sake of having a good time (Erikson, 1986).

Work

Perhaps the most common role that middle-age adults share is being workers. Much of their pride and sense of satisfaction is derived from their work. For middle-age working adults, work is equated with being "grown up"; one can easily recall the "What do you want to be when you grow up?" questioning of youth. Success and achievement are evaluated in terms of careers and family life. The work ethic still persists, especially with individuals born during the Great Depression. Much of their conversation evolves from what they do, such as, "My name is Leslie Smith. I am a real-estate agent." To be mature is to be a responsible, hard-working individual (Erikson, 1986). Research has shown older adults are more satisfied with their jobs than are younger adults (Mottaz, 1987; Zeitz, 1990).

Middle-age adults make up most of the work force of 110 million people. Vocations play a major role in their levels of wellness. Approximately 10 million injuries occur every year; 3 million of these are severe, including 3400 to 11,000 deaths and 1.8 million total disabling injuries (U.S. Department of Health and Human Services, 2000).

More than 22% of fatal occupational injuries involve motor vehicles; other injuries include falls, nonvehicular

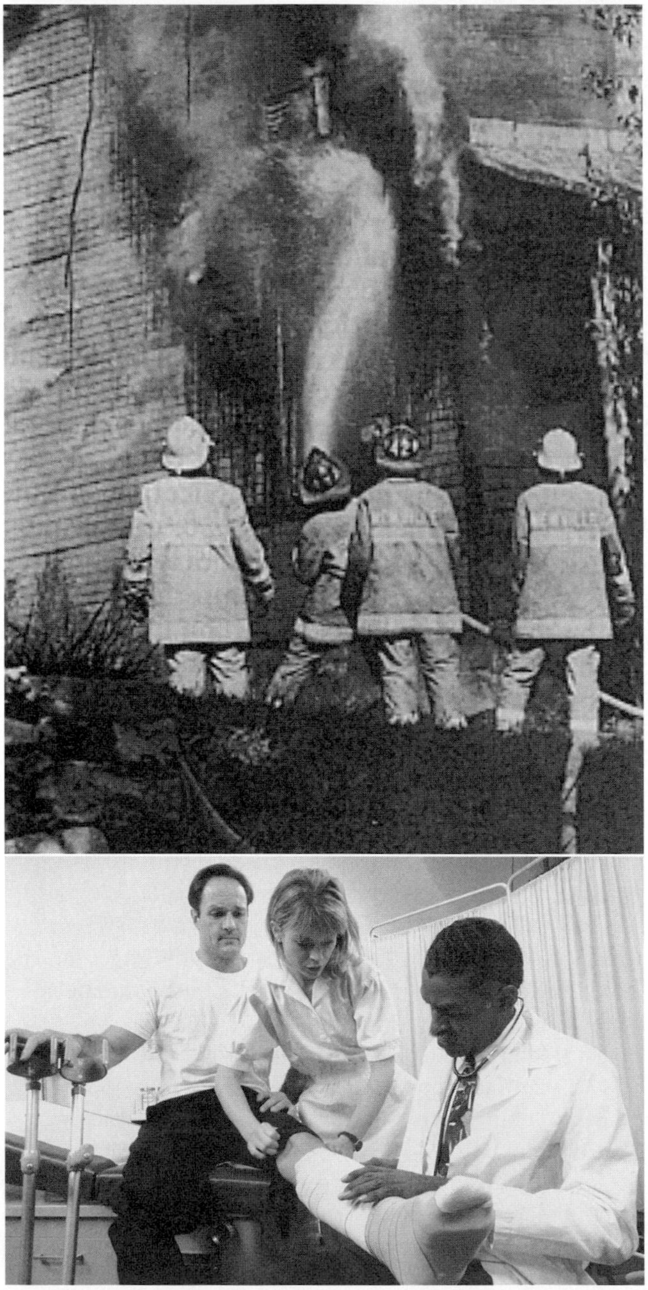

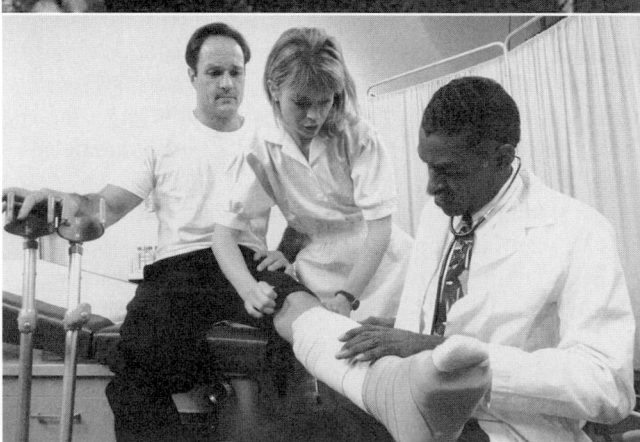

A

B

Fig. 23-2 **A,** Firefighters face a great risk for work-related injury or death. (Photograph by David S. Strickler.) **B,** On-the-job injuries may require rehabilitation and thus result in lost income, producing another stressor on middle-age workers.

injuries, blows, and electrocutions. Although the number of fatal occupations appears to be decreasing, work-related illness and injuries appear to be increasing (U.S. Department of Health and Human Services, 2000). Workers in mining, agriculture, fire fighting, transportation, and construction are at an increased risk of dying from a work-related injury (Fig. 23-2). Poor housekeeping and poor design predispose the worker to falls and other illnesses (U.S. Department of Health and Human Services, 2000).

Many injuries that contribute significantly to the morbidity and mortality of adults can be prevented. Fixing faulty steps, repairing faulty electrical wires, securing carpets, and using rubber mats in the bathtub are only a few of the many preventive measures.

Accidents are twice as high among smokers as compared with nonsmokers. Possible explanations include the loss of attention, the use of one hand for smoking, and irritation of the eyes (U.S. Preventive Services Task Force, 1996).

Other work-related problems include exposure to harmful substances resulting in lung diseases, cancers, and workplace violence (see Health Teaching box). Homicide remains the second leading cause of work-related injury deaths, accounting for 856 deaths in 1997 (U.S. Department of Health and Human Services, 1999).

The effect of life events on mental health depends on the personal strength of the individual, available supports, and the nature and number of events and their significance for the person. Three common examples of life events with potential disruptive effects are divorce, the increasing number of families with two or more jobs, and caring for aging parents. Their negative effects may be alleviated if assistance is provided early in the process of that change.

Two-or-More-Job Family: Family and Work Responsibilities

More and more women are in the workforce; many feel the necessity for financial gain, especially with the increased cost of living and college expenses. Other women, who are postmenopausal and have been separated from their last child, have a newfound freedom and begin or rediscover a career. The husband may be a support person in this venture or he may feel threatened by his wife's new pursuit. These role changes can be stressors to the family.

The relationship between marital status, with or without children at home, and employment status determines the psychological status of the woman in her middle years. The educated woman who is married, has children at home, and has not worked since her marriage is at an increased risk for psychological disturbances (McKinlay & McKinlay, 1988).

Historically, women have worked with their husbands within the family farm or business. Only in the few decades immediately after World War II did many middle-class White women stay at home while the husband went to work. Currently, women make up a significant portion of the workforce. Additionally, many women are able to become highly educated and motivated to pursue careers. Both men and women are increasingly taking jobs that do not end at 5:00 PM. The problems and challenges of the workplace are experienced at home as adults bring projects and problems home with them.

Job-related travel has also increased in the last few years for both men and women. Travel by either partner means additional responsibilities for the parent who remains at home. Additionally, if one spouse travels far more than the other travels, feelings of resentment may develop, or the common ground for discussion of work events may be altered. The one who stays at home may feel "put upon" when the spouse is perceived as having such fun. In contrast, travel is tiring and is not usually as exciting as it appears to observers. The traveling spouse can come home tired and irritable and desire peace and quiet, which may conflict with the expectations of other family members.

Men may feel threatened by highly successful and visible women. For some families, the postWorld War II prototype was for the husband to financially support the family and gain status through achievements of work outside the home. As women gain recognition and acclaim for their career accomplishments, even the most "enlightened" man may experience twinges of envy and discomfort. Men have few role models to which to turn in learning the ways to be a participant in a successful two-career family. Men may need as much, if not more, support than do women in adapting to contemporary family styles. Opportunities to discuss what it means to be a man in today's society can be helpful, such as in support groups with volunteers or professionals who provide services to various agencies and community resources (Real, 1997).

In addition to the changes in women and the effect on families of two-or-more-job adults, the nature of the parental work environment is critical to family coping

HEALTH TEACHING Workplace Violence Plan

- Establish workplace violence policy
- Define conflict resolution methods
- Establish and maintain communication between management and staff
- Establish threat-reporting process
- Manage specific cases
- Analyze the environment for potentials for violence
- Debrief after incidents
- Take corrective actions as soon as possible

From Hinojosa, I. (1996). Taking control of violence in the workplace. *Advances in Nursing Practice*, *11*, 36.

ability. Work that is emotionally draining, particularly when it is filled with conflict, poses special threats to family stability. When one or both parents come home tired, angry, or frustrated from their experiences at work, they likely have limited emotional support to share with other family members.

When people gain self-esteem from their jobs and generally enjoy going to work, they tend to experience less frustration and dissatisfaction with themselves and their positions, enabling them to give more of themselves to other members of the family (Reifman, Biernat, & Lang, 1991).

Middle age is important when looking at the career clock. Issues that need to be considered include midcareer changes in occupations and preretirement planning. Retirement is a major turning point; to many people, it is the transition from middle age to old age and the period of work to the period of leisure or different work.

Adults are working up to and beyond the age of retirement, and many are entering new careers later in life. As adults progress through the middle years, they become increasingly aware of the time remaining until retirement: "Can I readjust my goals?" "Is there disparity between where I am in my career and where I would like to be?" An example might be the 60-year-old veteran nightclub singer whose goal to cut a solo album remains to be achieved. The heightened awareness of age and the decreased likelihood of finding another suitable job can precipitate increased anxiety or depression in this singer.

Comprehensive health-promotion programs at the work site contain the following elements: "(1) health education that focuses on skill development and lifestyle behavior change in addition to information dissemination and awareness building, preferably tailored to employees' interests and needs; (2) supportive social and physical work environments, including established norms for healthy behavior and policies that promote health and reduce the risk of disease, such as work site smoking policies, healthy nutrition alternatives in the cafeteria and vending services, and opportunities for obtaining regular physical activity; (3) integration of the work site program into the organization's administrative structure; (4) related programs, such as employee assistance programs; and (5) screening programs, preferably linked to medical care service delivery to ensure follow-up and appropriate treatment as necessary and to encourage adherence. Optimally, these efforts should be part of a comprehensive occupational health and safety program" (U.S. Department of Health & Human Services, 2000, p. 7-28). The efficacy of these programs is beginning to be documented (Van der Hek & Plomp, 1997).

Caring for Aging Parents

The needs of aging parents and of the adult's own children can create additional demands in the middle years. The middle-age adult can feel "caught between one's children and one's parents." Both children and older parents can present unrealistic, excessive demands and be difficult to please (Fig. 23-3).

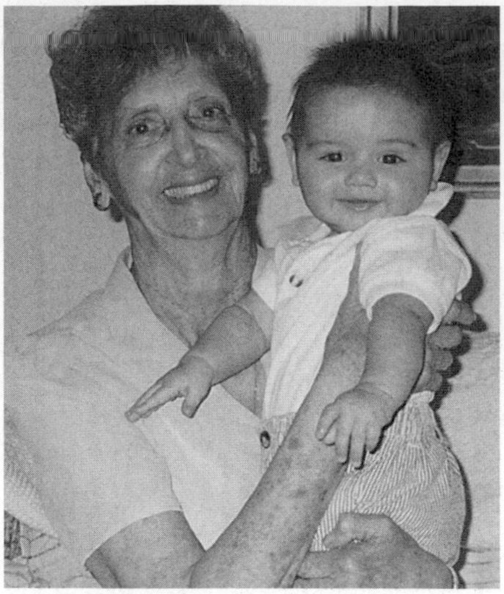

Fig. 23-3 Middle-age adults can be part of the "sandwich" generation and involved in meeting the needs of their older adult family members and their young children.

Middle-age adults may be faced with having frail and ill parents live within their own family unit or placing them into a nursing home (Fig. 23-4). These dilemmas are complicated by the reality that their parents are growing older and may not have long to live. The recognition of the parents' impending death heightens middle-age adults' awareness of their own aging and mortality.

Difficulties in caring for elderly parents can be somewhat lessened when potential situations are discussed before a crisis arises. This instance is particularly true when all members of the middle-adult family are working, space in their home is limited, and the community has few resources for the well or ill elderly adults. Although institutionalization is undesirable to many families, the care of ill, elderly parents may eventually require it. By anticipating these potential needs and dealing with them, middle-age children and their elderly parents can develop further meaningful relationships with one another.

Divorce

Divorce is a potentially major disruption of the marriage and family and to each individual's short- and long-term health. As the divorce rate has risen in recent years, individuals and families have been faced with new and frequently multiple problems. When a divorce occurs, each family member must confront the necessity to examine and, in many cases, modify an accustomed style of living and adapting. In a 5-year study of 60 families, with 131 children ranging from ages 3 to 18, Wallerstein and Kelly (1977) found the first year after a divorce to be the most

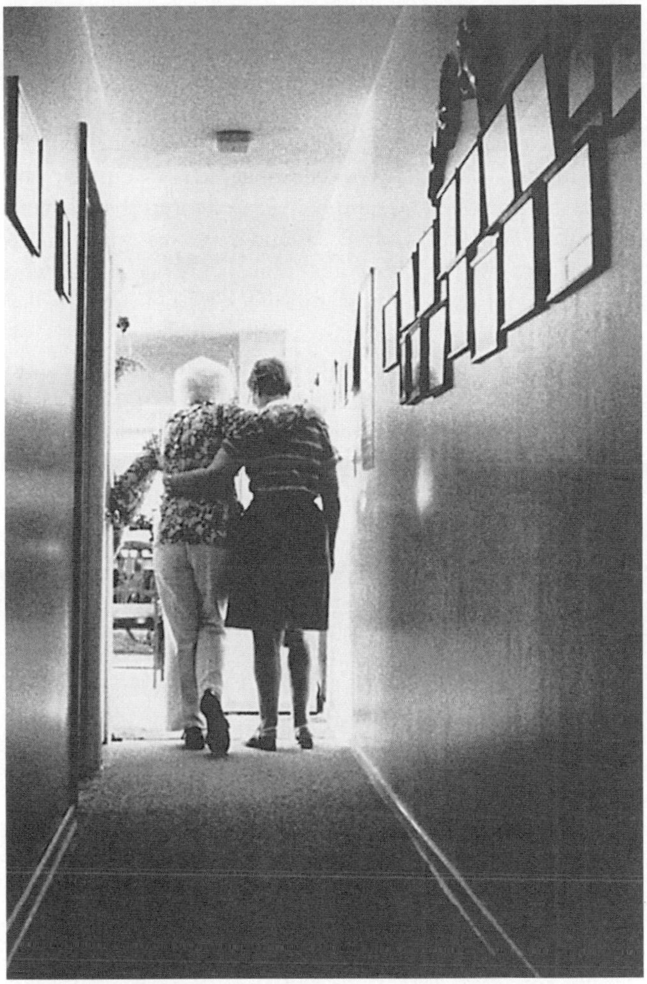

Fig. 23-4 A daughter helps her mother down the hallway of her home. (Courtesy Rod Schmall, West Linn, OR. From Lueckenotte, A. G. [1996]. *Gerontologic nursing.* St. Louis: Mosby.)

difficult and money constituted a major source of stress. The researchers initially thought that divorce is essentially a time-limited crisis for all involved that taxes the usual coping mechanisms to the extent particularly because adults have diminished abilities to parent effectively during the acute stage of adjustment. Wallerstein and her colleagues have also subsequently described long-term consequences of divorce (Wallerstein, 1991; Wallerstein & Johnston, 1990; Wallerstein, Lewis, & Blakeslee, 2000).

Death

Similar to divorce, death of a spouse can result in grieving for the loss of companionship and the lost "planned-for" future, free from the responsibilities of work and children. The surviving spouse may be unprepared to be "single again" and to live alone. The loneliness may be exacerbated by ill or dying peers or parents. Middle-age adults become increasingly aware of the finiteness of life, thinking not only of the number of years since birth, but also of the number of years left to live. The midlife review is a common outcome of this recognition.

Sexuality-Reproductive Pattern

Men and women can continue to have a satisfactory pattern of sexual functioning through out the middle and older adult years. As in any other developmental phase, middle-age adults need counseling to make health-promoting decisions with their sexual behaviors.

Unintended pregnancies are high in all ages of American women, but are the highest (77% of all pregnancies) in middle-age women. In contrast, women planning to have children in the fourth and fifth decades of life should know that fertility rates decrease and infant mortality rates increase, especially when mothers are age 44 years and older (U.S. Department of Health & Human Services, 2000). Additionally, maternal deaths in women 35 years and older are the highest rate of any developmental phase (16.1 per 100,000 live births) (U.S. Department of Health and Human Services, 2000).

Changes in the reproductive systems of men and women result in changes in sexual function throughout adulthood. During middle adulthood, sexual arousal is slower, orgasms are less intense, and a return to prearousal levels is more rapid, with men having longer refractory periods between erection and ejaculation. When a person continues to be sexually active, these functional changes occur over decades and are minimally noticeable until later in adulthood, unless external factors are present, such as the negative effects of some antihypertensive and antidepressant agents.

After menopause, many women enjoy sex more, especially because no risk of pregnancy exists. Conversely, menopause can bring many challenges to a woman. American culture values women largely for their youth, beauty, and childbearing ability (Roundtree, 1993). Middle-age women may confront their own aging for the first time and may be perplexed as to their symptomatic factors and possibly changing roles (Nachtigall, Nachtigall, & Heilman, 1999). Women can experience vaginal dryness, difficulty finding a partner, less interest in initiating sex, and longer instances to reach orgasm. No data exists that report decreases in postmenopausal women's interest in and physical capacity for sex.

Although men and women frequently enjoy satisfactory sexual relationships throughout the middle adult years, men in their middle age are more vulnerable to sexual dysfunction than are women. Frequently, middle-age men first experience problems with premature ejaculation, impotence, and retrograde ejaculation between ages 40 and 50 (Friedman, 1986; Rew, 1990).

Abnormal genital bleeding and secondary amenorrhea are common gynecological complaints that indicate serious physical problems. Abnormal genital bleeding is the most common reason for gynecological office visits by adult women. Although pregnancy and menopause are the most common causes of secondary amenorrhea, other conditions related to abnormal pregnancy, functional disorders, physiological changes, or pathological factors must be considered (Buttaro, Trybulski, Bailey, & Cook, 1999).

As in adolescents and young adults, sexually transmitted diseases (STDs) continue to be major public health problems in the middle-age adult. Women and children bear an inordinate share of the burden: sterility, ectopic pregnancy, fetal and infant deaths, birth defects, and mental retardation. Cancer of the cervix can be linked to the sexually transmitted herpes 2 virus. Similar to many other health behaviors and diseases, the full effect on the life of an individual and family may not be realized until middle age. "Americans 50 years of age and older are a forgotten population at risk for HIV infection and AIDS and presently comprise 10% of reported cases of AIDS in the United States" (Johnson, Haight, & Benedict, 1998, p. 8). As a result, nurses are increasingly aware of the importance of taking a comprehensive sexual history and not missing the diagnosis of HIV infection. Nurses also practice universal precautions, such as caring for older adults in all settings, including offices, nursing homes, and home care. Each nurse should develop appropriate strategies to enhance communication about sexuality throughout the adult years (MacLaren, 1995). Adults need accurate information about sexual health promotion, including developmental changes, STDs, and related treatment strategies to promote satisfying, responsible health behaviors (Flaskerud & Calvillo, 1991).

Coping–Stress-Tolerance Pattern

Long-held myths about women during and after menopause were dispelled in a 5-year study of 2500 middle-age Massachusetts women. The following percentages of these women reported stress from children away from home (8.5%); children living at home (20.3%); children recently returned home (23.6%); husbands away from home (3.6%); husbands living at home (6.3%); and parents or in-laws receiving no care (13%), being cared for outside the woman's home (49.1%), and being cared for in the woman's home (52.7%). This study also found that stress was reduced by one half when the woman had someone close who provided emotional support and practical help (McKinlay & McKinlay, 1988) (see Case Study and Care Plan box).

In a 45-year longitudinal study of 173 men, Vaillant and Vaillant (1990) found that the extent of tranquilizer use before age 50 was the most powerful negative predictor of both mental and physical health outcomes at age 65. Another important predictor for health outcomes was the maturity of defenses against stress (sublimation, anticipation, altruism, and humor).

CASE STUDY

Alan A.

Alan A., a 6-week-old infant, was brought to the hospital with multiple injuries resulting from repeated stabbings with a meat fork. He sustained a pneumo-hemo-thorax and liver lacerations, but was quickly stabilized. Mrs. Angie A., his mother, explained that she had been unable to quiet him. Alan had cried all morning, although she had fed him, changed him, and rocked him. He usually enjoyed his bath, and his mother had thought that might calm him. However, Alan's crying increased until it was intolerable. After she injured him, she called for an ambulance. The nursing history was obtained from Mrs. A. in the pediatric intensive care unit after the baby had been admitted.

What are some of the stresses on middle-age adults that make them feel part of the "sandwich" generation?

What resources are available to manage these stresses?

Describe the components of the health history the nurse will do with Mrs. A.?

From McFarland, G. K., & McFarlane, E. A. (1993). *Nursing diagnosis and intervention: Planning for patient care* (2nd ed.). St. Louis: Mosby.

Stress and Heart Disease

As reiterated throughout this chapter, heart disease is the leading cause of death in the middle-age adult. In landmark studies, Hayes, Feinlieb, and Kannel (1978) describe the relationship of psychosocial factors to coronary heart disease using the Framingham study (Hayes, Feinlieb, & Kannel, 1978, 1980). In the study, 24 measures of psychosocial stress (PSS) were used. In men, aging worries were significantly correlated with systolic and diastolic blood pressures. Marital disagreement and personal worries were significantly correlated with diastolic blood pressure. Both diastolic and systolic pressures were significantly correlated with work changes and anxiety in employed women between 45 and 64 years of age. Anger suppressed, anger discussed, tension, and anger symptoms were significantly correlated with diastolic blood pressure in this age group.

Among white-collar men in this age group, the Framingham type A and ambitiousness scales also were significantly correlated with elevated diastolic blood pressure. The correlation of anger symptoms and anger discussed with diastolic pressures was significant for white-collar women between ages 45 and 64. The initial findings by Haynes and her colleagues have been supported by many other studies, including Spielberger, Jacobs, Russell, and Crane (1983); Kawachi, Sparrow, and Spiro, Vokonas, and Weiss (1996); and Williams and her coinvestigators (2000).

The death of a parent enhances awareness of one's vulnerability to illness and death. The more opportunities and time people have to prepare for these stressful events, the more likely the person will be to feel more in control and less anxious and helpless. When an individual takes on more responsibility for one's own life, decisions lead to specific concrete behaviors, such as drafting a will or **advance directive,** appointing a **durable power of attorney,** and making funeral arrangements (Scharlach & Fredriksen,

1993). An advance directive is a legal document prepared when an individual is alive, competent, and able to make decisions to provide guidelines for health care providers in the future when the individual is not able to make decisions because of physical disability (being unconscious) or mental incompetence. By appointing a durable power of attorney, the individual designates another person (spouse, son, daughter, or friend) to make health care decisions (especially about how aggressive treatment should be in forestalling death) when an individual becomes unable to make such decisions.

The nurse helps middle-age adults anticipate stressors so they are better prepared to effectively cope and prevent additional physical, psychosocial, and spiritual stressors, thereby optimizing their health (Sachs, 1998).

Values-Beliefs Pattern

When adults make decisions affecting their lives, it is usually the result of a personal, complex pattern of values and beliefs (Amaro, 1988; Robertson, 1985; Smith, 1995; McFadden & Gerl, 1990). Much of what people value or believe to be true is formed early in life and can be the most difficult to alter (Rippe, 1996). Normally, people do not spend a great deal of conscious thought on abstract explanations of the meaning of life and why certain things are valued. During times of an illness or crisis, however, people frequently take time to review their value system and seek meaning about what is important (Spector, 2000; Stuart, Deckro, & Mandle, 1989).

A crisis at any age can be a turning point during which both increased vulnerability and increased potential are

CARE PLAN

Nursing Diagnosis: Altered Parenting Related to Unrealistic Expectations for Self, Inadequate Knowledge, Lack of Positive Parental Role Identity, and Lack of Adequate Social Support

Plan of Care for Mrs. Angie A.

EXPECTED PARENT OUTCOMES AND NURSING INTERVENTIONS:

Mrs. A. will provide a safe environment for the child, as evidenced by no further attempts to harm him.

- Provide for Alan's care while in hospital.
- Observe interaction between Mrs. A. and Alan to ensure safety.
- Follow hospital policy regarding the reporting of child injury.

Mrs. A. will develop parent-child attachment behaviors, as evidenced by appropriate touching and eye contact.

- Allow Mrs. A. to touch and hold Alan as soon as possible.
- Allow and encourage Mrs. A. to be involved in Alan's daily care as soon as possible.

Mrs. A. will have an adequate knowledge base for effective parenting, as evidenced by appropriate responses to Alan's crying.

- Identify Mrs. A.'s knowledge about why babies cry and caretaking strategies for crying; provide information on how to cope with her feelings when Alan cries.
- Provide opportunity for Mrs. A. to test new information.
- Create positive learning environment.

Mrs. A. will develop realistic expectations for herself, spouse, and child within the family, as evidenced by ability to verbalize needs and expectations.

- Help Mrs. A. identify expectations for herself, Mr. A., and Alan.
- Help Mrs. A. identify areas of failure to meet her expectations, such as her inability to understand Alan's needs or that her husband would be as available to help her as she believed her father had been.
- Provide Mrs. A. with an opportunity to express her feelings about unmet expectations.
- Encourage Mrs. A. to speculate about reasons for unmet expectations.
- Develop strategies to increase possibilities of having expectations met, such as discussing expectations with Mr. A., identifying steps that must occur to meet expectations.

Mrs. A. will develop role identity as parent, as evidenced by nurturing behaviors.

- Help Mrs. A. identify major components within role identity (child of own, parents, spouse, career), perceptions of specific parenting behaviors that are successful with crying babies, and source of "ideal" parenting behavior.
- Observe interactions between Mrs. A. and Alan for congruency between verbalized "ideal" and actual behavior when Alan is crying.
- Provide opportunity for Mrs. A. to observe and experience effective parent behaviors with crying babies.
- Provide opportunity for Mrs. A. to implement alternative parenting behaviors.

Mrs. A. will experience emotional, social, and physical support, as evidenced by decreased isolation and anxiety.

- Help Mrs. A. identify specific areas in which she needs additional emotional, social, or physical support.
- Help Mrs. A. identify her specific strengths and support systems.
- Provide Mrs. A. information about additional resources to meet needs.
- Act as liaison or advocate for Mrs. A. as needed in obtaining help from appropriate resources, such as contacting Mr. A. and arranging for his immediate return.

This care plan focuses on the parent (Mrs. A.) who has demonstrated "altered parenting" behaviors. Mr. A., as the spouse, is viewed as a part of her support system. If further assessment indicates that Mr. A. also needs help in developing appropriate parenting behaviors, then the plan should be altered.

From McFarland, G. K., & McFarlane, E. A. (1993) *Nursing diagnosis and intervention: Planning for patient care* (2nd ed.). St. Louis: Mosby.

present. When the crisis is successfully managed, a virtue of strength will evolve. Erikson names "caring" as a middle-age adult virtue that can be developed.

Committed responsibilities for the care and welfare of others promotes moral development. When middle age is lived with generativity, many opportunities to live life by one's higher principles is afforded. The middle adult can differentiate among personal wants and needs, duties demanded by society, and principles by which to live. Kohlberg's work on moral development delineated these phases as conventional and postconventional. His studies of men described stage 3 as an interpersonal definition of morality, whereas stage 4 is a societal definition, based on law and order. Kohlberg concludes that most American adults are in these phases of moral development. In contrast, stage 5 is the concern and willingness to sacrifice for the well being of others (Kohlberg & Lickona, 1986). Subsequent studies by Gilligan on moral development in women and men demonstrates gender differences in describing high morality. Women discussed issues of selfishness versus responsibility, of exercising care with and avoiding hurting. Men described terms of justice, fairness, and rights of individuals. Gilligan (1982, 1990) concludes that a different process of moral development exists in women in society.

Valuing others, having relationships, and being responsible to others enables middle-age adults to make the transitions of moral development. This process is accomplished through raising children, developing more junior employees, and serving the community. These commitments increasingly treat others as equals and gradually develop a sensitivity and desire to change barriers to human worth and equality, such as racial prejudice, homelessness, inadequate access to health care, and weapon stockpiles.

ENVIRONMENTAL FACTORS

Environmental factors are significant variables in health promotion. Placing the emphasis on sanitation, preventing pollution, and controlling sectors must continue. The complex interactions between physical, biological, and chemical agents threaten health. Additionally, "the monitoring of public exposure to increasing numbers of toxins and research into the relationship of toxic exposure to disease are important, but are confounded due to the complexities of measuring the level of toxins in the environment, the relative exposure of the population, and individual characteristics that mitigate the effects of the exposure" (U.S. Department of Health and Human Services, 1999, p. 116).

Because there are approximately 100 million workers in the United States, occupational hazards are a serious threat to national health. Exposures to toxic chemicals, asbestos, coal dust, cotton fiber, ionizing radiation, physical hazards, excessive noise, and stress can precipitate numerous health problems. For the middle-age worker, these problems include cancers, lung and heart diseases, decreased hearing, bodily injuries, and mental health problems (U.S. Department of Health and Human Services, 2000).

Physical Agents

Ionizing radiation is a prime example of a physical agent that can cause cancer. Among the best known examples of potential cancer from medical procedures include the use of x-ray films and radiation.

Water pollution has become another major concern. Many industrial and agricultural wastes, such as benzene and chlordane, have been recovered in rivers and lakes from which drinking water is obtained.

Air pollution from auto emissions, burning fuels, and industrial incineration have warranted smog alerts and air pollution indexes. These agents are especially important to the individual with chronic respiratory or cardiovascular disease (U.S. Department of Health and Human Services, 2000).

Noise pollution in industry is a potential problem for the middle-age adult worker. Hearing loss can be prevented if federal guidelines are followed with regard to noise exposure levels and hearing conservation programs.

Exposures to excessive noise, radiation, sunlight, and vibration can produce problems such as chronic obstructive lung disease (COLD), cancer, and degenerative diseases in the middle-age adult.

Biological Agents

As noted throughout this text, the occurrence of health or disease is influenced by the interaction among the agent, host, and environment. Agent factors can be biological, physical, chemical, or psychological in nature. Many of these agents are transmitted through the air or by contact with certain media, such as water or food. These agents enter through the respiratory or gastrointestinal tracts. The size of the agent is important; if it is extremely small, the portal of entry is the respiratory tract. Several of the categories merit special discussion in relation to middle adulthood.

Hepatitis A is caused by viral infection, with transmission occurring primarily through the fecal-oral route. This host-agent interaction typically occurs in the middle-age adult living in an environment with poor sanitation and having close contact with an infected person. The person may also be exposed through contaminated food and water. Hepatitis B is transmitted primarily in the blood or plasma of the infected individuals, which is particularly significant for the adult who is employed in health care settings. Routes of exposure include the following (U.S. Preventive Task Force, 1996):

1. Inoculation by contaminated needle (hospital employees, drug abusers)

2. Minute skin cuts or abrasions (laboratory workers)
3. Mucosal surfaces, such as in the mouth and eyes
4. Sexual contact (virus is carried in saliva and semen)
5. Indirect transfer via vectors (a carrier that transmits the causative organism of a disease) or inanimate environmental surfaces

Hepatitis B is an occupational hazard among medical and dental personnel, with surgeons, oral surgeons, and pathologists at the highest risk, six times higher than that of the general population.

The biological causes of diseases include bacteria, viruses, rickettsiae, fungi, parasites, and food poisoning. Because these causes are often limited to identifiable occupations, they can be readily diagnosed, treated, and prevented (Table 23-1).

Chemical Agents

Chemicals contain a wide variety of substances that increase the risk of morbidity and mortality in the middle-age adult. When the home of the middle-age adult is located near an industry, there is the risk of exposure to toxic chemicals that pollute the air. Contaminants can also be carried home on the clothing from the workplace.

Workers at increased risk include coal miners, wood handlers, and asbestos and coke workers. Pneumoconiosis is found in approximately 15% of coal miners, with black lung disease implicated in thousands of deaths per year. Wood handlers and asbestos workers have increased risk of certain cancers. The asbestos worker also has an increased risk of death from mesothelioma and asbestosis. Approximately 2 million workers each year have been exposed to benzene and vinyl chloride, which may be carcinogens (U.S. Department of Health and Human Services, 2000).

Nine out of ten American industrial workers may be inadequately protected from exposure to at least 10 of the 163 most common hazardous chemicals. More than 2000 of the 50,000 chemicals found in the workplace are suspected human carcinogens (U.S. Department of Health and Human Services, 2000).

Tobacco

Many 50-year-old adults have a 30-plus-year history of cigarette smoking. Cigarette smokers have nearly twice the heart disease death rates of nonsmokers, with the risk being proportional to the amount of smoke inhaled and the number of cigarettes smoked (Joint National Committee, 1997b). Smokers are at increased risks for colds, chronic bronchitis, emphysema, and cancers of the mouth, lungs, esophagus, pancreas, and bladder. More blue-collar workers smoke than do white-collar workers (Pierce, Fiore, Nouotny, Hatziandreu, & Davis, 1989; Centers for Disease Control and Prevention, 1999). A study of 2092 urban adults found that knowledge about the health effects of smoking was generally low among women, older adults, Blacks, those of lower education levels, and current smokers (Brownson et al., 1992).

Few smokers realize that cigarettes contain 2000 known chemicals, including tar, nicotine, hydrogen cyanide, formaldehyde, and ammonia. Cigarette smoking is, for most smokers, an addiction to nicotine, which is absorbed into the bloodstream. Nicotine acts in the two divisions of the nervous system to affect the central part of the brain and the spinal cord and the peripheral portion that controls the arms and legs. Effects of nicotine stimulation can be observed in both electroencephalographic changes and in hand tremors. Nicotine also acts to stimulate the heart, leading to an increased pulse and elevated blood pressure. Although smokers frequently believe that cigarettes have a calming effect, this notion is misleading. Nicotine stimulates the body, whereas increasing levels of carbon

Table 23-1 Examples of Occupational Biological Hazards and Preventive Measures

Disease	Target Organ	Occupational Source	Exposed Occupations	Preventive Measures
Fever (rickettsia)	Systemic	Placental tissue, excreta from infected cattle, sheep	Laboratory workers, farmers, slaughterhouse workers	Hygiene; immunization
Histoplasmosis (fungus)	Lung	Fowl droppings	Farmers, poultry workers, demolition workers	Dust control, environmental sanitation
Hookworm (parasite)	Small intestine	Larvae in human feces penetrating skin	Farmers, sewer workers, recreation workers	Environmental sanitation; use of shoes, boots, gloves
Tetanus (bacterium)	Nervous system	Soil	Construction workers, farmers	Immunization
Rabies (virus)	Central nervous system	Wild animals, cows	Laboratory workers, veterinarians, hunters	Immunization of humans in contact with dogs, cats, skunks, foxes, bats, raccoons

Modified from Cohen, R. (1990). Occupational biologic hazards. *Occupational Health Nursing, 28* (8), 20-24.

monoxide cause lethargy. Smokers may feel calm, although they are actually having their sensations dulled by the elevated level of carbon monoxide (Joint National Committee, 1997a).

Additive effects can lower midexpiratory flow values, as in those from chlorine, cotton dust, and beta-radiation. Profound effects can also be observed with asbestos interaction. In a 4-year study of 370 asbestos insulation workers, 24 of the 283 cigarette smokers died of bronchogenic carcinoma. None of the 87 nonsmokers died. Asbestos workers who smoke have eight times the risk of lung cancer compared with all other smokers. Workers exposed to asbestos have 92 times the risk of nonsmokers (U.S. Preventive Services Task Force, 1996).

SOCIAL PROCESSES

Culture and Ethnicity

Spector (2000) describes culture as the "sum of beliefs, practices, habits, likes, dislikes, norms, customs, rituals . . . we have learned from our families during the years of socialization" (p. 1). Spector further relates the ways in which one's cultural background is a component of one's ethnic background. The major ethnic groups of the United States are Asians, Blacks, Native Americans, and Hispanics.

Nurses must understand their own ethnic cultures and that of others, largely because differences in beliefs, practices, and rituals can exist (Brownson et al., 1992; Kerr & Ritchey, 1990; Duffy, Rossow, & Hernandez, 1996). The middle-age adult may not interpret dizziness as a possible symptom of hypertension, for example; it may be described simply as a "spell." What the Black adult defines as "health" may be completely different from that of the White health care provider or the Asian person. The obese adult who has received positive reinforcement throughout life for being pleasingly plump is less motivated to lose weight than is the adult who defines health as being "svelte" (Duffy, Rossow, & Hernandez, 1996; Roberson, 1985; Smith, 1995).

The current health problems of middle-age adults, even within major ethnic groups, are varied. Recent immigrants who live in crowded urban areas have higher mortality rates than do earlier immigrants of the same cultural group who live in healthier environments. Their working conditions continue to be poor, with long hours and minimal wages. Modern preventive health care is difficult, if not impossible, to obtain.

Hispanic subgroups comprise the largest minority group in the United States. The Hispanic American adult's primary health care problems, as identified by Spector (2000), are the barriers faced when they seek health care. These barriers include language, poverty, and time orientation. Few Spanish-speaking health care providers practice at this time. The problem is compounded by the Hispanic tendency to place little value on the exact time of day, which makes appointment-keeping frustrating for both the individual and the nurse. Poverty can predispose the middle-age Hispanic adult and any other group to tuberculosis, malnutrition, and delayed screening (mammography).

Poverty is also reported in approximately one third of Native Americans. The middle-age adult Native American is faced with a high rate of tuberculosis; alcohol abuse; inadequate immunization; mental health problems, such as depression; and dental problems (Spector, 2000; U.S. Department of Health and Human Services, 2000).

For many women in society, the cessation of menses is associated with aging; the role of the middle-age woman may be shaped by her culture. Some cultures afford menopausal women greater freedom, occasionally labeling them as witches with curative powers (Watson, 1989).

Cultural competency attainment by nurses can ensure the provision of appropriate health promotion, especially for vulnerable populations and those individuals, families, and communities who have special health care needs. Rorie, Paine, and Barger (1996) describe experiences that can hinder the development and delivery of culturally appropriate care.

Economics

Adults in the middle years are frequently at the peak of their careers. Although their net income may be greater than it was in early adulthood, middle-age adults frequently have significant additional financial expenditures. Children may be in college and need financial support, and preretirement planning can stress the budget. The care of an aging parent can be an additional financial burden and can be costly in terms of present lifestyle. When the adult or family members have ongoing health problems, the economic status of the family can be further compromised (see Multicultural Awareness box).

The individual's economic status also plays a role in the incidence of mental illness. Mental illness is increased in adults at the lower socioeconomic level, with higher rates of anxiety, depression, and phobias.

MULTICULTURAL AWARENESS

Single Mothers

Many women in midlife have inadequate economic resources. Black, Hispanic, and Native American women in particular have high rates of poverty, especially when they are single and heads of households. Increasingly, these women are being joined by White, middle-class women rearing children alone or living on small fixed incomes. Because of inadequate incomes and the high cost of health insurance, many women in this age group postpone obtaining adequate health care.

Data from National Clearinghouse for Women Workers, Policy Makers and Others, 320 East 43rd St., New York, NY 10017.

Health Care Delivery System

The nurse can contact numerous agencies that are geared to middle adulthood. These agencies can be categorized as official, voluntary, and service agencies (Box 23-6). Councils of community services frequently publish a directory of services that may be helpful. Official agencies include those that are state and federally funded, such as public health departments and drug treatment centers. Voluntary agencies include the American Cancer Society, the American Lung Association, and Alcoholics Anonymous. Many educational and self-help programs are sponsored by these organizations. The American Lung Association sponsors a "Stop Smoking" program, which can be conducted on a group basis in a work or community setting. Service agencies include professional organizations, such state nurses' associations, the American Medical Association (sponsor of the Tel-Med program), bar associations, YMCAs, hospice

Box 23-6 Examples of Community Resources for Health Promotion During Middle Adulthood

ADVOCACY
- Family and children's services
- Legal services

EDUCATION AND COMMUNITY CENTERS
- American Red Cross
- Community centers
- Public schools
- Young Women's Christian Association (YWCA)
- Young Men's Christian Association (YMCA)

ALCOHOL AND DRUG ABUSE TREATMENT AND REHABILITATION
- Alcoholics Anonymous
- Mental health centers
- Hospital alcohol and drug abuse programs
- Local council on alcohol and drugs
- Narcotics Anonymous
- State departments of mental health (alcohol and drug division)
- Veterans' hospitals (mental health unit)

CLINICS AND HEALTH CENTERS
- Community clinics
- Health departments
- Planned Parenthood clinics
- United Neighborhood Health Service

COMMUNITY PLANNING, ORGANIZATION, AND DEVELOPMENT
- Chambers of commerce
- Councils of community
- Metropolitan development and housing agencies
- Metropolitan planning commissions
- Metropolitan social service departments
- Urban League
- State commissions on the status of women
- State law enforcement planning agencies

CONSUMER AFFAIRS
- Better Business Bureaus
- State division of consumer affairs

COUNSELING
- American Red Cross
- State divisions of family services
- Rape and sexual abuse centers
- Social service departments
- YWCA

CRISIS INTERVENTION SERVICES
- Crisis hotlines
- Rape and sexual abuse centers

EMPLOYMENT COUNSELING, TRAINING, AND PLACEMENT
- Career counseling centers
- Employment security offices
- YWCA Displaced Homemakers Program

ENVIRONMENTAL PROTECTION
- State health departments
- State departments of conservation
- State departments of public health
- State environmental councils

HEALTH EDUCATION AND PROMOTION
- American Red Cross
- Arthritis Association
- American Cancer Society
- American Lung Association
- American Dietetic Association
- American Diabetes Association
- American Heart Association
- American Kidney Foundation
- Academy of Medicine
- Council on Alcohol and Drug Abuse
- Tel-Med (recorded messages)
- State dental associations

SPOUSE ABUSE
- Crisis intervention centers
- Legal services
- YWCA

WOMEN'S ORGANIZATIONS
- Homemakers Back to Work
- Junior League
- League of Women Voters
- National Council of Jewish Women
- YWCA Women's Resource Center

programs, and the Women's Occupational Health Resource Center.

NURSING INTERVENTIONS

The nurse must first understand the hazards to which the individual is exposed by listening, conferring with other individuals in the same environment, and reviewing available health and safety data.

As a health educator, the nurse then initiates programs that emphasize helping adults accept more responsibility for their own health. This effort can be provided on a one-to-one basis or in a seminar fashion. For example, with the goal of "early detection of high blood pressure," the nurse in the community or industry might increase consumers' knowledge of hypertension, screen people who have sought health care for any reason, set up mechanisms to screen people outside the health care system, and refer and follow up on all persons with blood pressure elevations (Joint National Committee, 1997a).

The target groups identified by the nurse should have common needs, such as individuals exposed to a particular chemical, smokers, substance abusers, women entering the workplace for the first time, or men nearing retirement. In a work environment, the occupational health nurse (OHN) can also assess absenteeism rates for any trends. In gathering data, the nurse can initiate research projects with multidisciplinary input.

The preemployment physical examination not only provides the employer with information about proper placement, but also provides a baseline health assessment (Lindsay, 1989). Frequently, this examination is the only assessment that the individual has had in years.

The Occupational Safety and Health Administration (OSHA) mandates that the employee have a healthy and safe work environment. Therefore a complete health history of the adult is essential. Is there a history of hypertension, arthritis, cancer, or hernia? Is there any significant family history? Is the person a smoker? How many packs per day? Is the person taking any medications? Medical limitations must be addressed; for example,

innovative practice

Mind/Body Medical Clinic Symptom Reduction Programs

Research demonstrates that 60% to 90% of health care visits are for symptoms such as headaches, insomnia, weakness or fatigue, and gastrointestinal symptoms, all of which are frequently stress related. The Mind/Body Medical Clinic Symptom Reduction Programs are designed to help patients with chronic illnesses (including life-threatening illnesses) or stress-related symptoms better manage their health problems and optimize their quality of life. The interventions combine conventional medical care with knowledge about the effects of behaviors and attitudes on health.

The biopsychosocial-spiritual approach of the assessment and treatment plans with patients includes:

- Eliciting the relaxation response—a state of deep rest that changes responses to stress (decreases vital signs and muscle tenseness, increased mindfulness)
- Enhancing coping skills through cognitive-behavioral strategies
- Encouraging exercise or physical activity
- Providing nutritional counseling
- Monitoring and adjusting medication, when necessary, in consultation with the patient's physician

Insurance claims for these outpatient visits are submitted directly to patients' insurance carriers. Because health insurance policies differ, coverage and reimbursement vary. A patient advocate (with a business degree) helps patients research their specific health insurance coverage and billing requirements.

Research demonstrates that after these interventions:

- Patients with pain reduced their physician visits by 36%.
- Visits to an HMO were reduced by approximately 50% after a relaxation response-based intervention, resulting in significant cost savings.
- Blood pressure was lowered and the use of medications was decreased in 80% of hypertensive patients; 16% of the patients were able to discontinue all of their medications.
- Sleep patterns were improved for 100% of patients with insomnia; 90% reduced or eliminated the use of sleep medication.
- Infertile women reported decreased levels of depression, anxiety, and anger, and a 35% conception rate.
- Women with severe premenstrual syndrome (PMS) experienced a 57% reduction in physical and psychological symptoms
- Health-promoting behaviors, such as nutrition, social supports, self-esteem, health responsibility, and exercise, increased after the program and were maintained in a 6-month follow-up.
- Six months after the program, 80% of patients continued to experience a decrease in their physical symptoms.
- Anxiety and depression normalized for most participants and were maintained 6 months following the program
- Women with menopause reported reduced "hot flashes," lower blood pressure, improved sleep, and decreased depression, anxiety, and anger.

Harvard Medical School
Beth Israel Deaconess Medical Center
Division of Behavior Medicine
Mind/Body Medical Clinic
Symptom Reduction Programs
Carol Lynn Mandle, PhD, RN, CS-FNP, Codirector
Website: www.mindbody.harvard.edu
Email: mbclinic@caregroup.harvard
Phone: 617-632-9530

Courtesy Carol Lynn Mandle, PhD, RN.

decreased visual acuity means no driving, and dermatitis means no oils, chemicals, or solvents. Removing a worker from a particular job may be indicated if the worker might endanger coworkers, has a disease condition that might be aggravated by the job, or if the worker is taking prescribed medications with potentially harmful side effects.

The nurse in the community and in industry should reiterate some key safety issues to the adult, such as wearing seat belts and observing speed limits. With a decrease in visual acuity, driving at night can be hazardous. The middle-age adult's reaction time is also decreasing, which reinforces the need to enforce recommendations by the National Highway Traffic Safety Administration for specific interval retesting.

With an increase in leisure time, the middle-age adult is at greater risk for recreational accidents. As noted, moderation should be stressed. Alcohol is a depressant and should be avoided in activities that require attentiveness.

Protection from burns is essential; 56% of fatal residential fires are cigarette related, such as from smoking in bed. Falls can occur at any age, and safety measures should be considered for the entire family, with preparatory planning for aging parents. A few suggestions to the adult might be to avoid highly waxed floors, poor lighting, high beds, and bathtubs without nonslip bottoms.

Handgun availability is controversial at best; however, approximately 20% of American households have them. When the person believes strongly about having a firearm, safety measures to avoid accidental injury should be discussed, such as security locks and proper storage.

The Occupational Safety and Health Act (1970) was designed to ensure that workers are employed under safe and healthy working conditions. The act is applicable to every employer who is engaged in a business that affects commerce. The employer must ascertain that the workplace is free from recognized hazards and must comply with the act. OSHA has offices in most major cities and can provide recommended standards for occupational agents.

Nurses can actively participate in the safety committee of the industry in which they are employed. When no similar committee exists, many protection measures will fall on the nurse. Suggestions include:

1. Tour the facilities on a regular basis. Be familiar with resource books, laws, and available codes.
2. Develop a toxicology chart with symptoms of overexposure and current treatment. Update this chart frequently.
3. Be a role model in safety issues; wear safety glasses, protective footwear, and gloves, and do not smoke.
4. Discuss the preemployment physical with the employee, with an emphasis on risk factors. Monitor health problems and exposure levels in the work setting.

The worker must be aware of the protective clothing that should be worn, sanitation measures for the work environment, general hygiene measures, and proper immunization. The food handler, for instance, should have an annual tuberculosis skin test, wear clean clothing and appropriate hair protection, and use good hand-washing techniques. The nurse should not assume that workers know how to protect themselves and others.

A major challenge for the nurse is to encourage workers to assume responsibility for protecting their own health. Increasingly, organizations are interested in promoting the health of their employees for many reasons, including enhancing their recruiting efforts and minimizing lateness, absenteeism, turnover, physical and emotional inabilities to work, disability costs, and health and life insurance costs. Health-promotion programs are increasingly recognized for their vital contributions to the financial viability of organizations (Hellings, 1989; O'Donnell, 1995; Pruitt, 1992; Weitzel & Waller, 1990).

Health-promotion programs within an organizational setting can be categorized in one of three levels: (1) awareness, (2) lifestyle change, and (3) supportive environment. The goal of a health program at the level of awareness is to increase the individual's knowledge or interest in a particular health issue, such as smoking cessation. Examples of awareness programs include special events, flyers, lunch seminars, meetings, and newsletters. Changing health behaviors or status are not the goals of awareness programs, but are goals of lifestyle change programs.

Lifestyle change programs last at least 8 to 12 weeks and include assessment, education, and evaluation components to help individuals implement long-term changes in health behavior and status. To maintain these long-term changes in health behavior and status and to develop a healthy lifestyle, a supportive organizational environment is needed. This type of environment includes health-promoting physical settings, corporate policies and culture, ongoing programs, and employee ownership of programs (U.S. Department of Health and Human Services, 2000).

Five models of nurse-managed primary health care delivery at the work site have recently been proposed as part of the American Nurses' Association's program for reform of this nation's health care system, known as "Nursing's Agenda for Health Care Reform." Each model is developed to enable employers to fulfill the goal of providing accessible, quality, and affordable care at locations that are familiar and convenient for employees. These designs assist employers in introducing or expanding health care services at the work site, controlling health care costs, and meeting the health care needs of their employees.

SUMMARY

Nurses are in a position to help the middle-age adult improve the quality of life, both for the present and for the future, through the identification of risk factors, health promotion, and other appropriate nursing interventions.

Nurses work in a variety of health care settings available to healthy middle-age adults: outpatient clinics, occupational health clinics, and private practice.

Health promotion and disease prevention are aimed at the personal habits and lifestyles of adults to improve their biological, spiritual, and psychosocial development. Strategies to help an adult achieve a higher level of health include individual or group counseling based on identified risk factors, providing self-help information that is most relevant to the middle-age adult, and describing available resources.

Through these strategies, the nurse is better able to motivate middle-age adults to assume more responsibility for their health behaviors. Changes may be effected after years of poor health practices, decreasing the adult's risk of disability from chronic disease.

REFERENCES

Amaro, H. (1988). Women in the Mexican-American community: Religion, culture and reproductive attitudes and experiences. *Journal of Community Psychology, 16*, 6-20.

Anonymous. (1998). Clinical guidelines on the identification, evaluation, and treatment of overweight and obesity in adults: Evidence report. *Obesity Research* (6 Suppl), 209S-251S.

Apter, T. (1991). *Altered loves: Mothers and daughters during adolescence*. New York: Ballantine.

Ben-Kiki, J. S., & Herman, R. S. (1998). *I love menopause because* . . . . Kansas City, MO: McMeel.

Benson, L., Nelson, E. C., Napps, S. E., Roberts, E., Kane-Williams, E., & Salisbury. (1989). Evolution of staying healthy after fifty educational program: Impact on course participants. *Health Education Quarterly, 16* (4), 485-508.

Berger, K. S. (1998). *The developing person through the life span* (4th ed.). New York: Worth Publishers.

Bischof, L. (1989). *Adult psychology*. New York: Harper & Row.

Bloom, B. S. (1984). *Taxonomy of educational objectives: Handbook I, cognitive domain*. New York: Longman.

Bonnick, S. L. (1997). *The osteoporosis handbook*. Dallas: Taylor.

Bronfman, D., & Bronfman, R. (1998). *CalciYum! Calcium-rich, dairy-free vegetarian recipes*. Toronto: Bromeda.

Browder, S. E. (1998). Attention, women over 50! The 3 health problems you have most to fear, and what to do now. *New Choices: Living Even Better After 50, 38* (1), 25-26.

Brown, W. J., Young, A. F., & Byles, J. E. (1999). Tyranny of distance? The health of mid-age women living in five geographical areas of Australia. *Australian Journal of Rural Health, 7* (3), 148-154.

Brownson, R. C., Jackson, T., Thompson, J., Wilkenson, J. C., Davis, J. R., Owens, N. W., & Fisher, E. B. (1992). Demographic and socioeconomic differences in beliefs about the health effects of smoking. *American Journal of Public Health, 82*, 99-103.

Brownson, R. C., Houseman, R. A., Brown, D. R., Jackson-Thompson, J., King, A. C., Malone, B. R., & Sallis, J. F. (2000). Promoting physical activity in rural communities: Walking trail access, use and effects. *American Journal of Preventive Medicine, 18* (3), 235-241.

Burgel, B. J. (1993). *Innovation at the work site: Delivery of nurse-managed primary health care services*. Washington, DC: American Nurses Publishing.

Buttaro, T. M., Trybulski, J., Bailey, P. P., & Sandburg-Cook, J. S. (1999). *Primary care: A collaborative practice*. St. Louis: Mosby.

Centers for Disease Control and Prevention. (1999). Prevalence of current cigarette and cigar smoking adults-United States, 1998. *Morbidity and Mortality Weekly Report, 48* (45), 1034-1039.

Cleeman, J. I., & Lenfant, C. (1998). The National Cholesterol Education Program: Progress and prospects. *Journal of the American Medical Association, 280*, 2099-2104.

Cohen, R. (1990). Occupational biologic hazards. *Occupational Health Nursing, 28* (8), 20-24.

Craig, C. J. (1989). *Human development* (5th ed.). Englewood Cliffs, NJ: Prentice Hall.

Duffy, M. E., Rossow, R., & Hernandez, M. (1996). Correlates of health promotion activities in Mexican American women. *Nursing Research, 45*, 18-24.

Dunn, A. L., Marcus, B. H., Kampert, J. B., Garcia, M. E., Kohl, H. W., & Blair, S. N. (1999). Comparisons of lifestyle and structured interventions to increase physical activity and cardiorespiratory fitness: A randomized trial. *Journal of the American Medical Association, 281*, 327-334.

Duvall, E. M., & Miller, B. (1984). *Marriage and family development* (6th ed.). New York: Harper Collins.

Erikson, E. H. (1986). *Childhood and society* (35th ed.). New York: W. W. Norton.

Flaskerud, J. H. & Calvillo, E. R. (1991). Beliefs about AIDS, health and illness among low income Latino women. *Research in Nursing & Health, 14*, 431-438.

Flowers, J. S., & McLean, J. E. (1996). Psychometric studies of the Flowers Midlife Health Questionnaire. *Journal of Nursing Science, 1* (3,4), 115-126.

Friedman, M. M. (1986). *Family nursing theory and assessment* (2nd ed.). New York: Appleton-Lange.

Futterman, L. A., & Jones, J. E. (1997). *The PMS and perimenopause sourcebook: A guide to the emotional, mental, and physical patterns of a woman's life*. Los Angeles: Lowell House.

Gilligan, C. (1982). *In a different voice: Psychological theory and women's development*. Cambridge, MA: Harvard University Press.

Gilligan, C. (1990). *Mapping the moral domain*. Cambridge, MA: Harvard University Press.

Hansen, J. P. (1986). Older maternal age and pregnancy outcomes: A review of the literature. *Obstetrical & Gynecological Survey, 41*, 726-742.

Hartweg, D. L., & Berbiglia, V. A. (1996). Determining the adequacy of a health promotion self-care interview guide with healthy, middle-aged, Mexican-American women: A pilot study. *Health Care for Women International, 17* (1), 57-68.

Havighurst, R. I., & Orr, B. (1956). *Adult education and adult needs*. Chicago: Center for Study of Liberal Education for Adults.

Hayes, S. G., Feinleib, M., & Kannel, W. B. (1978). The relationship of psychosocial factors to coronary heart disease in the Framingham Study. *American Journal of Epidemiology, 107* (5), 362-380.

Hayes, S. G., Feinleib, M., & Kannel, W. B. (1980). The relationship of psychosocial factors to coronary heart disease in the Framingham Study. *American Journal of Epidemiology, 111* (5), 37-58.

Haynes, S. G., Levine, S., Scotch, N., Feinleib, M., & Kannel, W. B. (1978). The relationship of psychosocial factors to coronary heart disease in the Framingham Study. *American Journal of Epidemiology, 107* (5), 362-383.

Hellings, P. (1989). *Using nursing research. Instructor's manual: Critiques of research on health promotion and primary care nursing* (Pub. no. 15). New York: National League for Nursing.

Hinojosa, I. (1996). Taking control of violence in the workplace. *Advances in Nursing Practice, 11*, 36.

Hornstein, G. (1986). The structuring of identity among mid-life women as a function of their degree of involvement in employment. *Journal of Personality, 54*, 551-575.

Jacobs, G. D. (1998). *Say goodnight to insomnia*. New York: Henry Holt.

Johnson, M., Haight, B. K., & Benedict, S. (1998). AIDS in older people. A literature review for clinical nursing research and practice. *Journal of Gerontological Nursing, 24*, 8-13.

Joint National Committee. (1997a). The 1984 report of the Joint National Committee on prevention, detection, evaluation and treatment of high blood pressure. *Archives of Internal Medicine, 114*, 1045-1057.

Joint National Committee. (1997b). The sixth report of the Joint National Committee on detection, evaluation and treatment of high blood pressure. *Archives of Internal Medicine, 157*, 2413-2446.

Kawachi, I., Sparrow, D., Spiro, A., Vokonas, P., & Weiss, S. T. (1996). A prospective study of anger and coronary heart disease: The Normative Aging Study. *Circulation, 94*, 2090-2095.

Kerr, M. J., & Ritchey, D. A. (1990). Health promoting lifestyles of English-speaking and Spanish-speaking Mexican-American migrant farm workers. *Public Health Nursing, 7*, 80-87.

Kohlberg, L., & Lickona, T. (1986). *The stages of ethical development: From childhood through old age*. New York: Harper Collins.

Kriketos, A. D., Sharp, T. A., Seagle, H. M., Peters, J. C., & Hill, J. O. (2000). Effects of aerobic fitness on fat oxidation and body fitness. *Medicine and Science in Sports & Exercise, 32* (4), 805-811.

Lancaster, J. B., & King, B. J. (1985). *An evolutionary perspective. In her prime: A new view of middle-aged women*. South Hadley, MA: Bergin & Garvey.

Landau, C., Cyr, M. G., & Moulton, A. W. (1995). *The complete book of menopause: Every woman's guide to good health*. New York: Perigree & Berkley.

Levinson, D. (1986a). A conception of adult development. *American Psychologist, 41*, 3-13.

Levinson, D. (1986b). *The seasons of a man's life*. New York: Ballantine.

Levinson, D. (1996). *The seasons of a women's life*. New York: Knopf.

Lindsay, R. (1989). Prevention of osteoporosis. *Clinical Orthopedics and Related Research, 222*, 44-59.

Lubkin, I. M. (1998). *Chronic illness-impact and interventions* (4th ed.). Boston: Jones & Bartlett.

MacLaren, A. (1995). Primary care for women: Comprehensive sexual assessment. *Journal of Nurse-Midwifery, 40*, 104-119.

McFadden, S., & Gerl, R. (1990). Approaches to understanding spirituality in the second half of life. *Generations, 14*, 35-38.

McKinlay, J., & McKinlay, S. (1988). *Massachusetts women's health study: 9th annual scientific sessions*. Boston: The Society of Behavioral Medicine.

Morgan, I. S. (1999). Health promotion in midlife women: A grounded theory of influencing processes. *Communicating Nursing Research, 32*, 61-68.

Mottaz, C. J. (1987). Age and work satisfaction. *Work and Occupations, 14*, 387-409.

Nachtigall, L. E., Nachtigall, R. D., & Heilman, J. R. (1999). *What every woman should know: Staying healthy after 40*. New York: Warner Books.

National Institutes of Health, National Heart, Lung, and Blood Institute. (1998). *Morbidity and mortality: 1998 chartbook on cardiovascular, lung, and blood diseases*. Washington, DC: The Author.

National Osteoporosis Foundation. (1998). *Boring up on osteoporosis: A guide to prevention and treatment*. Washington, DC: The Foundation.

National Sleep Foundation. (1998). *Women and sleep*. Washington, DC: The Foundation.

Nelson, M. E. (1997). *Strong women stay young*. New York: Bantam Books.

Nelson, M. E., & Wernick, S. (1998). *Strong women stay slim*. New York: Bantam.

Newman, D. K., & Dzurinko, M. K. (1997). *The urinary incontinence sourcebook*. Los Angeles: Lowell House.

North American Menopause Society. (1998). *Menopause guidebook*. Cleveland: The Society.

O'Donnell, M. P. (1995). *Design of workplace health promotion programs* (6th ed.). Rochester Hills, MI: American Journal of Health Promotion, Inc.

Pender, N. (1996a). *Health promotion in nursing practice*. Stamford, CT: Appleton-Lange.

Pender, N. (1996b). *Health promotion*. Norwalk. CT: Appleton-Lange.

Philipp, J. S. (1999). *An analysis of health status among diabetic and non-diabetic women at midlife*. Unpublished doctoral dissertation, University of South Dakota.

Piaget, J. (1970). *Structuralism*. New York: Basic Books.

Pierce, J. P., Fiore, M. C., Nouotny, T. E., Hatziandreu, E. J., & Davis, R. M. (1989). Trends in cigarette smoking in the United States: Projections to the year 2000. *Journal of the American Medical Association, 261*, 56-60.

Pruitt, R. H. (1992). Effectiveness and cost efficiency of interventions in health promotion. *Journal of Advanced Nursing, 17*, 926-932.

Ray, O. S. (1982). *Drugs, society, and human behavior* (4th ed.). St. Louis: Mosby.

Real, T. (1997). *I don't want to talk about it: Men and depression*. New York: Scribner.

Reifman, A., Biernat, M., & Lang, E. (1991). Stress, social support, and health in married professional women with small children. *Psychology of Women Quarterly, 15*, 431-445.

Rew, L. (1990). Correlates of health promoting lifestyles and sexual satisfaction in a group of men. *Issues in Mental Health Nursing, 11*, 283-295.

Rippe, J. M. (1996). *Fit over forty: A revolutionary plan to achieve lifelong physical and spiritual health and well-being*. New York: William Morrow.

Robertson, H. B. (1985). The influence of religious beliefs on health choices in Afro-Americans. *Advances in Nursing Science, 7*(3), 57-63.

Rorie, J. L., Paine, L. L., & Barger, M. K. (1996). Primary care for women: Cultural competence in primary care services. *Journal of Nurse-Midwifery, 41*, 92-100.

Roundtree, C. (1993). *On women turning 50-celebrating mid life discoveries*. New York: Harper Collins.

Rowe, J. W., & Kahn, R. L. (1998) *Successful aging*. New York: Dell.

Sachs, J. (1998). *Break the stress cycle! 10 steps to reducing stress for women*. Holbrook, MA: Adams Media.

Schaie, K. (1994). The course of adult intellectual development. *American Psychologist 49*, 304-343.

Scharlach, A., & Fredriksen, R. (1993). Reactions to the death of a parent during midlife. *Omega Journal of Death and Dying, 27*, 307-319.

Schiff, I., & Parson, A. B. (1996). *Menopause*. New York: Times Books.

Shandler, N. (1997). *Estrogen: The natural way*. New York: Villard Books.

Silverstein, O., & Rashbaum, B. (1995). *The courage to raise good men*. New York: Penguin.

Smith, C. A. (1995). The lived experience of staying healthy in rural African American families. *Nursing Science Quarterly, 8*, 17-21.

Spector, R. E. (2000). *Cultural diversity in health and illness* (5th ed.). East Norwalk, CT: Appleton-Lange.

Spielberger, C. D., Jacobs, G., Russell, S., & Crane, R. S. (1983). Assessment of anger: The state-trait anger scale. In J. N. Butcher, & C. D. Speilberger, *Advances in personality assessment: Vol. 2*. Hillsdale, NJ: Lawrence Erlbaum Associates.

Stuart, E., Deckro, J., & Mandle, C. L. (1989). Spirituality in health and healing: A clinical program. *Holistic Nursing Practice, 3*, 35-46.

Boston Women's Health Book Collective. (1999). *Our bodies, ourselves for the new century*. New York: Touchstone.

Thomas, S. P. (1995). Psychosocial correlates of women's health in middle adulthood. *Issues in Mental Health Nursing, 16*, 285-314.

U.S. Department of Health and Human Service, Centers for Disease Control and Prevention, National Center for Health Statistics. (1998). *Health, United States*. Hyattsville, MD: The Author.

U.S. Department of Health and Human Services. (1999). *Healthy people 2000 review*. Washington, DC: U.S. Government Printing Office.

U.S. Department of Health and Human Services. (2000). *Healthy people 2010*. Washington, DC: U.S. Government Printing Office.

U.S. Preventive Services Task Force. (1996). *Guide to clinical preventive services: An assessment of the effectiveness of 169 interventions* (2nd ed.). Baltimore: Williams & Wilkins.

Vaillant, G., & Vaillant, C. (1990). Natural history of male psychological health: A 45-year study of predictors of successful aging at age 65. *American Journal of Psychology, 147* (1), 31-37.

Van der Hek, H., & Plomp, H. N. (1997). Occupational stress management programs: A practical overview of published effect studies. *Occupational Medicine, 47* (3), 133-141.

Wallerstein, J. S. (1991). The long-term effects of divorce on children: A review. *Journal of the American Academy of Child and Adolescent Psychiatry, 30*, 349-360.

Wallerstein, J. S., & Johnson, J. R. (1990). Children of divorce: Recent findings regarding long-term effects and recent studies of joint and sole custody. *Pediatric Reviews, 11*, 197-204.

Wallerstein, J. S., & Kelly, J. B. (1977). Divorce counseling: A community service for families in the midst of divorce. *American Journal of Orthopsychiatry, 47*, 4-22.

Wallerstein, J. S., Lewis, J., & Blakeslee, S. (2000). *The unexpected legacy of divorce: A 25 year landmark study*. New York: Hyperion.

Watson, G. L. (1989). *Feminism and women's issues, 1974-1986: An annotated bibliography and research guide*. Hamden, CT: Garland.

Weitzel, M. H., & Waller, P. R. (1990). Predictive factors for health promotion behaviors in White, Hispanic and blue-collar workers. *Family & Community Health, 13*, 23-34.

Willett, W. H., Dietz, W. H., & Colditz, G. A. (1999). Primary care: Guidelines for healthy weight. *New England Journal of Medicine, 341*, 427-434.

Williams, J., Paton, C., Siegler, I. C., Eigenbrodt, M. L., Nieto, F. J., & Tyroler, H. A. (2000). Anger proneness predicts coronary heart disease risk: Prospective Analysis from the Atherosclerosis Risk in Communities (ARIC) Study. *Circulation, 101* (17), 2034-2039.

Zeitz, G. (1990). Age and work satisfaction. *Hum Relations, 43*, 419-438.

Chapter 24

TERRY FULMER
MEREDITH WALLACE
CAROLE LIUM EDELMAN

Older Adult

objectives

After completing this chapter, the nurse will be able to:

- Identify normal aging changes in the older adult.
- Evaluate morbidity data according to age, gender, and race.
- Discuss nutritional factors that affect the health promotion of the older adult.
- Analyze environmental factors that have an effect on older adults.
- Recognize risk factors that occur with activities of daily living in later adulthood.
- Enumerate the five most prevalent conditions and the five leading causes of mortality among older people.
- Discuss environmental, biological, physical, and mechanical agents that contribute to disability, morbidity, and mortality in later adulthood.
- Analyze political and social issues that influence the well being of the older adult.
- List the leading causes of injury among older adults and suggest preventive measures.
- Identify major resources that are available for health teaching for the older adult.

key terms

Alzheimer's Disease
Cogiation
Cognition
Constipation
Decubitus Ulcer
Dementia
Depression
Falls
Euthanasia or Physician-Assisted Suicide
Mini-Mental Status Examination
Multiinfarct Dementia
Osteoporosis
Overflow Incontinence
Stress Incontinence
Sundown Syndrome
Urge Incontinence
Urinary Incontinence

THINK About It

Older Adult Smokers

You are the director of a senior center in which 10 of your 40 members smoke. The smoking individuals currently experience many health problems. One older woman has chronic obstructive pulmonary disease (COPD) and avoids using her oxygen because she is not supposed to smoke while the oxygen tank is in the room. One older gentleman has high blood pressure; another one of the smokers has been diagnosed with lung cancer. As director of the center, you realize that these older adults should stop smoking, and you have referred them to their physicians to obtain assistance with smoking cessation. However, each of the participants, all of whom are Medicare recipients, receive their Medicare-entitled care through a health maintenance organization that offers no smoking-cessation programs and no payment for nicotine-replacement therapy. All of the older adults are on limited incomes and cannot afford to pay the charge of either a behavioral management class or nicotine-replacement therapy. Although your primary concern is for the health of the individuals who are smoking, you are also concerned about the effects of second-hand smoke on the other members of the senior center.

1. What types of resources are available to help you obtain the necessary assistance for these smokers?
2. What policy changes might be instituted within the senior center to prevent second-hand smoke from harming the older adults in the center's care?

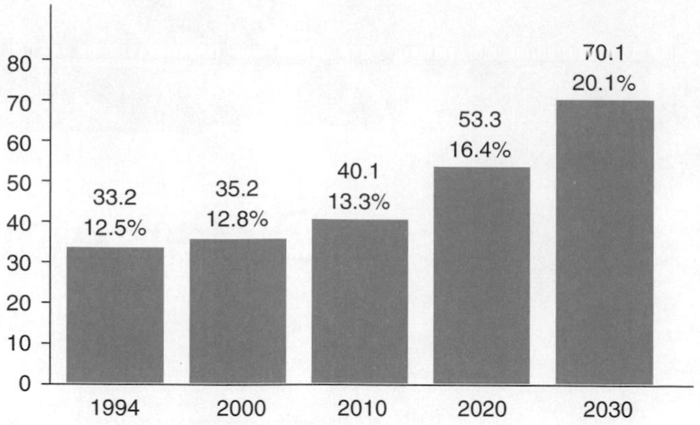

Fig. 24-1 Projected numbers of people in millions who are age 65 and older in the United States. These numbers are based on medium growth assumptions for fertility, mortality, and immigration. (Data from U.S. Department of Commerce, Bureau of Census. [1999]. *Statistical abstracts of the United States: National data book* [119th ed.]. Washington, DC: U.S. Government Printing Office.)

Box 24-1 Misconceptions About the Need for Health Promotion in the Older Adult

1. Disease is normal and unavoidable.
2. Older adults have no future for which health-promoting activities are relevant.
3. Damage to health resulting from inactivity or poor nutrition is irreversible.

From Kolcabar, K., & Wykle, M. (1994). Health promotion in long-term care facilities. *Geriatric Nursing, 15* (5), 266-269.

As a result of health promotion and technological advances, health care professionals now enjoy the gift of caring for an older population. To be caring for a population of human beings who were virtually nonexistent 100 years ago is truly extraordinary. The current standard of living, nutrition, prevention and treatment of infectious diseases, and progress in medical care have sharply increased the survival rate for people born in the United States. After these individuals reach adulthood, they are likely to survive to old age. In 1990 the number of Americans age 65 and older was approximately 28 million, or 12% of the population. By the year 2030 the percentage is projected to increase to more than 18% of the population. In fact, the fastest growing age group in the country is that of adults age 75 and older. One of the fastest-growing age groups within the older adult population is 85 years and older. According to *Healthy People 2010*, individuals age 65 years can be expected to live an average of 18 more years than they did 100 years ago, for a total of 83 years. Individuals age 75 years can be expected to live an average of 11 more years, for a total of 86 years (U.S. Department of Health and Human Services, 2000) (Fig. 24-1).

During the last few decades, mostly tertiary care has been provided for older adults. Health care providers waited until older adults became sick before providing needed nursing care. Insurance reimbursement and introduction into the health care system has come too late for many of these older individuals, resulting in a high prevalence of illness and limited health-promotion interventions. The misconceptions surrounding the older adult's need for health promotion are stated in Box 24-1. These misconceptions impede the ability of nurses to provide the best possible care for older adults. It is time to overcome these misconceptions and begin to promote the health of older adults rather than waiting until they are sick to affect the highest quality of life possible. Health promotion is as important in later adulthood as it is in childhood. Older adults can derive the same benefits from health-promotional activity as do their younger counterparts; they are not "too old" to stop smoking, start exercising, change their diet, or relinquish other bad health habits. The potential for improvement is great, and nurses have a key role in changing common societal misconceptions about this population and in creating new fields of knowledge surrounding health promotion and older adults.

AGE AND PHYSICAL CHANGES

Although the need to promote the health of the older population is great, numerous challenges are presented in fulfilling this need. As stated, one of the great challenges to health promotion among older adults lies in the misconceptions about the benefits of health promotion for this population. Another challenge in caring for the older population concerns separating the normal changes of aging from pathological processes and illness. Normal aging changes are frequently regarded as inevitable and irreversible, occurring with time. An extraordinary amount of variability exists in the age-related changes that occur in each individual. Exposure to environmental injury, illness, genetics, stress, and many other factors combine to influence the aging process. Most researchers agree that biological changes show growth and development peaking in the thirties, with subsequent linear decline until death. These normal changes must be distinguished from pathological changes to focus health-promotion interventions on behaviors that can and should be changed. For example, older adults experience a decline in their respiratory vital capacity. Therefore when recommending exercise programs to the older adult, the selected program must start gradually, allowing the individual to experience the exercise free from respiratory distress. Weinrich and Boyd (1992) report that teaching older adults can be ineffective when nurses do not adapt the teaching process to accommodate for normal aging changes. Specific normal age-related changes and their relationship to problems typical of older adults are summarized in Table 24-1. These changes will be discussed specifically under each section of the physiological and psychological processes of older adults.

Another challenge to promoting the health of older adults lies in the large prevalence of chronic illness among this population. Although chronic illness is not a normal change of aging, years of environmental assault, poor health behaviors, and stress have placed the older adult at a high risk for developing these illnesses. Generally, health deteriorates with aging through an accumulation of chronic disorders and disabilities. According to the Centers for Disease Control and Prevention (CDC), chronic conditions significantly limit daily activity for 39% of persons over 65 years of age. Although older Americans comprise 13% of the population, they account for nearly 36% of health care costs (CDC, 2001a). Box 24-2 lists the nation's leading causes of death and Table 24-2 lists the number of chronic conditions among older adults. The experience of illness among older adults impairs an individual's capacity and motivation to learn new health-promoting behaviors. This prevalence of illness clearly indicates that the older population has a great need for health promotion. However, this population is also one of the most difficult in which to effect change.

Goals of Health Promotion

The U.S. Department of Health and Human Services (2000) has developed *Healthy People 2010: National Health-Promotion and Disease-Prevention Objectives,* for health-promotion programs for the older population (Box 24-3, p. 715). These goals focus on increasing health-promotion programs and decreasing morbidity and mortality related to various disease states. The leading causes of death for people older than 65 years of age are shown in Box 24-2.

Approximately 13% of the total elderly population belongs to minority groups (Fig. 24-2, p. 716). Some of the common health problems among Blacks include higher incidences of stroke, cancer, diabetes, obesity, and hypertension. Hispanics have higher rates of hypertension, cancer, diabetes, arthritis, and high cholesterol than do their White counterparts. In the Native American population, an increased rate of diabetes and alcoholism is present, leading to accidents and cirrhosis of the liver. Asian Americans–Pacific Islanders battle with a higher incidence of cancer (Keating, 1995).

Theories of Aging

The study of how and why people age has continued over many years and has been the source of a great deal of debate. Despite this attention, the debates among biogerontological, psychogerontological, sociogerontological, and other theories of aging will continue through the next decade (Bengtson, Parrott, & Burgess, 1996). Age has been defined as a change in an organism that begins at conception and progresses through a series of stages until death (Mitchell, Gingrich, & Jones, 1994). Although heredity and genetics were once regarded as a major factor in the length of time that an individual lives, other influences on aging are as important. Today, heredity and genetics are considered as only part of a larger picture influencing the aging process. Mitchell, Gingrich, and Jones (1994) report that aging is influenced by heredity, lifestyle, behavior, nutrition, and education level.

Many different theories have been formulated to describe the phenomenon of aging (Knight, 1995). These theories are physical, physiological, spiritual, and sociological in nature. Each hypothesis has been supported by research (Mitchell, Gingrich, & Jones, 1994). However, no consensus has been reached that describes the entire aging process. Explanations of each of these theories is extremely interesting, but beyond the scope of this book. Some of the theories used to explain aging are listed in Box 24-4 (p. 716).

GORDON'S FUNCTIONAL HEALTH PATTERNS

Health Perception-Health Management Pattern

The most important factor is the older adult's motivation to promote one's own health; all the best nursing in the world cannot make an individual do something believed to be unnecessary. A primary factor in the older adult's motivation to promote personal health is the perception of health and its subsequent management.

In a study by Frenn (1994) that examines the health patterns of 80 adults over the age of 65, three patterns are identified that influence an older adult's perception of

Table 24-1 Basic Changes Accompanying Aging and Their Possible Extrapolation to Illnesses, Symptoms, Signs, and Problems Typical of the Elderly

Organ or System	Basic "Normal" Aging Change	Disease(s) or Problems
Arteries	Increased peripheral resistance; diminished aortic elasticity	Abdominal pulsation, bruits, and aneurysms
	Increased systolic and diastolic blood pressure	Positive correlation between blood pressure and morbidity: unclear if this is cause and effect or simply a correlation related to a third factor; possible protective effect on brain of moderately elevated blood pressure
	Arteriosclerotic and atherosclerotic changes in blood vessels	Occlusion of arteries leading to ischemia
Gastrointestinal tract	Diminished hydrochloric acid secretion (probable)	Association with increased iron deficiency anemia and possible association with gastric carcinoma and/or other absorption difficulties
	Diminished large bowel motility	Diminished frequency of bowel movements
	Diminished hepatic synthesis	Diminished serum albumin
	Decreased sensitivity to thirst	Constipation; dehydration
	Decreased absorption of calcium	Malabsorption; osteoporosis
Renal	Decreased in size of urinary bladder	Incontinence and frequency
	Decrease in size of kidneys and number of glomeruli; diminished renal blood flow, glomerular filtration rate, and tubular function	Drug toxicities when kidney is a major route of excretion; greater tendency toward at least transient, if not permanent, renal insufficiency in the presence of dehydration, diuretics, hypotension, or fever
Genital tract	Enlarged prostate gland	Prostatic obstruction
	Weakening of the pelvic floor	Stress incontinence, cystocele, and urethrocele
	Diminished vaginal and cervical secretions	Pruritus; dyspareunia
	Some, though not total, decrease in sexual function	Fear of impotence; embarrassment at sexual desires
Musculoskeletal system	Decreased synthesis and increased degradation of system bone	Osteoporosis and/or fracture
	Diminished muscle size and strength	Fatigue
Eyes	Decreased accommodation to light; decreased ability to distinguish between various intensities of light	Accidents
	Increased density of lens	Cataracts
	Loss of elasticity of lens	Presbyopia
	Change in aqueous kinetics	Glaucoma
Mouth and teeth	Resorption of gum and bony tissue surrounding teeth and bone of mandible	Loss of teeth and periodontal disease
	Decreased saliva flow	Malnutrition; disturbing symptom of "burning tongue" (glossopyrosis)
	Decreased number of taste buds	Weight loss
Ears	Anatomical change in inner ear and cochlea	Diminished hearing of high-pitched sounds (presbycusis)
Heart	Decreased cardiac muscle and catecholamine level	Diminished cardiac output (50% decrease by age 65); increased congestive heart failure
	Increased calcification of valves	Murmurs from aortic and mitral area and/or endocarditis; valve stenosis and/or insufficiency
	Calcification of the skeleton of the heart	Conduction defects; irritability of the cardiac muscle may result in alterations in rhythm
	Sclerosis of the conduction system	Most cases of complete heart block are of unknown origin

Modified from Libow, L., & Sherman, F. (1981). *The care of geriatric medicine*. St. Louis: Mosby. Prepared with the assistance of Rein Tidenksaar, P. A. C., Jewish Institute for Geriatric Care, New Hyde Park, NY, assistant professor of Allied Health, Health Sciences Center, State University of New York at Stony Brook, Stony Brook, NY; Resnik, N. M. (1997). *Geriatric medicine in current medical diagnosis and treatment*. Norwalk, CT: Lang.

Continued

Table 24-1 Basic Changes Accompanying Aging and Their Possible Extrapolation to Illnesses, Symptoms, Signs, and Problems Typical of the Elderly—cont'd

Organ or System	Basic "Normal" Aging Change	Disease(s) or Problems
Lungs	Decreased elasticity and increased size of alveoli	Changes in lung mechanics, such as decreased vital capacity, maximal voluntary ventilation (MVV), and increased closing volume
	Decreased diffusion and surface area across the alveolar-capillary membrane	Diminished Po_2
	Diminished activity of cilia and decreased cough reflex	Impaired bronchoelimination and increased incidence of pneumonia
Immunological status	Decreased T-cell function Maintenance of secondary immune response (B-cell antibody)	Increased negativity in skin tests such as purified protein derivative; possible relationship to increased prevalence for malignancies
Psychological status	Role changes	Retirement
	Losses	
	Physical	Correlation with increased death rate within year of loss of spouse
	Psychological	Depression
	Social	Loss of significant others, family, and friends
Hormones	Decreased metabolic clearance rate and plasma concentration of aldosterone	Decreased sodium reabsorption
	Decreased estrogen; diminished ovarian function	Postmenopausal decrease of secondary sex characteristics
	Decreased insulin response and peripheral effectiveness	Hyperglycemia
	Increased antidiuretic hormone (ADH) response to hyperosmolarity	Inappropriate ADH with hyponatremia
	Insensitivity of pituitary gland to thyrotropin-releasing hormone in older healthy men	Men less likely to develop hyperthyroidism
Brain	Probable decrease in brain weight and/or number of cells in specific areas	Memory loss and/or senile dementia
	Alteration in sleep patterns; older people tend to dream less and have increased periods of wakefulness	Increased complaints of insomnia
	Increased atherosclerosis of cerebral vessels	Multiinfarct dementia
	Increased activity of monoamine oxidase enzyme	Mental depression
	Decreased reaction time	Decrease in intelligence quotient (IQ) scores when speed of response is a factor; some aspects of IQ (verbal and vocabulary skills) increase in late life
Skin	Decreased response to pain sensation and temperature changes	Accidents
	Decreased response to temperature and vibration; increased pain threshold	Burns
	Decreased subcutaneous fat; loss of fat padding over bony prominences	Decubitus ulcers
	Atrophy of sweat glands	Difficulty in body temperature regulation
	Decreased ability of body to rid itself of heat by evaporation	Heat stroke

health: (1) maintaining relationships, (2) attending to health behaviors, and (3) remaining active. In another analysis by Ruffing-Rahal (1991), three patterns are identified that influence social integration. Research continues to explore what is important to older adults and will assist nurses to determine what is of value to the older individual's health behavior. Determining what motivates each older adult to commit to a healthy lifestyle is a large step in assisting older adults in adopting healthy behaviors.

Ideal health maintenance behaviors include exercise, good nutrition, sexual safety, and appropriate sleep-rest patterns. Health maintenance practices should also include regular health care checkups, which will provide early

Box 24-2 Top 10 Causes of Death in the United States

All cardiovascular diseases
All cancers
Unintentional injuries
Chronic obstructive pulmonary diseases
Pneumonia and influenza
Diabetes mellitus
HIV
Suicide
Homicide
Other

Reprinted from Centers for Disease Control and Prevention. (1998). *Chronic disease and their risk factors: The nation's leading causes of death*. Washington, DC: U.S. Department of Health and Human Services.

Table 24-2 Number of Chronic Conditions by Gender per 1000 Population

Chronic Condition	Men	Women
Arthritis	855.7	1118.0
Heart disease	749.2	612.2
Hearing impairment	745.9	491.1
High blood pressure	646.9	796.2
Orthopedic impairment	313.7	351.7
Cataracts	293.7	399.2

From Adams, P., & Marnao, M. (1995). Current estimates, national center for health statistics. *Vital Health Statistics, 10,* 1930.

detection and treatment for diseases that may occur (Box 24-5, p. 717).

Nutritional-Metabolic Pattern

In a secondary analysis of data from the U.S. Department of Agriculture's "Continuing Survey of Food Intake," a sample of 1113 people age 65 and older were surveyed to determine whether diets met the recommended daily allowance (RDA) and to examine the factors that contributed to dietary adequacy. The results showed that diets were inadequate in 16.7% of the older participants. Nutritional knowledge and the possession of positive attitudes and beliefs contributed to good diets in the older population (Howard, Gates, Ellersieck, & Dowdy, 1998). In a sample of Black adults, aged 74 years and older, Bernard, Anderson, and Forgey (1995) found that 20% of subjects had a relatively low serum albumin level, and 14% had cholesterol levels below 160 mg/dl. Many factors account for the high prevalence of nutritional deficiencies in older adults. Naturally, the normal changes of aging place the older adult at an increased risk for nutritional deficiencies. Keithley (1996) reports that the decline of organ function in the older adult can lead to changes in digestion metabolism and the absorption and elimination of nutrients. Additionally, a decrease in the smell, vision, and taste senses and the high frequency of dental problems makes maintaining adequate daily nutrition difficult for the older adult. Lifelong eating habits, such as a diet high in fat and cholesterol, are other obstacles to maintaining optimal nutrition. This type of diet is a leading cause of coronary artery disease. More recently, the dietary consumption of refined sugars has been implicated as a cause of coronary artery disease.

The environment in which the older adult lives affects the nutritional status. For community-dwelling older adults who live alone, eating foods that are easy to prepare with poor nutritional quality or lack of interest in food is frequently the outcome. A fixed income and inflation can leave the community-dwelling older adult with insufficient money to purchase food. The tendency in this case is to rely on what is considered "fast food." When institutionalized in either a hospital or a long-term care facility, availability of food is not a problem. However, some institutions are slow to respond to health-promotion trends, and the meals served in institutions frequently contain excessive fat, cholesterol, or salt and a lack of fiber. Additionally, the availability of fresh fruit and vegetables is diminished, and the nutritional value of produce is significantly reduced when the food is canned or cooked. Finally, institutional food has the tendency to be unappealing or culturally different to many older adults who are accustomed to preparing and eating their own food.

Anorexia or lack of appetite can accompany diseases that the older person experiences (Dudley-Brown, 1996). Medications or a lack of dentures can also cause the older person to eat less than is usual. Older individuals who are in acute care hospitals or long-term care facilities may experience a lack of appetite as a result of their illness. The hospital stay is a time during which good nutrition is most important to heal internal and external wounds and to restore energy. However, a lack of interest in or energy for eating during these stays places the older adult at a high risk of developing nutritional disorders.

Promoting good nutrition in the older adult helps prevent cancer, obesity, and gastrointestinal disorders. Good nutrition also provides older adults with the energy required to function in all activities of daily life. Good nutrition can be measured in the older adult by ascertaining whether the older adult is meeting the RDAs for caloric intake, established by the National Academy of Sciences and the National Research Council. The RDA identifies 2000 to 2800 calories for men ages 51 to 75 and 1650 to 2450 for men 76 years of age and older. The range for women 51 to 75 years of age is between 1400 and 2200 calories; for women 76 years of age and older, 1200 to 2000 calories are recommended.

The nurse assists the older adult in maintaining the highest possible nutritional level (see Hot Topics box, p. 717). Teaching an older adult about the food needed to maintain an optimal nutritional status is of utmost impor-

Box 24-3 Selected National Health-Promotion and Disease-Prevention Objectives for the Older Adult

1-4: Increase the proportion of persons who have a specific source of ongoing care.
1-9: Reduce hospitalization rates for three ambulatory-care-sensitive conditions (pediatric asthma, uncontrolled diabetes, and immunization-preventable pneumonia and influenza in older adults).
2-9: Reduce the overall number of cases of osteoporosis.
2-10: Reduce the proportion of adults who are hospitalized for vertebral fractures associated with osteoporosis.
3-12: Increase the proportion of adults who receive a colorectal cancer screening examination.
4-1: Reduce the rate of new cases of end-stage renal disease (ESRD).
4-5: Increase the proportion of dialysis patients registered on the waiting list for transplantation.
4-6: Increase the proportion of patients with treated chronic kidney failure who receive a transplant within 3 years of registration on the waiting list.
4-7: Reduce kidney failure from diabetes.
5-1: Increase the proportion of persons with diabetes who receive formal diabetes education.
5-2: Prevent new cases of diabetes.
5-3: Reduce the overall rate of diabetes that is clinically diagnosed.
5-4: Increase the proportion of adults with diabetes whose condition has been diagnosed.
5-5: Reduce the diabetes death rate.
5-6: Reduce diabetes-related deaths among persons with diabetes.
5-7: Reduce deaths from cardiovascular disease in persons with diabetes.
5-10: Reduce the rate of lower extremity amputations in persons with diabetes.
5-12: Increase the proportion of adults with diabetes who have a glycosylated hemoglobin measurement at least once a year.
5-13: Increase the proportion of adults with diabetes who have an annual dilated eye examination.
5-14: Increase the proportion of adults with diabetes who have at least an annual foot examination.
5-15: Increase the proportion of persons with diabetes who have at least an annual dental examination.
5-16: Increase the proportion of adults with diabetes who take aspirin at least 15 times per month.
5-17: Increase the proportion of adults with diabetes who perform self-blood glucose monitoring at least once daily.
6-3: Reduce the proportion of adults with disabilities who report feelings such as sadness, unhappiness, or depression that prevent them from being active.
6-4: Increase the proportion of adults with disabilities who participate in social activities.
6-5: Increase the proportion of adults with disabilities reporting sufficient emotional support.
6-6: Increase the proportion of adults with disabilities who report satisfaction with life.
6-7: Reduce the number of people with disabilities in congregate care facilities, consistent with permanency planning principles.
6-8: Eliminate disparities in employment rates between working-age adults with and without disabilities.
7-12: Increase the proportion of older adults who have participated during the preceding year in at least one organized health-promotion activity.
8-22: Increase the proportion of persons living in pre-1950s housing that have tested for the presence of lead-based paint.
10-1: Reduce infections caused by key food-borne pathogens.
12-6: Reduce hospitalizations of older adults with heart failure as the principal diagnosis.
14-5: Reduce invasive pneumococcal infections.
14-28: Increase hepatitis B vaccine coverage in high-risk groups.
14-29: Increase the proportion of adults who are vaccinated annually against influenza and were ever vaccinated against pneumococcal disease.
15-1: Reduce hospitalization for nonfatal head injuries.
15-15: Reduce deaths caused by motor-vehicle crashes.
15-16: Reduce pedestrian deaths on public roads.
15-25: Reduce residential fire deaths.
15-27: Reduce deaths from falls.
15-28: Reduce hip fractures among older adults.
17-3: (Developmental) Increase the proportion of primary care providers, pharmacists, and other health care professionals who routinely review with their patients aged 65 years and older and patients with chronic illnesses or disabilities all newly prescribed and over-the-counter medicines.
18-14: Increase the number of states, territories, and the District of Columbia with an operational mental health plan that addresses mental health crisis interventions, ongoing screening, and treatment services for elderly persons.
19-1: Increase the proportion of adults who are at a healthy weight.
19-2: Reduce the proportion of adults who are obese.
19-5: Increase the proportion of persons age 2 years and older who consume at least two daily servings of fruit.
19-6: Increase the proportion of persons age 2 years and older who consume at least three daily servings of vegetables, with at least one-third being dark green or deep yellow vegetables.
19-7: Increase the proportion of persons age 2 years and older who consume at least six daily servings of grain products, with at least three being whole grains.
19-8: Increase the proportion of persons age 2 years and older who consume less than 10% of calories from saturated fat.
19-9: Increase the proportion of persons age 2 years and older who consume no more than 30% of calories from fat.
19-11: Increase the proportion of persons age 2 years and older who meet dietary recommendations for calcium.
19-17: Increase the proportion of physician office visits made by patients with a diagnosis of cardiovascular disease, diabetes, or hyperlipidemia that includes counseling or education related to diet and nutrition.

From U.S. Department of Health and Human Services. (2000). *Healthy people 2010: National health promotion and disease prevention objectives*. Washington, DC: U.S. Government Printing Office. Available: http://www.health.gov/healthypeople.

Continued

Box 24-3 Selected National Health-Promotion and Disease-Prevention Objectives for the Older Adult—cont'd

19-18: Increase food security among U.S. households and, in so doing, reduce hunger.
21-4: Reduce the proportion of older adults who have had all their natural teeth extracted.
21-10: Increase the proportion of children and adults who use the oral health care system each year.
22-1: Reduce the proportion of adults who engage in no leisure-time physical activity.
22-2: Increase the proportion of adults who engage regularly, preferably daily, in moderate physical activity for at least 30 minutes per day.
22-3: Increase the proportion of adults who engage in vigorous physical activity that promotes the development and maintenance of cardiorespiratory fitness 3 or more days per week for 20 or more minutes per occasion.
22-4: Increase the proportion of adults who perform physical activities that enhance and maintain muscular strength and endurance.
22-5: Increase the proportion of adults who perform physical activities that enhance and maintain flexibility.
24-1: Reduce asthma deaths.
24-2: Reduce hospitalizations for asthma.
24-3: Reduce hospital emergency department visits for asthma.
24-9: Reduce the proportion of adults whose activity is limited because of chronic lung and breathing problems.
24-10: Reduce deaths from chronic obstructive pulmonary disease (COPD) among adults.
27-10: Reduce the proportion of nonsmokers exposed to environmental tobacco smoke.

From U.S. Department of Health and Human Services. (2000). *Healthy people 2010: National health promotion and disease prevention objectives*. Washington, DC: U.S. Government Printing Office. Available: http://www.health.gov/healthypeople.

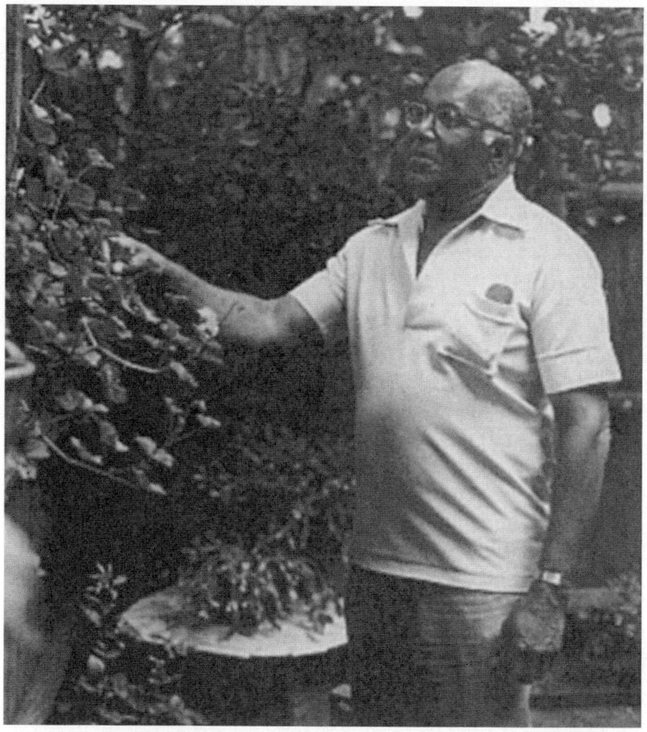

Fig. 24-2 Black adults who are 84 years of age and older tend to outlive White adults in this age group.

Box 24-4 Theories of Aging

- Growth Hormone Secretion Theory
- Waste Product Theory
- Cross-Linkage Theory
- Rate of Living Theory
- Wear and Tear Theory
- Social Theories of Aging
- Gene Regulation Theory
- Somatic Mutation Theory
- DNA Damage Theory
- Free Radical Theory
- Error Theory
- Programmed Cell-Loss Theory
- Neuroendocrine Theory
- Immunological Theory
- Autoimmune Theory

Modified from Mitchell, R. B., Gingrich, D., & Jones, R. L. (1994). The biology of aging. *Journal of the American Academy of Physician Assistants, 7* (3), 210-216; Kyriazis, M. (1994). Age and reason. *Nursing Times*, 90 (18), 61-63.

tance. In the community setting, the nurse assists the older adult in acquiring the transportation to obtain food, apply for food stamps at designated sites, or to eat at senior centers that provide daily meals or have Meals On Wheels. Nurses who work in institutional settings are charged with the difficult task of encouraging good nutrition in residents who frequently do not want to eat. These residents are encouraged to eat the types of food that they enjoy. Encouraging family members to bring in food that the resident enjoys is helpful. A pleasant setting with socialization can also enhance the older adult's desire to eat.

Elimination Pattern

Bowel and bladder functions in the older adult are altered by the normal changes of age. In the older adult, the bladder retains its tonus, but its volume capacity decreases. Large bowel motility also decreases as people age. In addition to some of the normal changes of aging, diet plays

Box 24-5 Recommended Health Screenings for Persons Age 65 and Older

HISTORY (SCREENING):
- Prior symptoms of transient ischemic attacks
- Dietary intake
- Physical activity
- Tobacco, alcohol, and drug use
- Functional status at home

PHYSICAL EXAMINATION (SCREENING):
- Height and weight
- Blood pressure
- Visual acuity
- Hearing and hearing aids
- Clinical breast exam

LABORATORY OR DIAGNOSTIC PROCEDURES (SCREENING):
- Nonfasting total blood cholesterol level
- Dipstick urinalysis
- Mammogram
- Thyroid function tests

DIET AND EXERCISE (COUNSELING):
- Fat, cholesterol, complex carbohydrates, fiber, sodium, and calcium
- Caloric balance
- Exercise program

SUBSTANCE USE (COUNSELING):
- Tobacco cessation
- Alcohol and other drugs
- Limiting consumption
- Driving or other dangerous activities under the influence
- Treatment for abuse

INJURY PREVENTION (COUNSELING):
- Prevention of falls
- Safety belts
- Smoke detectors
- Smoking near bedding or upholstery
- Water heater temperature
- Safety helmets

DENTAL HEALTH:
- Regular dental visits
- Tooth brushing and flossing

OTHER PREVENTIVE MEASURES:
- Glaucoma testing by eye specialist

IMMUNIZATIONS:
- Tetanus-diphtheria booster
- Influenza vaccine
- Pneumococcal vaccine

PROBLEMS FOR WHICH TO REMAIN ALERT:
- Depression symptoms
- Suicide risk factors
- Abnormal bereavement
- Changes in cognitive function
- Medications that increase risk of falls
- Signs of physical abuse or neglect
- Malignant skin lesions
- Peripheral arterial disease
- Tooth decay, gingivitis, loose teeth

Modified from Fisher, M. (1996). *Guide to clinical preventive services* (2nd ed.). Baltimore: Williams & Wilkins.

a significant role in problems with intestinal motility and constipation. Increased incidence of nutritional disorders, particularly decreased intake of fluids and fiber, contributes in large part to elimination problems in older adults. Many medications, frequently taken by older adults, cause elimination concerns. Lack of physical activity and changes in environment that decrease privacy also lead to elimination problems for the older adult. To maintain healthy bowel hygiene, the nurse encourages the older adult to have adequate fluids, roughage, and exercise.

Constipation is a major problem for older adults and has far-reaching effects on their quality of life. By encouraging older adults to exercise and change their fluid and dietary intake, nurses can help reduce their incidence of constipation. Exercise has a rapid and favorable effect on constipation. Dietary modifications, such as the increase of fiber and fluid, can stimulate the colon and resolve constipation (Dudley-Brown, 1996).

HOT topics

HERBAL AND NUTRITIONAL SUPPLEMENT USE IN OLDER ADULTS

The scientific study of herbs is a fairly new area of research in the United States. The first major U.S. study on unconventional therapy use was conducted in 1991. In this study, unconventional therapy was defined as medical intervention not widely taught at medical schools in the United States. In a sample of 1539 people age 18 years and older, 28% of individuals age 50 and older reported using unconventional therapies.

Are you, as the nurse counselor, prepared to include information about the use of herbal and nutritional supplements in your health assessment?

Why do older adults use herbs?

Are the alternatives used more for health promotion reasons or for chronic condition relief?

Adapted from Eisenberg, D. (1998). Unconventional medicine in the U.S. *North Carolina Medical Journal, 3328* (4), 246-252.

Box 24-6 Causes of Urinary Incontinence in Older Adults

DELIRIUM

New onset of urinary incontinence (UI) may be associated with delirium from acute underlying conditions requiring diagnosis and treatment.

RESTRICTED MOBILITY

Acute conditions causing immobility may precipitate UI; environmental manipulation and scheduled toileting are appropriate while rehabilitative efforts are undertaken.

INFECTION

Acute cystitis may precipitate urge UI. Asymptomatic bacteriuria, with or without pyuria, should not be treated in the absence of symptoms of acute UTI.

INFLAMMATION

Atrophic vaginitis and urethritis can cause irritative voiding symptoms, including UI.

IMPACTION

Fecal impaction may be associated with UI and fecal incontinence.

POLYURIA

Poorly controlled diabetes with glucosuria can contribute to urinary frequency and UI.
Excess intake of caffeinated beverages may exacerbate symptoms.
Edema from congestive heart failure and/or venous insufficiency can cause nocturia and exacerbate nocturnal UI.

PHARMACEUTICALS

Rapid-acting diuretics (urge UI)
Psychotropic drugs (sedation, immobility)
Anticholinergics, alpha-antagonists, calcium channel blockers, narcotics (urinary retention)
Alpha-antagonists (stress UI)
Alcohol (sedation, immobility, polyuria)

Adapted from Ouslander, J. G. (June, 2000). Incontinence management in LTC. *Annals of Long-Term Care*, 8 (6), 35-41.

Urinary incontinence affects 12 million Americans (Baum, Appell, & Moss, 1994). The causes of urinary incontinence are summarized in Box 24-6. Incontinence is recognized as a major risk factor associated with the alteration in skin integrity (Adamson, 1996). Despite the high prevalence of the problem, older adults frequently fail to report incontinence to their health care provider (Cohen et al., 1999). Lack of reporting may be a result of embarrassment or acceptance of incontinence as a normal aging change. Accepting incontinence as a manageable problem and seeking appropriate treatment is important for continued health and self-esteem.

Incontinent older adults tend to avoid physical and social activities because of this problem. The nurse implements many interventions in the community, hospital, or long-term care facility that help the older adult restore bladder function. The first intervention is to diagnose the type and cause of incontinence. Baum, Appell, and Moss (1994) report that three different types of incontinence exist. **Stress incontinence** is the most common and occurs during exercise, laughing, coughing, or sneezing. **Urge incontinence** is the inability to delay voiding after the bladder is full. **Overflow incontinence** is caused by an obstruction in the elimination system, such as an enlarged prostate gland or urethral stricture.

After a diagnosis is made, several interventions are available to help alleviate the symptoms of incontinence. The nurse practitioner or physician may prescribe a pessary to help an older woman retain her continence. Kegel exercises may be taught to improve the musculature of the urination system. To perform Kegel or pelvic floor exercises, the first step is to locate the muscle that requires strengthening. The individual is instructed to squeeze around the finger for 10 seconds. Repetitions of 10 cycles of 10 seconds each six times will result in fewer accidents in a period of approximately 2 weeks.

For some individuals, incontinence interventions are ineffective. However, effective ways to manage the incontinence are available. One way is to encourage regular toileting or habit training. This approach is most effective when the older adult can select specific times during the day for urination. After developing a schedule, the individual is instructed to use the toilet 30 minutes before this time each day. This technique may prevent incontinence. Prompted voiding is another method to decrease incontinent episodes. The older adult is reminded or asked about voiding. A more structured bladder-training program allows older individuals to develop a voiding schedule that is progressive by increasing the time between voids and ensuring that adequate fluids are taken from 7:00 AM to 7:00 PM. Postponing voids by using relaxation, imagery, or distraction is essential to the success of this management strategy. However, this type of training is difficult and relies on a good working relationship between the individual and the nurse.

Activity-Exercise Pattern

The benefits of regular exercise in promoting health and preventing disease are widely accepted. The overwhelming evidence of the positive effects of exercise has led the U.S. Department of Health and Human Services to develop within its program, *Healthy People 2010*, national objectives for increasing the numbers of adults who exercise regularly. The American College of Sports Medicine (1995) has made specific recommendations for exercise in the adult population. As life expectancy increases in the

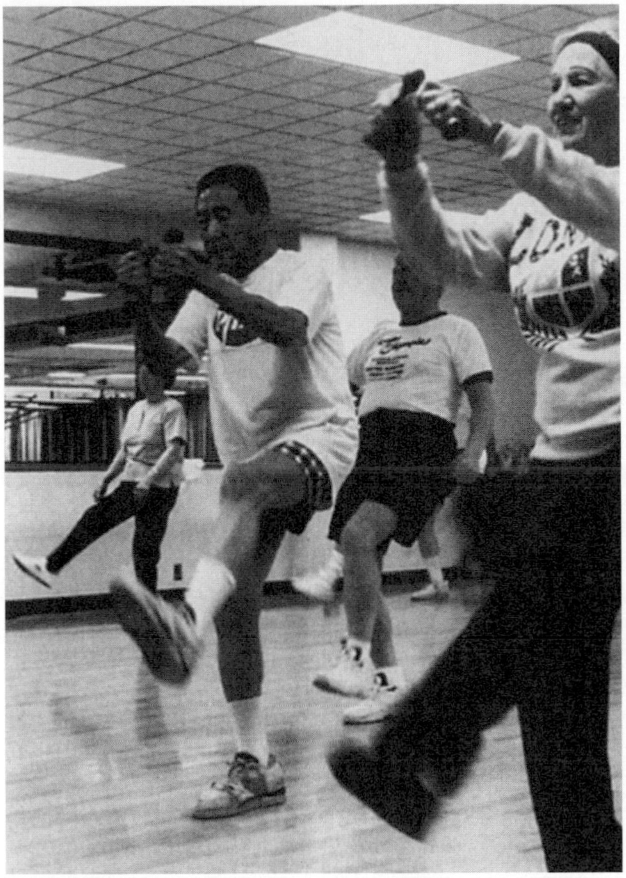

Fig. 24-3 Older adults practice health promotion by participating in an exercise class. (Courtesy Ursula Ruhl, St. Louis. From Lueckenotte, A. G. [1996]. *Gerontologic nursing.* St. Louis: Mosby.)

United States and the population over age 65 grows, exploring ways to maintain functional independence and general health and well being of older adults is especially important.

Investigation of older adults in industrialized countries reveals that the amount of physical exercise performed declines with age (Stephens & Capersen, 1994). However, although exercise tends to decrease in this age group, no physiological or psychological explanation has been found to explain this decline (Dishman, 1994) Normal changes of aging, pathological conditions, and environmental deterrents do not prevent older adults from exercising (Fig. 24-3). Nagler (1992) reports that although 30% of hip mobility is lost by age 40, exercise can improve the range of motion of any older adult. Nagler further notes that joint inflexibility and muscle shortening and weakening are associated more with lifestyle than with aging.

The nurse teaches the interventions necessary to help older adults participate in exercise programs (Dishman, 1994). Teaching the benefit of exercise is the first lesson in motivating the older adult to participate. Individual counseling is the second step, which helps the older person identify exercises that can be enjoyed and continued (Fig. 24-4). The nurse assists the older adult in designing an appropriate exercise program that will maintain strength, flexibility, and balance (Judge, 1993). Walking is broadly reported as the most widely accepted form of exercise among older adults. Siegel, Brackbill, and Heath (1995) found that 35.6% of the individuals who were tested revealed that they were walkers. Walking is an exercise that can occur in both community settings and health care facilities. A study by Lacroix, Leveille, Hecht, Grothaus, and Wagner (1996) indicated that walking more than 4 hours a week was significantly correlated with a decreased risk of hospitalization from cardiovascular disease. Krall and Dawson-Huges (1994) in a study of 239 White, postmenopausal female walkers, found that women who walk 7.5 miles or more per week had increased bone density in the entire body.

Other popular exercises for older adults include weight-bearing and aquatic exercises. Recent research shows that resistance or strength training improves strength and functional mobility for older adults (Fiatarone et al., 1994). Weight-bearing and muscle-building exercises help to maintain functional mobility, promote independence, and prevent falls (Connelly & Vandervoort, 1995, 1996). Weight-bearing exercises are shown to be highly effective in reducing bone wasting common to osteoporosis (Katz & Sherman, 1998). However, weight-bearing exercises may need to be avoided in individuals who have been already diagnosed with osteoporosis.

Older individuals who suffer from arthritis find aquatic exercise a pain-free way of promoting their health and increasing their functional ability. Exercising in the water is also an effective and enjoyable activity for older adults without arthritis (Stamford, 1994).

The effects of exercise on the older adult are extensive. Box 24-7 lists many benefits that the older adult can derive from participating in an exercise program.

Before beginning any exercise program, an older person who has not been exercising should consult a physician or nurse practitioner. After the program begins, activity levels should be increased gradually. Adherence to exercise is a major problem for all populations, including older adults. Dishman (1994) reports that only 50% of people who begin an exercise program will continue the program beyond 3 months. The best tools available to encourage continued exercise among older adults are to communicate the role of exercise in maintaining their quality of life and to help them choose an exercise that they enjoy and that is easily accessible.

Sleep-Rest Pattern

Inability to sleep well is one of the most frequent complaints of older adults. The high prevalence of sleep disorders in this population indicates that older adults are

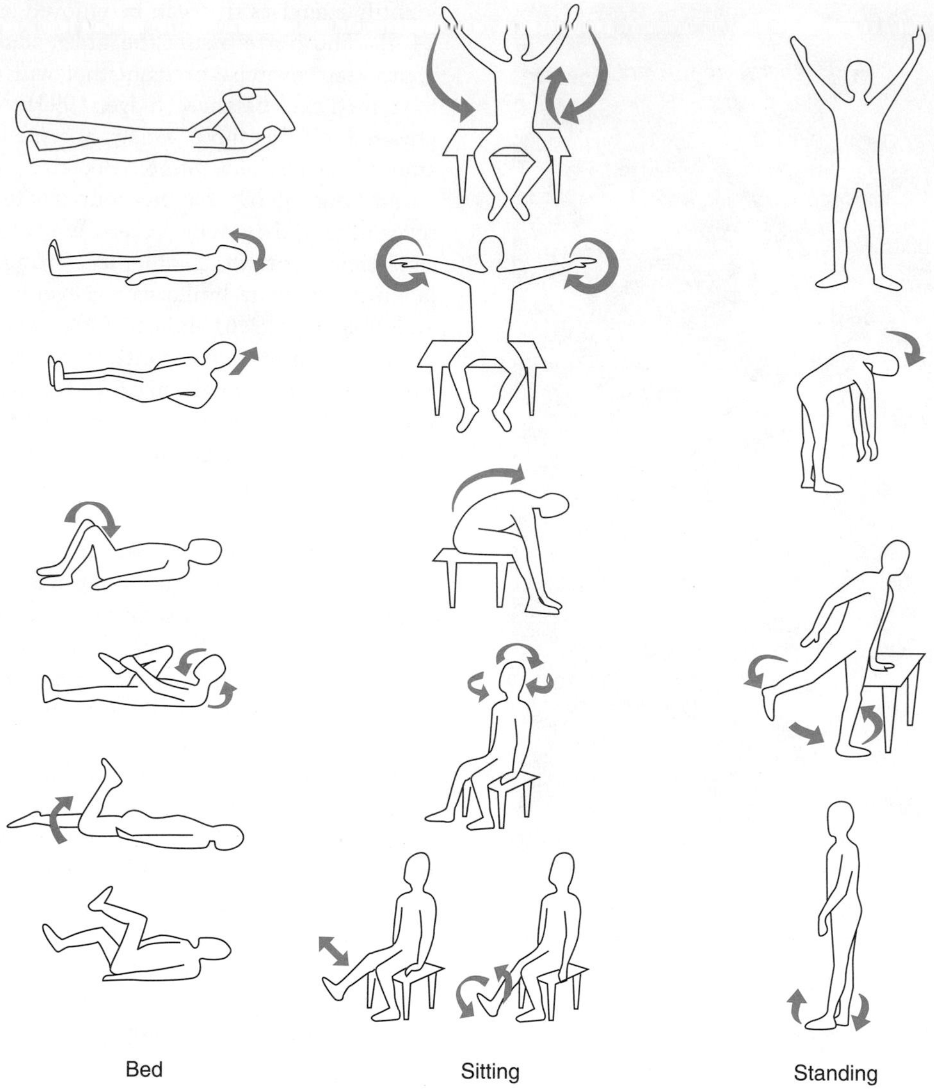

Fig. 24-4 Bed-lying, sitting, and standing exercises. (From Ebersole, P., & Hess, P. [1998]. *Toward healthy aging: Human need and nursing response* [3rd ed.]. St. Louis: Mosby.)

Box 24-7 Benefits of Exercise in the Older Adult

- Better sleep
- Reduced constipation
- Lower cholesterol level
- Lower blood pressure
- Better digestion
- Weight loss
- Socializing opportunities

experiencing a great need for assistance in getting to sleep and staying asleep. In a study by Floyd (1993), 50% of the 42 respondents reported one or more bothersome sleep characteristics. The older adult experiences several normal aging changes (Monk, Buysse, Reynolds, Jarrett, & Kupfer, 1992). Research on sleep in older adults shows a decrease in the total hours of sleep that is required, an increase in nocturnal awakenings and overall sleep efficiency (Floyd, 1993; Bliwise, 1993), shorter periods of sleep (Miceli, 1996), and a decrease in slow wave activity (Bliwise, 1993; Gorbein, 1993).

The benefits of a good night's sleep are numerous. Overall increases in energy, motivation to continue a high quality of life, and improved immune function are only a few of the many rewards of a good night's sleep. One sleep study that used quantitative and qualitative research methods developed four themes to help explain sleep disorders in older adults: (1) physical pain or bodily discomfort, (2) external environment, (3) emotional discomfort, and (4) sleep pattern changes (Floyd, 1993). The effect of aging on changes in sleep patterns are the subject of a great deal of

research highlights

Exercise and Older Adults

Little nursing research is available that describes the effects of exercise in older adults. One study by Dawe and Moore-Orr (1995) examined the effect of a single session of mild exercise on cognitive performance for a group of cognitively intact, institutionalized residents age 70 and over. The data revealed that even mild exercise, such as range-of-motion activities, improved the recall ability of the resident and that the effect remained for at least 30 minutes. The researchers recommend that mild exercise programs are a practical and low-cost nursing intervention that can be used to enhance memory and independence.

Data from Dawe, D., & Moore-Orr, R. (1995). Low-intensity, range-of-motion exercise: Invaluable nursing care for elderly patients. *Journal of Advanced Nursing, 21*, 675-681.

descriptive nursing research. Researchers have associated changes in sleeping patterns with circadian rhythm changes among older individuals (Bliwise, 1993). Minors, Atkinson, Bent, Rabbitt, and Waterhouse (1998) conducted a longitudinal study of 112 noninstitutionalized subjects from 53 to 82 years of age for a period of 10 years. At specified points throughout the study period, subjects recorded in their diary the times of going to bed, awakening, and eating, in addition to whether they lived alone or with another person or persons, during a "typical" week. The researchers assessed the diaries to determine the effects of living alone on the subjects' lifestyle. The results indicated that age was correlated with changes in the sleep-wake cycle and mealtimes and a decrease in lifestyle variability. When the changes were examined between subjects living alone and those living with another person, an increase was found in the amount of time spent in bed and a decrease was revealed in lifestyle variability for adults who were living alone. The researchers concluded that both a deteriorating body clock and an increasingly inflexible lifestyle explain some of the variability in circadian rhythm observed among older adults.

Nurses assist older adults in achieving good sleep habits through sleep assessment that might reveal possible causes of the sleep disturbances. For all older adults, teaching about the normal changes in the aging sleep system can provide reassurance that their sleep patterns have changed, but are not necessarily harmful. Having this information can decrease some of the worry that they have. Increasing physical activity can also help the older adult fall asleep more readily in the evening or night hours. Increased pain medication or alternative pain methods can help older adults who suffer from painful conditions obtain better rest at night. Residents of nursing facilities or persons in acute care facilities may have difficulty adjusting to the environment at night. Adjustments in noise and lighting can help these individuals sleep better. Frequently, emotional disorders can be identified and treated with therapy and medication during the day to help the older adult sleep peacefully at night. Finally, daytime napping has been viewed as inhibiting a good night's sleep for older adults. Floyd (1995) asserts that although this may be the case for some older adults, evidence is inconclusive.

The **sundown syndrome** has been a possible cause of sleep disruption in older adults with dementia, particularly in nursing facilities (Evans, 1986). Burney-Puckett (1996) defines the sundown syndrome as "behavior observed in patients with dementia associated with increased agitation and confusion that occurs in the late afternoon" (p. 40). The cause of sundown syndrome is not well understood. However, pathological changes in the older adult's physical or emotional status or facility schedules at odds with individual sleep-rest patterns may be to blame. Further explanations may include disturbance in rapid eye movement (REM) sleep, episodes of sleep apnea, and a deterioration of the suprachiasmatic nucleus of the hypothalamus (Burney-Puckett, 1996). Behaviors common to sundown syndrome occur generally between 3:00 PM and 7:00 PM and include verbal outburst, wandering, acts of violence, agitation, and resistance to or refusal of care (Wallace, 1994). The goal in managing sundown syndrome is to prevent residents from causing injury to themselves or others. Interventions to lessen the symptoms of sundown syndrome should include the specialized training of staff on the ways to deal with disruptive behaviors (Wallace, 1994) (see Health Teaching box).

Cognitive-Perceptual Pattern

Cognition

Thinking processes (**cognition**) in old age have been the subjects of intensive study over the last few decades. With aging, brain weight decreases, and a shift occurs in the proportion of gray matter to white matter. The ways in which these changes are manifested in individuals varies because of heredity, lifestyle, environmental exposures, and many other factors. Furthermore, no consensus has been reached as to the ways in which these changes translate into human behavior. The common belief is that the majority of older adults will develop dementia at some point in their lifetime. However, **dementia** is an illness of the cognitive system as a person ages and is not currently accepted as a normal change of aging. *The majority of older adults live without cognitive difficulties*. However, Shelkey (2000) reports that 15% of people over age 65 are estimated to have cognitive impairment. Additionally, cognitive alterations are a key symptom indicating changes in physiological function among the aged. Therefore incorporating cognitive assessment as part of the overall assessment of older adults is essential.

HEALTH TEACHING Sleep and the Older Adult

When you believe that you suffer from poor sleep, ask your health care provider about what is considered normal for adults your age. Follow these suggestions to improve your sleep:

- Plan a regular bedtime and wake-up schedule.
- Pursue activities and hobbies.
- Avoid daytime napping; consider any nap you take as part of your sleep total for the day.
- Exercise will help you fall asleep easily, but avoid exercise immediately before bedtime
- Avoid caffeine after 10:00 AM.
- Avoid drinking too much alcohol.
- Avoid some over-the-counter medications, such as cough syrup and allergy medicine.
- Avoid sleeping medications.
- Avoid tobacco products.

To further your getting a good night's sleep, your bedroom should include the following:

- Quiet surroundings
- Darkness
- Coolness and comfort
- A firm and comfortable mattress

Contact your health care provider if you are experiencing any of the following:

- Sleepiness while driving
- Depression, anxiety, or severe personal stress
- Trouble doing your usual daily activities

How will my health care provider find the cause of my sleep problem?

To find the cause of your sleep problem, your health care provider may:

- Ask you many questions about your and your family's health.
- Ask your sleep companion questions about your sleeping habits.
- Ask you to complete a sleep log; in the sleep log, you record whether you were tired during the day, when you fell asleep, how well you slept, and when you woke up.
- Perform tests, which may include a blood test or having you fall asleep in a laboratory so that your sleep can be observed.
- Refer you to a sleep specialist.

What usually causes sleep problems in older adults?

Sleep problems can be caused for different reasons, including certain medications you may be taking; certain medical conditions, such as angina, asthma, or anxiety; poor sleeping habits; and sleep disorders.

Adapted from Sleep and the older adult. (2000). *Nurse Practitioner, 25* (9), 36.

One tool that has been used successfully to measure the mental status of older adults is the **Mini-Mental Status Examination** (MMSE) (Folstein, Folstein, & McHugh, 1975) (Fig. 24-5). This instrument was developed to assess the baseline mental status of older adults accurately and to monitor progress or decline in mental functioning. The MMSE is based on a 30-point scale that measures level of awareness and orientation, appearance and behavior, speech and communication, mood and affect, disturbances in thinking, problems with perceptions, and abstract thinking and judgment. The higher the older adult scores are on the examination, the more intact the mental status is presumed to be. When the scale is 23 or lower, the individual is determined to have a problem with cognition.

The MMSE is relatively easy to perform after a little practice and has been used for initial and subsequent evaluation of older adults in a variety of settings. The most effective way to perform the assessment is to make the person comfortable and establish a rapport. Eliminating noise and promoting attention and concentration will allow individuals to answer questions to the best of their ability. After the examination, the score can be computed and used as a basis for care planning.

Although stereotypes suggest that old people are less capable of learning and lose their intellectual capacity, research has not supported this notion. Although studies indicate that older persons do not show a decrease in intellect (Shelkey, 2000), nurses are recommended to allow older individuals more time to process information. Therefore nurses should encourage older individuals to take classes, read, engage in stimulating conversation and entertainment, and keep their minds active and continue learning throughout their entire lives. Older adults are encouraged to continue with self-care activities rather than to relinquish them to caregivers. Because some memory impairment may be present in cognitively healthy older adults, memory aids and familiar environments should be encouraged (Wallace, 1994) (see Research Highlights box).

Dementia

Dementia is a pathological condition that affects cognition in old age. Two main types of dementia exist. The first type is **multiinfarct dementia**, which is caused by the death of brain tissue, diagnosed through a computerized axial tomography (CAT) scan of the brain. The death of the tissue may be caused by of a lack of blood flow to the brain from a cerebral vascular accident (CVA) or from another cause. The other type of dementia is **Alzheimer's disease** (AD). AD is one of the most devastating diseases of older people, affecting 3 to 4 million people. This number is expected to triple in the next 15 years. Because effective treatment methods are not readily available to date and research is ongoing, the disease accounts for a disproportionate share of this country's total expenditure. Although extensive research has been done on the cause of this disease (Morley & Solomon, 1994), the cause of this plaque

Mini Mental Status Examination Sample Items

Orientation to Time

"What is the date?"

Registration

"Listen carefully,

I am going to say three words.

You say them back after I stop.

Ready? Here they are...

HOUSE (pause), CAR (pause), LAKE (pause).

Now repeat those words back to me."

[Repeat up to 5 times, but score only the first trial.]

Naming

"What is this?"

[Point to a pencil or pen.]

Reading

"Please read this and do what it says."

[Show examinee the words on the stimulus form.]

CLOSE YOUR EYES

Fig. 24-5 Mini Mental State Examination Sample Items. (Reproduced by special permission of the Publisher, Psychological Assessment Resources, Inc., 16204 North Florida Avenue, Lutz, Florida 33549, from the Mini Mental State Examination, by Marshal Folstein and Susan Folstein, Copyright © 1975, 1998 by Mini Mental LLC, Inc. Published 2001 by Psychological Assessment Resources, Inc. Further reproduction is prohibited without permission of PAR, Inc. The MMSE can be purchased from PAR, Inc. by calling [800] 331-8378 or [813] 968-3003.)

formation is remains unknown. The disease cannot be diagnosed by a CAT scan, but rather, only by its symptoms. However, progress is being made in developing a laboratory test for the diagnosis of Alzheimer's disease, which examines spinal fluid for the presence of an amyloid beta-protein precursor (Morley & Solomon, 1994).

The symptoms of dementia include forgetfulness, inattentiveness, disorganized thinking, altered levels of consciousness, perceptual disturbances, sleep-wake disorders, psychomotor disturbances, and disorientation. Nurses who work with older adults are developing interventions to increase the quality of life for those who suffer from dementia. The Harvard Medical School (1996) states that caring for the Alzheimer's patient is difficult for the caregiver. The school suggests some techniques for managing these individuals, such as developing and keeping routines; working in a calm, gentle, and unhurried manner; encouraging self-care activity; and reducing sensory overload. Interventions to keep the older adult safe include curtailing wandering behavior and preventing falls, cuts, and bruises. Current research is being conducted on the effect of certain medications on cognitive processes.

research highlights

The ability of older adults to estimate their own memory, frequently referred to as "meta memory," has been evaluated. A sample of 5444 randomly selected, community-dwelling people over age 70 were asked whether they believed their memory was excellent, very good, fair, or poor. These residents were then administered a cognitive assessment derived from the Mini-Mental Status Examination. The older persons' assessment of their memory corresponded with their actual performance on cognitive measures. Persons who reported depressive symptoms and who had impairment in activities of daily living were more likely to state that their memory was impaired, although they performed well on cognitive measures.

Adapted from Turvey, C. L., Schiltz, S., Arndt, S., Wallace, R. B., & Herzog, R. (2000). Memory complaint in a community sample aged 70 and older. *Journal of the American Geriatrics Society, 48* (11), 1435-1441.

CASE STUDY

Larry Johnson

Larry Johnson, a 75-year-old healthy man, lives in his own apartment and is completely independent in ADLs and IADLs. Last Friday morning, Larry left his apartment complex at 8:09 AM to go to the store. While backing out of his driveway, he failed see a school bus passing on the intersecting street and his car struck the bus. Although no one was injured, this incident that Larry reports to his primary nurse indicated the need for a follow-up sensory and neurological assessment. The assessment revealed both hearing and visual deficits.

However, because of the inability to evaluate the effects of these medications directly on the brain, behavior-related outcomes remain inconclusive. Antidepressant medications have frequently been shown to enhance the functioning of Alzheimer's patients. Antianxiety and antipsychotic medications are also used to help reduce unsafe and disruptive behaviors in demented older adults, but only when all other medications are discontinued because of their negative side effects. (Harvard Medical School, 1996). Support groups, usually listed in telephone directories, can provide important peer understanding for families and victims.

Sensory Factors

Older adults experience several age-related changes in the five senses. Because of the normal and pathological changes associated with the older adult's senses, nursing interventions for individuals in all settings are needed. Because of a variety of structural changes, overall visual acuity decreases, color discrimination becomes less acute, pupil size and constriction ability decrease, and peripheral vision diminishes. The lens of the eye becomes yellow and predisposes older adults to the development of cataracts. The older adult is also at an increased risk for developing glaucoma (a group of eye disorders characterized by increased intraocular pressure). Because of the normal changes in the aging eye and the high risk for disease, older adults should have a baseline eye assessment early in this stage of life. Based on the normal changes and any disease processes assessed, follow-up eye appointments should be scheduled at least annually. Safety, particularly while driving, is a concern for society. Nurses should encourage older adults to take driving classes that will help them deal with the diminishment of certain senses and learn how to become a safer driver as these changes occur.

Hearing deficits are also common in old age, resulting from inner ear atrophy or sclerosis of the tympanic membrane. The inner ear can also undergo a number of changes, including those that are cell degenerative and nerve related. Sound threshold changes, with an associated difficulty in understanding what others are saying. Similar to the changes of the eye, changes in hearing and high risk for pathogenicity indicate that older adults should begin regular ear and hearing screening early in this stage of life. On the recommendation of the audiologist, subsequent hearing testing should be conducted at least annually. The appropriate use of hearing aids can assist older adults with hearing loss in communicating more effectively. The nurse assesses, on an ongoing basis, for the buildup of wax in the older person's ear to ensure good hearing (see Case Study and Care Plan boxes).

Taste changes with aging because of a loss of taste bud receptors. The flavors of sweet, sour, salty, and bitter become blurred with this bud loss (Ebersole & Hess, 1998). The sensations brought about by touch may also diminish with sensory nerve losses, especially in the presence of debilitating diseases such as diabetes, stroke, or Parkinson's disease. The ability to smell and the acuity of the olfactory nerve also decrease with age. Because of the loss of smell and taste sensations, older adults have the tendency to use unsafe amounts of salt and sugar in their food. Teaching about safe cooking and seasoning of food may be appropriate. Additionally, cognitive relations to common danger signals such as smoke or rotten food are impaired. Older adults should be taught to check the dates on their food packages frequently and be attentive when cooking and preparing meals.

The loss of taste and smell sensations, combined with the many other problems of an older adult in obtaining appropriate nutrition, makes dental care of vital importance to this population. Lack of preventive dentistry and nonfluoridated water during the developmental years have caused tooth and gum problems to prevail in the older population. Tooth loss among adults is a common contributor to decreased taste sensation. In fact, *Healthy People 2010* has established goal 21-4 to decrease the number of older adults who have had all their natural teeth extracted (U.S. Department of Health and Human Services, 2000). The inability to chew and swallow food in a comfortable manner works synergistically with decreased smell and taste sensations and other problems to inhibit

CARE PLAN

Nursing Diagnosis: Risk for Injury Related to Unsafe Driving

PLANNING

Larry will have no further automobile accidents.

IMPLEMENTATION

1. Assist Larry in registering for a renewal driving program.
2. Assist Larry in finding alternate modes of transportation until visual and hearing alterations are corrected and when driving in the evening.
3. Schedule hearing and vision appointments for Larry and assist in transportation to appointments.

EVALUATION

Larry remains accident-free.

Nursing Diagnosis: Alteration in Hearing Related to Presbycusis

PLANNING

Larry will be assessed and fitted for a hearing aide to wear when driving.

IMPLEMENTATION

1. Schedule hearing appointments for Larry and assist in transportation to appointments.
2. Reinforce the use of a hearing aide for Larry and provide follow-up teaching as needed.
3. Larry appropriately wears hearing aide while driving.

Nursing Diagnosis: Alteration in Vision Related to Decrease in Accommodation and Peripheral Fields

PLANNING

Larry will understand visual losses and will refrain from driving at night and in poor weather.

EVALUATION

Larry will understand effects of aging on vision and does not drive when conditions are unfavorable.

proper nutrition in the older adult. The American Dental Association recommends that adults be seen for oral hygiene and counseling at least twice a year (American Nurses' Association, 1994a). During the initial evaluation, follow-up visits should be scheduled to ensure that teeth and gums remain in good condition to chew food or that appropriate dental devices are being used.

Skin changes occur over time, becoming thinner, wrinkled, and more fragile. Although sweating decreases and injuries take longer to heal, the skin remains capable of sensing and carrying out its protective role. However, the presence of chronic disease can place an individual at risk for a decreased sense of feeling throughout the body. CVAs or neuropathies resulting from diabetes are two examples of diseases in older adults that disrupt the ability to feel pain and pressure through the skin. Resulting from the lack of sensation in the skin, the safety of older adults can be at risk. When older adults are homebound, information about cooking on a hot stove and bathing and showering should be provided to prevent these adults from burning themselves. The nurse should also perform frequent skin assessments to detect alterations in skin integrity at an early stage.

The potential for skin impairment is common for older adults who suffer sensory deprivation from physical disease or dementia. A pressure sore (**decubitus ulcer**) is a localized area of tissue necrosis that develops when soft tissue is compressed between two bony prominences or between a bony prominence and an external surface for a prolonged period. In addition to prolonged pressure on the skin, friction, moisture, shearing, and lack of nutrition place the older adult at risk of developing a decubitus ulcer, which is difficult to treat after it has developed. Preventing the ulcer is the best method for maintaining the intactness of the skin. People at risk for decubitus ulcers should shift their position at least every 2 hours to distribute pressure appropriately throughout all areas of the skin. Elevating the lower extremities and maintaining proper body alignment are imperative to prevent decubitus ulcers. Specialty beds are readily available in most care settings to decrease pressure and assist in positioning individuals at risk. Positioning pillows and other orthopedic devices provide ways to help maintain the proper support of body parts and body alignment. Proper nutrition, including zinc and vitamins C and E, will help prevent this skin disease.

Self-Perception–Self-Concept Pattern

The variability of self-concept in the older adult is similar to the variability that is seen in the general population. Similar to all aspects of health, the environment, the family, health and lifestyle factors, and heredity combine to form self-concept. Self-concept includes individual's attitudes, perception of abilities (cognitive, affective, or physical), body image, identity, general sense of worth, and general emotional pattern (Harper, 1995). Personality traits in individuals tend to remain constant throughout life.

Erikson's Theory

The prevailing belief holds that adults no longer grow either emotionally or physically in their later years. Although the rate of physical decline exceeds the rate of physical growth in the older adult, no evidence exists that emotional growth declines in any way. In fact, Erikson's theory of development (1982) asserts that older adults must pass through developmental stages as do infants, children, and younger adults. As in all stages of psychosocial development, unsuccessful passage through a stage yields psychological illness, and successful passage through the stage promotes health (Erikson, 1982).

Ego integrity versus despair and disgust is the developmental stage of older adults (Erikson, 1982). The quality associated with successful passage of this stage is integrity, defined as an honest acceptance of the life that has passed and the stage of life that is currently being lived. Individuals who have reached this stage are said to be at peace with themselves. The inability to reach this stage leads to fear of death and despair that life has been lived in vain (Erikson, 1982). Based on the expanding lifespan, this stage of development was expanded into three additional stages: (1) ego differentiation versus work role preoccupation, which involves achieving identity apart from work; (2) body transcendence versus body preoccupation, which focuses on adjusting to normal and aging changes; and (3) ego transcendence versus ego preoccupation, which involves accepting death.

Nurses working in all settings are charged with helping older adults successfully pass through Erikson's psychosocial stages, enabling them to reach ego integrity. One successful method of assistance for older adults at all cognitive levels is reminiscence (Nugent, 1995). Reminiscence is defined as "thinking about or relating past experiences, especially those personally significant" (McMahon & Rhudick, 1961, p. 292). Asking older adults about their memories of certain smells or photographs is one way to stimulate reminiscence. Butler (1963) recommends the following suggestions for stimulating reminiscence: writing about or tape recording memories of past events, developing a family tree, and encouraging the older adult to write to old friends (Soltys & Coats, 1994).

Cogiation

Nystrom (1995) developed a term known as **cogiation** to describe the experience of healthy withdrawal by residents of long-term care facilities. Studies have shown that residents who are recognized as possessing integrity by the nursing staff frequently withdraw from the daily activity of the long-term care facility to sit alone and consider how they and other people behaved, think about alternatives for life, and evaluate situations. This process might involve present or past events. Promoting cogiation among older adults can also be an effective method to promote ego integrity in this population (Nystrom, 1995).

Roles-Relationships Pattern

Although the general framework of self-perception remains constant throughout the lifespan, the source of an individual's self-perception often changes with older adulthood. The formation of the self that has focused on a person's role in the family changes when the children become independent or a spouse passes away. Roles such as daughter, son, sister, brother, wife, or husband may be lost because of death or illness. The loss of these roles can bring a great deal of sadness and possible depression to the older adult. However, with the loss of these roles, a new role, such as grandparenting, frequently evolves (Fig. 24-6). Furthermore, during the last decade, a sharp rise in the number of grandparents raising grandchildren has occurred, from 4.9% in 1992 to 5.5% in 1997 (U.S. Department of Commerce, 1999). The role of grandparent frequently brings great joy and happiness at a time when the older adult feels loss. However, grandparents who rear grandchildren raises several issues. Research conducted to date suggests that grandparents who rear grandchildren are at increased risk for poor health and increased psychological distress (Kelly, 2000). Encouraging and supporting older adults in this role is necessary to help them fill the void left by the loss of their parental, job, or spousal roles and to prevent the stress and strain of this caregiver role (see Multicultural Awareness box).

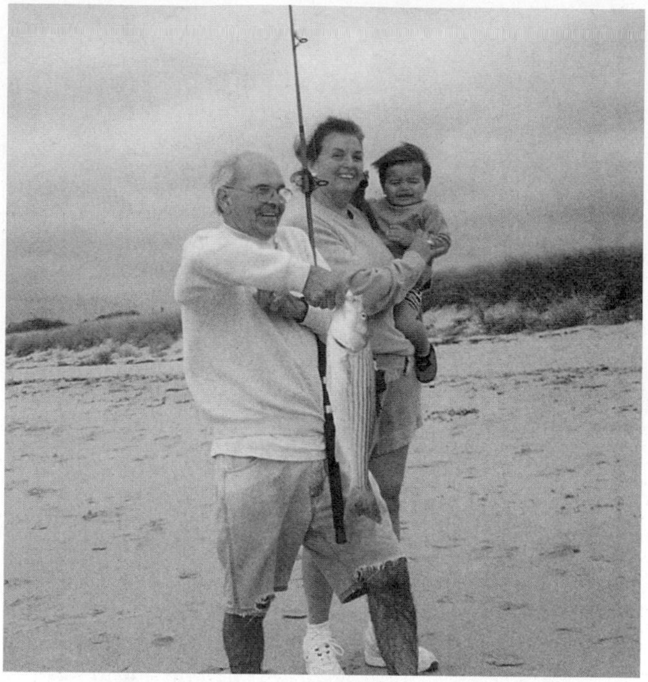

Fig. 24-6 Passing on traditions and skills by spending time with grandchildren fulfills a developmental task for older adults.

With the average lifespan increasing, older adults can spend a mean of 30 years in retirement. An estimated 27.2 million retirees were reported in December 1997, based on the number of people receiving retired-worker benefits (The Social Security Administration, 1998). Rosenkoetter (2000) offers several theories to help understand retirement. For people who view retirement in a positive light, it is a time that is peaceful and less stressful than the work years were for healthy individuals. For individuals who have an adequate amount of money, retirement can be a time for travel, golf, painting lessons, or other favorite hobbies and leisure activities for which time was previously unavailable. For other older adults, retirement can be a long void at the end of life that is full of ill health and financial difficulty. Further assaults on the individual's

MULTICULTURAL AWARENESS

How Different Cultures Care for Older Adults

How fortunate is today's society to enjoy the variety of many cultures? Individuals and families who immigrated to the United States in the early 1900s are now spending their later years as citizens of the United States. However, although many older adults have lived in the United States for many years, remembering the countries from where they came is of great importance. An understanding of the individual cultural backgrounds of older adults allows nurses to provide care that is respectful of the whole individual.

Schmall (1996) indicates that five major cultural groups in the United States have developed differing attitudes toward older adults. The majority White Anglo-Saxon Protestant culture shows less respect for older adults and their role in the family than do other cultures. Older men and women tend to share in the family structure more equally. Parents are expected to live away from their children and not be overly dependent on their adult children. Although this view represents the mainstream American culture, other distinct and important cultures within the United States should be recognized and respected.

The Black culture generally has a greater respect for older adults and their family role compared with White cultures. Black people also place a value on kinship and the extended family that is no longer present in White cultures. East Asians have a especially high level of respect for older adults: the older an individual is, the more respect that individual is given. Additionally, the oldest son in East Asian cultures assumes responsibility for the care of the aging parents. Hispanic cultures give more overt respect to older adults than do White cultures. In many families, aging parents live in households that consist of numerous extended family members. Finally, Native-American cultures have a high level of respect for older adults because of their years of accumulated wisdom and knowledge, and they are frequently sought out for their advice.

Acknowledgment of the different cultures in the United States provides the nurse with a broader understanding of the psychosocial mechanics underlying an individual's illness. Understanding the older adult's role within the family gives the nurse the information that is needed to develop an appropriate plan of care. Caring for older adults within their culture requires that the nurse understand that many of them will be well cared for by family members and others do not expect or value care from family members. Additionally, the role that older adults are expected to fulfill within their culture, such as grandparent, as primary caregiver, or family decision maker, must be considered when nurses are attempting to understand the value of health and illness to the older adult. Although nurses generally believe that the health of the individual should come first, an understanding of the culture can help a nurse understand that, for example, an aging Hispanic grandfather prefers to be home when his grandchildren return from school rather than at the clinic receiving dialysis treatments in the afternoon.

Data from Schmall, V. L. (1996). Family influences. In A. G. Lueckenotte, *Geronotologic nursing* (pp. 136 166). St. Louis: Mosby.

self-concept may include a lowered income, loss of friends, disease, and disability. Volunteering can be an effective method for these older adults to continue to feel engaged in the working environment as a productive contributing member of society. Older adults who volunteer have an external incentive for getting dressed in the morning; they take a great amount of pride in their work. Filling a volunteer position can remedy negative feelings about retirement and other role changes.

Federal and state funding has created a number of subsidized work programs for older adults. With the assistance of this funding through private agencies and the Area Agencies on Aging, older adults are given the opportunity to work for pay. Although the pay may not be comparable to what the older adult earned before retirement, the earnings can be a necessary supplement, after the age of 70, to Social Security benefits. These programs allow older adults to work with children in day care centers, disabled and ill older adults at home, and in administrative positions. Nurses should provide interested individuals with information on these programs.

Leaving home, widowhood, retirement, and relocation can illicit profound feelings of loss. Older adults who remain engaged in a variety of activities and relationships are happier and healthier. Personality, and its expression over time, is considered as a major determinant of how engaged or active a person will be late in life. Other variables such as health, bereavement, and habit affect activity as well.

Health-promotion activities center on an understanding of the individual's usual behavior and any unexpected or unexplained deviation in that behavior. Nurses help the older adult identify the meaning of their lost roles and the subsequent loss to work through any reaction to the loss. In the more traumatic cases, support groups, such as bereavement groups, can be helpful. The nurse supports older adults going through role changes by eliciting reactions and facilitating communication about these reactions. Significant others, such as children, neighbors, and friends, can provide important support in an ongoing way. The nurse is integral in helping older adults develop and explore their new role as grandparents.

Sexuality-Reproductive Pattern

A great deal of debate has taken place over the presence or absence of sexual desire among older adults. Society generally believes that older adults do not participate in sexual relationships. Kain, Reilly, and Shultz (1990) report that society's views about sex among older individuals is usually negative and that these views inhibit the expression of sexuality among the aging. The myths regarding sexual activity among older adults include the following (Wallace, 2000):

- Older adults are no longer interested in sex.
- Medical illnesses common to older adults prevent them from having sex.
- Impotence is a normal aging change.

The most accurate predictor of sexual interest in older adulthood is the enjoyment and frequency of sex at a younger age. No data are available that show that men or women lose interest in, or the ability toward, sexual activity as they age. The frequency of sexual activity has been positively related to competence in married men and women over 60 years of age (Marsiglio & Donnelly, 1991). *The Janus Report on Sexual Behavior* found that on a weekly basis, sexual activity for both men and women continues past middle age. (Janus & Janus, 1993). Current research supports that sexual interest among older adults exists and is active. Older adults must also fulfill the human need to touch and be touched (Fig. 24-7). Touch is an overt expression of closeness and an integral part of sexuality. Although the need to express sexuality continues, older adults are susceptible to many disabling medical conditions, such as cardiac problems, arthritis, and normal aging changes, and these can make the expression of sexuality difficult. In both genders, reduced availability of sex hormones results in less rapid and less extreme vascular responses to sexual arousal. The lack of circulating hormones in both men and women results in changes in four areas of the sexual system: arousal, orgasm, postorgasm, and extragenital changes. Additionally, the treatments for a medical condition can actually hinder sexual response.

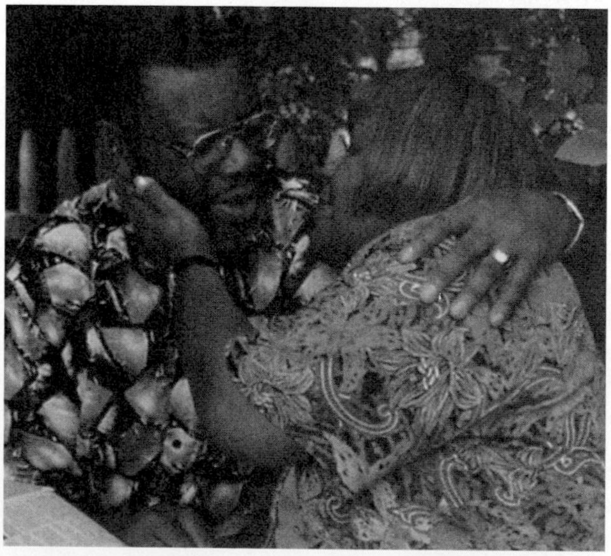

Fig. 24-7 Sexual feelings, such as the need for companionship, touch, and intimate communication, continue in older adults. (From Ebersole, P., & Hess, P. [1998]. *Toward healthy aging: Human need and nursing response* [3rd ed.]. St. Louis: Mosby.)

Nurses are in an ideal position to help older adults fulfill their sexual desires by enabling them to compensate for normal aging changes and disabling medical conditions and medications. After making a sexual assessment, nurses can intervene at an early point to prevent or correct sexual problems. However, nurses frequently choose not to consider older adult sexuality when planning care. One of the reasons for this refusal is that nurses believe the societal myths about older adults' sexuality. A nurse's basic discomfort with sexuality issues may actually distort perceptions of the needs of older adults (Drench & Losee, 1996). Hillman and Stricker (1994) report that nurses fail to intervene and facilitate the expression of sexuality among older adults because nurses lack the knowledge and training to do so. Without proper training and experience, nurses are not sufficiently confident to venture into this delicate area.

The expression of sexuality among older adults results in a higher quality of life achieved through fulfilling a natural desire. Butler and Lewis (1993) suggest that sexual orgasm relieves anxiety and contributes to the general well being of older adults. In long-term care facilities, the need to address the sexual needs of older adults is great because of the frequent experience of disabilities in these residences. In the community setting, nurses have access to the entire family unit in their natural surroundings. The information that is necessary to make a sexual assessment is readily accessible.

Many nurses believe that acquired immunodeficiency syndrome (AIDS) and other sexually transmitted diseases are not problems for older adults. However, this notion is no longer the case. The number of older adults with the human immunodeficiency virus (HIV) has risen sharply over the last decade. Older adults should use proper precautions, such as a barrier method, to prevent the spread of disease from one person to another. Nurses use universal precautions to protect themselves from HIV and other blood-borne pathogens. Older adults should follow the safer sex guidelines recommended by the CDC.

Coping–Stress-Tolerance Pattern

An individual's ability to cope with the common stresses of older adulthood is a key factor in maintaining self-concept and subsequent integrity. The nurse who cares for the older adult can be extremely helpful in the coping process. Moos and Billings (1986) have identified three ways in which older individuals can cope with stress: (1) appraisal-focused coping, which concerns defining the meaning of the situation; (2) problem-focused coping, which focuses on dealing with the reality of the situation by modifying the source of the threat, handling the consequences of the problem, or changing oneself; and (3) emotion-focused coping, which is aimed at managing emotions aroused by an event. After assessing the most appropriate way in which the individual desires to cope with a situation, the nurse helps create an appropriate environment for coping.

Depression

The rate of **depression,** symptoms of sadness, decreased ability to experience pleasure, pessimism, inhibition, retardation of action, and physical complaints (Wykle & Zauszniewski, 2000), rises sharply with age. According to *Healthy People 2010* (U.S. Department of Health and Human Services, 2000), adults and older adults have the highest rates of depression. Depression rates are especially high among older adults with coexisting medical conditions. Research further reports that 12% of older persons hospitalized for problems such as hip fracture or heart disease are diagnosed with depression. Rates of depression for older people in nursing homes range from 15% to 25%. The cause of this increase is not completely understood. The numerous losses experienced by older adults may be partly to blame for the onset of depression in this population. Depression is also caused by physiological changes in the aging body. As a manifestation of an individual's self-concept, depression has been the subject of detailed study. Although the illness appears to affect older adults in much the same way as it affects younger individuals, certain patterns of symptoms and older adult's overall susceptibility is different from those of younger counterparts.

Nurses are integral in helping to diagnose and treat depression in older adults. Depression can be found in all environments of care. Some of the behaviors common to depression include sullen affect, lack of appetite and weight loss, sleeplessness, fatigue, decreased ability to think or concentrate, psychomotor agitation, decreased participation in daily living activities and social activities, and suicidal ideation. Many instruments are available to assist nurses in assessing for this commonly occurring disorder among older adults. The Geriatric Depression Scale (Yesavage et al., 1983) is available in both a 15- and a 30-question format and is an easily administered instrument to screen for depression in older adults (Fig. 24-8). After the depression is diagnosed, successful treatment may include antidepressant medications and psychosocial therapy.

Suicide

According to the CDC and unpublished mortality data from the National Center for Health Statistics (CDC, 2001b), suicide rates increase with age and are highest among Americans age 65 years and older. Men accounted for 83% of suicides among persons age 65 years and older in 1997. From 1980 to 1997, the largest relative increases in suicide rates occurred among people 80 to 84 years of age. The rate for men in this age group increased 8% (from 43.5 to 47.0 per 100,000). Firearms were the most common method of suicide by both men and women age 65 years and older in 1997, accounting for 77.1% of male and 32.7% female suicides in this age group (CDC, 2001b). The reason for the high number of suicides in the older adult population continues to be explored. The elevated rate of depression helps the medical community understand the motive of many older adults. Many older adults have serious medical illnesses that provide an explanation for wanting to die. Risk factors for suicide include social isolation, alcohol abuse, psychosis, bereavement, serious medical illness, and depression (Casey, 1991). Grabbe, Demi, Camann, and Potter (1997) found that when other variables were accounted for, persons who had successfully committed suicide were significantly more likely than were those who had died from accidents to have a history of cancer, moderate or heavy alcohol use, and mental or emotional disorders. Older adults may visit a health care provider with a somatic complaint before the suicide attempt as, perhaps, a final call for help. Nurses working with the older population are aware of the high rate of suicide in this population and are alert for the risk factors. Suicide threats are taken seriously and interventions are implemented to keep the older adult safe.

The chronic illness that frequently accompanies old age raises a concern for ethical care for older adults. Many members of society believe that with the increased lifespan of older adults, individuals can be subjected to more suffering. A solution to ending the suffering of older adults with chronic illness has been **euthanasia,** or **physician-assisted suicide** (PAS). Many states are actively lobbying to legalize PAS in their states. The American Nurses' Association (1994b) believes that nurses should refuse to participate in assisted suicide. Nurses are subsequently charged with helping society to understand the many benefits of older adulthood and celebrating the extended lifespan rather than deeming it wasteful. Additionally, nurses caring for chronically ill older adults have the added burden of determining which older adults are at risk for wanting PAS and helping these older adults to live their extended lifespan free of pain and discomfort. Nurses are instrumental in ensuring that the older person experiences a pain-free death by advocating for the appropriate pain-management program and working with other health care professionals toward this end (see Hot Topics box).

Values-Beliefs Pattern

Every older adult for whom nurses have the opportunity to care will have a different sense of spirituality, which will have a profound influence on the person's motivation and ability to live a healthy lifestyle. Zorn and Johnson (1997) explored the role of spirituality among 114 younger, institutionalized rural women and reported a significant positive correlation between "religious well being" and social support and hope. Respondents scored higher on "religious well being" when they reported regular participation in religious activities, highly rated the value or influence of religious beliefs in their lives, and identified that religious beliefs were increasingly important with age.

The individual sense of spirituality is influenced by

Geriatric Depression Scale
– short form –

1. Are you basically happy with your life?	yes	no
2. Have you dropped many activities and interests?	yes	no
3. Do you feel that your life is empty?	yes	no
4. Do you often get bored?	yes	no
5. Are you in good spirits most of the time?	yes	no
6. Are you afraid that something bad is going to happen to you?	yes	no
7. Do you feel happy most of the time?	yes	no
8. Do you often feel hopeless?	yes	no
9. Do you prefer to stay home rather than go out and do new things?	yes	no
10. Do you feel you have more problems with memory than most people?	yes	no
11. Do you think it is wonderful to be alive now?	yes	no
12. Do you feel worthless the way you are now?	yes	no
13. Do you feel full of energy?	yes	no
14. Do you feel that your situation is hopeless?	yes	no
15. Do you think most people are better off than you are?	yes	no
Score:		

Score 1 for answer in shaded box.
0 to 5: not depressed
6 to 15: depressed

Fig. 24-8 Yesavage Geriatric Depression Scale: Short Form. (From Yesavage, J. A., Brink, T., Rose, T., Lum, O., Huang, V., Adey, M., & Leirer, V. [1983]. Development and validation of a geriatric depression screening scale: A preliminary report. *Journal of Psychiatric Research, 17,* 37-49.)

gender, past experiences, religion, economic status, ethnic background, and other beliefs (Brush, 2000). Although no universal sense of spirituality exists among older adults, many researchers (Morris, 1996; Stolley & Koenig, 1997; Musick, Koenig, Hays, & Cohen, 1998; Koenig, George, & Peterson, 1998) report that spiritual resources are related to mental health in this population.

Nurses who care for older adults may find themselves in a difficult position in attempting to promote the spiritual health of individuals. One reason for this perceived difficulty may be the nurse's discomfort with the older adult's belief system. A study by Forbes (1990) on older adults and their caregivers indicates a high correlation between the spiritual and religious well being of caregivers and older adults. Consequently, when nurses possess spiritual and religious well being, they can share this with older adults. Another reason nurses may not intervene to affect the spiritual well being of individuals is that they lack the knowledge on the best way to do so (Millison, 1995). Coming to terms with their own sense of spirituality for their own well being and for the well being of older adults is important for nurses.

There may be as many different spiritual values and beliefs as there are individuals. Varying spiritual values make helping older adults actualize their spirituality and thus acquire a high quality of life, difficult for nurses. Forbes

HOT topics

PHYSICIAN-ASSISTED SUICIDE

Assessing the Problem

Although a great deal of time has been spent celebrating the medical technology that has succeeded in expanding the lives of older adults, this longevity also causes a number of problems. With a longer lifespan, people may be subjected to more prolonged suffering. One solution to this problem is euthanasia or physician-assisted suicide (PAS). Older adults in the community or in acute-care or long-term care settings are all potential candidates for PAS because of the increased incidence of disability, chronic illness, and terminal disease. PAS may be viewed as the only way to escape pain and suffering for some older adults. In fact, several states are actively lobbying to legalize PAS.

The Nursing Position

The American Nurses' Association (ANA) developed a position statement on assisted suicide: "Nurses, individually and collectively, have an obligation to provide comprehensive and compassionate end-of-life care, which includes the promotion of comfort and the relief of pain, and at times, foregoing life-sustaining treatments. ANA believes that the nurse should not participate in assisted suicide. Such an act is in violation of the Code for Nurses with Interpretive Statements and the ethical traditions of the profession" (American Nurses' Association, 1994b, p. 45).

How Nurses Can Recognize and Intervene to Help Patients at Risk for PAS

Coyle (1992) reports that several factors make people vulnerable to requesting PAS. These factors include poorly relieved pain and other symptoms, advanced illness, depression, loss of self-esteem, delirium, a sense of losing control, fear of abandonment, fatigue and exhaustion (experienced by the individual, family, and health care providers), preexisting psychopathological conditions, and previous suicide attempts. Understanding these factors will help the nurse identify high-risk individuals. After determining that a person is at risk, interventions can be implemented to help older adults make appropriate decisions and live the rest of their lives comfortably. Coyle (1992) recommends that after determining that a person is at risk, a careful medical and psychosocial history can help identify the issues underlying the desire for PAS. A multidisciplinary plan of care can then be developed to help manage the issues, alleviate the factors underlying the desire for PAS, and assure the individual and family that they are not alone in their suffering.

What Do You Think?

1. When nurses believe that ending a person's suffering is necessary, should they participate in PAS?
2. Do you agree with the position of ANA on PAS? If not, then what is your position?

Data from American Nurses' Association. (1994b). *Position statement on assisted suicide.* Washington, DC: The Association; Coyle, N. (1992). The euthanasia and physician-assisted suicide debate: Issues for nursing. *Oncology Nursing Forum, 19* (7), 41-46.

(1990) reports that because of the highly personal quality of spirituality, an unobtrusive and sensitive presence by the nurse is needed to allow the person in any setting to achieve spiritual health. Additionally, spiritual assessment tools are available to guide nurses with the right questions to help get to the root of the person's spirituality. Open-ended questions, such as, "What is the individual's perception of God and spirituality?" can encourage discussions about the person's innermost spirituality with the nurse.

PATHOLOGICAL PROCESS

Accidents

The National Center for Health Statistics annual mortality data tapes for 1987 through 1996 indicate that fall-related deaths for older adults increased sharply with advancing age and were consistently higher among men in all age categories. Men were 22% more likely than women were to sustain fatal **falls.** A trend of increasing rates of fall-related deaths was observed from 1987 through 1996 in the United States, although rates were consistently lower for women throughout this period. Rates of hospitalizations for hip fracture differed by age and were higher for White women than they were for other groups. Rates increased with advancing age for both sexes, but were consistently higher for women in all age categories. Hospitalization rates for hip fracture increased for women from 1988 through 1996 and the rates for men remained stable (Stevens et al., 1999).

Some of the causes of falls in older adults are neuromuscular dysfunction, osteoporosis, stroke, and sensory impairment. Although a fall in a younger individual may not be problematic, a fall in an older adult can have devastating consequences. Because of the higher risk of osteoporosis in the older population, a fall can result in a fracture. **Osteoporosis** is a disease of bone loss common to women age 70 and older and men age 80 and older. The disease occurs six times more frequently in women than it does in men. The rapid decline in estrogen secretion at the onset of menopause signals the calcium in the bones to move into the bloodstream, which allows the bones to become weak and brittle. Because of this bone weakness, falls in older adults with osteoporosis frequently result in fractures, which places these individuals in a spiral of iatrogenesis beginning with weeks of immobilization and possibly resulting in decubitus ulcers, psychological trauma, pneumonia, and even death.

Risk factors for osteoporosis include a small, thin frame; Caucasian or Asian ancestry; family history; excessive thyroid medication or high dose of cortisonelike drugs for asthma, arthritis, or cancer; a diet low in dairy products and other sources of calcium; physical inactivity; smoking

HEALTH TEACHING Preventing Falls in the Older Adult

Injuries from a fall can limit an individual's ability to lead a healthy and happy life. Older individuals are at especially high risk for falls because of normal and pathological changes in their senses and neuromuscular status.

Do You Know?

- Falls are the greatest cause of injury in people over 70 years of age.
- Because of the increased risk of osteoporosis in this population, even minor falls can result in fractures.
- Fractures in older adults can result in immobilization, decubitus ulcers, psychological trauma, pneumonia, and death.

Guidelines for Preventing Falls

Although falls can result in serious injury and even death, an estimated two thirds of falls can be prevented. Nurses in all settings are in an ideal position to help older adults modify their environment to prevent falls.

- Incorporate hearing and vision testing into the older adult's annual physical examination.
- Discuss the side effects of medication with individuals, making them aware of periods during which they may be sedated or dizzy and at an increased risk of falls.
- Instruct the older adult who is on blood pressure medication, is hypotensive, or is experiencing orthostatic hypotension to rise slowly and stand still for a minute before attempting to move.
- Encourage the older adult to limit alcohol consumption.
- Encourage the use of a cane or walker, when necessary.
- Instruct the older adult to wear supportive, rubber-soled, low-heeled shoes.
- Help the older adult make other arrangements to obtain food and other supplies during icy weather to avoid outside falls.
- Encourage a program of regular exercise, particularly weight-bearing exercises, to build new bones.
- Assess the home environment and remove area rugs, electrical cords, and furniture that may contribute to falls.
- Assess bathrooms for grab bars and nonskid mats.
- Suggest the use of night lights or dimmer switches in hallways and bathrooms.

cigarettes; and drinking alcohol. Osteoporosis is typically diagnosed after an older adult sustains a fracture. However, bone density testing is available to diagnose individuals at risk before a fracture. Although estrogen replacement therapy with the synthetic hormone progestin prevents the development of osteoporosis in postmenopausal women, having sufficient calcium in the diet remains vitally important and will continue to reduce the normal bone loss of aging. Most women need 1000 mg a day before menopause and 1500 mg a day after menopause. Consuming this amount of calcium from today's average diet is nearly impossible; therefore a calcium supplement is essential. For the prevention of osteoporosis and the optimal health maintenance of both psychological and physical well being in the older adult, physical activity is necessary.

A program to prevent falls is essential in the care of older adults. Because many factors contribute to falls, assessment of the risk factors for falls is also essential. Recommendations for fall prevention are abundant within the literature. Tinnetti (1997) states that by identifying the risks for falls among the older adult population, falls can be prevented. A great deal has been written about predicting the older adult's risk for falls. By assessing an older adult's vision, hearing, medication usage, blood pressure, mobility, and other factors, falls can be successfully predicted and subsequently prevented. Steps to prevent falls are summarized in the Health Teaching box.

Several fall-risk assessments that identify these factors have been developed. These assessments are easy-to-use instruments that can be employed in acute or long-term care or in home settings to identify older adults at risk for falls. After completing the assessment, scores are obtained that can assist in care planning to prevent the older adult from sustaining a fall. Nurses in all settings will then be prepared to implement environmental, physiological, and psychological interventions to prevent falls.

Table 24-3 lists frequent causes of accidents in the home and specific nursing interventions to prevent accidents. Nurses in the home-care environment are in an ideal position to prevent injuries. During the initial and subsequent assessments, the nurse can evaluate individuals' homes for common factors leading to poisoning, fires, and falls. Determining the causes of potential injuries in homes, such as frayed wires on electrical appliances that can produce sparks and start fires or improperly labeled cleaning products that can be accidentally ingested, allows the nurses to intervene at an early point to prevent injuries. Health teaching should incorporate the concept of accident prevention to all older adults living not only in the community, but also in acute care and long-term care facilities.

The older adult's ability to feel changes in heat and cold may be impaired related to normal and pathological changes of aging. Because of this process, documented cases exist of older adults who died from the effects of heat waves or cold spells. During periods of heat and humidity, older people should increase fluid and salt intake; they should stay in cool quarters, remain quiet, have more rest periods, and refrain from going outdoors when the temperature goes above 90° F. Sweating, which tends to be delayed and reduced in older adults, can be facilitated by wearing light-colored, lightweight cotton clothing. If sweating ceases, then the older person can be at risk for heat stroke. Heat stroke can contribute to sepsis, myocardial infarction, and CVAs, particularly in patients with diabetes. Reduced

Table 24-3 Safety Risk Areas

Area of Attention	Intervention
Stairways	• Secure handrails • Stairways illuminated with light switches at both top and bottom • Nonskid treads for steps
Bedroom	• Night lights • Tacked-down carpet • Discourage use of throw rugs • Furniture securely placed that will not obstruct clear pathways • Extension cords and telephone wires secured and not in walking areas
Bathroom	• Handrails used near tub and toilet • Nonskid mats in tub area • Bath thermometer for tub hot water
Kitchen	• Nonflammable, lightweight, loose clothing when cooking • Dishes and cooking devices at reasonable heights • Use stepstools according to specifications and only when not alone • Keep off wet floor and refrain from using slippery wax • Never climb on chairs • Keep emergency numbers near the telephone • Locks should to be easy to open in times of emergency • Cook at front of the stove rather than at the back
Living room	• Furniture that is easy to get in and out of • Fire detectors installed at appropriate places
Outdoors	• Stairs free of breaks and cracks, clear of snow and ice • Safe handrails • Good lighting for stairs and walkways

body heat can also present problems in the older adult. Symptoms of and interventions for hypothermia are listed in Table 24-4.

Preventing Injury

Many causes of death by injury exist for older adults. Some of these causes are motor-vehicle accidents, falls, suffocation, fires, and poisoning. Because of normal age-related changes and the increased incidence of illness, older adults can experience a decrease in muscle strength and reaction time and may subsequently become more vulnerable to environmental hazards. Decreased sensory acuity and impaired balance further diminish an older person's ability to interpret the environment.

As the percentage of older adults living in the United States increases, the number of older drivers also increases (Burke, 1994). Older individuals are at a high risk for hospitalization and death from motor-vehicle injuries because of the many changes in their neuromuscular and sensory abilities. Consequently, the ability to respond to emergency driving situations may be slowed (Burke, 1994). According to the 1990-1997 National Highway Traffic Safety Administration's Fatality Analysis Reporting System and General Estimates System, rates of motor-vehicle-related injuries increased slightly from 1990 through 1997, and marked variations in state-specific death rates were observed; in most states, older men had death rates approximately twice those for older women. Older adults are encouraged to relearn to drive to adapt to their neuromuscular and sensory changes. Nurses working in the community setting with older adults who drive encourage them to contact American Association of Retired Persons (AARP) for driving classes specifically designed to meet the needs of the older driver (Burke, 1994). Attending these classes frequently allows savings on car insurance.

Table 24-4 Nursing Interventions for Hypothermia

Symptom	Interventions
Cold to touch	Warm hands and feet
Slow respirations	Cover with blanket
Bradycardia	Set room temperature to 70° F
Low blood pressure	Wear cap to bed at night
Slurred speech	Wear several layers of clothing
Drowsiness	Increase activity
Temperature 95° F rectally	Decrease alcohol intake

Biological Agents

A large emphasis is placed on immunizing young children against disease. However, older adults can also benefit from some commonly available vaccines that have been shown to lower both morbidity and mortality in this age group. In many cases, older adults failed to receive primary immunization against diphtheria and tetanus in their childhood years. Lack of immunization against these diseases leaves the older adult vulnerable to illness and possible death from these two toxoids. Table 24-5 lists appropriate immunization schedules for older adults.

Influenza

Influenza is a major cause of morbidity and mortality in older adults. The 65 and older population experiences an estimated 20,000 deaths per year from this preventable virus (Osguthorpe & Morgan, 1995). Influenza immunization rates doubled in adults age 65 and older, between the years 1989 and 1997 (U.S. Department of Health and Human Services, 2000). Despite the increase in immuni-

Table 24-5 Routine Adult Immunization for Influenza, Pneumococcal Disease, Tetanus, Diphtheria, Measles, Mumps, and Rubella, Based on Age and Risk Group

Vaccine or Toxoid	Timing of Administration	Dosage/Route	Risk Groups
Influenza	Yearly for people 65 and older	0.5 mL intramuscularly	People with chronic cardiac, metabolic, or respiratory disease
Pneumococcal	Generally every 7 years for people age 65 and older	0.5 mL intramuscularly	People with chronic cardiac, renal, or respiratory disease
Tetanus and diphtheria	Every 10 years	0.5 mL intramuscularly	Elderly people who were not in the military
Measles-mumps-rubella	Once or twice, depending on risk group and age	0.5 mL subcutaneously	College students and health care workers

From Zimmerman, R. K., & Clover, R. D. (1995). Adult immunizations: A practical approach for clinicians. *American Family Physician, 51* (4), 859.

zation rates and recent Medicare reimbursement for the vaccine, fewer than 50% of older adults receive it (Osguthorpe & Morgan, 1995). The influenza vaccine can markedly reduce the incidence of complications, hospitalizations, and death from the disease (CDC, 1995). The influenza vaccine, composed of inactivated whole virus or virus subunits grown in chick embryo cells, is given annually to all older adults, especially those with chronic conditions such as pulmonary or cardiac problems and those in long-term care facilities. Vaccination is contraindicated in people who have experienced a reaction to the vaccine in the past (CDC, 1995). Caution should be exercised in administering the vaccine to older adults who have allergies to eggs (CDC, 1995). A *Healthy People 2010* goal (#14-29 a-b) is to increase the number of older adults who are vaccinated annually against influenza and ever vaccinated against pneumococcal disease (U.S. Department of Health and Human Services, 2000).

Pneumonia

Estimates indicate that pneumococcal infections are responsible for approximately 40,000 deaths each year among older adults (Osguthorpe & Morgan, 1995). In 1997 only 43% of persons age 65 and older had ever received a pneumococcal vaccine (U.S. Department of Health and Human Services, 2000). The CDC recommends that older adults with normal immune systems who live with chronic illnesses (including cardiovascular disease, pulmonary disease, diabetes, alcoholism, cirrhosis, or cerebrospinal fluid leaks), immunocompromised older adults, and older adults with HIV should receive vaccination against pneumococcal disease. However, many barriers about pneumococcal vaccination, such as the prevailing lack of importance of the disease and vaccination and the myth that receiving the vaccination will result in the disease, prevent the older adults from receiving immunization. The vaccine should be given once during the lifespan to all individuals with chronic cardiac or pulmonary disease and conditions predisposing to pneumococcal infection and to all people over 65 years of age. Revaccination is recommended for individuals at high risk for fatal pneumococcal disease who have received the vaccination more than 6 years before. Pneumococcal vaccination is effective in providing some protection against pneumococcal disease 2 to 3 weeks after vaccination (CDC, 1995).

Tuberculosis

Commonly referred to as consumption, tuberculosis (TB) was the leading killer among infectious diseases from the nineteenth century into the midtwentieth century. The TB organism is usually inhaled and deposited in the lung, where it expands and causes morbidity and mortality in all populations, especially older adults. The TB epidemic was virtually wiped out with the introduction and appropriate use of various medications. However, in 1984 rates for TB began to rise again. The increase in poverty, homelessness, drug and alcohol abuse, and AIDS have produced multiple strains of drug-resistant TB. The CDC estimates that there are currently 17,528 active cases in of TB the United States (CDC, 1999b).

The chances of acquiring TB in public areas with adequate ventilation are not significant. In fact, ultraviolet rays of the sun kill the virus. The major risk comes from close contact with individuals who are carrying the TB virus. Nurses who suspect TB infection in older adults should look for the following signs and symptoms: cough, fatigue, anorexia, nausea, fever, night sweats, and weight loss. However, atypical symptoms frequently occur in older adults, including delirium, weight loss, and anorexia. A tuberculin skin test will indicate exposure to the TB organism, and a chest x-ray can confirm the presence of the disease in the person's lungs.

Current therapy for tuberculosis includes isoniazid (300 mg a day) and rifampin (600 mg a day) orally for 9 months (CDC, 1994). Unfortunately, because of the possibility of concomitant altered liver function in older adults, these medications can produce side effects after the therapy has killed the virus. However, people must be instructed to take the medications exactly as ordered and not to skip a dose, specifically because this leads to drug-resistant strains of TB.

Drug Use

Normal changes of aging have a significant influence on drug use in the older adult. The way in which medications are absorbed, distributed, metabolized, and cleared from the body are all subject to changing organ systems and illness. Even when medications are taken as prescribed by the physician, age-related changes and the presence of disease can increase the risk of undesirable side effects in the older adult. In addition to problems caused by the processing of drugs within the older adult's body, the use of drugs in the older adult is disproportionate to census findings. A study of 174 nursing home residents indicates that the residents were prescribed a mean of approximately eight different drugs (Horgas, 1992).

One problem that results from the large amount of drug usage among older adults is drug-drug interactions. Evidence suggests that as a person ages, the chance of experiencing a drug reaction is increased, and each prescribed or over-the-counter preparation that is taken multiplies the possibility of an adverse reaction. Horgas (1992) found that over 30% of the residents in the sample were exposed to at least one clinically significant drug-drug reaction. Federal government regulations (Omnibus Reconciliation Act) developed in 1987, implemented in 1990, and revised in 1997, have attempted to curtail the large use of unnecessary medications by older adults in long-term care facilities. As a rule, nurses should take a medication history of older adults to assess for past drug reactions. Medications should be started at their lowest effective dose and slowly increased as needed.

The use of illegal drugs among older adults is a problem that has been around since the 1960s, but remains not widely accepted by health care professionals (Kostyk, 1994). Because of this lack of emphasis, drug abuse is frequently overlooked as a problem of older adults (McMahon, 1993). Walker (1993) suggests that some of the problems of older adults, such as accidents, neglected personal hygiene, malnutrition, noncompliance, and memory loss, may actually be signs of substance abuse. New tools designed to detect the problems of substance abuse in the older adult are currently being developed that will help nurses assess this problem in older adults and refer them to appropriate treatment programs.

Alcohol Use

Current data indicate that alcohol problems among older adults have been underestimated and hidden. Alcoholism affects an estimated 2.5 million older adults (Mackel, Sheehy, & Badger, 1994). Similar to other substance abuse problems, alcohol abuse in seniors frequently goes unnoticed because the symptoms can be similar to those of other common problems of aging, and the affected individuals are no longer in the work force, where they can be observed. The longer the problem remains undetected, the greater the problem becomes (Mackel, Sheehy, & Badger, 1994). Older adults are also more vulnerable to the effects of alcohol because their systems do not detoxify and excrete as efficiently as do those of younger people. Alcoholism predisposes older adults to accidents, nutritional deficiencies, disease, and decreased functional ability (Mackel, Sheehy, & Badger, 1994). Interestingly, when older adults seek active treatment for their alcoholism, their prognosis is many times better than it is for their younger counterparts. When alcohol abuse is suspected in an older adult, referral to an appropriate treatment program will help the person conquer the problem and return to a higher degree of functioning.

Tobacco Use

Cigarette smoking causes heart disease, several kinds of cancer (lung, larynx, esophagus, pharynx, mouth, and bladder), and chronic lung disease. Cigarette smoking also contributes to cancer of the pancreas, kidney, and cervix (U.S. Department of Health and Human Services, 2000). Aging men of today are perhaps the first generation to smoke practically throughout their adult lives. The results of smoking occur slowly over time, and problems are usually not experienced until lung damage has occurred. Research demonstrates that because smoking can initiate and promote disease processes, it is one of the most important negative predictors of longevity. Other diseases common to smokers are chronic obstructive pulmonary diseases, including bronchitis, asthma, emphysema, and bronchiectasis. Because of the large number of medications and the potential for drug interactions, smoking is a particular problem for older adults. Nicotine-drug interactions can cause many problems for the older adult.

Older adults can experience the benefits of smoking cessation even after the age of 65 (CDC, 1993). In fact, older adults may be more motivated to quit smoking because they are likely to see some of the damage that smoking has caused and anticipate that smoking cessation will restore their health. Timmreck and Randolph (1993) report that smokers who survive heart attacks have a 50% cessation rate. Nurses in acute-care settings are in an ideal position to assist older adults in making the commitment to quit smoking while recovering from an acute illness. Nurses in long-term care and community settings also have the opportunity to motivate individuals to quit smoking and have access to resources to help older adults to quit. Smoking cessation in the form of behavioral management classes are available to community-dwelling older adults. Older adults may also be candidates for nicotine-replacement therapy and some nonmedical interventions to help them quit smoking.

Cancer

Cancer rates for older adults are disproportionate to census rates in the United States. Although only 12% of the population is considered as older adults, more than 50% of all diagnosed cancers are found in the older adult population. The reason for the large proportion of cancer in this country is unknown. Theories that have been postulated include longer exposure to carcinogens, increased susceptibility to cancer in the older body, decreased

Table 24-6 Three Leading Cancer Sites in the Elderly by Age, Subgroup, Race, and Sex

	Age Subgroup (in years)		
Sex	65 to 74	75 to 84	85 and Over
Men	(1) Prostate (2) Lung (3) Colon	(1) Prostate (2) Lung (3) Colon	(1) Prostate (2) Colon (3) Lung
Women	(1) Breast (2) Lung (3) Colon	(1) Breast (2) Colon (3) Lung	(1) Colon (2) Breast (3) Lung

Adapted from Boyle, D. M. et al. (1992). Oncology nursing society position paper on cancer and aging: The mandate for oncology nursing. *Oncology Nursing Forum, 19* (6), 913-33.

cellular healing ability, loss of tumor-suppressing genes, and decreased immune function. Although the exact cause cannot be determined, clearly, cancer is a large problem for older adults in the United States.

The type of cancers common to older adults are listed by age and race in Table 24-6. Prostate cancer is the leading cancer among men of all races and ages and is clearly the most common male cancer and the second leading cause of death from cancer in men in the United States. Current estimates are that 8% of all men in the United States will be diagnosed with prostate cancer during their lifetime. Early detection of prostate cancer allows treatment while it is still localized in the prostate gland and highly curable. Evidence suggests that by using a combination of screening techniques, more cases of prostate cancer can be detected earlier. A review of the literature identified the three key components of an appropriate prostate screen: (1) symptomatology, (2) prostate specific antigen (PSA), and (3) a digital rectal examination (DRE) (Poburksy, 1995).

Breast cancer is the most common cancer in older women of all ages and races in the United States. Reports suggest that one in nine women will develop breast cancer in her lifetime. Three quarters of all breast cancers occur in women over 50. The risk of breast cancer is increased in women whose close female relatives (mothers or sisters) have had the disease. Women who have never had children or had their first child after age 30 appear to have an increased risk for breast cancer. The causes breast cancer remains unclear. However, the best protection from breast cancer is early detection and prompt treatment. The American Cancer Society recommends that women have annual mammograms and breast examinations beginning at age 40 and practice monthly breast self-examinations.

Nurses help older adults change the habits that place them at a high risk for developing cancer. Following nutritional guidelines as suggested earlier in this chapter, reducing stress, adopting a program of regular exercise, and smoking cessation are a few of the approaches that nurses can help older adults take to promote individual wellness. Additionally, periodic monitoring and screening in the form of regular visits with a primary health care provider or community screening can alert older adults to early signs and symptoms of cancers that occur during the later years.

SOCIAL PROCESSES

Environments of Care

The incidence of chronic and acute illnesses, the subsequent decline in functional status, changes in economic status, and changes in family structure frequently place older adults in situations in which they are admitted to acute-care facilities or must make a temporary or permanent move into another housing situation or a long-term care facility. When providing health-promotion services to older adults, the fact that older adults might live in a number of different settings must be taken into consideration. However, the link between housing and health for the older adult is not well recognized (MacDonald, Remus, & Laing, 1994).

When older adults move to a variety of residences or permanently reside in an alternative setting, they enter a continuum of care extending from the acute-care facility to the long-term care or community setting (Fig. 24-9). Nurses who work in each of the different settings on the continuum can promote health to the older adult population in many ways. One consistent intervention that runs through the continuum of care is teaching. Weinrich and Boyd (1992) report that because older adults have more health problems, their education requirements tend to be many and complex. These researchers further report that teaching the older adult is also influenced by their developmental level, current lifestyle, role changes, and body image. One of the primary health-promotion priorities is to make an appropriate assessment of the older adult's readiness to learn in each environment and provide the necessary teaching on lifestyle changes.

From the acute-care setting through each stage of the continuum until the older adult returns home, opportunities are available for nurses to introduce older adults and their families to community resources (Table 24-7). The acute care nurse has the opportunity to present older adults with health-promotion strategies at a time during which they perceive the greatest need to change their lifestyle to return to a healthy status. In most cases, an acute-care admission is a perfect opportunity to introduce the older individual to health-promotion teaching. However, the acute-care nurse may feel frustrated by the inability to see the results of this teaching and may therefore give it a low priority in the person's plan of care.

Nevertheless, older adults will rapidly grasp material that they believe will prevent future hospital admissions and restore their health. Setting up visiting-nurse appointments, transportation, homemaking and chore services, adult day care, and assistance with grocery shopping or home-delivered meals will help the older adult return to the home care environment more readily prepared to

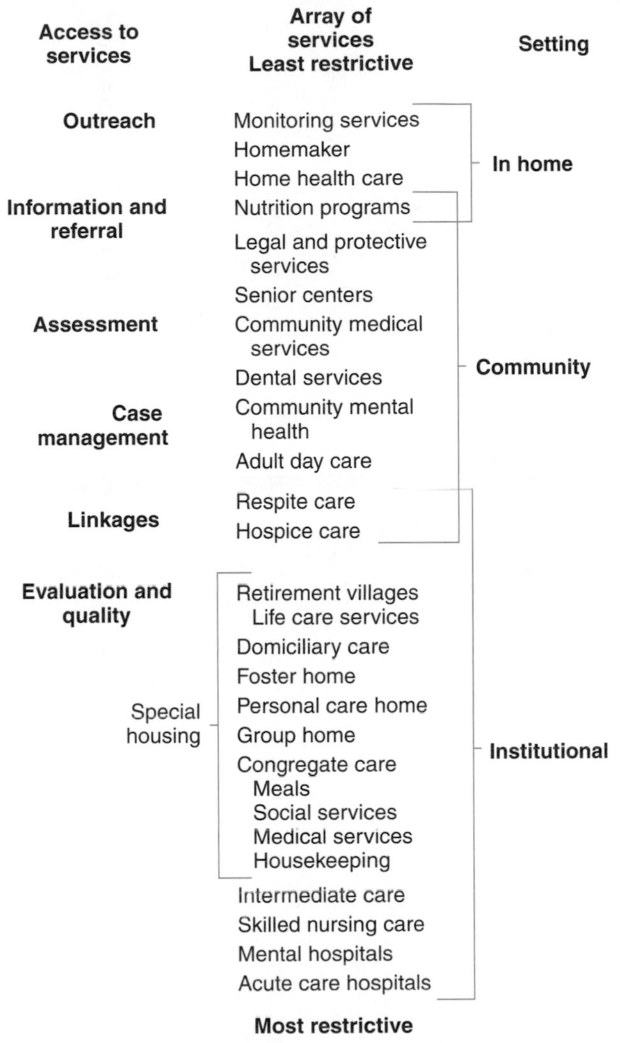

Fig. 24-9 Continuum of care for older adults. (From Wetle, T. [1982]. *Handbook of geriatric care.* East Hanover, NJ: Sandoz.)

recover from the illness. Additionally, helping older adults to locate smoking-cessation programs, stress-management workshops, or weight-loss and exercise programs during the hospitalization will encourage them to enter these programs immediately after discharge, while they are motivated.

Long-term care nurses are able to locate and plan community resources during the resident's stay. Researching some of the community services discussed will allow older individuals to return home to an environment in which their health can continue to be promoted. Additional community resources that may help older adults who are discharged from long-term care facilities include support groups and medical resources, telephone information, and referral services. In addition to individual care planning, long-term care nurses can be more involved in institutional policy changes. Recommendations about smoking policies and healthy diets may prompt interdisciplinary changes that will result in improved health for the entire institution.

The community health nurse or geriatric care manager who sees people in their original residences or in housing complexes may be charged with individual care planning of health promotion. Keating (1995) reports that nurses in the home care setting provide health care information and services to both individuals and their families. The resources available to community health nurses are frequently rich and enable the nurses to draw on a variety of sources to assist them in promoting the health of community-dwelling older adults. Procuring transportation, home-delivered meals, assistance with housekeeping, socialization, exercise programs, and self-help groups are only a few of the health-promotion resources available within the community. Nurses in all settings may take the opportunity to call the town or city older adult services office for information on the many resources available to help them access services to promote their health.

The AARP provides many services to people over age 55, including excellent educational materials and community program packages. The topics reflect a broad range of concerns that are common to older adults and are generally presented in a self-help manner. Among the topics covered are smoking, exercise, nutrition, and wellness. Each program serves as a guide as the older person tries to negotiate a system or learns more about a health problem. These topics are written in layperson's terms, are easily understandable, and they are printed in large letters to accommodate vision changes in the elderly population. This self-help method is especially important for older adults who feel uncomfortable addressing questions on finances or sexuality to nurses and physicians.

Two additional environments of care have emerged over the last half of the twentieth century in the United States: (1) Adult Day Programs and (2) Assisted Living Facilities. Adult Day Programs (ADPs) are defined as "a structured, community based, group program designed to meet the assessed physical, emotional, psychosocial needs of functionally limited older adults" (Abraham, 2000, p. 105). These programs are held in a variety of settings, including long-term care facilities or freestanding ADPs. Assisted Living Facilities (ALFs) are defined as a special combination of housing, supportive services, personalized assistance, and health care designed to respond to the individual needs of those who need help with activities of daily living (ADL) and instrumental activities of daily living (IADL) (Assisted Living Federation of America, 1997). Nurses play a large and important role in developing and operating both ADPs and ALFs. Further research in both environments of care has been indicated to clarify the nurse's role in these settings and the subsequent care that is provided to older adults.

Health Care Delivery System

This chapter has clearly brought the need for health-promotion services for older adults into the limelight.

Table 24-7 Long-Term Care Housing and Assessment Continuum

	Independent Living	Retirement Community	Assisted Living	Nursing Facility
Description	Covers a broad range of housing options (residential houses, apartments, condominiums, townhouses, subsidized senior housing) for older persons who are functionally and socially independent.	Provides a living arrangement, which integrates shelter and services for older persons who do not need 24-hour protective oversight.	Provides a living arrangement that integrates shelter and services for frail older persons who are functionally and/or socially impaired and require 24-hour protective oversight.	Provides a living arrangement that integrates shelter with medical, nursing, psychosocial, and rehabilitation services for older persons who require 24-hour nursing supervision.
Primary Services	-A- • Environmental security • Possibly coordination of resident services (transportation, activities, house-keeping) • Or no services are available	-B- "A" plus: • Meals (1-3 per day) • Transportation • Activities • Housekeeping assistance • Assistance with coordination of community-based services	-C- "A&B" plus: • Assistance with activities of daily living • Medication monitoring • 24-hour protective oversight	-D- "A&B&C" plus: • Medication administration • 24-hour nursing supervision
Mobility	Capable of moving about independently OR ambulatory with cane or walker. Independent with wheelchair, but needs help in an emergency.	Capable of moving about independently. Able to seek and follow directions. Able to evacuate independently in emergency OR ambulatory with cane or walker. Independent with wheelchair, but needs help in an emergency.	Mobile, but may require escort or assistance resulting from confusion, poor vision, weakness, or poor motivation OR requires occasional assistance to move about, but is usually independent.	May require assistance with transfers from bed, chair, toilet OR requires transfer and transport assistance. Requires turning and positioning in bed and wheelchair.
Nutrition	Able to prepare own meals. Eats meals without assistance.	Able to prepare own meals. Eats meals without assistance. Generally a minimum of one meal a day is available.	All meals and snacks provided. May require assistance getting to dining room and/or requires minimal assistance (opening cartons or other packages, cutting food, or preparing trays).	May be unable or unwilling to go to dining room. May be dependent on staff for eating or feeding needs OR fully dependent on staff for nourishment (includes reminders to eat and/or feeding).
Hygiene	Independent in all care, including bathing.	Independent in all care, including bathing and personal laundry.	May required assistance with bathing or hygiene OR may require assistance, initiation, structure, or reminders. Resident may be able to complete tasks.	May be dependent on staff for all personal hygiene.

Housekeeping	Independent in performing housekeeping functions (includes making bed, vacuuming, cleaning, and laundry).	Independent in performing housekeeping functions (includes making bed, vacuuming, cleaning, and laundry) OR may need assistance with heavy housekeeping, vacuuming, laundry, and linens.	Housekeeping and laundry services provided.	Housekeeping and laundry services provided.
Dressing	Independent and dresses appropriately.	Independent and dresses appropriately.	May require occasional assistance with shoelaces, zippers, etc., and/or medical appliances or garments OR may require reminders, initiation, or motivation.	May be dependent on staff for dressing.
Toileting	Independent and continent.	Independent and completely continent OR may have incontinence, colostomy, or catheter, but independent in caring for self through proper use of supplies.	Same as "retirement community" OR may have occasional problem with incontinence, colostomy, or catheter and may require assistance in caring for self through proper use of supplies.	May have problem with incontinence, colostomy/catheter and requires assistance OR may be dependent and unable to communicate needs.
Medications	Responsible for self-administration of all medications.	Responsible for self-administration of all medication OR may arrange for family or home health agency to establish a medication administration system.	Able to self-administer medications OR facility staff may remind or monitor the actual process OR facility staffed by RN or LPN who administers medications.	Medications administered by staff personnel or self if assessed as capable.
Mental Status	Oriented to person, place, and time. Memory intact, but has occasional forgetfulness AND able to reason, plan, and organize daily events. Mentally capable of identifying needs and meeting them.	Oriented to person, place, and time AND memory is intact, but has occasional forgetfulness without consistent pattern of memory loss, AND able to reason, plan, and organize daily events. Mentally capable of identifying environment needs and meeting them.	May require occasional direction or guidance in getting from place to place OR may have difficulty with occasional confusion that may result in anxiety, social withdrawal, or depression OR orientation to time or place or person may be impaired.	Judgment can be poor and may not attempt tasks that are not within capacities OR may require strong orientation and reminder program. May need guidance in getting from place to place OR disoriented to time, place, and person OR memory is severely impaired.
Behavioral Status	Deals appropriately with emotions and uses available resources to cope with inner stress.	Deals appropriately with emotions and uses available resources to cope with inner stress AND deals appropriately with other residents and staff OR may require periodic intervention from staff to resolve conflicts with others to cope with situational stress.	May require periodic intervention form staff to facilitate expression of feelings to cope with inner stress OR may require periodic intervention from staff to resolve conflicts with others to cope with situational stress.	May require regular intervention from staff to facilitate expression of feelings and to deal with periodic outbursts of anxiety or agitation OR maximal staff intervention is required to manage behavior.

Adapted from Steven Bender (geriatric social worker), Colorado Springs, CO.

However, few if any health care plans that pay for health-promotion services exist (Keating, 1995). Medicare (the primary health insurance coverage for older adult) offers little coverage for preventive services. Although older adults require a wide range of services that ideally exist on a continuum, not all services on this continuum are available to older adults in various care settings.

Medicare and other federal expenditures for older adults (direct or indirect) constitute a large part of the current federal budget. The majority goes to old age and retirement programs, disability, and Medicaid. Because of the large percentage of the federal budget consumed by Medicare, this insurance program is currently undergoing much scrutiny. Current legislature is being reviewed to save taxpayers on the Medicare budget. Lawmakers anticipate that approximately $49 billion of the savings would come from more effective use of health maintenance organizations and prospective payment systems instituted in the home. Regardless of the source of funding cuts, obviously, the more illness that can be prevented, the more financially stable the older adult will remain. Nurses will play a key role during the years of Medicare reform in promoting health not only to prevent illness, but also to prevent older adults from losing all their savings and entering poverty.

A current trend in the health care market is for Medicare beneficiaries to be managed by health maintenance organizations (HMOs) or other managed-care companies (MCCs). HMOs often provide a team of doctors, nurses, and health care professionals who will help the older adult to coordinate and manage care in the most fiscally responsible manner. MCCs can be in the form of HMOs, hospitals, or other insurance companies. Older adults are often faced with the decision of which HMO or MCC to choose to manage their Medicare benefits. Careful thought should go into this choice. Price, coverage, limitations, and exclusions should be explored before a decision is made. For traditional Medicare beneficiaries, Medigap policies have been encouraged for older adults to pay for the health care coverage not afforded by Medicare. There are currently approximately nine Medigap policies. Each one provides varying levels of coverage. Choices about whether to purchase coverage for durable health care supplies, prescription medications, and other medical charges must be made to appropriately select a Medigap policy. There is a charge for the policy that varies according to the level of coverage selected.

Unfortunately, many older adults have failed to prepare financially for older adulthood. Although some individuals receive supplemental incomes from pensions or individual retirement accounts, this situation is rare. The majority of older adults live on limited incomes. Several resources are available to help older adults with limited finances live quality lives. Medicaid, authorized by Title 19 of the Social Security Act, is a program designed to help older adults who are receiving public assistance to pay for medical expenses. Both federal and state governments fund the Medicaid program. To qualify for Medicaid, an individual must have limited income and assets. The coverage afforded by Medicaid is more extensive than that of Medicare. For example, Medicaid covers stays in long-term care facilities, transportation, and prescription drug services. Medicare covers these services only in limited and medically acute situations. Frequently, older adults and their caretakers desire coverage by Medicaid so that more extensive health coverage can be obtained. These individuals are required to "spend down" their assets, which enables them to be eligible for Medicaid.

Other resources are available to help older adults live this last stage of life in a high-quality manner. Food stamps are available to older adults who meet certain economic criteria. Food stamps can help the older adult obtain nutritious food at participating markets without depleting their limited budget. Supplemental medication payment programs assist older adults in purchasing their prescription medications. When income criteria are met, older adults may be entitled to purchase medications by paying only small copayments rather than the large amount of money that is frequently charged for their medication.

Careful financial planning before the onset of illness is ideal to avoid the need to spend down assets and to help the older adult live at a desirable income level. This task can be accomplished through meeting with lawyers and financial planners as early in life as 30 years of age. Completing advance directives, including naming a conservator in advance of illness, assists caregivers, physicians, clergy, and the family in making difficult decisions at the end of life, during which time the older person is no longer able to make them. The better prepared the older adult is, the easier it is to receive appropriate care and treatment during times of illness. Reverse Annuity Mortgages (RAMs) are one option for older adults to provide them with increased income during the later years of life. A RAM is obtained when a bank or private business purchases the home of an older adult. The bank pays the person a set amount of money each month until the house is paid for in its entirety. The older adult continues to remain in the home. This approach provides the person with necessary funds and negates the need to move and sell the house if an acute illness arises.

A newer option available to older adults to pay for the possibility of a long-term care admission is long-term care insurance. Similar to other insurance programs, older adults purchase a policy, now widely available from reputable insurance agents. A premium is paid each month that entitles the beneficiary to receive long-term care benefits at home or in a long-term care facility if an illness arises. Older individuals are cautioned to explore the many options available for long-term care insurance. The benefits and coverage vary, and exclusions are frequently written into the contract to prevent care in certain situations.

Fortunately, because of population shifts that have allowed for a large number of older adults in the United States, political movements toward protecting older adults' rights are abundant and strong. Nowhere is there more political activity than among the groups responsible for social policy and aging. However, this large number has created problems of consistency, equity, and authority. Several large programs, including the Social Security Administration, the Health Care Financing Administration, and the Department of Veterans Affairs, have difficulty with coordination because of their size and the large number of cases they handle.

The nurse who specializes in the care of older adults can do a great deal to promote their health and well being through education, research, and practice. In education, curricula should be continually evaluated to ensure that appropriate and accurate content related to aging is taught. The quality of care depends on the clinician's knowledge base in gerontological nursing. Education for the older person is equally important and begins with an assessment of the level of understanding that the individual has about health-promotion activities.

Research in the area of health promotion in older adults is only beginning. A great deal more remains to be done in exploring the concepts of health promotion, relating these concepts, and developing and testing hypotheses. Research may best begin with an attempt to debunk commonly held beliefs about older adults. Defining some of the concepts of health promotion, such as quality of life and functional ability, to the older adult will yield immeasurable amounts of information that can be tested. Eventually, with the commitment of qualified nurses, health promotion will be respected for the integral role it plays in the quality of life of older adults.

SUMMARY

Life expectancy is now beyond 70 years of age for both men and women, with the fastest-growing age group being those over 85. This phenomenon is indeed wonderful. However, aging causes physiological changes in many bodily

innovative practice

Geriatric Assessment

The present health care system, with its emphasis on acute care, busy office schedules, and fragmented delivery systems, often frustrates older persons and their families. The very old or frail person's health problems are frequently overlooked, ignored, or only partially treated. A health care service is currently available in many communities that uses a team approach to meet the special needs of older adults. This service is known as *Geriatric Assessment*.

GOALS OF GERIATRIC ASSESSMENT

- Maintain health and health maintenance practices.
- Minimize hospitalizations.
- Establish complete diagnoses that are frequently overlooked, including hearing impairment, vision deficits, early dementia, depression, poor nutrition and falls
- Decrease overprescription of medications.

Geriatric Assessment uses an interdisciplinary team consisting of a geriatric nurse practitioner, physical therapist, and a social worker. Each member of the team evaluates the person from a health care, functional, cognitive, or psychosocial point of view. Additional members of the team might include a geropsychiatrist, geriatrician, nutritionist, pharmacist, dentist, or podiatrist. The program team evaluates the home environment, advance directives, falls, incontinence, vision and hearing impairments, memory loss, depression and anxiety, functional decline, deconditioning, caregiver stress, economic resources, and quality-of-life issues. The team is coordinated by the geriatric nurse practitioner.

Geriatric Assessment is not meant for all older persons. The people who benefit are the "frail" older adult. A typical person who might benefit from Geriatric Assessment would be:

- Over age 80
- Falling frequently
- Losing weight because of poor nutrition
- Depressed because of loss of spouse and friends
- Has mild memory loss
- Hospitalized three times in 2 months
- Taking more than five medications regularly and frequently getting them confused
- Has no close family in the community
- Is in need of health teaching

Targeting Geriatric Assessment to these people usually identifies their strengths and weaknesses. Following this assessment, the geriatric nurse practitioner begins developing a plan of care to address usable strengths and assist with weaknesses.

The primary care physician, family physician, or internist is a key link between the Geriatric Assessment team and the individual, primarily because this provider must cooperate with the team's recommendation and monitor the person's progress. In most cases, the nurse practitioner coordinates between the team and the person's primary physician and family.

Geriatric Assessment clinics are available in many larger cities. As the U.S. health care system changes from its costly system of treating acute health problems with frequent office and hospital visits to a more cost-controlled coordinated, comprehensive health management system, Geriatric Assessment will play a key role in identifying individual strengths, correcting problems, and maintaining the health and quality of life of older citizens.

Courtesy Carole Lium Edelman.

functions. Although some of these changes are benign, the older adult has a higher frequency of illness compared with the younger population. With these physiological and pathological changes, health-promotion services are integral to helping older adults to lead high-quality lives throughout their expanded lifespan.

Many problems of old age are related to lifestyle. Changes in nutritional needs, sleep patterns, and activity level are required to adapt to normal and pathological processes. Psychological health depends on reassessing spirituality, self-concept, and role functions. Change and adaptation are possible. With the assistance of nurses and other health care professionals, older adults can be empowered to live their final years with integrity.

Some of the dysfunctional aspects of aging have extrinsic causes, such as environmental pollution. Older adults are as susceptible as any age group is to society's problems, such as homelessness, mistreatment, and drug and alcohol abuse. In conjunction with physiological and pathological changes, cancer, TB, and other disorders can result. Internal and public policy changes will continue to help older adults live in a world in which old age can be the most rewarding stage of life.

REFERENCES

Abraham, B. (2000). Adult Day Care. In J. Fitzpatrick, T. Fulmer, M. Wallace & E. Flaherty (Eds.), *Geriatric nursing research digest* (pp. 105-106). New York: Springer.

Adams, P., & Marnao, M. (1995). Current estimates, national center for health statistics. *Vital Health Statistics, 10,* 1930.

Adamson, G. M. (1996). The incontinence connection. *Contemporary Long-Term Care, 78,* 129.

American College of Sports Medicine. (1995). *American college sports medicine's guidelines for exercise testing and prescription* (5th ed.). Baltimore: Williams & Wilkins.

American Nurses' Association. (1994a). *Clinician's handbook of preventive services*. Waldorf, MD: The Association.

American Nurses' Association. (1994b). *Position statement on assisted suicide*. Washington, DC: The Association.

Assisted Living Federation of America. (1997). *The assisted living industry, 1996*. Fairfax, Virginia: The Author.

Baum, N., Appell, R. A., & Moss, H. (1994). Helping incontinent patients resume activity. *The Physician and Sportsmedicine, 22* (5), 70-80.

Bengtson, V. L., Parrott, T. M., & Burgess, E. O. (1996). Progress and pitfalls in gerontological theorizing. *Gerontologist, 36* (6), 768-772.

Bernard, M. A., Anderson, C., & Forgey, M. (1995). Health and nutritional status of old-old African Americans. *Journal of Nutrition for the Elderly, 14* (2-3), 55-67.

Bliwise, D. G. (1993). Sleep in normal aging and dementia. *Sleep 16* (1), 40-61.

Brocklehurst, J. C., Tallis, R. C., & Fillet, H. M. (1992). *Textbook of geriatric medicine and gerontology*. Edinburgh: Churchill Livingstone.

Brush, B. (2000). Spirituality. In J. Fitzpatrick, T. Fulmer, M. Wallace, & E. Flaherty, *Geriatric nursing research digest* (pp. 91-93). New York: Springer.

Burke, M. (1994). Motor vehicle injury prevention for older adults. *Nursing Practice, 5,* 26-28.

Burney-Puckett, M. (May, 1996). Sundown syndrome: Etiology and management. *Journal of Psychosocial Nursing & Mental Health Services, 34* (5), 40-43.

Butler, R. N., & Lewis, M. I. (1993). *Love and sex after 60*. New York: Ballantine Books.

Butler, R. (1963). The life review: An interpretation of reminiscence in the aged. *Psychiatry, 26,* 65-76.

Casey, D. A. (1991). Suicide in the elderly: A two-year study of data from death certificates. *Southern Medical Journal, 84* (10), 1185-1187.

Centers for Disease Control and Prevention. (1993). *Vital and health statistics*. Washington, DC: U.S. Department of Health and Human Services.

Centers for Disease Control (1994). Questions and Answers about TB [On-line]. Available: http://www.cdc.gov/nchstp/tb/faqs/qa.htm#disease_1.

Centers for Disease Control and Prevention. (1995). *Epidemiology & prevention of vaccine preventable diseases*. Washington, DC: U.S. Department of Health and Human Services.

Centers for Disease Control and Prevention. (1998). *Chronic disease and their risk factors: The nation's leading causes of death*. Washington, DC: U.S. Department of Health and Human Services.

Centers for Disease Control and Prevention. (1999a). *Prevention and control of tuberculosis in facilities providing long-term care to the elderly*. Washington DC: U.S. Department of Health and Human Services.

Centers for Disease Control (CDC) (1999b). *Reported tuberculosis in the United States* [On-line]. Available: http//www.cdc.gov/nchstp/tb/surv/surv99.htm.

Centers for Disease Control (CDC) (2001a). *Healthy aging: Preventing disease and improving quality of life among older Americans: At a glance* [On-line]. Available: http://www.cdc.gov/nccdphp/aag-aging.htm.

Centers for Disease Control (CDC) (2001b). *Suicide in the United States* [On-line]. Available: http://www.cdc.gov/ncipe/factsheets/suifacts.htm.

Cohen, S. J., Robinson, D., Dugan, E., Howard, G., Suggs, P. K., Pearce, K. F., Carroll, D. D., McGann, P., & Preisser, J. (1999, Jan.). Communication between older adults and their physicians about urinary incontinence. *Journal of Gerontology. Series A, Biological Sciences & Medical Sciences. 54* (1), M34-37.

Connelly, D. M., & Vandervoort, A. A. (1995). Improvement in knee extensor strength of institutionalized elderly women after exercise with ankle weights. *Physiotherapy Canada, 47,* 15-23.

Connelly, D. M., & Vandervoort, A. A. (1996). Improving muscle strength in the frail elderly. *Canadian Nursing Home, 7,* 26-30.

Coyle, N. (1992). The euthanasia and physician-assisted suicide debate: Issues for nursing. *Oncology Nursing Forum, 19* (7), 41-46.

Dawe, D., & Moore-Orr, R. (1995). Low-intensity, range-of-motion exercise: Invaluable nursing care for elderly patients. *Journal of Advanced Nursing, 21,* 675-681.

Dishman, R. K. (1994). Motivating older adults to exercise. *Southern Medical Journal, 87* (5), S79-S82.

Drench, M. E., & Losee, R. H. (1996). Sexuality and sexual capacities of elderly people. *Rehabilitation Nursing, 21* (3), 118-123.

Dudley-Brown, S. (1996). Gastrointestinal function. In A. Lueckenotte, *Gerontologic nursing* (pp. 644-692). St. Louis: Mosby.

Ebersole, P., & Hess, P. (1998). Toward healthy aging: Human need and nursing response (5th ed.). St. Louis: Mosby.

Eisenberg, D. (1998). Unconventional medicine in the U.S. *North Carolina Medical Journal, 3328* (4), 246-252.

Erikson, E. H. (1982). *The life cycle-review*. New York: W. W. Norton.

Evans, L. K. (1986). Sundown syndrome in institutionalized elderly. *Journal of the American Geriatrics Society, 35,* 101-108.

Fiatarone, M. A., O'Neill, E. F., Ryan, N. D., Clements, K. M., Solares, G. R., Nelson, M. E., Roberts, S. B., Kehayias, J. J., Lipsitz, L. A., & Evans, W. J. (1994). Exercise training and nutritional supplementation for physical frailty in very elderly people. *The New England Journal of Medicine, 330,* 1769-1775.

Fisher, M. (1996). *Guide to clinical preventive services* (2nd ed.). Baltimore: Williams & Wilkins.

Floyd, J. A. (1993). The use of across method triangulation in the study of sleep concerns in the older adult. *Advances in Nursing Science, 16* (2), 70-80.

Floyd, J. A. (1995). Another look at napping in older adults. *Geriatric Nursing, 16* (3), 136-138.

Folstein, M. E., Folstein, S. E., & McHugh, P. (1975). Mini-mental state: A practical method for grading the cognitive state of patients for the clinician. *Journal of Psychiatric Research 12,* 189-198.

Forbes, E. J. (1990). Spirituality, aging, and the community dwelling caregiver and care recipient. *Geriatric Nursing 15* (6), 297-302.

Frenn, M. (1994). Older adults' experience of health promotion: A theory for nursing practice. *Public Health Nurse, 13* (1), 65-71.

Gorbein, M. J. (1993). When your older patient can't sleep: How to put insomnia to rest. *Geriatrics, 48* (9), 65, 67-68.

Grabbe, L., Demi, A., Camann, M. A., & Potter. L. (1997). The health status of elderly persons in the last year of life: A comparison of deaths by suicide, injury, and natural causes. *American Journal of Public Health, 87* (3), 434-437.

Harper, M. S. (1995). Aging minorities. *Healthcare Trends & Transition,* 6 (4), 9.

Harvard Medical School. (1996). *Alzheimer's disease.* Boston: Health Publications Group.

Hillman, J. L., & Stricker, G. (1994). A linkage of knowledge and attitudes toward elderly sexuality: Not necessarily a uniform relationship. *The Gerontologist, 34* (2), 256-260.

Horgas, A. L. (1992). *Prescription drug use and drug-drug interactions in nursing homes: Prevalence, predictors and health outcomes.* (Unpublished doctoral dissertation). University Park: Pennsylvania State University.

Howard, J. H., Gates, G. E., Ellersieck, M. R., & Dowdy, R. P. (1998). Investigating relationships between nutritional knowledge, attitudes and beliefs, and dietary adequacy of the elderly. *Journal of Nutrition for the Elderly, 17* (4), 35-52.

Janus, S. C., & Janus, C. L. (1993). *The Janus report on sexual behavior.* New York: John Wiley & Sons.

Judge, J. O. (1993). Exercise programs for older persons: Writing an exercise prescription. *Connecticut Medicine, 57* (5), 269-275.

Kain, C. D., Reilly, N., & Schultz, E. D. (1990). The older adult: A comparative assessment. *Nursing Clinics of North America, 25* (12), 833-848.

Katz, W. A., & Sherman, C. (1998). Exercise is medicine. Osteoporosis: The role of exercise in optimal management. *The Physician and Sportsmedicine, 26,* 39-42.

Keating, S. B. (1995). Health promotion and disease prevention in home care. *Geriatric Nursing 16* (4), 184-186.

Keithley, J. K. (1996). Geriatrics. In K. A. Hennessy, & M. E. Orr, *Nutrition support nursing* (3rd ed.). Silver Spring, MD: American Society for Parenteral and Enteral Nutrition.

Kelly, S. (2000). Grandparents raising grandchildren. In J. Fitzpatrick, T. Fulmer, M. Wallace, & E. Flaherty, *Geriatric nursing research digest* (pp. 20-24). New York: Springer.

Knight, J. A. (Jan-Feb, 1995). The process and theories of aging. *Annals of Clinical & Laboratory Science, 25* (1): 1-12.

Koenig, H. G., George, L. K., & Peterson, B. L. (1998). Religiosity and remission of depression in medically ill older patients. *American Journal of Psychiatry, 155* (4), 536-542.

Kolcabar, K., & Wykle, M. (1994). Health promotion in long-term care facilities. *Geriatric Nursing, 15* (5), 266-269.

Kostyk, D., Lindblom, L., Fuchs, D., Tabisz, E., & Jacyk, W. R. (1994). Chemical dependency in the elderly: treatment phase. *Journal of Geriatric Social Work, 22* (1-2), 175-191.

Krall, E. A., & Dawson-Huges, B. (1994). Walking is related to bone density and rates of bone loss. *The American Journal of Medicine, 96,* 20-26.

Kyriazis, M. (1994). Age and reason. *Nursing Times,* 90 (18), 61-63.

Lacroix, A. Z., Leveille, S. G., Hecht, J. A., Grothaus, L. C., & Wagner, E. H. (1996). Does walking decrease the risk of cardiovascular disease hospitalizations and death in older adults? . . . including commentary by Wittinger, W. H. Jr. *Journal of the American Geriatric Society, 44*(2), 113-120, 207-208.

Libow, L., & Sherman, F. (1981). *The care of geriatric medicine.* St. Louis: Mosby.

Lueckenotte, A. G., (1996). *Gerontologic nursing.* St. Louis: Mosby.

MacDonald, M., Remus, G., & Laing, G. (1994). The link between housing and health in the elderly. *Journal of Gerontological Nursing, 20* (7), 5-10.

Mackel, C. L., Sheehy, C. M., & Badger, T. A. (1994). The challenge of detection and management of alcohol abuse among elderly. *Clinical Nurse Specialist,* 8 (3), 128-135.

Marsiglio, W., & Donnelly, D. (1991). Sexual relations in later life: A study of named persons. *Journal of Gerontology, 16,* S338-S344.

McMahon, A. L. (1993). Substance abuse among the elderly. *Nurse Practitioner Forum, 4* (4), 231-238.

McMahon, M., & Rhudick, P. (1961). Reminiscence. *Archives of General Psychiatry, 10,* 292-298.

Miceli, D. L. G. (1996). Sleep and activity. In M. Lueckenotte, *Gerontologic nursing* (pp. 224-243). St. Louis: Mosby.

Millison, M. (1995). A review of research on spiritual care and hospice. *The Hospice Journal, 10* (4), 3-18.

Minors, D., Atkinson, G., Bent, N., Rabbitt, P., & Waterhouse, J. (1998). The effects of age upon some aspects of lifestyle and implications for studies on circadian rhythmicity. *Age and Ageing 27,* 67-72.

Mitchell, R. B., Gingrich, D., & Jones, R. L. (1994). The biology of aging. *Journal of the American Academy of Physician Assistants, 7* (3), 210-216.

Monk, T. H., Buysse, D. J., Reynolds, C. F., Jarrett, D. B., & Kupfer, D. J. (1992). Rhythmic versus homeostatic influences on mood, activation and performance in the young and old men. *Journal of Gerontology, 47* (4), 221-227.

Moos, R., & Billings, A. (1986). Conceptualizing and measuring coping resources and processes. In L. Goldberger, & S. Breynitz, *Handbook of stress: Theoretical and clinical perspectives.* New York: Free Press.

Morley, J. E., & Solomon, D. H. (1994). Major issues in geriatrics over the last five years. *Journal of the American Geriatric Society, 42* (2), 218-223.

Morris, L. E. H. (1996). A spiritual well-being model: Use with older women who experience depression. *Issues in Mental Health Nursing, 17,* 439-455.

Musick, M. A., Koenig, H. G., Hays, J. C., & Cohen, H. J. (1998). Religious activity and depression among community-dwelling elderly persons with cancer: The moderating effect of race. *Journal of Gerontology, 53B* (4), 218-227.

Nagler, W. (1992). The case for exercise. *Update on Aging,* 8 (1), 3.

Nugent, E. (1995). Reminiscence as a nursing intervention. *Journal of Psychosocial Nursing and Mental Health Services, 33* (11), 7-11.

Nystrom, A. E. M. (1995). The concept of cogiation. *Journal of Advance Nursing, 21,* 364-370.

Osguthorpe, N. C., & Morgan, E. P. (1995). An immunization update for primary health care providers. *Nurse Practitioner, 20* (6), 52, 54, 60-65.

Ouslander, J. G. (June, 2000). Incontinence management in LTC. *Annals of Long-Term Care,* 8 (6), 35-41.

Pobursky, J. (May/June, 1995). Prostate cancer: Detection and treatment options. *Today's OR Nurse, 17* (3), 5-9.

Resnik, N. M. (1997). *Geriatric medicine in current medical diagnosis and treatment.* Norwalk, CT: Lang.

Rosenkoetter, M. (2000). Retirement. In J. Fitzpatrick, T. Fulmer, M. Wallace, & E. Flaherty, *Geriatric nursing research digest* (pp. 34-37). New York: Springer.

Ruffing-Rahal, M. A. (1991). Rationale and design for health promotion with older adults. *Public Health Nurse, 8* (4), 258-263.

Schmall, V. L. (1996). Family influences. In A. G. Lueckenotte, *Geronotologic nursing*. St. Louis: Mosby, 136-166.

Shelkey, M. (2000). Cognitive impairment. In J. Fitzpatrick, T. Fulmer, M. Wallace, & E. Flaherty, *Geriatric nursing research digest* (pp. 325-333). New York: Springer.

Siegel, P. A., Brackbill, R. M., & Heath, G. W. (1995). The epidemiology of walking for exercise: Implications for promoting activity among sedentary groups. *American Journal of Public Health, 85* (5), 706-710.

Social Security Administration (1998). Table 1. C3.-OASDI benefits: Number and average amount of retired-worker benefits in current-payment status with and without reduction for early retirement, by sex, 1993-1997. *Social Security Bulletin, 61*, 80.

Soltys, F. G., & Coats, L. (1994). The SolCos model: Facilitating reminiscence therapy. *Journal of Gerontological Nursing, 20*, 11-16.

Stamford, B. (1994). Making a splash. *The Physician and Sportsmedicine, 22* (6), 105-106.

Stephens, T., & Capersen, C. J. (1994). The demography of physical activity. In C. Bouchard, R. J. Shephard, & T. Stephens, *Physical activity, fitness and health*. Champaign, IL: Human Kinetics.

Stevens, J. A., Hasbrouck, L. M., Durant, T. M., Dellinger, A. M., Batabyal, P. K., Crosby, A. E., Valluru, B. R., Kresnow, M., & Guerrero, J. L. (1999). *Surveillance for injuries and violence among older adults* [On-line]. Available: http://www.cdc.gov/epo/mmwr/preview/mmwrhtml/ss4808a3.htm.

Stolley, J. M., & Koenig, H. G. (1997). Religion/spirituality and health among elderly African Americans and Hispanics. *Journal of Psychosocial Nursing, 35* (11), 32-38, 45-46.

Timmreck, T. C., & Randolph, J. F. (1993). Smoking cessation: Clinical steps to improve compliance. *Geriatrics, 48* (4), 69-70.

Tinnetti, M. (1997). Falls. In C. Cassell, *Geriatric medicine* (3rd ed., pp. 787-799). New York: Springer.

Turvey, C. L., Schultz, S., Arndt, S., Wallace, R. B., & Herzog, R. (2000). Memory complaint in a community sample aged 70 and older. *Journal of the American Geriatrics Society, 48* (11), 1435-1441.

U.S. Department of Commerce, Bureau of Census. (1999). *Statistical abstracts of the United States: National data book* (119th ed.). Washington, DC: U.S. Government Printing Office.

U.S. Department of Health and Human Services. (2000). *Healthy people 2010: National health promotion and disease prevention objectives*. Washington, DC: U.S. Government Printing Office. Available: http://www.health.gov/healthypeople.

Walker, N. V. (1993). Commentary on substance abuse among the elderly. *Nurse Practitioner Forum 4* (4), 231-238.

Wallace, M. (1994). The sundown syndrome. *Geriatric Nursing, 15* (3), 164-166.

Wallace, M. (2000). Sexuality and intimacy. In A.G. Lueckenotte, *Gerontologic nursing* (pp. 244-256). St. Louis: Mosby.

Weinrich, S. P., & Boyd, M. (1992). Education in the elderly: Adapting and evaluating teaching tools. *Journal of Gerontological Nursing, 18* (1), 15-20.

Wetle, T. (1982). *Handbook of geriatric care*. East Hanover, NJ: Sandoz.

Wykle, M. L., & Zauszniewski, J. (2000). Depression In J. Fitzpatrick, T. Fulmer, M. Wallace & E. Flaherty, Geriatric nursing research digest (pp. 199-204) New York: Springer.

Yesavage, J., Brink, T., Rose, T., Lum, O., Huang, V., Adey, M., & Leirer, V. (1983). Development and validation of a geriatric depression screening scale: A preliminary report. *Journal of Psychiatric Research, 17*, 37-49.

Zimmerman, R. K., & Clover, R. D. (1995). Adult immunizations: A practical approach for clinicians. *American Family Physician, 51* (4), 859-1147.

Zorn, C. R., & Johnson, M. T. (1997). Religious well-being in noninstitutionalized elderly women. *Health Care for Women International, 18* (3), 209-219.

Unit Five

Challenges As We Enter the New Millennium

25 Health Promotion in the Twenty-First Century: Throughout the Lifespan and Throughout the World

Chapter 25

KATHLEEN HUTTLINGER
CAROL LYNN MANDLE

Health Promotion in the Twenty-First Century: Throughout the Lifespan and Throughout the World

objectives

After completing this chapter, the nurse will be able to:

- Identify global trends and directions for health promotion and disease prevention.
- Discuss the values, goals, and targets of *Health for All* in the twenty-first century.
- Describe major health-promotion priorities for 2000 through 2010 that influence nursing practice, research, and health care policy.
- Summarize activities across public and private sectors that reflect the *Healthy People 2010* objectives.

key terms

Advocate
Ecological Model
Health for All
Ottawa Charter
Vulnerable Populations
World Health Organization

THINK About It

Nancy

Nancy is a fourth-year nursing student at the university and is completing her final clinical rotation in the emergency department at a local community hospital in a rural area in the South. She has been at this facility for a month and has been assigned to the 3:00 PM to 11:00 PM shift. Nancy has been amazed at the number of people who come to the emergency room for care for nonemergency illnesses. The vast majority of these people also do not appear to have a regular doctor or a means to pay for the hospital's services. Nancy has been struck by the number of people who exhibit poor health habits in terms of preventive activities, such as following a healthy diet, avoiding tobacco products, and getting adequate exercise. When discussing these concerns with the nursing staff, Nancy was told that many of the people who come to the emergency department wait until they are sick because, even when they are working, many cannot afford health insurance.

1. What activities can nurses do to be involved in policy decisions that assist people in making basic health improvements, including health-promotion and disease-prevention activities?
2. How are nurses able to influence health perceptions and practices of individuals, families, communities, and groups?

A number of changes have occurred at world and national levels over the last 30 years that have supported and encouraged more global and comprehensive approaches to health promotion and disease prevention. Many of these changes have focused on and assisted individuals and local communities in identifying their health-care needs. The ability to deal directly with people by providing information and technical assistance, at both personal and community levels, is a necessary approach to establishing good health and is vital to health promotion and all forms of prevention activities. The challenge that faces the health care community in the new millennium is for health care professionals, consumers, and communities to develop collaborative skills that foster partnerships with each other, which will allow all people and communities to make informed decisions about health and health care.

Since World War II, people throughout the world have experienced globalization-complex; that is, interrelated economic, political, social, and cultural processes (Berlinguer, 1999; Henry, 1998; Yach & Bettcher, 1998a, 1998b). A variety of changes at national and international levels have also proposed, encouraged, and supported more comprehensive and global approaches to health promotion.

As discussed in Chapters 1, 2, and 3 of this book, the most significant development to promote health in the second half of the twentieth century was the creation of the **World Health Organization,** an international agency founded immediately following World War II to promote health around the world. In defining health as a state of complete physical, mental, and social well being and not merely the absence of disease or infirmity, the founders of the constitution of the World Health Organization transformed the definitions for health throughout the world. Furthermore, the writers stated "The health of all people is fundamental to the attainment of peace and security and is dependent upon the fullest cooperation of individuals and states" (World Health Organization, 1998b, p. 4). This effort has been the world's challenge for over 50 years and continues as the twenty-first century begins.

This challenge requires individuals, families, groups, health care professionals, communities, and nations to develop collaborative skills that foster partnerships with each other, which will allow all people to make informed decisions about health and health care, including the many related processes.

Many examples of national and worldwide achievements illustrate this effort, such as women's health programs for disease prevention and health care, issues involving social health, networking projects that facilitate early detection and intervention with acquired immunodeficiency syndrome (AIDS), and child immunization projects (World Health Organization, 2000). However, many government-sponsored programs throughout the world have experienced setbacks, economic shortfalls, and disappointments because of economic rationing, lack of available technology, and marketing schemes that fall short of delivery.

In reshaping the national and the world's health care systems, questions arise, such as, "Can health outcomes be purchased from competing providers?" "Can communities combine their resources to act as providers of health promotion?" "Can the economic and technological environments mix community interest with an individualized customer approach in delivering health care as a commodity?" "How can future health care practitioners combine holistic views with the health marketplace to improve health?"

As a profession, nursing has enjoyed a long-standing interest and focus on health-promotion activities throughout the lifespan and has the reputation of serving as advocates for individuals, families, and communities. Recognition as an **advocate,** a person who supports and pleads for another, has served nursing well by providing opportunities for giving educational guidance and counseling in both institutional and community settings. In fact, education and teaching are considered an integral part of nursing's role (American Association of Colleges of Nursing, 1998).

The increased need for health-promotion and disease-prevention activities nationally and worldwide has generated many employment opportunities in the public and private sectors for a variety of health care workers, including nurses. Opportunities exist for teaching personal wellness at workplaces, advising national and local governments, and consulting with hospitals, schools, and health insurers (Catford & St. Leger, 1996). In doing so, health promotion and disease prevention has moved from the single realm of health education to modern health-policy-driven programs.

Nurses are in a significantly unique position among all health care professionals to act on the opportunities for promoting health care activities. With an enduring emphasis on health promotion and disease prevention, nurses function in a variety of roles, including primary health care practitioner, health advocate and enabler, educator, and researcher. Therefore nurses are critical links in the health care delivery system and function as change agents in the achievement of health for all in the new millennium (World Health Organization, 2000).

This chapter provides a description of national and international trends in health promotion and specifically revisits the philosophies, goals, and strategies of the World Health Organization's ***Health for All*** and the *Healthy People* initiatives from the U.S. Department of Health and Human Services. Examples of health problems and national health-promotion programs developed by many other countries around the world are also described. Examples of the many roles of nurses in health promotion in the next millennium are discussed from the dimensions of policy development and the advancement of practice, education, and research at both national and international levels. Nurses are challenged to provide experiences, vision, and leaderships to fulfill the goals of health for all.

HEALTH PROMOTION: PAST DEVELOPMENTS AND FUTURE DIRECTIONS

Although the world aspires to achieve health for all through health-advancing strategies, many challenges lie ahead. For example, although health promotion and disease prevention are now considered global terms, they are frequently misused, with the inherent values distorted (Lamarche, 1995; Lefebvre, 1996).

When considering future directions in health promotion and disease prevention, reviewing past achievements can be useful. During the 1950s, 1960s, and into the early 1970s the focus of many health-promotion activities was on the control and prevention of communicable diseases. This goal was achieved though mass immunization and education programs that emphasized major preventive and health-protection strategies. In the 1970s, tackling preventable diseases and reducing premature death and risky health behaviors through early identification and education formed a key strategy in many countries. Most noteworthy was the initiation of the goal *Health for All,* the health-promotion goal of the World Health Organization's strategies around the world (1978).

The decade of the 1980s saw the first U.S. Surgeon General's Report on Health Promotion and Disease Prevention (1981). Subsequently, the World Health Organization's European regional office published *Targets for Health for All* in 1985 and reissued this document in 1991 following input from representatives from many European countries. In 1988, Australia published its first set of national health goals and targets also based on the U.S. model. In addition to national objectives, countries such as Australia and the United States have encouraged their states and communities to develop objectives that are compatible with the national goals, but more specific to regional needs (U.S. Department of Health and Human Services, 2000).

Another worldwide event occurred in the 1980s that set the agenda for health promotion. A meeting was held in Ottawa, Canada in 1986 (World Health Organization, 1986) that was attended by health leaders from around the world. The outcome of this meeting was a set of health-promotion guidelines that can be used worldwide, known as the **Ottawa Charter.** A new health paradigm emerged with an increased focus on determinants and prerequisites outside the health care realm, such as adequate income, employment, housing, food, education, and a safe social and physical environment for health development. One example of the worldwide influence of this conference and charter was the International Conference for Health Promotion in Colombia in 1992 and the adoption of the 1993 Caribbean Charter for Health Promotion (Pommier, Deschamps, Romero, & Zubarew, 1997).

During the 1990s, the importance of reaching people through various settings and sectors, such as schools, cities, hospitals, and workplaces, and the development of needs-based programs, was initiated in many countries, including Canada, Australia, and the United States (Catford & St. Leger, 1996; Tsouros, 1996), and by the World Health Organization (1991; 1995; 1998).

The new millennium brings a need to sustain the momentum and add another dimension to health promotion and disease prevention. From a narrow point of view of disease control and prevention, health care delivery throughout the world has developed a broader agenda for health, wellness, and welfare. In the wake of massive demographic and social changes in global trade, migration, urbanization, transportation, and collaboration between countries in sharing and redistributing knowledge, a new health perspective must certainly be part of the vision (Huttlinger, 2000). For example, an unprecedented growth has occurred in the number of older adults in both developed and underdeveloped countries. "The total aged population (greater than 60 years old) worldwide will rise from 605 million in the year 2000 to 1.2 billion in 2025" (Kalache & Keller, 2000, p.33) because of longevity and decreased fertility. This one demographic example demonstrates the significant consequences that include shifts from infectious diseases to chronic diseases resulting in intergenerational, social, economic, cultural, health, and ethical challenges, to name only a few (Howson, 2000; Cohen, 2000; Kalache & Keller, 2000).

GLOBAL STRATEGY OF HEALTH FOR ALL

Health for All

As discussed, the World Health Organization has developed a series of global health initiatives to fulfill the goal of *Health for All* (1978, 1986, 1995, 1998a, 1998b) These initiatives continue to include "the right of all people to a standard of living adequate for health and well being, including the right to adequate food, water, clothing, housing, health care, education, reproductive health, and social services; and the right to security in the event of unemployment, sickness, disability, old age, or lack of livelihood in circumstances beyond an individual's control. Respect for human rights and the achievement of public health goals are complementary" (World Health Organization, 1998a, p. 3). *Health for All* continues to be a call for social justice, enabling all individuals to live economically and socially productive lives. Additionally, analytics of the World Bank recommend that governments invest in the health of the socially weak because decreases in the differences of income, in addition to strengthening of various forms of social cohesion, civic solidarity, legitimate equality, and ethical justice, can substantially improve the health status of populations and social conciliation" (Zacek, 2000, p. 163). More specifically, the World Health Organization proposes in its new program for Europe (*21 Goals for the 21st Century*) that "health status differences among the European states should diminish by one third by 2020" (Zacek, 2000, p. 163). "Furthermore *Health for All* acknowledges the uniqueness of each person and the need to respond to each individual's spiritual quest for meaning, purpose and belonging" (World Health Organization 1998b, p. 4).

Based on these values, *Health for All* proposes the following goals: (1) to provide the highest attainable standard of health as a fundamental right; (2) to strengthen the application of ethics to health policy, research, and service provision; (3) to implement equity-oriented policies and strategies that emphasize solidarity; and (4) to incorporate a gender perspective into health policies and strategies (World Health Organization, 1998a). From these goals, 10 global health targets have been prioritized (Box 25-1).

On May 16, 1998 the *World Health Declaration* was annexed to the constitution of the World Health Organization. The major components are described in Box 25-2.

Health Care Systems

Although a variety of health care strategies have been established and progress has been made in improving health and quality of life (decreased maternal and infant mortality rates, improved sanitation and drinking water, increased immunizations) (Brundtland, 2000; World Health Organization, 1995), great disparities and inequities continue to exist. More poignant are the injustices within the allocations of resources in industrialized countries. For example, although a wide variety of health-promotion strategies have been instituted in most industrialized countries, technology and expensive health care modalities appear to be the dominant and prevailing paradigm. Despite the evidence that health status cannot be determined by increasing health care resources (infrastructure and work force), for example, a large part of the U.S. health care budget has been used to provide expensive health care services and, in many cases, for only a few people. In this approach, emphasis is not given to other influences such as poverty, education, environment, and social well being. Additionally, a recent trend is the increasing privatization of health care with profit as the goal (Henry, 1998; Yach & Bettcher, 1998a, 1998b; Berlinguer, 1999; Navarro, 1999). In contrast to the industrialized countries, health-promotion initiatives throughout the world have emphasized the importance of ensuring financial and geographical access to health-promotion services and has become the preferred way to improve a population's health (Hassmiller, 2000).

Unfortunately, even in countries with universal access to health care, such as Canada, the following is evident:

- Health care expenditure has grown four to five times faster than the country's collective wealth. In contrast, in the United States, which does not have universal access, spending on health care reached 13.9% of the gross national product in 2000 (Mauer, 2000).
- Social health problems such as AIDS, single-parent families, and the growing number of elderly and minority population groups lead to increasing health care management problems.
- The diminishing effect of health care on health has been clear, because major indexes, such as life expectancy at birth, are not related to investment in health care.

In addition to actual costs of health care delivery services, the value of services being offered at cost is being

Box 25-1 *Health for All* Global Health: Targets for the Twenty-First Century

- Health equity: childhood stunting
- Survival: maternal mortality rates, childhood mortality rates, life expectancy
- Reverse global trends of five major pandemics: malaria, AIDS, tuberculosis, hepatitis, and influenza
- Eradicate and eliminate certain diseases (diseases related to malnutrition)
- Improve access to water, sanitation, food, and shelter
- Measures to promote health
- Develop, implement, and monitor national *Health for All* policies
- Improve access to comprehensive, essential, quality health care
- Implement global and national health information and surveillance systems
- Support research for health

From World Health Organization. (1998). *Health for all in the 21st century*. Geneva, Switzerland: The Organization.

Box 25-2 Major Components of the World Health Declaration Annexed to the World Health Organization Constitution, May 16, 1998

I affirmation (a) of the dignity and worth of every person, (b) that health is a fundamental right of every person, (c) the equal rights, equal duties, and shared responsibilities of all for health

II improvement of health is the ultimate aim of social and economic development by reducing social and economic inequities through commitment to equity, solidarity, and social justice and incorporation of a gender perspective

III strengthening, adapting, and reforming health systems, including the essentials of primary health care

IV in all nations, communities, families, and individual are interdependent

V full participation and partnership by all member states

questioned in many countries and must be rigorously debated. Historically, the nursing profession has helped the cost of delivery by serving as primary care providers for the urban poor and rural dwellers. In doing so, nurses have rendered a preventive-focused and individualized sickness-care service at low cost. The same initiative must now be taken in improving the health status of populations by promoting cooperation with other disciplines and encouraging them to be active participants in the provision of health care services for the more inaccessible populations.

New Public Health Movement

As noted, the *Ottawa Charter* (World Health Organization, 1986) is a major landmark for health promotion throughout the world that influences public health policy and initiatives in many countries. A growing movement toward redefining and resurrecting ideas that once formed the traditions of public health, but appeared to be forgotten serves as evidence of this trend. The initiative refocuses health and retrieves some of the most important basic elements of public health, including links to health promotion and disease prevention, that highlights a new way of considering health as one in which a sense that health is to be considered a human right, an investment in society, and a resource for everyday living (Kickbush, 1989; Thompson & Stachenko, 1994; O'Byrne, 2000).

Legge (1991), a critic of the old, or pre-*Ottawa Charter*, version of public health, asserts that a knowledge-action gap exists and that an important assumption that knowledge of health promotion and disease prevention must be made as a precondition before a behavior change is made. Additionally, according to Legge, the old public health system failed to provide guiding frameworks for health care interventions in which the inequalities of health care were addressed. The new public health effort shifts the focus from behavior change to healthy public policy and community empowerment.

Ecological Foundations of Health Promotion

One conceptual framework that has been advanced to assist the understanding of health promotion and disease prevention is the **ecological model** (Kulbok, 1985; Heiss & Walden, 2000). An ecological perspective or model has been one of the approaches used in public health theory, and many believe that this approach is central to understanding public health issues and concerns, including health promotion and disease prevention. The model describes health as a product of the interdependence between individuals and the subsystems of ecosystems, and it assumes a connectedness among human beings, their physical and social environment, and their health (Brown, 1992; Chu, 1994; Heiss & Walden, 2000). Therefore the thrust of action-oriented ecological health promotion is population-based approaches, such as healthy public policies and the integration of environment and health through interdisciplinary collaboration (Green, Richard, & Potvin, 1998). Brown (1992) has identified four major areas within the model that have health-promotion implications: equity, sustainability, conviviality, and preservation of the global environment. Ecological health promotion points to the role of various determinants of health, economic, and social conditions to assist people, for example, who are engaging in behaviors that are conducive to health.

Goals and Targets for Health Promotion

The concept of health for all by the year 2010 has proved attractive to nations that are committed to tackling the marked disparities in health status and access to health services and those that are interested in refocusing attention on social and economic determinants of health, including improving performance measures for all health systems (World Health Organization, 2000; Musich, Adams, & Edington, 2000). Goals and targets have been considered to be statements of direction and intent in relation to health, such as a specified percentage reduction in deaths because of cardiovascular disease or change in the social, economic, and physical environment by a certain year. The United States was the first country to develop goals and objectives in a comprehensive format in a document entitled *Promoting Health, Preventing Disease: Objectives for the Nation* (U.S. Department of Health and Human Services, 1990). During the same period, the health-for-all strategy focused on setting goals and targets that became the blueprint for all World Health Organization member nations. The framework proved to be a valuable resource for planning health-promotion programs and setting targets. However, different approaches for defining targets and differing strategies for achieving these goals have been adopted (Thompson & Stachenko, 1994). European countries accepted a common approach to health policy and grouped targets around four major issues: (1) lifestyle and health, (2) risk factors affecting health and the environment, (3) reorientation of the health care system, and (4) infrastructure support to implement changes (World Health Organization, 1985; Dekker, 2000; Zacek, 2000; Visschedijk & Simeant, 1998).

The Australian Report, *Health for All Australians* (Health Targets and Implementation Committee, 1988), was compiled to improve health and reduce inequalities in health status. This document was the result of a penetrating analysis of the Better Health Commission (1986) and contained a series of recommendations on priorities for national action. This effort led to the development of better health programs, with funding to establish programs with a focus on five major priority areas: (1) preventable cancers, (2) hypertension, (3) nutrition, (4) injury prevention, and (5) the health of elderly adults (Better Health Commission, 1986). These programs were reevaluated during the 1990s and most recently in 1998 (Farrell, 1998). The reviews indicated that an understanding of the social and environmental determinants of health is required to achieve greater equity and that the role of the mainstream health system must be articulated more clearly (Commonwealth Department of Health, Housing, and Community Services, 1993). Four groups of health targets were selected after a review in 1994: (1) preventable mortality and morbidity, (2) healthy lifestyles and risk factors, (3) health literacy and health skills, and (4) healthy environments. Principles of health promotion have been built into major national health strategies and programs in Australia, such as mental health, rural health, and the divisions of general practice (Farrell, 1998; Smith, 2000).

Other countries, such as New Zealand, England, Wales, and the United States, have also developed targets to raise the overall status of health. To evaluate progress, monitoring systems and accountability measures have been established for the use of resources and for achieving health care outcomes (Nutbeam, 1993). Conversely, Canada has developed a collaborative strategy in a partnership with interdisciplinary and intersectoral groups of many health professionals, including the Canadian Nurses Association. The strategy, known as "enhancing prevention practices of health professionals," involves a partnership-building process that uses networks to stimulate change to promote the concepts of participation, empowerment, and ownership of programs by the communities, thereby encouraging local action around health problems (Thompson & Stanchenko, 1994). Many other approaches to assessment and planning have been occurring in other countries, such as Brazil (Degani, 1999) and Jamaica (Figueroa, 1998).

The United States adopted a "life stage" approach to analyzing the health status of Americans and identified 15 priority issues using a "management by objectives" planning model (U.S. Department of Health and Human Services, 1990). A recent progress review in 1998 indicated a significant improvement, particularly with regard to infants and children (U.S. Preventive Services Task Force, 1996). The review indicated positive changes in human immunodeficiency virus (HIV) and AIDS control, but showed poor health in minority groups (U.S. Department of Health and Human Services, 1998). Additionally, in 1991 the American Public Health Association established criteria for the development of health promotion and education that offered five standards for program design and implementation, which remain a major focus for the organization today as well (Lissi, 2000). These standards indicated that a program should do the following:

1. Address one or more risk factors that are carefully defined, measurable, modifiable, and prevalent among the members of the target group.
2. Address special characteristics, needs, and preferences of the target group.
3. Include interventions that will effectively reduce a targeted risk factor.
4. Select interventions that make optimal use of available resources.
5. Select a program design that ensures continued operation and the ability to evaluate it.

Higgins and Green (1994) used these criteria for case analysis of four *Healthy Communities* projects in British Columbia, Canada, concluding that the American Public Health Association criteria would disqualify most of the *Healthy Communities* projects as worthy because the majority of these projects lack modifiable risk-factor targets of known epidemiological importance to health outcomes or interventions that effectively reduce the risks of evaluation.

Health Rather Than Health Care As a Starting Point

In 1974 the Canadian *Lalonde Report* (Department of National Health and Welfare, 1974) promoted the concepts of lifestyle and environment as two major determinants of health, leading to health-promotion programs. Following this report and the *Ottawa Charter* implementation, many initiatives were undertaken around the world that investigated the nature of funding disparities and service reimbursement (Smith, 2000).

Answers about social environment, human biology, and health care spending may lead to balance spending on health and health care policy and programs. Some industrialized countries, such as Denmark and Sweden, have changed "the mix" by balancing health care spending and health-promotion and disease-prevention spending (Musich, Adams, & Edington, 2000). The United States has continued to focus on health care alone, with an emphasis on health risks and disease-prevention strategies (U.S. Department of Health and Human Services, 2000; Catford & St. Leger, 1996).

Nursing's focus on disease prevention and health promotion is based on a tradition of providing holistic care to people in a variety of health care settings. Nursing is a profession that prides itself in considering all aspects of the social, physical, and spiritual domains rather than focusing on simply an individual's health status within the prevalent health care paradigm. This view is coherent and in step with a rapidly changing health care environment that is not confined to health care agencies and institutions. Although a majority of nurses are still employed in institutional care settings, many are seeking more nontraditional roles in many different community settings, such as in schools, in parish nursing programs, nurse-run clinics, and so on (Smith & Mauer, 2000).

Healthy lifestyles and risk factors, quality-of-life indicators, healthy environment, development of health literacy, and life skills link with the target group and relate to specific determinants and health-promotion strategies. However, addressing the social perspective within community and individual approaches is also important for the new millennium.

REFORM OF HEALTH PROMOTION AND HEALTH CARE

Clinical Effectiveness of Preventive Health Care

The U.S. Preventive Services Task Force (1989) was the first to identify the clinical effectiveness of preventive health care. This report provided specific age-, gender-, and risk-factor recommendations for the prevention of more than 60 major causes of morbidity and mortality. The methodology of the report involved a thorough examination of the quality of scientific evidence for the effectiveness of screening tests, immunizations, and counseling interventions. *Healthy People 2010* (U.S. Department of Health and Human Services, 2000) builds on this report and the document *Healthy People 2000* and strives to increase the years of healthy life and eliminate health disparities. A relevant implication for nursing in these publications is that education and counseling are needed to change personal health behaviors long before the onset of clinical disease and that this approach is a promising means of achieving health-promotion and disease-prevention practices. The task force report that was revised in 1996 (U.S. Department of Health and Human Services, 1996) continues to advise that all health care providers and individuals assume responsibility for health promotion (see Research Highlights). This premise, naturally, assumes that an individual will become self-empowered or highly motivated to make a needed health-related change in behavior. This effort requires a constant update on a variety of skills through education (see Hot Topic box).

Recent health care reform efforts at state and national levels reflect a gradual realization that the current system is costly and is grounded in acute hospital care rather than primary and preventive health care, which are delivered most frequently in community and public health agencies. Policy makers and the American public have come to realize that the ultimate solution to the current health care dilemma is a comprehensive reform in the financing, organization, and provision of health care services within an integrated and coordinated system. The concept of equitable access to preventive care for all Americans has been nourished in recent years by the demonstrated effectiveness of preventive services in reducing premature morbidity and mortality (U.S. Preventive Services Task Force, 1989, 1996). However, despite these efforts, an equal opportunity for health-promotion and disease-preventive care remains unrealized for many citizens (Lissi, 2000).

Current estimates indicate that at least 41 million American citizens have no health coverage (U.S. Department of Commerce, 1996) and that 10 to 20 million people are without health insurance at some time during a 12-month period (Employee Benefits Research Institute, 1996). Current health care reform proposals are investigating measures to control costs while promoting quality of care (Guico-Pabia & Endsley, 2000). Additionally, legislators are closely examining the rights of consumers and ways to improve access to many underserved populations (Lissi, 2000). Another effort is aimed at evaluating managed care to determine whether these organizations can provide care to everyone while remaining profitable (Mauer, 2000).

A more clinical approach to health promotion has served its purpose for primary and secondary disease-prevention efforts. Although this approach has been of some value to educated middle-class populations, it falls

research highlights

Health-Promotion Discharge Counseling

A two-group comparative study was conducted to examine the documentation of health risk factors and health-promotion discharge counseling in medical records by physicians and nurse practitioners in an emergency department. The study examined the medical records of 305 nonacute ambulatory patients for selected risk factors, including smoking, alcohol use, elevated blood pressure, obesity, and dental caries. The results of the study indicated that 59% of the study sample had one or more risk factors, and of these, only 22% received health-promotion counseling. An analysis revealed that the nurse practitioners were slightly more likely to provide counseling for health risks than did the physicians. Additionally, many of the recommendations for health-promotion and disease-prevention counseling that were recommended in *Healthy People 2010* were not documented. All health providers in all health care settings are encouraged to identify risk factors and document their health-promotion counseling during the course of every patient encounter.

Data from Sheahan, S. L. (2000). Documentation of health risks and health promotion counseling by emergency department nurse practitioners and physicians. *Image: Journal of Nursing Scholarship, 32* (3), 245-250.

HOT topics

HEALTH PROMOTION AND PEOPLE WITH DISABILITIES

Many people with disabilities experience multiple difficulties in obtaining access to health-promotion services. This lack of access is critical in light of the fact that people with physical disabilities have a high occurrence of suffering from secondary illnesses and acute health problems. People with disabilities must be made aware of the preventive and health-promotional services that are available to them and that barriers to these service are eliminated or minimized. Nurses can play important roles in assisting disabled people, particularly because nurses are frequently the first line of contact for them. These concerns are becoming increasingly significant global issues as the world's population is becoming older.

short of meeting the needs of many medically underserved and less well-educated groups. Many people in need of health care must first realize and obtain the basic necessities of life before they can appreciate the value of and be motivated to adopt healthy lifestyle behaviors. As advocates, nurses must focus on interventions that can address some of these concerns. Nursing's long-standing support of health promotion for underserved groups can play a major role in achieving equitable access to preventive health services for all Americans (Stanhope & Lancaster, 2000).

Cost-Effectiveness of Preventive Health Care

A belief exists that prevention should be judged by whether the gains in health are a reasonable return for the costs incurred, primarily because the nation continues to endure the economic burden of preventable illness and death. The portion of the gross national product in the United States spent on health care rose from 5.3% in 1960 to 13.9% in 1999 (National Center for Health Statistics, 2000). The diagnosis and treatment of diseases, including heart disease, cancer, injuries, and HIV and AIDS, have outstripped society's ability to pay for what are essentially preventable conditions. Although compiling the cost of preventable illness and premature death is certainly possible, determining the value of health-promotion programs and dollar savings is difficult. During the last 10 years, attempts have been made to develop health-promotion indicators, standards, and health outcomes (National Center for Health Statistics, 2000).

Generally, reported outcomes have been limited to aggregates of changes in health behavior or attitudes for which the cost can be estimated for professional time, materials, and so on, but that underestimate the gains made by the communities from interventions, involving processes such as empowerment or capacity-building to exercise health-related decision making (Smith & Mauer, 2000).

The reality of skyrocketing health care expenditures has ushered in cost-effectiveness analysis as a method for determining the way in which financial resources are being use and the way in which they should be used in health care. The specific purpose of cost-effectiveness analysis is to help clinicians and policy makers focus on investments that provide the most health for the required expenditure, with outcomes reported either as a single measure (years of life saved) or as several measures combined on a single scale (quality-adjusted life years) (Feldstein, 1993). Cost-effectiveness analyses of preventive services have included screenings for lead, cholesterol, breast cancer, and cervical cancer. The fact that most counseling interventions have not been analyzed for cost-effectiveness is consistent with the finding that primary care physicians spend less than 15% of their time counseling individuals on weight reduction, cholesterol reduction, smoking cessation, and breast self-examination (Woodwell, 1989). A primary care provider survey, sponsored by the Public Health Service to track provider-related *Healthy People 2010* objectives, should help determine the nature and amount of preventive health care delivered by primary health care providers, including nurse practitioners (see Health Teaching box).

Estimates indicate that providing coverage for preventive services is likely to increase costs in the short term (Mauer, 2000). Furthermore, preventive services vary in clinical and cost-effectiveness when performed by health care providers using different guidelines and methods. Another consideration involves the differential costs per year for services that have undergone cost-effectiveness analysis, suggesting that personal and social values may influence whether a preventive intervention is judged to be cost-effective.

Because the U.S. health care delivery system has evolved with a bias toward coverage for acute illness, providing coverage for preventive services in most public and private insurance plans has been difficult. At a time of heightened attention to health care reform, preventive services of known effectiveness must be incorporated into a comprehensive benefits package for all Americans. A core set of clinical preventive services, including immunizations, screening, and counseling, was recently prepared for inclusion in an overall benefits package. These services are specified according to age- and gender-specific periodic health examinations to ensure their economic efficiency in primary care settings (Kulbok, Laffrey, & Goeppinger, 2000). However, continued focus on clinical preventive

HEALTH TEACHING Smoking Cessation

Tobacco use is a risk factor for over 25 diseases, including lung cancer, which is one of the leading causes of cancer-related mortality throughout the world. Although smoking is on the decline in the United States, the smoking rates among residents of other countries (and American adolescents and school-age children) are rising at alarming rates. School-based interventions and personal contact with this age group by nurses can assist in preventing this potentially harmful activity. Conducting a thorough assessment of tobacco use during the health intake is a necessary part of recognizing a potential harmful risk for this age group.

services is a short-term solution and cannot assist in the long-term gains of health advancement of populations.

Health Promotion and Vulnerable Populations

In 1996 approximately 40 million Americans who might have been classified as medically indigent were without health insurance. Among the people most likely to be uninsured were Blacks (21%), people with incomes below the poverty line (42%), the unemployed (36%), and people with less than 12 years of education (30%). Many of these uninsured individuals and families received care, as needed at local emergency rooms, and those people with higher incomes were more likely to receive their care through ambulatory clinical and private physician's offices. In 1999, less than 1% of Medicaid funding was directed to early and periodic screening, rural health clinics, and family planning services (National Center for Health Statistics, 2000). Little has changed since the publication of a report by the National Medical Expenditure Survey (NMES) (Agency for Health Care Policy and Research, 1991) in 1987 that indicated that persons who are uninsured or who have inadequate coverage usually forego primary and preventive health care. Additional evidence of this primary care underservice is reflected in several reports by the Robert Wood Johnson Foundation's National Access to Care surveys (1978, 1983, 1987, 1997), which identify factors associated with utilization of health care services. One survey indicated that 40 million Americans had no health care provider, clinic, or hospital as a regular source of health care, representing a 7% increase over an earlier survey. Concurrently, the percentage of people who reported having no ambulatory visit in the prior 12 months rose significantly, from 19% to 33%. Underserved populations were affected disproportionately, with a significantly higher percentage of poor, uninsured, and ethnic minority individuals reporting no regular source of care, no ambulatory visits within the preceding 12 months, and fair or poor health status. Other indicators, such as high infant mortality rate, illnesses related to poor diet, inadequate housing, and lack of other basic necessities of life, are evident among the vulnerable groups (Agency for Health Care Policy and Research, 1991; U.S. Department of Health and Human Services, 2000) (see Case Study).

Groups are referred to as disadvantaged, at-risk, or vulnerable *minorities* who represent those with socioeconomic vulnerability factors that may include poverty, lack of education, and homelessness. Other vulnerable groups include people who have age-related vulnerability and include the youth, pregnant adolescents, and frail elderly (Aday, 1997). Providing a "band-aid" service when the needs are much greater constantly frustrates nurses. Questions may be raised as to whether the needs are adequately addressed and whether greater health risks, limited control, disenfranchisement, victimization, disadvantaged status, and powerlessness are ever understood when dealing with people's vulnerability.

Among all age groups, older adults and homeless people represent those who are most in need of clinical preventive services to offset disabling and life-threatening conditions (Aday, 1997). Examples of conditions in these people, which are frequently overlooked by clinicians, include numerous types of chronic infections, skin conditions, trauma, and malnutrition (Weinreb, 1998). McMurry (1994) contends that these groups need uplifts through nurses' mediation, social advocacy, supportive environments, political advocacy, and professional advocacy.

For some **vulnerable populations,** unstable or dangerous physical environments, isolation, and the lack of adequate and available health services exacerbate the already high rates of preventable illness and death. Perhaps for no other group is the convergence of economic hardship, social isolation, and physical and mental disability more apparent than for homeless individuals and families. For example, a report from the Institute of Medicine (1988) entitled *Homelessness, Health, and Human Needs,* revealed that families with young children were one of the fastest-growing groups among the American homeless. Since this publication, more recent data state that families with children comprise 36.5% of the homeless population; single men comprise 46%, single women 14%, and adolescents 3.5% (Waxman & Henderliter, 1996).

CASE STUDY

Derek

Derek is a 4-year-old Haitian-American boy who was brought to a rural health department clinic by his grandmother. Derek and his family are recent immigrants from Haiti, having lived in this area for less than 2 years. Derek has received all of his care since coming to the United States at the clinic and is up to date on his immunizations. His last visit to the clinic was 6 months ago when his grandmother brought him in with a low-grade fever and diarrhea. The problems were resolved and the clinic nurse discussed basic child care and health-promotion activities with his grandmother, including nutrition. For the past month, Derek has been attending preschool for the first time. Derek lives with his grandmother, a 14-year-old cousin, his 19-year-old mother, and 2-year-old brother. Derek's grandmother is concerned that Derek has been wetting the bed 2 out of 7 nights a week for the last 3 weeks and appears less interested in food than he was at the time of his last visit.

1. Given Derek's age and social situation, what types of health-promotion information might you want to make certain to discuss with Derek's grandmother?
2. What type of nutritional guidance should be shared with his grandmother?
3. What are some possible explanations for the bed wetting?

IMPLICATIONS OF NURSING LEADERSHIP IN HEALTH PROMOTION

Implications for Policy Development

The health-promotion priorities that have been presented in this chapter pose an interesting challenge for all nurses. This is an opportunistic time for nurses, as individuals and as a profession, to play a key role in a health system that must emphasize health promotion and disease prevention. Because nurses have long believed in and practiced the principles of primary prevention, their leadership and participation in health-promotion policy development is critical during an upcoming era that might bring dramatic changes in health care reform (Gullotta, 2000). Through a perspective on the development of community-based, health-promotion programs, nurses can bring a balance to decisions that will be made about the appropriate use of health care resources. In 1981, the World Health Organization presented a challenge of health for all by the year 2000 to nurses throughout the world through its proposal that nurses consolidate their resources and become a powerful influence in the world's health (World Health Organization, 1981). The report asserts that overall responses by nurses have been fragmented, sporadic, planned, inadequate, and coordinated, involving relatively few nurses practicing beyond their limited clinical paradigms. Since that time, new directions for nurses have been established at the World Health Organization (2000) that involve nurses in roles that incorporate the ability to affect social differences in terms of poverty, population displacement from rural to urban areas, and epidemiological and demographic transitions resulting in a growing number of elderly people (see Multicultural Awareness box).

MULTICULTURAL AWARENESS

Health and Health Promotion in a Native American Tribe: The Navajo

The Navajo people of the *Dine' Bike'yah* live on a vast land on which the four states of Arizona, Utah, New Mexico and Colorado intersect. The *Dine'* hold this land as sacred and as an integral part of their lives. The Navajo believe that health is a part of the *Hozho'*, which is a personal sense of well being and rightness with the world and is all inclusive. For the Navajo, health is not separate from the overall state of balance between the body, mind, spirit and the surrounding environment. When one of these is out of balance, *Hozho'* is not achieved. *Hozho'* is everything that a Navajo thinks of as being good, in terms of good and evil or favorable and unfavorable. The Navajo strive to maintain *Hozho'* and to live in harmony with all things that surround them. The goal of Navajo life in this world is to live to attain maturity with *Hozho'* and to die of old age, the result of which incorporates beauty, harmony, and happiness or *sa'ah naagha'ii bik'eh hozho'*. When the body, spirit, or mind fall out of *Hozho'*, a traditional healer or medicine man is sought. In many instances, the medicine man recommends that the individual seek Western Medicine and the traditional ways to cure the problem.

Since 1955, trends in Navajo health have demonstrated a progressive improvement, particularly in the areas of maternal and infant mortality. However, on the increase are lifestyle-related diseases and premature deaths for which health-promotion activities can have an effect. Among these lifestyle-related diseases include adult-onset diabetes, AIDS, and alcohol and substance abuse. Health care providers who work with the Navajo must address all health-promotion and disease-prevention activities in terms of an appreciation for the cultural and economic realities and the needs of this community.

Implications for Practice

Nurses have been challenged to use their capacity to bring about positive health gains. The preventive services delivered by nurses, including efforts such as health assessment, screening, and counseling, are necessary tools to empower individuals to promote and maintain optimal health and well being. Achieving the U.S. 2010 objectives is possible only by a comprehensive implementation of health-promotion activities at the community level, including work sites, schools, homes, and neighborhood settings. In collaboration with other professional and business groups, nurses can educate and empower individuals, families, and communities to become active participants in defining their health needs, in making informed decisions to meet these needs, and ultimately, in bringing about improvements in health status and quality of life. New models must be generated (Howson, 2000; Gebre-Medhim & Wekell, 1999), such as with creative inventions (telemedicine) to meet these complex needs (Hetherington, 1998).

Additionally, because individuals will be increasingly responsible for their own health, they will need access to quality information that has not been readily available in the past. For example, Marine et al. (1998) have developed *Net Wellness*, an electronic consumer health information service to provide the best possible health information to the broadest possible populations.

Implications for Education

The demand for primary health care providers will continue to spur the need for more advanced-practice nurses, including nurse practitioners and clinical nurse specialists. Meeting the demand can be accomplished if undergraduate students, indeed, pre-undergraduate students without specific career goals, are introduced to a global perspective and to the concepts of health promotion and disease prevention early in their education and personal lives. Then, health promotion, quality of life, and social-economic justice will become increasingly valued in cultures throughout the world.

Curricula with global frameworks (Brown, 1999; Pomrehn, Davis, Chen, & Barker, 2000) that develop concepts and experiences directed toward maximizing health for all, will enable nurses to fulfill innovative roles in reformed health care systems around the world. Faculty and students will work increasingly together in interdisciplinary teams with and in communities, using an expanding variety of health-promotion services. The team will be guided by national and international standards. For example, in 1997 the Bureau of Health Professions of the Health Resources and Services Administration and the Association of Teachers of Preventive Medicine convened a task force to update the 1984 *Inventory of Knowledge and Skills Relating to Disease Prevention and Health Promotion*. In addition to completing this objective, the task force created a list of competencies that are essential to all disciplines, which are described by Pomrehn, Davis, Chen, and Barker, (2000).

Nursing faculty will bring the strength of tested nursing theories to their teaching, practice, and research with students of nursing, faculty, and students in other disciplines throughout the university, not simply within health care. Nursing practice and literature will continue to demonstrate the limitations of the biomedical model in promoting health for all. Curricula that provide experiences directed toward maximizing health will enable nurses to fulfill innovative roles in a reformed health care system. Given the increasing focus on self-care in disease prevention and health promotion, nurses can respond directly to the health needs of individuals, families, communities, and groups by focusing on health promotion and by supporting new ways to work and live (see Innovative Practice box).

Implications for Research

In the area of research, a heightened need for nurses exists to test individual, family, community, and group interventions that optimize health and well being. Because of the evidence that maximal effectiveness in lifestyle modification occurs through a combination of educational and environmental interventions, future research will identify the most effective combinations of these interventions under different conditions. Additionally, nurse researchers will be testing these theories to examine the relationships between the delivery of health promotion interventions and cost, access, utilization, and health outcomes associated with this type of care (Badalik, Hegyi, Farkas, & Honza, 2000).

Given the acknowledged importance of health-promotion and disease-preventive care in health care reform deliberations, articulating an agenda that will ensure the nursing profession's role of leadership and active participation is critical. In 1991, the American Nurses' Association (ANA) issued a report entitled *Nursing's Proposal for Health Care Reform,* which offers a broad-based strategy that calls for a nationally defined standard package of primary and preventive health services. The ANA has continued this effort by promoting the development of relationships in health care that are targeted at activities that will improve health outcomes in a cost-effective manner of an individual, family group or community (American Nurses' Association, 2000). By acting on this agenda, nursing can assume a position of leadership in promoting the health of all. Nurses need to consider the following three principal goals:

1. Participate in health-promotion policy development. Cultivating nursing leadership in health policy development involves time, funds, expertise, authority, and education (American Nurses' Association, 2000). Although nurses continue to focus on the care of individuals in acute settings, equal support for altering the contexts that result in preventable illness and disability should be afforded. Professional attention to health-promoting environments and behaviors provides an entry point to the development of community-based models of primary care that emphasize health promotion and disease prevention.
2. Influence public expectations about health promotion. Presentations and other forms of public dialog and education will help raise awareness of the value of individual and community health promotion. Nurses have the collective capacity to change the philosophy of the system from selling health care in the marketplace to creating a milieu for changing health behavior. Encouraging meaningful community participation in addressing health issues provides a significant opportunity to narrow the gap between what is possible in terms of health promotion in this country and what is reality.
3. Increasing consumer demand for preventive health care and provider willingness to offer such care is largely influenced by the coverage of preventive services in health insurance plans. Nurses should participate in a broad range of activities that evaluate options for expanding coverage of preventive health care. Nurses should also lobby for equitable reimbursement of preventive services delivery. One approach might be to advocate a periodic preventive health visit fee, which would specify a package of preventive services for different population groups.
4. Promote equitable access to preventive health care. Given the higher rates of preventable conditions among underserved populations, a justified need to promote the distribution and utilization of preventive health services is apparent. Community-based efforts that combine public and private resources should be targeted to people most in need of preventive health care. Delivery models that focus on integrating preventive and primary care should be expanded into more areas.

Preventive health care delivery should be based on a broad research agenda that encompasses multiple health and social science perspectives. Nurses should participate

innovative practice

Parish Nursing and Health Promotion

Parish nursing provides a model for health promotion in a faith community context. Faith communities are ideal settings for health promotion for several reasons. First, they are intergenerational. In many cases, families of several generations are a part of the same congregation; but, even without family intergenerational contacts, singles and people of all ages come together in a community context. Life passages, such as births, deaths, marriages, and graduations, are all celebrated in the faith context. People in a new stage of life, such as new parents, have access to people who have successfully transitioned to that phase. As people age, younger members of the community can provide personal and functional support to maintain function.

Second, faith communities endure over time. People become known and valued for who they are. People experience illness and health and are supported in both aspects by members of staff or volunteers.

Finally, faith communities deal with the meaning of life on a regular basis. Health issues frequently challenge a person's faith. Spiritual support is useful for healthy lifestyle change and for facing life-threatening illness. Most faith traditions deal with health issues from ancient texts and scriptural traditions.

Parish nursing began as an idea of Granger Westburg, who was a hospital chaplain at Lutheran General in Chicago. With grant funding, a group of nurses from various denominations met and were supported in developing the new role. Today, parish nurses function in health care settings and congregations in many countries around the world.

Parish nurses function as integrators of faith and health, performing activities such as health teaching, personal health counseling, conducting blood pressure screening clinics, making home and hospital visits, leading or participating in healing services, making referrals to community agencies, and coordinating volunteers. These nurses do not duplicate services already provided by community agencies, but rather, they serve as a link to help people gain access to these services. Some parish nurses perform their responsibilities as volunteers, but many congregations are funding these positions because they see the value to members and to the congregation as a whole.

Activities at one congregation of approximately 300 members include monthly blood pressure screening, organizing a volunteer visiting program for shut-ins, leading educational programs, and arranging home and hospital visits. Many informal conversations arise in the church hallways. People have questions about their own conditions and about those of their friends. One woman recently asked why a friend's husband who was on oxygen had the annoying habit of blowing hard every time he breathed out, sometimes disturbing others at the table. After a few questions, the parish nurse was able to explain that people with chronic obstructive pulmonary disease frequently need to extend their expiration and that pursed-lip breathing can help keep airways open. Other conversations relate to ways of supporting aging parents who live in other states.

Educational programs can include general topics such as senior living options, end-of-life-treatment decision making with a physician guest speaker, or funeral decision making with a local funeral agent as speaker. Other educational programs can examine general healthy living choices, personal responsibility for societal health, and dealing with grief and loss.

The parish nurse works as a partner with the congregational clergy. In some denominations, clergy shortages prompt the sharing of ministry with lay parish nurses. In other denominations, Parish Nursing programs are supported because of a sense of mission of the congregation. Skills in leadership of prayer and discussing the theology of health and illness are the areas in which parish nurses often need the most support, because they are infrequently part of basic nursing curricula.

Preparation for parish nursing positions varies greatly. The International Parish Nurse Resource Center in Illinois (800-556-5368) has developed a curriculum for Basic Parish Nursing and for Parish Nurse Coordinators. The resource center maintains a list of course offerings around the country. Currently, no national certification is required for parish nurses, but qualification may come in the future. Community assessment and program development require skills similar to advanced-practice-level skills, but many parish nurses without advanced degrees maintain effective programs. The Health Ministries Association is a membership group for nurses, clergy, and other health professional members.

Because parish nurses frequently work alone or in small teams, they typically organize for regular meetings with other parish nurses in their area to obtain support, to develop ideas for programming, and to share resources. Other resources include an annual Westburg Symposium, sponsored by the International Parish Nurse Resource Center in Chicago, Illinois.

Parish nursing is a rewarding experience that allows the parish nurse to integrate body, mind, and spirit in offering health-promotion programming to people of all ages.

Courtesy Susan K. Chase, ED.D., R.N., C.S.; associate professor and chairperson, Adult Health Nursing; co-coordinator, Joint MS Nursing/MA Pastoral Ministry Program, Boston College; and health ministries coordinator, St. John Evangelical Lutheran Church, Sudbury, Massachusetts.

in areas of research that will influence both personal and community health in a cost-effective manner. Service delivery can also benefit from an expanded health services research agenda that fosters collaboration with other disciplines, such as nutrition and education. Most importantly, preventive health care should be adapted to the health and social problems of specific groups and supplemented as needed by the services of social workers, nutritionists, translators, and outreach workers. Alternative forms of health-promotion approaches and preventive-service delivery should also be examined, including mobile vans, schools and worksite clinics, and other community-based, intersectoral collaboration to reorient the health system beyond health care (see Innovative Practice box).

innovative practice

Haitian Health Foundation: A Charitable Outreach to Neighbors in Need

A volunteer effort of health professionals initiated in Haiti in 1982 by Dr. Jeremiah Lowny and his wife, Virginia, has grown into an outpatient health care facility supported by a nondenominational foundation called the Haitian Health Foundation, Inc. (HHF). In 1985, after working for 4 years in Port au Prince, HHF moved its outreach to Jeremie, Haiti, at the suggestion of Mother Teresa of Calcutta, to bring health care, hope, and opportunity to this especially poor and remote area. The clinic at Jeremie employs 105 people, including 2 full-time physicians, 1 full-time dentist, 10 registered nurses, 2 LPNs, a medical technician, a dental assistant, and 70 to 80 auxiliary personnel (all Haitians). The clinic provides health care to 350 to 400 Haitians daily.

The Haitian "Agents de Sante" program currently employs villagers in 936 villages surrounding Jeremie. This program was initiated by the work of a doctorally prepared nurse who enlisted an individual in each village who had a seventh grade education. After being educated in health promotion, the person became the Health Agent of that village. These Health Agents are trained by HHF to provide preventive and basic health care and education. Many villages have also begun Mothers Groups by which women can share experiences and knowledge relating to nutrition, health care, and other topics that have an effect on their quality of life. Breast feeding classes and immunization programs are available.

Another program was begun through the building of a Food Distribution Pavilion. This building will be used to store and distribute food to over 1000 children and prenatal women three times per week. The pavilion will also be used to educate participants in nutrition and preventative health care. Much of the education in these programs is accomplished through song, primarily because this approach appears to be a successful way to enable the Haitians to remember what is being taught.

For over 8 years, another education program has provided access to schools for poor children in a country in which education is neither free nor mandatory. Currently, 1250 students are attending school through this program. Tuition, uniforms, books, and shoes are provided by HHF funds or through the Save-a-Family Program.

The Haitian Health Foundation relies heavily on the generosity of donors and the many volunteers who donate their time and talents to supplement the staff in Haiti. Volunteers travel to Jeremie, at their own expense from America, Canada, and Europe to share their skills and resources with the poor. These volunteers include health care providers, electricians, plumbers, teachers, clergy, and students.

These programs are only a few examples of the health-promotion programs sponsored by the HHF. These efforts show, however, the way in which dedicated professionals can make a difference, even in third world countries in which health care resources are rare.

Courtesy Jeremiah Lowney, MD, MPH.

Box 25-3 Checklist for Review of Personal Influences

- Do you believe that a paradigm shift toward health promotion has actually been realized by health care professionals?
- What are the political implications of health promotion for the country of your residence?
- What does "determinants of health status" mean to you? How would you propose to serve as an advocate for them?
- What are some of the positive attributes of collaboration with other health care professionals that you have implemented, or might easily implement, in your practice? Which ones are most important to you?
- As a nurse working in acute-care hospital services, what does health promotion mean to you? Does an acceptance of being "doers" to "enablers" cause professional conflict with your values or belief system?
- What outcomes have been achieved by the implementation of *Healthy People 2010* or parallel policies that grab your attention?

Professional Perspective

- What lessons are to be learned from past approaches or the over-reliance on health care delivery to solve all health-promotion and disease-prevention problems?
- Have national or international public policy developments influenced any negative and positive views of health of people?
- If you have been involved in influencing contemporary policy at the local or national level, then what implications does this have for your work as a health-promotion practitioner?
- What are some of the obstacles that nurses must overcome with regard to their involvement in policy debate for social and health policies?
- To what extent have health rights and consumer perspectives been realized by health care professionals? Provide three examples from your practice.
- Do you believe that in the current economic climate, introduction of health-promotion principles is not a cost-effective exercise?
- Do you believe that clinical effectiveness through risk-factor identification is a cost-effective, population-oriented approach?
- Would you participate in encouraging community action for public awareness and lobbying against political issues, such as tobacco advertising in sports, the proposed development of a casino in your area, the development of an industry that will emit toxic wastes, and proposed discriminatory laws against certain minority groups?

SUMMARY

This chapter has described selected past developments and future directions in health promotion and disease prevention throughout the lifespan and throughout the world. After reading this chapter, it is quite apparent that health promotion as a field of practice is quite complex. For some people, the concept of health promotion dwells on idealism, and in the current climate of economic realities, health promotion requires a considerable shift of philosophy and resources. Jargon such as healthy public policy, healthy communities, and healthy people have been politicized and interpreted in different ways by different professionals and countries depending on their power base. Most counties have adopted some of the core concepts as a "health for all" strategy (Box 25-3).

In this chapter, priority issues and future directions for nursing in the area of health promotion have been presented. Current health care reform efforts pose significant opportunities and challenges for nurses, educators, and researchers. With an enduring emphasis on (1) individuals, families, communities, and the environments in which people live, work, and play and (2) health promotion and disease prevention, nurses are critical links for promoting the nation's health. As the twenty-first century begins, nurses have the vision, expertise, and experience to truly make a difference in the health of all women, men, and children. This chapter has demonstrated that the nursing profession can make a greater difference if a commitment can be made to realizing an equal opportunity for the improved health status of populations using a variety of investigated strategies. Through a combination of leadership, creativity, and determination, nurses can and will establish a healthier future for all people around the globe. These thoughts are best expressed in the poem *Prospective Into the 21st Century*.

REFERENCES

Aday, L. A. (1997). Vulnerable populations: A community-oriented perspective. *Family and Community Health, 19* (4), 1-18.

Agency for Health Care Policy and Research. (1991). *National medical expenditure survey: Health insurance, use of health services and health care expenditures*. Rockville, MD: Public Health Service.

American Association of Colleges of Nursing. (1998). *Essentials of baccalaureate education in professional practice*. Washington, DC: The Association.

American Nurses' Association. (1991). *Nursing's agenda for health care reform*. Kansas City, MO: The Association.

American Nurses' Association. (2000). *Achieving access for all Americans*. New York: The Association.

American Public Health Association. (1991). *Healthy communities 2000: Model standards for community attainment of the year 2000 national health objectives* (3rd ed.). Washington DC: The Association.

Badalik, L., Hegyi, L., Farkas, D., & Honza, Z. (2000). Research and knowledge for health-important part of the strategy: Health for all in the 21st century. *Eurorehab, 4*, 210-211.

Berlinguer, G. (1999). Globalization and global health. *International Journal of Health Services, 29* (3), 579-595.

Better Health Commission. (1986). *Looking forward to better health*. Canberra, Australia: Australian Government Publishing Service.

Bohm, D. (1992). On dialogue. *Noetic Sciences Review, 23*, 16-18.

Brown, G. (1999). A visit to the Republic of South Africa and Botswana: A modern country with a relic from the past. *Association of Black Nursing Faculty Journal, 10* (5), 116-118.

Brown, V. (1992). Health care policies, health policies or policies for health. In H. Gardiner, *Health policy development, implementation, and evaluation in Australia*. Melbourne, Australia: Churchill Livingstone.

Brundtland, G. H. (2000). *Fifth global conference on health promotion* [Online]. URL http://www.who.int/directorgeneralspeeches/2000/200000605_mexico.html [Retrieved June 5, 2000].

Catford, J., & St. Leger, L. (1996). Moving into a new decade and a new dimension. *Health Promotion International, 11* (1), 1-7.

Chu, C. (1994). Integrating health and environment: The key to an ecological public health. In K. Huttlinger, *Ecological public health: From vision to practice*. Brisbane, Australia: Griffith University Institute of Applied Environmental Research.

Cohen, G. D. (2000). Aging at a turning point in the 21st century. *American Journal of Geriatric Psychiatry, 8* (1), 1-3.

Commonwealth Department of Health, Housing and Community Services. (1993). *Towards health for all and health promotion*. Canberra, Australia: AGPS.

Degani, V. C. (1999). Health survey: A brief reflexion on individual and public health. *Revista Gaucha de Enfermagen, 20* (1), 49-57.

Dekker, E. (2000). Health policy in the Netherlands: Description and analysis of 10 years of national health policy development emphasizing the health of all strategy. *World Health Organization Regional Publications-European Series, 86*, 110-129.

Department of National Health and Welfare. (1974). *A new perspective on the health of Canadians (The Lalonde Report)*. Ottawa: Department of National Health and Welfare.

Employee Benefits Research Institute. (1996). A monthly newsletter. *Education and Research Fund, 17* (1), 1-7.

Farrell, M. (1998). Trends in global healthcare environment: The developed countries. *Contemporary Nurse, 7* (4), 180-189.

Feldstein, P. J. (1993). *Health Care Economics* (4th ed.). West Albany, NY: Delmar Publishers.

Figueroa, J. P. (1998). The new public health: A vision for the future. *West Indian Medical Journal, 47* (Supplement 4), 13-15.

Gebre-Medhin, M., & Wekell, P. (1999). Focus on children! A model for international development cooperation. *Lakartidningen, 96* (3), 188-193.

Goodman, J. (1979). *We are the earthquake generation*. New York: Berkley.

Green, L. W., Richard, L., & Potvin, L. (1998). Ecological foundations of health promotion. *American Journal of Health Promotion, 10* (4), 270-276.

Guico-Pabia, C. J., & Endsley, D. (2000). Lessons from a health promotion victory. *Business Health, 18* (8), 43-44.

Gullotta, T. P. (2000). How will we understand prevention in the 21st century? *Journal of Primary Prevention, 21* (2), 145-146.

Hassmiller, S. B. (2000). Public health and primary health care systems and health care transformations. In M. Stanhope, & J. Lancaster, *Community and public health nursing* (pp. 42-59). New York: Mosby.

Health Targets and Implementation Committee. (1988). *Health for all Australians: Report to the Australian Minister's Advisory Council and the Australian Health Ministers Conference*. Canberra, Australia: AGPS.

Heiss, G., & Walden, L. S. (2000). Health promotion and risk reduction in the community. In. C. M. Smith, & F. A. Maure, *Community health nursing* (pp. 447-476). Philadelphia: W. B. Saunders.

Henry, B. (1998). Globalization, nursing philosophy, and nursing science. *Image: Journal of Nursing Scholarship, 30*, 302.

Hetherington, L. T. (1998). High tech meets high touch: Telemedicine's contribution to patient wellness. *Nursing Administration Quarterly, 22* (3), 75-86.

Higgins, W. H., & Green, L. W. (1994). The APHA criteria for development of health promotion programs applied to four healthy community projects in British Columbia. *Health Promotion International*, 9 (4), 311-316.

Howson, C. P. (2000). Perspectives and needs for health in the 21st century: 20th century paradigms in 21st century science. *Journal of Human Virology, 3* (2), 94-103.

Huttlinger, K. (2000). Perspectives on international health. In M. Stanhope, & J. Lancaster, *Community and public health nursing* (pp. 60-77). New York: Mosby.

Institute of Medicine. (1988). *Homelessness, health and human needs*. Washington, DC: National Academy Press.

Kalache, A., & Keller, L. (2000). The graying world: A challenge for the twenty-first century. *Science Progress, 83* (Pt1), 33-54.

Kickbush, I. (1989). *Health in public health policy: A context for "new community health," a keynote address at Second Health Promotion Conference*. Sydney, Australia: AGPS.

Kulbok, P. (1985). Social resources, health resources and previous health behavior: Patterns and predictions. *Public Health Nursing, 2* (2), 67-81.

Kulbok, P., Laffrey, S. C., & Goeppinger, J. (2000). Community health promotion: An integrative model for practice. In M. Stanhope, & J. Lancaster, *Community and public health nursing* (pp. 284-303). New York: Mosby.

Lamarche, P. A. (1995). Our health paradigm in peril. *Public Health Reports, 110* (5), 556-562.

Land, G., & Jarman, B. (1992). *Breakpoint and beyond*. New York: Harper Business.

Lefebvre, C. (1996). Health reform in the United States: A marketing perspective. *Health Promotion International, 9* (4), 229-234.

Legge, D. (1991). Towards a politics of health. In H. Gardiner, *The politics of health: The Australian experience*. Melbourne, Australia: Churchill Livingstone.

Lissi, P. E. (2000). Setting goals in health promotion: A conceptual and ethical platform. *Medical healthcare philosophy, 3* (20), 169-173.

Marine, S., Guard, R., Morris, T., Haag, D., Kaya, B., Riep, J., Schick, L., Tsipis, G., & Shoemaker, S. (1998). A model for enhancing worldwide personal health and wellness. *MedInfo, 9* (2), 1265-1268.

Mauer, F. (2000). The U.S. health care system. In F. Mauer, & C. Smith, *Community health nursing* (pp. 107-139). Philadelphia: W. B. Saunders.

McMurry, A. (1994). *Community health nursing: Primary health care in practice*. Melbourne, Australia: Churchill Livingstone.

Musich, S. A., Adams, L., & Edington, D. W. (2000). Effectiveness of health promotion programs in moderating medical costs in the U.S.A. *Health Promotion International, 15* (1), 5-15.

National Center for Health Statistics, Centers for Disease Control and Prevention. (2000). *Health United States, 2000*. Hyattsville, MD: U.S. Public Health Service.

Navarro, V. (1999). Health and equity in the world in the era of "globalization." *International Journal of Health Services, 29* (2), 215-226.

Nutbeam, D. (2000). Health literacy as a public health goal: A challenge for contemporary health education and communication strategies into the 21st century. *Health Promotion International, 15* (3), 259-267.

Nutbeam, D. (1993). *Goals and targets for Australia's health in the year 2000 and beyond*. Canberra, Australia: Commonwealth Department of Health.

O'Byrne, D. (2000). Global conference on health promotion: Mexico 2000. *Promotion Education, 7* (3), 15-16.

Pommier, J., Deschamps, J. P., Romero, M. I., & Zubarew, T. (1997). Health promotion in adolescents in Latin America. *Promotion et Education, 4* (4), 29-31.

Pomrehn, P. R., Davis, M. V., Chen, D. W., & Barker, W. (2000). Prevention for the 21st century: Setting the context through undergraduate medical education. *Academic Medicine, 75* (Supplement 7), S5-S13.

Robert Wood Johnson Foundation. (1978). *A new survey on access to medical care*. Princeton, NJ: The Foundation.

Robert Wood Johnson Foundation. (1983). *Updated report on access to health care for the American people*. Princeton, NJ: The Foundation.

Robert Wood Johnson Foundation. (1987). *Access to health care in the United States: Results of a 1986 survey*. Princeton, NJ: The Foundation.

Robert Wood Johnson Foundation. (1997). *A survey to access medical care*. Princeton, NJ: The Foundation.

Smith, R. D. (2000) Promoting the health of people with physical disabilities: A discussion of public health services in Australia. *Health Promotion International, 15* (1), 79-86.

Smith, C. M., & Mauer, F. A. (2000). *Community health nursing: Theory and Practice* (2nd ed.). Philadelphia: W. B. Saunders.

Stanhope, M., & Lancaster, M. (2000). *Community and public health nursing*. New York: Mosby.

Thompson, P. R., & Stachenko, S. (1994). Building and mobilizing partnerships for health: A national strategy. *Health Promotion International*, 9 (3), 211-218.

Tsouros, A. D. (1996). World Health organization Healthy Cities Project: State of the art and future plans. *Health Promotion International, 10* (2), 133.

U.S. Department of Commerce, Bureau of Census. (1996). *Statistical abstracts of the United States: National data book* (116th ed.). Washington, DC: U.S. Government Printing Office.

U.S. Department of Health and Human Services. (1990). *Healthy people 2000: National health promotion and disease prevention objectives*. Washington, DC: U.S. Government Printing Office.

U.S. Department of Health and Human Services. (1996). *Healthy people 2000: Mid-course review*. Washington, DC: U.S. Government Printing Office.

U.S. Department of Health and Human Services. (1998). *Task force report on AIDS and HIV*. Washington, DC: U.S. Government Printing Office.

U.S. Department of Health and Human Services. (2000). *Healthy people 2010: Understanding and improving health*. Washington, DC: U.S. Government Printing Office.

U.S. Department of Health and Human Services, U.S. Public Health Service, Office of the Surgeon General. (1981). *Report on health promotion and disease prevention*. Washington, DC: U.S. Government Printing Office.

U.S. Preventive Services Task Force. (1989). *Guide to clinical preventive services: An assessment of the effectiveness of 169 interventions*. Baltimore, MD: Williams & Wilkins.

U.S. Preventive Services Task Force. (1996). *Guide to clinical preventive services: An assessment of the effectiveness of medical interventions*. Baltimore, MD: Williams & Wilkins.

Visschedijk, J., & Simeant, S. (1998). Targets for health for all in the 21st century. *World Health Organization Statistics Quarterly, 51* (1), 56-67.

Waxman, L., & Henderliter, S. (1996). *Status report on hunger and homelessness in America's cities*. Washington, DC: U.S. Conference of Mayors.

Weinreb, L. (1998). Health characteristics and medical service use patterns of sheltered homeless and low-income housed mothers. *Journal of General Internal Medicine, 13* (6), 389-393.

Woodwell, D. A. (1989). *Office visits to internists: Advance data, vital and health statistics*. Washington, DC: National Center for Health Statistics.

World Health Organization. (1978). *Primary health care. Report of the International Conference on Primary Health Care*. Alma Ata, USSR; Geneva, Switzerland: The Organization.

World Health Organization. (1981). *Global strategy for health for all by the year 2000*. Geneva, Switzerland: The Organization.

World Health Organization. (1985). *Targets for health for all*. Copenhagen, Denmark: The Organization.

World Health Organization. (1986). *Ottawa charter for health promotion*. Copenhagen, Denmark: The Organization, Regional Office for Europe.

World Health Organization. (1991). *World health progress report*. Geneva, Switzerland: The Organization.

World Health Organization. (1995). *The world health report 1999: Bridging the gaps*. Geneva, Switzerland: The Organization.

World Health Organization. (1998a). *Health for all in the twenty-first century*. Geneva, Switzerland: The Organization.

World Health Organization. (1998b). *World health report 1998: Life in the 21st century-a vision for all*. Geneva, Switzerland: The Organization.

World Health Organization. (2000). *World health report 2000*. Geneva, Switzerland: The Organization.

Yach, D., & Bettcher, D. (1998a). The globalization of public health, I: Threats and opportunities. *American Journal of Public Health*, 88 (5), 735-738.

Yach, D., & Bettcher, D. (1998b). The globalization of public health, II: The convergence of self-interest and altruism. *American Journal of Public Health*, 88 (5), 738-743.

Zacek, A. (2000). Determinants of health and health policy (Part 3): From intervention of quality of life. *Cas Lek Cesk*, 139 (6), 163-165.

Glossary

A

acculturation (Ch. 2) The process by which a cultural group adapts or learns how to take on the behaviors of another group. It is a necessary step, but not an adequate one in assimilation.

acculturation stress (Ch. 2) A psychological problem experienced by ethnic groups, including language barriers, culture shock, lack of social support, and discrepancies between expectations and achievements following immigration.

achievement-oriented stress (Ch. 22) The stress of an overachiever, deriving from internal pressures to succeed as measured by self-defined goals.

achievement tests (Ch. 20) Tests that measure the amount of information learned in a specific area.

acne (Ch. 21) The result of sebaceous follicles becoming clogged with sebum and debris, forming comedones (blackheads or whiteheads).

Acquired Immune Deficiency Syndrome (AIDS) (Ch. 16) A syndrome involving a defect in cell-mediating immunity that has a long incubation period, follows a protracted and debilitating course, and has a poor prognosis.

acquired lactase deficiency (Ch. 19) Intolerance to milk products, manifested by diarrhea.

active immunization (Ch. 17) A substance is introduced into the body that stimulates the production of antibodies to a specific antigen.

acupuncture (Ch. 14) A therapy that manipulates life energy by stimulating precisely mapped points on the skin surface.

acute lymphocytic leukemia (ALL) (Ch. 19) The most common cancer in children from infancy to 5 years of age.

adolescence (Ch. 21) The period characterized by the psychological, emotional, social, and spiritual changes that result in the transition from child to young adult.

advance directive (Ch. 23) A legal document prepared when an individual is alive, competent, and able to make decisions to provide guidelines for health care providers in the future when the individual is not able to make decisions because of physical disability (being unconscious) or mental incompetence.

advocate (Ch. 3, 25) One who brings awareness to certain issues.

aerobic exercise (Ch. 12, 22) Activity that uses large muscle groups over an extended time to improve the efficiency of the oxidative energy-producing system and to improve cardiorespiratory endurance; uses stored adipose tissue as the major fuel source.

affirmation (Ch. 13) A positive thought, in the form of a short phrase, that has meaning for the individual.

Alzheimer's disease (Ch. 24) A type of dementia or progressive mental deterioration thought to result from plaque formation. Its ultimate cause remains unknown.

amblyopia (Ch. 18, 19) The loss of vision or diminished vision caused by the disuse of an eye.

amenorrhea (Ch. 21) The absence of an expected menstrual period.

amniocentesis (Ch. 16) Diagnostic tool used to identify a number of fetal problems.

anaerobic exercise (Ch. 12) High intensity, short duration activity that improves the efficiency of the phosphocreatine and glycolytic energy-producing systems and increases muscle strength, power, and speed of reactivity; uses phosphagens and glucose/glycogen as major fuel sources.

anorexia nervosa (Ch. 21) A disorder of self-starvation characterized by significant weight loss, amenorrhea, compulsive physical activity, preoccupation with food, and a distorted body image.

antiviral drug (Ch. 2) A drug that is destructive to viruses.

Apgar scoring system (Ch. 16) The measure evaluating an infant's general condition at birth. The scoring, made at 1 minute and 5 minutes of age, may be repeated until the infant's condition has stabilized. Determination of the total score is accomplished by adding the values allotted to observations of heart rate, respiratory effort, muscle tone, reflex irritability, and color. The highest possible score is 10. A score of 8 to 10 indicates that the baby is adapting well.

argot (Ch. 21) Words devised and used by participants in a certain subculture.

aromatherapy (Ch. 14) The use of aromatic plant materials and essential oils in a therapeutic manner.

assertive communication (Ch. 13) Using nonjudgmental statements that express one's feelings and opinions and reaffirms one's rights.

asset planning (Ch. 1) A planning approach that focuses the family and the providers on the building blocks for their future, given the realities of the present.

assimilation (Ch. 2) A minority group conforming and modifying its ways of life to conform to the dominant group.

assimilation model (Ch. 2) A model of ethnic relations that maintains that cultural differences between groups disappear as generations pass.

asthma (Ch. 19) A chronic inflammatory disorder of the airways.

astigmatism (Ch. 20) Blurred vision caused by a poorly focused image on the retina.

attention deficit hyperactivity disorder (ADHD) (Ch. 20) A behavior disorder that reflects developmentally inappropriate degrees of inattention, impulsiveness, and hyperactivity.

B

basal metabolic rate (BMR) (Ch. 22) The rate of the amount of activity needed to maintain essential body functions.

behavior change (Ch. 10) Voluntary changes of behaviors to result in improved health status.

Bender Copy Forms (Ch. 19) A test giving an estimate of a child's visual-motor perception. The child responds to standard figures by reproducing the figures in a timed situation; scoring of the child's responses occurs against normative data supplied with the test.

birth defect (Ch. 17) An abnormality of structure, function, or metabolism. It may result from a genetic or environmental influence on the fetus, but is usually a combination of both.
body motion (Ch. 4) Also called *kinetic behavior.* Motions including facial expressions, eye movements, body movements, gestures, and posture.
braces (Ch. 20) Short-term orthodontic appliances.
bradycardia (Ch. 16) Fetal heart rate below 120 beats/min or below 60 beats/min in an adult.
breast self-examination (BSE) (Ch. 22) A procedure in which a woman examines her breasts and their accessory structures for evidence of change that could indicate a malignant process.
bulimia nervosa (Ch. 21) A disorder characterized by a pattern of binge eating followed by forced vomiting and/or laxative use, accompanied by a general feeling of lack of control over eating.

C

calcium (Ch. 23) A mineral essential in developing and maintaining bone mass.
cancer (Ch. 11) A neoplasm characterized by the uncontrolled growth of anaplastic cells that tend to invade the surrounding tissue and metastasize to distant body sites.
candida albicans (Ch. 16) Yeast present in a woman's vagina or cervix.
capitation system (Ch. 3) A system in which each provider, such as an HMO, receives a flat annual fee for each individual, regardless of how often services are used.
cardiac output (Ch. 23) The volume of blood expelled by the ventricles of the heart.
cardiorespiratory fitness (Ch. 12) The ability to deliver and use oxygen throughout the body to allow physical activity over an extended period without excessive fatigue.
cardiovascular disease (Ch. 11) Any abnormal condition characterized by dysfunction of the heart and blood vessels.
care-based reasoning (Ch. 5) Also known as *care ethics,* a reasoning process that includes identifying the moral conflict or problem in context, considering others who are involved in the conflict and how they are interrelated; feeling concern for relationships and individuals and identifying oneself in relation to the individuals and problems involved.
caries (Ch. 20) Dental cavities.
case-controlled study (Ch. 1) A study in which both the study group and the control group are selected on the basis of whether they have the disease rather than whether they have been exposed to a risk factor or a clinical intervention.
case management (Ch. 3) A method of coordinating care to improve continuity and quality of care and lower costs; it occurs across a continuum of care.
centering (Ch. 14, 19) The process of becoming calm, fully present in the moment, and connected to another individual.
cervix (Ch. 16) The lower portion of the uterus that protrudes into the vagina.
chi (qi) (Ch. 14) The energy that flows through the body, nourishing organs and promoting optimal functioning.
child abuse (Ch. 18) Intentional injury to a child.
chlamydia (Ch. 16) One of the most common sexually transmitted organisms in North America and a frequent cause of sterility.
chloroma (Ch. 19) A localized tumor mass that has a greenish appearance.
cholesterol (Ch. 11) A waxy lipid found only in animal tissues. It facilitates the absorption and transport of fatty acids.
chorionic and amniotic membranes (Ch. 16) The membranes that surround the fetus throughout gestation, supporting the developing infant and protecting it from injury.
chorionic villi (Ch. 16) Passages though which fetal circulation flows.
chronic serous otitis media (Ch. 20) Long-term fluid in the middle ear causing inflammation or infection.
clinical trial (Ch. 1) Experiments in which individuals are assigned into groups called *study* and *control* groups; the study group receives the intervention and the control group does not receive the intervention.
codes (Ch. 5) Statements developed by a profession that indicate the profession's acceptance of the responsibility and trust society invests in them. Their purpose is to serve as frameworks for each nurse to generate personal ethical decisions within the guidelines of the profession.
cogiation (Ch. 24) Term developed by Nystrom to describe the experience of healthy withdrawal by residents of long-term care facilities.
cognition (Ch. 24) Thinking processes.
cognitive restructuring (Ch. 13) A technique or series of strategies that help people evaluate their thoughts, challenge them, and replace them with responses that are more rational. It teaches people to recognize that negative thinking often causes emotional distress. This recognition, in turn, reduces the negative consequences of stress and enhances health.
cohort study (Ch. 1) A study in which the investigators do not determine at the outset which individuals receive the intervention.
collective monologs (Ch. 20) The instance when one child pursues a private conversation regardless of what another child says. The first child talks "at" rather than "to" the second child.
colostrum (Ch. 16) Breast milk that precedes mature breast milk.
communication process (Ch. 4) A process by which information is exchanged between individuals through a common system of symbols, signs, or behaviors.
community (Ch. 8) A specific group of people, often living in a defined geographical area, who share common culture, values, and norms and are arranged in a social structure according to relationships that have developed over time.
community-based care (Ch. 1) Care that is provided in nontraditional health care settings in the community.
community diagnosis (Ch. 8) Description of a community health problem that serves as the basis for planning and implementing interventions and nursing actions and making evaluative judgements about health concerns.
community evaluation (Ch. 8) Identification of a specific or potential health concern and planned actions to achieve the desired community outcome.

community health promotion (Ch. 8) A process including involved community participation with representatives from at least three of the following community sectors: government, education, business, faith organizations, health care, media, voluntary agencies, and the public; community assessment guided by a community assessment and planning model to determine community health problems, resources, perceptions, and priorities for action; targeted and measurable objectives to address any of the following: health outcomes, risk factors, public awareness, services, and protection; comprehensive, multifaceted, culturally relevant interventions that have multiple targets for change; and monitoring and evaluation of the processes to determine whether the objectives are reached.

community nursing intervention (Ch. 8) An action or behavior implemented by the nurse to fulfill a health goal of the community.

community outcome (Ch. 8) A goal that is projected before the actual implementation of planned actions and is stated in terms of the individual behaviors that are expected to result from nursing actions.

community pattern (Ch. 8) A clustering of information about a community obtained from assessment data.

community risk factors (Ch. 8) Characteristics that contribute to identified potential and existing health-related concerns.

concrete operations (Ch. 20) The stage within Piaget's stages of cognitive development in which a child is able to move from egocentric interactions to more cooperative interactions.

congenital defect (Ch. 16) An abnormality in structure and function occurring in the fetus when cells do not develop adequately at the necessary point in time and sequence.

conservation (Ch. 20) The concept that certain characteristics of objects remain constant.

constipation (Ch. 23, 24) A change in bowel habits characterized by decreased frequency and/or passage of hard, drier stools and difficult defecation.

contraception (Ch. 21) A drug or device that impedes conception.

conventional level (Ch. 20) The level of moral judgment in which a child looks to others for approval and to society to define rules.

cool-down period (Ch. 12) A period that allows the body to readjust gradually from the demands of exercise to baseline; it follows the endurance phase.

coping (Ch. 13) The ability to deal with difficulties by finding a balance between acceptance and action and between letting go and taking control.

coping strategies (Ch. 20) Behaviors intended to buffer perceived stressful events.

coronary artery disease (CAD) (Ch. 22) Any one of the abnormal conditions that may affect the heart's arteries and produce various pathological effects.

coronary heart disease (Ch. 11) A term formerly used for coronary artery disease.

cost-benefit ratio analysis (Ch. 9) An analysis that compares various outcomes in monetary terms.

cost-effectiveness analysis (Ch. 9) An analysis that determines the optimal use of available resources to reach a predetermined, constant end point—the desired health outcome.

cost-efficiency analysis (Ch. 9) An analysis whose purpose is to be efficient and budget a limited amount of money toward achieving as much of the preselected desired outcome as possible; the funds are the central issue, not the health benefit.

countertransference (Ch. 4) Transference—reacting to another as if that person were someone from the past—experienced by the health care professional.

cultural competence (Ch. 6, 7) Care given to an individual that demonstrates awareness of and sensitivity to the underlying personal and cultural reality of the individual by identifying and using cultural norms, values, and communication and time patterns in collecting and interpreting assessment information.

cultural focus (Ch. 6) One of the five areas of focus that characterize functional health patterns. It includes culturally-based age, developmental, and gender norms.

culture (Ch. 2) An element in ethnicity, consisting of shared patterns of values and behaviors that characterize a particular group.

cytomegalovirus (Ch. 16) A member of a group of large species-specific herpes-type viruses with a wide variety of disease effects. It is the most common infection that exerts possible serious complications for the fetus.

D

decidua (Ch. 16) Fetal nourishing cells in the uterus.

decubitus ulcer (Ch. 24) A localized area of tissue necrosis that develops when soft tissue is compressed between two bony promenences or between a bony prominence and an external surface for a prolonged period.

degenerative joint disease (Ch. 23) Deterioration of the joint(s).

dementia (Ch. 24) A pathological condition that affects cognition in old age. Symptoms include forgetfulness, inattentiveness, disorganized thinking, altered levels of consciousness, perceptual disturbances, sleep-wake disorders, psychomotor disturbances, and disorientation.

demography (Ch. 8) The study of a population. It provides information on population characteristics, such as size, age distribution, gender ratio, racial composition, marital status ratio, nationality, language, religious grouping, and educational and occupational distributions.

Denver Development Screening Test (DDST) and Denver II (Ch. 17, 18) A standardized tool that screens for developmental problems in children from birth to 6 years old.

deontology (Ch. 5) The ethical theory that the moral act does not depend entirely on the consequences of the act; there are duties or obligations affecting actions that have ethical validity independent of the consequences. Also called *formalism*.

depression (Ch. 20, 21, 24) A disorder characterized by an all-pervasive sadness that is present much of the time.

development (Ch. 15) Changes in skill and capacity to function. Qualitative in nature, development evolves from the maturation of physical and mental capacities and learning.

developmental pattern (Ch. 15) A pattern of development of physical and mental abilities showing certain common and predictable characteristics.

developmental periods (Ch. 15) Distinct stages over the lifespan that have unique developmental patterns.

developmental theory (Ch. 8) An explanation of the phases of human development—physical, psychosocial, cognitive, and spiritual dimensions—based on descriptive research studies.

dietary guidelines (Ch. 11) Federal government nutrition guidelines that form the foundation of the federal nutrition policy in the United States. They were first issued in 1980 in response to the public's desire for authoritative, consistent guidance on diet and health and are reviewed every 5 years.

disease (Ch. 1) The failure of a person's adaptive mechanisms to counteract stimuli and stresses adequately, resulting in functional or structural disturbances.

distress (Ch. 13) Stress that is chronic or excessive, resulting in the body being unable to adapt and maintain homeostasis, producing negative results.

dilemmas (Ch. 5) Questions of what is right or what should be done.

disease prevention (Ch. 10) Efforts that work to prevent disease and disability.

divergent family structures (Ch. 7) Nontraditional family structures. Three predominant types have been described: adolescent unwed mothers whose developmental needs and lack of parenting skills pose particular challenges; couples who, after widowhood or divorce, have remarried and merged two families; and older couples or older individuals (mostly women) living alone.

doll or puppet play (Ch. 19) Using toy objects to tell a personal story; it provides valuable insight into a child's sense of self.

Down Syndrome (Ch. 16) A genetic birth defect that results from the presence of an extra chromosome.

Draw-a-Person and Draw-a-Family Tests (Ch. 19) Psychological tests used to give estimates of intelligence and interpretations of a child's emotional development.

durable power of attorney (Ch. 23) The procedure in which an individual designates another person (spouse, son, daughter, or friend) to make health care decisions (especially about how aggressive treatment should be in forestalling death) when that individual becomes unable to make such decisions.

dyslexia (Ch. 20) The tendency to reverse the normal appearance of letters and numbers.

dysmenorrhea (Ch. 21) Side effects of menstruation including cramping and lower abdominal pain during menses often accompanied by nausea, vomiting, diarrhea, and headaches.

E

Early and Periodic Screening, Diagnosis, and Treatment (EPSDT) (Ch. 19) A health-screening program for children provided by Medicaid.

ecological model (Ch. 25) The model describing health as a product of the interdependence between individuals and the subsystems of ecosystems. It assumes a connectedness among human beings, their physical and social environment, and their health.

ecomap (Ch. 7) A form of documentation diagramming a family's social environment.

egocentric (Ch. 18, 19) An individual who sees everything through his or her own perspective and doesn't realize that other ways of viewing things may exist.

emancipated minor (Ch. 21) An adolescent who has not reached the standard legal age for certain activities, but who is permitted to take on full responsibility for decisions because he or she is economically separate from his or her family.

embryo (Ch. 16) The growing baby from 2 to 8 gestational weeks.

empathy (Ch. 4, 13) The ability to understand another's feelings without losing personal identity and perspective.

encopresis (Ch. 20) A condition in which a child over the age of 4 persistently passes stool in his or her underpants.

endometrium (Ch. 16) The inner lining of the uterus.

energy (Ch. 14) A life force present in all living and nonliving elements of the universe.

enuresis (Ch. 20) The involuntary passing of urine at an age when control should be present.

environmental tobacco smoke (ETS) (Ch. 22) Tobacco smoke that exposes individuals to nicotine and carbon monoxide, which causes endothelial injury, vasospasm, increased platelet aggregation, and atheroslerotic plaques that affect oxygenation of all body cells.

epidemiology (Ch. 1) The study of health and disease in society.

episiotomy (Ch. 16) A surgical incision into the perineum to assist in delivering a baby.

Epstein-Barr Virus (EBV) (Ch. 22) A herpes virus that causes mononucleosis. It resides in the salivary glands.

Erikson's Theory of Psychosocial Development (Ch. 15) The theory based on the need of each person to develop a sense of trust in self and others and a sense of personal worth.

estrogen (Ch. 16) A hormone influencing reproduction.

ethical issue (Ch. 9) A situation that presents a dilemma involving right and wrong.

ethics (Ch. 5) A search for what shapes the human being and contributes to the growth and development of the person. It is an attempt to discover all the elements required to make and keep life human so a person may achieve the goals of the humanization process and live as properly and well as possible.

ethnic group (Ch. 2) A collectivity within a larger society; a group whose markedly contrasting values, rituals, and maintenance of separate institutions differentiate it from the larger society. An involuntary group of people who identify themselves and/or are identified by others as belonging to the same involuntary group.

ethnic symbol (Ch. 2) Routine items that are internal to a culture and/or race; items that are emphasized by ethnic people to differentiate themselves.

ethnicity (Ch. 2) A group that shares kinship patterns, physical contiguity, religious affiliation, language or dialect forms, tribal affiliations, nationality, phenotypical features, or a combination of these; an involuntary group of people who identify themselves and/or are identified by others as belonging to the same involuntary group.

ethnocentric perspective (Ch. 2) A perspective that sees other ways as inferior, unnatural, or even barbaric.

eustress (Ch. 13) Stress that can be challenging and useful.

euthanasia or physician-assisted suicide (PAS) (Ch. 24) The painless ending of a person's life with the person's consent.

evidence-based practice (Ch. 1) The conscientious, explicit, and judicious use of current best evidence in making decisions about the care of individual patients.

exercise (Ch. 12, 13) Planned, structured, and repetitive bodily movement done to improve or maintain one or more components of physical fitness.

expected outcomes (Ch. 6) Goals set for a patient's behavior that, if achieved, reflect positive results from nursing interventions.

expressive language (Ch. 19) Language that is used to coherently express ideas and feelings.

extended kinship (Ch. 2) Three or more generations of a family, which is enlarged by membership of nonrelatives who are included through various religious ceremonies.

external locus of control (Ch. 20) The view that an outside force in the environment is the source of control over behavior, actions, or the results of a task.

F

fable of immunity (Ch. 21) The belief that an individual is immune to the consequences of risk-taking behavior because he or she is the "exception."

failure-to-thrive (FTT) syndrome (Ch. 17) The term used to describe infants who fail to gain weight, resulting from the failure to obtain or use necessary calories.

fall (Ch. 24) Collapse from loss of balance.

false negative (Ch. 9) Reports of a test that indicate that individuals *do not* have a condition when they actually *do* have it.

false positive (Ch. 9) Reports of a test that indicate that individuals *do* have a condition when they actually *do not* have it.

family developmental task (Ch. 7) Tasks for establishing a mutually satisfying adult relationship that fits into the kinship network.

family function (Ch. 7) The process of continual change in the system as information and energy are exchanged between the family and the environment.

family health status (Ch. 7) The status that is considered functional, potentially dysfunctional (potential problem), or dysfunctional (actual problem).

family nursing diagnosis (Ch. 7) A concise summary statement of a problem or potential problem. The diagnosis provides direction for outcomes and interventions by identifying the negative health state and the factors that must be changed to alleviate or prevent it.

family nursing intervention (Ch. 7) Actions aimed at assisting the family in carrying out functions that the members cannot perform for themselves.

family pattern (Ch. 7) Family developmental norms and age-specific risk factors.

family risk factor (Ch. 7) Factors that put the health of a family at risk. They can be inferred from lifestyle, biological factors, environmental factors, social and psychological dimensions, and the health care system.

family strength (Ch. 7) Factors or forces that contribute to family unity and solidarity and foster the development of inherent family potential.

family structure (Ch. 7) The family's roles and relationships.

fat (Ch. 11) A substance composed of lipids or fatty acids occurring in various forms or consistencies ranging from oil to tallow.

fee-for-service (Ch. 3) Individual health care payment arrangement in which the patient pays for each visit.

feedback (Ch. 4) A monitoring system through which a person (or group) controls the internal and external responses to behavior (output) and accommodates the responses appropriately.

fertilization (Ch. 16) The union of sperm and egg.

fetal heart monitor (Ch. 16) A machine monitoring fetal heart rate and activity during labor.

fetus (Ch. 16) An unborn offspring that has attained the particular form of the species.

fiber (Ch. 11) A generic term for nondigestible carbohydrate substances found in plant cell walls and surrounding cellular material.

first stage (of labor) (Ch. 16) The stage that begins with the regularity of uterine contractions and ends with complete dilation and effacement of the cervix.

flexibility (Ch. 12) Adequate muscle length and joint mobility to allow free and painless movement through a wide range of motion (ROM).

folk system (Ch. 2) A system that embodies the beliefs, values, and treatment approaches of a particular cultural group.

food guide pyramid (Ch. 11) A graphic representation of dietary balance and variety that classifies foods into six food groups, each of which contains a variety of nutritionally similar foods.

formal operations (Ch. 21) Piaget's stage of cognitive development in which thought processes develop into mature, adult-like patterns with specific traits that allow for adult accomplishments in thinking.

fourth stage (of labor) (Ch. 16) The first 2 hours after delivery when the mother faces the greatest danger of postpartum hemorrhage.

functional aerobic capacity (Ch. 23) Oxygen consumption capacity needed to maintain normal physical functioning.

function of a community (Ch. 8) The process of dynamic change or adaptation in the community system's parts and the way the community system and its subsystems interact.

functional focus (Ch. 6) One of the areas of focus characterizing functional health patterns, which refers to an individual's functional level.

functional health patterns (Ch. 6, 7, 8) An assessment framework of 11 health-related behaviors developed by Gordon. These patterns interact to make up an individual's lifestyle.

functioning (Ch. 1) The ability to perform desired or necessary tasks. Can be characterized as being present or absent, high level or low level. There are physical, mental, and social levels of function reflected in terms of performance and social expectations.

fundus (Ch. 16) The upper segment of the uterus.

G

gene therapy (Ch. 2) A procedure that involves the injection of healthy genes into the bloodstream of a person to cure or treat a hereditary disease or similar illness.

generativity (Ch. 23) A feeling of productivity and creativity as evidenced by reaching previously established goals.

genetic impairment (Ch. 22) Congenital defect caused by abnormal genes.

genital herpes virus (Ch. 22) A chronic infection caused by type 2 herpes virus, occurring in the genital area and usually transmitted by sexual contact.

genogram (Ch. 7) A family diagram that depicts each member of the family and shows connections between the generations.

Gilligan's Theory of Moral Development (Ch. 15) The theory suggesting that there is a different process of moral development in women than in men.

gingivitis (Ch. 23) Inflammation of the gums. Redness and swelling develops around the teeth. Bleeding of the gums while brushing the teeth is an early sign.

Gonococcus (Ch. 16) A microorganism that causes gonorrhea. It causes an infection that can infect a newborn's eyes and has been commonly prevented by treating all newborns with silver nitrate or erythromycin eye drops at birth.

goal setting (Ch. 13) A dynamic process that develops an action plan for change to work towards a more balanced health-promoting lifestyle consistent with an individual's values and beliefs.

group beta streptococcus (Ch. 16) A gram B strep infection.

group or mass screening (Ch. 9) A screening in which a target population is selected on the basis of an increased incidence of a condition or a recognized element of high risk within the group.

growth (Ch. 15) Changes in structure and size.

growth index (Ch. 17) Height and weight measurements plotted on a standard growth chart to assess for normal progression.

growth patterns (Ch. 15) Patterns of development for different age periods. Different parts of the body increase in size at different rates. There is rapid growth in the prenatal through the infancy period and the adolescence period, with the head growing the fastest during the infancy period. From age 1 to adolescence, the legs grow the fastest. There is also growth in the body organs and systems.

H

health (Ch. 1) A state of physical, mental, and social functioning that realizes the potential of which a person is capable.

health behavior (Ch. 10) Any activities that an individual undertakes to enhance health, prevent disease, and detect and control the symptomatic stage of a disease.

health belief model (Ch. 10) A paradigm used to predict and explain health behavior that is based on value-expectancy theory.

health counseling (Ch. 10) Referring people to health education resources or assisting them in acquiring health information pertinent to solving a health problem.

health department (Ch. 3) The local health unit of a town, city, county, township, or district; it is usually the first line of access and health responsibility for the population it serves.

health education (Ch. 10) The process of assisting individuals, acting separately or collectively, to make informed decisions on matters affecting individuals, family, and community health.

Health for All (Ch. 25) The health-promotion initiative of the World Health Organization, established in the late 1970s.

health maintenance organization (HMO) (Ch. 3) The prototypical managed care structure that encompasses two possibilities: (1) a health plan whose providers assume some of the financial risk and (2) a health plan that uses primary care providers as gatekeepers.

health officer (Ch. 3) The chief administrator of a health department appointed by the mayor, the board of health, or some other executive governing body.

health promotion (Ch. 1, 10) The science and art of helping people change their lifestyle to move toward a state of optimal health. The process of advocating health to enhance the probability that person (individual, family, and community), private (professional and business), and public (federal, state, and local government) support of positive health practices will become a societal norm.

health status (Ch. 6) The condition of an individual's physiological state and his or her interaction with the environment.

healthy diet (Ch. 13) Balanced food choices from the five food groups.

Healthy People 2010 (Ch. 1) The latest edition of the *Healthy People* documents, the U.S. federal government's health-promotion initiative, sets out 28 specific areas for health improvement in 467 objectives.

healthy pleasure (Ch. 13) Activities that bring feelings of peace, joy, and happiness.

helping relationship (Ch. 4) A process in which one person promotes the development of another by fostering the latter's maturation, adaptation, integration, openness, and ability to find meaning in the present situation.

Hepatitis B (Ch. 16, 22) An inflammatory condition of the liver caused by the hepatitis B virus.

Herpes Simplex Virus (Ch. 16) A virus that causes small, transient, irritating, and sometimes painful, fluid-filled blisters on the skin and mucous membranes.

heterophoria (Ch. 19) A tendency for a child's eyes to cross.

heterotropia (Ch. 19) A condition in which the child's eyes do not focus together to transmit good, coordinated binocular vision.

high-level wellness (Ch. 1) A sense of well being, life satisfaction, and quality of life.

hippocratic theory (Ch. 2) A theory that states that illness occurs when there is an imbalance.

holism (Ch. 1, 14) The theory that persons have an existence other than the mere sum of their parts.

holistic approach (Ch. 2) An approach that incorporates family and support systems, consideration of the individual's viewpoint, and caring.

homelessness (Ch. 2) The lack of a fixed, regular, and adequate residence.

homeostasis (Ch. 19) A relative constancy in the internal environment of the body, naturally maintained by adaptive responses that promote healthy survival.

human chorionic gonadotrophin (Ch. 16) A hormone of pregnancy produced by the placenta.

human immunodeficiency virus (HIV) (Ch. 11) A retrovirus that causes acquired immunodeficiency syndrome.

human papilloma virus (HPV) (Ch. 22) A virus that is the cause of common warts of the hands and feet and lesions of the mucous membranes of the oral, anal, and genital cavities. HPV is spread through sexual contact and some forms of the virus, in combination with smoking, are strongly related to the later development of cervical dysplasia and cancer.

humor (Ch. 13) Something comical or amusing that causes laughter.

hyperopia (Ch. 20) The condition in which an image falls behind the retina. Also known as farsightedness.
hypertension (Ch. 11, 22) High blood pressure.

I

identity (Ch. 21) A component of self-concept characterized by persisting consciousness of being an individual, separate and distinct from others.
illness (Ch. 1) A social construct where people are in an imbalanced, unsustainable relationship with their environment and are failing in the ability to survive and to create a higher quality of life.
imagery (Ch. 14) A practice in which a person relaxes and focuses attention on images chosen or presented.
individual screening (Ch. 9) A screening in which one person is tested by a health professional who has designated the individual as high risk.
inductive explanation (Ch. 19) Answer arrived at by examining specific data to determine a general concept.
Infant mortality (Ch. 2) Death within the first year of life.
infant mortality rate (Ch. 16) A statistical reflection of the number of infants dying before their first year of life and the leading indicator of a nation's health.
infertility (Ch. 22) The lack of conception in the presence of unprotected sexual intercourse for a period of at least 12 months.
input (Ch. 4) The act of taking in information from outside the individual or group.
insurance (Ch. 3) Individual payment to a fund to provide protection for each contributor against financial losses resulting from an unlikely, but possible, occurrence.
integrity-preserving compromise (Ch. 5) The settlement of differences by which each side makes concessions without violating important basic beliefs.
intelligence (Ch. 20) The quantity of information that people possess; their ability to think; and how they compare with others at the same time, chronological age, and experience level.
intelligence quotient (IQ) (Ch. 20) The ratio of a person's performance compared with other individuals, calculated by dividing maturational age (MA) by chronological age (CA) and multiplying by 100 (MA/CA × 100 = IQ).
internal locus of control (Ch. 20) The view that a person is the source of control over his or her behavior, actions, or the results of a task.
interobserver reliability (Ch. 9) The occurrence of the same result emerging from two individuals performing a test.
interview (Ch. 8) Person-to-person meeting to collect information.
interview data (Ch. 8) Verbal statements gathered during an interview.
intervillous spaces (Ch. 16) The spaces through which the placenta allows maternal blood to flow.
intraobserver reliability (Ch. 9) The occurrence in which an individual is able to reproduce a result several times in a test.
irreversibility (Ch. 19) The inability to connect a reversible situation.
Ishihara's Test (Ch. 19) A test for color blindness using a series of cards with color-tinted letters and figures.

J

journal writing (Ch. 13) Self-confessional writing.

K

kinetic behavior (Ch. 4) Also called *body motion.* Motions including facial expressions, eye movements, body movements, gestures, and posture.
Kohlberg's Theory of Moral Development (Ch. 15) The theory that responses to moral dilemmas indicate distinct sequential stages of moral thinking.
kyphosis (Ch. 23) An aggeration or angulation of the posterior spine (commonly known as "hunchback").

L

Lamaze (Ch. 16) A method of childbirth preparation developed in the 1950s. It requires classes, practice at home, and coaching during labor and delivery. The physiology of pregnancy and childbirth and exercises and techniques are taught to promote control and relaxation during labor.
Lanoue water survival technique (Ch. 19) A method of floating based on the principle that the body is naturally buoyant when the lungs are filled with air and that the natural floating position is face downward, beneath the surface of the water.
law (Ch. 3) A rule enforced by a ruling authority by which society is governed.
learning disabilities (Ch. 20) Learning impairments of individuals who have normal or above normal intelligence and do not have emotional problems or visual, hearing, or motor handicaps.
lecithin-spingomyelin ratio (Ch. 16) The ratio of two components of amniotic fluid used for predicting fetal lung maturity.
levels of prevention (Ch. 1) Primary, secondary, and tertiary means to avert the development of disease in the future.
life expectancy (Ch. 2) Expectancy for length of lifespan.
limit setting (Ch. 20) Teaching children what behaviors are acceptable in society.
lobbying (Ch. 3) The process of trying to persuade legislators to vote for or against measures important to the represented interest group.
lobbyist (Ch. 3) A registered representative of a special interest group.

M

magical thinking (Ch. 20) Beliefs inconsistent with reality.
managed care (Ch. 3) A system that seeks to manage the cost of health care, the quality of that health care, and access to care. It is based on the belief that health care costs can be controlled by "managing" the way in which health care is delivered.
maternal mortality (Ch. 2, 22) All deaths related to pregnancy, delivery, and the postpartum period.
measurement (Ch. 8) A method of data collection using instruments to quantify data in information collection.
meconium (Ch. 16) Fecal matter.
meditation (Ch. 14) A self-directed practice for relaxing the body and calming the mind that involves the focusing of concentration on a single point. When the mind wanders, the individual consciously brings the mind back to the point of concentration. The focus of concentration can be a burning candle, a word, a phrase, the breath, or simply a quiet awareness of what is happening in the present moment.
menarche (Ch. 20, 21) The advent of monthly bleeding or menses.

menopause (Ch. 23) The time in which production of ovarian estrogen and progesterone ceases; the remaining estrogen is produced by the adrenal glands, usually occurring between ages 45 and 55. As a result of the diminished estrogen level, a woman's secondary sex characteristics regress, such as loss of pubic hair and decrease in breast size. The female reproductive organs shrink in size and vaginal secretions decrease.

metacommunication (Ch. 4) A phenomenon that refers to a message about a message. Metacommunication is the relationship aspect of communication. It involves reading between the lines or going past the surface content of the message to glean nuances of meaning.

midlife crisis (Ch. 23) A time in middle age of reassessment, turmoil, and change.

Mini Mental Status Examination (MMSE) (Ch. 24) An instrument developed to accurately assess the baseline mental status of older adults and monitor progress or decline in mental functioning.

mini-relaxation (Ch. 13) Responses that can be used to help develop awareness and to counter the negative effects of stress on mind, body, and spirit. They can be anything from a few conscious, deep diaphragmatic breaths to several minutes of sitting quietly.

minority group (Ch. 2) A group that consists of people who receive less than their share of wealth, power, and/or social status. The identity of the minority group is tied in with the dominant group that is perceived to possess the authority to control the value system and the allocation of resources. A minority may consist of a particular racial, religious, or occupational group.

morality (Ch. 5) A synonym for ethics derived from the Latin *mosmoris,* which also signifies "the customary way of acting" in the sense of that which "customarily" brings about true humanization.

morbidity (Ch. 2) An illness or an abnormal condition or quality.

Moro reflex (Ch. 16) A normal mass reflex in a young infant elicited by a sudden loud noise. Usually consisting of a flexion of the legs, an embracing posture of the arms, and a brief cry.

mortality rates (Ch. 23) Rate of death in a certain population.

mnemonic strategies (Ch. 19) Techniques for remembering things.

multiinfarct dementia (Ch. 24) Dementia that is caused by the death of brain tissue, diagnosed through a computerized axial tomography (CAT) scan of the brain. The death of the tissue may be caused by of a lack of blood flow to the brain from a cerebral vascular accident (CVA) or from another cause.

multiple test screening (Ch. 9) The administration of two or more tests to detect more than one disease.

muscular fitness (Ch. 12) The strength and endurance of muscles that allows for participation in daily activities with low risk of musculoskeletal injury.

mutual storytelling (Ch. 19) A technique in which a nurse begins a story and the child finishes it.

myelinization (Ch. 20) Process of acquiring a myelin sheath for nerve fibers.

myopia (nearsightedness) (Ch. 20) The condition in which an image falls in front of the retina, causing difficulty in seeing distant objects.

myopic vision (Ch. 19) The condition of having myopia (nearsightedness).

N

natural history (Ch. 9) The progression of a specific disease from prepathogenesis to pathogenesis.

neuroblastoma (Ch. 19) A tumor in the sympathetic nervous system.

night terrors (Ch. 18, 19) The occurrence in which a child does not waken completely, but cries out, looks terrified, and cannot be aroused for several minutes.

nightmares (Ch. 19) Anxiety dreams.

nonverbal communication (Ch. 4) Any type of communication that is not verbal, including gestures, facial expressions, movements, body messages or signals, and artistic symbols.

nursing center (Ch. 3) An organization that gives the individual access to professional nursing services. The key components of a community nursing center include: a nurse as chief manager, nursing staff who are accountable and responsible for care and professional practice, and nurses as the primary providers of care.

nursing diagnosis (Ch. 6) The identification and naming of an individual's response to actual or potential health problems or life processes.

nursing intervention (Ch. 6) Actions taken by the nurse to promote the health of an individual.

nutrition screening (Ch. 11) The process of discovering characteristics or risk factors that are known to be associated with dietary or nutrition problems.

O

obesity (Ch. 11, 23) A Body Mass Index (BMI) of 30 kg/m^2 or more, or weight about 20% or more over what is considered a healthy weight for that individual.

object permanence (Ch. 18) The realization that an object exists, has permanence, and can be made visible once again.

observation data (Ch. 8) Data obtained by using sight, hearing, touch, smell, or taste.

one-test specific screening (Ch. 9) The administration of a single test that searches for a specific characteristic indicating a high risk of developing a disorder.

ossification (Ch. 20) Replacement of cartilage with bone.

osteoporosis (Ch. 11, 23, 24) Decreased bone mass, resulting in weak and brittle bones.

otitis media (Ch. 18, 19) Inflammation or infection in the middle ear resulting from a buildup of secretions in the middle ear chamber.

Ottawa Charter (Ch. 25) A set of health-promotion guidelines to be used worldwide. It was the outcome of a meeting of health leaders from around the world held in Ottawa, Canada in 1986. These guidelines put forth a new health paradigm with an increased focus on determinants and prerequisites outside the health care realm, such as adequate income, employment, housing, food, education, and a safe social and physical environment for health development.

output (Ch. 4) The outcome of information processing.

overflow incontinence (Ch. 24) Incontinence caused by an obstruction in the elimination system, such as an enlarged prostate gland or urethral structure.

overweight (Ch. 11) About 10% to 20% over healthy weight.

P

Papanicolaou (Pap) smear (Ch. 22) Screening test for cervical cancer.

paralanguage (Ch. 4) Vocalization other than the expression of words that includes many aspects of sound, such as tone, pitch, and tempo of speech.

parental divorce (Ch. 19) A final decision of the parents to divorce, usually culminating from a period of conflict, stress, and changing relationships.

passive immunization (Ch. 17) The injection of already-formed antibodies. After an individual has been exposed to a disease, a passive immunization is given to prevent contracting the disease. Passive immunizations provide a short immunity, usually 1 to 6 weeks, which will protect the person until the danger of contracting the disease from exposure is passed. Passive immunity occurs naturally in newborns by maternal antibodies passed through the placenta or breast milk.

pattern focus (Ch. 6) One area that characterizes functional health patterns. This focus explores patterns or sequences of behavior over time. The recognition of a pattern is a cognitive process that occurs during information collection. As information is collected, a pattern emerges that represents historical and current behavior over time. This pattern is easiest to recognize when behavior or information is quantifiable.

Peabody Picture Vocabulary Test (Ch. 19, 20) A test examining verbal intelligence.

pediculosis (Ch. 20) Infestation with scabies or lice.

periodontitis (Ch. 23) A gum disease involving tooth loss and bone destruction.

peers (Ch. 20) Persons of the same age, experience, and usually gender.

phonics (Ch. 20) Learning to read by sounding out the letters of a word.

physical activity (Ch. 12) Bodily movement that is produced by the contraction of skeletal muscle that substantially increases energy expenditure.

physical fitness (Ch. 12) A set of attributes that people have or achieve that relates to the ability to perform physical activity without undue fatigue or risk of injury.

Piaget's Theory of Cognitive Development (Ch. 15) The theory of mental processes that is concerned primarily with structure rather than content; that is, how the mind works rather than what it does.

pica (Ch. 16) The eating of nonfood substances.

placenta (Ch. 16) The vascular fetal organ that exchanges with maternal circulation. It provides the primary nourishment to the fetus and protects the fetus throughout the pregnancy process.

pluralistic (Ch. 2) The model of ethnic relations that maintains the need for continued persistence of the immigrant's culture. This position developed as a response to the question of the relationship between immigrant populations and host culture.

point-of-service (Ch. 3) A health care plan in which members decide how to receive services at the time of service; it combines HMO and indemnity features. As with HMOs, providers are paid through a capitation or risk-based system and, as with PPOs, individuals can choose a nonplan provider by paying extra.

policy decision making (Ch. 3) Involvement in decisions about health care policy.

politics (Ch. 3) The use of power to promote a needed change. The political process determines the decision makers who negotiate a desired outcome.

positive reinforcement (Ch. 20) A reward for good or positive behavior.

positive signs of pregnancy (Ch. 16) The signs that diagnose fetal existence.

postconventional level of moral reasoning (Ch. 22) The phase in which an individual is able to differentiate the self from the rules and expectations of others and to define principles regarding rights in terms of self-chosen principles.

prana (Ch. 14) The Hindu term for the energy that flows through the body, nourishing organs and promoting optimal functioning.

prayer (Ch. 14) A request for divine intervention, a type of meditation (centering prayer), or a form of intentionality useful in healing.

precede-proceed model (Ch. 10) A comprehensive planning guide for the administration of health education programs. The precede framework guides the planner to arrive at a highly focused subset of factors as targets for intervention and examines the multiple factors that shape health status and quality of life. The precede aspect helps generate specific objectives and criteria for evaluation. The proceed framework gives additional steps for developing policy and initiating the processes of implementation and evaluation. These two frameworks work in tandem, providing a continual series of steps or phases in planning, implementation, and evaluation. Precede guides the planner in identifying priorities and setting objectives and further provides the objectives and criteria for policy, implementation, and evaluation in the proceed phases.

preconceptual phase (Ch. 18) The phase heralding the beginning of symbolic thinking by which a word, gesture, or image (the signifier) stands for an object, person, or event (the significate).

preconventional level (Ch. 20) The level of moral judgment that depends on punishment and obedience, individualism, instrumental purpose, and exchange.

preferred provider organization (PPO) (Ch. 3) A network of providers who agree to deliver services for a discounted fee. The provider generally incurs no financial risk; the financial burden is on the patient rather than the provider.

preoperational stage (Ch. 19) The preconceptual substage that includes the ability to function symbolically using language.

presbycusis (Ch. 23) Impaired auditory acuity.

presbyopia (Ch. 23) Farsightedness.

Preschool Readiness Experimental Screening Scale (PRESS) (Ch. 19) A screening for developmental lags or abnormalities that would interfere with a child's ability to succeed in the academic and social world of school.

presence (Ch. 14) The act of being available in a situation with the wholeness of one's individual being; of "being with" rather than "doing to."

primary appraisal (Ch. 13) An appraisal of coping that includes descriptions of perceived actual and potential positive and negative outcomes.

primary care (Ch. 3) Basic health care that emphasizes general health needs rather than specialized care. It involves continual and comprehensive care that includes efforts to keep people as healthy as possible and to prevent disease. It is delivered in settings close to where people live and work.

primary care providers (PCP) (Ch. 3) Health care providers who provide care in the managed care arena. They can be physicians or midlevel practitioners (physicians' assistants, nurse practitioners, or nurse midwives) who provide basic health care services.

primary sex characteristic (Ch. 21) The physical organs necessary for reproduction.

probable signs of pregnancy (Ch. 16) Objective changes that carry a high degree of probability of pregnancy.

process of becoming an ethnic (Ch. 2) The identification of members of an ethnic group by other individuals.

progesterone (Ch. 16) The hormone that prepares the uterus for reception of the fertilized ovum.

proxemics (Ch. 4) The use of space between communicators.

puberty (Ch. 20, 21) The period that involves the development and maturation of the reproductive, endocrine, and structural systems.

Public Law 94-142 (Ch. 20) The law stating that all disabled children must receive appropriate public education. Each child with special needs has the right to have an evaluation by school and/or health professionals, who then develop an individualized educational plan (IEP) for that child.

punishment (Ch. 20) Negative reinforcement of problem behavior.

Q

Qi Gong (Ch. 14) A part of traditional Chinese medicine that combines relaxed movements with a meditative aspect and controlled breathing to move Qi energy through the energy channels. The goal of this technique is to balance, smooth, and strengthen the individual's Qi energy.

quickening (Ch. 16) Intrauterine movements of the fetus felt by the mother.

R

race (Ch. 2) A biological term that refers to a grouping of individuals with distinct physical characteristics, such as skin color, hair texture, or facial features.

racial group (Ch. 2) People of the same race who share common cultural characteristics.

randomized clinical trials (Ch. 1) Experiments in which individuals are randomly assigned into groups called *study* and *control* groups. The study group receives the intervention and the control group does not receive the intervention.

receptive language (Ch. 19) Language that retains information. Children can comprehend the meaning of words and phrases that are not a part of their expressive vocabulary and can make associations between concepts although they are unable to explain these concepts.

reflex (Ch. 17) A response that is normally exhibited after a particular type of stimulation.

reflexology (Ch. 14) A method of moving energy by applying hand pressure to mapped points on the feet and hands.

refractive errors (Ch. 19) Defects in the ability of the lens of the eye to focus an image accurately, as occurs in nearsightedness and farsightedness.

regression (Ch. 18) The act of reverting to an earlier, previously abandoned developmental stage of behavior to retain or regain mastery of a stressful situation.

regulations (Ch. 3) Agency or department rules developed for the implementation of laws.

rehearsal (Ch. 20) Repeating an item to be learned to help with memorization.

Reiki (Ch. 14) A Japanese holistic therapy that requires training by a Reiki Master. The Reiki Master teaches hand placements and symbolic gestures and attunes the student. Attunement, opening the energy channel, enables the student to bring universal energy through the body and to the recipient.

relationship stages (Ch. 4) Sequential phases in a therapeutic relationship. They may overlap, vary in length, or involve issues that appear over time rather than in a set sequence. Orientation (introductory), working, and termination phases have been identified by researchers and clinicians.

relaxation response (Ch. 12, 13) An inborn set of physiological changes that offset those of the fight-or-flight (stress) response.

reliability (Ch. 9) An assessment of the reproducibility of a test's results when the test is performed by different individuals with the same level of skill during different periods and under different conditions.

research utilization (Ch. 1) Reading and evaluating research that will contribute to building a sound knowledge base for developing nursing interventions and influencing policy formation.

resistance training (Ch. 12) Exercise designed primarily to increase strength.

retinoblastoma (Ch. 19) Cancer of the eye.

risk factors (Ch. 6) Circumstances or conditions that increase the risk of health problems.

risk factor theory (Ch. 7, 8) The theory that a risk estimate can be obtained by comparing the frequency of deaths, illnesses, or injuries from a specific cause in a group that has some specific trait or risk factor with the frequency in another group that does not have this trait or in the population as a whole. The identification of human characteristics and behaviors that increase the likelihood of the manifestation of health problems.

ritual (Ch. 18) Routine action.

role confusion (Ch. 21) Confusion that may be experienced by an adolescent during the establishment of identity about what roles he or she should adopt. It includes identity diffusion and negative identity.

rubella (Ch. 16, 22) German measles.

S

salary system (Ch. 3) A system involving a straight amount paid for services provided in a particular time frame.

santeria (Ch. 2) A Hispanic folk remedy practice. It is viewed as a link to the past and is used to cope with problems. A *santero* may be consulted in balancing or neutralizing various aspects of an illness.

sanitarians (Ch. 3) Persons who work to maintain a clean environment.

scoliosis (Ch. 21) A lateral s-shaped curvature of the spine.

second stage (of labor) (Ch. 16) The stage in which the baby descends into the birth canal.

secondary appraisal (Ch. 13) An appraisal that includes the individual's identification of available choices to cope with the actual or potential harm, threat, or challenge.

secondary sex characteristic (Ch. 21) An external feature that differentiates male from female, but is not essential for reproduction.

self-disclosure (Ch. 4) Sharing aspects of the self.

self-esteem (Ch. 20) The extent to which an individual believes oneself to be capable, significant, successful, and worthy.

self-insurance (Ch. 3) The instance in which an employer (or union) assumes the claims risk of its insured employees.

semantics (Ch. 20) Meaning of language.

sensitivity (Ch. 9) A measurement of the proportion of persons with a condition who correctly test positive when screened.

sensorimotor period (Ch. 17, 18) The period (up to age 18 months) describing the infant's involvement in mastering simple coordination activities to interact with the environment.

separation anxiety (Ch. 18) An infant's feelings of anxiety and sadness and not being in control when separated from familiar people, especially the mother and father.

serving size (Ch. 11) The recommended amount of food for one serving.

sexual abuse (Ch. 20) Use of a child for sexual, exploitative purposes. It includes any sexual contact with a child.

sexually transmitted disease (Ch. 2, 16, 21) A contagious disease usually acquired by sexual intercourse or genital contact.

shaman (Ch. 2) In Native American folk practice, a medicine man or woman called upon to affect cures. Usually, the shaman is a powerful individual in a tribe. They are treated with respect for their role in inculcating religious beliefs and promoting spirituality, good health, and good living for the people.

sleep hygiene (Ch. 13) Science and practice related to sleep and rest.

sleep talking (Ch. 20) Talking in one's sleep. Words tend to be simple, but difficult to understand, and the individual quickly falls back to sleep.

sleepwalking (Ch. 20) Complex motor activity during sleep, usually culminating in leaving the bed and walking about. The person has no recall of the incident upon awakening.

Snellen E Chart (Ch. 19) A test that can provide a reliable estimate of the actual visual acuity of a child.

social cognitive theory (SCT) (Ch. 10) A model developed by Bandera that emphasizes the influence of efficacy beliefs and outcome expectations on health behavior. Formerly known as *social learning theory*.

social learning theory (SLT) (Ch. 10) The old name for social cognitive theory (SCT).

social marketing (Ch. 10) The application of commercial marketing technologies to the analysis, planning, execution, and evaluation of programs designed to influence the voluntary behavior of target audiences to improve their personal welfare and that of their society.

social support (Ch. 13) A network of close family, friends, co-workers, and professionals.

socialization (Ch. 20) The process in which a child is exposed to a variety of social roles and interactions.

somatization (Ch. 20) The transfer of feelings to a physical problem.

specificity (Ch. 9) A measurement of a test's ability to recognize negative reactions or nondiseased individuals.

spiritual practice (Ch. 13) Activities that help people find meaning, purpose, and connection for their life.

spontaneous abortion (Ch. 16) Natural loss of conceptive products.

stagnation (Ch. 23) The result of a lack of accomplishment during developmental tasks in middle age.

Stanford-Binet Test (Ch. 20) An intelligence test with a heavy emphasis on abstract thinking.

strabismus (Ch. 18, 19) A deviation of the line of vision from the midline because of extraocular muscle weakness or imbalance.

stress (Ch. 13, 22) The negative physical, psychological, social, or spiritual effects of life's pressures and events.

stress incontinence (Ch. 24) Incontinence occurring during exercise, laughing, coughing, or sneezing.

stress management (Ch. 13) The process improving the quality of life by increasing healthy effective coping, thereby reducing the unhealthy consequences of distress.

stress warning signals (Ch. 13) The physical or emotional reaction to a particular stressful experience.

stressor (Ch. 13) Any experience that disrupts homeostasis, thereby requiring change or adaptation. They can be of a physical, psychological, social, spiritual, or environmental nature.

stroke (Ch. 11) An abnormal condition of the brain characterized by occlusion by an embolus, thrombus, or cerebrovascular hemorrhage, resulting in ischemia of the brain tissues normally perfused by the damaged vessels.

structure of a community (Ch. 8) A community system or subsystem that can be seen as the formal or informal arrangement of its parts at any given time, including animate and inanimate properties.

subtle energy (Ch. 14) The energy that flows through the body, nourishing organs and promoting optimal functioning.

Sudden Infant Death Syndrome (SIDS) (Ch. 17) The sudden and unexpected death of an infant who has been healthy; for whom the cause of death is unexplained after a thorough postmortem examination.

sugar (Ch. 11) Any of several water-soluble carbohydrates. It supplies calories, but is limited in nutrients.

sun exposure (Ch. 22) Exposure to natural radiation from sunlight.

sundown syndrome (Ch. 24) Behavior observed in patients with dementia associated with increased agitation and confusion that occurs in the late afternoon.

syntax (Ch. 20) Grammar of language.

syphilis (Ch. 16) A sexually transmitted disease caused by the spirochete *Treponema pallidum*.

systems theory (Ch. 7, 8) A theory that provides an overall framework in which otherwise unconnected parts can be integrated. A system is an entity composed of interrelated, interacting parts or components within a boundary that filters both the type and the rate of input and output.

T

tachycardia (Ch. 16) Fetal heart rate above 160 beats/min or above 100 beats/min for an adult.

tai chi (Ch. 14) A dancelike sequence of poses based on the movements of animals combining physical movement, breath control, and meditation. A holistic therapy that began as a Chinese martial art. It combines physical movement, breath control, and meditation. The slowness of movement and focus on breathing brings an awareness of the moment-to-moment state of the body and produces a meditative state.

Tao doctrine (Ch. 2) A doctrine that states that humans are microcosms within the universe and achieving harmony between the two is essential because the energies of both intertwine.

target population (Ch. 1) A collection of people to whom interventions are directed within the broader community population.

teleology (Ch. 5) An ethical theory that is concerned with what the act does rather than what the act is; it maintains that no action as such can be termed intrinsically evil; the principle determinant of the morality of any act is its consequences.
teratogen (Ch. 16) An agent that causes either a functional or structural disability to the organism based on exposure to that agent.
testicular self-examination (TSE) (Ch. 22) A procedure recommended for detecting tumors or other abnormalities in the male testes.
thalidomide (Ch. 16) A sedative-hypnotic drug that has been withdrawn from general use because it has potential to cause birth defects when taken during pregnancy.
therapeutic touch (TT) (Ch. 14) A touch therapy based on the idea that the ability to transmit universal energy is a natural ability of all humans. Three essential elements comprise TT practice: (1) centering, (2) assessment, and (3) treatment.
therapeutic use of self (Ch. 4) The application of cognitions, perceptions, and behaviors to create interpersonal encounters that promote health in another person, family, group, or community.
third stage (of labor) (Ch. 16) The stage that begins after the birth and lasts until placental expulsion.
toddler (Ch. 18) The age period of 18 to 36 months characterized by a child becoming secure in the ability to walk and run and achieving language ability sufficient to express most needs and desires.
toilet training (Ch. 18) Bowel and bladder training.
toxoplasmosis (Ch. 16) An infection resulting from the intracellular protozoan parasite *Toxoplasma gondii* that infects people through undercooked meat and the handling of cat feces. Although this infection is rare, if a pregnant woman is infected, the results to an infant can be severe.
transductive reasoning (Ch. 19) Moving only from particular to particular in making associations and solving problems.
transference (Ch. 4) Reacting to another person in an exchange as if that person were someone from the past.
trimester (Ch. 16) One of three equal time measurements.
tympanograms (Ch. 20) Tests used to measure the sensitivity of the tympanic membrane to vibrations induced by pressure and sound waves.
Type 2 Diabetes (Ch. 11) Noninsulin-dependent diabetes mellitus; also known as adult-onset diabetes.

U

ultrasound (Ch. 16) Sonogram testing that uses high-frequency sound waves that bounce off the fetus and are interpreted by a computer. It allows defined visualization of the fetus and gestational structures throughout pregnancy.
underweight (Ch. 11) Body mass index of less than 18.5.
urge incontinence (Ch. 24) The inability to delay voiding once the bladder is full.
urinary incontinence (Ch. 24) Decrease in control of urination.

V

validity (Ch. 9) A measurement of a test's ability to correctly distinguish between diseased and nondiseased clients.
value orientation (Ch. 2) Orientations that are learned and shared through the socialization process, reflecting the personality type of a particular society. The dominant value orientations are shared by the majority of the group. Kluckhohn's model of value orientations incorporates themes regarding basic human nature, the relationship of human beings to nature, human beings' time orientation, valued personality type, and relationships between human beings.
values clarification (Ch. 4, 13) A method whereby a person purposely seeks to discover what his or her values are and what importance these values have.
vegetarian (Ch. 11) One who eats no meat products.
Vineland Social Maturity Scale (Ch. 19) A test that provides an objective, standardized estimate of social maturity.
vulnerable population (Ch. 25) A population group that experiences factors that can cause or exacerbate health problems. Such factors may include poverty, lack of education, unstable or dangerous physical environments, isolation, and the lack of adequate and available health services.

W

warm-up period (Ch. 12) Physical activity that prepares both the musculoskeletal and cardiorespiratory systems for the transition from rest to exercise by increasing the blood flow, respiration, and body temperature and improving muscle flexibility.
weaning (Ch. 17) A gradual, caring process that introduces the infant to a cup that replaces the bottle or breast.
Wechsler Series (Ch. 20) A series of intelligence tests that emphasize aggregate, or global, knowledge.
wellness (Ch. 1) A state involving progression toward a higher level of functioning, an open-ended and ever-expanding future, with its challenge of fuller potential and the integration of the whole being.
wellness-illness continuum (Ch. 1) A paradigm that is a bipolar, interactive portrayal of health and illness in myriad configurations, ranging from high-level wellness to depletion of health (death).
Western health care (Ch. 2) Professional care that emphasizes approaches that are based on data from scientifically proven methods of research.
Wilms' tumor (Ch. 19) Cancer of the kidney.
windshield survey (Ch. 8) Obtaining data about a community through direct observation involving all of the senses.
World Health Organization (WHO) (Ch. 25) An international agency founded after World War II to promote health around the world.

Y

yoga (Ch. 12, 14) A form of spiritual practice involving mindful physical stretching that has Hindu origins. Awareness is focused on feeling the body as it moves.

Z

zygote (Ch. 16) The beginning of a human being, resulting from the successful penetration of a sperm cell into an egg in the fallopian tube. Additional division of zygotic cells results in more differentiated structures that eventually produce an embryo and a fetus.

Index

A

Abortion
spontaneous, 442
surgical, 127-128
Acculturation, 31
of Asian Americans–Pacific Islanders, 37
of Hispanic Americans, 30, 238
Acne, in adolescents, 620-621
Acquired immunodeficiency syndrome. *See* HIV and AIDS.
Acquired lactase deficiency, 535
Activity levels. *See* Exercise and physical activity.
Acupressure, 377f, 378
Acupuncture, 377-378, 377f
Adequate intake, 275b
Adipose tissue
and fat calories
during pregnancy, 433
exercise and, 327
growth changes of, 405t-406t
Adolescents, 401t, 617-646
accidents involving, 637
alcohol consumption by, 199, 640b
bacterial and biological agents affecting, 639
contraception for, 131-133, 132b, 632-634
developmental tasks vs wellness tasks for, 145t
family with, 189-190
functional health-pattern assessment of, 623-637
motor vehicle accidents of, 639
nursing interventions with, 646
pathological processes affecting, 637-643
peers of, 632, 632f
pressure from, 640b
physical changes in, 618-623
pregnant, 429b, 634-635
community coping regarding, 218
education intervention involving, 254
reproductive system in, 621-623
boys, 621-622, 622f
girls, 622-623, 622f
secondary sex characteristics, 621t
risk behaviors of, 617b
school for, 643
sexual practices of, 83, 624b
social processes affecting, 643-646
sports injuries of, 637-638
substance abuse by, 624b, 636, 639-641
alcohol, 199, 640b
marijuana, 640b
signs of, 639b
violence involving, 638-639, 638f

Page numbers followed by the letter f refer to figures, those followed by the letter t refer to tables, and those followed by the letter b refer to boxes.

Adult day programs, 737
Adults
middle-age. *See* Middle-age adults.
older. *See* Older adults.
young. *See* Young adults.
Advance directives, 125, 698-699
Advocates, nurses as, 21, 70, 134-135, 748
Aerobic capacity, exercise and, 329
Aerobic exercise, 321, 333-336
and relaxation response, 338-339
by young adults, 658
Affirmations, in stress management, 366
Affluence, and school-age children, 608-609
Aging. *See also* Older adults.
and exercise, 327-328, 330
and future population changes, 24-25
theories of, 711, 716b
AIDS. *See* HIV and AIDS.
Air pollution
infants affected by, 496
middle-age adults affected by, 700
school-age children affected by, 602
young adults affected by, 672
Alcohol abuse
by middle-age adults, 689-690
by older adults, 735
by women, 141
by young adults, 673-674
community-based action regarding, 220, 220b
homelessness and, 45
Alcohol consumption
and cancer risk reduction, 299
and diabetes diet intervention, 312b
by adolescents, 199, 640b
by middle-age adults, 687b
by young adults, 673-674
during pregnancy, 429b, 448-449
in healthy diets, 283t
Allocation of resources, 119, 134
Alzheimer's disease, 722-724
caregiver's stress in, 193
Amblyopia, in toddlers, 517
Ambulatory private care settings, 60
Amenorrhea, 622-623
American Nurses' Association
Code for Nurses, 114, 114b, 122, 123-124
on research, 123-124
politics of, 79
Americans with Disabilities Act (ADA), 65
Amniocentesis, 444b
Anaerobic exercise, 321
Anemia, iron-deficiency, 270t
Anorexia nervosa, 625-626, 626b
Antibiotics, used during pregnancy, 448

Anticonvulsants, used during pregnancy, 448
Anxiety
as communication barrier, 98
separation, 524
Anxiety dreams. *See* Nightmares.
Apgar score, 427, 428t
Appearance, in nonverbal communication, 90
Aromatherapy, 386-387, 387b
Arthritis, exercise and, 329-330
Artificial insemination, 130
Asian Americans–Pacific Islanders, 36-37, 36b
AIDS in, 48-49
higher education of, 36t
Assessment
in administration of health education programs, 258-261
of health status, 142t
functional health patterns in. *See* Functional health patterns.
of older adults, 741b
process of, 160-163
Assimilation, of ethnic relations, 31
Assisted living facilities, 737, 738t-739t
Assisted suicide, 133
Asthma, 561
Astigmatism, 580
Attention deficit hyperactivity disorder, 583-584, 584b
Attitudes, as communication barrier, 98
Autonomy, self-determination and, 119, 120

B

Bacteria
adolescents affected by, 639
as food contaminants, 285t, 286t
preschoolers infected by, 557-559
toddlers infected by, 527
Bacterial vaginosis, 667t
Balanced Budget Acts of 1997, 69, 74, 75, 77
Barbiturates, used during pregnancy, 448
Barriers
in language, 257, 500
to care, 33-35, 672
to heart disease compliance, 294
to learning, 260f, 262-263
Behavior(s)
health education and, 253-255, 260
in functional health patterns. *See* Functional health patterns.
kinetic, 89-90
moral, 593
of preschoolers, 536t
risk
of adolescents, 617b
of young adults, 655
stress and, 356-357
Behavioral health history, 652, 653f
Behavioral interventions, 23
Beliefs
during pregnancy, 431b, 442, 455b
functional health-pattern assessment of
during pregnancy, 431b, 442
of adolescents, 636-637
Beliefs—cont'd
functional health-pattern assessment of—cont'd
of communities, 210t, 213
of families, 185
of individuals, 160
of infants, 489-490
of middle-age adults, 699-700
of older adults, 729-731
of preschoolers, 553-554
of school-age children, 592-593
of toddlers, 524-525
of young adults, 670-672
health belief model, 25, 253-254
in stress management, 370
Bender-Gestalt test, 546, 583t
Beriberi, 270t
Bicycling
accidents involving
preschoolers in, 555, 557
school-age children in, 594b, 598-599, 599b
of young adults, 658f
Bioethics. *See* Ethics, health care.
Biological agents
fetus affected by, 443-447
infants affected by, 491-493
middle-age adults affected by, 700-701, 701t
preschoolers affected by, 557-559
school-age children affected by, 599-601
toddlers affected by, 527
Biomedical ethics. *See* Ethics, health care.
Biophysical profile, 444b
Birth control. *See* Contraception.
Black Americans, 39-41, 39b
AIDS in, 48, 49
child-rearing practices of, 412b, 606b
health problems of, 39-40, 684
higher education of, 36t
life expectancy of, 716f
middle-age, 684
older adults, 44
poverty among, 215
Bladder cancer, diet and, 298t
Bladder control. *See* Elimination pattern.
Blood pressure levels, 295t
achieving desirable, 293
high. *See* Hypertension.
screening of, 236t, 237t, 242
Blood work, Medicare benefits for, 73t, 774t
Blue Cross and Blue Shield, 71, 72
Body concept, 586
Body image, of adolescents, 630-631, 631b, 634b
Body mass index, 305f, 306f
for adults, 304-306
for children, 306
Body motion, in nonverbal communication, 89-90
Bodywork, 385-386
Borg scale, 335, 335f
Botulism, infant, 477b
Bovine spongiform encephalopathy, 284
Bowel function. *See* Elimination pattern.

Braille, 89
Brain, of older adults, 713t
Brain tumors
school-age children with, 603
warning signs in children, 560b
Breast cancer
decreasing risk for, 300b
diet and, 298t, 300b
in adolescents, 641-642, 642f
in middle-age adults, 687b
in older adults, 736, 736t
in young women, 675
screening for, 236t, 240, 240f, 300b, 687b
collaborative partnership community care plan for, 231, 232-233
of Hispanic women, 238
stress and, 356b
Breast examination
clinical, 236t
self-examination, 240, 241f
by adolescents, 641-642, 642f
by young adults, 652
Breast feeding, 473-474, 475b-476b
advantages of, 474b
dietary reference intakes during, 277t
hospitals and, 474b
incidence of, 460b
pacifiers and, 473b
recommended dietary allowance during, 278t
Brennan school, 379-380
Buddhists, food and, 281
Bulimia nervosa, 626, 626b
Burn injuries
preschoolers with, 555-556
school-age children with, 595, 596b
therapeutic touch for, 380b
toddlers with, 526

C

Caffeine, 688-689
used during pregnancy, 449
Calcium
foods containing, 303t
for middle-age adults, 687-688
in osteoporosis prevention, 302-303, 732
Calories
burning of
fat calories, 327
methods of, 334f
fat
burning of, 327
ingestion of during pregnancy, 433
Campylobacter jejuni, 285t
Canadian health care system, 77-78, 78b, 78f, 750
Cancer. *See also* specific types of cancer.
epidemiology of, 297-298
in adolescents, 641-643
in infants, 497-498, 498b
in older adults, 735-736, 736t
in preschoolers, 559-561
Cancer—cont'd
in school-age children, 603
in young adults, 674-675
risk reduction of
diet intervention for, 298-299, 298t, 300b
exercise in, 331-332
in infants, 498b
warning signs in children, 560b
Candida albicans, 667t
fetus affected by, 445
Capitation system, 62, 68
Carbohydrates
during pregnancy, 433
for infants, 473
Cardiopulmonary disease, 342b
Cardiorespiratory fitness, 321
Cardiovascular disease, 292-294
diet intervention in, 292-294
hypertension as. *See* Hypertension.
in middle-age adults, 687b
in pregnancy, 447
in women, 164, 447
myocardial infarction as, 11, 12-14
risk reduction in
for preschoolers, 561b
for school age children, 573b
stress and, 698-699
Cardiovascular system
growth of, 404t
of adolescents, 619
of middle-age adults, 682
of older adults, 712t
of preschoolers, 535
of school-age children, 568-570
Care managers, nurses as, 21
Care plan
community, 217-220
collaborative partnership, 231, 231f, 232-233
evaluation with community in, 221
implementation of, 219t, 220-221, 220t
evaluation of, 165
with community, 221
with family, 196
family, 192-194, 195-196
in altered family processes, 414b
following myocardial infarction, 13
for altered parenting
in child abuse by middle-age adult, 699b
with situational crisis, 524b
for childbearing preparation, 671b
for exercise program, 346b
for homeless infants, 488b
for ineffective coping skills, 359
during labor, 425b
of preschool child, 554b
regarding work stress, 371
for low self-esteem in adolescent, 631b
for older adults
in minority groups, 43
with hearing and vision loss, 724b, 725b

Care plan—cont'd
implementation of, 165
community, 219t, 220-221, 220t
family, 195-196
in nursing process, 164-165
Care-based reasoning and care ethics, 110, 112
Car-safety seats
for infants, 459b-460b, 490f, 497
for preschoolers, 557
for toddlers, 527
Case management, 69, 69b
Case-controlled studies, 23
Centering, 278
in Piaget's theory of cognitive development, 542
Cerebrovascular accident, 687b
Cervical cancer
in adolescents, 642-643, 643b
in young adults, 675
increased risk for, 643b
Native Americans and, 367
screening for, 231, 232-233, 236t, 240-241
Cesarean delivery, 429b
Chemicals
as food contaminants, 286t
fetus affected by, 447-449
infants affected by, 493-496
middle-age adults affected by, 701-702
preschoolers affected by, 559
school-age children affected by, 601-603, 603b
toddlers affected by, 527-528, 527f
Chi, 376, 377b
Child abuse
by middle-age adults, 698b, 699b
cultural awareness and, 523b
legislation regarding, 529
of infants, 483-485, 485b
of preschoolers, 551
of school-age children, 588, 589b
of toddlers, 522-523, 522b
Child-abuse syndrome, 483
Childbearing families. *See* Parenting.
Childproofing, 493b, 525-526, 527f
Children
adolescents. *See* Adolescents.
body mass index for, 306
culture and rearing of, 412b
developmental tasks vs wellness tasks for, 145t
dietary reference intakes for, 276t
fiber intake of, 298-299
gay or lesbian, 678b
high velocity grid for girls, 402f
homeless, 45, 46
infants, 486-487, 487b, 488b
school-age children, 608b
infants. *See* Infants.
lead intoxication of. *See* Lead levels, in children.
metacommunication and, 90
physical activity increases in, 347
preschool. *See* Preschool children.
prevention of injuries to, 204
Children—cont'd
recommended dietary allowance for, 278t
school-aged. *See* School-age children.
toddlers. *See* Toddlers.
type 2 diabetes in, 310
WIC Program for, 290-291, 453
Children's Health Insurance Program (CHIP), 77, 608
Chinese culture, food in, 281
Chlamydia, 445, 667t
Cholesterol
blood levels of. *See also* Lipoprotein levels.
achieving desirable, 293-294
and coronary heart disease, 323t
exercise and, 324
high, 272, 323t
screening of, 236t, 237t, 242, 242f, 293t
in diabetes diet intervention, 311b
in healthy diet, 283b
Chorionic villus sampling, 444b
Christianity
Catholicism. *See* Roman Catholicism.
morality in, 110-11
personal health in, 120-121
Protestantism. *See* Protestantism.
quality of life in, 121-122
Chronic disease(s)
in Hispanic Americans, 39
number of, 714t
progressive stages of, 175b
Cigarette smoking. *See* Smoking.
Circulatory system
during pregnancy, 421
during transition from fetus to newborn, 428b
growth changes of, 404t
of toddlers, 509
Civil law, and ethical issues, 118
Clarification
of patient's content and meaning, 96
of values, 84-87, 85b, 370
Cochlear implants, 133-134
Code for Nurses (ANA), 114, 114b, 122, 123-124
Code of Ethics for Nurses (International Council of Nurses), 114, 115b-116b
Codes of ethics, 113-114, 114b, 115b-116b, 122, 123-124
Cogiation, 726
Cognitive development, Piaget's theory of. *See* Piaget's theory of cognitive development.
Cognitive restructuring, 365-366, 365b, 366b
Cognitive skills
functional health-pattern assessment of
during pregnancy, 431b, 435-438
of adolescents, 628-630, 628f
of communities, 207t, 211-212
of families, 180
of individuals, 153-155
of infants, 480-482
of middle-age adults, 691-692
of older adults, 721-725
of preschoolers, 542-548
of school-age children, 578-584

Cognitive skills—cont'd
functional health-pattern assessment of—cont'd
of toddlers, 516-518
of young adults, 659-661
physical exercise of older adults and, 721b
testing of, 583t
Cohort studies, 23
Coining (cao gio), 523b
Collaborative partnership community care plan, 231, 231f, 232-233
College students
drinking behaviors of, 650b
health promotion needs of, 625b
Colorectal cancer
diet and, 298t
screening for, 236t, 237t, 241, 688b
Communication, 88
accepting, 97
assertive, 367-368
context of
multicultural, 99
situational, 88-89
effective
barriers to, 97-100
in stress management, 367-368
ethics in, 95, 96
functional health-pattern assessment of, 160-161
functionality of, 90-94
functions of, 88-89
meta, 90
nonverbal, 89-90
of listening, 92
via touch, 92-93, 93f
patient-centered, 88, 88b
process of, 88-94, 89f
purposeful, 94
verbal, 89
Community(ies), 199-222
and alcohol abuse, 220, 220b
and increased physical activity, 347
and nursing process, 200-201
and teen pregnancies, 218
assessment of, 178-179
using functional health patterns, 204-213
bargaining within, 207t
care plans for, 217-220
collaborative partnerships, 231, 231f, 232-233
implementation of, 219t, 220-221, 220t
coercion within, 207t
from developmental perspective, 200, 203-204
from risk factor perspective, 200, 204, 215
from systems perspective, 202-203
function of, 203
functional health-pattern assessment of, 204-213
interaction of, 203
preschoolers in, 561-562
school-age children in, 604-605
screening program resources in, 230-231
sources of information regarding, 202
stages of change in, 213t
Community(ies)—cont'd
strengths and concerns of, 215b
structure of, 202-203, 203f
young adults in, 675-676, 676f
Community nursing centers, 10-11, 60-61
Community partnership, 10
and aid to homeless persons, 47
collaborative partnerships community care plans, 231, 231f, 232-233
community nursing centers, 10
Community-based care, 20
Compromise, integrity-preserving, 133
Confidentiality, in research, 124
Confrontation, constructive, 97
Conscience, 524-525
Consequentialism, 111-112, 122
Constipation, 717
Consultant, nurses as, 21
Contraception, 666t
adolescents and, 131-133, 132b, 632-634
ethical issues involving, 124-127, 131-133, 132b
health education involving, 249-250, 250f
Contract theory, 111
Contraction stress test, 444b
Control, sense of, 586
Coping skills
and stress management. *See* Stress management.
effective, 371-372, 371b
functional health-pattern assessment of
during pregnancy, 431b, 441-442, 442b, 455b
of adolescents, 635-636, 635b
of communities, 209t-210t, 212-213, 218
of families, 184-185
of individuals, 158-160
of infants, 488-489
of middle-age adults, 698-699
of older adults, 728-729
of preschoolers, 551-553
of school-age children, 589-592, 590t
of toddlers, 523-524
of young adults, 669-670
ineffective, 359
by preschool child, 553b, 554b
during labor, 425b
related to work stress, 371
Coronary artery disease, 11, 12-14
in young adults, 654, 655
Coronary heart disease
exercise and, 323-326, 341-342
risk factors for, 323t
Costs
containment of, 68-69
of health care, 66, 68-69
of prescription medications, 74, 74f, 75
of preventive health care, 754-755
Coumadin, used during pregnancy, 448
Countertransference, as communication barrier, 98
Craniosacral therapy, 386
Cretinism, 270t
Creutzfeldt-Jacob disease, new variant, 284

Cross training, 333-334, 334f
Cultural diversity, 49-50
  as ethical issue, 120
  transcultural nursing. *See* Transcultural nursing.
Cultural values, 9, 33, 34t
  of Asian Americans–Pacific Islanders, 37b
  of Black Americans, 40-41
  of deaf persons, 133-134
  of Hispanic Americans, 38-39
  of Native Americans, 42
Culture, 33, 34f
  adolescents and, 643-644
  and caring for older adults, 727b
  and child-rearing practices, 412b
  and pregnancy, 451-452
  food and, 281
  infants and, 499-500, 499b
  middle-age adults and, 702
  preschoolers and, 562
  school-age children and, 605-607
  toddlers and, 528
  young adults and, 670-672, 676
Cupping (ventouse), 523b
Curandero, 380
Curative care, vs preventative care, 58-60
Cystic fibrosis, 510
Cytomegalovirus, 445

D

Dairy products
  for preschoolers, 539t
  in food guide pyramid, 280-281
  sodium content of, 296t
Data, 202
  analysis of
    in functional health-pattern assessment, 161-162, 185-191, 213-215, 213t
    in nursing process, 163
  collection of
    in functional health-pattern assessment, 161-162, 176-185, 201-202
    in nursing process, 163
Day care centers
  for infants, 498-499, 499b
  for preschoolers, 550b
  for toddlers, 528-529
  legislation regarding, 529
Death
  causes of, 682b, 714b
  of middle-age adults, 697
Decision-making
  by young adults, 655
  ethical, 95, 118-122
Decubitus ulcer, 725
Delirium, urinary incontinence with, 718b
Dementia
  in Alzheimer's disease, 193, 722-724
  in older adults, 721, 722-724
  multiinfarct, 722
Demography, 203
Dental caries, 569b, 570
Dental health
  of adolescents, 619-620, 624b
  of older adults, 712t, 724-725
  of preschoolers, 535, 535f, 563b
  of school-age children, 569b, 570-571, 570f
  of toddlers, 509, 510b
  orthodontic appliances in, 571
Denver Developmental Screening Test, 465, 466f, 467f, 518
Deontology, 110-111
Depression
  in adolescents, 635
  in older adults, 729, 730f
  in school-age children, 591-592
  maternal, and infants, 484b
Development, 399-415
  concept of, 402-403
  of fetus, 419, 419b
  patterns of, 403, 403b
  theories of. *See* Developmental theories.
Developmental crisis, of infants, 488-489
Developmental disabilities
  and forced sterilization, 126-127
  infants at risk for, 504b
Developmental levels
  of infants, 461b-462b
  of preschoolers, 536t, 546-548
Developmental periods, 400, 401t
Developmental tasks
  during pregnancy, 436-438
  family, 173, 173b
  of infants, 462-463, 463b
    parenting tasks during, 463t
    vs wellness tasks, 145t
  of middle-age adults, 691b
  of older adults, 726f
  wellness tasks vs, 145t-146t
Developmental theories, 4, 6, 411-415
  Erikson's theory of psychosocial development. *See* Erikson's theory of psychosocial development.
  in community assessment, 200, 203-204
  in family assessment, 173-175, 174t, 185-191
  Kohlberg's theory of moral development, 413, 414t, 465, 592-593
  of infancy, 463-465
  Piaget's theory of cognitive development. *See* Piaget's theory of cognitive development.
Diabetes, 308-313
  and coronary heart disease, 323t
  diet intervention for, 310-313
  exercise and, 342-343
    food adjustments in, 344t
    insulin adjustments in, 345t
    recommendations and precautions regarding, 344b
  in pregnancy, 447
  in young adults, 655
  prevalence and incidence of, 309
  screening for, 236t, 237t, 244

Diabetes, type 2, 309
ethnic groups and, 325
in children, 310
medical nutrition therapy for, 310-312, 311b-312b
desired outcomes of, 310t
registered dietitian referral for, 312f
Diagnosis, nursing. *See* Nursing diagnosis.
Diagnosis-related groups (DRGs), 68, 74
Diet. *See also* Nutrition.
excess and imbalance in, 270-271, 271t
fad weight loss, 309
functional health-pattern assessment of, 148-149
in HIV and AIDS, 314b
of toddlers, 511t
supplementation of. *See* Nutrient supplementation.
Dietary fiber
children's intake of, 298-299
fad diets high in, 309
foods containing, 299t
in diabetes diet intervention, 311b-312b
Dietary guidelines, 280, 282b-283b
Dietary reference intakes, 275-278, 275b, 276t-277t
Digestive system. *See* Gastrointestinal system.
Digital rectal exam, 236t, 237t, 241
Dignity, right to, 122-123
Dilantin, used during pregnancy, 448
Disabled persons
communication methods for, 89
education of, 529, 607
gender of, 510
Medicare benefits for, 72
tertiary prevention for, 20
Discipline, 587b
Disease(s), 6-7. *See also* specific diseases.
chronic
in Hispanic Americans, 39b
number of, 714t
progressive stages of, 175b
hot and cold concept of, 38-39
nutrition and, 292-313
screening for. *See* Screening.
significance of, 229
Distant healing, 384, 384f
Divorce
of young adults, 662-663
parental, 550-551, 590-591
Domestic violence, 174, 181, 182
and young adults, 663-664, 665b
during pregnancy, 456b
Down syndrome, 430
Draw-a-Person and Draw-a-family tests, 546-548, 583t
Drowning
of preschoolers, 556
of school-age children, 595
of toddlers, 526
Drug abuse. *See* Substance abuse.
Drug-resistant organisms, 58
Drugs
over-the-counter
infants affected by, 493-494
used during pregnancy, 448
prescription. *See* Prescription medications.
Dual careers, 677
middle-age adults with, 695-696
Durable power of attorney, 698-699
Dysmenorrhea, 623

E

Early and Periodic Screening, Diagnosis and Treatment, 562-563
Ears, of older adults, 712t
Eating disorders
diagnostic criteria for, 626b
of adolescents, 625-626
Eating patterns. *See* Diet.
Ecomaps, 182, 184f
Economic factors
ethical issues involving, 134, 234-235
for adolescents, 644
health care system influenced by, 58
in infant health, 502-504, 502b
in middle years, 702
in pregnancy, 453
in preschool health, 562
in school-age children's health, 607-609
in screening, 234-235
in toddler health, 529-530
young adults and, 677
Ecuador, 222
Education
Education of the Handicapped Act, 529
health. *See* Health education.
higher degrees of, 36t
of disabled persons, 529, 607
of nurses, 756-757
schools. *See* Schools.
Education of the Handicapped Act, 529
Egocentricity
of preschoolers, 542
of toddlers, 517
Elderly persons. *See* Older adults.
Elimination pattern
and encopresis, 577
functional health-pattern assessment of
during pregnancy, 431b, 434
of adolescents, 627
of communities, 206t, 211
of families, 179
of individuals, 149-150, 161b
of infants, 476-477
of middle-age adults, 690
of older adults, 716-718
of preschoolers, 539-540
of school-age children, 575-577
of toddlers, 512-513
of young adults, 658

Emergency room visits
counseling upon discharge, 753b
non-emergency, 747b
Emotions
during labor and delivery, 366-367
during pregnancy, 436
Empathy
in stress management, 368-369
in therapeutic relationship, 95
Employment. *See* Workplace.
Encopresis, 577
Endocrine system
during pregnancy, 422
growth of, 410t
hormones and
in middle age, 693
in older adults, 713t
of adolescents, 619f
of adolescents, 618, 619f
of toddlers, 508-509
Endometrial cancer, diet and, 298t
Energy work, 376-380, 377b
acupressure in, 377f, 378
acupuncture in, 377-378, 377f
reflexology in, 378
touch therapies in, 378-380, 378b
Enuresis, 576, 576b
Environment
and administration of health education program, 260
and developmental outcome, 411b
carcinogens in, 674-675
chemicals in, 449
Environmental health and protection, 239
teaching preschoolers about, 549b
Environmental Protection Agency (EPA), 65
Environmental services, 25
Epidemiological assessment, 259, 259f
Erikson's theory of psychosocial development, 411-412, 413t
adolescents in, 629-630
infants in, 464
middle-age adults in, 692
older adults in, 725-726
preschoolers in, 549
school-age children in, 584-585
toddlers in, 518-520
young adults in, 660
Escherichia coli, 285t
Esophageal cancer, diet and, 298t
Estimated average requirement, 275b
Ethical issues, 107-135
as to contraception, 124-127
as to HIV and AIDS, 131, 134, 243f
as to research, 122-124
as to screening, 229, 234-235
decision-making and, 95, 118-122
involving health education, 256-257
"is" and "ought" relationship, 109
principles currently stressed, 114-117
Ethics, 108
care. *See* Care-based reasoning.
code of, 113-114, 114b, 115b-116b
elements of, 110-111
feminist, 112
health care, 113-118
in communicating, 95, 96
situation, 112
types of, 110
Ethnic groups. *See* Minority groups.
Ethnicity, 31-33
adolescents and, 643-644
infants and, 499-500, 499b
middle-age adults and, 702
pregnancy and, 451-452
preschoolers and, 562
school-age children and, 605-607
toddlers and, 528
young adults and, 670-672, 676
Ethnocentric perspective, 35, 36
Eugenics, 128
Euphenics, 128
Euthanasia, 729
Euthenics, 128
Evidence-based practice, 22-24
Exercise and physical activity, 319-347
adherence and compliance with program of, 343-345
amount of, 332-337, 333b
and hydration, 340, 340t
and relaxation response, 337-339
and weight management, 282b
climate supporting, 345, 345b
clothing for, 340-341
definitions of, 321
foot wear for, 340
functional health-pattern assessment of
during pregnancy, 431b, 434-435
of adolescents, 627
of communities, 206t, 211
of families, 179, 179f
of individuals, 150-152, 150f, 161b
of infants, 477-478, 478f
of middle-age adults, 690-691
of older adults, 718-719, 719f, 720b, 720f
of preschoolers, 540
of school-age children, 577
of toddlers, 513-515, 514f
of young adults, 658-659, 658b, 658f
gift of, 320b
Healthy People 2010 on, 9-10, 320-322, 321-322, 322f
in HIV and AIDS, 314b
in stress management, 364, 364b
knowing vs doing, 319
medical examination prior to, 341-343, 341t
of adolescents, 624b, 627
of middle-age adults, 690-691
of older adults, 718-719, 719f
benefits of, 720b
cognitive performance improved with, 721b
specific exercises, 720f

Exercise and physical activity—cont'd
of preschoolers, 540, 563b
of school-age children, 577, 611t
of toddlers, 513-515, 514f
of young adults, 658-659, 658b, 658f
risk reduction via, 300b, 323-332
warm-up and cool-down periods in, 336
while ill, 339-340
Expanded Care for Healthy Outcomes (ECHO), 383b
Expenditures on health, 66, 66t, 78f
Experimentation, human, 122-123
Eyes
and vision. *See* Visual ability.
in nonverbal communication, 89-90
of older adults, 712t
retinoblastoma of
in infants, 497
in preschoolers, 560

F

Facilitators, to learning, 260f, 262-263
Failure-to-thrive syndrome, 485-486
family assessment in, 486b
mothers in, 485b
prevention of, 486b
Faith community
and aid to homeless persons, 47
as healthcare partner, 11-12
parish nursing and, 756b
Fall injuries
of infants, 490, 490f
of older adults, 731-732, 732b
Family(ies), 169-197
and increased physical activity, 346-347
care planning with, 192-194, 195-196, 414b
childbearing. *See* Parenting.
couple, 185-188
dual careers and, 677
development of, 172t, 174t
domestic violence in, 174, 181, 182
and young adults, 663-664, 665b
during pregnancy, 456b
from developmental perspective, 173-175, 174t, 185-191
from risk factor perspective, 173-175, 175b, 176t-177t
from systems perspective, 171-173
functional health-pattern assessment of, 176-185, 186b-187b
health teaching to, 251
single-parent, 181, 181f
and isolation of child, 610b
and poverty, 702b
structures of, 180-182, 180t
survival and continuity of, 173b
with adolescents, 189-190
with middle-age adults, 190-191, 693-694
with older adults, 191
with preschoolers, 189
with school-aged children, 189
with young adults, 190
Family and Medical Leave Act, 451
Family health, 171, 192b
Fasting, 309
Fat calories
during pregnancy, 433
exercise and, 327
Fat intake
cancer risk reduction and, 299
in diabetes diet intervention, 311b
in food guide pyramid, 281-282
in healthy diet, 283b, 284t
of infants, 473
of middle-age adults, 686-687
of preschoolers, 539t
Fecal occult blood test, in colorectal cancer screening, 236t, 237t, 241
Federal government. *See also* specific agencies.
and infant health care programs, 502b
food and nutrition programs by, 288t
public health services of, 63-65, 64b, 79
Feedback
and self-reflection, 86-87
as communication function, 88
in functional communication, 91
on health education instructor's performance, 264
Fee-for-service, 60
Feet
homelessness and problems of, 46
massage of, 385, 386f
Feminist ethics, 112
Fertilization, 418
Fetal heart rate monitoring, 444b
Fetus(es)
biological agents affecting, 443-447
chemical agents affecting, 447-449
death rate of, 429b
diagnostic tools for, 443
functional health-pattern assessment of, 434, 435
growth and development of, 419, 419b
mechanical forces affecting, 449-450
pathological processes affecting, 442-450
transitioning to newborn, 427-430
Fever, fetus affected by, 446
Fibrinolysis and platelet aggregability, 326
15-minute interviews, 102-104, 102b
Filipino community, 44
Financial factors, 66-77
costs. *See* Costs.
funding sources, 66-67, 67f
mechanisms in, 68-69
Firearms and firearm safety
preschoolers and, 555
school-age children and, 594b, 595-596
young adults and, 663, 663b
Fish, sodium content of, 296t
Fitness programs, at worksite, 55
Flexibility
and exercise, 321, 336-337
in functional communication, 92
Florence Nightingale Pledge, 113, 114b

Fluids
and exercise, 340, 340t
during infancy, 473
Fluoride requirements
of infants, 473
of toddlers, 509
Folk health care systems
of Asia, 37
of Hispanic Americans, 39
Western health care systems vs, 35-36, 35t
Food
culture and, 281
intake of. *See* Diet.
solids for infants, 474, 476b, 477b, 477t
Food additives, 688
infants affected by, 495
school-age children affected by, 601
Food and nutrition recommendations, 275-282
Food assistance programs, 289-291, 289t
Food diary, 512f
Food guide pyramid, 280-282, 511
Food safety, 283-288, 283b, 287b
and causes of food-borne illness, 284
at home, 287b
contaminants affecting, 285t-286t
food temperatures in, 287f
Food stamp programs, 289-290
Foreign objects, infants swallowing, 490-491, 492b
Foundations, philanthropic, 65-66
Fruits
for preschoolers, 539t
in cancer risk reduction, 298, 300b
in food guide pyramid, 280
in healthy diet, 282b-283b
sodium content of, 296t
Functional health patterns, 142-160
assessment process with, 160-163, 161b
communities and, 204-213
during adolescence, 623-637
during infancy, 472-490
during middle age, 685-700
during older adulthood, 711-731
during pregnancy, 430-442, 431b, 454, 455b
during preschool period, 537-554
during school-age years, 572-593
during toddlerhood, 511-525
during young adulthood, 651-672
families and, 176-185, 186b-187b
characteristics of, 143-144
framework of, 143-146
rationale for use of, 144-146
typology of, 143t
Functioning, 6
Funding sources, 66-67, 67f
Fungus, as food contaminant, 286t

G

Gastrointestinal system
during pregnancy, 421
during transition from fetus to newborn, 428b
Gastrointestinal system—cont'd
growth changes of, 405t
of middle-age adults, 682
of older adults, 712t
of preschoolers, 535
of school-age children, 599-600
of toddlers, 508
Gay and lesbian wellness series, 678b
Gemeinschaft, 207t
Gender
and infants, 465-470
and middle-age adult health, 684
and middle-age adults, 683-684, 684
and pregnancy, 427-428
and preschoolers, 535-537
and school-age children, 571-572, 588-589
and toddlers, 510
Genetic disorders
and pregnancy, 430, 471
in adolescents, 623
in middle-age adults, 685
in preschoolers, 537
in school-age children, 572
in toddlers, 510-511
values involving prenatal diagnosis and, 670
Genetic engineering, 128, 129
Genetic testing, 126
Genetic therapy, 128-129
Genital herpes, 667t
Genital warts, 667t
Genograms, 182, 183f, 184f
Geriatric assessment, 741b
Gilligan's theory of moral development, 415, 415t
Gingivitis, 690
Glaucoma screening, 236t, 237t, 242-243, 688b
Glucose intolerance
diabetes in. *See* Diabetes.
exercise and, 325-326
Goals
in family nursing diagnosis, 194, 194b
in stress management, 370
in therapeutic relationship, 95
of health education, 250-251, 263
of health promotion, 711, 751-752
of learning, 263
Goiter, 270t
Gonorrhea, 667t
fetus affected by, 445
screening for, 688b
Gordon's functional health patterns. *See* Functional health patterns.
Government. *See also* specific agency.
and prevention, 25
federal. *See also* specific agencies.
and infant health care programs, 502b
food and nutrition programs by, 288t
public health services of, 63-65, 64b, 79
legislation by. *See* Legislation.
politics and, 58, 62-63, 79

Government—cont'd
state
food assistance programs by, 290
Medicaid administered by, 75, 76
public health services of, 63
Grains, dietary, 282b
for preschoolers, 539t
in food guide pyramid, 280
sodium content of, 296t
Grief, of SIDS parents, 479-480, 480b
Group process, 90
Growth, 399-415
concept of, 400
during infancy, 461b-462b
of adolescents, 618-619
of fetus, 419, 419b
of school-age children, 568, 572
patterns of, 400-402, 403f
Growth retardation, 460b
Guidance, anticipatory, 400
Guided imagery, 384-385
Guns. *See* Firearms and firearm safety.
Guthrie test, 236t, 237t, 239-240, 240f

H

Haitian Health Foundation, 759b
Hand washing, 284
Head Start Program, 10
Healers, nurses as, 21
Healing touch, 378-379
Health
as value, 33-35
concepts of, 4-6
health care vs, 752
models of, 5-6
planning for, 7-8
stewardship of, 121, 124
"Health at any size," 307, 308
Health belief model, 25, 253-254
Health care delivery system
development of, 56-60
for adolescents, 644-646
for infant care, 504
for middle-age adults, 703-704, 703b
for older adults, 737-741
for preschoolers, 562-563
for school-age children, 609-610, 609t
for toddlers, 530
for young adults, 676, 677-678
growth of, 4-5
of Canada, 77-78, 78b, 78f
organization of, 60-66, 60t
personal cultural values and, 9b
pregnancy and, 453-454
Health care environment
for ill older adults, 736-737
healthy employment practices in, 11
sexual orientation and, 678b
Health care ethics. *See* Ethical issues.
Health care, health vs, 752
Health care professionals
and increased physical activity, 346
associations of, 66
competencies of, 24b
drug abuse by, 134
personal influences on, 759b
sexual orientation and, 678b
Health Care Promotion Model (Pender), 239
Health care proxy, 125
Health care reform, 62-63, 63, 63b, 753-755
Health departments, 12, 63
local, 64t
state, 63
Health disparities, 8-9, 58
elimination of, 238
in physical activity, 10
screening and, 237-238
Health education, 18, 247-266. *See also* Learning.
administering programs for, 258-261, 258f, 259f, 260f
and instructor performance feedback, 264
challenges regarding, 248
content of, 263
during school-age period, 611t
ethical issues involving, 256-257
goals of, 250-251, 263
influences of, 264
interventions in, 255-256
nurse's role in, 21, 244-245
organizing skills in, 265-266
regarding AIDS and HIV, 48
resource referrals in, 264
screening and, 244-245
social marketing and, 257-258
teaching plan in, 261-265
teaching skills in, 265-266
throughout pregnancy, 422-424
Health fairs, 645b
Health for All (WHO), 749-750, 750b
Health insurance, 70-77
and pregnancy, 452-453
private, 71-72
public, 72-76. *See also* Medicaid; Medicare.
Health Insurance Portability and Accountability Act, 77
Health maintenance organizations, 60, 61-62, 71, 72
capitation system in, 68
Medicare and, 740
Health officers, 63
Health policy
future of, 63
nurses influencing, 78-79, 501-502, 756
regarding infant health, 501-502
Health promotion, 16-20, 748-749
ecological foundations of, 751
for vulnerable populations, 755
goals and targets of, 711, 751-752
reform of, 753-755
strategies in, 16-18
Health Promotion Center, 10
Health Resources and Services Administration,
64, 64b

Health status
  assessment of, 142t
    functional health patterns in, 142-160. *See also* Functional health patterns.
    process of, 160-163
  nutrition-related, 271-274
  self-assessment by Hispanic Americans, 147
Healthy People, 7
Healthy People 2000, 8, 9
  Midcourse Review and 1995 Revisions, 8
Healthy People 2010, 8-14, 22, 49, 56
  focus areas in, 9, 9b, 14
  leading health indicators in, 9-10, 10b
  nutrition objectives of, 271-275, 272t, 273t-274t
  on adolescents, 248-249
  on diabetes, 308-309
  on exercise and physical activity, 9-10, 320-322, 321b, 322f
  on health education, 248-249
  on heart disease, 292
  on HIV and AIDS, 313
  on hypertension, 295
  on middle-age adults, 683b
  on obesity, 304
  on older adults, 715b-716b
  on osteoporosis, 301
  on prenatal period, 429b
  on preschoolers, 534b
  on school-age children, 569b
  on toddlers, 508b
  on young adults, 651b
Healthy pleasures, in stress management, 369
Hearing ability
  of infants, 481, 481f, 481t
  of middle-age adults, 692
  of older adults, 712t, 724, 724b, 725b
  of preschoolers, 544, 544b, 545t
  of school-age children, 580-581
  of toddlers, 517, 519t
Heart. *See* Cardio- *entries*.
Heart rate
  during aerobic exercise, 334-335
  fetal, 444b
Heimlich maneuver, on infants, 491, 492f
Helmets, motorcycle, 121
Helping relationships. *See* Therapeutic relationships.
Hepatitis A, 285t, 700
Hepatitis B
  fetus affected by, 446
  middle-age adults with, 700-701
  young adults with, 655-656
Hepatitis C, 656
Herbal medicines, 278-279
  for older adults, 717b
Herpes simplex virus
  fetus affected by, 445
  genital, 667t
Higher education degrees, 36t
High-level wellness, 4, 6, 6f
Hindus, food and, 281
Hip fractures, osteoporotic, 299-301
Hippocratic theory, of pathology, 38-39
Hispanic Americans, 37-39, 38b
  adolescent's body image, 634b
  AIDS in, 49
  and access to health care, 702
  breast cancer screening of, 238
  census survey of, 42
  chronic illness in, 39
  elderly, 44
  health care practices of, 30
  higher education of, 36t
  nutrition and, 292
  self-assessed health status of, 147
HIV and AIDS, 47-49, 47b, 313, 667t
  and access to reproductive technologies, 131
  confidentiality and, 134, 243f
  diet intervention in, 313, 314b
  exercise and, 331
  fetus affected by, 445-446
  in infants, 491-492
  in school-age children, 600, 600b
  in young adults, 668-669
  incidence and treatment of, 58
  screening for, 131, 236t, 237t, 243, 243f, 688b
Hodman Square Project, 530b
Holistic health, 375-393
  aromatherapy in, 386-387
  bodywork in, 385-386, 386t
  energy work and, 376-380
  folk systems of, 36
  guided imagery in, 384-385
  meditation and, 382-383, 382b
  movement arts, 380-382
    Qi Gong, 379, 380-381
    Tai Chi, 330b, 338, 381
    yoga, 336f, 337, 338, 381-382, 381b
  music therapy in, 385
  prayer and distant healing in, 383-384, 383b, 384f
  presence in, 387-393, 387t
  self-knowledge in, 388f-392f, 393
Home environment
  air pollution in, 496
  assessment of, 178
  childproofing of, 493b, 525-526, 527f
  poisonous houseplants in, 494-495, 494t, 495b
  preschoolers in, 556b
  safety risk areas in, 733t
Home health care, Medicare benefits for, 73t
Home visits, 170, 171b
Homeless persons, 44-47
  causes, 45
  children as, 45, 46
    infants, 486-487, 487b, 488b
    school-age children, 608b
  health problems of, 45-46
  numbers of, 45
  spiritual care for, 383b
  young adults as, 677
Honey, and infants, 477b

Hormones
in middle age, 693
in older adults, 713t
of adolescents, 619f
Hospice care, Medicare benefits for, 72, 73t
Hospitals
and breast feeding, 474b
early discharge after delivery, 452
healthy employment practices in, 11
Human Genome Project, 442, 443b
Human immunodeficiency virus. *See* HIV and AIDS.
Humor
in functional communication, 92, 92f
in stress management, 370, 371b
Humor Potential, Inc., The, 156
Hydantoin, used during pregnancy, 448
Hygiene
for school-age children, 611t
sleep. *See* Sleep hygiene.
Hyperinsulinemia
diabetes in. *See* Diabetes.
exercise and, 325-326
Hypertension, 242, 272, 294-297
and coronary heart disease, 323t
by age group, 570t
diet intervention for, 295-296
during pregnancy, 447, 457b
epidemiology of, 295
exercise and, 324-325
in adolescents, 619
in middle-age adults, 687b
in school-age children, 569-570
in young adults, 654-655
screening for, 687b
Hypothermia, 733t

I

"I" statements, 91
Illness, 6-7, 26
Immigration to U.S., 30-31
Immune function
exercise and, 331-332
in older adults, 713t
in preschoolers, 535
in toddlers, 509
Immunization
active, 492
and tetanus prophylaxis, 601
for HIV and AIDS, 48
of adolescents, 624b
of children, 460b
of infants, 488b, 492-493, 493t
of older adults, 734t
of pregnant women, 446
of preschoolers, 557, 558t, 563b
of school-age children, 600-601
of young adults, 655-656
passive, 493
Implantation, of fertilized egg, 418-419
In vitro fertilization, 108, 130-131
Incentive systems
for smoking cessation, 10
in health promotion, 19
Income level
low, 238
poverty. *See* Poverty.
screening and, 238
Independent living, for older adults, 738t-739t
Independent practice associations, 60
Infant mortality rate, 429, 429b, 501
Infants, 401t, 459-505
abuse of, 485b
and failure-to-thrive syndrome, 485-486, 485b, 486b
biological agents affecting, 491-493, 493b
cancer in, 497-498, 498b
car seats for, 459b-460b, 490f, 497
chemical agents affecting, 493-496, 494t, 495b, 496t
childproofing for, 493b
Denver Developmental Screening Test, 465, 466f, 467f
development of, 461b-462b, 463-465
developmental tasks of, 462-463, 463b
parenting tasks during, 463t
vs wellness tasks, 145t
dietary reference intakes for, 276t
feeding of
breast feeding. *See* Breast feeding.
solids, 474, 476b, 477b, 477t
weaning, 474-476
functional health-pattern assessment of, 472-490
growth of, 461b-462b
boys, 469f, 471f
girls, 468f, 470f
health care programs for, 502b
homelessness of, 486-487, 487b, 488b
in motor vehicles accidents, 490f, 496-497
nursing interventions for, 504
pathological processes affecting, 490-498
radiation exposure of, 497
recommended dietary allowance for, 278t
schedule of health care for, 503t
social processes in, 498-504
unintentional injuries of, 490-491, 490f, 491b, 492b, 493b
WIC Program for, 290-291, 453
Infectious diseases, of young adults, 655-656
Infertility, of young adults, 664
Influenza, older adults and, 733-734
Informed consent
as ethical issue, 119, 120
in HIV screening, 131
in human experimentation, 122, 123, 124
Input, as communication function, 88
Insurance, health. *See* Health insurance.
Integumentary system, 409t
Intelligence
of adolescents, 630
of middle-age adults, 691-692
of school-age children, 582
of young adults, 660
International Council of Nurses, 114, 115b-116b

Internet, 71
  and therapeutic relationships, 104
  as health education tool, 266
  for care managers, 21
  on cancer, 299
  on diabetes, 313
  on heart disease, 294
  on HIV and AIDS, 313
  on hypertension, 296-297
  on obesity, 307-308
  on osteoporosis, 303
Interventions
  in health education, 255-256
  nursing. *See* Nursing interventions.
  screening in absence of, 233-234
Interview data, 202
Iodine deficiency, 270t
Iron requirements
  of children, 460b
  of infants, 473
Islamic food laws, 281

J

Johari window, 86, 86f, 87f
Journal writing, in stress intervention, 363
Judaism
  food laws in, 281
  morality in, 110-11
  on abortion, 127
  on donor artificial insemination, 130
  personal health in, 120-121
  quality of life in, 121-122
Justice, role of, 117-118

K

Kantian system of morality, 111
Kidneys. *See* Renal *entries*.
Kinetic behavior, in nonverbal communication, 89-90
Klinefelter's syndrome, 623
Kohlberg's theory of moral development, 413, 414t, 465, 592-593, 637, 660

L

Labor and delivery, 418, 424-426
  emotional support during, 366-367
  ineffective coping during, 425b
  medications used during, 449
  newborn injuries during, 450
  nursing support during, 426-427
  signs of labor, 424b
Lactation. *See* Breast feeding.
Language, 89
  barriers to
    and health teaching, 257
    and infant care, 500
  para, 90
Language skills
  of adolescents, 630
  of infants, 481
Language skills—cont'd
  of preschoolers, 544, 545t, 546b
  of school-age children, 581-582
  of toddlers, 516, 518, 519t
Lanoue water survival technique, 556
Lead levels
  in children, 243-244, 460b
    infants, 495-496, 496t
    preschoolers, 557b
    school-age children, 602-603, 602f
    toddlers, 528
  screening for, 236t, 237t, 243-244
Lean body mass, in HIV and AIDS, 314b
LEARN, 307
Learning. *See also* Health education.
  assessing needs regarding, 261-263
  assumptions regarding, 251
  climate for, 264
  determining outcomes of, 263
  facilitation of, 251b
  goals of, 263
  levels of, 263
  objectives of, 263
  strategies of, 263-265
  three domains of, 263
Learning disabilities, 582-584
Legislation
  and adolescence, 644
  and infant health, 501-502
  and pregnancy issues, 452-453
  and preschool health, 562
  and toddler safety, 529
  for school-age children, 607
  young adults and, 676
Leukemia, preschoolers with, 559, 560b
Lice, 600
Lifestyle
  and pregnancy, 455b
  screening and, 238
  sedentary, 323t
Limit setting, for school-age children, 587
Lipoprotein levels. *See also* Cholesterol, blood levels of.
  high-density, 324
  in middle-age adults, 687b
Liquid diets, 309
Listening
  by toddlers, 517
  in functional communication, 91-92
Listeria monocytogenes, 285t
Liver cancer, 298t
Lobbying, 79
Long-term care housing
  for older adults, 738t-739t
  paying for, 740
Low back pain, exercise and, 330-331
Lung cancer, 175
  diet and, 298t
  in middle age, 681b
  in young women, 675

Lymphoid tissue
growth changes of, 406t
in school-age children, 570
Lymphoma
school-age children with, 603
warning signs in children, 560b

M

Mad cow disease, 284
Mammogram, 236t, 240, 240f
Managed health care organizations, 56-57, 61, 69-70, 71
and rights to health care, 117-118
cost containment by, 68-69
Medicaid and, 76
Medicare and, 740
perceptions about, 70
suing, 70
terminology of, 61b
Management of health
functional health-pattern assessment of
by communities, 204, 205t
by families, 177-179
by individuals, 147-148, 161b
by older adults, 711-714
by preschoolers, 537
by school-age children, 572-574
by toddlers, 511
by young adults, 651-656
during infancy, 472
during pregnancy, 430, 431b
Marijuana use, 640b
Marital status
and health, 683-684
divorce, 550-551, 590-591, 662-663
separation, 662-663
Massage therapy, 385-386, 386f
Swedish, 386t
Masturbation, by toddlers, 523
Maternal mortality, 651, 666
Maternal serum alpha-fetoprotein level, 444b
Meats
for preschoolers, 539t
in food guide pyramid, 280-281
sodium content of, 296t
Medicaid, 67-68, 75-76, 79
and pregnancy, 452, 453
and Prenatal Care Initiative, 424b
and preschool health, 562-563
Medicare compared, 75t
Medical ethics. *See* Ethics, health care.
Medical savings account, 74-75, 77
Medicare, 67, 72-75, 80, 740
cost containment by, 68-69
Medicaid compared, 75t
services covered by, 72-74, 73t-74t
universal, 77
Meditation, 382-383
breath, 382, 382b
mindfulness, 382
Meditation—cont'd
Transcendental, 382-383
walking, 382
Memory skills
of older adults, 724b
of preschoolers, 546
of school-age children, 582
of toddlers, 518
Men
dietary reference intakes for, 276t
health tests and screenings for, 237, 237t
mortality rates of, 683-684
recommended dietary allowance for, 278t
self-esteem in, 411b
Menarche, 622, 622f
Meningococcal disease, 656
Menopause, 682, 697-698, 702
Mental health
exercise and, 332
in middle age, 692-693
in older adults, 713t
Mental illness
and forced sterilization, 126-127
homelessness and, 45, 46, 47
touch as nonverbal communication in, 93
Meridians, 377f
Metabolic needs
during pregnancy, 422, 430-434, 431b
functional health-pattern assessment of
during pregnancy, 430-434, 431b
of communities, 204-211, 205t
of families, 179
of individuals, 148-149, 161b
of older adults, 714-716
of preschoolers, 537-539, 539t
of school-age children, 574-575
of toddlers, 511-512, 511b, 512f
of young adults, 656-658, 657b
Metacommunication, 90-91
Metaethics, 110
Metals exposure
in school-age children, 602-603
lead. *See* Lead levels.
Mexican Americans, 634b
Micronutrients, in diabetes diet intervention, 311b-312b
Middle-age adults, 401t, 681-706
biological agents affecting, 700-701, 701t
caring for aging parents, 169b, 696, 696f
community resources for, 703b
death of, 697
divorce of, 696-697
environmental factors affecting, 700-702, 701t
families with, 190-191
functional health-pattern assessment of, 685-700
in rural areas, 684b
in workplace, 694-696, 694f
lung cancer in, 681b
nursing interventions for, 704-705
obesity of, 685-686
physical agents affecting, 700

Middle-age adults—cont'd
physical changes in, 682-685
screening of, 686b-688b
social processes affecting, 702-704
Midlife crisis, 693
Mineral requirements
during pregnancy, 433
of infants, 473
Mini-Mental Status Examination, 722
Minority groups, 32. *See also* specific minority groups.
aging in, 43-44, 201
AIDS in, 47-48, 48b
and health care barriers, 672
and type 2 diabetes, 325
drug response variations in, 674b
health disparities among. *See* Health disparities.
screening of, 237-238
Mold, as food contaminant, 286t
Moral development
Gilligan's theory of, 415, 415t
Kohlberg's theory of, 413, 414t, 465, 592-593, 660
of young adults, 660-661
Morality, 108
Mortality rate
of middle-age adults, 683, 684f
Motion sensation, of infants, 481
Motivation, in health education, 262
Motor development
of school-age children, 571, 572t
of toddlers, 509-510
Motor vehicle accidents
adolescents in, 199, 639
and safety precautions, 497b
drinking while driving and, 199
infants injured in, 496-497
preschoolers injured in, 555, 557
school-age children injured in, 597-598
toddlers injured in, 526-527
Motorcycle helmets, 121
Mouth
and oral cancer screening, 688b
of older adults, 712t
teeth. *See* Dental health.
Movement arts, 380-382
Qi Gong, 379, 380-381
Tai Chi, 330b, 338, 381
yoga, 336f, 337, 338, 381-382, 381b
Mucus, in newborns, 427
Multicultural nursing. *See* Transcultural nursing.
Muscular fitness, 321
Muscular system
during pregnancy, 422
growth changes of, 408t
of adolescents, 619
of middle-age adults, 682
of older adults, 712t
of preschoolers, 535f
of school-age children, 571
of toddlers, 509
Music therapy, 385
Myocardial infarction, 11, 12-14
Myopia, in school-age children, 580, 580f

N

Narcotics, used during pregnancy, 448
National Center for Complementary and Alternative Medicine, 3
National Committee for Quality Assurance's Quality Compass, 70
National Institute of Nursing Research, 22, 22b, 64
National Institutes of Health, 64, 64b, 307
National School Lunch Program, 290
Native Americans and Alaskan Natives, 41-43, 41b, 702, 756b
cervical cancer and, 367
elderly, 44
health problems of, 42
higher education of, 36t
Neonates. *See* Newborns.
Nervous system
during transition from fetus to newborn, 428b
growth changes of, 408t
of preschoolers, 535f
of school-age children, 571
Neuroblastoma
in infants, 497-498
in preschoolers, 560-561
Newborns
gender of, 427-428
low birth weight, 429b
risk factors for, 501, 501b
siblings of, 439-440, 440b
transition of fetus to, 427-430, 428b
Niacin deficiency, 270t
Nicotine
middle-age adults affected by, 701-702
pregnancies affected by, 449
Night terrors, 515, 516, 541
Nightmares, 541-542
1990 Health Objectives for the Nation, The: A Midcourse Review, 8
Noise pollution
middle-age adults affected by, 700
young adults affected by, 672
Non–insulin-dependent diabetes mellitus. *See* Diabetes, type 2.
Nonpersonal services, 25
Nonstress test, 444b
Nontraditional therapies, 3-4
Nonverbal communication, 89-90
of listening, 92
via touch, 92-93, 93f
Norwalk-like virus, 286t
Not-for-profit health organizations. *See* Voluntary health organizations.
Nurse practitioners, 68, 756-757
Nurses
and transcultural nursing. *See* Transcultural nursing.
at schools, 611-613, 613f
education of, 756-757
transcultural nursing and, 50
independent practice of, 68

Nurses—cont'd
leadership role of, 756-758
payment of, 68
presence of, 387-393, 387t
role of, 20-24, 26, 748, 756-758
during labor and delivery, 426-427
in care of homeless, 46-47
in community health, 201
in screening, 244-245
with family members, 171
self-disclosure by, 87
stress management strategies for, 369b
Nursing centers, 10-11, 60-61
Nursing diagnosis
community, 216
family, 191-192, 192t, 194, 194b
in nursing process, 163-164
Nursing facilities, 738t-739t
Nursing interventions
community, 217
during pregnancy, 439, 442b, 454-456, 454f
during transition of fetus to newborn, 427, 428b
family, 195-196
for middle-age adults, 704-705
in infancy, 504
plan for. *See* Care plan.
with adolescents, 646
with preschoolers, 563
with school-age children, 610-611
with toddlers, 530-531
Nursing process, 163-165
communities and, 200-201
families and, 170-173
Nutrient supplementation, 278-279
during pregnancy, 433
for older adults, 717b
indications for, 279
Nutrient-deficiency diseases, 270, 270t
Nutrition. *See also* Diet.
and disease, 292-313
functional health-pattern assessment of
during infancy, 472-476
during pregnancy, 430-434, 431b
of adolescents, 624-627
of communities, 204-211, 205t
of families, 179
of individuals, 148-149, 161b, 162
of middle-age adults, 685-690
of older adults, 714-716
of preschoolers, 537-539, 539t
of school-age children, 574-575
of toddlers, 511-512, 511t, 512f
of young adults, 656-658
good, 18
in stress management, 363-364
of adolescents, 624b
of infants, 488b, 493
poor, 270-271, 271t
Nutrition counseling, 269-315
and food safety, 283-288, 283b
and poverty, 288-291
food and nutrition recommendations, 275-282
for preschoolers, 563b
for school-age children, 611t
Healthy People 2010 on, 271-275, 272t, 273t-274t
information sources regarding, 313-315
objectives for U.S., 274-275
screening and, 291-292
Nutrition Program for the Elderly, 291
Nutritional self-assessment, 269-270

O

Obesity, 303-308
diet intervention for, 306, 575b
epidemiology of, 303-304, 304t
exercise and, 326-327
Healthy People 2010 on, 9-10
of adolescents, 626-627, 627f
of middle-age adults, 685-686, 687b
of school-age children, 575
and cardiovascular disease, 573b
prevention of, 575b
of young adults, 657f
Object permanence, 516
Occupational Safety and Health Act, 705
Occupational Safety and Health Administration, on workplace violence, 216
Occupational setting. *See* Workplace.
Official agencies, 63-65
Oils, in food guide pyramid, 281-282
Older adults, 401t, 709-742. *See also* Aging.
accidents of, 731-733, 732b, 733t
alcohol abuse by, 735
assessment of, 741b
biological agents affecting, 733-736
cancer in, 735-736
caring for, 169
continuum of, 737f
culture and, 727b
environment of, 736-737
dementia in, 193, 721, 722-724
developmental tasks vs wellness tasks for, 146t
families with, 191
federal health insurance for. *See* Medicare.
from minority groups, 43-44, 201
functional health-pattern assessment of, 711-731
immunization of, 734t
influenza in, 733-734
numbers of, 710f
Nutrition Program for the Elderly, 291
pathological processes affecting, 731-736
physical changes in, 710-711, 712t-713t
pneumonia in, 734
prescription medications for, 734-735
costs of, 74, 74f, 75
urinary incontinence caused by, 718b
sensory changes in, 724-725, 724b, 725b

Older adults—cont'd
smoking by, 710, 735
social processes affecting, 736-741
tuberculosis in, 734
Omnibus Reconciliation Act, 74
Oral cancer screening, 688b
Orthodontic appliances, 571
Osteoarthritis, exercise and, 329-330
Osteoporosis, 272-274, 299-303
and older adults, 731-732
and young adults, 657-658
epidemiology of, 299-301
exercise and, 328-329
pathophysiology of, 301-302
prevention of, 302
risk factors for, 302b
Other-care cultures, 59
Otitis media, 527, 535, 580-581
Ottawa Charter (WHO), 749, 751
Output, as communication function, 88
Ovarian cancer
in middle-age adults, 687b
screening for, 687b-688b
Over-the-counter drugs
infants affected by, 493-494
used during pregnancy, 448
Overweight persons, 272, 303, 304t
type 2 diabetes and, 325
young adults as, 657f
Oxford Institutionalists, 111

P

Pacifiers, and breast feeding, 473b
Papanicolaou (pap) smear, 236t, 240-241
for adolescents, 642-643
Paralanguage, in nonverbal communication, 90
Parenting, 188, 662, 662f
values involved in, 670
Parish nursing, 756b
Patient Self-Determination Act, 65, 114, 125
Patient's Bill of Rights, 70
Payment systems, prospective, 68-69
Peabody Picture Vocabulary Test, 546, 582, 583t
Pellagra, 270t
Perceptions
about health
functional health-pattern assessment of
by adolescents, 623-624
by communities, 204, 205t
by families, 177-179
by individuals, 147-148
by middle-age adults, 685
by older adults, 711-714
by preschoolers, 537
by school-age children, 572-574
by young adults, 651-656, 659-661
during infancy, 472
during pregnancy, 430, 431b
of toddlers, 511
about managed health care organizations, 70
Perceptions—cont'd
functional health-pattern assessment of
by communities, 204, 207t, 211-212
by families, 180
by individuals, 153-155, 161b
during pregnancy, 431b, 435-438
of adolescents, 628-630, 628f
of infants, 480-482
of middle-age adults, 691-692
of older adults, 721-725
of preschoolers, 542-548
of school-age children, 578-584
of toddlers, 516-518
Personal health workbook, 388-392
Pesticides
as food contaminant, 286t
infants affected by, 495
Pets, and self-esteem, 585f
Pew Health Professions Commission, 24, 24b
Phenobarbital, used during pregnancy, 448
Phenylketonuria, 236t, 237t, 239-240, 240f
Philosophical ethics, 109
Physical activity. *See* Exercise and physical activity.
Physical fitness, 321, 322f
Piaget's theory of cognitive development, 412-413, 413t
adolescents in, 628-629
infants in, 464-465, 464t
middle-age adults in, 691
preschool children in, 542-543
school-age children in, 578-580
toddlers in, 516-517
young adults in, 660
Pica, 433
Placenta
detachment of, 426b
development and function of, 419-420
structure of, 420f
Plants, infants poisoned by, 494-495, 494t, 495b
Play
for preschoolers, 543b, 551-552, 551f
for toddlers, 513-515, 514f, 516-517
Pneumonia, older adults in, 734
Point-of-service plans, 62, 72
Poison control centers, 528
Poisoning
of children, 460b
of school-age children, 601
of toddlers, 527-528, 528b
Polarity Therapy, 379
Politics, 58, 62-63, 79
Polyuria, 718b
Pool safety
and school-age children, 594b, 595b
drowning and. *See* Drowning.
Populations
changes in, 24-25, 29-51
ethnicity and, 31-33
immigration to U.S., 30-31
special, 58
vulnerable, 755

Por Cristo–Boston College School of Nursing Health Project, 222
Positive reinforcement, 587
Postpartum period, 440t
Poultry, sodium content of, 296t
Poverty
among Black Americans, 215
and health care access, 40
and income distribution, 288-289
and preschoolers, 562
and school-age children, 607-608
food, nutrition, and, 288-291
screening and, 238
statistics regarding, 289t
Prana, 376
Prayer, 383, 384, 384f
Preconception care, 188
Preferred provider organizations, 60, 62, 71, 72
Pregnancy(ies), 420f
adaptive changes in other systems during, 421-422
adolescent, 429b, 634-635
community coping regarding, 218
education intervention involving, 254
alcohol use during, 85
and maternal mortality, 651, 666
biological agents affecting, 443-447
chemical agents affecting, 447-449
diagnostic tools used during, 421, 421f, 443, 444b
dietary reference intakes during, 277t
discomforts of, 422, 423t
duration of, 418
education intervention involving, 251
first, 440t
first trimester of
fetal growth and development during, 419b
first pregnancy, 440t
functional health-pattern assessment during, 430-442, 431b, 454, 455b
maternal changes in, 421-427
mechanical forces affecting, 449-450
nursing interventions during, 454-456, 454f
pathological processes during, 442-450
physical changes in, 418-427
preparing for, 671b
recommended dietary allowance during, 278t
second trimester of
fetal growth and development during, 419b
first pregnancy, 440t
signs of, 421, 421b, 421f
social processes during, 450-454
teaching throughout, 422-424
third trimester of
fetal growth and development during, 419b
first pregnancy, 440t
ultrasound used during, 421, 421f, 444b
unintended, 429b
of middle-age adults, 697
of young adults, 664-666
uterine enlargement during, 422f
weight gain during, 424, 429b
Prenatal care, 424b, 429b
guidelines for, 437
nursing interventions in, 439, 442b, 454-456, 454f
Prenatal Care Initiative, 424b
Prenatal period. *See* Pregnancy(ies).
Preschool, 558-559, 561-562
Preschool children, 401t, 533-564
aggressive behavior in, 534b
asthma in, 561
behavioral milestones in, 536t
biological and bacterial agents affecting, 557-559
chemical exposures of, 559
developmental milestones in, 536t
family with, 189
functional health-pattern assessment of, 537-554
injuries to, 555-556
literature regarding, 538b
mechanical forces affecting, 557
nursing intervention with, 563, 563b, 563t
pathological processes affecting, 554-561
physical changes of, 534-537
social processes affecting, 561-563
teaching health promotion to, 252
Preschool Readiness Experimental Screening Scale, 546, 547f-548f
Prescription medications. *See also* specific type of medication.
education interventions involving, 255-256
for older adults, 734-735
costs of, 74, 74f, 75
urinary incontinence caused by, 718b
infants affected by, 494
racial and ethnic variations in response to, 674b
used during pregnancy, 447-448
Presence
in holistic healing, 387t
Presence, in holistic healing, 387-393
Pressure sore, 725
Prevention
clinical effectiveness of, 753-754
cost-effectiveness of, 754-755
curative care vs, 58-60
in young adults, 652-656, 654t
levels of, 14-20, 15f
of childhood injuries, 204
of falls of older adults, 732b
of HIV and AIDS, 48-49
of obesity in school-age children, 575b
of osteoporosis, 302-303
primary, 15f, 16-19
screening in. *See* Screening.
secondary, 15f, 20
tertiary, 15f, 20
under Medicaid, 76
Primary care, 60
Primary care provider, 61
Privacy, right to, 122-123
Private sector health care, 60-62, 67
Problem-solving, promotion of, 96, 97
Procreate, right to, 125, 126, 127
Professional associations, 66

Professional oaths, 113-114, 114b, 115b-116b, 123-124
Prospective payment system, 68-69
Prostate cancer
diet and, 298t
in older adults, 736, 736t
screening for, 237t, 241, 245
Prostate specific antigen, 237t, 241
Protection, specific, 19
Protein
deficiencies of, 270t
fad diets high in, 309
in diabetes diet intervention, 311b
requirements for
during pregnancy, 433
for infants, 473
Protestantism
on abortion, 127-128
on donor artificial insemination, 130
Proxemics, 93
Psychosocial development, Erikson's theory of. *See* Erikson's theory of psychosocial development.
Public health, 62-66
development of, 57, 59
new movement for, 751
Public health officials, 12
Public Law 94-142, 607
Punishment, of school-age children, 587

Q

Qi Gong, 379, 380-381
Quality Compass, National Committee for Quality Assurance's, 70
Quality of life, 121-122
Questions, in functional communication, 91

R

Race
and adolescent health, 623
and future population changes, 24
and health disparities. *See* Health disparities.
and middle-age adult health, 684
and minority groups. *See* Minority groups.
and preschoolers, 537
and toddlerhood, 510
drug response variations and, 674b
fetal health and, 428-429
screening and, 237
young adults and, 670-672
Racial groups, 32, 32f
Radiation exposure
during pregnancy, 450
from excessive sun exposure, 658-659
of middle-age adults, 700
of school-age children, 603, 603b
Randomized clinical trials, 23
Rapport, in therapeutic relationship, 94
Rating perceived exertion, 335, 335f
Reciprocity, 87, 92
Recommended dietary allowance, 275b, 278t
Recreation
injuries of school-age children, 596, 596b
of families, 675-676, 676f
Reflection, in therapeutic communication, 96-97
Reflexology, 378
Registered dietitians
in diabetes, 310-312, 312f
in HIV and AIDS, 314b
Regression, upon new sibling's arrival, 521-522
Reiki healing, 379
Relational messages, 102
Relationships
functional health-pattern assessment of
of adolescents, 631-632
of communities, 208t, 212
of individuals, 156-158
of infants, 482-487
of middle-age adults, 693-697
of older adults, 726-727
of preschoolers, 549-551
of school-age children, 586-588
of toddlers, 520-523
of young adults, 661-664
Relaxation response, 360, 362f, 363
exercise and, 337-339
mini-, 363, 363b
Relaxation techniques
for young adults, 659b, 660b
learning and practicing, 360-363, 362f
Religion. *See also* specific religions.
and infant care, 500-501
food and, 281
Renal cancer
warning signs in children, 560b
Wilms' tumor as, 559-560
Renal system
during transition from fetus to newborn, 428b
of middle-age adults, 682
of older adults, 712t
of preschoolers, 535
Reproduction
functional health-pattern assessment of
during pregnancy, 431b, 441
of adolescents, 632-635
of communities, 209t, 212
of families, 182-184
of individuals, 158
of middle-age adults, 697-698
of young adults, 664-669
Reproductive system
contraception and. *See* Contraception.
during pregnancy, 422
growth changes of, 409t
of adolescents, 621-623
boys, 621-622, 622f
girls, 622-623, 622f
secondary sex characteristics, 621t
of middle-age adults, 682-683
of older adults, 712t

Reproductive system—cont'd
pregnancy and. *See* Pregnancy(ies).
young adult's problems with, 664
Reproductive technology, 129-131
Research
at National Institute of Nursing Research, 22, 22b
ethical issues regarding, 122-124
including women and minorities, 42
nurse's role in, 757-758
utilization of, 24
voluntary agencies and, 66
Researchers, nurses as, 21-24
Resistance, as communication barrier, 98
Resistance training, 337, 338b-339b, 339
Respiratory system
during pregnancy, 421-422
during transition from fetus to newborn, 428b
growth changes of, 407t
lung cancer. *See* Lung cancer.
of adolescents, 619
of older adults, 713t
of preschoolers, 535
of school-age children, 568
of toddlers, 508
Responsibility, personal, 10
Rest patterns
functional health-pattern assessment of
during pregnancy, 431b, 435
of adolescents, 627-628
of communities, 207t, 211
of families, 179
of individuals, 150-152
of infants, 478-480
of middle-age adults, 691
of older adults, 719-721
of preschoolers, 541-542
of school-age children, 578
of young adults, 659, 659b
Retinoblastoma
in infants, 497
in preschoolers, 560
Retirement communities, 738t-739t
Rh-blood-group incompatibility, 447
Rho (D) immune globulin (RhoGAM), 447
Rights, role of, 117-118
Risk behaviors
of adolescents, 617b
of middle-age adults, 685
of young adults, 655
Risk factor theory
in community assessment, 200, 204, 215
in family assessment, 173-175, 175b, 176t-177t
Risk factors
for coronary heart disease, 323t
for low birth weight newborns, 501, 501b
for middle-age adults, 685
for osteoporosis, 302b
screening to identify, 228
Role(s)
functional health-pattern assessment of
during pregnancy, 431b, 439-441
of adolescents, 631-632
of family members, 180-182, 183f, 184f
of individuals, 156-158
of infants, 482-487
of middle-age adults, 693-697
of older adults, 726-727
of preschoolers, 549-551
of school-age children, 586-588
of toddlers, 520-523
of young adults, 661-664
within communities, 208t, 212
maternal, 439
of justice, 117-118
of nurses. *See* Nurses, role of.
of schools, 611-613
Roman Catholicism
on abortion, 128
on donor artificial insemination, 130
RU 486, 127-128
Rubella
fetus affected by, 445
in young adults, 656
Rural areas
homeless persons in, 45
women in, 684b

S

Salary system, of payment, 68
Salmonella, 286t
Santeria, 39
Scabies, in school-age children, 600
School breakfast program, 290
School-age children, 567-613
accidents of, 593-597
after-school care for, 604-605, 605b
biological agents affecting, 599-601
cancer in, 603
chemical exposures of, 601-603
family with, 189, 401t
functional health-pattern assessment of, 572-593
latchkey, 605b
literature regarding, 591b
mechanical forces affecting, 597-599
nursing intervention for, 610-611
pathological processes affecting, 593-603
physical changes in, 568-572
radiological agents affecting, 603
social processes affecting, 603-610
teaching health promotion to, 252
television and, 605-606
Schools
adolescents and, 643
health care role of, 611-613
increased physical activity at, 347
isolation of child at new, 610b
nurses at, 611-613, 613f

Schools—cont'd
parent's concerns regarding, 676
pre-, 558-559, 561-562
Scientific advances, 57-58
Scoliosis, in adolescents, 620, 620f
Screening, 20, 227-245
advantages and disadvantages of, 228-229
conditions screened, 236t, 237t, 239-244
Denver Developmental Screening Test, 465, 466f, 467f, 518
group, 228
individual, 228
instruments for, 230
mass, 228
multiple-test, 229
nurse's role in, 244-245
nutrition, 291-292
of adolescents, 624b
of men, 236t
of middle-age adults, 686b-688b
of preschoolers, 544b, 562-563, 563b
of women, 236t, 675
one-test disease specific, 229
population selected for, 235-239
selection of diseases for, 229-234
Scurvy, 270t
Self
components of, 86, 86b, 86f, 87f
therapeutic use of, 85-87
Self-awareness, 86
development of, 359-363
of nurses, 87
Self-care activities, 135
Self-concept, 85-86
functional health-pattern assessment of
during pregnancy, 431b, 438-439
of adolescents, 630-631
of communities, 208t, 212, 212f
of families, 180
of individuals, 155-156
of infants, 482
of middle-age adults, 692-693
of older adults, 725-726
of preschoolers, 548-549
of school-age children, 584-586, 586b
of toddlers, 518-520
of young adults, 661
Self-determination
autonomy and, 119, 120
Code for Nurses on, 123-124
Self-disclosure, 87
Self-efficacy concept, 254, 254f
Self-esteem, 85
in school-age children, 585
men vs women, 411b
of adolescents, 631b
of school-age children, 585f
Self-funded insurance plans, 72
Self-insurance, 72
Self-knowledge, and holistic health, 388f-392f, 393
Self-perception
functional health-pattern assessment of
during pregnancy, 431b, 438-439
of adolescents, 630-631
of communities, 208t, 212, 212f
of families, 180
of individuals, 155-156
of infants, 482
of middle-age adults, 692-693
of older adults, 725-726
of preschoolers, 548-549
of school-age children, 584-586
of toddlers, 518-520
of young adults, 661
Self-reflection, 86-87
Sensory barriers, as communication barriers, 99
Sensory perception
of adolescents, 630
of older adults, 724-725
of preschoolers, 544
of school-age children, 581
Separation anxiety, 524
Serum lipids, 293t. *See also* Cholesterol.
Service delivery, nurse's role in, 21
Seventh Day Adventists, food and, 281
Sex characteristics
in adolescents, 621-623, 621t
primary, 621
secondary, 621, 621t
Sexual practices
of adolescents, 83, 624b
safe, 668b
unprotected, 83
Sexuality
and couples family, 187-188
and television, 185
functional health-pattern assessment of
during pregnancy, 431b, 441
of adolescents, 632-635
of individuals, 158
of infants, 487-488
of middle-age adults, 697-698
of older adults, 727-728, 728f
of preschoolers, 551, 551f
of school-age children, 588-589
of toddlers, 523
of young adults, 664-669
within communities, 209t, 212
within families, 182-184
health education for school-age children regarding, 611t
of aging women, 159
Sexually-transmitted diseases, 666-669, 667t. *See also* specific diseases.
fetus and newborns affected by, 443-446
in adolescents, 633, 639
in middle-age adults, 698
Shamanism, 43, 380
Shelters, for homeless persons, 46

Siblings
of newborns, 439-440
rivalries between, 521-522
SIDS. *See* Sudden infant death syndrome (SIDS).
Sigmoidoscopy, 236t, 237t, 241
Sign language, 89
Silence, in functional communication, 92, 97
Single-parent families, 181, 181f
and isolation of child, 610b
and poverty, 702b
Situation ethics, 112
Situational crisis
and altered parenting, 524b
of infants, 489
Skeletal system
building and maintaining health in, 301-302
during pregnancy, 422
growth changes of, 407t
of adolescents, 619
of middle-age adults, 682
of older adults, 712t
of school-age children, 571
of toddlers, 509
Skin
of adolescents, 620
of older adults, 713t, 725
Sleep disturbances
of preschoolers, 541
of school-age children, 578
of toddlers, 515
Sleep hygiene
functional health-pattern assessment of
during pregnancy, 431b, 435
of adolescents, 627-628
of communities, 207t, 211
of families, 179
of individuals, 150-152
of infants, 478-480, 478t
of middle-age adults, 691
of older adults, 719-721, 722b
of preschoolers, 541-542
of school-age children, 578
of toddlers, 515-516
of young adults, 659
in stress management, 364-365
strategies for, 365b
sudden infant death syndrome and sleep position, 479b
Smell sensation
of infants, 481
of older adults, 724
of toddlers, 518
Smoking
and coronary heart disease, 323t
and preschoolers, 563b
by adolescents, 641
by middle-age adults, 687b, 701-702
by older adults, 710, 735
by school-age children, 601-602
by young adults, 674
during pregnancy, 429b, 449
Smoking cessation, 675b, 754b
in young adults, 675b
personal incentives for, 10
workplace initiatives for, 11
Snellen E chart, 543
Social cognitive theory, 254-255, 345f
Social marketing, health education and, 257-258
Social Security Amendments of 1983, 68
Social support
during labor and delivery, 366-367
during pregnancy, 455b
in stress management, 366-367, 366b
Socioeconomic influences, of health care, 57
Sodium intake
and hypertension, 295-296
diets high in, 689
from specific foods, 296t
in diabetes diet intervention, 312b
in healthy diet, 283t
Somatization, in school-age children, 591-592
Space, in functional communication, 93-94, 93f
Special senses. *See also* specific senses.
growth changes of, 405t
Speech
of preschoolers, 545t
of toddlers, 519t
Spiritual distress, 157
stress and, 357
Spiritual practice
and toddlers, 525
in stress management, 369
of older adults, 729-731
Spores, as food contaminant, 286t
Sports activities, 659
Sports injuries
of adolescents, 637-638
of school-age children, 596, 596b
of toddlers, 526
Stanford-Binet Intelligence Scale, 583t
Staphylococcus aureus, 286t
State governments
food assistance programs by, 290
Medicaid administered by, 75, 76
public health services of, 63
Sterilization, forced, 126-127
Stewardship, of health, 121, 124
Stomach cancer, diet and, 298t
Strabismus, in toddlers, 517
Street-safety, 598b
Streptococcus infection, 445
fetus affected by, 445
school-age children with, 599
Stress
achievement-oriented, 669
and breast cancer, 356b
functional health-pattern assessment of
during pregnancy, 431b, 441-442
of adolescents, 635-636
of communities, 209t-210t, 212-213
of families, 184-185

Stress—cont'd
functional health-pattern assessment of—cont'd
of individuals, 158-160, 358-359
of infants, 488-489, 489b
of middle-age adults, 698-699
of older adults, 728-729
of preschoolers, 551-553
of school-age children, 589-592
of toddlers, 523-524
of young adults, 669-670
physiological effects of, 355, 356f
psychological effects of, 355-356
social-behavioral effects of, 356-357
sources of, 354-355
spiritual effects of, 357
warning signs of, 360, 361f
Stress management, 353-372
and breast cancer risk reduction, 300b
exercise and, 332
health benefits of, 357-358
interventions in, 359-370
of caregiver in Alzheimer's disease, 193
The Humor Potential, Inc. for, 156
Stress response, 356f
Stress-disinhibition effect, 357
Stroke, in middle-age adults, 687b
Structural hazards, for toddlers, 525-526
Substance abuse. *See also* specific substances.
by adolescents, 199, 624b, 636, 639-641, 639b, 640b
by health professionals, 134
by young adults, 673
during pregnancy, 429b, 448-449
health education for school-age children regarding, 611t
homelessness and, 45
Subtle energy, 376, 377b
Sudden infant death syndrome (SIDS), 460b, 478-480, 479b
Sugars. *See* Sweets.
Suicide
assisted, 133
of adolescents, 635-636, 636b
of older adults, 729
of young adults, 663, 664t, 669-670
physician-assisted, 729, 731b
Sundown syndrome, 721
Sweeteners, in diabetes diet intervention, 311b-312b
Sweets
in food guide pyramid, 281-282
in healthy diet, 283t
preschoolers and, 539t
Syphilis, 667t
fetus affected by, 443-445
screening for, 688b
Systems theory
in community assessment, 202-203
in family assessment, 171-173

T

Tai Chi, 330b, 338, 381
Talking Circle, 367
Tao doctrine, 37
Taste sensation
of infants, 481
of middle-age adults, 692
of older adults, 724
of toddlers, 518
Tattooing, by adolescents, 630b
Teaching, health. *See* Health education.
Team cooperation, within communities, 207t
Teenagers. *See* Adolescents.
Teeth. *See* Dental health.
Telehealth, 104
at rural schools, 612b
Telenursing, 104, 265
Teleology, 111-112
Television
and sex, 185
school-age children and, 605-607
Temperament
of preschoolers, 552b
of toddlers, 521b
Teratogens, 431, 432f, 442-443
Testicular cancer
in adolescents, 643
screening for, 688b
self-examination, 652
Tetanus prophylaxis, 601
Tetracycline, used during pregnancy, 448
Thalidomide, 447
Theological ethics, 109
"Therapeutic lifestyle changes" treatment plan, 294
Therapeutic relationships, 83-104
communication in. *See* Communication.
communication process in, 88-94
effectiveness in, 94, 101b
in brief interactions, 102-104
settings for, 100
stages of, 100-102, 100b, 102b
techniques in, 95-97
values clarification in, 84-87, 85b
Therapeutic touch, 378-379, 379b, 380
clinical evaluation of, 378b, 379f
for burn pain, 380b
Thiamin deficiencies, 270t
Time orientation, of adolescents, 630
Tobacco use. *See* Smoking.
Toddlers, 507-531
and new siblings, 521-522, 522f
and nursing interventions, 530-531
biological and bacterial agents affecting, 527
car seats for, 527
chemical exposures of, 527-528, 527f
childproofing for, 525-526, 527f
functional health-pattern assessment of, 511-525
grandparents providing care for, 524b
in motor vehicles accidents, 526-527
limit setting for, 507b
pathological processes affecting, 525-528
physical changes in, 508-511

Toddlers—cont'd
social processes affecting, 528-531
temperament of, 521b
unintentional injuries of, 525-526
Toilet training, 512-513, 513b
Tolerable upper intake level, 275b
Tolerance levels
functional health-pattern assessment of
during pregnancy, 431b, 441-442
of adolescents, 635-636
of communities, 209t-210t, 212-213
of families, 184-185
of individuals, 158-160
of infants, 488-489
of middle-age adults, 698-699
of older adults, 728-729
of preschoolers, 551-553
of school-age children, 589-592
of toddlers, 523-524
of young adults, 669-670
Touch
in functional communication, 92-93, 93f
therapeutic, 378-379, 379b, 380
clinical evaluation of, 378b, 379f
for burn pain, 380b
therapies utilizing, 378-380
Touch sensation, of infants, 481
Touch therapies, 378-380
Touchpoints Model Program, 504b
Toxins
and school-age children, 594b
infants affected by, 495-496, 496t
vitamins as, 279
Toxoplasmosis, 443
Toys, toddler trauma due to, 526
Trager therapy, 386
Trance surgery, 380b
Transcendental Meditation, 382-383
Transcultural nursing, 33, 50, 59, 144, 499b
and family health, 192
and health teaching, 257
and infant care, 499-500, 500b
and therapeutic communication, 99
in pregnancy, 451-452, 452b
Transference, as communication barrier, 98
Traumatic injuries
during pregnancy, 449-450
occupational, 694-695, 694f
to adolescents, 637-638
to infants, 490-491, 490f, 491b, 492b, 493b
to older adults, 732-733, 732b, 733t
to preschoolers, 555-556
to school-age children, 593-597, 597b, 611t
to toddlers, 525-526
to young adults, 672
Trichinella spiralis, 286t
Trichomoniasis, 667t
Tridione, used during pregnancy, 448
Triglyceride levels
exercise and, 293t
screening of, 293t
Trimethadione, used during pregnancy, 448
Trust, in therapeutic relationship, 94
Tuberculosis
homelessness and, 45-46
incidence of, 58
older adults and, 734
screening for, 688b
Turner's syndrome, 623

U

Ultrasound, during pregnancy, 421, 421f, 444b, 457b
Uninsured persons, 71, 76-77
Upper respiratory infections
exercise and, 331, 331f
of toddlers, 527
Urinary incontinence, 718, 718b
Urinary system
and elimination pattern. *See* Elimination pattern.
and enuresis, 576
during pregnancy, 421, 434
growth changes of, 404t
Urinary tract infections
during pregnancy, 434
urinary incontinence with, 718b
U.S. Department of Health and Human Services, 63-64, 64b
U.S. Preventative Services task Force, 250, 250b
Uterus
cancer screening, 688b
enlargement during pregnancy, 422f
fetal malpositioning in, 450
Utilitarianism, 111-112

V

Vaccines. *See* Immunization.
Validity, of screening instruments, 230
Values
functional health-pattern assessment of
during pregnancy, 431b, 442
of adolescents, 636-637
of communities, 210t, 213
of families, 185
of individuals, 160
of infants, 489-490
of middle-age adults, 699-700
of older adults, 729-731
of preschoolers, 553-554
of school-age children, 592-593
of toddlers, 524-525
of young adults, 670-672
nurse's conflicts with individual's, 83, 84
Values clarification, 84-87, 85b
in stress management, 370
Valuing process, 84, 85b
Vascular system
cardio-. *See* Cardiovascular system.
in older adults, 712t

Vegetables
for preschoolers, 539t
in cancer risk reduction, 298, 300b
in food guide pyramid, 280
in healthy diet, 282b-283b
sodium content of, 296t
Veterans Administration, 64
Vineland Social Maturity Scale, 550, 583t
Violence
adolescents and, 638-639, 638f
diffusion of, 216
domestic, 174, 181, 182, 456b, 663-664, 665b
workplace, 216, 695b
young adults at risk for, 663-664
Viruses, as food contaminants, 285t, 286t
Visual ability
of infants, 480-481, 480t
of middle-age adults, 692
of older adults, 724, 724b
of preschoolers, 543-544, 544b
of school-age children, 580, 580f
of toddlers, 517
Vitamin(s)
deficiencies of, 270, 270t
requirements for
during pregnancy, 433
of infants, 473
toxicity of, 279
Vitamin A
deficiencies of, 270t
toxicity associated with, 279
Vitamin C deficiencies, 270t
Vitamin D, and osteoporosis, 302
Voluntary health organizations, 65-66, 65t
and infant health, 502b
Voluntary motor movements, in toddlers, 509-510
Vulnerable populations, 755

W

Walking, as exercise, 336
Warfarin sodium, used during pregnancy, 448
Warts, genital, 667t
Water intake, by infants, 473
Water pollution
infants affected by, 496
middle-age adults affected by, 700
Water safety
and school-age children, 594b, 595b
drowning and. *See* Drowning.
Websites. *See* Internet.
Wechsler Intelligence Scale for Children, 582, 583t
Weight management, 293
and dietary guidelines, 282b
and obesity. *See* Obesity.
and overweight persons, 272, 303, 304t
type 2 diabetes and, 325
young adults as, 657f
by adolescents, 627b
during pregnancy, 424, 429b
fad diets for, 309
Weight management—cont'd
in cancer risk reduction, 299, 300b
in middle age, 682
Welfare reform bill, 76
Well child care, 609-610, 609t
Wellness communities, 196
Wellness tasks, developmental tasks vs, 145t-146t
Wellness-illness continuum, 4, 5-6, 5f, 7f
Western health care systems, folk systems vs, 35-36, 35t
Whites, higher education of, 36t
WIC (Women, Infants, and Children) Program, 290-291, 453
Wilms' tumor, 559-560
Windshield survey, 201-202
Women
aging and sexuality of, 159
AIDS in, 49
alcoholism assessment of, 141
and domestic violence. *See* Domestic violence.
and maternal mortality, 651, 666
and menopause, 682, 697-698, 702
cancer in
breast cancer. *See* Breast cancer.
cervical cancer. *See* Cervical cancer.
endometrial cancer, 298t
lung cancer, 675
ovarian cancer, 687b-688b
screening for, 675
uterine cancer, 688b
dietary reference intakes for, 276t
health tests and screenings for, 236t, 237
heart disease in, 164
in rural areas, 684b
in workplace. *See* Workplace.
mortality rates of, 683-684
recommended dietary allowance for, 278t
self-esteem in, 411b
WIC Program for, 290-291, 453
Women, Infants, and Children (WIC) Program, 290-291, 453
Workplace
as community partner, 10, 11
fitness programs at, 55, 347
for middle-age adults, 694-695, 694f
hazards and stressors in
biological hazards as, 701t
chemical agents as, 701
for middle-age adults, 694-695, 694f
for young adults, 672-673
nursing intervention in, 705
increased physical activity at, 347
occupational screening at, 239
sexual orientation and, 678b
smoking policy of, 17
violence in, 216, 695b
women in
and dual careers, 677, 695-696
and latchkey children, 605b
and pregnancy, 450-451
day care centers and. *See* Day care centers.
maternal return to work, 521, 604-605, 605b

World Health Declaration (WHO), 750, 750b
World Health Organization (WHO), 65, 748
  Health for All, 749-750, 750b
  World Health Declaration, 750, 750b

X

Xerophthalmia, 270t

Y

Yerkes-Dodson Law, 354-355, 355f
Yoga, 336f, 337, 338, 381-382, 381b
Young adults, 401t, 649-679
  accidents of, 672
  and firearm safety, 663, 663b
  and violence, 663-664
  behavioral health history of, 652
  cancer in, 674-675
  chemical exposures affecting, 673
  decision making by, 655
  excessive sun exposure by, 658-659
Young adults—cont'd
  families with, 190
  functional health-pattern assessment of, 651-672
  immunization of, 655-656
  in college
    drinking behaviors of, 650b
    health promotion needs of, 625b
  infectious diseases in, 655-656
  pathological processes affecting, 672-675
  physical changes in, 650-651
  pollution affecting, 672
  preventative care of, 652-656
  risk behaviors of, 655
  social processes affecting, 675-678
  sports for, 658f, 659
  workplace hazards and stressors for, 672-673

Z

Zygote, 418